DISEASES/CONDITIONS AND ICD-9-CM CODES

Abruptio placentae	641.2**
Acne vulgaris	706.1
Acromegaly	253.0
Actinic keratosis	702.0
Acute bronchitis	466.0
Acute and chronic viral hepatitis	070.9
Acute diarrhea (NOS)	787.91
Acute leukemia (plain leukemia)	208.0**
Acute myocardial infarction	410.9**
Acute otitis media	382.9
Acute pancreatitis	577.0
Acute peripheral facial paralysis (Bell's palsy)	351.0
Acute renal failure	584.9
Acute respiratory failure	518.81
Acute stress disorder	308.9
Adrenocortical insufficiency	255.4
Adverse reactions to blood transfusions	999
Alcoholism	303.9**
Allergic reactions to drugs	995.2
Allergic reactions to insect stings	989.5
Allergic rhinitis	477.8
Alopecia areata	704.01
Alzheimer's disease	331.0
Amebiasis	006.9
Amenorrhea	626.0
Anal fissure,	565.0
Anaphylaxis, NOS	995.0
Angina pectoris	413.9
Angioedema	995.1
Ankle fracture	824.8
Ankylosing spondylitis	720.0
Anorectal abscess	566.
Anorexia nervosa	307.1
Aortic aneurysm and dissection	441.00
Aplastic anemia	284.9
Asthma	493.9**
Atelectasis	518.0
Atopic dermatitis	691.8
Atopic fibrillation	427.31
Attention deficit/hyperactivity disorder	314.01
Autoimmune hemolytic anemia	283.0
Bacterial meningitis	320
Bacterial pneumonia	482.9
Bacterial vaginitis	616.1
Benign prostatic hyperplasia	600
Blastomycosis	116.0
Bleeding esophageal varices	456.0
Brain abscess	324.
Brain tumors	239.6
Breast cancer	174
Brucellosis	023
Bulimia nervosa	307.51
Bullous diseases	694
Burns	940-949
Bursitis	726-727
Cancer of the endometrium	182.0
Cancer of the skin	172-173
Cancer of the uterine cervix	180
Cardiac arrest, sudden cardiac death	427.5
Care after myocardial infarction	414.8
Cellulitis	682.
Chancroid	099.3
Chlamydia trachomatis infection	079.88
Cholelithiasis and cholecystitis	574.1-574.9
Cholera	001
Chronic fatigue syndrome	780.71
Chronic leukemia	208.1**
Chronic obstructive pulmonary disease	491.2**
Chronic pancreatitis	577.1
Chronic renal failure	585
Chronic serous otitis media	381.1**
Coccidioidomycosis	114*
Colorectal cancer	153
Concussion	850
Congenital heart disease	745-747
Congenital rubella	771.0
Congestive heart failure	428.0
Conjunctivitis, acute	372.0**
Connective tissue disease	710*
Constipation	564.0
Contact dermatitis	692
Cough	786.2
Cushing's syndrome	255.0
Delirium	780.0
Dementia, multi-infarct, uncomplicated	294.8
Depression psychosis	298.0
Depression with anxiety	300.4
Diabetes insipidus	253.5
Diabetes mellitus, I	250.01
Diabetes mellitus, II	250.02
Diabetic ketoacidosis	276.2**
Diphtheria	032*
Diseases of the mouth	528*
Disseminated intravascular coagulation	286.6
Diverticulitis	562.11
Drug abuse (nondependent)	305.9**
Dysfunctional uterine bleeding	626.6
Dysmenorrhea	635.5
Dysphagia and esophageal obstruction	530.3
Ectopic pregnancy	633*
Elbow dislocation	832.0**
Encephalitis	323*
Endometriosis	617*
Enuresis	786.30
Epididymitis	604**
Episodic vertigo	386.11
Erythema multiforme	695.1
Fetal lung immaturity	770.4
Fever	780.6
Fibrocystic diseases of the breast	610.1
Fibromyositis	729.1
Fifth disease	057.0
Finger dislocation, closed	834.0**
Finger fracture	816.0**
Fistula (anal)	565.1
Fitting of diaphragm	V25.02
Folliculitis	704.8
Food allergy	693.1
Food poisoning	005*
Foot fracture	825.2**
Frostbite	991*
Gangrene	785.4
Gastritis	535**
Gastroesophageal reflux disease (GERD)	530.81
Generalized anxiety disorder	300.02
Generalized epilepsy	345.1**
Genital warts (condylomata acuminata)	078.11
Giant cell arteritis	446.5
Giardiasis	7.1
Gilles de la Tourette syndrome	307.23
Glaucoma	365**
Gonorrhea	098.0
Gout	274.9
Granuloma inguinale (donovanosis)	099.2
Guillain-Barré syndrome	357.0
Headache.	784.0
Heart block	426.1**
Heat exhaustion	992.3
Heat stroke	992.0
Hemochromatosis	285.0
Hemolytic disease of the fetus and newborn	773.2
Hemophilia and related conditions	286.0
Hemorrhoids	455.6
Herpes gestationis	646.8**
Herpes simplex	054*
Herpes zoster	053*
Hiccups	786.8
High-altitude sickness	993.2
Histoplasmosis	115**
HIV-associated infections	042.0
HIV infection, asymptomatic	V08
HIV infection, early symptomatic	042
HIV infection, late symptomatic	042
Hyperlipoproteinemias	272*
Hyperparathyroidism	252.0
Hyperprolactinemia	253.1
Hypersensitivity pneumonitis	495
Hypertension (essential)	401*
Hyperthyroidism	242**
Hypertrophic cardiomyopathy	425.4
Hypoparathyroidism	252.1
Hypothyroidism	244*
Immunization practices	V03, VO4, VO5, VO6**
Impetigo	684
Impotence	302.72
Indigestion	536.8
Infectious diarrhea	009.2
Infectious mononucleosis	075
Infective endocarditis	424.9**
Influenza	487.2
Ingrowing nail	703.0
Insect and spider bite	989.5
Insertion of intrauterine device	V25.1
Insomnia (NOS)	780.52

DISEASES/CONDITIONS AND ICD-9-CM CODES *(Continued)*

Intracerebral hemorrhage 431
Iron deficiency anemia 280.0-280.9
Irritable bowel syndrome 564.1
Jellyfish sting 989.5
Juvenile rheumatoid arthritis 714.3**
Keloids 701.4
Laryngitis 464.00
Lead poisoning 984*
Legionnaires' disease 482.84
Leishmaniasis 085*
Leprosy 030*
Lichen planus 697.0
Low back pain 724.2
Lyme disease 088.81
Lymphogranuloma venereum 099.1
Malabsorption 579*
Malaria 084.6
Measles (rubeola) 055.9
Meconium aspiration 770.1
Melanoma, malignant 172*
Ménière's disease 386.0**
Meningitis 320-322
Menopausal. 627.2
Migraine headache 346**
Mitral valve prolapse 424.0
Monilial vulvovaginitis 121.1
Multiple myeloma 203.0**
Multiple sclerosis 340
Mumps 072.9
Myasthenia gravis 358.0**
Mycoplasmal pneumonias 483.0
Mycosis fungoides 202.1**
Nausea and vomiting 787.01
Neoplasm of the vulva 239.5
Neutropenia 288.0
Nevi 216*
Newborn physiologic jaundice 774.6
Nongonococcal urethritis 099.4**
Non-Hodgkin's lymphomas 202.8**
Non-autoimmune hemolytic anemia 283.1**
Normal delivery 650
Obesity 278.00
Obsessive-compulsive disorders 300.3
Onychomycosis 110.1
Optic neuritis 377.3**
Osteoarthritis 715**
Osteomyelitis 730**
Osteoporosis 733.00
Otitis externa 380.10
Paget's disease of bone 731.0
Panic disorder 300.01
Pap smear V72.3
Parkinsonism 332.0
Paronychia 681.0**
Partial epilepsy 345.4**
Patent ductus arteriosus 747.0
Pediculosis 132*
Pelvic inflammatory disease 614*
Peptic ulcer disease 533*
Pericarditis 432.9
Peripheral arterial disease 443.9
Peripheral neuropathies 356*
Pernicious anemia 281.0
Personality disorder 301**
Pheochromocytoma 227.0
Phobia 300.2**
Pigmentary disorders—vitiligo 709.01
Pinworms 127.4
Pityriasis rosea 696.3
Placenta previa 641**
Plague 020*
Platelet-mediated bleeding disorders 287.1
Pleural effusion 511.9
Polycythemia vera 238.4
Polymyalgia rheumatica 725
Porphyria 277.1
Postpartum hemorrhage 666.1**
Post-traumatic stress disorder 309.81
Pregnancy V22.2
Pregnancy-induced hypertension 642**
Premature beats 427.69
Premenstrual tension syndrome (PMS) 625.4
Prescribed oral contraceptive. V25.01
Pressure ulcers 707.0
Preterm labor 644.2**
Primary glomerular disease 581-583
Primary lung abscess 513.0
Primary lung cancer 162.9
Prostate cancer 185

Prostatitis 601*
Pruritus 698.9
Pruritus ani 698.0
Pruritus vulvae 698.1
Psittacosis (ornithosis) 073*
Psoriasis 696.1
Pulmonary embolism 415.1
Pyelonephritis 590**
Q fever 083.0
Rabies 071
Rat-bite fever 026*
Relapsing fever 087*
Renal calculi 592
Reye syndrome 331.81
Rheumatic fever 390
Rheumatoid arthritis 714.0
Rib fracture 807.0**
Rocky Mountain spotted fever 082.0
Rosacea 695.3
Roseola 057.8
Rubella 056*
Salmonellosis 003.0
Sarcoidosis 135
Scabies 133.0
Schizophrenia 295**
Seborrheic dermatitis 690.1**
Septicemia 038*
Sézary's syndrome 202.2**
Shoulder dislocation 831.0**
Sickle cell anemia 282.6**
Silicosis 502
Sinusitis, chronic 473*
Skull fracture 800, 801, 803
Sleep apnea 780.57
Sleep disorders 780.50
Snakebite 989.5
Stasis ulcers 454.0
Status epilepticus 345.3
Stomach cancer 151*
Streptococcal pharyngitis 034.0
Stroke 436
Strongyloides infection 127.2
Subdural or subarachnoid hemorrhage ..852**
Sunburn 692.71
Syphilis 090-097
Tachycardias 785.0
Tapeworm infections 123*
Telogen effluvium 704.02
Temporomandibular joint syndrome ...524.6**
Tendonitis 726.90
Tetanus 037
Thalassemia 282.4**
Therapeutic use of blood components ...V59.0**
Thrombotic thrombocytopenic purpura ...446.6
Thyroid cancer 193
Thyroiditis 245*
Tinea capitis 110.0
Tinnitus 388.3**
Toe fracture 826.0
Toxic shock syndrome 040.82
Toxoplasmosis 130*
Transient cerebral ischemia 435*
Trauma to the genitourinary tract 958,959
Trichinellosis 124
Trichomonal vaginitis 131.01
Trigeminal neuralgia 350.1
Tuberculosis, pulmonary 011**
Tularemia 021*
Typhoid fever 002.0
Typhus fevers 080, 081
Ulcerative colitis 556*
Urethral stricture 598*
Urinary incontinence 788.30
Urticaria 708*
Uterine inertia 661.0**
Uterine leiomyoma 218*
Varicella 052*
Venous thrombosis 453.8
Viral pneumonia 480.9
Viral respiratory infections 465.9
Vitamin deficiency 264-269
Vitamin K deficiency 269.0
Warts (verrucae) 078.10
Wegener's granulomatosis 446.4
Whooping cough (pertussis) 033*
Wrist fracture 814.0**

*4th digit needed
**5th (or 4th and 5th) digit needed

CONN'S
Current Therapy 2007

Provided as an
educational service by

Takeda Pharmaceuticals
and
TAP Pharmaceuticals Inc.

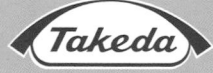

CONN'S
Current
Therapy
2007

Robert E. Rakel, MD

Professor, Department of Family and
  Community Medicine
Baylor College of Medicine
Houston, Texas

Edward T. Bope, MD

Director, Riverside Family Practice Residency Program
Clinical Professor, Department of Family Medicine
The Ohio State University College of Medicine
Columbus, Ohio

LATEST APPROVED METHODS
OF TREATMENT FOR
THE PRACTICING PHYSICIAN

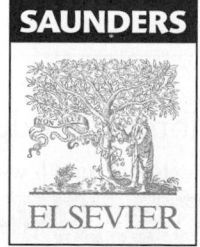

SAUNDERS

ELSEVIER

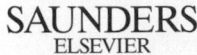

SAUNDERS
ELSEVIER

1600 John F. Kennedy Blvd.
Ste 1800
Philadelphia, PA 19103-2899

CONN'S CURRENT THERAPY 2007

ISBN-13: 978-1-4160-3281-6
ISBN-10: 1-4160-3281-9

Notice

Knowledge and best practice in this field are constantly changing. As new research and experience broaden our knowledge, changes in practice, treatment, and drug therapy may become necessary or appropriate. Readers are advised to check the most current information provided (i) on procedures featured or (ii) by the manufacturer of each product to be administered, to verify the recommended dose or formula, the method and duration of administration, and contraindications. It is the responsibility of the practitioner, relying on his or her experience and knowledge of the patient, to make diagnoses, to determine dosages and the best treatment for each individual patient, and to take all appropriate safety precautions. To the fullest extent of the law, neither the Publisher nor the Editor assumes any liability for any injury and/or damage to persons or property arising out of or related to any use of the material contained in this book.

The Publisher

Library of Congress Cataloging-in-Publication Data
Current therapy; latest approved methods of treatment for the practicing physician.
Editors: H. F. Conn and others
   v. 28 cm. annual
     ISBN 1-4160-3281-9
  1. Therapeutics.   2. Therapeutics, Surgical.   3. Medicine—Practice.
    I. Conn, Howard Franklin, 1908–1982 ed.

  RM101.C87   616.058   49–8328 rev*

Acquisitions Editor: Rolla Couchman
Developmental Editor: Heather Krehling
Publishing Services Manager: Frank Polizzano
Project Manager: Jeff Gunning
Design Direction: Karen O'Keefe-Owens

Printed in the United States of America

Last digit is the print number: 9 8 7 6 5 4 3 2 1

Contributors

Charles S. Abrams, MD
Associate Professor, University of Pennsylvania School of
Medicine; Staff Physician, Hospital of the University
of Pennsylvania, Philadelphia, Pennsylvania
Platelet-Mediated Bleeding Disorders

Mark J. Abzug, MD
Professor of Pediatrics (Infectious Diseases), University of
Colorado School of Medicine; Staff Pediatrician,
The Children's Hospital, Denver, Colorado
Viral Meningitis and Encephalitis

Tod C. Aeby, MD
Residency Program Director, Department of Obstetrics,
Gynecology, and Women's Health, University of Hawaii
John A. Burns School of Medicine, Honolulu, Hawaii
Uterine Leiomyomas

Marc E. Agronin, MD
Director of Mental Health Services, Miami Jewish Home
and Hospital for the Aged; Assistant Professor of Psychiatry,
Miller School of Medicine at the University of Miami,
Miami, Florida
Delirium

Carl M. Allen, DDS, MSD
Professor, Department of Oral Pathology, The Ohio State
University College of Dentistry; Director, Oral & Maxillofacial
Surgery and Pathology, University Hospital; Professor,
Department of Pathology, The Ohio State University College
of Medicine and Public Health, Columbus, Ohio
Diseases of the Mouth

Navin M. Amin, MD
Professor and Chairman, Department of Family
Medicine/Pediatrics, University of California, Irvine, School of
Medicine, Irvine; Associate Professor of Medicine, David Geffen
School of Medicine at UCLA, Los Angeles; Associate Professor
of Family Medicine, Stanford University School of Medicine,
Bakersfield, California
Infective Endocarditis

Robert J. Anderson, MD
Professor of Medicine, Creighton University School of
Medicine; Chief, Section of Endocrinology, Omaha Veterans
Affairs Medical Center, Omaha, Nebraska
Adrenocortical Insufficiency

Aydin Arici, MD
Professor, Department of Reproductive Endocrinology
and Infertility, Yale University School of Medicine,
New Haven, Connecticut
Dysfunctional Uterine Bleeding

Noel A. Armenakas, MD
Clinical Associate Professor, Department of Urology, Cornell
Weill Medical School; Attending Surgeon, Lenox Hill Hospital
and New York Presbyterian Hospital, New York, New York
Trauma to the Genitourinary Tract

Gopal H. Badlani, MD
Vice Chairman, Department of Urology, Long Island Jewish
Medical Center, New Hyde Park, New York
Benign Prostatic Hyperplasia

Adrianne Williams Bagley, MD
Clinical Associate, Johns Hopkins University School of
Medicine; Associate Staff, Johns Hopkins Hospital,
Baltimore, Maryland
Pelvic Inflammatory Disease

Ian M. Baird, MB, ChB
Clinical Associate Professor of Medicine, The Ohio State
University College of Medicine and Public Health; Senior
Attending Physician, Riverside Methodist Hospital,
Columbus, Ohio
Smallpox

David A. Baker, MD
Professor, Department of Obstetrics, Gynecology, and
Reproductive Medicine, State University of New York
at Stony Brook Health Sciences Center School of Medicine,
Stony Brook, New York
Vulvovaginitis

Robert A. Balk, MD
Director, Division of Pulmonary and Critical Care Medicine,
Rush University Medical Center; Rush Medical College,
Chicago, Illinois
Severe Sepsis and Septic Shock

David M. Bamberger, MD
Professor of Medicine and Vice-Chair of Educational Affairs,
Department of Medicine, University of Missouri–Kansas City
School of Medicine; Chief, Infectious Diseases Section,
Truman Medical Center, Kansas City, Missouri
Gonorrhea

Uriel S. Barzel, MD
Professor of Medicine, Albert Einstein College of Medicine
of Yeshiva University; Montefiore Medical Center, Bronx,
New York
Osteoporosis

Heidi M. Bauer, MD, MS, MPH
Chief, Office of Medical and Scientific Affairs, STD Control Branch, California Department of Health Services, Oakland, California
Nongonococcal Urethritis

David E. Beck, MD
Clinical Associate Professor of Surgery, F. Edward Hébert School of Medicine of the Uniformed Services University of the Health Sciences, Bethesda, Maryland; Chairman, Department of Colon and Rectal Surgery, Ochsner Clinic Foundation, New Orleans, Louisiana
Constipation

William S. Beckett, MD, MPH
Professor, Environmental Medicine and Medicine, University of Rochester School of Medicine and Dentistry, Rochester, New York
Silicosis and Asbestosis

Meg Begany, RD, CSP, LDN
Clinical Neonatal Dietitian, The Children's Hospital of Philadelphia, Philadelphia, Pennsylvania
Normal Infant Feeding

Nicholas P. Bell, MD
Clinical Assistant Professor, The University of Texas Medical School at Houston, Houston, Texas
Glaucoma

Pelayo C. Besa, MD
Radiation Oncology Head, Santiago, Chile
Hodgkin's Disease: Radiation Therapy

Karl R. Beutner, MD, PhD
Associate Clinical Professor of Dermatology, University of California, San Francisco, School of Medicine, San Francisco, California
Condyloma Acuminatum (Genital Warts)

Zulfiqar A. Bhutta, MB, BS, PhD
Husein Lalji Dewraj Professor of Pediatrics, Aga Khan University and Medical Center, Karachi, Pakistan
Typhoid Fever

Rodger L. Bick, MD, PhD
Clinical Professor of Medicine, University of Texas Southwestern Medical School, Dallas, Texas
Disseminated Intravascular Coagulation

Joseph Biederman, MD
Professor of Psychiatry, Harvard Medical School; Chief of Clinical and Research in Pediatric Psychopharmacology, Massachusetts General Hospital, Boston, Massachusetts
Attention Deficit Hyperactivity Disorder

John P. Bilezikian, MD
Professor of Medicine and Pharmacology, Columbia University College of Physicians and Surgeons; Attending Physician, New York–Presbyterian Hospital, New York, New York
Primary Hyperparathyroidism and Hypoparathyroidism

Jonathan Bond, MB, MRCPI
Specialist Registrar in Hematology, The Adelaide and Meath Hospital, Dublin, Ireland
Chronic Leukemias

William Z. Borer, MD
Professor, Department of Pathology, Jefferson Medical College at Thomas Jefferson University, Philadelphia, Pennsylvania
Reference Intervals for the Interpretation of Laboratory Tests

Patrick Borgen, MD
Chief, Breast Service, Department of Surgery, Memorial Sloan-Kettering Cancer Center, New York, New York
Diseases of the Breast

Harisios Boudoulas, MD, PhD
Professor of Medicine and Pharmacy Emeritus, The Ohio State University College of Medicine and Public Health, Columbus, Ohio; Director, Center of Clinical Research, Academy of Athens, Athens, Greece
Mitral Valve Prolapse: The Floppy Mitral Valve, Mitral Valve Prolapse, and Mitral Valvular Regurgitation

Louis-Philippe Boulet, MD
Professor of Medicine, Université Laval Faculty of Medicine; Pneumologist, Hôspital Laval, Quebec City, Quebec, Canada
Asthma in Adolescents and Adults

Kraig S. Bower, MD
Assistant Professor, Department of Surgery, F. Edward Hébert School of Medicine of the Uniformed Services University of the Health Sciences, Bethesda, Maryland; Director, Center for Refractive Surgery, Walter Reed Army Medical Center, Washington, DC
Vision Correction Procedures

Robert Bradsher, MD
Ebert Professor of Medicine, Director, Division of Infectious Diseases, Department of Internal Medicine, University of Arkansas for Medical Sciences; Director, Division of Infectious Diseases, Department of Medicine, Central Arkansas Veterans Healthcare System, Little Rock, Arkansas
Blastomycosis

Michael T. Brady, MD
Professor and Interim Chair, Department of Pediatrics, The Ohio State University College of Medicine and Public Health; Physician-in-Chief, Columbus Children's Hospital, Columbus, Ohio
Rubella and Congenital Rubella

Chad M. Braun, MD
Assistant Professor, Department of Family Medicine, University of Illinois at Chicago College of Medicine, Chicago, Illinois
Nausea and Vomiting

Maxime Breban, MD, PhD
Professor of Rheumatology, University Versailles-Saint-Quentin en Yvelines; Division of Rheumatology, Hospital Ambroise Paré, Boulogne-Billancourt, France
Ankylosing Spondylitis

Kenneth R. Bridges, MD
Founder, Joint Center for Sickle Cell and Thalassemic Disorders, Brigham and Women's Hospital; Associate Professor of Medicine, Partners in HealthCare, Harvard Medical School, Cambridge, Massachussetts
Management Issues in Sickle Cell Disease

Andrew R. Brown, MD
Clinical Instructor, Department of Internal Medicine and Fellow, Division of Gastroenterology, University of South Alabama, Mobile, Alabama
Irritable Bowel Syndrome

Richard L. Brown, MD, MPH
Associate Professor, Department of Family Medicine,
University of Wisconsin Medical School, Madison,
Wisconsin
Alcohol Use Disorders

J. James Bruno II, MD
Lenox Hill Hospital, New York, New York
Trauma to the Genitourinary Tract

John Brusch, MD
Assistant Professor of Medicine, Harvard Medical School,
Boston; Associate Chief of Medicine, Cambridge Health
Alliance, Cambridge, Massachusetts
Streptococcal Pharyngitis

Peter Buckley, MD
Professor of Psychiatry, Medical College of Georgia;
Staff Psychiatrist, MCG Medical Center, Augusta, Georgia
Schizophrenia

James J. Burke II, MD
Associate Professor of Obstetrics and Gynecology,
Mercer University School of Medicine–Savannah Campus;
Attending Physician, Memorial Health University Medical
Center, Savannah, Georgia
Endometrial Cancer

Kenneth D. Burman, MD
Chief, Endocrine Section, Washington Hospital Center;
Professor, Department of Medicine, Georgetown University
School of Medicine, Washington, DC
Hyperthyroidism

Kevin A. Bybee, MD
Assistant Professor of Medicine, University of Missouri–Kansas
City School of Medicine; Consulting Cardiologist;
Cardiovascular Consultants, P.A., at Mid-America Heart
Institute, Kansas City, Missouri
Acute Myocardial Infarction

John Byrne, MCH
Assistant Professor, The Vascular Group, Albany Medical
Center, Albany, New York
Acquired Diseases of the Aorta

Alexander Bystritsky, MD, PhD
Professor, Department of Psychiatry and Biobehavioral
Sciences, David Geffen School of Medicine at UCLA; Director,
Anxiety Disorders Program, Neuropsychiatric Institute and
Hospital, Los Angeles, California
Panic Disorder

Diego Cadavid, MD
Associate Professor, Department of Neurology and
Neuroscience, UMDNJ–New Jersey Medical School,
Newark, New Jersey
Relapsing Fever

Thomas R. Caraccio, PharmD
Associate Professor of Emergency Medicine, State University
of New York at Stony Brook Health Sciences Center School of
Medicine, Stony Brook; Assistant Professor of Pharmacology
and Toxicology, New York College of Osteopathic Medicine,
Old Westbury, New York
*Medical Toxicology: Ingestions, Inhalations, and Dermal and Ocular
Absorptions*

Enrique V. Carbajal, MD
Associate Clinical Professor of Medicine, University of
California, San Francisco, School of Medicine, San Francisco;
Staff Physician–Cardiology, Veterans Affairs Central California
Health Care System (VACCHCS), Fresno, California
Premature Beats

Serguei A. Castaneda, MD
Research Associate, Cancer Research Center, Boston University
School of Medicine, Boston, Massachusetts
Thalassemia

Daniel Cattran, MD
Senior Scientist, Division of Clinical Investigation and Human
Physiology, Toronto General Research Institute, Toronto,
Ontario, Canada
Primary Glomerular Disease

Frank R. Cerniglia, Jr., MD
Director of Pediatric Urology, Urologic Institute of
New Orleans, New Orleans, Louisiana
Childhood Enuresis

Santiago Chahwan, MD
Senior Vascular Surgery Resident, Jobst Vascular Center,
The Toledo Hospital, Toledo, Ohio
Venous Thrombosis

Sarah L. Chamlin, MD
Assistant Professor of Pediatrics and Dermatology,
Northwestern University Feinberg School of Medicine;
Staff Physician, Children's Memorial Hospital, Chicago, Illinois
Atopic Dermatitis

Miriam M. Chan, RPh, PharmD
Clinical Assistant Professor of Family Medicine, The Ohio
State University College of Medicine and Public Health, and
Clinical Assistant Professor of Pharmacy, The Ohio State
University College of Pharmacy, Columbus, Ohio; Adjunct
Assistant Professor of Pharmacy, Ohio Northern University,
Ada, Ohio, Affiliate Faculty of Pharmacy Pratice, Idaho State
University, Pocatello, Idaho; Director of Pharmacy Education,
Riverside Family Medicine Residency Program, Riverside
Family Practice Center, Riverside Methodist Hospital,
Columbus, Ohio
*Some Popular Herbs and Nutritional Supplements; New Drugs in 2005
and Agents Pending FDA Approval*

Ying Chan, MD
Attending Perinatologist, Englewood Hospital and Medical
Center, Englewood, New Jersey
Antepartum Care

Sam S. Chang, MD
Associate Professor of Urologic Surgery, Vanderbilt University
School of Medicine, Nashville, Tennessee
Malignant Tumors of the Urogenital Tract

Darren Chapman, MD
Resident, Urology, The Ohio State University College of
Medicine and Public Health, Columbus, Ohio
Epididymitis

Mahmoud Charif, MD
Transfusion Medicine Fellow, Hoxworth Blood Center,
University of Cincinnati Academic Health Center,
Cincinnati, Ohio
Therapeutic Use of Blood Components

Nadeem A. Chaudhary, MD
Staff Gastroenterologist, Regions Hospital/HealthPartners,
St. Paul, Minnesota
Malabsorption

Gary C. Chen, MD
Resident Physician of Internal Medicine, Cedars-Sinai
Medical Center, Los Angeles, California
Bleeding Esophageal Varices

R. Dale Childress, MD
Staff Physician, Division of Endocrinology and Metabolism,
Memphis Veterans Affairs Medical Center, Memphis,
Tennessee
Hyperosmolar Hyperglycemic Syndrome and Diabetic Ketoacidosis

Sandra Y. Cho, MD
Private Practice, Tarantino Eye Center, Glen Burnie, Maryland
Conjunctivitis

Stella T. Chou, MD
Clinical Instructor, University of Pennsylvania School of
Medicine; Attending Physician, The Children's Hospital of
Philadelphia, Philadelphia, Pennsylvania
Nonimmune Hemolytic Anemia

Julie Chuan, MD
Clinical Faculty, Department of Family and Preventive
Medicine, University of California, San Diego, School of
Medicine, San Diego; Staff Physician, Palomar Medical Center,
and Sports Medicine Physician, Neighborhood Healthcare
Clinic, Escondido, California
Common Sports Injuries

Claus-Frenz Claussen, MD
Professor Extraordinarius in Neuro-otology, Julius-Maximilaus
University Faculty of Medicine, Wuerzburg, Germany; Visiting
Professor, Charles University 3rd Medical Faculty, Prague,
Czechia; President, Neuro-otological Research Institute of 4GF,
Bad Kissingen, Germany; President, International Neuro-
otological and Equilibriometric Society (NES); Editor,
International Tinnitus Journal (ITJ)
Tinnitus

Harris R. Clearfield, MD
Professor of Medicine, Drexel University College of Medicine;
Section Chief, Gastroenterology, Hahnenann University
Hospital, Philadelphia, Pennsylvania
Diverticula of the Alimentary Tract

Donald Clemons, MD
Clinical Assistant Professor, Department of Family Practice,
Quillen School of Medicine, Johnson City, Tennessee
Premalignant Lesions

Keith K. Colburn, MD
Chief, Division of Rheumatology, Loma Linda University
Medical Center, Loma Linda, California
Bursitis, Tendinitis, Myofascial Pain, and Fibromyalgia

Anthony J. Comerota, MD
Adjunct Professor, University of Michigan Medical School,
Ann Arbor, Michigan; Director, Jobst Vascular Center,
The Toledo Hospital, Toledo, Ohio
Venous Thrombosis

Melanie W. Conway, MD
Assistant Professor, Department of Psychiatry, James H. Quillen
College of Medicine, East Tennessee State University, Johnson
City, Tennessee
Mood Disorders

Michael S. Cookson, MD
Associate Professor of Urologic Surgery, Vanderbilt University
School of Medicine, Nashville, Tennessee
Malignant Tumors of the Urogenital Tract

John F. Coyle II, MD
Clinical Professor, Department of Medicine, University of
Oklahoma College of Medicine–Tulsa, Tulsa, Oklahoma
Disturbances Caused by Heat

Gail Cresci, MD, RD
Assistant Professor of Surgery, Medical College of Georgia;
Director, Surgical Nutrition Service, MCG Medical Center,
Augusta, Georgia
Total Parenteral Nutrition in Adults

Nancy F. Crum-Cianflone, MD, MPH
Voluntary Assistant Professor, University of California,
San Diego, School of Medicine; Adjunct Professor, San Diego
State University College of Health and Human Services;
Staff Attending Physician in Infectious Diseases and Internal
Medicine, Naval Medical Center San Diego; HIV Research
Physician, Inservice AIDS Clinical Consortium, San Diego,
California
Coccidioidomycosis

Burke A. Cunha, MD
Professor of Medicine, State University of New York at Stony
Brook Health Sciences Center School of Medicine, Stony
Brook; Chief Infectious Disease Division, Winthrop-University
Hospital, Mineola, New York
Viral and Mycoplasmal Pneumonias; Urinary Tract Infections in Women

Stella Dantas, MD
Physician, Department of Obstetrics & Gynecology, Beaverton
Medical Office, Northwest Permanente PC, Physicians and
Surgeons, Beaverton, Oregon
Uterine Leiomyomas

Daniel F. Danzl, MD
Professor and Chair, Department of Emergency Medicine,
University of Louisville School of Medicine; Chair, Department
of Emergency Medicine, University of Louisville Hospital,
Louisville, Kentucky
Disturbances Caused by the Cold

R. Clement Darling III, MD
Professor of Surgery, Chief, Division of Vascular Surgery,
Albany Medical Center Hospital, The Vascular Group, PLLC,
Albany, New York
Acquired Diseases of the Aorta

Susan Davids, MD, MPH
Assistant Professor of Medicine, Medical College of Wisconsin;
Associate Program Director, Internal Medicine Residency,
Clement J. Zablocki Veterans Affairs Medical Center,
Milwaukee, Wisconsin
Acute Bronchitis

Susan A. Davidson, MD
Associate Professor, University of Colorado Health Sciences
Center School of Medicine; Chief, Gynecologic Oncology,
University of Colorado Hospital, Denver, Colorado
Neoplasms of the Vulva

Phillip J. DeChristopher, MD, PhD
Medical Director, Blood Bank/Transfusion Medicine, University
of Illinois–Chicago Medical Center, Chicago, Illinois
Adverse Effects of Blood Transfusion

Prakash C. Deedwania, MD
Professor of Medicine, University of California, San Francisco,
School of Medicine, San Francisco; Chief Cardiology Section,
Veterans Administration Central California Health Care
System, Fresno, California
Premature Beats

Albert A. Del Negro, MD
Clinical Assistant Professor of Medicine, Georgetown University
of School of Medicine, Washington, DC; Medical Director,
Cardiac Pacemaker Clinic, and Cardiac Electrophysiologist,
Inova Fairfax Hospital, Fairfax, Virginia
Heart Block

Alfred DeMaria, Jr. MD
Chief Medical Officer, State Epidemiologist, Center for
Laboratories and Disease Control, Massachusetts Department
of Public Health, Boston, Massachusetts
Giardiasis

Marie-France Demierre, MD
Associate Professor of Dermatology and Medicine, Boston
University School of Medicine; Director, Skin Oncology, Boston
Medical Center, Boston, Massachusetts
Cutaneous T Cell Lymphoma

Stephen R. Deputy, MD
Assistant Professor of Neurology, Louisiana State University
Health Sciences Center, Children's Hospital, New Orleans,
Louisiana
Traumatic Brain Injury in Children

Robert L. Deresiewicz, MD
Assistant Professor of Medicine, Harvard Medical School;
Associate Physician, Channing Laboratory and Infectious
Disease Division, Brigham and Women's Hospital, Boston,
Massachusetts
Toxic Shock Syndrome

Sarah E. Dick, MD
Senior Dermatology Resident, Hospital of the University
of Pennsylvania, Philadelphia, Pennsylvania
Bullous Diseases

Ram Dickman, MD
Research Fellow, Southern Arizona VA Health Care System,
Neuro-Enteric Clinical Research Group, Tucson, Arizona
Gaseousness and Indigestion

Pere Domingo, MD, PhD
Associate Professor of Medicine, Faculty of Medicine,
Autonomous University of Barcelona; Chairman, Department
of Internal Medicine, Hospital de la Santa Creu i Sant Pau,
Barcelona Spain
Q Fever

Alice N. Do, DO
Research Fellow, Solano Clinical Research, Division Dow
Pharmaceutical Sciences, Vallejo, California
Condyloma Acuminatum (Genital Warts)

Alan B. Douglass, MD
Assistant Director, Family Practice Residency Program,
Middlesex Hospital, Middletown, Connecticut
Pain

Douglas A. Drevets, MD, DTM&H
Associate Professor of Medicine, University of Oklahoma
School of Medicine; Staff Physician, Oklahoma City VA Medical
Center, Oklahoma City, Oklahoma
Plague

Andjela Drincic, MD
Assistant Professor of Medicine, Department of Medicine,
Endocrine Division,Creighton University School of Medicine;
Medical Director, Clinical Diabetes Program, Creighton
University Medical Center, Omaha, Nebraska
Adrenocortical Insufficiency

Lynne A. Eaton, MD, MS
Assistant Professor, Department of Obstetrics and Gynecology,
Division of Gynecologic Oncology, The Ohio State University
College of Medicine and Public Health; Staff Physician, James
Cancer Hospital and Solove Research Institute, Columbus, Ohio
Ovarian Cancer

Kamryn T. Eddy, MA
Doctoral Candidate, Boston University/Center for Anxiety
and Related Disorders, Boston, Massachusetts
Bulimia Nervosa

Libby Edwards, MD
Associate Clinical Professor of Dermatology, University of
North Carolina at Chapel Hill School of Medicine, Chapel Hill;
Chief, Division of Dermatology, Carolinas Medical Center and
Southeast Vulvar Clinic, Charlotte, North Carolina
Pruritus Ani and Vulvae

George E. Ehrlich, MD
Adjunct Professor, Department of Medicine, University of
Pennsylvania School of Medicine, Philadelphia, Pennsylvania;
Adjunct Professor of Clinical Medicine, New York University
School of Medicine, New York, New York
Osteoarthritis

Kimberly May Eickhorst, MD
Chief Resident, St. Lukes/Roosevelt Hospital, New York,
New York
Diseases of the Hair

Melto James Eliades, MD, MPH
Medical Epidemiologist, Division of Parasitic Diseases, Centers
for Disease Control and Prevention, Atlanta, Georgia
Malaria

Magda Elkabani, MD
Assistant Professor, Department of Hematology, University
of South Florida College of Medicine/Moffitt Cancer Center,
Tampa, Florida
Polycythemia Vera

C. Gregory Elliott, MD
Professor of Medicine, University of Utah School of Medicine;
Chief, Pulmonary and Critical Care Division, Los Hospital,
Salt Lake City, Utah
Pulmonary Embolism

Helen Enright, MD
Department of Haematology, Adelaide and Meath Hospitals, Tallaght, Dublin, Ireland
Chronic Leukemias

Per-Olaf Eriksson, DDS, PhD
Professor, Department of Odontology, Clinical Oral Physiology, Umeå University Faculty of Medicine, Umeå; Center for Musculoskeletal Research, Gävle University, Gävle and Umeå, Sweden
Cervico-Cranio-Mandibular Disorders

Chukwuemeka N. Etufugh, MD
Resident, Department of Pathology, Baylor University Medical Center, Dallas, Texas
Venous Stasis Ulcers

Ronnie Fass, MD
Professor of Medicine, University of Arizona School of Medicine; Director, GI Motility Laboratories, University of Arizona Health Sciences Center and Southern Arizona VA Health Care System, Tucson, Arizona
Gaseousness and Indigestion

Eve S. Ferdman, BA
Managing Editor, *Brachytherapy*, Memorial Sloan-Kettering Cancer Center, New York, New York
Brain Tumors

Jonathan F. Finks, MD
Assistant Professor of Surgery, University of Michigan Medical School, Ann Arbor, Michigan
Gastrointestinal Reflux Disease

L. Jaime Fitten, MDS
Professor of Psychiatry and Biobehavioral Sciences, David Geffen School of Medicine at UCLA; Director, Geriatric Psychiatry, Greater Los Angeles Veterans Administration, Sepulveda Campus, Los Angeles, California
Alzheimer's Disease

Adriana Foster, MD
Assistant Professor, Department of Psychiatry and Health Behavior, Medical College of Georgia; Staff Psychiatrist, MCG Medical Center, Augusta, Georgia
Schizophrenia

Melvin H. Freedman, MD
Professor Emeritus, Department of Pediatrics, University of Toronto Faculty of Medicine; Honorary Consultant, Hematology-Oncology; Senior Scientist Emeritus, Research Institute; and Chair, Reserarch Ethics Board (IRB), Hospital for Sick Children, Toronto, Ontario, Canada
Neutropenia

Liane K. Freels, MD, FAAP
Pediatrician, Columbia Pediatrics, Columbia, Tennessee
Rat-Bite Fever

Ellen W. Freeman, PhD
Research Professor, Department of Obstetrics/Gynecology and Department of Psychiatry, University of Pennsylvania School of Medicine, Philadelphia, Pennsylvania
Premenstrual Syndrome

Roger D. Freeman, MD
Clinical Professor Emeritus of Psychiatry and Associate Professor, Department of Pediatrics, University of British Columbia Faculty of Medicine, Vancouver, British Columbia, Canada
Gilles de la Tourette Syndrome

Faith Joy Frieden, MD
Director, Maternal-Fetal Medicine, Englewood Hospital and Medical Center, Englewood, New Jersey; Clinical Assistant Professor, Mount Sinai School of Medicine, New York, New York
Antepartum Care

Edward D. Frohlich, MD
Professor of Medicine and Physiology, Louisiana State University School of Medicine at New Orleans; Clinical Professor of Medicine and Adjunct Professor of Pharmacology, Tulane University School of Medicine; Alton Ochsner Distinguished Scientist, Ochsner Clinic Foundation New Orleans, Louisiana
Hypertension

Maisie M. Fung, MD
Attending Physician, Camino Medical Group, Sunnyvale, California
Peripheral Arterial Disease

Steven L. Galetta, MD
Ruth Wagner Van Meter and Ray Van Meter Professor of Neurology, University of Pennsylvania School of Medicine, Philadelphia, Pennsylvania
Optic Neuritis

R. Michael Gallagher, DO
Professor, Department of Family Medicine, University of Medicine and Dentistry of New Jersey, School of Osteopathic Medicine, Stratford, New Jersey
Headache

Donald G. Gallup, MD
Professor and Chairperson, Department of Obstetrics and Gynecology, Mercer University School of Medicine, Macon; Attending Physician, Memorial Health University Medical Center, Savannah, Georgia
Endometrial Cancer

Michael Thomas Gambla, MD
Urology Surgeon, Riverside Methodist Hospital; Urology Surgeons, Inc., Columbus, Ohio
Epididymitis

Bruce J. Gantz, MD
Professor of Otolaryngology, The University of Iowa Roy J. and Lucille A. Carver College of Medicine; Head, Department of Otolaryngology–Head and Neck Surgery, University of Iowa Hospitals and Clinics, Iowa City, Iowa
Acute Facial Paralysis (Bell's Palsy)

Juan Armando Garcia, MD
Staff-Intensivist, Cardiovascular ICU, The Methodist Hospital, Houston, Texas
Management of Chronic Obstructive Pulmonary Disease

James M. Gebel, Jr., MD
Medical Director, Jewish Hospital Emergency Stroke Center, Louisville, Kentucky
Intracerebral Hemorrhage

Roger L. Gebhard, MD
Professor of Medicine and Gastroenterology Training Program
Director, University of Minnesota Medical School, Minneapolis;
Staff Gastroenterologist, Regions Hospital/HealthPartners,
St. Paul, Minnesota
Malabsorption

Christopher S. George, MD
Attending Physician, Department of Hematology and Medical
Oncology, Riverside Methodist Hospital, Columbus, Ohio
Primary Lung Cancer

James N. George, MD
George Lynn Cross Professor of Medicine, University of
Oklahoma College of Medicine; Hematology-Oncology Section,
Department of Medicine, University of Oklahoma Health
Sciences Center, Oklahoma City, Oklahoma
Thrombotic Thrombocytopenic Purpura

Teresa M. George, MD
Assistant Program Director, Internal Medicine Residency
Program, Riverside Methodist Hospital, Columbus, Ohio
Primary Lung Cancer

Katherine G. Gerges, MS, CNP
Clinical Nurse Practitioner, Department of Family Medicine,
The Ohio State University, Columbus, Ohio
Travel Medicine

David B. K. Golden, MD
Associate Professor of Medicine, Johns Hopkins University
School of Medicine; Director, Allergy-Immunology, Sinai
Hospital, Baltimore, Maryland
Allergic Reactions to Insect Stings

Nora Goldschlager, MD
Professor of Clinical Medicine, University of California, San
Francisco; Co-Director, Division of Cardiology, San Francisco
General Hospital; Director, Coronary Care Unit, ECG
Laboratory and Pacemaker Clinic, San Francisco General
Hospital, San Francisco, California
Tachycardias

Michael H. Goldstein, MD
Assistant Professor of Ophthalmology, Tufts University School
of Medicine; Attending Surgeon, Cornea, Cataract, Refractive
Service, Tufts-New England Medical Center, Boston,
Massachusetts
Conjunctivitis

Monica Peterson Gordon, MD
Geriatric Psychiatry Fellow, David Geffen School of Medicine at
UCLA, Los Angeles, California
Alzheimer's Disease

E. Ann Gormley, MD
Professor of Surgery (Urology), Dartmouth Medical School;
Staff Urologist, Dartmouth-Hitchcock Medical Center,
Lebanon, New Hampshire
Urinary Incontinence

John E. Gough, MD, FACEP
Professor, Department of Emergency Medicine, East Carolina
University; Attending Physician, Emergency Department, Pitt
County Memorial Hospital, Greenville, North Carolina
Marine Trauma, Envenomations, and Intoxications

Marina Grandis, MD
Neurologist, Department of Neurosciences, Ophthalmology,
and Genetics, University of Genoa, Genoa, Italy
Peripheral Neuropathies

Mark A. Granner, MD
Associate Professor of Neurology, University of Iowa Carver
College of Medicine; Director, Iowa Comprehensive Epilepsy
Program, University of Iowa Hospitals and Clinics, Iowa City, Iowa
Seizures and Epilepsy in Adolescents and Adults

Joseph Greensher, MD
Professor of Pediatrics, State University of New York at Stony
Brook Health Sciences Center School of Medicine, Stony
Brook; Medical Director and Associate Chair, Department of
Pediatrics, Long Island Regional Poison and Drug Information
Center, Winthrop-University Hospital, Mineola, New York
*Medical Toxicology: Ingestions, Inhalations, and Dermal and Ocular
Absorptions*

Charles Grose, MD
Professor of Pediatrics, The University of Iowa Roy J. and
Lucille A. Carver College of Medicine; Director of Infectious
Diseases Division, Children's Hospital of Iowa, Iowa City, Iowa
Varicella (Chickenpox)

Hans W. Grünwald, MD
Associate Professor of Medicine, Division of Hematology-
Oncology, Department of Medicine, Mount Sinai School of
Medicine, New York; Attending Physician, Division of
Hematology-Oncology, Department of Medicine, Queens
Hospital Center, Jamaica, New York
Acute Leukemia in Adults

Joan Guitart, MD
Associate Professor of Dermatology and Pathology,
Northwestern University Feinberg School of Medicine, Chicago,
Illinois
Nevi

Abdo Haddad, MD
Fellow, Hematology and Medical Oncology, Cleveland Clinic
Foundation, Cleveland, Ohio
Aplastic Anemia

Frank G. Haluska, MD, Ph D
Tufts University School of Medicine; Deputy Director and
Clinical Director, Cancer Center, Tufts-New England Medical
Center, Boston, Massachusetts
Melanoma

Kerry Hammond, MD
Clinical Fellow, Department of Colon and Rectal Surgery,
Ochsner Clinic Foundation, New Orleans, Louisiana
Hemorrhoids, Anal Fissure, Perianal Abscess, and Fistula

Rashidul Haque, MB, PhD
Scientist, Laboratory Sciences Division, International Centre
for Diarrhoeal Disease Research, Bangladesh (ICDDR, B),
Dhaka, Bangladesh
Amebiasis

Rachel Haroz, MD
Assistant Professor of Emergency Medicine, University of
Medicine and Dentistry, New Jersey; Attending Physician,
Department of Emergency Medicine, Cooper University
Hospital, Camden, New Jersey
Spider Bites and Scorpion Stings

E. John Harris, Jr., MD
Professor of Surgery, Division of Vascular Surgery, Stanford
University School of Medicine, Stanford, Calfornia
Peripheral Arterial Disease

Adelaide A. Hebert, MD
Professor, Department of Dermatology, The University of Texas
Medical School at Houston, Houston, Texas
Fungal Diseases of the Skin

Nicholas J. Hegarty, MD, FRCS
Endourology Research Fellow, Glickman Urological Institute,
The Cleveland Clinic Foundation, Cleveland, Ohio
Renal Calculi

William Henderson, MD
Clinical Assistant Professor, University of British Columbia
Faculty of Medicine, Vancouver; Attending Physician, Royal
Columbia Hospital, New Westminister, British Columbia,
Canada
Acute Respiratory Failure

David B. Herzog, MD
Professor of Psychiatry (Pediatrics), Harvard Medical School,
Cambridge; Director, Eating Disorders Unit—Child Psychiatry
Service, and Director, Harris Center for Education and
Advocacy in Eating Disorders, Massachusetts General Hospital,
Boston, Massachusetts
Bulimia Nervosa

Camile Hexsel, MD
Research Fellow, Department of Dermatology, Henry Ford
Hospital, Detroit, Michigan
Sunburn

David G. Hill, MD
Waterbury Pulmonary Associates, Waterbury, Connecticut;
Yale University School of Medicine, New Haven, Connecticut
Cough

Brian D. Hoit, MD
Professor of Medicine, Physiology and Biophysics, Case School
of Medicine; Director, Echocardiography, University Hospitals
of Cleveland, Cleveland, Ohio
Pericarditis

Richard H. Hongo, MD
Cardiac Electrophysiologist, California Pacific Medical Center,
San Francisco, California
Tachycarditis

A. A. Hoosen, MSc, MB, ChB, MMed, FC Path
Professor and Head of Department, Department of
Microbiological Pathology, University of Limpopo Faculty of
Medicine, Medunsa Campus, Pretoria, South Africa
Granuloma Inguinale (Donovanosis) and Lymphogranuloma Venereum

Michael P. Hopkins, MD, MEd
Professor and Chair, Department of Obstetrics and Gynecology,
Northeastern Ohio Universities College of Medicine,
Rootstown; Director, Department of Obstetrics and
Gynecology, Aultman Health Foundation, Canton, Ohio
Cancer of the Uterine Cervix

Tamara Salam Housman, MD
Procedural Dermatology/Mohs Micrographic Surgery Fellow,
Dermatologic Surgery, University of Washington Medical
Center, Seattle, Washington
Warts (Verrucae)

Scott A. Hundahl, MD, FACS, FSSO, FAHNS
Professor of Clinical Surgery, University of California at Davis,
Davis; Chief of Surgery, Veterans Administration Northern
California Health Care System, Sacramento VA Medical Center,
Sacramento, California
Tumors of the Stomach

John G. Hunter, MD
Professor and Chairman, Department of Surgery, Oregon Health
& Science University School of Medicine, Portland, Oregon
Gastroesophageal Reflux Disease

Matilde Iorizzo, MD
Department of Dermatology, University of Bologna,
Bologna, Italy
Diseases of the Nails

Alan C. Jackson, MD, FRCPC
Professor of Medicine (Neurology) and Microbiology and
Immunology, Queen's University; Attending Staff, Kingston
General Hospital, Kingston, Ontario, Canada
Rabies

Robert M. Jacobson, MD
Professor of Pediatrics, Mayo Clinic College of Medicine; Chair,
Department of Pediatrics and Adolescent Medicine,
Mayo Clinic, Rochester, Minnesota
Office-Based Immunization Practices

James J. James, MD, DrPH, MHA
Director, Center for Disaster Preparedness and Emergency
Response, American Medical Association, Chicago, Illinois
*Toxic Chemical Agents Reference Chart: Symptoms and Treatment;
Biologic Agents Reference Chart: Symptoms, Tests, and Treatment*

Stephen G. Jenkinson, MD
Chief, Pulmonary Diseases Section, Audie Murphy VA
Medical Center, San Antonio, Texas
Management of Chronic Obstructive Pulmonary Disease

Gordon L. Jensen, MD, PhD
Director, Vanderbilt Center for Human Nutrition; Professor of
Medicine, Vanderbilt University Medical Center, Nashville,
Tennessee
Obesity

Candice E. Johnson, MD, PhD
Clinical Professor of Pediatrics, University of Colorado Health
Sciences Center School of Medicine; Volunteer Faculty, The
Children's Hospital, Denver, Colorado
Bacterial Infections of the Urinary Tract in Girls

Joseph L. Jorizzo, MD
Professor, Founding and Former Chair, Department of
Dermatology, Wake Forest University School of Medicine,
Winston-Salem, North Carolina
Cutaneous Vasculitis

Marc A. Judson, MD
Professor of Medicine, Division of Pulmonary and Critical Care
Medicine, Medical University of South Carolina, Charleston,
South Carolina
Sarcoidosis

Rome Jutabha, MD
Associate Professor of Medicine, David Geffen School of
Medicine at UCLA; Director, UCLA Center for Small Bowel
Diseases, UCLA Medical Center, Los Angeles, California
Bleeding Esophageal Varices

Tamilarasu Kadhiravan, MD
Senior Resident, Department of Medicine, All India Institute of Medical Sciences, New Delhi, India
Management of the Patient with HIV Disease

Matthew Karlovsky, MD
Staff Urologist (Voiding Dysfunction/Female Urology), Private Practice, Center for Urological Services, P.C., Phoenix, Arizona
Benign Prostatic Hyperplasia

Andreas Katsambas, MD, PhD
Professor and Chairman, 1st Department of Dermatology, University of Athens School of Medicine; Attending Physician, "Andreas Sygros" Hospital for Skin and Venereal Diseases, Athens, Greece
Parasitic Diseases of the Skin

David E. Katz, MD
Medical Director, Medical Affairs, Cubist Pharmaceuticals, Lexington, Massachusetts
Giardiasis

Andrew M. Kaunitz, MD
Professor, Department of Obstetrics and Gynecology, University of Florida College of Medicine, Jacksonville, Florida
Contraceptive Methods

Sean Keenan, MD
Clinical Assistant Professor of Medicine, University of British Columbia Faculty of Medicine, Vancouver; Head, Department of Critical Care Medicine, Royal Columbian Hospital, New Westminister, British Columbia, Canada
Acute Respiratory Failure

Jennifer Kelly, DO
Assistant Professor of Medicine, Division of Endocrinology, SUNY Upstate Medical University, Syracuse, New York
Diabetes Insipidus

Stephen F. Kemp, MD
Associate Professor of Medicine and Assistant Professor of Pediatrics, University of Mississippi School of Medicine; Director, Allergy and Immunology Fellowship Program, University of Mississippi Medical Center, Jackson, Mississippi
Anaphylaxis and Serum Sickness

James W. Kendig, MD
Professor of Pediatrics, Pennsylvania State University School of Medicine; Staff Pediatrician, Division of Newborn Medicine, Penn State Children's Hospital, Hershey, Pennsylvania
Hemolytic Disease of the Newborn

Ramesh K. Khurana, MD, FAAN
Chief of Neurology, Union Memorial Hospital, Baltimore, Maryland
Tetanus

Craig S. Kitchens, MD
Professor of Medicine, University of Florida College of Medicine; Associate Chief of Staff for Education, Malcolm Randall VA Medical Center, Gainesville, Florida
Snake Bite

Ira W. Klimbere, MD
Medical Director and Staff Physician, Florida Healthcare Research, Urology Center of Florida, Ocala, Florida
Prostatitis

Debra G. Koivunen, MD
Associate Professor of Surgery and Program Director, General Surgery Residency, University of Missouri–Columbia School of Medicine, Columbia, Missouri
Thyroid Cancer

Luciano Kolodny, MD
Endocrinologist, HealthPartners Medical Group, Woodbury, Minnesota
Erectile Dysfunction

Gerald B. Kolski, MD, PhD, FAAAAI, FAAP
Clinical Professor of Pediatrics, Temple University School of Medicine; Adjunct Clinical Professor of Pediatrics, Drexel University School of Medicine, Philadelphia; Chairman, Department of Pediatrics, Crozer Chester Medical Center, Upland, Pennsylvania
Asthma in Children

John Koo, MD
Professor and Vice Chairman, Department of Dermatology, University of California, San Francisco, School of Medicine; Director, UCSF Psoriasis Treatment Center, Phototheraphy Unit and Clinical Research Unit, University of California San Francisco Medical Center, San Francisco, California
Papulosquamous Disorders

Stephen L. Kopecky, MD
Professor of Medicine, Mayo Clinic College of Medicine, Rochester, Minnesota
Acute Myocardial Infarction

Katalin I. Koranyi, MD
Professor of Clinical Pediatrics, Department of Pediatrics, The Ohio State University College of Medicine and Public Health; Pediatrician, Columbus Children's Hospital, Columbus, Ohio
Measles (Rubeola)

Milind J. Kothari, DO
Professor of Neurology and Vice Chair of Education and Training, Pennsylvania State College of Medicine, Hershey, Pennsylvania
Myasthenia Gravis and Related Disorders

Carl A. Krantz, Jr., MD
Associate Program Director, Riverside Methodist Hospital; Clinical Assistant Professor, The Ohio State University College of Medicine and Public Health, Worthington, Ohio
Amenorrhea

Jeffrey A. Kraut, MD
Chief of Dialysis, Veterans Affairs Greater Los Angeles Healthcare System; Professor of Medicine, David Geffen School of Medicine at UCLA, Los Angeles, California
Chronic Renal Failure

Leonard R. Krilov, MD
Professor of Pediatrics, State University of New York at Stony Brook Health Sciences Center School of Medicine, Stony Brook; Chief, Pediatric Infectious Disease, and Vice-Chairman of Pediatrics, Winthrop-University Hospital, Mineola, New York
Infectious Mononucleosis

Paul Y. Kwo, MD
Associate Professor of Medicine, Division of Gastroenterology/Hepatology, Indiana University School of Medicine, Indianapolis, Indiana
Cirrhosis

Robert A. Kyle, MD
Professor of Medicine and Laboratory Medicine and Pathology,
Mayo Clinic College of Medicine, Rochester, Minnesota
Multiple Myeloma

Lori M.B. Laffel, MD, MPH
Associate Professor of Pediatrics, Harvard Medical School;
Chief, Pediatric, Adolescent, and Young Adult Section, and
Investigator, Section on Genetics and Epidemiology, Joslin
Diabetes Center, Boston, Massachusetts
Diabetes Mellitus in Children and Adolescents

Christopher J. Lahart, MD
Associate Medical Director, Hepatitis and Oncology, Gilead
Sciences, Inc., Foster City, California
Tuberculosis and Other Mycobacterial Diseases

Gabriella Lakos, MD, PhD
Associate Professor, University of Debrecen, Debrecen,
Hungary
Connective Tissue Disorders

Charles R. Lambert, MD, PhD
Dr. Kiran Patel Research Institute Professor of Medicine,
University of South Florida College of Medicine; Medical
Director, Pepin Heart Hospital, Tampa, Florida
Angina Pectoris

Paul R. Lambert, MD
Professor and Chairman, Department of Otolaryngology,
Medical University of South Carolina, Charleston, South Carolina
Ménière's Disease

Barbara A. Latenser, MD
Clara L. Smith Professor of Burn Treatment, Department of
Surgery, The University of Iowa Roy J. and Lucille A. Carver
College of Medicine; Director, Burn Treatment Center,
University of Iowa Hospitals and Clinics, Iowa City, Iowa
Burn Treatment Guidelines

Luca Lazzarini, MD
Department of Infectious Diseases and Tropical Medicine, San
Bortolo Hospital, Vicenza, Italy
Osteomyelitis

Andrew G. Lee, MD
Professor of Opthalmology, Neurology, and Neurosurgery, The
University of Iowa Roy J. and Lucille A. Carver College of
Medicine, Iowa City, Iowa
Optic Neuritis

Chai Sue Lee, MD
Assistant Professor, Department of Dermatology, University of
California, Davis, School of Medicine, Davis; Director, Psoriasis
and Phototherapy Treatment Center, UC Davis Medical Center,
Sacramento, California
Papulosquamous Disorders

Jason T. Lee, MD
Assistant Professor of Surgery, Division of Vascular Surgery,
Stanford University School of Medicine, Stanford, California
Peripheral Arterial Disease

Teofilo Lee-Chiong, Jr., MD
Associate Professor, University of Colorado Health Sciences
Center School of Medicine; Head, Section of Sleep Medicine,
National Jewish Medical and Research Center, Denver,
Colorado
Sleep Apnea

Julie Leegwater-Kim, MD, PhD
Fellow in Movement Disorders, Columbia University Medical
Center, Department of Neurology, New York, New York
Parkinsonism

Jacques W. M. Lenders, MD, PhD
Associate Professor of Vascular Medicine, Department of
Medicine, Division of Internal Medicine, Radboud University
Medical Center, Nijmegen, The Netherlands,
Pheochromocytoma

Norman Levine, MD (Retired)
Tucson, Arizona
Pigmentary Disorders

Eyal Levit, MD
Assistant Clinical Professor of Dermatology, Columbia
University College of Physicians and Surgeons; Director
of Dermatologic and Cosmetic Surgery, St. Lukes Hospital;
Director, Procedural Dermatology Fellowship, New York–
Presbyterian Hospital and St. Lukes/Roosevelt Hospital,
New York, New York
Diseases of the Hair

Phillip L. Lieberman, MD
Clinical Professor of Medicine and Pediatrics, Departments
of Internal Medicine and Pediatrics (Divisions of Allergy and
Immunology), University of Tennessee College of Medicine;
University of Tennessee Allergy and Asthma Care, Memphis,
Tennessee
Nonallergic Rhinitis

Henry W. Lim, MD
Chairman and Clarence S. Livingood Chair, Department of
Dermatology, Henry Ford Hospital, Detroit, Michigan
Sunburn

Gary H. Lipscomb, MD
Professor and Vice Chairman, University of Tennessee College
of Medicine; Director, Division of Gynecologic Specialties,
University of Tennessee Health Science Center, Memphis,
Tennessee
Ectopic Pregnancy

James A. Litch, MD, DTMH
Clinical Assistant Professor, University of Washington School of
Medicine and School of Public Health, Seattle, Washington
High-Altitude Illness

Virginia Litle, MD
Assistant Professor of Surgery, Mount Sinai School of Medicine;
Assistant Attending, Department of CT Surgery, Mount Sinai
Medical Center, New York, New York
Primary Lung Abscess

Dan L. Longo, MD
Scientific Director, National Institute on Aging, National
Institutes of Health, Baltimore, Maryland
Pernicious Anemia and Other Megaloblastic Anemias

Jonathan S. Lopresti, MD, PhD
Associate Professor of Clinical Medicine, Keck School of
Medicine at USC; Attending Physician, LAC/USC Medical
Center, Los Angeles, California
Hypothyroidism

Jacqueline M. Losi-Sasaki, MD
Chief Resident, Division of Dermatology, Department of
Medicine, University of Texas Health Science Center at
San Antonio, San Antonio, Texas
Viral Diseases of the Skin

Anthony A. Luciano, MD
Professor of Obstetrics and Gynecology, University of
Connecticut School of Medicine, Farmington; Director,
Center for Fertility and Women's Health,
New Britain, Connecticut
Hyperprolactinemia

Danielle E. Luciano, MD
Department of Obstetrics and Gynecology, University of
Connecticut School of Medicine, Farmington; Center for
Fertility in Women's Health, New Britain, Connecticut
Hyperprolactinemia

James M. Lyznicki, MS, MPH
Senior Scientist, Center for Disaster Preparedness and
Emergency Response, American Medical Association,
Chicago, Illinois
Toxic Chemical Agents Reference Chart: Symptoms and Treatment;
Biologic Agents Reference Chart: Symptoms, Tests, and Treatment

Jaroslaw P. Maciejewski, MD, PhD
Staff, Hematologic Oncology and Blood Disorders, Section
Head, Experimental Hematology and Hematopoiesis,
Associate Professor, Cleveland Clinic Lerner College of
Medicine, Cleveland, Ohio
Aplastic Anemia

Kelly Maloney, MD
University of Colorado Health Sciences Center School of
Medicine; The Children's Hospital, Denver, Colorado
Acute Leukemia in Children

Massimo Mannelli, MD
Full Professor in Endocrinology, University of Florence,
Florence, Italy
Pheochromocytoma

Woraphong Manuskiatti, MD
Associate Professor, Mahidol University School of Medicine;
Laser and Cutaneous Surgery Division, Department of
Dermatology, Siriraj Hospital, Bangkok, Thailand
Keloids

Susan M. Manzi, MD, MPH
Associate Professor of Medicine, University of Pittsburgh
School of Medicine, Pittsburgh, Pennsylvania
Connective Tissue Disorders

David A. Margolin MD
Director of Colon and Rectal Research, Department of Colon
and Rectal Surgery, Ochsner Clinic Foundation, New Orleans,
Louisiana
Hemorrhoids, Anal Fissure, Perianal Abscess, and Fistula

Ali J. Marian, MD
Associate Professor of Medicine, Baylor College of Medicine;
Staff Physician, The Methodist Hospital; Professional Staff,
St. Luke's Episcopal Hospital/Texas Heart Institute,
Houston, Texas
Hypertrophic Cardiomyopathy

Barry J. Marshall, MD
Clinical Professor, University of Western Australia; Senior
Principal Research Fellow, Sir Charles Gardner Hospital,
Nedlands, Western Australia, Australia
Gastritis and Peptic Ulcer Disease

Robert Martindale, MD, PhD
Chief, Gastrointestinal Surgery, MCG Medical Center;
Professor of Surgery, Medical College of Georgia,
Augusta, Georgia
Total Parenteral Nutrition in Adults

Pierre Marty, MD, PhD
Professor of Parasitology–Mycology, University of Nice–Sophia
Antipolis Faculty of Medicine; Staff Physician, Centre
Hospitalier L'Archet and Centre Hospitalier Universitaire
de Nice, Nice, France
Visceral Leishmaniasis

Maria Mascarenhas, MBBS
Associate Professor of Pediatrics, University of Pennsylvania
School of Medicine; Section Chief, Nutrition Division of
Gastroenterology and Nutrition; Director, Nutrition Support
Service, The Children's Hospital of Philadelphia, Pennsylvania
Normal Infant Feeding

Wissam E. Mattar, MD
Indiana University School of Medicine, Indianapolis, Indiana
Cirrhosis

Martin J. McCaffrey, MD
Director, Neonatal Intensive Care Unit, Naval Medical Center;
Specialty Advisor to the Navy Surgeon General for
Neonatology, San Diego, California
Resuscitation of the Newborn

Carol F. McCammon, MD
Assistant Professor, Department of Emergency Medicine,
Eastern Virginia Medical School, Virginia Beach, Virginia
Acute Pyelonephritis

Kurt A. McCammon, MD
Assistant Professor of Urology, Eastern Virginia Medical
School, Virginia Beach, Virginia
Acute Pyelonephritis

Michael T. McCann, MD
Clinical Assistant Professor, Baylor College of Medicine,
Houston, Texas
Spine Pain

Laura J. McCloskey, PhD
Clinical Assistant Professor of Pathology, Anatomy, and Cell
Biology, Jefferson Medical College of Thomas Jefferson
University; Associate Director of Clinical Laboratories, Director
of Clinical Immunology Laboratory, and Director of JHN
Laboratory, Thomas Jefferson University Hospital, Philadelphia,
Pennsylvania
Reference Intervals for the Interpretation of Laboratory Tests

Jacqueline Carinhas McGregor, MD
Director, Baylor Child Psychiatry Clinic; Associate Professor,
Menninger Department of Psychiatry and Behavioral Sciences,
Baylor College of Medicine, Houston, Texas
Anxiety Disorders

Michael McGuigan, MD
Medical Director, Long Island Regional Poison and Drug Information Center, Winthrop-University Hospital, Mineola, New York
Medical Toxicology: Ingestions, Inhalations, and Dermal and Ocular Absorptions

Dilcia McLenan, MD
Assistant Professor of Pediatrics, Baylor College of Medicine, Pearland, Texas
Care of the High-Risk Neonate

William S. McMahon, MD
Director, Pediatric Cardiac Catheterization Laboratory, Associate Professor of Pediatrics, Department of Pediatric Cardiology, University of Alabama-Birmingham, Birmingham, Alabama
Congenital Heart Disease

J. Scott McMurray, MD
Associate Professor, University of Wisconsin School of Medicine and Public Health, Madison, Wisconsin
Otitis Media

Donald McNeil, MD
Associate Professor of Clinical Medicine, Department of Immunology, The Ohio State University College of Medicine and Public Health, Columbus, Ohio
Allergic Reactions to Drugs

Anupama Menon, MD, MPH
Assistant Professor of Medicine, Department of Medicine, Division of Infectious Diseases, University of Arkansas for Medical Science; Assistant Professor of Medicine, Central Arkansas Veterans Healthcare System, Little Rock, Arkansas
Blastomycosis

Ted A. Meyer, MD, PhD
Assistant Professor, Department of Otolaryngology, Medical University of South Carolina, Charleston, South Carolina
Ménière's Disease; Acute Facial Paralysis (Bell's Palsy)

Maria D. Mileno, MD
Associate Professor of Medicine, Brown Medical School; Director, Travel Medicine Service, The Miriam Hospital, Providence, Rhode Island
Intestinal Parasites

Merry N. Miller, MD
Professor and Chair, Department of Psychiatry and Behavioral Sciences, James H. Quillen College of Medicine, East Tennessee State University, Johnson City, Tennessee
Mood Disorders

Paul D. Miller, MD
Distinguished Clinical Professor of Medicine, University of Colorado Health Sciences Center; Medical Director, Colorado Center for Bone Research, Lakewood, Colorado
Paget's Disease of Bone

Ayesha Mirza, MD
Assistant Professor, Department of Pediatric Infectious Diseases and Immunology, University of Florida; Pediatric Infectious Diseases and Immunology, Wolfson Children's Hospital and Shands Hospital, Jacksonville, Florida
Mumps

Shirwan A. Mirza, MD
Clinical Assistant Professor of Medicine, State University of New York Upstate Medical University College of Medicine, Syracuse; Chairman, Department of Medicine, Auburn Memorial Hospital, Auburn, New York
Diabetes Mellitus in Adults

William F. Miser, MD, MA
Associate Professor of Family Medicine, Department of Family Medicine, The Ohio State University College of Medicine, Columbus, Ohio
Travel Medicine

Howard C. Mofenson, MD
Professor of Pediatrics and Emergency Medicine, State University of New York at Stony Brook Health Sciences Center School of Medicine, Stony Brook; Professor of Pharmacology and Toxicology, New York College of Osteopathic Medicine, Old Westbury, New York
Medical Toxicology: Ingestions, Inhalations, and Dermal and Ocular Absorptions

Alladi Mohan, MD
Adjunct Professor, Department of Medicine, Sri Venkateswara Institute of Medical Sciences, Andhra Pradesh, India
Viral Upper Respiratory Tract Infections

Robert M. Moldwin, MD
Assistant Professort of Urology, Albert Einstein College of Medicine of Yeshiva University, Bronx; Director, Interstitial Cystitis Center, North Shore–Long Island Jewish Health Care System, New Hyde Park, New York
Bacterial Infections of the Urinary Tract in Males

Mark E. Molitch, MD
Professor of Medicine, Division of Endocrinology, Metabolism and Molecular Medicine, Northwestern University Feinberg School of Medicine; Attending Physician, Northwestern Memorial Hospital, Chicago, Illinois
Acromegaly

Eugene W. Monroe, MD
Assistant Clinical Professor of Dermatology, Medical College of Wisconsin; Advanced Healthcare, Milwaukee, Wisconsin
Urticaria and Angioedema

Angela Yen Moore, MD
Arlington Center for Dermatology, Arlington, Texas
Viral Diseases of the Skin

Terry L. Moore, MD
Professor of Internal Medicine, Pediatrics, and Molecular Microbiology and Immunology, Saint Louis University School of Medicine; Director, Division of Pediatric Rheumatology and Adult Rheumatology, Saint Louis University Medical Center, St. Louis, Missouri
Juvenile Idiopathic Arthritis

Arnold M. Moses, MD
Professor of Medicine, State University of New York Upstate Medical University College of Medicine; Attending Physician, University Hospital, Syracuse, New York
Diabetes Insipidus

Alan C. Moss, MD
Instructor, Harvard Medical School; Fellow in Gastroentrology, Beth Israel Deaconess Medical Center, Boston, Massachusetts
Inflammatory Bowel Disease

Kugathasan Mutalithas, MRCP
Medical Registrar, Department of Respiratory Medicine, Manchester Royal Infirmary, Manchester, United Kingdom
Psittacosis

Ashwatha Narayana, MD
Assistant Professor, Department of Radiation Oncology, Memorial Sloan-Kettering Cancer Center, New York, New York
Brain Tumors

Lisa R. Nash, DO
Assistant Professor, Department of Family Medicine, The University of Texas Medical Branch School of Medicine, Galveston, Texas
Postpartum Care

Laeth S. Nasir, MBBS
Professor, Department of Family Medicine, University of Nebraska College of Medicine; Staff Physician, University of Nebraska Medical Center, Omaha, Nebraska
Dysmenorrhea

David N. Neubauer, MD
Assistant Professor, Johns Hopkins University School of Medicine; Associate Director, Johns Hopkins Sleep Disorders Center, Baltimore, Maryland
Sleep Disorders

Ronald Lee Nichols, MD
William Henderson Professor of Surgery–Emeritus and Professor of Microbiology and Immunology, Tulane University School of Medicine, New Orleans, Louisiana
Bacterial Diseases of the Skin

Electra Nicolaidou, MD, PhD
Lecturer in Dermatology, 1st Department of Dermatology, University of Athens School of Medicine; Lecturer in Dermatology, "Andreas Sygros" Hospital for Skin and Venereal Diseases, Athens, Greece
Parasitic Diseases of the Skin

John T. Nicoloff, MD
Professor of Medicine and Senior Associate Chair for Research, Department of Medicine, Keck School of Medicine at USC; Attending Physician, LAC/USC Medical Center, Los Angeles, California
Hypothyroidism

Christopher O'Brien, MD
Professor of Clinical Medicine, Miller School of Medicine at the University of Miami; Attending Physician, Jackson Memorial Hospital and Miami VA Medical Center, Miami, Florida
Acute and Chronic Viral Hepatitis

Kevin W. Olden, MD
Professor, Division of Gastroenterology, Department of Medicine and Psychiatry, University of South Alabama, Mobile, Alabama
Irritable Bowel Syndrome

David L. Olive, MD
Professor of Obstetrics and Gynecology, University of Wisconsin School of Medicine and Public Health, Madison, Wisconsin
Endometriosis

Colm O'Loughlin, MB
Assistant Professor of Medicine, Division of Gastroenterology and Hepatology, Medical College of Wisconsin, Milwaukee, Wisconsin
Dysphagia and Esophageal Obstruction

Winnie W. Ooi, MD, MPH, DMD
Assistant Professor of Medicine, Tufts University School of Medicine, Boston; Medical Director, Travel and Tropical Medicine, Department of Infectious Diseases, Lahey Clinical Medical Center, Burlington, Massachusetts
Leprosy

Richard R. Orlani, MD
Associate Professor of Otolaryngology–Head and Neck Surgery, University of Utah School of Medicine, Salt Lake City, Utah
Sinusitis

Gary D. Overturf, MD
Professor of Pediatrics and Pathology, University of New Mexico School of Medicine; Director, Pediatric Infectious Diseases, Children's Hospital of New Mexico, Albuquerque, New Mexico
Bacterial Meningitis

Richard L. Page, MD
Robert A. Bruce Professor of Medicine and Head, Division of Cardiology, University of Washington School of Medicine, Seattle, Washington
Atrial Fibrillation

Paul M. Palevsky, MD
Professor of Medicine, University of Pitittsburgh School of Medicine; Chief, Renal Section, VA Pittsburgh Healthcare System, Pittsburgh, Pennsylvania
Acute Renal Failure

Biff F. Palmer, MD
Professor of Internal Medicine and Director, Renal Fellowship Program, Department of Internal Medicine, Division of Nephrology, University of Texas Southwestern Medical School, Dallas, Texas
Hyponatremia

Monica Parise, MD
Division of Parasitic Diseases, Centers for Disease Control and Prevention, Atlanta, Georgia
Malaria

Charles J. Parker, MD
Professor of Medicine, University of Utah School of Medicine, Salt Lake City, Utah
Autoimmune Hemolytic Anemia

Lorne S. Parnes, MD
Professor and Chairman, Department of Otolaryngology, The University of Western Ontario Faculty of Medicine, London, Ontario, Canada
Episodic Vertigo

Manisha J. Patel, MD
Department of Dermatology, Wake Forest University School of Medicine, Winston-Salem, North Carolina
Cutaneous Vasculitis

Ian M. Paul, MD, MSc
Assistant Professor of Pediatrics and Health Evaluation Sciences, Pennsylvania State College of Medicine, Hershey, Pennsylvania
Fever

Mark A. Peppercorn, MD
Professor of Medicine, Harvard Medical School; Senior Consultant, Center for Inflammatory Bowel Disease, Beth Israel Deaconess Medical Center, Boston, Massachusetts
Inflammatory Bowel Disease

Susan P. Perrine, MD
Associate Professor, Department of Medicine, Pediatrics, and Pharmacology and Experimental Therapeutics; Director, Hemoglobinopathy-Thalassemia Research Unit, Boston University School of Medicine, Boston, Massachusetts
Thalassemia

Petros Perros, BSc, MBBS, MD
Honorary Senior Lecturer, School of Clinical Medical Sciences, University of Newcastle upon Tyne; Consultant Endocrinologist, Freeman Hospital, Newcastle upon Tyne, United Kingdom
Thyroiditis

Andrew C. Peterson, MD
Assistant Professor of Surgery, F. Edward Hébert School of Medicine of the Uniformed Services University of the Health Sciences, Bethesda, Maryland; Urology Residency Program Director, Madigan Army Medical Center, Tacoma, Washington
Management of Urethral Stricture Disease

William A. Petri, Jr., MD, PhD
Department of Medicine, University of Virginia, Charlottesville, Virginia
Amebiasis

Tania J. Phillips, MD
Professor of Dermatology, Boston University School of Medicine; Consulting Dermatologist, Boston Medical Center, Boston, Massachusetts
Venous Stasis Ulcers

Michael E. Pichichero, MD
Professor of Microbiology and Immunology, Pediatrics, and Medicine, Department of Microbiology and Immunology, University of Rochester School of Medicine and Dentistry, Rochester, New York
Pertussis

Claus A. Pierach, MD
Professor of Medicine and History of Medicine, University of Minnesota Medical School, Minneapolis, Minnesota
The Porphyrias

Bianca Maria Piraccini, MD, PhD
Department of Dermatology, University of Bologna, Bologna, Italy
Diseases of the Nails

Michael J. Pollack, MD
Gastroenterology Fellow, University Hospitals of Cleveland, Cleveland, Ohio
Hiccups

Uday Popat, MD
Associate Professor of Medicine, University of Texas M.D. Anderson Cancer Center, Houston, Texas
Non-Hodgkin's Lymphoma

Lawrie W. Powell, MD, PhD
Professor Emeritus, School of Medicine, The University of Queensland Faculty of Health Sciences; Director of Research, Teaching and Research Unit, Royal Brisbane and Women's Hospitals, Brisbane, Queensland, Australia
Hemochromatosis

Richard A. Prinz, MD
Professor of Surgery, Rush Medical College; Chief, General Surgery, Rush University Medical Center, Chicago, Illinois
Acute and Chronic Pancreatitis

Beth W. Rackow, MD
Instructor, Department of Reproductive Endocrinology and Infertility, Yale University School of Medicine, New Haven, Connecticut
Dysfunctional Uterine Bleeding

S. Vincent Rajkumar, MD
Professor of Medicine, Mayo Clinic College of Medicine, Rochester, Minnesota
Multiple Myeloma

Mobeen H. Rathore, MD
Professor and Assistant Chairman, Department of Pediatrics, and Chief, Pediatric Infectious Diseases and Immunology, University of Florida; Chief, Pediatric Infectious Diseases, Wolfson Children's Hospital and Shands Hospital; Hospital Epidemiologist, Infection Control and Hospital Epidemiology, Wolfson Children's Hospital, Jacksonville, Florida
Mumps

Steven Reid, MD, PhD
Honorary Senior Lecturer in Psychological Medicine, Imperial College School of Medicine; Consultant Liaison Psychiatrist, St. Mary's Hospital, London, United Kingdom
Chronic Fatigue Syndrome

Martin Reite, MD
Professor of Psychiatry, University of Colorado Health Sciences Center School of Medicine; Medical Staff, University Hospital, Denver, Colorado
Treatment of Insomnia

Jordi Rello, MD, PhD
Professor, Rovira and Virgili Medical School, Joan XXIII University Hospital; Chief, Critical Care Department, Joan XXIII University Hospital, Tarragona, Spain
Legionellosis

Jeffrey Rentz, MD
Resident in Thoracic Surgery, Beth Israel Deaconess Medical Center, Boston, Massachusetts
Pleural Effusion and Empyema Thoracis

Robert W. Rho, MD
Assistant Professor of Medicine, Division of Cardiology, University of Washington School of Medicine, Seattle, Washington
Cardiac Arrest: Sudden Cardiac Death; Atrial Fibrillation

Lawrence Rice, MD
Professor of Medicine and Professor of Thrombosis Research, Baylor College of Medicine; Staff Physician, The Methodist Hospital, Houston, Texas
Non-Hodgkin's Lymphoma

James P. Richardson, MD, MPH
Chief, Geriatric Medicine, Union Memorial Hospital; Clinical Professor of Family Medicine, University of Maryland School of Medicine, Baltimore, Maryland
Tetanus

James R. Roberts, MD
Professor of Emergency Medicine, Senior Consultant of Medical Toxicology, Drexel University College of Medicine; Chairman of Emergency Medicine, Director, Division of Toxicology, Mercy Hospital of Philadelphia, Philadelphia, Pennsylvania
Spider Bites and Scorpion Stings

Jenice Robinson, MD
Assistant Professor of Neurology, Pennsylvania State College of Medicine, Hershey, Pennsylvania
Myasthenia Gravis and Related Disorders

Maria C. Rodriguez-Barradas, MD
Associate Professor, Baylor College of Medicine; Staff Physician, Michael E. DeBakey VAMC, Houston, Texas
Bacterial Pneumonia

Jorge Roig, MD, PhD, FCCP
Chief, Pulmonary Division, Hospital Nostra Senyora de Meritxell, Escaldes, Andorra
Legionellosis

Eric Rosenthal, MD, PhD
Professor of Internal Medicine, University of Nice–Sophia Antipolis Faculty of Medicine; Staff Physician, Centre Hospitalier l'Archet and Centre Hospitalier Universitaire de Nice, Nice, France
Visceral Leishmaniasis

Oscar Ruiz, MD
Program Director, General Surgery Residency, Riverside Methodist Hospital, Columbus, Ohio
Cholelithiasis and Cholecystitis

Louis J. Rusin, MD
Adjunct Assistant Professor, Department of Dermatology, University of Minnesota Medical School, Minneapolis; Staff Physician, Park Nicollet Clinic, St. Louis Park, Minnesota
Pruritus

Ronald A. Sacher, MD
Professor of Internal Medicine and Pathology, Division of Hematology/Oncology, University of Cincinnati College of Medicine, Cincinnati, Ohio; Adjunct Professor of Medicine, Oncology and Pathology, Georgetown University School of Medicine, Washington, DC
Therapeutic Use of Blood Components

Evangelista Sagnelli, MD
Full Professor of Infectious Diseases, Second University of Naples Faculty of Medicine; Attending Physician, Department of Public Health, Hospital Gésù e Maria, Naples, Italy
Food-Borne Illness

Eduardo Salazar-Lindo, MD
Pediatrician, Hospital Cayetano Heredia, Lima, Peru
Cholera

Karl J. Sandin, MD
Central Coast Physical Medicine and Rehabilitation Medical Group, Santa Barbara, California
Rehabilitation of the Stroke Patient

Robert Thayer Sataloff, MD, DMA
Professor and Chairman, Department of Otolaryngology–Head and Neck Surgery, and Associate Dean for Clinical Academic Specialties, Drexel University College of Medicine, Philadelphia, Pennsylvania
Hoarseness and Laryngitis

Wilson Sawa, MD
Instructor, Department of Obstetrics and Gynecology, Northeastern Ohio Universities College of Medicine, Rootstown, Ohio
Cancer of the Uterine Cervix

Peter C. Schalock, MD
Instructor in Dermatology, Harvard Medical School; Assistant in Dermatology, Massachusetts General Hospital, Boston, Massachusetts
Contact Dermatitis

Ralph M. Schapira, MD
Professor and Vice Chair, Department of Medicine, Medical College of Wisconsin; Staff Physician, Milwaukee Veteran Affairs Medical Center, Milwaukee, Wisconsin
Histoplasmosis; Acute Bronchitis

Randall T. Schapiro, MD
Director, The Schapiro Center for Multiple Sclerosis and the Minneapolis Clinic of Neurology, Minneapolis, Minnesota
Multiple Sclerosis

Isaac Schiff, MD
Joe Vincent Meigs Professor of Gynecology, Harvard Medical School; Chief, Vincent Memorial Obstetrics and Gynecology Service, Massachusetts General Hospital, Boston, Massachusetts
Menopause

Craig Michael Schramm, MD
Associate Professor, Department of Pediatrics, University of Connecticut Health Center, Farmington; Chief, Pediatric Pulmonary Division, Connecticut Children's Medical Center, Hartford, Connecticut
Atelectasis

Kathryn G. Schuff, MD
Associate Professor of Endocrinology and General Clinical Research Center, Clinical Research Compliance Manager, Oregon Health and Science University School of Medicine, Portland, Oregon
Cushing's Syndrome

Mrunal Shah, MD
Clinical Assistant Professor of Family Medicine, The Ohio State University College of Medicine and Public Health; Assistant Program Director, Riverside Family Practice Residency Program, Columbus, Ohio
Syphilis

Reza Shaker, MD
Professor of Medicine, Radiology, and Otolaryngology, Medical College of Wisconsin; Chief, Division of Gastroenterology and Hepatology, Froedtert and Medical College Clinics, Milwaukee, Wisconsin
Dysphagia and Esophageal Obstruction

Joseph C. Shanahan, MD
Assistant Professor of Medicine, Division of Rheumatology and Immunology, Duke University School of Medicine, Durham, North Carolina
Rheumatoid Arthritis

Surendra K. Sharma, MD, PhD
Chief, Division of Pulmonary and Critical Care Medicine, All India Institute of Medical Sciences, New Delhi, India
Management of the Patient with HIV Disease; Viral Upper Respiratory Tract Infections

Raj D. Sheth, MD
Director, Comprehensive Epilepsy Program; Professor, University of Wisconsin–Madison School of Medicine, Madison, Wisconsin
Epilepsy in Infancy and Childhood

Kenneth Shieh, MD
Gastroenterology Fellow, Brown Medical School/Rhode Island Hospital, Providence, Rhode Island
Intestinal Parasites

Jan L. Shifren, MD
Assistant Professor of Obstetrics, Gynecology, and Reproductive Biology, Harvard Medical School; Director, Menopause Program, Vincent Memorial Obstetrics and Gynecology Service, Massachusetts General Hospital, Boston, Massachusetts
Menopause

Michael E. Shy, MD
Professor of Neurology, and Molecular Medicine and Genetics, Wayne State University School of Medicine, Detroit, Michigan
Peripheral Neuropathies

Marc A. Silver, MD
Clinical Professor of Medicine, University of Illinois at Chicago College of Medicine, Chicago; Adjunct Professor, Department of Biomedical Engineering, Illinois Institute of Technology, Chicago; Chairman, Department of Medicine, and Director, Heart Failure Institute, Advocate Christ Medical Center, Oak Lawn, Illinois
Heart Failure

Kenneth J. Smith, MD, MSc
Assistant Professor of Medicine, University of Pittsburgh School of Medicine, Pittsburgh, Pennsylvania
Influenza

Michael J. Smith, MD
Instructor, Department of Pediatrics, University of Pennsylvania School of Medicine; Fellow, Division of Infectious Diseases, The Children's Hospital of Philadelphia, Philadelphia, Pennsylvania
Cat-Scratch Disease

Javier Solera, PhD
Associate Professor, Department of Medicine, Faculty of Medicine, University of Castilla–La Mancha—Albecete Campus; Chief, Internal Medicine Service, University General Hospital, Albacete, Spain
Brucellosis

Solomon S. Solomon, MD
Professor of Medicine and Pharmacology, University of Tennessee College of Medicine; Chief, Endocrinology and Metabolism, Memphis VA Medical Center, Tennessee
Hyperosmolar Hyperglycemic Syndrome and Diabetic Ketoacidosis

William B. Solomon, MD
Associate Professor of Medicine, Division of Hematology/Oncology, State University of New York Downstate Medical Center College of Medicine; Attending Physician, University Hospital of Brooklyn and Kings County Hospital Center, Brooklyn, New York
Iron Deficiency

Carmen C. Solorzano, MD
Assistant Professor of Surgery, Miller School of Medicine at the University of Miami; Department of Surgery, Chief Endocrine Surgery, University of Miami/Sylvester Cancer Center, Miami, Florida
Acute and Chronic Pancreatitis

Akshay Sood, MD, MPH
Associate Professor, Department of Medicine, University of New Mexico Health Sciences Center School of Medicine, Albuquerque, New Mexico
Silicosis and Asbestosis

Suman Sood, MD
Fellow, Hematology-Oncology Division, University of Pennsylvania School of Medicine, Philadelphia, Pennsylvania
Platelet-Mediated Bleeding Disorders

Thomas Spencer, MD
Associate Professor of Psychiatry, Harvard Medical School; Assistant Director of Clinical and Research Program in Pediatric Psychopharmacology and Director of Depression and Tourette's Clinic, Masschusetts General Hospital, Boston, Massachusetts
Attention Deficit Hyperactivity Disorder

Stanley M. Spinola, MD
David H. Jacobs Professor and Director, Division of Infectious Diseases, Indiana University School of Medicine, Indianapolis, Indiana
Chancroid

E. William St. Clair, MD
Professor of Medicine and Immunology, Division of Rheumatology and Immunology, Duke University School of Medicine, Durham, North Carolina
Rheumatoid Arthritis

Erik K. St. Louis, MD
Assistant Professor of Neurology, University of Iowa Carver College of Medicine; Co-Director, Iowa Comprehensive Epilepsy Program, University of Iowa Hospitals and Clinics, Iowa City, Iowa
Seizures and Epilepsy in Adolescents and Adults

Richard K. Sterling, MD
Professor of Medicine, Medical College of Virginia– Virginia Commonwealth University School of Medicine, Richmond, Virginia
Cirrhosis

Catherine Stevens-Simon, MD
Associate Professor of Pediatrics, Division of Adolescent Medicine, University of Colorado Health Sciences Center School of Medicine; Staff Physician, Children's Hospital, Denver, Colorado
Chlamydia trachomatis

Christopher D. Still, DO
Medical Director, Center for Nutrition and Weight Management, Department of Gastroenterology and Nutrition, Geisinger Health Care System, Danville, Pennsylvania
Obesity

John H. Stone, MD, MPH
Associate Professor of Medicine, Division of Rheumatology, Johns Hopkins School of Medicine; Director, The Johns Hopkins Vasculitis Center, Johns Hopkins Bayview Medical Center, Baltimore, Maryland
Giant Cell Arteritis and Polymyalgia Rheumatica

David J. Straus, MD
Attending Physician, Department of Medicine, Memorial Sloan-Kettering Cancer Center; Professor of Clinical Medicine, Joan and Sanford I. Weill Medical College of Cornell University, New York, New York
Hodgkin's Disease: Chemotherapy

Stevan B. Streem, MD*
Head, Section of Endourology and Stone Disease, Glickman Urological Institute, The Cleveland Clinic Foundation; Professor of Surgery, Cleveland Clinic Lerner College of Medicine/Case Western University School of Medicine, Cleveland, Ohio
Renal Calculi

Richard D. Stutzman, MD
Staff Physician, Cornea and External Diseases, Walter Reed Army Medical Center, Washington, DC
Vision Correction Procedures

Paniti Sukumvanich, MD
Fellow, Breast Service, Department of Surgery, Memorial Sloan-Kettering Cancer Center, New York, New York
Diseases of the Breast

Scott Swanson, MD
Professor of Surgery, Mount Sinai School of Medicine; Attending Surgeon, Mount Sinai Medical Center, New York, New York
Primary Lung Abscess

Misha F. Syed, MD
Assistant Professor, Department of Ophthalmology and Visual Sciences, University of Texas Medical Branch School of Medicine, Galveston, Texas
Glaucoma

James S. Tan, MD*
Department of Medicine, Summa Health System, Akron, Ohio
Necrotizing Skin and Soft-Tissue Infections

Kenneth S. Taylor, MD
Director, University of California–San Diego Sports Medicine Fellowship; Associate Professor, Department of Family and Preventive Medicine, University of California, San Diego, School of Medicine, San Diego, California
Common Sports Injuries

David R. Thomas, MD
Professor of Medicine, Saint Louis University School of Medicine, St. Louis, Missouri
Pressure Ulcers

Alan G. Thorson, MD, FACS
Associate Professor of Surgery and Program Director, Section of Colon and Rectal Surgery, Creighton University School of Medicine; Clinical Associate Professor of Surgery, University of Nebraska College of Medicine, Omaha, Nebraska
Tumors of the Colon and Rectum

Robert L. Thurer, MD
Associate Professor of Surgery, Harvard Medical School; Associate Chief of Thoracic Surgery, Beth Israel Deaconess Medical Center, Boston, Massachusetts
Pleural Effusion and Empyema Thoracis

Joyce A. Tinsley, MD
Associate Professor, Department of Psychiatry; Director of Psychiatric Residency Training and Director of Addiction Psychiatry Training, University of Connecticut School of Medicine, Farmington, Connecticut
Drug Abuse

Lama L. Tolaymat, MD, MPH
Assistant Professor, Department of Obstetrics and Gynecology, University of Florida College of Medicine, Jacksonville, Florida
Contraceptive Methods

Linus H. Santo Tomas, MD, MS
Assistant Professor of Pulmonary Critical Care Medicine, Medical College of Wisconsin, Milwaukee, Wisconsin
Histoplasmosis

Marcia G. Tonnesen, MD
Associate Professor of Dermatology and Medicine, State University of New York at Stony Brook Health Sciences Center School of Medicine, Stony Brook; Chief of Dermatology, Veterans Affairs Medical Center, Northport, New York
Erythema Multiforme, Stevens-Johnson Syndrome, and Toxic Epidermal Necrolysis

Peter P. Toth, MD, PhD
Chief of Medicine, CGH Medical Center; Visiting Clinical Associate Professor, University of Illinois at Chicago School of Medicine, Chicago; Director of Preventive Cardiology, Sterling Rock Falls Clinic, Sterling, Illinois
Dyslipoproteinemias

Raymond R. Townsend, MD
Professor of Medicine, University of Pennsylvania School of Medicine; Director, Hypertension Program, University of Pennsylvania Health System, Philadelphia, Pennsylvania
Primary Aldosteronism

Maria Trent, MD, MPH
Assistant Professor of Pediatrics, Johns Hopkins University School of Medicine; Active Staff, Johns Hopkins Hospital Children's Center, Baltimore, Maryland
Pelvic Inflammatory Disease

Penny Turner, MD
Assistant Clinical Professor, Department of Medicine, University of Alberta Faculty of Medicine and Dentistry; Edmonton, Alberta, Canada
Primary Glomerular Diseases

---

*Deceased.

Arvid E. Underman, MD, FACP, DTMH
Clinical Professor of Medicine and Microbiology, The Keck
School of Medicine, University of Southern California,
Los Angeles; Director of Graduate Medical Education,
Huntington Hospital, Pasadena, California
Salmonellosis

Mary Lee Vance, MA, MD
Professor of Medicine and Neurosurgery, University of Virginia
School of Medicine, Charlottesville, Virginia
Hypopituitarism

Brian A. VanderBrink, MD
Chief Resident, North Shore–Long Island Jewish Health Care
System, New Hyde Park, New York
Bacterial Infections of the Urinary Tract in Males

John Varga, MD
Professor of Medicine, Division of Rheumatology, Northwestern
University Feinberg School of Medicine, Chicago, Illinois
Connective Tissue Disorders

Todd W. Vitaz, MD
Assistant Professor, Department of Neurological Surgery,
University of Louisville School of Medicine; Director of
Neurosurgical Oncology; Co-Director, Neurosciences ICU,
Norton Hospital, Louisville, Kentucky
Management of Head Injuries

Jeffery T. Vrabec, MD
Associate Professor, Department of Otolaryngology–Head and
Neck Surgery, Baylor College of Medicine; Clinical Associate
Professor, Department of Head and Neck Surgery, MD
Anderson Cancer Center; Active Staff, Otolaryngology–Head
and Neck Surgery, The Methodist Hospital; Courtesy Staff,
Otolaryngology Service, Texas Children's Hospital, and Head
and Neck Surgery, MD Anderson Cancer Center, Houston,
Texas; Chair, Facial Nerve Disorders Committee, and Member,
SIPac Committee, American Academy of Otolaryngology–Head
and Neck Surgery; Chair, ByLaws Committee, American
Neurotology Society Membership Committee
Otitis Externa

Richard F. Wagner, Jr., MD
Professor, Department of Dermatology, The University of Texas
Medical Branch School of Medicine, Galveston, Texas
Cancer of the Skin

Laura Waikart, MD
Fellow (Allergy), University of Tennessee College of Medicine,
Knoxville, Tennessee
Nonallergic Rhinitis

David H. Walker, MD
Professor and Chairman, Department of Pathology, The
University of Texas Medical Branch School of Medicine,
Galveston, Texas
Rickettsial and Ehrlichial Infections

Shobha Wani, MD
Fellow, Section of Rheumatology, Washington Hospital Center,
Washington, DC
Lyme Disease

Thomas T. Ward, MD
Associate Professor of Medicine, Oregon Health and Science
University School of Medicine; Chief, Infectious Diseases,
Portland Veterans Affairs Medical Center, Portland, Oregon
Toxoplasmosis

Cheryl Waters, MD
Albert and Judith Glickman Professor, Department of
Neurology, Columbia University, New York, New York
Parkinsonism

Peter C. Weber, MD, MBA
Professor and Program Director, Department of
Otolaryngology, Cleveland Clinic, Cleveland, Ohio
Acute Facial Paralysis (Bell's Palsy)

Richard W. Weber, MD
Professor of Medicine, University of Colorado Health Sciences
Center School of Medicine and National Jewish Medical and
Research Center, Denver, Colorado
Allergic Rhinitis Caused By Inhalant Factors

Guy F. Webster, MD, PhD
Clinical Professor of Dermatology, Jefferson Medical College of
Thomas Jefferson University, Philadelphia, Pennsylvania
Acne and Rosacea

Arthur Weinstein, MD, FCAP, FCAR
Professor of Medicine, Georgetown University School of
Medicine; Associate Chairman, Department of Medicine, and
Director, Section of Rheumatology, Washington Hospital
Center, Washington, DC
Lyme Disease

Steven D. Weisbord, MD, MSc
Assistant Professor of Medicine, University of Pittsburgh School
of Medicine; Staff Physician, Renal Section, and Core Faculty
Member, Center for Health Equity Research and Promotion,
VA Pittsburgh Healthcare System, Pittsburgh, Pennsylvania
Acute Renal Failure

David G. Weismiller, MD
Associate Professor and Vice Chair for Academic Affairs,
Department of Family Medicine, The Brody School of Medicine
at East Carolina University, Greenville, North Carolina
Hypertensive Disorders of Pregnancy

Mitchell J. Weiss, MD, PhD
Associate Professor of Pediatrics, University of Pennsylvania
School of Medicine; The Children's Hospital of Philadelphia,
Philadelphia, Pennsylvania
Nonimmune Hemolytic Anemia

Thomas R. Welch, MD
Professor and Chair, Department of Pediatrics, State University
of New York Upstate Medical University College of Medicine,
Syracuse, New York
Parenteral Fluid Therapy for Infants and Children

Victoria Werth, MD
Professor, Department of Dermatology, University of
Pennsylvania School of Medicine; Chief, Dermatology,
Philadelphia VA Medical Center, Philadelphia, Pennsylvania
Bullous Diseases

Simon Wessely, MD, PhD
Professor of Liaison and Epidemiological Psychiatry, Guy's, King's, St. Thomas School of Medicine; Honorary Consultant Psychiatrist, King's College Hospital, London, United Kingdom
Chronic Fatigue Syndrome

Derek S. Wheeler, MD
Assistant Professor of Clinical Pediatrics, Division of Critical Care Medicine, Cincinnati College of Medicine; Staff Physician, Cincinnati Children's Hospital Medical Center, Cincinnati, Ohio
Resuscitation of the Newborn

Scott C. Wickless, DO
Clinical Faculty, Department of Dermatology, Northwestern University Feinberg School of Medicine, Chicago, Illinois
Nevi

Timothy Wilens, MD
Associate Professor of Psychiatry, Harvard Medical School; Director of Substance Abuse Services, Massachusetts General Hospital, Boston, Massachusetts
Attention Deficit Hyperactivity Disorder

Kira Williams, MD
Chief Resident in Psychiatry, Anxiety Disorders Clinic, Department of Psychiatry and Biobehavioral Sciences, Neuropsychiatric Institute and Hospital, Los Angeles, California
Panic Disorder

Steven R. Williams, MD
Clinical Assistant Professor, Department of Obstetrics and Gynecology, The Ohio State University College of Medicine and Public Health, Columbus, Ohio
Infertility

Phillip M. Williford, MD
Associate Professor of Dermatology and Director of Mohs Micrographic Surgery, Department of Dermatology, Wake Forest University, Winston-Salem, North Carolina
Warts (Verrucae)

Elzbieta Wirkowski, MD
Associate Professor of Clinical Neurology, SUNY at Stony Brook, Long Island; Director of Cerebrovascular Disorders and Co-Director of Neurological Intensive Care Unit, Winthrop University Hospital, Mineola, New York
Ischemic Cerebrovascular Disease

Martin S. Wolfe, MD
Clinical Professor of Medicine, George Washington University School of Medicine and Health Sciences; Clinical Professor of Medicine, Georgetown University School of Medicine, Washington, DC
Acute Infectious Diarrhea

Wing-Yen Wong, MD
Associate Professor of Pediatrics, Keck School of Medicine at USC; Director, Hemostasis and Thrombosis Center, Children's Hospital Los Angeles, Los Angeles, California
Hemophilia and Related Disorders

Jamie R. S. Wood, MD
Instructor in Pediatrics, Harvard Medical School; Research Associate, Sections on Genetics and Epidemiology and Vascular Cell Biology, and Staff Physician, Pediatric, Adolescent, and Young Adult Section, Joslin Diabetes Center, Boston, Massachusetts
Diabetes Mellitus in Children and Adolescents

Mark Woodhead, BSc, DM
Honorary Lecturer, University of Manchester; Consultant Physician, Department of Respiratory Medicine, Manchester Royal Infirmary, Manchester, United Kingdom
Psittacosis

Jon B. Woods, MD
Associate Professor of Pediatrics, Uniformed Services University of the Health Sciences, Bethesda, Maryland; Pediatric Infectious Diseases, Wilford Hall Medical Center, Lackland Air Force Base, San Antonio, Texas
Anthrax

Charles F. Wooley, MD
Professor of Medicine Emeritus, Division of Cardiology, Heart and Lung Research Institute/The Ohio State University School of Medicine and Public Health, Columbus, Ohio
Mitral Valve Prolapse: The Floppy Mitral Valve, Mitral Valve Prolapse, and Mitral Valvular Regurgitation

Kimberly Workowski, MD
Associate Professor of Medicine, Division of Infectious Diseases, Emory University School of Medicine; Division of STD Prevention, Centers for Disease Control and Prevention, Atlanta, Georgia
Nongonococcal Urethritis

Robert L. Wortmann, MD
Professor and C. S. Lewis, Jr., MD, Chair of Medicine, University of Oklahoma College of Medicine, Tulsa, Oklahoma
Gout and Hyperuricemia

Ronald F. Young, MD
Director of Neurosurgery, California Neuroscience Institute, St. John's Regional Medical Center, Oxnard, California
Trigeminal Neuralgia

Michael C. Zacharisen, MD
Associate Professor of Pediatrics and Medicine (Allergy/Immunology), Medical College of Wisconsin; Staff Physician, Children's Hospital of Wisconsin, Milwaukee, Wisconsin
Hypersensitivity Pneumonitis

Hamayun Zafar, PT, PhD
Assistant Professor, Department of Odontology–Clinical Oral Physiology, Umeå University Faculty of Medicine, Umeå; Center for Musculoskeletal Research, Gävle University, Gävle and Umeå, Sweden
Cervico-Cranio-Mandibular Disorders

Robert L. Zanni, MD
Associate Clinical Professor of Pediatrics, Drexel University
College of Medicine, Philadelphia, Pennsylvania; Director,
Pediatric Pulmonary Medicine, and Director, Cystic Fibrosis
Center, Saint Barnabas Health Care System, Monmouth
Medical Center, Long Branch, New Jersey
    Cystic Fibrosis

Jami Star Zeltzer, MD
Associate Professor, Department of Obstetrics and Gynecology,
Division of Maternal-Fetal Medicine, University of
Massachusetts Medical School, Worcester, Massachusetts
    Vaginal Bleeding in Late Pregnancy

Steven Zgliniec, MD
Fellow, Division of Pulmonary and Critical Care Medicine,
Rush Medical College/Rush University Medical Center,
Chicago, Illinois
    Severe Sepsis and Septic Shock

Kenneth S. Zuckerman, MD
Harold H. Davis Professor of Cancer Research and Professor
of Oncology, Internal Medicine, and Biochemistry/Molecular
Biology, University of South Florida School of Medicine,
Tampa, Florida
    Polycythemia Vera

Kathryn A. Zug, MD
Associate Professor of Medicine(Dermatology), Dartmouth
Medical School, Hanover; Staff Physician, Dartmouth Hitchcock
Medical Center, Lebanon, New Hampshire
    Contact Dermatitis

Preface

Starting in 1949, *Conn's Current Therapy* has provided a yearly update on the practical treatment of nearly 400 diseases and disorders. Howard Conn was the initial developer and author, who set out to provide a concise and up-to-date reference of the most recent advances in therapy for conditions most commonly encountered in practice. Some less common conditions also are included because certain disorders can have serious consequences if not diagnosed early and managed appropriately. Well-known scholar and clinician Robert Rakel, MD, took over editorship after Dr. Conn's death and remains today as the editor. Edward Bope, MD, joined him to share the editor responsibilities.

Each year, new experts are chosen to write on the topics. They are selected on the basis of recommendations from other authorities, or scholarly activity and/or research. Changing authors with each edition keeps the book crisp in coverage, fresh in tone, and brimming with the latest in practical advice. The authors give references for their discussions but also tell you how they manage the problem in their own clinical practice. Such practical wisdom is of immense value to today's physician, who typically is inundated with sometimes conflicting information from multiple sources. New topics are included every year, so the book remains current with the problems likely to be encountered in practice.

Now with the purchase of *Conn's Current Therapy 2007* you also can have your favorite or commonly referenced topics available on your computer or handheld device. In fact, you will have access to both the 2006 and 2007 editions for downloading your favorite articles from the book.

Conn's Current Therapy is indeed an international book. Contributing authors from around the world offer advice about the diagnosis and management of conditions not common to the United States. The contribution of these international experts adds greatly to the comprehensive nature of the book, and given the amount of international travel, it is quite possible to see unusual disorders far from the homeland of their origin.

Each chapter includes Key Diagnostic and Key Therapeutic boxes for quick reference. As always, tables, graphs, and figures are used when possible to present in-depth data in a convenient format. References for further reading provide some options for additional information if needed. In keeping with today's emphasis on evidence-based medicine, the clinician is pointed toward good evidence, when available, for treatment success. Careful attention is given to ensuring that the information included is correct and up to date. All of the material is reviewed by a pharmacist, Dr. Rakel or Dr. Bope, and multiple copy editors for accuracy and readability. Trade names are included alongside the generic drug name to help the clinician identify the medicines by whatever name is familiar.

We greatly appreciate the assistance of the very capable editorial staff at Elsevier and particularly the contribution of our pharmacist reviewers, Miriam Chan, RPH, PharmD, and Grace Kuo, PharmD. Special thanks go to Raegan Thompson, our editorial assistant, who keeps us all organized and focused on the tasks involved in producing this book.

Robert E. Rakel, MD
Edward T. Bope, MD

Contents

SECTION 3
Diseases of the Head and Neck

SECTION 4
The Respiratory System

SECTION 7
The Digestive System

SECTION 8
Metabolic Disorders

SECTION 9
The Endocrine System

SECTION 10
The Urogenital Tract

SECTION 17
Psychiatric Disorders

SECTION 18
Physical and Chemical Injuries

SECTION 19
Appendices and Index

Contents

XXXV

Symptomatic Care Pending Diagnosis

Pain

Method of
Alan B. Douglass, MD

Pain, an almost ubiquitous human condition, is a common reason for seeking medical care. Ninety percent of patients with advanced cancer, 45% to 80% of nursing home patients, and 25% to 50% of community adults report daily pain. Pain is a major cause of lost productivity, with United States (U.S.) annual costs of more than $60 billion in lost work alone. Improving pain assessment and management is currently a U.S. national priority.

The literature clearly documents that 90% of pain can be adequately controlled using standard techniques such as the World Health Organization (WHO) pain ladder and the Agency for Healthcare Policy and Research (AHCPR) (now known as the Agency for Healthcare Research and Quality [AHRQ]) guidelines. However, undertreatment is rife. More than 50% of patients, even those at the end of life, do not receive adequate analgesia.

Pain is defined by the International Association for the Study of Pain as "an unpleasant sensory and emotional experience associated with actual or potential tissue damage, or described in terms of such damage." Pain is a complex and subjective sensory, emotional, and cognitive phenomenon. The degree of pain experienced by a patient does not always correlate well with identifiable tissue injury, making assessment challenging.

Acute pain often follows an injury but may also arise de novo as the result of structural degeneration, infection, or metabolic changes. Acute pain tends to abate as tissues heal, and it generally responds well to analgesics and other therapies. Chronic pain persists over time and is generally defined as either lasting longer than 3 to 6 months or lasting 1 month longer than the usual time required for an injury to heal. The management of chronic pain is often complex.

Pain is generally divided into two broad categories: nociceptive and neuropathic. Nociceptive pain is induced when nociceptive receptors are stimulated by a tissue injury process and is further divided into visceral and somatic pain. Visceral pain originates in internal organs. It is often poorly localized and described as cramping, squeezing, or colicky, if originating from a hollow viscus, or aching and dull, if originating from a solid organ. Somatic pain is more easily localized and usually described as achy, throbbing, or dull.

Neuropathic pain is induced by pathophysiologic changes to the central and peripheral nervous systems. It is typically described as a sharp, tingling, burning, or electric sensation that often radiates. Pain of neuropathic origin may be associated with dysesthesias (unpleasant abnormal sensations), hyperalgesia (mildly painful stimuli perceived as very painful), or allodynia (nonpainful stimuli perceived as painful). Neuropathic pain usually requires a multimodal approach to therapy and tends to be more refractory to treatment than nociceptive pain.

Patient Assessment

Pain is a subjective, complex, multidimensional experience perceived only by the patient. Patient response to pain involves physical, psychologic, and cognitive facets. Pain assessment is always challenging for clinicians because no single objective measurement is available. Consequently, the patient's assessment of the severity and quality of the pain should be considered the best available assessment tool.

Pain reporting by patients can be subject to exaggeration, minimization, and misinterpretation. Many factors can influence the pain perception of others. Generally speaking, family members tend to overestimate, whereas health care professionals tend to underestimate. Reduced cognitive ability, reduced level of consciousness, and stoicism can result in under-reporting. Cultural, ethnic, and gender factors on the part of both patients and caregivers all can affect pain interpretation and communication.

Effective pain management begins with comprehensive patient assessment. A number of validated pain assessment tools of varying length and complexity are available. Simple examples include the numeric rating scale (1 to 10) and visual analogue scale. Special instruments, such as the faces scale, are available when language barriers are present and for rating discomfort in young children and the cognitively impaired. Frequent reevaluation is an essential part of effective pain management.

Pharmacologic Management

Medication is the mainstay of pain management. The pharmacologic management of pain is based on the WHO analgesic ladder, where the selection of agent depends on the severity and type of pain experienced. Patients with mild pain are treated with step 1 nonopioid agents such as acetaminophen or nonsteroidal anti-inflammatory drugs (NSAIDs), with or without the addition of adjuvant medications. Pain that is moderate in intensity is treated with step 2 weak opioids in addition to step 1 medications. Severe pain is treated with step 3 strong opioids, such as morphine, in addition to adjuvants and appropriate adjuvants. Some authors recommend a fourth step in the ladder, representing interventional pain management techniques. If pain is initially severe, the treating physician does not have to proceed up the ladder sequentially but may begin with either step 2 or step 3.

ACETAMINOPHEN OF PHARMACOLOGIC MANAGEMENT

Full-dose acetaminophen (Tylenol) is an effective, well-tolerated analgesic in a variety of pain scenarios. Although 4 g per day are listed as the maximal safe dosage, many experts advocate maximum dosages of 2 to 3 g per day. Furthermore, in alcoholism, fasting states, hepatic disease, the presence of certain medications (especially anticonvulsants), or in the frail elderly, liver toxicity can occur at recommended doses. Toxicity increases when acetaminophen is taken in conjunction with an NSAID. Particular care should be taken that daily dose limits are not exceeded inadvertently when patients are taking combination analgesics containing acetaminophen.

NONSTEROIDAL ANTI-INFLAMMATORY DRUGS OF PHARMACOLOGIC MANAGEMENT

Strong evidence indicates the efficacy of NSAIDs in acute and chronic pain. The efficacy of all NSAIDs appears roughly equivalent, but patient response to any particular agent is highly idiosyncratic.

Nonacetylated salicylates (choline magnesium trisalicylate [Trilisate], salsalate [Disalcid]), and cyclooxygenase (COX)-2-specific inhibitors are effective and may have fewer gastrointestinal side effects than traditional NSAIDs. Salicylates have the additional advantage of low cost. If traditional NSAIDs are chosen, gastric cytoprotection should be considered based on the patient's risk profile. Clinicians should also be aware of potential nephrotoxicity in the elderly and in patients with renal disease.

Recent research suggests that at least some NSAIDs may increase the risk of cardiovascular events. Care should be taken in prescribing to at-risk patients. NSAIDs should be particularly considered when inflammation is playing a substantial role in the production of the pain process.

OPIOIDS OF PHARMACOLOGIC MANAGEMENT

Opioids are an effective option in the management of moderate to severe pain. They are often the drug of choice in acute and chronic cancer pain. Opioids recently became more accepted in the long-term management of severe chronic noncancer pain, although concerns are raised about the safety and efficacy of prolonged high-dose opioid therapy.

Traditionally, opioids were thought superior to other agents because of the absence of a ceiling effect. Recent research suggests a ceiling may exist, but it is variable and often determined by side effects such as myoclonus. Doses can be escalated by 50% to 100% in a 24-hour period for severe uncontrolled pain. Increases of less than 25% are usually ineffective in this situation, but smaller increases may be effective for moderate pain.

Immediate-release opioids commonly prescribed orally in the ambulatory setting include codeine, hydrocodone, and oxycodone (Roxicodone). Codeine tends to be very constipating and should be used with care in the elderly. Propoxyphene (Darvon) has a limited analgesic effect and active metabolites accumulate over time. Its use should be limited to the short term. Partial agonists such as butorphanol (Stadol) are strongly discouraged as first-line agents. They should not be given to patients taking pure opioid agonists because they may precipitate withdrawal.

Morphine, the prototypical opioid, is available in a variety of dosage forms and widely used. Fentanyl (Duragesic) and hydromorphone (Dilaudid) are also commonly used. Hydromorphone is particularly useful because of its high potency but is available only in short-acting preparations. Methadone (Dolophine) is increasingly used in the management of chronic pain because of its low cost and beneficial side-effect profile. Because of its peculiar pharmacokinetics that can lead to drug accumulation and toxicity, however, it should be prescribed only after careful consideration and only by physicians experienced in its use. Meperidine (Demerol) is not recommended because of accumulation of active metabolites that can trigger neurotoxicity and seizures. In patients with renal failure fentanyl and methadone carry the least risk.

In patients with chronic pain, the use of sustained-release morphine and oxycodone should be considered. Once at steady state, sustained-release opioids are more convenient and prevent the peaks and valleys associated with short-acting agents. However, many patients, particularly those with cancer pain, require an additional short-acting agent to manage breakthrough pain.

The diversity of opioid receptors allows the transition from one opioid agonist to another when one agent ceases to be effective or side effects limit dose escalation. Opioid rotation must be done with care. Doses of different agents are not equivalent, so a conversion table (Table 1) should be used to calculate the equianalgesic doses. Alternatively, the

TABLE 1 Single-Dose Opioid Equianalgesic

Drug	Doses in Milligrams	
	Oral Dose	Parenteral Dose
Morphine	15	5
Meperidine (Demerol)	150	50
Hydromorphone (Dilaudid)	3.75	0.75
Oxycodone (Roxicodone)	10	NA
Hydrocodone	15	NA
Codeine	90	NA

dose of the original agent can be converted to oral morphine equivalents (Table 2) and then converted to the correct dosage of the new agent. To account for the phenomenon of incomplete cross-tolerance, the equianalgesic dose of the new agent should be decreased by 25% to 50%.

Opioids can be delivered by a variety of routes, including orally, rectally, intravenously, and subcutaneously. The intramuscular route is not recommended because of the pain associated with injections and wide fluctuations in blood levels. Fentanyl (Duragesic) is highly lipophilic and can be delivered transdermally through a 72-hour patch. Butorphanol (Stadol NS), a mixed agonist-antagonist, can be delivered intranasally. Interventional delivery of a variety of agents through the intrathecal or epidural route is also possible. Patient-controlled analgesia through the intravenous or epidural route can be very effective. When changing from one route to another, doses must be recalculated even if the same agent is used (see Table 1).

The most common side effect of opioid therapy is constipation, which, once established, can be severe and difficult to treat. All patients started on an opioid should receive a prophylactic bowel regimen with a stimulant laxative. Use of a stool softener alone is rarely effective. Nausea and vomiting are common but usually transient. Sedation and impaired psychomotor function occur in a dose-dependent fashion and are most common when initiating therapy. Symptoms typically dissipate over time, and patients on long-term opioid therapy are often capable of carrying out their usual daily activities, including working and driving.

The long-term use of opioids in the management of chronic noncancer pain is currently being debated. Some patients clearly can benefit from this approach.

TABLE 2 Oral Morphine Equivalents (OME)

Drug	OME
Morphine	1
Codeine, 30 mg	1-2
Hydrocodone, 5 mg	2
Oxycodone, 5 mg	5
Hydromorphone, 4 mg	15

Recent research on prolonged high-dose opioid therapy raises concerns of opioid-induced abnormal pain sensitivity, hormonal changes, including changes in libido and fertility, and immune suppression. Daily doses of more than 180 mg of daily morphine equivalent are not validated as effective in clinical trials and may present an increased risk of toxicity. The decision on an appropriate dose in a given patient should be individualized, with a focus on efficacy, avoiding potential toxicities, and functional improvement.

Both physicians and patients are often leery about using opioids because of fears of addiction and abuse. The nature of addiction and its risk in the use of opioids for pain management is frequently misunderstood, and confusion over definitions worsens the problem. The result often is undertreatment of pain.

Addiction is a primary, chronic, neurobiologic disease with genetic, psychosocial, and environmental risk factors. It is characterized by behaviors such as impaired control over drug use, cravings and excessive or compulsive drug use, and persistent use despite adverse consequences. Addiction occurs very infrequently in patients receiving opioid analgesia, and the risk is generally overrated. *Pseudoaddiction* is the manifestation of opioid-seeking behaviors that superficially appear similar to addiction but in reality are driven by undertreatment of pain. Unlike addiction, symptoms of pseudoaddiction disappear when pain is treated effectively.

Two terms describe the physiologic adaptation to chronic opioid therapy. Both are universal and predictable. *Dependence* is adaptation to a medication that results in a class-specific withdrawal syndrome if that medication is discontinued abruptly. This abstinence syndrome should not be confused with addiction. *Tolerance* is the development of diminution of drug effect over time, resulting in the need for increasing dosages to achieve the same analgesic effect. Tolerance occurs most commonly early in the course of opioid therapy. In cancer patients, an increasing need for opioid therapy usually reflects disease progression rather than tolerance.

ADJUVANT ANALGESICS OF PHARMACOLOGIC MANAGEMENT

Anticonvulsants are effective treatments for all types of neuropathic pain. Responses can be complete and dramatic in some patients. They are often used in combination with analgesics. All require gradual dose titration to maximize response while minimizing side effects. Pregabalin (Lyrica) has been recently approved and has a similar mechanism of action. Gabapentin (Neurontin)[1] is commonly prescribed and has few drug interactions, although sedation and ataxia can be problematic at higher doses. Topiramate (Topamax),[1] because of its several mechanisms of action, may be more effective than existing anticonvulsants but is not as well studied. Older anticonvulsants, such as carbamazepine (Tegretol), are as effective as and less expensive than newer agents but associated with more side effects and adverse reactions.

Tricyclic antidepressants can be effective adjuvants in the management of headache and neuropathic pain, although it is

---

[1]Not FDA approved for this indication.

unusual for responses to be complete. Amitriptyline (Elavil)[1] has been studied extensively. Secondary amines, such as nortriptyline (Pamelor)[1] and desipramine (Norpramin),[1] are also effective, however, and they have less anticholinergic side effects. Small doses (10 to 25 mg at bedtime) can be effective in some patients, but the response is generally dose dependent and greatest in the 100 to 150 mg per day range. Dose-limiting side effects include dry mouth, sedation, weight gain, constipation, and urinary retention. Serious side effects, including cardiac rhythm disturbances, are reported, so patients should be evaluated for cardiac abnormalities prior to initiating therapy.

Selective serotonin reuptake inhibitors have not been demonstrated to have an independent analgesic effect beyond their antidepressant action. However, the mixed serotonin and norepinephrine selective reuptake inhibitors Venlafaxine (Effexor) and Duloxetine (Cymbalta) have a clear analgesic effect in neuropathic pain, and the latter has been FDA approved for this indication.

Corticosteroids are highly useful agents in the management of a variety of painful cancer syndromes, including bone, visceral, and neuropathic pain, as well as headaches caused by increased intracranial pressure and soft tissue infiltration by tumor. In addition to their analgesic actions, they have a number of beneficial secondary effects, such as antiemetic activity, improved mood, energy, and sense of well-being, and appetite stimulation. Choice of agent is empirical. There is no therapeutic dose ceiling, but toxicities are related to dose and duration of therapy. To minimize problems, including hyperglycemia, immunosuppression, myopathy, osteoporosis, and gastrointestinal toxicity, short-term use at the lowest effective dose is recommended.

Topical anesthetics such as transdermal lidocaine (Lidoderm) are effective in neuropathic pain with minimal side effects.

Muscle relaxants can sometimes be helpful in acute musculoskeletal pain. Side effects, such as sedation and the potential for abuse of some agents, limit their use. They have a limited role in long-term pain management.

In addition to their role in the management of hypercalcemia, bisphosphonates can substantially reduce cancer-related bone pain caused by osteolytic metastases either alone or in combination with radiation therapy. Pamidronate (Aredia)[1] and zoledronic acid (Zometa)[1] are available only in intravenous form.

Nonpharmacologic Management

Although pharmacologic therapies are clearly a mainstay of pain management, optimal care often also involves the use of nonpharmacologic strategies that complement and supplement medications.

PHYSICAL MODALITIES OF PHARMACOLOGIC MANAGEMENT

Substantial high-quality evidence indicates that a variety of physical modalities can be effective in managing both acute and chronic pain. Physical rehabilitation, such

---

[1]Not FDA approved for this indication.

CURRENT DIAGNOSIS

- Pain, an almost ubiquitous human condition, is commonly underdiagnosed and undertreated.
- Acute, chronic, somatic, visceral, and neuropathic pain should be distinguished.
- Comprehensive patient assessment is critical.
- Pain is subjective and perceived only by the patient. The patient's perception should be considered the best available assessment tool.
- Factors that can affect symptom interpretation and communication should be carefully explored.
- Clinicians must differentiate addiction, pseudoaddiction, dependence, and tolerance.

---

as stretching, exercise, and ergonomic attention, is of benefit in many pain situations and can prevent maladaptive deconditioning. Thermotherapy and neurostimulatory approaches can have independent analgesic effects. In certain musculoskeletal problems, massage, mobilization, and manipulation can be helpful.

PSYCHOLOGIC METHODS OF PHARMACOLOGIC MANAGEMENT

In appropriate clinical settings, individual counseling, group therapy, relaxation training, biofeedback, and support groups all can be useful adjuncts. Treatment of coincident depression and anxiety is clearly shown to improve pain control, quality of life, and functionality.

ALTERNATIVE MODALITIES OF PHARMACOLOGIC MANAGEMENT

Americans are turning to alternative therapies in ever-increasing numbers. Studies of the treatment efficacy of a

CURRENT THERAPY

- Most pain can be adequately controlled using standard techniques, such as the WHO pain ladder.
- Acetaminophen and nonsteroidal anti-inflammatory drugs (NSAIDs) are effective analgesics, but clinicians should be mindful of their potential toxicities.
- Opioids in a variety of forms are an effective option in the management of moderate to severe pain. Constipation is common with opioid use and should be managed proactively. Other side effects, such as nausea and sedation, typically dissipate over time.
- For neuropathic pain, adjunctive agents, such as tricyclic antidepressants and anticonvulsants, should always be considered.
- Nonpharmacologic measures, such as physical modalities, psychologic methods, and alternative approaches supported by evidence of benefit, should be used whenever feasible.
- Referral for an interventional procedure should be considered if a structural lesion is likely and a potentially beneficial procedure is available.

variety of alternative modalities are ongoing, but strong evidence currently supports only a limited number of therapies. Physicians should discuss alternative therapies openly with patients and be knowledgeable about evidence of efficacy, side effects, and the potential for interactions with other conventional therapies.

INTERVENTIONAL APPROACHES OF PHARMACOLOGIC MANAGEMENT

Interventional pain specialists offer a variety of diagnostic and therapeutic techniques that can be helpful in the care of some patients. These include diagnostic facet and nerve blocks, therapeutic rhizotomies and nerve ablations, and selective joint and epidural injections. Referral to an interventionalist is appropriate if a structural defect is likely and a potentially beneficial procedure is available. Good communication between treating physicians is critical for overall treatment success.

REFERENCES

American Geriatrics Society Panel on Persistent Pain in Older Persons: The management of persistent pain in older persons. J Am Geriatr Soc 2002;50:S205-S224.
American Pain Society: Principles of Analgesic Use in the Treatment of Acute Pain and Cancer Pain, 5th ed. Glenview, IL: American Pain Society, 2003.
Ballantyne JC, Mao J: Opioid therapy for chronic pain. New Engl J Med 2003;349(20):1943-1953.
Dean M: Opioids in renal failure and dialysis patients. J Pain Symptom Management 2004;28(5):497–504.
Dworkin RH, Backonja M, Rowbotham MC, et al: Advances in neuropathic pain: Diagnosis, mechanisms, and treatment recommendations. Arch Neurol 2003;60(11):1524-1534.
Graham AW, Schultz TK, Mayo-Smith MF, et al: Principles of Addiction Medicine, 3rd ed. Chery Chase, MD, American Society of Addiction Medicine, 2003.
Levy MH: Pharmacologic treatment of cancer pain. N Engl J Med 1996;335(15):1124-1132.
Loeser JD, Butler SH, Chapman CR, Turk DC: Bonica's Management of Pain, 3rd ed. Philadelphia, Lippincott, Williams, & Wilkins, 2001.

Nausea and Vomiting

Method of
Chad M. Braun, MD

Nausea and vomiting are protective reflexes caused by a wide range of etiologies spanning from benign conditions to emergent disorders. Nausea and vomiting can occur independently but most often are associated. Usually nausea precedes vomiting and is often accompanied by skin pallor, increased sweating, and feeling flushed. It is also described as the urge to vomit. Vomiting (emesis) is the forceful oral expulsion of the contents of the stomach. Retching is the repetitive contraction of the muscles of the diaphragm and abdominal wall that often precede or accompany vomiting. Nausea and vomiting are mediated by efferent stimuli from the vomiting center in the brain to the musculature in the abdomen and chest. The neurotransmitters commonly associated with nausea and vomiting are acetylcholine, histamine, serotonin, and dopamine. These neurotransmitters are important in the treatment of persistent or severe nausea and vomiting. Most episodes of nausea and vomiting are acute, self-limited, and easily diagnosed based on the clinical picture. Chronic nausea and vomiting (1 month or more) is a diagnostic and therapeutic challenge for the clinician.

Differential Diagnosis

Causes of nausea and vomiting are numerous and varied (Table 1). Of these causes, one of the most common is an adverse reaction to a medication. Nonsteroidal anti-inflammatories, chemotherapeutic agents, antidepressants, narcotics, antibiotics, and oral contraceptives are all commonly associated with nausea and vomiting. It is important to note, however, that almost any medication can cause nausea. An accurate medication history thus is very important.

Viral and bacterial infections are another common cause of nausea and vomiting. This manifestation is often as an acute syndrome with fever and diarrhea. Common viral agents are rotavirus, enterovirus, and adenovirus. Bacterial causes such as *Salmonella, Campylobacter*, and *Shigella* are usually seen with the consumption of tainted food or water and can be associated with bloody diarrhea.

Disorders of the gastrointestinal tract can cause nausea and vomiting. Common examples of this are peptic ulcer disease, gastroparesis, dyspepsia, and irritable bowel disease. In addition, gastrointestinal emergencies such as acute appendicitis, acute cholecystitis, mesenteric ischemia, and intestinal obstruction can be associated with nausea and vomiting.

Nausea and vomiting are also exhibited during pregnancy. This is usually most frequent in the first trimester and manifested as "morning sickness." It is most common in the first pregnancy and is usually self-limited. Rarely seen is hyperemesis gravidarum, a condition characterized by intractable vomiting and weight loss that is often accompanied by fluid and electrolyte abnormalities.

Psychological disorders are also associated with nausea and vomiting. These can be seen in anxiety, depression, eating disorders such as anorexia and bulimia, and in psychogenic vomiting. Note that patients with psychogenic vomiting usually maintain a normal level of nutrition because they vomit only a small amount of the ingested food.

CURRENT DIAGNOSIS

- Acute and chronic nausea and vomiting must be differentiated.
- Nausea and vomiting have a wide range of possible causes.
- Control patient symptoms and then look for an underlying etiology.
- Few evidence-based therapy guidelines exist outside of postchemotherapy and postoperative nausea and vomiting.

TABLE 1 Differential Diagnosis of Nausea and Vomiting

Medications

Analgesics—acetaminophen, aspirin, nonsteroidal anti-inflammatory drugs (NSAIDs), rheumatologic and antigout drugs, opioids (codeine, morphine, oxycodone [Roxicodone])

Anesthetic agents—halothane, fentanyl (Sublimaze)

Antiasthmatics—theophylline

Anticonvulsants—phenobarbital, phenytoin (Dilantin)

Antidepressants—selective serotonin reuptake inhibitors (SSRIs)

Antimicrobials—acyclovir (Zovirax), erythromycin, itraconazole (Sporanox), metronidazole (Flagyl), sulfonamides, tetracycline

Antiparkinsonian drugs—levodopa (Dopar), carbidopa (Lodosyn)

Cancer chemotherapy—cisplatin (Platinol-AQ), cyclophosphamide (Cytoxan), dacarbazine (DTIC-Dome), nitrogen mustard

Cardiovascular agents—antiarrhythmics, antihypertensives, β-blockers, calcium channel antagonists, digoxin, diuretics

Corticosteroids—prednisone

Diabetic drugs—sulfonylureas, metformin (Glucophage)

Ergot alkaloids—dihydroergotamine (Migranal), ergotamine (Ergomar), methysergide (Sansert)

Gastrointestinal agents—azathioprine (Imuran), sulfasalazine (Azulfidine)

Hormonal agents—estrogen, progesterone, oral contraceptives

Iron replacement—ferrous sulfate

Substance abuse—alcohol, nicotine

Infectious Causes

Gastroenteritis—viral, bacterial, parasitic

Other—otitis media, systemic sepsis

Gastrointestinal Disorders

Functional disorders—chronic intestinal pseudo-obstruction, gastroparesis, irritable bowel syndrome, nonulcer dyspepsia

Mechanical obstruction—gastric outlet obstruction, small bowel obstruction

Organic gastrointestinal disorders

Appendicitis

Hepatobiliary disease—biliary colic, cholecystitis, hepatitis, neoplasia

Inflammatory bowel disease—Crohn's disease

Mesenteric ischemia

Peptic diseases—esophagitis, *Helicobacter pylori*, nonulcer dyspepsia, peptic ulcer disease

Pancreatic disease—pancreatitis, pancreatic adenocarcinoma

Paralytic ileus

Peritoneal irritation—peritonitis, metastases

Postoperative gastric surgery

Retroperitoneal fibrosis

Central Nervous System (CNS) Disorders

Increased intracranial pressure—abscess, hemorrhage, hydrocephalus, infarction, malignancy, meningitis, pseudotumor cerebri

Demyelinating disorders

Labyrinthine disorders—labyrinthitis, Méniére's disease, motion sickness

Migraine headaches

Parkinsonian disorders

Seizures—complex partial

Psychologic/Psychiatric Disorders

Anxiety

Depression

Eating disorders—anorexia nervosa, bulimia nervosa

Pain

Psychogenic vomiting

Medical Conditions

Cardiac—acute myocardial infarction, congestive heart failure

Genitourinary—acute nephritis, nephrolithiasis, ovarian torsion, pyelonephritis, testicular torsion

Endocrinologic and metabolic conditions—acute intermittent porphyria, Addison's disease, diabetic ketoacidosis, hypercalcemia, hyperparathyroidism, hyperthyroidism, hypoparathyroidism, uremia

Pregnancy—hyperemesis gravidarum, morning sickness

Postoperative Nausea and Vomiting

Radiation Therapy

Idiopathic Conditions

Cyclic vomiting syndrome

Gastric dysrhythmias

Other causes of nausea and vomiting not to be overlooked include central nervous system (CNS) disorders such as acute labyrinthitis, Ménière's disease, and motion sickness. In addition, any condition that causes increased intracranial pressure can cause nausea and vomiting. Further, approximately three fourths of all surgical procedures are complicated by postoperative nausea and vomiting. Most of this is thought to be anesthesia related.

Clinical Assessment

To narrow the wide differential associated with nausea and vomiting, it is important for the clinician to use a thoughtful approach to determine the underlying cause. Assessment begins with the differentiation of these symptoms from regurgitation (passive retrograde flow of gastric or esophageal contents into the mouth) and rumination (an effortless regurgitation of recently digested food into the mouth followed by spitting or reswallowing). With a thorough history and physical examination, the clinician can determine whether the patient can be effectively treated as an outpatient or requires hospitalization for treatment and further evaluation. To do this, the clinician must effectively characterize the patient's symptoms with special attention to the onset, duration, frequency, and severity of the symptoms. Some sample questions and scenarios follow.

When did the symptoms begin? How long have they been present? Acute causes of nausea and vomiting such as gastroenteritis or an adverse reaction to a medication has a much different course than chronic causes such as gastroparesis or irritable bowel syndrome. When does the vomiting occur? Is it in the morning or after meals? The temporal course is important. Early morning vomiting is often associated with pregnancy and uremia, whereas nausea and vomiting after meals can be seen with a motility disorder or an obstruction. It is also important to explore the character of the vomitus, specifically if it contains food, bile, or blood. In addition, the clinician should query the patient about any exacerbating or alleviating factors and whether or not the patient has experienced any weight loss or recently traveled.

After completing the history, the clinician should perform a focused physical examination. Here the key is to search for any consequences or complications of vomiting and to identify any signs that may point to the cause of the symptoms. Areas to be highlighted would be as follows. Vital signs, mucous membranes, and skin turgor should be examined for signs of dehydration. Bowel sounds should be quantified as normal, hyperactive, or hypoactive. The abdomen should be evaluated for distention and tenderness because specific sites of discomfort can give a clue to a diagnosis. Any visible hernias, surgical scars, or peristalsis should be noted. A neurologic exam should also be performed, including an assessment of the patient's optic fundus and gait. The teeth should be inspected for signs of enamel breakdown. A brief screening for any signs of psychological disease such as anxiety or depression should also be undertaken.

Diagnostic Testing

The history and physical examination guides the clinician to any further diagnostic testing that is required. Many cases of nausea and vomiting do not require any further testing. If necessary, screening laboratory testing should include serum chemistries, which may detect electrolyte abnormalities, dehydration or uremia, and a complete blood count, which may detect signs of infection. Depending on the clinical picture, an erythrocyte sedimentation rate (ESR), thyroid-stimulating hormone, and liver and pancreatic function testing can be considered. All women of childbearing age should have a pregnancy test. Stool studies can also be considered (e.g., giardiasis). Serum drug levels for toxicity should be considered in appropriate patients.

Further diagnostic testing is dictated by the patient presentation. If any obstruction or perforation is suspected, flat and upright abdominal radiographs can be obtained. Note that these can be normal in early or intermittent obstruction. Further studies such as an upper gastrointestinal barium study or a small bowel followthrough can be helpful if obstruction is considered. Esophagogastroduodenoscopy (EGD) is used to evaluate the mucosa of the esophagus, stomach, and duodenum for signs of inflammation. Additional testing that may be helpful depending on symptomatology includes an abdominal ultrasound, abdominal computed tomography (CT) scan, enteroclysis, and electrogastrography. For hypothesized gastric motility disorders, a gastric emptying study and antroduodenal manometry can be pursued.

If nausea and vomiting are persistent or severe and a gastrointestinal cause is not found, other etiologies such as systemic disease, CNS disorders, and psychological causes must be considered. CNS causes are best evaluated by head CT or magnetic resonance imaging (MRI). MRI provides better visibility of a posterior fossa lesion if that is of concern. Patients with chronic unexplained nausea and vomiting should also be screened for psychiatric disorders. If the clinician has pursued this diagnostic evaluation and is still unsure of the cause of persistent symptoms, consultation with a specialist should be obtained. Most often this would begin with a gastroenterologist but would depend on the symptom picture.

Treatment

Effective treatment of nausea and vomiting depends on identification and correction of the underlying cause. Most cases of nausea and vomiting require no specific treatment. However, patients may require evaluation for fluid and electrolyte disorders associated with nausea and vomiting. Symptomatic therapy should be based on symptom severity and the clinical presentation. Except in the case of pregnancy or drug overdose, antiemetic agents are often used empirically for relief. Oral rehydration, or intravenous if necessary, can then be pursued. If abdominal pain is also present, surgical consultation may be warranted.

With mild nausea and vomiting, dietary changes may be sufficient. Patients should be counseled to try small amounts (1–4 ounces/serving) of cool, clear liquids and advance as tolerated. A goal of 1 to 2 liters of fluid a day is a good one. If the patient successfully tolerates clear liquids, addition of small portions of easily digested foods such as bananas, rice, bouillon, and toast are in order. Dietary fat content should be reduced. Dairy products should be avoided. The diet can gradually be advanced with easily tolerated foods such as plain chicken or turkey and vegetables, bland soups, and fruit. Food should be consumed deliberately, and the patient should take care not to overeat. Increased physical activity around times of eating should be avoided. Note that nausea and vomiting associated with pregnancy can very often be treated with dietary changes alone.

With persistent or severe nausea and vomiting, antiemetic agents may be warranted. Most of these agents are centrally acting and can be divided into nine families (Table 2). By using medications from different families as needed or in combination, the likelihood of adverse drug reactions can be lessened. Because these agents work in the CNS, most adverse effects are also central, such as sedation, lethargy, and extrapyramidal effects. Outside of postoperative and postchemotherapy nausea and vomiting, there are few trials that identify an antiemetic of choice. Commonly used antiemetics are prochlorperazine (Compazine), promethazine (Phenergan), metoclopramide (Reglan), and trimethobenzamide (Tigan).

CURRENT THERAPY

- Most cases of nausea and vomiting do not require any therapy except dietary change.
- Hydration status must be monitored.
- Depending on symptom severity, antiemetics can be given by a variety of routes: oral, intravenous, and rectal.
- Use of medications is often limited by adverse effects.

TABLE 2 Commonly Used Medications for Nausea and Vomiting

Class/Medication	Usual Dosage	Route(s)	Adverse Effects
Anticholinergic			
Scopolamine (Transderm Scop)	1 patch every 3 d	Transdermal	Dry mouth, drowsiness, impaired eye accommodation; rare: disorientation, memory disturbance, dizziness, hallucinations
Antihistamines			
Diphenhydramine (Bendadryl)	25-50 mg q4-6h	IM, IV, PO	Sedation, dry mouth, constipation, confusion, blurred vision, urinary retention
Hydroxyzine (Atarax, Vistaril)	25-100 mg q6h	IM, PO	
Meclizine (Antivert)	25-50 mg q6h	PO	
Promethazine (Phenergan)	12.5-25 mg q4-6h	IM, IV, PO, PR	
Benzamides			
Metoclopramide (Reglan)	5-15 mg q6h	IM, IV, PO	Sedation, restlessness, diarrhea, agitation, central nervous depression, extrapyramidal effects, hypotension, neuroleptic syndrome, supraventricular tachycardia
Trimethobenzamide (Tigan)	250 mg q6-8h	IM, PO, PR	
Benzodiazepines			
Lorazepam (Ativan)[1]	0.5-2.5 mg q8-12h	IM, IV, PO	Sedation, amnesia, respiratory depression, ataxia, blurred vision, hallucinations, emotional reactions
Butyrophenones			
Droperidol (Inapsine)	0.625-1.25 mg q3-4h[3]	IM, IV	Sedation, hypotension, tachycardia, extrapyramidal effects, dizziness, blood pressure increase, hallucinations, chills, QT prolongation, torsade de pointes
Haloperidol (Haldol)[1]	05.-5 mg q8h	IM, IV, PO	
Cannabinoids			
Dronabinol (Marinol)	2.5-5 mg q8h	PO	Drowsiness, euphoria, vision difficulties, somnolence, vasodilation, abnormal thinking, dysphoria, diarrhea, flushing, tremor, myalgias
Corticosteroids			
Dexamethasone (Decadron)[1]	4 mg q6h	IM, IV, PO	Gastrointestinal upset, anxiety, insomnia, hyperglycemia, facial flushing, euphoria, peritoneal itching
Phenothiazines			
Chlorpromazine (Thorazine)	10-25 mg q4-6h	IM, PO, PR	Sedation, lethargy, skin irritation, cardiovascular effects, extrapyramidal effects, cholestatic jaundice, hyperprolactinemia, neuroleptic malignant syndrome, blood abnormalities
Prochlorperazine (Compazine)	5-10 (25PR) mg q6h	IM, IV, PO, PR	
Thiethylperazine (Torecan)	10-20 mg q6h[3]	IM, IV, PO	
5-HT3 Serotonin Antagonists			
Ondansetron (Zofran)	8 mg q8h	IV, PO	Headache, constipation, fever, asthenia, arrhythmias, diarrhea, dizziness, ataxia, tremor, somnolence, thirst, nervousness, elevated hepatic transaminases
Granisetron (Kytril)	2 mg per 24 h	IV, PO	
Dolasetron (Anzemet)	100 mg per 24 h	IV, PO	

[1]Not FDA approved for this indication.
[3]Exceeds dosage recommended by manufacturer.
Abbreviations: IM = intramuscular; IV = intravenous; PO = orally; PR = per rectum.

Antiemetic Drugs

SEROTONIN ANTAGONISTS

Ondansetron (Zofran), granisetron (Kytril), and dolasetron (Anzemet), especially when introduced prior to treatment, are effective in the prevention of chemotherapy- and radiation-associated emesis. They are also effective in postoperative nausea and vomiting, but less expensive options (e.g., droperidol [Inapsine] and dexamethasone [Decadron][1]) are equally effective. The serotonin antagonists are usually well tolerated.

DOPAMINE ANTAGONISTS

The phenothiazines, butyrophenones, and substituted benzamides are all examples of antiemetics that work

[1]Not FDA approved for this indication.

through dopaminergic blockade. Phenothiazines are often not effective for severe vomiting and have a high incidence of side effects including sedation, hypotension, and extrapyramidal effects. Metoclopramide (Reglan) is more effective for severe nausea and vomiting but again has a high incidence of adverse effects. This agent has been especially effective in treating gastroparesis. It should be noted that droperidol (Inapsine) has been associated with QT prolongation and electrocardiogram (EKG) monitoring is recommended with administration.

ANTIHISTAMINES AND ANTICHOLINERGICS

Antihistamines and anticholinergics are of value in the prevention of nausea and vomiting associated with inner ear disturbances, motion sickness, vertigo, and migraines. They often cause drowsiness.

BENZODIAZEPINES

These medications can be helpful in psychogenic and anticipatory vomiting.

CORTICOSTEROIDS

Dexamethasone (Decadron)[1] is commonly used in combination with other antiemetics. Use of steroids and serotonin antagonists is effective in chemotherapy-associated nausea and vomiting, and steroids and low-dose droperidol (Inapsine) is useful in postoperative nausea and vomiting.

CANNABINOIDS

Marijuana is used as an antiemetic and an appetite stimulant. Its efficacy is increased when combined with prochlorperazine (Compazine). Dronabinol (Marinol) is a synthetic cannabinoid available by prescription. CNS side effects are very common with these drugs.

NONPHARMACOLOGIC OPTIONS

Note that both ginger and acupressure are effective in the treatment of nausea and vomiting.

Special Circumstances

CHEMOTHERAPY INDUCED

Attempt to treat patients prophylactically to avoid nausea and vomiting. Use combination therapy. Try to avoid using medications from the same family to decrease the chance of adverse reactions. Note that chemotherapy-induced emesis may begin as long as 24 hours post treatment and may require therapy for 4 to 7 days.

DIABETES

Use promotility agents such as metoclopramide (Reglan) for gastroparesis-associated nausea and vomiting.

PREGNANCY

Morning sickness is common in the first trimester of pregnancy but usually resolves by the second. Reassurance, frequent small meals, and dietary changes are usually sufficient. For some patients, pyridoxine (vitamin B$_6$)[1] is helpful. In most cases, antiemetics are avoided in pregnancy. In severe cases involving protracted symptoms and fluid and electrolyte abnormalities (hyperemesis gravidarum), hospitalization and intravenous hydration may be required. No antiemetics are approved for use in pregnancy. Selection of any medication to be used in pregnancy should be with careful consideration of the severity of symptoms and potential risk to the fetus. Meclizine (Antivert) and promethazine (Phenergan) are used in pregnancy but neither is FDA-approved for this indication.

MOTION SICKNESS

Anticholinergics and antihistamines are effective here. Transdermal scopolamine patches (Transderm Scop) are convenient for those exposed to motion for long periods (cruise ships).

POSTOPERATIVE

Approximately 80% of patients who undergo anesthesia experience nausea and vomiting in the perioperative or postoperative period. Serotonin antagonists or combination therapy with dexamethasone (Decadron)[1] and droperidol (Inapsine) are effective here.

REFERENCES

American Gastroenterological Association: Medical position statement: Nausea and vomiting. Gastroenterology 2001;120(1):261-262.
Anthony L: Nausea and vomiting. Conn's Current Therapy, 2004.
Hasler WL, Chung O: Approach to the patient with gastrointestinal disease. Harrison's Principles of Internal Medicine, 16th ed. 2005.
McQuaid KR: Nausea and vomiting. Current Medical Diagnosis and Treatment. 2006.
Miser WF: Nausea and vomiting. Conn's Current Therapy. 2005.
Pasricha PJ: Treatment of disorders of bowel motility and water flux; antiemetics; agents used in biliary and pancreatic disease. Goodman and Gilman's The Pharmacological Basis of Therapeutics, 11th ed. 2005.

Gaseousness and Indigestion

Method of
Ram Dickman, MD, and Ronnie Fass, MD

Gaseousness

Gaseousness includes bloating, belching, and flatulence, which are among the most common gastrointestinal symptoms reported by patients who seek their physician's advice and especially by those with functional bowel disorders.

---

[1]Not FDA approved for this indication.

[1]Not FDA approved for this indication.

CURRENT DIAGNOSIS

Gaseousness

- History: drugs (narcotics, calcium channel blockers, anticholinergics), surgery (vagotomy, adhesions, Nissan fundoplication), diabetes, celiac sprue, intestinal myopathies, diet (consumption of starch, lactose, fructose, sorbitol, beans, cabbage, cauliflower, Brussels sprouts)
- Alarm symptoms: weight loss, anemia, anorexia, fever, and gastrointestinal bleeding
- Blood tests: complete blood count, glucose and electrolytes, thyroid-stimulating hormone
- Upper or lower endoscopy and/or 24-hour pH monitoring
- Breath testing for lactose and fructose intolerance

Indigestion

- Upper endoscopy with biopsies for *Helicobacter pylori*
- 24-hour pH monitoring
- Gastric emptying rate measurement
- Water-load test
- Psychological evaluation

Despite the clinical importance of gaseousness, the pathophysiology of this disorder is not fully understood. Bloating and flatulence are frequently attributed to excess gas within the gut lumen; however, gas transit studies in patients with bloating have not demonstrated an increased amount of gas within the gut. The current mainstays of treatment of gaseousness include lifestyle and diet modifications.

BLOATING

Abdominal bloating is a sensation of a swollen or distended abdomen. The term is sometimes used to describe a sensation of excess gas or a full belly.

Abdominal bloating may affect between 10% and 30% of the general population. Bloating is a very common complaint, especially in patients with functional bowel disorders, such as irritable bowel syndrome (IBS) and functional dyspepsia (FD).

Objective Evidence

The gastrointestinal lumen of a normal subject contains less than 200 mL of gas, which is a combination of swallowed air (N_2, O_2) and gases that are produced during acid neutralization (CO_2) and bacterial fermentation (H_2, methane, CO_2). Measurement of a patient's abdominal girth using abdominal impedance plethysmography allows objective assessment of reports of bloating.

Studies in IBS patients show a greater 24-hour fluctuation in abdominal girth as compared to healthy controls. Abdominal distention (objective parameter) peaks 4 to 6 hours before bedtime and was correlated with bloating (subjective parameter) only in the subgroup of patients with constipation-predominant IBS. However, in other subgroups of IBS patients, there was no association between symptoms and changes in abdominal girth.

Interestingly, studies that assessed intestinal gas dynamics found that IBS patients have delayed transit of gas along the gut and a significant increase in gas retention as compared to controls. Specifically, gas retention within the jejunum seems to be the main cause for the patients' symptoms. However, other studies found that the total amount of gas within the gut in symptomatic patients (mainly IBS) who complained of bloating was the same as in asymptomatic controls. In one study, for example, during gas infusion into the gut, patients with IBS and bloating complained of greater discomfort and gaseousness than did controls. Thus, it appears that the key mechanism for bloating in patients with functional bowel disorders is an abnormal perception of intestinal gas.

BELCHING

Belching is the expulsion of gas from the stomach while retaining solid and fluid material. Occasional belching is a normal physiologic process aimed to remove air from the stomach, typically during or after meals. The air is commonly swallowed during meals or introduced into the stomach through carbonated beverages and other food products. Repetitive belching not related to meals is secondary to esophageal air aspiration. Excessive belching is almost always associated with functional gastrointestinal disorders (functional dyspepsia and aerophagia) and with gastroesophageal reflux disease (GERD). Patients may also complain of an inability to belch. Common causes of the latter include esophageal achalasia and post-Nissan fundoplication ("gas-bloat syndrome"). In one large study, 17% of 8351 healthy subjects reported having excessive belching with a similar frequency in men and women.

Patient Evaluation

Evaluation of patients with excessive belching is appropriate only if an underlying organic cause is suspected and should include an upper endoscopy, esophageal pH monitoring, and esophageal manometry (the latter to rule out achalasia). Radiographic studies of the esophagus and stomach may also be helpful in patients with co-morbid factors.

FLATULENCE

Studies of healthy subjects found that the frequency of flatus passed per day ranges from 10 to 14 times. Flatus volume is difficult to measure in clinical practice. Thus, clinicians should rely on their patient's reported average frequency of flatus episodes per day over a predetermined period of time (1 to 2 weeks).

Increased flatus production (more than 22 times per day) may be caused by malabsorption of carbohydrates in patients with celiac sprue, pancreatic insufficiency, and short bowel syndrome. Additionally, in susceptible patients, malabsorption of lactose, fructose, sorbitol, and starch can result in excessive flatus production because of colonic bacterial fermentation of these unabsorbable carbohydrates.

CLINICAL ASSESSMENT

The clinical assessment of gaseousness is aimed to rule out more serious conditions that have clinical manifestations similar to benign functional bowel disorders.

TREATMENT

Treatment of gaseousness includes recommendations to reduce ingestion of gas-forming food products and drugs that facilitate intestinal passage. Patients need to reduce air swallowing (aerophagia) by avoidance of carbonated beverages, gum chewing, and smoking and by drinking from a straw. Dietary modifications include avoidance of dietary fibers, caffeine, cabbage, Brussels sprouts, beans, broccoli, and cauliflower. Loperamide (Imodium) may increase intestinal fluid absorption in patients with rapid transit. Tegaserod (Zelnorm) may improve bloating in constipation-predominant IBS patients. Antibiotics may be beneficial in the case of bloating caused by bacterial overgrowth.

CURRENT THERAPY

Gaseousness

- Bloating and flatulence
  - Reduce air swallowing (avoidance of carbonated beverages, gum chewing, smoking; drinking from a straw)
  - Dietary modifications (avoidance of dietary fibers, caffeine, beans, cabbage, broccoli, cauliflower)
  - Loperamide (Imodium), 2 mg PO 1–2/d, for malabsorption because of rapid transit
  - Tegaserod (Zelnorm), 6 mg PO 2/d, for constipation-predominant irritable bowel syndrome
  - Short courses of antibiotics for bacterial overgrowth
  - Simethicone (Mylicon)
- Belching
  - Reduce air swallowing

Indigestion

DYSPEPSIA

- Prokinetics
  - Metoclopramide (Reglan),[1] 10 mg PO 1–3/d
  - Tegaserod (Zelnorm),[1] 6 mg PO 3/d
  - Domperidone (Motilium),* 40 mg PO 3/d
- Proton pump inhibitors (PPIs)
  - Omeprazole (Prilosec),[1] 20 mg PO 1–2/d
  - Rabeprazole (AcipHex),[1] 20 mg PO 1–2/d
  - Pantoprazole (Protonix),[1] 40 mg PO 1–2/d
  - Lansoprazole (Prevacid),[1] 30 mg PO 1–2/d
  - Esomeprazole (Nexium),[1] 40 mg PO 1–2/d
- Combination PO therapy for *H. pylori* infection: 10–14 d: PPI 2/d + 1 g amoxicillin 2/d + 500 mg clarithromycin 2/d

FUNCTIONAL DYSPEPSIA

- Antidepressants
  - Nortriptyline (Aventyl/Pamelor),[1] amitriptyline (Elavil/Endep),[1] Doxepin (Sinequan), 50 mg PO qhs
  - Trazodone (Desyrel), 100–150 mg PO 1/d
- Hypnotherapy
- Psychological treatments

---

[1]Not FDA approved for this indication.
*Investigational drug in the United States.
Abbreviation: PO = orally.

Indigestion (Dyspepsia)

Dyspepsia is a persistent or recurrent pain or discomfort in the epigastrium associated with a feeling of fullness, early satiety, bloating, belching, and nausea. It is estimated that up to 40% of the adults in the United States experience dyspeptic symptoms at least once a year.

ETIOLOGY

In most of the patients with dyspepsia (60%), no significant organic finding underlies patients' symptoms. These patients are defined as having functional dyspepsia. Other causes include peptic ulcer disease (15% to 25%), *Helicobacter pylori* infection (30% to 60%), GERD, gastric cancer, and nonsteroidal anti-inflammatory drug (NSAID) use. The underlying mechanisms for functional dyspepsia include antral hypomotility, impaired gastric accommodation, disordered gastric electrical activity, and visceral hypersensitivity. Additionally, studies found that psychological co-morbidity (anxiety, neuroses, and depression) are more common in FD than in controls.

CLINICAL ASSESSMENT

Because of the many symptoms included in the category of dyspepsia, the clinical evaluation of dyspeptic patients implies that many other conditions are included in the differential diagnosis such as gastroesophageal reflux disease, *H. pylori* infection, and gastric cancer. Consequently, an appropriate workup for patients with dyspepsia may include upper endoscopy, 24-hour esophageal pH monitoring, *H. pylori* assessment, gastric emptying studies, and the water-load test. In patients with functional dyspepsia, psychological consultation is an important part of the patient's evaluation.

TREATMENT

Physicians should tailor their treatment approach to dyspepsia according to the severity and frequency of the patient's symptoms. Evaluation for psychosocial abnormalities may be essential in a significant subset of dyspeptic patients. Although not systematically validated, therapeutic recommendations include dietary and lifestyle modifications such as eating smaller and frequent meals and avoiding foods with high fat and fiber content. Antisecretory medications, promotility drugs, and pain modulators should be considered in the proper clinical scenario. Hypnotherapy is more effective in FD patients as compared to medical therapy. Psychological intervention is an essential therapeutic modality in patients with psychological disturbances.

REFERENCES

Kellow J, Lee OY, Chang FY, et al: An Asia-Pacific, double blind, placebo controlled randomised study to evaluate the efficacy, safety, and tolerability of Tegaserod in patients with irritable bowel syndrome. Gut 2003;52:671-676.

Mertz H, Fass R, Krodner A, et al: Effect of amitriptyline on symptoms, sleep, and visceral perception in patients with functional dyspepsia. Am J Gastroenterol 1998;93:160-165.

Moayyedi P, Forman D, Braunholtz D, et al: The proportion of upper gastrointestinal symptoms in the community associated with *Helicobacter pylori*, lifestyle factors, and nonsteroidal anti-inflammatory drugs. Leeds HELP Study Group. Am J Gastroenterol 2000;95:1448-1455.

Salvioli B, Serra J, Azpiroz F, et al: Origin of gas retention and symptoms in patients with bloating. Gastroenterology 2005;128:574-579.

Serra J, Azpiroz F, Malagelada JR, et al: Impaired transit and tolerance of intestinal gas in the irritable bowel syndrome. Gut 2001;48:14-19.

Talley NJ, Vakil NB, Moayyedi P: American Gastroenterological Association technical review on the evaluation of dyspepsia. Gastroenterology 2005;129:1756-1780.

Hiccups

Method of
Michael J. Pollack, MD

Hiccups are a common and usually benign phenomenon that affects nearly everyone at some time. It is more accurately termed *singultus*, derived from the Latin word *singult*, which means the act of catching one's breath while sobbing. Hiccups are caused by synchronous contractions of the diaphragmatic and intercostal muscles followed by the immediate and sudden closure of the glottis. The forcefully inspired air meeting the closed glottis creates the hiccup sound. Most episodes are transient and resolve without medical therapy. Rarely, hiccups are the only symptom of a serious systemic illness. The role of the practitioner is to know when to initiate the appropriate workup and how to treat the hiccups until the underlying problem, if identified, is resolved.

Classification

Hiccups can be classified as transient, persistent, or chronic. An episode of hiccups that lasts less than 1 day is transient. This type of episode is usually a benign, often physiologic phenomenon. An episode lasting up to 1 month is deemed persistent. Beyond this time it is considered chronic. Practically speaking, hiccups should be viewed as either transient or chronic. Most people experience some form of hiccups throughout their lives. The majority of these episodes are a transient nuisance. Chronic hiccups are quite rare with an estimated prevalence of approximately 1 in 100,000 people but can lead to significant adverse effects including malnutrition, weight loss, fatigue, and generalized debilitation. Those patients who present to their practitioner with hiccups most often experience them chronically. Hiccups can occur in utero, but they have no known physiologic function. Chronic hiccups occur more often in males, but transient hiccups affect both males and females equally.

Mechanism

The precise mechanism of hiccups is unknown. Three neural pathways are described in the hiccup reflex: afferent (phrenic and vagus nerves); a poorly characterized hiccup center in the brainstem; and efferent (phrenic, vagus, cervical,

TABLE 1 Selected Causes of Persistent Hiccups

Phrenic/Vagus Nerve Irritation	CNS Disorders	Toxic-Metabolic Disorders	Postoperative Factors	Drugs	Psychogenic Factors
Pharyngitis	Meningitis	Alcohol	General anesthesia	Barbiturates	Stress
Laryngitis	Encephalitis	Uremia	Tracheal intubation	Steroids	Excitement
Pneumonia	Cerebrovascular accident	Hypoglycemia	Neck extension	Benzodiazepine	Malingering
Esophagitis	Arteriovenous malformation	Hyponatremia	Gastric distention	Methyldopa	Conversion
Aortic aneurysm	Brain abscess	Hypocalcemia	Organ manipulation		
Mediastinal tumors	Neoplasms	Septicemia			
Pancreatitis	Trauma				
Peptic ulcer disease	Temporal arteritis				
Subphrenic abscess	Multiple sclerosis				
Myocardial infarction	Hydrocephalus				
Gallbladder disease	Ventriculoperitoneal shunts				
Gastric distention					

Abbreviation: CNS = central nervous system.

and thoracic nerves). The hiccup center is thought to involve a complex interaction among the brainstem, respiratory centers, phrenic nerve nuclei, the reticular activating center, and the hypothalamus. Theoretically, pathology in or around any of these areas can trigger hiccups. The frequency of hiccups is known to increase with a decline in arterial PCO_2 and to decrease as PCO_2 rises. This is the physiologic basis for the home remedy of breathing into a paper bag to stop hiccups.

Etiology

Transient hiccups are usually caused by overdistention of the stomach by air (such as during endoscopy), overeating, eating too fast, or alcohol or tobacco use; these typically resolve without medical therapy. Other benign causes include sudden changes in ambient or gastrointestinal temperature, sudden excitement, or emotional stress. Chronic hiccups may be caused by many underlying processes (Table 1). Processes affecting either the vagus or the phrenic nerve are the most common cause. Examples of precipitating irritants include foreign bodies in contact with the tympanic membrane (auricular branch of the vagus), pharyngitis, laryngitis or neck tumors (recurrent laryngeal nerve of the vagus), mediastinal masses, subdiaphragmatic abscesses, and gastroesophageal reflux (phrenic nerve).

Central nervous system (CNS) disorders, toxic-metabolic disorders, and psychogenic factors are also implicated, to some extent, in the etiology of hiccups. CNS disorders include structural, vascular, and infectious processes. Toxic-metabolic disorders include uremia, alcoholic intoxication, and general anesthetic agents. Psychogenic factors associated with both transient and persistent hiccups include stress, anxiety, and even malingering.

Medical Evaluation

The approach to the patient with an attack of hiccups depends on its duration. Transient hiccups are both common and benign and do not require investigation. However, chronic hiccups may be the only symptom of an underlying medical condition, and they require a thorough evaluation. The initial approach to identify the cause of chronic hiccups is a complete patient history and comprehensive physical examination, with a focus on the duration, frequency, alleviating factors, and aggravating factors.

Laboratory tests should start with a complete blood count and renal function with full electrolyte panel. A chest radiograph is important to aid in the detection of possible anatomic irritants to the phrenic or vagus nerves. An electrocardiogram helps detect pericardial disease or even pacemaker dysfunction. If the radiograph and electrocardiogram are unrevealing, second-level testing should be pursued guided by the relevant history and clinical findings, including a computed tomography of the head, chest, and abdomen; lumbar puncture; upper endoscopy; or bronchoscopy. Further testing, if required, would include magnetic resonance imaging of the head, an electroencephalogram, pulmonary function tests, and esophageal manometry.

Treatment

Because chronic hiccups are usually a sign of an underlying systemic disease, priority should be given to treating the condition. For example, proton pump inhibitors can be used if gastroesophageal reflux is implicated, or systemic chemotherapy can be administered if a neoplasm is detected.

When a cause cannot be determined and hiccups persist, empirical therapy is warranted. It can be used to palliate chronic, transient, or persistent hiccups while treatment of the underlying condition is ongoing. No single modality or agent is universally accepted as the treatment of choice.

Interventions can be divided into pharmacologic (Table 2) and nonpharmacologic therapies (Table 3). Examples of nonpharmacologic treatments include the age-old and well-known home remedies that include breath holding, breathing into a paper bag, swallowing a teaspoon of sugar, the Valsalva maneuver, and gargling with ice water.

TABLE 2 Pharmacotherapy for Persistent Hiccups

Antipsychotics	Anticonvulsants	Muscle Relaxants	Dopamine Antagonists	Antidepressants
Chlorpromazine (Thorazine) Haloperidol (Haldol)[1]	Phenytoin (Dilantin)[1] Carbamazepine (Tegretol)[1] Valproic acid (Depakene)[1] Gabapentin (Neurontin)[1]	Baclofen (Kemstro)[1] Cyclobenzaprine (Flexeril)[1]	Metoclopramide (Reglan)[1]	Amitriptyline (Elavil)[1]

[1]Not FDA approved for this indication.

CURRENT THERAPY

- Most transient hiccups resolve spontaneously.
- Numerous nonpharmacologic and pharmacologic therapies are proposed for treating chronic hiccups.
- Although symptom control is important, a search for an underlying etiology is essential.

Some of these maneuvers have a physiologic basis because they are based on an attempt to interrupt the vagally mediated afferent limb of the hiccup reflex arc.

Several drugs are successful anecdotally in the treatment of hiccups. The most widely used agent is chlorpromazine (Thorazine), a phenothiazine antipsychotic. It is the only agent that has achieved U.S. Food and Drug Administration (FDA) approval for treatment of hiccups. Chlorpromazine is a centrally acting agent whose precise mechanism in terminating hiccups is unknown. Intravenous administration is considered to be most effective and frequently used in an emergency department setting. Its side effects include hypotension, dystonic reactions, and excessive drowsiness. These are usually rare occurrences and avoidable if the drug is administered slowly. Oral formulations in doses of 25 to 50 mg three to four times daily as needed can be used up to 7 to 10 days. Metoclopramide (Reglan),[1] a dopamine antagonist and promotility agent, is often used when chlorpromazine does not alleviate the hiccups. It has a more favorable side-effect profile but is not as effective as chlorpromazine. The usual dose is 10 mg three to four times a day. Baclofen (Kemstro),[1] an analogue of γ-aminobutyric acid, has shown some success in limited case series, and it has fewer side effects than the other agents used to treat hiccups. The usual dosage is 10 mg three times a day. Various anticonvulsants, antidepressants, and CNS agents are all reported to terminate intractable hiccups. When the therapies just cited fail, both nonconventional and invasive modalities may be successful. Both hypnosis and acupuncture have been tried, and case reports laud their success. Phrenic nerve blocking and crushing are successful as well. Diaphragmatic pacing ameliorates those afflicted with chronic hiccups.

In summary, hiccups are a common annoyance that most people experience at some point in their lives. Their self-limiting nature usually obviates the need for

[1]Not FDA approved for this indication.

TABLE 3   Home Remedies to Treat Hiccups

Breath holding
Forcible traction on the tongue
Direct pharyngeal stimulation
Biting on a lemon
Valsalva maneuver
Ice-water gargles
Swallowing granulated sugar
Fright
Breathing into a bag
Rubbing back of neck (C5 dermatome)

medical intervention. Hiccups rarely are chronic and can be the sole symptom of a serious underlying condition. The approach to the management of patients with symptomatic hiccups is the search for and treatment of the underlying problem as well as the implementation of the numerous methods known to resolve hiccups.

REFERENCES

Friedman NL: Hiccups: A treatment review. Pharmacotherapy 1996;16:986-995.
Kolodzik PW, Eilers MA: Hiccups: Review and approach to management. Ann Emerg Med 1991;20:565-573.
Lewis JH: Hiccups: Causes and cures. J Clin Gastroenterol 1985;7: 539-552.
Rousseau P: Hiccups. South Med J 1195;88:175-181.
Souadjian J, Cain J. Intractable hiccups: Etiological factors in 220 cases. Postgrad Med 1968;43:72-77.

Acute Infectious Diarrhea

Method of
Martin S. Wolfe, MD

Acute infectious diarrhea is generally defined as the passage of three or more loose stools in a 24-hour period and continuing for less than 14 to 21 days. Associated symptoms may include nausea, vomiting, abdominal cramps, and fever. The occurrence of fever with blood or mucus in the stool indicates a more severe dysenteric syndrome related to infection with a more invasive organism.

The causative agents of acute infectious diarrhea include bacteria, viruses, parasites, and certain fungi. Incubation periods may vary from 1 to 48 hours for viruses and bacteria to 7 or more days for certain parasites. A very common bacterial agent, particularly in travelers, is enterotoxigenic *Escherichia coli*, which causes a relatively mild syndrome that is self-limited within a few days. Other types of *E. coli* causing diarrheal illness include enteroaggregative *E. coli*, enteroinvasive *E. coli*, and enterohemorrhagic *E. coli*. The latter two types can cause severe acute bloody diarrhea. Enterohemorrhagic *E. coli* is primarily contracted from eating undercooked infected beef. Potentially colonic tissue-invasive bacteria include *Shigella, Campylobacter*, and *Salmonella*, which can cause a more severe debilitating and often prolonged infection if left untreated. Less common bacterial causes in travelers include *Aeromonas* species, *Plesiomonas shigelloides*, and *Vibrio parahaemolyticus* and other *Vibrio* species. *Clostridium difficile* must be considered when an antimicrobial agent has been used recently. Food-borne bacterial infections, including such cosmopolitan organisms as *Clostridium* species, *Staphylococcus aureus*, and *Bacillus cereus*, are more often the cause of common-source diarrhea outbreaks. Most viral infections are caused by a rotavirus in infants and the Norwalk agent in older children and adults. The most common parasitic protozoal agents are *Cryptosporidium, Giardia lamblia, Entamoeba histolytica*, and *Cyclospora* with usual incubation periods of 2 to 10 days or more.

CURRENT DIAGNOSIS

- Immediate microscopic examination for fecal leukocytes or red blood cells.
- Culture identification for bacteria.
- When indicated, stool tested for *C. difficile* cytotoxin.
- Stool ova and parasite examination and stool antigen tests.

CURRENT THERAPY

- Replace fluid and electrolyte loss with oral rehydration solutions.
- Use antimotility agent or bismuth subsalicylate to improve symptoms of moderately severe diarrhea.
- While awaiting culture results, consider empirical antibiotic treatment in patients with fever and dysenteric stools.
- Treat pathogenic intestinal protozoa with appropriate antiprotozoal drugs.

Overgrowth of *Candida* species secondary to antibiotic use can be an essential factor in the development of both acute and chronic diarrhea not related to other causes. Noninfectious causes of acute diarrhea include laxatives, lactose intolerance, and as a side effect from particular drugs.

Diagnosis

Initial evaluation should be with an immediate microscopic examination for fecal leukocytes. The presence of many leukocytes indicates colonic inflammation and a high likelihood of invasive bacteria (*Shigella, Campylobacter, Salmonella*). With prior antibiotic use, *C. difficile* could possibly also be present. Acute amebiasis may cause blood in the stool but is usually not accompanied by leukocytes. *G. lamblia, Cryptosporidium,* and *Cyclospora* are only rarely associated with blood or mucus in the stool. Enterotoxigenic *E. coli* and other less common bacteria and viruses are noninvasive pathogens of the small bowel and do not lead to leukocytes or red blood cells in the stool. Cultural identification of a particular bacterial species should be made with standard techniques and with other specialized media for *Campylobacter* and *Vibrio* species. When indicated, stool can be tested for the presence of *C. difficile* cytotoxin. Only specialized laboratories can identify enterotoxigenic *E. coli*, and diagnosis is usually made from clinical features and exclusion of other organisms. An antigen test is available for rotavirus but not for the Norwalk agent. Standard procedures for ova and parasite detection should be performed on a series of preserved stool specimens. More sensitive stool antigen

tests are available for *E. histolytica, G. lamblia,* and *Cryptosporidium*. The most common fungal agents, *Candida* species, can be suspected on a stool smear and confirmed by a stool fungal culture.

Treatment

SYMPTOMATIC TREATMENT

An otherwise healthy individual with acute diarrhea is not likely to develop dehydration and can replace lost fluids and electrolytes with any beverage plus a source of sodium chloride (such as salted crackers). Young children, people greater than 60 years of age, and those individuals with certain underlying medical problems requiring diuretics who have severe diarrhea are more threatened by dehydration. With mild to moderate diarrhea, rehydration can be accomplished with flavored mineral water containing glucose and a salt solution. Packets of World Health Organization formula oral rehydration salts or rice-based oral electrolyte solutions (CeraLyte) may be used with more severe diarrhea. During the acute diarrheal episode, the diet should be modified. Milk and other dairy products should be avoided, and a bland diet emphasizing such foods as bananas, clear soups, juice, gelatin, and boiled vegetables should be consumed. As stools become formed, the diet can gradually return to normal as tolerated.

Antimotility agents such as loperamide (Imodium) or bismuth subsalicylate (Pepto-Bismol) can improve the symptoms of moderately severe diarrhea (Table 1).

TABLE 1 Symptomatic Therapy for Acute Diarrhea

Drug	Adult Dosage	Pediatric Dosage

Loperamide (Imodium)
Prescription (Imodium)
2-mg capsule OTC
  (Imodium A-D)
2-mg caplet
Liquid 5 mL,
  contains 1 mg
	4 mg; then 2 mg after each loose stool; not to exceed 16 mg/d (prescription) or 8 mg/d (OTC)	Use Imodium A-D (OTC)
		24–47 lb: 1 tsp initially, then 1 tsp after each loose stool; not to exceed 3 tsp/d
		48–59 lb: 2 tsp or 1 caplet initially, then 1 tsp or ½ caplet after each loose stool; not to exceed 4 tsp or 2 caplets/d
		60–95 lb: Same as 48–59 lb but not to exceed 6 tsp or 3 caplets/d

Bismuth subsalicylate	30 mL every 30 min for 8 doses	3–8 y: 5 mL 6–9 y: 10 mL 9–12 y: 15 mL Dose to be taken q30min for 8 doses

Abbreviation: OTC = over the counter.

Loperamide liquid and caplets are available as over-the-counter remedies. These products should not be administered to children younger than 2 years. If symptoms persist more than 48 hours or if fever or blood or mucus in the stool develops, these medications should be discontinued. Bismuth subsalicylate liquid taken as 1 oz every half hour for eight doses works somewhat more slowly but is also effective in moderately severe diarrhea. It may produce darkening of the stools and tongue, which is harmless. Other agents such as kaolin pectin and aciduric bacteria such as *Lactobacillus* were ineffective in clinical trials.

ANTIMICROBIAL TREATMENT

While awaiting culture results in patients with fever and dysenteric stools, empirical antimicrobial treatment can be directed against the most likely bacterial causes: *Shigella, Campylobacter,* or *Salmonella.* With appropriate treatment, symptoms are usually improved within the time required for culture confirmation. The only antimicrobials effective against all three of these invasive organisms are the quinolones (Table 2). I prefer ciprofloxacin, 500 to 750 mg twice daily for 3 to 5 days. Quinolones are contraindicated

in children, who could alternatively receive trimethoprim-sulfamethoxazole (TMP-SMX) (Bactrim, Septra) plus erythromycin because the former drug alone is not effective against *Campylobacter.*

Azithromycin (Zithromax) is another alternative for children and the drug of choice for travelers to areas with a high prevalence of quinolone-resistant *Campylobacter,* such as Thailand. In travelers' diarrhea, the most common agent is noninvasive enterotoxigenic *E. coli,* which causes a self-limited illness after a few days and usually can be managed with symptomatic treatment alone. However, moderate and distressing symptoms can be more quickly and dramatically improved with a 3-day course of TMP-SMX or a quinolone together with loperamide. Rifaximin (Xifaxan) is a new poorly absorbed antibiotic that is effective in the treatment of toxigenic *E. coli.* The role for antibiotic treatment for the other types of *E. coli* is uncertain. *Aeromonas* species and *Plesiomonas shigelloides* generally respond to TMP-SMX or a quinolone. *Vibrio parahaemolyticus* is self-limited, and most patients do not require antimicrobial therapy. Supportive therapy is adequate for food poisoning, which usually lasts less than 24 hours.

TABLE 2 Therapeutic Drugs for Acute Diarrhea

Drug	Indication	Adult Dosage	Pediatric Dosage
Trimethoprim-sulfamethoxazole (TMP-SMX) (Bactrim, Septra)	*Shigella,* invasive *Salmonella,*[1] toxigenic *Escherichia coli, Aeromonas,*[1] *Plesiomonas*[1]	TMP 160 mg, 800 mg SMX bid for 3–5 d	TMP 10 mg/kg/d, SMX 50 mg/kg/d in 2 divided doses for 3–5 d
Ciprofloxacin (Cipro)	*Campylobacter* (plus preceding bacteria)	500 or 750 mg for 3–5 d	Contraindicated in children
Erythromycin[1]	Drug of choice for *Campylobacter* in children and alternative for adults	250 mg qid for 5 d	40 mg/kg/d in 4 divided doses for 5 d
Azithromycin (Zithromax)	For quinolone-resistant *Campylobacter* or as alternative to ciprofloxacin for *Campylobacter* in children	500 mg once daily for 3 d	5–12 mg/kg/d for 3 d
Rifaximin (Xifaxan)	*E. coli,* toxigenic	200 mg bid for 3 d	Not recommended for children <12 y
Metronidazole (Flagyl)	Giardiasis[1] *Clostridium difficile* Amebiasis—moderate to severe	250 mg tid for 7 d 250 mg qid for 10–14 d 500–750 mg tid for 10 d	15 mg/kg/d in 3 divided doses for 7 d 20 mg/kg/d in 4 divided doses for 10–14 d 30–45 mg/kg/d in 3 divided doses for 10 d
Nitazoxanide (Alinia)	Giardiasis Cryptosporidiosis	500 mg bid for 3 d	1–3 y: 5 mL of suspension bid for 3 d 4–11 y: 10 mL of suspension bid for 3 d >12 y: as per adult dose
Paromomycin (Humatin)	Amebiasis follow-up to metronidazole; alone for mild amebiasis	500 mg tid for 7 d	25–30 mg/kg/d in 3 divided doses for 7 d
Iodoquinol (Yodoxin)	Same as for paromomycin	650 mg tid for 20 d	30–40 mg/kg/d in 3 divided doses for 20 d
Quinacrine (Atabrine)[1]*	Giardiasis	100 mg tid for 5 d	6 mg/kg/d in 3 divided doses for 5 d
Nystatin (Mycostatin)	Intestinal candidiasis	500,000 U tid for 7 d	250,000-500,000 U tid for 7 d

[1]Not FDA approved for this indication.
*Can be obtained from certain compounding pharmacists.

Acute diarrhea following antibiotic use could be caused by *C. difficile* or a *Candida* species. With a positive *C. difficile* cytotoxin test, treatment should initially be with metronidazole, 250 mg four times daily for 10 to 14 days. Persistent or very severe infections would require oral vancomycin, 125 mg four times daily for 10 to 14 days. In the absence of other causative agents or with a considerable amount of yeast found on a wet stool smear or stool fungal culture, treatment for *Candida* may be given with oral Mycostatin (nystatin), 500,000 U three times daily for 7 days.

For acute invasive amebic dysentery, initial treatment is with metronidazole (Flagyl), 750 mg three times daily for 10 days. This should always be followed with a course of a poorly absorbed luminal drug, either paromomycin (Humatin), 500 mg three times a day for 7 days, or iodoquinol (Yodoxin), 650 mg three times a day for 20 days. For moderate nondysenteric amebiasis, 500 mg of metronidazole, three times daily for 10 days, followed by a luminal drug should be adequate. For very mild amebiasis, a luminal drug alone is sufficient. Acute giardiasis can be treated with metronidazole, 250 mg three times daily for 7 days. Quinacrine (Atabrine) in a 5-day course of 100 mg three times daily is an even more effective treatment for giardiasis; albeit with potentially more troublesome side effects. However, this drug has to be obtained from a compounding pharmacy. Nitazoxanide (Alinia) is a new agent that is effective against *Giardia* and *Cryptosporidium* agent. It comes in a liquid formulation and in tablets for adults. A 3-day course is effective and well tolerated in all age groups. Cryptosporidiosis in a nonimmunosuppressed individual is self-limited within 3 or 4 weeks, and symptomatic treatment alone is generally sufficient because currently no reliable curative treatment is available.

Complications

Reactive arthropathies developing within 4 weeks of the primary infection are linked with *Yersinia, Campylobacter, Shigella, Salmonella*, and *Cryptosporidium* infections. Acute renal failure may occur after infection with certain strains of *E. coli* and *Salmonella*. A rare complication of infection with *Campylobacter* is an association with the delayed development of Guillain-Barré syndrome. Persistent gastrointestinal complaints including irritable bowel syndrome are common after acute or travelers' diarrhea and are not associated with a particular pathogen.

Prevention

The practice of appropriate food and water hygiene is the best preventive measure against infection with the agents causing acute diarrhea. Antimicrobial drug prophylaxis is generally not recommended for travelers because of resistance and potential side effects. In particular situations where antimicrobial drug prophylaxis is indicated, quinolones are considered to be most effective and safe. Bismuth subsalicylate, taken as two tablets chewed four times a day, gives approximately 65% protection against diarrhea. This should not be used for more than 3 weeks or by persons who either cannot take salicylates or are already taking salicylates for other purposes.

REFERENCES

Adachi JA, Ostrosky-Zeichner L, DuPont HL, et al: Empirical antimicrobial therapy for traveler's diarrhea. Clin Infect Dis 2000;31:1079-1083.

Allos BM: Campylobacter jejuni infections: Update on emerging issues and trends. Clin Infect Dis 2001;32:1201-1206.

Guerrant RL, Van Gilder T, Steiner TS, et al: Practice guidelines for the management of infectious diarrhea. Clin Infect Dis 2001;32:331-350.

Nitazoxanide (Alinia)—a new anti-protozoal agent. Med Lett Drugs Ther 2003;45:29-31.

Okhuysen RC: Traveler's diarrhea due to intestinal protozoa. Clin Infect Dis 2001;33:110-114.

Okhuysen RC, Jiang ZD, Carlin L, et al: GI complaints following traveler's diarrhea. Am J Gastroenterol 2004;99:774-1778.

Ortega YR, Sterling CR, Gilman RH, et al: Cyclospora species—a new protozoan pathogen of humans. N Engl J Med 1993;328:1308-1312.

Rees JH, Soudain SE, Gregson NA, et al: *Campylobacter jejuni* infection and Guillain-Barré syndrome. N Engl J Med 1995;333:1374-1379.

Steffen R, Sack DA, Riopel L, et al: Therapy of traveler's diarrhea with rifaximin on various continents. Am J Gastroenterol 2003;98:1073-1078.

Constipation

Method of
David E. Beck, MD

Constipation is a common and potentially distressing constellation of symptoms rather than a definable disease. The prevalence of constipation in Western countries ranges from 2% to 27%. Self-reported constipation is more prevalent in women, nonwhites, and those older than 65 years. It accounts for 2.5 million physician visits annually in the United States, 20,000 hospitalizations each year, and 3 million prescriptions for laxatives each year.

Defining constipation is challenging. From a medical standpoint, constipation is the inability to evacuate stool completely and spontaneously more than three times per week. Most patients define constipation as the passage of hard stools, a sense of incomplete evacuation, a sense of excessive straining, and excessive time spent in unsuccessful defecation. Most clinicians use a combination of subjective and objective criteria to address these complaints. Table 1 lists one standardized set of criteria developed in 1999.

Etiology and Pathophysiology

The causes of constipation are multifactorial and can result from neurologic or systemic disorders or as a side

TABLE 1 Rome II Criteria for Constipation

Straining in >25% of defecations
Lumpy or hard stools in >25% of defecations
Sensation of incomplete evacuation in >25% of defecations
Sensation of anorectal obstruction/blockade in >25% of defecation
Manual maneuvers to facilitate >25% of defecation
Fewer than 3 defecations per week

CURRENT DIAGNOSIS

- Adequate history to exclude treatable etiologies
- Anatomic evaluation of colon
- Functional study (colonic transit study) in refractory patients

effect of medications. To guide treatment, constipation is divided into three categories: normal-transit constipation, slow-transit constipation, and outlet obstruction. In normal-transit constipation (functional constipation), the patient's stool frequency and transit through the colon are normal, but patients have subjective symptoms. These patients usually respond to dietary fiber supplementation or osmotic laxatives. Slow-transit constipation (colonic inertia) is a motility dysfunction that often only responds to surgical treatment. Outlet obstruction or defecatory disorders include pelvic floor dyssynergia and structural abnormalities such as rectal intussusception and rectocele.

Evaluation

The initial evaluation should consist of a thorough history and physical examination. An important part of the medical history is establishing the nature and duration of the symptoms. Recent onset of changes in bowel habits increases the incidence of an identifiable cause. The use of medications associated with constipation (Table 2) as well as medical conditions such as hypothyroidism and diabetes (Table 3) must be considered. Patients without an identifiable cause of constipation, those who are refractory to dietary

TABLE 2 Medications Commonly Associated with Constipation

Anticholinergics
Antihistamines
Tricyclic antidepressants
Antipsychotics
Neuroleptic agents
Antiparkinsonian drugs
Antihypertensive
    Clonidine (Catapres)
    Calcium channel blockers
Cation-containing agents
    Iron supplements
    Calcium (antacids [Tums], supplements)
    Aluminum (antacids, sucralfate [Carafate])
    Bismuth
Diuretics
Opiates
Morphine
Diphenoxylate with atropine (Lomotil)
Codeine
Nonsteroidal anti-inflammatory agents
Resins
Cholestyramine (Questran)
Sympathomimetics
Serotonin type 3 antagonists
Ondansetron (Zofran)
Granisetron (Kytril)

TABLE 3 Systemic Diseases Associated with Constipation

Endocrine and Metabolic Disorders
    Diabetes mellitus
    Hypothyroidism
    Hypercalcemia
    Chronic renal failure
Central Nervous System Disorders
    Dementia
    Parkinson's disease
    Multiple sclerosis
    Spinal cord lesions
    Cerebrovascular disease
Neuromuscular Diseases
    Progressive systemic sclerosis
    Muscular dystrophy
    Hirschsprung's disease
    Chagas' disease
    Autonomic neuropathy
Others
    Amyloidosis
    Dermatomyositis
    Depression

modification with fiber, or those with risk factors for colorectal cancer (e.g., >35 years, family history) should have an anatomic evaluation of their colon. This can be accomplished with a colonoscopy or a barium enema. Because constipated patients often have difficulty with the cleansing required for a colonoscopy and can be difficult to colonoscope, a barium contrast study is usually the better option for evaluating chronic constipation. Additional studies, such as a colonic transit study to document slow colonic transit and studies of outlet function (defecogram, manometry, or balloon expulsion test), are indicated for refractory cases.

Colonic transit studies can be performed in a number of ways. The author's preference is to have the patient ingest a capsule with 24 radiopaque markers (commercially available as Sitz-Markers, Konsyl Pharmaceuticals, Fort Worth, Texas) and obtain abdominal radiographs on days 1, 3, and 5 after ingestion of the markers. Eighty percent of normal subjects pass 80% of the markers by day 3. An abnormal test suggestive of colonic inertia has 20 or more markers distributed throughout the colon on day 3 or 5. With outlet obstruction or rectal dysfunction, more than 20 markers have usually grouped in the distal sigmoid colon or proximal rectum on day 3 or 5.

Anatomic abnormalities such as strictures, cancers, or volvulus should be referred for appropriate surgical treatment. Colonic inertia is confirmed by an abnormal transit study and a normal outlet study. Selected patients with colonic inertia should be referred for colonic resections. Patients with outlet dysfunction are a more challenging problem.

Treatment

GENERAL MEASURES

Initial management includes patient education and an explanation of normal bowel habits. Medications known to

CURRENT THERAPY

- Medication adjustment and associated disease treatment
- Trial of daily fiber or laxatives
- Surgical referral for appropriate patients
- Colectomy and ileoproctostomy for colonic inertia

cause constipation should be minimized and metabolic abnormalities (e.g., hypothyroidism) should be corrected. Regular exercise and increases in fiber and oral fluids are encouraged.

FIBER

Dietary fiber increases stool bulk and water content and reduces colonic transit time. The goal is to increase fiber intake to 20 to 30 g daily, which can be achieved through diet and fiber supplements (Table 3). Patients are encouraged to increase their intake of fruits, vegetables, and high-fiber breakfast cereals or raw bran. High-fiber cereals contain 8 to 10 g of fiber per serving; 1 tablespoon of bran powder sprinkled over foods adds 2 g of fiber. Patients with lactulose intolerance or poor dietary compliance are better managed with dietary supplements such as psyllium (Metamucil) or methylcellulose (Citrucel) (Table 3). Patient compliance with fiber is often poor because of the side effects of bloating, flatulence, and distention. Different types and amounts of fiber affect patients differently. For this reason, patients are encouraged to start at a lower dose and slowly increase their intake. If one type of fiber does not improve symptoms, other types should be tried.

PHARMACOLOGIC

Osmotic laxatives, such as polyethylene glycol (MiraLax) or lactulose (Chronulac), can be used in patients with continuous symptoms who do not respond to fiber. These agents are safe to use long term and do not promote dependency. The different types of osmotic agents (unabsorbed agents or salts) all work by retaining or pulling fluid into the intestinal lumen. They should be titrated over several days to a dose that produces a semisolid to soft stool. Because excessive doses of some of these agents can produce fluid overload or electrolyte abnormalities, they must be used with care in patients with renal insufficiency or cardiac dysfunction.

Emollient laxatives soften stool by reducing surface tension, allowing intestinal fluids to penetrate the fecal mass. Mineral oil requires caution in the elderly (>60 years), neurologically impaired, and those with impaired swallowing on account of its risk of aspiration and the potential for interference with absorption of fat-soluble vitamins.

Stimulant laxatives are used in patients with severe constipation who do not respond to fiber or osmotic laxatives. These agents increase intestinal motility and stimulate fluid secretion into the bowel lumen. Despite folklore, no level 1 or 2 evidence indicates that chronic use of stimulants causes "cathartic colon" (dilated colon and loss of haustoria). Chronic use of anthraquinones (senna) can cause melanosis coli, a brown-black pigmentation of the colonic mucosa. This condition has no clinical consequence and regresses if the patient stops taking the laxative. Although anthraquinones were a common component of commercially available laxatives in the past, currently they are rarely seen except in so-called natural over-the-counter preparations. The goal with stimulants is to use the lowest and least expensive product to relieve the patient's symptoms. Different agents or combinations may be required.

Enemas can be self-administered to assist evacuation. Tap water is preferred for a small-volume stimulation. Oil-retention enemas are useful for hard or impacted stool. Small volumes or near normal osmolarity are preferred to prevent injury to the mucosa and fluid absorption.

Prokinetic agents have been approved for selective patient groups. Tegaserod (Zelnorm) is a serotonin receptor agonist that accelerates transit through the small bowel and colon. It is currently approved for short-term treatment of women with constipation-predominant irritable bowel syndrome.

Table 4 summarizes the pharmacologic options available to manage constipation. The therapeutic goal is to use the least expensive agent that relieves the patient's symptoms. Over time some medications may become less effective and may need to be altered or combined with other agents. Patients that remain refractory to maximal therapy may benefit from a surgical referral.

SURGICAL

A small group of patients who are refractory to these regimens may be considered for surgical treatment. Refinement of physiologic evaluations and experience has helped optimize patient selection. The two groups of patients who benefit from surgery are those with either an anatomic abnormality or a specific functional aberration such as colonic inertia. Surgery has a very limited role in treating outlet obstruction.

Several operations are used to treat colonic inertia. All involve a colonic resection and have varied from a segmental resection (left or right colectomy), to a subtotal colectomy with cecorectal or ileosigmoid anastomosis, to a total colectomy. The best results are obtained with colectomy and ileorectal anastomosis (ileoproctostomy). Performing a lesser operation leads to a high incidence of recurrent constipation. Overall, the more of the colon that is removed, the lower incidence of constipation and the higher number of bowel movements. As a compromise, most surgeons currently perform a total colectomy with an ileorectal anastomosis (ileoproctostomy) with the anastomosis at the level of the sacral promontory. This leaves the patient with 12 to 18 cm of rectum and allows a patient to average two to four bowel movements per day. The stool is looser than normal but becomes formed after a short period of adaptation. The patients have good control, and the incidence of recurrent constipation is very low. More than 95% of properly selected patients can be expected to be satisfied with their surgical treatment and experience long-term results.

Patients with outlet obstruction should be evaluated with a defecogram. If an anatomic problem is identified, a surgical option may be possible. Rectal prolapse can be corrected with a perineal procedure such as that of

TABLE 4 Pharmacologic Management of Constipation

Medication	Dosages
Bulk (Fiber) Laxatives	
Psyllium (Metamucil, Konsyl)	Titrate up to 12–20 g/d[3]
Methylcellulose (Citrucel)	
Polycarbophil (FiberCon)	
Gum (Benefiber)	
Bran	
Osmotic Laxatives	
Unabsorbed sugars or inert agents	15–30 mL qd or bid
Lactulose (Cephulac, Chronulac)	15–30 mL qd or bid
Sorbitol 70% (Cytosol)	17–36 g qd or bid[3]
Polyethylene glycol (MiraLax)	17–36 g qd or bid
Polyethylene glycol and electrolytes[1]	15–30 mL qd or bid
(GoLYTELY, NuLYTELY, Colyte)	150–300 mL as needed
Salts	15–30 mL qd[3] mixed with 1/2 glass of water
Magnesium hydroxide (Milk of Magnesia)	1–3 tablets qd or bid[3]
Magnesium citrate (Evac-O-Mag)	
Sodium phosphate	
Fleet Phospho-Soda	
Visicol	
Stimulant Laxatives	
Bisacodyl (Dulcolax)	5–10 mg suppository nightly
Senna (Senokot)	70–100 g qd[3]
Cascara sagrada (Colamin)*	2–5 mL qd
Aloe (casanthranol)	30–60 mg qd
Castor oil (Purge)	15–30 mL qd
Emollients or Stool Softeners	
Mineral oil	5–15 mL orally at night for children (6–12 y)
	15–45 mL for adults
Docusate sodium (Colace)	100 mg bid
Rectal Enemas or Suppository	
Glycerin, bisacodyl suppository (Dulcolax)	10 mg qd
Tap-water enema	500 mL qd
Phosphate enema (Fleet Enema)	120 mL qd
Mineral oil retention enema (Fleet Mineral Oil enema)	100 mL qd
Prokinetic Agent	
Serotonin receptor agonist (Tegaserod [Zelnorm])	6 mg bid

[1]Not FDA approved for this indication.
[3]Exceeds dosage recommended by the manufacturer.
*Available as a dietary supplement.

Altemeier or Delorme, and a symptomatic rectocele can be corrected with a transanal or transvaginal repair. Patients with normal colonic motility and outlet obstruction from a nonrelaxing puborectalis muscle should initially be offered biofeedback. The few patients not helped with this therapy may be considered for a botulinum A toxin injection (Botox)[1] into the puborectalis muscle.

Patients with colonic inertia and rectal dysmotility can be offered an ileostomy. A very select group of these patients is helped with a restorative proctocolectomy. The potential benefits of this procedure must be balanced against its functional limitations and its associated morbidity.

Fecal Impaction

Patients with fecal impactions can be managed by several maneuvers. Low impactions of hard stool often require digital disimpaction, which can be assisted by the administration of an oil retention enema (Fleet Mineral Oil) to soften the retained stool. An effective alternative in patients without an intestinal obstruction is the administration of an oral osmotic laxative. A polyethylene glycol solution (MiraLax) can be administered at a rate of 1 capful[3] in 4 oz of water every 15 minutes until stool evacuation occurs. After resolution of the impaction, patients who have not had a recent colonic evaluation should have

[1]Not FDA approved for this indication.

[3]Exceeds dosage recommended by the manufacturer.

one, and a maintenance program (daily fiber or laxative) should be initiated.

REFERENCES

Araghizadef F: Fecal impaction. Clin Colon Rectal Surg 2005;18:116-119.

Beck DE: Constipation. In Fazio VW (ed): Current Therapy in Colon and Rectal Surgery. Hamilton, Ontario, Canada, BC Decker, 1990, pp 339-343.

Beck DE: Initial evaluation of constipation. In Wexner SD, Bartolo DCC (eds): Constipation: Etiology, Evaluation, and Management. London, Butterworth-Heinemann, 1994, pp 31-38.

Beck DE: Surgical management of constipation. Clin Colon Rectal Surg 2005;18:81-84.

Camilleri M, von der Ohe M: Methods to measure small bowel and colonic transit. In Wexner SD, Bartolo DCC (eds): Constipation. London, Butterworth-Heinemann, 1994, pp 39-51.

Ellis CN: Treatment of obstructed defecation. Clin Colon Rectal Surg 2005;18:85-95.

Pikarsky AJ, Singh JJ, Weiss EG, et al: Long-term follow-up of patients undergoing colectomy for colonic inertia. Dis Colon Rectum 2001; 44:179-183.

Schmitt SL, Wexner SD, Bartolo DCC: Surgical treatment of colonic inertia. In Wexner SD, Bartolo DCC (eds): Constipation: Etiology, Evaluation, and Management. London, Butterworth-Heinemann, 1995, pp 153-159.

Stewart J, Kumar D, Keighley MR: Results of anal or low rectal anastomosis and pouch construction for megacolon and megarectum. Br J Surg 1994;81:1051-1053.

Takahashi T, Fitzgerald SD, Pemberton JH: Evaluation and treatment of constipation. Rev Gastroenterol Mex 1994;59:133-138.

Wexner SD, Daniel N, Jagelman DG: Colectomy for constipation: physiologic investigation is the key to success. Dis Colon Rectum 1991;34:851-856.

Fever

Method of
Ian M. Paul, MD, MSc

Fever is both sign and symptom of an underlying disease process that often produces anxiety for patients, parents, and health care providers. This so-called fever phobia can cause inappropriate management of the illness and fever. Fever is typically a transient phenomenon that only requires treatment when it is accompanied by discomfort or otherwise compromises a patient's health.

Definitions

Fever is characterized by an elevated core body temperature that occurs as a protective response to a pathogen. Observations by Wunderlich in 1868 defined normal body temperature at 37°C (98.6°F) and febrile temperature at 38°C (100°F) or higher. Studies also show diurnal variation and differences in temperature based on temperature site (mouth, rectum, ear, or temporal artery), but most clinicians classify a temperature of 38°C (100.4°F) or greater as fever.

Many clinicians, patients, and parents also use the term *high fever*, although this is not based on consistent objective criteria. Nonetheless, a temperature of 40°C (104°F) or greater is considered by many to be a high fever because

CURRENT DIAGNOSIS

- Temperatures taken by oral, rectal, tympanic, or temporal artery thermometers of 38.0°C (100.4°F) or more are consistent with fever.
- Fever is a normal physiologic response but can cause dehydration and increase metabolic rate. Benign febrile seizures can occur in young children with fevers.
- The other symptoms accompanying a fever help determine the severity of the febrile illness.
- Fever in infants younger than 3 months or in neutropenic patients is considered a medical emergency until proved otherwise.
- Fevers lasting 8 or more days without a clear cause are considered a fever of unknown origin (FUO). They may warrant more extensive evaluation.

nearly universally, patients are uncomfortable when experiencing a body temperature of this magnitude. Some worry that without treatment body temperature continues to rise during fever. This fear is unjustified, however, because only rarely do temperatures exceed 41.1°C (106°F), the temperature considered to be the physiologic limit of the febrile response. If a temperature recorded is greater than 41.1°C (106°F), superimposed hyperthermia is probable. Hyperthermia is distinguished from fever and characterized by a temperature above the hypothalamic set point. This is related to a hypothalamic insult or a disruption in normal homeostatic mechanisms that balance heat production and dissipation.

Two other definitions related to fever are fever without a source and fever of unknown origin (FUO). Both terms are used when no cause is determined for the fever and/or its associated illness. The majority of cases in both have infectious etiologies; the difference relates to duration of the fever. Fever without a source is used in the first week of an illness, whereas FUO is used for a fever lasting 8 or more days or occurring at intervals over weeks or months.

Physiology and Pathophysiology

Fever begins with an inciting stimulus that triggers an inflammatory response. Most often this stimulus is infectious and causes leukocytes to release cytokines including interleukin-1β, tumor necrosis factor-α, interleukin-6, and interferon-γ. These and other cytokines interact with the temperature regulatory tissues in the anterior hypothalamus and release prostaglandin E_2 (PGE_2). PGE_2 then alters the firing rate of neurons in the preoptic area of the anterior hypothalamus, increasing the thermoregulatory set point.

Other systems respond to increase body temperature as this set point rises. Examples of these responses include shivering to increase heat production and peripheral vasoconstriction to reduce heat loss. Behavioral responses such as wearing warm clothes or covering up with a blanket may also occur.

The febrile response to an antigenic challenge is a beneficial one. Numerous studies show improved outcomes in those who manifest proper febrile responses and that many components of the immune system function better at higher temperatures (e.g., enhanced neutrophil migration, increased T-cell proliferation, and production of interferon). Clinical studies supporting this concept show treatment with acetaminophen prolonged the duration of active varicella in children, and aspirin therapy prolonged the shedding of rhinovirus in adults.

Fever Phobia and the Complications of Fever

Fever phobia, the fear surrounding fever, termed by Dr. Barton Schmitt, has been recognized for several decades. Schmitt found some startling results when questioning parents about fever. His study shows that 56% of parents gave antipyretics for temperatures less than 37.8°C (100°F), and 58% thought temperatures less than 38.9°C (102°F) constituted a "high fever." Further, 62% thought fever caused permanent harm, with "brain damage" a common concern. In 2001, a similar study found equally troubling results. These authors found that 85% of parents woke their child to give antipyretics, 52% checked their child's temperature every hour or less, and most worrisome, 58% gave antipyretics too often.

Fever is the normal physiologic process previously described. Complications are rare and usually well tolerated. Common adverse events are dehydration and, in children 6 months to 6 years of age, benign febrile seizures, which are a common occurrence in young children without subsequent focal findings. The belief that seizures are caused by a rapid rise in temperature has been contradicted. In addition, no evidence suggests that aggressive use of antipyretics prevents a febrile seizure.

Fever is generally a protective physiologic response, but under some circumstances, it is harmful. For example, the metabolic rate steadily increases as body temperature rises. Further, myocardial depression, orthostatic dysfunction, and increases in oxygen consumption, respiratory minute volume, and respiratory quotient may not be tolerated by patients, especially those with chronic conditions. Severe complications such as death or so-called brain damage occurring during febrile illness are related to the underlying disease process, not fever.

Treatment of Fever

It is important to overcome the desire to focus on a thermometer's reading when treating a fever by evaluating and treating the underlying illness and treating the discomfort associated with the febrile illness. The underlying condition may be age or disease specific. For example, infants younger than 3 months and neutropenic patients with fever are considered medical emergencies and require aggressive evaluation. Fever in the absence of a condition like one of these requires treatment only when accompanied by discomfort or other morbidity.

ACETAMINOPHEN

Acetaminophen (Tylenol) is the most commonly used medication to treat fever. This drug is well absorbed from

CURRENT THERAPY

- Treat the underlying illness and the discomfort associated with the febrile illness, not the number on the thermometer.
- If antipyretic/analgesic medications are used, appropriate choices for *children* are:
  - Acetaminophen (Tylenol) 15 mg/kg every 4 to 6 hours up to five times per day as needed for children older than 3 months.
  - Ibuprofen (Motrin, Advil) 10 mg/kg every 6 hours as needed for children older than 6 months.
- If antipyretic/analgesic medications are used, appropriate choices for *adolescents and adults* are:
  - Acetaminophen (Tylenol), 650 to 1000 mg every 4 to 6 hours as needed (maximum 4000 mg per day).
  - Ibuprofen (Motrin, Advil), 200 to 400 mg every 6 hours as needed.
  - Aspirin, 325 to 650 mg every 6 hours as needed.
- Sponge bathing, if chosen, should use tepid water with an antipyretic medication and no alcohol.

oral and rectal routes and widely available in liquid and tablet preparations around the world. Acetaminophen produces its antipyretic effect by inhibiting the release of PGE_2 yet does not possess the anti-inflammatory properties of nonsteroidal anti-inflammatory agents. Children at least 3 months or older may be given acetaminophen at a dose of 15 mg/kg every 4 to 6 hours up to a maximum of 75 mg/kg per day. Remember that children less than 3 months of age require evaluation when presenting with fever, and acetaminophen should be used with caution so as not to miss a serious bacterial infection. Doses of 650 to 1000 mg every 4 to 6 hours with a maximum daily dose of 4000 mg may be given to adolescents and adults. An extended-release preparation of 1300 mg maximum every 8 hours is also available for adolescents and adults.

IBUPROFEN

Ibuprofen (Motrin, Advil) is a nonsteroidal anti-inflammatory drug (NSAID) that has analgesic and anti-inflammatory properties in addition to its antipyretic effects. This drug is highly effective and generally well tolerated with short-term administration when given orally. Ibuprofen's antipyretic mechanism of action blocks prostaglandin synthesis through inhibition of cyclooxygenase. This converts arachidonic acid to cyclic endoperoxides. Ibuprofen may be given to febrile children 6 months or older at a dose of 10 mg/kg every 6 to 8 hours. This dose has similar efficacy to that of acetaminophen. Adolescents and adults may take doses of 200 to 400 mg every 6 hours as needed.

ASPIRIN

Aspirin (acetylsalicylic acid) is used less than it was in recent years. This drug was the standard treatment of fever for many years but is no longer used with children because of an association with Reye's syndrome. It has anti-inflammatory, analgesic, and antipyretic properties similar to ibuprofen and remains an effective treatment for adults. Adults may be given doses of 325 to 650 mg every 4 to 6 hours as needed. Bleeding commonly occurs with aspirin therapy because of its antiplatelet effect (e.g., in the gastrointestinal tract).

MEDICATION COMBINATIONS

Combinations or alternating regimens of antipyretics should be used with caution, although studies show that aspirin and acetaminophen combinations are more effective. The American Academy of Pediatrics (AAP) cautions against using multiple antipyretics because of an increase in the likelihood of dosing errors. The AAP also cites a lack of evidence to support the joint use of acetaminophen with ibuprofen.

NONPHARMACOLOGIC TREATMENT

External cooling, most commonly sponge bathing, is used to reduce fever. Some have advised against its use because it can cause discomfort. Discomfort is less likely to occur during sponging when using tepid water and antipyretic administration, but the efficacy of this treatment is questioned. Alcohol should not be a component of the bath because it may cause dehydration and hypoglycemia.

REFERENCES

Acetaminophen toxicity in children. Pediatrics 2001;108(4):1020-1024.
Aronoff DM, Neilson EG: Antipyretics: Mechanisms of action and clinical use in fever suppression. Am J Med 2001;111(4):304-315.
Bouchama A, Knochel JP: Heat stroke. N Engl J Med 2002;346(25):1978-1988.
Crocetti M, Moghbeli N, Serwint J: Fever phobia revisited: Have parental misconceptions about fever changed in 20 years? Pediatrics 2001;107(6):1241-1246.
Doran TF, De Angelis C, Baumgardner RA, Mellits ED: Acetaminophen: More harm than good for chickenpox? J Pediatr 1989;114(6):1045-1048.
Kluger MJ: Fever: Role of pyrogens and cryogens. Physiol Rev 1991;71(1):93-127.
Kluger MJ: Fever revisited. Pediatrics 1992;90(6):846-850.
Mackowiak PA, Worden G: Carl Reinhold August Wunderlich and the evolution of clinical thermometry. Clin Infect Dis 1994;18(3):458-467.
Schmitt BD: Fever phobia: Misconceptions of parents about fevers. Am J Dis Child 1980;134(2):176-181.
Sharber J: The efficacy of tepid sponge bathing to reduce fever in young children. Am J Emerg Med 1997;15(2):188-192.
Simons SHP, Anderson BJ, Tibboel D: Analgesic agents. In Yaffe SJ, Aranda JV (eds): Neonatal and Pediatric Pharmacology: Therapeutic Principles in Practice, 3rd ed. Philadelphia, Lippincott Williams & Wilkins, 2005, pp 638-662.
Stanley ED, Jackson GG, Panusarn C, et al: Increased virus shedding with aspirin treatment of rhinovirus infection. JAMA 1975;231(12):1248-1251.

Cough

Method of
David G. Hill, MD

Cough is among the most common presenting complaints of outpatients in the United States. It serves as a protective reflex against foreign material and as a method to clear secretions from the airway. The cough center is located in the medulla, and the cough reflex is mediated by way of multiple nervous system pathways including the trigeminal, glossopharyngeal, vagus, and phrenic nerves. Cough is mediated by separate neural pathways from bronchoconstriction. When cough occurs there is a synchronized activation of muscles, the glottis opens, and the lungs expand. At the peak of inspiration the glottis closes and expiratory muscles contract. This results in increased intrathoracic pressure; when the glottis opens airflow can reach 500 miles per hour. The cough reflex varies in different patient populations. Women have a more sensitive cough reflex than men. Smokers' cough reflexes are depressed despite the increased frequency of cough in this population. Patients who have a decreased cough sensitivity following cerebral vascular accidents have an increased incidence of pneumonia. Angiotensin-converting enzyme (ACE) inhibitors increase cough reflex sensitivity and have been shown to decrease the risk of pneumonia in patients with cerebrovascular accidents. The evaluation of cough as a patient complaint may best be pursued by examining the duration of the symptoms. Cough can be subcategorized into acute and chronic cough. Cough that occurs following an acute respiratory infection may narrow the differential diagnosis and is addressed separately.

Acute Cough

Acute cough may be defined as cough that has been present for less than 8 weeks. Because all causes of chronic coughs initially cause acute symptoms, patients with acute cough may actually have cough caused by one of the etiologies discussed later in this section; however, acute cough more commonly is the result of a less indolent process (Box 1). Infectious etiologies are a frequent cause of acute cough. Most acute cough is the result of viral infections, specifically the common cold. Most cough resulting from the common cold is self-limited and lasts less than 3 weeks. Most episodes of sinusitis are of viral etiology; however, bacterial sinusitis can also result in acute cough. The presence of a significant smoking history raises the possibility of an acute exacerbation of chronic obstructive pulmonary

---

BOX 1 Causes of Acute Cough

- Viral upper respiratory infections (the common cold)
- Acute sinusitis (usually viral, occasionally bacterial)
- Exacerbation of chronic obstructive pulmonary disease
- Allergic rhinitis
- *Bordetella pertussis* infection

disease (COPD) as the cause of acute cough, especially in patients with previously documented COPD. *Bordetella pertussis* infection may also be the etiology of an acute episode of cough. Noninfectious processes that lead to acute cough include allergic rhinitis, congestive heart failure, asthma, and aspiration. The clinical history, physical exam, and diagnostic testing are of particular importance in differentiating these disease states and often point to the diagnosis.

Postinfectious Cough

Postinfectious cough begins with an acute upper respiratory tract infection but persists following the resolution of the other acute symptoms (Box 2). Postnasal drip syndrome may present following the common cold or sinusitis. Bronchospasm may lead to postinfectious cough either as a result of a single episode of postinfectious wheezing or an exacerbation of underlying asthma. Postinfectious cough may be the initial presentation of asthma. Recurrent episodes of airflow obstruction are required to confirm the diagnosis of this chronic illness. Because *B. pertussis* can present with an indolent course, this infection can be confused with a postinfectious cough. Similarly, bacterial sinusitis can be confused with postinfectious cough. Both of these etiologies of cough are the result of ongoing infection rather than true postinfectious cough. *Mycoplasma pneumoniae* and *Chlamydia pneumoniae* infections may also result in postinfectious cough likely because of persistent airway inflammation and increases in cough reflex sensitivity.

Chronic Cough

Chronic cough presents the most difficult diagnostic dilemma for the health care practitioner. Cough of greater than 8 weeks' duration can be considered chronic. Lesser duration of symptoms may still be indicative of one of the etiologies discussed in this section, but such cough is more likely the result of one of the infectious or postinfectious etiologies described previously. In patients who have never smoked, chronic cough is most likely the result of asthma, postnasal drip syndrome, or gastroesophageal reflux. These three etiologies are the most common cause of chronic cough regardless of patient age. In nonsmokers with a normal chest radiograph who are not taking an ACE inhibitor, these three etiologies alone or in combination are the cause of more than 85% of chronic cough (Box 3). Postnasal drip syndrome is the most common of these etiologies. Cough may be the sole presenting symptom of any of these conditions; they are not mutually exclusive and may coexist, particularly in the patient with troublesome, persistent symptoms. Most patients with problematic, persistent cough have multiple etiologies contributing to their symptoms. COPD must be considered in current smokers and in those patients with a significant smoking history. Smokers can have a cough of any etiology, however, and it should not be assumed that their cough is the result of smoking or COPD. Although smokers frequently admit to cough when a history is taken, they infrequently seek medical attention for this symptom. Cough resulting from the use of ACE inhibitors must be considered in all patients being treated with these medications. Less common, yet frequent causes of cough include chronic bronchitis from irritants other than tobacco smoke and eosinophilic bronchitis. Occasionally, chronic cough may be the result of:

- Bronchogenic carcinoma
- Metastatic carcinoma
- Bronchiectasis
- Sarcoidosis
- Pulmonary fibrosis
- Pneumoconiosis
- Hypersensitivity pneumonitis
- Congestive heart failure
- Chronic infection, such as tuberculosis or *Mycobacterium avium* complex
- Recurrent aspiration because of pharyngeal or esophageal abnormalities

Key Diagnostic Points

The evaluation of acute cough should focus on the history and physical exam. Most acute cough will be the result of self-limited viral upper respiratory infections. More thorough evaluation is necessary in the workup of cough of longer duration particularly if the cough has been present for more than 2 months. The history of onset of the cough and whether it was associated with an acute infectious episode should be elicited. Exposure to sick contacts particularly to a known case of *B. pertussis* are important historic considerations. The timing and nature of the cough and any associated sputum must be described. Factors that mitigate or worsen the cough should be examined, and prior history of episodic cough, allergies, wheezing, asthma, and gastroesophageal reflux should be questioned. A thorough medication history particularly regarding use of ACE inhibitors must be obtained. Environmental factors both at home and in the work place should be reviewed. Although smoking history is important, it is again noted that smoking-related cough is an infrequent reason for a patient to seek medical attention. The physical exam should focus most on the head, neck, and thorax with a thorough examination

---

BOX 2 Causes of Postinfectious Cough

- Postnasal drip syndrome
- Bronchospasm
- *Bordetella pertussis* infection
- Bacterial sinusitis
- *Mycoplasma pneumoniae/Chlamydia pneumoniae* infection

BOX 3 Causes of Chronic Cough

- Postnasal drip syndrome
- Asthma
- Gastroesophageal reflux disease (GERD)
- Eosinophilic bronchitis
- Angiotensin-converting enzyme inhibitors

of the upper respiratory tract including the auditory canal, nose, and oropharynx. The cardiopulmonary exam should also be thorough to elicit signs of less common illnesses.

Acute cough associated with an acute respiratory illness and prominent upper airway symptoms can be assumed to be secondary to the common cold. Diagnostic testing is not indicated in such patients; a chest radiograph would be normal and is thus not recommended. Patients who have abnormal sinus transillumination, purulent nasal secretions, sinus pain or tenderness, or maxillary toothache could possibly have bacterial sinusitis. Again, a viral etiology of sinusitis is more likely than bacterial sinusitis, and antibiotic therapy should be initiated only in patients with persistent symptoms despite symptomatic therapy. Patients with documented COPD who present with acute cough, purulent sputum, dyspnea, and wheezing have an exacerbation of their underlying COPD and should be treated appropriately. Allergic rhinitis usually presents with a clear clinical history of episodic nasal and other allergy symptoms, and allergen avoidance can be initiated. It is important to note that allergic rhinitis can present with perennial symptoms.

Postinfectious cough should be evaluated with thorough history and physical exams followed by limited diagnostic evaluation and empiric therapies. Patients should be treated for postnasal drip syndrome, particularly in the setting of described rhinitis, postnasal drip, or frequent throat clearing. The presence of nasal inflammation and congestion, cobblestoning of the pharyngeal mucosa, or mucus in the oropharynx should also lead to empiric therapy for postnasal drip syndrome. If cough persists in the patients with suspected postnasal drip syndrome, evaluation of the sinuses with imaging and treatment of those patients with evidence of bacterial sinusitis should be pursued. Computed tomography (CT) imaging of the sinuses is the gold standard for diagnosing bacterial sinusitis. Patients with postinfectious cough and an abnormal respiratory exam should have a chest radiograph. Patients with a normal radiograph and evidence of bronchospasm can be empirically treated for airway hyperreactivity. Again the diagnosis of asthma requires recurrent airflow obstruction and cannot be made on the basis of a single episode of postinfectious wheezing or airway hyperreactivity. In subjects with cough and vomiting, known exposure to a case of *B. pertussis*, or in the presence of a *B. pertussis* epidemic in the community, empiric therapy for this illness should be pursued.

Before the vaccine era, *B. pertussis* was an endemic disease, which occurred in cyclic epidemics. It has been documented that *B. pertussis* continues to circulate in the adult population despite control of the disease in the pediatric population by vaccination. Immunity to *B. pertussis,* whether as a result of primary infection or immunization, is shortlived. The longer the elapsed interval since prior infection or immunization and repeat infection, the more likely repeat infection will be symptomatic. Perhaps repeat adolescent and adult booster immunization programs should be implemented to effectively control or eliminate this infection.

History and physical exam remain paramount in the patient presenting with chronic cough. The majority of patients should have a chest radiograph obtained as part of their evaluation. If the history and physical exam suggest that postnasal drip, asthma, or gastroesophageal reflux is

the etiology of a patient's symptoms, empiric therapy for these conditions should be initiated. Cough triggered by environmental factors or changes may be secondary to rhinitis and postnasal drip or airway hyperreactivity and asthma. Substernal burning or a sour taste in the mouth, particularly when triggered by supine positioning or bending, should increase the suspicion of gastroesophageal reflux.

If asthma is suspected, spirometry should be performed to document whether airflow obstruction is present. Response to inhaled bronchodilator with normal spirometry is indicative of airway hyperreactivity. Improvement in symptoms and spirometry with empiric asthma therapy even in the setting of normal baseline flow rates also confirms an asthmatic etiology. A methacholine challenge can be performed to confirm airway hyperreactivity. If cough in the setting of a positive methacholine challenge shows absolutely no response to empiric asthma therapy with inhaled corticosteroids and bronchodilators, consider a trial of systemic steroids. If the cough does not respond to aggressive asthma therapy, the methacholine challenge test results were probably false positive; asthma therapy can be discontinued and diagnostic efforts focused elsewhere.

Cough patients being treated with ACE inhibitors should cease these medications. Up to 30% of patients treated with ACE inhibitors will develop a persistent cough, more commonly in women, nonsmokers, and patients of Chinese ancestry. It may take 4 weeks or more for cough caused by ACE inhibitors to resolve following cessation of these medications. In the presence of ACE inhibitor use, further evaluation of dry cough should not be pursued until the patient has been withdrawn from these medications for 1 month.

An abnormal chest radiograph can direct further diagnostic studies and therapies, whereas a normal chest radiograph makes less common etiologies of chronic cough such as carcinoma, congestive heart failure, sarcoidosis, or interstitial lung disease unlikely. Evidence of basilar infiltrates or fibrosis may suggest interstitial lung disease or chronic aspiration. Severe gastroesophageal reflux must be considered in those patients with radiographic evidence of chronic aspiration.

Chronic cough without a definitive etiology can be troubling to both patient and health care provider. A systematic approach can simplify both diagnosis and treatment (Figure 1). It is again stressed that such a cough may be the result of multiple etiologic factors. In the absence of specific factors that help to point to an etiology of chronic cough, empiric treatment for postnasal drip syndrome should be pursued. Methacholine challenge testing will rule out asthma if it is negative and should also be performed early in the evaluation of chronic cough. Cough may be the sole manifestation of asthma in nearly 60% of patients presenting with chronic cough. A positive methacholine challenge does not have 100% predictive value but should lead to empiric asthma therapy.

Empiric therapy for silent gastroesophageal reflux should be initiated in those who do not respond to treatment for postnasal drip syndrome and do not have evidence of or respond to treatment for asthma. Cough may be the only manifestation of gastroesophageal reflux up to 30% of the time. Definitive diagnosis of gastroesophageal reflux requires invasive testing and may require more than one testing modality. Therefore it is

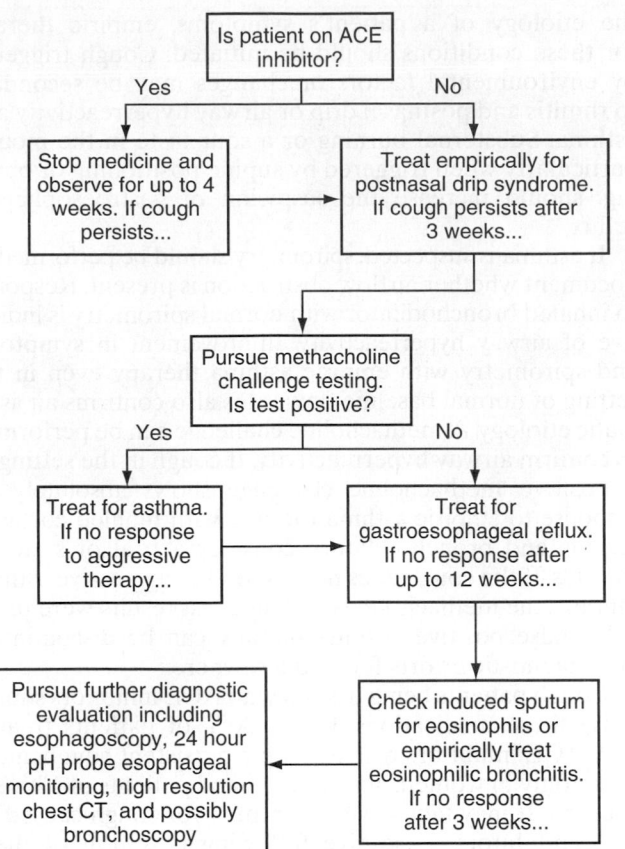

FIGURE 1. Approach to chronic cough of uncertain origin. ACE = angiotensin-converting enzyme; CT = computed tomography

 CURRENT DIAGNOSIS

All Patients Presenting With Cough

- Perform thorough history and physical examination.
- Review timing and nature of cough along with exacerbating or mitigating factors.
- Review prior history of cough, allergies, asthma, or gastroesophageal reflux.
- Take medication history, particularly use of ACE inhibitors.
- Focus physical exam on head, neck, and thorax.

Patients With Postinfectious or Chronic Cough

- Obtain chest radiograph, particularly in patients with an abnormal respiratory exam.
- Evaluate airflow obstruction with spirometry.
- Stop ACE inhibitors and assess for improvement.
- Administer empiric therapy for postnasal drip, asthma, or gastroesophageal reflux.
- Consider methacholine challenge testing to evaluate for airway hyperreactivity.
- Induce sputum for eosinophils or empiric trial of corticosteroids for eosinophilic bronchitis.
- If cough persists, consider esophagoscopy, 24-hour pH probe monitoring, high-resolution chest CT, or bronchoscopy.

Abbreviations: ACE = angiotensin-converting enzyme; CT = computed tomography.

recommended that empiric therapy for reflux be pursued before diagnostic testing. Reflux therapy should include conservative approaches such as dietary and lifestyle changes, bed positioning, and pharmacologic treatment. Gastroesophageal reflux–related cough can be particularly troublesome and persistent and may take weeks or months to respond to appropriate and intensive antireflux therapy. This may include higher-than-normal doses of proton pump inhibitors and promotility agents. Surgical treatment of reflux may be necessary to effectively treat reflux related cough in some patients. In patients with persistent cough, the common etiologies of cough often coexist and exacerbate one another. Therapy should often be additive, for instance treating both asthma and reflux, rather than mutually exclusive. Persistent cough should result in further diagnostic evaluation including sputum studies, esophagoscopy, 24-hour pH probe esophageal monitoring, high-resolution chest CT, and possibly bronchoscopy. In the presence of normal chest imaging, bronchoscopy is unlikely to yield beneficial diagnostic information in the patient with chronic cough.

Eosinophilic bronchitis in the absence of asthma is also a frequent cause (up to 13% of cases) of chronic cough. Patients with eosinophilic bronchitis will have normal spirometry and a negative methacholine challenge. The disease may be diagnosed by appropriate induced sputum analysis showing at least 3% eosinophils. Alternatively it can be empirically treated with a course of inhaled corticosteroids. Most patients appear to respond to inhaled corticosteroids

within 3 weeks. Systemic corticosteroids may be required to improve the symptoms in some cases. There may be an association of gastroesophageal reflux with eosinophilic bronchitis. Patients with gastroesophageal reflux have been found to have increased sputum eosinophilia.

Bronchiectasis may infrequently result in chronic cough. Bronchiectasis is characterized by the abnormal dilatation of one or more branches of the bronchial tree. It can effectively be diagnosed by high resolution CT scan of the thorax. Bronchiectasis may occur following a severe infection, distal to an area of airway obstruction, congenitally, from chronic inflammatory processes, and as a result of chronic parenchymal scarring and traction. Patients with bronchiectasis may present with productive or nonproductive coughs. They may have recurrent episodes of infection resulting from persistent colonization of the abnormal bronchial segment. Infectious agents may include routine bacterial organisms and typical or atypical mycobacterium. Bronchiectasis may be seen in a variety of chronic illnesses. The presence of bronchiectasis in a patient without a known predisposing cause should prompt the clinician to look for appropriate clinical states. such as:

- Primary or acquired immunodeficiencies
- Abnormalities of ciliary function, such as ciliary dyskinesia or cystic fibrosis
- Postinfectious inflammatory processes, such as allergic bronchopulmonary aspergillosis
- Collagen vascular diseases
- Inflammatory bowel disease
- Sarcoidosis
- Yellow nail syndrome

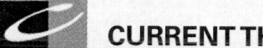
Treatment of Acute Cough

- Common cold: Supportive care with dexbromphenir-amine, 6 mg, and pseudoephedrine, 120 mg (Drixoral Cold and Allergy Tablets); or ipratropium nasal spray (Atrovent, 0.06%), two 42-mcg sprays in each nostril 3 times daily for 4 to 7 days depending on duration of symptoms.
- Acute sinusitis: Treat as a common cold. Add oxymetazoline (Afrin), two sprays twice daily for three days. If symptoms persist, consider antibiotic therapy directed against *Haemophilus influenzae* and *Streptococcus pneumoniae* such as azithromycin (Zithromax), 500 mg daily for 3 days.
- Exacerbation of chronic obstructive pulmonary disease: Antibiotics directed against *H. influenzae* and *S. pneumoniae* for 3 to 7 days such as clarithromycin (Biaxin), 500 mg twice daily for 7 days; systemic corticosteroids such as prednisone (Deltasone), 40 mg tapered over 10 days; inhaled anticholinergics such as tiotropium (Spiriva), one inhalation daily; and short-acting beta agonists such as albuterol (Proventil), two inhalations every 4 hours as needed; smoking cessation.
- Allergic rhinitis: Nasal corticosteroids such as mometasone (Nasonex), two sprays in each nostril daily; nonsedating antihistamines such as fexofenadine (Allegra), 180 mg daily; allergen avoidance if possible.
- *Bordetella pertussis*: Erythromycin 500 mg four times daily for 14 days or trimethoprim 160 mg/sulfamethoxazole (Bactrim DS),[1] 800 mg twice daily for 14 days. Other macrolide antibiotics such as azithromycin (Zithromax)[1] or clarithromycin (Biaxin)[1] are likely effective and may be better tolerated.

Treatment of Postinfectious Cough

- Postnasal drip syndrome: Dexbromphenir-amine, 6 mg, and pseudoephedrine (Drixoral Cold and Allergy Tablets), 120 mg for up to 3 weeks; ipratropium (Atrovent), 0.06% nasal spray for up to 3 weeks; azelastine (Astelin) nasal spray (137 mcg), two sprays each nostril twice daily for up to 3 weeks.
- Bronchospasm: Inhaled corticosteroid such as budesonide (Pulmicort),[1] two inhalations daily with or without inhaled long-acting beta agonist such as formoterol (Foradil), two inhalations twice daily; short-acting beta agonist such as albuterol (Ventolin), two puffs every 4 hours as needed. Oral steroids such as prednisone (Deltasone), 40 mg tapered over 10 days.
- *Bordetella pertussis*: Erythromycin, 500 mg four times daily for 14 days, or trimethoprim 160 mg/sulfamethoxazole, 800 mg (Bactrim DS)[1] twice daily for 14 days. Other macrolide antibiotics such as azithromycin (Zithromax)[1] or clarithromycin (Biaxin)[1] are likely effective and may be better tolerated.
- Bacterial sinusitis: Dexbrompheniramine, 6 mg, and pseudoephedrine (Drixoral Cold and Allergy Tablets), 120 mg for up to 3 weeks; oxymetazoline (Afrin), two sprays twice daily for 3 days; azithromycin (Zithromax), 500 mg daily for 3 days.
- Chlamydia/mycoplasma: Clarithromycin (Biaxin), 500 mg twice daily for 14 days.

Treatment of Chronic Cough

- Postnasal drip syndrome
    Nonallergic: Dexbrompheniramine, 6 mg, and pseudoephedrine (Drixoral Cold and Allergy Tablets), 120 mg for up to 3 weeks; ipratropium (Atrovent), 0.06% nasal spray for up to 3 weeks; azelastine (Astelin) nasal spray (137 mcg), two sprays each nostril twice daily for up to 3 weeks.
    Allergic: Fluticasone (Flonase) (50 mcg), two sprays each nostril daily; fexofenadine (Allegra), 180 mg daily; allergen avoidance.
- Asthma: Albuterol (Proventil), two puffs every 4 hours as needed; inhaled corticosteroid such as budesonide (Pulmicort), two inhalations daily with or without inhaled long-acting beta agonist such as formoterol (Foradil), two inhalations twice daily; combination of long-acting beta agonist and inhaled steroid such as fluticasone/salmeterol (Advair) (100/50 mcg), inhaled twice daily; montelukast (Singulair), 10 mg daily; prednisone (Deltasone), 40 mg daily with tapering dose over 10 days.
- Gastroesophageal reflux: Dietary and lifestyle modifications, lansoprazole (Prevacid), 30 mg daily for up to 3 months; metoclopramide (Reglan), 10 mg before meals and sleep.
- Eosinophilic bronchitis: Fluticasone (Flovent)[1] (110 mcg), two inhalations twice daily; prednisone (Deltasone), 30 mg daily for 3 weeks.
- ACE inhibitor: Discontinue medication.

[1]Not FDA approved for this indication.

The presence of localized bronchiectasis may be an indication to pursue flexible fiberoptic bronchoscopy to rule out an obstructing lesion and to obtain appropriate culture specimens. Treatment of bronchiectasis is aimed at the underlying disease state if one can be identified. Infections should be treated with appropriate antibiotics. Clearance of bronchial secretions can be aided with mucolytics and chest physiotherapy including use of percussive devices. In some cases surgical therapy to remove the bronchiectatic segment can be considered.

Treatment

The key treatments for cough are best described based on the suspected etiology. Acute cough therapy should focus on supportive treatment of the underlying suspected etiology, which will likely be a viral upper respiratory infection. Therapy for exacerbation of chronic obstructive pulmonary disease, allergic rhinitis, bacterial sinusitis, or *B. pertussis* infection is more specific. Postinfectious cough should focus on therapy for postnasal drip syndrome or airways reactivity if suspected. In chronic cough of uncertain etiology (see Figure 1), cough therapy should begin with empiric treatment of postnasal drip syndrome, evaluation and treatment of asthma, empiric treatment of gastroesophageal reflux syndrome, and finally evaluation or empiric therapy for eosinophilic bronchitis.

Cough is a frequent and troublesome symptom for both patient and health care provider. Acute cough although at times troubling is usually self-limiting. Postinfectious cough and chronic cough are more problematic, but can effectively be evaluated and treated by performing a thorough history and physical exam and pursuing a systematic approach to diagnostic evaluation and both empiric and guided therapies. The resolution of chronic troubling cough is a therapeutic relief for the patient and a gratifying experience for the caregiver.

REFERENCES

Barnes TW, Afessa B, Swanson KL, Lim KG: The clinical utility of flexible bronchoscopy in the evaluation of chronic cough. Chest 2004;126: 268-272.

Breitling CE, Ward R, Goh KL: Eosinophilic bronchitis is an important cause of chronic cough. Am J Respir Crit Care Med 1999; 160:406-410.

Cherry JD: Epidemiological, clinical, and laboratory aspects of pertussis in adults. Clin Infect Dis 1999;28(suppl2):S112-S117.

Cohen M, Sahn SA: Bronchiectasis in systemic diseases. Chest 1999; 116:1063-1074.

Irwin RS, Madison JM: Symptom research on chronic cough: A historical perspective. Ann Intern Med 2001;134:809-814.

Irwin RS, Madison JM: The diagnosis and treatment of cough. N Engl J Med 2000;343:1715-1721.

Irwin RS, Madison JM: The persistently troublesome cough. Am J Respir Crit Care Med 2002;165:1469-1474.

Kiljander TO: The role of proton pump inhibitors in the management of gastroesophageal reflux disease-related asthma and chronic cough. Am J Med 2003;115(3A):S65-S71.

Treatment of Insomnia

Method of
Martin Reite, MD

Three things should be remembered when considering treatment of an insomnia complaint. First, insomnia is more often a symptom, than a specific disorder. Second, it is important to perform a systematic differential diagnosis, keeping in mind the possibility that there will be very likely more than one cause of an insomnia complaint. Finally, the cause of the complaint usually can be determined, and most patients complaining of insomnia can be helped. Also, insomnia must not be trivialized.

Insomnia is among the most frequent complaints in the population; untreated insomnia is associated with increases in new-onset anxiety and depression, increased daytime sleepiness, and increased health-related concerns.

Insomnia can include difficulty in getting to sleep (sleep-onset insomnia), difficulty staying asleep (sleep-maintenance insomnia), or early morning awakening (terminal insomnia). Because such subtypes are not stable over time, this method of subtyping may have little clinical usefulness. As a rule, insomnia complaints are more frequent in women, elderly persons, and patients of lower socioeconomic status.

Screening for Sleep Complaints

Three routine questions, illustrated in Box 1, will detect most significant sleep problems. A positive answer to any of these questions merits consideration of a more detailed sleep history to determine whether in fact a sleep disorder is present. Box 2 outlines the items to be covered in a sleep history.

Sources of diagnostic information should include the bed partner whenever possible because many sleep-related symptoms are apparent only to the bed partner. A several-week daily sleep diary also can be useful at this stage of the evaluation because it can provide a detailed daily description of sleep/wake activity patterns.

Transient and Short-Term Insomnia

Transient (1 to several days) and short-term (up to 3 weeks) insomnias are typically stress related, and respond well to pharmacologic (short-term hypnotic) intervention. They should be considered for active treatment, because untreated short-term insomnia can lead to a state of "conditioned arousal" resulting in a chronic insomnia.

BOX 1 **Detection of Specific Sleep Disorders**

Are you content with your sleep? (identifies most insomnia complaints)
Are you excessively sleepy during the day? (identifies most disorders of excessive sleepiness)
Does your bed partner complain about your sleep? (identifies most parasomnia disorders)

BOX 2 **Sleep History Questionnaire**

When did the symptoms start, and what was going on at the time?
What has been the symptom pattern across time?
Are symptoms stress or situationally related?
What is your typical daily schedule, hour by hour?
What medications and treatments have been and are currently being used to date?
Is there a presence of familial sleep-related symptoms?

Differential Diagnosis of the Chronic Insomnia Complaint

The differential diagnosis of a chronic insomnia complaint can represent a more challenging task and requires a thorough differential diagnostic evaluation, which includes systematically considering the conditions or combinations of conditions that are most likely to result in insomnia complaints. General practice parameters for the evaluation of chronic insomnia complaints can be found at: http://www.aasmnet.org/PDF/ChronicParameter.pdf. Box 3 lists the common causes of insomnia (not necessarily listed in order of frequency). Each cause is briefly discussed.

MEDICAL CONDITIONS AND TREATMENT

Medical conditions, and in susceptible patients, many pharmacologic treatments of medical conditions, can result in insomnia complaints. The endocrinopathies are notorious for being associated with sleep-related complaints, as are conditions associated with chronic pain, breathing difficulties, cardiac arrhythmias, arthritis, renal failure, and central nervous system (CNS) disorders. Box 4 lists the more commonly used medications that can result in insomnia complaints.

The treatment of insomnia associated with medical conditions is first to isolate and appropriately treat the medical condition and the symptoms (e.g., pain) causing the insomnia. If the insomnia complaint persists, evaluate the possibility of an additional cause for the sleep complaint. Supplementary use of a short half-life hypnotic agent [e.g., zolpidem (Ambien), 5-10 mg at bedtime] may be helpful. Insomnia associated with fibromyalgia and chronic fatigue syndrome is frequently resistant

to treatment, although small doses of amitriptyline (Elavil)[1] (10-50 mg at bedtime) or cyclobenzaprine (Flexeril)[1] (10 mg three times a day) have been reported to be helpful; occasionally, zolpidem (5-10 mg) will help with the associated insomnia complaints.

Dementing illnesses are often associated with severe insomnia complaints that are quite disruptive to patients and families and often are the factors precipitating institutional care. Sleep is often disturbed in such disorders on the basis of disease-associated CNS lesions, and different specific pathophysiologies (not yet well understood) may respond to different treatments. Until such specific treatments can be based on specific pathophysiology, we should adhere to optimal environmental circadian principles (quiet, dark nocturnal environment; bright, socially stimulating daytime environment). Appropriate use of hypnotics may be helpful, although responses may be variable.

PSYCHIATRIC DISORDERS

Psychiatric disorders, especially those associated with anxiety or depression, frequently include insomnia (delayed sleep onset, frequent awakening, or early morning awakening) as an associated symptom. Effective treatment of the psychiatric condition will often relieve the insomnia complaint, although a supplemental hypnotic might be indicated early in treatment. Different antidepressant agents have quite different effects on sleep as illustrated in Table 1, and the initial choice of an antidepressant might profitably take such effects into account.

If, for a patient already complaining of insomnia, an antidepressant with a known high incidence of insomnia side effects is chosen, it may be useful to augment it with a hypnotic agent early in the course of treatment.

SUBSTANCE USE SLEEP DISORDERS

Alcohol abuse remains a significant problem in the etiology of sleep complaints, as do stimulants and other drugs of abuse. Treatment includes withdrawal of the offending substance, with long-term abstinence as the goal. Treatment of substance abuse-related insomnia should emphasize behavioral treatment strategies to the fullest extent possible, because psychoactive agents have already proved to be a problem.

CIRCADIAN RHYTHM DISORDERS

Disturbances in the regulation of the circadian system frequently present as sleep-related complaints, although the source of the problem lies in the circadian system rather than sleep pathology. Sleep per se may be adequate, but it occurs at the wrong time. Delayed sleep-phase syndrome (DSPS) is the most common, and is likely a genetically based disorder with frequent onset in adolescence or early adulthood. These individuals cannot get to sleep (because of phase delay in the body temperature rhythm) until 3 to 4 a.m., and if allowed to sleep, 8 to 9 hours may do well. If they have to arise at 7 a.m. for school or work, they will be sleep deprived and complain of insomnia.

Early morning bright-light exposure, with restriction of light exposure in the evening, has been found to be

[1]Not FDA approved for this indication.

TABLE 1 Effect of Antidepressants on Sleep Scale*

Drug	Trade Name	Effects on EEG Sleep Continuity	SWS	REM	Sedation Effects
TCAs					
Amitriptyline	Elavil	I (3)	I (1)	D (3)	4
Doxepin	Sinequan	I (3)	I (2)	D (2)	4
Imipramine	Tofranil	I (0-1)	I (1)	D (2)	2
Nortriptyline	Pamelor	I (1)	I (1)	D (2)	2
Desipramine	Norpramin	(0)	I (1)	D (2)	1
Clomipramine	Anafranil	I (0-1)	I (1)	D (4)	0
MAOIs					
Phenelzine	Nardil	D (1)	(0)	D (4)	0
Tranylcypromine	Parnate	D (2)	(0)	D (4)	0
SSRIs					
Fluoxetine	Prozac	D (1)	D (0-1)	D (0-1)	0
Paroxetine	Paxil	D (1)	D (0-1)	D (2)	0
Sertraline	Zoloft	(0)	(0)	D (2)	0
Citalopram	Celexa	D (1)	(0)	D (1)	ND
Fluvoxamine	Luvox	D (1)	(0)	D (1)	ND
Escitalopram	Lexapro	(0)	(0)	D (2)	0
Other					
Bupropion	Wellbutrin	D (0-1)	(0)	I (1)	0
Venlafaxine	Effexor	D (1)	D (1)	D (3)	2
Trazodone	Desyrel	I (3)	I (0-1)	D (1)	4
Mirtazapine	Remeron	I (3)	I (2)	(0)	3
Nefazodone	Serzone	I (1)	(0)	I (1)	1

Abbreviations: EEG = electroencephalogram; MAOIs = monoamine oxidase inhibitors; REM = rapid eye movement; SSRIs = selective serotonin reuptake inhibitors; SWS = slow-wave sleep; TCAs = tricyclic antidepressants.
*Scale 0-4: 0 = no significant effect; I = increase and D = decrease.

effective for phase-advancing the circadian system in DSPS. Evening bright-light treatment is effective in treating advanced sleep-phase syndrome. Low-dose (1-3 mg) melatonin[1],[*] at bedtime may help regulate circadian rhythms in some individuals.

Jet lag and shift-work–related sleep problems also fall in the category of circadian rhythm problems. A detailed discussion of these problem areas is beyond the scope of this article, but recently emerging data suggest that properly timed bright-light exposure, supplemented with melatonin[1],[*] administration and appropriate hypnotic use, can significantly reduce associated symptoms.

PERIODIC LIMB MOVEMENTS OF SLEEP AND RESTLESS LEGS SYNDROME

Both restless legs syndrome (RLS) and periodic limb movements of sleep (PLMS) are associated with a variety of medical conditions, including iron deficiency, but they may occur in otherwise healthy individuals (especially the elderly). A polysomnogram (PSG) is usually required for accurate diagnosis of a PLMS disorder, quantifying both the number of events and their association with awakenings or arousals. Table 2 lists the drugs currently used in the treatment of PLMS and RLS.

[1]Not FDA approved for this indication.
[*]Available as a dietary supplement.

CENTRAL SLEEP APNEA

Central sleep apnea with frequent arousals is a relatively rare cause of chronic insomnia except at higher altitudes, and may require a PSG for accurate diagnosis. Both oxygen and continuous positive airway pressure (CPAP) can be used in the treatment of central apnea in patients with medical disorders. The efficacy of pharmacologic agents in the treatment of central sleep apnea has yet to be clearly established in well-controlled studies. Acetazolamide (Diamox)[1] (250 mg twice a day) may be effective for the prevention of high altitude-induced central apnea.

THE PRIMARY INSOMNIA, CONDITIONED INSOMNIA, AND SLEEP-STATE MISPERCEPTION SYNDROME GROUP

Although there are several more rare causes of a chronic insomnia complaint, most often it is generally safe to assume that once the aforementioned specific causes have been systematically excluded or appropriately treated (and the insomnia complaints remain), we are in all probability left with either a primary insomnia disorder (DSM-IV 307.42), a conditioned insomnia, a sleep-state misperception syndrome (SSMS), or some combination thereof.

[1]Not FDA approved for this indication.

TABLE 2 Beginning Dose Schedules for PMLS and RLS

Drug	Dose (mg)	Administration
Dopa Agonists		
Carbidopa/Levodopa	25/100-50/200	Bedtime/(Sinemet)[1] symptom onset
Controlled-release	25/100-50/200	Bedtime/Carbidopa/Levodopa symptom onset (Sinemet CR)[1]
Bromocriptine (Parlodel)[1]	2.5-5	Bedtime
Baclofen (Lioresal)[1]	20-40	Bedtime
Pergolide (Permax)[1]	0.05	Bedtime/symptom onset
Pramipexole (Mirapex)[1]	0.125	Bedtime
Ropinirole (Requip)[1]	0.25	Bedtime
Other Agents		
Oxycodone (Roxicodone)[1]	5-15	Bedtime
Codeine[1]	10-60	Bedtime
Triazolam (Halcion)[1]	0.125-0.25	Bedtime
Temazepam (Restoril)[1]	15-30	Bedtime
Clonazepam (Klonopin)[1]	0.5-1.5	Bedtime
Gabapentin (Neurontin)[1]	100-300	Bedtime

[1]Not FDA approved for this indication.

A treatment approach that combines both behavioral and pharmacologic approaches is generally recommended. Such a combined treatment approach offers the advantage of a pharmacologic agent that can produce rapid relief of the sleep complaint, along with behavioral strategies, which take longer to become effective but provide long-term results that are under a patient's control. Active and continued involvement of the patient is important for any chronic insomnia treatment.

Sleep Laboratory Studies

All night PSGs, which monitor multiple physiologic variables during sleep, are rarely needed in the evaluation of insomnia complaints, except for symptoms associated with PLMS or for a sleep-related breathing disorder, where a PSG is usually required for accurate diagnosis. A recent review of the use of PSGs in the insomnia complaints can be found at: http://www.aasmnet.org/PDF/260616.pdf

The 24-hour recording of activity (Actigraphy) can also be useful in the diagnosis of circadian rhythm-based sleep complaints (e.g., see: http://www.aasmnet.org/PDF/260315.pdf

Treatment

After completing the evaluation of a chronic insomnia complaint and arriving at a diagnostic formulation, a treatment plan should be developed addressing all likely contributing causes. The treatment plan will likely include both behavioral and pharmacologic components, and should be discussed in detail with the patient. Patients might be encouraged to visit the web pages of the American Sleep Disorders Association (www.asda.org) and the National Sleep Foundation (www.nsf.org) to learn more about factors influencing sleep. Patient education facilitates effective treatment.

BEHAVIORAL TREATMENTS

Behavioral treatment strategies are aimed at (a) breaking bad sleep habits and replacing them with sleep-promoting habits; (b) directly decreasing physiologic arousal levels using cognitively based or learned strategies; and (c) providing the patient with several types of cognitive strategies to deal with sleep difficulties, thus promoting a sense of competence and diminishing anxiety about sleep. First and foremost among the behavioral strategies is good sleep hygiene—the behaviors and habits that foster good sleep. Box 5 highlights the principles of good sleep hygiene. It is helpful to prepare a handout for patients summarizing good sleep hygiene practices that they can take with them. Box 6 lists additional behavioral strategies.

BOX 5 Good Sleep Hygiene

Establish a regular sleep schedule that does not vary by more than 1 hour.
Maintain a state of good aerobic fitness with regular exercise (but not within 3 hours of sleep onset).
Do not use caffeine or alcohol to excess.
Ensure a quiet, dark, cool bedroom.
Provide a time to wind down in the evening before sleeping.
Consider a high-tryptophan snack (milk, cookies, banana) before bed.
Use the bedroom for sleep and sex but not for reviewing or thinking about the affairs of the day.
Minimize exposure to late evening bright light to avoid phase-delaying the circadian system.

PHARMACOLOGIC TREATMENTS

Benzodiazepine (BZ) compounds and newer nonbenzodiazepine agents active at the level of the BZ receptor are the most commonly used hypnotic agents. Older hypnotic agents (chloral hydrate, paraldehyde [Paral], barbiturates) may have limited usefulness for very short-term use in specific patients, but they cannot be recommended for the treatment of chronic insomnia.

BZ agents activate all BZ receptors (hypnotic, anxiolytic, muscle relaxant, anticonvulsant), and different agents demonstrate relatively little receptor specificity.

The BZ compounds differ substantially in terms of half-life and are illustrated in Table 3. The clinician can choose the agent with a half-life most appropriate for the clinical situation.

Long half-life BZ agents may be associated with residual daytime sedation and impairments in psychomotor performance. All BZ agents interfere with memory consolidation, the more potent agents (e.g., triazolam [Halcion]) most prominently. All BZ agents are prone to the development of tolerance, dependence, and rebound insomnia in response to rapid withdrawal. BZ agents also tend to decrease stages 3 to 4 sleep, and increase fast activity in the waking and sleeping electroencephalogram (EEG). These results may continue after drug discontinuation. Clearly useful for the treatment of insomnia associated with anxiety, the use of long-term BZ treatment of primary insomnia is problematic, especially in light of the research and development of new, apparently safe and effective nonbenzodiazepine agents designed to be selectively more active on the hypnotic receptor.

Newer non-BZ agents selectively active at the omega$_1$ BZ receptor include zolpidem and zolpidem-MR (Ambien and Ambien-CR), zaleplon (Sonata), and eszopiclone (Lunesta). These agents do not appear to alter sleep architecture, and appear less prone to induce significant tolerance, dependence, or withdrawal compared to conventional benzodiazepines. All have relatively rapid onset of action, but differ in half life and duration of action. Approximate half lives are zaleplon ~1 hr, zolpidem ~1-3 hr, zolpidem MR ~2-4 hr, and eszopiclone ~6 hr. Neither zolpidem-MR or eszopiclone have restrictions on duration of use.

The melatonin receptor agonist ramelteon (Rozerem) has also been recently released for the treatment of insomnia (possibly most effective in circadian regulation problems), and has no duration of use restriction.

Antidepressant agents, especially sedative tricyclics, are frequently used at low doses to manage chronic insomnia despite the relative lack of well-controlled double-blind studies demonstrating efficacy. These agents are clearly indicated in insomnia that accompanies depressive disorders, where their effectiveness is clear. These agents are normally taken about one hour before bedtime so their sedative effects have time to emerge. This effectively teaches the patient to take a pill to sleep, which is counterproductive for treating insomnia. The new non-BZ hypnotics with their rapid onset of action can be placed at the bedside and are taken if the patient has not fallen asleep within 30 minutes.

Several agents more directly involved in modulating γ-aminobutyric acid (GABA) activity, such as tiagabine (Gabitril)[1] and sodium oxybate (Xyrem),[1] have been used in limited studies to promote slow-wave sleep, but there are insufficient published data to make specific recommendations as to their potential usefulness in insomnia at this time.

LONG-TERM USE OF HYPNOTIC AGENTS

Current thinking suggests we might best conceptualize primary insomnia as a chronic disorder that will likely require long-term treatment. Considering the known adverse effects of chronic sleep loss, in the context of the present availability of relatively safe and effective hypnotic agents, there would appear to be no reason to withhold or severely limit pharmacologic

---

[1]Not FDA approved for this indication.

TABLE 3 Benzodiazepines

Name		Dose (mg)			
Generic	Trade Name	Adult	Elderly	Onset	Half-Life (Hours)
Triazolam	Halcion	0.125-0.25	0.125-0.25	Rapid	1.5-5.5
Estazolam	ProSom	1-2	0.5-1	Rapid	20-30
Temazepam	Restoril	15-30	7.5-15	Intermediate	8-20
Quazepam	Doral	7.5-15	7.5	Intermediate	15-120
Flurazepam	Dalmane	15-30	7.5	Intermediate	36-250

treatment in those responsible patients for whom a comprehensive and thorough diagnostic evaluation has established the presence of a primary insomnia disorder. It should go without saying, however, that behavioral treatment also should be actively implemented in those patients who are being considered for long-term pharmacologic management.

Pruritus

Method of
Louis J. Rusin, MD

For thousands of years itch has tormented humankind as well as the physicians from whom these patients have sought help. It is the sensation that provokes the desire to scratch and the most common patient symptom encountered by dermatologists. Itching can become severe, causing discomfort, frustration, agitation, difficulty concentrating, and loss of sleep for the patient (and the treating physician). Itching causes scratching, which creates inflammation, stimulates nerve fibers, and leads to more scratching. Scratching alters the integrity of the skin, damages the skin barrier, and causes changes in the skin such as redness, scaling, lichenification, excoriations, ulcers, prurigo nodules, and secondary infection. Successful treatment requires interruption of this cycle.

Etiology

Itching is a complex psychoneurodermatologic phenomenon involving peripheral sensory cutaneous nerve fibers and central nervous system (CNS) processes. The axons of neurons that conduct itch are unmyelinated C fibers that end at the dermoepidermal junction. Cutaneous nerve stimulation is mediated by several substances including histamine, neuropeptides such as substance P, and calcitonin gene-related peptide; and it is sensitive to inflammatory mediators. Most of the nociceptive afferents terminate in the superficial region of the dorsal horn of the spinal column. The pathway proceeds along the lateral spinothalamic tract to the thalamus and then to the sensorimotor and cingulate cortex. The sensation of itch is processed in the brain and causes the motor nerves to respond by scratching.

Causes of Pruritus

Itching is a symptom, not a disease. Clinically, it may be categorized as dermatologic, systemic, neuropathic, or psychogenic (Table 1).

Dermatologic causes of itching are myriad. Most commonly, itching can be related to dry skin but can also be related to atopic dermatitis, allergic contact dermatitis, psoriasis, asteatotic dermatitis, seborrheic dermatitis, fungal infection, irritant dermatitis, pruritus ani, kraurosis vulvae, scabies, or urticaria.

TABLE 1 Categories of Itch

- Dermatologic: related to skin diseases
- Systemic: related to diseases of organs other than skin
- Neuropathic: related to diseases or disorders of the peripheral or CNS
- Psychogenic: related to psychiatric or psychologic conditions

Abbreviations: CNS = central nervous system.

Systemic causes of itching account for up to 50% of generalized itching and may include the following:

- Infectious: viral disease such as HIV, varicella, rubella, fungal, trichinosis, intestinal parasites
- Drug eruptions: allergic reactions to drugs or chemotherapy with antineoplastic drugs
- Endocrine: hyperthyroidism, hypothyroidism, parathyroidism, diabetes
- Cirrhosis, intrahepatic or posthepatic biliary obstruction, cholestasia, renal disease: 70% to 90% of patients on hemodialysis
- Hematologic disease: Hodgkin's disease, polycythemia vera, iron deficiency, mast cell disease, myelomatosis leukemia, mycosis fungoides
- Occult malignancy
- Allergies to ingestants or inhalants
- Autoimmune disease

Neuropathic causes include diseases or disorders of the peripheral or CNS including multiple sclerosis, neuropathy, brain tumor, nerve compression, or irritation.

Psychogenic causes include neurotic excoriations, obsessive-compulsive disorder, and delusions of parasitosis. Stress intensifies all forms of pruritus.

Some patients may have multiple causes of their itching concomitantly.

Evaluation

Evaluation can be especially difficult if the itching is generalized, has been present for months to years, and has been treated with many over-the-counter products. All evaluations require a detailed history, physical exam, and appropriate laboratory studies.

HISTORY

The history is the most important part of the workup and needs to be accurate and thorough:

- Onset?
- Initial location?
- Course?
- Duration?
- Intermittent or persisting?
- Periodic or seasonal variation?
- Thorough review of systems?
- Relationship to occupation?
- Prescription medications?
- Over-the-counter medications including topicals, home treatments, and skin care practices?

CURRENT DIAGNOSIS

Causes of Pruritus

- Dermatologic diseases or disorders: atopic dermatitis, asteatotic dermatitis, allergic contact dermatitis, psoriasis, seborrheic dermatitis, scabies
- Systemic: infectious, drug eruptions, endocrine, hepatic disease, renal disease, hematologic disease, and occult malignancy
- Allergic: ingestants or inhalants, autoimmune disease
- Neuropathic: multiple sclerosis, neuropathy, brain tumor, nerve compression or irritation
- Psychogenic: neurotic excoriations, obsessive compulsive disorder, delusions of parasitosis

Answers to these questions may prompt more detailed questions regarding affected family members; exposures to plants, animals, or chemicals; history of recent travel; factors that make it worse or better; malignancy; chemotherapy; infection; and the patient's emotional state.

PHYSICAL EXAM

If the onset is recent, the involved areas may be localized, show a specific distribution, or primary lesions may be present, which may make the diagnosis easier.

LABORATORY TESTING

See Table 2.

Treatment

Treatment of pruritus is often difficult, exasperating, and frustrating for the patient and the provider. It consists of trying to identify and treat any underlying disease or external factors, topical therapy, systemic therapy, and patient education.

- Treat the underlying disease or disorder. If the history, exam, and laboratory findings identify a specific cause, treat accordingly.

CURRENT THERAPY

- Treat the underlying disease or disorder
- Stop aggravating products or behaviors
- Patient education
- Menthol or camphor creams or lotions
- "Soak and smear"
- Cortisone creams and ointments
- Topical immunomodulators
- Sedating oral antihistamines before bedtime
- CNS-specific medications
- Cortisone injection or tapering oral prednisone
- Gabapentin (Neurontin)[1]

[1]Not FDA approved for this indication.

TABLE 2 Laboratory Testing

- Routine chemistry profile including hepatic and renal function tests, fasting blood sugar, and thyroid screening
- Ferritin level
- Complete blood count with differential
- Stool for ova and parasites, chest radiograph, malignancy workup, and other appropriate tests if indicated by history and exam

- Topical therapy.
  - Ultraviolet light treatments.
  - Soak and smear. It is reported that soaking for 20 minutes in plain water followed by application of 0.1% triamcinolone ointment (Kenalog) cured more than 90% of itching patients in 2 weeks; 90% to 100% improvement.
  - Ultrapotent cortisone creams or ointments for 2 weeks followed by use of low- to medium-strength cortisone creams or ointments. *Not* to be used on the face or moist skin folds.
  - Menthol/camphor containing creams (Sarna Anti-Itch lotion).
  - Tacrolimus ointment (Protopic) or pimecrolimus cream (Elidel).
  - Capsaicin cream (Zostrix), doxepin cream (Zonalon), topical aspirin (Aspercreme).
- Systemic therapy.
  - Sedating antihistamines are helpful when given 1 hour before bedtime when the itching is usually most intense. Diphenhydramine (Benadryl) 25 to 100 mg,[3] hydroxyzine (Atarax, Vistaril) 25 to 50 mg, and cyproheptadine (Periactin) work well. The nonsedating antihistamines cetirizine (Zyrtec), fexofenadine (Allegra), loratadine (Claritin), and desloratadine (Clarinex) are ineffective for itching unless caused by urticaria.
  - CNS-specific medications. Doxepin (Sinequan)[1] 25 mg per day; alprazolam (Xanax)[1] 0.125 to 0.5 mg per day; buspirone (BuSpar)[1] 10 mg bid; pimozide (Orap)[1] 1 to 2 mg daily; clomipramine (Anafranil[1]) 25 mg per day; fluoxetine (Prozac)[1] 20 mg per day.
  - Occasionally, cortisone injection or a tapering course of oral prednisone is necessary to break the scratch-itch-scratch cycle so oral antihistamines and topical products are effective. Oral antibiotics may be necessary if excoriating has caused secondary infection, especially in patients with atopic dermatitis.
- Patient education.
  - This is the *most* important part of the treatment. Spend time discussing how the itching will take some time and effort to resolve so the patient has realistic expectations. Stress how scratching perpetuates and aggravates itching. Discuss specific factors to avoid that are aggravating (excessive bathing; extremely hot showers or baths; harsh or liquid soaps; dry environment; electric blankets; and avoiding topical diphenhydramine [Benadryl], lidocaine, neomycin, and botanical products,

---

[3]Exceeds dosage recommended by the manufacturer.
[1]Not FDA approved for this indication.

because many people develop contact dermatitis to them). Emphasize preventive measures such as using mild soaps, applying emollients after bathing, taking warm baths or showers, wearing wicking clothing when exercising, and using a humidifier.

Pruritus is a difficult but common presenting complaint of patients. They are often frustrated, uncomfortable, agitated, and tired because they have not been able to sleep. Oftentimes, they have tried numerous over-the-counter products and seen other providers without relief of their symptoms; may be skeptical yet hopeful you can help. There is relief for these patients, but the provider must *listen* to the patients, take a thorough and detailed history, do a physical exam, and order appropriate laboratory tests. Identifying a cause, eliminating irritating or aggravating external factors, and treating underlying skin or systemic disease are often curative. Symptomatic treatment or dealing with an underlying psychogenic etiology will still provide relief for these patients.

REFERENCES

Lotti T (ed.): Pruritus, itch mechanisms, and treatments. Dermatol Ther 2005;18(4):283–363.
Gutman AB, Kligman AM, Sciacca J, James WD: Soak and smear. Arch Dermatol 2005;141:1556–1559.
Rusin LJ: Pruritus (itching). In Rakel RE, Bope ET (eds.): Conn's Current Therapy. Philadelphia: Saunders, 2004, pp 37–39.
Yesudian PD, Wilson NJE: Efficacy of gabapentin in the management of pruritus of unknown origin. Arch Dermatol 2005;141:1507–1509.
Yosipovitch G, Hundley JL: Practical guidelines for the relief of itch. Medscape 2004;9.

Tinnitus

Method of
Claus-Frenz Claussen, MD

Tinnitus is noise(s) in the ear, which is usually subjective and can be extremely disturbing and frustrating to those affected. According to studies of the American Tinnitus Association, approximately 36 million Americans older than 40 years suffer from tinnitus.

Tinnitus has been regarded as a disease entity for many centuries. During the second half of the 20th century, physicians were able to discriminate among several different kinds of tinnitus including bruits, maskable tinnitus, and nonmaskable tinnitus. Under the influence of Shulman and his team, the term *tinnitology* was coined.

The present interest of researchers in the field of tinnitology is split into two fields of action: suggestions for improvement of objective and quantitative differential diagnostics in tinnitus and research and development to improve various types of treatment for different kinds of tinnitus.

General Phenomena of Tinnitus

A noise without any human information function, a tinnitus, can be a normal as well as a pathologic function of

CURRENT DIAGNOSIS

Irritating subjective or objective perception of irritating acoustic noise or sound in the ear, head, or body that may be described, for example, as:
- Pulsating
- Humming
- Roaring
- Whistling
- Hissing

human hearing. On the one hand, tinnitus can be regarded as a problem of acoustic resolution of the inner ear microphone, that is, the cochlear noise-to-signal ratio. In a well-dampened soundproof chamber, most normal-hearing persons experience a sizzling sound in their ears because of their perception of molecular vibrations from inner ear fluids (as known from thermodynamics). Yet this underlying percept is masked in everyday life by normal environmental noise.

On the other hand, tinnitus patients regularly tell their physicians about subjective ear noises that they describe, for example, as pulsating, humming, roaring, whistling, hissing, fullness of the ear, and pressure and pain in the ear.

Table 1 presents the subjective sensational qualities of tinnitus in 823 tinnitus patients (77.52% male and 22.48% female with a mean age of 50.87 years ± 8.68 years) from Bad Kissingen, Germany, who underwent clinical inpatient rehabilitation therapy for several weeks for severe disabling tinnitus.

In these same patients, we looked for descriptions of different time/intensity patterns of their tinnitus (Table 2), and the subjective background of discomfort was investigated as shown in Table 3. Additionally, the patients named the most irritating factors related to their tinnitus (Table 4).

Sleep disturbance is a common and frequent complaint. Scientific studies report decreased tolerance and increased discomfort when insomnia and depression are associated with tinnitus.

In 1991, a sample of 338 New Zealanders regularly experiencing tinnitus completed and returned questionnaires to associations for people with tinnitus or hearing impairment. Nearly half the sample was sometimes depressed because of tinnitus. Those reporting depression and those reporting more severe problems as a consequence of the tinnitus saw more health care professionals and used more coping strategies. Most respondents did

TABLE 1 Subjective Classification of Ear Noises in 823 (= 100%) Tinnitus Patients

Complaints	Right Ear (%)	Left Ear (%)
Pulsating	1.94	1.94
Humming	7.41	6.93
Roaring	14.10	14.22
Whistling	50.67	51.76
Hissing	9.96	10.81
Pressure in the ear	6.32	5.83
Pain in the ear	14.10	14.22

TABLE 2 Subjective Classification of Different Time/Intensity Patterns of Tinnitus in 823 (= 100%) Patients

Time/Intensity Patterns	%
Permanent	59.17
Intermittent	19.97
Swelling up and going down	43.26

TABLE 3 Subjective Classification of Subjective Background of Discomfort in 823 (= 100%) Patients

Subjective Complaints About Factors of Discomfort	%
Headache	69.02
Migraine	4.13
Exhaustion	59.99
Lacking in drive	42.16
Feeling of weakness	55.29
Forgetfulness	68.41
Disorientation	0.49
Daze	44.84
Tiredness	63.91
Insomnia	69.50

not remember exactly when they first noticed the tinnitus.

A questionnaire investigation comprising 1091 patients from Bispebjerg Hospital, Copenhagen (1993), concerning "tinnitus-incidence and handicap," was conducted at a hearing center. A majority of patients, 59%, claimed that they were troubled by tinnitus. Neither a greater degree of hearing loss nor a longer duration of tinnitus was associated with more severe tinnitus. Among patients with both subjective hearing loss and tinnitus, 23% stated that tinnitus was the greater problem, and 38% said that tinnitus and hearing loss were equally troublesome. The corresponding figures for patients with hearing impairment of such a degree that a hearing aid was deemed necessary were 9% and 41%, respectively. Stress symptoms such as headache, tension of facial muscles, and sleep disturbances were correlated to tinnitus. Of patients with tinnitus, 83% were interested in obtaining treatment for it.

TABLE 4 Subjective Classification of Most Irritating Factors Related to Their Tinnitus in 823 (= 100%) Patients

Most Irritating Factors Related to Tinnitus	%
All patients with specific additional statements	25.76
Difficulties in going to sleep	10.69
Difficulties in sleeping through the night	11.06
Depression	0.24
Abnormal sounds (also hallucinations)	2.67
Acute hearing loss	8.38

The so-called Copenhagen Male Study reported on the results from a 10-year follow-up examination concerning hearing and factors known to cause hearing problems. The original sample comprised 5050 subjects, and at the present examination, 3387 (67%) men at a median of 63 years of age (range, 53 to 75 years) participated. An increasing prevalence of 30% to 40% of hearing problems was demonstrated with increasing age. A prevalence of 17% of tinnitus of more than 5 minutes' duration was found; 3% indicated that tinnitus was so annoying that it interfered with sleep, reading, and/or concentration. The prevalence of tinnitus increased up to 70 years of age and seemed to remain constant thereafter.

In Norway, 15% of the adult population has experienced shorter or longer periods of tinnitus. Three percent of these, in total approximately 7000 to 10,000 persons, suffer from continuous tinnitus followed by symptoms that represent a handicap or occupational disability. Similar observations were reported from many other countries.

Clinical Types

Tinnitus is no longer considered to be a syndrome or a single disease. Because of improvements in neuro-otometry, several different types of tinnitus can be differentiated.

By means of modern audiometry, the framework for normal hearing can be described objectively and quantitatively. Therefore, in any tinnitus case, a thorough analysis of the hearing function and pathways needs to be performed including threshold audiometry, audiometric tinnitus masking (if possible), acoustic dynamics between the measurable thresholds of hearing and acoustic discomfort, speech audiometry, otoacoustic emissions, acoustic brainstem-evoked potentials, and acoustic late-evoked potentials. Thereby signs of pathology within the hearing pathways between the ear and the human brain cortex can be measured.

Thus, we know from thorough neuro-otologic studies that approximately 24% of cases of disabling tinnitus have their source within the otoacoustic periphery (i.e., inner ear and the eighth cranial nerve). Approximately 35% originate from the acoustic pathways within the brainstem. Approximately 41% have their cause within supratentorial structures and/or functions. These pathologies also should serve as basic information for planning systematic pharmacotherapy directed to the central nervous system (CNS) focus of dysfunction.

At least four different kinds of tinnitus (Figure 1) can be discriminated, which can be determined by the physician using a simple question-and-answer procedure as follows.

BRUITS

Q: Has someone informed you that he or she could hear a noise coming from your head?

A: Yes. Their description of what they heard listening from outside my head is similar to what I perceive.

By means of auscultation through a stethoscope or a microphone, a real sound can be objectively heard emanating

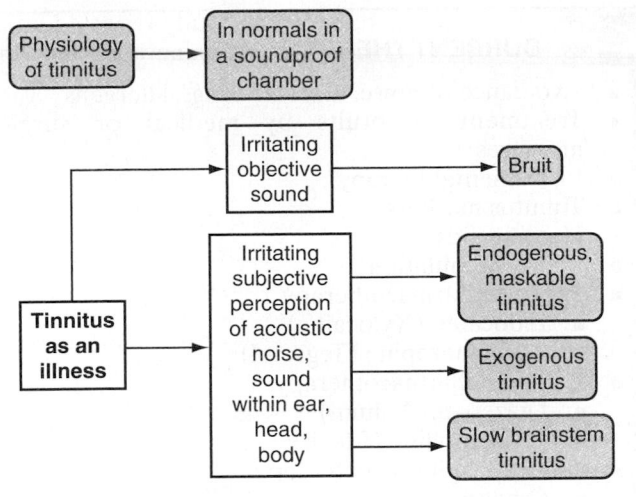

FIGURE 1. Categories of physiologic and clinical types of tinnitus.

from the patient's skull. Patients frequently report, for example, a bubbling, hissing, or pulsating sound.

The cause can be vascular in origin, that is, abnormal curling of blood caused by atheromas, vascular dissections, scars, compressions, or high blood pressure amplitudes, for example.

Bruits also can originate from the middle ear and its connections toward the epipharynx: middle ear inflammations with bubbling sounds of gas, whizzing middle ear muscles, or an open eustachian tube.

Cracking sounds, which are misinterpreted as tinnitus, are reported from arthritic and other mandibular joint disorders. Also, sounds can be transferred from the cervical spine and its joints as well as its vessels into the cranial structures so that they become misinterpreted as tinnitus.

ENDOGENOUS TINNITUS

Q: Where is your feeling of well-being better, in a busy and noisy environment or in cavelike silence?
A: I much prefer a busy and noisy environment.

The patient with a maskable or endogenous tinnitus prefers covering it with external sounds. When using masking procedures, easily three zones of tinnitus can be discriminated within the hearing field:

1. Low-tone tinnitus (at and below 750 Hz)
2. Middle-frequency tinnitus (1 to 2 kHz)
3. High-frequency tinnitus (above 2 kHz until 10 kHz or even 12 kHz)

Low-tone tinnitus is more frequently found in Ménière's disease and some other cochlear-apical disorders, and middle-tone tinnitus is more frequently found in diseases such as otosclerosis. Most frequently tinnitus is matched in the high-tone range and is related, for example, to noise trauma, whiplash, head and skull trauma, cardiovascular failure, stress, acoustic neuromas, and toxic events including those associated with pharmaceutical, nicotine, or drug abuse. Also, several masking points may exist simultaneously.

Dysfunctions of the inner ear contribute to the development of tinnitus. But tinnitus by itself depends on a cortical process of the human brain. A sleeping patient does not suffer from any kind of tinnitus.

Since approximately 1985, the Würzburg neuro-otology group of Claussen et al. has been able to detect by means of vestibular evoked potentials (VestEP) and brain electrical activity mapping (BEAM) groups of patients suffering from a maskable or endogenous tinnitus that respond cortically in a typical, reproducible, and measurable manner:

1. Location of the site of the potentials around the upper gyrus of the temporal lobe (Brodmann's area 41)
2. Typical shortening of the latencies of evoked quantitative electroencephalograms (QEEGs)
3. Enlarged DC shift of the evoked QEEGs
4. Typical cortical electrical burst expansion in three phases on the brain surface

Since approximately 1990, the New York group of Shulman, Strashun, and Goldstein has followed a neuro-radiologic path for deciphering the cortical modalities in tinnitus patients by using single-photon emission computer tomography (SPECT). They discovered remarkably elevated metabolic processes in the temporal lobes of patients suffering from a maskable tinnitus.

Thereafter we were able to prove in therapeutic trials with pharmacotherapy (e.g., extractum ginkgo biloba [EGB 761]*), as well as with physiotherapy (competitive kinesthetic interaction therapy [KKIT]), that the subjective reduction or abolition of tinnitus goes together with an electrophysiologic measurable normalization of the VestEP with BEAM or QEEG. So the endogenous tinnitus could be proven to be a CNS network phenomenon.

EXOGENOUS TINNITUS

Q: Where is your feeling of well-being better, in a busy and noisy environment or in cavelike silence?
A: I much prefer a cavelike silence because noise and/or a group of people speaking at the same time are most confusing. It provokes ringing and shrieking sounds within my ears.

Unlike endogenous tinnitus, patients suffering from exogenous tinnitus cannot benefit from masking noises from their surroundings. Some physicians wrongly call this condition *hyperacusis*, but these patients do not hear better as this term suggests. Seemingly better is the named syndrome of the hypersensitive ear.

In exogenous tinnitus, pure-tone audiometry may be normal or exhibit regular deficits of the hearing threshold, but there is no maskable tinnitus. However, when measuring the acoustic dynamics by adding the audiometrically recorded discomfort threshold, the discomfort level, which is usually between 1 and 8 kHz below 95 dB, rises below this level to values of 90 to 60 dB or even 50 dB. The person being exposed to sound exceeding the level of his low discomfort threshold experiences a loss of understanding together with subjective pain and noise in the ears accompanied by possible vegetative reactions.

Hearing aids can adjust the incoming sounds by filtering, peak clipping, and cleaning of the sound signals so they fit optimally into the remaining acoustic dynamics of the individually existing hearing field. Thus, hearing aids

---

*Available as dietary supplement.

are the first choice for treating exogenous tinnitus. Some other methods for treating this type of tinnitus are physiotherapy, psychotherapy, stress reduction, and supportive pharmacotherapy.

TINNITUS IN SLOW BRAINSTEM SYNDROME (CLAUSSEN)

Q: How would you best describe your tinnitus?

A: I am becoming increasingly more in a daze and more disoriented and hear ringing and other sounds, which I cannot really localize in my ears or my head. The noise disturbs me as much as my mental instability.

We regularly see older patients who complain about a hazy tinnitus in combination with vertigo, giddiness, and dizziness and also report a reduced state of alertness. These patients have a connected statoacoustic problem. Objectively, affected patients exhibit an increase in the latencies of the experimentally provoked vestibular nystagmus as well as of the acoustically evoked brainstem potentials.

Especially in this group, we have noted by evaluating our therapeutic responses that a combination of cocculus[†] (picrotoxin), conium[†] (coneine), amber and petrol oil (Vertigoheel[†]) has a so-called tuning-up effect on the brainstem. Then the typical symptoms also disappear.

COMBINED ENDOGENOUS AND EXOGENOUS TINNITUS

A combination of both types of subjective tinnitus, endogenous and exogenous, is also found in tinnitus patients. Affected patients report that the noise they hear is present during both the day and night; however, the noise fluctuates. Especially the intensity of the noise can be very increased, for example when the patient is in a noisy environment or busy place or in a conversation with several participants.

Even though patients with combined endogenous and exogenous tinnitus have maskable tinnitus, they report that therapeutic acoustic maskers do not reduce their symptoms. They need a thorough audiometric and neuro-otologic workup.

Contemporary and Practical Treatment

Modern therapy of tinnitus appears to be complex and sometimes incomprehensible. But when talking about therapy of disabling tinnitus, we emphasize a main therapeutic approach in the sense that we have to break and inhibit the psychosomatic cycle of deterioration from tinnitus to stress, to insomnia, to panic. Some aspects of this reactional behavior are similar to pain.

The steps for individual tinnitus therapy must be chosen according to the kind of tinnitus diagnosed. Tinnitus is frequently associated with conditions such as stress, hearing loss, noise trauma, otorhinolaryngologic disorders (e.g., Ménière's disease, otosclerosis, perilymphatic fistula,

---

[†]Available as homeopathic remedy.

CURRENT THERAPY

- Avoidance of noise, ototoxic drugs, allergens
- Treatment of bruits by medical or surgical measures
- Instrumental therapy
- Tinnitus maskers
- Hearing aids
- Electrostimulation
- Specific pharmacotherapy
  - Lidocaine (Xylocaine)[1]
  - Carbamazepine (Tegretol)[1]
- Calming pharmacotherapy
  - Diazepam (Valium)[1]
  - Amitriptyline (Elavil)[1]
- Nontropic pharmacotherapy
  - Gingko[*]
  - Flunarizine[2]
- Neurotransmitter-directed pharmacotherapy
  - Betahistine[*]
  - Gabapentin (Neurontin)
- Psychotherapy
  - Retraining therapy (TRT)
- Physiotherapy
  - Competitive kinesthetic interaction therapy (KKIT)
- Other therapies
  - Hypnotherapy
  - Counseling
  - Acupuncture

[1]Not FDA approved for this indication.
[2]Not available in the United States.
[*]Available as dietary supplement.

acoustic neuroma), high blood pressure, metabolic disorders, allergy, intoxications, whiplash and other head and neck traumas, functional disorders of the neck, burnout syndrome, mandibular joint problems, and extracranial and intracranial vascular problems.

The Current Therapy box lists different therapeutic approaches to tinnitus. These 10 therapies must be individually interrelated with the different types of tinnitus (see Figure 1). Besides the severe disabling types of tinnitus, minor forms of tinnitus also occasionally occur that may be event related or may be time limited.

NOISE AVOIDANCE AND BASICS OF THERAPY

Avoidance can help in noise-related tinnitus by the prevention of noise exposure or at least by wearing ear protection. The use of ototoxic drugs must be controlled and limited. Inflammatory ear disease needs specific treatment of the external and the middle ear with antibiotics and anti-inflammatory drugs. Control and maintenance of a satisfactory degree of aeration of the middle ear is necessary. Acoustic neuroma calls for surgical removal of the tumor. Surgery is also necessary in otosclerosis and perilymphatic fistula. Specific gnatholic therapy by a dentist is recommended in a temporomandibular joint syndrome.

INSTRUMENTATIONS FOR THERAPY

Instrumentations currently available and frequently used according to the type and the chronicity of tinnitus are as follows:

1. Tinnitus maskers/tinnitus instruments, tapes/CDs for masking and relaxation
2. Acoustic ultra-high-frequency stimulation
3. Hearing aids
4. External electrical stimulations

PHARMACOTHERAPY

Pharmacotherapy, that is, treatment with pharmaceutical agents, is important in the management of tinnitus. It may be the main therapy or may play only a supportive, palliative, or intermittent role. The four lines of therapeutic agents used in the treatment of tinnitus may overlap and may be combined.

First-Line Agents

First-line therapeutic agents can relieve tinnitus either slowly or quickly. Lidocaine (Xylocaine),[1] a local anesthetic drug, only has a temporary effect in suppressing tinnitus. It is an aminoethylamide, which is well soluble in water.

A daily intravenous dose of lidocaine of 1 mg per kg of body weight can temporarily alleviate the phenomenon of endogenous tinnitus. The duration, however, depends on the blood level. As soon as the level of lidocaine in the blood is lowered below a threshold, tinnitus returns.

In tinnitus, lidocaine is best applied by iontophoresis through an electrical field with an active electrode in the external ear and a passive electrode at an arm, after instillation of a solution of lidocaine (1:100,000) into the external meatus.

This therapy temporarily relieves the disturbing tinnitus, so that the patients at least get some hours of rest and sleep. However, the untoward side effects of lidocaine also have to be taken into consideration.

Some forms of tinnitus also have an acoustic hallucinatory component, as in epilepsy. Therefore, carbamazepine (Tegretol),[1] which is an important antiepileptic agent used for bipolar affective disorders, is also used in tinnitus with a supratentorial focus. We have seen beneficial effects in very specific cases of endogenous tinnitus. Chemically, carbamazepine belongs to the tricyclic antidepressants. In adults, we give a daily dose of 200 mg. However, renal, hepatic, and hematologic parameters have to be monitored thoroughly.

Second-Line Agents

This group of drugs is especially used to treat the emotional effects seen in endogenous tinnitus, exogenous tinnitus, and combined endogenous and exogenous tinnitus, which can lead via sleeplessness to anxiety and panic. Here we see an indication for alprazolam (Xanax)[1] and similar substances. Alprazolam is administered to tinnitus patients in a daily dosage of 0.75 to 1.5 mg. Also chlordiazepoxide (Librium)[1] can alternatively be applied in a

daily dosage of 15 to 30 mg. Even diazepam (Valium)[1] is used in a daily dosage of 4 to 30 mg.

The mood changes associated with tinnitus can lead to psychosis and insomnia. Here a tricyclic antidepressant such as amitriptyline (Elavil)[1] in a daily dosage of 75 to 150 mg can be helpful.

Additionally, this agent has a desired sedative component. Other sedatives and psychotropic drugs are also used to treat the psychologic effects associated with tinnitus, but they must be applied very carefully.

Third-Line Agents

Third-line therapeutic agents comprise the so-called nootropic drugs. These are pharmacologic agents that activate brain function through improved metabolism, leading to a better adaptation and interconnection. They were originally developed to treat senile dementia. Within this group, in Germany, we use piracetam (Nootrop, Normabraïn) in a daily dosage of 800 to 1200 mg.

We have seen very beneficial effects from extract of ginkgo biloba (EGB 761*) (Tebonin, Rökan), which is administered in a daily dosage of 120 mg.

We also use calcium channel antagonists, among which flunarizine (Sibelium),[2] in a daily dosage of 15 to 30 mg, is effective in tinnitus with irritative foci, especially in mesencephalic and diencephalic areas. Cinnarizin[2] was the predecessor. This holds especially for the endogenous tinnitus group.

Fourth-Line Agents

The fourth line of therapy involves neurotransmitter-directed pharmacotherapy. According to the chemical structures of the neurotransmitters, we mainly use one system of the amines (i.e., the histamine mechanism) and one system of amino acids (i.e., γ-aminobutyric acid [GABA]).

Because it is known that inner ear functions are regulated at the neurotransmission level of the histaminergic H_1, H_2, and H_3 receptors, betahistine (Serc)[2] plays an important role in inner ear receptor-targeted therapy. The daily dosage that we administer in peripheral cochlear tinnitus is 16 to 48 mg.

The inhibitory neurotransmitter GABA is extremely potent in its ability to alter neuronal discharges because of failures in the supratentorial CNS neurotransmission. According to recent findings, endogenous tinnitus with a supratentorial dysregulation can be influenced by gabapentin (Neurontin).[1] It is used in dosages starting with 300 mg daily and can be increased to 900 mg daily. Originally gabapentin was used as an additional therapy in partial epilepsia without secondary generalized seizures. Like with other antiepileptic drugs, the parameters from kidney, liver, and blood have to be supervised.

ADAPTED PSYCHOTHERAPY

Nowadays so-called tinnitus retraining therapy (TRT) is widely applied. It includes a therapeutic wide-band

[1]Not FDA approved for this indication.

[1]Not FDA approved for this indication.
*Available as dietary supplement.
[2]Not available in the United States.

low-level noise generator. It is based on habituation, which is defined as a reduced response to a stimulus after repeated exposure. It is a state in which the tinnitus signal no longer elicits any response. Resetting or reprogramming neuronal networks involved in subcortical signal detection brings about habituation.

Also, in cases with a known interrelation of stress and tinnitus, a stress–diathesis model for tinnitus was proposed by Shulman et al. Stress management techniques require a counselor and the close cooperation of the patient, physician, biofeedback therapist, and psychologist.

A cognitive therapy that provides significant support to the patient with severe disabling tinnitus, particularly for control of the effect, is strongly recommended and encouraged.

ADAPTED PHYSIOTHERAPY

A specific program of physiotherapy successfully applied in endogenous tinnitus is KKIT. This therapy uses expressive movements of body language. In a special rehabilitation program, different groups of muscles in the hand, arm, leg, foot, and body, rising from the feet up to the face, are activated, which guides the tinnitus patient into a situation of peaceful resting, reduction of tension, and finally into relaxation. This scheme was adapted from a program of treating pain. KKIT points toward mechanisms of interference of expressive gestural movements with facilitating tinnitus from around the basal ganglia of the brain.

OTHER METHODS OF THERAPY

Other methods of tinnitus therapy recommended in the literature include acupuncture, counseling, group therapy, and hypnotherapy.

REFERENCES

Alster J, Shemesh Z, Ornan M, Attias J: Sleep disturbance associated with chronic tinnitus. Biol Psychiatry 1993;34:84-90.

Arnesen AR, Engdahl B: Tinnitus—etiology, diagnosis and treatment. Tidsskr Nor Laegeforen 1996;116:2009-2012.

Bergmann JM, Bertora GO: Cortical and brainstem topodiagnostic testing in tinnitus patients—a preliminary report. Int Tinnitus J 1996;2: 151-158.

Bertora GO, Bergmann JM: Tinnitus: Supratentorial areas study through brain electric tomography (LORETA). ASN 2004;2:2, ISSN 1612-3352. Available at http://www.neurootology.org

Claussen CF: Treatment of the slow brainstem syndrome with Vertigoheel. Biol Med 1985;3:447-470, 4:510-514.

Claussen CF: Medical classification of tinnitus between bruits: Exogenous and endogenous tinnitus and other types of tinnitus. ASN 2004;2, ISSN 1612-3352. Available at http://www.neurootology.org

Claussen CF, Kolchev C, Schneider D, Hahn A: Neurootological brain electrical activity mapping in tinnitus patients. Proceedings of the 4th International Tinnitus Seminar, Bordeaux, 1991;1092:351-355.

Claussen CF, Schneider D, Koltchev C: On the functional state of central vestibular structures in monaural symptomatic tinnitus patients. Int Tinnitus J 1995:1:5-12.

George RN, Kemp S: A survey of New Zealanders with tinnitus. Br J Audiol 1991;25:331-336.

Jastreboff PJ, Hazell JWP: A neurophysiological approach to tinnitus: Clinical implications. Br J Audiol 1993;27:1-11.

Parving A, Hein HO, Suadicani P, et al: Epidemiology of hearing disorders. Some factors affecting hearing. The Copenhagen Male Study. Scand Audiol 1993;22:101-107.

Quaranta A, Assennato G, Sallustio V: Epidemiology of hearing problems among adults in Italy. Scand Audiol Suppl 1996;42:9-13.

Shulman A: A final common pathway for tinnitus—the medial temporal lobe system. Tinnitus J 1996;2:115-126.

Shulman A, Aran JM, Feldmann H, et al: Tinnitus diagnosis/treatment. Philadelphia, Lea & Febiger, 1991.

Shulman A, Strashun AM, Afriyie M, et al: SPECT imaging of brain and tinnitus—neurotologic/neurologic implications. Int Tinnitus J 1995:1:13-29.

ACKNOWLEDGMENT

Sponsored by grant Projekt D. 1417, durch die LVA Baden-Württemberg, Stuttgart, Germany.

Spine Pain

Method of
Michael T. McCann, MD

Back pain is one of the most common musculoskeletal complaints seen in primary care practices; empirical treatment is frequently based on conjecture. Our understanding of the pathophysiology of spine and radicular pain has increased dramatically over the last decade as a result of new technology and more advanced diagnostic testing. Early and accurate diagnosis is imperative if we are to provide specific lesion-based treatment to optimize patient outcomes and health care spending.

Although patients are satisfied with their care for most major illnesses, 20% to 25% of surveyed patients were dissatisfied with their care for back pain. Only headache treatment also received such poor scores. The top reason patients listed for dissatisfaction with their physician's care was inadequate explanation of why they hurt.

Although muscle strain is the most common reason given to patients as the cause of their back pain, it is actually highly unlikely to be the etiology for back pain severe enough for a patient to seek medical care or for pain that lasts more than 2 weeks. An underlying spinal disorder is usually present, leading to overlying myofascial tenderness and tightness. Isolated back pain is not a neurologic problem. Rather, it is an orthopedic problem, as will be evident from the following discussion.

Epidemiology

Eighty percent of the U.S. population develops back pain, limiting day-to-day activities, at some time in their lives. The peak incidence of such pain is between 35 and 65 years of age, declining thereafter. Based on radiographic degeneration alone, we would expect the incidence to increase linearly with age. In 80% of patients, episodes are self-limited, but in 15% to 20%, the pain chronically restricts function. Direct and indirect economical costs are estimated to be between $80 and $100 billion per year in the United States and, from an insurer's standpoint, costs may exceed expenditures on pediatric and obstetrical care combined. The majority of treatment expenditures are on the 20% of patients whose pain does not resolve spontaneously: recurrent or chronic back pain sufferers.

To limit expenditures and optimize patient outcomes, it is vital that we prevent progression to a chronic state. Such prevention can best be achieved by early and accurate diagnosis and treatment.

Pathophysiology

Somatic (nociceptive) pain is caused by noxious stimulation of nerve endings in the vertebrae, joints, ligaments and disks, whereas radicular (neuropathic) pain is produced by evoked ectopic impulses in the dorsal root ganglia (Figure 1).

Somatic Pain

In primary somatic back pain, we try diagnostically to separate the pain generators into two anatomic categories based on their relation to the spinal canal. Treatment is significantly different based on the site of the lesions. Note that primary spinal nerve or cord pathology does not in and of itself produce axial back pain.

Pain generators in the anterior column are the disks and vertebral bodies. Only the outer third of a disk's annulus is innervated. Tears of these outer annular fibers produce exquisite pain and back spasm even without complete disruption of the disk. This is a frequent missed cause of nonspecific back pain because these internal disk disruptions are rarely visualized on routine spine magnetic resonance imaging (MRI) or computer tomography (CT) scans. If noted on MRI, a high-intensity zone (HIZ) finding in a disk is highly suggestive of a painful internal annular tear. Definitive diagnosis is established with manometric provocative CT diskography. Diskitis, although rare, is also suggested by MRI findings, although aspiration may be necessary to establish an inflammatory or infectious etiology definitively.

Vertebral compression fractures, whether osteoporotic, traumatic, or pathologic, also contribute to anterior column primary axial pain. CT scanning or plain radiographs generally confirm the diagnosis; however, bone scanning may be necessary to confirm acuteness of a finding and to help rule out metastatic foci. Osteomyelitis should also be considered in any fracture with associated fever or a recent septic source.

The posterior column sources of back pain include the facet joints from the atlanto-occipital articulation caudad to the sacroiliac joints. All are true diarthrodial joints. The surfaces are capped with articular cartilage and lined with a synovial membrane. These paired innervated structures are subject to degeneration and painful traumatic injuries. In double-blind placebo controlled studies, the cervical facets appear to be the source of pain in 59% of patients with postwhiplash cervicalgia. Estimates regarding the lumbar spine place the incidence of facet-based low back pain between 15% and 40%, and the incidence increases significantly after 65 years of age.

Spondylolisthesis refers to a shift in the alignment between two vertebrae. With associated stress fractures of the pars interarticularis (spondylolysis), it is another posterior column source of pain. In chronic cases, instability leads to associated fibrosis under the pars fractures that produce radicular compression and neuropathic extremity pain. The slippage may also lead to central and foraminal stenosis with neurogenic claudication.

Neuropathic Pain

The most common cause of lumbar radicular pain in young patients is disk herniation (98%). Nerve compression alone, however, does not offer a satisfactory explanation for the pain produced. In human studies, root compression alone produces distal extremity paresthesias and numbness but no pain. Isolated lumbar radiculopathy does not cause significant back pain, and disk herniation size does not correlate with severity of pain on straight leg raise testing. Nucleus pulposus placed within the epidural space produces extreme inflammation with a 100,000-fold increase in phospholipase-A_2 immunoreactivity that can be directly correlated with mechanical hyperalgesia. In the complete absence of root compression, nucleus pulposus stimulates sustained discharges of $A\delta$ and $A\beta$ pain fibers in the dorsal root ganglia and causes a conduction delay in the roots. Intravenous methylprednisolone (Solu-Medrol)[1] prevents this conduction delay. Radicular pain appears to be caused by a combination of mechanical irritation in an otherwise chemically sensitized root.

Other sources of radicular pain include central spinal and lateral recess stenosis caused by facet arthropathies, ligamentous hypertrophy, and spondylolisthesis. Even more etiologies include neuromeningeal anomalies, neoplasms, infections, and vascular malformations. Peripheral neuropathies, including thoracic outlet, cubital and carpal tunnel syndromes, piriformis syndrome, tarsal tunnel, and other primary mononeuropathies, may also mimic or exist in conjunction with radiculopathies.

Assessment

The goal of the initial assessment is to screen for emergent causes of back or radicular pain including aneurysms,

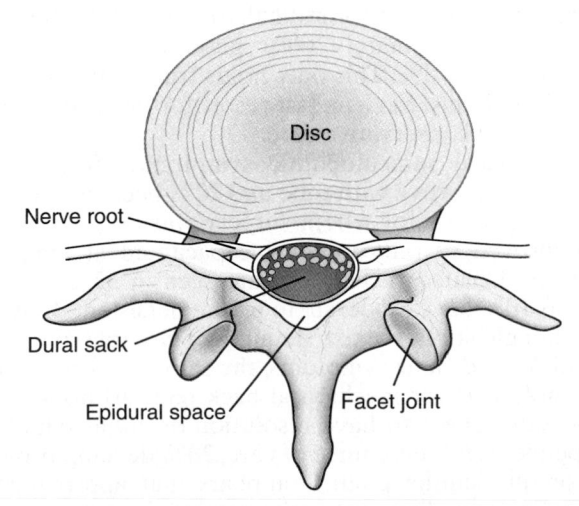

FIGURE 1. Spine cross section.

Disc

Nerve root

Dural sack

Epidural space

Facet joint

[1]Not FDA approved for this indication.

CURRENT DIAGNOSIS

Emergent or Urgent Conditions Associated with Back Pain (Red Flags)

ASSOCIATED SYMPTOMS	CONDITION
■ New onset bowel or bladder incontinence	Myelopathy
■ Balance difficulties	Myelopathy
■ Diffuse distal weakness or immobility	Myelopathy
■ Recent weight loss	Tumor
■ Severe chest or abdominal pain	Aortic aneurysm

HISTORY	CONDITION
■ Osteoporosis	Fracture
■ Recent trauma	Fracture
■ Intravenous drug use	Infection
■ Recent infection	Infection
■ Immunosuppressed state	Infection

AGE	CONDITION
■ <15 y or >60 y	Tumor suspicion
■ Male >55 y (M:F 4:1)	Aortic aneurysm

ASSOCIATED SIGNS	CONDITION
■ Tender abdomen	Aortic aneurysm
■ Saddle sensory loss	Cauda equina syndrome
■ Hyperreflexia with positive clonus, Babinski's sign, and Hoffmann's sign	Myelopathy

infections, segmental instability, fractures, tumors, and myelopathy. A careful history and examination should help delineate referred cardiac, pulmonary, gastrointestinal, urologic, gynecologic, and vascular sources.

History

For all patients presenting with back or radicular pain, the screening history should include weight loss, recent fevers or infections, and significant change in bowel or bladder function, including incontinence. For patients with cervicothoracic or upper extremity radicular pain, a cardiac history should be added. Abdominal symptoms, hematuria, dysuria, or vaginal discharge should be included for lumbar pain.

Radicular pain is lancinating with superficial and deep components that extend in distinct, but not necessarily dermatomal, distributions. Pain may extend partially or entirely in the distribution of the affected spinal nerve. Somatic referred pain is deep, aching, and diffuse. It can overlap with radicular symptoms in the proximal extremities. Proximal extremity pain can be radicular, whereas distal extremity pain is not necessarily always radicular.

Diffuse distal symptoms with dysesthesia, complaints of bowel or bladder urgency or incontinence, and a history of balance difficulties are red flags for myelopathy. Most patients also give a history of cervicothoracic or associated

radicular pain. If accompanied by severe low back pain and complaints of saddle numbness, consider cauda equina syndrome, a surgical emergency.

Claudication symptoms are suggestive of spinal stenosis and usually there is little pain at rest. Differentiation from vascular claudication is sometimes difficult, but pain with neurogenic claudication is usually not worsened with supine positioning and leg elevation.

Examination

Although clinical exam may establish the presence of a radiculopathy or localize the segmental pain level, etiology must be established by other means. Tumors, cysts, stenosis spondylolisthesis, and disk herniations may all cause very similar clinical signs.

Muscle pain and spasm should not be considered the primary source of the patient's back pain unless all other potential sources are ruled out and an objective rheumatologic etiology is identified pointing to a myositis. An antalgic gait from distal degenerative joint disease may cause lumbar muscular aching, but rarely is the back the site of greatest pain. This is not to say that muscles cannot be painful, but rather that in the majority of primary back pain cases, the muscles are simply reacting to an underlying derangement in the spine itself.

More specifically, examination should note hyperreflexia and clonus and test for Babinski's and Hoffmann's signs to note upper motor neuron irritability. Screening cardiovascular and abdominal examination helps rule out other sources of back pain.

Natural Course of the Disease

For lumbar radicular pain in patients treated conservatively, 50% of patients can expect to have resolution of radicular symptoms after 4 weeks. At 12 months, in 49% of males and 33% of females, radicular pain remains improved. Unfortunately, 60% to 70% of these patients developed back pain by 4 weeks that persisted at 12 months regardless of the radicular pain improvement.

For patients treated surgically versus conservatively, at 10 years there appears to be little statistically significant difference in outcome for radicular pain, with both groups achieving approximately 60% good results and poor results in 7% to 8%. This only holds true if surgery is not applied randomly, but as a last resort for patients who fail to respond to conservative care.

For cervical radiculopathic symptoms, 70% can be expected to improve with time and 20% become asymptomatic. In patients for whom surgery was an option, 90% are improved or only mildly incapacitated at long-term follow-up. Isolated recurrences are seen in 32% of cases, whereas 10% have moderate to severe persistent disability.

Although studies exist detailing favorable outcomes overall for radicular symptoms, the same does not necessarily hold true for mechanical back pain. Although 80% of patients appear to have resolution of initial symptoms independent of their course of care, 20% develop progressive or unrelenting pain. It appears that approximately 35% of persons have intermittent recurrences that limit their activities.

Management

Take an algorithmic approach to the patient presenting with back and/or radicular symptoms of new onset. If initial history and examination suggest an emergent cause for these symptoms, appropriate additional diagnostic testing and referral should be made. Indications for urgent surgical interventions are few but include progressive motor deficit and cauda equina syndrome—progressive neurologic deterioration with loss of bowel and bladder function.

Once an emergent source of pain is ruled out, studies show that primary care physicians who prescribe the least amount of analgesics and place the fewest restrictions on activities have the best patient outcomes. In many cases, a more aggressive approach may reinforce illness behavior and foster a fear of future debilitation.

Radicular Pain Predominating

If radicular pain predominates in a minimally distressed patient, simple reassurance and an explanation of the natural course of recovery may suffice. Avoiding bed rest and activity modification to prevent axial loading should be discussed (no lifting in a forward flexed position and no

CURRENT THERAPY

Acute Presentation without Red Flags: Treatment Ladders (Frequent Reassessment as Indicated)

BACK OR NECK PAIN PREDOMINATING

- Education, activity modification, and reassurance
- Limited course of analgesics dependent on stress
  - NSAIDs
  - Opioids
  - Muscle relaxants
  - Consider steroid taper regimen
- Physical therapy with spinal stabilization regimen
- Screening radiographs with flexion and extension views (rule out gross instability)
- Referral for spinal diagnostic assessment or orthopedic spine evaluation
- Fusion or disk replacement as indicated

RADICULAR PAIN PREDOMINATING

- Education, activity modification, and reassurance
- Early treatment of inflammation with steroid taper regimen
- Limited course of analgesics and muscle relaxants
- Early initiation of neuropathic pain medications
  - Gabapentin (Neurontin)[1]
  - Duloxetine (Cymbalta)[1]
  - Pregabalin (Lyrica)[1]
- Physical therapy guided by McKenzie assessment
- MRI (with gadolinium contrast for cancer, spinal cord pathology, and postoperative spine cases)
- Selective transforaminal steroid injection
- Surgical assessment for decompression

[1]Not FDA approved for this indication.
Abbreviations: NSAIDs = nonsteroidal anti-inflammatory drugs.

repetitive flexion activities). A 2-week reassessment allows any insidious red flag conditions to be picked up, provides reassurance, and allows adjustment of treatment.

For more significantly distressed patients with acute radicular pain, additional analgesics and more frequent follow-up may be required. Although no analgesic regimen alters the natural course of recovery, based on the inflammatory pathogenesis of radicular pain a pulse dose of prednisone or methylprednisolone with a taper can be considered over a week. However, in randomized controlled trials, the nonsteroidal anti-inflammatory drugs (NSAIDs) piroxicam (Feldene) and indomethacin (Indocin) did not offer any greater analgesia or enhance recovery more than placebo. A limited course of muscle relaxants and opioid analgesics may be prescribed but often provide little relief in cases of true neuropathic pain. The limited duration of these prescriptions should be explained to the patient at the outset. Despite ongoing pain, the goal is to avoid dependency and reliance on these medications for activities that may be detrimental to the natural course of the disorder.

Currently, greater success may be found with early initiation and titration of gabapentin (Neurontin)[1] for radicular pain. With low toxicity and few side effects, tolerance is usually good. Initiate dosing at night with 100 to 300 mg (lower dosing in patients >65 years old), escalating every 1 to 3 days as tolerated up to 1200 mg three times daily. If improvement is not obtained by 600 mg three times daily, further escalation is unlikely to be efficacious.

For distressed patients, duloxetine (Cymbalta)[1] may be efficacious while providing additional anxiolysis and antidepressive effects. Because nausea is a frequent side effect for the first few days upon initiation of dosing, we start with 30 mg every morning and advance to 60 mg every morning after 1 week. If sedation occurs, change to every-evening dosing. Symptomatic improvement is often seen by 7 to 10 days.

If at follow-up significant progress is not made and reassessment still lacks red flags, physical therapy with instructions for a McKenzie assessment and therapy over 2 weeks is indicated, with a home program to follow. Again, no scientific studies validate any particular regimen of therapy. However, from a spinal education standpoint, and as an impetus to maintaining function, an empirical recommendation can be made. Follow-up should be scheduled and if progress is partial, another 2 weeks of therapy could be considered.

Failure to improve or deterioration of function at any point would be an indication for additional imaging studies. An MRI provides the most comprehensive survey of causes for radicular symptoms. It does not, however, guarantee that anatomic changes are definitively the source for a patient's symptoms. In asymptomatic patients younger than 40 years, 30% had abnormal spine MRIs, whereas 60% to 70% of patients older than 40 years had abnormal MRIs. The prevalence of asymptomatic disk herniations alone ranged between 20% and 40% in patients between 40 and 60 years of age.

Evidence-based review of the literature currently does not support the use of electromyogram and nerve conduction velocity (EMG/NCV) studies) for diagnosis in cases of radiculopathic pain. Pain is mediated through Aδ

[1]Not FDA approved for this indication.

and C fibers, and an EMG tests activity in $A\alpha$ motor fibers. H and F reflexes similarly lack specificity in clinical trials with radiculopathy, despite proposed theoretical foundations. EMG/NCV testing would be indicated in cases where peripheral neuropathy or nerve entrapment is suspected and when objective muscle strength testing is suspect or primary myopathy may be present.

Recent prospective randomized blinded studies support selective nerve root injection (i.e., fluoroscopically guided transforaminal epidural steroid or epiradicular injections) as the next line of treatment. This highly selective procedure may reduce the need for surgical intervention in up to 59% of radicular cases and should be considered in cases where lack of improvement is noted as soon as 2 weeks. Serial MRI studies in humans show statistically significant improvement in the rate of disk reabsorption and symptoms in patients treated with transforaminal injections as compared to controls. The older regimen of translaminar epidural steroid injections is not nearly as efficacious and in some studies appears no more effective than placebo. Partial improvement at 10- to 14-day follow-up would be an indication for repeat injection. An automatic series of three injections is no longer considered standard of care, and response to a single transforaminal injection should guide additional treatment. Lack of improvement or further functional decline would lead to surgical assessment.

Long-term management of a patient with radicular pain either unrelieved with surgery or in the patient for whom surgical options do not exist falls into the realm of neuropathic pain control. Narcotic regimens should be avoided because long-term efficacy has never been demonstrated. Medications options are limited, but gabapentin (Neurontin)[1] and duloxetine (Cymbalta)[1] are efficacious in reducing pain for a large number of patients with both radicular and other sources of neuropathic pain. The newest drug with indications for neuropathic pain is pregabalin (Lyrica)[1]. Efficacy for radicular pain is as yet undetermined but is expected to approximate gabapentin with fewer dose-related side effects. Other drugs to be considered include mexiletine (Mexitil)[1], tricyclic antidepressants,[1] and some of the newer anticonvulsants including levetiracetam (Keppra),[1] oxcarbazepine (Trileptal),[1] zonisamide (Zonegran),[1] and tiagabine (Gabitril).[1] All modify neuropathic pain in the presence and absence of associated depression.

For patients in whom neuropathic extremity pain far exceeds any mechanical back pain, despite optimization of all conservative treatment and surgical options, spinal cord stimulation may be considered. This modality is efficacious in between 60% and 70% of patients with neuropathic extremity pain predominating. It is not indicated for mechanical back pain. For permanently implanted patients, 70% continue to have approximately 50% improvement in neuropathic pain at 5-year follow-up.

Axial Pain Predominating

For patients with nonurgent acute back or neck pain, again the level of distress helps guide care. Studies regarding early treatment and analgesic regimens for nociceptive

---

[1]Not FDA approved for this indication.

back pain lack validity and specificity because early diagnosis is not usually sought because of the high incidence of spontaneous improvement. Early treatment thus remains empirical.

In a minimally distressed patient, supportive education and activity modification support the natural course of recovery. For an initial episode, physical therapy with spinal stabilization exercises, followed by a home program, is recommended to provide back education and to help reduce recurrences.

For the more distressed patient, oral analgesics may be indicated. Because the source of axial pain is nociceptive, NSAIDs should be considered as a first-line analgesic, with opioids reserved for very severe pain and again only for a limited duration. Failure to improve is not an indication for continued daily use of opioids. For moderate to severe pain where a significant inflammatory component is suspected, a bolus/taper dose of steroids over 1 week is often efficacious, and risks are low with this regimen. Muscle spasms are best managed with gradual stretching and paced activities. In severe cases, however, muscle relaxants may be beneficial, and even a limited course of benzodiazepines can be considered.

If at 2-week reassessment progress is not seen, physical therapy over 1 month (usually 3 to 4 times per week) for range of motion and stabilization exercise should be considered. Partial improvement would be an indication for another month of therapy or, in the motivated patient, another month of a home exercise program.

The goal of therapy is to maintain range of motion, strengthen supportive musculature, and maintain activities of daily living without additional injury. To this end, almost all exercise regimens claim efficacy, although no valid studies as yet show that any specific therapy actually alters the natural history.

Should a patient with primary back or neck pain fail to improve with therapy, screening radiographs may be indicated. Plain radiographs for mechanical back pain should always be obtained with flexion and extension views to rule out gross instability as well as other mechanical derangements, including spondylolisthesis, spondylolysis, and compression fractures.

Unfortunately, although all radiographic studies of the spine demonstrate anatomic abnormalities, they cannot show whether these abnormalities are painful. With physical examination also notoriously unreliable for making a definitive diagnosis, referral for more advanced spinal diagnostic assessment may often be indicated in patients who fail to improve or who have frequent recurrences.

For the 20% of patients whose function remains limited by back pain despite maximized conservative care, identification of the exact pain source is imperative to improving outcomes. These patients are prone to seek numerous opinions, undergo fruitless operations, and pay for unproven modality-based treatments. Physicians tend toward making diagnoses based on response to treatment as opposed to the other way around. An early definitive diagnosis allows realistic treatment options and prognosis to be given. Patients can thus adjust their lifestyle to function within the limits imposed by their spinal condition.

Significant advances are being made in the field of diagnosing back pain. Select spinal injection techniques are refined to isolate the exact source of a patient's pain in the majority of cases. Validity testing can also determine if a patient's complaint has an anatomic basis or if symptom magnification is present.

CT-provocative diskography is the only test available to document internal disk anatomy precisely and to determine if a disk is the source of a patient's back pain. Studies show that compared with surgical findings, its anatomic accuracy exceeds MRI and CT myelography. With the use of manometry, intradiskal symptomatic pressures help determine the proper surgical technique to optimize patient outcomes. Diagnostic facet injections can also identify a symptomatic joint precisely, further helping determine options for treatment.

New nonsurgical or minimally invasive treatments are now validated, including radiofrequency thermocoagulation (RFTC) lesioning for desensitization of painful facet joint arthropathies, intradiskal electrothermal therapy (IDET) for treatment of painful disk lesions, and percutaneous disk decompression by both mechanical and laser techniques. For vertebral compression fracture, vertebroplasty and kyphoplasty may offer remarkable and rapid relief of associated fracture pain but do carry a risk of severe neurologic injury and embolism. Treatment outcomes for all of these procedures rely heavily on obtaining an exact diagnosis using the preceding tests.

Surgical assessment for nonemergent back pain should be reserved for those patients who fail conservative management and are not candidates for minimally invasive treatment or who have identifiable gross segmental spinal instability. Unlike radicular pain, decompression alone does not improve primary back pain. For mechanical back pain from segmental instability, the only surgical option is fusion. Poor pain relief is seen most frequently in patients who undergo fusion procedures for back pain based on radiographic findings alone. Provocative testing to isolate the actual pain generators and to determine the integrity of surrounding support structures maximizes the chances for success. For patients with isolated diskogenic pain, validated with manometric CT diskography, newer disk replacement techniques hold promise. Fusions cause a load shift to adjacent spinal motion segments causing degeneration. This leads to a 30% reoperation rate for fusion patients within 10 years. The hope is that disk replacements will prevent this transitional zone degeneration and lower the reoperation rate.

Not all patients are candidates for surgical reconstruction. In many cases, surgical intervention may only serve to worsen a patient's state. Tolerance of symptoms with acceptance of functional limitations is the preferred course.

To conclude, patients presenting with pain of spinal origin should be divided into those with predominantly radicular symptoms and those with primarily mechanical back or neck pain. In the vast majority of cases, back and neck pain originates from derangements of the facets, disks, or vertebrae, not the muscles. Radicular pain is most likely secondary to a compressive lesion with associated underlying inflammation.

TABLE 1 Clinical Pearls

Muscle strain is a very unusual cause of back pain severe enough to seek medical attention.

For back pain, think facets, disks, and vertebrae.

Referred back and neck pain can extend into the extremities and mimic radicular patterns.

Radicular pain does not always extend into the distal extremities (L5 radiculopathy can mimic hip trochanteric bursitis).

Magnetic resonance imaging (MRI) cannot tell you what hurts, only what might be causing pain.

MRI does not rule out all spinal pathology that can cause pain.

Order MRI with gadolinium contrast only if:
  You suspect cancer.
  You suspect a primary spinal cord lesion.
  Spine surgery was performed in the suspect region.

Laminectomy alone should not be used to treat predominant back pain (only radicular pain).

Fusions and disk replacements are for predominant back pain.

Only spinal diagnostic testing (selective computer tomography [CT] diskography, facet blocks, and transforaminal injections) can isolate the source of pain in refractory cases.

Electromyogram and nerve conduction velocity (EMG/NCV) studies should be used only if you:
  Suspect an underlying peripheral neuropathic process (double crush).
  Suspect lack of effort on motor testing.
  Suspect a primary myopathy.

Early referral for accurate diagnostic testing is the key to optimizing care: the more accurate the diagnosis, the more accurate the care.

Proper diagnosis is paramount to optimizing patient treatment (both conservative and surgical) and to prevention of progress to a chronic dysfunctional state. MRIs have limitations in what they are able to visualize and do not guarantee that anatomic derangements are actually the source of the patient's pain. For an accurate diagnosis in a patient who fails to respond to initial conservative care, more specialized interventional spinal diagnostic testing is indicated (Table 1).

Identification and isolation of specific spinal pain generators has allowed for the development of specific lesion-based minimally invasive treatments. These include transforaminal injections for radiculopathy, RFTC desensitization for facet-based pain, and percutaneous decompression for disk displacement pain. Decompressive surgery is very effective at relieving severe radicular pain unresponsive to conservative care and injections, but it is complicated by postlaminectomy spinal instability. Spinal fusion surgery for well-diagnosed painful segmental instability remains the definitive treatment for this disorder; newer disk replacement surgery may offer an alternative to fusion for primary diskogenic back or neck pain.

The Infectious Diseases

Management of the Patient with HIV Disease

Method of
Surendra K. Sharma, MD, PhD, and
Tamilarasu Kadhiravan, MD

AIDS was described initially in the United States in 1981 among several case clusters of previously healthy young men who had sex with men, presenting with unusual infections such as *Pneumocystis jiroveci* pneumonia (PCP), mucosal candidiasis, disseminated cytomegalovirus (CMV) disease, and Kaposi's sarcoma. The cause of AIDS remained elusive then, leading to several speculations. A few years later, amid much controversy, the causative agent was established as HIV, which has a predilection to infect and destroy the immune effector cells, primarily the CD4+ T lymphocytes. The discovery of HIV led to the development of definitive diagnostic tests that unearthed, to everyone's dismay, a widespread, hitherto invisible, smoldering pandemic in evolution.

Epidemiology

Since the beginning of the epidemic, approximately 25 million people have died of AIDS worldwide, making it one of the most devastating epidemics of all times. An estimated 40 million people are living with HIV/AIDS globally, including 17.5 million women and 2.3 million children younger than 15 years. In 2005 alone, an estimated 5 million people got newly infected, and approximately 3 million people died because of AIDS. More than half of the burden of HIV/AIDS is borne by sub-Saharan Africa, particularly the southern African nations. In countries such as Botswana, South Africa, Zimbabwe, Swaziland, and Namibia, the prevalence of HIV infection among expectant mothers is consistently in excess of 20%.

North America accounts for approximately 1.2 million people living with HIV/AIDS, most of them in the United States. Every year, more than 35,000 new cases are reported in the United States. Blacks and Hispanics are disproportionately represented among them, and pediatric AIDS accounts for approximately 1% of the cases. With the widespread implementation of preventive measures, a marginal but significant fall in HIV infection rates was observed for the first time among non-Hispanic blacks and injection drug users.

The Causative Agent

HIV is an enveloped single-stranded RNA virus (family: Retroviridae; subfamily: Lentivirinae). Embedded in its envelope are glycoprotein spikes (gp120, gp41) that are crucial for binding with the host cell surface receptors such as CD4, CCR5, and CXCR4 and subsequent entry into the host cell. HIV is a retrovirus that elaborates the enzyme reverse transcriptase. It enables transcription of genomic RNA to proviral DNA for integration into the host cell DNA. Host cells that bear CD4+ (helper T cells, macrophages, etc.) are the main targets of HIV infection. There are two human immunodeficiency viruses, HIV-1 and HIV-2. Compelling genetic evidence suggests that they originated from the simian immunodeficiency viruses, of the chimpanzee (SIVcpz) and the sooty mangabey monkeys (SIVsm), respectively, in Africa several decades back. HIV-1 is global in distribution, whereas HIV-2 is confined mainly to western Africa. HIV-2 infection is less effectively transmitted and results in lower levels of viremia and slower disease progression compared to HIV-1.

Isolates of HIV-1 across the globe exhibit marked genetic heterogeneity and are classified into three groups (M, O, and N) and several clades. Clade C is the most common form worldwide. In North America and Europe, clade B is the predominant subtype. Genetic recombination among co-circulating clades often occurs, and such a recombinant subtype AE is the most prevalent form in Southeast Asia. Clade AE viruses are transmitted more effectively by the heterosexual route than the clade B virus. The genetic heterogeneity of HIV has to be taken into consideration in the development and evaluation of HIV vaccines.

Modes of Transmission

Transmission of HIV occurs through contact with the body fluids of a HIV-infected person. The routes of transmission are sexual, both male to male as well as heterosexual contact; mother to child; transfusion of HIV-tainted blood and blood products; injection drug use; and occupational exposure in health care and laboratory workers. No evidence suggests that HIV is transmitted by casual contact and insect bites. Heterosexual transmission is the most prevalent route of HIV transmission worldwide, especially in developing countries. In the United States, male-to-male sexual contact is the most common route of transmission; however, the proportion of cases caused by heterosexual transmission is steadily increasing.

The average risk of HIV transmission per coital act in sero-discordant heterosexual couples is approximately 0.1%. Several factors, such as the presence of other sexually transmitted infections (ulcerative as well as nonulcerative) and higher viral load, increase the risk of transmission; condom use and male circumcision considerably reduce the risk. Female-to-male transmission is less effective than male-to-female transmission. Commercial sex is associated with a higher risk of transmission of approximately 5% to 10%. Receptive anal intercourse is associated with a higher risk of transmission as compared to vaginal intercourse. Even though the risk of transmission by oral sex is very low, it should not be considered completely safe.

Mother-to-child transmission of infection can occur during pregnancy, during delivery, or by breast-feeding. More than half of the transmissions occur intrapartum, mediated by direct contact of infant mucosa with HIV-laden maternal blood, amniotic fluid, and cervical/vaginal secretions. Placental microtransfusion also plays a role. High maternal plasma viremia, prolonged rupture of membranes, and chorioamnionitis increase the risk of mother-to-child transmission, whereas cesarean delivery and use of peripartum antiretroviral prophylaxis decrease the risk markedly.

With the implementation of mandatory testing practices, transmission through infected blood and blood products is almost eliminated in the developed world. However, despite using the highly sensitive nucleic acid-based tests, given the enormous number of transfusions in clinical practice, the risk of transfusion-transmitted HIV infection cannot be overlooked. It is estimated that each year 16 infectious donations are available for transfusion in the United States.

Although injection drug use is responsible for approximately 20% of HIV transmission in the United States, it is the driving force behind the HIV epidemic in Southeast Asian countries and China. Apart from direct transmission through sharing of contaminated needles and other paraphernalia, injection drug use also promotes risk-taking behavior and unsafe sexual practices. In developing countries, unsafe injections administered at health care facilities are a potential, but underappreciated, route of HIV transmission. Occupational transmission occurs through percutaneous needle stick injuries and after mucous membrane or nonintact skin exposure to infected body fluids. The risk of HIV infection following a contaminated needle stick injury is approximately 0.3% and is approximately 0.09% following mucous membrane exposure.

Pathogenesis and Natural History of HIV Infection

Following infection, HIV localizes to the lymphoid organs of the body where it productively infects the CD4+ helper T lymphocytes in the milieu provided by the dendritic cells and subsequently spills over into the circulation. In the absence of an immune response, this results in intense viremia in the early weeks following primary infection. During this phase, extensive dissemination of the virus occurs throughout the body. In approximately 50% to 70% of individuals, this might become clinically manifest as a self-limited, mononucleosis-like illness known as "acute HIV syndrome" (Table 1). Soon, with the elaboration of HIV-specific cell-mediated as well as humoral immune responses, viremia is brought under control albeit incompletely. A balance thus is struck between the opposing influences of viremia and the host immune response, establishing the viral load around a relatively low, stable level known as the virologic setpoint. The virologic setpoint is one of the important determinants of the pace of subsequent disease progression. Even if the viremia gets suppressed to below-detectable limits, despite the disease being clinically silent, active viral replication occurs throughout the course of HIV disease.

TABLE 1 Acute HIV Syndrome*

Clinical Features	Differential Diagnosis
Common (> 50%)	
Fever	Infectious mononucleosis
Malaise	Acute cytomegalovirus
Lymphadenopathy	infection
Pharyngitis	Secondary syphilis
Rash—erythematous,	Acute toxoplasmosis
maculopapular; urticarial;	Rickettsial infections
mucocutaneous ulcers	Rubella
Myalgia and arthralgia	Systemic lupus
	erythematosus
	Still's disease
Frequent (10%–50%)	
Diarrhea	
Headache	
Nausea and vomiting	
Hepatosplenomegaly	
Oral thrush	
Anorexia and weight loss	
Occasional (<10%)	
Aseptic meningitis	
Acute meningoencephalitis	
Guillain-Barré syndrome	
Myelopathy	
Brachial neuritis	
Facial palsy	
Peripheral neuropathy	
Opportunistic infections	

*Occurs approximately 3–6 wk following primary infection; symptoms last for 1 to several weeks, followed by gradual, spontaneous resolution; in a small proportion (approximately 10%), despite resolution of initial symptoms, rapid immunologic deterioration follows.

Some aspects of viral dynamics in vivo are important from a therapeutic point of view. An enormously large amount of virions (10^{10} to 10^{11}) are produced and cleared every day. Thus, the chances of a drug-resistant strain emerging under the selection pressure exerted by anti-retroviral therapy are very high. Even in patients who achieve undetectable viral loads for prolonged periods of time following treatment, ongoing active viral replication occurs. If therapy is stopped in these patients, viral load promptly bounces back. Further, antiretroviral therapy does not eliminate the large reservoir of latently infected cells that are capable of giving rise to replication-competent virus. Theoretically, it would take several decades of uninterrupted viral suppression for this reservoir to get depleted on its own.

During the phase of clinical latency, continuous viral replication leads to progressive depletion of CD4+ helper T cells, resulting from direct cytopathicity as well as by diverse indirect mechanisms. When the CD4+ cell count falls below 200 cells/μL, the risk of opportunistic infections (OIs) increases greatly, culminating in AIDS. The CD4+ cell count, as an index of immunosuppression because of HIV infection, predicts strongly the risk of OIs and thereby the risk of progression to AIDS and subsequent death (Table 2). However, when the CD4+ counts are above 350 cells/μL, their usefulness in predicting the risk of disease progression is limited. Conversely, the plasma viral load is a more robust predictor of the risk of AIDS,

independent of the CD4+ count at all levels (Table 2). The rate of decline in CD4+ count is highly variable among individuals. Some progress very rapidly, whereas a few others maintain normal levels of CD4+ counts and immuno-competence for prolonged periods without treatment. In Western populations, the median time to development of AIDS is approximately 10 years, and approximately 10% of patients remain asymptomatic beyond 20 years. The latter are known as long-term nonprogressors.

Apart from the viral load, several host-related factors also influence the rate of disease progression. It is well known that people who are homozygous for the deletion mutation *CCR5-Δ 32*, which codes for a nonfunctional CCR5, are highly resistant to HIV infection despite repeated exposure. HIV-infected individuals who are heterozygous for this allele have comparatively lower plasma viral loads and slower rate of progression to AIDS. Likewise, homo/heterozygosity for the mutant allele *CCR2 64I*, the product of which dimerizes with and decreases the expression of CXCR4 on the cell surface, results in slower disease progression. HLA alleles B*5701 and B*2705 also are strongly associated with long-term nonprogressor status. Conversely, individuals having the single nucleotide polymorphism at the promoter site of the inhibitory cytokine IL-10 (IL-10-5′-592A) are at a higher risk for HIV infection upon exposure, and they progress to AIDS more rapidly once infected. Certain exogenous

TABLE 2 Predicted 6-Month Risk of AIDS in the CASCADE Project, Based on Age, Current CD4+ Count, and Plasma Viral Load

Viral Load (copies/mL)	Predicted Risk at Current CD4+ Cell Count (cells/μL)									
	50	100	150	200	250	300	350	400	450	500
Age 25 y										
3,000	6.8	3.7	2.3	1.6	1.1	0.8	0.6	0.5	0.4	0.3
10,000	9.6	5.3	3.4	2.3	1.6	1.2	0.9	0.7	0.5	0.4
30,000	13.3	7.4	4.7	3.2	2.2	1.6	1.2	0.9	0.7	0.6
100,000	18.6	10.6	6.7	4.6	3.2	2.4	1.8	1.4	1.1	0.8
300,000	25.1	14.5	9.3	6.3	4.5	3.3	2.5	1.9	1.5	1.2
Age 35 y										
3,000	8.5	4.7	3.0	2.0	1.4	1.0	0.8	0.6	0.5	0.4
10,000	12.1	6.7	4.3	2.9	2.0	1.5	1.1	0.9	0.7	0.5
30,000	16.6	9.3	5.9	4.0	2.8	2.1	1.6	1.2	0.9	0.7
100,000	23.1	13.2	8.5	5.8	4.1	3.0	2.3	1.7	1.3	1.1
300,000	30.8	18.0	11.7	8.0	5.7	4.2	3.1	2.4	1.9	1.5
Age 45 y										
3,000	10.7	5.9	3.7	2.5	1.8	1.3	1.0	0.7	0.6	0.5
10,000	15.1	8.5	5.4	3.6	2.6	1.9	1.4	1.1	0.8	0.7
30,000	20.6	11.7	7.5	5.1	3.6	2.6	2.0	1.5	1.2	0.9
100,000	28.4	16.5	10.6	7.3	5.2	3.8	2.9	2.2	1.7	1.3
300,000	37.4	22.4	14.6	10.1	7.2	5.3	4.0	3.1	2.4	1.9
Age 55 y										
3,000	13.4	7.5	4.7	3.2	2.3	1.7	1.2	0.9	0.7	0.6
10,000	18.8	10.7	6.8	4.6	3.3	2.4	1.8	1.4	1.1	0.8
30,000	25.4	14.6	9.4	6.4	4.6	3.3	2.5	1.9	1.5	1.2
100,000	34.6	20.5	13.3	9.2	6.5	4.8	3.6	2.8	2.2	1.7
300,000	44.8	27.5	18.2	12.6	9.1	6.7	5.0	3.9	3.0	2.4

Abbreviation: CASCADE = Concerted Action on Seroconversion to AIDS and Death in Europe.
Reproduced with permission from Phillips A; CASCADE collaboration: Short-term risk of AIDS according to current CD4 cell count and viral load in antiretroviral drug-naïve individuals and those treated in the monotherapy era. AIDS 2004;18(1):51-58.

factors might also influence the course of HIV infection. The orphan virus GB virus C slows down disease progression and is associated with better survival in patients dually infected with HIV and GB virus C. CMV co-infection possibly augments the rate of HIV disease progression. Incident OIs, especially tuberculosis and deficiency of micronutrients, also accelerate disease progression.

Changing Face of HIV/AIDS

Highly active antiretroviral therapy (HAART) has dramatically changed the long-term outcome of patients with HIV/AIDS, which once was a rapidly fatal illness. HAART not only improves the CD4+ counts but also decreases the risk of OIs and reduces the mortality substantially. The benefit of HAART is evident even in those patients with advanced immunosuppression. From a public health perspective, HAART is a cost-effective intervention, in the developed world and the developing nations alike. In fact, HAART is comparatively more cost-effective than some of the widely accepted therapies for certain non-HIV diseases.

Since the introduction of HAART in 1995, AIDS-related mortality has declined considerably in the United States. With improved survival of patients with AIDS, noninfectious complications of AIDS such as AIDS-related malignancies and chronic renal failure are increasingly seen. Similarly, some novel problems of long-term antiretroviral therapy, such as lipodystrophy, insulin resistance syndrome, increased risk of cardiovascular events, and osteoporosis, are also being recognized. However, the changing face of AIDS is not a global phenomenon; paradoxically, the populations that need it the most are the ones with poor access to HAART.

Whom to Test for HIV Infection

HIV testing should be offered to all persons reporting any of the known risk factors for HIV acquisition and those requesting a HIV test on their own, irrespective of their risk behavior. Patients presenting with OIs and noninfectious illnesses possibly related to HIV, such as lymphoma, cervical cancer, and anal cancer, should also be tested for HIV infection. Subtle clinical clues of immunocompromise, such as oral thrush, herpes zoster in a young person, or failure to thrive in children, should alert the physician to the possibility of HIV infection. In developing nations, it is not uncommon for a young child to be the index case of a HIV-infected family. All women who are receiving antenatal care and, in underdeveloped nations, antenatal cases coming into contact with the health care system for the first time while in labor should be screened for HIV infection. In addition, patients seen in certain high-risk settings in which the prevalence of HIV infection is known to be high, such as sexually transmitted disease clinics, tuberculosis clinics, detoxification clinics, and correctional facilities, should also be offered HIV testing. HIV infection should be systematically excluded by testing while evaluating patients presenting with fever of unknown origin, autoimmune disorders such as Sjögren's syndrome, systemic lupus erythematosus, Reiter's syndrome, and polymyositis, and neurologic illnesses such as young-onset dementia and unexplained peripheral neuropathy. To say there are no contraindications for offering HIV testing to a patient is no overstatement.

It is estimated that every fourth HIV-infected person in the United States is not aware of his or her serostatus. This not only jeopardizes their own care but also places others at risk of potential transmission, which could be prevented if they are detected early. In recent times, the current trend of "HIV exceptionalism" has come under considerable criticism. This calls for a public health approach, based on standard principles of epidemic control, which encompasses a nonselective HIV testing strategy instead of the targeted-testing practices in vogue. Recent evidence suggests that nonselective HIV testing, in health care settings and possibly in the general population also, could be cost effective.

Diagnosis of HIV Infection

All persons who are offered HIV testing should receive appropriate pretest counseling, and their explicit consent must be obtained. Notification of the result must be confidential and has to be accompanied by post-test counseling. Post-test counseling should focus on behavior modification for persons who test negative and for persons who test positive as well.

Laboratory diagnosis of HIV infection is based on a sequential testing strategy for the detection of antibodies to HIV-specific antigens. The first test is a highly sensitive enzyme immunoassay (EIA) that contains antigens of both HIV-1 and HIV-2. If the test is negative, further testing is not warranted, unless the exposure was within the past 3 months, in which case it has to be repeated in 3 months. If the first test returns positive or indeterminate, the test is repeated in duplicate. If the repeat EIA tests are positive or indeterminate, the HIV-1 Western blot assay is needed for confirmation. A Western blot demonstrating antibodies to products of all three major genes of HIV (*gag*, *pol*, and *env*) is conclusive evidence of HIV infection (rare false-positives can occur with the conventional Centers for Disease Control and Prevention criterion that does not require reactivity to products of *pol*); a negative assay shows no bands. Patterns that fall in between are considered indeterminate and must be repeated after an interval of 1 month. Alternatively, one may proceed to a specific test such as the p24 antigen capture assay or HIV-1 RNA assay. If the HIV-1 Western blot result is discordant with that of EIA, the possibility of HIV-2 infection should be considered, and HIV-2-specific testing is warranted.

 CURRENT DIAGNOSIS

- Threshold to offer HIV testing to a patient should be low; nonselective HIV testing in health care settings could be cost effective.
- A repeatedly reactive enzyme immunoassay, rapid test, or nucleic acid-based test for HIV infection needs confirmation with a Western blot assay.
- Estimation of CD4+ count and plasma viral load should be performed to assess the need for antiretroviral therapy and the risk of opportunistic infections.

Four rapid tests—OraQuick Advance, Uni-Gold Recombigen, Reveal G2, and Multispot HIV-1/HIV-2—are approved by the U.S. Food and Drug Administration for point-of-care testing in acute care settings and for on-site testing at outreach testing sites. A positive result by any of these tests should be considered only as "preliminary positive," and further confirmatory testing is essential.

Management of the HIV-Infected Patient

Similar to any other disease, there seems to be a learning curve in the case of HIV care as well. It is well known that the outcome of patients with HIV/AIDS receiving treatment, at least to a certain extent, depends on the expertise of the care provider. However, this does not mean that all HIV-infected patients should be treated only by a specialist, which is not a feasible proposition. The sheer magnitude of the problem calls for greater participation on the part of the primary care physician. The U.S. Department of Health and Human Services panel recommends care by a physician with at least 20, preferably 50, HIV-infected patients. It is essential for a primary care physician to be familiar with the initial care of patients with HIV/AIDS. Primary care physicians who have not cared for a considerable number of patients with HIV/AIDS should liaise with a specialist in the field. Referral to a specialist is warranted in cases of treatment-failure and for the management of complications. Care of HIV-infected patients is multifaceted, and it needs a multidisciplinary approach. Such a comprehensive care is delivered better by the primary care physician.

INITIAL EVALUATION

Evaluation of the HIV-infected patient is carried out in several stages: assessment of the stage of disease and the need for antiretroviral therapy; symptom-oriented evaluation for opportunistic conditions; screening to assess the risk of opportunistic infections (OIs) in the future; screening for diseases that are co-transmitted, such as sexually transmitted infections and viral hepatitis; and prevention of further transmission of HIV infection.

History should be elicited with reference to the route and time of HIV acquisition. Time of exposure and earlier negative HIV tests are useful to assess reasonably the latter but may not be available in every case. More often than not, patients have multiple risk factors, and some patients may not report any of the known risk factors. A nonjudgmental approach is important while taking a sexual history. In addition, questions should focus on symptoms of other sexually transmitted infections such as urethral/vaginal discharge, genital ulcers, dysuria, dyspareunia in females, and perianal/oral ulcers and sore throat in those who report anal/oral sex. It is also important to elicit how the patient is coping with the diagnosis of HIV infection and the social and family support available to the patient. All patients have to be screened for depression and the presence of suicidal ideations, and they should be encouraged to inform their spouse/sexual partner of their HIV status. The physician has to be aware of the legal obligations regarding partner notification because they vary from place to place.

History should focus also on symptoms such as unexplained weight loss, prolonged fever, chronic diarrhea, recurrent oral ulcers, dysphagia, shortness of breath, cognitive decline, and new-onset seizures pointing toward the presence of opportunistic conditions that need further diagnostic evaluation. In treatment-experienced patients, details of previous antiretroviral treatment and the response to it should be meticulously looked into and properly recorded. This can be invaluable while changing the therapy in cases of treatment failure. Medication history should include details of allergic reaction to drugs such as cotrimoxazole (Bactrim), nevirapine (Viramune), and abacavir (Ziagen), and details of other drug-related adverse effects, such as pancreatitis, peripheral neuropathy, and hepatitis too. Details of past illnesses like tuberculosis and viral hepatitis, contact with cases of tuberculosis, and travel to areas endemic for certain infections such as histoplasmosis (Ohio and Mississippi river valleys), coccidioidomycosis (southwestern United States, northern Mexico), penicilliosis (Southeast Asia), and leishmaniasis (tropics, subtropics, and southern Europe) should be elicited.

A complete physical examination has to be performed at the time of initial evaluation and at subsequent visits. Attention should be paid to the presence of lymphadenopathy, hepatomegaly/splenomegaly, serosal effusions, and features of wasting or lipodystrophy. Examination of the nervous system should focus on possible peripheral neuropathy, proximal myopathy, focal neurologic signs, meningism, and cognitive impairment. If the latter is suspected, further neuropsychological testing is required. In patients presenting with OIs, skin lesions often hold the clue. Funduscopic examination should be done, and in patients with CD4+ less than 50 cells/μL, detailed examination by an ophthalmologist is needed to screen for cytomegalovirus (CMV) retinitis and other ocular manifestations of HIV. One should look for thrush, hairy leukoplakia, mucosal lesions of Kaposi's sarcoma, and aphthous ulcerations while examining the oral cavity. Diligent examination of the anogenital area for urethral discharge, genital/perianal ulcerations, condylomata, and adnexal tenderness in females is needed. Table 3 describes the laboratory evaluation of HIV-infected patients.

ANTIRETROVIRAL THERAPY

Antiretroviral drugs fall into four classes: nucleoside/nucleotide reverse transcriptase inhibitors (NRTIs), non-nucleoside reverse transcriptase inhibitors (NNRTIs), protease inhibitors (PIs), and fusion inhibitors (Table 4). HAART is a combination of at least three potent antiretroviral drugs, typically a combination of two NRTIs as the backbone, along with either a PI or an NNRTI. Antiretroviral drugs act by inhibiting the enzyme reverse transcriptase either competitively (NRTIs) or noncompetitively (NNRTIs) or by inhibiting the viral protease that is essential for virion assembly (PIs), or by causing functional inhibition of gp41 that is important for entry into the host cell (fusion inhibitors). NNRTIs are specific for the HIV-1 reverse transcriptase and have no activity against HIV-2. HIV-2 carries, constitutively, many of the mutations associated with PI resistance that might limit the activity of PIs against HIV-2.

The goal of treatment is to achieve maximal and sustained suppression of plasma viremia to undetectable levels

CURRENT THERAPY

- History of any AIDS-defining illness, CD4+ count <200 cells/µL, and symptomatic HIV disease warrant initiation of highly active antiretroviral therapy (HAART).
- HAART should be offered also to patients with CD4+ counts 200–350 cells/µL, irrespective of viral load and symptoms.
- HAART can be deferred if CD4+ count is >350 cells/µL with plasma viral load below 100,000 copies/mL.
- Once initiated, HAART has to be continued lifelong without interruption.
- Adherence is a very important determinant of virologic outcome.
- Regular monitoring of viral load should be done to diagnose treatment failure early.
- At least two fully active drugs, based on treatment history and resistance testing, should be included in the salvage regimen.

(less than 50 to 80 copies/mL for currently available tests). In this regard, HAART is far superior to dual and monotherapies and is the standard of care. Table 5 presents the regimens recommended currently for use in treatment-naïve HIV-1-infected patients. Selection among these regimens is made individually, taking into consideration factors such as pill burden, co-morbidities, potential drug interactions, and pregnancy. Triple NRTI regimens are inferior to PI- and NNRTI-based regimens in achieving durable viral suppression, and hence triple NRTI regimens are to be used only when PI/NNRTI-based regimens cannot be given. NNRTI-based regimens containing nevirapine (Viramune) should be avoided in females with CD4+ more than 250 cells/µL and in males with CD4+ more than 400 cells/µL because of the high risk of serious hepatotoxicity. Efavirenz (Sustiva) is the preferred NNRTI in such situations. Efavirenz-based regimens are equivalent to PI-based regimens in terms of efficacy and durability and have the advantage of low pill burden and limited long-term toxicity. Once initiated, for reasons mentioned earlier, HAART has to be continued lifelong. Structured treatment interruptions, aimed at preventing drug resistance, place the patient unduly at risk of disease progression and death during the period of interruption and are not recommended. Similarly, the strategy of withholding HAART once CD4+ counts improve following treatment (CD4+-guided therapy) is also inferior to uninterrupted treatment.

WHEN TO INITIATE HAART?

The decision to start HAART is a fine balance between the potential benefits of delaying the treatment and the risk of progression to AIDS and death. The patient has to be fully apprised of the benefits as well as the risks involved, and he or she has to play an active role in decision making. Initiation of HAART is warranted in patients with history of any of the AIDS-defining illnesses (irrespective of CD4+ count and viral load) and in those with

advanced immunosuppression (CD4+ less than 200 cells/µL, irrespective of viral load and symptoms). Conversely, initiation of HAART can be delayed safely in patients with CD4+ counts more than 350 cells/µL and plasma viral load less than 100,000 copies/mL. Data from randomized, controlled trials are lacking regarding the optimal time of initiating HAART in patients with CD4+ counts of 200 to 350 cells/µL. Observational data suggest that it is desirable to initiate HAART in these patients before their CD4+ counts drop below 200 cells/µL. Current consensus is that these patients should be offered treatment, especially if the viral load is more than 50,000 to 100,000 copies/mL or the decline in CD4+ count is rapid (more than 100 cells/µL per year). Treatment of patients having CD4+ more than 350 cells/µL with high viral loads (more than 100,000 copies/mL) is considered optional, and if treatment is deferred, CD4+ count and viral load should be monitored closely (every 3 months). Likewise, in the absence of supporting evidence, treatment of patients with acute HIV infection and those in whom seroconversion occurred within the past 6 months is considered optional.

MONITORING RESPONSE TO ANTIRETROVIRAL THERAPY

In a patient on treatment, CD4+ counts have to be monitored every 3 to 6 months and the viral load every 3 to 4 months. A reproducible change in absolute CD4+ count of at least 30% and/or 3 percentage point change in the CD4+ percentage are considered significant. Similarly, for viral load, a threefold or 0.5 $\log_{10}$ copies/mL change is deemed significant. It is important that these estimations are not performed during an episode of intercurrent infection or vaccination because transient fluctuations in viremia and CD4+ counts can occur during such episodes. Because of large variations in absolute CD4+ count estimations and interassay differences in estimating viral load, serial evaluations should be obtained from the same laboratory using the same assay. Before making any treatment change based on the laboratory results, they should be repeated and reconfirmed.

Following the initiation of effective antiretroviral therapy, CD4+ counts rapidly improve within a few weeks, largely as a result of redistribution of cells, and they subsequently improve at the rate of approximately 100 cells/µL per year over the subsequent years until a plateau is reached. Plasma viral load rapidly falls in the initial weeks and becomes undetectable in approximately 4 to 6 months. The rate of initial decline in viral load depends on the potency of the HAART regimen, and it predicts the durability of viral suppression. Determination of viral load at 2 to 8 weeks after the initiation or change in treatment thus is also recommended. An adequate response is defined as a decrease of at least 1.0 $\log_{10}$ copies/mL at 2 to 8 weeks after starting treatment; plasma viral load should become undetectable by 16 to 24 weeks.

DRUG RESISTANCE AND RESISTANCE TESTING

A patient may be infected with a drug-resistant virus to begin with (primary resistance) or else resistance can emerge as a result of treatment (secondary). The latter is more common. With widespread use of antiretrovirals,

TABLE 3 Initial and Subsequent Laboratory Evaluation of the HIV-Infected Patient

Baseline Testing	Follow-up Testing[a]
CD4+ count[b]	Once in 3–6 mo
Plasma HIV RNA load[c]	Once in 3–4 mo if not on treatment; at 2–8 wk after initiating/ changing treatment, then q3–4mo
Viral resistance testing[d]	Recommended in virologic failure
Complete blood count	q3mo, especially in patients taking zidovudine (Retrovir)
Blood urea, creatinine, electrolytes	q3–6mo, especially in patients taking indinavir (Crixivan) or other nephrotoxic drugs
Transaminases, alkaline phosphatase, bilirubin, albumin	q2wk in first month, monthly for next 3 mo, then once in 3 mo
Fasting blood glucose	If on PIs, at 1–3 mo after initiation, then q3–6mo
Fasting serum lipids	If on PIs, at 3–6 mo, then annually
Urinalysis—proteinuria, sediments	q3–6mo, especially in patients taking indinavir (Crixivan)
Chest radiograph	As clinically indicated
Electrocardiogram	As clinically indicated
Serologic Screening	
Antitoxoplasma IgG[e]	If seronegative, when CD4+ <100/μL and unable to take cotrimoxazole (Bactrim)
Syphilis serology (VDRL or RPR)	Annually, if sexually active[f]
Anticytomegalovirus IgG[g]	As clinically indicated
HBsAg, HBsAb, HCV-Ab, HAV-Ab[h]	As clinically indicated
Antivaricella IgG[i]	Not indicated
Tuberculin skin test[j]	Not indicated
Urine-based (first-void) NAAT for *Chlamydia* species, *Neisseria gonorrhoeae*[k]	Annually, if sexually active[f]
In Women	
Cervical Papanicolaou smear	Annually, if sexually active[f]
Vaginal secretions for *Trichomonas* species	Annually, if sexually active[f]
Cervical specimen for NAAT for *Chlamydia* species (if sexually active)	Annually, if sexually active[f]

[a]May be repeated more frequently if clinically indicated.
[b]Preferably 2 baseline values measured 1–4 wk apart; if discordant, repeat third time.
[c]Preferably 2 baseline values measured 1–4 wk apart.
[d]Optional in acute HIV infection and before starting treatment in chronic HIV infection.
[e]Seronegative patients should be counseled regarding proper preparation of meat and appropriate handling of cat feces.
[f]q3–6mo in asymptomatic persons at higher risk.
[g]Seronegative patients should be transfused CMV-negative or leukocyte-depleted blood products only.
[h]Vaccination recommended for hepatitis B and hepatitis A, if found susceptible; testing for antibody to hepatitis B core antigen is optional.
[i]May be tested if no history of chickenpox or shingles; if seronegative, postexposure prophylaxis with varicella zoster immune globulin is indicated.
[j]Unless a history of tuberculosis or positive test earlier.
[k]In men and women reporting receptive anal sex, culture rectal sample for *Chlamydia* species, and *N. gonorrhoeae*, and in those reporting receptive oral sex, culture pharyngeal sample for *N. gonorrhoeae*.
Abbreviations: HAV-Ab = hepatitis A antibody; HBsAb = hepatitis B surface antibody; HBsAg = hepatitis B surface antigen; HCV-Ab = hepatitis C antibody; NAAT = nucleic acid amplification test; PI = protease inhibitor; RPR = rapid plasma reagin test; VDRL = venereal diseases research laboratory test.

primary resistance is increasing. Most NNRTI-associated resistance mutations confer cross-resistance to all other NNRTIs as well. Among NRTIs, cross-resistance is common but varies by drug. Paradoxically, lamivudine(Epivir) resistance related to the M184V mutation enhances the susceptibility to zidovudine (Retrovir). With PIs, initial mutations might confer limited resistance only; however, accumulation of sequential mutations leads to broad cross-resistance. Tipranavir (Aptivus)/ritonavir (Norvir) is active against such strains of HIV-1 resistant to multiple PIs.

Drug-resistance testing is done by either genotypic or phenotypic assays. Overall, the resistance tests have a limited sensitivity. Resistance may not be detected if viremia is less than 1000 copies/mL or the frequency of resistant quasispecies is less than 10% to 20%. These tests are to be performed while the patient is still taking the failing regimen or within 4 weeks after discontinuation to avoid overgrowth of the resistant quasispecies by the wild strain.

The exact role of resistance testing in clinical practice is not yet clear. In patients receiving tailored regimens based on resistance testing, benefit in terms of improved virologic outcome is modest only. However, testing for drug resistance is indicated in patients failing treatment, those having suboptimal virologic response, and in those treated for acute HIV infection. Routine resistance testing in drug-naïve patients with chronic HIV infection may also be considered, especially if the prevalence of primary resistance is more than 4%. Failure to identify any resistance in a patient failing treatment points toward poor adherence.

TREATMENT FAILURE

Failure of treatment can be classified into virologic failure, immunologic failure, and clinical progression. Virologic failure is evidenced by repeated detection of viremia more than 400 copies/mL after 24 weeks or more than

TABLE 4 Currently Approved Antiretroviral Drugs

Drug	Dosage	Food/Fasting Requirement
Nucleoside/Nucleotide Reverse Transcriptase Inhibitors (NRTIs)		
Abacavir (Ziagen)	300 mg bid or 600 mg qd	No effect of meals
Didanosine (Videx)	400 mg qd or 200 mg bid (≥60 kg); 250 mg qd or 125 mg bid (<60 kg)	½ hr before or 2 hr after meals
Emtricitabine (Emtriva)	200 mg qd	No effect of meals
Lamivudine (Epivir)	150 mg bid or 300 mg qd	No effect of meals
Stavudine (Zerit)	40 mg bid (≥60 kg); 30 mg bid (<60 kg)	No effect of meals
Tenofovir (Viread)	300 mg qd	No effect of meals
Zalcitabine (Hivid)	0.75 mg tid	No effect of meals
Zidovudine (Retrovir)	300 mg bid or 200 mg tid	No effect of meals
Non-Nucleoside Reverse Transcriptase Inhibitors (NNRTIs)		
Delavirdine (Rescriptor)	400 mg tid	No effect of meals
Efavirenz (Sustiva)	600 mg qd	At or before bedtime; empty stomach
Nevirapine (Viramune)	200 mg qd for 14 d; then 200 mg bid	No effect of meals
Protease Inhibitors (PIs)		
Amprenavir (Agenerase)	1400 mg bid	No effect of meals; avoid high-fat meals[a]
Atazanavir (Reyataz)	400 mg qd	With meal[b]
Fosamprenavir (Lexiva)	1400 mg bid; 1400/rtv 200 mg qd[c]	No effect of meals
Indinavir (Crixivan)/rtv	800/100–200 mg q12h[d]	No effect of meals; if given unboosted, 1 hr before or 2 hr after meals
Lopinavir/rtv (Kaletra)	400/100 mg bid or 800/200 mg qd[e]	With meals
Nelfinavir (Viracept)	1250 mg bid or 750 mg tid[f]	With meal or snack
Ritonavir (Norvir)	100–400 mg/d[g]	With meals
Saquinavir hard gel (Invirase)/rtv	1000/100 mg bid	Within 2 hr of meals
Saquinavir soft gel (Fortovase)/rtv	1000/100 mg bid	With or up to 2 hr after meals
Tipranavir (Aptivus)/rtv	500/200 mg bid	With meals
Fusion Inhibitor		
Enfuvirtide (Fuzeon)	90 mg SC bid	Injectable only

Note: Fixed-dose combinations of various NRTIs with or without an NNRTI are also commercially available.
[a]Ritonavir, if given for boosting, should not be administered simultaneously.
[b]Not to be taken with antacids.
[c]Should be given only as 2 equally divided doses in PI-experienced patients.
[d]800 mg q8h if given unboosted.
[e]533/133 mg bid in patients taking nevirapine or efavirenz.
[f]In pregnant patients, 750 mg tid should not be used.
[g]Doses given for pharmacokinetic boosting.
Abbreviations: rtv = ritonavir-boosted; SC = subcutaneous.

50 copies/mL after 48 weeks of treatment in a drug-naïve patient or by persistent viremia after achieving complete suppression (virologic rebound). Inadequate CD4+ response (improvement of fewer than 25 to 50 cells/μL in the first year) or a fall below the pretreatment CD4+ level constitutes immunologic failure. Occurrence or recurrence of HIV-related events after the third month of HAART, in the absence of an alternative explanation, is considered indicative of clinical progression. Usually virologic failure is the first to occur, to be followed months to years later by immunologic failure, and finally by clinical progression. Sometimes discordant responses (i.e., immunologic failure and clinical progression despite suppressed viremia) may occur. Provided that viremia is well suppressed, changing the regimen may not be warranted in such settings.

In a patient with virologic failure, although drug resistance is the proximate cause of failure, one must carefully look for factors that contributed to the emergence of drug resistance in that particular patient and try to address them.

Otherwise, the new regimen is also bound to fail. Such factors include inadequate regimen potency, high baseline viral load, poor adherence, drug intolerance, preexisting resistance, and suboptimal pharmacokinetics because of malabsorption, noncompliance with food/fasting requirements, and drug interactions. Past-treatment experience of the patient should also be evaluated to inform them about further treatment choices (Table 6). In general, the new regimen should include at least two, preferably three, fully active drugs. A fully active drug is one that is likely to be effective based on both the treatment history and susceptibility on resistance testing. Addition of a single drug may be justified if substitution is being made to manage toxicity in a patient with otherwise good response or in a patient failing treatment where no resistance is identified, after ruling out poor adherence and improperly timed resistance testing. Although the goal of treatment remains complete suppression of viremia below detectable limits, in treatment-experienced patients

TABLE 5 First-Line Antiretroviral Regimens for Treatment-Naïve HIV-1-Infected Patients

Recommendation/Regimen Class	Antiretroviral Regimen
	Preferred
NNRTI-based	Efavirenz (Sustiva)* + (lamivudine [Epivir] or emtricitabine [Emtriva]) + (zidovudine [Retrovir] or tenofovir [Viread])
	I-based (Lopinavir + rtv [Kaletra]) + (lamivudine [Epivir] or emtricitabine [Emtriva]) + zidovudine (Retrovir)
	Alternative
NNRTI-based	Efavirenz (Sustiva)* + (lamivudine [Epivir] or emtricitabine [Emtriva]) + (abacavir [Ziagen] or didanosine [Videx] or stavudine [Zerit])
	Nevirapine (Viramune)† + (lamivudine [Epivir] or emtricitabine [Emtriva]) + (zidovudine [Retrovir] or stavudine [Zerit] or didanosine [Videx] or abacavir [Ziagen] or tenofovir [Viread])
PI-based	Atazanavir (Reyataz) + (lamivudine [Epivir] or emtricitabine [Emtriva]) + (zidovudine [Retrovir] or stavudine [Zerit] or didanosine [Videx] or abacavir [Ziagen] or tenofovir [Viread] + rtv])‡
	(Fosamprenavir [Lexiva] ± rtv) + (lamivudine [Epivir] or emtricitabine [Emtriva]) + (zidovudine [Retrovir] or stavudine [Zerit] or didanosine [Videx] or abacavir [Ziagen] or tenofovir [Viread])
	(Indinavir [Crixivan] + rtv or lopinavir + rtv [Kaletra] or saquinavir [Invirase/Fortovase]+ rtv) + (lamivudine [Epivir] or emtricitabine [Emtriva]) + (zidovudine [Retrovir] or stavudine [Zerit] or didanosine [Videx] or abacavir [Ziagen] or tenofovir [Viread])
	Nelfinavir (Viracept) + (lamivudine [Epivir] or emtricitabine [Emtriva]) + (zidovudine [Retrovir] or stavudine [Zerit] or didanosine [Videx] or abacavir [Ziagen] or tenofovir [Viread])
Triple NRTI§	Abacavir (Ziagen) + zidovudine (Retrovir) + lamivudine (Epivir)

Note: Once-daily regimens can be tailored by selecting the appropriate drug among the interchangeable choices presented here.
*Contraindicated in women who are pregnant, plan to conceive, or are not using effective contraception.
†Avoid in women with CD4+ >250/μL and men with CD4+ > 400/μL (see text).
‡If combined with tenofovir (Viread), atazanavir (Reyataz) should be boosted with rtv.
§Should be used only if NNRTI-based and PI-based regimens should not or cannot be given (see text).
Abbreviations: NNRTI = non-nucleoside reverse transcriptase inhibitor; NRTI = nucleoside reverse transcriptase inhibitor; PI = protease inhibitor; rtv = low-dose ritonavir (Norvir), 100–400 mg/d for pharmacokinetic boosting; not considered as fourth drug in the regimen; ritonavir (Norvir) alone should not be used as the sole PI.
Based on Guidelines for the use of antiretroviral agents in HIV-1-infected adults and adolescents, U.S. Department of Health and Human Services, October 2005.

with resistance to multiple drugs, this may not always be feasible. In such patients with limited options, even a 0.5 to 1.0 $\log_{10}$ reduction in viral load may be acceptable. In patients failing treatment with extensive prior treatment, if no fully active drug is available, continuing with the failing regimen might decrease the risk of clinical progression.

ADHERENCE TO TREATMENT

Adherence to prescribed treatment is a complex issue but of utmost importance. Antiretroviral treatment is very exacting in terms of adherence when compared to other chronic diseases; missing as little as 5% to 10% of doses is known to affect virologic outcome adversely. The natural tendency is to miss a few doses, and physician estimates of adherence are known to be unreliable. It is thus important to suspect noncompliance in every patient. Before initiating treatment, the patient must be counseled regarding medication requirements, and readiness to take the treatment has to be ensured. It has to be impressed on the patient that the first regimen has the best chance for long-term success. Adherence counseling and assessment of adherence should be done at each clinical encounter. Adherence is conventionally assessed by patient self-reports, pill counting, and a patient-recorded medication diary. Microelectronic monitoring systems like Medication Event Monitoring System (MEMS Track Cap) and therapeutic drug monitoring could provide more objective assessment of adherence. However, all these methods have their limitations, and it is preferable to use more than one method simultaneously.

Noncompliance with treatment has many causes. Patient-related factors, such as substance abuse, depression, lack of social support, and age; medication-related factors, such as dosing frequency, pill burden, food/fasting requirements, and adverse effects; and health care system–related factors, such as attitude of staff, communication, and accessibility, all operate in tandem to influence the adherence. Adherence can be improved by simplifying the dosage schedules, providing pillboxes, tailoring to suit the lifestyle, entrusting medication intake to a family member, using reminder calls and alarms and community-based case managers, alerting to adverse effects, providing patient education materials, making the clinic appointments convenient, and making the health system encounter pleasant. In patients found nonadherent, enough time should be spent to identify the responsible factors and to find acceptable solutions while involving the patient actively in the process.

TABLE 6 Salvage Therapy in Patients with Treatment Failure (Virologic Failure)

| Initial Regimen | First Virologic Failure | | Subsequent Virologic Failures |
	Resistance Identified	No Resistance Identified	
NNRTI-based (2 NRTIs + NNRTI)	2 NRTIs (based on resistance testing) + PI (unboosted or rtv-boosted)	Check adherence to treatment; if poor, address compliance. Was the resistance testing properly timed? (see text); if not properly timed, continue same regimen; repeat genotypic testing in 2–4 wk or start a new regimen; repeat genotypic testing in 2–4 wk.	Include at least 2, preferably 3, fully active drugs (see text); add a drug from new class, if available. If 3-class virologic failure, start > 1 NRTI (based on resistance testing) + a new boosted-PI (based on resistance testing) ± enfuvirtide (Fuzeon). If only 1 fully active agent available, add to failing regimen only if CD4+ <100/µL; otherwise, continue failing regimen. If no fully active agent available, continue failing regimen; do not interrupt.
PI-based (2 NRTIs + PI [unboosted or rtv-boosted])	2 NRTIs (based on resistance testing) + NNRTI or 2 NRTIs (based on resistance testing) + a new boosted PI (based on resistance testing) or 1 or more NRTI(s) (based on resistance testing) + NNRTI + a new boosted PI (based on resistance testing)	If adherence and timing of testing are acceptable, start a new regimen; repeat genotypic testing in 2–4 wk or intensify by adding 1 NRTI (tenofovir [Viread]) or boost the PI with rtv.	
Triple NRTI (3 NRTIs)	2 NRTIs (based on resistance testing) + NNRTI or PI (unboosted or rtv-boosted) or 1 or more NRTI(s) (based on resistance testing) + NNRTI + PI (unboosted or rtv-boosted) or NNRTI + PI (unboosted or rtv-boosted)		

Based on Guidelines for the use of antiretroviral agents in HIV-1-infected adults and adolescents, U.S. Department of Health and Human Services, October 2005.

Abbreviations: NNRTI = non-nucleoside reverse transcriptase inhibitor, NRTI = nucleoside reverse transcriptase inhibitor, PI = protease inhibitor, rtv = ritonavir (Norvir).

ADVERSE DRUG REACTIONS AND DRUG INTERACTIONS

Adverse drug reactions (ADRs) are common with antiretroviral therapy and an important cause of nonadherence. They also contribute to a significant proportion of clinic visits and mortality. ADRs can be idiosyncratic, dose related, time related (delayed), or dose and time related (cumulative). A particular ADR may be common to all drugs of the same class (e.g., lactic acidosis and fatty liver because of NRTIs, lipodystrophy because of PIs), or it might be drug specific (e.g., hypersensitivity to abacavir [Ziagen], nephrolithiasis because of indinavir [Crixivan]). The patient often is on other drugs as well, with overlapping ADR profiles, apart from antiretrovirals. A symptom-based approach is useful from a practical point of view (Table 7). Although many of the ADRs can be managed conservatively, some, such as symptomatic lactic acidosis, systemic hypersensitivity reactions, Stevens-Johnson syndrome, acute pancreatitis, and severe hepatotoxicity, are potentially life threatening. Serious ADRs necessitate withdrawal of the offending drug, and rechallenge of the drug should not be attempted in these situations.

Drug interactions are often the underlying cause of ADRs. PIs are metabolized by the hepatic cytochrome P450 (CYP) enzymes. At the same time, PIs are potent inhibitors of CYP. Conversely, NNRTIs, especially efavirenz (Sustiva), are a potent inducer of CYP. When antiretrovirals are co-administered with other drugs metabolized by or affecting CYP (antihistamines, prokinetics, lipid-lowering agents, antifungals, antitubercular drugs, anticonvulsants, etc.),

TABLE 7 Approach to Adverse Drug Reactions in the HIV-Infected Patient[a]

Adverse Effect	Manifestations	Causative Drug(s)		Stepwise Action
		Antiretroviral(s)	Other Drugs	
Stevens-Johnson syndrome/toxic epidermal necrolysis[b]	Rash, mucosal ulcerations, fever, hepatic dysfunction	NNRTIs most commonly NVP; rarely APV, LPV/r, ATV, ABC, ZDV, ddI	Cotrimoxazole, sulfadiazine, dapsone, atovaquone, voriconazole	Discontinue all ARVs and any other possible drug; manage like severe burns; do not rechallenge offending drug.
Hypersensitivity reaction[c]	Fever, diffuse rash, malaise, arthralgia, respiratory and GI symptoms, circulatory collapse	ABC, enfuvirtide (Fuzeon)	Cotrimoxazole, sulfadiazine, dapsone	Discontinue all ARVs and any other possible drug; rule out other causes; do not rechallenge ABC/enfuvirtide.
Skin rash	Maculopapular rash only; no blisters, skin tenderness, mucosal ulceration, or fever	DLV > EFV > APV, fAPV = ATV > NVP > ABC, TPV[d]	Cotrimoxazole, sulfadiazine, dapsone, atovaquone, voriconazole	Antihistamines; continue offending drug; watch for progression of rash; if so, discontinue.
GI intolerance[e]	Anorexia, nausea, vomiting, epigastric pain	PIs, ddI, ZDV	Isoniazid, rifamycins, pyrazinamide	Administer with food (not for ddI, unboosted IDV); antiemetics; switch to less emetogenic ARV.
	Diarrhea	PIs, especially NFV, LPV/r, and buffered ddI formulations	Clindamycin, atovaquone	Rule out OIs; antimotility agents, calcium salts, bulk forming agents; rehydration, if needed.
Hepatotoxicity[f]	Jaundice, fever, vomiting, hepatic necrosis, encephalopathy	NVP	Isoniazid, rifamycins, pyrazinamide	Discontinue all ARVs and any other possible drug; rule out viral hepatitis; supportive management; do not rechallenge NVP.
	Symptomatic or subclinical hepatic enzyme elevations	NNRTIs, d4T, ddI, ZDV, PIs, especially TPV	Isoniazid, rifamycins, pyrazinamide, azithromycin, clarithromycin, all azole antifungals	If symptomatic, discontinue all ARVs and switch to nonhepatotoxic ARVs after normalization; if asymptomatic, monitor closely.
Lactic acidosis, fatty liver[g]	Nonspecific GI symptoms, tachypnea, tachycardia, hepatomegaly, hyperlactatemia, multiorgan failure	NRTIs especially d4T, ddI, ZDV	Metformin	Discontinue all ARVs; hydration; supportive treatment; IV thiamine/riboflavin; switch to ABC/3TC/TDF or NRTI-sparing regimens.
Pancreatitis[g]	Epigastric pain-postprandial, vomiting, fever, elevated amylase, lipase	ddI, d4T, ddC, RTV; 3TC (in children)	Alcohol, cotrimoxazole, pentamidine	Discontinue offending drugs; manage like acute pancreatitis related to any other cause; do not rechallenge.
Peripheral neuropathy[g]	Numbness, paresthesia—often painful; recovery possibly incomplete	ddI, d4T, ddC	Isoniazid	Switch to ABC/3TC/TDF; gabapentin, tricyclic antidepressants, narcotic analgesics.
Myopathy[g]	Myalgia, muscle tenderness, proximal weakness, elevated creatine kinase	ZDV	Statins, fibrates, steroids	Switch to another NRTI; improves in 3–4 wk after discontinuation; coenzyme-Q, L-carnitine (unproven).

Continued

TABLE 7 Approach to Adverse Drug Reactions in the HIV-Infected Patient[a]—cont'd

Adverse Effect	Manifestations	Causative Drug(s)		Stepwise Action
		Antiretroviral(s)	Other Drugs	
Nephrolithiasis, crystalluria[h]	Flank pain, nondescript abdominal pain, dysuria, hematuria, renal dysfunction	IDV	Cotrimoxazole, sulfadiazine, acyclovir	Discontinue IDV; hydration and analgesics; IDV can be resumed with plenty of oral fluids; if recurs, consider switching.
Nephrotoxicity	Renal dysfunction; nephrogenic diabetes insipidus; Fanconi syndrome	IDV, TDF	Acyclovir, amphotericin B, cotrimoxazole, pentamidine	Discontinue offending drug; hydration; generally reversible.
Hematologic	Anemia, neutropenia[i]	ZDV	Cotrimoxazole, dapsone, sulfadiazine, pyrimethamine, flucytosine, trimetrexate, amphotericin B, ganciclovir, valganciclovir, rifabutin	Discontinue concomitant marrow suppressant, if any; exclude marrow involvement by OIs/malignancy; erythropoietin or filgrastim; switch to another NRTI.
	Bleeding tendency in hemophiliacs	PIs		Factor VIII infusion; consider NNRTI-based regimens.
	Eosinophilia	Enfuvirtide (Fuzeon)	Cotrimoxazole, dapsone, sulfadiazine	Exclude disseminated strongyloidiasis, malignancy; watch for hypersensitivity.
CNS symptoms[j]	Drowsiness, insomnia, vivid dreams, nightmares, hallucination, worsening of psychiatric disorders, suicidal ideation	EFV	Isoniazid, dapsone, steroids	Usually resolve in 2–4 wk; consider discontinuation, if persistent or exacerbates psychiatric illness.
Lipodystrophy	Loss of subcutaneous fat, buffalo hump, double chin, dyslipidemia, insulin resistance, diabetes mellitus	PIs (except ATV); NRTIs, especially d4T	Steroids	Assess cardiac risk factors; lifestyle modification; metformin, glitazones, statins, fibrates[k]; consider early switching to ATV- or NNRTI-based regimens.

[a]Only common and serious side effects are dealt with; side effects such as osteoporosis, avascular osteonecrosis (PIs), unconjugated hyperbilirubinemia, retinoid-like effects (IDV) and cranial malformations (EFV) are also known to occur.

[b]Approximately 0.3%-1% with NVP; a low dose, lead-in period for NVP (see Table 4) may decrease the risk; less common (0.1%) with DLV and EFV; occurs in the initial weeks after initiation; safety of replacing NVP with another NNRTI is unknown.

[c]Approximately 5% with ABC; once daily dosing possibly increases the risk; If ABC-related, symptoms resolve within 48 hrs after discontinuation of ABC.

[d]APV, fAPV, and TPV are sulfonamide derivatives; potential cross-hypersensitivity with sulfonamides.

[e]Symptoms begin with first doses; might abate with time.

[f]Low-dose, lead-in period for NVP might reduce the risk; monitoring: see Table 3; onset within the first few weeks with NNRTIs, after weeks to months with PIs, and after months to years with NRTIs; discontinuation of 3TC, FTC, or TDF in HBV co-infected patients might cause acute flare-up of hepatitis; safety of replacing NVP with another NNRTI is unknown.

[g]Class-specific adverse effect of NRTIs, because of mitochondrial toxicity; do not combine ddI/d4T/ddC; ABC, 3TC, and TDF are less prone; all 4 syndromes can occur in variable combinations; symptomatic lactic acidosis is rare but is associated with high mortality.

[h]Approximately 10% of patients taking IDV experience at least 1 episode of colic; monitoring: see Table 3; recurrence is seen in only 50%, if fluid intake is improved (at least 1.5–2 L of noncaffeinated fluid; water preferably).

[i]Almost all ZDV-treated patients have isolated macrocytosis; anemia and neutropenia occur in approximately 1%-4% and 2%-8% respectively; monitoring: see Table 3.

[j]Occurs during initial weeks of treatment; patients are to be warned to restrict risky activities.

[k]Only atorvastatin (Lipitor) and pravastatin (Pravachol) among statins, and gemfibrozil (Lopid) and fenofibrate (Triglide) among fibrates, can be co-administered with PIs.

Abbreviations: 3TC = lamivudine (Epivir); ABC = abacavir (Ziagen); APV = amprenavir (Agenerase); ATV = atazanavir (Reyataz); CNS = central nervous system; d4T = stavudine (Zerit); ddC = zalcitabine (Hivid); ddI = didanosine (Videx); DLV = delavirdine (Rescriptor); EFV = efavirenz (Sustiva); fAPV = fosamprenavir (Lexiva); FTC = emtricitabine (Emtriva); GI = gastrointestinal; IDV = indinavir (Crixivan); LPV/r = lopinavir/ritonavir (Kaletra); NFV = nelfinavir (Viracept); NNRTI = non-nucleoside reverse transcriptase inhibitor; NRTI = nucleoside reverse transcriptase inhibitor; NVP = nevirapine (Viramune), OI = opportunistic infection; PI = protease inhibitor; RTV = ritonavir (Norvir); TDF = tenofovir (Viread); TPV = tipranavir (Aptivus); ZDV = zidovudine (Retrovir).

Based on Guidelines for the use of antiretroviral agents in HIV-1-infected adults and adolescents, U.S. Department of Health and Human Services, October 2005.

complex pharmacokinetic interactions occur; this can lead to potentially toxic or subtherapeutic drug levels. In a patient on HAART, unnecessary prescriptions are to be avoided, and it is prudent always to check the compatibility and the dose modifications needed before prescribing.

Management of Opportunistic Conditions

GENERAL CONSIDERATIONS

OIs are the most common cause of disability and death in HIV-infected patients who are not receiving treatment. Hence, it is important that OIs are promptly recognized and treated. Different pathogens may cause similar disease patterns, and multiple OIs may occur concurrently. Although it is important to make a definitive diagnosis in these patients, diagnostic workup should not delay unduly the initiation of appropriate treatment. Empirical treatment based on clinical suspicion may be justified in acutely ill patients. In a patient with a severe OI as the initial manifestation of HIV disease, management of the OI takes precedence over immediate initiation of HAART. This avoids potential drug interactions and possibly decreases the occurrence of immune reconstitution inflammatory syndrome (IRIS). However, in patients with OIs for which no effective treatment is available (cryptosporidiosis, microsporidiosis, progressive multifocal leukoencephalopathy, and Kaposi's sarcoma), HAART itself can result in improvement and hence should be initiated as soon as possible.

IRIS manifests as the occurrence of a new OI or worsening of a preexisting OI following initiation of HAART, usually in the first 3 months. Symptoms include fever, lymphadenopathy, serosal effusions, worsening or fresh pulmonary infiltrates, vitreitis, uveitis, and intracranial lesions. Occasionally life-threatening complications like acute respiratory distress syndrome (ARDS) and acute renal failure develop. Most instances of IRIS respond well to nonsteroidal anti-inflammatory drugs. HAART and OI-specific treatment need to be continued without interruption. Steroids may be useful in patients with life-threatening complications.

OIs can be prevented by timely initiation of primary chemoprophylaxis (Table 8). It has to be stressed that OIs listed in the table can also occur, albeit less often, in patients with CD4+ counts above the cutoffs for initiation of prophylaxis. Following treatment for an episode of OI, lifelong secondary prophylaxis is needed to prevent relapse. However, if a sustained improvement in CD4+ count is achieved following HAART, secondary prophylaxis for most of the OIs and primary prophylaxis can be withdrawn safely. Table 9 presents the possible etiology of opportunistic conditions. Management of common potentially life-threatening OIs is presented next.

PNEUMOCYSTIS JIROVECI PNEUMONIA (PCP)

PCP is the most common OI in HIV-infected patients. Approximately 90% of cases occur among patients with CD4+ less than 200 cells/μL. Although the overall mortality is approximately 10% to 20%, it exceeds 50% in those requiring mechanical ventilation for respiratory failure. PCP manifests as a subacute febrile illness accompanied by nonproductive cough and progressive exertional dyspnea. In patients with mild disease, physical findings are often scanty, barring tachypnea and scattered so-called cellophane crackles. Hypoxemia is useful to assess the severity of disease, and moderate to severe hypoxemia (PaO_2 less than 70 mm Hg or $[A-a]DO_2$ more than 35 mm Hg while breathing ambient air) indicates severe disease. Chest radiograph demonstrates diffuse, bilateral, interstitial infiltrates in a perihilar distribution. Atypical radiographic appearances like upper lobe predominance (in patients on inhaled pentamidine [NebuPent] prophylaxis), nodular infiltrates, cysts, and pneumothorax are also seen. An apparently normal-looking radiograph in a patient with compatible clinical presentation does not rule out a diagnosis of PCP. Diagnosis is established by the demonstration of cysts and trophozoites of *Pneumocystis* in induced sputum (sensitivity, 50% to 90%), bronchoalveolar lavage (90% to 99%), and transbronchial lung biopsy (95% to 100%) specimens by Gomori methenamine silver, Giemsa, or calcofluor staining. Immunofluorescent staining has better sensitivity and specificity than the tinctorial stains. rRNA-PCR techniques are currently being evaluated and can be used on oral washings.

Cotrimoxazole (TMP-SMX, Bactrim) is the drug of choice. Mild to moderately severe cases can be managed with oral TMP-SMX (two double-strength tablets [Bactrim DS] three times daily for 21 days) on an ambulatory basis. Patients developing PCP despite TMP-SMX (Bactrim) prophylaxis can also be effectively treated with standard doses of TMP-SMX. Intravenous therapy (15–20 [TMP]/75–100 [SMX] mg/kg/day every 6 to 8 hours for 21 days) is indicated for patients with severe hypoxemia. In addition, steroids (prednisone,[1] 40 mg orally twice daily for days 1 to 5, 40 mg every day for days 6 to 10, and 20 mg every day for days 11 to 21) improve the mortality and reduce the need for mechanical ventilation in severe cases and should be started within 72 hours of starting anti-PCP treatment. Lack of clinical improvement or worsening hypoxemia after at least 4 to 8 days of anti-PCP treatment indicates failure and warrants changing of treatment. Serious ADRs related to TMP-SMX (Bactrim) also often necessitate a treatment change. The preferred alternative treatments are pentamidine (Pentam, 4 mg/kg intravenously [IV] every day) or clindamycin (Cleocin, 600 to 900 mg IV every 6 to 8 hours) plus primaquine[1] (15 to 30 mg [base] orally every day). Dapsone (100 mg orally every day) plus trimethoprim (Trimpex,[1] 15 mg/kg/day orally thrice daily), atovaquone (Mepron, 750 mg orally twice daily), or trimetrexate (Neutrexin, 1.2 mg/kg IV every day with leucovorin, 0.5 mg/kg IV every 6 hours) can be used also as alternatives in mild to moderately severe PCP. Following treatment, patients should be administered secondary prophylaxis, which has to be discontinued if the CD4+ counts improve to more than 200 cells/μL for 3 months after initiating HAART. However, in those who develop PCP while their CD4+ counts were more than 200 cells/μL, it is prudent to continue the secondary prophylaxis lifelong.

---

[1]Not FDA approved for this indication.

TABLE 8 Primary Chemoprophylaxis for Opportunistic Infections in the HIV-Infected Patient*,†

Opportunistic Pathogen	Criteria for Initiation	Preferred Regimen	Alternative Regimens	Criteria for Discontinuation‡
Pneumocystis jiroveci	CD4+ <200/μL; oropharyngeal candidiasis	TMP-SMX (Bactrim), 960 mg qd or 480 mg qd	TMP-SMX (Bactrim), 960 mg tiw, or dapsone, 100 mg qd, or aerosolized pentamidine (NebuPent), 300 mg monthly, or atovaquone (Mepron), 1500 mg qd	CD4+ >200/μL for ≥3 mo
Toxoplasma gondii	CD4+ ≤100/μL in IgG toxoplasma antibody-positive patients	TMP-SMX (Bactrim), 960 mg qd	TMP-SMX (Bactrim), 480 mg qd, or dapsone, 50 mg qd, + pyrimethamine, 50 mg qw, + leucovorin, 25 mg qw, or atovaquone (Mepron), 1500 mg qd	CD4+ > 200/μL for ≥3 mo
Mycobacterium avium-intracellulare	CD4+ <50/μL	Azithromycin (Zithromax), 1200 mg qw, or clarithromycin (Biaxin), 500 mg bid	Rifabutin (Mycobutin), 300 mg qd	CD4+ >100/μL for ≥3 mo
Mycobacterium tuberculosis§	TST ≥5 mm; positive TST in past without treatment; contact with active case, irrespective of TST	Isoniazid (Laniazid) + pyridoxine, 300 + 50 mg qd or 900 + 100 mg biw, for 9 mo	Rifampicin (Rifadin), 600 mg qd for 4 mo	Not applicable

*Apart from chemoprophylaxis, annual influenza immunization in all, pneumococcal vaccination in those with CD4+ ≥200/μL, and hepatitis A and hepatitis B vaccinations in susceptible patients are recommended.

†Primary chemoprophylaxis not recommended for cytomegalovirus, *Cryptococcus neoformans*, *Histoplasma capsulatum*, *Coccidioides immitis*, *Salmonella* species, herpes simplex, and *Candida* species

‡Primary prophylaxis to be restarted if CD4+ falls again below levels recommended for initiation.

§Not prophylaxis in strict sense. For isoniazid-susceptible *M. tuberculosis* only; if probability of exposure to isoniazid-resistant *M. tuberculosis* is high, rifampicin (Rifadin), 600 mg qd, or rifabutin (Mycobutin), 300 mg qd, for 4 mo.

Abbreviations: biw = twice weekly; TMP-SMX = cotrimoxazole (Bactrim); TST = tuberculin skin test; qw = once a week; tiw = 3 times a week.

Based on USPHS/IDSA guidelines for the prevention of opportunistic infections in persons infected with HIV, 2001.

CRYPTOCOCCOSIS

Cryptococcosis occurs mostly among patients with CD4+ less than 50 cells/μL. Although the route of infection is via the lungs, most often the disease manifests as meningitis. Disseminated infection is common in HIV-infected patients, and in fact approximately 60% of patients with AIDS-associated cryptococcal meningitis have fungemia. Pulmonary involvement occurs either as a part of disseminated disease or as primary pneumonia. Molluscoid skin lesions with central hemorrhagic crust may be seen. Patients typically present with subacute onset of fever, prominent headache, and vomiting. The classical signs of meningeal inflammation are often absent. Occasionally, cognitive decline and personality changes might be the only presenting symptoms. Cryptococcomas may present as a focal neurologic deficit.

Diagnosis is readily established by the demonstration of yeast cells by India ink staining of cerebrospinal fluid (CSF). Fungal culture and latex agglutination for cryptococcal antigen have better sensitivity than the India ink stain. The antigen can also be detected in the blood in most patients with meningitis. Untreated disease is uniformly fatal. Amphotericin B deoxycholate (Fungizone, 0.7 mg/kg IV every day for 2 weeks) is the preferred treatment. Infusion-related ADRs such as chills, rigors, and fever are common and can be reduced by premedicating with acetaminophen (Tylenol). Liposomal preparations of amphotericin B (AmBisome, 4 mg/kg/day) can be used also to reduce nephrotoxicity. Addition of flucytosine (Ancobon, 25 mg/kg orally four times a day for 2 weeks) sterilizes the CSF faster and reduces the rate of relapse but not mortality. Amphotericin B is to be followed by fluconazole (Diflucan, 400 mg orally every day) for at least 8 weeks or until the CSF cultures become sterile and then lifelong (200 mg every day) for secondary prophylaxis. In patients with immune recovery following HAART, secondary prophylaxis can be discontinued if the CD4+ count is more than 100 to 200 cells/μL for 6 months. Raised intracranial pressure is very common and associated with early deaths. If symptomatic, daily lumbar punctures to reduce the pressure are needed, and in refractory cases, CSF shunting should be performed.

TABLE 9 Etiology of Opportunistic Conditions in the HIV-Infected Patient

System Affected	Etiology (infectious as well as noninfectious)		
	Very common	*Somewhat common*	*Rare*

Pulmonary	PCP
	Streptococcus
	   pneumoniae
	Haemophilus
	   influenzae
	Myobacterium
	   tuberculosis[a]
		Pseudomonas aeruginosa
		Staphylococcus aureus
		Enteric GNB
		Histoplasma species
		Cryptococcus species
		Cytomegalovirus
		Kaposi's sarcoma
		Aspergillus species
		Pulmonary lymphoma
		Heart failure
			Nocardia species
			Legionella species
			Myobacterium avium complex
			Toxoplasma gondii
			Cryptosporidium
			Rhodococcus equi
			Strongyloides
			Primary pulmonary hypertension
			DILS

Central nervous system (CNS)	*Cryptococcus* species *Toxoplasmosis* ADRs Psychiatric illness HIV dementia PMLE CNS lymphoma	*M. tuberculosis*[a] Cytomegalovirus Bacterial brain abscess	*Nocardia* species *Histoplasma* species *Coccidioides immitis* *Aspergillus* species *Listeria monocytogenes* Varicella-zoster virus Herpes simplex virus *Treponema pallidum* *Acanthamoeba* species *Trypanosoma cruzi* DILS
Gastrointestinal (GI)	Cytomegalovirus *Clostridium difficile* *Salmonella* species *M. avium* complex *Giardia lamblia* ADRs	*Shigella* species *Campylobacter* species *Microsporum* *Cryptosporidium Isospora* *Cyclospora* *Cryptococcus* species *Histoplasma* species	Amebiasis *Strongyloides* GI lymphoma Kaposi's sarcoma Enteroaggregative *Escherichia coli* DILS
Undifferentiated fever	*M. avium* complex *M. tuberculosis** Cytomegalovirus ADRs Sinusitis Catheter-related Early PCP Acute HIV syndrome	Endocarditis Lymphoma	Extrapulmonary *Pneumocystis* *Bartonella henselae* *Coccidioides immitis* *Mycobacterium kansasii* *Penicillium marneffei* *Leishmania* species *Toxoplasma gondii*

*Incidence of tuberculosis varies greatly depending on the local prevalence.
Abbreviations: ADR = adverse drug reaction; DILS = diffuse infiltrative lymphocytosis syndrome; GNB = gram-negative bacilli; PCP = *Pneumocystis jiroveci* pneumonia; PMLE = progressive multifocal leukoencephalopathy.
Adapted from Sax PE: Opportunistic infections in HIV disease: Down but not out. Infect Dis Clin North Am 2001;15:433-455.

DISSEMINATED *MYCOBACTERIUM AVIUM* INFECTION

Like cryptococcosis and CMV disease, disseminated atypical mycobacterial infections occur more commonly in patients with CD4+ less than 50 cells/µL. Most infections are caused by *Mycobacterium avium-intracellulare*. Infections by *Mycobacterium kansasii* and *Mycobacterium haemophilum* are also known to occur. Symptoms are nonspecific and include fever, weight loss, diarrhea, and abdominal pain. Peripheral and axial lymphadenopathy, hepatosplenomegaly, anemia, elevated alkaline phosphatase, and bone marrow infiltration are common features. Localized manifestations occur commonly as a manifestation of IRIS. Pulmonary lesions in the form of miliary nodules and air-space infiltrates may be seen. Diagnosis is established by demonstrating mycobacteremia or by isolating the organism from involved tissue specimens.

Treatment should include at least two effective drugs, usually clarithromycin (Biaxin, 500 mg orally twice daily) and ethambutol (Myambutol,[1] 15 mg/kg orally every day). Addition of a third drug should be considered, especially when CD4+ is less than 50 cells/µL, effective HAART is unavailable, or the mycobacterial load is high (more than 2.0 $\log_{10}$ colony-forming units/mL of blood). Rifabutin (Mycobutin,[1] 300 mg orally every day) is the preferred third drug. Fluoroquinolones and amikacin (Amikin)[1] can be used as alternative agents. Generally, if possible, HAART should be initiated within 1 to 2 weeks after initiating antimycobacterial therapy. Lack of clinical improvement accompanied by persisting mycobacteremia after 4 to 8 weeks of treatment indicates failure, and further selection of drugs should be guided by susceptibility testing. Treatment has to be continued lifelong for secondary prophylaxis. However, if the CD4+ count improves to more than 100 cells/μL for 6 months, it can be discontinued, provided the patient is asymptomatic and treatment has been given for at least 12 months.

CYTOMEGALOVIRUS DISEASE

Retinitis is the most common manifestation of CMV disease. It presents as progressive painless loss of vision, and patients often experience floaters. Funduscopy reveals focal necrotizing retinitis, characterized by perivascular fluffy infiltrates with hemorrhages. Lesions spread centrifugally from the periphery, and those adjacent to the macula are sight threatening. Visual loss, if it occurs, is irreversible. Other manifestations include colitis, esophagitis, meningoencephalitis, and pneumonitis. Colitis causes persistent diarrhea and may result in extensive hemorrhage, perforation, and bacterial sepsis. CNS disease presents as dementia, ventriculoencephalitis, or ascending polyradiculomyelopathy. Viremia in the absence of end-organ disease may be seen but does not warrant immediate therapy.

Sight-threatening retinitis is treated with an intraocular ganciclovir implant (Vitrasert) along with valganciclovir (Valcyte, 900 mg orally every day) lifelong. For peripheral lesions, valganciclovir (Valcyte), 900 mg orally twice daily for 2 to 3 weeks is to be followed by 900 mg every day for life. Ganciclovir (Cytovene, 5 mg/kg IV every 12 hours), foscarnet (Foscavir, 60 mg/kg IV every 8 hours), or cidofovir (Vistide, 5 mg/kg IV every day) for 2 to 3 weeks can be used as alternatives. Colitis and esophagitis are treated with ganciclovir (Cytovene) or foscarnet (Foscavir) for at least 3 to 4 weeks or until symptoms resolve. A combination of ganciclovir (Cytovene) and foscarnet (Foscavir) until symptoms resolve is required for the treatment of neurologic disease. Secondary prophylaxis can be discontinued if CD4+ is more than 100 to 150 cells/μL for 6 months. However, regular ophthalmologic monitoring should be done to detect relapse early. IRIS occurs in most of the patients with CMV retinitis following initiation of HAART, resulting in vitreitis or uveitis. Periocular steroids or short courses of oral steroids often control the symptoms.

TUBERCULOSIS IN HIV-INFECTED PATIENTS

Tuberculosis is the most common OI in HIV-infected patients from developing countries. In contrast to other OIs, tuberculosis can occur at any level of CD4+ count. Extrapulmonary and disseminated forms become more common as the immunosuppression worsens. Meningeal and miliary dissemination often occurs. In advanced immunosuppression, typical cavitary and sputum-smear-positive pulmonary disease are seldom seen. Diagnostic and therapeutic approaches to tuberculosis remain the same as in a HIV-negative patient, except that once-weekly rifapentine (Priftin) and if CD4+ counts are less than 100 cells/μL, twice-weekly rifabutin (Mycobutin)[1] should not be used. Standard four-drug short-course regimens (see chapter on tuberculosis) are equally effective in HIV-infected patients with drug-susceptible tuberculosis. All patients should receive directly observed treatment, and thrice-weekly

---

[1]Not FDA approved for this indication.

intermittent regimens can be used. Extensive interactions occur between rifamycins, PIs, and NNRTIs. If the patient is already on HAART, rifabutin (Mycobutin) is the preferred rifamycin, and HAART has to be continued with appropriate changes (Table 10). If the patient is not on HAART, it is better started after the completion of the intensive phase in those with CD4+ more than 200 cells/μL. In those with CD4+ less than 200 cells/μL, it is preferable to initiate HAART early, after approximately 2 weeks of intensive-phase treatment.

Management of the Pregnant HIV-Infected Woman

Apart from the usual indications for initiating HAART, in a pregnant HIV-infected woman, an additional aim is to prevent perinatal transmission. This is most effectively achieved by suppressing viremia to undetectable levels with HAART. From this perspective, all pregnant HIV-infected women should be initiated on HAART, irrespective of the viral load, CD4+ count, and symptoms. Efavirenz (Sustiva), a combination of didanosine (Videx) and stavudine (Zerit), nevirapine (Viramune) in those with CD4+ more than 250 cells/μL, and oral liquid formulations of amprenavir (Agenerase) should be avoided. Although NRTIs and nevirapine (Viramune) can be administered in the usual adult doses, nelfinavir (Viracept) has to be given only twice daily (Table 4). Initiation is better timed at the second trimester, to improve the tolerability and to avoid early fetal exposure to antiretrovirals. A detailed second-trimester fetal survey is indicated.

The goal of treatment, follow-up assessment, and indications for resistance testing all remain the same as in a nonpregnant patient. HAART has to be continued without interruption through delivery. Intrapartum, zidovudine (Retrovir) has to be administered IV until the umbilical cord is clamped and other drugs can be continued by oral route. The option of elective cesarean delivery should be offered to patients with viral loads higher than 1000 copies/mL despite HAART. If opted for, elective cesarean delivery is performed at 38 weeks' gestation, avoiding an amniocentesis to document fetal lung maturity. Following delivery, the infant should receive zidovudine (Retrovir) for 6 weeks. To avoid transmission through breast milk, nursing the infant should be avoided completely, if resources permit. Where the sole indication for initiating HAART was the prevention of perinatal transmission, HAART may be discontinued (in a staggered fashion, if nevirapine [Viramune] was included) after delivery. All infants exposed to antiretrovirals in utero should be followed up for possible adverse effects, regardless of the HIV status. Combined together, these interventions, namely HAART, cesarean delivery, and avoidance of breast-feeding, have brought down the risk of mother-to-child HIV transmission from approximately 25% to 1% to 2% in developed countries. In resource-limited settings and for HIV-infected women without prior HAART presenting in labor, peripartum prophylaxis with zidovudine (Retrovir), zidovudine with lamivudine (Combivir), nevirapine (Viramune), or zidovudine with nevirapine are acceptable alternatives.

TABLE 10 Pharmacokinetic Interactions between Antiretrovirals and Rifamycins

Antiretroviral Drug	Compatibility with Rifampicin (Rifadin)		Compatibility with Rifabutin (Mycobutin)	
	Antiretroviral dose change	Rifampicin (Rifadin) dose change	Antiretroviral dose change	Rifabutin (Mycobutin) dose change
Saquinavir (Invirase, Fortovase)	Should not be used together		Should not be used together	
Saquinavir/ritonavir (Invirase Fortovase/Norvir)	(↓ 400/↑ 400) mg bid	None	None	↓ 150 mg qod*
Indinavir (Crixivan)	Should not be used together		↑ 1000 mg tid	↓ 150 mg qd†
Nelfinavir (Viracept)	Should not be used together		↑ 1000 mg tid	↓ 150 mg qd†
Amprenavir (Agenerase)	Should not be used together		None	↓ 150 mg qd†
Atazanavir (Reyataz)	Should not be used together	None	↓ 150 mg qod*	
Lopinavir/ritonavir (Kaletra)	(400/↑ 400) mg bid	None	None	↓ 150 mg qod*
Efavirenz (Sustiva)	↑ 800 mg qd	None	None	↑ 450 mg qd‡
Nevirapine (Viramune)	None	None	None	None
Delavirdine (Rescriptor)	Should not be used together		Should not be used together	

Note: Increase or decrease in the doses are indicated with appropriately directed arrows.
*Can be administered as 150 mg tiw.
†Can be administered as 300 mg tiw.
‡Can be administered as 600 mg tiw.
Based on Centers for Disease Control and Prevention: Updated guidelines for the use of rifamycins for the treatment of tuberculosis among HIV-infected patients, 2004.

Postexposure Prophylaxis of HIV Infection

The importance of adhering to universal precautions in preventing occupational transmission of HIV cannot be overstated. Administration of postexposure prophylaxis (PEP) can substantially reduce the risk of HIV transmission following accidental occupational exposure in the health care setting. However, PEP is associated with significant morbidity and potentially serious side effects. HIV testing of the health care personnel should be done at the time of exposure, at 6 weeks, 12 weeks, and 6 months after exposure. Generally, all grades of percutaneous, mucous membrane, and nonintact skin exposure to a known HIV-infected source warrant administration of PEP. In the case of mucosal or nonintact skin exposure to a small volume (a few drops) of body fluid from a known HIV-infected source, the decision to initiate PEP should be made on a case-to-case basis, after discussing with the exposed person the benefits as well as the risks of PEP.

PEP should be initiated as soon as possible, preferably within hours following the exposure. The basic prophylaxis is with a two-drug regimen, usually a combination of two NRTIs (zidovudine + lamivudine [Combivir] or emtricitabine + tenofovir [Truvada]). If the exposure is more severe, three-drug regimens containing a PI are recommended. PEP is to be given for 4 weeks. If the source serostatus is unknown, administration of basic prophylaxis should be considered if the source is likely to be HIV infected and the exposure was percutaneous or involved a large volume of potentially infectious body fluid.

The recommendations for PEP were extended recently to include nonoccupational exposures also (e.g., those reporting within 72 hours following an unanticipated sexual or injection drug use exposure to a known HIV-infected source).

REFERENCES

Aberg JA, Gallant JE, Anderson J, et al: Primary care guidelines for the management of persons infected with human immunodeficiency virus: Recommendations of the HIV Medicine Association of the Infectious Diseases Society of America. Clin Infect Dis 2004;39: 609-629.

Carr A, Cooper DA: Adverse effects of antiretroviral therapy. Lancet 2000;356:1423-1430.

Centers for Disease Control and Prevention: Treating opportunistic infections among HIV-infected adults and adolescents: Recommendations from CDC, the National Institutes of Health, and the HIV Medicine Association/Infectious Diseases Society of America. MMWR Morb Mortal Wkly Rep 2004;53(No. RR-15):1-112.

Centers for Disease Control and Prevention: Antiretroviral postexposure prophylaxis after sexual, injection-drug use, or other nonoccupational exposures to HIV in the United States: Recommendations from the U.S. Department of Health and Human Services. MMWR Morb Mortal Wkly Rep 2005;54(No. RR-2):1-19.

Centers for Disease Control and Prevention: Updated U.S. Public Health Service guidelines for the management of occupational exposures to HIV and recommendations for postexposure prophylaxis. MMWR Morb Mortal Wkly Rep 2005;54(No. RR-9):1-17.

Chesney MA: Factors affecting adherence to antiretroviral therapy. Clin Infect Dis 2000;30(Suppl 2):S171-S176.

Grinspoon S, Carr A: Cardiovascular risk and body fat abnormalities in HIV-infected adults. N Engl J Med 2005;352:48-62.

Hammer SM: Management of newly diagnosed HIV infection. N Engl J Med 2005;353:1702-1710.

Panel on clinical practices for the treatment of HIV infection, U.S. Department of Health and Human Services: Guidelines for the use of antiretroviral agents in HIV-1-infected adults and adolescents.

October 6, 2005. Available at http://AIDSinfo.nih.gov (accessed February 1, 2006).

Sax PE: Opportunistic infections in HIV disease: Down but not out. Infect Dis Clin North Am 2001;15:433-455.

Yeni PG, Hammer SM, Hirsch MS, et al: Treatment of adult HIV infection. 2004 recommendations of the International AIDS Society—USA panel. JAMA 2004;292:251-265.

Amebiasis

Method of
Rashidul Haque, MB, PhD, and
William A. Petri, Jr., MD, PhD

Amebiasis, a disease caused by the protozoan parasite *Entamoeba histolytica*, is estimated to be the third leading parasitic cause of deaths worldwide in humans. There are noninvasive species of ameba including *Entamoeba dispar* and *Entamoeba moshkovskii* that are morphologically indistinguishable from *E. histolytica* by traditional light microscopy. Amebiasis is distributed worldwide, but the majority of cases are found in developing countries. The World Health Organization estimates that approximately 50 million people suffer from invasive amebiasis each year, resulting in 40,000 to 100,000 deaths annually. For example, a prospective study of preschool children in an urban slum of Dhaka, Bangladesh, demonstrated a 39% incidence of *E. histolytica* infection during the first year of observation.

Human beings are the only known host of the parasite *E. histolytica*. Individuals become infected with *E. histolytica* when they ingest cysts in fecally contaminated food or water. When these cysts reach the intestine, they swell and release the motile, symptom-inducing form of *E. histolytica*, called the trophozoite. Trophozoites can remain in the intestine and even form new cysts without causing disease symptoms. They colonize the large intestine by adhering to colonic mucins via a galactose and *N*-acetyl-D-galactosamine (Gal/GalNAc)–specific lectin. Reproduction of trophozoites is without a recognized sexual cycle, and the overall population structure of *E. histolytica* appears to be clonal. Aggregation of amebae in the mucin layer likely signals encystation via the Gal/GalNAc lectin. Cysts excreted in stool perpetuate the life cycle by further fecal–oral spread. Invasive disease results when the trophozoite penetrates the intestinal mucus layer, which acts as barrier to invasion by inhibiting amebic adherence to the underlying epithelium and by slowing trophozoite motility. In addition, trophozoites can be carried through the blood to other organs, most commonly the liver, where they form life-threatening abscesses.

Intestinal Amebiasis

There are several clinical classifications of amebiasis based on the invasiveness and site of infection with different treatments. Intestinal amebiasis is a term that encompasses the entire spectrum of clinical intestinal disease, including amebic colitis. Patients with amebic colitis typically present with a several week history of cramping abdominal pain, weight loss, and watery or, less commonly, bloody diarrhea. The insidious onset and variable signs and symptoms make diagnosis difficult, with fever and grossly bloody stool absent in most cases. Differential diagnosis of a diarrheal illness with occult or grossly bloody stools should include *Shigella*, *Salmonella*, *Campylobacter*, and enteroinvasive and enterohemorrhagic *Escherichia coli*. Noninfectious causes include inflammatory bowel disease, ischemic colitis, diverticulitis, and arteriovenous malformation.

Unusual manifestations of amebic colitis include acute necrotizing colitis, toxic megacolon, ameboma, and perianal ulceration with potential fistula formation. Acute necrotizing colitis is rare (<0.5% of cases) and is associated with a greater than 40% mortality. Patients with acute necrotizing colitis are typically very ill-appearing with fever, bloody mucoid diarrhea, abdominal pain with rebound tenderness, and peritoneal signs of irritation. Surgical intervention is indicated if there is bowel perforation or if the patient fails to improve on antiamebic therapy. Toxic megacolon is rare (approximately 0.5% of cases) and typically is associated with corticosteroid use.

Amebic Liver Abscess

Amebic liver abscess is 10 times more common in men than women and is a rare disease in children. Approximately 80% of patients with amebic liver abscess present with symptoms that develop relatively acutely (typically <2 to 4 weeks in duration) with fever, cough, and a constant, dull, aching abdominal pain in the right upper quadrant or epigastrium. Involvement of the diaphragmatic surface of the liver may lead to right pleural pain or referred shoulder pain. Associated gastrointestinal symptoms occur in up to 10% to 35% of cases and include nausea, vomiting, abdominal cramping, abdominal distention, diarrhea, or constipation. Hepatomegaly with point tenderness over the liver, below the ribs, or in the intercostal spaces is a typical finding. Complications from amebic liver abscess may arise from rupture of the abscess with extension into the peritoneum, pleural cavity, or pericardium. Extrahepatic amebic abscesses have occasionally been described in the lung, brain, and skin, and presumably reach these sites hematogenously.

Diagnosis

Historically, diagnosis of amebiasis was complicated and often unreliable for various reasons. The signs and symptoms of amebiasis can provide means to obtain clinical diagnosis. However, the confirmation of an amebic infection rests with laboratory identification. Over the last 25 years, various molecular diagnostic tests have been developed to diagnose *E. histolytica*. The diagnosis of intestinal amebiasis must be based on tests that distinguish *E. histolytica* from *E. dispar*. *E. histolytica*-specific antigen detection test and polymerase chain reaction (PCR) tests are now available for specific diagnosis of *E. histolytica* (Table 1). Enzyme-linked immunoabsorbent assay–based antigen detection kits are now commercially available. Field studies that directly compared PCR to stool culture or antigen-detection

TABLE 1 Sensitivity of Laboratory Tests for the Diagnosis of Amebiasis

Laboratory Tests	Amebic Colitis	Amebic Liver Abscess
Microscopy (stool)*	25%–60%	8%–44%
Microscopy (abscess fluid)	N/A	<20%
Stool antigen detection†	>90%	40%
Serum antigen detection†	<65%	>90% (before therapy)
PCR/real-time PCR (stool)	>90%	>40%
PCR/real-time PCR (abscess fluid)	N/A	90%–100% (before therapy)
Serology		
Acute	50%–70%	70%–90%
Convalescent	>90%	>90%

*Does not distinguish *Entamoeba histolytica* from the commensal parasites *Entamoeba dispar* and *Entamoeba moshkovskii*.
†TechLab *E. histolytica* II antigen detection test.
Abbreviation: PCR = polymerase chain reaction.

tests for the diagnosis of *E. histolytica* infection suggest that these three different methods perform equally well. An important aid to antigen detection and PCR-based tests is the detection of serum antibodies to amebae, which are present in 70% to 90% of patients with symptomatic *E. histolytica* infection. A drawback of current serologic tests is that patients remain positive for years after infection, making it difficult to distinguish new from past infection in regions of the world where amebiasis is endemic. Colonic mucosal biopsies and exudates can reveal a range in histopathologic appearance and severity of intestinal lesions associated with amebic colitis.

Amebic liver abscess patients may reveal a mild to moderate leukocytosis and anemia. Patients with an acute presentation of amebic liver abscess tend to have a normal alkaline phosphatase and elevated aspartate transaminase with the opposite true for patients with a chronic presentation. Ultrasound, abdominal computed tomography scan, and magnetic resonance imaging of the liver are all excellent imaging modalities for detecting liver lesions (most commonly single and in the right lobe) but are not specific for amebic liver abscess. The differential diagnosis of a liver mass should include pyogenic liver abscess, necrotic hepatoma, and echinococcal cyst (usually an incidental finding that would not be the cause of fever and abdominal pain). Patients with amebic abscess are more likely than patients with pyogenic liver abscesses to be male and younger than age 50 years; have immigrated from or traveled to an endemic country; and lack jaundice, biliary disease, or diabetes mellitus. Fewer than half of patients with amebic liver abscess have parasites detected in their stool by antigen detection. Helpful clues to the diagnosis include the presence of epidemiologic risk factors for amebiasis and the presence of serum antiamebic antibodies (present in 70% to 80% of patients at the time of presentation; see Table 1). Occasionally, aspiration of the abscess is required to rule out a pyogenic abscess. Amebae are visualized in the abscess pus in a minority of patients with amebic liver abscess. Traditional PCR and real-time PCR tests can be used for the detection of *E. histolytica* DNA in the stool and liver abscess pus samples and have been found to be sensitive and specific (see Table 1).

Therapy

Therapy differs for invasive versus noninvasive infections (Table 2). Noninvasive infections can be treated with lumen active agents such as paromomycin (Humatin) to eradicate cysts and lumen-dwelling trophozoites. Nitroimidazoles, particularly metronidazole (Flagyl), are the mainstay of therapy for invasive amebiasis (see Table 2). Nitroimidazoles with longer half-lives (namely tinidazole [Tindamax], secnidazole,[2] and ornidazole[2]) are better tolerated and allow shorter duration of treatment; they are recently available in the United States. Approximately 90% of patients presenting with mild to moderate amebic colitis or dysentery respond to nitroimidazole treatment. In the rare case of fulminant amebic colitis, it is prudent to add broad-spectrum antibiotics to treat intestinal bacteria that may spill into the peritoneum, with patients occasionally requiring surgical intervention for acute abdomen, gastrointestinal bleeding, or toxic megacolon. Parasites persist in the intestine in as many as 40% to 60% of metronidazole (Flagyl)-treated patients. Therefore, metronidazole (Flagyl) treatment should be followed with paromomycin (Humatin) or the second-line agent diloxanide furoate (Furamide)[2] to cure luminal infection (see Table 2). Do not treat with metronidazole (Flagyl) and paromomycin (Humatin) at the same time because the diarrhea, a common side effect of paromomycin, (Humatin) may make it difficult to assess response to therapy.

Therapeutic aspiration of an amebic liver abscess is occasionally required as adjunctive treatment to antiparasitic therapy. Abscess drainage should be considered in patients who fail to clinically respond to drug therapy within 5 to 7 days or those with high risk of abscess rupture as defined by cavity size greater than 5 cm or location in the left lobe. Bacterial coinfection of amebic liver abscess has been occasionally observed (both prior to and as a complication of drainage), and it is reasonable to add antibiotics or drainage, or both, to the treatment regimen if a prompt response to nitroimidazole therapy is not observed. Imaging-guided percutaneous treatment (needle aspiration

[2]Not available in the United States.

TABLE 2 Drug Therapy for the Treatment of Amebiasis*

Type of Infection	Drug	Adult Dosage	Pediatric Dosage
Asymptomatic intestinal colonization	Paromomycin (Humatin) or Diloxanide furoate (Furamide)*	25–35 mg/kg/d in 3 doses × 7 d 500 mg tid × 10 d	25–35 mg/kg/d in 3 doses × 7 d 20 mg/kg/d in 3 doses × 10 d
Amebic liver abscess[†]	Metronidazole (Flagyl) or Tinidazole (Tindamax) *followed by luminal agent* Paromomycin (Humatin) or Diloxanide furoate (Furamide)[5]	750 mg tid × 7–10 d in 3 doses × 7–10 d 800 mg tid × 5 d[3] in 3 doses × 5 d 25–35 mg/kg/d in 3 doses × 7 d 500 mg tid × 10 d in 3 doses × 10 d	35–50 mg/kg/d 60 mg/kg/d[3] 25–35 mg/kg/d in 3 doses × 7 d 20 mg/kg/d
Amebic colitis[†]	Metronidazole (Flagyl) *followed by luminal agent (similar to amebic liver abscess)*	500–750 mg tid × 7–10 d in 3 doses × 7–10 d	35–50 mg/kg/d

*The information is updated annually by the Medical Letter on Drugs and Therapeutics at http://www.medletter.com/htmlprm.htm#Parasitic.
[†] Treatment of amebic liver abscess and amebic colitis should be followed by a treatment with a luminal agent.
[3] Exceeds dosage recommended by the manufacturer.
[5] Investigational drug in the United States.

or catheter drainage) has replaced surgical intervention over more recent years as the procedure of choice for therapeutically reducing abscess size.

REFERENCES

Diamond LS, Clark CG: A redescription of *Entamoeba histolytica* Schaudin 1903 (amended Walker 1911) separating it from *Entamoeba dispar* (Brumpt 1925). J Eukaryot Microbiol 1993;40:340–344.

Haque R, Mollah NU, Ali IKM, et al: Diagnosis of amebic liver abscess and intestinal infection with the TechLab *Entamoeba histolytica* II antigen detection and antibody tests. J Clin Microbiol 2000;38: 3235–3239.

Haque R, Ali IKM, Akther S, Petri WA Jr: Comparison of PCR, isoenzyme analysis, and antigen detection for diagnosis of *Entamoeba histolytica* infection. J Clin Microbio1998;36:449–452.

Haque R, Ali IKM, Sack RB, et al: Amebiasis and mucosal IgA antibody against the *Entamoeba histolytica* adherence lectin in Bangladeshi children. J Infect Dis 2001;183:1787–1793.

Haque R, Huston CD, Hughes M, et al: Current concepts: Amebiasis. N Engl J Med 2003;348:1565–1573.

Petri WA Jr, Haque R, Lyerly D, Vine RR: Estimating the impact of amebiasis on health. Parasitol Today 2000;16:320–321.

Petri, WA Jr, Singh U: State of the art: Diagnosis and management of amebiasis. Clin Infect Dis 1999;29:1117–1125.

Stanley SL Jr: Amoebiasis. Lancet 2003;22;361(9362):1025–1034.

Tanyuksel M, Petri WA Jr: Laboratory diagnosis of amebiasis. Clin Microbiol Rev 2003;16:713–729.

World Health Organization: Amoebiasis. Wkly Epidemiol Rec 1997;72: 97–100.

Giardiasis

Method of
*David E. Katz, MD, and
Alfred DeMaria, Jr., MD*

Background/Organism

Giardiasis is an intestinal infection caused by the protozoan parasite *Giardia lamblia* (also known as *Giardia intestinalis* and *Giardia duodenalis*). Giardiasis is the most common protozoal infection in humans. *Giardia* exists in two forms: The trophozoite is responsible for the clinical illness, and the environmentally resistant cyst is responsible for transmission of infection. Trophozoites are pear shaped, flagellated, and binucleate and contain a ventral disc thought to aid in attachment of the organism to small intestine villi. Trophozoites measure 9 μm to 15 μm long, 5 μm to 15 μm wide, and 2 μm to 4 μm thick. Cysts are oval, contain four nuclei, and are approximately 10 μm to 12 μm long.

Pathogenesis

Giardia cysts persist in the environment. After ingestion, excystation in the proximal small intestine is thought to be triggered by exposure to gastric acid in the stomach and/or the alkaline, protease-rich environment of the proximal duodenum. Excystation releases two mobile trophozoites, which replicate by binary fission. *Giardia* is not invasive but causes mucosal damage in the proximal small bowel, which leads to malabsorption and diarrhea. Trophozoites encyst in the jejunum, triggered by biliary secretions. Trophozoites and cysts are then passed intermittently in the stool.

Epidemiology

Giardiasis occurs worldwide. The prevalence of *Giardia* in stool ranges from 2% to 5% in industrialized countries to 20% to 30% in developing countries. However, patients are often asymptomatic or have nonspecific symptoms. In 1997 the incidence of reported disease in the United States was 9.5 cases per 100,000 population. It is estimated that nearly 5000 people are hospitalized annually in the United States with severe giardiasis. Reservoir hosts include human beings as well as farm, wild, and domesticated animals. Two major groups of *G. lamblia* organisms have been recognized as infecting humans worldwide. Although no consensus exists as to nomenclature, the term *assemblages* has been widely used. Current research endeavors to understand how genetic variability of the parasite is correlated with pathogenicity. Studies have shown that *G. lamblia* from certain animals can potentially infect humans. Although isolates of *G. lamblia* from humans and various animals are morphologically similar, the existence of distinct host-adapted genotypes has been demonstrated.

Transmission is via fecal–oral spread and can be person-to-person, food-borne, or waterborne. Waterborne transmission is the major source for epidemic spread. Because cysts are killed by cooking, food-borne spread is uncommon. The age distribution is bimodal, with peaks at ages 0 to 5 years as well as 31 to 40 years. The incidence of giardiasis is similar among men and women. Seasonal variation exists with most cases occurring in the summer. High-risk groups include:

- Diaper-age children
- Children in daycare settings
- Child-care workers
- Immunocompromised persons
- Institutionalized persons
- Foreign travelers
- Persons who drink untreated water from lakes, streams, and swimming pools
- Men who have sex with men
- Patients with intestinal metaplasia and/or hypochlorhydria

Studies of giardiasis in poorly nourished children in developing regions have demonstrated growth retardation, cognitive impairment, and delayed psychomotor development. Repeated or chronic low-level exposure to *Giardia* likely stimulates some protection from symptomatic infection. Children born to nonimmune mothers are significantly more likely to acquire *Giardia* infection and develop giardiasis with more severe symptoms compared with children of immune mothers. Antibodies in mother's milk may protect children against giardiasis.

Clinical Presentation

Clinical presentation can vary greatly and may depend on variations among strains of *Giardia*. Ingestion of as few as 10 to 25 cysts can lead to giardiasis. After an incubation period of 1 to 2 weeks, signs and symptoms may develop such as nausea, vomiting (less common), malaise, flatulence, cramping, diarrhea, steatorrhea, and weight loss. A history of gradual onset of diarrhea is characteristic. Symptoms lasting 2 to 4 weeks with weight loss are typical. Chronic giardiasis may follow an acute syndrome or present without severe antecedent symptoms. Chronic signs and symptoms such as loose stool, steatorrhea (with frothy, foul-smelling stools), a 10% to 20% weight loss, malabsorption (of fats, vitamin B_{12}, and D-xylose [D-XYL]), malaise, fatigue, and depression may wax and wane over many months in untreated individuals. Rash and urticaria may be present in a hypersensitivity reaction. Giardiasis may rarely be associated with reactive arthritis or asymmetric synovitis, usually of the lower extremities.

Approximately 60% of infected individuals may be asymptomatic. Even asymptomatic infection may lead to vitamin deficiencies (A, B_{12}, and folate) and hypoalbuminemia. Acquired lactose intolerance occurs in up to 20% to 40% of cases because of a transient lactase deficiency, which can take many weeks to normalize.

Diagnosis

Diagnosis is based on detection of trophozoites, or more commonly, cysts in the stool and is difficult because the number of cysts excreted varies from day to day. In addition, shedding occurs intermittently. Eosinophilia and fecal leukocytosis do not occur. Radiographic imaging is not useful. Stool microscopy (ova and parasite examination) may require three separate stool specimens collected on nonconsecutive days for maximum yield. The sensitivity of parasite identification is 50% to 70% with a single specimen and 90% after three specimens. Several commercial antigen detection immunoassays for stool exist, including counterimmunoelectrophoresis (CIE), enzyme-linked immunosorbent assay (ELISA), enzyme immunoassay (EIA; detects soluble antigens), direct fluorescent antibody (DFA; detects intact organisms), and the immunochromatographic lateral-flow immunoassay (rapid assay).

 CURRENT DIAGNOSIS

- Clinical presentation can vary greatly.
- More than half of infected individuals may be asymptomatic.
- Chronic infection can last for months and result in significant weight loss.
- Lactose intolerance may persist after symptoms resolve.
- Cyst excretion occurs intermittently.
- Diagnosis is optimized with three separate specimens for stool microscopy.
- Assays that detect soluble antigen may give false positives in individuals recently cured of infection.

Many of these tests have demonstrated sensitivities and specificities greater than 95%. However, sensitivity and specificity of diagnostic methods based upon *Giardia* antigen detection may be affected by genetic variability of *Giardia* isolates present in a given geographic area. Antigen assays are quick and are similar in cost to ova and parasite exam. Assays that detect *Giardia* antigen should be carefully interpreted because they might be positive even after a person stops shedding intact organisms, giving false-positive results in individuals who might actually be cured but still symptomatic because of disaccharidase deficiency. Serology is of limited value because IgG and IgM antibodies both persist after infection. Secretory antibodies found in saliva may be used for diagnosis in the future. Duodenal aspirates, biopsies, brush cytology, and the string test are invasive and/or costly procedures. Although biopsy is most sensitive, it should be reserved for confusing or refractory cases. Culture and polymerase chain reaction (PCR) tests are available only as research tools.

Treatment

Table 1 provides the current therapy for giardiasis. Metronidazole (Flagyl)[1] is the first-line agent for treatment of giardiasis in the United States, despite not being approved by the U.S. Food and Drug Administration (FDA). Reported cure rates range from 80% to 95%. Side effects are uncommon but include gastrointestinal upset, headache, nausea, leukopenia, a metallic taste in the mouth, and a possible disulfiram-like reaction with alcohol ingestion. Because metronidazole (Flagyl)[1] is reported to be carcinogenic, teratogenic, and mutagenic, it is contraindicated in pregnant women during the first trimester. Seizures, peripheral neuropathy, depression, irritability, restlessness, and insomnia are rarely reported. Drug resistance is not yet widespread but has been reported.

---

[1]Not FDA approved for this indication.

CURRENT THERAPY

- Metronidazole (Flagyl)[1] is the current first-line agent but cannot be used in the first trimester of pregnancy.
- Patients taking metronidazole (Flagyl)[1] should abstain from alcohol.
- Paromomycin (Humatin)[1] can be used in pregnancy.
- Nitazoxanide (Alinia) is available in suspension and tablet form and is approved for children greater than 1 year of age.
- Diet modification may reduce acute symptoms and promote host defenses.
- Asymptomatic carriers may need to receive treatment during an outbreak.

[1]Not FDA approved for this indication.

ALBENDAZOLE (ALBENZA)

Albendazole (Albenza)[1] is an antihelminthic used as an alternative treatment for giardiasis. It is a benzimidazole derivative comparable in efficacy to metronidazole (Flagyl).[1] Cure rates are reported as 62% to 95%. It is becoming a first-line drug for giardiasis and a variety of other parasitic gastrointestinal diseases. Side effects include gastrointestinal upset, abdominal pain, nausea, vomiting, diarrhea, dizziness, vertigo, fever, increased intracranial pressure, and variable increases in transaminases (seen in approximately 15% of patients and reversible). Discontinuation of the drug is usually not required for abnormal liver function tests. In vitro resistance has been reported.

PAROMOMYCIN (HUMATIN)

Paromomycin (Humatin)[1] is considered investigational for giardiasis by the FDA. It is a poorly absorbed aminoglycoside

---

[1]Not FDA approved for this indication.

TABLE 1 Common Current Therapies for Treating Giardiasis		
Drug	**Dose**	**Comment**
Metronidazole (Flagyl)[1]	Adult: 250 mg PO tid for 5d or 2 g qhs for 3d[3] Pediatric: 15 mg/kg/d PO divided into 3 daily doses for 5 days	Cost effective.
Albendazole (Albenza)[1]	Adult: 400 mg PO for 5d Pediatric: 10 mg/kg/d PO for 5d	Recommended dosages vary.
Paromomycin (Humatin)[1]	Adult: 500 mg PO qid for 7d Pediatric: 25–35 mg/kg/d PO divided into 3 daily doses	Useful in pregnancy.
Tinidazole (Tindamax)	Adult: 2.0 g PO for 1d Pediatric: 50 mg/kg PO for 1d (2 g max)	Tindamax FDA approved May 2004. For use in children ages >3 years.
Nitazoxanide (Alinia)	12–47 months: 100 mg (5mL) PO bid for 3d 4–11 years: 200 mg (10 mL) PO bid for 3d ≥12 years: 500 mg (25 mL) PO bid for 3d	Available in liquid and tablet form. Approved for children 1 year of age or older.

[1]Not FDA approved for this indication.
[3]Exceeds dosage recommended by the manufacturer.
Abbreviations: bid = twice daily; d = days; PO = by mouth; qhs = at bedtime; qid = four times daily; tid = three times daily.

and, therefore, is one of the only antigiardial medications recommended for symptomatic pregnant patients. Reported efficacy against giardiasis is 60% to 70%. Side effects include nausea, increased gastrointestinal motility, abdominal pain, and diarrhea.

FURAZOLIDONE (FUROXONE), QUINACRINE (ATABRINE), AND NITROIMIDAZOLE DERIVATIVES

Furazolidone (Furoxone)[2] and quinacrine (Atabrine)[2] have been used in the past but are no longer readily available in the United States and have been supplanted by other agents. Nitroimidazole derivatives include tinidazole (Tindamax), now available in the United States, and ornidazole (Tiberal).[2] Ornidazole (Tiberal)[2] is not approved in the United States, but it is used as a front-line agent in other countries. Advantages are a reported cure rate of 90% and less frequent dosing. Side effects include gastrointestinal upset, vertigo, and bitter taste.

NITAZOXANIDE (ALINIA)

Nitazoxanide (Alinia), a 5-nitrothiazole derivative, has activity against protozoans, helminths, and some aerobic and anaerobic bacteria. It is available in liquid or tablet form and is approved for the treatment of giardiasis in immunocompetent children (>1 year of age) and adults. Nitazoxanide (Alinia) has the advantages over metronidazole (Flagyl)[1] of a liquid formulation and shorter duration of treatment. Trials show nitazoxanide (Alinia) to be 83% to 100% effective (for giardiasis). Side effects include abdominal pain, diarrhea, nausea, vomiting, and headache similar to those for placebo; yellow sclera caused by drug deposition occurs rarely and resolves after discontinuation. Nitazoxanide (Alinia) should be taken with food. Caution is needed when adding nitazoxanide (Alinia) to regimens consisting of other highly plasma protein-bound medication (warfarin, valproic acid, carbamazepine, and aspirin). Metronidazole (Flagyl)[1]-refractory cases should be treated with nitazoxanide (Alinia), higher doses of metronidazole (Flagyl), or combination therapy (e.g., quinacrine [Atabrine][2] and metronidazole [Flagyl][1]).

SPECIAL PROBLEMS

Immunocompromised patients might experience relapses and require prolonged treatment or combination therapy. Patients with persistent symptoms after treatment, or for whom repeated treatment has failed, should be evaluated for lactose intolerance, underlying common variable immunodeficiency, and functional irritable bowel disease.

Prevention and Control Measures

Centers for Disease Control and Prevention (CDC) publishes recommendations for the prevention and control of giardiasis (http://www.cdc.gov/ncidod/dpd/parasites/giardiasis/factsht_giardia.htm). Prevention of giardiasis is accomplished through proper sewage disposal, water treatment, and hygiene. Water should be treated by flocculation, sedimentation, filtration, or chlorination. *Giardia* cysts can be inactivated by boiling water for at least 1 minute using filters (pore size less than 1 μm). Halogens, including chlorine and iodine, may not be effective in all circumstances. When traveling overseas, bottled beverages (preferably carbonated) are the safest. Raw food should be washed with uncontaminated water. Fecal exposure should be avoided during sexual activity. In daycare centers, strict hand washing and separate diaper-changing areas should be implemented. Symptomatic children, teachers, and family members should be treated. People with diarrhea should be excluded from child care. Individuals diagnosed with giardiasis should not swim in recreational water for at least 2 weeks after diarrhea stops.

Treatment of asymptomatic carriers is generally not recommended. Possible exceptions are carriers in households of patients with hypogammaglobulinemia or cystic fibrosis, diaper-age children in households with pregnant women, and food handlers, or in the presence of an outbreak. If a child does not have diarrhea but is experiencing nausea, fatigue, weight loss, or a poor appetite, treatment should be considered. If an outbreak is continuing to occur at a daycare center despite control efforts, screening and treating asymptomatic children should be considered.

REFERENCES

Adam RD: Biology of *Giardia lamblia*. Clin Microbiol Rev 2001;14:447-475.
Anonymous: Nitazoxanide (Alinia)—a new antiprotozoal agent. Med Lett Drugs Ther 2003;45(1154):29-31.
Bailey JM, Erramouspe J: Nitazoxanide treatment for giardiasis and cryptosporidiosis in children. Ann Pharmacother 2004;38:634-640.
Caccio SM, De Giacomo M, Pozio E: Sequence analysis of the β-giardin gene and development of a polymerase chain reaction-restriction fragment length polymorphism assay to genotype *Giardia duodenalis* cysts from human faecal samples. Int J Parasitol 2002;32:1023-1030.
Faubert G: Immune response to *Giardia duodenalis*. Clin Microbiol Rev. 2000;13:35-54.
Furness BW, Beach MJ, Roberts JM. Giardiasis surveillance—United States, 1992-1997. MMWR 2000;49(7):1-13.
Gardner TB, Hill DR: Treatment of giardiasis. Clin Microbiol Rev 2001;14:114-128.
Johnston SP, Ballard MM, Beach MJ, et al: Evaluation or three commercial assays for detection of *Giardia* and *Cryptosporidium* organisms in fecal specimens. J Clin Microbiol 2003;41:623-626.
Mineno T, Avery MA: Giardiasis: Recent progress in chemotherapy and drug development. Curr Pharm Des 2003;9:841-855.
Petri WA Jr: Therapy of intestinal protozoa. Trends Parasitol 2003;19(11):523-526.
Sulaiman IM, Fayer R, Bern C, et al: Triosephosphate isomerase gene characterization and potential zoonotic transmission of *Giardia duodenalis*. Emerg Infect Dis 2003;9(11):1444-1452.

---

[1]Not FDA approved for this indication.
[2]Not available in the United States.

Severe Sepsis and Septic Shock

Method of
Steven Zgliniec, MD, and Robert A. Balk, MD

Sepsis has been defined as the systemic inflammatory response to an infection. The true incidence of sepsis is unknown, in part related to the lack of a uniformly accepted definition. The Centers for Disease Control and Prevention (CDC) had previously reported a dramatic 139% increase in the septicemia discharge diagnosis over a decade of monitoring. Using discharge-coding data from seven states, it has been recently suggested that there are more than 750,000 episodes of severe sepsis each year in the United States. Severe sepsis accounts for 1 out of every 10 intensive care unit (ICU) admissions and represents 2% to 3% of all hospital admissions. Furthermore, incidence of sepsis in the United States is projected to rise at a rate of 1.5% per year. Factors responsible for this increase include the continued growth in the number of elderly patients, an increased number of immunocompromised patients, the increased use of invasive procedures and devices to care for patients, the growing problem with resistant microorganisms, and a greater awareness and recognition of this disorder.

Sepsis is now reported to be the tenth most common cause of death in the United States and is one of the two most common causes of death in the noncoronary ICU. Using the extrapolated annual incidence of 750,000 episodes of sepsis in the United States and a relatively conservative mortality estimate of 28%, there would be an annual mortality of greater than 220,000. This surprisingly high mortality rate has been projected despite our enhanced understanding of the pathophysiologic alterations that occur in sepsis, technologic improvements in monitoring and support of the critically ill patient, and use of more potent antibiotic therapy. There have also been multiple attempts to improve the outcome of the septic patient using innovative therapeutic strategies that are designed to target selected aspects of the pathophysiologic response to the causative microorganism(s).

A recent epidemiologic review of sepsis in the United States reported that sepsis is more common in males and in the nonwhite population. Over the past 22 years, gram-positive organisms have become the predominant cause of sepsis, but there has also been a dramatic increase in the number of episodes of fungal sepsis. During this observation period, the incidence and number of sepsis-related deaths have increased, whereas the actual sepsis mortality rate has improved.

Definitions of Systemic Inflammatory Response Syndrome and Sepsis

The approach to management of patients with severe sepsis and septic shock begins with prompt recognition of the septic process (Current Diagnosis box). As mentioned,

CURRENT DIAGNOSIS

Infection (documented or suspected) and some of the following:

General Variables

- Fever (core temperature >38.3°C [101°F]
- Hypothermia (core temperature <36°C [96.8°F]
- Heart rate >90/min or >2 SD above the normal value for age
- Tachypnea
- Altered mental status
- Significant edema or positive fluid balance (>20 mL/kg more than 24 h)
- Hyperglycemia (plasma glucose >120 mg/dL, or 7.7 mmol/L in the absence of diabetes)

Inflammatory Variables

- Leukocytosis (WBC count >12,000/μL)
- Leukopenia (WBC count <4000/μL)
- Normal WBC count with >10% immature forms (bands)
- Plasma C-reactive protein >2 SD above the normal value
- Plasma procalcitonin >2 SD above the normal value

Hemodynamic Variables

- Arterial hypotension (systolic BP <90 mm Hg, MAP <70, or a systolic BP decrease >40 mm Hg in adults or <2 SD below normal for age)
- SvO_2 >70%
- Cardiac index >3.5 L/min/m^2

Organ Dysfunction Variables

- Arterial hypoxemia (PaO_2/FiO_2 <300)
- Acute oliguria (urine output <0.5 mL/kg/h or 45 mmol/L for at least 2 h)
- Creatinine increase >0.5 mg/dL
- Coagulation abnormalities (INR >1.5 or aPTT >60s)
- Ileus (absent bowel sounds)
- Thrombocytopenia (platelet count <100,000/μL)
- Hyperbilirubinemia (plasma total bilirubin >4 mg/dL or 70 mmol/L)

Tissue Perfusion Variables

- Hyperlactatemia (>1 mmol/L)
- Decreased capillary refill or mottling

Abbreviations: aPTT = activated partial thromboplastin time; BP = blood pressure; INR = international normalized ratio; MAP = mean arterial pressure; SD = standard deviation; WBC = white blood cell.
From Levy MM, Fink MP, Marshall JC, et al: 2001 SCCM/ESICM/ACCP/ATS/SIS International sepsis definitions conference. Crit Care Med 2003;31:1250-1256.

in the past there has been difficulty in identifying septic patients, in part related to the lack of a uniformly accepted definition. In 1991 the American College of Chest Physicians and the Society of Critical Care Medicine convened a consensus conference to develop a set of definitions that would assist the medical community in communication about sepsis and provide for the early recognition of the septic patient. The definition would incorporate predominantly readily available clinical criteria that would facilitate patient identification and enrollment in investigational trials of innovative therapeutic agents. The consensus conference recognized that some patients with presumed sepsis based on their clinical presentation lacked a positive culture or other evidence of a documented infection. These individuals were classified as having the systemic inflammatory response syndrome (SIRS). SIRS can result from a diverse group of insults, such as trauma, burns, pancreatitis, and so forth. Sepsis was defined as the SIRS response to a documented infection.

Defined as a widespread systemic inflammatory response to a variety of insults, SIRS includes but is not limited to infection. SIRS was operationally defined by the presence of two or more of the following:

- Temperature greater than 38°C (100.4°F) or less than 36°C (96.8°F)
- Heart rate more than 90 beats per minute (bpm)
- Respiratory rate greater than 20 breaths per minute or $Paco_2$ less than 32 mm Hg
- White blood cell (WBC) more than 12,000 cells/mm^3, fewer than 4000 cells/mm^3, or greater than 10% immature band forms

Sepsis is the systemic inflammatory response to a documented infection. The diagnosis of sepsis requires the presence of at least two of the above SIRS criteria as a response to an infection. Signs of infection include an inflammatory response to the presence of microorganisms and the invasion of normally sterile host tissue by those organisms. There is a continuum of injury severity in SIRS and sepsis. Severe SIRS and severe sepsis are defined by the presence of organ dysfunction or hypoperfusion as a result of the inflammatory response. Hypoperfusion and perfusion abnormalities may include, but are not limited to, lactic acidosis, oliguria, or an acute alteration in mental status. Sepsis-induced hypotension occurs when systolic blood pressure (BP) falls to less than 90 mm Hg or there is a reduction of at least 40 mm Hg from baseline systolic pressure in the absence of other causes for hypotension.

Septic shock is a subset of severe sepsis with hypotension despite adequate fluid resuscitation, along with the presence of perfusion abnormalities. Patients receiving inotropic or vasopressor agents may no longer be hypotensive by the time they manifest hypoperfusion abnormalities or organ dysfunction, yet they would still be considered to have septic shock. Multiple organ dysfunction syndrome (MODS) is the alteration of organ function such that normal homeostasis cannot be maintained without intervention. Unfortunately, there is no consensus on how to define the dysfunction or failure of specific organ systems. However, most would agree that the need for organ support or replacement therapy signifies the presence of specific organ failure.

Validation of these conference definitions came from a prospective evaluation of University of Iowa patients who met the SIRS criteria, as well as sepsis, severe sepsis, and septic shock definitions. These patients demonstrated an increase in mortality as they moved down this continuum of injury severity.

In 2001 the International Sepsis Definitions Conference convened to revisit the American College of Chest Physicians/Society of Critical Care Medicine (ACCP/SCCM) Consensus Conference Definitions. Representatives from

TABLE 1 PIRO Staging of Sepsis

Predisposition: Premorbid conditions that influence likelihood of infection, sepsis, morbidity, survival (i.e., age, sex, hormonal state, genetic polymorphisms for TNF, IL-10, IL-6, IL-1ra, TLR)
Insult/Infection: Insult or organism associated with the sepsis response (i.e., type of organism, sensitivity pattern, community, or nosocomial acquisition)
Response: Clinical manifestations of the SIRS response (procalcitonin, IL-6, HLA-DR, TNF, PAF, CRP, etc.)
Organ dysfunction: Type and number of dysfunctional organs (reversible versus irreversible dysfunction) Severity of dysfunction (judged by scoring systems, e.g., MODS, LODS, SOFA)

Abbreviations: CRP = C-reactive protein; HLA-DR = human leukocyte antigen-D region–related; IL = interleukin; LODS = logistic organ dysfunction system; MODS = multiple organ dysfunction syndrome; PAF = platelet-activating factor; SOFA = sepsis-related organ failure assessment; TNF = tumor necrosis factor.
From Levy MM, Fink MP, Marshall JC, et al: 2001 SCCM/ESICM/ACCP/ATS/SIS International sepsis definitions conference. Crit Care Med 2003;31:1250-1256.

the SCCM, ACCP, European Society of Intensive Care Medicine, American Thoracic Society, and the Surgical Infection Society reaffirmed the basic validity of the 1991 definitions. To enhance the clinician's ability to recognize severe sepsis and to possibly enhance the specificity of the clinical diagnosis of sepsis, the conference provided a listing of common signs and symptoms of sepsis (see Current Diagnosis box). In addition, the International Sepsis Definitions Conference developed a classification scheme for sepsis modeled after the TNM system used in cancer staging (Table 1). The PIRO classification system hoped to aid in stratifying septic patients on the basis of the predisposing condition(s), the nature of the insult, the nature and magnitude of the host's response, and the degree of concomitant organ dysfunction. The potential utility of the proposed staging systems is the ability to discriminate the morbidity associated with the infection from the morbidity arising from the response to infection.

Pathogenesis of Sepsis

The septic response begins as a normal physiologic response to an infection that attempts to wall off and eliminate the offending microbiologic organism(s). The pathologic process clinically recognized as sepsis results from an excessive and uncontrolled physiologic response that may culminate in endothelial cell injury, MODS, or death. The normal response to infection involves a process that serves to localize and contain an invading organism, usually resulting in the initiation of repair of injured host tissue. When this inflammatory response to infection becomes generalized and extends to healthy host tissue, it becomes the SIRS. With the onset of SIRS, normal host tissue whether infected or not, becomes damaged. This results in the release of proinflammatory and anti-inflammatory molecules and mediators capable of producing injury and/or altering the host's immune response. These contrasting elements help facilitate host tissue repair and healing. When there is an

TABLE 2 The Five Stages of Sepsis

The infectious insult
Preliminary systemic response
Overwhelming systemic response
The compensatory anti-inflammatory reaction
Immunomodulatory failure

TABLE 3 Potential Molecules Involved in the Pathogenesis of Systemic Inflammatory Response Syndrome and Sepsis

Pro-inflammatory Molecules and Cells
PMNLs
Tissue macrophages and monocytes
Platelets
Arachidonic acid metabolites
Prostaglandins, prostacyclin, thromboxane, leukotrienes
Cytokines (interleukins 1, 2, 6, 8, 15, TNF, G-CSF)
Soluble adhesion molecules
PAF
Complement and activation of the complement cascade
Various kinins (e.g., bradykinin)
Endorphins
Histamine and serotonin
Proteolytic enzymes
Elastase and lysosomal enzymes
Protein kinase, tyrosine kinase
Toxic oxygen metabolites
Superoxide, hydroxyl radical, hydrogen peroxide, peroxynitrite, etc.
Endotoxin and other bacterial and microbial toxins
Activation of the coagulation cascade
Neopterin
PAI-1
CD14
Toll-like receptors 2 & 4
NF-κB
Vasoactive neuropeptides
MCP-1 and -2

Potential Anti-inflammatory Molecules
IL-1ra
Type II IL-1 receptor
IL-4, IL-10, IL-13
Transforming growth factor-β (TGF-β)
IκB
Glucocorticoid receptors
Epinephrine
sTNFr
Leukotriene B$_4$ receptor antagonist
Soluble CD14
LPS binding protein

Abbreviations: G-CSF = granulocyte colony-stimulating factor; IL = interleukin; IL-1ra = interleukin-1 receptor antagonist; LPS = lipopolysaccharide; MCP = monocyte chemoattractant protein; NF-κB = nuclear factor-kappa B; PAF = platelet-activating factor; PAI1 = plasminogen activator inhibitor-1; PMNL = polymorphonuclear leukocyte; sTNFr = soluble TNF receptor; TNF = tumor necrosis factor.

imbalance in the complex and intricate septic cascade, however, either a SIRS or a compensatory anti-inflammatory response syndrome (CARS) can predominate. If the SIRS response predominates, there is a predisposition for an exaggerated proinflammatory response that can culminate in the production of MODS. In contrast, when the CARS response predominates, there is a state of immune suppression that can result in secondary or nosocomial infections. These additional inflammatory insults may supply additional *hits* to the immune system; this pathomechanism has been termed the *multiple hits hypothesis* for the production of multiple organ dysfunction (MOD) or failure. The sepsis cascade has been categorized into five stages by Bone and colleagues (Table 2).

Host factors responsible for important first line of defense against the infectious insult include epithelial barriers, mucociliary flow, pH of body fluids, urine volume, and secretory immunoglobulins. Overall immune function of the host is also a key consideration. Chronic diseases such as diabetes mellitus, HIV infection, and chronic alcoholism commonly predispose the host to an infectious insult. The adaptive and innate immunity of the host also provide key defenses against infectious insults. The adaptive arm of host immunity is composed of specialized B cells and T cells. Receptors unique to each of these cell lines results in a proliferation of immune response when stimulated. The innate arm of the immune response uses receptors that recognize highly conserved antigenic regions in large groups of microorganisms. A group of cell surface receptors that have become of particular interest are the toll-like receptors (TLR). For example, activation of TLR-4 by circulating endotoxin from the gram-negative bacterial cell wall induces the transcription of a number of inflammatory and immune response genes. Gram-negative organisms contain a component of endotoxin within the cell wall that is responsible for many of the manifestations of sepsis. Gram-positive organisms produce exotoxins that may function as superantigens. The result is a massive activation of mononuclear cells and macrophages with an overproduction of cytokines and an out of control immune response.

Mediators of the host inflammatory response are initially found in high concentrations locally, at the nidus of infection. In severe infections proinflammatory cytokines will produce systemic symptoms. This usually becomes the telltale sign that the infection is unable to be contained locally. Some of the more common primary pro- and anti-inflammatory molecules and mediators are listed in Table 3. Included in the list of pro-inflammatory cytokines are tumor necrosis factor (TNF)-α, interleukin (IL)-1, IL-6, and interferon-γ.

An overwhelming systemic inflammatory response results when the host is unable to contain the pro-inflammatory response locally. The massive, uncontrolled production of pro-inflammatory molecules and cytokines produce

the SIRS. Endothelial dysfunction typically ensues from the inflammatory response coupled with the activation of the coagulation syndrome. The result is microvascular thrombi as well as upregulation of endothelial adhesion molecules causing increased microvascular permeability, vasodilatation, organ dysfunction, and shock.

The overwhelming pro-inflammatory response is then followed by CARS, which down-regulates the pro-inflammatory cascade. The balance that ensues during the mixed antagonistic response syndrome (MARS) will determine the clinical manifestations and outcome of the response to the infection. The principal mediators of the CARS response include IL-4, IL-10, and transforming growth factor (TGF)-β. In some cases the compensatory reaction can lead to excessive production of counterreg ulatory cytokines leading to immune suppression. This can be recognized by a decreased production of IL-6 and TNF-α by monocytes. The final result may be immunomodulatory failure, progression of infection, or superinfection along with coagulation activation or abnormalities of fibrinolysis leading to MODS and death.

Management of Severe Sepsis and Septic Shock

In 2003 critical care and infectious disease experts representing 11 international organizations developed management guidelines for severe sepsis and septic shock entitled the "Surviving Sepsis Campaign." These were published in 2004 in both *Critical Care Medicine* and *Intensive Care Medicine* journals. Management of sepsis and septic shock begins with prompt recognition of the process. Along with recognition and determination of a probable site and cause of the infection, the initial management begins with an assessment of the physiologic derangements. In critically ill patients the general management involves source control, restoration and maintenance of normal hemodynamic function, adequate oxygenation, ventilation, tissue oxygen delivery, and prevention of complications. The assessment of adrenal function and detection of occult adrenal insufficiency in vasopressor-dependent patients with septic shock is important for defining a role for physiologic adrenal replacement therapy. It is also imperative to evaluate for the presence of complications of critical illness and to administer preventive strategies where appropriate. The Current Therapy box outlines the general management principles.

SOURCE CONTROL

Prompt, effective management of the source of the infection is the cornerstone of sepsis management. Early initiation of appropriate, effective antimicrobial therapy is essential for a favorable outcome in the septic patient. Necessary specimens should be sent for culture and sensitivity testing as early as possible, because this information will guide subsequent antimicrobial therapy and allow for good antimicrobial stewardship. The initial antimicrobial therapy is empirical and should be directed toward the organisms likely to cause the infection giving rise to the septic response. A review of nosocomial infections suggests that the urinary tract (UT), respiratory system (RS), and bloodstream are the three most common sources of hospital-acquired infections.

Clinical trials of new agents for the treatment of sepsis have observed that the respiratory tract and the abdomen are the most common sources of infection. After identification of the likely site and cause of the infection, the initial antibiotic selection should be made taking into account the antibiogram of the institution or specific unit where the infection was acquired. When the results of the various cultures and their sensitivity pattern are available, the antimicrobial therapy should then be appropriately tailored. It has been well documented that the use of early effective antimicrobial therapy will decrease mortality,

CURRENT THERAPY

Identify the Cause and Source of Infection

Obtain suitable material for needed cultures, Gram stains, and diagnostic studies.
Implement surgical drainage where appropriate.

Initiate Appropriate Antibiotic Therapy

Initial therapy will be empirical, but tailored therapy may be started when more data are available.
Survival is improved when the initial antibiotic therapy is effective against the isolated organism(s) and started early.

Restore and Maintain Hemodynamic Function

Implement an early goal-directed therapeutic approach.
Fluids are the initial choice for volume resuscitation and may include crystalloids, colloids, volume expanders, or blood products.
If hypotension and poor perfusion persist, then vasoactive agents should be used as necessary to ensure adequate hemodynamic function.
Hemodynamic monitoring is frequently used to ensure the adequacy and effectiveness of therapy (i.e., arterial line, CVP, PA catheter).
Physiologic dose corticosteroid replacement therapy may be beneficial for vasopressor-dependent patients with inadequate cortisol response.

Support Oxygenation and Ventilation

Supplemental oxygen as needed to ensure the patient has adequate arterial oxygen saturation.
Ensure adequate tissue oxygen delivery.
Implement mechanical ventilation as necessary.
Use lung protective ventilator support.
Implement protocol-derived weaning.

Antithrombotic, Profibrinolytic, Anti-inflammatory Therapy

Use drotrecogin alfa (activated) (Xigris) as per package insert recommendations.

Metabolic Support

Maintain early nutritional support.
Maintain intestinal mucosa barrier function by enteral route, the preferred method.
Control hyperglycemia to decrease infectious complications, may need IV insulin therapy.

Prevent Complications of Critical Illness

Prevent DVT prophylaxis.
Prevent stress-related gastrointestinal bleeding.
Prevent organ system dysfunction.
Prevent nosocomial and secondary infections.
Recognize critical illness polyneuropathy/myopathy.
Anticipate anemia of critical illness.

Abbreviations: CVP = central venous pressure; DVT = deep vein thrombosis; IV = intravenous; PA = pulmonary artery.
Adapted from Balk RA: Optimum treatment of patients with severe sepsis and septic shock: Evidence in support of the recommendations. Dis Mon 2004;50:168-213.

particularly in patients with gram-negative bacteremia, elderly patients with *Streptococcus pneumoniae* pulmonary infection, and critically ill patients with bloodstream infections and/or hospital-acquired pneumonia. The use of early effective antibiotic therapy in critically ill patients is associated with significant reductions in infection-related and all-cause mortality rates. This benefit was present despite the addition of effective antibiotics once the culture and sensitivity data was available. This observation underscores the importance of initiating the correct initial empirical therapy. Correct antibiotic decisions are crucial in this era of increasing antibiotic resistance. It is important to know the ecology of organisms in your institution along with the antibiogram for the institution. Several recent reviews have been published to assist with the initial empirical antibiotic selection.

HEMODYNAMIC MANAGEMENT

Sepsis is characterized by vasodilatory or distributive shock, and there is an increase in vascular capacitance along with the decrease in the systemic vascular resistance. Septic patients are typically intravascularly volume depleted related to the presence of increased permeability as a result of endothelial cell injury and an increase in fluid loss coupled with a decrease in fluid replacement. Early recognition of significant hemodynamic derangements and restoration of normal organ perfusion are vital in preventing organ dysfunction and failure. The goal of hemodynamic resuscitation should be either to raise the mean arterial pressure above 60 to 65 mm Hg or to achieve a systolic BP of at least 90 mm Hg. The resuscitative efforts and the adequacy of tissue perfusion can be assessed at the bedside by monitoring heart rate, BP, orthostatic BP changes, mental status, hourly urine output, and skin perfusion.

The initial hemodynamic resuscitation should take the form of fluid for volume replacement. The fluid resuscitation can be accomplished with a variety of fluids including crystalloid, colloid, blood, synthetic starches, and hypertonic saline. Most clinicians accomplish the fluid resuscitation with intravenous (IV) infusion of either crystalloid or colloid. Bolus infusions are typically administered using the clinical response and/or measurements of central venous pressure (CVP) or pulmonary capillary wedge pressure (PCWP) as a guide. In many instances adequate volume resuscitation may be sufficient to restore normal perfusion pressure. The choice of crystalloids versus colloids for fluid resuscitation has been the subject of numerous studies and reviews. The Saline versus Albumin Fluid Evaluation (SAFE) trial, a large multicenter, prospective, randomized trial conducted by the Australia-New Zealand Critical Care Trials Group found that saline and 5% albumin (Albuminar-5) were equally effective for fluid resuscitation of the patient with shock. Currently there is no clear benefit of one fluid over the other. Crystalloids tend to be cheaper and more readily available, but a larger volume is required. Generally it may take significant liters of fluid to adequately resuscitate patients with severe septic shock. Colloids are typically more expensive and may be associated with coagulation abnormalities, but smaller volumes are needed.

Invasive vascular monitoring may be used to aid in the determination of adequate hemodynamic resuscitation. If a central venous catheter is present, the CVP can be measured to assess the adequacy of the intravascular volume status. In selected patients with hemodynamic insufficiency, the insertion of pulmonary artery catheters to measure the left-sided (and right-sided) filling pressures and the various hemodynamic parameters may be beneficial. A sphygmomanometer may be unreliable for BP measurement in hypotensive septic patients. Insertion of an arterial line may be required, especially if the patient is unresponsive to volume resuscitation and requires the addition of vasopressor therapy for hemodynamic resuscitation.

VASOPRESSOR MANAGEMENT

If adequate fluid resuscitation is insufficient to restore adequate hemodynamic function, then vasopressor and/or inotropic therapy will be necessary. There are a wide variety of vasoactive medications that are useful in the hemodynamic resuscitation of septic shock. Table 4 lists some of the more commonly used agents. Despite a wide range of possible agents, dopamine (Intropin) and norepinephrine (Levophed) are typically used in most clinical units. Some centers prefer to use phenylephrine (Neo-Synephrine) in patients with tachycardia or a history of arrhythmias because this pure alpha agent will cause less tachycardia and arrhythmias.

Unfortunately, there is a lack of large, prospective, randomized, protocol-controlled clinical trials that have compared dopamine (Intropin) to norepinephrine (Levophed) for the management of patients with septic shock. Therefore, until such data are available to guide the decision process, there is no clear benefit of one vasopressor strategy over the other, so either agent is acceptable in the management of hypotensive patients. Dopamine (Intropin) has been the preferred agent in many units, in part related to its ease of use, the concept that it improves splanchnic and renal perfusion, and its safety record. Recent clinical trial results have revealed that there is no specific beneficial effect of so called renal dose dopamine (Intropin) in preventing the development of renal failure or in decreasing the need for renal replacement therapy. In addition, the use of dopamine (Intropin) has been associated with an increase in the incidences of arrhythmias and a decrease in the gastric intramucosal pH (an indicator of splanchnic oxygen delivery and use). Norepinephrine (Levophed) is a potent vasoconstrictor that also has some increased inotropic and chronotropic effect on the heart. There is no decrease in renal or splanchnic perfusion as was once thought, and in fact there is an increase in the perfusion of these vascular beds as a result of the increased cardiac output and vasoconstriction. A large observational study of French septic shock patients who required high doses of vasopressor therapy, demonstrated a significant improvement in survival with the use of norepinephrine (Levophed) as compared to high doses of dopamine (Intropin) with or without the addition of epinephrine.

There has been renewed interest in the use of vasopressin in patients with vasodilatory shock. The initial release of stored vasopressin (Pitressin)[1] from the posterior pituitary during hypotension depletes the body's store of the hormone. As the shock state persists, there is a state of vasopressin deficiency, which some view as a hormone-deficiency state that is amenable to replacement therapy. Some centers are now infusing vasopressin (Pitressin)[1] as a

---

[1]Not FDA approved for this indication.

TABLE 4 Vasoactive Agents Commonly Used in the Management of Severe Sepsis[1]

Drug	Receptor Activity	Dose	Effect	Notes
Norepinephrine (Levophed)	α_1: 3+, α_2: 2+, β_1: 2+	0.03-1.5 µg/kg/min	Vasoconstriction	Little change in heart rate or CI. May decrease lactate.
Epinephrine	α_1: 3+, α_2: 3+, β_1: 3+, β_2: 2+	0.1-0.5 µg/kg/min	Increase stroke volume and CI	Unpredictable dose-response. Decrease splanchnic blood flow. Increase oxygen consumption and delivery.
Dopamine (Intropin)	α_1: 3+, α_2: 3+, β_1: 3+, β_2: 2+	<5. µg/kg/min	Vasodilation	Dopaminergic effects predominate. Dilation of renal, mesenteric, and coronary arteries. Increased GFR. Sodium excretion.
Dopamine (Intropin)	α_1: 3+, α_2: 3+, β_1: 3+, β_2: 2+	5-10 µg/kg/min	↑ Inotropy and chronotropy	β-adrenergic effects predominate. Increased CI primarily caused by increased stroke volume.
Dopamine (Intropin)	α_1: 3+, α_2: 3+, β_1: 3+, β_2: 2+	>10 µg/kg/min	Vasoconstriction	α-Adrenergic effects predominate.
Dobutamine (Dobutrex)	α_1: 1+, v_2: 1+, β_1: 3+, β_2: 2+	2-20 µg/kg/min	↑ Inotropy and chronotropy	25%-50% increase in CI. Decreases PAOP.
Phenylephrine (Neo-Synephrine)	α_1: 3v	0.5-8 µg/kg/min	Vasoconstriction	Increases MAP without change in heart rate. CI may decrease.
Vasopressin (Pitressin)[1]	V_1	0.01-0.04 U/min IV	Vasoconstriction	Hormone replacement therapy may potentiate the vasoconstrictor effect of endogenous catecholamines or act directly on a V_1 receptor.

[1]Not FDA approved for this indication.
Abbreviations: CI = cardiac index; GFR = glomerular filtration rate; IV = intravenous; MAP = mean aortic pressure; PAOP = pulmonary artery occluded pressure.
Modified from Steel A, Bihari D: Choice of catecholamine: Does it matter? Curr Opin Crit Care 2000;6:347-353.

hormone replacement therapy in a constant, nonescalating dose to augment dopamine (Intropin) or the pressor effects of norepinephrine (Levophed). The importance of early goal-oriented hemodynamic resuscitation was emphasized in a recent trial comparing this technique with more traditional resuscitation efforts. The early goal-oriented protocol was associated with significant improvement in ICU and hospital survival and significantly fewer deaths from sudden hemodynamic collapse.

Some patients with severe sepsis and septic shock have a reversible biventricular myocardial dysfunction, which has been attributed to circulating TNF-α, IL-1, and/or nitric oxide that are elaborated as part of the SIRS response. Ventricular dilatation and a reduced ejection fraction comprise this myocardial depression. Inotropic agents such as dobutamine (Dobutrex) or epinephrine can improve the myocardial contractility and hemodynamic function in these patients. By increasing stroke volume and heart rate, dobutamine (Dobutrex) increases the cardiac index. Although epinephrine can also increase the cardiac index, its use should be limited in the septic patient because it can impair splanchnic blood flow and increase systemic and regional lactate concentrations.

SUPPORT OXYGENATION AND VENTILATION

Abnormalities of the respiratory system are some of the most common evidence of organ systems involvement in sepsis. Septic patients should be assessed for adequacy of oxygenation, oxygen delivery, ventilation, and the ability to protect the airway. Septic patients commonly have abnormalities of oxygenation and increased work of breathing.

Patients who are hypoxemic should be given supplemental oxygen with a goal of achieving arterial oxygen saturation of at least 90%.

Another decision to make in caring for the septic patient is the need and timing for endotracheal intubation and ventilatory support. Acute lung injury (ALI) and ARDS are relatively common manifestations of pulmonary dysfunction in the patient with severe sepsis and septic shock. Up to 35% of septic patients may manifest ARDS. The goal of mechanical ventilation is to maintain the PaO_2 in the 55 to 70 mm Hg range while keeping the FiO_2 below 60% (0.6). The traditional approach to mechanically ventilating patients with ALI and ARDS has been to employ tidal volumes in the 10 to 15 mL/kg range. The Acute Respiratory Distress Syndrome Network (ARDSNet) trial of low tidal volume ventilation of 6 mL/kg ideal body weight, coupled with maintaining an end-inspiratory plateau pressure up to 30 cm H_2O and a nomogram for positive end-expiratory pressure (PEEP) titration based on FiO_2, and oxygenation goals demonstrated an overall decrease in hospital mortality along with an increase in ventilator-free and organ failure–free days.

The risk of infection and ventilator-associated complications increases with the duration of ventilatory support. Patients should be removed from the ventilator as soon as they no longer need mechanical ventilatory support. The use of weaning protocols implemented by trained ICU support staff have been shown to speed the weaning process and improve the overall process of extubating the critically ill patient. It is also important to use sedation and analgesia appropriately in this critically ill population. Excessive sedation and analgesia have been linked to prolonged stays on mechanical ventilatory support and increased complications.

In a large, multicenter, controlled trial conducted in critically ill patients without ischemic cardiac disease or acute blood loss, the restrictive practice of packed red blood cell (RBC) transfusions in the management of anemia and low hemoglobin (Hb) levels (between 7.0 and 9.0 g/dL) was shown to provide adequate oxygen delivery to the tissues and in a subgroup of younger patients and less ill patients was found to be associated with a lower mortality rate compared to a more liberal transfusion policy with Hb levels maintained between 10.0 and 12.0 g/dL. The use of weekly recombinant erythropoietin (Epogen)[1] has also been shown to reduce the need for transfusions in critically ill patients. Aggressive use of packed RBC transfusions in an effort to achieve super-normal oxygen delivery states should be discouraged.

SUPPORTIVE CARE FOR THE CRITICALLY ILL PATIENT

Patients with severe sepsis and septic shock are critically ill and susceptible to the multiple complications common in the critically ill population. These complications include deep vein thrombosis and pulmonary emboli, stress-related gastrointestinal (GI) bleeding, nosocomial infections, MODS, and critical illness polyneuropathy/myopathy. Patients in the ICU with sepsis or septic shock should receive prophylaxis for deep vein thrombosis with unfractionated heparin or low-molecular-weight heparin, unless they have contraindications for their use. Pneumatic compression devices can be used if they have a coagulopathy or increased risk of bleeding. Prophylaxis for stress-related GI bleeding may be accomplished with H_2-recoptor blockers, proton pump inhibitors,[1] sucralfate (Carafate)[1] or early enteral feeding.

Nutritional support of the patient with severe sepsis is important from multiple standpoints. Proper nutrition is important to maintain the necessary immune function during the catabolic septic metabolic process. Enteral administration of nutrition may prevent stress-related GI bleeding and may prevent the translocation of bowel organisms and/or endotoxin by maintaining the integrity of the GI tract's mucosal barrier function. Nutritional requirements during severe sepsis and septic shock have been addressed by numerous organizations and medical societies. Adequate nutrition is responsible for improved wound healing, decreasing susceptibility of critically ill patients to infection and optimizing immune function. The following nutritional guidelines have been recommended for patients with sepsis:

- Daily caloric intake: 25 to 30 kcal/kg per usual body weight per day
- Protein: 1.3 to 2.0 g/kg per day
- Glucose: 30% to 70% of total nonprotein calories to maintain serum glucose fewer than 150 mg/dL
- Lipids: 15% to 30% of total nonprotein calories
- Omega-6 polyunsaturated fatty acids: reduce in septic patients, maintaining that level, which avoids deficiency of essential fatty acids (7% of total calories—generally 1 g/kg per day)

Metabolic management also includes correction of electrolyte abnormalities as well as tight control of blood sugar, which may require constant insulin infusion. In a report of postsurgical predominantly ventilated patients, tight glucose control aimed at keeping the blood sugar between 80 and 110 mg/dL was associated with a significant improvement in ICU and hospital survival. There were four times more deaths from multiple organ failure secondary to a proven septic focus in the group that did not receive the tight glucose control.

Innovative Therapies in Severe Sepsis and Septic Shock

Severe sepsis and septic shock have continued to be associated with significant mortality despite the improvements in our understanding of the septic process, the use of powerful antibiotic agents, and the provision of basic sepsis management. Advances in technology have also brought forward antibodies, receptor blockers, and other innovative agents designed to interrupt or block aspects of the septic cascade. The majority of innovative experimental strategies were directed at various components of the proinflammatory response evident during the initial phases of SIRS and sepsis. Because most of these trials were unsuccessful, there has been a shift in the target for interruption toward a later stage aspect of the septic cascade. A number of these recent strategies have taken aim at the coagulation system to inhibit the generation of thrombin and fibrin, which may be instrumental in the disorder of the microcirculation that may be at least partially responsible for the organ system dysfunction and MODS seen in severe sepsis and SIRS.

CORTICOSTEROID THERAPY

Experimental studies in animal models of sepsis and septic shock have demonstrated improved survival with the pretreatment or early treatment with high doses of corticosteroids. Such doses in humans with severe sepsis and septic shock have not been associated with significant improvements in survival except for one study. As a result of multiple trials of high-dose steroids in patients with severe sepsis showing no benefit and potentially harm this practice has been abandoned. Recently, the observation that basal cortisol levels and the cortisol response to the administration of adrenocorticotropic hormone (ACTH) (Corticotropin)[1] could predict survival in patients with severe sepsis, and septic shock has drawn attention back to the use of steroid therapy. A French study of patients with septic shock demonstrated that a basal cortisol level of up to 34 µg/dL along with the ability to increase the cortisol level by at least 9 µg/dL was associated with a 74% survival rate. In comparison, patients who had a basal cortisol level of more than 34 µg/dL and were unable to increase their cortisol level by at least 9 µg/dL had an 18% survival rate. The investigators proposed that some patients with septic shock have a state of relative adrenal insufficiency or problems with their glucocorticoid receptors that can be improved with the use of more physiologic corticosteroid replacement therapy. A recent multicenter, prospective,

---

[1]Not FDA approved for this indication.

[1]Not FDA approved for this indication.

randomized, controlled trial of 300 patients with vasopressor-dependent septic shock who were all receiving mechanical ventilatory support and were resuscitated according to a defined protocol demonstrated an improved survival rate in patients who failed to increased their basal cortisol level by more than 9 μg/dL and were given physiologic corticosteroid replacement therapy. For this trial the physiologic corticosteroid replacement therapy consisted of 50 mg of IV hydrocortisone (Solu-Cortef)[1] every 6 hours for 7 days combined with once-daily fludrocortisone (Florinef)[1] given enterally at 50 μg per day. The authors of this trial concluded that physiologic corticosteroid therapy is beneficial and should be administered to vasopressor-dependent patients in septic shock who manifest relative adrenal insufficiency as defined by the failure to increase the cortisol level by more than 9 μg/dL after ACTH stimulation.

HIGH-VOLUME CONTINUOUS VENOVENOUS HEMOFILTRATION THERAPY

The use of high-volume, continuous hemofiltration (either continuous arteriovenous or venovenous) benefits the hemodynamic course and outcome in patients with intractable circulatory failure resulting from septic shock. The use of this form of management is expensive, requires defined expertise, and may be associated with metabolic and coagulation abnormalities. Further studies are needed to determine if this mode of therapy improves outcome in septic patients. Its use should probably be limited to patients with renal indications for hemofiltration.

ANTITHROMBOTIC THERAPY

Newer therapies have been directed toward inhibitors of the coagulation system as a potential therapeutic strategy for patients with severe sepsis and septic shock. Earlier therapies targeting the pro-inflammatory stage have shown little benefit in reducing mortality. Among the therapies that have been used are Antithrombin, tissue factor pathway inhibitor (TFPI),* and activated protein C replacement therapy.

Antithrombin (AT)* is an endogenous serine protease that has antithrombotic and anti-inflammatory properties. In an early trial in a small number of patients, the administration of AT to patients with septic shock and disseminated intravascular coagulation demonstrated a trend toward improved survival. Subsequently a large multicenter, prospective, randomized, double-blind, placebo-controlled trial was conducted, which unfortunately showed no difference in mortality compared to placebo at 30, 60, and 90 days.

TFPI* inhibits factor VIIa within the factor VIIa/tissue factor complex, after first binding and inactivating factor Xa. Recently, a phase 3 multicenter, prospective, randomized, double-blind, placebo-controlled trial has been completed and failed to demonstrate a significant benefit in the primary endpoint, which was 28-day all-cause mortality.

As with antithrombin, the protein C system is one of the endogenous antithrombotic agents. Drotrecogin alfa (activated) (Xigris) is recombinant human activated protein C. A recent phase 3 trial was stopped after the second interim analysis demonstrated a significant survival benefit associated with the use of activated protein C versus placebo in 1690 patients with severe sepsis and septic shock. Treatment with a 96-hour infusion of drotrecogin alfa (activated) (Xigris) produced a 6.1% absolute risk reduction and a 19.4% relative risk reduction in the 28-day all-cause mortality in patients with severe sepsis ($P = 0.005$) The drotrecogin alfa (activated) (Xigris)-treated population experienced more serious bleeding complications (3.5%) compared to the placebo group (2.0%), and this difference trended toward significance. These results suggest that for every 66 patients treated with drotrecogin alfa (activated) (Xigris), 1 additional serious bleeding event would occur. The number needed to treat to save an additional life was 16.

The Food and Drug Administration (FDA) and 19 other regulatory bodies in other countries (including the European Union) have approved the use of drotrecogin alfa (activated) (Xigris) for the treatment of severe sepsis in adult patients with a high risk of mortality. The FDA gives the example of using the Acute Physiology and Chronic Health Evaluation (APACHE) II to estimate the risk of death (APACHE II score ≥25) and other means such as the number of dysfunctional organs to determine the target population of patients. Currently, the safety and efficacy of drotrecogin alfa (activated) (Xigris) in pediatric patients has not been determined. Contraindications to the use of drotrecogin alfa (activated) (Xigris) include patients with known sensitivity to drotrecogin alfa (activated) (Xigris) and patients with a high risk of death from or significant morbidity associated with bleeding. This group would include patients with active internal bleeding, recent (within 3 months) hemorrhagic stroke, recent (within 2 months) intracranial or intraspinal surgery or severe head trauma, trauma with increased risk of life-threatening bleeding, the presence of an epidural catheter, an intracranial neoplasm, or mass lesion or evidence of cerebral herniation. Septic patients who have undergone surgery within the prior month were also found to have a higher mortality rate when given activated protein C and clinicians are warned about using this agent in this group of patients.

Prognosis

Despite the tremendous advances in our appreciation of the pathophysiologic processes that comprise the septic response coupled with improved antibiotics and technologic support of the critically ill, the mortality rate for patients with severe sepsis and septic shock remains high. Clinical trials have reported placebo-group mortality rates attributable to severe sepsis and septic shock of 20% to 50%, with mortality rates up to 80% to 85% with septic shock and multiple organ failure. This high rate of morbidity and mortality demands an aggressive approach for early diagnosis and treatment in an attempt to improve the outcome of these critically ill patients. A number of factors have been found to impact survival including, age, co-morbid condition, site and type of infection, severity of illness, the number, and specific organ system failures. In addition, a patient's genetic makeup and/or gender may have a dramatic impact on whether they develop sepsis, as well as the severity, clinical manifestations, and outcome of the sepsis. Also, survivors of sepsis have increased 6- and

---

[1]Not FDA approved for this indication.
*Investigational drug in the United States.

12-month mortality rates compared to nonseptic critically ill patients. There is a reduced quality of life and more health-related issues in patients who have survived an episode of sepsis. These observations underscore the importance of early aggressive management of the septic patient and suggest that our future focus should also be directed toward prevention of sepsis.

REFERENCES

Angus DC, Linde-Zwirble WT, Lidicker J, et al: Epidemiology of severe sepsis in the United States: Analysis of incidence, outcome, and associated costs of care. Crit Care Med 2001;29:1303-1310.

Annane D, Sebille V, Charpentier C, et al: Effect of treatment with low doses of hydrocortisone and fludrocortisone on mortality in patients with septic shock. JAMA 2002;288:862-871.

Balk RA: Optimum treatment of patients with severe sepsis and septic shock: Evidence in support of the recommendations. Dis Mon 2004; 50:168-213.

Bernard GR, Vincent J-L, Laterre P-F, et al: Efficacy and safety of recombinant human activated protein C for severe sepsis. N Engl J Med 2001;344:699-709.

Dellinger RP, Carlet JM, Masur H, et al: Surviving Sepsis Campaign guidelines for management of severe sepsis and septic shock. Crit Care Med 2004;32(3):858-873.

Levy MM, Fink MP, Marshall JC, et al: 2001 SCCM/ESICM/ACCP/ ATS/SIS International sepsis definitions conference. Crit Care Med 2003;31:1250-1256.

Martin GS, Mannino DM, Eaton S, et al: The epidemiology of sepsis in the United States from 1979 through 2000. N Engl J Med 2003;348: 1546-1554.

Rivers E, Nguyen B, Havstad S, et al: Early goal-directed therapy in the treatment of severe sepsis and septic shock. N Engl J Med 2001;345:1368-1377.

Steel A, Bihari D: Choice of catecholamine: Does it matter? Curr Opin Crit Care 2000;6:347-353.

The Acute Respiratory Distress Syndrome Network: Ventilation with lower tidal volumes as compared with traditional tidal volumes for acute lung injury and the acute respiratory distress syndrome. N Engl J Med 2000;342:1301-1308.

The SAFE Study Investigators: A comparison of albumin and saline for fluid resuscitation in the intensive care unit. N Engl J Med 2004; 350:2247-2256.

Van den Berghe G, Wouters P, Weekers F, et al: Intensive insulin therapy in critically ill patients. N Engl J Med 2001;345:1359-1367.

Brucellosis

Method of
Javier Solera, PhD

Human brucellosis is a zoonosis caused by facultative intracellular gram-negative bacteria of the genus *Brucella*. Six species exist, of which four cause disease in humans: *Brucella abortus, Brucella melitensis, Brucella suis,* and *Brucella canis;* animal reservoirs are cattle, sheep and goats, pigs, and dogs, respectively. More recently, marine mammals have been recognized as additional animal reservoirs for *Brucella* species; *Brucella cetaceae* and *Brucella pinnipediae* are the newly proposed species names.

In animals, brucellosis is a chronic infection resulting in abortion and sterility. A large bacterial load is present in milk, urine, and the products of pregnancy. Human beings may acquire the organism by ingesting unpasteurized dairy products, by inhaling infected aerosols, or from direct contact with secretions and blood of diseased animals.

Clinical Manifestations

Not everyone who has contact with *Brucella* specimens develops active brucellosis. For example, more than 50% of slaughterhouse workers and up to 33% of veterinarians have high anti-*Brucella* antibody titers but no history of recognized clinical infection. Persons who develop acute, symptomatic brucellosis may manifest a wide spectrum of symptoms including fever, sweats, malaise, anorexia, headache, arthralgias, myalgias, backache, and weight loss. Fever may become undulant if left untreated. Examination frequently shows nothing abnormal, apart from fever; however, lymphadenopathy, splenomegaly, or hepatomegaly are found in some cases. Complications of brucellosis may affect any organ and occur anywhere in the body. Apart from abscess formation complications include spondylitis, sacroiliitis, osteomyelitis, meningitis, and orchitis (Table 1). The main cause of mortality, however, is endocarditis. The most important factor in poor outcome is probably delay in initiating effective antibiotic treatment.

 CURRENT DIAGNOSIS

Initial Evaluation

- Seek a history of exposure to *Brucella* (jobs, travel, unpasteurized dairy products).
- Historic evaluation should include determination of the length of symptoms, and presence and character of focal disease.
- Seek underlying conditions that contraindicate certain specific antibiotics.

Laboratory Tests

- Blood cultures (maintain cultures for at least 30 days)
- Serologic test: standard tube agglutination (with or without 2-mercaptoethanol test), rose Bengal test, anti-*Brucella* Coombs test, or enzyme-linked immunosorbent assay, IgG, and IgM tests
- Complete blood count and erythrocyte sedimentation rate (or C-reactive protein)
- Chemistry profile including renal and liver function test

Special Tests if Focal or Complications Are Suggested by History or Physical Examination

- Magnetic resonance imaging or computerized tomography (if or when vertebral osteomyelitis, sacroiliitis, hip arthritis, or hepatic and/or splenic abscess is suspected)
- Echocardiogram (if or when endocarditis is suspected)
- Cerebrospinal fluid analysis (if neurobrucellosis is suspected), consisting of white cell and differential counts; measurements of protein and glucose; serologic test; Gram stain; and culture for bacteria

TABLE 1 Complications of Brucellosis

Complication	Type	Comment
Skeletal	Arthritis, spondylitis, sacroiliitis, osteomyelitis, bursitis, tenosynovitis	• Occur in approximately 20%–85% of patients • In children, arthritis of hip and knee joints most common • Unilateral sacroiliitis common in young adults • Spondylitis most serious complication; frequent paraspinal and epidural abscess
Neurologic	Meningoencephalitis, cerebral abscess, myelitis, neuritis, depression and psychosis, cerebral venous thrombosis	• Occur in approximately 2%–5% of patients • Cerebrospinal fluid examination reveals a lymphocytic pleocytosis with elevated protein and normal or low glucose levels • Gram stain and culture have low sensitivity • Computerized tomography may demonstrate basal ganglia calcification and abscesses
Genitourinary	Epididymo-orchitis, prostatitis, cystitis, interstitial nephritis, glomerulonephritis	Unilateral epididymo-orchitis frequent in young men
Cardiovascular	Endocarditis, myocarditis, and pericarditis, endarteritis, thrombophlebitis	• Occur in <2% of cases but are the most common cause of death • Common embolic phenomena • Valve replacement warranted in most cases • Mycotic aneurysms of the aorta and large vessels are rare
Hepatobiliary	Nongranulomatous and granulomatous hepatitis, hepatic abscess, cirrhosis, acute cholecystitis	• Abnormal liver function tests occur in 30%–90% of patients • Percutaneous drainage and prolonged course of antibiotics
Spleen	Splenomegaly, spleen abscess, splenic calcifications	Surgical drainage of localized suppurative lesions and splenectomy may be of value if antimicrobial treatment is ineffective
Pulmonary	Hilar adenopathy, perihilar infiltrates, nodular lesions, lung abscess, interstitial pattern, and pleural effusions	Cough and other pulmonary symptoms in approximately 15%–25% of patients
Hematologic	Anemia, leukopenias, thrombocytopenia and pancytopenia, hemophagocytosis, disseminated intravascular coagulation	• More common in patients with *Brucella melitensis* • Hemophagocytosis
Cutaneous	Rashes, papules, petechiae, purpura, cutaneous granulomatous vasculitis and erythema nodosum	• Occur in approximately 5% of patients • Many transient and often nonspecific skin lesions have been described
Other	Uveitis, thyroiditis, colitis	

Diagnosis

Diagnosis depends on keen awareness of possible infection and a thorough occupational and travel history. Definitive diagnosis requires isolation of the organism from blood culture or other clinical samples of infected patients. However, diagnosis of brucellosis is often made serologically, most frequently by standard tube agglutination (STA), measuring antibody to *B. abortus* antigen. A fourfold or greater rise in titer to 1:160 or higher is considered significant. This test equally detects antibodies to *B. abortus*, *B. suis*, and *B. melitensis* but not to *B. canis*. Diagnostic methods based on the polymerase chain reaction (PCR) have been developed in the past two decades to detect *Brucella* DNA in human samples. Proven more sensitive than culture in patients with relapse or focalized brucellosis, PCR is particularly useful when an antibiotic therapy has been administered before clinical specimen collection for *Brucella* culture.

Treatment

Antimicrobial therapy is useful for shortening the natural course of the disease, decreasing the incidence of complications, and preventing relapse. Appropriate antibiotics should have high in vitro activity and good intracellular penetration. Current treatment recommendations are based on the results of published scientific studies and clinical experience.

TREATMENT OF ACUTE BRUCELLOSIS IN ADULTS WITHOUT COMPLICATIONS OR FOCAL DISEASE

Adults without complications or focal disease should be treated as outpatients and, apart from microbiologic studies, do not require extensive workups to establish the diagnosis. The preferred regimen is combination therapy with doxycycline (Vibramycin) (100 mg orally, twice daily for 45 days) and streptomycin (1 g intramuscularly, once daily for the first 14 days). Gentamicin (Garamycin)[1] (5 mg/kg/day, once daily) may be substituted for streptomycin. In patients for whom tetracyclines are contraindicated, no other antibiotic combination is as effective as doxycycline-streptomycin or doxycycline-rifampin (Rifadin)[1] in the treatment of acute brucellosis.

---

[1]Not FDA approved for this indication.

Summary for patients with acute brucellosis according to quality of evidence.

DRUG REGIMENS	DOSAGE (DURATION)	STRENGTH OF RECOMMENDATION (GRADE OF EVIDENCE)*	COMMENT
Combination Regimens			
Doxycycline (Vibramycin) plus Streptomycin	• 100 mg/12 h (30–45 d) • 1 gm/24 h (14–21 d)	A (I)	Classic regimen, used widely and successfully since 1950s; >90% of patients cured
Doxycycline plus Gentamicin (Garamycin)[1]	• 100 mg/12 h (30–45 d) • 5 mg × kg/24 h IM (7–14 d)	B (II)	Gentamicin may be substituted for streptomycin
Doxycycline plus Rifampin (Rifadin)[1]	• 100 mg/12 h (45 d) • 600–900 mg/24 h (45 d)	B (I)	Recommended by World Health Organization Expert Committee on Brucellosis regimen 17% relapses versus 5% doxycycline + streptomycin
Rifampin (Rifadin) plus Ofloxacin (Floxin)[1]	• 600 mg/24 h (42 d) • 200 mg /12 h (42 d)	B (I)	• Only two small comparative open studies • Relapses 3.2% and failures 1.50%
Rifampin (Rifadin) plus Ciprofloxacin (Cipro)[1]	• 600 mg /12 h (30–45 d) • 500 mg/12 h (30–45 d)	C (I)	Clinical trials have produced conflicting results (relapses 15%)
Rifampin (Rifadin) plus Cotrimoxazole (TMP-SMZ,[1] Bactrim)[†‡]	• 15 mg × kg/24 h (45 d) • 240–1200 mg/12 h (45 d)	C (II)	Interaction of rifampin and cotrimoxazole has been described
Rifampin (Rifadin) plus Gentamicin (Garamycin)[†]	• 100 mg/12 h (30–45 d) • 5 mg × kg/24 h IM (5–7 d)	C (I)	Only one controlled trial
Cotrimoxazole (TMP-SMZ) plus Garamycin[†]	• 100 mg/12 h (30–45 d) 5 mg × kg/24 h IM (5–7 d)	C (I)	Clinical trials have produced conflicting results (relapses range 0%–60%)
Doxycycline plus TMP-SMZ	• 100 mg/12 h (60 d) • 240–1200 mg/12 h (60 d)	C (I)	Only a comparative open study
Monotherapy Regimens			
Doxycycline	100 mg/12 h (45 d)	C (I)	More relapses (14%) than combination regimen doxycycline plus streptomycin (5%)
Rifampin (Rifadin)[‡]	15 mg × kg/24 h (45 d)	D (II)	Emergence of rifampin-resistant strains Recommended for pregnant women by World Health Organization Expert Committee on Brucellosis regimen

DRUG REGIMENS	DOSAGE (DURATION)	STRENGTH OF RECOMMENDATION (GRADE OF EVIDENCE)*	COMMENT
Cotrimoxazole (TMP-SMZ)	240–1200 mg/ 12 h (45–180 d)	D (I)	Treatment during prolonged periods with cotrimoxazole has produced favorable results in children
Ciprofloxacin	500 mg/12 h (30–45 d)	E (II)	• Relapse rate, 21%–66% • Emergence of ciprofloxacin-resistant strains

*Strength of recommendation (quality of evidence supporting the recommendation).

†Recommended regimen for children younger than 8 y.

‡Recommended regimens for pregnant and nursing women.

1Not FDA approved for this indication.

Abbreviations: A = preferred (should generally be offered); B = acceptable alternative; C = offer when A or B regimens cannot be given; D = should generally not be offered; E = should never be offered; I = at least one randomized trial with clinical endpoints; II = nonrandomized clinical trials or conducted in other populations; III = expert opinion; TMP-SMZ = trimethoprim-sulfamethoxazole; IM = intramuscularly.

THERAPY IN PATIENTS WITH FOCAL DISEASE

The more common complications of brucellosis are summarized in Table 1. Except for a few localized complications for which surgery is necessary, antimicrobial agents constitute the basic treatment for focal brucellosis. The preferred regimen is the same as for uncomplicated brucellosis. However, duration of therapy must be individualized. Some patients, especially those with endocarditis, neurobrucellosis, or spondylitis, may require longer courses of treatment. Surgery should be considered for patients with endocarditis, cerebral or epidural abscess, spleen or hepatic abscess, or other antibiotic-resistant abscesses.

PREGNANCY

Increased rates of spontaneous abortion, premature delivery, and intrauterine infection with fetal death have been described among pregnant women with clinical evidence of brucellosis. Women who received early diagnosis and adequate treatment had successful maternal and fetal outcomes. Tetracyclines and streptomycin should be avoided during pregnancy. Rifampin (Rifadin)1 (900 mg, once daily for 6 weeks) is considered the regimen of choice. Cotrimoxazole (trimethoprim-sulfamethoxazole [TMP-SMZ]1 Bactrim) plus rifampin is an alternative regimen.

CHILDREN YOUNGER THAN 8 YEARS OLD

Children often have fewer or milder symptoms than adult patients. Tetracyclines are generally contraindicated for children younger than 8 years old. The preferred regimen is rifampin (Rifadin) with cotrimoxazole (TMP-SMZ)1 for 6 to 8 weeks. An alternative regimen is rifampin (Rifadin) or cotrimoxazole (TMP-SMZ) for 8 weeks with gentamicin (Garamycin)1 (5 mg/kg/day for the first 5 days). Treatment over prolonged periods (>6 months) with cotrimoxazole (TMP-SMZ) has produced favorable results in some clinical studies.

RISK FACTORS AND THERAPY FOR RELAPSES

Relapse occurs in 5% to 30% of patients, usually 1 to 6 months after initial infection, and tends to be milder than the original attack. The bacterial isolate from a relapsed patient usually demonstrates the same antibiotic-susceptibility pattern as the isolate obtained during the original episode. Consequently, nearly all relapse cases respond to a repeated course of antimicrobial therapy.

CONCLUSION

Therapy for human brucellosis should be prescribed with the following rules in mind. The diagnosis of brucellosis must be sound (clinical evidence of disease supported by bacteriologic or serologic tests), and focal disease or complications should be identified. The choice of regimen and duration of antimicrobial therapy should be based on the presence of focal disease and underlying conditions that contraindicate certain antibiotics (i.e., pregnant patients and children younger than 8 years old). Most individuals with acute brucellosis respond well to a combination of doxycycline plus aminoglycosides or rifampin for 6 weeks. Patients with focal disease (such as spondylitis) may require longer courses of antibiotics, depending on clinical evolution. Patients with persistent symptoms following extended antibiotic therapy for whom focal disease

1Not FDA approved for this indication.

1Not FDA approved for this indication.

or relapse have been ruled out, pose a difficult clinical management problem. This disabling syndrome, sometimes called *chronic brucellosis*, is similar to chronic fatigue syndrome and must be treated symptomatically.

REFERENCES

Colmenero JD, Reguera JM, Martos F, et al: Complications associated with *Brucella melitensis* infection: A study of 530 cases. Medicine (Baltimore) 1997;76(2):139.

Madkour MM: Brucellosis. In Fauci AS, et al (eds.): Harrison's Principles of Internal Medicine (14th ed.) 1998; pp 969–971.

Navarro E, Segura JC, Castaño MJ, Solera J: Use of quantitative real-time PCR to monitor the evolution of *B. melitensis* DNA load during therapy and post-therapy follow-up in patients with brucellosis. Clin Infect Dis (in press).

Solera J, Martinez-Alfaro E, Espinosa A: Recognition and optimum treatment of brucellosis. Drugs 1997;53(2):245–256.

Varicella (Chickenpox)

Method of
Charles Grose, MD

Chickenpox is caused by varicella zoster virus (VZV). After chickenpox occurs, VZV enters the sensory nerve and establishes latency in the dorsal root ganglia along the spinal cord. When VZV reactivates in late adulthood, the virus causes the disease known as shingles (herpes zoster).

Pathogenesis of Chickenpox

Chickenpox is an airborne infection. The virus first infects the mucosa tissues of the nose and subsequently establishes an infection in the tonsils or lymph nodes around the neck. After 4 to 6 cycles of replication, the primary viremia occurs (Figure 1). The virus then disperses to multiple organs in the body. After a second period of replication, the second viremia occurs. The virus is carried within lymphocytes in the bloodstream. The vesicular lesions occur after the virus exits the capillaries and enters the epidermis.

CURRENT DIAGNOSIS

- Diagnosis of chickenpox is usually made by observation or rash.
- Diagnosis is confirmed by a rapid viral diagnosis kit performed on a vesicle smear.
- Diagnosis of past varicella infection is made by serology.
- Commercial antibody kits may not be sensitive enough to detect serum antibody after varicella vaccination.

Epidemiology after Approval of the Vaccine

The varicella vaccine was approved for administration to children in the United States in 1995, and the vast majority of states have approved the administration of varicella vaccine to all young children. Approximately 4 million cases of chickenpox occurred annually in the United States prior to 1995. There were also approximately 100 deaths annually, the vast majority in otherwise healthy children, and more than 14,000 hospitalizations per year.

More than 10 years later, the effect of universal varicella immunization in the United States is dramatic. The number of hospitalizations and deaths was reduced by 75%. Similarly, the total number of cases of chickenpox in the United States has also decreased dramatically. Nevertheless, more than half a million cases of chickenpox will probably continue to occur annually. These cases will include many immunocompromised children who remain unimmunized.

ADMINISTRATION OF VARICELLA VACCINE

Varicella vaccine is a live attenuated virus. Each dose of vaccine (0.5 mL) is administered subcutaneously. The virus must replicate in the infected child for an immune response to occur (Figure 2). The initial virus replication can cause a few vesicles near the site of infection. The replication can also lead to a viremia with a short-lived rash anywhere on the body. The vaccine virus can, in very few cases, replicate to a sufficient extent that the infection transfers to another person who will subsequently develop a mild case of vaccine-related chickenpox. As of July 2005, a single dose of varicella vaccine was recommended for every child between 12 and 18 months of age. For catch-up immunizations of an older child who has never been immunized, one vaccination is recommended for any child up to 12 years of age. Two varicella vaccinations separated by 4 to 8 weeks are recommended for those 13 years and older.

RISK FACTORS FOR BREAKTHROUGH CHICKENPOX

Breakthrough chickenpox refers to a wild-type chickenpox that is usually a mild illness with less than 50 vesicles that occurs in children given varicella vaccine at least 42 days previously. Thus, breakthrough chickenpox is a form of vaccine failure. Breakthrough chickenpox was thought to be relatively uncommon during the prelicensure clinical studies. However, by 2000 it was apparent that breakthrough chickenpox was not a rare event. Several reports documented large outbreaks of wild-type chickenpox in immunized children who are attending large child care facilities or grade schools.

The most cited risk factors are twofold. The first risk factor is the number of years after vaccination, especially 5 or more years. The second risk factor is the age of immunization, namely 12 to 15 months. When children immunized at 12 to 15 months of age were compared with those immunized at 18 months or older, children in the younger age group were more likely to contract breakthrough chickenpox. Therefore, it is suggested that children younger than 15 months should not receive the varicella vaccination.

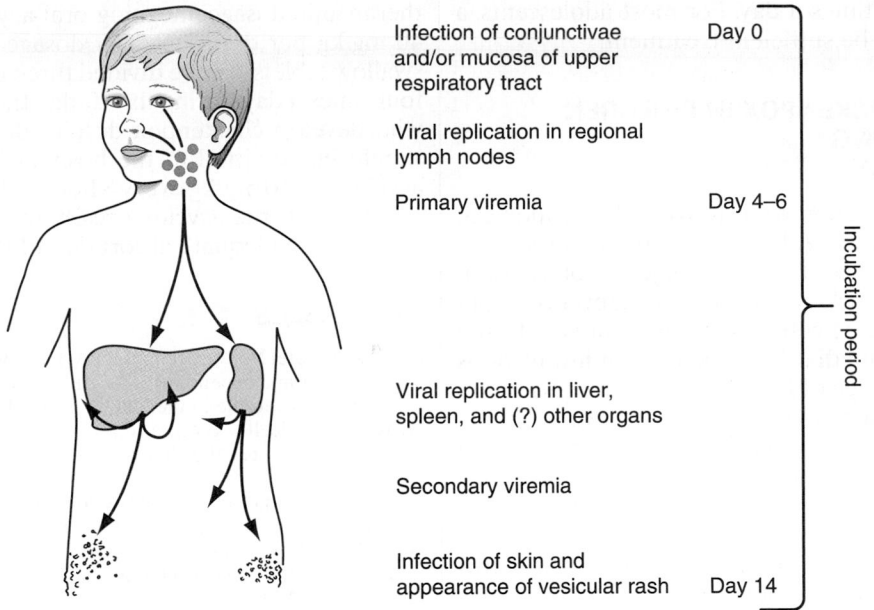

FIGURE 1. Diagrammatic representation of the pathogenesis of acute varicella infection. There are two viremias during the 14-day incubation period. The first viremia occurs after local replication at the site of infection. The typical chickenpox rash appears at the end of the second viremia. See Grose (2005) for a more detailed description.

Infection of conjunctivae and/or mucosa of upper respiratory tract — Day 0

Viral replication in regional lymph nodes

Primary viremia — Day 4–6

Viral replication in liver, spleen, and (?) other organs

Secondary viremia

Infection of skin and appearance of vesicular rash — Day 14

Incubation period

Treatment

TREATMENT OF SEVERE CHICKENPOX IN HEALTHY CHILDREN

Chickenpox is considered a more severe disease in children younger than 1 year and in postpubertal adolescents. VZV is highly susceptible to acyclovir and two second-generation antiviral agents: famciclovir (Famvir) and valacyclovir (Valtrex). Acyclovir is now a generic drug and very economical. Every case of chickenpox in a child younger than 1 year should be treated with acyclovir. The oral dosage is 20 mg/kg four times a day for 5 to 7 days. Chickenpox in children older than 1 year can also be treated with acyclovir to reduce the severity and duration of disease. The maximum dosage is 800 mg four times a day. Acyclovir is available in a liquid suspension and tablets containing 200, 400, or 800 mg. The 800-mg tablet is very large and may be difficult for some children to swallow.

Famciclovir (Famvir) or valacyclovir (Valtrex) are the preferred antiviral agents for adolescents because these are better adsorbed than acyclovir. However, they are much more expensive. The dosage of famciclovir (Famvir) is 500 mg orally three times a day. The dosage of valacyclovir

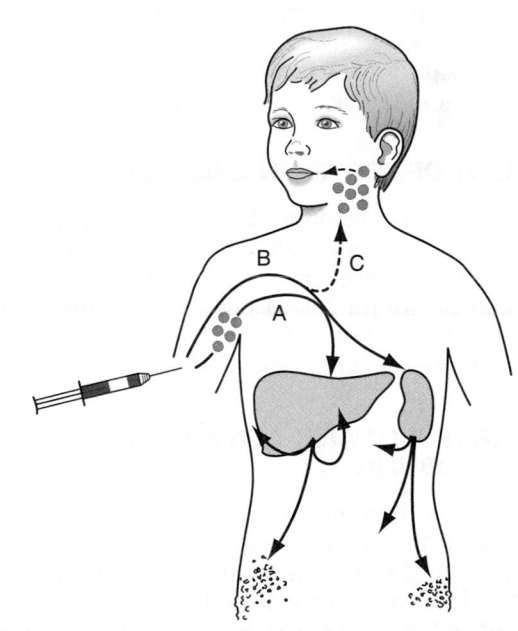

FIGURE 2. Pathways of infection following administration of varicella vaccine. Pathway A shows a rash that sometimes appears at the site of injection after local replication of the virus. Pathway B shows a viremia with appearance of a few small papulovesicular lesions on the skin distant from the site of injection. Pathway C shows the virus as it travels to the respiratory tract where infection can be spread on rare occasions to other individuals. See Grose (2005) for a more detailed description.

CURRENT THERAPY

- Severe chickenpox in infants and immunosuppressed children is treated with intravenous acyclovir (30 mg/kg/d).
- Severe chickenpox in healthy children is treated with oral acyclovir (80 mg/kg/d).
- Severe chickenpox in adolescents is treated with either famciclovir (Famvir) (500 mg tid) or valacyclovir (Valtrex) (1 g tid).
- Prophylaxis following exposure to chickenpox can be managed with a course of oral acyclovir (40 mg/kg/d).

(Valtrex) is 1 g three times a day. For most adolescents, a 5-day regimen should be sufficient treatment.

TREATMENT OF CHICKENPOX IN CHILDREN WITH AN UNDERLYING IMMUNODEFICIENCY

Children with HIV infection who contract chickenpox can usually be managed with oral acyclovir treatment as long as their HIV is under control. The majority of children diagnosed with acute chickenpox who have cancer or organ transplantation should be considered for admission to the hospital and begin immediate treatment with intravenous (IV) acyclovir. The dosage of IV acyclovir is 10 mg/kg every 8 hours. The dosage can be raised to 15 mg/kg every 8 hours in patients presenting varicella pneumonia or varicella encephalitis. The serum creatinine level should be monitored daily and the acyclovir dosage adjusted downward if the serum creatinine reaches 1 mg/dL.

The efficacy of oral famciclovir or valacyclovir is better than oral acyclovir, allowing older children with chickenpox and an immunosuppressive condition to be discharged more quickly from the hospital. Discharge is generally considered after no new vesicle formation is noted for 24 hours. Antiviral therapy (combined IV and oral) for 10 to 14 days is usually suggested, although each case must be assessed individually. Children who have varicella encephalitis or varicella pneumonia may require more than 2 weeks of antiviral therapy.

TREATMENT OF CHICKENPOX IN CHILDREN RECEIVING CORTICOSTEROIDS

Children receiving high-dose oral corticosteroid treatment for conditions such as acute asthma are also at high risk of severe chickenpox. These children should be treated with antivirals just as aggressively as those with cancer. Children receiving only intermittent inhaled corticosteroids do not appear to be at high risk of severe chickenpox.

TREATMENT OF ZOSTER IN CHILDREN

Zoster in otherwise healthy children is usually a benign illness. The disease is normally improving by the time the diagnosis is made. However, zoster in immunocompromised children may persist for 2 weeks or longer, requiring immediate treatment with one of the oral antiviral drugs recommended. The dosage is the same as for severe chickenpox.

ALTERNATIVES TO VARICELLA-ZOSTER IMMUNE GLOBULIN

Varicella-zoster immune globulin (VZIG) has been given in the past to infants and children with cancer who were exposed to chickenpox. VZIG has been discontinued after 2005. Physicians can consider the administration of IV gammaglobulin as a single infusion of 500 mg/kg for infants who are exposed to varicella shortly after birth. An alternative regimen is oral acyclovir suspension at 40 mg/kg per day divided every 6 hours. Acyclovir should be initiated on the day of exposure and continued for 10 days.

Prophylaxis with oral acyclovir also can be considered for VZV-nonimmune children with cancer after an exposure to chickenpox. The recommended dosage is half of the therapeutic dosage, meaning oral acyclovir can be given at 40 mg/kg per day. The daily dosage for children who can swallow tablets can be divided three times a day rather than four times a day during the 10-day therapy period. Children who develop chickenpox despite oral acyclovir treatment should be admitted to the hospital for treatment with IV acyclovir at 10 mg/kg every 8 hours. There are extremely few examples of true acyclovir-resistant VZV; most failures are caused by inadequate absorption of the oral formulation.

REFERENCES

Davis MM, Patel MS, Gebremariam A: Decline in varicella-related hospitalizations and expenditures for children and adults after introduction of varicella vaccine in the United States. Pediatrics 2004;114:786-792.

Grose C: Varicella vaccination of children in the United States: Assessment after the first decade, 1995–2005. J Clin Virol 2005;33:89-95.

Grose C, Widerman J: Generic acyclovir vs. famciclovir and valacyclovir. Pediatr Infect Dis J 1997;16:838-841.

Hay M, Kimura H, Oshiro M, et al: Varicella exposure in a neonatal medical center: Successful prophylaxis with oral acyclovir. J Hosp Infect 2003;54:212-215.

Nguyen HQ, Jumaan AO, Seward JF: Decline in mortality due to varicella after implementation of varicella vaccination in the United States. N Engl J Med 2005;352:450-458.

Takahashi M: Effectiveness of live varicella vaccine. Expert Opin Biol Ther 2004;4:199-216.

Cholera

Method of
Eduardo Salazar-Lindo, MD

Cholera is a life-threatening intestinal infectious disease caused by *Vibrio cholerae*, a noninvasive organism that colonizes the small bowel and elaborates the cholera toxin, a potent enterotoxin that induces an exceptionally profuse watery diarrhea and vomiting, rapidly progressing to severe dehydration, acidosis, and potassium depletion. Prompt and effective treatment is mandatory to rescue the patient from collapsing and dying or developing renal and other ischemic complications.

Although cholera toxin severely disturbs electrolyte and water transport in the small bowel mucosa, resulting in a hypersecretory condition, it spares other transport systems such as that of the coupled sodium-glucose absorption. The discovery of this fact was fundamental to the development of the modern concept of oral rehydration therapy (ORT), which denotes that, even in the face of a severe hypersecretory diarrhea, with the oral intake of an equimolar glucose-salt solution, it is possible to rehydrate a patient who is still able to drink. Given at an early stage of the disease, that is, at home, ORT could avoid the need for an intravenous (IV) resuscitation treatment in the hospital. Also, used as soon as the patient is again able to drink after being rescued from shock status, ORT could help avoid the more expensive and less available IV solutions. These attributes of ORT are particularly relevant during an outbreak of cholera when hundreds and eventually thousands of patients have to be treated at the same time, as was the experience during the huge cholera epidemic of 1991 in Peru.

Cholera is transmitted by fecally contaminated water or food and can thus spread rapidly among susceptible individuals, causing outbreaks and epidemics, particularly explosive in areas with poor sanitation. The current seventh pandemic of cholera, which started in 1961 in Indonesia, has since continued to spread around the globe, reaching West Africa in 1970, southern Europe in 1971, and Latin America in 1991. No cases of cholera are described in Latin America in the last 5 years, but outbreaks of the disease are still being reported from Africa and Asia.

Cholera should not be regarded as an exotic infectious tropical disease. It is endemic in many areas of the tropical region of the world and easily travels with people and trading products. It is believed, for instance, that cholera was introduced in Latin America from Indonesia via the bilge water of cargo vessels traveling with contaminated water uploaded in the port of origin and downloaded upon arrival at the destination port. Physicians from both industrialized and developing countries should be aware of the existence of cholera and learn how to recognize it and provide proper treatment.

Epidemiology and Transmission

A person contracts cholera by ingesting *V. cholerae* in contaminated water or food. Direct person-to-person transmission is rare because the infective dose is rather large (10^8 organisms as compared to 10^3 in shigellosis). Because the organism does not survive well in an acidic environment such as that in the stomach, people who have ingested the organism with a buffering meal, those with gastric hypoacidity from gastrectomy or chronic gastritis, or those who are on medication to neutralize gastric acidity are at increased risk of disease. For unknown reasons, severe disease occurs more frequently in people in blood group O than in those in other blood groups.

Clinical Features

Symptoms of cholera in its typical form include profuse watery diarrhea and vomiting. Fever, if present, is usually mild. The disease typically starts abruptly with abdominal discomfort that is relieved after passing a watery stool, then vomiting ensues and diarrheic stools continue. The diarrheic stool initially is a brownish fluid containing fecal matter; with the increasing high volume, stools soon progress to a whitish fluid resembling the water in which rice is washed. This so-called rice-water stool is rich in sodium, bicarbonate, and potassium. At the peak of the disease, which occurs within the first 24 hours, an individual with cholera could pass 500 to 1000 mL of liquid stools per hour, rapidly leading to dehydration and shock, severe metabolic acidosis, and arm and leg cramps from the loss of potassium.

Cholera patients are initially very thirsty and conscious, but as dehydration progresses, they become drowsy and disoriented, with weak pulse, low blood pressure, eyes deeply sunken, and skin pale, cold, and with no turgor (it remains folded after a skin fold is formed by examiner). At this stage, there is no urine output and patients may stop

passing stools because their body is literally empty of water. Hypoglycemia is often present as a result of poor or no food intake, consumption of glycogen stores, and insufficient gluconeogenic response. Death is imminent, and a vigorous resuscitation treatment is necessary to avoid it.

Diagnosis

Diagnosis of cholera is clinical. In endemic areas, mild cases of cholera can mimic diarrheal illness of other causes and are discovered only if a surveillance system is in place. Any case of severe watery diarrhea rapidly progressing to dehydration and shock, especially when an unusual number of similar cases are present, should be considered a suspected case of cholera, and a stool sample should be obtained and sent to a microbiology laboratory for analysis and confirmation.

Vibrios in stool specimens may not grow on routine enteric media but are easily isolated with a selective medium like thiosulfate-citrate-bile salts-sucrose (TCBS) agar. This medium inhibits growth of other enteric flora and contains 0.5% NaCl and sucrose. The former favors the growth of this salt-requiring organism, and the latter facilitates its recognition by sucrose fermentation. Determination of sensitivity/resistance to antimicrobials of the isolates is necessary because the organism is capable of developing resistance to the commonly used antibiotics.

Reliable methods for rapid diagnosis of cholera, such as monoclonal antibody-based coagglutination, are available. Darkfield examination of the stool is rapid and sensitive but requires experience and special equipment.

TREATMENT

The first aim of proper treatment of cholera is to restore and then maintain the normal volume and composition of

TABLE 1 Clinical Assessment of the Degree of Dehydration

Signs and Symptoms	Mild Dehydration	Moderate Dehydration	Severe Dehydration
Mental status and general appearance	Alert, thirsty	Restless or disoriented, thirsty	Drowsy or comatose, cold, cyanotic extremities
Respiration	Normal	Rapid	Deep and rapid
Radial pulse	Normal	Rapid	Feeble
Blood pressure	Normal	Normal, orthostatic hypotension	Low; may be imperceptible
Skin elasticity	Normal	Pinched skin retracts slowly	Pinched skin remains folded
Eyes	Normal	Sunken	Deeply sunken
Oral and eye membranes	Slightly dry	Dry	Very dry
Urine flow	Normal or slightly reduced	Reduced and darkened	None
Estimated fluid deficit	30–50 mL/kg	60–90 mL/kg	100 mL/kg

body fluids. Adjuvant therapies are aimed to reduce the severity and duration of the disease.

The first step is to assess rapidly the degree of dehydration (Table 1). Patients in severe dehydration should immediately receive IV isotonic fluids to replace the estimated deficit. Patients with moderate dehydration should be treated with oral rehydration unless they are vomiting excessively.

REPLACEMENT OF DEFICITS

With severe dehydration, the patient should receive 100 mL/kg of an isotonic solution IV: 50% of the calculated volume during the first hour and the remaining 50% during the following 2 hours. Suitable IV solutions are Lactated Ringer's, Dhaka solution,[2] and Peru polyelectrolyte solution[2] (Table 2). Normal saline, used alone in large volumes,

---

[2]Not available in the United States.

may hamper the correction of metabolic acidosis by lowering the strong ion difference and causing postresuscitation hyperchloremia. After these first 3 hours of rapid replacement of deficits, the patient's condition should be assessed to determine if an additional 1 or 2 hours of the same infusion rate may be necessary or if the patient is ready to continue treatment by the oral route.

REPLACEMENT OF ONGOING LOSSES

After replacement of deficits is achieved, ongoing losses should be replaced on a volume-to-volume basis to maintain hydration status. If the patient is able to drink, this replacement could be done effectively with an oral rehydration solution (ORS). The World Health Organization is currently promoting a reduced-osmolarity ORS (see Table 2) with the claim that this solution, although still effective to treat cholera cases, would be more effective than the previously promoted standard solution when used in noncholera cases. Rice-based ORS has the additional

TABLE 2 Composition of Cholera Stool and Intravenous and Oral Rehydration Solutions Used to Treat Cholera

Fluid	Sodium (mmol/L)	Potassium (mmol/L)	Chloride (mmol/L)	Base* (mmol/L)	Glucose (mmol/L)
Cholera stool					
Adults	135	20	100	45	—
Children	105	30	90	30	—
Intravenous fluids					
Lactated Ringer's	128	4	109	28	—
Dhaka solution[2]	133	13	98	48	111
Polyelectrolyte Peru solution[†,2]	90	20	80	30	—
Normal saline	154	—	154	—	—
ORS					
WHO standard	90	20	80	30	111
WHO low osmolality	75	20	65	30	75
Rice based	75	20	65	30	30[‡]

[2]Not available in the United States.
*Bicarbonate, lactate, acetate, or citrate.
[†]Used extensively in Peru during the cholera epidemic of 1991.
[‡]Contained in 30–50 g of rice depending on level of hydrolysis.
Abbreviations: ORS = oral rehydration solution; WHO = World Health Organization.

TABLE 3 Antimicrobials for Treatment of Cholera

| Antimicrobial | Dose and Administration* | |
	Children	Adults
Tetracycline (Sumycin)	12.5 mg/kg, qid for 3 d[1,3]	500 mg, qid for 3 d
Doxycycline (Vibramycin)	6 mg/kg, one single dose[1,3]	300 mg, one single dose
TMP-SMX (Bactrim)[1]	5 mg/kg TMP + 25 mg/kg SMX, bid for 3 d	160 mg TMP + 800 mg SMX, bid for 3 d
Furazolidone (Furoxone)*	1.25 mg/kg, qid for 3 d	100 mg, qid for 3 d
Norfloxacin (Noroxin)[1]	Not FDA approved	400 mg, qid for 3 d
Ciprofloxacin (Cipro)[1]	Not FDA approved	250 mg, qd for 3 d

[1]Not FDA approved for children <8 y.
[3]Exceeds dosage recommended by the manufacturer.
*Recommended in pregnant women.
Abbreviations: TMP-SMX = trimethoprim-sulfamethoxazole.

advantage of reducing the purging rate by approximately a third.

ANTIMICROBIALS

In contrast to other causes of infectious watery diarrhea, cholera patients may benefit from antimicrobials. With an effective antimicrobial given at an early stage of the disease, the severity and duration of the choleric diarrhea may be significantly reduced. Tetracycline, doxycycline (Vibramycin), trimethoprim-sulfamethoxazole (Bactrim),[1] furazolidone (Furoxone), norfloxacin (Noroxin), and ciprofloxacin (Cipro)[1] are the proven antimicrobial options (Table 3). The selection of an antimicrobial depends on the known resistance/sensitivity pattern of the cholera organism circulating in the community.

Prevention and Control

Handwashing, especially after defecation, continues to be the best measure to decrease the spread of *V. cholerae* into the environment. Disinfection of drinking water by chlorination, boiling, or sunlight treatment and sanitary treatment of wastewater before discharging into other bodies of water are important measures to control a cholera epidemic. Treatment of contacts with antimicrobials is not effective and promotes the emergence of antibiotic resistance. Vaccines are still in the process of development. Travelers to areas affected by cholera should avoid undercooked foods and untreated water or ice.

REFERENCES

Bhattacharya SK, Bhattacharya MK, Dutta P, et al: Double-blind, randomized, controlled clinical trial of Norfloxacin for cholera. Antimicrob Agents Chemother 1990;34:939-940.
Carpenter CCJ: The treatment of cholera: Clinical science at the bedside. J Infect Dis 1992;166:2-14.
Curtis V, Cairncross S, Youli R: Domestic hygiene and diarrhoea: Pinpointing the problem. Trop Med Int Health 2000;5:22-32.
Duggan C, Fontaine O, Pierce NF, et al: Scientific rationale for a change in the composition of oral rehydration solution. JAMA 2004;291: 2628-2631.
Gore SM, Fontaine O, Pierce NF: Impact of rice based oral rehydration solution on stool output and duration of diarrhoea: Meta-analysis of 13 clinical trials. BMJ 1992;304:287-291.
Gotuzzo E, Seas C, Echevarria J, et al: Ciprofloxacin for the treatment of cholera: A randomized, double-blind, controlled clinical trial of a single daily dose in Peruvian adults. Clin Infect Dis 1995;20:1485-1490.
Nalin DR, Hirschhorn N, Greenough W 3rd, et al: Clinical concerns about reduced-osmolarity oral rehydration solution. JAMA 2004; 291:2632-2635.
Skellett S, Mayer A, Durward A, et al: Chasing the base deficit: Hyperchloraemic acidosis following 0.9% saline fluid resuscitation. Arch Dis Child 2000; 83:514-516.
World Health Organization: Management of the patient with cholera. Geneva, Switzerland: WHO Programme for Control of Diarrhoeal Disease. Publication WHO/CDD/SER/91.15, 1991.

Food-Borne Illness

Method of
Evangelista Sagnelli, MD

Food-borne illnesses are defined by the World Health Organization as "diseases of an infectious or toxic nature caused by, or thought to be caused by, the consumption of contaminated food or water." In the United States, food-borne illnesses are considered responsible for approximately 76 million illnesses, 325,000 hospitalizations, and 5,200 deaths each year. Epidemiologic data from other countries are considered less accurate or insufficient or are unavailable.

Toxin-Related Food-Borne Illness

Several bacteria produce toxins that cause food poisoning characterized by symptoms ranging from gastrointestinal disorders to paralysis and may have a fatal outcome (Table 1).

---

[1]Not FDA approved for this indication.

TABLE 1 Bacterial Toxin-Related Diseases

Signs and Symptoms	Associated Foods	Incubation	Etiologic Agents	Treatment
Watery diarrhea, nausea, cramps, fever rare	Meats, poultry, often precooked	8–16 h	*Clostridium perfringens*	Fluids, supportive care.
	Meats, stews, gravies, often precooked	10–16 h	*Bacillus cereus* diarrheal toxin	
Sudden onset with severe nausea and vomiting ± diarrhea	Nonrefrigerated meat, potato and egg salad, cream pastries	1–6 h	Staphylococcal food poisoning	Fluids, supportive care.
	Improperly refrigerated/reheated cooked and fried rice	1–6 h	*B. cereus* emetic toxin	
Blurred vision, dysphagia, descending muscle weakness, vomiting ± diarrhea	Home-canned foods with low-acid content	12–72 h	*Clostridium botulinum*	Supportive care; botulinum antitoxin helpful if given early in course of illness.

Clostridium perfringens, one of the most common agents of food-borne illness in the United States, is an anaerobic, gram-positive, spore-forming rod widely disseminated in the environment that produces a heat-labile enterotoxin (Table 1). This toxin binds to a brush-border membrane receptor in the small bowel cells inducing loss of low molecular weight metabolites and ions, which are associated with morphologic cell damage and even cell lysis. Abdominal cramps and diarrhea are the most frequent symptoms, beginning 8 to 22 hours after the consumption of contaminated foods (meats or poultry, especially if precooked) and disappearing within 24 hours. Treatment includes the administration of fluids and supportive care.

Clostridium botulinum is an anaerobic, gram-positive, spore-forming rod; the spore is heat resistant and can survive in incorrectly processed foods. A potent neurotoxin is produced when incorrectly processed homemade or commercial foods lead to the growth of this microorganism (Table 1). The ingestion of foods with this toxin may cause botulism (severe food poisoning). The toxin is heat labile and can be destroyed if heated at 80°C (176°F) for 10 minutes or longer. The lethal dose is very low (a few micrograms). The onset of symptoms occurs 18 to 36 hours after ingestion. The toxin causes paralysis by blocking the motor nerve terminals at the myoneural junction; asphyxia induced by the neurotoxin or, in some cases, by superinfections may result in death. Treatment is based on the early administration of specific immunoglobulins that are usually available by contacting the health authorities in the different countries.

Staphylococcus aureus is a facultative anaerobic gram-positive coccus; some strains produce an enterotoxin responsible for staphylococcal food poisoning (Table 1). This agent is currently the most frequent cause of food-borne illness. *S. aureus* is responsible for a disease whose severity is related to three factors: toxin-mediated virulence, invasiveness, and antibiotic resistance of the agent. The onset is rapid (from 30 minutes to 8 hours) and characterized by abdominal cramps, nausea and vomiting, and sometimes followed by diarrhea; spontaneous remission usually occurs within 24 hours. Many foods provide a good growth medium for *S. aureus*, including milk, cream, cream-filled pastries, butter, ham, cheeses, and canned meat. However, the foods most often involved in staphylococcal food poisoning

differ largely from one country to another. The treatment of bacterial toxin-related illness usually includes only the replacement of fluids and supportive care.

Bacillus cereus is a gram-positive, facultative aerobic spore-forming rod. Two types of illness are caused by two distinct metabolites: high molecular weight heat-labile protein (diarrheal toxin) and low molecular weight heat-stable peptide (emetic toxin) (Table 1). The clinical forms most often related to diarrheal toxin (closely resembling the syndrome described for *C. perfringens*) are characterized by watery diarrhea, abdominal cramps, and pain starting 6 to 16 hours after consumption of the contaminated food and lasting 24 hours. The low molecular weight heat-stable peptide causes nausea and vomiting, a clinical syndrome resembling more a staphylococcal food-borne infection.

Other toxin-related syndromes are because of fish and shellfish poisoning (Table 2) or to mushroom poisoning (Table 3). Among fish poisonings, ciguatera poisoning is the most common in the United States; it is caused by polyether sodium channel activator toxins produced by dinoflagellates (*Gambierdiscus toxicus*) that may contaminate predacious tropical reef fish, such as barracuda, grouper, red snapper, and jack. Symptoms start 1 to 6 hours after the ingestion of the fish, with abdominal pain, nausea, vomiting, and diarrhea; a pathognomonic symptom is the reversal of hot and cold tactile perception, which develops after 3 to 5 days and persists for months. In severe cases, hypertension and tachycardia develop after a transient episode of serious hypotension and bradycardia. After the classic ciguatera syndrome, some patients may suffer a so-called second neurologic phase characterized by ataxia, dysmetria, and resting or kinetic tremor. These symptoms may persist for 2 to 6 weeks. A similar toxin-associated syndrome is described for histamine fish poisoning (see Table 2).

Paralytic, neurotoxin, and amnesic shellfish poisoning in humans is caused by the ingestion of mollusks that fed on dinoflagellates. Paralytic shellfish poisoning is characterized by paresthesia of the mouth, lips, face, and extremities. Dyspnea, dysphagia, muscle weakness or frank paralysis, ataxia, and respiratory insufficiency may occur in severe cases. This disease is caused by several toxins, one of which is known as saxitoxin, which is a water-soluble, heat- and

TABLE 2 Fish or Mollusk Toxin-Related Syndrome

Signs and Symptoms	Associated Foods	Incubation	Etiologic Agents	Treatment
Abdominal pain, nausea, vomiting, diarrhea; hypotension, and bradycardia in severe cases; ataxia, dysmetria, tremor	Large predacious tropical reef fish: barracuda, grouper, red snapper, jack	For gastrointestinal symptoms: 1–6 h; for neurologic symptoms: 12 h–5 d	Ciguatera fish poisoning	Supportive care; atropine and blood pressure support; in chronic cases amitriptyline (Elavil[1]) may be beneficial.
Flushing, rash; burning sensation of skin of the mouth	Improperly refrigerated "scombroid" fish	5 min–1 h	Histamine fish poisoning	Supportive care.
Paresthesias of the mouth, lips, face, and extremities	Mollusk feeding on dinoflagellates (*Gonyaulax catanella, Gonyaulax tamarensis*)	5 min–4 h	Paralytic shellfish poisoning	
Dyspnea, dysphagia, paralysis, ataxia in severe cases	Mollusk feeding on dinoflagellates (*Gymnodinium breve*)	5 min–4 h	Neurotoxic shellfish poisoning	Supportive care.
Vomiting, abdominal cramping, diarrhea; confusion, amnesia, coma, cardiovascular instability	Mollusk feeding on dinoflagellates (*Nitzschia pungens*)	15 min–6 h	Amnesic shellfish poisoning	Supportive care.

[1]Not FDA approved for this indication.

acid-stable toxin that is not destroyed by ordinary cooking; saxitoxin is believed to block sodium conductance by inhibiting neuromuscular transmission at the axonal and muscle membrane levels (Table 2).

The clinical features of neurotoxin shellfish poisoning are similar to those of paralytic shellfish poisoning, except for paralysis; several poorly characterized neurotoxins may be responsible for this syndrome. The symptoms correlated to amnesic shellfish poisoning are initially nonspecific (vomiting, abdominal cramping, and diarrhea), but within a few hours, confusion and amnesia, the most pathognomonic symptom, progressively increase and, in some cases, become severe. This syndrome is caused by domoic acid, a toxin that may cause bilateral destruction of the hippocampus with consequent persistent amnesia. The treatment of fish or mollusk toxin-related illness usually only includes the replacement of fluids and supportive care.

TABLE 3 Mushroom Toxin-Related Syndrome

Signs and Symptoms	Associated Mushrooms	Incubation	Toxins	Treatment
Parasympathetic hyperactivity (sweating, salivation, lacrimation, bradycardia, hypotension)	*Inocybe* spp.	30 min–2 h	Muscarine	Supportive care
Hallucination syndrome (hallucination, mood elevation)	*Psilocybe* spp.; *Panatelas* spp.	30–60 min	Psilocybin, psilocin	Supportive care
Disulfiram reaction (headache, nausea, vomiting)	*Coprinus* spp.	30 min after alcohol	Coprime	Supportive care
Delirium syndrome (dizziness, ataxia, hyperactivity)	*Clitocybe* spp; *Amanita* spp.	20–90 min	Ibotenic acid, muscimol isoxazole	Supportive care
Gastroenteritis, hepatorenal failure	*Amanita phalloides*	6–24 h	Amatoxins and phallotoxins	Hospitalization and treatment in ICU
Gastroenteritis, hepatic failure, hemolysis, seizures	*Gyromitra* spp.	2–12 h	Gyromitrin	Hospitalization and treatment in ICU
Thirst, nausea, headache, abdominal pain, renal failure	*Coronarius* spp.	3–5 d	Orellanine	Hospitalization and treatment in ICU

Abbreviations: ICU = intensive care unit.

Mushroom poisoning (Table 3) is characterized by at least four very short incubation syndromes starting within 2 hours of ingestion of the mushroom toxin or by at least three short incubation syndromes starting at least 6 hours after ingestion. The very short incubation syndromes are self-limited diseases lasting 24 hours and require only supportive care. They are characterized by parasympathetic hyperactivity (from mushrooms containing muscarine), hallucination syndrome (from mushrooms containing psilocybin and psilocin), or delirium syndrome (from mushrooms containing coprime). Patients poisoned by mushrooms containing coprime, a disulfiram-like substance, develop nausea, vomiting, headache, flushing, paresthesia, and tachycardia if they ingest alcohol within 48 hours of mushroom ingestion. The short-incubation mushroom syndromes are very severe (e.g., in *Amanita phalloides* poisoning, the mortality rate is 20% to 50%). Amanita poisoning is responsible for a biphasic illness; gastroenteritis characterizes the first period, which usually resolves within 24 hours. After a 24- to 48-hour asymptomatic period, severe hepatic and/or renal failure develop. Gyromitra poisoning syndrome is caused by the ingestion of the gyromitrin toxin, which causes gastroenteritis, hemolysis, seizures, and hepatic, but not renal, failure. Because of the severity of the short-incubation mushroom syndromes, all patients must be immediately hospitalized in intensive care units.

Treatment of Diarrhea

WATERY DIARRHEA

Watery diarrhea can occur with the ingestion of a large variety of foods (Table 4); it can be caused by one of several infectious agents, all showing a similar clinical presentation. The identification of the pathogen requires microbiologic and/or immunologic investigations, which are successful in only half of the cases.

Caliciviruses, including *Norwalk* and *Norwalk-like agents,* are responsible for approximately 80% of watery diarrhea cases and are usually self-limited. The action of the viruses on the mucosal cells is evident by the shortening of microvilli, whereas the cells appear intact.

The bacterium more frequently isolated in watery diarrhea is an enterotoxigenic *Escherichia coli* (ETEC), currently considered responsible for 85% of bacterial food-borne infections. ETEC produces a heat-labile toxin (adenylate cyclase-like cholera toxin) that induces a diarrheic syndrome of varying severity, from self-limited to life-threatening forms.

Another pathogenetic process causing watery diarrhea is entero-adherence, exerted by enteropathogenic *E. coli* (EPEC) and enteroaggregative *E. coli* (EaggEC) on enterocytes by a mechanism only in part clarified (see Table 2).

Listeria monocytogenes is an intracellular organism usually found in the gastrointestinal flora of healthy individuals. This agent has a surface protein called internalin, which interacting with E-cadherin, a receptor present on enteric cells, allows its introduction to the intestinal cells; *Listeria* is responsible for mild to severe forms of gastroenteritis in immunocompetent patients but can also be responsible for bacteremia and meningitis in immunocompromised hosts, children, and the elderly; in pregnant women, both a flulike syndrome and premature birth can occur.

Vibrio vulnificus is associated with a systemic syndrome characterized by acute gastroenteritis beginning 24 hours after the ingestion of raw oysters; it is self-limited in immunocompetent subjects but can be severe in the immunocompromised, with a lethality rate of approximately 1%.

Successful treatment of watery diarrhea includes preventing dehydration and reducing the symptoms and duration of the illness. Enteral or parenteral rehydration is the basic component of therapy; specific treatment is often unnecessary because watery diarrhea is self-limiting in a large percentage of cases. The World Health Organization suggests enteral rehydration with 3.5 g NaCl, 1.5 g KCl, 2.5g $NaCHO_3$ and 20 g glucose/L boiled water, but frequently intravenous (IV) rehydration is required. Antisecretory and antimotility drugs are highly effective in reducing the number of evacuations but not in curing the disease. Several studies showed that loperamide (Imodium), an antisecretory and antimotility drug, used in combination with an antibiotic is superior to either drug given alone. Antimicrobial therapy is not currently recommended in watery diarrhea because excessive prescribing of antibiotics contributes to the development of resistance to drugs previously considered of choice. This has occurred with cotrimoxazole (Bactrim), which is currently of limited use. In several studies, however, fluoroquinolones reduced the duration of diarrhea from 3 to 4 days to 1.5 days or less. A single oral dose of 750 mg is as effective as a 3-day treatment with 500 mg orally twice daily. In *V. vulnificus* infection, combination therapy with cefotaxime (Claforan[1]), 2 g IV every 8 hours, and minocycline (Minocin), 100 mg orally every 12 hours, is necessary.

BLOODY DIARRHEA

Bloody diarrhea characterizes inflammatory lower intestinal diseases caused by infective and noninfective agents, often associated with abdominal cramps and fever (Table 5). Most of the infective agents responsible for these clinical manifestations are bacterial, but some are protozoal. The pathogenic mechanisms are often represented by a lesion in the intestinal cells caused by the penetration of the etiologic agents in the mucous membrane, with subsequent enterorrhagia. *Campylobacter* and *Salmonella* are the bacteria generally implicated in inflammatory intestinal disease. Approximately 2 million food-borne *Campylobacter* infections occur each year in the United States. This infection has become one of the most common causes of infectious colitis in adolescents and young adults (18 to 30 years old) in the last decade.

Some etiologic agents responsible for bloody diarrhea (i.e., *Shigella species, Entamoeba histolytica, Campylobacter,* and *Salmonella species*) are increasingly recognized as possible causes of traveler's diarrhea. The role of other pathogens such as *Yersinia enterocolitica* was underestimated in the past because of the difficulty detecting the agent in feces.

The main components of successful treatment of bloody diarrhea include preventing dehydration and reducing the symptoms and duration of the illness. The decision to use

---

[1]Not FDA approved for this indication.

TABLE 4 Watery Diarrhea

Signs and Symptoms	Associated Foods	Geographic Areas	Etiologic Agents	Incubation Period	Pathogenesis	Treatment
Abdominal cramps, dehydration, ± fever, ± nausea and vomiting	Contaminated water, raw or undercooked meals, shellfish, meats, poultry often precooked	South and Central America, South and Southeast Asia, low income areas of Africa	Viral agents (rotavirus, Norwalk virus, etc.)	1–3 d	Unknown; probably toxin mediated or related to a lesion of gut cells	Fluids in severe cases (see text)
			EPEC, EaggEC	1–3 d	Entero-adhesivity	
			ETEC	1–3 d		
			Vibrio cholerae; see specific chapter	24–72 h		
	Raw oysters for *Vibrio vulnificus*		*Vibrio vulnificus*	1–4 d	Toxin-mediated secretory diarrhea	Fluids and antibiotics in severe cases (see text)
	Soft fresh cheeses and hot dogs for listeriosis		*Listeria monocytogenes*	9–48 h for GI symptoms; 2–6 wk for invasive disease	Tissue invasion (see text)	Fluids for gastroenteritis; for invasive disease, ampicillin, 3 g IV q4h, or TMP-SMX (Bactrim[3]) 5–25 mg/kg IV tid

[3]Exceeds dosage recommended by the manufacturer.
Abbreviations: EaggEC = enteroaggregative *Escherichia coli;* EPEC = enteropathogenic *Escherichia coli;* ETEC = enterotoxigenic *Escherichia coli;* GI = gastrointestinal; TMP-SMX = trimethoprim-sulfamethoxazole.

Food-Borne Illness

TABLE 5 Bloody Diarrhea

Signs and Symptoms	Associated Foods	Geographic Areas	Etiologic Agents	Incubation Period	Pathogenesis	Treatment
Dysentery with fever ± vomiting and cramps; fecal leukocytes	Undercooked bovine meat, poultry, nonpasteurized milk, eggs, contaminated water, unwashed raw vegetables, foods washed with contaminated water	Mediterranean countries, developing areas of Asia, Central and South America	*Escherichia coli* O157:H7; EHEC EIEC *Campylobacter jejuni*	1–8 d 1–3 d 2–5 d	Tissue invasion and toxin production	Antibiotics are contraindicated (see text).
			Salmonella spp. (see specific chapter)	12 h–2 d (*S. typhi,* 3–60 d)	Tissue invasion (inflammatory diarrhea)	Fluids and supportive care; in some cases antibiotics required.
			Entamoeba histolytica (see specific chapter)	Very long		
		United States, Northern Europe, and Canada	*Yersinia enterocolitica*	24–48 hr		

Abbreviations: EHEC = enterohemorrhagic *Escherichia coli*; EIEC = enteroinvasive *Escherichia coli.*

antibiotics should be made judiciously; recent studies suggest that the administration of antibiotics to children with *E. coli* O157:H7 infection currently increases the risk of hemolytic uremic syndrome. Cotrimoxazole was been the drug of choice for many years, but the increasing prevalence of resistance of several bacteria has progressively limited its use. Current studies suggest that erythromycin shortens the duration of illness if given early in the course of campylobacteriosis. Fluoroquinolones, however, remain the drug of choice because they reduce the duration of diarrhea from 3 to 4 days to 1.5 days or less. For the treatment of shigellosis or campylobacteriosis, a 3-day treatment with Ciprofloxin (Cipro) 500 mg orally twice daily is more effective than a large single dose (750 mg orally). However, the most recent data report shows that *Campylobacter* is now resistant to ciprofloxacin in 17% of patients. In these cases azithromycin was used instead of fluoroquinolones. Azithromycin[1] (Zithromax) (1000 mg orally as a single dose) is active against several enteric pathogens, being as effective as fluoroquinolones and even more effective in reducing the exacerbations of campylobacteriosis; it is usually safe and well tolerated in children.

Multidrug resistance is a serious problem for the treatment of shigellosis, particularly when it is caused by *Shigella dysenteriae* type 1; resistance to sulfonamides, tetracycline, ampicillin, and cotrimoxazole has strongly limited the use of these drugs. Nalidixic acid[1] (NegGram) showed encouraging results in the treatment of multiresistant *S. dysenteriae* type 1 infection, but resistance to this drug has emerged in several countries. After a short time in use, mecillinam still remains active in ciprofloxacin- and other fluoroquinolone-resistant *S. dysenteriae* type 1 infection, as observed in India, Bangladesh, and Nepal. However, the antimicrobial resistance pattern differs from country to country, and differences can even be seen between different regions in the same country.

CHRONIC DIARRHEA

Chronic diarrhea persists, by definition, for more than 2 weeks and is frequently associated with specific intestinal pathogens, particularly protozoa. *Entamoeba histolytica* and *Giardia species* account for 27% of cases. Currently agents like *Cryptosporidium*, *Cyclospora*, and *Isospora* were found responsible for chronic traveler's diarrhea in both immunocompetent and immunocompromised hosts.

Giardia lamblia is a protozoan of worldwide distribution that can frequently infect children in low-income geographical areas. The pathogenetic mechanism includes the disruption of the brush border, invasion of the mucous membrane, the elaboration of an enterotoxin, and a consequent inflammatory infiltration that leads to fluid and electrolyte secretion.

Aeromonas and *Plesiomonas* are increasingly associated with a diarrheic syndrome, almost always with other pathogens. *Aeromonas*, however, produces an enterotoxin that may cause diarrhea. Also *Plesiomonas shigelloides* was detected in patients with gastroenteritis, but the pathogenetic mechanism is still unknown. Chronic colitis following acute *Aeromonas* and *Plesiomonas* diarrheas is observed in adults, especially if HIV infected.

Cryptosporidium organisms are found in the microvillus layer of intestinal cells, in immunocompetent hosts in the distal small intestine and proximal colon tracts, and in immunodeficient hosts in all tracts of the intestine, biliary tract, and respiratory tract. The pathogenetic mechanisms responsible for watery diarrhea remain unclear, but the absence of morphologic lesions may suggest a toxin-related mechanism.

Cyclospora infection is found worldwide, even in immunocompetent subjects, but it is better known as an opportunistic infection in immunocompromised hosts. The parasite is found in epithelial cells of the small bowel, where it elicits a secretory diarrhea by unknown mechanisms; the absence of blood and leukocytes in the stools and the lack of cytopathic damage suggest a toxin-mediated mechanism.

The pathogenesis of isosporiasis is not yet clarified, but it is hypothesized that cell damage consequent to parasite invasion may be caused by the parasite itself, cell-mediated inflammation, or proteins and oxidants released from mast cells.

Clinical signs and symptoms do not distinguish cyclosporiasis from *Cryptosporidia* or *Isospora* infection. The organisms invade the intestinal epithelium and proliferate during an incubation period of 1 week. In immunocompetent individuals, a mild watery diarrhea is usually described, which is sometimes associated with abdominal cramps, nausea, vomiting, and fever. In HIV-infected patients, the clinical manifestations vary; in those with CD4 cell counts above 150 the disease is usually self-limited, whereas if the CD4 cell count is lower than 150, diarrhea often relapses. A chronic outcome with dehydration and significant weight loss is frequent.

Aeromonas and *Plesiomonas* infections are usually responsible for watery self-limited diarrhea, but in some cases chronic colitis develops, with fever, abdominal pain, and bloody stools. Infections with *Giardia species* include an asymptomatic disease, acute and self-limited diarrhea, and a chronic syndrome with malabsorption and weight loss. Although most patients with giardiasis have a mild disease, some subjects, more frequently children younger than 5 years and pregnant women, may develop severe dehydration requiring hospitalization. Table 6 shows the treatments for the diseases presented in this section.

Miscellanea

Trichinella spiralis infection occurs after the ingestion of raw or undercooked pork or wild boar or of other foods contaminated during their preparation. Because of the presence of adult organisms or larvae in the intestinal tract, the initial symptoms are abdominal pain, diarrhea in approximately 40% of cases, or constipation. Myalgias, periorbital edema, muscle tenderness, splinter hemorrhage, or central nervous system involvement come later and suggest the diagnosis. Treatment consists of albendazole (Albenza[1]), 400 mg orally twice daily for 8 days, plus glucocorticoids in severe cases.

Anisakiasis is an infection caused by nematodes that may be acquired by ingesting raw or undercooked fish such as salmon and herring; it is rare in the United States

---

[1]Not FDA approved for this indication.

[1]Not FDA approved for this indication.

TABLE 6 Chronic Diarrhea

Signs and Symptoms	Associated Foods;	Geographical Areas	Etiologic Agents	Incubation Period	Pathogenesis	Treatment
Lasting for >2 wk with fever, fatigue, bloated abdominal pain ± vomiting; often relapsing	Contaminated surface water; foods contaminated by water; food workers	South and Southeast Asia; frequent in immunocompromised hosts from all countries	*Cryptosporidium* spp.	2–28 d	Adherence, tissue invasion, toxin production	Supportive care
			Cyclospora spp.	1–11 d		TMP-SMZ (Bactrim[1]), 160/800 mg PO bid for 7-10 d, or Ciprofloxacin (Cipro[1]), 500 mg PO bid for 7 d
			Isospora belli	1 wk		TMP-SMZ (Bactrim[1]), 160/800 mg PO qid for 10 d and bid for 3 wk, or Ciprofloxacin, (Cipro[1]) 500 mg PO bid for 7 d
			Giardia lamblia (see specific chapter)	1–4 wk		Metronidazole (Flagyl[1]). 250 mg PO tid for 5 d, or Tinidazole (Tindamax), 2 g once
			Plesiomonas shigelloides	Unknown		TMP-SMZ (Bactrim), Cloranfenicol,[2] Ciprofloxacin (Cipro)
	Australia; more frequent in children		*Aeromonas* spp.	Unknown		TMP-SMZ (Bactrim[1]), Gentamicin[1] (Garamycin)

[1]Not FDA approved for this indication.
[2]Not available in the United States.

but very common in the Netherlands and Japan. An acute illness characterized by abdominal pain, nausea and vomiting starts a few hours after ingesting the infected food; a chronic disease resembling Crohn's disease follows 1 or 2 weeks later with fever, intermittent abdominal pain, nausea, and at times diarrhea. When possible, treatment consists of surgical or endoscopic removal of larvae.

Taenia solium is a tapeworm observed worldwide but is more frequent in Latin America, Africa, South and Southeast Asia, and Eastern Europe and causes two distinct forms of infection: the presence of the adult tapeworm in the intestine or the presence of larval forms in the tissues (cysticercosis). Cysticercosis occurs in industrialized countries largely as a result of the immigration of infected individuals from endemic areas. The intestinal infection may be asymptomatic, and nausea, weight loss, and diarrhea are rare. In cysticercosis, the clinical manifestations differ according to the number and location of the cysticerci; neurologic symptoms are the most common, with arachnoiditis that may cause hydrocephalus and an increase in intracranial pressure. The beef tapeworm *Taenia saginata* is found in all countries but is more frequent in the Middle East and sub-Saharan Africa. It is characterized by the presence of the adult tapeworm in the intestine. Humans are contaminated by ingesting raw or undercooked beef containing a cysticercus. Abdominal pain, nausea, changes in appetite, weakness, and weight loss are the most frequently recorded symptoms.

A single dose of praziquantel[1] (Biltricide) (5 to 10 mg/kg) or a single 2-g dose of niclosamide[2] (Niclocide, four 500-mg chewing tablets) is highly effective in eradicating the adult tapeworm infection. The management of neurocysticercosis requires symptomatic treatment of the neurologic signs and praziquantel[1] at a dose of 50 to 60 mg/kg divided in three doses daily for 15 days.

REFERENCES

Al-Abri SS, Beeching NJ, Nye FJ: Traveller's diarrhoea. Lancet Infect Dis 2005;5:349-360.

Allos BM, Moore MR, Griffin PM, Tauxe RV: Surveillance for sporadic foodborne disease in the 21st century: The foodNet perspective. Clin Infect Dis 2004;38:115-120.

Brett MM: Food poisoning associated with biotoxins in fish and shellfish. Curr Opin Infect Dis 2003;16:461-465.

Chiang SR, Chuang YC: *Vibrio vulnificus* infection: Clinical manifestation, pathogenesis and antimicrobial therapy. J Microbiol Immunol Infect 2003;36:81-88.

Diaz JH: Syndromic diagnosis and management of confirmed mushroom poisonings. Crit Care Med 2005;33:427-436.

Eberhard ML, Arrowood MJ: *Cyclospora* spp. Curr Opin Infect Dis 2002;15:519-522.

Huang DB, Okhuysen PC, Jiang ZD, DuPont HL: Enteroaggregative *Escherichia coli:* An emerging enteric pathogen. Am J Gastroenterol 2004;99:383-389.

Mangili A, Gendreau MA: Transmission of infectious diseases during commercial air travel. Lancet 2005;365:989-996.

Minenoa T, Avery MA: Giardiasis: Recent progress in chemotherapy and drug development. Curr Pharm Des 2003;9:841-855.

Smith HV, Corcoran GD. New drugs and treatment for cryptosporidiosis. Curr Opin Infect Dis 2004;17:557-564.

---

[1]Not FDA approved for this indication.
[2]Not available in the United States.

Necrotizing Skin and Soft-Tissue Infections

Method of
James S. Tan, MD

Necrotizing skin and soft-tissue infection is a rapidly progressive disease characterized by necrosis of skin and its underlying tissues including superficial and deep fascia, subcutaneous fat, nerves, arteries, veins, and muscles. In addition, thrombosis of cutaneous microcirculation is frequently observed. Although these infections are found in almost any anatomic area, the most frequently encountered sites are the abdomen, perineum, and lower extremities. In most cases, these infections are not recognized early in the course of illness because of their seemingly benign presentation. However, once established, the progression is often fulminant. The prognosis hinges on timely diagnosis and surgical intervention.

Etiology

These infections may be polymicrobial or monomicrobial. Approximately half of the patients have polymicrobial infection. The remaining half is divided between monomicrobial infection and no identifiable etiology. Polymicrobial infections are usually caused by a mixture of anaerobes and aerobes that may have originated from the intestinal flora. These organisms act synergistically to propagate the infection.

Streptococcus pyogenes and *Clostridium perfringens* are common causes of monomicrobial infections causing necrotizing disease. The most common monomicrobial infection associated with necrotizing disease is *S. pyogenes*. *Streptococcus agalactiae* and other streptococcal species are also associated with necrotizing infections. More recent reports show that community-associated methicillin-resistant *Staphylococcus aureus* (MRSA) causes necrotizing skin and soft-tissue disease. These isolates possess Panton-Valentine leukocidin, which is associated with the increase in pathogenicity. Aerobic gram-negative rods such as *Klebsiella pneumoniae* and *Pseudomonas aeruginosa* are also associated with monomicrobial infections. In addition, marine vibrios such as *Vibrio vulnificus* are also associated with necrotizing infections, especially among patients with advanced liver disease.

Pathogenesis

Most commonly, the pathogen is introduced locally into the soft-tissue space through any disruption of the overlying skin from blunt trauma, penetrating injuries such as cuts, abrasions, burns, lacerations, bites from insects or animals, injections (intravenous or subcutaneous drug injections), and postoperative complications. Less commonly the pathogen may be hematogenously introduced.

Clinical Manifestations

Initially, the patient presents with an erythematous hot, swollen, and tender area of cellulitis accompanied by exquisite local pain and fever. Wound pain is consistently encountered. On examination, the external appearance of the skin wound frequently appears misleadingly benign and is the reason for the delay in diagnosis. Although the presence of gas in the tissues is considered a classic sign both clinically and radiographically, it is only found in approximately a fifth of the cases. Hence, its absence does not exclude a necrotizing infection. As the disease progresses, wound pain continues to be out of proportion to the physical findings. The skin is erythematous, smooth, shiny, swollen, and tense. The margins of erythema and induration widen rapidly. Within a few days, the skin darkens with patchy areas that are dusky blue. In addition, blisters and bullae with serous fluid appear. Hemorrhagic bullae are seen within a few days. At this stage, the infection is well established in the soft tissues. The resulting necrosis of the soft tissues such as the superficial fascia and fat produces a watery, thin, often foul-smelling fluid when anaerobes are present. Thrombosis of the skin nutrient arteries occurs, resulting in focal areas of skin necrosis; the skin becomes purplish and even gangrenous. Destruction of the subcutaneous nerves results in anesthetic skin.

Diagnosis

The triad of severe pain, local skin swelling, and fever should raise the suspicion for necrotizing infection. Although the diagnosis may be obvious in the later stages of these diseases, these infections often appear more benign and are frequently mistaken for cellulitis during the initial presentation. The hard woody feel of the subcutaneous tissue extending beyond the area of apparent skin involvement, presence of blisters or bullae, rapid spread of disease, presence of gas, systemic toxicity, and leukocytosis are added evidence for a necrotizing infection. Because of the grave prognosis, the urgency for timely surgical intervention and the importance of prompt antimicrobial therapy cannot be overemphasized. At surgery, the fascia is swollen and dull gray in appearance with stringy areas of necrosis with thin brownish exudates and no true purulence. Foul-smelling discharge that is characteristic of mixed aerobic/anaerobic infection is not found in monomicrobial infections because of *Streptococcus* and *Clostridium* species. Blood, aerobic, and anaerobic cultures from the wound should be obtained prior to antibiotic therapy.

Gram stain of the exudates may be helpful. In patients with *Clostridium* infection, clumps of large gram-positive rods and at times gram-variable rods can be seen. Leukocytes are scant to none in spite of the severity of illness. *Clostridium* produces an alpha toxin that destroys cell membranes, accounting for the paucity of leukocytes and erythrocytes seen on Gram stain. In patients with streptococcal and staphylococcal infections, Gram stain shows leukocytes and the corresponding cocci in chains or clusters. In the case of mixed infection, both gram-positive cocci and gram-negative rods of varying sizes together with leukocytes are easily observed.

Plain radiographs, computed tomography (CT), and magnetic resonance imaging (MRI) are used to aid in diagnosing necrotizing soft-tissue infections. Plain radiography is more sensitive than physical examination in detecting soft-tissue gas. CT scans have improved sensitivity over plain radiographs, especially when detecting soft-tissue edema, the presence of gas, obliteration of muscle planes, asymmetric fascial thickening, and the extent of soft-tissue damage. CT scans cannot differentiate cellulitis from necrotizing infections. MRI has very high sensitivity (93% to 100%) for diagnosing necrotizing infections; it shows good tissue contrast, detects soft-tissue fluid, and visualizes the pathologic process. Differentiating necrotizing infection from severe cellulitis and noninfectious inflammatory diseases may also prove problematic based on MRI alone. The diagnostic gold standard for necrotizing fasciitis remains the finding of fascial necrosis at the time of surgery.

CURRENT DIAGNOSIS

Common clinical manifestations:

- Wound pain that is severe and out of proportion to the physical findings
- Blistering or bullous skin lesions because of occlusion of deep vessels
- Foul watery discharge
- Gas in the soft tissue that can be shown by radiography; in more severe cases, crepitus can be appreciated
- Rapid spread along the fascial plane
- Systemic toxicity manifested by fever, delirium, and rapid progression to septic shock; leukocytosis and renal failure are often present

Microscopy of exudates:

- Polymicrobial infections: abundance of leukocytes and presence of gram-positive and gram-negative organisms
- *Clostridium perfringens:* paucity of leukocytes and presence of gram-positive or gram-variable rods
- *Streptococcus pyogenes:* abundance of leukocytes and presence of gram-positive cocci in chains

---

Treatment

SURGERY

Necrotizing skin and soft-tissue infection is a surgical emergency. Prompt recognition and timely aggressive surgical intervention accompanied by appropriate antimicrobial treatment are essential to improve survival. Surgical removal of all necrotic tissues is of paramount importance because antibiotic delivery to the involved area is ineffective related to the thrombosis of the supplying blood vessels. All necrotic tissues including the overlying skin must be removed until healthy-appearing bleeding tissue is encountered at the margin of the wounds. A second look should be done within 24 to 48 hours to assess the progression of the condition and the need for further débridement. This process is repeated as frequently as is necessary until the infection is under control.

CURRENT THERAPY

- Prompt surgical exploration, débridement, and amputation if necessary.
- Start antimicrobial therapy:
    - Clindamycin (Cleocin), 600–900 mg q8h IV plus:
        - Piperacillin/tazobactam (Zosyn), 4.5 g q6-8h IV, or
        - Imipenem/cilastatin (Primaxin), 500–750 mg q6–8h IV, or
        - Meropenem (Merrem), 1 g q8h IV.
- If MRSA infection is suspected, vancomycin (Vancocin), 15 mg/kg q12h should also be included.
- Alternate drugs: Broad-spectrum cephalosporin plus clindamycin with or without gentamicin.
- For patients who are intolerant of β-lactam drugs, clindamycin, 600–900 mg q8h IV, plus ciprofloxacin (Cipro), 400 mg q8h IV, or aztreonam (Azactam), 1–2 g q6-8-h IV, may be used with or without gentamicin.
- Tetanus toxoid or human tetanus immunoglobulin (BayTet) depending on the history of immunization.
- Intravenous immunoglobulin[1] (Gamimune) for severe cases.
- Fluid and electrolyte replacement including correction of hypoglycemia.
- Hyperbaric oxygen is adjunctive and should not delay or interfere with surgical intervention.

[1]Not FDA approved for this indication.

ANTIMICROBIAL AGENTS

Because of the nonspecificity of the initial presenting symptoms, empirical antimicrobial therapy should be started when necrotizing disease is suspected. The antimicrobial regimen chosen should have activity against streptococci, *Clostridium*, gram-negative rods, and anaerobes (Table 1). The combination of a β-lactam/β-lactamase inhibitor such as piperacillin/tazobactam (Zosyn) or a carbapenem such as imipenem (Primaxin) or meropenem (Merrem) should provide the necessary coverage.

β-Lactam agents are ineffective for treating necrotizing infections in the presence of a large inoculum of bacteria during their stationary phase of growth cycle. Clindamycin (Cleocin) has a greater efficacy because it acts at the ribosome by inhibiting protein synthesis; hence, clindamycin blocks further synthesis of bacterial toxins.

The need to cover MRSA (both health care and community associated) is important in geographic areas where MRSA isolates are commonly and increasingly encountered.

In patients who cannot tolerate β-lactam agents, clindamycin, 600 to 900 mg every 8 hours intravenously (IV), plus ciprofloxacin (Cipro), 400 mg every 8 hours IV, or aztreonam (Azactam), 1 to 2 g every 6 to 8 hours IV, may be used with or without gentamicin.

Unquestionably, aggressive and timely surgical intervention and appropriate antimicrobial therapy are essential for improved prognosis. After starting empirical therapy (Table 1), targeted antimicrobial treatment should be considered.

MIXED INFECTION

Patients with mixed bacterial infection should continue to receive broad-spectrum antibacterial therapy. Because of increasing resistance to different antibacterial agents among *Staphylococcus*, *Enterococcus*, and gram-negative bacteria, adjustment of antimicrobial therapy may be necessary when the susceptibility reports are available.

High-dose IV penicillin G (4 million U every 4 hours IV) plus clindamycin (900 mg every 8 hours IV) are effective for treating *S. pyogenes* and other streptococcal infections including *S. agalactiae*. For penicillin-intolerant patients, clindamycin may be given alone. With the increasing resistance of *S. agalactiae*, clindamycin alone is not recommended unless the susceptibility is known. New antimicrobial agents such as vancomycin (Vancocin), linezolid (Zyvox), and daptomycin (Cubicin) may also be considered.

For methicillin-sensitive *Staphylococcus aureus* (MSSA), antistaphylococcal penicillin (e.g., nafcillin, 2 g every 4 hours) or first-generation cephalosporins are effective. Vancomycin, 15 mg/kg every 12 hours IV, is recommended for MRSA infections. The dose should be adjusted based on renal function. For example, younger patients may have high renal clearance for vancomycin and may need vancomycin at more frequent intervals, and older patients (especially those with impaired renal function) may require adjustment to less frequent intervals. Most MRSA isolates are also susceptible to trimethoprim-sulfamethoxazole (Bactrim) and tetracyclines, preferably minocycline (Minocin) and doxycycline (Vibramycin). Community-acquired MRSA may be susceptible to clindamycin and resistant to macrolides. Certain MRSA strains may be reported as susceptible to clindamycin but are really resistant when subjected to the D-test. Newer agents effective against MRSA include linezolid (Zyvox), daptomycin (Cubicin), and tigecycline (Tygacil).

The combination of penicillin and clindamycin is more efficacious than single antibiotic therapy against *C. perfringens* and other *Clostridium* species (*Clostridium septicum, Clostridium sordellii, Clostridium novyi*). In patients who are intolerant to penicillin, clindamycin, chloramphenicol (Chloromycetin), tetracycline, and vancomycin alone may be used as the alternative agent.

Many infections from *Pasteurella canis* and *Pasteurella multocida* may not be limited to *Pasteurella* species alone. Other mouth organisms from the animal may be present at the site of injury. Piperacillin/tazobactam (Zosyn), 4.5 g IV every 8 hours, is recommended. An alternate regimen is third-generation cephalosporin (Ceftriaxone or Rocephin, 1 to 2 g IV every 24 hours) plus metronidazole (Flagyl), 500 mg IV every 8 hours. For a penicillin-intolerant patient, clindamycin (Cleocin), 900 mg IV every 8 hours, plus levofloxacin (Levaquin), 750 mg IV every 24 hours, or trimethoprim-sulfamethoxazole (Bactrim), double strength IV or orally every 12 hours, may be given.

Aeromonas hydrophila infections may be treated with ciprofloxacin, 400 mg IV every 12 hours, or levofloxacin, 750 mg IV every 24 hours. Alternative therapy includes third-generation cephalosporins such as ceftriaxone or trimethoprim-sulfamethoxazole.

V. vulnificus and *Vibrio* species infections may be treated with minocycline (Minocin), 100 mg IV or every 12 hours orally, plus ceftriaxone, 1 to 2 g IV every 24 hours. Ciprofloxacin may be used as the alternate therapy.

TABLE 1 Microbiology and Recommended Antimicrobial Treatment for Necrotizing Soft-Tissue Infection

Suspected Pathogens	Recommended Treatment

I. Mixed aerobic/anaerobic infections	Piperacillin/tazobactam (Zosyn), 4.5 g q6h IV
	   or
	imipenem/cilastatin (Primaxin),
	500–750 mg q6–8h IV
	   or
	meropenem (Merrem), 1 g q8h IV
	For penicillin-intolerant patients, clindamycin (Cleocin), 900 mg q8h IV, plus
	   ciprofloxacin (Cipro), 400 mg q8h IV

II. Monobacterial infections	
A. *Clostridium perfringens* and other *Clostridium* species including *C. septicum*, *C. sordelli*, *C. novyi*	Penicillin G, 4 million U q4h, plus clindamycin, 900 mg q8h IV For penicillin-intolerant patients, clindamycin, 900 mg q8h IV
B. *Streptococcus pyogenes*	Penicillin G, 4 million U q4h, plus clindamycin, 900 mg q8h IV For penicillin-intolerant patients, clindamycin, 900 mg q8h IV
C. *Streptococcus agalactiae*	Penicillin G, 4 million U q4h, plus clindamycin, 900 mg q8h IV For penicillin-intolerant patients, clindamycin, 900 mg q8h IV Must check for clindamycin resistance. If resistant to clindamycin, may consider other alternatives such as vancomycin (Vancocin), 1 g q12h (adjust dose for those with renal impairment)
D. *Staphylococcus aureus*, methicillin resistant, community acquired	Vancomycin (Vancocin), 1–1.5 g q12h (check renal function and trough levels) Alternative agent: linezolid (Zyvox), 600 mg q12h IV (may switch to oral when patient is stabilized)
E. *Pasteurella canis* and *Pasteurella multocida*	Frequently associated with polymicrobial infection as well; piperacillin/tazobactam, 4.5 g q6h IV For penicillin-intolerant patients: clindamycin, 900 mg q8h, plus ciprofloxacin, 400 mg q12h

F. *Aeromonas hydrophila*	Ciprofloxacin, 400 mg q8h
	   or
	trimethoprim-sulfamethoxazole (Bactrim), 1 double-strength tab q12h
	   or
	ceftriaxone (Rocephin), 1 g q24h, cefotaxime (Claforan), 1 g q12h

G. *Vibrio vulnificus*	Minocycline (Minocin), 100 mg IV or oral q12h plus ceftriaxone, 1–2 g IV q24h Ciprofloxacin may be used as the alternate therapy

H. Other gram-negative aerobic bacteria
  1. *Klebsiella pneumoniae*
  2. *Escherichia coli*
  3. *Pseudomonas aeruginosa*
  4. Serratia marcescens
	Based on susceptibility

Abbreviations: IV = intravenous.

Other gram-negative rods include *Klebsiella*, *Escherichia coli*, *Pseudomonas aeruginosa*, and *Serratia marcescens* infections. Treatment should be based on susceptibility results.

ADJUNCTIVE TREATMENT

Attention must be placed on fluid and electrolyte replacement including blood sugar control. In severe cases, IV immunoglobulin[1] (Gamimune) may be considered. Hyperbaric oxygen is advocated by some authorities, but this modality of treatment must not delay or interfere with urgent surgical intervention.

In summary, necrotizing skin and soft-tissue infection when suspected is a medical and surgical emergency. Surgical consultation for intervention must be promptly instituted. Initial empirical antimicrobial therapy must include agents with spectrum for both aerobic and anaerobic bacteria and include clindamycin to provide activity against further protein synthesis and toxin production. Adjunctive supportive treatment is important but should be secondary to surgical and antimicrobial treatment.

REFERENCES

File TM, Jr: Necrotizing soft tissue infections. In Tan JS (ed): Expert Guide to Infectious Diseases. Philadelphia, American College of Physicians; 2002, pp 618-633.

Gorbach SI: Skin and soft tissue infections. In Gorbach SL, Bartlett JG, Blacklow NR (eds): Infectious Diseases, 3rd ed. Philadelphia, Lippincott, 2004, pp 836-845.

[1]Not FDA approved for this indication.

Vinh DC, Embil JM: Rapidly progressive soft tissue infections. Lancet Infect Dis 2005;5(8):501-513.

Wong CH, Wang YS: The diagnosis of necrotizing fasciitis. Curr Opin Infect Dis 2005;18(2):101-106.

Young MH, Aronoff DM, Engleberg NC: Necrotizing fasciitis: Pathogenesis and treatment. Expert Rev Anti Infect Ther 2005;3(2):279-294.

Toxic Shock Syndrome

Method of
Robert L. Deresiewicz, MD

Staphylococcal toxic shock syndrome (TSS) is an acute, severe, febrile illness characterized by fever, hypotension, rash, multiorgan dysfunction, and convalescent-stage desquamation. It results from intoxication by any of several related *Staphylococcus aureus* exotoxins, most commonly TSS toxin type-1 (TSST-1). A related and clinically indistinguishable illness, toxic shock–like syndrome (TSLS), may follow infection by toxigenic strains of *Streptococcus pyogenes*.

TSS was first described in a pediatric population but became widely known in 1980 following a large outbreak among young, menstruating women, the overwhelming majority of whom were tampon users. Menstrual cases presently account for about half of TSS cases reported in the United States. The remainder are attributable to staphylococcal colonization or infection of diverse body sites, and occur in patients of either gender and at any age. With prompt recognition and proper management the outcome is usually good; the principal challenge, as with many rare and severe diseases, is to recognize the illness and promptly intervene.

Etiology and Pathogenesis

Virtually all menstrual TSS cases and about 60% of nonmenstrual cases are caused by TSST-1. Most of the remainder are caused by staphylococcal enterotoxin B (SEB) and a small fraction by enterotoxin C. Coagulase-negative staphylococci do not produce TSS toxins and, therefore, cannot cause TSS. The TSS toxins are encoded by variable genetic elements, meaning that the genetic capability to produce one or more of the toxins is present in only a subset of strains. Approximately 10% to 20% of human *S. aureus* isolates produce TSST-1 and 7% to 14% produce SEB.

Necessary steps in the pathogenesis of TSS are colonization of a nonimmune host by a toxigenic strain, toxin production, toxin absorption, and intoxication. Approximately 4% to 10% of people harbor toxigenic staphylococci at any site at any given time, including approximately 1% to 4% of postmenarcheal women who carry TSST-1–producing staphylococci in the vagina. Most people acquire protective levels of antibodies to TSST-1 and SEB during youth and adolescence, presumably consequent to benign staphylococcal colonization or trivial infection. By adulthood, more than 90% of people are immune to each toxin.

Toxigenic staphylococci that have the genetic capability to produce a TSS toxin actually do so only at limited times. The risk of TSS associated with the use of tampons or certain surgical dressings likely results from changes that these products cause to the local microenvironment, and the stimulus to toxin production resulting therefrom. For example, tampon use introduces oxygen into the normally anaerobic vagina; oxygen is required for TSST-1 synthesis, at least in vitro. Once produced, TSST-1 is rapidly transported across the vaginal mucosa.

The TSS toxins are superantigens—restricted T-cell mitogens—whose toxicity to humans is thought to derive from their ability to stimulate certain immune cells and thereby provoke exuberant, dysregulated cytokine release. How cytokine release culminates in the various manifestations of TSS remains uncertain. An important sequela, however, is the development of capillary leak syndrome, which may be principally responsible for the hypotension and end-organ damage that occurs in TSS.

Epidemiology

TSS is principally a disease of the first three decades of life. As noted, cases may be classified as menstrual or nonmenstrual. Menstrual cases peak in incidence between the third and fifth days of menses. The vast majority are in tampon users. Nonmenstrual cases include those related to colonization or infection of the female genitourinary tract (e.g., puerperal cases and cases associated with barrier contraceptive use, septic abortion, and nonobstetric gynecologic surgery); those associated with skin or soft-tissue infections (including both primary staphylococcal infections such as folliculitis, cellulitis, and furunculosis, and secondary infections such as of burns, bites, varicella lesions, or surgical wounds); and those related to infections of the respiratory tract (e.g., staphylococcal pharyngitis, tracheitis, sinusitis, or pneumonia) the musculoskeletal system (e.g., osteomyelitis, septic arthritis), or, rarely, the bloodstream. In postoperative cases, the illness may manifest within hours of the surgical procedure or may be delayed for days or weeks.

The number of TSS cases reported annually to the Centers for Disease Control and Prevention (CDC) has dropped considerably since the early 1980s. The drop is partly attributable to the development of safer tampons and tampon usage practices, but likely also reflects substantial under-reporting. The true frequency of menstrual TSS is probably at least 1 per 100,000 women per year, and is likely higher among women in their teens and early twenties. According to a recent study, the incidence of postoperative (nonmenstrual) TSS is 3 cases per 100,000 women.

Mortality also appears to have diminished over time. For the 10 years ended in 1996, the minimum case fatality rate for definite or probable menstrual cases reported to the CDC was 1.8%; for nonmenstrual cases the minimum rate was 5.5%.

Clinical Manifestations

Mild prodromal, flu-like symptoms occur in a minority of patients. The acute illness begins precipitously, with high fever, chills, headache, severe myalgias, muscle tenderness, abdominal pain, nausea, vomiting, and profuse watery diarrhea. Oral, conjunctival, and vaginal mucosal irritation also typically occurs. Orthostasis or hypotension and the characteristic macular erythroderma develop during the next 2 days. The erythroderma is usually generalized, often intense, and blanches with pressure. However, it may be locally distributed, mild, or fleeting; and it may be subtle, particularly in the presence of severe hypotension. On admission patients appear toxic, with hypotension, tachycardia, and oliguria. Examination may reveal conjunctival suffusion; tender, beefy-red oral or vaginal mucosa; and a strawberry tongue. Peripheral cyanosis and edema are common, as is diffuse abdominal tenderness. Rales may be present. The liver, spleen, and lymph nodes are usually unremarkable. Encephalopathy as evidenced by confusion, disorientation, agitation, or somnolence is also common, but the neurologic examination is typically nonfocal. The site of staphylococcal toxin production may be purulent or erythematous, or it may appear entirely benign. Laboratory studies reflect multiorgan dysfunction. Frequent findings include leukocytosis, thrombocytopenia, coagulopathy, azotemia, transaminitis, hypoalbuminemia, hypocalcemia, hypophosphatemia, and pyuria. Disseminated intravascular coagulation is not a common feature of TSS.

Like many other toxin-mediated diseases, TSS follows a fairly predictable course. The early manifestations of fever, erythroderma, gastrointestinal distress, and blood chemistry abnormalities resolve within the first few days of illness. In severe cases, hypotension may persist and may be complicated by myocardial dysfunction, pulmonary edema, rhabdomyolysis, hepatic damage, renal failure, or peripheral gangrene.

Desquamation is a late event in TSS. Superficial flaking of the skin on the trunk and extremities begins about a week into the illness. The characteristic full-thickness desquamation of the palms, soles, and digits follows in the second week and may continue for up to 1 month. Late sequelae of TSS include postfebrile telogen effluvium (reversible loss of the hair and nails), prolonged weakness or fatigue, memory loss, emotional changes, and impaired ability to concentrate. Fatalities typically occur within the first few days of illness, most commonly from refractory shock, respiratory failure, or cardiac arrhythmia.

Although not included in the case definition of TSS, mild systemic intoxications by the TSS toxins probably occur. Such cases lack two or more criteria for TSS but have certain clinical or epidemiologic features suggestive of the diagnosis (e.g., erythroderma, severe gastrointestinal disturbance, and/or convalescent desquamation). The occurrence of such an illness during menses in a young tampon user should prompt a search for evidence of TSST-1 involvement, particularly if the illness is recurrent. Compatible findings include the isolation of TSST-1-producing S. aureus from the vagina, and the demonstration of a nonprotective titer of serum anti-TSST-1 antibodies. Although such findings do not prove that an illness was TSST-1-related (certainly most perimenstrual flu-like illness is not attributable to TSST-1), they should, nevertheless, prompt discontinuation of tampon use until seroconversion has been documented. An attempt to eradicate vaginal staphylococcal carriage in such circumstances is also reasonable.

Diagnosis

The diagnosis of TSS is made exclusively on clinical grounds (Table 1). A host of possibilities other than TSS should be considered in the patient acutely ill with fever, rash, and hypotension. These include severe group A streptococcal infections (scarlet fever, necrotizing fasciitis, streptococcal TSLS), Kawasaki disease (particularly in children younger than 4 years of age), staphylococcal scalded skin syndrome, Rocky Mountain spotted fever, leptospirosis, meningococcemia, exanthematous viral syndromes, and severe allergic drug reactions.

In menstrual TSS cases, particularly when a purulent vaginal discharge is present, the diagnosis may be readily apparent. The challenge is to recognize subtle cases including nonmenstrual cases and cases in which the rash is evanescent. A careful history with attention to past health, possible infectious exposures, travel, vocation, avocation, vaccination status, menstrual status, and medication usage often considerably narrows the diagnostic possibilities. Backdrops particularly suggestive of TSS include the menstruating or postpartum female, the female who uses barrier contraceptive methods, the postoperative patient, the patient with varicella-zoster infection, and the patient with chemical or thermal burns.

Laboratory evaluation should include a complete blood count and differential, serum electrolytes, calcium, phosphate, albumin levels, liver and renal function tests, creatine phosphokinase level, coagulation studies, and urinalysis. A chest radiograph and an electrocardiogram should also be obtained. In females, vaginal culture should be performed. Blood, urine, and respiratory tract cultures should also be obtained, as should cultures of all wounds, regardless of how benign they might appear. The laboratory should be instructed to speciate any staphylococci isolated from mucosal sites. S. aureus isolates (mucosal or otherwise) should be referred for TSST-1 testing, if possible.

Acute and convalescent sera should be tested for antibody to TSST-1, particularly in suspected menstrual cases. The absence initially of a protective titer to TSST-1 supports the clinical diagnosis of TSS, and seroconversion, if it occurs, confirms it. The majority of patients, however, do not seroconvert following TSS; such patients, particularly those whose illness occurred in the perimenstrual period, are at risk for recurrent disease.

Treatment

With prompt treatment, the serious consequences of TSS (organ failure, limb loss, death) can often be avoided. Treatment involves four components:

1. Decontamination of the site of toxin production
2. Administration of antistaphylococcal antibiotics
3. Fluid resuscitation
4. General supportive care

The nidus of toxin production should be carefully sought. If present, vaginal tampons or other types of foreign bodies should be removed. Purulent foci should be drained and débrided and cutaneous lesions copiously irrigated. Thorough lavage lowers the burden of organisms and potentially slows toxin accretion. For TSS occurring in

TABLE 1 Staphylococcal Toxic Shock Syndrome: Case Definition

Criteria	Definition
1. Fever	Temperature ≥38.9°C (102°F)
2. Rash	Diffuse macular erythroderma (sunburn rash)
3. Hypotension	Systolic blood pressure ≤90 mm Hg (adults) or <5th percentile for age (children younger than 16 years of age)
	Orthostatic hypotension (orthostatic drop in diastolic blood pressure ≥15 mm Hg, orthostatic dizziness, or orthostatic syncope)
4. Organ involvement (at least 3 of the defined organ systems)	**GI** (vomiting or diarrhea at onset of illness)
	Muscular (severe myalgias or serum creatine phosphokinase level at least twice the upper limit of normal)
	Mucous membranes (vaginal, oropharyngeal, or conjunctival hyperemia)
	Renal (blood urea nitrogen or creatinine at least twice the upper limit of normal, or pyuria [≥5 leukocytes per high-power field] in the absence of urinary tract infection)
	Hepatic (total serum bilirubin or transaminase level [alanine aminotransferase or aspartate aminotransferase] at least twice the upper limit of normal)
	Hematologic (thrombocytopenia [platelets ≤100,000 per μL])
	CNS (disorientation or alteration in consciousness in the absence of focal neurologic signs at a time when fever and hypotension are absent)
5. Desquamation	1 to 2 weeks after onset of illness (typically of palms and soles)
6. Evidence against alternative diagnosis	If obtained, negative cultures of blood, throat, or cerebrospinal fluid*; absence of a rise in antibody titers to the agents of Rocky Mountain spotted fever, leptospirosis, or rubeola

*Blood cultures may be positive for *Staphylococcus aureus*.
Abbreviations: CNS = central nervous system; GI = gastrointestinal.
Adapted from Reingold AL, Hargrett NY, Shands KN, et al: Toxic shock syndrome surveillance in the United States, 1980 to 1981. Ann Intern Med 1982; 96(Part 2):875-880.

the postoperative period, the surgical wound must be explored, even if it appears uninfected.

Antibiotic administration offers a second opportunity to interrupt intoxication. While β-lactamase- resistant semisynthetic penicillins or first-generation cephalosporins have historically been given for TSS, growing evidence suggests that clindamycin (Cleocin) is superior. Under conditions of saturating (stationary phase) growth, staphylococci produce only low levels of penicillin-binding proteins. Penicillin-binding proteins are the molecular targets of β-lactam antibiotics. beta lactams are, therefore, relatively ineffective against such cells. On the other hand, TSST-1 is essentially only produced under those saturating conditions. Organisms producing TSST-1 are likely to be relatively resistant to β lactams. In addition, β-lactam levels fluctuate widely during dosing, and may fall below the minimum inhibitory concentration for *S. aureus* toward the end of each dosing interval. Subinhibitory concentrations of β lactams may actually enhance TSST-1 production.

Clindamycin, on the other hand, is a protein synthesis inhibitor; its antistaphylococcal activity is independent of growth phase. Moreover, clindamycin potentially suppresses TSST-1 production in vitro, even at concentrations insufficient to inhibit staphylococcal growth. The great majority of *S. aureus* strains causing TSS, particularly menstrual TSS, remain susceptible to clindamycin (and to methicillin). I suggest clindamycin 900 mg intravenously every 8 hours for suspected cases of TSS. In the critically ill patient in whom clindamycin- or methicillin-resistant infection may be a concern, it is reasonable to co-administer vancomycin (Vancocin) 1 g intravenously every 12 hours until microbiologic data are available. If the diagnosis of TSS is initially uncertain, broader empiric coverage is prudent.

Antibiotics should be administered for at least 10 days but can be given orally once the patient has stabilized.

Aggressive fluid resuscitation should be initiated to reverse hypotension and forestall end-organ damage. Adult patients may require up to 10 liters of crystalloid for the first 24 hours to maintain adequate cardiac filling. The principal mechanism of hypotension in TSS is capillary leak syndrome. Fluid therapy is, therefore, typically complicated by massive weight gain and peripheral edema. Pressors and central hemodynamic monitoring may be useful in cases of refractory hypotension, particularly if oxygenation is impaired.

In addition to the specific interventions outlined above, intensive care should be provided. Metabolic abnormalities should be corrected, and potential complications should be diligently sought. A final therapeutic option, especially for refractory cases or cases associated with an undrainable purulent focus, is pooled human immunoglobulin.[1] All commercial preparations contain anti-TSST-1 at concentrations sufficient to generate protective titers after a single intravenous dose of 400 mg/kg. Evidence supporting this therapy in humans is strictly anecdotal, but the approach makes sense on theoretical grounds.

---

[1]Not FDA approved for this indication.

Influenza

Method of
Kenneth J. Smith, MD, MSc

Influenza occurs annually during winter months. It produces an upper respiratory infection that can lead to complications with significant morbidity and mortality, causing an average of 36,000 deaths per year in the United States. Two viruses, influenza A and B, cause the typical influenza syndrome in humans. Changes in two viral surface glycoproteins, hemagglutinin (H) and neuraminidase (N), the main sites of immunologic recognition, lead to changes in population susceptibility to infection over time. Influenza A is prone to minor or major changes in either glycoprotein, whereas influenza B has sustained only minor changes in hemagglutinin. Minor changes are termed *antigenic drift* and occur as often as yearly, leading to localized outbreaks of influenza. Major glycoprotein changes are called *antigenic shift* and occur at irregular intervals (9 to 50 years), leading to worldwide influenza outbreaks or pandemics.

Outbreaks of avian influenza, an influenza A subtype, have raised concerns about the next pandemic. Human cases of avian influenza, mainly resulting from close contact with infected poultry or contaminated surfaces, have been relatively rare, but more than half of those infected have died. However, person-to-person spread has been very uncommon and has not continued beyond one person. Nevertheless, given the potential for viral mutations that could allow greater human-to-human spread, research is ongoing to develop an effective vaccine for this possible threat.

Traditionally, influenza control efforts have centered on illness prevention by vaccinating persons most susceptible to influenza complications in addition to health care workers. Antiviral medication use for prophylaxis and treatment had a relatively minor role, and tests were unavailable to assist clinicians in diagnosing influenza. More recently, vaccination is being recommended for lower-risk groups, nasal vaccination and newer antiviral agents are available, and rapid influenza tests can now potentially assist decision-making.

Clinical Manifestations

Clinical features of influenza are nonspecific but mainly respiratory. Onset often is abrupt, with fever, myalgia, and cough, but influenza often resembles other upper or lower respiratory infections, with nasal congestion, sore throat, fatigue, and malaise. In uncomplicated cases, fever and other symptoms are classically described as lasting approximately 3 days or longer with a convalescent period of 1 to 2 weeks. Recent antiviral trials show illness of 4 to 5 days' median duration in placebo recipients, with 70% reaching full recovery within 9 days after illness onset. The most common physical findings besides fever are hyperemic, nonexudative nasal and pharyngeal mucosa and small, tender cervical nodes; chest findings are typically absent.

Influenza complications can occur in up to 10% or more of otherwise healthy persons and more frequently in high-risk groups (patients with cardiac, renal, or pulmonary disease, or with diabetes, hemoglobinopathy, or immunosuppression; residents of nursing homes or chronic care facilities; and persons older than 65 years). Common complications are sinusitis, otitis media, bronchitis, and pneumonia. Pneumonia causes most of the morbidity and mortality of influenza and can be caused by the influenza virus itself, a bacterial superinfection (most commonly), or a mix of viral and bacterial pathogens. Primary influenza pneumonia is rare, and it is often fatal. As a viral illness, it does not respond to antibiotics, and its response to antiviral agents is unknown. Secondary bacterial pneumonia often presents as recurrent fever and systemic symptoms after acute influenza symptoms have improved. *Streptococcus pneumoniae*, *Staphylococcus aureus*, and *Haemophilus influenzae* are often cited as the leading causes based on a 1971 study; more recent data are unavailable. Other complications include exacerbations of chronic obstructive pulmonary disease (COPD) and asthma, myositis, and central nervous system (CNS) involvement. Reye's syndrome, characterized by nausea, vomiting, and mental status changes caused by liver dysfunction, can be seen in children with influenza (most often influenza B) and is associated with aspirin use.

Diagnosis

Because its clinical manifestations can resemble those of many other respiratory infections, influenza is typically a clinical diagnosis based on the presence of fever, nasal congestion, cough, and myalgia when influenza is active in the community. In this situation, the diagnosis is correct in 60% to 70% of patients. Previously, if confirmation of the diagnosis was desired, viral culture or other research-based techniques (immunofluorescence or polymerase chain reaction assays) were needed, or acute and convalescent serologic tests were performed. Unfortunately, test results came too late to be of help.

Now enzyme immunoassay tests can be performed in the physician's office, with test procedures that take less than 30 minutes. Tests are available to detect either influenza A or B, with no differentiation between the two (Flu OIA, QuickVue Influenza Test, and ZstatFlu), or detect either one with the ability to tell which virus is present (BD Directigen Flu A+B). Test specificity is generally high at 90% or greater; however, test sensitivity is low (65% to 86%), which leads to many false-negative test results when influenza prevalence is high.

Decision and cost-effectiveness analyses have shown that rapid testing for influenza is reasonable when influenza is

CURRENT DIAGNOSIS

- Influenza is mainly diagnosed when fever, nasal congestion, cough, and myalgia are present during known influenza activity in the community.
- Available rapid influenza tests have low sensitivity, leading to many false-negative test results when influenza is prevalent. Testing is more reasonable in situations where influenza likelihood is lower.

relatively uncommon, such as early or late in the typical influenza season or during influenza seasons where prevalence is low. When influenza prevalence is high, however, testing before treatment is not recommended because high rates of false-negative test results can lead to patients with influenza going untreated. Hence this strategy is not worth the expense of testing ($15 to $20).

If avian influenza is suspected, a polymerase chain reaction assay is available from the Centers for Disease Control and Prevention (CDC).

Prevention and Treatment

VACCINE

Influenza vaccination prevents influenza illness, complications, and death in high-risk groups. Cost-effectiveness analyses show that vaccination is cost-saving compared to no vaccination. Based on worldwide surveillance data, vaccine composition is modified to match that year's predictions of circulating influenza viruses. The CDC recommends intramuscular administration of inactivated influenza virus vaccine to the following groups at increased risk for influenza complications:

- Persons older than 65 years
- Residents of nursing homes and other chronic care facilities
- Adults and children with chronic cardiac or pulmonary disorders or with chronic metabolic diseases (including diabetes), renal dysfunction, hemoglobinopathy, or immunosuppression (including AIDS)
- Children and adolescents on chronic aspirin therapy (because of Reye's syndrome risk)
- Women who will be pregnant during the influenza season (influenza complication rates increase during pregnancy)
- Children ages 6 to 23 months

Intramuscular vaccination is also recommended for persons 50 to 64 years of age because of their greater likelihood for having high-risk conditions and because of the proven benefits for persons of this age who are not at high risk. Persons who can transmit influenza to those at high risk should also be vaccinated, including all personnel who have contact with patients in hospitals, outpatient settings, nursing home or chronic care facilities, and assisted living or retirement communities; home care personnel; and household contacts of persons in high-risk groups.

CURRENT THERAPY

- Antiviral agents are an adjunct to, not a replacement for, influenza vaccination.
- Antiviral therapy is clinically and economically reasonable based on clinical features without confirmatory testing when fever and typical symptoms are present during influenza outbreaks.
- Amantadine and rimantadine are relatively inexpensive, but they only cover influenza A and are more prone to side effects and antiviral resistance development. Zanamivir and oseltamivir are reasonable, but more expensive, options.

Live attenuated influenza vaccine (LAIV; FluMist) administered via the nasal passages is available, but it is more expensive than the inactivated vaccine. It can be given to healthy children and adolescents 5 to 17 years of age and healthy adults 18 to 49 years of age. If LAIV is given to persons who have contact with severely immunosuppressed patients, the CDC recommends refraining from patient contact for 7 days after vaccination because of virus shedding associated with this vaccine. LAIV is not recommended for persons at high risk for influenza complications or for patients younger than 5 years or older than 49 years. No significant differences in vaccine efficacy have been shown between the two modes of vaccination in adults younger than 50 years.

Neither vaccine should be administered to persons with anaphylactic reactions to eggs or to other influenza vaccine components. If high risk of influenza complications exists, however, allergy evaluation and desensitization followed by vaccination can be considered.

Optimal time of vaccination is October or November, but vaccination can continue into December and beyond. According to the CDC, acute febrile or nonfebrile illnesses are not a contraindication to vaccination, particularly in children with mild upper respiratory infections or allergic rhinitis, but vaccination should usually be delayed until symptoms have diminished.

Vaccine Dosage

Dosage of intramuscular inactivated vaccine is 0.50 mL, except in children 6 to 35 months old, in whom the dose is 0.25 mL. In children younger than 9 years who have not previously received influenza vaccination, a second dose should be administered at least 1 month after the first dose, ideally before December. Adults and older children should be vaccinated in the deltoid muscle, infants and younger children in the anterolateral thigh.

The live vaccine dose is 0.5 mL, divided equally between each nostril. Children ages 5 to 8 years, who have not previously received influenza vaccination of either type, should receive two doses separated by 6 to 10 weeks. Persons ages 9 to 49 years should receive one dose.

Vaccine Side Effects

Intramuscular inactivated vaccine causes local pain at the injection site in 10% to 64% of patients. The pain lasts for less than 2 days and rarely interferes with daily activities. Systemic reactions with fever, malaise, and myalgia lasting 1 to 2 days can occur, mainly in young children with no prior exposure to antigens contained in the vaccine. Placebo-controlled trials in healthy young adults and the elderly show no difference in systemic symptoms between placebo and influenza vaccine injections. Inactivated vaccine, containing killed virus, cannot cause influenza.

Intranasal vaccination of live attenuated virus can lead to higher rates of nasal congestion, headache, fever, and other systemic complaints than those seen in placebo recipients, particularly after the first dose. These side effects are largely mild and self-limited. Serious adverse effects are reported in less than 1%, and the incidence of pneumonia or other possible influenza complications was not statistically different from controls.

Guillain-Barré syndrome (GBS) occurred in less than 10 per million persons receiving the 1976 swine influenza vaccination. Since then, no statistically significant association between influenza and GBS has been found. According to the CDC, the risk of GBS with vaccination is approximately one per million vaccinations, which is much less than the risk of severe influenza complications, particularly in high-risk groups.

ANTIVIRALS

Two of the four available antiviral medications for influenza management, amantadine (Symmetrel) and rimantadine (Flumadine), are active only against influenza A, whereas the neuraminidase inhibitors zanamivir (Relenza) and oseltamivir (Tamiflu) are active against both influenza A and B. When given to patients with illness caused by susceptible virus within 48 hours, all agents decrease illness duration by approximately 1 day. Whether these medications decrease the likelihood of influenza complications is unclear; however, recent studies of zanamivir and oseltamivir strongly suggest that an impact on complications is likely, particularly in high-risk adults.

Deciding which drug to use for influenza treatment is complicated (Table 1). Amantadine and rimantadine are less expensive than zanamivir and oseltamivir but are effective only for influenza A and are more prone to side effects and induction of viral resistance. Because of reports of resistance, the CDC recommended against using amantadine and rimantadine during the 2005 to 2006 influenza season; whether high levels of resistance against these agents will continue in the future is unclear. The likelihood of influenza being caused by influenza A varies greatly and unpredictably from year to year and within single influenza seasons. CNS side effects (nervousness, anxiety, insomnia, difficulty concentrating, and lightheadedness) have occurred with amantadine (13%) and rimantadine (6%) and at higher levels in older populations. More severe CNS effects (marked behavioral changes, delirium,

agitation, seizures) are rare; gastrointestinal (GI) side effects occur in 1% to 3% of patients. Zanamivir should not be used in patients with asthma or COPD because of reported induction of bronchospasm and worsening pulmonary function after its use; otherwise, systemic side effects with zanamivir are similar to those with placebo. Unlike the oral formulations of the other agents, zanamivir is inhaled nasally and could be difficult to administer for some individuals. Oseltamivir causes nausea or vomiting in approximately 10% of patients; taking the medication with food may decrease this effect. Drug-resistant viruses occur in approximately one third of patients receiving amantadine or rimantadine, appearing within 2 to 3 days of starting therapy. Viral resistance to zanamivir and oseltamivir appears to be infrequent; surveillance for resistant viruses is being conducted. When antiviral therapy of influenza is warranted, cost-effectiveness analyses have shown that treatment with zanamivir or oseltamivir is clinically and economically reasonable, with amantadine or rimantadine as lower-cost options when influenza B is uncommon.

Chemoprophylaxis with antiviral agents, as an adjunct to vaccination, should be considered in:

- High-risk patients who are vaccinated during an influenza outbreak
- Persons caring for high-risk patients
- Persons with immunodeficiency and inadequate response to vaccination
- High-risk patients who cannot be vaccinated

Amantadine and rimantadine are approved for influenza A prophylaxis in patients ages 1 year and older (see Table 1). Oseltamivir is approved for influenza A and B prophylaxis in patients ages 1 year and older. When used with vaccination, antiviral prophylaxis should be given for at least 2 weeks after vaccination is completed. Otherwise, chemoprophylaxis should be continued for the duration of influenza activity in the community, although cost-effectiveness analysis suggests use only during peak influenza activity. When live attenuated vaccine is used,

---

TABLE 1 Approved Indications for Influenza Antiviral Medications

Treatment	Spectrum	Duration	Age Group (y)				
			1–6	7–9	10–12	13–64	≥65
Amantadine (Symmetrel)	Influenza A	5 d	5 mg/kg/d*	5 mg/kg/d*	100 mg bid	100 mg bid	≤100 mg/d
Rimantadine (Flumadine)	Influenza A	5 d	Not approved	Not approved	Not approved	100 mg bid	100 mg/d
Zanamivir (Relenza)	Influenza A or B	5 d	Not approved	10 mg bid	10 mg bid	10 mg bid	10 mg bid
Oseltamivir (Tamiflu)	Influenza A or B	5 d	Varies by weight	Varies by weight	Varies by weight	75 mg bid	75 mg bid
Prophylaxis							
Amantadine	Influenza A	†	5 mg/kg/d*	5 mg/kg/d*	100 mg bid	100 mg bid	≤100 mg/d
Rimantadine	Influenza A	†	5 mg/kg/d*	5 mg/kg/d*	100 mg bid	100 mg bid	100 mg/d
Oseltamivir	Influenza A or B	†	Varies by weight	Varies by weight	Varies by weight	75 mg/d	75 mg/d

*Up to 150 mg/d in two divided doses.
†Duration of influenza activity.

antiviral agents should not be used for 2 weeks afterward, because antivirals interfere with viral replication and subsequent immunity.

Avian influenza is resistant to amantadine and rimantadine. According to the CDC, oseltamivir and zanamivir "would probably work to treat influenza … but additional studies still need to be done to demonstrate their effectiveness." Oseltamivir prophylaxis is recommended for persons involved in outbreak control of avian influenza among poultry.

REFERENCES

Bridges CB, Harper SA, Fukuda K, et al; Advisory Committee on Immunization Practices: Prevention and control of influenza: Recommendations of the Advisory Committee on Immunization Practices (ACIP) [published correction appears in MMWR Morb Mortal Wkly Rep 2003;52:526]. MMWR Recomm Rep 2003; 52(RR-8):1-34.

Centers for Disease Control and Prevention online: Avian influenza (bird flu). Available at http//www.cdc.gov/flu/avian/

Hayden FG, Osterhaus AD, Treanor JJ, et al: Efficacy and safety of the neuraminidase inhibitor zanamivir in the treatment of influenzavirus infections. N Engl J Med 1997;337:874-880.

Jefferson TO, Demicheli V, Deeks JJ, Rivetti D: Amantadine and rimantadine for preventing and treating influenza A in adults. Cochrane Database Syst Rev 2002;(3):CD001169.

Kaiser L, Wat C, Mills T, et al: Impact of oseltamivir treatment on influenza-related lower respiratory tract complications and hospitalizations. Arch Intern Med 2003;163:1667-1672.

Muennig PA, Khan K: Cost-effectiveness of vaccination versus treatment of influenza in healthy adolescents and adults. Clin Infect Dis 2001;33: 1879-1885.

Rothberg MB, Bellantonio S, Rose DN: Management of influenza in adults older than 65 years of age: Cost-effectiveness of rapid testing and antiviral therapy. Ann Intern Med 2003;139(5 Pt 1):321-329.

Smith KJ, Roberts MS. Cost-effectiveness of newer treatment strategies for influenza. Am J Med 2002;113:300-307.

Treanor JJ, Hayden FG, Vrooman PS, et al: Efficacy and safety of the oral neuraminidase inhibitor oseltamivir in treating acute influenza: A randomized controlled trial. JAMA 2000;283:1016-1024.

Visceral Leishmaniasis

Method of
Pierre Marty, MD, PhD, and
Eric Rosenthal, MD, PhD

Leishmaniases are vector-borne diseases transmitted by sandfly bite and characterized by diversity and complexity. Depending on virulence factors of the parasite and on the immune response established by the host, a spectrum of diseases can appear: visceral, cutaneous, and mucosal leishmaniasis, which results from obligated replication of the protozoa in macrophage in the mononuclear system. Visceral leishmaniasis (VL) is a disseminated infection, in which macrophages of the liver, spleen, and bone marrow are parasite preferential and support intracellular replication. Diagnosis of VL is clinically suspected. According to sanitary conditions, the diagnosis is confirmed using either serologic tests, parasite demonstration, or molecular tests. Most often, the response criteria to treatment are clinical without parasitologic confirmation. Once established, the clinical course of untreated VL exhibits high mortality.

Epidemiology

VL is present in 61 countries on four continents where approximately 200 million people are exposed. The incidence is 500,000 cases per year with 90% in only five countries (India, Nepal, Bangladesh, Sudan, and Brazil). Severe epidemics occurred in India, 300,000 cases between 1977 and 1980 in the Bihar state with 2% mortality, and in Sudan, 100,000 deaths between 1989 and 1994. In the Mediterranean Basin, three countries of North Africa (Morocco, Algeria, and Tunisia) are particularly concerned as 95% of cases are observed in the children younger than 5 years. On the north bank of the Mediterranean Sea, sporadic cases of VL are observed in children but also in adults with or without permanent immunosuppression. Since the 1980s, VL is an emerging opportunistic disease in southwestern Europe (Portugal, Spain, France, and Italy) where more than 2500 cases of HIV-*Leishmania* co-infections are reported. Although not recognized as AIDS-defining criteria, VL constitutes an opportunistic disease in HIV-infected patients. Several studies have demonstrated that HIV/AIDS patients living in *Leishmania*-endemic areas are at greater risk of developing VL and that dual infection accelerates the clinical course of HIV disease. Clinical presentations are often atypical with unusual parasite localizations and frequent relapses. The introduction of highly active antiretroviral therapy (HAART) as a standard treatment for HIV patients has resulted in a significant decrease in the incidence of VL in southern European cases. Finally, the number of asymptomatic carriers demonstrated by transitory parasitemia in the human population and the role of humans as reservoirs of *Leishmania infantum* because of syringe sharing of intravenous drug users raise new questions.

Two epidemiologic types of VL must be considered:

- Zoonotic visceral leishmaniasis (ZVL) caused by *L. infantum* (*Leishmania chagasi* in Latin America) with dog as reservoir. This animal is frequently killed by the disease, but asymptomatic forms are not rare. ZVL is observed in China, Pakistan, Latin America, the Middle East, and the Mediterranean Basin.
- Anthroponotic visceral leishmaniasis (AVL) with human as unique reservoir is because of *Leishmania donovani* and is an epidemic disease in Sudan, East Africa, India, Nepal and Bangladesh.

After contamination by the parasitic sandfly bite, the evolution of asymptomatic carrier to the stage of patent VL may occur if the following risk factors are present: genetic susceptibility, acquired or iatrogenic immunosuppression, and dose of inoculated parasites and virulence of the strain.

Diagnosis

The clinical signs of the classic Mediterranean ZVL occurring in young children are constant irregular fever persistent over several weeks and splenomegaly associated with hepatomegaly in 50% to 70% of cases. Pallor is almost constant and lymphadenopathies rare. Adult cases of ZVL are more and more frequent in southwestern Europe (two thirds of total cases), and characteristic clinical signs are less constant in this population than in children. In half of

CURRENT DIAGNOSIS

Suspicion of zoonotic visceral leishmaniasis:

- Clinical: irregular fever, pallor, splenomegaly, ± hepatomegaly
- Living or past travel in endemic area: Mediterranean Basin, Latin America (northeast Brazil), China (Xia Jiang, Sichuan, Gansu)
- Biology: anemia, leukoneutropenia, thrombopenia, hyperproteinemia, hypergammaglobulinemia
- Immunosuppression: HIV, corticotherapy, transplantation, very young children, malnutrition

Confirmation via blood:

- Serology
- Leukoconcentration and microscopic examination
- Culture on special medium
- Polymerase chain reaction (PCR)

Confirmation via bone marrow aspirate:*

- PCR
- Microscopic examination
- Culture on special medium

*If serology and PCR results are positive or negative and leukoconcentration and microscopic examination and cultured special medium are negative, confirmation using bone marrow aspirate is necessary.

adult cases, a permanent immunosuppression is present (HIV infection or immunosuppressive treatment for neoplastic disease or transplantation).

AVL is diagnosed whatever the age. Pallor, high irregular fever, and splenomegaly are almost constant. Lymphadenopathy and cutaneous manifestations such as darkening, even blackening, of the skin, affecting especially the face, hands, and upper torso, are frequently associated in India (AVL = *kala azar*, which means "black sickness" in Sanskrit).

Pancytopenia is present with anemia, leukoneutropenia, and thrombopenia and associated with an inflammatory syndrome (hyperproteinemia and polyclonal hypergammaglobulinemia).

Serologic tests allow diagnosis in almost all the cases. The gold standard test is the indirect fluorescent antibody test (IFAT), but enzyme-linked immunosorbent assay (ELISA) is becoming more frequently used. Specificity and sensitivity of ELISA tests depend on the antigens used. ELISA is especially useful for field work; samples may be collected on filter papers and eluted directly into microtiter walls. The direct agglutination test (DAT) of fixed parasites is an inexpensive test that is also useful in field conditions. The new generation of this test is very sensitive (97% to 100%) like the rapid immunochromatographic tests (dipstick with a band impregnated with recombinant protein antigen, especially rK 39). Western blotting is very specific and very sensitive but also extremely expensive. This test is able to discriminate patent VL against asymptomatic carriers and negative people. It is appealing for epidemiologic studies.

The parasitologic diagnosis is based on the visualization of amastigote forms of the parasite on bone marrow aspiration (Latin tradition) or spleen aspirate (British tradition, particularly in India). Parasites can be detected on peripheral blood after concentration, particularly in severe immunosuppressed patients. The culture of blood or bone

marrow on special medium (Schneider, Novy, McNeal, Nicolle) is useful, especially for the characterization of the strain. Fortuitous diagnosis of atypical localizations is possible with digestive or cutaneous biopsies or bronchoalveolar lavages in at least a third of the patients with HIV co-infection. The molecular diagnosis is very sensitive but again expensive. Polymerase chain reaction (PCR) is used to decrease the number of false-negative results obtained with parasitologic methods. PCR is particularly useful for post-therapeutical follow-ups and to diagnose relapses.

Available Drugs

PENTAVALENT ANTIMONY

Organic salts of pentavalent antimony have been the cornerstone of the treatment for all the leishmaniases for more than 60 years. Two major pentavalent antimonials are currently used: sodium stibogluconate (Pentostam[2]), containing 100 mg/mL of antimony, and meglumine antimonate (Glucantime[2]), containing 85 mg/mL of antimony. The drugs are given intravenously (IV) or intramuscularly (IM) and are equal in efficacy when used in equivalent doses. The recommended regimen consists of once-daily injections of the full-dose drug (20 mg/kg) for 30 days (Table 1). Disadvantages of antimonials include the parenteral

[2]Not available in the United States.

CURRENT THERAPY

- Two major pentavalent antimonials are currently used: sodium stibogluconate (Pentostam[2]) and meglumine antimonate (Glucantime[2]). The drugs are given intravenously or intramuscularly and are equal in efficacy when used in equivalent doses. Disadvantages of antimonials include the parenteral mode of administration, the long duration of therapy, and adverse reactions.
- Lipid derivatives of amphotericin B were developed to increase the therapeutic index. AmBisome is a lipid formulation of amphotericin B in which the drug is packaged along with cholesterol and other phospholipids within a small unilamellar liposome. The highly specialized liposomal formulation of AmBisome has several characteristics that increase its efficacy against visceral leishmaniasis (VL) while minimizing toxicity.
- Miltefosine is the first orally administered treatment effective for VL but has toxic effects on reproductive capacity in female animals (pregnancy should be avoided for 2 months after completion of therapy).
- Injectable paromomycin was tested by OneWorld Health as a treatment for VL.
- In antimonial-resistant VL, pentamidine isethionate[1] (Pentam) may be used.
- Recommendations in the treatment of VL may be differentiated according to the different settings.

[1]Not FDA approved for this indication.
[2]Not available in the United States.

TABLE 1 Key Treatment

Type of VL	First-line Drug	Total Dose (mg/kg)	Regimen	Primary or Secondary Unresponsiveness	Total Dose (mg/kg)	Regimen
Zoonotic VL	Liposomal amphotericin B	20	*10 mg/kg days 1, 2, or smaller divided doses, but initial dose of at least 5 mg/kg is recommended	Not documented		
Anthroponotic VL	Pentavalent antimony	600	Sb^V 20 mg/kg/d qd ≥30 d	Liposomal amphotericin B or combination regimen without antimonial drugs	10–20	Various short schedules For example, liposomal amphotericin B plus miltefosine, or liposomal amphotericin B plus paromomycin
HIV co-infection	Liposomal amphotericin B	20–40	†100 mg/d 21 days or †4 mg/kg days 1–5, 10, 17, 31, 38	Crossover with first-line regimen		
	Pentavalent antimony	600	Sb^V 20 mg/kg/d qd ≥30 d	Or miltefosine		In adults: 100 mg/d for 28 d or longer

*This schedule needs to be validated in adults.
†Higher daily doses with shorter schedule need to be evaluated.
Abbreviations: HIV = human immunodeficiency virus; Sb^V = pentavalent antimony; VL = visceral leishmaniasis.

mode of administration, the long duration of therapy, and adverse reactions. Systemic toxicity normally relates to total dose administrated. Secondary effects are frequent, albeit usually reversible (e.g., fatigue, body aches, electrocardiographic abnormalities, raised aminotransferase levels, chemical pancreatitis). Severe adverse events remain rare; however, sudden death because of arrhythmia and acute pancreatitis with a fatal evolution are reported.

LIPID-ASSOCIATED FORMULATIONS OF AMPHOTERICIN B

The antifungal agent amphotericin B (AmBisome, Abelcet, Amphotec) has long been recognized as a powerful leishmanicidal drug. Largely because of the decline and fall of antimonials in some areas and the failure of pentamidine as a satisfactory substitute, amphotericin B has been rediscovered as an effective treatment for VL. Infusion-related side effects and renal toxicity of conventional amphotericin B are major problems. Lipid derivatives of amphotericin B were developed to increase the therapeutic index. AmBisome is a lipid formulation of amphotericin B in which the drug is packaged along with cholesterol and other phospholipids within a small unilamellar liposome. The highly specialized liposomal formulation of AmBisome has several characteristics that increase its efficacy against VL while minimizing toxicity.

The small size of the liposome (<100 μm) promotes wide distribution and penetration into tissues. The high transition temperature (55°C [155°F] compared to 25°C [77°F] for an amphotericin B lipid complex formulation) ensures liposome stability, which minimizes the release of the drug until contact is made with the pathogen. Tissue penetration is highest in the liver and spleen, and therapeutic levels persist in these organs several weeks or more after receiving doses of AmBisome. Pharmacokinetic studies demonstrate that high initial doses (at least 5 mg/kg,[3] with doses up to 50 mg/kg[3] tested in animals) give better tissue penetration and longer persistence in viscera than frequent low doses, suggesting that initial loading doses may increase efficacy. In humans, the terminal elimination half-life after repeated administration of AmBisome is approximately 7 hours with a trough level in blood by 24 hours. Although transient rises in creatine can occur, acute and chronic toxicity from AmBisome is low even when doses up to 15 mg/kg are used.

First used in antimonial-resistant VL in 1991, lipid formulations of amphotericin B increase the efficacy and limit the toxicity of conventional amphotericin B. Thirteen clinical trials of AmBisome for treatment of VL have been published. One objective was to find the lowest total dose with acceptable efficacy because of affordability concerns.

[3]Exceeds dosage recommended by the manufacturer.

A single dose of 7.5 mg/kg gave a 90% cure rate at 6 months in a fairly large Indian trial. In Europe, clinical trials demonstrated 90% to 98% efficacy with a total AmBisome dose of 18 to 21 mg/kg in immunocompetent patients. A variety of regimens are currently in use: 3 mg/kg, days 1 to 5 and 10, for a total dose of 18 mg/kg, in Italy; 3 mg/kg, days 1 to 5, 14, and 21 for a total dose of 21 mg/kg, for imported cases in the United States; 1 to 1.5 mg/kg for 21 days or 3 mg/kg for 10 days, in New Zealand. Published case series and current pediatric practice in Southern Europe suggest good efficacy for a total dose of 20 mg/kg, with many pediatricians currently using a regimen of 10 mg/kg/day for 2 consecutive days.

In HIV co-infected patients, there have been no formal randomized clinical trials of AmBisome treatment and secondary prophylaxis regimens and only two open-label dose-finding studies. The efficacy of antimonials and AmBisome were comparable in most case series, but the lower rate of toxicity for AmBisome has caused most clinicians to consider it as the antileishmanial drug of choice in HIV co-infected patients. Secondary prophylaxis with doses of AmBisome or other antileishmanials every 2 to 4 weeks after initial clinical cure of VL is now the standard of care in Europe.

OTHER DRUGS

Miltefosine

Hexadecylphosphocholine (miltefosine[2]) is one of a series of alkylphosphocholines. It was developed as an antineoplastic agent. The mechanisms of action of miltefosine against *Leishmania* are not well determined, although miltefosine blocks the proliferation of *Leishmania* and alters both the phospholipid and sterol composition. In fact, the activity of miltefosine on *Leishmania* is because of a direct cytotoxicity and the activation of cellular immunity. Miltefosine was the first orally administered treatment that proved effective for VL including those with antimony-resistant infections. The treatment is 100 mg per day for 28 days in adults and children older than 10 years. Vomiting and diarrhea are the most frequent side effects. Unfortunately, miltefosine has toxic effects on reproductive capacity in female animals, and pregnancy should be strictly avoided while on the drug and for 2 months after completion of therapy. Because of the long half-life, subtherapeutic levels of miltefosine may remain for some weeks after a 4-week course, and it is feared that this characteristic might encourage the emergence of resistance in the future.

Paromomycin

Paromomycin (Humatin) is an aminoglycoside antibiotic with antiparasitic activity. Injectable paromomycin was tested in India as a treatment for VL. The doses of 12 mg/kg/day, 16 mg/kg/day, and 20 mg/kg/day for 21 days were tested alone or in combination with antimony. The drug was well tolerated except for a few cases of hearing disturbance. OneWorld Health in collaboration with the World Health Organization (WHO) completed a phase 3 clinical trial of 667 patients in November 2004. This was the largest trial ever performed for this disease. Beginning in June 2003, the phase 3 trial enrolled patients in Bihar, India, with VL that was confirmed by the presence of the parasite in the spleen or bone marrow. They were randomized in a ratio of 3:1 to receive either paromomycin or the current standard therapy in India, amphotericin B.

Diamidine

In antimonial-resistant VL, pentamidine isethionate[1] (Pentam), 4 mg/kg (IM), was used three times weekly for 6 weeks. However, side effects (myalgia, nausea, headache, and hypoglycemia) were common at this dose including exceptional risks of irreversible diabetes. At present in antimonial-resistant areas, second-line treatment with pentamidine alone achieves poor response rates, which limits interest in pentamidine use.

Therapeutic Strategies

The declining activity and the toxicity of traditional leishmanicidal drugs stress the need for alternative compounds and for the optimization of therapeutic protocols. Recommendations in the treatment of VL may be differentiated according to the different settings.

ZOONOTIC VISCERAL LEISHMANIASIS

In 1995, the WHO agreed that four first-line regimens were acceptable for the management of VL in immunocompetent patients. However, AmBisome has been used with increasing frequency to treat VL over the past decade. Compared to existing antileishmanial drugs, AmBisome has the highest therapeutic index, confirming its use as first-line therapy. A total AmBisome dose of 20 mg/kg is adequate to treat immunocompetent children and adults. According to the recent recommendations of the WHO, the exact dosing schedule can be flexible (divided into doses of 10 mg/kg[3] on 2 consecutive days or in smaller divided doses), but AmBisome pharmacokinetics suggest that the initial dose provides better tissue levels if at least 5 mg/kg[3] is given. The schedule of 10 mg/kg[3] on 2 consecutive days needs to be validated in adults with zoonotic visceral leishmaniasis.

ANTHROPONOTIC VISCERAL LEISHMANIASIS

The first-line treatment remains antimonial pentavalent compounds with a minimal dose of 20 mg/kg/day for 28 days. Suboptimal doses, incomplete treatment, and substandard drugs may lead to clinical resistance. When unresponsiveness (primary and secondary) to antimonial drugs exceeds 10% in an area, policymakers should strongly consider a shift to an alternative first-line regimen. According to current WHO recommendations, two possible alternatives are an amphotericin B formulation (AmBisome at a total dose of 20 mg/kg) or a combination regimen that does not

---

[2]Not available in the United States.

[1]Not FDA approved for this indication.
[3]Exceeds dosage recommended by the manufacturer.

include antimonial drugs. Use of combination antileishmanial drug regimens should be promoted to prevent the development of resistance to existing drugs. With respect to AmBisome, AmBisome-miltefosine, AmBisome-paromomycin, and (in areas with less than 10% primary unresponsiveness to Sb^V) AmBisome-Sb^V combinations should be evaluated.

HIV CO-INFECTION

Access to HAART is high priority for co-infected patients. For HIV patients whose immune reconstitution is incomplete, data are insufficient to make firm recommendations regarding the best regimens for primary treatment and secondary prophylaxis of VL. Multicenter trials of first-line treatment and secondary prophylaxis of visceral leishmaniasis in HIV-infected patients are needed, and AmBisome regimens should be included in these trials.

REFERENCES

Adler-Moore J, Proffitt RT: AmBisome: Liposomal formulation, structure, mechanism of action and preclinical experience. J Antimicrob Chemother 2002;(Suppl 1.):21-30.

Alvar J, Canavate C, Guttierez-Solar B, et al: *Leishmania* and human immunodeficiency virus coinfection: The first ten years. Clin Microbiol Rev 1997;10:298-319.

Bern C, Adler-Moore J, Berenguer J, et al: WHO informal consultation on liposomal amphotericin B (AmBisome) in visceral leishmaniasis treatment. Clin Infect Dis 2006;43:917-924.

Bryceson A: A policy for leishmaniasis with respect to the prevention and control of drug resistance. Trop Med Int Health 2001;6:928-934.

Deniau M, Canavate C, Faraut-Gambarelli F, Marty P: The biological diagnosis of Leishmaniasis in HIV-infected patients. Ann Trop Med Parasitol 2003;97:S115-S133.

Desjeux P: Leishmaniasis: Current situation and new perspectives. Comp Immunol Microbiol Infect Dis 2004;27:305-318.

Kafetzis DA, Velissariou IM, Stabouli S, et al: Treatment of paediatric visceral leishmaniasis: Amphotericin B or pentavalent antimony compounds? Int J Antimicrob Agents 2004;25:26-30.

Le Fichoux Y, Quaranta JF, Aufeuvre JP, et al: Occurrence of *Leishmania infantum* parasitemia in asymptomatic blood donors living in an area of endemicity in southern France. J Clin Microbiol 1999;37:1953-1957.

Rosenthal E, Marty P, Del Giudice P, et al: HIV and *Leishmania* coinfection: A review of 91 cases with focus on atypical locations of *Leishmania*. Clin Infect Dis 2000;31:1093-1095.

Singh S, Dey A, Sivakumar R: Applications of molecular methods for *Leishmania* control. Expert Rev Mol Diagn 2005;5:251-265.

Sundar S, Jha TK, Thakur CP, et al: Oral miltefosine for Indian visceral leishmaniasis. N Engl J Med 2002;347:1739-1746.

Sundar S, Jha TK, Thakur CP, et al: Single-dose liposomal amphotericin B in the treatment of visceral leishmaniasis in India: A multicenter study. Clin Infect Dis 2003;37:800-804.

Leprosy

Method of
Winnie W. Ooi, MD, MPH, DMD

In May 1991, the World Health Organization (WHO) adopted a resolution establishing a goal of "the elimination of leprosy as a public health problem by the year 2000." Elimination was defined as a prevalence of one case or fewer per 10,000 population, with a case being defined as a patient receiving or requiring chemotherapy. Implementation of a short course of multiple drug therapy (MDT) worldwide since 1982 had resulted in many patients completing treatment and being removed from global case registers. Significant declines in incidence had also occurred in some countries, such as China and Mexico, before the introduction of MDT. This decline was thought to be secondary to better nutrition and living conditions, although widespread Bacille Calmette-Guérin (BCG) vaccination, which is protective against leprosy in Africa, may have played a role. This target for elimination was reached in 2000, but the major endemic countries such as Brazil and India did not reach the elimination goal. At the beginning of 2005, the global registered prevalence of leprosy was 286,063 cases, and the number of new cases detected during 2004 was 407,791. The number of new cases therefore fell by approximately 21% during 2004 compared with 2003. This decrease was mainly a result of the reduction in the number of new cases detected in India.

Epidemiology

Leprosy now remains a public health problem in Angola, Brazil, Central African Republic, Democratic Republic of the Congo, India, Madagascar, Mozambique, Nepal, and the United Republic of Tanzania.

This disease is rare in the United States, with 85% of detected cases occurring in immigrants. The diagnosis of leprosy is usually made during the first year after entry into the United States, but no evidence indicates that the imported cases resulted in local transmission. Small numbers of endemic cases are reported from Texas and Louisiana, possibly from exposure to the local wild armadillos, up to half of which have naturally acquired leprosy.

Diagnosis

Anesthetic skin or mucous membrane lesions in the presence of thickened nerves (Figure 1) are the hallmarks of leprosy. Acid-fast bacilli in slit-skin smears or skin biopsies, which should include subepidermal tissue, confirm the diagnosis. Patients with leprosy were classified as having paucibacillary (PB) disease and multibacillary (MB) disease based on slit-skin smears. In the field and when no laboratory facilities are available, a clinical classification is used: patients with two to five lesions (combination of skin lesions and palpable nerves) are described as having paucibacillary disease, and those with more than five lesions as having multibacillary disease. Acid-fast staining with Fite stain in skin biopsies is used for detecting *Myobacterium leprae*, and the density of bacilli is recorded logarithmically as the bacterial index (BI). Pure neural leprosy is characterized by the presence of a neurologic deficit and nerve thickening (with or without tenderness) in the absence of skin involvement. It is seen in up to 10% of patients with leprosy who present to treatment centers in India.

Serologic methods using antibodies to species-specific lipid antigens of *M. leprae*, such as phenolic glycolipid 1(PGL-1), are not sensitive enough to use for diagnosis in the individual patient. The majority of patients with paucibacillary disease do not have a detectable humoral

CURRENT DIAGNOSIS

WHO Classification	Ridley & Jopling Classification	Character of skin lesions	Modified Ziehl-Nielsen (Fite) stain	Nerve involvement
	Indeterminate (I)	Hypopigmented macular lesions	Negative	None
	Tuberculoid (TT)	Hypopigmented annular lesions	Negative	Localized, involving one or more large nerves around the skin lesions Asymmetric involvement
Paucibacillary (PB)	Borderline tuberculoid (BT)	Annular lesions with less distinct borders	Negative	Similar to tuberculoid disease
	Borderline (BB)	Spectrum between borderline tuberculoid and	Negative or Positive	Spectrum between tuberculoid disease and lepromatous disease
	Borderline (BB)	Borderline lepromatous		
Multibacillary (MB)	Borderline lepromatous (BL)	Infiltrated patches	Positive	Tends to be diffuse and may be asymmetrical
	Lepromatous (LL)	Diffuse, symmetrical skin infiltration	Positive	Diffuse and symmetrical, relatively slow and progressive distal polyneuropathy

Abbreviation: WHO = World Health Organization.

response, although there is a high rate of seropositivity in patients with multibacillary disease when studied in endemic populations.

In regions with low endemicity such as the United States, other methods of diagnosis, such as polymerase chain reaction (PCR), are positive only in biopsy specimens that have detectable organisms on Fite staining. As such, PCR is only useful clinically to support a diagnosis of leprosy if atypical clinical or histologic features are present.

Pathogenesis

The etiologic agent *M. leprae* is an obligate intracellular parasite that grows best at 27°C to 30°C (81°F to 86°F) in the experimental mouse footpad model and in humans but has not been cultured in vitro. Although humans are considered the major host and reservoir, the disease may be found in armadillos and primates. The mode of transmission of leprosy is not well understood: Transmission may occur primarily by direct contact with ulcerated skin lesions and sneeze aerosols. Consequently, household contacts of patients with borderline leprosy and lepromatous leprosy whose nasal mucosae are heavily infected with bacilli are at much higher risk of acquiring the disease.

The large variation of the host response to infection with *M. leprae* and therefore the clinical features are genetically influenced. Familial clustering is well documented, and concordance rates in identical twins are high. Susceptibility of leprosy is linked to the NRAMP1 gene, which in mice controls innate susceptibility to mycobacterial infections.

Clinical Features

The incubation period ranges from 3 months to 40 years, with an average of 7 years. The disease has an insidious onset and affects primarily the skin and peripheral nerves.

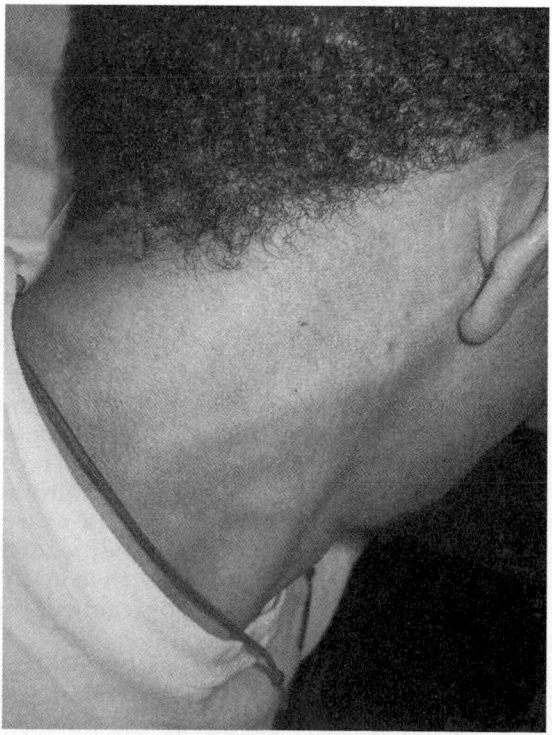

FIGURE 1. Enlarged nerve in borderline tuberculoid disease

The disease manifestations result from the interaction between the organism and the immune system of the infected host. Most infected individuals have an effective immunity without disease, whereas others have a spectrum of clinical manifestations on presentation that correlates with the cell-mediated immunity of the patient (Ridley-Jopling classification). This spectrum ranges from patients with tuberculoid leprosy (TT) who exhibit a relatively good cell-mediated immunity against *M. leprae* to lepromatous (LL) patients who are anergic to *M. leprae*, leading to a widespread systemic disease developing that involves not only the skin and upper respiratory tract but also the anterior chamber of the eye, the testes, lymph nodes, periosteum, and superficial sensory and motor nerves. Immunodeficiency associated with HIV-1 infection has not affected the case detection rate or the outcome of treatment for patients with leprosy. However, pregnancy, which causes a relative decrease in cellular immunity, may precipitate new reactions or relapses in patients with leprosy.

The bacilli favor the cooler areas of the body, such as the chin and malar areas of the face, earlobes, buttocks, knees, and distal extremities. Skin lesions range from the asymptomatic, ill-defined, slightly hypopigmented macule of indeterminate leprosy to the diffuse infiltration of the skin seen in lepromatous leprosy that causes thickening of the skin of the face and earlobes and produces the classic leonine facies. Eyebrows and eyelashes can be lost (madarosis), and anesthesia of affected areas is .extensive and accompanied by anhydrosis in lepromatous leprosy.

Drug Treatment

Until 1980 the treatment of patients with leprosy consisted of dapsone monotherapy. Multiple drug therapy was recommended by the World Health Organization (WHO) in 1982 because of increasing resistance (primary and secondary) to dapsone, approaching 40% in some countries.

Rifampin is by far the most effective bactericidal drug against *M. leprae*, rendering patients with lepromatous leprosy noninfectious within 2 days. The standard dose of 600 mg monthly of rifampin in multiple drug therapy regimens is relatively nontoxic, although rare instances of renal failure, thrombocytopenia, hemolytic anemia, and hepatitis are reported. Dapsone is a slow-acting bacteriostatic drug with a short half-life. Side effects include mild hemolysis (severe if the patient is glucose-6-phosphatase deficient [G6PD]), allergic rashes, methemoglobinemia, and agranulocytosis. Clofazimine has equal activity to dapsone but has additional anti-inflammatory activity. It commonly causes skin pigmentation and concentrates in areas with high bacterial loads. Gastrointestinal side effects are not uncommon, and small bowel obstruction is described with high doses.

Patients with paucibacillary disease were initially treated with rifampin and dapsone for 6 months. Patients with multibacillary disease also received rifampin, dapsone, and clofazimine for 24 months. Relapse rates after therapy were considered low enough in 1988 for the WHO to recommend decreasing the duration of therapy for patients with multibacillary disease to 12 months. The recommendations of American authorities on leprosy differ from the

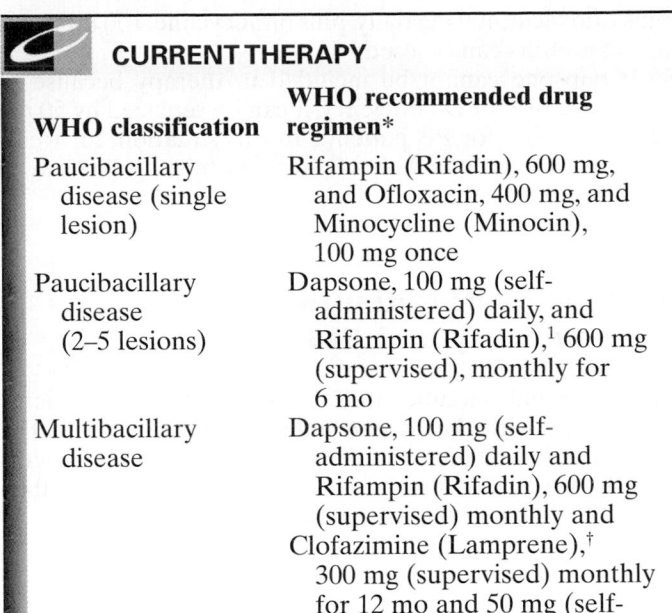

WHO classification	WHO recommended drug regimen*
Paucibacillary disease (single lesion)	Rifampin (Rifadin), 600 mg, and Ofloxacin, 400 mg, and Minocycline (Minocin), 100 mg once
Paucibacillary disease (2–5 lesions)	Dapsone, 100 mg (self-administered) daily, and Rifampin (Rifadin),[1] 600 mg (supervised), monthly for 6 mo
Multibacillary disease	Dapsone, 100 mg (self-administered) daily and Rifampin (Rifadin), 600 mg (supervised) monthly and Clofazimine (Lamprene),[†] 300 mg (supervised) monthly for 12 mo and 50 mg (self-administered) daily for 12 mo.

Note: PB patients who relapse are treated with regimens appropriate for MB. PB patients who relapse with MB disease or MB patients who relapse should have a mouse footpad sensitivity study carried out or PCR done on a skin biopsy for sensitivity testing, after which they should be treated with one of the MB regimens for 2 years.

[1]Not FDA approved for this indication.

*The recommendations of American authorities on leprosy differ from the WHO regimens in that 300 mg rifampin is often administered daily, and the length of treatment is 6 months for PB disease and 24 months for MB disease. Follow-up is also longer because of concerns about relapses.

[†]Not commercially available in the United States after July 2004; only available through the National Hansen's Disease Program by calling 1-800-642-2477 or visit their Web site at http://bphc.hrsa.gov/nhdp.

Abbreviation: WHO = World Health Organization.

WHO regimens in that 300 mg of rifampin is administered daily; and the length of treatment remains at 24 months for MB disease. The detection of viable *M. leprae* in tissues after 12 months of MDT in patients with a high BI (3+ or more) in some studies and the absence of long-term follow-up data for this limited duration of therapy would support this more cautious approach.

Ofloxacin, minocycline (Minocin), and clarithromycin also display modest bactericidal effects but much less than those of rifampin. All three drugs are usually well absorbed and associated with few significant side effects. Three bactericidal agents, rifampin (600 mg), ofloxacin (400 mg), and minocycline (100 mg) (ROM), in single doses were used successfully in clinical trials for single-lesion paucibacillary disease with success rates estimated at 99%. ROM was less efficacious than the standard PB drug therapy in one large Indian study, and long-term (more than 10 years) relapse rates are not yet reported. Many leprologists therefore prefer to give the standard PB treatment for single-lesion disease.

Alternative Treatment

For patients who cannot take clofazimine, 12 monthly (observed) doses of ROM for 24 months is recommended. In patients intolerant of rifampin, clofazimine, 50 mg daily, plus ofloxacin, 400 mg daily, plus minocycline, 100 mg daily, for 24 months can be used.

If dapsone cannot be included in therapy because of resistance or G6PD deficiency, it can be replaced by 50 mg of clofazimine for PB patients. In this situation, for treatment of MB patients, daily ofloxacin or minocycline can be substituted.

Treatment of Patients with Leprosy and HIV

No treatment modifications are suggested for patients co-infected with the human immunodeficiency virus. The reconstitution phenomenon has been observed for patients with HIV who are also infected with *M. leprae* when they first received antiviral medications.

Duration of Multidrug Therapy and Relapse Rates

The annual rates of relapse after stopping multiple drug therapy ranges from 0.01% to 0.14% and are higher in patients with high pretreatment bacterial load (3+ or more). Relapses generally occur late, in at least 5 (±2) years. In a prospective Filipino study, 217 MB patients treated for 24 months and then followed for 12 years or until relapse had relapse rates of 9%, with the latest relapse detected 11 years after treatment. Reversal reactions can also occur during the first year after stopping multiple drug therapy at a rate of 4.8% to 9.0%. Patients should therefore be checked every 3 months after discontinuing multiple drug therapy to detect late reactions or relapses. It may be difficult clinically to distinguish relapses from reversal reactions after multiple drug therapy, especially in paucibacillary disease, unless skin smears have become positive.

Persisters are viable, physiologically dormant bacilli that remain fully drug susceptible and survive for many years despite the use of MDT. The eyes and peripheral nerves may be common locations of persisters and may be the source of relapses. Most of these relapses occurred 6 to 9 years after therapy. Therefore, long-term follow-up of these patients, especially those with multibacillary disease, is believed to be crucial.

The prevalence of resistance to the three drugs used in MDT is unknown but appears to be low. Primary and secondary resistance to rifampin is reported but rare. PCR techniques have been used successfully to diagnose drug resistance to current and future drugs. Lesion material from relapses after multiple drug therapy in large prospective studies usually contain *M. leprae* that is rifampin and clofazimine sensitive (with small numbers showing partial or full dapsone resistance), and retreatment with multiple drug therapy is usually successful.

Patients with lepromatous disease who have previously had erythema nodosum leprosum (ENL), significant nerve damage, or eye involvement should be considered for long-term dapsone suppression after MDT unless dapsone resistance is documented.

Leprosy Reactions

Leprosy reactions are immunologically mediated episodes of acute or subacute superimposed inflammation that may occur before, during, or after chemotherapy. They continue to be important causes of disability despite successful chemotherapy and occur in up to a third of patients. Tumor necrosis factor-α, which is overproduced, is a key mediator of systemic symptoms and tissue damage during both reversal reactions and ENL. Recurrences of both reversal reactions and ENL are common.

Type 1 reactions consist of upgrading or reversal reactions. Reversal reactions are seen typically in the borderline forms of leprosy (BT, BB, or BL). This reaction usually includes a worsening of the signs and symptoms of the existing disease and the occurrence of new skin and nerve damage thought to be related to augmented cell-mediated immunity.

Type 2 reactions (ENL) occur almost exclusively at the lepromatous end of the spectrum. Clinically this presents as crops of painful erythematous papules (Figure 2) associated with fever, fatigue, acute neuropathy, lymphadenopathy, and uveitis. Anemia, leukocytosis, and abnormal liver function tests may be seen. ENL may be associated with the formation of immune complexes that are responsible for some of the clinical manifestations.

Treatment of Reactions

TYPE 1 REACTIONS

Mild reactions may be treated with nonsteroidal anti-inflammatory agents. Neural involvement requires the use of prednisone at 1 mg/kg/day instituted early in the course and continued until the reaction is controlled. Steroids should be continued for a period of at least 4 months or more to prevent relapse of neuritis. Other useful agents include cyclosporine (Neoral) and azathioprine (Imuran).

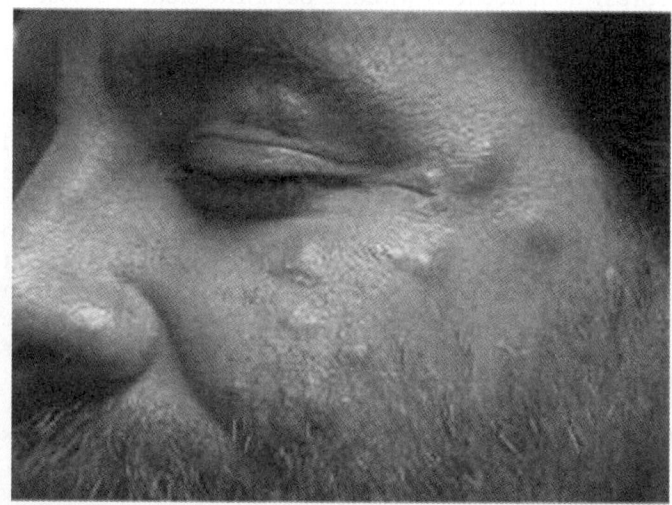

FIGURE 2. Tender nodules in erythema nodosum leprosum (ENL) in borderline lepromatous disease.

Specific treatment of pain syndromes may require a low dose of amitriptyline (Elavil), 10 to 25 mg, or gabapentin (Neurontin), 300 to 900 mg.

TYPE 2 REACTIONS

Thalidomide (Thalomid) remains the drug of choice for treatment of severe ENL but cannot be used for women of childbearing age.

Depending on the severity of the reaction, a total dosage of 100 to 300 mg per day is indicated. This is slowly tapered over 1 to 4 months. It is often used in combination with higher doses of clofazimine (100 mg/day) because of its anti-inflammatory effect. Maintenance long-term therapy with thalidomide may be necessary to prevent the constitutional symptoms and cutaneous lesions of ENL because of a high rate of recurrence of 45%. Thalidomide-induced peripheral neuropathy is rare (less than 1%) in patients with ENL and depends on the daily dose used. It is most frequent when this exceeds 75 mg a day. It may also be difficult to detect clinically unless nerve conduction studies are performed but is usually reversible when the drug is discontinued.

Unfortunately, thalidomide does not help appreciably in the treatment of the peripheral neuritis, iritis, and orchitis associated with ENL. Moderate doses of steroids remain more effective. Other steroid-sparing drugs to treat ENL are cyclosporine, azathioprine (Imuran), and pentoxifylline (Trental).

Treatment and Prevention of Nerve Damage

Even with effective antibacterial therapy, nerve lesions, often progressive and irreversible, may develop in a third of patients with leprosy. Prevention of permanent nerve damage is extremely important in the management of patients with leprosy because irreversible progressive damage to peripheral nerves and the tissue damage secondary to motor and sensory impairments are the most important consequences of this disease. Testing muscle function in hands and feet and assessing sensory loss with monofilaments at every visit should be done routinely because nerve damage can occur secondary to the disease process and during reactions. Patients with new sensory loss or muscle weakness or significant tenderness of enlarged nerves should be treated promptly with prednisolone at 40 mg per day, increasing the doses to 1 mg/kg/day if there is no response within 24 to 48 hours. Steroid therapy should be tapered slowly and not stopped before 20 weeks to reduce the risk of relapse of the neuritis.

Patients with BL (Figure 3) have the most extensive large nerve involvement, and their predisposition to reactions puts them at risk for the most severe nerve damage. Damage to nerves results in anesthesia, impaired sweating, dryness, and muscle paralysis. The lack of sensation and dryness of the skin predispose to injuries, with complicating infections producing osteomyelitis and ulcerations of digits. Because early steroid treatment of neural involvement was demonstrated to decrease disability, all newly diagnosed patients should be warned of the signs and symptoms of neuritis during therapy and the importance

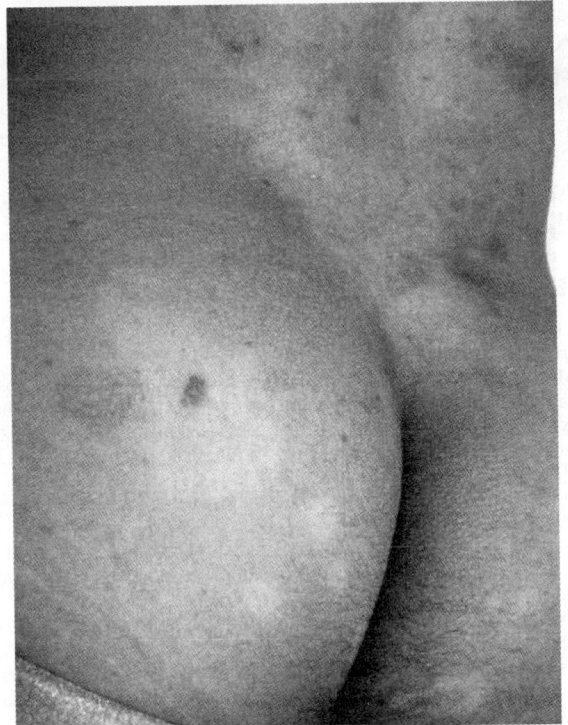

FIGURE 3. Hypopigmented macules in borderline lepromatous disease.

of prompt steroid treatment. An inflamed facial patch near the eye is associated with a high risk for the development of facial nerve damage, and consequently prophylactic steroid therapy is recommended for this particular problem. Other prophylactic uses for prednisolone cannot currently be routinely recommended. A prospective study using low-dose prophylactic prednisolone (20 mg per day) during the first 4 months of MDT for MB leprosy found that reactions and nerve function impairment were reduced in the short term but the effect was not sustained at 1 year.

In some instances, despite adequate chemotherapy, asymptomatic nerve damage progresses insidiously for prolonged periods ("silent" neuritis) without other features of typical reversal reactions. Although cell-mediated inflammation is probably the major etiologic factor, Schwann cell dysfunction and postinflammatory fibrosis may also contribute to this silent neuropathy. If the loss of function has not exceeded 3 months, it may improve with systemic steroids.

Prevention and Control Measures

Prevention of disease with vaccines based on *M. leprae* or other mycobacteria has thus far not proved effective. Repeated doses of BCG vaccine appear to be more effective, but this approach may have limited usefulness because of cost and potential adverse reactions in the immunosuppressed patient.

Multidrug therapy does not eliminate transmission in households. The early detection of subclinical leprosy or the carrier state is also difficult. *M. leprae* can be detected by PCR in nasal swabs from unaffected individuals exposed to leprosy, but the infectivity and risk of disease in these patients remain to be defined. Dapsone prophylaxis of high-risk contacts of index cases has not proved successful. In 2005, prevention of this disease depends on early detection, prompt treatment with MDT, and clinical evaluation of contacts.

REFERENCES

Abel L, Sanchez FO, Oberti J: Susceptibility to leprosy is linked to the human NRAMP1 gene. J Infect Dis 1998;177:133-145.

Becx-Bleumink M, Berhe D: Occurrence of reactions, their diagnosis and management in leprosy patients treated with multidrug therapy: Experience in the leprosy control program of the All Africa Leprosy and Rehabilitation Training Center (ALERT) in Ethiopia. Int J Lepr Other Mycobact Dis 1992;60:173-184.

Britton WJ: The management of leprosy reversal reactions. Lepr Rev 1998;9:225-234.

Lienhardt C, Kamate B, Jamet P: Effect of HIV infection on leprosy: A three-year survey in Bamako, Mali. Int J Lepr Other Mycobact Dis 1996;64:383-391.

Lockwood DN, Sinha HH: Pregnancy and leprosy: A comprehensive literature review. Int J Lepr Other Mycobact Dis 1999;67:6-12.

Parkash O, Chaturvedi V, Girdhar BK, Sengupta U: A study on performance of two serological assays for diagnosis of leprosy patients. Lepr Rev 1995;66:26-30.

Randomized controlled trial of single BCG, repeated BCG, or combined BCG and killed *Mycobacterium leprae* vaccine for prevention of leprosy and tuberculosis in Malawi. Karonga Prevention Trial. Lancet 1996;348:17-24.

Ridley DS, Job CK: The pathology of leprosy. In Hastings RC (ed): Leprosy. New York, Churchill Livingstone, 1985, p 129.

Ridley DS, Jopling WH: Classification of leprosy according to immunity. Int J Lepr 1966;31:255.

Sampaio EP, Hernandez MO, Carvalho DS, Sarno EN: Management of erythema nodosum leprosum by thalidomide: Thalidomide analogues inhibit *M. leprae*-induced TNF-alpha production in vitro. Biomed Pharmacother 2002;56:13-19.

Saunderson P, Gebre S, Desta K: The pattern of leprosy-related neuropathy in the AMFES patients in Ethiopia: Definitions, incidence, risk factors and outcome. Lepr Rev 2000;71:285-308.

Scollard DM, Gillis TP, Williams DL: Polymerase chain reaction assay for the detection and identification of *Mycobacterium leprae* in patients in the United States. Am J Clin Pathol 1998;109:642-646.

Malaria

Method of
Monica Parise, MD, and
Melto James Eliades, MD, MPH

Malaria is caused by infection with one or more of four species of *Plasmodium* (i.e., *P. falciparum, P. vivax, P. ovale,* and *P. malariae*) that can infect humans. The infection is transmitted by the bite of an infective female *Anopheles* mosquito. Almost all malaria cases reported each year in the United States are imported. In addition, a few reported cases (less than 10 per year) are likely acquired through local mosquito-borne transmission. Malaria should be considered in the differential diagnosis of any patient with fever who has returned from a malarious area in the previous year or who has fever of unknown origin regardless of travel history. Early diagnosis and treatment are imperative because untreated *P. falciparum* infections can rapidly progress to coma, renal failure, pulmonary edema, and death. Appropriate chemoprophylaxis and the use of personal protective measures are important in preventing malaria infection.

Description of Organism

TRANSMISSION

Malaria is most commonly transmitted though the bite of an infective female *Anopheles* mosquito. Transmission can also occur through direct inoculation of infected red blood cells congenitally, through blood transfusion, or by contact with contaminated needles.

LIFE CYCLE

Sporozoites from an infective female mosquito are injected into the bloodstream as the mosquito takes a blood meal. They are present in the peripheral blood for a very short period of time (approximately 30 minutes) before entering liver parenchymal cells. Here they undergo asexual multiplication and mature into tissue schizonts with thousands of merozoites. Within 6 to 16 days of initial infection, the hepatic cells containing the schizonts rupture and the merozoites are released into the bloodstream. In *P. falciparum* and *P. malariae* infection, the tissue schizonts release all their merozoites into the bloodstream and none persist in the liver. In *P. vivax* and *P. ovale*, there are two exoerythrocytic forms, one that ruptures into the bloodstream and another that remains dormant in the liver. These dormant cells, called hypnozoites, can rupture weeks, months, or years later and are responsible for relapsing infections. In contrast, recurrent parasitemia with *P. falciparum* or *P. malariae* is caused by the proliferation of persistent erythrocytic forms and is known as recrudescence. Long-term persistent infections may be seen with *P. malariae*, which can remain in the bloodstream for 20 to 30 years.

Merozoites released into the blood invade red blood cells, and depending on the species, they typically release from 6 to 32 new merozoites in 48 (*P. falciparum, P. vivax, P. ovale*) to 72 (*P. malariae*) hours. This process continues until contained by the host's immune system or antimalarial medication. Subpopulations of merozoites develop into sexual forms, gametocytes, which are ingested by the female anopheline mosquito during feeding. Sporozoites are formed, which migrate to the salivary gland of the mosquito, and can reinfect humans when the next blood meal is taken.

Epidemiology

Malaria transmission occurs in approximately 25% of the earth's land area, mostly in tropical regions including parts of Africa, Asia, the Middle East, Central and South America, Hispaniola, and Oceania, leaving approximately 41% of the world's population at risk. Malaria is a common illness for up to 3 billion people worldwide. The World Health Organization estimates that 300 to 500 million people become acutely ill and more than 1 million die from malaria each year. Ninety percent of deaths related to malaria occur in Africa south of the Sahara mostly among young children. *P. falciparum* and *P. malariae* have a worldwide distribution. *P. vivax* is endemic in most malarious areas but predominates in the Indian subcontinent, the Central Asian republics, Eastern Europe, and Central and most of South America. *P. ovale* is most common in West Africa. Transmission is also possible in temperate areas where *Anopheles* mosquitoes are present, such as the United States. Although most of the 1200 cases per year reported in the United States occur in travelers returning from malarious areas, local mosquito-borne outbreaks have occurred. Drug resistance has increasingly become a problem in the treatment of malaria. *P. falciparum* strains remain sensitive to chloroquine in only a limited number of regions including Central America north/west of the Panama Canal, Haiti, the Dominican Republic, and most of the Middle East. In addition, resistance to other antimalarial drugs including sulfadoxine-pyrimethamine (Fansidar) and mefloquine (Lariam) has developed. Chloroquine-resistant *P. vivax* is common in Papua New Guinea and Indonesia, and case reports from other parts of the world are described.

Clinical Manifestations

Clinical signs and symptoms of malaria result from schizont rupture and the release of merozoites into the bloodstream and the destruction of parasitized and unparasitized red blood cells. Semi-immune individuals from malaria endemic areas are at lower risk for complications and serious disease.

SYMPTOMS

Malaria causes an acute febrile illness characterized by periodic paroxysms. The typical paroxysm begins abruptly with chills followed by fever, diaphoresis, and often myalgias, malaise, and headache. The fever is often followed by a period of defervescence when the patient breaks out into a profuse sweat, the fever declines, and symptoms diminish. Nausea, vomiting, and cough may also occur. In primary attacks, this periodicity often requires days to develop. Many patients have asynchronous infections and this periodicity never becomes clinically apparent. Other symptoms associated with malaria may include abdominal pain, back pain, and diarrhea. Although the initial presentation of *P. falciparum* and non–*P. falciparum* infections are indistinguishable, *P. falciparum* infections have the potential to progress rapidly to severe illness or death.

SIGNS

Patients may by tachycardic, jaundiced, febrile, confused, and hepatosplenomegaly may be detected.

LABORATORY FINDINGS

Anemia, thrombocytopenia, and leukopenia are common. Serum transaminases, as well as both direct and indirect bilirubin, may be elevated. Serum creatinine and blood urea nitrogen may be elevated, and hypoglycemia often complicates falciparum malaria. Disseminated intravascular coagulation is reported, although laboratory evidence of coagulation abnormalities without bleeding is much more common. Parasites are detected on blood film (see Diagnosis section).

P. falciparum Malaria

The incubation period of *P. falciparum* is at least 7 days, and clinical malaria occurs in approximately 90% of infected individuals within 1 month of their return from a malarious area. It is responsible for almost all deaths attributed to malaria worldwide. *P. falciparum* can progress to serious disease and death because it invades erythrocytes of all ages, producing high-level parasitemias. In addition, it can adhere to endothelial cells causing microvascular obstruction and subsequent tissue damage that is not observed with the other three species.

COMPLICATIONS OF P. FALCIPARUM

Cerebral Malaria

The strict definition of cerebral malaria requires the presence of unarousable coma in a patient with *P. falciparum* parasitemia and no other obvious cause of their symptoms. However, any neurologic dysfunction or impaired consciousness should be treated aggressively. Mortality rates are typically between 15% and 25%. Most people recover completely, but approximately 10% are discharged with neurologic sequelae.

Convulsions

Convulsion in association with *P. falciparum* malaria can occur as a sign of cerebral malaria or because of hypoglycemia.

Severe Anemia

Severe anemia can develop rapidly in nonimmune individuals as a result of overwhelming parasitemia and hemolysis. In endemic areas, it is particularly common in children younger than 2 years and pregnant women.

Metabolic Complications

Hypoglycemia (blood glucose is 2.2 mmol/L or 40 mg/dL or less) is a frequent complication of *P. falciparum* infection and may also be associated with treatment with the cinchona alkaloids, quinine and quinidine (insulin secretagogues). Hypoglycemia is a poor prognostic factor in children and associated with increased mortality and neurologic sequelae. Metabolic acidosis (blood pH less than 7.3 or plasma lactate more than 5 mmol/L) is associated with severe disease and poor outcomes.

Renal Failure

Mild proteinuria, azotemia, and oliguria occur frequently in uncomplicated *P. falciparum* infection. Approximately a third of nonimmune adults with severe malaria develop biochemical evidence of renal dysfunction, although in only a minority of cases is there progression to acute renal failure. Acute renal failure is more common in adults, often reversible, and typically oliguric.

Respiratory Failure

Noncardiogenic pulmonary edema most commonly occurs late in the course of the infection in adults. The clinical picture is that of adult respiratory distress syndrome (ARDS) with normal right heart pressures. Patients are tachypneic, dyspneic, and have crepitations on examination. Mechanical ventilation may be necessary.

Algid Malaria

A minority of patients with severe malaria may develop signs of shock and circulatory collapse including hypotension, cold and clammy extremities, hypoglycemia, and metabolic acidosis.

Hemoglobinuria/Blackwater Fever

Severe intravascular hemolysis and hemoglobinuria may occur in patients with malaria and was historically attributed to sensitization of red blood cells to quinine after intermittent use as prophylaxis. It may be seen in a few different patient scenarios, including patients with G6PD deficiency who have received oxidant drugs or foodstuffs, those with G6PD deficiency who have acute malaria and have received treatment with antimalarial drugs, or those with normal levels of G6PD but who have acute and often severe malaria. The urine becomes mahogany colored or black, and the patient may have fever, tachycardia, tender hepatosplenomegaly, profound anemia, and jaundice. Impaired renal function and, less commonly, oliguric renal failure can occur.

Non–*P. falciparum* Malaria

P. VIVAX AND *P. OVALE*

Approximately 40% of *P. vivax* and *P. ovale* cases in the United States develop clinical malaria within 1 month of return from a malarious area, but the incubation period may be prolonged for months. Relapses are common within 6 months unless specific treatment to eradicate hypnozoites is given. Parasitemia is often lower than in *P. falciparum* infections. Splenic rupture is more commonly reported with *P. vivax*, carries a high mortality rate, and results from acute rapid enlargement of the spleen.

P. MALARIAE

P. malariae is the most chronic form of malaria. Parasites invade older erythrocytes. Symptoms can develop within weeks but may develop months or years later. Recrudescence of disease can also occur after months, years, or even decades after initial infection. In endemic areas *P. malariae* may be a cause of nephrotic syndrome with a histologic picture of glomerulosclerosis. Antimalarial treatment does not reverse the lesions, and few patients respond to corticosteroids. Some response to azathioprine

(Imuran[1]), and cyclophosphamide (Cytoxan[1]) has been demonstrated.

Hyperreactive Malarial Syndrome (Tropical Splenomegaly)

This syndrome is characterized by splenomegaly, which may be massive, in a person who has resided in a malarious area with an elevation of IgM antibodies (both polyclonal and malaria-specific). There is generally a past history of repeated infections, although parasitemia is usually not detectable when the patient presents. The syndrome is associated with severe anemia and increased susceptibility to infection, and patients can develop peritoneal signs on examination from splenic infarction. Untreated mortality is high.

Malaria in Special Populations

MALARIA IN PREGNANCY

Malaria infection during pregnancy can have adverse effects on both mother and fetus, including maternal anemia, fetal loss, premature delivery, intrauterine growth retardation, and delivery of low birth weight infants (less than 2500 g or 5.5 pounds). It is a particular problem for women in their first and second pregnancies and for women who are HIV positive.

CONGENITAL MALARIA

Congenital malaria can be caused by all four species of *Plasmodium* causing human infections, and the incubation period is typically between 2 and 8 weeks. The clinical signs and symptoms often mimic neonatal sepsis: The infant feeds poorly and is irritable, drowsy, and sometimes lethargic; hepatosplenomegaly and anemia are common. Initial blood smears may be negative.

Pathogenesis

Malaria parasites invade red cells, degrading hemoglobin and altering the cell membrane. The red cell becomes irregular in shape, more antigenic, and less deformable. In *P. falciparum* infections, membrane protuberances extrude an adhesive protein (PfEMP1) that mediates cytoadherence, or attachment to venular and capillary endothelium. Infected red cells may also adhere to uninfected cells. The result of these processes is sequestration in vital organs with interference of microcirculatory flow and metabolism. As a consequence, only the younger ring forms of the asexual parasites are seen on peripheral blood smear. Sequestration does not occur with the other three species of malaria, and all stages of parasites are evident on peripheral blood smear. Because *P. vivax*, *P. ovale*, and *P. malariae* have a predilection for either reticulocytes or older red cells, levels of parasitemia rarely exceed 2%.

---

[1]Not FDA approved for this indication.

CURRENT DIAGNOSIS

- Blood smear is the gold standard for the diagnosis of malaria.
- Thin and thick Giemsa-stained blood smears should be obtained on all patients with suspected malaria and examined immediately.
- A negative smear should be repeated every 12 to 24 hours for a 72-hour period.

Diagnosis

Malaria should be considered a potential medical emergency and treated accordingly. Delay in diagnosis and treatment is a leading cause of death in malaria patients in the United States. The diagnosis should be considered in any traveler returning from a malarious area with fever or in fever of unknown origin in any patient. The early signs and symptoms of malaria are nonspecific and found in many diseases. Furthermore, the typical malarial paroxysms are not usually observed. Therefore, for a definitive diagnosis to be made, laboratory tests must demonstrate the malaria parasites or their components.

MICROSCOPY

The gold standard for the diagnosis of malaria is the blood smear, although its accuracy depends on both the quality of the reagents and the microscope and on the experience of the laboratorian. Both thin and thick Giemsa-stained blood smears should be obtained on all patients with suspected malaria and examined immediately for the presence of parasites. Parasites are more easily identified on thick smear, although speciation and level of parasitemia are best determined on the thin smear. If the initial smear is negative, it should be repeated every 12 to 24 hours for a 72-hour period.

DIAGNOSTIC ALTERNATIVES

Assays Based on Polymerase Chain Reaction

Although polymerase chain reaction (PCR) is highly sensitive and species specific, because it requires sophisticated laboratory support and is not available in most centers, it is not used as an initial diagnostic modality. PCR is most effective in detecting low levels of parasitemia or identifying the infecting species if direct microscopy is inconclusive or a mixed infection is suspected.

Antigen Detection Techniques

Dipstick antigen-capture assays have been developed for P. falciparum and P. vivax. This technique is useful in the field where other resources are scarce; none are currently approved for use in the United States.

Malarial Antibody Testing

Serologic tests are useful in providing retrospective confirmation of malaria infection and for epidemiologic purposes. However, because of the acute nature of P. falciparum infections, they have limited value in diagnosis and in guiding treatment.

Treatment

GENERAL CONSIDERATIONS

Any person suspected of having malaria should have a blood smear done and examined immediately by a qualified laboratory technician or the pathologist or microbiologist on call. Any delay in the diagnosis of P. falciparum can lead to the rapid development of severe disease and death. Treatment should not be initiated until the diagnosis is confirmed. Presumptive treatment without the benefit of laboratory confirmation should be reserved for extreme circumstances (strong clinical suspicion in the face of severe disease and impossibility of obtaining prompt laboratory confirmation). Once the diagnosis of malaria is confirmed, appropriate antimalarial therapy must be initiated immediately.

Treatment should be guided by the infecting *Plasmodium* species, the clinical status of the patient, and the drug susceptibility of the parasite based on the geographic area where the infection was acquired.

Patients with malaria are generally categorized as having uncomplicated or severe malaria. Those with uncomplicated malaria can be treated with oral medications if they are able to take them. It is recommended that all patients with P. falciparum be admitted to the hospital for at least initial monitoring of their response to treatment both clinically and parasitologically. Clinical criteria indicating severe disease include one or more of the following listed in Table 1. These complications are most common with P. falciparum, and patients with one or more of these manifestations require immediate treatment with parenteral antimalarial drugs. Blood smears should be repeated in P. falciparum infections every 12 to 24 hours to evaluate treatment response and again after a full course of treatment is given.

UNCOMPLICATED MALARIA

P. falciparum or Species Not Identified

P. falciparum infections acquired in areas where the parasite is sensitive to chloroquine should be treated with oral chloroquine (Aralen). These areas include Central America west of the Panama Canal, Haiti and the Dominican Republic, and most of the Middle East (except Iran, Oman, Saudi Arabia, and Yemen).

Three treatment options are available for P. falciparum infections acquired in areas with reported chloroquine resistance: quinine sulfate plus doxycycline[1] (Vibramycin), tetracycline[1] (Sumycin), or clindamycin[1] (Cleocin); atovaquone-proguanil (Malarone); or mefloquine (Lariam). The first two options are preferred because of a higher rate of severe neuropsychiatric reactions seen at treatment doses with mefloquine. Mefloquine is recommended as a second-line agent if neither of the first two options can be used. Doxycycline and tetracycline are generally preferred

---

[1]Not FDA approved for this indication.

Clinical Diagnosis/ *Plasmodium* Species	Region Where Infection Acquired	Recommended Drug: Adult Dose[a,b]	Recommended Drug: Pediatric Dose[a,b,c]
Uncomplicated malaria/ *P. falciparum* (or species not identified[d])	Chloroquine sensitive (Central America west of Panama Canal; Haiti; the Dominican Republic; and most of the Middle East).	Chloroquine phosphate (Aralen and generics): 600 mg base (= 1000 mg salt) PO immediately, followed by 300 mg base (= 500 mg salt) PO at 6, 24, and 48 h. Total dose: 1500 mg base (= 2500 mg salt).	Chloroquine phosphate (Aralen and generics): 10 mg base/kg PO immediately, followed by 5 mg base/kg PO at 6, 24, and 48 h. Total dose: 25 mg base/kg. Quinine sulfate[e] plus one of the following: doxycycline[1,3] tetracycline[1,3] or clindamycin.[1]
	Chloroquine resistant or unknown resistance[a] (all malarious regions except those specified as chloroquine sensitive listed earlier. Middle Eastern countries with chloroquine-resistant *P. falciparum* include Iran, Oman, Saudi Arabia, and Yemen. Note: Infections acquired in the newly independent states of the former Soviet Union and Korea to date are uniformly caused by *P. vivax* and should therefore be treated as chloroquine-sensitive infections.)	Quinine sulfate[e] plus one of the following: doxycycline[1], tetracycline,[1] or clindamycin[1] (Cleocin). Quinine sulfate: 542 mg base (= 650 mg salt) PO tid × 3 to 7 d. Doxycycline: 100 mg PO bid × 7 d. Tetracycline: 250 mg PO qid × 7 d. Clindamycin: 20 mg base/kg/day PO divided tid × 7 d. Atovaquone-proguanil (Malarone)[g]: Adult tab = 250 mg atovaquone/100 mg proguanil; 4 adult tabs PO qd × 3 d.	Quinine sulfate: 8.3 mg base/kg (= 10 mg salt/kg) PO tid × 3 to 7 d. Doxycycline: 4 mg/kg/d PO divided bid × 7 d. Tetracycline: 25 mg/kg/d PO divided qid × 7 d. Clindamycin: 20 mg base/kg/day PO divided tid × 7 d. Atovaquone-proguanil (Malarone)[g]: Adult tab = 250 mg atovaquone/100 mg proguanil. Peds tab = 62.5 mg atovaquone/25 mg proguanil. 5–8 kg: 2 peds tabs PO qd × 3 d. 9–10 kg: 3 peds tabs PO qd × 3 d. 11–20 kg: 1 adult tab PO qd × 3 d. 21–30 kg: 2 adult tabs PO qd × 3d. 31–40 kg: 3 adult tabs PO qd × 3d. >40 kg: 4 adult tabs PO qd × 3d.
		Mefloquine (Lariam and generics)[h]: 684 mg base (= 750 mg salt) PO as initial dose, followed by 456 mg base (= 500 mg salt) PO given 6–12 h after initial dose. Total dose = 1250 mg salt.	Mefloquine (Lariam and generics)[h]: 13.7 mg base/kg (= 15 mg salt/kg) PO as initial dose, followed by 9.1 mg base/kg (= 10 mg salt/kg) PO given 6–12 h after initial dose. Total dose = 25 mg salt/kg.
Uncomplicated malaria/ *P. malariae*	All regions.	Chloroquine phosphate: Treatment as above.	Chloroquine phosphate: Treatment as above.
Uncomplicated malaria/ *P. vivax* or *P. ovale*	All regions.[b] Note: For suspected chloroquine-resistant *P. vivax*, see below.	Chloroquine phosphate plus primaquine phosphate[i]: Chloroquine phosphate: Treatment as above.	Chloroquine phosphate plus primaquine phosphate[i]: Chloroquine phosphate: Treatment as above.

Clinical Diagnosis/ *Plasmodium* Species	Region Where Infection Acquired	Recommended Drug: Adult Dose[a,b]	Recommended Drug: Pediatric Dose[a,b,c]
		Primaquine phosphate: 30 mg base[3] PO qd × 14 d.	Primaquine phosphate: 0.6 mg base/kg[3] PO qd × 14 d.
Uncomplicated malaria/*P. vivax*	Chloroquine resistant[b] (Papua New Guinea and Indonesia).	Quinine sulfate[e] plus either doxycycline[1] or tetracycline[1] plus primaquine phosphate[i]: Quinine sulfate: Treatment as above. Doxycycline or tetracycline: Treatment as above. Primaquine phosphate: Treatment as above. Mefloquine plus primaquine phosphate:[i] Mefloquine: Treatment as above. Primaquine phosphate: Treatment as above.	Quinine sulfate[e] plus either doxycycline[1,3] or tetracycline[1,3] plus primaquine phosphate[i]: Quinine sulfate: Treatment as above. Doxycycline or tetracycline: Treatment as above. Primaquine phosphate: Treatment as above. Mefloquine plus primaquine phosphate[i]: Mefloquine: Treatment as above. Primaquine phosphate: Treatment as above.
Uncomplicated malaria: alternatives for pregnant women[j,k,l,m]	Chloroquine-sensitive[m] (see uncomplicated malaria sections above for chloroquine-sensitive *Plasmodium* species by region).	Chloroquine phosphate: Treatment as above.	Not applicable.
	Chloroquine resistant *P. falciparum*[j,k,l] (see uncomplicated malaria sections above for regions with known chloroquine resistant *P. falciparum*).	Quinine sulfate[e] plus clindamycin[1]: Quinine sulfate: Treatment as above. Clindamycin: Treatment as above.	Not applicable.
	Chloroquine-resistant *P. vivax*[j,k,l,m] (see uncomplicated malaria sections above for regions with chloroquine-resistant *P. vivax*).	Quinine sulfate: 650 mg salt PO tid × 7 d.	Not applicable.
Severe malaria[n,o,p,q]	All regions.	Quinidine gluconate[o] or quinine dihydrochloride (not available in United States) plus one of the following: doxycycline,[1] tetracycline,[1] or clindamycin.[1]	Quinidine gluconate[o] or quinine dihydrochloride (not available in United States) plus one of the following: doxycycline,[1,3] tetracycline,[1,3] or clindamycin.[1] Quinidine gluconate: Same mg/kg dosing and recommendations as for adults.

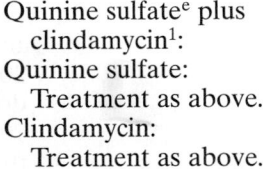

Continued

Clinical Diagnosis/ *Plasmodium* Species	Region Where Infection Acquired	Recommended Drug: Adult Dose[a,b]	Recommended Drug: Pediatric Dose[a,b,c]
		Quinidine gluconate: 6.25 mg base/kg (= 10 mg salt/kg) loading dose IV over 1–2 h, then 0.0125 mg base/kg/min (= 0.02 mg salt/kg/min) continuous infusion for at least 24 h. An alternative regimen is 15 mg base/kg (= 24 mg salt/kg) loading dose IV infused over 4 h, followed by 7.5 mg base/kg (= 12 mg salt/kg) infused over 4 h q8h, starting 8 h after loading dose (see package insert). Once parasite density <1% and patient can take oral medication, complete treatment with oral quinine, dose as above. Quinidine/quinine course = 7 d in Southeast Asia; = 3 d in Africa or South America. Quinine dihydrochloride: 20 mg salt/kg loading dose diluted in 10 mL/kg isotonic fluid IV over 4 h then, beginning 8 h after start of loading dose, 10 mg salt/kg over 4 h q8h until patient can take oral medication. Patient can then complete treatment with 10 mg salt/kg (maximum 600 mg) q8–12h. Quinine/quinidine course = 7 d in Southeast Asia; = 3 d in Africa or South America. Doxycycline: Treatment as above.	Quinine dihydrochloride: 20 mg salt/kg loading dose diluted in 10 mL/kg isotonic fluid IV over 4 h then, beginning 12 h after start of loading dose, 10 mg salt/kg over 2 h q12h until patient can take oral medication. Patient can then complete treatment with 10 mg salt/kg q8h. Quinine/quinidine course = 7 d in Southeast Asia; = 3 d in Africa or South America. Doxycycline: Treatment as above. If patient not able to take oral medication, may give IV. For children <45 kg, give 4 mg/kg IV q12h and then switch to oral doxycycline (dose as above) as soon as patient can take oral medication. For children >45 kg, use same dosing as for adults. For IV use, avoid rapid administration. Treatment course = 7 d. Tetracycline: Treatment as above. Clindamycin: Treatment as above. If patient not able to take oral medication, give 10 mg base/kg loading dose IV followed by 5 mg base/kg IV q8h. Switch to oral clindamycin (oral dose as above) as soon as patient can take oral medication. For IV use, avoid rapid administration. Treatment course = 7 d.

Clinical Diagnosis/ Plasmodium Species	Region Where Infection Acquired	Recommended Drug: Adult Dose[a,b]	Recommended Drug: Pediatric Dose[a,b,c]
		If patient not able to take oral medication, give 100 mg IV q12h and then switch to oral doxycycline (as above) as soon as patient can take oral medication. For IV use, avoid rapid administration. Treatment course = 7 d. Tetracycline: Treatment as above. Clindamycin: Treatment as above. If patient not able to take oral medication, give 10 mg base/kg loading dose IV followed by 5 mg base/kg IV q8h. Switch to oral clindamycin (oral dose as above) as soon as patient can take oral medication. For IV use, avoid rapid administration. Treatment course = 7 d.	

[1]Not FDA approved for this indication.

[3]Exceeds dosage recommended by the manufacturer.

[a]Note: Three options (A, B, or C) are available for treatment of uncomplicated malaria caused by chloroquine-resistant *P. falciparum*. Options A and B are equally recommended. Because of a higher rate of severe neuropsychiatric reactions seen at treatment doses, we do not recommend option C (mefloquine) unless options A and B cannot be used. For option A, because there are more data on the efficacy of quinine in combination with doxycycline or tetracycline, these treatment combinations are generally preferred to quinine in combination with clindamycin.

[b]Note: Two options (A or B) are available for treatment of uncomplicated malaria caused by chloroquine-resistant *P. vivax*. High treatment failure rates because of chloroquine-resistant *P. vivax* are well documented in Papua New Guinea and Indonesia. Rare case reports of chloroquine-resistant *P. vivax* is also documented in Burma (Myanmar), India, and Central and South America. Persons acquiring *P. vivax* infections outside of Papua New Guinea or Indonesia should be started on chloroquine. If the patient does not respond, the treatment should be changed to a chloroquine-resistant *P. vivax* regimen and the Centers for Disease Control and Prevention should be notified. (Malaria Hotline number 770-488-7788). For treatment of chloroquine-resistant *P. vivax* infections, options A and B are equally recommended.

[c]Pediatric dose should *never* exceed adult dose.

[d]If "species not identified" is subsequently diagnosed as *P. vivax* or *P. ovale*, see *P. vivax* and *P ovale* (later) regarding treatment with primaquine

[e]For infections acquired in Southeast Asia, quinine treatment should continue for 7 d. For infections acquired in Africa and South America, quinine treatment should continue for 3 d.

[f]Doxycycline and tetracycline are not indicated for use in children <8 y. For children <8 y with chloroquine-resistant *P. falciparum*, quinine (given alone for 7 d or given in combination with clindamycin) and atovaquone-proguanil are recommended treatment options; mefloquine can be considered if no other options are available. For children <8 y with chloroquine-resistant *P. vivax*, quinine (given alone for 7 d) or mefloquine are recommended treatment options. If none of these treatment options are available or are not being tolerated and if the treatment benefits outweigh the risks, doxycycline or tetracycline may be given to children <8 y.

[g]Give atovaquone-proguanil with food. If patient vomits within 30 min of taking a dose, repeat the dose.

[h]Treatment with mefloquine is not recommended in persons who have acquired infections from the Southeast Asian region of Myanmar, Thailand, and Cambodia because of resistant strains.

[i]Primaquine is used to eradicate any hypnozoite forms that may remain dormant in the liver, and thus prevent relapses, in *P. vivax* and *P. ovale* infections. Because primaquine can cause hemolytic anemia in persons with G6PD deficiency, patients must be screened for G6PD deficiency prior to starting treatment with primaquine. For persons with borderline G6PD deficiency or as an alternate to the above regimen, primaquine may be given 45 mg orally 1 time per wk for 8 weeks; consultation with an expert in infectious disease and/or tropical medicine is advised if this alternative regimen is considered in G6PD-deficient persons. Primaquine must not be used during pregnancy.

[j]For pregnant women diagnosed with uncomplicated malaria caused by chloroquine-resistant *P. falciparum* or chloroquine-resistant *P. vivax* infection, treatment with doxycycline or tetracycline is generally not indicated. However, doxycycline or tetracycline may be used in combination with quinine (as recommended for nonpregnant adults) if other treatment options are not available or are not being tolerated and the benefit is judged to outweigh the risks.

[k]Because there are no adequate, well-controlled studies of atovaquone and/or proguanil hydrochloride in pregnant women, atovaquone-proguanil is generally not recommended for use in pregnant women. For pregnant women diagnosed with uncomplicated malaria caused by chloroquine-resistant *P. falciparum* infection, atovaquone-proguanil may be used if other treatment options are not available or are not being tolerated, and if the potential benefit is judged to outweigh the potential risks. There are no data on the efficacy of atovaquone-proguanil in the treatment of chloroquine-resistant *P. vivax* infections.

[l]Because of a possible association with mefloquine treatment during pregnancy and an increase in stillbirths, mefloquine is generally not recommended for treatment in pregnant women. However, mefloquine may be used if it is the only treatment option available and if the potential benefit is judged to outweigh the potential risks.

Continued

[m]For *P. vivax* and *P. ovale* infections, primaquine phosphate for radical treatment of hypnozoites should not be given during pregnancy. Pregnant patients with *P. vivax* and *P. ovale* infections should be maintained on chloroquine prophylaxis for the duration of their pregnancy. The chemoprophylactic dose of chloroquine phosphate is 300 mg base (= 500 mg salt) orally once per wk. After delivery, pregnant patients who do not have G6PD deficiency should be treated with primaquine.

[n]Persons with a positive blood smear *or* history of recent possible exposure and no other recognized pathology who have one or more of the following clinical criteria (impaired consciousness/coma, severe normocytic anemia, renal failure, pulmonary edema, acute respiratory distress syndrome, circulatory shock, disseminated intravascular coagulation, spontaneous bleeding, acidosis, hemoglobinuria, jaundice, repeated generalized convulsions, and/or parasitemia of >5%) are considered to have manifestations of more severe disease. Severe malaria is practically always caused by *P. falciparum*.

[o]Patients diagnosed with severe malaria should be treated aggressively with parenteral antimalarial therapy. Treatment with IV quinidine should be initiated as soon as possible after the diagnosis is made. Patients with severe malaria should be given an IV loading dose of quinidine unless they have received more than 40 mg/kg of quinine in the preceding 48 h or if they have received mefloquine within the preceding 12 h. Consultation with a cardiologist and a physician with experience treating malaria is advised when treating malaria patients with quinidine. During administration of quinidine, blood pressure monitoring (for hypotension) and cardiac monitoring (for widening of the QRS complex and/or lengthening of the QTc interval) should be monitored continuously, and blood glucose (for hypoglycemia) should be monitored periodically. Cardiac complications, if severe, may warrant temporary discontinuation of the drug or slowing of the IV infusion.

[p]Consider exchange transfusion if the parasite density (i.e., parasitemia) is >10% *or* if the patient has altered mental status, nonvolume overload pulmonary edema, or renal complications. The parasite density can be estimated by examining a monolayer of red blood cells (RBCs) on the thin smear under oil immersion magnification. The slide should be examined where the RBCs are more or less touching (approximately 400 RBCs per field). The parasite density can then be estimated from the percentage of infected RBCs and should be monitored q12h. Exchange transfusion should be continued until the parasite density is <1% (usually requires 8–10 U). IV quinidine administration should not be delayed for an exchange transfusion and can be given concurrently throughout the exchange transfusion.

[q]Pregnant women diagnosed with severe malaria should be treated aggressively with parenteral antimalarial therapy.

Abbreviations: IV = intravenous; PO = orally.

to clindamycin in combination with quinine sulfate because more data on the efficacy of this regimen are available. For infections acquired in Southeast Asia, quinine treatment should continue for 7 days. For infections acquired in any other geographic area, quinine treatment for 3 days is usually sufficient.

Treatment options for pediatric patients are the same, except the drug dose is adjusted by weight and should never exceed the adult dose. Doxycycline and tetracycline should not be used in children younger than 8 years because of discoloration of teeth, hypoplasia of tooth enamel, and impaired bone growth; instead, quinine for a full 7 days or in combination with clindamycin should be used. Atovaquone-proguanil and mefloquine are both options as well; atovaquone-proguanil is not recommended for treatment in children weighing less than 5 kg. In rare circumstances when none of these treatment options are available or are not being tolerated, and if the treatment benefits outweigh the risks, doxycycline or tetracycline may be given in combination with quinine.

Infections in which the species is not initially identified should be treated as *P. falciparum* until the infecting species is confirmed.

P. malariae

Although there are a few possible case reports of chloroquine-resistant *P. malariae* from Indonesia, chloroquine (Aralen) remains the therapeutic drug of choice for all *P. malariae* infections.

P. vivax and P. ovale

Oral chloroquine (Aralen) is the treatment of choice for all *P. vivax* and *P. ovale* infections except for *P. vivax* infections acquired in Papua New Guinea (PNG) and Indonesia where a high prevalence of chloroquine resistance is documented. Rare case reports of chloroquine resistance are reported from Myanmar (Burma), India, and Central and South America. Persons acquiring *P. vivax* infection from any area outside PNG or Indonesia should initially be treated with chloroquine. If the patient does

not respond, treatment should be switched to a chloroquine-resistant regimen.

Infections acquired in PNG and Indonesia should be treated with a regimen effective against chloroquine-resistant *P. vivax*, either quinine sulfate plus doxycycline[1] or tetracycline[1], or mefloquine alone.

Infections with *P. vivax* and *P. ovale* can relapse because of hypnozoites in the liver. In addition to treatment of the blood stage parasites, persons with these infections also require a 14-day course of primaquine phosphate (30 mg/day[3]) to treat the liver stage hypnozoites. Primaquine phosphate can cause hemolytic anemia in patients with glucose-6-phosphate-dehydrogenase (G6PD) deficiency, and thus all persons must be screened prior to receiving this medication. An alternative primaquine dosing regimen of 45 mg weekly for 8 weeks[3] may be considered in persons with mild G6PD deficiency.

Alternatives for Pregnant Women

Treatment for pregnant woman with uncomplicated malaria infections acquired in areas with only chloroquine-sensitive strains of *P. falciparum* or *P. vivax* is similar to that for nonpregnant adults with chloroquine phosphate. Infections caused by *P. falciparum* or *P. vivax* acquired in areas of chloroquine resistance should be treated with the combination of quinine sulfate and clindamycin[1] (Cleocin). Current data are insufficient to recommend atovaquone/proguanil (Malarone) in pregnant woman. A possible association with mefloquine (Lariam) treatment during pregnancy and an increase in stillbirths is reported. Thus, mefloquine should only be used if no other treatment options are available and if the potential benefit is judged to outweigh the potential risks. Pregnant patients with severe malaria should be treated aggressively with parenteral antimalarial therapy as indicated for nonpregnant adults. To prevent congenital malaria, newborns of mothers who are parasitemic at the time of delivery should optimally be

---

[1]Not FDA approved for this indication.
[3]Exceeds dosage recommended by the manufacturer.

treated presumptively with an antimalarial medication effective against the infecting species in the mother, regardless of the results of the infant's blood smear.

SEVERE MALARIA

Patients with a positive blood smear who have one or more of the criteria for severe disease (Table 1) should have treatment with intravenous (IV) quinidine or IV quinine[2] initiated immediately after diagnosis. (Although IV quinine is used elsewhere, it is not available in the United States.) Although artemisinins[2] generally clear parasitemia more quickly than quinine, they are not yet available in the United States. A loading dose of quinidine should be given unless the patient has received more than 40 mg/kg of quinine in the preceding 48 hours or if he or she has received mefloquine in the previous 12 hours. The patient should be admitted for continuous cardiac monitoring (e.g., widening of the QRS complex or lengthening of the QTc interval can occur). Blood pressure and glucose levels should be monitored frequently. Exchange transfusion is recommended if the parasite density is more than 10% or if the patient has altered mental status, ARDS, or renal failure. Blood smears should be monitored every 12 hours, and transfusion should be continued until the parasite density is less than 1% (usually 8 to 10 U).

Prevention

Both chemoprophylaxis and personal protection should be used for the optimal prevention of malaria in persons visiting malarious areas.

CHEMOPROPHYLAXIS

The choice of antimalarial drug depends on where the person is traveling, resistance patterns, and contraindications to each medication (Table 2). Antimalarial drugs are most effective if taken exactly on schedule without skipping doses and if the drug is continued for the recommended duration of time after travel. Antimalarial drugs should be purchased before travel. Drugs purchased

---

[2]Not available in the United States.

TABLE 1 Severe Manifestations of *Plasmodium falciparum* Malaria

Impaired consciousness or coma
Severe normocytic anemia
Renal failure
Pulmonary edema
Acute respiratory distress syndrome
Circulatory shock
Disseminated intravascular coagulation
Spontaneous bleeding
Hemoglobinuria
Jaundice
Repeated generalized seizures
Parasitemia >5%

overseas may not be protective and may be dangerous because they were produced using substandard manufacturing practices, may be counterfeit, or may contain contaminants. Current information regarding country-specific risks and recommendations for travelers can be found at the Centers for Disease Control and Prevention's Web site at http://www.cdc.gov/travel/malariadrugs2.htm. Prophylaxis refers to the strategy of using medications before, during, and after exposure to prevent initial infection. Presumptive antirelapse therapy (PART) (also known as terminal prophylaxis) refers to the strategy that uses medications toward the end of the exposure period to prevent relapse or delayed onset of initial infection caused by *P. vivax* and *P. ovale*.

TRAVEL TO AREAS WITHOUT CHLOROQUINE-RESISTANT *P. FALCIPARUM*

For travel to areas without documented chloroquine-resistant *P. falciparum*, once a week use of chloroquine is recommended for prophylaxis. Chloroquine should be started 1 week before departure and continued for 5 weeks after return. Reported side effects include gastrointestinal disturbance, headache, dizziness, blurred vision, insomnia, and pruritus. Overdose may lead to arrhythmias. Patients who cannot tolerate chloroquine (Aralen) may take mefloquine (Lariam), atovaquone-proguanil (Malarone), or doxycycline[1] (Vibramycin) for prophylaxis.

TRAVEL TO AREAS WITH CHLOROQUINE-RESISTANT *P. FALCIPARUM*

For travel to areas with documented chloroquine-resistant *P. falciparum*, one of three options, listed here alphabetically, is recommended:

1. Atovaquone-proguanil (Malarone). Atovaquone-proguanil is a daily medication that should be started 1 to 2 days before travel and continued for 7 days after return. Reported side effects include headache, abdominal pain, nausea, and vomiting. It is not recommended in children weighing less than 5 kg.
2. Doxycycline[1] (Vibramycin). Doxycycline is a daily medication that should be started 1 to 2 days before travel and continued for 4 weeks after return. Doxycycline should be avoided in children younger than 8 years. It may cause gastrointestinal side effects (which may be lessened by taking the drug with a meal), photosensitivity, and increase the risk of monilial vaginitis.
3. Mefloquine (Lariam). Mefloquine is a weekly medication that should be started 1 to 2 weeks before travel and continued for 4 weeks after return. If there is concern about adverse events, most of these will occur within 3 to 4 weeks of beginning the drug, and thus clinicians may consider this alternative.

Mefloquine should not be used for travel to regions where mefloquine-resistant *P. falciparum* is reported (Thailand–Myanmar and Thailand–Cambodian borders). Mefloquine is contraindicated in persons allergic to

---

[1]Not FDA approved for this indication.

TABLE 2 Drugs Used in Prophylaxis of Malaria

Drug	Adult Dose	Pediatric Dose	Comments
Areas with Chloroquine-Sensitive *Plasmodium falciparum*			
Chloroquine phosphate (Aralen and generic)	300 mg base (500 mg salt) orally, once/wk.	5 mg/kg base (8.3 mg/kg salt) orally, once/wk, up to maximum adult dose of 300 mg base.	Begin 1–2 wk before travel to malarious areas. Take weekly on the same day of the week while in the malarious area and for 4 wk after leaving such areas. May exacerbate psoriasis.
or			
Hydroxychloroquine sulfate (Plaquenil)	310 mg base (400 mg salt) orally, once/wk.	5 mg/kg base (6.5 mg/kg salt) orally, once/wk, up to maximum adult dose of 310 mg base.	An alternative to chloroquine. Begin 1–2 wk before travel to malarious areas. Take weekly on the same day of the week while in the malarious area and for 4 wk after leaving such areas.
Chloroquine-Resistant Areas with Chloroquine-Resistant *Plasmodium falciparum*			
Atovaquone/proguanil (Malarone)	Adult tablets contain 250 mg atovaquone and 100 mg proguanil hydrochloride. 1 adult tablet orally, daily.	Pediatric tablets contain 62.5 mg atovaquone and 25 mg proguanil hydrochloride. 5–8 kg: ½ tablet 9–10 kg: ¾ tablet 11–20 kg: 1 tablet 21–30 kg: 2 tablets 31–40 kg: 3 tablets 41 kg or more: 1 adult tablet daily	Begin 1–2 d before travel to malarious areas. Take daily at the same time each day while in the malarious area and for 7 d after leaving such areas. Contraindicated in persons with severe renal impairment (creatinine clearance <30 mL/min). Atovaquone/proguanil should be taken with food or a milky drink. Not recommended for children <5 kg, pregnant women, and women breast-feeding infants weighing <5 kg.
or			
Doxycycline[1] (many brand names and generic)	100 mg orally, daily.	≥8y: 2 mg/kg up to adult dose of 100 mg/d.	Begin 1–2 d before travel to malarious areas. Take daily at the same time each day while in the malarious area and for 4 weeks after leaving such areas. Contraindicated in children <8 y and pregnant women.
or			
Mefloquine (Lariam and generic)	228-mg base (250 mg salt) orally, once/wk.	≤9 kg: 4.6 mg/kg base (5 mg/kg salt) orally, once/wk 10–19 kg: 1/4 tablet once/wk 20–30 kg: 1/2 tablet once/wk 31–45 kg: 3/4 tablet once/wk 46 kg and more: 1 tablet once/wk.	Begin 1–2 wk before travel to malarious areas. Take weekly on the same day of the week while in the malarious area and for 4 wk after leaving such areas. Contraindicated in persons allergic to mefloquine or related compounds (e.g., quinine and quinidine) and in persons with active depression, a recent history of depression, generalized anxiety disorder, psychosis, schizophrenia, other major psychiatric disorders, or seizures. Use with caution in persons with psychiatric disturbances or previous history of depression. Not recommended for persons with cardiac conduction abnormalities.

TABLE 2 Drugs Used in Prophylaxis of Malaria—cont'd

	Drug	Adult Dose	Pediatric Dose	Comments
Alternatives	*Usage*			
Primaquine[1]	An option for prophylaxis when none of the other medications for primary prophylaxis can be used.	30-mg base (52.6 mg salt) orally, daily.	0.5 mg/kg base (0.8 mg/kg salt) up to adult dose orally, daily.	Begin 1–2 d before travel to malarious areas. Take daily at the same time each day while in the malarious area and for 7 d after leaving such areas. Contraindicated in persons with G6PD deficiency. Also contraindicated during pregnancy and lactation unless the infant being breast-fed has a documented normal G6PD level. Use in consultation with malaria experts.
Primaquine	Used for presumptive antirelapse therapy (terminal prophylaxis) to decrease risk of relapses of *P. vivax* and *P. ovale*.	30-mg base (52.6 mg salt[3]) orally, once/d for 14 d after departure from the malarious area.	0.5 mg/kg base (0.8 mg/kg salt[3]) up to adult dose orally, once/d for 14 d after departure from the malarious area.	Indicated for persons who have had prolonged exposure to *P. vivax* and *P. ovale* or both. Contraindicated in persons with G6PD deficiency. Also contraindicated during pregnancy and lactation unless infant being breast-fed has documented normal G6PD level.

[1]Not FDA approved for this indication.
Abbreviation: G6PD = glucose-6-phosphate dehydrogenase.

Malaria

125

mefloquine and in persons with active depression, a recent history of depression, generalized anxiety disorder, psychosis, schizophrenia, other major psychiatric disorders, or seizures. It is not recommended for people with cardiac conduction abnormalities. Reported side effects include gastrointestinal disturbance, headache, insomnia, abnormal dreams, visual disturbances, depression, anxiety disorder, and dizziness. Other more severe neuropsychiatric disorders occasionally reported include sensory and motor neuropathies (including paresthesia, tremor, and ataxia), agitation or restlessness, mood changes, panic attacks, confusion, forgetfulness, hallucinations, aggression, paranoia, and encephalopathy.

PRESUMPTIVE ANTIRELAPSE THERAPY FOR *P. VIVAX* AND *P. OVALE*

PART with primaquine to treat the liver stages (hypnozoites) of *P. vivax* and *P. ovale* is generally indicated for persons who have had prolonged exposure in malaria-endemic areas such as missionaries, Peace Corp volunteers, and the military. PART is administered for 14 days after the patient has left the malarious area. It is best if the primaquine is taken in conjunction with the blood schizonticide. Therefore, if the patient is taking chloroquine, doxycycline, or mefloquine for primary prophylaxis, the primaquine should be taken during the last 2 weeks of postexposure prophylaxis. If the person is taking atovaquone-proguanil, the primaquine should be started during the first 7 days of the person's return. All individuals receiving primaquine should first be tested for G6PD deficiency because of the risk of acute hemolysis when the drug is administered to G6PD-deficient persons.

CHEMOPROPHYLAXIS FOR INFANTS, CHILDREN, AND ADOLESCENTS

In the United States, antimalarial drugs are available only in tablet form and may taste bitter. Pediatric dosages should be carefully calculated based on the child's current weight; children's dosages should never exceed adult dosage. Full-service (compounding) pharmacists can pulverize tablets, weigh out the precise dose, and place the dose in a gelatin capsule. Advise parents to open the gelatin capsule and mix the drug with something sweet and to give the drug on a full stomach to minimize stomach upset and vomiting. Parents should allow sufficient time before travel to allow preparation of these dosages.

CHEMOPROPHYLAXIS DURING PREGNANCY AND LACTATION

Pregnancy

Chloroquine phosphate (Aralen) or hydroxychloroquine sulfate (Plaquenil) is recommended for pregnant women traveling to areas with chloroquine-sensitive *P. falciparum*. Mefloquine (Lariam) is currently the only medication recommended for prophylaxis during pregnancy in areas with chloroquine-resistant *P. falciparum*. Studies indicate that prophylactic use during the second and third trimesters, as opposed to the dose used for treatment, is not associated with adverse fetal or pregnancy outcomes. More limited data suggest it is also safe during the first trimester.

Lactation

Very small amounts of chloroquine and mefloquine are excreted in breast milk; the amount of the drug is not sufficient to harm the infant, nor is the quantity sufficient to protect the child from malaria. Very limited data are available on the use of doxycycline in lactating women; most experts consider the theoretical possibility of adverse events to be remote. Primaquine should only be given to lactating women if both the woman and her infant were tested for G6PD deficiency and have documented normal enzyme levels.

PERSONAL PROTECTIVE MEASURES

Travelers to malarious areas should use personal protective measures in addition to chemoprophylactic medication including wearing protective clothing (particularly at dusk or dawn), using insecticide-treated bed nets, staying in well-screened areas, and using insect repellent containing diethyltoluamide (DEET).

PRESUMPTIVE SELF-TREATMENT

Persons traveling to remote areas where medical care is not available within 24 hours, even if they are taking effective prophylaxis, may decide, in consultation with their health care provider, to carry a dose of antimalarial medication to take if they develop fever, chills, or influenza-like illness. The medication taken for self-treatment should be different from the medication being taken for prophylaxis. Travelers should be advised that self-treatment is only a temporary measure and prompt medical care is still needed. The medication most commonly prescribed is atovaquone-proguanil (Malarone).

REFERENCES

Blumberg L: Severe malaria. In Feldman C, Sarosi GA (eds): Tropical and Parasitic Infections in the Intensive Care Unit. New York, Springer, 2005, pp 1-16.

Centers for Disease Control and Prevention: Health Information for the International Traveler 2003–2004. Atlanta, U.S. Department of Health and Human Services, Public Health Service, 2003.

Coatney GR, Collins WE, Warren M, Contacos PG: The Primate Malarias. Bethesda: U.S. Department of Health, Education, and Welfare, 1971.

Gilles HM, Warrell DA (eds): Essential Malariology, 4th ed. London, Arnold, 2002.

Malaria Surveillance—United States, 2003. MMWR Morb Mortal Wkly Rep, 2005;54(SS-2):25-30.

Nosten F: The effects of mefloquine treatment in pregnancy. Clin Infect Dis 1999;28(4):808-815.

Parise M, Lewis LS: Severe malaria: North American perspective. In Feldman C, Sarosi GA (eds): Tropical and Parasitic Infections in the Intensive Care Unit. New York, Springer, 2005, pp 17-38.

Strickland GT: Malaria. In Strickland GT (ed): Hunters Tropical Medicine and Emerging Infectious Diseases, 8th ed. Philadelphia, WB Saunders, 2000, pp 614-642.

Tran TH, Day NP: Blackwater fever in southern Vietnam: A prospective descriptive study of 50 cases. Clin Infect Dis 1996;23(6):1274-1281.

World Malaria Report, 2005. WHO and UNICEF.

Bacterial Meningitis

Method of
Gary D. Overturf, MD

Acute bacterial meningitis occurs at all age groups, but predominantly in children younger than 2 years and the elderly (older than 60 years). With the introduction of effective protein conjugate vaccines for *Haemophilus* and pneumococcal infection, the incidence of bacterial meningitis is rapidly declining in children, and adults are now the major population affected. Bacterial meningitis is a medical emergency requiring rapid and decisive action to prevent death or neurologic sequelae. Since the introduction of chloramphenicol (Chloromycetin) in the early 1950s, the mortality has remained between 5% and 40% depending on the age of the patient and the etiology. Of the survivors, 10% to 30% suffer permanent neurologic deficits. Prognosis is affected by the timeliness of therapy, the age of the patient, and the etiology. Presumptive diagnosis and administration of therapy are critical.

Diagnosis

Acute bacterial meningitis must be considered in the differential diagnosis of persons of any age presenting with fever and headache or signs of meningeal irritation or acute central nervous system dysfunction. Presentations can be subtle at the extremes of age or in patients who have received partially effective antibiotic therapy. The diagnosis of bacterial meningitis requires the examination of the cerebrospinal fluid (CSF), which must be performed as expeditiously as possible. Studies indicate that lumbar puncture may be safely performed on patients who have normal mental status or are without focal neurologic signs or papilledema; clinical impression was predictive of the computed tomography (CT) findings. If there are signs or symptoms suggesting the presence of an intracranial mass (e.g., tumor, cerebral hematoma, or brain abscess), blood cultures should be obtained and empirical antibiotics should be administered prior to the performance of a CT scan.

The CSF findings in bacterial meningitis include a cell count of greater than 500 to 1000 white blood cells

CURRENT DIAGNOSIS

- Patient age and epidemiology:
  - Clinical symptoms: Fever, headache, meningeal signs
  - CSF examination: High opening pressure >300 mm Hg
  - Elevated white blood cell count (>10–>5000)
  - >60% polymorphonuclear cells
- Low CSF glucose (<40 mg/dL or <50% serum glucose)
- High CSF protein (>50–>1.0 g/dL)
- Bacteria present on gram stain of CSF

Abbreviation: CSF = cerebral spinal fluid.

(WBC) per mm^3 with a predominance of neutrophils, a protein concentration of greater than 150 mg/mL, and a low glucose (e.g., less than 35 to 40 mg/dL). No single value is absolute, and a single value may be normal in up to a third of the cases. The Gram-stained sediment of centrifuged CSF is the critical examination leading to a specific diagnosis. In patients who have not received antibiotics capable of reaching the CSF, the Gram stain is positive in 80% to 90% of culture-confirmed cases. In persons previously treated with antibiotics (e.g., beta-lactam antibiotics, tetracycline, fluoroquinolones), the frequency of positive Gram stains is much reduced (e.g., 60% to 70%), but the cells, cell type, protein, and glucose concentrations are not significantly affected. CSF antigen tests are not reliable, and high false-positive and false-negative rates direct against relying on the use of such tests. Clinical judgment is paramount, and antibiotics should be given in situations of ambiguous results of the CSF examination.

Antibiotic Selection

The outcome of bacterial meningitis is closely related to the timely use of antibiotics. Hypotension, seizures, an altered mental status, and hypoglycorrhachia at the time of initial antibiotic administration are predictive of higher case fatality and neurologic sequelae. Because prompt administration of antibiotics is critical, the choice of antibiotics usually is made before results of the CSF cultures are known. If organisms are seen on Gram stain, therapy may be directed by the probable bacterial etiology (Table 1). In the event the CSF Gram stain fails to reveal a possible pathogen, empirical antibiotic therapy should be begun based on the age of the patient for those persons who have

---

 CURRENT THERAPY

- Neonates <2 mo
  - Group B streptococcal infection: cefotaxime (Claforan) or ampicillin
  - Gram-negative rods, other than *Pseudomonas*: cefotaxime
  - *Pseudomonas*: cefepime (Maxipime) or ceftazidime (Fortaz)
  - *Listeria*: Ampicillin + gentamicin (Garamycin)
- Children >2 mo
  - Empirical for unknown etiology: cefotaxime or ceftriaxone (Rocephin)
  - *Streptococcus pneumoniae*: cefotaxime or ceftriaxone
  - *Haemophilus influenza*: cefotaxime or ceftriaxone
  - *Neisseria meningitidis*: ampicillin or cefotaxime
- Older children and adults
  - Empirical for unknown etiology: cefotaxime or ceftriaxone
  - *S. pneumoniae*: cefotaxime or ceftriaxone
  - *N. meningitidis:* ampicillin or cefotaxime
  - Gram negative, postoperative, or *Staphylococcus aureus* (see Tables 1–4)
  - Add vancomycin if at risk for infection with resistant pneumococcus

---

acquired their infection in the community (Table 2). For those persons who are members of special risk groups, empirical therapy should be based on the likely etiology (Table 3). Once the CSF cultures are completed, therapy can be modified according to results of the culture and sensitivity data.

Antibiotics used in bacterial meningitis should be rapidly bactericidal and achieve high concentrations in the CSF. Antibiotics should be given in maximal doses (Table 4). Because the bactericidal activity of antibiotics in CSF is dose dependent, the fractional CSF-to-serum ratio is very small. Finally, the use of combinations of antibiotics should be minimized to avoid antagonizing the bactericidal activity.

Special Considerations for Antibiotic Therapy

During the past two decades, resistance to penicillin and some third-generation cephalosporins (e.g., ceftriaxone [Rocephin], cefotaxime [Claforan]) has steadily increased among strains of *Streptococcus pneumoniae*. Currently, approximately 30% to 50% of isolates are either intermediately (inhibitory concentration, 0.1 to 1.0 µg/mL) or fully (inhibitory concentration more than 2.0 µg/mL) resistant to *Penicillin* G and ampicillin. Resistance to ceftriaxone (Rocephin) and cefotaxime (Claforan) may occur as well in 10% to 15% of strains. Vancomycin (Vancocin) is recommended in those regimens for meningitis when pneumococci are considered. However, higher maximal doses are required for vancomycin because of its relatively poor penetration into the CSF. In general, lumbar puncture with CSF culture should be repeated in 48 hours in those cases where vancomycin therapy is the primary drug because of demonstrated penicillin or cephalosporin resistance.

Meningitis caused by gram-negative bacilli such as *Pseudomonas aeruginosa, Escherichia coli,* or *Enterobacter cloacae* should be treated with a cephalosporin with an extended spectrum of gram-negative activity, such as ceftazidime (Fortaz) or cefepime (Maxipime). Carbapenem, such as imipenem (Primaxin) or meropenem (Merrem), can also be used for antibiotic-resistant gram-negative enteric and pseudomonas meningitis. Meropenem is associated with less risk of drug-induced seizures and may be a better choice for bacterial meningitis.

Patients with ventriculoatrial- and ventriculoperitoneal shunt–associated meningitis and ventriculitis usually require removal of the shunt for cure, as well as the administration of antibiotics to clear the infection. Certain patients with infections caused by organisms of reduced virulence, such as coagulase-negative staphylococci, or those with exquisitely antibiotic-susceptible infections, can be treated with a trial of antibiotics alone.

Because of the extreme sensitivity of *Neisseria meningitidis* to antibiotics, uncomplicated meningitis may be treated with as little as 5 to 7 days of antibiotics. Pneumococcal meningitis may be treated with 10 to 14 days of antibiotics and haemophilus infections are treated successfully with 7 to 10 days of antibiotics. Gram-negative meningitis was treated in the past with 3 weeks of aminoglycosides, but current experience with newer

TABLE 1 Cerebrospinal Fluid Gram Stain Morphology and Antibiotic Recommendations

Morphology	Possible or Probable Pathogens	Treatment Options	Alternative Therapies
Gram-positive cocci, short chains or pairs	*Streptococcus pneumoniae, Streptococcus agalactiae* (group B streptococci)	Ceftriaxone (Rocephin) or cefotaxime (Claforan) plus vancomycin (Vancocin)	Chloramphenicol (Chloromycetin)
Gram-positive cocci, clusters; or gram-positive bacilli	*Staphylococcus aureus, Listeria monocytogenes*	Vancomycin, ampicillin plus gentamicin (Garamycin)	Nafcillin (Unipen) or Oxacillin, trimethoprim-sulfamethoxazole (Bactrim)
Gram-negative diplococci	*Neisseria meningitidis*	Ceftriaxone or cefotaxime	Ampicillin, Penicillin G, or chloramphenicol
Gram-negative coccobacilli	*Haemophilus influenzae*	Ceftriaxone or cefotaxime	Chloramphenicol
Gram-negative bacilli	*Escherichia coli, Klebsiella* species, *Pseudomonas aeruginosa*	Cefepime (Maxipime) or ceftazidime (Fortaz)	Imipenem (Primaxin) or meropenem (Merrem)

extended-spectrum cephalosporins (ceftriaxone, cefotaxime, carbapenems) suggests that 2 weeks of therapy is often sufficient in neonates as well as in some elderly patients and postoperative infections.

All patients with bacterial meningitis should be monitored carefully throughout the treatment period. Infectious disease consultation is recommended for most infections of the central nervous system. Repeated lumbar punctures are not routinely recommended for patients with fully susceptible bacterial isolates or in those who show good response to therapy. Repeated sampling of the CSF with lumbar puncture or, when appropriate, shunt or ventricular reservoir puncture should be performed in those with known resistant bacterial isolates, in patients who have an inadequate response, in those patients who deteriorate on therapy, or in those for whom clinical response may correlate poorly with the microbiologic response (shunt infections, neonates, and elderly patients).

Adjunctive Therapy

Corticosteroids reduce the incidence of permanent neurologic sequelae in children with bacterial meningitis, particularly when caused by *Haemophilus influenza* type b. Data in

support of steroids in either pneumococcal or meningococcal infections are less robust. Dexamethasone (Decadron[1]), 0.15 mg/kg every 6 hours for the first 2 to 4 days of treatment, was evaluated in children older than 2 months with bacterial meningitis. The first dose of dexamethasone should be given before, at the start, or within no later than 12 hours after beginning antibiotics.

Use of corticosteroids in adults is more controversial. Although doses of dexamethasone are recommended by some experts for adults with bacterial meningitis, its efficacy in adult meningitis has not been evaluated in a well-designed prospective trial. A recent study in adults found that corticosteroids significantly reduced the risk for unfavorable outcomes, particularly in patients with pneumococcal meningitis. There has been concern that the anti-inflammatory properties of dexamethasone may decrease the penetration of antibiotics, especially vancomycin, into the CSF. One study in children did not show this to be the case. Dexamethasone[1] should be administered in adults with proven or suspected pneumococcal meningitis, only if it can be given prior to the first dose of antibiotics in a dose of 10 mg every 6 hours for 4 days. In patients with meningitis

---

[1]Not FDA approved for this indication.

TABLE 2 Antibiotic Recommendations for Bacterial Meningitis Acquired in the Community, by Age Group and Probable Pathogen

Age Group	Probable Pathogens	Empirical Therapy
Neonate <1 mo	Group B streptococcus; *Escherichia coli*, or other gram-negative enteric rod; occasionally *Listeria monocytogenes*	Ampicillin plus cefotaxime (Claforan)
Infants 1–3 mo	*H. influenzae, N. meningitidis, S. pneumoniae,* Group B streptococci	Ceftriaxone (Rocephin) or cefotaxime (Claforan)
Children 3 mo–7 y and older children and adults 7–50 y	*H. influenzae, S. pneumoniae, N. meningitidis*	Ceftriaxone or cefotaxime plus vancomycin (Vancocin)
Older adults >50 y	*S. pneumoniae, N. meningitidis,* and *L. monocytogenes*	Ceftriaxone plus ampicillin

TABLE 3 Antibiotic Recommendations for Presumed Bacterial Meningitis in Persons with Special Risks

Condition or Risk Factor	Common Pathogens	Antibiotic Recommendations
Impaired immunity (e.g., HIV, early complement deficiency, agammaglobulinemia)	*Listeria monocytogenes, Streptococcus pneumoniae Haemophilus influenzae*	Ampicillin plus ceftriaxone (Rocephin) or cefotaxime (Claforan)
Closed head trauma with CSF leak	*S. pneumoniae, H. influenzae*	Ceftriaxone or cefotaxime plus vancomycin (Vancocin)
Asplenia	*S. pneumoniae, H. influenzae*	Ceftriaxone or cefotaxime plus vancomycin
Terminal complement deficiency	*Neisseria meningitidis*	Ceftriaxone or cefotaxime
Neurosurgical procedures	*Staphylococcus aureus*	Vancomycin plus ceftriaxone or cefotaxime
CSF shunt infections	Coagulase-negative staphylococci, gram-negative bacilli	
Elderly patients (>65 y)	*S. pneumoniae, Listeria monocytogenes*	Ceftriaxone or cefotaxime plus vancomycin
Recurrent bacterial meningitis (see CSF leak)	*Streptococcus pneumoniae*	Ceftriaxone or cefotaxime plus vancomycin
Alcoholic patients	*Streptococcus pneumoniae* and gram-negative bacilli	Ceftriaxone or cefotaxime plus vancomycin

Abbreviation: CSF = cerebrospinal fluid.

caused by *Streptococcus pneumoniae* highly resistant to penicillin (minimum inhibitory concentration [MIC] >2.0 µg/mL) or cephalosporins (MIC >4.0 µg/mL), vancomycin should not be used as a single agent if corticosteroids are used. The addition of rifampin (Rifadin[1]) is often recommended in these situations; other alternative is gentamicin.

Chemoprophylaxis for Bacterial Meningitis

Prophylactic antibiotics are recommended in case of meningitis caused by *Neisseria meningitidis* and *Haemophilus influenzae* type b. Prophylaxis is provided to eliminate the carriage of organisms among contacts and prevent spread to hosts susceptible to invasive disease. In cases of meningococcal meningitis, prophylaxis is indicated only for those with household or close intimate contact with the index case. Administration of prophylaxis to large groups (e.g., college students, schoolchildren, or preschool classes) is usually a special assessment and a recommendation of local or regional health departments. Chemoprophylaxis is not necessary for casual contacts or medical personnel unless there is a direct exposure to respiratory secretions. The recommended dose of rifampin (Rifadin) is 10 mg/kg (600 maximal, adults) twice a day for 2 days; ciprofloxacin (Cipro[1]), 500 mg as single dose, is also effective for adults. Third-generation cephalosporins used in treatment of the

[1]Not FDA approved for this indication.

[1]Not FDA approved for this indication.

TABLE 4 Antibiotic Doses for Adults and Children for Treatment of Bacterial Meningitis

Antibiotic	Daily Adult Dose	Daily Pediatric Dose	Dose Interval
Amikacin (Amikin)	15 mg/kg	15–20 mg/kg	8 h
Ampicillin	12 g	200–400 mg/kg	4–6 h
Cefotaxime (Claforan)	12 g	200–300 mg/kg	4–6 h
Ceftriaxone (Rocephin)	4 g	100 mg/kg	12 h
Ceftazidime (Fortaz)	6 g	150–200 mg/kg	8 h
Cefepime (Maxipime)	6 g	100–150 mg/kg	8 h
Gentamicin (Garamycin)	5 mg/kg	7.5 mg/kg	8 h
Meropenem (Merrem)	6 g	120 mg/kg	8 h
Nafcillin (Unipen)	12 g	200 mg/kg	4–6 h
Penicillin G	24 million U	250,000 units/kg	4 h
Tobramycin (Nebcin)	5 mg/kg	6–7.5 mg/kg	8 h
Trimethoprim-sulfamethoxazole (Bactrim)	10-15 mg/kg	10–20 mg/kg	8 h
Vancomycin (Vancocin)	2 g	60 mg/kg	12 h

Adapted from Bradley JS, Nelson JD: 2002–2003 Nelson's Pocket Book of Pediatric Antimicrobial Therapy, 15th ed. Philadelphia and New York, Lippincott Williams & Wilkins, 2002.
Gilbert DN, Moellering RC, Sande MA: The Sanford Guide to Antimicrobial Therapy 2005. Hyde Park, Antimicrobial Therapy Inc., 2005.

index case of meningitis are sufficient to eliminate carriage of the organism.

Chemoprophylaxis for *H. influenzae* type b is recommended for all household contacts of an index case if one of the contacts is an unvaccinated child younger than 4 years. If the index case is treated with ceftriaxone (Rocephin) or cefotaxime (Claforan), prophylaxis is not required, but if treated with ampicillin or chloramphenicol (Chloromycetin), prophylaxis is recommended to eliminate carriage. The recommended regimen for prophylaxis is rifampin,[1] 20 mg/kg (or 600 mg in adults) once a day for 4 days. With the near elimination of invasive infections caused by *Haemophilus influenzae* type b, with the use of routine immunization of children with conjugate haemophilus vaccines, *Haemophilus influenzae* types A, F, and rarely other serotypes have emerged, and the use of prophylaxis is not recommended in these situations because sufficient data are not available to support its efficacy, nor has spread within contacts been documented with any frequency.

Vaccines for Bacterial Meningitis

The universal recommendation for the use of protein-polysaccharide conjugate *Haemophilus influenzae* type b (HIB) vaccines in 1987 reduced the incidence of bacterial meningitis by this organism by greater than 97%. Three HIB vaccines (PedvaxHIB, ActHIB, HibTITER), licensed in the United States, are routinely given to children in dosage schedules employing three to four doses by 12 to 18 months of age (see www.cdc.gov).

A pneumococcal protein-polysaccharide conjugate vaccine (Prevnar) licensed in 2000 is routinely recommended for children and has markedly reduced the incidence of invasive infections with seven serotypes of pneumococci in children. This vaccine is also recommended for children at high risk of pneumococcal infections (e.g., HIV infection, asplenia, sickle cell disease, and others). A pneumococcal polysaccharide vaccine (Pneumovax 23) is recommended for adults older than 65 years or for those younger than 50 years with risk factors (e.g., alcoholism, diabetes or other metabolic or renal disease, chronic pulmonary or cardiac disease). Although clear evidence for prevention of bacterial meningitis is lacking, evidence supports its efficacy against invasive pneumococcal diseases, many of which are the preceding infections leading to bacteremia and meningitis.

Currently two vaccines remain available for prevention of meningococcal disease caused by four serotypes, A, C, Y, and W-135. The meningococcal polysaccharide vaccine (Menomune) is recommended for persons older than 2 years at high risk for severe meningococcal infections including adolescents and college students (particularly those residing in dormitories), military recruits, and those with complement deficiencies and asplenia. A quadrivalent protein-polysaccharide conjugate vaccines (Menactra) was licensed in 2005. This vaccine is recommended for routine immunization of all children 11 to 12 years of age and adolescents and college students at high risk as well as those more than 11 to 55 years of age with high-risk factors for meningococcal infection.

REFERENCES

Anderson EJ, Yogev LR: A rational approach to the management of ventricular shunt infections. Pediatric Infect Dis J 2005;24:557-558.

Andes DR, Craig WA: Pharmacokinetics and pharmacodynamics of antibiotics in meningitis. Infect Dis Clin North Am 1999;13(2):595-618.

De Gans J, van de Beek: Dexamethasone in adults with bacterial meningitis. N Engl J Med 2002;347:1549-1546.

Gray LD, Fedorko DP: Laboratory diagnosis of bacterial meningitis. Clin Microbiol Rev 1992;5:130-145.

Hussein AS, Shafran SD: Acute bacterial meningitis in adults: A 12-year review. Medicine (Baltimore) 2000;79:360-368.

Klinger G, Chin C-Y, Beyene J, et al: Predicting the outcome of neonatal bacterial meningitis. Pediatrics 2000;106:477-482.

Klein JO: Bacterial sepsis and meningitis. In Remington JS, Klein JO (eds): Infectious Diseases of the Fetus and Newborn Infant, 5th ed. New York and Saint Louis, WB Saunders, 2002, pp 943-998.

Odio CM, Faingezicht I, Paris M, et al: The beneficial effects of early dexamethasone administration in infants and children with bacterial meningitis. N Engl J Med 1991;324:1525-1531.

Ronan A, Hogg GG, Klug CL: Cerebrospinal fluid shunt infections in children. Pediatr Infect Dis J 1995;14:782-786.

Schuchat A, Robinson K, Wenger JD, et al: Bacterial meningitis in the United States in 1995. N Engl J Med 1997;337:970-976.

Unhanand M, Mustapha MM, McCracken GH, et al: Gram-negative enteric bacillary meningitis: A twenty-one year experience. J Pediatr 1993;122:15-17.

Van de Beek D, de Gans J, Spanjaard L, et al: Clinical features and prognostic factors in adults with bacterial meningitis. N Engl J Med 2004;351:1849-1858.

Infectious Mononucleosis

Method of
Leonard R. Krilov, MD

Infectious mononucleosis is a clinical illness characterized by fever (typically not higher than 39.5°C [103°F]), sore throat, tender cervical lymphadenopathy, fever, malaise, and anorexia; it occurs most commonly in adolescence and young adulthood. Initially described in the 19th century as glandular fever, the characteristic mononuclear response with atypical-appearing lymphocytes led to the name infectious mononucleosis.

Etiology

Epstein-Barr virus (EBV) was recognized as the primary cause of infectious mononucleosis in 1968. Other infectious agents such as cytomegalovirus (CMV), toxoplasma, or adenoviruses may cause a minority of cases of mononucleosis (or mononucleosis-like illness).

Epstein-Barr virus is an enveloped, double-stranded DNA virus of the Herpesviridae family. After primary EBV infection, as with other herpesviruses, the virus persists in a latent state throughout the patient's lifetime in a few B lymphocytes and is shed in saliva intermittently.

---

[1]Not FDA approved for this indication.

The virus has also been associated with African Burkitt's lymphoma, nasopharyngeal carcinoma, lymphoproliferative diseases after organ and bone marrow transplantation, and hairy leukoplakia and lymphocytic interstitial pneumonitis in HIV-infected patients. X-linked proliferative disease (Duncan syndrome) is a rare condition in which affected boys develop fulminant uncontrolled lymphoproliferation after acute infectious mononucleosis. Survivors develop severe chronic hypogammaglobulinemia, chronic EBV and enteroviral infections and B-cell lymphomas.

Epidemiology

Epstein-Barr virus infections occur at a younger age in lower socioeconomic groups; 70% to 90% of such children developing EBV antibodies by age 5 years compared to only 40% to 50% of those from higher socioeconomic groups. For unknown reasons primary infections occurring in adolescence and young adulthood are more likely to manifest as infectious mononucleosis than when initial infection occurs at a younger age. In younger children acute EBV infection is usually clinically inapparent or manifested by a nonspecific, uncomplicated upper respiratory tract infection or pharyngitis. Thus, infectious mononucleosis occurs most commonly among white high school and college students with an annual incidence of approximately 1 in 2500 among such individuals aged 15 to 25 years.

EBV transmission occurs through intimate sharing of saliva (thus, its description as the *kissing disease*) with an incubation period of 20 to 30 days (range 2 to 6 weeks). The efficiency of transmission is low, and outbreaks of disease are rare. Epstein-Barr virus' viral load in whole blood in the acute phase correlates with the severity of symptoms; but viral load in oral secretions is independent of symptoms. There is no seasonality or sex predilection to EBV infections. Post-transfusion development of symptoms of mononucleosis is most often associated with CMV infection.

Clinical Manifestations

The classic manifestations of infectious mononucleosis are fever, painful exudative pharyngitis, and lymphadenopathy. The enlarged nodes may be limited to the cervical regions (including posteriorly) or generalized. Splenomegaly and frequently hepatomegaly are the other hallmark findings of the illness. Elevated liver function tests are common in the acute phase of disease, but symptomatic jaundice is rare. Eyelid edema (Hoagland sign) has been reported in approximately 25% of cases. The acute symptoms typically resolve over 1 to 4 weeks, but lymphadenopathy and fatigue may last for 2 to 3 months.

Less common clinical manifestations include autoimmune hemolytic anemia (approximately 3%), severe neutropenia to less than 1000/mm^3 (approximately 3%), and neurologic involvement in up to 5% of cases. The reported neurologic manifestations of acute EBV infection include meningoencephalitis, Guillain-Barré syndrome, transverse myelitis, facial paralysis, optic neuritis, and metamorphopsia or Alice in Wonderland syndrome with altered perception of sizes, shapes, and spatial relationships.

CURRENT DIAGNOSIS

The clinical triad of fever, exudative pharyngitis, and lymphadenitis in association with atypical lymphocytosis and a positive heterophil response makes the diagnosis of infectious mononucleosis. Epstein-Barr virus serologies should be reserved for uncertain cases or to confirm the diagnosis in younger children who may not mount a heterophil response.

Most cases of mononucleosis resolve uneventfully. Splenic rupture and the previously cited neurologic complications are the most frequent serious complications of mononucleosis with rare deaths reported.

Diagnosis

In the presence of the clinical features noted earlier, infectious mononucleosis is diagnosed by the presence of atypical lymphocytosis (>5% to 10% of all leukocytes) frequently in association with a decline in the number of granulocytes and platelets. Additionally, among school-age children and young adults, heterophil or Paul-Bunnell antibodies are detectable in 80% to 90% of cases beginning in the second week of illness and can be detected for up to 6 to 9 months after resolution of symptoms. These IgM antibodies react with horse, sheep, and beef erythrocytes but not guinea pig red cells. They are not EBV-specific and are present in only 50% or fewer of children younger than 4 years of age. Office-based commercial rapid slide kits for detecting heterophil response are 96% to 99% sensitive and give a result in 2 minutes.

Measurement of specific antibodies to EBV can be used to confirm the diagnosis. In the acute phase of illness, IgM and IgG antibodies to the viral capsid antigen (VCA) of EBV are detectable. The IgM response persists for approximately 4 months, whereas the IgG antibodies remain for life. Although the height of the VCA-IgG response decreases as the acute infection resolves, serial measurements of antibody titers are not clinically beneficial as a rule. Antibodies to the EBV nuclear antigen (EBNA) appear several weeks to months after a primary infection and are considered a marker for a past or convalescent infection, but 10% to 20% of individuals never develop detectable levels of EBNA antibodies. More than 80% of patients develop transient antibodies to the early antigen (EA) of the virus as the VCA-IgM clears and EBNA responses develop (Table 1).

CURRENT THERAPY

Rest and supportive care with limitation of physical activity during the first 1 to 4 weeks of illness are the mainstays of managing infectious mononucleosis. Corticosteroids are reserved for severe illness, especially with upper airway obstruction because of tonsillar hypertrophy.

TABLE 1 Infectious Mononucleosis Serological Response Patterns (Typical Patterns)

	Heterophil Antibody	EBV VCA-IgM	EBV VCA-IgG	EBV EA	EBV EBNA
No Infection	−	−	−	−	−
Acute Infection	+	+	+/+	+/−	−
Past Infection	−	−	+	+/−	+

Abbreviations: EA = early antigen; EBNA = Epstein-Barr (virus) nuclear antigen; EBV = Epstein-Barr virus; VCA = viral capsid antigen.

Treatment

There is no effective antiviral therapy for EBV-associated infectious mononucleosis. Rest and supportive care are mainstays of therapy. Corticosteroids are frequently prescribed for severe cases, but critical evaluation of this modality is lacking. Indications include marked tonsillar hypertrophy with upper airway obstruction, neurologic manifestations, and hemolytic anemia. High-dose, short-term courses of steroids (dexamethasone [Decadron][1] [0.25 mg/kg every 6 hours]; methylprednisolone [Solu-Medrol][1] [1 mg/kg every 6 hours]; oral prednisone[1] [40 mg/day]) have been used with dramatic improvement typically noted over 24 to 72 hours.

REFERENCES

Ambinder RF, Lin L: Mononucleosis in the laboratory. J Infect Dis 2005; 192:1503–1504.

Balfour HH Jr, Holman CJ, Hokanson KM, et al: A prospective clinical study of Epstein-Barr virus and host interactions during acute infectious mononucleosis. J Infect Dis 2005;192:1505–1512.

Barone SR, Krilov LR: Infectious mononucleosis and other Epstein-Barr virus infections. In Hoekelman RA (ed.): Primary Pediatric Care (4th ed.). St. Louis, Mosby, 2001, pp 1573–1577.

Fafi-Kremer S, Morand P, Brion J-P, et al: Long-term shedding of infectious Epstein-Barr virus after infectious mononucleosis. J Infect Dis 2005;191:985–989.

Giffen BE, Xue S: Epstein-Barr virus infections and their association with human malignancies: Some key questions. Ann Med 1998;30: 249–254.

Henle G, Henle W, Diehl V: Relation of Burkitt's tumor-associated herpes-type virus to infectious mononucleosis. Proc Natl Acad Sci U S A 1968;59:94–101.

McGowan JE, Chesney PJ, Crossley KB, et al: Guidelines for the use of systemic glucococorticosteroids in the management of selected infections. Working group on steroid use, Antimicrobial Agents Committee, Infectious Diseases Society of America. J Infect Dis 1992;165:1–13.

Paul JR, Bunnell WW: Classics in infectious diseases. The presence of heterophile antibodies in infectious mononucleosis by John R. Paul and W. W. Bunnell. American Journal of the Medical Sciences, 1932. Rev Infect Dis 1982;4:1062–1068.

Sumaya CV, Ench Y: Epstein-Barr virus infectious mononucleosis in children. I. Clinical and general laboratory findings. Pediatrics 1985; 75:1003–1010.

Sumaya CV, Ench Y: Epstein-Barr virus infectious mononucleosis in children. II. Heterophil antibody and viral-specific responses. Pediatrics 1985;75:1011–1019.

---

[1]Not FDA approved for this indication.

Chronic Fatigue Syndrome

Method of
Steven Reid, MB, PhD, and
Simon Wessely, MD, PhD

Chronic fatigue syndrome (CFS) denotes an illness of uncertain etiology characterized by severe, disabling physical and mental fatigue made worse by minimal activity and not relieved by rest. In recent years it has attracted a resurgence of interest, at the same time becoming the subject of controversy regarding its cause and management. Along with fatigue, CFS is typically associated with other symptoms, including musculoskeletal pain, sleep disturbance, impaired concentration, and headaches. Together, these form the basis of the widely used case definition developed by the Centers for Disease Control and Prevention (CDC) (see Current Diagnosis box). The severity and duration of CFS varies considerably from patient to patient, but many experience a substantial decline in physical and cognitive functioning. Those who do not meet the fatigue severity or symptom criteria are given a diagnosis of idiopathic chronic fatigue.

Epidemiology

Fatigue is a common medical complaint, reported on one in five primary care visits. A smaller number suffer from idiopathic chronic fatigue, and studies based on community and primary care report the prevalence of CFS as 0.007% to 2.8%, depending on the definition and exclusion criteria used. Most studies show an increased prevalence of CFS in women, with a relative risk of 1.3 to 1.7. In contrast to those patients attending specialist clinics, community samples show an association with lower socioeconomic status and certain ethnic groups: Latinos, African Americans, and Native Americans are at increased risk. Most of those who fulfill the criteria do not use the term *chronic fatigue syndrome* to describe their illness, however.

Etiology

Despite considerable research effort and several hypotheses, the cause of CFS remains elusive. Hypercortisolism and a blunted adrenal response to stress are found in many patients, leading to a disturbance of the hypothalamic-pituitary-adrenal (HPA) axis posited as a cause of

CURRENT DIAGNOSIS

International Consensus Definition of Chronic Fatigue Syndrome

1. Clinically evaluated, unexplained, persistent or relapsing chronic fatigue (lasting more than 6 months) that is of new or definite onset (has not been lifelong); is not the result of ongoing exertion; is not substantially alleviated by rest; and results in substantial reduction in previous levels of occupational, educational, social, or personal activities.

2. Four or more of the following symptoms are concurrently present for more than 6 months:
   - Impaired memory or concentration
   - Sore throat
   - Tender cervical or axillary lymph nodes
   - Muscle pain
   - Multijoint pain
   - New headaches
   - Unrefreshing sleep
   - Postexertion malaise

3. Exclusionary clinical diagnoses:
   - Any active medical condition that could explain the chronic fatigue
   - Any previously diagnosed medical condition whose resolution has not been documented beyond reasonable clinical doubt and whose continued activity may explain the chronic fatiguing illness
   - Psychotic major depression; bipolar affective disorder; schizophrenia; delusional disorders; dementias; anorexia nervosa; bulimia nervosa
   - Alcohol or other substance abuse within 2 years prior to the onset of the chronic fatigue and at any time afterward

Adapted from Fukuda K, Straus SE, Hickie I, et al: The chronic fatigue syndrome: A comprehensive approach to its definition and study. Ann Intern Med 1994;121:953-959.

CFS symptoms. These abnormalities of HPA function are the most consistent and reproducible to date, but whether they are causal or epiphenomenal is yet to be established. Alterations in immune function are found in some patients, but many of the findings are inconsistent and nonspecific. One replicated finding is that of chronic low-level immune system activation, with increased expression of activation markers on the surface of T cells. Again, the significance of this abnormality in the development of CFS remains unclear.

CFS is frequently attributed to viral infection, but epidemiologic studies do not demonstrate any association with common infective agents. Certain infections, such as Epstein-Barr virus, toxoplasmosis, cytomegalovirus, and Q fever, can precipitate prolonged periods of fatigue, however. Clinical and laboratory evidence suggests a single infectious agent is unlikely to be responsible for CFS. Rather, a number of infections may act as triggers in predisposed individuals and perpetuate CFS symptoms.

The relationship between depression and CFS is complex. Many depressed patients complain of prolonged fatigue, and depression is very common in CFS populations.

As well as similarities, significant differences exist between the two illnesses. Patients with CFS often do not show the cognitions typically associated with depression—low self-esteem, hopelessness, suicidal ideation—and studies of neurotransmitter and neuroendocrine function in the two conditions emphasize a distinction. Depression is an indicator of poorer outcome in CFS.

CFS shares many similarities with other medically unexplained syndromes, such as fibromyalgia, irritable bowel syndrome, and multiple chemical sensitivities. Of particular importance in all of these illnesses are patients' health beliefs and attributions. Evidence suggests these factors have a significant role in influencing outcome. What is less clear is their role in symptom development.

Assessment

The management of CFS is by necessity collaborative, and establishment of a positive relationship with the patient, beginning at the assessment, is key. Unfortunately, many patients with chronic fatigue are confronted with disbelief when they consult medical practitioners, or they may be reassured nothing is physically wrong and their symptoms are "all in the mind." This interpretation understandably leads to resentment and a distrust of the medical profession, with the patient seeking alternatives either within the general medical sphere or in more unorthodox circles. So an important first step in management is to validate the patients' symptoms and allow them to ventilate the difficulties they may have experienced with previous medical encounters.

Fatigue is a common feature of a wide range of medical disorders, but most can be excluded on clinical grounds and with the use of simple screening tests. The need to rule out an organic disorder must also be balanced with the potential adverse consequences of continued investigation. The importance of an adequate history cannot be overemphasized. As well as detailing the nature and development of the presenting complaint, the history should include a comprehensive account of the patient's background, including family history, past medical and psychiatric history, employment, and financial situation. The mental state and physical examinations are both of central importance to making a diagnosis. The aim of the mental state examination, as well as excluding clearly distinguishable diagnoses such as psychotic illness, is to identify disorders such as anxiety and depression, which have significant implications for treatment. It is also important to identify potential obstacles to recovery by exploring the patient's illness beliefs, coping strategies, and prior experience of medical care, as well as the attitude of caregivers or family members. A thorough physical examination is essential, and abnormal findings such as pyrexia or persistent lymphadenopathy merit further investigation and should not be ascribed to CFS. There may be evidence on examination of prolonged physical inactivity, such as muscle wasting and postural hypotension, which indicate the severity of the illness.

A careful history and examination should be linked with appropriate use of investigations in patients presenting with chronic fatigue (Box 1). No diagnostic test is available for CFS, and laboratory tests are generally unremarkable. More detailed investigations should also be

CURRENT THERAPY

General
- Help patient accept illness.
- Educate patient about the illness.
- Encourage self-help and normal activity.
- Treat co-morbid psychiatric illness.

Pharmacologic
- Consider antidepressant medication.
- Avoid untested treatments.

Nonpharmacologic
- Set goals.
- Explain sleep hygiene.
- Suggest graded activity schedule.
- Refer for cognitive behavior therapy.
- Refer for other psychotherapies if indicated.

considered in the following circumstances: extremes of age, recent foreign travel, or absence of mental fatigue. Weight loss in particular is unusual in CFS and needs careful inquiry. Likewise, absence of any evidence of mental fatigue should increase suspicion of a primary neuromuscular disorder because the fatigue in CFS is of central origin and associated with both physical and mental fatigability.

A diagnosis of CFS should be made pragmatically (i.e., the patient complains of chronic physical and mental fatigue; fatigability manifests substantial disability in the absence of identifiable organic disease). A diagnosis provides patients with a coherent (although simply descriptive) label for their illness. It should be given in the context of understanding that the cause of the illness is poorly understood but treatment is available and recovery possible. The acronyms ME (myalgic encephalomyelitis) and CFIDS (chronic fatigue and immune dysfunction syndrome) should be avoided because myalgic encephalomyelitis is a misleading term that implies a known disease process, and no consistent evidence justifies the addition of "immune dysfunction" to the diagnosis. There will also be patients with idiopathic chronic fatigue (not quite meeting the case definition for CFS) who may still benefit from this approach to treatment.

Treatment

The principal aim of treatment is a reduction in functional disability, and the emphasis should be on rehabilitation rather than cure. Management follows a few basic principles, but the CFS population includes many people with differing needs. Treatments should be broadly divided into general and specific areas and tailored to the individual patient.

General education about CFS is necessary for most patients, and for some may be all that is required. The reality of the illness and its associated symptoms should be firmly acknowledged while emphasizing there is no specific underlying, ongoing disease process (i.e., it is not like HIV). The next step is to agree on a model for thinking about the illness that encompasses the many factors, both physical and psychological, involved in its development, but especially its persistence. Thus, patients learn how they can influence the outcome of their illness by modifying these factors. A helpful analogy is being involved in a hit-and-run accident, emphasizing the futility of searching for a cause but the importance of rehabilitation. Patients may also be reassured that CFS is not associated with mortality and people can improve and recover, but they have a significant role to play. For most patients, this involvement includes a gradual and monitored increase in activity levels, linked to overcoming previous and present avoidance behavior where relevant. Advice also needs to be offered on the importance of reducing stressors from employment or lifestyle that may be contributing to symptoms and hindering recovery.

PHARMACOLOGIC TREATMENTS

Patients who have a co-morbid depressive illness, whether it is considered a primary or secondary problem, should be offered treatment with antidepressants. For patients who are not depressed, the evidence for the use of antidepressants is unclear. Tricyclic antidepressants do have analgesic properties, however,[1] and they may also be beneficial in patients complaining of insomnia.[1] To minimize side effects (commonly dry mouth, constipation, postural hypotension), the patient should be started at the lowest possible dose, such as 10 mg of amitriptyline (Elavil) or imipramine (Tofranil), which may be increased incrementally. For depressed patients, the ideal dosage is 150 to 300 mg daily (divided if necessary). In nondepressed patients complaining of myalgia or insomnia, lower dosages are often effective. Selective serotonin reuptake inhibitors and other more recently developed antidepressants are more easily tolerated and may also have an alerting effect, but their analgesic properties are less clear.[1] Although many other drug treatments are being evaluated in the management of CFS, there is as yet insufficient evidence to recommend their use.

---

[1]Not FDA approved for this indication.

NONPHARMACOLOGIC TREATMENTS

Nonpharmacologic treatments consist of a combination of educational and behavioral interventions, which can be used without recourse to a special clinic. Graded activity is central to the treatment of CFS. As part of the assessment, patients should record levels of activity in a diary. Many patients with CFS initially overdo attempts to exercise, become severely fatigued, and develop a pattern of over- and underactivity (sometimes called "boom and bust"). Other patients avoid all levels of exercise and may develop features of deconditioning. So before any exercise plan is advised, current activity levels should be stabilized, which may even mean an overall reduction at the start of treatment. The aim is to produce consistency in activity before embarking on any program of gradually increasing activity. Activities should be set at an attainable level, and the patient should be made aware that initially symptoms may worsen but subsequently will improve. The first steps may involve simple tasks such as getting out of bed or going to the toilet unaided, and at this stage involvement of a partner or caregiver in supervising management can be helpful. Periods of adequate rest should also be included in the activity schedule. This treatment approach benefits children and adolescents as well as adults.

Sleep disturbance occurs commonly in CFS and may have a considerable impact on the patient's ability to participate in daily activities. A number of measures can be taken to correct abnormal sleep patterns. Daytime naps should be avoided; so should stimulants such as caffeine or nicotine in the evening. The bedroom should be used only for sleep and intimacy and not for other activities such as eating or watching television. Time spent in bed should be curtailed to the actual time spent sleeping, with the goal to build up a mild sleep debt that increases the patient's ability to stay asleep. Should these measures not prove sufficient, it may be necessary to consider a sedative antidepressant.

For some patients, their interpersonal problems and psychosocial difficulties may make progress with treatment difficult. In such cases, supportive therapy and graded activity may be insufficient, and referral to a specialist is required. Considerable research now backs the effectiveness of cognitive behavioral therapy, which include the principles of treatment already discussed and also places an emphasis on the reappraisal of illness beliefs. Other psychotherapies, such as family therapy and psychodynamic therapy, may have a role in the management of some patients, if specifically indicated.

In patients with a long history of severely impaired functioning or who prove consistently resistant to treatment, management is essentially supportive with infrequent but regular contact. This approach provides emotional support, reduces further deterioration, and assists in mobilizing social support.

Prognosis

Most studies of prognosis in CFS focus on people attending special clinics, who are likely to have a poorer prognosis. Outcome appears to be influenced by the presence of psychiatric disorders and beliefs about causation and treatment (Box 2). Approximately 20% to 50% of adults with

BOX 2 Perpetuating Factors in Chronic Fatigue Syndrome

- Depression and anxiety
- Lack of physical fitness
- Sleep disorder
- Chronic life stresses and difficulties
- Inaccurate or unhelpful illness beliefs
- Avoidance of activities

the disorder show some improvement in the medium term, but few return to their previous level of functioning. Conversely, children and adolescents appear to have a better outlook, with the majority showing definite improvement when followed up in the longer term.

Mumps

Method of
Mobeen H. Rathore, MD, and Ayesha Mirza, MD

Mumps or *parotitis epidemica* is an acute viral infection primarily affecting the parotid glands. Infection generally results in a mild, self-limited illness, but complications may occur. In most parts of the world, the annual incidence of mumps is in the range of 100 to 1000 per 100,000 population with epidemic peaks every 2 to 5 years. Because of highly successful immunization strategies, there has been a steady decline in reported cases in the United States from 5712 in 1989 to 221 cases in 2004. There has also been a shift in the number of reported cases since 1990, persons age 15 years and older have accounted for 30% to 40% of cases annually. A goal of elimination of indigenous mumps by the year 2010 has been established.

Pathogenesis

The causative agent of mumps, Rubulavirus belongs to the Paramyxoviridae family. Infection is spread via direct contact or by airborne droplets from the upper respiratory tract. Humans are the only known natural host for the mumps virus. Incubation period averages 16 to 18 days with a range of 2 to 4 weeks. Mumps virus replicates in the nasopharynx and regional lymph nodes. After 12 to 25 days viremia occurs, lasting 3 to 5 days. During this time, the virus spreads to various tissues including the meninges and glands such as the salivary, pancreas, testes, and ovary.

Clinical Features

Illness is characterized by nonspecific symptoms including myalgia, headache, malaise, and low-grade fever.

Within 1 to 2 days the characteristic unilateral or bilateral swelling of the parotid glands occurs. Other salivary glands are involved in approximately 10% of cases. Fever and glandular swelling disappear in approximately 1 week, and the illness resolves completely unless complications occur. In approximately 30% of cases, infection occurs with nonspecific symptoms, or there may be no symptoms at all. Natural infection confers lifelong immunity against the virus in most cases; however, recurrent attacks may occur.

Complications

Complications such as meningitis, encephalitis, or orchitis may occur. They occur more often in males than females, and adults are at a higher risk than children. Asymptomatic cerebrospinal fluid pleocytosis (>5 leukocytes/mm^3) is found in 50% to 60% of patients with mumps, whereas symptomatic meningitis is reported in up to 15% of cases. Mumps encephalitis is rare. Acquired sensorineural deafness in affected children may occur.

Orchitis occurs in 20% to 50% of postpubertal males; however, mumps orchitis is rarely associated with permanent infertility. Acquisition of mumps during the first 12 weeks of pregnancy is associated with a high (25%) incidence of spontaneous abortions, but malformations following mumps infection during pregnancy have not been reported. Pancreatitis is also reported as a complication, but the relationship of mumps disease to diabetes mellitus remains speculative. Other rare complications include thyroiditis, arthritis, mastitis, myocarditis, and thrombocytopenia (Table 1).

Diagnosis

Mumps virus replicates in a variety of cell cultures. Mumps virus has been isolated from the saliva, cerebrospinal fluid, urine, blood, breast milk, and other tissues of an infected person. If a viral culture is done, specimens should be collected within 5 days of the onset of the illness.

CURRENT DIAGNOSIS

- Lack of history of immunization (applicable to adults born after 1957)
- Unilateral or bilateral swelling of the parotid gland with or without involvement of the other salivary glands
- Resolution of illness within a week without intervention
- Marked tenderness with expression of pus from Stensen duct differentiates suppurative parotitis from mumps
- Onset of complications with preceding parotitis such as meningitis, deafness, orchitis (may depend on age)
- Blood count if indicated in sicker patients will show predominant lymphocytosis
- Presence of mumps-specific IgM by EIA or fourfold rise in antibody titer between acute and convalescent sera

Abbreviation: EIA = enzyme immunoassay.

TABLE 1 Complications Associated with Mumps

Aseptic meningitis	10%–15% of clinical cases
Encephalitis	2/100,000
Orchitis	20%–50% of postpubertal males
Mastitis	≤31% of females younger than 15 years
Pancreatitis	2%–5%
Deafness	5/100,000
Abnormal ECG findings (compatible with myocarditis)	3%–15%

Abbreviation: ECG, electrocardiogram.

Only one serotype of the mumps virus exists. Serology is the most common method used to diagnose mumps. Presence of a greater than fourfold rise in antibody titer between acute and convalescent serum samples or the presence of mumps-specific IgM antibody by enzyme immunoassay is the most reliable way to confirm the diagnosis. Several rapid diagnostic methods using real-time RT-PCR (reverse transcriptase polymerase chain reaction) assays have been developed but are not commercially available.

Treatment

There is no specific treatment available for mumps. Administration of fluids and analgesics to alleviate pain and discomfort are the mainstay of therapy in symptomatic patients.

Prevention

Mumps vaccine is routinely used in only 53% of countries, and importation of mumps into the United States is now increasingly recognized. Mumps epidemic was reported in the United Kingdom in 2005, most likely related to decreased rates of immunization. Even in countries where mumps vaccine is given, efficacy may vary. In unvaccinated communities, almost every person can get infected. Therefore, vaccination is highly recommended.

The protective efficacy of the live attenuated Jeryl Lynn strain used in the United States is approximately 95% after a single dose of the vaccine. The duration of vaccine-induced immunity is believed to be more than 25 years and is probably lifelong in most vaccine recipients. Although available as a single antigen preparation, the combined mumps-measles-rubella (MMR) vaccine is recommended when any of the individual components are required. Two doses are recommended in children, the first at 12 to 15 months of age and the second at 4 to 6 years of age. Immunization is also recommended for older children and adults, particularly those born after 1957 if they have not had mumps or have never been vaccinated.

Adverse reactions to vaccination are rare and mild. Mumps vaccine is very safe; and any symptoms such as fever, rash, or joint pains are attributable to the measles or rubella components. Immunization given to a person already immune to one or more of the viruses is not harmful. Pregnancy should be avoided for the first 30 days after vaccination, and individuals with known anaphylactic reactions to the vaccine, advanced immunodeficiency, or immunosuppression should not receive the vaccine. In their latest report, the Institution of Medicine of the National Academies in the United States concludes that neither the MMR vaccine nor the organic mercury compound thimerosal (used as a preservative in the vaccine until 1991) is associated with autism.

It is important to note that although the risk of mumps does seem to increase with the number of years following vaccination, suggesting some waning of protective immunity, most cases of parotitis in immunized persons are because of causes other than infection with the mumps virus.

Infection Control

Children should be excluded from school for 9 days after the onset of parotid swelling. Standard as well as contact precautions for the same time period are also recommended for hospitalized patients.

REFERENCES

American Academy of Pediatrics: Mumps. In Pickering L (ed.): Red Book: 2003 report of the Committee on Infectious Diseases (26th ed.). Elk Grove Village, IL, American Academy of Pediatrics, 2003: 439–443.

CDC: Measles, mumps and rubella-vaccine use and strategies for elimination of measles, rubella and congenital rubella syndrome and control of mumps. Recommendation of the Advisory Committee on Immunization Practices (ACIP). MMWR Recomm Rep 1998; 47(RR-8):1–57.

CDC: A detailed review of the epidemiology, pathogenesis, clinical features and management of mumps; February 2003 www.cdc.gov/nip/publications/pink/mumps.pdf/

CDC: Summary of provisional cases of selected notifiable diseases, United States, cumulative, week ending December 11, 2004 (49th week). MMWR Morb Mortal Wkly Rep 2004; 53(49):1161–1070.

Gupta RK, Best J, MacMahon E: Mumps and the UK epidemic 2005. BMJ 2005;330:1132–1135.

McCormick M, Bayer R, Berg A, et al: MMR vaccine and thimerosal-containing vaccines are not associated with autism, IOM report says. The National Academies, May 18, 2004. Available at http://www4.nationalacademies.org/news/

United States Department of Health and Human Services: Healthy people 2010: With understanding and improving health. Washington, DC, U.S. Government Printing Office, 2000.

Zimmerman l, Reef S, Wharton, M: VPD Surveillance Manual (3rd ed.). 2002, pp 7–12.

Plague

Method of
Douglas A. Drevets, MD, DTM&H

Plague caused by *Yersinia pestis* is an ancient disease, and historical descriptions indicate that it probably caused Justinian's Plague (AD 541) that led into the first plague pandemic. The second plague pandemic, also known as the Black Death, began in Central Asia in 1347 and then spread to Europe, Asia, and Africa. It killed an estimated 50 million persons. The third and current plague pandemic began in China and then disseminated throughout the world by shipping routes in 1899–1900. *Y. pestis* is a gram-negative, nonmotile, facultatively anaerobic, non-spore-forming coccobacillus that is approximately 0.5 to 0.8 μm in diameter and 1 to 3 μm in length. Genomic sequencing shows that *Y. pestis* is a recently emerged clone of *Y. pseudotuberculosis*.

Epidemiology

Plague is a zoonosis that is usually spread between mammalian hosts by the bite of infected fleas. The most important enzootic reservoirs are urban and sylvatic rodents; however, domestic cats and dogs also are linked to human disease. Human plague occurs in North and South America, Asia, and Africa. An average of 2547 cases of human plague were reported yearly to the World Health Organization between 1988 and 1997, 76% of which were from Africa, with an overall case fatality rate of 7.1%. In North America, 82% of 295 indigenous cases were from Arizona, Colorado, and New Mexico. Bubonic plague is the most common form in humans, accounting for 97% of cases in a recent outbreak in Madagascar. Similarly, 84% of U.S. cases reported between 1947 and 1996 were the bubonic form, with septicemic and pneumonic plague accounting for 13% and 2%, respectively.

Modes of Transmission

Most human infections are transmitted from rodent to humans via the bite of an infected flea. Infection also can be acquired by contact with body fluids from infected animals, such as during field dressing of game or by inhalation of respiratory droplets from animals, particularly cats, or humans with pneumonic plague.

Bioterrorism Threat

Plague was used as an agent of biowarfare by the Japanese in World War II and was a focus of intensive research and development in the former Soviet Union during the Cold War. Primary pneumonic plague is the most likely form of exposure because of biowarfare or bioterrorism.

Pathogenesis and Clinical Syndromes

Transdermal inoculation of bacilli from the bite of an infected flea ultimately leads to infection of the regional lymph nodes in which massive replication of bacteria creates the bubo (derived from the Greek "bubon" or "groin"), a swollen, erythematous, and painful lymph node in the groin, axilla, or cervical region. Bacteremia and septicemia frequently develop and lead to secondary infection of other organs including lungs, spleen, and the central nervous system. Primary pneumonic plague is a rare natural occurrence and results from the inhalation of respiratory droplets containing *Y. pestis* bacilli from another case of pneumonic plague, usually in humans or in cats. Secondary pneumonic plague results from seeding of the lungs by blood-borne bacteria in the setting of either bubonic or septicemic plague. Septicemic plague also begins with a transdermal exposure but manifests as primary bacteremia/septicemia without the bubo. Less common manifestations include meningitis, pharyngitis, and gastroenteritis.

Bubonic plague is an acute febrile lymphadenitis that develops 2 to 8 days after inoculation. Inflamed lymph nodes are usually 1 to 6 cm and painful. Abrupt onset of fever is an almost universal finding and occurs simultaneously with, or up to 24 hours before, the appearance of the bubo. Headache, malaise, and chills are frequent, along with nausea, vomiting, and diarrhea. Most patients are tachycardic, hypotensive, and appear prostrate and lethargic with episodic restlessness. Leukocytosis with a left shift is typical. Complications include pneumonia, shock, disseminated intravascular coagulation, purpuric skin lesions, acral cyanosis, and gangrene. The differential diagnosis of bubonic plague includes tularemia and Group A β-hemolytic streptococcal adenitis with bacteremia.

The symptoms of septicemic plague are not distinct from those caused by other gram-negative bacteria, and they are very similar to those of bubonic plague except that abdominal pain is more common in septicemic plague. Septicemic plague must be differentiated from fulminate septicemia caused by other gram-negative bacteria. Primary pneumonic plague has an abrupt onset of fever and influenza-like symptoms 1 to 5 days after inhalation exposure. Symptoms include shortness of breath, cough, chest pain, and bloody sputum with rapid progression to fulminate pneumonia and respiratory failure. Patients with secondary pneumonic infection show respiratory symptoms in addition to those attributed to the bubo or sepsis. Radiographic findings include patchy bronchopneumonia, multilobar consolidations, cavitations, and alveolar hemorrhage and are not pathognomonic of *Y. pestis*. Plague pneumonia must be differentiated from severe influenza, inhalation anthrax, and overwhelming community-acquired pneumonia.

Diagnosis

Plague is diagnosed by demonstrating *Y. pestis* in blood or body fluids such as a lymph node aspirate, sputum, or cerebrospinal fluid. A tentative diagnosis of bubonic plague can be made rapidly with fluid aspirated from a bubo showing gram-negative coccobacilli with bipolar staining. Serology showing a fourfold rise in antibody titers to F1 antigen or a single titer of more than 1:128 is also diagnostic.

CURRENT DIAGNOSIS

- Travel to a plague endemic area or contact with a case of animal or human plague.
- Abrupt onset of fever and prostration.
- Bubo in groin, axillae, or cervical areas.
- Gram-negative coccobacilli with bipolar staining identified in aspirate from bubo, on blood smear, or from blood-tinged sputum.

CURRENT TREATMENT

- Prompt administration of gentamicin or ciprofloxacin.
- Aggressive supportive care.
- Respiratory isolation of hospitalized cases.
- Postexposure prophylaxis to close contacts.

Treatment

The aminoglycosides gentamicin (Garamycin) and streptomycin, the fluoroquinolones ciprofloxacin (Cipro), levofloxacin (Levaquin), and ofloxacin (Floxin), and tetracyclines (i.e., doxycycline [Vibramycin]) are the first-, second-, and third-line classes of antibiotics, respectively. Typical minimal inhibitory concentrations for 90% (MIC$_{90}$) of tested strains for the fluoroquinolones are less than 0.03 to 0.25 µg/mL compared with less than 1.0 µg/mL and less than 1.0 µg/mL to 4.0 µg/mL for gentamicin and streptomycin, respectively, and less than 1.0 µg/mL for doxycycline. Streptomycin (15 mg/kg up to 1 g intramuscularly [IM] every 12 hours) and gentamicin (5 to 7 mg/kg/day intravenously [IV]/IM in one or two doses daily) are the drugs of choice for severe infection. Standard doses for the fluoroquinolones include ciprofloxacin, 400 mg IV/500 mg orally every 12 hours; levofloxacin, 500 mg IV/orally daily; and ofloxacin, 400 mg IV/orally every 12 hours. Doxycycline is administered at 100 mg IV/orally every 12 hours. Chloramphenicol (25 mg/kg IV/orally every 6 hours) can be used in select circumstances. Antibiotic therapy should be continued for a total of 10 days.

Prevention and Control

Standard infection control procedures that should be used when caring for patients with suspected plague include a disposable surgical mask, latex gloves, devices to protect mucous membranes, and good hand washing. Hospitalized patients with known or suspected pneumonic plague should be placed in strict isolation for at least 48 hours after appropriate antibiotics are initiated. Postexposure prophylaxis should be given to individuals with close contact (defined as less than 2 meters) with an infectious case or who have had a potential respiratory exposure. The recommended adult antibiotics for prophylaxis are doxycycline or ciprofloxacin in the same doses used for treatment. Postexposure prophylaxis can be given orally and should be continued for 7 days following exposure. Currently, there is no licensed plague vaccine.

REFERENCES

Butler T: A clinical study of bubonic plague. Observations of the 1970 Vietnam epidemic with emphasis on coagulation studies, skin histology and electrocardiograms. Am J Med 1972;53:268-276.

Boulanger LL, Ettestad P, Fogarty JD, et al: Gentamicin and tetracyclines for the treatment of human plague: Review of 75 cases in New Mexico, 1985–1999. Clin Infect Dis 2004;38:663-669.

Cler DJ, Vernaleo JR, Lombardi LJ, et al: Plague pneumonia disease caused by *Yersinia pestis*. Semin Respir Infect 1997;12:12-23.

Gage KL, Dennis DT, Orloski KA, et al: Cases of cat-associated human plague in the Western US, 1977–1998. Clin Infect Dis 2000;30:893-900.

Hull HF, Montes JM, Mann JM: Septicemic plague in New Mexico. J Infect Dis 1987;155: 113-118.

Inglesby TV, Dennis DT, Henderson DA, et al: Plague as a biological weapon: Medical and public health management. Working Group on Civilian Biodefense. JAMA 2000;283: 2281-2290.

Perry RD, Fetherston JD: *Yersinia pestis*—etiologic agent of plague. Clin Microbiol Rev 1997;10: 35-66.

Ratsitorahina M, Chanteau S, Rahalison L, et al: Epidemiological and diagnostic aspects of the outbreak of pneumonic plague in Madagascar. Lancet 2000;355: 111-113.

Wong JD, Barash JR, Sandfort, RF, Janda JM: Susceptibilities of *Yersinia pestis* strains to 12 antimicrobial agents. Antimicrob Agents Chemother 2000;44:1995-1996.

Anthrax

Method of
Jon B. Woods, MD

Anthrax has been a significant disease for both humans and their livestock for millennia. It was the first disease to fulfill Koch's postulates in 1876, as well as the first bacterial disease for which an effective vaccine was developed, for livestock, in 1880. This gram-positive rod-shaped bacillus species differs from the more benign members of its genera in containing two additional plasmids, one encoding for an antiphagocytic poly-D-glutamic acid capsule and the other encoding for two toxins. Three distinct toxin components combine to form two toxins, edema toxin and lethal toxin; the common component, protective antigen (PA), forms a pore through eukaryotic cell walls that allows the other two toxin components, edema factor (EF) and lethal factor (LF), to enter affected host cells. EF is an adenylate cyclase affecting many cell types and is responsible for the edema associated with anthrax infections. LF is a zinc metalloprotease that seems to have its greatest affect on macrophages; within the cells it cleaves mitogen-activated protein kinase and disrupts the cellular response to infection.

Background

Anthrax is an enzootic, and occasionally epizootic, disease of grazing animals worldwide. The incredibly durable spores of this bacillus can persist in soil for decades. These spores, when inadvertently ingested by herbivores while grazing, can germinate and then replicate in a rapid progression to bacteremia and subsequent death of the animal. At the time of death these animals can have as many as 10^8 vegetative bacilli per milliliter of blood. Those bacilli, which are exposed to oxygen upon the animal's death, can sporulate and then reenter the soil to begin the cycle anew.

Human anthrax can take several forms, most commonly cutaneous, but also intestinal, oropharyngeal, and inhalational disease. Naturally occurring human anthrax disease has typically been the result of exposure to infected animals or contaminated animal products such as hair or wool, bone meal, hides, or meat. Less commonly, human cutaneous anthrax has resulted from the bites of flies that have recently fed on infected animals. Gastrointestinal and oropharyngeal anthrax can result from ingestion of the raw or inadequately cooked flesh of an animal infected with anthrax. Endemic inhalational anthrax, or woolsorter's disease, results from inhalation of anthrax spores aerosolized during the manipulation of contaminated animal products, especially hair or wool; this was an exceedingly rare form of disease even prior to the institution of more stringent control measures and closure of most of the U.S. textile mills processing foreign-acquired goat hair by the 1970s. More recently, inhalational anthrax and cutaneous cases have resulted from exposure to spores intentionally processed and disseminated as biologic weapons. The extreme environmental stability of the spores, their ease of production, and their infectivity via the aerosol route are some features that have made *Bacillus anthracis* a top candidate for both nations and terrorists seeking biologic weapons. An apparently accidental aerosol release of dried anthrax spores from a biologic weapons facility in the Soviet city of Sverdlovsk in 1979 resulted in as many as 68 deaths because of inhalational anthrax. More recently, anthrax spores intentionally sent through the U.S. postal system resulted in 11 cases of inhalational anthrax and perhaps as many as 11 cases of cutaneous anthrax.

Clinical Features

Cutaneous anthrax represents approximately 95% of naturally occurring human anthrax cases. It typically occurs 1 to 7 days after exposure to infected livestock or contaminated livestock products, but rarely it is transmitted to humans by the bites of flies that have recently fed on infected animals. The lesion begins as a painless or mildly pruritic papule at the site of spore inoculation, progressing into an expanding round ulcer by the following day. Over the following several days the ulcer dries to a dark, almost black eschar, which resolves over the ensuing 1 to 2 weeks. The lesion can be surrounded by significant local edema and may be accompanied by regional lymphadenopathy. Treated, cutaneous anthrax is rarely fatal, although without antibiotics, progression to bacteremia and ultimately death can occur in up to 10% to 20% of cases.

Both forms of gastrointestinal anthrax are acquired via ingestion of insufficiently cooked meat from infected animals. The infectious dose is unknown. Intestinal anthrax may be initially misdiagnosed as either gastroenteritis or acute abdomen, typically presenting 1 to 6 days following contaminated meat consumption with fever, nausea, vomiting, and focal abdominal pain. Without prompt initiation of antibiotic therapy, disease can progress to hematemesis, hematochezia or melena, massive serosanguineous or hemorrhagic ascites, and sepsis, with mortality rates greater than 50%. Oropharyngeal anthrax typically presents after a 1- to 6-day incubation period with severe pharyngitis and fever, followed by appearance of pharyngeal or tonsillar ulcers. Gray or tan pseudomembranes can form over the ulcers, which are often accompanied by significant cervical lymphadenopathy and unilateral neck edema. Mortality of oropharyngeal anthrax varies from 10% to 50%.

Inhalation of aerosolized anthrax spores into the pulmonary alveoli can result in inhalational anthrax. The lethal dose via inhalation for 50% of humans (LD_{50}) is thought to be between 8000 and 55,000 spores. The alveolar spores are ingested by macrophages and carried to regional lymphatics, where they can germinate and replicate, eventually leading to hemorrhagic mediastinitis. The incubation period is presumably dose dependent, and although typically 1 to 6 days was suspected in at least one human case to be 43 days. Early inhalational anthrax presents suddenly as a nonspecific syndrome consisting of fever, malaise, headache, fatigue, and drenching sweats. Other common symptoms include nausea, vomiting, confusion, a nonproductive cough, and mild chest discomfort. Upper respiratory symptoms are notably absent. Physical findings are nonspecific in the early phase of the disease, but tachycardia is common. Auscultatory lung exam is typically normal at this stage, but dullness to percussion can develop over time in the lower lung fields as hemorrhagic pleural effusions accumulate. These early findings generally persist for 2 to 5 days before progressing fulminantly to tachypnea, cyanosis, shock, and multiorgan system failure. These late findings typically herald impending death within 24 to 36 hours. Gastrointestinal hemorrhage and hemorrhagic meningitis are common at autopsy. Prognosis is poor in the absence of intensive supportive care and early initiation of appropriate antibiotic combinations. Mortality ranges from 45% to more than 85% historically.

Diagnosis

None of the forms of human anthrax disease can be diagnosed on the basis of clinical findings alone (Table 1). For example, diagnosis of cutaneous anthrax requires the presence of a compatible skin lesion accompanied by confirmatory laboratory studies; an exposure history, or a known risk may also be present. Both forms of gastrointestinal anthrax are typically accompanied by a history of ingestion of the meat of anthrax-infected animals. Early intestinal anthrax can be difficult to differentiate clinically from other causes of gastrointestinal illness to include acute gastroenteritis, dysentery, or even peritonitis. Later in the course of intestinal disease, surgical or autopsy findings may include ileal or cecal ulceration, and bowel edema and necrosis is associated with hemorrhagic mesenteric adenitis and serosanguineous to hemorrhagic ascites. Oropharyngeal anthrax can clinically resemble diphtheria, with pharyngeal lesions and an edematous so-called bull neck. Early inhalational anthrax is a nonspecific febrile syndrome that may be difficult to distinguish clinically from many other infectious diseases. However, the presence of mental status changes, profuse sweating, and absence of upper respiratory symptoms or pneumonia in inhalational anthrax may aid in differentiating it from influenza-like respiratory illnesses.

TABLE 1   Empirical Antibiotic Therapy for Anthrax*

Cutaneous Anthrax (without Systemic Symptoms)	Inhalational, Gastrointestinal, or Cutaneous Disease with Systemic Symptoms
Ciprofloxacin (Cipro[1]) <ul><li>500 mg PO twice daily (adults)</li><li>15 mg/kg (up to 500 mg/dose) PO twice daily (children)</li></ul> *or* Doxycycline (Vibramycin) <ul><li>100 mg PO twice daily (adults)</li><li>2.2 mg/kg (up to 100 mg/dose) PO bid (children <45 kg)</li></ul> *or (if strain susceptible):* Penicillin G procaine (Bicillin C-R) <ul><li>1,200,000 U IM q12h (adults)</li><li>25,000 U/kg (maximum 1,200,000 U) q12h (children)</li></ul> *or* Penicillin V Potassium (Veetids) <ul><li>500 mg PO q6h (adults)</li></ul> *or* Amoxicillin (Amoxil[1]) <ul><li>500 mg PO q8h (adults and children >40 kg)</li><li>15 mg/kg q8h (children <40 kg)</li></ul> According to CDC recommendations, amoxicillin prophylaxis is appropriate only after 14–21 d of fluoroquinolone or doxycycline and only for populations with relative contraindications to the other drugs (children, pregnancy)	Ciprofloxacin (Cipro IV[1]) <ul><li>400 mg IV q12h (adult)</li><li>15 mg/kg/dose (up to 400 mg/dose) q12h (children)</li></ul> *or* Doxycycline (Vibramycin IV) <ul><li>200 mg IV, then 100 mg IV q12h (adults)</li><li>2.2 mg/kg (100 mg/dose maximum) q12h (children <45 kg)</li></ul> *or (if strain susceptible):* Penicillin G (Pfizerpen) <ul><li>4 million U IV q4h (adults)</li><li>50,000 U/kg (up to 4M U) IV q6h (children)</li></ul> *plus* One or two additional antibiotics with activity against anthrax. Clindamycin (Cleocin[1]) plus rifampin (Rifadin[1]) may be a good empiric choice, pending susceptibilities. Potential additional antibiotics include one or more of the following: clindamycin (Cleocin), rifampin (Rifadin), gentamicin[1] (generic), macrolides (erythromycin [generic], vancomycin (Vancocin[1]), imipenem (Pimaxin[1]), and chloramphenicol[1] (generic). Convert from IV to oral therapy when patient is stable, to complete at least 60 d of antibiotics. **Meningitis** Add Rifampin (Rifadin[1]) 20 mg/kg IV once daily or vancomycin (Vancocin[1]) 1 g IV q12h Oral dosing may be necessary for treatment of systemic disease in a mass casualty situation.

[1]Not FDA approved for this indication.
*Should be adjusted for susceptibilities.
Abbreviations: CDC = Centers for Disease Control and Prevention; IV = intravenous; PO = orally.
Adapted from Woods JB (ed): USAMRIID's Medical Management of Biological Warfare Casualties Handbook, 6th ed. 2005.

CURRENT DIAGNOSIS

Cutaneous/Oropharyngeal

- Painless or pruritic lesion beginning 1–7 d after exposure
  - Typical lesion progression from papule to ulcer to dark eschar (see text), often with significant edema

Plus

- Lesion gram stain, culture usually positive if patient has not received antibiotics
  - If negative, punch biopsy of lesion margin for IHC may still be positive
- Blood culture rarely positive in absence of systemic symptoms

Acute and convalescent serology or may give evidence of infection.

Gastrointestinal

- Gastrointestinal symptoms (variable) beginning 1–6 d after ingestion exposure.
  - Focal abdominal pain with hematochezia or melena common.
  - Nonspecific bowel wall edema, air–fluid levels, and ascites on radiographs.

Plus

- Stool culture (variably +).
- Blood culture (variably +).
- Acute and convalescent serology or blood sample for PCR may give evidence of infection.
- Ascites: often hemorrhagic.
  - Gram stain and culture, and IHC or PCR, if available, may be positive.

Surgical findings: hemorrhagic mesenteric adenitis, bowel edema, ileal and/or cecal ulcerations.

Inhalational

- Nonspecific febrile syndrome beginning abruptly 1–6 (but up to 43) d after aerosol exposure (see text).
  - Absence of upper respiratory findings, no pneumonia.
  - Widened mediastinum ± effusions on CXR or chest CT in *all* cases.

Plus

- Blood culture often positive if patient has not received antibiotics.
- Acute and convalescent serology or blood sample for PCR may give evidence of infection.
- Laboratory studies show hemoconcentration, mildly increased WBC with left shift, mildly increased AST and ALT, hypoalbuminemia.
- CSF (if meningitis) and pleural effusions are hemorrhagic.
- Gram stain and culture often positive.

If negative, IHC or PCR may be positive.

Abbreviations: AST = serum aspartate aminotransferase (level); ALT = serum alanine aminotransferase (level); CSF = cerebrospinal fluid; CXR = chest radiograph; CT = computed tomography study; IHC = immunohistochemical staining; PCR = polymerase chain reaction (study); WBC = white blood count.

Gram stain and culture of skin lesions are ideally performed on the fluid of an unopened vesicle and are often positive in the cutaneous anthrax patient who has not received antibiotics. Tissue biopsy can be performed on lesions for immunohistochemical staining in culture-negative patients. Blood culture should be collected in any systemically ill patient suspected of having any form of anthrax disease. *B. anthracis* grows quickly in standard laboratory culture media. Paired acute and convalescent serologic studies may suggest infection in patents that have negative cultures, albeit these studies are not well validated. Stool culture can be positive in intestinal anthrax, although it is only variably so. Peritoneal fluid, pleural effusions, or cerebrospinal fluid (CSF) (when meningitis is present) can potentially demonstrate organisms on Gram stain and culture or may be positive via immunostaining or polymerase chain reaction (PCR) studies.

For patients with inhalation anthrax during the attacks of 2001, the complete blood count (CBC) revealed a mean white blood cell count of 9800/μL, with a predominance of neutrophils and a mildly elevated hematocrit. Mildly elevated serum sodium, aspartate transaminase (AST), and alanine aminotransferase (ALT) were common, as was hypoalbuminemia.

A widened mediastinum caused by adenitis, as well as pleural effusions, may be visible on chest radiograph in patients with inhalational anthrax. Negative chest radiograph in a patient suspected of inhalational anthrax should prompt a chest computerized tomography (CT) scan. In the 2001 attacks, either the chest radiograph or CT was abnormal in all cases of inhalational disease. Abdominal radiographs in intestinal anthrax may demonstrate any number of nonspecific findings, to include ascites, diffuse air–fluid levels, and bowel edema.

Treatment

Patient survival for all forms of severe anthrax disease hinges on prompt initiation of appropriate antibiotics. Initial empirical therapy for patients with inhalational anthrax, gastrointestinal anthrax, or cutaneous anthrax with systemic symptoms should include intravenous (IV) ciprofloxacin (Cipro IV) or doxycycline (Vibramycin IV) combined with one or two additional antibiotics effective against anthrax (Table 2). One suggested combination includes a quinolone (ciprofloxacin [Cipro IV]), clindamycin (Cleocin[1]), and rifampin (Rifadin[1]). Antibiotic choices should be adjusted to reflect the specific susceptibilities of the infecting strain. Rifampin (Rifadin[1]), vancomycin (Vancocin[1]), or chloramphenicol[1] (generic) should be added if meningitis is suspected. IV antibiotics can be switched to oral treatment

[1]Not FDA approved for this indication.

TABLE 2 Anthrax Aerosol Postexposure Prophylaxis*

Immunized†	Not Immunized and Vaccine Available	Not Immunized and Vaccine Not Available

Ciprofloxacin (Cipro)
- 500 mg PO bid for adults
- 10–15 mg/kg PO twice daily (up to 1 g/d) for children

or

Doxycycline (Vibramycin)
- 100 mg PO bid for adults or children >8 y and >45 kg
- 2.2 mg/kg PO bid (up to 200 mg/d) for children <8 y

If antibiotic susceptibilities allow, patients who cannot tolerate tetracyclines or quinolone antibiotics can be switched to amoxicillin (Amoxil[1]), 500 mg PO tid for adults and 80 mg/kg divided tid (≥1.5 g/d) in children.

| Continue antibiotics for *at least* 30 d. | Receive at least 3 doses of anthrax vaccine[1] (BioThrax) at 2-wk intervals, and then continue antibiotics for *at least* 1–2 wk after receipt of 3rd dose of vaccine. | Continue antibiotics for *at least* 60 d. |

Patients should be closely observed after discontinuation of antibiotics.
If suspected clinical signs of anthrax disease occur, then resume empirical antibiotics.

[1]Not FDA approved for this indication.
*Unknown antibiotic susceptibilities.
†Immunized = completed 6 doses of anthrax vaccine and up to date on boosters, or minimum of 3 doses within past 6 mo. Those who have already received 3 doses within 6 mo of exposure should continue with their routine vaccine schedule.
Abbreviation: PO = orally.
Adapted from Woods JB (ed): USAMRIID's Medical Management of Biological Warfare Casualties Handbook, 6th ed. 2005.

as the patent's clinical condition improves, to complete at least 60 days of total antibiotic therapy. Specific antidotes for anthrax toxins are in development, including human anthrax immune globulin, which may be available as an investigational therapy for severe anthrax disease through the Centers for Disease Control and Prevention (CDC).

Patients with systemic anthrax disease often require aggressive supportive therapy, including fluid resuscitation, blood products, vasopressor agents, and airway management. Patients may also benefit from drainage of large hemorrhagic pleural or peritoneal fluid accumulations.

Although clinical data are lacking, severe edema or meningitis in anthrax disease may benefit from administration of corticosteroids.

Uncomplicated naturally acquired cutaneous anthrax should be treated empirically with 7 to 10 days of either oral ciprofloxacin (Cipro[1]) or doxycycline (Vibramycin). For cutaneous disease thought to have been acquired via exposure to an anthrax aerosol, at least 60 days of antibiotics is recommended.

[1]Not FDA approved for this indication.

CURRENT THERAPY

Cutaneous Anthrax (without Systemic Symptoms)

- Oral antibiotics (see Table 2 for details)
  - Doxycycline (Vibramycin), or
  - Ciprofloxacin (Cipro[1])
- Consider nonsteroidal anti-inflammatory agents (NSAIDS) or corticosteroids for severe edema
- Infection control:
  - Contact precautions

Do not debride lesions

Inhalational, Gastrointestinal, or Cutaneous Disease with Systemic Symptoms

- Supportive care
  - May need assisted ventilation and/or vasopressors
  - Drain pleural effusions and large peritoneal fluid collections
- Combination IV antibiotics (see Table 2 for details)
  - Doxycycline (Vibramycin IV), or
  - Ciprofloxacin (Cipro IV[1])

Plus

- One or two additional antibiotics
- Consider corticosteroids for severe edema or meningitis
- Consider human anthrax immune globulin (investigational), if available
- Infection control:
  - Contact precautions (not transmitted by droplet or aerosol)

Avoid autopsy or invasive procedures prior to receipt of antibiotics.

[1]Not FDA approved for this indication.

A licensed anthrax vaccine (BioThrax) has been available in the United States to the armed forces, veterinarians, and textile and laboratory workers since 1970. It is derived from the sterile supernatant of a liquid culture of an attenuated (nonencapsulated) strain of *B. anthracis* and is administered subcutaneously in a six-shot primary series over 18 months followed by annual boosters. The vaccine is licensed only for preexposure prophylaxis of persons 18 to 65 years of age but is available investigationally for postexposure and pediatric use.

Individuals exposed to aerosolized anthrax spores should immediately receive postexposure prophylaxis consisting of both oral antibiotics and anthrax vaccine. Oral doxycycline (Vibramycin) or ciprofloxacin (Cipro) are the preferred empiric antibiotics for postexposure prophylaxis. Antibiotics should be continued for variable lengths of time depending on the patient's anthrax immune status and the suspected inhaled dose of anthrax (Table 2). Exposed individuals should also receive the anthrax vaccine[1] (BioThrax) to counter delayed incubation of residual alveolar anthrax after discontinuation of antibiotics.

REFERENCES

Beatty ME, Ashford DA, Griffin PM, et al: Gastrointestinal anthrax, a review of the literature. Arch Intern Med 2003;163:2527-2531.

Centers for Disease Control and Prevention: Notice to readers: Use of anthrax vaccine in response to terrorism: Supplemental recommendations of the Advisory Committee on Immunization Practices. MMWR 2002;51(45);1024-1026.

Inglesby TV, O'Toole T, Henderson DA, et al: Anthrax as a biological weapon 2002: Updated Recommendations for Management. JAMA 2002;287(17):2236-2252.

Jernigan JA, Stephens DS, Ashford DA, et al: Bioterrorism-related inhalational anthrax: The first 10 cases reported in the United States. Emerg Infect Dis 2001;7:933-944.

Kuehnert MJ, Doyle TJ, Hill HA, et al: Clinical features that discriminate inhalational anthrax from other acute respiratory illnesses. Clin Infect Dis 2003;36:328-336.

Turnbull PCB: Guidelines for the Surveillance and Control of Anthrax in Humans and Animals, 3rd ed. World Health Organization Report WHO/EMC/ZDI/98.6, 1998.

Woods JB (ed): USAMRIID's Medical Management of Biological Warfare Casualties Handbook, 6th ed. 2005.

---

[1]Not FDA approved for this indication.

Psittacosis

Method of
*Mark Woodhead, BSc, DM, and
Kugathasan Mutalithas, MRCP*

Chlamydophila psittaci (formerly known as *Chlamydia psittaci*) causes disease in both humans and birds. In humans, it is the cause of psittacosis, also known as parrot fever and ornithosis. This is a zoonotic infection with transmission occurring mostly from infected birds. Although the original cases of human psittacosis had been traced to birds of the psittacine family (parrots, parakeets, and budgerigars), the organism has now been isolated in more than 130 bird species including pigeons, poultry, and turkeys. Transmission from other animals to humans is uncommon.

At present the disease has a worldwide distribution and usually occurs sporadically. In the United States where psittacosis is a notifiable disease, the Centers for Disease Control and Prevention received reports of 935 cases of psittacosis between 1988 and 2003. This may be an underestimation because seroprevalence studies suggest that the disease is much more common.

Microbiology

C. psittaci is one of two *Chlamydophila* species known to cause illness in humans within the newly classified Chlamydiaceae family (Figure 1). They are obligate intracellular bacteria and require the host for replication.

Transmission

Infection usually occurs when the organism is inhaled from aerosolized dried excreta and respiratory tract secretions from infected birds. Only a brief exposure is needed to allow transmission, and not all patients are able to recall contact with birds. Persons at risk include those exposed to pet birds, pigeon fanciers, employees in poultry processing plants, pet store employees, veterinarians, farmers, and zookeepers. Although most infected birds exhibit features of illness, some may not, and a seemingly healthy bird may be excreting organisms.

Clinical Features

Psittacosis is equally common in either sex and usually affects those in the 30 to 60 age group. Childhood infection is uncommon and mild. The spectrum of illness ranges from a mild unapparent illness to a fulminant illness with multiorgan involvement (Table 1). The incubation period typically ranges between 5 and 14 days. Disseminated infection may occur to include arthritis, endocarditis, myocarditis, glomerulonephritis, and meningoencephalitis. Pregnant women may have a severe illness with hepatitis, respiratory failure, and fetal death.

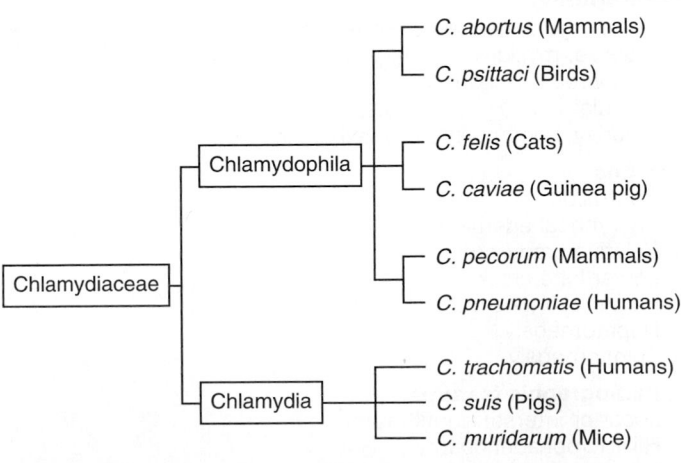

FIGURE 1. The Chlamydiaceae family with their usual hosts.

CURRENT DIAGNOSIS

- Flulike illness with a history of exposure to birds.
- Radiographic features may be more florid than anticipated by clinical features.
- No unique clinical or radiographic features.
- Detection of antibodies necessary to confirm diagnosis.

CURRENT THERAPY

- Doxycycline, 100 mg bid, or tetracycline, 500 mg qid.
- In those severely ill:
  - Doxycycline infusion at a dose of 4.4 mg/kg/d in divided doses.
  - Minimum duration of therapy: 2 wk.
  - Fluid balance and gas exchange should be managed according to illness severity.

Diagnosis

History of exposure to birds in a person with flulike illness or a chest radiograph that shows infiltrates more extensive than anticipated by clinical findings suggests the diagnosis. Psittacosis has no unique clinical, radiographic, or laboratory features. Serodiagnosis is the investigation of choice. Serum antibodies against *C. psittaci* are detected using complement fixation (CF) or microimmunofluorescence (MIF) methods. The MIF method is preferred to CF because of increased sensitivity and specificity. Antibodies that usually appear in the second week of illness may be delayed by antimicrobial treatment, and a late convalescent serum specimen may be required. In patients with suggestive clinical features, confirmed and probable cases are established as shown in Table 2.

Treatment

Assessment of illness severity and management of fluid balance and gas exchange are the same as for other causes of community-acquired pneumonia. Before the era of antibiotics, mortality with psittacosis was up to 20%. Death from psittacosis is now rare. The recommended antibiotics for the treatment of psittacosis are tetracyclines. Most patients require oral therapy only.

Macrolides are the best alternative for those for whom tetracyclines are contraindicated. Improvement is usually seen within 3 days of commencing treatment. Standard infection control precautions are sufficient for patients with psittacosis. Masks and isolation cubicles are not necessary. Reinfection can occur.

In the United States where psittacosis is a reportable disease, cases should be reported to the appropriate state or public health authorities. Local and state authorities may conduct epidemiologic investigations and institute additional disease control measures.

TABLE 2   Laboratory Confirmation of Psittacosis

Confirmed case of psittacosis (one of the following three):
  Chlamydophila psittaci is cultured from respiratory secretions.
  Fourfold increase in antibodies against *C. psittaci* between paired acute and convalescent- phase serum samples with at least a 1:32 titer in the convalescent sample.
  Single estimation of IgM against *C. psittaci* using MIF to ≥1:16 titer.
Probable case of psittacosis:
  Epidemiologically linked to a confirmed human case of psittacosis or
The patient has supportive serology of one antibody titer of ≥1:32 obtained after onset of symptoms.

Abbreviation: MIF = microimmunofluorescence.

TABLE 1   Clinical Features

Symptoms
Fever, rigors, headache, sore throat
Malaise, myalgia
Nonproductive cough
Macular rash (Horder spots)
Pleurisy, hemoptysis, epistaxis (uncommon)

Signs
Confusion
Pharyngeal edema
Relative bradycardia
Lower lobe crackles
Pleural rub (uncommon)
Hepatomegaly
Splenomegaly

Radiographic features
Lobar or interstitial infiltrates
Hilar lymphadenopathy
Pleural effusion and cavitation (rare)

REFERENCES

Couts I, Mackenzie I, White R: Clinical and radiographic features of psittacosis infection. Thorax 1985;40:530-532.
Cotton M, Partridge M: Infection with feline *Chlamydia psittaci*. Thorax 1998;53:75-76.
Crosse B: Psittacosis: A clinical review. J Infect 1990;21;251-259.
Gregory G, Schaffner W: Psittacosis. Semin Respir Infect 1997;12(1):7-11.
Hammers-Berggren S, Granath F, Julander M, Kalin M: Erythromycin for treatment of ornithosis. Scand J Infect Dis 1991;23:159-162.
Macfarlane J, Macrae A: Psittacosis. Br Med Bull 1983;39(2):163-167.
Smith K, Bradley K, Stobierski M, Tengelsen L: Compendium of measures to control *Chlamydophila psittaci* infection among humans (psittacosis) and pet birds. J Am Vet Med Assoc 2005;226.
Wainwright W, Beaumont A, Fox W: Psittacosis: Diagnosis and management of severe pneumonia and multiorgan failure. Intensive Care Med 1987;13:419-421.

Q Fever

Method of
Pere Domingo, MD, PhD

Epidemiology

Q fever is a zoonosis with a worldwide distribution that may present in humans with acute or chronic manifestations. It is caused by *Coxiella burnetii*, a gram-negative bacterium previously classified in the Rickettsiales order, but now considered as belonging to the gamma subdivision of Proteobacteria. The Q fever reservoir includes many wild and domestic mammals, birds, and arthropods such as ticks, although domestic ruminants represent the most common source of human infection. The aerosol route (inhalation of infected fomites) is the primary mode of human contamination with *C. burnetii*, whereas ingestion (mainly drinking raw milk) and person-to-person transmission (transplacental, during autopsies, via intradermal inoculation, or via blood transfusion) are extremely rare. The primary mode of transmission of Q fever has recently raised concern about the potential use of *C. burnetii* as an agent of bioterrorism. The true incidence of Q fever is unknown, because *C. burnetii* infection in humans is usually asymptomatic or manifests as a mild disease with spontaneous recovery, and it is rarely a notifiable disease. However, current epidemiologic studies indicate that Q fever should be considered a public health problem in France, the United Kingdom, Italy, Spain, Germany, Israel, Greece, and Canada (Nova Scotia).

Clinical Features

C. burnetii infection may present with acute or chronic clinical manifestations. The incubation period may last from 2 to 3 weeks. The most frequent clinical manifestation of acute Q fever is a self-limited febrile illness associated with severe headache. Other major clinical presentations include atypical pneumonia and hepatitis, and, more rarely, myocarditis, pericarditis, maculopapular or purpuric rashes, and meningoencephalitis. Less common manifestations of acute Q fever include hemolytic anemia, mediastinal lymphadenopathy, erythema nodosum, thyroiditis, pancreatitis, mesenteric panniculitis, epididymitis, orchitis, priapism, inappropriate secretion of antidiuretic hormone, optic neuritis, Guillain-Barré syndrome, extrapyramidal neurologic disease, and splenic rupture. During pregnancy, *C. burnetii* infection may result in miscarriage, neonatal death, premature birth, or death in utero. Chronic Q fever represents 0.2% of all the cases of *C. burnetii* infection and most commonly presents as culture-negative endocarditis. It supervenes almost exclusively in patients with previous cardiac valve defects. Its diagnosis is often delayed because of the negativity of conventional blood cultures and because cardiac vegetations are small and visible on echocardiography in only 12% of patients. Other, less common manifestations of chronic Q fever include vascular infections (aneurysms and vascular grafts), osteoarticular infections (osteomyelitis and osteoarthritis), chronic hepatitis, chronic pulmonary infections, amyloidosis, mixed cryoglobulinemia,

malignancy-like presentations (such as pseudotumor of the lung), and central nervous system manifestations. These presentations occur months or years after the acute disease, and they represent long-term sequelae of untreated (and possibly undiagnosed) acute Q fever infection.

Diagnosis

Q fever diagnosis is based on serologic methods because culture and molecular biology techniques are available only in reference laboratories. Serologic diagnosis is easy to establish, although antibodies are mostly detected only after 2 to 3 weeks from the onset of the disease. Thus, serologic tests should be performed on both acute- and convalescent-phase sera, and serology allows the differentiation[1] of acute and chronic *C. burnetii* infections. Seroconversion or a fourfold rise in antibody titers can be diagnostic of Q fever. The immunofluorescent assay (IFA) is the reference technique for Q fever diagnosis. During acute Q fever, seroconversion is usually detected from 7 to 15 days after the onset of clinical symptoms and antibodies are detected by the third week in approximately 90% of cases. An IgG anti–phase II antibody titer of 1:200 and an IgM anti–phase II antibody titer of 1:50 are diagnostic of acute infection. However, such results are observed only in 10% of patients during the second week following the onset of symptoms, with 50% observed during the third week, and 70% during the fourth week. Antibody titers reach their highest levels approximately 4 to 8 weeks after the onset of acute Q fever, with gradually decreasing levels over the subsequent 12 months. A persistence of high levels of anti–phase I antibodies despite therapy, or the reappearance of antibodies in a high titer after previously being undetectable or only present in low titers, may herald the development of chronic Q fever infection. If acute Q fever has been diagnosed, recommendations are for repeat serologic testing, monthly, for at least 6 months. An IgG anti–phase I antibody titer of 1:800 is highly predictive (98%) of chronic infection. Phase I IgA, which was first considered useful for the diagnosis of chronic Q fever, is now used only for serologic follow-up. Cross-reactions are the biggest source of confusion when interpreting serologic results, and have been described between *C. burnetii* and *Legionella pneumophila*, *Legionella micdadei*, and *Bartonella quintana* or *Bartonella henselae*. PCR-based methods are commonly applicable

---

[1]Not FDA approved for this indication.

 CURRENT DIAGNOSIS

- *Acute Q fever:* A flu-like illness together with atypical pneumonia, hepatitis, or both, accompanied by disproportionate headache and seroconversion or a fourfold rise in IgG anti–phase II antibody titers against *Coxiella burnetii*.
- *Chronic Q fever:* Intermittent fever, cardiac failure, hepatomegaly, and splenomegaly, together with an IgG anti–phase I antibody titer against *C. burnetii* of 1:800.

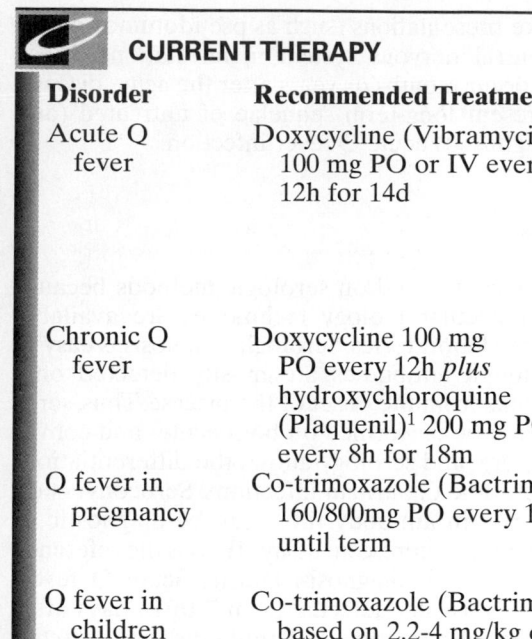

CURRENT THERAPY

Disorder	Recommended Treatment	Alternative Treatment*	Comments
Acute Q fever	Doxycycline (Vibramycin) 100 mg PO or IV every 12h for 14d	■ Ofloxacin (Floxin)[1] 200 mg PO every 8h for 14d ■ Pefloxacin (Pefocin)[2] 400 mg PO or IV every 12h for 14d ■ Erythromycin[1] 500 mg PO every 6h for 14d	Erythromycin is not recommended for severe cases. Corticosteroids may be used in Q fever hepatitis unresponsive to antibiotics alone.
Chronic Q fever	Doxycycline 100 mg PO every 12h *plus* hydroxychloroquine (Plaquenil)[1] 200 mg PO every 8h for 18m	Doxycycline 100 mg PO every 12h *plus* ofloxacin 200 mg PO every 8h for approximately 4y	Valvular replacement frequently required.
Q fever in pregnancy	Co-trimoxazole (Bactrim)[1] 160/800mg PO every 12h until term	Rifampicin (Rifampin)[1] 600 mg PO four times per day (length not known)	Doxycycline and fluoroquinolones are contraindicated in pregnancy.
Q fever in children	Co-trimoxazole (Bactrim)[1] based on 2.2-4 mg/kg of trimethoprim IV or PO every 12h for 14d	Chloramphenicol (Chloromycetin)[1] 25 mg/kg PO every 12h	Recommendations for treatment of chronic Q fever in children have not been established.

*In cases where more than one treatment is listed, choose only one.
[1]Not FDA approved for this indication.
[2]Not available in the United States.
Abbreviations: d = days; IV = intravenously; h = hours; m = months; PO = by mouth; y = years.`

only to tissue samples, especially cardiac valve specimens, and are not usually necessary for routine diagnosis. Nonspecific laboratory findings of Q fever include leukocytosis, elevated erythrocyte sedimentation rate, elevated creatine kinase, thrombocytopenia, moderate hepatic transaminase elevations (2 to 10 times normal values), and autoantibodies (antiphospholipid antibodies, anti–smooth muscle antibodies, antimitochondrial antibodies).

Treatment

Acute Q fever is most often a mild disease that resolves spontaneously within 2 weeks. Thus, clinical assessment of pharmacologic treatment is difficult. Doxycycline (Vibramycin) at 100 mg every 12 hours for 14 days is the current recommended regimen for acute Q fever. Fluoroquinolones are considered to be a reliable alternative and have been advocated for patients with Q fever meningoencephalitis, because they penetrate the cerebrospinal fluid. Although a macrolide compound or cotrimoxazole (Bactrim)[1] may be effective alternatives, no reliable antibiotic regimen can be currently recommended for children and pregnant women. Anecdotal reports indicate that lincomycin (Lincocin)[1], co-trimoxazole (Bactrim)[1], and chloramphenicol (Chloromycetin)[1] may be effective in the treatment of Q fever pneumonia. Erythromycin is ineffective in vitro against *C. burnetii*, but in vivo clinical efficacy has been suggested. The slow regression of

symptoms in patients with Q fever hepatitis has led to anecdotal reports of the benefit of a short, tapering, 1-week course of prednisone therapy together with antibiotic therapy. Adjunctive prednisone therapy may be considered in patients with Q fever hepatitis who have persistent fevers, persistent high elevations of erythrocyte sedimentation rate, and high titers of autoantibodies, especially when these occur despite adequate antibiotic therapy.

Combination antibiotic therapies are the most effective therapy for Q fever endocarditis. Combination regimens include lincomycin (Lincocin)[1], rifampin (Rifadin)[1], pefloxacin (Pefocin),[2] or ofloxacin (Floxin)[1] plus doxycycline. The combination of doxycycline with an alkalinizing agent of phagolysosomes, such as hydroxychloroquine (Plaquenil),[1] is bactericidal in vitro. In a comparison with doxycycline-ofloxacin, the doxycycline-hydroxychloroquine combination significantly diminished the relapse rate; patients improved more rapidly, and treatment duration could be shortened to 18 months (compared to 3 years with doxycycline-ofloxacin) to prevent most relapses. The optimum duration of antibiotic therapy cannot be accurately determined because no definite criteria for a Q fever cure are currently available. Suggestions have ranged from 1 year to indefinite administration of antibiotics. The surveillance of chronically infected patients should include titration of phase I IgG and IgA antibodies, and its decrease to a titer to 1:200 or less is the main predictive

---

[1]Not FDA approved for this indication.

[1]Not FDA approved for this indication.
[2]Not available in the United States

criterion of a clinical cure. Clinical and laboratory evaluation, including Q fever serology, should be performed monthly for the first 6 months of therapy, then every 3 months to assess the duration of treatment. An echocardiogram should be performed every 3 months. For patients on chloroquine therapy, regular ophthalmologic examination are warranted, and chloroquine serum levels should be regularly monitored. Valve replacement has been proposed in Q fever endocarditis as a result of hemodynamic failure.

Chemoprophylaxis

Postexposure prophylaxis after a biological attack might be considered for individuals or groups who have essential roles, and for those classified as being at high risk of acute disease in epidemiologic analyses, but is not recommended for the general public. Chemoprophylaxis is effective if begun 8 to 12 days after exposure and should be performed with tetracycline (Sumycin), 500 mg every 6 hours, or doxycycline (Vibramycin), 100 mg every 12 hours, for 5 to 7 days. Chemoprophylaxis is not effective and may prolong the onset of disease if given earlier than 7 days after exposure.

REFERENCES

Domingo P, Muñoz C, Franquet T, et al: Acute Q fever in adult patients. Report on 63 sporadic cases from an urban area. Clin Infect Dis 1999;29:874-879.
Madariaga MG, Rezai K, Trenholme GM, Wienstein RA: Q fever: A biological weapon in your backyard. Lancet Infect Dis 2003; 3:709-721.
Maurin M, Raoult D: Q fever. Clin Microbiol Rev 1999;12:518-553.
Raoult D, Houpikian P, Dupont HT, et al: Treatment of Q fever endocarditis. Comparison of 2 regimens containing doxycycline and ofloxacin or hydroxychloroquine. Arch Intern Med 1999; 159:167-173.
Raoult D, Tissot-Dupont H, Foucault C, et al: Q fever 1985-1998. Clinical and epidemiologic features of 1,383 infections. Medicine (Baltimore) 2000;79:109-123.

Rabies

Method of
Alan C. Jackson, MD, FRCPC

Rabies is an acute infection of the nervous system caused by rabies virus, which is a member of the family Rhabdoviridae in the genus *Lyssavirus*. Other lyssaviruses have only very rarely caused rabies in Europe, Africa, and Australia.

Pathogenesis

Rabies virus is usually transmitted by bites from rabid animals. Transmission has rarely occurred through an aerosol route (in a laboratory accident or bat cave containing millions of bats) or by transplantation of infected organs and tissues. The virus is in the saliva of the rabid animal and inoculated into subcutaneous tissues or muscles.

During most of the long incubation period (lasting 20 to 90 days or longer), the virus is close to the site of inoculation. The virus binds to the nicotinic acetylcholine receptor at the postsynaptic neuromuscular junction and travels toward the central nervous system (CNS) in peripheral nerves by retrograde fast axonal transport. There is rapid dissemination throughout the CNS by fast axonal transport. Under natural conditions, degenerative neuronal changes are not prominent, and it is thought that the rabies virus induces neuronal dysfunction by mechanisms that are not well understood. In rabies vectors, the encephalitis is associated with behavioral changes that lead to transmission by biting. After the CNS infection is established, the virus spreads by autonomic and sensory nerves to multiple organs, including the salivary glands in which the virus is secreted in high titer.

Clinical Features

In North America, where the bat is the most common rabies vector, a history of an animal bite is usually absent, and there may be no known contact with animals. The incubation period is usually between 20 and 90 days, but it may occasionally last 1 or more years. Prodromal features are nonspecific and include malaise, headache, and fever, and patients may also have anxiety or agitation. Approximately half of patients may experience pain, paresthesias, or pruritus at the site of the wound, which has often healed; this may reflect involvement of local sensory ganglia. Approximately 80% of patients with rabies have encephalitic rabies; approximately 20% have paralytic rabies. In encephalitic rabies, there are characteristic periods of generalized arousal or hyperexcitability separated by lucid periods. Autonomic dysfunction occurs frequently and includes hypersalivation, gooseflesh, cardiac arrhythmias, and priapism. Hydrophobia is the most characteristic feature of rabies and occurs in 50% to 80% of patients; contractions of the diaphragm and other inspiratory muscles occur on swallowing. This may become a conditioned reflex, and even the sight or thought of water can precipitate the muscle contractions. Hydrophobia is thought to be caused by inhibition of inspiratory neurons near the nucleus ambiguus.

In paralytic rabies, prominent muscle weakness usually begins in the bitten extremity and progresses to quadriparesis; typically there is sphincter involvement. Patients have a longer clinical course than in encephalitic rabies. Paralytic rabies is frequently misdiagnosed as the Guillain-Barré syndrome. Coma subsequently develops in both clinical forms. With aggressive medical therapy, a variety of medical complications develop, and multiple organ failure is a frequent occurrence. Survival is very rare and has usually occurred in the context of incomplete postexposure rabies prophylaxis that included administration of some rabies vaccine.

Epidemiology

Worldwide more than 55,000 human deaths per year are attributed to rabies. The impact is particularly significant in terms of years of life lost because children are frequently the victims. Most human rabies cases occur through transmission from dogs in developing countries with endemic dog rabies, particularly in Asia and Africa. In the United States and

Canada, the most common human cases are from insect-eating bats, and often, there is no known history of a bat bite or exposure to bats. A bat bite may not be recognized. The rabies virus variant responsible for most human cases is found in silver-haired bats and eastern pipistrelle bats. These are small bats not frequently in contact with humans. There are a variety of other rabies vectors in North American wildlife, including skunks, raccoons, and foxes, but these species are rarely responsible for transmission to humans. This is likely because of effective postexposure rabies prophylaxis.

Diagnosis

Most cases of rabies can be diagnosed clinically or the diagnosis strongly suspected, which is particularly important to initiate appropriate barrier nursing techniques and prevent exposures of many health care workers. Some cases may be candidates for an aggressive therapeutic approach. A serum neutralizing titer can be useful in a previously unimmunized individual, but a positive titer may not develop until the second week of clinical illness, and the result of the test may not be readily available. Detection of rabies virus antigen on a skin biopsy obtained from the nape of the neck using a fluorescent antibody technique is a useful diagnostic test. Detection of rabies virus ribonucleic acid (RNA) in saliva using reverse transcription polymerase chain reaction (RT-PCR) amplification is an important recent advance in rapid rabies diagnosis. Rabies virus antigen can be detected in brain tissue obtained by brain biopsy or postmortem.

Prevention

After recognition of a rabies exposure, rabies can be prevented with initiation of appropriate steps, including wound cleansing and active and passive immunization. After a human is bitten by a dog, cat, or ferret, the animal should be captured, confined, and observed for a period of at least 10 days. The animal should also be examined by a veterinarian prior to its release. If the animal is a stray, unwanted, shows signs, or develops signs of rabies during the observation period, the animal should be killed immediately, and its head should be transported under refrigeration for a laboratory examination. The brain should be examined via an antigen-detection method using the fluorescent antibody technique and viral isolation using cell culture or mouse inoculation.

The incubation period for animals other than dogs, cats, and ferrets is uncertain; these animals should be killed immediately after an exposure, and the head submitted for examination. If the result is negative, one may safely conclude that the animal's saliva did not contain rabies virus and, if immunization has been initiated, it should be discontinued. If an animal escapes after an exposure, it should be considered rabid unless information from public health officials indicates this is unlikely, and rabies prophylaxis should be initiated. The physical presence of a bat may warrant postexposure prophylaxis when a person (such as a small child or sleeping adult) is unable to reliably report contact that could have resulted in a bite.

Local wound care should be given as soon as possible after all exposures, even if immunization is delayed, pending the results of an observation period. All bite wounds and scratches should be washed thoroughly with soap and water. Devitalized tissues should be débrided.

Purified chick embryo cell culture vaccine (RabAvert), rabies vaccine absorbed (RVA), and human diploid cell vaccine (Imovax) are licensed rabies vaccines in the United States and Canada. Other vaccines grown in either primary cell lines (hamster or dog kidney) or continuous cell lines (Vero cells) are also satisfactory and available in other countries. A regimen of five 1-mL doses of rabies vaccine should be given intramuscularly (IM) in the deltoid area (anterolateral aspect of the thigh is also acceptable in children). Ideally, the first dose should be given as soon as possible after exposure, but failing that, it should be given regardless of the length of a delay. Four additional doses should be given on days 3, 7, 14, and 28. Pregnancy is not a contraindication for immunization. Live vaccines should not be given for 1 month after rabies immunization. Local and mild systemic reactions are common. Systemic allergic reactions are uncommon, and anaphylactic reactions may be treated with epinephrine and antihistamines. Corticosteroids may interfere with the development of active immunity. Immunosuppressive medications should not be administered during postexposure therapy unless they are essential. The risk of developing rabies should be carefully considered before deciding to discontinue vaccination because of an adverse reaction. A serum neutralizing antibody determination is necessary only after immunization of immunocompromised patients. Less expensive vaccines, derived from neural tissues, are still used in some developing countries; these vaccines are associated with serious neuroparalytic complications.

Human rabies immune globulin (Imogam or BayRab) should also be administered as passive immunization for protection before the development of immunity from the vaccine. It should be given at the same time as the first dose of vaccine and no later than 7 days after the first dose. Rabies vaccine and human rabies immune globulin should never be administered at the same site or in the same syringe. The recommended dose of human rabies immune globulin is 20 international units (IU)/kg; larger doses should not be given because they may suppress active immunity from the vaccine. After wounds are washed, they should be infiltrated with human rabies

- Details of an exposure determine whether postexposure rabies prophylaxis should be initiated.
- Wound cleansing is very important after a potential rabies exposure.
- Active immunization with a schedule of 5 doses of rabies vaccine at intervals is recommended.
- Passive immunization (if previously unimmunized) consists of human rabies immune globulin infiltrated into the wound and the remainder of the 20 IU/kg dosage given intramuscularly.

immune globulin (if anatomically feasible), and the remainder of the dose should be given IM in the gluteal area. If the exposure involves a mucous membrane, the entire dose should be administered IM. With multiple or large wounds, the human rabies immune globulin may need to be diluted for adequate infiltration of all of the wounds. Adverse effects of human rabies immune globulin include local pain and low-grade fever.

After an exposure, a previously immunized patient should receive two 1-mL doses of rabies vaccine on days 0 and 3, but the patient should not receive human rabies immune globulin.

Management of Human Rabies

Only six people have survived rabies, and five received rabies vaccine prior to the onset of their disease. The possibilities for an aggressive approach were recently reviewed (see Jackson et al., 2003). There was one survivor in Wisconsin in 2004 who did not receive rabies vaccine. It is not yet clear whether the therapy she received played a significant role in her favorable outcome. Palliation is an alternative approach and may be appropriate for many patients who develop rabies.

REFERENCES

Centers for Disease Control and Prevention: Human rabies prevention—United States, 1999: Recommendations of the Advisory Committee on Immunization Practices (ACIP). MMWR 1999;48 (No. RR-1):1-21.
Jackson AC: Human disease. In Jackson AC, Wunner WH (eds): Rabies. San Diego, Academic Press, 2002, pp 219-244.
Jackson AC: Rabies. Curr Treat Options Infect Dis 2003;5:35-40.
Jackson AC: Rabies: New insights into pathogenesis and treatment. Curr Opin Neurol 2006;19(3):267-270.
Jackson AC, Warrell MJ, Rupprecht CE, et al: Management of rabies in humans. Clin Infect Dis 2003;36:60-63.
Jackson AC, Wunner WH: Rabies. San Diego, Academic Press, 2002.
World Health Organization: WHO expert consultation on rabies: First report (First Report Edition). Geneva, WHO, 2005.

Rat-Bite Fever

Method of
Liane K. Freels, MD, FAAP

Rat-bite fever is a rare but potentially fatal disease characterized by the abrupt onset of fever, rash, and arthralgias that carries a mortality of 13% if left untreated. The responsible organisms are harbored in the upper respiratory tracts of rodents as well as animals who consume those rodents such as cats or dogs. Infection is typically transmitted via a bite or scratch from a colonized animal but may also be acquired by simply handling the animal or cage materials. Children account for more than 50% of documented cases. Any person exposed to rodents, for example, children living in rat-infested areas or laboratory workers, are at risk. Although there have been only 200 cases reported in the United States, one must consider the possibility of misdiagnosis as well as underreporting because it is not a reportable disease.

Rat-bite fever can be divided into three clinical syndromes. The first is rat-bite fever caused by *Streptobacillus moniliformis* infection, which is the predominant form seen in the United States. The second is caused by *Spirillum minus*, seen primarily in Asia and also known as Soduku (rat poison). When the clinical syndrome follows *S. moniliformis* ingestion via contaminated food, it is called Haverhill fever, so named for the first outbreak in 1926 at a boarding school in Haverhill, Massachusetts. Rat-bite fever can be an elusive diagnosis because of its clinical presentation with associated wide differential diagnoses and the difficulty recovering an organism. However, the growing popularity of rats and other rodents as pets, together with the risk of severe complications or invasive disease if unrecognized, demands our increased attention to rat-bite fever as a potential diagnosis.

Rat-Bite Fever Caused by *Streptobacillus Moniliformis*: Streptobacillary Fever

CLINICAL FEATURES

Rat-bite fever is a systemic illness characterized by abrupt onset of fever and chills, headache, myalgias, nausea, and vomiting 3 to 21 (usually less than 10) days after inoculation. If there is a bite, it usually heals quickly and does not exhibit significant inflammation or regional lymphadenopathy.

Fevers begin abruptly and usually resolve in 3 to 5 days but can relapse. The rash occurs in roughly 75% of patients and develops 2 to 4 days after the fever resolves. It may be maculopapular, petechial, or purpuric, but hemorrhagic pustules or vesicles may also be seen. It often involves the extremities, especially the hands and feet including the palms and soles, and may last up to 3 weeks. Approximately 20% of rashes caused by *S. moniliformis* desquamate. Within the first week, more than 50% of patients develop arthritis, which may be migratory polyarticular, sterile effusions or septic arthritis. Any joint may be involved, and migratory arthritis may persist for years despite appropriate treatment. Up to 25% of patients have false-rapid plasma reagent/positive venereal disease research laboratories (RPR/VDRL).

If infection with either organism goes unrecognized, there can be serious sequelae, including arthritis, endocarditis, myocarditis, pericarditis, pneumonia, amnionitis, pericardial effusion, hepatitis, nephritis, and meningitis. Abscesses are documented in nearly every organ, including skin, liver, kidney, spleen, and brain. Weight loss related to severe diarrhea may also be present in infants or small children.

DIAGNOSIS AND BACTERIOLOGY

Rat-bite fever must be suspected in any patient with the clinical symptomatology just described. Patients should be questioned carefully because often the history of a bite or contact with a potential animal vector is not immediately obvious. *S. moniliformis* is a pleomorphic, nonencapsulated gram-negative bacillus. It is an extremely fastidious organism that needs microaerophilic conditions to grow. Blood culture isolation is the gold standard, but *S. moniliformis* may also be isolated from abscess aspirates, synovial fluid, or wound cultures. Amplification in the laboratory is usually difficult secondary to the specific growth requirements. Optimal growth requires a trypticase soy agar or broth enriched with 20% blood, serum, or ascitic fluid. The sodium polyethylene sulfonate (SPS) added to most aerobic blood culture bottles inhibits the growth of *S. moniliformis*. However, the organism may grow in anaerobic culture bottles because SPS is not added. Laboratory personnel should always be notified of suspected rat-bite fever to optimize chances of organism recovery. Enzyme linked immunosorbent assays have been used with some success in laboratory rodents and may have some use in human disease. Polymerase chain reaction (PCR) amplification has also been used in laboratory animals, and a recent report demonstrated success in recovering *S. moniliformis* RNA from human blister fluid using PCR techniques. This technique may allow for more accurate diagnosis when blood cultures are negative, but it is not readily available.

 CURRENT DIAGNOSIS

- Rat-bite fever is characterized by abrupt onset of fever, chills, headache, vomiting, and myalgias, usually following a bite from an infected animal.
- Rash may be maculopapular, petechial/purpuric, hemorrhagic, or vesicular and involves the palms of hands and soles of feet.
- >50% of patients develop arthritis (any type).
- >25% have false-positive RPR/VDRL.
- Blood culture growth requires anaerobic culture bottles and careful communication with laboratory personnel to maximize the chances of recovery.

Abbreviation: RPR/VDRL = rapid plasma reagent/venereal disease research laboratories.

 CURRENT THERAPY

- Adult dosing: penicillin, 1.2 million U IV q6h
- Pediatric dosing: 20,000–50,000 U/kg/day
- IV therapy for 5–7 d
- May switch to oral penicillin/amoxicillin if patient appears well after initial IV course.

Abbreviation: IV = intravenous.

TREATMENT

Penicillin is the treatment of choice despite rare reports of penicillin-resistant strains. Current recommended treatment is 5 to 7 days of intravenous (IV) penicillin (Penicillin G) at doses of 1.2 million U IV every 6 hours (20,000 to 50,000 U/kg/day for pediatric dosing) followed by 7 days of oral Penicillin V (Veetids)[1] or Amoxicillin (Amoxil).[1] Patients usually respond quickly to therapy, and those who appear well after 5 to 7 days may complete therapy with a week of oral penicillin. One may consider treating mild cases with oral penicillin alone at doses of 1 to 2 g/day in divided doses for the entire course.

More severe infections (cardiac involvement, meningitis, intraabdominal abscesses) are so rare that the optimal therapy is unclear. It is reasonable to treat with higher doses and for an extended time (4 to 6 weeks). Penicillin-allergic patients may be given erythromycin (E-Mycin),[1] tetracycline (Sumycin),[1] clindamycin (Cleocin),[1] or chloramphenicol (Chloromycetin),[1] although the efficacy of these antimicrobials is not well established. There are no placebo-controlled trials to evaluate alternative therapies.

Any identified bite wounds should have thorough cleansing and tetanus prophylaxis if appropriate.

Rat-bite Fever Caused by *Spirillum Minus*: Spirillary Fever

CLINICAL FEATURES

After a longer incubation (1 to 36 days), *S. minus* infection is usually heralded by an indurated lesion at the site as symptoms become obvious. The area may ulcerate and there may be regional lymphadenopathy. In *S. minus* infection, the fevers are frequently relapsing separated by afebrile periods lasting 3 to 7 days. Approximately 50% of patients develop a violaceous red-brown rash that usually consists of large macules with occasional erythematous plaques or urticarial type lesions. Unlike *S. moniliformis*, joint manifestations are rare. The mortality with *S. minus* infection is slightly lower than that seen with *S. moniliformis* and approaches 6.5%.

DIAGNOSIS AND BACTERIOLOGY

Spirillum minus is a tightly coiled, spiral gram-negative rod. There are no serologic or molecular tests available for diagnosis, and isolation of the organism requires darkfield

[1]Not FDA approved for this indication.

microscopy of blood or ulcer/wound aspirate or from secondary inoculation of an animal with infected blood. Blood or wound aspirates are injected intraperitoneally into guinea pigs or mice, and darkfield exam of the animal's blood shows the spirochetes in 5 to 15 days.

TREATMENT

The treatment of choice for spirillary fever remains penicillin in the same doses as streptobacillary fever. Although *S. minus* is sensitive to alternative drugs (tetracycline,[1] chloramphenicol,[1] aminoglycosides[1]), there are no placebo-controlled studies to evaluate their efficacy.

REFERENCES

Azimi P: Pets can be dangerous. Pediatr Infect Dis J 1990;9(9):670-84.

Byington C, Basow, RD: *Streptobacillus moniliformis* (rat-bite fever). In Feigin R, Cherry JD (eds): Textbook of Pediatric Infectious Diseases, 4th ed. Philadelphia, WB Saunders, 1998, pp 1509-1511.

Byington C, Basow RD: *Spirillum minus* (rat-bite fever). In Feigin R, Cherry JD (eds): Textbook of Pediatric Infectious Diseases, 4th ed. Philadelphia, WB Saunders, 1998, pp 1542-1543.

Cunningham B, Paller A, Katz B: Rat bite fever in a pet lover. J Am Acad Dermatol 1998;38(2 Pt 2):330-332.

Elliott S, Freels L: Rat bite fever—three cases and literature review. Clin Pediatr 2004;43(3):291-296.

Glaser C, Lewis P, Wong S: Pet-, animal-, and vector-borne infections. Pediatr Rev 2000;21(7):219-232.

Rat-bite fever—New Mexico, 1996. MMWR Morb Mortal Wkly Rep 1998;47(5):89-91.

Rubin L: *Streptobacillus moniliformis* (rat-bite fever). In Long S, Pickering, LL, Prober CG (eds): Principles and Practice of Pediatric Infectious Diseases. New York: Livingstone; 1997, pp 1046-1047.

Washburn R: Rat bite fever. In Mandell GL, Bennett JE, Dolin R (eds): Principles and Practice of Infectious Diseases, 6th ed. Philadelphia, Churchill Livingstone, 2005, 2708-2710.

---

[1]Not FDA approved for this indication.

Relapsing Fever

Method of
Diego Cadavid, MD

Relapsing fever is one of several diseases caused by spirochetes. Other human spirochetal diseases are syphilis, Lyme disease, and leptospirosis. Notable features of spirochetes are wavy and helical shapes, length-to-diameter ratios of as much as 100 to 1, and flagella that lie between the inner and outer cell membranes. The spirochetes that cause relapsing fever are in the genus *Borrelia*. Other *Borrelia* species cause Lyme disease, avian spirochetosis, and epidemic bovine abortion. Table 1 shows the main *Borrelia* species of relapsing fever, their vectors, and an estimate of their geographic ranges. In the United States relapsing fever was considered a disease endemic only in the West. However, the recent finding of relapsing fever–like *Borrelia* in ticks and dogs in the eastern United States suggests the risk that relapsing fever may extend into the East.

Epidemiology

There are two forms of relapsing fever: epidemic transmitted to humans by the body louse *Pediculus humanus* (louse-borne relapsing fever, LBRF) and endemic transmitted to humans by soft-bodied ticks of the genus *Ornithodoros* (tick-borne relapsing fever, TBRF). In LBRF itching caused by skin infestation with lice leads to scratching, which may result in crushing of lice and release of infected hemolymph into areas of skin abrasion. Louse infestation is associated with cold weather and a lack of hygiene. Migrant workers and soldiers at war are particularly susceptible to this infection. Historically, massive outbreaks of LBRF occurred in Eurasia, Africa, and Latin America, but currently the disease is found only in Ethiopia and neighboring countries. However, immigrants can spread LBRF to other parts of the world.

The main risk factor for TBRF is exposure to endemic areas (Table 1). The risk of infection increases with outdoor activities in areas where rodents nest, like entering caves or sleeping in rustic cabins. *Ornithodoros* ticks are soft-bodied and feed for short periods of time (minutes), usually at night. They can live many years between blood meals and may transmit spirochetes to their offspring transovarially. Infection is produced by regurgitation of infected tick saliva into the skin wound during tick feeding. There are several natural vertebrate reservoirs for TBRF, but most common are rodents (deer mice, chipmunks, squirrels, and rats). In contrast, the body louse *Pediculus humanus* is a strict human parasite, living and multiplying in clothing.

Clinical Diagnosis

Relapsing fever should be suspected in any patient presenting with two or more episodes of high fever and constitutional symptoms spaced by periods of relative well-being. The index of suspicion increases if the patient has been exposed to endemic areas for TBRF or to countries where LBRF still occurs (Table 1). Whereas LBRF is usually associated with a single febrile relapse, TBRF usually has multiple relapses (up to 13). In LBRF the second episode of fever is typically milder than the first; in TBRF the multiple febrile periods are usually of equal severity. The febrile periods last from 1 to 3 days, and the intervals between fevers last from 3 to 10 days. During the febrile periods, numerous spirochetes are circulating in the blood. This is called spirochetemia and is sometimes unexpectedly detected during routine blood smear examinations. Between fevers, spirochetemia is not observed because the numbers are low. The fever pattern and recurrent spirochetemia are the consequences of antigenic variation of abundant outer membrane lipoproteins of relapsing fever *Borrelia* species that are the target for serotype-specific antibodies.

The mean latency between exposure to ticks in the endemic form or to lice in the epidemic form and onset of symptoms is 6 days (range, 3 to 18 days). Because *Ornithodoros* ticks feed briefly and painlessly at night, patients with TBRF may not be able to recall having been bitten by a tick. The clinical manifestations of TBRF and LBRF are similar, although some differences do exist. Table 2 lists the frequency of the most common manifestations of TBRF. The usual initial presentation is sudden

TABLE 1 Relapsing Fever *Borrelia* Species Pathogenic to Humans

Relapsing Fever	*Borrelia* Species	Arthropod Vector	Distribution of Disease
Endemic	*B. hermsii*	*Ornithodoros hermsi*	Western North America
	B. turicatae	*O. turicata*	Southwestern North America and northern Mexico
	B. venezuelensis	*O. rudis*	Central America and northern South America
	B. hispanica	*O. marocanus*	Iberian peninsula and northwestern Africa
	B. crocidurae	*O. erraticus*	North and East Africa, Middle East, southern Europe
	B. duttoni	*O. moubata*	Sub-Saharan Africa
	B. persica	*O. tholozani*	Middle East, Greece, Central Asia
	B. uzbekistan	*O. pappilipes*	Tajikistan, Uzbekistan
Epidemic	*B. recurrentis*	*Pediculus humanus*	Worldwide (recently only in East Africa including immigrants to Europe)

onset of chills followed by high fever, tachycardia, severe headache, vomiting, myalgia and arthralgia, and often delirium. In the early stages, a reddish rash may be seen over the trunk, arms, or legs. The fever remains high for 3 to 5 days, and then it clears abruptly. After an asymptomatic period of 7 to 10 days, the fever and other constitutional symptoms can reappear suddenly. The febrile episodes gradually become less severe, and the person eventually recovers completely. As the disease progresses, fever, jaundice, hepatosplenomegaly, cardiac arrhythmias, and cardiac failure may occur, especially with LBRF. Jaundice is more common at times of relapses. Patients with LBRF are more likely to develop petechiae on the trunk, extremities, and mucous membranes; epistaxis; and blood-tinged sputum. Rupture of the spleen may rarely occur. Multiple neurologic complications can occur as a result of disseminated intravascular coagulation in LBRF and as a result of infection of the meninges and cranial and spinal nerve roots by spirochetes in TBRF. The most common neurologic complications of TBRF are aseptic meningitis and facial palsy. Relapsing fever in pregnant women can cause abortion, premature birth, and neonatal death. Sometimes patients can have nonfebrile relapses, consisting of periods of severe headache, backache, weakness, and other constitutional symptoms without fever that occur at the time of expected relapses. Delirium may persist for weeks after the fever resolves, and rarely symptoms may be protracted.

Relapsing fever may be confused with many diseases that are relapsing or cause high fevers. These include typhoid fever, yellow fever, dengue, African hemorrhagic fevers, African trypanosomiasis, brucellosis, malaria, leptospirosis, rat-bite fever, intermittent cholangitis, cat-scratch disease, echovirus 9 infection, among others. Relapsing fever *Borrelias* have antigens that are cross reactive with Lyme disease *Borrelias* and inasmuch as the endemic areas of relapsing fever and Lyme disease overlap to some extent, confusion between the two infections can be expected.

Laboratory Diagnosis

Although the pattern of recurring fever is the clue to diagnosing relapsing fever, confirmation of the diagnosis requires demonstration of spirochetes in peripheral blood taken during an episode of fever. The comparatively large number of spirochetes in the blood during relapsing fever provides the opportunity for the simplest method for laboratory diagnosis of the infection, light microscopy of Wright or Giemsa stained thin blood smears or darkfield or phase-contrast microscopy of a wet mount of plasma. The blood should be obtained during or just before peaks of body temperature. Between fever peaks, spirochetes often can be demonstrated by inoculation of blood or cerebrospinal fluid (CSF) into special culture medium (BSK-H with 6% rabbit serum available from Sigma) or experimental animals. Enrichment for spirochetes is achieved by using the platelet-rich fraction of plasma or the buffy coat of sedimented blood. In the United States the most common causes of relapsing fever are *Borrelia hermsii* and *Borrelia turicatae*; both grow in BSK-H medium and in young mice or rats. Whereas direct visual detection of organisms in the blood is the most common method for laboratory confirmation of relapsing fever, immunoassays

TABLE 2 Frequent Clinical Manifestations of Tick-Borne Relapsing Fever

Sign or Symptom	Frequency (%)
Headache	94
Myalgia	92
Chills	88
Nausea	76
Arthralgia	73
Vomiting	71
Abdominal pain	44
Confusion	38
Dry cough	27
Ocular pain	26
Diarrhea	25
Dizziness	25
Photophobia	25
Neck pain	24
Rash	18
Dysuria	13
Jaundice	10
Hepatomegaly	10
Splenomegaly	6

CURRENT DIAGNOSIS

- There are two forms of relapsing fever: epidemic and endemic.
- Epidemic relapsing fever is transmitted from person to person by the body louse *Pediculus humanus*.
- Endemic relapsing fever is transmitted from rodent reservoirs to humans exposed to endemic areas by soft-bodied ticks of the genus *Ornithodoros*.
- The hallmark of relapsing fever is two or more febrile episodes separated by periods of relative well-being.
- The diagnosis is confirmed by visualization of the etiologic spirochetes in thin peripheral blood smears prepared at times of febrile peaks by phase-contrast or darkfield microscopy or light therapy microscopy after Wright or Giemsa staining.

CURRENT THERAPY

- The antibiotic of choice for treatment of relapsing fever is doxycycline (Doryx) except in children or pregnant women. In children <8 y, erythromycin (E-Mycin)[1] or oral penicillin[1] is used instead of tetracycline (Table 3).
- Relapsing fever if severe or complicated with neuroborreliosis requires treatment with the intravenous antibiotics ceftriaxone (Rocephin) or penicillin G (Table 3).
- The louse-borne epidemic form is treated with a single dose, whereas the endemic tick-borne form is treated with multiple doses for at least 1 week (Table 3).
- Antibiotic treatment of relapsing fever results in the Jarisch-Herxheimer reaction in as many as 60% of cases, more often in the epidemic than in the endemic form. It is characterized by the sudden onset of tachycardia, hypotension, chills, rigors, diaphoresis, and high fever. To reduce the risk of the JHR, antibiotics should be started between but not at times of febrile peaks.

[1]Not FDA approved for this indication.

for antibodies are the most common means of laboratory confirmation for Lyme disease. Although serologic assays have been developed for the agents of relapsing fever, these are not widely available and of dubious utility. The antigenic variation displayed by the relapsing fever species means there are hundreds of different "serotypes." If a different serotype or species is used for preparing the antigen, only antibodies to conserved antigens may be detected. For this reason, a standardized enzyme-linked immunosorbent assay (ELISA) with Lyme disease *Borrelia* as antigen may be the best available serologic assay for relapsing fever. ELISA for *Borrelia burgdorferi* antibodies is routinely done across the United States and Europe. If a positive result for IgM or IgG antibodies is obtained, the Western blot for antibodies to *B. burgdorferi* antigens would be expected to discriminate current or past Lyme disease from relapsing fever, as well as from syphilis, another cause of false-positive Lyme disease ELISA results. Other frequent laboratory abnormalities can occur in relapsing fever but are not diagnostic. These include elevated white blood cell count with increased neutrophils, thrombocytopenia, increased serum bilirubin, proteinuria, microhematuria, prolongation of the prothrombin time (PT) and partial thromboplastin time (PTT), and elevation of fibrin degradation products.

Treatment

Relapsing fever *Borrelias* are very sensitive to several antibiotics, and antimicrobial resistance is rare. Table 3 summarizes the treatment options for adults and children younger than 8 years. Children older than 8 years can be treated with the same antibiotics as adults, but the doses should be adjusted by weight. Before antibiotics are given, the possibility of causing the Jarisch-Herxheimer reaction should be considered (see later). The tetracycline antibiotics are most commonly used for treatment of LBRF and TBRF. The first antibiotic of choice in adults and children older than 8 years is doxycycline (Doryx). In general, shorter treatments are needed for LBRF than for TBRF. Single-dose therapy is usually recommended for LBRF.

TABLE 3 Treatment Options for Tick-Borne Relapsing Fever*

Adults
Nonsevere forms

1. Doxycycline (Doryx oral), 100 mg PO bid for 1–2 wk[†]
2. Tetracycline (Tetracyn), 500 mg PO qid for 1–2 wk
3. Erythromycin (Erythrocin),[1] 500 mg PO tid for 1–2 wk

Severe forms

1. Ceftriaxone (Rocephin),[1] 2g IV qd for 1–2 wk
2. Penicillin G parenteral aqueous (Pfizerpen),[1] 4 million U IV q4h for 1–2 wk

Children (≤8 y)
Nonsevere forms

1. Erythromycin suspension oral (EryPed),[1] 30–50 mg/kg/d divided tid for 1–2 wk
2. Azithromycin oral suspension (Zithromax),[1] 20 mg/kg on the first day followed by 10 mg/kg/d for 4 more days
3. Penicillin V (Pen-Vee K),[1] 25–50 mg/kg/d divided qid for 1–2 wk
4. Amoxicillin (Amoxil),[1] 50 mg/kg/d divided tid for 1–2 wk

Severe forms

1. Ceftriaxone (Rocephin),[1] 75–100 mg/kg/d IV for 1–2 wk
2. Penicillin G parenteral aqueous (Pfizerpen),[1] 300,000 U/kg/d given IV in divided doses q4h for 1–2 wk

[1]Not FDA approved for this indication.
*The same oral agents are used for treatment of louse-borne (epidemic) relapsing fever but given as a single dose.
[†]In general, treatment for 1 wk is recommended in early/milder cases and for up to 2 wk for more severe cases.
Abbreviations: IV = intravenous; PO = orally.

In contrast, in TBRF even multiple doses of tetracyclines for up to 10 days may fail to prevent relapses, and retreatment can be required. Alternative oral antibiotics to the tetracyclines are erythromycin (E-Mycin),[1] azithromycin (Zithromax),[1] amoxicillin (Amoxil),[1] penicillin,[1] and chloramphenicol (Chloromycetin).[1] However, oral chloramphenicol is no longer available in the United States. Erythromycin, azithromycin, and penicillin do not appear as effective as the tetracyclines; however, they are recommended for children younger than 8 years and for pregnant women. Amoxicillin is another alternative for young children with early Lyme disease; however, it is ineffective for human granulocytic ehrlichiosis, which sometimes occurs as a co-infection with Lyme disease.

Although treatment with antibiotics is usually given orally, they may need to be given intravenously if severe vomiting makes swallowing impractical. If there are symptoms and signs of meningitis or encephalitis without clinical and/or radiologic signs of increased intracranial pressure, the CSF should be examined to rule out central nervous system (CNS) infection. The finding of elevation of CSF cells and protein demands the use of parenteral antibiotics, such as penicillin G or ceftriaxone (Rocephin). Optimally, antibiotic treatment should be started during afebrile periods when the spirochetemia is low. Starting therapy near the peak of a febrile period may induce the Jarisch-Herxheimer reaction, in which high fever and a rise and subsequent fall in blood pressure, sometimes to dangerously low levels, may occur. Dehydration should be treated with fluids given intravenously. Severe headache can be treated with pain relievers such as codeine, and nausea or vomiting can be treated with prochlorperazine.

Jarisch-Herxheimer Reaction

Antibiotic treatment of relapsing fever causes the Jarisch-Herxheimer reaction (JHR) in as many as 60% of cases. The JHR is more common in LBRF than in TBRF. It is characterized by the sudden onset of tachycardia, hypotension, chills, rigors, diaphoresis, and high fever. Patients with the JHR have said that they felt as if they were going to die. The JHR is caused by the rapid killing of circulating spirochetes 1 to 4 hours after the first dose of antibiotic, which results in the release of large amounts of *Borrelia* lipoproteins in the circulation followed by massive release of tumor necrosis factor and other cytokines. If possible, patients with the JHR should be transferred to an intensive care unit for close monitoring and treatment. During several hours, the temperature declines and the patient feels better. Large amounts of intravenous fluids (0.9% sodium chloride solution) may be required to treat hypotension. Steroids and nonsteroidal anti-inflammatory agents have no effect on the frequency or severity of the JHR. One study found that pretreatment with anti-TNF-alpha monoclonal antibody (Humira)[1] suppressed the JHR after penicillin treatment for LBRF and reduced the associated increases in plasma cytokines. Death can occur as a result of the JHR secondary to cardiovascular collapse in up to 5% of patients with treated LBRF and much less frequently in TBRF.

Outcome

Complete recovery occurs in 95% or more of adequately treated patients. The prognosis for untreated cases or if treatment is delayed varies. Mortality as high as 40% is reported in untreated epidemics of LBRF. Relapsing fever also has a high mortality in neonates. Some neurologic sequelae can occur in patients with TBRF complicated with neuroborreliosis.

Prevention

Prevention of TBRF involves avoidance of rodent- and tick-infested dwellings such as animal burrows, caves, and abandoned cabins. Wearing clothing that protects skin from tick access (e.g., long pants and long-sleeved shirts) is also helpful. Repellents and acaricides provide additional protection. Diethyltoluamide (DEET) repels ticks when applied to clothing or skin, but it must be used with caution. It loses its effectiveness within 1 to several hours when applied to skin and must be reapplied; it is absorbed through the skin and may cause CNS toxicity if used excessively. Picaridin (KBR 3023), which has been used as an insect repellent for years in Europe and Australia, is now available in the United States in 7% solution as Cutter Advanced Repellent (Spectrum Brands). The U.S. Centers for Disease Control and Prevention (CDC) is recommending it as an alternative to DEET. Permethrin Insect Repellent, an acaricide, is more effective than DEET but should not be applied directly to skin. When applied to clothing, it provides good protection for 1 day or more. In LBRF, prevention can be achieved by promoting personal hygiene and by dusting undergarments and the inside of clothing with malathion[1,2] or lindane powder[2] when available. Widespread antibiotic use may be necessary to control epidemics of LBRF, using one or two doses of 100 mg doxycycline given within 1 week of exposure.

REFERENCES

Barbour AG, Hayes SF: Biology of *Borrelia* species. Microbiol Rev 1986;50:381-400.

Bryceson AD, Parry EH, Perine PL, et al: Louse-borne relapsing fever. Q J Med 1970;39:129-170.

Cadavid D, Barbour AG: Neuroborreliosis during relapsing fever: Review of the clinical manifestations, pathology, and treatment of infections in humans and experimental animals. Clin Infect Dis 1998;26:151-164.

Fekade D, Knox K, Hussein K, et al: Prevention of Jarisch-Herxheimer reactions by treatment with antibodies against tumor necrosis factor alpha. N Engl J Med 1996;335:311-315.

Kazragis RJ, Dever LL, Jorgensen JH, Barbour AG: In vivo activities of ceftriaxone and vancomycin against *Borrelia* spp. in the mouse brain and other sites. Antimicrob Agents Chemother 1996;40:2632-2636.

Melkert PW: Fatal Jarisch-Herxheimer reaction in a case of relapsing fever misdiagnosed as lobar pneumonia. Trop Geogr Med 1987;39: 92-93.

Southern P, Sanford J: Relapsing fever. Medicine 1969;48:129-149.

Taft W, Pike J: Relapsing fever. Report of a sporadic outbreak including treatment with penicillin. JAMA 1945;129:1002-1005.

---

[1]Not FDA approved for this indication.

---

[1]Not FDA approved for this indication.
[2]Not available in the United States.

Lyme Disease

Method of
*Arthur Weinstein, MD, FACP, FACR,
and Shobha Wani, MD*

Epidemiology

Lyme disease, or borreliosis, is a tick-transmitted infection caused by *Borrelia burgdorferi*. It is the most common insect-borne illness in the United States with more than 20,000 new cases reported annually. It occurs worldwide with hyperendemicity in temperate regions. In the United States, most cases originate from states in the Northeast, mid-Atlantic, upper Midwest, and Pacific coast regions. The life cycle of the Ixodes tick ensures that most cases of human borrelial infection occur from spring to fall. Three genospecies of *B. burgdorferi* account for human disease: *B. burgdorferi sensu stricto*, *B. garinii*, and *B. afzelii*. Although all three are found in Europe and the latter two in Asia, *B. burgdorferi sensu stricto* is the only cause of Lyme disease in the United States. Lyme disease occurs in all age groups with highest frequencies in young children and adults older than 30 years and is equally common in men and women. It often manifests clinically in stages, with exacerbations and remissions in each stage.

Clinical Features

EARLY LYME DISEASE

Localized skin infection and early disseminated infection occur within days to weeks after the bite of an infected tick. Erythema migrans (EM) rash, the hallmark of early Lyme disease, occurs in up to 70% to 80% of patients at the site of the tick bite. It usually is macular and asymptomatic but may burn or itch, and it is commonly found at the belt line, inguinal area, or in and around the axilla. It expands over days, often to a very large circumference and with central clearing, giving a bull's-eye appearance. Approximately 10% of patients have multiple skin lesions (disseminated EM), a sign of hematogenous spread of the borrelia. At this early stage, patients may have nonspecific flulike complaints, namely fever, fatigue, myalgia, arthralgia, and headache, resembling a viral syndrome. These symptoms occasionally occur without the rash. In untreated patients, EM resolves spontaneously within days to several weeks after onset, but treatment often accelerates its resolution.

Early disseminated disease occurs days to weeks after the tick bite and may occur without preceding localized EM. Certain subtypes of *B. burgdorferi* are associated with higher frequency of spirochetemia and dissemination to other organs. For instance, in Europe, EM is often an indolent, localized infection, whereas in the United States, it is associated with more intense inflammation and signs that suggest dissemination of the spirochete. The clinical manifestations of dissemination can be highly variable and may include disseminated EM rash and neurologic, cardiac, and musculoskeletal features either alone or in combination. Neurologic features (neuroborreliosis) are seen in approximately 10% of patients and include acute lymphocytic meningitis, cranial neuropathy, especially facial paresis, which may be bilateral, and radiculoneuritis. Neuroborreliosis is more common in Europe where neurotropic subspecies of borrelia (*B. garinii*, *B. afzelii*) are found. Meningitis usually resolves spontaneously, whereas treatment of other neurologic features can hasten recovery and prevent progression to the later stages of Lyme disease. Carditis, which includes varying degrees of atrioventricular block or mild myopericarditis, may develop in approximately 8% of untreated patients, but early treatment can prevent its occurrence. In more recent series, the incidence of Lyme carditis was reported as less than 1% in the United States. Rheumatic features at this stage consist of migratory, episodic joint, tendon, or bursal pains with or without objective signs of inflammation. Typically there is acute localized pain that lasts days to weeks, remits spontaneously, and then recurs in another region. Inflammatory polyarthritis is not a feature of early or late Lyme disease.

The diagnosis of early Lyme disease relies to a great degree on the clinical presentation. In an endemic area, with a history of possible tick exposure, the presence of a classical EM lesion is sufficient for the diagnosis. With very early infection and isolated EM, laboratory tests for antibodies to *B. burgdorferi* may be negative. Conversely, with disseminated early Lyme disease, antibody testing is frequently positive.

LATE LYME DISEASE

Late Lyme disease occurs months to years after initial infection (mean, 6 months) and may present de novo without prior features of early Lyme disease. Systemic symptoms are generally minimal or absent. Musculoskeletal complaints, the most common manifestation, are seen in 80% of untreated patients and include intermittent oligoarthritis (50%) and acute or subacute inflammatory arthritis that most often affects one or both knees. This arthritis may begin abruptly with knee pain and a large joint effusion. Synovial fluid is inflammatory with white

CURRENT DIAGNOSIS

- Erythema migrans is usually asymptomatic and expansile.
- Lyme disease can present with only flulike symptoms: fever, arthralgia, myalgia.
- Antibody testing for borrelial infection is often negative during early infection.
- A two-test strategy (serum ELISA, immunoblot) is recommended for diagnosis.
- IgM antibodies are commonly seen in early infection (4–8 wk) but may persist for many months.
- IgG antibodies are characteristic of late Lyme disease, especially Lyme arthritis.
- Intrathecal antibody synthesis is an important diagnostic marker for neuroborreliosis.
- Clinical symptoms combined with antibody status are of diagnostic importance.

Abbreviation: ELISA = enzyme-linked immunosorbent assay.

counts ranging in the thousands or tens of thousands. Radiographs may be normal except for soft-tissue swelling and joint effusion but may also demonstrate osteopenia, bone cysts, and even mild cartilage loss with small erosions. Untreated, these attacks of arthritis generally last many months, recur for several years but eventually may remit. *B. burgdorferi* is not culturable from the synovial fluid of patients with Lyme arthritis, but borrelial DNA can be detected by polymerase chain reaction (PCR) in over 80% of untreated patients. The PCR test is generally negative after appropriate antibiotic therapy.

Neurologic features of late Lyme disease are seen more frequently in Europe because *B. garinii* is the most neurotropic subspecies. There are a wide range of neurologic abnormalities, especially encephalomyelitis and radiculoneuropathy. In the United States, Lyme encephalopathy or polyneuropathy is described with subtle disturbances of memory and concentration, spinal radicular pain, or distal paresthesias. Nerve conduction studies reveal axonal polyneuropathy. Pleocytosis of the cerebrospinal fluid (CSF) is unusual in late neurologic Lyme disease. High CSF protein may be seen, but borrelial organisms by culture or PCR are not commonly found. Important to the diagnosis of neuroborreliosis is the demonstration of increased intrathecal synthesis of borrelia-specific antibodies.

A chronic skin lesion, acrodermatitis chronica atrophicans, caused by *B. afzelii*, is seen most commonly in Europe.

Laboratory Testing in Lyme Disease

Lyme disease should not be diagnosed purely on serologic tests because false-positive tests are common. Instead, serologic tests should be used to confirm the diagnosis in the appropriate clinical setting. Even a true positive test only confirms recent or past exposure to *B. burgdorferi*, but this must be evaluated in the context of the patient's past and current symptoms.

Despite these methodologic and diagnostic issues, measurement of antibodies to *B. burgdorferi* by enzyme-linked immunoassay (ELISA) is a useful screening test for early and late Lyme disease. This so-called Lyme test is positive in most cases of late Lyme disease and virtually always positive in late Lyme arthritis. It may be negative very early after infection or in those individuals who receive early antibiotic therapy. However, the high rate of false positivity has led to a two-test strategy whereby all sera that show positive or equivocal ELISA tests for borrelial antibodies are tested again by more specific Western (immuno) blotting. In patients with CNS disease, demonstration of intrathecal antibodies by ELISA in relatively higher concentration than serum antibodies is suggestive of neuroborreliosis.

Immunoblotting is usually performed for both IgM and IgG antibodies to borrelial proteins. Although this technique is not as automated or quantitative as ELISA, it is more specific because it identifies the borrelial antigens to which the antibodies are directed. There are recommendations for standardized testing and interpretation of Western blot results. IgM antibodies usually appear 2 to 4 weeks after EM, peak at 6 to 8 weeks, and decline thereafter, although IgM reactivity may occasionally persist for many years. An IgM blot is considered to be positive if two of three specified bands (23, 39, 41 kd) are present. The results of an IgM blot are best interpreted in the first weeks after symptom onset when the true positive rate exceeds the false-positive rate. A positive IgM blot found in a patient with long-standing symptoms should be interpreted with caution because it likely represents a false-positive result. IgG antibodies appear after 4 to 6 weeks, peak at 4 to 6 months, and then remain positive for many years, even decades. An IgG immunoblot is considered to be positive if 5 of 10 specified bands (18, 23, 28, 30, 39, 41, 45, 58, 66, 93 kd) are present. IgG seroconversion, with or without IgM seroconversion, can be taken as presumptive evidence of exposure to *B. burgdorferi* and in the proper clinical context supports the diagnosis of Lyme disease. However, a positive IgG immunoblot does not necessarily mean current or ongoing borreliosis. Conversely, a negative IgG immunoblot is presumptive evidence against the diagnosis of late Lyme disease. An ELISA assay for antibodies to a borrelial-specific surface protein (C6 peptide of VlsE) was demonstrated to be a sensitive and specific single test for the diagnosis of Lyme disease and is commercially available.

Culture of *B. burgdorferi* requires special medium and conditions and takes many weeks. Even so, in expert laboratories the organism can be recovered from the EM lesion in a high percentage of patients and from the blood in patients with disseminated early Lyme disease. Risk for spirochetemia starts the day the patient notices the rash and continues for 2 weeks.

B. burgdorferi is cultured only rarely from the CSF of patients with neuroborreliosis.

PCR to detect borrelial DNA is also positive with the same or higher frequency as culture from the skin, blood, and CSF. However, it is most useful in the synovial fluid of patients with suspected and untreated Lyme arthritis where it can be positive in more than 80% of patients despite universally negative cultures. PCR analysis of synovial tissue may be more likely to yield positive results than synovial fluid because *B. burgdorferi* associates with connective tissue. However, because virtually all cases of Lyme arthritis are strongly positive by ELISA and immunoblotting for IgG antibodies to *B. burgdorferi*, the diagnosis can usually be made with reasonable certainty using these tests alone.

Treatment

The goals of treatment of Lyme disease are to resolve the clinical symptoms by eradication of the organism and to prevent late stage disease with early therapy. Although most manifestations resolve spontaneously without treatment, clinical trials demonstrated that treatment with antibiotics hastens resolution and prevents late manifestations of Lyme borreliosis. In most of the trials, treatment of 3 weeks' duration was effective. Generally, early Lyme disease is treated with antimicrobials for 2 to 3 weeks, although studies showed that EM treatment with oral doxycycline for 10 days is as effective as treatment for 20 days. Effective oral medications include doxycycline (Vibramycin),[1] tetracycline, second-generation

---

[1]Not FDA approved for this indication.

CURRENT THERAPY

- Early antibiotic therapy hastens resolution of symptoms and prevents late complications.
- In adults, oral therapy with doxycycline (Vibramycin)[1] is preferred for most features of Lyme disease.
- Neuroborreliosis is usually treated with IV ceftriaxone.
- Duration of therapy is generally 2–4 wk.
- Lyme disease is cured after antibiotic treatment (one or two courses) in most patients.
- Some patients with Lyme arthritis develop persistent antibiotic-resistant synovitis, which may be autoimmune and is treated with antirheumatic drugs.
- Patients with chronic fatigue, arthralgia, and myalgia that begins, persists, or recurs after antibiotic treatment for Lyme disease generally have a post–Lyme disease syndrome and not ongoing infection.
- There is no scientific support for prolonged courses of oral or IV antibiotics for Lyme disease.

[1]Not FDA approved for this indication.
Abbreviation: IV = intravenous.

cephalosporins such as cefuroxime axetil (Ceftin), and amoxicillin (Amoxil).[1] Erythromycin (E-Mycin)[1] and azithromycin (Zithromax)[1] are somewhat less effective. Doxycycline and tetracycline should not be used in children younger than 8 years or in pregnant women. Oral therapy is sufficient for certain clinical features: EM, facial palsy without signs of meningitis, and first-degree heart block. Oral therapy with doxycycline (Vibramycin) is associated with fewer side effects and is much less expensive than the also employed intravenous (IV) therapy with

[1]Not FDA approved for this indication.

ceftriaxone (Rocephin).[1] Although amoxicillin and doxycycline appear to be equally efficacious, doxycycline has the distinct advantage of also being effective in treating *Anaplasma phagocytophila* infection, which causes human granulocytic ehrlichiosis (HGE) and is also transmitted by the Ixodes tick. In general, patients with neurologic manifestations, either early or late, other than isolated facial palsy, are treated de novo with IV ceftriaxone (Rocephin)[1] for 3 to 4 weeks, although aqueous penicillin (Penicillin G)[1] is also effective. Carditis with heart block may resolve spontaneously, but patients with higher grades of heart block and with cardiomyopathy are generally treated with IV antibiotics. If the oral regimen fails, as may occur with 20% of patients, parenteral therapy with ceftriaxone or cefotaxime (Claforan)[1] is warranted. In patients with persistent symptoms, a second parenteral regimen is usually administered. There is no need to change the medication because *B. burgdorferi* does not show resistance to any of the antimicrobials recommended.

Oral and parenteral therapies are both used with success in treating Lyme arthritis with treatment duration of 3 to 4 weeks. Occasionally a second month of treatment is needed to eradicate the organism from the joint. Even with successful treatment, the arthritis may resolve quite slowly with synovitis persisting over several months (Table 1).

PERSISTENT (TREATMENT-RESISTANT) LYME ARTHRITIS

Approximately 10% of patients with Lyme arthritis in the United States are treatment resistant, with recurrent inflammatory effusions, usually in one knee, for months to several years despite appropriate antibiotic therapy.

[1]Not FDA approved for this indication.

TABLE 1 Suggested Treatment of Lyme Disease

| Clinical Features/Indication | Antibiotic regimen | Regimen | | Duration of Therapy |
		Adults	Children	
Early Infection (Local and Disseminated Disease)	Doxycycline (Vibramycin)[1]	100 mg bid	<8 y: not recommended >8 y: 1–2 mg/kg bid; maximum 100 mg	2–3 wk
	Tetracycline[1]	500 mg qid	Not for pregnant women	2–3 wk
	Amoxicillin[1]	500 mg tid	As above	2–3 wk
	Cefuroxime axetil (Ceftin)	500 mg bid	50 mg/kg/d in 3 divided doses	2–3 wk
	Azithromycin (Zithromax)[1]	500 mg daily	30 mg/kg/d in 2 divided doses	7–10 d
	Erythromycin[1]	500 mg qid	50 mg/kg/d	2–3 wk
Neuroborreliosis Failure to Respond to Oral Therapy	Ceftriaxone (Rocephin)[1] Cefotaxime (Claforan)[1]	2 g IV daily	75–100 mg/kg/d	2–4 wk
	Penicillin G[1]	2 g IV tid	90–180 mg/kg/d in 3–4 divided doses	2–4 wk
Carditis	Oral or IV regimen	4–5 million U IV q4h	2–4 million U IV q4 h	2–4 wk
Late Lyme Arthritis	Oral or IV regimen Amoxicillin			2–3 wk
	Penicillin G			3–4 wk
Pregnancy	Ceftriaxone			2–4 wk
	Cefotaxime			

[1]Not FDA approved for this indication.
Abbreviation: IV = intravenous.

This antibiotic-resistant Lyme arthritis is thought to be related to an intra-articular autoimmune response in predisposed individuals. There is no evidence for persistent infection because borrelial DNA by PCR in synovial fluid or synovial tissue is not found in these individuals. A genetic predisposition is suggested by the increased frequency of HLA-DR4 and HLA-DRB1*0401, 0101, and related alleles, similar to that seen in rheumatoid arthritis. In this situation, treatment consists of nonsteroidal anti-inflammatory drugs, intraarticular steroid injections, and antirheumatic agents such as hydroxychloroquine (Plaquenil),[1] sulfasalazine (Azulfidine),[1] and even methotrexate (Rheumatrex).[1] In some cases, arthroscopic synovectomy proves effective. This arthritis usually remits after several years.

POST–LYME DISEASE SYNDROME

Although the long-term prognosis of treated Lyme disease is excellent, some patients develop arthralgia, myalgia, and fatigue, during or soon after infection, which persists despite adequate courses of antibiotics. Other features of this symptom complex include memory and concentration difficulties, neuropathic pains, headache, and unrefreshed sleep. This condition is often called post–Lyme disease syndrome, post-treatment chronic Lyme disease, or chronic Lyme disease. The actual frequency of this condition after Lyme disease is unclear but is likely no more than 5%. Some studies suggested that delay in initiating antibiotic treatment for borrelial infection is more likely to result in post–Lyme disease syndrome. In none of these studies did current serologic status correlate with persistent symptoms. Although these patients have significant somatic complaints and functional disability, they lack objective findings of an inflammatory condition. Although virtually all patients with this syndrome complain of problems with memory and concentration, demonstrable abnormalities on neurocognitive testing are not universally present. The pathogenesis of this chronic post-treatment symptomatic state and its relationship to Lyme disease are unclear. Patients may feel better during antibiotic therapy, but the effect is not durable and relapse is common when antibiotics are discontinued. The symptoms wax and wane, but the overall course is chronic. Controversy has raged as to whether chronic, relatively resistant borrelial infection plays a role and hence whether chronic antibiotic therapy is warranted. However, an important study on post–Lyme syndrome patients failed to document the presence of *B. burgdorferi* in the plasma or spinal fluid of these patients by culture or PCR. In addition, a controlled trial failed to show a response to a 3-month course of antibiotics (1 month of IV ceftriaxone [Rocephin][1] followed by 2 months of oral doxycycline[1]). This suggests that chronic infection is not the cause of post–Lyme disease syndrome, that the condition spontaneously waxes and wanes, and that prolonged antibiotic treatment does not result in long-term symptom remission.

Prevention

The best currently available method for preventing infection with *B. burgdorferi* and other tick-transmitted infections is to avoid tick infested areas through the summer. If exposure is unavoidable, use of protective clothing (shirt tucked into pants and pants tucked under socks) may interfere with attachment by ticks. Wearing light-colored clothing makes it easier to identify ticks. Daily inspection of the entire body to locate and remove ticks also decreases the transmission of infection. Attached ticks should promptly be removed with fine-toothed forceps, if possible. Tick and insect repellent applied to the skin and clothing provides additional protection. The most effective repellent is DEET (diethyltoluamide). Permethrin, a pesticide that kills ticks and mites when applied to clothing, decreases the risk of tick bite. Strategies to reduce the number of ticks may be somewhat effective in decreasing tick-borne illnesses, including the application of acaricides and landscaping to provide desiccating barriers. Although vaccination is available for dogs and a recombinant outer surface protein A (OspA)-based vaccine (LYMErix) is effective and relatively safe in humans, currently no marketed vaccine is available to prevent Lyme disease in humans.

AFTER TICK BITE

It is not recommended to treat all patients after a tick bite because several prospective studies demonstrated that the risk of drug-associated rash is as great as the risk of developing Lyme disease. Conversely, it may be reasonable to treat persons believed to be at higher risk for the development of borrelial infection prophylactically. Studies showed that transmission of *B. burgdorferi* from tick to host occurs with greater frequency when there has been tick attachment for more than 48 hours resulting in a blood-engorged tick. Because a controlled study demonstrated that a single 200-mg dose of doxycycline[1] effectively prevents Lyme disease when given within 72 hours of a tick bite, the threshold for treating patients after tick bites with this benign regimen is lower than in the past.

REFERENCES

Klempner MS, Hu LT, Evans J, et al: Two controlled trials of antibiotic treatment in patients with persistent symptoms and a history of Lyme disease. N Engl J Med 2001;345:85-92.

Nadelman RB, Nowakowski J, Fish D, et al: Prophylaxis with single dose doxycycline for the prevention of Lyme disease after an Ixodes scapularis tick bite. N. Engl J Med 2001;345:79-84.

Recommendations for test performance and interpretation from the Second National Conference on Serologic Diagnosis of Lyme Disease. MMWR 1995;44:590-591.

Steere AC: Lyme disease. N Engl J Med 2001;345:115-125.

Steere AC, Dhar A, Hernandez J, et al: Systemic symptoms without erythema migrans as the presenting picture of early Lyme disease. Am J Med 2003;114:58-62.

Steere AC, Sikand VK, et al: The presenting manifestations of Lyme disease and the outcomes of treatment. N Engl J Med 2003;348:2472-2474.

Treatment of Lyme disease. The Medical Letter 2005;47:41-43.

Tugwell P, Dennis DT, Weinstein A, et al: Clinical guideline 2: Laboratory evaluation in the diagnosis of Lyme disease. Ann Intern Med 1997;127:1109-1123.

Weinstein A, Britchkov M: Lyme arthritis and post-Lyme disease syndrome. Curr Opin Rheum 2002,14:383-387.

Wormser GP, Nadelman RB, Dattwyler RJ, et al: Practice guidelines for the treatment of Lyme disease. The Infectious Disease Society of America. Clin Infect Dis 2000;31(Suppl 1):S1-S14.

Wormser GP, Ramanathan R, Nowakowski J, et al: Duration of antibiotic therapy for early Lyme disease. A randomized, double-blind, placebo-controlled trial. Ann Intern Med 2003;138: 697-704.

[1]Not FDA approved for this indication.

Rubella and Congenital Rubella

Method of
Michael T. Brady, MD

Background and Epidemiology

Rubella is a mild, self-limited viral exanthem with a potential to cause serious disease in the fetus. In 1962, Parkman and Weller first isolated the rubella virus. This was the first step in the development of a live attenuated virus vaccine. The timing of the first isolation of the rubella virus was remarkable because it shortly predated one of the most devastating worldwide pandemics of rubella in 1964–1965. In the United States alone, this pandemic was responsible for more than 12.5 million cases of rubella with more than 20,000 cases of congenital rubella syndrome (11,800 deaf; 3,580 blind; 1,800 mentally retarded; 2,100 neonatal deaths, and 11,250 miscarriages/abortions). The licensure of the first rubella vaccine in 1969 with subsequent improvements in the vaccine (RA 27/3 was licensed in 1979) has resulted in dramatic reductions in rubella cases and congenital rubella in the United States (annual cases of rubella since 2001: 23 in 2001; 18 in 2002; 7 in 2003; and 9 in 2004) and in other countries with successful rubella immunization programs. Unfortunately, many developing nations are yet to benefit from the rubella vaccine where resources are not available to allow universal routine immunizations.

Postnatally acquired rubella is transmitted through direct or droplet contact. The virus is shed primarily in respiratory secretions (nasopharyngeal and to a lesser degree oropharyngeal). Efficient transmission of infection to susceptible persons requires prolonged and intimate contact. Individuals infected with rubella are contagious from a few days before the onset of symptoms (7 days before a rash) until 7 to 14 days after the rash. Children with congenital rubella shed virus from both respiratory secretions and the urine. Children with congenital rubella should be considered to be contagious until 1 year or more of age, unless they have repeated negative virus cultures of the nasopharynx and urine.

Before the widespread use of rubella vaccine, rubella was an epidemic disease occurring in 6- to 9-year cycles. Almost all clinically identified cases occurred in school-age (5-14 years) and preschool-age (1-5 years) children. The peak incidence of rubella infection in the prevaccine era was in late winter and early spring. Since the availability of the rubella vaccine in 1969, widespread rubella outbreaks have been prevented. However, in areas with low levels of vaccine use, low level of rubella transmission occurs year round.

Clinical Manifestation

POSTNATAL RUBELLA

Postnatally acquired rubella, or German measles, has an incubation period of 14 days (range, 12 to 23 days). Following exposure, initial virus replication occurs in the upper respiratory tract with subsequent viremia 5 to 7 days later. Postnatal rubella begins with a prodrome consisting of malaise, headache, low-grade fever, mild conjunctivitis, and lymphadenopathy. The prodrome may be so mild that it goes unnoticed. The rash follows the prodrome. Respiratory tract symptoms, constitutional symptoms, and rash are quite variable in presentation (25% to 50% of individuals with rubella are asymptomatic). Not all individuals who have symptomatic disease with acute rubella infection have a discernible rash. The rash has both scarlatiniform and morbilliform characteristics. Rubella should be suspected in susceptible individuals who develop a fine macular papular rash and lymphadenopathy following a possible rubella exposure. Arthritis, arthralgia, or both occur in up to a third of adolescent and adult women infected with rubella. Thrombocytopenia (1 in 3000 cases), encephalitis (1 in 6000 cases), neuritis, and orchitis occur very rarely. There is very little risk for morbidity or mortality following rubella infection.

CONGENITAL RUBELLA

The greatest risk for morbidity and mortality associated with rubella infection occurs when rubella virus is transmitted to the fetus. This intrauterine infection occurs following maternal viremia or placental infection during the entire gestational period. However, the risk for fetal damage and long-term sequelae is primarily seen following transmission that occurs early in gestation. The risk for the congenital rubella syndrome by gestational age is as follows: first month, 45%; second month, 25%; third month, 15%; fourth month, 10%; and minimal risk during all later months in gestation. Rubella infection in a susceptible mother after the 12th week of gestation is not likely to cause adverse consequences to either the fetus or the mother.

Infection of the fetus may lead to miscarriage, stillbirth, or the congenital rubella syndrome. The newborn with congenital rubella syndrome may be asymptomatic at birth and may subsequently develop clinical manifestations later in life. However, most children who are born with the congenital rubella syndrome exhibit some or many of the following findings: intrauterine growth retardation, petechiae/purpura, mental retardation, anemia, hepatosplenomegaly, congenital heart defect (particularly patent ductus arteriosus and peripheral pulmonary branch stenosis), radiolucent bone disease, cataracts, glaucoma, retinitis, failure to thrive, and occasionally postnatal death. The most common manifestations that may be identified later in life include hypogammaglobinemia, endocrine manifestations (diabetes, thyroiditis, hypothyroidism, and growth hormone deficiency), and progressive panencephalitis. The most significant of the long-term sequelae associated with the congenital rubella syndrome are permanent neurologic sequelae, including microcephaly, behavior problems, developmental delay, and chronic encephalitis.

Medical/Laboratory Diagnosis

Because most rubella infections are asymptomatic or associated with mild nonspecific symptoms, a clinical diagnosis of rubella is difficult, particularly during nonepidemic periods or in nonendemic locations. The rash of rubella has characteristics that are similar to both scarlet fever and measles and may be confused with mild forms of either of these infections. Other infections that need to be included in the differential diagnosis include Epstein-Barr virus (EBV), cytomegalovirus (CMV), roseola infantum (human herpesvirus 6), human herpesvirus 7, erythema infectiosum (parvovirus B19), numerous enteroviral infections, and toxoplasmosis.

Infants with congenital rubella may present with clinical manifestations that are indistinguishable from perinatally acquired CMV and toxoplasmosis. Thrombocytopenia, petechiae/purpura, anemia, hepatomegaly, splenomegaly, retinopathy, bone abnormalities, eighth nerve deafness, and intrauterine growth retardation may be seen with each of these congenital infections. Congenital heart defects, particularly patent ductus arteriosus and pulmonary artery branch stenosis, cataracts, and congenital glaucoma would be more common in the congenital rubella syndrome.

Nonspecific laboratory testing is usually not helpful in the diagnosis of rubella infection whether it be postnatally or perinatally acquired. Therefore, laboratory diagnosis of rubella depends on specific viral diagnostic studies. Rubella virus can be grown in a variety of primary and continuous cell culture lines. Virus isolation from a number of body sites (throat, urine, synovial fluid, amniotic fluid, cerebrospinal fluid) confirms the diagnosis of rubella infection. Virus excretion by individuals with postnatal rubella is transient and occurs from up to 10 days before the onset of symptoms (usually when the rash is noted) until 15 days after the onset of rash. Individuals with congenital rubella infection may excrete virus for many months and even years.

Serology has now become the more convenient and available method for establishing both postnasal and congenital rubella infections. Currently, a number of serologic assays can detect either rubella-specific IgG or rubella-specific IgM antibodies. Acute postnatal rubella infection can be presumed by the demonstration of rubella-specific IgM antibody on a single acute serum. A fourfold rise or seroconversion of rubella antibody (either IgG or IgM) in paired acute and convalescent specimens (minimum of 7 days apart; optimally 14 to 21 days after the acute sera) assayed by the same test in the same laboratory would also establish a diagnosis of acute rubella infection. A single positive rubella-specific IgG antibody merely verifies infection with rubella, either from a past or present infection. Rubella-specific IgM antibody results may be confounded by the fact that a false positive may occur as a result of problems with the assay (poor specificity) or

associated with other clinical conditions such as recent infections with parvovirus B19 or heterophile-positive EBV or persons with positive rheumatoid factor.

Serologic diagnosis of congenital infection with rubella may be established by a positive rubella-specific IgM antibody in the affected newborn (not in cord blood) or persistence of rubella-specific IgG antibodies beyond 9 months of age in an infant with compatible clinical syndrome who has not received the rubella vaccine and who is not from an endemic area. Intrauterine infection with rubella may be detected by the presence of rubella-specific IgM antibody in fetal blood.

Placental biopsy, cordocentesis with detection of rubella RNA by in situ hybridization and polymerase chain reaction (PCR), and detection of rubella antigen with monoclonal antibody are used for the diagnosis of congenital rubella infection.

Treatment and Management

Postnatal rubella is mild and self-limited. Treatment is supportive and usually only indicated for the uncommon occurrence of fever and joint complaints (arthralgia or arthritis). Nonsteroidal anti-inflammatory agents are adequate in most symptomatic patients.

Routine screening of pregnant women with rubella-specific IgG antibodies should be performed at the first prenatal visit. Women who have evidence of rubella-specific IgG antibodies should be considered immune with little risk to their fetus, even following a rubella exposure. Women who lack rubella-specific antibodies at their first prenatal visit should receive the rubella vaccine (Meruvax II) shortly after their delivery. Nonimmune women who are exposed to rubella while pregnant may benefit from passive immunization. Immune seroglobulin (ISG) was evaluated in exposed susceptible pregnant women and found to reduce symptoms in the infected women but did not consistently prevent viremia. Intravenous immunoglobulin (IVIG) theoretically could provide significantly higher levels of rubella-specific antibodies but its ability to prevent viremia needs to be established. Although efficacy is not yet established, IVIG might still be considered in the management of an exposed susceptible pregnant woman in the first 4 months of pregnancy if termination of the pregnancy is not an option.

Prevention

VACCINE

The currently licensed rubella vaccine is a live attenuated rubella strain (RA 27/3) (Meruvax II) prepared in human diploid cell cultures. The vaccine was licensed in the United States in 1979, and it replaced the previous live attenuated vaccine strains (e.g., HPV-77 and Cenderhill). The RA 27/3 vaccine induces an increased and more durable antibody response with fewer side effects than prior rubella vaccines. In the United States, the rubella vaccine is usually administered in combination with measles and mumps as the MMR vaccine (M-M-R-II). Ninety-five percent of persons older than 12 months receiving a single dose of the rubella vaccine develop serologic evidence of rubella immunity.

Available data suggest that one dose of rubella vaccine provides long-term and probably lifelong immunity. However, because there are still a significant number of individuals who did not respond to the first rubella vaccine, the current recommendation for rubella immunization in the United States is a two-dose MMR vaccine schedule (separated by at least 28 days) with the first dose to be given at 12 months of age and the second dose to be given prior to entry to school at 4 to 6 years of age. Adverse reactions following administration of the rubella vaccine occur primarily in susceptible vaccinees. These adverse events are similar to, although less severe than, those of natural rubella. Most frequent adverse events following rubella vaccine include fever, rash, and lymphadenopathy. These occur in 5% to 15% of susceptible individuals who receive the MMR vaccine approximately 5 to 12 days after vaccination. Transient joint complaints (arthralgia or even transient arthritis) may occur 7 to 21 days after vaccination, and these are more common in adult women (approximately 25% of susceptible adult women have these complaints). There does not appear to be any correlation with rubella immunization and development of chronic arthritis. Thrombocytopenia, parotitis, deafness, and encephalopathy are extremely rare events that occur following receipt of rubella vaccine.

Rubella vaccine is contraindicated during pregnancy or for women who are considering pregnancy within 3 months of vaccine administration. From 1971 until 1989, the Centers for Disease Control and Prevention (CDC) monitored 321 known rubella-susceptible pregnant women who had inadvertently been vaccinated with rubella vaccine within 3 months before or up to 3 months after conception (94 received HPV-77 or Cinderhill vaccine; 226 received RA 27/3 vaccine, and one was unknown). None of the 324 offspring had malformations compatible with congenital rubella. However, five infants (three exposed to HPV-77 or Cinderhill and two exposed to RA 27/3) had persistent serologic evidence consistent with subclinical infection. Thus, the current vaccine poses a negligible risk of vaccine-associated malformations (estimated risk is from 0% to 1.2%; 95% confidence levels). Vaccination during or just before pregnancy is normally not an indication for elective abortion.

Individuals with altered immunity (primary or secondary immune deficiency) could be at increased risk for complications following receipt of live virus vaccines. Rubella vaccine is contraindicated in individuals with B-lymphocyte (humoral), T-lymphocyte (cell mediated), and combined (cell mediated and humoral) immunodeficiencies. Children with complement deficiencies, phagocytic function deficiencies, or HIV-infected children who are not severely immunocompromised (immunologic categories 1 or 2) may receive the live rubella vaccine.

Health care workers, child care workers, and college students should be screened for rubella immunity, and those who are found to be susceptible should be vaccinated to prevent possible infection with congenital rubella. All instances of suspected or proven congenital rubella infection should be investigated and reported to local or state health departments or to the CDC.

ISOLATION

For postnatal rubella, droplet precautions in addition to standard precautions are required for 7 days after the onset of the rash. A single (private) room, if available, is preferred, but special air handling and ventilation are not necessary. The door may remain open. Masks are required for droplet precautions if patient contact is within 3 feet of the patient. Gowns and gloves should be worn for patient contacts if required for standard precautions.

Contact precautions are required for infants with or suspected of having congenital rubella. Infants with congenital rubella should be maintained in contact precautions until they are 1 year of age. Repeated negative cultures of the nasopharynx and urine of congenitally infected infants after 3 months of age would suggest that the infant has a low likelihood of transmission.

REFERENCES

Bosma TJ, Corbett KM, Eckstein MB, et al: Use of PCR for prenatal and postnatal diagnosis of congenital rubella. J Clin Microbiol 1995;33:2881-2887.

Centers for Disease Control and Prevention: Revised ACIP recommendations for avoiding pregnancy after receiving rubella-containing vaccine. MMWR 2001;50:1117.

Centers for Disease Control and Prevention: Achievements in Public Health: Elimination of Rubella and Congenital Rubella Syndrome—United States, 1969–2004. MMWR 2005;54:279-282.

Centers for Disease Control and Prevention: Available at www.cdc.gov/ncidod/diseases/submonus/sub_rubella.htm

Cooper LZ, Alford CA: Rubella. In Remington JS, Klein JO (eds): Infectious Diseases of the Fetus and Newborn Infant, 5th ed. Philadelphia, WB Saunders, 2001, pp 347-388.

Frenkel LM, Nielsen K, Garakian A, et al: A search for persistent rubella virus infection in persons with chronic symptoms after rubella and rubella immunization and in patients with juvenile rheumatoid arthritis. Clin Infect Dis 1996;22:287-294.

Reef SE, Frey TK, Theall K, et al: The changing epidemiology of rubella in the 1990s: On the verge of elimination and new challenges for control and prevention. JAMA 2002;287:464.

Report of the Committee on Infectious Diseases. Rubella. 2003 Red Book, 26th ed. Evanston, Ill, American Academy of Pediatrics, 2003, pp 536-541.

World Health Organization. Available at www.who.int/health_topics/rubella/en

Measles (Rubeola)

Method of
Katalin I. Koranyi, MD

Measles is a highly communicable, viral illness that can cause pneumonia, diarrhea, encephalitis, and death. In the United States rubeola was an almost universal infection of childhood until an effective measles vaccine became available. In recent years most cases of measles are imported from other countries. Measles continues to be a major cause of mortality and morbidity of children in the countries where vaccination is unavailable.

Rubeola (measles) virus is antigenically related to canine distemper. It is a member of the genus *Morbillivirus* of the Paramyxovirus family. Measles virus contains six structural proteins and surface envelope glycoproteins. The hemagglutinin (H) protein, the fusion (F) protein, and the surface envelope glycoproteins are important in the development of neutralizing antibodies. Neutralizing antibodies confer lifelong immunity to measles. Measles virus grows well in primary human and monkey kidney cultures. Although monkeys can be infected with measles virus, humans are the only natural hosts.

Epidemiology

The first measles vaccine became available in the United States in 1963, and universal vaccination began in 1965. Previously—the entire cohort of birth, estimated at 3.5 million individuals—usually children got measles. By 1968 the number of cases in the United States fell to 22,231. Since 1986 the number of measles cases increased again with more than 27,000 cases reported in 1990. The administration of a second dose of measles vaccine and high vaccination coverage rate have resulted in steady decline in the incidence of measles since that time, with an all-time low of 100 cases in 1998. Intermittent outbreaks of measles still occur because of the introduction of the virus from endemic regions. The seriousness and the economic impact of contracting measles in unvaccinated individuals traveling abroad is illustrated by the case of one college student exposed to measles while on a trip to India who returned to the United States during his infectious period. The containment effort by his state Department of Public Health was estimated at $142,452.

Pathogenesis

Measles is a highly communicable infection transmitted by aerosolized particles from the respiratory secretions of infected individuals. The measles virus enters the nasopharynx, invades the respiratory epithelium, and replicates in the local lymph nodes. The virus replicates in both local and distant reticuloendothelial sites, with secondary viremia that occurs between 5 and 7 days after infection. This is then followed by active replication of measles virus throughout the body and clinical manifestations of cough, coryza, conjunctivitis, and fever begin. Measles causes hyperplasia of the lymphoid tissues and the formation of multinucleated giant cells, especially in the respiratory tract.

The immune response to measles virus includes both humoral and cellular responses. Neutralizing antibodies confer lifelong immunity to measles. Cellular immune response is important in terminating the clinical symptoms during acute infection. Individuals with cellular immune deficiency will have severe or fatal infection with measles. Transient anergy is characteristic with measles occurring both after infection and vaccination.

Clinical Findings

The incubation period is 8 to 12 days, and individuals are contagious 1 to 2 days before onset of symptoms to 4 days after appearance of the rash. In the hospitalized patient airborne transmission precautions are indicated for 4 days after onset of the rash in the healthy child and for the duration of illness in the immunocompromised host. The initial phase or prodromal period is characterized by fever, conjunctivitis, coryza, and cough. Koplik's spots appear on

CURRENT DIAGNOSIS

Measles
- Prodrome
  - Cough, coryza, conjunctivitis, fever, and Koplik's spots
- Rash
  - Diffuse, erythematous maculopapular
- Leukopenia and lymphopenia
- Measles IgM titer elevated
- Measles IgG paired sera; fourfold rise
- Culture of measles virus from throat, blood, or CSF

Abbreviation: CSF = cerebral spinal fluid.

the buccal mucosa 2 days before the onset of the rash. These tiny bluish spots disappear by the end of the second day of the rash. The rash of measles appears on the third to fourth day after the onset of symptoms. It begins as an erythematous maculopapular eruption at the hairline and behind the earlobes and spreads centrifugally, reaching the hands and feet by the third day. The rash becomes confluent on the face and the upper chest, subsides in approximately 4 days, and is followed by fine desquamation. Other common manifestations of measles include malaise, decreased appetite, and diarrhea. Immunodeficient individuals may have a prolonged course oftentimes complicated by pneumonia. Modified measles, a generally milder disease, may occur in children who have received immunoglobulin after exposure to measles, or in infants who still have maternal measles antibody present.

Otitis media, croup, bronchiolitis, and viral pneumonia (giant cell pneumonia) and secondary bacterial pneumonia are the most common complications. Diarrhea occurring in already malnourished children adds to the morbidity and mortality of measles. Acute encephalomyelitis is a rare but serious complication and has a mortality rate of 15%, with 25% of the survivors suffering permanent neurologic sequelae. Subacute sclerosing panencephalitis (SSPE), a late complication of measles, is a slowly progressing viral infection of the brain characterized by progressive neurologic and intellectual deterioration. Death occurs within 6 months of the onset of symptoms. In children with vitamin A deficiency, corneal ulcerations may cause blindness.

Laboratory Tests

Leukopenia and lymphopenia are hallmarks of infection with measles. An elevated serum measles IgM antibody establishes the diagnosis. Paired sera demonstrating at least a fourfold rise of measles IgG antibody is also diagnostic. Measles virus can be isolated from urine, nasopharyngeal secretions, or blood. Suspected cases of measles must be reported to the local health department.

Treatment

Treatment of measles is mostly supportive. In severe cases of measles in immunocompromised patients,

CURRENT THERAPY

Vitamin A (Aquasol and others)[1]

- Recommended if hospitalized, malnourished, immunodeficient, with ophthalmologic evidence of vitamin A deficiency, malabsorption, or immigrant from areas with high measles mortality
- 6 months to 1 year: 100,000 IU once
- 1 to 2 years: 200,000 IU once

[1]Not FDA approved for this indication.

ribavirin (Virazole)[1] has been used. Vitamin A (Aquasol A)[1] is recommended to all children with measles living in parts of the world where vitamin A deficiency is frequent, or where the case fatality for measles is 1% or greater. In the United States vitamin A[1] is recommended for children between the ages of 6 months and 2 years hospitalized with complicated measles and in children with vitamin A deficiency, malnutrition, or recent immigrants from areas of the world with high mortality rate by measles. Children ages 6 months to 1 year should receive a single dose of 100,000 IU; for children older than 1 year of age, 200,000 IU orally is recommended. In children with ophthalmologic evidence of vitamin A deficiency a second dose is given the following day and again in 4 weeks.

Prevention

Prophylaxis with the administration of immunoglobulin (IGIM, BayGam) can prevent or modify measles when administered within 6 days of exposure. Measles vaccine when given within 3 days of exposure can also prevent or modify the disease. Measles vaccine alone (Attenuvax) or in combinations such as measles, mumps, and rubella virus vaccine (MMR) is safe and effective with a seroconversion rate of 95%. The first dose of MMR is given at or after 12 months of age and the second dose around 4 to 5 years. A new combination vaccine measles-mumps-rubella-varicella (MMRV) (ProQuad) was approved by the FDA in 2005. Measles vaccination is contraindicated in individuals who are significantly immunocompromised. The vaccine is recommended for those affected with HIV but without severe depression of CD4 count. Low-grade fever and a mild rash occur in a small proportion of children several days after immunization. For infants 6 to 11 months of age traveling to areas where measles is endemic, vaccine should be given before travel. These children should receive the MMR vaccine at 12 to 15 months of age and again at 4 to 5 years of age.

REFERENCES

Bellini WJ, Rota JS, Katz RS, et al: Subacute sclerosing panencephalitis: More cases of this fatal disease are prevented by measles immunization than was previously recognized. J Infect Dis 2005:10;1686–1693.
Campbell C, Levin S, Humphreys P, et al: Subacute sclerosing panencephalitis: Results of the Canadian Paediatric Surveillance Program and review of the literature. BMC Pediatr 2005:5;47.

[1]Not FDA approved for this indication.

Cherry JD. Measles virus. In Feigin RD et al (eds.): Textbook of Pediatric Infectious Diseases 5th ed.) pp 2283–2303.
Dayan GH, Ortega-Sanchez IR, LeBaron CW, et al: The cost of containing one case of measles: The economic impact on the public health infrastructure—Iowa, 2004. Pediatrics 2005:1;e1–4.
Yeung LF, Lurie P, Dayan G, et al: A limited measles outbreak in a highly vaccinated US boarding school. Pediatrics 2005:6;1287–1291.

Tetanus

Method of
Ramesh K. Khurana, MD, FAAN, and
James P. Richardson, MD, MPH

Tetanus, one of the oldest and most preventable afflictions of humankind, results from infection by the anaerobic gram-positive organism *Clostridium tetani*. Tetanospasmin, the neurotoxin produced by the organism, blocks spinal and brainstem inhibitory pathways, leading to localized or generalized muscle spasms. It often presents itself as the increased tone of the masseter muscles, or trismus—hence the former name *lockjaw*.

Etiology

The causative organism of tetanus, *C. tetani,* exists as spores that are resistant to boiling for 20 minutes and to disinfectants, and, hence, it is nearly ubiquitous. Spores have been found in animal and human feces, as well as soil, dust, human dwellings, and hospitals. Vegetative cells, however, are susceptible to heat, antiseptics, and several antibiotics.

Epidemiology

Tetanus is a rare disease in the United States, with an annual incidence of approximately 0.02 per 100,000 people. Less than 50 cases are reported to the Centers for Disease Control and Prevention (CDC) each year. However, many cases of tetanus probably go unreported. In recent cases reported to the CDC, 55% of the patients were 20 to 59 years old; 36% were 60 years old and older. There is a slightly higher incidence of tetanus in men, older adults, recent immigrants, and parenteral drug users. Serologic surveys document lower levels of protective antibody levels in older adults, women, Hispanic Americans, and those with lower incomes and educational levels. Untreated, tetanus is usually fatal. Even with treatment, the overall case-fatality rate is greater than 10%, increasing with age to 40% in those older than 60 years in the most recent report from the CDC. It is well worth noting, however, that in the United States since 1989, no deaths have occurred in individuals with current tetanus immunization.

The disease is much more common worldwide because of lower levels of immunization. The World Health Organization (WHO) estimates that in the year 2000, 309,000 people died of tetanus, including 200,000 neonates.

Pathogenesis

Tetanus spores gain entrance to the body through skin injuries. These injuries are often so minor that they do not result in any medical attention (e.g., a prick from a thorn bush or a minor puncture wound). Because *C. tetani* is an obligate anaerobe, the spores will grow only in areas of low oxygen tension, such as occurs with pressure sores, puncture wounds, or gangrene. Reports of tetanus following abortion, animal bites and stings, splinters, and body piercing are documented. The portal of entry in the newborn is usually through the contaminated umbilical stump. Growing or vegetative *C. tetani* organisms produce tetanospasmin, one of the most potent neurotoxins known, which reaches the nervous system via two routes: blood-borne delivery to peripheral nerves and retrograde intraneuronal transport. The toxin exerts its effects on the peripheral nerves, neuromuscular junction, muscle, spinal cord, brainstem, and possibly the hypothalamus.

Tetanospasmin is recognized by high-affinity receptors located on the surface of the peripheral nerve endings, is internalized and retrogradely transported to the neurons in the spinal cord and brainstem. The toxin then migrates transsynaptically to presynaptic terminals and blocks the release of the inhibitory neurotransmitters gamma-aminobutyric acid (GABA) and glycine. Loss of inhibition affects the alpha motor neurons and preganglionic sympathetic neurons, producing muscle spasms and autonomic hyperactivity, respectively. Recovery involves synthesis of new presynaptic components and their transport to the distal axons.

Clinical Presentation

The incubation period of tetanus is usually from 3 days to 3 weeks, but tetanus can occur several months after an injury. Cases with shorter incubation periods and rapid generalization of spasms tend to be the most severe. There are three clinical forms of tetanus based on the site of toxin action and the age of the patient: generalized, localized, and neonatal.

Generalized disease is the most common of the forms (Box 1). Typical presenting complaints include trismus, neck rigidity, stiffness, dysphagia, restlessness, and reflex spasms. Tetanus patients may display risus sardonicus (a characteristic grimace manifested as raised eyebrows and a wrinkled forehead with the corners of the mouth pulled up). Muscle rigidity usually starts with the jaw and facial muscles and then spreads to the trunk (opisthotonos) and extensor muscles of the limbs. Hands and feet are relatively spared. Spasms may occur spontaneously or may be provoked by external stimuli such as noise, touch, lights, and parenteral injections. Tetanic spasms differ from grand mal seizures in that patients with tetanic spasms remain conscious. These spasms affect agonist and antagonist muscle groups together and are extremely painful. Violent paroxysms of generalized spasms may result in fractures, muscle rupture and rhabdomyolysis, and laryngospasm and apnea, both of which preclude ventilation and feeding.

Autonomic dysfunction usually complicates severe cases, occurring some days after spasms. This dysfunction may be one of overactivity or underactivity of the sympathetic and parasympathetic nervous systems. Sympathetic disturbances

may manifest as labile or sustained hypertension, tachycardia, dysrhythmia, peripheral vasoconstriction, profuse sweating, glycosuria, and elevated plasma and urinary catecholamines. Parasympathetic manifestations include profuse salivation, increased bronchial secretions, gastric stasis, and ileus. Hypotension, bradycardia, and cardiac arrest may occur.

Two less common types of tetanus are localized tetanus and cephalic tetanus. Localized tetanus is characterized by painful spasms of muscles near the site of injury. This disorder is usually self-limiting and lasts less than 2 weeks, but progression to generalized disease can occur if untreated. Cephalic tetanus is a frequently severe form of localized tetanus. The bacillus enters through minor head trauma or chronic otitis media. Cephalic tetanus may present as single or multiple, often unilateral, cranial nerve palsies before the development of trismus, dysphagia, dysarthria, head tilt, and possible generalization.

Neonatal tetanus presents as an inability to suck and irritability 3 to 10 days after birth. It is usually a generalized form characterized by muscle rigidity, opisthotonos, apnea, and cyanosis.

Diagnosis

Tetanus is a clinical diagnosis; there is no specific confirmatory laboratory test. A history of a predisposing injury

CURRENT DIAGNOSIS

- The diagnosis is clinical; laboratory tests are not helpful, except in eliminating other diagnoses.
- A history of adequate tetanus immunization makes the diagnosis much less likely.
- Involuntary biting of a spatula because of masseter muscle spasm is highly suggestive.
- Generalized disease is the most common form of tetanus and may present as trismus, neck rigidity, stiffness, dysphagia, restlessness, reflex spasms, and risus sardonicus.

in an inadequately immunized host is helpful. As noted earlier, however, a history of injury is not always present. A well-documented history of primary immunization and a booster immunization within the last 10 years makes the diagnosis of tetanus less likely. The diagnosis is based on the observation of characteristic clinical features. Apte and colleagues, in administering a spatula test to diagnose tetanus, observed that 94% of 359 patients with tetanus involuntarily bit the spatula because of the reflex spasm of masseter muscles, instead of gagging and expelling it. Absence of sensory deficits and a clear sensorium supports the diagnosis of tetanus. Laboratory tests such as complete blood counts and routine blood chemistry tests are not helpful. Creatine kinase may be elevated. Cultures are positive in only 32% to 50% of patients, and, in any event, treatment cannot wait for their completion. Tetanus antitoxin antibody levels are not usually available quickly and are not reliable after the administration of human tetanus immune globulin (HTIG). Electromyography of the involved muscles, or the masseter muscle, shows continuous motor unit discharge. Laboratory tests can, however, be useful in excluding other conditions. For example, a urine screen may be positive in cases of strychnine poisoning.

Established generalized tetanus is easily recognized, whereas the diagnosis of cephalic tetanus can pose some difficulty. Cranial nerve involvement is common and may confuse the physician. Trismus may result from intraoral disease or an acute dystonic reaction to phenothiazines or metoclopramide (Reglan). Muscular stiffness can also be a manifestation of strychnine poisoning, meningitis, hepatic encephalopathy, rabies, hypocalcemic tetani, stiff-man syndrome, and conversion reaction. A delay in the diagnosis of tetanus has occurred in patients presenting with dysphagia. Rigid abdominal muscles may simulate an acute abdomen.

Treatment

Whenever possible, patients with suspected tetanus should be transferred to a facility that has experience with this disease. Patients should be kept in a quiet and dark environment to minimize sensory stimulation. Treatment has the following goals:

- Neutralization of the circulating toxin that has not yet entered the nervous system
- Elimination of the source of the toxin by careful surgical débridement and by antibiotic administration to inhibit growth of the bacilli
- Prevention of respiratory and metabolic complications
- Prevention of muscle spasms
- Management of cardiovascular complications caused by autonomic instability

Tetanus antitoxin should be given to prevent further fixation of the toxin to the central nervous system, although it will not reduce manifestations already present. Between 3000 and 6000 units of HTIG (or Hyper-Tet) should be given intramuscularly as soon as possible and definitely before manipulating the wound. Some authorities recommend giving some of the HTIG near the site of the wound. Tetanus does not confer immunity. Therefore, active immunization with tetanus and diphtheria toxoid (Td)

CURRENT THERAPY

- Tetanus antitoxin[2] and/or human tetanus immune globulin (BayTet) should be given immediately, followed by débridement and appropriate antibiotic therapy (e.g., metronidazole [Flagyl]).
- Tetanus immunization with tetanus and diphtheria toxoid (Td) should also be given.
- Tetanic spasms should be controlled with benzodiazepines.
- Fentanyl (Sublimaze)[1] may help control autonomic cardiovascular instability (manifested as hypertension and tachycardia) by attenuating the sympathetic efferent discharge.
- Supportive care includes protection of the airway, management of fluids and electrolyte balance, nutrition, bowel and bladder functions, skin care, deep venous thrombosis prophylaxis, and physiotherapy.

[1]Not FDA approved for this indication.
[2]Not available in the United States.

or diphtheria toxoid–pertussis vaccine–tetanus toxoid (DPT) or DTaP, as appropriate, also should be given, at a site contralateral from that for tetanus immune globulin (TIG) (Table 1).

Débridement is important for several reasons. It removes live organisms, creates an aerobic environment unfavorable for further growth, and secures specimens for culture. Débridement should be delayed until several hours after the administration of antitoxin because tetanospasmin may be released into the bloodstream. Antibiotic therapy is essential to sterilize the wound and eradicate the bacilli in their vegetative form. The antibiotic of choice is metronidazole (Flagyl), given at a dose of 7.5 mg per kg every 6 hours up to a maximum of 500 mg. Acceptable alternatives are doxycycline (Vibramycin) and imipenem cilastatin (Primaxin).[1] Penicillin, once the drug of choice, should not be used because it acts as a competitive antagonist to GABA and promotes hyperexcitability and convulsions.

[1]Not FDA approved for this indication.

TABLE 1 **Routine Diphtheria and Tetanus Immunization Schedule for Persons 7 Years of Age and Older**

Dose	Age/Interval	Product
Primary 1	First dose	Td
Primary 2	4–8 weeks after the first dose*	Td
Primary 3	6–12 months after second dose*	Td
Boosters	Every 10 years after last dose	Td

*Prolonging the interval does not require restarting series.
Abbreviation: Td = tetanus and diphtheria toxoid.
From Immunization Practices Advisory Committee: Diphtheria, tetanus, and pertussis: Recommendations for vaccine use and other preventive measures-recommendations of the Immunization Practices Advisory Committee (ACIP). MMWR 1991;40(No. RR-10).

Oxygenation is ensured by protecting the airway. In all but the mildest of cases, prophylactic intubation should be initiated early. Intubation will usually require sedation with a benzodiazepine (e.g., lorazepam [Ativan],[1] 2 mg intravenously) and neuromuscular blockade (e.g., vecuronium [Norcuron], 0.08 to 0.1 mg per kg). Patients in whom orotracheal intubation precipitates laryngeal spasms, require more than 10 days of intubation, or have generalized seizures should undergo elective tracheostomy. An oropharyngeal airway will allow removal of secretions and prevent biting in mild cases that do not require intubation.

Control of tetanic spasms and rigidity is best achieved with the benzodiazepines. Additional benefits are that these drugs produce sedation and amnesia. Diazepam (Valium)[1] can be given at a large dose of 0.5 mg per kg to 15 mg per kg per day[3] intravenously. Alternatively, continuous infusions of lorazepam (Ativan) at a dose of 0.1 to 2.0 mg per kg per hour,[3] midazolam (Versed)[1] at a dose of 0.01 to 0.10 mg per kg per hour, or propofol (Diprivan)[1] at a dose of 3.5 to 4.5 mg/kg per hour can be given. The intrathecal administration of baclofen (Lioresal)[1] has been found useful, but it is both costly and invasive.

In patients whose muscle spasms do not respond to sedation, neuromuscular blocking agents, such as vecuronium (Norcuron),[1] are often necessary. The patients will require assisted ventilation, often for several days or weeks. Because neuromuscular agents prevent skeletal muscle movements only and do not reduce pain or provide sedation, it is essential that patients be monitored very closely for adequate pain relief.

Later in the course of the disease, autonomic cardiovascular instability may develop. Both morphine[1] and fentanyl (Sublimaze)[1] may control hypertension and tachycardia by attenuating the sympathetic efferent discharge. Fentanyl (Sublimaze)[1] is considered superior because it does not depress myocardium. Previously used agents phentolamine (Regitine) and metoprolol (Lopressor) for treatment of hypertension and tachycardia are no longer recommended. Hypotension induced by phentolamine may be difficult to reverse, and β-adrenergic blockers may contribute to cardiac failure and high mortality. Hypotension may require monitoring of cardiac output and intravenous fluids or pressor agents. Bradycardia may develop, requiring placement of a pacemaker.

Complications

Supportive care is critical to the prevention of complications. It includes management of fluids and electrolyte balance, nutrition, bowel and bladder functions, skin care, and physiotherapy. Most of the complications are those that are common to immobile patients. Frequent turning of the patient will prevent pressure sores. Low-dose heparin or enoxaparin (Lovenox) should be administered to prevent deep venous thrombosis and formation of pulmonary emboli. Physical therapy should be given as soon as possible to prevent contractures. Orthopedic management may be required for fractures and dislocations resulting from tetanic seizures.

[1]Not FDA approved for this indication.
[3]Exceeds dosage recommended by the manufacturer.

Prognosis

The severity of illness, age of the patient, and the facilities available are the most important factors determining prognosis. In the developing world where mechanical ventilation is unavailable, asphyxia is the most common cause of death. Those who survive the acute phase may succumb to autonomic dysfunction. With expanding facilities for intensive care, most patients eventually make a full recovery over 4 to 6 weeks, but some patients remain hypertonic; some patients remain amnestic for the event, whereas others have unpleasant memories of painful tetanic spasms, physiotherapy to the chest, and tracheal suction. Tracheal stenosis as a sequel to prolonged intubation and tracheostomy is common. It is important that recovering patients complete a primary series of immunizations because having had the disease does not confer immunity (Table 2).

Prevention

Prevention of tetanus through immunization is the key to the elimination of tetanus. It is useful to distinguish between primary and booster immunization. A patient 7 years old or older who has never been immunized requires two additional doses of Td beyond that given when the wound is treated (see Table 2). Wounded patients who have never been immunized may require HTIG (see Table 1). The elderly are particularly susceptible if they have never been immunized or if their immunity has lapsed. The American Academy of Pediatrics now recommends that adolescents 11 to 18 years of age receive a single dose of Tdap (tetanus toxid, reduced diphtheria toxid, acellular pertussis vaccine) for booster immunization

TABLE 2 Guide to Tetanus Prophylaxis in Routine Wound Management

History of Adsorbed Tetanus Toxoid (doses)	Clean, Minor Wounds		All Other Wounds*	
	Td[†]	TIG[†]	Td[†]	TIG[†]
Unknown or <Three[‡]	Yes	No	Yes	Yes
≥Three[‡]	No[§]	No	No[‖]	No

*Such as, but not limited to, wounds contaminated from dirt, feces, soil, saliva; puncture wounds; avulsions; and wounds resulting from missiles, crushing, burns, or frostbite.
[†]For children under 7 years old, DTaP, DTP, or DT if pertussis vaccine is contraindicated is preferred to TT alone. For persons 7 years of age and older, Td is preferred to TT alone.
[‡]If only three doses of fluid toxoid have been received, a fourth dose of toxoid, preferably an adsorbed dose, should be given.
[§]Yes, if more than 10 years since last dose.
[‖]Yes, if more than 5 years since last dose. (More frequent boosters are not needed and can accentuate side effects.)
Abbreviations: DT = pediatric diphtheria and tetanus toxoid; DTaP = diphtheria and tetanus toxoid and acellular pertussis vaccine; DTP = diphtheria and tetanus toxoid and whole-cell pertussis vaccine; Td = tetanus and diphtheria toxoid; TIG = tetanus immune globulin; TT = tetanus toxoid.
From Immunization Practices Advisory Committee: Diphtheria, tetanus, and pertussis: Recommendations for vaccine use and other preventive measures—recommendations of the Immunization Practices Advisory Committee (ACIP). MMWR 1991;40(No. RR-10).

to prevent pertussis (in addition to tetanus and diphtheria) in this population. Those adolescents who have received Td but not Tdap should receive a single dose of Tdap after a suggested interval of at least 5 years to reduce the risk of adverse reactions.

Physicians should use a case-finding approach to increase tetanus immunization rates. System changes (such as clinical pathways that allow immunization without a physician's order) are the most effective means of increasing immunization rates. Reminders placed at physicians' desks or computer-generated reminders attached to charts or patients' bills have also increased immunization rates. Td should be given whenever tetanus immunization is necessary to ensure immunity to diphtheria as well as to tetanus.

Td is a safe vaccine. Adverse reactions consist primarily of local edema, tenderness, and fever. Anaphylactoid reactions are rare. Most adverse reactions occur in persons with evidence of hyperimmunization. The only contraindications of Td are a history of a neurologic sequela or a severe hypersensitivity reaction following a previous dose.

To reduce neonatal tetanus and protect the mother, pregnant women who are due for a booster should receive Td, preferably during the last two trimesters. HTIG should be given to pregnant women only when clearly indicated. The WHO recommends that women attending prenatal clinics in developing countries be given two doses:

- During the first pregnancy
- In the third trimester at least 4 weeks before delivery

These should be followed by one dose in each subsequent pregnancy, up to a total of five doses. Needless to say, promoting clean delivery and hygienic cord care practices constitutes a key element in the prevention of neonatal tetanus.

REFERENCES

Apte NM, Karnad DR: Short report: The spatula test: A simple bedside test to diagnose tetanus. Am J Trop Med Hyg 1995;53(4):386-387.

Borgeat A, Popovic V, Schwander D: Efficiency of a continuous infusion of propofol in a patient with tetanus. Critical Care Medicine 1991; 19(2):295-297.

Committee on Infectious Diseases. Prevention of pertussis among adolescents: recommendations for use of tetanus toxoid, reduced diphtheria toxoid, and acellular pertussis (Tdap). Pediatrics 2006;117:965-978.

Cook TM, Protheroe RT, Handel JM. Tetanus: A review of the literature. Br J Anaesth 2001;87(3):477-487.

Farrar JJ, Yen LM, Cook T, et al: Tetanus. J Neurol Neurosurg Psychiatry 2000;69:292-301.

Hsu SS, Groleau G. Tetanus in the emergency department: A current review. J Emerg Med 2001;20(4):357-365.

Moughabghab AV, Prevost G, Socolovsky C: Fentanyl therapy controls autonomic hyperactivity in tetanus. Br J Clin Practice 1996; 50(8):477-478.

Pascual FB, McGinley EL, Zanardi LR, et al: Tetanus surveillance—United States, 1998-2000. MMWR 2003;52(No. SS-3):1-8.

Richardson, JP, Knight AL: The management and prevention of tetanus. J Emerg Med 1993;11:737-742.

Schon F, O'Dowd L, White J, Begg N: Tetanus: Delay in diagnosis in England and Wales. J Neurol Neurosurg Psychiat 1994;57: 1006-1007.

Vandelaer J. Birmingham M, Gasse F, et al: Tetanus in developing countries: An update on the maternal and neonatal tetanus elimination initiative. Vaccine 2003;21:3442-3445.

Pertussis

Method of
Michael E. Pichichero, MD

Pertussis, or whooping cough, is a highly contagious acute respiratory tract infection caused by *Bordetella pertussis*. It causes prolonged cough illness, without associated fever, characterized by paroxysms of coughing, inspiratory "whoops," and post-tussive vomiting in severe cases and persistent intermittent staccato cough episodes in teenagers and adults. The incidence of pertussis is rising in the United States despite record-high vaccination coverage. In 2004, more cases occurred in adolescents and in adults than children.

Microbiology and Pathophysiology

B. pertussis is a gram-negative coccobacillus that is difficult to grow with standard media. *B. pertussis* does not invade the human host; bacteremia does not occur. The systemic effects of illness are produced by the organism's toxins, especially pertussis toxin. *B. pertussis* attaches to the nasopharynx and tracheobronchial tree with adhesins such as fimbriae, filamentous hemagglutinin, and pertactin where it produces toxins such as pertussis toxin, adenylate cyclase toxin, and tracheal cytotoxin that paralyze the respiratory cilia, resulting in inflammation of the respiratory tract.

Epidemiology

B. pertussis is a human pathogen transmitted from person to person via aerosolized droplets. Pertussis is highly contagious, similar to varicella, infecting 80% to 90% of susceptible contacts. Persons with pertussis are most contagious in the 2 weeks before cough onset and during the first 2 weeks of cough, typically a time frame before medical care is sought or clinicians consider the possibility of the diagnosis.

In 2004, approximately 20,000 cases of pertussis were reported to the Centers for Disease Control and Prevention (CDC); because substantial underreporting is a recognized problem, current estimates of true pertussis incidence per year in the United States probably is in the range of 1 to 3 million cases. A new development is the recognition that pertussis is a disease of adolescents and adults as well as children. Several studies showed that among teenagers and adults who seek care for cough illness of more than 1 week duration, approximately 20% have pertussis.

Immunity

It has been known for decades that immunity to tetanus wanes over time and boosters are needed approximately every 10 years to sustain protective antibody levels. The phenomenon of waning immunity to pertussis is a newer observation and one of the explanations of the rising incidence of pertussis in the United States. Apparently boosters of pertussis vaccines are also needed, perhaps, like tetanus, approximately every 10 years. Two new adolescent/adult pertussis vaccine formulations that are combined with tetanus and diphtheria vaccines (Boostrix, Adacel) were licensed and recommended for universal use in 2005 to address this problem.

Clinical Symptoms

Classic pertussis is a 30- to 90-day illness that presents in three stages: catarrhal, paroxysmal, and convalescent. The stages may be shorter in immunized children, adolescents, and adults. Pertussis is most severe when it occurs during the first 6 months of life.

In the catarrhal stage, nonspecific symptoms similar to the common cold predominate. The paroxysmal stage is characterized by a persistent cough, sometimes with bursts of numerous rapid coughs. A long inspiratory effort sometimes causes a high-pitched whoop. Typically, the patient is afebrile and, between coughing attacks, usually appears normal. The paroxysmal stage usually lasts 6 weeks. The cough gradually lessens over 2 to 3 weeks during the convalescent period. Milder paroxysms may recur with subsequent respiratory infections for many months following a pertussis infection. Infants may appear very ill and distressed during the paroxysmal stage and require close observation and supportive care. Older children, adolescents, and adults have a prolonged cough with paroxysms but no whoop.

Complications

Complications occur most commonly among young infants with pertussis. The most common complication is secondary bacterial pneumonia. Hypoxia or effects of pertussis toxin may contribute to neurologic complications including seizures and encephalopathy. In the United States, 90% of deaths occur in children younger than 6 months. Complications from pertussis in adolescents and adults are not uncommon (Table 1).

Diagnosis

A clinical diagnosis of pertussis is typically made based on the characteristic cough, although patients are often seen several times before the correct diagnosis is considered. Absolute lymphocytosis (>10,000 lymphcytes/mm^3) may be seen during the late catarrhal and paroxysmal stages but is less common among adults and immunized children. Chest radiographs may show peribronchial consolidation, interstitial edema, or variable atelectasis. The presence of

TABLE 1 Complications from Pertussis in Adolescents and Adults

Symptoms/Signs	Minnesota	Massachusetts	
		Adolescents	Adults
Paroxysmal cough	100%	85%	87%
Whooping	26%	30%	35%
Post-tussive emesis	56%	45%	41%
Apnea	—	19%	37%
Cyanosis	—	6%	9%
Hospitalization	0%	1.4%	3.5%

fever and consolidation with pertussis suggests a secondary bacterial pneumonia.

Isolation of *B. pertussis* from a culture of nasal secretions remains the gold standard for laboratory diagnosis. A nasopharyngeal specimen is obtained by inserting a small flexible Dacron or calcium alginate swab through the nose to the posterior nasopharynx (attempting to touch the adenoids) where it is held for a few seconds, perhaps inducing a cough. The specimen is transferred to *Bordetella*-specific transport media and subsequently plated on Regan-Lowe charcoal agar or Stainer-Scholte agar. Cultures are usually positive if obtained in the catarrhal or early paroxysmal stage of disease. Success in isolating *B. pertussis* diminishes if patients have received pertussis vaccine or recent antimicrobials or if specimens are obtained beyond the first 2 weeks of cough.

Polymerase chain reaction (PCR) is more sensitive among persons with mild or atypical symptoms and those who have received prior antimicrobial therapy. The CDC recommends using PCR as a presumptive assay in conjunction with culture. Direct fluorescent antibody (DFA) testing has a low sensitivity and variable specificity, requiring experienced laboratory personnel for consistent results. DFA testing should only be performed as a adjunct to culture or PCR. Serologic testing methods have recently emerged as a very valuable diagnostic tool. Single samples of 100 μL of blood can be used to measure pertussis antibodies that are compared to age-specific standards to confirm a clinical diagnosis. These methods are not widely available in hospitals or private laboratories, but state laboratories often can provide this testing.

Treatment

Infants and children with severe cough paroxysms associated with cyanosis or apnea require hospitalization and intensive care. Infants younger than 3 months should be

CURRENT DIAGNOSIS

- An illness marked by a staccato cough lasting >7 d in the absence of fever in an adolescent or adult may be pertussis.

CURRENT THERAPY

- Early treatment of pertussis not only eliminates contagion, it also shortens the illness.
- Macrolides are the treatment of choice; azithromycin (Zithromax) is preferred for ease of dosing, tolerability, and short duration of treatment.

TABLE 2 Licensed Vaccines for the Prevention of Pertussis in Infants, Children, Adolescents, and Adults

Indicated Age Group	Sanofi Pasteur Tripedia infants/children[†]	GlaxoSmithKline Infanrix* infants/children[†]	Sanofi Pasteur Daptacel infants/children[†]	GlaxoSmithKline Boostrix adolescents[‡]	Sanofi Pasteur Adacel adults/adolescents[‡]
Antigens					
PT (µg)	23.4	25	10	8	2.5
FHA (µg)	23.4	25	5	8	5
PRN (µg)	—	8	3	2.5	3
FIM 2 + 3 (µg)	—	—	5	—	5
D (Lf)	6.7	25	15	2.5	2
T (Lf)	5	10	5	5	5

*PEDIARIX also contains these DTaP components.
†6 wk to <7 y.
‡Boostrix is indicated for 10–18 y; Adacel is indicated for 11–54 y.
Abbreviations: D = diphtheria toxoid; FHA = filamentous hemagglutinin; FIM 2 + 3 = fimbrial agglutinogen 2 and 3; PRN = pertactin; PT = pertussis toxoid;
   T = tetanus toxoid.

admitted routinely for observation of their paroxysmal episodes, their need for supportive interventions, and their ability to feed appropriately. Continuous monitoring of heart rate, respiratory rate, and oxygen saturation is indicated.

All patients should receive antibiotics. Macrolides are the treatment of choice: erythromycin, clarithromycin (Biaxin),[1] azithromycin (Zithromax),[1] or telithromycin (Ketek).[1] Fluoroquinolones are also effective therapy for pertussis. Trimethoprim-sulfamethoxazole (Bactrim)[1] is an alternative choice although less effective.

Prevention

Pertussis is a preventable disease by vaccination. Vaccines are available and recommended for universal use in infants, children, adolescents, and selected adult populations (health care workers, adults caring for infants younger than 6 months, and those with chronic respiratory conditions, e.g., chronic obstructive pulmonary disease). Table 2 lists the vaccines licensed in the United States.

REFERENCES

Farizo KM, Cochi SL, Zell ER, et al: Epidemiological features of pertussis in the United States, 1980–1989. Clin Infect Dis 1992;14(3):708-719.

Lee LH, Pichichero ME. Costs of illness due to *Bordetella pertussis* in families. Arch Fam Med 2000;9(10):989-996.

Pichichero ME, Rennels MB, Edwards KM, et al: Combined tetanus, diphtheria, and 5-component pertussis vaccine for use in adolescents and adults. JAMA 2005;293(24):3003-3011.

Purdy KW, Hay JW, Botteman MF, et al: Evaluation of strategies for use of acellular pertussis vaccine in adolescents and adults: A cost-benefit analysis. Clin Infect Dis 2004;39:20-28.

Skowronski DM, De Serres G, MacDonald D, et al: The changing age and seasonal profile of pertussis in Canada. J Infect Dis 2002;185(10): 1448-1453. Epub 2002 Apr 22.

Strebel P, Nordin J, Edwards K, et al: Population-based incidence of pertussis among adolescents and adults, Minnesota, 1995–1996. J Infect Dis 2001;183(9):1353-1359. Epub 2001 Mar 30.

Yih WK, Lett SM, des Vignes FN, et al: The increasing incidence of pertussis in Massachusetts adolescents and adults, 1989–1998. J Infect Dis 2000;182(5):1409-1416. Epub 2000 Oct 09.

[1]Not FDA approved for this indication.

Office-Based Immunization Practices

Method of
Robert M. Jacobson, MD

Routine immunizations represent the cutting edge for consensus-driven, evidence-based practice guidelines in the care of children and adults. Perhaps no other office-based task is so universally accepted and practiced as well as evidenced as immunizations. We should be modeling the rest of our practices on the success that we have enjoyed with immunizations.

That is not to say that we are providing immunizations as well as we should; the practice of immunization is difficult, complex, and evolving. Other chapters deal with the specific diseases to which we direct our vaccines. Office practitioners must consider a variety of aspects that go beyond the understanding of the individual vaccine-preventable diseases. These include the adoption of a comprehensive immunization schedule, using a number of immunization-specific practices, and the understanding of common problems associated with immunization in the office.

The Adoption of a Comprehensive Immunization Schedule

In recent years, we have benefited from efforts made at the national level to harmonize and systematically update recommended schedules for routine immunizations.

CURRENT DIAGNOSIS

- At each patient contact, practitioners should review the patient's immunization record for vaccines due and overdue.

The Advisory Committee on Immunization Practices (ACIP), sponsored by the Centers for Disease Control and Prevention (CDC), works closely with the American Academy of Pediatrics (AAP) and the American Academy of Family Physicians (AAFP) to publish a single set of recommendations for routine immunizations for infants, children, and adolescents younger than 18 years. The Recommended Adult Immunization Schedule is similarly approved by the ACIP, the American College of Obstetricians and Gynecologists (ACOG), and the AAFP. These are published widely in a number of journals as well as on the Internet. The harmonized schedules address the use of both individual vaccine components as well as all licensed combinations species vaccines. The vaccine schedules give ranges of target age ranges for immunization rather than prescribe individual ages. For example, the measles-mumps-rubella combination is to be given from 12 to 15 months of life rather than either 12 months or 15 months. Furthermore, the pediatric schedule includes catch-up schedules for children who did not receive immunizations at the recommended ages. The adult schedule includes common conditions with vaccine-specific recommendations (such as for pregnancy).

Each of the 50 states in the United States has specific immunization requirements for day care, school, and even college attendance. These vary state by state and in some states affect not only initial enrollment but also continued participation in schools. Furthermore, the harmonized schedule mentioned previously has state-specific recommendations for the hepatitis A vaccine recommended for 11 of the 50 states where endemic rates of hepatitis A disease occur at more than 20 cases per 100,000 people.

For your office practice, you are encouraged to adopt a more specific schedule. For example, where the harmonized schedule might give you some latitude with what age to give the dose for the measles-mumps-rubella vaccine, it would be more appropriate for you and your colleagues to pick either 12 or 15 months. When all practitioners sharing an office adopt a uniform practice, they prevent parental and staff confusion and misunderstanding as well as mistakes in vaccine administration and patient scheduling.

Adoption of Immunization-Specific Practices

EDUCATION OF SELF AND STAFF

Immunization practices certainly have evolved over the last century, and much of the development has accelerated since the enactment of the National Childhood Vaccine Injury Act of 1986 (PL 99-660), which established the national Vaccine Injury Compensation Program (VICP),

a no-fault alternative to the tort system for resolving vaccine injury claims. This legislation protects vaccine providers and manufacturers from frivolous lawsuits directed against routine childhood immunization. Although in the 1980s it was routine for a child in the first year of life to receive three injections and three oral doses of polio, now the typical infant at 12 months of age may receive 20 separate injections against vaccine-preventable disease. In 2005, two new vaccines were added to the routine childhood schedule: the meningococcal conjugated vaccine (Menactra) and the tetanus-diphtheria-reduced-dose-acellular pertussis (Tdap) vaccine (Boostrix) that replaces the adolescent tetanus-diphtheria (Td) vaccine. Both are to be given routinely at 11 years of age. Such changes require a practitioner's continuing education and practice advancement.

A number of electronic Web sites provide announcements and updates of vaccines in form delivered for health care practitioners; the CDC's National Immunization Program (NIP) provides a Web site (www.cdc.gov/nip) with information resources for both parents and health care practitioners including sections on updates. In addition, the Immunization Action Coalition, a not-for-profit group dedicated to the dissemination of scientifically correct immunization information, also has a very useful Web site (www.immunize.org). The latter invites practitioners to sign up for routine mailings of updates on immunization practices. Similarly, providers can access the CDC's Morbidity and Mortality Weekly Report (MMWR) online. These provide updates and statements from ACIP. Furthermore, the AAP publishes on its Web site (www.pediatrics.org) its policy statements and recommendation online for members and nonmembers alike.

Paper-based resources are more difficult to keep up to date, but important ones include the paper-based publication *MMWR* published by the CDC and the *Red Book* published by the AAP. The *Red Book* not only does an outstanding job with vaccine-related issues but also includes a host of information for a general practitioner on pediatric and adolescent infectious diseases. The CDC publishes the "Pink Book" both in paper and online. It is formally entitled *Epidemiology and Prevention of Vaccine Preventable Diseases*.

The CDC's NIP and the Medical University of South Carolina have sponsored the development of an electronic-based educational program called Teaching Immunization Delivery and Evaluation (TIDE). Its Web site is http://www2.edserv.musc.edu/tide/menu.lasso, and the program is endorsed by the Ambulatory Pediatric Association and the Society of Adolescent Medicine. It is a flexible tool to teach immunization delivery, and it uses clinical scenarios that inspire problem solving. Self-contained modules are available that provide continued education credit.

ASSESSMENT OF INDIVIDUAL NEEDS

Each patient is unique, but the success of the routine immunization schedule depends on its universality. Precautions and contraindications exist, and the children and adults who most frequently attend health care providers' offices have relatively higher rates of chronic conditions than the general population. These conditions raise questions of contraindications and precautions. Therefore, individuals must be assessed for their individual needs. Even misperceptions of contraindications can lead to delays and require

CURRENT THERAPY

- Providing routine immunizations requires a practice to organize its educational activities, practice standards, communication methods, and documentation strategies.

catch-up. Practitioners should be familiar with the routine schedules (Tables 1 and 2) as well as the general precautions of contraindications associated with each vaccine.

One of the most important resources available for the busy practitioner is a chart developed by NIP organized by condition that specifies which vaccines are contraindicated by that condition. This chart is on the NIP Web site under the tab of Healthcare Professionals. It is entitled "Guide to Contraindications" (http://www.cdc.gov/nip/recs/contraindications_vacc.htm).

The NIP has developed survey tools that are available freely to download from its Web site (www.cdc.gov/nip). The practitioner can use this with the individual patient to assess vaccine needs. Assessment tools are available online for both adults and children.

PATIENT EDUCATION

Patient and parent education is incredibly important in applying immunizations. After all, we are giving a form of a biologic with known rates and associations with adverse events to large numbers of persons who are often well and without a medical need or condition. We should inform the patient, and, in the case of a child or adolescent not yet at the age of majority, the parent as best we can about the immunizations, the diseases for which we are vaccinating, the nature of the benefits from the vaccines, as well as the common adverse reactions and possible severe adverse reactions that might occur. The patients and parents should learn for whom the vaccines should be received as well as for whom the vaccines not be received and what they should do in case of an adverse event. This information is complex in depth and breadth, but the National Childhood Vaccine Injury Act of 1986 that created protection for vaccine providers and manufacturers at the same time created regulations with a uniform system of vaccine information statements to be provided. The National Immunization Program publishes brief vaccine-specific statements for all of the routine vaccines given to children and adults. These Vaccine Information Statements (VISs) are published in a highly readable format (www.cdc.gov/nip) and are required by U.S. law to be provided to the parent and recipient before each dose of certain vaccines including those on a routine childhood vaccine schedule. VISs also exist for some of the more exotic vaccines, such as the Japanese encephalitis vaccine, the smallpox vaccine, the typhoid vaccines, the yellow fever vaccine, as well as for the rabies vaccines. The Immunization Action Coalition (www.immunize.org) has partnered with the CDC and has translated the VISs for each vaccine into more than 20 different languages. More detailed information for the vaccines can be obtained from the statements from the ACIP (www.cdc.gov/nip/publications/acip-list.htm), the Food and Drug Administration–approved package inserts, and the AAP's *Red Book*.

PREVACCINATION PREPARATION

Not only should the parent and recipient of the vaccine be provided the VIS, but efforts should be taken to minimize the discomfort of the recipient. Information plays a large role. A study done at the Mayo Clinic demonstrated that informing the child prior to the visit actually decreased the amount of distress observed at the time of the visit.

Furthermore, efforts at the time of the visit including distraction or relaxation techniques can prevent or reduce distress associated with the vaccine. Office staff should learn methods of successful communication, distraction, and relaxation techniques to facilitate routine immunizations.

For some of the vaccines, antipyretics such as acetaminophen (Tylenol) or ibuprofen (Advil) might be administered at the time of immunization and then at regular intervals specific to that drug for the following 24 hours to reduce the occurrence and the severity of fever as well as the local injection pain that might occur with immunization.

The *Red Book* Committee, the Committee on Infectious Diseases of the AAP, recommends that practitioners consider a variety of efforts to minimize the discomfort of immunization including specific injection techniques, the use of multiple vaccinators to immunize simultaneously rather than serially, as well as possible local anesthetics and nonpharmacologic agents.

VACCINE DELIVERY

Vaccines may be given intramuscularly (IM) or subcutaneously (SC); for some travel conditions, oral vaccines exist. IM vaccines should be given deep into a muscle mass. Practitioners should use the anterolateral thigh muscle injections for children younger than 18 months and then move to the deltoid muscle in children older than 18 months when the muscle mass of the deltoid is large enough. SC injections should be given in subcutaneous fat of the anterolateral thigh or triceps with a shorter needle inserted at an angle.

PREVENTION OF NEEDLE INJURY

For the safety of the patient, parent, and provider, efforts should be made to minimize the exposure to an accidental needle stick. Although the risk of accidental inoculation with the patient's blood is minimal in immunization, as with the use of sharps in any office, employees should examine the safety needles available and choose a safety needle appropriate for minimizing accidental needle sticks. The office should provide a child-proof sharps container that allows for rapid disposal of the needle with a minimal amount of effort. The container should be checked regularly for function and emptied frequently to avoid overfilling during the workday.

DOCUMENTATION AND RECORDS

All offices should adopt a standard of documentation of immunizations. The physician's or nurse's order for a vaccine should not be used in place of documentation that the vaccine was given. Documentation of the vaccine administered should include the species and the brand name given as well as the lot number. The patient record should also include the location, date, and time. Such a record would be made more useful if all the vaccine-antigens could be viewed at once with regard to series and dates. To best manage combinations currently available as well as future possibilities, the record should be organized by vaccine-antigen and not common vaccine combinations. This requires that a combination vaccine then appear in several antigen categories. Furthermore, the record would be enhanced by clarification when vaccines were

Text continues on p. 179

TABLE 1 Recommended Childhood and Adolescent Immunization Schedule

DEPARTMENT OF HEALTH AND HUMAN SERVICES • CENTERS FOR DISEASE CONTROL AND PREVENTION
RECOMMENDED CHILDHOOD AND ADOLESCENT IMMUNIZATION SCHEDULE • UNITED STATES • 2006

Vaccine ▸ Age	Birth	1 month	2 months	4 months	6 months	12 months	15 months	18 months	24 months	4–6 years	11–12 years	13–18 years
Hepatitis B[1]	HepB	HepB	HepB	HepB[1]		HepB	HepB				HepB Series	
Diphtheria, tetanus, pertussis[2]			DTaP	DTaP	DTaP		DTaP	DTaP		DTaP	Tdap	Tdap
Haemophilus influenzae type b[3]			Hib	Hib	Hib[3]	Hib	Hib					
Inactivated poliovirus			IPV	IPV	IPV	IPV	IPV	IPV		IPV		
Measles, mumps, rubella[4]						MMR	MMR			MMR	MMR	MMR
Varicella[5]						Varicella	Varicella	Varicella	Varicella	Varicella	Varicella	Varicella
Meningococcal[6]									MPSV4		MCV4	MCV4
Pneumococcal[7]			PCV	PCV	PCV	PCV	PCV	PCV	PCV	PCV / PPV	PPV	
Influenza[8]					Influenza (Yearly)	Influenza (Yearly)	Influenza (Yearly)			Influenza (Yearly)	Influenza (Yearly)	Influenza (Yearly)
Hepatitis A[9]									HepA Series	HepA Series	HepA Series	HepA Series

Vaccines within broken line are for selected populations.

Legend: ▨ Range of recommended ages   ▨ Catch-up immunization   ▨ 11–12 year old assessment

This schedule indicates the recommended ages for routine administration of currently licensed childhood vaccines, as of December 1, 2005, for children through age 18 years. Any dose not given at the recommended age should be given at any subsequent visit when indicated and feasible. ▨ Indicates age groups that warrant special effort to administer those vaccines not previously given. Additional vaccines may be licensed and recommended during the year. Licensed combination vaccines may be used whenever any components of the combination are indicated and the vaccine's other components are not contraindicated and if approved by the Food and Drug Administration for that dose of the series. Providers should consult the respective ACIP statement for detailed recommendations. Clinically significant adverse events that follow immunization should be reported to the Vaccine Adverse Event Reporting System (VAERS). Guidance about how to obtain and complete a VAERS form is available at **www.vaers.hhs.gov** or by telephone, **800-822-7967**.

The Childhood and Adolescent Immunization Schedule is approved by:

Advisory Committee on Immunization Practices www.cdc.gov/nip/acip • American Academy of Pediatrics www.aap.org • American Academy of Family Physicians www.aafp.org

Footnotes
Recommended Childhood and Adolescent Immunization Schedule
United States • 2006

1. **Hepatitis B vaccine (HepB).** *AT BIRTH:* **All newborns** should receive monovalent HepB soon after birth and before hospital discharge. **Infants born to mothers who are HBsAg-positive** should receive HepB and 0.5 mL of hepatitis B immune globulin (HBIG) within 12 hours of birth. **Infants born to mothers whose HBsAg status is unknown** should receive HepB within 12 hours of birth. The mother should have blood drawn as soon as possible to determine her HBsAg status; if HBsAg-positive, the infant should receive HBIG as soon as possible (no later than age 1 week). **For infants born to HBsAg-negative mothers,** the birth dose can be delayed in rare circumstances but only if a physician's order to withhold the vaccine and a copy of the mother's original HBsAg-negative laboratory report are documented in the infant's medical record. *FOLLOWING THE BIRTHDOSE:* The HepB series should be completed with either monovalent HepB or a combination vaccine containing HepB. The second dose should be administered at age 1–2 months. The final dose should be administered at age ≥24 weeks. It is permissible to administer 4 doses of HepB (e.g., when combination vaccines are given after the birth dose); however, if monovalent HepB is used, a dose at age 4 months is not needed. **Infants born to HBsAg-positive mothers** should be tested for HBsAg and antibody to HBsAg after completion of the HepB series, at age 9–18 months (generally at the next well-child visit after completion of the vaccine series).

2. **Diphtheria and tetanus toxoids and acellular pertussis (DTaP) vaccine.** The fourth dose of DTaP may be administered as early as age 12 months, provided 6 months have elapsed since the third dose and the child is unlikely to return at age 15–18 months. The final dose in the series should be given at age ≥4 years. **Tetanus and diphtheria toxoids and acellular pertussis vaccine (Tdap – adolescent preparation)** is recommended at age 11–12 years for those who have completed the recommended childhood DTP/DTaP vaccination series and have not received a Td booster dose. Adolescents 13–18 years who missed the 11–12-year Td/Tdap booster dose should also receive a single dose of Tdap if they have completed the recommended childhood DTP/DTaP vaccination series. Subsequent **tetanus and diphtheria toxoids (Td)** are recommended every 10 years.

3. *Haemophilus influenzae type b conjugate vaccine (Hib).* Three Hib conjugate vaccines are licensed for infant use. If PRP-OMP (PedvaxHIB or ComVax [Merck]) is administered at ages 2 and 4 months, a dose at age 6 months is not required. DTaP/Hib combination products should not be used for primary immunization in infants at ages 2, 4 or 6 months but can be used as boosters following any Hib vaccine. The final dose in the series should be given at age ≥12 months.

4. **Measles, mumps, and rubella vaccine (MMR).** The second dose of MMR is recommended routinely at age 4–6 years but may be administered during any visit, provided at least 4 weeks have elapsed since the first dose and both doses are administered beginning at or after age 12 months. Those who have not previously received the second dose should complete the schedule by the visit at age 11–12 years.

5. **Varicella vaccine.** Varicella vaccine is recommended at any visit at or after age 12 months for susceptible children (i.e., those who lack a reliable history of chickenpox). Susceptible persons aged ≥13 years should receive 2 doses, given at least 4 weeks apart.

6. **Meningococcal vaccine (MCV4).** Meningococcal conjugate vaccine (MCV4) should be given to all children at the 11–12 year old visit as well as to unvaccinated adolescents at high school entry (15 years of age). Other adolescents who wish to decrease their risk for meningococcal disease may also be vaccinated. All college freshmen living in dormitories should also be vaccinated, preferably with MCV4, although **meningococcal polysaccharide vaccine (MPSV4)** is an acceptable alternative. Vaccination against invasive meningococcal disease is recommended for children and adolescents aged ≥2 years with terminal complement deficiencies or anatomic or functional asplenia and certain other high risk groups (see *MMWR* 2005;54 [RR-7];1-21); use MPSV4 for children aged 2–10 years and MCV4 for older children, although MPSV4 is an acceptable alternative.

7. **Pneumococcal vaccine.** The heptavalent **pneumococcal conjugate vaccine (PCV)** is recommended for all children aged 2–23 months. It is also recommended for certain children aged 24–59 months. The final dose in the series should be given at age ≥12 months. **Pneumococcal polysaccharide vaccine (PPV)** is recommended in addition to PCV for certain high-risk groups. See *MMWR* 2000;49(RR-9):1–35.

8. **Influenza vaccine.** Influenza vaccine is recommended annually for children aged ≥6 months with certain risk factors (including but not limited to asthma, cardiac disease, sickle cell disease, HIV, and diabetes), health care workers, and other persons (including household members) in close contact with persons in groups at high risk (see *MMWR* 2005;54[RR-8]: 1–55) and can be administered to all others wishing to obtain immunity. In addition, healthy children aged 6–23 months and close contacts of healthy children aged 0–23 months are recommended to receive influenza vaccine, because children in this age group are at substantially increased risk for influenza-related hospitalizations. For healthy persons aged 5–49 years, the intranasally administered live, attenuated influenza vaccine (LAIV) is an acceptable alternative to the intramuscular trivalent inactivated influenza vaccine (TIV). See *MMWR* 2005;54(RR-8):1–55. Children receiving TIV should be administered a dosage appropriate for their age (0.25 mL if 6–35 months or 0.5 mL if ≥3 years). Children aged ≤8 years who are receiving influenza vaccine for the first time should receive 2 doses (separated by at least 4 weeks for TIV and at least 6 weeks for LAIV).

9. **Hepatitis A vaccine.** Hepatitis A vaccine is recommended for children and adolescents in selected states and regions and for certain high-risk groups; consult your local public health authority. Children and adolescents in these states, regions, and high-risk groups who have not been immunized against hepatitis A can begin the hepatitis A immunization series during any visit. The 2 doses in the series should be administered at least 6 months apart. See *MMWR* 1999;48(RR-12):1–37.

Continued

TABLE 1 Recommended Childhood and Adolescent Immunization Schedule—cont'd

RECOMMENDED IMMUNIZATION SCHEDULE FOR CHILDREN AND ADOLESCENTS WHO START LATE OR WHO ARE MORE THAN 1 MONTH BEHIND
UNITED STATES • 2006

The tables below give catch-up schedules and minimum intervals between doses for children who have delayed immunizations. There is no need to restart a vaccine series regardless of the time that has elapsed between doses. Use the chart appropriate for the child's age.

CATCH-UP SCHEDULE FOR CHILDREN AGED 4 MONTHS THROUGH 6 YEARS

Vaccine	Minimum age for dose 1	Minimum interval between doses			
		Dose 1 to dose 2	Dose 2 to dose 3	Dose 3 to dose 4	Dose 4 to dose 5
Diphtheria, tetanus, pertussis	6 weeks	4 weeks	4 weeks	6 months	6 months[1]
Inactivated poliovirus	6 weeks	4 weeks	4 weeks	4 weeks[2]	
Hepatitis B[3]	Birth	4 weeks	8 weeks (and 16 weeks after first dose)		
Measles, mumps, rubella	12 months	4 weeks[4]			
Varicella	12 months				
Haemophilus influenzae type b[5]	6 weeks	4 weeks if first dose given at age <12 months / 8 weeks (as final dose) if first dose given at age 12–14 months / No further doses need if first dose given at age ≥15 months	4 weeks[6] if current age <12 months / 8 weeks (as final dose)[6] if current age ≥12 months and second dose given at age <15 months / No further doses need if first dose given at age ≥15 months	8 weeks (as final dose) This dose only necessary for children aged 12 months–5 years who received 3 doses before age 12 months	
Pneumococcal[7]	6 weeks	4 weeks if first dose given at age <12 months and current age < 24 months / 8 weeks (as final dose) if first dose given at age ≥12 months or current age 24–59 months / No further doses needed for healthy children if first dose given at age ≥24 months	4 weeks if current age <12 months / 8 weeks (as final dose) if current age ≥12 months / No further doses needed for healthy children if previous dose given at age ≥24 months	8 weeks (as final dose) This dose only necessary for children aged 12 months–5 years who received 3 doses before age 12 months	

CATCH-UP SCHEDULE FOR CHILDREN AGED 7 YEARS THROUGH 18 YEARS

Vaccine	Minimum interval between doses		
	Dose 1 to dose 2	Dose 2 to dose 3	Dose 3 to booster dose
Tetanus, diphtheria[8]	4 weeks	6 months	6 months if first dose given at age <12 months and current age <11 years; otherwise 5 years
Inactivated poliovirus[9]	4 weeks	4 weeks	IPV[2,9]
Hepatitis B	4 weeks	8 weeks (and 16 weeks after first dose)	
Measles, mumps, rubella	4 weeks		
Varicella[10]	4 weeks		

Footnotes

Children and Adolescents Catch-up Schedules • United States • 2006

1. **DTaP.** The fifth dose is not necessary if the fourth dose was given after the fourth birthday.
2. **IPV.** For children who received an all-IPV or all-oral poliovirus (OPV) series, a fourth dose is not necessary if third dose was given at age ≥4 years. If both OPV and IPV were given as part of a series, a total of 4 doses should be given, regardless of the child's current age.
3. **HepB.** Administer the 3-dose series to all children and adolescents <19 years of age if they were not previously vaccinated.
4. **MMR.** The second dose of MMR is recommended routinely at age 4–6 years but may be given earlier if desired.
5. **Hib.** Vaccine not generally recommended for children aged ≥5 years.
6. **Hib.** If current age <12 months and the first 2 doses were PRP-OMP (PedvaxHIB or ComVax [Merck]), the third (and final) dose should be administered at age 12–15 months and at least 8 weeks after the second dose.
7. **PCV.** Vaccine is not generally recommended for children aged ≥5 years.
8. **Td.** Adolescent tetanus, diphtheria, and pertussis vaccine (Tdap) may be substituted for any dose in a primary catch-up series or as a booster if age appropriate for Tdap. A five-year interval from the last Td dose is encouraged when Tdap is used as a booster dose. See ACIP recommendations for further information.
9. **IPV.** Vaccine is not generally recommended for persons aged ≥18 years.
10. **Varicella.** Give 2-dose series to all susceptible adolescents aged ≥13 years.

Report adverse reactions to vaccines through the federal Vaccine Adverse Event Reporting System. For information on reporting reactions following immunization, please visit www.vaers.hhs.gov or call the 24-hour national toll-free information line at 800-822-7967. Report suspected cases of vaccine-preventable diseases to your state or local health department.

For additional information about vaccines, including precautions and contraindications for immunization and vaccine shortages, please visit the National Immunization Program Web site at www.cdc.gov/nip or contact
800-CDC-INFO (800-232-4636)
(In English, En Español – 24/7)

Office-Based Immunization Practices

TABLE 2 Recommended Adult Immunization Schedule

RECOMMENDED ADULT IMMUNIZATION SCHEDULE BY VACCINE AND AGE GROUP
UNITED STATES, OCTOBER 2005–SEPTEMBER 2006

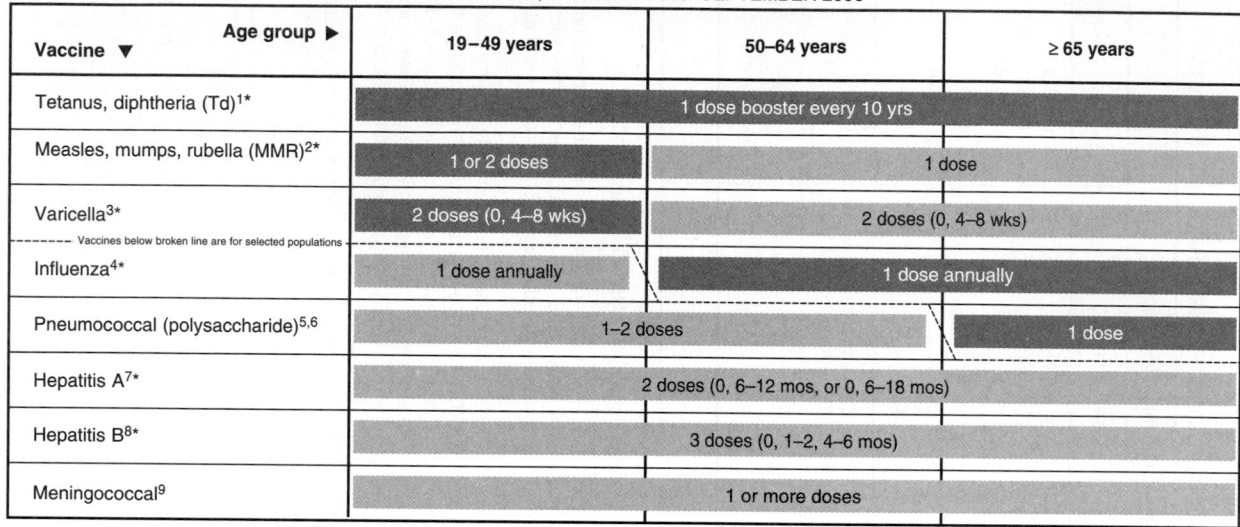

Vaccine ▼ Age group ▶	19–49 years	50–64 years	≥ 65 years
Tetanus, diphtheria (Td)[1]*	1 dose booster every 10 yrs		
Measles, mumps, rubella (MMR)[2]*	1 or 2 doses	1 dose	
Varicella[3]*	2 doses (0, 4–8 wks)	2 doses (0, 4–8 wks)	
Influenza[4]*	1 dose annually	1 dose annually	
Pneumococcal (polysaccharide)[5,6]	1–2 doses		1 dose
Hepatitis A[7]*	2 doses (0, 6–12 mos, or 0, 6–18 mos)		
Hepatitis B[8]*	3 doses (0, 1–2, 4–6 mos)		
Meningococcal[9]	1 or more doses		

Vaccines below broken line are for selected populations

NOTE: These recommendations must be read along with the footnotes.
*Covered by the Vaccine Injury Compensation Program.

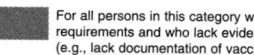

For all persons in this category who meet the age requirements and who lack evidence of immunity (e.g., lack documentation of vaccination or have no evidence of prior infection)

Recommended if some other risk factor is present (e.g., based on medical, occupational, lifestyle, or other indications)

This schedule indicates the recommended age groups and medical indications for routine administration of currently licensed vaccines for persons aged ≥19 years. Licensed combination vaccines may be used whenever any components of the combination are indicated and when the vaccine's other components are not contraindicated. For detailed recommendations, consult the manufacturers' package inserts and the complete statements from the ACIP (www.cdc.gov/nip/publications/acip-list.htm).

Report all clinically significant postvaccination reactions to the Vaccine Adverse Event Reporting System (VAERS). Reporting forms and instructions on filing a VAERS report are available by telephone, 800-822-7967, or from the VAERS website at www.vaers.hhs.gov.

Information on how to file a Vaccine Injury Compensation Program claim is available at www.hrsa.gov/osp/vicp or by telephone, 800-338-2382. To file a claim for vaccine injury, contact the U.S. Court of Federal Claims, 717 Madison Place, N.W., Washington D.C. 20005, telephone 202-357-6400.

Additional information about the vaccines listed above and contraindications for vaccination is also available at www.cdc.gov/nip or from the CDC-INFO Contact Center at 800-CDC-INFO (232-4636) in English and Spanish, 24 hours a day, 7 days a week.

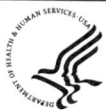

Department of Health and Human Services
Centers for Disease Control and Prevention

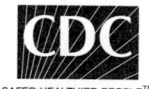

SAFER•HEALTHIER•PEOPLE™

Recommended Adult Immunization Schedule, by Vaccine and Medical and Other Indications
UNITED STATES, OCTOBER 2005–SEPTEMBER 2006

Vaccine ▼ / Indication ►	Pregnancy	Congenital immunodeficiency;[10] leukemia;[10] lymphoma; generalized malignancy; cerebrospinal fluid leaks; therapy with alkylating agents, antimetabolites, radiation, or high-dose, long-term corticosteroids	Diabetes; heart disease; chronic pulmonary disease; chronic liver disease, including chronic alcoholism	Asplenia[10] (including elective splenectomy and terminal complement component deficiencies)	Kidney failure, end-stage renal disease, recipients of hemodialysis or clotting factor concentrates	Human Immunodeficiency virus (HIV) infection[2,10]	Healthcare workers
Tetanus, diphtheria (Td)[1]*	1 dose booster every 10 yrs →						
Measles, mumps, rubella (MMR)[2]*	Contraindicated	Contraindicated	1 or 2 doses →			Contraindicated	
Varicella[3]*	Contraindicated	Contraindicated	2 doses (0, 4–8 wks) →			Contraindicated	2 doses
Influenza[4]*	1 dose annually			1 dose annually			
Pneumococcal (polysaccharide)[5,6]	1–2 doses			1–2 doses →			1–2 doses
Hepatitis A[7]*	2 doses (0, 6–12 mos, or 0, 6–18 mos) →						
Hepatitis B[8]*	3 doses (0, 1–2, 4–6 mos) →					3 doses (0, 1–2, 4–6 mos) →	
Meningococcal[9]	1 dose →			1 dose		1 dose	

NOTE: These recommendations must be read along with the footnotes.
*Covered by the Vaccine Injury Compensation Program.

Legend:
- For all persons in this category who meet the age requirements and who lack evidence of immunity (e.g., lack documentation of vaccination or have no evidence of prior infection)
- Recommended if some other risk factor is present (e.g., based on medical, occupation, lifestyle, or other indications)
- Contraindicated

Approved by the Advisory Committee on Immunization Practices (ACIP),
the American College of Obstetricians and Gynecologists (ACOG), and the American Academy of Family Physicians (AAFP)

Office-Based Immunization Practices

Continued

TABLE 2   Recommended Adult Immunization Schedule—cont'd

Recommended Adult Immunization Schedule, United States, October 2005–September 2006

Footnotes

1. **Tetanus and diphtheria (Td).** Adults with uncertain histories of a complete primary vaccination series with diphtheria and tetanus toxoid–containing vaccines should receive a primary series using combined Td toxoid. A primary series for adults is 3 doses; administer the first 2 doses at least 4 weeks apart and the 3rd dose 6–12 months after the second. Administer 1 dose if the person received the primary series and if the last vaccination was received ≥10 years previously. Consult ACIP statement for recommendations for administering Td as prophylaxis in wound management (www.cdc.gov/mmwr/preview/mmwrhtml/00041645.htm). The American College of Physicians Task Force on Adult Immunization supports a second option for Td use in adults: a single Td booster at age 50 years for persons who have completed the full pediatric series, including the teenage/young adult booster. A newly licensed tetanus-diphtheria-acellular pertussis vaccine is available for adults. ACIP recommendations for its use will be published.

2. **Measles, mumps, rubella (MMR) vaccination.** *Measles component:* adults born before 1957 can be considered immune to measles. Adults born during or after 1957 should receive ≥1 dose of MMR unless they have a medical contraindication, documentation of ≥1 dose, history of measles based on healthcare provider diagnosis, or laboratory evidence of immunity. A second dose of MMR is recommended for adults who 1) were recently exposed to measles or in an outbreak setting, 2) were previously vaccinated with killed measles vaccine, 3) were vaccinated with an unknown type of measles vaccine during 1963–1967, 4) are students in postsecondary educational institutions, 5) work in a healthcare facility, or 6) plan to travel internationally. Withhold MMR or other measles-containing vaccines from HIV-infected persons with severe immunosuppression. *Mumps component:* 1 dose of MMR vaccine should be adequate for protection for those born during or after 1957 who lack a history of mumps based on healthcare provider diagnosis or who lack laboratory evidence of immunity. *Rubella component:* administer 1 dose of MMR vaccine to women whose rubella vaccination history is unreliable or who lack laboratory evidence of immunity. For women of childbearing age, regardless of birth year, routinely determine rubella immunity and counsel women regarding congenital rubella syndrome. Do not vaccinate women who are pregnant or might become pregnant within 4 weeks of receiving the vaccine. Woman who do not have evidence of immunity should receive the healthcare MMR vaccine upon completion or termination of pregnancy and before discharge from the healthcare facility.

3. **Varicella vaccination.** Varicella vaccination is recommended for all adults without evidence of immunity to varicella. Special consideration should be given to those who 1) have close contact with persons at high risk for severe disease (healthcare workers and family contacts of immunocompromised persons) or 2) are at high risk for exposure or transmission (e.g., teachers of young children; child care employees; residents and staff members of institutional settings, including correctional institutions; college students; military personnel; adolescents and adults living in households with children; nonpregnant women of childbearing age; and international travelers). Evidence of immunity to varicella in adults includes any of the following: 1) documented age-appropriate varicella vaccination (i.e., receipt of 1 dose before age 13 years or receipt of 2 doses [administered at least 4 weeks apart] after age 13 years); 2) born in the United States before 1966; 3) history of varicella disease based on healthcare provider diagnosis or self- or parental report of typical varicella disease for non–U.S.-born persons born before 1966 and all persons born during 1966–1997 (for a patient reporting a history of an atypical, mild case, healthcare providers should seek either an epidemiologic link with a typical varicella case or evidence of laboratory confirmation, if it was performed at the time of acute disease); 4) history of herpes zoster based on healthcare provider diagnosis; or 5) laboratory evidence of immunity. Do not vaccinate women who are pregnant or might become pregnant within 4 weeks of receiving the vaccine. Assess pregnant women for evidence of varicella immunity. Women who do not have evidence of immunity should receive dose 1 of varicella vaccine upon completion or termination of pregnancy and before discharge from the healthcare facility. Dose 2 should be given 4–8 weeks after dose 1.

4. **Influenza vaccination.** *Medical indications:* chronic disorders of the cardiovascular or pulmonary system, including asthma; chronic metabolic diseases, including diabetes mellitus, renal dysfunction, hemoglobinopathies, or immunosuppression (including immunosuppression caused by medications or by human immunodeficiency virus [HIV]); any condition (e.g., cognitive dysfunction, spinal cord injury, seizure disorder or other neuromuscular disorder) that compromises respiratory function or the handling of respiratory secretions or that can increase the risk of aspiration; and pregnancy during the influenza season. No data exist on the risk for severe or complicated influenza disease among persons with asplenia; however, influenza is a risk factor for secondary bacterial infections that can cause severe disease among persons with asplenia. *Occupational indications:* healthcare workers and employees of long-term care and assisted living facilities. *Other indications:* residents of nursing homes and other long-term care and assisted living facilities; persons likely to transmit influenza to persons at high risk (i.e., in-home household contacts and caregivers of children born through

23 months of age, or persons of all ages with high-risk conditions); and anyone who wishes to be vaccinated. For healthy nonpregnant persons aged 5–49 years without high-risk conditions who are not contacts or severely immunocompromised persons in special care units, intranasally administered influenza vaccine (FluMist®) may be administered in lieu of inactivated vaccine.

5. **Pneumococcal polysaccharide vaccination.** *Medical indications:* chronic disorders of the pulmonary system (excluding asthma); cardiovascular diseases; diabetes mellitus; chronic liver diseases, including liver disease as a result of alcohol abuse (e.g., cirrhosis); chronic renal failure or nephrotic syndrome; functional or anatomic asplenia (e.g., sickle cell disease or splenectomy [if elective splenectomy is planned, vaccinate at least 2 weeks before surgery]); immunosuppressive conditions (e.g., congenital immunodeficiency, HIV infection [vaccinate as close to diagnosis as possible when CD4 cell counts are highest], leukemia, lymphoma, multiple myeloma, Hodgkin disease, generalized malignancy, organ or bone marrow transplantation); chemotherapy with alkylating agents, antimetabolites, or high-dose, long-term corticosteroids; and cochlear implants. *Other indications:* Alaska Natives and certain American Indian populations; residents of nursing homes and other long-term care facilities.

6. **Revaccination with pneumococcal polysaccharide vaccine.** One-time revaccination after 5 years for persons with chronic renal failure or nephrotic syndrome; functional or anatomic asplenia (e.g., sickle cell disease or splenectomy); immunosuppressive conditions (e.g., congenital immunodeficiency, HIV infection, leukemia, lymphoma, multiple myeloma, Hodgkin disease, generalized malignancy, organ or bone marrow transplantation); or chemotherapy with alkylating agents, antimetabolites, or high-dose, long-term systemic corticosteroids. For persons aged ≥65 years, one-time revaccination if they were vaccinated ≥5 years previously and were aged <65 years at the time of primary vaccination.

7. **Hepatitis A vaccination.** *Medical indications:* persons with clotting factor disorders or chronic liver disease. *Behavioral indications:* men who have sex with men or users of illegal drugs. *Occupational indications:* persons working with hepatitis A virus (HAV)–infected primates or with HAV in a research laboratory setting. *Other indications:* persons traveling to or working in countries that have high or intermediate endemicity of hepatitis A (for list of countries, visit www.cdc.gov/travel/diseases.htm#hepa) as well as any person wishing to obtain immunity. Current vaccines should be given in a 2-dose series at either 0 and 6–12 months, or 0 and 6–18 months. If the combined hepatitis A and hepatitis B vaccine is used, administer 3 doses at 0, 1, and 6 months.

8. **Hepatitis B vaccination.** *Medical indications:* hemodialysis patients or patients who receive clotting factor concentrates. *Occupational indications:* health-care workers and public-safety workers who have exposure to blood in the workplace; and persons in training in schools of medicine, dentistry, nursing, laboratory technology, and other allied health professions. *Behavioral indications:* injection-drug users; persons with more than one sex partner during the previous 6 months; persons with a recently acquired sexually transmitted disease (STD); and men who have sex with men. *Other indications:* household contacts and sex partners of persons with chronic hepatitis B virus (HBV) infection; clients and staff of institutions for the developmentally disabled; all clients of STD clinics; inmates of correctional facilities; or international travelers who will be in countries with high or intermediate prevalence of chronic HBV infection for >6 months (for list of countries, visit www.cdc.gov/travel/diseases.htm#hepa).

9. **Meningococcal vaccine.** *Medical indications:* adults with anatomic or functional asplenia, or terminal complement component deficiencies. *Other indications:* first-year college students living in dormitories; microbiologists who are routinely exposed to isolates of *Neisseria meningitidis*; military recruits; and persons who travel to or reside in countries in which meningococcal disease is hyperendemic or epidemic (e.g., the "meningitis belt" of sub-Saharan Africa during the dry season [Dec–June]), particularly if contact with the local populations would be prolonged. Vaccination is required by the government of Saudi Arabia for all travelers to Mecca during the annual Hajj. Meningococcal conjugate vaccine is preferred for adults meeting any of the above indications who are aged ≤55 years, although meningococcal polysaccharide vaccine (MPSV4) is an acceptable alternative. Revaccination after 5 years may be indicated for adults previously vaccinated with MPSV4 who remain at high risk for infection (e.g., persons residing in areas in which disease is epidemic).

10. **Selected conditions for which *haemophilus influenzae type b* (Hib) vaccine may be used.** *Haemophilus influenzae* type b conjugate vaccines are licensed for children aged 6 weeks–71 months. No efficacy date are available on which to base a recommendation concerning use of Hib vaccine for older children and adults with the chronic conditions associated with an increased risk for Hib disease. However, studies suggest good immunogenicity in patients who have sickle cell disease, leukemia, or HIV infection, or have had splenectomies; administering vaccine to these patients is not contraindicated.

not given because of precaution or contraindication as the basis. We have an ongoing problem with the adoption of chickenpox vaccine (Varivax). Those children who previously acquired chickenpox do not need the chickenpox vaccine, but we need to document the occurrence of that disease and its date to prevent overvaccination.

RECORD SHARING AND REGISTRIES

Vaccine registries at the community level or regional level dramatically reduce the miscommunication and the need for occurrence of both overimmunization as well as empowering physicians and nurses to feel better about taking advantage of missed opportunities in vaccinating children. Most parents whose children are undervaccinated report that their children are "up to date." Records that accurately reflect the child's full vaccine record would better equip the practitioner in best managing those patients.

VACCINE STORAGE

Storage requirements are much more complex than traditionally practiced. Offices must provide proper refrigeration as well as freezers for vaccines. Certain vaccines require refrigeration, other vaccines require freezing, and some vaccines are more heat labile or cold labile than others. Proper care and maintenance of refrigerator includes the purchase of appropriate dedicated equipment, the monitoring of the temperatures, the purchase of proper containers to be used on the shelves, and adequate space to allow for prevention of errors with storage. Furthermore, the staff must be trained and scheduled to provide oversight in the case of a power or equipment failure.

ASSESSMENT OF THE OVERALL PROCESS AND ITS OUTCOMES

Assessing an individual's immunization needs, providing the vaccines, and recording them properly in the individual's record is no longer adequate for the assessment of the overall process. Each office should make efforts to assess its overall practice. Each office must monitor the rates of on-time immunizations as well as up-to-date immunization and look for opportunities to improve these metrics. The effort of collecting this information has led to improvements in rates of on-time vaccination. Immunization practices are evolving and the maintenance of quality as well as the rapid adoption and improvement of practices require regular office meetings of staff. Physicians, nurses, and receptionists must be aware of new changes. Receptionists' misunderstanding of the vaccine needs frequently leads to missed opportunities to vaccinate. Misunderstanding between physicians and other clinicians can also lead to failed attempts. Regular office meetings should occur throughout the year to evaluate the vaccine schedule, the success of vaccinating the panel of patients, and considerations for practice improvements.

STANDING ORDERS

One of the most successful approaches in the office to make real efforts to improve immunization rates above and beyond that driven by the well child care schedule is to create standing orders that permit nursing staff to provide vaccines to patients without a doctor visit. This is particularly helpful with flu season and with acute care contacts with the patient. Such standing orders need to be written in such a way that they meet state law, facilitate nurse assessment of the patient's vaccine needs, as well as rule out any precautions or contraindications for the child's immunization. Materials exist online at the Immunization Action Coalition (www.immunize.org) that can help in writing such standing orders.

RECALL REMINDERS AND TRACKING

A second method for improving office vaccination rates are recall reminders and tracking. Providers should develop proactive approaches toward their patient panels to ensure compliance with the routine childhood schedule. Offices should contact patients when vaccines are due. Additional efforts should be made for those subjects who are behind in immunizations. Finally, offices should have systems to identify those children in families for whom the flu vaccine is indicated and make efforts every autumn to contact the families proactively and schedule immunization visits. The broadening of the flu vaccine indications has made this a major issue for office practices who care for either children or adults or both.

REPORTING ADVERSE EVENTS

The same laws that created the vaccine information statements and the protection for vaccine providers from frivolous lawsuits have also created the Vaccine Adverse Events Reporting System (VAERS). This system, set up by the federal government, collects information on adverse events believed to be related to immunization. These include certain ones required by regulation as well as those temporally associated with the immunizations that strike the provider or family as potentially significant. Vaccine manufacturers and providers are in fact required to report certain adverse events occurring after immunization whether or not they were caused by the immunization.

VAERS has actually led to the discontinuation of certain office-based immunization practices including the use of the tetravalent oral rhesus rotavirus vaccine (RotaShield). It has also helped to protect vaccines from unwarranted claims of harm. Although it has its weaknesses, statistical approaches have made it a powerful tool. Participation for providers of vaccines is required. All office staff, including receptionists, must understand the legal requirements of reporting.

VACCINES FOR CHILDREN

The U.S. government set up a program entitled Vaccines for Children (VFC) that enables providers to receive free-of-charge vaccines that can be given to patients with certain conditions including those who are younger than 18 years and are Medicaid eligible, uninsured, American Indian or Alaska Native, or whose health insurance benefit plan does not include vaccinations. Some recipients may be charged a vaccine provider fee, which is a limited amount. The federal government purchases vaccine for the VFC program and then distributes it to the state's health departments, which redistributes to the qualified providers. To learn how an office can participate, the VFC program can be contacted at NIP through its Web pages (www.cdc.gov/nip/vfc/).

Common Problems

Offices that provide vaccines to their patients struggle with common problems in immunization practice. These include missed or delayed vaccinations, vaccine shortages, catch-up, change-ups, decisions not to vaccinate, true and false contraindications, multiple providers, and incomplete records. One cannot make these problems disappear, but one can prepare for them, prevent them from happening in many cases, and minimize the harm when they do occur.

MISSED OR DELAYED VACCINATIONS

Although daycare and school-based requirements have resulted in very high vaccine rates by school entry, on-time immunization is tragically low. Many children do not get their vaccines when due and are left at risk. Although this occurs more frequently among those with multiple providers and those who do not have health insurance available, practitioners can change their office practices to reduce the problems in delayed immunizations. First of all, do not relegate routine immunization to the well child visit. Second, be assertive in obtaining the complete vaccine records from your patient's previous providers of health care. Third, create standing order policies to facilitate your office staff providing vaccines without a physician visit.

Furthermore, the practitioner should have charts available in the office explaining how to proceed with a child who has not received vaccines on time. Practitioners cannot be expected to memorize this information. It is complex, age dependent, and vaccine specific. The information must be available for ready reference. With the American Academies of Pediatrics and Family Practitioners, the ACIP has created catch-up schedules (http://www.cdc.gov/nip/recs/child-schedule.htm#catchup). There are two catch-up schedules: one for children 4 months to 6 years of age and one for 7 to 18 years of age.

LOCUS OF RESPONSIBILITY

Providers cannot expect their patients or their patients' parents, to take responsibility for timely vaccination. Patient-held immunization records have failed to improve vaccination rates. Office practitioners must also consider that even in a specialty practice their patients may be expecting them to monitor their immunization needs along with providing them the vaccines that they need. Providers, whether of specialty or primary care, must assess their individual patients and determine who is monitoring the patients' vaccination status and needs. Specialists must never assume that the patient is cognizant of the need or that a primary care provider is actively playing that role. All too often, patients relinquish their relationships with primary care providers once they begin an ongoing relationship with a specialist.

VACCINE SHORTAGES

Ongoing shortages do occur with vaccine supplies. Most famously were the shortages with the influenza vaccine, but we have shortages with vaccines when there have been changes in use or recommendations such as the adoption of the adolescent diphtheria/tetanus (Td) at 11 years of age and the rapid acceptance of the pneumococcal conjugate vaccine (Prevar). Manufacturers struggle to produce adequate supplies knowing the expense of creating inadequate supplies actually leads to distrust and anger directed toward the manufacturer as well as difficulties in completing on-time immunizations. Manufacturing too much vaccine can lead to unusable stockpiles of expired vaccine product. Therefore manufacturers seek to reach a balance. Shortages are communicated best to office practices in the United States through the online Web site at the National Immunization Program where information is provided for the basis of shortages as well as explanations for what the practitioners should do during this time. In most situations the vaccine providers are expected to record those people who have not received the vaccine on time because of the shortage and are to be called back in a timely manner when vaccine supplies are available.

CATCH-UP

Catching children up on missed or delayed vaccinations is a major problem. This activity results not just because of shortages but because of parents' delays in immunization. The third and four child in a family often suffer delays in immunizations because of parents' issues with the organization and scheduling of appropriate on-time well child visits. Offices that rely on the well child visit schedules as the only basis for immunization have higher rates of vaccine delays and more problems with catch-up than those who use every opportunity of every visit to assess vaccine status of the child and to vaccinate on time. To make matters worse, the current schedule when on time can call for five injections at once. Imagine the child who has accumulated significant delays and now needs to be caught up. One of the major difficulties of catch-up is the problem of information. I previously mentioned the chart that all vaccine providers should have available to facilitate on-time immunizations.

CHANGE-UPS

Change-ups are also difficult because the new adoption of a vaccine can lead to some confusion for those who previously received an older moiety. For example, the recipients of the meningococcal polysaccharide vaccine (Menomune) are not due for the meningococcal conjugate vaccine (Menacta), but those who previously received the adolescent tetanus-diphtheria (Td) vaccine may certainly benefit from the new adolescent tetanus-diphtheria-reduced-dose-acellular pertussis vaccine (Tdap, Boostrix).

DECISIONS NOT TO VACCINATE

There are many reasons why patients may fail to be vaccinated. Common reasons include misunderstandings by the practitioner or parent of contraindications regarding vaccines. These are vaccine specific and complex in language in application. Many more people fail to get vaccines because of contraindications than those who truly have them. Other common reasons include parents' failure to attend to the well-visit schedule and the practitioners' failures to use other visits as the basis for immunization.

Some parents, however, actually consider immunization and choose to refuse. They are suspicious that the vaccines do not work, are not necessary or at least no longer necessary, are not safe, weaken the immune system, provide a poorer immunity than the actual diseases they target, that children receive too many vaccines, and that some vaccine lots are contaminated. Practitioners should be familiar with these concerns and their rebuttals. Two good sources for information on these include NIP (www.cdc.gov/nip) and the Immunization Action Coalition (www.immunize.org). The latter organization has actually collected stories of parents who chose not to vaccinate their children and then suffered the consequences of vaccine-preventable disease.

TRUE AND FALSE CONTRAINDICATIONS

Perhaps one of the most common problems with immunization delivery in the United States with regard to the failure of the provider stems from common misconceptions regarding the presence or absence of contraindication to immunization. Although some contraindications are vaccine specific, certain principles apply. First, family histories of adverse events are never contraindications to immunization. Second, household pregnancy or breastfeeding is never a contraindication to immunization. Third, the presence of an illness or injury by itself is not a contraindication. If the illness is moderate or severe, with or without a fever, then a vaccine's administration may be contraindicated. Although local and systemic adverse reactions do occur with vaccines, these are in general not contraindications to further doses.

It would be impossible for a practitioner to memorize contraindications. NIP (www.cdc.gov/nip) has prepared a user-friendly online table that is indexed by disease and condition to guide the practitioner. This table should be available for ready use throughout the day.

MULTIPLE PROVIDERS AND INCOMPLETE RECORDS

Both under- and overimmunization occur much more frequently among patients who use more than one provider. Regional registries that allow practitioners to share their vaccine records greatly reduce both missed opportunities to vaccinate as well as the inadvertent administration of unnecessary doses. Practitioners should work with their local and state health departments to develop regional vaccine registries.

For all of the problems we face, for all of the intricacies of practice we must adopt, there is perhaps no one practice more important to the health of the community than the delivery of routine immunizations. Although it is worth the effort, it requires an ongoing commitment to continuing education, practice assessment, and evidence-based improvement of the office practice.

REFERENCES

American Academy of Family Physicians: AAFP Clinical Recommendations. http://www.aafp.org/x132.xml. Accessed August 7, 2006. This web site provides links to specific AAFP recommendations for immunizations.

American Academy of Pediatrics: American Academy of Pediatrics Policy Statements. http://aappolicy.aappublications.org/. Accessed August 7, 2006. This web site provides links to the AAP policies including its online Red Book with its recommendations regarding vaccines and immunizations.

Centers for Disease Control and Prevention: Recommendations of the ACIP (Advisory Committee on Immunization Practices). http://www.cdc.gov/nip/publications/acip-list.htm. Last modified on July 27, 2006. Accessed August 7, 2006. This web site provides links to the ACIP recommendations, which are updated annually as new data dictate. All of the documents listed on this page are current, regardless of their publication dates.

Centers for Disease Control and Prevention: Recommended Childhood and Adolescent Immunization Schedule, United States, 2006. http://www.cdc.gov/nip/recs/child-schedule.htm. Last updated April 18, 2006. Accessed August 7, 2006. This web site provides the harmonized 4-page schedule for children and adolescents with informative footnotes and two additional charts for catch-up for children between the ages of 4 months through 6 years and between 7 through 18 years.

Centers for Disease Control and Prevention: Recommended Adult Immunization Schedule by Vaccine and Age Group, United States, October 2005–September 2006. http://www.cdc.gov/nip/recs/adult-schedule.htm. Last updated April 18, 2006. Accessed August 7, 2006. Recommended immunizations for anyone older than 18 years.

Centers for Disease Control and Prevention: Vaccine Information Statements (VIS). http://www.cdc.gov/nip/publications/VIS/. Last updated July 12, 2006. Accessed August 7, 2006. This web page lists links to all of the federally mandated Vaccine Information Statements that practitioners must use in informed parents of the recommended vaccines.

Centers for Disease Control and Prevention: Vaccine Management: Recommendations for Storage and Handling Selected Biologicals. Revised June 2005. http://www.cdc.gov/nip/publications/vac_mgt_book.pdf. Accessed August 10, 2006. This document provides vaccine-specific instructions on storage of vaccines.

Immunization Action Coalition: State Mandates on Immunization and Vaccine-Preventable Disease. http://www.immunize.org/laws/. Last updated May 31, 2006. Accessed August 7, 2006. This web site provides specific state-by-state rules for school and day-care attendance.

Pickering LK, Baker CJ, Long SS, McMillan JA (eds): Red Book: 2006 Report of the Committee on Infectious Diseases, 27th ed. Elk Grove Village, IL, American Academy of Pediatrics, 2006.

Shefer A, Briss P, Rodewald L, et al: Improving immunization coverage rates: An evidence-based review of the literature. Epidemiol Rev 1999;21(1):96-142. A systematic review of the published studies of interventions to improve vaccines uptake.

Travel Medicine

Method of
William F. Miser, MD, MA, and
Katherine G. Gerges, MS, CNP

Since commercial air travel began decades ago, continental borders have become less and less restrictive, and worldwide exploration is possible. This freedom to travel worldwide exposes travelers to conditions not commonly found in the Western world. Of the 50 million or more Americans who travel abroad each year, more than 10 million travel to remote, exotic, and/or developing countries. Up to half

TABLE 1 Frequent Causes of Illness and Death in U.S. Travelers Abroad

Causes of Death (Most deaths occur in men older than 55 years.)
- Cardiovascular events (49%)
- Unintentional injuries (22%)—motor vehicle accident, drowning, homicide, airplane accident, poisoning, burn, suicide, electrocution, natural disaster (e.g., earthquake, tsunami), other (animal mauling, falls from heights, etc.)
- Infections (1%)—malaria, typhoid, hepatitis B

Causes of Illness
- Acute (traveler's) diarrhea #1
- Acute respiratory infections, influenza
- Other viral syndromes
- Skin conditions (rash, cutaneous leishmaniasis, cutaneous larva migrans)
- Parasitic infestation (e.g., *Ascaris lumbricoides*, *Giardia lamblia*, *Entamoeba histolytica*, hookworm, tapeworms)
- Malaria
- Hepatitis A, B, and C
- Other infections (African trypanosomiasis, amebic meningoencephalitis, cholera, dracunculiasis, leptospirosis, meningococcal meningitis, plague, schistosomiasis, sexually transmitted diseases, typhoid, yellow fever, visceral leishmaniasis, other)

of those who travel become ill while abroad, and more than 6000 die annually on foreign soil (Table 1). Most of the morbidity that occurs during international travel is a result of common preventable problems, not rare diseases. These apparently minor diseases can inconvenience or ruin vacations. Despite these statistics, less than one third of travelers seek pretravel advice. The goals of physicians who provide travel advice are **prevention** of both rare and common conditions, so that health is maintained during travel, and **preparedness** for those circumstances when prevention fails.

As changes in world health occur frequently, those who provide travel advice must have available resources that provide current information about regional and country-specific disease risks and emerging infectious diseases. The Centers for Disease Control and Prevention Web site (www.cdc.gov/travel) provides excellent up-to-date information for both providers and travelers. Additional sources of travel information are listed in the References of this article. Other necessities for those who provide travel care include an adequate supply of necessary vaccines, a pharmacy that carries specific travel medications, a reliable laboratory that can perform travel-related tests, and a consultant in infectious disease who is available to offer advice for those puzzling post-travel conditions.

Travel medicine involves more than just providing immunizations, and consists of both pretravel and post-travel care. Ideally, the traveler should seek pretravel care at least 4 to 6 weeks prior to departure. This allows time for routine medical and dental examinations, pretravel counseling, and pretravel immunization. Travelers should be encouraged to return to the office after the trip to review potential health problems and to update their medical records.

Pretravel Care—More Than Just Shots

The consultation prior to travel is designed primarily to assess potential health threats and to identify required preventive measures. Physicians should ideally plan on spending 30 to 45 minutes with the traveler during the pretravel visit. Essential questions for the traveler should focus on the five W's and an H (Table 2). A preprinted travel questionnaire can be quite helpful to obtain this information, especially if the traveler is not well known to the provider. This information allows the provider to determine what medicines, immunizations, and laboratory tests may be required for the trip, and to provide specific counseling based on identified risks.

Regardless of the traveler's destination, several issues should be addressed during the pretravel visit (Table 3). Well-written patient-care handouts and referral to quality Web sites such as those listed in the References should complement the physician's discussion with the patient. This advice can be categorized into general advice applicable to all travelers, advice on avoiding infections, which includes proper vaccinations, and specific advice as determined by the traveler's health.

TABLE 2 Questions to Ask During Pretravel Visit (5 Ws and an H)

Who?—Gather information about travelers.
- How old are they? (Children and elderly are more likely to become ill while abroad.)
- Are they pregnant? (Certain medications and immunizations are contraindicated.)
- How is their general health? Do they have chronic medical problems?
- How is their immune status? (Those immunocompromised are at risk for disease.)
- What immunizations have they received in the past?
- What medications are they on?
- Do they have any allergies (medicines, vaccines, foods, insects)?

What?—Gather information about the trip.
- How long is the trip?
- What are the potential insect and animal exposures?
- What food and water sources will be available?

Where?—Get detailed information about the itinerary.
- What countries will they be visiting, and in what order?
- Where will they be staying (hotel, hut, tent)?
- What access will they have to quality medical care?
- What is the climate and altitude of their destination?
- Will they be traveling "off the beaten path"?

When?—Obtain detailed information about when they will be leaving (to time immunizations), determine whether it will be the rainy or dry season at their destination, and assess how much time will be spent outdoors during the early evening hours.

Why?—Find out the purpose of the trip—business, pleasure, or a combination.

How?—Determine how they will be traveling—by air, train, sea, and/or automobile.

TABLE 3 Topics to Discuss During Pretravel Visit

Accidents (second most common cause of death in travelers)
- Use common sense—wear seat belts in all vehicles (when available), don't drink alcohol and drive or get into the water, become familiar with local motor vehicle laws and customs, try to avoid nighttime travel by car, avoid the use of motorbikes and motorcycles.
- As a pedestrian, be aware of traffic patterns.
- Limitations exist for coverage outside of the United States, especially with Medicare—consider purchasing travel health care insurance if not provided by one's own plan
- Emergency evacuation to another country may be necessary or preferable—consider purchasing special evacuation insurance when visiting remote or developing countries.
- Try to avoid injections while abroad, because needles and syringes are often reused and are a major cause of hepatitis B and HIV transmission.

Sun Protection
- Sunburn and photoallergic reactions are common skin conditions reported by travelers.
- Certain medications, such as doxycycline (Vibramycin), may result in phototoxicity.
- Avoid sun exposure from 10:00 AM to 3:00 PM and use sunscreen with a SPF of at least 30.

Food and Water Hygiene (see Table 9)

Proper Clothing
- Wearing shoes prevents many parasitic infestations.
- Lightweight cotton fabrics absorb perspiration and light colors reflect sunlight.
- Wearing long-sleeved shirts and pants protects the skin from insect bites, stings, and sun.

Insect Repellent (see Table 10)
- DEET-containing products are effective and safe insect repellents.
- Permethrin-containing products are effective insecticides for clothing but not skin.

Sexually Transmitted Diseases
- STDs, including HIV, are a risk worldwide.

Abbreviation: DEET = diethyltoluamide.

General Advice

PREVENTION OF ACCIDENTS

Most travelers are adventurous and take risks that normally would be avoided while at home. An emphasis on the importance of accident prevention is key, as accidents are the second most common cause of death in travelers of all ages, and the most common cause in younger travelers. Travelers should be encouraged to use common sense while traveling. Seat belts should be worn, when available. The use of alcohol increases the risk of accidents and should be avoided when driving or swimming. Nighttime driving is particularly dangerous because roads may not be well lit or marked. Motorbikes and motorcycles are a major cause of death among young travelers. Be aware of local traffic patterns, and pedestrians should be particularly cautious when crossing the road, especially in countries where traffic comes from a direction opposite of what is customarily encountered in the United States.

HEALTH CARE AND EVACUATION INSURANCE

Limitations exist in coverage by standard health care policies when travel takes the individual outside the United States. For example, Medicare does not cover medical expenses outside the United States. As a general rule, no coverage is available at the time of service, and the traveler often is responsible for payment of all bills. Likewise, evacuation by air to a quality health care facility may be required, and can be quite costly. Most health care plans fail to provide coverage for emergency evacuation. Encourage travelers to read their policies carefully, and to consider purchasing additional health care and evacuation coverage for their travel, especially if going to remote areas. Medical assistance companies exist that can help travelers obtain competent local medical care and to coordinate services. Likewise, the U.S. embassy in each country, although not able to provide direct health care, can direct travelers to appropriate medical facilities in the local area.

PERSONAL MEDICAL KIT

Travelers should take with them a medical problem list that identifies their major health conditions and prior surgeries, blood type (if known), allergies, and medicines, by generic drug name, dosage, and indications. Include on this list your name, address, phone number, and e-mail address so that other health care providers can contact you if necessary. Travelers should take an extra pair of glasses or contact lenses, and have a refraction prescription. Because hearing aid batteries are hard to find in many countries, having replacements is essential. For travelers with known heart disease, a copy of their last electrocardiogram (ECG) is valuable. Prescription drugs should be carried by hand, not placed in checked luggage. These medicines should be in the original pharmacy bottle with printed label, and the traveler should have enough to last for the entire trip. Table 4 lists other useful items to consider.

SUN PROTECTION

For those traveling to tropical areas, sunburn is the most common problem skin condition reported. Certain agents enhance the skin's sensitivity to sunlight, whereas others may predispose one to photoallergic reactions. Although most travel to the tropical regions for the sun, the physician should still counsel the traveler to be smart about sun exposure. The most intense times for sunlight is typically midday, and travelers should avoid sun exposure from 10:00 AM to 3:00 PM. Wearing lightweight cotton, light-colored, long-sleeved shirts and pants protects against intense sun exposure. Sunscreens that contain benzophenones or anthranilates absorb both ultraviolet A (UVA) and ultraviolet B (UVB) light, and are protective against sunburns, phototoxicity, and photoallergic reactions.

AIR TRAVEL

The cabin of an airliner is usually kept at a pressure equivalent to 6000 to 8000 feet. As such, it is important to know the absolute and relative contraindications to air travel (Table 5). **Jet lag** is caused by an imbalance between one's biologic clock and the destination's time clock, and usually

TABLE 4 Symptom-Oriented Medical Supply Kit

Pack all ingredients in a self-sealing bag for organization, neatness, and protection against humidity; use plastic, rather than glass; Tupperware-type containers are tough and waterproof.

Pain Relief
- Aspirin, acetaminophen (Tylenol), or ibuprofen (Motrin); codeine if severe pain is anticipated. (Keep all drugs, especially narcotics, in their originally labeled containers to avoid problems at borders.)

Cold or Rash Symptoms
- Antihistamine—diphenhydramine (Benadryl 25-75 mg every 4 hours)[3] or nonsedating antihistamine as needed for insect bite, runny nose, itching, bee sting, and mild poison ivy.
- Decongestants.
- Disposable thermometer.

Infection-Specific
Product to use depends on the individual traveler and his or her past history of susceptibility to certain infections.
- **Skin**—topical mupirocin ointment (Bactroban); clotrimazole cream (Lotrimin).
- **Mouth**—Zilactin (topical oral formulation of tannic acid and boric acid for canker sores, which covers them with an adherent material that lasts 2-3 hours (stings when applied).
- **Eye/Ear**—simple eyewash or "liquid tears" for dust, irritated eyes; antibiotic eye drops for eye infection (especially for contact lens wearers) and antibiotic ear drops for "swimmer's ear."
- **Upper/Lower Respiratory**—erythromycin, amoxicillin, azithromycin (Zithromax); asthma inhaler (Proventil or Ventolin) for asthma or asthmatic bronchitis.
- **GI**—a fluoroquinolone for traveler's diarrhea; bismuth subsalicylate (Pepto-Bismol liquid and tablets), and/or loperamide (Imodium AD) for diarrhea; antacids; laxative for constipation.
- **GU**—trimethoprim/sulfamethoxazole (Bactrim), amoxicillin, or ciprofloxacin for UTIs; clotrimazole (Gyne-Lotrimin) or miconazole (Monistat) vaginal cream or fluconazole. (Diflucan), 150 mg tablet for yeast infections.

Dental Kit
First aid supplies for common dental emergencies—oil of cloves for dental pain.

First Aid Supplies
Packed individually or purchased in kit form:
- Nonstick bandages
- Tape
- Eyeglass repair kit
- Mole skin!)
- Pins/needles
- Band-Aids
- Fine tweezers (to remove splinters, ticks)
- Sterile gauze
- First aid manual

Miscellaneous
Supplies such as sanitary napkins and tampons may be difficult to find.

Destination-Specific
- Sunscreen for tropical or sunny destinations (#30 SPF, with oxybenzone for additional UVA protection); lip balm.
- Insect repellent—permethrin for clothing, polymer DEET for skin; permethrin aerosol 0.5% for clothing (active for 4-6 weeks or longer, even with laundering); new polymer DEET formulations such as Hour Guard by Amway (35% DEET), DEET Plus (25% DEET mixture), Skedaddle (10% DEET) allow for much lower concentrations of DEET without much skin absorption.
- Acetazolamide (Diamox) 125 mg twice a day (for use in acute mountain sickness).

Skin Care
- StokoGard cream (a fatty acid ester) applied to skin protects against plant dermatitis.
- Calamine lotion and 1% hydrocortisone cream relieves mild dermatitis and itching.

[3]Exceeds dosage recommended by the manufacturer.
Abbreviations: DEET = diethyltoluamide; GI = gastrointestinal; GU = genitourinary; SPF, sun protection factor; UTIs = urinary tract infections; UVA = ultraviolet A.

occurs during travel that involves five or more time zones in a short time. Symptoms typically involve fatigue, headache, anorexia, daytime sleepiness, nighttime insomnia, irritability, and difficulty concentrating. There is no easy solution for the problem of jet lag. Often the best advice is for travelers to adopt local time as soon as possible. Table 6 shows other recommended measures recommended. **Barotrauma** of the middle ear is a result of ambient pressure changes during air travel, and occurs most commonly in those with concurrent upper respiratory infections. Chewing or swallowing during ascent and descent can prevent barotrauma. Infants should be fed during these times. The use of pseudoephedrine slow-release (120 mg)[1]

[1]Not FDA approved for this indication.

TABLE 5 Contraindications to Air Travel

Absolute Contraindications
- Traveler who is unlikely to survive the flight
- Pneumothorax and/or pneumomediastinum
- Active contagious disease (such as active tuberculosis, varicella)
- Complete immobility

Relative Contraindications
- Cardiac—myocardial infarction within the past month, uncontrolled hypertension, severe congestive heart failure, cardiothoracic surgery within the past 3 weeks, symptomatic valvular disease, uncontrolled arrhythmia, unstable angina
- Pulmonary—hypoxic with room air, severe restrictive lung disease, active thrombophlebitis, pulmonary hypertension, active bronchospasm, congenital pulmonary cysts, sickle cell disease
- Ear-Nose-Throat—recent eye or middle ear surgery, acute sinusitis, acute otitis media, recent mandibular fracture
- Neuropsychiatric—recent stroke, brain tumor, recent skull fracture, uncontrolled seizure disorder, uncontrolled violent behavior, psychosis
- Other—pregnancy beyond 35 weeks, severe anemia with hemoglobin less than 7.5 g/dL, newborns younger than 2 weeks old

TABLE 6 Measures to Counteract Jet Lag

Change the Circadian Rhythm
- Adapt local meal and sleep times on arrival.
- Avoid large meals before, during, and immediately after long flights.

Stay Hydrated
- Because humidity on commercial airlines is low, drink large quantities of fluids such as water or apple juice; avoid alcohol and caffeinated beverages, which lead to dehydration.

Consider Taking Melatonin*
- If traveling eastward, take 3-5 mg daily at destination's bedtime (10 PM to midnight) on day of travel, and then nightly for 3-5 nights.
- If traveling westward, omit the dose on the day of travel, then take 3-5 mg at destination's bedtime (10 PM to midnight) nightly for 3-5 nights.

As a Last Resort, Try a Short-Acting Hypnotic
- May be helpful if the flight is long and several hours of uninterrupted sleep can be obtained.
- Possibilities include eszopiclone (Lunesta),[1] diphenhydramine (Benadryl),[1] zaleplon (Sonata),[1] zolpidem (Ambien).[1]
- Triazolam (Halcion)[1] may cause transient global amnesia.
- If used, test the medicine at home prior to traveling to ensure no unwanted side effects.

*Melatonin (N-acetyl-5-methoxytryptamine) is not FDA-approved, and is available as a dietary supplement.
[1]Not FDA-approved for this indication.

TABLE 7 Strategies to Prevent Motion Sickness

- Sit in the most stable part of the vehicle with the best view of the horizon (front seat of the car, on the deck amidships on water, over the wings on a plane).
- Minimize head and neck movements by reclining or by leaning back against a firm surface.
- Minimize activities such as reading or playing video games.
- Avoid strong odors such as tobacco smoke, perfumes, and colognes.
- Avoid large meals.
- Consider taking prophylactic medication before the trip.*
  - Dimenhydrinate (Dramamine) 50-100 mg q4-6hr, 2 hr before the flight.
  - Diphenhydramine (Benadryl) 25-50 mg q4-6hr.
  - Promethazine (Phenergan) 25 mg 30-60 min before travel, repeated every 8-12 hr as needed.
  - Meclizine (Antivert) 25-50 mg 1 hr before travel, repeated every 24 hr
  - Scopolamine (Transderm-Scop) adhesive patch, which is applied behind the ear 4 hr before travel and lasts up to 3 d. It is usually very well tolerated, but side effects could include dry mouth, dilated pupil (if hands are not washed), memory disturbance, hallucinations. Wash hands after applying patch to avoid a unilateral dilated pupil; avoid in those travelers who are on anticholinergic medicines, children, and those with glaucoma or prostate problems.
- Try alternatives such as ginger root and elastic wrist bands that apply acupressure at the P6 point above the wrist (Neiguan).

*Adjust dosage for children.

or oxymetazoline (Afrin)[1] nasal spray (Sudafed Non-Drowsy 12 Hour Long Acting) 30 minutes prior to flight departure decreases the risk of barotrauma in those with sinus or middle ear conditions. **Deep venous thrombosis (DVT)**, also known as Economy Class syndrome, may occur in those at high risk during prolonged flights because of venous pooling and dehydration. Encourage travelers to stretch their legs frequently by moving about the cabin every hour, to do isometric leg exercises, to stay well hydrated, and to avoid alcohol. For those at high risk, the use of elastic support stockings is warranted. **Motion sickness** can occur in anyone, but most often affects children and women. Table 7 shows strategies used to prevent motion sickness.

HIGH-ALTITUDE EXCURSIONS

Travelers who plan to be at altitudes greater than 6000 feet should take precautions to avoid high altitude illness, which includes acute mountain sickness (AMS), high-altitude cerebral edema (HACE), and high-altitude pulmonary edema (HAPE) (Table 8). The three general rules travelers planning on high altitude excursions must follow are:

1. Learn the early symptoms of AMS and be willing to recognize them when they are present (denial is a problem).

[1]Not FDA approved for this indication.

TABLE 8 Lake Louise Consensus on Definition of Altitude Illness

Acute mountain sickness (AMS)	In the setting of a recent gain in altitude, the presence of headache and at least one of the following symptoms: • Gastrointestinal upset (anorexia, nausea, vomiting) • Fatigue or weakness • Dizziness or lightheadedness • Difficulty in sleeping (more than just fitful rest)
High-altitude cerebral edema (HACE)	Can be considered "end stage" or severe AMS. In the setting of a recent gain in altitude, its symptoms are either: • The presence of a change in mental status and/or ataxia in a person with AMS, or • The presence of both mental status changes and ataxia in a person without AMS.

High-altitude pulmonary edema (HAPE)	In the setting of a recent gain in altitude, suspect in presence of the following:
	• Symptoms—at least two of the following:
	  • Shortness of breath at rest
	  • Cough
	  • Weakness or decreased exercise performance
	  • Chest tightness or congestion
	• Signs—at least two of the following:
	  • Rales or wheezing in at least one lung field (usually RML)
	  • Central cyanosis
	  • Rapid breathing
	  • Rapid heart rate

Adapted from The Lake Louise Consensus on the Definition and Quantification of Altitude Illness. In Sutton JR, Coates G, Houston CS (eds): Hypoxia and Mountain Medicine. Burlington, Vermont: Queen City Printers, 1992.

2. Ascend gradually to allow for acclimatization, usually climbing no more than 1000 feet per day when above an altitude of 10,000 feet.
3. Descend if symptoms of AMS occur.

Further advice can be found at the Web site *http://www.high-altitude-medicine.com/*.

Advice on Avoiding Infections

SEXUALLY TRANSMITTED DISEASES

Nearly a quarter of overseas travelers have sexual relations with someone they meet en route. All travelers should be cautioned that sexually transmitted diseases (STDs), including HIV and hepatitis B and C, might be contracted throughout the world. Abstinence outside of a mutually monogamous relationship is best, and if not possible, condoms and safe sex practices should be practiced.

UNSAFE INJECTIONS

Therapeutic injections are rarely necessary, but in most developing countries more than half of visits to physicians result in an injection being given. As needles and syringes are often reused in developing countries and are a major source of transmission of HIV and hepatitis B, warn travelers to avoid injections if at all possible.

FRESH WATER SWIMMING

Many infectious diseases, such as schistosomiasis and leptospirosis, are contracted through exposure to fresh water found in lakes, rivers, and streams. Travelers should be advised not to swim in fresh water and to wear shoes when walking through fresh water. Instead, they should only swim in well-maintained chlorinated pools or ocean water known to be free from pollution.

TRAVELER'S DIARRHEA

Traveler's diarrhea is the most common ailment encountered while abroad. The traveler should be counseled about proper food and water hygiene (Table 9). Traveler's diarrhea results in a twofold or greater increase in the frequency of unformed stools, associated with abdominal cramps, fecal urgency, bloating, nausea, fever, and malaise. It usually occurs during the first week of travel and is usually self-limited, lasting 3 to 7 days, which, although mild, may ruin a trip.

Prevention of traveler's diarrhea is best. Although the CDC no longer recommends antibiotic prophylaxis because it can lead to drug-resistant organisms, those traveling to remote areas with limited medical access may require it. If desired, bismuth subsalicylate (Pepto-Bismol),[1] two 262-mg tablets or 2 fluid ounces (60 mL) four times daily, can be used for chemoprophylaxis for up to 3 weeks. This agent should be avoided in those allergic to aspirin, are pregnant, or are on an anticoagulant, probenecid (Benemid), doxycycline (Vibramycin), or methotrexate (Rheumatrex). A quinolone taken once daily—such as ciprofloxacin (Cipro),[1] 500 mg, norfloxacin (Noroxin)[1] 400 mg, ofloxacin (Floxin)[1] 300 mg, or levofloxacin (Levaquin)[1] 500 mg—is

---

[1]Not FDA approved for this indication.

TABLE 9 Prevention of Traveler's Diarrhea

- In areas of poor sanitation, only the following are safe to drink:
  - Boiled water, or water that has been disinfected with iodine or chlorine tablets
  - Hot beverages such as tea or coffee, if made with boiled water or disinfected water
  - Canned or bottled water, carbonated beverages, fruit juices, beer, and wine
- Avoid ice unless sure it was made from "safe" water.
- Avoid tap water for drinking and brushing teeth.
- Small-pore (0.1 to 0.3 μm) filters can remove bacteria and protozoa, but not viruses.
- Regarding food, "boil it, peel it, cook it, or forget it!"
- All food, especially meat, should be well cooked and served hot.
- Avoid these foods:
  - Salads
  - Uncooked vegetables and fruit (that cannot be peeled)
  - Condiments
  - Unpasteurized milk and milk products, including ice cream
  - Shellfish
  - Certain fish such as red snapper, amberjack, grouper, sea bass, barracuda, and puffer fish may cause ciguatera poisoning due to toxin.
- Avoid food sold by street vendors.
- Chemoprophylaxis is generally not recommended.

TABLE 10 Personal Protection Against Insect Bites

- Cover skin with tightly woven fabrics that are light in color (tan, khaki, pale green), and:
  - Avoid sheer fabrics and tight clothing.
  - Tuck pant legs into socks and tuck shirttails into pants.
  - Avoid sandals and open-toe shoes.
- Avoid use of colognes and perfumes, which may attract insects.
- Check skin daily for insects.
- Avoid walking in tall grass and lying directly on the ground.
- Never dry clothing on the ground.
- Check inside footwear and sleeping bags for insects.
- Avoid outdoor activity during the twilight periods of dusk and dawn.
- Use air conditioning when available and keep windows closed.
- Sleep under insect netting of good quality with small mesh impregnated with permethrin.
- Choose camping areas that are high, dry, and away from food or rotting wood.
- Apply an insecticide such as permethrin to clothing and bedding.
- Apply an insect repellent containing 35% or less DEET to the skin

effective but is contraindicated in children and women who are pregnant.

If a traveler does develop diarrhea, early empiric self-treatment can shorten the course of symptoms. The traveler should replace fluids lost with an oral rehydration solution, reliable bottled water, or caffeine-free carbonated beverages. An antimotility agent such as loperamide (Imodium AD) or bismuth subsalicylate (Pepto-Bismol) combined with an antibiotic for 3 days effectively reduces symptoms and shortens the diarrhea course. Options for antibiotics include the quinolones mentioned previously, rifaximin (Xifaxan), 200 mg three times daily, and azithromycin (Zithromax),[1] 500 mg daily. Azithromycin is preferable for children and pregnant women, and in those traveling to areas where quinolone-resistant *Campylobacter* is present. Providers should review the information from the CDC's Web site for latest recommendations regarding treatment.

PREVENTING INSECT BITES

A number of parasitic and viral diseases that afflict travelers are caused by a mosquito or insect bite. Travelers need to take personal protective measures to avoid these ailments (Table 10). Permethrin repellent is an effective insecticide that can be sprayed on clothing, knapsacks, tents, and netting, but not directly on skin. It offers protection for approximately 2 weeks, even when laundered up to 20 times. Rooms can be sprayed 1 hour before bedtime, but travelers should stay out of the room for 30 minutes after spraying. Diethyltoluamide (DEET) is the most effective and best studied insect repellent currently on the market, with a safety profile of more than 40 years. It is applied to exposed skin and is effective for up to 4 hours. Adults should use a formula with 35% or less concentration, and children should use a concentration of 10% or less. It should be used sparingly in children 2 to 6 years old, and avoided in children younger than 2 years. Pregnant women can safely use DEET sparingly in a low concentration.

MALARIA PROPHYLAXIS

Malaria is a major international public health problem. Transmission of the disease occurs in Central and South America, Hispaniola, sub-Saharan Africa, the Indian subcontinent, Southeast Asia, the Middle East, and Oceania. Risk and need for prophylaxis depends on the itinerary, length of stay, and activities planned. Health care providers advising international travelers should consult a reputable resource before prescribing a prophylactic antimalarial, because chloroquine-resistant *Plasmodium falciparum* is increasing worldwide. The CDC Web site is an excellent resource.

Several prophylactic antimalarials are available (Table 11). Generally, when traveling to areas without resistance, **chloroquine** (Aralen) remains a good first agent, if not contraindicated. This medication is generally well tolerated with occasional mild adverse effects such as nausea, dizziness, or headache. It should be avoided in travelers with a history of psoriasis as it may exacerbate the condition.

---

[1]Not FDA approved for this indication.

TABLE 11 Chemoprophylaxis of Malaria

Malaria Risk	Drugs	Adult Dosage	Pediatric Dosage
Chloroquine-sensitive *P. falciparum* *P. vivax*	Chloroquine (Aralen)* *or* Chloroquine *plus*	300 mg base (500 mg salt) PO once/wk 300 mg base (500 mg salt) PO once/wk	5 mg base/kg (8.3 mg salt/kg) PO once/wk (max 300 mg base) 5 mg base/kg (8.3 mg salt/kg) PO once/wk (max 300 mg base)
P. ovale *P. malariae*	Proguanil (Paludrine)†	200 mg PO qd	PO once daily: <2 y, 50 mg; 2-6 y, 100 mg; 7-10 y, 150 mg; >10 y, 200 mg
Chloroquine-resistant *P. falciparum* *P. vivax*	Mefloquine* *or*	228 mg base (250 mg salt) PO once/wk	<15 kg, 4.6 mg base (5 mg salt)/kg/wk; 15-19 kg, 0.25 tablet/wk 20-30 kg, 0.5 tablet/wk; 31-45 kg, 0.75 tablet/wk; >45 kg, 1.0 tablet PO once/wk
	Doxycycline *or*	100 mg PO qd	≤8 y, contraindicated; >8 y, 2 mg/kg (max 100 mg) PO qd
	Atovaquone/Proguanil (Malarone)	1 tablet qd	11-20 kg: 1 pediatric tablet qd; 21-30 kg, 2 pediatric tablets qd; 31-40 kg, 3 pediatric tablets qd; >40 kg, 1 adult tablet qd
Mefloquine-resistant Quinine-resistant *P. falciparum*	Doxycycline* *or* Atovaquone/Proguanil	100 mg PO qd 1 tablet qd	≤8 y, contraindicated; >8 y, 2 mg/kg (max 100 mg) PO qd; 11-20 kg, 1 pediatric tablet daily; 21-30 kg, 2 pediatric tablets daily; 31-40 kg, 3 pediatric tablets daily; >40 kg, 1 adult tablet daily
Terminal prophylaxis of relapsing hypnozoites *P. vivax* *P. ovale*	Primaquine*,‡	15 mg base (26.3 mg salt) PO qd for 14 d after departure from malarious area	0.3 mg base/kg (0.5 mg salt/kg) PO once/d for 14 d after departure from malarious area

*Drug of choice.
†Not licensed in the U.S.; available in Canada, Europe, and many African countries.
‡Check G6PD levels before prescribing.
- No chemoprophylactic drug is absolutely safe or effective in preventing malaria.
- Begin chemoprophylaxis 1 week before travel (except doxycycline—start 1-2 days before travel) and continue for 4 weeks after return.
- Some prefer chloroquine 600 mg base PO once weekly or 150 mg base PO once daily in adults. Chloroquine with proguanil is ineffective in Africa, Thailand, Southeast Asia, and Oceania and should be used for travel to countries with chloroquine-resistant malaria only when mefloquine or doxycycline is contraindicated.
- Mefloquine rarely causes neuropsychiatric toxicity (1 in 10,000 patients); so can chloroquine (1 in 13,600 patients); doxycycline can cause photosensitivity.
- Keep chloroquine (and all medications) out of the reach of small children—one dose is enough to kill an infant.
- All patients must be screened for G6PD deficiency before treatment with primaquine. The dose of primaquine in Southeast Asia, Oceania, and the Amazon basin should be 22.5–30 mg PO qd for 14 days.
- Chloroquine, proguanil, mefloquine, and probably atovaquone/proguanil are safe in pregnancy. Doxycycline is contraindicated in pregnancy and in children younger than 8 years.
- Pregnant women, children, and patients unwilling or unable to take atovaquone/proguanil or mefloquine or doxycycline should not travel to chloroquine-resistant areas. If travel is unavoidable and malarial exposure is likely, the risks of malaria far exceed the potential toxicity of mefloquine or atovaquone/proguanil.
- Up-to-date malaria treatment recommendations and case management advice may be obtained from the CDC using the malaria hotline: (770) 736-7060.
Abbreviations: G6PD = glucose-6-phosphate dehydrogenase; PO = orally.
Data from Stanley J: Malaria. Emerg Med Clin North Am 1997;15(1):134-137; Juckett G: Malaria prevention in travelers. Am Fam Phys 1999;59:2523-2530.

It can be safely used in children and during pregnancy. Presently, chloroquine-resistant malaria has been reported in Southeast Asia, Indonesia, and Latin America. When traveling to areas of resistance, other prophylactic options must be considered.

The drug of choice for travelers going to areas of chloroquine-resistant *P. falciparum* is **mefloquine (Lariam)**. It is generally well tolerated, with occasional adverse effects of nausea, loss of appetite, diarrhea, dizziness, fatigue, and insomnia. Rarely (1 in 10,000), individuals may develop severe adverse reactions such as confusion, memory loss, nightmares, hallucinations, depression, paranoia, and agitation. Its use should be avoided in those with a history of heart conduction problems, epilepsy, depression or anxiety, and in those taking calcium channel blockers, beta-blockers, or quinidine. Mefloquine can be prescribed for children. However, because it cannot be made into a suspension, parents should crush the medication and place it into a very sweet juice or food. Parents should also be reminded to keep medications away from children, as overdoses of antimalarials can be fatal. Clinical trials and reports of inadvertent use of mefloquine during pregnancy suggest that its use during the second and third trimesters pose no threat of adverse outcomes. It can be considered for women in their second or third trimesters when exposure to chloroquine-resistant *P. falciparum* is unavoidable.

Another possible prophylactic antimalarial is **doxycycline**. As most adverse effects are gastrointestinal in nature, it is best taken with food. Concomitant use of antacids should be avoided because they may interfere with absorption of doxycycline. Photosensitivity may also occur, so travelers should use a sunscreen with an SPF of 15 or greater. Doxycycline cannot be used in children younger than 8 years and is contraindicated in pregnancy.

A combination antimalarial composed of **atovaquone** and **proguanil (Malarone)**, is another option that is generally well tolerated. It should be taken with food, as nausea is the most common adverse effect. It should be avoided in those taking tetracycline, metoclopramide (Reglan), rifampin (Rifadin), or rifabutin (Mycobutin). Although approved for use in children, it currently is not recommended in pregnancy.

It should be stressed to all travelers that despite the use of personal protective measures, repellents, and chemoprophylaxis, they still could develop malaria. Travelers should be advised that symptoms generally occur 10 to 14 days after an exposure and include high fever, severe myalgias, headache, nausea, and vomiting. These symptoms may abate and then return. If these symptoms are experienced, the traveler should seek health care immediately.

Malaria can be particularly severe in pregnant women, with a high risk of preterm delivery, miscarriage, and stillbirth. Because no chemoprophylactic regimen is 100% effective, travel to endemic areas should be avoided or postponed until after delivery. If the woman cannot be dissuaded from traveling to endemic areas, she should at least postpone travel until the second trimester (18 to 24 weeks), a time when there is less risk and when an antimalarial can be prescribed. Pregnant women considering travel should consult their family doctor or obstetrician before international departures to discuss individual risk factors.

PROPER IMMUNIZATION

The reason most travelers seek pretravel care is to make sure they are properly immunized. Vaccinations fall into three general categories (Table 12):

1. Routine immunizations everyone should have, regardless of destination
2. Immunizations required by law in some countries
3. Immunizations that are medically recommended based on destination and traveler's proposed activities, but not required

Immunizations should be properly documented on an approved International Certificate of Vaccination (PHS-731). Live virus vaccinations should either be given simultaneously or separated by 3 weeks, and should be avoided if at all possible in pregnant women and those who are immunocompromised. Because tuberculosis is a major problem worldwide, consider tuberculin (purified protein derivative [PPD]) skin testing for individuals who do not have a prior positive test, and repeat testing 1 to 2 months upon return from their trip.

Many countries only require **yellow fever** vaccination. Yellow fever vaccination should only be given at designated yellow fever sites and documented on the PHS-731. Evidence suggests that individuals 65 years and older are at increased risk for adverse events following administration of the vaccine. In this case, the elderly traveler and health care provider should weigh carefully the risks and benefits. For those unable to receive this vaccination because of contraindications, an exemption letter can be written using official letterhead and bearing an official stamp. Although cholera vaccine is no longer commercially available in the United States, some countries may still want to see proof of **cholera** vaccination. Prior to travel, one should ensure that cholera vaccination is not required; if it is, efforts should be made to obtain the vaccine from another country before travel.

When deciding what other vaccinations should be given, the risk of exposure should be weighed against the risk of the vaccination. For example, most people would feel it is better not to pet stray dogs in the street than it is to receive a rabies vaccination. Vaccinations recommended for most individuals, depending upon destination, include those to prevent **hepatitis A** (Havrix, Vaqta, and Twinrix), **immunoglobulin** (if the hepatitis A vaccine cannot be given), and **typhoid**. Other vaccinations such as those for **hepatitis B**, **Japanese encephalitis**, and **rabies** depend upon the traveler's proposed activities and are rarely needed.

AWARENESS OF CURRENT EPIDEMICS

Periodically epidemics occur worldwide that concern travelers. A recent example is **avian influenza A (H5N1)**. This virus, which normally affects wild birds, has caused serious disease in the poultry of Asia and Europe, and has spread to humans in several Asian countries. There is currently no vaccine for H5N1. Antiviral drugs such as oseltamivir (Tamiflu) may effectively treat H5N1, but not enough data exist to fully support its use as an effective agent. The best advice that can currently be offered to travelers is to avoid open-air markets where poultry or birds are displayed for purchase. All poultry that are consumed must be well cooked. Keeping the hands as clean as possible with alcohol-based hand rubs is also very good advice. H5N1 continues to be an emerging infectious disease of interest. Primary care providers should stay as up to date as possible regarding H5N1 by continuing to monitor postings of the CDC (*www.cdc.gov*) and the World Health Organization (WHO) (*http://www.who.org/*).

Post-Travel Care

Providers offering care to travelers should be able to recognize, diagnose, and treat unusual conditions acquired during travel. Not all persons who travel need a post-travel evaluation, especially for those who are healthy and had a short-term trip. Those returning from long trips (30 days or more) and expatriates from developing countries should undergo evaluation even if asymptomatic. At a minimum, a history and physical examination, complete blood count, chemistry profile, PPD, and stool examination should be performed. Every traveler who develops a fever or flulike symptoms should be considered to have malaria unless proved otherwise.

Resources for Health Care Providers and Travelers

1. **http://www.cdc.gov/travel**. Web site maintained by the CDC that is a must for those involved in travel medicine. It contains the latest blue sheet (cholera and yellow fever information); Yellow Book; green pages (cruise sanitation information); and the latest, updated information on vaccination requirements.
2. **Health Information for International Travel (Yellow Book)**. This outstanding resource is usually published

TABLE 12   Immunizations for International Travel

Vaccine	Type	Schedule	Children's Dose	Booster	Indications	Precautions
Routine Immunizations Everyone Should Have, Regardless of Destination						
Influenza (Fluzone)	Inactivated viral whole split cell influenza A and B virus	One dose (0.5 mL IM or SQ)	Two doses for those <8 y: 6 mo - 3 y: 0.25 mL 3 - 8 y: 0.5 mL 8 y: 0.5 mL (1 dose)	Annually	>64 y old. Traveling to tropics or Southern Hemisphere Apr- Sep. Immunocompromised.	Egg allergy (anaphylaxis).
Tetanus-diphtheria (Td)	Bacterial toxoid	Three doses at 0, 1, and 6-12 mo (0.5 mL SQ or IM)	Same as adult dosage Recommended 11-18 y	q10 y	Those who have never received the primary series, or have not received a booster in the last 10 y.	Give during the 2nd or 3rd trimester of pregnancy, if possible.
DTaP (Boostrix)		One dose	Approved up to age 65	q10 y		
Measles	Attenuated live viral monovalent or combined MMR (measles-mumps-rubella)	Two doses on or after 1st birthday (0.5 mL SQ)	Same as adult dosage	None after completing primary series	Adults born after 1956 who were never immunized and children who have not completed the primary series.	Immunocompromised. Pregnancy. Neomycin allergy. Avoid 2 wk before or 12 wk after SIG (serum immunoglobulin).
Pneumococcus (Pneumovax 23)	Bacterial polysaccharide	One dose (0.5 mL SQ)	Same as adult dosage	5 y after 1st dose, once	>64 y old. COPD. Functional asplenia. Immunocompromised.	None.
Poliomyelitis (IPOL)	Inactivated viral IPV: injectable – the preferred route (oral polio – OPV - no longer available in the US)	IPV: four doses at 0, 1-2, and 6-12 mo (for those not properly immunized). (0.5 mL SQ)	Same as adult dosage	Once when >18 y old (provides lifelong immunity after age 18 if primary series given)	Travel to polio endemic countries of South Asia, sub-Saharan Africa, and New Independent States.	Avoid during pregnancy if at all possible.

Immunizations Required by Law in Some Countries

	Type	Dose	Schedule	Interval	Indications	Contraindications/Comments
Meningococcal (Quadrivalent) A/C/Y/W-135)	Menomune: Inactivated bacterial Polysaccharide Menactra: Inactivated bacterial Conjugate	One dose (0.5 mL SQ) One dose (0.5 mL IM)	0.5 mL Age 11 and up only	q3-5 y Unknown	Travel to sub-Saharan Africa from Dec–Jun. Functional asplenia. Required for those traveling to Mecca for Islamic pilgrimage.	Not recommended in those < 2 y. Menactra is indicated for ages 11–55 y.
Yellow Fever (YF-VAX)	Attenuated live viral	One dose (0.5 mL SQ)	6 months of age (delay until 9 months if possible); 0.5 mL SQ	q10y	Travel to equatorial Africa and S. America. Required by some countries.	Egg allergy. Pregnancy. Age < 6 months. Immunocompromised.

Immunizations Recommended Based on Destination and Proposed Activities

	Type	Dose	Schedule	Interval	Indications	Contraindications/Comments
Hepatitis A (Havrix) (Vaqta)	Inactivated viral Inactivated viral	Two doses (1440 EL.U) at 0 & 6-12 mo (1.0 mL IM) Two doses (50 U) at 0 & 6-12 mo (1.0 mL IM)	12mo–18 y: two doses (720 EL.U) at 0 and 6-12 mo (0.5 mL IM) 12mo–17 y: two doses (25 U) at 0 and 6-18 mo	q20y q20y	Travel to endemic areas, 4 wk before travel. Travel to endemic areas.	Not recommended for age <12 mo. Age <12 mo.
Hepatitis B (Engerix-B, Recombivax)	Inactivated viral yeast-derived recombinant surface antigen	Three doses at 0, 1, 6 mo, or accelerated: 0, 1, 2 mo Energix: 20 µg Recombivax: 10 µg	Engerix-B:<10 y: 10 µg 10 y: 20 µg Recombivax: <11 y: 2.5 µg 11-19 y: 5 µg	If given via accelerated schedule, repeated at 12 mo; otherwise, none	Child, adolescent, sexually active or travel > 6 mo to endemic area. Health care workers who may be exposed to blood products.	None.
Hepatitis A/B combined vaccine (Twinrix)	Combination of Havrix (720 EI U) and Engerix-B (20 µg/mL)	Three doses at 0, 1, 6 mo (1.0 mL IM)	Not recommended	Not yet determined	Same as hepatitis A & B.	Not approved for children < 19 y.
Serum immune globulin (BayGam)	Fractionated immunoglobulins	One dose: 0.02 mL/kg IM for 3 mo protection 0.06 mL/kg IM for 5 mo protection	Same as adult dosage (minimum dose 0.5 mL)	3–5 mo intervals, as per initial dose	Single visit of < 3 mo to endemic area.	Give live virus vaccines >2 wk before or >3 mo after SIG (yellow fever unaffected).

Continued

TABLE 12   Immunizations for International Travel—cont'd

Vaccine	Type	Schedule	Children's Dose	Booster	Indications	Precautions
Japanese B encephalitis (JE Vax)	Inactivated viral	Three doses at 0, 7, and 30 d (1 mL SQ) Accelerated: 0, 7, 14	1-2 y: 0.5 mL ≥2 y: 1.0 mL	q2y (1 mL)	> 30-d stay to SE Asia, India, or China/Korea, especially visits to rice paddies and pig farms.	Pregnancy. Age < 1 y. Departure less than 10 d after vaccination.
Rabies (Imovax)	Inactivated viral HDCV (Imovax), or RVA, or PCEC (RabAvert)	Three doses at 0, 7, and 21–28 d (1 mL IM deltoid; 0.1 mL ID for HCDV only)	Same as adult dosage	1 y after completing series for those at risk; 3 y if antibodies decline	> 30 d in SE Asia. Potential close exposure to animals.	HDCV - do not begin chloroquine/mefloquine until 30 d after series is completed.
Typhoid	Oral live attenuated Ty21a vaccine (Vivotif)	1 capsule every 48 hr for four doses; not given concomitantly with antibiotics or antimalarials	Same as adult dose 2 y: 0.5 mL	5 y 2–3 y	>2 wk in developing country. Same as Vivotif.	Impaired gastric defenses. Pregnancy. Immunocompromised. Age < 6 y. Pregnancy. Age < 2 y.
	Bacterial polysaccharide ViCPS (Typhim Vi)	One dose (0.5 mL IM)				

Abbreviations: COPD = chronic obstructive pulmonary disease; HDCV = human diploid cell vaccine; IM = intramuscular; IPV = inactivated poliomyelitis (virus) vaccine; PCEC = purified chick embryo cell (culture); RVA = rabies vaccine adsorbed; SIG = serum immunoglobulin; SQ = subcutaneous;
Data from Advice for Travelers. Medical Letters 1998;40:47-50; Thanassi WT, Weiss EL: Immunizations and travel. Emerg Med Clin N Am. 1997;15(1):43-70; and Foster JA, Watson B, Bell LM: Travel with infants and children. Emerg Med Clin N Am 1997;15(1):71-92; Thompson RF: Travel & Routine Immunizations: A Practical Guide for the Medical Office. Milwaukee, WI: Shoreland, 2001.

every 2 years by the CDC and contains a list of all countries, with their requirements for immunizations and risk for malaria and other diseases. This is a good resource for those who don't have access to the CDC Web site.

3. **International Travel and Health.** A convenient country-by-country list of required vaccinations, along with pertinent information about the malaria situation in every country in the world. This can be downloaded from the Web site of the World Health Organization (WHO) at *http://www.who.int/*.

4. **International Association for Medical Assistance to Travelers (IAMAT)** (http://www.iamat.org/). A nonprofit organization that provides assistance to travelers. Information available to members includes a worldwide directory of English-speaking physicians trained in the United States, Canada, and the United Kingdom, and who have agreed to a set fee schedule (IAMAT does not credential or certify the competency of these physicians). Other information includes an immunization chart, malaria risk chart, world climate charts, and other useful information.

5. **The U.S. Department of State** (*http://travel.state.gov*). Travel warnings, tips for safe travel, and consular information sheets.

6. **International Society of Travel Medicine** (*http://www.istm.org*). The largest organization of professionals dedicated to the advancement of travel medicine. The Web site contains a directory of travel medicine clinics in more than 40 countries that assist travelers in locating health care professionals with expertise in travel medicine.

7. **Needle Tips & the Hepatitis B Coalition News** (*http://www.immunize.org*). Information published by the Immunization Action Coalition for individuals and organizations concerned about vaccine-preventable diseases.

8. **Travel & Routine Immunizations—A Practical Guide for the Medical Office.** Published annually by Shoreland (*http://www.shoreland.com*), this guide provides general information, health precautions, immunizations, disease risk summary, and current health concerns for each country. *Travel Medicine Monthly* is a compendium of travel medicine abstracts and original articles.

9. **The CIA World Factbook** (*http://www.odci.gov/cia/publications/factbook/index.html*). A good overview on each country, including its geography, weather, politics, economy, and other facts about the populace.

10. **Passport Information** (*http://travel.state.gov/passport*). The latest information needed for passports.

11. **High Altitude Medicine** (*http://www.high-altitude-medicine.com/*). Home page for the Himalayan Rescue Association that provides an excellent source of information on high altitude medicine for both patients and physicians.

Toxoplasmosis

Method of
Thomas T. Ward, MD

Toxoplasmosis is the disease caused by infection with the obligate intracellular protozoan *Toxoplasma gondii*. Toxoplasmosis is a worldwide zoonosis and causes infection in both birds and mammals. Cats, the definitive hosts for *T. gondii*, are the animals in which the parasite maintains an enteroepithelial sexual cycle. Human beings and domestic animals are secondary hosts and are important in maintaining an extraintestinal asexual cycle of transmission. Although most human infection is asymptomatic, self-limited clinical disease can infrequently occur after primary infection in immunocompetent persons. Because of the persistence of dormant cyst forms, all infection becomes chronic and latent. Primary infection during pregnancy can result in transplacental transmission of infection to the fetus; resultant congenital toxoplasmosis has varied clinical manifestations. Reactivation of dormant cysts is an important cause of infection in immunocompromised patients with defective T-cell–mediated immunity, including those patients with advanced HIV infection, hematologic malignancies, and bone marrow and solid-organ transplants.

T. gondii exists in three forms: the oocyst, the tissue cyst, and the tachyzoite. Oocysts are formed only in infected felines; these cats excrete large numbers of cysts for approximately 2 weeks after infection. Oocysts may remain viable in the soil for months and are an important environmental reservoir for infection of incidental hosts. Tachyzoites occur with acute infection in incidental hosts; their presence is required for the histologic confirmation of active disease. Tissue cysts occur after replication of tachyzoites and likely persist for the life of the incidental host. Dormant cysts are most commonly located in skeletal and smooth muscle, heart, brain, and eye. The presence of tissue cysts in histologic sections is indicative of past infection, but by itself it does not signify active infection.

The human incidence of seropositivity for *T. gondii* antibody varies greatly throughout the world. Within the United States, seropositivity increases with age, and the overall seroprevalence is approximately 15%. Within Western Europe, seroprevalence ranges between 50% and 70%. Human transmission occurs by oral exposure to oocysts that have contaminated water sources, vegetables, or other food products or, even more commonly, by ingesting poorly cooked or raw meat that contains tissue cysts. As many as 25% of lamb or pork samples contain tissue cysts.

After human ingestion of either oocysts or tissue cysts, specialized forms of *T. gondii* emerge that penetrate the intestinal mucosa, establish intracellular infection within white blood cells, and enter the blood and lymphatic circulations to result in widespread dissemination throughout the body. Intact cell-mediated immunity leads to clearance of intracellular tachyzoites and the formation of dormant tissue cysts. Impaired cell-mediated immunity leads to either uncontrolled, primary infection (as in the fetus) or reactivation of infection later in life (as in AIDS and other immunosuppressed conditions).

Diagnosis

The diagnosis of *T. gondii* infection can be established by serologic tests, amplification of specific nucleic acid sequences, or histologic demonstration of the parasite or its antigens. Rarely employed reference or research methods for diagnosis include isolation of the organism, specific IgG avidity tests, various antigen detection tests, and lymphocyte transformation tests.

IgG antibodies appear in immunocompetent individuals within 2 to 3 weeks after infection. A negative IgG test essentially excludes previous or past infection with *T. gondii*. IgG antibody may persist in high titers for years after infection; therefore, a single positive IgG titer does not differentiate whether infection is recently acquired, chronic and latent, or chronic and reactivated. Sequential IgG antibody tests that increase by more than two tube dilutions are consistent with recent infection. Specific IgM and IgA antibody tests are usually positive during the first 6 months after acquisition of infection, and negative tests have a high predictive value for excluding recent infection. A positive IgM test can indicate recent onset of infection; however, both false-positive results and persistently positive IgM antibody test results in chronically infected individuals can occur. When therapeutic decisions will be based on the interpretation of a positive IgM antibody test, confirmatory testing by a reference laboratory should be performed if feasible. Serologic tests can be more difficult to interpret in immunocompromised patients.

Polymerase chain reaction (PCR) for detection of specific *T. gondii* nucleic acid sequences has been successfully employed using vitreous and aqueous humor, bronchoalveolar lavage fluid, peripheral blood buffy coat preparations, cerebrospinal fluid, and amniotic fluid after 18 weeks of gestation. False-positive results on brain tissue PCR tests may occur in patients with HIV infection and suspected toxoplasmic encephalitis.

Specific histopathologic findings on resected lymph nodes can be strongly suggestive of the diagnosis of toxoplasmosis in immunocompetent patients. Demonstration of tachyzoites in tissue is invariably diagnostic of active infection. Although the presence of a single cyst does not differentiate between active and chronic or latent infection, multiple cysts present on cytopathologic examination suggest the presence of active disease. Staining for specific antigens (e.g., immunoperoxidase techniques) is highly specific for active infection when positive, and it is much more sensitive than hematoxylin and eosin or Wright-Giemsa staining alone. Tests employing direct fluorescent antibody tests can be nonspecific and are best avoided.

Clinical Manifestations

Most patients with acute *T. gondii* infection do not have symptomatic disease. Clinical manifestations of acute infection occasionally occur in immunocompetent adults, as does reactivation of infection within the retina of the eye. Infection during pregnancy results in congenital toxoplasmosis at an incidence of approximately 1 in 8000 live births in the United States; the frequency in which *T. gondii* causes spontaneous abortion is unknown. Reactivation infection from dormant cysts is the cause of toxoplasmic infections in patients with AIDS, patients with bone marrow or solid-organ transplants, and other immunosuppressed hosts. The clinical syndromes in each of the foregoing settings are sufficiently distinct to warrant separate comment.

ACUTE INFECTION IN IMMUNOCOMPETENT PATIENTS

Approximately 15% of immunocompetent patients who become infected have either regional lymphadenopathy or a mononucleosis-like syndrome characterized by generalized adenopathy and constitutional symptoms. Toxoplasmic lymphadenopathy is largely a self-limited disease in immunocompetent patients, and it rarely requires therapy. Epstein-Barr virus and cytomegalovirus infections are much more common causes of the mononucleosis syndrome. Other causes of lymphadenopathy that need to be considered include cat-scratch disease, lymphoma or metastatic malignancy, sarcoidosis, tuberculosis, and the deep mycoses. Serologic testing and lymph node biopsy are most beneficial in establishing a diagnosis. Infections acquired by blood transfusion or through a laboratory accident may be severe and should be treated.

OCULAR TOXOPLASMOSIS IN IMMUNOCOMPETENT PATIENTS

Approximately 33% of all cases of chorioretinitis within the Unites States are caused by *T. gondii*. Most cases are believed to result from unrecognized congenital infection that reactivates, most commonly during the second and third decades of life. Retinal clinical findings are highly suggestive of *T. gondii* infection when evaluated by ophthalmologists experienced in managing this infection. Serologic testing is usually positive for prior exposure to toxoplasmosis, but in difficult cases, PCR testing may be performed on samples of aqueous or vitreous humor to confirm the diagnosis. Control of the host inflammatory response by the concomitant use of corticosteroids may be required in some patients receiving therapy for toxoplasmosis. Relapse of infection requiring repeated treatment is not uncommon.

CONGENITAL TOXOPLASMOSIS

Congenital toxoplasmosis results from transplacental spread of *T. gondii* infection that is asymptomatically acquired either during pregnancy or shortly before the onset of gestation. The risk of fetal infection varies with the stage of trimester; it is highest during the second and third trimesters. Approximately 60% of maternal infections acquired during the third trimester will result in fetal infection. Fetal infection occurring during the first trimester is believed to result frequently in spontaneous abortion. Clinical manifestations of congenital toxoplasmosis are varied. There may be no sequelae, or clinical disease may become manifest at birth or at various times after birth. Children may be born with the nonspecific manifestations of the TORCH (toxoplasmosis, other infections, rubella, cytomegalovirus, and herpes simplex) syndrome, including chorioretinitis, hydrocephalus, intracranial calcifications, hepatosplenomegaly, rash, anemia, and/or jaundice. Other infectious causes such as herpes simplex, cytomegalovirus infection, rubella, and syphilis should be considered and excluded. In those infants born with subclinical congenital infection, studies suggest that most will eventually demonstrate evidence of clinical disease even though they appear normal at birth. Years or decades later, previously subclinically infected children may develop chorioretinitis, seizure disorders, or psychomotor and mental retardation. Early recognition and treatment of congenital infection reduce the likelihood of subsequent sequelae; therefore, congenital *T. gondii* infection should always be treated regardless of whether there are symptoms at birth. Treatment of acute maternal infection diagnosed during pregnancy reduces the risk of fetal infection by approximately 60%.

Because congenital toxoplasmosis occurs almost exclusively in women infected during pregnancy, it is important that such infection be recognized and treated aggressively. In some countries where there is a higher seroprevalence of *T. gondii* infection (e.g., France), routine screening for acquisition of infection during pregnancy is performed. Routine pregnancy screening is not currently advocated in the United States. Women who have IgG antibody but who lack specific IgM antibody are believed to have evidence of past, chronic infection and are not at risk of transmitting congenital infection. A positive IgM test requires further confirmatory testing through a reference laboratory to determine whether infection has been recently acquired. Confirmation of acutely acquired maternal infection during pregnancy mandates testing during and after pregnancy to determine whether fetal or congenital infection has occurred. PCR testing of amniotic fluid at 18 weeks of gestation and beyond is approximately 60% sensitive and 100% specific in diagnosing fetal infection. Diagnosis of congenital toxoplasmosis at birth is usually confirmed by the presence of specific IgA (or IgM) in fetal serum, with careful attention to exclusion of maternal contamination of fetal blood. In children with suspected congenital toxoplasmosis, it is important to perform ophthalmologic evaluation and neuroimaging studies and to examine the cerebrospinal fluid for pleocytosis or elevated protein concentrations.

TOXOPLASMOSIS IN AIDS AND IMMUNOCOMPROMISED PATIENTS

In immunocompromised patients, toxoplasmosis almost always occurs as reactivation infection. One exception is infection after heart transplantation, in which primary infection can occur when a seronegative host receives a donor heart from a seropositive donor. The central nervous system is the most commonly affected site, resulting in necrotizing focal or multifocal encephalitis and, less frequently, focal spinal cord involvement. Other forms of infection include chorioretinitis, myocarditis, and pneumonia. Active toxoplasmosis in immunodeficient patients can cause significant morbidity and mortality and always requires therapy. The duration of therapy is largely dependent on the degree of chronic immunosuppression, and, on occasion, lifelong maintenance therapy is indicated.

In natural history studies of HIV infection performed before effective antiretroviral therapy, it was observed that approximately one third of toxoplasmosis-seropositive patients with AIDS developed toxoplasmic encephalitis before death. Daily receipt of one tablet of double-strength trimethoprim (160 mg)-sulfamethoxazole (800 mg) (Bactrim DS) largely eliminates the risk of disease. Most episodes of toxoplasmic encephalitis complicating AIDS occur in patients with $CD4^+$ counts of less than 100 cells/mm^3, and infection is uncommon if the $CD4^+$ count exceeds 200 cells/mm^3. Patients with toxoplasmic encephalitis most commonly present with focal neurologic abnormalities of subacute (weeks) onset, often with fevers, headache, or subtle mental status or memory changes. Motor palsies are the most common focal abnormalities, although cranial nerve abnormalities, visual field defects, and seizure disorders can be the major presenting symptoms. Neuroradiologic imaging is best performed using magnetic resonance imaging, with the most common finding being multiple, ring-enhancing cerebral lesions. Involvement of the basal ganglion area is common. Computed tomography is, in general, less sensitive in defining disease and its extent. Single lesions on magnetic resonance imaging are unusual in toxoplasmic encephalitis and suggest possible central nervous system lymphoma. Multifocal leukoencephalopathy resulting from JC virus can also cause neuroradiologic findings that resemble toxoplasmosis. PCR can be performed on cerebrospinal fluid for Epstein-Barr virus, JC virus, and toxoplasmosis.

A definitive diagnosis of toxoplasmic encephalitis is made by brain biopsy and by the histologic demonstration of tachyzoites. However, to avoid the morbidity associated with brain biopsy, in patients with HIV infection who are toxoplasmosis seropositive and who have consistent neuroradiologic findings, it is now standard practice to treat these patients for toxoplasmosis empirically and to observe the clinical response. Although neuroradiologic resolution is delayed, most patients with toxoplasmic encephalitis demonstrate clinical improvement within 7 days of initiating therapy. Failure to respond clinically to empirical therapy, seronegativity to *T. gondii* antibody, and the presence of a single lesion on magnetic resonance imaging all are findings that suggest the possibility of an alternative diagnosis and warrant consideration of performing a brain biopsy.

Tissue biopsies with histologic examination are usually necessary for diagnosing toxoplasmosis at other sites in immunocompromised patients. PCR testing on bronchoalveolar lavage fluid can be positive in cases of pneumonitis. Endomyocardial biopsy should be performed if toxoplasmosis is a consideration in the seronegative heart recipient of a seropositive donor.

Therapy

Treatment of toxoplasmosis is summarized in Table 1. Most infections in immunologically normal adults are self-limited and do not require therapy. In ocular, central nervous system, and congenital toxoplasmosis, first-line therapy is the combination of pyrimethamine (Daraprim), and sulfadiazine, with folinic acid (leucovorin, not folic acid). Treatment duration is based on time of clinical resolution, but it is usually approximately 6 weeks in ocular and central nervous system infections and 12 months in congenital infection. In patients with AIDS who have persistently low $CD4^+$ counts (less than 200 cells/mm^3), and in other patients with continued profound immunosuppression, long-term maintenance therapy with

TABLE 1 Therapy of Toxoplasmic Infection

	Adult Doses	Pediatric Doses
Immunologically Normal		
Acute lymphadenopathy	No treatment	No treatment
Acute chorioretinitis	Pyrimethamine (Daraprim) 100 mg PO bid on day 1, then 25 mg PO qd + sulfadiazine 1 g PO qid + folinic acid (leucovorin) 5 mg PO qd	
Pregnancy	Spiramycin* 1.0 g PO q8h (see text)	
Congenital toxoplasmosis		Pyrimethamine 2 mg/kg for 2 d, then 1 mg/kg PO qd + sulfadiazine 50 mg/kg PO bid + folinic acid 10 mg 3 × wk PO
AIDS and Immunologically Impaired		
Encephalitis and other tissue sites of infection	Pyrimethamine 200 mg PO × one dose, then 75 mg PO qd + sulfadiazine 1 g PO qid ?+ folinic acid 5-10 mg PO qd	

*Not available in the United States except from the FDA (call 301-827-2335).
Abbreviations: bid = twice daily; PO = orally; q = every; qd = every day; qid = four times daily.

pyrimethamine–sulfadiazine–folinic acid should be continued at the same doses used for primary therapy. Spiramycin[1],* (3 g per day) is the drug of choice for pregnant women with acquired primary *T. gondii* infection. Spiramycin should be continued until term if there is no evidence of fetal infection. Spiramycin does not cross the placenta and will not treat infection in the fetus. If fetal infection is demonstrated to be present by amniotic fluid PCR, pyrimethamine–sulfadiazine–folinic acid should be administered during the second and third trimesters. Pyrimethamine is potentially teratogenic and should not be administered during the first 16 weeks of pregnancy.

Allergic reactions to sulfonamides are common in patients with HIV infection. Alternative drugs to sulfadiazine that may be employed in combination therapy include clindamycin (Cleocin),[1] 600 to 1200 mg every 6 hours intravenously or orally; clarithromycin (Biaxin),[1] 1 g every 12 hours orally; atovaquone (Mepron),[1] 750 mg every 6 hours orally; azithromycin (Zithromax),[1] 1200 to 1500 mg per day orally; and dapsone,[1] 100 mg per day orally. Alternatively, increasing experience suggests that trimethoprim-sulfamethoxazole (Bactrim, Septra),[1] 5 mg/kg trimethoprim component every 6 hours orally or intravenously (20 mg/kg per day total), is as effective as the pyrimethamine-containing combination regimens in patients who are not allergic to sulfa agents.

Corticosteroids can be administered to patients with ocular toxoplasmosis in whom a brisk inflammatory response is believed to be contributing to ocular pathology. Similarly, in toxoplasmic encephalitis with cerebral edema or significant mass effect, short-duration corticosteroids may be concomitantly employed with antitoxoplasmic antimicrobial therapy.

Prevention

Prevention of *T. gondii* infection is of major importance in pregnant women and immunodeficient patients who have not been previously exposed. Risk of primary infection can be reduced by not eating undercooked meat and by taking proper precautions when disposing of or cleaning cat litter material. Cysts in meat are killed at 60°C (140°F) or higher. Hands should be thoroughly washed after soil contamination, and all fruits and vegetables should be washed before they are eaten.

Primary prophylaxis should be administered in patients with AIDS who have CD4+ counts of less than 100 cells/mm^3 and who are seropositive for toxoplasmosis antibody. Trimethoprim (160 mg)-sulfamethoxazole (800 mg),[1] one double-strength tablet daily, is highly effective for prevention of toxoplasmosis infection. Alternative prophylactic regimens include either (a) pyrimethamine, 50 to 75 mg orally per week, plus dapsone,[1] 50 mg per day or 200 mg per week; or (b) pyrimethamine-sulfadoxine (Fansidar),[1] three tablets every 2 weeks. Dapsone alone is not effective at preventing toxoplasmosis.

[1]Not FDA approved for this indication.
*Not available in the United States except from the FDA (call 301-827-2335).

[1]Not FDA approved for this indication.

Cat-Scratch Disease

Method of
Michael J. Smith, MD

Cat-scratch disease (CSD), regional lymphadenopathy following a cat scratch or bite, has been described since the 1950s. *Bartonella henselae*, a pleomorphic, facultative intracellular gram-negative bacillus, was not identified as the etiologic agent until 40 years later. As the laboratory detection of *B. henselae* has improved, it has become associated with an increasing number of clinical entities. These have traditionally been divided into typical CSD, the classic finding of unilateral regional lymphadenopathy following a cat scratch or bite, and atypical CSD, which includes all other presentations.

Epidemiology

As CSD is not a reportable disease, the true incidence remains unknown. However, there are an estimated 24,000 cases in the United States each year. Predominantly a disease of childhood and adolescence, CSD has the highest age-specific incidence rate occurring in children younger than 10 years of age. Although less frequent, CSD does occur in older individuals as well. A recent study found that 6% of patients with confirmed CSD were older than the age of 60 years.

Nearly 90% of patients with CSD have exposure to cats and approximately half recall a definitive scratch or bite. Early epidemiologic evidence suggested an increased risk of CSD in patients with kittens as compared to patients with adult cats. It was subsequently shown that kittens have a higher rate of *B. henselae* bacteremia than adult cats. In contrast, adult cats are more likely to have antibodies indicative of past infection. Most bacteremic cats are asymptomatic, so even a healthy-appearing animal can transmit disease.

The cat flea, *Ctenocephalides felis*, has been implicated in the transmission between cats. Consequently, CSD is more prevalent in warm and humid environments that support the growth of fleas with infection occurring primarily in the fall and winter months. To date, no evidence exists for human to human transmission.

Clinical Manifestations

Typical CSD is the most common form of CSD in immunocompetent patients. Initially, papules develop at the site of inoculation within the first week after a cat scratch or bite. This is followed by the gradual onset of unilateral regional lymphadenopathy over the next several weeks. Occasionally these lymph nodes may suppurate. The location of lymphadenopathy depends on the site of inoculation but most commonly occurs in the axillary, inguinal or cervical chains. In contrast to bacterial lymphadenitis, the lymph nodes are not inflamed. Patients are usually well-appearing and afebrile. Lymphadenopathy gradually resolves over several months without specific therapy.

The most common form of atypical CSD is Parinaud's oculoglandular syndrome (POGS), which occurs when bacteria are inoculated directly into the eye or eyelid. Small papules develop, almost always in the palpebral conjunctiva, in association with ipsilateral preauricular lymphadenopathy. There is also a painless, nonpurulent conjunctivitis. Similar to typical CSD, these symptoms resolve without antimicrobial therapy over several weeks.

Typical CSD and POGS share a similar pathophysiology; direct inoculation followed by a local immune response. In contrast, the other types of atypical CSD are due to systemic infection with *B. henselae*. These include hepatosplenic CSD, osteomyelitis, endocarditis, encephalitis, and neuroretinitis. *Bartonella* has also been implicated in the etiology of fever of unknown origin (FUO). One recent study revealed that 5% of all children with FUO of infectious etiology had antibodies against *B. henselae* indicative of current or recent infection.

In immunocompromised individuals, *B. henselae* can cause life-threatening invasive disease. Bacillary angiomatosis (BA), which is also caused by other *Bartonella* species, is caused by the angioproliferative effects of *Bartonella* and results in multiple vascular tumors in the skin and subcutaneous tissues. Bacillary peliosis (BP) is another form of vasoproliferative disease that leads to the development of blood-filled cysts in the reticuloendothelial element of the liver, spleen, and bone marrow of severely immunocompromised patients.

Diagnosis

A detailed history and physical examination are essential for the diagnosis of CSD. Any contact with cats or kittens, especially if bites or scratches occurred, should raise suspicion for CSD, regardless of the patient's age and clinical presentation.

Bartonella is a fastidious organism that takes several weeks to grow, making culture impractical. Therefore, serologic testing has become the mainstay of diagnosis. Indirect fluorescent antibody testing for IgM and IgG against *B. henselae* is performed by most commercial laboratories as well as the Center for Disease Control. A single elevated titer or a fourfold or greater increase between acute and convalescent titers is diagnostic of CSD.

The combination of history, physical examination, and serologic testing may obviate the need for biopsy in cases

---

CURRENT DIAGNOSIS

- Suspect CSD in any patient with lymphadenopathy and a history of cat exposure, regardless of age.
- Serologic testing can confirm the diagnosis.
- If biopsy is performed, specimens should be sent for pathology as well as fungal, mycobacterial, and routine bacterial cultures.
- Granulomas with central necrosis are characteristic of CSD but are not specific. When available, PCR is highly specific for CSD.

Abbreviations: CSD = cat-scratch disease; PCR = polymerase chain reaction.

of typical CSD. If a node is removed, the characteristic histopathologic finding is the formation of granulomas with microabscesses and central necrosis. Rarely, gram-negative bacilli may be identified using the Warthin-Starry silver stain. These are both nonspecific findings, and any patient undergoing biopsy should have samples sent for fungal and mycobacterial cultures in addition to standard bacterial culture and sensitivity. Polymerase chain reaction (PCR) testing of tissue is emerging as a highly specific diagnostic tool. Sensitivity of PCR testing varies with the specific DNA target used but is usually quite high. It is becoming increasingly available in commercial laboratories.

Treatment

Treatment of typical CSD is supportive and mainly consists of needle aspiration of suppurative lymph nodes when required. There is no evidence to suggest that treatment with antibiotics significantly alters the course of disease. In the only prospective, randomized, double blinded study of typical CSD, a 5-day course of azithromycin (Zithromax) or placebo was given to 29 patients with clinical CSD. Although the subjects who received azithromycin had a more rapid reduction in lymphadenopathy as measured by ultrasound at 30 days, the long-term outcomes were identical for both groups.

Evidence for the treatment of atypical CSD in immunocompetent patients is limited to case reports and retrospective reviews. Success has been reported using a range of oral antibiotics including trimethoprim-sulfamethoxazole[1] (Bactrim, Septra), rifampin (Rifadin),[1] azithromycin (Zithromax),[1] doxycycline (Vibramycin), and ciprofloxacin (Cipro[1]), as well as intravenous gentamicin (Garamycin).[1] Nevertheless, most cases of atypical CSD are thought to resolve without antibiotic therapy. A notable exception is endocarditis, which requires surgical replacement of the damaged valve in addition to antibiotic therapy. One retrospective review found that treatment of endocarditis with

----

[1]Not FDA approved for this indication.

a regimen that included an aminoglycoside for at least 14 days was significantly associated with a higher rate of survival.

Immunocompromised patients with BA or BP warrant antimicrobial treatment. There have been no controlled studies to determine optimal therapy, but either erythromycin (E.E.S.)[1] or doxycycline (Vibramycin) is effective. Most experts recommend a treatment course of at least 3 months to prevent relapse.

Prevention

Cat owners should avoid activities that may result in a cat scratch or bite, and should promptly wash any cat-inflicted wounds. Appropriate flea control will also reduce the likelihood of CSD. Because of the risk for invasive disease caused by *B. henselae*, immunocompromised individuals should be specifically warned of the risks of cat exposure. If possible, they should avoid purchasing or adopting kittens.

REFERENCES

American Academy of Pediatrics: Cat-scratch disease. In Pickering LK (ed.): Red Book: 2003 Report of the Committee on Infectious Diseases (26th ed.). Elk Grove Village, IL, American Academy of Pediatrics, pp 232–234.

Bass JW, Freitas BC, Freitas AD, et al: Prospective randomized double blind placebo-controlled evaluation of azithromycin for treatment of cat-scratch disease. Pediatr Infect Dis J 1998;17:447–452.

Batts S, Demers DM: Spectrum and treatment of cat-scratch disease. Pediatr Infect Dis J 2004;23:1161–1162.

Ben-Ami R, Ephros M, Avidor B, et al: Cat-scratch disease in elderly patients. Clin Infect Dis 2005;41:969–974.

Hansmann Y, DeMartino S, Piemont Y, et al: Diagnosis of cat scratch disease with detection of *Bartonella henselae* PCR: A study of patients with lymph node enlargement. J Clin Microbiol 2005;43:3800–3806.

Jacobs RF, Schutze GE: *Bartonella henselae* as a cause of prolonged fever and fever of unknown origin in children. Clin Infect Dis 1998;26:80–84.

Massei F, Gori L, Machhia P, Maggiore G, et al: The extended spectrum of Bartonellosis in children. Infect Dis Clin North Am 2005;19:691–711.

Raoult D, Fournier PE, Vandenesch F, et al: Outcome and treatment of *Bartonella* endocarditis. Arch of Int Med 2003;163:226–230.

Rolain JM, Brouqui P, Koehler JE, et al: Recommendations for treatment of human infection caused by *Bartonella* species. Antimicrob Agents Chemother 2004;48:1921–1933.

Zangwill KM, Hamilton DH, Perkins BA, et al: Cat scratch disease in Connecticut: Epidemiology, risk factors, and evaluation of a new diagnostic test. N Engl J Med 1993;329:8–13.

CURRENT THERAPY

Immunocompetent Patients
- Typical CSD only requires supportive treatment.
- No antibiotics are indicated.
- For atypical CSD there are no definitive treatment recommendations.
- Endocarditis requires surgery and antibiotic therapy, which should include at least 14 days of an aminoglycoside.

Immunocompromised Patients
- BA or BP treatment for at least 3 months with either
  - Erythromycin (E.E.S.)[1] 500 mg PO qid or
  - Doxycycline (Vibramycin) 100 mg PO bid.

----

[1]Not FDA approved for this indication.
Abbreviations: BA = bacillary angiomatosis; BP = bacillary peliosis; CSD = cat-scratch disease.

----

[1]Not FDA approved for this indication.

Salmonellosis

Method of
Arvid E. Underman, MD, FACP, DTMH

Salmonellosis refers to a group of infections caused by members of the genus *Salmonella*. This genus is named after Salmon, a pathologist who first isolated the organism, later designated as *Salmonella choleraesuis*, from the intestine of pigs with diarrhea. *Salmonellae* are widely distributed throughout nature and are adapted to a myriad of warm and cold-blooded hosts. In humans there are four main clinical presentations:

1. Acute gastroenteritis
2. Bacteremia
3. Focal extraintestinal infection
4. Chronic carriage (Table 1)

Microbiology

Salmonellae are motile, Gram-stain negative, nonspore-forming bacilli that are differentiated from other *Enterobacteriaceae* by inability to ferment lactose and sucrose while producing acid, hydrogen sulfide, and gas (except *Salmonella typhi*). Members of the genus were more accurately classified into serotypes using the Kauffman-White schema that differentiated and grouped them serologically dependent on their lipopolysaccharide somatic (O) and flagellar (H) antigens.

More recently, DNA analysis has divided the genus into two species. Initially the first of the two species was named *Salmonella choleraesuis* and was divided into six subspecies, each of which was then divided into more than 2400 serotypes (serovars) by Kauffman-White methodology. The second species, *Salmonella Bongori*, is inconsequential.

Serotypes were named historically from the host or the geographic locale of the first isolate, such as *Salmonella typhimurium* or *Salmonella dublin*. However, under the new DNA division, *choleraesuis* was both a species and a serotype. To avoid confusion the name *Salmonella enterica* has been widely adopted. The first of the six subspecies (Group I) is also named *enterica*. It contains the more than 1400 serotypes that occur in warm-blooded animals. Using nomenclature employed by the United States Centers for Disease Control and the World Health Organization (WHO), the species and subspecies name is understood; and the serotype is capitalized. Thus, the formal *S. enterica* subspecies *enterica* serotype *typhimurium* becomes simply *S.* Typhimurium, which except for the capital T is where we started!

Epidemiology

In the last 25 years, the incidence of nontyphoid salmonellosis has increased two- to threefold with approximately 1.5 million cases occurring annually in the United States. This is an underestimate because most cases are sporadic (endemic) and go unreported. Children younger than 5 years of age have the highest incidence of gastroenteritis and constitute the greatest number of cases.

Animals are the source of nontyphoid salmonella infection in humans. Infection occurs from food of animal origin such as meat, poultry, eggs, and dairy products. Contamination may occur during the production, slaughter, processing, or distribution of these products. Outbreaks have been associated with eggs, ice cream, and processed meats. Increasingly there have been outbreaks associated with raw vegetables (e.g., scallions) that are crosscontaminated during growth and distribution. Restaurant or home outbreaks occur in the context of improper preparation, cooking, and refrigeration. Most of the outbreaks can be attributed to centralized mass production and preparation of food along with globalization of the food trade. Novel sources of human salmonella include pet turtles, lizards, iguanas, African hedgehogs, rattlesnakes, and even marijuana contaminated by manure.

Emergence of antibiotic resistant species is a formidable problem. It is believed that resistance is driven worldwide by improper antibiotics use. However, in developed countries it is attributable to widespread use in animal feeds. Large numbers of transferable resistance plasmids have been described. Resistance rates of more than 50% to ampicillin, chloramphenicol (Chloromycetin), and trimethoprim-sulfamethoxazole (TMP-SMZ) (Bactrim) occur in parts of Asia, Africa, and Latin America. One strain of *S.* Typhimurium (DT104) is resistant to five antimicrobials; the three mentioned previously plus tetracycline and streptomycin. This organism has spread widely in livestock throughout the United States, Canada, United Kingdom, Europe, and the Middle East. Likewise, resistance to third-generation cephalosporins is increasing and is mediated by plasmids producing both regular and extended-spectrum beta-lactamases (ESBLs). Even more disturbing is fluoroquinolone resistance caused by mutated DNA gyrase, topoisomerase IV, or efflux pumps. The latter literally expel the quinolone from the bacterium before it can act on its target. Fluoroquinolone resistance is most pronounced in Southeast Asia, Europe, and the Middle East.

TABLE 1 Clinical Presentations of Salmonellosis

Acute gastroenteritis (90%–95% of cases)
Bacteremia (<5% of cases)
- Transient during acute gastroenteritis
- Enteric fever (nontyphoid)
- Persistent or recurrent (especially HIV)
Focal complications following bacteremia
- Bronchopneumonia, empyema, chest wall abscess
- Aortitis with mycotic aneurysm
- Prosthetic graft or valve infection
- Endocarditis, endarteritis
- Osteomyelitis (especially with sickle cell anemia)
- Septic arthritis
- Soft tissue abscess
- Hepatic or splenic abscess
- Meningitis or brain abscess
- Suppurative urogenital disease
Carriage (asymptomatic)
- Convalescent excretors (<2 mo)
- Convalescent carriers (2–12 mo)
- Chronic carriers (>12 mo)

Pathogenesis

Human infection usually requires 10^6 organisms. Fewer organisms may cause disease in patients who have hypochlorhydria or achlorhydria, have impaired cellular immunity, are at the extremes of age, or are taking certain drugs (Table 2). *Salmonellae* predominately infect the terminal ileum and proximal colon through attachment. Initially host response is by neutrophils followed by lymphocytes and macrophages. Strains vary genetically in their virulence and invasiveness. The organisms can survive intracellularly, thus avoiding antibiotic agents that lack intracellular penetration. Bacteria that are not contained regionally in the gut or lymph nodes may enter the blood. There are many predisposing factors associated with this and subsequent focal complications (see Table 2).

Clinical Presentation

GASTOENTERITIS

Acute gastroenteritis is by far the most common clinical presentation of salmonellosis. It should be emphasized that there is considerable overlap in its presentation with other infectious intestinal pathogens such as *Campylobacter* species. Given this, the incubation ranges from 6 to 96 hours but most commonly occurs between 12 and 48 hours. Initial symptoms include nausea and vomiting, followed by headaches, myalgias, malaise, chills, low-grade fever, abdominal cramps, and diarrhea. High temperatures (40°C [104°F]) should alert the clinician to invasive disease. Stools may be merely loose or profuse and watery. On direct examination, they may or may not contain polymorphonuclear

TABLE 2 Predisposing Factors for Salmonellosis

Gastrointestinal
- Achlorhydria
- Gastric surgery
- Inflammatory bowel disease

Immune or structural compromise
- Age (<6 mo, >60 y)
- Lymphoma
- Splenectomy
- Cirrhosis with portal hypertension
- Diabetes mellitus
- Chronic uremia
- Hemolytic anemia (iron overload)
- Sickle cell (bone infarct, autosplenectomy)
- Systemic lupus
- Atheromata, aortic aneurysm

Infections
- HIV/AIDS (decreased T-cells)
- Malaria
- Bartonellosis
- Schistosomiasis

Drugs
- H_2-blockers, H^+ proton pump inhibitors
- Antibiotic administration
- Antimotility agents
- Chemotherapy
- Corticosteroids
- Transplant antirejection agents

CURRENT DIAGNOSIS

- More than 95% of nontyphoid Salmonellosis presents as uncomplicated acute gastroenteritis.
- The clinical presentation of different causes of gastroenteritis and diarrhea overlaps significantly.
- The physician should be familiar with groups of patients at risk for complicated Salmonellosis.
- Specific diagnosis requires culture of the stool or blood.
- Focal complications are always suspect in high-risk patients who are blood culture positive for nontyphoid *Salmonellae* (e.g., aortitis or mycotic aneurysm in patients older than age 60 years with atherosclerosis).

leukocytes or occult blood. The presence of mucus or gross blood in the absence of hemorrhoids or fissures should alert the clinician to organisms causing dysentery such as *Shigella* species. The white count is most often normal or slightly elevated, with a left shift containing 10 to 15 bands. Low white counts with greater numbers of bands should alert the clinician to possible bacteremia or enteric fever. The diagnosis can be confirmed only by stool or blood culture. Serum serology examinations are not helpful. Most healthy adults have a self-limited, uncomplicated course, with resolution of symptoms without treatment within 48 to 72 hours.

Treatment

FLUID AND ELECTROLYTE REPLACEMENT

The sine qua non in the treatment of diarrhea is fluid and electrolyte replacement. In most cases increased oral intake of bland juices coupled with clear broth and temporary

CURRENT THERAPY

- Fluid and electrolyte replacement is of paramount importance.
- The physician should avoid routine empiric antibiotic in acute uncomplicated patients.
- The physician should avoid antimotility agents for diarrhea presenting with fever or with mucus and blood present.
- More than 95% of patients with nontyphoid salmonellosis *will get better* on their own.
- Fluoroquinolone antibiotics should be reserved for when they are truly indicated clinically.
- Increasing resistance mandates sensitivity testing (including tests for ESBL) to guide therapy of bacteremia and its complications.
- Do not prescribe *prophylactic* antibiotics to prevent diarrhea in travellers.
- Stress personal hygiene and prudent food choice with proper preparation.

Abbreviation: ESBL = extended spectrum beta lactamases.

elimination of lactose-containing foods will suffice. Commercial electrolyte solutions (Pedialyte) may be useful. Although not readily available in the United States, rehydration salts are widely employed in many developing countries. WHO distributes packets containing its recommended formula of 90 mmol of sodium, 20 of potassium, 80 of chloride, 30 of bicarbonate, along with 111 mmol of glucose to dissolve in 1 L of sterile or boiled water. This mixture should be consumed at a rate sufficient to compensate for diarrheal losses while maintaining an adequate output of dilute appearing urine. Within 24 to 48 hours, the diet can be supplemented with bland, soft foods given in small, frequent feedings. If the patient has profuse vomiting or severe dehydration as determined by orthostatic changes in blood pressure, parenteral rehydration should be used. Frequently, this can be accomplished as an outpatient in an infusion room or with a home agency rather than through admission to hospital. When there is persistent emesis, profuse diarrhea, systemic toxicity, or abnormalities in serum electrolytes, parenteral rehydration in hospital is prudent.

ANTIMOTILITY AND ANTINAUSEA AGENTS

The use of agents such as atropine-diphenoxylate (Lomotil) or loperamide (Imodium) should be discouraged. Although they may result in symptomatic improvement in cramps and diarrhea, they can increase complications and even predispose to bacteremia. In general, if the patient has a fever and the diarrhea contains blood or mucus, their use should be eschewed. Most pediatricians feel they should never be used in children younger than 5 years of age. An alternative is bismuth subsalicylate (Pepto-Bismol). The adult dose is 1 ounce (2 tablespoons) or 2 tablets (262.5 mg) every 30 minutes for 8 hours. The pediatric dose is 1.1 mL/kg at 4-hour intervals for up to 5 days. Although nausea and vomiting are occasional presenting symptoms with enterocolitis, they rarely persist. Prochlorperazine (Compazine) or trimethobenzamide (Tigan) may be helpful. Both are available in oral, suppository, or parenteral form, even though injectable prochlorperazine (Compazine) has been in short supply. Suppositories usually stimulate further diarrhea. Vomiting may preclude oral administration. A singular muscular injection of prochlorperazine (Compazine) 5 to 10 mg, is often all that is needed. This may be repeated every 4 to 6 hours as needed. Promethazine hydrochloride (Phenergan) is more frequently used in children and may be used orally (0.5 mg/pound or 1 mg/kg every 6 hours) or intramuscularly in the same doses. A 5-HT$_3$ receptor antagonist such as ondansetron (Zofran)[1] is expensive and inefficacious.

ANTIBIOTICS

The routine empiric use of antibiotics, especially fluoroquinolones, for any and all cases of diarrhea is not only unjustifiable but should be decried. Certainly antibiotics are not needed in the treatment of uncomplicated *Salmonella* gastroenteritis in otherwise healthy children or adults. Studies have shown that they neither shorten the course nor improve symptoms. No doubt some of this usage is patient driven. However, overuse is contributing to the emergence of resistance, and may increase risk of symptomatic and bacteriologic relapse. Indeed antibiotic use may actually prolong the convalescent excretion or contribute to chronic carriage of the organism. Postponing antibiotic therapy until the return of a stool culture often provides the physician with a way to avert the frequent demand for antibiotic therapy. Often patients are better by the time results become available. Nevertheless, high-risk patients, as previously identified (see Table 2), should receive treatment to prevent potential complications from bacteremia. Additionally, if patients are sick enough to require hospitalization, antibiotic therapy should be considered.

Appropriate antibiotic therapy should be guided by susceptibility testing. Initially, TMP-SMZ (cotrimoxazole, Bactrim, or Septra)[1] may be administered to the nonsulfonamide-sensitive patient. The dose is 5 to 8 mg/kg trimethoprim every 12 hours for children or 1 double-strength tablet (160 mg trimethoprim/800 mg sulfamethoxazole) every 12 hours for adults. Although widely used, trimethoprim-sulfamethoxazole has not yet received FDA approval. If the organism is susceptible, ampicillin, 50 mg/kg orally to 100 mg/kg/day intravenously, each in four divided doses for children, or 2 to 4 g/day in four divided doses for adults, may be administered. Amoxicillin (Amoxil)[1] in equivalent oral dosage may be substituted. The duration of therapy is generally 5 days.

Newer fluoroquinolone antibiotics, such as ciprofloxacin,[1] ofloxacin,[1] and norfloxacin,[1] are among the most effective agents with excellent oral bioavailability and intracellular concentration. They are contraindicated in prepubertal children and pregnant women. Adult doses are ciprofloxacin (Cipro), 500 mg twice daily; ofloxacin (Floxin), 400 mg twice daily; or norfloxacin (Noroxin), 400 mg twice daily. It must be emphasized that the trend in the United States to use these agents empirically for all suspected bacterial diarrhea should be vigorously resisted by the thoughtful clinician.

Bacteremia and Focal Infection

Bacteremia in acute uncomplicated *Salmonella* gastroenteritis is infrequent. Therefore, blood cultures are not routinely necessary except for patients who are in high-risk categories. Shaking chills or high fever (40°C [104°F]) should alert the clinician to possible bacteremia. Focal suppurative infection following bacteremia is also infrequent but may occur at any site. Thus, *Salmonella* has been associated with bronchopneumonia, soft tissue infection, aortic mycotic aneurysms, endocarditis, septic arthritis, splenic or hepatic abscesses, meningitis, and osteomyelitis. The clinician should suspect an endovascular mycotic aneurysm in all blood culture positive patients older than 50 years of age. *Salmonella* should always be suspected in individuals with sickle cell disease in whom bone and joint infection is the most frequent cause of extraintestinal infection. Meningitis occurs primarily in infants younger than 5 months of age. The diagnosis of a *Salmonella* bacteremia in HIV patients will almost always be accompanied by recurrent episodes.

---

[1]Not FDA approved for this indication.

[1]Not FDA approved for this indication.

Treatment

ANTIBIOTICS

Bacteremia and localized suppurative infection require antibiotic therapy. The choice of effective treatment is less predictable with the emergence of resistance. Therapy must be altered according to the results of susceptibility testing. Therefore the recovery of the organism is extremely important, and adequate cultures of blood or infected material must be obtained before initiation of therapy.

Parenteral ampicillin, 100 to 200 mg/kg/day divided into four doses, or TMP/SMZ,[1] 8 to 10 mg/kg of trimethoprim per day in three divided doses, may be used. In the case of resistance or allergy to the foregoing, third-generation cephalosporins such as cefotaxime (Claforan) or ceftriaxone (Rocephin) have reasonable activity, but intracellular concentrations are not optimal. Cefotaxime, 1 to 2 grams every 6 to 8 hours for adults, or 100 to 200 mg/kg/day in three or four divided doses for children, has been found effective in bacteremia, osteomyelitis, septic arthritis, and a variety of other focal *Salmonella* infections. The use of chloramphenicol (Chloromycetin) is not recommended but a preparation of it in oil (Typhomycine)[2] is in use in developing countries. Ciprofloxacin (Cipro)[1] 7.5 mg/kg intravenously twice daily is becoming a favored agent; not only is it effective but oral bioequivalence facilitates the change to 500 to 750 mg by mouth twice daily. If fluoroquinolone resistance is encountered, imipenem (Primaxin)[1] may be tried. Efficacy data for it or other agents such as azithromycin (Zithromax)[1] are scant.

SURGERY

Focal infection often requires surgery. Often this is as simple as the drainage of localized suppuration or lavage of a septic joint. However, in the case of infected aortic aneurysms, extensive resection and vascular reconstruction are required. Infected prosthetic grafts must be removed in nearly all cases with courses of antibiotics before and after surgery.

The duration of therapy for simple bacteremia is 10 to 14 days. Septic arthritis is usually treated 4 weeks whereas osteomyelitis and endovascular infections require 6 weeks. Oral fluoroquinolones such as ciprofloxacin (Cipro), 500 mg twice daily, may be helpful in treating osteomyelitis. TMP-SMZ (Bactrim)[1] can also be used in this manner. Both have adequate blood levels after oral administration. I have had to use continuous prophylaxis of either TMP-SMZ or ciprofloxacin in several HIV patients to prevent recurrent bacteremia. Because prophylactic TMP-SMZ is used chronically for *Pneumocystis,* it may be preferred.

Enteric Fever

The clinical picture of nontyphoid *Salmonella* enteric fever is indistinguishable from that of typhoid fever, which is discussed elsewhere in this publication. However, the following discussion also applies to enteric fever caused by nontyphoid *Salmonellae.*

TREATMENT

The adjunct and antibiotic therapy of nontyphoid enteric fever parallels that of the treatment of typhoid. Antibiotics should be adjusted and altered once the results of susceptibility testing are available. Acceptable regimens include ampicillin, amoxicillin,[1] and TMP-SMZ (Bactrim),[1] along with third-generation cephalosporins and fluoroquinolone antibiotics. My preference was cefotaxime (Claforan)[1] in the same doses as for bacteremic salmonellosis. The duration is 10 to 14 days. Relapse rates are low and is seen within 2 to 6 weeks. Relapse requires an equivalent course of therapy in both dose and duration. Currently, I prefer ciprofloxacin (Cipro)[1] intravenously 7.5 mg/kg every 12 hours continued until the patient is afebrile and clinically able to start it orally. Comparative studies are ongoing using both third-generation cephalosporins, such as ceftriaxone (Rocephin)[1] or cefixime (Suprax),[1] and oral fluoroquinolones in short-course therapy of typhoid as well as nontyphoid enteric fever. Although these show some promise, they are currently not the standard of practice in the United States. Nevertheless, a strong case can be made for oral fluoroquinolones use, with obvious cost saving. Otherwise healthy young adults may be treated orally as outpatients. This advantage, if for no other reason, should *prevent* the physician from prescribing quinolones for uncomplicated gastroenteritis or other self-limited diarrheas of bacterial origin.

Adjunctive measures are of importance, including attention to fluid and electrolyte balance and nutrition. As in typhoid the routine use of corticosteroids is controversial. Use in patients who are steroid dependent or believed to be hypoadrenal is indicated. In those who are delirious, obtunded, comatose, or in shock it may be warranted; but there are little supportive data. It has been my overall impression that nontyphoid enteric fever is somewhat milder than typhoid itself, and complications such as gastrointestinal bleeding or ileal perforation are exceedingly rare.

Carrier State

Asymptomatic excretion of organisms invariably occurs following clinical *Salmonella* gastroenteritis. It exceeds 8 weeks in 5% to 10% of patients. Chronic carriage, either in the stool or urine, is defined as excretion of the organism for more than 1 year. Its incidence is stated to be 1% in adults and 5% in children younger than 5 years of age. This is somewhat less than that seen with *S. typhi.* Convalescent excreters need only maintain strict personal hygiene to prevent transmission of the organism. Those involved in food preparation or in child and health care should be kept off work until three successive cultures are negative at intervals required by the public health department. It goes without saying that all positive cases of salmonellosis are reportable by law to local public health authorities.

Recently, oral quinolones have been used (ciprofloxacin [Cipro],[1] 500 to 750 mg twice daily for 5 to 14 days), to curtail institutional outbreaks, as in nursing homes or

[1]Not FDA approved for this indication.
[2]Not available in the United States.

[1]Not FDA approved for this indication.

psychiatric facilities. Although this may be expeditious, eliminating or preventing the source of the outbreak in a prospective fashion is preferable. In the case of food handlers and health or child care workers, some feel that quinolone therapy eliminates the problem of convalescent excretion, hence individuals may return to work without delay. The data are debatable and the successive negative stool requirement will not be obviated.

The management of the chronic carriage of nontyphoidal salmonellosis is the same as that of *S. typhi*, which is discussed in detail elsewhere. A 4- to 6-week course of oral antibiotics may be tried when no evidence of gallbladder disease exists. However, if chronic cholecystitis and/or cholelithiasis are present, cholecystectomy is almost always necessary. Despite cholecystectomy, a certain number of individuals will continue to excrete organisms thought to be of hepatobiliary origin. Chronic carriage is seen, albeit rarely, in the United States with either *Schistosoma mansoni* or *Schistosoma haematobium*. When these parasites are treated, subsequent therapy of the *Salmonella* results in termination of the stool or urinary carrier state.

Prevention

Prevention of salmonellosis has both personal and public health dimensions. Food and leftovers should be rapidly refrigerated. I recommend separate plastic (not wood) cutting boards for meats and vegetables that are washed after each use. Spillage of raw animal juices should be immediately cleaned. All preparation surfaces should be washed and dried after each meal. Detergent rather than antibacterial cleaners should be used; bleach is beautiful.

Public health surveillance is essential with regular inspection of restaurants, food retailers, and industrial food processors. National efforts to coordinate and computerize surveillance systems such as FoodNet should be expanded and fully funded so as to guarantee our food supply. Preservation technologies including irradiation need study.

Finally, the practicing physician should take the time to reiterate to patients with HIV, malignancies or other immune compromised patients (see Table 2) how they can avoid food-borne pathogens.

REFERENCES

Brenner FW, Villar RG, Angulo FJ, et al: Salmonella nomenclature. J Clin Microbiol 2000;38: 2465–2465.

Fierer J, Swancutt M: Non-typhoid *Salmonella*: A review. In Remington, JS, Swartz, MN (eds.): Current Clinical Topics in Infectious Diseases 20. Boston, Blackwell Science, 2000, pp 134–157.

Heriksstad H, Hayes P, Mokhtar M, et al: Emerging quinolone-resistant Salmonella in the United States. Emerg Infect Dis 1997;3:371–372.

Molbak K: Human health consequences of antimicrobial drug resistant *Salmonella* and other foodborne pathogens. Clin Infect Dis 2005;41:1613–1620.

Sirinivan S, Garner P: Antibiotics for treating Salmonella gut infections. Cochrane Database Sys Rev 2000;93:CD001167.

Su LH, Chiu CH, Chu CS, et al: Antimicrobial resistance in nontyphoid *Salmonella*: A global challenge. Clin Infect Dis 2004;39:546–551.

Voetsch AC, Van Gilder TJ, Angulo FJ, et al: FoodNet estimate of the burden of illness caused by nontyphoidal Salmonella infections in the United States. Clin Infect Dis 2004;38(Suppl 3):S127–134.

Typhoid Fever

Method of
Zulfiqar A. Bhutta, MB, BS, PhD

Despite vast advances in public health and hygiene in much of the developed world, typhoid fever remains endemic in many developing countries. Probably because of the ease of modern travel, cases are also reported in most developed countries.

Etiology

Typhoid fever is caused by *Salmonella typhi*, a gram-negative bacterium. A very similar but often less severe disease is caused by *Salmonella* serotype *paratyphi* A. The ratio of disease caused by *S. typhi* to that caused by *S. paratyphi* is approximately 10:1, although the proportion of *S. paratyphi* infections is increasing in some parts of the world. Although *S. typhi* shares many genes with *Escherichia coli* and at least 90% with *Salmonella typhimurium*, several unique gene clusters known as pathogenicity islands and others were acquired during evolution. One of the specific genes is for the polysaccharide capsule Vi. This is present in approximately 90% of all freshly isolated *S. typhi* organisms and has a protective effect against the bactericidal action of the serum of infected patients.

Epidemiology

Although accurate community-based figures are unavailable, an estimated 16 million cases occur annually, with more than 0.6 million deaths. The vast majority of cases occur in Asia. Given the paucity of microbiologic facilities in developing countries, these figures may largely represent the clinical syndrome. Regional incidence rates vary from 100 to 1000 cases per 100,000 population, and there may be differences in the spectrum of the disorder. Recent population-based studies from south Asia also indicate that, contrary to previous views, the disease may largely affect children younger than 5 years of age. In contrast, data from sub-Saharan Africa and HIV-endemic areas indicate that nontyphoidal *Salmonella* bacteremia far outstrips typhoid fever as a cause of community-acquired bacteremia.

In recent years, typhoid fever is notable for the emergence of drug resistance. Following sporadic outbreaks of chloramphenicol-resistant typhoid, many strains of *S. typhi* developed plasmid-mediated multidrug-resistance to all of the three primary antimicrobials (ampicillin [Chloromycetin], chloramphenicol, and trimethoprim-sulfamethoxazole [Septra]). More troubling, chromosomally acquired quinolone resistance in *S. typhi* was recently described in various parts of Asia and may be a consequence of widespread and indiscriminate use of these agents.

Pathogenesis

Typhoid fever occurs by the ingestion of the organism, and a variety of sources of fecal contamination are reported, including street vendor foods and contamination of water reservoirs. A larger infecting dose leads to a shorter incubation period and more severe infection. The organism crosses the intestinal mucosal barrier after attachment to the microvilli by an intricate mechanism involving membrane ruffling, actin rearrangement, and internalization in an intracellular vacuole. Once inside the intestinal cells, *S. typhi* find their way into the circulation and reside within the macrophages of the reticuloendothelial system. The clinical syndrome is produced by a release of proinflammatory cytokines (interleukin [IL]-6, IL-1β, and tumor necrosis factor [TNF]-α) from the infected cells. Some 1% to 5% of patients with acute typhoid infection may become chronic carriers of the infection in the gallbladder, depending on age, sex, and treatment regimen.

Clinical Features

Patients with typhoid fever usually present with high-grade fever and a wide variety of associated symptoms, such as abdominal pain, hepatosplenomegaly, diarrhea, and constipation. In the absence of localizing signs, the early stage of the disease may be difficult to differentiate from other endemic diseases including malaria and dengue fever. The classic stepladder rise of fever is relatively rare, but the presentation of typhoid fever may be tempered by coexisting morbidities and early administration of antibiotics. In malaria-endemic areas and in parts of the world where schistosomiasis is common, the presentation of typhoid may also be atypical.

Although data from South America and parts of Africa suggest typhoid may present as a mild illness in young children, this may vary in different parts of the world. Emerging evidence from south Asia indicates the presentation of typhoid may be more dramatic in children younger than 5 years of age, with comparatively higher rates of complications and hospitalization. Diarrhea, toxicity, and complications such as disseminated intravascular coagulopathy are also more common in infancy, with higher case fatality rates. Some of the other features of typhoid fever seen in adults, however, such as relative bradycardia, are rare, and rose spots may be visible only at an early stage of the illness in fair-skinned children.

It is also recognized that multidrug-resistant (MDR) typhoid is a more severe clinical illness with higher rates of toxicity, complications, and case fatality rates. This may be related to the increased virulence of MDR *S. typhi* as well as a higher number of circulating bacteria. These findings may have implications for treatment algorithms, especially in endemic areas with high rates of MDR typhoid.

Diagnosis

The mainstay of the diagnosis of typhoid fever is a positive culture from the blood or another anatomic site. But the sensitivity of blood cultures in diagnosing typhoid fever in many parts of the developing world is limited because

CURRENT DIAGNOSIS

- In the absence of localizing signs, the early stage of the disease may be difficult to differentiate from other endemic diseases such as malaria or dengue fever.
- The presentation and diagnosis of typhoid fever may be tempered by coexisting morbidities and early administration of antibiotics.
- The presentation of typhoid may be more dramatic in children younger than 5 years of age, with comparatively higher rates of complications and hospitalization.
- The sensitivity of blood cultures in diagnosing typhoid fever may be limited in many developing countries because of antibiotic prescribing.
- Multidrug-resistant (MDR) typhoid is a more severe clinical illness with higher rates of toxicity and complications. In particular, recent cases of quinolone-resistant typhoid may be more severe.

widespread use of antibiotics may render bacteriologic confirmation difficult. Although bone marrow cultures may increase the likelihood of bacteriologic confirmation of typhoid, these are difficult to obtain and relatively invasive.

The serologic diagnosis of typhoid is also fraught with problems because results of a single Widal test may be positive in only 50% of cases in endemic areas, and serial tests may be required in cases presenting in the first week of illness. Newer serologic tests such as a dot enzyme-linked immunoabsorbent assay (ELISA) (TyphiDot) and the TUBEX tests are promising but require further evaluation in large-scale studies in community settings. In much of the developing world, the mainstay of diagnosis of typhoid remains clinical, and several diagnostic algorithms are being evaluated in endemic areas.

Therapy

An early diagnosis of typhoid fever and institution of appropriate treatment are essential. The vast majority of typhoid patients can be managed at home with oral antibiotics and close medical follow-up for complications or failure to respond to therapy. But patients with persistent vomiting, severe diarrhea, and abdominal distention may require hospitalization and parenteral antibiotic therapy. These are the general principles of typhoid management:

- Adequate rest, hydration, and attention to correction of fluid-electrolyte imbalance
- Antipyretic therapy (acetaminophen, 120 to 750 mg orally every 4 to 6 hours[3]) as required
- Soft, easily digestible diet unless the patient has abdominal distention or ileus

[3]Exceeds dosage recommended by the manufacturer.

CURRENT THERAPY

- The vast majority of typhoid patients can be managed at home with oral antibiotics and close medical follow-up for complications or failure to respond to therapy.
- Although newer quinolones are associated with better cure rates and clinical outcomes, there is insufficient evidence to recommend them as first-line agents in children.
- Recent emergence of quinolone resistance among *S. typhi* isolates requires treatment with alternatives such as third-generation cephalosporins and azithromycin.

- Antibiotic therapy (the right choice, dosage, and duration)
- Traditional therapy with either chloramphenicol (Chloromycetin) or amoxicillin,[1] associated with relapse rates of 5% to 15% and 4% to 8%, respectively; newer

___
[1]Not FDA approved for this indication.

quinolones and third-generation cephalosporins associated with higher cure rates

Some authorities recommend treatment with second-line agents in all cases of typhoid. Others questioned this on the basis of adequate response to therapy among sensitive cases with first-line agents. Blanket administration of second-line agents such as fluoroquinolones and third-generation cephalosporins in all cases of suspected typhoid is expensive and may lead to the rapid development of further resistance. Table 1 gives the recommended therapy for typhoid fever based on a recent consensus document by the World Health Organization (2003).

Preventive Strategies for Typhoid

Of the major risk factors for outbreaks of typhoid, contamination of water supplies with sewage is the most important. During outbreaks, therefore, a combination of central chlorination and domestic water purification is important. In endemic situations, consumption of street vendor foods, especially ice cream and cut-up fruit, is recognized as an important risk factor. The human-to-human spread by chronic carriers is also important, and attempts should be made to target food handlers and high-risk groups for *S. typhi* carriage screening.

TABLE 1 Treatment of Typhoid Fever Based on Diagnosis, Treatment, and Prevention

Susceptibility	Optimal Therapy			Alternative Effective Drugs		
	Antibiotic	Daily Dose (mg/kg)	Days	Antibiotic	Daily Dose (mg/kg)	Days
Uncomplicated Typhoid Fever						
Fully sensitive	Fluoroquinolone (e.g., ofloxacin [Floxin][1] or ciprofloxacin [Cipro])	15	5-7*	Chloramphenicol (Chloromycetin) Amoxicillin[1] TMP-SMX (Bactrim)[1]	50-75[3] 75-100[1] 8/40	14-21 14 14
Multidrug resistance	Fluoroquinolone or Cefixime (Suprax)[1]	15 15-20[3]	5-7 7-14	Azithromycin (Zithromax)[1] Cefixime	8-10[3] 15-20[3]	7 7-14
Quinolone resistance[†]	Azithromycin (Rocephin)[1] or Ceftriaxone (Rocephin)[1]	8-10[3] 75[3]	7 10-14	Cefixime[1]	20[3]	7-14
Severe Typhoid Fever						
Fully sensitive	Fluoroquinolone (e.g., ofloxacin)[1]	15	10-14	Chloramphenicol Ampicillin[1] TMP-SMX	100[3] 100[3] 8/40	14-21 14 14
Multidrug-resistant	Fluoroquinolone	15	10-14	Ceftriaxone[1] or Cefotaxime (Claforan)[1]	60[3] 80[3]	10-14
Quinolone-resistant	Ceftriaxone[1] or cefotaxime[1]	60[3] 80[3]	10-14	Fluoroquinolone	20[3]	14

[1]Not FDA approved for this indication.
[3]Exceeds dosage recommended by the manufacturer.
*Three-day courses are also effective and are particularly so in epidemic containment.
[†]The optimum treatment for quinolone-resistant typhoid fever is not determined. Azithromycin, the third-generation cephalosporins, or a 10- to 14-day course of high-dose fluoroquinolones is effective.
Abbreviation: TMX-SMZ = trimethoprim-sulfamethoxazole.
From World Health Organization (WHO)/Vaccines and Biologicals/03.07.

The classic heat-inactivated whole cell vaccine is associated with an unacceptably high rate of side effects. Two newer vaccines that offer protection for school-age children and for adults are the Vi polysaccharide vaccine (Typhim Vi) and the orally administratable, attenuated Ty21a vaccine (Vivotif Berna). Both offer a protective efficacy of 70% to 80% for at least 3 to 5 years. In younger children, the experimental Vi-conjugate vaccine has a protective efficacy exceeding 90% and may offer protection in parts of the world where a large proportion of preschool children are at risk for the disease.

REFERENCES

Bhutta ZA: Impact of age and drug resistance on mortality in typhoid fever. Arch Dis Child 1996;75:214-217.

Chinh NT, Parry CM, Ly NT, et al: A randomized controlled comparison of azithromycin and ofloxacin for treatment of multidrug-resistant or nalidixic acid-resistant enteric fever. Antimicrob Agents Chemother 2000;44:1855-1859.

Communicable Disease Surveillance and Response Vaccines and Biologicals, World Health Organization: Treatment of Typhoid Fever. Background Document: The Diagnosis, Prevention and Treatment of Typhoid Fever, 2003, pp. 19-23. Available online at http://www.who.int/entity/vaccine_research/documents/en/typhoid_diagnosis.pdf)

Crump JA, Luby SP, Mintz ED: The global burden of typhoid fever. Bull World Health Organ 2004;82:346-353.

Gasem MH, Keuter M, Dolmans WM, et al: Persistence of salmonellae in blood and bone marrow: Randomized controlled trial comparing ciprofloxacin and chloramphenicol treatments against enteric fever. Antimicrob Agents Chemother 2003;47:1727-1731.

Luby SP, Faizan MK, Fisher-Hoch SP, et al: Risk factors for typhoid fever in an endemic setting, Karachi, Pakistan. Epidemiol Infect 1998;120:129-138.

Parry CM, Hien TT, Dougan G, et al: Typhoid fever. N Engl J Med 2002; 347:1770-1782.

Sinha A, Sazawal S, Kumar R, et al: Typhoid fever in children aged less than 5 years. Lancet 1999;354:734-737.

Thaver D, Zaidi AK, Critchley J, et al: Fluoroquinolones for treating typhoid and paratyphoid fever (enteric fever) (CD004530.pub2). Cochrane Database Syst Rev 2005;2.

Rickettsial and Ehrlichial Infections

Method of
David H. Walker, MD

Vector-borne transmission of obligately intracellular bacteria occurs in persons exposed to infected ticks, mites, fleas, and lice in endemic areas of the United States, as well as in returning international travelers (Table 1).

Rocky Mountain Spotted Fever and Other Rickettsioses

Rocky Mountain spotted fever (RMSF) is the most severe rickettsiosis, with a case-fatality rate of 23% unless treated with an appropriate antimicrobial agent sufficiently early in the course. Infection is highly seasonal (May through September) according to the activity of the American dog tick in the Eastern and Pacific coastal United States and the wood tick in the Rocky Mountain states. Because the tick bite is painless, a history of tick attachment is often not available.

After inoculation of *Rickettsia rickettsii* in tick saliva into the skin during feeding, the organisms spread hematogenously and enter endothelial cells throughout the body where they grow and spread contiguously from cell to cell. Rickettsial infection injures endothelial cells, particularly in the microcirculation, leading to increased vascular permeability, edema, hypovolemia, acute renal failure, noncardiogenic pulmonary edema, and meningoencephalitis. Host factors including age, glucose-6-phosphate dehydrogenase (G6PD) deficiency, alcohol use, and underlying diseases such as diabetes mellitus are associated with enhanced severity of rickettsial disease. Delay in treatment with a tetracycline or chloramphenicol (Chloromycetin) greater than 5 days worsens the outcome dramatically.

After an incubation period of 2 to 14 days days, the onset is characterized by fever, headache, myalgia, nausea, vomiting, and often abdominal pain. Rash usually does not appear until the third to fifth day of illness, and in 10% of cases there is no rash. Cough, confusion, ataxia, focal neurologic signs, stupor, coma, and seizures reflect life-threatening pulmonary edema and encephalitis.

Clinical laboratory data usually include a normal white blood cell count, progressive thrombocytopenia, hyponatremia, and elevated serum transaminases and urea. True disseminated intravascular coagulation is rare.

The differential diagnosis of RMSF and other rickettsioses and ehrlichiosis in the absence of a rash includes influenza, enteroviral infection, infectious mononucleosis, viral hepatitis, leptospirosis, typhoid fever, bacterial sepsis, toxic shock syndrome, and malaria. Bacterial and viral enterocolitis, acute surgical abdomen, bronchitis, pneumonia, meningitis, or encephalitis may be suspected with prominent gastrointestinal, respiratory, or

CURRENT DIAGNOSIS

- Because diagnostic antibodies are not present during the first week of illness in rickettsioses, ehrlichioses, and anaplasmosis, a presumptive diagnosis must be made and empirical treatment given on a clinical and epidemiologic basis.
- For RMSF, HME, and HGA, the possibility of tick exposure and presence of thrombocytopenia are useful clues. Patients frequently do not recall a tick attachment but are more often aware of exposure to ticks.
- A rash will seldom be present early in RMSF and is usually absent in HME and HGA. Never wait for rash involvement of the palms and soles or the appearance of petechiae to consider RMSF.
- Always collect acute and convalescent sera, test for antibodies against *Rickettsia rickettsii*, *Rickettsia typhi*, *Ehrlichia chaffeensis*, and *Anaplasma phagocytophilum*, and report the case to the state health department.

Abbreviations: HGA = human granulocytotropic anaplasmosis; HME = human monocytotropic ehrlichiosis; RMSF = Rocky Mountain spotted fever.

TABLE 1 Diseases, Etiologic Agents, Geographic Distribution, Ecology, and Transmission of Rickettsioses and Ehrlichioses Presenting for Medical Care in the United States

Disease	Agent	Geographic Distribution	Natural Cycle	Transmission to Humans
Rocky Mountain spotted fever	*Rickettsia rickettsii**	47 states, especially southeastern, south central, and mid-Atlantic states; Mexico; Central and South America	Transovarian maintenance in *Dermacentor variabilis* and *Dermacentor andersoni* ticks and horizontal from rickettsemic rodents	Tick bite
Murine typhus	*Rickettsia typhi**	Tropical and subtropical coastal regions; in U.S., particularly Texas and California	*Ctenocephalides felis* (cat flea)–opossum and *Xenopsylla cheopis* (rat flea)–rat cycles	Flea feces
Typhus	*Rickettsia prowazekii**	Eastern U.S.; Andes and other poverty-burdened highlands	Flying squirrel species-specific flea and louse cycle; human–body louse cycle	Flea feces; louse feces
Rickettsialpox	*Rickettsia akari*	New York City and other urban and rural foci	*Liponyssoides sanguineus* (mite)–domestic mouse	Feeding mite
American tick-bite fever	*Rickettsia parkeri*	Southern U.S. to Uruguay	Transovarian maintenance in *Amblyomma* ticks	Tick bite
African tick-bite fever[†]	*Rickettsia africae*	Sub-Saharan Africa; French West Indies	Transovarian maintenance in *Amblyomma* ticks	Tick bite
Flea-borne spotted fever	*Rickettsia felis*	Worldwide	Transovarian maintenance in *C. felis* fleas	Unknown
Scrub typhus[†]	*Orientia tsutsugamushi*[†]	Eastern Asia, Northern Australia	Transovarian in trombiculid mites	Feeding mite
Human monocytotropic ehrlichiosis	*Ehrlichia chaffeensis*	47 states, predominantly south central and southeastern U.S.	Tick (mainly *Amblyomma americanum*)–vertebrate host (mainly white-tailed deer) cycles	Tick bite
Ehrlichiosis ewingii	*Ehrlichia ewingii*	South central and southeastern U.S.	Tick (mainly *Amblyomma americanum*)–vertebrate host (mainly white-tailed deer) cycles	Tick bite
Human granulocytotropic anaplasmosis	*Anaplasma phagocytophilum*	Northeastern, upper Midwest, Pacific coast of U.S.; Eurasia	Tick (*Ixodes scapularis, Ixodes pacificus, Ixodes ricinus*), rodent and ruminant cycles	Tick bite

*Agents potentially dispersed as low-dose stable aerosol by bioterrorists.
[†]Diseases occurring in international travelers after return.

neurologic manifestations. When a rash is observed, the differential diagnosis often includes drug eruption, measles, rubella, meningococcemia, disseminated gonococcal infection, secondary syphilis, idiopathic or thrombotic thrombocytopenic purpura, Kawasaki syndrome, immune complex disease, dengue, and arenaviral or filovirus hemorrhagic fever.

In most cases, patients are treated empirically for RMSF if the clinical manifestations and likelihood of tick exposure suggest the possibility of the disease. Laboratory testing that is effective in the acute stage when therapeutic decisions are made (e.g., immunohistochemical detection of rickettsiae in biopsy of a rash lesion) is often inconvenient and unavailable. Immunohistochemical diagnosis has 70% sensitivity and 100% specificity. Polymerase chain reaction detection of rickettsial DNA has been applied as an investigative diagnostic method, and rickettsial isolation is performed only in research centers. Antibodies are detected by indirect immunofluorescence or enzyme immunoassay in the second week of illness or later and are unreliable for diagnosis at the time of presentation.

The drug of choice for RMSF in nonpregnant adults and children of all ages, who do not have hypersensitivity to tetracyclines, is doxycycline (Vibramycin). Doxycycline (Vibramycin), 100 mg, is given orally every 12 hours, for adults and children weighing more than 45 kg. If the patient is vomiting or in a coma, the same dosage is administered intravenously. Children weighing less than 45 kg are given 2.2 mg/kg body weight of doxycycline (Vibramycin) twice daily. Although no studies of the optimal duration of study have been published, doxycycline (Vibramycin) treatment is usually continued for 5 to 10 days or until the patient has been clinically improved and afebrile for at least 48 hours. The risk of dental staining with short courses of doxycycline (Vibramycin) in children younger than 8 years of age[1] is minimal and does not justify use of the less effective antibiotic chloramphenicol (Chloromycetin). However, pregnant women should be treated with chloramphenicol (Chloromycetin), 500 mg intravenously every 6 hours.

---

[1]Not FDA approved for this indication.

CURRENT THERAPY

- Treat RMSF, HME, HGA, and *Ehrlichia ewingii* infections in nonpregnant persons of all ages with doxycycline (Vibramycin), 100 mg orally every 12 hours for adults. Children less than 45 kg body weight are given 2.2 mg/kg body weight of doxycycline (Vibramycin) twice daily.
- Treat pregnant women with RMSF with chloramphenicol (Chloromycetin), 500 mg every 6 hours.
- In pregnant women with HGA or HME, consider treatment with rifampin unless the severity is life-threatening, in which case doxycycline (Vibramycin) should be used.

Abbreviations: HGA = human granulocytotropic anaplasmosis; HME = human monocytotropic ehrlichiosis; RMSF = Rocky Mountain spotted fever.

RMSF is prevented by avoidance of tick bites by tucking pants into boots; permethrin treatment of clothing; and daily bodily tick search. Ticks are removed with tweezers or fingers protected by a cloth, tissue paper, or paper towel using firm traction to avoid leaving tick mouth parts in the skin.

Murine typhus, flying squirrel–associated typhus, rickettsialpox, American and African tick-bite fevers and scrub typhus are distinguished by the epidemiology of exposure including travel history and, for the latter four diseases, the potential presence of an eschar. Antigenic cross-reactivity between *Rickettsia typhi* and *Rickettsia prowazekii* and among *Rickettsia akari, Rickettsia africae, Rickettsia parkeri,* and *R. rickettsii* impedes a specific serologic diagnosis. The treatment for all is the same with the reservation that scrub typhus resistant to doxycycline (Vibramycin) and chloramphenicol (Chloromycetin) has been observed in northern Thailand.

Ehrlichiosis

Ehrlichia are obligately intracellular bacteria that grow within a cytoplasmic vacuole in monocytes or macrophages (*Ehrlichia chaffeensis*) or neutrophils (*Ehrlichia ewingii* and *Anaplasma phagocytophilum*). They have evolved to manipulate their phagocytic host cells to their advantage. Transmitted by ticks, these organisms are not maintained transovarially from one generation to the next in ticks, but their survival requires horizontal transmission by ticks and persistent infection in a wild vertebrate host to survive (see Table 1).

Infection by *E. chaffeensis,* human monocytotropic ehrlichiosis (HME), has an incidence as high as 100 cases per 100,000 people in areas where white-tailed deer and Lone Star ticks are abundant. Infection is highly seasonal with 68% of cases occurring from May through July. Patients usually manifest headache, myalgia, and malaise. Less than 40% have rash, gastrointestinal, respiratory, or central nervous system (CNS) abnormalities. Leukopenia, thrombocytopenia and mildly to moderately elevated hepatic transaminases are frequently observed. Half of the patients are hospitalized. Severely ill patients may develop

meningoencephalitis, toxic shock–like syndrome, respiratory insufficiency, and acute renal failure. The case-fatality rate is 3%. Immunocompromised patients are prone to develop overwhelming fatal infection. It is unclear whether in the rural southeastern and south central states this highly prevalent life-threatening infection is being treated empirically with doxycycline (Vibramycin), possibly as suspected RMSF, and thus aborting severe disease, or not.

Infection with *E. ewingii* is milder than HME and has been diagnosed mainly in immunocompromised patients.

Infection by *A. phagocytophilum,* human granulocytotropic anaplasmosis (HGA), has an incidence greater than 50 cases per 100,000 population in the upper Midwest and southern New England. Most cases occur between May and July when nymphal *Ixodes scapularis* ticks are active. HGA is usually an undifferentiated febrile illness with headache, myalgias, rigors, and malaise. Rash is rare. Leukopenia, thrombocytopenia, and elevated serum hepatic transaminases occur frequently. Severely ill patients may develop shock, confusion, pneumonitis, acute renal failure, hemorrhages, and opportunistic infections, which are the major cause of death. CNS infection is rare, and the case-fatality rate is less than 1%.

Diagnosis generally relies on indirect fluorescent antibody serology, which should test with both antigens in regions where both *E. chaffeensis* and *A. phagocytophilum* are circulating. Cross-reactive antibodies occur in some patients with the higher titer directed against the causative organism. Seroconversion or a fourfold rise in titer in a patient with a consistent illness is supportive of the diagnosis. Authorities' opinions of the value for a diagnostic single titer vary between 1 in 64 and 1 in 256. In most cases, the acute serum does not contain antibodies. *E. chaffeensis* serves as a surrogate antigen for *E. ewingii,* which has never been cultivated. Polymerase chain reaction assay is a relatively sensitive diagnostic test in the acute stage, is highly specific, and can distinguish *E. chaffeensis, E. ewingii,* and *A. phagocytophilum.* Microcolonies of organisms are seldom observed in peripheral blood monocytes (*E. chaffeensis*) and neutrophils (*E. ewingii*) except in some immunocompromised patients, but vacuoles containing *A. phagocytophilum* are observed in many patients with HGA.

The drug of choice for HME, HGA, and *E. ewingii* infections in adults and children weighing more than 45 kg is doxycycline (Vibramycin) given orally or intravenously in doses of 100 mg twice daily. Children weighing less than 45 kg are given doxycycline (Vibramycin) orally or intravenously at a dose of 2.2 mg/kg body weight twice daily. Defervescence usually occurs within 24 to 48 hours after starting this treatment. Treatment is continued for at least three days after defervescence. The organisms have been demonstrated to be resistant to chloramphenicol (Chloromycetin) in vitro. Pregnant women with life-threatening HME or HGA should be treated with doxycycline (Vibramycin).[1] Although there are no clinical trials to support the use of rifampin (Rifadin),[1] it has been used to treat HGA in pregnancy with a favorable outcome and could be used if the patient was only mildly ill and had an absolute contraindication against doxycycline (Vibramycin).[1]

---

[1]Not FDA approved for this indication.

In vitro testing has shown that *E. chaffeensis* is also sensitive to rifampin.

Prevention relies on protection from transmission by ticks as for RMSF.

REFERENCES

Bakken JS, Dumler JS: Human granulocytic ehrlichiosis. Clin Infect Dis 2000;31:554.

Buller RS, Arens M, Hmiel SP, et al: *Ehrlichia ewingii*, a newly recognized agent of human ehrlichiosis. N Engl J Med 1999;341:148.

Dumler JS, Taylor JP, Walker DH: Clinical and laboratory features of murine typhus in South Texas, 1980 through 1987. JAMA 1991; 266:365.

Elghetany MT, Walker DH: Hemostatic changes in Rocky Mountain spotted fever and Mediterranean spotted fever. Am J Clin Pathol 1999;112:159-168.

Fishbein DB, Dawson JE, Robinson LE: Human ehrlichiosis in the United States, 1985 to 1990. Ann Intern Med 1994;120:736.

Helmick CG, Bernard KW, D'Angelo LJ: Rocky Mountain spotted fever: Clinical, laboratory, and epidemiological features of 262 cases. J Infect Dis 1984;150:480.

Holman RC, Paddock CD, Curns AT, et al: Analysis of risk factors for fatal Rocky Mountain spotted fever: Evidence for superiority of tetracyclines for therapy. J Infect Dis 2001;184:1437.

Kaplowitz LG, Fischer JJ, Sparling PF: Rocky Mountain spotted fever: A clinical dilemma. Curr Clin Top Infect Dis 1981;2:89.

Olano JP, Masters E, Hogrefe W, et al: Human monocytotropic ehrlichiosis, Missouri. Emerg Infect Dis 2003;9:1579.

Paddock CD, Childs JE: *Ehrlichia chaffeensis*: A prototypical emerging pathogen. Clin Microbiol Rev 2003;16:37.

Raoult D, Ndihokubwayo JB, Tissot-Dupont H, et al: Outbreak of epidemic typhus associated with trench fever in Burundi. Lancet 1998;352:353.

Walker DH: Principles of the malicious use of infectious agents to create terror: Reasons for concern for organisms of the genus *Rickettsia*. Ann N Y Acad Sci 2003;990:1.

Watt G, Walker DH: Scrub typhus. In Guerrant RL, Walker DH, Weller PF (eds): Tropical Infectious Diseases: Principles, Pathogens, & Practice, 2nd ed. Philadelphia, Elsevier.

Smallpox

Method of
Ian M. Baird, MB, ChB

At the beginning of the 21st century, following the events of September 11, 2001, and the realization that terrorism can result in major human tragedy, we must be concerned about the possibility of bioterrorism and the use of biologic agents to cause illness and death in our population. The historical disease smallpox is an infection which if unleashed on humanity would have the potential for producing immense tactical and strategic damage. With a mortality rate of approximately 30% in a large mobile and susceptible population, the disease could spread throughout the world and cause death and disease, the likes of which would be unprecedented.

History

Smallpox has been a scourge of humanity for a millennium. It probably existed in Central Africa as early as 10,000 BC and from there traveling to Asia and the Pacific Rim. The first European epidemic occurred around 1350 BC. Thereafter the disease occurred throughout the development of the Old World with an estimated mortality between 20% and 40%. Smallpox during this time had a significant impact on the development of the human race, and by its constant pressure, it resulted in major erosions in population growth. When smallpox was introduced into the New World by Spanish explorers, the mortality was often very high with many populations of aboriginals eliminated from the North American continent.

So significant was this disease and so devastating the effects on survivors, the early attempts to prevent the disease unwittingly had some scientific background. In 17th-century China, the process of variolization, or the intentional exposure of susceptible hosts to infected material from a person who had a mild case of smallpox, was widely practiced. Variolization became redundant in 1796 when the English physician Edward Jenner demonstrated that infection with material from a cowpox lesion rendered the "vaccinated" person protected from subsequent infection with smallpox. Cowpox virus is no longer used for vaccinations, but vaccinia virus, a similar virus of low pathogenic potential, is used when vaccination is required. This is a laboratory virus that belongs to the same orthopoxvirus family of smallpox and cowpox but has no naturally occurring host.

Widespread use of vaccination resulted in significant decline of the disease until smallpox was eventually eliminated. The final bastion of disease was Somalia where the last case was recognized in 1977. Elimination of smallpox came about for a number of unique reasons, not the least of which was an intense psychological desire to be rid of the disease and to use the necessary resources to do so. This was a major undertaking by the World Health Organization (WHO) that was embarked on and ultimately successful. Other factors unique to the smallpox virus, however, are equally important. It has a relatively long incubation period, an average of 12 days with a range of 7 to 17 days and a relatively low level of communicability. Smallpox has no animal reservoir in which the virus can persist during endemic periods and from which it could cause epidemic human disease. Importantly, we have an effective method of immunization so that contacts, immunized shortly after exposure, are protected from the infection.

The program of elimination of smallpox led by Henderson and his colleagues began in 1967 and was completed in 1977. In 1980, it was certified that the world was free of naturally occurring smallpox, and worldwide immunization was discontinued. Many developed countries, including the United States, had stopped civilian vaccination as early as 1972.

Smallpox as a Biologic Weapon

Although naturally occurring smallpox no longer exists, there remains a nagging fear that the virus has the potential to be used as an agent in biologic warfare. Following the eradication of naturally occurring smallpox, much discussion ensued concerning the destruction of the remaining stocks of virus known to exist in both the United States and in Russia. There was intense debate concerning this matter, but ultimately a recommendation was made to maintain stocks of smallpox virus for the purpose of antiviral and vaccine development. Initially it was felt that the possibility of reappearance of smallpox was minuscule. However, with the events of September 11, 2001, and those that followed, such fears have risen in our consciousness, and there is a great deal of concern that rogue governments and the terrorists they support might, given the opportunity, use this agent in warfare. Certainly Cold War scientists from the Eastern bloc may share their expertise in the management of smallpox virus with such groups.

Deliberate reintroduction would be an international crime of unprecedented proportion. Because there is an average incubation period of 12 days, the possibility of worldwide spread is extremely high, and limitation or confinement of the infection to a given population or ethnic or religious group would be almost impossible. Developing countries would be much more seriously affected by an outbreak of smallpox than developed countries because of their lack of resources to provide medical care and to provide prompt widespread immunizations in the event of epidemic disease.

Virology

Smallpox is caused by the variola virus, a large DNA virus that belongs to the Orthopoxvirus family. It is unique to humans with no known animal reservoir. To sustain and maintain itself, it must be transmitted from person to person. The mechanism of spread is by droplet aerosol or direct person-to-person contact. Indirect contact is also a route of transmission, including contact with contaminated clothing or bed linens. Outbreaks are characterized by seasonal distribution seen most commonly in late winter and early spring, at a time that coincides with the appearance of chickenpox in most communities. There appear to be two strains of smallpox virus, variola major and variola minor, also known as Alastrim. Whereas the former has a mortality of 30% or higher, alastrim has a mortality of 1% or lower and hence is designated variola minor.

Epidemiology

Smallpox typically affected children, with the overwhelming majority of cases in the former epidemic situation occurring in individuals younger than 14 years. However, in rural communities where vaccination was less common, disease incidence paralleled the age of the population. Sexes are equally affected. Smallpox is seen with a higher incidence in lower economic groups, presumably the result of overcrowding. Because almost the entire population is now susceptible to smallpox, in the event of a terrorist-produced outbreak, illness would occur in all age groups with the highest mortality rates seen at the extremes of age.

Clinical Manifestations

The infection begins with multiplication of the virus within the respiratory system. The illness begins with high fever and accompanying intense malaise and prostration. The virus localizes to small blood vessels of the dermis, where it produces the typical deep indurated nodular lesions. The rash commonly is more marked on the face, forearms, and hands and then the lower limbs and, to a lesser extent, the trunk. They begin as macules, quickly evolve to papules, and then to vesicles. By day 8 of the illness, the lesions are pustular. These lesions are deeply embedded within the dermis. The pustules are followed by scabs, which may leave pitted, depigmented, and unsightly scars.

Patients suffering from smallpox are most infectious during the first 7 to 10 days after the onset of lesions. Persons with smallpox are not contagious during the intense prodromal, prerash illness when high fever, malaise, and myalgias are striking. This tends to keep patients confined to their homes, and therefore as the rash develops, they present risk mostly to their caregivers.

The most common differential diagnosis for smallpox is chickenpox, and during the early days of the rash it may be difficult to distinguish the two. Chickenpox is characterized by the development of a rash that involves all the typical lesions of maculopapules, vesicles, pustules, and scabs, but they tend to appear in crops with lesions appearing at different ages. The lesions of smallpox tend to evolve simultaneously. The patient remains contagious until the lesions crust and desquamate.

Because of the availability of antibiotic therapy, secondary bacterial infections are less important as a cause of associated morbidity and mortality. Death when it occurs does so secondary to massive viremia and is the result of multiple organ failure.

Diagnosis and Treatment

The identification of even a single suspected case of smallpox should be treated as a major health emergency. State and local health departments should be notified immediately, who will notify national health officials at the Centers for Disease Control and Prevention (CDC). Laboratory confirmation of the diagnosis in a smallpox outbreak is important. Specimens should be collected only by an individual who was vaccinated successfully within the preceding

---

 CURRENT DIAGNOSIS

- Incubation period is 12–14 d (range, 7–17 d).
- Severe nonspecific prodrome is 2–4 d.
- Development of centrifugal rash:
  - Lesions are palpable and intradermal.
  - Mucous membranes are involved.
  - All lesions appear simultaneously (compare to chickenpox).
  - Lesions evolve from vesicles to pustules to scabs.
  - Scabs desquamate in 2–3 wk with much scarring.
- Diagnosis confirmed by laboratory with high containment facilities.
- Specimens handled only by experienced vaccinated personnel.
- Diagnostic methods include electron microscopy, polymerase chain reaction, and isolation in cell culture.

36 months. Throat swabs and pustular or vesicular fluid should be harvested and transmitted immediately to state or local health laboratories for confirmation. Laboratory evaluation requires fastidious containment facilities and should be undertaken only by experienced personnel. Methods of definitively identifying smallpox virus include electron microscopy, isolation in cell culture, and identification by polymerase chain reaction methods. The diagnosis of chickenpox versus smallpox can be determined by identifying varicella zoster virus using monoclonal antibody techniques.

At the present time, there is no approved antiviral drug for treatment of smallpox. Cidofovir (Vistide[1]) is an antiviral drug licensed for the management of CMV retinitis in immunocompromised hosts. This agent has in vitro activity against vaccinia and variola, as well as other pox viruses. This drug has significant nephrotoxicity and is available currently only for intravenous (IV) administration. It should be administered only by physicians experienced with its use.

Postexposure prophylaxis is the ideal method for prevention of this disease. However, as noted later, certain groups of individuals may not receive this agent (immunocompromised hosts), and the vaccine is certainly not without complications, such as myocarditis and encephalitis. For individuals in whom the vaccine is contraindicated, the use of a limited supply of vaccinia immunoglobulin* is available through the CDC and should be used judiciously.

Postexposure Management and Vaccination

In the United States, vaccination against smallpox was discontinued in 1972 and has not been used worldwide since the disease was eradicated in 1979. Persistence of antibodies may be found for up to 10 years, but humoral immunity does wane. The persistence and protective effects of cellular immunity are not known.

Vaccination consists of administering vaccinia virus harvested from tissue monolayers.[†] It is applied with a bifurcated needle using a scarification technique. A successful take results in the appearance of a vesicle with associated erythema, which goes on to scab and then desquamates in 2 to 3 weeks.

---

[1]Not FDA approved for this indication.
*Investigational drug in the United States.
[†]Available only from the CDC.

Vaccination is not without complications. It is a live virus, and therefore no immunocompromised individual should ever be vaccinated. There is a recognized rate of postvaccinia encephalitis, approximately 2.5 cases per million vaccines administered. In addition, extensive cutaneous involvement, either as generalized vaccinia, eczema vaccinatum, or vaccinia gangrenosa, can result in serious illnesses. The overall mortality rate of vaccination in previously unvaccinated persons is estimated to be 2 or 3 per million recipients.

Between January 2003 and April 30, 2005, several thousand health care workers were vaccinated in a government program to establish a core group of workers who would be in a recently vaccinated state and thus appropriate for a first line of defense should an outbreak occur. In that population, the most common adverse effect was inadvertent inoculation of the individuals themselves or inadvertent transmission to close contacts. However, there was an unexpected incidence of myocarditis or pericarditis occurring approximately 1 in 1000 among this highly select group of civilian recipients and approximately 1 in 10,000 among a much larger group of military personnel. Consequently, individuals with known heart disease were also added to the exclusionary groups for vaccination.

Management of a Smallpox Outbreak

Should there be a situation where smallpox is suspected, involved individuals should be isolated, and all household and work contacts should be vaccinated. Currently the CDC states that they have among their resources enough vaccine to vaccinate the entire U.S. population. Because of the potential for aerosol transmission, individuals suspected of having smallpox should be managed at home rather than admitted to the hospital. In the event of confirmation of the diagnosis, if at all possible, patients should be kept at home in an attempt to contain the disease. If contacts can be vaccinated within 4 days of exposure, there will likely be prevention or significant amelioration of any subsequent illness. Should there be a very large outbreak, it is highly likely that within any given community, one or more hospitals would be designated as smallpox hospitals, and patients requiring more routine medical care would be transferred to other area hospitals.

The success of these programs would be proportional to the organizational and functional capability of the Public Health Service to distribute the vaccine to the sites of greatest need. Widespread dissemination of information to the public would be mandatory to reduce the strategic damage that such an occurrence could evoke.

Since the early 1970s, smallpox had been a disease of historical importance only. But in 2001 with the acute realization of the many faces of terrorism, including the dissemination of anthrax via the U.S. Postal Service, the specter of the use of smallpox virus as a bioterrorist weapon has been brought to the surface of our consciousness. Although smallpox is less likely to be used in this situation than agents such as anthrax and plague, we must be aware that the possibility of dissemination worldwide to huge susceptible populations is real. The effects could be devastating, but the same widespread surveillance, isolation, and vaccination that eliminated naturally occurring disease in 1978 will once again result in containment of a terrorist-induced epidemic.

REFERENCES

Blendon RJ, DesRoches CM, Benson JM, et al: The public and the smallpox threat. N Engl J Med 2003;348:426-432.

Breman J, Henderson DA: Diagnosis and management of smallpox. N Engl J Med 2002;346:1300-1308.

Lane JM, Goldstein J: Evaluation of 21st-century risks of smallpox vaccination and policy options. Ann Intern Med 2003;138:488-493.

Smallpox vaccination and adverse reactions. MMWR Morb Mortal Wkly Rep, February 21, 2003/52(RR04);1-28. Available at www.cdc.gov/mmwr/preview/mmwrhtml/rr5204al.htm.

Weiss MM, Weiss PD, Mathisen G, Guze P: Rethinking smallpox. Clin Infect Dis 2004;39(11):1668-1673.

Diseases of the Head and Neck

Vision Correction Procedures

Method of
Kraig S. Bower, MD, and
Richard D. Stutzman, MD

Refractive errors are the most frequent eye problems in the United States. Nearly half of the U.S. population requires vision correction of some kind at a cost of more than $15 billion annually. Since the Food and Drug Administration (FDA) approved the first excimer laser for refractive surgery in 1995, laser eye surgery has been performed on more than 6 million people worldwide. Almost 2 million more are expected to undergo treatment in the coming year. This chapter describes the different refractive problems and various surgeries used to treat them.

Corneal Anatomy

The cornea is 550 ± 50 mm thick and has five distinct layers. The outermost layer is stratified squamous epithelium, approximately five cell layers thick, coated by a thin tear film. It provides a smooth optical surface and barrier against infection. Beneath the epithelium, Bowman's membrane serves as a barrier and for structural purposes. The stroma, which accounts for 90% of the corneal thickness, is made up of uniform and regularly spaced collagen fibrils. The endothelium and its basement membrane (Descemet's membrane) form the innermost layers. Endothelial cells remove fluid from the cornea via an active sodium-potassium-adenosine-triphosphatase (ATPase) pump. Corneal dehydration, lack of vascularity, and regular collagen arrangement provide corneal transparency.

Optics, Refraction, and Vision

Refraction refers to the way the eye focuses light, the source of vision. Three elements determine the eye's ability to focus: the shape of the cornea, the power of the lens, and the length of the eyeball. The cornea is responsible for two thirds of the total focusing power. The lens, which lies behind the pupil, accounts for one third and can change its shape to adjust focusing power.

In an eye with normal vision, the power of the cornea and lens perfectly matches the length of the eye. Light rays from a distant object are focused precisely on a light-sensitive membrane called the retina, and a clear image is perceived. Objects viewed up close require additional focusing power by the lens in a process known as accommodation.

Refractive Error

Refractive errors occur when light entering the eye does not focus on the retina. They are normal differences in visual ability rather than true diseases. The three basic types of refractive errors are myopia, hyperopia, and astigmatism.

In myopia, the cornea and lens are too powerful for the length of the globe. Distant objects cannot be seen clearly because light rays are focused in front of the retina. However, because the myopic eye has a focal point close to the eye, near objects can be seen clearly without corrective lenses, hence the term *nearsighted*.

In hyperopia, the cornea and lens are too weak or the eyeball is too short. Light rays reach the retina before they are focused to a single point, resulting in a blurry image. Accommodation may bring a distant object into focus but may be inadequate for near vision, hence the term *farsighted*.

Astigmatism often occurs with either myopia or hyperopia. It is an irregular curvature of the cornea in which the refractive power of the eye varies in different meridians. Light rays cannot be brought to a single point, and objects are blurry at any distance.

Another refractive problem, presbyopia, occurs as the aging lens loses its ability to accommodate. This change occurs in everybody, usually around age 45 years, resulting in eyestrain with prolonged near work. Myopes frequently notice that it is easier to remove their glasses to read. Hyperopes who rely on accommodation have increasing difficulty focusing. Once presbyopia develops, additional focusing power is necessary in the form of reading glasses or bifocals.

Corrective lenses alter the path of light rays entering the eye. Myopia is treated with concave lenses with minus (divergent) power. Hyperopia requires convex lenses with plus (convergent) power. Astigmatism is corrected with cylindrical lenses. Glasses have been used for centuries and are simple, relatively inexpensive, and safe. Contact lenses are an option for those who find glasses unacceptable. Problems with contacts, such as intolerance, infection, inconvenience, and cost, limit their use in some people.

Refractive Surgery

Refractive surgery is a modern alternative to glasses or contact lenses. Procedures are generally permanent and irreversible. They are performed in otherwise healthy eyes and do not treat reduced vision from cataract, glaucoma, macular degeneration, and other disorders that may require other medical or surgical treatments. Myopia, hyperopia, and astigmatism are the refractive problems most commonly treated with surgery. Table 1 lists the indications and contraindications for refractive surgery.

All patients require a complete eye examination by a provider experienced in refractive surgery. Evaluation includes refraction, slit-lamp examination, intraocular

TABLE 1 Eligibility Criteria for Refractive Surgery

Indications
Age ≥ 18 y
Myopia ≤ 14.00 D
Astigmatism ≤ 4.00 D
Hyperopia ≤ +6.00 D
Stable refraction at least 1 y*
Reasonable expectations
Medical Contraindications
Uncontrolled vascular disease
Autoimmune disease
Immune suppressed/immune compromised
Pregnant or nursing
Keloid formation[†]
Diabetes[†]
Isotretinoin (Accutane), sumatriptan (Imitrex),
   or amiodarone
Ocular Contraindications
Keratoconus
Herpetic keratitis
Progressive myopia
Cataract
Corneal disease[‡]
Glaucoma[‡]
Amblyopia[‡]

---

*No more than a 0.5 D change in the 12 mo preceding surgery.
[†]Relative contraindications. Well-controlled diabetes mellitus is not an absolute contraindication to surgery, but fluctuating refractions caused by uncontrolled blood sugar levels, diabetic cataract, or diabetic retinopathy may recommend against refractive surgery.
[‡]Other eye problems including previous infections, scarring, surgery, trauma, glaucoma, dry eye, or blepharitis must be carefully evaluated to determine whether they pose an increased risk or will significantly alter the results of refractive surgery.
Abbreviation: D = diopter.

pressure testing, and a dilated examination to rule out cataracts or retinal abnormality. Computerized videokeratography and wavefront aberrometry, measurements of corneal curvature, shape and thickness, and the pupil size are also needed for a successful visual outcome. Patients must review information about the surgery and discuss risks, benefits, alternatives, expected outcomes, and potential complications with their surgeon before deciding to have surgery. Based on the patient's expectations and examination findings, the surgeon and patient must select the correct surgical procedure to maximize results while minimizing risks.

Excimer Laser Procedures

Lasers have been used in medicine and surgery for decades. One of the most important advances in refractive surgery is the excimer laser. In 1995, the FDA approved the first excimer laser to treat mild and moderate myopia. Since then, additional lasers have been approved for an expanded therapeutic range.

The excimer laser combines argon (Ar) and fluoride (F) gases to generate a beam of ultraviolet light with a 193-nm wavelength. This has sufficient energy to break molecular bonds within corneal collagen in a process called ablative photodecomposition, or photoablation. The laser removes microscopic amounts of corneal tissue with little risk of thermal damage to surrounding tissues. A computer programmed with the patient's prescription controls the laser beam to reshape the cornea with great precision. In myopia, the laser flattens the central cornea to decrease its focusing power. In hyperopia, the laser indirectly steepens the central cornea by flattening the periphery. Astigmatism is treated with an elliptical or cylindrical beam to flatten the steepest corneal meridian.

PHOTOREFRACTIVE KERATECTOMY

Excimer laser photorefractive keratectomy (PRK) is approved for myopia and hyperopia. The desired correction is programmed into the laser's computer, and the patient is given topical anesthetic drops (0.5% proparacaine [Alcaine]). The eyelids are swabbed with 1% povidone iodine solution and draped with adhesive plastic drapes. A speculum gently retracts the eyelids. The corneal epithelium is removed using a soft-bristled rotary brush, the laser, or an instrument that resembles a spatula. The patient views a fixation target while the surgeon aligns the laser and delivers the laser treatment. Immediately after treatment the cornea is irrigated with chilled saline, and a contact lens is placed to protect the cornea. After surgery, the patient uses topical nonsteroidal anti-inflammatory drugs (NSAIDs) for 48 hours, antibiotic drops for 1 week, steroid drops for 1 month, and oral analgesics as needed.

For the first few days, patients experience blurred vision and moderate discomfort as the corneal surface heals. The contact lens is removed after the epithelium has healed, usually in 3 to 5 days. Mild blurriness is common for several weeks as the cornea heals. Once the healing process is complete, 96% of treated eyes are 20/40 or better—sufficient to drive legally without corrective lenses.

TABLE 2 Complications of Refractive Surgery

Excimer Laser Procedures	Nonexcimer Corneal Procedures	Intraocular Procedures
Possible with All	**Laser Thermal Keratoplasty**	**Phakic Intraocular Lenses**
Overcorrection	Overcorrection/undercorrection	*Angle supported*
Undercorrection	Astigmatism	Endophthalmitis
Astigmatism	Regression	Uveitis
Central island	Infection	Glaucoma
Decentration	Corneal scarring	Cystoid macular edema
Regression	Corneal edema	Decentration
Infection	**Conductive Keratoplasty**	Pupillary changes
Dry eye	Overcorrection/undercorrection	Corneal decompensation
Glare/halos	Astigmatism	*Iris supported*
More Likely with PRK	Regression	Endophthalmitis
Delayed epithelial healing	Infection	Uveitis
Corneal haze	Corneal abrasion	Dislocation
Scarring	Corneal scarring	Iris atrophy
Recurrent erosion	Corneal edema	Corneal decompensation
Steroid-induced glaucoma	**Intacs**	Cystoid macular edema
More Likely with LASIK	Intolerance/foreign-body sensation	Glare and edge effects
Intraoperative flap complications	Infection	*Posterior chamber*
Ocular penetration	Overcorrection/undercorrection	Endophthalmitis
Recurrent erosion	Astigmatism	Pupillary block
Traumatic flap dislocation	Glare/halos	Anterior subcapsular cataract
Epithelial ingrowth	Abnormal wound healing	Pigment dispersion
Interface debris	**Radial Keratotomy**	Iris atrophy
Flap striae	Wound leak, ocular penetration	Open-angle glaucoma
Diffuse lamellar keratitis	Infection	Edge effect and glare
More Likely with LASEK	Overcorrection/undercorrection	**Clear Lens Extraction**
Same as PRK	Astigmatism	Endophthalmitis
Sloughed flap	Glare and starburst effects	Glaucoma
	Fluctuating vision	Corneal decompensation
	Ocular rupture with blunt trauma	Retinal detachment
	Progressive hyperopia	

Two thirds have unaided vision of 20/20 or better. Potential problems include over- or undercorrection, astigmatism, scarring, glare, and corneal haze (Table 2). The latter is more common after treating higher degrees of myopia.

LASER-ASSISTED IN SITU KERATOMILEUSIS

Laser-assisted in situ keratomileusis (LASIK) is an effective treatment for myopia and hyperopia. After topical anesthesia and lid preparation similar to PRK, the surgeon uses an instrument called a microkeratome to create a hinged corneal flap 8.5 to 9.5 mm in diameter with a thickness of 130 to 180 mm (average, 160 mm). The flap is folded back to expose the underlying tissue to the laser. After ablation the surgeon returns the flap to its original position and irrigates under the flap with saline solution. The flap seals without the need for sutures. Topical antibiotic, an NSAID, and steroid drops are applied, and the eyelid speculum and drapes are carefully removed. The flap is inspected by slit-lamp examination to confirm good position and stability before the patient leaves the office.

Visual results are comparable with PRK. Advantages of LASIK include quicker postoperative visual recovery with less discomfort and lower risk of corneal haze. A disadvantage is the potential for corneal flap complications (Table 2). Although such complications may result in the loss of vision, they are, fortunately, rare (less than 0.1% of surgeries).

LASER EPITHELIAL KERATOMILEUSIS

Laser epithelial keratomileusis (LASEK) is a modification of the PRK technique that may address the shortcomings of LASIK and PRK. In LASEK, a 20% alcohol solution is applied for 25 to 35 seconds to separate the epithelium from Bowman's membrane. The loosened epithelium is retained as an intact flap that is returned to position after the laser ablation is complete. The early postoperative course is similar to PRK. LASEK may result in less corneal haze than PRK and offers an alternative for patients with high myopia who are unable or unwilling to undergo LASIK. This typically includes patients with thin corneas and patients at increased risk of flap trauma, such as athletes in contact sports and military personnel.

WAVEFRONT-GUIDED SURGERY

Since the 1800s, doctors have described optical imperfections (aberrations) in terms of myopia, hyperopia, and astigmatism and used simple letter charts to measure and express vision (e.g., 20/20, 20/40, etc.). Using modern diagnostic tools that allow analysis of the visual system in more detail, we now know that simple refractive errors are not the only optical aberrations. Higher-order aberrations may be associated with night vision difficulties or reduced contrast sensitivity despite eye chart vision of 20/20 or better.

An exciting advance in ophthalmology is wavefront technology. Astronomers use wavefront technology to identify atmospheric distortions (aberrations) of incoming light and to correct these aberrations to produce clear images of distant stars and other celestial bodies beyond the earth's atmosphere. In the same way, a wavefront capture device, called an aberrometer, analyzes light rays reflected from the retina to identify all aberrations, lower and higher order, of the eye. These aberrations are then displayed as a three-dimensional wavefront map.

Wavefront-guided (WFG) surgery makes it possible to address higher-order aberrations while treating lower-order refractive errors with the excimer laser. In clinical trials for myopia without astigmatism, WFG LASIK reduced higher-order aberrations, improved contrast sensitivity, and resulted in a quality of vision superior to conventional LASIK. Several wavefront-guided laser systems have FDA approval for LASIK and others are currently under investigation. Additional clinical trials will determine the effectiveness of WFG PRK, WFG treatment for hyperopia, and customized treatment of eyes with special visual disorders.

Intraocular Procedures

Excimer laser procedures have limits in treating high myopia and high hyperopia, which require removal of significantly more corneal tissue to achieve the desired treatment effect. Although the FDA approved a therapeutic range of −14.00 to +6.00 D (diopters), in most cases the realistic limits of laser keratectomy are −10.00 D of myopia to +5.00 D of hyperopia. One must look beyond the cornea to treat refractive errors outside of this range.

CLEAR LENS EXTRACTION

The success of modern cataract surgery has resulted in interest in lens extraction as a means of treating refractive error. Predictability and stability of results are the chief advantages. There is a significant risk of retinal detachment after intraocular surgery in the highly myopic eye, and this procedure is not generally recommended. Results of clear lens extraction for high hyperopia have been promising, with significant improvement in unaided vision and few complications. Current formulas for calculating intraocular lens (IOL) power allow most patients to achieve a postoperative refraction within 1.00 D of the refractive goal. A drawback to refractive clear lens extraction in younger patients is the loss of accommodation that comes with removal of the crystalline lens.

PHAKIC INTRAOCULAR LENS

Phakic IOLs are implanted in the eye without removing the patient's natural lens. They may prove to be a powerful surgical option for individuals with refractive errors not amenable to laser treatment. Unlike clear lens extraction, the patient keeps the natural lens, allowing accommodation.

There are three lens types based on their location in the eye: angle supported (in front of the iris), iris supported, and posterior chamber. Most phakic IOLs provide good short-term results, but long-term safety data are lacking. All are intraocular procedures with a higher risk profile than the excimer laser. Most significant is the risk of postoperative endophthalmitis. Table 2 lists additional complications.

Surgery for Hyperopia

The excimer laser is approved for hyperopia up to +6.00 D with up to 4.00 D of astigmatism. The technique is the same as for myopic PRK and LASIK, but a larger ablation is required and, therefore, a larger epithelial defect or flap, respectively, is possible. Surgery is safe and effective, although results are generally not as good as those seen with myopic treatments. Higher levels of hyperopia are better addressed with clear lens extraction.

Thermal keratoplasty offers an alternative to the excimer laser for hyperopia. A series of thermal spots tightens the peripheral cornea, which, in turn, leads to central corneal steepening. Treatment occurs outside of the visual axis with risk of no flap complications or compromise of the structural integrity of the cornea. The FDA has approved two systems for the treatment of low-to-moderate hyperopia.

LASER THERMAL KERATOPLASTY (LTK)

The Hyperion LTK system uses a holmium: YAG laser as a heat source to treat low hyperopia without astigmatism. After topical anesthetic drops, an eyelid speculum is placed and the cornea carefully dried. The patient is positioned at the laser console and instructed to view a fixation light during the treatment, which takes less than 5 seconds. Following surgery, the patient is treated with a topical NSAID for 48 hours, topical antibiotic drops for a week, and oral analgesics as needed. The most common complication is hyperopic regression. This can be retreated with LTK, CK, or the excimer laser.

CONDUCTIVE KERATOPLASTY

Conductive keratoplasty (CK) uses a radiofrequency probe that is inserted into the peripheral corneal stroma.

Resistance to current along the probe results in localized heat and collagen shrinkage. The Refractec ViewPoint CK System is approved for the treatment of mild-to-moderate hyperopia. The eye is anesthetized with 0.5% proparacaine (Alcaine) drops, and the cornea is marked for the treatment. The treatment pattern, determined by the patient's preoperative refraction, takes 8 to 32 spots. Additional spots can be placed to steepen the flattest meridian in astigmatic eyes. The treatment takes approximately 5 minutes to perform. Postoperative topical antibiotics, topical NSAIDs, and oral analgesics are given. Results are promising, with 51% of eyes demonstrating uncorrected visual acuity (UCVA) 20/20 or better and 91% 20/40 or better at 12 months postoperatively. Importantly, there is less hyperopic regression than with LTK.

Surgery for Presbyopia

As Benjamin Franklin remarked (in a letter to Jean-Baptiste Leroy, November 13, 1789), "in this world nothing can be said to be certain, except death and taxes." Franklin, the inventor of bifocal glasses, no doubt suffered from another certainty in this world, presbyopia. Dependence on reading glasses remains a potential source of dissatisfaction in older patients following otherwise successful refractive surgery. A cure for presbyopia is a highly sought-after goal.

One approach is monovision, which intentionally creates mild myopia in one eye to achieve reading vision. This was traditionally done with contact lenses and can be the target correction with the laser as well, but not all patients tolerate monovision.

Another approach is to increase accommodation through surgery to the sclera. Scleral expansion surgeries are under continued investigation, but at the present time do not offer a safe, reproducible, effective, and stable alternative.

Multifocal lenses mimic accommodation by allowing for both distance and near vision at the same time. They tend to compromise the quality of both and continue to have limited acceptance. Accommodating IOLs are designed to increase their optical power by shifting position as the patient attempts to accommodate. They have a promising future but are not presently approved or readily available in the United States.

Other Procedures

INTRASTROMAL CORNEAL RINGS (INTACS)

Intacs are clear plastic rings threaded into the outer part of the cornea to alter its shape. Potential advantages include avoidance of the visual axis and reversibility by removing the rings. FDA clinical trials demonstrated efficacy equal to PRK and LASIK after 12 months; however, long-term results and safety are unknown. Intacs have not gained widespread acceptance by patients or surgeons as an alternative to excimer laser surgery. Currently, Intacs are primarily being used for the off-label treatment of keratoconus.

TABLE 3 Evaluating the Results of Refractive Surgery

Term	Definition/Measurement
Predictability	Ability to achieve target of emmetropia (0.50 or 1.00 D)
Efficacy	Percentage that meet UCVA goal (±20/20, 20/25, or 20/40)
Stability	Long-term maintenance of the surgical effect over time
Safety	Preservation of preoperative BSCVA
	Side Effects and Complications
Patient satisfaction	Patient expectations and how well the outcome matches those expectations

Abbreviations: BSCVA = best spectacle-corrected visual acuity; UCVA = uncorrected visual acuity.

INCISIONAL SURGERY

Radial keratotomy (RK) uses radial or spokelike corneal incisions to alter corneal curvature. Although more than 1 million Americans have had this procedure since the late 1970s, RK has significant limitations (Table 2) and has been abandoned since the advent of the excimer laser. Astigmatic keratotomy (AK) and limbal relaxing incisions (LRI) use transverse or arcuate incisions in the peripheral cornea to flatten the steep corneal meridian. Indications include isolated astigmatism, often in association with cataract surgery or following corneal surgery.

The excimer laser has revolutionized ophthalmology and is the procedure of choice for most patients desiring refractive surgery. Current and emerging procedures must be evaluated in terms of predictability, efficacy, stability, and safety (Table 3) before they find their place in the refractive surgery armamentarium.

Conjunctivitis

Method of
Sandra Y. Cho, MD, and Michael H. Goldstein, MD

Anatomy

The conjunctiva is a thin, transparent membrane that covers both bulbar and palpebral structures of the eye. It extends from the corneal limbus to the mucocutaneous junctions of the upper and lower lid margins. The epithelium contains goblet cells for mucin secretion, and the underlying substantia propria contains lymphocytes, vessels, nerves (from V1), and lymphatics that drain toward the preauricular and submandibular lymph nodes.

History

Patients with conjunctivitis complain of nonspecific symptoms such as redness, foreign body sensation, tearing, discharge, itching, lid swelling, and burning. Symptoms not usually associated with conjunctivitis include severe pain, photophobia, or marked changes in vision. In any patient presenting with these symptoms, other causes of a red eye should be considered.

In addition to noting the past medical, ocular, family, and social history, as well as medications, eye drops, allergies, and a review of systems, some key questions can give clues to the etiology of the conjunctivitis: Have there been any sick contacts or "red eye" contacts? Does the patient have any children in daycare? Has there been a recent upper respiratory tract infection? Is the patient a contact lens wearer? Is there a history of skin rashes or eczema? Does the patient have seasonal or contact allergies? Has the patient had any recent cold sores? Is the patient sexually active? Does the patient have any genitourinary symptoms?

Examination

Check the vision in each eye. Inspect the skin and eyelids for rashes, vesicles, or chronic inflammation. Palpate the preauricular node for lymphadenopathy. Examine the lower palpebral conjunctiva by pulling down the lower lid and asking the patient to look up. If possible, flip the upper lid. Infection and inflammation cause conjunctival hyperemia, chemosis, and thickening of the epithelium. Lymphocytes in the substantia propria can be stimulated to form follicles and papillae that can be seen clinically on the inferior or superior palpebral conjunctiva and occasionally on the bulbar conjunctiva. Note whether one or both eyes are involved.

It can be difficult even for the experienced practitioner to differentiate the various types of conjunctivitis, although some characteristics may be helpful. These include the following:

- Adnexa
  - Preauricular lymphadenopathy: viral, severe hyperacute bacterial, chronic bacterial
  - Discharge:
    - Ropy white mucoid discharge: allergic
    - Serous discharge: Viral>allergic>toxic, bacterial
    - Scant purulent discharge: Bacterial
    - Gross purulent discharge: Gonococcal
- Timing
  - Hyperacute: *Neisseria gonorrhoeae* or *meningitidis*
  - Acute: Viral, bacterial
  - Chronic (over 4 weeks): *Chlamydia trachomatis*, toxic; molluscum contagiosum, toxic, allergic; blepharoconjunctivitis (rosacea, blepharitis)
- Unilateral or bilateral:
  - Unilateral: Often bacterial or toxic (if using medication in one eye)
  - Bilateral: Often viral (adenovirus), allergic, toxic (if using medication in both eyes)

Viral

ADENOVIRUS

A common cause of conjunctivitis, adenoviral conjunctivitis is characterized by a history of a recent upper respiratory tract infection or a sick contact. Patients may be exposed by unaffected children. Patients complain of burning, foreign body sensation, itching, redness, lid swelling, serous discharge and tearing, and eyelids that stick together upon awakening. It frequently starts in one eye and affects the second eye several days later. On examination, look for inferior palpebral follicles and a palpable preauricular lymph node. Cultures are not necessary. Treatment is supportive and consists of frequent artificial tears (four to eight times a day) and cool compresses. There are currently no FDA-approved medications to treat adenoviral conjunctivitis. If itching is severe, topical antihistamines can be used. Patients should be counseled that the symptoms often get worse before they get better in the following 1 to 2 weeks, and the virus is very contagious for 10 to 12 days from onset. Patients should avoid direct contact with others, wash their hands frequently, and clean shared surfaces such as towels, computer keyboards, and so on.

Routine use of topical antibiotics and steroids is discouraged. Viral conjunctivitis is usually benign and self-limited, and bacterial superinfection is not typical. Topical steroids can be used for severe adenoviral conjunctivitis in the case of subepithelial infiltrates or pseudomembrane formation. However, given the risk of worsening other similar eye diseases, the adverse effects of steroids such as glaucoma and cataracts, and the possibility of prolonging the disease course, steroids should only be given under the supervision of an ophthalmologist.

HERPES SIMPLEX CONJUNCTIVITIS

Herpes simplex (most commonly type 1) affects the eye in a variety of ways including eyelid dermatitis, conjunctivitis,

---

CURRENT DIAGNOSIS

- The history provides the main clues to the type of conjunctivitis. Other clues are the type of discharge, duration of symptoms, presence of preauricular lymphadenopathy, and periocular skin and lid abnormalities.
- Conjunctival cultures are rarely needed to make the diagnosis but may be helpful in specific situations: hyperacute conjunctivitis, chronic conjunctivitis (>4 wk), epidemics, health care workers, newborns, and immunocompromised patients.
- Viral conjunctivitis is more common than bacterial conjunctivitis.
- Itching is typically noted with allergic conjunctivitis. If the patient has no itching, consider another diagnosis.
- Pain is typically not a feature of conjunctivitis. If the patient has pain, consider another diagnosis.

keratitis, and uveitis. Keratitis is the most devastating visually and beyond the scope of this chapter. Unilateral eye redness, a palpable preauricular lymph node, and vesicular lesions on the eyelid margin are suggestive of HSV conjunctivitis. The virus establishes latent infection in the trigeminal nerve and may reactivate to cause recurrent disease. When vesicular lesions are very close to the lid margin, or if the conjunctiva is already inflamed without corneal involvement, prophylactic topical trifluridine 1% (Viroptic) should be used five times a day. Discontinue after 7 to 14 days to avoid surface toxicity. Alternative therapies include acyclovir (Zovirax), 200 to 400 mg[3] orally five times a day. Topical steroids are contraindicated.

MOLLUSCUM CONTAGIOSUM

Molluscum lesions are domed, umbilicated, cream-colored nodules that can cause a chronic unilateral follicular conjunctivitis if located close to the eye. This is a relatively uncommon cause of conjunctivitis. At-risk groups are immunocompromised patients and children. Viral particles from lesions cause a toxic reaction in the conjunctiva. Treatment is by excision of the lesion(s).

Bacterial

ACUTE BACTERIAL

The organisms most commonly responsible for bacterial conjunctivitis are staphylococcal species, *Streptococcus pneumoniae*, and *Haemophilus influenzae* (especially in children). The incidence is relatively low compared with other causes of conjunctivitis. Patients complain of burning, tearing, mucopurulent or purulent discharge, and they often report that their eyelids stick together in the morning. On examination the conjunctiva is injected and mucopurulent discharge can be seen in the fornices. Preauricular lymphadenopathy is typically absent. Cultures are rarely necessary unless severe, unresponsive to treatment, chronic, or recurrent.

The course is self-limited and resolves in days to 1 to 2 weeks without treatment. However, empirical antibiotic therapy can shorten the course of the infection and decrease morbidity. Broad-spectrum antibiotic drops (e.g., polymyxin/trimethoprim [Polytrim], fluoroquinolones), four times daily, or ointments (e.g., erythromycin, bacitracin/polymyxin B), four times daily for 5 to 7 days, are well tolerated and provide excellent coverage for the pathogens responsible for bacterial conjunctivitis. Sulfacetamide is also a broad-spectrum bacteriostatic agent but has the rare complication of Steven-Johnson syndrome. The aminoglycosides are less appropriate given their primarily gram-negative coverage and the incidence of surface toxicity and allergy. *Haemophilus influenzae* conjunctivitis in children should also be treated with oral amoxicillin/clavulanate (Augmentin), 20 to 40 mg/kg/day in three divided doses because of associated otitis media, pneumonia, and meningitis.

[3]Exceeds dosage recommended by the manufacturer.

NEISSERIA GONORRHOEAE OR MENINGITIDIS (HYPERACUTE)

A true ocular emergency, it is critical that gonococcal conjunctivitis be recognized and treated without delay. *Neisseria gonorrhoeae* (occasionally *meningitidis*), a gram-negative diplococcus, has the ability to penetrate an intact epithelium and can cause corneal ulcers and perforation in a short amount of time. It is seen most frequently in sexually active adults in their teens to thirties.

Patients describe a hyperacute onset of purulent discharge, photophobia, redness, and eyelid swelling in one or both eyes. On exam there are follicles, frequently a preauricular lymph node, and characteristically a massive purulent discharge. The cornea should be examined carefully for infiltrates (white opacities). Conjunctival scraping for immediate Gram stain, cultures, and sensitivities should be obtained. If the cornea is not involved, ceftriaxone (Rocephin), 1 g intramuscularly for one dose, is given. If the cornea is involved or cannot be excluded, the patient should receive ceftriaxone, 1 g intravenously every 12 to 24 hours for 3 days. Topical fluoroquinolone eyedrops are given every 1 to 2 hours, and saline is used for frequent irrigation to remove the discharge. Concomitant sexually transmitted diseases should be treated. Sexual partners should be treated as well.

CHLAMYDIA TRACHOMATIS (CHRONIC)

Adult chlamydial inclusion conjunctivitis is caused by *Chlamydia trachomatis* serotypes D through K (serotypes A through C cause trachoma). It is sexually transmitted and frequently occurs with concomitant genital infection. It is a common cause of chronic follicular conjunctivitis (more than 4 weeks' duration). Giemsa stain, direct immunofluorescent monoclonal antibody staining of conjunctival smears, and McCoy cell cultures can help establish the diagnosis. Erythromycin ointment is used twice daily for 2 to 3 weeks. Azithromycin (Zithromax), 1 g orally in a single dose, treats the infection. Patients can also be treated with oral doxycycline (Vibramycin), 100 mg orally twice a day for 1 week. Sexual partners should also be evaluated and treated.

Blepharoconjunctivitis

A common condition, blepharitis is a chronic bilateral inflammation of the eyelids because of meibomian gland dysfunction. Patients present with irritation, tearing, crusting, itching, and foreign body sensation. The lids are thickened and erythematous with telangiectatic vessels at the margins. There can be a loss of lashes, crusting, and chronic injection of the bulbar conjunctiva. Blepharitis is associated with rosacea (commonly missed), seborrheic dermatitis, staphylococcal colonization, chalazia, and dry eyes. Treatment consists of artificial tears, warm compresses, lid scrubs with a mild detergent (e.g., infant shampoo). For more severe cases, doxycycline, 100 mg orally two times a day, or flaxseed oil*[1]

*Herbal supplement.
[1]Not FDA approved for this indication.

capsules, 2000 to 3000 mg per day, are effective. Antibiotic ointments (erythromycin, bacitracin) can be used on the lids. Topical metronidazole (Flagyl) can help with rosacea.

Allergy

SEASONAL/PERENNIAL

The hallmark of allergic conjunctivitis is itching. Seasonal and perennial allergic conjunctivitis is associated with a personal or family history of atopy, allergy, asthma, and environmental triggers. In addition to itching, common symptoms include lid swelling, chemosis, injection, and watery or mucoid discharge. Papillae are seen on the palpebral conjunctiva. Treatment is aimed at reducing symptoms with artificial tears, topical antihistamines, and mast cell stabilizers. Topical nonsteroidal anti-inflammatory drugs (NSAIDs) are reported to be effective in reducing symptoms. Also helpful are cold compresses, artificial tears, and allergen avoidance.

VERNAL AND ATOPIC

Vernal and atopic keratoconjunctivitis are more severe forms of allergy. Both are associated with atopic manifestations of eczema, rhinitis, and asthma. Symptoms are intense itching, tearing, photophobia, and stringy mucous discharge. Vernal conjunctivitis is more common in boys in their first and second decades, with a higher incidence in the spring and fall. The hallmark is giant papillae on the upper palpebral conjunctiva that lead to corneal irritation and occasionally a corneal abrasion or a "shield" ulcer as well as upper lid ptosis. Atopic keratoconjunctivitis can occur in patients with a history of atopic dermatitis. The eyelids have a thick, erythematous, scaly, and leathery appearance. Papillae are small. Corneal neovascularization and opacification, conjunctival scarring, and cataracts can occur as sequelae. There is a higher incidence of staphylococcal and herpes simplex virus ocular infections. Treatment for both vernal and atopic keratoconjunctivitis consists of topical and oral antihistamines, mast cell stabilizers (cromolyn sodium [Crolom], 4% four times daily; olopatadine [Patanol], 0.1% twice daily), and topical steroid drops (fluorometholone, prednisolone acetate, 1% four times daily). Skin changes should be treated with mild topical steroid creams or steroid-sparing agents (e.g., tacrolimus[1] [Protopic] 0.03% and 0.1%). Treatment time is lengthy and requires follow-up with an ophthalmologist.

Toxic/Medication

Eyedrops may cause toxicity to the conjunctiva, especially if used for long periods of time. Most notable are aminoglycoside antibiotics, antivirals (trifluridine [Viroptic]), certain glaucoma medications (brimonidine [Alphagan], pilocarpine, etc.), eyedrop and contact lens solution preservatives (thimerosal, benzalkonium chloride), and topical anesthetics. Over-the-counter (OTC) antihistamine/vasoconstrictor preparations may also cause chronic conjunctival injection and irritation. Symptoms rebound if stopped. A careful history is crucial. There is a follicular

CURRENT THERAPY

- Most cases of viral or bacterial conjunctivitis are self-limited and require supportive care.
- Viral conjunctivitis is particularly contagious and patients should be advised of such. Good handwashing is essential.
- Steroids are rarely a first-line treatment for any type of conjunctivitis. Any patient on topical steroids should be followed by an ophthalmologist.
- All toxic or allergic exposures should be eliminated. Stop contact lens use, preserved over-the-counter artificial tears, and over-the-counter topical vasoconstrictors.
- Refer to an ophthalmologist: any patient not responding in the expected manner, symptoms >4 wk, hyperacute conjunctivitis, loss or change in vision, pain, or those with photophobia.

reaction in the inferior fornices and occasionally corneal involvement, especially with topical anesthetic abuse. Patients should be instructed to stop their medications, discontinue contact lens wear, and use preservative-free artificial tears frequently.

REFERENCES

Jackson WB: Differentiating conjunctivitis of diverse origins. Surv Ophthalmol 1993;38:91-104.

Krachmer JH, Mannis MJ, Holland EJ: Cornea, 2nd ed. Philadelphia, Elsevier Mosby, 2005:37-43, 601-613.

Kunimoto D, Kanitkar K, Makar M (eds): Wills Eye Manual, 4th ed. Philadelphia, Lippincott Williams & Wilkens, 2004, pp 89-95.

Ono SJ, Abelson MB: Allergic conjunctivitis: Update on pathophysiology and prospects for future treatment. J Allergy Clin Immunol 2005;115(1), 118-122.

Rikkers SM, Holland GN, Drayton GE, et al: Topical tacrolimus treatment of atopic eyelid disease. Am J Ophthamol 2003;135(3): 297-302.

Romanowski EG, Roba LA, Wiley L, et al: The effects of corticosteroids of adenoviral replication. Arch Ophthalmol 1996;114(5):581-585.

Sheikh A, Hurwitz B: Antibiotics versus placebo for acute bacterial conjunctivitis. Cochrane Database Syst Rev 2006 April 19; (2): CD001211.

Soparkar CN, Wilhemus KR, Koch DD, et al: Acute and chronic conjunctivitis due to over-the-counter ophthalmic decongestants. Arch Ophthalmol 1997;115(1):34-38.

Optic Neuritis

Method of
Andrew G. Lee, MD, and Steven L. Galetta, MD

Optic neuritis (ON) is the most common cause of acute loss of vision caused by an optic neuropathy in a young adult. In this chapter we use the term *ON* to refer to cases that are idiopathic or demyelinating.

Clinical Features of Demyelinating Optic Neuritis

The typical patient with ON is a young adult woman presenting with acute, unilateral visual loss associated with pain worsened by eye movement. ON can occur in patients of any age and in either gender, however. The examination shows variable loss of visual acuity (20/20 to no light perception), visual field, or color vision, and an ipsilateral relative afferent pupillary defect (RAPD). The optic nerve typically appears normal at onset (i.e., retrobulbar optic neuropathy) but may be swollen (i.e., papillitis). Optic atrophy may develop over time in a sector or diffuse pattern. In cases with papillitis, the disc edema is typically mild. The presence of retinal hemorrhages, exudates, or cotton wool patches should suggest an alternative optic neuropathy (e.g., anterior ischemic optic neuropathy, inflammatory or infiltrative optic neuropathy).

The Optic Neuritis Treatment Trial (ONTT) was a randomized, controlled clinical trial in the United States that has provided excellent clinical information on ON. Table 1 summarizes the typical features, and Table 2 summarizes the atypical features of ON. Table 3 summarizes the recommendations for ON.

Clinical Course

The majority (95%) of cases of ON recover vision (20/40 or better). Recurrence of ON is seen in up to 19% of patients in the affected eye and 17% in the fellow eye over a 10-year period. Patients with ON are at risk for the development of multiple sclerosis (MS), and that risk may be predicted by the findings on brain magnetic resonance imaging (MRI). Those patients with white matter lesions typical of demyelinating disease on a

CURRENT DIAGNOSIS

- Young (<40 years, often female) patient
- Acute loss of vision
- Pain with eye movement
- Relative afferent papillary defect
- Normal-appearing optic nerve common (retrobulbar optic neuropathy)
- Improvement over time
- Associated with multiple sclerosis

TABLE 1 Features of Typical Optic Neuritis in Adults

Acute to subacute onset
Usually unilateral loss of visual acuity, contrast, color, or visual field
An ipsilateral relative afferent pupillary defect (RAPD)
Periocular pain (90%), especially with eye movement
Normal (65%) or swollen (35%) optic nerve head
A young adult patient (usually <40 y) but may occur at any age
Eventual visual improvement in majority of patients
Absence of anterior or posterior segment inflammation

Modified with permission from Lee AG, Brazis PW: Clinical Pathways in Neuro-ophthalmology: An Evidence-based Approach, 2nd ed. New York, Thieme, 2003.

CURRENT THERAPY

- Intravenous methylprednisolone (1000 mg/d) for 3 d followed by oral taper speeds rate of visual recovery but does not change final visual outcome versus placebo.
- Oral steroids in conventional doses (e.g., prednisone, 60 mg/d) increased the rate of new attacks and are contraindicated.
- Immunomodulatory therapy (e.g., interferon β-1a) may reduce the development of clinically definite multiple sclerosis in patients with monophasic neurologic events including optic neuritis with demyelinating lesions on magnetic resonance imaging studies.

baseline MRI have a 56% chance of developing clinically definite MS, whereas those with a normal scan have a 22% chance over a 10-year period.

REFERENCES

Beck RW: The optic neuritis treatment trial: Three-year follow-up results. Arch Ophthalmol 1995;113:136-137.

Beck RW, Arrington J, Murtagh FR, et al: Brain magnetic resonance imaging in acute optic neuritis: experience of the optic neuritis study group. Arch Neurol 1993;50:841-846.

Beck RW, Cleary PA, Anderson MA, et al: A randomized, controlled trial of corticosteroids in the treatment of acute optic neuritis. N Engl J Med 1992;326:581-588.

Beck RW, Cleary PA, Trobe JD, et al: The effect of corticosteroids for acute optic neuritis on the subsequent development of multiple sclerosis. N Engl J Med 1993;329:1764-1769.

Galetta SL, Markowitz C, Lee AG: Immunomodulatory agents for the treatment of relapsing MS: A systematic review. Ann Intern Med 2002;162:2161-2169.

Jacobs LD, Beck RW, Simon JH, et al: Intramuscular interferon beta-1a therapy initiated during a first demyelinating event in multiple sclerosis. CHAMPS Study Group. N Engl J Med 2000; 343:898-904.

Kaufman DI, Trobe JD, Eggenberger ER, Whitaker JN: Practice parameter: The role of corticosteroids in the management of acute monosymptomatic optic neuritis. Report of the Quality Standards Subcommittee of the American Academy of Neurology. Neurology 2000;54:2039-2044.

TABLE 2 Features of Atypical Optic Neuritis in Adults

Bilateral simultaneous onset of optic neuritis in an adult patient
Painless visual loss
Unusual intraocular findings
    Anterior uveitis*
    Posterior uveitis*
    Retinal exudates (e.g., macular "star figure")
    Retinal infiltrates or retinal inflammation
Markedly swollen optic nerve
Marked retinal hemorrhages (e.g., 360 degrees of peripapillary hemorrhages)
Lack of significant improvement or worsening of visual function after 30 d
Age >50 y
Diagnosis or evidence of other systemic conditions other than multiple sclerosis that might cause an optic neuropathy
Extremely steroid-sensitive or steroid-dependent optic neuropathy
No light perception vision

---

*Anterior uveitis, pars planitis, and retinal periphlebitis may be seen in optic neuritis associated with multiple sclerosis but should be considered as unusual findings.
Modified with permission from Lee AG, Brazis PW: Clinical Pathways in Neuro-ophthalmology: An Evidence-based Approach, 2nd ed. New York, Thieme, 2003.

All patients in the Optic Neuritis Treatment Trial (ONTT) underwent brain MR scan, laboratory testing (e.g., antinuclear antibody (ANA) for systemic lupus erythematosus, serologic testing for syphilis), and a chest radiograph for sarcoidosis. A lumbar puncture however was optional. None of the laboratory testing proved to be helpful in the diagnosis of ON in typical cases. The lumbar puncture only showed demyelinating disease in cases where the cerebrospinal fluid was abnormal. The cranial MR scan however is a powerful predictor for the development of demyelinating disease.

Treatment of Optic Neuritis

In the ONTT, there were three treatment groups: oral prednisone, intravenous (IV) methylprednisolone followed by oral prednisone, and oral placebo. The final visual outcome was the same in all of the treatment groups, although IV steroids sped the rate of visual recovery. Oral steroids alone, however, at least in conventional doses, increased the rate of new attacks and therefore are not currently recommended in conventional doses for ON.

The Controlled High-Risk Subject Avonex Multiple Sclerosis Prevention Study

The Controlled High-Risk Subject Avonex (i.e., interferon β-1a) Multiple Sclerosis Prevention Study (CHAMPS) was a randomized, double-blind, placebo-controlled, clinical trial ($n = 383$). All patients had an acute clinical demyelinating event (e.g., ON) and demyelinating white matter lesions on brain MR scan. All patients received IV methylprednisolone followed by treatment in one of two treatment arms: weekly intramuscular (IM) injections of 30 μg of IFN β-1a ($n = 193$) and placebo ($n = 190$). The treatment group had a 44% reduction in the rate of clinically definite MS after 3 years compared to placebo ($p = 0.002$); a relative reduction in the volume of brain lesions ($p < 0.001$); fewer new or enlarging MR lesions ($p < 0.001$); and fewer gadolinium-enhancing lesions ($p < 0.001$).

The Early Treatment of Multiple Sclerosis (ETOMS) study was a randomized, placebo-controlled trial ($n = 308$) of interferon β-1a (Rebif) 22 μg subcutaneously weekly. As in CHAMPS, patients had an initial demyelinating event and demyelinating lesions on MRI. There was a decreased rate of progression to clinically definite MS and a reduction in MRI abnormalities in the treatment group.

TABLE 3 Summary of Recommendations for Optic Neuritis

Cranial MRI scan should be strongly considered for all patients with ON.
The cranial MR scan is the most powerful predictor for clinically definite MS.
Even a single attack of ON is a risk factor for developing clinically definite MS.
Neurologic consultation should be considered to discuss the risks of MS and the options for treatment (e.g., interferon β-1a).

Abbreviations: MRI = magnetic resonance imaging; MS = multiple sclerosis; ON = optic neuritis.

Glaucoma

Method of
Misha F. Syed, MD, and Nicolas P. Bell, MD

Glaucoma is a group of disorders with various manifestations linked by a common optic neuropathy, resulting in characteristic, progressive optic nerve atrophy, and visual field loss. Glaucoma was once defined simply as intraocular pressure (IOP) greater than 21 mm Hg, but now this is recognized as only a risk factor. Elevated IOP dilates the optic cup, which subjects the ganglion cells to ischemic pressure forces. Peripheral visual field defects emerge in the areas subtended by the damaged retinal ganglion cells. Central vision loss is typically a late finding.

Glaucoma is classified by the anatomy of the anterior chamber angle, which may be *open* or *closed*. Gonioscopy, a detailed evaluation of the angle using a mirrored lens, is required to differentiate types of glaucoma. Childhood glaucoma may be primary or secondary to developmental ocular abnormalities. Patients who do not meet criteria for diagnosis within one of these groups are followed as glaucoma suspects.

Regardless of etiology, glaucoma is a leading cause of irreversible blindness. Of the 67 million people with glaucoma worldwide, 7 million are bilaterally blind. In the United States, more than 2.5 million people are diagnosed with glaucoma, and it is estimated that as many are undiagnosed. Glaucoma is the second leading cause of blindness in the United States; it is the most frequent cause among African Americans, in whom there is an earlier onset and more aggressive course. In 2000 the prevalence of blindness from glaucoma in the United States was greater than 1:130,000 people.

Types of Glaucoma

PRIMARY OPEN-ANGLE GLAUCOMA

The most common glaucoma is primary open-angle glaucoma (POAG). Increased resistance to outflow of the aqueous humor through the trabecular meshwork leads to gradual and painless elevation of IOP; hence, it is typically asymptomatic. It is bilateral but can be asymmetric. The existence of a subgroup of POAG patients without elevated IOP (normal-pressure glaucoma) suggests that other factors may be significant,

CURRENT DIAGNOSIS

- The most common form of glaucoma in the United States is POAG.
- Risk factors for POAG include increasing age, African American race, and a positive family history.
- Screening for POAG is recommended every 2 to 4 years after age 40 years and every 1 to 2 years after age 65 years.
- If risk factors for POAG are present, screening is recommended every 2 to 4 years after age 30 years and every 1 to 2 years after age 65 years.
- 95% of patients with POAG and 5% of normal patients may experience IOP elevation >15 mm Hg while taking steroids; therefore, patients with known glaucoma on long-term steroids (>1 month) need close follow-up with an ophthalmologist.
- Primary angle-closure glaucoma has an acute onset with pain, haloes, red eye, decreased vision, and nausea and/or vomiting. Emergent ophthalmologic referral is required.

Abbreviations: IOP = intraocular pressure; POAG = primary open-angle glaucoma.

such as insufficient vascular flow to the optic nerve head, accelerated programmed cell death (apoptosis), diurnal fluctuations of IOP, and autoimmunity.

Diseases such as diabetes mellitus, systemic hypertension, and vasospastic disorders have been associated with glaucoma but are not clearly linked to the disease. Increasing age is a risk factor, because 8% of the population older than 70 years old and only 0.1% of those younger than 40 years of age are affected. African American patients have a 5 to 15 times greater risk than white patients. Immediate family members of glaucoma patients have a 10- to 15-fold increased risk for developing glaucoma.

The prolonged asymptomatic phase of POAG can only be discovered by ocular evaluation. Complete eye examination is recommended every 2 to 4 years for patients older than 40 years of age and every 1 to 2 years for those older than 65 years. Patients with risk factors (age, race, family history) should be evaluated earlier and more frequently.

Screening in the primary care setting can include a family and medical history, vision (and possibly IOP) screening, and examination of the optic nerve head by direct ophthalmoscopy. Clinical findings may be subtle. Visual acuity is often normal, and decreased central vision secondary to glaucoma suggests advanced disease. Normal confrontation fields do not exclude glaucoma because this examination technique has a very low yield in identifying glaucomatous visual field loss. Formal visual field testing is preferred. Although not diagnostic, intraocular pressure greater than 21 mm Hg warrants thorough evaluation. Dilated fundus examination shows enlarged cupping of the optic nerve head and/or asymmetry between the optic nerves. Focal loss of neural rim tissue (notching) may occur, and flame hemorrhages may be seen at the disc margin, especially in actively progressing disease. If glaucoma is suspected, a patient should be referred for further ophthalmologic evaluation.

Patients with suggestive findings but no definitive glaucomatous damage are classified as glaucoma suspects. The Ocular Hypertension Treatment Study, a recent multicenter randomized, controlled clinical trial, conducted a long-term follow-up of glaucoma suspects with elevated IOP, normal optic nerve appearance, and no visual field defects. This study found that over 5 years, maintaining IOP 20% below baseline reduced the rate of progression to POAG from 9.5% to 4.4%.

SECONDARY OPEN-ANGLE GLAUCOMA

Secondary open-angle glaucomas result from increased resistance to outflow through the trabecular meshwork because of a preexisting or underlying condition. Examples include pigmentary, pseudoexfoliative, traumatic, and steroid-induced glaucoma.

In pigment dispersion syndrome and pseudoexfoliation syndrome, deposition of iris pigment and fibrillar protein, respectively, in the trabecular meshwork may obstruct aqueous outflow and secondarily elevate IOP, leading to glaucoma. Blunt ocular trauma (often remote) is a common cause of unilateral glaucoma because of structural changes in the trabecular meshwork.

Chronic use of glucocorticosteroids can create resistance to trabecular outflow and IOP elevation, resulting in a glaucoma resembling POAG. Steroid-induced pressure elevation generally correlates with the dose and length of administration. Although most often seen with topical and periocular use, it can also result from systemic or inhaled administration. Steroid responses of greater than 15 mm Hg IOP elevation can develop in 95% of patients with POAG and in only 15% of patients without glaucoma. All patients with a known diagnosis of glaucoma should be evaluated by an ophthalmologist within 1 month of initiating a long-term steroid regimen for systemic diseases.

PRIMARY ANGLE-CLOSURE GLAUCOMA

Primary angle-closure glaucoma can have an acute, subacute, intermittent, or chronic presentation. Attacks of acute angle closure are ocular emergencies, because irreversible vision loss can occur within hours. Those at risk have an anatomic predisposition with narrow anterior chamber angles. If the pupillary margin of the iris contacts the lens for 360 degrees, which may occur in susceptible eyes when the iris is mid-dilated, flow of the aqueous humor from the posterior to the anterior chamber is blocked. The peripheral iris bows anteriorly and apposes the trabecular meshwork, obstructing outflow. The IOP may rise rapidly to greater than 60 mm Hg.

In Asian populations primary angle-closure glaucoma is more common than open-angle glaucoma. The risk increases with age, with most cases occurring during the sixth and seventh decades. Women have primary angle-closure glaucoma attacks 2 to 4 times as often as men. Environmental circumstances may trigger an acute attack of angle closure in predisposed eyes; these include movie theaters or dark rooms (physiologic mydriasis), sudden anxiety or pain (sympathetic stimulation causing pupil dilation), or medications causing mild mydriasis (anticholinergics and adrenergic stimulants such as sleep and cold medications).

The diagnosis of an acute angle-closure glaucoma attack requires gonioscopic evidence of a closed anterior chamber angle preventing aqueous flow into the trabecular meshwork. Patients may complain of ocular pain, brow ache, rainbow-colored halos around lights, and/or blurred vision. They may experience intense nausea and vomiting, bradycardia, and sweating. Ocular exam reveals elevated IOP, conjunctival vascular injection, a cloudy cornea (if IOP rose acutely and recently), a shallow anterior chamber, a closed angle by gonioscopy, and a globe, which is firm to palpation.

SECONDARY ANGLE-CLOSURE GLAUCOMA

Scarring and adhesions between the peripheral iris and the anterior chamber angle may block outflow of aqueous. Diabetes mellitus may result in neovascularization of the retina, which can progress to neovascularization of the anterior segment including the iris and angle, blocking aqueous outflow and/or closing the angle. The resultant neovascular glaucoma can be devastating and refractory to treatment. Central retinal vein occlusion, a vascular accident closely linked to uncontrolled hypertension and diabetes, can also lead to retinal neovascularization and a similar process. Uveitis from systemic diseases such as sarcoidosis or autoimmune arthropathies can produce

CURRENT THERAPY

- Although POAG is typically treated first medically, in select circumstances laser and incisional surgery may be appropriate first-line interventions.
- Glaucoma medications lower IOP by either decreasing production of aqueous humor or increasing its outflow.
- Topical β-blockers have been the traditional primary medical therapy for POAG, but prostaglandin analogues are now emerging as the first-line choice.
- Laser trabeculoplasty increases aqueous outflow through the trabecular meshwork.
- Incisional filtering surgery creates a new outflow drain, which bypasses the dysfunctional trabecular meshwork.
- Primary angle closure attacks require emergent treatment both medically and with laser iridotomy.
- Secondary angle closure glaucoma may be difficult to manage medically and often requires surgery.

Abbreviations: IOP = intraocular pressure; POAG = primary open-angle glaucoma.

intraocular scarring and secondary angle closure if not controlled.

Sulfonamide-based systemic medications can rarely cause swelling of the ciliary body, which anteriorly displaces the lens and iris. This can produce a secondary acute angle-closure glaucoma, which requires discontinuation of the medication and urgent lowering of the IOP. This phenomenon has also been reported with topiramate (Topamax).

CHILDHOOD GLAUCOMA

Congenital or childhood glaucoma develops from aqueous outflow obstruction because of abnormal anatomical development of the angle, ocular inflammation, or trauma. Primary congenital glaucoma often presents in infancy with the classic triad of photophobia, epiphora (tearing), and blepharospasm, but these signs are unnecessary for diagnosis. Buphthalmos (enlarged eye) may occur secondary to increased IOP if the glaucoma develops during the first 3 years of life. Juvenile glaucoma is similar in etiology to POAG and has been linked to several specific genetic loci. Enlargement of the cornea and sclera is not seen in this subtype.

Treatment

The Glaucoma Preferred Practice Pattern Committee of the American Academy of Ophthalmology suggests a target of 20% to 30% reduction of IOP from the untreated levels. Medical treatment is usually attempted first. Parameters that factor into selection of medications include efficacy in lowering IOP, systemic and localized side effect profiles, ease of compliance, and cost (Table 1). Noncompliance with treatment regimens may be responsible for 10% of visual loss in glaucoma; and in one study, approximately

TABLE 1

Topical Medications	Efficacy	Local Side Effects	Systemic Side Effects	Dosing	Cost
Prostaglandin analogues	+++	++	none to +	Once daily	+++
β-Blockers	+++	+	+++	bid	++*
α₂ Agonists	++	++	++	bid–tid	+++*
Carbonic anhydrase inhibitors	++	++	+ to ++	bid–tid	+++†

+++ = high
++ = moderate
+ = low
* = generic available
† = systemic form less costly

60% of patients failed to use eyedrops as prescribed. If medications fail to control IOP, changes in optic nerve structure and visual field function may occur. Surgical treatment may become necessary to slow the progression of glaucomatous damage.

PROSTAGLANDIN ANALOGUES

This newest class of antiglaucoma agents has become a popular initial medical treatment because of the efficacy and lack of major systemic side effects. These medications reduce IOP by increasing aqueous humor outflow. Latanoprost (Xalatan), bimatoprost (Lumigan), and travoprost (Travatan) require only once daily dosing, whereas unoprostone (Rescula) is administered twice daily. Side effects include conjunctival hyperemia during the first several weeks of therapy, eyelash lengthening and thickening, occasional iris and periocular skin hyperpigmentation, and rarely, exacerbation of ocular inflammation.

BETA-ADRENERGIC ANTAGONISTS

Beta-adrenergic antagonists lower IOP by decreasing the production of aqueous humor. They are very effective at lowering IOP and include timolol (Timoptic, Betimol, Istalol), carteolol (Ocupress), metipranolol (OptiPranolol), and levobunolol (Betagan). Topical formulations may be absorbed into the bloodstream, and potential side effects are similar to systemic β-blockers, including exacerbation of chronic obstructive or reactive pulmonary disease, worsening of heart block or heart failure, bradycardia, systemic hypotension, mood effects/altered mental status, decreased libido, and masking of hypoglycemic symptoms in diabetic patients. Care should be taken in patients already taking systemic β-blockers, because additive side effects may develop. Betaxolol (Betoptic) is a selective β₁ antagonist, which may minimize the pulmonary side effects, but still must be used cautiously in patients suffering from asthma or COPD. Topical β-blockers are dosed once or twice daily, depending on the formulation of the eyedrop.

α₂ AGONISTS

α₂ Adrenergic agonists such as apraclonidine (Iopidine) and brimonidine (Alphagan) lower IOP by decreasing aqueous humor production. They are dosed 2 to 3 times daily. Major systemic side effects include somnolence and dry mouth. These medications should be used cautiously in infants and young children because of the risk of respiratory depression. α₂ Agonists are contraindicated in patients taking monoamine oxidase (MAO) inhibitors because of potential systemic hypertension. Ocular side effects include allergic follicular conjunctivitis, which may necessitate discontinuation.

CARBONIC ANHYDRASE INHIBITORS

Carbonic anhydrase inhibitors decrease production of aqueous humor. Systemic carbonic anhydrase inhibitors such as acetazolamide (Diamox) and methazolamide (Neptazane) have been used to treat glaucoma for decades, but up to 60% of patients are intolerant of the side effects. These include metallic taste alteration, loss of appetite, fatigue, confusion, nausea and vomiting, paresthesias, polyuria, urolithiasis, and hearing dysfunction or tinnitus. Rare side effects include Stevens-Johnson syndrome (in patients with sulfonamide allergies) and idiosyncratic aplastic anemia. Oral agents may also lower serum potassium levels, and patients on diuretics or digoxin should be monitored closely. Dorzolamide (Trusopt) and brinzolamide (Azopt) are topical preparations of carbonic anhydrase inhibitors dosed 2 to 3 times daily. Systemic side effects are minimized, but ocular stinging, localized allergic responses, and metallic taste alteration may occur. Systemic carbonic anhydrase inhibitors are more efficacious, but the improved tolerability of the topical agents has made them popular.

NONSPECIFIC SYMPATHOMIMETICS AND PARASYMPATHOMIMETICS

Nonspecific sympathomimetic and parasympathomimetic drugs have historically been used for the treatment of glaucoma, but with the newer agents available these are no longer commonly prescribed. The mechanism for both classes involves increasing aqueous humor outflow. The sympathomimetic agents include epinephrine (Epifrin) and dipivefrin (Propine). Potential adverse effects include systemic hypertension, headache, cardiac arrhythmias including premature ventricular contractions and tachycardia, and anorexia. Parasympathomimetic medications such as pilocarpine (Pilocar) can cause gastrointestinal cramping, diarrhea, vomiting, syncope, hypotension, increased sweating, and pupillary constriction.

ACUTE ANGLE CLOSURE

Acute angle closure patients require emergent ophthalmologic referral and treatment to prevent severe permanent sequelae. If this is not immediately possible, treatment should be initiated promptly with a topical β-blocker and a topical $α_2$ agonist every 30 minutes and a single dose of oral acetazolamide (Diamox) (250 mg × 2 tablets). Oral glycerin (Osmoglyn) or intravenous mannitol (Osmitrol) (1.0 to 1.5 g/kg) may be used if necessary. Pilocarpine should be used cautiously because it may worsen underlying inflammation. Once the attack has been broken medically, the corneal edema will clear and a laser peripheral iridotomy can be made to prevent future attacks. This opening in the peripheral iris allows aqueous flow to bypass any obstruction caused by pupillary block. Prophylactic iridotomy of the other eye is recommended if anatomically at risk. The management of *chronic* angle-closure glaucoma is generally similar to that for POAG.

LASER

Laser may also be used to treat open-angle glaucomas. Argon laser trabeculoplasty (ALT) or the newer selective laser trabeculoplasty (SLT) lowers IOP by facilitating aqueous outflow. For pigmentary, pseudoexfoliative, and select POAG patients, this may be an effective adjunct to medical therapy.

SURGERY

Surgical measures to control glaucoma include filtering procedures such as trabeculectomy or aqueous shunt placement, which increase aqueous outflow by creating alternative filtration pathways. After trabeculectomy, patients are warned of an increased lifetime risk for serious ocular infection and must report to an ophthalmologist immediately for any changes, including redness, pain, and/or decrease in vision. For poor surgical candidates with severely advanced disease, cyclodestructive procedures can be performed in the office to decrease aqueous production by ablating the ciliary body.

If glaucomatous damage has left an eye with no vision, the only reason to treat IOP is to control pain. In most cases, topical agents will suffice. If pain becomes frequent and severe, injections of retrobulbar absolute alcohol or even enucleation of the blind, painful eye may be offered.

REFERENCES

Allingham RR: Shields' Textbook of Glaucoma, 5th ed. Philadelphia, Lippincott Williams & Wilkins, 2005.

American Academy of Ophthalmology Online: Preferred practice patterns: Primary angle Closure glaucoma, primary open angle glaucoma, primary open angle glaucoma suspect 2003. Available at http://www.aao.org/

Kass MA, Heuer DK, Higginbotham EJ, et al: The ocular hypertension treatment study: A randomized trial determines that topical ocular hypotensive medication delays or prevents the onset of primary open-angle glaucoma. Arch Ophthalmol 2002;120:701–713.

Morrison JC, Pollack IP: Glaucoma: Science and Practice, New York, Thieme, 2003.

Tsai JC, Forbes M: Medical Management of Glaucoma, 2nd ed. West Islip, NY, Professional Communications, 2004.

Otitis Externa

Method of
Jeffrey T. Vrabec, MD

Otitis externa is defined as an acute infection originating in or limited to the external auditory canal. This common affliction may occur in any age group and may be caused by a variety of infectious agents.

Anatomy and Physiology

Functionally, the ear canal serves two purposes. It is important for sound localization and because of resonance effects it improves sound perception in the frequency range from 2500 to 4000 hertz (Hz). The ear canal is approximately 25 mm in length and has a diameter of approximately 7.5 mm. The medial half is an osseous channel formed by the merger of the tympanic bone with the mastoid posteriorly and the squamous portion of the temporal bone superiorly. The lateral half of the canal wall is cartilaginous with a thick squamous epithelium that contains sebaceous glands, sweat glands, and hair follicles. The medial skin covering the bony canal is quite thin, measuring only 0.2 mm in thickness. The medial skin lacks a subcutaneous layer and is in continuity with the outermost layer of the tympanic membrane.

The external canal receives its blood supply from the superficial temporal and posterior auricular branches of the external carotid artery. Venous drainage is to the external jugular vein. The external canal receives sensory innervation via multiple cranial nerves. The trigeminal nerve supplies sensation to the superior and anterior aspect of the canal, the facial nerve supplies the anterior inferior area, and the glossopharyngeal and vagus nerves innervate the inferior and posterior regions. Because of the diverse nerve supply, otalgia may often reflect referred pain from oral cavity, nasal, or pharyngeal sources.

Several anatomic features serve to protect the external canal and tympanic membrane (TM) from injury or infection. The gentle curvature of the canal and the narrowing at the bone–cartilage junction (the isthmus) reduce the probability of large objects penetrating the TM. The hair and cerumen also protect the canal, trapping airborne particles that enter the external meatus. Cerumen has the additional benefit of repelling water. The acidic composition of cerumen lowers the ambient pH of the external canal, making it less hospitable to infectious organisms. The phenomenon of epithelial migration is documented in the ear canal. Surface epithelium moves laterally from the umbo to the annulus of the TM and then laterally to the external meatus. Epithelial movement on the TM proceeds at a rate of 0.05 mm per day and is typically slower in the external canal. Lateral migration helps clear the medial canal of surface epithelium and attached debris. This migratory pattern is arrested in chronic infection of the external canal.

Diagnosis

Infections develop in the external canal when organisms breach the anatomic barriers. Trauma to the canal skin, excessive removal of the cerumen, and excessive moisture in the canal may all facilitate otitis externa. Presenting symptoms of an external ear infection include pain, itching, and hearing loss. Pain develops rapidly, is typically constant, and may be quite severe. Manipulation of the ear or jaw movement exacerbates the pain. Conductive hearing loss occurs because of accumulation of debris in the external canal and is exacerbated by concurrent edema. Persistent symptoms despite treatment are a matter of great concern and may indicate a developing osteitis. Cranial nerve deficits are ominous symptoms and indicate an advanced osteitis of the temporal bone.

Physical examination findings typically include erythema, edema, and drainage. Differences in examination findings can help distinguish bacterial from fungal infections. Bacterial infections usually produce marked edema of the canal skin, especially in the lateral cartilaginous canal. Drainage is usually scant and may have a mucoid or mucopurulent consistency and often has a foul odor. In contrast, fungal infections typically involve the medial canal skin and produce little edema. Drainage is thick and surface spore formation is evident. Focal granulation tissue develops in areas with invasive disease and TM perforations are occasionally present. Bloody drainage can be seen with either bacterial or fungal infections because of maceration of the canal skin or from granulation tissue formation.

Regional or systemic symptoms are uncommon in otitis externa. Periaural erythema, mild lymphadenopathy, and low-grade fever are possible. The presence of regional symptoms indicates a more virulent infection.

Treatment

The initial approach to outer ear infections involves aural toilet and avoidance of further trauma or moisture. Topical antibiotics are prescribed in accordance with the likely infectious organism. Many preparations have a rather broad spectrum of efficacy so routine culture of aural discharge is not performed. It is prudent to obtain culture and sensitivity data in recalcitrant cases. Analgesics are prescribed as necessary to control pain. Narcotics are occasionally required. Patients are instructed to avoid or minimize water exposure. With appropriate treatment, symptoms improve rapidly, and complete healing is seen in 2 weeks or less.

The most common organism identified in routine cases of external otitis is *Pseudomonas aeruginosa*. Staphylococcal species are the next most common. Topical fluoroquinolone or aminoglycoside antibiotics are the most appropriate choice for treatment. Preparations that include a steroid are recommended. Drops are instilled three times daily until resolution of the infection, usually 7 to 10 days. When severe edema of the canal skin is

CURRENT DIAGNOSIS

Presenting symptoms include:
- Pain: develops rapidly, typically constant; exacerbated by movement of ear or jaw
- Itching
- Hearing loss: exacerbated by concurrent edema

Exam findings include:
- Erythema
- Edema
- Drainage: sometimes bloody
- Bacterial infections: often have edema of the canal skin with minimal drainage that has foul odor
- Fungal infections: involve the medial canal skin with slight edema, thick drainage, evident surface spore formation

present, a wick is inserted into the canal to facilitate drug delivery. Persistent symptoms indicate inadequate treatment, although this may also be because of inappropriate antibiotic, inefficient drug delivery, noncompliance, or progressive infection.

Differential Diagnosis and Treatment

There are many other infectious disorders of the external canal, although each can usually be distinguished by characteristic clinical findings. Malignancy may also mimic chronic infection. Biopsy is recommended for abnormal tissue that does not quickly resolve with treatment.

ACUTE INFECTIONS

Furuncles occur at the external meatus in the hair-bearing skin. Erythema and edema are localized, and skin a few millimeters away from the infection has a healthy appearance. Pain can be severe and is exacerbated by pressure or manipulation of the auricle. Furuncles are caused by staphylococcal infection. Spontaneous rupture of the lesion leads to resolution of the infection and pain. If fluctuance is present at presentation, the lesion is drained under local anesthesia. Topical antibiotics (bacitracin, neomycin, or mupirocin [Bactroban] ointment or solution) are a useful adjunct.

The physical findings in otomycosis were outlined earlier. The predominant organisms are *Aspergillus* and *Candida* with considerable variation in prevalence according to geographic region. Fungal infections produce more destruction of the canal skin but less edema. Granulation tissue and TM perforations are not uncommon, although most perforations heal spontaneously after eradication of the infection. Treatment requires meticulous cleaning of debris and topical antifungals. Clotrimazole (Lotrimin) solution is effective

CURRENT THERAPY

- Provide aural toilet and encourage avoidance of further trauma and water exposure.
- Obtain culture and sensitivity data in recalcitrant cases.
- Prescribe topical antibiotics that include a steroid and analgesics (for pain) as needed.

for *Candida* species, but eradication of *Aspergillus* species is most efficient with ketoconazole (Nizoral) cream applied directly to the affected skin.

Bullous external otitis is diagnosed based on the characteristic finding of hemorrhagic vesicles in the external canal. Spontaneous rupture of the lesions produces bloody otorrhea. The lesions are quite painful, and lancing the bullae to drain the fluid does not provide relief as is seen in bullous myringitis. Involvement of the medial canal skin is typical. The etiology of this infectious process is unclear. However, the disease responds to a broad spectrum of topical antibiotics. Topical or oral analgesics are a useful adjunctive treatment.

Herpes zoster oticus, or Ramsay Hunt syndrome, occurs because of reactivation of latent varicella zoster virus in the geniculate ganglion. Vesicles may develop in the sensory distribution of the facial nerve. The appearance of skin lesions is characteristic of zoster eruptions. Initially, the vesicles are erythematous with a straw-colored fluid. Spontaneous rupture results in a crusted ulcer that may take several weeks to heal. Facial paralysis, dysgeusia, dizziness, and sensorineural hearing loss are typical in herpes zoster oticus but extremely rare in other infectious diseases of the external ear canal. Treatment of the facial paralysis is the primary objective, necessitating systemic steroids and antivirals. The skin lesions of the ear canal usually heal without incident, but secondary bacterial otitis externa is possible.

CHRONIC INFECTIOUS DISORDERS

Skull base osteitis occurs when disease extends from soft tissues of the canal into the temporal bone. Elderly patients, diabetics, and immunocompromised individuals are at increased risk of developing osteitis. The diagnosis is suspected when pain, discharge, fever, and/or granulation tissue persist despite treatment. Progressive involvement of the skull base may lead to cranial nerve palsies, vascular thrombosis, and intracranial infection. Laboratory testing reveals a markedly increased sedimentation rate. Technetium-99m bone scan displays increased uptake throughout the course of the disease and is useful for initial diagnosis. Computed tomography (CT) of the temporal bone displays bone erosion in advanced cases. Magnetic resonance imaging (MRI) is useful to detect soft-tissue and dural involvement. Biopsy of infected tissue or bone may be necessary to identify the responsible organism. Systemic antibiotics are selected according to culture and sensitivity data and should be continued until the sedimentation rate returns to normal. This may require months of treatment.

Osteoradionecrosis is a late complication of temporal bone irradiation. Contemporary stereotactic techniques should significantly reduce the incidence of this problem. The process is typically limited, and symptoms are much less severe than in skull base osteitis. Exposed necrotic bone with slight granulation and purulent drainage is seen on examination. Local débridement and topical antibiotics are usually sufficient to control the infection. Recurrence is common because the irradiated ear canal is highly susceptible to infection after exposure to water or minor trauma.

MISCELLANEOUS

With the exception of herpes zoster oticus, none of the entities just described typically involves the pinna. Inflammation of the external canal in conjunction with pinna involvement may signify dermatologic disease. Some common entities include eczema, neomycin allergy, relapsing polychondritis, and erysipelas.

REFERENCES

Clark WB, Brook I, Bianki D, Thompson DH: Microbiology of otitis externa. Otolaryngol Head Neck Surg 1997;116:23-25.

Hawke M, Wong J, Krajden S: Clinical and microbiological features of otitis externa. J Otolaryngol 1984;13:289-295.

Hurst WB: Outcome of 22 cases of perforated tympanic membrane caused by otomycosis. J Laryngol Otol 2001;115:879-880.

Litton WB: Epithelial migration over tympanic membrane and external canal. Arch Otolaryngol 1963;77:254-257.

Lucente FE: Fungal infections of the external ear. Otolaryngol Clin North Am 1993;26:995-1006.

Sreepada GS, Kwartler JA: Skull base osteomyelitis secondary to malignant otitis externa. Curr Opin Otolaryngol Head Neck Surg 2003;11:316-323.

Sweeney CJ, Gilden DH: Ramsay Hunt syndrome. J Neurol Neurosurg Psychiatry 2001;71:149-154.

Otitis Media

Method of
J. Scott McMurray, MD

Ear infections, their complications and sequelae, comprise most patient-clinician interactions. Estimates suggest nearly $3 billion in direct and indirect cost for acute otitis media (AOM) and otitis media with effusion were spent in 1995 alone. In 2000 more than 16 million office visits were made for otitis media and 802 prescriptions per 1000 visits were written for a total of more than 13 million prescriptions. As common as the problem may be, it continues to be a source of confusion and controversy in terms of its diagnosis, treatment, and expectation for outcomes. Recently, there has been a renewed interest in determining the appropriate evaluation and management of these afflicted children, based on evidence-based medicine.

Along with new diagnostic protocols and realigned treatment strategies, there is a realization that children may fall into different at-risk groups and will therefore benefit from different treatment options. In his recent editorial in the International Journal of Pediatric Otolaryngology on a practical classification of otitis media subgroups, Richard Rosenfeld quoted Stanley Hoerr saying, "It is difficult to make the asymptomatic patient feel better." Yet, he added, much of the research on which we base our decisions to treat or not to treat children with otitis media has been formulated on those who would otherwise do well without treatment, the so-called innocent bystander. Children in the at-risk or suffering groups have been excluded from research trials for ethical reasons against withholding treatment. It is possible to group children into four subgroups with otitis media:

1. Innocent bystander
2. Susceptible child
3. At-risk child
4. Suffering child

These different subgroups imply different treatment limbs. The innocent bystander may do well without any therapy and may tolerate careful observation, whereas the suffering child with a similar disease process deserves rapid and intensive medical or surgical treatment or both.

The stratification of children into different subgroups may appear daunting at first glance but after closer reflection answers the problem of conflicting research data and perhaps uses more common sense (confirmed by clinical trials) in determining treatment. Otherwise developmentally and physically healthy children may be closely observed rather than treated medically or surgically for their acute ear infection or middle ear effusion (MEE). Other children who are at risk for developmental delays, physically challenged, or suffering from the effects or side effects of AOM or otitis media with effusion should be treated more aggressively with either the appropriate medical or surgical plan of care. Unfortunately, this increases the number of possible permutations when determining the appropriate treatment for the afflicted child. Fortunately, however, this new paradigm allows more freedom in determining the appropriate treatment option to be followed. Our challenge lies in honing our abilities to make a correct diagnosis and an accurate assessment of risk so that an appropriate treatment protocol with adequate follow-up can be implemented.

In 2004, the American Academy of Pediatrics, the American Academy of Family Practice, and the American Academy of Otolaryngology Head and Neck Surgery combined forces to create two separate clinical guidelines for AOM and otitis media with effusion. These guidelines serve as an excellent frame on which to build a knowledge base and understanding for the treatment of all children with AOM or otitis media with effusion. These references are invaluable and are recommended reading for all who treat children with ear pathology.

Definitions

Acute otitis media is defined as an abrupt onset of inflammation of the middle ear space. This contrasts with otitis media with effusion, which is fluid in the middle ear without signs and symptoms of inflammation. Otitis media with effusion is much more common than AOM but may be seen as a residual finding of a recently resolved infection. The distinction between the two and the ability of the clinician to distinguish between these disease entities is paramount to decision making and appropriate treatment.

The signs and symptoms of AOM are found in an abrupt onset of fluid in the middle ear with redness or distinct pain. Children suffering with AOM may or may not also exhibit systemic signs of infection, such as fever. Fever, pain, and irritability are seen in 90% of children with AOM, but it is also seen in 76% of children with upper aerodigestive tract viral illnesses as well. History alone may lead to an erroneous conclusions and unnecessary treatment. The distinction lies in the physical findings of MEE with inflammation. Fullness or bulging of the tympanic membrane, air fluid levels, opacification of the tympanic membrane, or bullous vesicles on the tympanic membrane are signs suggesting AOM when associated with acute inflammation. Visualization of the tympanic membrane and the use of pneumatic otoscopy should confirm the presence of a MEE and inflammation. Tympanometry can confirm suspicion of a MEE, but the clinician should work to be proficient with pneumatic otoscopy.

Otitis media with effusion alone may result from a resolved infection or from eustachian tube dysfunction alone. The physical findings are similar to those described but without the signs of acute inflammation. Although the tympanic membrane may be red in the otherwise healthy child crying at the displeasure of being examined, pain and an effusion are not generally associated with normal health.

Treatment Recommendations

Children with AOM should have adequate pain management. Acetaminophen, ibuprofen, and occasionally narcotics are useful in treating the pain of AOM. Rarely, myringotomy is required to relieve the discomfort of an acute ear infection.

If an acute bacterial infection in the middle ear is recognized, antibacterial therapy may be used in all age groups. If the diagnosis is uncertain, antibacterial therapy is recommended in the very young, younger than age 6 months. Antimicrobials may also be administered if one is uncertain of the diagnosis, if the illness is severe in those from 6 months to 2 years of age. If the child is older than age 2 years and the diagnosis is uncertain, observation and close follow-up is recommended.

If antibacterial treatment is instituted, amoxicillin at 80 to 90 mg/kg/day is used as a first line of therapy. If severe illness is encountered or if coverage for beta-lactamase–positive organisms such as *Haemophilus influenzae* or *Moraxella catarrhalis* is required, amoxicillin-clavulanate (Augmentin) is suggested (90 mg/kg/day of the amoxicillin component).

Children who are allergic to amoxicillin, but not with urticaria or anaphylaxis, may be given cefdinir (Omnicef),

CURRENT THERAPY

- Adequate pain management is key in treating AOM.
- If a child has an acute bacterial otitis media, antibiotics are indicated.
- Amoxicillin at 80 to 90 mg/kg/day is the first therapy of choice in nonallergic children.
- Children older than age 2 years may be observed without antibiotic therapy if the diagnosis is uncertain.
- Children younger than age 2 years may be treated with antibiotics if the diagnosis is uncertain.

Abbreviation: AOM = acute otitis media.

cefpodoxime (Vantin), or cefuroxime (Ceftin). Children with type-1 hypersensitivity to amoxicillin may be given azithromycin (Zithromax), clarithromycin (Biaxin), erythromycin-sulfisoxazole (Pediazole), or sulfamethoxazole-trimethoprim (Bactrim). In AOM where the organism is thought to be penicillin resistant *Streptococcus pneumoniae*, clindamycin is a reasonable choice.

Patients who fail to respond within 48 to 72 hours, whether in the observation or antibacterial therapy group, should be reassessed and treatment changed depending on the findings. Reduction of risk factors for AOM is encouraged for everyone. No recommendations were made regarding the efficacy of complementary and alternative medicine for the treatment of AOM.

Otitis media with effusion is common after resolution of acute otitis. Some children also present with asymptomatic otitis media with effusion as well. Treatment of children with persistent middle effusion depends on their at-risk grouping. Children at risk for speech, language, or other learning problems should be treated more promptly than other children not at risk. The at-risk groups include children with a permanent hearing loss independent of the otitis media, suspected or known speech and language delays, autism-spectrum disorder or other pervasive developmental disorder, syndromes or craniofacial disorders, blindness or uncorrectable visual impairment, cleft palate with or without associated syndrome, or developmental delay. The management of the child with otitis media with effusion in these at-risk groups should include hearing tests, speech and language assessment and therapy,

hearing aids or other amplification devices for hearing loss independent of the otitis media, tympanostomy tube placement, and assessment of hearing after resolution of the otitis media with effusion to detect underlying hearing loss independent of the middle ear fluid.

Children who do not fall in the at-risk group may be watched for 3 months before intervention. If the MEE persists for longer than 3 months, audiometric assessment of hearing should be obtained. Intervention is then based on the presence of a hearing loss of generally greater than 20 decibels, suspicion of language development delay, or other impending complications related to the MEE. If the hearing loss is mild (21 to 39 decibels), strategies to optimize the listening and learning environment and/or surgical intervention should be suggested. If the hearing loss is greater than 40 decibels, surgical intervention to correct the MEE is indicated and most efficacious.

Initial surgical treatment of a problematic persistent MEE as described earlier is tympanostomy tube placement. Adenoidectomy is reserved for children who have other distinct indications, such as nasal airway obstruction or chronic adenitis, or in whom another set of pressure equalization tubes are necessary. Approximately 20% to 50% of children relapse after their tympanostomy tubes extrude and will require additional tubes. When adenoidectomy is performed with the second set of tubes, the rate of recidivism is decreased by 50%. This advantage is seen in children as young as age 2 years, with the greatest effect seen in children aged 3 years and older, regardless of adenoidal size. Children older than age 4 years may also benefit from adenoidectomy and myringotomy without tube placement. Myringotomy alone without tympanostomy tube insertion and/or tonsillectomy alone solely for the treatment of otitis media with effusion has not been found to be efficacious.

Conclusion

The key to successful management of a child with AOM or otitis media with effusion, as it is with any medical problem, is based on the clinician's ability to correctly diagnose and stratify at-risk groups. The new recommended clinical pathways developed by the AAP, AAFP, and AAO-HNS for AOM and otitis media with effusion may at first seem to increase complexity of treatment because it increases the number of pathways possible. Closer reflection, however, will reveal an easier paradigm. It is the clinician's responsibility to attain the skills and knowledge set to make the correct initial diagnosis and assessment of risk for the patient. The support from the evidence-based-medicine clinical pathways will then help in the decision making and treatment formulation.

REFERENCES

American Academy of Family Physicians, American Academy of Otolaryngology Head and Neck Surgery, American Academy of Pediatrics Subcommittee on Otitis Media with Effusion: Otitis media with effusion. Pediatrics 2004; 113(5):1412-1429.

American Academy of Pediatrics Subcommittee on Acute Otitis Media: Diagnosis and management of acute otitis media. Pediatrics 2004; 113(5):1451-1465.

Bell LM: The new clinical practice guidelines for acute otitis media: An editorial. Ann Emerg Med 2005; 45(5):514-516.

CURRENT DIAGNOSIS

- The diagnosis of AOM requires acute signs of illness such as fever and pain along with signs of middle ear inflammation such as fluid and erythema.
- Associated symptoms of AOM include fever, pain, and irritability.
- Visualization of the tympanic membrane and pneumatic otoscopy are required to confirm the diagnosis of AOM.
- Fluid behind the tympanic membrane does not necessarily indicate an infection in the middle ear space.

Abbreviation: AOM = acute otitis media.

Bluestone CD: Epidemiology and pathogenesis of chronic suppurative otitis media: Implications for prevention and treatment. Int J Pediatr Otorhinolaryngol 1998; 42(3):207-223.

Ohlms LA, Chen AY, Stewart MG, Franklin DJ: Establishing the etiology of childhood hearing loss. Otolaryngol Head Neck Surg 1999; 120(2):159-163.

Paradise JL, Campbell TF, Dollaghan CA, et al: Developmental outcomes after early or delayed insertion of tympanostomy tubes. N Engl J Med 2005;353(6):576-586.

Rosenfeld RM: A practical classification of otitis media subgoups. Int J Pediatr Otorhinolaryngol 2005; 69(8):1027-1029.

Rosenfeld RM, Culpepper L, Doyle KJ, et al: Clinical practice guideline: Otitis media with effusion. Otolaryngol Head Neck Surg 2004; 130(5 Suppl):S95-118.

Rosenfeld RM, Lous J, Bluestone CD, et al: Recent advances in otitis media. 8. Treatment. Ann Otol Rhinol Laryngol Suppl 2005; 194: 114-139.

Episodic Vertigo

Method of
Lorne S. Parnes, MD

For many, if not most, clinicians, assessing a patient with episodic vertigo, which is defined as episodic misperception of the self moving relative to the environment or vice versa, can be daunting. Much of the angst stems from the difficulties and inconsistencies patients have in describing their symptoms, leaving the clinician without a path to follow in corroborating a diagnosis. If given a chance, patients will often interchange the term dizziness for vertigo. Dizziness is a much more non-specific symptom, and is used to describe many varied sensations including vertigo. Thus, obtaining an accurate history is by far the most important but also the most challenging aspect of assessing these patients; however, it gets easier with practice. For many patients, vertigo often is described as a frightening experience. Thus, for those who have recurrent, episodic vertigo, the first bout is often the most memorable because many think they have experienced a graver event, such as a stroke. The term *vertigo* is merely a descriptor, with its physiologic or pathologic source in any part of the nervous system that contributes to spatial orientation. The major contributors to these neurologic signals are the vestibular, visual, and proprioceptive systems, all of which integrate at several levels throughout the brainstem, cerebellum, and cortex.

Everyone experiences normal physiologic bouts of vertigo. One example is the optokinetic-induced vertigo induced by the IMAX theater experience. The visual-vestibular mismatch creates the false perception of the self moving, and the nervous system treats the conflicting signals as a noxious stimulus, resulting in heightened vagal tone with nausea and even vomiting. Another example of vertigo occurs with the common childhood game of spinning around and around and then stopping suddenly. The resulting vestibular-induced vertigo is the sensation of the environment turning around, when of course neither it nor the self is moving at all.

Pathophysiology

There are many physiologic and pathologic causes of vertigo. For a better understanding of the pathophysiology of vestibular-induced vertigo, it is best to think of vertigo as resulting from a steady-state malfunction. The normal physiologic vestibular receptors in the bony labyrinth monitor the motion and position of the head in space by detecting angular and linear acceleration forces. Inside the bony labyrinth is the perilymphatic space, within which there is the membranous labyrinth and its contained endolymphatic space. The two otolith organs, one in the utricle and one in the saccule, in each inner ear monitor linear acceleration forces, including gravity, whereas the three semicircular canals in each inner ear detect angular acceleration. The canals are positioned at near right angles to each other so that they sense movements in any and all planes in space, with the left and right sides complementing each other. Thus, there is redundancy built into this system, which, as will be discussed later in this article, is an important concept in the outcome and treatment of the disease state. Each canal is filled with endolymph and has a swelling at the base that is called the ampulla. The ampulla contains the cupula, a gelatinous mass with the same density as endolymph, which is attached to polarized hair cells.

With the head at rest, the hair cells from both labyrinths emit a steady baseline rate of discharges that induces a steady rate of vestibular nerve impulses. As long as the nerve input at the level of the vestibular nuclei is equal from both labyrinths, the perception will be one of no (head) movement. It is the function of the vestibular end organs to modulate these steady-state signals and interact with the ocular motor system, the locomotive system, and the cognitive region of the brain to stabilize vision with head movements, maintain a stable upright posture against gravity and movement, and produce a conscious three-dimensional awareness of where the head and body are in space. As always, there are feedback loops from each of these systems, and the signals are modulated further by the cerebellum.

Displacement of the neutrally positioned cupula by head turning (an angular acceleration or deceleration) causes either a stimulatory or an inhibitory response of any or all semicircular canals bilaterally, depending on the direction and plane of the motion (Figure 1). It should be noted that the cupula forms an impermeable barrier across the lumen of the ampulla. The term *utriculofugal* refers to cupular movement away from the utricle, whereas *utriculopetal* refers to cupular movement toward the utricle. In the superior and posterior semicircular canals, utriculofugal deflection of the cupula is stimulatory and utriculopetal deflection is inhibitory. The opposite is true for the lateral semicircular canal.

Nystagmus, one of the key manifestations and signs of vertigo, is defined as the repeated and rhythmic oscillation of the eyes. Stimulation (or inhibition) of the semicircular canals most commonly causes jerk nystagmus, which is characterized by a slow phase (slow movement in one direction) followed by a fast phase (rapid movement in the other direction). Although it is the modulated vestibular signal that induces the slow phase, the nystagmus is named according to the direction of the fast phase. The fast phase

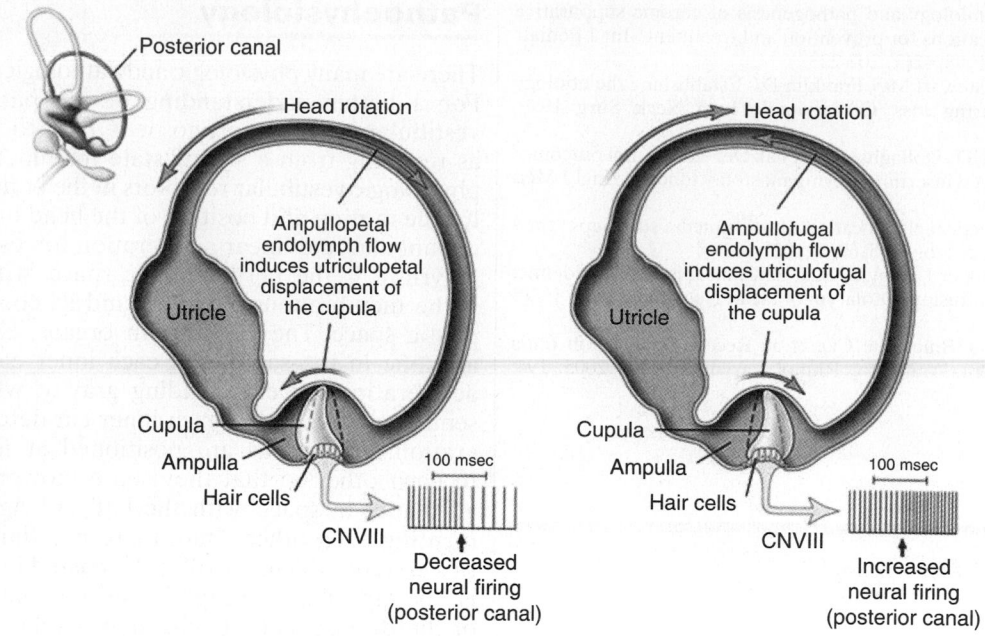

FIGURE 1. Semicircular canal physiology (posterior canal example). (From Parnes LS, Agrawal SK, Atlas J: Diagnosis and management of benign paroxysmal positional vertigo (BPPV). CMAJ 2003;169(7):681-693. Used with permission.)

is in fact a saccade generated by the reticular activating system; this is why nystagmus is more evident during states of heightened consciousness. Nystagmus can be horizontal, vertical, oblique, torsional (rotatory), or any combination and may be induced by vestibular signal asymmetries or disturbances that arise more centrally. The Current Diagnosis section summarizes the important key clinical features that help differentiate peripheral (inner ear) from central causes of vertigo.

Disorders

There are a host of peripheral, central, and other disorders that can cause vertigo (Table 1). Although there is some controversy about whether clinicians should make this differentiation, it is a useful exercise to help make the differential diagnosis. This will help direct the workup, guide the treatment, and, if indicated, direct the patient to the proper specialist. Peripheral disorders induce vertigo through their evoked, nonphysiologic asymmetric central input. Therefore, not surprisingly, the peripheral disorders listed in Table 1 are all typically unilateral.

Ultimately, these disorders resolve with time, returning the system to the normal steady state; alternatively, if the vestibular end organ remains dysfunctional, the system (brain) adjusts to a new norm (vis-à-vis the new steady state). This process is mediated by the cerebellum and brainstem and occurs automatically in most individuals as long as the contralateral vestibular organ remains normal (the redundancy described earlier in this article). The process is facilitated greatly by head, visual, and body motion/stimulation and can be inhibited by vestibular

suppressant medication and immobility. Thus, even though patients favor sedentary activity because it tends to minimize the vestibular "asymmetry," anyone with an acute vestibular disorder should be encouraged to ambulate as much and as soon as possible and avoid taking vestibular suppressants such as the benzodiazepines. For many individuals, a formal course of vestibular rehabilitation physiotherapy greatly facilitates the process.

As a result of impaired central compensation, virtually all these acute or episodic inner-ear disorders can become chronic. It therefore is important for the clinician to differentiate between cases of "true" episodic vertigo brought on by head movement (as in benign paroxysmal positional vertigo [BPPV]) and the dysequilibrium arising from the asymmetry of an uncompensated loss that is aggravated by motion.

In addition to an uncompensated unilateral vestibular loss, chronic (vestibular) dysequilibrium may result from bilateral vestibular hypofunction (Box 1). Bilateral disorders provide no backup, without any future possibilities for vestibular compensation. When both sides are affected simultaneously, as is often the case, there is no resultant vestibular asymmetry and thus no initial period of vertigo. The hallmark features, all of which are derived from the absent vestibular input, are gait ataxia, oscillopsia (visual blurring with head movement), and the absence of symptoms with the head at rest. The hallmark vestibular-ocular test findings include reduced caloric responses and abnormal lateral head thrusts bilaterally. Unfortunately, there are few treatments to offer these patients; however, their long-term safety should be considered when they are advised about the operation of heavy machinery and automobiles and counseled on assistive living devices

TABLE 1 Causes of Vertigo

	Peripheral	Central	Mixed/other

Single vertigo attack > 24h	• Vestibular neuronitis
	• Viral labyrinthitis
	• Bacterial labyrinthitis
	• Trauma
	• Surgically destructive procedure
		• Vertebrobasilar infarct
		  PICA
		  AICA
		• Cerebellar/brainstem hemorrhage
		• Multiple sclerosis
		• Trauma	

Recurrent (episodic) vertigo	• BPPV • Ménière's disease • Recurrent vestibulopathy • Perilymphatic fistula • Oval/round window • Semicircular canal erosion from cholesteatoma • Dehiscent superior semicircular canal syndrome • Autoimmune inner-ear disease • Large vestibular aqueduct syndrome and other inner-ear malformations	• Migraine (may have peripheral component) • Benign paroxysmal vertigo of childhood • Vertebrobasilar TIAs • Multiple sclerosis • Seizures • Familial periodic ataxia • Arnold-Chiari malformation	• Psychogenic • Cardiac • Cervicogenic • Microvascular eighth nerve compression

Abbreviations: AICA = anterior inferior cerebellar artery; BPPV = benign paroxysmal positional vertigo; PICA = posterior inferior cerebellar artery; TIAs = transient ischemic attacks.

(canes, walkers, and railings). They also must learn to rely more on their visual and proprioceptive systems.

Assessment and Management

The article by Eggers and Zee provides a review of bedside and laboratory assessment of patients with vestibular disorders. Box 2 and the Current Therapy box list the important overall and specific medical treatment considerations.

Among all the disorders listed in Table 1 that can cause episodic dizziness and/or vertigo, BPPV is by far the most common, accounting for approximately 20% of patients seen in specialized dizziness clinics. The two other most common disorders that cause episodic vertigo, Ménière's disease and migraine, both have articles in this edition and will not be discussed here. Most of the other listed disorders are uncommon, and in those cases, imaging can be helpful in making a diagnosis. For example, high-resolution temporal bone computed tomography (CT) is useful in the diagnosis of perilymph fistula or large vestibular aqueduct syndrome, whereas magnetic resonance imaging (MRI) is more helpful with central disorders such as multiple sclerosis and vertebrobasilar artery disease.

BOX 1 Causes of Chronic Vestibular Dysequilibrium

• Uncompensated unilateral loss
• Vestibulotoxicity (aminoglycosides)
• Congenital/hereditary
• Bilateral Ménière's disease
• Autoimmune disorders
• Meningitic labyrinthitis
• Trauma
• Presbyastasis (aging)
• Chronic radiation effects
• Bilateral acoustic neuromas (neurofibromatosis type 2)
• Idiopathic

BOX 2 Key Considerations in Treatment of Vertigo

• Psychologic (common)
  Stress
  Anxiety
• Lifestyle (common)
  Sleep
  Diet
  Exercise
• Other coexisting illnesses
• Physical therapy (very common)
  Vestibular rehabilitation
  Repositioning maneuvers
• Medication (common)
  Oral
  Intratympanic
  Intravenous (rarely)
• Devices (see Ménière's disease article)
• Surgery
  Nondestructive
  Destructive

Recurrent vestibulopathy is relatively common and is essentially a diagnosis of exclusion. These patients have recurrent bouts of vertigo that each last less than 24 hours, similar to Ménière's disease vertigo attacks but without any associated hearing loss, tinnitus, aural fullness, or any other symptoms aside from the vegetative response. This is usually a self-limited disorder, and there is no treatment except symptomatic relief of the acute attacks.

Benign Paroxysmal Positional Vertigo

BPPV is a condition that usually is easy to diagnose and, more important, is readily treated with a simple office-based procedure. BPPV can be caused by either canalithiasis (free-floating endolymph debris) or cupulolithiasis (debris stuck to the cupula) and can affect each of the three semicircular canals, though the vast majority of cases are of the posterior canal variant. Most posterior canal BPPV cases result from canalithiasis because free-floating endolymph debris tends to gravitate to the posterior canal, which is the most gravity-dependent part of the vestibular labyrinth in both the upright and supine positions. Once debris enters the posterior canal, the cupular barrier at the shorter, more dependent end of the canal blocks the exit of the debris. Therefore, the debris becomes "trapped" and can exit only at the nonampullated end. Once in the canal, the canalith mass moves to a more dependent position when the orientation of the semicircular canal is modified in the gravitational plane. The drag that is created must overcome the resistance of the endolymph in the semicircular canal and the elasticity of the cupular barrier to deflect the cupula. The time needed for this to occur, plus the original inertia of the particles, explains the latency seen during the Dix-Hallpike maneuver.

In the head-hanging position, the canalith mass will move away from the cupula to induce utriculofugal cupular deflection. In the vertical canals, utriculofugal deflection produces an excitatory response. This causes an abrupt onset of vertigo and the typical torsional nystagmus in the plane of the posterior canal. In the left head-hanging position (left posterior canal stimulation), the fast component of the nystagmus beats clockwise as viewed by the examiner. Conversely, the right head-hanging position (right posterior canal stimulation) results in counterclockwise nystagmus. These nystagmus profiles correlate with the known neuromuscular pathways that arise from stimulation of the posterior canal ampullary nerves in an animal model.

This nystagmus is of limited duration because the endolymph drag ceases when the canalith mass reaches the limit of descent, and the cupula then returns to its neutral position. Reversal nystagmus occurs when the patient returns to the upright position; the mass moves in the opposite direction, thus creating a nystagmus in the same plane but in the opposite direction. The response is fatigable because the particles are dispersed along the canal and become less effective in creating endolymph drag and cupular deflection.

LATERAL CANAL BPPV

There is no doubt that by far BPPV most commonly affects the posterior semicircular canal. However, reports on the frequency of the horizontal canal variant vary. The posterior canal hangs inferiorly and has its cupular barrier at its shorter, more dependent end. Any debris that enters the canal essentially becomes trapped within it. Conversely, the lateral canal slopes upward and has its cupular barrier at the upper end. Therefore, free-floating debris in the lateral canal tends to float back out into the utricle with natural head movements, and this probably accounts for the quicker resolution of lateral canal BPPV. By the same token, its incidence probably is underestimated because usually it has resolved by the time the patient is examined.

Although cupulolithiasis is thought to play a greater role in lateral canal BPPV, canalithiasis is still more common. The vertigo is more intense, leading to more nausea, and the induced nystagmus is purely horizontal. Testing for lateral canal BPPV is done with the patient supine, turning the head to one side for a minute or two and then to the other. Depending on the underlying mechanism (cupulolithiasis or canalithiasis), the induced nystagmus can be apogeotropic (fast phase away from the ground) or geotropic (toward the ground), with one side producing a stronger response. Lateral canal testing, diagnosis, and treatment should be carried out in a specialized vestibular clinic.

ETIOLOGY

In most cases, BPPV is found in isolation and is termed primary or idiopathic BPPV, accounting for approximately 50% to 70% of cases. Secondary BPPV can result from head trauma, vestibular neuronitis, Ménière's disease, and migraine and as a complication of inner-ear surgery.

SYMPTOMS

Patients describe sudden, severe attacks of either horizontal or vertical vertigo or a combination of both that is precipitated by certain head positions and movements. The most common movements include rolling in bed, extending the neck to look up, and bending forward. Patients often can identify the affected ear by stating the direction of movement that precipitates the majority of the attacks (e.g., when rolling in bed to the right but not the left precipitates the dizziness, that indicates right ear involvement). The attacks of vertigo typically last less than 30 seconds, but some patients overestimate the duration by several minutes. The reasons for this discrepancy may include the fear associated with the intense vertigo and the nausea and disequilibrium that may follow the attack. Most patients experience several attacks per day.

In addition to vertigo, many patients complain of light-headedness, nausea, imbalance, and, in severe cases, sensitivity to all directions of head movement. Many patients also become extremely anxious for two main reasons: Some fear that the symptoms may represent a sinister underlying disorder such as a brain tumor; for others, the symptoms can be so unsettling that they go to great lengths to avoid the movements that bring on the vertigo. Some may not realize when the condition has resolved, as it often does over time without any treatment. BPPV can be described as self-limited, recurrent, or chronic.

As the name implies, BPPV is most often a benign condition. However, in certain situations it can be dangerous.

For example, a painter looking up from the top of a ladder may suddenly become vertiginous and lose his or her balance, risking a bad fall. The same is true for underwater divers, who may get very disoriented from acute vertigo. Heavy machinery operators should use great caution, especially if the job involves significant head movement. Most people can drive a car safely as long as they are careful not to tip the head back when checking the blind spot.

The diagnostic maneuver for posterior canal BPPV was described by Dix and Hallpike in 1952 (Figure 2). The patient is seated and positioned so that the head will extend over the edge of the table in the supine position. The head is turned 45 degrees toward the ear that is being tested, and the patient quickly is lowered into the supine position with the head extending below the level of

the table. The patient's head is held in this position, and the examiner observes the eyes for nystagmus. After lowering of the head, the typical nystagmus onset has a brief latency (1 to 5 seconds) and a limited duration (typically less than 30 seconds). With the eyes in the midposition (neutral), the nystagmus has a slight vertical component, the fast phase of which is upbeating. There is a stronger torsional component, in the fast phase of which the superior pole of the eye beats toward the affected (dependent) ear. The direction of the nystagmus reverses when the patient is brought into the upright position, and the nystagmus will fatigue with repeat testing. Along with the nystagmus, the patient will describe feeling vertiginous; the intensity of that symptom parallels the nystagmus response. It should be emphasized that the two posterior canals are tested independently, the right with the head turned right and the left with the head turned left. Overall, the history and eye findings during positional testing are the gold standards for diagnosing BPPV and additional testing is not normally necessary.

MANAGEMENT

The management of BPPV has changed dramatically in the last 20 years as understanding of the condition has progressed. Because medications were found to be largely ineffective, traditionally patients were instructed to avoid positions that induced the vertigo. Although BPPV is usually self-limited, with most cases resolving within 6 months, as the theories of cupulolithiasis and canalithiasis emerged, several noninvasive techniques were developed to correct the pathology directly. Figure 3 demonstrates a maneuver that is called the particle repositioning maneuver (PRM), a variant of the so-called Epley maneuver. With proper understanding of inner-ear anatomy and the pathophysiology of BPPV, appropriately trained health professionals, including family doctors and physiotherapists, should be able to carry out the PRM in most straightforward cases. Atypical cases, nonresponders, and patients with presumed lateral or anterior canal variants should be referred to a tertiary care "dizzy" clinic.

Overall, the PRM should take less than 5 minutes to complete. Studies using the repositioning maneuvers are difficult to compare because they vary considerably in terms of the technique, length of follow-up, number of treatment sessions, number of maneuvers per session, use of sedation, and use of mastoid vibration, but the overall response rate is on the order of 90% to 95%. In the author's clinic, physicians normally do not use sedation and typically perform only one maneuver per session as long as the nystagmus response is favorable (see Figure 3). Contrary to the original recommendations, recent studies suggest that the use of mastoid (skull) oscillation or postmaneuver head movement limitation is unnecessary. Recent evidence suggests that as many as 50% of patients will have at least one long-term recurrence.

For those with troublesome symptoms who have frequent recurrences or do not respond initially to the PRM, surgical occlusion of the posterior semicircular canal is a safe, reliable alternative. Before the institution of the PRM, free-floating endolymph debris often was seen during these operations, and in one instance it was removed and subjected to electron microscopy and found to be consistent with degenerating otoconia.

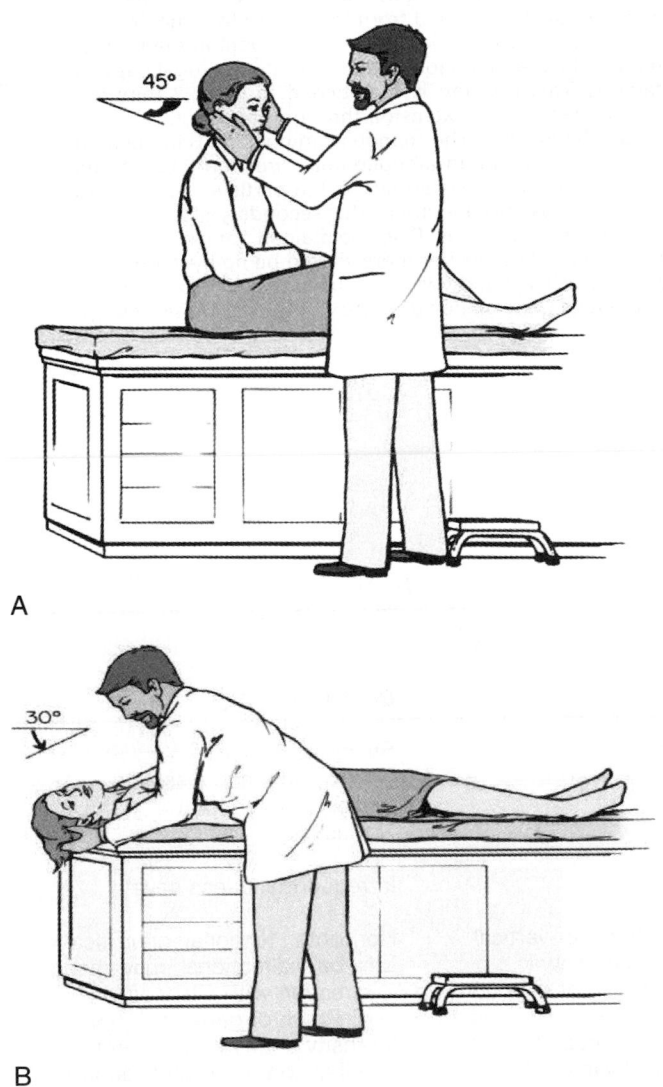

A

B

FIGURE 2. Dix-Hallpike maneuver (right ear). In this case, with the right side being tested, in position B the examiner should expect to see a fast-phase counterclockwise nystagmus. To complete the maneuver, the patient is returned to the seated position (position A) and the eyes are observed for reversal nystagmus, in this case a fast-phase clockwise nystagmus. (From Parnes LS, Agrawal SK, Atlas J: Diagnosis and management of benign paroxysmal positional vertigo (BPPV). CMAJ 2003;169(7):681-693. Used with permission.)

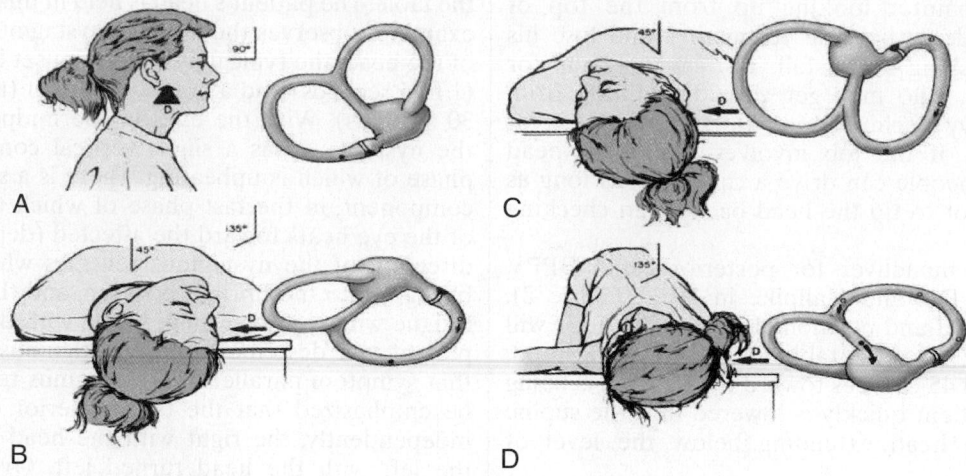

FIGURE 3. Particle repositioning maneuver (right ear). Schema of patient and concurrent movement of posterior and superior semicircular canals and utricle. The patient is seated on a table as viewed from the right side (**A**). The remaining parts show the sequential head and body positions of a patient lying down as viewed from the top. Before moving the patient into position B, turn the head 45° to the side being treated (in this case the right side). The patient in the normal Dix-Hallpike head-hanging position (**B**). Particles gravitate in an ampullofugal direction and induce utriculofugal cupular displacement and subsequent counterclockwise rotatory nystagmus. This position is maintained for 1 to 2 minutes. The patient's head then is rotated toward the opposite side with the neck in full extension through position C and into position D in a steady motion by rolling the patient onto the opposite lateral side. The change from position B to position D should take no longer than 3 to 5 seconds. Particles continue to gravitate in an ampullofugal direction through the common crus into the utricle. The patient's eyes are observed immediately for nystagmus. If the particles continue to move in the same ampullofugal direction, that is, through the common crus into the utricle, this secondary-stage nystagmus should beat in the same direction as the primary-stage nystagmus. Position D is maintained for another 1 to 2 minutes, and then the patient sits back up to position A. With a successful maneuver there should be no nystagmus or vertigo when the patient returns to the sitting position because the particles already will have been repositioned into the utricle. (From Parnes LS, Agrawal SK, Atlas J: Diagnosis and management of benign paroxysmal positional vertigo (BPPV). CMAJ 2003;169(7):681-693. Used with permission.)

 CURRENT DIAGNOSIS

	Peripheral	Central
Onset of vertigo	Usually sudden	Sudden or gradual
Severity of vertigo	Often intense and disabling	Less distinct and disabling
Pattern of vertigo	Single self-limited or episodic	Episodic or constant
Vertigo aggravated by head movement	Yes	Not usually
Associated nausea, vomiting, diaphoresis	Frequent and prominent	Infrequent and less severe
Nystagmus type	Horizontal or torsional (or mixed); never vertical	Horizontal, torsional, or vertical
Nystagmus direction	Unidirectional with fast phase usually away from the affected ear (irrespective of direction of gaze)	May be bidirectional; may change direction with changes in direction of gaze
Nystagmus intensity affected by fixation	Intensity decreased or totally suppressed by visual fixation (except torsional variant)	Intensity unaffected or, rarely, enhanced by visual fixation
Nystagmus intensity affected by direction of gaze	Nystagmus intensity may be increased when patient looks in direction of fast phase	Nystagmus intensity usually not affected by direction of gaze
Hearing loss and facial weakness	May be present	Very uncommon
Central nervous system symptoms/signs	Absent	Often present
Gait	Mild to moderate ataxia with tendency to fall toward side of lesion	Moderate to severe ataxia with tendency to fall to either side

CURRENT THERAPY

Target symptom	Medication type
Motion sickness prevention	• Motion sickness medications
Vertigo prevention	• Diuretics
	• Vasodilators
	• Vestibular suppressants
Nausea and vomiting	• Antiemetics
	• Vestibular suppressants
Co-morbid conditions, symptoms	• Anxiolytics
	• Antidepressants
	• Sedatives
Autoimmune, inflammatory	• Corticosteroids—oral and intratympanic
Destructive	• Aminoglycosides—intratympanic (rarely intramuscular)

Presumably, then, multiple otoconia become detached from the otolithic membrane in the utricle and migrate downward into the posterior canal, resulting in a case of canalithiasis. This mechanism can result from trauma, Ménière's disease, and even migraine. Usually it occurs spontaneously, which accounts for the vast majority of cases.

REFERENCES

Dieterich M: Dizziness. Neurologist 2004;10(3):154-164.
Eggers SD, Zee DS: Evaluating the dizzy patient: Bedside examination and laboratory assessment of the vestibular system. Semin Neurol 2003;23(1):47-58.
Minor LB: Labyrinthine fistulae: Pathobiology and management. Curr Opin Otolaryngol Head Neck Surg 2003;11(5):340-346.
Neuhauser H, Lempert T: Vertigo and dizziness related to migraine: A diagnostic challenge. Cephalalgia 2004;24(2):81-82.
Parnes LS, Agrawal SK, Atlas J: Diagnosis and management of benign paroxysmal positional vertigo (BPPV). CMAJ 2003;169(7):681-693.
Ruckenstein MJ: Autoimmune inner ear disease. Curr Opin Otolaryngol Head Neck Surg 2004;12(5):426-430.
Strupp M, Zingler VC, Arbusow V, et al: Methylprednisolone, valacyclovir, or the combination for vestibular neuritis. N Engl J Med 2004;351(4):354-361.
Welling DB, Parnes LS, O'Brien B, et al: Particulate matter in the posterior semicircular canal. Laryngoscope 1997;107(1):90-94.

Ménière's Disease

Method of:
Ted A. Meyer, MD, PhD, and Paul R. Lambert, MD

Ménière's disease is a disorder of fluid balance of the endolymph of the peripheral auditory and vestibular systems. The inner ear contains an endolymph-filled membranous labyrinth housed inside the perilymph-filled bony labyrinth. The sensory receptor cells of the inner ear are contained in the membranous labyrinth. The composition of perilymph is very similar to cerebrospinal fluid (CSF) (high sodium, low potassium), whereas the composition of endolymph is like intracellular fluid (high potassium, low sodium). The uniqueness of endolymph lies in its high positive resting potential (+80 mV). Disturbances in the fluid dynamics of the endolymph appear to be involved in the hearing loss and peripheral vestibular disorders associated with Ménière's disease. The exact mechanism or mechanisms involved in Ménière's disease are not completely understood, but it appears that an overabundance of endolymph, either through overproduction and/or underabsorption, is the pathologic basis of the disease.

Clinical Presentation

The symptomatology of Ménière's disease was first described almost 150 years ago by the French physician for whom it is named, Prosper Ménière. Patients with Ménière's disease present with unilateral fluctuating sensorineural hearing loss, aural fullness, tinnitus, and spells of disabling vertigo that typically last between 20 minutes and 24 hours. Many patients with Ménière's disease have nonspecific dizziness and imbalance in between spells of vertigo as well. A small percentage of patients develop or present with drop attacks, or spells of Tumarkin. These attacks occur when a patient's vestibular system goes into a crisis and the patient loses extensor tone. Patients often describe an aura followed by a feeling that they are going to fall. Patients do not lose consciousness unless they hit their head. Patients with Ménière's disease may not present with all symptoms, and the severity and progression of hearing loss, tinnitus, and vertigo are variable. For the majority of patients, Ménière's disease occurs in a single ear; however, if patients are followed for a long enough time, the literature reports bilateral Ménière's disease in a wide percentage of patients. Patients with bilateral Ménière's disease whose hearing loss progresses to profound levels are excellent candidates for a cochlear implant.

Office Evaluation

The majority of patients with dizziness or vertigo present to their primary care physician (PCP) or to the emergency room. Many of these patients are given 25 mg of meclizine (Antivert) and are instructed to take it up to three times a day as needed. When the vertigo spells continue, they are often then referred to an otolaryngologist or otologist.

CURRENT DIAGNOSIS

- Severe and often disabling vertigo lasting minutes to hours
- Fluctuating and progressive sensorineural hearing loss, often low-frequency
- Tinnitus: often low-pitched with roaring quality
- Aural fullness
- Complete neurologic evaluation
- Complete audiometric evaluation
- Consider further testing (MRI, FTA-ABS, tests for autoimmune disorders)

Abbreviations: FTA-ABS = fluorescent treponemal antibody absorption (test); MRI = magnetic resonance imaging.

Patients who are regularly taking meclizine as a prophylactic should stop the medication as quickly as possible.

When the patient with dizziness or vertigo presents to the clinic, the diagnosis of Ménière's disease can usually be obtained through the history and physical examination. The patient should give a history of disabling spells of vertigo, aural fullness or a "stuffy ear," fluctuating and progressive hearing loss, and tinnitus. The nature of the vertigo and the duration of the spells aids in the diagnosis. The vertigo is usually severe and can last between 20 minutes and 24 hours. Rarely does a Ménière's attack last longer than 24 hours. Longer attacks (days) are more consistent with vestibular neuritis. The attacks are not provoked by specific movements, such as the brief spell of benign paroxysmal positional vertigo (BPPV) that lasts seconds to a few minutes often after rolling over in bed. Aural fullness is variable, but when present it is often more pronounced during the attack. The sensorineural hearing loss associated with Ménière's disease is often a low-frequency loss that is fluctuant and progressive. The hearing loss is often worse during the attack; however, some patients are so vertiginous and nauseated during an attack that characteristics of their hearing loss or aural fullness are not appreciated. Tinnitus with Ménière's disease is variable, but many patients describe a low-pitched roaring sound, "like a refrigerator running."

A complete and thorough physical examination should be performed on all patients who present with dizziness or vertigo. The background and expertise of the PCP is different from that of the otologist, and the PCP should evaluate the patient for other causes of dizziness or lightheadedness. The physician should then perform a complete head and neck examination. Otoscopy is usually unremarkable unless the patient has a history of eustachian tube disease. Pneumatic otoscopy should be performed and should not be associated with any vertigo or nystagmus suggestive of a perilymphatic fistula. The cranial nerves and cerebellar function should be assessed. At a minimum, the patient should be evaluated for spontaneous and gaze-evoked nystagmus, and the Dix-Hallpike, Romberg, and Fukuda step tests should be performed. Tuning fork tests should be performed to determine the nature of the hearing loss. Assuming that hearing in the ear not in question is relatively normal, the sound from a tuning fork placed on the center of the head (Weber test) should lateralize to the normal ear. The Rinne test should confirm that hearing by air conduction is louder than bone-conduction hearing.

AUDIOMETRIC AND VESTIBULAR TESTING

Formal pure-tone and speech audiometry should be obtained on all patients with suspected Ménière's disease. Tympanometry and acoustic reflexes should be obtained as well. Patients usually present with a characteristic asymmetric low-frequency sensorineural loss that may recover to some degree between attacks. Patients with long-standing diagnoses of Ménière's disease rarely demonstrate normal and symmetric hearing. They often present with pure-tone thresholds in the 60-dB range, with diminished word recognition scores.

Vestibular testing is often performed on patients with Ménière's disease. Patients may have relatively normal responses to caloric irrigations in the affected ear; however

with long-standing Ménière's disease, caloric responses are usually reduced. The patient should not have spontaneous, positional, or gaze-evoked nystagmus, and ocular motor testing should be unremarkable. Electrocochleography is rarely performed for patients with suspected Ménière's disease anymore.

LABORATORY AND RADIOLOGIC TESTING

Some otologists believe that Ménière's disease is a clinical diagnosis and when they are confident in the diagnosis, they perform few other tests. With concerns about the exponential increase in the cost of health care, we as health care providers must have accurate data to justify this approach. Other clinicians feel that a battery of tests is warranted for patients who present with the clinical and audiologic manifestations of Ménière's disease, including a magnetic resonance imaging (MRI) scan to search for an acoustic neuroma or other retrocochlear pathology, fluorescent treponemal antibody absorption (FTA-ABS) test for syphilis, and the anti68-kD protein test for autoimmune inner ear disease. The clinician may take a prudent approach when ordering tests for patients with classic symptoms and signs of Ménière's disease and consider ordering more tests when the diagnosis is less clear.

Treatment

The therapeutic goal of treating patients with Ménière's disease is to prevent or minimize the disabling spells of vertigo. The mainstay of modern treatment for patients is management of dietary sodium intake and the use of a diuretic. Patients should be instructed to minimize the sodium in their diet. Patients should typically restrict their sodium intake to 1500 mg per day. Many patients consume 5 to 10 g of sodium per day, and a reduction to 1.5 g per day requires a major change in lifestyle. Patients are also asked to decrease their caffeine and alcohol input, and if they smoke, they are told to stop and given information on different options available for smoking cessation.

 CURRENT THERAPY

Medical

- Low sodium diet (<1500 mg/d)
- Smoking cessation
- Caffeine restriction
- Alcohol restriction
- Diuretic (hydrochlorothiazide, 25 mg, plus triamterene, 37.5 mg qd [Dyazide, Maxzide-25], may increase to bid)
- Vestibular suppressants for acute attacks

Surgical

- Hearing preservation:
  - Intratympanic gentamicin
  - Endolymphatic sac decompression/shunt
  - Vestibular nerve section (three approaches)
- Hearing ablative:
  - Labyrinthectomy

If the patient is not allergic, and there are no medical contraindications, the diuretic of choice is a combination of 25 mg hydrochlorothiazide and 37.5 mg of triamterene (Dyazide, Maxzide-25). Although triamterene is a potassium-sparing diuretic, patients are still encouraged to eat foods containing potassium (bananas, oranges, potatoes) and watch for signs of hypokalemia.

Low-salt diet and diuretic therapy successfully control the spells of vertigo in the majority of patients with Ménière's disease. Before considering another treatment option when low-salt diet and diuretic therapy are not effective, patients should be counseled on maintaining an even more restrictive diet (1000 mg of sodium per day) and if not medically contraindicated, the diuretic can be increased from once to twice daily. For patients who continue to have spells of vertigo despite aggressive medical therapy, other treatment options should be discussed.

MENIETT

A mechanical device that delivers low-pressure bursts of air to the external auditory canal is now available and shows some promising early results. Patients who consider the Meniett (Xomed) device first undergo a myringotomy and placement of a tympanostomy tube. In an adult, this can often be performed under local anesthesia in the clinic. The Meniett is an expensive device, and many insurance providers do not cover it. However, Medicare currently reimburses for the device.

OTOTOXIC ANTIBIOTICS

Injecting gentamicin into the middle ear to create a partial chemical labyrinthectomy has become popular in recent years, and it is performed by many general otolaryngologists as well as otologists. The procedure is performed in the office under topical anesthesia. Most otologists use a low-dose titration method in hopes of damaging the vestibular system while causing as little hearing loss as possible. Patients often have vague dizziness or balance problems several days after the procedure, and they normally compensate for this partial chemical labyrinthectomy. Gentamicin is helpful in reducing or halting the disabling spells of vertigo in the majority of patients who undergo the procedure. The risk of profound hearing loss after a single gentamicin injection is low, but it can occur.

SURGERY

Three procedures are used for patients with Ménière's disease: endolymphatic sac decompression/shunting, vestibular nerve section, and labyrinthectomy. The procedure is chosen based on the patient's age, overall health, and hearing status. If the patient has good hearing, then an endolymphatic sac decompression/shunt is recommended as the primary surgical procedure. In this outpatient surgery, a mastoidectomy is completed, and the endolymphatic sac is identified. The bone covering the sac is removed to decompress the sac. The sac is opened, and a silastic stent is placed in the sac. The risks of major complications such as facial paralysis or hearing loss are minimized with this procedure. Approximately 65% to 75% of patients undergoing an endolymphatic sac procedure receive substantial benefit.

If the patient continues to have spells of vertigo, the endolymphatic sac decompression can be repeated, or if the hearing is still good, the patient may opt for a vestibular nerve section. The vestibular nerve may be sectioned by one of three approaches (middle fossa, retrosigmoid, or retrolabyrinthine) depending on the surgeon's training and expertise and the age and health status of the patient. These procedures are more involved and in general require an overnight stay in the intensive care unit. There is a slight risk of hearing loss with these procedures from disruption of the blood supply to the cochlea or from damage to the cochlear nerve. More than 90% of patients who undergo vestibular nerve section receive substantial benefit.

If a patient has poor hearing, then a labyrinthectomy is the procedure of choice. A labyrinthectomy is performed via a mastoidectomy. The three semicircular canals are removed and the vestibule is opened to remove the neuroepithelium of the utricle and saccule. Operative risks such as damage to the facial nerve and a CSF leak are low with this procedure. A somewhat less-complete labyrinthectomy can be performed through the external auditory canal. This procedure is typically reserved for an elderly patient. It can be performed while the patient is awake. After a labyrinthectomy, the patient loses all hearing in that ear. Patients undergoing a labyrinthectomy are often acutely vertiginous and many require overnight observation. Control of vertigo after a labyrinthectomy is excellent. Approximately 95% of patients are free from spells of vertigo following this procedure, and the vast majority of patients, even the elderly, recover from this total unilateral vestibular loss quite well.

In summary, Ménière's disease is often misdiagnosed, and despite a great deal of research, it remains poorly understood. Patients must receive proper treatment and be educated about simple methods that can be used to prevent their symptoms. When sodium restriction and diuretics do not control the severe disabling spells of vertigo, patients should be offered one of the treatment options described here.

REFERENCES

Gates GA Green D: Intermittent pressure therapy of intractable Ménière's disease using the Meniett device: A preliminary report. Laryngoscope 2002;112:1489-1493.

Graham MD, Kemink JL: Transmastoid labyrinthectomy: Surgical management of vertigo in the nonserviceable hearing ear. A five-year experience. Am J Otol 1984;5:295-299.

Harner SG, Driscoll CL, Facer GW, et al: Long-term follow-up of transtympanic gentamicin for Ménière's syndrome. Otol Neurotol 2001;22:210-214.

Lustig LR, Yeagle J, Niparko JK, Minor LB: Cochlear implantation in patients with bilateral Ménière's syndrome. Otol Neurotol 2003;24:397-403.

Schessel DA, Minor LB, Nedzelski J: Ménière's disease and other peripheral disorders. In Cummings CW (ed): Cummings Otolaryngology Head and Neck Surgery. Philadelphia, Mosby, 2005, pp 3209-3253.

Welling DB, Pasha R, Roth LJ, Barin K: The effect of endolymphatic sac excision in Ménière disease. Am J Otol 1996;17:278-282.

Sinusitis

Method of
Richard R. Orlandi, MD

Classification and Etiologic Factors

Sinus inflammation is reported by more than 30 million adults in the United States and generates nearly 12 million office visits per year and at least $2.4 billion annually in direct medical costs. Loss of productivity likely has an even larger economic impact, with these patients reporting a quality-of-life impairment that is worse than patients with congestive heart failure.

The sinuses are air-filled chambers lined by respiratory epithelium that communicate with the nasal cavity through narrow openings or ostia. Mucus is produced by goblet cells within the respiratory mucosa and is propelled toward the ostia by the surface cilia. This mucociliary clearance is a self-cleaning mechanism for the nose and sinuses. Mucus and trapped particulate matter are transported into the nasopharynx and from there swallowed and eliminated via the gastrointestinal tract. The mucus blanket moves at approximately 8 mm per minute, resulting in a complete turnover every 10 minutes.

The anterior ethmoid and maxillary sinuses drain into a narrow trough within the middle meatus called the ethmoid infundibulum. This narrow system of drainage channels, called the ostiomeatal complex, can become easily blocked if the sinus and nasal mucosa swell because of inflammation, whatever the source. Mucociliary transport is then interrupted, trapping secretions and particulate matter, which can worsen the inflammation. This intensified inflammation can then spread to the frontal sinuses, as well as to the posterior ethmoid and sphenoid sinuses.

Inflammation within the nose has been traditionally referred to as *rhinitis*, whereas that in the paranasal sinuses has been called *sinusitis*. As understanding of the physiology and pathophysiology of the nose and sinuses has improved, it has become clear that the two conditions are interrelated and the term *rhinosinusitis* has been proposed. This disease has been categorized into a number of entities, including acute rhinosinusitis, where signs and symptoms last less than 4 weeks and chronic rhinosinusitis, where they are present for more than 12 weeks. Recurring acute rhinosinusitis, acute exacerbation of chronic rhinosinusitis, and subacute rhinosinusitis are also recognized subcategories.

Rhinosinusitis is an inflammatory condition with multiple etiologic factors. Anatomic variations, allergy, viruses, reflux, chronic bone inflammation (osteitis), fungi, and bacterial superantigens have all been postulated to play a role. Some of these factors, such as allergy or reflux, may create a background inflammation that makes patients more prone to an acute bacterial infection when another etiologic factor is introduced, such as a viral upper respiratory infection (URI). Other factors, such as osteitis, fungi, or bacterial superantigens, may perpetuate inflammation in a positive feedback loop and lead to chronic sinus and nasal inflammation. Rarer underlying conditions, such as immunodeficiency, granulomatous diseases, cystic fibrosis, and immotile cilia syndromes, also may predispose patients to acute and chronic rhinosinusitis.

Rhinosinusitis may be a final common pathway of inflammation with multiple etiologies, a constellation of signs and symptoms comprising a syndrome rather than a disease. Acute rhinosinusitis is often a bacterial infection that follows the inflammation of a viral upper respiratory illness. Conversely, chronic rhinosinusitis appears to be a primarily inflammatory condition with acute bacterial exacerbations. Long-term treatment should therefore be anti-inflammatory with antibiotics reserved for acute flares.

Diagnosis

Diagnosing rhinosinusitis can be challenging. Headache syndromes, allergic and nonallergic rhinitis, nasal septal deviation, esophageal and laryngopharyngeal reflux, and temporomandibular joint disease all share signs and symptoms with rhinosinusitis. Multiple attempts to define one or two key diagnostic criteria have failed, and it appears that the diagnosis of rhinosinusitis rests, instead, on a constellation of signs or symptoms. Some more common ones include facial pain or pressure, a sense of nasal obstruction or congestion, altered sense of smell, discolored nasal discharge, and fever (in acute cases). Minor symptoms include headache, cough, halitosis, fatigue, dental pain, and ear pressure or pain. In children, irritability, fatigue, congestion, and nighttime cough may be the more prominent symptoms.

In differentiating viral upper respiratory infections from acute bacterial rhinosinusitis, the timing and severity of symptoms may be most important. Viral URIs are common in children and adults, and only 1 in 200 such infections progress to acute bacterial rhinosinusitis.

CURRENT DIAGNOSIS

- Acute rhinosinusitis lasts less than 4 weeks whereas chronic rhinosinusitis is primarily an inflammatory condition, lasting more than 12 weeks.
- Rhinosinusitis shares symptoms with headache syndromes, allergic and nonallergic rhinitis, nasal septal deviation, esophageal and laryngopharyngeal reflux, and temporomandibular joint disease, making diagnosis challenging.
- There are not one or two defining diagnostic characteristics for acute or chronic rhinosinusitis. Instead, the diagnosis is often made using the physician's overall impression.
- Discolored nasal discharge does not necessarily indicate a bacterial infection.
- Imaging cannot differentiate between viral and bacterial rhinosinusitis, making it less helpful in acute disease.
- Symptoms of a viral URI typically resolve within 5 to 7 days. Severe or worsening symptoms during this period, or failure of symptoms to resolve within 7 to 10 days, are more likely to represent an acute bacterial rhinosinusitis.

When this does occur, symptoms of congestion, facial discomfort, and fever may persist longer than 10 days or worsen within 5 to 7 days of onset. Discolored discharge may be present from the start of the viral URI and does not necessarily correlate with bacterial infection, but rather is a sign of inflammation.

Because the symptoms of rhinosinusitis are nondescript, radiologic imaging may be called upon to make the diagnosis. Plain films of the sinuses have been all but supplanted by computed tomography (CT) because of the much greater information this modality affords. Nevertheless, the CT must be interpreted within the context of the patient's symptoms and prior treatment. Viral upper respiratory conditions generate inflammation within the nasal cavity as well as the sinuses, and CT during a URI will demonstrate changes consistent with "sinusitis." CT does not, therefore, play a prominent role in the diagnosis of acute rhinosinusitis, as it is unable to differentiate viral from bacterial disease. CT is more effective in diagnosing patients with chronic symptoms of rhinosinusitis, especially when performed after a trial of medical therapy and between acute exacerbations. Under these conditions, CT can determine the degree of inflammation and guide additional therapy. Unusual findings on CT mandate further evaluation, including unilateral disease, bone erosion, or sinus expansion. These findings may indicate neoplasia or an impending orbital or intracranial complication. In these cases, magnetic resonance imaging (MRI) may be helpful, but this modality is rarely indicated in uncomplicated rhinosinusitis because of its increased expense and lack of specificity.

Treatment Strategies

Whether the inflammation is acute or chronic, treatment is directed at diminishing the inflammation and re-establishing ostial patency and mucociliary clearance. Antibiotics form the mainstay for treatment of acute bacterial rhinosinusitis. Community-acquired acute bacterial rhinosinusitis is commonly caused by *Streptococcus pneumoniae* or *Haemophilus influenzae* in adults, with the addition of *Moraxella catarrhalis* in children. In acute exacerbations of chronic rhinosinusitis, *Staphylococcus aureus* and other staphylococcal species, as well as gram-negative enteric organisms, play a larger role.

Nearly 70% of patients with acute bacterial rhinosinusitis will improve without antibiotics, but that number goes up to 85% with appropriate antibiotics. The incidence of severe complications from acute rhinosinusitis is low and is not influenced by antibiotic use. Consequently, antibiotics should be prescribed for moderate to severe cases of acute bacterial rhinosinusitis or in immunocompromised individuals who may be more at risk for complications. Uncertain or mild cases of acute bacterial rhinosinusitis may be observed for spontaneous resolution, especially early in the course of disease.

Once the decision is made to prescribe antibiotics, the next complexity is which one to choose. Numerous studies and reviews still support the use of amoxicillin, either in standard or high doses (depending on local resistance patterns). Addition of clavulanate appears to improve the symptom resolution rate but is associated with increased gastrointestinal side effects. Second-line treatment for

amoxicillin failures or allergic patients includes respiratory quinolone or ketolide antibiotics.

Adjunctive treatments to reduce inflammation and symptoms include mucolytics/expectorants, nasal saline spray, anticholinergics, and decongestants (both topical and systemic). Topical decongestant therapy should not be continued for more than 5 days because of its propensity to cause a rebound rhinitis medicamentosa. Antihistamines are also indicated in patients with an underlying allergic component. Despite their anti-inflammatory effect, nasal steroid sprays have not been shown to have a clear impact on acute disease.

Because chronic rhinosinusitis is primarily an inflammatory condition with periodic acute bacterial exacerbations, antibiotics play a much smaller role. Nasal corticosteroids instead form the mainstay of treatment for chronic rhinosinusitis. Treatment of underlying allergy, when present, typically also improves the patient's overall sinus and nasal inflammation. Leukotriene inhibitors, effective in treating asthma and allergic rhinitis, may play a role in patients with chronic rhinosinusitis, especially those with nasal polyps. Patients who are not sufficiently responsive to medical therapy often benefit from surgical intervention to widen the sinus drainage pathways, followed by continued medical management.

Complications of Sinusitis

Complications of sinus disease are rare but potentially serious. The sinuses are separated from the orbit and intracranial cavity by thin bone perforated by venous and lymphatic channels, which can act as conduits for the spread of infection. Intracranial abscess, cerebritis, venous sinus thrombosis, or meningitis may complicate acute sinusitis, typically involving the frontal or sphenoid sinuses. Orbital cellulitis or abscess typically results from ethmoid or maxillary sinusitis and is more common in children. High fever, severe or worsening headache, meningeal signs, altered mental status, infraorbital hypesthesia, significant facial swelling, diplopia, ptosis, chemosis, proptosis, or pupillary or extraocular movement abnormalities should prompt a thorough evaluation, including dedicated imaging and more intensive therapy and observation.

Immunocompromised patients are at special risk for invasive fungal rhinosinusitis, a rare but lethal condition, where weakened host defenses allow tissue invasion and rapid spread of fungus. This disease has a predilection for neutropenic patients, poorly controlled diabetics (particularly during ketoacidosis), and patients undergoing hemodialysis. Early signs may be as subtle as a low-grade fever of unknown origin and can rapidly progress to orbital or cerebral symptoms as a result of extension of the disease to these areas. Therapy is directed toward swift reversal of the underlying immunocompromise, systemic antifungal therapy, and debridement of affected necrotic tissues, which can be disfiguring. Outcomes for this rare condition correlate with the ability to reverse the underlying immunocompromise.

Summary

Rhinosinusitis represents inflammation of the nose and paranasal sinuses and has many etiologies. The symptoms of rhinosinusitis overlap with many other conditions, making diagnosis somewhat difficult. Imaging may be helpful but must be interpreted in the context of the patient's symptoms. Acute bacterial rhinosinusitis typically follows a viral URI and is an infectious process while chronic rhinosinusitis is primarily an inflammatory process with infrequent bacterial exacerbations. Treatment is therefore primarily anti-infectious in acute disease and anti-inflammatory in chronic disease. As the etiologies and pathophysiology of acute and chronic rhinosinusitis are better defined, improved therapy will likely result.

REFERENCES

Benninger MS, Ferguson BJ, Hadley JA, et al: Adult chronic rhinosinusitis: definitions, diagnosis, epidemiology, and pathophysiology. Otolaryngol Head Neck Surg 2003;129(3 Suppl):S1-S32.

Lau J, Zucker D, Engels EA, et al: Diagnosis and Treatment of Acute Bacterial Rhinosinusitis. Evidence Report/Technology Assessment No. 9 (Contract 290-97-0019 to the New England Medical Center). Rockville, Md, Agency for Health Care Policy and Research, March 1999.

Orlandi RR, Kennedy DW: Surgical management of rhinosinusitis. Am J Med Sci 1998;316:29-38.

Sinus and Allergy Health Partnership: Antimicrobial treatment guidelines for acute bacterial rhinosinusitis. Otolaryngol Head Neck Surgery 2004;130(1 Suppl):1-45.

Nonallergic Rhinitis

Method of
Laura Waikart, MD, and Phillip L. Lieberman, MD

Epidemiology

Rhinitis is defined as inflammation of the membranes lining the nose. The symptoms include sneezing, nasal congestion, postnasal drainage, and anterior rhinorrhea. Chronic rhinitis may be either allergic or nonallergic in origin. Nonallergic rhinitis is distinguished from its allergic counterpart by the absence of a clinically relevant IgE antibody response to aeroallergens. Thus, the diagnosis of chronic nonallergic rhinitis is one of exclusion. Nonallergic rhinitis is not a single disorder; it consists of a variety of syndromes that manifest the above-mentioned symptoms and share a single characteristic: the absence of allergy.

The frequency of nonallergic rhinitis and of the various syndromes that make up this broad class of disease is estimated to be 17% to 57% of all rhinitis patients worldwide (Table 1). Based on the findings of one of the studies conducted by the National Rhinitis Classification Task Force, a nationwide epidemiologic survey of patients in the outpatient setting is currently underway. This survey, which uses a patient-screening tool for rhinitis, is being conducted in 25,000 office-based nonallergy practices nationwide. The goal of this study is to develop better epidemiologic data on the incidence of allergic, nonallergic, and mixed (allergic and nonallergic) disease and to assess the diagnostic usefulness of the rhinitis screening tool. Interim data in 3500 patients show that 32% of patients have allergic rhinitis, 22% have nonallergic rhinitis, and 46% have mixed rhinitis.

Nonallergic rhinitis is more prevalent in adults older than the age of 20 years (approximately 70%), whereas allergic disease is more common in patients younger than 20 years of age. Female gender may also be a risk factor for nonallergic rhinitis.

Pathophysiology and Classification

VASOMOTOR RHINITIS

Nonallergic rhinitis is classified into distinct syndromes based on etiologic and cytologic features (Table 2). Vasomotor rhinitis (VMR), or idiopathic perennial nonallergic rhinitis, is the most common of these syndromes (61%). The term *vasomotor* implies a vascular or neurologic dysfunction but is perhaps a misnomer because no mechanism of production has been established. The syndrome is unrelated to allergy, infection, structural lesions, systemic disease, or drug use. VMR probably results from multiple causes. The symptoms are similar to those of allergic rhinitis without the pruritus. VMR is characterized by nonspecific nasal hyperreactivity on exposure to nonimmunologic stimuli. Mucosal biopsy may reveal an increase in mast cells similar to allergic rhinitis but without an increase in goblet cells. Stimuli include changes

TABLE 1 Frequency of Occurrence of Rhinitis

Investigator (year)	N	Allergic Rhinitis	Nonallergic Rhinitis	Mixed Rhinitis
Mullarkey (1980)	142	48%	52%	Not studied
Enberg (1989)	152 (128)	54%	30%	16%
Togias (1990)	362	83%	17%	Not studied
ECRHS (1999)	1412	75%	25%	Not studied
NRCTF (1999)	975	43%	23%	34%

Abbreviations: N = Number of patients.

in temperature or relative humidity, ingestion of alcohol, strong odors (perfumes, hair spray, paint products), and airborne irritants (chemical cleaning products, tobacco smoke, and automobile exhaust fumes). Hyperreactivity of the nasal mucosa to capsaicin (Zostrix), histamine, and methacholine in vivo has been demonstrated.

NONALLERGIC RHINITIS EOSINOPHILIA SYNDROME

Nonallergic rhinitis with eosinophilia syndrome (NARES), first described in 1981, is characterized by increased nasal eosinophilia and makes up 15% to 20% of nonallergic rhinitis cases. The pathophysiology is unknown. Patients present with profuse watery rhinorrhea and nasal pruritus. Patients may also report hyposmia or anosmia. Eosinophilia, the hallmark of this syndrome, may contribute to nasal mucosal dysfunction owing to the release of major basic protein and eosinophil cationic protein. These toxins damage nasal ciliated epithelium and prolong mucociliary clearance. Nasal polyps are often associated with nasal eosinophils; consequently, concerns have been raised that nasal eosinophilia may be a precursor to the aspirin-induced tetrad syndrome (NARES, asthma, sinusitis, and nasal polyps). Blood eosinophilia nonallergic rhinitis syndrome (BENARS), a related disorder that accounts for approximately 4% of all nonallergic rhinitis cases, is associated with an increase in blood eosinophils.

BASOPHILIC/METACHROMATIC NASAL DISEASE

A subcategory of nonallergic rhinitis is basophilic/metachromatic cell nasal disease, or nasal mastocytosis. Mast cell infiltration ($>2000/mm^3$) requires, like NARES, a histologic diagnosis. Likely symptoms include profuse rhinorrhea and congestion without significant sneezing or pruritus. The cause of this syndrome is unknown.

TABLE 2 Classification of Nonallergic Rhinitis Based on Etiologic and Cytologic Features

Nonallergic Rhinitis, Inflammatory	Nonallergic Rhinitis, Noninflammatory	Nonallergic Rhinitis, Structurally Related
Eosinophilic nasal disease (NARES, BENARS)	Rhinitis medicamentosa	Septal deviation
Basophilic/metachromatic nasal disease	Topical decongestants	Septal perforation
Infections (viral, bacterial)	Systemic medications	Foreign body
Nasal polyps	Vasomotor rhinitis	Obstructive adenoid hyperplasia
Aspirin intolerance	Physical rhinitis	Nasal valve dysfunction
Chronic sinusitis	(Cold air or bright-light induced)	Trauma
Churg-Strauss syndrome		Malformation
Young's syndrome (sinopulmonary disease,	Gustatory rhinitis	Tumors/neoplasms
azoospermia)	Irritant rhinitis	CSF leak
Cystic fibrosis	Rhinitis sicca	
Kartagener's syndrome (bronchiectasis, chronic	Endocrine/metabolic	
sinusitis, nasal polyps)	Pregnancy or estrogen-related	
Atrophic rhinitis	rhinitis	
Immunologic nasal disease (non-IgE mediated or	Hypothyroidism	
secondary to systemic immunologic disorders)	Acromegaly	
Sjögren's syndrome		
Systemic lupus erythematosus		
Relapsing polychondritis		
Churg-Strauss syndrome		
Sarcoidosis		
Wegener's granulomatosis		

Abbreviations: BENARS = blood eosinophilia nonallergic rhinitis syndrome; CSF = cerebral spinal fluid; NARES = nonallergic rhinitis with eosinophilia syndrome.

DRUG-INDUCED RHINITIS

Multiple drugs can cause nonallergic rhinitis symptoms (Box 1). Rhinitis medicamentosa commonly describes the rebound nasal congestion that occurs with overuse of decongestant nasal sprays as well as cocaine abuse. Underlying rhinitis can lead to this type of overuse. The rebound swelling of this disorder can be the result of interstitial edema without vasodilation. A number of oral agents, such as antihypertensives, hormones, and other drugs, also can cause rhinitis. In addition, eyedrops, via transit through the nasal-lacrimal duct, also can produce this syndrome.

ENDOCRINE-INDUCED OR HORMONALLY INDUCED RHINITIS

Oral contraceptives, estrogen replacement therapy, pregnancy, hypothyroidism, and acromegaly can cause rhinitis. Pregnancy can produce rhinitis characterized mainly by congestion because of increased blood volume in combination with hormonally induced vasodilation. Rhinitis has been estimated to affect up to 30% of pregnant women. It most commonly develops at approximately the second month of pregnancy and frequently persists until after delivery or the cessation of breast-feeding. Hypothyroidism and acromegaly both can cause turbinate hypertrophy.

GUSTATORY RHINITIS OR PHYSICAL RHINITIS

Rhinitis can be caused by exposure to certain triggers including eating (gustatory rhinitis), cold air (skier's or jogger's nose), or sunlight. This form of rhinitis is characterized by profuse, watery rhinorrhea because of an overly sensitive cholinergic reflex. It begins within minutes of eating or exposure to cold air; spicy foods and alcoholic beverages are frequent culprits.

ATROPHIC RHINITIS

Atrophic rhinitis is more common in elderly patients, but it can occur at any age. Symptoms may include dryness of the nasal mucosa, a sensation of nasal congestion, and a bad smell (ozena) in the nose. In industrialized countries this condition is rare and mostly associated with complications of an overly aggressive removal of nasal tissue during surgery. In other areas of the world, atrophic rhinitis is frequently associated with *Klebsiella* colonization, and the symptoms of epistaxis, crusting, stuffiness, and a foul odor are more prominent.

RHINITIS ASSOCIATED WITH AUTOIMMUNE OR GRANULOMATOUS DISEASES

Rhinitis can occur with systemic autoimmune diseases such as Churg-Strauss vasculitis, Sjögren's syndrome, systemic lupus erythematosus, and relapsing polychondritis. Wegener's granulomatosis and sarcoidosis also can cause upper airway symptoms including rhinitis.

GASTROESOPHAGEAL REFLUX DISEASE–ASSOCIATED RHINITIS

Upper airway symptoms, including rhinitis, have recently been associated with gastroesophageal reflux disease (GERD). This association was confirmed in a study by Theodoropoulos and colleagues. Interestingly, rhinitis and other upper airway symptoms occurred even when the GERD was limited to the distal esophagus. This finding implies direct contact with the upper airway or occult aspiration is not required. The pathogenesis is not currently understood but may involve a neurogenic mechanism.

Diagnosis

The differential diagnosis of rhinitis can be difficult given the often indistinguishable symptoms of nonallergic and allergic rhinitis, the number of patients presenting with mixed rhinitis, and the multiple syndromes that make up nonallergic rhinitis (see Box 1).

Although historically classic physical examination findings are described with several forms of rhinitis, these are nonspecific findings. For example, allergic rhinitis is frequently characterized by pale, boggy turbinates; infectious rhinitis is suspected by the presence of purulent nasal discharge; and rhinitis medicamentosa may have erythematous or hemorrhagic mucosa. However, NARES, nasal polyposis, and nasal mastocytosis frequently appear indistinguishable from allergic rhinitis. The appearance of vasomotor rhinitis can vary and often overlaps with several other types of rhinitis. As a result, physical examination is generally unhelpful in distinguishing between allergic and nonallergic disease, but it is essential in the evaluation of structural problems such as septal deviations, septal perforations, polyps, and tumors.

Anatomic abnormalities represent approximately 5% to 10% of chronic nasal disorders. Nasal septal deviation is common and often aggravated by other coexisting forms of rhinitis. Nasal polyps may be associated with other disorders including the aspirin tetrad syndrome (nasal polyposis, aspirin intolerance, sinusitis, and asthma), cystic fibrosis, Kartagener's syndrome, Churg-Strauss syndrome, or chronic sinusitis. Very rare structural causes of rhinitis include tumors and neoplasms such as chordoma, neurofibroma, angiofibroma, squamous cell carcinoma, sarcoma, lymphoma, teratoma, encephaloceles, meningoceles, and

TABLE 3 Differential Diagnosis of Rhinitis

Manifestation	Allergic Rhinitis	Chronic Nonallergic Rhinitis
Age of onset	<20 years of age	>20 years of age
Seasonality	Seasonal variations: spring and fall	Usually perennial, but can be worse with weather changes
		Irritant exposure, weather changes
Exacerbating factors	Allergen exposure	Rare
Nature of symptoms		
Pruritus	Common	Common
Congestion	Common	Usually not prominent, but dominant in some cases
Sneezing	Prominent	
Postnasal drainage	Not prominent	Prominent
Other related manifestations (e.g., allergy, conjunctivitis, atopic dermatitis)	Often present	Absent
Family history	Usually present	Usually absent
Physical appearance	Variable, classically described as pale, boggy, swollen mucosa but may appear normal	Variable, erythematous
Allergy testing	Allergy testing always positive	Allergy testing negative or not clinically significant
Nasal eosinophilia	Usually present	Present 15%-20% of the time (NARES)

Abbreviations: NARES = nonallergic rhinitis with eosinophilia syndrome.

inverting papilloma. Another rare but serious cause of rhinorrhea is a cerebral spinal fluid (CSF) leak, which can occur as a result of trauma, surgical complications, or even spontaneously. CSF leaks occur after approximately 5% of all basilar skull fractures. The diagnosis requires a high index of suspicion and can be confirmed by the detection of β_2-transferrin in the fluid.

The features that distinguish nonallergic from allergic disease in terms of the history are seen in Table 3. The definitive diagnosis rests on the presence or the absence of clinically important IgE-mediated reactions to aeroallergens. The test of choice in this regard is the allergy skin test; however, a positive test does not rule out the presence of nonallergic disease and must be evaluated for significance in light of the history. However, negative tests establish the presence of nonallergic rhinitis by exclusion.

Management

Management of chronic nonallergic rhinitis can be difficult because some cases are relatively resistant to therapy. The mainstay of treatment is pharmacologic, but of course avoidance of triggers is helpful. Two pharmacologic approaches can be taken to treat vasomotor rhinitis: nonspecific, broad-based therapy aimed at multiple symptoms or therapy tailored to specific symptoms (Table 4). Owing to the variability of vasomotor symptoms, nonspecific treatment may be preferable.

NONSPECIFIC, BROAD-BASED TREATMENT

Broad-based treatment includes the topical antihistamine azelastine (Astelin) or topical corticosteroids, the only

TABLE 4 Examples of Some Typical Medications Used to Treat Nonallergic Rhinitis

Generic Name	Trade Name(s)	Dosage
Broad-Based Treatments		
Azelastine*	Astelin	2 sprays each nostril qd-bid
Fluticasone*	Flonase	2 sprays each nostril qd or 1 spray each nostril bid
Budesonide*	Rhinocort AQ	1 spray each nostril bid to 4 sprays each nostril qd
Beclomethasone*	Beconase AQ	1-2 sprays each nostril bid
	Vancenase AQ	1-2 sprays each nostril qd
Symptom-Specific Treatments		
Ipratropium bromide*	Atrovent	0.03%, 2 sprays each nostril bid-qid
Decongestants[†]		
Pseudoephedrine	Multiple formulations	varies
Phenylephrine	Multiple formulations	varies
Saline nasal spray	SeaMist, Ocean, Pretz	1-3 sprays each nostril prn

*Examples provided are typical adult dosages.
†There are multiple formulations and dosage schedules for the decongestants.
Abbreviations: bid = twice daily; prn = as needed; qd = every day.

two forms of therapy demonstrated to be of use for the management of nonallergic rhinitis. Azelastine is the only antihistamine approved for use in both allergic and nonallergic rhinitis. The antihistamine and anti-inflammatory activities of azelastine produce a high response rate (82% to 85%) in vasomotor rhinitis, improve all associated rhinitis symptoms (congestion, rhinorrhea, postnasal drainage, and sneezing), and have a rapid onset of action. In addition, three topical corticosteroids have been approved for use in the treatment of nonallergic rhinitis: budesonide (Rhinocort Aqua),[1] fluticasone (Flonase), and beclomethasone (Beconase AQ). Budesonide has only been approved for this condition in its aerosol form, which is no longer available. However, it is not unreasonable to assume that the aqueous form would also be effective. There are no comparative studies that assess the relative efficacy of any of these drugs, and the choice of therapy remains speculative. Possible side effects are generally mild and include local irritation, mucosal bleeding, and, rarely, septal perforation. Long-term treatment with beclomethasone dipropionate was shown to be safe and did not produce nasal atrophy after 5 years of continuous treatment. Using the proper technique for administration of nasal steroids can minimize the risk of any significant side effects.

SYMPTOM-SPECIFIC THERAPY

For treatment tailored to specific symptoms, decongestants are first-line therapy for patients whose symptoms are obstructive. Decongestants, however, have no effect on other manifestations such as rhinorrhea or sneezing. Commonly used oral decongestants include pseudoephedrine[1] and phenylephrine.[1] Potential side effects include insomnia, nervousness, urinary hesitancy, palpitations, and elevated blood pressure. They are generally considered safe to use in patients with stable, controlled hypertension. However, they are contraindicated in patients taking MAO-inhibitors. Relative contraindications include thyroid disease, glaucoma, and coronary artery disease. They are not recommended for use during pregnancy. Topical decongestants such as oxymetazoline (Afrin)[1] and phenylephrine (Neo-Synephrine)[1] can be used effectively in certain situations as a temporary measure. However, their use should be strictly limited to less than 3 to 5 days to avoid the rebound symptoms of rhinitis medicamentosa.

The topical anticholinergic agent ipratropium bromide (Atrovent) is first-line treatment for vasomotor rhinitis with a predominant symptom of rhinorrhea. Anticholinergics primarily affect rhinorrhea with only modest effects on congestion. The only intranasal anticholinergic agent available in the United States is ipratropium bromide in a 0.03% solution for use in chronic nonallergic rhinitis. An anticholinergic agent is a particularly effective choice of therapy for physical rhinitis symptoms (gustatory or cold induced rhinitis) requiring treatment. It can be used approximately 1 hour prior to exposure to cold air or eating. Ipratropium bromide can be used alone or in combination with topical nasal corticosteroids. The benefits of this particular therapeutic combination appear to

CURRENT DIAGNOSIS

- The diagnosis of nonallergic rhinitis encompasses a variety of syndromes that share common symptoms, such as sneezing, nasal congestion, postnasal drainage, and anterior rhinorrhea.
- Nonallergic rhinitis is distinguished from allergic rhinitis by the lack of a clinically relevant IgE response to aeroallergens.
- Nonallergic rhinitis is a diagnosis of exclusion. To distinguish this condition from allergic rhinitis the diagnostic test of choice is allergy skin testing. However, results must be properly interpreted and clinically correlated with the patient's history.
- Physical examination findings are nonspecific in nonallergic rhinitis and cannot be used exclusively to distinguish between allergic and nonallergic rhinitis.
- Mixed rhinitis (allergic and nonallergic) occurs in a significant number of patients.
- Vasomotor rhinitis or idiopathic perennial nonallergic rhinitis is the most common subtype of nonallergic rhinitis, approximately 61% of nonallergic rhinitis syndromes.
- Vasomotor rhinitis is characterized by nasal hyperreactivity on exposure to nonimmunologic stimuli including temperature or humidity changes, strong odors, and airborne irritants.
- Nonallergic rhinitis with eosinophilia syndrome (NARES) represents approximately 15% to 20% of nonallergic rhinitis and is characterized by increased nasal eosinophilia. The pathophysiology of this disorder is poorly understood.
- Multiple drugs can cause rhinitis, especially antihypertensive medications, hormones, and cocaine.
- The overuse of topical nasal decongestants is a common cause of rebound nasal congestion, rhinitis medicamentosa.
- Endocrine disorders can lead to rhinitis, including hypothyroidism and acromegaly.
- Rhinitis of pregnancy is a common condition affecting up to a third of pregnant women.
- Many autoimmune or granulomatous diseases can be associated with rhinitis.
- Rhinitis symptoms can be related to multiple structural problems. A deviated septum, turbinate deformation, nasal valve dysfunction, or obstructive adenoid hypertrophy may be identified as the cause of rhinitis symptoms.
- Other rare, but serious, conditions can cause rhinitis symptoms including tumors, neoplasms, and trauma.

be additive compared with the use of either drug alone. Ipratropium has minimal side effects (infrequent episodes of nasal dryness and minor epistaxis).

Topical saline solution alone or in combination with other therapies may provide additional relief from the symptoms of postnasal drainage, sneezing, and congestion in vasomotor rhinitis. In patients who do not respond to pharmacotherapy, several surgical approaches have been tried successfully.

OTHER THERAPEUTIC APPROACHES AND CONSIDERATIONS

Surgical approaches that divide the parasympathetic supply to the nasal mucosa, thereby reducing nasal secretion, are endoscopic vidian nerve section and electrocoagulation of the anterior ethmoidal nerve. In cases in which the predominant symptom is congestion, turbinectomy is a treatment option. However, there may be a recurrence of symptoms after surgery.

Rhinitis of pregnancy is a particularly challenging therapeutic problem. The major principle that guides therapy for this disorder is caution in medication use. First-line treatment should include the safest therapies, such as steam inhalation, saline solution nasal sprays, and avoidance of irritants. Unfortunately, rhinitis of pregnancy can often be recalcitrant, responding only to topical corticosteroids. At present there are two class B antihistamines, cetirizine (Zyrtec) and loratadine (Claritin); one class B topical nasal steroid, budesonide (Rhinocort AQ); and one class B leukotriene modifier, montelukast (Singulair) approved for use in allergic rhinitis. Only one of these, budesonide (Rhinocort AQ),[1] has shown efficacy in nonallergic rhinitis.

Treatment of rhinitis medicamentosa requires withdrawal from the topical decongestant, the oral agent, or the eyedrops as well as treatment of the underlying rhinitis.

[1]Not FDA approved for this indication.

 CURRENT THERAPY

- Treatment for nonallergic rhinitis can be generally divided into nonspecific broad-based treatment or symptom-specific treatment options.
- Nonspecific broad-based options include topical corticosteroids and azelastine (Astelin).
- Topical corticosteroids shown to be effective in nonallergic rhinitis include budesonide (Rhinocort),[1] fluticasone (Flonase), and beclomethasone (Beconase AQ).
- Obstructive symptoms can be treated symptomatically with decongestants. These agents do not affect rhinorrhea or sneezing.
- The topical anticholinergic, ipratropium bromide (Atrovent) can be used to treat rhinorrhea, with minimal effect on congestion.
- Topical saline solution can provide some benefit in the treatment of postnasal drainage, sneezing, and congestion because of vasomotor rhinitis.
- Rhinitis of pregnancy can be resistant to therapy. Treatment options are often limited by safety concerns.
- Surgical options exist for nonallergic rhinitis but are mainly reserved for those patients who do not respond to pharmacotherapy.

[1]Not FDA approved for this indication.

This is often best accomplished with a 1-week tapering course of an oral glucocorticoid, with gradual discontinuation of the decongestant spray beginning on the second or third day of treatment. Administration of a topical corticosteroid spray also can begin on the third day of treatment and should be maintained subsequently. Oral decongestants can be used as needed.

The presence of nasal eosinophilia in patients with chronic nonallergic rhinitis is generally regarded as a good prognostic indicator for response to treatment with topical corticosteroids. Patients with NARES and massive eosinophilic infiltration also may require intermittent use of oral glucocorticoids to control symptoms.

TREATING MIXED RHINITIS

Once a differential diagnosis of mixed rhinitis has been confirmed, empirical treatment with a topical broad-based agent effective in both allergic and nonallergic rhinitis (e.g., azelastine or an intranasal corticosteroid) is a reasonable choice for first-line therapy. Other agents such as oral decongestants or ipratropium (Atrovent) can be used adjunctively as indicated.

REFERENCES

Banov C, Laforce C, Lieberman P: Double-blind trial of Astelin nasal spray in the treatment of vasomotor rhinitis. Ann Allergy Asthma Immunol 2000;84:138.

Dockhorn R, Aaronson D, Bronsky E, et al: Ipratropium bromide nasal spray 0.03% and beclomethasone nasal spray alone and in combination for the treatment of rhinorrhea in perennial rhinitis. Ann Allergy Asthma Immunol 1999;82:349-359.

Dykewicz MS, Fineman S, Skoner DP, et al: Diagnosis and management of rhinitis: Complete guidelines of the Joint Task Force on Practice Parameters in Allergy, Asthma, and Immunology. American Academy of Allergy, Asthma and Immunology. Ann Allergy Asthma Immunol 1998;81:478-518.

Graf P, Hallen H, Juto JE: The pathophysiology and treatment of rhinitis medicamentosa. Clin Otolaryngol 1995;20:224-229.

Incaudo GA, Schatz M: Rhinosinusitis associated with endocrine conditions: Hypothyroidism and pregnancy. In Schatz M, Zeigler RS, Settipane GA (eds.): Nasal Manifestations of Systemic Diseases. Providence, RI, OceanSide Publications, 1991, p 54.

Moneret-Vautrin DA, Hsieh V, Wayoff M, et al: Nonallergic rhinitis with eosinophilia syndrome a precursor of the triad: Nasal polyposis, intrinsic asthma, and intolerance to aspirin. Ann Allergy 1990;64:513-518.

Settipane RA, Lieberman PL: Update on nonallergic rhinitis. Ann Allergy Asthma Immunol 2001;86(5):494-507.

Theodoropoulos DS, Ledford DK, Lockey RF, et al: Prevalence of upper respiratory symptoms in patients with symptomatic gastroesophageal reflux disease. Am J Respir Crit Care Med 2001;164(1):72-76.

Togias A: Age relationships and clinical features of nonallergic rhinitis. J Allergy Clin Immunol 1990;85:182.

Turkeltaub PC, Gergen PJ: The prevalence of allergic and nonallergic respiratory symptoms in the U.S. population: Data from the second national health and nutrition examination survey 1976-1980 (NHANES II). J Allergy Clin Immunol 1988;81:305.

Zeiger RS: Differential diagnosis and classification of rhinosinusitis. In Schatz M, Zeiger RS, Settipane GA (eds.): Nasal Manifestations of Systemic Diseases. Providence, RI, OceanSide Publications, 1991.

Zlab MK, Moore GF, Daly DT, Yonkers AJ: Cerebrospinal fluid rhinorrhea: A review of the literature. Ear Nose Throat J 1992;71:314-317.

Hoarseness and Laryngitis

Method of
Robert Thayer Sataloff, MD, DMA

Until the 1980s, most physicians who cared for patients with voice disorders asked only a few basic questions, such as: How long have you been hoarse? Do you smoke? The physician's ear was the sole instrument routinely used to assess voice quality and function. Visualization of the vocal folds was limited to indirect examination using regular light and looking through a mirror placed inside the patient's mouth, or by direct laryngoscopy with anesthesia in the operating room. Treatment of patients generally was limited to administration of medicines for infection or inflammation, surgery for masses, and no treatment if the vocal folds looked normal. Occasionally, voice therapy was recommended, but the specific nature of the therapy was not well defined or controlled, and results were often disappointing. Since the early 1980s, the standard of care for the diagnosis and treatment of voice disorders has changed dramatically.

What Kinds of Questions Should Be Asked?

Good medical diagnosis in all fields often hinges on asking the right questions, and listening carefully to the answers. This process is known as taking a history. Recently, medical care for voice problems has made use of a markedly expanded, comprehensive history that reflects new knowledge supporting the premise that there is more to the voice than simply the vocal folds. Virtually any body system may be responsible for voice complaints. In fact, problems outside the larynx often cause voice dysfunction in persons whose vocal folds appear fairly normal but function abnormally. These patients would have received no effective medical care for their voice problems just a few years ago.

WHAT IS HOARSENESS?

Most people with voice problems complain of hoarseness or laryngitis. A more detailed description of the problem (or the patient's chief complaints) is often helpful in identifying the cause. Hoarseness is a coarse, scratchy sound caused most commonly by abnormalities on the vibratory margin of the vocal fold. These may include swelling, roughness from inflammation, growths, scarring, or anything that interferes with symmetrical, periodic vocal fold vibration. Such abnormalities produce turbulence, which we perceive as hoarseness.

Breathiness is caused by abnormalities that keep the vocal folds from closing completely, including vocal fold paralysis, muscle weakness, cricoarytenoid joint injury or arthritis, vocal fold masses, or atrophy of the vocal fold tissues. These abnormalities permit air to escape when the vocal folds are supposed to be closed tightly. The air escape is perceived as breathiness.

Fatigue of the voice is the inability to continue to phonate for extended periods of time, with change in vocal quality.

Often it is caused by misuse of abdominal and neck musculature, or overuse (singing or speaking too loudly or too long). Vocal fatigue may be a sign of general tiredness or serious illnesses such as myasthenia gravis.

Volume disturbance may appear as inability to speak or sing loudly or inability to phonate softly. Most volume problems are secondary to intrinsic limitations of the voice or technical errors in voice production, although hormonal changes, aging, superior laryngeal nerve paresis, and neurologic disease are other causes.

Even nonsingers normally require only 10 to 30 minutes to warm up the voice. Prolonged warmup time, especially in the morning, is caused most often by reflux laryngitis. Tickling or choking during speech or singing is associated with laryngitis or voice abuse. Often a symptom of pathology of the vocal fold's leading edge, this symptom requires that voice use be avoided until vocal fold examination has been accomplished. Pain while vocalizing can indicate vocal fold lesions, laryngeal joint arthritis, infection, or gastric (stomach) acid irritation of the posterior portion of the larynx; however, it is much more commonly caused by voice abuse with excessive muscular activity in the neck, rather than acute pathology on the leading edge of a vocal fold, and it does not usually require immediate cessation of phonation pending medical examination.

WHAT IS INVOLVED IN A PHYSICAL EXAMINATION OF A PERSON WITH VOICE PROBLEMS?

Physical examination of a person with voice complaints involves a complete ear, nose, and throat assessment by an otolaryngologist and examination of other body systems. Subjective examination is supplemented by technologic aids that improve our ability to "see" the vocal mechanism, and allow quantification of aspects of its function. With phonation at middle C, the vocal folds come together and separate approximately 250 times per second. Strobovideolaryngoscopy uses a laryngeal microphone to trigger a strobe light that illuminates the vocal folds, allowing the examiner to assess them in slow motion. This technology allows visualization of small masses, vibratory asymmetries, adynamic segments caused by scar or early cancer, and other abnormalities that were simply missed under continuous light. The instruments typically found in a well-equipped clinical voice laboratory assess six categories of vocal function: vibratory, aerodynamic, phonatory, acoustic, electromyographic, and psychoacoustic. State-of-the-art analysis of vocal function is extremely helpful in diagnosis, therapy, and evaluation of progress during treatment of voice disorders (outcomes assessment).

Common Diagnoses and Treatments

After a thorough history has been obtained, and after physical examination and clinical voice laboratory analysis have been performed, it is usually possible for the physician to arrive at an accurate explanation for voice dysfunction. Treatment, of course, depends on the etiology. Fortunately, because technology has improved voice medicine, the need for laryngeal surgery has diminished. In a great many cases, voice disorders result from respiratory,

CURRENT DIAGNOSIS

- "Hoarseness" is a term used commonly to describe any voice abnormality. Dysphonia should be described more specifically because hoarseness, breathiness, voice fatigue, and other voice disturbances have diagnostic significance.
- Laryngopharyngeal reflux is associated commonly with voice disorders. This diagnosis is often missed because typical symptoms do not include heartburn or epigastric discomfort.
- Systemic diseases are reflected often as voice disturbances. Hormone imbalances typically cause voice changes.
- Sudden voice change necessitates prompt examination of the vocal folds. In addition to being caused by infectious laryngitis, sudden voice change may be a result of vocal fold hemorrhage, which may necessitate prompt prescription of voice rest, or to more serious problems including neoplasm.

 CURRENT THERAPY

- Vocal nodules should be treated with expert voice therapy. Approximately 90% resolve or become asymptomatic without surgery.
- Laryngopharyngeal reflux requires prolonged treatment with high-dose proton pump inhibitor therapy.
- Vocal fold hemorrhage and mucosa disruption should be treated with absolute voice rest (silence), but rarely for more than approximately 1 week.
- Treatment for dysphonia depends upon accurate diagnosis, which often requires strobovideolaryngoscopy, and in some cases, laboratory and imaging studies. However, dysphonia is a symptom, not a disorder, and the etiology should be determined accurately in all cases so that appropriate treatment can be rendered.

neurologic, gastrointestinal, psychologic, or endocrine causes, or from some other treatable medical etiology.

DOES AGE AFFECT THE VOICE?

Age affects the voice substantially, especially during childhood and older age. Children's voices are particularly fragile. Voice abuse during childhood may lead to problems that persist throughout a lifetime. Any child with unexplained or prolonged hoarseness should undergo prompt, expert medical evaluation performed by a laryngologist who specializes in voice care.

In geriatric patients, vocal unsteadiness, loss of range, and voice fatigue may be associated with typical physiologic aging changes, such as vocal fold atrophy. In routine speech, such vocal changes are the reason a person can be identified as old even over the telephone. With appropriate muscular conditioning of the body and voice, many of the characteristics associated with vocal aging can be eliminated, and a more youthful sound can be restored. Occasionally, surgery also may be useful.

DO ALLERGY AND POSTNASAL DRIP BOTHER THE VOICE?

Allergies and postnasal drip alter the viscosity of secretions and the patency of nasal airways, and have other effects that impair voice function. Many of the medicines used commonly to treat allergies (such as antihistamines) also have undesirable effects on the voice. If allergies are severe enough to cause persistent throat clearing, hoarseness, and other voice complaints, a comprehensive allergy evaluation and treatment by an allergy specialist is advisable. Postnasal drip, the sensation of having excessive secretions, may or may not be caused by allergy. Contrary to popular opinion, the condition usually involves secretions that are too thick rather than too abundant. If postnasal drip is not caused by allergy, it is usually managed best through hydration and by mucolytic agents such as guaifenesin (Mucinex). Reflux laryngitis can cause

symptoms very similar to those of postnasal drip, and this diagnosis should always be considered in persons who have the sensation of throat secretions, and in those who feel a lump in the throat or who clear their throat excessively.

WHAT IS THE EFFECT OF AN UPPER RESPIRATORY TRACT INFECTION WITHOUT LARYNGITIS?

Although mucosal irritation usually is diffuse, patients sometimes have marked nasal obstruction with little or no soreness of the throat and a normal voice. If the laryngeal examination shows no abnormality, a person with a head cold should be permitted to speak or sing, but advised not to try to duplicate his or her usual sound.

HOW ABOUT LARYNGITIS WITH SERIOUS VOCAL FOLD INJURY?

Serious vocal fold injuries, such as hemorrhage in the vocal folds and mucosal disruption (a tear), are contraindications to voice use. When these are observed, the therapeutic course of treatment includes strict voice rest (silence) in addition to correction of any underlying disease. Vocal fold hemorrhage is most common in premenstrual women who are using aspirin products or nonsteroidal medicines for cramps. Severe hemorrhage or mucosal scarring may result in permanent alterations in vocal fold vibratory function. In rare instances, surgical intervention may be necessary.

WHAT ABOUT LARYNGITIS WITHOUT SERIOUS VOCAL FOLD INJURY?

Mild to moderate edema and erythema of the vocal folds may result from infection or from noninfectious causes. In the absence of mucosal disruption or hemorrhage, these disorders are not absolute contraindications to voice use. If no pressing professional need for voice use exists, inflammatory conditions of the larynx are treated best with relative voice rest in addition to other modalities. However, in some instances speaking or singing may be permitted. The more good voice training a person has had, the safer it is to use the voice under adverse circumstances.

DOES VOICE REST HELP LARYNGITIS?

Voice rest (absolute or relative) is an important therapeutic consideration in any case of laryngitis. When no professional commitments are pressing, a short course (up to a few days) of absolute voice rest (silence) may be considered because it is the safest and most conservative therapeutic intervention. Absolute voice rest is necessary only for serious vocal fold injury such as hemorrhage or mucosal disruption. Even then, it is virtually never indicated for more than 7 to 10 days. Other patients with vocal problems should also be instructed to speak softly and as infrequently as possible, often at a slightly higher pitch than usual, and with a slightly breathy voice; to avoid excessive telephone use; and to speak with abdominal support as they would in singing. This is relative voice rest, and it is helpful in most cases. It should be noted that voice rest is used based on anecdotal evidence, and evidence-based studies to confirm or refute its efficacy have not been performed.

WHAT ARE THE HAZARDS OF LARYNGEAL TRAUMA?

The larynx can be injured easily during altercations and motor vehicle accidents. Blunt anterior neck trauma may result in laryngeal fracture, dislocation of the arytenoid cartilages, hemorrhage, and airway obstruction. Late consequences, such as narrowing of the airway, also may occur. Hoarseness or other changes in voice quality after neck trauma should call laryngeal trauma to mind, with the first priority being the safety of the airway. Prompt evaluation by visualization and radiologic imaging should be performed. In many cases, surgery is needed.

DO LUNG PROBLEMS CAUSE VOICE DISORDERS?

Respiratory problems are especially problematic to singers and other voice professionals, but they may cause voice problems in anyone. Respiratory support is essential to healthy voice production. Obstructive pulmonary disease is the most common culprit in voice dysfunction. Even mild obstructive lung disease can impair support enough to cause compensatory increased neck and tongue muscle tension and abusive voice use, capable of producing vocal nodules and other structural lesions. Treatment of the underlying pulmonary disease to restore effective support is essential to resolving the vocal problem. Treating asthma is rendered more difficult in professional voice users because of the need in some patients to avoid not only oral steroid inhalers but also any bronchodilator medications that produce even a mild tremor.

HOW ABOUT SMOKE AND POLLUTION?

Exposure to environmental irritants is a well-recognized cause of voice dysfunction. Smoke, dehydration, pollution, and allergens may produce hoarseness, frequent throat clearing, and voice fatigue. These problems can generally be eliminated by environmental modification, medication, or simply breathing through the nose rather than the mouth as the nose warms, humidifies, and filters incoming air.

The deleterious effects of tobacco smoke on the vocal folds have been known for many years. Smoking not only causes chronic irritation, but cancer as well.

In addition to pollution-related voice disorders that may affect factory workers and the general population, singers, actors, and other performers may be exposed to a great many environmental irritants and pollutants and are at special risk for developing environmentally induced dysphonias. Some of these irritants and pollutants are encountered by almost all performers at some time during their careers. For example, theatrical halls are commonly not cleaned adequately. Consequently, actors, singers, dancers, and others are exposed to dust and mold in high concentrations during rehearsals and performances. These conditions are aggravated if set construction is carried out coincident with rehearsals. Sawdust (often from wood treated with chemicals), fumes from oil-based paints, and other noxious substances are generated, frequently only a few feet from performers. These exposures may result in mucosal and respiratory changes that affect voice performance adversely, and even may aggravate or cause health problems such as acute allergic episodes, asthma, and cough.

Performers may be exposed to even greater hazards if they work around artificial fogs and smokes, or around pyrotechnic effects. Artificial fogs and smokes may be created using a variety of substances, including glycol-based products, oil-based products, organic chemicals, and inorganic chemicals. Often the situation is aggravated by the addition of dyes or fragrances that are included for theatrical effect. Guidelines regarding use of artificially created smokes and fogs are controversial. Unfortunately, some of the substances still in common use contain materials that are toxic and can create substantial health problems. Pyrotechnic effects may be similarly troublesome. The explosives and colorants used to create pyrotechnic effects are potentially hazardous and include substances such as toxic metals (mercury and lead) and known carcinogens.

CAN FOODS OR DRUGS AFFECT THE VOICE?

The use of various foods and drugs also may affect the voice. Some medications may even permanently ruin a voice, especially androgenic hormones, such as those given to women with endometriosis. Similar problems occur with use of anabolic steroids (also male hormones) that are used for postmenopausal loss of libido; these drugs are also used illicitly by body builders. More common drugs, including antihistamines, oral steroid inhalers, and many neurologic, psychologic, and respiratory medications, also have deleterious vocal effects. Some foods may also be responsible for voice complaints in people with normal vocal folds. Milk products are particularly troublesome to some people because the casein they contain increases and thickens mucosal secretions.

WHAT ABOUT HORMONES?

Endocrine problems have marked vocal effects, many by causing accumulation of fluid in the superficial layer of the lamina propria, altering the vibratory characteristics. Mild hypothyroidism typically causes a muffled sound, slight loss of range, and vocal sluggishness. Similar findings may be seen in pregnancy, during use of oral contraceptives (in approximately 5% of women), for a few days before menses, and at the time of ovulation. However, male hormones may actually cause laryngeal growth in women (as they do in boys at the time of puberty), permanently altering laryngeal structure and sound.

DO STOMACH PROBLEMS OR HIATAL HERNIA AFFECT THE VOICE?

Gastrointestinal disorders commonly cause voice complaints. In gastroesophageal reflux laryngitis, stomach acid refluxes into the throat, allowing droplets of the irritating gastric juices to come in contact with the vocal folds, and even to be aspirated into the lungs. Reflux can occur with or without a hiatal hernia. Common symptoms are hoarseness, especially in the morning, prolonged vocal warmup time, bad breath, sensation of a lump in the throat, chronic sore throat, cough, and a dry or "coated" mouth. Typical heartburn is frequently absent. Over time, uncontrolled reflux may cause cancer of the esophagus and larynx. Thus this condition should be treated conscientiously.

DOES ANXIETY HAVE ANYTHING TO DO WITH THE VOICE?

When the principal cause of vocal dysfunction is anxiety, the physician often can accomplish much by assuring the patient that no organic difficulty is present and by stating the diagnosis of anxiety reaction. Tranquilizers and sedatives are rarely necessary and are undesirable because they may interfere with fine motor control, affecting voice adversely. Recently, β-adrenergic blocking\agents such as propranolol hydrochloride (e.g., Inderal) have achieved some popularity in the treatment of preperformance anxiety in singers and instrumentalists. β-Blockers should not be used routinely for voice disorders and preperformance anxiety. If anxiety or other psychological factors are the cause of a voice disorder, their treatment by a psychologist or psychiatrist with special interest and training in arts medicine is extremely helpful. This therapy should occur in conjunction with voice therapy.

CAN ABUSING THE VOICE CREATE PROBLEMS?

Voice abuse through technical dysfunction is an extremely common source of hoarseness, vocal weakness, pain, and other complaints. It is seen routinely in vocally untrained singers, teachers, clergy, politicians, salespeople, secretaries, and others. In some cases, voice abuse can even create structural problems such as vocal nodules, cysts, and polyps. Now that the components of voice function are better understood, techniques have been developed to rehabilitate and train the voice for speech and singing. Voice therapy with a certified, licensed, speech-language pathologist who specializes in voice is invaluable.

WHAT ARE VOCAL NODULES?

Small, callus-like bumps on the vocal folds called nodules are caused by voice abuse. Occasionally, laryngoscopy reveals asymptomatic vocal nodules that do not appear to interfere with voice production; in such cases, the nodules need not be treated. However, in most cases, nodules are associated with hoarseness, breathiness, loss of range, and vocal fatigue. Voice therapy always should be tried as the initial therapeutic modality and often cures the majority of patients, even if the nodules look firm and have been present for many months or years. Even in those who eventually need surgical excision of the nodules, preoperative voice therapy is essential to prevent recurrence.

WHAT ARE VOCAL FOLD CYSTS?

Submucosal cysts of the vocal folds are usually also traumatic lesions that result from blockage of a mucus gland duct, although they may also occur for other reasons and may even be present at birth. They often cause contact swelling on the opposite vocal fold and are usually misdiagnosed initially as nodules. Often, they can be differentiated from nodules by strobovideolaryngoscopy revealing a mass that is obviously fluid-filled. They require voice therapy and usually surgery.

WHAT ARE VOCAL FOLD POLYPS?

These lesions are generally the result of trauma. In some cases, even sizable polyps resolve with relative voice rest, voice therapy, and a few weeks of low-dose corticosteroid therapy. However, many require surgical removal. If unilateral polyps are not treated, they may produce contact injury on the contralateral vocal fold. Voice therapy should be used.

WHAT ABOUT VOCAL FOLD PARALYSIS?

Paralysis or paresis may involve one or both vocal folds, and one or both nerves to each vocal fold. When paralysis/paresis is limited to the superior laryngeal nerve, the patient loses his or her ability to control longitudinal tension (stretch) in the vocal fold. Although superior laryngeal nerve paresis involves only one muscle (cricothyroid), the problem is difficult to overcome. The vocal fold sags at a lower level than normal, and the patient notices difficulty controlling pitch, controlling sustained tones, and projecting the voice. The recurrent laryngeal nerve controls all the other intrinsic laryngeal muscles. When it is injured, the vocal fold cannot move toward or away from the midline, although longitudinal tension is preserved and the vocal fold remains at its appropriate vertical level if the superior laryngeal nerve is not paretic. Compensation often occurs spontaneously during the first 6 to 12 months after paralysis, with the paralyzed vocal fold moving closer to the midline. At least 6 months (and preferably 12 months) of observation are needed prior to surgical intervention, unless it is absolutely certain that the nerve has been cut and destroyed, because spontaneous recovery of neuromuscular function is common. Laryngeal electromyography (EMG) is helpful in establishing the diagnosis and prognosis. Vocal fold paralysis should be treated initially with voice therapy. If voice therapy fails, vocal fold motion remains impaired, and voice quality or ability to cough or swallow normally is unsatisfactory to the patient; surgical treatments are generally quite satisfactory.

WHAT IS SPASMODIC DYSPHONIA?

Spasmodic (or "spastic") dysphonia is a diagnosis given to patients with specific kinds of voice interruptions. These patients may have a variety of diseases that produce the same vocal result, which is termed a laryngeal dystonia. There are also many interruptions in vocal fluency that are incorrectly diagnosed as spasmodic dysphonia. This error should be avoided because different types of dysphonia require different evaluations and treatments, and carry different prognostic implications. Spasmodic dysphonia is subclassified into adductor and abductor types.

ARE THERE OTHER NEUROLOGIC VOICE DISORDERS?

Many other neurologic problems commonly cause voice abnormalities, including myasthenia gravis, Parkinson's disease, essential tremor, and numerous other disorders. In some cases, voice abnormalities are the first symptoms of a systemic problem.

WHAT ABOUT CANCER OF THE LARYNX?

Cancers of the larynx are common and are usually associated with smoking, although cancers also occur occasionally in nonsmokers, especially in persons with laryngopharyngeal reflux. Persistent hoarseness is one of the most common symptoms. Laryngeal cancers may also present with throat pain or referred ear pain. If diagnosed early, these cancers respond to therapy particularly well and often are curable. Treatment usually requires radiation, surgery, or a combination of the two modalities. It is usually possible to preserve or restore voice, especially if the cancer is detected early.

WHAT SHOULD BE CONSIDERED WHEN VOICE SURGERY IS CONTEMPLATED?

Principles

Scar tissue occurs in response to trauma, including surgery. If scar tissue replaces the normal anatomic layers, the vocal fold becomes stiff and adynamic (nonvibrating). This results in asymmetrical, irregular vibration with air turbulence that we hear as hoarseness, or it results in microscopically incomplete vocal fold closure, allowing air to escape, which makes the voice sound breathy. Such vocal folds may look normal on traditional examination, but can be seen as abnormal under stroboscopic light. Conveniently, most benign pathology (e.g., nodules, polyps, or cysts) is superficial. Consequently, surgical techniques have been developed to permit removal of lesions from the epithelium or superficial layer of the lamina propria without disruption of the intermediate or deeper layers in most cases, thus reducing the risk of scar formation. All of these delicate microsurgical techniques are commonly referred to as phonomicrosurgery. Vocal fold "stripping" has not been an acceptable technique for more than a decade. Otolaryngologists with training in the new subspecialty of laryngology should be sought to provide patients with optimal results.

Precautions

A detailed discussion of laryngeal surgery is beyond the scope of this article. However, a few points are worthy of special emphasis. Surgery for vocal nodules should be avoided whenever possible and should almost never be performed without an adequate trial of expert voice therapy, including patient compliance with therapeutic suggestions. In most cases, a minimum of 6 to 12 weeks of observation should be allowed while the patient is using therapeutically modified voice techniques under the supervision of a certified speech-language pathologist and possibly a singing or acting voice teacher. Proper voice use rather than voice rest (silence) is the correct therapy.

WHAT CAN BE DONE ABOUT A VOICE THAT IS WORSE AFTER SURGERY?

Too often, the physician is confronted with a desperate patient whose voice has been "ruined" by vocal fold surgery, recurrent or superior laryngeal nerve paralysis, trauma, or some other tragedy. Occasionally, the cause is as simple as a recently dislocated arytenoid cartilage that can be reduced. However, if the problem is an adynamic segment, decreased bulk and pliability of one vocal fold after "stripping," bowing caused by superior laryngeal nerve paralysis, or some other serious complication in a mobile vocal fold, great expertise is needed. Voice therapy is nearly always helpful in optimizing compensatory strategies and minimizing fatigue, but it usually will not restore the patient's normal voice. None of the available surgical procedures for these conditions is consistently effective in restoring normal voice, although improvements are obtained routinely. Tertiary subspecialty consultation should be obtained for such patients.

ARE THERE OTHER NEW DEVELOPMENTS IN SURGICAL TECHNIQUE?

New techniques of external laryngeal surgery to modify the laryngeal skeleton have become extremely useful in treatment of vocal fold paralysis, a common consequence of viral infection, surgery, and cancer. Until the late 1980s, vocal fold paralysis was managed most often by endoscopic injection of polytef (Teflon) into the tissues adjacent to the paralyzed vocal fold. This pushed the paralyzed side toward the midline, allowing the normal vocal fold to meet it, thus permitting glottic closure and improving voice. Although polytef is relatively inert, granulomatous reactions to the foreign body are not uncommon, and stiffness of the vocal fold edge frequently impairs voice quality. Polytef infiltrated into tissues is hard to remove if the results are unsatisfactory, and injection of it has been replaced by autologous fat or fascia injection, hydroxyapatite, or thyroplasty, which are better techniques. Thyroplasty is a technique in which a window is cut in the laryngeal skeleton, and tissues are depressed inward and held in place with a silicone block or Gore-Tex strip. This pushes the vocal fold toward the midline fairly reversibly, without injecting a foreign body into the tissues.

WHAT ABOUT SINGERS, ACTORS, AND OTHER VOICE PROFESSIONALS?

Professional singers, actors, announcers, politicians, and others put "Olympic" demands on their voices. These patients are often best managed by subspecialists familiar with the latest concepts in professional voice care.

HOW CAN THE VOICE BE KEPT HEALTHY?

Preventive medicine is always the best medicine. The more people understand about their voices, the more they will appreciate their importance and delicacy. Education helps us understand how to protect the voice, train and develop it to handle our individual vocal demands, and keep it healthy. Even a little bit of expert voice training can make a big difference. Avoidance of abuses, especially smoking, is paramount. If voice problems occur, expert medical care should be sought promptly. Interdisciplinary collaboration among family physicians, internists, laryngologists, speech-language pathologists, singing teachers, acting teachers, many other professionals, and especially voice users themselves, has revolutionized voice care since the early 1980s. Technologic advances, scientific revelations, and new medical techniques inspired originally by interest in treating professional opera singers have brought a new level of expertise and concern to the medical profession and improved dramatically the level of care available for all patients with voice dysfunction.

REFERENCES

Rosen DC, Sataloff RT: Psychology of Voice Disorders. San Diego, Calif, Singular Publishing, 1997.

Sataloff RT: Professional Voice: The Science and Art of Clinical Care, 3rd ed. San Diego, Calif, Plural Publishing, 2005.

Sataloff RT, Brandfonbrener A, Lederman R (eds): Performing Arts Medicine, 2nd ed. San Diego, Calif, Singular Publishing, 1998.

Sataloff RT, Castell DO, Katz PO, Sataloff DM: Reflux Laryngitis, 3rd ed. San Diego, Calif, Plural Publishing, 2006.

Sataloff RT, Mandel S, Heman-Ackah YD, et al.: Laryngeal Electromyography, 2nd ed. San Diego, Calif, Plural Publishing, 2006.

Sataloff RT, Rubin J, Korovin G: Diagnosis and Treatment of Voice Disorders, 3rd ed. San Diego, Calif, Plural Publishing, 2006.

Streptococcal Pharyngitis

Method of
John Brusch, MD

The pharyngitis syndrome (sore throat) is characterized primarily by sore throat with associated fever and myalgias; occasionally with cough. It is responsible for 10% of outpatient visits and an estimated 50% of ambulatory care antibiotic usage. Of adult patients who receive treatment for a sore throat, 73% receive antibiotic treatment when at least 50% of these cases are of viral etiology. The increase in the overall resistance to antibiotics of the oral pharyngeal flora is due, in great part, to this overprescribing of antimicrobial agents. A variety of bacteria and viruses may produce this syndrome. Group A β-hemolytic streptococci (GABHS) is the most common bacterial cause of acute pharyngitis. The diagnosis of "strep throat" has long been a concern of the physician because of its suppurative and nonsuppurative complications. There is such a great deal of overlap in their clinical presentations that the clinician must rely on the laboratory to diagnose GABHS from both other bacteria and viruses as the cause of the sore throat of his/her patient. The correct interpretation of the available diagnostic tests adds to the clinician's burden. For more than 50 years, the appropriate choice of antibiotic and duration of treatment of GABHS pharyngitis has been established. The real challenge of treating streptococcal pharyngitis lies not in the selection of treatment, but in deciding when to institute antibiotic therapy.

Microbiology

Most sore throats are viral in origin. GABHS is responsible for 10% of cases of adult pharyngitis. Its importance lies in the fact that its treatment can prevent the development of rheumatic fever and local complications. Gonorrheal pharyngitis primarily arises from oral sex, but may be a complication of disseminated gonorrhea. It is usually asymptomatic but may produce a typical sore throat. *Yersinia* pharyngitis, like that of groups C and G streptococci, is foodborne. In United States, *Corynebacterium diphtheriae* pharyngitis occurs primarily among the homeless often in outbreaks. It may not be associated with any systemic symptoms. *Arcanobacterium haemolyticum* is a true mimic of GABHS pharyngitis. This organism is more common in Scandinavia and in the United Kingdom than in other parts of the world. It produces a scarlatiniform rash involving the trunk and extremities (50% of cases) with a vesicular component. Occasionally a membranous exudate, resembling that of diphtheria, occurs. Anaerobic oral pharyngeal overgrowth can produce a severe sore throat (Plaut-Vincent or fusospirochetal angina). It is caused by an anaerobic, nonsporulating gram-negative rod. Infection with this organism classically results in an ulceration of the throat or tonsils that is covered by a grayish membrane. Widespread necrosis of surrounding tissue and sepsis may ensue. The presence of fusospirochetal angina may be a clue to a severe leukopenic state in the host. Cases of *Chlamydia pneumoniae* and *Mycoplasma pneumoniae* sore throat are usually seen with concurrent lung infection. The clinical courses may be quite prolonged. Unresponsiveness to the penicillins provides a useful clue to their presence. Many species of bacteria are commonly cultured from the upper airway. *Staphylococcus aureus*, *Streptococcus pneumoniae*, and *Haemophilus influenzae* are part of the normal pharyngeal flora, especially during the winter. They seldom cause pharyngitis. Their isolation from symptomatic individuals usually represents colonization.

Epstein-Barr virus (EBV) infections of the throat are marked by an exudate pharyngitis with palatal petechiae and a gelatinous uvula. In patients older than 30 years of age, only 25% of EBV pharyngitis presents with the classic picture of diffuse cervical adenopathy, diffuse adenopathy, lymphocytosis, and splenomegaly. These patients often develop a diffuse scarlatiniform rash approximately 5 days into a course of ampicillin or other β-lactam antibiotics ("fifth-day rash"). The pharyngitis of *Cytomegalovirus* and herpesvirus type 6 may present in similar fashion to that of EBV without the fifth-day rash. Primary human immunodeficiency virus (HIV) infection may cause a sore throat that is characterized by a nonexudate pharyngitis fever, diffuse lymphadenopathy, and a

CURRENT DIAGNOSIS

Organism	% of Cases	Comments
Viral organisms	Total = 40%	Often associated with coryza, laryngitis, and diarrhea
Rhinovirus	20%	
Coronavirus	5%	
Herpes simplex	2%	
Retroviruses	?%	Present in 70% of cases of primary HIV infection
Primary Epstein-Barr	?%	Only 25% exhibit other manifestations of mononucleosis viral infection
Coxsackievirus	?%	Concurrent findings of herpangina and hand, foot, and mouth disease
Adenovirus	?%	Concurrent conjunctivitis
Bacterial organisms	Total = ?%	
GABHS	30%-50% in children; 10% in adults	1%-5% of adults are carriers of GABHS
Groups C, G streptococci	10%	Often foodborne
Nonstreptococcal bacteria	10%	
Neisseria gonorrhoeae	1%	May be the only manifestation of gonorrhea; associated with oral sex
Yersinia enterocolitica	?%	Often foodborne
Corynebacterium diphtheriae	?%	Seen in the homeless; often pharyngitis is the only manifestation
Arcanobacterium hemolyticum	0.4%	Causes a diffuse scarlatiniform rash; it is indistinguishable from GABHS pharyngitis

Abbreviations: GABHS, group A β-hemolytic streptococci.

maculopapular rash within 1 to 5 weeks of acquisition. Acute retroviral infection is truly a "cannot miss" diagnosis.

Epidemiology

GABHS pharyngitis primarily affects individuals 5 to 15 years of age. Up to 20% of these are carriers of GABHS. Infection is most commonly spread from human to human by large airborne droplets. The cold weather of winter and early spring produces the highest attack rates as a consequence of the indoor crowding that occurs during these seasons. Symptomatic patients, closeness of contact, and virulent strains are factors that promote spread of the disease. Transmission by both food and water is well documented.

During the acute phase of the illness, M-type streptococci are frequently isolated from the nares and oropharynx. Colonization of the upper airway with these strains can last for several months. Gradually, the streptococci lose their M proteins and with this loss their infectivity. Antibody to the M protein confers type-specific immunity to the host. The carrier state results from the ability of particular strains to penetrate the interior of respiratory epithelial cells. In this location, GABHS is protected from type-specific M protein antibody, from the suppressive effects of the host's oral flora, and from the actions of many types of antibiotics. In the developed world, both suppurative and nonsuppurative complications of GABHS pharyngitis have greatly lessened. This is a result of an overall improvement in living conditions (less crowding) and to the disappearance of M protein from many isolates of GABHS. This decreased pathogenicity has to be factored into any treatment strategy for "strep throat." However, the inner cities of the United States still provide conditions

that are conducive to the development of poststreptococcal rheumatic fever.

Clinical Manifestations

Fever (>100.4°F [38°C]) and sore throat are invariably present in GABHS pharyngitis. The presence of rhinitis, laryngitis, diarrhea, conjunctivitis and bronchitis are inconsistent with this diagnosis and are more characteristic of a viral etiology. Examination reveals pharyngeal erythema or exudative pharyngitis, with or without palatal petechiae, that is associated with significant anterior cervical adenopathy. Untreated, 75% of patients defervesce within 3 days unless there is a local suppurative complication. This may include peritonsillar abscess, suppurative adenitis, and otitis media. Over a few more days, the individual's other signs and symptoms resolve. In the absence of antibiotic therapy, most patients carry streptococci for many months. With appropriate treatment, the carrier state is reduced to between 6% and 29% of patients.

Diagnosis

Although the diagnosis of GABHS pharyngitis cannot be based solely on clinical signs and symptoms, they have been quite useful in establishing the likelihood of streptococcal infection; especially in adults with an extremely low incidence of "strep throat." Determining the probability of GABHS pharyngitis is essential for establishing indications for diagnostic testing, as well as for interpreting the results of these tests. Several such scoring systems stratifying the importance of physical findings and symptoms have been developed. All are quite similar and include the presence of (a) fever higher than 99.9°F (37.7°C), (b) tonsillar exudate, and (c) anterior cervical adenopathy, and (d) absence of cough. The presence of all four makes the probability of GABHS 56%. When three conditions exist, the likelihood decreases to 32% and plummets to 15% and 6% when there are two and one positive indicators, respectively. If there are no positive indicators, the probability of a positive culture is less than 2.5%. At this level of risk, diagnostic testing is usually not required.

The throat culture remains the diagnostic gold standard. The throat should be swabbed under direct visualization in repeated sweeps extending from each tonsillar fossa and involving the posterior pharynx but avoiding any other area of the mouth. The swabs should be immediately cultured on sheep blood agar incubated in 10% CO_2. If there is no growth at 24 hours, the plate is re-incubated for another 24 hours. Sampling errors may cause false negatives in 9% to 12% of patients. Rarely, GABHS will not produce β hemolysis. False positives may be due to β hemolysis produced by non-GABHS organisms. The use of the bacitracin disk controls for this by inhibiting GABHS but not other types of β hemolytic flora. The specificity of the throat culture ranges from 95% to 99% with 88% to 91% sensitivity. When obtained in physicians' offices, the throat cultures are much less sensitive (<75%). The major disadvantage of the throat culture is the diagnostic delay. In adults, this may not be all that significant (see below).

Rapid antigen detection tests (RADTs) were developed to provide useful probability information at the time of the patient's visit. RADTs employ either enzyme or acid techniques to extract streptococcal antigen from the swabs, which is then measured by latex agglutination, coagglutination, or enzyme-linked immunosorbent assay (ELISA) techniques. Overall, the sensitivity of RADTs ranges from 77% to 95%. The higher range of values is associated with the newer optical immunoassay technique, which may approach the sensitivity of a well-performed throat culture. The specificity of the RADT is as high as that of the throat culture. Because of its low sensitivity, a negative RADT in any child or adolescent should be followed by a throat culture. In adults, this approach is not thought to be necessary because of the low incidence of GABHS pharyngitis and rheumatic fever in this population. However, when only an RADT is performed, the opportunity to detect a treatable non-GABHS cause of bacterial pharyngitis is lost.

Both throat culture and RADT are unable to distinguish streptococcal carriers from those whose symptoms are caused by GABHS and not by another organism. Of symptomatic adult patients with positive diagnostic tests, 30% to 50% are not infected with GABHS. Measurement of antibody titers against streptolysin O (ASL-O) or other streptococcal products is the most specific way to diagnose GABHS pharyngitis. Their levels require 2 to 4 weeks to peak and thus are not available to the clinician in a timely fashion.

Treatment

In the developed world, the reasons why we treat GABHS pharyngitis have markedly changed since the landmark

CURRENT THERAPY

- Empirically treat all patients with 3 or more clinical predictors of GABHS pharyngitis.
- Optimal treatment still remains 10 days of oral penicillin or one injection of Bicillin.
- Avoid 3-day treatment regimens.
- Avoid trimethoprim-sulfamethoxazole and the tetracyclines (doxycycline). They have little effect on eradicating GABHS.
- Always keep in mind that culture of GABHS from an adult may represent a carrier state and that the pharyngitis is produced by another organism.
- Do not reculture at the end of clinically successful therapy unless the patient has an above-average risk for developing rheumatic fever.
- Always keep in mind the possibility of primary HIV infection as the cause of the pharyngitis.
- Do not culture family members unless there is an epidemic situation of or recurrence of proven GABHS pharyngitis in the family.
- Do not give prophylactic antibiotics to exposed family members.

studies that demonstrated such a significant drop in the incidence of poststreptococcal rheumatic fever. This is attributable to the change in epidemiology of the streptococcus (Table 1). In the early days of antimicrobial therapy, it was established that 10 days of treatment with oral penicillin or one intramuscular injection of penicillin G was effective in preventing rheumatic fever if begun within 5 to 9 days after the onset of clinical symptoms of GABHS pharyngitis. It was also demonstrated that for those

TABLE 1 Reasons for Treating Streptococcal Pharyngitis

Item	Rationale
Preventing rheumatic fever	Rheumatic fever occurs in 2.1% of untreated patients and in 0.3% of treated patients
Preventing streptococcal glomerulonephritis	No evidence that treatment of streptococcal pharyngitis is effective
Preventing scarlet fever	Extremely rare in the antibiotic era
Reducing suppurative complications	They accounted for 13% of hospitalizations in the pre-antibiotic era; currently quite unusual
Reducing duration and severity of disease	Antibiotics have some mild effect when started early
Reducing spread of GABHS	Quite effective in preventing spread; patients become noncontagious after 24 hours of treatment

Abbreviation: GABHS, group A β-hemolytic streptococci.

TABLE 2 Management Strategies for GABHS Pharyngitis

Number of Positive Features	Action
0	No culture; no treatment
1	Culture; treat positive cultures
2	Culture; treat positive cultures
3	No culture or treatment
4	No culture or treatment

Abbreviation: GABHS, group A β-hemolytic streptococci.

patients in whom penicillin failed to eradicate GABHS, the risk of developing rheumatic fever was the same as that of an untreated patient. Table 2 presents the clinical indications for obtaining a throat culture/RADT and beginning antibiotic treatment. I prefer a culture over RADT as it is generally more sensitive and detects other possible pathogens. Its 1- to 2-day delay in receiving final results has little clinical significance. It was recently demonstrated that culture is the most effective and least expensive approach when the prevalence of GABHS pharyngitis is 10% or less. Empirical antibiotic treatment was found to be neither the most clinically useful nor cost-effective strategy for any degree of risk. This stepped approach holds true only for adults in the developed world who have no history of rheumatic fever, immunosuppression, or chronic pharyngitis. It is not applicable during an epidemic of GABHS/rheumatic fever. Eradication of the carrier state is not an indication for treatment unless the patient has a history of rheumatic fever. It is unnecessary to do sensitivity testing of GABHS for any of the β-lactam antibiotics. GABHS remains quite sensitive to penicillin. The administration of oral penicillin for 10 days achieves almost 100% effectiveness in eradicating GABHS. In those who have been treated for 7 days or 5 days, the cure rate decreases to 89% and 50%, respectively.

In penicillin-allergic patients, erythromycin has traditionally been the alternative drug of choice. In the United States, 4% to 5% of isolates are resistant to erythromycin. Resistance to erythromycin is significantly higher in those countries where it is more commonly used as a first-line drug. The other macrolides hold no therapeutic advantage over erythromycin, but are much better tolerated, especially as regards the gastrointestinal tract. In my opinion, clindamycin (Cleocin) rarely should be used because of the significant risk of developing *Clostridium difficile* colitis. The most desirable treatment regimen remains 10 days of

TABLE 3 Current Therapy

Drug	Dose	Duration of Therapy
Penicillin V (Pen-Vee K)	1000 mg bid,[3] 25 mg/kg bid*	10 d
Benzathine penicillin (Bicillin)	1.2 million U, 2500 U/kg*	1 dose
Cephalexin (Keflex)	500 mg bid, 25 mg/kg bid	10 d
Cefadroxil (Duricef)	1 g/d, 30 mg/kg/d*	5 d[†]
Cefuroxime (Ceftin)	250 mg bid, 10 mg/kg bid*	5 d[†]
Amoxicillin-clavulanate (Augmentin)[‡,1]	250 mg tid, 15 mg/kg tid*	10 d
Azithromycin (Zithromax)	500 mg first day, then 250 mg qd; 12 mg/kg qd	5 d[†]
Clarithromycin (Biaxin)	500 mg bid, 8 mg/kg bid*	10 d

*For children who weigh less than 40 kg (88 lb).
[†]Only azithromycin is approved by the Food and Drug Administration for less than 10 days of therapy.
[‡]Useful for recurrent GABHS pharyngitis or treatment of the carrier state if necessary.
[1]Not FDA approved for this indication.
[3]Exceeds dosage recommended by the manufacturer.
Abbreviation: GABHS, group A β-hemolytic streptococci.

TABLE 4 Reasons for Apparent Recurrent GABHS Pharyngitis

Cause	Solution
Not truly a GABHS pharyngitis (most likely to be of viral origin)	Document infection by culture or RADT (see text)
Poor compliance (most frequent cause of recurrence)	Choose 5-day antibiotic regimen or intramuscular benzathine penicillin
Repeated exposure to GABHS, especially in families (ping-pong phenomenon)	Culture samples from all family members and treat culture-positive individuals
Decreased host immunity to GABHS because of initiation of antibiotic therapy within 48 hours of the onset of symptoms	Delay antibiotic treatment for 48 hours; this does not increase the risk for suppurative or nonsuppurative complications
Coexistence of β lactamase-producing bacteria (becoming a more common problem)	Use a β lactamase-resistant antibiotic (cephalosporin or amoxicillin-clavulanate)
Patient is carrier for GABHS and pharyngitis is caused by another organism, usually a virus	Confirm by positive culture or RADT in asymptomatic period; also obtain ASL-O titer for weeks after infection (should not show rise in the carrier state); generally no need to treat; if necessary to intervene, use a macrolide or amoxicillin-clavulanate
Deep-seated GABHS infection (i.e., tonsillar crypts)	Use intraleukocytic-active antibiotic such as a quinolone or a macrolide
Inadequate dose of penicillin	Increase dose or use better-absorbed form (amoxicillin)

Abbreviations: ASL-O, antistreptolysin O; GABHS, group A β-hemolytic streptococci; RADT, rapid antigen detection test.

penicillin therapy. If compliance is in doubt, one dose of Bicillin is next best. The other β-lactams offer little advantage except for 5-day courses. There is some indication that they may have a somewhat higher clinical and bacteriologic success rate because of their resistance to breakdown by penicillinase-producing oral pharyngeal flora. They have as yet not stood the test of time. Three-day regimens should be avoided because of unacceptably high rates of failure and recurrence. More complete discussions of antibiotic therapy of GABHS pharyngitis are available in the referenced sources (Table 3).

Recurrence of GABHS has increased in the last 20 years from 9% of cases to greater than 30% currently. This has been paralleled by a slight decline in the bacteriologic and clinical success rates, currently 84% and 89%, respectively. Table 4 presents several possible reasons for these trends.

After a successful clinical result, there is no need to repeat the throat culture unless during an outbreak of rheumatic fever or in an individual who has already been stricken by the disease. In the antibiotic era, tonsillectomy for preventing relapse or recurrence is rarely necessary.

REFERENCES

Bisno AL: Acute pharyngitis. N Engl J Med 2001;344:205.
Bisno JL, Gerber MA, Gwaltney JM, et al: IDSA practice guidelines for the diagnosis and management of group A streptococcal pharyngitis. Clin Infect Dis 2002;35:113.
Gerber MA, Shulman ST: Rapid diagnosis of pharyngitis caused by group A streptococci. Clin Microbiol Rev 2004;17:571.
Komaroff AL: Pharyngitis coryza and related infections in adults. In: Branch WT Jr (ed): Office Practice of Medicine. Philadelphia, WB Saunders, 2003, p. 153.
Stollerman GH: Global changes in group A streptococcal diseases and strategies for their prevention. Adv Intern Med 1982;27:373.

The Respiratory System

Acute Respiratory Failure

Method of
William Henderson, MD, and Sean Keenan, MD

The maintenance of normal respiration requires adequate oxygen and carbon dioxide (CO_2) exchange at the alveolar-capillary interface. For this to occur, there must be adequate minute ventilation, perfusion to capillaries, and appropriate delivery and distribution of gas within the lungs. Failure to properly regulate any of these facets of normal respiration will lead to respiratory failure and, if uncorrected, death.

Respiratory failure is characterized by a failure of oxygenation or ventilation. Therefore, acute respiratory failure is commonly divided into hypoxemic and hypercapnic etiologies.

Causes of Hypoxic Respiratory Failure

HYPOVENTILATION

Hypoventilation occurs when there is a central decrease in the drive to breathe, most commonly secondary to medications (e.g., morphine, benzodiazepines). As minute ventilation drops, increased alveolar CO_2 displaces oxygen, decreasing the oxygen available for capillary uptake. This occurs because the combined partial pressures of all of the gases within an alveolus must equal atmospheric pressure.

VENTILATION-PERFUSION MISMATCH

Ventilation-perfusion mismatch is caused by imperfect matching of ventilated and perfused lung units, usually secondary to alveolar injury, infection, or fluid.

SHUNTS

Shunts may be intracardiac or intrapulmonary. Intracardiac shunts are usually through a patent foramen ovale, but atrial and ventricular septal defects are occasionally seen. Intrapulmonary shunting occurs when blood flows past unventilated alveoli. Whatever the etiology of the shunt, it can be differentiated from ventilation-perfusion mismatching, because it is refractory to increasing alveolar oxygen tension (the application of supplemental oxygen does not relieve the hypoxemia).

IMPAIRMENT OF DIFFUSION

Impairment of diffusion is caused by short red blood cell transit time through the pulmonary vasculature or because of thickening of the endothelial barrier in the lungs. Diffusion impairment rarely causes hypoxia at rest but can cause hypoxia during exercise.

DECREASED INSPIRED OXYGEN CONCENTRATION

Decreased inspired oxygen concentration, whether because of high altitude or the presence of other gases, decreases alveolar oxygen tension.

Most patients with hypoxic respiratory failure have a right-to-left intrapulmonary shunt with some ventilation-perfusion mismatch.

Hypercapnic Respiratory Failure

Arterial CO_2 concentrations are inversely proportional to alveolar minute ventilation and are determined by tissue CO_2 production and alveolar elimination. Alveolar minute ventilation can be impaired in two ways. First, total minute ventilation can be decreased by extrapulmonary diseases; and second, dead space ventilation may be increased because of lung disease. Dead space ventilation is defined as ventilation that is not delivered to alveoli; in other words it is the ventilation to portions of the airway, such as the trachea, bronchi, and unperfused alveoli, that are not involved in gas exchange.

Primary pulmonary diseases are the most common causes of hypercapnic respiratory failure and are the single greatest cause of admission to the intensive care unit.

Clinical Presentation

Although dyspnea is the most common symptom associated with acute respiratory failure, the presentation to some degree depends on the precipitating problem. Patients who develop acute hypoxemic respiratory failure will usually have a clear recent history that points to a precipitating cause, such as trauma, pneumonia, sepsis, or pulmonary embolism. Typically, these patients demonstrate significant distress, with tachypnea and agitation as prominent symptoms. Physical examination may reveal signs consistent with the inciting disease, and chest examination will often reveal inspiratory crackles and decreased air entry in affected lung portions.

Patients with predominantly hypercapnic respiratory failure will also exhibit signs and symptoms consistent with the precipitating disease. Patients with recent opioid or benzodiazepine use as a cause of hypoventilation may exhibit a clear troxidone. Those with neuromuscular diseases will typically have a past medical history that points to the cause of their respiratory failure. Most patients with an exacerbation of chronic obstructive respiratory disease (COPD) or of asthma will have a medical history that points to these diseases, and will typically have a recent history that is significant for a gradual and steady worsening of their bronchospastic symptoms. Many of these patients will describe steady and increasing use of bronchodilators over the several days prior to presentation. Physical examination in hypercarbic respiratory failure patients is often helpful in narrowing the differential diagnosis. Patients with a central or toxicologic cause of hypercarbic respiratory failure usually have clear lungs on auscultation and will not exhibit intercostal in drawing or accessory muscle use. Those with an exacerbation of COPD or asthma will often have both of these signs.

Diagnosis

Initial investigations in the diagnosis of acute respiratory failure include physical examination, pulse oximetry, arterial blood gas analysis and chest radiograph. In some situations, it may be necessary to investigate further through the use of computerized tomography or lung biopsy to establish a diagnosis.

Arterial blood gas analysis is central to the diagnosis and management of acute respiratory failure. Accepted normal values for PaO_2 decline with age because of structural changes in the lungs and may be calculated using the formula:

$$PaO_2 = 100.1 - 0.323 \times age$$

While breathing room air, a PaO_2 of 55 mm Hg or less is consistent with significant hypoxemic respiratory failure. However, when patients receive supplemental O_2, PaO_2 may be significantly elevated. It is useful in this situation to calculate a PaO_2 to FIO_2 ratio (P/F) to account for this increase in alveolar O_2 concentration. Patients with normal gas exchange demonstrate a P/F of greater than 500, whereas a P/F of less than 300 is consistent with significant oxygen exchange abnormalities, and less than 200 is consistent with acute respiratory distress syndrome (ARDS).

In healthy patients, the normal range for PCO_2 is 35 to 45 mm Hg. Levels higher than this are seen in both chronic and acute hypercarbic respiratory failure. In chronic conditions compensatory reactions increase serum bicarbonate levels to decrease the drop in pH caused by hypercarbia. It is therefore often possible to determine the acuity of the hypercarbia by evaluating the serum bicarbonate level; in chronic hypercarbia, bicarbonate levels will be elevated beyond the normal range, whereas in acute hypercarbia, compensation will not yet have occurred, and bicarbonate levels will be normal.

The chest radiograph is an invaluable tool in the diagnosis of respiratory failure. In patients with hypoxic respiratory failure, chest radiography often allows the clinician to rapidly narrow the differential diagnosis based on whether the chest radiograph shows normal lung parenchyma, focal abnormalities or diffuse bilateral abnormalities. In hypercarbic respiratory failure, the chest radiograph allows the clinician to appreciate the degree of hyperinflation present during exacerbations of COPD or asthma and may help determine whether an infection has precipitated this exacerbation. In patients with hypercarbic respiratory failure caused by abnormalities of the central nervous system, the chest radiograph may allow the diagnosis of complicating aspiration pneumonitis.

Management

The goals of management in acute respiratory failure are to support oxygenation and ventilation, diagnose and treat the underlying cause, and avoid iatrogenic injury.

Maintenance of oxygenation may initially be achieved through the application of supplemental oxygen in an

---

 CURRENT DIAGNOSIS

- Acute respiratory failure is divided into hypoxemic and hypercapnic etiologies.
- Initial investigations in the diagnosis of acute respiratory failure include physical examination, pulse oximetry, arterial blood gas analysis and chest x-ray.
- Normal values for PaO_2 can be calculated using the formula: $PaO_2 = 100.1 - 0.323 \times age$
- On breathing room air, a PaO_2 of 55 mm Hg or less is consistent with significant hypoxemic respiratory failure
- In healthy patients, the normal range for PCO_2 is 35 to 45 mm Hg. Levels higher than this are seen in both chronic and acute hypercarbic respiratory failure
- In patients with hypoxic respiratory failure, chest radiography often allows the clinician to rapidly narrow the differential diagnosis based on whether the chest x-ray shows normal lung parenchyma, focal abnormalities or diffuse bilateral abnormalities.
- In hypercarbic respiratory failure, the chest x-ray allows the clinician to appreciate the degree of hyperinflation present during exacerbations of COPD or asthma, and may help determine whether an infection has precipitated this exacerbation.

attempt to maintain a PaO$_2$ greater than 65 to 70 mm Hg (SaO$_2$ > 92%). If this provides insufficient support, consideration should be given to noninvasive positive-pressure ventilation (NPPV) or intubation and mechanical ventilation.

Noninvasive positive-pressure ventilation may be suitable for properly selected patients suffering from acute hypoxic respiratory failure and may decrease the need for mechanical ventilation and decrease morbidity in these patients. However, great caution must be used in the selection of hypoxic patients for NPPV, because it is not an appropriate therapy to use in unstable patients or those with impaired airway protection. Tolerance for NPPV may be improved by using a nasal mask and starting with low inspiratory pressure (e.g., 5 cm H$_2$O). For patients who are too unstable or who are unable to tolerate NPPV, intubation and mechanical ventilation may be necessary.

In patients with hypoxic respiratory failure secondary to ARDS, careful attention to how ventilatory support is supplied may prevent further lung injury from iatrogenic causes. Recent evidence demonstrates that overly aggressive tidal volumes during mechanical ventilation worsen lung injury and survival in ARDS patients. It is prudent to target a tidal volume of no more than 4 to 6 cc/kg predicted body weight in these patients, and to tolerate lower PaO$_2$ and higher PCO$_2$ than normal in these patients.

Concurrent with support of oxygenation, the treatment of acute hypoxic respiratory failure requires the diagnosis and treatment of the underlying disease. In cases of pneumonia or aspiration, early antibiotic use is recommended, whereas in pulmonary edema, the use of afterload reducing agents (nitroglycerin- or angiotensin-converting enzyme inhibitors) and diuretics such as furosemide (Lasix 20 to 60 mg IV every 6 hours) may be needed. The medical care of patients with pulmonary contusions or alveolar hemorrhage is largely supportive, whereas the management of pulmonary embolism requires anticoagulation, and occasionally, the use of fibrinolytics.

During the treatment of hypercarbic respiratory failure, maintenance of oxygenation is usually less difficult than the maintenance of adequate minute ventilation, clearance of CO$_2$, and prevention of muscular fatigue.

β-Adrenergic bronchodilators such as albuterol (Ventolin) help decrease bronchospasm in patients with acute exacerbations of COPD or asthma. The addition of anticholinergic bronchodilators to β-agonists such as ipratropium bromide (Atrovent) may produce added benefit. Corticosteroids such as hydrocortisone sodium succinate (Solu-Cortef) are used to treat significant exacerbations of diseases associated with bronchospasm and inflammation. These may be given orally (prednisone) or intravenously (methylprednisolone [Solu-Medrol]). Patients with symptoms suggestive of an infectious etiology (e.g., increased sputum, fever, chest radiograph changes) may benefit from antibiotic therapy. NPPV has a clear role in the treatment of stable, alert patients with hypercarbic respiratory failure. When used in this population, NPPV can reduce rates of intubation and intensive care unit (ICU) length of stay. Like other patients who are not adequately supported by or who do not tolerate NPPV, consideration should be given to intubation and mechanical ventilation.

CURRENT THERAPY

- Maintain oxygenation with supplemental oxygen in an attempt to maintain a PaO$_2$ greater than 65-70 mm Hg (SaO$_2$ >92%).
- β-adrenergic bronchodilators such as albuterol (Ventolin) may decrease bronchospasm in patients with acute exacerbations of COPD or asthma.
- Anticholinergic bronchodilators such as ipratropiurn bromide (Atrovent) may produce added benefit.
- Corticosteroids are used to treat significant exacerbations of diseases associated with bronchospasm and inflammation
- NIPPV has a clear role in the treatment of stable, alert patients with hypercarbic respiratory failure.
- Indications for intubation and mechanical ventilation include: failure of ventilation, failure of oxygenation, failure of airway protection, and inability to manage secretions or pulmonary toilet
- Large tidal volumes during mechanical ventilation worsen lung injury and survival in ARDS patients. In these patients a target tidal volume of no more than 4 to 6 cc/kg predicted body weight may prevent ventilator induced lung injury.
- In hypercarbic respiratory failure caused by exacerbations of COPD or asthma, low levels of PEEP can decrease the work of breathing performed by patients, allowing them to decrease their CO$_2$ production, and decreasing their propensity to develop respiratory muscle failure.
- High levels of PEEP are also associated with barotraumas such as pneumothorax and pneumomediastinum

Mechanical Ventilation

Mechanical ventilation is a powerful tool in the management of acute respiratory failure because it allows the control of minute ventilation, offers opportunities to support oxygenation, and facilitates patient recovery from muscular fatigue. It is important to bear in mind, however, that it does not replace accurate diagnosis and aggressive treatment of the underlying disease.

Indications for intubation and mechanical ventilation include: failure of ventilation, failure of oxygenation, failure of airway protection, and inability to manage secretions or pulmonary toilet. Typically, ventilators in North American ICUs are programmed to deliver a predetermined tidal volume. This occurs unless a clinician-determined airway pressure is exceeded. This mode is called *assist-control* or *volume-control* ventilation. The patient is able to trigger the ventilator, at which time the predetermined tidal volume is delivered. If the patient does not attempt to trigger the ventilator within a specified time period, or is unable to generate sufficient air flow to cause triggering, the ventilator will deliver a minimum number of *mandatory* breaths.

Other less frequently used modes of ventilation include pressure control ventilation, synchronized intermittent mandatory ventilation, bilevel ventilation, and APRV. There is no convincing evidence that one mode improves patient outcomes more than another, but clinical experience suggests that different patients may *prefer* certain modes in terms of comfort and ventilator synchrony.

Positive end-expiratory pressure (PEEP) is a controllable characteristic of both invasive and noninvasive ventilation that is useful in the management of both hypoxic and hypercarbic respiratory failure. During normal breathing in the healthy patient, there is minimal residual pressure (above atmospheric pressure) in the airways at end expiration. The use of mechanical ventilation allows the clinician to artificially exert continuous pressure into the airway and lungs throughout the respiratory cycle, including end expiration. The benefits depend on the clinical scenario. In patients with hypoxic respiratory failure the alveoli are often collapsed because of surfactant abnormalities (ARDS) or flooded with inflammatory cells (pneumonia), edema (left heart failure), blood (alveolar hemorrhage and trauma) or exudates and transudates (ARDS). In these situations PEEP can reinflate atelectatic alveoli and improve oxygenation. In hypercarbic respiratory failure caused by exacerbations of COPD or asthma, low levels of PEEP can decrease the work of breathing performed by patients, allowing them to decrease their CO_2 production and their propensity to develop respiratory muscle failure.

Positive end-expiratory pressure, although helpful in acute respiratory failure, may create complications. By increasing intrathoracic pressure, PEEP can impair venous return to the heart and decrease cardiac output, which can cause overt hypotension, or, more subtly, interfere with adequate tissue perfusion (thus preventing the initial purpose of PEEP—improved tissue oxygen delivery). High levels of PEEP are also associated with barotraumas such as pneumothorax and pneumomediastinum.

Atelectasis

Method of
Craig Michael Schramm, MD

The term *atelectasis* refers to the consolidation of an area of lung because of loss of inflating air, rather than displacement by alveolar fluid. It is one of the most common pulmonary abnormalities in patients of all ages. Atelectasis may be characterized by the duration of its presence (i.e., acute or chronic), its location within the lung (central or peripheral, lobar or segmental), or its etiologic mechanisms (Table 1). The term *lobar atelectasis* refers to complete or incomplete collapse of a lobe of lung. *Subsegmental, discoid,* and *platelike atelectasis* are synonymous terms indicating collapse at a subsegmental level within a lobe. The presentation and treatment of atelectasis are related to the etiologies involved in its pathogenesis.

Pathogenesis

The most frequent cause of loss of alveolar gas volume is *resorption atelectasis*, which develops when air is blocked

TABLE 1 Etiologies of Atelectasis

Resorption Atelectasis
Intrinsic—airway obstruction
Mucus plug
Foreign body aspiration
Bronchial granuloma
Bronchial adenoma/tumor
Bronchial stenosis

Extrinsic airway obstruction
Hilar adenopathy
Left atrial enlargement
Mediastinal mass
Lung cyst
Airway torsion
Malpositioned endotracheal tube

Passive Atelectasis
Intrapleural—lesions
Pneumothorax
Pleural effusion or empyema
Diaphragmatic hernia
Chest wall masses

Hypoventilation
Postoperative
Neuromuscular weakness
Diaphragm dysfunction

Dependent Atelectasis

Compression Atelectasis
Peripheral lung mass or cyst
Air trapping in adjacent lung
Bronchial obstruction
Lobar emphysema
Extensive interstitial disease

Adhesive Atelectasis
Inadequate surfactant production
Premature infant
Prolonged shallow breathing
Pulmonary embolism
Surfactant destruction
Adult respiratory distress syndrome (ARDS)
Toxic aspiration or inhalation

Cicatrization Atelectasis
Pulmonary fibrosis
Pulmonary granulomatous disease

to a lobe, lobar segment, or individual acini. The airway obstruction may result from intrinsic airway lesions such as mucus plugs, foreign bodies, and tumors, extrinsic airway compression, or airway torsion. Alveoli distal to the site of obstruction lose volume because of the passive diffusion of gases from higher partial pressures in the alveoli to lower partial pressures in mixed venous blood. The extent of the resorption atelectasis and the rate by which it develops depend on several factors, including the extent of collateral ventilation in the lung region and the composition of the trapped gas. Complete volume loss occurs within 18 to 24 hours of airway obstruction in a previously healthy lung inflated with room air but within minutes of obstruction during ventilation with 100% oxygen. The loss is also accelerated in the presence of lung disease. In contrast, postobstructive atelectasis is attenuated by collateral ventilation between the obstructed segment and neighboring areas of lung, through accessory ventilatory pathways such as the channels of Martin and pores of Kohn. Obstruction of these pathways by inflammation or lung disease or their incomplete development at birth predisposes an obstructed lung region to develop resorptive atelectasis.

Another common cause of alveolar volume loss is *passive atelectasis* because of the natural propensity of the lung to collapse. Normally, the inward elastic recoil forces of the lung are balanced by the outward elastic forces of the chest wall. When these opposing forces are uncoupled, as occurs when the intrapleural space is filled with air or fluid, the adjacent lung volume diminishes. Young children are more prone to passive atelectasis than adults because their more compliant chest walls exert less outward forces to balance their lung elastic recoil force. In contrast, adults demonstrate more gravity-dependent effects because of their larger chest dimensions. The weight of blood and tissue in dependent lung regions adds to the opposition of chest wall recoil forces and thereby decreases regional lung volumes. Such gravity-dependent atelectasis may be potentiated by prolonged recumbency as can occur postoperatively or by processes that promote shallow breathing, such as postoperative pain and analgesia or neuromuscular disease. *Compression atelectasis* occurs by a similar mechanism when the expanding forces of the chest wall are countered by compressive forces of a parenchymal lesion, causing the adjacent lung volume to diminish.

Other types of atelectasis include *adhesive atelectasis* and *cicatrization atelectasis*. Alveoli are lined with surfactant to reduce the surface tension at the air–tissue interface. In the absence of surfactant, high surface tensions cause the luminal surfaces of alveolar walls to adhere together. Adhesive atelectasis may result from inadequate surfactant secretion or from excessive surfactant destruction. *Cicatrization atelectasis* refers to the loss of lung volume accompanying pulmonary interstitial fibrosis. Fibrous tissue retracts with time, reducing the compliance of the lung region and resulting in loss of affected lung volume.

Diagnosis

The clinical signs of atelectasis depend on its location, extent, and duration. Because of compensatory overdistention of surrounding lung regions, chronic atelectasis presents with fewer signs and symptoms than acute atelectasis. Acute atelectasis of a lobe or lung often is accompanied by tachypnea and dyspnea. Rapid losses of volume may elicit pain in the affected side. Physical examination findings may include ipsilateral shifts in the apical cardiac impulse or the lower extrathoracic trachea because of displacement of the heart and mediastinum to the affected side and dullness to percussion because of increased density in the atelectatic region. Vocal fremitus and breath sounds may be absent when atelectasis is caused by bronchial obstruction but are enhanced when the atelectatic lung is in contact with a patent bronchus. Pectoriloquy and bronchophony may also be appreciated in cases of nonobstructive atelectasis. To be detected, these auscultatory findings usually require at least lobar consolidation to be present, and they are frequently absent in young children because of transmission of sounds from adjacent lung areas. Cyanosis and arterial hypoxemia may be present if there is ventilation–perfusion mismatching in a large area of atelectatic lung.

Although a suspicion of atelectasis may be raised by any of the findings just described, its presence is typically confirmed by chest radiograph. Radiologic signs of atelectasis are variable but include pulmonary opacification, ipsilateral shift of the mediastinum, elevation of the hemidiaphragm, crowding of bronchi and pulmonary vessels, crowding of ribs, displacement of lobar fissures, and compensatory overinflation of the normal lung. Airlessness of an involved lung region usually presents as radiographic opacification; however, some patients with *microatelectasis* have diffuse, distal, passive atelectasis but normal-appearing radiographic lung density. Another type of peripheral lobar collapse can cause *rounded atelectasis*, which is manifest by a round subpleural density often mistaken for a tumor. Air bronchograms within the opacified region are commonly present in atelectasis of all causes other than resorption, where their absence indicates large airway obstruction.

Specific areas of involvement in atelectasis result in distinct radiographic patterns. The right upper lobe tends to collapse superiorly and medially, causing elevation of the right hilum and minor fissure, anterior displacement of the major fissure, and tenting of the juxtaphrenic peak of the diaphragmatic pleura. The left upper lobe usually collapses more anteriorly and superiorly, resulting in anterior displacement of the major fissure and a poorly delineated left perihilar opacity. Compensatory hyperinflation of the superior segment of the left lower lobe may result in an air crescent between the opacified left upper lobe and the mediastinum (the so-called Luftsichel sign). The right middle lobe collapses medially, obscuring the right heart border on a posteroanterior radiograph and resulting in a wedge-shaped triangle or linear band on lateral radiograph demarcated by an inferiorly displaced minor fissure and a superiorly displaced major fissure. Lingular atelectasis obscures the left heart border and has a lateral wedge shape with a more irregular or poorly defined superior border because of the absence of a left minor fissure. Both lower lobes collapse posteriorly and inferiorly, resulting in downward displacement of the hilum, an inferior and medial shift of the major fissure, and blurring of the posterior third of the ipsilateral hemidiaphragm.

Treatment

The longer that a region of lung remains unexpanded, the more likely it may become infected and eventually develop fibrotic and/or bronchiectatic changes. Successful treatment of atelectasis requires the reestablishment of normal gas volume in the collapsed lung region. In large part, this must entail treating the underlying etiology, ranging from removing an aspirated foreign body in resorptive atelectasis to promoting deep breathing and early ambulation in postoperative passive atelectasis or to administering surfactant in some cases of adhesive atelectasis.

In addition, a number of treatment modalities assist in the recruitment of lung volume, either by direct or collateral routes.

Principal among these volume recruitment methods are various types of chest physiotherapy, the most traditional of which are incentive spirometry and chest percussion and postural drainage. Incentive spirometry combines deep inspirations with voluntary coughing. Patients who are unable to perform effort-dependent maneuvers may benefit from administered chest percussion and postural drainage. The delivery of positive pressure either intermittently during inhalation (as with intermittent positive-pressure breathing, or IPPB) or continuously (as with continuous positive airway pressure, or CPAP) may augment lung volume in patients with passive atelectasis because of postoperative sedation, neuromuscular disease, or diaphragmatic dysfunction. Intra- or extrapulmonary applied oscillations may help displace inspissated mucus and reopen plugged airways, particularly if coupled with positive expiratory pressure. Aerosolized β-adrenergic agonists are often administered prior to chest physiotherapy to dilate any constricted airways and facilitate mucociliary clearance, but the efficacy of this practice is unproven. Some patients with mucus plugging may also benefit from mucolytic agents (such as N-acetylcysteine [Mucomyst] or recombinant human DNase[1] [Pulmozyme]) delivered either by aerosol or direct intrabronchial lavage.

Flexible bronchoscopy is indicated in patients with respiratory compromise from their atelectasis, in patients with acute atelectasis lasting more than 24 to 48 hours, and in patients with chronic atelectasis refractory to 1 to 2 months of medical management. The bronchoscopy is diagnostic, to look for causes of central airway obstruction. It may be also therapeutic if mucus plugs can be removed by bronchoalveolar lavage; however, nonresorptive types of atelectasis are usually not responsive to lavage. In intubated patients, the bronchoscope may be used as a guide to position the endotracheal tube above the area of atelectasis so that gentle manual insufflation can be delivered directly to the atelectatic region in an attempt to reinflate it.

Occasionally, chronically atelectatic lobes reexpand and function after atelectatic periods of 1 to 2 years. More commonly, however, chronic atelectasis of any etiology progresses to adhesive atelectasis and eventually to a permanently fibrotic lung region. Bronchiectasis may develop in such chronically atelectatic areas, leading to chronic or recurrent purulent infection. If this pattern occurs, surgical resection of the atelectatic lobe may be needed.

REFERENCES

Fraser RS, Muller NL, Colman N, Pare PD (eds): Fraser and Pare's Diagnosis of Diseases of the Chest, 4th ed. Philadelphia, WB Saunders, 1999, pp 513-562.

Oberwaldner B: Physiotherapy for airway clearance in paediatrics. Eur Respir J 2000;15(1):196-204.

Wallis C, Prasad A: Who needs chest physiotherapy? Moving from anecdote to evidence. Arch Dis Child 1999;80(4):393-397.

Woodring JH, Reed JC: Radiographic manifestations of lobar atelectasis. J Thorac Imaging 1996;11(2):109-144.

[1]Not FDA approved for this indication.

Management of Chronic Obstructive Pulmonary Disease

Method of
Juan Armando Garcia, MD, and
Stephen G. Jenkinson, MD

Chronic obstructive pulmonary disease (COPD) is characterized by airflow limitation that is not fully reversible. The airflow limitation is usually both progressive and associated with an abnormal inflammatory response of the lungs to noxious particles of gases. Under the direction of the National Heart, Lung, and Blood Institute (NHLBI) and the World Health Organization (WHO), collaborative guidelines on the diagnosis and management of chronic obstructive pulmonary disease (COPD) have been assembled by an expert panel: the Global Initiative for Chronic Obstructive Lung Disease (GOLD). These guidelines define the classifications of COPD on the basis of both severity and type of symptoms and explore all new information on the diagnosis and treatment of COPD. The GOLD initiative aims to improve prevention and management of COPD through a concerted worldwide effort of people involved in all facets of health care policy and to encourage a renewed research interest in this extremely prevalent disease.

To assure that recommendations for management of COPD are based on current scientific literature, the GOLD program established a science committee to update the sections of the report on recommendations for management of COPD each year. Although the update of these sections will occur each year and will be posted on the Web site (http://www.goldcopd.com), the full report will be updated and printed every 5 years. The latest update, including new modifications of management, was published in late 2003.

Pathophysiology

The pathophysiology of COPD is somewhat different in various patients, and the terms *emphysema* or *chronic bronchitis* were used in the past. Both of these disorders cause airway obstruction. Emphysema is defined pathologically as abnormal permanent enlargement of airspaces distal to the terminal bronchioles, accompanied by destruction of their walls and without obvious fibrosis. This tissue destruction results in enlargement of proximal and distal airspaces and can ultimately form bullae in the lung parenchyma. These bullae result in loss of surface area for gas exchange in the involved lungs. There is also a genetically inherited form of emphysema which is caused by the α_1-antitrypsin (AAT) deficiency. This disorder accounts for less than 1% of COPD cases in the United States. AAT is a protease inhibitor produced by the liver that circulates into tissues. Active proteases are released into the lung by lung macrophages, which can contribute to the development of emphysema. When patients smoke cigarettes, they also recruit a neutrophil population into their lungs. These neutrophils release neutrophil elastase (another type of protease) and other toxic molecules, which can destroy alveolar walls and may also contribute to the production of emphysema. AAT offers protection from these effects, but the protection found in normal people is inadequate in patients with AAT deficiency. Patients who develop emphysema despite normal levels of AAT usually develop emphysema in the fifth or sixth decades of life, whereas patients with AAT deficiency can develop emphysema as early as the third or fourth decades of life, depending on the extent of their deficiency and smoking history.

All patients developing emphysema who form bullae before the age of 45 years should be evaluated for AAT deficiency. A normal serum level of AAT is greater than 11 mmol/L (>80 mg/dL). Patients with low levels of AAT should be evaluated by a pulmonologist and may be candidates for AAT replacement therapy.

Chronic bronchitis is defined clinically as the presence of chronic, productive cough for 3 months during each of 2 consecutive years, and for which other causes of chronic cough are excluded. The other most common causes of chronic cough include asthma, gastric reflux, or postnasal drip secondary to sinus disease. The pathologic findings of chronic bronchitis are enlargement of tracheobronchial mucus glands, variable amounts of airway smooth-muscle hyperplasia, inflammation, and bronchial wall thickening. Abnormalities of small airways may be present as well and are accompanied by fibrosis and the presence of a mononuclear inflammatory process. The forced expiratory volume at 1 second (FEV_1) of a COPD patient is inversely proportional to the number of inflammatory cells in the airways. Patients with chronic bronchitis also have increased mucus hypersecretion, goblet cell metaplasia, increased submucosal gland formation, and abnormal matrix deposition.

The use of the terms *emphysema* or *chronic bronchitis* is no longer specified in the GOLD definition of COPD. The inflammation seen in COPD is different from that seen in asthma, but some obstructive lung disease patients do have pathologic changes that can be seen in both diseases, so some overlap does occur.

Epidemiology and Risk Factors

In the United States COPD is presently the fourth leading cause of death and affects more than 21 million people. Death rates have risen more than 22% in the last decade and the disease is responsible for approximately 700,000 hospital stays each year. The disease is now almost equal in men and women because of increasing amounts of tobacco in the female population. The primary risk factor associated with the development of COPD, cigarette smoking increases the death rate and disability caused by COPD and causes lung function to deteriorate over time much more rapidly than in a nonsmoker. Cigar and pipe smokers have greater COPD incidence than nonsmokers. Approximately 20% of smokers will develop COPD. The risk of development of COPD is increased in first-degree relatives of patients with COPD, which suggests the importance of genetic factors, but AAT deficiency is the only proved genetic risk factor in COPD. Exposures other than smoking that have been associated with COPD development include passive smoking, ambient air pollution, occupational dust and chemical exposure, and severe respiratory childhood infections.

Diagnosis

The diagnosis of COPD is suggested on the basis of symptoms, which may include those caused by the airway irritation (cough and sputum production) and those reflecting altered lung mechanics (dyspnea, wheezing, and occasionally chest pain). Individuals usually experience cough and sputum production years before the development of airflow limitation, while not all individuals with cough and sputum production go on to develop COPD.

Physical examination of individuals with COPD can reveal hyperinflation, wheezing, diminished breath sounds, hyperresonance, or prolonged expiration. Visual inspection during an examination can reveal signs of increased respiratory rate, increased anteroposterior (AP) chest diameter, hyperresonance to chest percussion, and impaired respiratory muscle function. Patients with COPD commonly have a respiration rate greater than 16 breaths per minute, and often this is proportional to disease severity; patients with COPD severe enough to exhibit hypercapnia (partial pressure of arterial carbon dioxide [$PaCO_2$] greater than 45 mm Hg) may have breathing rates of greater than 25 breaths per minute. Absence of wheezing does not exclude COPD. Patients with end-stage COPD may adopt body positions that help relieve dyspnea, such as leaning forward or expiring through pursed lips. Use of accessory muscles for respiration, such as the use of the abdominal rectus muscle on expiration, is a sign of advanced disease. Other signs of hyperinflation may include decreased diaphragm movement, tracheal tug, or pulsus paradoxus greater than 20 mm Hg.

Patients with advanced COPD may also have central cyanosis, peripheral edema, and signs of cor pulmonale associated with right heart failure. Other objective findings often include arterial blood gas changes demonstrating hypercapnia, severe hypoxemia, compensated respiratory acidosis with elevated carbon dioxide (CO_2), tension and a normal pH, and elevated serum bicarbonate level. Morning headaches in COPD patients may be indicative of hypercapnia.

The diagnosis of COPD is confirmed by spirometry. The standard pulmonary function test used to measure airway obstruction is the forced expiratory spirogram. This test assesses the rate of change in volume that occurs as a function of time. Pulmonary functions useful in the evaluation of patients presenting with symptoms of COPD include FEV_1, the forced vital capacity (FVC), and the ratio of FEV_1/FVC, which is also called the *timed vital capacity*. The FVC provides a measure of lung volume and the FEV_1 and FEV_1/FVC both provide a measure of obstruction. In most of these patients, other abnormal lung volumes that may exist include increases in both the total lung capacity (TLC) and the residual volume (RV). These increases in lung volumes are caused by hyperinflation of the lungs.

An FEV_1/FVC less than 70% of predicted confirms the presence of airflow obstruction. The FEV_1 serves as a marker of severity of the airflow obstruction. Other pulmonary function tests such as the flow volume loop or diffusing capacity for carbon monoxide (DL_{CO}) can help rule out other types of airway obstruction or help quantitate a patient's risk for surgery. Chest radiographs are only helpful for diagnosis in COPD if there are signs of bullous disease or severe hyperinflation or loss of vascular markings.

Computed tomography (CT) scanning can show the location of bullous disease which can be helpful in narrowing the differential diagnosis of a patient with airway obstruction and also may be used to help determine if a patient is a candidate for lung reduction surgery.

COPD Classification

The GOLD committee presented a new classification of COPD. The management of COPD is largely symptom driven, and there is only an imperfect relationship between the degree of airflow limitation and the presence of symptoms. The staging therefore is aimed at practical implementation and should be only regarded as an educational tool, and a general indication of the approach to management. All FEV_1 values refer to postbronchodilator FEV_1.

This classification includes stages 0 to IV (Figure 1).

Stage 0: At Risk—Characterized by chronic cough and sputum production. Lung function, as measured by spirometry, is still normal.

Stage I: Mild COPD—Characterized by mild airflow limitation (FEV_1/FVC <70% but FEV_1 >80% predicted) and usually, but not always, chronic cough and sputum production. At this stage, the individual may be unaware of abnormal lung function.

Stage II: Moderate COPD—Characterized by worsening airflow limitation (<50% FEV_1 <80% predicted) and usually the progression of symptoms, with shortness of breath typically developing on exertion. This is the stage at which most patients typically first seek medical attention because of dyspnea or an exacerbation of their disease.

Stage III: Severe COPD—Characterized by further worsening of airflow limitation (<30% FEV_1 <50% predicted), increased shortness of breath, and repeated exacerbations which have an impact on the patient's quality of life.

Stage IV: Very Severe COPD—Characterized by severe airflow limitation (FEV_1 <30% predicted) or the presence of chronic respiratory failure. Patients may have very severe (Stage IV) COPD even if the FEV_1 is greater than 30% predicted, if respiratory failure is present. At this stage, quality of life is appreciably impaired and exacerbations may be life-threatening.

Management of Stable COPD

The general guidelines to management of COPD include the avoidance of risk factors to prevent disease progression and pharmacotherapy as needed to control symptoms. In addition, patient education including counseling about smoking cessation, instruction in physical exercise, and nutritional advice are necessary components of a comprehensive COPD management plan. The goals of management are to relieve symptoms, increase exercise tolerance, improve quality of life, prevent and treat complications, and decrease disease progression.

Smoking cessation is the single most effective (and cost-effective) intervention to reduce the risk of developing COPD and stop its progression. Comprehensive tobacco elimination policies and programs with clear and repeated nonsmoking messages should be delivered through every feasible system possible. Legislation to establish smoke-free schools, public facilities, and work environments should be encouraged by working with government officials, public health workers, and the public. Guidelines for smoking cessation were published by the U.S. Agency for Health Care Policy and Research (AHCPR) in 2000.

There are numerous effective pharmacotherapies for smoking cessation. Except in the presence of special circumstances, pharmacotherapy is recommended when counseling is insufficient. Nicotine replacement therapy in any form (nicotine gum, inhaler, nasal spray [Nicotrol NS], transdermal patch [Nicoderm], sublingual tablet

THERAPY AT EACH STAGE OF COPD

	0: At risk	I: Mild	II: Moderate	III: Severe	IV: Very severe
Characteristics	• Chronic symptoms • Exposure to risk factors • Normal spirometry	• FEV_1/FVC < 70% • $FEV_1 \geq 80\%$ • With or without symptoms	• FEV_1/FVC < 70% • $50\% \leq FEV_1 < 80\%$ • With or without symptoms	• FEV_1/FVC < 70% • $30\% \leq FEV_1 < 50\%$ • With or without symptoms	• FEV_1/FVC < 70% • $FEV_1 < 30\%$ or $FEV_1 < 50\%$ predicted plus chronic respiratory failure
	Avoidance of risk factor(s); influenza vaccination				
		Add short-acting bronchodilator when needed			
			Add regular treatment with one or more long-acting bronchodilators *Add* rehabilitation		
				Add inhaled glucocorticosteroid if repeated exacerbations	
					Add long-term oxygen if chronic respiratory failure. Consider surgical treatments

FIGURE 1. Therapy for different stages of COPD.

[Nicorette Microtab],[2] or lozenge [Commit]) reliably increases long-term smoking abstinence rates. The antidepressants bupropion (Zyban) and nortriptyline (Pamelor)[1] have also been shown to increase long-term quit rates. The antihypertensive drug clonidine (Catapres)[1] can also be used to help a patient quit smoking, but side effects should be carefully reviewed with each patient. Special consideration should be given before using pharmacotherapy in selected populations including patients smoking fewer than 10 cigarettes per day, pregnant patients, and adolescent smokers.

The overall approach to managing stable COPD should be characterized by a stepwise increase in treatment, depending on the severity of the disease. The management strategy is based on an individualized assessment of disease severity and response to various therapies. Disease severity is determined by the severity of symptoms and airflow limitation (using pulmonary function measurements) and other factors such as the frequency and severity of exacerbations, complications, respiratory failure, co-morbidities (cardiovascular disease and sleep-related disorders), and the general health status of the patient. Different types of pharmacologic agents treat patients with COPD (Box 1). Pharmacologic therapy is used to prevent and control symptoms, reduce the frequency and severity of exacerbations, improve health status, and improve exercise tolerance. Initial use should decrease airway obstruction and decrease dyspnea. None of the existing medications for COPD had been shown to alter the inevitable long-term

---

[1]Not FDA approved for this indication.
[2]Not available in the United States.

BOX 1   Current Drugs Used to Manage Chronic Obstructive Pulmonary Disease

- SABAs
- Albuterol (salbutamol) (Proventil)
- LABAs
- Formoterol (Foradil)
- Salmeterol (Serevent)
- Short-acting anticholinergics
- Ipratropium (Atrovent)
- Long-acting anticholinergics
- Tiotropium (Spiriva)
- Combination SABA + anticholinergic in 1 inhaler
- Albuterol/ipratropium (Combivent)
- Methylxanthines
- Theophylline (Theo-Dur)
- Inhaled corticosteroids
- Beclomethasone (QVAR)
- Budesonide (Pulmicort)
- Fluticasone (Flovent)
- Triamcinolone (Azmacort)
- Combination LABA + ICS in 1 inhaler
- Formoterol/budesonide (Symbicort)
- Salmeterol/fluticasone (Advair)
- Systemic corticosteroids
- Prednisone
- Methylprednisolone (Medrol)

Abbreviations: LABAs = Long-acting β_2 agonists; SABAs = short-acting β_2 agonists.

decline in lung function that occurs with COPD; however, they can decrease morbidity and may also delay disability and mortality in some patients. Medications may also decrease the number of exacerbations of COPD occurring per year.

Bronchodilators are primary medications for symptomatic management of COPD. Bronchodilator drugs commonly used include anticholinergics (short and long acting), β_2 agonists (short and long acting), and long-acting methylxanthines. All of these medications have been shown to improve exercise capacity in COPD patients even if the FEV_1 is insignificantly changed. Inhaled drugs tend to have fewer side effects than oral drugs. Short-acting bronchodilators on an as-needed basis are recommended for mild (Stage I) COPD. The GOLD guidelines recommend the use of regular daily treatment with bronchodilators for moderate (Stage II) or severe (Stages III and IV) COPD and long-acting bronchodilators are preferred to short-acting drugs because of better compliance because of longer duration of action (Box 1). Regular use of a long-acting anticholinergic (tiotropium [Spiriva]) or a long acting β_2-agonist (salmeterol [Serevent] or formoterol [Foradil]) improves health status. Theophylline (Theo-Dur) is effective in COPD, but because of its potential toxicity, inhaled bronchodilators are preferred when available. All studies that have shown efficacy of theophylline (Theo-Dur) in COPD were done with slow-release preparations (theophylline [Theo-Dur]). Each of the inhaled bronchodilators requires a delivery device which must be used correctly. Each type of device requires patient education and monitoring, and the GOLD guidelines recommend consideration of the delivery device as part of the selection process for drug treatment in a single patient. As symptoms of COPD worsen, several different types of COPD therapy are given simultaneously, and deletion of drug therapy is usually not possible. In general nebulized therapy for a stable patient is unnecessary unless it has been demonstrated to be more effective than conventional metered dose or dry powder inhaler dose therapy in that patient.

Combinations of bronchodilators with different mechanisms and durations of action tend to increase the degree of bronchodilation in COPD patients with increases in FEV_1, FEV_1/FVC, and peak expiratory flow (PEF). Changes in pulmonary function are indirectly additive with increasing the number of bronchodilators being administered, but combinations usually increase pulmonary function more than each agent alone. Short-acting β_2 agonists (SABAs) are quick-relief medications for use only when necessary rather than on a daily, regular schedule. The regular use of a SABA results in twice as much β_2 agonist use without any noted clinical benefits. Increasing use or daily use of a SABA for rescue indicates the need for additional therapy to achieve long-term control. Inhaled SABAs include albuterol (Proventil, Ventolin), bitolterol (Tornalate), pirbuterol (Maxair), and terbutaline (Brethaire). These medications are effective for 4 to 6 hours after use. Adverse effects of SABAs include palpitations, chest pain, tachycardia, tremor, unstable coronary artery disease or nervousness. Patients with coronary artery disease or cardiac dysrhythmias should also be monitored closely. Use caution in giving these medications to patients receiving monoamine oxidase inhibitors or tricyclic antidepressants. The short-acting anticholinergic agent, ipratropium bromide (Atrovent), causes bronchodilation by competitive inhibition of muscarinic receptors. This agent reverses cholinergically mediated bronchospasm and may decrease mucus-gland secretions. It is effective for 4 to 6 hours after use.

The most recent addition to the long-acting bronchodilators is tiotropium (Spiriva), a long-acting anticholinergic agent that lasts 24 hours, allowing for once-daily administration. Tiotropium (Spiriva) has shown in several recent studies with COPD patients to result in significant improvement in lung function compared with ipratropium (a short-acting anticholinergic) or salmeterol (Serevent, a long-acting β_2 agonist [LABA]). Inhaled LABAs are highly preferred than the extended-release oral formulation because of longer action and fewer side effects. Salmeterol (Serevent) and formoterol (Foradil) are both long-acting, inhaled β_2 agonists, and extended-release albuterol (Proventil Repetabs) are long-acting, β_2 agonists available as oral agents. The long-acting inhaled agents have a slower onset of action and longer duration of action, remaining active for more than 12 hours. The onset of action of formoterol (Foradil) is more rapid than salmeterol (Serevent), but it should not be used for rescue during episodes of acute shortness of breath. It remains a chronic bronchodilator therapy. Like the short-acting inhaled β_2 agonists, the long-acting agents produce bronchodilation by smooth muscle relaxation as a result of adenylate cyclase activation and increasing cyclic AMP in smooth muscle cells. Combining β_2 agonists and anticholinergics may increase the effects of these agents. Several studies have shown superior efficacy for either a SABA or LABA in combination with an anticholinergic.

Theophylline (Theo-Dur) inhibits phosphodiesterase action, which causes smooth muscle relaxation and leads to bronchodilation. It also increases central respiratory drive, diaphragm strength, promotes venous pooling in the legs, and may have some mild anti-inflammatory activity. Therapy with theophylline (Theo-Dur) should be individualized, taking into account such factors as drug interactions, current smoking, the patient's age, and the presence of congestive heart failure or liver disease. Serum theophylline (Theo-Dur) concentrations should be maintained at levels between 5 and 15 μg/mL. Dosage adjustment is based on the patient's clinical response, tolerance to the agent, and serum theophylline (Theo-Dur) levels. Some patients metabolize theophylline (Theo-Dur) very rapidly. Although theophylline (Theo-Dur) is not a preferred first line agent in the management of COPD, it may be a second-line agent in patients with severe COPD.

Inhaled corticosteroids (ICSs) are not recommended as single agents for chronic use in COPD management, which is quite different from the recommendations in asthma. They are recommended in combination therapy with other bronchodilators in severe COPD, and the only Food and Drug Administration (FDA)-approved combinations of ICS and a LABA are fluticasone plus salmeterol (Advair) or formoterol (Foradil) plus budesonide (Symbicort)[4] (see Box 1). Systemic steroids are clinically beneficial to patients hospitalized with COPD exacerbations and maximum effects of oral steroids after 3 days of intravenous (IV) steroids are achieved by 2 weeks of therapy.

Longer use of oral steroids increases side effects without increasing pulmonary functions. Long-term treatment with oral glucocorticosteroids is not recommended in COPD. There is no evidence of a long-term benefit from this treatment. Moreover, a side effect of long-term treatment with systemic glucocorticosteroid is steroid myopathy, which contributes to muscle weakness, decreased functionality, and respiratory failure in patients with advanced COPD. Oral glucocorticosteroid use for long periods of time can also complicate control of diabetes and hypertension as well as causing bone demineralization.

Other pharmacologic treatments have been evaluated by the GOLD committee with some being beneficial. Use of influenza vaccines can reduce serious illness and death in COPD patients by approximately 50%. Use of the influenza vaccine has also been shown to reduce outpatient visits for influenza and reduces both hospital costs and death. Vaccines containing killed (Fluzone) or live, inactive viruses (FluMist)[1] are recommended and should be given once (in autumn) or twice[3] (in autumn and winter) each year. A pneumococcal vaccine containing 23 virulent serotypes (Pneumovax-23) has been used in an effort to decrease the number of cases of pneumococcal pneumonia in COPD patients but evidence supporting its effectiveness in COPD patients is lacking. An oral vaccine* using a strain of nontypeable *Haemophilus influenzae* has been shown to produce short-lived reduction in the number of exacerbations in some groups of COPD patients. The use of antibiotics, other than in treating infectious exacerbations of COPD or other bacterial infections such as pneumonia, is not recommended. Although a few patients with viscous sputum may benefit from mucolytics, the overall benefit is small. Therefore, the widespread use of these agents cannot be recommended.

Cough, although sometimes a troublesome symptom in COPD, has a significant protective role and the regular use of antitussives is contraindicated in stable COPD. The use of doxapram (Dopram), a nonspecific respiratory stimulant available as an intravenous formulation, is not recommended in stable COPD. Almitrine bismesylate (Duxil) also is not recommended for regular use in stable COPD patients. Narcotics are contraindicated in COPD because of their respiratory depressant effects and potential to worsen hypercapnia. Clinical studies suggest that morphine use to control dyspnea may have serious adverse effects, but it may provide benefits to a few select limited patients. Codeine and other narcotic analgesics should be avoided. Nonsteroidal anti-inflammatory agents (Nedocromil [Tilade]) and leukotriene modifiers have not been adequately tested in COPD patients and are not recommended for use. Alternative healing methods including herbal medicine, acupuncture, and homeopathy are not recommended for treatment in COPD.

Nonpharmacologic management of COPD patients includes pulmonary rehabilitation and long-term oxygen therapy. The principal goals of pulmonary rehabilitation are to improve quality of life, decrease symptoms, and increase physical participation in everyday activities. To accomplish these goals, pulmonary rehabilitation addresses

---

[4]Not yet approved for use in the United States.

*Investigational drug in the United States.
[1]Not FDA approved for this indication.
[3]Exceeds dosage recommended by the manufacturer.

a range of nonpulmonary problems, including exercise deconditioning, relative social isolation, altered mood states (especially depression), muscle wasting, and weight loss. COPD patients at all stages of disease benefit from exercise training programs and improve with respect to both exercise tolerance and symptoms of dyspnea and fatigue. These benefits can be sustained even after a single pulmonary rehabilitation program. Benefits have been reported from rehabilitation programs conducted in inpatient, outpatient, and home settings. Ideally, a comprehensive pulmonary rehabilitation program includes exercise training, nutrition counseling, and education. Baseline and outcome assessments of each participant in a pulmonary rehabilitation program should be made to quantify individual gains and target areas for improvement and include a detailed medical history and physical exam; measurement of spirometry before and after a bronchodilator drug; assessment of exercise capacity; measurement of the impact of breathlessness and/or health status; and assessment of inspiratory and expiratory muscle strength and lower limb strength (e.g., quadriceps) in patients who suffer from muscle wasting.

The long-term administration of oxygen (more than 15 hours per day) to COPD patients with chronic respiratory failure has been shown to increase survival. In studies done in Britain by the Medical Research Council Trial and in the United States in the Nocturnal Oxygen Therapy Trial, patients receiving continuous oxygen therapy had increased survival as compared with patients that did not receive oxygen or received oxygen only at night. Oxygen also has a beneficial impact on hemodynamics, hematologic characteristics, exercise capacity, lung mechanics, and mental state. Oxygen therapy also should be used if the patient has evidence of pulmonary hypertension, peripheral edema suggesting either right- or left-sided heart failure or evidence of polycythemia (hematocrit greater than 55%). Therapy can be given continuously, acutely to combat acute dyspnea, or intermittently during exercise. It is recommended to perform arterial blood gas measurement in patients with FEV_1 less than 40% predicted or with clinical findings suggestive of respiratory failure or cor pulmonale.

Management of Exacerbations

Patients with COPD will have usually two to three exacerbations of symptoms of their disease each year with some requiring hospitalization. The economic and social burden of COPD exacerbations is extremely high. The most common causes of an exacerbation are pulmonary infections (acute bacterial bronchitis) and air pollution. The exact cause of approximately one-third of severe exacerbations cannot be identified and may be related to reactive airway disease. Other conditions that may produce the symptoms of an acute exacerbation of COPD include pneumonia, myocardial ischemia, congestive heart failure, pneumothorax, formation of a pleural effusion, pulmonary embolism, cardiac arrhythmias, esophageal reflux, or noncompliance with medications. The clinical diagnosis of a COPD exacerbation is an increase in amount of sputum production, change in color of sputum, or increase in dyspnea. Exacerbations may also be accompanied by a number of nonspecific complaints such as malaise, insomnia, sleepiness, fatigue, anxiety, depression, confusion, or panic attacks. Patients with exacerbations of COPD may require hospital admission, and some patients will require ICU admission. There is a high incidence of *H. influenzae* infections in patients with a COPD exacerbation caused by infection. Other important bacterial causes include *Streptococcus pneumoniae, Moraxella catarrhalis,* and *Pseudomonas aeruginosum.* Hospital admission must be considered in COPD with an exacerbation if they have marked increase in symptoms, failure to respond to outpatient treatment, confusion, lethargy and coma, worsening oxygenation, or development of respiratory acidosis. Oxygen therapy is usually required in a hospitalized patient with an acute exacerbation of COPD; but this may lead to CO_2 retention and acidosis, which in turn could lead to either noninvasive mechanical ventilation, or mechanical ventilation depending on the cause of the exacerbation and the patient's wishes. Hospital mortality for patients with COPD admitted for an acute exacerbation is approximately 10%. Ventilator associated pneumonia is also an important risk in a COPD patient treated with invasive mechanical ventilation.

The primary objectives of mechanical ventilatory support in patients with acute exacerbations of severe COPD are to decrease mortality and morbidity and relieve symptoms. Ventilatory support can be given through an orotracheal or nasotracheal tube or tracheostomy connection, which is referred to as invasive (conventional) mechanical ventilation and is particularly suitable in severe acute exacerbations occurring in patients with end-stage disease. Ventilatory support can also be given through a noninvasive means using either negative or positive pressure devices. Fewer complications occur with noninvasive ventilation, but many patients presenting with severe exacerbations of COPD, including respiratory acidosis, may not be candidates for noninvasive ventilation. Noninvasive positive-pressure ventilation (NPPV) involves using a mechanical ventilator connected by tubing to an interface that allows airflow into the nose or the nose and mouth by using a mask or a mouthpiece. Head straps are used to secure the mask tightly to the patient. NPPV allows ventilation without the use of an endotracheal tube. Use of NPPV in acute respiratory failure has been studied in both uncontrolled and randomized controlled trials. The studies show consistently positive results with success rates of 80% to 85%. Taken together they provide evidence that NPPV increases pH, reduces $PaCO_2$, reduces the severity of breathlessness in the first 4 hours of treatment, and decreases the length of hospital stay. More importantly, mortality and intubation rates are reduced by this intervention. However, NPPV is not appropriate for all patients and invasive mechanical ventilation may still be needed to maximize arterial blood gases values. NPPV can be delivered by different types of ventilators: volume-controlled, pressure-controlled, bilevel positive airway pressure, or continuous positive airway pressure. The use of NPPV together with long-term oxygen therapy has been shown to result in a significant improvement in daytime arterial blood gases, total sleep time, sleep efficiency, quality of life, and overnight $PaCO_2$.

Other treatments that can be useful in COPD patients who must be hospitalized include fluid administration as needed to keep the patient normovolemic; nutrition supplementation as needed with careful attention to the amount of carbohydrates given because excessive amounts can increase CO_2 production; and the use of low molecular weight heparin in immobilized patients with or without a history of thromboembolic disease. Manual or mechanical chest percussion and postural drainage may also be beneficial in patients producing greater than 25 mL sputum per day or those with lobar atelectasis.

Surgical Options

Surgical treatments of COPD include bullectomy, lung volume reduction surgery, and lung transplantation. In carefully selected patients, bullectomy can be effective in reducing dyspnea and improving lung function. A thoracic CT scan, arterial blood gases measurement and comprehensive respiratory function tests are essential before making a decision regarding a patient's suitability for resection of a bulla. Specific large bullae may be removed if they are compressing significant amounts of normal lung tissue.

Lung volume reduction surgery (LVRS) is another option for COPD patients and involves removing 20% to 30% of the upper lobes to improve airway mechanics and increase FEV_1. The National Emphysema Treatment Trial (NETT) study was a randomized controlled trial in 1218 patients with severe emphysema who received either LVRS or medical therapy. The results showed no overall survival benefit with LVRS compared with medical therapy, but improved exercise capacity and quality of life. The best outcome of this surgery was in patients with predominantly upper lobe emphysema and initial low exercise capacity. The surgery was prohibitive in patients with an FEV_1 of up to 20% and either a homogeneous distribution of emphysema or a concomitant diffusing capacity of lung for carbon monoxide (DL_{CO}) of up to 20%.

In appropriately selected patients with very advanced COPD, lung transplantation has been shown to improve quality of life and functional capacity. The average 3-year survival rate is approximately 60% when performed by highly skilled medical or surgical teams that specialize in lung transplantation. Appropriate criteria for lung transplantation recipients include FEV_1 of up to 35% of predicted, $PaCO_2$ greater than 55 mm Hg, PaO_2 less than 60 mm Hg on room air, or the presence of secondary pulmonary hypertension.

Cystic Fibrosis

Method of
Robert L. Zanni, MD

Cystic fibrosis (CF) is a complex, multisystem clinical syndrome involving exocrine glands, including sweat glands, the pancreas, and mucous glands of the respiratory, gastrointestinal, and reproductive tracts. It is characterized by elevated sweat electrolyte content, chronic obstructive pulmonary disease, and exocrine pancreatic insufficiency.

CF is the most common lethal genetic disease among the white population. The disorder is autosomal recessive, and the incidence is 1 in 3000 in the caucasian population. CF is less common in African Americans with an incidence of 1 in 10,000, in Asian Americans with an incidence of 1 in 31,000, and in Hispanic Americans with an incidence of 1 in 6000. Initially CF was thought to be a rare and invariably fatal disease. As a result of refined diagnostic techniques and improved therapeutic approaches, however, there has been an increase in life expectancy. Emphasis on early diagnosis, prevention of lung disease, and improving nutrition are the current areas of concentration on diagnosis and therapy. The median predicted survival is currently 36.8 years.

Pathophysiology

The isolation and cloning of the gene mutation causing CF occurred in 1989. The CF gene is located on the long arm of human chromosome 7. The CF gene codes for the production of a membrane transport protein termed cystic fibrosis transmembrane regulator (CFTR). This protein is expressed in all the epithelial cells affected in CF. This includes the lung, pancreas, sweat glands, liver, large intestine, and testes. CFTR acts as an apical chloride conductance channel resulting in reduced activation of chloride ion transport. CFTR is important in controlling other ions as well. It has been shown that CFTR secondarily regulates sodium absorption in the CF airways. The combined function of CFTR as a chloride channel and regulator of sodium channels suggests that CFTR is the trigger that balances the rates of chloride secretion and sodium absorption to properly hydrate airway secretions in normal airway epithelial cells.

To date, more than 1000 mutations have been identified to cause CF. Progress has been made in understanding the molecular mechanisms by which CF-associated mutations cause dysfunction of the CFTR protein. Depending on the type of mutation, one of five mechanisms may come into play. Five different class mutations result in different degrees of chloride channel defects causing different degrees of disease severity. Class I mutations are associated with defective CFTR production resulting in a lack of production of full length or functional protein. In class II mutations, the protein is not correctly processed and unable to progress through the biosynthetic pathway to the cell membrane. Class III mutations cause defects in chloride channel regulation. Class IV mutations result in reduced flow of chloride through the channel. Class V mutations result in decreased amounts of functional CFTR. In general, individuals with class I and II mutations are pancreatic insufficient, whereas classes III, IV, and V are pancreatic sufficient.

PULMONARY MANIFESTATIONS

As a result of the dysfunctional CFTR, the secretions of the airway become abnormally thick and tenacious. This situation leads to chronic obstruction of the bronchial airways. The inspissation of secretions causes chronic infection and inflammation to progress. This cyclic process progresses to bronchiectasis, fibrosis, and eventual respiratory failure (Figure 1). Infection is initially caused by

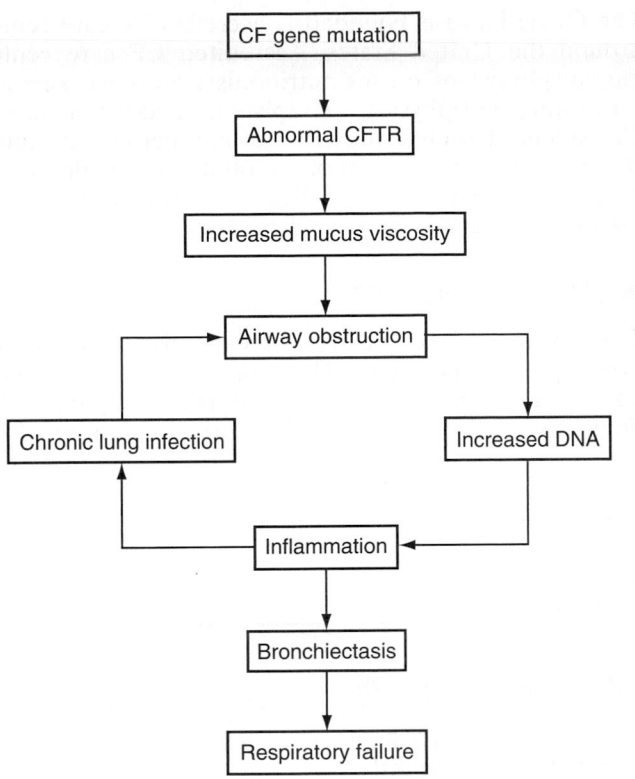

FIGURE 1. A vicious cycle of chronic airway obstruction, infection, and inflammation leads to progressive pulmonary damage. *Abbreviations:* CF = cystic fibrosis; CFTR = cystic fibrosis transmembrane regulator.

Staphylococcus aureus and *Haemophilus influenzae.* As patients age, infection with *Pseudomonas aeruginosa* becomes most prominent. The rate of progression of lung disease is variable among patients. Factors associated with acceleration in decline of lung function are poor nutritional status, infection with *P. aeruginosa*, tobacco exposure, pancreatic insufficiency, and lack of consistent medical care. The key clinical manifestation of the upper respiratory tract is pansinusitis. Approximately 25% of patients with CF will develop nasal polyps.

GASTROINTESTINAL/NUTRITIONAL MANIFESTATIONS

As many as 90% of patients with CF are pancreatic insufficient. Inspissation of thick secretions within the pancreatic ducts causes insufficient or total absence of secretion of pancreatic enzymes, which leads to maldigestion and malabsorption of fats and protein. This is clinically manifested by steatorrhea and failure to thrive.

There are other manifestations of CF related to the gastrointestinal (GI) tract. CF-related diabetes mellitus occurs in approximately 17% of patients. Approximately 20% of infants with CF present at birth with meconium ileus. This is an obstruction of the distal small bowel with viscous, thick meconium. Children, adolescents, and adults with CF may suffer from distal small bowel obstruction (distal intestinal obstruction syndrome [DIOS]). Approximately 5% of CF patients develop liver disease characterized by focal biliary cirrhosis.

 CURRENT DIAGNOSIS

Diagnosis is Based on:

- Presence of one or more characteristic phenotypic features or
- A history of CF in a sibling or
- Positive newborn screening test

  Plus

- Elevated sweat chloride concentrations (chloride > 60 mmol/L) or
- Identification of two CF mutations or
- Characteristic abnormalities in ion transport across the nasal epithelium

Characteristic Phenotypic Features:

1. Chronic sinopulmonary disease
   - Chronic cough and sputum production
   - Clinical findings consistent with airway obstruction (wheezing, air trapping)
   - Pansinusitis, nasal polyps
   - Persistent pulmonary infection with typical CF pathogens (*Staphylococcus aureus, Haemophilus influenzae, Pseudomonas aeruginosa*)
   - Persistent chest radiograph abnormalities (bronchiectasis, atelectasis, infiltrates, hyperinflation)
   - Digital clubbing
2. Gastrointestinal and nutritional abnormalities
   - Intestinal: Meconium ileus, DIOS, rectal prolapse
   - Pancreatic: Pancreatic insufficiency, recurrent pancreatitis
   - Hepatic: Focal biliary cirrhosis
   - Nutritional: Protein-calorie malnutrition; hypoproteinemia and edema; complications secondary to fat-soluble vitamin deficiency
3. Salt loss syndrome
   - Acute salt depletion
   - Chronic metabolism alkalosis
4. Male urogenital abnormalities resulting in obstructive azoospermia

Abbreviations: CF = cystic fibrosis; DIOS = distal intestinal obstructive syndrome.

Diagnosis

Approximately 50% of patients are diagnosed by 6 months of age and 68% by the age of 1 year. The key to diagnosing patients with CF is to have a high index of suspicion based on presenting symptoms. Classic clinical features include chronic sinopulmonary disease and GI symptoms. A small percentage of patients present with less-than-classic symptoms. These patients tend to be pancreatic sufficient.

Confirmation of the diagnosis can be obtained through a sweat test. To avoid false-positive or false-negative results, the sweat test should be performed by experienced laboratory personnel using the iontophoresis pilocarpine technique (Gibson-Cooke method). Positive sweat tests yield sweat chlorides of more than 60 mmol/L. Diagnosis also can be confirmed through DNA analysis by finding two known CF mutations. Difficult diagnostic cases may require testing by nasal transepithelial potential difference.

Prenatal and carrier testing may be offered where there is a family history. More states have mandated newborn screening for CF by measuring immunoreactive trypsinogen (IRT) in a dried blood sample. An elevated IRT is then followed by CF mutation analysis. When the newborn screen is positive, confirmation of the diagnosis is recommended by sweat testing.

Management

GENERAL

A comprehensive, multidisciplinary approach to the care of CF patients improves their health and life expectancy.

The Cystic Fibrosis Foundation accredits CF care centers around the United States. Accredited CF care centers employ physicians, nurses, nutritionists, social workers, and respiratory and physical therapists trained in the care of CF patients. Patients who enter comprehensive treatment programs before the onset of symptomatic lung disease do better than patients who begin treatment after lung disease has manifested itself clinically.

PULMONARY DISEASE

The prognosis of patients with CF depends on the progression of pulmonary disease. The main goals of therapy focus on efforts to reduce the frequency of pulmonary exacerbations, prevent the decline in pulmonary function, and delay

CURRENT THERAPY

Drug	Dosage
Antibiotics: Oral	
Amoxicillin/clavulanate (Augmentin)	45 mg/kg/d divided q 12h
Azithromycin (Zithromax)	10 mg/kg/d on day 1
	5 mg/kg/d on days 2–5
Cephalexin (Keflex)	25–100 mg/kg/d divided q 6h
Cefuroxime (Ceftin)	30 mg/kg/d divided q 6h
Ciprofloxacin (Cipro)	30–40 mg/kg/d divided q12h
Levofloxacin (Levaquin)	500 mg/d
Tetracycline (Sumycin)	25–50 mg/kg/d divided q 12h
Trimethoprim/sulfamethoxazole (Bactrim)	8–10 mg/kg/d of trimethoprim divided q 12h
Antibiotics: Aerosolized*	
Tobramycin for inhalation (TOBI)	300 mg bid
Colistin (Coly-Mycin M)[1]	150 mg bid
Antibiotics: Parenteral	
β-lactam penicillins	
Nafcillin (Nafcil)	50–100 mg/kg/d divided q 6h
Piperacillin (Pipracil)	400–500 mg/kg/d divided q 6h
Piperacillin/tazobactam (Zosyn)	400–500 mg/kg/d divided q 6h
Ticarcillin (Ticar)	200–400 mg/kg/d divided q 6–8h
Other β-lactams	
Ceftazidime (Fortaz)	150–200 mg/kg/d divided q 6–8h
Meropenem (Merrem)	120 mg/kg/d divided q 8h
Aztreonam (Azactam)	150-200 mg/kg/d divided q 6–8h
Aminoglycosides[†]	
Amikacin (Amikin)	15 mg/kg/d divided q 8–12h
Gentamicin (Garamycin)	7.5–15 mg/kg/d divided q 8–12h
Tobramycin (Nebcin)	7.5–10 mg/kg/d divided q 8–12h
Mucolytics	
Dornase alfa (Pulmozyme)	Inhalation of 2.5 mg per dose once daily
Anti-inflammatory	
Azithromycin (Zithromax)[1]	Ages 6 years and older
	<40 kg, 250 mg tiw
	>40 kg, 500 mg tiw
Pancreatic Enzymes	
Pancrelipase (Creon, Pancrease, Ultrase)	1000–2000 lipase U/kg/meal
Nutritional	
Multivitamins (A, D, E, K [ADEK]; Vitamax; A, B, D, E, K [ABDEK])	Dose varies according to age

[1]Not FDA approved for this indication.
*Aerosolized antibiotics may be used for 2 to 3 weeks for acute exacerbation or for 28 days on, 28 days off as chronic therapy.
[†]Monitor serum peak and trough levels and for renal toxicity and ototoxicity.
Abbreviations: d = daily; h = hour; q = every; tid = three times a day; tiw = three times a week; U = unit.

irreversible lung damage. Clinically these goals can be achieved by controlling pulmonary infection, relieving airway obstruction through various modalities, and minimizing inflammation of the airway epithelium. The progression of pulmonary disease can be monitored by serial pulmonary function testing, yearly chest radiographs, and routine clinical follow-up of the patient.

ANTIBIOTICS

Antibiotics are used to treat pulmonary exacerbations. A pulmonary exacerbation for CF is defined as a change in respiratory signs and symptoms from one's baseline. Commonly these can be an increase in chest congestion, a decrease in exercise tolerance, and the onset of new or an increase in crackles on chest examination. Patients may experience an increase in frequency or duration in cough, an increase in sputum production, and a change in sputum color. Dyspnea, decreased appetite, and hemoptysis may also herald a pulmonary exacerbation.

Most patients require antibiotics intermittently for treatment of exacerbations; few require continuous antibiotic therapy. The choice of antibiotics is based on sputum or oropharyngeal culture and sensitivities. The most common organisms are *S. aureus,* generally found in younger patients, and *P. aeruginosa,* which predominates in older patients.

The treatment of a mild exacerbation can be achieved with the use of an oral antibiotic, an inhaled antibiotic, or both. Generally patients will return to their baseline within 14 days. If patients fail to improve or if the exacerbation is more complex, intravenous antibiotic therapy is advised. Intravenous therapy and frequent airway clearance should be continued until the patient reaches his or her best pulmonary function. This is generally achieved within 14 days. When intravenous antibiotics are used, a combination of an aminoglycoside with an antipseudomonal penicillin, cephalosporin, or antistaphylococcal agent is recommended. The choice of intravenous antibiotics also is based on culture and sensitivity results. Combination therapy helps to avoid the development of bacterial resistance.

Recent evidence supports the use of inhaled tobramycin (TOBI) in patients who are chronically infected with *P. aeruginosa.* TOBI is used on a cycle of 28 days on, 28 days off. Its use can minimize pulmonary exacerbations and improve lung function.

BETA 2 AGONISTS

Although not all patients with CF have airway hyperreactivity, it has become accepted practice to use aerosolized bronchodilators prior to the initiation of airway clearance techniques. Albuterol (Proventil) or levalbuterol (Xopenex) are commonly used.

MUCOLYTICS

The airway secretions of CF patients are extremely thick, tenacious, and viscous. This is because of the increased amount of DNA present from neutrophils. Inhaled dornase alfa (Pulmozyme) is a purified solution of recombinant human deoxyribonuclease I (DNAse I). This enzyme cleaves extracellular neutrophil-derived DNA resulting in the thinning of airway secretions allowing them to be expectorated more easily. Studies support that the once-daily use of dornase alfa (Pulmozyme) preserves lung function and decreases pulmonary exacerbations.

ANTI-INFLAMMATORY THERAPY

Chronic infection is associated with chronic inflammation. Inhaled anti-inflammatory agents such as cromolyn (Intal), nedocromil (Tilade), and inhaled corticosteroids have been used but not studied adequately. Use of alternate day oral corticosteroids and ibuprofen (Motrin) has been studied sufficiently and shows improvement in lung function. Serious side effects have limited their widespread use in CF patients. A recent trial of azithromycin (Zithromax)[1] given three times per week has shown pulmonary benefits. Although the use of azithromycin (Zithromax)[1] for this purpose is off-label, it is a recommended therapy for CF patients 6 years of age and older who have chronic infection with *P. aeruginosa.*

AIRWAY CLEARANCE

Daily airway clearance is recommended for all CF patients. There are various techniques that can be offered to patients. Chest physical therapy using percussion and postural drainage is effective for infants and young children. Older children, adolescents, and adults mostly prefer the various mechanical devices that are available. These devices offer levels of independence for the patients. Examples of such devices are positive expiratory pressure devices (Flutter, Therapep), vibratory positive expiratory pressure devices (Acapella), and high-frequency, chest wall oscillation devices (Vest).

NUTRITIONAL MANAGEMENT

The basis for malnutrition in CF patients is multifactorial. The majority of patients with CF are pancreatic insufficient and unable to digest fats and proteins. CF patients also have increased caloric needs because of an increase in metabolism. The increased metabolic state results from chronic pulmonary infection and increased work of breathing.

Pancreatic enzyme replacement, along with high-calorie, high-fat diets and fat-soluble vitamins, provides adequate nutrition for many patients with CF. If the patient fails to gain weight, high-calorie oral supplements or enteral feeds at nighttime are helpful.

COMPLICATIONS

Respiratory, gastrointestinal, and other organ system complications can occur in patients with CF. Box 1 lists the more common complications encountered in the care of patients with CF.

Research

As the understanding of the genetic and molecular basis for the disease increases, new therapeutic approaches will become available. Current therapeutic approaches involve correcting the genetic defect (gene therapy); regulation of

---

[1]Not FDA approved for this indication.

BOX 1   Clinical Complications

Pulmonary
- Hemoptysis
- Pneumothorax
- Allergic bronchopulmonary aspergillosis

Gastrointestinal/Nutritional
- Distal intestinal obstructive syndrome
- Protein-caloric malnutrition
- Pancreatitis
- Focal biliary cirrhosis

Endocrine
- Cystic fibrosis-related diabetes mellitus (CFRDM)
- Osteopenia/osteoporosis

Rheumatologic
- Arthropathy
- Arthritis

Urogenital
- Congenital bilateral absence of vas deferens
- Male infertility

Abbreviations: CF = cystic fibrosis; DM = diabetes mellitus.

ion transport, which will affect abnormal mucus production; and novel anti-infective and anti-inflammatory therapies. An unprecedented number of therapies for CF are being tested in well-designed clinical trials.

REFERENCES

Boat T, Cantin A, Cutting G, et al: The diagnosis of cystic fibrosis: Consensus statement. Consensus Conferences, Concepts in Care, Cystic Fibrosis Foundation, Bethesda, MD, March 25, 1996; Volume VII, Section 1, 1-15.

Borowitz D, Baker R, Stallings V: Consensus report on nutrition for pediatric patients with cystic fibrosis. J Pediatr Gastroenterol Nutr 2002;35:246-259.

Cystic Fibrosis Foundation: Cystic Fibrosis Foundation Patient Registry, annual data report to the center directors for 2003. Cystic Fibrosis Foundation, Bethesda, MD, 2004.

Farrell P, Korosok M, Rock M, et al: Early diagnosis of cystic fibrosis through neonatal screening prevents severe malnutrition and improves long term growth. Pediatrics 2001;107:1-13.

Farrell P, Zanhai L, Korosok M, et al: Bronchopulmonary disease in children with cystic fibrosis after early and delayed diagnosis. Am J Respir Crit Care Med 2003;168:1100-1108.

Gibson R, Burns J, Ramsey B: Pathophysiology and management of pulmonary infections in cystic fibrosis. Am J Respir Crit Care Med 2003;168:918-951.

Gross S, Boyle C, Batkin J, et al: Newborn screening for cystic fibrosis. MMWR 2004;53:1-36.

Sleep Apnea

Method of
Teofilo Lee-Chiong Jr., MD

In an adult, obstructive apnea is generally defined as a cessation of nasal and oral airflow, despite the persistence of ventilatory efforts, for at least 10 seconds. The definition of obstructive hypopnea is less established; hypopnea is considered a reduction of airflow or amplitude of thoracoabdominal movement by at least 30% from baseline, of at least 10 seconds in duration, and accompanied by oxyhemoglobin desaturation of 4% or more. Obstructive apnea or hypopnea occurs when the forces that maintain upper airway patency, such as activation of dilator muscles, are insufficient to counteract the factors that promote upper airway closure during sleep (e.g., negative intraluminal pressure).

The severity of obstructive sleep apnea (OSA) can be classified based on the apnea index (number of apneas per hour of sleep) or the apnea–hypopnea index (AHI). This is the number of apneas plus hypopneas per hour of sleep: mild AHI is 5 to 15; moderate AHI is 16 to 30; and severe AHI is greater than 30. The respiratory disturbance index (RDI) represents the mean hourly frequency of apneas plus hypopneas plus respiratory event-related arousals (RERAs, or reduction in airflow that does not meet the criteria for either apnea or hypopnea and is not associated with significant oxygen desaturation).

Demographics and Essential Features

OSA is a major public health concern. It is estimated to affect 24% of middle-age males and 9% of middle-age females; in the general population, 4% of men and 2% of women have an AHI greater than 5 and complain of daytime sleepiness. OSA has been associated with greater mortality and significant adverse cardiovascular and cerebrovascular consequences, including hypertension, and insulin resistance. As a result of increased sleepiness, OSA is known to increase driving- and work-related accident rates, and to impair performance and neurocognitive functions. Risk factors for OSA include obesity, increasing age, untreated hypothyroidism, and male gender. Prevalence in women increases with menopause.

Clinical manifestations that should alert the clinician to the presence of OSA include complaints of daytime sleepiness or fatigue, bed partner accounts of witnessed apneas and snoring, awakenings with a sensation of gasping or choking, nocturnal diaphoresis, morning headaches, nocturia, and alterations in mood. Physical examination may be entirely unremarkable. Common physical findings consist of obesity, a large neck circumference, nasal septal deviation or turbinate hypertrophy, retro- or micrognathia, macroglossia, enlarged tonsils (especially among children), and a crowded and narrow oropharynx. Because clinical and physical examination features are neither sufficiently sensitive nor specific, a polysomnogram (PSG) is required for the diagnosis of OSA.

CURRENT DIAGNOSIS

- A polysomnogram is required to document the presence and severity of OSA because clinical and physical examination features are neither sufficiently sensitive nor specific for the diagnosis of OSA.

Therapy

Patients should be advised to achieve and maintain optimal weight, to exercise regularly, and to avoid alcohol, smoking, and the use of sedative-hypnotics and narcotic analgesics. In selected patients in whom respiratory events occur exclusively or predominantly during a supine sleep position, elevation of the head or restricting sleep to lateral recumbency might be tried. This could be accomplished by attaching a tennis ball-filled pocket to the back of a pajama top, or by sleeping with a Styrofoam-filled backpack. Reversible causes of upper airway obstruction, such as nasal mucosal swelling, enlarged turbinates, nasal polyps, and enlarged tonsils, should be addressed. Issues regarding sleep hygiene (getting adequate sleep each night and maintaining regular bedtime and waking time), as well as safety counseling to not operate motor vehicles or engage in other potentially dangerous activities unless fully alert, should be discussed with the patient.

POSITIVE AIRWAY PRESSURE THERAPY

Administration of positive airway pressure (PAP) is the treatment of choice for most patients with OSA. It is generally held that continuous positive airway pressure (CPAP) functions as a pneumatic splint for the vulnerable portions of the nasopharyngeal airway. Treatment modalities currently available for positive airway pressure therapy include CPAP, bilevel positive airway pressure, autotitrating positive airway pressure, and nocturnal noninvasive positive pressure ventilation.

A variety of methods have been used to determine the single, optimal CPAP level, such as laboratory-attended polysomnographically guided CPAP titration (either full-night studies or split-night studies that consist of an initial diagnostic portion and a subsequent CPAP titration on the same night), unattended laboratory or home titration, or using autotitrating devices. The current standard of practice involves a technician-attended pressure titration during a laboratory PSG. Sleep stages and respiratory variables are monitored to obtain a fixed, single pressure that eliminates apneas, hypopneas, snoring, and RERAs, maintains adequate oxyhemoglobin saturation, and improves

sleep architecture and quality in all body positions and all sleep stages. It is generally accepted that higher pressures are required to prevent airway occlusion during rapid eye movement (REM) sleep and during sleep in a supine position. The patient is then administered this fixed, single CPAP pressure nightly.

PAP therapy has salutary effects on mortality, cardiovascular profiles (e.g., blood pressure and heart rate), and cardiac function in patients with OSA and congestive heart failure (CHF), daytime alertness, functioning and well-being, and sleep quality (e.g., number of arousals). Treating patients with OSA is also associated with significant reduction in health care utilization, including physician claims and hospitalizations. Thus, CPAP is an effective treatment in patients with moderate and severe OSA; less certain is whether patients with mild OSA obtain benefit from CPAP as well. The minimal severity of OSA at which patients benefit from CPAP treatment is not well characterized. Additionally, patients with mild OSA might have a higher rate of CPAP discontinuation. Patients should be cautioned against intermittent use of CPAP, as virtually all of the sleep and daytime alertness gains derived from sleeping with CPAP are rapidly reversed with CPAP discontinuation.

Optimal CPAP utilization is a significant problem in clinical practice. Subjective reports of CPAP use may overestimate actual use. Reasons for nonadherence to PAP therapy include patient perception of lack of benefit, discomfort with its use, noise from the device, and inconvenience. Common complaints reported by patients on CPAP therapy consist of nocturnal awakenings and nasal problems. Long-term adherence to CPAP use may be inferred by the patterns of CPAP use in the first few days of treatment. Adherence can be improved with CPAP education (e.g., additional home visits, participation in group clinics, periodic phone calls to uncover any problems and to encourage use, and even simple written information on the importance of regular CPAP use), airway humidification, proper selection of the CPAP mask interface, and prompt management of adverse effects. Nasal symptoms that are complained about include nasal dryness, rhinorrhea, nasal congestion, sneezing, and epistaxis. Nasal resistance is affected by both mouth leakage and the use of humidification. Mouth leakage might influence nasal resistance by causing high unidirectional airflows in the nasal passages. As a result of the high incidence of nasal symptoms, humidification has become an important adjunct to CPAP therapy. Humidifying the inspired air can help minimize the drying effect on the nasal passages and might enhance compliance with CPAP use.

If dissatisfaction with CPAP use is related to complaints of mouth air leakage, a full-face mask or chinstrap can be provided. A full-face interface may also be tried for patients who are unable to tolerate nasal masks. The use of a ramp mechanism has been proposed to improve patient comfort. By resetting the pressure to 3 cm H_2O and then slowly increasing to the prescribed pressure over a period of up to 45 minutes, the ramp device theoretically allows the patient sufficient time to fall asleep before the higher and, likely, more uncomfortable prescribed pressure is reached. Bilevel PAP may be tried with patients who complain of dyspnea or discomfort, especially during expiration against the continuous pressure (because expiratory pressure is lower with bilevel positive airway pressure),

CURRENT THERAPY

- CPAP improves sleepiness and quality of life in symptomatic patients with moderate or severe OSA. Further studies are needed to assess the benefits of CPAP therapy for patients with less severe OSA, especially on secondary outcomes of treatment, such as cardiovascular risk.
- The effectiveness of CPAP is compromised because a large proportion of patients cannot tolerate the devices. Compliance can be improved by proper selection of the device interface, patient education, and prompt correction of adverse effects such as nasal dryness.
- Oral devices and upper airway surgery may be considered in patients who are either unwilling or unable to use PAP therapy.

and with those in whom oxygen desaturation because of hypoventilation persists despite CPAP therapy. The use of hypnotic agents has been suggested to assist patients during the acclimatization phase of initial CPAP use. Caution should be taken whenever benzodiazepines are used for this purpose as they have the potential to increase the arousal threshold to airway occlusion, prolong apnea duration, and worsen desaturation.

OTHER MODES OF POSITIVE AIRWAY PRESSURE

The optimal CPAP pressure may have significant intranight and internight variability, and the needed CPAP pressure can differ considerably with sleeping posture and sleep stages. Using a fixed, single CPAP pressure based on parameters obtained during REM-supine sleep (when CPAP pressure requirements may be greater) for the entire night might increase the tendency to develop mask and mouth leaks, as well as pressure intolerance; these, in turn, might reduce CPAP acceptance and use. Autotitrating PAP devices automatically and continuously adjust the delivered pressure, as needed, to maintain airway patency. The mean pressure required is generally lower during autotitrating PAP than during constant CPAP. These devices can be used to identify a fixed, single pressure for subsequent treatment with a conventional CPAP device (autotitrating PAP titration) or used in a self-adjusting mode for nightly therapy of OSA (autotitrating PAP treatment).

Not all autotitrating PAP systems are comparable in efficacy, and certain systems might be less useful with mild to moderate OSA. In an American Academy of Sleep Medicine report on the efficacy of autotitrating PAP for treatment of OSA, it noted insufficient evidence that autotitrating PAP can be used to treat patients with significant CHF, chronic obstructive pulmonary disease (COPD), or significant amounts of central apnea. Autotitrating PAP titration and treatment are not currently recommended for patients with daytime hypoxemia and respiratory failure from any cause, or for patients with prominent nocturnal arterial oxygen desaturation caused by conditions other than OSA (e.g., obesity hypoventilation syndrome), or for use in split-night sleep studies.

ORAL DEVICES

Oral devices worn during sleep can be considered in the management of patients with mild to moderate OSA who are intolerant of CPAP therapy or when upper airway surgery for OSA has failed. With these devices, the mandible and tongue are repositioned to improve the upper airway dimensions during sleep. There are two types of oral devices currently available for the management of OSA: tongue-retaining devices that hold the tongue in an anterior position, and mandibular repositioners that advance the mandible. A third device, palatal lifters, is not currently used. Complications from the use of oral devices include a dry mouth sensation related to mouth breathing, excessive salivation, undesirable dental movements associated with mandibular repositioning devices, and jaw or temporomandibular joint pain. Mandibular repositioners are contraindicated in patients with compromised dentition (i.e., loose, broken, or diseased teeth), inadequate

dentition to support the oral device, or significant temporomandibular joint dysfunction. Tongue-retaining devices are preferred for edentulous patients and patients with compromised dentition. Oral devices should be avoided in patients unable to breathe nasally or who have high resistance to nasal airflow.

UPPER AIRWAY SURGERY

Surgical procedures for OSA are designed to increase the dimensions of the retropalatal airspace (e.g., uvulopalatopharyngoplasty [UPPP] or transpalatal advancement pharyngoplasty); retrolingual airway (e.g., genioglossal advancement, hyoid myotomy and suspension, or mandibular advancement); or both (e.g., maxillomandibular advancement). In rare instances of severe OSA, a tracheostomy, which uses a percutaneous tracheal opening to bypass the area of airway collapse, might be necessary. Many surgeons perform upper airway surgery in sequential phases with an initial stage consisting generally of various combinations of UPPP, genioglossal advancement, and hyoid myotomy and suspension followed by a maxillomandibular advancement if symptoms persist. Data on long-term surgical effectiveness are limited. Surgical procedures may be particularly useful for patients with definitive craniofacial or upper airway abnormalities.

MANAGEMENT OF RESIDUAL SLEEPINESS

Occasionally, complaints of excessive daytime sleepiness may persist despite regular use of CPAP in patients with OSA. Coexisting sleep disorders, such as narcolepsy (if present), should be appropriately treated. Modafinil (Provigil), a wake-promoting agent, may be considered as an adjunct therapy for enhancing wakefulness and alertness in patients with residual sleepiness.

REFERENCES

American Academy of Sleep Medicine Task Force: Sleep-related breathing disorders in adults: Recommendations for syndrome definition and measurement techniques in clinical research. The Report of an American Academy of Sleep Medicine Task Force. Sleep 1999;22(5):667-689.

Bailey DR: Dental therapy for obstructive sleep apnea. Semin Respir Crit Care Med 2005;26(1):89-95.

Black JE, Hirshkowitz M: Modafinil for treatment of residual excessive sleepiness in nasal continuous positive airway pressure-treated obstructive sleep apnea/hypopnea syndrome. Sleep 2005;28(4):464-471.

Littner M, Hirshkowitz M, Davila D, et al: Practice parameters for the use of auto-titrating continuous positive airway pressure devices for titrating pressures and treating adult patients with obstructive sleep apnea syndrome: An American Academy of Sleep Medicine report. Sleep 2002;25(2):143-147.

Meoli AL, Casey KR, Clark RW, et al: Hypopnea in sleep-disordered breathing in adults. Sleep 2001;24(4):469-470.

Naughton MT, Bradley TD: Sleep apnea in congestive heart failure. Clin Chest Med 1998;19(1):99-113.

Partinen M, Jamieson A, Guilleminault C: Long-term outcome for obstructive sleep apnea syndrome patients. Mortality. Chest 1989;96(3):703-704.

Peppard PE, Young T, Palta M, Skatrud J: Prospective study of the association between sleep-disordered breathing and hypertension. N Engl J Med 2000;342(19):1378-1384.

Punjabi NM, Shahar E, Redline S, et al: Sleep-disordered breathing, glucose intolerance, and insulin resistance: The Sleep Heart Health Study. Am J Epidemiol 2004;160(6):521-530.

Shahar E, Whitney CW, Redline S, et al: Sleep-disordered breathing and cardiovascular disease: Cross-sectional results of the Sleep Heart Health Study. Am J Respir Crit Care Med 2001;163(1):19-25.

Sher AE: Upper airway surgery for obstructive sleep apnea. In: Lee-Chiong T (ed): Sleep: A Comprehensive Handbook. New York, Wiley, 2006, pp 365-372.

Young T, Palta M, Dempsey J, et al: The occurrence of sleep-disordered breathing among middle-aged adults. N Engl J Med 1993; 328(17):1230-1235.

Primary Lung Cancer

Method of
Christopher S. George, MD, and
Teresa M. George, MD

Lung cancer is a significant health problem in the United States. It is the second most commonly diagnosed cancer in both men and women. Despite not being the most common form of cancer, it has the highest mortality rate of all malignancies, and tumors of the lung and bronchus account for 32% of all cancer deaths in males and for 25% of all cancer deaths in females. In 2005, it was estimated that 79,560 patients would develop lung cancer and that 73,020 deaths would occur. Both men and women have seen increases in mortality over the last 100 years. The mortality in males is finally starting to decrease; in females, there has been a steady rise in mortality over the last 40 years. Only in recent years has this started to level off. Despite advances in diagnosis and treatment, the overall 5-year survival rate is low at 15%.

Risk Factors

Cigarette smoking remains the major risk factor for the development of lung cancer. It is associated with pulmonary malignancies in more than 80% of cases. The incidence and mortality trends of lung cancer are reflective of the trends of tobacco use of males and females over the last several decades. Both active and passive tobacco exposure have been implicated in the development of lung cancer. Exposure to tobacco other than in cigarettes (e.g., cigar and pipe smoking) has also caused an increase in the incidence of pulmonary cancers, although to a lesser degree than cigarettes. The smoking of marijuana and cocaine has not been studied as much as cigarette use, but it is believed that use of these substances probably increases the risk of lung cancer.

In addition to tobacco, many other environmental and occupational toxins are associated with the development of respiratory cancers. High levels of prolonged exposure to radon, asbestos, haloethers, polycyclic aromatic hydrocarbons, arsenic, and nickel cause lung cancer. Although these increase lung cancer in nonsmokers, the risk appears to be magnified in smokers, demonstrating a synergy between these carcinogens.

Other risk factors for the development of pulmonary malignancies include genetic or familial risk factors. First-degree relatives of patients with lung cancer have a 1.5- to 5-fold increased risk themselves. It should be noted that the exact molecular basis accounting for the increased risk is not well understood.

Patients with certain benign underlying lung diseases may also be at increased risk for the development of lung cancer. In particular, there is an increased risk in patients with pulmonary fibrosis, asbestosis, and possibly even chronic obstructive pulmonary disease (COPD). Increasing numbers of nonsmokers are developing non–small cell lung cancer in this country.

Clinical Manifestations

Occasionally lung cancer is discovered incidentally with bronchoscopy or chest x-ray; in the majority of cases, patients present with signs and symptoms. The exact clinical presentation depends on the site and spread of the primary tumor (Table 1). Many of the symptoms are nonspecific and may be seen more often in other disease entities. Most commonly, patients present with cough, dyspnea, chest pain, or hemoptysis. Fatigue, weight loss, and bone pain are also seen in patients, especially those with metastatic disease.

There are several distinct syndromes that can be seen with pulmonary malignancies. Some of these are caused by the tumor's spread into the mediastinum or surrounding structures. In the superior vena cava syndrome, patients may exhibit periorbital and facial edema and headaches. In later stages, this may be accompanied by a

TABLE 1 Clinical Manifestations

Associated with Primary Lesion	Associated with Intrathoracic Spread	Secondary to Metastases	Paraneoplastic Syndromes
Cough	Pleural effusion	Bone pain	Hypercalcemia
Dyspnea	Pericardial effusion	Generalized weakness	Hypertrophic osteoarthropathy
Hemoptysis	Hoarseness	Weight loss	SIADH
Chest pain	Superior vena cava syndrome	Headache	Cushing's syndrome
Weight loss	Pancoast syndrome	Nausea	Eaton-Lambert syndrome
Unilateral wheezing	Horner syndrome	Vomiting	Cerebellar ataxia
Fever secondary to pneumonia		Neurologic symptoms	Dementia
		Abdominal pain	Sensorimotor neuropathies

Abbreviation: SIADH, syndrome of inappropriate secretion of antidiuretic hormone.

bluish discoloration and new vessel formation on the anterior chest. Pancoast syndrome results from involvement of the brachial plexus by superior sulcus tumors. Patients may present with shoulder and arm pain with associated sensorimotor changes. If the sympathetic trunk is involved, patients may have Horner syndrome, which is characterized by ptosis, miosis, facial flushing, and anhidrosis on the side affected by the tumor.

In addition to syndromes caused by direct extension of the tumor, patients may also present with syndromes caused by the production of biologically active substances. Some of these are better understood than others. These are collectively referred to as the paraneoplastic syndromes. Examples of paraneoplastic syndromes observed in lung cancer include hypercalcemia from the production of parathyroid hormone-related peptide, hypertrophic osteoarthropathy, syndrome of inappropriate secretion of antidiuretic hormone (SIADH), Cushing's syndrome, and Eaton-Lambert syndrome.

Diagnosis

Once lung cancer is suspected, pathologic diagnosis must be made (Table 2). The diagnosis can be established based on cytologic specimens or histologic biopsy. Cytologic specimens may consist of sputum, bronchial washings or brushings, transbronchial or transthoracic needle aspirates, or bronchoalveolar lavage. Histologic biopsy can be from endobronchial, transbronchial, transthoracic, or open biopsy procedures. Generally, if the lesion is central, bronchoscopy is recommended for evaluation. If the abnormality is peripheral, use of computed tomography (CT)-guided transthoracic needle aspiration or biopsy is recommended. If the diagnosis is still equivocal, a more definitive open procedure may be needed.

Pretreatment Evaluation

After a pathologic diagnosis is established, the pretreatment evaluation must be done. This consists of two main parts: complete staging of the tumor so that treatment recommendations can be made (Table 3), and if surgery is a consideration, a preoperative assessment. The primary care physician can take the initial role in both of these evaluations.

CURRENT DIAGNOSIS

- Lung cancer is the second most common cancer in the United States, but has the highest mortality
- Cigarette smoking is the major risk factor
- Most common symptoms are cough, dyspnea, chest pain, and hemoptysis
- Diagnosis is made by cytologic specimen or histologic biopsy
- Staging must be done on all patients and should consist of history, physical examination, laboratory studies, and radiographic examinations
- Preoperative evaluation must be done in patients who are considered for surgery

TABLE 2   World Health Organization Histologic Classification of Epithelial Bronchogenic Carcinoma

Malignant	
Squamous cell (epidermal) and spindle cell carcinoma	
Small cell	Oat cell carcinoma (lymphocytic-like) Intermediate cell type Combined oat cell carcinoma (mixed histologic types, small with squamous cell carcinoma or adenocarcinoma)
Adenocarcinoma	Acinar Papillary Bronchoalveolar Mucinous secreting
Large cell	Giant cell Clear cell
Adenosquamous carcinoma	Carcinoid Bronchial gland carcinoma Adenoid cystic Mucoepidermoid
Others	

Adapted from World Health Organization: Histologic Typing of Lung Tumors, 2nd ed. Geneva, WHO, 1981.

Evaluation is needed to determine the stage of the tumor (staging systems for small cell lung cancer [SCLC] and non–small cell lung cancer [NSCLC] are discussed later). A good history and physical examination is the first step in any staging process. Then laboratory studies, including complete blood count, electrolytes, creatinine, calcium, alkaline phosphatase, aspartate aminotransferase (AST), alanine aminotransferase (ALT), bilirubin, and albumin should be done in all patients. The American Thoracic Society recommends that all patients receive CT of the chest with inclusion of liver and adrenals. If pleural effusions are present, patients should undergo evaluation with thoracentesis. Patients with SCLC should also receive bone scan and either CT or magnetic resonance imaging (MRI) of the brain. In patients with NSCLC, a bone scan should only be done in those with bone pain or elevated serum calcium or alkaline phosphatase from the bone. Neuroimaging is only recommended in NSCLC patients with signs or symptoms of neurologic disease. Select patients with suspected mediastinal lymph node involvement may require additional procedures such as mediastinoscopy, mediastinotomy, or thoracoscopy for staging. Over the last decade, positron emission tomography (PET) has also become more commonly used in staging. It has been approved by Medicare for the diagnosis, staging, and restaging of NSCLC. The American Society of Clinical Oncologists (ASCO) recommends it for locoregional staging in patients with NSCLC without distant metastatic disease on CT. PET scanning is less clear in the staging of SCLC.

If the patient has limited disease and is recommended for surgery, preoperative assessment must be done. In addition to normal preoperative assessment of cardiovascular risks, pulmonary assessment must be performed as well.

TABLE 3 International Staging System for Lung Cancer

Primary Tumor (T)	Nodal Involvement (N)	Distant Metastasis (M)	Stage Groupings of TNM Subsets
Tx—Primary tumor cannot be assessed or tumor proven by the presence of malignant cells in sputum or bronchial washings but not visualized by imaging or bronchoscopy	Nx—Regional lymph nodes cannot be assessed	M0—No distant metastasis	Occult carcinoma Tx, N0, M0
T0—No evidence of primary tumor	N0—No regional lymph node involvement	M1—distant metastasis present *or* separate tumor nodules in a different lobe	Stage 0 Tis, N0, M0
Tis—Carcinoma in situ	N1—Ipsilateral peribronchial or hilar nodes involved		Stage IA T1, N0, M0
T1—Tumor ≤3 cm in greatest dimension, surrounded by lung tissue *and* no bronchoscopic evidence of tumor proximal to the lobar bronchus	N2—Ipsilateral mediastinal or subcarinal nodes involved		Stage IB T2, N0, M0
T2—Tumor >3 cm in greatest dimension, *or* tumor of any size that involves the visceral pleura or is associated with atelectasis extending to the hilum (but not involving the entire lung) and must be ≥2 cm from the carina	N3—Contralateral mediastinal or hilar nodes *or* scalene or supraclavicular nodes involved		Stage IIA T2, N1, M0
T3—Tumor involves the chest wall, diaphragm, mediastinal pleura or pericardium, *or* is <:2 cm from the carina (but does not involve it)			Stage IIB T2, N1, M0 T3, N0, M0
T4—Tumor involves the carina or trachea *or* invades the mediastinum, heart, great vessels, esophagus *or* vertebrae, *or* malignant pleural effusion is present, *or* separate tumor nodules in the same lobe			Stage IIIA T3, N1, M0 T1-T3, N2, M0
			Stage IIIB Any T, N3, M0 T4, Any N, M0 Stage IV Any T, Any N, M1

Adapted from Mountain CF: Revisions in the international staging system for lung cancer. Chest 1997;111:1710-1717.

The single most useful test is the measurement of forced expiratory volume in 1 second (FEV_1). Guidelines from the American College of Chest Physicians state that patients with FEV_1 of greater than 2 L generally tolerate pneumonectomy. For lobectomy, an FEV_1 of 1 to 1.5 L is recommended. If preoperative FEV_1 is less than 2 L, further evaluation with measurement of carbon monoxide diffusion in the lung (DL_{CO}), quantitative split perfusion lung scanning, or cardiopulmonary exercise testing may be considered.

Prognostic Factors

There are several factors that may indicate poorer prognosis in patients with lung cancer. Extent of disease portrays prognosis with those with advanced stages faring worse. Baseline poor performance status and weight loss are also signs of worse prognosis. In SCLC, for an unknown reason, women tend to do better. The presence of paraneoplastic syndromes is a poor prognostic sign. Race, age, and histologic subtype are less important in determining prognosis.

Treatment

NON–SMALL CELL LUNG CANCER

Stage I

Stage I includes T1 and T2 tumors (see Table 3) without lymph node involvement or distant metastases. Patients undergo mediastinoscopy with frozen section analysis of lymph nodes, followed by resection of the primary tumor. Lobectomy is the typical surgical procedure performed; more proximal tumors may require a pneumonectomy or sleeve resection. Limited surgery, such as a wedge resection, has been associated with inferior results in some series and is generally reserved only for elderly, frail patients, or those with less cardiopulmonary reserve. In these patients,

CURRENT THERAPY

Non–Small Cell Lung Cancer

Stage IA

- Surgery

Stage IB

- Surgery and chemotherapy

Stage II

- Surgery and chemotherapy

Stage IIIA

- Surgery ± chemotherapy ± radiation

or

- Chemoradiation ± surgery

Stage IIIB

- Chemoradiation ± surgery

Stage IV

- Chemotherapy ± VEGF inhibitor, EGFR tyrosine kinase inhibitor, supportive care

Small Cell Lung Cancer

Limited Stage

- Concurrent chemoradiation ± prophylactic cranial irradiation

Extensive Stage

- Chemotherapy
- Palliative radiation
- Clinical trial participation preferred in all stages.

Abbreviations: EGFR, epidermal growth factor receptor; VEGF, vascular endothelial growth factor

video-assisted thoracic surgery (VATS) may be performed with decreased perioperative morbidity and less postoperative pain. The expected 5-year survival following a lobectomy is 60% to 70% in most series. It has been noted that survival rates are better for patients who have their surgery performed at hospitals that perform higher volumes of this surgery. Also, patients with no or minimal comorbid conditions have better survival rates.

At present, there are limited data for induction or neoadjuvant chemotherapy before surgical resection, and this should be considered experimental. Primary radiation therapy can be used for nonsurgical patients, including those with very poor cardiopulmonary reserve or those who refuse surgery. However, the results are clearly inferior to surgery, with only 15% of patients enjoying long-term survival, as 24% die of other illnesses and 60% succumb to progression of lung cancer. As such, newer radiation techniques are being investigated, such as hyperfractionation and stereotactic radiosurgery.

Postoperative radiation therapy (PORT) remains of unproven benefit. The PORT meta-analysis noted a decrease in survival compared with surgery alone despite potentially reducing local recurrence rates. The cause of this finding is uncertain, but higher rates of cardiopulmonary failure and infections were noted. Outdated radiation therapy

techniques may have also contributed. Currently, the routine use of PORT is discouraged as a standard approach. The use of adjuvant chemotherapy was previously thought to be unhelpful, likely because of ineffective chemotherapy developed in the 1980s. Several meta-analyses have shown only 4% to 5% survival benefit. However, two current, well-conducted North American trials have yielded significant results that have changed the standard of care. The Cancer and Leukemia Group B (CALGB) 9633 trial was presented in abstract form in 2004. Three hundred forty-four patients with stage IB were randomized to surgery alone or surgery followed by four cycles of adjuvant carboplatin (Paraplatin[1]) and paclitaxel (Taxol). The 4-year overall survival rate was 59% for the surgery-alone group and 71% for the chemotherapy group. The lung cancer mortality rate decreased from 19.9% to 11%. Importantly, no treatment-related deaths were noted. In 2005, the National Cancer Institute of Canada (NCIC) trial JBR10 was published in the *New England Journal of Medicine*. This study included 482 patients randomized to surgery alone or adjuvant cisplatin (Platinol AQ[1]) and vinorelbine (Navelbine) for four cycles. The patient population was different with both stages IB and II (excluding T3 N0) included. Despite only 50% of patients completing chemotherapy, there was a significant improvement in 5-year overall survival rates of 54% surgery alone compared to 69% surgery plus chemotherapy (p = 0.03). Two treatment-related deaths were noted (0.8%). Median survival was also prolonged at 73 months surgery alone compared to 94 months surgery plus chemotherapy (p = 0.04). Four cycles of adjuvant chemotherapy has become the standard of care in this country. The Japanese have investigated oral uracil plus tegafur (UFT) with a meta-analysis of their six trials showing a 5-year survival benefit of 5%. This drug is currently not available in the United States.

Stage II

Stage II cancers include those with spread to ipsilateral hilar lymph nodes but no mediastinal nodes or distant metastases. It also includes T3N0 tumors (see Table 3). This stage is the least-common stage. Long-term survival is uncommon without surgical intervention. As with stage I, lobectomy is the standard approach except for proximal tumors that require pneumonectomy. Mediastinal lymph node dissection is associated with a small to moderate survival advantage. The 5-year overall survival rate is 30% to 45% in most studies. Hospital volume appears to influence survival rates. Squamous cell cancers may do better than other tumors. Neoadjuvant chemotherapy studies show encouraging results. Those unfit for surgery have been treated with radiation therapy with 5-year survival rates of 19% to 25%. PORT has not been proven to be helpful in improving long-term survival rates. Adjuvant chemotherapy is the standard approach following surgery as described above.

Stage III

Stage III is a heterogeneous group that includes patients with ipsilateral or subcarinal nodes (N2) and T3 tumors

---

[1]Not FDA approved for this indication.

with N1 nodes for stage IIIA, as well as patients with contralateral nodes (N3) or T4 lesions for stage IIIB (see Table 3). In 1997, the International Staging System removed T3N0 tumors from this group and changed them to stage IIB, making it difficult to interpret results of older studies. The application of prior studies' results to current practice is also limited because of inadequate staging by modern standards.

The treatment of stage III tumors is one of the most controversial aspects of lung cancer care; enrollment in clinical trials is of paramount importance. Patients with nonbulky stage IIIA tumors are generally resected with curative intent. The role of PORT is again unclear. Although no improvement in survival has been noted, radiation can decrease local recurrence (which can be a devastating occurrence) and may be reasonable. The recent adjuvant chemotherapy data from stages I and II combined with the 1995 meta-analysis and recent International Adjuvant Lung Cancer Trial (IALT), suggesting 5% improvement in 5-year survival, also make postoperative chemotherapy a reasonable consideration (whether chemotherapy should be concurrent or sequential is an area needing further investigation). Given the high risk of distant metastases in stage III, induction or neoadjuvant chemotherapy has appeal. The theoretical benefits include decreasing tumor volume, earlier treatment of micrometastatic disease, and better tolerance to the drugs. With all tumors, chemotherapy response rates for the primary tumor is generally higher than with metastatic disease, presumably as a result of less-resistant clones having developed.

PORT alone has been abandoned in favor of chemotherapy or combination radiation and chemotherapy. A recent phase III study by the North American Intergroup reported a significant improvement in progression-free survival with surgery following induction concurrent chemoradiation. The 2005 abstract update also showed no improvement in overall survival as a result of the higher death rate from postoperative complications, including a 29% operative mortality in patients who required a complex pneumonectomy. Despite even trimodality therapy, the 5-year survival rates remain 20% to 25% at most.

Patients with bulky stage IIIA and stage IIIB tumors are generally unresectable and do quite poorly with 5-year survival rates around 5% to 10%. Radiation therapy has been used as a single agent, with local control being a significant problem. Only 17% obtain a complete remission on x-ray. Induction chemotherapy has been repeatedly studied, and has an approximately 10% relative reduction in death or an absolute survival advantage of 2% to 3%. The benefit of this approach seems to disappear after the second year of follow-up. Local failure within the chest remains a significant problem with this approach. Concurrent chemotherapy with radiation offers the potential benefit of improved local and distant control, with chemotherapy adding to local control as a radiation sensitizer and distant control with treatment of micrometastatic disease. The optimal regimen is uncertain and the subject of active investigation. A regimen from the Southwest Oncology Group (SWOG) employing cisplatin (Platinol AQ[1]) and etoposide (VePesid[1]) with radiation followed by docetaxel (Taxotere) has yielded a 5-year overall survival

rate of 15%. A regimen with weekly carboplatin (Paraplatin[1]) and paclitaxel (Taxol) is popular in the United States, with phase II data yielding a 4-year survival rate of 16%.

Stage IIIB with Malignant Pleural Effusion and Stage IV

With rare exceptions, stage IV (see Table 3) patients are incurable with currently available modalities, and the treatment goals are palliation of symptoms and prolongation of survival. Occasionally patients with an isolated metastasis, such as that involving the brain, may be cured with surgical resection followed by whole-brain radiation therapy. In the 1970s, when response rates with all chemotherapy were quite low, it was widely held that chemotherapy held no value in the treatment of advanced lung cancer. With the advent of potentially more effective therapies, it has been shown that chemotherapy offers not only some improvement in survival, but also a better quality of life and economic savings because of fewer hospitalizations for symptom management. Although the median survival rates are improved by only 2 to 3 months, with modern therapies, it is expected that 30% to 45% of patients live beyond 1 year, approximately 20% live beyond 2 years, and an occasional patient lives 5 years or longer with metastatic disease. This is in stark contrast to the historical 1-year survival rate of 15% with essentially no 5-year survivors.

The cornerstone of current therapy is platinum-based doublets (two drugs), which is the preferred approach in otherwise healthy patients with preserved functional performance status. Meta-analyses show improved median and 1-year survival response rates compared with single-agent drugs. A large randomized trial comparing four different platinum-containing regimens showed no clear advantage to any. Paclitaxel (Taxol), gemcitabine (Gemzar), vinorelbine (Navelbine), docetaxel (Taxotere), and irinotecan (Camptosar[1]) are among the drugs that can be combined with carboplatin (Paraplatin[1]) or cisplatin (Platinol AQ[1]). The choice of the second agent is somewhat arbitrary at this point, and the decision is often based on the side-effect profile relative to the patient's other medical problems and physician's bias toward a particular regimen. Treatment is generally four to six cycles for those who tolerate the regimen and show clinical and radiographic response. Patients with a poor functional status have (for the most part) been excluded from clinical trials making the optimal treatment of this patient population uncertain. One approach might be to treat those patients debilitated from their cancer with aggressive combination chemotherapy. Those patients disabled by comorbid illnesses may tolerate single-agent chemotherapy better.

Second-line therapy is now available for patients who have progressed after initial treatment. The FDA has approved the single-agent chemotherapy drugs docetaxel (Taxotere) and pemetrexed (Alimta) based on improvement in survival and quality of life.

Recently, there has been a movement toward more targeted drugs in the treatment of lung cancer. Examples are the small-molecule tyrosine kinase-inhibitor erlotinib

---

[1]Not FDA approved for this indication.

[1]Not FDA approved for this indication.

(Tarceva) and gefitinib (Iressa). Lung cancer growth is dependent on cell surface membrane receptors that regulate intracellular signal transduction pathways. These can affect cell proliferation, apoptosis (programmed cell death), angiogenesis, cell-to-cell adhesion, and motility. In normal cells, these mechanisms are tightly controlled. The malignant cell has transformed and evades these controls allowing uncontrolled malignant growth. One such tyrosine kinase receptor is the epidermal growth factor receptor (EGFR), otherwise known as erbB-1 or HER-1. These inhibitors were developed to regain control of the discussed pathways as mutations in the adenosine triphosphate (ATP)-binding site cleft of the tyrosine kinase domain results in prolonged expression of tyrosine kinase activity in response to the epidermal growth factor. Overall response rates are 10% as second-line therapy. However, certain subgroups appear to have a more favorable response, with bronchoalveolar cell carcinoma patients responding 38% of the time. Women, Asians, and nonsmokers appear to also have a higher response rate. Recently, activating somatic mutations in the tyrosine kinase domain of the EGFR gene have been found to highly correlate to responsiveness to erlotinib (Tarceva) and gefitinib (Iressa). Several studies have addressed the issue of combination therapy with small-molecule tyrosine kinase inhibitors and chemotherapy, but no clinical benefit was found. Consequently, these drugs are currently used as single agents. The vascular endothelial growth factor (VEGF) receptor antagonist bevacizumab (Avastin[1]) provides a survival benefit when combined with carboplatin (Paraplatin[1]) and paclitaxel (Taxol). Lung cancer treatment will probably move further away from traditional nonselective chemotherapy drugs and continue to become more refined with molecularly targeted therapies such as these.

SMALL CELL LUNG CANCER

Small cell lung cancer accounts for approximately 15% of lung cancers and occurs exclusively in smokers. This malignancy is characterized by rapid growth and early development of widespread metastatic disease. In the 1970s, it was hoped that it would be curable with chemotherapy as most tumors are very sensitive to treatment. Overall, 60% to 80% respond well to chemotherapy, but there is often a concern that tumor lysis syndrome may develop.

Although the primary tumor, regional nodes, metastases (TNM staging system as used in NSCLC) also applies (see Table 3), from a practical standpoint patients are classified as limited stage or extensive stage. Patients who have disease that can be encompassed in a single radiation port are classified as limited stage; extensive stage covers those who have widespread disease. The current treatment for limited stage disease involves four cycles of cisplatin (Platinol AQ[1]) and etoposide (VePesid) with concurrent radiation therapy starting with cycle one. The addition of more drugs to the chemotherapy mixture has not resulted in higher cure rates and more toxicity is seen. With the standard approach, 20% to 40% of patients are alive at 2 years; the long-term survival rate is only 10% to 15%. Patients cured of their small cell cancer are at risk for developing non–small cell lung cancers, as well as head and neck malignancies.

Isolated brain metastases can also be seen in patients in remission, leading to the concept of prophylactic cranial irradiation. No convincing data exist to definitively prove the benefit of this approach. If offered to patients, a thorough discussion of potential long-term cognitive and neurologic side effects must occur before proceeding.

Patients with extensive stage disease are incurable, but chemotherapy doubles survival with most living 8 to 12 months. A platinum drug (carboplatin or cisplatin) with etoposide (VePesid) for four cycles is first-line therapy. There is no demonstrated benefit to maintenance therapy. Triplet and quadruplet drug therapies have been evaluated but not commonly used because of significant toxicity with minimal benefit. Irinotecan (Camptosar[1]) with cisplatin (Platinol AQ[1]) has shown a survival benefit in a Japanese study, but a recent U.S. study failed to confirm those results. Patients who obtain a radiographic response that is durable beyond 6 months can be retreated with the same regimen on relapse. Other second-line drugs include topotecan (Hycamtin) and paclitaxel (Taxol[1]), but participation in a clinical trial is preferred.

Surgery usually has no role in small cell lung cancer except in the rare patient with a small, solitary, pulmonary nodule. If extensive staging, including mediastinoscopy and bone marrow biopsies, fails to demonstrate widespread disease, the approach includes resection followed by adjuvant chemotherapy.

Screening

The purpose of any lung cancer screening is to identify asymptomatic individuals with the disease in hopes that screening will detect the cancer at an earlier stage and, as a result, improve overall survival. There have been multiple studies that have looked at lung cancer screening involving thousands of patients. All of these studies were done in males, prior to the lung cancer epidemic in females. Numerous modalities, including plain chest radiography, sputum cytology, and computed tomography, have been evaluated. Despite some suggestion of improvement in stage distribution and resectability, there has been no improvement in mortality. As a result, all of the major advisory organizations have recommended against routine screening for lung cancer even in patients at high risk. In particular, the United States Preventive Services Task Force (USPSTF) states that "the evidence is insufficient to recommend for or against screening in asymptomatic persons for lung cancer." This position statement is also upheld by the American Academy of Family Physicians. The case of lung cancer screening is not closed; there are two very large studies under way that may change these recommendations in the future.

Lung cancer remains a major public health problem in the United States. Despite recent advances in treatment, the mortality rate remains quite high. Further research and patient participation in clinical trials will undoubtedly lead to continued progress. Greater impact could be achieved by prevention through smoking cessation programs and by preventing our youth from starting tobacco use in the first place.

---

[1]Not FDA approved for this indication.

[1]Not FDA approved for this indication.

REFERENCES

Albain KS, Swann RS, Rusch VR, et al: Phase III Study of concurrent chemotherapy and radiotherapy (CT/RT) vs CT/RT followed by surgical resection for stage IIIA (pN2) non-small cell lung cancer (NSCLC): Outcome update of North American Intergroup 0139 (RTOG 9309) (abstract 7014). Proc Am Soc Clin Oncol 2005.

Jemal A, Murray T, Ward E, et al: Cancer statistics, 2005. CA Cancer J Clin 2005;55:10.

Lung cancer screening: Recommendation statement. Ann Intern Med 2004;140:738.

Lynch TJ, Bell DW, Sordella R, et al: Activating mutations in the epidermal growth factor receptor underlying responsiveness of non-small cell lung cancer to gefitinib. N Engl J Med 2004;350:2129-2139.

Mulshine JL, Sullivan DC: Lung cancer screening. N Engl J Med 2005;2714-2720.

Sandler AR, Gray R, Brahmer J, et al: Randomized phase II/III Trial of paclitaxel (P) plus carboplatin (C) with or without bevacizumab (NSC # 704865) in patients with advanced non-squamous non-small cell lung cancer (NSCLC): An Eastern Cooperative Oncology Group (ECOG) Trial—E4599 (abstract 4). Proc Am Soc Clin Oncol 2005.

Shepherd FA, Pereira JR, Ciuleanu T, et al: Erlotinib in previously treated non-small-cell lung cancer. N Engl J Med 2005;353:123-132.

Spira A, Ettinger DS: Drug therapy: Multidisciplinary management of lung cancer. N Engl J Med 2004;350:379-392.

Strauss GM, Herndon J, Maddaus MA, et al: Randomized clinical trial of adjuvant chemotherapy with paclitaxel and carboplatin following resection in Stage IB non-small cell lung cancer (NSCLC): Report of Cancer and Leukemia Group B (CALGB) Protocol 9633. J Clin Oncol 2004;22(Suppl 14):7019.

Winton T, Livingston R, Johnson D, et al: Vinorelbine plus cisplatin vs. observation in resected non-small cell lung cancer. N Engl J Med 2005;352:2589-2589.

Coccidioidomycosis

Method of
Nancy F. Crum-Cianflone, MD, MPH

Coccidioidomycosis ("Valley Fever") is a re-emerging fungal disease that causes approximately 150,000 infections annually in the United States. The incidence of coccidioidomycosis has risen in the last decade as a result of increasing population of endemic areas and tourism. Until recently, the causative agent of coccidioidomycosis was assumed to be *Coccidioides immitis*. A second species, *C. posadasii*, has now been described with similar clinical manifestations.

Coccidioides is a dimorphic fungus that exists in two forms: a mycelium form in the environment that separates into arthroconidia and a spherule containing endospores in the host. Arthroconidia are the infective form of the fungi and may become airborne when the soil is disrupted. Natural events (e.g., dust storms and earthquakes) as well as human activities (e.g., archaeologic digs and recreational activities) increase the risk of infection. Heavy winter rains followed by a hot, dry summer also increase the number of infections; most cases are noted during the summer and fall. Infection typically occurs after inhalation of arthroconidia; rare cases have occurred in association with organ transplantation or primary skin inoculation. Person-to-person transmission via the respiratory route does not occur.

The geographic distribution of *Coccidioides* includes the southwestern United States (Arizona, California, and parts of Nevada, Utah, New Mexico, and Texas), Mexico (semiarid areas near the U.S. border), and Central and South America (Argentina, Colombia, Paraguay, Venezuela, and Brazil). Coccidioidomycosis is an infection of worldwide importance despite these limited areas of endemicity. Cases may present in nonendemic locations as a result of travel or reactivation of disease.

Clinical Manifestations

Infection is asymptomatic in two-thirds of cases. Symptomatic disease typically manifests as a respiratory infection 1 to 3 weeks after the inhalation of arthroconidia. Manifestations of coccidioidomycosis are usually indistinguishable from other common pulmonary infections; rash, travel to an endemic area, and failure to respond to conventional antibiotic therapy may suggest coccidioidomycosis. The most common presenting symptoms include fever (76%), cough (73%), chest pain (44%), and dyspnea (32%); fatigue, weight loss, headache, chills, night sweats, and myalgias are also common. Rashes may occur in the setting of acute coccidioidomycosis and include toxic erythema (a fine, pruritic, erythematous rash), erythema multiforme, and erythema nodosum; the latter two rashes are hypersensitivity phenomena occurring most often in females. The triad of erythema nodosum, fever, and arthralgias is commonly referred to as "desert rheumatism" and suggests a favorable prognosis. Symptoms last several days to a few weeks; however, fatigue may persist for months after resolution.

Physical examination findings may include fever, pulmonary rales, and rash. The most common laboratory finding is an elevated erythrocyte sedimentation rate. Leukocytosis, eosinophilia, anemia, and hypergammaglobulinemia may also be noted; some patients have normal laboratory studies. Chest radiography typically shows an infiltrate; hilar, paratracheal, and/or mediastinal adenopathy occurs in 20% of cases and effusions in 6%. The presence of mediastinal adenopathy is associated with a high risk for disseminated disease. A miliary pattern on chest radiograph is a sign of severe disease, which most often occurs in immunocompromised hosts.

Although pulmonary coccidioidomycosis typically resolves in weeks to months without specific therapy, complicated infections may occur. Patients may present with respiratory failure or shock; both are associated with high mortality rates. Patients who develop pneumonia may fail to resolve and develop chronic fibrocavitary pulmonary infection characterized by prolonged cough, hemoptysis, dyspnea, fevers, and weight loss. Other potential complications are residual nodules (5% of cases), which may prompt biopsies to exclude malignancy. Thin-walled cavities occur in 5% of pneumonias; these may self-resolve within 2 years or may rupture, forming a pneumothorax. Extrapulmonary *Coccidioides* infections represent disseminated disease and develop in 1% to 5% of patients. The risk for dissemination is elevated among patients with cellular immunosuppressive conditions (e.g., acquired immune deficiency syndrome [AIDS]; cancer such as Hodgkin's lymphoma; treatment with chemotherapy, corticosteroids, or tumor necrosis factor inhibitors) and during late pregnancy and the postpartum period. In addition, males and specific racial groups (e.g., African

Americans, Filipinos, and Hispanics) have a higher risk. Persons presenting with coccidioidomycosis with any of these risk factors and those with a complement fixation (CF) titer of greater than 1:16 should be carefully evaluated for the presence of disseminated disease.

Coccidioides can infect nearly every organ in the body, although the lymph nodes, skin, bones/joints, and central nervous system are the most common sites involved. Dissemination typically occurs a few weeks to months after the initial pulmonary infection; the chest radiograph may have normalized by this time. A high index of suspicion is often necessary as coccidioidomycosis is a "great imitator." The most common presenting symptoms of disseminated disease are fevers, night sweats, and localizing symptoms to the area of dissemination.

Cutaneous disease accounts for 15% of disseminated cases and manifests as nodules, papules, abscesses, ulcers, plaques, or draining sinuses. Any chronic, nonhealing skin lesion should prompt consideration of coccidioidomycosis. Diagnosis can be rapidly established by obtaining a punch biopsy of the lesion for fungal culture and histopathology.

Bone and/or joint disease occurs in approximately 20% of disseminated cases and most frequently involves the axial skeleton (e.g., vertebrae, ribs, skull, sternum), the ends of long bones and bony prominences. The knee is the joint most often affected. Plain radiographs may demonstrate marginated, punched-out lytic lesions. A bone scan is the test of choice to rule out bony disease; this test is important as many patients with bone/joint disease have multiple sites of involvement. Areas of abnormal uptake on bone scan should be evaluated by computer tomography (CT) or magnetic resonance imaging (MRI) scans, which provide more information regarding soft-tissue involvement and bony destruction.

Central nervous system (CNS) disease is the most serious form of coccidioidomycosis. Any patient with a headache or neurologic signs should be evaluated with a CT or MRI of the brain and a lumbar puncture. Basilar meningitis, parenchymal lesions, and hydrocephalus are the classic CNS findings. Cerebrospinal fluid (CSF) analysis shows an elevated white blood cell count, elevated protein, depressed glucose, and/or a predominance of lymphocytes and sometimes eosinophils.

Diagnosis

A high index of suspicion for the diagnosis of coccidioidomycosis is needed among residents or recent travelers to endemic areas. The diagnosis is established by culture, histopathology, or serologic tests. Fungal cultures, especially of the skin or bone, may yield the organism in 3 to 5 days; special care must be taken to prevent *Coccidioides* from being transmitted to laboratory personnel. Histopathology may demonstrate *Coccidioides* spherules (pathognomonic for the disease) as well as granulomas. Serologic tests are commonly used to diagnosis coccidioidomycosis and include enzyme immunoassay (EIA), CF titer, and immunodiffusion. The EIA serology tests for both IgM and IgG; a positive IgM and seroconversion of the IgG from a negative to a positive test suggest acute disease. Of note, the EIA IgM is occasionally falsely positive because of the high sensitivity of the test; therefore, a positive IgM should be confirmed with a concurrent

CURRENT DIAGNOSIS

High index of suspicion among travelers or residents of an endemic area
- Diagnostic Tests:
  - Positive culture
  - Histopathology showing *Coccidioides* spherules
  - Serology: enzyme immunoassay, complement fixation titer, immunodiffusion

positive IgG or CF test. An isolated positive IgG suggests a prior infection. CF titers greater than 1:16 strongly suggest the possibility of disseminated disease. CF titers are helpful for following the disease activity, as rising titers suggest disease progression and falling titers suggest clinical response.

Treatment

Management of all coccidioidomycosis cases includes patient follow-up for at least 2 years to document resolution of the infection and to identify the development of complicated disease as early as possible. Treatment of coccidioidomycosis is dependent on the form of disease, the severity and site(s) of infection, and the immune and demographic characteristics of the patient. Guidelines have been published by the Infectious Disease Society of America and were recently updated.

Specific antifungal medications active against *Coccidioides* include amphotericin B deoxycholate (Fungizone), amphotericin B lipid formulations (Amphotec, Abelcet, AmBisome), fluconazole (Diflucan), itraconazole (Sporanox), and ketoconazole (Nizoral) (Table 1). Ketoconazole is rarely used today. Voriconazole (Vfend), posaconazole (Noxafil[4]), and caspofungin (Cancidas[1]) are novel antifungal agents with activity against *Coccidioides*, but further clinical data are needed.

Treatment is debatable as primary pneumonias typically resolve without antifungal therapy. Specific clinical and demographic factors that prompt consideration for therapy have been identified. These include risk factors for dissemination or severe disease such as the following:

- AIDS, organ transplant, and cancer patients
- Systemic corticosteroids and tumor necrosis factor inhibitors
- Pregnancy/immediate postpartum period
- African Americans, Filipinos, Hispanics
- Diabetes, preexisting cardiopulmonary disease, age >55 years
- Significant symptoms (weight loss >10%, night sweats >3 weeks, inability to work, or symptoms >2 months)
- Radiographic findings with infiltrates involving more than half of one lung or portions of both lungs or prominent hilar or mediastinal adenopathy
- CF titer >1:16

Most experts recommend an oral azole (fluconazole 400 mg daily or itraconazole oral solution 200 mg twice daily)

[1]Not FDA approved for this indication.
[4]Investigational drug in the United States.

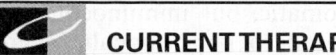
CURRENT THERAPY

Site of Infection	Management
Primary Pulmonary Infection	
No risk factors for dissemination and no prolonged symptoms*	Observe or fluconazole 400 mg qd for 3–6 months or itraconazole 200 mg bid for 3–6 months
Risk factors or prolonged symptoms*	Fluconazole 400 mg/d for 3–6 months or itraconazole 200 mg bid for 3–6 months
Diffuse pneumonia (miliary), respiratory failure, septic shock	Amphotericin B 1 mg/kg IV daily or lipid formulation of amphotericin 5 mg/kg daily; after clinical improvement, switch to azole; treat for at least 1 year
Chronic fibrocavity pulmonary disease	Azole therapy for at least 1 year
Disseminated Disease	
Nonmeningeal—immediately life-threatening†	Amphotericin B 1 mg/kg IV daily or lipid formulation of amphotericin 5 mg/kg daily; after clinical improvement, switch to azole for at least 1–2 years
Nonmeningeal—slowly progressive, stable disease	Azole therapy for at least 1–2 years; itraconazole is preferable for bony disease.
Meningeal or CNS	Fluconazole 400-2000 mg[3] daily or Itraconazole 600 mg daily or azole plus intrathecal amphotericin B. Requires lifelong azole therapy.

*See text for specific details.
†Some experts also begin with amphotericin B for patients with multifocal disease or with lesions in critical locations such as the vertebrae.
[3] Exceeds dosage recommended by the manufacturer.

for 3 to 6 months in patients with one or more of these factors. During pregnancy, amphotericin B is the treatment of choice since azoles are teratogenic.

Patients presenting with a miliary infiltrate or with respiratory failure should initially be treated with amphotericin B (Fungizone). An oral azole may be used to complete at least 1 year of therapy after clinical improvement, which usually happens after several weeks. Chronic fibrocavitary disease cases are usually treated with oral azoles for at least 1 year. Asymptomatic lung nodules or cavities do not require antifungal therapy.

Disseminated disease requires prompt antifungal medications in all cases and consultation with an infectious disease specialist. Therapy for nonmeningeal disseminated disease should be administered for a minimum of 1 to 2 years, including at least 6 months after disease is inactive. Patients with localized skin or bone/joint infections can typically be managed with oral azoles (fluconazole 400 to 800 mg qd[3] or itraconazole 200 mg oral solution bid-tid[3]).

The oral itraconazole solution is superior to fluconazole when treating bony disease. The oral solution of itraconazole is preferable to capsules because of improved bioavailability; however, itraconazole absorption can be erratic necessitating monitoring of serum drug levels. Some experts recommend that disease in multiple sites and/or in critical locations, such as the vertebrae, receive amphotericin B; an azole can be substituted after clinical, radiographic and laboratory improvement. Those patients who fail to respond or progress on azole therapy should be treated with amphotericin B.

Amphotericin side effects include rigors and fevers; these can be managed with acetaminophen (Tylenol) 650 mg, diphenhydramine (Benadryl) 50 mg, and/or meperidine (Demerol) 25 mg. Nausea may be treated with prochlorperazine (Compazine) 5 to 10 mg or other antiemetics. Renal dysfunction with associated hypokalemia, hypomagnesemia and a metabolic acidosis may occur. Electrolytes should be monitored daily and replaced via oral or intravenous route. Amphotericin should be held when the creatinine reaches 2.5 to 3.0 mg/dL and a lipid formulation of amphotericin considered as these agents are associated with a lower risk of nephrotoxicity.

Meningitis is treated with fluconazole 400 to 1600 mg daily.[3] Alternatives include oral itraconazole or intrathecal amphotericin B (intravenous amphotericin is ineffective at treating central nervous system infections). A few clinical reports have found voriconazole useful, but further studies are needed. The presence of hydrocephalus often requires placement of a shunt. Patients with CNS disease require lifelong azole therapy.

In addition to antifungal agents, surgery may be useful to remove pulmonary cavities at risk for rupture. In addition, patients with bone/joint disease often benefit from surgical debridement, especially those with a poor response to antifungal agents and with nonviable tissue or sequestra.

TABLE 1 Antifungal Medications for Coccidioidomycosis

Antifungal Agent	Dose	Route
Ketoconazole (Nizoral)*	200–400 mg	PO
Fluconazole (Diflucan)	200–1600† mg	PO, IV
Itraconazole (Sporanox)	200–600 mg	PO, IV
Amphotericin B deoxycholate (Fungizone)	0.6–1.5 mg/kg	IV
Lipid complex amphotericins	3–6 mg/kg	IV

*Ketoconazole is rarely used as newer azoles with fewer adverse effects are available.
†Exceeds the recommended dose by the manufacturer. Doses >1000 mg may be associated with dry skin, alopecia, chapped lips, and balanitis. Azoles are not FDA approved for this indication, but clinical trials support their use.

[3]Exceeds dosage recommended by the manufacturer.

All cases of coccidioidomycosis should be carefully monitored for disease relapse, especially among those with cellular immunodeficiencies or nonwhite race. Clinical visits and CF titers are recommended at a minimum of every 3 to 6 months; patients with evolving disease require more frequent evaluations. Patients with persistent immunocompromising conditions should continue on azoles to prevent relapse.

Prevention of infection may be possible with a polyvalent vaccine; human trials are underway. Prophylaxis studies employing fluconazole among high-risk groups, such as organ transplant recipients, are also ongoing.

REFERENCES

Chiller TM, Galgiani JN, Stevens DA: Coccidioidomycosis. Infect Dis Clin North Am 2003;17:41-57.

Cole GT, Xue JM, Okeke CN, et al: A vaccine against coccidioidomycosis is justified and attainable. Med Mycol 2004;42:189-216.

Crum NF, Lederman ER, Stafford CM, Parrish JS, Wallace MR: Coccidioidomycosis: A descriptive survey of a reemerging disease. Clinical characteristics and current controversies. Medicine (Baltimore) 2004;83:149-175.

Crum NF, Wallace MR: Laboratory values are predictive of disseminated coccidioidomycosis. Infect Dis Clin Pract 2005;13:68-72.

Desai SA, Minai OA, Gordon SM, et al: Coccidioidomycosis in nonendemic areas: A case series. Respir Med 2001;95:305-309.

Deresinski SC: Coccidioidomycosis: Efficacy of new agents and future prospects. Curr Opin Infect Dis 2001;14:693-696.

Galgiani JN: Coccidioidomycosis: A regional disease of national importance. Rethinking approaches to control. Ann Intern Med 1999;130:293-300.

Galgiani JN, Ampel NM, Blair JE, et al: Coccidioidomycosis. Clin Infect Dis 2005;41:1217-1223.

Galgiani JN, Catanzaro A, Cloud GA, et al: Comparison of oral fluconazole and itraconazole for progressive, nonmeningeal coccidioidomycosis: A randomized, double-blind trial. Ann Intern Med 2000;133:676-686.

Johnson RH, Einstein HE: Coccidioidal meningitis. Clin Infect Dis 2006;42:103-107.

Pappagianis D: Serologic studies in coccidioidomycosis. Semin Respir Infect 2001;16:242-250.

Stevens DA: Coccidioidomycosis. N Engl J Med 1995;332:1077-1082.

Histoplasmosis

Method of
*Linus H. Santo Tomas, MD, MS, and
Ralph M. Schapira, MD*

Etiology and Epidemiology

The causative organism of histoplasmosis, *Histoplasma capsulatum*, is found worldwide, but thrives best in moist acidic soil with high organic content. In the United States, infection is highest in areas of the Ohio, Mississippi, and Missouri River valleys. Bat and avian droppings enhance soil characteristics that augment sporulation. Bats can also be infected, thereby transmitting the fungus in their droppings. *H. capsulatum* is a dimorphic fungus that exists in mycelial form in the environment. The infective spores are introduced to the lungs via inhalation and the organism is transformed to a yeast form in the mammalian host.

Most infections are asymptomatic, but immunocompromised hosts and those exposed to large inoculums are more likely to develop progressive or severe disease.

Pathogenesis

Inhaled spores transform to the yeast form in the alveoli within hours to days. This leads to bronchopneumonia. The organism is ingested by macrophages and may be disseminated hematogenously to regional lymph nodes, liver, spleen, and other organs. Neutrophils, which can also phagocytose the organism and release antifungal proteins and granules, are thought to play an important role in limiting the initial phase of the infection. Yeasts may continue to multiply intracellularly within alveolar macrophages. Maturation of cell-mediated immunity is critical to effective control of the disease. The inflammatory response leads to the development of caseating lesions that heal, forming fibrotic lesions with granulomas. The dense fibrotic lesions frequently calcify. Yeast forms have been identified in these calcified lesions, and although attempts to culture the fungus from these lesions have been unsuccessful, the recrudescence of disease in immunocompromised individuals who are no longer in endemic areas suggests that some organisms may remain viable for years.

Clinical Manifestations

Most infections are asymptomatic, and in endemic areas it is not unusual for radiologic studies to show evidence of previous infection in the chest and abdomen, which most commonly appear as calcified granulomas in the lung parenchyma or spleen. The incubation period is from 3 to 21 days after exposure. The development of clinical disease is mainly dependent on the immune status of the host and the inoculum load. The more common presentations of the disease are discussed in the following section.

ACUTE PULMONARY HISTOPLASMOSIS

Localized Pulmonary Disease

Sixty percent of those who develop clinical disease present with acute pulmonary histoplasmosis. Initial symptoms are usually nonspecific and consist of fever, chills, fatigue, and cough. The chest radiograph may reveal mediastinal and hilar adenopathy accompanied by patchy pneumonic infiltrates, but may also be normal in some cases. Limited exposure in an immunocompetent host may manifest with a localized pneumonia that may be mistaken for a bacterial pneumonia. Most do not require antifungal treatment unless there is no improvement after a month.

Diffuse Pulmonary Involvement

More intense exposure, even in an immunocompetent host, can lead to diffuse pulmonary histoplasmosis. The typical chest radiograph may show bilateral reticulonodular or miliary-type infiltrates. Aside from fever, cough, chest pain, and chills, affected patients can have clinically significant hypoxemia that may require ventilatory support.

CHRONIC PULMONARY HISTOPLASMOSIS

In persons with underlying pulmonary disease, especially emphysema, the acute exposure can eventually lead to chronic pulmonary histoplasmosis that is characterized by fibrocavitary lesions on chest radiographs. Symptoms include cough, fatigue, fever, weight loss, and night sweats. Patients can also present with hemoptysis and progressive dyspnea. Chronic pulmonary histoplasmosis may mimic progressive mycobacterial disease, particularly tuberculosis.

GRANULOMATOUS MEDIASTINITIS

Occasionally, lymphadenopathy associated with histoplasmosis may be severe enough to cause compression of the airways, mediastinal vascular structures, and the esophagus. This can lead to cough, chest pain, hemoptysis, dysphagia, and signs of superior vena cava syndrome. Granulomatous mediastinitis has to be distinguished from fibrosing mediastinitis, a rare long-term sequelae of infection. Granulomatous mediastinitis can improve significantly with antifungal and corticosteroid treatment.

DISSEMINATED HISTOPLASMOSIS

Immunocompromised individuals, whether from extremes of age, debilitating comorbid disease, immunosuppressive medications, or immune deficiency syndromes, are at greater risk for disseminated disease. Symptoms may be nonspecific, and can include fever, chills, and weight loss. Physical examination may reveal pneumonitis, hepatosplenomegaly, and lymphadenopathy. Other manifestations depend on specific organs that may be involved. Five percent to 20% of cases may have central nervous system involvement.

OTHER MANIFESTATIONS

Less common manifestations of histoplasmosis include pericarditis, rheumatologic syndromes, broncholithiasis, and fibrosing mediastinitis. Pericarditis is thought to be caused by local immunologic response to release of inflammatory substances from adjacent necrotizing lymph nodes. Arthritis or arthralgia is usually polyarticular and symmetric, and is thought to be secondary to a systemic inflammatory response to the infection rather than actual joint invasion.

DIAGNOSIS

The nonspecific clinical manifestations of histoplasmosis can make diagnosis difficult, and maintaining a high clinical suspicion in the appropriate setting is important. It should be considered as a possible cause of nonresolving pneumonia and fever of unknown origin, especially in endemic areas. A high index of suspicion is also appropriate in immunocompromised hosts. A number of laboratory tests are available for confirmation of suspected disease, each with its own advantages and disadvantages. A combination of these laboratory tests may be needed to maximize the yield of diagnostic tests in less florid infections. Obtaining specimens from respiratory secretions, bronchoalveolar lavage, tissue biopsy, blood, and urine can also increase the overall yield.

CURRENT DIAGNOSIS

- Because clinical presentation is usually nonspecific, a high index of suspicion is needed to arrive at the diagnosis.
- Histoplasmosis should be considered in nonresolving pneumonia and fever of unknown etiology, especially in endemic areas and immunocompromised hosts.
- For rapid diagnosis, the urine *Histoplasma* polysaccharide antigen detection test has good sensitivity (89%) in disseminated histoplasmosis.
- A combination of tests using different specimen types may be needed to maximize the diagnostic yield and confirm the diagnosis.

FUNGAL STAINING

Rapid diagnosis of histoplasmosis can be made with identification of *H. capsulatum* with silver-methenamine stain of biologic specimens. The organism may also be identified by Wright stain of peripheral blood smears in individuals with severe disseminated disease. However, these have lower sensitivity compared to antigen detection and culture.

FUNGAL CULTURE

Blood and bone marrow culture can be positive in 85% to 90% of patients with disseminated and chronic pulmonary disease. The lysis-centrifugation method is best for blood cultures. Analyzing multiple specimens may improve yield. Bronchoalveolar lavage cultures should also be analyzed in patients with pulmonary involvement. The relatively long duration to obtain positive growth on culture limits its usefulness in an acute setting.

DETECTION OF SERUM ANTIBODIES

Serologic testing for antibodies to histoplasma antigen are positive in 80% to 90% of patients with diffuse pulmonary involvement and disseminated disease. Complement fixation and immunodiffusion assays are available. Precipitins to the M or H antigen may be detected but both have significant false positives as a consequence of cross-reactivity with other fungal infections. Other limitations of the test include false negatives early in the course of disease and reduced sensitivity in immunocompromised hosts.

POLYSACCHARIDE ANTIGEN DETECTION

The *Histoplasma* polysaccharide antigen can be detected by conventional radioimmunoassay (RIA) or enzyme immunoassay (EIA) in the urine of up to 92% of patients with disseminated disease and in 37% to 39% with self-limited disease. The same test can be used on serum and other body fluids, but the sensitivity may be lower. It is most useful when serologic tests are less likely to be positive, such as in the early phase of an infection or in immunocompromised hosts. Antigen levels correlate with treatment response and recrudescence and can be used to guide treatment of disseminated histoplasmosis.

Treatment

Most patients who have histoplasmosis recover without treatment. The need for treatment is determined by the type of involvement, the severity and duration of the disease, and the immune status of the patient. Treatment is generally reserved for chronic pulmonary involvement, disseminated disease, or severe acute infections. Such infections most commonly occur in immunocompromised hosts or in those exposed to a large infectious inoculum. Table 1 summarizes the treatment recommendations.

In general, severe disease is initially treated with intravenous deoxycholate amphotericin B (Fungizone) at a dose of 0.7 mg/kg per day. The cumulative dose of amphotericin B depends on the clinical response, but for *Histoplasma* meningitis, completion of a 35-mg/kg course given over 3 to 4 months is recommended. The same cumulative dose of amphotericin B is recommended for other severe forms of histoplasmosis if the patient is unable to take oral medications. A shift from intravenous amphotericin to oral itraconazole (continuation phase) can be considered if there is clinical improvement (i.e., when the patient becomes afebrile, hemodynamically stable, or no longer requires ventilatory support) and is able to take

CURRENT THERAPY

- Treatment is indicated in severe acute (diffuse or localized) pulmonary disease, chronic pulmonary disease, granulomatous mediastinitis with obstructive or invasive symptoms, and disseminated infection.
- Mild to moderate acute pulmonary involvement that persists beyond 4 weeks also warrants treatment.
- Intravenous deoxycholate amphotericin B (Fungizone) is the drug of choice for initial treatment of severe disease. Although more expensive, liposomal amphotericin B (AmBisome)[1] may lead to better outcomes in AIDS patients with moderate to severe disease.
- Oral itraconazole (Sporanox) is the drug of choice for initial treatment of mild to moderate disease and in continuation phase therapy of severe disease that has improved after intravenous amphotericin treatment.
- Fluconazole (Diflucan),[1] which is less active than itraconazole against *H. capsulatum*, has special usefulness in continuation phase therapy of meningitis because of its good cerebrospinal fluid penetration.

[1]Not FDA approved for this indication.

TABLE 1   Recommendations for Treatment of Histoplasmosis

Type of Histoplasmosis	Treatment Regimen
Acute Pulmonary Disease	
Mild to moderate, >4 weeks	Itraconazole (Sporanox) 200 mg, once to twice daily for 6–12 weeks*
Severe	Amphotericin B (Fungizone) 0.7 mg/kg/d,[†] then itraconazole 200 mg once to twice daily for 12 weeks
	Consider corticosteroids (effectiveness not proven)
Chronic Pulmonary Disease	
Mild to moderate	Itraconazole 200 mg once to twice daily for 12–24 months
Severe	Amphotericin B 0.7 mg/kg/d,[†] then itraconazole 200 mg once to twice daily for 12–24 months
Granulomatous Mediastinitis	
Mild to moderate	Itraconazole 200 mg once to twice daily for 6–12 months
Severe	Amphotericin B 0.7 mg/kg/d,[†] then itraconazole 200 mg once to twice daily for 6–12 months
Disseminated Disease (without AIDS)	
Mild to moderate	Itraconazole 200 mg once to twice daily for 6-18 months
Severe	Amphotericin B 0.7 mg/kg/d,[†] then itraconazole 200 mg once to twice daily for 6–18 months[‡]
Disseminated Disease (with AIDS)	
Mild to moderate	Itraconazole 200 mg once to twice daily for life
Severe	Amphotericin B 0.7 mg/kg/d,[†] then itraconazole 200 mg once to twice daily for life
Meningitis	Amphotericin B 0.7 mg/kg/d[†] to total 35 mg/kg over 3–4 months, then fluconazole (Diflucan)[1] 800 mg daily[3] for 9–12 months

*Blood levels may be checked if poor absorption or increased metabolism is suspected.
[†]If amphotericin B is used exclusively, a total course dose of ≤35 mg/kg is recommended. Lipid preparation of amphotericin may be given at 3 mg/kg/d; recent studies in AIDS patients suggest better outcomes compared to deoxycholate amphotericin B (see text).
[‡]Continue treatment until *Histoplasma* urine and serum antigen concentrations <4 units.
[1]Not FDA approved for this indication.
[3]Exceeds dosage recommended by the manufacturer.

oral medications. The duration of itraconazole (Sporanox) treatment also varies according to the type and severity of histoplasmosis (see Table 1). Monitoring of itraconazole blood levels should be considered if there is concern about absorption or use of medications that may reduce its bioavailability.

The lipid formulations approved for use with invasive fungal infections include amphotericin lipid complex (Abelcet), amphotericin B colloidal dispersion (Amphotec), and liposomal amphotericin B (AmBisome), but only the latter has been studied with histoplasmosis. Recent studies involving AIDS patients suggest that liposomal amphotericin B may lead to better clinical outcomes, including earlier clearance of the fungal burden, as well as improved survival, when compared to deoxycholate amphotericin B and itraconazole for treatment of moderate to severe histoplasmosis. Thus, although liposomal amphotericin B[1] may be more costly, it should be considered as an alternative first-line drug for AIDS patients who have moderate to severe disease, especially for those who are at risk for, or who already have, renal insufficiency.

Among the oral agents itraconazole (Sporanox) has the greatest activity against *H. capsulatum*. Ketoconazole (Nizoral) is also active against *Histoplasma* but is less well tolerated than itraconazole. Although fluconazole (Diflucan)[1] is the least active against *Histoplasma*, it has special usefulness in meningitis because of its ability to reach 80% of the blood concentration in the cerebrospinal fluid. To reduce the relapse risk of meningitis, fluconazole 800 mg PO daily[3] is recommended for 9 to 12 months after the full course of intravenous amphotericin is completed. Itraconazole does not enter the cerebrospinal fluid.

Anti-inflammatory treatment, as an adjunct to antifungal therapy, may be considered in certain forms of histoplasmosis. The inflammatory response in diffuse pulmonary histoplasmosis is thought to add to the severity of respiratory dysfunction. In addition to antifungal treatment, a 2-week course of prednisone at 60 mg daily can be considered. Pericarditis may also respond to treatment with corticosteroids or nonsteroidal anti-inflammatory agents. For rheumatologic manifestations, nonsteroidal anti-inflammatory agents can be given for 2 to 12 weeks.

REFERENCES

Durkin MM, Connolly PA, Wheat LJ: Comparison of radioimmunoassay and enzyme-linked immunoassay methods for detection of *Histoplasma capsulatum* var. *capsulatum* antigen. J Clin Microbiol 1997;35(9):2252-2255.

Johnson PC, Wheat LJ, Cloud GA, et al: Safety and efficacy of liposomal amphotericin B compared with conventional amphotericin B for induction therapy of histoplasmosis in patients with AIDS. Ann Intern Med 2002;137(2):105-109.

Newman SL, Bucher C, Rhodes J, Bullock WE: Phagocytosis of *Histoplasma capsulatum* yeasts and microconidia by human cultured macrophages and alveolar macrophages. Cellular cytoskeleton requirement for attachment and ingestion. J Clin Invest 1990; 85(1):223-230.

Newman SL, Gootee L, Gabay JE: Human neutrophil-mediated fungistasis against *Histoplasma capsulatum*. Localization of fungistatic activity to the azurophil granules. J Clin Invest 1993;92(2):624-631.

Sathapatayavongs B, Batteiger BE, Wheat J, et al: Clinical and laboratory features of disseminated histoplasmosis during two large urban outbreaks. Medicine (Baltimore) 1983;62(5):263-270.

---

[1]Not FDA approved for this indication.
[3]Exceeds dosage recommended by the manufacturer.

Wheat J: Histoplasmosis. Experience during outbreaks in Indianapolis and review of the literature. Medicine (Baltimore) 1997;76(5): 339-254.

Wheat J, Sarosi G, McKinsey D, et al: Practice guidelines for the management of patients with histoplasmosis. Infectious Diseases Society of America. Clin Infect Dis 2000;30(4):688-695.

Wheat LJ, Cloud G, Johnson PC, et al: Clearance of fungal burden during treatment of disseminated histoplasmosis with liposomal amphotericin B versus itraconazole. Antimicrob Agents Chemother 2001;45(8):2354-2357.

Wheat LJ, Connolly-Stringfield P, Kohler RB, et al: *Histoplasma capsulatum* polysaccharide antigen detection in diagnosis and management of disseminated histoplasmosis in patients with acquired immunodeficiency syndrome. Am J Med 1989;87(4):396-400.

Wheat LJ, Kauffman CA: Histoplasmosis. Infect Dis Clin North Am 2003;17(1):1-19, vii.

Williams B, Fojtasek M, Connolly-Stringfield P, Wheat J: Diagnosis of histoplasmosis by antigen detection during an outbreak in Indianapolis, Ind. Arch Pathol Lab Med 1994;118(12):1205-1208.

Blastomycosis

Method of
Robert Bradsher, MD, and
Anupama Menon, MD, MPH

Epidemiology

Blastomycosis is caused by infection with the thermally dimorphic fungus *Blastomyces dermatitidis*. The organism grows as a yeast form at 98.6°F (37°C) and as a mycelial form at room temperature. In the environment, the fungus is thought to exist in warm, moist soil associated with decomposing vegetation and decaying wood. In North America, *B. dermatitidis* is endemic along the Mississippi and Ohio River basins, in the regions that surround the Great Lakes, and in a small area of New York and Canada along the St. Lawrence River. Hyperendemic areas with very high rates of blastomycosis have been reported within these endemic regions. Cases outside North America have been described most commonly in Africa, but there have been reports of blastomycosis on several continents.

Infection with *B. dermatitidis* usually occurs via inhalation of aerosolized conidia. Cutaneous inoculation has been reported after inadvertent exposure in the laboratory, at autopsy, and after dog bites. Person-to-person transmission has been described in rare cases of sexual and perinatal transmission. The median incubation period is approximately 30 to 45 days.

Clinical Manifestations

Approximately 50% of infected individuals may be asymptomatic. Pulmonary disease may be acute or chronic. Acute pulmonary blastomycosis presents similarly to bacterial pneumonia with abrupt onset of fever, chills, pleuritic chest pain, myalgias, arthralgias, and cough that is initially nonproductive but later becomes productive of purulent sputum. Chest radiography demonstrates lobar or segmental consolidation; pleural effusion and hilar adenopathy are unusual. Patients diagnosed with blastomycosis may develop progressive, chronic disease that may involve pulmonary and numerous extrapulmonary sites. Patients with chronic pulmonary blastomycosis present with productive cough, hemoptysis, weight loss, pleuritic chest pain, and low-grade fever. Alveolar or fibronodular infiltrates, mass lesions, nodular lesions, and cavitation are seen on chest radiography. Findings may mimic tuberculosis, other endemic mycoses, or bronchogenic carcinoma. Acute respiratory failure may be seen with miliary disease or diffuse pneumonitis and is associated with a very high mortality.

Hematogenous dissemination to almost any other organ may occur. Manifestations in the skin, bone, or genitourinary tract are the most common and may be seen after clearance of pulmonary manifestations. The skin is the most frequently encountered extrapulmonary site of infection. Lesions are usually characterized as verrucous or ulcerative; they may be mistaken for squamous cell carcinoma, atypical mycobacterial infection, pyoderma gangrenosum, or keratoacanthoma. After the skin, bone is the most frequent site of dissemination. Manifestations include osteolytic lesions with associated soft-tissue abscesses or chronic draining sinuses. Genitourinary disease occurs in some male cases, affecting the prostate and epididymis. Although central nervous system (CNS) infection is reported in only a small number of normal hosts, it is a relatively common complication in immunocompromised patients, in whom it may present as an abscess or meningitis. In a review of AIDS patients with blastomycosis, 40% had CNS involvement. Indeed, blastomycosis is more often disseminated and fulminant in patients with AIDS and other types of chronic immunosuppression; mortality rates of 30% to 40% have been reported in these groups.

Diagnosis

The definitive diagnosis of blastomycosis is based on isolation of the organism from cultures of clinical specimens. Mycologic media usually demonstrate growth after an incubation period of 2 to 4 weeks. Conversion from the mycelial form to the yeast phase is required for confirmation.

Because isolation of the organism may take weeks, presumptive diagnosis of blastomycosis is established by identification of the characteristic yeast form in clinical specimens. With a compatible clinical picture, treatment should be initiated if round, broad-based budding yeasts with thick, doubly refractile cell walls are seen on a wet

mount preparation with addition of 10% potassium hydroxide to digest mammalian cells. In histopathologic specimens, acute suppurative and granulomatous inflammation are found. Visualization in tissue is improved by the use of special stains, such as the Gomori methenamine silver and periodic acid-Schiff stains. Nucleic acid hybridization tests are now commercially available and significantly shorten identification time. Most serologic tests are neither adequately sensitive nor specific to be useful in diagnosing blastomycosis, although newer antigen assays may be more reliable. A recently developed assay detects *Blastomyces* antigen in urine, serum, and other body fluids, including cerebrospinal fluid. The test is most sensitive in urine samples, in which 70% to 80% are positive in disseminated blastomycosis, and almost 100% are positive in pulmonary disease. Antigen is detected in serum in approximately 50% of cases. Cross-reactivity can occur in patients with other endemic mycoses. The assay may be used to monitor response to therapy and to detect recurrence.

Treatment

Although spontaneous resolution of acute blastomycotic pneumonia has been reported in immunocompetent hosts, most patients with blastomycosis require treatment. Treatment is indicated in all immunocompromised individuals and in all patients with progressive pulmonary disease or extrapulmonary disease. Factors to consider when initiating therapy include the severity and extent of disease, the immune status of the patient, and the toxicities of the antifungal agents.

PULMONARY DISEASE

For mild to moderate lung disease, itraconazole (Sporanox) is the preferred oral agent because it is efficacious and well tolerated. The initial dose should be 200 to 400 mg daily.

CURRENT DIAGNOSIS

- Because colonization with *B. dermatitidis* does not occur, identification by culture or histology confirms infection.
- The gold standard for diagnosis is culture of the organism from clinical specimens, which may take up to 4 weeks.
- A presumptive diagnosis may be made by visualization of the typical yeast from clinical specimens in the appropriate setting

CURRENT THERAPY

- Itraconazole (Sporanox) is the agent used most commonly to treat blastomycosis. It is administered in an oral dose of 200 to 400 mg daily for 6–12 months, depending on the site of infection.
- For life-threatening pulmonary disease (adult respiratory distress syndrome [ARDS]) or severe disseminated disease, amphotericin B (Fungizone) is the drug of choice. After initial improvement, itraconazole may be substituted.
- For CNS blastomycosis, amphotericin is used because itraconazole does not adequately penetrate the CNS. Liposomal amphotericin is used when high doses are needed or adverse effects from amphotericin B are encountered.
- Fluconazole (Diflucan),[1] ketoconazole (Nizoral), and IV itraconazole have lesser roles in the treatment of blastomycosis. Voriconazole (Vfend)[1] has not been studied adequately, but it may hold promise for CNS disease.

[1]Not FDA approved for this indication.

Treatment should continue for at least 6 months. Bioavailability of itraconazole capsules is enhanced with food, whereas the oral suspension should be taken while fasting. Attention should be given to the patient's concurrent medications because of the potential for drug–drug interactions. Intravenous itraconazole has not been studied in blastomycosis and has no major benefits to offer. Ketoconazole (Nizoral) at 400 to 800 mg daily is an alternative agent to itraconazole, but it is associated with significant adverse effects, serious drug interactions, and higher rates of relapse. Clinical experience with fluconazole (Diflucan)[1] indicates that this agent is as efficacious as ketoconazole at doses of 400 to 800 mg daily. In patients with life-threatening pulmonary disease, progression of disease while on an azole or inability to tolerate an azole, amphotericin B (Fungizone) remains the agent of choice. A dose of 0.7 to 1.0 mg/kg daily should be administered until a cumulative dose of 1.5 to 2.5 g is completed. Some patients may be switched to oral itraconazole at 200 to 400 mg daily after clinical stabilization with amphotericin B. Lipid formulations of amphotericin B have not been adequately studied, but have been used in patients unable to tolerate conventional amphotericin B.

NERVOUS SYSTEM DISEASE

CNS infection should be treated with amphotericin B at a dose of 0.7 to 1.0 mg/kg daily to complete a total dose of 2.0 to 2.5 g. Itraconazole and ketoconazole are not recommended because of inadequate CNS penetration; fluconazole at 800 mg daily may be considered if amphotericin B is not tolerated.

EXTRAPULMONARY DISEASE (WITHOUT CNS INVOLVEMENT)

For mild to moderate disease, itraconazole at 200 to 400 mg daily is recommended for a minimum of 6 months. Patients whose disease progresses on this agent should be switched to amphotericin B to complete at least 1.5 g. Bone disease should be treated for at least 1 year. For life-threatening disease, amphotericin B at 0.7 to 1.0 mg/kg daily should be administered for a total dose of 2.0 to 2.5 g. In immunocompromised individuals, many authorities recommend long-term suppressive therapy with itraconazole after a treatment course of amphotericin B. Pregnant women should be treated with amphotericin B because the azoles are teratogenic. Data on blastomycosis in children are sparse, but some authorities suggest initial amphotericin B because of a potential unfavorable response to azoles.

NEW ANTIFUNGAL AGENTS

Voriconazole (Vfend)[1] is active in vitro and in animal models of pulmonary blastomycosis; the in vitro activity against *B. dermatitidis* is similar to itraconazole. Although clinical data in treating blastomycosis in humans are inadequate, voriconazole has good CNS penetration based on reports of successful treatment of CNS aspergillosis. Posaconazole (Noxafil),[4] which is not yet licensed in the

United States, is also active in vitro and in animal models. Further data are needed before these agents may be recommended for use in blastomycosis. The echinocandin class of antifungal agents shows variable activity against *B. dermatitidis* and there are no clinical data to support their use.

REFERENCES

Bradsher RW: Clinical features of blastomycosis. Semin Respir Infect 1997;12:229-234.

Bradsher RW, Chapman SW, Pappas PG: Blastomycosis. Infect Dis Clin North Am 2003;17:21-40.

Chapman SW. *Blastomyces dermatitidis*. In: Mandell GL, Bennett JE, Dolin R (eds): Principles and Practice of Infectious Diseases. New York, Churchill Livingstone, 2005, pp. 3026-3040.

Chapman SW, Bradsher RW, Campbell GD, et al: Practice guidelines for the management of patients with blastomycosis. Clin Infect Dis 2000;30:679-683.

Chapman SW, Lin AC, Hendricks KA, et al: Endemic blastomycosis in Mississippi: Epidemiological and clinical studies. Semin Respir Infect 1997;12:219-228.

Lemos LB, Guo M, Baliga M: Blastomycosis: organ involvement and etiologic diagnosis. A review of 123 patients from Mississippi. Ann Diagn Pathol 2000;4:391-406.

Pappas PG: Blastomycosis in the immunocompromised patient. Semin Respir Infect 1997;12:243-251

Schutze GE, Hickerson SL, Fortin EM, et al: Blastomycosis in children. Clin Infect Dis 1996;22:496-502.

Sugar AM, Liu X-P: Efficacy of voriconazole in treatment of murine pulmonary blastomycosis. Antimicrob Agents Chemother 2001;45:601-604.

Pleural Effusion and Empyema Thoracis

Method of
Jeffrey Rentz, MD, and Robert L. Thurer, MD

The pleural space normally contains 0.1 to 0.3 mL/kg of serous fluid. Each day, the parietal pleura produces 0.25 mL/kg of fluid, essentially all of which is absorbed by the pleural lymphatics. Because the normal pleura and lungs have a large absorptive capacity (approximately 5-10 mL/kg/day), any fluid collection in the pleural space is abnormal. When effusions do occur, patients may have symptoms such as dyspnea, chest pain, fatigue, and cough. Fever and weight loss are symptoms of pleural space infection.

Pleural effusions are categorized as transudates or exudates. Altered osmotic or hydrostatic forces cause transudative effusions. Notably, transudates contain low protein. Treatment of transudative effusions is initially directed toward correction of the causative disorder. Exudative effusions develop from alterations in lymphatic drainage or abnormalities of the capillary permeability of the pleura itself. These effusions contain higher levels of protein. Treatments of exudative effusions also may deal with the underlying disorder, but pleural interventions are necessary more often. Common causes of both transudates and exudates are shown in Box 1.

Various imaging studies are appropriate for evaluating a patient with suspected or known pleural effusion.

---

[1]Not FDA approved for this indication.

[4]Investigational drug in the United States.

BOX 1 Common Etiologies of Transudative and Exudative Effusions

Transudates

Congestive heart failure
Renal disease
Nephrotic syndrome
Uremia
Peritoneal dialysis
Cirrhosis
Myxedema

Exudates

Malignancy
Infection
Pancreatitis
Subphrenic abscess
Collagen vascular diseases
Methotrexate exposure
Asbestos exposure
Postcardiotomy and post infarction syndromes
Hemothorax
Chylothorax

Upright posterior-anterior and lateral chest radiographs should be always obtained but do not reliably identify pleural fluid collections of less than 500 mL. Lesser amounts of fluid may be detected as blunting of the costophrenic angle on the lateral film. Decubitus films are more sensitive for identifying minimal effusions and can help determine whether the fluid is loculated. Thoracic ultrasound is useful to define loculated collections and is associated with a reduction in complications during thoracentesis. Chest computed tomography (CT) scans are relied on to define and characterize fluid collections and assess the underlying lung. They are very helpful in following the course of treatment of patients with pleural effusions or empyema. Magnetic resonance imaging (MRI) offers little more information than chest CT.

Thoracentesis is typically performed for initial evaluation of patients with pleural effusion. As much fluid as possible should be drained because adequate drainage may be therapeutic as well as diagnostic. CT scanning provides better visualization of the lung parenchyma and pleural process when done after rather than before initial drainage. Thoracentesis is the simplest method of pleural drainage and can be performed at the bedside with or without image guidance. Proper fluid analysis begins with gross observation (for clarity, cloudiness, blood, or foul smell), Gram stain, culture with sensitivity, pH, cell count and differential, cytology, protein, lactate dehydrogenase (LDH), and glucose. Bilirubin levels are appropriate when hepatic diseases are suspected. Elevated amylase is present in patients with effusions related to pancreatic disorders.

If targeted treatments fail or if symptoms require management before those treatments are effective, therapeutic drainage of the pleural space is required. For most patients, bedside or ultrasound-guided thoracentesis will suffice. Video-assisted thoracentesis allows a thorough examination of the lung and pleural space with biopsies if necessary as well as enhanced drainage of loculated effusions. Patients usually require general anesthesia and single lung ventilation, whereas diagnostic thoracoscopy can be done with conscious sedation and local anesthesia in good-risk patients. Chemical pleurodesis is appropriate for patients with recurrent effusions (especially malignant effusions) as long as the lung expands well following drainage. We typically use talc (Sclerosal) introduced as an aerosol (5 g) during thoracoscopy or as a *slurry* (5 g suspended in 100 mL normal saline) placed through chest drains for patients with malignant effusions. Diluted doxycycline (Vibramycin)[1] (10 mg/kg diluted in 100 mL normal saline) is appropriate for patients with benign disorders because the incidence of late fibrothorax may be less with doxycycline (Vibramycin)[1] than with talc. For patients with lung entrapment because of malignancy, an indwelling silastic catheter that can be intermittently drained as an outpatient (Pleurx) may help control dyspnea. Hepatic hydrothorax is difficult to treat with pleurodesis unless the underlying disease has been treated. Reexpansion pulmonary edema occurs if more than 1.5 L are drained at one time, however, this is uncommon.

Empyema

Empyema refers to infected pleural fluid or frank pus in the pleural space. It is related usually to bacterial pneumonia, but other causes include chest trauma, esophageal perforation, seeding from systemic infection, and complications of thoracic procedures. Parapneumonic effusions frequently are present in patients hospitalized for pneumonia. Most are uninfected *sympathetic* effusions, but up to 20% progress to empyema. Light has described criteria that define empyema based on pleural fluid analysis (Box 2).

Although generally divided into three phases, the pathophysiology of empyema should be thought of as a continuum. The first or acute exudative phase is characterized by thin, purulent fluid and expandable underlying lung. During the second transitional or fibrinopurulent phase, fibrin organizes on the lung. The fluid is more turbid and the cellularity increases. A thick, organized fibrous peel that envelops the visceral pleura and effectively *traps* the lung typifies the third or chronic organizational phase.

The principles of management for patients with empyema are drainage of the infected fluid, reexpansion of the underlying lung with obliteration of free spaces in the pleura (no space—no problem) as well as systemic administration of appropriate antibiotics. Percutaneous drains (small *pigtail* catheters or larger chest tubes) adequately treat most early stage patients. No further instrumentation is needed if the fluid is removed, the lung expands, and there is no additional fluid accumulation. Tube thoracostomy with a 28-F to 32-F chest tube is preferable to a small catheter when the fluid is thick or turbid.

---

[1]Not FDA approved for this indication.

BOX 2 Light's Criteria for Exudative Effusions

Pleural fluid protein to serum protein ratio greater than 0.5
Pleural LDH greater than 200 or pleural LDH/serum LDH greater than 0.6

Abbreviations: LDH = lactate dehydrogenase.

CURRENT DIAGNOSIS

- Transudates are characterized by low protein and low LDH.
- Exudates are characterized by high protein and high LDH.
- Chest CT scans should be obtained after therapeutic thoracentesis.
- Direct observation of the pleural fluid is important for diagnosis.

Abbreviations: CT = computed tomography; LDH= lactate dehydrogenase.

During the transitional phase, the fluid becomes loculated and more complicated to drain. Tubes may be placed using image guidance and fibrinolytics can be instilled to promote drainage. The majority of patients in this stage are best treated by video-assisted decortication and drainage. With this method, loculations can be lysed, the fluid drained completely and lung expansion improved by debridement of the visceral pleura. Video-assisted drainage has a higher rate of success, and results in fewer intensive care unit days and fewer hospital days of care than treatment with fibrinolytics. Mortality increases with delays in drainage.

When an empyema progresses to the organized stage with *trapped* lung, thoracoscopic surgery is difficult, and open thoracotomy is needed for adequate decortication. If the lung expands well and there is only a small residual effusion, the chest tubes may be removed in 3 to 4 days. If the lung fails to expand, the residual space can be managed by removing the tubes slowly over several weeks or by daily irrigation with anti-biotic solution followed by primary closure (Clagett procedure). For patients unable to tolerate thoracotomy, open drainage by rib resection and marsupialization (Eloesser flap) is preferable to prolonged closed drainage.

Special consideration is needed for patients with empyema and bronchopleural fistula. Initial therapy requires drainage of the infected fluid to prevent aspiration of purulent material through the fistula. Definitive treatment ranges from open repair with vascularized flap coverage (chest wall muscle or omentum), if the fistula is discovered promptly, to open drainage with an Eloesser flap. This may be followed by a Clagett procedure if the fistula heals.

The authors wish to thank Dr. David Feller-Kopman for his helpful review of the manuscript.

CURRENT THERAPY

- Thoracentesis always should remove as much fluid as possible.
- Early drainage is indicated for patients with parapneumonic effusions.
- Video assisted procedures are more effective than drainage with small or large bore tubes.
- Prompt decortication is more effective than lesser operations.

REFERENCES

Clagett OT, Geraci JC: A procedure for the management of postpneumonectomy empyema. J Thorac Cardiovasc Surg 1963;45:141.

Erickson KV, Yost M, Bynoe R, et al: Primary treatment of malignant pleural effusions: video-assisted thoracoscopic surgery poudrage versus tube thoracostomy. Am Surg 2002;68(11):955-959.

Hasley PB, Albaum MN, Li YH, et al: Do pulmonary radiographic findings at presentation predict mortality in patients with community-acquired pneumonia? Arch Intern Med 1996;156(19):2206-2212.

Kennedy L, Rusch VW, Strange C, et al: Pleurodesis using talc slurry. Chest 1994;106(2):342-346.

Light RW, MacGregor MI, Luchsinger PC, et al: Pleural effusions: The diagnostic separation of transudates and exudates. Ann Int Med 1972;77:507.

Yim AP, Chan AT, Lee TW, et al: Thoracoscopic talc insufflation versus talc slurry for symptomatic malignant pleural effusions. Ann Thorac Surg 1996;62:1655.

Primary Lung Abscess

Method of
Scott Swanson, MD, and
Virginia Litle, MD

Definition

A primary lung abscess is defined as a localized collection of pus within the lung parenchyma with associated pulmonary necrosis. Empyema is an extraparenchymal collection of pus within the pleural space. A primary lung abscess can progress to an empyema with a bronchopleural fistula. A secondary lung abscess develops from airway obstruction and suppuration or from extension of another localized infection.

An acute lung abscess has been present for fewer than 6 weeks. An abscess with a longer duration is considered chronic. Most lung abscesses are solitary; but multiple abscesses can occur, especially in immunocompromised patients or in the setting of septic emboli. Primary lung abscesses are more common in the right lung because of the bronchial anatomy and in the posterior segments of the upper lobes and superior segments of the lower lobes of the lungs because they are the dependent segments in the supine patient.

Cause

The most common cause of a primary lung abscess is aspiration and occurs in patients with impaired level of consciousness from acute alcoholism, drug overdose, seizures, or cerebrovascular accidents. Poor oral hygiene and dentition is a risk factor for primary lung abscess. A necrotizing pneumonia essentially progresses to a primary lung abscess. Cancer, HIV, diabetes mellitus, or organ transplant patients are also at risk of developing a primary lung abscess, as are malnourished and debilitated intensive care unit patients (Table 1).

The secondary lung abscess results from airway obstruction from a benign or malignant tumor, a broncholith, or a foreign body such as an aspirated tooth. A pulmonary

TABLE 1 Risk Factors for Primary Lung Abscess

- Neurologic impairment
- Alcoholism
- Seizures
- Cerebrovascular accident
- Poor oral hygiene and dentition
- Pneumonia
- Immunodeficiency
- HIV
- Organ transplantation
- Diabetes mellitus
- Chemotherapy
- ICU patient
- Esophageal dysfunction
- Gastroesophageal reflux disease
- Zenker's diverticulum
- Achalasia
- Presbyesophagus
- Esophageal cancer/stricture
- Anemia

Abbreviation: ICU = intensive care unit.

infarct can become secondarily infected and result in a secondary lung abscess, whereas an intra-abdominal abscess also can infect the lung across the diaphragm. Infected bronchogenic cysts and bullae are not considered true lung abscesses but radiographically resemble them.

Signs and Symptoms

A patient typically presents with fever, cough, fatigue, and night sweats. Hemoptysis may be present. An anaerobic infection produces foul-smelling sputum. The patient occasionally has new-onset dyspnea with or without exertion. On exam the patient is tachycardic, tachypneic, and often hypoxemic. Altered mental status, poor dentition, and decreased unilateral breath sounds are common. Erythema or fluctuance of the chest wall suggests an empyema necessitatis, which is not typically associated with a lung abscess.

Diagnosis and Treatment

The workup involves routine blood work, sputum cultures, blood cultures, and broad-spectrum antibiotics. The degree of leukocytosis will depend on the patient's underlying disease state, but a left shift is present. There will be an air fluid level on plain chest radiograph. An infected bulla or previously undiagnosed bronchogenic cyst may have similar presentation and study results.

The organisms involved are listed in Table 2. If the specific organism is unknown, empiric intravenous antibiotics traditionally included high-dose penicillin; but with current antibiotic resistance patterns, better choices include single-agent therapy with cefoxitin (Mefoxin), imipenem-cilastatin (Primaxin), piperacillin-tazobactam (Zosyn), or ampicillin-sulbactam (Unasyn).

A noncontrast chest computed tomography (CT) scan is indicated to define the size of the abscess and degree of lobar involvement. A loculated hydropneumothorax on

CURRENT DIAGNOSIS

Neurologic impairment
- Alcoholism
- Stroke
- Seizure

Poor dentition/oral hygiene
Immunocompromised patient
- Transplant
- Cancer
- HIV
- Diabetic

Fever, productive cough, malaise
Air-fluid level on chest radiograph
CT scan of chest: hydropneumothorax within lung

Abbreviation: CT = computed tomography.

radiographs can also be seen with an empyema with a bronchopleural fistula. The CT may reveal an associated foreign body including a tooth or neoplasm causing obstruction. If the patient has positive blood cultures and multiple, peripheral lung abscesses, an echocardiogram is done to look for an intracardiac source of septic emboli to the lung. Any intravenous or dialysis catheters or chemotherapy ports should be removed.

Flexible or rigid bronchoscopy may then be necessary to relieve airway obstruction, to obtain tissue diagnosis of a neoplasm, or for pulmonary toilet and good sputum samples for culture. Hemoptysis is also an indication for bronchoscopy because the bleeding may be from an endobronchial malignancy, which could be controlled with extraction of the cancer with a rigid bronchoscope or with laser therapy. If there is no endobronchial lesion on bronchoscopy, massive hemoptysis (>600 mL/24 hours) from the abscess requires bronchial artery embolization by the interventional radiologists or lung resection to control bleeding.

After initiation of broad spectrum antibiotics, most patients improve. If clinical signs of sepsis continue, more than 90% of cases are successfully treated with CT- or ultrasound-guided drainage of the lung abscess with placement of a pigtail catheter into the cavity and confirmation of the culprit organism to guide antibiotic therapy. Chest tube placement should be avoided because a bronchopleural fistula results.

Risk factors for medical failure include an abscess greater than 6 cm; an immunocompromised patient; or infection with *Staphylococcus aureus, Klebsiella pneumoniae,*

CURRENT THERAPY

Broad-spectrum IV antibiotics
- Second-generation cephalosporin
- A carbapenem
- Third- or fourth-generation penicillin

Continued sepsis
- Percutaneous pigtail drain in abscess
- No chest tube

Persistent abscess after 6 weeks
- Lung resection or rib resection and cavernostomy

Abbreviation: IV = intravenous.

TABLE 2 Organisms Causing Primary or Secondary Lung Abscess

Anaerobic
- *Bacteroides*
- *Peptococcus*
- *Peptostreptococcus*
- *Fusobacterium*
- *Prevotella*
- *Clostridium*

Aerobic
- *Staphylococcus aureus*
- *Klebsiella pneumoniae*
- *Pseudomonas aeruginosa*
- *Streptococcus*
- *Escherichia coli*

or *Pseudomonas aeruginosa*. When the abscess persists after 6 weeks of medical treatment or in cases of massive hemoptysis, surgical exploration is indicated. Lung resection can range from a wedge resection to a lobectomy to remove all grossly infected tissue. A pneumonectomy is associated with a high mortality and is rarely indicated or necessary. If lung resection will result in excessive pulmonary compromise, a surgical cavernostomy with rib resection and debridement of infected lung tissue and wound packing with gauze is done. After an average of 2 weeks of dressing changes and optimization of nutrition, the patient undergoes placement of a muscle flap into a clean lung bed and chest closure.

Prevention

Prevention of impaired consciousness and good oral hygiene prevents development of most primary lung abscesses, especially in the immunocompromised population of cancer, transplant, and HIV patients. Lung abscess incidence should decrease for the patient by maintaining adequate nutrition, elevating the head of the bed more than 30 degrees, and attentive oral care in the intensive care unit (ICU). In ICU patients requiring prolonged endotracheal intubation (>10 days), a tracheostomy and percutaneous feeding tube also will improve oral hygiene and nutrition and assist with pulmonary toilet to reduce lung abscess risk. Routine pulmonary toilet for all patients with pulmonary abscesses includes chest physiotherapy, postural drainage, incentive spirometry, expectorants, and ambulation.

REFERENCES

Mansharamani N, Balachandran D, Delaney D, et al: Lung abscess in adults: Clinical comparison of immunocompromised to non-immunocompromised patients. Respir Med 2002;96(3):178–185.

Postma MH, Le Roux RT: The place of external drainage in the management of lung abscess. S Afr J Surg 1986;24(4):156–158.

Refaely Y, Weissberg D: Gangrene of the lung: Treatment in two stages. Ann Thorac Surg 1997;64:970–974.

Rice TW, Ginsberg RJ, Todd TR: Tube drainage of lung abscesses. Ann Thorac Surg 1987;44(4):356–359.

Rowe S, Cheadle WG: Complications of nosocomial pneumonia in the surgical patient. Am J Surg 2000;179(2A):63S-68S.

Tan TQ, Seilheimer DK, Kaplan SL: Pediatric lung abscess: Clinical management and outcome. Pediatr Infect Dis J 1995;14(1):51–55.

Weissberg D: Percutaneous drainage of lung abscess. J Thorac Cardiovasc Surg 1984;87(2):308–312.

Acute Bronchitis

Method of
Susan Davids, MD, MPH, and
Ralph M. Schapira, MD

Acute bronchitis is one of the most common diagnoses made by primary care physicians in the United States and accounts for nearly 10 million office visits per year. Acute bronchitis is a transient, self-limited inflammatory process of the upper respiratory tract, specifically the trachea and bronchi. Antibiotics are overprescribed to patients with acute bronchitis; this practice has raised significant concern related to the worldwide rise of antibiotic resistance, which is viewed as one of the world's most pressing public health problems.

Acute bronchitis manifests as an acute respiratory illness of less than 3 weeks' duration, with or without sputum production. Acute bronchitis is a clinical diagnosis and must be distinguished from other respiratory diseases, such as pneumonia, acute exacerbation of chronic bronchitis (episode of worsening of symptoms and expiratory airflow obstruction in patients with chronic obstructive pulmonary disease), and the onset of asthma. Most cases of acute bronchitis occur in the fall and winter. The etiology of acute bronchitis is infectious, and viruses appear to be the cause of most cases. Influenzas A and B are the most common viruses isolated, although a wide variety of infectious agents have been identified, such as adenovirus, coronavirus, parainfluenza virus, respiratory syncytial virus, coxsackievirus, *Mycoplasma pneumoniae*, *Bordetella pertussis*, and *Chlamydia pneumoniae*.

Diagnosis of acute bronchitis is based on findings of a prominent cough that may be accompanied by wheezing and sputum production. Most patients are otherwise healthy and without preexisting respiratory disease. Nonspecific constitutional symptoms may also be part of acute bronchitis. Appropriate management of acute bronchitis is essential because it is one of the most common illnesses that present to physicians in the outpatient setting. Antibiotics are often prescribed unnecessarily for acute bronchitis and other respiratory tract illnesses; these prescriptions may potentially lead to adverse events (i.e., allergic reactions and gastrointestinal side effects) and bacterial resistance. Other medications, such as inhaled bronchodilators and antitussives, are often prescribed for acute bronchitis despite questionable evidence to support their routine use.

Pathophysiology of acute bronchitis involves an acute inflammatory response involving the mucosa of the trachea and bronchi, resulting in injury to the respiratory tract epithelium. Sputum production is increased and bronchoconstriction (potentially resulting in airflow obstruction and wheezing) can occur. Positron emission tomography (PET) of a patient with acute bronchitis confirms that the primary inflammatory changes occur in the trachea and bronchi and not the remainder of the lower respiratory track.

Diagnosis

Cough, phlegm (which may be purulent as both bacteria and viruses can cause purulent sputum), and wheezing

CURRENT DIAGNOSIS

- Normal healthy adult with cough
- Predominance of cough
- Lasts 1 to 3 weeks
- With or without sputum
- Can be accompanied by other respiratory and constitutional symptoms
- Absence of abnormal vital signs and physical exam suggesting pneumonia, particularly
  - Heart rate >100 beats per minute
  - Respiratory rate >24 breaths per minute
  - Temperature >100.4°F (38°C)
  - Lung findings suggest a consolidation process

CURRENT THERAPY

- Antibiotics not routinely recommended
- If influenza is highly probable and patient is presenting within the first 48 hours, consider treatment with
  - Oseltamivir (Tamiflu) 75 mg PO bid with food for 5 days (influenza A/B)
  - Zanamivir (Relenza) 10 mg bid by inhalation for 5 days (influenza A/B)
  - Amantadine (Symmetrel) 100 mg bid or 200 mg once daily for 5 days (influenza A)
  - Rimantadine (Flumadine) 100 mg bid for 5 days (influenza A)
- In patients with evidence of bronchial hyperresponsiveness, consider treatment with
  - β_2-agonists for 1 to 2 weeks
  - Antitussives in those with cough for 2 to 3 weeks
  - Antipyretics and analgesics as needed
  - Smoking cessation
- Education: cough most likely to last up to 3 weeks.

help differentiate acute bronchitis from upper respiratory infections such as pharyngitis and sinusitis. Acute bronchitis must be differentiated from acute bacterial pneumonia. The absence of abnormalities in vital signs (heart rate >100 bpm, respiratory rate >24 breath/min, oral temperature >100.4°F [38°C] and physical examination of the chest) supports the diagnosis of acute bronchitis and makes the need for chest radiography unnecessary in most cases. The treatment and outcome of acute bronchitis and pneumonia are very different; a chest radiograph should always be obtained if there is uncertainty about the diagnosis. Chest radiography will demonstrate no lung infiltrates in a patient with acute bronchitis. In contrast, lung infiltrates are present in pneumonia. Pertussis or whooping cough should be considered in adults with cough in the setting of what appears to be an upper respiratory infection, even in those previously immunized. Typically, the cough of pertussis, unlike acute bronchitis, lasts for longer than 3 weeks. Other respiratory diseases, such as previously undiagnosed asthma, can also mimic acute bronchitis, although several features differentiate asthma from acute bronchitis (see Section 12). Rapid testing to diagnose influenza viruses A and B (the most common causes of acute bronchitis) as a cause of acute bronchitis should be considered given the availability of effective treatment if initiated in the first 48 hours.

Treatment

ANTIBIOTICS, INHALED BRONCHODILATORS, AND ANTITUSSIVES

Existing evidence does not support the routine use of antibiotics for uncomplicated cases of acute bronchitis. Although most cases of acute bronchitis are caused by viral infections, upwards of 60% of patients are prescribed antibiotic therapy, which is contributing to the rise of bacterial resistance to commonly used antibiotics. Meta-analyses examining the effectiveness of antibiotic therapy in patients without underlying lung disease suggest no consistent effect of antibiotics on the severity or duration of acute bronchitis. A recent study evaluated children and patients with colored sputum and found that they also did not benefit from antibiotics. This study also found that compared to other populations, the elderly were less likely

to benefit from antibiotics. Smokers with acute bronchitis are even more likely to be prescribed antibiotics. Their response to antibiotics was either equal to or worse than that of nonsmokers.

One possible reason for overuse of antibiotics is the concern by physicians about patient satisfaction. Studies show that patients presenting to the doctor expecting antibiotics were more likely to be prescribed antibiotics; studies also suggest that satisfaction is more related to appropriate patient education than to receiving antibiotics. Patient education should include information regarding the duration of symptoms associated with acute bronchitis. It was found that patients presented on average after 9 days of cough and that the cough persisted for an additional 12 days after the physician visit. This information can impart a realistic expectation of illness duration to the patient.

If influenza is highly suspected and the patient presents within 48 hours of the onset of symptoms, rapid diagnostic testing and treatment should be considered. Both amantadine (Symmetrel) and rimantadine (Flumadine) are effective for influenza A, and neuraminidase inhibitors, inhaled zanamivir (Relenza), and oral oseltamivir (Tamiflu) are effective for influenzas A and B. If these medications are initiated within the first 48 hours of symptoms (and ideally within 30 hours), the duration of illness can be shortened.

The evidence supporting the use of inhaled bronchodilators for the treatment of the symptoms has been variable. Two small trials reported a shorter duration of cough with the use of inhaled β-agonists; another study reported benefit in those with evidence of bronchial hyperresponsiveness. Current recommendations support the use of β-agonists only in patients with evidence of bronchial hyperresponsiveness (wheezing or spirometry demonstrating a forced expiration volume in 1 second [FEV_1] <80% of predicted).

Antitussive agents have not been shown to improve the acute or early cough but did show some improvements in cough lasting longer than 3 weeks. The current recommendations are to use antitussives, namely dextromethorphan (Benylin) or codeine, in patients with cough of 2 to 3 weeks' duration.

Acute uncomplicated bronchitis is most often a viral illness in which antibiotics are not routinely indicated. Patients presenting with an acute respiratory illness, who are younger than 65 years old without existing pulmonary disease or other significant comorbid illness, should have a thorough physical examination, including vital signs. If the vital signs are normal and physical examination of the chest is clear, pneumonia can most likely be ruled out. In patients who present within 48 hours of onset of symptoms, influenza should be considered as effective therapy is available for acute bronchitis caused by influenzas A or B. Otherwise, the evidence for treatment with antibiotics does not support their routine use. Bronchodilators should be considered in those with evidence of bronchial hyperresponsiveness; cough suppressants should be considered in those with 2 to 3 weeks of cough. Patient education is an integral part of the treatment, and patients should receive information that provides realistic expectations regarding the duration of cough.

REFERENCES

Aagaard E, Gonzales R: Management of acute bronchitis in healthy adults. Infect Dis Clin North Am 2004;18:919-937.

Ebell MH: Antibiotic prescribing for cough and symptoms of respiratory tract infection. JAMA 2005;294(3):3062-3064.

Fahey T, Smucny J, Becker L, Glazier R: Antibiotics for acute bronchitis. Cochrane Database Syst Rev 2004;(4):CD000245.

Gonzales R, Sande M: Uncomplicated acute bronchitis. Ann Intern Med 2000;133:981-991.

Kicska G, Zhuang H, Alavi A: Acute bronchitis imaged with F-18 FDG positron emission tomography. Clin Nucl Med 2003;28(6):511-512.

Little R, Rumsby K, Kelly J, et al: Information leaflet and antibiotic prescribing strategies for acute lower respiratory tract infection. JAMA 2005;293(24):3029-3035.

Linder JA, Sim I: Antibiotic treatment of acute bronchitis in smokers. J Gen Intern Med 2002;17:230-234.

Martinez FJ: Acute bronchitis: State of the art diagnosis and therapy. Compr Ther 2004;30(1):55-59.

Smucny J, Flynn C, Becker L, Glazier R: Beta$_2$-agonists for acute bronchitis. Cochrane Database Syst Rev 2004;(1):CD001726.

Bacterial Pneumonia

Method of
Maria C. Rodriguez-Barradas, MD

Bacterial pneumonia is a common cause of hospitalization among ambulatory adults, a serious complication among hospitalized patients, and associated with important morbidity, mortality, and health care costs.

Bacterial pneumonias are classified as community- or hospital-acquired based on where the patient is coming from; they are discussed separately because of the differences in clinical presentation, microbiologic etiology, and therapeutic approach that applies to each category. Different scientific and government bodies have issued recommendations on the management and treatment of community-acquired and hospital-acquired pneumonias. The recommendations generally cited and followed in the United States are those made by the American Thoracic Society (ATS) and the Infectious Diseases Society of America (IDSA). These societies, which previously issued separate guidelines, are providing a consensus set of recommendations in 2006. Other countries have recently issued updated or new guidelines, to which we will refer. Why is this much effort being placed in *guidelines*? Because studies have shown that implementation of guidelines has consistently improved pneumonia-related outcomes, such as decreased mortality rate, decreased hospitalization for low-mortality risk patients, decreased length of stay, and decreased (intravenous) IV antibiotic use.

We review here the principles for the management and treatment of bacterial pneumonias using the published guidelines as a reference.

Community-Acquired Pneumonia

CLINICAL EVALUATION

Diagnosis of pneumonia is based on the presence of fever, cough, pleuritic chest pain, and the presence of a pulmonary infiltrate. Clinicians are not good at predicting pneumonia solely by physical exam, and radiologic evaluation is frequently required but not uniformly recommended by all published guidelines. After a diagnosis of pneumonia is made, the next step is to assess the severity of the process and the need for hospitalization. Clinicians generally overestimate the severity of disease and need for inpatient management. Furthermore, among patients hospitalized with community-acquired pneumonia (CAP), the need for admission to an intensive care unit (ICU) is underestimated; patients admitted to the wards who later require transfer to an ICU setting have a concomitant increased rate of poor outcome associated with the delayed ICU admission. Hence, severity of pneumonia is better assessed by validated scoring systems, such as the Pneumonia Severity Index (PSI) and CURB-65 (confusion, *u*remia [urea > 20 mg/dL], *r*espiratory rate ≥ 30 breaths/min, *b*lood pressure systolic < 90 or diastolic ≤ 60 mm Hg, *65*—age ≥ 65). The PSI (also called PORT [Pneumonia Outcomes Research Team]) score includes items that cannot always be applied in an office practice or may even be too demanding for the busy emergency room clinician. The CURB-65 is recommended by most of the guidelines because of its simplicity (one point for each item present; score is 0 to 5). Oxygenation level, as measured by pulse oximetry or arterial blood gases, is by itself a good predictor of severity of disease and needs to be obtained on all patients. When systematically used, systems that stratify patients into risk categories decrease the rate of hospitalization for patients at low risk of mortality without increasing rate of complications, and they increase the rate of ICU admission for those with more severe disease. Absolute indications for ICU admission are respiratory distress or hypotension or both; other parameters that may influence the decision on ICU admission include multilobar pneumonia, the presence of marked electrolyte or hematologic abnormalities, or concomitant uncontrolled co-morbidities that may require intensive care.

Although guidelines help determine the need for admission to the hospital or to the ICU, physicians must use their best clinical judgment and consider factors that can affect the ability to properly treat as an outpatient (ability to take oral medications, social support system, substance use, among other considerations) or to properly treat in the ward (ability to manage other co-morbidities, risk factors for impending deterioration).

MICROBIOLOGIC EVALUATION

The microbiology of CAP has been extensively studied; *Streptococcus pneumoniae* is the most frequently isolated pathogen, followed by *Haemophilus influenzae*, and the so-called atypical pathogens: *Mycoplasma pneumoniae*, *Chlamydophila pneumoniae*, and *Legionella pneumophila*, *Moraxella catarrhalis*, the Enterobacteriaceae, *Pseudomonas aeruginosa*, and *Staphylococcus aureus*. Among different geographic areas and patient populations, the relative frequency of the different microorganisms is variable, and specific pathogens are more frequently associated with certain underlying diseases; however, *S. pneumoniae* is, across the board, the most prevalent cause of pneumonia (Table 1).

For a variety of reasons in routine clinical practice a microbiologic etiology is never established in most patients with pneumonia. Consequently, for most patients with mild to moderate disease treated as outpatients, microbiologic evaluation (sputum and blood cultures) is

---

TABLE 1 Microbiologic Etiology of CAP According to Risk Factors and/or Underlying Diseases

- *Streptococcus pneumoniae* is the most frequently isolated pathogen among all populations, followed by nontypeable *Haemophilus influenzae*.
- *Moraxella catarrhalis* causes disease mostly in patients with COPD.
- The atypical pathogens, *Mycoplasma pneumoniae* and *Chlamydophila pneumoniae* are common, especially among younger adults (<age 60 years old). Other atypical pathogens are infrequent and associated with specific exposures (birds for *C. psittaci*, parturient cats for *Coxiella brunetti*, and rabbits for *Francisella tularensis*).
- *Legionella pneumophila* is more prevalent among patients admitted with severe pneumonia. COPD, smoking, and immunosuppression are risk factors for legionellosis.
- Staphylococcal pneumonia is seen more frequently following influenza infection.
- Enterobacteriaceae cause pneumonia among debilitated patients, patients with underlying diseases, patients with prior antibiotic use and nursing home residents.
- *Klebsiella pneumoniae* infection is associated with alcoholism.
- *Pseudomonas aeruginosa* infection is associated with cystic fibrosis, bronchiectasis, COPD, debilitating diseases, and prior antibiotic use.
- Anaerobic infections are more frequent among patients at risk for aspiration and with periodontal disease.
- HIV infection is associated with pneumococcal pneumonia as well as with nonbacterial causes of pneumonia (*Pneumocystis jiroveci*, tuberculosis, and endemic fungi).

Abbreviations: CAP = community-acquired pneumonia; COPD = chronic obstructive pulmonary disease.

---

not usually recommended. For inpatients, the ATS/IDSA guidelines recommend that blood cultures be performed when indicated by certain parameters (underlying diseases, severity of disease, presence of complicating features) and sputum cultures be performed only when a good-quality specimen and good-quality processing can be guaranteed. Those experts that recommend routine microbiologic evaluation reason that the results may assist in the evaluation of the specific patient and provide the required local epidemiologic information. Because the yield of cultures is highly dependent on the quality of the specimen and the timing of sample collection, careful attention should be given to obtaining good-quality samples (purulent sputum, adequate amount of blood) before antibiotics are administered (but treatment should not be delayed for the purpose of obtaining samples; see the following text). A test for pneumococcal urine antigen can be used. *Legionella* urine antigen and *Legionella* cultures should be obtained in patients with severe pneumonia, especially in those with negative gram-stain of a purulent sputum.

ANTIMICROBIAL TREATMENT

For purposes of antibiotic choice, most guidelines classify patients in the following categories:

- Nonsevere pneumonia (CURB 0-1)
- Severe pneumonia requiring non-ICU hospital admission (CURB 1-3)
- Severe pneumonia requiring ICU admission (CURB 4-5)

Antibiotic recommendations are based on the following factors:

- Microbiology of CAP is fairly predictable.
- Coinfection with atypical pathogens (*M. pneumoniae* and *C. pneumoniae*) is common.
- The response rate in patients with pneumonia caused by penicillin nonsusceptible *S. pneumoniae* is not affected by the choice of β-lactam antibiotics.
- Patients with bacteremic pneumococcal pneumonia may have a better outcome when treated with combination antibiotic therapy.
- Risk factors for less-common pathogens have been relatively well established and can be assessed at initial evaluation.
- Patients with severe pneumonia have a higher frequency of less-common pathogens.

The ATS/IDSA guidelines recommend that a previously healthy individual, with no co-morbidities, no prior antibiotic use, and in a setting of known low rate (<25%) of high-level community macrolide resistance should be treated with a macrolide or doxycycline (Vibramycin); in the presence of any of the parameters listed, the recommendation is to treat with either respiratory fluoroquinolone, β-lactam plus a macrolide, or telithromycin (Ketek) (the latter to be used only if the risk for infection with gram-negative organisms is low) (Table 2). For patients admitted to the hospital ward, the recommended regimens are a respiratory fluoroquinolone or a beta-lactam plus a macrolide. For the patient admitted to the ICU with severe pneumonia, the recommended regimens

TABLE 2 Recommended Antibiotics for the Treatment of Community- and Hospital-Acquired Pneumonia (CAP and HAP, Respectively) (Adapted from the ATS/IDSA Guidelines and the British Guidelines)

Assessment	Special Considerations	Recommended Antibiotics
Nonsevere CAP: Outpatient Rx	• No risk factors for atypical or less usual pathogens • Suspected atypical pathogens • Presence of co-morbidities or prior antibiotic use	• Amoxicillin (Amoxil) high dose • Macrolide or doxycycline (Vibramycin) • Respiratory fluoroquinolone
Severe CAP: Ward admission	• Evaluate closely for any signs of impending deterioration	• β-lactam **plus** a macrolide or β-lactam **plus** respiratory fluoroquinolone
Severe CAP: ICU admission	• Dual antibiotics may be beneficial for bacteremic pneumococcal pneumonia • If suspected *Pseudomonas* infection • If suspected MRSA	• β-lactam **plus** a macrolide or • β-lactam **plus** respiratory fluoroquinolone • Antipseudomonal, antipneumococcal β-lactam **plus** an antipseudomonal quinolone or • Antipseudomonal, antipneumococcal β-lactam **plus** an aminoglycoside **plus** azithromycin (Zithromax) or quinolone • β-lactam **plus** macrolide or quinolone **plus** vancomycin (Vancocin) or linezolid (Zyvox)
HAP (including VAP): Any disease severity	• Early onset (<5 days) and no risk factors for MDR gram-negative bacilli • Risk factors for MDR gram-negative bacilli • If suspected MRSA	• Ceftriaxone (Rocephin) or • Ampicillin/sulbactam (Unasyn) or • Respiratory quinolone or • Ertapenem (Invanz) • Antipseudomonal β-lactam **plus** antipseudomonal quinolone or aminoglycoside • Add vancomycin or linezolid to previous
Aspiration pneumonia	• Risk factors for anaerobic infection	• β-Lactam/β-lactamase inhibitor or • Carbapenem or • Clindamycin (Cleocin) ± quinolone

ATS = American Thoracic Society; HAP = hospital-acquired pneumonia; ICU = intensive care unit; IDSA = Infectious Diseases Society of America; MDR = multidrug-resistant; MRSA = Methicillin-resistant *Staphylococcus aureus;* Rx = prescription; VAP = ventilator-associated pneumonia.

include a β-lactam together with either a macrolide or a respiratory fluoroquinolone. When *Pseudomonas* infection is suspected, the β-lactam should be an antipneumococcal, antipseudomonal agent; and the regimen should also include an antipseudomonal fluoroquinolone (ciprofloxacin [Cipro] or high-dose levofloxacin [Levaquin]) or an aminoglycoside plus a macrolide or respiratory quinolone. For suspected community-acquired MRSA the regimen should include vancomycin (Vancocin) or linezolid (Zyvox).

There are caveats to some of the considerations on which the treatment recommendations are made:

• The rate of dual infection may be overestimated (based on the diagnostic methods used).
• Some studies suggest that not treating the atypical bacteria in cases of nonsevere pneumonia does not affect outcome.
• The frequency of legionnaires' disease is highly variable and mostly low among cases of nonsevere pneumonia.
• The rate of infection with gram-negative organisms among patients with co-morbid conditions may be overestimated; most of these patients will have pneumonia caused by pneumococci.

These considerations have led to differences in the antibiotic recommendations between the North American and European guidelines. In general the ATS/IDSA guidelines have a broader approach in the empirical treatment of nonsevere CAP than their European counterparts. For example, the Swedish and British guidelines recommend, respectively, to use penicillin or amoxicillin (Amoxil) for CAP treated in the community, regardless of the presence or absence of co-morbidities.

Regardless of the choice of antibiotics, all the guidelines agree that antibiotic therapy should be started as soon as possible on patients with severe pneumonia and if at all possible within 4 to 8 hours of presentation. Patients seen at the doctor's office or in the emergency room should receive their first antibiotic dose before transfer to the hospital or during the admission process, respectively.

Once the etiology of the pneumonia has been established, the antibiotic treatment can be tailored to the identified organism(s). Treatment can also be switched from intravenous to oral antibiotics as soon as patients are clinically improving, able to tolerate medications by mouth, and in the absence of impaired absorption (i.e., ongoing diarrhea). Discharge can be considered for patients without fever who have stable vital signs and oxygen saturation. The concept of clinical stability is important, because patients discharged, whereas having more than one unstable clinical parameter (temperature >37.8°C [101.7°F], heart rate > 100 beats/min, respiratory rate > 24 breaths/min, systolic blood pressure < 90, arterial oxygen saturation < 90% or pO$_2$ < 60) have a higher rate of readmission.

Duration of treatment will depend on the suspected or proven pathogen. Patients with uncomplicated pneumonia that clinically improves within 48 to 72 hours can be treated for 5 to 10 days. Patients with severe or complicated pneumonia or pneumonia caused by pathogens other than pneumococci may need a longer course (14 days or longer).

In summary, once CAP has been diagnosed, assessment of severity of disease will indicate the setting in which the patient can or should be treated. For patients admitted to the hospital, appropriate sputum and blood samples should be obtained, and antibiotic treatment should be started promptly. Patients with severe pneumonia should be reassessed frequently for the first 24 hours and undergo further testing, including *Legionella* cultures, urine *Legionella* antigen (which only detects infection caused by serogroup 1), and any other test that may be indicated by the patient's condition or prior exposures, or both. Those that improve can be switched to oral antibiotics and discharged. Those lacking improvement require more intensive diagnostic evaluation for complications and other potential etiologies. Many patients admitted with an initial diagnosis of CAP have other diagnoses such as pulmonary tuberculosis or cancer. HIV testing should be considered in all patients admitted with pneumonia, especially those with bacteremic pneumococcal disease.

NONANTIBIOTIC INTERVENTIONS

Two other interventions must be considered in all patients with severe CAP admitted to the ICU:

1. Administration of immunomodulator agents (drotrecogin alfa activated [Xigris][1])
2. Screening for adrenal insufficiency

The use of drotrecogin alfa activated has shown benefit in this patient population, especially among patients with severe pneumococcal pneumonia when administered within 24 hours of admission. Administration of stress doses of hydrocortisone (Solu-Cortef) has shown beneficial effects on patients with bacterial pneumonia who have laboratory evidence of adrenal insufficiency.

Hospital-Acquired Pneumonia

Hospital-acquired pneumonia (HAP) includes patients who develop pneumonia while hospitalized. This is not a uniform population, because patients who acquire pneumonia soon after hospitalization tend to have better prognosis and have microbiology that more closely resembles that of CAP than those who acquire pneumonia after more prolonged hospitalization. The population is also heterogeneous because HAP includes pneumonia acquired in wards and intensive care units, as well as pneumonia among ventilated patients (ventilator-associated pneumonia [VAP]). In addition, some of the same considerations given to HAP apply to patients admitted from chronic health care facilities, such as nursing homes or patients receiving medical care at home; hence, the broader term *health care–associated pneumonias* is frequently used. Pneumonias associated with health care settings can be caused by a wide spectrum of bacterial pathogens. Most concerning are infections caused by multidrug-resistant (MDR) gram-negative or gram-positive pathogens. Among the MDR gram-negatives, *P. aeruginosa* is one of the most prevalent, but *Klebsiella*, *Enterobacter*, *Serratia*, and *Acinetobacter* species can also be seen in endemic or epidemic patterns. When evaluating and treating HAP, it is of the utmost importance to be familiar with the microbiology of the particular health care facilities, because the most frequently isolated pathogens, as well as the susceptibility profiles, can differ from place to place (i.e., a resistant *Acinetobacter* species may be the MDR problem in one ICU, whereas a resistant *Klebsiella* or *Pseudomonas* may be the problem at the facility across the street). Risk factors for MDR organisms include prolonged hospitalization, intubation, prior antibiotic use, and underlying, debilitating diseases.

DIAGNOSIS

Hospital-acquired pneumonia should be suspected in a hospitalized patient with a new or worsening radiographic infiltrate, fever, leukocytosis or leukopenia, and purulent secretions. The presence of these criteria is highly specific for pneumonia but low in sensitivity. In addition, the picture can be confounded in patients with a baseline abnormal chest roentgenogram because of other etiologies (i.e., congestive heart failure) in which the presence of a new or worsening infiltrate is difficult to evaluate. This difficulty is particularly pertinent for the diagnosis of VAP. In some ventilated patients, the presence of fever, leukocytosis, and purulent secretions (even in the presence of a pulmonary infiltrate) is because of purulent tracheobronchitis and not pneumonia; in others, unexplained hemodynamic instability or deterioration of blood gases, or both, during mechanical ventilation are manifestations of the lung infection.

Because of the difficulty in making an accurate clinical diagnosis, efforts have been made to pursue a microbiologic diagnosis of HAP; this approach has its own caveats. Sputum cultures should be obtained; however, organisms cultured from the sputum could represent colonization and not necessarily lung infection. A lower respiratory tract specimen (obtained through bronchoscopy or tracheal aspirate) is a more representative sample but is seldom obtained in nonintubated patients. When lower respiratory tract secretions (bronchoalveolar lavage [BAL], endotracheal aspirates or protected brush specimen) are obtained, the sample can be processed as qualitative or quantitative cultures. Quantitative cultures have the advantage of increased specificity for the diagnosis of pneumonia, resulting in fewer patients treated and narrower spectrum antibiotics used. It has the disadvantage of requiring more specialized and time-consuming laboratory techniques, and is not available at all centers. Given the difficulty in making the diagnosis of VAP, and the lack of specificity of routine microbiology testing, researchers have studied other diagnostic tools, such as immunologic markers on lower respiratory tract samples (BAL), for differentiating true infection from colonization; these tests may have clinical applications in the future.

ANTIMICROBIAL TREATMENT

Antibiotic selection for the treatment of HAP depends on the clinical setting, the length of hospital stay, and the presence or absence of risk factors for MDR (Table 3).

---

[1]Not FDA approved for this indication.

TABLE 3 Initial Doses of Antibiotics for Empiric Therapy of Community- and Hospital-Acquired Pneumonia

Class/Properties	Drugs	Dose
	Oral	
β-Lactams	• Amoxicillin (Amoxil)	• 1 g tid
	• Amoxicillin/clavulanate (Augmentin)	• 2 g bid
Macrolides	• Azithromycin (Zithromax)	• 250 mg qd
	• Clarithromycin (Biaxin)	• 500 mg bid
Tetracyclines	• Doxycycline (Vibramycin)	• 100 mg bid
Ketolides	• Telithromycin (Ketek)	• 800 mg qd
Respiratory quinolone	• Gatifloxacin (Tequin)	• 400 mg qd
	• Moxifloxacin (Avelox)	• 400 mg qd
	• Levofloxacin (Levaquin)	• 500 mg qd
	Intravenous	
β-Lactam	• Ampicillin (Principen)	• 1 g q6h
	• Ampicillin/sulbactam (Unasyn)*	• 1.5 g q6h
	• Ceftriaxone (Rocephin)	• 1–2 g qd
	• Cefotaxime (Claforan)	• 1 g q8h
	• Ertapenem (Invanz)**	• 1 g qd
Antipseudomonal β-lactam	• Piperacillin/tazobactam (Zosyn)*	• 4/0.5 g q6h
	• Cefepime (Maxipime)	• 1–2 g q8–12h
	• Imipenem (Primaxin)**	• 500 mg q6h
	• Meropenem (Merrem)**	• 1 g q8h
Respiratory quinolones	Same as oral	Same as oral
Antipseudomonal quinolones	• Ciprofloxacin (Cipro)	• 400 mg q8h
	• Levofloxacin (Levaquin)	• 750 mg qd
Aminoglycosides	• Gentamicin (Garamycin)	• 5–7 mg/kg qd
	• Amikacin (Amikin)	• 15–20 mg/kg qd
Anaerobic coverage	• β-Lactam/β-lactamase inhibitor	• See previous*
	• Carbapenem	• See previous**
	• Clindamycin (Cleocin)	• 300–450 mg q6h
Anti-MRSA coverage	• Vancomycin (Vancocin)	• 15 mg/kg q12h
	• Linezolid (Zyvox)	• 600 mg q12h

Abbreviation: MRSA: Methicillin-resistant *Staphylococcus aureus*.
*β-lactam/β-lactamase inhibitor.
**Carbapenem.

The prevalence of MDR in nursing homes and other nonhospital, health care–associated settings may be overestimated by the clinician; in most instances patients will have pneumonia caused by the most common pathogens for CAP (*S. pneumoniae, H. influenzae*). However, studies done among patients in ICU settings have shown that patients who receive initial appropriate antimicrobial therapy for HAP had lower mortality than those who did not. For this reason, guidelines recommend that when risk factors for MDR are present, to start broad-spectrum empiric treatment and simplify or de-escalate treatment when microbiologic results (culture and sensitivities) become available. Because bacterial ecology differs among hospitals, each hospital should have its own antibiogram readily available to unit and ward physicians and antibiotic selection for empiric initial treatment should be based on the local pattern of MDR infections. One controversial issue in the treatment of gram-negative pneumonias is that of mono versus combination therapy. The rationale for combination therapy directed against a specific pathogen is to provide synergistic effect and to avoid the emergence of resistance. Although supported by in vitro data, clinical studies have failed to consistently show any advantage of combination therapy except possibly when treating *Pseudomonas* infection (pneumonia or bacteremia). The recommendation for empirical combination therapy for HAP is solely to broaden the coverage for MDR. Once an organism is identified, treatment should be continued with the most appropriate drug. In addition, if MDR infection is not documented, treatment should also be simplified. When combination therapy is prescribed, the combination should be that of a β-lactam with a quinolone or aminoglycoside. The aminoglycosides have the advantage of conserved activity against most MDR pathogens. However, clinicians are usually concerned with associated toxicities. To minimize toxicity, once-daily dosing is preferred and short courses (3 to 5 days) should be considered. Quinolones are associated with less toxicity; however, MDR pathogens (especially *P. aeruginosa*) tend to have higher rate of resistance to these drugs, minimizing their potential advantage for combination therapy. Adjunctive therapy with inhaled antibiotics (aminoglycosides or polymyxin) for the treatment of MDR–gram-negative pneumonia can be considered for selected cases. Another more recent controversial subject has been that of duration of therapy. Traditionally, the recommendation has been to treat gram-negative pneumonia and staphylococcal pneumonia with prolonged courses (2 to 3 weeks) of antibiotics. However, recent studies have shown that for most patients with suspected VAP that improve after 3 to 5 days of antibiotic therapy, a shorter course of antibiotics can be given; thus, except when clinically indicated (delayed response, lack of response, complicating features, *Pseudomonas* infection) treatment for VAP can be stopped after 8 to 10 days. This approach minimizes the risk of superinfection with MDR and other complications associated with antibiotic use, such as *Clostridium difficile* colitis. Clinical improvement in patients with HAP can be as difficult to assess as it was to make the diagnosis, given all the concurrent factors that may interplay, especially in ventilated patients. In general, improvement occurs after the first 48 to 72 hours of antimicrobial therapy and is usually manifested by decreased fever and leukocytosis. Radiologic improvement commonly lags after clinical improvement. However, any patient with deteriorating clinical or radiologic parameters beyond 48 to 72 hours must be re-evaluated for complications of pneumonia (cavitation, empyema), other causes of pulmonary infiltrates (congestive heart failure, pulmonary emboli, pulmonary hemorrhage, atelectasis), unsuspected or drug-resistant organisms, and other sites of infection. Remember that lack of response is not always an MDR or antibiotic problem but has to do with the patient's underlying co-morbidities. Mostly for this reason, despite attempts to reduce the pneumonia-attributable mortality, HAP continues to be associated with a high mortality rate.

Aspiration Pneumonia

Aspiration pneumonia is a misnomer in that aspiration is the underlying pathogenic mechanism for most pneumonias. However, aspiration pneumonias refer to those situations in which relatively larger amounts of oropharyngeal secretions or gastric contents are aspirated into the respiratory tract and/or the bacterial concentration of the oropharyngeal content is markedly increased and/or the host defense mechanisms to these insults are impaired. For patients at risk for aspiration of gastric contents, the distinction with chemical pneumonitis needs to be made; however, this distinction may not be easy to make solely on clinical grounds. The microbiology of aspirated material depends importantly on host parameters. Patients with periodontal disease will have predominantly normal oral flora including anaerobes; those coming from health care settings or treated with antibiotics will have a predominance of gram-negative bacteria, MRSA, or both. In general, it has been recommended that when treating aspiration pneumonia, an antibiotic with anaerobic activity needs to be included; however, recent studies have suggested that this may not need to be the case, and coverage of usual pathogens along with gram-negative pathogens when indicated will suffice. Treatment recommendations for aspiration pneumonia are included in Table 2.

Pneumonia in Immunocompromised Hosts

When evaluating immunocompromised patients (because of HIV infection, malignancy, immunosuppressive treatment, or other etiologies) with pneumonia, the differential diagnosis includes all the pathogens and situations discussed earlier plus the pathogens to which this host is susceptible because of underlying diseases or treatments. It is not possible in many situations to differentiate bacterial from nonbacterial causes of pneumonia in these patients. When evaluating immunocompromised patients, it is useful to assess which arms of the immune system are predominantly affected to infer which are the most likely pathogens responsible for the infection. Patients with impaired humoral immunity (multiple myeloma, CLL) and neutropenia are more prone to bacterial infections than patients with defective cellular immunity. Although HIV infection is the prototype for impaired cellular immunity, pneumococcal disease is 30 to 100 times more frequent in this patient population. Epidemiologic risk factors need to be carefully evaluated among immunosuppressed patients with pneumonia because in many cases pneumonia is caused by reactivation of an endemic disease. Although endemic infections of mycobacterial and fungal etiologies usually have subacute to chronic presentations, in the immunosuppressed patient they can present relatively acutely. In these patients initial evaluation must be more aggressive, empirical coverage may need to be broader, and invasive diagnostic evaluation (CT, bronchoscopy) must be pursued sooner. For patients that undergo bronchoscopy, BAL and biopsy, when possible, must be obtained.

CURRENT DIAGNOSIS

- The diagnosis of pneumonia is based on the presence of consistent clinical symptoms and signs (fever, chills, cough, pleuritic chest pain, purulent sputum production, and/or rales) and a radiologic infiltrate.
- The microbiologic etiology of CAP is fairly predictable. *Streptococcus pneumoniae* is the most frequent causative agent among all populations.
- Severity of disease at presentation will indicate the setting in which the patient can or should be treated: outpatient, hospital ward, or ICU; and the most appropriate initial empiric antibiotic choice.
- HAP within a few days of hospitalization tends to resemble CAP in its microbiology. Pneumonia among nursing home residents tends to behave as HAP.
- Prolonged hospitalization, prior antibiotic use, and ventilator use are risk factors for infection with resistant gram-negative and gram-positive organisms.
- Among ventilated patients with abnormal chest roentgenograms, the distinction between colonization, purulent tracheobronchitis, pneumonia, and other pulmonary processes is difficult to make.
- All patients admitted to the hospital with a diagnosis of CAP and all patients with presumptive HAP should have sputum and blood cultures obtained. Additional testing, including *Legionella* antigen and cultures, bronchoscopy, pleural tap, further imaging, and other diagnostic serologies will be done as indicated by the patient's underlying diseases, exposures and clinical course, or both.
- Among immunocompromised patients presenting with pneumonia, nonbacterial pathogens are more frequently encountered, empirical coverage may need to be broadened, and more aggressive testing may need to be pursued sooner.
- HIV testing should be considered in patients presenting with pneumonia, especially those with bacteremic pneumococcal disease.

Abbreviations: CAP = community-acquired pneumonia; HAP = hospital-acquired pneumonia; ICU = intensive care unit.

Bronchoalveolar lavage has a lower sensitivity for identifying fungi and mycobacteria, and in these cases histologic examination of lung tissue may give an earlier diagnosis until culture results become available. In addition, other diagnostic tests such as serology (serum and urine antigen test), biopsy of extrapulmonary tissues with disease manifestations (skin, lymph node) should be actively pursued. In this patient population viral etiologies, which are not as prevalent among CAP and HAP, other than for seasonal influenza, are frequent culprits; and PCR techniques applied to proper samples will provide the diagnosis.

Summary

Bacterial pneumonia, whether acquired in the community or in health care settings, is associated with significant morbidity and mortality. Despite published guidelines based on the medical literature, there are some relevant differences in the recommendations for evaluation and treatment of pneumonia issued by the different bodies, suggesting that some degree of subjectivity operates among the committees generating them. These differences emphasize that at all times, clinicians should use their best clinical judgment when making decisions. Guidelines are meant to improve clinical outcomes; however, this has not been proved for all recommendations. Guidelines can also be misused or used for purposes other than for what they were initially intended and for which they may have not been validated. As long as sound reasoning is used and documented, the process followed when evaluating and treating a patient with bacterial pneumonia may differ from what the guidelines recommend. As worded by an IDSA spokesperson, "If patients are always being treated 100% according to the guidelines, they're probably being inappropriately treated."

Because prevention may be the most effective intervention to decrease the morbidity associated with pneumonia, every opportunity should be used to administer proper immunizations that include yearly influenza vaccination to patients at risk as well as their family members, and pneumococcal immunization.

REFERENCES

American Thoracic Society; Infectious Diseases Society of America: Guidelines for the management of adults with hospital-acquired, ventilator-associated, and healthcare-associated pneumonia. Am J Respir Crit Care Med 2005;171:388–416.

American Thoracic Society; Infectious Diseases Society of America: Guidelines for the management of adults with community-acquired pneumonia. Clin Infect Dis 2006 (in press).

British Thoracic Society Standards of Care Committee: BTS guidelines for the management of community acquired pneumonia in adults. Thorax 2001;56 Suppl IV:IV1–64.

British Thoracic Society Standards of Care Committee: BTS Guidelines for the management of community acquired pneumonia in adults—2004 update. Available at www.brit-thoracic.org.uk/

Centers for Disease Control and Prevention: Guidelines for preventing health-care-associated pneumonia. 2003. Atlanta, GA, US Department of Health and Human Services, 2004. Available at http://www.cdc.gov/ncidod/hip/pneumonia/default.htm/

El-Solh AA, Pietrantoni C, Bhat A, et al: Microbiology of severe aspiration pneumonia in institutionalized elderly. Am J Respir Crit Care Med 2003;167:1650–1654.

Hutt E, Kramer AM: Evidence-based guidelines for management of nursing home-acquired pneumonia. J Fam Pract 2002;51:709–716.

Marik PE: Aspiration pneumonitis and aspiration pneumonia. N Engl J Med 2001;344:665–671.

Mills GH, Oehley MR, Arrol B: Effectiveness of β lactam antibiotics compared with antibiotics active against atypical pathogens in non-severe community acquired pneumonia: meta-analysis. BMJ 2005;330:456–462.

Mylotte JM: Nursing home-acquired pneumonia. Clin Infect Dis 2002;35:1205–1211.

Hedlund J, Stralin K, Ortqvist A, et al: Swedish guidelines for the management of community-acquired pneumonia in immunocompetent adults. Scand J Infect Dis 2005;37:791–805.

Shefet D, Robenshtok E, Paul M, Leibovici L: Empirical atypical coverage for inpatients with community-acquired pneumonia. Systematic review of randomized controlled trials. Arch Intern Med 2005;165:1992–2000.

Soo Hoo GW, Wen Ye, Nguyen TV, Goetz M: Impact of clinical guidelines in the management of severe hospital-acquired pneumonia. Chest 2005;128:2778–2787.

CURRENT THERAPY

- The selection of antibiotic therapy is based on the setting where the pneumonia is acquired (community versus health care setting), the severity of the disease, and the presence of risk factors for less usual pathogens.
- Patients with nonsevere community-acquired pneumonia and no other indications for hospital admission can be treated as outpatients with oral antibiotics. Total duration of treatment is 5 to 10 days.
- Patients with severe pneumonia require treatment as inpatients. Antibiotics should be started promptly (within 4 to 8 hours); first dose should be given at the doctor's office (before transfer) or in the emergency room (while waiting for admission). Efforts should be made to obtain samples for cultures before antibiotics are administered.
- Patients critically ill with pneumonia require combination treatment. Those with hypotension, respiratory distress, or uncontrolled underlying conditions require ICU admission.
- Once a pathogen is identified, antibiotic treatment can be simplified and tailored to the culprit. Antibiotics can be switched to oral once patient has been afebrile and is clinically stable. Stable patients can be discharged as soon as switched to oral drugs.

Abbreviation: ICU = intensive care unit.

Viral Upper Respiratory Tract Infections

Method of
Surendra K. Sharma, MD, PhD, and Alladi Mohan, MD

Upper respiratory tract infections (URTIs) caused by viruses ("common cold") are one of the most common infectious diseases in humans. Although rarely fatal, they are an important cause of morbidity, economic loss, and an important contributor to disability-adjusted life years

(DALYs) lost globally. In the United States, viral URTIs account for approximately 22 million absences from school in children and 20 million absences from work annually, and $2 to $3 billion are spent on over-the-counter preparations for relief from cold symptoms.

Nearly 200 viruses are implicated as causes of viral URTIs of which rhinovirus, coronavirus, respiratory syncytial virus (RSV), influenza virus (types A and B), parainfluenza virus, adenovirus, enteroviruses, and human metapneumovirus are the most frequent causes. Disease transmission occurs by droplet infection (large and small particle aerosols), droplet nuclei via the inhalation route, and direct contact. Spread of infection from hand-to-hand contact with contaminated nasal secretions and self-inoculation from eye rubbing or nose picking is common. Once contact is made between the virus and nasal mucosa, infection is initiated. Immunity against some of the viruses (e.g., rhinovirus and enteroviruses) is persistent and serotype-specific, whereas some of the other viruses are capable of reinfection in spite of the presence of neutralizing antibodies. Given that there are more than 100 serotypes of rhinovirus and more than 70 serotypes of enteroviruses, reinfection is common. Salient pathophysiologic mechanisms include selective neutrophil recruitment and increase in cytokine concentrations that orchestrate chemotaxis, transmigration, and activation of inflammatory and immunocompetent cells. Clinical manifestations occur as a result of a combination of viral cytopathic effect and the activation of inflammatory pathways. Superadded bacterial infections may further complicate the course of the disease.

Clinical Presentation

Subjects with viral URTIs often present with rhinorrhea, nasal congestion, and sore throat. Other common presenting symptoms include nonproductive cough, sneezing, pain in the eyes, and headache. Rarely, constitutional symptoms such as malaise and myalgias may be prominent (influenza and parainfluenza virus infection). Infants and children may manifest a high-grade fever. In adults, fever is uncommon and is low grade when present. The nasal discharge is clear and watery initially and may become white later because of the presence of leukocytes. In adults, a change in the color of rhinorrhea to a greenish tinge may suggest secondary bacterial infection. Sometimes conjunctivitis (adenovirus), laryngitis (parainfluenza virus) and skin rash (enteroviruses) may also be present. However, it is impossible to distinguish various viral etiologic causes on clinical manifestations alone. Moreover, these symptoms mimic the clinical presentation of a bacterial URTI, and it is indeed a challenge for clinicians to differentiate viral from bacterial URTIs because the therapeutic options are different.

Physical examination of the nasal cavity may reveal postnasal discharge and erythema around the nose and nasal mucosa. The nasal mucous membranes may appear glassy because of the presence of proteinaceous exudates and increased mucus secretion. Pharynx may appear congested, and exudates may be present on the tonsils. Jugulodigastric lymph nodes may be enlarged and tender. Pharyngeal pain, odynophagia, and presence of exudates may indicate secondary bacterial infection. Otoscopic examination may reveal a bright red, bulging, opaque tympanic membrane and the presence of fluid in the middle ear suggestive of otitis media.

Because the clinical presentation of common cold may mimic the initial presentation of some of the more serious life-threatening conditions such as influenza (flu), avian influenza (bird flu), or severe acute respiratory syndrome (SARS), clinicians must have an open mind to recognize and distinguish the innocuous viral URTIs from these life-threatening disease mimics.

Unless complications develop, viral URTIs run a self-limited course and resolve in approximately a week's time. In infants and preschool children, the symptoms may persist up to 2 weeks. Complications of viral URTIs include superadded bacterial infection, sinusitis, otitis media, acute exacerbations of asthma, chronic obstructive pulmonary disease (COPD), and cystic fibrosis.

Diagnosis

Viral URTIs often get treated empirically because of the paucity and expense involved in laboratory testing for viruses. Virus isolation performed with cell cultures is highly specific and constitutes the gold standard for the diagnosis. However, cultures take 3 days to 1 week to yield results and are technically difficult. Serodiagnosis requires paired specimens and are therefore not useful for early diagnosis at the time of initial presentation. More recent methods of direct testing of patient specimens with simplified antigen assays and molecular methods such as reverse transcriptase polymerase chain reaction (RT-PCR) and ligase chain reaction (LCR) are being explored.

Management

Symptomatic and supportive treatment is the mainstay of management. Therapy is therefore directed to alleviate the symptoms of common cold rather than address the

---

CURRENT DIAGNOSIS

- Subjects with common cold present with rhinorrhea, nasal congestion, and sore throat, cough, scanty sputum, sneezing, and headache. Rarely, constitutional symptoms such as fever, malaise, and myalgias are prominent. Sometimes conjunctivitis, laryngitis, and skin rash may also be present.

- Unless complications develop, viral URTIs run a self-limited course and resolve in approximately 1 week's time. In infants and preschool children, the symptoms may persist up to 2 weeks.

- Complications of viral URTIs include secondary bacterial infection, sinusitis, otitis media, acute exacerbations of asthma, chronic obstructive pulmonary disease (COPD), and cystic fibrosis.

- *It is impossible to distinguish various viral etiologic causes on clinical manifestations alone.* Viral URTIs often get treated empirically because of the paucity, expense involved, and nonavailability of laboratory testing and isolation of viruses.

Abbreviation: URTI = upper respiratory tract infection.

CURRENT THERAPY

TARGET SYMPTOM	MEDICATION TYPE
Rhinorrhea	■ Anticholinergics 0.06% Ipratropium bromide (Atrovent) nasal spray: adults and children ≥5 y, two sprays of the nasal solution into each nostril tid or qid ■ First-generation antihistamines Diphenhydramine (Benadryl): children >6 y and adults, 25–50 mg tid or qid Chlorpheniramine (Chlor-Trimeton): adults, 4-mg regular-release tablet bid or qid
Nasal Obstruction: Caused by secretions	Nasal saline drops (0.7% Otrivin saline pediatric nose drops)
Caused by mucosal swelling	Topical decongestants: ■ Children 2–12 y: 0.05% xylometazoline (Otrivin), 2–3 drops or sprays of 0.05% solution in each nostril q8–10h for 4–5d ■ Adults and children >12 y: 0.1% xylometazoline (Otrivin), 1–3 drops or sprays of 0.1% solution in each nostril q8–10h for 4–5d
Sore Throat	Warm saline gargles (half teaspoon of salt in 4 oz warm water) NSAIDs: acetaminophen (Tylenol): children, 10–15 mg/kg, up to 650 mg/d; adults, 650 mg, q4–6h; ibuprofen (Advil): children, 10 mg/kg, up to 200–400 mg q6–8h; adults, 400–600 mg, given q6–8h
Constitutional Symptoms (e.g., fever, myalgias, malaise)	■ NSAIDs: acetaminophen (Tylenol): children, 10–15 mg/kg, up to 650 mg/d; adults, 650 mg, q4–6h; ibuprofen (Advil): children, 10 mg/kg, up to 200–400 mg q6–8h; adults, 400–600 mg, given q6–8h
Cough: Caused by nasal obstruction/postnasal drip	Nasal saline drops (0.7% Otrivin saline pediatric nose drops)
Caused by reactive airways disease Nonspecific cough	Topical decongestants ■ Children 2–12 y: 0.05% xylometazoline (Otrivin), 2–3 drops or sprays of 0.05% solution in each nostril q8–10h for 4–5d ■ Adults and children >12y: 0.1% xylometazoline (Otrivin), 1–3 drops or sprays of 0.1% solution in each nostril q8–10h for 4–5d Bronchodilator therapy sometimes helpful Cough suppressants: Dextromethorphan (Benylin), codeine: children, 1 mg/kg up to 60 mg; adults, 15–60 mg, q4–6h Levodropropizine syrup (Levotuss[2]) (6 mg/mL): adults, 10 mL tid

[2]Not available in the United States.
Abbreviations: NSAIDs = nonsteroidal anti-inflammatory drugs.

etiologic cause. Perhaps no other diseases have so many ineffective therapeutic options ranging from anecdotal and ancient folk remedies to well-researched and designed drugs. Not surprisingly, the tendency for overmedication and inappropriate use of antibiotics is rampant.

Adequate bed rest and fluid intake should be ensured. Anticholinergic nasal sprays (ipratropium [Atrovent 0.06%]) reduces rhinorrhea. Saline nasal drops (Nasal Mist, Ocean) can be helpful in nasal obstruction by liquefying the thick nasal secretions. When nasal obstruction is caused by mucosal swelling, nasal decongestants like xylometazoline nasal spray (Otrivin) are used to obtain temporary relief. These agents improve cold symptoms in adults. However, their use is associated with adverse drug reactions such as supraventricular tachycardia (especially in children), rebound obstruction, and nasal epithelial drying. These agents should not be used for more than 3 to 4 days and must be used with caution in infants, children, and in patients receiving monoamine oxidase (MAO) inhibitors. Oral decongestant formulations do not offer any additional advantage over topical preparations, and adverse drug reactions are more frequent with the oral formulations.

Antihistamines are often used as cold remedies even though no evidence implicates histamine in the pathogenesis of viral URTIs. Although there are anecdotal reports of efficacy of first-generation antihistamines in alleviating the symptoms, definitive evidence is not available from published controlled studies to endorse their routine use in the common cold. Warm saline gargles are helpful in relieving sore throat. Sometimes, acetaminophen (Tylenol) or ibuprofen (Motrin) may be needed to provide adequate relief from throat pain. There is concern regarding the use of salicylates because of the risk of occurrence of Reye's syndrome. Nonsteroidal anti-inflammatory drugs (NSAIDs) such as acetaminophen, naproxen (Aleve), and ibuprofen are also useful for relief from constitutional symptoms such as fever, myalgias, and malaise.

No evidence suggests that antibiotics alter the course or outcome in patients with viral URTIs. Antibiotic treatment is potentially hazardous, promotes evolution of drug-resistant strains, and does not prevent complications associated with the condition; thus irrational antibiotic prescription practices should be discouraged. When cough is severe and disturbs sleep, cough suppressants such as codeine, dextromethorphan (Benylin), or levodropropizine (Levotuss[2]) may be tried. Use of these agents is associated with adverse drug reactions such as drowsiness and bronchoconstriction, and they should not be used in children younger than 5 years and in patients receiving MAO inhibitors. When nasal obstruction or postnasal drip are the cause of cough, nasal decongestants may be beneficial. If reactive airways disease is the cause of cough, bronchodilator therapy may have to be administered. In some patients, cough caused by reactive airways disease may not respond to any form of treatment and may persist for 4 to 6 weeks.

Antiviral drugs available for the treatment of influenza virus infection include amantadine (Symmetrel), rimantadine (Flumadine), oseltamivir (Tamiflu), and zanamivir (Relenza). Pleconaril,* a specific inhibitor of human picornaviruses, was effective in community-acquired colds caused by rhinoviruses in two placebo-controlled trials. However, enough evidence is not available to endorse its use in viral URTIs. There is little objective published evidence to support the use of second-generation antihistamines, corticosteroids, zinc, or echinacea as treatment for the common cold.

Prevention

Avoiding exposure to infected persons, prompt hand washing, and avoiding direct contact of ocular and nasal mucous membranes appear to be the most useful measures to prevent the transmission of the common cold. The usefulness of other measures such as use of tissues coated with antiviral drugs, oral vitamin C, zinc lozenges,[1] and echinacea[1] in the prevention of viral URTIs is yet to be proved. Other investigational agents, such as intranasal interferon-α2, interferon-γ, capsid-function inhibitors such as pleconaril, RNA inhibitors such as enviroxime, and 3C protease inhibitors such as AG7088, are being studied for prevention and treatment of viral URTIs.

REFERENCES

Arroll B: Non-antibiotic treatments for upper-respiratory tract infections (common cold). Respir Med 2005;99:1477-1484.

Anzueto A, Niederman MS: Diagnosis and treatment of rhinovirus respiratory infections. Chest 2003;123:1664-1672.

Charles CH, Yelmene M, Luo GX: Recent advances in rhinovirus therapeutics. Curr Drug Targets Infect Disord 2004;4:331-337.

Mossad SB: Current and future therapeutic approaches to the common cold. Expert Rev Anti Infect Ther 2003;1:619-626.

Wat D: The common cold: A review of the literature. Eur J Intern Med 2004;15:79-88.

West JV: Acute upper airway infections. Br Med Bull 2002;61:215-230.

---

[1]Not FDA approved for this indication.
[2]Not available in the United States.
*Investigational drug in the United States.

Viral and Mycoplasmal Pneumonias

Method of
Burke A. Cunha, MD

Influenza pneumonia is the most important cause of viral pneumonia in adults. Influenza A is the predominant type of influenza found in adults, and influenza B is more common in children. Influenza A has the potential for severe disease, occurs seasonally, and is the predominant type involved in influenza pandemics. *Mycoplasma pneumoniae* community-acquired pneumonia (CAP) was first recognized decades ago as distinctive from bacterial and viral pneumonias. It was originally described by Eaton as "Eaton agent" pneumonia caused by a pleuropneumonia-like organism (PPLO), later shown to be caused by *M. pneumoniae*. *M. pneumoniae* is a common cause of pneumonia in all age groups, but the peak incidence of *M. pneumoniae* CAP is in young adults. *M. pneumoniae* CAP is a common cause of ambulatory CAP.

The term *atypical pneumonia* was first applied to viral pneumonias because the clinical laboratory and radiologic findings were different from those caused by typical bacterial pulmonary pathogens. In influenza pneumonia, the clinical findings are confined to the trachea, bronchi, lung parenchyma, and central nervous system. *M. pneumoniae* CAP is a systemic infection with a pulmonary component. Over the years, atypical pneumonia has come to refer to pneumonia caused by systemic nonviral/nonbacterial pathogen agents that have a pulmonary component. Viral pneumonias are no longer considered atypical pneumonias. Atypical pneumonias may be divided into nonzoonotic and zoonotic atypical CAPs. Nonzoonotic CAPs are most commonly caused by *M. pneumoniae, Chlamydia pneumoniae,* or *Legionella* species; whereas the three most common zoonotic atypical pneumonias are caused by *Chlamydia psittaci* (psittacosis), *Francisella tularensis* (tularemia), or *Coxiella burnetii* (Q fever). All of the atypical pneumonias are distinct clinical entities that may be differentiated on the basis of their characteristic pattern of extrapulmonary organ involvement. Although some viruses may occasionally have extrapulmonary manifestations (i.e., influenza, adenovirus with viral pneumonias), the primary clinical features are confined to the lungs. *M. pneumoniae* is a critical cause of nonzoonotic atypical CAP, particularly in the ambulatory setting. *M. pneumoniae* CAP may be severe in patients with impaired host defenses or those with severe, preexisting cardiopulmonary disease.

Viral Influenza Pneumonia

Viral influenza pneumonia affects children and adults. Influenza B is the primary type, causing mild influenza in children and adults. Influenza A is primarily an infection of adults that may be mild to severe. Influenza A has the potential for pandemic spread.

Influenza occurs during the winter months, usually peaking in February. Influenza is spread by aerosolized droplet infection from person to person and via fomites.

Viral influenza A is classified into subtypes based on neuramidase (N) [YG1] and hemagglutinin (H) surface proteins. An important characteristic of influenza A virus is antigenic drift, which refers to a change in surface protein shift in the neuramidase or hemagglutinin receptors. With influenza A, these surface receptor proteins are important in cellular adherence of the influenza virus and the spread of influenza from respiratory epithelial cells. The vaccine for the flu season most often includes the influenza hemagglutinin and neuramidase types seen at the end of the preceding year's season. Prevention of attachment and spread of the virus is helpful to controlling the spread of influenza; vaccine protection conferred by specific antibody response to influenza A is highly protective (approximately 80% in noncompromised hosts).

During the years when influenza B has been important, vaccines for the subsequent year contain an influenza B component. The prophylactic effects of amantadine (Symmetrel) and rimantadine (Flumadine) are based on preventing viral adherence, thus preventing entry and infection of respiratory epithelial cells. Neuramidase inhibitors have anti-influenza activity.

Clinical manifestations of influenza A in adults varies considerably from mild to fatal infection. Mild infection is usually manifested as an acute febrile illness characterized by headache and myalgias with dry unproductive cough, rhinorrhea, and tracheobronchitis. Mild viral influenza may be a result of influenza A or B and usually resolves in a few days without complications in normal hosts who have good cardiopulmonary function.

Severe viral influenza A occurs in normal healthy adults and may be fatal. The onset of severe influenza A is sudden, and the patient often recalls the exact hour of onset. The patient is febrile with early/extreme prostration rendering the patient bedridden. Fever rapidly rises and may be accompanied by chills. Neck soreness, severe headache, and myalgias are typical. Sore throat, eye pain, conjunctival injection, and hemoptysis are frequently present. Chest pain worsened by deep inspiration is not truly pleuritic but rather reflects influenza A myositis of the intracostal muscles. Shortness of breath is related to the degree of hypoxemia. Severe influenza A causes an oxygen diffusion defect as manifested by an increased A-a gradient (>35). Profound hypoxemia may be accompanied by cyanosis. Hypotension caused by hypoxemia and vascular collapse may follow. The course of severe viral influenza A is fulminant and of short duration.

Physical findings are few in viral influenza (i.e., conjunctival suffusion). Auscultation reveals absolutely quiet lungs because the infectious process is interstitial and not alveolar. Routine blood tests are usually unremarkable except for leukopenia/lymphopenia and, less commonly, thrombocytopenia. Few atypical lymphocytes may be noted, and low titers of cold agglutinins may be present. Cold agglutinins (if present) have low titers less than or equal to 1:16. In severe cases, a pale bluelike hue of the skin may be noted, and there may be bleeding from diffuse intravascular coagulation (DIC) from multiple orifices preterminally. The chest radiograph in uncomplicated viral influenza A is unremarkable or may have minimal perihilar bilateral increased prominence of interstitial markings. In severe influenza A pneumonia, the chest radiograph shows bilateral symmetrical perihilar infiltrates without pleural effusions.

Patients may die from severe influenza A without superimposed bacterial pneumonia. Most deaths during the 1918 pandemic were young military recruits who died of influenza A pneumonia without bacterial superinfection. Viral influenza may be complicated by bacterial pneumonia. Bacterial pneumonias complicating viral influenza may occur concurrently at presentation or may present 1 to 2 weeks after the presentation of viral influenza. Viral influenza A presenting concurrently with a bacterial pneumonia is usually caused by *Staphylococcus aureus*. In contrast to uncomplicated viral influenza, bacterial superinfection is manifested by an increase in fever, shaking chills, leukocytosis, purulent sputum, localized rales on auscultation, bacteremia, and focal/segmental infiltrates on chest radiograph. Alternately, patients with viral influenza A may develop a secondary bacterial infection (same manifestations as noted previously) 1 to 2 weeks later. Secondary bacterial pneumonia is less severe than with concurrent *S. aureus* and is usually caused by *Streptococcus pneumoniae* or *Haemophilus influenzae*.

ANTI-INFLUENZA THERAPY

Therapy of viral influenza is directed at inhibiting viral replication and preventing further infection of respiratory epithelial cells. The neuramidase inhibitors zanamivir (Relenza) and oseltamivir (Tamiflu) have anti-influenza A and B activity. Neuramidase inhibitors decrease the severity and duration of influenza symptoms by 1 to 2 days. Amantadine (Symmetrel) and rimantadine (Flumadine) are useful prophylactically and therapeutically in influenza. Amantadine and rimantadine have anti-influenza A activity, but no influenza B activity. Amantadine and rimantadine inhibit early M2 protein-dependent replication and prevent adherence of the influenza virus to respiratory epithelial cells, thus preventing progression of infection and minimizing further cell to cell spread. Amantadine and rimantadine also affect peripheral airway dilatation and oxygenation is improved, which is of critical importance because patients with severe influenza A uncomplicated by bacterial superinfection die of severe hypoxemia. Mild influenza A/B may be treated with neuramidase inhibitors. Mild cases of influenza A should be treated at the onset of the illness. For severe influenza A, amantadine or rimantadine in combination[1] with neuramidase inhibitors provide optimal anti-influenza therapy (Table 1). For avian influenza (H_5N_1), these antiviral drugs may be ineffective.

Mycoplasma pneumoniae Pneumonia

M. pneumoniae is a common cause of ambulatory CAP. It affects all age groups, and in normal hosts with intact cardiopulmonary function, *Mycoplasma* CAP is usually a mild, self-limiting infection. However, *M. pneumoniae* derives its importance from difficulty in diagnosis, the necessity for non–β-lactam therapy, and because of its effect on peripheral airways.

Mycoplasma CAP is one of the nonzoonotic causes of CAP (the others being *Legionella* and *Chlamydia pneumoniae*). *M. pneumoniae* is an atypical pneumonia that is a

---

[1]Not FDA approved for this indication.

TABLE 1   Adult Anti-Influenza Antivirals

Antiviral	Treatment Dose	Prophylactic Dose
Mild Influenza A/B		
Zanamivir (Relenza)	2 inhalations (5 mg per inhalation) q12h × 5d	No FDA indication
Severe Influenza A		
Amantadine (Symmetrel)	200 mg (PO) q24h Persons age 65: 100 mg	200 mg (PO) q24h Persons age 65: 100 mg
	or	
Rimantadine (Flumadine)	100 mg (PO) q12h Persons with hepatic/renal failure (CrCl <10 mL/min) or elderly 100 mg (PO) q24h	100 mg (PO) q12h Persons with hepatic/renal failure (CrCl <10 mL/min) or elderly 100 mg (PO) q24h
	plus	
Oseltamivir[1] (Tamiflu)	75 mg (PO) q12d × 5d*	75 mg (PO) q24h × 7d

[1]Not FDA approved for this indication.
*For avian influenza, 150 mg (PO) q12h may be more effective.

systemic infectious disease with a pulmonary component. It may be distinguished from other atypical pneumonias by its characteristic pattern of extrapulmonary organ involvement. *M. pneumoniae* CAP most closely resembles *C. pneumoniae* CAP clinically, but is very different from Legionnaires' disease in terms of its epidemiology, age distribution, pattern of extrapulmonary organ involvement, and severity.

Clinically, *M. pneumoniae* presents as a subacute febrile illness. Temperatures rarely exceed 102°F (38.9°C). Rigors are not a feature of *M. pneumoniae* CAP, but patients may complain of chilly sensations. Mild headache and/or myalgias are not uncommon. The most common presenting symptom in *Mycoplasma* CAP is the prolonged, nonproductive dry cough. Patients with *Mycoplasma* CAP often complain of or have mild nonexudative pharyngitis. Rhinorrhea and conjunctivitis are not features of *M. pneumoniae* CAP. Watery diarrhea is commonly present in *Mycoplasma* CAP, but abdominal pain is not a clinical finding. Other extrapulmonary manifestations are uncommon or rare (e.g., meningoencephalitis, pericarditis, hemolytic anemia, glomerular nephritis, Guillain-Barré syndrome, erythema multiforme). *M. pneumoniae* has a distinctive pattern of extrapulmonary organ involvement that does not include cardiac involvement (relative bradycardia) or hepatic involvement, including normal serum glutamate-oxaloacetate transaminase (SGOT) or serum glutamate-pyruvate transaminase (SGPT). The distinguishing laboratory feature of *M. pneumoniae* CAP is elevated cold agglutinin titers. Although a variety of infectious and noninfectious diseases are associated with cold agglutinin elevations, they are usually of low titer (i.e., <1:16). There are no pulmonary infections presenting as CAP that are associated with high elevations of cold agglutinin titers (i.e., ≥1:64). Although elevated cold agglutinins occur early in up to 75% of patients with *M. pneumoniae* CAP, they are still diagnostically important when present. In a patient with CAP and a cold agglutinin titer greater than or equal to 1:64, the diagnosis of *M. pneumoniae* CAP is very likely.

M. pneumoniae may be differentiated from the typical bacterial pneumonias because of the presence of extrapulmonary findings, including nonexudative pharyngitis, loose stools or watery diarrhea, erythema multiforme, and high cold agglutinin. Patients with typical bacterial CAP usually have a more acute onset of presentation, a productive cough, and temperatures that may exceed 102°F (38.9°C), often accompanied by chills. Patients with typical pneumonia often have pleuritic chest pain, which is not a feature of *M. pneumoniae* CAP. Among the atypical pneumonias, the zoonotic pneumonias (i.e., tularemia, psittacosis, Q fever) may be eliminated from consideration if there is a recent zoonotic contact history with the appropriate vector.

C. pneumoniae resembles closely *M. pneumoniae* CAP. *C. pneumoniae* may be distinguished by the absence of cold agglutinins and the presence of hoarseness, which is a feature of *C. pneumoniae* but not *M. pneumoniae* CAP. Loose stools or watery diarrhea are not usual features of *C. pneumoniae* CAP. The most common clinical problem is differentiating *Legionella* from *Mycoplasma* CAP; this may be done by appreciating the differences in the pattern of extrapulmonary organ involvement with each of these pathogens. *Legionella* may be clinically differentiated from *Mycoplasma* by acuteness of onset or severity, the presence of relative bradycardia, temperatures greater than 102°F (38.9°C), and the presence of abdominal pain. From a laboratory standpoint, highly elevated cold agglutinin titers argue strongly against the diagnosis of *Legionella* and point to *M. pneumoniae*. Nonspecific laboratory tests in a patient with CAP that suggest *Legionella* and argue against *M. pneumoniae* include otherwise unexplained hypophosphatemia, hyponatremia, microscopic hematuria, and increased creatinine. *Legionella* does not affect the upper respiratory tract as does *Mycoplasma* (e.g., nonexudative pharyngitis). Ear findings are not a feature of Legionnaires' disease but are common in *M. pneumoniae* CAP. The finding most likely to cause confusion between *M. pneumoniae* and *Legionella pneumophila* is the presence of loose stools or watery diarrhea, which is found in both.

M. pneumoniae may be cultured from the throat in viral culture media, but the diagnosis is usually made serologically. An elevated enzyme-linked immunosorbent assay (ELISA) or enzyme immunoassay (EIA) IgM titer suggests acute or recent infection, but an elevated IgG titer indicates past exposure but not acute infection. Elevated IgG titers regardless of degree of elevation are not diagnostic of current infection with *M. pneumoniae* and only indicate previous antigenic exposure. *M. pneumoniae* ELISA IgM levels may take up to 3 months to decrease. Therefore, clinicians should take into account recent antecedent respiratory illness in order to properly interpret elevated IgM titers, including patients with nonexudative pharyngitis within 3 months prior to the presentation of CAP. The combination of an increased *M. pneumoniae* IgM titer and highly elevated cold agglutinin titers is virtually diagnostic of acute infection. Cold agglutinin titers are elevated transiently early and rapidly fall; the simultaneously elevated cold agglutinins and IgM titers of *M. pneumoniae* indicate active or current infection. In patients with CAP caused by another organism (e.g., *S. pneumoniae*), the presence of elevated *Mycoplasma* IgG titers does not indicate co-infection but only preexisting serologic exposure to *M. pneumoniae*.

THERAPY

M. pneumoniae has a predilection for the respiratory epithelial cells and resides literally on their surface. Mycoplasmas have no definite cell wall like the typical pathogens causing CAP. Their position on the surface of the respiratory epithelium and their absence of a cell wall necessitates the therapeutic approach, which includes non–β-lactam antibiotics with the capacity to penetrate into the *Mycoplasma* organisms. Traditionally, macrolides and tetracyclines have been used successfully to treat *M. pneumoniae*. Both CAP tetracyclines and macrolides are effective against *Mycoplasma* because they interfere with intracellular protein synthesis at the ribosomal level. Tetracyclines penetrate intracellularly better than macrolides, with the exception of penetration into the alveolar macrophage, which is relevant in *Legionella*, but

CURRENT DIAGNOSIS

Viral Influenza
- Mild influenza A or B presents acutely with headache, fever, sore throat, plus/minus rhinorrhea.
- Severe influenza A presents with an acute onset (patients often able to name the hour the influenza began) and rapidly become bed bound.
- Headache, myalgias, and prostration are severe.
- Auscultation of the lungs is quiet, disproportionate to the degree of respiratory distress. Influenza is an interstitial process and not alveolar, which explains the absence of rales.
- With severe influenza, patients rapidly become hypoxemic. Hypoxemia is accompanied by an AA gradient (>35), which suggests an interstitial oxygen diffusing defect typical of severe viral influenza pneumonia.
- Severe tracheobronchitis is common and is manifested by hemoptysis.
- Leukopenia/lymphopenia is typical; thrombocytopenia may occur. Low titer elevations of cold agglutinins are not infrequent (≥1:16).
- Patients may have chest pain exacerbated by breathing mimicking pleuritic chest pain. This is the result of direct intracostal muscle involvement with the influenza virus, which results in myositis and pain on inspiration.
- The chest radiograph in early viral influenza, in mild to moderate cases, is normal or near normal, with minimal, if any, increase in perihilar interstitial markings. The chest radiograph in fulminant cases shows symmetrical bilateral patchy infiltrates without pleural effusion in 24 to 48 hours.
- Severe viral influenza A is accompanied by severe hypoxemia or cyanosis, which may be followed by a fatal outcome.
- Influenza pneumonia may present alone without bacterial superinfection. Bacterial infection may accompany or follow.

- Purulent sputum with viral influenza indicates concurrent bacterial pneumonia usually caused by *S. aureus*. Bacterial pneumonia following influenza (after 1 to 2 weeks), is suggested by leukocytosis, focal or segmental pulmonary infiltrates, and purulent sputum; the pathogens are not *S. aureus*, but most commonly are *S. pneumoniae* or *H. influenzae*.
- A laboratory diagnosis may be made by DFA staining of respiratory secretions, viral influenza titers, or viral cultures.

Mycoplasma pneumoniae
- In a patient with CAP and a dry nonproductive cough, without severe headache or myalgias, the most likely diagnosis is *M. pneumoniae*. *M. pneumoniae* CAP is commonly accompanied by nonexudative pharyngitis and/or loose stools or watery diarrhea.
- The temperature is usually less than 102°F (38.9°C) and is not accompanied by frank rigors or pleuritic chest pain.
- Relative bradycardia and elevations in the serum transaminases are not features of *M. pneumoniae* CAP.
- Respiratory viruses are often associated with mild elevations of cold agglutinins (≤1:16) but *M. pneumoniae* is the only pathogen causing CAP associated with highly elevated cold agglutinin titers (≥1:64). Elevated cold agglutinin titers occur in up to 75% of patients with *M. pneumoniae*, and occur early and transiently.
- In a patient with CAP, elevated cold agglutinin titers (>1:8) effectively rule out the typical pathogens, as well as *Legionella* species and *C. pneumoniae*.
- Elevated *M. pneumoniae* ELISA IgG titers indicate past exposure/infection and not current infection or co-infection with another pathogen.
- In the absence of an antecedent respiratory tract infection (e.g., nonexudative pharyngitis, otitis, etc., in the preceding 3 months), the presence of an increased *M. pneumoniae* ELISA IgM titer is diagnostic of acute infection.

not *M. pneumoniae*, infections. Macrolides and tetracyclines are both active against *Mycoplasma*; the relative lack of penetration by macrolides into respiratory epithelial cells accounts for differences in therapeutic response. Patients treated with macrolides or tetracyclines defervesce rapidly over 24 to 48 hours. Clinical defervescence manifests by an increased feeling of well-being and a decrease in fever. The dry cough persists during and after therapy regardless of the anti-*Mycoplasma* antimicrobial used.

There are important differences in the shedding rates of *Mycoplasma* from respiratory epithelial cells posttherapy when using tetracyclines instead of macrolides.

 ## CURRENT THERAPY

Viral Influenza
- The aim of therapy is to inhibit the influenza virus and prevent its attachment/spread to uninfected respiratory epithelial cells.
- The neuramidase inhibitors shorten the course of influenza by 1 to 2 days and have antiviral activity. These agents are active against both influenza A and B.
  - Amantadine (Symmetrel) or rimantadine (Flumadine) do not have antiviral properties but are important in prevention/therapy.
  - Amantadine and rimantadine prevent the adherence of influenza virus to uninfected upper respiratory epithelial cells, thereby limiting the extent of the infection.
  - Amantadine and rimantadine also have an important therapeutic effect in influenza A by increasing distal airway dilation and increasing oxygen action; their effect on peripheral airways is important in severe influenza A. Amantadine and rimantadine are not active against influenza B.
  - Amantadine and rimantadine should be given for the duration of viral influenza. Used prophylactically, amantadine and rimantadine should be given before, during, and following an outbreak of influenza A.

Mycoplasma pneumoniae
- The agents active against *M. pneumoniae* are macrolides, tetracyclines, quinolones, and ketolides. β-Lactam antibiotics are not active against *M. pneumoniae* because the organisms do not contain a bacterial cell wall.
- Goals of therapy of *M. pneumoniae* CAP are to eradicate the infection, decrease the shedding of *Mycoplasma* in respiratory secretions posttherapy, and to prevent posttreatment asthma.
- Therapy is equally efficacious with macrolides, doxycycline (Vibramycin), respiratory quinolones, or telithromycin (Ketek) intravenously, orally, or in combination for 1 to 2 weeks.
- The mode of administration is determined by the severity of the CAP and the setting. Outpatients are usually treated orally. Patients hospitalized with severe CAP are initially treated intravenously and then changed to an oral agent.
- Resistance to *M. pneumoniae* with antimicrobials has not been described and is not a clinical consideration.

Tetracycline therapy is associated with a more rapid decrease in shedding. Tetracyclines with better ability to penetrate intracellularly, such as doxycycline (Vibramycin), are the most rapid at decreasing *Mycoplasma* shedding, which is an important public health consideration. Mycoplasmas are transmitted by aerosolized droplet infection. Because patients with *Mycoplasma* have a prolonged cough, organisms not eliminated from respiratory epithelial cells may be aerosolized during coughing for weeks following the acute infection, spreading the infection to susceptible individuals via aerosolized droplets. The aim of therapy is to rapidly treat the patient's pneumonia and extrapulmonary sites of involvement. The secondary goal is to rapidly decrease shedding and aerosolization to prevent the spread of *Mycoplasma* to other individuals. An additional therapeutic goal is to decrease the incidence of post-*Mycoplasma* asthma seen in some patients. *M. pneumoniae* CAP may exacerbate preexisting asthma, but may also cause permanent post-CAP asthma in some individuals.

Until recently, doxycycline was the most active antimicrobial to use against *M. pneumoniae*. Currently, the "respiratory quinolones," levofloxacin (Levaquin), gatifloxacin (Tequin), moxifloxacin (Avelox), and gemifloxacin (Factive), are all highly active anti-*M. pneumoniae* antimicrobials. Telithromycin (Ketek), a ketolide antibiotic, also has a high degree of anti-*M. pneumoniae* activity. The respiratory quinolones and telithromycin all penetrate cells efficiently and interfere with intracellular enzymes or protein synthesis of intracellular organisms. Respiratory quinolones and telithromycin are highly effective anti-*Mycoplasma* agents and rapidly decrease shedding of *M. pneumoniae* in respiratory secretions.

Therapy for *M. pneumoniae* is ordinarily 1 to 2 weeks. Patients who have impaired cardiopulmonary disease or compromised host may require 2 full weeks of therapy. In patients with borderline cardiopulmonary function, *M. pneumoniae* as with other relatively low virulence

TABLE 2　Antibiotics Effective Against *M. pneumoniae*

Antibiotic	Dose (Adult)
Mild/Moderate CAP	
Erythromycin	500 mg (base, estolate, stearate) (PO) q6h
Erythromycin lactobionate	1 g (IV) q6h
Clarithromycin (Biaxin)	500 mg (PO) q12h
Azithromycin (Zithromax)	500 mg (IV) q24h × 2 doses, followed by 500 mg (PO) q24h
Gemifloxacin (Factive)	320 mg (PO) q24h
Telithromycin (Ketek)	800 mg (PO) q24h
Severe CAP	
Doxycycline	100 mg (IV/PO) q12h
Levofloxacin (Levaquin)	500 mg (IV/PO) q24h, or 750 mg IV/PO q24h (may allow for shorter duration of therapy)
Gatifloxacin (Tequin)	400 mg (IV/PO) q24h
Moxifloxacin (Avelox)	400 mg (IV/PO) q24h

pathogens may present as severe CAP. Antimicrobial therapy for typical or atypical CAP should be directed against the presumed pathogen and not based on co-morbidities. Normal healthy hosts are treated with the same antimicrobial as patients hospitalized with severe CAP. Patients hospitalized with compromised cardiopulmonary function severe *Mycoplasma* CAP are most often initially treated intravenously with doxycycline (Vibramycin), a macrolide, or a respiratory quinolone. Most patients with *M. pneumoniae* CAP present in the ambulatory setting, which permits therapy with oral doxycycline, macrolide, a respiratory quinolone, or telithromycin (Ketek) (Table 2).

REFERENCES

Ali NJ, Sillis M, Andrews BE, et al: The clinical spectrum and diagnosis of *Mycoplasma pneumoniae* infection. Q J Med 1986;58:241-251.

Cunha BA: Influenza and its complications. Emerg Med 2000;2:56-67.

Cunha BA: Hepatic involvement in *Mycoplasma pneumoniae* community-acquired pneumonia. J Clin Microbiol 2003;3:385-386.

Cunha BA: Influenza: Historical aspects of epidemics and pandemics. Infect Dis Clin North Am 2004;18:141-155.

Cunha BA: Pneumonia Essentials. Royal Oak, MI, Physicians' Press, 2006.

Debré R, Couvreur J: Influenza: Clinical features. In: Debré R, Celers J (eds): Clinical Virology: The Evaluation and Management of Human Viral Infections. Philadelphia, WB Saunders, 1970, pp 507-515.

File TM, Tan JS: *Mycoplasma pneumoniae* pneumonia. In: Marrie TJ (ed): Community-Acquired Pneumonia. New York, Kluwer Academic/Plenum Publishers, 2001, pp 487-500.

Hammerschlag MR: *Mycoplasma pneumoniae* infections. Curr Opin Infect Dis 2001;14:181-186.

Louria DB, Blumenfield HL, Ellis JT: Studies on influenza in the pandemic of 1957-1958. II. Pulmonary complications of influenza. J Clin Invest 1959;38:213-265.

Marrie TJ: Empiric treatment of ambulatory community-acquired pneumonia: Always include treatment for atypical agents. Infect Dis Clin North Am 2004;18:829-841.

Murray HW, Masur H, Senterfit LS, Roberts RB: The protean manifestations of *Mycoplasma pneumoniae* infection in adults. Am J Med 1975;58:229-242.

Schmidt AC: Antiviral therapy for influenza: A clinical and economic comparative review. Drugs 2004;6:2031-2046.

Waites KB, Talkington DF: *Mycoplasma pneumoniae* and its role as a human pathogen. Clin Microbiol Rev 2004;17:697-728.

Legionellosis

Method of
Jorge Roig, MD, PhD, FCCP, and
Jordi Rello, MD, PhD

In most series of severe community-acquired pneumonia (CAP), *Legionella* usually ranks second to pneumococcus in the list of most common etiologic agents. However, the real incidence of pneumonia caused by the genus *Legionella* remains to some extent unknown because many of the *Legionella* species and serogroups cannot be properly diagnosed by the current commercially available microbiologic tests.

Legionella pneumophila serogroup 1 is the predominant identified cause of legionellosis worldwide. The usual mechanism of transmission in humans is the inhalation of contaminated aerosols, although aspiration of contaminated water is also often reported. Legionellosis prevention is based on eradication of *Legionella* from water reservoirs.

Cigarette smoking, elderly (more than 65), and many underlying diseases are the usual predisposing factors to legionellosis. However, legionnaires' disease, even with a severe clinical presentation, may also occur in previously healthy people.

Legionellosis may range from mild respiratory illness to fulminating pneumonia. Pontiac fever, an acute, usually self-limited, flulike illness, is a benign form of legionellosis. Numerous comparative studies of both community acquired and nosocomial legionellosis have shown that the clinical, radiologic, and laboratory features of legionellosis are not specific. A few clinical data, such as fever greater than 39°C (102°F), diarrhea, confusion, creatine phosphokinase (CPK) increase, or hyponatremia, are considered suggestive of *Legionella* infection. However, many prospective studies confirm that these data are not distinctive of legionellosis and their absence does not exclude this diagnosis.

Isolation of *Legionella* by culture in specific media continues to be the gold standard for diagnosing *Legionella* infection (Table 1). The progressive use of rapid, easier tests to detect *Legionella pneumophila* serogroup 1 antigen in urine samples parallels a worrying trend to decrease the number of cultures that eventually would permit the identification and isolation of other *Legionella* species different from *L. pneumophila* serotype 1.

Treatment

In patients with CAP who require admission to hospital, especially the elderly and those fulfilling severity criteria, clinical criteria are not predictive of the

CURRENT DIAGNOSIS

- Clinical, radiologic, and laboratory features are often indistinguishable from other bacterial pneumonias.
- In the setting of outbreaks, a positive *Legionella* antigen result in urine may be associated with more severe cases.
- Performance of specialized cultures from clinical samples is mandatory because usually antigenuria only detects *Legionella pneumophila* serogroup 1 infection.
- Progression of radiologic infiltrates is a negative predictive factor.
- A positive *Legionella* urine antigen test may last from many weeks to 1 year.
- Serology is widely used, but its sensitivity is <80% for *L. pneumophila* serogroup 1.
- Early diagnosis leads to prompt therapy and low mortality.

CURRENT THERAPY

- Early administration of effective therapy is a crucial, favorable prognostic factor, especially in severe pneumonia.
- Short-course oral therapy (7–10d) is feasible in mild-to-moderate cases
- In pregnancy, azithromycin (Zithromax)[1] and erythromycin (E-Mycin)[1] are the safest options
- Use of fluoroquinolones should be avoided in children.
- Eradication failures, poor clinical resolution, or relapse of pneumonia are not caused by the development of resistance to antimicrobial agents.
- A short course of therapy in immunocompromised patients must be avoided.
- More prolonged treatment (3 wk) is needed for the severe immunocompromised.
- Longer than usual treatment is needed for patients with heart valve endocarditis.
- Any purulent collection (sometimes unsuspected) should be drained.
- Consider dual infection, particularly in the immunocompromised patient.
- Acute lung injury in pneumonia may itself cause a poor clinical response.
- Combined therapy is not proven to be superior to monotherapy.
- If combined therapy is considered, the association of azithromycin (Zithromax) and a newer fluoroquinolone is recommended.
- Rifampin (Rifadin) should not be administered alone; its use is associated with reversible hepatic cholestasis.

[1]Not FDA approved for this indication.

pathogen involved. Consequently, the initial empirical therapeutic approach of many cases of CAP should include a therapeutic agent that is effective against *Legionella*. Therapeutic approach remains an important goal because the case-fatality rate is 5% to 30%, with elderly and immunocompromised patients at the greatest risk of death.

ANTIBIOTICS

In vitro susceptibility studies do not correlate with clinical efficacy because *Legionella* is an intracellular pathogen. Treatment guidelines are supported by data obtained from in vitro studies, experimental studies with the animal model, and observational studies, some of which come from prospective clinical studies in CAP. Optimal therapy against *Legionella* infection is then based on agents with high intrinsic activity; an appropriate pharmacokinetic and pharmacodynamic profile, including the ability to penetrate phagocytic cells; a low incidence of adverse reactions; and an advantageous cost–efficacy relationship. The treatment of choice has changed from erythromycin (E-Mycin) to the newer macrolides and fluoroquinolones (Table 2). Duration of therapy has to be decided individually. Combined therapy may be recommended for severe episodes by some guidelines, but no evidence supports this suggestion.

Extrapulmonary manifestations of legionellosis are uncommon and tend to occur in patients with immunocompromise (Table 3). Suppurated focus of infection should be drained by means of catheter insertion or a surgical procedure.

DUAL INFECTION

Mixed infection by more than one pathogen should not be neglected, particularly in the immunocompromised host (Table 4). Fatalities were reported when clinicians failed to be aware of some of these dual infections.

ADULT RESPIRATORY DISTRESS SYNDROME

Adjunctive measures are the cornerstone of therapy for ARDS. Respiratory failure with progressive hypoxemia is a significant cause of death. In patients undergoing intubation, the goal is to improve gas interchange and avoid producing ventilatory-induced lung injury, maintaining plateau pressures under 25. A protective strategy of ventilation with low tidal volumes (less than 7 mL/kg) protects the lung in ARDS. FIO_2 should be minimized to target an acceptable Sao_2 up to 90%. Recruitment maneuvers may prevent alveolar collapse and improve oxygenation.

TABLE 1 Noninvasive Diagnostic Tests for Detection of *Legionella*

Tests	Sensitivity	Specificity	Time Required
Sputum culture	10%–80%	100%	2–7 d
Serology	40%–70%	95%–99%	1–6 mo
DFA of sputum	33%–70%	95%–99%	2–4 h
Urinary Antigen Assay			
ELISA	>90%	99%–100%	2–3 h
IC*	>90%	99%–100%	15 min if NCU
PCR (serum, urine, respiratory samples)	33%–70%	98%–100%	2–6 h

Abbreviations DFA = direct fluorescent antibody staining; ELISA = enzyme-linked immunoabsorbent assay; NCU = nonconcentrated urine; PCR = polymerase chain reaction.
*IC = immunochromatography: 2 h more if urine is concentrated as advised.
Modified from Roig J, Rello J: Legionnaire's disease: A rational approach to therapy. JAC 2003;51:1119-1129.

TABLE 2 Recommended Therapy in Legionellosis

Antimicrobial Agent		Dosage	Route
Macroazalides	Azithromycin* (Zithromax)[1]	500 mg q24h	IV, PO
	Clarithromycin (Biaxin)[1,2]	500 mg q12h	IV, PO
Tetracyclines	Doxycycline (Vibramycin)[1]	100 mg q12–24h	IV, PO
Fluoroquinolones	Levofloxacin* (Levaquin)	500–750 mg q24h	IV, PO
	Moxifloxacin*(Avelox)[1]	400 mg q24h	IV, PO
	Gemifloxacin† (Factive)[1]	320 mg q24h	PO
	Gatifloxacin†(Tequin)[1]	200–400 mg q24h	IV, PO
	Ciprofloxacin (Cipro)	400–750 mg q12h	IV, PO
Ketolides	Telithromycin† (Ketek)[1]	800 mg q24h	PO

*Recommended in the more severe cases, particularly in the immunocompromised.
†Because of short accumulated clinical experience, their use is recommended only in mild to moderate cases.
[1]Not FDA approved for this indication.
[2]IV form not available in the United States.
Abbreviations: IV = intravenous; PO = orally.

TABLE 3 Extrapulmonary Manifestations of Legionellosis

Cardiovascular	Pericarditis, myocarditis,* endocarditis, aortic graft involvement
Neurologic	Encephalitis that may mimic that caused by herpes, brain abscess, cerebellar ataxia,* corpus callosum involvement
Digestive	Colon involvement that may mimic ulcerative colitis, pancreatitis, digestive tract abscess, liver involvement, spleen rupture, severe diarrhea*
Renal	Kidney abscess, acute renal failure, interstitial nephritis*
Blood*	Thrombopenia, disseminated intravascular coagulation (DIC)
Joint and bone	Arthritis,* osteomyelitis
Miscellaneous	Wound infection, cellulitis, rhabdomyolysis, posttraumatic stress disorder

*Some of these manifestations are just reactive and they do not mean real local infection. A short course of steroid therapy may then be useful.

TABLE 4 Polymicrobial Infection* in Legionellosis

Other *Legionella* species	Dual infections by different species of *Legionella* and different serotypes of *Legionella pneumophila*
Other bacteria	*Streptococcus pneumoniae, Proteus mirabilis, Staphylococcus aureus, Escherichia coli, Prevotella intermedia, Enterococcus faecium, Enterobacter cloacae, Klebsiella pneumoniae, Haemophilus influenzae, Streptococcus mitis, Listeria monocytogenes, Nocardia asteroides*
Mycobacteria	*Mycobacterium tuberculosis*
Virus	Herpesvirus, influenza, cytomegalovirus
Fungus	Aspergillus, cryptococcus
Parasites	*Pneumocystis jiroveci, Leishmania*

*Alleged mixed infections with *Mycoplasma pneumoniae, Chlamydia pneumoniae,* and *Coxiella burnetii* are reported on the basis of serology, which raises much concern on specificity.

Positioning patients in the prone position may be used as rescue therapy for the most severe episodes. Preliminary studies in the animal model raise some concern about the risk of hyperoxia in severe legionellosis. Extracorporeal membrane oxygenation (ECMO) is reported anecdotally as a successful therapeutic option in treating severe *Legionella*-associated ARDS. Hemodynamic control must be another priority when linked to severe sepsis or septic shock.

STEROIDS

Table 5 lists the potential indications of steroid therapy in legionellosis. Figure 1 suggests an algorithmic approach to

TABLE 5 Potential Role of Steroid Therapy in Legionellosis

Proliferative phase of diffuse alveolar damage (ARDS)	Controversial use, as happens in other types of pneumonia with adult respiratory distress syndrome
Reactive extrapulmonary manifestations	Arthritis Myocarditis Some neurologic manifestations Some renal manifestations Some hematologic
Inflammatory pattern in lung tissue biopsy*	Plasma-cell interstitial pneumonia Chronic interstitial pneumonia Lymphocytic interstitial pneumonia Nonspecific interstitial pneumonia Bronchiolitis obliterans–organizing pneumonia (BOOP)

*These diagnoses should be based on representative samples of lung biopsy. When these findings are just observed in small samples, such as those usually provided by transbronchial biopsy, they may not be extrapolated to the whole lung.
Abbreviation: ARDS = adult respiratory distress syndrome.

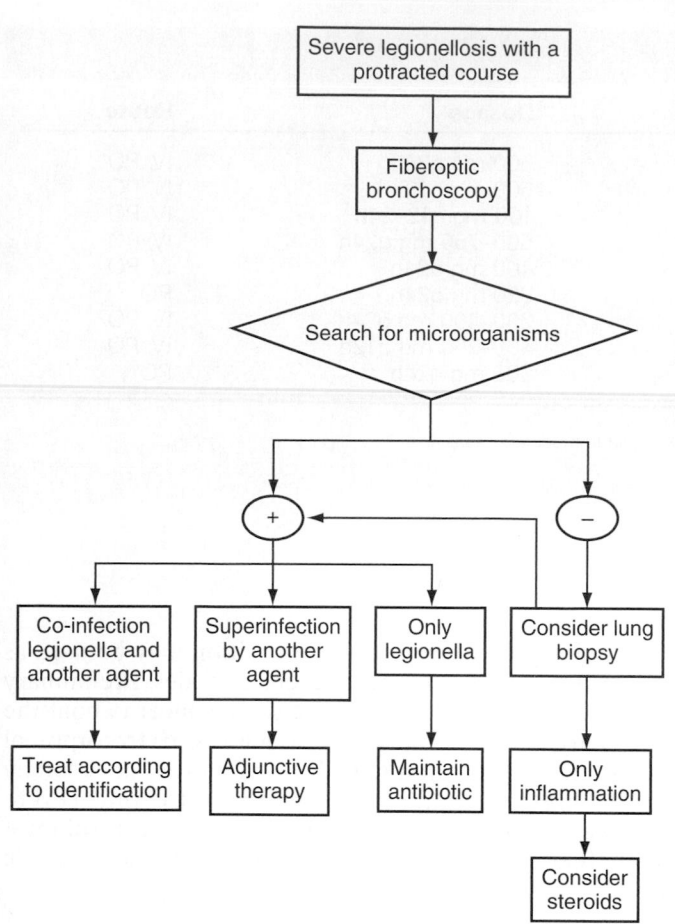

FIGURE 1. Proposal for algorithmic approach to management of intubated patients with nonresolving legionellosis. Modified from Roig J, Rello J: Legionnaire's disease: A rational approach to therapy. JAC 2003;51:1119-1129.

severe legionellosis with poor clinical resolution. In patients with delayed resolution, superinfection by *Pseudomonas aeruginosa* should be suspected early.

REFERENCES

Baltch AL, Bopp LH, Smith RP, et al: Antibacterial activities of gemifloxacin, levofloxacin, gatifloxacin, moxifloxacin and erythromycin against intracellular *Legionella pneumophila* and *Legionella micdadei* in human monocytes. J Antimicrob Chemother 2005;56(1):104-109.

Blázquez RM, Espinosa FJ, Martínez-Toldos CM, et al: Sensitivity of urinary antigen test in relation to clinical severity in a large outbreak of *Legionella* pneumonia in Spain. Eur J Clin Microbiol Infect Dis 2005;24:488-491.

Edelstein PH: Antimicrobial chemotherapy for legionnaires' disease: Time for a change. Ann Intern Med 1998;129:328-330.

Fernandez-Sabe N, Roson B, Carratala J, et al: Clinical diagnosis of *Legionella* pneumonia revisited: Evaluation of the Community-Based Pneumonia Incidence Study Group scoring system. Clin Infect Dis 2003;37:483-489.

Kraus CN, Zalkikar J, Powers JH: Levofloxacin and macrolides for treatment of legionnaires' disease. Multiple comparisons give few answers. Clin Infect Dis 2005;41:416.

Nara C, Tateda K, Matsumoto T, et al: Legionella-induced acute lung injury in the setting of hyperoxia: Protective role of tumour necrosis factor-a. J Med Microb 2004;53:727-733.

Reilly KM, Urban MA, Barreiro T, et al: Persistent culture-positive *Legionella* infection in an immunocompromised host. Clin Infect Dis 2005;40:e87-e89.

Roig J, Rello J: Legionnaires' disease: A rational approach to therapy. JAC 2003;51:1119-1129.

Roig J, Sabria M, Pedro-Botet ML: *Legionella* spp.: Community-acquired and nosocomial infections. Curr Op Infect Dis 2003;16:145-151.

Sabria M, Yu VL: Hospital-acquired legionellosis: Solutions for a preventable infection. Lancet Infect Dis 2002;2:368-373.

Stout JE, Sens K, Mietzner S, et al: Comparative activity of quinolones, macrolides and ketolides against *Legionella* species using in vitro broth dilution and intracellular susceptibility testing. Int J Antimicrob Agents 2005;25:302-307.

Yu VL, Greenberg RN, Zadeikis N, et al: Levofloxacin efficacy in the treatment of community-acquired legionellosis. Chest 2004;125:2135-2139.

Pulmonary Embolism

Method of
C. Gregory Elliott, MD

Diagnosis

The diagnosis of acute pulmonary embolism (PE) remains a challenge, in spite of numerous technical advances. The decision to order diagnostic studies and the quantification of the clinician's suspicion that the patient has pulmonary embolism are both critical steps (Figure 1). It is well recognized that patients die from PE that was never suspected by their physicians. Conversely, many patients present with symptoms, signs, and laboratory abnormalities caused by diseases that mimic PE. A low threshold for ordering screening studies is important when the clinical presentation suggests PE in patients who have risk factors (Table 1). Even when risk factors are not present, the common symptoms of sudden dyspnea, unexplained pleuritic chest pain with or without hemoptysis, and hypotension with or without syncope should lead the physician to consider PE. The clinician must also be aware of uncommon presentations of PE, such as abdominal pain, cough, fever, wheezing, sudden unexplained arrhythmia, or oxygen desaturation in the hospitalized patient.

Once the physician suspects acute PE, it is important to estimate how likely this diagnosis is before performing diagnostic tests. The prior probability influences the likelihood that PE can be confirmed or excluded by a diagnostic test. Both physician empirical assessment (gestalt) and formalized clinical prediction rules may be used to assess the pretest probability of PE. Both approaches depend on key elements of the history, physical examination, and basic laboratory tests to assign a probability of high, intermediate (moderate), or low. The prior probability alters the probability that a given test result correctly confirms or rules out PE.

D-DIMER

Enzyme-linked immunoabsorbent assays (ELISA) for d-dimer fragments of cross-linked fibrin are sensitive tests for acute deep vein thrombosis and PE in outpatients. In this group of patients, a negative ELISA d-dimer assay excludes acute PE when the pretest clinical estimate is low. Conversely, a positive test does not confirm the diagnosis of PE. Instead, it confirms the need for additional tests.

CURRENT DIAGNOSIS

- The decision to order diagnostic studies and the quantification of the clinician's suspicion of acute PE are critical steps.
- A low threshold for ordering screening studies is important.
- Even when risk factors are not present, the common symptoms of sudden dyspnea, unexplained pleuritic chest pain, and hypotension, with or without syncope, should lead the physician to consider PE.
- ELISA d-dimer assays are sensitive tests for acute PE in outpatients.
- A normal perfusion lung scan excludes clinically important PE.
- A negative CT pulmonary arteriogram may not exclude acute PE, and additional tests such as duplex (compression) ultrasonography of the legs may be needed.

Abbreviations: CT = computed tomography; ELISA = enzyme-linked immunoabsorbent assay; PE = pulmonary embolism.

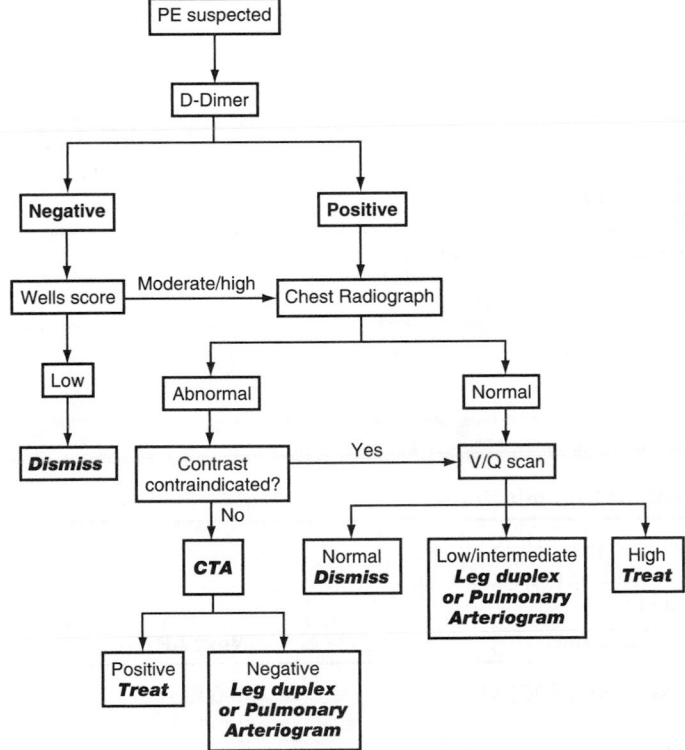

FIGURE 1. This is one of the several possible algorithms for the evaluation of outpatients with suspected PE. This approach to the diagnosis of acute PE emphasizes an estimate of the clinical probability for PE, the use of rapid ELISA assays of d-dimer, the appropriate use of CT pulmonary angiography, and duplex studies of the legs. CT = computed tomography; CTA = computed tomographic angiography; ELISA = enzyme-linked immunoabsorbent assay; PE = pulmonary embolism.

ELISA d-dimer assays are not useful for patients who have undergone major surgery recently.

LUNG SCANS

A normal lung perfusion scan excludes clinically important PE and eliminates the need for anticoagulant therapy. However, an abnormal perfusion scan alone is not sufficiently specific to confirm the diagnosis of acute PE. When combined with ventilation scanning and a clinical estimate of prior probability, the likelihood that the patient has PE can be estimated (Table 2). In general, additional testing is needed to confirm a diagnosis of PE if the perfusion and ventilation scans are abnormal but not high probability or the physician's estimate of the presence of PE was not high and the scan pattern suggests a high probability for PE. Most patients with abnormal perfusion lung scans require additional diagnostic tests before a management strategy is chosen.

COMPUTED TOMOGRAPHIC PULMONARY ANGIOGRAPHY

CT pulmonary angiography is now ordered routinely to investigate clinical findings that suggest acute PE. At present,

TABLE 2 Influence of Prior Probability on the Likelihood That Ventilation and Perfusion Lung Scan Patterns Are Related to Acute Pulmonary Embolism

	Prior Probability for PE		
	High	*Intermediate*	*Low*
Scan pattern	80–100	20–79	0–19
High	96	88	56
Intermediate	66	28	16
Low	40	16	4

Prior probability for pulmonary embolism (PE) was determined from clinical information by experienced clinicians who estimated the likelihood of PE (high = 80%–100%, intermediate = 20%–79%, and low = 0%–19%). Data express the likelihood (expressed as percentage) for identifying acute PE on pulmonary angiograms. Modified from the PIOPED Investigators: JAMA 1990;263:2753-2759. Copyright 1990, American Medical Association.

negative CT pulmonary angiography alone may be insufficient to exclude acute PE. The combination of negative duplex ultrasonography studies of the deep veins in both legs and negative CT pulmonary angiography provides the evidence necessary to withhold anticoagulants safely (i.e., with a very low rate of subsequent venous thromboembolism) when a clinical presentation suggests acute PE.

PULMONARY ANGIOGRAPHY AND LEG DUPLEX

Pulmonary angiography remains the gold standard for the diagnosis of acute PE. However, angiography is invasive, expensive, and not always readily available. These limitations have led to the development of alternative diagnostic strategies. Serial duplex ultrasonography with compression of the leg veins relies on the knowledge that proximal deep venous thrombosis of the lower extremities underlies the majority of PE. Therefore, positive studies confirm the diagnosis of venous thromboembolism, and negative studies of the leg veins over a 2-week period allow the clinician to withhold anticoagulation because the risk for recurrent PE is low (less than 3%). This strategy should not be applied to patients who have serious cardiopulmonary compromise. Whenever possible, these patients should undergo pulmonary angiography, as should patients at increased risk for venous thrombi in other locations (e.g., upper extremities, renal veins, or the right heart).

Treatment

Unfractionated heparin (UFH) or low molecular weight heparin (LMWH) followed by warfarin (Coumadin) is highly efficacious therapy for the majority of patients with PE. When using UFH, rapid achievement of an adequate anticoagulant effect is crucial to prevent recurrent venous thromboembolism. An initial bolus of 5000 U of heparin followed by a constant intravenous infusion should be initiated when the diagnosis is confirmed or when clinical suspicion is high and bleeding risk is low (Table 3).

CURRENT THERAPY

- Either UFH or LMWH followed by warfarin is highly efficacious therapy for the majority of patients with acute PE.
- When using UFH, rapid achievement of an adequate anticoagulant effect is crucial to prevent recurrent venous thromboembolism. Emphasis should be placed on rapidly exceeding the lower threshold of the targeted therapeutic range.
- UFH or LMWH should be continued for a minimum of 5 days.
- Measurement of the APTT is not necessary when LMWH is given.
- UFH is preferred in patients with renal failure (creatinine clearance <30 mL/h or extremes of body weight (<40 kg or >150 kg).
- Platelet counts should be monitored daily during initial heparin therapy.
- Major bleeding complications are more likely to occur in patients who have identifiable risks for bleeding.
- Warfarin should be continued for at least 3 mo for PE after major surgery or trauma and at least 6 mo when there was no or minimal provocation.
- Patients with active cancer are less likely to experience recurrence when LMWH rather than warfarin is provided for long-term management.
- Removable vena cava filters offer a therapeutic alternative when anticoagulants are contraindicated or when anticoagulants must be discontinued because of bleeding.
- Patients are more likely to die when PE causes hypotension or right ventricular dysfunction. In this setting, thrombolysis or embolectomy must be considered.

Abbreviations: LMWH = low molecular weight heparin; PE = pulmonary embolism; UFH = unfractionated heparin.

TABLE 3 Protocols for Initial Heparin Therapy

Reference	Initial Bolus	Constant Unit Infusion		
Hull et al.,1992*	5000 U	1680 U/h (low risk to bleed) 1240 U/h (high risk to bleed)†		
Raschke et al.,1993‡	80 U/kg	18 U/kg/h		
APTT (sec)	**Dose Change (U/h)**	**Additional Action**		**Next APTT**
≤45	+240	Re-bolus with 5000 U		4–6 h
46–54	+120	None		4–6 h
55–85	0	None		
86–110	−120	Stop infusion for 1 h		4–6 h after restart
>110	−240	Stop infusion for 1 h		4–6 h after restart

*Hull RD, et al: Optimal therapeutic level of heparin therapy in patients with venous thrombosis. Arch Intern Med 1992;152:1589-1595.
†High risk to bleed in the judgment of the attending physician; common criteria include surgery or trauma within 2 wk, thrombocytopenia, thrombotic stroke, or history of peptic ulcer.
‡Raschke RA, et al: The weight-based heparin dosing nomogram compared with a "standard care" nomogram. Ann Intern Med 1993;119:874-881.
Abbreviation: APTT = activated partial thromboplastin time.

An initial heparin infusion of 1000 U per hour is not sufficient for most patients. The constant infusion should deliver either 1240 U per hour to patients with a high risk for bleeding complications or 1680 U per hour for those without identifiable risks for bleeding complications. Alternatively, the initial infusion may be weight adjusted at 18 U per kg (actual body weight) per hour. Measurement of the activated partial thromboplastin time (APTT) approximately 4 to 6 hours later permits adjustment of the heparin dose to achieve APTT results in the targeted therapeutic range. Emphasis should be placed on rapidly exceeding the lower threshold of the targeted therapeutic range because persistently subtherapeutic heparin levels permit recurrent venous thromboembolism. Heparin should be continued for a minimum of 5 days, and it may be continued for 7 to 10 days for more seriously affected patients (e.g., patients with massive PE).

Rarely, therapeutic prolongation of the APTT cannot be used to guide heparin therapy. When patients with the lupus anticoagulant have PE or when pseudo-heparin resistance caused by increased factor VIII levels leads to persistently "subtherapeutic" APTT results in spite of large (more than 50,000 U per 24 hours) heparin doses, heparin levels may be used to guide therapy. The target therapeutic range is 0.2 to 0.4 U/mL using protamine titration or an antifactor Xa level of 0.35 to 0.70 U/mL.

Subcutaneous LMWH provides an acceptable alternative to UFH (Table 4). Measurement of the APTT is not necessary when LMWH is given. This strategy may also be used for compliant outpatients with deep venous thrombosis, asymptomatic PE, and those at low risk for bleeding complications. UFH is preferred in patients with renal failure (creatinine clearance less than 30 mL/hour) or extremes of body weight(less than 40 kg or more than 150 kg). For such patients without venous access, subcutaneous LMWH provides an alternative to UFH. However, monitoring the anticoagulant effect on the anti-Xa level is advisable.

HEPARIN-INDUCED THROMBOCYTOPENIA

Platelet counts should be monitored daily during initial heparin therapy. When the platelet count falls abruptly, or when the platelet count falls below 100,000/μL, heparin should be discontinued and alternative treatment should be begun (Table 5), with heparin-induced thrombocytopenia

diagnosed presumptively. Heparin-induced thrombocytopenia is caused by heparin-induced immune complexes, and it may cause life-threatening arterial or venous thrombi. The diagnosis may be confirmed by normalization of the platelet count after discontinuing heparin, exclusion of other causes of thrombocytopenia, and a positive heparin-induced platelet aggregation test.

Fondaparinux (Arixtra) is a new synthetic anticoagulant with anti-Xa activity that provides effective treatment for PE. Fondaparinux is given as a subcutaneous injection once daily. The dose is based on the patient's weight. Avoidance of heparin-induced thrombocytopenia appears to be an important potential advantage of fondaparinux.

BLEEDING

Bleeding and heparin-induced thrombocytopenia with or without thrombosis are the major early complications of heparin treatment. Major bleeding complications that require blood transfusion and discontinuation of heparin are more likely to occur in patients who have identifiable risks for bleeding, such as thrombocytopenia, surgery or trauma within the past 2 weeks, or a history of peptic ulcer disease. In the absence of such risks, an excessively prolonged APTT is not a strong predictor of major bleeding. Most major

TABLE 4 Guidelines for Anticoagulation with Low Molecular Weight Heparin

Low Molecular Weight Heparin	Dose
Dalteparin sodium[1] (Fragmin)	200 anti-Xa U/kg/d SC (not >18,000 U in 1 dose)
Enoxaparin sodium (Lovenox)	1 mg/kg q12h SC or 1.5 mg/kg qd SC (single daily dose not >180 mg)
Nadroparin calcium[2] (Fraxiparine)	86 anti-Xa U/kg bid SC or 171 anti-Xa U/kg qd SC
Tinzaparin sodium[1] (Innohep)	175 anti-Xa U/kg qd SC

[1]Not FDA approved for this indication.
[2]Not available in the United States.
Abbreviation: SC = subcutaneous.

TABLE 5 Treatment of Heparin-Induced Thrombocytopenia

Drug	Dose	Half-life	Comment
Argatroban	2 μg/kg/min (no initial bolus) Target APTT 1.5–3.0 × baseline (mean of normal range for your laboratory)	40–50 min	Excreted by the liver. Preferred for patients with renal failure. Prolongs the prothrombin time, making transition to warfarin a challenge. Not associated with allergic reactions
Lepirudin	0.4 mg/kg over 15–20 s as bolus dose, followed by 0.15 mg/kg/h as continuous infusion Target APTT 1.5 to 2.5 × baseline (mean of normal range for your laboratory)	80 min	Excreted by the kidney. Preferred for patients with liver failure. Prolongs the prothrombin time. Anaphylactoid reactions can occur. Death occurs rarely.

Abbreviation: APTT = activated partial thromboplastin time.

bleeding episodes can be managed by discontinuing heparin, but when bleeding is life-threatening, the anticoagulant effects of heparin can be reversed more rapidly by protamine. The dose should be estimated (i.e., 1.0 mg of protamine for 100 U of heparin bolus, or 0.5 mg of protamine for the number of heparin units given by constant infusion during the past hour), and protamine should be given (2 mg/mL in saline) slowly—no more than 50 mg in 10 minutes—to avoid hypotension and anaphylactoid reactions.

WARFARIN

Warfarin (Coumadin) usually can be initiated on the first full hospital day. An initial dose of 5 or 10 mg is appropriate for most patients. Subsequent doses depend on the prothrombin time (PT) response. Because there is a delay between warfarin administration and its antithrombotic effect, a prolonged PT during the first 4 days of warfarin therapy does not always indicate that an antithrombotic effect was achieved. For this reason, heparin and warfarin are overlapped for approximately 4 days, and heparin is discontinued when the anticoagulant effect, as measured by the international normalized ratio (INR), is between 2.0 and 3.0 on 2 consecutive days. Warfarin should be continued for a minimum of 3 months for patients who have had a PE after major surgery or trauma and 6 months when there was no or minimal provocation. Longer courses of warfarin are warranted for patients with continuing risk factors, such as anticardiolipin antibodies. Indefinite treatment is appropriate for patients who have had more than one objectively documented venous thromboembolism. Recurrent thromboembolism is more likely when warfarin dosing is inadequate, and serious bleeding complications are more likely when the anticoagulant effect of warfarin is excessive. Therefore, weekly or biweekly measurements of PT are appropriate initially to guide dosage adjustment for most patients. Monthly measurements of PT are appropriate when the PT response to warfarin stabilizes. Excessively prolonged PT results can be treated with oral or subcutaneous vitamin K, fresh-frozen plasma, or prothrombin complex concentrate (Table 6).

Patients with active cancer are less likely to experience recurrent thromboembolism when LMWH is continued for 6 months or more rather than when they receive extended treatment with warfarin.

Pregnant patients or those who may become pregnant during anticoagulant therapy cannot receive warfarin because of the risk of teratogenicity. In this situation, heparin must be continued either as a constant infusion (UFH) or subcutaneously (UFH or LMWH). Severe osteopenia is a potential complication of prolonged (more than 4 months) heparin administration.

VENA CAVA FILTER

Vena cava filters offer a therapeutic alternative when anticoagulants are contraindicated or when anticoagulant therapy must be stopped. Newer vena cava filters often can be removed when anticoagulant therapy can be resumed. A vena cava filter also should be placed when massive PE requires surgical embolectomy, when objectively documented recurrent PE occurs in spite of adequate anticoagulant treatment, or in selected circumstances in which thromboembolism may prove fatal, such as extensive unattached large vein thrombi or smaller thrombi in patients who have had hemodynamically significant PE. Anticoagulant therapy should be resumed when possible after vena cava filter insertion to prevent further morbidity from deep vein thrombi in the legs.

MASSIVE PULMONARY EMBOLISM

Patients with massive PE—that is, PE that causes hypotension or cardiac arrest—are more likely to die from acute PE. For this reason, more aggressive management options must be considered. These options include insertion of a vena cava filter to prevent recurrence, administration of thrombolytic drugs to dissolve the thrombus more rapidly than endogenous fibrinolysis, use of catheters to fragment the thrombus, and embolectomy performed either with a catheter or surgically. The choice of intervention(s) depends on available resources and expertise. Furthermore, well-designed clinical trials have not been conducted to prove the efficacy of any of these methods, although the absence of such trials should not preclude judicious use of these therapies.

THROMBOLYSIS

Thrombolytic therapy accelerates the dissolution of clot when compared with heparin. Thus, thrombolysis may be lifesaving for those few patients with acute PE that

---

TABLE 6   Management of High International Normalized Ratio (INR)

INR	Clinical State	Action
<5.0	No bleeding	Hold warfarin or lower dose.
>5.0 and <9.0	No bleeding	Hold warfarin and give vitamin K1 (1–2 mg orally)
>9.0	No bleeding	Hold warfarin and give vitamin K1 (3–5 mg orally)
>10	Serious bleeding	Hold warfarin and give fresh-frozen plasma or prothrombin complex concentrate and vitamin K1, 10 mg by slow IV infusion.
>10	Life-threatening bleeding	Hold warfarin and give prothrombin complex concentrate supplemented by vitamin K1, 10 mg by slow IV infusion.

Abbreviations: INR = international normalized ratio. IV = intravenous.

produces hypotension, cardiac arrest, or profound arterial hypoxemia refractory to supplemental oxygen. Unlike other treatments for massive PE, thrombolysis can cause serious bleeding by dissolving hemostatic plugs. For this reason, absolute and relative contraindications to thrombolytic therapy must be considered before administering any thrombolytic drug (Table 7). If available, alternative treatment such as embolectomy or catheter fragmentation should be used when relative or absolute contraindications exist. If therapeutic alternatives are not available, thrombolysis may be given in the face of relative contraindications when survival is unlikely without such treatment, such as cardiac arrest or shock refractory to medical management.

A number of thrombolytic agents and dosing regimens are available (Table 8). The selection of the agent and dosing regimen must take into consideration drug availability and cost, as well as the benefits and risks. Shorter infusions of recombinant tissue-type plasminogen activator (rt-PA) (Activase) or urokinase (Abbokinase) are more rapidly efficacious than FDA-approved regimens for urokinase and streptokinase that are infused over 12 and 24 hours, respectively.

EMBOLECTOMY

Pulmonary embolectomy is appropriate for patients who have large, centrally located thromboembolisms accompanied by circulatory shock that is unresponsive to medical therapy. In my opinion, surgical embolectomy is also the treatment of choice for patients with intracardiac thrombi. Pulmonary embolectomy can be performed with a suction catheter or surgically with cardiopulmonary bypass. When selected patients undergo this procedure, approximately 80% survive to hospital discharge, and their long-term function is usually excellent. The prognosis is poorer for patients who suffer cardiopulmonary arrest, but reported survival of patients undergoing cardiopulmonary resuscitation makes emergency cardiopulmonary bypass and surgical embolectomy appropriate for some patients in this situation.

When surgical or catheter embolectomy is not available and thrombolysis is contraindicated, catheter fragmentation can be attempted. Standard cardiac catheters with

---

TABLE 7 Contraindications to Thrombolytic Therapy

Absolute
Active internal bleeding (gastrointestinal, genitourinary, central nervous system, etc.)

Relative
Major surgery, trauma, or internal bleeding within past 10 d
Cerebrovascular disease
Uncontrolled hypertension (systolic blood pressure >180 mm Hg and/or diastolic BP >110 mm Hg
Hemostatic defects (thrombocytopenia, renal failure, liver failure, anticoagulant therapy)
Pregnancy
Pericarditis
Diabetic hemorrhagic retinopathy
Advanced age (>75 y)

TABLE 8 Thrombolytic Therapy for Acute Pulmonary Embolism

Discontinue heparin*	
Streptokinase (Streptase)	250,000 U bolus 100,000 U/h infused for 24 h
Urokinase (Abbokinase)	4400 U/kg loading dose 4400 U/kg/h infused for 12 h or 3×10^6 U infused over 2 h
Tissue plasminogen Activator (Activase)	100 mg infused over 2 h or 0.6 mg/kg bolus infused over 2 min[†]

*Heparin should be reinstituted approximately 3–4 h after the thrombolytic infusion ends and when the thrombin time is < 2 × baseline.
[†]Heparin infusion can continue during bolus infusion of tissue plasminogen activator.

---

or without guidewires can be used to fragment large proximal PE.

REFERENCES

Ansel J, Hirsh J, Dalen J, et al: Managing oral anticoagulant therapy. Chest 2003;119:22S-38S.
Bates SM, Greer I, Hirsh J, Ginsberg JS: Use of antithrombotic agents during pregnancy. Chest 2004;126:627S-644S.
Buller HR, Agnelli G, Hull RD, et al: Antithrombotic therapy for venous thromboembolic disease. Chest 2004;126:401S-428S.
Fedullo PF, Tapson VF: The evaluation of suspected pulmonary embolism. N Engl J Med 2003;349:1247-1256.
Lee AYY, Levine MN, Baker RI, et al: Low-molecular-weight heparin versus a coumarin for the prevention of recurrent venous thromboembolism in patients with cancer. N Engl J Med 2003;349:146-153.
Perrier A, Roy PM, Sanchez O, et al: Multidetector-row computed tomography in suspected pulmonary embolism. N Engl J Med 2005;352:1760-1768.
Stein PD, Hull RD, Patel KC, et al: D-dimer for the exclusion of acute venous thrombosis and pulmonary embolism. Ann Intern Med 2004;140:589-602.
The Matisse Investigators: Subcutaneous fondaparinux versus intravenous unfractionated heparin in the initial treatment of pulmonary embolism. N Engl J Med 2003;349:1695-1702.
van Belle A, Buller HR, Huisman MV, et al: Effectiveness of managing suspected pulmonary embolism using an algorithm combining clinical probability, d-dimer testing, and computed tomography. JAMA 2006;295:172-179.

Sarcoidosis

Method of
Marc A. Judson, MD

Sarcoidosis is a multisystem, granulomatous disease of unknown cause. The lung is most commonly affected, but any organ may be involved. The clinical presentation of sarcoidosis is variable for two main reasons. First, the manifestations of pulmonary sarcoidosis are variable and may range from an asymptomatic state to significant pulmonary dysfunction. Second, extrapulmonary manifestations of sarcoidosis are common and may cause the prominent symptoms of the disease. This variability in disease presentation often makes the diagnosis of sarcoidosis problematic.

Epidemiology

Sarcoidosis occurs worldwide and affects all races and ages. Although the disease shows a predilection for the third decade of life, a smaller second peak in diagnosis occurs in people older than 50. There is a slightly higher disease rate in women. The highest prevalence of sarcoidosis is found in whites in Scandinavia and in persons of African descent in the United States. In the United States, the lifetime risk of sarcoidosis is 0.85% in whites and 2.4% in African Americans, with an age-adjusted incidence rate of 10.9 per 100,000 people for the white population and 35.5 per 100,000 people for African Americans. The relative risk for having sarcoidosis increases significantly if a family member has it as well. In the United States, nearly 20% of African Americans with sarcoidosis have an affected first-degree relative compared with 5% in whites.

The clinical presentation and severity of sarcoidosis varies among racial and ethnic groups. The disease tends to be more severe in African Americans, whereas whites are more likely to be asymptomatic at presentation. Extrathoracic manifestations are more common in certain populations, such as ocular and cardiac sarcoidosis in Japanese populations, chronic uveitis in African Americans, and erythema nodosum in Europeans. There is increasing evidence that genetic polymorphisms affect the risk and manifestations of the disease. This is consistent with the current theory that sarcoidosis does not have a single cause but is the result of an abnormal host (granulomatous) response to one of many potential antigens in a genetically susceptible individual.

Immunopathogenesis

The exact immunopathogenesis of sarcoidosis is unknown, but it is thought to be similar to other granulomatous diseases. That is, antigen-presenting cells (APCs), usually either macrophages or dendritic cells, process and present an antigen via a human leukocyte antibody (HLA) class II molecule to T lymphocytes and their receptors. These T lymphocytes are usually of the CD4 T-helper 1 (Th1) class. The antigen involved in this reaction is unknown; and as previously mentioned, there may be many putative antigens that are each associated with a specific HLA class II molecule and T cell receptor. This may explain the inability to determine one specific cause of sarcoidosis and the varied phenotypic expression of the disease. The interaction of APCs and T lymphocytes activates the APCs to produce tumor necrosis factor-α (TNF-α), and other cytokines. A proliferation of CD4 Th1 lymphocytes also ensues that results in the secretion of interferon gamma (INF-γ), interleukin (IL)-2, IL-12, and other cytokines. These cytokines activate and recruit monocytes and macrophages and transform them into giant cells, which are important building blocks of the granuloma.

The typical sarcoidosis lesion is a noncaseating (nonnecrotic) granuloma. The sarcoid granuloma consists of a compact core of macrophage-derived epithelioid and multinucleated giant cells surrounded by a perimeter of monocytes, lymphocytes, and fibroblasts. Granulomas may resolve spontaneously or with therapy; however, they may also persist and lead to peripheral hyalinization and fibrosis. The development of such fibrosis may cause permanent organ damage and in large part determines the prognosis.

Clinical Features/Clinical Course

PULMONARY SARCOIDOSIS

Between 30% and 60% of patients with pulmonary sarcoidosis are asymptomatic, such that sarcoidosis is detected as an incidental chest radiographic finding. Patients may also present with nonspecific pulmonary symptoms, such as dyspnea, cough, wheezing, and chest pain. Respiratory failure from sarcoidosis is extremely rare at presentation. Unlike many other interstitial lung diseases, crackles are rarely heard on chest auscultation.

Abnormalities on the chest radiograph occur in more than 90% of patients with pulmonary sarcoidosis. Bilateral hilar adenopathy occurs in 50% to 85% at disease presentation, and 25% to 50% have parenchymal infiltrates. Sarcoid granulomas have a predilection for the bronchovascular bundles, subpleural locations, intralobular septa, and the airways. A radiographic staging system was developed several decades ago (Table 1). Groups of patients with higher radiographic stages have more severe pulmonary dysfunction, lower remission rates, and greater mortality. However, there is significant overlap between these groups such that predictions concerning individual patients based on stage are highly inaccurate.

Advanced pulmonary stage IV sarcoidosis displays destruction of the lung architecture with upward traction of the hila, lung distortion, upper lobe volume loss, fibrocystic disease, honeycombed cysts, and decreased lung volumes. Aspergillomas may develop in these large cystic lesions and may be associated with life-threatening hemoptysis. Bronchiectasis from airway distortion also may occur and is an additional potential cause of hemoptysis.

The majority of patients with pulmonary sarcoidosis have a vital capacity of greater than 70% of predicted at diagnosis. There is frequently discordance between pulmonary function and the chest radiographic findings. In pulmonary sarcoidosis patients with a normal lung parenchyma (stage 1), the vital capacity, diffusing capacity, partial pressure of oxygen, arterial (PaO_2) at rest, PaO_2 with exercise, and lung compliance are abnormal in 20% to 40% of cases. Patients with abnormal lung parenchyma have abnormal pulmonary function tests 50% to 70% of

TABLE 1 Chest Radiograph Stages of Sarcoidosis

Stage	Lymph node Enlargement	Parenchymal Disease
0	No	No
1	Yes	No
2	Yes	Nonfibrotic
3	No	Nonfibrotic
4	No or yes	Fibrotic

Adapted from Judson MA, Baughman RP: Sarcoidosis. In Diffuse Lung Disease: A Practical Approach. London: Arnold, 2004, pp 109-129.

the time. Patients with stage IV fibrocystic sarcoidosis tend to have the most severe pulmonary dysfunction.

Sarcoidosis is an interstitial lung disease with a restrictive ventilatory defect often found on spirometry. It is underappreciated, however, that endobronchial involvement is common in sarcoidosis; and therefore airflow obstruction may be the major abnormality found on pulmonary function testing. Wheezing may be the prominent presenting symptom of sarcoidosis, and many sarcoidosis patients are misdiagnosed as having asthma. Airflow obstruction is also common in chronic pulmonary sarcoidosis, where it is caused by airway distortion from fibrosis.

The cause of dyspnea in pulmonary sarcoidosis is multifactorial. It may be the result of abnormalities of gas exchange or lung mechanics, weakness of the respiratory muscles, obesity from corticosteroid therapy, pulmonary hypertension or sarcoidosis involvement of the heart.

Only 3% to 5% of patients die of sarcoidosis. In the United States, 75% of these deaths are the result of pulmonary involvement. Death from pulmonary involvement is rarely acute but an insidious process that develops over 5 to 25 years with the development of progressive pulmonary fibrosis. Several studies have suggested that pulmonary hypertension is a major risk factor for death from pulmonary sarcoidosis. Patients with aspergillomas and stage IV fibrocystic sarcoidosis are also at risk of death from episodes of life-threatening hemoptysis. Other organs that result in fatalities from sarcoidosis include the heart and the central nervous system (CNS). In Japan death from sarcoidosis is more commonly caused by cardiac rather than pulmonary involvement.

EXTRAPULMONARY SARCOIDOSIS

Sarcoidosis is a multisystem disease that may affect any organ in the body. The extrapulmonary manifestations of sarcoidosis may predominate in many patients. The presence of extrapulmonary disease may affect the prognosis and treatment options for sarcoidosis. The eye and skin are the most common extrapulmonary organs involved with sarcoidosis. Ocular manifestations occur in 25% to 50% of patients; anterior uveitis is the most common manifestation. Symptoms of anterior uveitis include red eyes, painful eyes, and photophobia. However, in one-third of patients with anterior uveitis from sarcoidosis, the eye is *quiet,* and without symptoms. In addition, an intermediate or posterior uveitis may cause vision problems or be asymptomatic. For this reason, all patients diagnosed with sarcoidosis should undergo an eye examination by an ophthalmologist. Other ocular manifestations of sarcoidosis include conjunctivitis, keratoconjunctivitis sicca (dry eyes), scleritis, and optic neuritis.

Skin lesions in sarcoidosis can be classified into two categories: specific lesions that demonstrate noncaseating granulomas on biopsy and nonspecific lesions that do not. The specific skin lesions are often papular and have a predilection for areas of previous scars and tattoos. Lupus pernio is a type of specific skin lesion causing disfiguring lesions on the face, often with erythema and significant induration. These lesions have a predilection for the nose, cheeks, medial and lateral sides of the eyes, and lateral sides of the mouth. Lupus pernio lesions are relatively recalcitrant to therapy and often respond only partially to corticosteroids. The most common nonspecific skin lesion is erythema nodosum that is often seen with an acute sarcoidosis presentation of fever, arthritis (especially in the ankles), pulmonary symptoms, and bilateral hilar adenopathy on chest radiograph. This syndrome is known as *Löfgren's syndrome* and tends to have a good long-term prognosis.

Cardiac and neurologic sarcoidosis can be life-threatening and is therefore important to recognize. Cardiac involvement is detected clinically in 5% of sarcoidosis patients premortem but in 25% at autopsy. Cardiac sarcoidosis may cause left ventricular dysfunction and cardiac arrhythmias possibly resulting in sudden death. All patients with sarcoidosis are recommended to have a 12-lead electrocardiogram; and if this test is abnormal it should prompt further evaluation. The diagnosis of cardiac sarcoidosis is problematic because the disease is patchy and diagnosed less than 25% of the time by endomyocardial biopsy because of sampling error. Often the diagnosis is made noninvasively, if a typical clinical presentation is coupled with detection of abnormalities on echocardiography, gallium scanning, thallium scanning, or cardiac magnetic resonance imaging (MRI), or positron emission tomography (PET) scanning.

Clinically apparent neurosarcoidosis occurs in less than 10% of sarcoidosis patients. Palsy of the seventh cranial nerve is the most common manifestation of neurosarcoidosis, and it often predates the diagnosis of the disease. Sarcoidosis can affect any part of the peripheral nervous system (PNS) and CNS and may cause a cranial nerve palsy, mononeuropathy or polyneuropathy, aseptic meningitis, seizures, mass lesions in the brain and spinal cord, and encephalopathy.

Sarcoidosis causes clinically apparent peripheral lymphadenopathy in more than 10% of patients. Splenic involvement may be present in up to 50% of patients, but it is usually asymptomatic and rarely causes hypersplenism. Bone involvement is occasional, usually presenting as small cysts or cortical defects found in the small bones of the hands and feet. An acute sarcoid arthritis often is present at disease onset and has a good prognosis. This is commonly found in the ankles of patients who present with Löfgren's syndrome. Chronic sarcoid arthritis is rare. It is usually a nondestructive arthropathy of the shoulders, wrists, knees, ankles, and small joints of the hands and feet. Sarcoidosis of the sinuses is underappreciated. It may occur in the nasopharynx, hypopharynx, larynx, or any of the sinuses and is known as *sarcoidosis of the upper respiratory tract* (SURT). SURT is often relatively recalcitrant to therapy. Histologic evidence of hepatic sarcoidosis is present in 50% to 80% of sarcoidosis patients, although most are asymptomatic and have normal liver function blood tests. Hepatomegaly, abdominal pain, and pruritus are the most common symptoms associated with hepatic sarcoidosis but are present only in 15% to 25% of patients with hepatic involvement. Elevation of the serum alkaline phosphatase is the most common liver function test abnormality. Hypercalcemia or hypercalciuria leading to nephrolithiasis and renal dysfunction may occur with sarcoidosis. These phenomena are the result of the enzyme, 1-α hydroxylase in activated macrophages that convert 25-hydroxyvitamin D to 1,25-dihydroxyvitamin D, the active form of the vitamin. This results in increased gut absorption and increased renal

African American race
Extrathoracic disease
Stage II-III versus stage I CXR
Age older than 40
Splenic involvement
Lupus pernio
Disease duration >2 years
FVC <1.5 L
Stage IV CXR/aspergilloma

Abbreviations: CXR = chest radiograph; FVC = forced vital capacity.
From Judson MA, Baughman RP: Sarcoidosis. *In* Diffuse Lung Disease: A Practical Approach. London: Arnold, 2004, pp 109-129. (Used with permission.)

excretion of calcium that can cause nephrolithiasis. Sarcoidosis rarely involves the thyroid, renal parenchyma, and GI tract.

Constitutional symptoms such as fever, night sweats, weight loss, malaise, and fatigue may occur at presentation. These symptoms occasionally are associated with hepatic sarcoid involvement but together may be a sign of the systemic nature of the disease, presumably from cytokine release, rather than specific organ involvement.

Patients who present with Löfgren's syndrome or with asymptomatic bilateral hilar adenopathy on chest radiograph have a good prognosis. African Americans tend to have a worse prognosis than whites with lower forced vital capacity and more new organ involvement within 2 years of diagnosis. Box 1 lists risk factors associated with a poor prognosis.

Diagnosis/Initial Workup

The diagnosis of sarcoidosis requires a compatible clinical picture, histologic demonstration of noncaseating granulomas, and exclusion of other diseases capable of producing a similar histologic and clinical picture. Mycobacterial and fungal diseases always must be considered as alternative diagnoses. Therefore, stains and cultures of tissue specimens for mycobacteria and fungi always should be obtained when the diagnosis of sarcoidosis is considered.

Because sarcoidosis is a diagnosis of exclusion (granulomatous inflammation of unknown cause), bear a healthy degree of skepticism in the diagnosis and follow the patient closely for additional clues supporting an alternate diagnosis. Sarcoidosis is a systemic disease, so the signs or symptoms of extrathoracic disease such as uveitis, skin lesions, or an elevated serum alkaline phosphatase should be sought. The diagnosis in a patient with granulomas on lung biopsy who has interstitial infiltrates without adenopathy on radiographic studies is suspect. In this situation, granulomatous infections and bioaerosol exposure causing hypersensitivity pneumonitis should be strongly considered.

Because of the varied clinical presentation of sarcoidosis, there is no single diagnostic algorithm. It is prudent to select a biopsy site associated with less morbidity, such as the skin if a lesion is present. Transbronchial lung biopsy has a diagnostic yield of 40% to more than 90% in pulmonary sarcoidosis. It is recommended that at least four lung biopsy specimens be collected to maximize the diagnostic yield. Endobronchial biopsy has 40% to 60% sensitivity and adds to the yield of transbronchial biopsy. Bronchoalveolar lavage (BAL) with examination of lymphocyte populations has been used in the evaluation of possible pulmonary sarcoidosis. In sarcoidosis, there is an increased number of BAL lymphocytes, and these are predominantly CD4 positive. It has been proposed that an increase in BAL lymphocytes and a BAL CD4/CD8 ratio of greater than 3.5 make the diagnosis of sarcoidosis highly likely. Although serum angiotensin-converting enzyme (SACE) often is elevated in active sarcoidosis, the specificity and sensitivity of this test is inadequate for it to be used diagnostically. SACE may be used as supportive evidence for the diagnosis, and it also may be used in some instances to follow disease activity. Gallium-67 (67Ga) scanning is cumbersome because it takes several days to complete and is infrequently used as a diagnostic test. However, bilateral hilar uptake and right paratracheal uptake (lambda sign) coupled with lacrimal and parotid uptake (panda sign) with 67Ga strongly suggest a diagnosis of sarcoidosis.

Ideally, the diagnosis of sarcoidosis requires demonstration of noncaseating granulomas in at least one organ. However, certain clinical presentations are so specific for the diagnosis of sarcoidosis that the diagnosis may be accepted without tissue biopsy. Extreme caution must be taken in these situations to ensure that there is no clinical information that would suggest an alternative diagnosis that should prompt a tissue biopsy. Clinical or laboratory findings that would strongly support the diagnosis of sarcoidosis without a tissue biopsy are listed in Box 2.

Treatment

Therapy is not mandated for sarcoidosis because the disease may remit spontaneously. Therapy is indicated for potentially dangerous disease that includes neurosarcoidosis, cardiac sarcoidosis, hypercalcemia that does not respond

CURRENT DIAGNOSIS

- The diagnosis of sarcoidosis is one of exclusion.
- Tissue biopsy, confirming noncaseating granulomatous inflammation, is required in most cases.
- Efforts should be made to search for the least invasive biopsy site.

Löfgren's syndrome
Heerfordt's syndrome (uveoparotid fever)
Asymptomatic bilateral hilar adenopathy on chest radiograph
67Ga scan showing a lambda sign and panda sign

Abbreviation: 67Ga = Gallium-67.

CURRENT THERAPY

- Many cases of sarcoidosis do not require treatment.
- All patients should be evaluated for possible pulmonary, eye, and cardiac disease.
- When therapy is indicated, corticosteroids are most commonly used.
- Topical corticosteroids should be given whenever possible.

to dietary measures, ocular sarcoidosis that does not respond to topical (eyedrop) therapy, and other life- or organ-threatening disease. Therapy also should be considered when the disease is progressive. Relative indications for therapy include arthritis that fails to respond to nonsteroidal, anti-inflammatory agents; a systemic inflammatory response syndrome of fever, night sweats, fatigue, and arthralgias; and symptomatic hepatic disease.

In general, treatment is discouraged for asymptomatic elevations of serum liver function tests, specific levels of angiotensin converting enzyme, or asymptomatic uptake on 67Ga scan (except if found in the heart or brain).

The decision to treat sarcoidosis can be problematic, because the disease has a variable prognosis that must be weighed against the potential side effects of therapy. It is often most prudent to monitor patients without therapy if they are asymptomatic or have only mild organ dysfunction.

For pulmonary sarcoidosis, asymptomatic patients and those with mild disease that may spontaneously remit usually are not treated. For patients with clinical findings that predict spontaneous remission (e.g. erythema nodosum), the benefits of treatment often are exceeded by the toxicity of therapy. Often these patients can be managed with palliative therapy such as nonsteroidal anti-inflammatory agents for arthralgias and fever, and bronchodilators and inhaled corticosteroids for wheezing and cough. It is recommended that patients with mild to moderate pulmonary sarcoidosis be observed for 2 to 6 months, if possible. Patients who improve will have avoided the toxicity of corticosteroids, whereas patients who deteriorate over this period should be considered for treatment. Patients with pulmonary dysfunction who neither improve nor deteriorate during the observation period often are given a corticosteroid trial, or they may be observed further. Patients with severe pulmonary dysfunction or pulmonary symptoms causing significant impairment should be treated.

Corticosteroids often are used to treat sarcoidosis, but the dose, duration of therapy, and method by which one can assess effectiveness have not been standardized. Topical corticosteroid therapy should be used whenever possible in an attempt to minimize systemic complications. This would include corticosteroid eyedrops for anterior sarcoid uveitis and corticosteroid creams and injections for localized skin lesions.

Pulmonary sarcoidosis usually is treated initially with 20 to 40 mg per day of prednisone or its equivalent. Higher doses may be required for neurosarcoidosis and cardiac sarcoidosis. The patient usually is evaluated within 2 to 12 weeks for a response. Patients failing to respond to therapy within 3 months are unlikely to respond to a more protracted course of therapy or a higher dose. Among the responders, the corticosteroid dose is tapered to 5 to 10 mg/day of prednisone equivalent or an every-other-day regimen. Treatment is usually continued for 12 months. The relapse rate after corticosteroid therapy is withdrawn may be as high as 70%, and therefore patients need to be followed closely as the corticosteroid dose is tapered and discontinued. In some patients, there may be recurrent relapses requiring long-term, low-dose therapy. On occasion the chronic prednisone dose needed to prevent relapse may be less than 5 mg per day.

Patients who relapse after corticosteroids have been withdrawn should be retreated with corticosteroids. In addition, alternative agents should be considered *corticosteroid-sparing agents* to control the patient on a chronic low dose of prednisone. On occasion, alternative agents may completely replace corticosteroid therapy. In general, corticosteroid-sparing agents should not be considered unless the patient requires more than 7.5 mg per day of daily prednisone to control the disease.

Methotrexate (Rheumatrex)[1] and hydroxychloroquine (Plaquenil)[1] are the most studied alternative sarcoidosis medications. They are usually used as corticosteroid-sparing agents but at times can be used as replacement therapy. Methotrexate is most useful for pulmonary, skin, joint, and eye sarcoidosis. Hydroxychloroquine is used often for skin, joint, neurosarcoidosis, and hypercalcemia from sarcoidosis. Azathioprine (Imuran)[1] may be useful for sarcoid uveitis, but usually it is added to corticosteroid plus methotrexate in this instance. Monocycline (Minocin)[1] and doxycycline (Vibramycin)[1] may be useful for skin sarcoidosis. Cyclophosphamide (Cytoxan)[1] is used occasionally and seems to have a potential role for neurosarcoidosis. Recently anti–TNF-α therapies have shown promise in the treatment of sarcoidosis. Such agents include pentoxifylline (Trental),[1] thalidomide (Thalomid),[1] and monoclonal antibodies against TNF-α, such as infliximab (Remicade).[1]

REFERENCES

Baughman RP, Teirstein AS, Judson MA, et al: Clinical characteristics of patients in a case control study of sarcoidosis. Am J Respir Crit Care Med 2001;164:1885-1889.

Gibson GJ, Prescott RJ, Muers MF, et al: British Thoracic Society Sarcoidosis study: Effects of long term corticosteroid treatment. Thorax 1996;51:238-247.

Hunninghake GW, Costabel U, Ando M, et al: ATS/ERS/WASOG statement on sarcoidosis. Am J Respir Crit Care Med 1999;160:736-755.

Hunninghake GW, Gilbert S, Pueringer R, et al: Outcome of treatment for sarcoidosis. Am J Respir Crit Care Med 1994;149:893-898.

Judson MA: An approach to the treatment of pulmonary sarcoidosis with corticosteroids. Chest 1999;111:623-631.

Judson MA, Baughman RP: Sarcoidosis. In Diffuse Lung Disease: A Practical Approach. London: Arnold, 2004, pp 109-129.

Judson MA, Baughman RP, Teirstein AS, et al: Defining organ involvement in sarcoidosis: The ACCESS proposed instrument. Sarcoidosis Vasc Diffuse Lung Dis 1999;16:75-86.

Lower EE, Baughman RP: Prolonged use of methotrexate in refractory sarcoidosis. Arch Intern Med 1995;155:846-851.

Lynch JP, Kazerooni EA, Gay SE: Pulmonary sarcoidosis. Clin Chest Med 1997;755-785.

Newman LS, Rose CS, Maier LA: Sarcoidosis. N Engl J Med 1997;1224-1234.

Sharma OP: Pulmonary sarcoidosis and corticosteroids. Am Rev Respir Dis 1993;147:1598-1600.

---

[1]Not FDA approved for this indication.

Silicosis and Asbestosis

Method of

Akshay Sood, MD, MPH, and
William S. Beckett, MD, MPH

Silicosis

Silicosis, an interstitial fibrotic lung disease caused by inhaled silica dust, is one of the most common occupational lung diseases worldwide. Silica (silicon dioxide, quartz), the main compound in sand, is present in most rocks and encountered in mining and construction and as a raw material in many manufacturing processes.

Inhalation of silica dust in a form that is crystalline (as opposed to amorphic, such as common glass) and not bound to other minerals (free silica as opposed to silicates such as asbestos or kaolin) causes silicosis and its associated diseases and complications. Silica dust is nonirritating to breathe, and most individuals are entirely asymptomatic during heavy clinically significant exposure. Still, it may cause disabling or fatal lung disease, with onset occurring within a few months to more than a decade after exposure.

All forms of silicosis are associated with increased risk for pulmonary tuberculosis (TB). At the time of diagnosis, if the patient is not a known positive tuberculin reactor, a purified protein derivative (PPD) skin test should be performed. If the PPD skin test has an area of induration greater than 9 mm in diameter and the patient has no findings of active TB, then treatment of latent infection (also known as prophylaxis) should be offered irrespective of status with regard to bacille Calmette-Guérin (BCG) and regardless of patient age. Treatment is with isoniazid (Nydrazid), 300 mg tablets, one tablet daily for 1 year.

Patients with silicosis should also receive an annual influenza immunization (0.5 mL intramuscular) and pneumococcal immunization (Pneumovax) (0.5 mL intramuscular) every 6 years.[3]

Whenever a diagnosis of silicosis is made, the patient, employer, and local health department should be notified in writing because of its occupational nature and the potential for prevention of disease in others. Case reporting of silicosis to the local or state health department is required by law in 23 states. If an ongoing hazard is suspected, with the patient's permission, the regional office of the Occupational Safety and Health Administration (OSHA) should be notified to perform testing for dangerously high air levels of silica. OSHA can be found under the Department of Labor in the federal government pages of the telephone directory, and state offices are listed on the OSHA Web site, www.OSHA.gov.

BRONCHITIS

The earliest manifestation of high inspired concentrations of silica dust may be acute or chronic bronchitis (without interstitial lung disease) from large airway inflammation. The resulting daily cough with expectoration of mucus can

CURRENT DIAGNOSIS

- Silicosis is usually an interstitial nodular lung disease with biapical nodules in the setting of a significant occupational exposure history to rock or mineral dust.
- Asbestosis can usually be diagnosed by the presence of very slowly progressive interstitial changes appearing at first at both lung bases, often with the presence of pleural plaques, in the context of heavy occupational asbestos exposure 10 or more years preceding diagnosis. The predominant pattern is restriction with decreased diffusing capacity.

be treated with removal of the offending dust inhalation and inhaled ipratropium bromide[1] (Atrovent), 18 µg per puff by metered-dose inhaler, two puffs four times a day, or tiotropium[1] (Spiriva HandiHaler), 18 µg per puff, one puff daily. If this is ineffective, an inhaled corticosteroid such as beclomethasone[1] (QVAR), 40 µg per puff, two puffs four times a day, may be tried.

NODULAR SILICOSIS

Nodular or "simple" silicosis consists of multiple discrete small nodules seen on chest radiograph. The nodules are seen more frequently at the lung apices. When this diagnosis is made, attention must first be turned to preventing further exposure to silica (if exposure is ongoing) because disease may progress with further exposure. Progression may also occur even after exposure ceases. Therapy consists of treatment of associated respiratory symptoms and prevention or treatment of associated TB.

No specific treatment to reverse or slow the progression of silicosis has been found, although rapid advances in understanding the pathophysiology of pulmonary fibrosis mean that specific treatment may become available. In its milder forms, nodular silicosis may be asymptomatic. If dyspnea on exertion or at rest is present, pulmonary function testing may show whether a potentially treatable obstructive abnormality is present. If chronic airflow obstruction is present, a therapeutic trial of bronchodilator medication, as would be used in smoking-related chronic obstructive pulmonary disease (COPD), may be made. Inhaled β-agonists for occasional symptoms and oral theophylline,[1] 300 mg extended-release preparation (Slo-bid) every 12 hours or the long-acting inhaled β-agonist salmeterol (Serevent Diskus), 50 µg per puff, 1 puff every 12 hours, may be tried. If the patient has no symptomatic or significant improvement in lung function after a 2-week trial, these medications should be discontinued.

In the case of advanced disease, evaluation is needed to determine whether continuous low-flow oxygen (1 to 2 L per minute by nasal or trans-tracheal cannula) is needed to prevent the complications of pulmonary hypertension. Supplemental oxygen is indicated when pulmonary hypertension is present or when oxygen saturation is below approximately 85%. Oxygen should be given continuously if pulmonary hypertension or oxygen desaturation at rest

---

[3]Exceeds dosage recommended by the manufacturer.

[1]Not FDA approved for this indication.

is present, or it should be given during exercise or sleep if desaturation only occurs with those activities. Supplemental diuretics may also be needed to manage dependent edema associated with right heart failure.

ACUTE AND ACCELERATED SILICOSIS

Heavier exposure to silica dust or exposure to the more biologically active forms of silica (tridymite and cristobalite) may be associated with more severe rapidly progressing interstitial disease. Recommended therapy is the same as for nodular silicosis. Whole lung lavage under anesthesia through a divided endotracheal tube is now an investigational treatment. Patients with acute and accelerated silicosis are at highest risk for developing concurrent pulmonary or extrapulmonary infection with *Mycobacterium tuberculosis* or with nontuberculous mycobacteria (see silicotuberculosis). Patients likely to progress to respiratory failure should be referred early to a lung transplantation center; lung transplantation is effective in prolonging life in silicosis.

SILICOPROTEINOSIS (PULMONARY ALVEOLAR PROTEINOSIS)

Silicosis in individuals with heavy silica dust exposure may be complicated when type II alveolar cells produce a thick, tenacious liquid that fills the alveoli and prevents gas exchange. This life-threatening form of silicosis is difficult to distinguish from idiopathic alveolar proteinosis but is associated with very heavy dust exposures. Removal of the liquid by whole lung lavage can be an effective treatment. In some cases, this therapy has to be repeated after some years to remove reaccumulated material. Referral of patients to a center with previous experience in this technique is advisable.

SILICOTIC LYMPH NODE DISEASE

Inhalation of silica dust may cause enlargement of mediastinal, other pulmonary lymph nodes, or lymph nodes distant from lung (e.g., nodes of the celiac axis or porta hepatis). Invasive procedures should be avoided because biopsy or removal does not benefit the patient unless relieving symptomatic obstruction of a vital structure such as the trachea.

SILICOTUBERCULOSIS

Silicotuberculosis is pulmonary or extrapulmonary infection caused by *Mycobacterium tuberculosis* or nontuberculous mycobacteria (e.g., *Mycobacterium kansasii* and *Mycobacterium intracellulare*) in a patient with silicosis. In any patient with silicosis and a positive tuberculin test, it is important to make sure the patient does not have active TB before giving isoniazid prophylaxis alone. Management of TB in patients with silicosis is the same as for other patients with TB (see article on tuberculosis). When cultures of nontuberculous mycobacteria are consistently grown from sputum, treatment needs to be modified according to the organism and its sensitivities.

BRONCHOGENIC CARCINOMA

Patients with pulmonary silicosis are at increased risk for developing bronchogenic carcinoma. Because a new bronchogenic carcinoma may appear identical on the chest

CURRENT THERAPY

- Because of the higher risk of reactivation of tuberculosis (TB) in silicosis, purified protein derivative (PPD) skin testing should be done in all patients with silicosis, and treatment for latent TB should be given if the skin test is positive.
- Oxygen is used to prevent cor pulmonale in those with advanced asbestosis and arterial desaturation. No medication has yet been found that affects the progression of asbestosis.

radiograph to a silicotic nodule or to a conglomerate mass of complicated silicosis, an increased index of suspicion is needed to detect a malignancy. Treatment of bronchogenic carcinoma in patients with silicosis is the same as for other patients with bronchogenic carcinoma.

Asbestos-Related Diseases

Asbestos is a general term for hydrated magnesium silicate minerals that tend to separate into fibers. Asbestos fibers have great tensile strength, heat resistance, and acid resistance. Asbestos fibers are classified as serpentine (chrysotile) and amphiboles (of which there are five types: crocidolite, amosite, anthophyllite, actinolite, and tremolite). All forms of asbestos fibers are associated with a spectrum of diseases (Table 1).

ASBESTOS EXPOSURE

Asbestos use is now severely restricted or banned in many Western countries. In the developing world where the use of asbestos continues and may even be increasing, workers and their families continue to be exposed. Table 2 outlines the selected occupational and environmental sources of asbestos exposure in the United States. When taking a detailed asbestos exposure history, it is essential to emphasize exposures that occurred 10 years and more before symptom presentation. Prolonged exposure (more than 10 to 20 years) is more important to the individual's history, yet short, intense exposure ranging from several months to

TABLE 1 Nonmalignant and Malignant Asbestos-Related Diseases

Nonmalignant Lung Diseases
Parenchymal diseases
- Asbestosis

Airway diseases
- Chronic airflow obstruction

Pleural diseases
- Circumscribed pleural thickening (parietal pleural plaques)
- Diffuse pleural thickening
- Benign pleural effusion
- Rounded atelectasis

Malignant Lung Diseases
- Bronchogenic carcinoma
- Diffuse malignant mesothelioma

TABLE 2   Selected Occupational and Environmental Exposures to Asbestos

Extraction and Transportation of Asbestos	Mining, Milling, Packing and Handling
Manufacture and end use of products made from asbestos	Friction products (brake linings) Textiles (fireproof clothing and gas masks) Asbestos cement products (water pipes, tiles) Heating trades (boilermakers, heating mechanics, furnace builders) Construction trades (electricians, plumbers, carpenters, roofers) Railroads and shipyards Glass factories Pipe fitting
Contemporary occupational exposures to asbestos	Workers in building and equipment maintenance, in asbestos-abatement activities
Environmental exposures to asbestos	Tailings of asbestos mines Prolonged exposure in buildings with exposed sources of asbestos contamination (undisturbed and nonfriable asbestos insulation in buildings not a hazard) Passive exposure occurring in families of workers carrying home asbestos on their clothing

1 year may also be sufficient when diagnosing asbestos-related diseases.

ASBESTOSIS

Asbestosis is the interstitial pneumonitis and fibrosis caused by inhalation of asbestos fibers. The latency period is often 2 decades from the start of exposure. Asbestosis is more prevalent and more advanced in cigarette smokers, presumably because of reduced clearance of asbestos fibers from the lung. Asbestosis is usually associated with dyspnea, bibasilar rales, and restrictive changes in pulmonary function. It is associated with bilateral small, primarily irregular parenchymal opacities in the lower lobes on chest radiograph. A profusion of irregular opacities at the level of 1/0 under the *International Classification of Radiographs of Pneumoconiosis* (ILO classification) is used as the boundary between normal and abnormal in the evaluation of the film. When the abnormalities are indeterminate, high-resolution computed tomography (CT) scanning is often useful.

Asbestosis may remain static or progress; regression is rare. Asbestosis may resemble idiopathic pulmonary fibrosis on presentation but is much less rapid in its progression. The presence of pleural plaques on imaging and asbestos bodies (asbestos fibers that were coated with an iron-rich proteinaceous concretion) in tissue sections may be useful to differentiate asbestosis from other forms of interstitial fibrosis.

CIRCUMSCRIBED PLEURAL THICKENING (PLAQUES)

Pleural plaques are the most common manifestation of the effect of asbestos. They are usually seen after 20 years following first exposure. Smoking plays no role in the prevalence of pleural plaques. They are usually bilateral, but not symmetric, lesions of the parietal pleura. Characteristically, they are found following the ribs on the lower posterior thoracic wall and over the central tendons of the diaphragm. Plaques generally spare the costophrenic angles and apices. Differentiation of subpleural

fat from pleural plaques may sometimes be difficult but is readily made by CT scan.

Slow progression of plaques is typical. The presence of plaques is associated with a greater risk of mesothelioma and lung cancer related to greater asbestos exposure or retained body burden, not malignant degeneration. Plaques are also indicators of increased risk for the future development of asbestosis. Plaques result in a small reduction in lung function, averaging approximately 5% of forced vital capacity (FVC), even when asbestosis is absent on the radiograph.

DIFFUSE PLEURAL THICKENING

Diffuse pleural thickening affects the visceral pleural surface and may be extensive. Those with diffuse pleural thickening may have a significantly greater decrement in FVC (by a factor of two or more) than those with circumscribed pleural thickening; this is primarily a result of adhesions of the parietal with the visceral pleura. Ventilatory failure leading to carbon dioxide (CO_2) retention, cor pulmonale, and death is described in some patients. Decortication may be beneficial. The major differential diagnostic consideration with diffuse pleural thickening is mesothelioma, which is rapidly progressive and more likely to be symptomatic at the time of detection.

BENIGN PLEURAL EFFUSION

Asbestos may cause an acute pleural exudative effusion that is often hemorrhagic with variable numbers of erythrocytes, neutrophils, lymphocytes, and often eosinophils. It may occur early (within 10 years, unlike other asbestos-related diseases) or late after the onset of asbestos exposure. Although it is usually asymptomatic, it may occasionally be exuberant with fever and severe pleuritic pain. The effusion may persist for months. The diagnosis is made by exclusion of other causes of acute pleuritis, mesothelioma, and pleural extension of a pulmonary malignancy.

ROUNDED ATELECTASIS

Rounded atelectasis is usually an incidental radiographic finding of a pleural-based lung mass and may be mistaken for a tumor. The lesion is thought to develop when thickened visceral pleura folds into collapsed intervening lung parenchyma. The classic comet sign is pathognomonic and often more readily seen on a CT scan than on plain films. Signs that indicate rounded atelectasis include a band connecting the mass to an area of thickened pleura and a slower evolution than that of a lung cancer.

CHRONIC AIRWAY OBSTRUCTION

Asbestos-related chronic airway obstruction may result in reduction in expiratory flow rates. Changes of chronic inflammation, fibrosis, and smooth muscle hyperplasia in the walls of small airways form the anatomic basis of this airflow limitation. Effects on airflow begin before the development of asbestosis. In general, the magnitude of the asbestos effect on airway function is relatively small.

LUNG CANCER

All forms of asbestos have equal carcinogenic potency with a three- to fourfold increase in risk for lung cancer after heavy and prolonged occupational exposure. The peak incidence of lung cancer occurs 30 to 35 years after the initial exposure to asbestos. Asbestos exposure favors an upper lobe location of tumor and does not influence the histology of lung cancer. The clinical presentation and management of asbestos-related lung cancer is not distinct from lung cancer from other causes.

Whether asbestos acts directly as a carcinogen or through indirect mechanisms such as causing chronic inflammation remains uncertain. It seems likely that asbestosis is an indicator of higher exposure and contributes additional risk to lung cancer beyond that conferred by asbestos exposure alone. The presence of pleural plaques is similarly associated with a greater risk for lung cancer, likely because of greater exposure or retained body burden of asbestos. Although both asbestos and cigarette smoking are independent causes of lung cancer, they act synergistically in combination. This may result from the enhanced retention of asbestos fibers by cigarette smokers. Homozygous deletion of the glutathione S-transferase M1 (GSTM1) gene, or an N-acetyltransferase 2 (NAT2) slow acetylator genotype, may confer an additional risk of lung cancer among persons exposed to asbestos. Periodic health surveillance for lung cancer is not currently recommended in asbestos-exposed individuals.

DIFFUSE MALIGNANT MESOTHELIOMA

Diffuse malignant mesothelioma is also caused by asbestos, but the risk is not affected by smoking. Crocidolite appears to be more potent than other asbestos varieties in its capacity to induce mesothelioma. The mean latency period is typically longer than 30 years. Some research suggests that asbestos and simian virus SV-40 can function as cocarcinogens. Mesothelioma has a molecular pathology characterized by the loss of tumor suppressor genes. Familial clustering is also described with an autosomal dominant pattern of inheritance with incomplete penetration.

Mesothelioma is usually diagnosed in those 50 to 70 years of age with a strong predominance in men. Patients typically present with breathlessness and chest pain with bloody pleural effusions that are usually unilateral. Cytologic diagnosis from pleural fluid may be helpful, although histologic assessment of samples obtained by CT-guided or thoracoscopic pleural biopsy is usually necessary. Immunocytochemical stains and electron microscopy can help differentiate mesothelioma from adenocarcinoma in difficult cases. This is an aggressive, treatment-resistant tumor with a median survival time of approximately 1 year from symptom onset, although chemotherapy may provide some palliation.

REFERENCES

Beckett W, Abraham J, Becklake M, et al: Respiratory effects of inhaled crystalline silica. American Thoracic Society Official Statement. Am J Respir Crit Care Med 1997;155:761-765.

Guidtotti TL, Miller A, Christiani D, et al: Diagnosis and initial management of nonmalignant disease related to asbestos. Am J Respir Crit Care Med 2004;170:641-675.

Hessel PA, Gamble JF, McDonald JC: Asbestos, asbestosis, and lung cancer: A critical assessment of the epidemiological evidence. Thorax 2005;60(5):433-436.

Robinson BW, Musk AW, Lake RA: Malignant mesothelioma. Lancet 2005;366(9483):397-408.

Ziskind M, Jones RN, Weill H: Silicosis. Am Rev Respir Dis 1976;13(5):643-665.

327

Hypersensitivity Pneumonitis

Method of
Michael C. Zacharisen, MD

Hypersensitivity pneumonitis (HP), or extrinsic allergic alveolitis, is an uncommon non-IgE-mediated immunologic inflammatory interstitial pulmonary disease caused by the inhalation of small organic antigens. This disease is seen primarily in adults in relation to occupations or hobbies, but it is reported in children when exposures occur in the residential environment.

Etiology

Small (less than 5 μm) organic airborne antigens inhaled into the distal lower respiratory tract can activate alveolar macrophages and induce a cascade of inflammatory cytokines with features of both type III and type IV (antigen-antibody and delayed or cellular type) hypersensitivity reactions. This culminates in an interstitial inflammatory cell infiltration comprised of lymphocytes, plasma cells, and the formation of noncaseating granulomas. The inflammatory cytokines involved are typical of a T helper 1 (TH1) pattern such as γ-interferon, tumor necrosis factor-α (TNF-α), and interleukin-1 (IL-1).

Antigens capable of inducing HP are derived from microorganisms (actinomycetes, bacteria, fungi, amoebae), animal (primarily avian) and plant products, low molecular weight chemicals, and various drugs (Table 1).

TABLE 1 Antigens Capable of Inducing Hypersensitivity Pneumonitis

Antigen	Exposure	Dust Source
Avian	Pigeon, parakeet, dove, duck, chicken, lovebird, goose, owl	Feather bloom or excrement from cage, nest, or coop
Bacteria		
Thermophilic	Farming, compost, building ventilation systems	Moist grain, hay, compost, heating, ventilating and air-conditioning (HVAC) system
Nonthermophilic	Machinists	Metal working fluids*
Chemicals	Epoxy resin, plastic, paint	Diisocyanate*
Fungi		
Outdoor	Farmers, peat moss workers, woodworkers, grain loaders	Compost, hay, grain, peat moss, wood, bark, sawdust
Indoor	Greenhouse, mushroom pickers, sauna water	Moldy airborne mists or disturbed moist soil
	Salami, cheese, mushroom, and malt industries	Aerosol mists in food preparation
Japan	Trichosporum	Moldy house dust in summer
Amoebae	Contaminated water	Residential humidifier
Medications	Amiodarone (Cordarone), clozapine (Clozaril), gold, nitrofurantoin (Macrodantin), β-blocker	Oral administration
Unknown	Pet fish food, tap water, mummy wrappings	

*Also responsible for occupational asthma.

Cigarette smoking appears to be protective from acute HP by affecting alveolar macrophage function but may worsen the prognosis for chronic HP. Genetic susceptibility is linked to polymorphisms in the promoter region of the TNF-α gene on chromosome 6, and a concomitant viral infection may increase the risk of developing HP.

Clinical Presentation

Despite the wide variety of causative antigens, clinical presentation is similar and classified as acute, subacute, or chronic. Acute disease is characterized by abrupt onset of nonproductive cough, dyspnea, chest pain, chills, fever, and malaise 4 to 8 hours after exposure. This is typical of occupational HP occurring with exposures at the workplace and is also seen with certain hobbies. The subacute form is characterized by gradual progressive cough and dyspnea without fever and is related to frequent antigen exposure. The chronic form presents with insidious onset of dyspnea with exertion with nonproductive cough and occasional wheezing related to prolonged but low-grade antigen exposure. Fever is lacking, but weakness and weight loss are more common.

Diagnosis

Acute HP is frequently diagnosed erroneously as infectious pneumonia, and chronic HP may be diagnosed as idiopathic pulmonary fibrosis because of the overlap in clinical findings. No single diagnostic test is available to confirm HP. A combination of elements from the history, physical examination, and basic laboratory, radiographic, and pulmonary function tests establish the diagnosis. Inquiry about home and occupational exposures most often uncovers the sources and nature of the offending antigen.

CURRENT DIAGNOSIS

- History (acute, subacute, chronic):
  - Recurrent or chronic dry cough, dyspnea, chest pain
  - Poor response to asthma therapy and antibiotics
  - Improves with avoidance of offending antigen
- Environment: occupation, home, and hobby
  - Presence of dust, fumes, chemicals, fungi, bacteria, or birds
- Pulmonary function: restrictive defect with or without obstruction with decreased DLCO
- Exercise challenge: hypoxemia with exercise
- Radiologic: chest radiograph and high-resolution computed tomography
  - Interstitial ground glass, reticulonodular, bilateral diffuse infiltrates without lymphadenopathy or pleural fluid
- Laboratory:
  - Precipitating antibodies (indicate significant exposure, not disease)
  - Elevated inflammatory markers: ESR, CRP, LDH, and quantitative immunoglobulins (except IgE)
- Bronchoscopy with alveolar lavage
  - Lymphocytic alveolitis with T-cell subsets CD8+>CD4+ and negative cultures
- Histology: lung biopsy (not required)
  - Noncaseating granulomas and foamy alveolar macrophages, consistent with nonspecific interstitial pneumonitis (NSIP). No vasculitis demonstrated.

Abbreviations: CRP = C-reactive protein; DLCO = diffusing capacity of lung for carbon monoxide; ESR = erythrocyte sedimentation rate; LDH = lactate dehydrogenase.

Diagnostic criteria include the following:

- Symptoms compatible with HP
- Known exposure to an offending antigen
- Recurrent episodes of symptoms 4 to 8 hours after exposure
- Evidence of exposure to the offending antigen by serum precipitins and/or bronchoalveolar lavage fluid (BALF) antibody
- Findings compatible with HP on chest radiograph or high-resolution chest computed tomography (HRCT) scan
- BALF lymphocytosis (if bronchoalveolar lavage [BAL] performed)
- Lung histologic changes compatible with HP
- A "natural challenge" with reproduction of symptoms and laboratory abnormalities after exposure to the suspected environment

Minor criteria include bibasilar rales or crackles, restrictive ventilatory defect on lung function testing, decreased diffusing capacity, and arterial hypoxemia at rest or with exercise. Weight loss is a common finding, especially in children and in the chronic form. Invasive procedures including BAL and open lung biopsy are reserved for difficult cases.

Treatment

Complete and indefinite avoidance of the causative antigen is most important. Treatment for acute HP includes oxygen, systemic corticosteroids, and antipyretics. For subacute HP, long-term alternate-day steroid therapy may be helpful. A trial of oral steroids for chronic HP is indicated and continued if clinical, radiologic, and pulmonary function parameters improve.

The most important aspect of treatment is avoidance of the offending antigen, whether it is specifically identified or suspected in the environment. Depending on the circumstances (industry versus home environment), intervention may entail personal respiratory protection, enclosing machining processes, changes in the heating, ventilation, air-conditioning process, or even a change of job duties. Changes in occupations and retraining, however, can lead to financial hardship.

 CURRENT THERAPY

- Avoid offending antigen:
  - Remove/isolate antigen from environment
  - Example: Enclose machining processes, fungicides, biocides, improve ventilation, clean regularly, introduce air purifiers
  - Remove patient from environment
  - Example: change in occupation or hobby
  - Personal respiratory protection
- Oxygen
- Systemic corticosteroids
- Prednisone, 40–80 mg/d with a gradual taper
- Asthma therapy (if obstructive airway defect)

Pharmacologic treatment for chronic or recurrent disease is less defined. There are insufficient data on using inhaled corticosteroids at this time. However, one case demonstrated successful treatment with beclomethasone in hydrofluoroalkane (HFA) propellant (QVAR[1]) likely with peripheral airway deposition because of its extrafine aerosol characteristics. Also, a teenager improved with pulse therapy using methylprednisolone (Solu-Medrol) in combination with budesonide inhalation (Pulmicort[1]).

When an obstructive defect is identified, treatment with inhaled corticosteroids, with or without long-acting inhaled bronchodilators, can be started. In challenge studies, albuterol (Proventil) was helpful when there was an acute fall in forced expiratory volume in 1 second (FEV_1). Similarly, inhaled cromolyn sodium (Intal[1]) prevented symptoms in the laboratory, but no evidence indicates that it prevents disease during times of natural exposure.

Experimental treatments include cyclosporin A[1] (Neoral) because of its anti-inflammatory effect on inflammatory cytokines produced by alveolar macrophages. Although there are promising in vitro effects of pentoxifylline[1] (Trental) on cytokine production from alveolar macrophages in patients with HP, clinical trials will be necessary to determine clinical efficacy.

Prognosis

Early treatment of acute and subacute diseases typically results in complete recovery. Patients with the chronic form may experience permanent and progressive symptoms, especially if antigen exposure continues. Although oral steroids may decrease acute symptoms and improve pulmonary function, they do not appear to change the long-term outcome. Findings of pulmonary fibrosis with severe restrictive lung changes portend a poor prognosis. Depending on the antigen, fatalities range from 1% to 10%.

REFERENCES

Fink JN, Ortega HG, Reynolds HY, et al: Needs and opportunities for research in hypersensitivity pneumonitis. Am J Respir Crit Care Med 2005;71:792-798.

Fink JN, Zacharisen MC: Hypersensitivity pneumonitis. In Adkinson NF, Yunginger JW, Busse WW, et al (eds): Allergy: Principles and Practice, 6th ed. St. Louis, Mosby, 2003, pp 1373-1390.

Jacobs RL, Andrews CP, Coalson JJ: Hypersensitivity pneumonitis: Beyond classic occupational disease-changing concepts of diagnosis and management. Ann Allergy Asthma Immunol 2005;95:115-128.

Kokkarinen JI, Tukiainen HO, Terho EO: Effect of corticosteroid treatment on the recovery of pulmonary function in farmer's lung. Am Rev Respir Dis 1992;145:3.

Lacasse Y, Selman M, Costabel U, et al: Clinical diagnosis of hypersensitivity pneumonitis. Am J Respir Crit Care Med 2003;168:952-958.

---

[1]Not FDA approved for this indication.

Tuberculosis and Other Mycobacterial Diseases

Method of
Christopher J. Lahart, MD

Tuberculosis (TB) is a curable and preventable disease, but it is the cause of more deaths each year worldwide than any other infectious disease. Although apparently contradictory, both of these statements about TB are accurate and, unfortunately, will remain accurate for years to come. The World Health Organization (WHO) estimates that during 2001 there were 8.5 million new cases of TB with 1.9 million deaths. The vast majority of these cases and deaths occur in the developing world. In the United States, the Centers for Disease Control and Prevention (CDC) reported a total of 14,874 cases in 2003 and 802 deaths in 2002. Within the United States TB cases are unevenly distributed, with a concentration in urban and medically underserved areas. The top five states in numbers of TB cases (California, Texas, New York, Florida, and Illinois) account for more than 53% of the national cases, whereas the five states with the lowest occurrence have less than 1%. There are fewer than 50 cases in each of 15 states. In 2002, for the first time since nation-of-birth data were collected, persons born outside of the country accounted for more than 50% of the TB cases in the United States. This highlights the worldwide issues of resource distribution and the ability of infectious diseases to transcend national borders and natural boundaries. In recognition of this, CDC has increased efforts of collaboration with international organizations to improve TB control in countries heavily impacted by the disease.

Case identification and treatment are essential elements of TB control efforts. Another is identification of individuals with latent TB infection who are at high risk of progressing to active disease. With an estimated 25% of the human population infected by *Mycobacterium tuberculosis,* this is an enormous task. It is even more important in areas with a low prevalence of active TB, such as the United States, where a high percentage of the annual cases arise from these latently infected people. Approximately 10% of the U.S. population has latent TB infection, providing a reservoir of more than 25 million individuals from which active cases may arise. Primary care physicians are on the front line of this challenge and must learn to assess a patient's risk and then test for latent TB infection when warranted.

An additional challenge to TB control in the United States is presented by the increasing infrequency of the disease itself. Fewer cases mean fewer physicians familiar with the disease's presentation, complications, and treatment. Despite a decreasing chance of encountering TB, practitioners must remind themselves to *think TB* when confronted with patients who have symptoms and signs suggestive of TB.

Pathogenesis of Tuberculosis

The human disease termed *tuberculosis* is caused by the organism *M. tuberculosis.* Archeologic findings have determined the presence of this disease since before recorded history, and it is more prevalent now than ever before. Transmission of *M. tuberculosis* is from person to person with no intermediate host or environmental reservoir. A person with respiratory tract TB expels airborne particles that contain *M. tuberculosis* during coughing and sneezing but also during normal speech and respiration. The particles of greatest importance are generally only 1 to 5 μm in size and can remain suspended in air for a considerable period of time. Another individual inhales them along with ambient air. After inhalation, organism-containing particles of appropriate size come to rest in pulmonary alveoli where the organisms are promptly ingested by alveolar macrophages. *M. tuberculosis* can survive and multiply within macrophages, is released with cell death, and spreads to regional lymph nodes and hematogeneously to other well-perfused organ systems. The resulting immune response from this initial infection induces cell-mediated immunity as well as granuloma formation. Delayed-type hypersensitivity reaction is developed to certain tuberculin antigens and forms the basis of tuberculin skin testing. Latent TB infection (LTBI) is thus established. This is the condition present in 25 million persons in the United States and 1.5 billion persons worldwide.

The immune response generated by this initial infection is able to perpetuate this latency as a lifelong condition in 90% of those infected. Only 10% will progress from latent infection to active disease. Half of this progression (5% of the infected total) will occur within the first 2 years following initial infection. The other half will occur during the remaining lifetime, often associated with the development of other medical complications such as diabetes, malignancy, renal failure, or immunosuppressive diseases or therapy. The proportions progressing to active disease and the time course of progression are dramatically altered by HIV infection. This interaction between TB and HIV is a critical driving force of the TB epidemic in the developing world, but also of major importance in the United States. This is elaborated on in a separate section of this article, highlighting the recommendations for HIV testing and special considerations for both TB and HIV therapy.

Diagnosis of Latent Tuberculosis Infection

TUBERCULIN SKIN TESTING

Although 25 million persons in the United States have LTBI, mass screening is not recommended. Rather, practitioners must assess the risk an individual has to progress to active disease if latently infected and then test for latent infection in those at high risk. The diagnosis of LTBI is based on purified protein derivative (PPD) tuberculin skin testing to elicit the delayed-type hypersensitivity reaction. This reaction is usually present within 2 to 12 weeks following infection. Tuberculin is injected intradermally on the volar aspect of either forearm, and the intensity of the reaction is assessed within 48 to 72 hours by measuring the amount of induration around the injection site. Prior vaccination with bacille Calmette-Guérin (BCG) is not a contraindication to tuberculin skin testing, and a significant reaction should not be ascribed to such vaccination. Persons receive this vaccination because they reside in a country with a high burden of TB, and the significant tuberculin reaction is more likely a reaction to LTBI than to BCG.

Because of the sensitivity and specificity of the tuberculin skin test, as well as the prevalence of LTBI in different groups, the interpretation of the skin test reaction incorporates three different cutpoints for significance of reaction (Table 1). For those at highest risk of developing active TB and those with immunosuppressive conditions that may impair their response, 5 mm of induration indicates a significant reaction. Persons with an increased likelihood of recent infection or other social or clinical conditions associated with higher risk of progression exhibit a significant reaction at the 10 mm level. For those

TABLE 1 Targeted Skin Testing to Identify Persons With Latent Tuberculosis Infection Who Would Benefit From Treatment: Criteria for Purified Protein Derivative Positivity for Specific Disease Risk Factors

Positive Result	Risk for Disease After Infection*
5 mm	HIV infection
5 mm	Fibrotic changes on chest radiograph consistent with old healed TB
5 mm	Recent contact with infectious TB case
5 mm	Organ transplantation or other immunosuppression†
10 mm	Medical conditions Diabetes mellitus End-stage renal disease Silicosis Immunosuppressive therapy Hematologic or reticuloendothelial diseases Cancers of the head, neck, and lung Intestinal bypass or gastrectomy Chronic malabsorption Body weight 10% or more below ideal
10 mm	History of inadequately treated TB in the past
10 mm	TB infection within 2 y (skin test increase by ≥10 mm)
10 mm	Illicit injection of drugs or cocaine use
10 mm	Children age <4 y, children and adolescents exposed to high-risk adults
10 mm	Foreign individuals from high-prevalence countries who have resided in the United States <5 y
10 mm	Prolonged travel/residence in a high-prevalence region
10 mm	Residents or employees of high-risk group settings‡
10 mm	Health care workers serving high-risk persons
10 mm	Mycobacteriology laboratory personnel
15 mm	No risk factors§

*Includes individuals with a high likelihood of recent infection and thus more at risk for disease.
†Prednisone doses of ≥15 mg/d for ≥1 mo.
‡Prisons, jails, shelters, health care facilities, nursing homes; low-risk individuals being tested for the first time for longitudinal screening programs are not included.
§Includes those being tested for the first time as part of a longitudinal screening program.
Abbreviations: TB = tuberculosis.

with no perceived risk factors or who are entering into a longitudinal screening program such as for employment, 15 mm is a significant reaction size. Results of tuberculin skin testing should be recorded in millimeters of induration and not as positive or negative. Depending on certain life events, what was once considered to be an insignificant reaction could be significant with the development of a new clinical diagnosis (e.g., HIV infection).

If sequential tuberculin skin testing is anticipated, such as annual screening in the health care industry, special consideration must be given to the boosting phenomenon. In some individuals the cellular immune response to tuberculin may be lost over a period of years. The initial application of tuberculin may not elicit a significant response but the second application may. If this second tuberculin exposure is part of the annual re-examination, it may be misinterpreted to signify recent TB infection during the past year of employment. Repercussions of such a misinterpretation include investigations of lapses in TB control within the facility and placement of the individual in a high-risk category for progression because of recent infection. However, the infection may have been remote, the risk of progression low, and there may have been no TB transmission in the facility. To prevent this mishap, a two-stage approach to the initial tuberculin screening needs to be used. A second tuberculin test should be done shortly following the initial one to assess the presence or absence of boosting.

CHEST RADIOGRAPHS

Once the diagnosis of LTBI has been considered, care must be taken to not miss a diagnosis of active disease. A missed diagnosis can have serious consequences; the treatment regimens for LTBI are inadequate for active disease and would foster drug resistance. All persons diagnosed with LTBI in whom treatment is being considered should have a chest radiograph performed. A single posterior-anterior exposure is appropriate for children older than 5 years of age. For those younger than 5 years the only manifestation of active TB may be small pleural effusions or adenopathy, so a lateral projection of the chest also should be obtained. Pregnant women with LTBI or with recent contact with active TB cases are at risk for progression to active disease and congenital TB in the infant. Chest radiography should be performed with the use of proper shielding in the radiology suite.

SPUTUM EXAMINATION

In a person with LTBI and a chest radiograph that is clear of changes for TB, no sputum examination for mycobacterial smear or culture is necessary. However, a special consideration is the HIV-infected person with or without respiratory symptoms. If symptoms are present, sputum specimens from 3 consecutive days should be submitted unless the respiratory symptoms are explained by an alternate diagnosis and resolve with treatment. If no symptoms are present but the HIV infection is advanced, as indicated by an AIDS diagnosis, sputum should be examined if recent contact with a TB case is suspected.

Persons with chest radiographs that are suggestive of prior or healed TB infection, but with no history of prior TB treatment, should have sputum samples sent for examination on 3 consecutive days. Initiation of treatment for LTBI can await the results of these examinations, or treatment for active TB disease can be initiated and subsequently tapered to treatment of LTBI once results are final and negative.

Treatment of Latent Tuberculosis Infection

Because the decision to test for LTBI should be based on the identification of those at high risk of progression to active disease, the decision to test is also a decision to treat those in whom LTBI is diagnosed. The primary contraindication to the treatment of LTBI with a recommended single-drug regimen is the inability to rule out active TB disease. If active TB remains a clinical consideration, multidrug therapy should be initiated and maintained until active disease is no longer a consideration. Other contraindications to treatment are the presence of active hepatitis or end-stage liver disease.

PRETREATMENT EVALUATION

The major pretreatment evaluation is to eliminate active disease from consideration. The evaluation in preparation of LTBI treatment is an assessment of the risk of hepatic disease. Persons with a history or physical examination indicative of liver disease or regular excessive use of alcohol should have baseline liver function tests (LFTs). The presence of risk factors for hepatitis B or C infection or diagnosed HIV infection also should prompt baseline LFTs. Pregnant women and those in the immediate postpartum period also should undergo such testing. Routine baseline testing is not indicated. If rifampin (Rifadin) is to be used, a baseline complete blood count (CBC) should be obtained.

TREATMENT REGIMENS

A common misunderstanding is that isoniazid (INH) therapy for LTBI is not recommended for persons older than 35 years of age. Current recommendations do not include consideration of age. Individuals at high risk of progression, regardless of age, should receive treatment of LTBI because the risk of active TB is higher than the risk of treatment-related complications. Practitioners must assess individual patients for their risk of a treatment-related complication.

There are four recommended regimens for treatment of LTBI. Medications used to treat LTBI are the same as those used to treat active TB. The preferred regimen consists of INH given daily for 9 months (which can be self-administered by the patient), or alternately, the drug may be taken on a twice-weekly dosing schedule given as part of a directly observed protocol. It should be emphasized that because of the concern for the development of drug resistance, any intermittent therapy, whether for latent or active TB, should be only prescribed as part of a directly observed therapy. A second but less preferred regimen is INH given for 6 months. This also can be given daily or twice weekly but should be reserved for those unable to complete a full 9-month course. It also is not preferred for those with HIV infection or fibrotic lesions on chest radiograph. The 6-month regimen results in slightly higher rates of active disease despite treatment of LTBI.

A third regimen, better studied in the HIV-infected population, consists of rifampin (Rifadin) plus pyrazinamide administered for 2 months. This also can be prescribed as daily therapy or twice weekly. Caution must be taken with this regimen because of its higher rate of hepatotoxicity, especially in the non–HIV-infected patient. This regimen can be considered for patients who are close contacts with a person who has INH-resistant TB. Patients should be evaluated every 2 weeks while on this regimen to minimize the chance of continued treatment administration during development of hepatitis. Although well studied in the HIV infected, the use of rifampin (Rifadin) can complicate treatment of HIV infection because of the significant drug–drug interactions between rifampin (Rifadin) and many HIV medications. The fourth regimen consists of rifampin (Rifadin) alone, administered for 4 months as daily therapy.

MONITORING DURING TREATMENT OF LATENT TUBERCULOSIS INFECTION

After the initial clinical evaluation and the initiation of treatment for LTBI, patients should receive monthly follow-up evaluations if they are receiving INH or rifampin (Rifadin) alone. If they are receiving rifampin (Rifadin) and pyrazinamide, they should be evaluated at weeks 2, 4, 6, and 8. The evaluation should include examination for symptoms and signs of hepatitis. Routine laboratory monitoring is not recommended. Only patients with abnormal baseline LFTs or those at risk for hepatic disease should be retested routinely during therapy. Follow-up chest radiographs are not indicated.

Diagnosis of Active Tuberculosis Disease

Control of TB depends on the prompt recognition of active TB disease and the initiation of effective therapy. Because TB is generally a slowly progressive disease of an indolent nature, it is uncommon for the individual suspected of TB to require hospitalization. Patients suspected of infectious TB should preferably be evaluated as outpatients, remaining in the environment in which they have resided instead of bringing them into a new environment with potential new contacts, many of whom may be immunosuppressed. Should a patient suspected of having TB need hospitalization because of the severity of illness, co-morbidities, or to facilitate evaluation, he or she should be placed in strict respiratory isolation until three sputum specimens are smear negative for acid-fast bacilli. Unfortunately, studies show significant delays in the diagnosis of active TB in hospitalized patients with up to 50% of the cases unsuspected at admission. Consideration of TB must remain prominent in clinicians' minds.

CLINICAL FEATURES

Active TB typically presents as a chronic illness with progression of symptoms occurring over a period of weeks to months. Symptoms often include chronic cough, fever, night sweats, and weight loss. Some patients may minimize these symptoms, but will present themselves within days of the development of hemoptysis. Roughly 80% of TB cases have pulmonary involvement; 72% have pulmonary alone and 8% have both pulmonary and extrapulmonary. Approximately 20% have only extrapulmonary disease, which is characterized by constitutional symptoms plus symptoms referable to the organ system involved. Many of the so-called extrapulmonary cases actually involve intrathoracic sites that are separate from the pulmonary parenchyma, such as mediastinal lymph nodes and pleural disease. Other sites include bones and joints, the genitourinary system, the central nervous system (CNS), the meninges, and peritoneal TB. Granulomas may be seen in the liver or spleen.

RADIOGRAPHS

The typical chest radiograph of active TB shows unilateral or bilateral upper lobe involvement with fibronodular disease and/or cavitation. Such findings should always raise suspicion of TB. Although this is the typical appearance of adult reactivation disease from the latent state, TB disease caused by progression of initial infection may be seen in children or the immunosuppressed, especially advanced HIV infection. This picture includes middle and lower lobe infiltrates, pleural effusions, and hilar adenopathy.

SPUTUM EXAMINATION

In pulmonary TB, sputum specimens have positive acid-fast bacilli (AFB) smears in 45% of the cases and cultures positive for *M. tuberculosis* in 70% of the cases. When pulmonary TB is considered, sputum should be submitted for examination. Because of specimen quality issues and test sensitivity, a sputum specimen from each of 3 consecutive days is recommended. The initial culture-positive specimen should have drug susceptibility testing performed as a routine procedure. Most mycobacteriology laboratories will do this without a specific request, but the practitioner must confirm this. Up to 17% of TB cases in the United States are based on clinical and radiographic suspicions when sputum specimens remain smear and culture negative. In these instances, appropriate diagnostic studies should be performed to evaluate other possible diagnoses; however, if TB remains the leading diagnostic concern, therapy should be initiated. Clinical and radiographic responses to TB treatment at 2 months should be assessed to provide further support for the TB diagnosis.

Treatment of Active Tuberculosis

Current regimens for treatment of active TB have a 97% success rate in the initial treatment and less than a 5% relapse rate. The success of these regimens depends on the use of appropriate multidrug therapy to eliminate the emergence of drug-resistant organisms, the extended duration of therapy to reach the slowly replicating mycobacteria and to prevent later relapse, and maximum adherence to the regimen dosing and duration. Adherence is best

addressed through the use of directly observed therapy. Directly observed therapy uses the resources of the local public health authority to deliver therapy to the patient with the public health worker observing the patient taking the medication. In addition to verifying treatment administration, the worker also inquires about potential side effects and serves as a resource for the patient, further enhancing adherence.

PRETREATMENT EVALUATION

Much like treatment of LTBI, active TB patients must be assessed for the presence or potential for hepatic disease. Baseline LFTs should be obtained along with a CBC and platelet count. Most patients also receive ethambutol (Myambutol) as part of their initial regimen, so testing of visual acuity and color vision should be performed and recorded.

TREATMENT REGIMENS

There are four recommended regimens for treating active TB. Three of the regimens use typical four-drug therapy, including INH, rifampin (Rifadin), pyrazinamide, and ethambutol (Myambutol). The fourth regimen is for patients who are unable to take pyrazinamide (severe liver disease, gout, and pregnancy) and includes the remaining three drugs. Each regimen has a 2-month initial phase followed by a 4- or 7-month continuation phase. The minimal acceptable duration of treatment for any case of culture-positive TB is 6 months. The differences between the regimens are how intermittent some of the dosing frequencies are and how soon in the course of treatment the intermittent administration begins. For all treatment, directly observed therapy is recommended, but for any intermittent therapy it is absolutely necessary.

Regimen 1 is the daily administration of all four drugs for the initial 2 months of treatment. In regimen 2 the same medications are administered daily for the first 2 weeks, followed by twice-weekly dosing for 6 weeks. Regimen 3 consists of the same four drugs administered three times weekly for 8 weeks. Regimen 4 is INH, rifampin (Rifadin), and ethambutol (Myambutol) administered daily for 8 weeks. Patients with advanced HIV infection are an exception. These patients should never receive medications less than three times per week because of the higher rate of relapse seen in that setting. The usual prescription for these patients is daily therapy for 2 weeks followed by thrice-weekly dosing to completion.

After the initial 2-month phase there is a second decision point. By this time drug susceptibility results should be known and if the organism is pansensitive, both pyrazinamide and ethambutol (Myambutol) should be discontinued. Pyrazinamide is used to hasten early sterilization, and the early phase is completed. Ethambutol (Myambutol) is used to protect the other medications in the setting of possible drug resistance and actually can be discontinued as soon as susceptibility results demonstrate no resistance. Most patients will continue therapy for 4 additional months (regimens 1, 2, and 3). Those who should continue for 7 months include persons with cavitary disease whose sputum culture obtained at the 2-month interval remains positive and those who did not receive pyrazinamide (regimen 4). For all four regimens, the continuation phase can consist of INH and rifampin (Rifadin) given daily, twice weekly, or thrice weekly; the exceptions are regimen 3, which continues on the thrice-weekly schedule, and the patient with advanced HIV infection who should never receive twice-weekly dosing.

Rifapentine (Priftin) is a recently approved anti-TB medication that allows for once-weekly dosing in the continuation phase of therapy. Rifapentine (10 mg/kg, 600 mg maximum) can be given with INH (900 mg) once per week for the final 4 months in persons known to be HIV-negative, AND with noncavitary pulmonary disease, AND with negative sputum cultures after the initial 2 months. This can be only done via directly observed therapy.

MONITORING THERAPY

Therapy is often initiated before culture results are finalized. Drug susceptibility results will further lag the culture results. A sputum specimen for AFB smear and culture should be submitted at monthly intervals until two consecutive cultures are negative. If a culture obtained after 3 months of treatment is reported as positive, drug susceptibility testing should be repeated on that isolate to assess acquired drug resistance. If AFB cultures have been negative throughout the evaluation, a repeat chest radiograph at 2 months should be done to check for response to therapy. No other chest radiographs are needed during the course of therapy. A chest radiograph at the time of completion of therapy should be done to serve as the new baseline study with which future radiographs will be compared.

PARADOXICAL REACTIONS

Although more typically seen in the current era with HIV co-infection, paradoxical reactions had been described with anti-TB therapy before the HIV epidemic. A paradoxical reaction appears to indicate a worsening of the disease or failure of treatment when in actuality it is occurring during adequate therapy. Symptoms occur weeks into therapy and may include a return of cough or fever, enlarging lymph nodes, a chest radiograph with worsening of prior infiltrates or development of new infiltrates, effusions, or adenopathy. In the HIV-infected TB case, paradoxical reactions are related to the initiation of effective anti-HIV therapy. They may occur in the early, middle, or late stages of TB treatment but are more common when HIV therapy initiation is closer to the initiation of TB therapy. In the more advanced HIV infected, care must be taken not to assume these symptoms are related to TB. They also may signify an immune reconstitution reaction to other disseminated infections such as histoplasmosis, *Cryptococcus,* or *Mycobacterium avium* complex (MAC). These events should prompt a review of all data, including laboratory results of cultures and sensitivities, and assessment of adherence to therapy. In patients with no prior HIV testing, it should be recommended again at this time. Records of adherence from public health administered directly observed therapy are invaluable to evaluate the possibility of treatment failure. If all other etiologies are ruled out, consideration may be given to administration of steroids to moderate the reaction.

Tuberculosis and HIV Co-Infection

HIV infection alters the natural history and presentation of TB. In the non–HIV-infected person there is a 10% lifetime risk of developing TB after infection. If a person with LTBI becomes infected with HIV, the risk for active TB approaches 7% per year. A person without HIV who is newly infected by TB has a 5% risk of developing TB in the next 1 to 2 years. Depending on the degree of immunosuppression, an HIV-infected person has up to a 40% risk of developing active TB within the first year after infection. Additionally, HIV-related TB is more likely to present as primary infection with noncavitating pulmonary infiltrates in the middle and lower lobes, pleural effusions, and hilar adenopathy. Because of this dramatic alteration of ability to control TB infection, many active cases of TB are in persons with HIV infection. Thus, all patients with active TB should be tested for HIV infection. In many U.S. urban areas, the HIV rate in TB cases may be 20%. Also, to properly interpret a tuberculin skin test, a person's risk for HIV needs to be assessed. As noted in Table 1, a 5-mm reaction is significant if HIV infection is known but is insignificant for the majority of those tested.

Performing HIV testing in TB cases can help make an earlier diagnosis of HIV infection, preventing an opportunistic infection in the future. Should a person with TB be diagnosed with HIV, a question about the timing of therapy for HIV arises. The therapies for HIV and TB have multiple drug–drug interactions. If a person with HIV/TB does not have an imminent need for HIV therapy, it likely is best to complete treatment of TB prior to starting HIV therapy. If it is determined that HIV therapy is necessary before the completion of TB therapy, treatment should be done in consultation with a health care provider experienced in such dual therapy. The primary concern in dual therapy is the interaction of rifampin (Rifadin) with HIV medications in the protease inhibitor and non-nucleoside reverse transcriptase inhibitor classes. Rifampin (Rifadin) induces the hepatic cytochrome P450 metabolic pathway, which results in accelerated metabolism and reduced drug levels of these HIV medications. Such lowered drug levels can result in treatment failure because of HIV drug resistance. In general, rifabutin (Mycobutin)[1] can be substituted for rifampin (Rifadin) without altering the anti-TB efficacy, but it greatly reduces the degree of enzyme induction. There is still much to be learned about these drug interactions; the practitioner supervising the treatment of either TB or HIV, or both, needs to consult the most recent guidelines available through the CDC or the AIDS Treatment Information Service of the National Institutes of Health (NIH) at www.AIDSinfo.nih.gov/.

Disease Caused by Nontuberculous Mycobacteria

Once considered the realm of pulmonary consultants, nontuberculous mycobacteria (NTM) are becoming more important causes of pulmonary disease, especially as TB

---

[1]Not FDA approved for this indication.

CURRENT THERAPY

(First-Line Antituberculosis Drugs)

Drug	Form	Dose: mg/kg (Maximum)*					
		Daily		2×/wk†		3×/wk†	
		Adults	Children	Adults	Children	Adults	Children
Isoniazid	100-, 300-mg tablets Intramuscular syrup, 50 mg/5 mL	5 (300 mg)	10-20**	15 (900 mg)	20-40	15 (900 mg)	20-40
Rifampin (Rifadin)	150-, 300-mg capsules Intravenous syrup, 50 mg/5 mL	10 (600 mg)‡§	10-20‡	10 (600 mg)‡§	10-20‡	10 (600 mg)‡	10-20‡
Rifabutin (Mycobutin)[1]	150-mg capsules Intravenous[2]	5 (300 mg)‡	10-20‡	5 (300 mg)‡	10-20‡	5 (300 mg)‡	Unknown
Pyrazinamide	500-mg tablets	15-30 (2 g)	15-20	50-70 (4 g)	50-70	50-70** (4 g)	50-70
Rifamate	Fixed-combination capsules containing 150 mg Isoniazid, 300 mg rifampin (Rifadin)	2 capsules					
Rifater	Fixed-combination capsules containing 50 mg Isoniazid capsules containing 120 mg Rifampin (Rifadin) capsules containing 150 mg isoniazid, 50 mg isoniazid, 300 mg pyrazinamide, 300 mg rifampin	<45 kg: 4 tablets 45-54 kg: 5 tablets >54 kg: 6 tablets					
Ethambutol (Myambutol)	100-, 400-mg tablets 300 mg pyrazinamide	15-25	15-25** (1 g) 20-40 (1 g)	50	50 (4 g**)	25-30	25-30
Streptomycin	Intramuscular 100-, 400-mg tablets Intravenous	15 (1 g) Age >60 y	10 (750 mg)	25-30 (1.5 g)	25-30 (1.5 g)	25-30 (1.5 g)	25-30 (1.5 g)

*Maximal doses for children are the same as those for adults.

**Exceeds manufacturer's recommended dose.

†Directly observed therapy should be used with intermittent dosing.

‡Complex drug interactions occur with many medications, including those used for HIV infection; refer to the text.

[1] Not FDA approved for this indication.

[2] Not available in the United States.

becomes less common, the general population ages, and the prevalence of chronic obstructive pulmonary disease (COPD) increases. Many of the NTM are ubiquitous in the environment and can colonize airways, may cause transient infection, or even contaminate clinical specimens. A decision to make a diagnosis of disease caused by NTM involves an analysis of symptoms, radiographic findings, and culture data.

CLINICAL AND RADIOGRAPHIC FEATURES

Much like TB, disease caused by NTM is characterized by a slow progression over time and is symptomatic with chronic cough, fever, night sweats, and weight loss. Hemoptysis also may occur. Radiographic findings also are similar to TB with the most common finding being upper lobe pulmonary disease that is fibrotic and/or cavitary. There is often evidence of underlying pulmonary disease such as COPD, healed TB, silicosis, or even malignancy. Tuberculin skin tests may exhibit some cross-reactivity to NTM, but the recommended cutpoints (see Table 1) take this into consideration. A significant reaction to tuberculin skin testing should be interpreted to indicate LTBI, even in the setting of confirmed NTM. On presentation NTM and TB usually are indistinguishable. In the interest of the patient and public health, anti-TB therapy often is initiated before receiving the laboratory report of the final culture results. Respiratory isolation should be maintained in institutional settings until TB is ruled out.

TREATMENT REGIMENS

Like the treatment of active TB, treatment of NTM requires prolonged multidrug therapy. Because of the lack of person-to-person transmission and thus any public health concerns, there is no option for directly observed therapy via local public health authorities. Often, TB is initially suspected and such therapy will be initiated; this can be done through directly observed therapy. Once NTM is the final diagnosis, directly observed therapy will no longer be available. The two most common disease-causing NTM are MAC and *Mycobacterium kansasii*. Both can be successfully controlled by any of the four-drug anti-TB regimens, but therapy can be tailored to the causative organism once it is identified. MAC therapy uses a macrolide antibiotic, either clarithromycin (Biaxin) (500 mg twice daily) or azithromycin (Zithromax) (250 mg once daily), plus ethambutol (Myambutol) (25 mg/kg once daily) plus either rifampin (Rifadin) (600 mg once daily) or rifabutin (Mycobutin)[1] (300 mg once daily). In HIV-infected patients with disseminated MAC, effective therapy has been only a macrolide plus ethambutol (Myambutol), which allows for the more important anti-HIV therapy to continue without the drug interactions of the rifamycins. *M. kansasii* is treated with antituberculous doses of INH[1] plus rifampin (Rifadin)[1] plus ethambutol (Myambutol).[1]

Duration of therapy is generally recommended to be for 12 months after culture conversion, which often occurs around month 6. Thus, 18 months of therapy is usually taken as a full course. With the amount of underlying lung

CURRENT DIAGNOSIS

Mycobacteria* in HIV-Positive and HIV-Negative Individuals

Symptoms
- Cough, fatigue, sputum, weight loss, hemoptysis not solely explained by an underlying condition.

Radiographic Abnormalities
- Cavities, infiltrates, nodules.
- High-resolution computed tomography, and multifocal bronchiectasis and/or multiple tiny nodules.
- Radiographic findings not explained by another condition.

Sputum
- 3 sputum/bronchial washing specimens from previous 12 months *and*
- 3 washings grow positive cultures, but AFB smears are NTM negative *or*
- 2 cultures are positive and 1 AFB smear is positive *or*
- 1 bronchial washing is available *and* culture is positive with a 2+, 3+, or 4+ AFB smear *or* 2+, 3+, or 4+ growth on solid media.

Lung Biopsy
- Culture positive for NTM *or*
- Lung biopsy shows granulomas *and/or*
- Positive AFB and one or more sputum/bronchial washing is culture-positive for NTM.

*These criteria best apply to disease caused by MAC, *Mycobacterium kansasii*, and *Mycobacterium abscessus*.
Abbreviations: AFB = acid-fast bacillus; NTM = nontuberculous mycobacteria.

disease present in many patients, therapy is often extended because of persistent positive cultures. In patients with advanced HIV infection, lifelong therapy formerly was considered likely. The increasing efficacy of anti-HIV therapy has allowed recovery of some immune function and these relatively low-grade pathogens are often contained by the reconstituted immunity. Still, therapy is continued as long as cultures are positive; discontinuation is considered after at least 12 months of therapy, with negative cultures, and on recovery of the CD4+ lymphocyte count.

REFERENCES

Blumberg HM, Burman WJ, Chaisson RE, et al: American Thoracic Society/Centers for Disease Control and Prevention/Infectious Diseases Society of America: Treatment of tuberculosis. Am J Respir Crit Care Med 2003;167:603-662.

Centers for Disease Control and Prevention: Targeted tuberculin testing and treatment of latent tuberculosis infection. MMWR Recomm Rep 2000;49(No. RR-6):1-51.

Centers for Disease Control and Prevention: Updated guidelines for the use of rifabutin or rifampin for the treatment and prevention of tuberculosis among HIV-infected patients taking protease inhibitors or nonnucleoside reverse transcriptase inhibitors. MMWR Morb Mortal Wkly Rep 2000;49:185-189.

National Center for HIV, STD, and TB Prevention at the Centers for Disease Control and Prevention. Available online at http://www.cdc.gov/nchstp/tb/. This Web site posts information as soon as it is released.

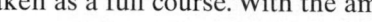

[1]Not FDA approved for this indication.

The Cardiovascular System

Acquired Diseases of the Aorta

Method of
John Byrne, MCh, and
R. Clement Darling III, MD

The management of aortic diseases continues to evolve. The certainties of a decade or two ago have been replaced by questions about new technology. The paradigm shift in general surgery from open to minimally invasive therapy has been mirrored in aortic surgery. Diagnosis now depends more on computed tomography (CT) and magnetic resonance scanning than catheter-based angiography. Treatment has also changed: At the Albany Medical Center, 65% of patients now undergo stenting of their aortic aneurysms; no such stenting was done in 1997. Acquired aortic diseases fall into three categories: aneurysmal disease, occlusive disease, and aortic dissection.

ANEURYSMAL DISEASES OF THE AORTA

According to Sir William Osler, Canadian physician and educator (1849–1919), "There is no disease more conducive to clinical humility than aneurysm of the aorta." Abdominal aortic aneurysms (AAAs) continue to be a major cause of death. Their first manifestation may be circulatory collapse. They are no respecters of social position or standing: both Charles de Gaulle and Albert Einstein succumbed to ruptured aneurysms. Mortality for elective repair is 2% to 5%. The mortality rate for patients with ruptured AAAs who make it to hospital is 40% or greater. The goal, therefore, is to prevent rupture.

Definitions

An aneurysm is a permanent focal swelling of an artery. By consensus, an artery is considered to be *aneurysmal* when its diameter increases by 50%. The normal diameter of the male infrarenal aorta is 2.1 cm; the normal female aorta is 1.9 cm. *Ectasia* is diffuse dilation, whereas *arteriomegaly* refers to arteries that are enlarged but not aneurysmal. *Small* AAAs are 3.0 to 5.5 cm by ultrasound; *large* ones are those more than 5.5 cm.

Inflammatory aneurysms are AAAs characterized by an intense sterile fibrosis around the aorta and surrounding tissues, often with ureteric obstruction. Mycotic aneurysms are those caused by bacterial infection, most commonly Salmonella. They are never caused by a fungus, despite their name.

Epidemiology

Approximately 15,000 people die annually in the United States from ruptured AAAs. The incidence of abdominal aortic aneurysms is 36.5 to 49.3 per 100,000 person-years with a male-to-female ratio of 4:1. In men 65 to 80 years of age, 4.3% to 7.1% have an AAA. Thoracic aneurysms have an incidence of 5.9 per 100,000 person-years. They affect the ascending aorta in 40% to 50%, the aortic arch in 10% to 15%, and the descending aorta (including thoracoabdominal) in 35% to 45%.

Natural History

Aortic aneurysms usually grow at 2 to 3 mm per year. Approximately 20% grow at more than 4 mm per year. There is no means of identifying "rapid growers." The only factor that independently increases growth rate is cigarette smoking. Risk of rupture is directly related to sac diameter. The "small aneurysm" trials have confirmed that the risk of rupture for AAAs less than 5.5 cm in size is 1% or less per annum. Large AAAs measuring 5.5 to 7.0 cm have an annual rupture risk of 6.6%. For an aneurysm larger than 7 cm, the risk rises to 20%. Perhaps owing to their smaller aortas, women have a four times' increased risk of rupture in the 5.0 to 5.9 cm range compared to men, so there may be good reason to intervene at 5 cm in women.

For thoracic aortic aneurysms (TAAs) less than 6 cm in size, the rupture rate at 3 years is 16%. For TAAs larger than 7 cm, the risk is 31%.

Etiology

AAAs are not simply atherosclerotic, although these patients often have atheroma-related diseases. Patients with low ankle-brachial pressure indexes (ABPIs) indicating peripheral vascular disease have lower rates of expansion than those with normal ABPIs. The two main pathologic processes are proteolysis and inflammation. In AAAs, the adventitia has an intense lymphocytic infiltration, whereas the media is thin with elastin fragments. A subset of enzymes called matrix metalloproteinases (MMPs) are implicated in expansion, specifically MMP-2, MMP-3, and MMP-9. MMPs are normally involved in connective tissue repair. There is also an inherited component to AAAs, as the incidence in first-degree male relatives is six times greater than expected.

Thoracic aortic aneurysms are related to previous aortic dissection, atherosclerosis, collagen vascular diseases (e.g., Marfan's syndrome, autoimmune disorders, Takayasu's arteritis), and syphilis. In some series, chronic dissection accounts for a third of all thoracic aneurysms.

Diagnosis

Abdominal aortic aneurysms are usually asymptomatic. Back pain indicates either acute expansion of an existing AAA or an inflammatory aneurysm. Rupture is indicated by severe abdominal and back pain and shock. Clinical examination in a thin patient with a large aneurysm is frequently diagnostic. In overweight patients, however, clinical examination can be negative even in the presence of sizable aneurysms. Ultrasound is a reliable and inexpensive diagnostic tool. Many AAAs are picked up incidentally on ultrasound or CT scanning. In patients in whom intervention is planned, a spiral CT scan gives essential additional information.

With thoracic and thoracoabdominal aortic aneurysms, rupture may also be the first indication. Many are discovered incidentally on chest CT or suspected on the basis of an abnormal chest radiograph. Chest, back, and abdominal pain are the most common symptoms. Aortic root dilation may lead to symptoms of congestive heart failure because of aortic insufficiency.

Treatment

MEDICAL MANAGEMENT

If risk of rupture of an AAA is related to size, then limiting expansion should prevent rupture. Controlling blood pressure was thought, at one stage, to prevent expansion. However, the only trial of the effects of β-blockers (propranolol) showed no effect on AAA expansion, and there was a large dropout rate because of side effects of the medication. If enzymatic or inflammatory processes are involved, inhibition of these processes ought to

CURRENT DIAGNOSIS

Abdominal Aortic Aneurysms

- Men >60 y are most at risk.
- AAAs are usually asymptomatic and often clinically undetected.
- Ultrasound is the test of choice for screening for abdominal aortic aneurysms.

Aortoiliac Occlusive Disease

- History and clinical examination are usually diagnostic.
- Pulse volume recordings (PVRs) are usually confirmatory.
- Magnetic resonance angiography (MRA) or contrast angiography is confirmatory.

Acute Aortic Dissection

- Awareness of the condition is essential.
- Chest radiographs can point to the diagnosis but are normal in up to 20% of patients.
- Computed tomography and transesophageal echocardiography are the gold standards in diagnosis.

prevent expansion. Currently, doxycycline[1] is being evaluated because it is a potent inhibitor of all MMPs.

SURGICAL TREATMENT

Operative mortality rates are 2% to 5%. The most common approach is a transperitoneal approach to the aorta via a

CURRENT THERAPY

Abdominal Aortic Aneurysms

- There are no proven treatments to prevent AAA expansion.
- Traditional open repair of AAAs has a 2%–5% mortality rate.
- Early data comparing endovascular aneurysm repair (EVAR) with open surgery show EVAR has a significantly lower perioperative mortality.

Aortoiliac Occlusive Disease

- Angioplasty and stenting is a good option for high-risk patients or iliac lesions.
- Aortobifemoral bypass is the gold standard treatment but carries a 4%–6% operative mortality.
- Axillobifemoral bypass is reserved for high-risk patients who require surgical bypass.

Acute Aortic Dissection

- Stanford type A dissections are treated surgically.
- Medical therapy is preferred for Stanford type B dissections.
- Endovascular therapy is increasingly being used for type B dissections.

---

[1]Not FDA approved for this indication.

vertical laparotomy incision. A transverse laparotomy incision is sometimes used in patients with pulmonary compromise. An alternative approach, and the one we prefer, is retroperitoneal repair through a left flank incision through the left tenth intercostal space. This affords better access to the proximal neck, results in less pulmonary compromise, and, being extraperitoneal, reduces postoperative ileus. Despite the morbidity involved, open repair is durable and the need for reintervention rare.

Surgery for isolated thoracic aneurysms depends on location and extent. Aneurysms involving the ascending aorta and transverse aorta require cardiopulmonary bypass. The aortic valve is usually replaced with ascending aortic aneurysms, and the arch vessels require implantation with aneurysms of the transverse aorta. Aneurysms confined to the descending aorta traditionally were repaired using a standard Gore-Tex or Dacron tube with reimplantation of the intercostal vessels to reduce the risk of paraplegia. Many of these descending aneurysms are now stented.

Surgery for thoracoabdominal aortic aneurysms is complex and challenging. It is usually performed through a posterolateral thoracotomy incision (fifth and sixth intercostal spaces) using partial cardiopulmonary bypass. Operative mortality is 5% to 10% with paraplegia rates from 5% to 15%.

ENDOVASCULAR TREATMENT

Endovascular repair involves exposure of the femoral arteries under local, spinal, or general anesthesia. An endograft is then introduced through these groin incisions under radiographic guidance and deployed just distal to the renal arteries. The stent-graft device is then fixed distally in the iliacs. The requirements for stenting are a good proximal aortic neck of 1.5 cm or more to fix the device proximally and healthy iliacs to fix the device distally. Exclusion criteria are extreme angulation of the proximal neck or lack of a good proximal neck (juxtarenal AAAs), occluded iliacs precluding delivery of the device to the aorta, or tortuosity of the iliacs. Endovascular aneurysm repair (EVAR) also mandates close CT follow-up to detect graft migration or leakage around the stented graft ("endoleaks"). Approximately 6% of patients per annum require secondary interventions for graft-related problems with current technology. In 2004 and 2005, the results of the first randomized control trials were reported. There were significantly lower mortality rates in patients undergoing EVAR (1.2% to 1.7%) versus open repair (4.6% to 4.7%).

Given the morbidity from open surgery for thoracic aneurysms, EVAR has potential advantages. At our institution, most descending thoracic aneurysms are treated this way. Reported mortality rates are 0% to 4% with a 0% to 1.6% paraplegia rate. Thoracoabdominal aneurysms are more difficult to treat, and despite some reports of endovascular treatment, their complexity has led some to question whether they are a "bridge too far" for endoluminal therapy.

SCREENING

As a screening tool, clinical examination is not useful. Ultrasound is highly sensitive and specific, noninvasive, and cheap—the ideal screening tool. Does it reduce mortality? The largest study enrolled more than 27,000 male patients and showed a 53% reduction in AAA-related mortality in screened versus nonscreened patients. Despite the absence of a national screening program, deaths from ruptured AAAs are decreasing in the United States despite operative mortality remaining constant. This is probably because of the number detected "incidentally" on routine scanning.

OCCLUSIVE DISEASE OF THE AORTA

René Leriche, a French surgeon (1879–1955), wrote this in 1923: "The ideal treatment [of occlusion of the aortic bifurcation] would be the excision of the occluded part.... and re-establishment of arterial continuity.... This ideal will never be achieved."

Atherosclerosis affects both the thoracic and abdominal aorta. When it affects the abdominal aorta, it is primarily occlusive, producing symptoms because of low perfusion. When atherosclerosis affects the thoracic aorta, it is primarily ulcerative and produces embolic disease.

Definitions

Aortoiliac occlusive lesions are classified according to the TransAtlantic Inter-Society Consensus (TASC) document as types A to D. Type A lesions are single focal stenoses affecting a single iliac artery. The focus of this section is type D lesions, which are those affecting the aorta and usually both iliacs.

Ulcerative atherosclerotic plaques of the thoracic aorta are classified as 1 to 5, with 1 being normal and 5 being the presence of a mobile plaque.

Epidemiology

Peripheral vascular disease affects 5 million Americans. It is difficult to estimate how many have aortoiliac occlusive disease.

In contrast, the prevalence of aortic atheroma among patients undergoing transesophageal echocardiography (TEE) for routine clinical indications is 8%. It is 38% in those with known carotid disease, and with coronary disease as many as 90% are affected.

Natural History

From the few natural history studies, patients with lesions confined to the aortic bifurcation tend to be female and have a longer life expectancy than those with more extensive disease.

However, there are many prospective studies of thoracic plaques. High-grade lesions are particularly dangerous. In one study, the risk for cerebral or peripheral events was 33% at 14 months.

Etiology

As with atherosclerosis elsewhere, the major risk factors are male gender, advancing age, smoking, dyslipidemia, diabetes mellitus, and hypertension. Hyperhomocysteinemia is also now recognized as a significant factor in disease progression. Of these factors, smoking is the factor that is most modifiable.

Diagnosis

Patients with aortoiliac occlusive disease (AIOD) complain of buttock or thigh claudication or occasionally rest pain. In men, a history of impotence may also point to the diagnosis (Leriche syndrome). Femoral pulses are absent or markedly reduced. Pulse volume recordings (PVRs) show damped or monophasic signals over the femoral arteries. Magnetic resonance angiography (MRA) is noninvasive and accurate and avoids use of nephrotoxic dye. Aortic surgery can be planned on the basis of good-quality MRA images. Formal angiography has long been the gold standard of investigation of occlusive disease. However, in the presence of severe occlusive disease of the aorta and iliacs, patients may need a transaxillary or transbrachial approach. Rarely, AIOD is a source of peripheral atheroemboli producing "blue-toe syndrome."

Thoracic plaques may be asymptomatic or produce emboli resulting in stroke, mesenteric ischemia, or acute extremity ischemia. These lesions are also a source of cerebral emboli when the aorta is manipulated during cardiac surgery. Diagnosis is made by TEE.

Treatment

MEDICAL MANAGEMENT

Smoking cessation is key to successful management. All patients should be on low-dose aspirin, and after the Clopidogrel versus Aspirin in Patients at Risk of Ischemic Events (CAPRIE) trial, there is evidence for the addition of clopidogrel (Plavix). All patients should be placed on a statin regardless of cholesterol level. Exercise regimens and oral agents like cilostazol (Pletal) are beneficial. However, aortic disease responds less well to these regimens than infrainguinal disease.

ENDOVASCULAR TREATMENT

Balloon angioplasty of the abdominal aorta has always been a concern in case of aortic rupture. However, stenting of isolated aortic lesions can be performed safely in selected patients using smaller stents to reduce trauma to the aortic wall. Lesions at the aortic bifurcation and proximal common iliacs have been safely stented for many years using the so-called kissing-stent technique.

SURGICAL OPTIONS

In patients with aortic atherosclerosis, surgery is often required. The options are aortobifemoral bypass, endarterectomy of the aorta and iliacs, or extra-anatomic bypass with an axillobifemoral bypass or femoro-femoral bypass. Rarely, the thoracic aorta can be used as an inflow source to perform a thoracofemoral bypass. Mortality rates for aortobifemoral bypass are 4% to 6%. This is higher than AAA repair because of coexisting cardiopulmonary and cerebrovascular disease. Patency rates for aortobifemoral bypass are superb, however, with 10-year patency rates in the order of 90%. Axillobifemoral bypass and femoro-femoral bypass have lower morbidities than aortic bypass, but patency rates are only 60% to 80% at 5 years. Therefore, it is reserved for high-risk patients with lower life expectancy.

AORTIC DISSECTION

"The diagnosis [of aortic dissection]...chiefly depends upon recognition and interpretation of the facts... together with an ever alert suspicion on the part of the physician" (Willius FA, Cragg RW: Mayo Clin Proc, 1941). Acute aortic dissection (AAD) is a catastrophic event. It can be a difficult diagnosis in the emergency setting. In an autopsy study in 2000, acute aortic dissection was the initial clinical impression in only 15% of patients dying from AAD. Awareness of the condition is still paramount in making the diagnosis.

Definitions

An aortic dissection occurs when an intimal tear allows blood to enter the media. Blood then propagates along the aorta. There are two classification systems: the Stanford and the DeBakey. The Stanford system classifies dissections as type A if the ascending aorta is involved; type B if the descending aorta is affected. In the DeBakey system, type 1 involves the whole aorta and originates in the ascending aorta, type 2 is confined to the ascending aorta, and type 3 includes those distal to the left subclavian artery.

Epidemiology

Approximately 2000 cases of aortic dissection occur annually in the United States. It is often stated that AAD is the most common aortic catastrophe. This is not quite accurate. Population studies from the Mayo Clinic show the incidence of AAD is 3.5 per 100,000 people. This is identical to that of ruptured thoracic aneurysm but less than that for ruptured AAA (9/100,000). Males are three times more likely than females to have AAD. Half the females affected by AAD are younger than 40 years and often in the third trimester of pregnancy. Interestingly, AAD exhibits chronobiologic variations with a peak onset in the morning and in winter.

Natural History

Contemporary data show that 21% of patients with aortic dissections die before admission to the hospital. Most natural history studies come from the "pretreatment" era. Untreated type A dissections have a 25% mortality at

24 hours, 70% mortality at 1 week, and 80% mortality at 2 weeks.

Etiology

The key predisposing factor for AAD is *cystic medial necrosis*, which makes the layers of the aorta less cohesive. Approximately 5% to 10% of AAD patients have an underlying connective tissue disease such as Marfan's or Ehlers-Danlos syndrome. Intimal tears are more likely at points of increased wall stress. The repetitive pulsation of the ascending aorta with each ventricular contraction makes it the most vulnerable area of the aorta. Accordingly, most AADs occur in the ascending aorta (65%). The transverse aorta is affected in 10% and the descending aorta in 25%. Almost 90% of patients are hypertensive. Approximately 15% of patients have no intimal tear but have a spontaneous intramural hematoma because of rupture of vasa vasorum in the aortic wall.

Diagnosis

Osler stated in 1910 that "a spontaneous tear of the arterial coats is associated with atrocious pain, with symptoms, indeed, in the case of the aorta, of angina pectoris and many instances have been mistaken for it." This remains true. However, if dissection of the transverse aorta occurs, stroke or arm ischemia may be a symptom because of carotid or subclavian occlusion. Involvement of the mesenteric or renal vessels may lead to bowel ischemia or renal failure, and extension to the aortic bifurcation may result in leg ischemia. CT scanning with intravenous contrast is diagnostic. Magnetic resonance angiography and conventional angiography are also useful. TEE determines the site of origin of the dissection, which guides therapy.

Treatment

MEDICAL TREATMENT

The goal of medical therapy is to reduce mean arterial blood pressure to 60 to 75 mm Hg. The drugs most frequently used are sodium nitroprusside (Nitropress) and labetalol (Trandate), a combined α- and β-blocker. Patients with Stanford B dissections not involving any of the major aortic branches have a 75% survival rate whether treated medically or surgically. Because many patients with type B dissections are older, medical therapy is more commonly employed. For type A, medical therapy is of little help because of the likelihood of retrograde dissection and cardiac tamponade.

SURGICAL TREATMENT

For type A dissections, surgery is mandatory. Surgery aims to excise and replace the segment of aorta containing the intimal dissection rather than replace the entire dissected aorta. Even in expert hands, this is associated with mortality rates of up to 20% at 30 days. With type B dissections, emergency surgery is reserved for those patients with visceral, renal, or extremity ischemia.

ENDOVASCULAR TREATMENT

Because surgery for type B dissections carries at least 11% mortality and the goal of therapy is to seal the "entry point" of the dissection, treatment of AAD by a covered stent-graft seems a plausible idea. Closure of the primary entry tear produces thrombosis of the false lumen that ought to produce a good long-term outcome. However, the walls of freshly dissected aortas are not robust. Despite the absence of controlled trials, initial reports suggest endovascular stenting is at least as good as medical therapy. However, evidence on long-term outcomes is lacking.

The management of acquired aortic diseases is changing. "Doubt is not a pleasant condition, but certainty is absurd," commented Voltaire (1694–1778), the French author and philosopher. The future may bring about advances in medical treatment of AAAs and atherosclerotic disease. Advances in molecular biology may allow for specific targeting of enzymatic defects underlying aneurysmal disease as well as identification of those most at risk. Although there is still a role for open surgery in the management of aortic disease, endovascular therapy will continue to evolve and play an increasing role. There will be further controversies along the way. The only certainty is that the journey is not yet complete.

REFERENCES

Ashton HA, Buxton MJ, Day NE, et al: Multicentre Aneurysm Screening Study Group. The Multicentre Aneurysm Screening Study (MASS) into the effect of abdominal aortic aneurysm screening on mortality in men: A randomised controlled trial. Lancet 2002;360:1531-1539.

Blankensteijn JD, de Jong SE, Prinssen M, et al: Dutch Randomized Endovascular Aneurysm Management (DREAM) Trial Group. Two-year outcomes after conventional or endovascular repair of abdominal aortic aneurysms. N Engl J Med 2005;352:98-405.

Brewster DC, Cronenwett JL, Hallett JW Jr, et al: Joint Council of the American Association for Vascular Surgery and Society for Vascular Surgery. Guidelines for the treatment of abdominal aortic aneurysms. Report of a subcommittee of the Joint Council of the American Association for Vascular Surgery and Society for Vascular Surgery. J Vasc Surg 2003;37:1106-1117.

CAPRIE Steering Committee: A randomised, blinded trial of Clopidogrel versus Aspirin in Patients at Risk of Ischaemic Events (CAPRIE). Lancet 1996;348:1329-1339.

Clouse WD, Hallett JW Jr, Schaff HV, et al: Acute aortic dissection: Population-based incidence compared with degenerative aortic aneurysm rupture. Mayo Clin Proc 2004;79:176-180.

Collins R, Armitage J, Parish S, et al: Heart Protection Study Collaborative Group. MRC/BHF Heart Protection Study of cholesterol-lowering with simvastatin in 5963 people with diabetes: A randomised placebo-controlled trial. Lancet 2003;361:2005-2016.

Dormandy JA, Rutherford RB: Management of peripheral arterial disease (PAD). TASC Working Group. TransAtlantic Inter-Society Concensus (TASC). J Vasc Surg 2000;31(1 Pt 2):S1-S296.

Greenhalgh RM, Brown LC, Kwong GP, et al: Comparison of endovascular aneurysm repair with open repair in patients with abdominal aortic aneurysm (EVAR trial 1), 30-day operative mortality results: Randomised controlled trial. Lancet 2004;364:843-848.

Johnston KW, Rutherford RB, Tilson MD, et al: Suggested standards for reporting on arterial aneurysms. Subcommittee on Reporting Standards for Arterial Aneurysms, Ad Hoc Committee on Reporting Standards, Society for Vascular Surgery and North American Chapter, International Society for Cardiovascular Surgery. J Vasc Surg 1991;13:452-458.

Khan IA, Nair CK: Clinical, diagnostic, and management perspectives of aortic dissection. Chest 2002;122:311-328.

Meszaros I, Morocz J, Szlavi J, et al: Epidemiology and clinicopathology of aortic dissection. Chest 2000;117:1271-1278.

Angina Pectoris

Method of
Charles R. Lambert, MD, PhD

Evaluation of the Patient With Chest Pain

Evaluation of the patient with chest pain is a common task for the practicing physician, whether generalist or specialist. Differentiation of cardiac from noncardiac pain is of primary importance in such situations. Angina pectoris is usually described as a heavy chest pressure with a squeezing or burning characteristic that can be associated with difficulty breathing. It can be associated with radiation to the neck, left shoulder, arm, or jaw. Typical stable angina builds over several minutes and is usually associated with physical activity or psychologic stress. This type of angina is usually caused by a mismatch between myocardial oxygen supply and demand and is most commonly secondary to significant obstructive atherosclerotic coronary artery disease. The principal clinically measurable determinants of myocardial oxygen demand are heart rate and blood pressure. The importance of these simple physiologic parameters in treatment of patients with myocardial ischemia cannot be overestimated. Myocardial oxygen supply is determined primarily by coronary blood flow and the oxygen-carrying capacity of blood.

Characteristics of chest pain not usually related to myocardial ischemia include a pleuritic nature, primary localization to the abdomen with radiation to the chest, and radiation to the lower extremities. Pain that can be localized with a single finger over the left ventricular apex or that is present and persists for many hours or lasts for seconds is usually not caused by myocardial ischemia. It should be noted, however, that many episodes of ischemia in patients with documented coronary artery disease occur without symptoms and that even myocardial infarction can occur without symptoms. Indeed, the most significant litigation issue in emergency room evaluation of patients with myocardial ischemia is missed myocardial infarction.

Several grading systems have been developed to characterize angina pectoris; the most commonly used was developed by the New York Heart Association and the Canadian Cardiovascular Society (Table 1). These are very useful in describing the clinical status of a patient and documenting any changes that occur with natural history of the disease or with therapy. The differential diagnoses of chest pain include esophageal motility disorders, biliary colic, costosternal syndromes, severe pulmonary hypertension, pulmonary embolism, aortic dissection, myocardial infarction, and pericarditis.

Evaluation of the patient with chest pain of unknown cause or established angina pectoris begins with a complete and thorough physical examination as well as electrocardiogram (ECG) and chest radiograph. A resting ECG during an episode of chest pain can be particularly useful in establishing a diagnosis. Biochemical testing is done to define risk factors for development of coronary artery disease including hypercholesterolemia, other dyslipidemias, carbohydrate intolerance, and insulin resistance. Other markers such as C-reactive protein are also useful in clinical management of patients with coronary artery disease.

Echocardiography is performed in patients with stable angina who have a systolic murmur suggestive of aortic stenosis, mitral regurgitation, or hypertrophic cardiomyopathy. Echocardiography or radionuclide angiography is used to assess left ventricular function in patients with a history of prior myocardial infarction, pathologic Q waves, symptoms or signs of heart failure, or complex ventricular arrhythmias. Exercise ECG testing, with or without an imaging modality, is used for diagnostic purposes in patients with an intermediate pretest probability of coronary artery disease based on age, gender, and symptoms. It is also used for risk assessment and prognosis in patients undergoing initial evaluation. Stress testing is less useful in patients with either a high– or low–pretest probability of coronary artery disease. Dipyridamole (Persantine) or adenosine (Adenocard) myocardial perfusion imaging or exercise echocardiography is used in patients with left-bundle-branch block, a paced rhythm, and inability to exercise or with other baseline electrocardiographic abnormalities.

Direct referral for coronary angiography is appropriate when noninvasive imaging is contraindicated or unlikely to be adequate, when patients' occupations could pose a risk to themselves or others, or when the pretest probability of coronary artery disease is high. Patients who are in Canadian Cardiovascular Society classes III and IV, despite medical therapy, should undergo coronary angiography, as should patients who have survived sudden cardiac death or who have angina with associated congestive heart failure. Coronary angiography is also considered for patients with an uncertain diagnosis after noninvasive testing in whom the possible benefits of a certain diagnosis outweigh the risks of catheterization. Coronary angiography is also considered in patients with inadequate prognostic information after diagnostic testing or who cannot undergo such testing because of disability, illness, or body habitus. The extent and severity of coronary artery disease and left ventricular dysfunction identified during cardiac catheterization remain the most powerful predictors of long-term outcome for patients with coronary atherosclerosis and angina pectoris.

Medical Management

Once clinical evaluation of the patient with angina is complete, a treatment strategy is individualized for each patient that includes reduction of risk factors, treatment of exacerbating diseases, pharmacologic therapy, revascularization, and alterations related to general psychosocial and lifestyle issues. Associated diseases or conditions that can exacerbate angina pectoris include anemia, thyroid disease, fever, infections, tachycardia, and weight gain. These generally alter the myocardial oxygen supply–demand ratio, as do sympathomimetic drugs. Any condition that increases left ventricular wall stress such as worsening heart failure, valvular dysfunction, or tachyarrhythmias can also worsen anginal symptoms through increasing myocardial oxygen demand in the face of limited supply.

Risk factor reduction and associated education should be stressed to all angina patients. Hypertension is a

TABLE 1 Grading Systems for Angina Pectoris

Class	New York Heart Association Functional Classification	Canadian Cardiovascular Society Functional Classification	Specific Activity Scale
I	Patients with cardiac disease but without resulting limitations of physical activity. Ordinary physical activity does not cause undue fatigue, palpitation, dyspnea, or anginal pain.	Ordinary physical activity, such as walking and climbing stairs, does not cause angina. Angina with strenuous or rapid or prolonged exertion at work or recreation.	Patients can perform to completion any activity requiring ≤7 metabolic equivalents (e.g., can carry 24 lb up eight steps; carry objects that weigh 80 lb; do outdoor work [shovel snow, spade soil]; do recreational activities [skiing, basketball, squash, handball, jog/walk at 5 mph])
II	Patients with cardiac disease resulting in slight limitation of physical activity. They are comfortable at rest. Ordinary physical activity results in fatigue, palpitation, dyspnea, or anginal pain.	Slight limitation of ordinary activity. Walking or climbing stairs rapidly, walking uphill, walking or stair climbing after meals, in cold, in wind, or when under emotional stress, or only during the few hours after awakening. Walking more than two blocks on the level and climbing more than one flight of ordinary stairs at a normal pace and in normal conditions.	Patients can perform to completion any activity requiring ≤5 metabolic equivalents (e.g., have sexual intercourse without stopping, garden, rake, weed, roller skate, dance fox trot, walk at 4 mph on level ground) but cannot and do not perform to completion activities requiring ≥7 metabolic equivalents.
III	Patients with cardiac disease resulting in marked limitation of physical activity. They are comfortable at rest. More than ordinary physical activity causes fatigue, palpitation, dyspnea, or anginal pain.	Marked limitation of ordinary physical activity. Walking one to two blocks on level ground and climbing more than one flight of stairs in normal conditions.	Patients can perform to completion any activity requiring ≤2 metabolic equivalents (e.g., shower without stopping, strip and make bed, clean windows, walk 2.5 mph, bowl, play golf, dress without stopping) but cannot and do not perform to completion any activities requiring ≥5 metabolic equivalents
IV	Patient with cardiac disease resulting in inability to carry on any physical activity without discomfort. Symptoms of cardiac insufficiency or of the anginal syndrome may be present even at rest. If any physical activity is undertaken, discomfort is increased.	Inability to carry on any physical activity without discomfort; anginal syndrome *may be* present at rest.	Patients cannot or do not perform to completion activities requiring ≥2 metabolic equivalents. *Cannot* carry out activities listed above (Specific Activity Scale, class III).

From Goldman L, Hashimoto B, Cook EF, Loscalzo A: Comparative reproducibility and validity of systems for assessing cardiovascular functional class: Advantages of a new specific activity scale. Circulation 1981;64:1227. Copyright 1981, American Heart Association.

well-established effector linked to coronary heart disease mortality and severity. Left ventricular hypertrophy is an even stronger predictor of adverse outcome in hypertensive patients. Rigorous blood pressure control is essential in management of patients with coronary artery disease and angina pectoris. Tight diabetes control is also essential in managing the patient with coronary artery disease. Weight reduction should be stressed and pursued in obese patients. Cigarette smoking is one of the most powerful predictors for the development of coronary artery disease in all age groups. In patients with coronary artery disease, smoking is associated with a higher 5-year risk of sudden death, myocardial infarction, and all-cause mortality than patients who have quit smoking. Smoking appears to increase myocardial oxygen demand, decrease coronary blood flow, stimulate progression of atherosclerosis, and reduce the efficacy of drug therapy. Clearly, discontinuation of smoking should be a primary target of antianginal therapy.

The National Cholesterol Education program guidelines suggest use of cholesterol-lowering therapy in all patients with coronary artery disease to 100 mg/dL or less. Most cardiologists target levels less than 80 mg/dL supported by other clinical studies. Lipid-lowering therapy with statins reduces the level of circulating C-reactive protein, improves endothelial responses, and favorably influences the composition of atheroma. Lipid-reduction therapy is associated with a reduction in coronary events and improvement in survival for patients with coronary artery disease and is a mainstay of therapy in patients with angina pectoris. Low HDL cholesterol represents an additional risk factor for coronary events. Therapy includes diet and exercise with LDL-cholesterol reduction in patients with concomitant elevation. The Veterans Affairs High Density Lipoprotein Cholesterol Intervention Trial demonstrated a 24% reduction in death, nonfatal myocardial infarction, and stroke with gemfibrozil therapy in patients with low HDL but no elevation in LDL cholesterol. Lipid-lowering therapy also improves outcome after coronary artery bypass surgery where LDL cholesterol is a risk factor for development of graft-occlusive disease.

Although past studies are conflicting, current evidence does not suggest using hormone replacement therapy in women for cardiovascular prevention. However, it is generally suggested that exercise is beneficial in patients with angina pectoris if begun under supervision and increased gradually. Exercise improves cardiopulmonary conditioning, aids in weight loss and cigarette discontinuation, and supplies other pathophysiologic benefits in patients with coronary artery disease and angina pectoris.

Aspirin therapy is associated with reductions in acute myocardial infarction and sudden death in patients with coronary artery disease. In the absence of contraindications, 75 to 325 mg of aspirin should be given every day to patients with stable angina pectoris and/or coronary artery disease. Clopidogrel (Plavix) can be substituted for aspirin in patients with aspirin hypersensitivity or intolerance. This agent offers additional long-term benefit in patients with non–sinus tachycardia (ST) elevation coronary syndromes or who underwent percutaneous coronary intervention.

In the absence of contraindication, β-adrenergic blockers are generally considered first-line therapy for treatment of patients with coronary artery disease. They are effective in prevention or delay of exercise-induced angina pectoris and reduce death and recurrent myocardial infarction in patients who sustained a previous myocardial infarction. β-Blockers also have beneficial effects on certain arrhythmias and in patients with left ventricular dysfunction. They are also very effective agents in management of hypertension. β-Blockers exert their favorable effects in angina pectoris primarily by reducing heart rate, blood pressure, myocardial contractile state, myocardial wall stress, and subsequently myocardial oxygen demand. Patients with obstructive coronary artery disease can exercise longer and at a higher level before reaching the double product of heart rate and blood pressure that precipitates angina without therapy.

Calcium antagonists are used in combination with β-blockers when the efficacy of the former is incomplete or as a substitute for β-blockers when they are not tolerated because of adverse effects. Although verapamil (Calan) has the most negative chronotropic and inotropic effects of the class, the dihydropyridines such as nifedipine (Procardia) and nicardipine (Cardene) have the most vascular selective and least chronotropic and inotropic effects. Diltiazem (Cardizem) lies between these classes. When combined with β-blocker therapy, the least adverse effects are usually seen when using the dihydropyridines.

A reflex tachycardia is seen when the latter are used alone without β-blockade.

Sublingual nitroglycerin should be given to all patients with angina pectoris with appropriate education on how and when to use it for treatment of acute angina episodes. Long–acting nitrates—oral, sublingual, or topical—can be used either in addition to β-blockers and calcium antagonists, or as monotherapy in patients with coronary artery disease and angina pectoris.

Angiotensin-converting enzyme (ACE) inhibitors are not indicated specifically for the treatment of angina pectoris; however, they appear to have very beneficial effects in reducing the incidence of future ischemic events in coronary artery disease patients. They are currently indicated in patients with left ventricular systolic dysfunction and/or diabetes. Data clarified after development of these guidelines, we feel, support treating most coronary artery disease patients with ACE inhibitors even in the absence of left ventricular dysfunction if no contraindications exist.

Although conflicting evidence was presented in the past, current recommendations do not include therapy with supplemental vitamin E, vitamin C, chelation therapy, or beta carotene for treating coronary artery disease. However, treatment of depression, including pharmacotherapy, should be considered integral to management of patients with coronary artery disease and angina pectoris. Changes in lifestyle with respect to both work and recreation in association with education, weight loss, stress reduction therapy, and structured exercise can all benefit the angina patient. Often, the best place to start such an effort is not in a busy physician's office but in a good cardiac rehabilitation program. It is not rare to see a patient who underwent hundreds of thousands of dollars' worth of interventional procedures without ever having any exposure to the basic educational programs and support available in cardiac rehabilitation.

Percutaneous Coronary Intervention

Percutaneous coronary intervention (PCI) therapy for coronary artery disease has changed dramatically since the initial introduction of balloon angioplasty. Advances in technology, pharmacotherapy, and stent development along with formal training programs, augmented–quality management, and adjunctive therapies have fueled dramatic expansion in the number of procedures performed. Conversely, a reduction in the number and increase in the complexity of cardiac surgical revascularization has emerged, especially with the advent of drug eluting stents with their associated lower restenosis rate. Interventional cardiology is a recognized subspecialty of cardiology, and it is beyond the scope of this article to explore the many criteria for selection of patients and lesions, as well as performance of interventions and probable outcomes. In general, however, it can be stated that patients with chronic stable angina who are ideal for PCI have symptoms or objective evidence for ischemia despite intensive medical therapy, are at low risk of complications, and have anatomy associated with high technical success.

Current guidelines recommend PCI for patients with stable angina pectoris with double- or triple-vessel disease including proximal left anterior descending (LAD) involvement with suitable anatomy, normal left ventricular function, and no diabetes. PCI is also suitable for single- or double-vessel disease without LAD involvement but with a large area of myocardium at risk and high-risk criteria on noninvasive testing. PCI is indicated for recurrent stenosis with a significant area of myocardium at risk and for patients who have failed medical therapy and can undergo intervention with acceptable risk. PCI is also used for patients with focal-vein-graft stenosis where the area of myocardium at risk is significant, and medical therapy is ineffective. PCI is not indicated in borderline lesions (50% to 60%) without evidence of ischemia. PCI is not yet established as primary therapy for left main coronary artery disease in patients who are candidates for coronary artery bypass surgery.

Coronary Artery Bypass Graft Surgery

Coronary artery bypass graft (CABG) surgery is a mainstay of therapy for patients with chronic stable angina as well as other coronary syndromes. Currently, CABG is considered to be primary therapy for patients with left main coronary artery disease although increasing evidence suggests that PCI with drug-eluting stents offers comparable efficacy and durability. CABG is indicated for patients with triple-vessel disease and offers an additional survival benefit in such patients with impaired left ventricular function. In other patient subsets, as listed earlier for PCI, CABG offers an alternative revascularization therapy and must be individualized with respect to risk of the respective procedure, the probability of achieving complete revascularization, the expected durability of the result, and informed patient preference. Revascularization therapy is not considered in patients with hemodynamically insignificant lesions (<50%) and where there is a small area of viable myocardium supplied by the target artery.

Patient Follow-Up

Coronary artery disease is a chronic condition, and patient follow-up with careful attention to the measures reviewed under medical management earlier are very important. In general, patients with chronic stable angina should have follow-up evaluations every 4 to 6 months during the first year and at least annually thereafter. Patients need to understand that more frequent evaluation must occur should symptoms change. The guidelines for use of testing during follow-up are generally conservative. We individualize stress testing and echocardiographic or radionuclide testing based on clinical status, the severity of underlying disease, the presence of stents and whether they are drug eluting, also considering risk factors and general patient compliance. For patients who had PCI, we generally do yearly functional assessments with stress testing for a period after initial treatment. For CABG patients, the initial interval is generally 1 year as well. If patients have other confounding conditions, such as valvular dysfunction, hypertrophic cardiomyopathy, severe hypertension, or arrhythmias, more frequent follow-up and testing are needed.

Unstable Angina

In contrast with stable angina pectoris, unstable angina pectoris is characterized by one or more of the following clinical characteristics:

- Symptoms occurring at rest or with minimal exertion
- New onset
- A crescendo pattern

Symptoms in unstable angina are often more severe than for stable angina and often persist until nitroglycerin is administered. Patients with unstable angina comprise a very heterogeneous population, and classification schemes are useful in considering pathophysiology and treatment. The progression or transition of stable angina to unstable angina and myocardial infarction occurs because of a number of processes. The most common of these is probably plaque erosion or rupture with superimposed nonocclusive thrombus. This can be associated with dynamic coronary vasoconstriction such as that seen in Prinzmetal's angina. Unstable angina develops with a simple progression of obstructive coronary artery disease, inflammation, or with factors affecting the demand side of myocardial energetics such as anemia, tachycardia, hypertension, or hyperthyroidism. The line between unstable angina and non–ST elevation myocardial infarction is thin and defined by the presence of infarction. It is not surprising that these patients share many clinical characteristics.

Unstable angina patients frequently have ST-T changes on the electrocardiogram. Continuous monitoring shows labile ST segments even in the absence of symptoms indicating ongoing ischemia and is in general an indicator of poor outcome. In general, patients with unstable angina have severe coronary artery disease, although nonobstructive disease can be seen and can implicate dynamic coronary constriction or microvascular dysfunction.

Treatment goals for patients with unstable angina are to stabilize the unstable nature of the clinical syndrome, presumably by "passivating" the unstable coronary lesion and exacerbating conditions. Ischemia should be alleviated followed by appropriate invasive or noninvasive testing and then institution of revascularization, if indicated, and secondary presentation measures. A mainstay of initial therapy in unstable angina is antithrombotic and includes aspirin, clopidogrel (Plavix), unfractionated or fractionated heparin, and platelet glycoprotein IIb/IIIa receptor antagonists.

Anti-ischemic therapy not only serves to review ongoing ischemia but also to stabilize the unstable atherosclerotic plaque. With active pain, nitrates are initially given by sublingual administration followed by intravenous infusion. Care is taken to avoid hypotension that can compromise coronary perfusion pressure. Early intravenous administration of β-blockers is used to optimize heart rate and blood pressure while reducing contractile state. Care should be taken in patients with significant reduction in left ventricular function and bradycardia or conduction disturbances. β-Blockers such as pindolol (Visken), with intrinsic sympathomimetic activity, should be avoided.

After nitrates, β-blocker, and anticoagulation therapy is instituted, calcium antagonists can be used for adjunctive antithetic therapy or for rhythm control if indicated. These agents are also useful in patients who do not tolerate β-blockers. Short-term acute use of ACE inhibitors does not seem to add significant benefit in unstable angina therapy, although later chronic therapy as discussed in the stable angina section earlier is indicated. Lipid-lowering therapy should be started as initial therapy in unstable angina and can be associated with improved outcome most probably because of stabilization of the evolving atherosclerotic lesion.

Two strategies have evolved involving evaluation of patients with unstable angina. These include an aggressive or invasive strategy with early angiography and revascularization with PCI or CABG and a conservative strategy with medical management followed by noninvasive risk stratification. These strategies have been tested in multiple clinical trials with current recommendations for an early invasive strategy when feasible in high-risk patients. These include individuals with ST changes, positive troponin, recurrent ischemia, or congestive heart failure. An invasive strategy is also advised in patients who have a history of PCI or CABG or an earlier episode of unstable angina or myocardial infarction within 6 months. Noninvasive testing is generally used to stratify patients who are at low risk, to guide conservative strategy, to assess prognosis and residual ischemia and left ventricular function, and to direct chronic management and cardiac rehabilitation.

In general, the same considerations apply to selection of revascularization strategies in unstable angina as in stable angina. Technical and procedural factors in these cases differ because of the high prevalence of thrombus in these lesions and frequent active ongoing ischemia. Adjunctive pharmacotherapy, device therapy such as aspiration thrombectomy or distal protection, and intraaortic balloon counterpulsation are more commonly used in the catheterization laboratory treatment of patients with unstable ischemic syndromes when compared to more stable patients.

Therapy of the patient with angina pectoris requires coordination of noninvasive and invasive diagnostic strategies, medical therapy, lifestyle, risk factor modification, revascularization, support, and education. The goals are to minimize myocardial ischemia and maximize long-term clinical outcomes and quality of life. Although tremendous advances have been made in all of these areas, our efforts remain lifelong and palliative.

REFERENCES

Gibbons RJ, Abrams J, Chatterjee K, et al: ACC/AHA 2002 guideline update for the management of patients with chronic stable angina—summary article: A report of the American College of Cardiology/American Heart Association Task Force on Practice Guidelines (Committee on the Management of Patients with Chronic Stable Angina). J Am Coll Cardiol 2003;41:159-168.
Hamm CW, Braunwald E: A classification of unstable angina—revisited. Circulation 2000;102:118.

Cardiac Arrest: Sudden Cardiac Death

Method of
Robert W. Rho, MD

Sudden cardiac arrest is the cause of death in up to 250,000 people per year in the United States. This accounts for more than 50% of all cardiovascular deaths. Sudden cardiac arrest is responsible for more deaths in the United States than stroke, breast cancer, and lung cancer combined. Approximately 1 sudden cardiac arrest occurs every 1.5 minutes in the United States. Unfortunately, 80% of cardiac arrests occur outside of the hospital and resuscitation is only attempted in approximately two thirds of these patients. Even in most urban communities, where an organized emergency medical system (EMS) is available, the survival rate of patients who suffer an out-of-hospital cardiac arrest is less than 10%. Approximately 10% to 40% of these patients have severe neurologic impairment at the time of discharge. This chapter provides a contemporary overview of the epidemiology, mechanism, diagnosis, and treatment of cardiac arrest.

Definitions

- Cardiac arrest: A primary cardiac disorder that results in sudden loss of cardiac output and a resultant loss of end-organ perfusion resulting in death unless the primary cardiac disorder is corrected.
- Sudden death: Death that occurs unexpectedly within a short interval of time from the onset of symptoms. (Definition varies in the literature from 1 hour to 24 hours from the onset of symptoms.)
- Aborted sudden cardiac death: An intervention or spontaneous event that reverses a life-threatening but modifiable cardiac process (malignant arrhythmia, pump failure, or ischemia) that would have otherwise resulted in sudden death.

Epidemiology

Approximately 250,000–400,000 patients suffer a cardiac arrest annually in the United States. The incidence of cardiac arrest in the United States is estimated to be approximately 1.5 to 2.0 per 1000 subject-years. The incidence of cardiac arrest based on a retrospective review of death certificates in Multnomah County, Oregon, was 1.5 per 1000 subject-years. The incidence of cardiac arrest reported in a population based case-control study in Seattle was 1.9 per 1000 subject-years. The incidence varies across clinical subsets known to be at greater risk of cardiac arrest. In the Seattle study, the incidence in patients with prior myocardial infarction was 13.7 per 1000 subject-years and in those with a history of heart failure was 21.9 per 1000 subject-years.

Prognosis

Patients who suffer an out-of-hospital cardiac arrest have a poor prognosis. Survival depends on the availability and quality of bystander cardiopulmonary resuscitation (CPR), early defibrillation, and the availability of EMS. In many densely populated urban communities (such as Chicago and New York City), survival to hospital discharge is less than 5%. In smaller urban communities with well-coordinated EMS systems, survival can approach 15% to 20% (Rochester, Minnesota, and Seattle, Washington). The initial rhythm when a defibrillator is available for monitoring has significant prognostic implications. Among patients who have ventricular fibrillation (VF) as their initial rhythm, 10% to 40% survive to hospital discharge. In contrast, patients who are found to be in asystole or pulseless electrical activity (PEA) have a grim prognosis, and less than 5% survive to hospital discharge.

Etiology

Cardiac arrhythmias account for the vast majority of all causes of cardiac arrests. The remaining minority of patients have cardiac arrest due to nonarrhythmic mechanisms such as left ventricular pump failure and cardiac tamponade.

The majority of patients suffering a cardiac arrest have coronary artery disease (CAD), but other conditions that predispose to cardiac arrest include hypertrophic cardiomyopathy, dilated cardiomyopathy, arrhythmogenic right ventricular cardiomyopathy, myocarditis, drug toxicities (antiarrhythmic agents, cocaine, amphetamines), congenital heart disease (especially tetralogy of Fallot and transposition of the great vessels [after a Mustard or Senning procedure]), ion-channel disorders such as long QT syndrome, Brugada syndrome, and short QT syndrome (Table 1).

Patients with abnormalities in myocardial substrate are predisposed to ventricular tachycardia because of a reentry mechanism. Most patients who suffer a cardiac arrest develop a rapid monomorphic ventricular tachycardia that degenerates to ventricular fibrillation and then ultimately (after 8 to 10 minutes) to asystole (Figure 1).

Management of Cardiac Arrest

The International Liaison Committee on Resuscitation (ILCOR) published its most recent recommendations for management of patients of cardiac arrest in November 2005. The recommendations from 2000 were updated based on an up-to-date review of resuscitation science between 2000 and 2005. Figure 2 shows the ILCOR universal cardiac arrest algorithm.

The initial rhythm encountered by EMS in patients suffering a cardiac arrest are ventricular fibrillation, pulseless ventricular tachycardia (VT), asystole, and PEA. Most patients who suffer an out-of-hospital cardiac arrest are found to be in ventricular fibrillation, but asystole or PEA has been found to be the initial rhythm in increasing frequency in the more recent literature.

TABLE 1 Causes of Cardiac Arrest

1. **Coronary Artery Disease**
   a. Atherosclerotic coronary artery disease
   b. Nonatherosclerotic coronary artery disease
      - Anomalous coronary origin
      - Acute coronary spasm
      - Coronary vasculitis (Kawasaki's disease, connective tissue disease)
      - Aortic dissection
      - Embolic coronary obstruction

2. **Structural Heart Disease**
   a. Ischemic cardiomyopathy
   b. Idiopathic dilated cardiomyopathy
   c. Hypertrophic cardiomyopathy
   d. Arrhythmogenic right ventricular cardiomyopathy
   e. Myocarditis
   f. Prior myocardial infarction
   g. Heart failure exacerbation

3. **Ion Channel Abnormality**
   a. Brugada syndrome
   b. Congenital or acquired long QT syndrome
   c. Short QT syndrome
   d. Idiopathic ventricular fibrillation

4. **Drug Toxicity**
   a. Cocaine
   b. Amphetamines
   c. Antiarrhythmic agents
   d. Digoxin toxicity
   e. Drug-induced long QT syndrome

5. **Metabolic Abnormalities**
   a. Severe hypokalemia or hyperkalemia
   b. Severe hypomagnesemia
   c. Severe acidosis

Acute Management of Cardiac Arrest

Survival from a cardiac arrest depends critically on what the American Heart Association describes as the "chain of survival." The chain of survival includes early recognition and initiation of bystander CPR, activation of the EMS system, early defibrillation (which may include automated external defibrillators), and advanced cardiac life support. Because a bystander may provide three of the four links to the chain of survival, community awareness and education in basic life support is a key element in increasing the likelihood of survival of cardiac arrest victims.

RECOGNITION

The initial management of patients experiencing cardiac arrest should be focused on the patient's ABCs: airway, breathing, and circulation. Delay in the recognition that a patient is experiencing cardiac arrest can waste critical minutes in initiating CPR and providing timely defibrillation. Rescuers should suspect cardiac arrest in any individual who is not moving, not breathing, and unresponsive. Involuntary gasps for air should not be confused for spontaneous respiration because agonal breathing patterns can

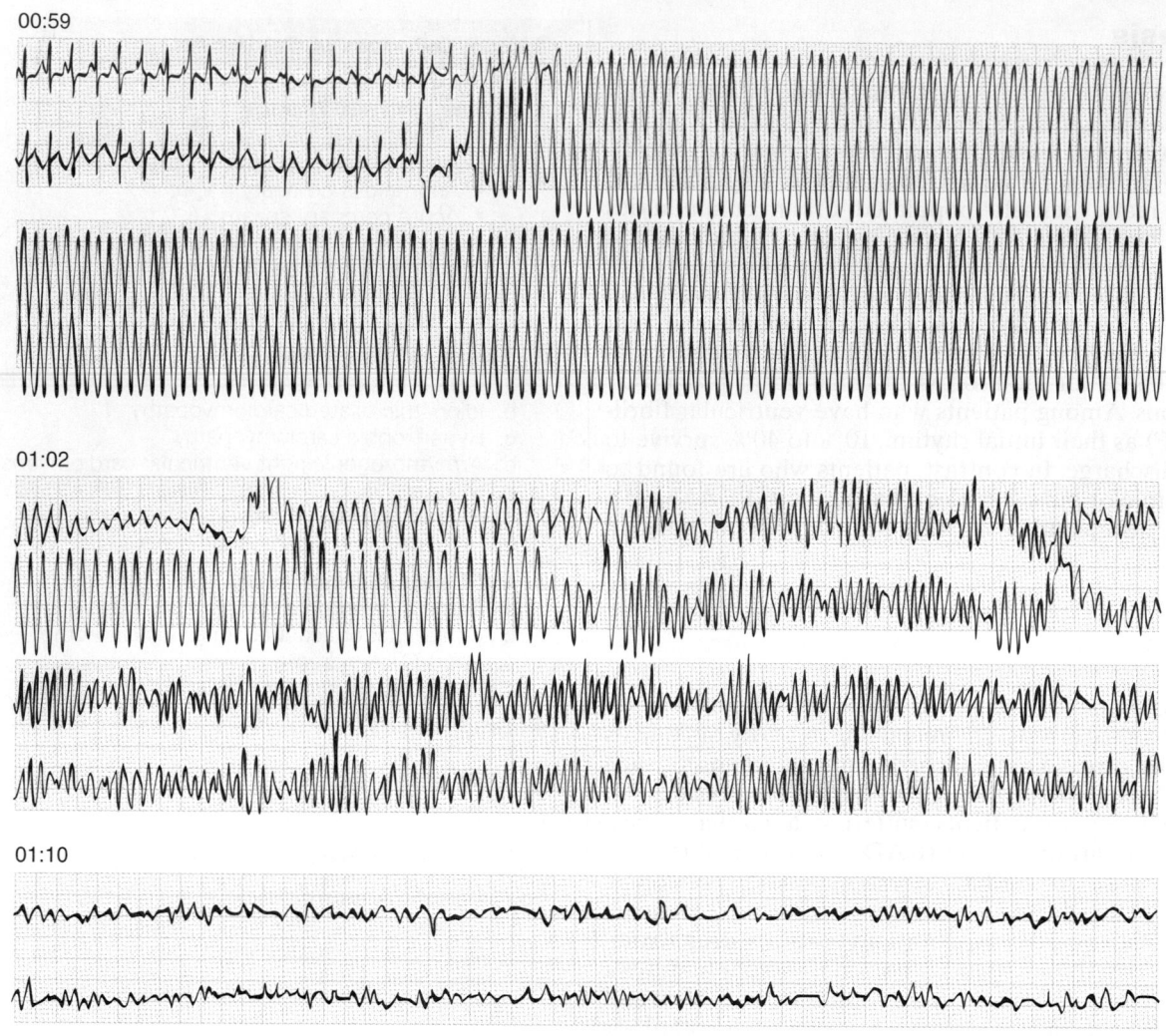

FIGURE 1. A Holter tracing of sudden death starting with monomorphic ventricular tachycardia and degenerating into ventricular fibrillation. (From Aziz S, McMahon RF, Garratt CJ: Images in cardiovascular medicine. Sudden cardiac death in arrhythmogenic right ventricular dysplasia. Circulation 2000;101:825-827. Reprinted with permission.)

be present in the early phases of 40% of all cardiac arrests and should not delay initiation of CPR.

ACTIVATION OF THE EMS SYSTEM

As soon as a patient is recognized to be experiencing a cardiac arrest, the EMS system should be activated. In most communities the system can be activated by calling the universal emergency number 911. The interval of time from onset of the cardiac arrest to arrival of EMS is critical. The shorter this interval of time, the more likely the patient will survive without neurologic injury. Survival is improved in those communities that have a well-organized and well-trained EMS system. Response times can be shortened when other professionals (e.g., firefighters or police officers) trained in CPR and equipped with a defibrillator are employed as first responders.

AIRWAY

The airway should be opened using a head-tilt, chin-lift technique. If a foreign object is visible, a finger sweep of the oropharynx may be performed. Endotracheal intubation

is the optimal means to establish control of the airway. Care must be taken to rule out esophageal intubation once the tube is inserted. While performing intubation, interruption of CPR must be minimized. Other invasive airway adjuncts have been developed and have proven field success. These include the Combitube and the laryngeal mask airway (LMA).

BREATHING (VENTILATION)

Ventilation can be achieved by mouth-to-mouth or bag-valve-mask. Each breath should be given a 1-second inspiratory time to achieve a chest rise. A tidal volume of approximately 500 mL to 750 mL should be delivered with a ventilatory rate of 8 to 10 breaths per-minute. When an advanced airway is in place (endotracheal tube or LMA), the rescuer should provide ventilation without interruption in CPR.

CIRCULATION

The quality of CPR and minimizing interruption of CPR received significant emphasis in the 2005 ILCOR

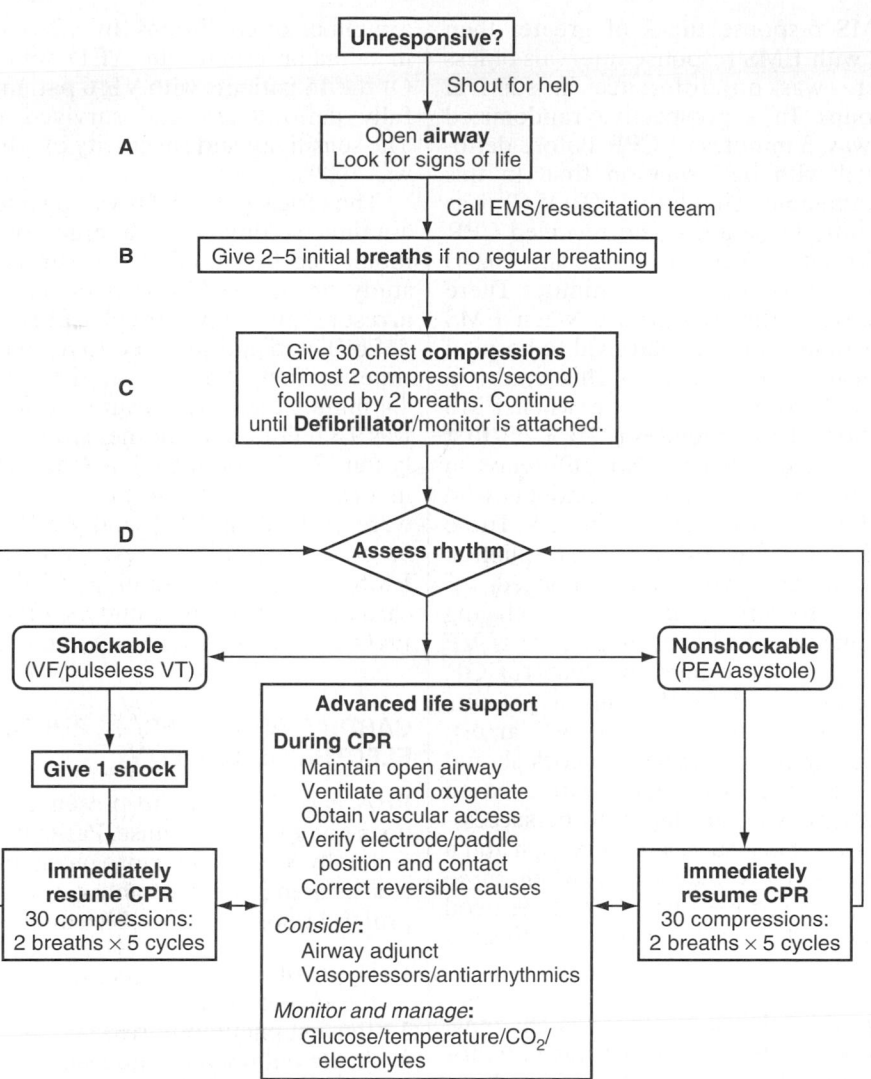

FIGURE 2. 2005 ILCOR universal cardiac arrest algorithm. CPR = cardiovascular resuscitation; PEA = pulseless electrical activity; VF = ventricular fibrillation; VT = ventricular tachycardia. (From Circulation 2005;112:1-11. Reprinted with permission.)

guidelines. Even with optimal chest compressions, the maximum cardiac output achieved is only a third of normal. Chest compressions should be performed with the patient on the floor or with a backboard placed under the patient. The rescuer should place the dominant hand on the lower half of the sternum with the nondominant hand placed over the lower hand. The rescuer should use the weight of his or her torso to compress the chest by 1.5 to 2 cm. After each compression, adequate decompression should be allowed while maintaining a compression-decompression rate of 100 compressions per minute. The ratio of time for decompression should be at least 50% of the total compression-decompression cycle. Several studies have demonstrated that chest compression rate, depth, and decompression are inadequate even among trained professionals. Inadequate chest compressions may not provide satisfactory hemodynamic support and result in worse survival and neurologic outcome. The quality of CPR (compression, decompression, rate, and depth) should be monitored by all rescuers involved in the

resuscitative effort. During prolonged resuscitation, a fatigued rescuer performing CPR should be replaced by a fresh rescuer.

DEFIBRILLATION

The most critical intervention in patients who have cardiac arrest during ventricular fibrillation or pulseless VT is immediate initiation of chest compressions by a bystander and early defibrillation. In patients with VF, every 1-minute delay in defibrillation reduces the chance of survival by approximately 8% to 10%. The priority of defibrillation and CPR is time dependent. Several studies have demonstrated that when myocardial energy supplies are depleted from prolonged ischemia, coronary perfusion must be achieved before defibrillation. In a study conducted in Seattle, patients who received 90 seconds of CPR before defibrillation had significantly better survival to hospital discharge compared to patients who received defibrillation first. This finding was only significant among patients who had EMS response times of greater than 4 minutes. In patients with EMS response intervals of less than 4 minutes, there was no difference in survival between the two groups. In a prospective randomized study from Oslo, Norway, 3 minutes of CPR before defibrillation was compared with defibrillation first. In this study, return of spontaneous circulation (ROSC) was observed more frequently in patients who received CPR first compared to defibrillation first (58% vs. 38%; p <0.04) if the EMS response time was more than 5 minutes. There was no difference between the two groups when EMS response time was less than 5 minutes. Survival to hospital discharge was significantly improved in this study in patients who had CPR before defibrillation when EMS response times were more than 5 minutes (22% CPR first vs. 4% defibrillation first; p = 0.006). No difference in survival to hospitalization was observed in patients who had EMS response times of less than 5 minutes. These studies demonstrated that CPR prior to defibrillation improved survival in patients who had prolonged VF arrests and did not seem to worsen survival (by delaying defibrillation) in patients who had shorter periods of VF arrest. Based on these data and others, the 2005 ILCOR recommends CPR preceding defibrillation in patients who have an unwitnessed out-of-hospital VF arrest. Furthermore, ILCOR recommends that one shock should be given rather than three successive shocks. This is based on the fact that, in patients who are likely to be successfully defibrillated, the first shock success is very high and a significant interruption in CPR may occur when three successive shocks are delivered because of the time need to charge the defibrillator, deliver the shock, and check a pulse three times.

When a defibrillator becomes available, the rescuer should continue CPR while the defibrillator is charging. The rescuer should give one shock and continue CPR for five cycles before checking for a pulse. The initial shock energy should be 200 J for a biphasic defibrillator and 360 J for a monophasic defibrillator.

AUTOMATED EXTERNAL DEFIBRILLATORS

The automated external defibrillator (AED) is a portable device with a battery, capacitor, and a processor that provides an accurate analysis of the cardiac rhythm and an algorithm that instructs the operator if a shock is indicated. The arrhythmia analysis algorithm in the AED has the capacity to interpret complicated cardiac rhythms and to recommend appropriate therapy with a high degree of accuracy. Several studies have demonstrated that AED arrhythmia detection for VF has a 100% sensitivity and specificity. The operation of the AED is simple and involves four steps:

1. Turn on the AED.
2. Connect the pads to the patient.
3. Wait for the AED to analyze cardiac rhythm.
4. Press the shock button (if shock is advised by the AED).

The AED uses voice and text prompts to guide the user through these steps. Because of ease of use, the AED can be safely and reliably operated by a nonmedically trained person.

Since the majority of cardiac arrests occur out of the hospital, the efficacy of AEDs has been tested in a number of conditions. In a 2-year study of AEDs used in a major airline, an AED was used in 200 patients. Of the 15 patients with VF, 6 patients (40%) were successfully defibrillated and survived to hospital discharge. The sensitivity and specificity of VF detection by the AED was 100%.

The efficacy of AEDs was also tested in casinos. This is a unique setting where a large population of patients are monitored by closed-circuit surveillance cameras. In this study, 56 of 105 (53%) patients who suffered a cardiac arrest because of ventricular fibrillation were successfully defibrillated and survived to hospital discharge. The mean time to first shock from the AED in this study was 4.4 minutes, and the mean time for arrival of paramedics was 9.8 minutes. In another study of public access defibrillation (PAD) conducted in Seattle; 475 AEDs were placed in a variety of public settings, and more than 4000 persons were trained in CPR and AED operation. A total of 50 cases of cardiac arrest were treated by PAD before EMS arrival, representing 1.33% of all EMS-treated cardiac arrests in the county. Of the 50 patients treated by PAD, 25 (50%) patients survived to hospital discharge.

CARDIAC ARREST FROM PULSELESS ELECTRICAL ACTIVITY

PEA is defined by the presence of a heart rhythm that does not generate a pulse. Patients who are found in PEA generally have a poor prognosis but may be successfully resuscitated if a correctable cause is identified and treated promptly. Some correctable causes of PEA include:

1. Hypovolemia
2. Exsanguination
3. Tension pneumothorax
4. Acute pulmonary embolism
5. Cardiac tamponade from a pericardial effusion
6. Hypothermia
7. Hyperkalemia
8. Metabolic acidosis (preexisting)

Patients suspected to be hypovolemic from obvious bleeding should be resuscitated with volume expanders (normal saline, lactated Ringer's) and transfused as soon as blood is available. O negative blood (universal donor) may be transfused in patients in extremis. A tension pneumothorax results from a tear in the pleura that serves as a one-way valve, allowing air to enter but not leave the pleural space. This results in significant increase in pleural pressure and intrathoracic pressures. It should be suspected in patients with absence of breath sounds and a deviated trachea toward the contralateral lung. A large-bore needle may be inserted at the midclavicular line over the second rib to decompress the affected lung rapidly, followed by insertion of a chest tube. In selective cases an acute pulmonary embolism may be successfully treated with thrombolytic medication. Cardiac tamponade should be treated with a pericardiocentesis. Hypothermia may be treated with rewarming. Hyperkalemia should be treated with intravenous (IV) calcium, insulin and glucose, or sodium bicarbonate. Rapid assessment of these secondary causes and immediate treatment may be life saving in some patients who present with reversible causes of PEA.

CARDIAC ARREST CAUSED BY ASYSTOLE

Asystole is usually a terminal rhythm in cardiac arrest victims who have had a prolonged episode of hypoxia and ischemic injury. External pacing has demonstrated no improvement in survival in patients who present in the field with asystole. Hyperkalemia is a reversible cause of asystole. Patients who present with asystole because of hyperkalemia may be successfully resuscitated with early bystander CPR and rapid treatment of hyperkalemia.

Pharmacologic Treatment in Cardiac Arrest

The primary goals in the successful resuscitation of a patient with cardiac arrest is to restore a rhythm that results in adequate perfusion of the two most vulnerable organs to hypoxemia, the heart and the brain, and maintain adequate perfusion to the heart and brain to prevent irreversible injury during the arrest until a rhythm and adequate hemodynamics are restored. To date, no randomized clinical trials have demonstrated an improvement in survival to hospital discharge among patients who have suffered a cardiac arrest attributable to any drugs currently used in advanced cardiac life support.

Drugs Used to Restore Rhythm

No randomized human studies have demonstrated that the use of antiarrhythmic agents in cardiac arrest improves survival to hospital discharge. Despite the lack of evidence supporting the role of antiarrhythmic agents, these agents are used routinely in shock refractory ventricular arrhythmias.

AMIODARONE

A randomized, double-blind, placebo-controlled study of IV amiodarone (Cordarone) in out-of-hospital cardiac arrest demonstrated an improvement in survival to hospitalization in patients treated with IV amiodarone versus placebo (44% vs. 34%; $p = 0.03$). This study demonstrated no difference in survival to hospital discharge (13.4% vs. 13.2%) but was not powered to evaluate this endpoint. Furthermore, there was no difference among survivors in the ability to resume independent living activities (55% vs. 50%). In another randomized, controlled study of amiodarone versus lidocaine in out-of-hospital cardiac arrest, amiodarone was superior to lidocaine in survival to hospitalization (22.8% vs. 12%; $p = 0.009$), but there was no difference in survival to hospital discharge.

LIDOCAINE

No randomized, placebo-controlled studies of lidocaine have been performed in out-of-hospital cardiac arrest. In one study with historical controls, lidocaine was associated with an improvement in return of spontaneous circulation and survival to hospitalization but not in survival to discharge. However, other studies have demonstrated no benefit in survival with lidocaine.

Drugs Used to Support Blood Pressure

Despite the standard use of vasopressors in cardiac arrest, there is a lack of clinical evidence demonstrating improved survival with these interventions.

EPINEPHRINE

Epinephrine is a mixed adrenergic agonist and acts on α-1, α-2, β-1 and β-2 adrenergic receptors. It is the α actions of epinephrine that provide the most benefit during resuscitation. Through its α actions, epinephrine increases coronary perfusion pressure and maintains peripheral vascular tone. The beta-adrenergic effects of epinephrine may be detrimental in patients during cardiac arrest. Stimulation of β-1 receptors results in an increase in myocardial oxygen consumption and decreases subendocardial perfusion.

There are no randomized trials of standard dose epinephrine versus placebo in cardiac arrest. Herlitz et al. compared 417 patients with out-of-hospital VF who received epinephrine (1 mg every 3 to 5 minutes) with 786 patients (historical control) who did not receive epinephrine. Although more patients had return of spontaneous circulation and survived to hospitalization when treated with epinephrine, there was no significant difference in survival to hospital discharge.

Evidence on high-dose epinephrine (5 to 15 mg) in cardiac arrest did not show a benefit in survival in out-of-hospital arrest. Although high-dose epinephrine is associated with a higher rate of return of spontaneous circulation, there is no difference in survival to discharge. These patients who survive to hospitalization are likely to have significant neurologic injury. Most of these patients do not survive to hospital discharge.

Despite the lack of clinical data demonstrating an improvement in survival with epinephrine in cardiac arrest, the ILCOR recommends the continued use of epinephrine at standard dose (1 mg every 3 to 5 minutes) on a routine basis for cardiac arrest. High-dose epinephrine is not recommended.

VASOPRESSIN

Vasopressin (Pitressin) is an endogenous vasopressor that causes selective vasoconstriction of resistance vessels. Although vasopressin appears to have pharmacologic properties well suited for cardiac arrest (increases vascular tone without β-adrenergic stimulation), clinical trials comparing vasopressin to epinephrine showed no difference in outcomes. However, in a study of vasopressin versus epinephrine in 1186 patients with cardiac arrest because of VF, PEA, or asystole, vasopressin was superior to epinephrine with the endpoint of survival to discharge in the subset of patients who had asystole (4.7% vs. 1.5%; $p = 0.04$). This study, like others, demonstrated no difference in survival to hospital discharge in the subset of patients who presented with VF or PEA.

The ILCOR concluded that "There is insufficient evidence to support or refute the use of vasopressin as an alternative to, or in combination with, epinephrine in any cardiac arrest rhythm." For the management of cardiac arrest because of VF refractory to defibrillation, asystole, or PEA, a dose of epinephrine (1 mg) IV may be repeated every 3 to 5 minutes. Vasopressin may substitute for the first or second dose of epinephrine. In patients who present with asystole, vasopressin may be preferred over epinephrine. Drugs should be administered without interruption of CPR.

Alternative Routes for Drug Administration

IV access cannot always be established during a resuscitation attempt. CPR and defibrillation should not be delayed to establish IV access. As an alternative to IV access, resuscitative drugs may be given via the endotracheal tube. Drugs that are absorbed via the trachea can be remembered by the mnemonic *navel*: *n*aloxone, *a*tropine, *v*asopressin, *e*pinephrine, and *l*idocaine. When drugs are administered via the endotracheal tube, two to three times the usual IV dose should be given to achieve the same serum levels.

Management and Evaluation of Survivors of Cardiac Arrest

The management of survivors of cardiac arrest begins with a continuous effort to identify the cause of the cardiac arrest at the onset of the resuscitation. After return of spontaneous rhythm and circulation, the patient should be monitored in an intensive care setting. During the initial period of hospitalization, the patient is vulnerable to cardiac arrhythmias and hemodynamic and respiratory instability. Patients are also prone to ongoing ischemic neurologic injury. Other issues encountered in the postarrest period include acute renal failure, shock liver, ischemic bowel, sepsis, and acute respiratory distress syndrome. The patients may require antiarrhythmic agents, inotropic support, and ventilatory support during the early period after a cardiac arrest. Frequent monitoring of arterial blood gas and electrolytes should be performed, and abnormalities should be corrected. Recent studies showed an improvement in neurologic outcomes in patients treated with hypothermia (32° to 34° C [90° to 93°F]) for 12 to 24 hours postresuscitation. The ILCOR recommends therapeutic hypothermia in all patients who are unconscious for a period of 12 to 24 hours after a cardiac arrest.

The physician should begin a detailed history and physical examination. Family members should be contacted to see whether the patient had an advance directive. A myocardial infarction should be ruled out with an electrocardiogram (EKG) and serial cardiac enzymes, and a thorough review of available medical records including a complete review of current medications should be performed. Minimum initial workup should include a chest radiograph and laboratory evaluation (electrolytes, arterial blood gas, liver and renal function tests, and toxicology screening). An echocardiogram should be performed to assess the presence or absence of structural heart disease. Because the majority of all cardiac arrests occur in patients with significant coronary artery disease, coronary angiography should be performed in most patients who have suffered a cardiac arrest.

HISTORY

It is often difficult to obtain any history from the patient. If the patient is awake, he or she may have significant neurologic impairment and retrograde amnesia of events preceding the arrest. History taken from witnesses to the cardiac arrest and family members and friends close to the victim may be valuable. Important information gained from the history would include any recent medications, heart failure symptoms preceding the arrest, angina preceding the arrest, illicit drug use, and a family history of sudden death.

12-LEAD ELECTROCARDIOGRAM

A 12-lead EKG may demonstrate signs of myocardial ischemia or injury. Other findings on the 12-lead EKG include the presence of epsilon waves suggesting arrhythmogenic right ventricular cardiomyopathy; incomplete right bundle branch block with ST-segment elevations in the right precordial leads (suggestive of Brugada syndrome); a prolonged or abnormally short (<300 ms) QT segment, which may suggest long QT syndrome or short QT syndrome, respectively; ventricular pre-excitation because of a bypass tract; and severe conduction system disease (bifascicular block or evidence of heart block). The 12-lead EKG should be screened carefully for these abnormalities.

LABORATORY EVALUATION

Laboratory evaluation should include electrolytes, arterial blood gas, liver and renal function tests, serial cardiac enzymes, complete blood count, and a toxicology screen. The causal role of the abnormalities detected should be interpreted carefully. Hypokalemia may occur because of intracellular shifting of potassium secondary to endogenous catecholamines or epinephrine given during the cardiac arrest. Elevations in myocardial band enzymes of creatine phosphokinase (MB CK) and troponins indicate myocardial infarction; however, mild elevations in cardiac enzymes may result from prolonged CPR and defibrillation and may not be indicative of a primary myocardial infarction.

Other laboratory findings may be helpful in screening for end organ damage. Significant elevations in transaminases and elevated protime may be evidence of ischemic liver injury. Bloody stools and persistent lactic acidosis should increase the suspicion for ischemic bowel. Acute renal failure is commonly seen after an arrest.

ECHOCARDIOGRAM

An echocardiogram is essential in the workup of patients who have survived a cardiac arrest. The echocardiogram may detect evidence of hypertrophic cardiomyopathy, left ventricular dysfunction, regional wall motion abnormalities, abnormalities in the RV that might be suggestive of arrhythmogenic right ventricular cardiomyopathy, significant valvular disease, and other structural cardiac abnormalities. The presence of left ventricular dysfunction early postarrest may be because of "stunning" (caused by ischemia and defibrillation) and may not be representative of the patient's true left ventricular function.

CARDIAC CATHETERIZATION

Coronary angiography should be performed in most patients who have suffered a cardiac arrest to rule out significant epicardial coronary artery disease or congenital coronary anomalies.

ELECTROPHYSIOLOGIC STUDY

Currently, the electrophysiologic study in cardiac arrest victims has a limited role. However, an electrophysiologic study may be useful in a select group of patients: those with ventricular preexcitation (Wolff-Parkinson-White [WPW] pattern) on the EKG because the electrophysiologic study will allow characterization of the anterograde conduction properties of the bypass tract and may offer a curative strategy; patients with suspected bundle branch reentry ventricular tachycardia, which occurs in patients with dilated cardiomyopathy; and provocative drug testing for concealed long QT syndrome (epinephrine), Brugada syndrome (sodium channel blocker), or significant His-Purkinje disease. The electrophysiologic study is not routinely indicated in patients who have suffered a cardiac arrest.

Neurologic Assessment

Patients who are unconscious after cardiac arrest require an assessment of the degree of irreversible global neurologic injury. Patients should be assessed while normothermic and after all sedation is withheld. Assessment of neurologic status in a comatose patient includes apnea testing and assessment of brainstem reflexes. Absence of reflexes and abnormal apnea testing is associated with a grim prognosis. Additional neurologic testing with excellent predictive accuracy includes a median nerve somatosensory evoked potential (SSEP) and an electroencephalogram (EEG). An abnormal SSEP assessed at 72 hours postresuscitation predicts a poor outcome with 100% specificity. An EEG may also be a useful prognostic tool.

Patients who are conscious may still suffer from varying degrees of amnesia, short term memory loss, and from motor or sensory deficits. They may require physical therapy, occupational therapy, speech therapy, and rehabilitation.

ROLE OF IMPLANTABLE CARDIAC DEFIBRILLATORS

Currently, most patients who are survivors of a ventricular fibrillation or ventricular tachycardia–related cardiac arrest are treated with an implantable cardiac defibrillator (ICD) even if there is an identifiable reversible cause. A randomized controlled study of amiodarone versus implantable cardiac defibrillator among cardiac arrest survivors (Antiarrhythmics Versus Implantable Defibrillators [AVID]) demonstrated a survival advantage in patients treated with an ICD. A subset analysis revealed that survival benefit was observed only in patients with ejection fraction (EF) less than 35%. Patients with EF more than 35% had no difference in survival whether treated with an ICD or amiodarone. Patients in AVID with reversible or correctable causes were excluded from and

followed in a registry. The mortality among the 278 patients followed in the registry at 3 years was found to be higher than in patients who did not have transient or reversible causes. Contemporary practice is that most patients who have suffered a VT/VF cardiac arrest are treated with an ICD regardless of whether their arrest was because of a transient or reversible cause and regardless of their EF. An important exception are patients with preserved left ventricular function who had a VT/VF arrest within 72 hours of an acute transmural myocardial infarction. These patients have a low recurrence rate of cardiac arrest if they have no evidence of residual ischemia and preserved left ventricular function. Amiodarone is a reasonable option for patients with preserved EF with contraindications for an ICD.

Some situations where an ICD may not be appropriate are patients who have a cardiac arrest less than 72 hours after a transmural myocardial infarction, patients who do not wish to have an ICD, patients who had a cardiac arrest because of rapidly conducting atrial fibrillation via a bypass tract (WPW) that was treated successfully with a radiofrequency ablation procedure, and patients of advanced age and significant co-morbidities (the risks and benefits of ICD implantation should be carefully considered in such patients).

Cardiac arrest is a major public health concern killing hundreds of thousands of people annually in the United States. The cornerstone of treatment of patients suffering a cardiac arrest is early recognition, early activation of EMS, early bystander CPR, early defibrillation, and advanced cardiac life support. Despite our best efforts, the prognosis of cardiac arrest victims remains poor. Recent advances in the science of resuscitation have provided grounds to make some significant changes to the guidelines for resuscitation of cardiac arrest. Communities with a well-established EMS system, public access defibrillation programs, and citizens who are well educated in basic life support have the highest rates of survival for cardiac arrest victims.

REFERENCES

Antiarrhythmics versus implantable defibrillators (AVID) investigators: A comparison of antiarrhythmic-drug therapy with implantable defibrillators in patients resuscitated from near-fatal ventricular arrhythmias. N Engl J Med 1997;337:1576–1583.

Cobb LA, Fahrenbruch CE, Walsh TR, et al: Influence of cardiopulmonary resuscitation prior to defibrillation in patients with out-of-hospital ventricular fibrillation. JAMA 1999;281:1182–1188.

Connolly SJ, Hallstrom AP, Cappato R, et al: Meta-analysis of the implantable cardioverter defibrillator secondary prevention trials. Eur Heart J 2000;21:2071–2078.

Cully CL, Rea TD, Murray JA, et al: Public access defibrillation in out-of hospital cardiac arrest. Circulation 2004;109:1859–1863.

Dorian P, Cass D, Schwartz B, et al: Amiodarone as compared with lidocaine for shock-resistant ventricular fibrillation. N Engl J Med 2002;346:884–890.

2005 International consensus on cardiopulmonary resuscitation (CPR) and emergency cardiovascular care (ECC) science with treatment recommendations. Circulation 2005;112:1–11.

Kudenchuk PJ, Cobb LA, Copass MK, et al: Amiodarone for resuscitation after out-of-hospital cardiac arrest due to ventricular fibrillation. N Engl J Med 1999;341:871–878.

Page RL, Joglar JA, Kowal RC, et al: Use of automated external defibrillators by a US airline. N Engl J Med 2000;343:1210–1216.

Pepe PE, Fowler RL, Roppolo LP, et al: Clinical review: Reappraising the concept of immediate defibrillatory attempts for out-of-hospital ventricular fibrillation. Crit Care 2004;8:41–45.

Rea TD, Eisenberg MS, Sinibaldi G, et al: Incidence of EMS-treated out-of-hospital cardiac arrest in the United States. Resuscitation 2004; 63:17–24.

Wyse DG, Friedman PL, Brodsky MA, et al: Life threatening ventricular arrhythmias due to transient or correctable causes: high risk for death in follow-up. J Am Col Cardiol 2001;38:1718–1724.

Zhong J, Dorian P: Epinephrine and vasopressin during cardiopulmonary resuscitation. Resuscitation 2005;66:263–269.

Atrial Fibrillation

Method of
Robert W. Rho, MD, and Richard L. Page, MD

Atrial fibrillation (AF) is the most common arrhythmia requiring treatment. Many patients with AF suffer from impaired quality of life, heart failure, stroke, and at times significant symptoms. Every year more than 70,000 patients in the United States die from stroke or heart failure that occurs as a consequence of AF. Significant advancements in treatment options and understanding of appropriate strategies for the long-term management of AF have been made in recent years.

Epidemiology

An estimated 2.2 million individuals suffer from AF in the United States. The incidence of AF increases with age and with the presence of structural heart disease. The prevalence of AF is 2% to 3% in patients older than 40 years, 6% in patients older than 65 years, and 9% in patients older than 80 years. With the aging of the population in the United States, the prevalence of AF is increasing at an alarming pace. It is estimated that by the year 2050, more than 5 million Americans will suffer from AF.

Definitions

- *Paroxysmal atrial fibrillation:* AF that starts and terminates spontaneously without any intervention.
- *Persistent atrial fibrillation*: AF that continues for more than 7 days or requires pharmacologic or electrical cardioversion to sinus rhythm.
- *Permanent atrial fibrillation*: AF that has been present for more than 1 year and in which attempts at cardioversion either were not attempted during this time interval or failed.
- *Lone atrial fibrillation:* Patients younger than 65 years with AF who have no clinical evidence of cardiovascular disease and are at low risk for thromboembolism.

Mechanism

AF results from triggers that initiate multiple wavelets of reentry within the left atrium. Triggers responsible for initiation of AF are usually atrial premature depolarizations (APDs) that originate from the pulmonary veins, but other supraventricular tachycardias, including atrial flutter, may also serve as triggers that initiate AF. These triggers initiate wavelets of reentry that may spin randomly around islands of functionally refractory tissue and around fixed anatomic obstacles. These wavelets of reentry are facilitated by the following left atrial characteristics: short refractory periods, regional heterogeneity of atrial refractory periods, regions of slow conduction velocities, and increased left atrial size. Exposure of the atria to AF or other rapid atrial arrhythmias can lead to electrophysiologic and structural changes (electrophysiologic remodeling) that result in a more favorable environment for the perpetuation of AF. Furthermore, structural and electrophysiologic changes may occur from the hemodynamic consequences of structural heart abnormalities (i.e., left ventricular dysfunction and mitral regurgitation) resulting in left atrial enlargement and fibrosis. The frequency of triggers and the electrophysiologic characteristics of the atrium determine the clinical burden (frequency and duration) of AF. Because continued exposure to AF itself causes electrophysiologic and structural remodeling, the natural history of paroxysmal AF is to become persistent, then permanent.

Clinical Consequences

SYMPTOMS

AF may be symptomatic or asymptomatic. Symptoms are generally caused by a combination of irregularity of the heart rhythm, rapid ventricular rate, and loss of atrial contribution to ventricular filling. Symptomatic patients may complain of palpitations, shortness of breath, lightheadedness, chest pressure, weakness, and fatigue. Symptoms of AF are not a reliable indicator of the clinical burden of AF. In one study of patients with symptomatic paroxysmal AF, asymptomatic episodes occurred 12 times more frequently than symptomatic recurrences. In another study of patients with AF who had an implantable atrial recording device, 60% of patients had asymptomatic AF. These studies highlight how unreliable symptoms may be in assessing the duration of an episode and the efficacy of treatments aimed at rhythm control. The absence of symptoms does not mean absence of AF (or absence of the risk of stroke).

QUALITY OF LIFE

Patients with AF have a significantly impaired quality of life. In a study of patients referred for electrophysiologic procedures, patients with AF had lower SF-36 scores (a measure of quality of life) compared to those with heart failure or a history of myocardial infarction. A quality of life substudy of the Canadian Trial of Atrial Fibrillation demonstrated an improvement in quality of life measures with treatment of AF.

STROKE

Patients with AF have a significantly higher risk of stroke than patients in sinus rhythm. The annual risk of stroke in patients with AF is 3% to 5% (or even higher in certain groups). The risk of stroke increases with age, history of hypertension, history of congestive heart failure, a prior history of stroke, and diabetes (Table 1). In the Stroke

TABLE 1 Risk Factors for Stroke (Nonvalvular Atrial Fibrillation)

Age >65 y
History of hypertension
History of congestive heart failure or left ventricular dysfunction
Prior history of stroke or systemic embolus
Diabetes

Prevention in Atrial Fibrillation (SPAF) study, prior thromboembolism, a systolic blood pressure of greater than 160 mm Hg, female sex, age greater than 75 years, recent stroke, and left ventricular fractional shortening of less than 25% were independent risk factors for stroke. Patients with paroxysmal AF are at the same risk as patients with chronic AF. In a subanalysis of the SPAF study, no significant difference in stroke rate was observed between patients with paroxysmal AF versus permanent AF (3.2% vs 3.3%; p = NS). Stroke may be the first presentation of patients suffering from AF. In a study of patients with cryptogenic stroke, 24% of these individuals were found subsequently to have asymptomatic bouts of AF. In contrast, patients with lone AF (i.e., without any risk factors for stroke, including no prior history of hypertension and younger than 65 years) have a low annual stroke risk (less than 1%).

CONGESTIVE HEART FAILURE

AF and heart failure often coexist. The incidence of AF in patients with heart failure ranges from 10% to 50% with the highest incidence in patients with the most severe heart failure symptoms. In patients with heart failure, AF may be either the consequence or the cause of decompensated heart failure. Patients with AF and poor ventricular rate control may suffer acute hemodynamic decompensation because of abbreviated filling times and loss of atrial contribution to ventricular filling. Furthermore, prolonged exposure to rapid rates may contribute to a chronic deterioration in left ventricular function. This phenomenon, called tachycardia-mediated cardiomyopathy, is a common cause of reversible left ventricular dysfunction. In general, patients who have an average heart rate of greater than 100 to 120 bpm are at risk of developing a tachycardia-mediated cardiomyopathy. This may be the primary etiology of newly diagnosed left ventricular dysfunction or may contribute to the worsening of a preexisting cardiomyopathy. The development of heart failure in patients with AF is associated with a higher mortality.

SICK SINUS SYNDROME

A strong association exists between sinus node dysfunction and AF. Patients with sinus node dysfunction may be completely asymptomatic or may have significant postconversion pauses resulting in presyncope, syncope, or rarely cardiac arrest. Sinus node dysfunction may result directly from the same myopathic process affecting the atrium, predisposing it to AF. Additionally, sinus node dysfunction may result from electrical remodeling from the chronic bombardment of electrical activity during repetitive bouts of AF. The contribution of the latter etiology may be reversible. In a study in which electrophysiologic study of sinus node function was assessed before and after AF ablation, significant improvement in sinus node function 6 months after successful ablation of AF was observed.

Significant sinus node dysfunction should be suspected in all patients with advanced age and in those individuals with AF conducting with a slow ventricular rate. These patients are more likely to experience significant postcardioversion pauses. Antiarrhythmic agents may further exacerbate sinus node dysfunction after cardioversion and suppress any atrial, junctional, or ventricular escape mechanisms. Sinus node dysfunction must be considered when performing electrical or pharmacologic cardioversion or when antiarrhythmic agents are employed for maintenance of sinus rhythm. Elective cardioversion and antiarrhythmic agents should be used cautiously in patients with a history of sinus node dysfunction, advanced age, slow ventricular response without atrioventricular AV nodal agents, or history of presyncope or syncope. Temporary pacing may be necessary in such patients following elective cardioversion. In some patients, permanent pacing may be necessary to allow up-titration of rate-control medications and to prevent symptomatic pauses following spontaneous conversion to sinus rhythm.

Diagnosis and Evaluation

Patients with AF may be completely asymptomatic or may complain of fatigue, lack of energy, dyspnea on exertion, palpitations, chest pressure, lightheadedness, and lower extremity edema. Findings on physical examination include absence of the A-wave on the jugular venous pulse, irregularly irregular ventricular rate, slight variations in the intensity of the first heart sound, and a weak, rapid, and irregularly irregular pulse. The radial pulse may not reflect the true apical pulse, and therefore auscultation of the apical pulse provides a more accurate assessment of the ventricular rate (pulse deficit). In patients with evidence of heart failure, an S3 gallop may be auscultated, but an S4 will be absent during AF.

The 12-lead electrocardiogram will show absence of P-waves and irregular R-to-R intervals. Occasionally, a wide QRS complex may be observed following a long-short R-to-R interval sequence, which is the manifestation of aberrancy, usually in the right bundle, and is known as Ashman's phenomenon. At times, AF may appear similar to atrial flutter in lead V1. An irregular R-to-R interval and absence of flutter waves in the inferior leads are clues that the rhythm is AF and not atrial flutter (Figure 1).

Patients with asymptomatic AF may escape diagnosis for years. In some patients, asymptomatic AF may be discovered incidentally on routine examination or after presenting with congestive heart failure or stroke. AF should be suspected in all patients presenting with cryptogenic stroke or in patients who present with new-onset

 CURRENT DIAGNOSIS

- Detailed history and physical examination
- 12-lead electrocardiogram (Figure 1)
- Echocardiogram
- 24-hour Holter monitor or loop recorder
- Laboratory tests including thyroid function test

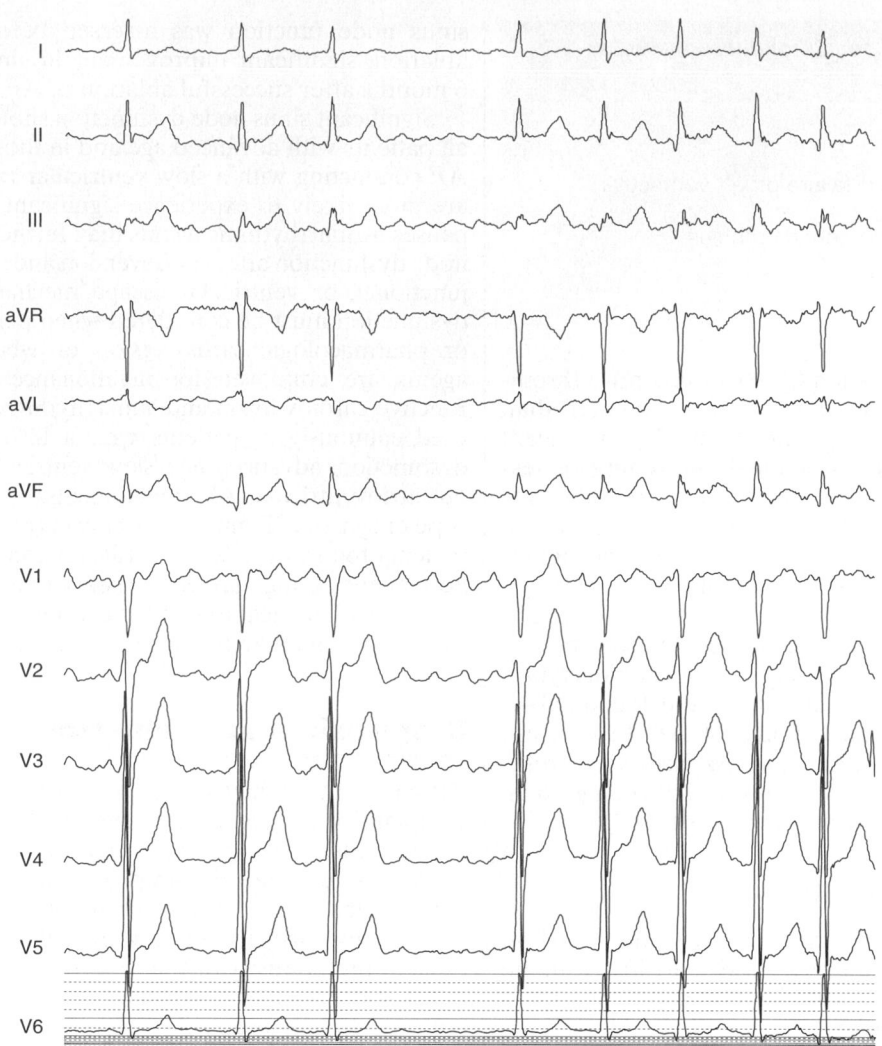

I

II

III

aVR

aVL

aVF

V1

V2

V3

V4

V5

V6

FIGURE 1. Atrial fibrillation mimicking atrial flutter. Atrial fibrillation may look "regular" in lead V1; however, the "irregularly irregular" R-to-R intervals and absence of flutter waves in the inferior leads are clues that this is atrial fibrillation and not atrial flutter

heart failure or acute decompensation of previously controlled heart failure. In such individuals, continuous telemetry monitoring during their hospitalization followed by frequent and random transmissions from an external loop recorder may lead to the diagnosis of AF. Patients with existing pacemakers or implantable defibrillators should have programmed diagnostic features optimized to capture episodes of asymptomatic AF.

In all patients with new-onset AF, causes of secondary AF should be sought (Table 2). Clinical evidence of thyrotoxicosis should be ruled out. Patients who have a pulmonary embolism may present with new-onset AF as their only clinical sign. In such cases, a careful history and high index of suspicion will lead to the appropriate diagnosis. After a careful history and physical examination, additional tests for new-onset AF should include pulse oximetry and laboratory assessment with a complete blood count, electrolytes, and thyroid function test. An echocardiogram should be performed to assess left ventricular function, valvular morphology and function, and left atrial size. In patients with pacemakers or implantable defibrillators (especially with atrial leads present), diagnostic information may be stored in the device and can be analyzed with an interrogator.

Treatment

When approaching a patient with AF, four general questions should be asked: Should the patient be acutely cardioverted? What is the patient's stroke risk, and is aspirin or warfarin indicated to mitigate the risk? Is the patient's rate adequately controlled while in AF? Is a rate or rhythm control strategy most appropriate? Once each question has been answered, treatment options for patients with AF (Table 3) include electrical cardioversion or pharmacologic cardioversion; stroke prevention with heparin (short term), warfarin, or aspirin; rate control with pharmacologic AV node blocking agents or by radiofrequency ablation of the AV junction and implantation of a pacemaker; and rhythm control with antiarrhythmic drugs, percutaneous catheter-based AF ablation, or surgical maze procedure. Selection of the appropriate treatment options for patients with AF depends on age, presence or degree of symptoms, assessment of stroke risk, co-morbid conditions, and hemodynamic effects of AF.

TABLE 2 Secondary Causes of Atrial Fibrillation

Cardiac	Noncardiac
Ischemia	Thyrotoxicosis
Hypertension	Electrolyte abnormalities
Mitral valve disease	Drugs (sympathomimetics)
Heart failure	Ethyl alcohol
Pericarditis	Hypothermia
Endocarditis	Pneumonia
Myocarditis	Pulmonary embolism
Wolff-Parkinson-White syndrome	Trauma
	Pheochromocytoma
Cardiac tumor	Noncardiac surgery
Congenital heart disease	Lung cancer
Postcardiac surgery	

SHOULD THE PATIENT UNDERGO CARDIOVERSION?

Patients should undergo immediate cardioversion if they are clinically unstable, as with hypotension, worsening heart failure, or ongoing ischemia. In all other situations, cardioversion is elective, and careful consideration of stroke risk must accompany all decisions to perform cardioversion. Patients who have been in AF for less than 48 hours can be safely cardioverted without anticoagulation. Patients who have been in AF for an unknown period of time or who have been in AF greater than 48 hours have two options: transesophageal echocardiogram-guided cardioversion while anticoagulated with heparin or warfarin, and treatment with warfarin for at least 3 to 4 weeks before cardioversion (we recommend at least weekly laboratory tests targeting an international normalized ratio [INR] more than 2 with a goal of 2 to 3). In patients who have been in AF for more than 48 hours, cardioversion is associated with a 5% to 7% risk of stroke without anticoagulation and a 1% risk of stroke with anticoagulation. This risk is irrespective of the method of cardioversion (electrical or pharmacologic). Patients

CURRENT THERAPY

- Rhythm control
  - DC cardioversion
  - Pharmacologic cardioversion
  - Antiarrhythmic agents
  - Atrial fibrillation ablation
  - Surgical maze procedure
- Rate control
  - Digitoxin
  - β-Blocker
  - Nondihydropyridine calcium channel blockers
    - Diltiazem
    - Verapamil
  - AV junction radiofrequency ablation and implantation of a permanent pacemaker
- Stroke prevention
  - Aspirin
  - Coumadin

TABLE 3 Treatment Options

Cardioversion
Electrical cardioversion
External (biphasic or monophasic waveforms)
Internal
Pharmacologic cardioversion
Ibutilide (Corvert), 1 mg IV
Propafenone (Rythmol), 450–600 mg PO
Flecainide (Tambocor), 300 mg PO

Rate Control
Pharmacologic rate control
β-Blockers
    Atenolol[1] (Tenormin) (PO)
    Metoprolol[1] (Lopressor) (PO or IV)
    Esmolol (Brevibloc) (IV; IV drip available)
Calcium channel blockers
    Diltiazem (Cardizem) (PO[1] or IV; IV drip available)
    Verapamil (Calan) (PO[1] or IV)
Digoxin

Nonpharmacologic rate control
AV node ablation and pacemaker

Rhythm Control
Antiarrhythmic drugs (Vaughn-Williams classification)

Amiodarone (Cordarone) (I, II, III)	100–400 mg/d (qd)
Propafenone (Rythmol) (IC)	450–900 mg/d (tid)
Flecainide (Tambocor) (IC)	100–300 mg/d (bid)
Sotalol (Betapace) (III, II)	160–320 mg/d (bid)
Dofetilide (Tikosyn) (III)	500–1000 µg/d (bid)
Procainamide (Pronestyl) (IA)	1000–4000 mg/d (qid)
Quinidine (IA)	600–1500 mg/d (tid)
Disopyramide (Norpace) (IA)	400–750 mg/d (qid)

Nonpharmacologic treatments
Atrial fibrillation ablation
Surgical maze procedure

Stroke prevention
Aspirin (325 mg/d)
Warfarin (Coumadin) (dosed for target INR of 2–3)

[1]Not FDA approved for this indication.
Abbreviations: INR = international normalized ratio; IV = intravenous; PO = orally.

should remain anticoagulated for a minimum of 4 weeks after cardioversion because mechanical activity may not resume immediately after sinus rhythm is reestablished. This period of 4 weeks is the absolute minimum, and we often recommend long-term anticoagulation in patients who have risk factors for stroke associated with AF.

Patients with symptomatic AF who have not converted spontaneously within 24 to 36 hours may be candidates for cardioversion. We typically perform cardioversion once before initiating an antiarrhythmic agent. Cardioversion should be discouraged in patients with frequent paroxysms of AF without the aid of an antiarrhythmic agent because their risk of recurrence after cardioversion is high. Patients with structural heart disease and AF of longer duration are less likely to remain in sinus rhythm after cardioversion, whereas patients who have structurally normal hearts and AF duration of less than 7 days are more likely to remain in sinus rhythm after cardioversion. In patients with AF for greater than 3 months, prior failed cardioversion, structural heart disease, or increased left atrial size, an appropriate antiarrhythmic agent (Table 4) may be necessary to maintain sinus rhythm successfully after cardioversion.

TABLE 4 Guidelines for Choosing Antiarrhythmic Drugs

Underlying Disorder	First Line	Second Line
No structural heart disease	Flecainide (Tambocor) Propafenone (Rythmol) Sotalol (Betapace)	Amiodarone (Cordarone) Dofetilide (Tikosyn)
Left ventricular dysfunction	Amiodarone Dofetilide	
Coronary artery disease	Sotalol	Amiodarone Dofetilide
Hypertension with left ventricular hypertrophy <1.4 cm	Flecainide Propafenone	Amiodarone Dofetilide Sotalol
Hypertension with left ventricular hypertrophy >1.4 cm	Amiodarone	

Electrical Cardioversion

Although some studies demonstrated a failure rate in more than 20% of patients, with meticulous technique, success rates of 95% can be achieved. Studies of biphasic shock waveforms have demonstrated higher success rates with less energy and less evidence of skin burns in comparison to conventional monophasic waveforms. Electrical cardioversion requires anesthesia and should be performed with an initial synchronized shock energy of 300 J when performed with monophasic shock and 150 J when performed with a biphasic shock. For best results, the shock electrodes should be placed in an anterior–posterior configuration.

Pharmacologic Cardioversion

Advantages of antiarrhythmic agents for cardioversion are convenience and not requiring anesthesia. Disadvantages include modest efficacy and the risk of proarrhythmia. Antiarrhythmic agents demonstrating efficacy in cardioversion include ibutilide (intravenous [IV]) (Corvert), amiodarone (IV or oral) (Cordarone), flecainide (Tambocor), and propafenone (oral) (Rythmol). Ibutilide, flecainide, and propafenone should not be used in patients with structurally abnormal hearts or coronary artery disease. Ibutilide is associated with a risk of torsades de pointes, and therefore careful monitoring in an intensive care unit (ICU) setting is warranted for 4 hours after administration. The risk of torsades de pointes is low in patients with no structural heart abnormalities, no coronary disease, and normal baseline QT interval.

WHAT IS THE PATIENT'S STROKE RISK AND SHOULD WARFARIN OR ASPIRIN BE INITIATED?

Patients with AF and rheumatic mitral valve disease have an 18-fold increased risk of stroke, and therefore they should be anticoagulated with warfarin. Risk factors for stroke are identified in patients with nonvalvular AF, and include age greater than 65 years, prior history of stroke, history of hypertension (even if currently well treated), history of heart failure or LV dysfunction, and diabetes. Pooled data from studies comparing warfarin and aspirin to placebo demonstrated a 62% and 22% reduction in the risk of stroke with warfarin and aspirin, respectively. Furthermore, patients who have strokes while being treated

with warfarin have smaller strokes and suffer less morbidity from their strokes. Despite the abundance of data on the beneficial effects of warfarin in stroke prevention, warfarin is underused in clinical practice. Studies of patients with AF reveal that only half of patients eligible for anticoagulation are prescribed warfarin. This is especially true in patients >65 years old who are at greatest risk for stroke and who would benefit the most from anticoagulation. Based on available clinical evidence, patients with no risk factors for stroke have a low risk of stroke (less than 1%) and may be treated with aspirin, 325 mg per day. Patients with one or more risk factors for stroke should be anticoagulated with warfarin for a target INR of 2 to 3 (Figure 2).

IS THE PATIENT ADEQUATELY RATE CONTROLLED?

Goals of rate control are to manage symptoms and to prevent tachycardia-mediated cardiomyopathy. It is important to control rate, not only at rest, but also with exercise.

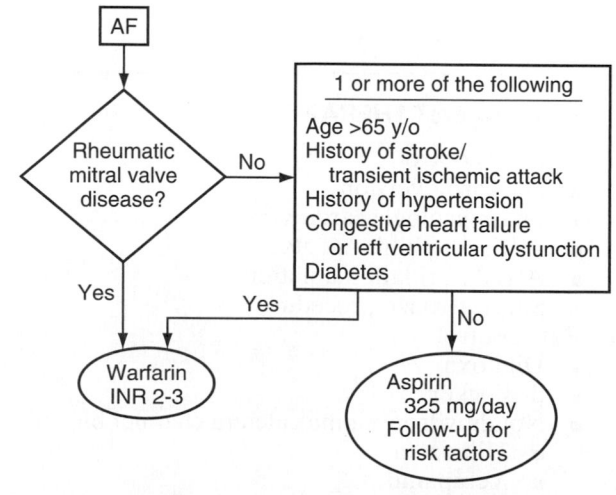

ANTICOAGULATION FOR ATRIAL FIBRILLATION

FIGURE 2. A suggested algorithm for stroke prevention with the use of aspirin or warfarin. All patients with rheumatic heart disease (especially with rheumatic mitral valve disease) should be anticoagulated. In patients with one or more risk factors, warfarin is the most effective treatment to prevent stroke. AF = atrial fibrillation; INR = international normalized ratio.

Current guidelines recommend a goal of 60 to 80 bpm at rest and 90 to 115 bpm with exercise.

Pharmacologic Treatment Strategies

Several pharmacologic agents are effective in achieving ventricular rate control. These drugs include β-blockers, calcium channel blockers (nondihydropyridine), and digoxin. Digoxin generally should not be used alone for rate control because its efficacy is poor during periods of exercise or emotional excitement. However, digoxin is effective in combination with a β-blocker or a calcium channel blocker. The two calcium channel blockers used for ventricular rate control are diltiazem (Cardizem) and verapamil. Diltiazem has the added benefit of being available as a continuous infusion for patients hospitalized with hemodynamic compromise because of excessive ventricular rates. β-Blockers, as a class, are also effective agents for rate control in patients with AF, and they may be the first choice in patients with coronary artery disease and left ventricular dysfunction.

Nonpharmacologic Rate-Control Strategies

Rate control may not be able to be achieved in some patients despite maximal doses of AV nodal agents. Furthermore, it may be difficult to treat patients who are hypotensive or in those who have paroxysmal AF with rapid ventricular response but significant sinus bradycardia (tachy-brady syndrome). Percutaneous radiofrequency ablation of the atrioventricular node is an effective means to achieve rate control in patients with drug-refractory rate control. This procedure causes complete heart block, and therefore a permanent pacemaker is required and depended on. Patients remain in AF after the procedure, and therefore lifelong anticoagulation is required after the procedure. Several observational clinical studies have shown improvement in symptoms and quality of life after the procedure. We reserve this procedure for patients >65 year old after all other means of rate control have been exhausted. In patients with tachybrady syndrome, implantation of a pacemaker may allow treatment with AV nodal agents that could not be used previously because of bradycardia.

IS A RATE-CONTROL OR RHYTHM-CONTROL STRATEGY MOST APPROPRIATE?

Recent randomized trials comparing the strategy of rate control versus rhythm control in patients with AF showed no difference in mortality or stroke risk. AFFIRM (Atrial Fibrillation Follow-Up Investigation of Rhythm Management) was the largest of the studies and randomized 4060 patients with one or more risk factors for stroke to a strategy of rate control or rhythm control. Physicians were given the option of discontinuing anticoagulation in the rhythm control group. Over a 5-year follow-up period, 63% of patients in the rhythm control group were in sinus rhythm, and more than 80% of patients in the rate-control group had adequate rate control. Although no significant difference in cumulative mortality was observed between groups, there was a trend toward reduced survival in the rhythm control group. An important finding in AFFIRM was that ischemic stroke was observed in 5.5% of the rate control and 7.1% of the rhythm control arm. Most of these strokes occurred in patients who were not anticoagulated or who were subtherapeutic on warfarin. Important conclusions from AFFIRM are that a rhythm-control strategy does not protect patients from stroke, and that a rate-control strategy is a reasonable treatment strategy for patients with AF. Important limitations in the ability to generalize this study into clinical practice is that the average age of patients in AFFIRM was approximately 70 years of age, and the majority of patients were asymptomatic. Furthermore, antiarrhythmic agents were employed for rhythm control, and it is not known whether similar conclusions can be drawn about nonpharmacologic rhythm control treatments (e.g., AF ablation, surgical maze). Therefore, it is difficult to apply these results to symptomatic patients ≤65 years old with paroxysmal AF in whom rhythm control may be more appropriate. Based on the data available, the preferred treatment strategy for asymptomatic patients >65 years old is rate control and chronic anticoagulation. Patients who have symptoms despite adequate rate control are not likely to tolerate a rate-control strategy and may be treated with antiarrhythmic agents and cardioversion if necessary. If antiarrhythmic drugs are ineffective, AF ablation may be considered in select individuals. It is important to stress that in patients with one or more risk factors for stroke, continued anticoagulation is recommended even if the patient has no symptomatic evidence of recurrent AF.

Rhythm-Control Strategies

Antiarrhythmic Drugs

Table 4 provides a list of antiarrhythmic agents. Most antiarrhythmic drugs carry a risk of serious adverse effects. These toxicities relate to the underlying cardiac condition; therefore selection of antiarrhythmic drug therapy should be made after evaluation for structural heart disease and coronary disease. The physician must carefully consider co-morbidities (especially renal and liver function), current medications, and the patient's compliance history. The long-term efficacy for maintaining sinus rhythm with antiarrhythmic agents is modest. The 1-year efficacy for maintaining sinus rhythm with antiarrhythmic drugs is approximately 40% to 60%, with 30% to 40% of patients stopping medications because of side effects or adverse effects. Amiodarone is the most effective in maintaining sinus rhythm but is associated with a number of serious side effects, including pulmonary fibrosis, hepatotoxicity, and thyroid abnormalities. Toxicity from amiodarone is proportional to cumulative doses, and therefore it is a good option at the low doses used to treat AF (typically 200 mg per day) in patients older than 65 years. Amiodarone should not be used for lifelong therapy in patients younger than 60 years. Table 4 shows a suggested algorithm for the selection of antiarrhythmic agents.

Nonpharmacologic Treatment Strategies for AF Rhythm Control

Radiofrequency Ablation

Over the last decade, percutaneous catheter-based radiofrequency ablation has emerged as a viable option for patients with paroxysmal AF. Ideal candidates for AF ablation are young patients with symptomatic paroxysmal

AF and structurally normal hearts. Complications of catheter ablation include pulmonary vein stenosis, cardiac perforation and tamponade, atrial-esophageal fistula, and stroke.

Surgical Maze Procedure

In the surgical maze procedure, lines of conduction block are strategically created in atrial tissue to create a pathway for conduction from the sinus node to the AV node. As a result, the atria are compartmentalized and propagation of multiple wavelets of reentry is prevented. The original maze procedure was performed by cutting and sewing to create these lines of conduction block. Other intraoperative methods to create these conduction barriers are now used, such as radiofrequency, microwave, and cryoablation. Currently, this procedure should be reserved for patients with AF with other indications for cardiac surgery, but a number of minimally invasive techniques for AF surgery are under investigation.

AF is a common arrhythmia associated with significant co-morbidities. Effective treatment strategies for stroke prevention, rate control, and rhythm control are available to physicians caring for patients with AF. With a thorough understanding of the mechanisms, clinical issues, and treatment options, along with careful consideration of the patient's individual clinical presentation, physicians may now make evidence-based decisions for the management of patients with AF.

REFERENCES

American College of Cardiology/American Heart Association Task Force on Practice Guidelines and the European Society of Cardiology Committee for Practice Guidelines and Policy Conferences.

Dorian P, Jung W, Newman D, et al: The impairment of health-related quality of life in patients with intermittent atrial fibrillation: Implications for the assessment of investigational therapy. J Am Coll Cardiol 2000;36:1303-1309.

Go AS, Hylek EM, Phillips KA, et al: Prevalence of diagnosed atrial fibrillation in adults: National implications for rhythm management and stroke prevention: The anticoagulation and risk factors in atrial fibrillation (ATRIA) study. JAMA 2001;285:2370-2375.

Hocini M, Sanders P, Jais P, et al: Techniques for curative therapy of atrial fibrillation. J Cardiovasc Electrophys 2004;15:1467-1471.

Hylek EM, Go AS, Chang Y, et al: Effect of intensity of oral anticoagulation on stroke severity and mortality in atrial fibrillation. N Engl J Med 2003;349:1019-1026.

Israel CW, Gronefeld G, Ehrlich JR: Long-term risk of recurrent atrial fibrillation as documented by an implantable monitoring device: Implications for optimal patient care. J Am Coll Cardiol 2004;43:47-52.

Klein AL, Grimm RA, Murray RD, et al: Assessment of cardioversion using transesophageal echocardiography. Use of transesophageal echocardiography to guide cardioversion in patients with atrial fibrillation. N Engl J Med 2001;344:1411-1420.

Page RL, Wilkinson WE, Clair WK, et al: Asymptomatic arrhythmias in patients with symptomatic paroxysmal atrial fibrillation and paroxysmal supraventricular tachycardia. Circulation 1994;89:224-227.

The atrial fibrillation follow-up investigation of rhythm management (AFFIRM) investigators: A comparison of rate control and rhythm control in patients with atrial fibrillation. N Engl J Med 2002; 347:1825-1833.

Van Gelder IC, Hagens Ve, Bosker HA, et al: A comparison of rate control and rhythm control in patients with recurrent persistent atrial fibrillation. N Engl J Med 2002;347:1834-1840.

Wang TJ, Larson MG, Levy D: Temporal relations of atrial fibrillation and congestive heart failure and their joint influence on mortality. The Framingham Heart Study. Circulation 2003;107:2920-2925.

Premature Beats

Method of
Prakash C. Deedwania, MD, and
Enrique V. Carbajal, MD

Premature beats are the most common form of cardiac arrhythmia encountered in clinical practice. Premature beats are one of the most common causes of irregular pulse and palpitations. In many instances, premature beats are not associated with any symptoms. They result from electrical depolarization of myocardium that occurs earlier than the sinus impulse. Premature beats have been referred to by a variety of names, including premature contractions, premature complexes, ectopic beats, and early depolarizations. Although no single term is ideal, most electrophysiologists refer to them as premature complexes because although the term *ectopic beat* denotes the abnormal site of origin of the depolarization, it does not necessarily require the beat to be premature, and, in some cases, ectopic rhythm indeed occurs as an escape phenomenon.

Although premature beats generally occur in patients with organic heart disease, they frequently can be seen in the absence of any structural heart disease, especially in elderly patients. Premature beats can be triggered by, or increase in frequency with, myocardial ischemia and heart failure. Premature beats can be provoked by, or occur in association with, a variety of systemic abnormalities, including electrolyte disturbances, acid-base imbalance, toxins from recreational drug and/or alcohol abuse, metabolic perturbations, systemic illnesses such as thyroid disorders, pulmonary disease, infections, and febrile illnesses, and any condition associated with increased catecholamine levels.

Most premature beats occur as a result of enhanced automaticity, but other electrophysiologic mechanisms, including reentry and triggered activity, might play a role. Based on the corresponding site of origin, premature electrical depolarizations are called *premature atrial complexes* (PACs), *premature junctional complexes* (PJCs), and *premature ventricular complexes* (PVCs). Morphologic features and timing of the premature beat on electrocardiographic (ECG) recording(s) help determine the site of origin and the nature of premature complexes. Premature beats can occur in a repetitive fashion as *bigeminy* (after every other normal beat), *trigeminy* (after each sequence of two normal beats), or *quadrigeminy* (after each sequence of three normal beats). They also can occur as two or three successive premature beats, defined as *couplets* and *triplets*, respectively. In this article, the primary focus is on single premature beats.

Premature Atrial Complexes

PACs are the most common form of atrial arrhythmias that can originate at any site in the atria. The exact morphology of the atrial activation (P wave) varies depending on the site of origin of the PAC. Careful and systematic examination of the ECG features of PACs usually can distinguish them from PVCs.

ELECTROCARDIOGRAPHIC FEATURES

The cardinal features of PACs include their prematurity with reference to sinus beats, abnormal P wave morphology, and, in most cases, QRS morphology that is similar to that of sinus beats. The P wave morphology of the PAC generally differs from the sinus P wave unless the premature complex originates in the high right atrial area adjacent to the sinus node, in which case distinguishing PACs from sinus arrhythmia may be difficult. Although sinus arrhythmias are generally phasic in nature, being influenced by the respiratory cycle, this feature would be helpful in differentiating from high right atrial PACs only when the PACs are frequent and repetitive. When the PAC occurs quite early in the diastolic phase, the P wave may not be obvious on surface ECG because it is often hidden in the preceding T wave and would be evident only by watching carefully for the notched or peaked T wave.

If the PAC is too premature, it might fail to conduct to the ventricles if the atrioventricular (AV) node is refractory owing to conduction of the preceding sinus impulse. Such nonconducted PACs are called *blocked PACs*, and they are important because they can be confused with instances of AV block. Such erroneous interpretation can be avoided by simply remembering a common rule of thumb that requires normal successive P-P intervals for all sinus beats, including the interval for a blocked P wave, before considering the diagnosis of AV block. Although most PACs have a normal or prolonged PR interval, the relationship of the PAC to the subsequent QRS complex depends on the site of origin of the PAC and the prematurity index. For example, a PAC originating in the lower atrial area near the AV node generally has a shorter PR interval, whereas a PAC that is quite premature and originates in the upper left atrial area might have a longer than usual PR interval. In general, the PR interval of a PAC is inversely related to its prematurity.

Because most PACs are able to depolarize the sinus node, they usually can reset the sinus automaticity; therefore, the subsequent pause following most PACs is generally less than compensatory because the sinus node fires earlier than expected. In this case, measurement of the P-P interval between the sinus P wave preceding the PAC and the P wave following the PAC is generally less than twice the basic sinus cycle length. This is in contrast to the full compensatory pause often observed in conjunction with PVCs. In some cases, the PAC collides with the sinus impulse in the perinodal tissue and thus fails to reset the sinus node, thereby resulting in a full compensatory pause.

In general, electrical depolarization below the AV node is normal with PAC and results in an unchanged (baseline) QRS complex. Aberrant conduction, however, may be encountered when the PAC reaches the infranodal tissue during the period when it is still partially refractory. Most frequently, the aberrant conduction usually occurs when a short coupled PAC follows a long pause in patients with sinus bradycardia (long-short cycle). This usually results in a right bundle-branch block pattern and is commonly referred to as the *Ashman phenomenon*.

CLINICAL FEATURES

Although PACs can occur in normal individuals of all ages, they are quite infrequent except in the elderly. Their frequency increases with age; as many as 50% to 70% of the elderly may have occasional PACs. Some elderly individuals without organic heart disease have frequent PACs and occasionally atrial bigeminy or two to three PACs in a row. Whether the increased frequency of PACs in these individuals is secondary to senile amyloidosis, myocardial fibrosis, or diastolic dysfunction secondary to aging-related changes in the heart is not known. PACs are extremely common in patients with heart disease and in patients with acute as well as chronic respiratory failure. The frequency of PACs can increase markedly during periods of acute febrile illness, shock states, and metabolic disorders, especially in patients with hyperthyroidism and conditions associated with increased catecholamine levels. Use of excessive caffeine, alcohol, tobacco, and recreational drugs can increase the frequency of PACs. In patients with acute myocardial infarction (MI), frequent PACs usually are precursors of atrial fibrillation and occur in association with ventricular failure. In general, the presence of frequent PACs in the setting of acute MI is an indicator of poor prognosis.

In general, PACs are benign except when they are a marker of an underlying cardiopulmonary disorder(s). The major clinical importance of PACs is related to the increased risk of atrial tachyarrhythmias in patients with an established history of such arrhythmias as well as in the elderly who are generally at high risk for atrial fibrillation. As indicated earlier, in rare instances the blocked PACs may be confused with episodes of AV nodal block; however, careful examination of the ECG features described previously easily establishes the correct diagnosis and avoids unnecessary pacemaker implantation.

TREATMENT

The correction of an underlying structural cardiopulmonary disorder and other precipitating factors (e.g., electrolyte or metabolic abnormalities) usually is all the treatment that is needed. No specific treatment is generally required in most patients because PACs usually are benign except in patients with a history of recurrent atrial tachyarrhythmias, for example, atrial flutter/fibrillation. In such patients, specific treatment may be indicated and could include a β-blocker or a heart rate-modulating calcium channel blocking agent such as verapamil (Calan) or diltiazem (Cardizem). Recent studies have shown that verapamil is quite effective in patients with frequent PACs

CURRENT THERAPY

- In general, premature beats in patients without evidence of organic heart disease do not require any specific antiarrhythmic therapy because generally there is no significant increased risk of life-threatening arrhythmia.
- Correction of any underlying structural cardiopulmonary disorder and other precipitating factors (e.g., electrolyte or metabolic abnormalities).
- Suppression of PVCs using currently available antiarrhythmic drugs (except for amiodarone) is not advisable for most patients primarily because of the increased risk of proarrhythmic effects of these drugs.
- In the occasional patient who is disabled by annoying symptoms due to PVCs, a trial of β-blocker therapy should be considered and often is effective in many patients.

and multifocal atrial tachycardia in the setting of acute or chronic ventilatory insufficiency. In patients who are at risk for recurrent atrial fibrillation, treatment with a specific antiarrhythmic agent, such as propafenone (Rythmol) or flecainide (Tambocor), may be beneficial; however, these drugs should be used only when the patient has a history of recurrent atrial flutter/fibrillation because of the increased risk of proarrhythmia, especially in the presence of organic heart disease such as recurrent ischemia or heart failure.

Premature Junctional Complexes

PJCs are rarely seen in normal individuals and are infrequently encountered even in patients with organic heart disease. When present, PJCs can occur due to abnormal automaticity or reentry phenomenon. Although digitalis toxicity is cited as a common etiologic factor, PJCs also can occur in the setting of MI, myocarditis, and electrolyte/metabolic disturbances.

ELECTROCARDIOGRAPHIC FEATURES

The ECG characteristics of PJCs are distinct from those of PACs in that the P wave usually is inverted in the inferior leads (II, III, and aVF) because of retrograde conduction to the atria from the ectopic foci in the junctional area. The second feature of PJCs is that the PR interval almost always is shorter than the normal PR interval because of the proximity of ectopic foci to the AV node and bundle of His. In most cases, the P wave might not even be visible on surface ECGs because it lies hidden within the QRS complex. Rarely, the P wave precedes the QRS complex when the ectopic impulse traverses to the atria before traveling down to depolarize the ventricle. In general, the infranodal conduction of PJCs is normal, and thus the QRS morphology of the conducted PJCs is similar to that noted during sinus rhythm. When the PJC is closely coupled to the preceding sinus beat, aberrant conduction might occur if the impulse traverses down the bundle

branch during the relative refractory period (most frequently manifesting as a right bundle-branch block pattern). Because in many instances no obvious P wave accompanies a PJC, aberrantly conducted PJCs may be hard to differentiate from PVCs.

In some instances when PJCs occur during the period when the AV node as well as the infranodal conduction systems both are refractory, the PJC may encounter both retrograde and antegrade blocks for impulse propagation. In such situations, no P wave or QRS complex is related to the PJC. Although the ectopic impulse would be invisible on a surface ECG, it would penetrate a portion of the conduction system and thus make it partially or completely refractory to conduction of the subsequent sinus impulse. This would be manifested as a sudden prolongation of subsequent PR interval in case of partial refractoriness or as an episode of "pseudo AV nodal block" due to the blocked sinus beat if the infranodal tissue were unable to conduct the sinus impulse. Thus, even though some PJCs might not have any surface ECG complexes, their presence can be suspected based on their influence on the conduction of the following sinus beat owing to the electrophysiologic phenomenon described as "concealed conduction."

CLINICAL FEATURES

PJCs usually are not seen in normal persons and are rarely encountered in cardiac patients except in the setting of digitalis intoxication and infrequently in the setting of MI or myocarditis. In patients with digitalis toxicity, PJCs may lead to junctional tachycardia, occasionally resulting in palpitation, but are rarely associated with hemodynamic compromise. Because in some cases concealed conduction of PJCs might result in periods of varying degrees of pseudo AV blocks, it is clinically important to recognize their presence in order to prevent undue concern and avoid inappropriate pacemaker implantation.

Premature Ventricular Complexes

PVCs are the most common form of arrhythmia and can be encountered frequently in both healthy individuals as well as in patients with a variety of cardiac disorders. PVCs are often triggered by electrolyte abnormalities, acid-base imbalance, metabolic perturbations, hypoxia, and ischemia.

ELECTROCARDIOGRAPHIC FEATURES

PVCs occur as a result of premature depolarization of the ventricles due to ectopic foci in the ventricular myocardium or Purkinje fibers. In general, PVCs result in wide QRS complexes with the T wave axis usually opposite to that of the QRS. In the vast majority of cases, PVCs do not conduct retrogradely and thus do not result in a distinct P wave. The sinus beats may, however, continue uninterrupted and thus manifest as an instance of AV dissociation in conjunction with PVCs. For the same reason, because PVCs usually do not conduct retrogradely and depolarize the atrium and the sinus node, there usually is a full compensatory pause in contrast to the partial compensatory pause generally seen with PACs. In patients with slow sinus rates, however, interpolated PVCs might occur. If the ectopic foci for PVCs are located high in the His-Purkinje system, the resulting premature complexes may have a narrow QRS morphology quite similar to that seen during sinus rhythm. Additionally, if the PVCs occur rather late, in close proximity to the sinus impulse, there may also be a narrow complex QRS because of fusion between the normal depolarization due to sinus impulse and the abnormal activation sequence from the ectopic foci. In the instance of fusion beats, a normal P wave precedes the QRS. The PR interval is shorter, and the QRS morphology may be only partially altered. In some cases, this might give the appearance of an intermittent bundle-branch block or preexcitation (Wolff-Parkinson-White syndrome) pattern.

Based on the morphologic features of PVCs, they have been classified as *uniform* or *multiform;* they also have been referred to as *unifocal* or *multifocal.* Also recommended is classification of PVCs based on their coupling interval with the preceding sinus beat. PVCs with a short coupling interval near or on the previous T wave have been described as showing R-on-T phenomenon; alternatively PVCs may have long coupling intervals. Based on the underlying electrophysiologic mechanism responsible for PVCs, the coupling interval may be *fixed*, as in reentrant beats, or *variable*, as seen with ventricular parasystole. PVCs may have a repetitive pattern, for example, bigeminy or trigeminy, or they may occur in pairs. It is now believed that repetitive PVCs, such as couplets and triplets, are prognostically more important than just the frequency of isolated PVCs.

CLINICAL FEATURES

PVCs can be recorded frequently in normal individuals, and, similar to PACs, their frequency increases with age. In patients without organic heart disease or without prior evidence of sustained ventricular tachyarrhythmias, the mere presence of frequent PVCs is not considered prognostically important. However, individual exceptions do exist, and the clinician is advised to evaluate each given patient accordingly. In patients with organic heart disease, PVCs are the most common form of arrhythmia and carry significant prognostic importance, especially in survivors of acute MI and patients with recurrent ischemia and advanced heart failure. It has been well established during the past 2 decades that frequent PVCs occurring during the acute phase of MI are associated with an increased risk of sustained ventricular arrhythmias in the initial 48 hours, but they do not predict long-term outcome or risk of arrhythmic events. More recently, it has been shown in patients receiving thrombolytic therapy that PVCs, particularly episodes of nonsustained ventricular tachycardia, increase in frequency but are generally short-lived and represent a sign of myocardial reperfusion. However, the presence of frequent PVCs during the postdischarge evaluation of survivors of MI is indicative of a poor prognosis.

Although as many as 80% to 90% of patients with chronic heart failure have frequent PVCs, the results of several recent studies have shown that only the presence of nonsustained ventricular tachycardia (defined as three or more PVCs in a row) at a rate greater than 100 bpm is strongly predictive of an increased risk of sudden cardiac death in these patients. This is in clear contrast to the findings of several large clinical trials, which showed that more than 10 PVCs per hour in post-MI patients are predictive of a poor prognosis and an increased risk of arrhythmic death.

Overall, the association between PVCs and an increased risk of ventricular tachyarrhythmias and sudden cardiac death appears to be related not only to the frequency and complexity of PVCs but also to the severity of underlying structural heart disease. For example, a patient with mitral valve prolapse and frequent PVCs would be at relatively lower risk for arrhythmic events compared to a patient with advanced heart failure who has repetitive PVCs and episodes of nonsustained ventricular tachycardia. Proper evaluation of the risk of PVCs has become more crucial than ever because most currently available antiarrhythmic drugs have the potential for causing serious adverse reactions, including proarrhythmias, in patients with advanced cardiac disorders.

TREATMENT

In general, PVCs in patients without evidence of organic heart disease do not require any specific antiarrhythmic therapy because generally there is no significantly increased risk of life-threatening arrhythmia. However, when PVCs are associated with disabling palpitations, reassurance and treatment with β-blockers (atenolol [Tenormin], metoprolol [Toprol-XL]) may help in relieving symptoms. In patients with systemic illness or other provoking factors (e.g., electrolyte abnormalities or acid-base imbalance), immediate correction of the underlying abnormality usually is associated with beneficial effects.

Because of the associated poor prognosis with PVCs in the setting of acute MI, common practice in the past consisted of routine administration of intravenous lidocaine (Xylocaine) in an effort to suppress PVCs during the initial phase of acute MI. However, because recent data suggest that the routine use of lidocaine is not necessary and often can be harmful, lidocaine should be avoided because of the risk of serious adverse reactions, especially central nervous system side effects such as seizures in the elderly. With the ready availability of cardiac monitoring, it now is possible to accurately identify a harbinger of ventricular tachyarrhythmias early in the coronary care unit, so prophylactic use of lidocaine is generally not recommended. Furthermore, results from several studies and their meta-analyses have demonstrated that routine use of prophylactic lidocaine during the acute or healing phase of MI does not alter the overall mortality in patients with acute MI.

In contrast, it is well established that the presence of frequent PVCs (≥10 per hour) during the postdischarge evaluation of survivors of acute MI predicts an increased risk of arrhythmic death and overall cardiac mortality. Numerous trials have been conducted with a variety of different antiarrhythmic drugs. Many of the studies demonstrated that suppression of PVCs with most currently available antiarrhythmic drugs is not beneficial in reducing the increased risk associated with PVCs. The Cardiac Arrhythmia Suppression Trials (CAST I and II) clearly demonstrated that, compared to placebo, treatment with class Ic antiarrhythmic drugs (which primarily work by slowing conduction) was associated with an increased risk of arrhythmic death despite adequate suppression of PVCs. The findings from CAST I and II, as well as several other clinical trials, indicate that although frequent PVCs may be a marker for an adverse event, suppression of PVCs with type I antiarrhythmic agents does not favorably influence the associated increased risk of death. Results from the Canadian Amiodarone Myocardial Infarction Arrhythmia Trial (CAMIAT) and the European Myocardial Infarct Amiodarone Trial (EMIAT) suggest that in patients with frequent PVCs in the post-MI setting, use of amiodarone (Cordarone), a complex drug with predominantly class III antiarrhythmic properties, in combination with β-blockers is associated with improved outcome. However, because of the associated drug toxicity with long-term amiodarone use, it is generally considered suitable only for the high-risk cohort (although many patients with low left ventricular ejection fraction now undergo implantation of an automatic internal cardiac defibrillator).

In general, suppression of PVCs using currently available antiarrhythmic drugs (except for amiodarone) is not advisable for most patients, primarily because of the increased risk of proarrhythmic effects of these drugs. In the occasional patient who is disabled by annoying symptoms due to PVCs, an initial trial of β-blocker therapy should be considered and is effective in many patients. Correction of the provoking factors and appropriate management of any underlying heart disease often are beneficial in managing patients with frequent PVCs.

REFERENCES

Barrett PA, Peter CT, Swan HJ, et al: The frequency and prognostic significance of electrocardiographic abnormalities in clinically normal individuals. Prog Cardiovasc Dis 1981;23:299.

Boutitie F, Boissel J-P, Connolly SJ, et al, EMIAT and CAMIAT Investigators: Amiodarone interaction with β-blockers: Analysis of the merged EMIAT (European Myocardial Infarct Amiodarone Trial) and CAMIAT (Canadian Amiodarone Myocardial Infarction Trial) databases. Circulation 1999;99:2268.

Brodsky M, Wu D, Denes P, et al: Arrhythmias documented by 24 hour continuous electrocardiographic monitoring in 50 male medical students without apparent heart disease. Am J Cardiol 1977;39:390.

Cairns JA, Connolly SJ, Roberts R, et al: Randomised trial of outcome after myocardial infarction in patients with frequent or repetitive ventricular premature depolarisations: CAMIAT. Lancet 1997;349:675.

Echt DS, Liebson PR, Mitchell B, et al: Mortality and morbidity in patients receiving encainide, flecainide, or placebo. N Engl J Med 1991;324:781.

Fleg J, Kennedy H: Cardiac arrhythmias in a healthy elderly population. Chest 1982;81:302.

Julian DG, Camm AJ, Frangin G, et al: Randomised trial of effect of amiodarone on mortality in patients with left-ventricular dysfunction after recent myocardial infarction: EMIAT. Lancet 1997;349:667.

Morganroth J: Premature ventricular complexes. Diagnosis and indications for therapy. JAMA 1984;252:673.

Romhilt D, Chaffin C, Choi S, et al: Arrhythmias on ambulatory electrocardiographic monitoring in women without apparent heart disease. Am J Cardiol 1984;54:582.

Rosen KM, Rahimtoola SH, Gunnar RM: Pseudo A-V block secondary to premature nonpropagated His bundle depolarizations: Documentation by His bundle electrocardiography. Circulation 1970;42:367.

Ruskin JN: Ventricular extrasystoles in healthy subjects. N Engl J Med 1985;312:238.

Simpson RJ Jr, Cascio WE, Schreiner PJ, et al: Prevalence of premature ventricular contractions in a population of African American and white men and women: The Atherosclerosis Risk in Communities (ARIC) study. Am Heart J 2002;143:535.

Heart Block

Method of
Albert A. Del Negro, MD

The general term *heart block* refers to a group of electrophysiologic disturbances of atrioventricular (AV) conduction. The causes are many, and clinical clues to the significance of AV block as well as mandates for therapy often are deduced from surface electrocardiography (ECG). In other cases, only invasive characterization of heart block with electrophysiologic study provides the direction for therapy.

Starting with Wenckebach and Mobitz, AV block in all its forms remained a descriptive phenomenon until the advent of invasive testing in the 1960s and 1970s; such testing refined our understanding of the significance of the various forms of AV block. In this article, we necessarily start with the anatomy and physiology of the AV conduction system, which serve as a basis for understanding treatment rationales.

Functional Anatomy of the Atrioventricular Conduction System

The AV node lies at the apex of Koch's triangle, the limits of which in the right heart are the septal portion of the tricuspid valve anteriorly, the ligament of Todaro posteriorly, and the subeustachian isthmus from the inferior septal aspect of the tricuspid valve to the coronary sinus. The AV node itself consists of a mixture of atrial muscle cells, stellate P cells, and transitional cells imbedded in a collagen matrix. On the left side of the ventricular septum, it lies just under the noncoronary sinus of the aortic valve.

The proximal portion of the AV node receives impulses from internodal tracts connecting with the sinus node. These tracts convey impulses using the sodium fast channel. However, in the AV node, conduction is slowed as the sodium fast channel gives way to slow calcium channel-mediated conduction. Sympathetic as well as parasympathetic influences are richly present in the AV node, and these influences have profound effects on automaticity as well as on conduction. The distal portion of the AV node, also known as the *compact AV node*, is somewhat insulated from electrical influences by the surrounding collagen matrix. As the node passes into the transitional area from the atrium to the ventricle, it gives rise to the bundle of His. Data from invasive electrophysiologic testing suggest that the bundle of His is the origin of nodal or junctional rhythm. Furthermore, sympathetic and parasympathetic influences remain strong within this area. Therefore, AV nodal block is not usually associated with cardiovascular collapse because default to the lower-order idiojunctional pacemaker usually sustains cardiac output with a satisfactory heart rate. Furthermore, parasympathetic withdrawal and sympathetic stimulation can speed idiojunctional rhythm and satisfactorily support the heart rate.

Below the area of the bundle of His, however, the major fascicules arise and form the bundle branches. Whereas the right bundle branch fans out throughout the right septum, in most individuals the left bundle branch has at least two major subdivisions. These are the left anterior superior division, a slender division that originates along with the right bundle branch, and the left posterior inferior division, a stout division that originates separately from the right bundle branch and superior division of the left bundle branch. Of major importance is that although sympathetic influences still may have some limited effect on automaticity below the bundle of His, parasympathetic influences that mediate conduction and automaticity are absent. The result of heart block at this level is reliance on idiofascicular or idioventricular pacemakers, which usually are too slow to support the heart rate and hemodynamics satisfactorily. Because of this situation, it is convenient to divide the AV conduction system into two generally different areas: a proximal area (AV node) and a distal area (His bundle, bundle branches, and their divisions).

From the aspect of coronary anatomy, the body of the AV node before the bundle branches (proximal area) is supplied by a branch of the right coronary artery in 90% of individuals, whereas the area of the conduction system below the His bundle (distal area) is fed by branches from the left anterior descending coronary artery in almost 100% of individuals. These facts have implications for the significance of AV block associated with inferior myocardial infarction and anterior myocardial infarction.

Electrocardiographic Classification of Heart Block

For the purposes of ECG interpretation, the three patterns of AV block are first-, second-, and third-degree AV block. *First-degree AV block* occurs when there is prolongation of the PR interval without failure of conduction of each atrial impulse or P wave. The upper limit of PR conduction time is 0.21 seconds measured in the limb leads of the scalar ECG. Although PR prolongation to greater than 0.21 seconds is generally thought to reflect prolongation of conduction through the AV nodal portion of the conduction system, in reality this may not be the case because PR interval prolongation may reflect delay within the AV node, His bundle, proximal bundle branches, or a combination of the three.

Second-degree AV block occurs when some or any P waves fail to propagate to the ventricle. As with first-degree AV block, this pattern does not clearly imply the locus of the block. Second-degree AV block is further divided. In *type I block*, first described by Wenckebach in 1899, there is gradual prolongation of the PR interval until a P wave fails to conduct to the ventricle. This pattern retains his name: *Wenckebach block*. (Part of Wenckebach's genius is that he theorized the electrophysiologic happenings of failed AV conduction without the use of an ECG recording. He used a smoked-drum recorder to record the jugular venous and carotid waves from an individual with second-degree AV block.) Some years later, Mobitz described a second form of second-degree AV block, in which there is no prolongation of the PR interval before loss of conduction. This form is called *Mobitz II*, or *type II*, *block*. Necessary to the diagnosis of both type I and type II second-degree AV block is the occurrence of at least relatively regular atrial timing, because multiple closely coupled premature atrial beats may fail to conduct even with normal AV conduction.

Although type I second-degree AV block usually implies that the AV node is the locus of the block, especially if the QRS is narrow (<0.120 second), this may not always be the case because the block may occur instead within the bundle of His. If the QRS is wide (bundle branch block), there is at least a 25% to 30% chance that type I block occurs within or below the His bundle.

High-grade AV block is a general term for sequentially nonconducted P waves but with some P waves having the ability to conduct; thus, it is a form of second-degree AV block. The diagnosis, as for type I and type II second-degree AV block, requires relatively regular atrial activity. The term implies that fewer than 50% of P waves are able to conduct to the ventricle.

Third-degree AV block occurs when no atrial activity is capable of conduction. This results in AV dissociation with the ventricles and atrial beating at different and unrelated rates. Generally speaking, the atrial rate should be faster than the ventricular rate for the diagnosis to be made, because junctional tachycardia (arising from the His-bundle area) may occur at a rate faster than normal sinus rhythm. In such a case, there is AV dissociation but not necessarily AV block because P waves have no chance for conduction owing to the faster usurping junctional rate. Third-degree AV block can occur at the AV nodal level or at the His-Purkinje level; that is, it may be due to either proximal or distal block.

CLINICAL ASPECTS OF HEART BLOCK

The AV node and the His-Purkinje system have separate embryologic origins, and their failure to unite in development results in congenital AV block. Originally thought to be a benign entity not necessarily requiring pacemaker therapy, the contemporary view is that pacing at an early age is desirable to prevent the development of cardiomyopathy.

Several acquired forms of heart block have varied significance for therapy. Table 1 lists several of the more common causes of AV block. Heart block associated with use of medications generally is reversible with discontinuation of therapy. AV block that is confined to the AV node usually is reversible with time and the course of the clinical entity responsible for it. Even temporary pacing is rarely required because this form of "proximal" block results in preservation of responsive escape mechanisms from the distal AV node and proximal bundle of His that will support the heart rate at physiologic levels. Furthermore, withdrawal of parasympathetic influences with atropine will speed idiojunctional rhythm to which proximal AV block patients default.

Diseases such as acute diphtheria and acute rheumatic fever provoke first- or second-degree block that resolves with the acute illness. The appearance of AV nodal block in an otherwise healthy young patient without structural heart disease should always suggest the possibility of Lyme disease, a reversible infectious cause of AV block. Often the telltale fever and rash are absent, and AV block may be the first manifestation of the illness. Serologic studies can

TABLE 1 Clinical Presentation and Indications for Pacing in Acquired Atrioventricular Block

Etiologies	Locus	Pacing Therapy
Idiopathic (aging) fibrosis	Distal	Always
Sarcoidosis	Proximal	Usually
Hemochromatosis	Proximal and distal	Always
Lyme disease	Proximal	Always unless reversible
β-Blockers, Ca^{2+} channel blockers	Proximal	Never if reversible
Na^+ channel blockers	Distal	Never if reversible
Calcific aortic stenosis	Distal	Always
Anterior infarction	Distal	Always
Inferior infarction	Proximal	Almost never
Neuromuscular disorders	Unclear—likely proximal	Always

confirm the diagnosis, and antibiotics can reverse AV block if started early enough. Thiamine deficiency (beriberi), which results in AV nodal block, may not be reversible because scarring within the AV node may permanently impair AV nodal function. Infiltrative diseases causing AV nodal block may cause permanent AV block and lead to the need for permanent pacing. These diseases include sarcoidosis, rheumatoid arthritis, and hemochromatosis, the last of which can also create delay and conduction impairment below the His bundle.

HEART BLOCK IN ACUTE MYOCARDIAL INFARCTION

Few events in clinical cardiology are more threatening than AV block in acute myocardial infarction. AV block, either second degree or complete third degree, complicates inferior myocardial infarction in approximately 30% of cases. However, because the condition is due to AV nodal block, it almost always is reversible and very rarely requires permanent pacing. Cautious use of atropine can reverse AV block or at least speed idiojunctional rhythm that results from AV nodal block in this setting. Aminophylline[1] also may speed such rhythms and even abolish AV block in this setting because AV block in acute infarction seems to be due to local elaboration of adenosine for which aminophylline is the antidote and not due to the AV nodal infarction itself.

Unlike inferior infarction, acute anterior myocardial infarction rarely provokes AV block. The mechanism of AV block in anterior infarction is necrosis of the proximal fascicles arising from the bundle of His. This is not completely reversible even if conduction block resolves, in marked contrast to inferior infarction. Block at this level results in default of rhythm to so-called idiofascicular or idioventricular rhythm, usually with an inadequate heart

rate (20–35 per minute) and subsequent hemodynamic collapse.

An antecedent clue to impending AV block in anterior infarction is the development of bifascicular block (right bundle-branch block and left anterior fascicular block) or new left bundle-branch block. Data suggest the incidence of acute AV block in such patients is upward of 40%. The appearance of such a new conduction abnormality in acute anterior myocardial infarction mandates at least temporary transvenous pacing even before AV block occurs. AV block occurring in anterior infarction with or without antecedent conduction delay, even if transient, also mandates prophylactic temporary transvenous pacing followed by eventual permanent pacing because the natural history of this form of AV block is malignant, and progression to permanent complete AV block is the rule.

Use of positive chronotropic agents for heart rate support in patients with heart block has no role in acute infarction. In the patient with unstable infarction, agents such as dopamine, isoproterenol (Isuprel), and epinephrine have the potential to induce life-threatening tachycardia. Furthermore, prophylactic use of antiarrhythmic agents such as lidocaine and amiodarone (Cordarone) for suppression of potential ventricular arrhythmias in patients with heart block can only worsen AV block in acute infarction. These antiarrhythmic drugs, if necessary for arrhythmia suppression, should be used only after temporary transvenous ventricular pacing has been established.

ADDITIONAL DIAGNOSTIC AIDS

Table 1 lists the indications for permanent pacing in heart block. Note that type II AV block is an absolute indication for permanent pacing. This is the case because all examples of type II AV block reported in the contemporary medical literature are due to block within or below the His bundle. Invasive cardiac electrophysiologic testing can assist in the differential diagnosis of AV block, that is, whether proximal (potentially not requiring permanent pacing) or distal (permanent pacing absolutely required). Such testing involves positioning a temporary recording electrode via the femoral transvenous route within the area of the His bundle. Unique ECG recordings from this area easily identify the level of AV block, which has enormous significance for therapy. Furthermore, the recording electrode thereafter can provide temporary transvenous pacing when positioned within the right ventricle. Stressing the conduction system by atrial pacing during invasive electrophysiologic testing in ambiguous cases adds to the clinical decision-making process.

The finding of reversible proximal block does not rule out the use of temporary or even permanent ventricular pacing. Good clinical judgment should assist in the decision about pacing. Pacing is indicated if the heart rate is chronically below 35 bpm or if pauses of 2 seconds or longer occur while the patient is awake, irrespective of the locus of block. Distal block, irrespective of symptoms, should always prompt pacing. In 2002, a joint committee of the American Heart Association, the American College of Cardiology, and the North American Society of Pacing and Electrophysiology (now named the Heart Rhythm Society) set standards for temporary and permanent pacing.

---

[1]Not FDA approved for this indication.

TABLE 2 Indications for Temporary Pacing in Atrioventricular Block

Symptomatic second-degree degree AV block
Hemodynamically significant bradycardia due to AV block
Anterior myocardial infarction with new or age-
  indeterminate right bundle-branch block
Third-degree AV block with bradycardia-induced ventricular
  tachycardia/ventricular fibrillation

Abbreviation: AV = atrioventricular.

Pacing Modalities

TEMPORARY CARDIAC PACING

Table 2 lists the indications for temporary cardiac pacing. Several modalities of temporary pacing exist, and they all are useful. Their utility and applicability depend somewhat on the immediacy of the need for pacing as well as the expertise of the physician in attendance; however, properly executed, each can provide heart rate support for the profoundly bradycardic patient.

TEMPORARY TRANSCUTANEOUS PACING

Temporary transcutaneous pacing can be a lifesaving temporary treatment of sudden and unanticipated hemodynamically deleterious bradycardia of any mechanism, including heart block. Passage of current applied from cutaneous large-surface-area electrodes positioned so that the heart is in the path of the current flow will result in cardiac excitation and contraction. Energies of at least 40 to 60 mA are required, but care must be taken not to mistake the contraction of intercostal and pectoral muscles associated with device discharge for cardiac contraction. Verification of a palpable pulse coincident with electrical stimulation is essential. The ECG recorded from modern stimulation devices is filtered to dampen the stimulus of pacing, enabling accurate assessment of cardiac response to the pacing stimulus. Sedation plays an important role in the patient so treated, because associated intercostal or diaphragmatic stimulation can be uncomfortable.

TEMPORARY PERCUTANEOUS TRANSTHORACIC PACING

In the author's experience, temporary percutaneous transthoracic pacing is little used because it is invasive, involves cardiac puncture, and is seldom effective because it is commonly a last resort applied late in the resuscitative effort. The technique involves passage of a needle from the subxiphoid area aiming for the left shoulder until right ventricular blood is aspirated. A J-shaped electrode wire is passed into the right ventricle, and the needle is withdrawn. Recording a unipolar ECG from the needle can verify contact with the right ventricle instead of the right atrium.

TEMPORARY TRANSVENOUS ENDOCARDIAL PACING

The preferred temporary pacing modality for heart block is temporary transvenous endocardial pacing. Placed from the percutaneous transfemoral, subclavian, or internal jugular route, this technique requires use of fluoroscopy. Complications of the technique include cardiac perforation and the risk of cardiac tamponade. Electrode dislodgment is common unless a temporary active-fixation electrode with a helical coil on the distal portion of the electrode that worms its way into the ventricular wall with rotation of the temporary pacing electrode is used. Currently available electrodes are very flexible and require introduction through a guiding catheter that itself is relatively rigid and that can easily perforate the thin-walled right ventricle. This technique requires an experienced practitioner for safe use.

Positioned from the femoral route, passage into the right ventricular apex is relatively easy. Positioned from the internal jugular or subclavian route, inadvertent passage into the coronary sinus is relatively simple. This is not a satisfactory position from which to pace the heart. This pitfall can be avoided by first passing the pacing catheter from above into the right ventricular outflow tract and into the pulmonary artery, thereafter withdrawing it into the body of the right ventricle and to the right ventricular apex.

After acceptable placement of the temporary pacing electrode, satisfactory parameters of pacing and sensing should be ensured. If the parameters are suitable, 0 silk sutures should be used to secure the electrode to the adjacent skin, coiling the electrode to inhibit traction and dislodgment. Placing a sterile barrier over the assembly at the insertion site will help to ensure impediment to infection. Changing the insertion site at least every 5 days also will prevent problems with infection and venous thrombosis.

Once placed, a temporary pacemaker electrode can facilitate entry of stray electrical currents to the patient's heart. Modern coronary care units are carefully constructed to ensure safe grounding of all electrical devices in the environment. However, the additional measure of placing the connection between the temporary pacing electrode and the temporary pacer cable within a latex or nitrile glove and sealing it with tape will ensure protection against stray currents that can inadvertently induce ventricular fibrillation.

Most patients endure temporary right ventricular pacing well, but those with reduced left ventricular compliance, right ventricular infarct, or postoperative coronary artery bypass surgery may actually deteriorate hemodynamically. The condition results from loss of regular association of the atrium with the ventricle. Temporary dual-chamber pacing will restore hemodynamic balance to such patients. Temporary atrial pacing as well as ventricular pacing is required, and special temporary pacemakers capable of this task are readily available.

Spontaneous electrode dislodgment of temporary pacer electrodes occurs in upward of 20% of patients. This percentage is lower with use of temporary active-fixation electrodes. A rising threshold may be the first clue to impending loss of pacing from dislodgment. The appearance of ventricular ectopy similar in configuration to paced beats signals mechanical stimulation of the myocardium from electrode dislodgment. These events should alert the clinician to re-establish satisfactory parameters of pacing and sensing by repositioning or replacing the pacing electrode.

Table 3 Indications for Permanent Pacing in Atrioventricular Block

Symptomatic second-degree AV block at any level
Second-degree AV block within the His-Purkinje system
Third-degree AV block
Mobitz II (type II) AV block
AV block in anterior infarction even if transient
Bilateral bundle branch block (likely distal)

Abbreviation: AV = atrioventricular.

PERMANENT PACING

Table 3 lists the indications for permanent cardiac pacing. Percutaneous access of subclavian or axillary veins easily facilitates permanent pacemaker implantation. Cutdown to access the cephalic vein is less common today because the percutaneous route in experienced hands is simple and quick, and the complication of pneumothorax is infrequent and, if promptly recognized, causes little morbidity. Currently, implanters more frequently are cardiologists rather than surgeons because, as devices have become more sophisticated and complicated, the intricacies of pacemaker programming and follow-up are more in the cardiologic than the surgical realm.

After achievement of satisfactory electrode placement verified by measures of sensing and pacing, the operator creates a subcutaneous pocket to accommodate the pacer and its electrode(s). Pacing at high outputs usually confirms the absence of diaphragmatic or intercostal stimulation, which would necessitate electrode repositioning. Individual patient clinical profiles and needs determine programming parameters. These include voltage outputs, parameters of sensing P waves and R waves, and programmed schemes to detect and potentially treat arrhythmias. Modern pacers have the ability to alert the monitoring physician about occult arrhythmias (e.g., ventricular tachycardia or atrial fibrillation) that have a major impact on treatment.

Following implantation, observation in a monitored setting can ensure normal and satisfactory pacemaker function. Early problems include sensing failure, induction of mechanically induced ventricular ectopy, and failure of pacing to capture the heart. Pacing electrode dislodgment is the most frequent cause of these postoperative problems. Although pacemaker programming can overcome several problems, a thorough evaluation postimplantation can assure that repeat surgery to reposition the electrodes is not necessary.

Follow-up of patients with pacemakers has the aim of reducing the energy required of pacing based on office or clinical evaluation of the minimum energy requirement for successful and consistent cardiac pacing (threshold determination). This conservation of battery energy lengthens battery life and reduces the need for frequent surgeries to replace depleted pacer batteries. Frequency of office visits depends on prior performance history and the patient's condition, but visits once yearly are adequate for patients with single-chamber pacers and twice yearly for patients with dual-chamber pacers. Transtelephonic monitoring on a regular basis detects arrhythmias if patients are symptomatic and provides assessment of battery function by recording and verifying pacing rates. A rate reduction when a magnet is placed over the pacer signals the need for device replacement.

PACING DEFIBRILLATORS

The choice of pacing therapy now embraces an entirely new modality of therapy. The implantable cardiac pacer/defibrillator provides heart rate support with atrial and ventricular pacing, arrhythmia monitoring with reports, and stored and real-time electrograms available to the monitoring physician during clinical interrogation. These devices also provide therapy in the form of antitachycardia pacing and cardioversion/defibrillation shock therapy. These devices not only can treat ventricular arrhythmias, but some models also deliver therapy for atrial arrhythmias. Recent studies of patients with depressed left ventricular function document survival improvement in patients with poor left ventricular function (ejection fraction <35%) treated with implantable cardioverter-defibrillators. This constitutes therapy for primary prevention of sudden cardiac arrest in a highly vulnerable population. These facts make it imperative that preoperative assessment of pacemaker candidates with heart disease, especially those with congestive heart failure, include estimations of ejection fraction. Those on a stable and standard regimen for treatment of heart failure, including β-blockers, angiotensin-converting enzyme inhibitors, or angiotensin receptor blockers and spironolactone (Aldactone) when appropriate, with ejection fractions less than 35% should receive a pacing defibrillator rather than a pacemaker alone even in the absence of demonstrable ventricular arrhythmias.

Chronic cardiomyopathy of any etiology results in suboptimal systolic effort of the left ventricle. Magnifying this problem is the frequent association of cardiomyopathy with left bundle-branch block. Because activation of the left ventricle begins at the interventricular septum and spreads outward to activate the basal-posterior portion of the left ventricle last, the presence of left bundle-branch block results in markedly delayed posterolateral wall activation. This considerable delay promotes left ventricular dyssynchrony, in which two already impaired walls move not as a unit but separately. In patients with left ventricular dysfunction and class II or III heart failure and bundle-branch block, cardiac function and clinical class improve with pacing and cardiac resynchronization therapy. Right ventricular stimulation occurs at the right ventricular apex via the traditionally implanted right ventricular electrode. Left ventricular activation timed with right ventricular activation occurs from an electrode placed within the coronary sinus and advanced through the coronary venous system to the lateral wall on the left ventricular epicardial surface. Resynchronization occurs by attachment of right and left ventricular electrodes to a cardiac resynchronization therapy device that delivers separate but simultaneously timed stimuli to these two places and resynchronizes ventricular activation and contraction.

Studies of heart block and its treatment have progressed considerably in the last several years. The parallel growth in the technology of pacing and the several scientific studies evaluating the natural history of cardiomyopathy of any etiology have resulted in the application of pacing therapy coupled with defibrillator therapy to an increasing number of patients. As time passes and our understanding of conduction system disease increases, the number of patients treated with the various forms of pacing therapy likely will grow exponentially.

REFERENCES

Bardy GH, Lee KL, Mark DB, et al: Amiodarone or an implantable-cardioverter defibrillator for congestive heart failure. N Engl J Med 2005;352:225-2237.

Bristow MR, Saxon LA, Boehmer J, et al; for the Comparison of Medical Therapy, Pacing, and Defibrillation in Heart Failure (COMPANION) Investigators: Cardiac resynchronization therapy with or without an implantable defibrillator in advanced chronic heart failure. N Engl J Med 2004;350:2140-2150.

Gregoratos G, Abrams J, Epstein AE, et al: ACC/AHA/NASPE 2002 guideline update for implantation of cardiac pacemakers and antiarrhythmia devices. Circulation 2002;106:2145-2161.

Moss AJ, Zareba W, Hall WJ, et al; Multicenter Automatic Defibrillator Implantation Trial II Investigators: Prophylactic implantation of a defibrillator in patients with myocardial infarction and reduced ejection fraction. N Engl J Med 2002;346:877-883.

Young JB, Abraham WT, Smith Al, et al: Combined cardiac resynchronization and implantable cardioversion defibrillation in advanced chronic heart failure: The MIRACLE ICD Trial. JAMA 2003;289:2685-2694.

Tachycardias

Method of
Richard H. Hongo, MD, and
Nora Goldschlager, MD

Tachycardia in the adult is defined as a heart rate of more than 100 beats per minute (bpm) and can be characterized as either supraventricular or ventricular. *Supraventricular* tachycardias (SVTs) are abnormal rhythms that originate from structures above the ventricles, including the atria, the sinoatrial nodal tissue, and the atrioventricular (AV) node. SVTs also involve accessory pathways that are abnormal electrical connections between supraventricular and ventricular tissue separate from the AV node left behind during embryonic development. *Ventricular* tachycardias (VTs) originate in, and involve, either the His-Purkinje conduction system or the ventricular myocardium.

There are three electrophysiologic mechanisms of tachycardia:

1. Abnormal Automaticity: An abnormal increase in depolarization rate of pacemaker cells, or spontaneous depolarization of non-pacemaker cells.
2. Reentry: A repetitive loop of electrical activation around a circuit formed by barriers to rapid conduction (such as scar tissue).
3. Triggered Activity: An abnormal cell depolarization triggered by oscillations in membrane potential during, or immediately following, normal depolarization (early or delayed "after depolarizations").

A tachycardia is generally described as *focal* when the mechanism is either abnormal automaticity or triggered activity; however, reentry can also appear focal if the activation circuit is small.

Tachycardias present clinically as palpitations, dizziness, presyncope, or frank syncope. Sudden cardiac death (SCD) can be the presenting manifestation of ventricular tachyarrhythmias, and much more rarely, of supraventricular tachycardia. Patients can also be asymptomatic, and the tachycardia is discovered incidentally.

The analysis of a 12-lead electrocardiogram (ECG) obtained during tachycardia, when available, is the first step in defining the tachycardia mechanism (Figure 1). The tachycardia is first assessed as regular or irregular. An irregular rhythm to the QRS complexes without a pattern to the irregularity (called an *irregularly irregular rhythm*) is the hallmark of atrial fibrillation (AF). If the tachycardia is regular, the next step is assessing the QRS complex duration as narrow or wide. A narrow (<120 milliseconds) QRS complex tachycardia is invariably supraventricular in origin. A wide (≥120-millisecond) QRS complex tachycardia can be either ventricular or supraventricular with preexisting bundle branch block, aberrant conduction, or preexcitation.

Approximately 80% of wide QRS complex tachycardias are VT. A history of heart disease in a patient with wide QRS complex tachycardia has a positive predictive value of 95% for VT. Typical bundle branch block patterns are observed in patients with SVT when there is a fixed or aberrant (rate-related) conduction block within the Purkinje system. Although a QRS morphology atypical for bundle branch block, or a QRS duration of more than 160 milliseconds makes VT more likely, these findings can be seen in patients with SVT who have hyperkalemia or severe dilated cardiomyopathy. AV dissociation, established by identifying either P waves dissociated from QRS complexes, capture beats, or fusion beats, is diagnostic of VT. A *capture beat* is a sinus beat that conducts down the AV node and captures (depolarizes) the entire ventricle before its depolarization from the VT source. It appears as a narrow QRS complex in the midst of wide complexes. A *fusion beat* is a sinus beat that conducts down the AV node and fuses with depolarization from the VT source, resulting in a beat intermediate in width and morphology between normal and wide complexes. A preexcited SVT is suspected when a slurred upstroke of QRS complexes resulting in shortened PR interval (delta waves) is present during sinus rhythm.

Hemodynamic stability must be established in patients with sustained tachycardia. Any tachyarrhythmia should be immediately treated with electrical cardioversion if the blood pressure is excessively low or consequences of hypoperfusion (cognitive impairment, chest pain, heart failure) are present. VT tends to lead to hemodynamic instability because it generally occurs in patients with structural heart disease. Because a delay in treating VT can be life threatening, a wide QRS complex tachycardia of unclear origin should be considered VT until proved otherwise. Antiarrhythmic drugs can be administered as initial therapy to stable patients (Table 1).

Adenosine (Adenocard) is an especially useful drug in managing narrow QRS complex tachycardia because of its selective blocking effect on the AV node and its elimination by cellular uptake within seconds. AV nodal reentrant tachycardia (AVNRT) and AV reciprocating tachycardia (AVRT) (see later) are reliably terminated by adenosine (Adenocard) because the AV node is critical to the circuit of these tachycardias (Table 2). Some types of

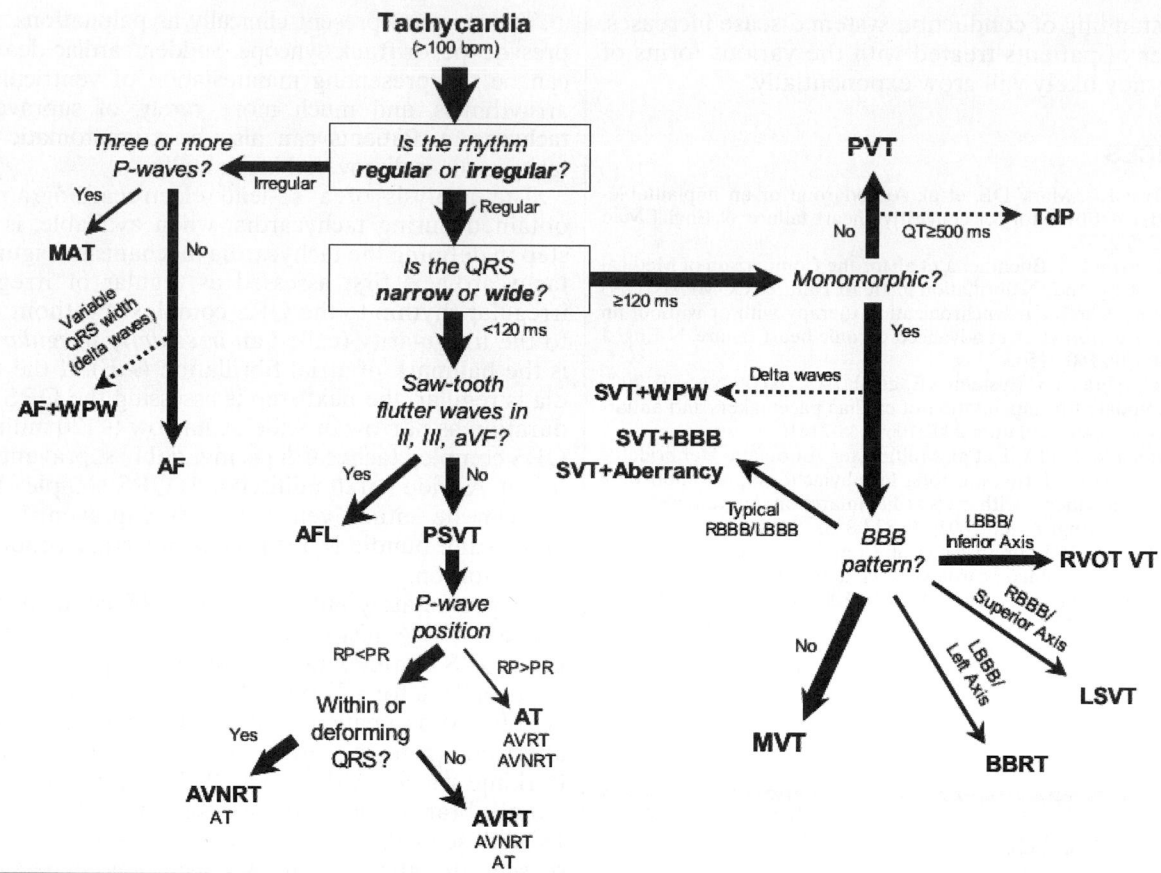

FIGURE 1. General algorithm for diagnosing tachycardias by electrocardiographic criteria. The relative weight of the arrows approximates the frequency of arrhythmias. AF = atrial fibrillation; AFL = atrial flutter; AT = atrial tachycardia; AVNRT = atrioventricular nodal reentrant tachycardia; AVRT = atrioventricular reciprocating tachycardia; BBB = bundle branch block; BBRT = bundle branch reentry tachycardia; LBBB = left bundle-branch block; LSVT = left septal ventricular tachycardia; MAT = multifocal atrial tachycardia; MVT = monomorphic ventricular tachycardia; PSVT = paroxysmal supraventricular tachycardia; PVT = polymorphic ventricular tachycardia; RBBB = right bundle-branch block; RVOT = right ventricular outflow tract; SVT = supraventricular tachycardia; TdP = torsades de pointes; VT = ventricular tachycardia; WPW = Wolff-Parkinson-White syndrome.

TABLE 1 General Guide to Antiarrhythmic Therapy

Vaughn Williams Class	Specific Agent	Preparation/Dosage	Typical Use	Comments
Class IA Na$^+$ channel blockade (prolongs RP, QT)			Prevention of SVT in patients without SHD	Rarely used to prevent VT; increased mortality in patients with SHD
	Procainamide (Pronestyl)	IV: load = 1 g IV: infusion = 1-4 mg/min PO: 250-500 mg q6h	Termination of VT or AF; prevention of SVT	Especially appropriate for stable preexcited AF
	Quinidine (Quinaglute)	PO: 324-648 mg q8-12h	Prevention of SVT	
	Disopyramide (Norpace)	PO: 200-400 mg bid	Prevention of SVT	
Class IB Na$^+$ channel Blockade	Lidocaine (Xylocaine)	IV: load = 1 mg/kg IV: infusion = 1-4 mg/min	Termination of VT; prevention of VT	Probably less effective than amiodarone or procainamide except during active ischemia
	Mexiletine (Mexitil)	PO: 200-300 mg q8h	Prevention of VT	Contraindicated in heart block

TABLE 1 General Guide to Antiarrhythmic Therapy—cont'd

Vaughn Williams Class	Specific Agent	Preparation/Dosage	Typical Use	Comments
Class IC Na$^+$ channel Blockade			Prevention of SVT in patients without SHD	Increased mortality in patients with SHD or ischemia
	Flecainide (Tambocor)	PO: 50-150 mg q12h	Prevention of SVT	Contraindicated in heart block
	Propafenone (Rythmol)	PO: 150-300 mg q8h	Prevention of SVT	May be used prn to terminate AF or AFL
Class II β-Blockade	Metoprolol (Lopressor)	PO: 25-100 mg bid	Decreases VR in SVT; prevention of SVT	Multiple oral β-blockers available. Metoprolol is shown as an example
	Esmolol (Brevibloc)	IV: load = 500 μg/kg IV: infusion = 50-200 μg/kg/min	Decreases VR in SVT	Preferred IV preparation because of short half-life
Class III K$^+$ channel blockade (prolongs RP, QT)	Sotalol (Betapace)	PO: 80-160 mg bid	Prevention of SVT or VT	Dosage interval decreased with renal failure
	Amiodarone (Cordarone)	IV: load = 150 mg, then 1 mg/min × 6 h, then 0.5 mg/min × 18 h PO: 200-400 mg qd	Termination of VT; prevention of SVT or VT	Often started with an oral load (800-1200 mg qd)
	Dofetilide (Tikosyn)	PO: 125-500 μg bid	Prevention of AF	Dosage decreased with renal failure
	Ibutilide (Corvert)	IV: 0.01 mg/kg up to 1 mg over 10 min	Cardioversion of AF, AFL	
Class IV Ca^{++} channel blockade				Dihydropyridines have no significant AV nodal blocking effect
	Verapamil (Calan)	PO: 120-240 mg bid	Decreases VR in SVT; prevention of SVT	Should be avoided in patients with WPW
	Diltiazem (Cardizem)	IV: infusion = 5-15 mg/h PO: 120-360 mg qd	Decreases VR in SVT; prevention of SVT	Should avoid if tachycardia is possibly VT
Miscellaneous	Digoxin (Lanoxin)	IV: load = 0.5 mg, then 0.25 mg q6h × 2 doses PO: 0.25-0.625 mg qd	Decreases VR in SVT	Should be avoided in patients with WPW
	Adenosine (Adenocard)	IV: 6-12 mg rapid bolus	Termination of SVT	Diagnostically useful

Abbreviations: AF = atrial fibrillation; AFL = atrial flutter; AV = atrioventricular; RP = refractory period; SHD = structural heart disease; SVT = supraventricular tachycardia; VR = ventricular rate; VT = ventricular tachycardia; WPW = Wolff-Parkinson-White syndrome.

VT, especially right ventricular outflow tract (RVOT) VT, are also adenosine (Adenocard) sensitive (Table 3). Termination of a tachycardia with adenosine (Adenocard) is not always diagnostic of the type of arrhythmia because of the wide range of adenosine-sensitive rhythms. Transient AV nodal block with continuation of an atrial arrhythmia, such as atrial flutter or atrial tachycardia, however, is diagnostic (Figure 2).

Ongoing advances in catheter ablation of tachyarrhythmias and establishment of the efficacy of implantable cardioverter defibrillators (ICDs) has changed the chronic management of tachycardias. Whereas the mainstay

TABLE 2 Electrocardiographic Features of Supraventricular Tachycardia

Tachycardia	P Morphology	AV Relationship	RP Interval*	AV Node Dependence[†]	Response to Adenosine (Adenocard)[‡]
Sinus tachycardia	Same as sinus	1:1	Long RP	No	Transient suppression of sinus and/or AV block
Atrial tachycardia	Different from sinus	Usually 1:1 or 2:1	Long RP, can be short RP	No	Transient suppression, termination, or AV block
MAT	≥3 different P waves	Usually 1:1	Long RP, variable	No	Transient AV block
Atrial fibrillation	No discrete P waves	Variable	Not applicable	No	Increased AV block
Atrial flutter	Flutter, sawtooth	Usually 2:1, variable	Not applicable	No	Flutter waves with AV block
AVNRT	Retrograde[§], within, or distorting QRS	Usually 1:1, may be 2:1 AV or VA block	Very short RP	Yes	Usually terminates with AV block
AVRT	Retrograde[§]	1:1	Short RP	Yes	Usually terminates with AV block

*The RP interval is termed long RP if RP > PR, and short RP if RP > PR.
[†]AV node dependence indicates that the AV node is an obligate component of the tachycardia mechanism.
[‡]Adenosine (Adenocard) is not FDA approved for diagnosing supraventricular tachycardia.
[§]A retrograde P wave, caused by retrograde conduction from either the AV node or an accessory pathway, is negative in leads II, III, aVF.
Abbreviations: AV = atrioventricular; AVNRT = atrioventricular nodal reentrant tachycardia; AVRT = atrioventricular reciprocating tachycardia; MAT = multifocal atrial tachycardia; VA = ventriculoatrial.

of tachycardia management has been suppression with antiarrhythmic drugs, most tachycardias are now amenable to cure with catheter ablation. Patients with severe dilated cardiomyopathy are at increased risk for SCD and can be protected with ICD implantation. Recurrent VT, requiring frequent ICD shocks, is treated with antiarrhythmic drug suppression. Catheter ablation, aimed at disrupting reentry circuits within a ventricular scar, also can be performed to decrease VT episodes and thus the frequency of ICD shocks.

TABLE 3 Electrocardiographic Features of Ventricular Tachycardia

Tachycardia	QRS Morphology	RS Interval	QT Interval	Response to Adenosine (Adenocard)	Response to Verapamil (Calan)
Scar-related VT	Variable, not typical BBB pattern, multiple morphologies common	>100 msec	Normal	−	−
BBRT	LBBB/LAD		Normal	−	−
LS VT	RBBB/superior axis	60-80 msec	Normal	−	+
RVOT VT	LBBB/inferior axis		Normal	+	+
ARVC VT	Usually LBBB pattern, multiple morphologies common		Normal	−	−
Polymorphic VT	Variable amplitude		Normal	−	−
Torsades de pointes	Variable amplitude, "turning on point"		Prolonged	−	−

Abbreviations: + = sensitive; − = no response; ARVC = arrhythmogenic right ventricular cardiomyopathy; BBB = bundle branch block; BBRT = bundle branch reentry tachycardia; LAD = left axis deviation; LBBB = left bundle-branch block; LS = left septal; RBBB = right bundle-branch block; RVOT = right ventricular outflow tract; VT = ventricular tachycardia.

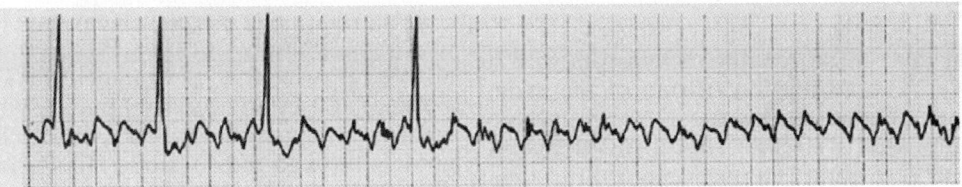

FIGURE 2. Adenosine (Adenocard)-induced atrioventricular block revealing an underlying atrial flutter.

Supraventricular Tachyarrhythmias

SINUS TACHYCARDIAS

Enhanced automaticity of the sinus node appropriate to physiologic demand results in physiologic sinus tachycardia. The P-wave morphology and frontal plane axis is that of sinus rhythm, and gradual (rather than abrupt) changes in heart rate are characteristic of normal sinus node function. Sinus tachycardia is not an arrhythmia, and therapy is thus directed toward the underlying cause, such as fever, anemia, hypotension, hypoxemia, thyrotoxicosis, myocardial ischemia, and pain.

In contrast, increase in sinus node automaticity disproportionate to the level of exertion can be caused by inappropriate sinus tachycardia, of which the mechanism is not fully understood. Treatment can be attempted with beta- or calcium channel blockers but is often inadequate despite large doses. Modification of the sinus node region with catheter ablation is occasionally effective (<25% of cases), but the recurrence of symptoms is high and thus the procedure has been virtually abandoned. The diagnosis of inappropriate sinus tachycardia should be made only after other causes of tachycardias that originate in and around the sinus node, such as sinus node reentry tachycardia, are excluded. Sinus node reentry tachycardia is diagnosed by its abrupt onset and reproducibility with pacing during electrophysiology (EP) study, and it can be cured with catheter ablation in the majority of cases. Calcium channel blockers and digoxin (Lanoxin) may prevent sinus node reentry tachycardia; beta-blockers have been reported to be less effective.

ATRIAL TACHYCARDIAS

In focal atrial tachycardia, the impulse originates from a location within the atria separate from the sinus node (called "ectopic"). The underlying mechanism can be abnormal automaticity, reentry using a discrete but small circuit, or triggered activity. The P wave morphology differs from that of sinus rhythm and depends on the location of the focus. The PR interval is normal (unless there is associated AV block), and thus a long RP interval, relative to the PR interval, is present during tachycardia. The demonstration of atrial tachycardia during induced AV block (e.g., by carotid sinus massage, Valsalva maneuver, adenosine [Adenocard]) is diagnostic. Digoxin toxicity can cause a unique combination of AT and AV block, which is rarely seen today because of the decreasing use of digoxin (Lanoxin).

The management of atrial tachycardias can be challenging. Class IC[1] and III[1] antiarrhythmic drugs can be tried, but suppression of atrial tachycardia is often difficult. Even without complete suppression of the atrial arrhythmia, AV nodal blocking agents can be used to try and control ventricular rate and symptoms. The success of catheter ablation of a focal atrial tachycardia ranges between 70% and 90% and depends on the ability to reproduce the tachycardia and localize the atrial focus during EP study.

The presence of multiple active atrial foci results in multifocal atrial tachycardia (MAT). This arrhythmia is an irregularly irregular rhythm with three or more discrete P wave morphologies and PR intervals; nonconducted P waves are common. MAT frequently occurs in the setting of severe pulmonary disease, and therapy is directed toward the underlying disease because the arrhythmia itself is generally not destabilizing hemodynamically. AV nodal blocking agents can be used to slow an excessively rapid heart rate; reactive airway disease often limits the use of beta-blockers.

ATRIAL FIBRILLATION

Atrial fibrillation (AF) is an atrial arrhythmia that lacks organized atrial activity or organized input into the AV node His-Purkinje system, resulting in an irregularly irregular QRS rhythm without discrete P waves. The clinical presentation of AF varies and depends on an interplay between focal atrial triggers and diseased atrial myocardium. In younger (e.g., age <75), more symptomatic patients, the suppression of AF with antiarrhythmic drugs is initially pursued. Catheter ablation techniques that can isolate electrically the regions within the atria that are important to the initiation and maintenance of AF are available, and they have demonstrated success rates of up to 90% in selected patients. In older (e.g., age >65), less symptomatic patients, ventricular heart rate control with AV nodal blocking agents may be the preferred approach. If adequate rate control cannot be achieved, catheter ablation of the AV node with implantation of a permanent ventricular pacemaker can be performed. Warfarin (Coumadin) is recommended for all patients with risk factors for thromboembolic stroke: congestive heart failure, hypertension, age 75 years or older, diabetes, and history of transient ischemic attack or stroke.

---

[1]Not FDA approved for this indication.

ATRIAL FLUTTER

Atrial flutter is an intra-atrial reentry tachycardia with a circuit that involves a large portion of one of the atria. Typical (right atrial) flutter is the most common type of atrial flutter and uses a circuit around the tricuspid annulus. Continuous activation of a portion of the atria via this reentry circuit results in a characteristic undulating baseline likened to a sawtooth pattern (see Figure 2) in ECG leads II, III, and aVF. In other forms of atrial flutter (atypical atrial flutters), the undulations are less distinct and the classic sawtooth pattern may be absent.

The atrial rate in flutter is 250 to 300 bpm; the ventricular rate depends on the degree of AV conduction block (e.g., 2:1, 3:1, etc.). Ventricular rate control can be achieved with AV nodal blocking agents, but unlike AF, good control is often difficult. As with AF, the risk of a thromboembolic stroke is a concern if the arrhythmia persists beyond 48 hours. Unless cardioversion is urgently indicated because of hemodynamic instability, the patient should be anticoagulated for more than 3 weeks (international normalized ratio [INR] of 2 to 3) or have intracardiac thrombus excluded by transesophageal echocardiogram before cardioversion. Cardioversion can be performed either by external shock or with medications such as ibutilide (Corvert) infusion. The risk of postconversion stroke is considered the same with either modality.

In typical flutter, the reentry circuit passes through an isthmus of atrial tissue bordered by the inferior vena cava and tricuspid annulus. This isthmus is readily accessible during EP study, and catheter ablation of the isthmus has become the mainstay of therapy for typical flutter with success rates exceeding 90% and the need for a repeat procedure is rare (<5%). Atypical atrial flutters involve less well-defined reentry circuits, and thus catheter ablation success is variable.

PAROXYSMAL SUPRAVENTRICULAR TACHYCARDIAS

Episodes of paroxysmal supraventricular tachycardia (PSVT) have abrupt onset and termination. The sudden onset of palpitations, difficulty breathing, and anxiety in PSVT not infrequently leads to an erroneous diagnosis of panic attacks. Because the episodes can be transient and PSVT typically occurs in patients without structural heart disease or an abnormal ECG, the arrhythmia may remain undiagnosed for years. PSVT typically is a regular, narrow QRS complex tachycardia with a rate between 150 and 250 bpm.

Atrioventricular nodal reentrant tachycardia (AVNRT) is the most common PSVT (approximately 60%), and the number of women affected is twice that of men. AVNRT is a reentry tachycardia that involves a slow and fast conducting pathway connecting the AV node to the atrium. The central location of the AV node results in simultaneous, or near-simultaneous, excitation of the atria and ventricles. Although the P waves are most commonly obscured and buried within the QRS complexes, at times the P waves can deform the QRS morphology, manifesting as pseudo R′ waves in lead V_1 or as pseudo S waves in leads II, III, and aVF. The complaint of neck pounding is a sensitive (93%) and specific (100%) symptom of AVNRT and is caused by right atrial contraction occurring against a closed tricuspid valve during ventricular systole.

Atrioventricular reentry tachycardia (AVRT) accounts for approximately 30% of PSVTs the number of men affected is twice that of women. AVRT is a reentry tachycardia that uses an accessory pathway between atrium and ventricle. Approximately 90% of AVRT conducts antegradely through the AV node His-Purkinje system (orthodromically) and retrogradely through the accessory pathway to the atrium; this results in a narrow QRS complex tachycardia with P waves distinct from the QRS complexes. Conduction over the accessory pathways is typically rapid, and therefore the RP interval is short relative to the PR interval. Reverse activation of the reentry circuit, or antidromic (retrograde conduction through AV node) AVRT, results in a wide QRS complex tachycardia with maximal delta waves because of exclusive excitation of the ventricles through the accessory pathway. Because both the atrium and ventricle are part of the reentry circuit, loss of 1:1 AV relationship during tachycardia excludes AVRT as the diagnosis. Most of the remaining 10% of patients with PSVT have atrial tachycardias.

When medical management is preferred for the treatment of PSVTs, AV nodal blocking agents can be used. Digoxin[1] and verapamil (Calan)[1] should be avoided in the chronic management of patients with AVRT and preexcitation because these drugs are associated with serious hemodynamic decompensation during preexcited AF, should this occur. Both class I and III antiarrhythmic drugs can be used to treat AVNRT and AVRT. Infrequent episodes of AVNRT that are well tolerated and responsive to vagal maneuvers can be observed without chronic therapy.

Currently, fewer patients with PSVT are managed with chronic drug therapy. Catheter ablation of SVT is a safe and curative procedure that can be offered as first-line therapy. The slow pathway in AVNRT and the accessory pathway in AVRT are targeted for ablation with a success rate between 95% and 98%. Major complications are rare and include complete AV block (1%), pericardial tamponade (0.6%), and stroke (0.2%).

WOLFF-PARKINSON-WHITE SYNDROME

In Wolff-Parkinson-White (WPW) conduction, ventricular preexcitation (early activation of the ventricle) occurs over an accessory pathway that electrically connects the atrium directly to the ventricle. This results in a loss of the isoelectric PR segment and in a slurring of the initial portion of the QRS complex that is termed the delta wave (Figure 3). Ventricular preexcitation appears to be a benign condition in asymptomatic patients. But patients with symptoms of palpitations, dizziness, or syncope have an approximate 1 in 1000 annual risk of SCD. The diagnosis of WPW syndrome is ventricular preexcitation accompanied by symptoms, thus implying a SCD risk.

In addition to orthodromic and antidromic AVRT, other SVTs can occur in WPW syndrome. The most concerning, and a cause of SCD, is preexcited AF, an arrhythmia recognized by an irregularly irregular rhythm with varying QRS width (Figure 4). The width of the QRS complex reflects the degree of ventricular preexcitation relative to normal AV nodal His-Purkinje conduction. Antegrade conduction over the accessory pathway can result in AF-inducing ventricular

---

[1]Not FDA approved for this indication.

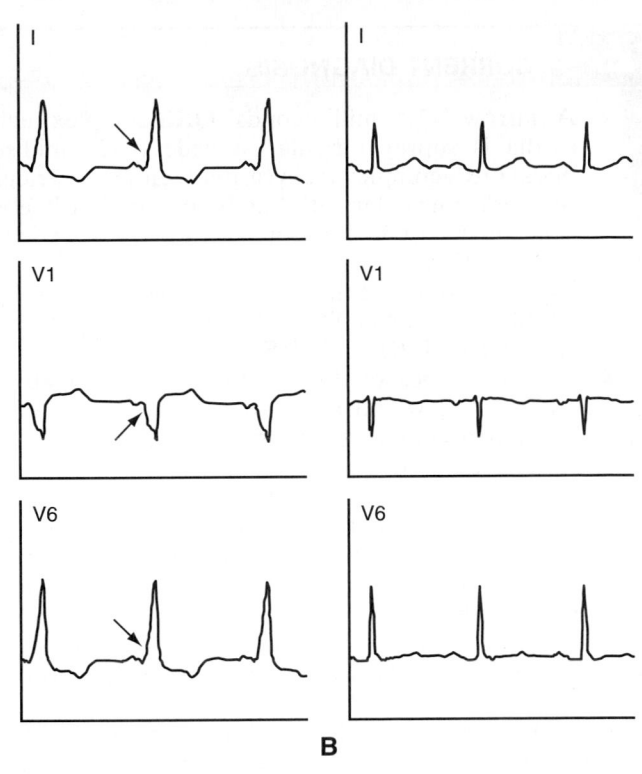

FIGURE 3. Electrocardiogram leads I, V₁, and V₆, before and after catheter ablation of an atrioventricular accessory pathway. **A,** Arrows indicate delta waves. **B,** Delta waves no longer present.

fibrillation (VF). The risk of VF is higher with more rapid antegrade accessory pathway conduction; an accessory pathway is characterized as malignant if the shortest RR interval during preexcited AF is less than 250 milliseconds. In contrast, the loss of delta waves during sinus rhythm, either spontaneously or with treadmill testing, is evidence of a poorly conducting accessory pathway that is benign.

Hemodynamic instability during preexcited AF should prompt immediate external cardioversion. The use of AV nodal blocking agents can be deleterious because they do not slow conduction over the accessory pathway. Verapamil and digoxin have been associated with precipitation of hemodynamic collapse and death, and should

be avoided. Intravenous procainamide (Pronestyl)[1] is the pharmacologic treatment of choice because of its ability to block conduction in the accessory pathway. EP study with catheter ablation of the accessory pathway is recommended for patients with WPW and AF. Catheter ablation of the accessory pathway eliminates the risk of SCD, and can cure the AF, in some (<5%) patients. EP study and prophylactic ablation of the accessory pathway should also be considered in patients with WPW syndrome if the occurrence of an arrhythmia during performance of their occupation poses a hazard (such as pilots, bus drivers, and professional athletes).

Ventricular Tachyarrhythmias

VENTRICULAR ARRHYTHMIAS AND STRUCTURAL HEART DISEASE

In both ischemic and nonischemic dilated cardiomyopathy, ventricular scar-related reentry tachyarrhythmias are a major cause of death. Ventricular tachycardia, defined as three or more ventricular beats at a tachycardia rate, is considered sustained when persistent for longer than 30 seconds. The QRS complex morphology can be unchanging (monomorphic) or variable (polymorphic). VF is chaotic ventricular activity recognized by variable ventricular undulations. Self-limited VT or VF results in dizziness or syncope; sustained tachyarrhythmias can result in SCD. Antiarrhythmic drugs are ineffective in improving survival in patients at risk for SCD, but multiple studies have established the efficacy of ICDs in preventing death in cardiac arrest survivors. Recent trials also demonstrate the effectiveness of ICDs in primary prevention of SCD in patients with depressed left ventricular ejection fraction (≤35%) due to either ischemic or nonischemic heart disease.

When patients with structural heart disease present with ventricular tachyarrhythmia, the general approach is to recommend ICD implantation to prevent SCD. Antiarrhythmic drugs, such as amiodarone (Cordarone), are used in patients who experience frequent ICD shocks. Although amiodarone (Cordarone) does not improve overall survival, it can decrease the number of arrhythmic events. Catheter ablation can target and disrupt VT

---

[1]Not FDA approved for this indication.

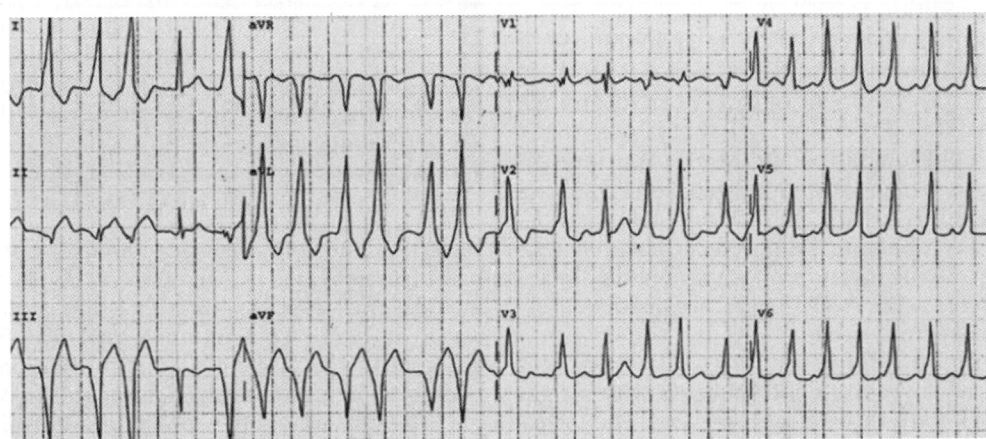

FIGURE 4. Twelve-lead electrocardiogram, preexcited atrial fibrillation. The arrhythmia is characterized by an irregularly irregular rhythm with variable QRS width.

reentry circuits in and around a scar. Although the elimination of all reentry circuits is not usually a realistic goal because of the complex nature of cardiomyopathic scars, catheter ablation can be effective in decreasing the number of VT episodes in selected cases.

Sustained monomorphic VT in nonischemic dilated cardiomyopathy frequently turns out to be *bundle branch reentry tachycardia*. This form of reentry tachycardia involves diseased bundle branches and most commonly manifests as a left bundle-branch block pattern with left axis deviation. Catheter ablation targeting one of the involved bundle branches can be performed with relative ease, curing a tachycardia that is typically rapid and recurrent. ICDs should still be considered in these patients since they are still at risk for SCD because of underlying cardiomyopathy.

IDIOPATHIC VENTRICULAR TACHYCARDIA

VT occurring in the absence of structural heart disease is termed idiopathic. In general, the risk of SCD is low. More than 80% of idiopathic VT originates from the RVOT and characteristically has a left bundle branch block pattern with an inferior mean frontal plane QRS axis. RVOT VT presents either as repetitive bursts of nonsustained VT or episodes of sustained VT brought about by physical or emotional stress. In most patients, the mechanism is catecholamine-induced cyclic adenosine monophosphate (cAMP)-mediated intracellular calcium increase, resulting in triggered activity. Because adenosine (Adenocard) decreases cAMP levels in ventricular cells and is effective in terminating RVOT VT, response to adenosine is useful in distinguishing RVOT VT from other forms of idiopathic VT.

RVOT VT is responsive to a wide range of antiarrhythmic drugs. Beta-blockers are usually tried first, and effectiveness of therapy can be assessed with treadmill testing. Diltiazem (Cardizem)[1] and verapamil[1] appear equally effective. The accessibility of the RVOT makes RVOT VT amenable to catheter ablation as well. The focus is usually found just below the pulmonary valve on the septal aspect of the RVOT, but variant foci can be found in the left ventricular outflow tract or epicardium. The success rate of catheter ablation exceeds 90%. Sotalol (Betapace) or flecainide (Tambocor) can also be considered in patients unresponsive to beta-blockers or calcium channel blockers who are not amenable to catheter ablation.

An important condition to exclude in patients presenting with a right ventricular (RV) VT is arrhythmogenic right ventricular cardiomyopathy (ARVC). In ARVC there is gradual fibrofatty displacement of the RV myocardium, resulting in scar-facilitated reentrant VT that is potentially life threatening. A gold standard diagnostic test currently is lacking; the diagnosis is made from multiple clinical criteria and results from various tests, which include echocardiography looking for RV dilation, and gated cardiac magnetic resonance imaging looking for intramyocardial fat. ICDs are considered in patients with ARVC who are inadequately treated with antiarrhythmic drugs.

The most common idiopathic left VT originates from the left ventricular septum and presents with a right bundle branch block pattern with superior axis. The tachycardia mimics a focal tachycardia with an origin in the

CURRENT DIAGNOSIS

- A narrow (<120 milliseconds) QRS complex tachycardia is supraventricular; a wide (≥120 milliseconds) QRS complex tachycardia is either ventricular or supraventricular with bundle branch block, aberrant intraventricular conduction, or ventricular preexcitation.
- Typical right atrial flutter is recognized by a unique undulating baseline likened to a sawtooth pattern in ECG leads II, III, and aVF.
- Transient block of the AV node (vagal maneuvers, adenosine [Adenocard]) with continuation of an atrial arrhythmia, such as atrial flutter or atrial tachycardia, is diagnostic.
- Multifocal atrial tachycardia is defined as an irregularly irregular rhythm, more than 100 beats per minute, with three or more discrete P wave morphologies and PR intervals. These features distinguish it from atrial fibrillation.
- The sensation of neck pounding is a sensitive (93%) and specific (100%) symptom of atrioventricular nodal reentrant tachycardia.
- Distortion of the terminal portion of the QRS complex during supraventricular tachycardia, by negative P waves in ECG leads II, III, aVF (pseudo S waves) or upright P waves in V_1 (pseudo R′ waves), is highly suggestive of atrioventricular nodal reentry tachycardia.
- Preexcited atrial fibrillation is associated with induction of ventricular fibrillation and recognized by an irregularly irregular rhythm with varying QRS width because of delta waves of varying duration. An accessory pathway is malignant when it conducts rapidly (shortest RR interval during atrial fibrillation less than 250 milliseconds). Catheter ablation of the accessory pathway is thought to eliminate the risk of sudden death.
- A history of heart disease in a patient with wide QRS complex tachycardia has a positive predictive value of 95% for ventricular tachycardia.
- Ventricular-atrial dissociation, established by dissociated P waves, capture beats, or fusion beats, is diagnostic of ventricular tachycardia.
- Right ventricular outflow tract ventricular tachycardia characteristically has a left bundle branch block pattern with inferior frontal plane QRS axis and is distinguishable from other idiopathic ventricular tachycardias by its sensitivity to adenosine (Adenocard).

region of the left posterior fascicle, but the mechanism has been revealed to be reentry involving a circuit that includes the left posterior fascicle and abnormal verapamil-sensitive tissue (presumably Purkinje fibers) that runs adjacent to the fascicle. Catheter ablation of the diseased Purkinje fibers is curative. Although this VT is sensitive to intravenous verapamil,[1] less data are available on chronic oral verapamil for long-term arrhythmia suppression.

---

[1]Not FDA approved for this indication.

[1]Not FDA approved for this indication.

CURRENT THERAPY

- For any tachyarrhythmia, if the blood pressure is excessively low or consequences of hypoperfusion (cognitive impairment, chest pain, heart failure) are evident, immediate electrical cardioversion should be performed.
- Because a delay in therapy of ventricular tachycardia can be life threatening, a wide QRS complex tachycardia should be considered ventricular tachycardia until proved otherwise.
- Persistence of atrial fibrillation or atrial flutter for more than 48 hours is associated with an increased risk for thromboembolic stroke, and exclusion of intracardiac thrombus should precede cardioversion unless hemodynamic instability dictates urgent therapy.
- Adenosine (Adenocard) reliably terminates atrioventricular nodal reentry tachycardia and atrioventricular reciprocating tachycardia.
- Infrequent episodes of atrioventricular nodal reentry tachycardia that are well tolerated and responsive to vagal maneuvers can be managed with observation. Episodes that are frequent and/or poorly tolerated are best treated with catheter ablation.
- Verapamil and digoxin have been associated with precipitating hemodynamic collapse and death when administered during preexcited atrial fibrillation. Intravenous procainamide is the treatment of choice because of its ability to block the accessory pathway.
- Fewer patients with supraventricular tachycardias are chronically managed with drugs. Catheter ablation is effective in curing atrial flutter, atrioventricular nodal reentry tachycardia, atrioventricular reciprocating tachycardia, some forms of atrial tachycardia, Wolff-Parkinson-White syndrome, and selected patients with atrial fibrillation.
- Implantable cardioverter defibrillators are effective in preventing sudden cardiac death in patients with depressed left ventricular function.
- Frequent implantable cardioverter defibrillator shocks resulting from recurrent ventricular tachycardia can be treated with antiarrhythmic drugs, which reduce the number of tachycardia episodes. Catheter ablation can target and disrupt ventricular tachycardia reentry circuits in and around scar tissue, and can decrease ventricular tachycardia episodes in selected patients.
- Intravenous magnesium[1] is the initial treatment of choice for nonsustained torsades de pointes.

[1]Not FDA approved for this indication.

LONG QT SYNDROMES AND TORSADES DE POINTES

Prolongation of the QT interval denotes an abnormality in ventricular repolarization that can lead to triggered activity. This can result in torsades de pointes, a polymorphic VT with continuously changing QRS amplitude and polarity that has the appearance of "twisting around a point" along the isoelectric baseline. Long QT syndrome (LQTS) encompasses congenital and acquired forms. An extensive list of drugs is recognized to cause QT prolongation and includes class IA and III antiarrhythmic drugs, various antipsychotic agents, and some antibiotics. Continually updated lists of QT prolonging drugs are available for reference (e.g., http://www.torsades.org).

Intravenous magnesium[1] is the initial treatment for nonsustained torsades de pointes. Lidocaine (Xylocaine)[1] infusion can also be effective. To suppress further episodes of tachycardia, the heart rate can be increased with temporary atrial or ventricular pacing; the increase in heart rate is accompanied by shortening of the QT interval. Isoproterenol (Isuprel)[1] can also be used for this purpose, but exacerbation of ventricular arrhythmia can occur, especially in patients with ischemic heart disease. Any potential causes for QT prolongation must be identified and eliminated. Certain types of congenital LQTS can be treated chronically with beta-blockers. ICDs are employed in patients at high risk for SCD (e.g., syncope, aborted SCD).

A growing number of other genetic tachyarrhythmia syndromes are recognized. These syndromes are relatively rare, but their unique presentations aid in diagnosis and management. Genetic testing is increasingly available for definitive diagnosis, as well as for risk assessment of family members.

REFERENCES

Akhtar M, Shenasa M, Jazayeri M, et al: Wide QRS complex tachycardia: Reappraisal of a common clinical problem. Ann Intern Med 1988;109:905-912.

Baerman JM, Morady F, DiCarlo LA, et al: Differentiation of ventricular tachycardia from supraventricular tachycardia with aberration: Value of the clinical history. Ann Emerg Med 1987;16:40-43.

Bardy GH, Lee KL, Mark DB, et al: Amiodarone or an implantable cardioverter-defibrillator for congestive heart failure. N Engl J Med 2005;352:225-237.

Calkins H, Yong P, Miller JM, Olshansky B, et al: Catheter ablation of accessory pathways, atrioventricular nodal reentrant tachycardia, and the atrioventricular junction: Final results of a prospective, multicenter clinical trial. The Atakr Multicenter Investigators Group. Circulation 1999;99:262-270.

Echt DS, Leibson PR, Mitchell LB, Peters RW, et al: Mortality and morbidity in patients receiving encainide, flecainide, or placebo. The Cardiac Arrhythmia Suppression Trial. N Engl J Med 1991; 324:781-788.

Ferguson JD, DiMarco JP: Contemporary management of paroxysmal supraventricular tachycardia. Circulation 2003;107:1096-1099.

Gürsoy S, Steurer G, Brugada J, Andries E, et al: The hemodynamic mechanism of pounding in the neck in atrioventricular nodal reentrant tachycardia. N Engl J Med 1992;327:772-774.

The Antiarrhythmics versus Implantable Defibrillators (AVID) Investigators: A comparison of antiarrhythmic-drug therapy with implantable defibrillators in patients resuscitated from near-fatal ventricular arrhythmias. N Engl J Med 1997;337:1576-1583.

Wellens HJ: Contemporary management of atrial flutter. Circulation 2002;106:649-652.

Wellens HJ: Cardiac arrhythmias: The quest for a cure: A historical perspective [Review]. J Am Coll Cardiol 2004;44:1155-1163.

Wellens HJ: Catheter ablation for cardiac arrhythmias. Circulation 2004;351:1172-1174.

[1]Not FDA approved for this indication.

Congenital Heart Disease

Method of
William S. McMahon, MD

Congenital heart disease occurs in approximately 0.8% of live newborns, but there is a wide spectrum of specific anatomic and physiologic anomalies. Significant advances in medical and surgical therapy over the past half-century have allowed many affected individuals who previously died during infancy or childhood to survive into adulthood. More recent advances in interventional cardiac catheterization techniques and devices have allowed less invasive treatment of some forms of congenital heart disease. Most recently, prenatal diagnosis of congenital heart disease offers the possibility that initial forays into treatment options for fetuses with some forms of congenital heart disease will offer a real chance of palliation or treatment before birth.

Clinical Evaluation

The challenge to the primary care physician is identifying those individuals who would benefit from further evaluation by a congenital heart disease specialist. Children with congenital heart defects may present from the first day of life throughout childhood and then into adulthood. The most common presenting signs and symptoms of children with congenital heart disease are cardiac murmurs, cyanosis, and the signs and symptoms of congestive cardiac failure.

By far, most cardiac murmurs in infants and children are benign and are not associated with any cardiac anomaly. Benign, or innocent, murmurs commonly identified in childhood include the pulmonary flow murmur of the newborn, pulmonary outflow murmur in older children,

---

CURRENT DIAGNOSIS

- Most common forms of congenital heart disease, approximate order of incidence, and most common presenting signs or symptoms

■ Ventricular septal defect	Murmur/CHF
■ Atrial septal defect	Murmur
■ Patent ductus arteriosus	Murmur/CHF (infant)
■ Pulmonary stenosis	Murmur
■ Tetralogy of Fallot	Cyanosis
■ Coarctation of aorta	Diminished lower-extremity pulse
■ Transposition of the great arteries	Cyanosis
■ Aortic stenosis	Murmur
■ Atrioventricular septal defect	Murmur/CHF
■ Hypoplastic left heart syndrome	Cyanosis/CHF

Abbreviation: CHF = congestive heart failure.

---

the vibratory innocent (Still's) murmur, supraclavicular bruit, and venous hum. These murmurs are typically quiet, grade 1 to 2 on a scale of 6, but frequently are as loud as grade 3/6, especially the vibratory murmur. An important identifying feature of the innocent murmur is the absence of other abnormal findings on physical examination, such as an ejection click, wide and fixed split of the second heart sound (S_2), palpable thrill, increased precordial activity, or abnormal pulses. Additionally, with the exception of the venous hum, a continuous murmur or a murmur with a prominent diastolic component is not likely to be benign.

The clinical finding of cyanosis results from desaturated hemoglobin and therefore is greatly dependent on the hemoglobin level. Central cyanosis occurs as a result of reduced arterial oxygen saturation and has respiratory system, central nervous system, hematologic, and cardiac causes. Peripheral cyanosis results from hemoglobin desaturation in the peripheral blood, frequently due to increased oxygen extraction at the tissue level. Severe hypoxemia due to intracardiac right-to-left shunt caused by congenital heart disease will fail to respond to a hyperoxia challenge test, with the partial pressure of oxygen on an arterial blood gas sample usually remaining less than 50 mm Hg. Perioral cyanosis without central cyanosis is a common benign finding in otherwise healthy children.

Clinical manifestations of congestive cardiac failure are similar in different age groups throughout childhood, but the most common causes of heart failure in children change significantly with age. Tachypnea and tachycardia are the cardinal signs of congestive heart failure (CHF) in childhood. Increased perspiration, poor feeding, and poor weight gain are common in infants with CHF. Dyspnea on exertion is common in older children. Cardiomegaly by chest radiography is almost always present in CHF, but other signs common in adults, such as lower-extremity edema, jugular venous distention, and rales on pulmonary auscultation, are not commonly encountered in children.

Congenital cardiac abnormalities can be categorized into simple and complex anomalies, and by the basic physiologic changes caused by the anomaly. *Left-to-right shunt* lesions cause increased pulmonary blood flow. *Obstructive* lesions cause right or left ventricular pressure overload. *Right-to-left shunt* lesions cause systemic arterial hypoxemia and cyanosis.

Left-to-Right Shunt Lesions

VENTRICULAR SEPTAL DEFECT

Ventricular septal defect (VSD) is the most common congenital cardiac defect, constituting 25% to 30% of all congenital heart lesions. It is the most common isolated lesion. It commonly occurs as part of more complex lesions, such as tetralogy of Fallot and double-outlet right ventricle. VSD causes a harsh, commonly grade 2/6 to 4/6 holosystolic murmur, usually best heard at the mid and lower left sternal border. The manifestations of VSD and the volume of left-to-right shunt depend primarily on the defect size. Small defects cause no significant hemodynamic consequences and, thus, no important symptoms. Large defects cause important pulmonary overcirculation and congestive cardiac failure, typically beginning at 1 to 2 months of age. Small muscular VSD is a common source of holosystolic murmur heard in the first few days of life in a healthy newborn. The murmur of the VSD may disappear, as 30% to 40% of all VSDs close spontaneously. The murmur of the VSD occurs most frequently with small defects and in the first year of life.

Anatomic subtypes of VSD include the *perimembranous VSD*, anatomically related to the aortic and tricuspid valves; the *muscular VSD*, within the muscle of the septum and not related to valve structures; the *inlet VSD*, anatomically related to the atrioventricular valves and commonly part of an atrioventricular septal defect (AVSD); and the *supracristal*, or *subarterial, VSD*, anatomically related to the aortic and pulmonic valves. Perimembranous VSD is by far the most common.

Individuals with a small VSD present with an asymptomatic murmur, are normally grown, and have normal exercise tolerance. A moderate to large VSD causes symptoms of CHF. Tachypnea and difficult feeding with subsequent slow weight gain are common early signs of CHF in infants. Patch closure of large VSD with cardiopulmonary bypass is indicated in infants with symptomatic heart failure unresponsive to medical therapy. Medical therapy is indicated to treat CHF prior to surgery or to palliate mild to moderate symptoms in infants with a moderate or large VSD without pulmonary hypertension, as even some large defects will become smaller to the point of being hemodynamically and symptomatically insignificant. Pulmonary artery banding as an initial alternative to intracardiac repair is rarely necessary unless specifics of associated anatomy or patient-specific complicating factors are present. Children without symptoms of pulmonary hypertension, but with a large left-to-right shunt, should undergo operation after infancy. Asymptomatic small VSDs with minimal increase in pulmonary blood flow as indicated by a ratio of pulmonary blood flow to systemic blood flow (Qp/Qs) less than 1.5 do not require closure. Medical prophylaxis against infective endocarditis should be instituted following the recommendations of the American Heart Association in all patients with VSD.

Children with perimembranous VSD should be reevaluated periodically because of the risk for progressive aortic insufficiency, right ventricular (RV) outflow

obstruction, and subaortic stenosis. The supracristal VSD is least common but is frequently complicated by aortic cusp prolapse and aortic insufficiency. Most cardiologists recommend closure of this type of defect upon diagnosis.

Advances have been made in transcatheter device closure of VSD. One device currently is approved for use in muscular defects thought to be high risk for surgical repair. Other devices, specifically designed for perimembranous or muscular defects, are under investigation. These devices show promise for being clinically useful and may allow routine, less invasive closure of VSD in the near future.

ATRIAL SEPTAL DEFECT

Atrial septal defect (ASD) is the second most common congenital cardiac defect. It is the most common defect to persist undetected into young adulthood and older age groups, so it is the most common form of congenital heart disease diagnosed in adults.

Infants and children with ASD are almost exclusively asymptomatic. Physical findings include a systolic murmur at the left upper sternal border, representing increased flow across the right ventricular outflow tract (RVOT). Therefore, the murmur may be quite similar to the innocent pulmonary flow murmur. The characteristic abnormal finding is a widely split and fixed S_2. With a large left-to-right shunt, a mid-diastolic rumble may be audible at the left lower sternal border.

Anatomic subtypes of ASD affect the management options. Secundum ASD is by far the most common, is centrally located at the fossa ovalis, and may have associated anomalies of pulmonary venous return (<10%). Ostium primum ASD occurs as part of partial or complete AVSD (endocardial cushion defect). In partial AVSD, there is primum ASD, located low in the atrial septum and closely related to the atrioventricular valves, and deformity of the anterior mitral leaflet (anterior septal leaflet cleft). Primum ASD usually is large and does not close spontaneously. Surgical repair, preferably performed during early childhood, involves patch closure of the ASD and mitral valve repair. Sinus venosus ASD occurs at the superior vena cava–right atrial junction and almost always includes anomalous drainage of the right pulmonary veins to the right atrium or superior vena cava. Repair is accomplished by patch closure. The patch is fashioned so that it will close the defect and direct anomalous pulmonary vein flow to the left atrium. Coronary sinus ASD is rare; it involves a defect, or "unroofing" of the coronary sinus so that left atrial blood has access to the right atrium through the coronary sinus. Closure of the coronary sinus abolishes the left-to-right shunt, leaving the coronary sinus draining into the left atrium.

The natural history of ASD in infants and young children includes the possibility of spontaneous closure. The probability of spontaneous closure is greatest for small defects with diameters 5 mm and less. Defects that persist and are associated with a significant left-to-right shunt (Qp/Qs >1.5) cause increased pulmonary blood flow, and right atrial and right ventricular enlargement. Symptoms and complications of heart failure, pulmonary hypertension, and atrial arrhythmias occur in adulthood. Cerebrovascular accident due to paradoxical embolism across an ASD is rare. Endocarditis associated with secundum ASD is thought to be extremely

CURRENT THERAPY

- Recent established and investigational advances in therapeutic options for treatment of congenital heart disease
- Atrial septal defect—Percutaneous device closure, secundum atrial septal defect
- Ventricular septal defect—Percutaneous device options
- Coarctation of aorta—Stent angioplasty
- Fetal intervention—Balloon aortic and pulmonic valvuloplasty
- Pulmonic insufficiency—Percutaneous valve/stent implantation
- Aortic valve disease—Ross procedure for valve replacement
- Hybrid surgical/interventional catheterization procedures

rare, and subacute bacterial endocarditis (SBE) prophylaxis is generally not advised. Closure of ASD in childhood prevents the development of late complications and early death. Surgical closure of ASD by suture or patch technique is associated with very low mortality (<1%) but moderate morbidity. Transcatheter closure of ASD has rapidly become the procedure of choice for patients with appropriate secundum ASD anatomy in most pediatric heart centers since approval of the Amplatzer ASO device in 2001.

PATENT DUCTUS ARTERIOSUS

The ductus arteriosus is an important part of normal fetal circulation, directing RV flow from the pulmonary artery to the aorta. In premature infants, left-to-right shunt with ductal patency complicates lung disease. Pharmacologic treatment with prostaglandin inhibitor agents frequently is successful in prompting ductal closure, although surgical ligation is sometimes necessary.

In older infants and children, patent ductus arteriosus (PDA) usually presents as a continuous "machinery" murmur, best heard in the left infraclavicular space. Symptoms of CHF may occur in infants with large PDA. Bounding peripheral pulses and wide pulse pressure may be present. The natural history of large PDA includes frequent respiratory infections due to pulmonary congestion, symptoms of CHF, and pulmonary vascular obstructive disease. Small PDA presents an increased risk of infectious endocarditis. Surgical ligation by left thoracotomy has largely been supplanted in the past 10 to 15 years by percutaneous coil embolization for occlusion of small to moderate PDA. A duct occluder device, specifically designed for PDA closure, now is available and allows more routine transcatheter closure of moderate to large PDA.

ATRIOVENTRICULAR SEPTAL DEFECT

Atrioventricular septal defect, also known as *endocardial cushion defect*, presents as partial and complete forms. The *complete form*, which includes common atrioventricular valve, large primum ASD, and large inlet VSD, is common in children with trisomy 21. The *partial forms* generally have separate atrioventricular valves, primum ASD, and no or a small ventricular defect component. For the complete form, signs and symptoms are similar to those of large VSD, with heart failure in infancy. Complete AVSD should be repaired in early infancy. Repair includes reconstruction of the atrioventricular valves and patch closure of the associated ASDs and VSDs. Successful closure of the VSD and repair of the mitral valve component without important residual mitral regurgitation are the primary determinants of long-term outcome.

Obstructive Lesions

Obstructive congenital cardiac lesions include obstruction of right or left ventricular outflow and obstruction of the pulmonary artery or aorta. Branch pulmonary artery stenosis, as part of more complex congenital heart disease (e.g., tetralogy of Fallot) or as part of a syndrome (e.g., Alagille or Williams syndrome), is less common.

PULMONARY STENOSIS

Isolated pulmonary stenosis (PS) is most commonly valvar. The affected leaflets are typically thin, with commissural fusion and a dome or windsock appearance on opening. Dysplastic abnormally thickened pulmonary valve leaflets as the cause of stenosis is less common and may be associated with Noonan's syndrome. Individuals with mild PS are asymptomatic. Easy fatigability and exertional symptoms may occur with moderate to severe PS, and heart failure may develop with long-standing severe PS. Valvar PS is associated with an audible systolic ejection click. A systolic ejection quality murmur is present over the left upper sternal border. Murmur intensity ranges from grade 2 to 4, and stenosis severity generally varies with murmur intensity. The natural history of PS depends on the severity of stenosis. Infective endocarditis may occur, but PS is said to be a low-risk lesion. Severity of PS is based on the pressure gradient across the stenosis. In infants and young children, the ratio of right ventricular pressure to aortic pressure (RV/Ao) is also useful. *Mild PS* is defined as a peak pressure gradient less than 30 mm Hg, and RV/Ao less than 0.5. Beyond infancy, mild PS is unlikely to progress in severity, and only intermittent follow-up evaluation is required. Sports participation is permitted. *Moderate PS* is associated with a pressure gradient 30 to 80 mm Hg, and RV/Ao between 0.5 and 0.8. Symptoms are more common, as is progression to more severe PS. *Severe PS* is associated with a high pressure gradient greater than 80 mm Hg, and RV pressure approximates the aortic pressure. Symptoms are expected, and athletic participation should be withheld.

Percutaneous balloon valvuloplasty during cardiac catheterization has been the treatment of choice for PS since the first reports of the procedure performed in children and young adults 25 years ago. Reduction of the pressure gradient to the mild range is associated with a good long-term prognosis. Recurrence of moderate to severe stenosis uncommonly warrants follow-up valvuloplasty. Patients with thick dysplastic valves or an important subvalvar or supravalvar component of the stenosis are more likely to have inadequate relief of pressure gradient by balloon valvuloplasty and may require surgical treatment.

AORTIC STENOSIS

Aortic stenosis is more common in males than females by a 4:1 ratio. The anatomy is most commonly bicuspid aortic valve with commissural fusion. Subvalvar aortic stenosis may be caused by a discrete membrane protruding into the left ventricular outflow tract or by a long segment, tunnel-like narrowing of the left ventricular outflow tract. Supravalvar AS is the least common form. It typically is caused by discrete narrowing at the junction of the aortic valve sinuses and the ascending aorta. This anatomy is associated with Williams syndrome and with a "nonsyndromic" form of autosomal-dominant familial supravalvar AS. Children with mild AS are generally asymptomatic. Many children with moderate AS are asymptomatic, but some children exhibit exertional symptoms. Children with severe AS may exhibit exertional chest pain and syncope. As in adults, these symptoms suggest an increased risk of sudden death. CHF symptoms may predominate in newborns and young infants with critical AS and limited cardiac output. On examination, a systolic thrill is typically present in the suprasternal notch, even in many cases of mild AS. More moderate or severe cases will also have an upper sternal border thrill. An ejection click is typically heard with valvar AS and is absent when subvalvar or supravalvar AS is present. The murmur of AS is typically harsh, grade 2/6 to 4/6, depending on stenosis severity. It is best heard at the right upper sternal border or left midsternal border and radiates to the carotid arteries. As with PS, the natural history of AS is dependent on the severity of obstruction, but mild or moderate AS is more likely than is PS to increase in severity as the child grows. In addition, the risk of sudden death (1%–2% per year) and infective endocarditis is substantial in AS compared to PS of similar severity. Pressure gradients that define mild, moderate, and severe categories of AS are similar to those of PS. *Mild AS* typically presents with a peak pressure gradient less than 30 to 40 mm Hg, no symptoms, and no changes on electrocardiogram. It typically requires no specific therapy except for SBE prophylaxis. Close follow-up for evidence of increasing gradient, development of left ventricular hypertrophy, onset or increase in aortic insufficiency, or development of important aortic root dilation is important. *Moderate AS* typically presents with a pressure gradient of 40 to 70 mm Hg. In this group, the presence of exertional symptoms, exertional chest pain or syncope, ischemic electrocardiographic changes, or important left ventricular hypertrophy indicates the need for invasive treatment. Severe AS presents with a higher peak pressure gradient, with or without symptoms, and requires treatment.

Percutaneous balloon aortic valvotomy has several advantages over surgical valvotomy or valve replacement and, therefore, is the initial treatment of choice for most patients with congenital aortic stenosis in most congenital heart centers in the United States. Development of valvar insufficiency is more problematic for aortic valve than for the pulmonic valve, so children with moderate or greater pre-existing aortic insufficiency are not good candidates for balloon valvotomy. Balloons with smaller diameters are used, and higher residual gradients are accepted in order to prevent development of severe insufficiency. Mechanical aortic valve replacement is avoided when possible in small children. In some centers, the Ross pulmonary autograft operation for aortic valve replacement has been used with good results.

COARCTATION OF THE AORTA

Coarctation results from thickening of the aortic wall in the aortic isthmus and proximal descending aorta, resulting in luminal obstruction. In severe cases, the obstruction may extend proximally into the transverse aortic arch. Associated defects such as VSD are common. Bicuspid aortic valve is present in approximately 50% of patients. Coarctation is more common in males. Approximately 30% of females with Turner's syndrome have coarctation. Infants with critical coarctation present at the time of ductal closure with heart failure and shock. Older children presenting with coarctation are generally asymptomatic and are identified by upper-extremity hypertension or by absent or weak and delayed lower-extremity pulses. Because severe primary hypertension is uncommon in children, the finding of hypertension should prompt evaluation of the lower-extremity pulses to rule out coarctation.

Murmur of VSD, or murmurs and ejection click due to bicuspid aortic valve, may be present. Untreated coarctation results in long-standing hypertension, left ventricular hypertrophy, and late CHF. More than 90% of untreated individuals with coarctation die by 50 years of age. Coarctation associated with symptoms, hypertension, left ventricular hypertrophy, or a peak pressure gradient greater than 15 to 20 mm Hg should be treated. Treatment options are surgical repair and balloon and/or stent angioplasty. Resection of the coarctation segment and direct or extended reanastomosis is the usual surgical technique of choice. Use of the left subclavian artery or of other material as an aortic patch is an alternative or complementary technique. Recurrent coarctation after primary surgical repair is a problem primarily after operation in infants. Balloon angioplasty is the treatment of choice for recurrent coarctation. Primary balloon angioplasty is a less invasive alternative to primary surgical repair. Balloon angioplasty in young infants is associated with a higher recurrence rate and the need for reintervention; therefore, surgical repair is generally the procedure of choice in this age group. Balloon angioplasty with stent implantation has become the treatment of choice in selected patients at some centers, but intermediate- and long-term follow-up for this approach currently are not available. The optimal treatment method for children and young adults with coarctation remains a topic of investigation.

Regardless of the treatment method, residual hypertension and the long-term effects of aortic wall intervention require lifelong follow-up and periodic imaging of the aortic arch. Cardiovascular magnetic resonance imaging and fast computed tomography provide good images for this purpose. Residual hypertension requiring ongoing treatment despite adequate relief of the aortic obstruction may occur more commonly following later initial diagnosis and treatment.

Right-to-Left Shunt Lesions, Cyanotic Defects

TETRALOGY OF FALLOT

Tetralogy of Fallot is the most common cyanotic congenital heart defect. The original pathologic description of large VSD combined with RVOT obstruction, RV hypertrophy, and overriding aorta describes most cases of tetralogy of Fallot. In most cases, cyanosis is present early, although young infants may not initially display obvious cyanosis. In some cases, a lesser degree of RV outflow obstruction does not significantly limit pulmonary blood flow, and cyanosis does not develop. This results in the so-called *acyanotic form*, or *pink tetralogy*. In these infants, the physiology of left-to-right shunt, with CHF symptoms, may predominate. In less than 10% of cases, the RVOT is completely atretic. These cases generally present with severe cyanosis in the newborn period when the ductus arteriosus closes, but patients may present later if aortic collateral vessels provide sufficient pulmonary blood flow.

Severe signs and symptoms of cyanosis, including clubbing, squatting, and hypercyanotic spells, are less frequently encountered in the current era of early palliative and corrective surgery. However, the hypercyanotic spell, or "tet spell," commonly occurs at age 2 to 4 months, so this emergency of severe cyanosis is still encountered. These spells can occur in any patient with a large VSD or single ventricle and obstruction to pulmonary blood flow. Spells are marked by severe and increasing cyanosis, irritability, prolonged crying, paroxysmal hyperpnea (rapid, deep breathing), and decreased intensity of the murmur during the spell due to decreased flow across the RVOT obstruction. Severe spells can result in stroke or death. Emergent treatment is necessary for prolonged spells, and further medical, or preferably surgical, treatment is indicated to prevent further spells. Auscultation reveals a long, loud, grade 3/6 to 4/6 systolic murmur at the left middle and upper sternal border, radiating to the lung fields. The murmur is shorter in duration with more severe RV outflow obstruction.

Most routine cases of tetralogy of Fallot are treated by surgical repair in early infancy. Patch closure of the VSD and relief of the RVOT obstruction are performed with the child on cardiopulmonary bypass. Morbidity and mortality are low for good surgical candidates. Children with more complex anatomy, including tetralogy of Fallot with pulmonary atresia or severely diminutive pulmonary arteries, usually require initial palliation with an aortopulmonary shunt prior to operation for repair at a later age.

The postoperative course and intermediate- to long-term prognosis are quite good for most patients. Some patients will have a late course complicated by residual VSD or residual RVOT obstruction, pulmonary artery stenosis (particularly left pulmonary artery stenosis), long-term consequences of pulmonary insufficiency, RV dysfunction, ventricular arrhythmia, or sudden death.

TRANSPOSITION OF THE GREAT ARTERIES

Transposition of the great arteries is more common in males than females by a 3:1 ratio. It is the most common form of cyanotic congenital heart disease in newborns. The aorta and main pulmonary artery are transposed so that the aorta arises directly from the RV and the pulmonary artery from the left ventricle. This situation results in two circulations in parallel rather than in series, with desaturated blood remaining in the systemic circulation and oxygenated blood remaining in the pulmonary circulation. Some mixing between the two circulations is necessary for survival; therefore, newborns present with cyanosis before ductal closure or with very severe cyanosis with acidosis when the ductus arteriosus closes. Additional defects, such as VSD and PS, are present in about 40% of cases. Infants with a large VSD or PDA are less cyanotic, but they develop CHF. Examination reveals a single, loud S_2 due to the anterior location of the aorta. Typically, there is no important heart murmur in cases with uncomplicated transposition of the great arteries with intact ventricular septum. A murmur of VSD or PS may be present when these complicating lesions are present.

In newborns without an adequate anatomic atrial or ventricular level site for mixing, severe cyanosis ensues with ductal closure. Prostaglandin E_1 or alprostadil (Prostin VR Pediatric) infusion will open the ductus arteriosus and improve mixing and oxygenation. In many cases, an additional source of mixing may be necessary or desired to improve oxygenation. Rashkind balloon atrioseptostomy was the first interventional cardiac catheterization procedure. In this percutaneous procedure, a balloon inflated on the tip of a catheter passed through a patent foramen ovale into the left atrium is forcefully and rapidly pulled into the right atrium to create an ASD adequate for mixing of venous blood and for relief of severe cyanosis.

For almost all patients, definitive treatment of transposition of the great arteries is the arterial switch operation. In most cases, this operation is performed in the first 2 weeks of life and allows anatomic and physiologic correction. The great vessels are transected above the aortic and pulmonic valves, respectively, and moved to the appropriate semilunar valve. The coronary arteries are moved individually, to stay with the aorta. VSD closure is performed if necessary. Specific associated anatomic problems, including some anomalies of coronary artery origin and course, and important left ventricular outflow obstruction or native pulmonary valve stenosis may complicate routine repair.

Prior to the current era of complete repair by arterial switch in neonates, an atrial switch repair was the common mode of surgical treatment. Two similar but separate techniques, the Senning and Mustard operations, were used to direct systemic venous blood via an intraatrial baffle to the mitral valve and the pulmonary venous blood to the tricuspid valve and thus to the RV and the aorta. The youngest of the large group of patients who were routinely treated by these surgical techniques now are approximately 20 years old. Most patients have done well through childhood, but late postoperative problems related to poor RV function (the RV functions as the systemic ventricle in this anatomy) and subsequent heart failure as well as atrial and ventricular arrhythmias are increasingly common.

REFERENCES

Allen HD (ed): Moss and Adams' Heart Disease in Infants, Children, and Adolescents, Including the Fetus and Young Adult, 6th edition. Baltimore, Lippincott Williams & Wilkins, 2000.

Garson A, Bricker TJ, Fisher DJ, Neish SR (eds): The Science and Practice of Pediatric Cardiology, 2nd ed. Baltimore, Williams & Wilkins, 1998.

Graham TP: The year in congenital heart disease. J Am Coll Cardiol 2005;45:1887-1899.

Johnson WH, Moller JH: Pediatric Cardiology. Philadelphia, Lippincott Williams & Wilkins, 2001.

Hypertrophic Cardiomyopathy

Method of
Ali J. Marian, MD

Definition

Hypertrophic cardiomyopathy (HCM) is a primary disease of the myocardium characterized by unexplained cardiac hypertrophy, a hyperdynamic left ventricle with a small cavity, and often dynamic outflow tract obstruction. The pathologic features of HCM include myocyte hypertrophy, disarray, and interstitial fibrosis. Myocyte disarray is considered the pathologic hallmark of HCM.

The current clinical diagnosis of HCM is neither specific nor highly sensitive. For example, the presence of systemic hypertension, per convention, excludes the diagnosis of HCM, despite the possibility of concomitant HCM in hypertensive individuals. "Unexplained cardiac hypertrophy" also can occur in storage diseases, mitochondrial disorders, and triplet repeat syndromes. The presence of a hyperdynamic left ventricle, outflow tract obstruction, and asymmetric hypertrophy favors the diagnosis of true HCM. In contrast, depressed global cardiac systolic function, conduction defects, neurologic abnormalities, and skeletal myopathy favor the possibility of a phenocopy.

Prevalence

The prevalence of HCM, defined as a wall thickness of 15 mm or greater on echocardiogram in the absence of a secondary cause, is estimated to be 1:500 in individuals 23 to 35 years old. However, the disease probably is more common, as expression of cardiac hypertrophy is age dependent. Many young individuals with the disease-causing mutation may exhibit mild hypertrophy or express cardiac hypertrophy late in life.

Clinical Manifestations

Clinical manifestations of HCM are variable, ranging from an asymptomatic course to that of severe heart failure and sudden cardiac death (SCD). The majority of patients with HCM are asymptomatic or minimally symptomatic. The most common symptoms are dyspnea, chest pain, palpitations, and lightheadedness. Syncope is an infrequent symptom that often indicates serious cardiac arrhythmias. Atrial fibrillation and nonsustained ventricular tachycardia are the most common cardiac arrhythmias in patients with HCM.

HCM is the most common cause of SCD and often is the first manifestation of the disease in young competitive athletes, accounting for almost half of cases. A history of SCD, syncope, a strong family history of SCD, serious ventricular arrhythmias including frequent episodes of nonsustained ventricular tachycardia, severe cardiac hypertrophy, exertional hypotension, and genetic factors are considered risk factors for SCD. None of the risk factors alone is a reliable predictor; hence, the global risk, which is derived from a combination of multiple risk factors, should be assessed. The overall estimated annual mortality rate of patients with HCM is about 1% in the adult population.

Molecular Genetics

HCM is a genetic disease with an autosomal dominant mode of inheritance. A family history of HCM can be elicited in approximately half to two thirds of cases. The seminal report by Seidman and colleagues in 1999 of the R403Q mutation in the β-myosin heavy chain (β-MyHC) led to elucidation of the molecular genetic basis of HCM. To date, more than 400 causal mutations in more than a dozen different genes, all encoding the sarcomeric proteins, have been identified. Accordingly, HCM is considered a disease of mutant sarcomeric proteins (excluding HCM phenocopy). Mutations in *MYH7* and *MYBPC3*, which encode β-MyHC and myosin-binding protein-C (MyBP-C), respectively, are the most common, each accounting for approximately 30% of HCM cases. Mutations in *TNNT2* and *TNNI3*, which encode cardiac troponin T and cardiac troponin I, respectively, each accounts for 3% to 5% of HCM cases. The vast majority of causal mutations are missense and private mutations; hence, the frequency of each specific mutation is low.

There is considerable variability in the phenotypic expression of HCM, even among patients with similar or identical causal mutations. Multiple mutations are often associated with more severe phenotypes but are present in only a small fraction of cases. The genetic background of individuals, defined by the presence of single nucleotide polymorphisms, is considered an important determinant of phenotypic variability of HCM. In addition, environmental factors, such as isometric exercises, are expected to affect phenotypic expression of HCM.

GENETIC SCREENING

There is considerable interest in genetic testing for the diagnosis and prognostication of HCM patients. Currently, the primary utility of genetic testing is in families in which the causal mutation is already known, which makes possible the accurate diagnosis of mutation carriers from noncarriers. In families in which the causal mutation is unknown, initial genetic linkage mapping could help to identify the putative candidate gene, followed by mutation screening. Genetic testing in isolated cases of HCM is complicated by the need for extensive genetic screening of a large number of genes and a 30% to 40% chance of not finding the causal mutation. However, advances in rapid and high-throughput screening techniques are expected to change the current approach. The significance of genetic testing in clinical prognostication and identification of individuals at risk for SCD remains to be established. In general, information on the causal genes as well as the modifier genes and the environmental factors will be necessary for accurate prognostication and genetic counseling of HCM patients.

Pathogenesis

Elucidation of the molecular genetic basis of HCM has provided significant clues to its pathogenesis. The evolution of phenotype can be categorized into three sets: the initial functional phenotype, the intermediary molecular phenotype, and the final morphologic phenotype. The collective results of a large number of in vitro and in vivo mechanistic studies indicate that the initial defects are diverse and encompass reduced ATPase activity of the myofibrils, impaired actomyosin cross-bridging, and enhanced Ca^{2+} sensitivity of myofibrils. The intermediary molecular phenotype occurs in response to the functional phenotype and is largely unknown but is expected to include expression and activation of intracellular signaling molecules. The morphologic and histologic phenotypes are the consequence of the intermediary molecular phenotype and, hence, are considered secondary and potentially reversible.

Treatment

The goals in the management of patients with HCM are fourfold: to determine the risk of SCD, to reduce the risk of SCD, to alleviate symptoms, and to provide genetic counseling to patients and family members.

MANAGEMENT ACCORDING TO THE RISK OF SUDDEN CARDIAC DEATH

There is no close correlation between the risk of SCD and the presence of symptoms. Overall, the majority of patients with HCM are at low risk for SCD and are asymptomatic or minimally symptomatic. These individuals require periodic evaluation to determine risk of SCD and to assess symptoms. Accordingly, history, physical examination, electrocardiography, Holter monitoring, and two-dimensional and Doppler echocardiography are performed at least annually. Asymptomatic individuals at high risk for SCD should undergo internal cardioverter-defibrillator (ICD) implantation. Otherwise, no pharmacologic or nonpharmacologic intervention is necessary in asymptomatic patients who are at low risk for SCD.

MANAGEMENT OF SYMPTOMATIC PATIENTS

Therapeutic options in symptomatic patients include pharmacologic therapy, surgical myectomy, and transcatheter septal ablation; the latter two are options for those with significant outflow tract obstruction. Symptomatic patients at high risk for SCD should undergo ICD implantation in addition to medical therapy. Medical treatment of symptomatic patients is largely empiric and limited to β-blockers, verapamil hydrochloride[1] (Calan and Verelan), disopyramide[1] (Norpace), low-dose diuretics, and amiodarone[1] (Cordarone and Pacerone[1]). The goals are to improve diastolic function, reduce outflow tract obstruction, and prevent cardiac arrhythmias. β-Blockers such as atenolol (Tenormin[1]) and metoprolol (Lopressor and Toprol XL[1]) are the first line of therapy and are generally well tolerated. β-Blockers with intrinsic sympathetic activity are avoided. β-Blockers are also the preferred choice in patients with sympathetic-driven symptoms, such as exercise-induced dyspnea, outflow tract obstruction, and chest pain. The most common side effect of β-blocker therapy is easy fatigability. Other side effects include excess bradycardia, hypotension, and bronchospasm.

Verapamil and, to lesser extent, diltiazem (Cardizem, Cartia XT, Dilacor, Tiazac[1]) are the most commonly used calcium channel blockers in patients with HCM. They are commonly used in conjunction with β-blockers.

CURRENT THERAPY

Asymptomatic

- Periodic follow-up for symptoms and risk factors assessment for SCD
- ICD implantation in patients at high risk for SCD

Symptomatic

- ICD implantation in patients at high risk for SCD
- Medical therapy with β-blockers and calcium channel blockers
- Surgical myectomy, transcoronary septal ablation, and dual-chamber pacing in patients refractory to medical therapy, septal thickness >15 mm, and outflow tract obstruction >50 mm Hg
- Atrial fibrillation
  1. Acute: Cardioversion
  2. Chronic: β-Blockers and amiodarone (Cordarone), anticoagulation, and radiofrequency ablation if refractory to medical therapy
- Syncope
  1. β-Blockers and clonidine in patients with inappropriate vasodilatory response
  2. ICD and antiarrhythmic drugs in patients with ventricular arrhythmias
  3. Antiarrhythmic drugs in patients with supraventricular arrhythmias and radiofrequency ablation for refractory cases
  4. Myectomy or transcoronary septal ablation in patients with severe outflow tract obstruction

Abbreviations: ICD = internal cardioverter-defibrillator; SCD = sudden cardiac death.

Symptomatic relief with calcium channel blockers presumably is achieved through improving left ventricular relaxation and reducing left ventricular filling pressure. Calcium channel blockers impart a negative inotropic effect, which could contribute to reduction of outflow tract obstruction. Nonetheless, the use of verapamil is primarily restricted to patients without an outflow tract obstruction because of concern about the vasodilatory effect inducing hypotension, syncope, and rarely death. The most common side effect of verapamil is constipation. Nifedipine (Adalat and Procardia) is avoided because of its potent vasodilatory effect.

Disopyramide is commonly reserved for patients who do not respond to β-blockers and/or calcium channel blockers, because of the relatively higher rate of anticholinergic side effects with disopyramide. The beneficial effect of disopyramide is mediated through its negative inotropic effect, which results in a significant reduction in left ventricular outflow tract gradient and symptomatic improvement. Diuretics are used judiciously to relieve dyspnea while avoiding intravascular volume depletion. Rapid changes in intravascular volume should be avoided because of enhanced susceptibility to hypotension. Mineralocorticoid receptor blockers may be preferable because of their antihypertrophic and antifibrotic effects in addition to their diuretic effects. Angiotensin-converting enzyme inhibitors and angiotensin-II receptor blockers

---

[1]Not FDA approved for this indication.

are not conventionally used. However, experimental data favor their use because of their antihypertrophic and antifibrotic effects.

In a small fraction of patients, HCM evolves into advanced heart failure with systolic dysfunction and a congestive state. These patients are treated, as are those with other forms of systolic heart failure, with β-blockers, angiotensin-converting enzyme inhibitors, angiotensin-II receptor blockers, digoxin, and diuretics.

MANAGEMENT OF CARDIAC ARRHYTHMIAS

Patients with palpitations should undergo 12-lead electrocardiography, Holter monitoring, and electrophysiologic studies, if needed, to delineate the etiology and to provide appropriate therapy. Chronic or intermittent atrial fibrillation occurs in approximately 20% of patients. Atrial fibrillation with a fast ventricular rate is not well tolerated and often results in severe dyspnea and hypotension, particularly in those with severe cardiac hypertrophy or left ventricular outflow tract obstruction. Electrical cardioversion is indicated in such patients. Electrical or chemical cardioversion is also warranted in patients with new-onset atrial fibrillation (<48 hours in duration) if they are at low risk for intracardiac thrombus. Otherwise, transesophageal echocardiography should be performed to exclude intracardiac thrombi prior to cardioversion. Patients with chronic or intermittent atrial fibrillation require chronic anticoagulation. Medical treatment of atrial fibrillation includes use of β-blockers, verapamil, diltiazem, and amiodarone. Amiodarone is the most effective, but its long-term use is associated with considerable toxicity; therefore, only low-dose amiodarone (up to 200 mg daily) is recommended. Experience with other antiarrhythmic agents, such as flecainide (Tambocor), for treatment of arrhythmias in patients with HCM is limited. Radiofrequency ablation is reserved for patients refractory to medical therapy.

Patients with frequent nonsustained ventricular tachycardia or sustained ventricular tachycardia should undergo ICD implantation because they are considered at high risk for SCD. In addition, medical treatment with antiarrhythmic drugs such as amiodarone or β-blockers is recommended. Patients with rare episodes of nonsustained ventricular tachycardia should undergo further evaluation to assess the risk of SCD and then treated according to the risk of SCD.

MANAGEMENT OF SYNCOPE

Recurrent syncope is a serious event in patients with HCM because it often heralds SCD. The most common causes of syncope are malignant ventricular or supraventricular arrhythmias, exercise-induced hypotension, severe outflow tract obstruction, and neurally mediated syncope (vasodepressor syncope). Evaluation of patients with syncope includes Holter monitoring, exercise test, tilt-table testing, and, if needed, electrophysiologic studies. Patients with repetitive bursts of nonsustained ventricular tachycardia and those with sustained ventricular tachycardia are candidates for ICD implantation. Ventricular arrhythmia is the main cause of SCD in individuals with HCM. Implantation of an ICD as a preventive measure reduces the risk of SCD.

Patients with syncope due to supraventricular arrhythmias are treated with antiarrhythmic drugs, and those refractory to medical therapy are treated with radiofrequency ablation. Surgical myectomy and transcoronary septal ablation are considered in patients with syncope due to severe outflow tract obstruction. Treatment of patients with syncope due to an inappropriate peripheral vascular response to exercise includes propranolol (Inderal[1]), clonidine (Catapres[1]), and sometimes paroxetine (Paxil[1]).

MANAGEMENT OF OUTFLOW TRACT OBSTRUCTION

Left ventricular outflow tract obstruction is a dynamic phenotype that is associated with symptoms of heart failure, but its contribution to the risk of SCD is not well established. Most patients with outflow tract obstruction respond well to medical therapy and remain asymptomatic or mildly symptomatic. Treatment with β-blockers alone may suffice. A subset of patients who exhibit significant resting or exercise-induced outflow tract obstruction (>50 mm Hg) remain in New York Heart Association functional class III and IV despite optimal medical therapy. These patients are candidates for percutaneous transcoronary septal ablation or surgical myectomy. The prerequisite for invasive interventions is an interventricular septal thickness of 15 mm and greater. Otherwise, invasive procedures are not warranted because of a potentially excessive risk-to-benefit ratio. Instead, treatment should focus on diastolic dysfunction.

No prospective randomized studies have compared clinical outcomes after surgical myectomy and percutaneous transcoronary septal ablation. Several observational studies suggest the two interventions are equally effective in reducing the left ventricular outflow tract gradient and alleviating symptoms. However, neither is a curative intervention, and additional treatment usually is necessary.

A. *Surgical Myectomy (Myomectomy):* Surgical myectomy involves resection of a small portion of the interventricular septum, commonly at the base, through a transaortic approach (Morrow procedure). It reduces outflow tract obstruction and results in significant improvement of heart failure symptoms. It is best reserved for symptomatic patients with significant outflow tract obstruction at rest who are refractory to pharmacologic therapy.

It is the procedure of choice in patients with concomitant valvular disease and/or coronary artery disease. The recurrence rate of outflow tract obstruction is low, and a second intervention is seldom required. The overall mortality rate of surgical myectomy in experienced centers is 1% to 5%, but the rate is higher among the elderly and those with concomitant cardiac surgeries. Surgical myectomy is associated with excellent short-term and long-term symptomatic relief and survival, and it has a favorable impact on the risk of SCD.

B. *Transcoronary Septal Ablation:* The procedure is performed through percutaneous coronary catheterization and injection of 1 to 3 mL of pure ethanol

---

[1]Not FDA approved for this indication.

into the main septal perforators of the left anterior descending artery. Accordingly, focal myocardial necrosis, emulating surgical myectomy, is induced. It reduces the outflow tract gradient significantly and improves symptoms. It is indicated in symptomatic patients who are refractory to medical therapy, have an interventricular septal thickness of 15 mm and greater, and have a significant resting left ventricular outflow tract gradient. In those with significant exertional dyspnea, a provoked exercise-induced gradient can be used as a surrogate phenotype for septal ablation.

Overall, the procedure is well tolerated and has relatively low perioperative morbidity and mortality. The most common complication is the development of advanced atrioventricular (AV) conduction defect requiring permanent pacemaker placement in 15% to 20% of patients. There is a small risk of ventricular arrhythmias arising from the localized myocardial necrosis. Progressive left ventricular remodeling occurs predominantly within the first 6 months. Short-term and intermediary follow-up data show favorable outcome that is largely comparable, but probably not equal, to that of surgical myectomy.

C. **Dual-Chamber Pacing:** Dual-chamber pacing is designed to reduce outflow tract obstruction by inducing dyssynchronized left ventricular contraction. Thus, optimal timing of the AV interval is considered essential. Randomized clinical studies show no significant direct benefit to pacing strategy but rather a considerable placebo effect and no discernible improvement in exercise tolerance. Accordingly, dual-chamber pacing is reserved for occasional symptomatic patients who are refractory to medical therapy and are not candidates for either surgical or transcatheter septal ablation.

Experimental Pharmacologic Agents

Recent experimental studies have suggested the potential utility of β-hydroxy-β-methylglutaryl-coenzyme A (HMG-CoA) reductase inhibitors (statins), angiotensin-II receptor blockers, aldosterone blockers, and antioxidants in the prevention, attenuation, and reversal of cardiac phenotype in patients with HCM. Clinical studies testing the potential utility of these agents for treatment of patients with HCM are ongoing.

REFERENCES

Cannan CR, Reeder GS, Bailey KR, et al: Natural history of hypertrophic cardiomyopathy. A population-based study, 1976 through 1990. Circulation 1995;92:2488-2495.

Geisterfer-Lowrance AA, Kass S, Tanigawa G, et al: A molecular basis for familial hypertrophic cardiomyopathy: a beta cardiac myosin heavy chain gene missense mutation. Cell 1990;62:999-1006.

Hess OM, Sigwart U: New treatment strategies for hypertrophic obstructive cardiomyopathy: Alcohol ablation of the septum: the new gold standard? J Am Coll Cardiol 2004;44:2054-2055.

Marian AJ: Pathogenesis of diverse clinical and pathological phenotypes in hypertrophic cardiomyopathy. Lancet 2000;355:58-60.

Marian AJ: Recent advances in genetics and treatment of hypertrophic cardiomyopathy. Future Cardiol 2005;1:341-353.

Maron BJ, Gardin JM, Flack JM, et al: Prevalence of hypertrophic cardiomyopathy in a general population of young adults. Echocardiographic analysis of 4111 subjects in the CARDIA Study. Coronary Artery Risk Development in (Young) Adults. Circulation 1995;92:785-789.

Maron BJ, Shen WK, Link MS, et al: Efficacy of implantable cardioverter-defibrillators for the prevention of sudden death in patients with hypertrophic cardiomyopathy. N Engl J Med 2000;342:365-373.

Maron BJ, Shirani J, Poliac LC, et al: Sudden death in young competitive athletes. Clinical, demographic, and pathological profiles. JAMA 1996;276:199-204.

Ommen SR, Maron BJ, Olivotto I, et al: Long-term effects of surgical septal myectomy on survival in patients with obstructive hypertrophic cardiomyopathy. J Am Coll Cardiol 2005;46:470-476.

Woo A, Williams WG, Choi R, et al: Clinical and echocardiographic determinants of long-term survival after surgical myectomy in obstructive hypertrophic cardiomyopathy. Circulation 2005;111:2033-2041.

Mitral Valve Prolapse: The Floppy Mitral Valve, Mitral Valve Prolapse, and Mitral Valvular Regurgitation

Method of
Charles F. Wooley, MD, and
Harisios Boudoulas, MD, PhD

The floppy mitral valve (FMV) is the central theme in the mitral valve prolapse (MVP) narrative. It has taken 6 decades to reconcile the observations by the pathologists who described the FMV morphology in the 1940s with the role of the FMV in clinical mitral valvular regurgitation (MVR). When the early cardiac surgeons encountered floppy, myxomatous mitral valves at open heart surgery, they described prolapse (MVP) of the FMV into the left atrium and used the FMV terminology for descriptive purposes, a term also used by the early cardiac pathologists. The clinicians initially described, and later recorded, apical systolic clicks and late systolic murmurs, but with a few exceptions they tended to regard these auscultatory findings as extracardiac in origin. When left ventricular angiography became feasible, the pathologic, surgical, and auscultatory phenomena were reconciled and came into clear focus. The nonejection systolic clicks were clearly related to prolapse (MVP) of an FMV into the left atrium, and the mid to late apical systolic murmurs represented a unique form of MVR. At this stage of clinical understanding, the auscultatory, angiographic, surgical, and pathologic correlates were quite distinct.

When the M-mode echocardiogram came into clinical usage, the result was a mixed blessing for diagnostic accuracy in patients with the FMV–MVP–MVR triad. Clinical auscultatory findings were ignored, and the nonspecific echocardiographic criteria produced a prolonged period of diagnostic confusion, elements of which persist to the present. This era was characterized by the separation of MVP from FMV, and the result was grossly exaggerated estimates of the incidence and prevalence of MVP. Gradually, however, with the use of the evolving technologic advances in multidimensional echo-Doppler transthoracic

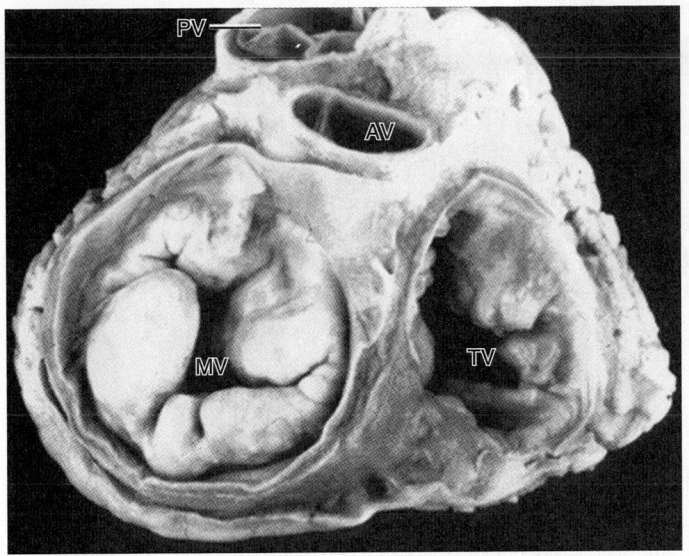

FIGURE 1. Floppy mitral valve. *Abbreviations:* AV = aortic valve; MV = mitral valve; PV = pulmonic valve; TV = tricuspid valve. (Photograph courtesy of Dr. William D. Edwards, Mayo Clinic.)

Surgical Observations

Open heart surgery allowed cardiac surgeons to visualize the mitral valve in the beating heart. In 1965, Read and colleagues used the term *floppy valve syndrome* to describe patients with significant mitral and aortic valvular regurgitation due to myxomatous transformation of the mitral and aortic valves. Valvular regurgitation was related to "valve prolapse" because of loss of valve integrity from structural fatigue, ruptured chordae, or interference with valvular coaptation. Their report was marked by descriptive language—floppy valve for myxomatous changes in valve tissue; dynamic terminology—valve prolapse as a mechanism for valvular regurgitation; and the recognition of connective tissue disorders as the etiology for valvular disease. Subsequently, cardiac surgeons developed FMV reconstructive procedures from careful analysis of FMV morphology and dynamics.

Clinical Observations

During the 1960s, the clinicians' approach to FMV and MVR, in particular by Barlow, Criley, and their coworkers, resulted from auscultatory–phonocardiographic, hemodynamic, and angiographic studies of patients with apical systolic clicks and apical mid and late systolic murmurs. Apical systolic clicks were shown to be of intracardiac origin, distinct from aortic and pulmonary ejection clicks, and were classified as nonejection clicks; apical mid and late systolic murmurs were related to a unique anatomic type of MVR associated with FMV prolapse into the left atrium (i.e., MVP); and bulging of the mitral leaflets was identified as the angiographic counterpart of the balloon deformity seen at necropsy by Bailey and Hickam in 1944.

MVP postural auscultatory phenomena (i.e., postural exercise hemodynamic abnormalities and changes in timing and intensity of the systolic click–apical systolic murmur) were explained in hemodynamic terms as changes in the timing and extent of MVP, and the time of onset and duration of MVR were related to postural changes in left ventricular volume and contractility (Figure 2). Thus, by the 1970s and 1980s, clinical auscultatory observations, postural auscultatory dynamics, and angiographic definition of FMV characteristics with established pathologic correlates provided a reasonable clinical diagnostic profile for the FMV–MVP–MVR triad.

A number of events transpired that obscured this relatively simple diagnostic profile. Clinical phonocardiography virtually disappeared as remuneration for phonocardiograms was halted and production of phonocardiographic equipment ceased. This was followed by an auscultatory "silent spring" phenomenon, when physicians in training were not exposed to the self-critique that phonocardiography imposed on the discipline of auscultation.

Sensitivity and specificity diagnostic criteria suffered, as studies that relied on unproven M-mode echocardiographic criteria proliferated, FMV was uncoupled from MVP, and estimates of MVP incidence and prevalence reached epidemic proportions. Patients or individuals with small, hyperdynamic left ventricles were placed into the same category as patients with the FMV–MVP–MVR triad. When the M-mode echocardiographic prolapse

and esophageal techniques, close attention to in vivo mitral valve anatomy, and rigorous clinical conference, reason was restored to the diagnostic process. Revised imaging diagnostic criteria once again were based on fundamental FMV morphology, the mechanisms of MVP, and precise identification and quantification of MVR.

These developmental observations are highly significant because no other valvular lesion has a lineage similar to that of FMV. Thus, recognition and definition of an FMV as a discrete pathologic entity producing mitral valvular dysfunction was the key step to our current understanding (Figure 1). Essential steps in comprehending the clinical significance of the FMV–MVP–MVR triad was the recognition that the mitral valve dysfunction associated with FMV resulted in prolapse of the mitral valve into the left atrium (MVP) and that FMV/MVP resulted in a specific form of mitral valvular regurgitation (MVR).

Pathologic Observations

Early cardiac pathologists also called attention to the long natural history of patients with FMVs. In 1944 Bailey and Hickam pointed out the discrete nature of FMV and emphasized that this type of valve was a nonrheumatic entity. They noted fibrosis of the mitral valve without rheumatic stenosis, increased valve thickness with histologic evidence of dense acellular connective tissue thickening and basophilic areas of degeneration. The long natural history of the disorder, the susceptibility to infectious endocarditis, and the late onset of rapidly progressive congestive heart failure were important clinical correlates. Subsequent studies of FMV incidence, pathobiology, and complications by Davies and other cardiac pathologists provided clinicians with a new chapter in valvular heart disease. Thus, the natural history of patients with FMVs was reasonably well defined early on; however, the translation of these early observations into the clinical realm took much longer than generally appreciated.

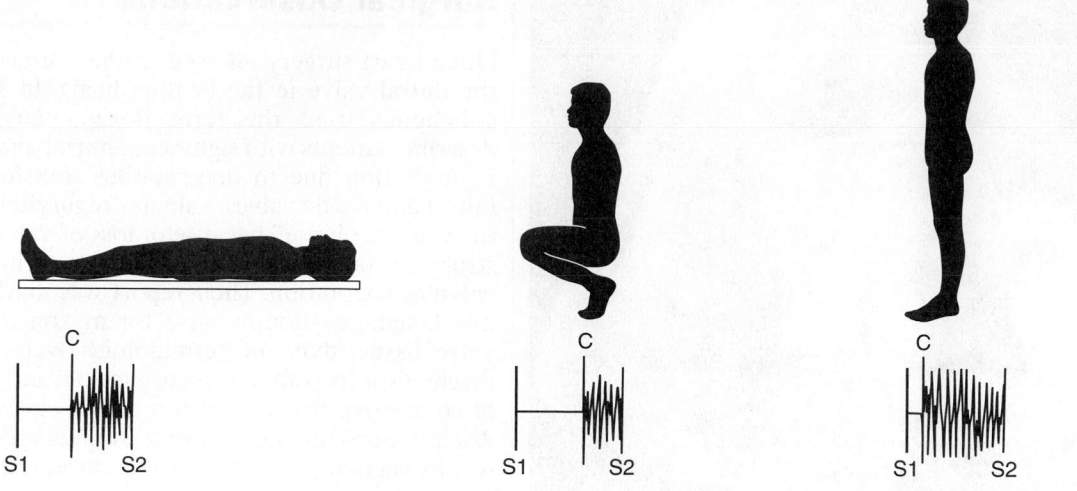

FIGURE 2. Floppy mitral valve–mitral valve prolapse–mitral valvular regurgitation: Postural auscultatory complex. *Abbreviations:* C = systolic click; S₁ = first heart sound; S₂ = second heart sound.

comet swept across psychiatry, individuals with anxiety and panic syndromes were engulfed, and the epidemic became pandemic.

Historical Perspective

Why introduce the historical perspective? First, recalling the ways in which MVR, FMV, and MVP diagnostic criteria evolved during the past 50 years helps us understand that these clinical entities were moving targets, constantly being defined and redefined by pathologists, surgeons, auscultors, imagers, and epidemiologists, and hence the multitude of names for the clinical entities and the variability of diagnostic criteria. Second, when the FMV–MVP–MVR clinical auscultatory–phonocardiographic–angiographic profile was separated from the prolapse imaging diagnosis that ignored FMV morphology and focused on a 1- to 2-mm disputed zone, cardiologists wandered into areas fraught with difficulties. As the MVP pendulum moved away from the exaggerated incidence/prevalence figures of the past 2 decades, it is apparent that the FMV occupies the high ground and is the central issue in the FMV–MVP–MVR triad (see Figure 1).

Heritable Disorders of Connective Tissue

FMV may be an inherited lesion, either as an isolated event or as part of the recognized or incompletely defined heritable disorders of connective tissue. FMV–MVP inheritance and phenotypic features have been well described. FMV has gradually become recognized as a common cardiac lesion in the Marfan syndrome. Although FMV–MVP may be genetically determined, clinical manifestations do not usually become evident before childhood. Although children and adolescents with FMV–MVP may have the same symptoms as adults, the frequency of symptoms appears to be less in children. At present, the family history remains the cornerstone in clinical genetic

analysis, as FMV genetic diagnostic testing has not entered clinical practice.

DIAGNOSTIC CONSIDERATIONS

FMV is a common mitral valve abnormality with a broad spectrum of structural and functional changes. Although the pathobiology of FMV has been, and continues to be, re-examined in contemporary terms, we are still dealing with gross structural and morphologic characteristics at the clinical level. Distinguishing between a normal mitral valve with its minor variants and an FMV mitral valve with an intrinsic structural derangement remains a central issue. Thus, it is important to emphasize the necessity for clinical coherence in the FMV–MVP–MVR dialogue.

Tic-tac-toe has its origins in the ancient "three in a row" category of games of strategy. Diagnostic tic-tac-toe avoids the pitfalls of a diagnosis based on a single phenomenon and places emphasis on a multidimensional approach to FMV–MVP–MVR diagnostics similar to our diagnostic approach to any complex cardiac disorder or disease (Figure 3).

We are more comfortable with the FMV–MVP–MVR diagnosis when (1) the clinical auscultatory phenomena

MEDICAL HISTORY,
PHYSICAL EXAMINATION,
LABORATORY

Diagnostic tic-tac-toe

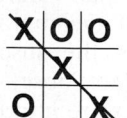

Multidimensional approach
to FMV, MVP, MVR diagnosis

FIGURE 3. Diagnostic tic-tac-toe. Emphasis is placed on a multidimensional approach to the diagnosis. *Abbreviations:* FMV = floppy mitral valve; MVP = mitral valve prolapse; MVR = mitral valvular regurgitation.

CURRENT DIAGNOSIS

- Clinical coherence should exist among the medical history, the physical examination, and the imaging procedure.
- Because the floppy mitral valve–mitral valve prolapse–mitral valvular regurgitation triad is accompanied by dynamic clinical phenomena, dynamic examination procedures may be indicated in individual situations.
- A family pedigree is a vital part of the clinical evaluation.

TABLE 1 Classification of Floppy Mitral Valve–Mitral Valve Prolapse–Mitral Valvular Regurgitation (FMV-MVP-MVR)

FMV-MVP-MVR
Common mitral valve abnormality with a spectrum of structural and functional changes, mild to severe

The Basis for
Systolic click; mid-late systolic murmur
Mild or progressive mitral valve dysfunction
Progressive mitral regurgitation, atrial fibrillation, congestive heart failure
Infectious endocarditis
Embolic phenomena
Characterized by long natural history
May be heritable or associated with heritable disorders of connective tissue
Conduction system involvement possibly leading to arrhythmias and conduction defects

FMV-MVP-MVR Syndrome
Patients with mitral valve prolapse
Symptom complex; chest pain, palpitations, arrhythmias, fatigue, exercise intolerance, dyspnea, postural phenomena, syncope-presyncope, neuropsychiatric symptoms
Neuroendocrine or autonomic dysfunction (high catecholamine levels, catecholamine regulation abnormality, hyperresponse to adrenergic stimulation, parasympathetic abnormality, baroreflex modulation abnormality, renin-aldosterone regulation abnormality, decreased intravascular volume, decreased ventricular diastolic volume in the upright posture, atrial natriuretic factor secretion abnormality) may provide explanation for symptoms
Mitral valve prolapse—a possible marker for autonomic dysfunction

are precisely described, preferably recorded, and dynamic auscultation has been performed; (2) the clinical auscultatory phenomena are matched with an imaging procedure that captures and quantitates FMV morphology and function; and (3) the imaging procedure demonstrates MVP and the presence, absence, or quantification of MVR.

Postural auscultation, electrocardiogram, and echocardiogram with Doppler, assessment of orthostasis, dynamic exercise testing, ambulatory electrocardiographic or blood pressure monitoring, and dynamic interventional imaging or hemodynamic studies may be required, depending on the patient's symptoms or the specific clinical situation.

FLOPPY MITRAL VALVE—MITRAL VALVE PROLAPSE—MITRAL VALVULAR REGURGITATION: CLASSIFICATION

The classification of cardiovascular diseases is in constant evolution, and our textbooks and literature do not always reflect the dynamics of this process. At present, we classify patients with the FMV–MVP–MVR triad into two general categories (Table 1). The first category places emphasis on the FMV anatomy and pathobiology and includes patients whose symptoms, physical findings, laboratory abnormalities, and clinical course are directly related to the progressive mitral valve dysfunction and complications associated with the FMV–MVP–MVR triad. The second category includes FMV–MVP patients whose symptoms cannot be explained on the basis of the valvular abnormality alone but result from the occurrence, or coexistence, of various forms of neuroendocrine or autonomic nervous system dysfunction. We refer to this group as patients with the FMV–MVP syndrome.

We have found this to be a clinically useful classification, but one that should be subject to revision or modification as we better understand the pathogenesis and mechanisms of symptoms in patients with the FMV–MVP–MVR triad.

FLOPPY MITRAL VALVE—MITRAL VALVE PROLAPSE—MITRAL VALVULAR REGURGITATION: COMPLICATIONS AND NATURAL HISTORY

Profiles of the natural history of the FMV–MVP–MVR triad have been limited by variations in diagnostic criteria, the nature of the populations studied, and the duration of clinical follow-up.

The FMV–MVP association has well-defined clinical auscultatory correlates; however, the sensitivity and specificity of these clinical phenomena have not been determined with contemporary objective methods. Similarly, the FMV–MVP association has specific imaging correlates, yet these are being constantly redefined as echo-Doppler, magnetic resonance imaging, and angiographic technologies improve and diagnostic criteria are reassessed.

The FMV–MVP association may lead to progressive mitral valvular dysfunction and severe MVR over time; however, the individual patient's natural history may not fully develop for 7 to 8 decades. Hence, studies or evaluations at one point in time have limitations (Figure 4).

Valve surface phenomena occur in patients with FMVs. A FMV is particularly vulnerable to infection and may be a site for infective endocarditis. The pathogenesis is poorly understood, and we currently mask our lack of understanding by using incident-related antibiotic prophylaxis prior to dental, gastrointestinal, and genitourinary procedures. Although guidelines have been evolving, simply stated, infectious endocarditis prophylaxis is indicated for patients with FMVs. Thromboemboli are additional valve surface complications of FMV; however, this is an area that is not well defined.

Chordal rupture, progressive MVR, left atrial and left ventricular failures, and atrial and ventricular arrhythmias occur in varying combinations and permutations, usually

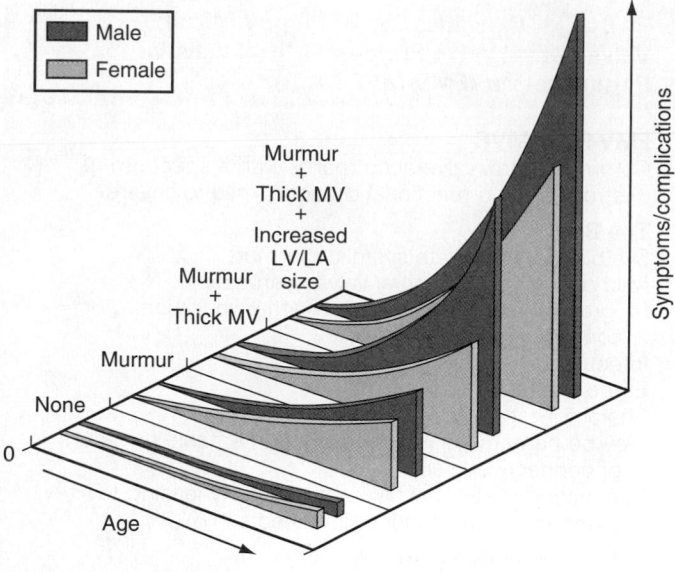

FIGURE 4. Floppy mitral valve–mitral valve prolapse–mitral valvular regurgitation: High-risk patient. Symptoms and complications plotted against age. *Abbreviations:* LA = left atrium; LV = left ventricle; MV = mitral valve.

as late complications in certain patients with FMV. FMVs have been documented as being one of the leading causes of MVR requiring mitral valve surgery. Sudden cardiac death has been reported in a small subset of patients with FMV.

Therapeutic Implications

Each of the FMV–MVP–MVR complications has implications involving prevention, recognition, and treatment. Individual patient evaluation and management are fundamental considerations, as is the necessity of regular, long-term clinical follow-up.

Individuals with progressive mitral valvular dysfunction require initial and periodic assessment of their hemodynamic status. Individuals with the MVP syndrome as defined earlier whose symptoms may be related to autonomic dysfunction, neuroendocrine abnormalities, volume depletion, or vasoconstriction require investigation and therapeutic approaches aimed at these pathogenetic mechanisms. Both groups require careful explanations of their individual situation, the rationale for regular follow-up, and infective endocarditis prophylaxis.

High-risk Patients

Individuals with FMV–MVP and thick, redundant mitral valve leaflets are at high risk for developing complications; those older than 50 years with arterial hypertension are at particularly high risk (see Figure 4). A mitral systolic murmur also is a risk factor for complications. Left atrial and left ventricular enlargement and dysfunction in patients with FMV–MVP–MVR have been used as predictors for the need for mitral valve surgery. When two or more of these abnormalities coexist, the possibility of

complications increases. In contrast, the absence of all three of these features identifies patients at low risk (see Figure 4). These individuals, whether or not they are symptomatic, may require more sophisticated imaging studies, exercise testing, or hemodynamic and angiographic assessment. Individuals with a history of atrial or ventricular arrhythmias should be evaluated with contemporary electrophysiologic monitoring or testing. Patients who have a history of syncope, lightheadedness, or unexplained collapse or who are postresuscitation require further diagnostic testing.

SURGICAL CONSIDERATIONS

Decisions regarding surgical intervention (mitral valve repair or replacement) in symptomatic FMV patients have been based on the impact of MVR on left atrial and left ventricular functions expressed in both hemodynamic terms and echocardiographic measurements. Improvements in FMV repair techniques and intraoperative imaging coupled with better echo-Doppler methods of quantitating MVR severity prompted recommendations for earlier intervention extending into the asymptomatic state. This is another moving target in the FMV–MVP–MVR lineage that requires careful assessment and analysis by thoughtful clinicians.

Patients with MVP syndrome are sensitive to volume depletion and increased adrenergic activity. Thus, prophylaxis for volume depletion before, during, or immediately after physical exercise may be particularly beneficial to patients with low intravascular volume. Removing catecholamine and cyclic adenosine monophosphate stimulation by abstaining from caffeine, tobacco, alcohol, and prescription or over-the-counter drugs containing epinephrine may help. Low doses of β-blocking drugs administered for a short time during stressful periods or in a single dose may be beneficial. Exercise programs are frequently beneficial in patients with the MVP syndrome.

Summing up, the concept of a triad, a group of three closely related things, as expressed in the floppy mitral valve–mitral valve prolapse–mitral valvular regurgitation triad, emphasizes the central role of the FMV in the MVP–MVR lineage. A recent in-depth review of the subject by Hayek, Gring, and Griffin contains clinical wisdom for clinicians involved in the diagnosis, care, and management of patients with the FMV–MVP–MVR triad.

CURRENT THERAPY

- Guidelines for surgical intervention in patients with floppy mitral valve–mitral valve prolapse–mitral valvular regurgitation should include the feasibility of floppy mitral valve repair, surgical competence, low operative mortality and morbidity, and long-term clinical results.
- Careful explanation of the clinical findings and the nature of mitral valve prolapse will help reassure the anxious patient with the mitral valve prolapse syndrome.
- As is always the case, individual patient evaluation and diagnostic certainty precede rational therapy.

REFERENCES

Bailey OT, Hickam JB: Rupture of mitral chordae tendineae. Am Heart J 1944;28:578-600.

Barlow JB, Pocock WA, Marchand P, et al: The significance of late systolic murmurs. Am Heart J 1963;66:443-452.

Bashore TM, Grines CL, Utlak D, et al: Postural exercise abnormalities in symptomatic patients with mitral valve prolapse. J Am Coll Cardiol 1988;3:499-507.

Boudoulas H, Wooley CF: Mitral Valve: Floppy Mitral Valve, Mitral Valve Prolapse, Mitral Valvular Regurgitation. Armonk, NY, Futura, 2000.

Carpentier A: Cardiac valve surgery: The "French correction." J Thorac Cardiovasc Surg 1983;3:323-337.

Criley JM, Lewis KB, Humphries JO, et al: Prolapse of the mitral valve: Clinical and cineangiographic findings. Br Heart J 1966;28:488-496.

Davies MJ, Moore BP, Braimbridge MV: The floppy mitral valve. Study of incidence, pathology, and complications in surgical, necropsy and forensic material. Br Heart J 1978;40:468-481.

Enriquez-Sarano M, Avierinos JF, Messika-Zeitoun D, et al: Quantitative determinants of the outcome of asymptomatic mitral regurgitation. N Engl J Med 2005;352:875-883.

Fontana ME, Wooley CF, Leighton RF, Lewis RP: Postural changes in left ventricular and mitral valvular dynamics in the systolic click-late systolic murmur syndrome. Circulation 1975;1:165-173.

Glesby MJ, Pyeritz RE: Association of mitral valve prolapse and systemic abnormalities of connective tissue. JAMA 1989;262:523-528.

Hayek E, Gring CN, Griffin BP: Mitral valve prolapse. Lancet 2005;365:507-518.

Otto CM, Salerno CT: Timing of surgery in asymptomatic mitral regurgitation. N Engl J Med 2005;352:928-929.

Read RC, Thal AP, Wendt VE: Symptomatic valvular myxomatous transformation (the floppy valve syndrome). A possible forme fruste of the Marfan syndrome. Circulation 1965;32:897-910.

Heart Failure

Method of
Marc A. Silver, MD

Heart failure is an epidemic in the United States. Every day, clinicians face the task of caring for more patients with heart failure in all its forms. Heart failure is the primary reason for hospitalization of Americans older than 65 years, and although 6 million Americans are estimated to have symptomatic heart failure, that number is expected to double over the next 7 years. Many millions more have asymptomatic left ventricular dysfunction or existing medical conditions that make it quite likely heart failure will develop and they will die.

It is truly in the hands of primary care physicians, who care for most heart failure patients, as well as those with common precursors of heart failure, to understand heart failure and its natural history better and thereby make an impact on this challenging epidemic. With this concept in mind, heart failure is discussed here from the perspective of understanding its natural history or stages, as well as a chronic disease process amenable to strategic planning.

Definitions

All clinicians define heart failure differently. Some choose to think about heart failure only when the patient has advanced disease characterized by significant volume overload and exercise limitation. Others consider heart failure to be present only when the left ventricle is dilated. Although broad by intent, *heart failure* is usually defined as a complex clinical syndrome that affects cardiac function (its ability to fill and/or eject blood) and is often preceded by and certainly accompanied by systemic neurohormonal abnormalities that participate in and perpetuate the dysfunction of the heart as well as other target organs, including the vasculature and muscles.

Although a wide range of signs and symptoms may accompany the heart failure syndrome of whatever cause, once symptomatic, patients usually have evidence of dyspnea, fatigue, and sodium and water retention manifested as congestion in the lungs, legs, and gut. It is useful, however, to think about heart failure not only as a symptomatic disease but also as a disease whose development begins decades before the patient crosses the threshold of clinical symptoms.

Classification and Stages of Heart Failure

Although many clinicians bristle at the concept of prescribed sets of recommendations or guidelines applied to a diverse disease process such as heart failure, these guidelines are frequently a place where available evidence is evaluated in a critical way and balanced with consensus to provide a distillation of what might work when caring for a patient with a disease process.

One of the well-accepted standard guidelines for heart failure recently was revised. Within the 2001 Revision of the American College of Cardiology/American Heart Association Guidelines for the Evaluation and Management of Chronic Heart Failure for the Adult (executive summary and full text available online at http://www.acc.org/clinical/guidelines/failure/ hf_index.htm), aside from detailed information on the testing and therapies currently supported by evidence, appears a new classification for heart failure (Table 1). The classification most clinicians are familiar with is that of the New York Heart Association (NYHA) (Box 1). The NYHA classification is generally applied to patients who at some point become symptomatic. Although they may revert to a symptom-free status (NYHA functional class I), it is still implied the patient has overt heart failure. Even though the NYHA classification is of great value and carries prognostic value, it also tends to allow us to think of a patient with mild or moderate symptoms (i.e., NYHA functional class II to III) as having a mild or moderate disease, but indeed, patients in this category have a markedly shortened life span and by definition less than optimal functional status.

The new classification (Box 2), in contrast, identifies four stages of heart failure based on the spectrum of common clinical syndromes from which they have evolved. By so doing, it is hoped the clinician recognizes the patient's increased risk for the clinical syndrome and then acts aggressively to reduce the risk and/or intervene earlier just as one would with a patient at risk for cancer.

The classification addresses four stages. Unlike the NYHA classification, in which a patient may easily pass back and forth through several functional classes over a period of days to weeks, as the patient passes through each stage of the new classification, there is no longer any hope

TABLE 1 Common Heart Failure Drugs and Their Therapeutic Targets

Drug	Dose	Comment
Loop diuretics (expressed as furosemide [Lasix] equivalent units)	40-100 mg once or twice daily	Many factors affect the doses required, such as patient compliance with dietary restrictions, fluid intake, and associated titration of other medication, including ACE inhibitors and β-blockers.
ACE inhibitors (expressed as enalapril [Vasotec] equivalent units)	10-20 mg twice daily	Higher doses seem to have an impact on hospitalization rates. Be aware of adverse events that will limit use, including hyperkalemia. To allow adequate titration of β-blockers, reduced doses may be used.
β-Blockers (expressed as carvedilol [Coreg] equivalent units)	25-50 mg twice daily	Dependent on body size. Although data suggest clinical improvement and decreased mortality with smaller doses, the target remains full dose.
Digoxin	0.125-0.25 mg daily	Adjustment needed for renal function. Routine measurement of serum levels is not required unless done to confirm toxicity.

Abbreviation: ACE = angiotensin-converting enzyme.

of reverting to an earlier stage, which should act as an impetus to capture the patient at the earliest stage and prevent progression to the next stage by using the proper diagnostics and therapeutics.

Stage A refers to patients who by virtue of having other common clinical conditions are at increased risk of heart failure ultimately developing. These conditions include hypertension, diabetes mellitus, and coronary artery disease. Similarly, patients with a family history of heart failure have an increased risk. The heart failure syndrome clearly does not develop in all these patients, but acknowledging their at-risk status gives the clinician and the patient fair warning of the potential risk of development of heart failure and may serve as an early warning detection system for the insidious progression to more advanced heart failure. Progression to the next stage is preventable, and disease progression is usually measured in years or decades.

Stage B refers to patients in whom structural and even functional abnormalities in heart function are already developed, but because of enormous cardiac reserve, the signs or symptoms that usually bring these patients to medical attention are not yet developed. This stage has also been referred to as "asymptomatic left ventricular dysfunction." Progression to the next stage may be slowed and again may be measured in years.

Stage C represents most of what is called heart failure today: specifically, a patient who has structural and

functional disease but who has now progressed and used up enough cardiac reserve actually to have signs and symptoms of the disease. By looking at heart failure in this perspective, it becomes clear that any symptomatic heart failure indeed represents a serious condition that the clinician must diagnose and treat accordingly. In this stage of the disease, clinicians can intervene to improve symptoms

---

BOX 2 Stages of Heart Failure

Stage A
- Patients who are at increased risk for heart failure because of associated medical conditions (e.g., hypertension, coronary artery disease, or diabetes mellitus).
- Heart structure and function: Not yet affected.
- Potential therapies: Treatment of hypertension, smoking cessation, and weight loss; ACE inhibitors in appropriate patients.

Stage B
- Patients who have abnormal heart structure and/or function but who have not manifested signs or symptoms.
- Heart structure and function: Abnormal.
- Potential therapies: Same as for stage A, plus ACE inhibitors and β-blockers in all appropriate patients.

Stage C
- Patients with symptomatic heart failure. These patients indeed have advanced heart failure. Note that signs and symptoms develop as late phenomena after significant perturbation of many homeostatic mechanisms and the consumption of large cardiac reserves.
- Heart structure and function: Abnormal.
- Potential therapies: Same as for stages A and B, plus ACE inhibitors, β-blockers, and digoxin and diuretics in most patients; also, coronary revascularization and repair of mitral regurgitation in select patients.

Stage D
- Patients with extremely advanced heart failure.
- Heart structure and function: Extremely abnormal.
- Potential therapies: Same as for stages A, B, and C, plus consideration of advanced therapies including investigational therapies, consideration for left ventricular assist devices, heart transplantation for appropriate patients, as well as end-of-life counseling and hospice.

Abbreviation: ACE = angiotensin-converting enzyme.

BOX 1 New York Heart Association Functional Classification of Heart Failure*

I. Symptoms occur only at a level that would cause normal individuals to become symptomatic.

II. Symptoms occur with ordinary exertion or moderate levels of activity.

III. Symptoms occur with less than ordinary degrees of activity.

IV. Symptoms occur even at rest.

*This classification scheme is generally applied to patients once they are or have been symptomatic with heart failure (stages C and D). Note: In general, the classification implies the patient's worst level of functioning related to a heart failure symptom (e.g., fatigue, dyspnea, exercise intolerance).

and quality of life, as well as improve, but not completely abolish, the increased mortality. Progression to the next stage is quite variable but is usually measured in months to years.

Stage D represents very advanced disease in which even standard measures cannot overcome its severity and advanced measures need to be undertaken. During this stage, despite best efforts, patients usually have increased use of resources, decreased quality of life, and progressive limitation. Although many advanced resources are applied during this stage, including heart transplantation and ventricular restraint and assist devices, generally these patients ultimately die of either progressive heart failure or sudden cardiac death.

Steps for Appropriate Heart Failure Management

Physicians often take a reflex approach to initiating drug therapy in a patient with symptomatic heart failure. For example, a patient who is volume overloaded might be treated with diuretics as monotherapy while overlooking the need not only to treat the current symptoms but also plan a strategy to limit progression of disease. Thus a useful approach in planning patient care involves two broad steps. The first is assessing the information needed to create a management plan, and the second is understanding the therapeutic targets in heart failure treatment.

An assessment of what is known or yet needed to be known to best make the diagnosis and treat a patient with heart failure is a very useful step. This assessment generally involves an understanding of the etiology of the heart failure, the current stage or functional class, and so forth. Even after a detailed history and physical examination and collection of some diagnostic data, however, a gap can remain in the information needed to complete the therapeutic plan. Generally, the clinician can group the areas that need to be completed into three main categories: diagnostics, therapeutics, and prognostics. In fact, these three areas are useful to consider each time a patient is seen in the office or hospital. Even though treatment is often initiated without complete information in each of these areas, not asking what other information is needed often leads to an incomplete understanding of the disease syndrome, as well as suboptimal therapy.

Diagnostics refers to any additional information that allows a better understanding of the etiology, status, degree of limitation, and signs and symptoms of a patient. For example, an echocardiogram allows assessment of the nature and degree of left ventricular function and may lead to consideration of myocardial ischemia (wall motion abnormalities) or valvular disease (valvular regurgitation or stenosis) as a therapeutic target. Often in this category are tests that might reveal an easily addressable cause of the heart failure and even a form of heart failure that is potentially reversible (such as hyperthyroidism).

Therapeutics refers to the design of the treatment strategy based on what is currently known about the patient and that patient's disease. It is also useful to write down a therapeutic plan, including the one or two next steps that might be taken should the patient's signs or symptoms not abate with the current regimen. For example, the clinician might begin with using angiotensin-converting enzyme (ACE) inhibitors but indicate that if the patient is found to have underlying coronary artery disease, the addition of long-acting nitrates should be considered.

Prognostics refers to focusing in on what is known about the patient's heart failure in terms of predicting what might be the path of progression in the near future. Although imperfect, many pieces of information are closely linked to survival and disease progression, including functional status, exercise tolerance, and left ventricular ejection fraction. In considering any additional prognostics, the clinician should always ask what might be done differently given the result. Over the years we have become more willing to intervene earlier with therapeutics, which can alter progression of the disease, and therefore we depend less on a bad set of prognostic markers to make these decisions. Nevertheless, awareness of a low peak oxygen consumption, a low right ventricular ejection fraction, or a markedly elevated neurohormonal marker often serves to alert the physician and the patient and family to review the current therapeutic plan and broaden considerations to include the next level of care and treatment, which might consist of investigational therapies and evaluation for heart transplantation. The role of measurement of B-type natriuretic peptide in this regard is of some interest and may prove to be a prognostic marker against which to target our therapies.

TREATMENT TARGETS

In designing the drug treatment plan, the following treatment targets for patients with heart failure should be considered: improved survival, improved symptoms, slowing and/or reversal of disease progression, improved functional status and quality of life, avoidance of troublesome adverse events, and decreased use of resources, including hospitalization. With the recognition that not all these targets are concordant or attainable, the drug regimen reflects these targets and our understanding of the ability of drugs to address them.

In general, patients with symptomatic heart failure are managed with a core group of four drug classes, including diuretics, an ACE inhibitor, a β-blocker, and, usually, digoxin. The former and the latter are generally applied to relieve symptoms or to improve functional status or exercise tolerance, whereas the middle two are also administered with the specific intention of altering disease progression, reversing the structural and/or functional abnormalities of the heart and other target organs, and improving medium- and long-term survival.

Increasing evidence supports the initiation of ACE inhibitors and β-blocker jointly when caring for a symptomatic patient. Diuretics often need to be adjusted up or down, depending on a patient's level of compensation, as well as where they are in terms of other (β-blocker) titration. Target doses for most of the commonly used drugs come from clinical trials suggesting their benefit (ACE inhibitors) or from tradition, as well as from attempts to balance drug efficacy with drug safety (digoxin and diuretics). Target doses are listed in Table 1. Excellent details and practical considerations of implementing and titrating heart failure drugs can be found in recent guidelines (http://www.acc.org/clinical/guidelines/failure/hf_index.htm).

NONPHARMACOLOGIC MEASURES

An enormous armamentarium outside routine drug therapy is available to clinicians caring for patients with heart failure. In general, most nonpharmacologic measures should be used in a simultaneous fashion with the initiation and titration of drug therapy. Although most of these therapies either have not or will not undergo rigorous clinical investigation, they nonetheless remain therapeutic cornerstones of complete heart failure care. Dramatic functional improvement can often be observed with more careful attention to nonpharmacologic therapies. Of particular interest is an understanding that sleep-disordered breathing (including obstructive and central forms of sleep apnea) may be present in nearly 40% of heart failure patients. Increasing evidence suggests therapy that includes continuous positive airway pressure may alter symptoms, disease progression, and even survival (Box 3). As far as dietary advice, generally admonitions for avoidance of excessive sodium intake and fluid are given along with specific information on lowering dietary saturated fat. Emerging information is that the patient with heart failure suffers a significant energy imbalance, however, and may well benefit from nutritional assessment, including measurement of nitrogen balance.

Use of Disease Management and Other Resources

Perhaps one of the greatest tools at hand for clinicians caring for patients with heart failure, as well as for their families, is providing a thorough understanding of the heart failure syndrome and how self-empowered actions may have a significant impact on how they feel, what they can do, and how long they might live. Studies have repeatedly demonstrated the benefits of a structured disease management program in reducing symptoms, improving functional status, and, in particular, reducing heart failure hospitalizations. The clinician frequently can best serve the patient by fostering and supporting a heart failure disease management program. Although not present in all communities yet, the resources required (a physician and/or a nurse champion) are often accessible. Abundant educational patient-oriented books and materials are available to support these programs.

Disease management programs are often part of a larger specialized heart failure center. Within these structures are advanced strategies, including investigational therapies. It is incumbent on clinicians to be aware of these local and regional resources and refer patients when appropriate. Even with advanced disease, these centers can often offer improved outcomes and strategies not available to all clinicians.

Another area within the disease management spectrum is the home care programs that exist in most communities. These services frequently provide a link between intensive hospital-based care and infrequent, less intensive office-based care. In addition, for many patients with advanced disease, home care meets the constraints of patients and families.

For patients with advanced disease, physicians often begin discussions surrounding end-of-life issues too late. Patients who have advanced disease requiring frequent hospitalization and treatment generally are aware of their likelihood of death and, in fact, they value regaining some control of their lives through discussion of end-of-life planning and preferences. For some, hospice care is the choice made, whereas for others, referral to specialized centers and participation in emerging therapies through clinical trials might be the correct choice. Understanding comes only with an open and frank discussion with each patient and family.

Emerging and Emerged New Therapeutic Areas

Because of the intense interest in heart failure, a variety of important additional therapies are undergoing clinical investigation. These therapies include new application of biventricular pacemakers, aggressive mitral valve repair for patients with ongoing mitral valve regurgitation, and the use of left ventricular assist devices as bridges to heart recovery, as well as destination or permanent therapies.

CURRENT DIAGNOSIS

- Determine the etiology. It is critical to determine the underlying cause of a patient's heart failure; common clinical conditions including hypertension, diabetes mellitus, and coronary artery disease increase the risk of developing heart failure.
- Assess a patient's stage and functional class (see text). These are good guides to help recognize disease severity and guide treatment. Symptoms include evidence of dyspnea, fatigue, and sodium and water retention as congestion in the lungs, legs, and gut; these are usually late symptoms.
- Assess the volume status on every patient at every visit. Inability to assess volume carefully often leads to errors in therapeutics.
- Use additional tests and biomarkers such as peak oxygen consumption, ventricular ejection fraction, and elevated neurohormonal markers (B-type natriuretic peptide), which may provide early clues to disease severity.

CURRENT THERAPY

Targets

- Improved survival
- Improved symptoms
- Slowing and/or reversal of disease progression
- Improved functional status, quality of life
- Avoidance of adverse events
- Decreased use of resources including hospitalization

Care for Patients With Heart Failure

- Treatment of hypertension
- Smoking cessation
- Dietary counseling
- Exercise
- Weight loss
- Treatment of sleep-disordered breathing
- Angiotensin-converting enzyme (ACE) inhibitors (at target doses)
- β-Blockers (at target doses)
- Digoxin and diuretics
- Coronary revascularization
- Repair of mitral regurgitation
- Investigational therapies
- End-of-life counseling and hospice

Moreover, several new cardiac restraint devices are being applied with some success. Within years, genomic therapies will broaden, as will areas of vascular and myogenic regeneration. Again, although most clinicians are not aware of all these newly emerging therapies, they can offer their patients referrals to specialized centers where suitable therapies can be sought.

REFERENCES

Gattis WA, O'Connor CM, Gallup DS, et al: Predischarge initiation of carvedilol in patients hospitalized for decompensated heart failure: Results of the Initiation Management Predischarge: Process for Assessment of Carvedilol Therapy in Heart Failure (IMPACT_HF) trial. J Am Coll Cardiol 2004;43:1534-1541.

Hunt SA, Baker DW, Chin MH, et al: ACC/AHA guidelines for the evaluation and management of heart failure in the adult: A report of the American College of Cardiology/American Heart Association Task Force on Practice Guidelines (Committee to Revise the 1995 Guidelines for the Evaluation and Management of Heart Failure), 2001. American College of Cardiology Web site. Available online at http://www.acc.org/clinical/guidelines/failure/hf_index.htm

Konstam MA: Systolic and diastolic dysfunction in heart failure? Time for a new paradigm. J Card Fail 2003;9:1-3.

Pitt B, Remme W, Zannad F, et al: Eplerenone, a selective aldosterone blocker in patients with left ventricular dysfunction after myocardial infarction. N Engl J Med 2003;348:1309-1321.

Poole-Wilson PA, Swedberg K, Cleland JG, et al: Comparison of carvedilol and metoprolol on clinical outcomes in patients with chronic heart failure in the Carvedilol or Metoprolol European Trial (COMET): Randomized controlled trial. Lancet 2003;362:7-13.

Redfield MM: Heart failure—an epidemic of uncertain proportions. N Engl J Med 2002;347:1442-1444.

Infective Endocarditis

Method of
Navin M. Amin, MD

Epidemiologic Changes

Infective endocarditis denotes microbial infection of the cardiac valves and, less frequently, infection of the mural endocardium or of septal defects. At present, infective endocarditis accounts for 1 case per 1000 hospital admissions. The age of patients with endocarditis has increased. In the preantibiotic era, the average age of patients with endocarditis was 32 to 39 years old; currently more than half the cases occur in patients older than 60 years of age. Men are affected twice as often as women; the ratio increases to 5:1 in men older than 60 years of age.

Three major epidemiologic changes are observed in endocarditis:

1. The pattern of infective organisms has changed. Early in the antibiotic era, group A *Streptococci* (β hemolyticus), *Pneumococci, Gonococci,* and *Meningococci* were the predominant pathogens. *Streptococcus viridans, Staphylococcus aureus* (methicillin-sensitive [MSSA] or methicillin resistant [MRSA]), coagulase—negative *Staphylococcus epidermidis* or *lugdunensis*—and gram-negative organisms are more common today.
2. Certain signs and symptoms, once characteristic of endocarditis, are seen in less than 5% of cases today: peripheral lesions involving skin, nails, and eyes— petechiae, subungual hemorrhage, Janeway lesions, Osler nodes, or Roth's spots.
3. Surgical procedures can be both a cause and a cure of endocarditis. Prosthetic valves inserted to improve mechanically malfunctioning valves can predispose recipients to endocarditis. But surgery can be lifesaving in patients with refractory congestive heart failure (CHF) or resistant infections.

Forms of Endocarditis

Endocarditis is classified as acute or subacute on the basis of its clinical course. The acute form, which evolves over days to weeks, is diagnosed within 2 weeks. Invasive organisms such as *Staphylococcus aureus, Streptococcus pneumoniae,* group A streptococci, *Neisseria gonorrhoeae, Haemophilus influenzae, Salmonella,* other Enterobacteriaceae, and *Pseudomonas aeruginosa* are usually the cause. Clinically acute endocarditis is associated with high fever, systemic toxicity, and leukocytosis with rapid destruction of the valves. It carries high morbidity and mortality.

Subacute endocarditis has a duration of more than 6 weeks and an indolent course. The most common agents are streptococcal species, with *Streptococcus viridans* the most predominant: *Enterococcus,* HACEK (*Haemophilus, Actinobacillus, Cardiobacterium, Eikenella, Kingella*) organisms, fungi, and *Coxiella burnetii.* Clinically subacute endocarditis is associated with prolonged low-grade fever (fever of unknown origin [FUO]), night sweats, weight loss, and vague symptoms such as generalized weakness, lethargy, and myalgia.

Infective endocarditis can also be grouped into three categories:

1. *Native valve endocarditis* usually develops when there is structural damage to the heart valve. Rheumatic/syphilitic valvular disease is responsible in 20% to 40% of the cases. The mitral valve is involved in 85%, and the aortic valve is affected in 50% of the cases. In patients older than age 60 years, 30% of cases occur with degenerative cardiac lesions such as calcified mitral valve annulus and calcified nodular lesions secondary to atherosclerosis or postmyocardial infarction thrombus. Twenty percent of cases with mitral valve prolapse (with thickened leaflets or significant mitral regurgitation) and obstructive cardiomyopathy can predispose to endocarditis. In 6% to 25% of cases, congenital heart disease is a risk factor as is evident in ventricular septal defect (VSD), patent ductus arteriosus (PDA), tetralogy of Fallot, or coarctation of the aorta. It can also occur with a stenotic or regurgitant valve such as bicuspid aortic valve and pulmonary stenosis. Endocarditis is rare in patients with atrial septal defect (secundum type) because of the low-pressure gradient between the atria. Finally is a group of patients without any structural defect who are susceptible to endocarditis. Tricuspid valve endocarditis can develop in intravenous drug abusers and immunocompromised patients (with chronic renal failure, severe burns, chronic active hepatitis, collagen vascular disease, or neoplasm involving the pancreas, lung, or stomach).

2. *Prosthetic valve endocarditis* (PVE) at present constitutes 20% of all cases of endocarditis. It occurs in 2% to 4% of patients with a prosthetic valve. It can be early or late. Early PVE occurs within 60 days of the valve replacement, and predominant organisms are *Staphylococcus epidermidis* and *S. aureus* (MSSA or MRSA). In the case of late-onset endocarditis, which occurs after 2 months, *Streptococcus viridans* is the main offending pathogen.

3. *Nosocomial endocarditis* commonly affects patients older than age 60 years and seriously ill hospitalized patients. These individuals are subjected to invasive procedures such as insertion of central venous pressure, monitoring lines, hyperalimentation catheters, or intracardiac pacemaker wires that represent nidus of infection. Box 1 summarizes the factors predisposing to endocarditis.

Microbiology

Any microorganism can cause endocarditis (Table 1). Certain pathogens have increased ability to adhere to valvular leaflets, thereby establishing infection. Approximately 70% of the cases are caused by streptococci and staphylococci.

Staphylococci (MSSA or MRSA) are encountered predominantly in intravenous drug abuse (IVDA), in early PVE, in an immunocompromised host, and in nosocomial endocarditis. *S. viridans* is more commonly seen in native valve endocarditis and in late PVE. Gram-negative bacilli

---

BOX 1   Factors Predisposing to Endocarditis

Native Valve Endocarditis
- Structural Damage
    Rheumatic valvular disease
    Syphilitic valvular disease
    Degenerative
        Calcified mitral/aortic valve
        Calcified post-MI thrombus
    Mitral valve prolapse
    IHSS
    Congenital heart disease
        Regurgitant or stenotic valve, bicuspid aortic valve, PS, Ebstein's anomaly, Marfan's syndrome
        High-pressure shunt, VSD, PDA, coarctation of the aorta, tetralogy of Fallot
- No Structural Damage
    IVDA
    Immunocompromised

Prosthetic Valve Endocarditis
- Early (<2 mo)
    Staphylococcus epidermidis
    Staphylococcus aureus
- Late (>2 mo)
    Staphylococcus viridans

Nosocomial Endocarditis
- Invasive procedures

Abbreviations: IHSS = idiopathic hypertrophic subaortic stenosis; IVDA = intravenous drug abuse; MI = myocardial infarction; PDA = patent ductus arteriosus; PS = pulmonary stenosis; VSD = ventricular septal defect.
Adapted with permission from Amin NM: Infective endocarditis. Consultant 1994;34(3):319-343.

---

commonly cause right-sided endocarditis as in IVDA and in patients with intravascular catheters.

Approximately 10% of patients with endocarditis have a negative blood culture after 48 to 72 hours of incubation. Factors that produce culture-negative endocarditis are (1) antibiotic therapy before cultures are obtained; (2) a low level of bacteremia (common with right-sided and mural endocarditis); (3) infection with fastidious or nutritionally deficient bacteria that require prolonged cultures (2 to 3 weeks) or additional supplements (e.g., pyridoxine) for growth; this group includes HACEK organisms, *Brucella*, and nutritionally deficient streptococci; (4) nonbacterial infectious agents such as fungi, viruses, spirochetes, *Rickettsia*, *Chlamydia*, or parasites; and (5) noninfectious causes: left atrial myxoma, Libman-Sacks endocarditis, systemic lupus erythematosus, Löffler's hypereosinophilic endocarditis, carcinoid syndromes, and marantic endocarditis associated with malignancies of the pancreas, stomach, or lung.

Clinical Manifestations

The clinical manifestations of infective endocarditis are extremely diverse and can mimic pulmonary, neurologic, renal, or bone and joint disease. The classic manifestations of fever, heart murmur, splenomegaly, and petechiae of the skin and the mucous membranes help establish the diagnosis.

TABLE 1 Microbiology of Infective Endocarditis

Type of Infection	Specific Associated Risk Factors
Bacterial	
Gram Positive	
Streptococci (40%-60%)	
S. viridans, S. pneumoniae, S. bovis, S. pyogenes,	NVE, late-onset PVE
S. sanguis	
Enterococci (Group D) (5%-20%)	
S. faecalis, S. faecium, S. durans	Gastrointestinal malignancies
Staphylococci (17%-40%)	IVDA, early PVE
S. aureus, S. epidermidis, S. lugdunensis	
Diphtheroids	
Listeria	IVDA, early PVE
Gram Negative	
Cultured easily	
Pseudomonas aeruginosa, Serratia marcescens,	IVDA, immunocompromised, nosocomial endocarditis
Salmonella, Proteus mirabilis, Shigella, Providencia,	
Enterobacter, Neisseria gonorrhoeae, Escherichia coli	
Difficult to culture	
(HACEK) (1%-10%)	
Haemophilus, Actinobacillus, Cardiobacterium,	
Eikenella, Kingella	
(not HACEK)	
Brucella, Legionella	
Nonbacterial	
Fungi (2%-4%)	
Candida, Aspergillus, Histoplasma, Coccidioides,	IVDA, PVE, cardiac surgery, IV catheters,
Blastomyces	immunosuppressed
Viruses	
Coxsackie B, adenovirus	
Spirochetes	
Borrelia burgdorferi	Tick bite
Spirillum minus	Rat bite
Rickettsiae	
Coxiella burnetii	Infected livestock or unpasteurized milk
Chlamydia	
C. psittaci	Infected birds
Parasites	
Trypanosoma cruzi (Chagas' disease)	Kissing bug bite

Abbreviations: IVDA, intravenous drug abuse; NVE, native valve endocarditis; PVE, prosthetic valve endocarditis.
Modified from Amin NM: Infective endocarditis. Consultant 1994;34(3):319-343.

The onset may be abrupt or insidious. The early manifestations may be vague flulike symptoms that occur within 3 weeks after an invasive procedure. The patient may complain of malaise, fatigue, weakness, myalgia, arthralgia, low-grade fever, night sweats, or weight loss. Anorexia is almost universal. When the onset is acute, as in intravenous (IV) drug abuse, PVE, or nosocomial endocarditis, there may be evidence of severe infection heralded by high fever (90% to 95%), shaking chills and rigors, or, more ominous, symptoms of frank heart failure or embolic phenomena.

In patients older than age 60 years, diagnosis is often delayed because 5% may not have fever or are admitted with diagnosis of cerebral vascular accident (CVA), pneumonia, occult neoplasm, degenerative joint disease, or osteomyelitis. Infective endocarditis should always be considered in patients older than age 60 years who have fever and associated unexplained CHF, CVA, renal failure, weight loss, anemia, new-onset murmur, or confusional state.

In 85% of the cases, cardiac manifestations include a heart murmur. In right-sided endocarditis and mural infection, murmur is absent. A new or changing murmur (usually of aortic regurgitation) occurs in 5% to 10% of patients and is a very helpful diagnostic sign. Persistent or progressive CHF is indicative of a serious complication that carries a high mortality rate.

Peripheral cutaneous manifestations take a variety of forms: skin pallor caused by secondary anemia; petechiae found in 20% to 40% of cases concentrated on the conjunctiva, palate, buccal mucosa, and distal extremities; clubbing of nails in 10% to 20% if infection is long-standing; splinter hemorrhages as linear red-to-brown streaks in the middle of the nail bed of fingers and toes; Osler nodes (5% to 20% cases), which are small painful, tender, purplish subcutaneous nodules in the pads of fingers and toes; and Janeway lesions, which are small macular, painless, erythematous or hemorrhagic plaques on the palms or soles.

Ocular manifestations include Roth's spots, which occur in 5% of the patients and appear as oval or boat-shaped white or pale retinal lesions surrounded by hemorrhage and located near the optic disk. In a few cases there may be presence of cotton-wool exudates, petechiae, or flame-shaped hemorrhages.

Embolization can occur in 15% to 35% of cases. A cerebral emboli may produce hemiplegia, monoplegia, aphasia, or unilateral blindness. Mesenteric emboli can result in acute abdominal pain, ileus, or melena. Splenic emboli may cause left upper quadrant pain that radiates to the left shoulder of the chest with a small pleural effusion or splenic frictional rub. Flank pain with hematuria indicates a renal infarction. Peripheral arterial emboli may produce pain or gangrene. Large arterial occlusions are frequently seen with fungal endocarditis. Very rarely, emboli to coronary arteries cause acute myocardial infarction, myocardial abscess, or mycotic aneurysm.

Neurologic complications (30% to 40%) include CVA from embolization, mycotic aneurysm causing cerebral of subdural hemorrhage and seizure, and brain abscess or toxic encephalopathy with confusion and nonspecific obtundation.

Renal manifestations are accompanied by microscopic or frank hematuria secondary to renal infarct, diffuse membranoproliferative glomerulonephritis, focal embolic glomerulonephritis, or renal abscess.

Splenomegaly occurs in 25% to 45% of the patients and is more common in subacute than in acute endocarditis.

Diagnosis

Infective endocarditis may mimic any systemic disorder. For this reason and because of its high morbidity and mortality, the diagnosis should be kept in mind whenever a high-risk patient has an unexplained fever, constitutional symptoms, or multiple systemic involvement with a changing or new heart murmur. A high index of suspicion for endocarditis in certain clinical situations is very helpful:

- Intravenous drug abusers with high fever
- Patients older than age 60 years with nonspecific vague symptoms with a calcified mitral valve annulus
- Unknown source of embolization
- Certain virulent infections caused by organisms such as *Staphylococcus* or *Enterococcus*

A thorough history, complete examination, and laboratory tests should establish the correct diagnosis. Box 2 outlines the various laboratory abnormalities in infective endocarditis.

A baseline electrocardiogram (ECG) is helpful to detect chamber enlargement or possible conduction defect that may indicate underlying valvular or congenital anomalies. Later development of first-degree atrioventricular (AV) block, new bundle branch block, or new ectopic beats may indicate a myocardial abscess, especially in aortic valve endocarditis.

Echocardiography (transesophageal [TEE], M mode, two-dimensional, or Doppler) can confirm the diagnosis, detect complications, and help assess the prognosis. The echocardiogram can detect vegetations larger than 2 to 3 mm on mitral or aortic valves. Sensitivity in detecting

---

BOX 2   Laboratory Abnormalities in Endocarditis

- Hematologic
  - Leukocytosis
  - Anemia of chronic disorder
  - Thrombocytopenia (10% SBE)
  - Elevated ESR
- Urinalysis
  - Hematuria, microscopic
  - Proteinuria
- Cardiac abnormality
  - ECG: chamber enlargement, conduction defect
- Chest radiograph
  - Cardiomegaly
  - Evidence of congestive heart failure
  - Nodular infiltrate (staphylococcal endocarditis)
- Diagnostic gold standards
  - Echocardiography (transesophageal [TEE] preferred)
  - Three sets of blood (embolus) cultures
- Immunologic abnormalities
  - Rheumatoid factor (disappears after treatment)
  - Hypergammaglobulinemia
  - Cryoglobulinemia
  - Circulating immune complexes
  - Low complement levels

Abbreviations: ECG = electrocardiogram; ESR = erythrocyte sedimentation rate; SBE = subacute bacterial endocarditis.

---

vegetations is approximately 87% to 90% with TEE, 30% to 75% with M-mode, 40% to 50% with two-dimensional, and 50% with Doppler echocardiography. False-positive results are seen with old healed vegetations, myxomatous valvular degeneration, arterial myxoma, or a thrombus.

Echocardiogram can detect complications such as torn or perforated valves, ruptured chordae tendineae, myocardial abscess, or pericardial effusion that may require surgical intervention. Large-sized vegetations in the left side of the heart or in the aortic valve, or myocardial abscess, suggest a relatively poor prognosis, and surgery may be indicated.

Serial blood cultures are required to establish the diagnosis by isolating the offending bacterium or fungus. A minimum of three blood samples should be drawn 30 to 60 minutes apart before initiating empiric antibiotic therapy. If the patient has taken antibiotics in the preceding 2 weeks, two or three additional sets of blood cultures should be taken. Cultures of arterial blood offer no additional advantage over venous blood. Ninety percent of the blood cultures become positive within 7 days of incubation. Negative blood cultures are likely seen in patients who have received prior antibiotics or who have endocarditis caused by fastidious gram-negative (HACEK) bacilli, fungi, or nutritionally deficient streptococci. The microbiology laboratory should be alerted to the suspected endocarditis, and a report for prolonged incubation for 2 weeks included.

In fungal endocarditis, in which there is embolization of large arteries, a culture of the removed embolus can establish the diagnosis. Serologic studies can be helpful in fungal infection (histoplasmosis or coccidioidomycosis) or when rickettsial (Q fever) *Legionella* or *Chlamydia* infections are suspected.

Treatment of Infective Endocarditis

The main goal is eradicating the infecting pathogens as quickly as possible to reduce the risks of morbidity and mortality. This can be achieved with antibiotic therapy, surgical intervention, or both.

ANTIBIOTIC THERAPY

In using antibiotics to treat infective endocarditis, the following guidelines are helpful:

- Parental antibiotics are used to sustain bactericidal activity.
- Bactericidal antimicrobials are used for complete eradication of the pathogens. Synergistic bactericidal activity is achieved with combination therapy such as ampicillin and aminoglycosides in treatment of enterococcal endocarditis.
- The drug regimen and appropriate duration of course, 2 to 6 weeks, must be tailored to prevent relapse.
- The bactericidal activity of the antibiotic is monitored by determining the minimum inhibitory concentration (MIC) and the minimum bactericidal concentration (MBC) against the infecting organisms.
- Antibiotic therapy is initiated as quickly as possible. When endocarditis is severe and/or complicated, empiric treatment should be instituted immediately with antibiotics effective against *S. aureus* and enterococci. A combination of vancomycin (Vancocin) and gentamicin (Garamycin) is recommended. Once a specific organism is identified, appropriate bactericidal antibiotics should be used.

Most streptococci other than enterococci are exquisitely sensitive to penicillin. If MIC is less than 0.2 µg per mL, high-dose penicillin alone or in combination with either gentamicin (Garamycin) or streptomycin or ceftriaxone (Rocephin) can be used for 4 weeks. If the MIC is below 0.1 µg per mL, treatment should be for 2 weeks. If MIC is greater than 0.2 µg per mL or the MBC to MIC ratio exceeds 10:1, as it occurs in 15% to 20% of cases with *S. viridans* infection, higher dose of penicillin with aminoglycoside should be used. In penicillin-allergic patients, vancomycin is the best alternative with or without aminoglycoside (Table 2).

In enterococcal endocarditis, ampicillin is recommended in combination with an aminoglycoside. Gentamicin is

TABLE 2 Antibiotic Regimens for Bacterial Endocarditis

Infecting Organism	Antibiotic	Dosage, Route, and Frequency	Duration in Weeks
Penicillin susceptible *Streptococcus viridans*, and *S. bovis* (MIC <0.2 µg/dL)	*Preferred Regimen* Penicillin G or	12-16 million U/d IV in 6 divided doses	4
	Penicillin G PLUS	12-16 million U/d IV in 6 divided doses	4
	Gentamicin or	1 mg/kg IM or IV q8h	2
	Penicillin G PLUS Gentamicin or	Dosages same as above regimen	2
	Ceftriaxone	2g IV or IM q24h	4
	Alternative Regimen Vancomycin	0.5 g IV q6h	4
Relative penicillin-resistant streptococci (MIC >0.2 µg/dL)	*Preferred Regimen* Penicillin G PLUS	20-30 million U/d IV in 6 divided doses	4
	Gentamicin	1 mg/kg IV or IM q8h	4
	Alternative Regimen Vancomycin	0.5 g IV q6h	4
Staphylococcus epidermidis	*Native Valve* Vancomycin	0.5 g IV q6h	4
	Prosthetic Valve Vancomycin PLUS	0.5 g IV q6h	4-6
	Gentamicin or	1 mg/kg IV or IM q8h	2
	Rifampin	300 mg PO/IV q12h	2
Enterococcus (S. faecalis, S. faecium, S. durans)	*Preferred Regimen* Penicillin G PLUS	20-30 million U/d IV in 6 divided doses	4-6
	Gentamicin or	1 mg/kg IM or IV q8h	4-6
	Ampicillin PLUS	2g IV q4h	4-6

Continued

TABLE 2 Antibiotic Regimens for Bacterial Endocarditis—cont'd

Infecting Organism	Antibiotic	Dosage, Route, and Frequency	Duration in Weeks
	Gentamicin *Alternative Regimen*	1 mg/kg IM or IV q8h	4-6
	Vancomycin *PLUS*	0.5 g IV q6h	4-6
	Gentamicin *Preferred Regimen*	1 mg/kg IM or IV q8h	4-6
Staphylococcus aureus (methicillin sensitive)	Nafcillin or Oxacillin or	2 g IV q4h	4-6
	Oxacillin *PLUS*	2 g IV q4h	4-6
	Gentamicin *OR/PLUS*	1 mg/kg IM or IV q8h	2
	Rifampin *Alternative Regimen*	300 mg PO/IV q12h	2
	Cefazolin or	2 g IV q6h	4-6
	Vancomycin	0.5 g IV q6h	
S. aureus (methicillin resistant [MRSA])	Vancomycin *PLUS*	0.5 g IV q6h	4-6
	Gentamicin *OR/PLUS*	1 mg/kg IM or IV q8h	2
	Rifampin[1]	300 mg PO/IV q12h	2
HACEK group (*Haemophilus, Actinobacillus, Cardiobacterium, Eikenella, Kingella*)	Ampicillin or	2 g IV q6h	4
	Ampicillin *PLUS*	2 g IV q6h	4
	Gentamicin or	1 mg/kg IM or IV q8h	4
	Ceftriaxone	2 g IV q24h	4
Culture negative	Vancomycin *PLUS*	0.5 g IV q8h	6
	Gentamicin	1 mg/kg IM or IV q8h	6

Abbreviations: MIC = minimum inhibitory concentration
Modified from Amin NM: Infective Endocarditis. Consultant 1994;34(3):319-343.
[1]Not FDA approved for this indication

preferred because 40% of the isolates are resistant to streptomycin. In penicillin-allergic patients, vancomycin with an aminoglycoside is the best choice.

In *S. aureus* infection, semisynthetic penicillin or first-generation cephalosporins are the agents of first choice. Addition of gentamicin or rifampin (Rifadin)[1] during the first few days rapidly reduces bacteremia. Vancomycin is recommended for patients allergic to penicillin or if the organism is methicillin resistant (MRSA). Addition of rifampin, although controversial, is recommended in patients demonstrating poor bactericidal activity during therapy with beta-lactams or vancomycin and for patients with suppurative complication, such as a valve ring abscess.

Endocarditis with *S. epidermidis*, which commonly develops on prosthetic valves, is ideally treated with vancomycin and rifampin.[1] An aminoglycoside may be added for 2 weeks.

Gram-negative infections causing high mortality are best treated with broad-spectrum penicillin or, preferably, a third-generation cephalosporin with an aminoglycoside. In most of these patients, valve replacement is necessary.

SURGICAL INTERVENTIONS

Approximately 25% of patients with severe or complicated endocarditis undergo surgery. The chief indications for surgery are refractory moderate or severe CHF; perivalvular invasion or myocardial abscess as evident by persistent fever despite antibiotics or electrocardiographic changes of conduction defects; systemic or arterial embolization; fungal endocarditis; PVE of early onset; large bulky vegetations that increase risk of CHF; persistent infection (particularly with gram-negative bacilli) that does not respond to 7 to 10 days of antibiotic therapy; and staphylococcal endocarditis in IV drug abusers that does not respond to antimicrobials.

PREVENTION OF BACTERIAL ENDOCARDITIS

Transient bacteremia that develops after a variety of manipulations or surgical procedures in patients with structural heart defects causes endocarditis. Prophylactic antibiotics

[1]Not FDA approved for this indication.

in this situation can be highly effective when given before the procedure. Administration of these agents only once is required 30 minutes to 2 hours before the procedure (Table 3).

In choosing prophylactic therapy, the following questions (Table 4) are useful:

- Is the patient at increased risk for endocarditis with underlying structural defect?
- Is there a high risk the procedure will produce bacteremia with organisms that cause endocarditis, such as *S. viridans* infection with oral cavity procedures or enterococcal with gastrointestinal or genitourinary procedures?

Antibiotic prophylaxis is recommended for patients with VSD, PDA, pulmonary or aortic stenosis, tetralogy of Fallot, or coarctation of the aorta. Such therapy is needed for patients with rheumatic or syphilitic valvular defects, prosthetic valves, calcified valves, obstructive cardiomyopathy, or mitral valve prolapse with either regurgitant murmur or with thickened mitral valve leaflets.

Endocarditis prophylaxis is not advised for patients with isolated secundum atrial septal defect or those who have undergone surgical repair for VSD or PDA and have no residual defect beyond 6 months. The same is true for those who have coronary artery bypass graft, previous rheumatic fever, or Kawasaki disease without any valve dysfunction. Prophylaxis is not recommended for those who have mitral valve prolapse (MVP) without mitral regurgitation (MR) and for persons with a cardiac pacemaker or implanted defibrillator (Table 5).

Procedures for which antibiotic prophylaxis is needed are those in which transient bacteremia develops when mucosal surfaces colonized with microorganisms are traumatized. For example, bacteremia may occur following dental manipulation in 80% of cases or in 20% of patients after urethral instrumentation. Prophylactic antimicrobials are recommended for high-risk patients who are

TABLE 3 Preprocedural Antibiotic Prophylaxis for At-Risk Patients

Type of Procedure and Situation	Antibiotic	Dosage, Route, and Frequency
Dental, oral respiratory tract, and esophageal procedures		
Standard prophylaxis	Amoxicillin	2 g PO 1 h before procedure
Patient unable to take oral medication	Ampicillin	2 g IM/IV within 30 min before procedure
Patient allergic to penicillin	Clindamycin (Cleocin*)	600 mg PO 1 h before procedure
	or	
	cefadroxil (Duricef*)	2 g PO 1 h before procedure
	or	
	cephalexin (Keflex*)	2 g PO 1 h before procedure
	or	
	azithromycin (Zithromax*)	500 mg PO 1 h before procedure
	or	
	clarithromycin (Biaxin*)	500 mg PO 1 h before procedure
Patient allergic to penicillin and unable to take oral medication	Clindamycin (Cleocin*)	600 g IV within 30 min of starting procedure
	or	
	cefazolin (Ancef)	1 g IV within 30 min of starting procedure
	or	
	vancomycin (Vancocin)	1 g IV over 1-2 h within 60 min of starting procedure
Genitourinary/gastrointestinal procedures		
Moderate-risk patient	Amoxicillin	2 g PO 1 h before procedure
	or	
	ampicillin	2 g IM/IV within 30 min of starting procedure
Moderate-risk penicillin-allergic patient	Vancomycin	1 g IV over 1-2 h infusion completed within 30-60 min of starting procedure
High-risk patient	Ampicillin	2 g IM/IV given within 30 min of starting procedure
	PLUS	
	gentamicin	1.5 mg/kg IV given within 30 min of starting procedure
	6 h later	
	Ampicillin	1 g IM or IV
	or	
	amoxicillin	1 g PO
High-risk penicillin-allergic patient	Vancomycin	1 g IV over 1-2 h
	PLUS	
	gentamicin	1.5 mg/kg IV given within 30 min of starting procedure

Modified from Dajani AS, Taubert KA, Wilson W, et al: Prevention of bacterial endocarditis: Recommendation by the American Heart Association. JAMA 1997;277(22):1794-1801.
*Not FDA approved for this indication

TABLE 4 Indications for Endocardial Prophylaxis

Cardiac Conditions	Procedures

High-risk category
Prosthetic valve
Previous endocarditis
Complex cyanotic disease
   Tetralogy of Fallot, single ventricle
Surgically conducted systemic-pulmonary shunt
 	
Moderate-risk category
Congenital heart disease: VSD, PDA, AS, PS
Acquired valvular dysfunction
   Rheumatic/syphilitic
Hypertrophic cardiomyopathy
MVP with MR or thickened leaflets
	Dental
	Dental extraction
	Periodontal procedures: surgery, scaling, root planing
	Dental implant replacement
	Subgingival placement of antibiotic fibers
	Intraligamentary local anesthetic injection
	Cleaning of teeth or implants
	
	Respiratory
	Tonsillectomy/adenoidectomy
	Rigid bronchoscopy
	
	Gastrointestinal
	Sclerotherapy
	Esophageal stricture dilation
	ERCP with biliary obstruction
	Biliary tract surgery
	Surgery involving intestinal mucosa
	
	Genitourinary
	Prostatic surgery
	Cystoscopy
	Urethral dilation
	Septic abortion

Abbreviations: AS = aortic stenosis; ERCP = endoscopic retrograde cholangiopancreatography; MVP = mitral valve prolapse; MR = mitral regurgitation; PDA = patent ductus arteriosus; PS = pulmonary stenosis; VSD = ventricular septal defect.
Modified from Dajani AS, Taubert KA, Wilson W, et al: Prevention of bacterial endocarditis: Recommendations by the American Heart Association. JAMA 1997;277(22):1794-1801.

TABLE 5 Endocardial Prophylaxis Not Recommended

Cardiac Conditions	Procedures
Isolated secundum ASD Surgical repair of ASD, VSD, PDA (without residue > 6 mo) Previous CABG surgery MVP without valvular dysfunction Functional murmur Kawasaki disease without valvular dysfunction Previous rheumatic fever without valve dysfunction Cardiac pacemaker and implanted defibrillators Cardiac catheterization, balloon angioplasty Coronary stent placement	**Dental** Restorative dentistry Local anesthetic injections Intracanal treatment Postoperative suture removal Oral impression/radiograph Fluoride treatment Shedding of primary teeth **Respiratory** Endotracheal intubation Fiberoptic bronchoscopy Tympanostomy tube insertion **Gastrointestinal** TEE* Endoscopy with/without biopsy* **Genitourinary** Vaginal delivery/hysterectomy* Cesarean section Urethral catheterization Uterine dilation and curettage Insertion/removal of IUD Circumcision

*Prophylaxis optional for high-risk category.
Abbreviations: ASD = atrial septal defect; CABG = coronary artery bypass graft; IUD = intrauterine device; MVP = mitral valve prolapse; PDA = patent ductus arteriosus; TEE = transesophageal echocardiogram; VSD = ventricular septal defect.
Modified from Dajani AS, Taubert KA, Wilson W, et al: Prevention of bacterial endocarditis: Recommendations by the American Heart Association. JAMA 1997;277(22):1794-1801.

CURRENT DIAGNOSIS

- High index of suspicion
- Febrile patient (temperature >38°C [100.4°F]) with
  Valvular or congenital heart defects
  Intravenous drug abuse
  Prosthetic or vascular access
  New onset or changing cardiac murmur
  Unknown source of embolization
- Positive blood cultures on at least two different specimens.
- Presence of vegetation detected on echocardiography (transesophageal [TEE] preferred)

scheduled to have certain dental, oropharyngeal, gastrointestinal, or genitourinary manipulations.

Standard antibiotic prophylaxis for patients undergoing oral, dental, or upper respiratory tract manipulations include oral amoxicillin. Clindamycin (Cleocin),[1] cefadroxil (Duricef),[1] cephalexin (Keflex),[1] or azithromycin (Zithromax)[1] or clarithromycin (Biaxin)[1] should be given to those who cannot tolerate or are allergic to penicillin.

Parenteral ampicillin is recommended for patients who cannot take oral antibiotics and for those at high risk for infective endocarditis, such as patients with a prosthetic valve, previous endocarditis, or surgical systemic pulmonary shunts. Clindamycin[1] or cefazolin (Ancef) can be used as an alternative. Patients undergoing gastrointestinal or genitourinary instrumentation should be given vancomycin.

As recommended by the American Heart Association, all prophylactic antibiotics should be used only once before the procedure. There is no need for additional antibiotic administration except in high-risk patients who are undergoing gastrointestinal or genitourinary manipulation and who are given an ampicillin and gentamicin combination.

---

[1]Not FDA approved for this indication.

CURRENT THERAPY

- Empiric antibiotics should be started immediately with vancomycin and gentamicin.
- Specific therapy should be started once the pathogen is identified:
  Use combination therapy for synergetic activity.
  Monitor MIC/MBC level whenever possible.
  Administer therapy for 2 to 6 weeks.
- Surgical interventions should be undertaken for severe, refractory, and complicated endocarditis.
- Prophylactic antibiotics are recommended in patients with structural heart defects undergoing surgical procedures or manipulations that can cause transient bacteremia, as recommended by the American Heart Association.
- Administration of antibiotic is usually once and 30 minutes to 1 to 2 hours before the procedure.

Abbreviations: MBC = minimum bactericidal concentration; MIC = minimum inhibitory concentration.

REFERENCES

Amin NM: Infective endocarditis. Consultant 1994;34(3):319-343.

Bansal RC: Infective endocarditis. Med Clin North Am 1995;79:1205-1220.

Bayer AS, Bolger AF, Taubert KA, et al: Diagnosis and management of infective endocarditis and its complications. Circulation 1998;98:2936-2948.

Bayer AS, Ward JI, Ginzton LE, Shapiro SM: Evaluation of new clinical criteria for diagnosis of infective endocarditis. Am J Med 1994;96:211-219.

Cunha BA, Gill MV, Lazar JM: Acute infective endocarditis. Infect Dis Clin North Am 1996;10(4):811-834.

Dajanai AS, Taubert KA, Wilson W, et al: Prevention of bacterial endocarditis. Recommendations by American Heart Association. JAMA 1997;277:1794-1801.

Giessel BE, Koenig CJ, Blake RL: Management of bacterial endocarditis. Am Fam Physician 2000;61:1725-1732.

Karchner AW: Infections on prosthetic valves and intravascular infections. In Mandell GL, Bennett JE, Dolin R (eds): Mandell, Douglas and Bennett's Principles and Practice of Infectious Diseases, 5th ed. Philadelphia, Churchill Livingstone, 2000, pp 903-917.

Li JS, Sexton DJ, Mick N, et al: Proposed modification to Duke criteria for diagnosis of infective endocarditis. Clin Infect Dis 2000;30:633-638.

Mylonakis E, Calderwood SB: Infective endocarditis in adults. N Engl J Med 2001;345(18):1318-1330.

Hypertension

Method of
Edward D. Frohlich, MD

Hypertension is a major disease that affects approximately one billion people worldwide. In the United States, it affects more than 20% of adult whites, 40% of adult blacks, more than 50% of those older than 65 years, and about 90% of those older than 80 years. It is the most common risk factor accounting for deaths from stroke, cardiac failure, coronary heart disease, and end-stage renal disease. The higher the blood pressure (systolic or diastolic), the higher the morbidity and mortality. Most important from these dramatic statistics, this risk can be reversed dramatically with effective control of arterial pressure, although many authorities believe that some forms of antihypertensive pharmacologic therapy may be more effective than others in controlling elevated pressure as well as morbid and mortal events in certain demographic or clinical groups of patients. This latter point is covered in some detail in this discussion, and all authorities emphasize the great importance of blood pressure control (Table 1). The final shocking statistic from the National Health and Nutrition Survey in the United States revealed that only 34% of all adults with hypertension had their blood pressure under control. These data, which are perhaps the best in the world, reflect a National High Blood Pressure Education Program effort of 35 years' duration. However, a much better job must be done by all who provide health care. After all, we know from the earliest of the multicenter trials and from public health records that if blood pressure can be effectively controlled, deaths from stroke and coronary heart disease can be reduced by more than 72% and 55%, respectively, and deaths from hypertensive emergencies can be prevented.

TABLE 1 Trends in Awareness, Treatment, and Control of High Blood Pressure 1976–2000 National Health and Nutrition Examination Survey (expressed as percentage)

	1976–1980	1988–1991	1991–1994	1999–2000
Awareness	51	73	68	70
Treatment	31	55	54	59
Controlled*	10	29	27	34

Percentage of adults aged 18–74 years with systolic pressure ≥140 mm Hg and/or diastolic pressure ≥90 mm Hg or taking antihypertensive medication.
*Systolic pressure <140 mm Hg and diastolic pressure <90 mm Hg and on antihypertensive treatment.

Classification of Blood Pressure Levels

TECHNIQUE

Over the years, the severity of hypertension in adults has been classified with respect to the height of the measured blood pressure. Of course, the reliability of this index is determined primarily with respect to accuracy measurement, and guidelines have been published in each of the Joint National Committee (JNC) reports; the most recent is the seventh (JNC-7). The most important features involved in taking the blood pressure are: the patient should be seated and relaxed for at least 5 minutes, the patient should be cautioned beforehand to refrain from smoking or caffeine ingestion for at least 30 minutes, the patient's arm should be bare in order to obviate arterial constriction by clothing, and pressures should be obtained two or more times at each visit and measurements obtained on at least three occasions before diagnosis or treatment is made. If clinical circumstances are such that therapy must be instituted immediately (e.g., if the repeated pressures are inordinately elevated), then clearly therapy also is recommended. In the earliest classifications, severity was based on the height of diastolic pressure; however, in more recent years, both systolic and diastolic pressures are necessary for classification, and the systolic reading probably is more significant, especially in the elderly patient.

Several changes were instituted with publication of JNC-7, including use of the term *prehypertension* instead of *high normal* in the definition of normal pressure, and the reduction of the number of severity stages from three to two (Table 2). Based on this classification, the report recommends specific lifestyle modifications (for prevention as well as treatment) and guidelines for selection of pharmacologic therapy.

TABLE 2 Classification of Blood Pressure for Adults

Hypertension Classification	Systolic Pressure (mm Hg)	Diastolic Pressure (mm Hg)
Normal	<120	And <80
Prehypertension	120–139	or 80–89
Stage 1 hypertension	140–159	or 90–99
Stage 2 hypertension	≥160	or ≥100

CONCERNS

Because this discussion reflects some personal biases of the author, I shall offer certain aspects of my thinking, but, when offered, they will be indicated clearly in the text. My first personal comment relates to what I believe is the very controversial term *prehypertension*, which was introduced in JNC-7 to include those adults whose blood pressures ranged from 120 to 139 mm Hg systolic and from 80 to 89 mm Hg diastolic. Although these individuals do not yet have "true" hypertension, such values had been termed as *high normal* pressures since JNC-3. The rationale for this most recent change in terminology is related to the greater likelihood and risk of these people eventually developing sustained hypertension later in life; and this potential eventuality may be prevented by instituting specific lifestyle measures (discussed later). To my way of thinking, the earlier term *high normal* was more appropriate because not all of these people will eventually develop outright hypertension, and some of these individuals (many) may be inappropriately rated for higher insurance premiums (especially because this new term is to receive a diagnostic code); already some have been denied the opportunity to serve as kidney donors. In these respects, however, we must be hopeful that the noble wishes of our colleagues to promote this new and more evangelistic term are appropriate in order to stimulate established lifestyle recommendations and, thus, prevent later development of hypertension.

SELF-MEASUREMENT AND AMBULATORY MONITORING

A brief discussion is appropriate concerning the use techniques for ambulatory and self-measurement of blood pressure. The ambulatory and portable techniques are useful and valid; however, in my opinion, diagnosis of hypertension should not be based on these measurements because normative data are not yet available. In contrast, self-measurement techniques have been used for many years to help guide selection and dosing of therapy and to obviate overmedication. I, personally, have been using this approach of self-measurement of home pressures to manage patients and their therapy for many years. On the other hand, the use of ambulatory monitoring has several useful indications, which include selection and dosing of drug therapy, consideration of the so-called patient with "white coat hypertension," relating blood pressure levels to specific clinical "spells" (e.g., nocturnal angina, suspected pheochromocytoma, postural hypotension associated with meals, exercise), and for research purposes to obtain data to determine efficacy of therapy, to evaluate cost and reimbursement issues, and to develop new concepts for overall clinical management.

Evaluation of the Hypertensive Patient

SIGNS AND SYMPTOMS

Most patients with hypertension have no clinical manifestations of the disease other than the elevated pressure. Therefore, unless blood pressure is measured in all adult patients, the disease will remain unrecognized and, regrettably, untreated. Consequently these individuals will be predisposed to the end-organ outcomes of the disease. Thus, the most common complaints in hypertension relate to target organ involvement: for cardiac involvement, reduced exercise tolerance, easy fatigability, chest discomfort, and cardiac awareness (e.g., palpitations, ectopic beats, feelings of abnormal cardiac rate or rhythm); for renal involvement, nocturia, proteinuria, and hematuria; and for brain involvement, dysarthria or signs of sensory or motor deficit. Of course, at that later time, the disease will have progressed to greater severity of cardiovascular and other organ involvement. Hence, once again, management of the disease begins with the earliest evidence of risk, and that is early detection of the elevated arterial pressure.

FUNDUSCOPIC CHANGES

Additional physical findings are associated with hypertension, including ophthalmologic findings (Table 3). Small-vessel constriction of both arterioles and venules, either generalized or focal, may be detected early (group I of Keith, Wagener, and Barker). Coexisting arteriolosclerotic changes are also manifested by discontinuity of the arterioles at arteriovenous crossings (i.e., arteriovenous "nicking" in group II). Later, evidence of more accelerated

CURRENT DIAGNOSIS

Cardiac Involvement

- Reduced exercise tolerance
- Easy fatigability
- Chest discomfort
- Cardiac awareness

Renal Involvement

- Nocturia
- Proteinuria
- Hematuria

Brain Involvement

- Dysarthria
- Signs of sensory or motor deficit

Funduscopic Changes

- See Table 3
- Laboratory studies

TABLE 3 Classification of Hypertensive Retinopathy

Keith-Wagener-Barker Classification
Group I—Tortuosity, minimal constriction
Group II—Above + arteriovenous nicking
Group III—Above + hemorrhages and exudates
Group IV—Papilledema

American Ophthalmological Society Committee Classification (Wagener-Clay-Gipner)

Generalized arteriolar constriction
Grade 1—Arterioles ¾ of normal caliber; A/V ratio 1:2
Grade 2—Arterioles ½ or normal caliber; A/V ratio 1:3
Grade 3—Arterioles ⅓ of normal caliber; A/V ratio 1:4
Grade 4—Arterioles threadlike or invisible

Focal arteriolar constriction or sclerosis
Grade 1—Localized arteriolar narrowing to ⅔ caliber of proximal segment
Grade 2—Localized arteriolar narrowing to ½ caliber of proximal segment
Grade 3—Localized arteriolar narrowing to ⅓ caliber of proximal segment
Grade 4—Arterioles invisible beyond focal constriction

Generalized sclerosis
Grade 1—Increased light-striping; mild arteriovenous nicking
Grade 2—Coppery arteriolar color; moderate arteriovenous nicking veins almost completely invisible below arteriolar crossing
Grade 3—Silver arteriolar color; severe arteriovenous nicking
Grade 4—Arterioles visible only as fibrous cords without bloodstreams
Hemorrhage and exudates—Grades 1–4 (based on number of affected quadrants divided by 2)
Papilledema—Grades 1–4 (based on diopters of elevation)

Abbreviation: A/V = Arteriovenous.

disease can be seen with the appearance of exudates and hemorrhages (group III) and with full-blown malignant hypertension with papilledema (group IV). Careful search for cholesterol and other emboli should be made in patients suspected of having transient ischemic attack. In addition, because diabetes mellitus frequently coexists with hypertension, it is important to carefully search funduscopically for microaneurysms and more characteristic exudates associated with diabetes on all office visits.

PERIPHERAL ARTERIES

Intensity and propagation of the femoral and brachial arterial pulsations should be checked carefully for delay and diminution (especially in younger patients) in order to exclude the possibility of aortic coarctation. These signs are also important in older patients and in those with occlusive peripheral arterial disease. In addition, careful auscultation of the carotid and other arteries (including abdominal) should be performed to detect bruits suggesting neural or renal involvement. With respect to the latter, it is especially important to note the timing of the arterial bruit because systolic as well as diastolic timing is even more suggestive of renal arterial occlusive disease.

TABLE 4 Abnormal Diagnostic Electrocardiographic Criteria of Left Atrial Abnormality

P wave in lead II ≥0.3 mV and ≥0.12 sec
Bipeak interval in notched P wave ±0.04 sec
Ratio of P-wave duration to PR segment ≥1.6 (lead II)
Terminal atrial forces (in lead V_1) ≥0.04 sec

CARDIAC EXAMINATION

Even before left ventricular hypertrophy (LVH) is detectable, palpation of a hyperdynamic apical cardiac impulse early in the disease should suggest a hyperkinetic circulatory state. Later, with development of LVH, the apical impulse is more sustained and lifts the palpating hand. The earliest clinical evidence of LVH is demonstrable by left atrial enlargement and by the presence of an atrial diastolic gallop (fourth heart sound) rhythm, findings that are highly concordant with electrocardiographic evidence of left atrial abnormality (Table 4). Hemodynamic and echocardiographic studies have clearly demonstrated that when these findings are present, LVH has already occurred and is associated with impaired left ventricular (LV) function. Thus, these abnormal atrial findings reflect impaired LV filling during diastole as a result of a less distensible hypertrophying LV. In addition, a functional "click" may be audible in patients with a hyperkinetic circulation if the posterior leaflet of the mitral valve is everted as a consequence of increased adrenergic drive to the heart. With auscultatory appearance of a third heart sound, there is further impairment of LV function and decompensation. Although cardiac murmurs specifically related to hypertensive disease are rare, a systolic hemic flow murmur may be present early with a hyperdynamic circulation, and an aortic systolic ejection-type murmur may be present in older patients with a sclerotic or calcific aortic valve. In addition, the murmur of aortic insufficiency may be present if the arterial pressure is markedly elevated, thereby everting the aortic valve.

LABORATORY STUDIES

Guidelines sometimes neglect the rationale and necessity for obtaining certain laboratory studies, so for this reason we include a brief discussion. Remember, if a patient is already receiving diuretic therapy, hypokalemia may obscure the possibilities of adrenal (including primary hyperaldosteronism, Cushing's disease or syndrome, or other) cortical diseases or renal arterial disease. Thus, it is worthwhile to have the patient discontinue the diuretic, if at all possible, for at least 2 weeks prior to initial evaluation. Furthermore, it is wise to consider that hypokalemia may also be encountered in patients with laxative abuse, chronic vomiting or diarrhea, or with a large colonic adenoma.

Other laboratory studies that I consider important initially are a complete blood count without necessity for differential count, determination of renal function (serum creatinine concentration is the more important), fasting blood glucose level, and serum uric acid concentrations, as well as a full lipid profile. Not infrequently, patients with hypertension have a higher hematocrit or hemoglobin concentration as a consequence of plasma volume contraction as arterial pressure (and total peripheral resistance) increases. However, if anemia coexists with hypertension, one must always consider renal involvement if there is no suggestion of a hemoglobinopathy or blood loss (overt or occult). Not infrequently, a panel of automated chemical tests is much less expensive than ordering these or other studies individually. In the chemistry panel, inclusion of hepatic function tests may be of value because the physician eventually may order a multiplicity of drugs if hepatic involvement occurs. Remember that most patients take two or more medications for treatment of hypertension, and other agents are frequently prescribed for comorbid diseases, including hyperlipidemia, gout, and type 2 diabetes mellitus.

Other important studies are urinalysis, 12-lead electrocardiography, hemoglobin A_{1c} value if the patient has diabetes, and more specific endocrinologic studies if an endocrinopathy is suspected (e.g., hyperthyroidism or hypothyroidism, parathormone in the case of elevated calcium concentration, and others for adrenal steroid tumors or pheochromocytoma). An echocardiogram is not usually indicated, particularly if the presence of LVH is already established by electrocardiography, but this technique is valuable for assessing ventricular function or coexistent valvular heart disease.

Treatment

LIFESTYLE (NONPHARMACOLOGIC) THERAPY

A number of lifestyle modifications have been demonstrated to be effective for control of arterial pressure. Indeed, they have been shown to be particularly useful (and even preventive) in patients with "prehypertension," who may be particularly predisposed to later development of established hypertension. Interventions that have been shown to be particularly effective are weight control, reduction of excessive alcohol intake, sodium restriction, maintenance of an adequate potassium intake, and a regular isometric exercise program. Less emphasized, but to my

---

 CURRENT THERAPY

Nonpharmacologic

- Weight control
- Alcohol restriction
- Sodium restriction
- Smoking cessation
- Isometric exercise

Pharmacologic

- Diuretics
- α-Adrenergic receptor blockers
- β-Adrenergic receptor blockers
- α-/β-Adrenergic receptor blockers
- Angiotensin-converting enzyme inhibitors
- Angiotensin II (type 1) receptor blockers
- Calcium antagonists

thinking an equally (or more) important antihypertensive measure, is smoking cessation. The national guidelines emphasize the importance of smoking cessation as a general cardiovascular measure. A number of multicenter trials have demonstrated clearly that the smoker who takes a β-adrenergic receptor–blocking agent, and who has as effective control of pressure as a similar patient taking a diuretic, will not have the same protection against death from stroke or coronary heart disease as does the patient taking the diuretic. A trial of lifestyle interventions is always in order, but if they are not effective in controlling pressure, I then institute antihypertensive drug treatment. This, however, does not mean that the lifestyle measures that had already been initiated should be discontinued. Therefore, a few words are in order with respect to these interventions.

WEIGHT CONTROL

Overweight (or obesity) is exceedingly common in hypertensive patients and, for that matter, in our general population (but more so with hypertension). Many studies have demonstrated that weight reduction may be associated with a decline in arterial pressure as well as a decrease in the number of drugs (or dose requirements) taken by a given patient with hypertension. Moreover, this reduction in body weight may be independent of the dietary sodium intake, and it may also be associated with a reduction in serum lipid levels. Nevertheless, this behavior modification is exceedingly important in reducing the morbidity and mortality associated with hypertension and other cardiovascular diseases. It is well acknowledged that recidivism is a characteristic of this and other desired lifestyle changes; however, certain dietary measures have been documented to be particularly successful in providing the necessary positive feedback necessary for sustained weight reduction. Specifically, the Dietary Approaches to Stop Hypertension (DASH) diet, which is high in fruits, vegetables, and low-fat dairy products, has been particularly helpful. Personally, I have found that prescription of a diet in which bread, cake, and cookies with no fried chicken or fish but with careful selection of beef, pork, or veal without fat graining, is particularly acceptable. Thus, the patient is not restricted in consuming these meats, fowl, and fish, but substituting cooking methods may be quite helpful.

Alcohol Restriction

Many studies have demonstrated clearly that the quantity of alcohol (i.e., ethanol) consumption is directly related to the height of arterial pressure. For this reason, the national guidelines have recommended restriction of ethanol intake to no more than 1 oz (or its equivalent) daily.

Sodium Restriction

Sodium restriction continues to be a subject of great controversy, primarily because even though restriction of sodium may be effective in reducing the doses or number of antihypertensive drugs, only about 35% of patients with essential hypertension have been shown to be "sodium" or "salt dependent." More recently, however, our

experimental studies have shown that even though further increase of arterial pressure may be minimal, dietary salt excess also promotes profound structural and functional alterations of the heart, aorta and large vessels, and kidneys. These experimental studies are now being supported by additional clinical reports, and hence I believe it is essential to be more vigorous in counseling salt (i.e., sodium)-restricted diets. One must remember that, in doing so, about half of the daily sodium dietary intake is derived from salt; the remainder is in the form of food additives such as preservatives and taste enhancers. With these thoughts, the national recommendation of restricting daily sodium intake to no more than 100 mEq (2.3 g) is not only reasonable but is eminently "doable." In this consideration, potassium intake of approximately 90 mmol daily has also been found to be effective in reducing pressure. However, one should realize that consumption of fruit juices and uncooked vegetables will add to this effectiveness. Moreover, remember that prolonged boiling can leach out necessary potassium content.

Exercise

A regular program of aerobic (isometric) exercise has been shown to be of value in reducing arterial pressure. This involves walking, jogging, bicycling, treadmill exercise, or swimming. Such a program not only can reduce pressure, but it may augment the effectiveness of antihypertensive drug therapy. In contrast, isotonic exercises such as weight lifting and rowing can add to the increased total peripheral resistance that is already present with the hypertensive disease; therefore, I do not encourage the isotonic form of exercise.

PHARMACOLOGIC THERAPY

In discussing pharmacologic therapy, there are eight classes of antihypertensive drugs presently used in daily practice, but for the sake of brevity I exclude the centrally acting adrenergic inhibitors and the direct-acting vascular smooth muscle relaxants. In this discussion, I include primarily a consideration of each of the other six classes: their overall clinical mechanisms of action, hemodynamic effects, side effects, and some personal considerations about each of their merits for selection as initial antihypertensive therapy for specific patients with hypertension (whether or not the indications are termed "compelling"). With respect to each of these six antihypertensive drug classes, many authorities believe that the most important consideration is their ability to reduce and control arterial pressure. However, I believe that in addition to lowering arterial pressure, other important features of these agents relate to their specific intraorgan protective effects on the target organs of the disease. Thus, my discussion also emphasizes this aspect of the efficacy of each of the drug classes.

Efficacy

Controlled clinical trials, and almost 50 years of clinical experience, have demonstrated incontrovertibly the overall efficacy, safety, and feasibility of antihypertensive therapy. In addition, this vast clinical track record has shown through the intrinsic ability of antihypertensive therapy not only that it is possible to control arterial pressure but that it is possible to prevent and reverse many of the complications of hypertensive cardiovascular disease on the heart, kidneys, and brain.

Initial Options

As indicated, eight classes of antihypertensive agents can be considered as options for the initial therapy for hypertension: diuretics, β-adrenergic receptor–blocking agents, α-adrenergic and α-/β-adrenergic blockers, centrally acting adrenergic inhibitors, angiotensin-converting enzyme (ACE) inhibitors, angiotensin II (type 1) receptor blockers (ARBs), and calcium antagonists. I discuss each of these classes of antihypertensive agents with respect to their side effects with the exception of the centrally acting adrenergic inhibitors. These compounds, although still used around the world, are no longer recommended by the JNC or the World Health Organization (WHO) guidelines because of their side effects. I agree with this action, although methyldopa and clonidine occasionally may be prescribed for patients with more severe hypertension or in hypertensive emergencies (see Table 11). Other pharmacologic classes are under study at this time (e.g., renin inhibitors and blockers of the synthesis of endothelin or an ACE inhibitor with a neutral endopeptidase inhibitor).

Diuretics

The thiazide diuretics (including their chemical congeners) are as close to the "ideal" as any of the agents that are available. They have withstood the test of time as effective monotherapy for a large percentage of the essential hypertensive population. They are well tolerated and have a relatively low incidence of side effects, particularly if lower recommended doses are used. They can be administered once daily (or even less frequently in some circumstances). By definition, they will not produce pseudotolerance (i.e., expansion of intravascular [plasma] volume as pressure is reduced, thereby detracting from blood pressure control). They are relatively inexpensive, particularly when they may not require additional potassium supplements, potassium-retaining agents, or other drugs that have hypouricemic, hypoglycemic, or hypolipidemic actions.

Over the years, a large number of chemical formulations of the thiazides and their congeners have been introduced (Table 5). Unfortunately, few studies have included sufficient patient numbers demonstrating the clinical, biochemical, and physiologic equivalence of these agents in generally accepted doses. Nevertheless, they are listed with putatively equivalent dosages based on their marketed doses. Unfortunately, these equivalent dosages have been extrapolated for use in multicenter studies,

TABLE 5   Diuretic Agents

Generic Name	Proprietary Name	Dose Range (mg/day)	Frequency (times/day)
Thiazides			
Bendroflumethiazide	Naturetin	5.0–20.0	1–2
Benzthiazide[2]	Aquatag, Exna	125–500	2
Chlorothiazide	Diuril	125–500	1–2
Chlorthalidone	Hygroton	12.5–50.0	1
Hydrochlorothiazide	Hydro-DIURIL, Esidrix	12.5–50.0	1
Indapamide	Lozol	1.25–5.0	1
Methyclothiazide	Enduron	2.5–10.0	1–2
Metolazone	Zaroxolyn	2.5–5.0	1
	Mykrox	0.5–1.0	1
Trichlormethiazide	Naqua	2–4	1
Loop Diuretics			
Bumetanide	Bumex	0.5–2.0	1
Ethacrynic acid	Edecrin	25–100	1
Furosemide	Lasix	20–80	1
Torsemide	Demadex	2.5–10.0	1
Potassium-sparing Agents			
Amiloride	Midamor	5–10	1–2
Triamterene	Dyrenium	50–100	1–2
Aldosterone Antagonists			
Eplerenone	Inspra	50–100	1
Spironolactone	Aldactone	25–100	1

[2]Not available in the United States.
[3]Exceeds dosage recommended by the manufacturer.
Adapted from JNC-5 through JNC-7.

and making inferences from their statistically significant clinical effects when comparing them with other formulations may be fraught with unfounded conclusions. For example, the equivalence of hydrochlorothiazide doses with chlorthalidone in the doses used in major trials has not been tested prospectively.

CLINICAL MECHANISMS. Fifty years of successful use for the initial treatment of hypertension have attested to the rationale for using diuretic agents and to their safety and efficacy. They reduce arterial pressure initially by contracting intravascular and extracellular fluid volume through their natriuretic and diuretic actions. However, these initial actions do not explain their long-term antihypertensive mechanisms. Thus, associated with the initial diuresis is a reduction in cardiac output and arterial pressure; however, soon (after about 8 weeks) intravascular (i.e., plasma) volume and cardiac output return to pretreatment levels and total peripheral resistance decreases. Additionally, there is an immediate attenuation of the pressor responses to endogenous circulating pressor substances (e.g., norepinephrine, angiotensin II), a modification in adrenergic function, and an enhanced vascular responsiveness to therapeutic and naturally occurring depressor substances. This explains their usefulness in enhancing or potentiating other antihypertensive compounds added to the therapeutic program.

PATIENT SELECTION. Abundant evidence clearly demonstrates that diuretic agents are appropriate for initially selected antihypertensive therapy for most patients with uncomplicated essential hypertension. Nevertheless, it must be remembered that more than 85% of these patients will require more than one class of agents to achieve optimal control of pressure, and, in these patients, the diuretic will enhance the efficacy of the additionally selected agent(s).

It can be reasoned, therefore, that the diuretics would be of greater value as monotherapeutic agents for those patients whose hypertension is more volume dependent. This includes patients with renal parenchymal disease even if their renal excretory function is normal, individuals whose pressure is more steroid dependent (e.g., primary aldosteronism), those with suppressed plasma renin activity, black patients, women who have fluid retention at different times during the menstrual cycle, and the elderly. These patients respond well to thiazide therapy (e.g., hydrochlorothiazide or its congeners initially in doses from 12.5–25.0 mg once daily, which can be increased to 50–100 mg daily). In general, the "loop"-acting agents are not necessary. These latter agents are best selected for patients who cannot take the thiazides or their congeners for one reason or another, who have impaired renal function, or who require a rapidly acting agent (see Table 5).

SIDE EFFECTS. Biochemical or metabolic side effects may complicate therapy, particularly when the daily dose of hydrochlorothiazide (or equivalent) exceeds 50 mg. To protect against hypokalemia and its complications, it is wise to control dietary sodium intake, prescribe potassium supplements, or add potassium-retaining agents (i.e., spironolactone or eplerenone, triamterene, amiloride). Perhaps the most common cause of hypokalemia is encountered in patients who ingest a high-sodium diet while taking a diuretic. In these patients, the diuretic induces a state of secondary hyperaldosteronism, and when the high sodium load is presented to the distal renal tubule, the sodium/potassium exchange mechanism is facilitated, thereby promoting kaliuresis and the resulting state of hypokalemia. Therefore, in these patients, reduction of dietary sodium intake should rectify the hypokalemia.

Other metabolic side effects induced by the thiazide diuretics include hyperuricemia, hyperglycemia, hypercholesterolemia, or a slight rise in serum creatinine or calcium levels. Most of these alterations can be reduced markedly, if not prevented, by using the lower doses of thiazides. Early multicenter studies used higher doses of hydrochlorothiazide (50–100 mg or more; usually 100 mg), and, as a result, hypokalemia was encountered more frequently. However, more recent studies (e.g., Systolic Hypertension in the Elderly Program [SHEPS]) used lower doses, with equal efficiency but fewer biochemical alterations. However, data from the Antihypertensive and Lipid-Lowering Treatment to Prevent Heart Attack Trial (ALLHAT) suggested that more patients receiving diuretics developed carbohydrate intolerance while receiving these lower doses, but their long-term implications (i.e., >4 or even 7 years) was not established. After all, diabetes mellitus and its complications require a longer duration, and the thiazide congener chlorthalidone (and not hydrochlorothiazide) was used. Furthermore, in other studies involving patients with diabetes mellitus or experimental studies of spontaneously hypertensive rats, the diuretics seemed to be associated with deleterious intrarenal effects. It is of importance to note that these adverse effects can be prevented by adding an ACE inhibitor, an ARB, or both. Whether these negative alterations were associated with use of higher doses of the thiazides or whether chlorthalidone may be more potent is not clear. Nevertheless, it is important that the patient receiving diuretics (especially in the higher doses) be followed periodically for development of hypokalemia, carbohydrate intolerance, or any of the other metabolic side effects.

In some patients with renal parenchymal disease, particularly when renal function is so impaired that a thiazide diuretic is ineffective in exerting its natriuretic action, an agent that acts at the loop of Henle (e.g., furosemide) is necessary. The loop-acting agents have a more linear dose-response relationship, and, as long as there are functioning nephrons, a natriuretic response may be expected. Other patients with volume-dependent secondary forms of hypertension may respond better to other diuretics that inhibit the mechanism responsible for the hypertension. For example, spironolactone (or eplerenone) may be more appropriate for the patient with primary aldosteronism because it specifically antagonizes aldosterone's action at its receptor site.

β-Adrenergic Receptor–Blocking Agents

CLINICAL MECHANISMS. The β-adrenergic receptor–blocking agents have been used for initial therapy for hypertension for more than 4 decades (Table 6). Their precise mechanism of antihypertensive action remains unresolved. We know that they inhibit β-adrenergic receptor–mediated functions and suppress the release of renin from the kidney; hence, they involve possible participation of the systemic renal renopressor system. The β-blockers reduce arterial pressure associated with decreased cardiac output

TABLE 6 β-Adrenergic Receptor–blocking Agents

Generic Name	Proprietary Name	Dose Range (mg/day)	Frequency (times/day)
β-Blockers			
Atenolol*	Tenormin	25–100	1
Betaxolol*	Kerlone	5–20	1
Bisoprolol*	Zebeta	2.5–10.0	1
Metoprolol*	Lopressor	50–100	1 or 2
Metoprolol* Toprol-XL (extended-release)	Toprol	50–300	1
Nadolol	Corgard	40–120	1
Propranolol	Inderal	40–240	1–2
Propranolol	Inderal LA (long acting)	60–180	1
Timolol	Blocadren	20–60	1–2
α-/β-Blockers			
Carvedilol	Coreg	12.5–50.0	2
Labetalol	Normodyne, Trandate	200–800	2

*Cardioselective.
Adapted from JNC 5 through JNC 7.

and heart rate (although those compounds with intrinsic sympathomimetic activity exert these actions less). Consequently, there is a paradoxical increase in calculated total peripheral resistance associated with the pressure reduction. However, a decrease in the total peripheral resistance does not imply an increase in all organ vascular resistances with treatment because most β-blockers decrease renal vascular resistance in patients with uncomplicated essential hypertension. Vascular smooth muscle responses of organs depend on β-receptor density of their circulations. Moreover, a more recently introduced group of β-blockers (e.g., exemplified by carvedilol) possesses multiple actions: β-adrenergic receptor–blocking properties, α-adrenergic receptor–blocking effects (but not as potent as labetalol), and a third anti-inflammatory effect. Consequently, they may immediately decrease total peripheral as well as organ vascular resistances associated with antioxidative actions. Yet another compound (i.e., celiprolol, which is not in use today) had cardiac β_1-receptor–blocking effects and peripheral β_2-receptor agonistic (i.e., vasodilating) effects.

PATIENT SELECTION. Some authorities have recently challenged the initial use of β-adrenergic receptor–blocking drugs because they believe efficacy has not been adequately demonstrated. However, in general, it is clear that patients who respond better to β-adrenergic receptor–blocking drugs appear to be younger, male, with a hyperdynamic circulation, white patients, or those who have higher plasma renin activity. Clinically, these patients may also demonstrate greater lability of arterial pressure, a faster resting heart rate, increased force of cardiac contraction, and postural hypertension, and they may present with symptoms of cardiac awareness and adrenergically mediated cardiac dysrhythmias. Patients who have certain cardiac dysrhythmias (e.g., supraventricular tachycardia) or have sustained a prior myocardial infarction should benefit from a β-blocker, as many trials have demonstrated the efficacy of β-adrenergic–blocking agents (without intrinsic sympathomimetic activity) in preventing a second infarction.

The β-adrenergic receptor–blocking drugs have also been shown to be effective in other diseases. They have been used for the long-term management of patients with previous myocardial infarction, angina pectoris, cardiac dysrhythmias, migraine headaches, and even glaucoma (in the latter case as eyedrops). Indeed, those β-blockers without intrinsic sympathomimetic activity have secondary protective effects on death from coronary heart disease. Should any of the foregoing conditions coexist in a patient with hypertension, a β-blocking drug may be a wise initial selection to obviate the need for a second (antihypertensive) agent. Clearly, using one agent is more rational than using two or more. It is worth a try. Such therapeutic simplicity favors overall adherence, is more cost effective, and reduces the likelihood of side effects and problems stemming from drug–drug interactions.

In recent years, the β-blocking drugs have been shown to be effective for the treatment of cardiac failure. This subject is discussed in the Heart Failure article starting on page 391; however, a word of caution may be worth noting with respect to hypertension. Those multicenter trials demonstrating the efficacy of β-blockers for treatment of patients with cardiac failure included few patients with hypertension. Hypertension remains the most common cause of cardiac failure; however, to my way of thinking, it is difficult to extend the value of the β-blockers to patients with hypertension and cardiac failure because use of β-blockers remain contraindicated for that complication of hypertension. Clearly, this subject requires immediate clarification, particularly with the introduction of the newer β-blockers that possess not only additional α-adrenergic receptor– blocking action but also an anti-inflammatory action (e.g., carvedilol).

A variety of β-blocking drugs are currently being used (see Table 6), and each may be associated with its own side effects. No one agent should be considered identical to any other. The antihypertensive action of β-blockers will be augmented by a diuretic. Pseudotolerance has not been a problem, particularly in individuals with mild to moderately severe hypertension. Also, they can be used in conjunction with ACE inhibitors or a calcium antagonist; however, with respect to the latter class of drugs, care must be taken to prevent unwanted negative chronotropic and inotropic cardiac effects (e.g., with verapamil).

SIDE EFFECTS. In general, the β-blockers are contraindicated in patients with a history of asthma, chronic obstructive lung disease, heart block (greater than first degree), or cardiac failure. They are relatively contraindicated in patients with a history of depression, insulin-dependent diabetes mellitus, peripheral arterial insufficiency, or hyperlipidemia. The side effects produced by one compound may not necessarily be produced by another. For example, if maximum dosages of a lipid-soluble agent provide suboptimal control of arterial pressure, switching to a more water-soluble agent may provide more optimal control without the necessity to withhold agents from the entire class. This is particularly important because this class of agents is deemed essential to preventing a second myocardial infarction or cardiac dysrhythmias.

α-Adrenergic and α-/β-Adrenergic Receptor–Blocking Agents

CLINICAL ASSESSMENT. These agents still have an important place in overall modern antihypertensive treatment. The *α-adrenergic blocking agents* do so by inhibiting the post-synaptic α-adrenergic receptors on vascular smooth muscle. Thus, arterial pressure is reduced by decreasing vascular smooth muscle tone and consequently total peripheral resistance and the organ vascular resistances. Although their effect on venular tone is minimal, not infrequently there may be an initial "first-dose" effect so that postural hypotension may be produced as a result of venous pooling of blood upon immediate assumption of upright posture. This initial postural hypotensive effect is usually short lived, disappearing with prolonged treatment. Nevertheless, it is important to advise patients, particularly the elderly, of this potential effect so that falls and bone fractures can be prevented by carefully assuming upright posture, especially when arising from bed and the supine position. In general, there is little effect on heart rate or cardiac output, although heart rate may reflexively increase, particularly with first dosing. Furthermore, there are no unusual hemodynamic responses in individual organ circulations. Changes in renal function are not a problem; and preglomerular and postglomerular arteriolar resistances as well as glomerular hydrostatic pressure have been reported to be reduced experimentally. As a result of the reduced arterial pressure and precapillary vascular resistance, intravascular (plasma) volume may expand, sometimes offsetting the controlled arterial pressure. In elderly patients, particularly if cardiac function is impaired, the resulting dependent edema, weight gain, and further impaired cardiac function can suggest cardiac failure. These latter circumstances most likely account for the greater incidence of cardiac failure than that experienced with diuretics, thereby explaining the withdrawal of prazosin by the monitoring committee of ALLHAT.

In contrast to the α-adrenergic receptor blockers, the α-/β-adrenergic receptor blockers (e.g., labetalol) are more potent, markedly reducing arterial pressure as a result of reduced total peripheral resistance and organ vascular resistances (see Table 6). This compound is also available as an intravenous preparation. Following intravenous administration, it will promptly reduce arterial pressure through a fall in vascular resistance without changing heart rate or cardiac output. Consequently, this formulation has been of great value in certain hypertensive emergencies and urgencies.

Another action of this class of α-adrenergic blockers is inhibition of α-adrenergically medicated tone of the bladder and urinary excretory muscles. The obvious beneficial effect of this action is a reduction in urinary frequency and nocturia, thereby imparting its value to men with benign prostatic hyperplasia. In order to obviate an unwanted fall in blood pressure, an α_{1A}-adrenergic inhibitor can be prescribed.

PATIENT SELECTION. The α-adrenergic receptor–blocking agents may be ideal for initial selection in those patients whose hypertensive disease is associated with benign prostatic hyperplasia. As described earlier, control of pressure may be lessened with expansion of intravascular (plasma) volume, and it may then be restored with the careful introduction of a diuretic so that undesired symptomatic postural hypotension does not complicate treatment. The α-/β-adrenergic receptor–blocking agent (e.g., labetalol) has been most useful for initial therapy in patients with higher levels of arterial pressure, especially in hypertensive urgencies and emergencies. If necessary, in these situations, the agent can be administered intravenously for initial control of pressure and then prescribed in the oral formulation for maintenance therapy. This application of therapy has been of particular value in black patients, who seem to respond well. Moreover, if additional therapy is indicated, pressure reduction can be enhanced with the addition of a diuretic and later perhaps with a calcium antagonist (if necessary).

SIDE EFFECTS. As a result of the potential hemodynamic changes, the more common side effects of α-blockers may include postural hypotension (particularly with the initial dosing), falls, and bone fractures. As stated previously, patients should be cautioned about the potential for falls when assuming the upright posture. This caution is particularly important in men with benign prostatic hyperplasia because they frequently arise from the supine position for nocturia, and thigh and hip fractures can be a major complication. For this reason, when the male patient is referred for urologic consultation, he should be asked to report to his primary care physician for the results of that consultation in order to re-evaluate the antihypertensive therapeutic program and dosing of medications so that potential overdosing and undesired excessive pressure reduction are obviated. These agents have no undesirable metabolic side effects, so they may be useful for patients who have certain side effects with the β-receptor blockers. The α-blockers have no central brain side effects, so they may be of value for the depressed patient who may not be able to take a β-blocker even though adrenergic inhibition may be desired.

Angiotensin-Converting Enzyme Inhibitors

CLINICAL ASSESSMENT. This class of antihypertensive agents inhibits the action of ACE by cleaving the terminal two peptides of the decapeptide angiotensin I to form the octapeptide angiotensin II. As a result, the natural endogenous production of the vasoactive octapeptide angiotensin II is inhibited. When initially introduced, these agents were recommended for patients whose hypertension was dependent on the renopressor system (i.e., angiotensin II), but it was soon learned that ACE inhibitors were also useful in treating less severe hypertensive patients with mild to moderately severe hypertension with normal or low plasma renin activity (even some individuals who were anephric).

In addition to inhibiting the generation of angiotensin II, these agents have secondary actions. Thus, because ACE is the same enzyme that inactivates the potent naturally occurring vasodilator bradykinin, there may be an additional effect by the augmented amount of available kinins. Moreover, there is diminished generation of angiotensin II available for interaction with other vasoactive substances. Thus, autocrine/paracrine nerve actions may amplify the actions of norepinephrine at central and peripheral nerve endings, with prostaglandins intrarenally, or in other tissues. Furthermore, there is less stimulation of aldosterone in the adrenal cortex.

The ACE inhibitors reduce arterial pressure associated with a reduction in total peripheral and organ vascular resistances. There is no compensatory or reflex cardiac stimulation, and, as a result, heart rate, cardiac output, and myocardial contractility are not increased. This most likely can be attributed to the reduced angiotensin II available centrally in the brain or at the postganglionic nerve endings. Related to the reductions in organ and intraorgan vascular resistance are reductions in renal vascular resistance and both afferent and efferent glomerular arteriolar resistances. The latter glomerular dynamic changes are responsible for a decrease in the glomerular hydrostatic pressure, protein ultrafiltration in the glomerulus, and consequently a reduction (or even prevention) of arteriolosclerosis. These changes have been demonstrated experimentally by renal micropuncture studies and subsequently confirmed by a number of studies involving a variety of ACE inhibitors, each of which demonstrated a reduction in the progression of renal functional impairment and the resultant progression to end-stage renal disease. For these reasons, the ACE inhibitors (and ARBs) are recommended for use in all patients with evidence of end-stage renal disease with hypertension, especially those with or without diabetes mellitus, in addition to more stringent goal of blood pressure control (to levels <130 mm Hg systolic and <70 mm Hg diastolic).

With respect to autocrine/paracrine actions of ACE inhibitors, the recently described action that is no longer controversial relates to the existence of local renin-angiotensin systems (RASs) in specific organs (e.g., heart, vessel wall, brain, liver, ovary, uterus). There is a classic endocrine RAS, whereby angiotensinogen is formed in liver and is acted upon by the enzyme renin released from the macula densa of the kidney. Renin generates the decapeptide angiotensin I from its protein substrate, that is then acted upon by ACE to remove a terminal dipeptide to form the octapeptide angiotensin II. Angiotensin II is responsible for the foregoing system of generation in brain, adrenal cortex, adrenal medulla, and of course vascular smooth muscle and heart. Therefore, in addition to the classic RAS, angiotensin II is formed locally in the organs noted, and each of the RAS components is produced locally in these organs (with the possible exception of renin generation itself). (Several authorities believe that renin is actually produced in the heart and vessel wall, although others believe that it may be taken up by these organs from circulating blood.) Nevertheless, locally produced angiotensin II is responsible for several important local cardiac and vascular actions, including myocytic hypertrophy (over and above the hypertrophy that is stimulated by pressure overload), collagen synthesis and fibrosis in the extracellular matrix and perivascularly, apoptosis, and proinflammatory cytokine changes in these organs. This then explains the untoward role of the RAS in remodeling with postmyocardial infarction and with cardiac failure. These effects can be prevented by ACE inhibitors or ARBs. This exciting and important new area of investigation has provided new insight into our understanding of the overall benefit of these agents clinically.

Currently, a variety of ACE inhibitors is available (Table 7). A small initial dose of ACE inhibitor followed by observation of the blood pressure response will provide insight into drug efficacy. Control of arterial pressure with ACE inhibitors may be expected, and the incidence of side effects appears to be low. Because of their effects on reducing LV preload and in antagonizing the effects of hyperaldosteronism, the ACE inhibitors are very useful in hypertensive (and for that matter normotensive) patients with cardiac failure. Moreover, because these drugs have

TABLE 7 Angiotensin-Converting Enzyme Inhibitors

Generic Name	Proprietary Name	Dose Range (mg/day)	Frequency (times/day)
Benazepril	Lotensin	10.0–40.0	1
Captopril	Capoten	25–100	2–3
Cilazapril	Inhibace	5.0–75.0	1–2
Enalapril	Vasotec	5.0–40.0	1–2
Fosinopril	Monopril	10.0–40.0	1–2
Lisinopril	Zestril, Prinivil	10–40	1
Moexipril	Univasc	7.5–30.0	1
Perindopril	Aceon	4–8	1
Quinapril	Accupril	10–80	1
Ramipril	Altace	2.5–20.0	1
Trandolapril	Mavik	1–4	1

Adapted from the JNC 5 through JNC 7.

been shown to reduce cardiac mass and remodel cardiovascular structure, they may be extremely valuable in preventing cardiac failure complicating myocardial infarction. Pseudotolerance generally is not a problem with the ACE inhibitors, and further control of pressure will be enhanced with an added diuretic.

PATIENT SELECTION. When first introduced, the ACE inhibitors were recommended for patients with severe hypertension associated with markedly elevated arterial pressure, high plasma renin activity, bilateral occlusive renal arterial disease, or congestive heart failure, or for those whose arterial pressure was unresponsive to other antihypertensive therapy. More recently, these agents have been shown to be of value in patients with uncomplicated hypertension, whether the circulating plasma renin activity is high, normal, or low. In addition, because many studies of a variety of ACE inhibitors have found that they prevent subsequent cardiac failure or death complicating recent myocardial infarction, these agents are of particular value in patients who have associated hypertension. These agents are also of value in patients in whom the epiphenomena of the LVH are associated with ischemia, fibrosis, and inflammatory responses. Moreover, ACE inhibitory treatment is not complicated with metabolic side effects. However, the ACE inhibitors may be associated with an undesired dry cough, and an ARB should be prescribed in their place; however, an ARB is not indicated if there is a history of angioneurotic edema. Personally, I have found that an ACE inhibitor has been of value for patients with hypertension associated with a collagen vascular disease (although this use is not specified in package inserts and does not have Food and Drug Administration approval). Finally, as discussed earlier, the ACE inhibitors are clearly indicated to prevent stroke as well as following stroke, and they are indicated for all patients with diabetes mellitus or hypertension to prevent progression of end-stage renal disease or to control arterial pressure at a goal lower (<130 mm Hg systolic and <80 mm Hg diastolic) than in other patients with hypertension.

SIDE EFFECTS. ACE inhibitors may produce proteinuria and leukopenia. Laboratory studies probably should be obtained during the first 3 months of therapy to inform the clinician whether patients with renal disease or those receiving immunosuppressive therapy may progress. Of particular note, this class of agents is absolutely contraindicated in women who are pregnant or who intend to be pregnant and in patients with a solitary kidney who have bilateral renal arterial disease or unilateral renal arterial disease.

Of particular concern in patients with renal disease who have impaired renal function is possible progression of functional impairment with treatment and hyperkalemia if potassium supplements or potassium-retaining agents are concomitantly prescribed with the ACE inhibitor. Less severe side effects include rash, ageusia, and a chronic dry cough, which are all reversible with cessation of therapy.

Angiotensin II (Type 1) Receptor Blockers

CLINICAL MECHANISMS. There are at least four types of angiotensin II receptors; however, the type 1 receptor is the only one that is targeted therapeutically with specific agents. This class of agents inhibits the angiotensin II (type 1) receptor. An experimental agent is available for the inhibition of the angiotensin II (type 2) receptor, but at present there are no clinical indications for its use, and no trials on its clinical application are anticipated. The type 1 angiotensin II receptor mediates vasoconstriction, adrenal cortical release of aldosterone, and, in part, catecholamine release from the adrenal medulla. Unlike the ACE inhibitors, kinin degeneration is not inhibited; hence, the dry cough related to ACE inhibition (attributed to the kinins) is not produced. Several ARBs are clinically available (Table 8). With angiotensin II type 1 receptor antagonism, ACE levels are not affected, the receptor may be up-regulated, and circulating levels of angiotensin II may increase slightly. Their hemodynamic effects are very similar to those of the ACE inhibitors, including its renal effects. Coronary hemodynamics are improved in association with reversal of LVH.

This class of agents that inhibit the RAS do so by antagonizing angiotensin II at the receptor level independent of the ACE. However, chymase is another important enzyme that converts angiotensin I to angiotensin II, especially in human myocardium. As a result, the ARB acts not only to antagonize that angiotensin II that escapes the action of an ACE inhibitor but also whatever angiotensin II is formed via the action of chymase. For this reason, an ARB has been used alone and in conjunction with an ACE inhibitor. Thus, the two types of RAS inhibitors have been shown to be of value in patients with prior myocardial infarction and cardiac failure (i.e., Candesartan in Heart failure Assessment of Reduction Mortality and morbidity [CHARM] study). However, at the present time, there are no formulations consisting of a combination of an ARB and an ACE inhibitor.

PATIENT SELECTION. The ARBs, in general, are of value in all patients in whom an ACE inhibitor is indicated but in

TABLE 8 Angiotensin II (Type 1) Receptor Antagonists

Generic Name	Proprietary Name	Dose Range (mg/day)	Frequency (times/day)
Candesartan	Atacand	8–32	1
Eprosartan	Teveten	400–80	1–2
Irbesartan	Avapro	150–300	1
Losartan	Cozaar	25–100	1–2
Olmesartan	Benicar	20–40	1
Telmisartan	Micardis	20–80	1–2

Adapted from JNC-5 through JNC-7.

whom the chronic cough associated with ACE inhibition has not been reported. Thus, these agents are of particular value in hypertensive patients with recent myocardial infarction, cardiac failure, long-standing hypertension complicated by impaired renal function, and end-stage renal disease. In the latter respect, they are likewise of great value in patients with diabetes mellitus in whom the goal of blood pressure reduction is still lower (<130 mm Hg systolic and <80 mm Hg diastolic) than in the patients whose hypertension is not complicated by diabetes.

SIDE EFFECTS. Because ACE is not inhibited, cough is not a side effect produced by the ARBs, making them of particular value in those patients who have experienced a disturbing cough. On the other hand, agents of this class are contraindicated for use in pregnant women or women who may become pregnant; they are at the same risk for teratogenetic defects. These agents have the same potential for producing angioneurotic edema as the ACE inhibitors and thus are contraindicated in these patients, especially if the condition has occurred with the ACE inhibitors. Furthermore, the ARBs are contraindicated in patients with bilateral occlusive renal arterial disease and in patients with only one kidney who have occlusive renal arterial disease. Care must be maintained whenever these agents are prescribed for patients with renal functional impairment, particularly when potassium supplements are prescribed or when these agents are simultaneously used with agents that actively retain potassium.

Calcium Antagonists

Calcium antagonists have been used widely for treating hypertensive patients for many years. The general term commonly used for this group of agents is *calcium channel blockers*, although the preferred term used by the International Union of Pharmacology is *calcium antagonists*. In reality, the latter term is more precise because at least four different calcium channel receptor sites have been cloned, and the agents that are prescribed may have variable (or even multiple) sites. Thus, most of the L-channel agents belong to the dihydropyridine receptor class; but even in that class, nifedipine also possesses additional α-adrenergic receptor–blocking properties. Moreover, some L-channel agents can be increased in dose without elevating pressure (or ameliorating angina pectoris) further when the dosage is increased; however, when a different calcium antagonist is added to the treatment along with the initial agent, pressure (or angina) control can be improved. Moreover, T-channel and N-channel calcium antagonists have been introduced clinically, although the T-channel compound (i.e., mibefradil) marketed in the United States has been withdrawn from the market. An N-channel inhibitor (i.e., cilnidipine) is clinically available in Japan; and both the T-channel and N-channel "blockers" also possess L-channel–blocking ability. Also important in their action, some calcium antagonists promote intramyocytic protein binding or release of the calcium ion from bound stores in the sarcoplasmic reticulum or the mitochondria. Hence, it is far too simplistic to conceive of these agents as being just "calcium channel blockers."

Nevertheless, each of the calcium antagonists decreases arterial pressure through a potent vasodilating mechanism that reduces the availability of calcium ions from interaction with the contractile machinery in the vascular smooth muscle cell or cardiomyocyte. The result is decreased total peripheral and organ (particularly of the target organs) vascular resistances. Some of these agents (e.g., diltiazem, nitrendipine, verapamil) increase renal blood flow without also increasing glomerular filtration rate, thereby reducing the renal filtration fraction. These effects have been confirmed by a decreased glomerular hydrostatic pressure, suggesting their potential value for patients with diabetes mellitus or other protein-losing nephropathic states. The net effect of this action is similar to that of the ACE inhibitors: dilation of afferent as well as efferent glomerular arterioles. Most of these compounds also have been used for angina pectoris resulting from occlusive, atherosclerotic epicardial coronary arterial disease as well as for coronary artery spasm. It follows then that these compounds can be used to treat hypertensive patients who have coronary arterial insufficiency and who may have suboptimal control of arterial pressure with a β-adrenergic receptor–blocking drug. Calcium antagonists may be of value for older patients who have coronary artery disease and who have diabetes mellitus, hyperlipidemia, or side effects associated with other antihypertensive drugs because calcium antagonists do not produce these adverse effects.

Several calcium antagonists are available (Table 9), and new compounds are under active clinical investigation. They exhibit considerable heterogeneity chemically, pharmacologically, physiologically, and clinically. For example, verapamil not only dilates arterioles but also slows cardiac rate. Nifedipine does not share that action, but it reduces arterial pressure without direct cardiac effects. Diltiazem produces both vascular and cardiac effects, although its cardiac slowing is less than that produced by verapamil. Another calcium antagonist, nimodipine, is used by neurosurgeons to control pressure in patients with cerebral bleeding; and this compound has little effect on arterial pressure. As suggested previously, some of these agents have been shown under controlled experimental conditions of renal micropuncture to dilate afferent as well as efferent glomerular arterioles and to reduce glomerular hydrostatic pressure, protein ultrafiltration, and hence glomerulosclerosis.

CLINICAL ASSESSMENT. These agents are well tolerated and produce a low incidence of adverse effects. Their dosage may be increased easily without symptoms or pseudotolerances; the latter may be explained by the intrinsic natriuretic property of these compounds. Some calcium antagonists must be given more than once daily, whereas others (most) have sustained once-daily action. Although they cost more than the thiazides and β-blockers, they are not prohibitively expensive; also, they do not require additional prescriptions for metabolic side effects.

INITIAL SELECTION. The calcium antagonists are of particular value for the initial selection of therapy when the arterial pressure is elevated and there is a need for more immediate reduction of pressure; for promotion of coronary vasodilation in patients with a history of angina pectoris unresponsive to a β-adrenergic receptor blocker; and when an ACE inhibitor or an ARB is contraindicated because of occlusive bilateral renal arterial disease or unilateral arterial disease in a solitary kidney. Large antihypertensive

TABLE 9 Calcium Antagonists

Drug (Proprietary Name)	Usual Dose Range (mg/day)	Usual Daily Frequency
Nondihydropyridines		
Diltiazem extended-release (Cardizem CD) Dilacor XR, Tiazac)	180–420	1
Diltiazem extended-release (Cardizem LA)	120–420	1
Verapamil immediate-release (Calan, Isoptin)	90–480	2
Verapamil (Covera HS, Verelan)	120–360	1
(Mibefradil, T-channel—removed from U.S. market)		
(Cilnidipine, N-channel inhibitor—available in Japan)		
Dihydropyridines		
Amlodipine (Norvasc)	2.5–10	1
Felodipine (Plendil)	2.5–20	1
Isradipine (DynaCirc-CR)	2.5–10	2
Nicardipine sustained-release (Cardene-SR)	60–120	2
Nifedipine long-acting (Adalat-CC, Procardia-XL)	30–90	1
Nisoldipine (Sular)	10–40	1

Adapted from the JNC-5 through JNC-7.

trials have shown that the calcium antagonists (i.e., dihydropyridines) reduce fatal and nonfatal strokes. The Systolic Hypertension in Europe (Syst-Eur) study was conducted with nitrendipine, an agent that is not available in the United States, so for this reason, the JNC report recommended use of the entire chemical group of dihydropyridine agents. One Veterans Administration Cooperative Study showed these agents to be of greater value in black than in white patients with hypertension. Their use certainly is of value in patients with diabetes mellitus or hypertension with renal functional impairment or end-stage renal disease, particularly if the ACE inhibitor or ARB does not achieve goal blood pressure reduction. Furthermore, these agents are of particular value in patients who cannot take other antihypertensive drugs because of undesired side effects.

SIDE EFFECTS. In general, the calcium antagonists have been shown to be relatively free of side effects. In the earlier days of their use when they were used in short-acting formulations, there were instances of unwanted reflexive cardiac stimulation including chest discomfort and flushing of the skin. However, these adverse experiences have not been as frequent in recent years with the longer-acting formulations. Clearly, as indicated previously, one of the more common side effects has been dependent peripheral edema. This effect is not related to fluid retention but to potent precapillary arterial dilation associated with reflexive postcapillary constriction that, in the upright position, favors increased capillary hydrostatic pressure and edema. These agents, to the contrary, promote sodium/calcium exchange at the distal renal tubule and hence do not promote fluid retention per se. Nevertheless, the postural edema may be helped by the addition of a short-acting (loop) diuretic during awake hours to prevent daytime postural edema when the patient is upright. It is of particular interest that none of the calcium antagonists has been formulated with a diuretic to enhance their antihypertensive action. In my personal experience, I have found that rather than increasing the dose of these compounds to promote better control of arterial pressure and thereby promote postural edema, the addition of a second calcium antagonist may obviate production of edema. Other disturbing side effects include constipation, bradycardia (both of which are particularly associated with verapamil), and gingival hyperplasia.

Hypertensive Emergencies

Hypertensive emergencies have been encountered far less frequently in recent years, but when they do occur, they are far easier to treat by control of arterial pressure. There is a relatively large variety of hypertensive emergencies (Table 10), and control of arterial pressure is eminently achievable given the variety of agents presently available for treatment of these situations (Table 11). However, in general, more than two or three agents are necessary to

TABLE 10 Hypertensive Emergencies

Hypertensive encephalopathy
Hypertension and intracranial hemorrhage
Malignant (and accelerated) hypertension
Hypertensive cardiac failure
Hypertension and dissecting aortic aneurysm
Severe hypertension associated with myocardial infarction
Hypertension (systolic pressure 160–170 mm Hg) following vascular surgery and/or vessel grafting
Pheochromocytoma crisis
Hypertensive crisis during cardiovascular catheterization procedure
Clonidine-withdrawal hypertension
Foodstuff-related hypertension associated with monoamine oxidase–inhibiting drugs
Hypertension (in child) with acute glomerulonephritis
Eclampsia

From JNC-7.

TABLE 11 Drugs Useful for Treatment of Hypertensive Emergencies

Agent	Proprietary Name	Dosage	Prime Indication Emergencies
Parenteral Agents			
Cryptenamine[2]	Unitensen	2 mg in 1000-mL isotonic saline infusion (IV)	Eclampsia
Diazoxide	Hyperstat	150 mg (IV), bolus	Hypertensive encephalopathy Intracranial hemorrhage
Enalaprilat	Vasotec	0.625–1.25 mg q6h (IV)	Cardiac failure
Furosemide	Lasix	40 mg (IV) or higher q4h, q6h, or q8h (as necessary)	Hypertensive heart failure
Guanethidine or Bethanidine	Ismelin	25–50 mg (PO) initially, one dose daily 0.25–0.50 mg/kg (PO) q6–8h (repeat to achieve effects eventually)	Malignant (and accelerated) hypertension Oral therapy to replace IV drugs (for emergency)
Hydralazine	Apresoline	10–20 (IV or IM) q4–6h	Eclampsia
Labetalol	Normodyne, Trandate	20–80 mg IV bolus 10 min and then 2 mg/min IV infusion	Malignant (and accelerated) hypertension Hypertension with glomerulonephritis
Methyldopa	Aldomet	250–500 mg (IV or IM) q1–6 h, prn	Malignant (and accelerated) hypertension
Nitroprusside or	Nitropress	0.25–10.0 µg/kg/min	Most hypertensive emergencies except myocardial ischemia, cardiac failure, and dissecting aneurysm
Trimethaphan[2] or	Arfonad	1000 mg/L IV infusion	Hypertension and aortic dissection
Nitroglycerin	Tridil	5–100 µg/min IV infusion	Hypertensive crisis during catheterization Malignant (and accelerated) hypertension Hypertension after vascular reconstructive surgery
Phentolamine	Regitine	5–10 mg (IV) bolus or 5–15 mg (IV), then infusion	Pheochromocytoma crisis Pressor crisis during catheterization Clonidine-withdrawal hypertension Foodstuff-related hypertension associated with monoamine oxidase–inhibiting drugs
Reserpine	Serpasil*	1.0–5.0 mg (IM) q6h	Malignant (and accelerated) hypertension
Orally Administered Agents			
Captopril	Capoten	12.5–25.0 mg (repeat as necessary)	Congestive heart failure, hypertensive pressor urgencies
Clonidine	Catapres	0.1–0.2 mg hourly as necessary	Clonidine withdrawal, hypertensive pressor urgencies, for diagnostic tests that suppress excessive circulating catecholamines in patients with pheochromocytoma
Labetalol	Normodyne	200–400 mg q2–3h	Most hypertensive emergencies (except cardiac failure)
Minoxidil	Loniten	2.5–5.0 mg q2–3h	Hypertensive pressor urgencies
Nifedipine	Procardia, Adalat	10 mg q20min as necessary[3]	Hypertensive pressor urgencies

[2]Not available in the United States.
[3]Exceeds dosage recommended by the manufacturer.
*No longer available under this name in the United States.
From JNC 7.

TABLE 12 Adrenergic Inhibitors

Generic Name	Proprietary Name	Dose Range (mg/day)	Frequency (times/day)
α_1-Receptor Blockers			
Doxazosin	Cardura	1–16	1
Prazosin	Minipress	1.0–30	2–3
Terazosin	Hytrin	1.0–20	1
α_1-/α_2-Receptor Blockers			
Phentolamine	Regitine	5–10 (IV)	prn
Phenoxybenzamine	Dibenzyline	10–40	bid, tid, or qid as indicated by pressure measurements
Centrally Acting α_2 Agonists			
Clonidine	Catapres	0.1–1.2	2
Clonidine (patch)	Catapres (TTS)	0.1–0.3	1 weekly
Guanabenz	Wytensin	8–32	2
Guanfacine	Tenex	1–3	1
Methyldopa	Aldomet	250–3000	1–2
Peripherally Acting Adrenergic Antagonists			
Reserpine	Serpasil	0.1–0.25	1
Rauwolfia serpentina	Raudixin	50–100	1
Alseroxylon fraction[2]	Rauwiloid	2–4	1
Rescinnamine[2]	Moderil	0.25–0.50	1
Deserpidine[2]	Harmonyl	0.25–0.50	1
Syrosingopine[2]	Singoserp	1–2	1
Guanadrel	Hylorel	10–75	2
Guanethidine	Ismelin	10–100	1

[2]Not available in the United States.
Adapted from JNC-5.

maintain pressure control, and from the previous discussion of the various agents, their selection should reflect thought. Thus, by understanding the underlying mechanisms associated with the pressure elevation and the mechanisms of action of the number of drugs that are available, a positive outcome of treatment should be expected (Table 11).

Table 12 provides additional information on adrenergic-blocking compounds.

REFERENCES

Frohlich ED: Corcoran Lecture: Influence of nitric oxide and angiotensin II on renal involvement in hypertension. Hypertension 1997;29:188-193.

Frohlich ED: Hypertension: Evaluation and Treatment. Baltimore, Williams & Wilkins, 1998:212.

Frohlich ED: Risk mechanisms in hypertensive heart disease. Hypertension 1999;34:782-789.

Frohlich ED: Treating hypertension. What are we to believe? [editorial] N Engl J Med 2003;348:639-641.

Frohlich ED (ed): Medical Clinics of North America, vol 88. Philadelphia, WB Saunders, 2004.

Frohlich ED: Clinical classifications of hypertensive diseases. In Fuster V, Topol EJ, Nabel EG, (eds): Atherothrombosis and Coronary Artery Disease, 2nd ed. Philadelphia, Lippincott Williams & Wilkins, 2005:99-216.

Frohlich ED, Varagic J: Sodium directly impairs target organ function in hypertension. Curr Opin Cardiol 2005;20:424-429.

Major outcomes in high-risk hypertensive patients randomized to angiotensin-converting enzyme inhibitor or calcium channel blocker vs diuretic. The Antihypertensive and Lipid-Lowering Treatment to Prevent Heart Attack Trial (ALLHAT). JAMA 2002;288:2981-2997.

The Seventh Report of the Joint National Committee on Prevention, Detection, Evaluation, and Treatment of High Blood Pressure (JNC-7). Hypertension 2003;42:1206-1252.

Vogel JHK, Bolling SF, Costello RB, et al: Integrating complementary medicine into cardiovascular medicine. J Am Coll Cardiol 2005:49:184-221.

Whelton PK, He J, Appel LJ, et al: Primary prevention of hypertension: Clinical and public health advisory from the National High Blood Pressure Education Program. JAMA 2002;288:1882-1888.

Acute Myocardial Infarction

Method of
Kevin A. Bybee, MD,
and Stephen L. Kopecky, MD

During the 20th century, acute myocardial infarction (AMI) became the leading cause of death in the United States and in other developed regions of the world including Europe. Individual mortality rates from AMI have recently decreased in both men and women because of modern therapeutic advances and increasing public awareness of AMI symptoms and the need for emergent evaluation. Despite advances in the diagnosis and treatment of AMI, however, it will likely remain the leading cause of death well into the future, given the aging of the population and the increasing prevalence of type II diabetes mellitus. Information obtained from clinical trials has revolutionized the modern approach to patients with AMI, emphasizing early and accurate diagnosis, early risk stratification, and prompt reperfusion therapy in those with ST-segment-elevation myocardial infarction (STEMI).

Diagnosis

In 2000 the American College of Cardiology (ACC) and the European Society of Cardiology (ESC) issued a joint recommendation that redefines the diagnosis of AMI, thus replacing the World Health Organization definition. The ACC/ESC definition requires the typical rise and fall of troponin or more rapid rise and fall of creatinine kinase myocardial band (CK-MB) in addition to one of the following:

- Symptoms consistent with myocardial ischemia
- Electrocardiogram (ECG) changes indicating myocardial ischemia (ST-segment depression or elevation)
- New pathologic Q waves
- Percutaneous coronary intervention (PCI)

Pathologic findings of AMI at autopsy are also considered diagnostic. Additionally, any patient presenting with a clinical history consistent with AMI and new left bundle branch block should be triaged as STEMI. Based on the ACC/ESC guidelines, as well as recommendations issued by the ACC and American Heart Association (AHA) in 2002, differentiating between unstable angina (UA) and non-ST-segment-elevation myocardial infarction (NSTEMI) is based on whether biomarkers of myocardial injury are elevated, denoting myocardial necrosis. Detectable elevations of troponin and CK-MB may not be apparent in those who present within the first 4 to 6 hours following symptom onset. Thus distinguishing between UA and NSTEMI may not be possible at the time of initial evaluation and may require serial measurements of cardiac biomarkers.

PATHOPHYSIOLOGY

AMI occurs when myocardial necrosis results from prolonged myocardial ischemia. Acute coronary syndromes (ACS) represent a spectrum of clinical presentations including UA, NSTEMI, and STEMI. Despite this spectrum of presentations, the underlying pathophysiologic mechanisms are similar in most cases. The most common initiating mechanism responsible for AMI is acute plaque rupture, with subsequent exposure of thrombogenic substances with the lipid-laden plaque core to circulating blood and consequent coronary thrombus formation. STEMI is almost always a result of complete thrombotic coronary occlusion. Subtotal coronary occlusion often results in UA or NSTEMI. Myocardial necrosis in the setting of NSTEMI may result from transient complete coronary occlusion with spontaneous partial recanalization, persistent near-complete coronary occlusion, and distal embolization of plaque debris and platelet-rich thrombi with associated vascular spasm. Most plaque ruptures involve relatively small, vulnerable nonobstructive coronary plaques. Studies using intravascular ultrasound document the presence of multiple ruptured plaques in many patients presenting with AMI. AMI can also result from endothelial erosion and in situations of prolonged increases in myocardial oxygen demand in the setting of a stable, yet high-grade coronary lesion. Other rare mechanisms of AMI include coronary artery spasm, coronary artery embolism, coronary artery dissection, and coronary injury from trauma.

HISTORY

Initial assessment of patients with suspected ACS should begin with a focused history, physical examination, and 12-lead ECG (Figure 1). Patients with AMI can present with a variety of symptoms—from crushing substernal chest pain to no pain at all. This variability in symptoms can make initial diagnosis challenging in some patients and reinforces the importance of physicians remaining astute. The discomfort classically associated with AMI is described as a crushing, squeezing, or tightness in the anterior left chest. These symptoms can radiate to the jaw, teeth, shoulders, arms, and back and usually last for at least 20 minutes. Older (age >75 years) patients, diabetics, and female patients are more likely to present with dyspnea as their primary symptom. Patients with AMI usually do not have pleuritic chest pain, which suggests an alternative diagnosis such as pericarditis, pulmonary embolism, pneumothorax, or pneumonia. Patients with tearing pain may have aortic dissection.

PHYSICAL EXAMINATION

The physical examination usually does not help significantly in the diagnosis of AMI, but it does it aid in the risk stratification of patients with suspected AMI and in an evaluation for non-AMI etiologies responsible for patient symptoms. Hemodynamic stability should be assessed. Evaluation of jugular venous pressure and wave form can give clues to right ventricular infarction and right atrial pressure as well as indirect information about left heart function and intravascular volume status. Lung evaluation should note the presence of rales, indicating left heart failure. Cardiac palpation can give clues to underlying cardiomyopathy. A soft S_1 suggests reduced left ventricle (LV) systolic function or first-degree atrioventricular (AV) block. A holosystolic murmur could indicate mitral regurgitation resulting from ischemic papillary muscle dysfunction or ventricular septal defect. An S_4 gallop is often present, indicating abnormal left ventricular relaxation, whereas an S_3 gallop suggests elevated left ventricular end-diastolic pressure. Hypotension at the time of presentation is usually caused by large areas of ischemic myocardium. Hypotension and rales greater than one third of the lung field are indicators of increased morbidity and mortality during hospitalization. Unstable patients should also be assessed for mechanical complications of AMI such as papillary muscle rupture, ventricular septal defect, and left ventricular free-wall rupture.

Alternative etiologies responsible for the patient's presentation should also be sought during the physical examination. Symmetry of pulses in all extremities and symmetry of blood pressure in both arms should be assessed in evaluating for aortic dissection. A pericardial rub suggests pericarditis, whereas a pleural rub suggests pulmonary embolism or pneumonia. Palpation of the chest wall may be helpful in identifying musculoskeletal etiologies. However, for unclear reasons, patients with documented AMI may have increased pain with chest wall palpation.

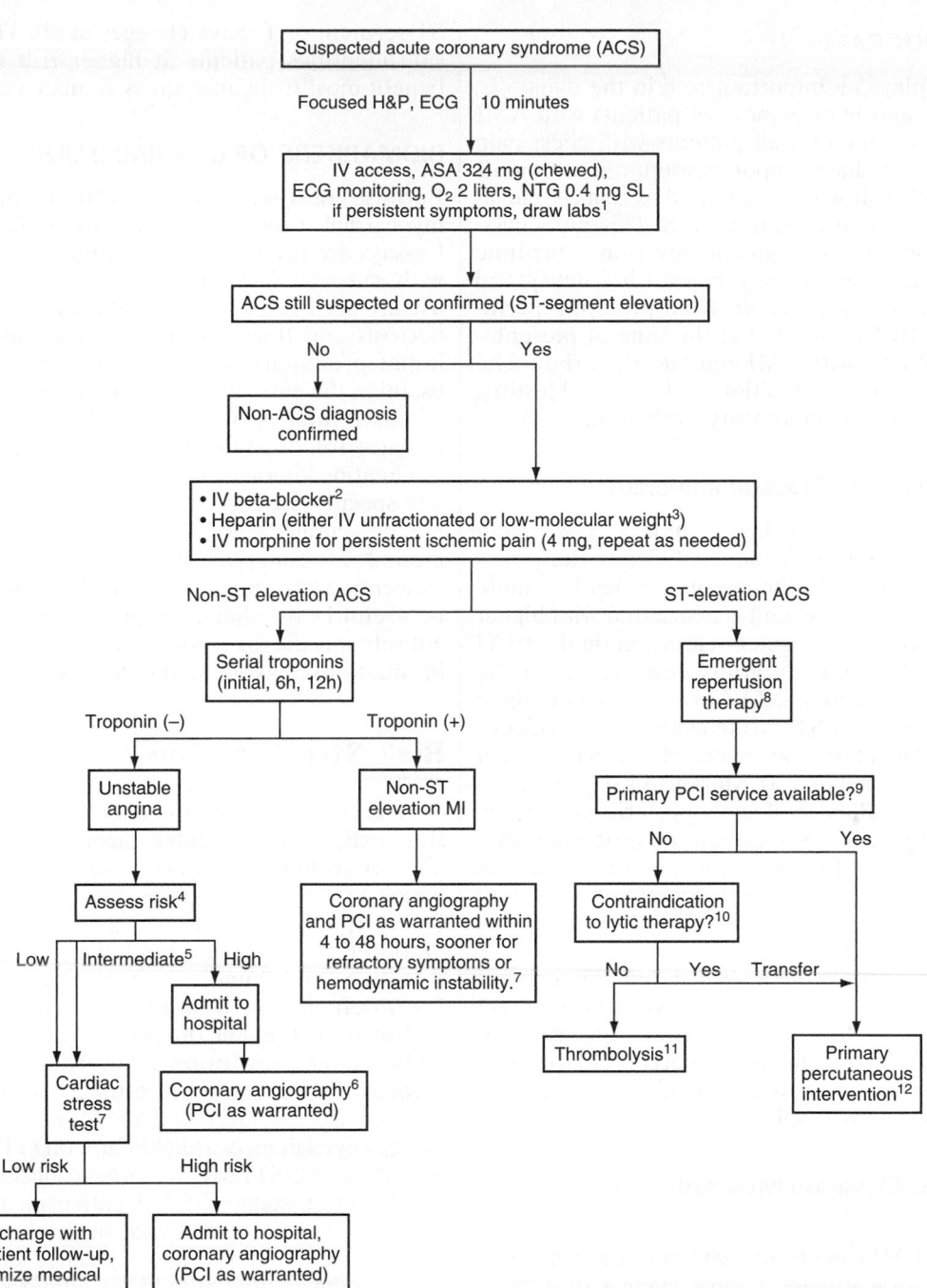

FIGURE 1. Algorithm for evaluation and treatment of patients with suspected acute coronary syndromes. ACS = acute coronary syndrome; ALT = alanine amino transferase; ASA = aspirin; CBC = complete blood count; CXR = chest radiograph; ECG = electrocardiogram; H&P = history and physical; IV = intravenous; MI = myocardial infarction; NSTEMI = non-ST-segment-elevation myocardial infarction; NTG = nitroglycerin; PCI = percutaneous coronary intervention; SL = sublingual.
[1]Troponin, CBC , electrolytes, creatinine, ALT, CXR.
[2]Metoprolol, 5 mg IV × 3 every 5 minutes, until heart rate 55 to 65 bpm; hold for hypotension or pulmonary edema.
[3]Low-molecular-weight heparin appears superior to IV unfractionated heparin in patients with unstable angina with high risk features and those with NSTEMI. Some interventionists prefer IV unfractionated heparin in patients undergoing coronary angiography/PCI.
[4]See Table 1 for risk assessment.
[5]For intermediate-risk patients, consider risk stratification if the chest pain unit is available.
[6]Consider addition of glycoprotein (GP) IIb/IIIa inhibitor. GP IIa/IIIb inhibitor can be initiated upon admission or just prior to PCI in the cardiac catheterization laboratory.
[7]Exercise electrocardiogram preferred; exercise imaging study if baseline ST changes present or if patient is on digoxin; pharmacologic imaging study if unable to walk on treadmill to acceptable workload.
[8]Administer reperfusion therapy if symptom onset within 12 hours. Refer for coronary angiography if symptom onset more than 12 hours and persistent chest symptoms or hemodynamic instability.
[9]Can consider transport to primary PCI facility if door-to-balloon time still less than 90 minutes.
[10]See Table 2 for absolute and relative contraindications to thrombolytic therapy.
[11]Door-to-needle time should be less than 30 minutes.
[12]Door-to-balloon time should be less than 90 minutes; goal is less than 60 minutes.

ELECTROCARDIOGRAM

The initial ECG plays an important role in the diagnosis, risk stratification, and management of patients with AMI and should be performed on all patients with chest pain and/or dyspnea immediately upon presentation. Patients presenting with AMI should be classified as non-ST-elevation ACS or ST-segment-elevation ACS. This nomenclature is preferred because ST-segment elevation at the time of presentation indicates ongoing myocardial injury and identifies patients who can benefit from prompt reperfusion therapy. The ECG is normal at the time of presentation in 10% of patients with AMI and therefore should be used as a supportive tool in addition to the clinical history, physical examination, and laboratory evaluation.

ST-Segment-Elevation Myocardial Infarction

STEMI is characterized by at least 1 mm of ST-segment elevation in two or more contiguous ECG leads. Reciprocal ST-segment depression may be present in leads remote from those with ST elevation and is associated with higher risk. The distribution of ST-segment elevation on the ECG can give clues to the coronary artery responsible for the ischemia (Table 1). A right-sided ECG should be obtained in all patients with inferior STEMI to evaluate for evidence of right ventricular infarction manifest by ST-segment elevation in lead V_3R and/or V_4R. Marked ST depression in leads V_1 to V_3 is the hallmark of acute posterior infarction, which can be confirmed by ST-segment elevation in posteriorly placed leads (V_7R to V_9R), and should be treated as an STEMI. Patients presenting with symptoms consistent with AMI and a new left bundle branch block should be triaged and managed as an STEMI.

Other disease entities with associated ST-segment elevation should be kept in mind when assessing a patient with suspected STEMI. These include pericarditis, myocarditis, left ventricular aneurysm, early repolarization, coronary artery spasm, intracranial bleeding, head trauma, and transient left ventricular apical ballooning syndrome.

Non-ST-Segment-Elevation Myocardial Infarction

Patients with NSTEMI can present with marked or minimal ST-segment depression, isolated T wave changes, or with no ST-segment or T wave changes at all. ST-segment depression identifies patients at higher risk who subsequently benefit most from an aggressive management strategy.

BIOMARKERS OF CARDIAC INJURY

Because of their high sensitivity and specificity for myocardial necrosis, cardiac troponin T and troponin I assays are preferred in the initial evaluation of patients with suspected AMI. Detectable troponin elevations usually occur 3 to 6 hours following onset of myocardial necrosis and thus may not be abnormal at the time of initial presentation. As a result, troponin may not be useful in the early diagnosis of STEMI and is most helpful in discerning UA and NSTEMI. Troponin remains elevated for 7 to 14 days following AMI.

Creatine kinase (CK) and CK-MB are less sensitive and less specific for myocardial necrosis. Elevated CK levels are detectable 4 to 6 hours following AMI and peak around 24 hours following the onset of necrosis. CK concentrations return to normal by 72 hours and thus may be useful in the diagnosis of reinfarction. CK-MB is not entirely specific for myocardial muscle and can be elevated in situations of skeletal muscle, bowel, and prostate injury.

Risk Stratification

Several characteristics are associated with a worse prognosis in patients with unstable angina (Table 2), NSTEMI, and STEMI, including advanced age, female gender, hemodynamic alterations (hypotension, tachycardia), left heart failure (pulmonary rales, S3 gallop, elevated BNP [brain natriuretic peptide]), cumulative extent of ST-segment deviation, new bundle branch block, proximal or mid-LAD (left anterior descending coronary artery) occlusion, aspirin use at the time of AMI, elevated C-reactive protein, diabetes mellitus, prior myocardial infarction or prior coronary artery bypass grafting, concomitant peripheral vascular disease, and underlying renal insufficiency. The thrombolysis in myocardial infarction (TIMI) risk scores for STEMI and NSTEMI are prognostically useful (Tables 3 and 4). Intermediate-risk UA patients may be risk stratified over 6 to 9 hours with serial biomarkers and an exercise ECG. If biomarkers become positive or the stress test is positive, the patient should be admitted. If negative, the

---

TABLE 1 Infarct-Related Artery and Associated Distribution of Electrocardiographic ST-Segment Elevation

Location of Coronary Occlusion	Distribution of ST-Segment Elevation	30-Day Mortality with Successful Reperfusion*
Proximal LAD (proximal to first septal perforator)	V_1-V_6, aVL, I, new LBBB common	19.6%
Mid-LAD (distal to first septal perforator and proximal to first large diagonal branch)	V_1-V_6, aVL, I,	9.2%
Distal LAD (distal to first large diagonal branch) or diagonal branch	V_1-V_4, or aVL, I, V_{5-6}	6.8%
Right coronary artery	II, III, aVF, V_{5-6} (V_3R, V_4R with RV infarction)	6.4%
Left circumflex	V_{5-6}, III, II, aVF (can have minimal ECG changes)	4.5%

*Derived from Global Utilization of Streptokinase and t-PA for Occluded Coronary Arteries-I (GUSTO-I) cohort population of patients receiving successful reperfusion therapy.

Abbreviations: ECG = electrocardiogram; LAD = left anterior descending; LBBB = left bundle branch block; RV = right ventricle.

TABLE 2 Risk Stratification in Patients With Unstable Angina

High Risk (20% Event Rate*)	Intermediate Risk (~6% Event Rate*)	Low Risk (~<1% Event Rate*)
Presence of at least one of the following:	No *high-risk* features but at least one of the following:	No *high intermediate risk* features but may present with one of the following:
- Acceleration of ischemic symptoms in last 48 h - Ongoing rest pain > 20 min - Age >75 y - New or worsening MR murmur - Pulmonary edema or evidence of worsening heart failure. - Hemodynamic instability - Rest angina associated with dynamic ST-segment deviation >0.05 mV - New bundle branch block - Ventricular tachycardia	- Known atherosclerotic vascular disease (prior MI/PCI/CABG, peripheral, cerebrovascular) - Rest pain (>20 min) now resolved with moderate or high likelihood of CAD - Rest angina <20 min relieved with NTG - Age >70 y - Prior aspirin usage - T wave inversions > 0.2 mV - Q waves	- New-onset angina within 2 wk to 2 mo - Increasing frequency of exertional angina without rest pain. - Normal or unchanged ECG

*Risk for death, unfatal MI at 6 months.
Abbreviations: CABG = coronary artery bypass graft; CAD = coronary arterial disease; ECG = electrocardiogram; MI = myocardial infarction; MR = mitral regurgitation; MV = millivolt; NTG = nitroglycerin; PCI = percutaneous coronary intervention.

patient should be dismissed with follow-up in 72 hours for re-evaluation and coronary artery disease (CAD) risk factor modification.

Treatment

The goals of initial treatment of patients presenting with AMI are:

- Obtain intravenous (IV) access and stabilize hemodynamics if unstable.
- Relieve ischemic discomfort using IV morphine and sublingual or IV nitroglycerin.
- Minimize myocardial oxygen supply-and-demand mismatch with IV β-blockers (goal: heart rate less than 70 beats per minute as blood pressure tolerates) and supplemental oxygen.
- Maintain or restore myocardial perfusion using aspirin and heparin (either IV unfractionated or subcutaneous low molecular weight).

Patients with STEMI should receive prompt reperfusion therapy (thrombolysis or primary percutaneous intervention). Table 5 outlines the recommended dosing regimens of medications commonly used in ACS.

Aspirin

All patients presenting with a proved or suspected AMI should receive 324 mg of aspirin (four 81 mg tablets chewed and swallowed or as a rectal suppository if unable to take orally) and continue at 81 mg daily thereafter. Aspirin significantly reduces mortality in AMI. In patients with STEMI, aspirin reduces mortality to a similar extent as thrombolytic therapy, with additive benefits of both. Aspirin-allergic patients should receive 300 mg of clopidogrel (Plavix).

Clopidogrel

Clopidogrel (Plavix) blocks the platelet ADP receptor and can be given in place of aspirin in aspirin-allergic patients. A 300-mg loading dose is administered with 75 mg daily administered thereafter. Clopidogrel is as efficacious as aspirin in AMI. Clopidogrel is beneficial in those undergoing primary percutaneous intervention for STEMI.

TABLE 3 TIMI Risk Score for Unstable Angina/Non-ST-Segment-Elevation Myocardial Infarction

One Point for Each of the Following:	Score	Risk of Adverse Event*
Age ≥65 y	0/1	4.7%
Presence of ≥3 CV risk factors†	2	8.3%
Recent (<24 h) severe angina	3	13.2%
Known coronary stenosis ≥50%	4	19.9%
ST-segment deviation on admission ECG ≥0.5 mm	5	26.2%
Use of aspirin within past 7 d	6/7	40.9%
Elevated biomarkers of cardiac injury (troponin, CK-MB)		

*Death, MI, or urgent revascularization within 14 days.
†Family history of premature coronary artery disease, hypertension, hyperlipidemia, diabetes mellitus, active smoker.
Abbreviations: CV = cardiovascular; ECG = electrocardiogram.

TABLE 4 TIMI Risk Score for ST-Segment-Elevation Myocardial Infarction

Risk Factor	Points	Score	30-Day Mortality (%)
Age ≥75 y	3	0	0.8
Age 65-74 y	2	1	1.6
Systolic BP <100 mm Hg	3	2	2.2
Heart rate >100 beats/min	2	3	4.4
Killip class >1	2	4	7.3
Anterior MI or LBBB	1	5	12.4
Diabetes mellitus, HTN, or angina	1	6	16.1
Weight <67 kg	1	7	23.4
Symptom onset to treatment >4 h	1	8	26.8
		>8	35.9

Abbreviations: BP = blood pressure; HTN = hypertension; LBBB = left bundle branch block; MI = myocardial infarction.

Clopidogrel in addition to aspirin, compared with aspirin alone, reduces the risk of cardiovascular death, myocardial infarction, or stroke in patients with NSTEMI who do not undergo percutaneous revascularization (CURE [Clopidogrel in Unstable Angina to Prevent Recurrent Events] trial) and in those who do undergo percutaneous revascularization (PCI-CURE [Percutaneous Coronary Intervention-Clopidogrel in Unstable Angina to Prevent Recurrent Ischemic Events] and CREDO [Clopidogrel for the Reduction of Events During Observation] trials). The decision to give clopidogrel prior to coronary angiography in patients with AMI should take into account the ultimate requirement of coronary artery bypass graft (CABG) in some patients, which would delay CABG for 5 to 7 days following the administration of clopidogrel. Clopidogrel, 75 mg daily, should be continued for at least 6 and preferably 12 months following percutaneous coronary revascularization in the setting of AMI. If coronary angiography is not anticipated, clopidogrel should be initiated and also continued for 9 to 12 months. A recent study suggests that clopidogrel imparts incremental benefit when given in combination with thrombolytic therapy in the setting of STEMI.

Heparin

Patients presenting with AMI should be treated with either IV unfractionated heparin (IVUFH) (60 IU/kg bolus, then 12 IU/kg per hour infusion) or subcutaneous low-molecular-weight heparin (LMWH), except for STEMI patients receiving streptokinase. In STEMI, IVUFH is required to maintain vessel patency in those receiving a

TABLE 5 Dosage of Medications Commonly Used in the Treatment of Myocardial Infarction

Medication	Dosing and Administration
Aspirin	• 324 mg chewed and swallowed (81 mg × 4) upon presentation, then 81 to 325 mg daily. • If unable to take PO, crush and administer via NG tube or as 325-mg rectal suppository.
Clopidogrel (Plavix)	• 300-mg oral loading dose, then 75 mg PO daily for 9 to 12 mo or indefinitely in high-risk patients.
Heparin	
• IV unfractionated	• 60 U/kg IV bolus (max: 5000 U), then 12 U/kg/h (max: 1000 U/h) for 48 h or PCI (goal aPTT 1.5 = 2.5 × control).
• Low-molecular-weight Enoxaparin (Lovenox)	• 1 mg/kg SC Q12 h for 48 to 72 h or until PCI. Initial 30-mg IV bolus can be given.
(Dalteparin (Fragmin)	• 120 IU/kg SC (max 10,000 IU) Q12 h.
β-Blockers	
• Metoprolol (Lopressor)	• 5 mg IV Q5 min × 3 to goal heart rate 60-65/min or hypotension, then 50 mg PO Q12 h.
• Atenolol (Tenormin)	• 5 mg IV Q5 min × 3 to goal heart rate 60-65/min or hypotension, then 50-100 mg PO daily.
• Esmolol (Brevibloc)	• 500 µg/kg IV bolus, then 50 µg/kg/min titrating to HR.
Nitroglycerin	0.4 mg sublingual Q5 min × 3 for persistent ischemic pain or IV infusion starting at 5-10 µg/min with up titration for persistent ischemic pain.
Morphine sulfate	4 to 6 mg IV; repeat as needed.
GP IIb/IIIa inhibitors	
• Eptifibatide (Integrelin)	• 180 µg/kg IV bolus, then infuse at 2.0 µg/kg/min × 72 h to 96 h
• Tirofiban (Aggrastat)	• 0.4 µg/kg/min IV for 30 min, then 0.1 µg/kg/min × 48 to 96 h
• Abciximab (ReoPro)	• Use ony if PCI planned or likely; 0.25 mg/kg bolus followed by infusion at 0.125 µg/kg/min (max 10 µg/min) for 12 to 24 h.

Abbreviations: IV = intravenous; HR = heart rate; NG = nasogastric; PCI = percutaneous coronary intervention; PO = by mouth; SC = subcutaneous.

fibrin-specific thrombolytic agent (alteplase, reteplase, and tenecteplase). The use of LMWH in combination with thrombolytic therapy is still being evaluated in clinical trials and is not currently recommended. Administration of LMWH reduces the risk of death and ischemic events compared with IVUFH in patients with NSTEMI and in unstable angina when high-risk features are present (see Table 2). LMWH appears safe when continued up until the time of coronary angiography and percutaneous intervention; however, individual PCI operator preference should be taken into account. LMWH should not be given to patients with significant renal insufficiency (creatinine clearance less than 30 mL per minute) or morbid obesity.

β-Blockers

β-Blockers should be given to all patients presenting with AMI unless hypotension, bradycardia, or other contraindications exist. Metoprolol (Lopressor) or atenolol (Tenormin), 5 mg IV, should be given every 3 to 5 minutes to achieve a resting heart rate of less than 70 beats per minute (bpm). Oral metoprolol (Lopressor) or atenolol (Tenormin) should then be administered 30 minutes following the last IV dose and continued indefinitely. β-Blockers reduce oxygen supply-and-demand mismatch in the setting of AMI by lowering heart rate, reducing myocardial contractility, and reducing afterload through systemic blood pressure reduction. In addition to reducing mortality in AMI, β-blockers also reduce the risk of atrial and ventricular arrhythmias and free wall rupture. If a patient's tolerance of β-blockers is uncertain, short-acting IV esmolol (Brevibloc) may be used initially.

Nitroglycerin

Nitroglycerin can be administered as a sublingual formulation or as an IV infusion and is given if symptoms of ongoing myocardial ischemia persist. Nitroglycerin does not improve prognosis in AMI and should be used with caution in patients with right ventricular infarction that could result in hypotension. Nitroglycerin should not be administered to patients who have taken Viagra or other phosphodiesterase inhibitor within 24 hours.

Glycoprotein IIb/IIIa inhibitors

Glycoprotein (GP) IIb/IIIa inhibitors block the GP IIb/IIIa platelet receptor, which functions as the receptor for fibrinogen adherence. GP IIb/IIIa inhibitors reduce ischemic complications associated with PCI and should be administered in patients for whom an early invasive strategy is planned. It is not clear if upstream GP IIb/IIIa administration upon admission is superior to initiation in the catheterization laboratory just prior to PCI. Benefit is shown with eptifibatide (Integrilin) and tirofiban (Aggrastat) in patients with non-ST-elevation ACS who do not undergo early PCI. This benefit appears isolated to high-risk patients including those with troponin elevation, ST-segment depression more than 0.5 mV, diabetes mellitus, and LV ejection fraction less than 40%. Post hoc analyses suggest a potential differential benefit of GP IIb/IIIa therapy in men versus women, and it is an area of continued investigation.

REPERFUSION THERAPY IN ST-SEGMENT-ELEVATION MYOCARDIAL INFARCTION

Patients presenting with STEMI represent a true medical emergency and require accurate, yet expeditious evaluation and treatment directed at reperfusion of ischemic myocardium. Regardless of the modality of reperfusion used, the time from symptom onset to establishment of myocardial reperfusion is the strongest predictor of myocardial salvage, recovery of myocardial function, and reperfusion-mediated improvements in mortality. Patients receiving successful reperfusion within 2 hours of symptom onset derive the greatest benefit from reperfusion therapy.

Thrombolysis

Thrombolytic therapy is the most commonly utilized method of reperfusion worldwide. The fibrin-specific t-PA derived thrombolytic agents (alteplase [Activase], reteplase [Retavase], and tenecteplase [TNKase]) have proved superior but significantly more expensive than the fibrin-nonspecific agents such as streptokinase. The fibrin-specific agents reduce 30-day mortality rates by 15% compared with streptokinase and appear to provide similar rates of successful reperfusion and mortality reduction. They differ primarily in the manner in which they are given and subsequently the ease of administration (Table 6). Clinically, successful thrombolysis is associated with resolution of chest symptoms and reduction of ST-segment elevation by at least 50%. Patients with persistent symptoms, persistence of ST-segment elevation, and/or hemodynamic instability following thrombolysis should be referred for emergent

TABLE 6 Thrombolytic Agents

Thrombolytic	Dosing/Administration	Fibrin Specific
Alteplase (t-PA) (Activase)	15 mg IV bolus, then 0.75 mg/kg over 30 min (max 50 mg), then 0.5 mg/kg over 60 min (max 35 mg)	Yes
Reteplase (rPA) (Retavase)	10 U IV bolus over 2 min, then second 10-U IV bolus 30 min later	Yes
Tenecteplase (TNK) (TNKase)	0.5 mg/kg single IV bolus (max 50 mg), or weight <60 kg, 30 mg; 60-69 kg, 35 mg; 70-79 kg, 40 mg; 80-89 kg, 45 mg; ≥90 kg, 50 mg	Yes
Streptokinase (Streptase)	1.5 million U IV over 60 min	Yes

Abbreviation: IV = intravenous.

coronary angiography. The absence of contraindications to thrombolytic therapy should be assured prior to administration (Box 1).

The benefit of routine predischarge coronary angiography in patients with apparent successful thrombolysis has been shown to be beneficial in a recent randomized trial. Patients who successfully reperfuse following thrombolysis and do not undergo in-hospital coronary angiography should undergo a submaximal exercise stress test or pharmacologic stress test prior to hospital discharge. Patients with an abnormal predischarge stress test, recurrent symptoms, or ECG changes, and those with an LV ejection fraction less than 40%, should undergo coronary angiography with PCI as warranted prior to discharge.

Early Invasive Versus Conservative Therapy in Unstable Angina/Non-ST-Segment-Elevation Myocardial Infarction

Patients with NSTEMI usually do not have complete occlusion of the culprit coronary artery. Thus emergent revascularization is generally not indicated except in patients with hemodynamic instability or persistent symptoms despite initial medical therapy. Whether or not patients with UA/NSTEMI benefit from an early invasive approach (i.e., routine coronary angiography and PCI as indicated during hospitalization) was evaluated in three studies using modern antithrombotic/antiplatelet therapy and current PCI technology. The FRISC II (Fragmin and Fast Revascularization During Instability in Coronary Artery Disease), TACTICS-TIMI 18 (Treat Angina With Aggrastat and Determine Cost of Therapy With Invasive or Conservative Strategy-Thrombolysis in Myocardial Infarction), and RITA 3 (Randomized Intervention Trial of Unstable Angina 3) trials demonstrate improved outcomes with an early invasive strategy in intermediate- and high-risk patients with unstable angina and in patients with NSTEMI. In response to the accumulating data demonstrating a benefit from an early invasive approach using contemporary medical management and modern interventional techniques, the ACC/AHA guidelines now recommend an early invasive approach in patients with NSTEMI.

ELECTRICAL COMPLICATIONS ASSOCIATED WITH ACUTE MYOCARDIAL INFARCTION

Conduction abnormalities are common in patients with AMI and should be assessed in all patients. Ischemia-mediated alterations in cardiac conduction can manifest as AV block (first, second, and third degree), bundle branch block, and fascicular block. Conduction abnormalities at the AV node level in the setting of inferior AMI are usually transient and usually do not require transvenous pacing, even in the setting of high-grade AV block. AV block as well as new bundle branch block in patients with anterior STEMI portends a worse prognosis and is associated with a high risk of progression to complete heart block. Temporary transvenous pacing should be considered in those with anterior myocardial infarction (MI) and Mobitz 2 AV block, third-degree AV block, or new left bundle-branch block (LBBB).

Ventricular fibrillation can complicate myocardial infarction and should be treated promptly with unsynchronized electrical shock as per current ACLS guidelines. Table 7 lists recommendations for the approach and treatment of ventricular tachycardia in the setting of AMI.

ADJUNCTIVE THERAPY/HOSPITAL DISCHARGE MEDICATIONS

Aspirin, 81 mg to 325 mg, should be continued indefinitely in all ACS patients. An angiotensin-converting enzyme inhibitor (ACEI) should be started within 24 hours in all hemodynamically stable patients with large anterior infarctions and in patients with LV ejection fraction less than 40%. We prefer starting with a short-acting ACEI such as captopril (Capoten), 3.125 mg by mouth every 8 hours, with titration upward as tolerated. Upon discharge, a longer acting ACEI can be substituted. Statin therapy in the setting of ACS improves short- and long-term outcomes and should be initiated before discharge in all ACS patients regardless of cholesterol levels. The recent PROVE-IT (Pravastatin or Atorvastatin Evaluation and Infection Therapy) trial showed that intensive statin therapy (mean LDL [low-density lipoprotein]: 62 mg/dL) following ACS reduces adverse cardiac events compared with less intensive statin therapy (mean LDL: 95 mg/dL). All patients with ACS should be discharged on a β-blocker unless a contraindication exists. One randomized trial (COMET [Carvedilol Or Metoprolol European Trial]) suggests that carvedilol (Coreg) at optimal doses is superior to short-acting metoprolol tartrate (Lopressor) in patients with symptomatic chronic heart failure and LV ejection fraction of less than 35%.

TABLE 7 Treatment of Ventricular Arrhythmias Associated With Acute Myocardial Infarction

Arrhythmia	Electrical Shock*	Other Therapeutic Measures
Sustained polymorphic VT	Yes, 200 J, 300 J, 360 J	As per current ACLS recommendations Normalize electrolyte abnormalities
Sustained monomorphic VT: with symptoms or hemodynamic compromise	Yes, 100, 200, 300, 360	As per current ACLS recommendations
Sustained monomorphic VT: without symptoms or hemodynamic compromise	No	Amiodarone (Cordarone), 150 mg IV infused over 10 min, then 360 mg over 6 h (1 mg/min), then 540 mg over 18 h (0.5 mg/min) (max 2.2 g over 24 h)
Nonsustained VT (within 48 h of MI)	No	No treatment recommended unless symptomatic or associated with hemodynamic compromise
Nonsustained VT (>48 h following MI)	No	Electrophysiology study with programmed stimulation. If sustained VT inducible, then insertion of AICD.
Accelerated idioventricular rhythm	No	None

Abbreviations: ACLS = Advanced Cardiac Life Support; AICD = Automatic Implantable Cardioverter Defibrillator; MI = myocardial infarction; VT = ventricular tachycardia.
*Energy is for monophasic defibrillators.

CARDIAC REHABILITATION/SECONDARY PREVENTION/RISK FACTOR MODIFICATION

All patients should undergo cardiovascular risk factor assessment and modification during and following hospitalization. Blood pressure readings should ideally be lower than 120/80 mm Hg. Smoking cessation should be addressed and glycemic control optimized in diabetic patients. Patients should be instructed on an AHA step II low-fat diet, and statin therapy should be initiated and/or modified to achieve an LDL lower than 70 mg/dL. The goal of cardiac rehabilitation is to help the patient safely return to and maintain normal daily activities and promote secondary prevention measures. This generally includes a staged approach with patients attending monitored exercise sessions for the first 6 to 8 weeks following MI during which levels of exercise are gradually increased. Following an uncomplicated MI, patients are instructed to return to work in 14 to 28 days, with driving allowed within 7 to 14 days. Patients with complicated MI, including those with significant ventricular arrhythmias, require a more gradual return to normal daily activities.

HOSPITAL FOLLOW-UP VISIT

Patients should generally be seen in follow-up between 3 and 6 weeks following hospital discharge. They should be evaluated for recurrence of symptoms, evidence of heart failure, and medication intolerance or noncompliance. Medications should be reviewed individually and the rationale for each discussed. Modification of cardiovascular risk factors should continue. A transthoracic echocardiogram should be obtained to assess LV function 4 to 6 weeks following discharge. Patients with an LVEF of less than 30% should be considered for prophylactic internal defibrillator insertion. Patients with an LVEF between 31% and 40% should undergo 48-hour Holter monitoring

CURRENT DIAGNOSIS

Acute myocardial infarction is defined as the typical rise and fall of cardiac troponin or creatine kinase myocardial band in addition to one of the following:
- Symptoms consistent with myocardial ischemia
- Electrocardiogram changes indicating myocardial ischemia (ST-segment depression or elevation)
- New pathologic Q waves
- Percutaneous coronary intervention

CURRENT THERAPY

- All patients with suspected AMI should immediately receive aspirin, 324 mg chewed and swallowed, with subsequent administration of β-blockers, heparin, and nitrates as indicated.
- Administration of adjuvant antithrombotic therapy using low molecular weight heparin, clopidogrel, and GP IIb/IIIa inhibitors should be used in high-risk patients including those with NSTEMI.
- Those with STEMI should receive either thrombolysis (if within 12 hours of symptom onset) or undergo emergent primary percutaneous intervention (if within 24 hours of symptom onset).
- Patients with NSTEMI and those with unstable angina with high-risk features benefit from an early invasive treatment strategy that includes coronary angiography and percutaneous coronary intervention as warranted.
- Patients younger than age 75 years presenting with AMI and cardiogenic shock should preferentially undergo emergent coronary angiography with percutaneous coronary intervention.

Abbreviations: AMI = acute myocardial infarction; GP = glycoprotein; MI = myocardial infarction; NSTEMI = non-ST-segment-elevation myocardial infarction; STEMI = ST-segment-elevation myocardial infarction.

with subsequent referral to an electrophysiologist if nonsustained ventricular tachycardia (VT) is present.

REFERENCES

Antman EM, Anbe DT, Armstrong PW, Bates ER, et al: ACC/AHA guidelines for the management of patients with ST-elevation myocardial infarction: A report of the American College of Cardiology/American Heart Association Task Force on Practice Guidelines, 2004. Available at www.acc.org/clinical/guidelines/stemi/index.pdf

Boersma E, Harrington RA, Moliterno DJ, et al: Platelet glycoprotein IIb/IIIa inhibitors in acute coronary syndromes: A meta-analysis of all major randomized clinical trials. Lancet 2002;359:189-198.

Braunwald E, Antman EM, Beasley JW, Califf RM, et al: ACC/AHA 2002 guideline update for the management of patients with unstable angina and non-ST-segment elevation myocardial infarction: Summary article: A report of the American College of Cardiology/American Heart Association Task Force on Practice Guidelines (Committee on the Management of Patients with Unstable Angina). J Am Coll Cardiol 2002;40:1366-1374.

Cannon CP, Weintraub WS, Demopoulos LA, et al: Comparison of early invasive and conservative strategies in patients with unstable coronary syndromes treated with the glycoprotein IIb/IIIa inhibitor tirofiban. N Engl J Med 2001;344:1879-1887.

Cohen M, Demers C, Gurfinkel EP, et al: A comparison of low-molecular-weight heparin with unfractionated heparin for unstable coronary artery disease. Efficacy and Safety of Subcutaneous Enoxaparin in Non-Q-Wave Coronary Events Study Group. N Engl J Med 1997; 337:447-452.

Fox KA, Poole-Wilson PA, Henderson RA, et al: Interventional versus conservative treatment for patients with unstable angina or non-ST-elevation myocardial infarction: The British Heart Foundation RITA 3 randomised trial. Randomized intervention trial of unstable angina. Lancet 2002;360:743-751.

Hochman JS, Sleeper LA, Webb JG, et al: Early revascularization in acute myocardial infarction complicated by cardiogenic shock. N Engl J Med 1999;341:625-634.

Schwartz GG, Olsson AG, Ezekowitz MD, et al: Effects of atorvastatin on early recurrent ischemic events in acute coronary syndromes: The MIRACL study: A randomized controlled trial. JAMA 2001; 285:1711-1718.

Yusuf S, Zhao F, Mehta SR, et al: Effects of clopidogrel in addition to aspirin in patients with acute coronary syndromes without ST-segment elevation. N Engl J Med 2001;345:494-502.

Pericarditis

Method of
Brian D. Hoit, MD

Although the diagnosis and treatment of pericardial disease is often simple and rewarding, it may offer unexpected challenges and frustrations to both clinician and patient for several reasons. First, the presence of pericardial heart disease may escape detection, often remaining clinically silent, being apparent only during the evaluation of unrelated complaints. In addition, pericardial disease may complicate, and be overshadowed by, extracardiac manifestations from a number of systemic disorders. Second, although guidelines for the diagnosis and management of pericardial diseases are now available, there are few randomized, placebo-controlled trials from which appropriate therapy may be selected and important clinical decisions supported. The physician thus often must rely heavily on clinical judgment because most data originate from small uncontrolled trials and anecdotal experience. Finally, therapeutic options in most cases are limited to nonspecific anti-inflammatory agents, drainage of pericardial fluid, and pericardiectomy. Although there is general agreement on how these measures should be applied in the patient with either very mild or severe disease, there is little consensus on how the large number of cases encountered with clinical manifestations between these two extremes should be managed. With these important caveats in mind, the options available for treating pericardial heart disease are reviewed here.

Acute Pericarditis

Hospitalization is warranted for most, if not all, patients who present with an initial episode of acute pericarditis to determine an etiology and to observe for the development of cardiac tamponade; close, early follow-up is critically important in the remainder. Table 1 lists the major definable causes of pericardial heart disease; however, in many cases, the etiology of pericardial heart disease is never identified..Features indicative of high-risk pericarditis that warrants hospitalization include fever higher than 38°C (100°F), subacute onset, an immune depressed state, trauma, oral anticoagulant therapy, myopericarditis, large pericardial effusion, cardiac tamponade, and aspirin failure. Establishing the exact cause of acute pericarditis is an important part of management in the high-risk case, but considerable judgment must be exercised when deciding whether and how to investigate suspected acute viral and idiopathic pericarditis.

Acute pericarditis usually responds to oral nonsteroidal anti-inflammatory drugs (NSAIDs), such as ASA, 650 mg every 4 to 6 hours, or ibuprofen, 300 to 800 mg every 6 to 8 hours. Gastrointestinal (GI) prophylaxis with H_2 blockers or proton pump inhibitors is often warranted, particularly in those at high risk or who require longer durations of treatment. Selective COX-2 inhibitors are NSAIDs with few adverse GI effects, but they are implicated in adverse cardiovascular events; moreover, they have not been tested in acute pericarditis. Cumulative anecdotal data suggest that colchicine[1] (1 mg/day, with or without a 2 mg loading dose), either as a supplement to the use of NSAIDs or as monotherapy, is effective for the acute episode, well tolerated, and may prevent recurrences. A recent prospective randomized, open-label trial found that colchicine[1] (1 to 2 mg for the first day, followed by 0.5 to 1 mg/day for 3 months) in addition to aspirin was more effective than aspirin alone in reducing symptoms and recurrences. Side effects (diarrhea and nausea) are usually mild and most often do not necessitate withdrawal of the drug.

Chest pain is often alleviated in 1 to 2 days, and the friction rub and ST segment elevation resolve shortly thereafter. The duration of therapy is controversial; a month of NSAIDs (e.g., high-dose aspirin for 7 to 10 days followed by a taper over 3 to 4 weeks) and 3 months of colchicine[1] is a regimen based on evidence. The intensity of therapy is dictated by the distress of the patient, and intravenous (IV) ketorolac (Toradol), 30 mg every 6 hours, or narcotics

---

[1]Not FDA approved for this indication.

CURRENT DIAGNOSIS

	Acute Pericarditis	Acute Myocardial Infarction
History	Sharp, retrosternal pain, pleuritic, radiates to trapezius ridge	Dull, precordial chest pain, radiates to neck/arm
Physical	Friction rub; may be fever, signs of inflammation, signs of underlying associated diseases	May be murmurs, ventricular gallops; signs of pulmonary congestion
EKG	Diffuse; characteristic evolutionary pattern; PR depression; absent Q waves pattern	Indicative ST and Q waves; characteristic evolutionary pattern
CXR	May be normal in uncomplicated cases May be signs of effusion, associated diseases	May be normal in uncomplicated cases May be large heart, signs of pulmonary congestion
Echo	Pericardial effusion confirms clinical suspicion May be normal	Regional wall motion abnormalities May identify mechanical complications
Laboratory	Nonspecific markers of inflammation; With extensive pericarditis may see isoenzyme changes characteristic of acute MI	Characteristic CK and troponin isoenzymes

Abbreviations: CK = creatine kinase; CXR = chest radiograph; EKG = electrocardiogram; MI = myocardial infarction.

may be required for severe pain. Although some cases necessitate steroid therapy (prednisone, 60 to 80 mg/day) for a week to control pain (with the dosage tapered carefully on an individual basis thereafter), corticosteroids should be avoided unless there are specific indications (such as connective tissue disease, autoreactive, or uremic pericarditis) because they enhance viral multiplication and may result in recurrences when the dosage is tapered; colchicine[1] may be particularly useful in this situation. Importantly, tuberculous and pyogenic pericarditis should be excluded before steroid therapy is initiated. Intrapericardial instillation of triamcinolone (Kenalog), 300 mg/m², avoids systemic side effects and is highly effective. Patients in whom pericarditis represents one manifestation of systemic illness (such as sepsis, uremia, connective tissue disease, or neoplasia) should receive therapy directed toward the primary disorder in addition to palliative and supportive treatment.

[1]Not FDA approved for this indication.

TABLE 1 Etiology of Pericardial Heart Disease

Idiopathic
Infectious (viral, bacterial, mycobacterial, fungal, protozoal, AIDS)
Neoplastic (breast, lung, melanoma, lymphoma, leukemia; mesothelioma)
Post myocardial infarction
Radiation induced
Nephrogenic (dialytic and uremic)
Traumatic (blunt and penetrating, chylopericardium)
Connective tissue diseases and arteritides (rheumatoid arthritis, systemic lupus erythematosus, scleroderma, polyarteritis nodosa, Takayasu's arteritis, Wegener's granulomatosis)
Myxedema
Iatrogenic (diagnostic and therapeutic procedures, drugs)
Miscellaneous (sarcoidosis, amyloidosis, Whipple's disease, dissecting aortic aneurysm)

Reproduced with permission from Hoit BD: Pericarditis. In Rakel RE, Bope ET (eds): Conn's Current Therapy 2002. Philadelphia, Elsevier, 2002.

Recurrent Pericarditis

Recurrent or relapsing acute pericarditis is one of the most distressing disorders of the pericardium for both patient and physician. Atypical features, such as the absence of physical findings, offer challenges for diagnosis and management and often necessitate close follow-up and rigorous emotional support. Recurrences occur with highly variable frequency over a course of many years; although they may be spontaneous, occurring at varying intervals after discontinuation of drug (i.e., "recurrent"), they are more commonly associated with either discontinuation or tapering of anti-inflammatory drugs (i.e., "incessant").

Painful recurrences of pericarditis may respond to NSAIDs but commonly require additional therapy. A recent prospective, randomized open-label trial compared aspirin (or steroids when necessary) and colchicine[1] (0.5 to 1 mg/day after a 1- to 2-mg load for 6 months) with aspirin alone. This study suggests that colchicine[1] is both efficacious and safe for the prevention of recurrences; moreover, corticosteroid use was an independent risk factor for further recurrences. When necessary, prednisone is begun at a high dose (1 to 1.5 mg/kg/day) for at least 4 weeks and tapered slowly (approximately 5 mg every 3 days) over the next 2 to 3 months. Azathioprine[1] (Imuran) and cyclophosphamide[1] (Cytoxan) are used to prevent recurrent episodes in patients who fail to respond to high-dose corticosteroids or who experience severe corticosteroid side effects; pericardiectomy should be considered only when repeated attempts at medical treatment have clearly failed, especially when there is evidence (e.g., from serial bone density scans) of steroid-induced complications.

[1]Not FDA approved for this indication.

Treatment of Specific Causes of Pericarditis

PURULENT PERICARDITIS

The incidence and bacterial spectrum of purulent pericarditis have changed because of the increasing frequency of cardiac surgery and instrumentation, selection-induced changes in the flora responsible for hospital-acquired infections, and the prolonged survival of immunocompromised hosts. Bacterial pericarditis is treated with surgical exploration and drainage (pericardiectomy is preferable) and appropriate systemic antibiotics. A high index of suspicion is critical because in the appropriate setting, pericardial involvement is often unrecognized when it complicates systemic infection, and the characteristic features of acute pericarditis are frequently absent. The threshold for echocardiography in the septic patient should be low, and whenever purulent pericarditis is suspected, the pericardial space should be explored. Fibrinolytics may be used to lyse fibrous adhesions, liquefy purulent exudates, and prevent constrictive pericarditis.

MYCOBACTERIAL AND FUNGAL PERICARDITIS

Tuberculosis is a major cause of pericarditis in nonindustrialized countries but is an uncommon cause of pericarditis in the United States. Nevertheless, its incidence is increasing because of HIV infection. Pericardial fluid should be removed, cultured, and antituberculous therapy begun. Depending on the echocardiographic appearance, subxiphoid drainage may be necessary. Some recommend early pericardiectomy in all cases of tuberculosis pericarditis, but the long-term (16 years) prognosis of patients without cardiac compression during the acute illness who are treated with medical therapy alone is excellent. Multiple drug therapy and corticosteroids are effective in tuberculous pericarditis, whereas atypical mycobacterial infections (especially *Myobacterium avium intracellulare*) may be resistant to treatment. Patients with tuberculous pericarditis should receive triple drug therapy (isoniazid, 5 mg/kg to a maximum of 300 mg; rifampin [Rifadin], 10 mg/kg to a maximum of 600 mg; and either streptomycin, 15 mg/kg to a maximum of 1 g, or ethambutol [Myambutol], 5 to 25 mg/kg to a maximum of 2.5 g) for a minimum of 9 months. Corticosteroids (prednisone, 1 to 2 mg/kg/day) may be useful if pericardial effusion persists or recurs during therapy, and they appear beneficial acutely in reducing morbidity and mortality. Pericardiectomy may be necessary for recurrent cardiac tamponade.

Patients should be observed for constriction because up to half of patients require pericardiectomy; failure to improve or worsening over 1 to 2 months, pericardial thickening, or evidence of constriction requires urgent pericardiectomy. In patients with hemodynamics consistent with effusive-constrictive pericarditis, plans for visceral and parietal pericardiectomy after a few weeks of chemotherapy are advisable.. Persistent hypotension may signify tuberculous adrenal insufficiency.

Pericarditis complicating deep fungal infection with histoplasma or coccidiomycosis may be immunologic, resolve spontaneously, and not require specific therapy. Amphotericin B (up to 2.5 g total), itraconazole (Sporanox), 200 to 400 mg/day, ketoconazole (Nizoral), 200 to 400 mg/day, and fluconazole (Diflucan), 200 to 400 mg/day, are rarely required. Tamponading effusion and constriction require decompression. Surgical decompression and specific antifungal or antimicrobial therapy may be necessary for disseminated infection with *Candida, Aspergillus, Actinomycetes,* and *Nocardia.*

NEOPLASTIC PERICARDITIS

Metastatic neoplasia remains the leading cause of pericardial disease in hospitalized patients, most often in patients with lung or breast cancer, melanoma, lymphoma, and acute leukemia. Many cases are asymptomatic and found only incidentally at autopsy, but others cause symptoms and may progress to cardiac tamponade. The pericardium may be thickened and cause constriction; less commonly, effusive-constrictive pericarditis occurs.

In almost every case, fluid should be removed if large effusions are refractory or if tamponade ensues. The specific approach depends on the patient's expected longevity and medical condition. Pericardiocentesis is associated with a high recurrence rate and does not provide tissue for biopsy. Sclerosing agents, such as tetracycline (500 to 1000 mg in 20 mL of sterile saline), reduce recurrences and can be considered for patients with a poor prognosis. However, sclerosis is painful, does not improve prognosis, and may not be superior to an indwelling catheter alone. Subtotal pericardiectomy is most effective but should only be performed in carefully selected patients. Balloon pericardiotomy avoids the discomfort and risk of surgery in critically ill patients with predictably limited survival.

CURRENT THERAPY

Type	Therapy
Acute viral/nonspecific pericarditis	ASA, NSAIDS, colchicine
Recurrent pericarditis	Colchicines in addition to ASA/NSAIDs; prednisone*
Purulent pericarditis	Specific systemic antibiotics; drainage; fibrinolytics
TB pericarditis	Antituberculous therapy; steroids; May require pericardiectomy
Neoplastic pericarditis	May require drainage; recurrences reduced by sclerosis, pericardiectomy
Postinfarction pericarditis	ASA
Nephrogenic pericarditis	Intensification of dialysis; drainage for tamponade and large resistant chronic effusions; instillation of steroids

---

*Prednisone should be avoided if possible.
See text for details, specific indications, and doses.
Abbreviations: ASA = aspirin; NSAIDS = nonsteroidal anti-inflammatory drugs; TB = tuberculosis.

PERICARDITIS COMPLICATING MYOCARDIAL INFARCTION

Pericarditis is common in the first few days after myocardial infarction, occurring in as many as 28% to 43% of fatal infarctions, but it is clinically apparent in as few as 7% of cases. Pericardial involvement is related to infarct size and associated with a poor prognosis. An important clinical issue is the extent to which acute pericarditis in myocardial infarction influences management with anticoagulants. A pericardial friction rub occurring in the first 2 or 3 days without an associated pericardial effusion should not influence clinical decisions, but pericarditis occurring later in the course or accompanied by pericardial effusion or tamponade is a contraindication to anticoagulant therapy. Cardiac tamponade seldom occurs, except in patients who receive systemic anticoagulants or have cardiac rupture.

Treatment of infarct pericarditis is seldom indicated, but when symptomatic it responds to ASA; corticosteroids should be avoided because of concerns of impaired infarct healing, steroid dependency, and toxic side effects.

RADIATION-INDUCED PERICARDIAL DISEASE

Acute pericarditis occurring early during radiation therapy is uncommon and most likely the result of the radiation-induced effects on the tumor rather than a direct toxic effect of the radiation on the pericardium. In this instance, therapy should not be disrupted, although a reduction in dose may be necessary. A delayed (usually less than 1 year, but highly variable) form of pericardial injury may present as acute pericarditis or effusion (often with some degree of cardiac compression); constrictive and effusive-constrictive pericarditis may become manifest only after many years.

Acute radiation-induced pericarditis can be managed symptomatically as acute idiopathic pericarditis. Hemodynamically insignificant pericardial effusion can also be managed conservatively because spontaneous resolution is the rule; however, pericardiectomy should be offered to symptomatic patients with large recurrent pericardial effusions. Constrictive pericarditis requires pericardiectomy unless otherwise contraindicated.

PERICARDIAL DISEASE IN PATIENTS WITH RENAL FAILURE

Pericarditis complicates both uremia and dialytic therapy (hemo- and peritoneal), and may be clinically silent. The clinical manifestation of nephrogenic pericardial disease may be acute fibrinous pericarditis, pericardial effusion, or cardiac tamponade; classic constrictive pericarditis is rare.

Although intensification of dialysis is an accepted treatment modality for hemodynamically insignificant disease, considerable controversy exists regarding the optimal management of large, persistent, or recurrent pericardial effusion. Tamponade is an indication for pericardial drainage, and large resistant, chronic effusion warrant pericardiocentesis, but a conservative approach—that is, intensification of dialysis and NSAIDs—may suffice in less severe cases. The instillation of nonabsorbable steroids (triamcinolone, 50 mg every 6 hours[3] for 2 to 3 days) directly into the pericardial space is advocated, but randomized controlled data are absent. If needle drainage is necessary, an indwelling catheter should be left in the pericardial space for at least 2 to 3 days. Dialysis-associated effusive pericarditis usually responds to intensification of dialysis and regional heparinization or by changing to peritoneal dialysis. Pericardiectomy may be necessary for intractable effusions.

Other Causes of Pericardial Disease

Pericarditis may accompany virtually any connective tissue disease and may present as either acute or chronic pericarditis with or without an effusion.. However, most cases are subclinical and in many instances are recognized only at autopsy. In the absence of tamponading or secondarily infected effusions, NSAIDs and corticosteroids are useful. Myxedema-associated effusions develop slowly and may grow very large; slow resolution usually follows institution of thyroid replacement therapy.

Iatrogenic pericardial disease results from both the calculated complications and the unanticipated misadventures of diagnostic and therapeutic procedures. Importantly, a wide variety of drugs and toxins may cause pericardial heart disease by producing drug-induced lupus (e.g., procainamide, hydralazine, isoniazid), a hypersensitivity or idiosyncratic reaction (e.g., penicillins, thiazides, anthracyclines), pericardial irritation, or hemorrhage (e.g., anticoagulants). Chylous pericardial effusions generally follow traumatic or surgical injury to the thoracic duct but may result from neoplastic obstruction of the thoracic duct, or they may be idiopathic. Failure to respond to either ligation of the thoracic duct and partial pericardiectomy or to a diet rich in medium chain triglycerides warrants implantation of a valved pericardioperitoneal conduit.

Pericardial Effusion and Tamponade

In the absence of tamponade or suspected purulent pericarditis, there are few indications for pericardial drainage. Persistent large and unexplained effusions (especially when tuberculosis is suspect or when present for more than 3 months) may warrant pericardiocentesis. Occasionally, suspected malignancy or systemic disease may necessitate pericardial drainage and biopsy. However, routine drainage of large effusions (20 mm echo-free space in diastole) has a very low diagnostic yield (7%) and no therapeutic benefit. Figure 1 presents an approach to the management of moderate and large pericardial effusions.

It is important to remember that tamponade is a clinical diagnosis and "echocardiographic signs of tamponade" is not by itself an indication for pericardiocentesis. Although the absence of any cardiac chamber collapse has a high negative predictive value (92%), the positive predictive value is substantially reduced (58%).

Removal of small amounts of tamponading pericardial fluid (approximately 50 mL) produces considerable

---

[3]Exceeds dosage recommended by the manufacturer.

MANAGEMENT OF MODERATE-LARGE PERICARDIAL EFFUSIONS

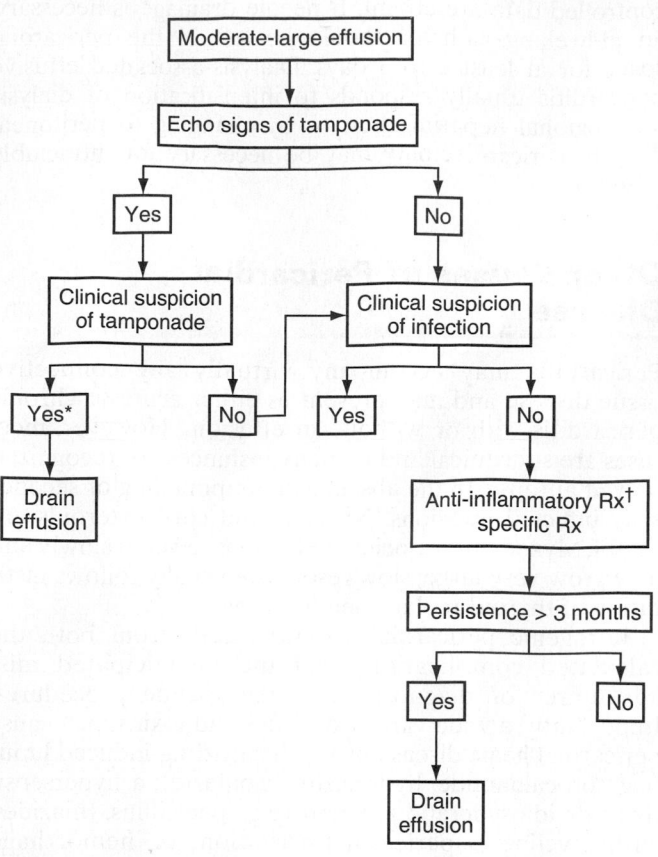

FIGURE 1. Algorithm for the management of moderate to large pericardial effusions. *Right heart catheterization may be required. †Anti-inflammatory treatment if there are signs of pericarditis. (Reprinted with permission from Hoit BD: Management of effusive and constrictive pericardial heart disease. Circulation 2002;105: 2939-2942.)

symptomatic and hemodynamic improvement because of the steep pericardial pressure–volume relation. Unless there is concomitant cardiac disease or coexisting constriction (i.e., effusive-constrictive pericarditis), removal of all of the pericardial fluid normalizes pericardial, atrial, ventricular diastolic and arterial pressures, and cardiac output. Mild or low-pressure tamponade (i.e., when the venous pressure is less than 10 cm of water, arterial blood pressure is normal and pulsus paradoxus is absent), particularly when the etiology is idiopathic, viral, or when responsive to specific therapy (e.g., thyroid hormone), does not require pericardiocentesis. At the other extreme, hyperacute tamponade (usually resulting from cardiac trauma) necessitates immediate pericardiocentesis as an initial triage measure. However, the majority of patients fall between these two extremes and require pericardial drainage. Either surgical means (via subxiphoid incision, video-assisted thoracoscopy, or thoracotomy) or percutaneously (with a needle or balloon catheter) accomplishes pericardial drainage. The choice between needle pericardiocentesis and surgical drainage depends on institutional resources and physician experience, the etiology of the effusion, the need for diagnostic tissue samples, and the prognosis of the patient. Unless the situation is

immediately life threatening, experienced staff should perform pericardiocentesis in a facility equipped with radiographic, echocardiographic, and hemodynamic monitoring to optimize the success and safety of the procedure. The safety of the procedure is increased by using 2D echo guidance. Pericardiocentesis is ill advised when there is less than 1 cm of effusion, loculation, or evidence of fibrin and adhesion.

Recurrent effusions may be treated by either repeat pericardiocentesis, sclerotherapy with tetracycline, surgical creation of a pericardial window, or pericardiectomy. Subtotal pericardiectomy is preferred when the patient is expected to survive greater than 1 year. A pleuropericardial window provides a large area for fluid to be reabsorbed and is often performed in patients with malignant effusions. Pericardiectomy may be required for recurrent effusions in dialysis patients. In critically ill patients, a pericardial window may be created percutaneously with a balloon catheter.

Constrictive Pericarditis

Constrictive pericarditis is a condition in which a thickened, scarred, and often calcified pericardium limits diastolic filling of the ventricles. Although acute pericarditis from most causes may eventuate in constrictive pericarditis, the most common antecedents are idiopathic, cardiac trauma and surgery, mediastinal irradiation, tuberculosis and other infectious diseases, neoplasms (particularly lung and breast), renal failure, and connective tissue diseases. Although it is commonly thought that a normal pericardial thickness excludes the diagnosis of constrictive pericarditis, 28% of 143 surgically confirmed cases had normal pericardial thickness on CT scan, and 18% had normal thickness on histopathologic examination.

Classic chronic constrictive pericarditis is less frequently encountered than in the past, whereas subacute constrictive pericarditis (weeks to months after the inciting injury, e.g., after cardiac surgery) is becoming more common. In this latter group of patients, constriction may be transitory, with a course that may span a matter of weeks to a few months; not surprisingly, pericardial calcification is uncommon. Doppler-detected constrictive physiology resolved without pericardiectomy in 36 of 212 patients studied retrospectively at Mayo Clinic after an average of approximately 8 weeks.

Pericardiectomy is the definitive treatment for constrictive pericarditis but is unwarranted either in very early constriction (occult and functional class I) or in severe, advanced disease (functional Class IV) when the risk of surgery is excessive (operative mortality 30% to 40% vs. 6% to 19%) and the benefits are diminished. It is prudent to give hemodynamically stable patients with subacute constrictive pericarditis a trial of conservative management for 2 to 3 months until it is clear that the constrictive process is permanent before recommending pericardiectomy. Complete or extensive pericardial resection is desirable.

Medical therapy of constrictive pericarditis has a small but important role. In some patients, constrictive pericarditis resolves either spontaneously or in response to various combinations of NSAIDs, steroids, and antibiotics; in the remaining patients, medical therapy is adjunctive.

REFERENCES

Haley JH, Tajik AJ, Danielson GK, et al: Transient constrictive pericarditis: Causes and natural history. J Am Coll Cardiol 2004;43:271-275.

Imazio M, Bobbio M, Cecchi E, et al: Colchicine as first-choice therapy for recurrent pericarditis: Results of the CORE (COlchicine for REcurrent pericarditis) trial. Arch Intern Med 2005;165:1987-1991.

Imazio M, Bobbio M, Cecchi E, et al: Colchicine in addition to conventional therapy for acute pericarditis: Results of the COlchicine for acute PEricarditis (COPE) trial. Circulation 2005;112:2012-2016.

Imazio M, Demichelis B, Parrini I, et al: Day-hospital treatment of acute pericarditis: A management program for outpatient therapy. J Am Coll Cardiol 2004;43:1042-1046.

Maisch B, Ristic AD, Pankuweit S: Intrapericardial treatment of autoreactive pericardial effusion with triamcinolone; the way to avoid side effects of systemic corticosteroid therapy. Eur Heart J 2002;23:1503-1508.

Maisch B, Seferovic PM, Ristic AD, et al: Guidelines on the diagnosis and management of pericardial diseases executive summary: The task force on the diagnosis and management of pericardial diseases of the European society of cardiology. Eur Heart J 2004;25:587-610.

Merce J, Sagrista-Sauleda J, Permanyer-Miralda G, Soler-Soler J: Should pericardial drainage be performed routinely in patients who have a large pericardial effusion without tamponade? Am J Med 1998;105:106-109.

Talreja DR, Edwards WD, Danielson GK, et al: Constrictive pericarditis in 26 patients with histologically normal pericardial thickness. Circulation 2003;108:1852-1857.

Peripheral Arterial Disease

Method of
Jason T. Lee, MD, Maisie M. Fung, MD, and E. John Harris Jr., MD

Peripheral arterial disease (PAD) encompasses a wide spectrum of disease entities involving blood vessels outside of the heart and the brain. This includes blood vessels of the upper and lower extremities, the carotid artery, and the aorta. The majority of the clinical manifestations of PAD occur as a consequence of progressive atherosclerotic narrowing of these vessels. Other acquired diseases of arteries are related to aneurysm formation, inflammation, or degenerative disorders. Significant morbidity and mortality results from PAD, and patients

CURRENT DIAGNOSIS

- Routine examination including palpation of extremity pulses and auscultation for bruits of the carotid artery and abdominal aorta should be performed during all health maintenance examinations.
- Duplex ultrasound by an accredited vascular laboratory can accurately measure the degree of carotid disease and determine which patients will benefit from carotid intervention.
- Vascular claudication is described as reproducible pain in the lower extremities brought on by exertion that is relieved by rest and should be evaluated by lower extremity duplex ultrasound evaluation of arterial waveforms with ankle-brachial indexes.

CURRENT THERAPY

- Carotid endarterectomy is a durable and safe procedure that is indicated for symptomatic carotid stenosis >70% and asymptomatic carotid stenosis >80% to reduce future stroke risk.
- Symptomatic patients who are deemed high risk can be considered for carotid stenting at a high-volume vascular center.
- Aggressive medical management and risk factor modification with a supervised exercise regimen should be instituted for all patients with claudication.
- Critical limb ischemia is a progressive process that requires urgent referral to a vascular surgeon for revascularization by open surgical or endovascular techniques.

can present in very acute or chronic settings. Recognizing the signs and symptoms of these diseases is paramount for the primary care physician to formulate an accurate differential diagnosis. Prompt diagnostic testing and appropriate referral to a vascular surgeon are necessary to provide definitive management and optimize patient outcomes. In the past decade, there have been numerous advances in the diagnosis, management, and treatment of PAD. Less invasive screening tests are supplementing and even replacing traditional angiography, and treatment options with endovascular approaches such as angioplasty and stenting are increasingly available and being shown to be feasible. In this chapter we focus on the most commonly encountered PADs including carotid artery stenosis and lower extremity occlusive disease.

Carotid Artery Disease

Carotid artery disease most commonly involves atherosclerotic changes in the carotid arteries resulting in stenosis of the vessels around the carotid bifurcation. Diminished flow and irregular plaque formation of the common and internal carotid arteries can lead to embolic or thrombotic events that may cause transient ischemic attacks (TIAs), amaurosis fugax, or stroke. Carotid occlusive disease accounts for 30% to 40% of all reported strokes. Stroke remains the third leading cause of death in the United States (only behind heart disease and cancer). According to the American Heart Association (AHA), 700,000 people in the United Stares experienced a stroke in 2001, with nearly a third being recurrent. One in 15 deaths in the United States in 2001 was from a cerebrovascular accident. On a positive note, there was a 63% decrease in stroke/death rates from 1970 to 2002. There remains, however, high cost associated with the care of stroke survivors in terms of long-term rehabilitation, diminished productivity, chronic medications, and other co-morbid medical conditions. Risk factors for carotid artery disease include smoking, diabetes, hypertension, high cholesterol, and family history of disease. Prevention strategies focus on the use of antiplatelet agents, smoking cessation, hypertension control, lipid-lowering medications, diabetes control, and screening for carotid artery disease.

Carotid artery disease can be symptomatic or asymptomatic. Asymptomatic patients may be diagnosed by the primary care physician after a carotid bruit is detected on physical examination, but more commonly no bruit is auscultated and risk factors and/or family history lead to a screening duplex ultrasound. Recently, patients are seeking consultation for confirmation of a carotid duplex examination done as part of a vascular screening series or total body scan outside of the physician's office. Symptomatic patients present with symptoms of stroke or TIAs. TIAs differ from strokes in that they are acute, focal neurologic deficits that resolve completely within 24 hours, whereas strokes involve incomplete recovery. A classic type of ocular TIA is amaurosis fugax, where there is a painless monocular loss of vision caused by retinal artery embolus or thrombus. Patients classically describe a curtain being drawn over the eye that appears and resolves suddenly and completely. Other symptoms associated with TIAs or strokes include motor, sensory, or speech defects. Global symptoms such as dizziness, syncope, or altered mentation are less clearly associated with carotid occlusive disease.

Patients with suspected carotid artery disease should undergo a thorough physical examination including pulse examination, listening for bruits, and neurologic examination. Diagnosis can be confirmed via duplex ultrasound scan of both carotid arteries (Figure 1). This can quantify the degree and location of the stenosis. The degree of stenosis is typically reported as a percentage of narrowing and is based on velocity criteria standardized and validated for each vascular laboratory. Computed tomography (CT) scan or magnetic resonance imaging (MRI) of the brain is necessary when stroke or TIA is suspected. Positive imaging findings within brain parenchyma indicate that an acute event has occurred. The advantage of MRI is that imaging of the neck and brain with magnetic resonance angiography (MRA) can be performed simultaneously to give details regarding carotid and vertebral artery anatomy as well as the intracranial circulation. The degree of stenosis seen on MRA is often overestimated and should be corroborated by a duplex ultrasound. Cerebral arteriography is currently used infrequently in the preoperative phase and reserved for cases in which questions remain unresolved with the other imaging modalities. Improvements in imaging technology also are allowing CT angiography to become more widely available.

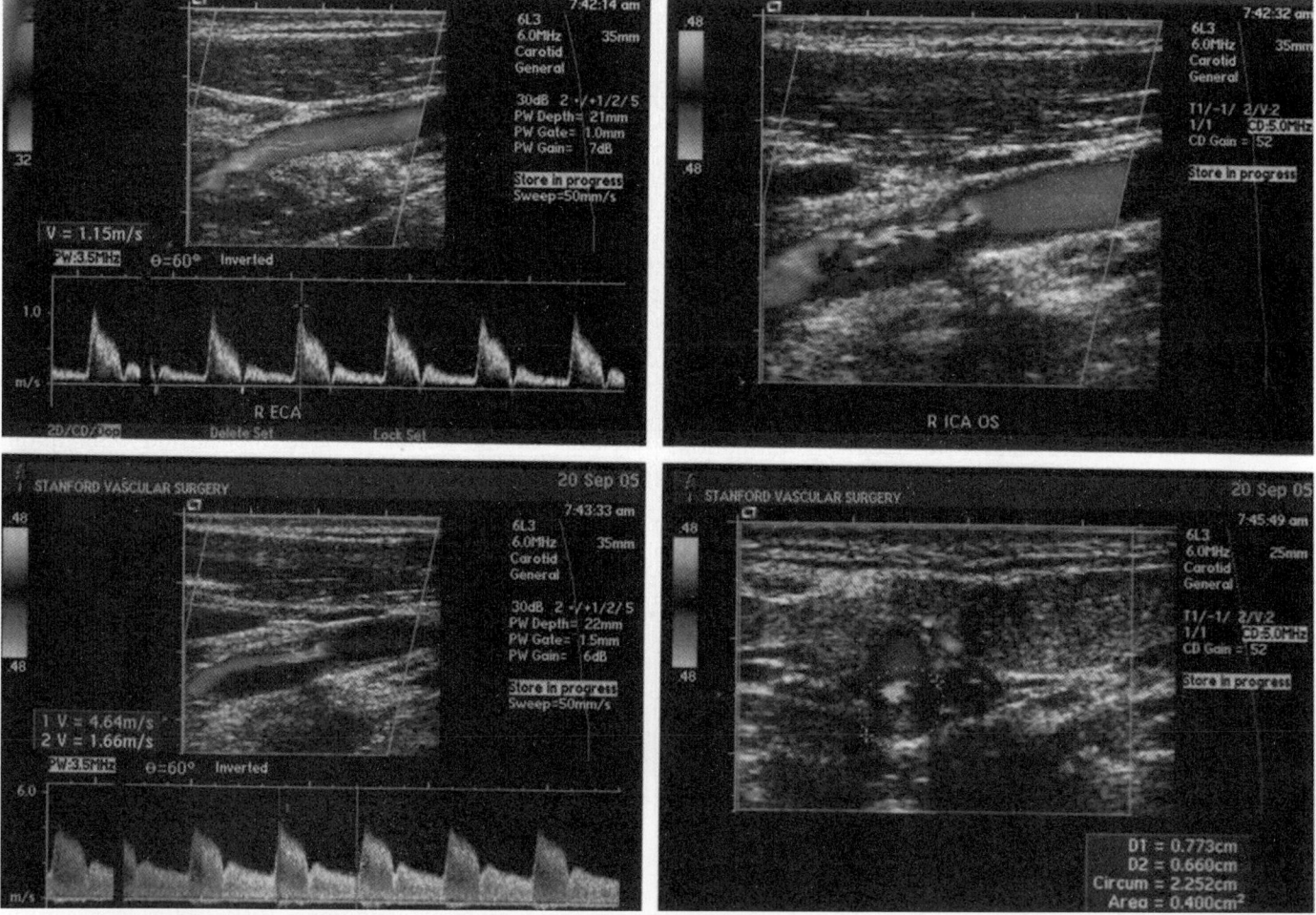

FIGURE 1.   Duplex ultrasound scan of 51-year-old man with hypercholesterolemia and hypertension found to have a right carotid bruit on examination. Note the severe narrowing of the right internal carotid artery orifice (evidenced by a peak systolic velocity of 4.64 m/s, which corresponds to a stenosis of 80%–89% by velocity criteria). He underwent successful right carotid endarterectomy.

Management of carotid artery disease is based on the degree of carotid stenosis measured by the various imaging modalities. Carotid endarterectomy (CEA) remains the most common procedure performed by vascular surgeons in the United States and is one of the most extensively studied operative procedures in the medical literature. Randomized, prospective trials including the North American Symptomatic Carotid Endarterectomy Trial (NASCET), European Carotid Surgery Trial (ECST), and the Veterans Affairs (VA) trial showed an approximately 50% relative risk reduction in symptomatic patients with more than a 70% stenosis who underwent surgery compared with medical treatment with aspirin. In the NASCET trial, the ipsilateral stroke rate at 2-year follow-up was reduced to 9% in the surgically treated patients as opposed to 26% in the medically treated patients, and the study was halted with all patients in the medical arm then offered CEA. The VA trial and ECST provide similar data documenting the benefit of surgical intervention in symptomatic patients with greater than 70% stenosis.

For asymptomatic patients, the Asymptomatic Carotid Atherosclerosis Study (ACAS) showed a 53% relative risk reduction of ipsilateral stroke at 5 years from 11.0% to 5.1% in surgically treated patients with greater than 60% stenosis. This represents, however, only a 1% absolute risk reduction per year, which is certainly less dramatic than the protective effects of intervention on a symptomatic patient. For this reason and with the development of newer antiplatelet agents like clopidogrel (Plavix), surgery at our institution is offered to asymptomatic patients only when they have reached 80% stenosis. Potential complications of surgery for either symptomatic or asymptomatic patients include myocardial infarction, stroke, bleeding, infection, cranial nerve injury, and recurrent stenosis. The possibility of recurrent disease highlights the importance of long-term follow-up after CEA that should include yearly duplex examination.

With the advent of endovascular techniques being driven by industry and patient desires for more minimally invasive interventions, it is no surprise that carotid angioplasty and stenting (CAS) has emerged as an alternative therapy. Recently published data, although sparse, suggests that in high-risk patients, CAS is not worse than traditional open surgery in terms of stroke and death rates. However, the best candidates for these procedures and long-term durability of these approaches are yet to be delineated. High-risk patients are defined differently at various institutions, but typically include those with severe uncontrolled co-morbid coronary symptoms, recurrent disease after previous endarterectomy, or irradiated necks. Currently there are only two FDA-approved devices for use (RX ACCULINK, manufactured by the Guidant Corporation, Indianapolis, Indiana; and Xact, manufactured by Abbott Laboratories, Abbott Park, Illinois). We believe carotid angioplasty and stenting should only be performed in high-volume centers with multidisciplinary expertise and the desire to track patients long term.

For patients who do not yet meet the criteria for surgery as determined by percentage of carotid stenosis, daily aspirin and aggressive risk factor reduction are indicated. These patients should be followed by duplex ultrasounds every 6 months and seen regularly by the vascular surgeon. Any new symptoms or progression of disease to a critical stenosis warrants a more aggressive approach to intervention.

Lower Extremity Arterial Occlusive Disease

Lower extremity peripheral arterial disease is a broad category of clinical entities that includes aortoiliac occlusive disease and femoropopliteotibial occlusive disease. The most common etiology of these diseases is atherosclerosis causing narrowing within these blood vessels. Risk factors again include smoking, hypertension, diabetes, elevated cholesterol, and family history. Up to 40% of patients also have coexisting coronary artery disease (CAD). Patients typically present with claudication, defined as pain in the lower extremities brought on by a reproducible amount of exercise and relieved only by a short period of rest. Depending on the location of the occlusion, symptoms may involve the buttocks, hip, thigh, or calf, and they can include impotence in men.

Lower extremity claudication is a significant health care issue, with studies documenting that 12% of the population experience claudication. Patients typically describe the pain as a sensation of muscle cramps or fatigue. This leads to chronic pain and health care provider visits, decreased productivity at work, and the possible progression toward a more sedentary lifestyle. The presence of claudication doubles age-specific mortality and decreases life expectancy on average by 10 years, and for this reason, patients should be aggressively managed medically with selective surgical intervention. It is important to note that the rate of limb loss in patients with claudication is approximately 3% to 6% over 10 years, so preventive care measures instituted by the primary care physician are a vital adjunct to vascular consultation.

Approximately 15% of mild cases of claudication progress to more significant lower extremity ischemia manifested by rest pain and tissue loss; typically seen in diabetic patients who continue to smoke. This indicates more severe atherosclerotic narrowing and the need for more aggressive and urgent management. Patients typically describe pain in the front of the foot occurring at night that is relieved by hanging the foot over the edge of bed or getting out of bed. Careful physical inspection looking for tissue changes is also important to document the severity of lower extremity occlusive disease. Skin atrophy with thickened nails, loss of hair on dorsum of the foot, shiny skin, and toe or heel ulcerations are all signs of significant atherosclerotic disease.

Documentation of pulses is important and can be graded as diminished or absent. Pulse palpation, however, is quite subjective and predisposed to error. When pulses are not easily palpable, a handheld Doppler in the clinic can be used objectively to assess blood flow, especially when ankle blood pressures are obtained. The ankle-brachial index (ABI) is obtained by dividing the systolic pressure at the ankle into that of the arm. Normal ABIs range from 1.0 to 1.2. Patients with claudication usually have an ABI less than 0.7, and patients with tissue loss have an ABI less than 0.5. An ABI less than 0.3 suggests critical ischemia and warrants urgent evaluation and intervention. Caution must be used in interpreting ABIs from diabetic patients because their arteries may be calcified, which leads to falsely elevated ABIs.

The vascular laboratory can provide useful diagnostic information regarding lower extremity blood flow.

Referral for formal duplex ultrasound with arterial waveform analysis is extremely helpful in determining the degree and location of stenosis. It is appropriate to obtain vascular consultation for patients with diminished ABIs and symptoms of lower extremity arterial occlusive disease. The decision to obtain more invasive and expensive studies should be made in consultation with the vascular surgeon. Recent advances in imaging technology have allowed CT angiography (Figure 2) and MRA to be a less invasive method of determining the extent of aortic, iliac, and distal occlusive changes. Traditional diagnostic angiography can be performed to delineate further the extent of disease, and it has the advantage of allowing access for percutaneous endovascular treatment of focal occlusive disease in the same setting.

Patients with mild claudication should be treated medically with aggressive risk factor reduction. Emphasis should be placed on smoking cessation, increasing exercise, weight loss, and controlling diabetes, hypertension, and high cholesterol. A strictly supervised exercise regimen is the only consistent therapy that increases pain-free walking distance and maximal walking distance. Numerous studies have looked at various medications for the treatment of

claudication, all with conflicting and often short-term success. FDA-approved medications include pentoxifylline (Trental) and cilostazol (Pletal), yet only a 30% response rate is observed in typical claudicants. These agents help lower blood viscosity and inhibit platelet aggregation. Although results with these medications are variable, a trial of 6 to 8 weeks of therapy should be attempted along with the exercise regimen. Long-term population studies have found that approximately 75% of patients experience improvement in symptoms with medical management alone. Sustained symptom relief requires a regular walking regimen.

Patients who do not respond to medical management alone may be candidates for revascularization. Indications for revascularization include claudication that significantly interferes with lifestyle, rest pain, nonhealing wounds, and tissue loss or necrosis. Open surgical options include aortofemoral reconstruction for aortoiliac occlusive disease and femoral-tibial bypasses for more distal disease. Long-term results from these operations are excellent in terms of relief of symptoms and wound healing. Morbidity rates from open surgery are in the range of 2% to 6% with possible complications including myocardial infarction, bleeding, wound infections, graft infection or thrombosis, and limb loss. Careful graft surveillance after bypass with duplex ultrasound is an important adjunct to maintain long-term patency of grafts.

Endovascular interventions of the lower extremities typically include angioplasty, stenting, and atherectomy. These procedures are most successful in cases involving short stenoses of the iliac arteries. As the disease enters the more distal vessels, there is a significant decrease in the durability of traditional angioplasty and stenting. Future improvements in the technology and developments such as drug-eluting stents may improve future use of endovascular interventions in the lower extremities. As with open surgical revascularization, the importance of long-term surveillance with duplex ultrasound allows reintervention when restenosis occurs. In contrast to failed surgical revascularization, failed endovascular revascularizations can lead to worsened and more acute limb ischemia. Although percutaneous methods appear to be less invasive, they are clearly not less risky, and ideally should be performed by vascular specialists dedicated to caring for all aspects of patients with lower extremity occlusive disease.

REFERENCES

Jemal A, Ward E, Hao Y, Thun M: Trends in the leading causes of death in the United States, 1970–2002. JAMA, 2005;294:1255-1259.

Moore WS, Barnett MJ, Beebe HE, et al: Guidelines for carotid endarterectomy: A multidisciplinary consensus statement from the Ad Hoc Committee, American Heart Association. Stroke 1995;26:188-201.

The Executive Committee for the Asymptomatic Carotid Atherosclerosis Study: Endarterectomy for asymptomatic carotid artery stenosis. JAMA 1995;273:1421.

TransAtlantic Inter-Society Consensus (TASC): Management of peripheral arterial disease (PAD). J Vasc Surg 2000;31:3-9.

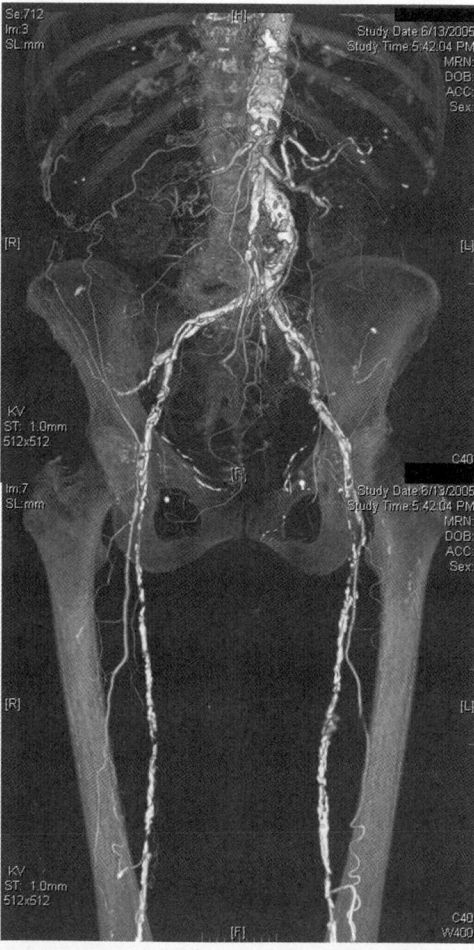

FIGURE 2. Computed tomographic (CT) angiography of an 81-year-old woman with severe thigh, buttock, and leg claudication and rest pain and a nonhealing left foot wound demonstrating severe calcified disease of her abdominal aorta and occluded iliac vessels and superficial femoral vessels. She underwent open aortofemoral bypass, which resulted in significant improvement in her walking and healing of her wound.

Venous Thrombosis

Method of
Anthony J. Comerota, MD, and
Santiago Chahwan, MD

It is estimated that in the United States 2 million patients are diagnosed with deep vein thrombosis (DVT) each year. Approximately 30% to 50% of these patients have concurrent pulmonary embolism (PE), of which 10% are fatal within the first hour. Furthermore, up to 90% of patients with iliofemoral DVT develop significant symptoms of the postthrombotic syndrome despite therapeutic anticoagulation. This debilitating condition has major medical, social, and economic consequences.

Although DVT and PE were once considered different clinicopathologic entities, numerous autopsy studies have demonstrated a strong association between them. Almost half of the patients with proven DVT have PE (often silent), and in patients with proven PE, 70% have demonstrable DVT of the lower extremities. Substantial evidence indicates that DVT and PE should be considered as the same medical problem, albeit at different stages of the disease process. For the purpose of this discussion, our focus is DVT of the lower extremities.

Acute DVT ranges from asymptomatic calf vein thrombosis to venous gangrene. Many physicians choose to treat the entire range of DVT similarly, with anticoagulation alone, beginning with heparin followed by oral anticoagulation with warfarin. Numerous studies have expanded our knowledge of the natural history of DVT as well as our understanding of the effects of early and therapeutic anticoagulation, the proper duration of oral anticoagulation, and selected fibrinolysis on the treatment of DVT. During the last two decades, the technique of venous thrombectomy has been refined and improved, and the results of a prospective clinical trial have put operative intervention into proper perspective.

Diagnosis

The clinical features of acute DVT occur because of obstruction of the deep venous system, an associated inflammatory response of the vessel wall and surrounding tissues, or fragmentation of the thrombus with concomitant embolization to the pulmonary vasculature. Unfortunately, the history and physical examination of patients with acute DVT and PE are insensitive and nonspecific. Swelling, tenderness, erythema, and pain with dorsiflexion of the foot (Homans' sign) are not always present. Patients with risk factors for DVT and nonspecific leg signs and symptoms should undergo objective diagnostic testing because DVT can neither be excluded nor confirmed on clinical grounds alone.

Venous duplex is the most commonly used diagnostic test for acute DVT. D-dimer (a breakdown fragment of complexed fibrin) is helpful when negative because it excludes DVT or PE, especially when associated with a low clinical suspicion. Elevated d-dimer levels are often not helpful, other than to raise concern that venous

CURRENT DIAGNOSIS

- Objective diagnosis of deep venous thrombosis (DVT) is mandatory.
- Venous duplex imaging is diagnostic in the majority of patients.
- D-dimer is helpful when it is negative (high negative predictive value) but of little assistance when positive.
- Phlebography is reserved for patients in whom a diagnosis cannot be made (or excluded) with venous duplex and d-dimer testing.
- A thrombophilia evaluation is indicated in patients:
    - Spontaneous DVT
    - Patients <50 y without a risk factor
    - Patients whose risk is only oral estrogen
    - Recurrent DVT
    - Recurrent superficial phlebitis without cancer
    - DVT at unusual sites (e.g., cerebral venous sinus, mesenteric venous thrombosis)
    - Warfarin-induced skin necrosis
    - Asymptomatic first-degree relatives of patients with symptomatic thrombophilias
    - Two consecutive or three nonconsecutive spontaneous abortions
    - Severe preeclampsia
    - Children with venous thromboembolism

thrombosis may be present. Ascending phlebography is now reserved for the few patients who cannot be diagnosed with less invasive methods. Once acute DVT is diagnosed, treatment decisions can have a major impact on both short- and long-term outcomes.

This chapter provides an overview of the natural history of acute DVT with information on anticoagulation, thrombolytic therapy, and operative venous thrombectomy. The final section reviews treatment strategies determined by the location and severity of the venous thrombosis as well as the patient's clinical characteristics.

Natural History

The complications of DVT, PE, and the postthrombotic syndrome are a source of substantial morbidity and mortality. Understanding the pathophysiology and natural history of DVT offers insight regarding appropriate prophylaxis, diagnosis, and treatment. Additionally, understanding of the pathophysiology of the postthrombotic syndrome can offer significant insight regarding the initial treatment of acute DVT. Ambulatory venous hypertension is the underlying pathophysiology of the postthrombotic syndrome. The two components causing ambulatory venous hypertension are residual venous obstruction and valvular incompetence. Partial patency of thrombosed veins may occur by recanalization as a result of spontaneous lysis involving cellular and humoral processes. Unless full patency is restored, some degree of residual venous obstruction persists. The additive effect of venous obstruction and valvular incompetence on ambulatory venous hypertension is well established. Patients who have both obstruction and valve incompetence have the highest ambulatory venous pressures and suffer the most severe postthrombotic sequelae. Therefore, if either obstruction or incompetence can be decreased or avoided, the severity of the postthrombotic syndrome can be reduced. Natural history studies of DVT treated with anticoagulation alone show progressive valvular dysfunction in most patients. However, if spontaneous lysis occurs within 2 to 3 months, patients are likely to preserve or regain normal valvular function. These observations dispel the previously erroneous concept that valves are irreparably destroyed within 3 to 5 days after the onset of venous thrombosis and suggest that treatment strategies designed to eliminate thrombus and effectively prevent recurrence reduce postthrombotic morbidity.

Anticoagulation

HEPARIN (UNFRACTIONATED HEPARIN)

Anticoagulation by unfractionated heparin (UFH) followed by oral warfarin compounds has been the mainstay of therapy for acute DVT. Anticoagulation is essentially prophylactic because these agents interrupt thrombus formation but do not actively dissolve the thrombus. However, effective anticoagulation prevents clot propagation and allows the body's endogenous

CURRENT THERAPY

- Early and persistent anticoagulation is important. Patients treated with UFH who become subtherapeutic (APTT <1.5× control) have a 15-fold increased risk of recurrence.
- Low molecular weight heparin has improved bioavailability compared to UFH and does not require monitoring (except in the pregnant and morbidly obese patient).
- Heparin anticoagulation (UFH or LMWH) should be continued for at least 5 days and the INR is therapeutic (2.0–3.0).
- Patients with iliofemoral DVT should be considered for a treatment strategy that includes thrombus removal.
- All patients with HIT should be treated with a direct thrombin inhibitor until their platelet count normalizes. At that point they can be converted to vitamin K antagonists for long-term anticoagulation if needed to treat an established thrombotic disorder.
- The proper duration of oral anticoagulation is determined by the characteristics of the patient and generally falls into one of five categories:
  - First DVT with transient risk factor
  - First DVT with no apparent risk factor (idiopathic)
  - First DVT with concurrent cancer
  - First DVT with a thrombophilia
  - Recurrent DVT

Abbreviations: APTT = activated partial thromboplastin time; DVT = deep venous thrombosis; HIT = heparin-induced thrombocytopenia; INR = international normalized ratio; LMWH = low molecular weight heparin; UFH = unfractionated heparin.

fibrinolytic system the opportunity to reduce the thrombus burden and recanalize the occluded vein.

Heparin was discovered to have antithrombotic properties approximately 90 years ago by McLean. It is an indirect anticoagulant; that is, it requires the plasma cofactors antithrombin III and antithrombin II for its action. Heparin binds to lysine sites on antithrombin, converting it from a slow thrombin inhibitor to a rapid inhibitor, irreversibly inhibiting their procoagulant activity. Heparin then dissociates and is reused. It was discovered that heparin binds to antithrombin III (ATIII) through a glucosamine unit that has contained within it a pentasaccharide sequence. This sequence was synthesized and developed as a low molecular weight heparin (LMWH) in the 1980s. Only a third of a dose of heparin binds to ATIII, and only its pentasaccharide fraction is responsible for its action. Heparin induces antihemostatic effects through three mechanisms: It binds to ATIII and inactivates factors IIa, Xa, IXa, and XIIa; it binds to cofactor II and inactivates factor IIa; and it binds to factor IX and inhibits factor Xa activation. The major mechanism for the anticoagulation effect is the first one.

The two routes for administration of UFH are continuous infusion and subcutaneous injection. Heparin is cleared through a combination of a rapidly saturable cellular mechanism and a slower, first-order, nonsaturable, dose-independent mechanism of renal clearance. At therapeutic doses, heparin is cleared through the rapid, saturable, dose-dependent mechanism. These pharmacokinetics make the heparin anticoagulation response nonlinear at therapeutic doses, with both the intensity and duration of effect increasing disproportionately with increasing dose. The initial dose of heparin for treatment of venous thrombosis is weight based (80 U/kg bolus followed by 18 U/kg/hour continuous infusion). The anticoagulant effect of heparin is monitored by the activated partial thromboplastin time (APTT) when the usual therapeutic dose is used. An APTT of 1.5 to 2.5 times the control value is associated with a decreased risk of recurrent thromboembolism. The APTT should be measured no earlier than 6 hours after the bolus dose, and the continuous infusion should be adjusted accordingly.

Some believe that the hemorrhagic risk of heparin anticoagulation increases as the dose increases and that patients with an increased bleeding risk can be identified by in vitro anticoagulation tests used to monitor heparin therapy. There is some merit to this observation in patients who have co-morbid risk factors, which can identify this high-risk group. However, in patients without co-morbid risk factors, whether a therapeutic or supratherapeutic APTT is targeted does not appear to be related to an increased risk of clinically important bleeding complications. Despite the importance of continuous therapeutic anticoagulation from the initiation of therapy, audits of heparin anticoagulation indicate that large numbers of patients continue to be inadequately treated. Investigators have repeatedly confirmed that a prescriptive approach to heparin administration is more effective than the subjective, individual approach attempted by most clinicians. This assumes clinical importance considering that a subtherapeutic APTT (less than 1.5× control) early in the course of treatment is associated with a 15-fold risk of recurrence.

To avoid undertreatment, we prefer supratherapeutic heparin anticoagulation during the initial 4 to 5 days of

TABLE 1 Prescriptive Approach to Intravenous Heparin Therapy

APTT*	Intravenous Infusion		Additional Action
	Rate Change (mL/h)	Dose Change (units 24 h)†	
≤45	+6	+5760	Repeat APTT in 4–6 h.
46–54	+3	+2880	Repeat APTT in 4–6 h.
55–85	0	0	None.‡
86–110	−3	−2880	Stop heparin sodium treatment for 1 h; repeat APTT 4–6 h after restarting heparin treatment.
>110	−6	−5760	Stop heparin sodium treatment for 1 h; repeat APTT 4–6 h after restarting heparin treatment.

*Activated partial thromboplastin time.
†Heparin sodium concentration, 20,000 U/500 mL = 40 U/mL.
‡During the first 24 h, repeat APTT in 4–6 h. Thereafter, the APTT will be determined once daily, unless subtherapeutic.

therapy in patients who do not have co-morbidities for bleeding. A 10,000-U heparin bolus is given intravenously (IV) and is followed by 2000 U per hour, checking the APTT 8 hours after the bolus. The goal is to maintain the APTT longer than 90 seconds. If the APTT is supratherapeutic (more than 100 seconds), the dose is continued. Although this varies from most protocols, it is effective in maintaining therapeutic anticoagulation without added bleeding. Using the prescriptive approach summarized in Table 1 is a good option and favored by most physicians. However, even with the prescriptive protocol, one must be cautious in patients with co-morbidities for bleeding.

Heparin resistance is the term used to define patients who need unusually large doses of heparin to achieve an anticoagulation effect. Several mechanisms are identified for heparin resistance, including ATIII deficiency, increased heparin clearance, elevations in heparin-binding proteins, factor VII, and fibrinogen levels. A large thrombus burden also requires higher heparin concentrations for therapeutic effectiveness. Randomized trials showed that oral anticoagulation alone, without initial and concomitant heparin anticoagulation, is associated with a significantly higher risk of recurrent venous thrombosis.

Heparin-induced thrombocytopenia (HIT) is a well-recognized and feared complication of heparin therapy caused by heparin-specific antibodies binding to the platelet membrane, stimulating platelet aggregation. It is usually recognized 2 to 10 days after heparin therapy is initiated, is reported in 2% to 10% of patients receiving heparin, and is more frequent with bovine heparin than with porcine heparin. Heparin-induced thrombocytopenia is an antigen-antibody immunologic response that is not dose related. Platelet counts should be monitored in all patients receiving heparin, regardless of the route of administration or the dose prescribed. A drop in platelet count by more than 30% indicates a high likelihood of HIT, and appropriate diagnostic tests should be obtained. If the platelet count drops 30%, heparin should be discontinued. When HIT is diagnosed, alternative antithrombotic therapy should be initiated in all patients. Lepirudin (Refludan) and argatroban, direct thrombin inhibitors proven to reduce the risk of serious consequences of HIT, are indicated in patients with HIT to prevent thromboembolic complications. Patients should be treated with direct thrombin inhibitors until their platelet counts return to normal. Warfarin compounds must be avoided early in the treatment of HIT patients because they can be a procoagulant, stimulating additional thrombosis and warfarin-induced skin necrosis. Vitamin K antagonists can be started after the platelet count returns to normal if additional anticoagulation is required.

WARFARIN COMPOUNDS

The coumarins, or vitamin K antagonists, are the basis of oral anticoagulation. They inhibit the vitamin K–dependent clotting factors II, VII, IX, and X. They also inhibit vitamin K–dependent carboxylation of proteins C and S. Because proteins C and S are naturally occurring anticoagulants that function by inhibiting activated factors V and VIII, any vitamin K antagonist can transiently cause a hypercoagulable state before achieving its anticoagulant effect because the half-life of proteins C and S is shorter than the half-life of the clotting factors. Vitamin K antagonists require careful monitoring in clinical practice for several reasons: They have a narrow therapeutic window; they have considerable variability in dose effect among subjects; their activity is influenced by a large number of drugs as well as diet; and miscommunication or misunderstanding of dose by physician and patient or noncompliance of patient alters outcome.

Evidence suggests that the anticoagulant and antithrombotic effects of warfarin can be dissociated and the reduction of factors II and X are required for effective anticoagulation. Studies showed that warfarin produces its antithrombotic effect by reducing factor II levels, which is consistent with observations that clot-bound thrombin is an important mediator of clot growth, and reduction in prothrombin levels reduces the generation of thrombin, thereby reducing thrombus formation. This is the pharmacologic basis for overlapping the administration of heparin with warfarin for at least 4 to 5 days and until the prothrombin time/international normalized ratio (INR) is therapeutic. Because the half-life of factor II is approximately 60 to 72 hours, at least 4 days of overlap are necessary to ensure a proper anticoagulant effect, even if the INR reaches therapeutic levels sooner.

The prothrombin time (PT) test is the proper test to monitor vitamin K antagonist therapy. The PT reflects the reduction of three of the four vitamin K–dependent factors that are affected by warfarin. Although the PT test reflects warfarin effect, it is not standardized when expressed in seconds or as a simple ratio of the patient's plasma effect compared to normal individuals. A calibration model is now common and used to standardize the therapeutic effect of warfarin. Several randomized studies have compared an INR between 2.0 and 3.0 to a higher intensity adjusted dose. An INR of 2.0 to 3.0 gave the best antithrombotic effect at the lowest risk of bleeding. The recommendations for initiation of oral anticoagulation suggest that doses between 5 to 10 mg for the first 1 or 2 days followed by dosing according to the INR response is the most appropriate. Monitoring is performed daily starting after the second or third dose until the therapeutic range is achieved and maintained for at least 2 days.

The management of patients whose INR is outside the therapeutic range is controversial because of the lack of comparison studies. Our approach is to monitor more frequently and adjust the dose appropriately or, if the INR is higher than 4.0, hold warfarin for a period of time and monitor more frequently to adjust the dose. Treatment directed at reversing the anticoagulant effect with vitamin K, fresh-frozen plasma, or recombinant factor VIIa is based on clinical judgment.

Warfarin compounds cross the placenta and are associated with teratogenic effects when given during the first trimester of pregnancy. Because there are similar concerns in the second trimester as well as the risk of fetal bleeding during and after delivery, warfarin compounds are generally avoided when treating all pregnant women. Women who are of childbearing potential and taking warfarin compounds should avoid pregnancy and receive contraceptive counseling. If anticoagulation is indicated during pregnancy, subcutaneous heparin or LMWH is recommended.

LOW MOLECULAR WEIGHT HEPARIN

LMWHs are derived from UFH through chemical or enzymatic depolymerization. The LMWHs have several advantages compared to UFH, including a reduced antifactor IIa activity relative to Xa activity, a greater benefit/risk ratio in animal studies, superior pharmacokinetic properties (better bioavailability when injected subcutaneously), no need for monitoring (except in pregnant and morbidly obese patients), and less risk of HIT. Compared with UFH, LMWHs have a longer plasma half-life and substantially higher plasma levels after subcutaneous injection. As a result of improved bioavailability, they have less variability in anticoagulant response to a fixed dose. The reduced binding to plasma proteins is responsible for the more predictable dose-response relationship of LMWHs.

Low molecular weight heparins are approved in the United States for DVT prophylaxis in general surgical and orthopedic patients, for the treatment of acute DVT and PE, and for prevention of ischemic complications of unstable angina and non-Q-wave myocardial infarction. The evidence that these newer anticoagulants are safe and effective for the treatment of acute DVT is impressive. Randomized trials evaluating the treatment of acute DVT with subcutaneous LMWH versus standard IV UFH demonstrated better thrombus resolution and fewer bleeding complications with LMWHs. In two trials, mortality was significantly reduced in those randomized to LMWH, the reduction in mortality occurring in patients with malignancy.

In the pregnant and morbidly obese patients being treated for acute DVT with LMWH, monitoring of the mid-interval Xa level is required to ensure therapeutic anticoagulation is achieved and maintained. The target Xa level depends on the frequency of dosing. The target Xa levels are 0.6 to 1.0 and 0.8 to 1.5 for every 12-hour and 24-hour dosing, respectively.

DIRECT THROMBIN INHIBITORS

Thrombin can be inhibited directly or indirectly. Direct inhibitors bind directly to the thrombin molecule, blocking its interaction with other substrates and reducing additional thrombus formation. Indirect inhibitors (i.e., heparin) act by catalyzing antithrombin or heparin cofactor II. In the growing population of patients with HIT, direct thrombin inhibitors offer valuable therapeutic alternatives. Three IV direct thrombin inhibitors (hirudin, argatroban, and bivalirudin) are licensed in North America.

Hirudin

Hirudin (Lepirudin [Refludan]) is available in its recombinant form. It is a 65-amino acid polypeptide that was originally isolated from salivary glands of the leech *Hirudo medicinalis*. Hirudin irreversibly binds to thrombin, which is one of its potential disadvantages because there is no specific antidote. The plasma half-life is approximately 60 minutes after IV injection. It is cleared by the kidneys and therefore must be used with caution in anyone with compromised renal function. The anticoagulation effect can be monitored by the APTT. Hirudin is indicated for anticoagulation in patients with HIT and associated thromboembolic disease to prevent further thromboembolic complications. It is particularly useful in patients with HIT associated with hepatic dysfunction because argatroban is contraindicated in these patients. As with other anticoagulants, bleeding is the most common adverse side effect. Serious anaphylactic reactions are reported.

Greinacher et al. conducted two prospective, multicenter, historically controlled clinical trials (HAT-1 and HAT-2) in 113 patients with confirmed HIT. It was concluded that by day 35 in the HAT-1 study, the group treated with hirudin showed a relative reduction of the cumulative risk for combined clinical endpoints (death, limb amputation, and new thromboembolic complications) by 73% versus historical controls. The same author published a meta-analysis of the HAT-1 and HAT-2 studies confirming that a statistically significant difference in the combined incidence of death, new thromboembolic complications, and amputations in patients treated with hirudin was seen versus historical controls in patients with thromboembolic complications. Relative risks for individual events also decreased.

When starting hirudin, an initial APTT is obtained. If 2.5, hirudin is held to avoid initial overdosing. The initial dose is a bolus of 0.4 mg/kg over 15 to 20 seconds followed by a continuous infusion of 0.15 mg/kg/hour. The duration of the therapy is generally 5 to 10 days.

Argatroban

Argatroban is a competitive inhibitor of thrombin that binds noncovalently to form a reversible complex. Its half-life is 45 minutes. Because it is metabolized in the liver, it must be used with caution in patients with compromised hepatic function. Argatroban nearly meets the requirements of the ideal anticoagulant for both the prophylaxis and treatment of HIT and associated thrombotic complications. As the first direct thrombin inhibitor approved for both the prophylaxis and treatment of thrombosis in HIT, argatroban is an effective anticoagulant that does not interact with heparin-dependent antibodies, offers a predictable dose-response relationship, and requires minimal monitoring. Therefore, it is frequently chosen to manage HIT.

Before initiating argatroban, heparin is discontinued, allowing the APTT to return to baseline. The initial dose of argatroban for adults without hepatic impairment is 2 μg/kg/minute administered as a continuous IV infusion. The APTT should be rechecked 2 hours after initiation and the dose should be adjusted until the target APTT value of 1.5 to 3.0 times baseline is attained (not to exceed 100 seconds). Concomitant use of argatroban with warfarin results in prolongation of the INR beyond that produced by warfarin alone. When patients are being converted to a vitamin K antagonist, at least 4 days of overlap is given. After this period, argatroban can be discontinued when the INR is more than 4. After stopping argatroban, a repeat INR is obtained in 4 to 6 hours. If the repeat INR is below the desired therapeutic range, infusion of argatroban is resumed and the procedure repeated daily until the desired INR is achieved with warfarin alone.

Bivalirudin

Bivalirudin (Angiomax) is an analogue of hirudin that binds reversibly to the active form of thrombin. Once bound, thrombin cleaves the bond within the amino terminal of bivalirudin, allowing the recovery of thrombin activity and making it a potentially safer drug than hirudin. Bivalirudin is cleared from plasma by a combination of renal mechanisms and proteolytic cleavage, with a half-life in patients with normal renal function of 25 minutes. It is a convenient drug to use because of its short half-life and its predictable anticoagulation response in patients undergoing percutaneous coronary interventions.

The recommended dose of bivalirudin is an initial bolus of 1 mg/kg IV, followed by a 4-hour IV infusion at a rate of 2.5 mg/kg/hour. If necessary, bivalirudin may be continued for an additional 20 hours at a rate of 0.2 mg/kg/hour. Bivalirudin is predominantly used as an alternative to heparin during percutaneous endovascular procedures. Other uses are being investigated.

Thrombolytic Therapy

Dissolution of thrombus from the deep venous system is an ideal goal of treatment that has the potential of eliminating venous obstruction and maintaining valvular function. Practical questions regarding thrombolysis for DVT are these: Can venous thrombi be lysed? and Is lysing venous clot important in preserving long-term valvular function?

Studies comparing anticoagulation therapy to systemic thrombolysis for acute DVT, documented phlebographically, showed that 45% had significant or complete clearing of their clot compared with only 4% of those treated with heparin. Although the precise level of venous occlusion was not known in each case, a reasonable number of patients were expected to have had iliofemoral DVT. Considering that patients treated with lytic therapy were given a systemic IV infusion and that systemic thrombolysis is generally inadequate for iliofemoral DVT, patients with femoropopliteal DVT likely had a better response. Prospective studies of systemic lytic therapy showed that patients successfully lysed have fewer postthrombotic symptoms and are more likely to retain normal valve function.

Patients with iliofemoral DVT represent a subset of patients who are not likely to respond to systemic lytic therapy. Because occlusive thrombus in the iliofemoral system has limited exposure to any circulating plasminogen activator, and because the thrombus burden is large, it is understandable why these patients are unlikely to respond to the systemic administration of plasminogen activators.

A number of reports indicated improved success with the delivery of a thrombolytic agent directly into the iliofemoral clot through the catheter-directed approach. A number of reported series in addition to a prospective venous registry observed an 85% to 90% success rate, with patency being maintained in 60% to 80% at 1 year. Identifying and correcting an underlying iliac venous stenosis significantly improved long-term patency. Bleeding complications can be expected in 6% to 10% of patients. A randomized trial of catheter-directed thrombolysis versus anticoagulation showed significant benefit of lysis in restoring venous patency and maintaining valve function. It is apparent that clinical sequelae of iliofemoral DVT are related to the patency of the iliofemoral venous segment.

Venous Thrombectomy

Operative venous thrombectomy plus long-term anticoagulation is more effective than anticoagulation alone for patients with acute iliofemoral DVT. Large case series, literature reviews, and a contemporary randomized trial show improved vein patency, better valve function, and reduced postthrombotic morbidity. Unfortunately, many continue to believe that there is no place for operative thrombectomy because of the high rates of rethrombosis observed in early reports. There has been marked improvement in the contemporary technique (Table 2),

Table 2 Venous Thrombectomy: Old versus Contemporary

Procedure	Old	Contemporary
Pre-Rx phlebography	Occasionally	Always
Venous thrombectomy catheter	No	Yes
Infrainguinal thrombectomy	No	Yes
Arteriovenous fistula	No	Yes
Operative fluoroscopy/ phlebography	No	Yes
Correct iliac vein stenosis	No	Yes
Post-Rx anticoagulation	Occasionally	Yes
Intermittent pneumatic compression postoperative	No	Yes

beginning with the preoperative assessment of the patient, intraoperatively guided thrombectomy with fluoroscopy, the addition of infrainguinal thrombectomy, an arteriovenous fistula, completion phlebography, correction of residual iliac vein lesions, early postoperative catheter-directed anticoagulation, and long-term oral anticoagulation.

Although it is not within the scope of this article to review the details of the operative technique, a thorough description of operative thrombectomy has been recently published.

Treatment Strategies for Acute DVT

Patients with acute DVT should be managed according to their clinical presentation, level of thrombus, associated co-morbidities, and duration of thrombotic risk. The following treatment strategies are recommended according to the level and extent of venous thrombosis. They are proposed based on the known natural history of the disease, the benefits of therapy, and published guidelines for care.

CALF VEIN THROMBOSIS

Calf vein thrombosis is not a benign disease. Calf vein thrombus can embolize and propagate to large veins, and it is associated with postthrombotic symptoms. A number of studies reviewing isolated calf vein thrombosis observed that propagation of up to 30% occur in postoperative and hospitalized patients. If untreated, recurrent venous thromboembolic complications were observed in up to 29% of patients.

In light of this information, anticoagulation of patients with isolated calf vein thrombosis is indicated, especially in patients in whom the etiology of their DVT is unclear and in those whose thrombotic risk continues. Symptomatic calf DVT and patients with ongoing thrombotic risk should be treated with 3 to 6 months of anticoagulation. In patients with a high risk of bleeding from anticoagulation, effective compression stockings (30 to 40 mm Hg) should be used and patients monitored with duplex ultrasound imaging at 3- or 4-day intervals until the high-risk period has passed to ensure that extension into the proximal veins has not occurred. If propagation to the popliteal vein is demonstrated, the patient must be reevaluated for definitive therapy.

FEMOROPOPLITEAL VENOUS THROMBOSIS

A ventilation-perfusion scan or helical computerized tomography (CT) scan of the chest should be considered part of the routine initial evaluation of patients with proximal DVT. Approximately 40% of these patients have an asymptomatic PE. Up to 25% of these patients subsequently experience signs or symptoms of PE while being anticoagulated. If unaware of the existing PE, physicians might interpret these new symptoms as recurrent venous thromboembolism because of failure of anticoagulation. A repeat CT scan that fails to identify a new PE indicates that the symptoms are related to the previous PE, and therefore vena cava filtration is not indicated because there is not a failure of anticoagulation.

All patients with proximal DVT should be treated with anticoagulation, assuming no contraindication. DVT involving the femoral and popliteal veins is the most common presentation. As previously stated, anticoagulation does not resolve the thrombus in the deep venous system but allows physiologic fibrinolysis to recanalize the occluded veins. If thrombus does not extend beyond the femoral vein, ligation of the femoral vein below the origin of the profunda femoris causes minimal morbidity because of adequate collateral drainage and prevents the clot from embolizing, although this is rarely recommended today.

Treatment with IV UFH is often recommended for hospitalized patients, beginning with a heparin bolus and followed by a continuous infusion. A prescriptive approach similar to the one described in Table 1 is frequently recommended. The importance of sustained early anticoagulation is underscored by the fact that an episode of subtherapeutic anticoagulation (APTT less than 1.5× control) increases the risk of recurrent venous thromboembolism 15-fold. Supratherapeutic anticoagulation with UFH is often preferred, giving the patient a 10,000-U bolus followed by 2000 U/hour. This generally keeps the APTT more than 100, maintains therapeutic anticoagulation, reduces the frequency of blood tests, and is not associated with increased bleeding complications in patients without known co-morbidities for bleeding.

Oral anticoagulation is started immediately after heparin is given and is continued over the long term, maintaining an INR of 2.0 to 3.0. Patients are allowed to ambulate normally after being fully anticoagulated with a snug elastic wrap on their legs until their 30 to 40 mm Hg elastic stockings become available. The appropriate duration of anticoagulation is under study; however, in most patients, longer durations of oral anticoagulation (1 year) are more effective than shorter courses of therapy. Longer therapy should be considered for patients with extensive DVT at the outset and those who have persistent venous obstruction on repeat duplex imaging when discontinuation of anticoagulation is being considered. Elevated d-dimer levels (250 µg/mL) at termination of anticoagulation are also associated with an increased risk of recurrence. If observed, continued anticoagulation should be considered. Maintaining the INR between 2.0 and 3.0 is associated with minimal bleeding complications, yet patients are effectively protected from recurrent thrombosis.

LMWHs are now the preferred initial treatment of most patients with acute DVT. As stated earlier, a weight-adjusted subcutaneous injection of 1 mg/kg of enoxaparin (Lovenox) every 12 hours or 1.5 mg/kg subcutaneously daily is recommended. This is continued until the patient has received oral anticoagulants for 4 or more days and the INR is therapeutic. Because LMWH is given subcutaneously and does not require monitoring, hospitalization is not mandatory for safe and effective treatment. An initial hospitalization period of 24 hours may be required for patients requiring instruction for self-injection and for planning the logistics of ongoing care.

Special considerations in the treatment of acute DVT are required in patients with compromised renal function, the morbidly obese, and the pregnant patient. Those with compromised renal function are generally treated with UFH acutely because LMWHs are renally excreted. Similarly, we favor UFH for the acute phase of anticoagulation in the morbidly obese to ensure therapeutic anticoagulation during the early phase of therapy while converting to oral agents.

Pregnant women requiring anticoagulation for venous thromboembolism are preferably treated with LMWH (enoxaparin, 1 mg/kg every 12 hours) injected subcutaneously. Mid-interval factor Xa levels are targeted at 0.6 to 1.0. Warfarin compounds are avoided in pregnant patients. Women can be converted to vitamin K antagonists during the postpartum period and continued for the appropriate duration of treatment, even in mothers who wish to breast-feed.

ILIOFEMORAL VENOUS THROMBOSIS

The most extensive DVT is iliofemoral thrombosis, associated with the most severe postthrombotic sequelae. Eliminating the thrombus from the iliofemoral system significantly improves short- and long-term venous function and reduces morbidity.

Once the diagnosis of iliofemoral DVT is established, a rapid CT scan with contrast is performed of the chest, abdomen, and pelvis, evaluating for associated pulmonary emboli and intraabdominal or pelvic pathology. At least 50% of these patients have pulmonary emboli, and a significant percentage have unexpected abdominal or pelvic pathology etiologically linked to their aggressive thrombotic disorder. Unexpected findings on abdominal and pelvic CT scans have included renal cell carcinoma, lymphoma, liver metastases, adrenal tumors, vena caval atresia, and iliac vein aneurysm. The CT scan also allows evaluation of the proximal extent of the thrombus.

Patients who are physically active and have a reasonable life expectancy (more than 2 years) are evaluated for a treatment strategy of thrombus removal, correcting any underlying venous pathology (such as an iliac vein stenosis, May-Thurner lesion) followed by long-term anticoagulation with vitamin K antagonists (Figure 1).

In patients without contraindications to thrombolysis, catheter-directed thrombolysis is the preferred method, using multi-sidehole catheters positioned into the thrombus from the ipsilateral popliteal or posterior tibial vein accessed under ultrasound guidance. Tissue plasminogen activator (t-PA) alteplase (Activase) is most frequently used, infusing a bolus of 4 to 8 mg, followed by a continuous infusion of 1 to 2 mg/hour. Phlebograms are repeated every 12 hours, and the catheters are repositioned if needed to maximize intrathrombus infusion. With the recent advances in technology, combined pharmacomechanical techniques, such as rheolysis, segmental pharmacomechanical thrombolysis with the Trellis catheter, or intrathrombus ultrasound accelerated thrombolysis, have shortened treatment times. A residual stenosis in the common iliac vein is frequently encountered, particularly on the left. If one exists, balloon angioplasty is performed. If recoil is observed, a venous stent is deployed, attempting to approximate the size of the native iliac vein and restoring unobstructed venous drainage into the vena cava.

If contraindication to thrombolysis exists or if the catheters cannot be positioned within the thrombus, an operative venous thrombectomy under fluoroscopy with construction of an arteriovenous fistula (AVF) should be performed. Once patency is restored, full anticoagulation is required to prevent rethrombosis. In patients with compromised arterial inflow because of massive edema of the

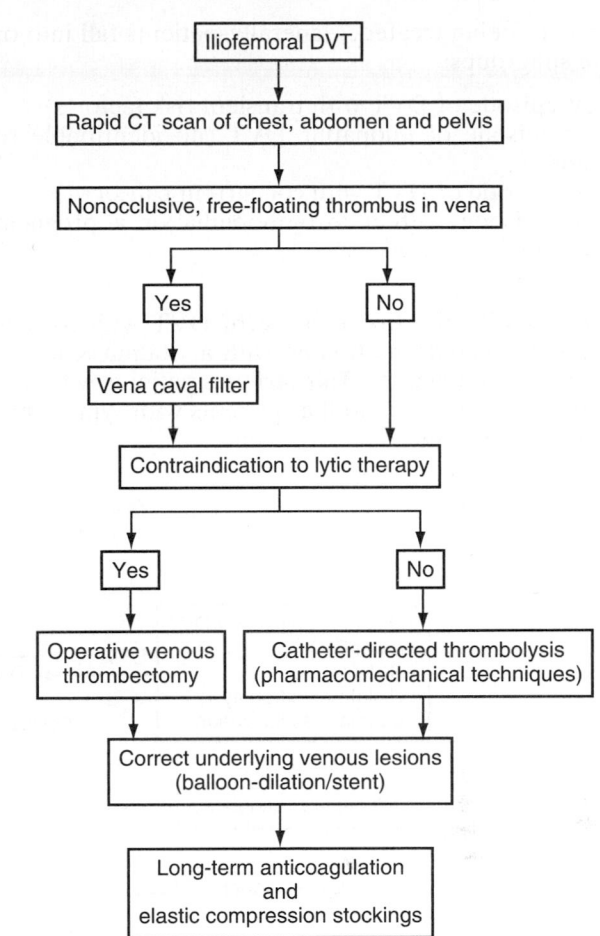

FIGURE 1. Algorithm for the management of patients with iliofemoral deep venous thrombosis. CT = computed tomography.

lower extremities, a compartment syndrome may develop. In such cases, patients may require fasciotomy, although after successful lysis or thrombectomy, fasciotomy is rarely required.

DURATION OF ORAL ANTICOAGULATION

The duration of anticoagulation is still somewhat controversial. The advantages of prolonging the duration of treatment must be weighed against the risk of bleeding complications. A number of randomized, controlled trials have been performed that uniformly demonstrate that the longer the duration of anticoagulation, the less the risk is for recurrent venous thromboembolic events. The risk of bleeding complications is not directly correlated to duration of anticoagulation because many patients who bleed do so early in the course of treatment because of their associated co-morbidities for bleeding.

A meta-analysis examining randomized trials demonstrated that patients receiving extended anticoagulation are protected from recurrent venous thromboembolic events. Clinical benefit is maintained after anticoagulation is discontinued; however, the magnitude of benefit is reduced.

Current guidelines suggest that the duration of anticoagulation should be determined by the characteristics of the patient being treated. Generally, patients fall into one of five subgroups:

1. First episode of DVT with transient risk factor(s)
2. First episode of idiopathic DVT (no identifiable risk factor)
3. First episode of DVT with concurrent cancer
4. First episode with a thrombophilia or a prognostic marker of increased risk
5. Recurrent DVT

Patients with the first episode of DVT with transient risk factor(s) should be treated with a vitamin K antagonist for at least 3 months. This includes patients with proximal vein thrombosis as well as patients with symptomatic calf vein thrombosis.

Patients who have the first episode of idiopathic DVT should be treated with a vitamin K antagonist for at least 6 to 12 months, with serious consideration being given to indefinite anticoagulation.

Those with DVT and concurrent cancer are treated with LMWH for the first 3 to 6 months, after which they are converted to oral anticoagulation with vitamin K antagonists. These patients should remain anticoagulated indefinitely or until the cancer is resolved.

Patients who have the first episode of DVT associated with a thrombophilic state or a prognostic marker of increased risk are treated for at least 12 months and should be considered for indefinite anticoagulation. Those patients with an antiphospholipid antibody or those who have two or more thrombophilic conditions (factor V

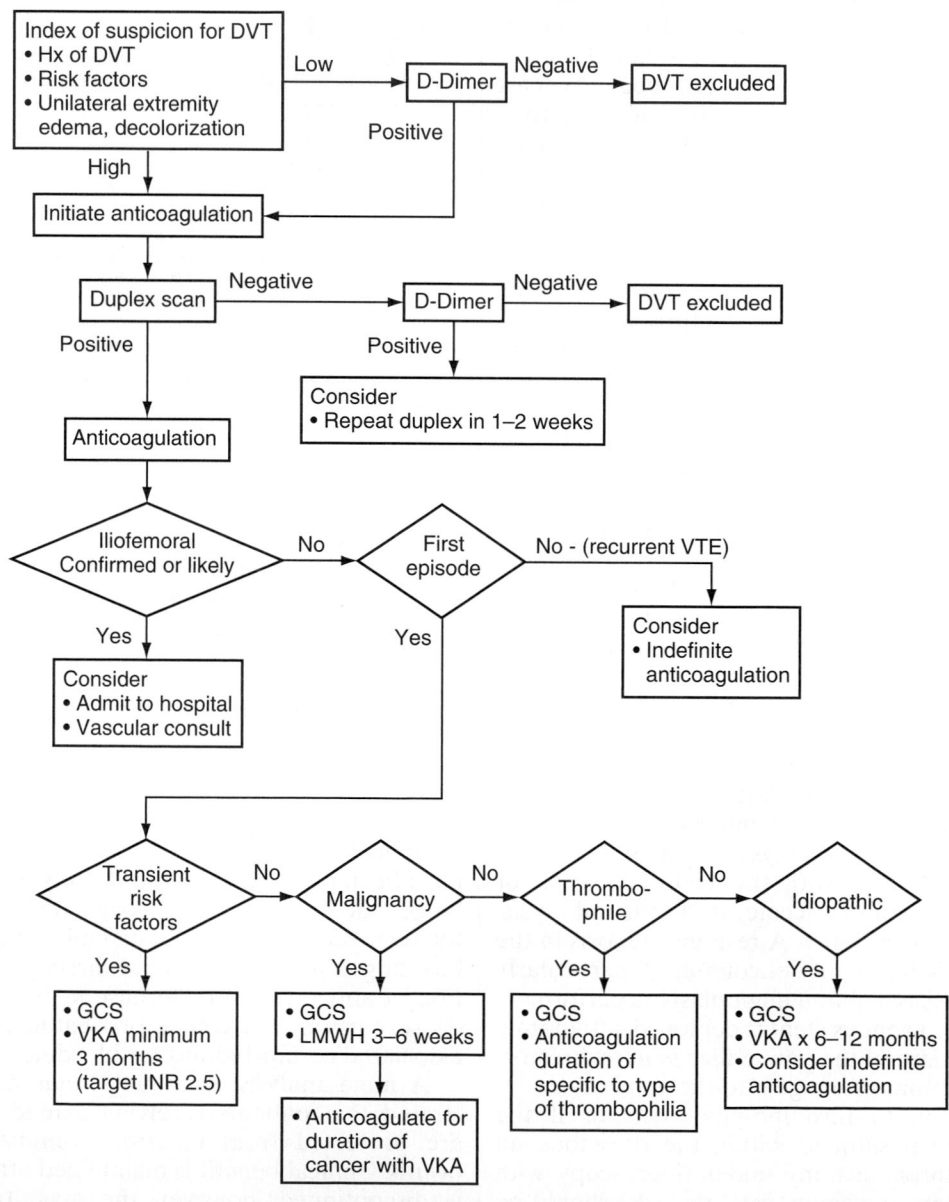

FIGURE 2. Recommendations for the diagnosis and treatment of acute DVT. DVT = deep venous thrombosis; GCS = graduated compression stockings; INR = international normalized ratio; LMWH = low molecular weight heparin; VKA = vitamin K antagonist [warfarin]; VTE = venous thromboembolism;

Leiden and prothrombin 20210 gene mutation) are treated indefinitely.

Patients with a recurrent venous thromboembolic event are treated indefinitely.

The dose of vitamin K antagonist should be adjusted to maintain a target INR of 2.5 (INR range, 2.0 to 3.0). Patients who receive indefinite anticoagulation therapy should be reassessed periodically regarding the risk-benefit ratio of continued treatment.

Venous duplex compression ultrasonography can be used to assess ongoing risk of recurrence. If the duplex examination normalizes, patients are at reduced risk of recurrence compared to those with ongoing venous abnormalities. Similarly, patients whose d-dimer levels are elevated are at increased risk for recurrence compared to those who do not have evidence of increased thrombus activity. Figure 2 summarizes the diagnostic and therapeutic approach to patients with venous thromboembolism.

Vena Caval Filters

Patients who are at high risk for PE despite anticoagulation or cannot receive anticoagulation are considered for vena caval filters. The indications for vena caval filtration fall into three categories: absolute, relative, and prophylactic. The absolute indications include patients in whom a DVT or PE has occurred and who have a contraindication to anticoagulation, a documented failure of anticoagulation, or complications of anticoagulation requiring transient or permanent discontinuation.

Relative contraindications include those patients who have DVT or PE and their physicians are concerned that the risk of PE is high despite therapeutic anticoagulation. The third category of prophylactic filters refers to those patients who do not have established DVT or PE, but the perceived risk of PE is high and the efficacy of standard DVT prophylaxis is considered poor.

Until 2003, only permanent vena caval filters were available. Since then, nonpermanent (retrievable) filters have been approved in the United States.

Nonpermanent filters can be considered in patients who require only temporary protection from PE. Additionally, the benefit of removal of the filter should outweigh the harm of permanent caval filtration. Important in this consideration is the fact that the majority of temporary filters remain as permanent filters. A small percentage of patients who have temporary filters removed require reinsertion of a caval filter because of recurrent risk of PE. Additionally, temporary filters appear to have a 3-month caval thrombosis rate of approximately 5%, which is the 5-year caval thrombosis rate reported with the permanent Greenfield filter.

Used appropriately, vena caval filtration provides a valuable adjunct to patients with venous thromboembolic disease. Figure 3 describes our decision matrix regarding vena caval filters.

Indications for Thrombophilia Evaluation

An underlying thrombophilia (coagulation disorder) is associated with an increased risk of thrombosis, usually venous thrombosis. However, in rare cases, arterial thrombosis occurs. Table 3 lists the prevalence of the various thrombophilias and their associated relative risk of a thrombotic complication. Patients who reasonably should be tested for thrombophilia include:

1. All patients with a first episode of spontaneous venous thromboembolism (VTE).

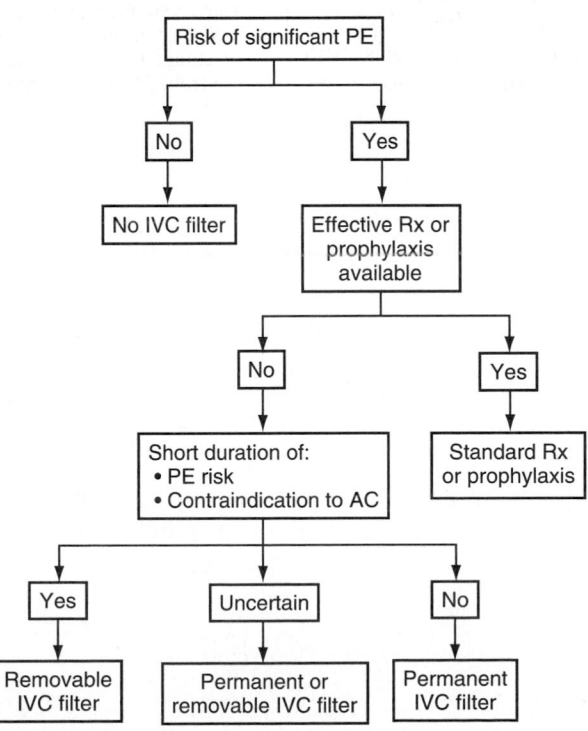

FIGURE 3. Decision matrix for vena caval filters. AC = anticoagulant; IVC = inferior vena cava.

Table 3 Prevalence of Inherited Thrombophilias and Associated Relative Risk for Venous Thromboembolism

Inherited Thrombophilia	Prevalence (%) in General Population	in Patients with VTE	Relative Risk of VTE
AT deficiency	0.07–0.16	1–3	20
Protein C deficiency	0.2–0.4	3–5	10
Protein S deficiency	0.03–0.13	1.5	10
Factor V Leiden mutation	3–15	20	5
Prothrombin mutation	1–2	4–7	2–3
Hyperhomocysteinemia	5	10	2.5
Elevated factor VIII	11	25	5

Abbreviations: AT = antithrombin; VTE = venous thromboembolism.

2. Patients younger than 50 years with VTE even with a transient predisposing factor.
3. Patients with VTE whose only risk factor is oral contraceptive therapy, estrogen replacement therapy, or pregnancy. However, screening with other than the molecular (polymerase chain reaction [PCR]) tests should be performed at least 2 months after delivery or hormone therapy cessation.
4. Patients with recurrent VTE irrespective of the presence of risk factors.
5. Patients with recurrent superficial thrombophlebitis without cancer and in the absence of varicose veins.
6. Patients with VTE at unusual sites such as cerebral venous sinus, mesenteric or hepatic veins, and retinal vein occlusion, and in patients younger than 21 years.
7. Patients with warfarin-induced skin necrosis and neonates with purpura fulminans not related to sepsis.
8. Asymptomatic first-degree relatives of individuals with proven symptomatic thrombophilia. This is particularly important for women of childbearing age.
9. Two consecutive or three nonconsecutive spontaneous abortions at any gestational age, or one fetal death after the 20th week.
10. Severe preeclampsia.
11. Children with VTE.

There is no point in screening for thrombophilia for patients in whom the decision has been made for prolonged or indefinite anticoagulation, such as those patients with cancer and VTE. Also, routine preoperative thrombophilia screening is not recommended because the result will not alter the thromboprophylactic strategy in the majority of patients. Preoperative thrombophilia screening should be reserved for patients with a personal or family history of VTE of unknown etiology who have not been investigated.

REFERENCES

Akesson H, Brudin L, Dahlstron JA, et al: Venous function assessed during a 5-year period after acute ilio-femoral venous thrombosis treated with anticoagulation. Eur J Vasc Surg 1990;4(1):43-48.

Buller HR, Agnelli G, Hull RD, et al: Antithrombotic therapy for venous thromboembolic disease: The Seventh ACCP Conference on Antithrombotic and Thrombolytic Therapy. Chest 2004;126:401S-28S.

Comerota AJ, Gale SS: Technique of contemporary iliofemoral and infrainguinal venous thrombectomy. J Vasc Surg 2006;43(1):185-191.

Comerota AJ, Thromb RC, Mathias S, et al: Catheter-directed thrombolysis for iliofemoral deep venous thrombosis improves health-related quality of life. J Vasc Surg 2000;32:130-137.

Eichinger S, Minar E, Bialonczyk C, et al: D-dimer levels and risk of recurrent venous thromboembolism. JAMA 2003;290:1071-1074.

Hann CL, Streiff MB: The role of vena caval filters in the management of venous thromboembolism. Blood Rev 2005;19:179-202.

Ost D, Tepper J, Mihara H, et al: Duration of anticoagulation following venous thromboembolism: A meta-analysis. JAMA 2005;294:706-715.

Plate G, Eklof B, Norgren L, et al: Venous thrombectomy for iliofemoral vein thrombosis—10-year results of a prospective randomized study. Eur J Vasc Endovasc Surg 1997;14:367-374.

Prandoni P, Lensing AW, Prins MH, et al: Below-knee elastic compression stockings to prevent the postthrombotic syndrome: a randomized, controlled trial. Ann Intern Med 2004;141:249-256.

The Blood and Spleen

Aplastic Anemia

Method of
Abdo Haddad, MD, and
Jaroslaw P. Maciejewski, MD, PhD

Historically, aplastic anemia (AA) has been the subject of intense investigations that have resulted in the assignment of bone marrow as a site of blood cell production, facilitated the concept of the hematopoietic stem cell, and led to the introduction of allogeneic bone marrow transplantation (BMT) as a therapeutic modality for human hematologic disorders. AA is defined as peripheral blood pancytopenia with obligatory hypocellular bone marrow. The current definition includes a decrease in at least two of three peripheral blood cell lineages. The current definition of AA incorporates severity of blood count depression that clearly correlates with prognosis. If not treated, severe AA is invariably fatal, whereas moderate AA has a good long-term prognosis.

The incidence of AA is estimated to be between two and five cases per million in the West but may be two to five times more frequent in the Far East. Typically, AA is a disease of the young, but the incidence has two peaks: one between the ages of 15 and 25 years and the other after the sixth decade of life. Whether the often described second peak is the result of diagnostic overlap of AA and myelodysplastic syndrome (MDS), which affects older individuals and can mimic AA, especially if marrow is hypocellular, is unclear.

Pathogenesis

CLASSIFICATION BASED ON PATHOGENESIS

Based on pathogenesis, AA can be classified as either inherited or acquired. Inherited forms of AA include Fanconi anemia and variants of dyskeratosis congenita, which are related to various mutations in the telomerase complex. Conceptually, acquired AA may evolve as a primary disease,

occurring in the form of idiopathic AA, or as a secondary condition related to iatrogenic use of ionizing radiation and cytotoxic therapy, idiosyncratic drug reactions, certain viruses, or in association with autoimmune conditions (Figure 1). Of note, the term "idiopathic" refers to the inability to identify a cause. It is possible that some unknown etiologic agents, such as viruses and certain chemicals, also serve as triggers in idiopathic AA. When iatrogenic causes are excluded, most cases of AA are idiopathic (Table 1).

ETIOLOGIC FACTORS AND THEIR INVOLVEMENT IN THE PATHOPHYSIOLOGY OF APLASTIC ANEMIA

Injury to the stem cell compartment with a qualitative and quantitative stem cell defect is the ultimate result of various and diverse pathophysiologic mechanisms. Idiopathic AA is likely mediated by the autoimmune attack of T cells leading to proliferation block and apoptosis of progenitor and stem cells. Apart from any infectious and systemic diseases that must be excluded before the diagnosis of idiopathic AA is made, direct or indirect causes of AA include direct chemical hematopoietic injury (see Figure 1). Treatment with cytotoxic chemotherapeutic drugs or irradiation causes direct injury to the bone marrow cells, which may lead to AA. However, a patient with acquired AA rarely has a history of such exposures.

Direct Chemical Hematopoietic Injury

Treatment with cytotoxic chemotherapeutic drugs can cause direct injury to the bone marrow cells, but a typical patient with acquired AA rarely has a history of such exposures, which would preclude the diagnosis of idiopathic AA.

Radiation

Both chronic and acute radiation exposure results in dose- and duration-dependent injury to the stem cell compartment. The lethal dose is dependent upon the level of supportive care. If the patient survives the acute phase, bone marrow hypoplasia may be the predominant factor influencing long-term prognosis.

TABLE 1 Etiology of Aplastic Anemia

Acquired Aplastic Anemia	Inherited Aplastic Anemia
Idiopathic aplastic anemia	Fanconi anemia
Pregnancy	Dyskeratosis congenita
Paroxysmal nocturnal hemoglobinuria	Reticular dysgenesis
	Shwachman anemia
Secondary	Genetic primary nonhematologic syndromes
Drugs	
Iatrogenic/cytotoxic	
Idiosyncratic	
Chloramphenicol	
Nonsteroidal anti-inflammatory drug	
Gold	
Antiepileptics	
Others	
Radiation	
Iatrogenic	
Accidental	
Viruses	
Epstein-Barr virus	
Non-A, non-B, non-C, non-G hepatitis	
Parvovirus	
HIV	
Pancytopenia of autoimmune diseases	

Direct Effects of Viruses

Viral infections, which include human cytomegalovirus and Epstein-Barr virus, have been implicated in rare cases of AA but do not constitute a typical cause of idiopathic AA.

Drug-related Aplastic Anemia

Medications may induce AA in the form of an idiosyncratic reaction. Various epidemiologic studies have implicated many drugs. Historically, chloramphenicol was considered the most notorious agent in AA. However, the etiologic fraction of AA attributed to drugs is low, and for most agents the odds ratio shows only a marginally increased risk of AA (i.e., between onefold and 10-fold). Of note, drug-related AA may display a similar course to the typical immune-mediated AA and often responds to immunosuppressive agents (Table 2).

Immune-Mediated Marrow Failure

Immune-mediated bone marrow failure is the most common cause of idiopathic AA. This process likely is triggered by viruses (e.g., AA/hepatitis syndrome is likely caused by a currently hypothetic non-A, B, C, D, E hepatitis virus) or by chemicals of altered proteins (e.g., resulting from transcription of mutated genes). Regardless of the inciting agents, the subsequent immunologic reaction may be uniform for various etiologies and includes an autoimmune T cell–mediated attack on hematopoietic progenitor and stem cells.

PATHOPHYSIOLOGY OF APLASTIC ANEMIA

The pathophysiology of idiopathic AA includes two major components: the stem cell compartment and immune effector mechanisms. Despite intense investigation, bone marrow stroma has not been identified as an important factor in the pathophysiology of AA. Aplastic stroma supports the growth of normal hematopoietic progenitors, and BMT is a successful therapeutic modality in AA, thus favoring the argument that patient's stromal cells can support the maintenance, proliferation, and differentiation of transplanted hematopoietic stem cells of the donor.

Stem Cells in Aplastic Anemia

A profound defect in the hematopoietic stem cell compartment has been consistently found in AA, as measured by colony-forming assays, long-term culture-initiating cell assays, and flow cytometry. It has been estimated that in AA the number of hematopoietic stem cells is decreased between 10-fold and 1000-fold. Hematopoietic suppression involves all stages of hematopoietic development. Apoptosis of hematopoietic progenitor and stem cells represents the final pathway; it has been consistently found in AA and is thought to be the result of immune effector mechanisms, including direct cell-mediated toxicity and inhibitory cytokines.

Autoimmune Mechanisms in Aplastic Anemia

Polyclonal T cell responses and increased frequency of activated cytotoxic T (Tc) cells and products, including interferon-γ and Fas ligand, have been found in AA. Although the initial inciting events may be diverse, the subsequent pathophysiologic mechanisms involve expansion of autoimmune clones recognizing antigens displayed by hematopoietic progenitor and stem cells. The effector pathways include direct killing via perforin/granzyme secretion, Fas-mediated killing, as well as effects of cytokines with inhibitory properties on hematopoiesis. Increased levels of interferon γ have been found in AA, likely as a result of altered Th1/Th2 and Tc1/Tc2 balances. Whereas principally T cell responses are polyclonal in AA,

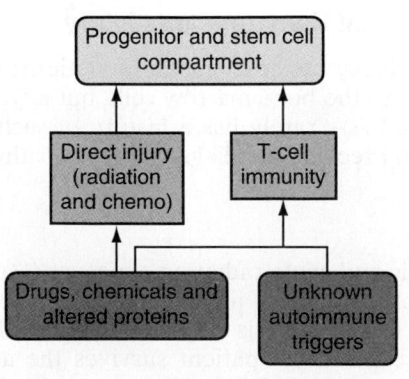

FIGURE 1. Stem cell injury in aplastic anemia.

TABLE 2 Drugs Most Commonly Implicated in Aplastic Anemia

Dose-Dependent Marrow Cytopenia	Drug That May Associate with Cytopenia	Drugs That Rarely Associate with Cytopenia
Chemotherapy	Chloramphenicol Nonsteroidal anti-inflammatory drugs Carbamazepine (Tegretol) Antithyroids Gold, penicillamine (Cuprimine) Sulfonamides Antidiabetics	Antibiotics Allopurinol (Zyloprim) Amiodarone (Cordarone), methyldopa (Aldomet), quinidine Lithium Chlorpromazine Antihistamine

immunodominant cytotoxic T cell clones can be detected and can serve as markers of the autoimmune process. Of note, inflammatory signs and markers, such as elevated erythrocyte sedimentation rate or C-reactive protein level, are consistently negative in AA. Patients with AA do not show hypoglobulinemia or hyperglobulinemia. Pathologic B cell responses and humoral immunity have not been conversely implicated in the pathophysiology of AA.

Target Antigens

Target antigens are not known, but from the spectrum of hematopoietic inhibition it can be concluded that they are located on immature hematopoietic stem cells. Specific autoantibodies have been only rarely described in AA, and their role remains unclear. The targets of immune recognition of antigens may be altered proteins, autoantigens, or cross-reactive antigens.

Clinical Presentation and Diagnostic Considerations

CLINICAL PRESENTATION

Pancytopenia and hypocellular bone marrow are the hallmarks of AA. The most common initial presentation is bleeding (serious bleeding, easy bruisability, petechiae, gum and nose bleeding, and, in females, heavy menstrual flow). Patients are rarely infected at presentation despite a low absolute neutrophil count (ANC). If patients with pancytopenia show systemic symptoms, such as fever, weight loss, pain, anorexia, and night sweats, then the possibility of alternative diagnoses should be entertained. Fatigue, lightheadedness, and shortness of breath are symptoms of anemia. AA patients can present with very low hemoglobin levels that are remarkably well tolerated but suggestive of the gradual decline in hemoglobin value.

PHYSICAL EXAMINATION

Patients with severe disease may look remarkably well given the levels of cytopenia. Petechiae usually occur over the pretibial surfaces, arm wrists, and occasionally in the oral area. Ecchymoses may present secondary to minor trauma. Retinal hemorrhage, gingival oozing, traces of heme in stool, and vaginal bleeding may occur in AA.

Hepatomegaly and splenomegaly are unusual in AA. The examiner should look for physical stigmata of hereditary conditions, such as Fanconi anemia or dyskeratosis congenita. Icterus may indicate an ongoing hemolysis and point toward a diagnosis of paroxysmal nocturnal hemoglobinuria (PNH) or suggest the possibility of hepatitis.

DIAGNOSIS AND DIFFERENTIAL DIAGNOSIS

Diagnosis of AA requires exclusion of systemic diseases that could mimic AA. The most common causes of cytopenia and marrow hypocellularity are obvious (e.g., history of cytotoxic drug usage); many other possible differential diagnostic considerations are rare (Table 3). All potentially offending medications should be discontinued. Blood cell count may be depressed to various extents; patients show low numbers of reticulocytes. Relative lymphocytosis is common, and most patients show a decrease in ANC and monocyte counts. Hypocellularity of the marrow is an obligatory finding for establishing the diagnosis of AA.

TABLE 3 Differential Diagnosis of Pancytopenia

Hypocellular Marrow	Hypercellular Marrow
Acquired aplastic anemia	**Primary Bone Marrow Disease** Myelodysplastic syndrome
Inherited aplastic anemia	Paroxysmal nocturnal hemoglobinuria
Myelodysplastic syndrome	Myelofibrosis
Rare aleukemic leukemia	Aleukemic leukemia
	Bone marrow lymphoma
	Hairy cell leukemia
Acute lymphoblastic leukemia	**Secondary to Systemic Disease** Systemic lupus erythematosus
Lymphomas of the bone marrow	Hypersplenism
	Vitamin B_{12}, folic acid deficiency
	Overwhelming infection
	Alcohol
	Brucellosis
	Ehrlichiosis
	Sarcoidosis
	Tuberculosis

TABLE 4 Severity Classification of Aplastic Anemia by Laboratory

Severe Aplastic Anemia	Moderate Aplastic Anemia
Bone marrow cellularity <10% Depression of at least two of three hematopoietic lineages: Absolute neutrophil count <500/μL Transfusion dependence with ARC <40,000/μL Platelet count <20,000/μL	Decreased bone marrow cellularity Depression of at least two of three hematopoietic lineages not fulfilling the criteria for severe aplastic anemia

Megaloblastic changes in erythroid series are common. The presence of even a few blasts indicates that the diagnosis of AA is unlikely. In typical cases, megakaryocytes are absent or severely diminished. The severity of AA can be described based on peripheral parameters (Table 4). The determination of a reticulocyte count is important for the diagnosis of bone marrow failure and the assessment of the severity of AA. The cytogenetic evaluation should show a normal karyotype. Although it is rational to assume that abnormal karyotyping precludes the diagnosis of AA (is consistent with myelodysplasia), the presence of some unbalanced translocations may be compatible with AA. In children and younger adults, Fanconi anemia should be excluded by appropriate tests. The diagnostic algorithm is outlined in Figure 2. PNH flow cytometry (detection of granulocytes and erythrocytes missing otherwise constitutive glycosylphosphatidylinositol (GPI)-anchored proteins) should be performed to establish baseline levels and rule out AA/PNH syndrome. Of note, 30% of AA patients may harbor subclinical levels of GPI-deficient cells. It is important to distinguish some of the common forms of AA.

Pregnancy-Associated AA

Pregnancy seems to predispose women to AA, but the mechanism remains unclear, making the nature of the association controversial. AA often resolves with termination of the pregnancy but can recur during subsequent pregnancies. Even if the initial presentation of AA was not associated with pregnancy, women with a recent history of successfully treated AA should be counseled not to get pregnant. Successful pregnancies have been described, and in the majority of cases most women had positive outcomes.

Seronegative Hepatitis/Aplastic Anemia Syndrome

From 2% to 9% of AA patients have a history of preceding hepatitis. In typical cases, AA evolves 3 to 6 months following a latency interval after initially severe and often fulminant non-A, B, C, D, and E hepatitis. At the time of AA presentation, transaminases may normalize.

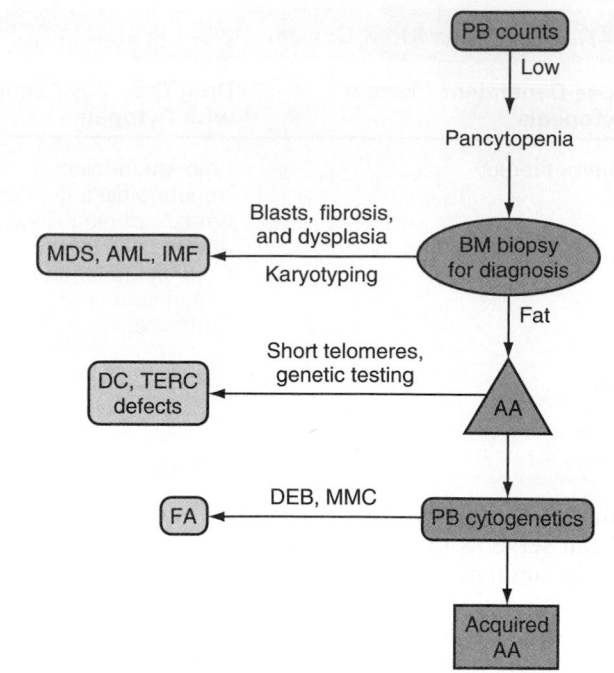

FIGURE 2. Diagnostic algorithm in aplastic anemia (AA). *Abbreviations:* AML = acute myeloid leukemia; BM = bone marrow; DC = dyskeratosis congenita; DEB = diepoxybutane; FA = Fanconi anemia; IMF = idiopathic myelofibrosis; MDS = myelodysplastic syndrome; MMC = mitomycin C; PB = peripheral blood; TERC = telomerase RNA component.

Post-Mononucleosis Aplastic Anemia

In rare instances, Epstein-Barr virus infections are associated with AA. The usual course is severe, and most of the described cases showed negative outcomes. Infectious mononucleosis may present with neutropenia and is clearly distinct from Epstein-Barr virus–associated AA.

Paroxysmal Nocturnal Hemoglobinuria/ Aplastic Anemia Syndrome

There is a strong association between AA and PNH. Manifest PNH can evolve in up to 15% of patients with AA, and GPI anchor–deficient clones are present in a significant proportion of patients with AA. However, AA/PNH syndrome usually displays higher percentages of GPI anchor–deficient blood cells and concomitant bone marrow suppression as indicated by depressed platelet count, ANC, and reticulocyte counts with frequently hypocellular bone marrow. Whereas moderate cytopenia may be consistent with the diagnosis of PNH, AA/PNH syndrome displays a clear crossover between the two diseases.

Chronic Moderate Aplastic Anemia

Moderate AA may serve as a transition stage of severe AA. However, some patients will maintain moderately depressed blood counts over extended periods (>3 months). Chronic moderate AA may constitute a separate entity, and some inherited marrow failure syndromes likely fall into this category. The response rates to immunosuppressive agents are not established and may be lower than those in severe AA. The therapies may include cyclosporine A (CsA; (Sandimmune[1]), antithymocyte globulin (ATG; Atgam), or anti–interleukin-2 receptor monoclonal antibody (daclizumab [Zenapax[1]], basiliximab [Simulect][1]), especially if patients are transfusion dependent. However, the prognosis is favorable if blood counts remain stable. Many hematologists may elect to approach moderate AA expectantly and treat only if counts worsen.

Therapy of Aplastic Anemia

SUPPORTIVE CARE

Consequences of pancytopenia can be life-threatening. AA can be cured by BMT or by immunosuppressive therapy (IS). Advances in supportive care likely are reflected in the improved survival rates of patients with AA in general, but especially patients who are refractory to therapies now can survive for extended periods.

Blood product transfusions have improved survival in patients with AA. Modern technology has made red blood cells and platelets available and fairly safe for transfusion. Alloimmunization is a major problem related to platelet transfusion. Alloimmunization can be prevented or delayed by the use of single donor–donor platelet transfusion and leukocyte depletion. The trigger values for platelet transfusions are a subject of controversy, but most hematologists transfuse platelets when levels fall below 10,000 to 20,000/μL. If a transplant from a related donor is planned, transfusions of blood from relatives should be avoided. Individuals who are physically fit may be asymptomatic, with a hemoglobin level higher than 7 g/dL. AA patients with ANC less than 500/μL are at increased risk for infection, and the recommendations for starting an empirical antibiotic therapy are the same as for other causes of prolonged neutropenia. Hematopoietic growth factors usually are ineffective for typical AA. Clearly, a broad-spectrum antibiotic and novel antifungal agent improve outcomes in patients with neutropenic fever.

CONSERVATIVE THERAPIES

IS with horse or rabbit ATG followed by CsA is the first-line, conservative therapy for severe AA (see Figure 3). Response rates are between 60% and 90%, with long-term survival in 60% to 70% of patients. ATG alone and CsA alone are inferior to the ATG/CsA combination. Refractory patients have poor prognosis. Repeated cycles of ATG/CsA can salvage up to 50% of initial nonresponders. Relapses are common (35%), but they can also be salvaged with repeated cycles of IS. In some patients, the counts remain dependent on chronic CsA therapy. In general, patients with HLA-DR1501 and those with the presence of PNH clones show higher rates of responsiveness to IS. Growth factors such as granulocyte colony-stimulating factor (filgrastim [Neupogen]), erythropoietin,[1] or granulocyte-macrophage colony-stimulating factor (sargramostim [Leukine][1]) do not appear to improve the response rate, and their benefit in conjunction with intense IS is questionable. Typical AA patients will not show

---

[1]Not FDA approved for this indication.

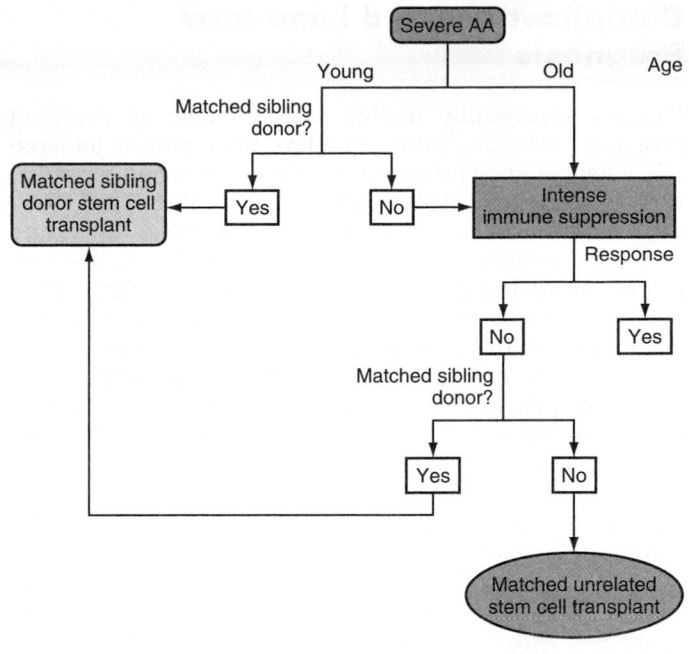

FIGURE 3. Severe aplastic anemia (AA) management.

response to granulocyte colony-stimulating factor and erythropoietin.

However, prolonged therapy with granulocyte colony-stimulating factor and erythropoietin has been applied as salvage therapy for patients refractory to IS. Corticosteroids are used to alleviate the side effects of serum sickness with ATG but should not be used as the sole agent in severe AA. Historically, androgens have been used as therapy for AA and show significant response rates, but they are clearly inferior to IS and consequently have a role only as a salvage modality.

BONE MARROW TRANSPLANTATION

Allogeneic BMT can cure AA (see Figure 3). Best results are achieved in children and young adults transplanted with grafts derived from matched sibling donors; survival rates range from 80% to 90%. Most common regimens use bone marrow as a source of stem cells along with cyclophosphamide (Cytoxan)/ATG–based conditioning regimens. BMT remains the treatment of choice for children with severe AA, if an appropriate family donor is available. Patients younger than 20 years have a 20% chance of developing acute graft-versus-host disease (GVHD). The risk of GVHD can be as high as 40% in patients older than 40 years. Methotrexate/CsA combination is used for GVHD prophylaxis. In general, for older patients the resulting overall survival from sibling–donor BMT as a first-line therapy is comparable or even superior to that from IS. Patients refractory to IS will be considered for BMT as second-line therapy. BMT results from a matched unrelated donor are less favorable, with survival ranging between 40% and 60%. Nonmyeloablative approaches are currently under development to improve BMT results in older patients and in those without a matched related donor.

Complications and Long-term Prognosis

Patients successfully treated with IS have an excellent prognosis, whereas nonresponders who cannot undergo BMT have a poor prognosis. However, in recent years the survival of chronically pancytopenic patients has improved due to advances in supportive care. Conversion of severe AA into moderate disease appears to be sufficient in significantly improving the long-term prognosis of patients. Thus, partial remissions of severe AA are compatible with long-term survival. The most common complications of conservatively treated AA include a high relapse rate, which can be as high as 37% in 10 years, and evolution of clonal disease, including MDS and PNH. The prognosis of relapse is good, with a high rate of success for reinduction IS. Evolution to MDS has poor prognosis, especially if accompanied by aberrations of chromosome 7 or complex cytogenetic abnormalities. The evolution rate is 10% to 20% in 15 years. Manifest hemolytic PNH may develop in another 10% to 20% of patients with AA. Although PNH may be associated with severe morbidity, most patients will show a good long-term survival. Recipients of allogeneic grafts show a different set of long-term complications, including chronic GVHD, cataracts, thyroid disorders, secondary cancers, and avascular bone necrosis.

REFERENCES

Bacigalupo A, Brand R, Oneto R, et al: Treatment of acquired severe aplastic anemia: Bone marrow transplantation compared with immunosuppressive therapy—The European group for blood and marrow transplantation experience. Semin Hematol 2000;37:69-80.

Bottiger LE: Epidemiology and aetiology of aplastic anemia. Haematol Blood Transfus 1979;24:27-37.

Hoffman R, Benz EJ, Shattil SJ: Hematology Basic Principles and Practice, 4th ed. Philadelphia, Churchill-Livingstone, 2005.

Maciejewski JP, Risitano A: Hematopoietic stem cells in aplastic anemia. Arch Med Res 2003;34:520-527.

Maciejewski JP, Rivera C, Kook H, et al: Relationship between bone marrow failure syndromes and the presence of glycophosphatidyl inositol-anchored protein-deficient clones. Br J Haematol 2001;115:1015-1022.

Maciejewski JP, Selleri C: Evolution of clonal cytogenetic abnormalities in aplastic anemia. Leuk Lymphoma 2004;45:433-440.

Margolis DA, Casper JT: Alternative-donor hematopoietic stem-cell transplantation for severe aplastic anemia. Semin Hematol 2000; 37:43-55.

Rosenfeld S, Follmann D, Nunez O, Young NS: Antithymocyte globulin and cyclosporine for severe aplastic anemia: Association between hematologic response and long-term outcome. JAMA 2003;289: 1130-1135.

Young NS: Acquired aplastic anemia. Ann Intern Med 2002;136:534-546.

Young NS, Gerson ST, High K: Clinical Hematology, 1st ed. Philadelphia, Mosby-Elsevier, 2006.

Young NS, Maciejewski J: The pathophysiology of acquired aplastic anemia. N Engl J Med 1997;336:1365-1372.

Iron Deficiency

Method of

William B. Solomon, MD

Iron, the fourth most abundant element in the earth's crust and the most abundant transition metal in living organisms, is required for oxygen transport, electron transfer reactions, and deoxynucleotide synthesis. Ironically, molecular iron is poorly absorbed in the gastrointestinal (GI) tract, making iron deficiency the most common cause of anemia in the world. In the United States, the National Health and Nutrition Examination Survey of 1999 to 2000 estimated the prevalence of iron deficiency to be 7% in toddlers ages 1 to 2 years, 9% to 16% in women of childbearing age, and 2% to 3% in men and women older than 50 years.

Mechanisms of Iron Deficiency

Depletion of iron stores is usually defined as a serum ferritin level less than 15 ng/mL. When this serum ferritin level is accompanied by a hemoglobin level less than 10.5 g/dL in children and in women of childbearing age or a hemoglobin level less than 13.5 g/dL in adult males, the criteria for diagnosis of iron-deficiency anemia are met. When iron depletion is sufficient to cause anemia, erythrocytes are *hypochromic*, as evidenced by a decreased mean cell hemoglobin level; *microcytic*, with a decreased mean cell volume of less than 80 fL; and *anisocytotic*, with an increased range distribution of width to more than 16%.

In infants and toddlers, iron depletion, even in the absence of anemia, may lead to psychomotor retardation. When deficiency of iron leads to a hemoglobin level less than 9 g/dL, there is accelerated production of blood lactate and tachycardia, leading to a decrease in exercise capacity and work performance. The impairment in performance, and the anemia, can be reversed by repletion of iron stores.

In infants, iron depletion and iron-deficiency anemia are usually caused by poor intake of dietary iron. Multiparous women, vegetarians, athletes, frequent blood donors, persons experiencing GI blood loss, patients who have undergone gastric surgery, users of antacid medications or nonsteroidal anti-inflammatory drugs (NSAIDs), and recent immigrants from hookworm-endemic regions have an increased risk of iron-deficiency anemia. In adults older than 50 years, iron-deficiency anemia is frequently secondary to blood loss in the lower or upper GI tract, necessitating investigation to locate the bleeding site(s).

Body Iron Stores, Daily Utilization, and Dietary Requirements

The total quantity of tissue iron in the average adult is 3800 mg. About two thirds, 2500 mg, is found in the red cell mass as the iron atoms that carry oxygen within the heme moieties of hemoglobin. The muscle masses contain myoglobin, the resident oxygen transport molecule, which in total contains about 500 mg of iron. The mitochondrial heme-containing enzymes account for about 50 mg, and other iron-containing enzymes account for about 200 mg. The major iron storage protein ferritin, which is synthesized in all cells, and its lysosomal breakdown product hemosiderin, contain approximately 750 mg of iron in adult men and 250 mg in adult women. Each nanogram per milliliter of serum ferritin is equivalent to body stores of approximately 8 mg of elemental iron. About 15 mg of iron is found on transferrin, which is the only circulating iron transport molecule.

Because iron is always tightly bound to proteins and is otherwise highly insoluble, there is no mechanism for excretion of iron except for the normal loss of about 1 mg/day occurring with exfoliation of cells from GI mucosae and skin. The development of iron-deficiency anemia requires a deficit of greater than 1500 mg of iron and is almost always the consequence of blood loss. Blood loss produces lost iron; in females of childbearing age, an additional 1.5 mg/day (on average) is lost, because the average monthly loss in menstrual blood is 40 ± 20 mL (about 0.5 mg of iron is lost for every milliliter of blood loss). Each full-term pregnancy results in a net utilization of about 800 to 1000 mg of iron.

The daily utilization of iron is about 35 mg. Almost all of this requirement is supplied from endogenous sources. About 25 mg is obtained from macrophages that remove senescent red cells from the circulation, thereby releasing iron from the heme moieties of hemoglobin. An additional 5 to 7 mg of iron is obtained after its release from ferritin storage. Therefore, there is a requirement for absorption of 1 to 2 mg of dietary iron each day. Because adequate delivery of iron to the tissues is maintained across a wide variety of iron intakes, the rate-limiting step in iron delivery to the cells appears to be its absorption. In iron-depleted states caused by chronic insidious blood loss, the increase in oral iron absorption does not compensate, and anemia results.

Absorption of Food Iron and Heme, and Iron Homeostasis

Food contains two sources of iron: ferric iron and iron incorporated into heme. The primary site of absorption of both forms of iron is the proximal duodenum. The duodenum provides an acid milieu and cells that express proteins specifically required for iron absorption.

There are distinct pathways for molecular iron and heme iron absorption in the duodenum. A specific receptor molecule for duodenal heme absorption called heme carrier protein-1 (HCP1) transports heme iron from the gut lumen into duodenal epithelial cells where iron is then released from heme.

The acid milieu of the duodenum causes free ferric iron to become soluble. It is further solubilized by reduction to ferrous iron by a ferrireductase called *duodenum-specific cytochrome b-like protein*, which is expressed on the luminal side of the duodenal cells. Soluble ferrous iron then is absorbed across the polarized cell by the divalent metal atom transporter DMT-1, also called *natural resistance-associated macrophage protein-2* (Nramp-2). The protein ferroportin, which is highly expressed in the duodenum, placenta, and macrophages, then pumps iron from the

duodenal cells into the blood, where ferrous iron is reoxidized to ferric iron by hephaestin, thus permitting ferric iron to be bound to the iron transport molecule transferrin. Transferrin, which bears two atoms of ferric iron, then circulates to all tissues, where it binds to the dimeric transferrin receptor that is synthesized by all cells. The transferrin receptor is subject to proteolytic cleavage, resulting in the soluble transferrin receptor that circulates in the blood.

The master regulator for excretion of iron atoms from duodenal cells and from macrophages is the hormone hepcidin. Hepcidin, which is synthesized in the liver, binds to ferroportin, causing it to be internalized and degraded; loss of ferroportin attenuates iron export from cells. Hepcidin expression is decreased in iron-deficient states and hypoxia, thus permitting increased iron absorption, and is highly increased by cytokines such as tumor necrosis factor-α and interleukin-6, cytokines expressed as a consequence of chronic infection, rheumatologic disease, inflammatory bowel disease, multiple myeloma, and other malignancies. Overexpression of hepcidin results in sequestration of iron in the liver, macrophages, and the reticuloendothelial cells of the bone marrow. This process starves erythroid precursor cells of iron, producing a functional iron deficiency, otherwise called the *anemia of chronic inflammatory disease* (ACD).

Diagnosis of Depleted Iron Stores or Iron-Deficiency Anemia

The serum ferritin level is the single best measure of total body iron stores. Expression of ferritin is regulated by body iron stores as well as levels of inflammatory cytokines. When body stores of iron are low, the conformation of cytosolic aconitase changes, permitting it to bind to an iron response element located at the 5' end of the ferritin mRNA. Binding of aconitase to the ferritin mRNA iron response element inhibits translation of the ferritin mRNA. Thus, in iron-deficient states the amount of ferritin is decreased; conversely, in states of iron overload, ferritin is increased. Measurements of serum iron level and total iron-binding capacity (TIBC; transferrin) also are helpful in making the diagnosis of iron-deficiency anemia.

There are three levels of iron deficiency. The first level, *depletion of iron stores*, is detected by a decreased serum

CURRENT DIAGNOSIS

- Hemoglobin:
  Children or women: <10.5 g/dL
  Men: <13.5 g/dL
  AND
- Mean cell volume <80 fL
  AND
- Serum ferritin level <15 ng/mL
  OR
- Increased serum soluble transferrin receptor
  OR
- Absent stainable iron stores in macrophages obtained from bone marrow aspirate

ferritin level to below 15 ng/mL. Persons with *decreased iron stores*, although they may not be anemic, will very probably benefit from increased iron intake. As the level of iron stores continues to drop to below 30 µg/dL, the amount of transferrin increases so that the TIBC increases to more than 400 µg/dL. Finally, there is the development of a *hypochromic, microcytic anemia*. A complete blood count demonstrates a decreased mean cell hemoglobin level and a decreased mean cell volume to less than 80 fL. With iron deficiency, hemoglobinization of each erythrocyte is quite variable, resulting in anisocytosis, which on a complete blood count is demonstrated by an elevated range distribution of width to more than 16%.

Establishing a diagnosis of iron-deficiency anemia is difficult because not all cases of anemia that are hypochromic and microcytic are secondary to iron deficiency. Two other common causes of hypochromic and microcytic anemias must be distinguished from iron-deficiency anemia, and occasionally they coexist with iron-deficiency anemia.

The *thalassemias* are a group of anemias characterized by a deficiency of globin chain synthesis, either α or β, which leads to cells that have decreased hemoglobinization. The consequence is a decrease in both mean cell hemoglobin level and mean cell volume. However, the defect appears to affect every red cell equally, leading to a normal range distribution of width. Furthermore, the absorption of iron may be increased in these disorders, often leading to a serum ferritin level above 50 ng/mL. Perhaps the most important laboratory finding that distinguishes the thalassemias from iron-deficiency anemia is a normal or elevated red blood cell count. Therefore, it is said that microcytosis in the presence of a red blood cell count greater that 5.0×10^6 per microliter is diagnostic for thalassemia and essentially rules out iron-deficiency anemia. A diagnosis of β-thalassemia can be confirmed by hemoglobin electrophoresis demonstrating an elevated hemoglobin A_2 level (and also by column chromatography for hemoglobin A_2). The diagnosis of α-thalassemia, which is common in African Americans and Asian Americans, can be confirmed, when warranted, by Southern blot analysis of the α-globin gene domain, which most often will detect deletions of one or both of the two α-globin genes located on one or both arms of chromosome 16.

Also difficult to distinguish from iron-deficiency anemia is ACD. Most often, ACD is a normochromic, normocytic anemia, although occasionally the erythrocytes are frankly hypochromic and microcytic. Furthermore, individuals with chronic inflammatory diseases, such as rheumatoid arthritis, often take aspirin or other NSAIDs, which can lead to GI blood loss, so that ACD can coexist with iron-deficiency anemia.

Certain findings are useful for distinguishing from among iron-deficiency anemia, ACD, and a combination of iron-deficiency anemia and ACD. In healthy individuals, a serum ferritin level of 15 ng/mL and less is considered evidence of iron deficiency. Because serum ferritin is an acute-phase reactant, in patients with a chronic disease such as a collagen vascular disorder, cancer, or rheumatoid arthritis, a serum ferritin level less than 40 ng/mL should be considered evidence of iron depletion; these patients may receive a trial of iron supplementation to determine whether they can benefit from iron treatment.

Some patients with ACD coexistent with iron-deficiency anemia have a serum ferritin level greater than 40 ng/mL. To help confirm that these persons indeed have iron-deficiency anemia, a soluble transferrin receptor assay can be performed. The transferrin receptor is found on all cells; by far the great mass of soluble transferrin receptor is produced by the erythroid component of the bone marrow. Therefore, any disorder that increases the amount of erythroid precursor cells in the bone marrow, such as a hemolytic anemia or thalassemia, will increase the amount of serum soluble transferrin receptor. If there is no increase in the number of erythroid bone marrow cells, then the other mechanism of increasing the amount of serum soluble transferrin receptor is via iron deficiency. In iron-deficient individuals there is an increase in the activity of the iron-binding protein, leading to increased stability and translation of the mRNA encoding for the transferrin receptor, with a consequent increase in the amount of serum soluble transferrin receptor protein produced by each erythroid bone marrow cell.

There is no increase in the soluble transferrin receptor in individuals with ACD (i.e., no increase in erythroid compartment mass and no change in the activity of the iron-binding protein). However, there is an increase in the binding activity of the iron-binding protein in patients with iron-deficiency anemia and in those with ACD combined with iron-deficiency anemia, leading to increased amounts of serum soluble transferrin receptor to more than 28 nM. It should be noted that each clinical laboratory may express the amount of soluble transferring receptor in different units. A more sensitive test for distinguishing ACD from iron-deficiency anemia is the ratio of the soluble transferrin receptor to ferritin level.

Another feature distinguishing iron-deficiency anemia from ACD is that, in most cases, ACD responds to erythropoietin. A series of erythropoietin (Epogen) injections can be used to raise red cell mass in persons with ACD in whom the hematocrit is low, particularly those who have cardiopulmonary diseases. In contrast, iron-deficiency anemia does not respond to erythropoietin.

To further complicate matters, the entity deemed "iron-deficient erythropoiesis" seen in iron-replete patients is frequently found in patients with the anemia of renal failure who receive erythropoietin injections. Individuals in whom hematocrit levels fail to increase after erythropoietin injections may benefit from the addition of supplemental iron, often given parenterally, resulting in a hematocrit increase.

Etiology, Symptoms, and Signs of Iron-Deficiency Anemia

Deficiency of iron in children and adolescents of both sexes is almost always secondary to inadequate intake. In adults, iron deficiency is both an illness and a sign of blood loss. In menstruating women, especially those who have had full-term pregnancies, iron deficiency is common and is almost always secondary to menstrual blood loss or the transfer, on average, of 800 mg of iron to the fetus. In adult males, iron deficiency is considered to be a herald sign of blood loss, and in the absence of an easily identifiable source of blood loss such as hemorrhoids, it is a mandate

TABLE 1 Risk Factors for Development of Iron-Deficiency Anemia

Demographic Factors
Age
    Infants, especially premature
    Adolescents
    Elderly
Females
    Menorrhagia
    Multiparity
Recent immigrants from hookworm-endemic regions
    (hookworm infestation is the most common cause
    of iron deficiency worldwide)

Diet
Vegetarian diet
Excess tannins (tea/coffee)
Excess phytates (brans and cereals)
Alcohol abuse

Gastrointestinal Diseases
Blood loss
Celiac disease
Atrophic gastritis
Helicobacter pylori infection

Drug History
Aspirin
Nonsteroidal anti-inflammatory drugs

Iron-deficiency anemia is most often found in persons with at least two risk factors.

CURRENT THERAPY

- Oral therapy, start with:
  Ferrous sulfate 325 mg PO, one per day with a meal
  If tolerated, then can increase to two or three per day with meals
      Concomitant vitamin C may increase iron absorption; drinking tea and eating bran/cereals may decrease iron absorption.
- If ferrous sulfate is not tolerated, can use:
  Niferex-150 capsule one per day or
  Chromagen Forte capsule one per day or
  Nu-Iron 150 capsule one or two per day
- If parenteral iron therapy is required:
  Venofer 200 mg of elemental iron (each milliliter of Venofer has 20 mg of elemental iron) diluted into 250 mL of normal saline, infuse over 1 hour. Give a total of 1–2 g over the course of 2–4 weeks.

for a GI blood loss workup. In all men, and in women older than 50 years, iron-deficiency anemia requires a full workup even in the face of an obvious site of GI blood loss because of the increased incidence of colorectal adenocarcinoma (Table 1).

Symptoms of iron deficiency include fatigue, lack of energy, and limited work performance. A rather specific symptom, although not universal, is pagophagia (ice eating). When patients are asked whether they go to the freezer and eat ice directly from the icebox, a typical response is "how did you know?"

Signs of iron deficiency include koilonychias (brittle spooning of the nails), atrophic glossitis, and esophageal webs. Iron-deficient children may have retarded skeletal growth or skeletal deformities.

Treatment

Once the diagnosis of iron-deficiency anemia is established, treatment is initiated with oral iron supplements. The standard oral preparation for iron replacement therapy is ferrous sulfate 325-mg (5-grain) tablets. Each ferrous sulfate tablet contains 65 mg of elemental iron. At best, an individual with iron-deficiency anemia will absorb (on average) no more than 20 mg of elemental iron per day. Thus, treatment can begin with just one ferrous sulfate 325-mg tablet per day. Although best absorbed when the stomach is empty, GI discomfort caused by each tablet can be ameliorated when the tablet is taken with food. Ideally,

the tablet should be taken with a meal containing foods rich in animal proteins and vitamin C, which promote iron absorption. The tablet should not be taken with meals rich in cereals or calcium, or with tea or coffee, all of which inhibit iron absorption. If one tablet per day is well tolerated, the dose of iron supplementation can be increased during the second week of treatment to two per day and then to three per day in the subsequent weeks of treatment. If ferrous sulfate tablets cannot be tolerated, an alternative oral treatment is a polysaccharide–iron complex capsule that contains elemental iron. Preparations are marketed under a number of names, including Niferex-150 and Nu-Iron 150; each capsule contains 150 mg of elemental iron and is taken once daily.

The response to treatment with oral iron can be ascertained by following the patient's reticulocyte count. Within 7 to 10 days after commencement of supplemental iron by mouth, the reticulocyte count increases. A twofold to fourfold increase above the baseline reticulocyte count is considered evidence of a response. To further confirm the reticulocyte response, hemoglobin and hematocrit levels are monitored and should be increased by at least 2 g/dL at 1 month following commencement of therapy. To confirm that iron stores are increased, there should be an increase in serum ferritin levels and a decrease in serum TIBC (transferrin) levels.

Treatment with oral iron preparations should be continued for 4 to 6 months after return of hematocrit levels to normal so that iron stores are replenished. To confirm that iron stores are adequate, a serum ferritin level can be obtained and should be greater than 20 ng/mL.

What if there is no response to oral iron supplementation after 1 month of compliance with therapy? The response to iron can be inhibited with ongoing GI blood loss, an acute inflammatory process (e.g., urinary tract infection or renal insufficiency), or excessive removal of calcium phytates or tannins with the iron. Lack of response to oral iron usually indicates persistent blood loss or true oral iron malabsorption secondary to atrophic/achlorhydric gastritis, *Helicobacter pylori*–induced gastritis, nontropical sprue, and other abnormalities of the proximal small bowel.

Patients who do not respond to oral iron therapy will require parenteral treatment, as will severely iron-deficient pregnant women who require certainty regarding an increase in hemoglobin level. Parenteral iron therapy is also used for hemodialysis patients receiving erythropoietin who develop functional iron deficiency.

Venofer, an iron sucrose, can be given via intravenous infusion at a dose of 200 mg of elemental iron (each milliliter of Venofer contains 20 mg of elemental iron) diluted into 250 mL of normal saline and infused over 1 hour. A total cumulative dose of 1 to 2 g of intravenous Venofer can be given over the course of 2 to 4 weeks. Within 1 week of treatment, the reticulocyte count will increase, with a subsequent increase in the hemoglobin level of 1 to 2 g/dL within 2 to 3 weeks. In contrast to other parenteral preparations of iron, the incidence of life-threatening reactions to Venofer is quite low.

REFERENCES

Bailie GR, Clark JA, Lane CE, Lane PL: Hypersensitivity reactions and deaths associated with intravenous iron preparations. Nephrol Dial Transplant 2005;20:1443-1449.

Beguin Y: Soluble transferrin receptor for the evaluation of erythropoiesis and iron status. Clin Chim Acta 2003;329:9-22.

Cook JD: Diagnosis and management of iron-deficiency anaemia. Best Pract Res Clin Haematol 2005;18:319-332.

Hershko C, Lahad A, Kereth D: Gastropathic sideropenia. Best Pract Res Clin Haematol 2005;18:363-380.

Weiss G, Goodnough LT: Anemia of chronic disease. N Engl J Med 2005;352:1011-1023.

Autoimmune Hemolytic Anemia

Method of
Charles J. Parker, MD

There are three general categories of autoimmune hemolytic anemia (AIHA), and each group has idiopathic and secondary forms (Table 1). In this review, drug-induced immune hemolytic anemia is treated as a subcategory of warm-antibody AIHA.

Warm-Antibody Autoimmune Hemolytic Anemia

Immune hemolytic anemia should be included in the differential diagnosis of patients with laboratory evidence of hemolysis (Table 2). The criteria for diagnosis of warm-antibody AIHA are shown in Table 3. In addition to the general laboratory signs of hemolysis (see Table 2), patients with warm-antibody AIHA present with two other important laboratory features. First, the peripheral blood film shows microspherocytes; and second, the direct antiglobulin (Coombs) test is positive (see Table 3). In approximately 67% of patients, the Coombs test is positive for both

---

TABLE 1   Classification of Autoimmune Hemolytic Anemias

Warm-Antibody Autoimmune Hemolytic Anemia (Accounts for Approximately 80% of Cases)
Idiopathic
Secondary (found in association with chronic lymphocytic leukemia, lymphoma [Hodgkin's and non-Hodgkin's], connective tissue diseases (primarily systemic lupus erythematosus), ulcerative colitis, ovarian cysts, immunodeficiency syndromes [including AIDS], antiphospholipid syndrome)
Drug-induced

Cold Agglutinin Syndrome (Accounts for Approximately 18% of Cases)
Idiopathic
Secondary (found in association with *Mycoplasma pneumoniae* infection, infectious mononucleosis, lymphoreticular malignancy, viral infections)

Paroxysmal Cold Hemoglobinuria (Accounts for Approximately 2% of Cases)
Idiopathic (associated with a chronic autoimmune disease in adults)
Secondary (found in association with viral illnesses, typically in children; also associated with syphilis)

---

immunoglobulin G (IgG) and complement, in 20% the test is positive for IgG but not complement, and in the remaining 13% the test is positive for complement but not IgG. The indirect Coombs test is positive in approximately 60% of cases. It is uncommon, but not rare, to have cases of "Coombs negative" warm-antibody AIHA (≈5% of cases are Coombs negative). In these cases, patients have laboratory evidence of hemolysis, and the peripheral blood film shows microspherocytes and polychromasia, but the standard Coombs test is negative. The presence of IgG, complement, or both, however, can often be demonstrated using more sensitive assays available in reference

---

TABLE 2   Laboratory Values That Suggest Hemolysis

Reticulocytosis >125,000/μL of blood*
Indirect bilirubin concentration between 1 and 5 mg/dL†
Haptoglobin concentration <50 mg/dL‡
Elevated lactic dehydrogenase concentration§

*If automated determination of reticulocyte concentration is unavailable, the value can be derived by multiplying the reticulocyte count (reported in percent) by the red blood cell (RBC) concentration (RBC/μL) and dividing the total by 100. For example, if the reticulocyte count is 1 and the RBC concentration is 5 × 10⁶/μL, the number of reticulocytes per microliter of blood is 50,000.
†Patients with Gilbert disease have an increased indirect bilirubin level in the absence of hemolysis. Unless the patient has underlying liver disease, the direct bilirubin level is rarely elevated in association with hemolysis.
‡Haptoglobin is an acute-phase reactant. When hemolysis occurs in association with inflammatory processes or with steroid administration, haptoglobin levels may be within the normal range.
§The normal range for lactate dehydrogenase (LDH) depends on the assay and the units of measurement and, therefore, varies among laboratories. LDH is mildly to moderately elevated in cases of extravascular hemolysis. Values are much higher in cases of intravascular hemolysis.

TABLE 3 Key Diagnostic Points for Warm-Antibody Autoimmune Hemolytic Anemia and Cold Agglutinin Syndrome

Warm-Antibody Autoimmune Hemolytic Anemia
Patient has not been transfused during previous 4 months*
Laboratory evidence of hemolysis[†]
Peripheral blood film shows microspherocytes and polychromasia
Positive direct Coombs test for IgG, complement C3, or both
Absence of a cold agglutinin of high thermal amplitude[‡]
Patient has a warm antibody with broad reactivity in the serum or eluted from the red cell[§]

Cold Agglutinin Syndrome
Clinical evidence of hemolytic anemia[†]
Agglutination of erythrocytes observed on blood film or when anticoagulated blood sample is collected at room temperature
Positive Coombs test for complement C3
Negative Coombs test for IgG**
Presence of a cold agglutinin with reactivity up to at least 30°C[¶]

---

*Patient may still have autoimmune hemolytic anemia, but delayed transfusion reaction should be excluded.
[†]See Table 2.
[‡]Reactivity up to 30°C.
[§]If the antibody is not present in the plasma (indirect Coombs test is negative), it can be eluted from the red cell membrane and its reactivity subsequently characterized.
**Cold agglutinins are almost invariably immunoglobulin M (IgM) antibodies that activate complement.
[¶]The antibody causes agglutination at temperatures up to 30°C.
Abbreviation: IgG = immunoglobulin G.

TABLE 4 Summary of Current Therapy for Warm-Antibody Autoimmune Hemolytic Anemia

Prednisone (1.0–1.5 mg/kg/day)*
Splenectomy[†]
Immunosuppressive therapy[‡]
Other[§]

---

*Patients who do not respond after 3 weeks are considered treatment failures. If patients respond, steroids should be tapered gradually over 3–4 months.
[†]Indications: (1) failure to respond to steroids; (2) steroid dose required to maintain remission is unacceptably high (10 mg/day or 15 mg/qod).
[‡]Indications: (1) failure to respond to splenectomy (or a combination of splenectomy and low-dose prednisone); (2) patients who cannot tolerate splenectomy. Cyclophosphamide (Cytoxan; 1.5–2.0 mg/kg/day) or azathioprine (Imuran; 2.0–2.5 mg/kg/day) is recommended. Treatment should continue for at least 3 months. Rituximab (anti-CD20), mycophenolate mofetil (CellCept), alemtuzumab (Campath), and cyclosporin A (Seromycin) have also shown efficacy.
[§]Plasmapheresis with plasma exchange may be beneficial in emergency situations. Intravenous immunoglobulin G produces a transient response in ≈ 30% of patients. Responses to danazol (Danocrine) and immunoadsorption columns have been reported. Patients should be supplemented with folate 1 mg/day.

laboratories (e.g., radioimmunobinding assays using monoclonal antibodies or enzyme-linked antiglobulin tests). The clinical diagnosis of Coombs negative AIHA is also supported by observing a response to an empirical trial of corticosteroids (see later).

The anti–red blood cell (RBC) antibodies of warm-antibody AIHA are almost invariably classified as panagglutinins because they cause agglutination of all of the erythrocytes that are part of the standard test panel used by the blood bank to characterize the reactivity of anti-RBC antibodies. More detailed analysis often shows that the antibodies are directed against antigenic determinants within the Rh system (although many other specificities have been reported).

MANAGEMENT OF IDIOPATHIC WARM-ANTIBODY AUTOIMMUNE HEMOLYTIC ANEMIA

An approach to treatment of warm-antibody AIHA is given in Table 4. All patients should receive folate supplementation to compensate for the increased utilization resulting from the compensatory enhancement of erythropoiesis. Approximately 80% of patients with warm-antibody AIHA will respond to steroids, and the response is usually rapid (within a few days); however, permanent remissions are observed in less than 20% of cases. The decision to recommend splenectomy should be based on

clinical criteria (see Table 4) because splenic sequestration studies using radiolabeled erythrocytes have not proved to be predictive of a response to splenectomy. In patients who relapse after splenectomy, low doses of steroids (≤5 mg/day) may be effective in controlling the hemolytic process. Immunosuppressive therapy (see Table 4) is often beneficial in patients who have not responded to splenectomy. Plasmapheresis with plasma exchange is unconventional therapy but offers the possibility of rapidly ameliorating the hemolysis in emergency situations. In contrast to its effectiveness in the management of immune thrombocytopenia, intravenous immunoglobulin therapy appears to be significantly less efficacious as treatment for AIHA. Approximately 30% of patients respond to intravenous immunoglobulin G, but responses are not durable, and maintenance therapy given every 3 to 4 weeks is usually required. Occasionally patients respond to the synthetic androgen danazol (Danocrine). Anecdotal reports suggest that some patients with AIHA may respond to immunoadsorbent therapy using immobilized protein A from *Staphylococcus aureus*. Response of refractory warm-antibody AIHA to rituximab (Rituxan) has been observed anecdotally and reported in small series.

MANAGEMENT OF SECONDARY WARM-ANTIBODY AUTOIMMUNE HEMOLYTIC ANEMIA

The approach to management of patients with secondary AIHA is similar to that described for patients with idiopathic AIHA. In the case of patients with chronic lymphocytic leukemia (CLL), it is particularly important to emphasize that treating the underlying disease is unlikely to ameliorate immune-mediated processes (e.g., AIHA or immune thrombocytopenic purpura [ITP]). In fact, treatment of CLL with purine nucleoside analogues, particularly fludarabine, has been associated with the development of AIHA and ITP. Patients who develop AIHA or ITP following fludarabine therapy should never receive additional fludarabine or other purine nucleoside analogues because of reports suggesting that such treatment may exacerbate AIHA or ITP, causing these processes to become intractable. Under these circumstances, morbidity and mortality rates are alarmingly high.

In general, for patients with secondary warm-antibody AIHA, the decision to treat the primary disease should be made separately from the decision to treat the hemolytic anemia. For example, a patient with Rai stage 0 CLL who has AIHA but no other symptoms should receive treatment for AIHA but not for CLL. In some instances, however, secondary AIHA may respond to treatment of the primary disease (e.g., treatment of lymphoma with combination chemotherapy). In other instances, treatment of the primary disease overlaps with treatment of AIHA (e.g., steroid therapy for systemic lupus erythematosus).

RESPONSE TO THERAPY

A normal hematocrit level is not necessary in order for the patient to be classified as a treatment success. The goal of therapy is to restore the hematocrit to a level that provides adequate oxygen transport capacity (usually >30% unless there are attendant problems). Furthermore, although the titer of the direct antiglobulin (Coombs) test may decrease in response to therapy, it is unusual for the test to become negative. Thus, a goal of therapy should not be normalization of the Coombs test.

It is important to keep in mind that idiopathic warm AIHA is a chronic disease and that relapses are common. Steroids should be tapered very slowly (over several months); however, disease exacerbations during the taper are frequently observed and are frustrating for both patient and physician. Patients requiring more than 10 mg of prednisone every day or more than 15 mg of prednisone every other day for more than a few months are candidates for splenectomy. Patients undergoing splenectomy should receive preoperative vaccinations against pneumococcal and meningococcal disease and against *Haemophilus influenzae* type B. Management of chronic AIHA is challenging, and not unusually patients require a combination of steroids, splenectomy, and immunosuppressive therapy. Patients should be informed that the disease is usually chronic and that relapses are common. Physicians should be prepared to monitor the patient frequently so that relapses can be treated promptly and therapy-related problems prevented. Prolonged use of steroids at unacceptably high levels is the most frequent cause of iatrogenic problems associated with treatment of chronic warm-antibody AIHA.

If the dose of prednisone required to maintain an appropriate hematocrit is unacceptably high after splenectomy, then immunosuppressive therapy should be initiated. In patients younger than 70 years, azathioprine (Imuran) is preferred over cyclophosphamide (Cytoxan) because the former is less leukemogenic than the latter. During the course of treatment, the hematocrit level, reticulocyte count, and lactate dehydrogenase (LDH) should be monitored regularly. A rising hematocrit in association with a falling reticulocyte count and LDH is consistent with a response to therapy. On the other hand, a falling hematocrit in association with a falling reticulocyte count suggests a superimposed bone marrow problem (e.g., parvovirus infection or megaloblastic crisis associated with folate deficiency) that requires further evaluation.

TRANSFUSION

Transfusion of patients with warm-antibody AIHA should be undertaken with caution. It is important to remember that response to steroid therapy is usually rapid (within a few days). Therefore, in most instances, transfusion can be avoided by reducing oxygen demand, which is accomplished by placing the patient at rest. Nonetheless, in cases of fulminant hemolysis or when a patient at rest becomes symptomatic while awaiting a response to therapy, transfusion can be lifesaving. Careful consideration should be given to the volume of blood infused because overtransfusion can be dangerous for two reasons. First, patients may become volume overloaded, causing further cardiopulmonary embarrassment. Second, the rate of hemolysis of donor red cells is exponentially related to the amount of blood infused. Consequently, problems associated with acute hemolysis are more likely to occur in patients who have received relatively large amounts of blood. Accordingly, the minimum amount of blood required to control the patient's symptoms should be transfused (e.g., 100 mL of packed cells twice per day may be effective in preventing high-output heart failure).

Because the autoantibody is almost always a panagglutinin, it is virtually impossible to find donor cells that are not recognized by the patient's antibody. Therefore, the goal of the blood bank staff is not to find donor cells that are unreactive in the cross-matching studies but rather to ensure that the patient's ABO and Rh phenotypes are properly determined and that the patient does not have an alloantibody in addition to an autoantibody. A detailed history of previous pregnancies and transfusions is important because patients with warm-antibody AIHA who have never been pregnant or been transfused likely would not have become alloimmunized. A number of assays are available that allow identification of a concurrent alloantibody, but these types of studies are not performed routinely. Accordingly, it is important that the blood bank have a level of sophistication and experience that ensures competence in the performance and interpretation of these critical studies.

Some immunohematologists advocate that studies be undertaken to determine the relative specificity of the autoantibody so that donor cells lacking the antigen can be transfused. For example, the antibody may react more strongly with cells that have the "little e" antigen than with those that have the "big E" antigen (E and e are part of the Rh antigen system). In this case, the antibody is said to have relative specificity for "little e." However, data from limited studies suggesting a clinical benefit from transfusing cells that lack the antigen of relative specificity are not compelling. Nonetheless, it seems prudent to determine the relative specificity of the antibody and to avoid transfusing cells that express the antigen, especially if in vitro studies indicate a strong degree of specificity (e.g., if the antibody induces hemolysis of antigen-positive but not antigen-negative cells).

Patients with AIHA who are being transfused should be monitored closely both during and after the infusion. Laboratory studies to document the extent of hemolysis (e.g., LDH, haptoglobin, plasma free hemoglobin, and hemoglobinuria) and the development of renal compromise should be obtained.

Drug-Induced Immune Hemolytic Anemia

In reviews of drug-induced hemolytic anemia from 30 years ago, methyldopa (Aldomet) was reported to be the responsible agent in the majority of cases. Because the use of methyldopa (Aldomet) as an antihypertensive has markedly declined over the last 20 years, the incidence of drug-induced hemolytic anemia has probably fallen. Nonetheless, drug-induced hemolytic anemia continues to account for a significant proportion of all cases of acquired immune hemolytic anemia, with cefotetan (Cefotan) and ceftriaxone (Rocephin) currently the drugs most commonly involved. At least 12 cyclosporins have been reported to cause drug-induced immune hemolytic anemia.

When evaluating patients with evidence of immune hemolysis, eliciting a detailed drug history is essential. In addition, a temporal relationship between drug administration and the development of hemolysis should be sought. Unfortunately, such relationships are often rendered inconclusive because patients are taking multiple drugs. Although some drugs induce immune hemolytic anemia more frequently than do others, in any one patient, any drug must be considered potentially culpable.

There are three basic mechanisms by which drugs can induce immune hemolytic anemia (Table 5). Prototypic drugs are included for each mechanism, but it is important to keep in mind that these drugs represent the best-characterized examples and that other drugs may induce hemolysis by the same mechanisms. For example, levodopa (Larodopa) and procainamide (Procan) have been reported to induce immune hemolytic anemia in a manner analogous to that of methyldopa (Aldomet). A detailed review of all of the drugs that have been implicated in the production of AIHA is beyond the purview of this article.

Recent reports strongly suggest that quinine can induce the hemolytic uremic syndrome (HUS). Patients present with chills, sweats, nausea and vomiting, abdominal pain, oliguria, and petechiae following exposure to quinine in the form of medications or beverages. Laboratory studies show anemia, severe thrombocytopenia, markedly elevated serum LDH level, and azotemia. Drug-dependent antibodies reactive with platelets, erythrocytes, and granulocytes have been identified. These patients have a favorable outcome when treated with plasmapheresis with plasma exchange and dialysis as indicated. Thus, prompt recognition and appropriate treatment of this clinical entity are imperative.

In an individual patient, almost any drug can produce an idiosyncratic reaction resulting in immune hemolytic anemia. Therefore, for patients with newly diagnosed acquired immune hemolytic anemia, all drugs that are not absolutely essential should be discontinued. Furthermore, any drug implicated by temporal events (and particularly any drug that has been reported to induce immune hemolysis) should be stopped and alternative therapy using a structurally unrelated compound initiated. A causal role for a particular drug can be established by using an in vitro assay. The basis of these types of assays is the indirect Coombs test modified to determine if antibody binding to the red cell is drug dependent. The technical aspects of the test (particularly the concentration of drug to use) can be obtained from published reports if studies of a particular drug have been performed. If a drug that has not been shown to induce immune hemolysis is suspected, experiments to establish the optimal conditions for testing are required. Unfortunately, drug-related antibodies cannot be conclusively demonstrated in many cases in which the clinical suspicion is strong. Adding to the problem is the fact that antibodies may be directed against metabolites rather than to the whole drug. In these cases, ex vivo antigens (present in the serum or urine of the patient) may be required to demonstrate the drug-dependent nature of the antibody.

Cold Agglutinin Syndrome

Whereas the presence of cold agglutinins in the plasma is relatively common, cold agglutinins that produce clinically significant hemolysis are relatively uncommon. A cold agglutinin titer of less than 1:64 is normal. Patients with cold agglutinin syndrome may complain of Raynaud's phenomenon or of acrocyanosis of the ears, nose tip, fingers, and toes that occurs at cold temperatures and vanishes quickly upon warming. These symptoms arise because as the blood flows through skin capillaries, the intravascular temperature drops to levels at which the cold agglutinin is functional. As a consequence of the agglutination, blood flow through the small vessels is restricted. Hemoglobinuria following exposure to cold may be part of the history, but, in general, this symptom is unusual. Hepatosplenomegaly is not usually prominent, and lymphadenopathy is uncommon. Agglutination of the red cells at room temperature is an obvious consequence of the disease.

The criteria for diagnosis of cold agglutinin syndrome are given in Table 3. It should be emphasized that mere observance of cold agglutination is not diagnostic of cold agglutinin disease. The antibodies of cold agglutinin disease are almost invariably immunoglobulin M (IgM), and, in the vast majority of cases, they are directed against determinants of the I antigen system. In most instances, the cold agglutinin titer in cold agglutinin syndrome is greater than 1:1000, but the titer at 4°C does not correlate well with the hemolytic potential of the antibody. A more useful characterization is determination of the thermal amplitude of the antibody (defined as the highest temperature at which the antibody causes agglutination). The majority of cold agglutinins that produce clinically significant hemolysis have a thermal amplitude of at least 30°C (if the thermal amplitude is <30°C, the antibody will not fully activate the complement system).

MANAGEMENT OF COLD AGGLUTININ SYNDROME

Treatment of cold agglutinin syndrome is notoriously difficult because currently available therapeutic modalities (i.e., corticosteroids, splenectomy, and alkylating agents) are relatively ineffective. Fortunately, most patients have a low-grade, compensated anemia that is best managed by

TABLE 5   Characteristics of Drug-Induced Hemolytic Anemias

Quinidine/Quinine Prototype

Proposed mechanism

The drug acts as a hapten after binding to a cell membrane protein. Consequently, antibodies against constituents of the drug–membrane protein complex arise.

Clinical characteristics

Small doses of drug induce the process.
Intravascular hemolysis is common; hemolysis may be severe and life-threatening. Can produce HUS.

Laboratory findings

Direct Coombs test positive for complement but not IgG.
Antibody may be IgG or IgM.
Positivity of the indirect Coombs test depends on the presence of the drug in the reaction mixture, thus demonstrating the drug-dependent nature of the antibody.

Therapy

Discontinue drug.
Supportive care (maintain renal blood flow, transfuse as needed).
In patients with severe hemolysis, an empirical trial of steroids is warranted.
Patients with HUS appear to benefit from plasma exchange. Dialysis is often required.

Penicillin Prototype

Proposed mechanism

Drug binds tightly to red cell. Antidrug antibody binds to drug on red cell surface.

Clinical characteristics

Large doses of drug required (10 million units or more per day).
Hemolysis is usually subacute, developing over 1–2 weeks.
Patients may have positive Coombs test without clinical evidence of hemolysis.
In rare instances, the process may be life-threatening.

Laboratory findings

Direct Coombs test positive for IgG, rarely positive for complement.
Patient's serum will react in indirect Coombs test with red cells coated with drug.

Therapy

Discontinue drug in cases of overt hemolysis.
If hemolysis is clinically insignificant, the drug can be continued while the patient is monitored closely.

Methyldopa (Aldomet) Prototype*

Proposed mechanism

Speculative but may alter the immune system, resulting in a pathophysiologic process similar to that observed in idiopathic autoimmune hemolytic anemia.

Clinical characteristics

Dose and time dependent (patient will have taken drug for at least 3 months).
Hemolysis is usually mild and resolves gradually over several weeks after cessation of the drug.
Patients may have positive Coombs test without clinical evidence of hemolysis.

Laboratory findings

Direct Coombs test positive for IgG, rarely for complement. When hemolysis is present, indirect Coombs test is invariably positive.
Positivity of Coombs test is not dependent on having the drug in the reaction mixture.
Coombs test may be positive for months after cessation of drug.

Therapy

Discontinue drug in cases of overt hemolysis.
If hemolysis is clinically insignificant, the drug can be continued while the patient is monitored closely. However, the availability of other effective agents makes prudent the switch to a structurally unrelated alternative antihypertensive agent.

*Methyldopa (Aldomet) is rarely used in current practice, but the mechanism of drug-induced hemolytic anemia may be applicable to other currently used agents, including levodopa (Larodopa) and procainamide (Procan)
Abbreviations: HUS = hemolytic uremic syndrome; IgG = immunoglobulin G; IgM = immunoglobulin M.

general supportive measures (avoiding cold exposure, transfusion if necessary). A minority of patients may benefit from chlorambucil (Leukeran; 0.1–0.2 mg/kg/day) or cyclophosphamide (Cytoxan; 1.5–2.0 mg/kg/day), and these agents should be prescribed if the disease is complicated by severe anemia. Several case reports and a few small series suggest that patients refractory to other treatments may respond to rituximab (Rituxan). This treatment is particularly attractive because of its favorable therapeutic index (generally well tolerated and associated with relatively few adverse effects). In situations where the cold agglutinin syndrome arises in association with an underlying neoplasia, the hemolytic process often ameliorates in response to treatment of the underlying disease.

Patients should avoid cold conditions, and in some instances patients may have to move to a warm climate. Inasmuch as the antibody is IgM, plasmapheresis offers the opportunity to lower the antibody concentrations in emergency situations.

TRANSFUSION

The I antigen is present on all adult red cells. Thus, it is not possible to transfuse nonreactive donor cells. Difficulties in establishing ABO and Rh phenotypes and in identifying alloantibodies are usually not encountered, however, because tests can be performed at a temperature above that at which the cold agglutinin is active. The clinical benefit of using in-line blood warmers during transfusion of patients with cold agglutinin disease (or with paroxysmal cold hemoglobinuria [PCH], see later) has not been clearly established. In general, properly crossed-matched blood can be transfused safely if it is warmed to room temperature and infused slowly. In cases of particularly severe cold agglutinin syndrome or PCH, however, use of an in-line warmer seems prudent.

SECONDARY COLD AGGLUTININ SYNDROME

Although the finding of cold agglutinins in association with infectious processes is relatively common (particularly for *Mycoplasma pneumoniae* infection and infectious mononucleosis), clinically significant hemolysis in this setting is unusual. The association of cold agglutinin disease with lymphoproliferative neoplasias is also uncommon. Some features of secondary cold agglutinin disease are given in Table 6.

TABLE 6 Secondary Chronic Cold Agglutinin Disease

Mycoplasma pneumoniae Infections
Approximately 50% of patients have elevated cold agglutinin titers, but overt hemolysis is rare.
When it does occur, the hemolytic process begins in the second or third week of the infection and onset is rapid. Fatalities have been reported.
Characteristically the cold reacting antibody is an IgM that recognizes I antigens.
The antibody may cross-react with mycoplasmal antigens.
The hemolysis is self-limited and steroids are ineffective.

Infectious Mononucleosis
Clinically significant hemolysis occurs infrequently.
Hemolysis occurs 1–2 weeks after onset of infection.
The antibody may be IgM anti-i, IgM anti-I, or IgG anti-i.*
Hemolysis is usually self-limited, but steroids may be of benefit.
Association with reticuloendothelial neoplasia is unusual.

---

*The I antigen is found predominantly on adult red cells, whereas the i antigen is found primarily on fetal red cells. In primary cold agglutinin disease, the antibody is almost invariably IgM anti-I. The cold agglutinins associated with infectious mononucleosis are unusual in that they may have specificity for the i antigen, and they may be IgG.
Abbreviations: IgG = immunoglobulin G; IgM = immunoglobulin M.

Paroxysmal Cold Hemoglobinuria

PCH is an uncommon disease that can be dramatic in presentation. Patients with PCH (usually children) experience acute attacks of shaking chills, fever, malaise, and aching pains involving the abdomen, back, and legs. Hemoglobin is usually present in the first urine passed after the attack. A history of exposure to cold is usually elicited, although the extent of the exposure may be modest. In rare instances, cold exposure is not part of the presenting history. Often there is a history of a flulike prodromal illness. The anemia is usually moderate to severe at the time of presentation and may be progressive despite keeping the patient warm.

The diagnosis of PCH is made by finding the Donath-Landsteiner antibody in the patient's plasma. This IgG antibody is directed against the P blood group antigen and is identified by using a bithermal assay. First, the patient's serum is incubated with erythrocytes at 4°C. Under these conditions, the cold reacting antibody binds to the red cells. Subsequently, the reaction mixture is warmed to 37°C, and the cells hemolyze as a result of complement activation initiated by the Donath-Landsteiner antibody.

MANAGEMENT OF PAROXYSMAL COLD HEMOGLOBINURIA

Most patients with PCH require only supportive care because the process is usually transient. The patient should be kept warm at all times. Guidelines for transfusion are the same as those for patients with cold agglutinin syndrome (see earlier). In severe cases, an empiric trial of corticosteroids is warranted. Although the association is now rare, patients with PCH should be evaluated for evidence of syphilis. PCH has also been reported as part of a chronic autoimmune process in adults.

REFERENCES

Arndt PA, Garratty G: The changing spectrum of drug-induced immune hemolytic anemia. Semin Hematol 2005;42:137-144.

Berentsen S, Ulvestad E, Gjertsen BT, et al: Rituximab for primary chronic cold agglutinin disease: A prospective study of 37 courses of therapy in 27 patients. Blood 2004;103:2925-2928.

Gottschall JL, Elliot W, Lianos E, et al: Quinine-induced immune thrombocytopenia associated with hemolytic uremic syndrome: A new clinical entity. Blood 1991;77:306-310.

Rosse WF, Hillmen P, Schreiber AD: Immune-mediated hemolytic anemia. Hematology (Am Soc Hematol Educ Program) 2004:48-62.

Shanafelt TD, Madueme HL, Wolf RC, Tefferi A: Rituximab for immune cytopenia in adults: Idiopathic thrombocytopenic purpura, autoimmune hemolytic anemia, and Evans syndrome. Mayo Clin Proc 2003;78:1340-1346.

Nonimmune Hemolytic Anemia

Method of
Stella T. Chou, MD, and
Mitchell J. Weiss, MD, PhD

The hemolytic anemias (HAs) are a heterogeneous group of disorders characterized by accelerated erythrocyte destruction. Intrinsic causes of hemolysis are usually inherited and include abnormalities in the erythrocyte membrane, metabolic defects, and altered hemoglobin structure. Extrinsic causes include erythrocyte-directed antibodies, trauma, infections, and toxins. Within these categories, there are virtually hundreds of specific etiologies. Here we address the most common and clinically significant disorders, focusing mainly on the congenital HAs.

Diagnosis

Anemia with reticulocytosis, hyperbilirubinemia, and an elevated lactate dehydrogenase (LDH) level strongly suggests hemolysis. The family history is often helpful for diagnosis. In particular, the clinician should inquire about ethnic background and family members with anemia, splenectomy, early gallstones/cholecystectomy, or significant neonatal jaundice. Several forms of HA confer protection against *Plasmodium falciparum* malaria. Accordingly, these disorders are relatively common in malaria endemic regions such as Africa, the Mediterranean basin, and Asia because of positive selective genetic pressure. Assessment of erythrocyte indexes and morphology are critical and frequently reveal distinct diagnostic clues (Table 1). Together, these initial data usually point to a specific diagnosis that can be confirmed by directed specialized testing that includes more detailed examination of erythrocytes and DNA analysis.

In addition, patients with primary hemolytic disorders may present during an aplastic episode, most typically from Parvovirus B19 infection. In this case, erythrocyte production stops temporarily resulting in reticulocytopenia and declining hemoglobin.

Management

Folate replacement is recommended for most patients with moderate to severe congenital hemolytic anemia. Iron from hemolyzed erythrocytes is usually reabsorbed, and supplementation is not necessary. Formation of gallstones is a common complication of HA, and therefore periodic screening abdominal ultrasounds are warranted. Concomitant Gilbert's syndrome, caused by a variant in the uridine diphosphoglucuronate glucuronosyltransferase 1A (UGT1A) gene promoter, increases the propensity for gallstones. Neonatal jaundice is common in many of the inherited disorders and may necessitate exchange transfusion for severe hyperbilirubinemia. Parvovirus B19–induced aplastic crisis is a life-threatening complication of congenital HA that frequently requires blood transfusion. Therefore, it is essential that patients with known hemolytic disorders be counseled to seek medical attention if they experience symptoms of viral illness, increased pallor, and lethargy.

Splenectomy is an effective treatment for many forms of severe congenital HA. The most significant problem from splenectomy is increased risk of life-threatening infections from encapsulated organisms. Prior to splenectomy, patients should be vaccinated against *Streptococcus pneumoniae, Haemophilus influenzae* type B, and *Neisseria meningitidis*. Daily penicillin prophylaxis is recommended

---

CURRENT DIAGNOSIS

- Anemia, reticulocytosis and hyperbilirubinemia suggest hemolytic anemia (HA).
- Reticulocytopenia in the context of chronic HA suggests a Parvovirus-induced aplastic crisis.
- Erythrocyte-intrinsic etiologies for HA are usually inherited abnormalities affecting the erythrocyte membrane, enzymes, or hemoglobin structure.
- Congenital HA can present with severe neonatal jaundice.
- Extrinsic causes for HA include antierythrocyte antibodies, trauma, infection, and toxins.
- History, physical examination, and examination of erythrocyte morphology combined with more specialized testing usually provides a specific diagnosis.
- Paroxysmal nocturnal hemoglobinuria is a clonal somatically acquired hematopoietic disorder characterized by intravascular hemolysis, thromboses, and sometimes cytopenias. Diagnosis is made by flow cytometry demonstrating a population of cells that lack glycosyl phosphatidylinositol (GPI)-anchored membrane proteins.

CURRENT THERAPY

- Many forms of congenital severe HA are ameliorated by splenectomy.
- Long-term risks of splenectomy include susceptibility to sepsis from encapsulated organisms and possibly increased risk of thrombosis.
- Splenectomized patients should be immunized against *Streptococcus pneumoniae, Haemophilus influenzae* type B, and *Neisseria meningitidis*. Daily penicillin prophylaxis is recommended for children.
- Splenectomized patients presenting with fever should receive appropriate parenteral antibiotics until a negative blood culture is documented.
- Aplastic crisis and hyperhemolytic episodes associated with HA are managed with erythrocyte transfusion.
- Folate (folic acid) replacement, 1 mg/d, is recommended for moderate to severe HA.

TABLE 1 Causes of Nonimmune Hemolytic Anemia

Type of Defect	Disease Mechanism	Example	Erythrocyte Morphology
Intrinsic erythrocyte defect	Membranopathy	Hereditary spherocytosis	Spherocytes
		Hereditary elliptocytosis	Elliptocytes
		Hereditary stomatocytosis	Stomatocytes
		Hereditary xerocytosis	Target cells, echinocytes
		Hereditary pyropoikilocytosis	Micropoikilocytes, microspherocytes, fragmented erythrocytes
		Paroxysmal nocturnal hemoglobinuria	Macrocytosis
	Enzymopathy	G6PD deficiency	Heinz bodies, bite cells, blister cells, anisocytosis, poikilocytosis
		Pyruvate kinase deficiency	Echinocytes
	Hemoglobinopathy	Sickle cell disease	Sickle cells
		Thalassemia	Microcytosis, target cells
		Unstable hemoglobinopathies	Heinz bodies
Extrinsic erythrocyte defect	Trauma	Heart valve hemolysis (macrovascular)	Schistocytes
		DIC/TTP/HUS (microvascular)	Schistocytes
	Thermal injury	Severe burns	Schistocytes
	Chemicals	Arsenic, lead, copper, and chlorates	Varied
	Toxins	Bee and wasp stings, spider bites, and snake venom	Schistocytes
	Infections	Malaria, *Babesia*, *Bartonella*, clostridia, streptococci, staphylococci, enterococcus, salmonella, mycoplasma, EBV, CMV, HSV, rubeola, influenza A	Intraerythrocytic parasites
			Schistocytes with bacterial infections

Abbreviations: CMV = cytomegalovirus; DIC = disseminated intravascular coagulation; EBV = Epstein-Barr virus; HSV = herpes simplex virus; HUS = hemolytic uremic syndrome; TTP = thrombotic thrombocytopenic purpura.

postsplenectomy, particularly for children. Splenectomized patients presenting with fever should be managed promptly with physical examination, blood culture, and appropriate parenteral antibiotics.

Congenital Hemolytic Anemias

ERYTHROCYTE MEMBRANE ABNORMALITIES

The erythrocyte membrane must be flexible and strong enough to withstand multiple passages through small capillary beds. A specialized membrane composed of a lipid bilayer, integral membrane proteins, and an underlying skeletal network formed by numerous proteins supports these requirements. Erythrocyte membrane proteins include alpha and beta spectrin, ankyrin, protein 4.1, and actin. Inherited mutations in these proteins disrupts the integrity of the membrane to cause HA.

Hereditary Spherocytosis

Hereditary spherocytosis is the most common cause of nonimmune HA in populations from Northern Europe and North America, with a prevalence of approximately 1 in 2000.

Pathophysiology

Hereditary spherocytosis is caused by varying degrees of spectrin loss, usually from deficient or dysfunctional ankyrin, band 3 and/or protein 4.2, or, less frequently, a primary spectrin defect. Disruption of the membrane skeleton destabilizes the lipid bilayer causing splenic removal of microvesicles and subsequent spherocyte formation. The molecular basis of hereditary spherocytosis is heterogeneous. Approximately two thirds of cases are autosomal dominant, with the remaining one third being autosomal recessive or arising from new mutations.

Clinical Manifestations and Diagnosis

The severity of hereditary spherocytosis varies from asymptomatic to severe and typically correlates with the degree of spectrin deficiency. Most diagnoses of hereditary spherocytosis are made in childhood, from a positive family history or a clinical presentation of anemia, jaundice, and splenomegaly. New patients occasionally present with a Parvovirus-induced aplastic crisis. In these clinical contexts, an elevated mean corpuscular hemoglobin concentration (MCHC) strongly indicates hereditary spherocytosis. This value reflects a decreased surface-to-volume ratio caused by splenic removal of the erythrocyte membrane. In addition, the red cell distribution width

(RDW) reflecting size variation, is elevated. The blood smear demonstrates spherocytes (erythrocytes lacking central pallor). A positive incubated osmotic fragility test, which demonstrates increased susceptibility to hypotonic lysis, supports the diagnosis. However, it is important to note that osmotic fragility is normal in 10% to 20% of hereditary spherocytosis cases. Moreover, other disorders, most notably immune HAs, are also characterized by spherocytes with increased osmotic fragility. A positive direct antiglobulin test (Coombs test) usually distinguishes immune HA from hereditary spherocytosis.

Patients with mild hereditary spherocytosis may have normal or near normal hemoglobin levels, mild reticulocytosis and hyperbilirubinemia, and typically have an uncomplicated course. More severely affected patients experience additional complications including severe neonatal hyperbilirubinemia and hyperhemolytic episodes later in life. The latter are frequently precipitated by viral illness and are characterized by worsening anemia, signs of accelerated hemolysis, and often, splenic enlargement. Rare complications of severe hereditary spherocytosis include leg ulcers, gout, and extramedullary hematopoiesis.

Management

Aplastic and hyperhemolytic episodes are supported with erythrocyte transfusions. Although splenectomy improves the anemia and reduces the risk of gallstones by removing the site of erythrocyte destruction, splenectomy should be reserved for patients with severe hemolysis, recurrent life-threatening hyperhemolytic episodes, or growth failure. Most clinicians prefer to treat as needed with transfusions until after 5 years of age when the postsplenectomy infection risk declines. In less severely affected patients, the threshold for recommending splenectomy varies among clinicians. In most centers, splenectomy is performed laparoscopically with very low morbidity and rapid recovery times. Moreover, improved vaccines, particularly pneumococcal, reduce the risk for postsplenectomy sepsis. However, some data indicate that splenectomy increases the long-term risk for venous and arterial thromboses, cardiovascular disease, and pulmonary hypertension. Accessory spleens are relatively common and should be searched for at the time of surgery.

Hereditary Elliptocytosis and Pyropoikilocytosis

The hereditary elliptocytoses are a heterogeneous group of inherited HAs with oval-shaped erythrocytes. Hereditary elliptocytosis is relatively common in African, Mediterranean, and Asian populations. Hereditary pyropoikilocytosis is a more rare and severe form of HA with erythrocyte fragmentation in which one parent usually has hereditary elliptocytosis.

Pathophysiology

Most forms of hereditary elliptocytoses are inherited in an autosomal dominant fashion and are relatively mild. The underlying molecular defects are usually mutations in genes encoding alpha or beta spectrin, band 3, or protein 4.1. These mutations all destabilize the latticework of spectrin organization underlying the plasma membrane to induce an oval or elliptical shape. Assorted hereditary elliptocytoses mutations that qualitatively alter membrane proteins produce subtle variations in cell shape that distinguish different clinical subtypes, which are categorized according to erythrocyte morphology. In hereditary pyropoikilocytosis, the patient usually inherits a common hereditary elliptocytosis mutation from one parent and a milder subclinical defect in spectrin synthesis from the other parent.

Clinical Manifestations and Diagnosis

Hereditary elliptocytosis is classified into three subtypes according to morphology: common hereditary elliptocytosis, the most prevalent form, which is characterized by biconcave elliptocytes; spherocytic hereditary elliptocytosis, a phenotype between hereditary spherocytosis and hereditary elliptocytosis; and Southeast Asian ovalocytosis, characterized by oval erythrocytes. Most patients are asymptomatic and diagnosed incidentally with minimal or mild compensated hemolysis. The peripheral smear demonstrates more than 30% elliptocytes. Patients who are homozygous or compound heterozygous have more severe HA. The peripheral blood smear also has budding erythrocytes, fragments, and other poikilocytes. Hereditary pyropoikilocytosis, at the extreme end of this spectrum, causes bizarre fragmented erythrocytes with microspherocytosis and micropoikilocytosis. The mean corpuscular volume is very low (25 to 75 fL), the osmotic fragility is abnormal, and erythrocytes characteristically demonstrate thermal instability. Hereditary pyropoikilocytosis typically presents in newborns or infants with jaundice and anemia.

Management

Most hereditary elliptocytoses patients have a mild course and do not require treatment. In cases of severe hemolysis because of homozygous or compound heterozygous hereditary elliptocytosis or hereditary pyropoikilocytosis, splenectomy is indicated.

Hereditary Stomatocytosis and Xerocytosis

Hereditary stomatocytosis and xerocytosis are rare inherited causes of hemolytic anemia associated with abnormal erythrocyte cation permeability and volume (increased in stomatocytosis and decreased in xerocytosis). Both disorders are autosomal dominant. Hereditary stomatocytosis patients have erythrocytes with a mouth-shaped (stoma) area of central pallor, whereas hereditary xerocytosis patients demonstrate target cells and echinocytes. The clinical courses of these diseases are highly variable, ranging from asymptomatic to moderate hemolysis and subsequent anemia. Most patients do not require treatment. Importantly, splenectomy is contraindicated in hereditary stomatocytosis because of an increased incidence of life-threatening thrombosis.

ERYTHROCYTE METABOLISM ABNORMALITIES

Erythrocytes rely on two major biochemical pathways: glycolysis for energy to maintain metabolic needs and the hexose-monophosphate shunt for antioxidant pathways. More than 20 enzymes are involved in these two pathways, and defects in each one are associated with various forms of HA. The two most common enzymopathies are deficiencies in glucose-6-phosphate dehydrogenase (G6PD) and pyruvate kinase (PK).

Glucose-6-Phosphate Dehydrogenase Deficiency

G6PD deficiency is the most common erythrocyte metabolism disorder, affecting as much as 3% of the world's population.

Pathophysiology

G6PD is the first enzyme in the hexose-monophosphate pathway, which is required to maintain a high level of reduced glutathione, an important antioxidant. G6PD-deficient erythrocytes undergo increased hemoglobin oxidation leading to hemolysis. G6PD deficiency is an X-linked recessive disorder. More than 300 G6PD genetic variants affect enzyme activity to different extents that determine the severity of HA. Type A$^-$ is a genetic variant seen in 10% to 15% of African American males and is associated with mild to moderate G6PD deficiency. Variants causing more severe HA are more prevalent in Mediterranean and Asian populations.

Clinical Manifestations and Diagnosis

G6PD deficiency is an X-linked disorder; therefore, hemizygous males and homozygous females are typically affected. Many G6PD variants are associated with neonatal jaundice. Severe forms of G6PD deficiency can cause chronic ongoing HA, but most commonly, affected individuals are asymptomatic in between hemolytic episodes. However, anemia develops rapidly following a precipitating event related to oxidative stress that induces acute intravascular hemolysis with the severity determined by the G6PD variant and the offending agent. Drugs are the most common inciting event in Africans with the A$^-$ variant (Table 2). Other precipitating events include mothball (naphthalene) exposure and infections. In some Mediterranean and Asian variants, ingestion of fava beans can cause acute life-threatening hemolysis. Symptoms can include fever, abdominal pain, nausea, diarrhea, and impressive hemoglobinuria, frequently described as Coca-Cola colored. The spleen is often enlarged and tender. Anemia ranges from mild to life-threatening and is normocytic and normochromic. Morphologic abnormalities include anisocytosis, poikilocytosis, "bite cells" (erythrocytes that are partially destroyed in the spleen), and "blister cells" (a thin strip of membrane overlying a bleb of clear cytoplasm). A methyl violet stain to detect Heinz bodies, indicative of denatured hemoglobin, is typically positive. Immediately after an acute hemolytic event, G6PD levels can be deceptively normal because of an elevated reticulocyte count, which can express significant enzymatic activity in some variants. Therefore, G6PD levels should be tested weeks to months later to obtain a true baseline level.

TABLE 2 Drugs Capable of Precipitating Hemolysis in G6PD Deficiency

Analgesics and Antipyretics	Acetanilid* Acetylsalicylic acid (aspirin)
Antibacterials	Chloramphenicol Furazolidone (Furoxone)* Nalidixic acid (NeGram)* Nitrofurantoin (Furadantin)* Sulfonamides* Trimethoprim-sulfamethoxazole (Bactrim)
Antimalarials	Pamaquine* Pentaquine* Primaquine* Quinacrine
Miscellaneous	Dimercaptosuccinic acid (Succimer) Methylene blue* Phenazopyridine (Pyridium)* Urate oxidase* Vitamin K

*These drugs have an increased tendency to cause clinically significant hemolysis. Most patients with mild G6PD deficiency alleles tolerate drugs that are not marked by the asterisk. For a more comprehensive list of drug–G6PD interactions, see reading by Beutler.
Abbreviation: G6PD = glucose-6-phosphate dehydrogenase.

Management

Treatment of the A$^-$ variant of G6PD deficiency is mostly preventive by avoiding oxidant stresses. When acute hemolytic episodes result in symptomatic anemia, erythrocyte transfusions are indicated. Rarely, acute renal failure develops secondary to severe intravascular hemolysis. This is managed by vigorous hydration, alkalinization, electrolyte monitoring, and occasionally hemodialysis.

Pyruvate Kinase Deficiency

Pyruvate kinase (PK) deficiency, which is most commonly seen in Northern European populations, accounts for more than 80% of the HAs due to glycolytic disorders.

Pathophysiology

PK deficiency is genetically heterogeneous, with many different mutations impairing enzyme activity to different extents. Pyruvate kinase deficiency causes decreased production of ATP, impairing erythrocyte survival. Inheritance is usually autosomal recessive; simple heterozygotes with 50% enzyme activity are unaffected.

Clinical Manifestations and Diagnosis

PK deficiency is extremely heterogeneous, ranging from life-threatening HA to asymptomatic compensated hemolysis. Erythrocyte morphology may be normal or show echinocytes (small dense crenated erythrocytes). Quantitation of erythrocyte enzyme activity is usually diagnostic.

Management

General supportive care for chronic hemolysis and supportive erythrocyte transfusions when needed are the mainstays of therapy. Patients with severe hemolysis may benefit from splenectomy, although the response is variable and unpredictable.

HEMOGLOBINOPATHIES

HA can be caused by mutations that alter the α- or β-like globin proteins that contribute to hemoglobin structure. Quantitative defects that impair globin gene expression comprise the thalassemia syndromes, discussed in the article on thalassemia. Qualitative defects are usually caused by missense mutations that alter hemoglobin structure and stability. The most important examples are the sickle syndromes, discussed in the article on sickle cell disease. Numerous other missense mutations that destabilize hemoglobin also cause HA. In these cases, hemoglobin precipitates may be detected by a Heinz body stain. Unstable hemoglobins can also be detected by hemoglobin electrophoresis or increased precipitation upon exposure to heat or isopropanol. If any of these tests are positive in the context of hemolysis, direct globin gene sequencing can provide a definitive diagnosis.

Acquired Nonimmune Hemolytic Anemias

PAROXYSMAL NOCTURNAL HEMOGLOBINURIA

Paroxysmal nocturnal hemoglobinuria (PNH) is a rare acquired disease with chronic HA, thrombosis, and often pancytopenia. The hemolytic anemia results from increased erythrocyte sensitivity to complement-mediated hemolysis.

Pathophysiology

PNH is an acquired clonal disorder caused by a somatically acquired inactivating mutation in the X-linked phosphatidylinositol glycan, class A (PIGA) gene, which encodes an enzyme involved in the synthesis of glycosyl phosphatidylinositol (GPI) anchor proteins. All blood cells derived from the abnormal clone lack surface proteins that require the GPI anchor. Hemolysis occurs from the deficiency of specific GPI-linked surface proteins that inhibit complement activation. The hypercoagulable state seen in PNH is most likely related to complement-mediated platelet activation and elevated levels of ADP from lysed erythrocytes, leading to platelet aggregation. For unknown reasons, PNH commonly progresses to aplastic anemia.

Clinical Manifestations and Diagnosis

PNH can present as a primary hemolytic syndrome with chronic intravascular HA, a thrombotic event, or with pancytopenia. Few patients exhibit the classic nocturnal hemoglobinuria, reporting red or brownish urine in the morning. In most patients hemoglobinuria occurs irregularly and is often precipitated by infection or stress. Iron deficiency can occur from urinary loss. Associated thromboses may be venous or arterial and can involve extremities, the hepatic vein (Budd-Chiari syndrome), other intraabdominal veins, and cerebral veins. Hence, PNH can present as severe abdominal pain or headaches. The majority of patients have defective hematopoiesis, ranging from a macrocytic anemia to severe aplastic anemia and pancytopenia. Rarely, PNH can also evolve into a myelodysplastic syndrome or acute leukemia. The median survival for patients diagnosed with PNH is 10 to 15 years.

Laboratory findings include anemia, variable reticulocytosis, leukopenia, and thrombocytopenia. The bone marrow examination typically reveals erythroid hyperplasia or, in the case of associated aplastic anemia, hypocellularity. Urine hemosiderin is typical. Laboratory diagnosis of PNH previously relied on assays that demonstrated abnormal erythrocyte sensitivity to complement (Ham test, sucrose hemolysis test). The current standard is flow cytometry demonstrating the absence of hematopoietic GPI-linked proteins, typically CD55 and CD59, on some or all circulating cells.

Management

Oral iron supplementation is recommended to replace the urinary losses associated with intravascular hemolysis. Corticosteroids can sometimes improve the hemolysis in the first 24 to 72 hours of a hemolytic episode. Anticoagulation is indicated for documented thromboses, and thrombolytic therapy can be effective for patients with hepatic vein thrombosis or massive thrombotic events. Short-term prophylactic therapy should be used in the setting of surgery or prolonged immobilization, even if there is no history of thrombosis. HLA-identical bone marrow transplantation is indicated for bone marrow failure associated with PNH. Alternatively, immunosuppressive therapy with antithymocyte globulin and cyclosporine is used for patients without a suitable bone marrow donor. Recent preliminary studies suggest that hemolysis of PNH can be alleviated by treatment with eculizumab,* a monoclonal antibody that inhibits activation of the terminal complement complex.

Hemolytic Anemia Caused by Erythrocyte Fragmentation

Erythrocyte fragmentation can occur in the macrovascular or microvascular circulations. Shear stress produces fragmented erythrocytes (schistocytes). Macroangiopathic hemolysis can occur with prosthetic surfaces, large thromboses, and aged or damaged heart valves, but it is usually mild. Microangiopathic causes of hemolysis include disseminated intravascular coagulation, thrombotic thrombocytopenic purpura, and hemolytic uremic syndrome, which are discussed in their respective articles.

*Orphan drug in the United States.

Hemolytic Anemia Caused by Chemical and Physical Agents

Arsenic, lead, copper, and chlorates can cause hemolysis through numerous mechanisms. Most notably, hemolytic anemia may be the presenting feature of the copper toxicity of Wilson's disease. Animal toxins associated with intravascular hemolysis include bee and wasp stings, brown recluse spider bites, and snake venom. Severe burns can also cause fragmentation hemolysis from the thermal injury.

Hemolytic Anemia Caused by Infection

Infections cause hemolysis by direct invasion of the erythrocyte, toxin production, or by immune-mediated mechanisms. Malaria is the most common infectious cause of hemolytic anemia worldwide. *Plasmodium falciparum* invades erythrocytes and is associated with severe hemolysis and hemoglobinuria (blackwater fever). Other parasitic infections associated with hemolysis are *Babesia microti* and *Bartonella bacilliformis*. Bacterial organisms that cause hemolysis via erythrocyte membrane injury and toxins include clostridia, streptococci, staphylococci, enterococcus, and salmonella. Immune hemolysis is associated with *Mycoplasma pneumoniae*, Epstein-Barr virus, cytomegalovirus, herpes simplex, rubeola, and influenza A (see topic in Section 2). Hemolysis improves once the underlying infection resolves.

REFERENCES

Beutler E: Glucose-6-phosphate dehydrogenase deficiency and other red cell enzyme abnormalities, in Beutler E, et al. (eds): Williams Hematology. New York, McGraw-Hill, 2001, pp 527-545.

Bolton-Maggs PH, Stevens RF, Dodd NJ, et al: Guidelines for the diagnosis and management of hereditary spherocytosis. Br J Haematol 2004;126(4):455-474.

Gallagher P, Lux S: Disorders of the erythrocyte membrane, in Nathan D, et al (eds): Nathan and Oski's Hematology of Infancy and Childhood. Philadelphia, WB Saunders, 2003, pp 560-684.

Hill A, Hillmen P, Richards SJ, et al: Sustained response and long-term safety of eculizumab in paroxysmal nocturnal hemoglobinuria. Blood 2005;106(7):2559-2565.

Parker C, Omine M, Richards S, et al: Diagnosis and management of paroxysmal nocturnal hemoglobinuria. Blood 2005;106(12): 3699-3709.

Tse WT, Lux SE: Red blood cell membrane disorders. Br J Haematol 1999;104(1):2-13.

Zanella A, Fermo E, Bianchi P, Valentini G: Red cell pyruvate kinase deficiency: Molecular and clinical aspects. Br J Haematol 2005;130(1):11-25.

Pernicious Anemia and Other Megaloblastic Anemias

Method of
Dan L. Longo, MD

Megaloblastic anemia is the name used to describe anemias in which the red blood cells (RBCs) are larger than normal, usually greater than 100 fL (10^{-15} L) in mean corpuscular volume (MCV). The term *megaloblastic* is from the Greek words *megas* meaning large and *blastos* meaning germ or bud. Megaloblastic anemias are caused by impaired DNA synthesis. Historically, 95% of cases of megaloblastic anemia were caused by folate and/or vitamin B_{12} deficiency. Since the advent of folate food supplementation in January 1998, however, the incidence of folate deficiency has declined (current incidence is estimated at 4 per 100,000 population). Precise incidence figures for pernicious anemia, the most common form of vitamin B_{12} deficiency, are lacking; however, the condition increases in incidence with age, and estimates are as high as 2% of people older than age 60 years. When asymptomatic patients older than age 65 years are screened, 10% to 15% or more may have biochemical evidence for vitamin B_{12} deficiency in the absence of anemia. Box 1 lists the causes of megaloblastic anemia.

Clinical Presentation

Anemia is associated with weakness, fatigue, shortness of breath, headache, exercise intolerance, or palpitations. On physical examination, the patient may have pallor or even a lemon-yellow cast from the combination of anemic pallor and low-grade icterus from the destruction of megaloblastic erythroid precursors in the marrow. The pulse is rapid and increases with even mild exertion. The effects of the nutritional deficiency may be manifest in the gastrointestinal (GI) tract in approximately 25% of patients; such symptoms may include a smooth or sore tongue (glossitis) and diarrhea.

The pattern of clinical presentation from vitamin B_{12} deficiency seems to have changed in the last 30 years. Classically, vitamin B_{12} deficiency was caused by pernicious anemia and patients presented with anemia. However, 75% to 89% of patients also had neurologic signs and symptoms including paresthesias, peripheral neuropathy, unsteady gait, and balance problems because of posterior column dysfunction called *combined systems disease*. Patients often had loss of vibration sense on physical examination. In addition, vitamin B_{12} deficiency was found to be associated with memory impairment or even frank dementia, irritability, personality change, depression, and psychosis. In series beginning in the late 1960s, however, neurologic signs and symptoms have accompanied the anemia in only approximately 44% of patients. In part this may be because of earlier diagnosis of anemia. Other evidence supporting a change in pattern is the occurrence of vitamin B_{12}-deficiency neurologic symptoms in the absence of anemia. Up to 25% of patients with

BOX 1   Causes of Megaloblastic Anemia*

Cobalamin Deficiency

1. Inadequate ingestion: Strict vegetarian
2. Malabsorption
   - Gastric disorders
     Pernicious anemia: Atrophic gastritis type A, antibodies to parietal cells or intrinsic factor
     Achlorhydria: Defective release of cobalamin from food
     Partial or total gastrectomy
   - Terminal ileum disorders
     Tropical and nontropical sprue
     Regional enteritis
     Bowel resection
     Tumors or granulomatous disorders (rare)
   - Pancreatic disease
     Trypsin and bicarbonate essential for absorption
     ZES: pH too acidic for absorption
   - Competition for cobalamin
     Blind loop/bacterial overgrowth syndromes
     Fish tapeworm (*Diphyllobothrium latum*)
   - Drug-induced malabsorption (see following text)
   - Inherited defects in absorption (see following text)
3. Congenital defects (rare)
   - Imerslund-Graesbeck syndrome (inherited selective B_{12} malabsorption)
   - Transcobalamin II deficiency
   - Intrinsic factor defects
4. Drug effects
   - **Block acid secretion:** Proton pump inhibitors such as omeprazole and H_2 blockers to a lesser degree
   - Block absorption at terminal ileum: Metformin, calcium channel blockers, para-aminosalicylate, colchicine
   - Destroy cobalamin: Nitrous oxide, large doses of ascorbic acid
5. Increased requirements: Hyperthyroidism

Folic Acid Deficiency

1. **Inadequate ingestion:** Malnutrition, alcoholism, imbalanced diet (no vegetables)
2. Increased requirements
   - Pregnancy
   - Increased hematopoiesis in chronic RBC disorders like sickle cell anemia, hemolytic anemia
   - Hemodialysis
   - Malignancy
   - Growing children
3. Malabsorption
   - Tropical and nontropical sprue
   - Drug effects (see text following)
4. Drug effects
   - Antifols: Methotrexate, trimethoprim pentamidine, sulfasalazine, triamterene
   - Block absorption in proximal small intestine: Phenytoin, barbiturates, ethanol, oral contraceptives, metformin
5. Congenital defects (rare)

Other Causes

1. Drug effects
   - Inhibitors of DNA synthesis
     Purine inhibitors: Thioguanine, azathioprine, 6-mercaptopurine
     Pyrimidine inhibitors: Azidothymidine, 5-fluorouracil, capecitabine
     Ribonucleotide reductase inhibitors: Cytosine arabinoside, hydroxyurea
     Other mechanisms: Procarbazine,
   - Other mechanisms: L-asparaginase, protein synthesis inhibitor; benzene, unknown mechanism
2. Congenital defects (rare)
   - Orotic aciduria/Lesch-Nyhan syndrome
3. Megaloblastic anemia of unknown etiology
   - Refractory megaloblastic anemia
   - Congenital dyserythropoietic anemia

*The more common causes are in **bold type.**
Abbreviations: RBC = red blood cell; ZES = Zollinger-Ellison syndrome.

B_{12} neuropathy are not anemic. Because a mechanism for the neurologic damage has not been defined, the reasons for the differential manifestations of vitamin B_{12} deficiency are unknown.

Vitamin B_{12} and folate deficiency differ in several respects. Because the body stores sufficient folate reserves to last approximately 3 to 4 months, if intake ceases completely anemia usually develops over a period of 10 to 15 weeks. By contrast, the body stores sufficient vitamin B_{12} that depletion does not occur for 4 or more years. If enterohepatic circulation is normal, the manifestations of vitamin B_{12} anemia may not occur for 20 years. Because the anemia may develop slowly, low levels of hemoglobin may be tolerated. Another important clinical difference between folate and vitamin B_{12} deficiency is that neurologic symptoms are an uncommon feature of folate deficiency. However, folate deficiency may occur in the setting of alcoholism, which can cause neurologic symptoms from thiamine deficiency that can mimic vitamin B_{12} deficiency. In addition, diabetic patients who develop folate deficiency may have neurologic manifestations of their diabetes that confuse the diagnosis. Thus, the differential diagnosis of megaloblastic anemia rests with laboratory testing or a therapeutic trial rather than clinical signs and symptoms. The important distinguishing features are based on understanding folate and B_{12} biochemistry and the physiology of their absorption.

Biochemistry and Physiology of Folate and Vitamin B_{12}

Folate and vitamin B_{12} biochemistry overlap in the de novo thymidylate synthesis pathway (Figure 1). Deoxyuridylate (deoxyuridine [dU] monophosphate) is converted to deoxythymidylate by the action of thymidylate synthase. A reduced folate, 5,10-methylene tetrahydrofolate (5,10-methylTHF), is the methyl donor, and dihydrofolate is a product of the reaction. The supply of reduced folate is replenished by the action of dihydrofolate reductase to form tetrahydrofolate (THF), and the methyl donor form of folate (5,10-methylene THF) is regenerated by the action of serine hydroxymethyl transferase, an

DE NOVO THYMIDYLATE SYNTHESIS

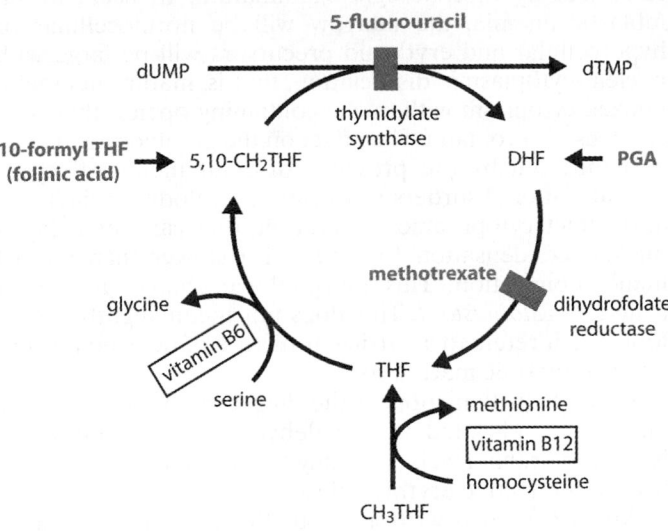

FIGURE 1. Vitamin B_{12} deficiency and folate deficiency both produce anemia by causing a cellular deficiency of thymidylate that inhibits DNA synthesis. The major food form of folate, methyl folate (CH_3THF), requires demethylation in order to enter cells and this step requires vitamin B_{12}. Thus, large amounts of folate can overcome the hematologic effects of vitamin B_{12} deficiency. Folate cannot correct the neurologic effects of vitamin B_{12} deficiency.

enzymatic reaction that requires pyridoxal phosphate (vitamin B_6). The predominant form of folate in food is methylTHF polyglutamate. Conjugases in the gut remove the extra glutamates and the methylTHF is absorbed. After absorption methylTHF requires vitamin B_{12} to enter cells; methylTHF is demethylated to THF by methionine synthase in a reaction that converts homocysteine to methionine and depends on the action of methylcobalamin (vitamin B_{12}). In reactions not shown in Figure 1, 5,10-methenylTHF participates in chemical reactions that contribute the 2 and 8 carbons to the purine rings of guanine and adenine.

Nearly all the manifestations of folate deficiency and the hematologic manifestations of vitamin B_{12} deficiency are because of an inadequate supply of reduced folate for thymidylate synthesis. In the absence of thymidylate, DNA synthesis slows and deoxyuridylate may be incorporated in its place. This can lead to abnormal base pairing (uridylate binding to cytosine residues instead of adenine residues) and mutations.

Figure 1 also illustrates where 5-fluorouracil and methotrexate act on this pathway and how folinic acid and pteroylglutamic acid can overcome blocks in the pathway. The dependence of the methylTHF demethylation step on vitamin B_{12} also illustrates how homocysteine levels can increase in vitamin B_{12} deficiency. In the absence of vitamin B_{12}, methylTHF levels in the serum usually increase (so-called methyl folate trap).

The second biochemical pathway involving vitamin B_{12} is the synthesis of succinyl CoA (coenzyme A) from methylmalonyl CoA in a reaction that requires adenosylcobalamin. Because neurologic dysfunction is more commonly associated with vitamin B_{12} than with folate deficiency, it has been hypothesized that a deficiency

in adenosylcobalamin underlies the neurologic symptoms in vitamin B_{12} deficiency, which are characterized by demyelination and axon loss. However, evidence for a role for a defect in fatty acid synthesis because of inadequate levels of succinyl CoA or excess levels of methylmalonyl CoA in the pathogenesis of vitamin B_{12}–deficiency-associated neuropathy has been inconsistent. The pathogenesis of the neurologic disease is undefined.

Nearly all folate deficiency is caused by inadequate dietary intake of vegetables and fruit. In patients with malabsorption syndromes because of small intestinal disease, other symptoms (diarrhea, weight loss) are more prominent before folate deficiency appears. After ingestion, food folate polyglutamates are deconjugated down to one glutamate group by intestinal enzymes and absorbed in the proximal third of the small intestine. Phenytoin (Dilantin) blocks folate absorption in the gut. After absorption, the monoglutamate form is taken up by cells in a vitamin B_{12}-dependent process and glutamates are added again; they aid in keeping the folate in the cell.

By contrast, most vitamin B_{12} deficiency is caused by inadequate absorption. Because vitamin B_{12} is in meats, milk, and eggs, dietary deficiency is rare. Food vitamin B_{12} is generally protein bound. Gastric acid releases it from food, and it is bound by R proteins (cobalophilins) in saliva and gastric juice. In the duodenum, the cobalamin-R binder complex is digested by pancreatic enzymes, and cobalamin is bound to intrinsic factor, a 60 kD protein made by gastric parietal cells. This cobalamin-intrinsic factor complex travels to the terminal ileum where it is absorbed by cells bearing specific receptors for the complex. Inside the intestinal mucosa, the intrinsic factor is degraded and cobalamin is bound to transcobalamin II, which transports the cobalamin through the blood to the liver for storage and marrow for use.

The most common causes of vitamin B_{12} deficiency are related to gastric disorders. Pernicious anemia is a familial autoimmune disease that attacks the parietal cells of the gastric fundus and body. H^+/K^+ ATPase is the most common target. Approximately 20% of the relatives of people with pernicious anemia have pernicious anemia. The gastric mucosa is infiltrated with inflammatory cells and the consequence of the chronic inflammation is atrophic gastritis. Atrophic gastritis is of two types, the antral-sparing type A associated with antibodies to parietal cells and intrinsic factor that cause achlorhydria and elevated gastrin levels, and the pangastritis (antrum involved) type B that occurs as a consequence of *Helicobacter pylori* infection associated with hypogastrinemia. Vitamin B_{12} deficiency is infrequent in type B gastritis, occurring only after many years of achlorhydria. Pernicious anemia may be associated with other autoimmune disorders including Hashimoto's thyroiditis, diabetes, Addison's disease, primary ovarian failure, Graves' disease, vitiligo, myasthenia gravis, Eaton-Lambert syndrome, and primary hypoparathyroidism. Patients are also at risk for gastric cancer and gastric carcinoid tumors. Chronic use of proton pump inhibitors (omeprazole [Prilosec]) and H_2 blockers to control gastroesophageal (GE) reflux is an increasingly common cause of achlorhydria and the inability to release vitamin B_{12} from food.

The recommended daily allowance for food folate is 400 μg (600 μg in pregnancy, 500 μg during lactation) and for vitamin B_{12} is 2.4 μg. Total body stores of folate are normally around 5 mg; vitamin B_{12} stores amount to approximately 4 mg.

Laboratory Testing in the Differential Diagnosis of Megaloblastic Anemia

The laboratory feature that most often identifies a patient with megaloblastic anemia is an elevated MCV on the automated complete blood count (CBC) in the setting of anemia. It is important to examine a peripheral blood smear in this setting. Macrocytosis is said to occur in two morphologic varieties: Megaloblastic erythropoiesis produces macro-ovalocytes (oval-shaped, large RBCs), but the presence of large RBCs of normal round shape is associated with alcoholism, renal or liver disease, or hypothyroidism in the absence of megaloblastic erythropoiesis. In megaloblastic anemia, anisocytosis and poikilocytosis are common. Another important reason for routinely examining the peripheral blood smear of an anemic patient is that 25% or greater of patients with vitamin B_{12} or folate deficiency may have concurrent iron deficiency. In this setting, the RBCs may be normal in size (the inhibition of hemoglobin synthesis compensates for the slow DNA synthesis), but a clue to the correct diagnosis will be apparent in the presence of hypersegmented neutrophils. Neutrophil hypersegmentation can be discerned in several ways: counting the lobes of 100 cells and dividing by 100 (level >3.5 is abnormal), finding 5% of the cells with five lobes (*rule of fives*), or finding a single cell with six or more lobes. Because folate deficiency and vitamin B_{12} deficiency are generally systemic problems affecting all dividing cells, patients with vitamin B_{12}- or folate-deficiency anemia have coincident pancytopenia in approximately 40% of cases. Furthermore, megaloblastic changes are apparent in the intestinal mucosa, oral mucosa, and cervical epithelium.

The first set of tests in the setting of a megaloblastic anemia is a serum vitamin B_{12} level, a red cell folate level, and a reticulocyte count. Folate and vitamin B_{12} deficiency states develop over time with tests becoming abnormal before the actual onset of anemia (Tables 1 and 2). Serum folate is a poor measure of tissue folate stores; RBC folate is a more reliable measure of folate availability for DNA synthesis. Folate deficiency is ruled out by an RBC folate level higher than 160 ng/mL, and folate deficiency is confirmed by levels less than 120 ng/mL. Vitamin B_{12} deficiency is ruled out by a serum level greater than 300 pg/mL and confirmed by levels less than 200 pg/mL. Reticulocyte counts are low. Marrow examination is generally not indicated unless folate and vitamin B_{12} levels are normal; in such a setting, a myelodysplastic syndrome must be ruled out by morphologic examination. In usual megaloblastic anemia, the marrow will be normocellular or hypercellular and erythroid precursors will be large with nuclear-cytoplasmic dissociation; that is, mature hemoglobinized cytoplasm with nuclei containing open rather than condensed chromatin. The effect on the granulocyte lineage is manifested by the presence of giant metamyelocytes. In maturation disorders (leukemias, myelodysplasias) that also affect cytoplasmic maturation, one can get delayed nuclear condensation together with slower than normal hemoglobinization. This morphologic change has been called *megaloblastoid*. This does not mean slightly megaloblastic; it refers to a particular picture of delayed nuclear and cytoplasmic maturation.

Other tests that support the diagnosis of megaloblastic anemia are elevated lactate dehydrogenase (LDH) and indirect bilirubin levels reflecting the intramedullary hemolysis of ineffective erythropoiesis.

Much has been written about the value of measuring homocysteine and methylmalonic acid levels in settings where the results of the vitamin measurements are equivocal. It is said that both of these metabolites are elevated in cobalamin deficiency whereas folate deficiency is more likely if homocysteine levels are elevated (>14 μM) and methylmalonic acid levels are normal (<270 nM or 0.4 μmol/L). However, in one study, 63% of cobalamin responsive patients did not have low cobalamin and high homocysteine and methylmalonic acid levels. Thus, as in many areas of medicine, clinical judgment is an important component of interpreting the laboratory tests.

Patients with cobalamin deficiency require additional testing to discern the cause. Antibodies to intrinsic factor that block binding to cobalamin are specific for pernicious anemia but are insensitive (positive in 70% of patients); antibodies to parietal cells are sensitive (positive in 90%) but not specific.

Unfortunately, the three most useful tests for diagnosing cobalamin deficiency and determining its cause are not routinely performed or available. The most sensitive indicator of cobalamin deficiency is serum levels of holo-transcobalamin II (transcobalamin II bound to vitamin B_{12}). Levels below 40 pg/mL are the first indication of vitamin B_{12} deficiency (see Table 2). Another extremely useful diagnostic test is the dU suppression test performed on bone marrow in vitro. As in Figure 1, for exogenously added dU to be able to suppress the incorporation of radiolabeled thymidine into DNA, the folate and vitamin B_{12} pathways need to be intact. In the setting of megaloblastic anemia, dU fails to optimally block thymidine incorporation. The particular nutrient that is lacking can be directly

---

TABLE 1 Laboratory Features of Folate Deficiency

	Normal	Folate Depletion	Folate Deficient Hematopoiesis	Folate Deficient Anemia
RBC folate (ng/ml)	>200	<160	<120	<100
PMN lobe average	<3.5	<3.5	>3.5	>3.5
RBC morphology	Normal	Normal	Normal	Macroovalocytes
MCV	Normal	Normal	Normal	>100 fL
Hemoglobin	Normal	Normal	Normal	<12 g/dL

TABLE 2 Laboratory Features of Vitamin B_{12} Deficiency

	Normal	Vitamin B_{12} Depletion	Vitamin B_{12} Deficient Hematopoiesis	Vitamin B_{12} Deficient Anemia
Holotranscobalamin II (pg/mL)	>50	<40	<40	<40
Serum B_{12} level (pg/ml)	>300	<300	<300	<150
Serum homocysteine	Normal	Normal or elevated	Elevated	Elevated
PMN lobe average	<3.5	<3.5	>3.5	>3.5
RBC morphology	Normal	Normal	Normal	Macroovalocytes
MCV	Normal	Normal	Normal	>100 Fl
Hemoglobin	Normal	Normal	Normal	<12 g/dL
Serum methylmalonate (µmol/L)	<0.4	<0.4	>0.4	>0.4

assessed in vitro by adding back either vitamin B_{12} or folate. The nutrient that restores the capacity of dU to inhibit thymidine incorporation is the deficient nutrient.

The third valuable and therapeutic diagnostic test is the Schilling test. This test and its variations can determine the mechanism of cobalamin malabsorption. The test involves injecting the cobalamin-deficient patient with a large dose of cobalamin intravenously or intramuscularly. The patient is then fed a radiolabeled dose of cobalamin (usually Co^{57} labeled). If less than 8% of the oral dose of radioactivity appears in the urine within 24 hours, the patient has a defect in absorption. If the feeding of intrinsic factor together with the labeled cobalamin results in an increased urinary excretion of labeled cobalamin (>8% in 24 hours), the patient has pernicious anemia. If not, the patient can be treated with antibiotics for 10 days to treat bacterial overgrowth. If this does not correct the malabsorption, ileal causes must be ruled out. Patients with the inability to release cobalamin from food may have normal excretion of oral labeled vitamin B_{12}. A variation on this test has been devised—but not yet clinically validated—in which one looks for a defect in releasing cobalamin from food by adding labeled vitamin B_{12} to a scrambled egg and assessing urinary excretion. People with achlorhydria excrete less than 8% in 24 hours.

Because of the unavailability of labeled vitamin B_{12} and the difficulty of 24-hour urine collections, the Schilling test is rarely performed. As a consequence of the general inadequacy of diagnostic tests, many clinicians favor an empirical therapeutic trial to confirm the diagnosis.

CURRENT DIAGNOSIS

- RBC morphology: macro-ovalocytes and hypersegmented neutrophils
- Vitamin levels assessment: Serum B_{12}, RBC folate
- Measurement of homocysteine and methylmalonic acid levels if vitamin levels are equivocal:
  If both are elevated, probably cobalamin deficiency
  If only homocysteine is elevated, probably folate deficiency
- Diagnosis of PA: In cobalamin deficiency, serum-blocking antibodies to intrinsic factor
- Empirical clinical trial may be indicated

Abbreviations: PA = pernicious anemia; RBC = red blood cell.

Treatment of Megaloblastic Anemia

An empirical therapeutic trial involves administering replacement doses of vitamin B_{12}[1] for 10 days while following the reticulocyte count. If daily intramuscular (IM) injections of 100 µg of cyanocobalamin[1] fail to produce a reticulocytosis, the process is repeated with oral folic acid in daily doses of 1 to 5 mg. If reticulocytosis is undocumented after the second 10 days, a bone marrow is performed looking for an alternative diagnosis such as myelodysplasia. Rare patients may have deficits in both nutrients (but it would be very unusual for none of the lab tests to suggest this possibility). Another cause of failure to respond might be inadequate levels of iron or erythropoietin to support vigorous red blood cell production.

For chronic replacement therapy in cobalamin deficiency, use either monthly IM injections of 1 mg[3] of

---

[1]Not FDA approved for this indication.
[3]Exceeds dosage recommended by the manufacturer.

CURRENT THERAPY

Cobalamin Deficiency
- Replenishment of stores: Cyanocobalamin 1 mg IM daily × 7, weekly × 3
- Chronic therapy: Cyanocobalamin 1 mg IM monthly or 2 mg PO daily or 500 µg intranasally weekly

Folate Deficiency
- Oral folate 1-5 mg per day until full recovery
- Prophylaxis in:
  Women contemplating pregnancy or lactating
  Women who have had a child with neural tube defects in the past
  People with hemolytic anemia or hemoglobinopathy
  People on renal dialysis
  Patients on methotrexate for a chronic inflammatory or autoimmune condition
- General Consideration
- Adequate iron stores and erythropoietin to support erythropoiesis
- Monitoring for hypokalemia and thrombocytosis

Abbreviations: IM = intramuscular injection; PO = orally.

cyanocobalamin (after initial daily therapy for 1 week and weekly therapy for 3 weeks) or daily oral administration of 2 mg. Oral therapy works because even without the normal mechanism of absorption, a small amount of a large dose will be absorbed by diffusion. Each approach has advantages and disadvantages; intramuscular injection is painful but reliable, oral medication is easier to take but adherence may be more erratic. Either approach should be monitored with serum B_{12} levels to assure compliance. A new alternative to these two approaches is the weekly administration of 500 µg (1 puff) intranasally. Lifelong treatment is essential unless a reversible cause is detected. Neurologic symptoms usually resolve over several months. Those that have not improved after one year are unlikely to be reversed.

Oral folate supplementation (1- to 5-mg tablet daily) should be provided until complete hematologic recovery is confirmed. Women who may become pregnant should take at least 400 µg of folate daily to prevent neural tube defects in the first trimester; usually pregnancy is not detected until after the risk period for these defects. Lactating women and people with hemolytic anemias, hyperproliferative hematologic states, or on dialysis and those on methotrexate for chronic inflammatory diseases like rheumatoid arthritis and psoriasis may need supplementation.

Replenishment of the deficient nutrient will produce a reticulocytosis in 3 to 7 days. During recovery of hematopoiesis, the rapid synthesis of new cells can produce hypokalemia. Therefore, serum K^+ should be followed and potassium supplements provided as needed. A more unusual response to therapy is thrombocytosis, which can lead to thrombotic complications in patients with other predisposing factors if the platelet count exceeds 1 million/µL.

Patients with pernicious anemia should be monitored for the development of other autoimmune diseases and should have stool guaiac tests at least annually to screen for gastric cancer.

REFERENCES

Baik HW, Russell RM: Vitamin B_{12} deficiency in the elderly. Annu Rev Nutr 1999;19:357-377.
Carmel R (ed.): Beyond megaloblastic anemia. Semin Hematol 1999;36:1-100.
Klee GG: Cobalamin and folate evaluation: Measurement of methylmalonic acid and homocysteine vs vitamin B_{12} and folate. Clin Chem 2000;46:1277-1283.
Solomon LR: Cobalamin-responsive disorders in the ambulatory care setting: Unreliability of cobalamin, methylmalonic acid, and homocysteine testing. Blood 2005;105:978-985.
Toh B-H, van Driehl IR, Gleeson PA: Pernicious anemia. N Engl J Med 1997;337:1441-1448.

Thalassemia

Method of
Susan P. Perrine, MD, and
Serguei A. Castaneda, MD

Pathophysiology: Basic Mechanisms of Hemoglobin Synthesis

The sequential expression of the globin genes results in production of specific types of hemoglobins at different stages of development. At 12 weeks of gestation, a transition from embryonic to fetal hemoglobin ($\alpha_2\gamma_2$) occurs, and at 28 weeks of gestation, increasing amounts of β-globin and of adult hemoglobin A (Hb A, $\alpha_2\beta_2$) are produced. α-Like globin protein must equal β-like globin proteins for intact hemoglobin tetramers to form. Thalassemia syndromes result from deficiencies in either α-globin (α-thalassemia) or β-like globin (β-thalassemia) chains. The diseases become apparent when the deficient globin is required during development. During gestation, α-thalassemia is symptomatic because α-globin is required for fetal hemoglobin (Hb F, $\alpha_2\gamma_2$). Because β-globin is not required in large amounts before birth, β-thalassemia is asymptomatic until approximately 6 months after birth. Mutations that cause prolonged production of fetal γ-globin chains may present later, at 2 to 4 years of age.

The major pathologic process in thalassemia is the imbalance of α- and non–α-globin chain accumulation. The unaffected chains, produced in normal amounts, precipitate during erythropoiesis. In β-thalassemia, the precipitated α-globin chains are particularly toxic, damaging cell membranes and causing rapid cell death (apoptosis). Red blood cell life span is further shortened by removal of abnormal cells in the reticuloendothelial system. Erythropoietin levels increase, causing erythroid hyperplasia. Hypersplenism causes more severe anemia.

In α-thalassemic fetuses, the unbalanced fetal (γ)-globin chains form tetramers (γ_4, hemoglobin Bart's); excess β-globin (β_4, hemoglobin H) accumulates after birth. Hemoglobin Bart's and hemoglobin H result in milder ineffective erythropoiesis but have abnormal oxygen binding. If all four α-globin genes are deleted, only hemoglobin Bart's is formed, with a massively left-shifted oxygen dissociation curve that provides no oxygen delivery to tissues and results in a lethal intrauterine condition, hydrops fetalis. Decreased production of α-globin from three or four abnormal α-globin genes causes moderate hemolytic anemia, hemoglobin H disease. Deletion of one (α-thalassemia-2) or two (α-thalassemia-1) loci is asymptomatic.

Thalassemia syndromes are graded according to severity of the anemia. Thalassemia major, in which severe anemia manifests during infancy, is caused by inheritance of two severely impaired β-globin alleles. Such homozygous or doubly heterozygous conditions have milder manifestations when there is an increase in fetal globin chain production or when the co-inheritance of α-thalassemia decreases the net imbalance of α-globin to β-globin. Thalassemia trait (inheritance of a single defective allele) is characterized by mild hypochromic, microcytic anemia and does not require treatment. Thalassemia intermedia causes moderate anemia with total hemoglobin levels of 6.0 to 10.0 g/dL. These patients require occasional transfusions with infections but do not require regular transfusions during childhood. Many thalassemia intermedia patients deteriorate later in life and develop similar complications as in thalassemia major.

Diagnosis

The diagnosis of severe thalassemia is usually straightforward in ethnic groups at risk (Mediterranean, African, Asian, Middle Eastern, East Indian) but occurs in any group. Thalassemia major and intermedia are marked by severe microcytic anemia; hyperbilirubinemia, elevated lactate dehydrogenase levels, and splenomegaly appear in the first few years of life. Hemoglobin A is absent on hemoglobin electrophoresis in β°-thalassemia and decreased in β+-thalassemia. Hydrops fetalis (α-thalassemia with classic four-gene deletions) presents as polyhydramnios and fetal distress during the second trimester. β-Thalassemia trait is characterized by mild anemia (hematocrit more than 30), low mean corpuscular volume (less than 75 fL), and erythrocytosis (red blood cell [RBC] count usually more than 5×10^6 per mm³) with elevated hemoglobins A_2 ($\alpha_2\delta_2$) and/or F. α-Thalassemia is most easily diagnosed by the presence of hemoglobin Bart's in cord blood. Hemoglobin H is unstable, and electrophoresis of fresh blood is required for its detection. Basophilic stippling, target cells, fragmented cells (schistocytes), and nucleated RBCs are typical of the severe thalassemias. The reticulocyte count may be relatively low because of ineffective erythropoiesis, and mean cell volume (MCV) may become high through skipped cell divisions. Prenatal diagnosis of thalassemia is performed by direct polymerase chain reaction (PCR) analysis of fetal DNA obtained by amniocentesis or chorionic villus sampling.

CURRENT DIAGNOSIS

- Microcytic anemia (MCV <80 fL)
- Blood smear: hypochromia, microcytes, target cells, nucleated RBCs
- (Hemoglobin H inclusion bodies) in α-thalassemia
- Quantitative hemoglobin electrophoresis
- α-Thalassemia: Hb Bart's (γ_4) in cord blood or Hb H (β_4) in fresh (not stored) blood specimens
- β-Thalassemia: elevated Hb F ($\alpha_2\gamma_2$), Hb A_2 ($\alpha_2\delta_2$), or both
  - β⁰⁰-Thalassemia: absence of Hb A ($\alpha_2\beta_2$)
  - β++-Thalassemia: decreased Hb A
- Hb E/β-thalassemia: Hb E and decreased or absent Hb A
- Molecular mutation analysis demonstrates two mutations in β-thalassemia major or thalassemia intermedia, and specific deletions in α-thalassemia
- Normal iron levels

Abbreviations: MCV = mean cell volume; HB = hemoglobin; RBC = red blood cell.

CURRENT THERAPY

Thalassemia Major

- Transfusions: 15 mL/kg PRBCs q3–4wk (to maintain total hemoglobin 10.5–13 g/dL)
- Splenectomy after 4–5 y of age, antibiotic prophylaxis
- Iron chelation: deferoxamine + deferiprone* + deferasirox†

*Orphan drug in the United States.
†FDA approved deferasirox in 2005.
Abbreviation: PRBC = packed red blood cell.

Transfusion Therapy

In β-thalassemia major, RBC transfusion is the mainstay of supportive therapy. Transfusions should maintain a hemoglobin level ideally above 10.5 to 11 g/dL (range, 10.5 to 13 g/dL) to suppress endogenous erythropoiesis, with the least amount of transfused blood required. Regular transfusions are begun for a persistent hemoglobin level below 7 g/dL in children with two β-thalassemic mutations or with severe α-thalassemia diagnosed in utero. A complete genotype of the patient's RBCs should be performed before transfusions are begun, to facilitate identification of involved antigens in the event of isoimmunization. Transfusions of 15 mL/kg of packed RBCs should be given at 3- to 4-week intervals using compatible blood from a limited donor pool and filtered to remove white blood cells. Cytomegalovirus (CMV)-negative preparations should be used for transplantation candidates. Acetaminophen and diphenhydramine before transfusions prevent febrile reactions. Transfusion records should be meticulously maintained to assess mean pre- and posttransfusion hemoglobin levels and annual blood consumption. An increase in transfusion requirements suggests hypersplenism, isoimmunization, or an accessory spleen.

Transfusions can transmit infections, including hepatitis viruses, human immunodeficiency virus (HIV), CMV, and other pathogens. Hepatitis C develops in 30% to 90% of transfused patients and advances to cirrhosis in 85%. Patients should be vaccinated against hepatitis A and B and monitored for elevated transaminase levels and hepatitis C antibodies. Combined treatment with PEG interferon alfa-2a or -2b and ribavirin produces sustained responses in hepatitis C. HIV testing should be performed annually.

Partial exchange transfusion by erythrocytapheresis, in which older red blood cells are exchanged for fresh packed red cells by pheresis, reduces iron accumulation compared to simple transfusion with iron chelation. Partial exchange transfusion by erythrocytapheresis does expose patients to more units of packed RBCs, minor side effects related to citrate, and requires two large vascular catheters for each monthly procedure, which can be limiting.

SPLENECTOMY

Splenectomy should be performed if a 40% or greater increase in the transfusion requirement occurs during a 1-year period, for a transfusion requirement greater than 200 mL/kg/year of packed RBCs without isoimmunization, or for thrombocytopenia. Splenectomy increases the risk of overwhelming sepsis with encapsulated organisms and *Yersinia* species, especially in young children, and, ideally, is deferred until children are 4 to 5 years of age. New infectious pathogens are a concern. Polyvalent pneumococcal vaccine should be given at least 1 month before splenectomy. Prophylactic oral Penicillin VK should be used in children younger than 10 years and for invasive (dental) procedures. Immediate medical attention should be sought and broad-spectrum antibiotics given emergently for significant fever (more than 38°C [101°F]) because patients are at risk for a fulminant course and death within hours.

COMPLICATIONS OF TRANSFUSION THERAPY

Approximately 1 mg of iron per mL of packed RBCs is administered in packed RBC transfusions, with no mechanism for elimination. Iron deposition causes dysfunction in the heart, liver, and endocrine organs. Glucose intolerance with insulin-dependent diabetes mellitus, primary hypothyroidism, hypoparathyroidism, delayed puberty, amenorrhea, and osteopenia are common; arrhythmias are often precipitated by cardiac hemosiderosis and hypocalcemia secondary to hypoparathyroidism. Growth retardation may respond to growth hormone before age 13 years. Hepatic iron and hepatitis C lead to fibrosis and cirrhosis.

Cardiac dysfunction is detectable early by cardiovascular magnetic resonance and effective transverse relaxation time (T2*) measurements less than 20 milliseconds (ms) as well as reduced ejection fractions. Presenting symptoms are fatigue, arrhythmias, or pericarditis, advancing to congestive heart failure (CHF), and arrhythmias. Cardiac events are the major cause of death in transfused patients (60%). Other causes are infections (13%) and liver disease, notably hepatitis C complications including hepatocellular carcinoma (6%). Pulmonary hypertension develops in both transfused thalassemia major and untransfused intermedia patients with hemolysis; a tricuspid regurgitation (TR) jet velocity less than 2 is associated with 25% mortality.

Osteopenia occurs in approximately 55% of thalassemia major and intermedia patients, may be severe and cause fractures, and even occurs in transfused patients in early childhood. Affected patients should be maintained on elemental calcium (1500 mg/day) and vitamin D (400 IU per day). Osteoporosis should be treated with bisphosphonates such as pamidronate (Aredia, 30 to 60 mg/month intravenous [IV]) or alendronate (Fosamax, 70 mg/week orally [PO]) and monitored with calcium, phosphate, 1,25-hydroxyvitamin D levels, 24-hour urinary calcium and hydroxyproline, and bone mineral density or dual-energy X-ray absorptiometry (DEXA) measurements annually.

MONITORING AND TREATMENT OF IRON OVERLOAD (see Table 1)

Although the parenteral iron chelator deferoxamine mesylate (Desferal) was the only first-line iron chelator available for many years, compliance is difficult, and oral iron chelators are better tolerated. Recently, the oral chelator deferiprone (L1) was definitively shown to provide superior chelation of cardiac iron, and it eliminated all cardiac events in patients treated over 8 years. Another oral iron chelator, deferasirox, was approved by the Food and Drug Administration (FDA) in 2005. Deferoxamine can maintain negative iron balance relative to the transfusion burden when administered five to seven times per week as a continuous subcutaneous or IV infusion, or as twice-daily bolus subcutaneous (not intramuscular) injections of the same total dose. Urinary iron excretion is used to adjust the dosage to maintain negative iron balance with deferoxamine. Although deferoxamine has been the only iron chelator available, cardiac failure has been the leading cause of death in thalassemia in the United States. Cardiac failure was eliminated from patients treated with deferiprone (L1) in seven thalassemia centers in Italy. Deferiprone has improved cardiac function in asymptomatic patients with impaired myocardial function and cardiac siderosis.

Iron overload should be documented by a challenge test after 12 to 18 months of regular transfusions because children require iron for growth, and chelation is detrimental for non-iron-overloaded patients. To begin chelation, iron in a 24-hour urine sample after 500 mg of deferoxamine subcutaneously should exceed 1 mg, or the serum ferritin level should consistently exceed 1000 µg/mL. Small infusion pumps are used for deferoxamine (20 to 60 mg/kg/day subcutaneously for 8 to 12 hours per night for 5 to 7 days per week), and it should be infused particularly at the time of blood transfusions, when significant iron is released from older transfused blood cells. Irritation and local reactions can be prevented by increasing the diluent to 2 mL per 500 mg of deferoxamine, hydrocortisone (2 mg/mL), or with topical diphenhydramine. A topical anesthetic cream should be applied 30 to 60 minutes before insertion of the needle. IV administration through an indwelling port device is often more tolerable because such devices can be accessed once weekly without repeated needle sticks. IV chelation is more effective, so fewer treatment days may suffice.

Arrhythmias and congestive heart failure have been reversed with high-dose deferoxamine in some patients (15 mg/kg/hour maximum for 24 hours per day, 7 days per week); the most effective treatment for cardiac iron overload is the combination of deferiprone and deferoxamine. Anaphylactic reactions can be treated with desensitization; idiosyncratic acute respiratory distress syndromes are rare but life-threatening, necessitating rapid recognition and intensive care. Excessive doses of deferoxamine can cause optic and acoustic neuritis, so ophthalmologic and hearing evaluations should be performed annually.

Iron overload causes depletion of vitamin C, which inhibits iron release from reticuloendothelial cells. Sudden availability of vitamin C can cause a massive release of iron and serious cardiotoxicity. Vitamin C (60 to 100 mg per day, to a maximum of 2 mg/kg/day PO) should be given only after the first cycle of deferoxamine in patients with reduced ascorbate levels. Despite deferoxamine therapy, 50% to 60% of transfused thalassemia patients have died of cardiac disease before 35 years of age.

New oral iron chelators offer major advantages. The oral chelator deferiprone (L1, Ferriprox,* 75 to

---

*Orphan drug in the United States.

100 mg/kg/day PO) has been approved in 47 countries outside North America and can be obtained on an individual treatment investigational new drug (IND) basis through the FDA (at the time of this submission) and ideally will be approved in North America soon as a first-line iron chelator.

Deferiprone crosses cell membranes more readily than deferoxamine does and selectively chelates cardiac iron, improves cardiac function, and prevents cardiac events. An international trial demonstrated that deferiprone does not promote hepatic fibrosis.

Another oral chelator deferasirox (Exjade) has shown efficacy in reducing hepatic iron overload at doses of 20 to 30 mg/kg/day PO, taken once daily, and was recently approved in the United States.

The most promising approach to managing iron overload is combined use of two chelators to produce a shuttle effect, using a bi- or tridentate chelator, such as deferiprone* that crosses membranes to mobilize iron from tissue compartments into the bloodstream, to exchange with a hexadentate "sink" such as deferoxamine. Combined use of deferiprone (75 mg/kg/day for 4 days per week) followed by deferoxamine (2 weekend days) produced greater iron excretion and reduced hepatic damage compared to deferoxamine alone and was accepted by patients who refused deferoxamine for 5 to 6 days per week. Other chelators in trials include 40SD02 (S-Desferal[4]), deferoxamine attached to a starch polymer, which can be given once per week IV, and deferritin (GT56-252). Deferasirox, deferiprone,[4] GT56-252,[4] and HBED[4] should all be useful in combination with deferoxamine because individual patients may respond differently to select chelators.

Serial ferritin levels should be followed every 3 to 6 months but *not correlated directly with cardiac iron*. Liver biopsy is used to assess hepatic iron and fibrosis but does not correlate with *cardiac* iron burden. Magnetic resonance imaging is available in selected centers. Myocardial T2* relaxation measurements less than 20 ms indicate ventricular dysfunction and impending failure. R2* correlates inversely with hepatic iron burden. Regularly updated information on medical centers that perform noninvasive imaging, deferiprone (L1) FDA Individual Treatment Use program, and open clinical trials is provided by the Cooley's Anemia Foundation (800-522-7222 or www.cooleysanemia.org).

THALASSEMIA INTERMEDIA

Patients with β-thalassemia who do not develop debilitating anemia should usually not be committed to a lifelong transfusion regimen, particularly when the hemoglobin levels remain above 8 g/dL. These patients generally have good exercise tolerability and feel well unless there is significant facial deformity from marrow expansion or other serious complication. Most specialists avoid regular transfusions at hemoglobin levels above 7 g/dL, particularly when the blood supply predictably transmits hepatitis C.

Intermittent transfusions are often necessary with infections and pregnancy and with increasing age.

Hypertransfusion can often be avoided by splenectomy. Patients should be monitored for marrow expansion, facial deformity, splenomegaly, growth retardation, endocrinopathies, and osteopenia. Pulmonary hypertension is a recently recognized risk, related to chronic hemolysis in untransfused patients. Tricuspid regurgitation (TR jet of less than 2 ms) is associated with a 25% mortality, for which transfusions should be instituted. Anemia, particularly in patients with high baseline Hb F levels (more than 65%) and erythropoietin levels (more than 130 mU/mL), often responds to experimental therapies to stimulate fetal globin production. Patients with β+ thalassemia and baseline erythropoietin levels less than 130 mU/mL require erythropoietin and a fetal globin stimulant.

The hyperplastic marrow in thalassemia intermedia stimulates intestinal iron absorption, and eventually, iron overload and endocrine deficiencies occur as in thalassemia major, although more slowly. Cardiomyopathy does not typically develop in untransfused patients. Avoidance of iron-rich meats and regular consumption of tea can reduce iron absorption. Osteopenia occurs in 55% of major and intermedia patients. Hypercoagulability and thromboembolic events may occur particularly in splenectomized patients, with conditions predisposing to thrombosis such as postoperative bedrest. This tendency is likely related to thrombocytosis, abnormalities in levels of coagulation factors, red cell membrane abnormalities that contribute to hypercoagulability, and hepatic dysfunction. Folic acid and antioxidant supplements should be used supportively.

Spinal cord compression syndromes from thoracic or vertebral paraspinal bone marrow masses should be suspected with acute or increasing weakness, numbness, and diminished reflexes in the lower extremities, and it constitutes a medical emergency. Diagnosis is made by magnetic resonance imaging (MRI) or computed tomography (CT); radiation therapy and steroids should be instituted emergently.

α-THALASSEMIA

The homozygous form of α-thalassemia is classically lethal in utero. Prenatal diagnosis and milder variants have enabled affected fetuses to be supported to term with intrauterine transfusions, followed by regular postnatal transfusions. For milder hemoglobin H disease, only folic acid, antioxidants, and monitoring for severe anemia during infections or with increasing splenomegaly are necessary. Because hemoglobin H is sensitive to oxidant stress, drugs such as sulfonamides should be avoided, particularly with coexistent glucose-6-phosphate dehydrogenase (G6PD) deficiency. Iron status should be monitored.

TRANSPLANTATION

Allogeneic bone marrow or stem cell transplantation is curative by replacing the patient's hematopoietic stem cells with normal stem cells, which contain normal β-globin genes or one normal and one thalassemic globin gene. Transplantation from a histocompatibility leukocyte antigen (HLA)-identical related donor in patients younger than 8 years, without hepatic fibrosis, and good iron chelation (risk class 1) has an excellent prognosis. The overall mortality rate of transplantation in experienced centers is still approximately 15%, and significant morbidity can

*Orphan drug in the United States.
[4]Not yet approved for use in the United States.

TABLE 1 Recommended Monitoring of Thalassemia Patients

Monitoring of Patients Undergoing Regular Transfusions	Cardiac Monitoring After 5 Years of Transfusions	Monitoring of Endocrine and Osteoporosis	Monitoring of Effects of Deferoxamine Therapy
Red blood cell phenotype (before transfusions)	Echocardiogram, ECG annually	TSH, free T_4 parathormone, calcium, inorganic	Ophthalmologic and hearing evaluation annually
History, monthly physical examination	T2* (cardiac MRI)	phosphorus, growth hormone levels annually	Sitting and standing height, weight q4–6mo until 18 y
Pre- and post-transfusion CBC and record of amounts of each transfusion	24-hour Holter or event monitor (for patients >12 y)	Glucose tolerance test, Cortrosyn stimulation test annually	of age
Indirect antibody screen twice annually or with a positive Coombs test result on crossmatch	Cardiology consultation, stress test (for patients >18 y)	Gonadotropins and estradiol or testosterone after 12 y of age	Zinc, copper, selenium, vitamin C, and vitamin E levels q4–6mo
Liver function studies (ALT, AST, bilirubin, LDH, alkaline phosphatase, albumin, total protein, and ferritin q3mo)		Bone mineral density test or DEXA, bone age annually	Urinary iron excretion annually or biannually and dose adjustment
Hepatitis A and B panels (before vaccine)		24-h urine calcium, creatinine, hydroxyproline annually	
Hepatitis C antibody (mRNA by PCR if antibody positive) and HIV test annually		Serum calcium, phosphorus, alkaline phosphatase, 1,25-hydroxyvitamin D level twice annually	
INR and PTT annually			
Liver biopsy, after 5 y of transfusions or with hepatomegaly, to assess iron content and fibrosis			
T2* and R2* MRI of hepatic and cardiac iron			

Abbreviations: ALT = alanine aminotransferase; AST = aspartate aminotransferase; CBC = complete blood cell count; ECG = electrocardiogram; GGT = gamma-glutamyltransferase; HIV = human immunodeficiency virus; INR = international normalized ratio; LDH = lactate dehydrogenase; MRI = magnetic resonance imaging; PCR = polymerase chain reaction; PT = prothrombin time; PTT = partial thromboplastin time; TSH = thyroid-stimulating hormone.

result from graft-versus-host disease (GVHD). Unrelated donors and cord blood as sources of donor cells have increased risks of GVHD and graft rejection but provide broader availability. Relapses (graft rejection) occur in 8% of patients receiving related donor transplants.

Because many patients do well clinically even with mixed chimeric states, less myeloablative preparative regimens are being evaluated in patients of higher risk classes to reduce morbidity. The serious risks of this curative treatment modality must be weighed against the lifelong burden of transfusion and chelation. This balance may be shifted with the approval of oral iron chelators.

STIMULATION OF FETAL GLOBIN GENE SYNTHESIS AND ERYTHROPOIESIS

A large body of evidence shows that reactivating fetal globin to approximately 60% to 70% of α-globin chain synthesis ameliorates anemia in β-thalassemia enough to eliminate transfusion requirements. Chemotherapeutic agents (hydroxyurea and 5-azacytidine or decitabine), short chain fatty acid (SCFA) derivatives, and rHu

erythropoietin (EPO) are being evaluated in clinical trials with the highest hematologic responses observed in patients with baseline (untransfused) Hb F levels greater than 50% and erythropoietin levels greater than 130 mU/mL. Combinations of these agents will likely be required to eliminate regular transfusion requirements in severe β-thalassemia patients. Nonmutagenic, noncytotoxic agents are preferable over chemotherapy for lifelong treatment. Sodium phenylbutyrate (Buphenyl*) and arginine butyrate* have increased total hemoglobin by 1 to 4 g/dL above baseline in untransfused patients but require large numbers of tablets or IV infusion, respectively. Patients with β^+ thalassemia and baseline EPO levels less than 80 mU/mL have responded best to combined therapy with butyrate and EPO. The long-acting EPO preparation darbepoetin (Aranesp) increases hemoglobin in some. These therapies require supplementation with oral iron to be effective, even in the presence of elevated ferritin levels, because stored iron may not be available for erythropoiesis, and several months of treatment are

*Orphan drug in the United States.

often required. New oral SCFA derivatives under evaluation appear more tolerable.

Gene Transfer

Gene therapy for β-thalassemia requires transfer of the fetal (γ) or a normal β-globin gene into repopulating hematopoietic stem cells and high-level expression of transferred genes with their regulatory elements, solely in erythrocytes. This transgene must be integrated at sites that allow high-level expression throughout life, a formidable challenge. Problems that must be surmounted include production of safe, effective vectors for long-term treatment, prevention of silencing of transduced genes, difficulty in transducing rare pluripotent repopulating stem cells, selective expansion of transduced stem cells, and ablative chemotherapy prior to infusion of transfected cells to create space for expansion of transduced stem cells. Progress is being made in all these areas. Clinical trials of gene therapy with limited endpoints, such as mobilization and harvesting of stem cells, are projected to begin in 2006–2007.

REFERENCES

Aessopos A, Farmakis D, Deftereos S, et al: Thalassemia heart disease: A comparative evaluation of thalassemia major and thalassemia intermedia. Chest 2005;127:1523-1530.

Anderson LJ, Wonke B, Prescott E, et al: Comparison of effects of oral deferiprone and subcutaneous desferrioxamine on myocardial iron concentrations and ventricular function in beta-thalassaemia. Lancet 2002;360:516-520.

Borgna-Pignatti C, Cappellini MD, DeStefano P, et al: Cardiac morbidity and mortality in deferoxamine- or deferiprone-treated patients with thalassemia major. Online first edition paper in Blood, December 22, 2005.

Cohen AR, Galanello R, Piga A, et al: Safety profile of the oral iron chelator deferiprone: A multicentre study. Br J Haematol 2000;108(2):305-312.

Cunningham MJ, Macklin EA, Neufeld EJ, Cohen AR: Complications of beta-thalassemia major in North America. Blood 2004;104:34-39.

Eldor A, Rachmilewitz EA: The hypercoagulable state in thalassemia. Blood 2002;99:36-43.

Giardina PJ, Grady RW: Chelation therapy in beta-thalassemia: An optimistic update. Semin Hematol 2001;38:360-366.

Hershko C, Cappellini MD, Galanello R, et al: Purging iron from the heart. Br J Haematol 2004;125:545-551.

Pennell DJ, Berdoukas V, Karagiora M, et al: Randomized controlled trial of deferiprone or deferoxamine in beta thalassemia major patients with asymptomatic myocardial siderosis. Online first edition paper in Blood, December 13, 2005.

Piga A, Gaglioti C, Fogliacco E, Tricta F: Comparative effects of deferiprone and deferoxamine on survival and cardiac disease in patients with thalassemia major: A retrospective analysis. Haematologica 2003;88:489-496.

Schrier SL, Angelucci E: New strategies in the treatment of the thalassemias. Annu Rev Med 2005;56:157-171.

Voskaridou E, Terpos E, Spina G, et al: Pamidronate is an effective treatment for osteoporosis in patients with beta-thalassaemia. Br J Haematol 2003;123:730-737.

Wonke B: Clinical management of beta-thalassemia major. Semin Hematol 2001;38:350-359.

Management Issues in Sickle Cell Disease

Method of
Kenneth R. Bridges, MD

Sickle cell disease (SCD) reflects substitution of a valine residue for glutamic acid at position 6 in the beta subunit of hemoglobin. With a few minor exceptions, people with one gene for hemoglobin S (Hb S) are phenotypically normal (sickle trait). Two Hb S genes produce sickle cell disease. Two important compound heterozygous states, sickle–β-thalassemia and sickle/hemoglobin C, also produce sickle disease pathology.

The mechanism by which these changes in the physical properties of the hemoglobin molecule produce the clinical manifestations of the disease is not unequivocally proven. The most widely accepted hypothesis is that erythrocytes deform as they release their oxygen in the capillaries and are trapped in the microcirculation. The blockade of blood flow produces areas of tissue ischemia, leading to the myriad of clinical problems seen with sickle cell disease.

Other cells in the circulation probably moderate the severity of sickle cell disease manifestations. High neutrophil counts correlate with a worse prognosis in sickle cell disease. Platelets and abnormally circulating endothelial cells might also adversely affect severity. Chronic damage to endothelial cells lining vessel walls could increase the risk of injury because of erythrocyte adhesion. Inflammatory cytokines also seem to mediate some problems in sickle cell disease.

Sickle cell disease is extremely varied in its manifestations. A study of the natural history of the disorder indicated that approximately 5% of patients account for nearly 33% of hospital admissions. Although the disease can be incapacitating, many people have few admissions and live productive and relatively healthy lives. The average life expectancy with sickle cell disease is below normal for the population, however, reflecting increased mortality attributed to the complications of the disease. Fortunately, improved care is lengthening life span.

Clinically, sickle cell disease is best thought of as two disorders, one involving children and one involving adults. With the exception of acute crisis pain, the manifestations of the two are largely different. Pediatric sickle cell disease is more of a purely hematologic disorder in which the pathophysiology derives directly from erythrocyte sickling. Because sickling is reversible, many of the associated problems are reversible, including vaso-occlusive pain episodes, splenic sequestration, and aplastic crisis. Chronic, fixed-organ damage comes to dominate the adult clinical picture. Renal dysfunction, avascular necrosis of bone, and chronic lung disease are gargantuan issues reflecting chronic injury. Therapeutic approaches must factor in these differences.

The advent of therapies that can significantly ameliorate the clinical course of sickle cell disease opens the possibility of early intervention. Multivariate clinical analysis of nearly 400 children followed at comprehensive sickle cell centers between infancy and 10 years of age

TABLE 1   Hydroxyurea Therapy in Sickle Cell Disease

Eligibility for Hydroxyurea	Clinical Indications for Hydroxyurea
Five years of age or older	Recurrent vaso-occlusive pain crises. Patients with three or more pain crises per year should be considered for hydroxyurea management.
Not pregnant	Recurrent acute chest syndrome Frequent or chronic transfusion requirement

uncovered several factors that augured a severe clinical course (Box 1). Children who manifest these characteristics should be considered for aggressive early treatment of their sickle cell disease. The special relationship of stroke risk to high blood velocity in the intracranial arteries is discussed later.

The Hydroxyurea Era of Sickle Cell Disease Management

Hydroxyurea (Hydrea) is the most important advancement in the care of people with sickle cell disease since the 1986 introduction of prophylactic penicillin. No message is more important than the need to assess *all* patients for possible treatment with hydroxyurea. The drug is neither investigational nor an esoteric intervention that is the province of sickle cell disease specialists. Hydroxyurea therapy is not appropriate for all people with sickle cell disease nor is it effective in everyone for whom it is tried. The medication can dramatically alter the clinical course of many patients, however. No vaticinator can augur which patients will respond to hydroxyurea. Consequently, the clinician is obliged to affirm that no patient who might benefit from hydroxyurea is neglected.

Every physician who cares for people with sickle cell disease must freshly visit the broad clinical picture of their patients with an eye toward a possible trial of hydroxyurea. Only when every patient has been considered for hydroxyurea, whether the drug is eventually used or not, will management attain standard-of-care status. The facts are that in a cohort of patients:

- Hydroxyurea reduces painful crises by half.
- Hydroxyurea reduces hospital stays for painful crises by half.
- Hydroxyurea reduces acute chest syndrome (ACS) by half.
- Hydroxyurea reduces transfusion requirements.

Hydroxyurea seems to lower mortality in sickle cell disease. Table 1 is a broad template against which each patient should be compared. For patients not needing hydroxyurea, the issue should be reviewed yearly. Pediatric studies confirm hydroxyurea safety in children 5 years of age and older. The drug seems more efficacious in children than in adults, and hydroxyurea should be a major focus in the management of pediatric sickle cell disease.

Although thrombocytopenia and/or neutropenia are relative contraindications, close monitoring allows nearly all patients to tolerate the medication. Bimonthly blood counts are required when patients are started on hydroxyurea. Occasionally, the hematocrit increases to the high 30s or even low 40s in response to hydroxyurea therapy necessitating dose reduction. No conclusive evidence exists to support hydroxyurea as prophylaxis against stroke, chronic leg ulcers, priapism, or other complications of sickle cell disease.

The dose of hydroxyurea needed to prevent painful crises is unknown. In the Multicenter Study of Hydroxyurea in Sickle Cell Anemia (MSH), patients received the maximum tolerated dose (MTD). The dose administered was increased stepwise until signs of toxicity, such as mild neutropenia, developed. The dose of hydroxyurea was then reduced slightly. Whether such intense treatment is required is unknown. Some specialists use lower doses of hydroxyurea (e.g., 25 mg/kg/day) with good success. Most patients treated with hydroxyurea develop macrocytosis (e.g., mean corpuscular volume = 110). Fleetingly few patients have thrombocytopenia or neutropenia at this medication dose. The therapeutic window is excellent for hydroxyurea in sickle cell disease.

Management of Acute Problems

PAIN

Vaso-occlusive pain episodes experienced by patients with sickle cell disease vary tremendously in frequency and severity. The cooperative study of the natural history of sickle cell disease showed that approximately 5% of patients accounted for 33% of hospital days devoted to pain control. To complicate matters further, the pattern of pain varies over time, so that a patient who has particularly severe problems one year might later have a prolonged period characterized by only minor pain.

The onset of sickle cell pain crises likewise varies in pattern. Patients can develop agonizingly severe pain in as little as 15 minutes without prevenient problems. In other cases, the pain gradually evolves over hours or even days. Patients manage most episodes of pain at home. Oral analgesics along with rest and fluids often allow people to "ride out" the pain episode. Some patients report that warm baths or warm compresses applied to aching joints ameliorate the severity of the pain.

The sites affected in acute painful crises vary. Pain usually occurs in the extremities, thorax, abdomen, and back. Pain tends to recur at the same site for a particular person. For each person, the quality of the crisis pain is usually similar from one crisis to another. During the evaluation, the provider should inquire whether the pain feels like "typical" sickle cell pain. Most patients can distinguish back pain caused by pyelonephritis or abdominal pain caused by cholecystitis, for instance, from their typical sickle cell pain. If the quality of the pain is not typical of their sickle cell disease, other causes should be investigated before ascribing it to vaso-occlusion.

No reliable objective index of pain exists. The provider depends solely on the patient's report. One of the most difficult problems that patients with sickle cell disease face is seeking treatment for pain in a setting in which they are unknown. Some providers mistakenly believe that the number of deformed sickle cells on the peripheral blood smear reflects the degree of patient pain. Other providers look to parameters such as blood pressure and heart rate. Although the latter measures provide more information than the peripheral smear, they do not reliably reflect pain severity. Trust in the patient report is key to the management of sickle cell pain crises.

Opioids

Vaso-occlusive sickle pain typically is severe in character. Most patients describe a major crisis as the most intense pain that they have ever experienced relative even to childbirth, the general touchstone of pain intensity. Pain control often requires large quantities of opioid analgesics. The exact amount varies, and depends in part on the frequency with which the person requires opioids. For many patients, 4 to 8 mg[3] of hydromorphone (Dilaudid) can be given as an intravenous bolus over 15 to 20 minutes followed by another 4 mg in 30 minutes if pain control is inadequate. More restrained dosing of opioids is indicated for patients naive to this class of drug. Two to four milligrams of hydromorphone every 30 to 45 minutes often suffices.

Pain relief occurs more slowly with intramuscular injections, and the injections themselves can produce substantial discomfort. Consequently, intravenous administration of analgesics is usually preferable. As pain control improves, the analgesia should be maintained to prevent symptom rebound. "PRN" (as needed) analgesic administration should be avoided. After stabilization of the emergency situation with intravenous boluses of opioids, the patient should be transferred to the floor and prescribed a maintenance regimen. Patient-controlled analgesia (PCA) often works well for pain relief. Patients can become drowsy as their pain is controlled. Often, this reflects the fatigue that comes with one or more sleepless nights with pain at home. The analgesics should not be discontinued automatically for somnolence as long as the patient is easily aroused. In addition to analgesia, patients with painful crises should also receive supplemental oxygen and intravenous fluids. Once the pain is under control, oral hydration can replace the intravenous fluids.

Meperidine (Demerol) can present problems for pain control with sickle cell disease. The half-life of the drug in the circulation is approximately 4 hours. The liver converts meperidine to normeperidine, a derivative that has analgesic activity but which also is toxic. Grand mal seizure is a particularly serious complication that occurs with the administration of large amounts of meperidine. Normeperidine likely is the primary culprit. Other opioid analgesics, therefore, are preferable to meperidine. The American Pain Society recommends that meperidine no longer be used to control pain requiring long-term or recurrent opioid analgesic treatment.

Eventually the patient should be switched to oral opioid analgesics, which might be necessary for a week or more after discharge. The parenteral analgesics should be tapered after the oral medication starts. Abrupt termination of parenteral analgesics when oral medications are begun can cause resurgence in sickle cell crisis pain. Patients should have a supply of analgesics at home (that might include opioids) to control less severe episodes of pain.

Epidural analgesia clearly controls acute sickle cell crisis pain. This approach is most effective when the major discomfort is below chest level. Although some patients receive good relief with epidural analgesia alone, others continue to require systemic analgesics, albeit at lower doses. Some patients have a psychological aversion to having infusion hardware introduced into their backs and balk at epidural analgesia, despite its superior pain relief relative to systemic analgesics.

Undermedication in emergency care settings is the most prevalent problem with respect to sickle cell disease pain management. Further antagonizing matters, patients often wait hours for attention before receiving inadequate doses of analgesics. Health care providers must guard against this fault and provide timely and adequate analgesic care to these vulnerable patients.

Nonsteroidal Anti-Inflammatory Drugs (NSAIDs)

Recently, NSAIDs have been added to the management algorithm of acute sickle cell pain with ketorolac tromethamine[1] (Toradol) occupying a prominent place. Existing clinical reports are largely anecdotal. Although some are positive, others show no effect of ketorolac in the treatment of acute vaso-occlusive pain crises. Ketorolac can produce gastritis and bleeding. The drug should be used cautiously in patients with peptic ulcer disease or a history of gastrointestinal bleeding. NSAIDs can impair kidney function and accelerate the renal injury intrinsic sickle cell disease. Consequently, an increasing number of specialists eschew NSAIDs in sickle cell disease management.

Transfusion

The complex pathophysiology of sickle cell disease confounds this intuitively rational approach to a problem deriving from deformed erythrocytes. Vaso-occlusive sickle cell crises are probably fueled, at least in part, by sluggish blood flow through the microcirculation. Slow blood flow promotes deoxygenation of hemoglobin and exacerbates red cell deformation. Although the oxygen-carrying capacity of blood increases with hematocrit, so does viscosity. As the hematocrit increases beyond the range of the low 30s, increased viscosity might outweigh enhanced oxygen delivery conferred by allogeneic blood transfusion and swing the dynamics toward sickling.

---

[3]Exceeds dosage recommended by the manufacturer.

[1]Not FDA approved for this indication.

Sporadic transfusion is not an effective intervention for the management of acute painful episodes in patients with sickle cell disease. Exchange transfusion has been used in attempts to alleviate bouts of severe, intractable pain with better effect, overall. Chronic transfusion for pain is more effective in children, for whom erythrocyte sickling is the dominant issue, than among adults, for whom fixed-organ damage is often a primary cause of pain.

Corticosteroids[1]

Reports exist of significant improvement in pain profile among children receiving large doses of intravenous steroids on each of the first 2 days of their painful sickle crises. Opioid analgesic requirements halved. The rate of pain relapse was significantly higher among patients who received steroid treatment, however. This intriguing observation awaits confirmation, particularly in adults with sickle cell disease. The observation is consistent with the idea that inflammatory cytokines are important in the pathophysiology of sickle cell disease.

ACUTE CHEST SYNDROME

ACS is difficult to diagnose because its etiology varies and its manifestations are variegated. Common characteristics include fever, dyspnea, cough, and pulmonary infiltrates. The infiltrates can have a lobar distribution, but often are bilateral. Sometimes, the pulmonary picture is one of diffuse, hazy opacities that resemble adult respiratory distress syndrome. In other cases, ACS looks like a simple pneumonia. This problem in diagnosis is aggravated by the fact that infectious agents such as viruses, bacteria, and mycoplasma can trigger the syndrome. Bone marrow infarction with secondary pulmonary fat emboli also can trigger the acute chest syndrome. In most instances, the etiology of ACS is a mystery.

The arterial blood oxygen saturation is key to the diagnosis of acute chest syndrome. Values often decrease to a greater degree than occurs with a simple pneumonia of the same magnitude. Patients with acute chest syndrome often have progressive pulmonary infiltrates despite treatment with antibiotics. Infection can set off a wave of local ischemia that produces focal sickling, deoxygenation, and additional sickling.

The microcirculatory vessels in the lung tend to constrict with hypoxia rather than dilate, as occurs with vessels in other parts of the body. Regions of vascular constriction can worsen microcirculatory occlusion. Consequently, bronchodilators are important components of the treatment regimen. Unchecked, ACS can produce cardiovascular collapse and death. ACS occurs more often in children than adults. People who survive an episode of ACS have a high propensity for future attacks. Patients who have recurrent episodes of ACS are prone to develop chronic lung insufficiency.

The most important step in the treatment of ACS is to recognize the disorder. Potential pneumonia in sickle cell patients should be treated with appropriate antibiotics. When symptoms progress, particularly in concert with

---

[1]Not FDA approved for this indication.

decreasing arterial oxygen saturation and worsening of the chest roentgenogram, acute chest syndrome must be considered. Blood gases are vital. Pulse oximetry provides limited information and particularly lacks crucial data on blood carbon dioxide levels and pH. A relentless decrease in arterial oxygenation is a harbinger of acute chest syndrome and demands urgent action.

Transfusion is key to the treatment of acute chest syndrome. Exchange transfusion is one option. The procedure involves exchange of the total blood volume and is done most efficiently using a pheresis machine. When a pheresis setup is not available, sequential transfusion/phlebotomy can be performed. A hemoglobin electrophoresis should be sent before the exchange transfusion. A second should be sent after the procedure. The object is to ensure that the exchange has reduced the percentage of Hb S cells to less than 30%. Patients can improve substantially within hours of an exchange.

Increasing arterial oxygenation and decreasing dyspnea usually augur recovery. The chest roentgenogram typically lags behind the clinical status. Because a bacterial pneumonia rarely can be excluded in these patients, most receive concomitant broad-spectrum antibiotics. Simple transfusion works as well, particularly with low starting hemoglobin values, which often exist. Simple transfusion alone decreases the fraction of sickle cells in the circulation.

Delayed transfusion reaction is a serious potential problem with exchange transfusion. Most patients with sickle cell disease are of African ancestry. Most of the blood available for transfusion comes from people of European descent. A number of minor red cell antigens are expressed at different frequencies in these two groups. Repeated transfusion of any African American can induce antibodies directed against these minor antigens. Transfusion with blood containing the offending antigen often rekindles formerly undetectable antibody production. With exchange transfusion, a large fraction of the circulating red cells can be destroyed in a deadly delayed transfusion reaction. Antibody screening should be repeated 3 to 4 weeks after the exchange transfusion to look for new alloantibodies to minor antigens.

INFECTION

Patients with sickle cell disease are susceptible to overwhelming infection. The most significant factor is splenic autoinfarction during childhood that leaves patients vulnerable to infections with encapsulated organisms such as *Streptococcus pneumoniae* and *Haemophilus influenzae*. Furthermore, some studies suggest that neutrophils do not function properly in patients with sickle cell disease. How the hemoglobin mutation might produce neutrophil dysfunction is unclear.

Patients with sickle cell disease and unexplained fever should be cultured thoroughly. If the scenario suggests septicemia, the best action is to start broad-spectrum antibiotics after complete culturing. Signs of systemic infection include fever, shaking chills, lethargy, malaise, and hypotension. A high baseline WBC is common in sickle cell disease. An increase above that baseline is concerning. Large numbers of bands means infection until proven otherwise. Patients with septicemia can expire in only a few hours.

ACUTE BONE MARROW NECROSIS

Acute bone marrow necrosis is recognized more often as a complication of sickle cell disease, in part because of improved methods of detection. Magnetic resonance imaging (MRI) techniques are most important in this regard. Bone marrow should have the density of other body tissues on MRI scans. With bone marrow necrosis, marrow liquefaction is easily detected on scan.

Patients with bone marrow necrosis often have excruciatingly severe pain. Some patients require drastic measures, such as epidural anesthesia to control wrenchingly intense pain. Acute bone marrow necrosis, frequently involving marrow of the ribs, femur, or tibia, produces "the worst pain I've ever experienced."

A decreasing hemoglobin level caused by marrow injury and the explosive release of immature cells into the circulation, including a plethora of nucleated red blood cells, are key findings. Exchange transfusion has been used with success in some patients with acute bone marrow necrosis. The experience is anecdotal, because the ability to document bone marrow necrosis is a relatively recent development. Pulmonary fat emboli can complicate bone marrow necrosis. Fat emboli can trigger respiratory insufficiency or even acute chest syndrome.

STROKE

Strokes are much more common in children than in adults, with an average age of approximately 4 years. The process that occludes large arteries such as the internal carotid or the middle cerebral remains mysterious in nature. Imaging procedures such as angiography and noninvasive magnetic resonance angiography (MRA) frequently show arterial narrowing near sharp vessel bends. Paradoxically, the higher rate of blood flow produced by arterial narrowing is believed to contribute to the risk of complete arterial occlusion. A complete occlusion at critical locations produces massive strokes. Erythrocyte sickling is not the cause of occlusive stroke because well-oxygenated regions of arterial circulation with high rates of blood flow are the key sites.

The Stroke Prevention Trial in Sickle Cell Anemia (STOP) enrolled 130 subjects, 2 to 16 years of age, who were at high risk for stroke on the basis of increased cerebral blood flow rates measured by transcranial doppler (TCD) screening tests (≥200 cm/second time averaged mean velocities). Children were randomized to receive either standard supportive care or periodic blood transfusions. The primary endpoint was stroke incidence in the treated and control groups. A 90% relative decrease in the stroke rate in the transfused patients prompted early termination of the investigation.

The STOP trial confirmed that TCD can identify children with sickle cell anemia at high risk for first-time stroke and that prophylactic transfusion reduces stroke risk. Because the greatest risk of stroke occurs in early childhood, children 2 to 16 years of age should be considered for TCD screening. Standardization issues involving TCD approaches and proper technical training remain major obstacles to the widespread use of this screening technique. Screening should be conducted at a site where clinicians have been trained to provide TCDs of comparable quality and information content to those used in the STOP trial.

Stroke in SCD is a medical emergency. The deficits are often profound, although many children recover substantial function. Exchange transfusion followed by maintenance hypertransfusion is mandatory. This action improves recovery and reduces the risk of recurrent stroke. In the absence of this intervention, as many as 66% of children will have subsequent events. The optimal duration of therapy is unclear. Several studies have shown that as many as 50% of children on maintenance therapy for as long as 5 years have new strokes within months of stopping treatment.

In adults, hemorrhagic stokes are more common than arterial occlusive strokes. Subarachnoid hemorrhages are most prevalent. The pathophysiology of thrombotic stroke in adults is as mysterious as in children. Nonetheless, exchange transfusion followed by maintenance hypertransfusion is a prudent course of action. No existing data address duration of therapy in adults.

SPLENIC SEQUESTRATION CRISIS

Splenic sequestration crisis is an almost exclusively pediatric issue that reflects acute splenic entrapment of a large blood volume. The manifestations are left upper quadrant pain and exacerbated anemia. In children, a large fraction of the circulating blood volume is frequently sequestered, making cardiovascular collapse a risk. Splenic sequestration crisis is a medical emergency that demands prompt and appropriate treatment. Parents should be familiar with the signs and symptoms of splenic sequestration crisis and know the basic techniques of splenic palpation. Children should be seen as speedily as possible in the emergency room. Circulatory collapse and death can occur in less than 30 minutes.

The treatment of splenic sequestration crisis entails intravenous fluids and transfusion as necessary to maintain the intravascular volume. A child who has one episode of splenic sequestration crisis is at greater risk of a second attack. Specialists debate whether children who survive an episode of splenic sequestration crisis should undergo splenectomy after their recovery. Consensus favors splenectomy after a second event.

APLASTIC CRISIS

Aplastic crisis is a potentially deadly complication primarily in pediatric sickle cell disease that develops when erythrocyte production temporarily decreases. Infection with parvovirus B-19 frequently is the culprit in aplastic crises. This adeno-associated virus causes "fifth disease," a normally benign childhood disorder associated with fever, malaise, and a mild rash. The virus has a tropism for erythroid progenitor cells and impairs cell division for a few days during the infection. Normal people experience, at most, a slight decrease in hematocrit because the half-life of erythrocytes in the circulation is 40 to 60 days. People with hemolytic anemias maintain reasonable hematocrits only through prodigious production of new red cells. Diminished erythroid production for a few days in these patients can produce potentially deadly decreases in hematocrit. Often, but not always, aplastic crises coincide with painful crises. The reticulocyte count of patients with sickle cell disease should be checked on admission to the emergency room or to the hospital. The treatment of aplastic crisis is purely supportive, with transfusions to maintain an acceptable hematocrit until marrow activity resumes.

HEPATIC SEQUESTRATION CRISIS

Sickled cells can lodge in the liver, obstructing blood flow through the organ. Painful hepatic enlargement accompanied by an increase in the plasma levels of hepatic synthetic enzymes (e.g., alanine aminotransferase, aspartate transaminase) is the result. The serum bilirubin levels often skyrocket to levels in the range of 30 to 40 mg/dL. Acute hepatic failure can ensue. Fluids, oxygen, and analgesia are the management interventions frequently undertaken. The benefit of more aggressive measures such as exchange transfusion is unknown.

MULTIORGAN FAILURE SYNDROME

Multiorgan failure syndrome is one of the most deadly complications of sickle cell disease, occurring both in children and adults. Pain frequently brings the victim to immediate attention where clinical events quickly highlight the gravity of the situation vis-à-vis "ordinary" sickle cell disease crisis. Decreasing arterial oxygen saturation accompanied by patchy lung opacities shows the condition to be more akin to acute chest syndrome. Decreasing hemoglobin values are typical. Decreasing renal function manifested by increasing blood urea nitrogen (BUN) and serum creatinine values along with oliguria bodes ill. Mental status changes often manifested as somnolence and confusion punctuate the dire nature of the condition. Exchange transfusion along with other supportive measures such as ventilator support and antibiotics early in the course sometimes reverses an otherwise grim scenario.

PRIAPISM

Priapism is a potentially serious problem for young men with sickle cell disease. The condition is believed to result from impaired blood egress from the corpus spongiosum of the penis, leading to prolonged painful erections. The affliction often occurs in association with spontaneous nocturnal erections. Episodes of priapism can last from several hours to several days. One group of investigators reported a 90% actuarial probability of at least one episode of priapism by age 21 years.

The most frequently used intervention in the past was irrigation of the ventral vein of the penis by a urologist in an attempt to alleviate blocked blood flow. This approach generally produced poor results because the problem is one of microvascular occlusion. More recently, exchange transfusion has been used in some of these patients with mixed results. Nonacute cases of priapism are sometimes treated with vasodilators such as pseudoephedrine[1] (Sudafed) or etilefrine hydrochloride[2] (Effortil). No overall consensus exists on a treatment algorithm for this debilitating complication of sickle cell disease.

---

[1]Not FDA approved for this indication.
[2]Not available in the United States.

Management of Chronic Problems

PAIN

Chronic pain is a central problem for many patients with sickle cell disease. The etiology of chronic pain in sickle cell disease is uncertain. Organ injury and necrosis produced by years of intermittent ischemia from vaso-occlusion likely have a large role. The severity of the pain varies greatly and can change over time. No universally applicable formula exists for management of chronic pain. Physicians frequently face the greatest management challenges from patients with persistent severe pain controlled by chronically administered opioid analgesics.

Nonsteroidal Anti-Inflammatory Drugs

NSAIDs can control chronic pain in many patients with sickle cell disease. The agents can be used alone or in conjunction with opioid analgesics. Most often, NSAIDs are used intermittently to control flares of pain. Awareness of the issue of renal dysfunction and associated complications makes most specialists chary of chronic NSAID use. Patients with sickle cell disease are more susceptible to renal injury, and the downhill slope to frank renal failure is steep. Physicians who opt for NSAID-based pain management *must closely monitor renal function*. Equally important is awareness that the clinical chemical profile of renal function in sickle cell disease differs importantly from that seen in normal people (see later). Cyclooxygenase-2 inhibitors allegedly produce less nephrotoxicity than do standard NSAIDs. Limited experience exists with these agents in sickle cell disease.

Opioid Analgesics

Most patients who require large or frequent doses of opioids to control pain are not seeking drugs for recreational purposes. Often, they become tolerant to opioids. Consequently, the quantity of medication needed to control severe pain exceeds that associated with a severe but self-limited painful episode, such as torn knee ligaments. Unfortunately, no objective measure of pain exists. Appropriate treatment of pain irrespective of the cause requires an ongoing dialog between the doctor and patient.

Whenever possible, patients should start taking their analgesics before the pain crescendos. Maintaining pain at a tolerable level is easier than reducing it from an intense apogee. Control of a typical episode of severe sickle pain can require 4 to 8 mg of oral hydromorphone every 3 hours to achieve relief. Many "severe" sickle crises can be managed at home with analgesics, fluids, and rest. If the pain progresses despite the use of reasonable quantities of medication, emergency medical care is the next option.

Health care providers often view sickle cell disease pain as episodic bouts secondary to occlusion of the microcirculation. Absent is the realization that severe chronic pain more loosely associated with vaso-occlusion also occurs. Chronic sickle cell pain is more common in adults than in children, reflecting permanent damage to the microcirculation secondary to years of recurrent sickle injury.

The short duration of action common to many analgesics, such as hydromorphone and meperidine, is a significant obstacle to adequate control of chronic pain. One of the most effective long-acting drugs for the control of chronic sickle cell pain is methadone (Phenadone). Although best known for its use in narcotic detoxification programs, methadone is a highly effective analgesic when given three times per day. Methadone can be dispensed only at certified detoxification centers for narcotic addiction control. Methadone for pain control can be given at other facilities in accordance with the guidelines for use of any opioid. Long-acting formulations of morphine sulfate (MS Contin) are effective long-acting analgesics but often produce debilitating somnolence. Oxycodone (OxyContin) is excellent for long-term pain control that recently fell victim to recreational use and abuse. Methadone is not immune to these issues, but poses fewer difficulties.

Drug-Seeking Behavior

Addiction is a concern both for medical providers and patients when chronic pain control requires long-term opioid use. The magnitude of the problem is less than is often imagined, however. People who develop addiction or drug-seeking behavior disproportionately frequent emergency rooms and hospital floors. This overrepresentation of a small number of patients leads some providers to conclude that drug-seeking behavior is a problem for most people with sickle cell disease. Opioids used for pain control, even when given in relatively high doses, do not produce addiction automatically.

An important first step in managing this problem is to define drug-seeking behavior. The use of large quantities of oral opioids or frequent visits to the emergency room do not de facto signify drug-seeking behavior. Drug-seeking behavior is the use of opioids in the absence of pain sufficiently severe to justify these medications. Reaching this conclusion is difficult without an objective yardstick for pain. Drug-seeking behavior can be established only by getting to know the patient and by observing the pattern of drug use. This means that over a period of months, tolerance of frequent and heavy use of opioids by a patient may be necessary to establish the pattern of drug consumption. Only then can the medical care providers reasonably say that drug-seeking behavior is likely. At this point, the patient can be approached to discuss what seems to be unwarranted use of drugs.

Patients can respond positively. Drug-seeking behavior can be a very psychologically painful experience. Many patients are relieved when they are confronted and given an option of help. Counseling or sessions with a psychologist or social worker can be useful. In establishing drug-seeking behavior, allowing a few patients to succeed in taking extra medication for a time outweighs punishing patients who have a legitimate need by imposing arbitrary limits on everyone.

Some patients demonstrate incorrigible and sometimes frankly sociopathic behavior. In these instances, the best approach is to limit opioid availability. The patient should be informed that a limit is being imposed and the reason for its implementation. The limit should be followed strictly. Tracking patterns of medication use is aided by logging all opioid prescriptions. Photocopies of prescriptions provide excellent documentation. If possible, a single provider should write the prescriptions and maintain the record. Covering staff and emergency room physicians should be alerted to the arrangement and should not supply additional prescriptions. The arrangement is not punitive. Rather, it allows the staff to better assess and treat legitimate sickle cell pain. Furthermore, this approach lifts a tremendous psychological burden from emergency or covering staff, permitting overall improved patient care. Health care providers should document their efforts to monitor and control excess use of opioids by their patients. Scrupulous record keeping also helps avoid entanglements with medical practice oversight agencies.

ANEMIA

Vitamin Supplementation

Patients with sickle cell disease, similar to other people with hemolytic anemias, require daily folic acid replacement. Folate is rapidly consumed by proliferating erythroid precursors. One milligram of supplemental folate per day is more than enough to satisfy the needs of the erythron. A patient with sickle cell disease whose hematocrit begins to decrease unexpectedly should be checked for folate deficiency as a part of the general workup.

Sporadic Transfusion

Patients with sickle cell disease are anemic, by definition. Baseline hematocrit values vary between patients but are stable for a particular individual. Most patients are conditioned to tolerate their degree of anemia, and routine transfusion is not necessary. Increasing the hematocrit provides no clinical benefit, unless the baseline value has decreased into the midteens, at which point oxygen-carrying capacity is seriously compromised. Also, hematocrits in such a low range leave little leeway for further decrease. However, transfusing patients with sickle cell disease to hematocrits in the mid- to upper-30s can be dangerous, because blood viscosity increases substantially at higher hematocrits with secondary vaso-occlusion possibly resulting.

Chronic Transfusion Therapy

The efficacy of chronic transfusion therapy is best documented for stroke victims. Chronic transfusion therapy is less well established for other issues in sickle cell disease including recurrent severe episodes of sickle pain, acute chest syndrome, priapism, and prophylaxis of pregnancy complications. The utility of chronic transfusion therapy is limited by complications, most notably alloimmunization and iron overload.

Alloimmunization

Alloimmunization against minor red cell antigens is a major problem for patients with sickle cell disease who receive frequent transfusions (see "Acute Chest Syndrome"). Kell, E, and C are the most problematic minor antigens. The rate of alloimmunization approaches 40% in some reports of chronic transfusion in sickle cell disease. Occasionally, patients develop such severe

---

problems with alloantibodies that transfusion becomes nearly impossible. Phenotype matching for these antigens markedly reduces the incidence of alloimmunization (Box 2). Routine use of blood from black donors for black patients with sickle cell disease is not warranted, however. The likelihood of finding matched units for patients with sickle cell disease is greater when black people are in the donor pool. Matching is necessary, nonetheless, because antigen variation among black people, as with all other humans, is great. An expanded donor pool substantially improves the chance of a match with antigen testing.

Age and Severity of Anemia

The severity of the anemia in sickle cell disease sometimes increases gradually with age. The basis of this marrow exhaustion phenomenon is unknown. Many patients have end-organ damage, such as a dilated cardiomyopathy, that can limit tolerance of severe anemia. Recombinant human erythropoietin[1] (rHuEPO; Procrit, Epogen) and hydroxyurea can improve the hemoglobin picture for some patients. Dosing can be adjusted from starting levels of 1000 mg daily of hydroxyurea and 40,000 U weekly of rHuEPO depending on patient response.

INFECTION PROPHYLAXIS

Antibiotics

The penicillin[1] prophylaxis trial completed in 1986 prompted the recommendation that all children be given prophylactic penicillin[1] (or equivalent) at a dose of 250 mg twice a day. A second study involving older children showed no difference in the incidence of severe infection among 5- to 12-year-olds. The role of prophylactic penicillin[1] in adults with sickle cell disease is undocumented, but the intervention is probably superfluous.

Immunization

Immunization with pneumococcal vaccine (Pneumovax 23) is standard practice both in adults and children with sickle cell disease. Several studies suggest that immunization provides some protection, although incomplete, against

---

[1]Not FDA approved for this indication.

---

pneumococcal infection. The vaccine seems to be effective even in adults whose splenic function is lost. The more recently available 7-valent vaccine provides improved coverage of specifically problematic bacterial subtypes relative to the earlier 23-valent vaccine. Although the duration of protection is unknown, most specialists reinoculate patients once every 5 to 7 years.

More recently, a vaccine against *H. influenzae* Type b (HibTITER) entered the clinical arena. The efficacy of this vaccine in sickle cell disease is unknown. Given the serious nature of *H. influenzae* infections in these patients, many specialists, particularly pediatricians, now routinely immunize patients against this organism.

Viral influenza is potentially deadly for older people and those with several chronic illnesses including sickle cell disease. Because bacterial infection and other problems often complicate influenza, prevention of the disease by immunization is a practical intervention (FLUMIST).

The need for hepatitis B immunization (Engerix-B vaccine) for patients with sickle cell disease reflects the high likelihood of transfusion at some point.

AVASCULAR NECROSIS OF BONE

Avascular necrosis of bone is a common and debilitating problem in sickle cell disease. This process differs totally from the acute bone marrow necrosis discussed earlier. With acute bone marrow necrosis, the pathology involves damage to hematopoietic elements within the bone marrow cavity. Bone is living tissue that can die as a result of poor blood circulation within the wall of the bone itself. The areas of bone most frequently affected are the acetabulum and the head of the humerus. The etiology of avascular necrosis of bone is unknown. One hypothesis posits that marrow hyperplasia in the femoral head crowds tissue and secondarily reduces blood flow through bony trabeculae.

The quality of the pain associated with avascular bone necrosis differs substantially from sickle cell pain. The articular cartilage thins and often disappears as the process progresses. The joints can deteriorate producing a bone-on-bone interface. Movement then becomes wrenchingly painful. Early on, nonsteroidal anti-inflammatory agents can be useful. With more severe situations, particularly those that involve the shoulder, corticosteroid injection into the joint articular space can relieve symptoms. Finally, decompression of the marrow tissue in the head of the humerus or the head of the femur is used by some orthopedic surgeons. This invasive procedure should be reserved for patients with more advanced avascular necrosis. No definitive data address the efficacy of the procedure.

These interventions slow osteonecrosis without halting the process, leading sometimes to joint replacement. Some patients with sickle syndromes tolerate artificial joints poorly. As many as 33% of patients require a second surgery within 4 years of joint replacement. Also, these patients, for unclear reasons, are vulnerable to infections of their orthopedic hardware. The unfortunate result can be a destroyed articular interface and a flail joint that, in the case of the femur, produces wheelchair confinement.

MR imaging is a promising addition to the diagnostic armamentarium that exceeds by far the sensitivity of plain bone films. The technique detects very early evidence of damage and holds the hope of earlier detection and improved management of this most debilitating of sickle cell disease complications.

OSTEOMYELITIS

Nearly three quarters of cases of osteomyelitis with sickle cell disease are attributed to *Salmonella* species. Local pain and fever are the most common indicators of chronic osteomyelitis. In the early stages of the disorder, bone roentgenograms and even bone scans frequently are unrevealing. Gallium scans can provide early evidence of the condition. The addition of MRI to the diagnostic arsenal is a promising development. Bone biopsy gives the definitive diagnosis. This procedure sometimes is not an option, depending on the location of the infection, however. Once the diagnosis is made, 4 to 6 weeks of intravenous antibiotic therapy are needed.

SKIN ULCERS

The 1% incidence of skin ulcers in the United States is low relative to the 30% reported incidence in Jamaica. The basic of the strikingly different figures is unknown. The most common site of skin ulceration is over the lateral malleoli. The ulceration often lacks clear-cut antecedent trauma and progresses over a period of weeks to the point that the lesions penetrate into the dermis and often into the underlying subcutaneous tissue. Breakdown in protection provided by the integument leaves patients susceptible to infections and other complications.

Treatment of ankle ulcers should be conservative. Rest, elevation, and dry dressings with antimicrobial ointments by far are the best approaches to this problem. Attempts at skin grafting are frequently frustrated by poor blood flow to the affected region. Healing usually requires weeks to months. The area should be protected against trauma when the patient is up and about. Socks or other clothing that cover the area should be avoided, to reduce friction injury. A simple dry dressing provides additional protection. Reports of enhanced healing of ulcers associated with chronic transfusion therapy are anecdotal.

RENAL DYSFUNCTION

The most common renal defect in sickle cell disease is impaired urine-concentrating ability (hyposthenuria) that often appears by 2 or 3 years of age. The condition can produce bedwetting in children or embarrassing wetting in public places such as classrooms. Hyposthenuria also occurs with compound heterozygous states (e.g., sickle-β-thalassemia). The extremely high osmolality in the distal tubule produces renal medullary sickling even in people with sickle trait. Consequently, hyposthenuria is the most common abnormality associated with sickle cell trait.

Medullary ischemia and papillary necrosis occur frequently. Sometimes, the necrotic papillae slough into the collecting system, obstructing the outflow tract. No effective specific intervention exists for this problem. Increasing BUN and creatinine values herald sickle glomerulonephropathy. The most important intervention is limiting protein consumption, as is recommended for many types of renal dysfunction including that associated with diabetic nephropathy. One report suggested that angiotensin-converting enzyme inhibitors[1] (e.g., enalapril [Vasotec]) might retard nephropathy progression in sickle cell disease. Unfortunately, confirmatory studies were never conducted.

Patients with sickle cell disease usually have *low* serum creatinine and BUN levels. This reflects the high glomerular filtration rate along with a high rate of creatinine secretion in the distal tubule. BUN values of 7 mg/dL and creatinine values of 0.5 mg/dL are typical for patients with sickle cell disease. Creatinine clearance often exceeds 150 mL/minute/1.73 m^2 surface area. A formal evaluation of glomerular filtration should be considered for patients in whom the serum creatinine increases above the level of approximately 1.0 mg/dL.

Limited experience exists on the efficacy of dialysis with sickle cell disease. Reports that hemodialysis is problematic in patients with sickle cell disease are anecdotal. Every effort should be undertaken to prevent renal deterioration. Microscopic hematuria is common with sickle cell disease (as well as some patients with sickle cell trait). Hematuria per se requires no intervention unless blood loss is massive. Some patients with sickle cell disease and renal failure have successfully received renal allografts.

Massive hematuria occasionally develops in people with sickle cell trait. Interestingly, the bleeding often comes from the left kidney. Hydration and alkalization of the urine are frequently used interventions. Anecdotal reports of the use of desmopressin[1] (DDAVP) in this situation are encouraging. Epsilon aminocaproic acid[1] (Amicar) has been used in some patients with refractory bleeding from the kidney. Bleeding can continue for weeks. Iron replacement may be necessary as treatment interventions continue. Nephrectomy has been performed, but this frightful intervention should be a last-ditch approach to a life-threatening situation.

RETINOPATHY

Retinopathy is a significant problem for 10% to 20% of people with sickle cell disease. The peak age of onset is in the 20s. For unknown reasons, the condition develops more frequently with hemoglobin sickle cell disease than with homozygous sickle cell disease. The problem resembles diabetic retinopathy both clinically and pathologically with retinal thinning and neovascularization. The areas affected, at least initially, are in the periphery of the retina with indirect ophthalmoscopy required for detection. Laser photocoagulation has been used in an effort to prevent retinal hemorrhage. A retina specialist is the preferred provider, particularly if diabetic retinopathy is a practice focus. Annual evaluation is key to early detection of lesions and prevention of complications. Retinopathy has no correlation with sickle cell disease pain profile. All patients must have retinal examination irrespective of clinical status.

HEART

Cardiomegaly is often caused by a sustained high cardiac output state. Whereas high output failure occurs in some patients with sickle cell disease, the heart usually is hyperdynamic. Pulmonary congestion caused by fluid overload

---

[1]Not FDA approved for this indication.

CURRENT DIAGNOSIS

Problem	Manifestation	Treatment
Acute chest syndrome	Decreasing oxygen saturation with partial pressure of oxygen less than 80 mm Hg on room air	Simple transfusion
		Exchange transfusion
	Chest radiograph infiltrates	Antibiotics
	Fever	Ventilation support
	Leukocytosis	Bronchodilators
Splenic sequestration crisis	Enlarging spleen on examination	Simple transfusion
	Left upper quadrant pain	
	Decreasing hemoglobin	
Stroke	Acute hemiplegia/hemiparesis	Exchange transfusion
	Severe headache	
	Nausea, vomiting	
Aplastic crisis	Reticulocyte count low or zero	Simple transfusion
	Decreasing hemoglobin	
	Fever, vaso-occlusive pain	
Septicemia	Fever	Cultures
	Leukocytosis	Broad-spectrum antibiotics
	Peripheral blood bands	
	Lethargy	
	Confusion	

during hydration for painful crisis is uncommon in young patients, but can be an issue in older adults. Careful monitoring of cardiovascular status can prevent serious problems with pulmonary congestion.

PREGNANCY

Women with sickle cell disease can carry pregnancies to term, but the process sometimes is complicated. The frequency of painful crises usually increases during pregnancy. Women who have painful crises during pregnancy should receive analgesics as necessary, including narcotics. The newborns with intrauterine opioid exposure must undergo opioid withdrawal. Warned of this issue, neonatologists can easily manage the problem. Routine transfusion is not indicated during pregnancy.

CURRENT THERAPY

- Hydroxyurea—Daily oral administration in children older than 5 years of age and adults who fit the appropriate treatment profile
- Penicillin prophylaxis—Daily penicillin or equivalent in children from ages 6 months to 7 years
- Pneumococcal immunization—Children and adults. Repeat every 5 to 7 years
- Hepatitis B immunization—Children and adults
- Viral influenza immunization—Adults every year
- Limited phenotype matched red cell transfusion—Children and adults when transfusion is needed
- Severe acute pain crisis—Parenterally administered, short-acting opioids
  - Patient-controlled analgesia (PCA)
  - Avoid meperidine

BONE MARROW TRANSPLANTATION

Bone marrow transplantation can cure SCD. This promising but complex intervention remains in the domain of highly specialized care groups who manage many such patients. The intervention is far more effective in children than in adults.

Without major breakthroughs in gene therapy or bone marrow transplantation that make these treatments applicable to many patients, drug intervention will remain the major therapeutic option for sickle cell disease. Currently, all patients must be assessed for possible treatment with hydroxyurea.

REFERENCES

Adamkiewicz T, Sarnaik S, Buchanan G, et al: Invasive pneumococcal infections in children with sickle cell disease in the era of penicillin prophylaxis, antibiotic resistance, and 23-valent pneumococcal polysaccharide vaccination. J Pediatr 2003;143:438-444. Pneumococcal sepsis remains a problem despite penicillin prophylaxis and vaccination with the 23-valent vaccine. Early aggressive treatment of suspected sepsis is vital.

Charache S, Terrin M, Moore R, et al: Effect of hydroxyurea on the frequency of painful crises in sickle cell anemia. Investigators of the Multicenter Study of Hydroxyurea in Sickle Cell Anemia. N Engl J Med 1995;332:1317-1322. The article presents the data on hydroxyurea for prophylactic treatment of sickle cell disease. This remains the only intervention proven to prevent problems, specifically acute vaso-occlusive pain crisis, crisis-related hospitalization, and acute chest syndrome. The drug also lowers transfusion requirements.

Falletta J, Woods G, Verter J, et al: Discontinuing penicillin prophylaxis in children with sickle cell anemia. Prophylactic Penicillin Study II. J Pediatr 1995;127:685-690. Penicillin prophylaxis can be safely stopped at 5 years of age.

Kinney T, Helms R, O'Branski E, et al: Safety of hydroxyurea in children with sickle cell anemia: Results of the HUG-KIDS study, a phase I/II trial. Pediatric Hydroxyurea Group. Blood 1999;94:1550-1554. This Phase I/II trial shows that hydroxyurea therapy is safe for children with sickle cell disease when treatment is directed by a pediatric hematologist.

Quinn C, Rogers Z, Buchanan G: Survival of children with sickle cell disease. Blood 2004;103:4023-4027. Childhood mortality from SCD is decreasing, the mean age at death is increasing, and a smaller proportion of deaths is from infection.

Scothorn D, Price C, Schwartz D, et al: Risk of recurrent stroke in children with sickle cell disease receiving blood transfusion therapy for at least five years after initial stroke. J Pediatr 2002;140:348-354. The absence of an antecedent or concurrent medical event associated with an initial stroke is a major risk factor for subsequent stroke while receiving regular transfusions.

Tahhan H, Holbrook C, Braddy L, et al: Antigen-matched donor blood in the transfusion management of patients with sickle cell disease. Transfusion 1994;34:562-569. Approximately 33% of patients who received chronic transfusion with blood that was not matched for extended phenotype developed alloantibodies. None of the matched patients developed alloantibodies. A cost saving also existed with the extended phenotype-matched blood because of lower subsequent laboratory testing expenses.

Vichinsky E, Neumayr L, Earles A, et al: Causes and outcomes of the acute chest syndrome in sickle cell disease. N Engl J Med 2000;342:1855-1865. The article provides the most extensive information available on the causes and treatment of acute chest syndrome. In particular, the study shows that although infection and fat emboli are the leading proven causes of acute chest syndrome, the etiology is mysterious in more than 33% of patients. Transfusions and bronchodilators are keys to treatment.

Zimmerman R: Pneumococcal conjugate vaccine for young children. Am Fam Physician 2001;63:1991-1998. The American Academy of Family Physicians recommends routine vaccination of infants, catch-up vaccination of children younger than 24 months, and catch-up vaccination of children 24 to 59 months of age with high-risk medical conditions such as sickle cell disease and congenital heart disease.

Neutropenia

Method of
Melvin H. Freedman, MD

TABLE 1 Classification of Neutropenia

Acquired or Extracellular Causes
Viral-induced marrow suppression
Nonviral infection or sepsis
Drug induced:
    Chemotherapy
    Other drugs
Immune mediated:
    Autoimmune disease at all ages
    Neonatal isoimmune
Neonatal neutropenia/maternal hypertension
Neonatal neutropenia/organic acid disorders
Hypersplenism
Nutritional deficiencies (vitamin B_{12}, folate, copper)
Pure white cell aplasia
Idiopathic neutropenia

Congenital, Inherited, or Intracellular Causes
Congenital neutropenia (agranulocytosis)/Kostmann's syndrome
Cyclic neutropenia
Autosomal dominant familial neutropenia
Dysgamma-/agammaglobulinemia, cellular immunodeficiency syndromes
Shwachman-Diamond syndrome
Glycogen storage disease type 1b
Barth syndrome

Other Causes
Fanconi anemia
Myelokathexis
Lazy leukocyte syndrome
Reticular dysgenesis
Cartilage-hair hypoplasia
Dyskeratosis congenita
Pseudo-neutropenia

An absolute neutrophil count (ANC) is equal to the total white blood cell count per microliter multiplied by the combined percentage of neutrophils and bands. Neutropenia is defined as an ANC below two standard deviations of the normal mean. Normal neutrophil levels can be stratified for age and race. For whites beyond infancy, the lower limit for normal neutrophil counts is 1500/µL. Blacks have somewhat lower neutrophil counts; the lower limit of normal is approximately 1200/µL. Individual patients may be characterized as having mild neutropenia with cell counts of 1000 to 1500/µL, moderate neutropenia with cell counts of 500 to 1000/µL, or severe neutropenia with cell counts less than 500/µL. This stratification is useful for predicting risk because patients with severe neutropenia have increased susceptibility to life-threatening infections.

Classification

Table 1 is a classification for formulating an informative clinical and laboratory assessment that leads to a specific diagnosis of neutropenia. There are some general points to consider when using this table. Unlike anemia and thrombocytopenia, which can be categorized as being caused by decreased production or increased destruction using marrow morphology and specific laboratory indicators, neutropenia is much more complex to define kinetically and laboratory testing is not as refined. Thus, for practical reasons, the classification in Table 1 is based on the *cellular basis* for neutropenia: either an acquired extracellular cause or a congenital, inherited, or intracellular cause.

Many of the diagnoses are age related. Most of the congenital or inherited diagnoses are detected early in infancy or childhood. In adolescence and adulthood, most of the disorders are acquired, but there is obviously some overlap. Some neutropenic conditions are common, others are rare. Viral-induced marrow suppression is the most common cause of childhood neutropenia, whereas congenital or inherited disorders are very rare. Drug-induced, autoimmune, and nutritional deficiency neutropenias are encountered more frequently in adult patients. There is also a clinical distinction between acute-onset and severe chronic neutropenia. Acute neutropenia can develop if neutrophils are used rapidly when marrow production is impaired.

Drugs used for chemotherapy are particularly likely to induce neutropenia because of their cytotoxic effect on the high proliferative rate of neutrophil precursors and the relatively short half-life of blood neutrophils. Other nonchemotherapeutic drugs can induce severe neutropenia by idiosyncratic or hypersensitivity reactions. These drugs include analgesics, antipsychotic agents, anticonvulsants, antithyroid drugs, cardiovascular drugs, the sulfas, and antibiotics.

Severe chronic neutropenia is a general term that describes ANCs less than 500/μL on serial testing for at least 3 months. Because neutrophils are crucial in protecting the body against invasion by bacteria, severe chronic neutropenia regularly predisposes a patient to pyogenic infections. Chronic neutropenia is caused by a variety of hematologic disorders as well as immunologic, metabolic, and infectious diseases. Congenital neutropenia, cyclic neutropenia, and idiopathic neutropenia are three major diagnostic categories of severe chronic neutropenia that respond to granulocyte colony-stimulating factor (G-CSF) therapy (see later).

Some neutropenias are serious with overt symptomatology, whereas others are clinically silent and are discovered in the context of a routine medical examination. Most severe forms of neutropenia ultimately present with one or more of the following: fever of unknown origin (so-called fever neutropenia), chronic oropharyngeal ulcers, gingivitis, periodontal disease, bacterial or fungal septicemia, cellulitis of the skin or perirectal area, abscesses despite the absence of true pus, and other life-threatening infections.

Clinical and Laboratory Evaluation

A complete medical history is an essential first step. Key historical information about previous blood cell counts may require some detective work. These counts are routinely performed in other physicians' offices for evaluation of other medical problems. This information can provide immediate confirmation that an episode of neutropenia is acquired or of recent onset. By using Table 1, other useful historical data can be generated. A detailed evaluation of infections is needed to determine the type, severity, duration, and recurrences, as well as the age at onset of symptoms to document whether the disorder is congenital or acquired. Antecedent viral infection should be noted; this is by far the most common explanation for neutropenia in young children. Medication usage, including that of nonprescription drugs, should be elicited. Symptoms of other systemic disorders such as autoimmune disease or chronic liver dysfunction that could produce splenomegaly must also be reviewed. The nutritional history should include symptomatology of vitamin B_{12} or folic acid deficiency.

For infants and children with neutropenia, the historical questions are more specific. In neonatal neutropenia, failure to thrive is suggestive of a metabolic disorder. A maternal history of hypertension is an important explanation for neonatal neutropenia. Similarly, in neonates, a family history of previously affected siblings but with non-neutropenic parents suggests an autosomal recessive inheritance pattern as seen in some Kostmann's syndrome patients, some immune deficiency disorders, Shwachman-Diamond syndrome, glycogen storage disease type 1b, and metabolic disorders. A history of a parent with neutropenia with one or more affected offspring implies an autosomal dominant mode of transmission as seen in one form of cyclic neutropenia and in a type of noncyclic severe chronic neutropenia. This history for classic cyclic neutropenia is that of mouth ulcers, periodontal complaints, cervical lymphadenopathy, fever, malaise, or infections every 21 days.

The physical examination is directed to sites of current or recent infections, especially the oral cavity, skin, perineum, and perirectal area. In adults, the focus should also be for signs of nutritional deficiency, collagen vascular disease, and splenomegaly, as well as pallor, bruises, or petechiae, which suggest a more generalized marrow disorder because of replacement or a myelodysplastic syndrome. In infants and children, particular attention is paid to growth and developmental parameters. A detailed evaluation is also performed for the presence of phenotypic abnormalities and skeletal anomalies, which are seen in Fanconi anemia, in Shwachman-Diamond syndrome, and in some of the other disorders listed in Table 1.

In infants and young children, the workup also includes blood cell counts on parents and siblings to unmask an inherited cause; testing for antineutrophil antibodies to diagnose autoimmune neutropenia of infancy; serologic studies for collagen vascular disorders; immunoglobulin quantitation and cellular immunity screening for diagnosis of an immunodeficiency syndrome; serial blood cell counts two to three times a week for 4 to 8 weeks to determine a predictable cyclic pattern; bone marrow aspiration and biopsy for diagnostic morphology coupled with cytogenetic studies on marrow cells to exclude a malignant clonal change; and a polymerase chain reaction molecular analysis of the cells for Epstein-Barr virus, cytomegalovirus, and herpes simplex virus. The marrow morphology can be very specific in diagnosing congenital neutropenia/Kostmann's syndrome (maturation arrest at the myelocyte stage) and myelokathexis (myeloid hypercellularity with degenerative, pyknotic granulocytes).

Specific syndromes listed in Table 1 such as Shwachman-Diamond syndrome, glycogen storage disease type 1b, neutropenia associated with metabolic disorders, and Fanconi anemia require highly specialized diagnostic testing at a subspecialty center. Many of the investigations for infants and younger children are also pertinent for older children and adults. Additional testing for older patients, however, should include determination of serum copper, serum vitamin B_{12}, and red blood cell folate levels; an HIV detection study in the appropriate clinical setting; and, if hypersplenism is present, imaging and other diagnostic testing to determine the cause.

CURRENT DIAGNOSIS

- Confirm a sustained ANC below lower limit of normal by serial testing.
- Establish cause by history, physical examination, and laboratory testing in context of *extracellular* versus *intracellular* etiologies (see Table 1).
- Severe chronic neutropenia (ANC <500/μL for >3 mo) requires urgent investigation and close supervision.

Abbreviation: ANC = absolute neutrophil count.

CURRENT THERAPY

- Fever of >38.5°C (101.3°F) with an ANC < 500/μL is a medical emergency and requires immediate blood and urine cultures and stat IV antibiotics based on the following considerations (see text):
  - Start an IV line; give standard fluids at 1.5 times maintenance.
  - If taking medications, stop them.
  - Consider past history of antibiotic resistance of previously cultured organisms.
  - Consider patient's clinical stability or instability or shock.
  - Determine if a significant β-lactam allergy exists or not.
  - Choose appropriate antibiotic combinations based on above.
  - Give IV G-CSF, 5–10 μg/kg (maximum dose, 300 μg)[3] once daily.

[3]Exceeds dosage recommended by the manufacturer.
Abbreviations: ANC, absolute neutrophil count; G-CSF = granulocyte colony-stimulating factor; IV = intravenous.

Therapy

GENERAL MEASURES

Management depends on the degree of the neutropenia, its etiology, and the patient's previous history of infections. In healthy-appearing asymptomatic adults and older children with isolated neutropenia and cell counts greater than 750/μL, clinical observation only without further diagnostic study may be warranted. Medications that may account for the neutropenia should be stopped, if possible. Serial blood cell counts can determine if the neutropenia is transient or persistent. If it persists longer than 4 to 8 weeks, additional workup is needed. If anemia or thrombocytopenia is present at any time, however, bone marrow aspiration or biopsy is the next diagnostic test. Infants, younger children, and patients of all ages with a history of chronic, recurrent, or severe infection with neutrophil counts less than 750/μL, especially less than 500/μL, require further diagnostic testing and a decision about medical intervention.

General preventive measures should include good hand washing, meticulous skin care, and good oral hygiene with regular dental checkups and professional cleaning. For neutropenic mouth ulcers, a "magic mouthwash" can be prepared by a pharmacist containing equal parts of 2% viscous lidocaine (Xylocaine) and diphenhydramine (Benadryl) in normal saline. A peroxide-based mouthwash can also be used for oral hygiene. Rectal examinations and rectal temperature taking, as well as suppositories and enemas, should be avoided if possible.

Patients who are neutropenic but with ANCs greater than 1000/μL generally exhibit normal defense against infection and can be regarded in the same manner as non-neutropenic patients. For patients with ANCs greater than 500/μL but less than 1000/μL who have recurrent infections, preventive medical therapy is an option.

Before the cytokine era, prophylactic antibiotics were sometimes used. The most popular agents were the penicillins and trimethoprim-sulfamethoxazole (Bactrim, Septra). These antibiotics may be effective in diminishing the frequency of infections and can be tried, but there may be significant problems associated with their continuous use. These include gastrointestinal complaints, "selection," and then overgrowth of antibiotic-resistant organisms and allergic reactions.

Patients whose ANC is less than 500/μL are at serious risk of bacterial infection, particularly from pathogens such as *Staphylococcus aureus* and gram-negative organisms. These are often of endogenous origin in the neutropenic host. The onset of fever of greater than 38.5°C (101.3°F) in these patients should be regarded as a medical emergency. By virtue of the low neutrophil counts, they may have few signs of inflammation but they must be hospitalized and empirically treated with antibiotics while awaiting culture results. In my clinic and emergency department, we immediately activate a treatment protocol before admission to avoid any delay in antibiotic therapy. The protocol was developed in our institution for management of patients on chemotherapy who develop fever-neutropenia, but it is equally suitable for any patient with a neutrophil count of less than 500/μL.

EMERGENCY DEPARTMENT MANAGEMENT

Stop all medications. Start an intravenous (IV) line and give standard fluids at 1.5 times maintenance. Order a chest film, a serum creatinine study, a urinalysis, and obtain cultures of blood and urine and from any apparent focus of infection. When selecting antibiotics, always consider the patient's past history regarding antibiotic resistance of previously cultured organisms as well as the patient's clinical stability. Standard initial antibiotics for the stable patient as described later may not be appropriate for a patient who has had previous serious infection from an antibiotic-resistant organism.

Administer the following antibiotics stat (i.e., they should be given before patient transfer from a clinic or emergency department to a hospital ward and before administration of any blood product):

For stable patients with no significant beta-lactam allergy, give:

- Piperacillin-tazobactam (Tazocin): children: 80 mg piperacillin/kg IV every 8 hours; adolescents and adults: maximum dose, 4 g IV every 8 hours
- Gentamicin: children younger than 9 years, 10 mg/kg IV every 24 hours; from 9 to younger than 12 years, 8 mg/kg IV every 24 hours; 12 years or older, 6 mg/kg IV every 24 hours; adults, 1 to 2 mg/kg IV every 8 hours or 4 to 6 mg/kg IV every 24 hours

If a significant β-lactam allergy exists, give:

- Ciprofloxacin (Cipro): children, 10 mg/kg IV every 12 hours; adults, 400 mg IV every 12 hours
- Clindamycin (Cleocin): children, 10 mg/kg IV every 8 hours; adults, 600 mg IV every 8 hours
- Gentamicin: dose as above

If the patient is unstable or in septic shock with no significant beta-lactam allergy, give:

- Meropenem (Merrem IV): children, 20 mg/kg IV every 8 hours; adults, 1 g IV every 8 hours
- Vancomycin (Vancocin): children, 15 mg/kg IV every 6 hours; adults, 1 g IV every 6 hours
- Gentamicin, dose as above

If a significant β-lactam allergy exists, give

- Ciprofloxacin: dose as above
- Vancomycin: dose as above
- Amikacin (Amikin): children, 20 mg/kg[3] IV every 24 hours; adults, 500 mg IV every 12 hours.

MANAGEMENT AFTER ADMISSION

Vital signs are measured hourly until the patient's condition stabilizes and then every 4 hours or as indicated. If blood cultures are subsequently positive, repeat cultures should be drawn when this result becomes known. Antibiotics specifically directed toward the identified organism should be added to the broad-spectrum therapy if the initial antibiotics do not provide adequate coverage. Broad-spectrum coverage must not be replaced by specific, narrow-coverage antibiotics alone in the neutropenic patient.

For patients who become afebrile, with an ANC of greater than 500/μL and with negative cultures, antibiotics can be stopped. For patients who become afebrile and with negative cultures but with neutrophils less than 500/μL, antibiotics can usually be stopped after 48 hours of therapy.

Patients who are persistently febrile but stable should continue to receive the initial empirical antibiotic regimen as described. If the patient's condition indicates an evolving infection at a particular site (e.g., abdominal pain, severe mucositis, pneumonia), antibiotics directed toward possible causative organisms should be added to the broad-spectrum coverage. After 5 to 7 days of persistent fever, consider the addition of amphotericin (Amphocin): for children, 1 mg/kg once a day IV, or, if older than 2 years, caspofungin (Cancidas), 50 mg/m² once a day IV. For adults, give amphotericin, 3 to 4 mg/kg once a day IV, or caspofungin, 70 mg IV once on day 1 followed by 50 mg IV once a day thereafter.

SPECIFIC AND GROWTH FACTOR TREATMENT

Referring to Table 1, there are several diagnoses of acquired neutropenia that respond to specific treatment. Excluding chemotherapy-induced neutropenia, when a drug is suspected as causing the problem, the product should be stopped and general supportive measures instituted. If neutropenia is severe, administration of growth factor (cytokine therapy) should be started (see later). Autoimmune neutropenia of infancy occurring in the first 3 years of life is clinically benign and self-limited, but the spontaneous resolution may take months to years. No therapy is needed unless a bacterial infection ensues, at which

point cytokine therapy is initiated in combination with antibiotics.

Treatment of chronic autoimmune neutropenia in older children and adults is usually supportive if the neutropenia is an isolated manifestation. Cytokine therapy and antibiotics should be used, however, if infection is a problem. A more generalized multisystem autoimmune disorder usually requires specialized management, conventionally starting with corticosteroids. One of these disorders, Felty's syndrome (rheumatoid arthritis, splenomegaly, and neutropenia), is managed with options ranging from splenectomy, antirheumatic therapy, immunosuppression, plasmapheresis, IV immunoglobulin (IVIG), and cytokine therapy.

Isoimmune neonatal neutropenia is the neutrophil equivalent of Rh hemolytic disease of the newborn and lasts an average of 7 weeks postnatally. Therapy is supportive with antibiotics as necessary, but in life-threatening infections, plasma exchange to remove antineutrophil antibodies, transfusion of maternal neutrophils that lack the immunogenetic antigen, IV immunoglobulin, and cytokine therapy can be used individually or in combination. In neutropenic neonates born to mothers with pregnancy-induced hypertension, the condition is characteristically limited to the first 72 hours of life and seldom requires treatment.

"Hypersplenic" neutropenia is seldom severe enough to cause serious infection. Therapy should be directed at correcting the underlying cause of splenomegaly if possible. Splenectomy is a last resort. Replacement therapy for nutritional deficiencies of vitamin B_{12} and folic acid specifically and promptly correct the associated neutropenia. Pure white cell aplasia, in which the bone marrow morphology shows absence of myeloid precursors, occurs in most cases with a thymoma and occasionally with ibuprofen therapy. Thymectomy may be effective in the former situation but usually also requires immunosuppression and/or IV immunoglobulins. With ibuprofen-induced neutropenia, stopping the drug corrects the problem.

For many of the congenital or inherited neutropenias, cytokine therapy is extremely effective in reversing the abnormal hematology. Severe chronic neutropenia was targeted in 1987 for clinical trials with G-CSF (filgrastim [Neupogen]), and more than 95% of patients with congenital, cyclic, and idiopathic forms of neutropenia responded completely. Based on data compiled by the Severe Chronic Neutropenia International Registry (University of Washington, Seattle), G-CSF is now considered the standard first-line treatment for these conditions. A second product, granulocyte-macrophage colony-stimulating factor (GM-CSF, sargramostim [Leukine]), is second-line therapy for severe chronic neutropenia in North America because of less predictable neutrophilic responses. For adults on chemotherapy for nonmyeloid malignancies, pegfilgrastim (Neulasta) can be used to offset severe neutropenia. The product is a long-lasting form of G-CSF that is indicated to decrease the incidence of infection in patients receiving marrow-suppressive antineoplastic agents (see later).

For patients with a neutrophil count of less than 500/μL with congenital neutropenia (encompassing Kostmann's syndrome, Shwachman-Diamond syndrome, glycogen storage disease type 1b, and Fanconi anemia), and for the cyclic and idiopathic forms, G-CSF is started

---

[3]Exceeds dosage recommended by the manufacturer.

at 5 µg/kg/day subcutaneously. If the ANC rises to 1000 to 5000/µL and plateaus, the same G-CSF dosage is maintained. If the ANC exceeds 5000/µL, the dose is reduced to 3 µg/kg to bring the count to 1000 to 5000/µL. If the ANC still exceeds 5000/µL, the dose is lowered further to 1 µg/kg or to alternate-day dosing, for example, 1 to 2 µg/kg every second day.

If there is no response to the starting dose, the G-CSF is increased to 10 µg/kg/day. If there is still no effect, increments are continued every 2 to 4 weeks to 20 µg/kg/day,[3] then 30 µg/kg/day,[3] and so on, up to a maximum of 120 µg/kg/day[3] (which would require a twice-daily administration or multiple subcutaneous injections at the same time). A patient who fails to respond to 120 µg/kg/day is defined as being refractory to G-CSF treatment. A trial of GM-CSF would then be warranted using a starting dose of 3 to 15 µg/kg/day (250 µg/m^2/day) subcutaneously. Another option is a hematopoietic stem cell transplantation if there is an HLA-matched donor.

G-CSF, 5 to 10 µg/kg/day, either IV or subcutaneously, is also indicated for other forms of severe neutropenia, especially those associated with chemotherapy, using the following guidelines that we developed at the Hospital for Sick Children, Toronto:

- For febrile neutropenic patients who have positive blood cultures, have an identified focus of infection, and/or whose vital signs are unstable
- For patients receiving chemotherapy protocols that predictably induce severe neutropenia to increase safety and to ensure that the full course of chemotherapy is administered and given on time. G-CSF should be administered after the first and subsequent cycles of the chemotherapy in these patients
- With antineoplastic dose-escalation protocols that predictably induce severe neutropenia
- For patients enrolled in multicenter chemotherapy protocols that specify the use of G-CSF
- For patients receiving antineoplastic agents in conjunction with large-volume irradiation involving bone marrow

In this setting as a preventive agent, G-CSF can be stopped when neutrophils are more than 1500 µL for 2 consecutive days. When G-CSF is given for fever-neutropenia, or to patients whose condition is unstable or who have a focus of infection or a positive culture, it can be stopped when neutrophils are greater than 1000/µL for 2 days if the patient is clinically improved, the focus has resolved, and the cultures are negative.

For adults receiving Neulasta, the recommended dosage is a single subcutaneous injection of 6 mg administered once per cycle of chemotherapy. It should not be given in the interval between 14 days before and 24 hours after chemotherapy because of the potential for an increase in sensitivity of rapidly dividing myeloid to cytotoxicity.

REFERENCES

Dinauer MC: The phagocyte system and disorders of granulopoiesis and granulocyte function. In Nathan DG, Orkin SH, Ginsburg D, Look AT (eds): Hematology of Infancy and Childhood, 6th ed. Philadelphia, WB Saunders, 2003, pp 923-1010.

Kowalczyk A (ed): 2005–2006 Drug Handbook and Formulary, Hospital for Sick Children, 24th ed. pp 178-185. To order or for drug information: Telephone: 416-813-6703; e-mail: druginfo@sickkids.ca

Watts RG: Neutropenia. In Greer JP, Foerster J, Lukens JN, et al (eds): Wintrobe's Clinical Hematology, 11th ed. Philadelphia, Lippincott, Williams & Wilkins, 2004, pp 1777-1800.

Hemolytic Disease of the Newborn

Method of
James W. Kendig, MD

Hemolytic disease of the fetus and newborn refers to a spectrum of problems that were formerly classified as four separate entities: erythroblastosis fetalis, congenital anemia, icterus gravis neonatorum, and hydrops fetalis. Further studies demonstrated that these entities are all manifestations of a single disease caused by red blood cell isoimmunization (alloimmunization).

The major red blood cell surface antigen responsible for this process is the $Rh_o(D)$ antigen. Because there is no corresponding "d" antigen, the term "d" refers only to the absence of the $Rh_o(D)$ antigen. $Rh_o(D)$-negative individuals (dd) have no $Rh_o(D)$ antigens on their red blood cells. $Rh_o(D)$-positive individuals may be homozygous (DD) or heterozygous (Dd) for the $Rh_o(D)$ gene, which is located on the short arm of chromosome 1. In addition to the $Rh_o(D)$ gene, the Rh blood group system includes the related Cc Ee structural gene, which encodes four specific antigens (C, c, E, and e) on the red blood cell surface. Zygosity for $Rh_o(D)$ may be predicted on the basis of classic serologic tests for the antigens C, c, D, E, e, and the known incidence of various phenotypes in different racial and ethnic groups.

$Rh_o(D)$ alloimmunization occurs when fetal $Rh_o(D)$-positive red blood cells (inherited from the father) cross the placenta and enter the circulation of an $Rh_o(D)$-negative (dd) mother. The maternal immune system is stimulated to produce $Rh_o(D)$ antibodies (IgG). ABO incompatibility (mother 0 and fetus A or B) helps to protect against the $Rh_o(D)$ sensitization of the $Rh_o(D)$-negative mother.

The maternal $Rh_o(D)$ antibodies cross the placenta of the current or a subsequent pregnancy and cause the destruction of the $Rh_o(D)$-positive fetal red blood cells. The fetus responds to this hemolytic anemia with extramedullary hematopoiesis involving the liver and spleen. The hepatic production of fetal albumin is compromised, leading to hydrops with edema, ascites, and pericardial and pleural effusions. Bilirubin, produced by the hemolysis of fetal red blood cells, readily crosses the placenta and is excreted by the maternal liver. After delivery, however, neonatal hyperbilirubinemia develops, which may lead to an acute encephalopathy (kernicterus). Other red blood cell antigen–antibody systems (Kidd, Kell, Duffy, the C/c and E/e alleles of the Rh system, and, rarely, the ABO system) may occasionally result in hemolytic disease of the fetus and newborn. In the case of anti-Kell isoimmunization, fetal

---

[3]Exceeds dosage recommended by the manufacturer.

anemia is caused by a suppression of erythropoiesis in addition to hemolysis.

Prevention of Rh$_o$(D) Alloimmunization

The development, commercial production, and widespread use of commercially prepared Rh$_o$(D) immunoglobulin (RhoGAM) for the prevention of Rh$_o$(D) alloimmunization are among the greatest scientific and medical achievements of the 20th century. This is an example of passive immunization preventing active immunization, but the precise mechanism by which the administration of the Rh$_o$(D) antibody blocks the mother's production of the same antibody is still not fully understood. RhoGAM is not beneficial to the Rh$_o$(D)-negative woman after alloimmunization has taken place, and it does not prevent sensitization because of the C/c and E/e antigens of the Rh blood group system. Box 1 gives a list of events and procedures that may lead to the Rh$_o$(D) alloimmunization of the Rh$_o$(D)-negative woman. An intramuscular dose of RhoGAM (300 μg) should be administered after these events and procedures. In the event of a severe fetal-to-maternal hemorrhage at delivery, more than 300 μg of RhoGAM may be required.

Blood type (ABO and Rh$_o$(D)) and an antibody screen (the indirect Coombs test) should be obtained on the first prenatal visit. The antibody screen detects Rh$_o$(D) antibodies as well as antibodies directed against the other red blood cell antigens, such as Kell, Duffy, C/c, and E/e. If the antibody screen is positive, alloimmunization has already occurred, and serial titers should be obtained. If the antibody titer is 1:16 or greater by 20 weeks' gestation, further testing is necessary.

ANTEPARTUM PREVENTION

At 28 weeks' gestation, all Rh$_o$(D)-negative mothers should have an antibody screen (indirect Coombs test).

> **BOX 1   Reproductive Events and Procedures That Can Lead to Alloimmunization of the Rh$_o$(D)-Negative Woman**
>
> **Events**
> - Threatened abortion and antepartum hemorrhage
> - Spontaneous abortion
> - Delivery at any gestational age
> - Ectopic pregnancy
> - Hydatidiform molar pregnancy
> - Abdominal trauma and motor vehicle accidents during pregnancy
> - Inadvertent transfusion with Rh-positive blood
>
> **Procedures**
> - Cordocentesis
> - Chorionic villous sampling
> - Induced abortion
> - Amniocentesis any time during pregnancy
> - External cephalic version
> - Delivery at any time

If the test is negative, a prophylactic intramuscular dose of RhoGAM (300 μg) should be administered, unless the father of the infant is definitely known to be Rh$_o$(D)-negative (dd). The purpose of this prophylactic antepartum dose is to prevent alloimmunization during the pregnancy. The half-life of this dose is 12 weeks. This antepartum dose may lead to a weakly positive indirect Coombs test in the mother at the time of delivery and a weakly positive direct Coombs test in the infant.

POSTPARTUM PREVENTION

Every Rh$_o$(D)-negative mother who has not undergone Rh$_o$(D) alloimmunization should receive an intramuscular dose of *at least* 300 μg of RhoGAM after the delivery of an Rh$_o$(D)-positive newborn. This critical step in the prevention of Rh$_o$(D) disease requires careful communication among the labor and delivery area, the hospital blood bank, and the postpartum floor. These communication issues are particularly important when early discharge from the hospital is being considered and when the birth has occurred outside the hospital.

A single dose of RhoGAM (300 μg) neutralizes approximately 30 mL of Rh$_o$(D)-positive fetal whole blood or 15 mL of packed fetal red blood cells. If a large fetal-to-maternal transfusion should occur at the time of delivery, a single dose of RhoGAM may be inadequate to prevent alloimmunization. Because of this possibility, the hospital blood bank should check the mother's blood after delivery to determine the presence and the magnitude of a fetal-to-maternal bleed. The rosette test is used to screen maternal blood for the presence of fetal red blood cells, and the Kleihauer-Betke stain is used to evaluate the magnitude of a fetal-to-maternal bleed. This information is used to determine the need for a larger (more than 300 μg) dose of intramuscular RhoGAM. RhoGAM should be administered within 72 hours of delivery. If administration has been inadvertently omitted, it may still be given up to 4 weeks after delivery. The Rh$_o$(D)-negative mother who is already Rh$_o$(D) alloimmunized at the time of delivery will not benefit from the administration of RhoGAM.

Obstetric Management of the Mother With a Positive Initial Antibody Screen

All pregnant women should have an antibody screen (indirect Coombs test) at the first prenatal visit. If the result is positive, the blood bank identifies the antibody and determines its titer. The blood bank examines the father's red blood cells for the corresponding antigen. If the father's result is negative for the antigen, and if the mother has absolutely no doubts regarding paternity, no further studies are required. If the father's result is positive for the involved antigen, the mother should have serial antibody titers at 1-month intervals. Early ultrasonography should also be done for gestational age assessment. If a critical antibody titer of 1:16 is reached, there is a risk of the development of erythroblastosis fetalis and hydrops, and further investigation and interventions are required (Figure 1).

The Rh$_o$(D)-alloimmunized mother with a history of a previous pregnancy requiring an intrauterine transfusion

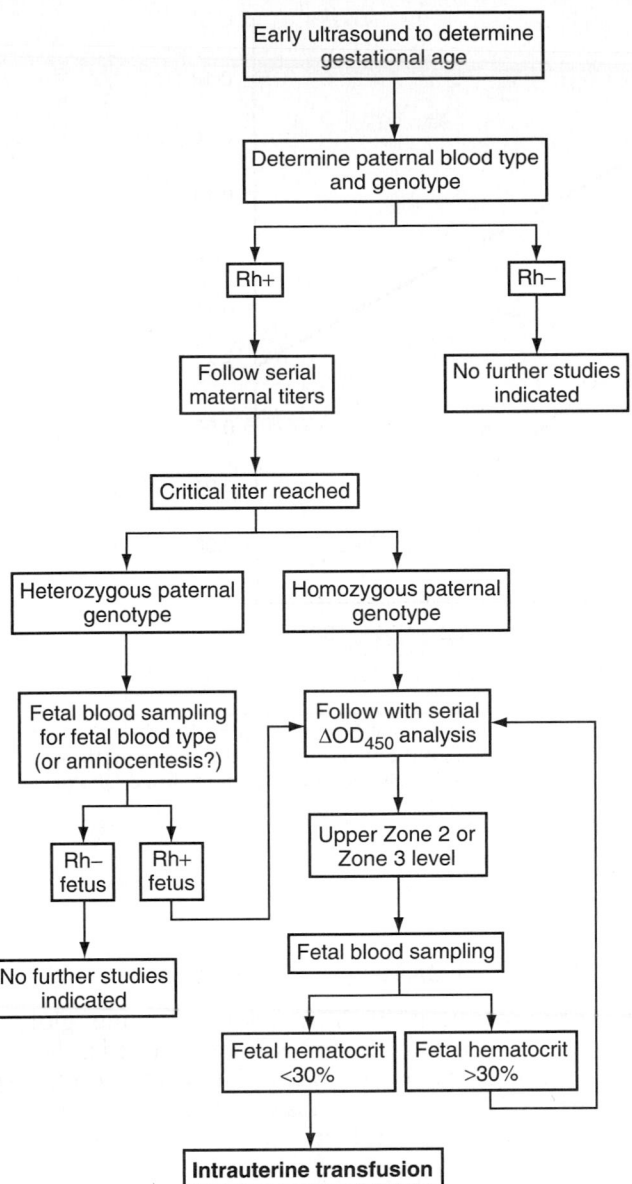

FIGURE 1. Algorithm used at Baylor College of Medicine, Houston, for the management of newly diagnosed, red blood cell $Rh_o(D)$ alloimmunization in pregnancy. (From Moise KJ: Changing trends in the management of red blood cell alloimmunization in pregnancy. Arch Pathol Lab Med 1994;118:421-428. Copyright 1994, American Medical Association. Used with permission.)

or a neonatal exchange transfusion is at a high risk for hydrops. With this history, serial ΔOD_{450} (optical density at 450 nm) evaluations of amniotic fluid are recommended, starting at 20 to 22 weeks' gestation, even if the antibody titer has not reached the critical level of 1:16.

PATERNAL ZYGOSITY

If the maternal antibody is $Rh_o(D)$, and the father has the corresponding $Rh_o(D)$ antigen, the blood bank determines whether he is homozygous (DD) or heterozygous (Dd). This prediction is based on the classic serologic tests for the C, c, E, and e antigens and the known incidence of various phenotypes in different racial and ethnic groups. If the

father is heterozygous, there is a 50% chance that the fetal red blood cells are $Rh_o(D)$-negative (dd) and that the fetus is not at risk for the development of erythroblastosis fetalis. If the father is heterozygous, it is useful to determine the fetal blood type.

DETERMINATION OF FETAL BLOOD TYPE

Techniques for obtaining samples of fetal blood from the umbilical vessels, using ultrasound guidance, have been perfected and are available at large regional perinatal centers. This procedure, known as cordocentesis, involves obvious risks and should be performed only by specialists experienced in fetal and maternal medicine. Several centers have used the polymerase chain reaction (PCR) to identify the fetal $Rh_o(D)$ genotype. This new technique is based on the amplification of the DNA from a few fetal red blood cells found in a centrifuged sample of amniotic fluid. If the mother has $Rh_o(D)$ antibodies and the fetus is $Rh_o(D)$-negative (by cordocentesis of a fetal blood sample or by PCR of fetal red blood cells from amniotic fluid), no further studies are indicated.

AMNIOTIC FLUID ΔOD_{450} MEASUREMENTS

If the maternal antibody titer reaches a critical titer of 1:16 and if there is a possibility that the fetal red blood cells are positive for the corresponding antigen, serial measurements of amniotic fluid ΔOD_{450} should be done every 10 to 14 days to evaluate the level of bilirubin in the amniotic fluid. These values are plotted on the modified Liley curve (Figure 2).

INTRAUTERINE FETAL TRANSFUSION

When ΔOD_{450} values climb to the upper indeterminate zone or anywhere in the $Rh_o(D)$-positive (affected) zone on the modified Liley curve, cordocentesis should be done to measure the fetal hematocrit. If this value is less than 30%, an intravascular fetal transfusion (via cordocentesis) of packed red blood cells should be carried out at a regional perinatal center by specialists experienced in maternal and fetal medicine. For severe hydrops, more than one intrauterine transfusion may be required. The timing of delivery should be based on gestational age estimates and the determination of fetal lung maturity.

Management of the Newborn With Erythroblastosis Fetalis

DELIVERY ROOM MANAGEMENT

With advances in the field of maternal–fetal medicine and the use of intravascular fetal transfusions, it is unusual for an infant to be delivered with severe erythroblastosis and hydrops secondary to $Rh_o(D)$. When this does occur, however, three teams of neonatologists, pediatricians, and nurse practitioners must be immediately available to initiate multiple interventions.

One team is responsible for airway management, including intubation, and the initiation of positive-pressure ventilation. This team also monitors the heart rate and initiates chest compressions, if needed. A second team

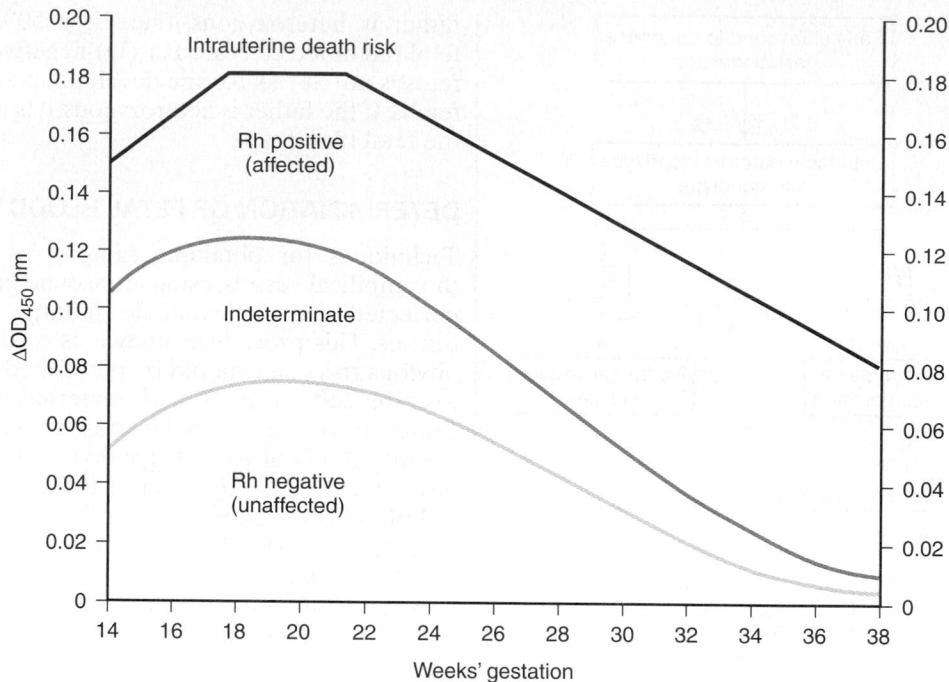

FIGURE 2. Amniotic fluid optical density (ΔOD_{450}) zones for management of pregnancy complicated by $Rh_o(D)$ alloim-munization. (From Queenan JT, Tomai TP, Ural SH, King JC: Deviation in amniotic fluid optical density at a wavelength of 450 nm in Rh-immunized pregnancies from 14 to 40 weeks' gestation: A proposal for clinical management. Am J Obstet Gynecol 1993;168:1370-1376. Used with permission.)

is responsible for securing immediate intravascular access, usually via the umbilical vein. A hematocrit value is obtained immediately, and if it is less than 30%, a partial exchange transfusion using 25 to 80 mL per kg of packed red blood cells is carried out within 30 minutes of birth to raise the hematocrit to 40% or higher. A third team should be available to perform paracentesis and thoracentesis, if needed. With severe hydrops, effective pulmonary ventilation frequently cannot be achieved until large collections of pleural and ascitic fluid have been removed.

Immediately after umbilical cord clamping, the obstetric team should obtain a sample of cord blood, which is sent to the laboratory for a direct Coombs test and determination of hematocrit, reticulocyte count, total and direct bilirubin levels, cord pH, and blood gas tension values.

INTENSIVE PHOTOTHERAPY

Upon admission to the neonatal intensive care nursery, the infant with erythroblastosis fetalis should be placed immediately under intensive phototherapy. This can be achieved by using multiple banks of special blue fluorescent tubes (e.g., F20T12/BB manufactured by General Electric, Westinghouse, and Sylvania).

Place the full-term infant in a bassinet rather than an incubator, and line the sides of the bassinet with white linens or aluminum foil to maximize surface area exposure.

Obtain serial serum bilirubin values (total and direct) at 2- to 3-hour intervals to establish the rate of rise under intensive phototherapy, and plot the levels, as shown in Figure 3.

INTRAVENOUS GAMMA GLOBULIN

The administration of intravenous immune globulin (IVIG) (0.5 g/kg over 2 hours) is recommended if the total serum bilirubin is rising in spite of intensive phototherapy or if the total serum bilirubin is within 2 to 3 mg/dL of the exchange level shown in Figure 3.

NEONATAL DOUBLE-VOLUME EXCHANGE TRANSFUSION

With the widespread use of RhoGAM to prevent the alloimmunization of $Rh_o(D)$-negative women, coupled with advances in fetal intravascular transfusion therapy, neonatal double-volume exchange transfusions are becoming rare procedures. When neonatal exchange transfusions are required, they should be done by experienced neonatologists and pediatricians working in neonatal centers that are prepared to deal with the various complications of the procedure, which include hypoglycemia, thrombocytopenia, necrotizing enterocolitis, and infection.

After the delivery of an infant with erythroblastosis fetalis, serial serum bilirubin values (total and direct) should be obtained at 2- to 3-hour intervals to establish the rate of rise. A serum indirect bilirubin level that is climbing by more than 0.5 mg per dL per hour indicates that there is a relatively brisk hemolytic process that may require a double-volume exchange transfusion within the first 12 hours after birth. Recently published guidelines for exchange transfusions are shown in Figure 3. In addition to lowering the serum bilirubin level, an early double-volume

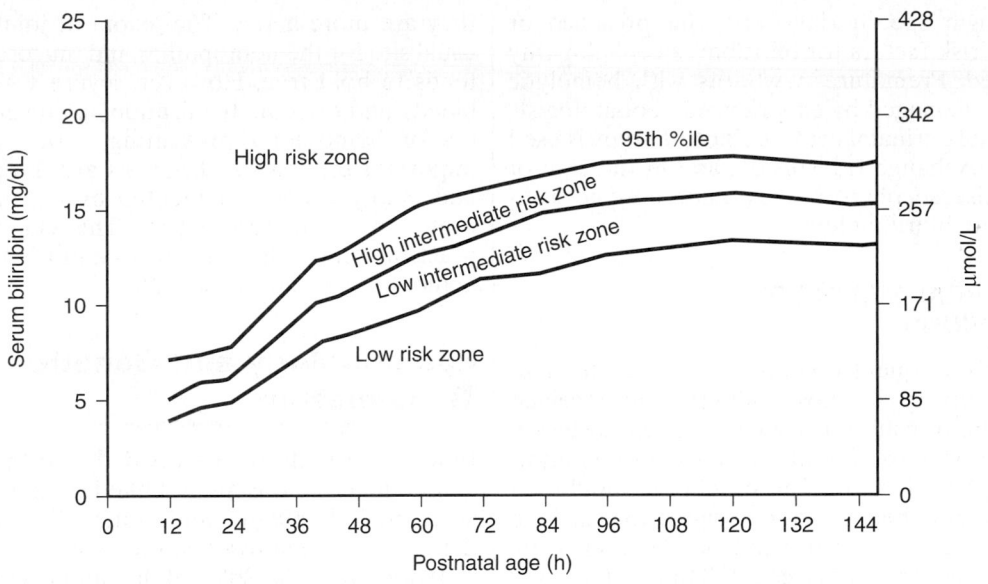

FIGURE 3. Nomogram for designation of risk in 2840 well newborns at 36 or more weeks' gestational age with birth weight of 2000 g or more, or 35 or more weeks' gestational age and birth weight of 2500 g or more based on the hour-specific serum bilirubin values. The serum bilirubin level was obtained before discharge, and the zone in which the value fell predicted the likelihood of a subsequent bilirubin level exceeding the 95th percentile (high-risk zone). (From Pediatrics 2004;114(1):297-316, American Academy of Pediatrics. Used with permission.)

exchange transfusion helps to correct the fetal anemia and removes a significant portion of the antibody-coated red blood cells before they hemolyze. The blood sample for routine metabolic screens for hypothyroidism, inborn errors of metabolism, and hemoglobinopathies should be drawn before the exchange transfusion is performed.

 CURRENT DIAGNOSIS

■ Blood type—ABO and Rh₀(D)—and an antibody screen (the indirect Coombs test) should be obtained on the first prenatal visit. If the antibody screen is positive, alloimmunization has already occurred, and serial titers should be obtained. If the titer reaches a critical level of 1:16 or greater, additional testing such as determination of paternal zygosity, amniocentesis, and cordocentesis will need to be done by a specialist in maternal–fetal medicine.

■ All Rh₀(D)-negative mothers who deliver an Rh₀(D)-positive infant should be screened with a rosette test or a Kleihauer-Betke test to detect an excessive fetal–maternal hemorrhage. Those mothers with evidence of an excessive fetal–maternal hemorrhage may need more than the standard 1 vial of Rh₀(D)-immunoglobulin (RhoGAM).

■ There is no single simple test to tell what level of bilirubin is dangerous to any given infant at any given time.

■ Following intensive phototherapy and/or exchange transfusion for moderate to severe erythroblastosis fetalis, serial hematocrit values must be followed carefully for 4 to 8 weeks to determine the need for a top-up transfusion of packed red blood cells.

Serial serum bilirubin levels should be continued even if an early double-volume exchange transfusion is not mandated by the rate of rise. It is impossible to determine exactly what level of indirect bilirubin constitutes a risk for encephalopathy (kernicterus on neuropathology) in any given infant at any given time. Prematurity, hypoxia, asphyxia, acidosis, sepsis, and hypoalbuminemia may increase the risk of bilirubin encephalopathy. Various drugs, such as the sulfa preparations and ceftriaxone, displace bilirubin from albumin-binding sites and increase the risk for encephalopathy.

In the otherwise healthy, full-term newborn with hemolytic disease, the indirect bilirubin level should not be permitted to climb above 20 mg per dL. With prematurity and hemolytic disease, lower threshold levels for exchange transfusion, based on gestational age, birth

 CURRENT THERAPY

■ The unsensitized, Rh₀(D)-negative patient should receive prophylactic anti-D immunoglobulin (RhoGAM) at 28 weeks' gestation and again post-delivery at any gestational age if newborn infant is Rh₀(D) positive.

■ The unsensitized, Rh₀(D)-negative patient should receive prophylactic RhoGAM after any of the following events and procedures: Ectopic gestation, abruption of placenta, abortion, abdominal trauma, amniocentesis, cordocentesis, chorionic villous sampling, and external cephalic version.

■ The combined use of intensive phototherapy and intravenous immunoglobulin may reduce the need for an exchange transfusion.

weight, chronologic age in days, and the presence or absence of other risk factors for bilirubin encephalopathy are recommended. Premature newborns with hemolytic disease should be managed by experienced neonatologists working in regional perinatal centers. Phototherapy is used as an adjunct to exchange transfusion, and in the case of mild hemolytic disease, phototherapy alone may be sufficient to control the bilirubin level.

DELAYED NEONATAL RED BLOOD CELL TRANSFUSIONS

A slow hemolysis frequently continues for up to 6 to 8 weeks after delivery in those infants who received a fetal intravascular transfusion or an exchange transfusion after delivery and in those infants with a mild hemolysis requiring only phototherapy. These infants should be followed up with serial hematocrit determinations at 1- to 2-week intervals during the first 6 to 8 weeks after birth. A transfusion of packed red blood cells (10 to 15 mL per kg) may be necessary to correct severe anemia. With severe hemolytic anemia, particularly in infants who received intrauterine transfusions, fetal and neonatal iron stores are elevated. Neonatal iron therapy should be withheld until the serum ferritin level returns to normal.

REFERENCES

American Academy of Pediatrics: Clinical practice guidelines for management of hyperbilirubinemia in the newborn infant 35 or more weeks of gestation. Pediatrics 2004;114(1):297-316.

American College of Obstetricians and Gynecologists: Prevention of RhD Alloimmunization. ACOG Practice Bulletin 4. Washington, DC, ACOG, 1999.

Gottstein R, Cooke RWI: Systematic review of intravenous immunoglobulin in haemolytic disease of the newborn. Arch Dis Child Fetal Neonatal Ed 2003;88:F6-F10.

Harkness UF, Spinnato JA: Prevention and management of RhD isoimmunization. Clin Perinatol 2004;31(4):721-742.

Maisels MJ: Why use homeopathic doses of phototherapy? Pediatrics 1996;98:283-287.

McKenna DS, Nagaraja HN, O'Shaughnessy R: Management of pregnancies complicated by anti-Kell isoimmunization. Obstet Gynecol 1999;93:667-673.

Hemophilia and Related Disorders

Method of
Wing-Yen Wong, MD

Hemophilia A and B and von Willebrand's disease (vWd) are the most common causes of bleeding. Less common bleeding disorders also need to be considered in the orderly workup of any coagulopathy. The newborn with prolonged bleeding after circumcision, the toddler with bruises not only on the shins and arms but also in areas not usually subject to direct trauma such as the torso and neck, and the teenager with more than 5 to 7 days of heavy menstrual bleeding all deserve attention. Moderately affected children may not present until toddler age when they are more active. The axiom of joint bleeding as the usual site for the hemophilias and mucosal bleeds for vWd tends to hold true. However, severe vWd can have joint bleeds, and extreme lyonization can result in female carriers of hemophilia presenting with menorrhagia. The important criteria for diagnosis are the patient's medical and family history augmented by age-appropriate interpretation of laboratory tests. This chapter focuses on a practical approach to diagnosis and treatment choices for hemophilia A and B, and vWd.

Epidemiology and Genetic Transmission

Inheritance patterns are divided into three main groups: hemophilia A and B are X-linked recessive, vWd is usually autosomal dominant, and some vWd and other factor deficiencies are autosomal recessive.

Approximately 30% of hemophilia in boys presents with new mutations and negative family histories. Incidence of hemophilia A is estimated at 1 in 5000 male births and 1 in 30,000 for hemophilia B. There are no geographic or racial differences. Mild hemophilia is often misdiagnosed and therefore may be underrepresented. Carrier and prenatal testing from blood and amniotic samples has more than 90% accuracy if performed at established laboratories, particularly if blood samples from various affected family members are available for DNA linkage studies.

Inversion within intron 22 of the FVIII gene is found in more than 45% of severely affected hemophilia A patients. DNA analysis for this and other mutations is available at certain research laboratories. Testing from chorionic villus sampling can be done at 10 to 12 weeks' gestation if the specific genetic mutation is known, but sampling of fetal blood for FVIII activity cannot be done prior to 16 weeks' gestation.

The incidence of vWd is unknown, and estimates vary from 0.2% to 2.0%. There are no gender or racial differences. The complexity of the various vWd subtypes and the generally mild nature of vWd has not lent itself to easy prenatal testing and hence is not usually performed. A large number of vWd molecular gene defects are identified. The information can be obtained from online databank sites. DNA testing can be helpful for vWd subtypes such as type 2N, which can be misdiagnosed as hemophilia A because both disorders have low levels of FVIII. In vWd type 2A, both vWf (von Willebrand's factor) and ristocetin cofactor (RCoF) are decreased, whereas hemophilia A has normal vWf and RCoF levels. People with blood type O have slightly lower baseline levels of vWd than type AB.

FXI deficiency is the most common hereditary coagulopathy in patients of Jewish descent. The degree of bleeding is highly variable.

Disease Classification and Laboratory Testing

The activated partial prothrombin time (APTT) measures most common clotting factor abnormalities associated with bleeding diatheses except for FVII and FXIII. Hemophilia A and B patients with inhibitors have

Bleeds/Procedures	Hemophilia A	Hemophilia B	Type 1 vWd
Minor	20–30 U/kg/12–24 h × 1–3 doses	30–50 U/kg/24-48 h × 1–3 doses	Stimate, 1–2 s/d × 1–2 d
Major*	40–50 U/kg /8–12 h	60–100 U/kg/12–24 h	Humate-P, 30–60 RCoF U/kg/12–24 h
Continuous infusion	Load with bolus as above; then 2–5 U/kg/h	Load with bolus as above; then 5–10 U/kg/h	

*Major bleeds/surgeries: levels should be monitored and maintained at 100% for at least 72 h.
Abbreviations: RCoF = ristocetin cofactor; vWd = von Willebrand's disease.

prolonged APTT uncorrected by a 1:1 mixing ratio with normal plasma. FVII deficiency is associated with a prolonged PT, whereas FXIII deficiency has normal prothrombin time (PT), APTT, and thrombin time (TT). Some causes of a prolonged APTT not associated with significant bleeding even with major trauma or surgery include deficiencies of high molecular weight kininogen (HMWK), prekallikrein, and FXII. Exclusion of an inhibitor such as antiphospholipid antibody should also be considered in the face of a prolonged APTT and a benign bleeding history. Excessive fibrinolysis such as α-2-antiplasmin deficiency also causes increased bleeding, but these disorders are rare.

The mechanism of disease in the coagulopathies may involve failure of synthesis of the necessary coagulation factor or synthesis of abnormal proteins with impaired activity. Hence, the functional protein activity may differ from the amount of protein measured.

Hemophilia A and B result in inadequate generation of thrombin for clot formation. The degree of disease severity and onset of symptoms vary with plasma FVIII or FIX activity levels. Boys with less than 1% factor activity have severe disease with early onset of joint and muscle bleeds. Those with hemophilia A have bleeding symptoms earlier in life, usually within the first year, compared to hemophilia B. Moderate and mild disease correlate to factor activity levels of 1% to 5% and more than 5%, respectively. Carrier females have factor levels ranging from 30% to 70%.

In vWd, the mechanism of disease is associated with failure to form an effective primary platelet plug. There are three main types of vWd and numerous subtypes. Type 1 vWd is caused by a partial quantitative deficiency of vWf, type 2 has qualitative variants, and type 3 has marked, sometimes complete, deficiency of vWf. Overall, types 1 and 2 tend to have mild to moderate severity of bleeding, whereas the rarer type 3 tends to have severe disease.

Type 2N has a defective affinity for FVIII, and both FVIII and vWf are markedly decreased. It is critical that physicians, especially gynecologists and obstetricians, consider the workup and diagnosis for vWd in any female with menorrhagia. Diagnosis of vWd can be difficult to ascertain with some affected individuals having near normal or fluctuating von Willebrand's factor antigen (vWf:Ag) and RCoF levels and significant clinical bleeding. Table 1 outlines the main characteristics of hemophilia A and vWd.

Treatment Options

HEMOPHILIA A AND B

The hallmark to effective treatment remains replacement of the deficient or abnormal factor as early as possible, at the appropriate dosage and frequency. The ability to self-infuse or have a caregiver administer the factor at home at the first sign of any bleeding has a positive impact on disease outcome. For this approach to be effective, early recognition of bleeding is required. Early symptoms for joint or muscle bleeds include increased warmth, tingling sensations, or a vague feeling at the affected or target joint. Increased irritability in the infant or young child often heralds the onset of a bleed. Patients should not wait for swelling or discoloration to infuse.

Care at a specialty hemophilia treatment center (HTC) significantly improves disease outcome. These facilities have the necessary expertise to coordinate all aspects of diagnosis and care, acute and chronic, as well as a multifaceted team approach. Close telephone contact should be maintained between the family and HTC personnel in the event of any bleeding episode, even when home therapy has been initiated successfully.

TABLE 1 Key Diagnostic Comparison of Hemophilia A and von Willebrand's Disease

	Hemophilia A	vWd*
Inheritance	X-linked	Autosomal
Bleeding pattern	Mainly joint, muscle bleeds	Mainly mucous membrane bleeds (e.g., epistaxis, menorrhagia)
PTT	↑	Nl or ↑
FVIIIa	↓	Nl or ↓
vWf:Ag	Nl	↓ or Nl
RcoF	Nl	↓ or Nl
Ivy bleeding time	Nl	↑

*Modifying factors include blood type (type O has decreased vWf), stress, physical activity, estrogen use, and pregnancy. Normal values do not definitively exclude diagnosis of vWd and can vary from time to time within the same individual.
Abbreviations: PTT = partial thromboplastin time; RCoF = ristocetin cofactor; vWd = von Willebrand's disease; vWf = von Willebrand's factor; vWf:Ag = von Willebrand's factor antigen.

For mild hemophilia A, desmopressin (Stimate), a concentrated form of desmopressin acetate (DDAVP), can be used without exposure to blood products. This is particularly helpful in persons avoiding blood products for religious reasons and in decreasing the risk of infectious transmissions. Details of this treatment option are covered later in the section on the treatment of vWd. Stimate should not be used for FIX-deficient patients.

The current treatment of choice for newly diagnosed severely affected individuals with hemophilia A or B is recombinant FVIII or FIX. New products within this category are being added to our armamentarium. Choice of treatment product for previously treated patients largely depends on patient preference and prior rating of clinical efficacy. Studies showed that infusion of ultra-high-purity products is associated with preservation of CD4 counts in HIV-infected individuals.

Table 2 lists the replacement factor choices for hemophilia A and B in categories of purity. With established efficacy, random changes are not advisable unless otherwise clinically indicated. However, because of intermittent product shortages, physicians and patients are sometimes required to substitute proprietary factor concentrates. I attempt to keep within a similar category if at all possible. A product may have two different brand names but can be interchangeable (e.g., Helixate and Kogenate). ReFacto is a recombinant FVIII product that has the B domain deleted and is a slightly smaller molecule. A new longer-acting liposomal-pegylated rFVIII is currently undergoing clinical trials.

TREATMENT DOSAGE AND FREQUENCY

Dosing regimens are targeted to maintain replacement plasma factor at certain levels based on the severity and site of bleed. FVIII has a shorter half-life than FIX and should be infused every 8 to 12 hours for an acute bleed compared to every 12 to 24 hours for FIX. FXIII has the longest half-life T_{12} and can be replaced monthly for most patients. Mild muscle and soft-tissue bleeds require 30% factor plasma level for 1 to 2 days. Major hemorrhage,

surgeries, and gastrointestinal (GI) or central nervous system (CNS) bleeds require more than 90% to 100% levels for at least 72 hours. Continuous infusions are often employed for major surgeries or severe bleeds to achieve consistent plasma factor levels.

Here are the calculations to achieve these targeted levels:

FVIII infusions: number of units required per dose = weight (kg) × % factor level desired × 0.5 (e.g., to achieve 100% in a 50-kg person, number of units required per dose = 50 × 100 × 0.5 = 2500 U)

However, wastage of extra factor above the calculated range is discouraged. Hence, the amount actually given is often rounded up to the closest vial size:

FIX infusions: number of units required per dose = weight (kg) × % factor level desired × 1

BeneFix infusion: number of units required per dose = weight (kg) × % factor level desired × 1.2

Monitoring of plasma levels (at 1 hour pre- and postinfusion) with initial infusions and at times of dosage change would guide dosage adjustment needs.

TREATMENT IN THE PRESENCE OF INHIBITORS

Inhibitory antibodies to FVIII arise in 30% of those with severely affected hemophilia A and 3% to 5% of children with hemophilia B during the first 15 to 30 infusion exposures. These antibodies develop after exposure to the exogenous protein and therefore tend to occur in those with large gene deletions and severe disease. The presence of inhibitors should be suspected when failure to achieve adequate hemostasis with routine replacement therapy is observed. Inhibitors are measured by the Bethesda assay in Bethesda units (BUs). High-titer or high-responding inhibitors are more than 5 BU. The level of inhibitor activity determines the choice of appropriate management options. Low-titer or low-responding FVIII inhibitors can be managed by using higher doses of factor concentrate. For mild to moderate bleeds, a dose of twice the routine amount usually suffices. For major bleeds, a bolus of 100 to 150 U/kg[3] followed by continuous infusion at 15 to 20 U/kg/hour for 3 to 4 days may be required. Inhibitor titers may rise sharply because of an anamnestic response and need to be monitored for optimum care.

High-responding inhibitors pose a difficult therapeutic challenge. Often continuous infusions fail to achieve and maintain hemostasis, particularly in major bleeds or surgery. Porcine FVIII at a 100 to 150 U/kg starting dose is successful in hemophilia A inhibitor patients. Monitoring antiporcine FVIII antibodies should be performed. Prothrombin complex concentrates (PCCs), a pool of FII, FIX, X, and FVII, can be used at 75 to 100 U/kg of FIX for minor bleeds. The dose can be repeated once or twice every 12 hours. If bleeding is not controlled within two to three doses, alternate treatment should be used.

TABLE 2   FVIII and FIX Concentrates

Factor Type	FVIII	FIX
Recombinant	Helixate FS/ Kogenate-FS ReFacto Recombinate Advate	BeneFix
Ultra high purity Plasma derived	Hemofil M Monark M Monoclate-P	AlphaNine SD Mononine
Other plasma derived	Alphanate* SD Humate-P*† Koate-DVI*	Bebulin VH Profilnine SD Proplex-T

*Contains varying amounts of von Willebrand's factor.
†FDA approved for von Willebrand's disease.

___

[3]Exceeds dosage recommended by the manufacturer.

Heparin should be added at 5 to 10 U/mL of the reconstituted PCC. The mechanism of action is unclear. Activated prothrombin complex concentrates (APCCs) can be similarly applied at 50 to 75 U/kg FIX. Both PCCs and APCCs have increased thrombogenic potential, and myocardial infarcts are reported with their use.

However, frequent monitoring of fibrin-split products or d-dimers as signals of thrombosis is of questionable value. The PCCs (Konyne, Proplex-T) and APCCs (FEIBA) are plasma-derived pooled concentrates. They have been the mainstay of inhibitor therapy and demonstrate good efficacy. Recombinant FVIIa (NovoSeven) is available with less thrombogenic effects. Dosage for rFVIIa is recommended at 90 μg/kg for 2 to 4 hours, but optimum dosing is not known. rFVIIa can be used either in the home or hospital setting. PCCs or APCCs should not be administered in close temporal proximity to rFVIIa because that would potentiate the danger of thrombosis, although there are instances of life-threatening bleeds or surgeries in high-titer inhibitor patients where combination of both were used under close monitoring at a HTC setting.

A specific group of FIX inhibitor patients develop anaphylactoid reactions upon infusion of concentrates containing any amount of FIX. The reactions vary from feeling flushed with chest discomfort to coughing, wheezing, and frank hypotension and shock requiring intubation and resuscitative efforts. Vigilance to possible anaphylactoid reactions in hemophilia B patients should be exercised. PCCs and APCCs should be avoided when detected. The use of rFVIIa is a proven safe and effective recourse for these patients.

Long-term management of hemophilia A and B inhibitor patients includes immune tolerance induction (ITI) to eradicate the antibody completely. There are numerous approaches involving the use of an immunosuppressant and daily FVIII. These methods vary with the dose of FVIII, use of intravenous immunoglobulin (IVIg) and/or cyclophosphamide, antibody adsorption column, or steroids. The decision to initiate such therapy should only be taken after serious consideration of the risks of failure (10% to 30%), intercurrent bleeding, and the enormous commitment required. Low pre-ITI inhibitor titer and early intervention is associated with a higher success rate. ITI should be performed under the care of an experienced HTC. As such, specific protocols are not outlined in this chapter.

Acquired Hemophilia

Acquired inhibitors occur later in life and are autoantibodies, predominantly to FVIII. Risk factors include diseases such as systemic lupus erythematosus (SLE), rheumatoid arthritis, malignancies, inflammatory bowel disease, and peripartum. More than 50% of cases have no identifiable cause. An estimated 30% to 40% remit spontaneously, and heroic interventions may not be necessary. When needed, the management of such patients can be difficult, with mortality rates exceeding 20%. A similar approach as outlined earlier for congenital hemophilia patients can be used, including ITI. rFVIIa has had more than 90% efficacy in the surgery setting for this high-risk group.

Preventive Measures

The primary focus of early intervention is to prevent the onset of chronic sequelae associated with bleeds. To that aim, primary and secondary prophylaxis are advocated. The success of prophylaxis is evidenced by the marked decline in arthropathies and hospitalizations in the past 5 years. Factor infusion at 20 to 40 U/kg two to three times a week, particularly prior to organized sports or physical activity, reduces bleeds. Plasma factor level should be kept within the 1% to 2% range for effective prophylaxis, although beneficial effects are seen even when these levels are not strictly enforced. In the infant and young child, primary prophylaxis is started prior to chronic arthropathy or co-morbidities. This often requires placement of a central venous access with associated risks of infection and thrombosis. Secondary prophylaxis should be encouraged in the older child or teenager and adult. The benefits of decreased bleeds, increased school or work attendance, and general quality of life is well documented.

Routine well child immunizations including hepatitis A and B vaccines should be given. Regular exercise and development of good muscle tone and strength decreases joint and muscle bleeds, not to mention optimizing the development of self-esteem and social interaction. Affected children are encouraged to participate in activities such as swimming and group sports with the proviso of consistent use of protective gear such as helmets and knee/elbow pads.

Adjunctive Therapy

Antifibrinolytics such as ε-aminocaproic acid (εACA) (Amicar) or tranexamic acid (Cyklokapron) decrease clot lysis. εACA is available in liquid, tablet, and IV forms. The liquid preparation comes in 250 mg/mL, and 50 mg/kg can be used four times daily[1] for 5 to 7 days. It should be used with extreme caution, if at all, in GI or renal bleeds. Antifibrinolytics are used with rFVIIa. Other agents include fibrin sealants, topical thrombin, and microfibrillar collagen, especially in the presence of mucosal bleeds. Adequate analgesia, for example, acetaminophen (Tylenol) with codeine or morphine, may be necessary for pain relief. Anti-inflammatory medications such as steroids are used in some cases to reduce edema in acute hemorrhage or synovitis. However, medications affecting platelet function such as aspirin or ibuprofen should be avoided. The mnemonic RICE—Rest, Ice, Compression, Elevation—should be applied to joint bleeds, although ice is often difficult to maintain on an irritable child. Oral contraceptives may reduce menorrhagia and also increase plasma FVIII and FIX levels.

GENE TRANSFER

Preliminary clinical trials of various FVIII and FIX gene transfer modalities can produce the target factor but are unable to maintain a sustained factor level. More studies are ongoing, but a detailed discussion is beyond the scope of this article.

---

[1]Not FDA approved for this indication.

VON WILLEBRAND'S DISEASE

DDAVP (Stimate) is effective in raising FVIII and vWf levels three to four times that of baseline levels in most individuals with mild to moderate hemophilia and vWd. It can be used for dental extractions and minor procedures. Stimate does not raise the level in severely affected individuals adequately to achieve hemostasis (e.g., a 1% baseline vWf level would only increase to 3% to 4% postadministration). Stimate can be administered IV or intranasally. IV dosage is 0.3 μg/kg. Intranasal dosage is 1 squirt (approximately 150 μg) for those less than 50 kg and 2 squirts for patients more than 50 kg. Intranasal administration is more convenient for most patients with faster access to treatment because they can carry the dispenser with them at all times. Side effects include facial flushing, transient blood pressure increases, and fluid retention. Fluid restriction is required to decrease the risk of hypertension, hyponatremia, and seizures. Stimate is contraindicated in neonates and the elderly (older than 75 years). Average time to peak level of FVIII and vWf is 45 minutes after IV and 90 minutes after intranasal administration. With its rapid response, it is most likely that the mechanism of action of Stimate is release of the premanufactured FVIII and vWf from storage sites. Because of depletion of stores from frequent use, Stimate should only be given one to two times a day for a maximum of 3 days consecutively. A trial dose is given at the HTC, and pre- and postdose levels are measured to document an adequate response prior to prescription of the drug for use. Educational sessions on its appropriate use and possible side effects have to be given *prior* to dispensing Stimate. A few patients may respond to the IV route of administration after failing the intranasal trial.

Key points in the use of DDAVP for mild hemophilia A and type 1 vWd are as follows:

- Only the concentrated form (1.5 mg/mL) of DDAVP should be used. The trade name is Stimate. Reference should be made only to Stimate as the appropriate medication to avoid prescription and dispensing errors. DDAVP used for enuresis is ineffective in achieving hemostatic control.
- Fluid should be restricted just prior to and for 12 to 24 hours postadministration.
- The treating physician should be notified if hemostasis is not achieved after the first two doses. Tachyphylaxis and concomitant side effects should be considered.

Treatment for patients with type 2s and 3 vWd require IV factor concentrate replacements containing adequate amounts of vWf. Table 2 lists these preparations that include Humate-P and Alphanate. Dosage for Humate-P can be calculated based on the vWf activity expressed as ristocetin cofactor (vWf:RCoF) units. For minor procedures and bleeding, 40 to 50 IU/kg every 8 to 12 hours for one to two doses is usually sufficient. However, major surgeries and bleeds including suspected intracranial hemorrhage (ICH) would require a loading dose of 60 to 80 IU/kg, then 40 to 60 IU/kg every 8 to 12 hours for a minimum of 5 to 10 days, keeping the vWf:RCoF activity more than 50%. Stimate is used as adjunctive therapy in type 3 vWd but should be avoided in most type 2 and platelet-type vWd patients. Recombinant and high-purity FVIII and FIX concentrates should *not* be used for vWd.

Recombinant vWF is available only at a research level and is being developed for future clinical trials. Adjunctive therapy as listed for hemophilia applies generally to vWd as well, including oral progesterone-containing contraceptives.

Other Related Disorders

Deficiencies of the other factors are often diagnosed by the APTT, PT, and TT. There are rare cases of familial combined factor deficiencies (e.g., FV + FVIII, FVIII + FIX, FII + VII + IX + X). In the latter case, high doses of vitamin K may be helpful.

Severe FVII deficiency (prolonged PT, less than 1% FVII) can vary in presentation, although most neonates succumb to intracranial hemorrhage (ICH). It would seem rational that the principle of replacing the deficient factor applies in this disease as in hemophilia A and B. rFVII is efficacious in maintaining hemostasis at 20 to 30 μg/kg every 6 to 12 hours. For the rest of the factor deficiencies that present with bleeding, fresh-frozen plasma (FFP) is often effective. Specific factor replacement is usually not available in the United States (e.g., FXI). Fibrinogen (Factor I) abnormalities require cryoprecipitate for effective hemostasis. FXIII deficiency can be treated with FFP or cryoprecipitate. Prophylactic treatment with FFP uses 10 mL/kg, or 1 to 2 U in adults every 4 to 6 weeks, or cryoprecipitate, 1 bag/10 kg body weight. The amount of each factor in FFP and cryoprecipitate varies according to the donor pool. Dosage varies according to the severity of bleeds and the half-life of the plasma factor involved. It is advisable for the overall treatment of any patient with a bleeding diathesis to be carried out at or under the guidance of a HTC.

REFERENCES

Ewing NP, Sanders NL, Dietrich SL, et al: Induction of immune tolerance of factor VIII in hemophiliacs with inhibitors. JAMA 1988;259:65-68.

Fuente B, Kasper CK, Rickles FR, et al: Response of patients with mild and moderate hemophilia A and von Willebrand disease to treatment with desmopressin. Ann Intern Med 1985;103:6-15.

Lusher JM, Arkin S, Abildgaard CF, et al: Recombinant factor VIII for the treatment of previously untreated patients with hemophilia. N Engl J Med 1993;328:453-459.

Manco-Johnson MJ, Nuss R, Geraghty S, et al: Results of secondary prophylaxis in children with severe hemophilia. Am J Hematol 1994;47:113-117.

Roth DA, Tawa NE, O'Brien J, et al: Non-viral gene transfer of blood coagulation factor VIII in patients with severe hemophilia A. Blood 2000;96:2532 [abstract].

Souci JM, Nuss R, Evatt B, et al: Mortality among males with hemophilia: Relations with source of medical care. Blood 2000;96:437-442.

Tuddenheam EGD, Schwabb R, Seehafer J, et al: Haemophilia A: Database of nucleotide substitutions, deletions, insertions and rearrangements of the factor VIII gene, second edition. Nucleic Acid Res 1994;22:3511-3533.

Warrier I, Koerper MA, DiMichele D, et al: Factor IX inhibitors and anaphylaxis in hemophilia B. J Pediatr Hematol Oncol 1997;19:23-27.

Platelet-Mediated Bleeding Disorders

Method of
Suman Sood MD, and Charles S. Abrams, MD

Both quantitative and qualitative platelet defects may result in bleeding. These situations are encountered frequently in clinical practice and in consultation.

Elements of Platelet Function

The vascular endothelium separates platelets from adhesive substrates in the subendothelial connective tissue. Platelet-mediated hemostasis is initiated by adherence to exposed collagen, fibronectin, and laminin following a breach to the vessel wall. Intracellular signaling cascades lead to secretion of thromboxane A2 platelet granules, and a conformational change in platelet surface complex GPIIb/IIIa that enables it to bind soluble fibrinogen or von Willebrand's factor (VWF). Release of thromboxane A2, or agonists contained within secretion granules such as adenosine phosphate (ADP) and serotonin activate

neighboring platelets to perpetuate the process. Fibrinogen binding to GPIIb/IIIa crosslinks the platelets into a hemostatic plug, resulting in platelet aggregation and accumulation at the site of injury. Other signaling pathways initiated by agonists such as thrombin, thromboxane A_2, and collagen help promote the process of aggregation. Additionally, activated platelet plasma membrane interacts with circulating coagulation factors and provides a surface for assembly and generation of active Factor X and thrombin. Secondary hemostasis occurs when the platelet plug is stabilized further by a thrombin-mediated fibrin mesh. The arrest of bleeding in a superficial wound almost exclusively results from the primary hemostatic plug. Platelet-mediated bleeding disorders are characterized by a prolonged bleeding time, mucocutaneous bleeding, petechiae, and purpura. In contrast, deficiencies in secondary hemostasis result in delayed deep bleeding, such as bleeding into muscles and joints.

CURRENT DIAGNOSIS

- Platelet-mediated bleeding disorders are characterized by a prolonged bleeding time, mucocutaneous bleeding, petechiae, and purpura.
- Thrombocytopenia can result from decreased platelet production, accelerated platelet removal, or platelet sequestration in an enlarged spleen.
- In an otherwise hemostatically normal patient, significant spontaneous bleeding generally does not occur until the platelet count declines to <5,000–10,000/µL. A prolonged bleeding time does not predict clinical bleeding.
- Medications are frequent causes of quantitative and qualitative platelet defects.
- Heparin-induced thrombocytopenia must always be considered when thrombocytopenia is detected in a hospitalized patient.
- Idiopathic thrombocytopenic purpura presents as otherwise unexplained spontaneous mucocutaneous bleeding or asymptomatic thrombocytopenia and is a diagnosis of exclusion.
- Although many medications impair platelet function *in vitro*, only a few, including aspirin, the thienopyridines ticlopidine (Ticlid) and clopidogrel (Plavix), and the GPIIb/IIIa antagonists, induce clinically significant bleeding.
- Although hereditary disorders of platelet adhesion and aggregation are rare, hereditary disorders of platelet secretion are not uncommon causes of easy bruising, menorrhagia, and excessive postoperative and postpartum blood loss. Platelet aggregation studies are helpful for diagnosis.

CURRENT THERAPY

- In the absence of bleeding, platelet counts of 5,000–10,000/µL are used as the threshold for prophylactic transfusion. Single-donor apheresis platelets should be considered to prevent alloimmunization.
- For hemorrhaging patients or patients scheduled to undergo delicate operations such as neurosurgery, maintaining the platelet count >75,000–100,000/µL is recommended.
- When heparin-induced thrombocytopenia is a possibility, all heparin administration must be stopped and alternative anticoagulation instituted, at least until the platelet count returns to normal.
- Because bleeding in patients with ITP is usually minimal to absent until platelet counts decline to below 30,000/µL, asymptomatic patients with platelet counts >30,000 can be followed without treatment.
- Treatment for ITP is initiated with prednisone (1 mg/kg); patients who fail to enter clinical remission are candidates for splenectomy or treatment with immunosuppressive agents including rituximab (Rituxan)[1] and azathioprine (Imuran).[1]
- High doses of corticosteroids (methylprednisolone 1g/d × 3 d) and/or intravenous immunoglobulin (IVIG, 1 g/kg/d × 2 d) are indicated for the emergent treatment of ITP. Platelet transfusion given concurrently with IVIG can be effective for critical bleeding. Anti-D immune globulin (WinRho) may be used instead of IVIG.
- The platelet dysfunction of uremia is usually corrected by dialysis. IV desmopressin (DDAVP), given at a dose of 0.3 µg/kg IV over 15–30 min shortens the bleeding time in most patients with uremia for approximately 4 h.
- When necessary, treatment of hereditary disorders of platelet adhesion and aggregation usually requires platelet transfusion.

[1]Not FDA approved for this indication.
Abbreviations: ITP = idiopathic thrombocytopenic purpura; IV = intravenous.

Quantitative Bleeding Disorders

Adequate numbers of platelets are required to achieve primary hemostasis. Thrombocytopenia may result from decreased platelet production by bone marrow megakaryocytes, accelerated platelet removal, or platelet sequestration in an enlarged spleen. The clinical context is essential because there is no easy test to differentiate among these possibilities. Most commonly, thrombocytopenia is caused by accelerated platelet removal.

Hemorrhage following trauma or surgery generally does not occur if the platelet count is more than 50,000/μL. In an otherwise hemostatically normal patient, significant spontaneous bleeding usually does not occur with a platelet count more than 5,000 to 10,000/μL. However, there is no absolute threshold for spontaneous bleeding caused by thrombocytopenia and it may occur at higher counts when fever, sepsis, severe anemia, and other hemostatic defects are present or when platelet function is impaired by medication. Notably, a prolonged cutaneous bleeding time does not accurately predict clinical bleeding.

THROMBOCYTOPENIA CAUSED BY DECREASED PLATELET PRODUCTION

Decreased platelet production occurs in primary diseases of the bone marrow such as acute leukemia and aplastic anemia; myelophthisic processes in which marrow is replaced by metastatic carcinoma, fibrosis, or multiple myeloma; following chemotherapy and/or radiation therapy; with ethanol toxicity; and during infections with viruses such as HIV, cytomegalovirus (CMV), Epstein-Barr virus (EBV), and varicella. Thrombocytopenia also occurs when megakaryocyte proliferation is impaired by myelodysplasia.

Overt bleeding in these disorders, when clearly caused by thrombocytopenia, is treated by platelet transfusion. Prophylactic platelet transfusion, however, is an area of controversy and is complicated by the short life span of platelets (10 days), the 5-day shelf life of stored platelets, and platelet immunogenicity. In patients undergoing treatment for acute leukemia, outcome is unchanged when platelet counts of 5,000 to 10,000/μL are used as the threshold for prophylactic transfusion. Single-donor apheresis platelets and/or platelet donors who are HLA identical to the recipient should be considered to prevent alloimmunization. The multicenter Platelet Dosing trial is currently accruing patients and should help clarify these issues.

THROMBOCYTOPENIA CAUSED BY INCREASED PLATELET DESTRUCTION

Nonimmune and immune processes can lead to a shortened platelet life span. Nonimmune causes include sepsis, disseminated intravascular coagulation (DIC), thrombotic thrombocytopenic purpura/hemolytic uremic syndrome (TTP/HUS), preeclampsia/eclampsia, cardiopulmonary bypass, and giant cavernous hemangiomas. The thrombocytopenia resolves with treatment of the underlying disorder, and platelet transfusion is rarely necessary. In TTP/HUS, thrombocytopenia is associated with thrombosis rather than bleeding and controversial reports of clinical deterioration following platelet transfusion exist.

Immune-mediated platelet destruction can be related to medication, alloimmune sensitization, or autoimmunity. Medications should always be considered as a possible etiology for thrombocytopenia. The potential list is long, but drugs with strong evidence of antibody-mediated platelet destruction include quinine, quinidine, sulfonamides, and gold salts. Besides stopping the offending medication, emergent treatment for severe thrombocytopenia with bleeding includes platelet transfusion and corticosteroids ± intravenous immunoglobulin (IVIG).

Heparin-induced thrombocytopenia (HIT) is a special case of drug-induced thrombocytopenia associated with arterial and venous thrombosis rather than bleeding. HIT occurs in 2% to 5% of patients given unfractionated heparin by any route for 5 to 10 days. Antibodies develop to a heparin platelet factor 4 (PF4) complex. HIT must always be considered when thrombocytopenia is detected in a hospitalized patient. If a patient has HIT, all heparin administration should be stopped and alternative anticoagulation such as the direct thrombin inhibitors recombinant hirudin and argatroban instituted, at least until the platelet count normalizes. Warfarin (Coumadin) should not be used in acute HIT because of its delayed therapeutic effect and association with a syndrome of venous limb gangrene.

Alloimmune thrombocytopenia related to sensitization to alloantigens such as PI^{A1} can result from transfusion (post-transfusion purpura, PTP) or maternal sensitization during pregnancy (neonatal alloimmune thrombocytopenia, NAIT). PTP causes profound thrombocytopenia 7 to 10 days after transfusion and can be treated with IVIG or plasma exchange. NAIT can cause severe thrombocytopenia and bleeding in neonates and is treated with platelet transfusion, corticosteroids, and IVIG.

Autoimmune thrombocytopenia, also known as idiopathic thrombocytopenic purpura (ITP), is caused by circulating antiplatelet autoantibodies. An ITP-like picture can also occur in autoimmune diseases such as systemic lupus erythematosus, in patients with low-grade lymphoproliferative disorders such as chronic lymphocytic leukemia, and in patients with HIV infections. ITP can occur at any age in both sexes and presents with either mucocutaneous bleeding or unexplained asymptomatic thrombocytopenia. The complete blood count (CBC) is otherwise normal, splenomegaly is absent, and peripheral blood smears are only remarkable for a decreased number of platelets, some of which may be larger than normal. Megakaryocytes are present in an ITP bone marrow, but marrow examination is usually not necessary in the absence of other findings suggesting myelodysplasia.

Management of ITP is guided by symptoms and platelet count. Asymptomatic patients with platelet counts higher than 30,000/μL can be followed without treatment. With bleeding and/or a platelet count lower than 30,000/μL, treatment with prednisone is initiated. Refractory patients are referred for splenectomy; 60% to 75% of patients enter remission following this procedure. Patients who fail splenectomy may require other forms of immunosuppression. Emergent presentation with severe thrombocytopenia (less than 5,000/μL) and/or internal bleeding should be treated with high doses of pulse corticosteroids and/or IVIG. Platelet transfusion may be given concurrently with the IVIG for critical bleeding. Anti-D immune globulin

(WinRho SDF) may be substituted for IVIG in Rh-positive patients who have not undergone splenectomy.

THROMBOCYTOPENIA CAUSED BY HYPERSPLENISM

Approximately 30% of the circulating platelet mass is normally present in the spleen. Additional platelets may be sequestered when the spleen enlarges because of portal hypertension or infiltrative diseases. Platelet counts in patients with hypersplenism generally are not lower than 40,000 to 50,000/μL. Consequently, bleeding caused by thrombocytopenia from hypersplenism alone is unusual.

Qualitative Platelet Disorders

ACQUIRED QUALITATIVE PLATELET DISORDERS

Acquired disorders of platelet function are relatively common but are usually asymptomatic or mild. Nonetheless, they can be of substantial clinical importance when engrafted on another hemostatic abnormality. They are subclassified as resulting from drugs, hematologic diseases, and systemic disorders. Drugs are the most frequent cause of dysfunction, most notably aspirin, which irreversibly inactivates the enzyme cyclooxygenase-1 (COX-1), thus inducing a permanent blockade in platelet prostaglandin synthesis. Although the antihemostatic effect is minimal in healthy individuals, it may be quite prominent in an individual with an underlying bleeding disorder. Nonsteroidal anti-inflammatory medications reversibly inhibit platelet prostaglandin synthesis and generally have little effect on hemostasis. Other medications that interfere with platelet function include clopidogrel (Plavix), ticlopidine (Ticlid), and GPIIb/IIIa receptor antagonists. Numerous other drugs are implicated in platelet dysfunction in case reports, but the evidence for most of these medications is less well established.

Bone marrow processes that may produce intrinsically abnormal platelets include myeloproliferative disorders, acute and chronic leukemias, myelodysplastic syndromes, and dysproteinemias such as multiple myeloma and Waldenström's macroglobinemia, in which abnormal plasma proteins impair platelet function. In addition, acquired forms of von Willebrand's disease, a rare disorder that may arise secondary to critical aortic stenosis, multiple myeloma, or other clonal hematologic disorders, may lead to a bleeding diathesis.

Renal failure is the most prominent systemic disorder associated with abnormal platelet function. The hemostatic defect is generally mild and corrects rapidly with the initiation of dialysis. Intravenous 1-deamino [8-D-arginine] vasopressin (DDAVP), a vasopressin analogue that causes release of VWF from tissue stores, is helpful in uremia, shortening bleeding time in 50% to 75% of patients. Dosing may be repeated, although tachyphylaxis may occur. Liver disease and DIC can also lead to impaired platelet function. Thrombocytopenia is a consistent feature of cardiopulmonary bypass surgery, typically secondary to hemodilution, platelet membrane activation from interaction with the bypass circuit, and fragmentation from hypothermia.

It generally resolves spontaneously within several days after bypass, but platelet transfusions may be helpful if bleeding persists.

HEREDITARY QUALITATIVE PLATELET DISORDERS

Bernard-Soulier syndrome (BSS) and Glanzmann's thrombasthenia (GT) are rare autosomal recessive disorders of the platelet membrane glycoproteins GPIb/IX and GPIIb/IIIa, respectively. They present with mucocutaneous bleeding in infancy or childhood. Patients with BSS are also thrombocytopenic and have very large platelets that do not agglutinate when exposed to ristocetin. Platelet counts and morphology are normal in GT, but the platelets cannot aggregate in response to ADP or thrombin. Reliable treatment of bleeding in both conditions requires platelet transfusion.

Hereditary disorders of platelet secretion are not infrequent causes of mucocutaneous bleeding and can be caused by α granule deficiency (gray platelet syndrome), the more common dense granule deficiency (delta storage pool disease [δSPD]), or to aspirin-like defects resulting from abnormalities of the platelet secretory mechanism. δSPD may be associated with albinism (Hermansky-Pudlak and Chediak-Higashi syndromes) or occur in otherwise normal individuals. Patients with δSPD have normal platelet counts with prolonged bleeding times and abnormal platelet aggregation studies with a diagnostic increased ATP/ADP related to the absence of platelet-dense granule ADP. Although bleeding in patients with secretion disorders can be controlled by platelet transfusion, DDAVP sometimes shortens the bleeding times and improves hemostasis.

REFERENCES

Bennett JS: Novel platelet inhibitors. Ann Rev Med 2001;52:161-184.

Cines DB, Blanchette VS: Immune thrombocytopenic purpura. N Engl J Med 2002;346:995-1008.

George JN, Caen JP, Nurden AT: Glanzmann thrombasthenia: The spectrum of clinical disease. Blood 1990;75:1383-1395.

Lind SE: The bleeding time does not predict surgical bleeding. Blood 1991;77:2547-2552.

Lopez JA, Andrews RK, Afshar-Kharghan V, et al: Bernard-Soulier syndrome. Blood 1998;91:4397-4418.

Mannucci PM: Desmopressin (DDAVP) in the treatment of bleeding disorders: The first 20 years. Blood 1997;90:2515-2521.

Nurden AT: Qualitative disorders of platelets and megakaryocytes. J Thromb Hemostasis 2005;3:1773-1782.

Patrono C: Aspirin as an antiplatelet drug. N Engl J Med 1994;330: 1287-1294.

Stanworth SJ, Hyde C, Brunskill S, et al: Platelet transfusion prophylaxis for patients with haematological malignancies: Where to now? Br J Haematol 2005;131:588-595.

Tefferi A, Nichols WL: Acquired von Willebrand disease: Concise review of occurrence, diagnosis, pathogenesis, and treatment. Am J Med 1997;103:536-540.

van den Bemt PM, Meyboom RH, Egberts AC: Drug-induced immune thrombocytopenia. Drug Saf 2004;27:1243-1252.

Warkentin TE: Heparin-induced thrombocytopenia: Pathogenesis and management. Br J Haematol 2003;121:535-555.

Disseminated Intravascular Coagulation

Method of
Rodger L. Bick, MD, PhD

Disseminated intravascular coagulation (DIC) is complex, with pathophysiology that is variable and dependent on the triggering event(s), host response(s) and co-morbid conditions. As a result of these complicated interactions, the clinical and laboratory findings are varied. DIC is an intermediary mechanism of disease usually seen in association with well-defined clinical disorders. The pathophysiology of DIC serves as an intermediary mechanism in many disease processes, which sometimes remain organ specific. This catastrophic syndrome spans all areas of medicine and presents a broad clinical spectrum that is confusing to many. Often not appreciated is the profound microvascular thrombosis and, sometimes, large vessel thrombosis. The hemorrhage is often simple to contend with in patients; it is the small and large vessel thrombosis, with impairment of blood flow, ischemia, and associated end-organ damage, that often leads to irreversible morbidity and mortality.

Etiology

DIC is usually seen in association with well-defined clinical entities. Table 1 summarizes those clinical disorders and circumstances most commonly associated with DIC. On very rare occasions, patients may develop DIC in which no apparent etiology is defined. Figure 1 illustrates the mechanisms by which a broad spectrum of unrelated pathophysiologic insults can give rise to the same common ultimate pathway, the syndrome of DIC. Figure 2 illustrates the pathophysiology of DIC.

Clinical Findings

The systemic signs and symptoms of DIC are variable, but the specific signs, which include petechiae and purpura (found in most patients), hemorrhagic bullae, acral cyanosis, and, sometimes, frank gangrene should immediately forewarn one to the probable diagnosis of DIC. Other symptoms include fever, hypotension, acidosis, proteinuria, hypoxia; wound bleeding, especially oozing from a surgical or traumatic wound is common in patients who have undergone surgery or suffered trauma. Oozing from venipuncture sites or intraarterial lines is another common finding. Large subcutaneous hematomas and deep tissue bleeding are also often seen. The average patient with DIC usually bleeds from at least three unrelated sites, and any combination may be seen. A remarkable volume of microvascular and large vessel thrombosis may occur that is not clinically obvious, unless and until looked for. Those organ systems having a high chance of microvascular thrombosis associated with dysfunction include cardiac, pulmonary, renal, hepatic, and central nervous system (CNS). Thrombotic thrombocytopenic purpura (TTP) is commonly associated with CNS dysfunction; however, it should be realized that this is observed just as commonly in DIC.

Laboratory Diagnosis

Because of the complex pathophysiology described earlier, many laboratory findings of DIC may be quite variable, complex, and difficult to interpret unless the pathophysiology is clearly understood and appropriate tests are performed. Fortunately, many newer modalities are now available to the routine clinical laboratory for easily assessing patients with DIC.

PERIPHERAL BLOOD SMEAR FINDINGS

Morphologic findings in DIC consist of characteristic peripheral smear findings and hemorrhage or thrombosis in any organ(s). Peripheral blood smear red cell fragments

TABLE 1 Accepted Disease Entities Generally Associated with Disseminated Intravascular Coagulation

Fulminant DIC	Low-Grade DIC
Obstetric accidents	Cardiovascular diseases
Amniotic fluid embolism	Autoimmune diseases
Placental abruption	Renal vascular disorders
Retained fetus syndrome	Hematologic disorders
Eclampsia	Inflammatory disorders
Abortion	
Intravascular hemolysis	
Hemolytic transfusion reactions	
Minor hemolysis	
Massive transfusions	
Septicemia	
Gram-negative (endotoxin)	
Gram-positive (mucopolysaccharides)	
Viremias	
HIV	
Hepatitis	
Varicella	
Cytomegalovirus	
Metastatic malignancy	
Leukemia	
Acute promyelocytic (M-3)	
Acute myelomonocytic (M-4)	
Burns	
Crush injuries and tissue necrosis	
Trauma	
Acute liver disease	
Obstructive jaundice	
Acute hepatic failure	
Prosthetic devices	
LeVeen or Denver shunts	
Aortic balloon assist devices	
Vascular disorders	

Abbreviation: DIC = disseminated intravascular coagulation.

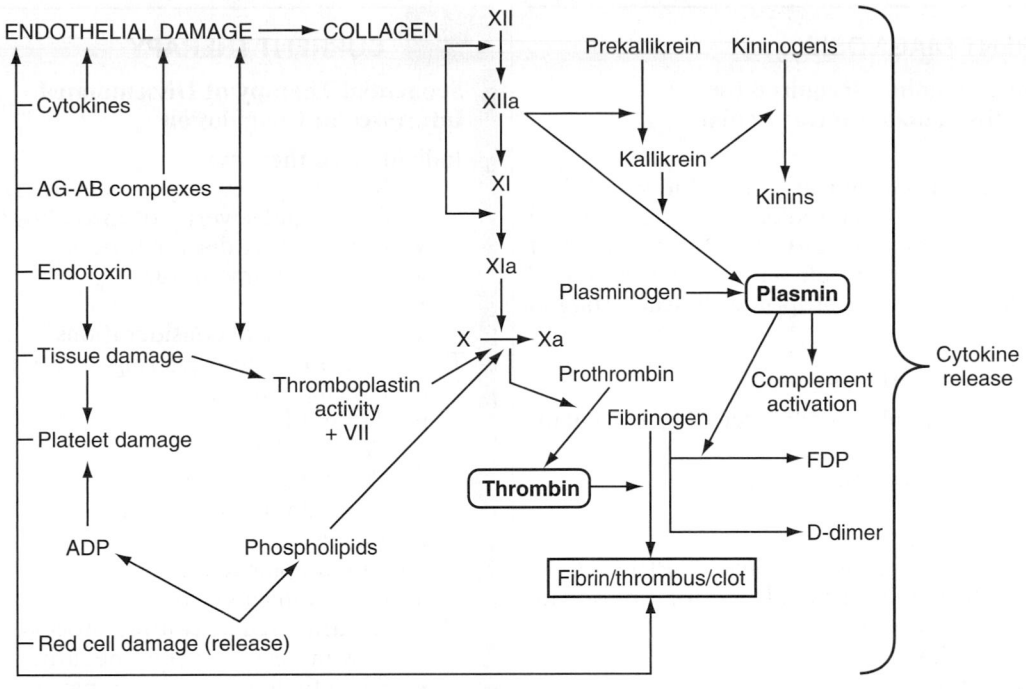

FIGURE 1. Triggering mechanisms for disseminated intravascular coagulation. *Abbreviations:* ADP = adenosine diphosphate; FDP = fibrin degradation product.

(schistocytes) are seen in approximately 50% of individuals with fulminant DIC. Most patients with fulminant DIC present with a mild reticulocytosis and a mild leukocytosis, usually associated with a mild to moderate shift to immature forms. Thrombocytopenia is usually present and often obvious by examination of the peripheral blood smear. Also, large platelets are usually seen on the peripheral smear, representing an increased population of young platelets resulting from increased platelet turnover and decreased platelet survival because of platelet entrapment in microthrombi.

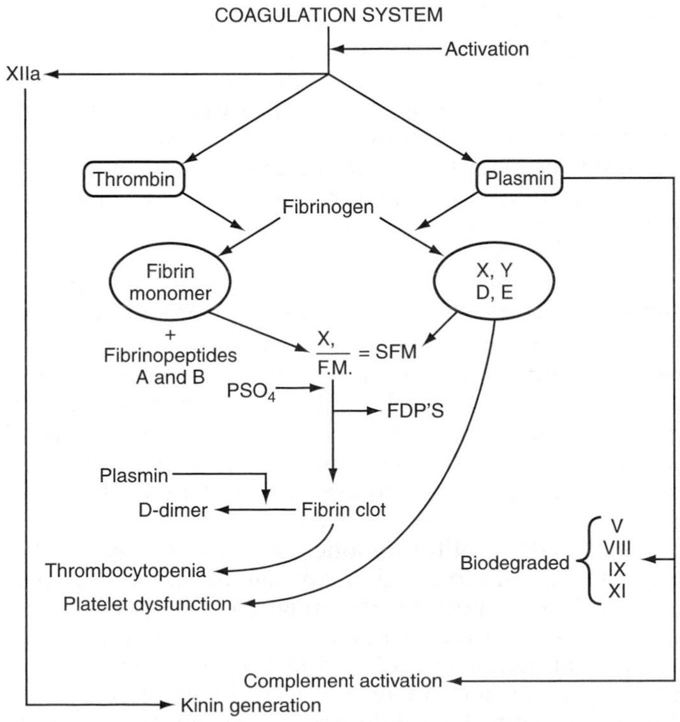

GLOBAL COAGULATION TESTS IN DISSEMINATED INTRAVASCULAR COAGULATION

The Current Diagnosis box lists the tests useful for aiding in a diagnosis of DIC. Most molecular markers for DIC are very sensitive to hemostasis activation, and careful phlebotomies are necessary. The laboratory diagnosis of DIC requires documentation of procoagulant system activation (group I tests), fibrinolytic system activation (group II tests), inhibitor consumption (group III tests), and end-organ damage (group IV tests). The Current Therapy box summarizes the manner in which these tests are used to provide documentation of these four requirements.

FIGURE 2. Pathophysiology of disseminated intravascular coagulation. *Abbreviations:* FDP'S = fibrin degradation products; PSO_4 = protamine sulfate; SFM = soluble fibrin monomer; X = fragment X.

Therapy of Disseminated Intravascular Coagulation

The treatment of DIC must be highly individualized, given the diverse etiologies and clinical manifestations. If logical, aggressive, and sequential therapy is undertaken, morbidity and mortality rates are excellent, with more than 75% of patients surviving with little or no morbidity from DIC itself.

As a guiding principle, therapy must be individualized for each patient, depending on clinical findings and manifestations of the process.

CURRENT DIAGNOSIS

Minimal Clinical Findings Required for Diagnosis of Disseminated Intravascular Coagulation

Understanding the usual clinical manifestations of DIC allows for minimal criteria required for the clinical component of a diagnosis of DIC. Clinical evidence of hemorrhage, thrombosis, or both should be present *and* should be occurring in the appropriate clinical setting as defined in the text.

LABORATORY DIAGNOSTIC CRITERIA*

- Tests currently suitable for evidence of procoagulant activation (*group I tests*):
    - Elevated prothrombin fragment 1+2
    - Elevated TAT
    - Elevated d-dimer
    - Elevated soluble fibrin monomer (TPP) ELISA
- Tests currently suitable as evidence for fibrinolytic activation (*group II tests*):
    - Elevated d-dimer
    - Elevated FDP
    - Elevated plasmin
    - Elevated PAP
    - Elevated soluble fibrin monomer (TPP) ELISA
- Tests currently suitable as evidence for inhibitor consumption (*group III tests*):
    - Decreased AT-III
    - Decreased α-2-antiplasmin
    - Decreased heparin cofactor II
    - Decreased protein C OR S
    - Elevated TAT complex
    - Elevated PAP complex
- Tests currently suitable as evidence for end-organ damage or failure (*group IV tests*):
    - Elevated LDH
    - Elevated creatinine
    - Decreased pH
    - Decreased PaO_2

*Only one abnormality each is needed in groups I, II, and III, and at least two abnormalities are needed in group IV tests to satisfy criteria for a laboratory diagnosis of DIC.
Abbreviations: ELISA = enzyme-linked immunoabsorbent assay; FDP = fibrin degradation product; LDH = lactate dehydrogenase; PAP = plasmin-antiplasmin complex; TAT = thrombin-antithrombin complex.

Therapy should be based on etiology of the DIC, age, hemodynamic status, site and severity of hemorrhage, site and severity of thrombosis, and other relevant clinical factors. The essential therapeutic modality to be delivered to a patient with fulminant DIC is an aggressive approach to eliminate or treat the triggering disease process responsible for DIC. Treatments removing or blunting the underlying disease process may attenuate the intravascular clotting process. If, however, control of the triggering event and pathophysiology is not achieved, later attempts at anticoagulant therapy, including heparin, low molecular weight heparin (LMWH), or antithrombin concentrate, rarely alleviate the process. Sometimes it is impossible or unlikely that the underlying disease can be alleviated.

 CURRENT THERAPY

Sequential Therapy of Disseminated Intravascular Coagulation

Individualize therapy:
- Site(s) and severity of hemorrhage
- Site(s) and severity of thrombosis
- Precipitating disease process
- Hemodynamic status
- Age
- Other clinical considerations

Treat or remove the triggering process:
- Evacuate uterus
- Antibiotics
- Control shock
- Volume replacement
- Maintain blood pressure
- Steroids?
- Antineoplastic therapy
- Other indicated therapy

Stop the intravascular clotting process:
- Low molecular weight heparin
- Subcutaneous porcine heparin
- *Antithrombin concentrates*
- Intravenous heparin?
- Antiplatelet agents?

However, often the removal of the triggering pathophysiology stops the DIC process; the classic example of this is an obstetrical accident, and another is septicemia. In cases of obstetrical accidents of any type (except amniotic fluid embolism), antithrombotic therapy, especially heparin/LMWH, is rarely needed. Simply evacuating the uterus or, in rare instances, hysterectomy, usually rapidly stops the intravascular clotting process. In septicemia, specific antibiotic therapy, alleviation of shock, volume replacement, and other specific therapy to stabilize hemodynamics often cause significant blunting of the intravascular clotting process and sometimes may stop the DIC process altogether.

The second principle is to treat the intravascular thrombotic process, recalling that thrombosis, usually of small vessels, is the process that most impacts morbidity and mortality in patients—not hemorrhage! Most patients, except those suffering from DIC secondary to obstetrical accidents or massive liver failure, next usually need antithrombotic therapy of some form to stop the intravascular clotting process. The use of subcutaneous low-dose heparin appears highly effective in mild and (sometimes) moderate DIC. Antithrombotic therapy is indicated if the patient continues to bleed or clot significantly for approximately 4 to 6 hours after the initiation of supportive therapy and therapy to stop or blunt the triggering event. When the patient continues to bleed in this situation, subcutaneous porcine heparin or LMWH (Fragmin) (at 80 to 100 U/kg every 4 to 6 hours as the clinical situation, site and severity of bleeding and thrombosis, and patient size dictate) is begun. Low-dose subcutaneous heparin appears to be as effective or possibly more effective than larger doses of intravenous (IV) heparin in DIC. With this approach, one often notes cessation of antithrombin consumption, lowering of fibrin degradation product (FDP), and increases in fibrinogen levels and slow or rapid correction of other abnormal laboratory modalities of acute DIC in 3 to 4 hours, followed shortly by blunting or cessation of clinically significant hemorrhage and thrombosis. LMWH appears as efficacious as large-dose heparin therapy and is associated with high patient survival when used with other therapeutic modalities. The contraindications of subcutaneous heparin, or heparin in any dose, would be in patients with fulminant DIC and CNS insults of any type, DIC associated with fulminant liver failure, and, usually, obstetrical accidents. Fulminant DIC is successfully treated with antithrombin concentrates in small groups of patients and in randomized trials, and evidence suggests these are quite effective. Antithrombin concentrates have become this author's treatment of choice for most patients with fulminant moderate and severe DIC. The dose needed is calculated as follows: Total units needed = (Desired level – Initial level) × 0.6 × Total body weight (Kg). The desired level should always be 125% or greater, and this calculation should be performed and the derived antithrombin dose delivered every 8 hours. Approximately 75% of patients respond to the two earlier outlined sequential therapeutic steps.

If patients continue to bleed after beginning reasonable attempts to treat the triggering pathophysiology responsible for DIC and anticoagulant therapy has been initiated, the most probable cause of continued bleeding is component depletion. In this instance, the precise components missing and thought to be contributing to hemorrhage should be defined and administered. The delivery of certain components is associated with potential hazards in patients with *ongoing* DIC, and as a general guideline, only concentrates and components void of fibrinogen should be delivered to a patient with ongoing DIC. Generally, the only components considered safe in patients with active, uncontrolled DIC are packed red cells, platelet concentrates, antithrombin concentrates, and nonclotting protein containing volume expanders, such as plasma protein fraction, albumin, and hydroxyethyl starch.

In those rare instances where bleeding continues after the three sequential steps previously described are instituted, in conjunction with aggressive supportive therapy, the fourth step in the therapy of fulminant DIC is to consider inhibition of the fibrinolytic system. This is rarely needed and only called for in approximately 3% of patients.

In summary, the pathophysiologic mechanisms, clinical, and laboratory manifestations of DIC are complex in part because of interrelationships within the hemostasis system. Only by clearly understanding these extraordinarily complex pathophysiologic interrelationships can the clinician and laboratory scientist appreciate the divergent and wide spectrum of often confusing clinical and laboratory findings in patients with DIC. Many therapeutic decisions to be made are controversial and lack validation. Nevertheless, newer antithrombotic agents and agents that can block, blunt, or modify cytokine activity and the activity of vasoactive substances appear to be of value. The complexity and variable degree of clinical expression suggest that therapy should be individualized depending on the nature of DIC, age, etiology of DIC, site and severity of hemorrhage or thrombosis, and hemodynamics and other appropriate clinical parameters. At the present time, treatment of the triggering event, low-dose heparin/LMWH or antithrombin concentrate, and the wise choice of components when indicated appear to be the most effective modes of therapy.

REFERENCES

Bick RL: Disseminated intravascular coagulation. In Bick RL (ed): Disorders of Thrombosis & Hemostasis: Clinical & Laboratory Practice. Philadelphia, Lippincott Williams & Wilkins, 2002, p 139.

Bick RL: Disseminated intravascular coagulation: Etiology, pathophysiology, diagnosis and management guidelines for care. Clin Appl Thromb Hemost 2002;8:1-32.

Bick RL: Disseminated intravascular coagulation. In Rakel RE, Bope ET (eds): Conn's Current Therapy. Philadelphia, WB Saunders, 2003, p 442.

Bick RL: Disseminated intravascular coagulation: Current concepts of etiology, pathophysiology, diagnosis, and management. Hematol Oncol Clin North Am 2003;17:149-176.

Thrombotic Thrombocytopenic Purpura

Method of
James N. George, MD

Thrombotic thrombocytopenic purpura (TTP) is a multisystem disorder defined pathologically by platelet thrombi occluding arterioles and capillaries of nearly all organs. A review of all patients reported until 1964 described a characteristic pentad of abnormalities: thrombocytopenia, microangiopathic hemolytic anemia, neurologic and renal abnormalities, and fever. In 1991, the Canadian Apheresis Study Group documented the effectiveness of plasma exchange treatment; mortality was 22% compared to 90% in patients reported before 1964. The availability of effective therapy created the urgency for diagnosis; urgency for diagnosis required more limited diagnostic criteria. Current diagnostic criteria are only thrombocytopenia and microangiopathic hemolytic anemia without another apparent etiology.

Etiologies and Associated Conditions

TTP is a syndrome with multiple etiologies. *Hemolytic uremic syndrome* (HUS), also diagnosed by thrombocytopenia and microangiopathic hemolytic anemia, is the term applied to the childhood illness caused by Shiga toxin-producing bacteria, such as *Escherichia coli* 0157:H7, and manifesting predominant renal failure. Most children with HUS following a prodrome of diarrhea survive with only supportive care. In adults, syndromes described as TTP or HUS are not distinct. Although it is commonly stated that patients with TTP have predominant neurologic abnormalities, whereas patients with HUS have predominant renal failure. Some patients may have neither neurologic abnormalities nor renal failure or both.

TABLE 1 Clinical Categories of Acquired TTP

Category	Comments
Idiopathic	Defined by absence of the associated conditions described below. Many patients may have severe ADAMTS13 deficiency. Immunosuppressive treatment, in addition to plasma exchange, is appropriate.
Shiga toxin	Follows enterohemorrhagic infection with *Escherichia coli* 0157:H7 or other Shiga toxin–producing organism. The etiology for the typical HUS of children, who are treated only with supportive care. In adults, plasma exchange is appropriate. Immunosuppressive treatment unnecessary.
Drug-induced immunologic	Quinine most common etiology; may also occur with ticlopidine or clopidogrel. Plasma exchange may be beneficial; immunosuppressive treatment unnecessary.
Drug-induced, dose-dependent toxicity	May occur with cancer chemotherapeutic agents (e.g., mitomycin C [Mutamycin], gemcitabine [Gemzar]) or immunosuppressive agents (cyclosporine [Sandimmune], tacrolimus [Prograf]). Insidious onset, often after etiologic agent discontinued. Benefit of plasma exchange uncertain.
Hematopoietic stem cell transplantation	A syndrome with clinical features of TTP may occur after allogeneic transplants. In most patients, initially unrecognized systemic infection is the cause of signs that suggested TTP. Benefit of plasma exchange doubtful.

Abbreviations: TTP = thrombotic thrombocytopenic purpura.

Therefore, among adults a distinction of TTP from HUS has no importance for initial diagnosis and management; the author uses the term TTP for all of the adult syndromes.

Table 1 describes clinical categories of TTP. Among patients with no preceding illness or apparent associated condition, termed *idiopathic TTP*, many have a deficiency of ADAMTS13, a plasma enzyme required for normal processing of von Willebrand's factor to smaller multimers. Acquired deficiency is caused by an autoantibody that inhibits ADAMTS13 activity; absence of ADAMTS13 activity results in abnormally large von Willebrand factor's multimers that facilitate formation of platelet thrombi. Deficiency of ADAMTS13 may not be sufficient to cause an acute episode of TTP. Acute episodes are often triggered by inflammatory conditions or pregnancy. The etiology of idiopathic TTP in patients without severe ADAMTS13 deficiency is not known. Congenital deficiencies of ADAMTS13 are very rare and not addressed here.

Drug-dependent antibodies can cause acute TTP as a result of diffuse endothelial damage resulting in microvascular thrombi. Quinine is the most common etiology. In addition to the characteristic features of TTP, including acute renal failure, quinine-dependent antibodies to diverse tissues can also cause liver toxicity, neutropenia, and disseminated intravascular coagulation. Ticlopidine (Ticlid) and clopidogrel (Plavix) are also associated with TTP. Other drugs, notably cancer chemotherapeutic and immunosuppressive (cyclosporine [Sandimmune], tacrolimus [Prograf]) agents, can cause a chronic, progressive, dose-dependent disorder similar to TTP. Syndromes similar to TTP may also occur in patients following allogeneic hematopoietic stem cell transplantation, but in many patients signs suggesting TTP following stem cell transplantation may actually be caused by systemic infections.

Diagnosis

The unexpected observation of thrombocytopenia and microangiopathic hemolytic anemia initiates consideration of TTP. However, these minimal criteria are not specific.

The most important diagnostic criterion is to exclude alternative etiologies. Thrombocytopenia and microangiopathic hemolytic anemia may also be caused by systemic infections, such as cytomegalovirus, Rocky Mountain spotted fever, and aspergillosis. Disseminated carcinoma causing occlusion of small vessels may mimic TTP. Malignant hypertension can cause all clinical features of TTP. The obstetric disorders of severe preeclampsia, eclampsia, and HELLP (*h*emolysis, *e*levated *l*iver function tests, *l*ow *p*latelets) syndrome may be initially indistinguishable from TTP. Acute flares of autoimmune disorders such as systemic lupus erythematosus may also be indistinguishable from TTP.

Because there are no conclusive diagnostic criteria, the decision to initiate plasma exchange treatment often

CURRENT DIAGNOSIS

- Suspicion for the diagnosis of TTP
- Unexplained thrombocytopenia and anemia
- Support for the diagnosis of TTP:
  - Evidence for microangiopathic hemolysis: fragmented red cells on the peripheral blood smear, elevated levels of serum bilirubin and lactate dehydrogenase (LDH)
  - Presence of neurologic or renal function abnormalities
  - (High fever and chills are evidence against the diagnosis of TTP)
- Confirmation of the diagnosis of TTP:
  - Exclusion of alternative etiologies
    - Malignant hypertension
    - Systemic infection
    - Systemic neoplasm
    - Preeclampsia, eclampsia, HELLP syndrome
    - Autoimmune disorders, such as systemic lupus erythematosus

Abbreviations: HELLP = hemolysis, elevated liver enzymes, and low platelets; TTP = thrombotic thrombocytopenic purpura.

depends on the severity of illness, progression of the patient's course, and confidence that other etiologies were excluded.

Treatment

PLASMA EXCHANGE THERAPY

Plasma exchange is the only treatment with effectiveness documented by a randomized clinical trial. The presence of severe acquired ADAMTS13 deficiency in some patients with TTP leads to the hypothesis that plasma exchange is effective because of removal of anti-ADAMTS13 antibodies and replacement of ADAMTS13 enzyme activity. However, plasma exchange treatment also appears to be effective in patients without ADAMTS13 deficiency. Although plasma exchange is not the standard treatment for children who have a diarrhea prodrome and the suspected etiology of E. coli 0157:H7, it may be beneficial in adults with TTP caused by E. coli 0157:H7. Plasma exchange may also be beneficial for patients with acute immune-mediated drug-induced TTP. Plasma exchange may not benefit patients whose syndromes are caused by dose-dependent drug toxicity or follow allogeneic hematopoietic stem cell transplantation.

Plasma exchange requires placement of a central venous catheter, similar to the catheters used for hemodialysis. There is substantial risk for critical complications caused by catheter insertion, catheter-related sepsis, and allergic reactions to plasma (Table 2). Therefore, the initial management decision regarding plasma exchange must balance the confidence in the diagnosis of TTP with the risks of the procedure. Plasma exchange is initially

TABLE 2 Complications of Plasma Exchange Treatment for TTP

Complication	Approximate Frequency
Death	2%
Sepsis	15%
Venous thrombosis requiring anticoagulant treatment	2%
Hypotension or hypoxia requiring intensive care	7%

Abbreviations: TTP = thrombotic thrombocytopenic purpura.
Data adapted from Howard MA, Williams LA, Terrell DR: Complications of plasma exchange in patients treated for clinically suspected thrombotic thrombocytopenic purpura-hemolytic uremic syndrome. III. An additional study of 54 consecutive patients. Transfusion 2006;46(1):154-156.

performed once daily, exchanging one plasma volume. In patients who are not initially responsive, or who deteriorate after beginning plasma exchange, higher volumes of plasma exchange may be more effective. Cryoprecipitate-poor plasma and routine fresh-frozen plasma are equally effective. Daily plasma exchange is continued until the platelet count returns to normal; further plasma exchange may have no benefit for residual renal or neurologic abnormalities. When plasma exchange is stopped, the signs of TTP may promptly recur, indicating an exacerbation of continued active TTP. In these patients, daily plasma exchange is resumed and adjunctive immunosuppressive therapy is appropriate.

IMMUNOSUPPRESSIVE THERAPY

Patients with idiopathic TTP related to the frequent autoimmune etiology causing ADAMTS13 deficiency should receive immunosuppressive therapy initially with glucocorticoids. A standard regimen is oral prednisone, 1 mg/kg/day. For more critically ill patients, intravenous methylprednisolone in higher doses, such as 1000 mg/day for 3 days, may be appropriate as initial therapy. Treatment with glucocorticoids may diminish the duration of required plasma exchange and diminish the risk for subsequent exacerbations. In patients who require prolonged and repeated courses of plasma exchange, more intensive immunosuppressive therapy is appropriate, with agents such as cyclophosphamide (Cytoxan[1]) or rituximab (Rituxan[1]). Cyclophosphamide is typically given intravenously in a dose of 1000 mg/m², repeated in 3 to 4 weeks as needed. Rituximab is given intravenously in the standard dose of 375 mg/m²/week for 4 weeks.

MANAGEMENT DURING REMISSION

Remission of TTP is achieved when there is no evidence of disease for 30 days after plasma exchange treatment is stopped. No treatment has documented effectiveness for maintaining remission and preventing relapses.

CURRENT THERAPY

- Plasma exchange:
  - Principal treatment for TTP.
  - Initial regimen: one plasma volume exchanged per day. For refractory patients increased exchange volume (1.5 plasma volumes) or increased frequency (one plasma volume twice daily) may be appropriate.
  - Fresh-frozen plasma and cryoprecipitate-poor plasma are equivalent as replacement fluid.
- Glucocorticoids:
  - Indicated for patients with idiopathic TTP and for patients who require prolonged plasma exchange.
  - Regimen may be oral prednisone, 1 mg/kg/d. For severely ill patients, IV methylprednisolone, 250–1000 mg/d for 3 d, may be appropriate.
- Intensive immunosuppression:
  - Indicated for patients with recurrent exacerbations or relapses
  - Regimen may be IV cyclophosphamide (Cytoxan[1]), 1000 mg/m² repeated at 3–4 wk intervals as needed, or rituximab (Rituxan[1]), 375 mg/m²/wk for 4 wk.

[1]Not FDA approved for this indication.
Abbreviations: IV = intravenous; TTP = thrombotic thrombocytopenic purpura.

[1]Not FDA approved for this indication.

Relapses may occur in as many as 50% of patients whose TTP is associated with severe ADAMTS13 deficiency; patients with other etiologies have a negligible risk for relapse. Appropriate management is only careful follow-up, with prompt evaluation, including a complete blood count, for any acute symptoms. If TTP recurs, daily plasma exchange is resumed and intensive immunotherapy is appropriate, ideally to achieve a more durable remission. Because pregnancy is associated with the occurrence of acute episodes of TTP and TTP occurs most commonly in young women, the risk of a future pregnancy is a common and serious concern. But in spite of the association of TTP and pregnancy, most subsequent pregnancies are uncomplicated.

Prognosis

Complete hematologic recovery is expected. In patients with acute renal failure, persistent renal insufficiency is common. Although most patients recover completely with no evidence of sequelae, many patients describe continuing subtle cognitive difficulties. Physicians should be aware of these potential difficulties to counsel and support their patients appropriately.

REFERENCES

Allford S, Hunt BJ, Rose P, Machin S; Haemostasis and Thrombosis Task Force: Guidelines on the diagnosis and management of the thrombotic microangiopathic haemolytic anemias. Br J Haematol 2003;120:556-573.

Amorosi EL, Ultmann JE: Thrombotic thrombocytopenic purpura: Report of 16 cases and review of the literature. Medicine 1966;45: 139-159.

George JN: The association of pregnancy with thrombotic thrombocytopenic purpura-hemolytic uremic syndrome. Curr Opin Hematol 2003;10:339-344.

George JN: Clinical practice. Thrombotic thrombocytopenic purpura. N Engl J Med 2006;354(18):1927-1935.

George JN, Li X, McMinn JR, et al: Thrombotic thrombocytopenic purpura-hemolytic uremic syndrome following allogeneic hematopoietic stem cell transplantation: A diagnostic dilemma. Transfusion 2004;44:294-304.

Howard MA, Williams LA, Terrell DR: Complications of plasma exchange in patients treated for clinically suspected thrombotic thrombocytopenic purpura-hemolytic uremic syndrome. III. An additional study of 54 consecutive patients. Transfusion 2006;46(1): 154-156.

Kojouri K, Vesely SK, George JN: Quinine-associated thrombotic thrombocytopenic purpura-hemolytic uremic syndrome: Frequency, clinical features, and long-term outcomes. Ann Intern Med 2001;135: 1047-1051.

McMinn JR, George JN: Evaluation of women with clinically suspected thrombotic thrombocytopenic purpura-hemolytic uremic syndrome during pregnancy. J Clin Apheresis 2001;16:202-209.

Moake JL: Thrombotic microangiopathies. N Engl J Med 2002;347: 589-600.

Rock GA, Shumak KH, Buskard NA, et al: Comparison of plasma exchange with plasma infusion in the treatment of thrombotic thrombocytopenic purpura. N Engl J Med 1991;325:393-397.

Vesely SK, George JN, Lammle B, et al: ADAMTS13 activity in thrombotic thrombocytopenic purpura-hemolytic uremic syndrome: Relation to presenting features and clinical outcomes in a prospective cohort of 142 patients. Blood 2003;101:60-68.

Vesely SK, Li X, McMinn JR, et al: Pregnancy outcomes after recovery from thrombotic thrombocytopenic purpura-hemolytic uremic syndrome. Transfusion 2004;44:1149-1158.

Hemochromatosis

Method of
Lawrie W. Powell, MD, PhD

When von Recklinghausen coined the name *hemochromatosis* in 1889 (because he believed the pigment in tissues was derived from the blood), he described the advanced disease with gross iron deposition in tissues and organ damage. Cirrhosis, diabetes mellitus, arthritis, cardiomyopathy, and hypogonadotrophic hypogonadism were the classical features. In his definitive monograph of the disease in 1935, Sheldon confirmed and extended this description, concluding that "in spite of its implicit but unproven assumptions it is the best name for the disease." Numerous large series and reviews were subsequently published leading to widespread acceptance of the concept of hemochromatosis as a disease of iron storage in which an inappropriate increase in intestinal iron absorption leads to excessive quantities of iron in tissues with eventual functional impairment of the organs involved, especially the liver, pancreas, heart, and pituitary. Simon and associates' discovery that the inheritance of HH is closely linked to the human leukocyte antigen (HLA)-A locus on chromosome 6 made definite identification of homozygous relatives of affected probands possible, and it eventually led to the identification of the two most common missense mutations, C282Y and H63D, of the major histocompatibility complex (MHC) class I gene on 6p, designated the hemochromatosis gene (HFE).

It is now established that 90% or more of cases of hemochromatosis in subjects of northern European extraction are because of homozygosity for the C282Y mutation in this gene. This is one of the most common genetic mutations in white populations (see later). It is probable, therefore, that von Recklinghausen and Sheldon were referring to this form of HFE-associated hemochromatosis. However, more recently additional mutations in other molecules involved in iron metabolism, notably hepcidin, hemojuvelin, and ferroportin, have been identified, and with the exception of the iron overload disorder resulting from mutations in the cellular iron transporter ferroportin, the resultant clinicopathologic syndrome closely resembles HFE-associated hemochromatosis. This has led to a new classification of iron overload and hemochromatosis that encompasses these newly described forms (Table 1).

Although a very similar clinicopathologic syndrome occurs with iron overload secondary to iron-loading anemia such as thalassemia major or sideroblastic anemia, the term *secondary* or *acquired hemochromatosis* has largely been abandoned in favor of defining the primary disease, that is, thalassemia major with secondary iron overload.

Iron Homeostasis

Despite the abundance of iron in nature, the solubility of its stable ferric form is extremely low. Living organisms hence were compelled to develop efficient mechanisms for iron transport and storage. There is no mechanism for excreting excess iron, and the inevitable end result of

TABLE 1 Classification of Iron Overload and Hemochromatosis

1. Primary hereditary hemochromatosis
   HFE-associated hereditary hemochromatosis (type 1)
      C282Y homozygosity
   C282Y/H63D compound heterozygosity
   Non-HFE associated hereditary hemochromatosis
      Juvenile hemochromatosis (type 2) (2A, hepcidin
      mutations; 2B, hemojuvelin mutations)
   Transferrin receptor 2 mutations hemochromatosis
      (type 3)
   Ferroportin mutations (autosomal dominant
      hemochromatosis) (type 4)
2. Acquired (secondary) iron overload
   Iron-loading anemias
      Thalassemia major
      Sideroblastic anemia
      Chronic hemolytic anemia
   Dietary iron overload (African)
   Parenteral iron overload (including multiple blood
      transfusions)
3. Other causes of iron overload (but rarely to the degree
      seen in hemochromatosis)
   Long-term hemodialysis
   Chronic liver disease
      Hepatitis C
      Alcoholic liver disease
   Nonalcoholic steatohepatitis
      Porphyria cutanea tarda
   Dysmetabolic iron overload syndrome
   Post-portacaval shunting
   Iron overload in sub-Sahara Africa
   Neonatal iron overload
   Aceruloplasminemia
   Congenital atransferrinemia

iron absorption exceeding physiologic needs is iron overload.

In recent years a number of key mechanisms have been described that are responsible for adaptation to changing environmental conditions. Production of the iron storage protein ferritin and the transferrin receptor (TfR) protein is reciprocally regulated by a translational mechanism in which the iron regulatory protein (IRP) is reversibly bound to the iron response elements (IRE) of their respective mRNAs. A similar iron-dependent translational mechanism may be responsible for the production of divalent metal transporter 1 (DMT1), which is responsible for the uptake of ferrous iron from the brush border of duodenal enterocytes (Figure 1), and ferroportin (IREG1), which is responsible for the export of ferrous iron through the basolateral members of the same cells. The brush border ferric reductase converts ferric to ferrous iron for use by DMT1, and hephaestin, a transmembrane-bound ferroxidase, converts ferrous to ferric iron, creating a concentration gradient of ferrous iron across the cell membrane facilitating iron egress. At low iron conditions the translation of TfR, DMT1, and ferroportin is enhanced, with the opposite occurring at high iron conditions. In addition, a new protein, hepcidin, was described recently and is probably the most important regulator of iron homeostasis. Hepcidin functions as an inhibitor of iron absorption and release from macrophages. Its production is increased by iron overload and inflammation and is suppressed by iron deficiency.

Genetics of Hereditary Hemochromatosis

The inheritance of the disease follows classical Mendelian genetics as an autosomal recessive trait. The most common scenario is thus two parents are heterozygous for the C282Y mutation and 25% of offspring are either normal or homozygous and 50% are heterozygous. Approximately 90% to 95% of HFE-related hemochromatosis in people of northern European extraction can be attributed to homozygous mutations of C282Y. C282Y/H63D compound heterozygotes contribute 4%, whereas H63D homozygotes may have elevated transferrin saturation or serum ferritin levels but do not develop serious iron overload. Rarer forms of non-HFE-linked hemochromatosis are not discussed further here but are well described in a recent review by Pietrangelo (2004).

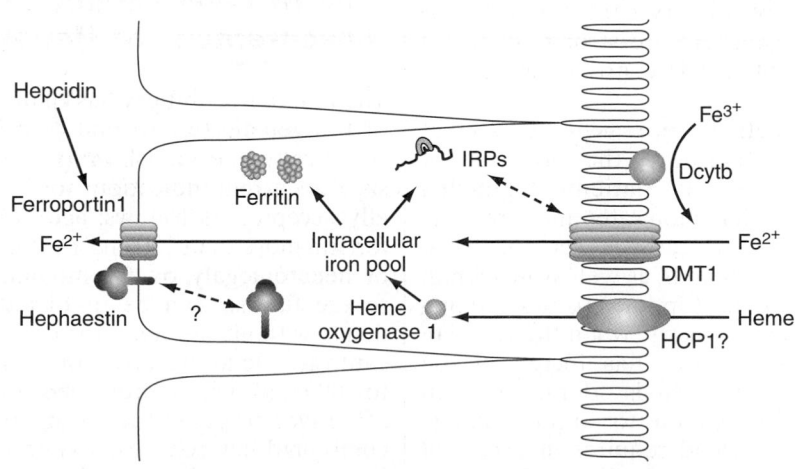

FIGURE 1. Cellular control of iron transport in the duodenal enterocyte. Dcytb = duodenal cytochrome b, DMT1 = divalent metal transporter 1, IRPs = iron regulatory proteins, HCP1 = haem carrier protein 1.

Early Clinical Presentation and Diagnosis

Compelling evidence indicates that the classic clinical manifestations of hemochromatosis such as cirrhosis, diabetes, and so on are related to tissue damage by iron because they occur in HFE-associated hemochromatosis, other forms of hemochromatosis described earlier, and also in gross iron loading secondary to the iron-loading anemias. However, with increased clinical awareness and improved diagnostic methodology, hemochromatosis is now frequently recognized at a much earlier stage before complications arise (latent or precirrhotic hemochromatosis). This is best seen in cascade screening in families after the diagnosis of an index case and in population screening. As a result it is perhaps not surprising that the clinical penetrance and frequency of complications of hemochromatosis is a subject of much current controversy. One recent controlled population study concluded that less than 1% of homozygotes for C282Y have advanced disease. Similarly, in the large Hemochromatosis and Iron Overload Screening (HEIRS) population study of 100,000 North Americans, self-reported symptoms of hemochromatosis were not more common in C282Y homozygous subjects than controls except for self-reported liver disease. However, both of these studies were based on self-reported questionnaires and did not include liver biopsy. A study of 672 C282Y homozygotes incorporating detailed clinical evaluation and liver biopsy in approximately 50% of individuals concluded that cirrhosis was present in 5.8% of homozygous men and 1.9% of homozygous women, and all of these subjects were asymptomatic. Further, advanced hepatic fibrosis was present in 25% of subjects and significantly improved after phlebotomy therapy. The logical conclusion is that a significant proportion of C282Y homozygous individuals are asymptomatic but have hepatic fibrosis. The factors that determine whether this progresses to cirrhosis are not well understood, but heavy alcohol intake is identified as a significant factor.

The association of hepatomegaly, skin pigmentation, diabetes mellitus, heart disease, arthritis, and hypogonadism should suggest the diagnosis. A high index of suspicion is needed to make the diagnosis early. Indeed, increasingly, the diagnosis of early hemochromatosis is made at health checkups by primary care physicians or by cascade family screening. There are strong advocates of population screening, but this is controversial at the present time.

As many as 30% of patients are asymptomatic at the time of diagnosis. Furthermore, the presence of asymptomatic cirrhosis in 5% of patients highlights the importance of improving detection rates and screening strategies. The development of cascade screening for family members of affected probands, as well as incidental findings of abnormal iron studies (opportunistic screening often performed to investigate lethargy when the clinician expects to detect iron deficiency), has increased the number of asymptomatic individuals identified with early hemochromatosis. Progression to organ damage as a consequence of iron overload requires in excess of 10 g of parenchymal iron storage and usually occurs after 40 years of age, but heavy alcohol intake substantially increases the risk of cirrhosis at lower body iron levels.

Laboratory Testing

In the absence of a consensus for population screening, a variety of indications for testing for hemochromatosis currently exist. Clearly patients with symptoms of liver disease and abnormal iron studies should be tested using genetic mutation analysis. In addition, those with type 2 diabetes, early-onset cardiac disease, premature sexual dysfunction, and atypical arthropathy require further evaluation. In the asymptomatic population, first-degree relatives of probands, individuals with abnormal iron studies detected incidentally, and those with clinical, biochemical, or radiologic evidence of liver disease should all be tested for hereditary hemochromatosis.

The transferrin saturation is the best initial phenotypic screening test. It is accepted as an accurate phenotypic marker of the genetic defect in HFE-associated hemochromatosis, but the level at which it should prompt further testing for hemochromatosis is controversial. A fasting transferrin saturation of 45% detected virtually all affected homozygotes, but the specificity increases with higher values.

The serum ferritin concentration is a good index of body iron stores. An increase of 1 µg/L in serum ferritin level reflects an increase of approximately 7 mg in body stores. In most untreated patients with hemochromatosis, the serum ferritin level is greatly increased. However, in patients with inflammation and hepatocellular necrosis, serum ferritin levels may be elevated out of proportion to body iron stores because of increased release from tissues. Importantly, in these situations the transferrin saturation is usually normal. In contrast, the serum ferritin in the absence of inflammation is a good guide to the degree of iron overload. A repeat determination of serum ferritin should, therefore, be carried out after acute hepatocellular damage has subsided (e.g., in drug- or alcohol-induced liver disease). Ordinarily, the combined measurements of the percentage of transferrin saturation and serum ferritin level provide a simple and reliable screening test for hemochromatosis, including the precirrhotic phase of the disease. If either of these tests is abnormal, genetic testing for hemochromatosis should be performed.

Role of Liver Biopsy and Measurement of Hepatic Iron

The role of liver biopsy has changed since the introduction of the genetic test to one of primarily prognostic value specifically to establish or exclude the presence of cirrhosis. The current indications for liver biopsy are now generally accepted as follows: age older than 40 years, serum ferritin more than 1000 µg/L, abnormal liver function tests, or hepatomegaly, or a combination of these. Absence of severe fibrosis can be predicted with reasonable confidence without the need for liver biopsy. The most significant variable for negative prediction is serum ferritin equal to 1000 µg/L with a prevalence of severe fibrosis of 1% to 3%. Liver biopsy in the setting of C282Y homozygosity or compound heterozygosity is now considered unnecessary if the serum ferritin level is less than 1000 µg/mL and the serum transaminase levels are normal. Similar guidelines cannot be used in the absence of C282Y homozygosity. The serum ferritin level is elevated in iron-loading anemias, chronic hemolysis, blood transfusions, hepatitis C, alcoholism, and steatohepatitis because of hepatic inflammation and also secondary iron overload. Liver biopsy should be considered even in C282Y or H63D heterozygotes with these disorders. Although transferrin saturation is significantly increased in individuals with either homozygosity or heterozygosity of the H63D mutation regardless of gender, serum ferritin is not usually affected and progressive iron overload does not develop. Liver biopsy should also be utilized in those individuals with clinical iron overload and uninformative genetic mutation analysis to firmly establish their diagnosis.

Comparison of usefulness of MRI for the assessment of liver iron burden with liver biopsy was undertaken in recent studies. Use of a highly T2-weighted protocol comparing liver and muscle (L/M) signal intensity produced a 89% sensitivity and 80% specificity using a threshold L/M ratio below 0.88. The investigators were able to detect liver iron concentration down to a threshold of 1.8 mg Fe/g dry tissue. In a second study, the ratio between iron concentration and signal intensity on magnetic resonance imaging (MRI) was calculated and an inverse linear relationship was found. The normal value for liver iron is less than 36 mol/g. The positive predictive value for hemochromatosis and iron overload, respectively, was more than 85 mol/g and more than 58 mol/g, whereas the negative predictive value was 100% at concentrations less than 40 mol/g and less than 20 mol/g, respectively.

Several attempts have been made to define serum markers of fibrosis and to determine whether it is possible to stratify subjects further with genetic hemochromatosis who may require liver biopsy. Serum type IV collagen concentrations are significantly increased in hemochromatosis patients when compared with healthy controls. Additionally, correlations between degree of fibrosis and serum type IV collagen concentrations are shown. In contrast, markers such as serum laminin, which is 81% accurate for detecting cirrhosis in alcoholics and those with chronic viral hepatitis, are not as useful in hemochromatosis. Recent claims that a panel of markers can accurately predict hepatic fibrosis are yet to be substantiated.

Treatment

Hemochromatosis should be treated with once to twice weekly phlebotomy in the first instance. Approximately 1 g of iron is removed with four phlebotomies. Hemoglobin monitoring as well as assessment of serum ferritin after each 1 to 2 g of iron is removed is required. In the absence of contraindications, venesection should be continued until serum ferritin is less than 50 µg/L. Individuals who commence treatment prior to the development of cirrhosis or diabetes have normal survival, and even in the setting of cirrhosis, patients with hemochromatosis have improved survival.

Some manifestations are improved by phlebotomy, including fatigue, malaise, elevated serum transaminase levels, and insulin requirements in diabetes. In addition, exercise tolerance and cardiac function can improve with aggressive iron depletion in patients with cardiac complications. In such cases chelation therapy with desferrioxamine is indicated. Although its progression can be slowed, diabetes is not completely reversed. Hypogonadism, arthropathy,

and cirrhosis do not resolve with venesection, and arthropathy may progress after complete iron removal. Treatment is symptomatic, although hip and knee replacement may be required. Hypogonadotrophic hypogonadism may be treated successfully with gonadotrophin therapy with or without parenteral testosterone therapy.

Chelation therapy is only used in rare circumstances when contraindications to venesection exist or in rare instances of cardiac disease as mentioned earlier. Subcutaneous desferrioxamine is the agent used for chelation when it is required. A typical regimen would be 1 to 2 g desferrioxamine in 100 to 200 mL water or saline infused over 10 to 12 hours during sleep. Patients should restrict their intake of iron-rich food and vitamin C. Obviously they should not be prescribed iron supplementation.

Liver Transplantation and Hemochromatosis

Much recent interest has been expressed in liver transplantation in subjects with hemochromatosis, both from the viewpoint of effective therapy for end-stage disease but also as to whether it sheds light on the basic pathophysiology of the disease. The results of orthotopic liver transplantation for end-stage hemochromatosis are less impressive than for other liver diseases. This is attributed to late diagnosis (often at the time of transplantation) or the concurrence of primary hepatocellular carcinoma, but also to a high infection rate, possibly related to the effects of gross hepatic iron deposition. Thus, if possible, subjects with end-stage liver disease because of hemochromatosis should undergo intensive deironing by phlebotomy and possibly desferrioxamine before transplantation.

The available evidence indicates that the fundamental metabolic abnormality in hemochromatosis is reversed by successful liver transplantation. Patients do not reaccumulate iron if transplanted with a donor liver from an HFE normal subject, and the transferrin saturation and the serum ferritin levels remain normal in the absence of inflammation. This strongly suggests that the basic defect responsible for HFE-associated hemochromatosis lies within the liver. This is consistent with the findings of Bridle et al., who found that hepcidin RNA levels were low, but not absent functionally, in C282Y homozygous patients with hemochromatosis whether treated or untreated. Gehrke et al. subsequently published similar observations. HFE thus appears to interact with hepcidin within the liver, probably in the hepatocyte, and the C282Y mutation interferes with this, resulting in low hepcidin levels and consequently inappropriately increased intestinal iron absorption leading to progressive hepatic iron overload. The precise elucidation of this interaction will be of great interest.

REFERENCES

Adams PC, Reboussin DM, Barton JC, et al:. Hemochromatosis and iron-overload screening in a racially diverse population. N Engl J Med 2005;352(17):1769-1778.

Bacon BR, Powell LW, Adams PC, et al: Molecular medicine and hemochromatosis: At the crossroads. Gastroenterology 1999;116(1):193-207.

Beutler E, Felitti VJ, Koziol JA, et al: Penetrance of 845G-A (C282Y) HFE hereditary haemochromatosis mutation in the USA. Lancet 2002;359:211-218.

Bridle KR, Frazer DM, Wilkins SJ, et al: Disrupted hepcidin regulation in HFE-associated haemochromatosis and the liver as a regulator of body iron homoeostasis. Lancet 2003;361(9358):669-673.

Feder JN, Gnirke A, Thomas W, et al: A novel MHC class I-like gene is mutated in patients with hereditary haemochromatosis. Nat Genet 1996;13(4):399-408.

Guyader D, Jacquelinet C, Moirand R, et al: Noninvasive prediction of fibrosis in C282Y homozygous hemochromatosis. Gastroenterology 1998;115(4):929-936.

Pietrangelo A: Hereditary hemochromatosis—a new look at an old disease. N Engl J Med 2004;350(23):2383-2397.

Powell LP, Dixon JL, Ramm GA, et al: The penetrance of HFE-associated hemochromatosis as assessed by clinical evaluation and liver biopsy in subjects identified by health checks, family screening or population screening. Hepatology 2004;40:74A.

Sheldon J: Haemochromatosis. London, Oxford University Press, 1935, p 339.

Simon M, Alexandre JL, Fauchet R, et al: The genetics of hemochromatosis. Prog Med Genet 1980;4:135-168.

St Pierre TG, Clark PR, Chua-anusorn W, et al: Noninvasive measurement and imaging of liver iron concentrations using proton magnetic resonance. Blood 2005;105(2):855-861. Epub 2004 July 15.

Tavill AS: Diagnosis and management of hemochromatosis. AASLD practice guidelines. Hepatology 2001;33(5):1321-1328.

von Recklinghausen F, Taggeblet de: Versainumlung Deutsch Naturforsch Arzt Heidelberg 1889;62:324-325.

Hodgkin's Disease: Chemotherapy

Method of
David J. Straus, MD

The use of radiotherapy and chemotherapy for Hodgkin's disease is one of the major success stories in medical oncology. An understanding of the clinical features and course of the disease aided this success. Extended field radiation therapy (EF RT), introduced nearly 40 years ago by Kaplan, was a major advance in the treatment of patients with early-stage Hodgkin's disease. DeVita and colleagues introduced combination chemotherapy to the treatment of advanced stages of Hodgkin's disease in the mid-1960s, which was the second major advance in treatment. Combinations of chemotherapy with radiation therapy were widely used during the past 20 years, and further improvements in outcome were seen with this approach, particularly in patients with early stages of Hodgkin's disease. More recently, chemotherapy alone has been employed for many patients with excellent results. Less late toxicity may be seen in patients cured of their Hodgkin's disease with reduction in the amount of radiation therapy in combination with chemotherapy or its complete elimination when it is not required.

Histopathology

Currently, the Rye modification of the Lukes and Butler classification is in use throughout the world. The lymphocyte-predominant subtype is characterized by an abundance of small lymphocytes with occasional, often atypical, Reed-Sternberg (R-S) cells of lymphocytic-histiocytic variety (L and H, or so-called popcorn cells) with vesicular, polylobulated nuclei and small nucleoli. Unlike the other forms of Hodgkin's disease, the atypical cells usually have B-cell antigens (CD19, 20, 22, 79a). The growth pattern is usually nodular, although less commonly a diffuse pattern is seen. The classic presentation is in a high cervical node in a young asymptomatic male. It is associated with a favorable prognosis, although late recurrences are reported in some series.

Nodular sclerosis is the most common subtype in North America and Western Europe. There is often abundant fibrosis in the node dividing tumor nodules containing inflammatory cells and the "lacunar cell" variant of R-S cells with a clear area surrounding the cells. The typical presentation is in a young female with mediastinal involvement with or without symptoms. Although it was classically believed to carry a relatively favorable prognosis, this seems to depend on the stage of the disease, the bulkiness of the tumor masses, and the presence or absence of systemic symptoms. The new World Health Organization (WHO) classification of neoplastic diseases of the hematopoietic and lymphoid tissues adds two histologic grades of nodular sclerosis Hodgkin's disease according to the British National Lymphoma Investigation criteria (grade 1, few R-S cells; grade 2, many R-S cells). Some studies demonstrated a worse outcome associated with grade 2 cases, and others showed no difference in outcome. For now, the grading is not required for clinical purposes but should be the subject of future investigations.

Mixed cellularity is characterized by a pleomorphic cellular infiltrate of plasma cells, eosinophils, lymphocytes, histiocytes, and R-S cells. Subdiaphragmatic and extranodal presentations and the presence of B systems may be somewhat more frequent than with the nodular sclerosis subtype. It is the second most common histologic subtype in North America and Western Europe and more common in the poorer parts of the world and among indigent populations. It is also somewhat more common among older patients. It is associated with a worse prognosis than nodular sclerosis, but this may be because of the association of this subtype with the unfavorable clinical prognostic features.

The lymphocyte-depletion subtype has a paucity of cellular elements and an increased reticular network. It is associated with advanced age, systemic symptoms, retroperitoneal lymphadenopathy, and extranodal involvement. It is a diagnosis that is now made infrequently because modern immunophenotyping and molecular genetic studies have demonstrated that many cases formerly thought to be lymphocyte-depletion Hodgkin's disease are actually T-cell non-Hodgkin's lymphomas. Lymphocyte-depletion Hodgkin's disease has the worst prognosis of the four histologic subtypes.

The R-S cells, in the cases of nodular sclerosis, mixed cellularity, and lymphocyte-depletion Hodgkin's disease, carry the CD30 surface antigen, an antigen that is expressed on activated and proliferating lymphocytes. They also stain with antibodies to CD15, more commonly a myeloid marker. Recent cloning of this molecule has enabled its identification as a new member of the tumor necrosis factor (TNF) receptor superfamily. Single cell polymerase chain reaction (PCR) of classic R-S cells literally scraped from slides shows a follicular center B-cell origin for these cells with clonally rearranged but crippled V heavy chain genes presumably leading to a block in apoptosis.

The R-S–like cells in the nodular variant of lymphocyte-predominant Hodgkin's disease are weakly reactive or nonreactive with antibodies to CD30, and, unlike those in the other Hodgkin's disease subtypes, demonstrate a mature B-cell marker phenotype with CD20 and also pan-lymphocyte antigen (CD45, leukocyte common antigen) expression. Molecular genetic studies also have demonstrated the clonal B-cell origin of the nodular variant of lymphocyte-predominant Hodgkin's disease. The R-S cells of the diffuse variant of lymphocyte-predominant Hodgkin's disease have the phenotypic features of classic R-S cells.

Staging

The current staging classification was established by the Ann Arbor Workshop in 1971. There is both clinical staging (CS), which consists of all staging procedures short of staging laparotomy, and pathologic staging (PS), which refers to the findings at staging laparotomy during which liver biopsies, splenectomy, and excisional biopsies of retroperitoneal nodes are performed. Staging laparotomies are performed infrequently at the present time because fewer patients are treated with radiation therapy alone and more patients with systemic treatment with chemotherapy alone or in combination with radiation therapy.

The Ann Arbor classification divides Hodgkin's disease into four stages: Stage I refers to disease limited to a single lymph node or lymph node group. Stage II refers to disease in two or more noncontiguous lymph node groups and/or spleen on the same side of the diaphragm. Stage III refers to disease in two or more lymph node groups and/or spleen on both sides of the diaphragm. Stage IV refers to disease in extranodal sites, usually lung, liver, bone or bone marrow, and more rarely other sites. Extranodal involvement by extension from lymph node disease to such sites as the lung, bone, pleura, or skin may occur in stages I_E and is not considered to increase the stage to IV. Such disease is designated by a subscript E (I_E, II_E, III_E). For each stage, the absence of systemic symptoms is designated by the suffix A, whereas the presence of unexplained fevers to 38°C (100.4°F) or higher, night sweats, and/or weight loss greater than 10% over 6 months is designated by a B suffix. In general, the prognosis worsens with higher stage, and, within each stage, the presence of symptoms (B) carries a worse prognosis than absence of such symptoms (A). A mediastinal tumor greater than a third of the thoracic diameter or lymph node disease greater than 10 cm is defined as bulky; a subscript X is added to the numerical stage if such disease is present (e.g., I_xB, II_xA, II_xB, III_xA, III_xB). Stage IIIA1 refers to subdiaphragmatic disease in spleen and/or high abdominal node, whereas IIIA2 indicates disease in lower retroperitoneal nodes.

Staging procedures include chest radiograph, computerized tomography (CT) of the chest, abdomen, and pelvis with oral and intravenous contrast, complete blood counts with platelet and differential counts, bone marrow aspiration and biopsy, serum liver biochemistries including alkaline phosphatase, and erythrocyte sedimentation rate. The latter test carries prognostic significance. A CT of the abdomen and pelvis will show enlarged retroperitoneal, mesenteric, and pelvic lymph nodes that are involved by disease.

If there are masses in the liver on CT scan, a positron emission tomography (PET) scan or liver-spleen scintigram or, if there are gross abnormalities of serum liver biochemical studies, a liver biopsy should be performed under CT-guided or laparoscopic visualization if the masses are accessible. Slight elevations of serum alkaline phosphatase may be seen without liver involvement.

Gallium-67 scanning is a useful imaging procedure for following mediastinal disease, but it can be associated with false negatives and false positives. It is of value in the decision of whether to biopsy a residual mass following treatment to determine the presence or absence of residual disease. A PET scan provides similar and even more detailed information. [18F]fluoro-2-deoxy-D-glucose (FDG) PET scanning is useful in predicting recurrences in residual masses following treatment for Hodgkin's disease. False-negative studies are less common (the negative predictive value is 95%) than false-positive studies (the positive predictive value is 60%).

A CT scan of the chest may show disease, particularly retrosternal disease, missed by a plain chest radiograph. Also, some patients with bulky mediastinal and hilar nodal disease have peripheral lung nodules that can only be

CURRENT DIAGNOSIS

- History: Enlarged lymph nodes, fevers to 38°C (100.4°F) (27% of patients), drenching night sweats, weight loss, pruritus, alcohol-induced pain in areas of enlarged lymph nodes (10% of patients), chest pain, cough, dyspnea
- Physical examination: Enlarged nontender lymph nodes (neck, supraclavicular, axillary, inguinal regions), palpable enlarged spleen and liver, signs of pleural effusion
- Laboratory: Anemia (usually normochromic, normocytic), granulocytosis, eosinophilia, thrombocytosis, elevated erythrocyte sedimentation rate, elevated alkaline phosphatase without other indications of liver involvement (other liver enzymes, bilirubin can be elevated in addition with liver involvement), low albumin
- Imaging: Superior or anterior mediastinal mass on chest radiograph, enlarged axillary, supraclavicular, mediastinal, retroperitoneal, inguinal nodes, liver and spleen on computerized tomography, increased radioactive nuclide uptake on gallium or positron emission scans
- Diagnosis: Tissue biopsy (fine-needle aspirate cytology rarely adequate)
- Classic Hodgkin's lymphoma: Reed-Sternberg cells CD30+, CD15+, usually CD20–
  - Nodular sclerosis
  - Mixed cellularity
  - Lymphocyte rich
  - Lymphocyte depleted (rare)
- Nodular lymphocyte-predominant Hodgkin's lymphoma: Reed-Sternberg morphologic variants ("L & H," "popcorn" cells) CD20+, CD30–, CD15–

CURRENT THERAPY

- Clinical stages I and II without bulky disease: Four cycles of ABVD with IF RT or six cycles of ABVD alone would both be acceptable. Although the equivalence of the outcome of chemotherapy alone to chemotherapy plus RT is not yet proven definitively, chemotherapy alone would probably reduce the late toxicities of treatment, most of which are related to RT.
- Clinical stages II$_x$A/II$_x$B: Six cycles of ABVD plus IF RT or Stanford V.
- Clinical stage IIIA: Six cycles of ABVD.
- Clinical stages IIIB and IV: Six cycles of ABVD, Stanford V, or BEACOPP regimens.
- Relapsed/refractory disease: Salvage chemotherapy followed by high-dose chemotherapy with peripheral blood stem cell support for most cases.

Abbreviations: ABVD = doxorubicin, bleomycin, vinblastine, and dacarbazine; BEACOPP = bleomycin, etoposide, doxorubicin, cyclophosphamide, vincristine, and prednisone; IF RT = involved field radiation therapy; RT = radiation therapy; Stanford V = 12-week chemotherapy program consisting of doxorubicin, vinblastine, bleomycin, nitrogen mustard, vincristine, etoposide,[1] and prednisone followed by RT to bulky sites (adenopathy = 5 cm, macroscopic splenic nodules).
[1]Not FDA approved for this indication.

detected by chest CT. Although traditional radiotherapy treatment seems rarely affected by these findings, CT does allow for refinements in radiotherapy treatment planning.

Treatment

STAGES IA/B AND IIA/B, NONBULKY

The work of Gilbert, Peters, and, later, Kaplan demonstrated that recurrences rarely occur within the treated lymph node areas with doses of radiation therapy (RT) to 3500 to 4500 cGy. The use of the linear accelerator made it possible to deliver these doses to large fields. The mantle port (cervical, supraclavicular, mediastinal, and axillary regions—an area like the mantle on a suit of armor) and the inverted Y port (para-aortic nodes, spleen [if not removed], splenic pedicle, and iliac, inguinal, and femoral nodes) and combinations of the two were developed in the 1960s. Total lymphoid irradiation (TLI) refers to combinations of the two that have also at times included low-dose irradiation of liver and lung. Subtotal lymphoid irradiation (STLI) includes the mantle port with irradiation of para-aortic nodes, splenic pedicle, and spleen if it was not removed.

Local irradiation is probably adequate for high-cervical-stage IA disease and lymphocyte-predominant or nodular sclerosis histology in a young patient. Lymphocyte-predominant Hodgkin's disease is often clinically localized, is usually effectively treated with irradiation alone, and may relapse late (a clinical feature reminiscent of low-grade lymphoma). The 15-year disease-specific survival is excellent (more than 90%).

There is also general agreement that bulky mediastinal disease with a mediastinal mass diameter more than a third of the chest diameter should be treated with combined modality treatment with chemotherapy and RT. Recently some groups have treated selected patients with bulky mediastinal masses whose disease is well defined on CT scan with RT only using ports designed with the aid of the CT scan.

The prognostic importance of contiguous extension of disease from hilar nodes into the lung parenchyma is controversial. Some centers employing radiotherapy only report good results using low-dose irradiation also administered to the entire affected lung aided by thin lung blocks. However, these patients are usually treated with combined chemotherapy and less complex involved field RT (IF RT).

The European Organization for Research and Treatment of Cancer (EORTC) found elevations of the erythrocyte sedimentation rate (ESR) (more than 50 mm/hour for stages IA and IIA, more than 30 mm/hour for stages IB and IIB) to be a powerful adverse prognostic factor among patients treated with RT only. However, this is not an adverse prognostic factor for patients treated with chemotherapy or combined modality treatment.

There are several treatment options for the majority of patients with stages IA and IIA Hodgkin's disease. Subtotal lymphoid irradiation, which can include the spleen, to doses of at least 3500 cGy in 3.5 weeks has resulted in a complete remission (CR) percentage in excess of 90% with a 20% to 40% relapse rate in pathologically staged patients, probably depending on radiotherapy technique and/or patient selection. The likelihood of salvage of these patients into a second durable CR may be in excess of 50%. This approach is rarely employed because of the long-term potential toxicities of extensive RT and the lower relapse rates seen after treatment with combined modality treatment or chemotherapy alone.

Combination chemotherapy alone and when combined with radiotherapy has resulted in a CR percentage greater than 90% with a relapse rate of approximately 10% or less. This was achieved in the past with six cycles of chemotherapy with MOPP (mechlorethamine [nitrogen mustard], vincristine [Oncovin], procarbazine, and prednisone) or similar regimens.

When radiotherapy is also used, fewer cycles of chemotherapy may give similar results. A protocol at Memorial Hospital randomized patients to four cycles of either MOPP or thiotepa, bleomycin, and vinblastine (TBV) combined with modified extended-field RT. The results with a median follow-up time of 65 months (7 to 96 months) were similar in both arms of this trial and also similar to the results achieved with six cycles of MOPP and similar radiotherapy.

Two French studies suggest that three cycles of MOPP may be sufficient in combination with radiotherapy. The H8-F trial of the EORTC demonstrated the superiority of three cycles of a MOPP/Adriamycin (doxorubicin), bleomycin, and vincristine/vinblastine (ABV) hybrid plus IF RT (36 to 40 Gy) (4-year treatment failure-free survival [TTFS] rate 99%) to EF RT at the same dose (TTFS rate 77%; $p < 0.001$) in favorable early-stage Hodgkin's disease.

The Southwest Oncology Group (SWOG) demonstrated a superior failure-free survival for three cycles of doxorubicin and vinblastine plus STLI (94%) as compared to STLI alone (81%; $p < .001$). The German Hodgkin's Lymphoma Study Group HD-7 study compared two cycles of doxorubicin, bleomycin, vinblastine, and dacarbazine (ABVD) plus EF RT (30 Gy)/IF RT boost (10 Gy) to EF RT (30 Gy)/IF RT (10 Gy) in favorable stage I and II patients. The freedom from treatment failure was 96% for combined modality treatment compared to 84% for EF RT alone.

From February 1990 to July 1996, in a randomized trial of patients with clinically staged early Hodgkin's disease (I bulky and/or B; IIA, IIA bulky, and IIEA), a comparison was made of four cycles of ABVD followed by STLI versus the same regimen followed by IF RT. There were 136 patients assessable, with the main characteristics fairly well balanced between the two arms. After a median follow-up of 87 months (range, 8 to 123), treatment outcome was as follows: complete remission 100% after ABVD plus STLI versus 97% after ABVD plus IF RT; FFP 97% versus 94%, and total survival 93% versus 94%, respectively. These results indicate that four cycles of ABVD followed by IF RT can achieve results comparable to the same regimen followed by extensive RT. This effective and safe regimen can be considered to be a standard option for most patients with early-stage Hodgkin's disease.

The results of a randomized trial from Memorial Hospital of chemotherapy with ABVD alone or combined with RT in clinical stages I, II, and IIIA disease without bulky mediastinal or peripheral nodal involvement were reported recently. Although this trial was not statistically powered to show equivalence of the two treatment approaches, no differences in CR percentage, freedom from progression, or overall survival were seen. The results of a randomized phase III trial of standard treatment (STLI, favorable; two cycles of ABVD plus STLI, unfavorable) versus experimental treatment (four to six cycles of ABVD alone) in stage IA and IIA patients without high-risk factors were recently reported from the National Cancer Institute of Canada Clinical Trial Group (NCIC-CTG) and the Eastern Cooperative Oncology Group (ECOG). The estimated progression-free survival (PFS) was 93% for the patients on the standard treatment arm and 87% for those in the experimental treatment arm, a statistically significant result. There was no difference in overall survival. Somewhat less than 30% of patients on the experimental arm received four cycles of ABVD alone, although it is not clear that an excess of relapses were seen in this group. In view of the high rate of salvageability of patients who might relapse after this type of chemotherapy, and the late morbidity of treatment that is mostly attributable to RT, the clinical meaning of a 6% difference in PFS is unclear. On the basis of these results, chemotherapy alone with six cycles of ABVD alone, which is more standard than four cycles, for nonbulky early-stage Hodgkin's disease, is also a treatment option, although, as mentioned earlier, there may be a slightly higher risk of relapse.

STAGES II$_X$, III, AND IV

The major advance for patients with advanced Hodgkin's disease came from the use of MOPP by DeVita and colleagues. Eighty-four percent of 188 patients achieved a CR, and 66% of these were free of disease for more than 10 years. Ninety percent of these patients had stage IIIB or IVB disease. There are many modifications of the MOPP regimen that achieved similar results.

The groups at Memorial Hospital and at the National Tumor Institute in Milan pioneered the use of alternating potentially non-cross-resistant drug combinations and low-dose RT. Santoro, Bonadonna, and their colleagues developed the ABVD combination and demonstrated similar CR percentages as seen with MOPP. Also, it was demonstrated that at least some patients relapsing after MOPP could be put into second remissions, although the duration of these remissions is not as long as with primary treatment. They suggested that the ABVD combination might be potentially non-cross-resistant with MOPP in that tumors resistant to MOPP might be sensitive to ABVD.

Following this suggestion, a program of alternating monthly MOPP and ABVD combined with reduced-dose RT was developed at Memorial Hospital. Adjuvant reduced-dose RT to the initially involved bulky lymph node regions was employed to prevent relapses in these areas. A protocol was designed in 1975 in which MOPP and ABVD were alternated monthly for eight cycles in combination with reduced-dose RT to bulky sites. In 1979, a new trial was started in which MOPP/ABVD/RT (eight-drug regimen) was randomized against three alternating potentially non-cross-resistant combinations (ten-drug regimen) and RT. The third combination was lomustine (CCNU), melphalan (Alkeran), and vindesine (DVA), following the demonstration of activity of vindesine alone and in this combination for relapsed patients. The same reduced-dose RT was administered as in the initial trial.

The results for the initial eight-drug/RT protocol and the subsequent eight-drug/RT versus ten-drug/RT protocol were the same. Between 1975 and 1988, 270 patients were treated with either two or three alternating drug combinations and low-dose RT. Two hundred twenty-two patients (82%) achieved a CR, 38 (14%) a PR, and 10 (4%) progressed. At 10 years, the relapse-free survival for the patients achieving a CR was 80%, overall survival was 74%, and progression-free survival was 70%. The relapse-free survival for CS IIB patients was 89% and at 10 years was 73% each for CS IIIB and IV patients.

Similar results were achieved in a number of trials with alternating monthly chemotherapy with or without RT. The cancer and acute leukemia group B (CALGB) conducted a randomized trial in patients with stages IIIA2, IIIB, and IV disease with assignment to MOPP, ABVD, or alternating MOPP/ABVD. Response and failure-free survival rates were superior for both MOPP/ABVD and ABVD as compared with MOPP alone. Similar results were also achieved using a compressed schedule hybrid approach in which the nitrogen mustard and vincristine are given on day 1 along with oral procarbazine, prednisone, doxorubicin, bleomycin, and vinblastine on day 8 (MOPP/ABV hybrid). Recently, the results of an intergroup (CALGB, Southwest Oncology Group [SWOG], ECOG, NCIC-CTG) randomized trial established ABVD as equivalent in treatment outcome to MOPP/ABV hybrid with less acute toxicity, myelodysplastic syndrome, and leukemia.

A number of short-course, dose-intense chemotherapy regimens combined with RT were introduced over the past decade. The Stanford V is a 12-week chemotherapy program consisting of doxorubicin, vinblastine, bleomycin, nitrogen mustard, vincristine, etoposide,[1] and prednisone followed

---

[1]Not FDA approved for this indication.

by RT to bulky sites (adenopathy = 5 cm, macroscopic splenic nodules). In a phase 2 trial conducted by ECOG in 47 patients with bulky mediastinal stage I/II or stages III/IV disease, the FFP was 85% and overall survival 96% at 5 years. Grade 3 or 4 neutropenia was seen in 59% of patients, and there was one acute monocytic leukemia. This regimen is strongly dependent on the RT to achieve maximal results.

The German Hodgkin's Lymphoma Study Group conducted a three-arm randomized trial, using a combination of bleomycin, etoposide, Adriamycin (doxorubicin), cyclophosphamide, vincristine, and prednisone (BEACOPP) versus dose-escalated BEACOPP with the aid of granulocyte colony-stimulating factor (G-CSF) versus cyclophosphamide, Oncovin (vincristine), procarbazine, and prednisone (COPP)/ABVD (∞ 8). After chemotherapy, RT was administered to initially bulky nodal sites or sites of residual disease. The freedom from treatment failure rates at 5 years were 69% for COPP/ABVD, 76% for standard BEACOPP, and 87% for dose-escalated BEACOPP ($p < 0.001$ for COPP/ABVD vs. dose-escalated BEACOPP). The 5-year survival rates were 83% for COPP/ABVD, 88% for standard BEACOPP, and 91% for dose-escalated BEACOPP ($p = 0.002$ for COPP/ABVD vs. dose-escalated BEACOPP). There was a considerable amount of acute toxicity including grade 4 neutropenia in 90% of patients and grade 4 thrombocytopenia in 47% with dose-escalated BEACOPP. The rate of secondary acute leukemias at 5 years was 2.5%, significantly higher than in the other two arms of the trial. The toxicity of this regimen and the possibility of successful salvage of resistant or relapsed patients after ABVD have somewhat tempered the enthusiasm for its use in this country.

However, another randomized trial showed a benefit for a conventional hybrid regimen over a shortened dose-intensified regimen using doxorubicin, cyclophosphamide, etoposide, vincristine, bleomycin, and prednisone (VAPEC-B) versus chlorambucil, vinblastine, procarbazine, prednisone/etoposide, vinblastine, and doxorubicin (ChlVPP/EVA) hybrid: A British and Italian cooperative trial of 225 patients with bulky or stage B I and II or stages III and IV were randomized to either 11 weekly cycles of VAPEC-B or ChlVPP/EVA hybrid. This trial also included RT to initial bulky nodal sites or sites of residual disease after chemotherapy. At a median follow-up time of 25 months, there was almost a three times increased progression rate in the VAPEC-B arm as compared with the ChlVPP/EVA hybrid arm.

Until recently, our policy was to administer adjuvant RT to all initially involved lymph node sites, whether or not they are bulky, in combination with alternating chemotherapy regimens for patients with advanced stages of Hodgkin's disease. The results of a large definitive randomized trial conducted by the EORTC showed no benefit to IF RT in patients achieving a CR after six to eight cycles of MOPP/ABV hybrid in patients with stages III and IV Hodgkin's disease, although a benefit for RT was seen in patients who only achieved a PR. At a median follow-up time of more than 6 years, there was an excess of deaths because of other causes including secondary malignancies approaching statistical significance in the group of patients in CR who received IF RT.

The issue of combined modality treatment as opposed to chemotherapy alone in most patients is being further addressed in a phase III randomized trial of short-course, intensive chemotherapy combined with involved field RT with the Stanford V regimen versus ABVD with RT only to bulky mediastinal sites in patients with locally extensive or stages III/IV Hodgkin's disease that is being conducted by ECOG and CALGB.

Based on the results with alternating chemotherapy with CS IIB, IIIB, and IV patients, a prognostic model was constructed in which five pretreatment characteristics emerged as having adverse prognostic importance in a multivariable analysis:

1. Low hematocrit
2. High-serum lactic acid dehydrogenase (LDH)
3. Older than 45 years
4. Inguinal node involvement (a reflection of extensive subdiaphragmatic disease)
5. Bulky mediastinal disease greater than 0.45 of the thoracic diameter

Approximately 60% of the patients had none or only one of these adverse factors, and their survival was greater than 95%. Patients with two or more of these factors had a dramatically inferior survival rate. The utility of this model has been confirmed by others.

Hasenclever and Diehl for the International Prognostic Factors Project on advanced Hodgkin's disease published a prognostic model based on a retrospective analysis of 1618 patients from 25 centers. In the final model, seven factors were used:

1. Albumin less than 4 g/dL
2. Hemoglobin (Hgb) less than 10.5 g/dL
3. Male sex
4. Stage IV
5. 45 years of age
6. White blood cell (WBC) count = 15,000 mm^3
7. Lymphocyte count less than 600 mm^3 or less than 8% of WBC

The worst prognostic group (7% = five, six, or seven factors) had a 5-year overall survival (OS) of 56% and a FFP of 42%. This model does not separate out a group with a very poor prognosis. A recently made comparison of seven prognostic models for Hodgkin's disease was retrospectively applied to 516 patients with advanced Hodgkin's disease. Three models were found to be the most predictive of outcome: the International Prognostic Factors Project Index (employing albumin, hemoglobin, gender, stage, age, WBC, and lymphocyte count); the Memorial Sloan-Kettering Cancer Center model (employing age, L-lactate dehydrogenase [LDH], hematocrit, inguinal nodal involvement, and mediastinal mass bulk); and the International Database on Hodgkin's disease (employing stage, age, B symptoms, albumin, and gender). Integration of the three models in a linear model improved their predictive power: Between 19% and 25% of patients fell into groups with either a 10% or a 50% risk of failure.

Salvage Treatment

Because of the high relapse rates seen following conventional salvage chemotherapy after primary chemotherapy, most groups are using high-dose chemotherapy with or without RT depending on the prior treatment with autologous bone marrow or peripheral stem cell rescue. The results are promising in selected patients with more than half the patients achieving remission of varying durations transplanted in second or subsequent remission. Results of high-dose chemoradiotherapy with autologous stem cell transplantation in 65 patients with relapsed or refractory Hodgkin's disease treated between 1994 and 1998 at Memorial Sloan-Kettering Cancer Center were recently reported. At a median follow-up time of 43 months, estimates of the proportion of patients alive are 73% and event free are 58% by intent-to-treat analysis. In a multivariable logistic regression model, there were three adverse prognostic factors: extranodal sites of relapse or refractory disease, complete remission duration of less than 1 year, or refractory disease and B symptoms. Patients with zero or one adverse factor had an OS of 90% and an event-free survival (EFS) of 83%. Patients with two adverse factors had an OS of 57% and an EFS of 27%, and those with three adverse factors had an OS of 25% and an EFS of 10%.

Toxicity

Most long-term toxicity of chemotherapy seems to be related to alkylating agent and procarbazine-containing regimens of the MOPP type. There is approximately a 3% lifetime risk of acute leukemia following MOPP-type chemotherapy. Among solid tumors, only alkylating agent-based regimens are associated with an increased risk of lung cancer. Azoospermia occurs in approximately 80% of men treated with six cycles of MOPP, and another 10% are rendered oligospermic. Sperm banking with cryopreservation is encouraged for male patients who may wish to have children in the future. Female patients younger than 30 years are less likely to become permanently infertile than those older than 30 years. The risks of infertility and secondary myelodysplastic syndromes or acute leukemias are less with ABVD than with MOPP-type regimens.

Vascular damage to coronary and peripheral arteries is a concern with RT. Carotid stenosis risk is increased after cervical RT. Patients who receive mantle field RT have a threefold increased risk of fatal myocardial infarction. Heart-valve fibrosis requiring surgical replacement and more subtle abnormalities, such as restrictive cardiomyopathy and conduction abnormalities, were also reported following mediastinal RT. The actuarial risk of second malignancies is 22% to 27% at 25 to 30 years following treatment for Hodgkin's disease. Most of this risk seems to be related to RT.

Neuromuscular problems are another late complication related to RT. Neck muscle atrophy resulting in neck pain and difficulty in neck extension occurs in some patients. Symptomatic radiation pulmonary and pericardial fibrosis and brachial plexopathies occur with current RT techniques but less frequently than in the past. Secondary hypothyroidism is usually manageable with thyroid replacement therapy.

Pulmonary toxicity from bleomycin treatment is a problem with the ABVD regimen. The major nonhematologic toxicity is pulmonary and related to bleomycin. In the trial conducted at Memorial Hospital, 33 patients (22%) discontinued bleomycin because of a decrease in DLCO. Ten of the symptomatic patients received brief courses of corticosteroids, and there was one death because of bleomycin during treatment.

REFERENCES

Adams MJ, Lipsitz SR, Colan SD et al: Cardiovascular status in long-term survivors of Hodgkin's disease treated with chest radiotherapy. J Clin Oncol 22(15);2004:3139-3148.

Aleman BM, Raemaekers JM, Tirelli V, et al: Involved-field radiotherapy for advanced Hodgkin's lymphoma. N Engl J Med 348(24);2003: 2396-2406.

Bhatia S, Yasui Y, Robison LL, et al: High risk of subsequent neoplasms continues with extended follow-up of childhood Hodgkin's disease: Report from the Late Effects Study Group. J Clin Oncol 21(23);2003: 4386-4394.

Bonadonna G, Bonfante V, Viviani S, et al: ABVD plus subtotal nodal versus involved-field radiotherapy in early-stage Hodgkin's disease: Long-term results. J Clin Oncol 22(14);2004:2835-2841.

Diehl V, Franklin J, Pfreundschuh M, et al: Standard and increased-dose BEACOPP chemotherapy compared with COPP-ABVD for advanced Hodgkin's disease. N Engl J Med 348(24);2003:2386-2395.

Hasenclever D, Diehl V: A prognostic score for advanced Hodgkin's disease. International Prognostic Factors Project on Advanced Hodgkin's Disease. N Engl J Med 339(21);1998:1506-1514.

Horning SJ, Hoppe RT, Breslin S, et al: Stanford V and radiotherapy for locally extensive and advanced Hodgkin's disease: Mature results of a prospective clinical trial. J Clin Oncol 20(3);2002:630-637.

Hull MC, Morris CG, Pipine CJ, et al: Valvular dysfunction and carotid, subclavian, and coronary artery disease in survivors of Hodgkin lymphoma treated with radiation therapy. JAMA 290(21); 2003:2831-2837.

Radford JA, Rohatiner AZ, Ryder WD, et al: ChlVPP/EVA hybrid versus the weekly VAPEC-B regimen for previously untreated Hodgkin's disease. J Clin Oncol 20(13);2002:2988-2994.

Straus DJ, Gaynor JJ, Myers J, et al: Prognostic factors among 185 adults with newly diagnosed advanced Hodgkin's disease treated with alternating potentially noncross-resistant chemotherapy and intermediate-dose radiation therapy. J Clin Oncol 8(7);1990:1173-1186.

Straus DJ, Portlock CS, Qin J, et al: Results of a prospective randomized clinical trial of doxorubicin, bleomycin, vinblastine, and dacarbazine (ABVD) followed by radiation therapy (RT) versus ABVD alone for stages I, II, and IIIA nonbulky Hodgkin disease. Blood 104(12);2004:3483-3489.

Hodgkin's Disease: Radiation Therapy

Method of
Pelayo C. Besa, MD

Hodgkin's disease is a malignancy of lymph nodes with a predictable pattern of spread. Advances in treatment have made Hodgkin's disease a highly curable cancer with a long-term survival rate of more than 90%. Cure rate, defined as 10-year freedom from relapse, for early-stage disease is in the range of 80% to 90%; for intermediate-stage disease, 70% to 80%; and for advanced disease, 30% to 50%.

Radiation therapy plays a major role in the management of Hodgkin's disease. Treatment planning and patient selection are based on thorough clinical staging and review of the pathology. Most patients afflicted with Hodgkin's disease are less than 30 years old and will be cured; therefore, they will be at risk of late toxicity from treatment. Ideal therapy should provide the highest cure rate with minimal long-term toxicity. With this goal, treatment programs have gradually adjusted therapy to the different clinical settings.

Adequate radiation therapy requires pretreatment simulation and therapy with a linear accelerator with a minimal photon beam energy of 6 MV through parallel opposed fields that deliver a tumoricidal dose in a fractionated fashion. Treatment reproducibility is verified periodically with portal films. After completion of therapy, the patient is observed regularly to detect early relapse and evaluate treatment-related toxicity.

Patient Evaluation and Staging

To determine the best treatment approach, the patient needs to undergo disease staging. A complete medical history is obtained with special attention to the tumor history, presence of B symptoms (unexplained fever, drenching night sweats, and unexplained weight loss), and general performance status. The physical examination should be thorough, with special attention to all nodal areas, Waldeyer's ring, liver, and spleen. When a single nodal site is involved, the low neck or supraclavicular area is involved in 60% of the cases, the mediastinum in 15%, axillae in 10%, and the inguinal-femoral regions in 10%. The disease progresses with involvement of contiguous nodal regions. Upper abdominal nodes are considered contiguous to the supraclavicular nodes through the thoracic duct. A biopsy must be performed, preferably with sampling from the most clinically suspicious node.

The hematologic assessment should include complete blood cell and platelet counts, erythrocyte sedimentation rate, and screen chemistries, including lactate dehydrogenase and thyroid function studies. An elevated erythrocyte sedimentation rate is associated with high risk of subclinical disease in the abdomen. An abnormal blood cell count and an elevated lactic dehydrogenase level suggest bone marrow involvement. Thyroid function testing must be done as a follow-up study because of a substantial risk of late dysfunction caused by radiation therapy.

Routine imaging studies include chest radiographs and computed tomography (CT) of the chest, abdomen, and pelvis. Magnetic resonance imaging (MRI) is used occasionally to better delineate hilar adenopathy and chest wall and pericardial extension and, in the abdomen, to distinguish unfilled bowel and vessels from adenopathy. Positron emission tomography fused with computed tomography (PET-CT) scans are most useful for distinguishing active disease in enlarged lymph nodes. Treatment response is evaluated with repeated PET-CT.

Bone marrow biopsies are performed in all patients except those with early stage (stage I or II) disease and no B symptoms. The overall frequency of bone marrow involvement in Hodgkin's disease is only 5%. Hodgkin's disease is staged according to the Ann Arbor staging classification system (Table 1). Figure 1 shows the lymphoid regions used in this system. Note that the infraclavicular, cervical occipital, and preauricular areas are a single region.

Radiation Treatment Technique

Treatment planning starts by reviewing the staging evaluation and pathology report. Clinical and radiologic studies are used to outline the extent of disease. The treatment fields include the known disease areas and adjacent nodal regions. Treatment volume varies according to the treatment plan. The *treatment volumes* are defined as involved field, extended field, and subtotal nodal irradiation. *Involved field irradiation* includes the entire nodal area in which nodes with Hodgkin's disease are noted; for example, if a low neck node is involved, the entire neck and supraclavicular areas are treated. *Extended field irradiation*

CURRENT DIAGNOSIS

History	Tumor history
	B symptoms (unexplained fever, drenching night sweats, unexplained weight loss)
Physical	All nodal areas
	Waldeyer's ring
	Liver/spleen
Laboratory tests	Complete CBC
	Erythrocyte sedimentation rate
	LDH
	Screen chemistries
Radiologic studies	CT chest/abdomen/pelvis
	PET-CT
Pathology	Lymph node or extranodal site
	Bone marrow

Abbreviations: CBC = complete blood count; CT = computed tomography; LDH = lactate dehydrogenase; PET-CT = positron emission tomography fused with computed tomography.

TABLE 1   Ann Arbor Staging Classification System

Stage I
Involvement of single lymph node region (I) or localized involvement of an extralymphatic organ or site (IE)

Stage II
Involvement of two or more lymph node regions on the same side of the diaphragm (II) or localized involvement of an extra lymphatic organ or site and one or more nodal regions on the same side of the diaphragm (IIE)

Stage III
Involvement of lymph node regions on both sides of the diaphragm (III), which may be accompanied by localized involvement of an extralymphatic organ or site (IIIE)

Stage IV
Diffuse involvement of one or more extralymphatic organs with or without associated lymph node involvement

Systemic Symptoms
A: Absence of systemic symptoms defined as B.
B: Unexplained fever with temperatures above 38°C (100°F), unexplained weight loss >10%, body weight, or drenching night sweats

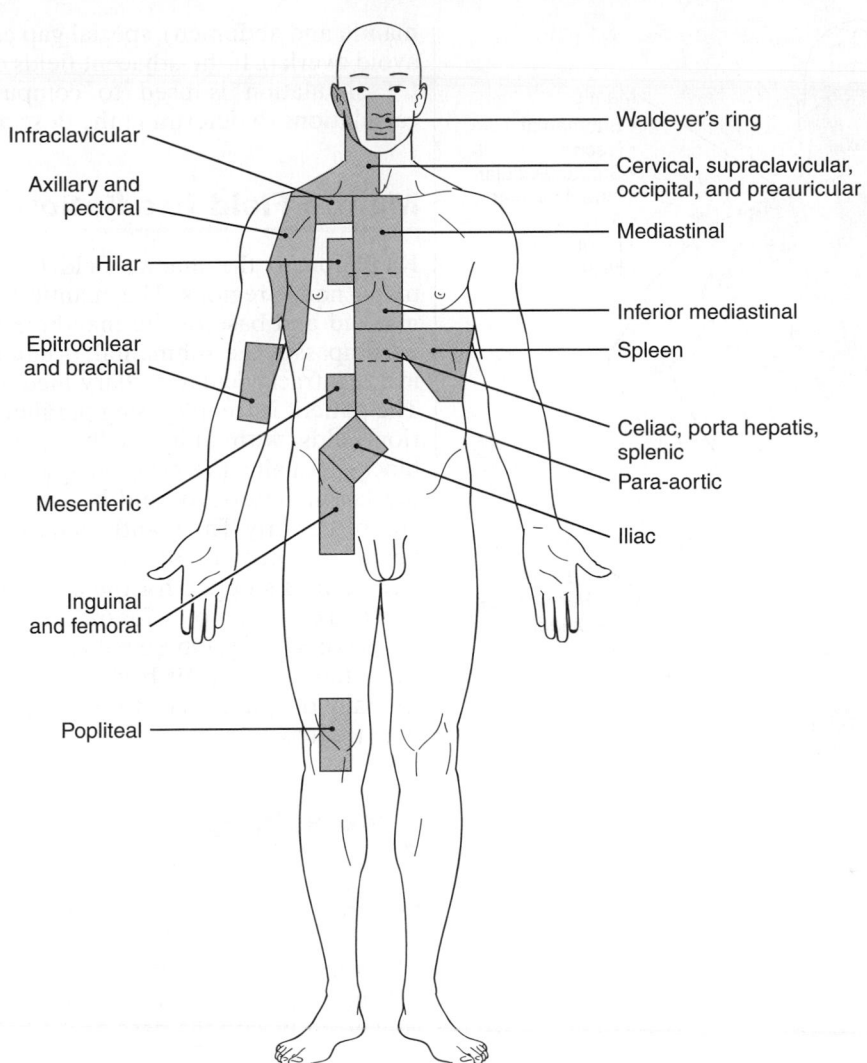

Infraclavicular

Axillary and pectoral

Hilar

Epitrochlear and brachial

Mesenteric

Inguinal and femoral

Popliteal

Waldeyer's ring

Cervical, supraclavicular, occipital, and preauricular

Mediastinal

Inferior mediastinal

Spleen

Celiac, porta hepatis, splenic

Para-aortic

Iliac

FIGURE 1. Lymphoid regions for Ann Arbor staging of Hodgkin's disease.

treats the entire nodal region. *Subtotal nodal irradiation* includes all the regions at risk: the supradiaphragmatic area including neck, supraclavicular, infraclavicular, axillary, mediastinal, and hilar nodes, and the infradiaphragmatic area, including para-aortic nodes, spleen, pelvic, and inguinal-femoral nodes. The nodal areas not included are mesenteric, presacral, popliteal, brachial, and epitrochlear nodes because they are only rarely involved with Hodgkin's disease. These regions are treated in three areas: the mantle for the supradiaphragmatic region, the abdomen, and the pelvis, including inguinal and femoral nodes (Figure 2). The junction between the fields must be placed away from the tumor to prevent underdosing, and normal tissue tolerance must be considered to avoid organ toxicity.

After the treatment plan is determined, the radiation field is simulated and marked on the patient. The simulator is a diagnostic radiography unit that reproduces the geometry of the therapy machine and takes verification films of the treatment fields. CT simulation is used to better outline the treatment areas and protect the normal tissue. CT cuts are used to outline the areas at risk, treatment volume, and the organs. Digital reconstructed images from CT simulation match the verification films from the simulator. To optimize reproducibility of the daily setup, patient immobilization devices are used; for example, a face mask of low-temperature thermal plastic (polycarbolactone) or vacuum body mold can be used for the mantle. Treatment fields include lymphoid regions, and to encompass all these areas, large and irregular fields are necessary.

The treatment volume generated with the CT simulation is used to outline the field to be treated and to design the blocks for the areas to be protected from irradiation. Divergent blocks are constructed from the drawings on the digital reconstructed images using either a low-melting-point alloy such as Lipowitz metal (Cerrobend) or a multi-leaf collimator, a machine device that shapes the beam with small movable leaves. Typically, the dose is prescribed to be delivered along the central axis at the midplane. The dose is higher for thin areas where diameters are small. To calculate the dose in the different areas, the three-dimensional reconstruction from the CT simulation is used and a dose distribution is obtained. Partial transmission blocks or shrinking field technique are used to compensate for the

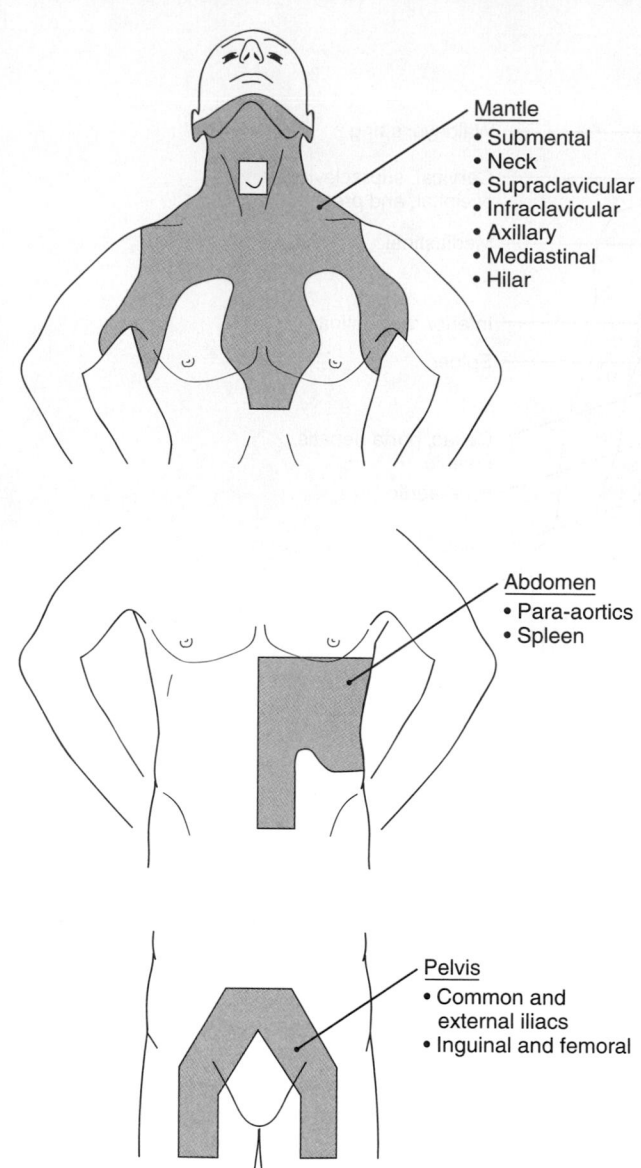

Mantle
• Submental
• Neck
• Supraclavicular
• Infraclavicular
• Axillary
• Mediastinal
• Hilar

Abdomen
• Para-aortics
• Spleen

Pelvis
• Common and external iliacs
• Inguinal and femoral

FIGURE 2. Radiation therapy extended fields: supradiaphragmatic: mantle; infradiaphragmatic: abdomen and pelvis.

difference in the diameters and to make the dose homogeneous throughout the treatment field. Better dose distributions are obtained with intensity modulated radiation therapy, using an electronic compensator, which modifies the beam moving the multileaf collimator to block the areas when they reach the prescribed dose.

Patients are treated on a linear accelerator at a 100-cm source-to-surface distance, usually using 6-MV photons for the upper torso and 18-MV photons for the abdomen and pelvis. The patient is seen on the treatment table by the radiation oncologist to verify the proper location of the fields. Machine portal films for verification are taken at the beginning of treatment and weekly thereafter. The dose delivered to the visible tumor areas is 39.6 Gy in 22 fractions over 4.5 weeks. The nodal areas treated prophylactically receive 30.6 Gy in 17 fractions over 3.5 weeks. In general, the treatment field is arranged with parallel opposed fields, using even-weighted beams, and all fields are treated daily. When two fields are matched (e.g.,

mantle and abdomen), special gap calculations are used to avoid overlap. If the adjacent fields overlie the spinal cord, CT simulation is used to computer-generated isodose calculations to determine the dose at the cord.

Mantle Field Irradiation

Radiation to the mantle field treats the supradiaphragmatic nodal regions. The mantle field extends from the mastoid and base of the mandible to the diaphragm and encompasses the submental, occipital, cervical, supraclavicular, infraclavicular, axillary, mediastinal, and hilar nodes. The patient is treated using parallel opposed anteroposterior fields, with individually contoured lung and heart blocks. Usually, the cervical spine is blocked posteriorly, the larynx anteriorly, and both humeral heads anteriorly and posteriorly. The mantle is treated with equally loaded beams to a dose of 30.6 Gy in 17 fractions. At this point, treatment is stopped for the areas of prophylactic irradiation and continues only for the areas of gross involvement to a dose of 39.6 Gy. Obese patients have a wide mediastinum when they lie on their back and can be treated sitting in a specially designed chair to decrease the amount of normal lung treated.

Subdiaphragmatic Irradiation

Subdiaphragmatic nodal areas are usually divided into two treatment fields: the abdomen, which includes the para-aortic nodes and spleen, with or without the pelvis, which includes the common and external iliac nodes and the inguinal-femoral regions. If the pelvic field is treated concurrently with the para-aortic field, the term *inverted Y* is used.

The field encompassing the para-aortic and spleen areas extends from the diaphragm to the bottom of the fourth lumbar vertebra; field edges are matched with those of the mantle with an appropriate skin gap; to encompass the para-aortic nodes, the field is drawn to the width of the transverse processes of the lumbar vertebral bodies, provided that the abdominal CT scan does not show nodes in a more lateral position. Radiation is delivered using parallel opposed anteroposterior fields with equally loaded beams that deliver a dose of 30.6 Gy in 17 fractions. An additional 9-Gy boost in five fractions is given to areas with tumor involvement. Individually contoured blocks are made to protect the kidneys and bowel. Often, it is not necessary to treat the pelvic lymph nodes and the radiation treatment stops at the level of the fourth lumbar vertebra. If needed, pelvic treatment is given through parallel opposed anteroposterior fields with 6-MV photons from the front (because the inguinal-femoral nodes are superficial) and 18-MV photons from the back. The pelvic field matches the abdomen field at the level of the fourth lumbar vertebra and extends to encompass the femoral lymph nodes. The nodal areas must be evaluated on the CT scan.

Careful blocking is used to spare the bone marrow as much as possible and, in young women, the ovaries. The ovaries are transposed medially and placed as low as possible behind the uterus to avoid radiation-induced amenorrhea and sterility. The ovaries are marked with radiopaque clips to aid in the placement of a double-thickness block. At a distance of 2 cm from the edge of the block, the ovaries receive approximately 8% of the pelvic dose.

Combined Modality Therapy

Many patients with intermediate or advanced Hodgkin's disease benefit from combined chemotherapy and radiation therapy. To reduce the toxicity from the combined modality approach, treatment must be tailored to the extent of disease and the risk of normal tissue injury. Special attention must be paid to the chemotherapy drugs, the number of cycles, the total dose, the time frequency between cycles or intensity, the radiation fields, the volume of tissue irradiated, and doses. Both the medical oncologist and the radiation oncologist must work together from the beginning to tailor the treatment plan.

Most patients with Hodgkin's disease treated with combined modality receive initially four or six cycles of a combination of doxorubicin (Adriamycin), bleomycin (Blenoxane), vinblastine (Velban), and dacarbazine (DTIC), the ABVD regimen, followed by radiation therapy to the involved areas. For patients with advanced Hodgkin's disease (stage IIIB or IV) or mediastinal masses larger than 15 cm, six cycles of chemotherapy are given, followed by radiation therapy to the involved sites.

PET-CT is used to evaluate the treatment response to chemotherapy. The test is done before chemotherapy begins and, if positive, repeated before radiation is delivered. Patients who become negative have a lower relapse rate.

Treatment Recommendations and Results

SUPRADIAPHRAGMATIC FAVORABLE STAGES I AND IIA

Upper torso presentation in patients younger than 40 years, with three or fewer sites of involvement, no large mediastinal mass, no B symptoms, and erythrocyte sedimentation rate less than 50 mm/hour should be treated with radiation therapy alone. Radiation is given to the mantle field and the para-aortic and spleen areas (Figure 2). Patients with mediastinal disease are excluded because they benefit from induction chemotherapy, which reduces

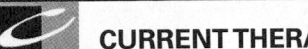

CURRENT THERAPY

Disease Extension	Treatment
Favorable I–IIA	XRT
Unfavorable I–IIB and favorable III	ABVD + IF-XRT
Advanced III–IV	ABVD or ABVD + IF-XRT
Relapse or refractory	High-dose chemotherapy + IF-XRT

Abbreviations: ABVD = doxorubicin/bleomycin/vinblastine/dacarbazine; IF = Involved field. XRT = radiotherapy.

the mediastinal mass and decreases radiation to normal lung. Freedom from relapse for this group of patients is 80% to 90% (Table 2).

Patients with stage IA nodular lymphocyte predominant Hodgkin's disease are a special subgroup who tend to have disease localized and have a late relapse pattern similar to low-grade nodular lymphomas. These patients must be treated to the involved field (Figure 3).

SUPRADIAPHRAGMATIC UNFAVORABLE STAGES I THROUGH IIA AND IIB

This group includes all patients with stages I and II disease who do not meet the so-called favorable criteria. These patients have an increased risk of abdominal involvement, approaching 30% according to the laparotomy data. Treatment is with combined modality therapy. Chemotherapy (four or six cycles of ABVD) is given first, followed by radiation therapy to the involved fields. The radiotherapy dose varies according to the chemotherapy response: For complete response 30 Gy is used, and for partial response, 40 Gy. Patients in this group, treated with chemotherapy followed by radiation therapy, have a disease-free survival between 80% and 90% and a survival rate of 90% at 6 years (Table 2).

STAGES I AND II WITH MEDIASTINAL INVOLVEMENT

Mediastinal involvement in very common in Hodgkin's disease and presents a special challenge to the radiation

---

TABLE 2 Treatment Results for Hodgkin's Disease

Series	Stage	Treatment	Survival % (y)	Freedom from Relapse % (y)
EORTC	I—IIA Favorable	XRT	96 (6)	81 (6)
EORTC	I—II Unfavorable	MOPP/ABV-XRT	89 (6)	94 (6)
JCRT	I—II large mediastinal mass	MOPP-XRT	88 (10)	89 (10)
MDACC	III (except III$_3$)	MOPP-XRT	87 (10)	83 (10)
EORTC	IIIB—IV	MOPP/ABV	85 (5)	85 (5)

Abbreviations: ABV = doxorubicin, bleomycin, vinblastine; EORTC = European Organization for Research and Treatment of Cancer; JCRT = Joint Center for Radiation Therapy; MDACC = MD Anderson Cancer Center; MOPP = mechlorethamine, vincristine, procarbazine, prednisone; XRT = radiotherapy.

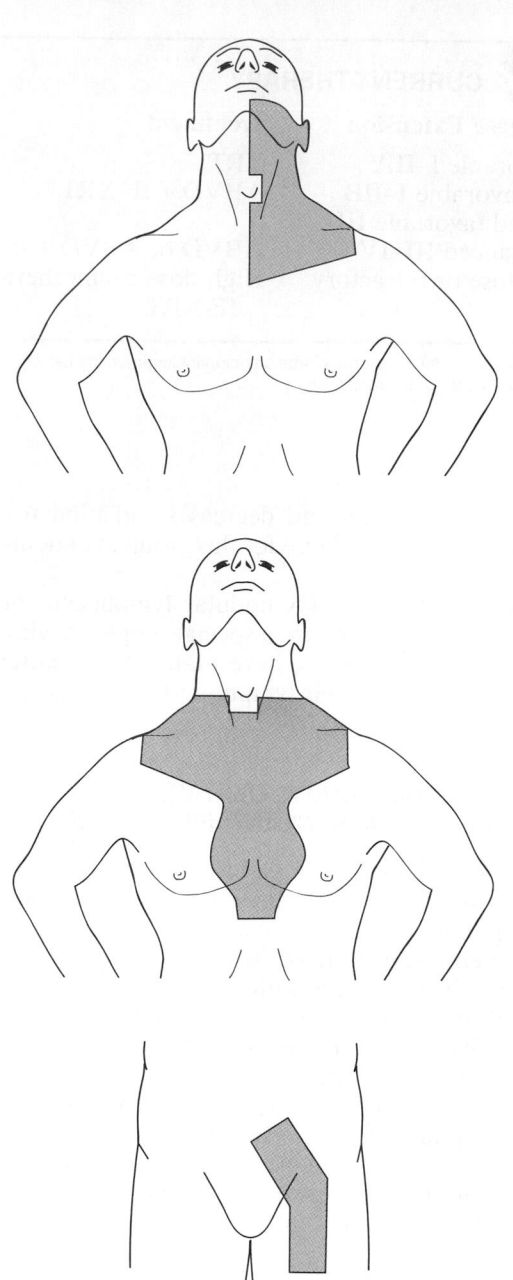

FIGURE 3. Radiation therapy involved field examples: neck, mediastinum, and inguinal-femoral.

oncologist because toxicity to the lungs and heart must be avoided. The extent of mediastinal tumor involvement is determined by measuring the maximum single horizontal width of the mediastinum on a standing posteroanterior chest radiograph. Three categories are defined as follows: Tumors less than 7.5 cm are small, those larger than 7.5 cm to less than 15 cm are large or bulky, and those larger than 15 cm are massive.

Patients with mediastinal involvement mass are treated with combined modality therapy. Chemotherapy is administered first to decrease the size of the mediastinal tumor. Patients receive six cycles of combination chemotherapy followed by radiation therapy to the involved field. Bleomycin is stopped after the fourth cycle if mediastinal irradiation is planned. Patients in this group, treated with combination chemotherapy followed by radiation therapy,

have a disease-free survival of 80% and an 89% survival rate at 10 years (see Table 2).

STAGES I AND II: SUBDIAPHRAGMATIC INVOLVEMENT

Fewer than 10% of patients with stage I or II Hodgkin's disease present with disease limited to the subdiaphragmatic areas. CT of the abdomen and pelvis is used to evaluate nodal and spleen involvement, and treatment is adjusted to the extent of tumor involvement.

For stage IA inguinal presentation, radiation is delivered to the involved field. More advanced cases receive combined modality therapy. Radiation therapy fields include the para-aortic nodes, the spleen, the common and external iliac nodes, and the inguinal-femoral regions. Treatment results for these patients are similar to those with supradiaphragmatic presentations.

FAVORABLE STAGE III

Nodal involvement in patients with stage III disease varies greatly. This heterogeneous group of patients is divided into subgroups according to extent of abdominal disease. Stage III_1 includes patients with disease limited to the upper abdomen (involving the celiac region, splenic hilum, and spleen). When the disease extends to the para-aortic region, it is classified as stage III_2; and if the pelvis or inguinal region is involved, the classification is stage III_3. With the exception of patients presenting with stage III_3 disease or IIIB, all patients with stage III receive six cycles of combination chemotherapy (ABVD), followed by radiation therapy to the involved areas (Figure 3). The relapse-free rate for this group is 85% with a cause-specific survival of 80% at 10 years.

ADVANCED STAGES III AND IV

The majority of patients with stage III_3 and many with stage IV receive combined modality therapy. Radiotherapy can be omitted for the patients that achieve a complete response to chemotherapy. Only approximately 35% of patients with advanced-stage disease treated with chemotherapy alone are alive and well at 10 years. Patterns of failure after chemotherapy show that recurrence overwhelmingly occurs in previously involved areas. Patients with stage III_3 ant IV Hodgkin's disease are treated initially with six cycles of combination chemotherapy (ABVD), followed by irradiation to the involved sites. With combined modality therapy, relapse-free survival of 85% and overall survival of 85% at 5 years is reported (see Table 2).

For relapsed or refractory Hodgkin's disease, involved field radiotherapy is used after high-dose chemotherapy and autologous bone marrow transplantation, with better local control and probable improved survival. The disease-free survival at 3 years is 66% and the survival is 57%.

Complications

Complications are classified as acute or late. Acute complications occur during or shortly after the course of radiation therapy; they are treated symptomatically and resolve quickly after the completion of treatment.

Acute complications include mild skin reactions and hair loss in the irradiated areas, dysphasia, dry cough, nausea, and diarrhea. These complications are treated symptomatically with skin ointments, analgesics, cough suppressants, and antinausea and antidiarrheal agents.

Late complications occur after treatment is complete, months or years later, and tend to be permanent. Late complications include pneumonitis, pericarditis, hypothyroidism, dental caries, and second malignancies. These reported toxicities observed in long-term survivors are clearly associated with treatment techniques that are different from the ones used today; therefore, in the future a decrease in these toxicities is expected.

Radiation pneumonitis occurs infrequently, and its risk is proportional to the volume of lung irradiated, the total dose, and the fraction size. The patient typically presents 6 to 12 weeks after the completion of the radiation therapy with dry cough, shortness of breath, pleuritic chest pain, and fever. The chest radiograph reveals interstitial infiltrates. Severe cases require treatment with high doses of corticosteroids for 4 to 6 weeks, with gradual tapering to avoid recurrence of symptoms.

Pericarditis is rare, occurring 6 to 12 months after treatment and usually after irradiation of the entire heart. Pericarditis presents as an acute episode of chest pain, fatigue, fever, and friction rubs or sometimes with decreased heart sounds because of pericardial effusion. Patients with mild pericarditis are managed with nonsteroidal anti-inflammatory agents, and for severe cases corticosteroids are used. Constrictive pericarditis and pericardial tamponade are rare complications that require surgical correction.

Subclinical hypothyroidism develops in a third of patients treated with mantle field irradiation. Patients are asymptomatic, and the physician is alerted by the elevation in the thyroid-stimulating hormone seen on the routine yearly blood measurement. Thyroid hormone replacement is necessary to avoid development of symptomatic hypothyroidism with weight gain, lethargy, temperature intolerance, irritability, and changes in skin and hair.

Xerostomia (mouth dryness) develops during irradiation of the mantle field that treats a portion of the salivary glands. There is minimal risk of clinically significant xerostomia, but partial decrease in saliva produces a favorable environment for dental caries. This complication can be prevented with pretreatment dental evaluation, careful dental care, and the daily use of fluoride.

Serious abdominal complications are extremely rare. An occasional gastric ulcer may occur. Bowel obstruction is related to prior laparotomy. In men, pelvic irradiation with adequate testicular shielding produces only temporary azoospermia. In women, ovariopexy is needed before pelvic irradiation to preserve fertility. The ovaries are meticulously shielded, but even this may not preserve ovarian function, especially in women older than 30 years.

The improved survival of patients with Hodgkin's disease is associated with an increase in the frequency of second malignancies. Leukemias are associated with the use of alkylating agents, and solid tumors are associated with radiation therapy. The most common cancers seen are breast cancer that occurs at a younger age, lung cancer in smokers, thyroid cancer, and non-Hodgkin's lymphoma. Shrink in the irradiation volume, with the use of involved fields, and the decrease in the total dose delivered should reduce the incidence of solid tumors in the future. Workup for early detection of cancer must be included in the yearly follow-up, and recommendations to avoid smoking given to all patients.

REFERENCES

Berthe MP, Aleman MD, John MM, et al: Involved-field radiotherapy for advanced Hodgkin's lymphoma. N Engl J Med 2003;348;24.

Eich H, Mueller R, Engert A, et al: Comparison of 30 Gy versus 20 Gy involved field radiotherapy after two versus four cycles ABVD in early stage Hodgkin's lymphoma: Interim analysis of the German Hodgkin Study Group Trial HD10. Int J Radiat Oncol Biol Phys 2005; 63(S1):S1-S2. Proceedings of the 47th Annual ASTRO meeting.

Hughes-Davies L, Tarbell NJ, Coleman CN, et al: Stage IA-IIB Hodgkin's disease: Management and outcome of extensive thoracic involvement. Int J Radiat Oncol Biol Phys 1997;39(2):361-369.

Noordijk EM, Carde P, Dupouy N, et al: Combined-modality therapy for clinical stage I or II Hodgkin's lymphoma: Long-term results of the European Organisation for Research and Treatment of Cancer H7 randomized controlled trails. J Clin Oncol 2006;24(19):3128-3135.

Poen JC, Hoppe RT, Horning SJ: High-dose therapy and autologous bone marrow transplantation for relapsed/refractory Hodgkin's disease: The impact of involved field radiotherapy on patterns of failure and survival. Int J Radiat Oncol Biol Phys 1996;36(1):3-12.

Acute Leukemia in Adults

Method of
Hans W. Grünwald, MD

Key Diagnostic Points

The prognosis of acute leukemia in adults is not yet as good as that achieved by newer treatments in children. However, enormous strides have been made in adults in the last few years with intensive induction and postremission combination chemotherapy (CT) and the use of stem cell transplantation in selected patients. With currently available therapeutic measures, the projected cure rate of acute leukemia (predicted from the freedom from relapse rate in the first 3 years) is expected to be 30% to 40% of all adults, and in selected subsets of patients with good prognostic features the cure rate may be as high as 50% to 60%. In addition to more intensive regimens of treatment, the reason for improved results can be ascribed to better supportive care and the increasing use of newer methods for the identification of characteristics of the disease,

CURRENT DIAGNOSIS

- Presentation with bleeding and/or infections
- Blood count shows anemia, neutropenia, and thrombocytopenia
- Presence of immature cells (blasts) in peripheral blood smear
- Bone marrow usually hypercellular and replaced by immature cells (blasts)

which better guide therapeutic decisions. Currently, it is essential to obtain cytochemical markers of the leukemic cells as well as their biochemical, immunologic, and especially cytogenetic characteristics. These may frequently be complemented by the investigation of molecular alterations at the DNA level using well-defined probes.

The use of growth factors (colony-stimulating factors [CSFs]) in the management of patients with acute leukemia helps shorten hospital stays by enhancing recovery from severe cytopenias induced by cytotoxic CT. They have been shown not to stimulate the regrowth of the leukemic cells that carry receptors for such growth factors, which is a concern in the acute myeloid leukemias (AMLs). Other major scientific advances that may yield a higher proportion of cures of acute leukemia in the future include the identification of minimal residual disease after completion of intensive postremission therapy using immunologic and/or molecular markers, and the potential for eradication of the residual disease by the use of biologic response modifiers (monoclonal antibodies, interleukins, and other cytokines) singly, in combination, or even combined with cytotoxic chemotherapeutic agents, or by the use of monoclonal antibodies either alone or attached to either toxins or radioisotopes. These investigational advances require that as many patients as possible participate in clinical trials. All new patients with acute leukemia should first be evaluated for entry eligibility on investigational protocols. They can be treated off-protocol if proved ineligible or if the patient refuses to participate. The intensive therapy needed both during remission induction and during postremission consolidation is associated with a high rate of complications and even a significant mortality. Therefore, all such patients should be treated in a major medical center capable of providing the needed supportive measures for such critically ill patients.

Acute Myeloid Leukemia

PRESENTATION

The clinical manifestations of AML are related mostly to bone marrow failure. The lack of erythropoietic activity manifested by anemia of varying severity causes fatigue, palpitations, lightheadedness, and dyspnea on exertion. The lack of megakaryocytic activity, manifested by thrombocytopenia, leads to purpura and mucosal bleeding. The lack of normal myeloid maturation, manifested by granulocytopenia, frequently leads to infections, which are often life-threatening. Common infections at presentation include pneumonia, perirectal abscesses, sinusitis, and otitis; however, fever and bacteremia without a localizing site of infection are common.

Some patients with hyperleukocytosis (>80,000 $M_1/\mu L$) can have mental symptoms characterized by confusion and even loss of consciousness (cerebral leukostasis) or pulmonary symptoms characterized by dyspnea and inadequate gas exchange (pulmonary leukostasis). Caution must be used in the interpretation of the results of an arterial blood gas specimen obtained in a patient with high leukocyte counts: The laboratory report may suggest extreme hypoxia in the patient; this pseudo-hypoxia is because of in vitro oxygen consumption by the white cells (*leukocyte oxygen larceny*). This laboratory abnormality

can be avoided by adding fluoride to the heparin in the syringe loaded with arterial blood, thus arresting glycolysis. Many patients with high leukocyte counts have been inappropriately intubated and placed on respirators for this reason.

Some patients with the myelomonocytic or monocytic variety of AML may present with severe gingival hyperplasia, marked tendency to gum bleeding, and skin and/or subcutaneous (SC) infiltrates.

Patients with the promyelocytic variant of AML frequently present with serious hemorrhagic manifestations and are found to have consumption coagulopathy (disseminated intravascular coagulation [DIC]) because of release of proteolytic (thrombin-like) enzymes into the circulation. These patients require close monitoring including all their coagulation parameters. Such patients may benefit from the administration of heparin in addition to fresh-frozen plasma (FFP) and/or cryoprecipitate until the coagulopathy is arrested by the treatment of the leukemia.

PROGNOSTIC FACTORS

Patients with a history of cytopenias caused by marrow dysplasia (myelodysplastic syndrome), exposure to aromatic hydrocarbons such as benzene, or treatment with alkylating and/or topoisomerase inhibitory chemotherapeutic agents (secondary myeloid leukemias) have a low remission induction rate (approximately half the complete remission [CR] rate of comparable patients with de novo AML). These remissions, when achieved, are rarely durable. Thus, in patients younger than 40 years of age with secondary AML and an HLA-matched sibling donor, early bone marrow transplantation should be considered.

Age is the second important prognostic feature in AML. The CR and the cure rates are higher in patients younger than age 40 years. In spite of the poorer prognosis of AML in the elderly, CR can be achieved even in the eighth and ninth decades of life, and treatment with curative intent should always be offered to the elderly provided they understand the risk involved. The risk-to-benefit ratio must be clearly presented to the patient to allow an informed decision to be made concerning treatment.

Certain subsets of patients with AML using the French-American-British (FAB) classification of leukemias (based on morphology and cytochemical features of the leukemic cells) are associated with a better prognosis (M4 with marrow eosinophilia, M3 hypergranular promyelocytic, etc.). These rare patients can often be better identified by their characteristic cytogenetic abnormality. Therefore, it is better to rely on the karyotype for therapeutic decisions after CR has been achieved (postremission therapy). The chromosome analysis (karyotype) is one of the best methods to identify subsets of AML that have a higher probability of prolonged remissions and cures. Such subsets include chromosomal inversions (inv) and translocations (t) such as inv(16), t(15;17), t(8;21). Chromosome analysis is also the best method to identify subsets of AML with a poor prognosis such as trisomy 8, abnormalities or loss of chromosome 5 or 7, abnormalities of chromosome 11q, or multiple translocations or trisomies. These abnormalities not only predict a short remission duration but also refractoriness to standard remission induction CT. More intensive regimens incorporating high-dose cytarabine (Cytosar-U) may be warranted for such patients, and allogeneic stem cell transplantation may be considered once a remission is attained.

Finally, immunophenotypic markers can identify patients with poorer prognosis. Patients whose blasts have the CD34 antigen on their surface (an antigen of early hematopoietic progenitors) have a high probability of being refractory to conventional induction CT, and warrant trials with a more intensive regimen.

Acute Lymphoblastic Leukemia

PRESENTATION

Most patients with acute lymphoblastic leukemia (ALL) present with manifestations of bone marrow failure: anemia, thrombocytopenia (with the characteristic purpura and mucosal bleeding), and granulocytopenia (with infections of all kinds). In addition, such patients often have bone pain and tenderness, generalized lymphadenopathy, and/or splenomegaly. Fever at presentation can be because of the high leukemic cell turnover but should always be considered to be of infectious origin until exhaustive investigations prove negative.

PROGNOSTIC FACTORS

Age is a very important prognostic factor in ALL. Young adults have a cure rate of approximately 70%, whereas in the elderly the prognosis of ALL is not much better than for AML (i.e., 20%).

The initial white blood cell (WBC) count is a major prognostic factor in ALL. Patients with leukocytosis above 50,000/μL readily achieve a CR but usually have an early relapse. Such patients warrant more intensive postremission therapy or stem cell transplantation.

The morphology of the leukemic blasts in peripheral blood and bone marrow smears can identify the Burkitt's type (FAB L3) of ALL. Such blasts are characteristically large with deep blue cytoplasm and with cytoplasmic vacuoles. This type of leukemia has a much lower CR rate than the L1 and L2 varieties of ALL and warrants the use of different, more intensive, therapeutic regimens. The Burkitt's type of leukemia can also be identified by the surface immunoglobulin of the blast cells, a characteristic of B cells, and by the characteristic chromosomal translocations [t(8;14) or t(8;22)] involving the c-myc oncogene on chromosome 8.

Chromosome analysis in ALL also can yield important prognostic clues. One or more translocations, especially t(4;11) and t(9;22), predicts for a high probability of early relapse after a remission has been attained. This justifies more intensive postremission CT or allogeneic stem cell transplantation if a suitable donor is available.

Initial Evaluation of the Patient with Acute Leukemia

Initial evaluation of the patient begins with a complete history and physical examination. Next is a careful and accurate evaluation of the peripheral blood and bone marrow smears for the morphology and classification of the leukemia. The bone marrow aspirate and biopsy stained with Wright or Giemsa yield the exact cytologic type and subtype (AML or ALL and its FAB class) in 80% to 90% of patients. It is also essential to perform a full cytochemical panel on the blood and marrow smears, assay for terminal deoxynucleotidyl transferase (TDT), immunophenotyping, and cytogenetic analysis on the bone marrow cells. This not only confirms the morphologic classification but also identifies the prognostic subtypes mentioned previously.

Also part of the initial evaluation of the patient is a careful analysis of the coagulation system, including prothrombin time (PT), activated partial thromboplastin time (APTT), plasma fibrinogen level and serum fibrin degradation product (FDP), or d-dimer assay. These tests can identify the DIC present in most patients with acute promyelocytic leukemia (AML FAB M3) and in some patients with myelomonocytic and monocytic leukemia (FAB M4 and M5).

Renal, hepatic, pulmonary, and especially cardiac function should also be assessed. Most antileukemic drugs are excreted by the kidneys and/or detoxified by the liver and are potentially toxic to these organs. Cardiac dysfunction diagnosed before treatment is begun can obviate the use of anthracyclines, which may lead to potentially fatal cardiac insufficiency in patients with poor cardiac function.

Multiple cultures should be obtained from blood and excreta and also from various mucosae prone to colonization by bacteria, fungi, and viruses (pharynx, nose, and rhinopharynx). Such cultures should be obtained not only in patients with suspected infection and fever but also in asymptomatic and afebrile patients to predict the possible microorganism responsible for an infection occurring later in the patient's course (*surveillance cultures*).

Finally, histocompatibility leukocyte antigen (HLA) typing should be performed in every new patient to identify potential stem cell donors among the patient's siblings (or even from the unrelated donor data banks) as well as to provide HLA-matched platelet transfusions if and when the patient becomes refractory to unmatched platelet transfusions because of alloimmunization. It is usually impossible to HLA-type the patient at the time alloimmunization is detected because there usually are few or no leukocytes in the peripheral blood to type as a result of the cytotoxic CT.

TREATMENT

Chemotherapeutic drugs should be started as soon as possible after diagnosing AML or ALL. There is rarely a need to initiate such treatment as an emergency, and there is usually sufficient time to perform all the aforementioned pretreatment evaluations. Biochemical, hemostatic, or other abnormalities should be corrected before initiation of cytotoxic CT. Hyperleukocytosis (>80,000 blast cells/μL), however, constitutes a medical emergency requiring immediate leukapheresis (removal of leukocytes by blood centrifugation at the bedside) and the rapid initiation of the cytotoxic CT to avoid pulmonary and/or cerebral leukostasis, which may be fatal.

Before CT, patients with acute leukemia should be hydrated and given allopurinol (Zyloprim) oral doses of 300 mg/day to avoid the development of hyperuricemia and urate nephropathy. Optimally, the allopurinol (Zyloprim) should be started 36 hours before the initiation of cytotoxic CT and continued for a total of 10 days. Thereafter, the risk

CURRENT THERAPY

- Correction of anemia and thrombocytopenia by transfusion of red cells and platelets
- Treatment of (presumed) infections with bactericidal antibiotics, antifungals and antivirals
- Induction CT based on cell of origin (myeloid or lymphoid)
- Consolidation CT also based on cell of origin
- Allogeneic stem cell transplantation in selected patients having a matched donor and high risk for relapse

Abbreviation: CT = chemotherapy.

of urate nephropathy is minimal, and the frequency of cutaneous hypersensitivity to the drug increases.

Venous access for the duration of treatment and the period of severe cytopenias that follows should be assured prior to initiation of the treatment. Many patients have adequate peripheral veins to permit administration of all required drugs and blood products. However, many patients eventually develop venous access problems during induction CT. Therefore, it is common to centrally implant a Silastic catheter (Hickman or Broviac) that is exposed to the outside. Alternatively, a port may be attached to the catheter and remain permanently under the skin (requiring a noncoring needle to access). Another method of achieving venous access is by means of a peripherally inserted central catheter (PICC) line, which does not require use of operating room facilities for insertion but can only remain in place for 3 to 6 weeks.

Another important issue before the initiation of cytotoxic CT is infection control. Appropriate bactericidal antibacterial, antiviral, and/or antifungal agents are used as needed. The use of bacteriostatic antibiotics (macrolides, etc.) must be avoided because they are ineffective in a granulocytopenic patient and may antagonize bactericidal antibiotics.

Finally, severe anemia and thrombocytopenia are corrected by packed red blood cell (RBC) and platelet transfusions, and FFP and heparin are given to correct the hemostatic abnormalities of the consumption coagulopathy. All blood cell transfusions (RBC and platelets) should incorporate a WBC-retaining filter to minimize the exposure to allogeneic HLA antigens and reduce the risks of eventual platelet refractoriness and presensitization for an eventual allogeneic stem cell transplant. For the same reason, family members of a patient deemed suitable for allogeneic stem cell transplantation should not be used as donors for RBC or platelet transfusions.

If evidence of a consumption coagulopathy is detected (prolonged PT and PTT; increased fibrin degradation products or d-dimers; prolonged thrombin time; decreased factors I, II, V, and VIII), prompt initiation of differentiation agent therapy (all-trans-retinoic acid [ATRA]), and/or heparinization in addition to administration of FFP and/or cryoprecipitate reduces the incidence of fatal hemorrhage. Heparin can be started with a bolus of 8 to 10,000 intravenous (IV) units, followed by a continuous IV infusion of 1000 U/hour during the first 48 hours, thereafter reduced

to 700 U/hour until correction of the coagulopathy (rise in fibrinogen is the best marker for this).

Acute Myeloid Leukemia

Most patients with AML of all types (FAB M1 through M7) respond to the standard induction combination CT of cytarabine (Cytosar-U) and an anthracycline given in the 7+3 regimen. Cytarabine (Cytosar-U) is given as a continuous IV infusion of 100 to 200 mg/m^2/day for 7 days, and daunorubicin (Cerubidine) is administered in doses of 45 mg/m^2/day as a slow IV bolus for the first 3 days. An alternative anthracycline, with similar therapeutic spectrum to daunorubicin (Cerubidine), is idarubicin (Idamycin) given at a dose of 12 mg/m^2/day as a slow IV bolus for 3 days. These doses are given irrespective of the initial blood count, because the goal is to achieve temporary marrow aplasia followed by normal marrow regeneration (achievement of a CR). However, if initial liver function tests demonstrate major impairment (bilirubin >3 mg/dL, ALT >3 times normal), the doses of both drugs should be reduced to half and the cytarabine (Cytosar-U) infusion stopped after 5 days if the liver function tests have not improved. Antiemetics such as ondansetron (Zofran), metoclopramide (Reglan), or prochlorperazine (Compazine) may be used liberally.

Patients older than 70 years of age should have the anthracycline dose decreased by 33% (30 mg/m^2/day for 3 days of daunorubicin [Cerubidine] or 8 mg/m^2/day for 3 days of idarubicin [Idamycin]). Patients with a history of coronary artery disease, heart failure, or who have a decreased cardiac ejection fraction on multigated angiogram (MUGA) scan can be given mitoxantrone (Novantrone) instead of daunorubicin (Cerubidine) (lower risk of heart failure) at a dose of 12 mg/m^2/day, given as a 1-hour IV infusion for the first 3 days, together with the 7-day cytarabine (Cytosar-U) infusion. An alternative for such high-risk patients is the use of continuous IV cytarabine (Cytosar-U) (100 mg/m^2/day) plus daily oral thioguanine (Tabloid) (2 mg/kg/day) until marrow aplasia is achieved. A bone marrow examination is performed on the day immediately following the conclusion of the cytarabine (Cytosar-U) infusion to assess the extent of cytoreduction. If the marrow cellularity on biopsy has not decreased to 20% or less and the proportion of leukemic blasts has not decreased by 80% or more, it is improbable that a CR will result. Additional CT consisting of 3 days of mitoxantrone (Novantrone), etoposide (VePesid), or high-dose cytarabine (Cytosar-U) (at dosages discussed in this article for refractory or recurrent AML) may then be considered but at the cost of increased toxicity (mucositis, pancytopenia of greater duration, etc.). An exception to the discussed recommendations is acute promyelocytic leukemia (FAB M3) with the t(15;17), where the ability of the leukemic blast cells to differentiate when exposed to retinoids has led to the use of ATRA as the mainstay of remission induction therapy. This has yielded not only an increase in the rate of CRs but also a dramatic prolongation of survival and a significant increase in the number of long-term, disease-free surviving patients (projected to be more than 75%). The treatment with tretinoin (Vesanoid) (ATRA) is given orally, 45 mg/m^2/day (in 2 doses) in addition to the standard 7+3 induction treatment with cytarabine

(Cytosar-U) and daunorubicin (Cerubidine) (or idarubicin [Idamycin]) as described previously for myeloblastic leukemia. A not uncommon complication of ATRA administration is the development of the retinoic acid syndrome, consisting of dyspnea, fluid retention, pleural and/or pericardial effusions, and occasionally even pulmonary edema. The retinoic acid syndrome usually improves with the administration of corticosteroids. Dexamethasone (10 mg orally twice daily for 3 to 5 days) should be initiated as soon as the first symptoms of the syndrome appear.

Daily blood count monitoring during and after induction CT is essential as a measure of the cytoreduction induced. Close platelet count monitoring guides the administration of platelet transfusions. Hemoglobin levels guide the administration of packed RBC transfusions. Frequent monitoring of serum electrolyte levels is needed to detect the occurrence (fortunately rare) of a tumor lysis syndrome.

A second postinduction bone marrow aspiration and biopsy should be performed 1 week after completion of the course of CT to help make the decision regarding need for a second course of induction CT. If the proportion of leukemic blasts in the aspirate remains above 5% and the cellularity on biopsy is more than 10%, a second course of the same drugs used initially should be given. However, the duration of the second CT course should be shorter, with a 5-day infusion of cytarabine (Cytosar-U) and two daily doses of the anthracycline at the same daily doses given for the first course (5+2). If the bone marrow shows a cellularity of less than 10%, but most cells are blasts, it is advisable to wait 3 to 5 days and repeat the bone marrow aspiration and biopsy, because it is virtually impossible to differentiate between residual leukemia and very early marrow regeneration. A subsequent marrow can reveal further lineage differentiation (appearance of promyelocytes, myelocytes, and even metamyelocytes) if it is early regeneration. A persistently leukemic marrow shows a further increase in blasts. If, after a second course of cytarabine (Cytosar-U) plus anthracycline (5+2) the marrow remains leukemic, characterize the patient as refractory to the induction CT.

Refractory or Relapsed Acute Myeloid Leukemia

Patients who are refractory to induction CT or who relapse after having attained a CR require more intensive induction CT, usually the high-dose cytarabine (HiDAC) (Cytosar-U) regimen consisting of 1 to 3 g/m^2 of cytarabine (Cytosar-U) every 12 hours for 6 days (a total of 12 doses) given as a 75-minute infusion each. Because HiDAC (Cytosar-U) concentrates in tears and can cause keratitis, it is important to wash the eyes with saline or artificial tears at least six times each day. Patients must also be closely monitored for cerebellar toxicity involving coordination and speech. The drug must be discontinued at the first sign of ataxia or slurred speech. Less-common toxicities of HiDAC (Cytosar-U) include hemorrhagic enterocolitis and noncardiac pulmonary edema (acute respiratory distress syndrome [ARDS]).

After the 6 days of cytarabine (Cytosar-U) infusions have been completed, bone marrow aspiration and biopsy are performed. If the marrow still shows more than 20%

leukemic blasts, it is advisable to give 3 days of mitoxantrone (Novantrone), 12 mg/m^2/day as a 1-hour infusion.

An alternative regimen for refractory or relapsed AML is the use of mitoxantrone (Novantrone) and etoposide (VePesid)[1]; etoposide (VePesid)[1] is given as a 5-day infusion of 150 mg/m^2/day, mitoxantrone (Novantrone) is given as a 1-hour IV infusion of 12 mg/m^2/day for the first 3 days. If, after completing this 5-day regimen, the marrow shows reduction but not disappearance of the leukemic blasts, a second 5-day course of these two drugs can be administered. These drugs require hepatic function for detoxification and should thus not be used if the patient has abnormal liver function tests (ALT > 3 times normal, bilirubin >3 mg/dL).

For elderly (over 60 years old) or poor-performance status patients with refractory or relapsed AML, an alternative regimen consists of the administration of gemtuzumab ozogamicin (Mylotarg) 9-mg/m^2/dose for two IV doses 14 days apart as a single agent. This drug, a monoclonal anti-CD33 antibody linked to the cytotoxic antibiotic calicheamicin, can induce remissions in refractory AML but usually of only short duration; so this therapy must be followed by some other antileukemic regimen, usually a nonmyeloablative allogeneic stem cell transplant.

Patients with relapsed or refractory acute promyelocytic leukemia (APL) (no longer responding to ATRA) can be treated with arsenic trioxide (Trisenox) at a daily IV dose of 0.15 mg/kg/day (most often given 5 days per week to allow ambulatory administration in units open only Monday through Friday) until a remission is achieved.

POSTREMISSION CONSOLIDATION

Once CR has been achieved (normal bone marrow, reticulocyte, platelet, and granulocyte counts) and the patient is deemed free of infections and aftereffects of the induction CT (attainment of a near-normal performance status), postremission therapy is planned. A significant advance in recent years is the attainment in a significant proportion of patients of long relapse-free survival (and thus possible cure of the leukemia), by the institution of intensive postremission consolidation CT. The intensity of treatment is similar or greater than that used for remission induction. Such treatment, however, may produce life-threatening toxicities. Most patients can be treated on an ambulatory basis (provided they live at a reasonable distance from the hospital). The regular need for platelet transfusions requires an ambulatory transfusion center. Furthermore, because most patients remain markedly neutropenic for periods ranging from 10 to 30 days following each consolidation course, they are advised to avoid external sources of infection (crowds, animals, vases with stagnant water, etc.) and to come to the hospital for prompt initiation of antibiotic therapy at the first evidence of chills, fever, or infection. Complete blood counts (CBCs) to monitor hemoglobin, leukocyte, and platelet counts are performed every other day (until recovery of adequate granulocyte and platelet counts), and blood biochemical monitoring is done weekly.

Drugs used for consolidation are the same as those used in induction and at doses similar to or higher than those

---

[1]Not FDA approved for this indication.

used for induction. Patients with the better prognostic karyotypes (core binding factor defects such as t;8:21 or inv;16) should receive at least 3 courses of HiDAC (Cytosar-U) 1 to 3 g/m^2 every 12 hours for a total of 6 to 10 doses per course. Patients with the less favorable karyotypes who are not scheduled to receive a stem cell transplant are usually given consolidation courses, which may consist of cytarabine (Cytosar-U) and an anthracycline used in the 7+3 induction regimen followed by at least one course of the HiDAC (Cytosar-U) regimen, and a third consolidation course, which might consist of the combination of etoposide (VePesid)[1] and mitoxantrone (Novantrone)[1] (as described previously for refractory or relapsed AML). The total number of consolidation courses ranges between three and six, depending on the patient's tolerance to the drugs, the rate of recovery from each course of consolidation (if the hematologic depression from a course is greater than 3 weeks, the probability for prolonged or even irreversible cytopenias after an ensuing course increases), and the initial prognostic category (patients with high relapse risk should receive the highest possible number of consolidation courses).

Patients at high risk for early relapse (high initial WBC count or other sign of high leukemic burden such as very high LDH, trisomy 8, abnormalities of chromosome 5 or 7, etc.) should be considered for a stem cell transplant if they attain a CR. Patients younger than 45 years of age with an HLA-matched sibling should receive an allogeneic stem cell transplant from that sibling. If an HLA-matched sibling is unavailable, a search for a voluntary unrelated donor (VUD) should be initiated through the National Marrow Donor Registry. For patients between 45 and 60 years of age, a nonmyeloablative allogeneic stem cell transplant should be considered.

Patients with less-than-optimal performance status or who are older than the age of 70 years should be considered for an autologous stem cell transplant; this procedure involves harvesting bone marrow or peripheral blood stem cells shortly before a planned intensive consolidation CT course. The marrow or peripheral blood stem cells may be subjected to in vitro purging (either using drugs or antibodies with complement) and frozen. Thereafter, the patient is given the preparative regimen of high-dose cyclophosphamide (Cytoxan)[1] plus total body irradiation (or busulfan) followed by infusion of the thawed marrow or peripheral blood cells.

Patients with APL who attained a remission with ATRA, cytarabine (Cytosar-U), and daunorubicin (Cerubidine) are given consolidation with cytarabine (Cytosar-U) and daunorubicin (Cerubidine) as for patients with AML without the t;15:17. However, the HiDAC, etoposide (VePesid),[1] and mitoxantrone (Novantrone) consolidations are omitted, and the patients are given maintenance oral ATRA on alternating weeks for at least 1 year at a dose of 45 mg/m^2 daily (the addition of methotrexate and mercaptopurine [Purinethol] to this maintenance is currently being evaluated).

Patients with relapsed or refractory APL who responded to arsenic trioxide (Trisenox) as second-line therapy are given a second consolidation course of IV arsenic trioxide (Trisenox) 0.15 mg/kg/day for 25 doses more than 5 weeks

(5 days per week). Thereafter, they should be considered for a possible allogeneic stem cell transplant.

ACUTE LYMPHOBLASTIC LEUKEMIA

Most patients with ALL achieve a remission following vincristine (Oncovin) and prednisone induction therapy. Significant increases in both remission rates and their duration can be attained by the addition of anthracyclines, L-asparaginase (Elspar), and alkylating agents. The presently recommended remission induction regimen for adults with ALL consists of the following drugs:

- One dose of cyclophosphamide (Cytoxan) 1 g/m^2 by slow IV injection
- Vincristine (Oncovin) 2 mg by slow IV injection weekly for 4 doses
- Prednisone 100 mg/day orally for 21 days (no need to taper)
- Daunorubicin (Cerubidine) 45 mg/m^2/day by slow IV injection for 3 days
- L-asparaginase (Elspar) 6000 U/m^2 intramuscularly (IM) (SC if the platelet count is below 50,000/µL) every 4 days for six doses

For patients older than the age of 65 years, the cyclophosphamide (Cytoxan) dose is reduced to 700 mg/m^2, the daunorubicin (Cerubidine) to 30 mg/m^2, and the duration of prednisone administration is reduced to 10 days. The administration of filgrastim (Neupogen), a granulopoiesis stimulant, at the dose of 5 µg/kg body weight, should be initiated on day 5 and continued until a granulocyte count of 10,000/µL is attained. Blood counts are performed daily to monitor cytoreduction and to evaluate the need for RBC and platelet transfusions. Bone marrow aspiration and biopsy are performed 4 weeks after the start of CT. If the leukemic blasts have not disappeared, an alternative induction regimen with teniposide, cytarabine (Cytosar-U), and prednisone should be initiated. If the marrow on day 28 shows disappearance of the leukemic blasts, but is not yet normal, an additional 7 to 10 days of CT may lead to the signs of remission (normalization of marrow, reticulocyte, granulocyte, and platelet counts).

Once remission has been documented, central nervous system (CNS) prophylaxis is given with 15 mg of intrathecal methotrexate (be careful to use preservative-free drug) every week for 4 weeks combined with cranial radiation (24 Gy). During this 4-week period, the patient is also given 6-mercaptopurine (6-MP) (Purinethol) 60 mg/m^2 daily by mouth and methotrexate 20 mg/m^2 weekly by mouth. Blood counts are done at least twice weekly, and the dosage of 6-MP (Purinethol) and methotrexate is reduced if cytopenias occur. Liver function tests should also be closely monitored and the dosage of both drugs reduced if abnormalities occur.

After completion of the CNS prophylaxis, and only if and when the blood counts and blood chemistries are normal, an intensive 2-month consolidation CT is initiated as follows:

- Cyclophosphamide (Cytoxan) 1 g/m^2 IV on weeks 1 and 5
- Cytarabine (Cytosar-U) 75 mg/m^2/day SC for 4 days on weeks 1, 2, 5, and 6
- 6-MP (Purinethol) 60 mg/m^2/day orally during weeks 1, 2, 5, and 6

---

[1]Not FDA approved for this indication.

- Vincristine (Oncovin) 2 mg IV/week on weeks 3, 4, 7, and 8
- L-Asparaginase (Elspar) 6000 U IM (SC if platelet count is below 50,000/μL) twice weekly on weeks 3, 4, 7, and 8

Patients usually require frequent platelet and occasional RBC transfusions during this period of consolidation, but the treatment can be accomplished on an ambulatory basis if an ambulatory transfusion and CT unit is available. If at the start of week 5 there is persistent thrombocytopenia and/or neutropenia (below 50,000 and 1000/μL), the scheduled CT should be postponed for 1 week. For patients with Ph+ ALL (t;9:22), the addition of imatinib (Gleevec)[1] is currently being evaluated as an additional agent during consolidation to eliminate minimal residual disease.

After completion of this intensive consolidation CT, repeat bone marrow aspiration and biopsy are performed to confirm continued remission. Then the 2-year maintenance phase is initiated, consisting of 6-MP (Purinethol) 60 mg/m^2 by mouth daily, methotrexate 20 mg/m^2 by mouth weekly, vincristine (Oncovin) 2 mg IV monthly, and prednisone 80 mg/day for 5 days every month (starting on the day of vincristine [Oncovin] administration). Blood counts are performed weekly and blood chemistries biweekly. If significant cytopenias and/or liver dysfunction occur, the maintenance CT is dose reduced or temporarily withheld until acceptable values are achieved.

Patients with prognostic indicators for early relapse (initial WBC count of 50,000/μL or higher, t(9;22) or t(4;11) translocations, etc.) may be considered for allogeneic bone marrow transplantation after achieving a remission if an HLA compatible sibling is available.

Patients with B-cell ALL (Burkitt's cell leukemia, FAB = L3) may be treated with a more intensive, shorter, aggressive lymphoma-like induction CT followed by CNS prophylaxis, without a prolonged maintenance phase. The regimen includes the use of high doses of cyclophosphamide (Cytoxan) and methotrexate (with leucovorin reversal) plus vincristine (Oncovin), dexamethasone,[1] cytarabine (Cytosar-U), etoposide (VePesid),[1] and doxorubicin.

SUPPORTIVE CARE

In addition to the proper chemotherapeutic agents, all other aspects of the patient's care must be optimal. The major reason for failure to achieve CR is the death of the patient because of complications of the disease and/or the CT. Primary resistance to CT is infrequent.

A most important clinical consideration is the assurance of adequate hemostasis; thrombocytopenia associated with acute leukemia and that resulting from the use of cytotoxic drugs is the most common cause of hemorrhage. Platelet transfusions have markedly reduced morbidity and mortality from bleeding. Platelets should be given whenever the platelet count is 10,000/μL or fewer, but hemorrhage can occur even with higher levels. Some patients may have very low platelet counts (below 10,000/μL) without bleeding. Patients who require an invasive intervention (insertion of a Hickman catheter, performance of a spinal tap, etc.) should have their platelet count increased to 50,000/μL with platelet transfusions. The presence of signs of DIC as manifested by prolonged PT, PTT, elevated FDP, and/or decreased fibrinogen in addition to thrombocytopenia mandates the administration not only of platelet transfusions (to increase the platelet count to greater than 30,000/μL) but also of FFP and/or cryoprecipitate to restore the hemostatic function to normal. In addition, heparin given to such patients (as described previously) has sometimes proven helpful in this situation. Finally, prolongation of PT and/or PTT well into the course of treatment may occur in some patients as a consequence of vitamin K deficiency. The latter may be because of poor oral food intake and prolonged antibiotic therapy that alters the intestinal flora. Hemostatic function must thus be monitored and supplementary vitamin K given as needed.

After a few weeks of treatment, some patients may become totally refractory to platelet transfusions as shown by a lack of increase in platelet count 1 hour after completion of the transfusion. This situation is usually because of HLA alloimmunization and can be overcome by obtaining HLA-matched platelets for transfusion. The use of filters, which remove WBCs from all transfused blood products (red cells and platelets) from the start, reduces (but does not eliminate) the incidence of HLA alloimmunization. This benefit not only decreases the incidence of platelet refractoriness, but also reduces the risk of an eventual graft rejection after bone marrow transplantation.

The main cause of morbidity and mortality in patients with acute leukemia is infection, both during induction CT and later during the intensive consolidation phases of treatment. Prophylactic antibacterial therapies with a quinolone such as ciprofloxacin (Cipro) or with trimethoprim-sulfamethoxazole (Bactrim),[1] and/or antifungal prophylaxis with fluconazole (Diflucan)[1] have not yet been proven to decrease the risk of such infections. However, it is advisable to initiate antibiotic and/or antifungal therapy as soon as fever occurs, especially if the granulocyte count is less than 500/μL. Fever in the neutropenic patient requires prompt and intensive attention: cultures for bacteria, fungi, and viruses should be obtained from all potential sites of infections. Immediately thereafter, treatment with broad-spectrum bactericidal antibiotics such as a semisynthetic penicillin like piperacillin (Pipracil)[1] and an aminoglycoside such as gentamicin (Garamycin)[1] should be initiated. For the possible cutaneous entry of hospital bacteria such as methicillin-resistant *Staphylococcus aureus*, or for catheter colonization by *Corynebacterium* of the JK subtype, the addition of vancomycin (Vancocin)[1] is recommended. If the patient remains febrile after 72 hours of such triple antibiotic therapy, antifungal therapy with amphotericin B (Fungizone)[1] should be started on an empiric basis. Therapy of infections is guided and modified according to results of cultures obtained prior to the initiation of the antibiotic therapy.

Although uncommon, viral infections must also be addressed. Serology for herpes simplex virus (HSV) and cytomegalovirus (CMV) should be obtained prior to the start of induction CT. Changes are then monitored during febrile episodes if mucosal lesions suggesting herpes simplex appear. Treatment with IV acyclovir (Zovirax)[1]

---

[1]Not FDA approved for this indication.

[1]Not FDA approved for this indication.

may be highly effective. Cytomegalovirus can cause interstitial pneumonia as well as esophagitis, enterocolitis and hepatitis, all of which can be treated with ganciclovir (Cytovene).

PSYCHOSOCIAL ASPECTS

Caution must be used in addressing the patients with acute leukemia and their families. They may not be prepared for the major lifestyle alterations that the disease and its treatment will require. In addition to calm counseling and explanation of all planned phases of treatment, it is important to reinforce these concepts repeatedly. An excellent source of information for both patient and family is a patient with a similar diagnosis who has already undergone a treatment similar to the one planned and can provide the information in terms easily understood by laypersons.

Once the induction CT has led to a CR and the patient has returned home, the availability of a group of patients with successfully treated hematologic neoplasms (such as *Candlelighters*) has proven helpful to make the adjustments required by the disease and its therapy more tolerable. These groups are led by a trained professional, and provide the wherewithal for physical and psychologic adjustment. The availability of a social worker and a psychiatrist with oncologic orientation as team members helps greatly in patient management.

REFERENCES

Byrd JC, Ruppert AS; Mrézek K, et al: Repetitive cycles of high-dose cytarabine benefit patients with acute myeloid leukemia and inv(16)(p13;q22) or t(16;16)(p13;q22): Results from CALGB 8461. J Clin Oncol 2004;22(6):1087-1094.

Carey RW, Ribas-Mundo M, Ellison RR, et al: Comparative study of cytosine arabinoside therapy alone and combined with thioguanine, mercaptopurine, or daunorubicin in acute myelocytic leukemia. Cancer 1975;36(5):1560-1566.

Daenen S, Löwenberg B, Sonneveld P, et al: Efficacy of etoposide and mitoxantrone in patients with acute myelogenous leukemia refractory to standard induction therapy and intermediate-dose cytarabine with Amsidine. Dutch Hematology-Oncology Working Group for Adults (HOVON). Leukemia 1994;8(1):6-10.

Herzig RH, Wolff SN, Lazarus, HM, et al: High-dose cytosine arabinoside therapy for refractory leukemia. Blood 1983;62(2):361-369.

Larson RA, Dodge RK, Linker CA, et al: A randomized controlled trial of filgrastim during remission induction and consolidation chemotherapy for adults with acute lymphoblastic leukemia: CALGB study 9111. Blood 1998;92(5):1556-1564.

Larson RA, Boogaerts M, Estey E, et al: Antibody-targeted chemotherapy of older patients with acute myeloid leukemia in first relapse using Mylotarg (gemtuzumab ozogamicin). Leukemia 2002;16(9):1627-1636.

Preisler H, Davis RB, Kirshner J, et al: Comparison of three remission induction regimens and two postinduction strategies for the treatment of acute nonlymphocytic leukemia: A cancer and leukemia group B study. Blood 1987;69(5):1441-1449.

Shen ZX, Chen GQ, Ni JH, et al: Use of arsenic trioxide (As2O3) in the treatment of acute promyelocytic leukemia (APL): II. Clinical efficacy and pharmacokinetics in relapsed patients. Blood 1997;89(9):3354-3360.

Tallman MS, Andersen JW, Schiffer CA, et al: All-trans retinoic acid in acute promyelocytic leukemia: Long-term outcome and prognostic factor analysis from the North American Intergroup protocol. Blood 2002;100(13):4298-302.

Yates J, Glidewell O, Wiernik P, et al: Cytosine arabinoside with daunorubicin or Adriamycin for therapy of acute myelocytic leukemia: A CALGB study. Blood 1982;60(2):454-462.

Acute Leukemia in Children

Method of
Kelly Maloney, MD

The acute leukemias are the most common malignancy of childhood, accounting for approximately 35% of all malignant diseases diagnosed in children younger than 15 years. Acute lymphoblastic leukemia (ALL) is the most common malignancy of childhood, accounting for approximately 25% of all cancer diagnosis in children younger than 15 years. The worldwide incidence of ALL is 1:25,000 children per year, including 3000 children per year in the United States. Acute myelogenous leukemia (AML) occurs less often than ALL, accounting for 800 to 900 cases per year in children and adolescents. Both disease processes continue to be the subject of intense biologic and epidemiologic studies. As well, clinical trials are available to continue to search for optimal therapy for both AML and ALL in childhood.

Patients with ALL and AML often have similar, nonspecific presenting symptoms. These presenting symptoms are often related to decreased bone marrow production of red blood cells (RBCs), white blood cells (WBCs), or platelets and to leukemic infiltration of extramedullary (outside the bone marrow) sites. Common presenting signs and symptoms include fever, anemia, fatigue, bleeding, petechiae, purpura, infection, bone and joint pain, lymphadenopathy (including mediastinal), hepatosplenomegaly, cranial nerve palsies, and testicular enlargement. Physical examination at diagnosis can range from virtually normal to highly abnormal. Hepatosplenomegaly occurs in approximately 60% of patients with ALL but to a lesser degree in AML. As well, lymphadenopathy, either localized or generalized, occurs in approximately 50% of patients with ALL but less in patients with AML. Most diagnosis of leukemia can be made with a complete blood count (CBC) and a chest radiograph. Most commonly, the CBC shows at least one

CURRENT DIAGNOSIS

Acute Leukemias

- Presenting signs and symptoms: fever, pallor, fatigue, bruising, bleeding, infection, bone and joint pain, lymphadenopathy
- Presenting physical findings: pallor, petechiae, purpura, bruising, lymphadenopathy, hepatosplenomegaly, cardiac murmurs, limited movement of extremities; more rarely: cranial nerve palsies, testicular enlargement, chloromas
- Laboratory findings:
  - Anemia
  - Thrombocytopenia
  - Low, normal, or high white blood cell count with presence of blasts
  - Elevated lactate dehydrogenase
  - Possibly elevated uric acid and creatinine

cytopenia (anemia, leukopenia, thrombocytopenia). If two or more blood cell cytopenias are observed, a bone marrow aspirate and possibly a bone marrow biopsy are the appropriate next step. The bone marrow aspirate typically reveals displacement of normal hematopoietic precursors by leukemic blast cells, which generally have a high nuclear-to-cytoplasmic ratio, often exhibit nucleoli, and more rarely may have vacuoles in the cytoplasm. Lymphoblasts are typically small, with cell diameters of approximately two erythrocytes, have scant cytoplasm, and are usually without granules. Myeloblasts are larger, with more cytoplasm. The nuclei typically have one or more nucleoli. The bone marrow sample is usually required for definitive diagnosis (peripheral blood can be used if the patient is too ill for a bone marrow aspirate/biopsy). The bone marrow sample is studied for morphology, flow cytometry, cytogenetics, and molecular techniques to further classify the type of leukemia in order to provide the appropriate therapy. Once leukemia is confirmed, additional tests include examination of the cerebrospinal fluid (CSF) for leukemic blasts, a chest radiograph to evaluate for a mediastinal mass, serum chemistries including blood urea nitrogen (BUN), creatinine, electrolytes, calcium, and phosphorus to assess for tumor lysis syndrome, and coagulation studies to rule out a coagulopathy, particularly in AML.

CLASSIFICATION

The acute leukemias of childhood are initially separated into two broad categories, ALL and AML. Morphologic examination of the smear is the traditional diagnostic study, along with special stains such as myeloperoxidase (MPO), and the esterase stains. The definition of acute leukemia is based on the percentage of blasts in the bone marrow being greater than 30% of the nucleated cells. Other criteria can be used in addition if there are less than 30% blasts, which may occur in AML. In the last two decades, immunophenotyping of leukemic blasts by flow cytometry has become standard in the classification. The technique uses specific monoclonal antibodies conjugated with fluorochromes to label various cellular antigens. The antigens were given cluster designation (CD) nomenclature to allow for consistency in analysis and in reporting results (Table 1). The results of flow cytometry help determine the type of leukemia immunologically, differentiating between AML and ALL:

ALL: T-cell origin: CD2, CD5, CD7; pre-B and B-cell origin: CD10, CD19, CD20, CD22
AML: CD13, CD33, CD65

The combined approach of using blast cell morphology and blast cell immunophenotype has facilitated the delivery of specific treatments to children with each of the major subtypes of acute leukemia; it has also augmented the application of risk-directed therapies to patients with subclasses of ALL and AML.

Also very important in the modern-day risk classification is cytogenetics and molecular classification of acute leukemias. Several well-described cytogenetic changes in blast cells are associated with important prognostic implications. For precursor-B ALL, certain translocations are known to predict a better outcome, whereas others would predict a worse outcome. The translocation t(12;21) found by fluorescence in situ hybridization (FISH) and molecular techniques imparts a better prognosis to children whose blasts express this translocation. As well, children whose blasts have trisomies of chromosomes 4, 10, and 17 have a very good prognosis. In contrast, the translocation t(9;22) or Philadelphia translocation imparts a poor prognosis to children whose blasts contain this translocation. Hypodiploidy (fewer than 44 chromosomes) is also associated with a poor prognosis. Another recurring chromosomal finding in ALL are translocations involving chromosome 11q23. Rearrangements in this part of the chromosome disrupt the MLL gene. MLL rearrangements are more often found in infants with ALL and impart a poor prognosis, which has partially been overcome in older children with more aggressive therapy. Recurring chromosomal rearrangements are also found in AML. As with ALL, some of the chromosomal abnormalities help predict outcome. More favorable outcomes are predicted in the presence of t(8;21), inv 16, t(15;17), whereas less favorable outcomes are predicted with monosomy 7, monosomy 5, or deletion of the long arm of chromosome 5, and 11q23 abnormalities. In summary, the classification of childhood acute leukemias is accomplished using morphology, immunophenotypic features, and blast cell cytogenetic and molecular features. The result of this classification impacts both choice of treatment and outcome.

SUPPORTIVE CARE

Improvements in supportive care have vastly contributed to improved outcomes for patients with acute leukemias. Anti-infective drugs developed for bacteria resistant to conventional antibiotics have made significant improvements in the treatment of both gram-positive and gram-negative infections. New antifungal drugs have improved survival from fungal infections in the immunocompromised patient. A new drug designed to reduce uric acid levels has found a place in the management of fulminant tumor

TABLE 1 Immunophenotypes of Major Categories of Acute Leukemia

Phenotype	Antigens Expressed	Frequency
Acute Lymphoblastic Leukemias		
B precursor	CD19, CD20, CD22, CD24, CD10	65%
Pre–B cell	As above plus cytoplasmic Ig	20%
Mature B cell	CD19, CD20, CD21, surface Ig	2%
T cell	CD2, CD5, CD7, CD1, CD4, CD8, CD3	13%
Acute Myelogenous Leukemia		
Myeloid	CD11, CD13, CD15, CD33, CD34, CD65	

lysis syndrome. Improvements in transfusional products provide much needed support while minimizing the transmission of infectious agents.

HYPERLEUKOCYTOSIS

At presentation, children with acute leukemia can have WBC counts greater than 100,000/μL. Hyperleukocytosis occurs in 9% to 13% of children with ALL and 5% to 20% of children with AML. Hyperleukocytosis is associated with a high circulating blast count and with a high viscosity. Clinical manifestations may include neurologic symptoms (headache, confusion, agitation, blurred vision, stupor), dyspnea, and hypoxia. Hyperleukocytosis may cause death by CNS thrombosis and/or hemorrhage, pulmonary insufficiency, and metabolic derangements associated with tumor lysis syndrome. Management of high WBC counts can range from single-agent therapy with corticosteroids to leukophoresis, both aimed at rapidly reducing the WBC count and the number of circulating leukemic blasts. Intensive monitoring, careful hydration, alkalinization, and administration of allopurinol or uric acid oxidase are recommended. Leukophoresis is usually considered when the WBC count is greater than 200,000 and the patients are symptomatic from their leukostasis. It is used more often in the setting of AML. The platelet count should be monitored carefully and platelet transfusions given as needed.

TUMOR LYSIS SYNDROME

The tumor lysis syndrome (TLS) consists of the metabolic triad of hyperuricemia, hyperkalemia, and hyperphosphatemia. Secondary renal failure and symptomatic hypocalcemia can also occur. The syndrome occurs before therapy or 1 to 5 days after the start of specific cytotoxic therapy. It occurs most commonly in Burkitt's (mature B-cell) leukemia/lymphoma and T-cell leukemia. It occurs infrequently in AML. TLS is caused by the release of intracellular uric acid, potassium and phosphate. The uric acid may then precipitate in the renal collecting ducts, resulting in a nephropathy. Hyperkalemia can also result from secondary renal failure. Hydration is the mainstay of therapy for TLS, and patients should receive two to four times the maintenance fluid with alkalinization. Allopurinol (Zyloprim), 10 mg/kg given two to three times per day, maximum dose 600 mg/day, or uric acid oxidase, 2.5 mg/kg intravenously daily for 2 to 5 days, should be given to decrease the uric acid. Hyperkalemia should be treated emergently, if necessary, and supplemental potassium should be avoided. Oral phosphate binders may be necessary. If hyperkalemia and renal failure cannot be controlled, then dialysis should be started; however, it is rare to need dialysis.

INFECTION

Infection remains the primary cause of death in patients with acute leukemia undergoing chemotherapy. The child with leukemia is immunocompromised because of both the underlying leukemia as well as the antileukemic therapy. When patients present with fever (usually defined as temperature higher than 38.3°C [100.9°F] once or higher than 38°C [100.4°F] repeatedly in the past 24 hours) and neutropenia (usually defined as a neutrophil count less than 500/μL), they require a rapid and meticulous physical examination, blood cultures from their central lines (if present), or peripheral blood cultures if no central line present, and they should be promptly started on broad-spectrum antibiotics. Cultures should be obtained from areas with localized signs of infection. Routine chest radiographs should not be done but are indicated when the patient has pulmonary symptoms. Many institutions obtain a urinalysis and culture but do not withhold antibiotics until the sample is obtained. In general, initial evaluation of the febrile neutropenic patient yields a defined source of infection in less than half of the patients. Broad-spectrum antibiotics should be chosen to cover both gram-negative and gram-positive organisms. Broadening coverage with a second gram-negative agent or a better gram-positive agent may be done based on the patient's appearance, history of past infections, or type of chemotherapy recently given. Monotherapy with a third-generation cephalosporin such as Cefepime (Maxipime), 50 mg/kg per dose, maximum dose 2000 mg, or ceftazidime (Fortaz), 50 mg/kg per dose, maximum dose 2000 mg, is the standard of care at many institutions and often used initially in the emergency department or clinic where the patient presents. The febrile neutropenic patient usually is managed as an inpatient with continued antibiotic coverage until the patient is afebrile, cultures are negative, and the absolute neutrophil count (ANC) is rising. Newer strategies are being developed and tested for outpatient management or rapid discharge once cultures are negative and the patient is afebrile. When specific organisms are identified, the therapy should be refined to provide for the most active antibiotics for the identified organism. In the face of continued fevers (usually greater than 5 days) and neutropenia without positive culture results or an identified source of fever, empirical antifungal agents, often amphotericin-B (Amphocin) or the lipid derivatives, are started. Newer antifungal agents are available (azoles that include fluconazole [Diflucan], voriconazole [Vfend], or echinocandins that include caspofungin [Cancidas]) and may be used in this setting. Identification of a fungal infection requires prolonged therapy with an antifungal. Fever during non-neutropenic periods also requires careful management because most patients have poor cell-mediated immunity. Because most pediatric patients have a central line, blood cultures should be obtained and a thorough physical examination performed. The determination of whether antibiotics are started should be based on the appearance of the patient or any concerns identified on exam or in the histroy.

Patients being treated for leukemia have a higher incidence of *Pneumocystis jiroveci* infection. This risk can be effectively reduced by administering trimethoprim-sulfamethoxazole (TMP/SMX). All patients who are not allergic should be placed on TMP/SMX at 5 mg/kg/day in two divided doses for 2 to 3 consecutive days per week. For intolerance to TMP/SMX, other alternatives include inhalation or intravenous pentamidine (Pentam) or dapsone. Prophylactic nystatin (Mycostatin) or fluconazole (Diflucan) is sometimes used during induction for ALL and for AML therapy to prevent or reduce the incidence of candidal infections.

TRANSFUSION THERAPY

Support of the plasma hemoglobin level and the platelet count are essential for successful management of patients with acute leukemia. All transfusions should be irradiated to prevent transfusion-associated graft-versus-host disease and leuko-depleted to decrease the exposure to cytomegalovirus and to prevent sensitization. Packed red blood cell (PRBC) transfusion is usually given when the patient's hemoglobin has fallen to less than 8 g/dL. However, young children may tolerate lower levels of hemoglobin before a PRBC transfusion is necessary. Symptoms of anemia including headache, dizziness, fatigue, and shortness of breath may lead to a lower threshold for transfusion. To prevent bleeding in a patient with thrombocytopenia, platelet transfusions are also given when the platelet count is less than 10,000/μL. When a patient is thrombocytopenic and bleeding, platelets should be administered despite the platelet count.

Treatment

ACUTE LYMPHOBLASTIC LEUKEMIA

The treatment of ALL is typically divided into several phases: induction of remission, consolidation/reintensification of remission, and maintenance of remission. Table 2 presents the schema used by the Children's Oncology Group (COG). With modern therapy, the overall 5-year event-free survival (EFS) is approximately 80% for children with B-precursor high-risk ALL and approximately 85% for children with B-precursor standard-risk ALL, with a distinct subset of low-risk ALL patients with an EFS of approximately 90%. Patients with T-cell ALL have an EFS of 70% to 75%. Infants are treated on a separate protocol and have a worse prognosis overall.

Risk group classification plays a major role in the treatment of B-precursor ALL. Initial risk group is defined by the patient's age and presenting WBC count (Table 3).

TABLE 2 Treatment Approach for Acute Lymphoblastic Leukemia

Risk Group	Induction	Consolidation	Interim Maintenance
Standard risk	VCR, DEXA, ASPARA IT, ARA-C/MTX	CYCLO, ARA-C, TG, MP, VCR, PRED/DEXA, IT MTX	VCR, DEXA, MP, MTX, IT MTX
High risk	VCR, PRED or DEXA, ASPARA, DAUNO, IT ARA-C/MTX	CYCLO, ARA-C, TG, MP, VCR, PRED/DEXA, IT MTX	VCR, PRED/DEXA, MP, MTX, IT MTX or IDMTX
Very high risk	VCR, PRED or DEXA, ASPARA, DAUNO, IT ARA-C/MTX	IFOS[1], ETOP[1], IT MTX, ± ST1571, HDARA-C, HDMTX	(Proceed to HSCT or to reinduction)
T Cell	VCR, PRED, DAUNO, ASPARA, MP, ARA-C, CYCLO, ± 506U78, IT MTX	MP, HDMTX, IT MTX	(Proceed to reinduction)

Risk Group	Reinduction/Reintensification	Maintenance	
Standard risk	VCR, DEXA, ASPARA, DOXO, IT MTX, CYCLO, ARA-C, TG	VCR, DEXA, MP, MTX, IT MTX	
High risk	VCR, DEXA, ASPARA, DOXO, IT MTX, CYCLO, ARA-C, TG	VCR, PRED/DEXA, MP, MTX, IT MTX	
Very high risk	VCR, DEXA, DAUNO, PEG-ASPARA, CYCLO, IT MTX, ±ST1571, HDMTX, ETOP[1], HDARA-C, ASPARA	HDMTX, VCR, DEXA, MP, IT MTX, MTX, ETOP[1], CYCLO, ± ST1571, ± CRXRT	
T cell	VCR, DEXA, DOXO, ASPARA, TG, CYCLO, ARA-C, ± 506U78, IT MTX, CR XRT	VCR, PRED, MP, MTX, ± 506U78	

Risk Group		Induction/Intensification	Reinduction/Reintensification
Infants		VCR, DEXA, DAUNO, CYCLO, ASPARA, ITT, HDMTX, ETOP	VCR, DEXA, DAUNO, CYCLO, ASPARA, ITT, IT ARA-C, VHDMTX, ETOP
	Consolidation	**Intensification/Maintenance**	**Maintenance**
	ARA-C, ASPARA, VHDMTX, VCR, IT ARA-C	VCR, DEXA, MTX, MP, IT ARA-C, ETOP, CYCLO	VCR, PRED, MTX, MP

*Recommendations are based on the following protocols: B-precursor standard risk = Children's Oncology Group (COG) AALL0331; B-precursor high risk = COG AALL0232; B-precursor very high risk = COG AALL0031; infants = CCG 1953; and T cell = COG AALLOOPZ.

Abbreviations: ARA-C = cytosine arabinoside (Cytosar-U); ASPARA = L-asparaginase (Elspart) or PEG (Oncaspar); CRXRT = cranial radiation therapy; CYCLO = cyclophosphamide (Cytoxan); DAUNO = daunorubicin (Cerubidine); DEXA = dexamethasone; DOXO = doxorubicin (Adriamycin); ETOP = etoposide (VePesid)[1]; HDARA-C = high-dose cytosine arabinoside; HDMTX = high-dose methotrexate; HSCT = hematopoietic stem cell therapy; IDMTX = intermediate-dose methotrexate; IFOS = ifosfamide (Ifex)[1]; IT = intrathecal; ITT = triple drug intrathecal (methotrexate, hydrocortisone, cytosine arabinoside); MP = 6-mercaptopurine (Purinethol); MTX = methotrexate; PEG-ASPARA = PEG asparaginase (Oncaspar); PRED = prednisone; ST1571 = imatinib (Gleevec)[1]; TG = 6-thioguanine (Tabloid); VCR = vincristine (Oncovin); VHDMTX = very-high-dose methotrexate.
[1]Not FDA approved for this indication.

CURRENT THERAPY

Acute Lymphoblastic Leukemia

- Induction: 3 or 4 drugs: vincristine (VCR), corticosteroid, PEG asparaginase (PEG), ± anthracycline, intrathecal chemotherapy
- Consolidation: Intrathecal chemotherapy with either mercaptopurine (MP), VCR or cyclophosphamide (CPM), MP, VCR, cytarabine (AraC), PEG
- Interim maintenance: Methotrexate (MTX), VCR, intrathecal chemotherapy, ± corticosteroid, PEG, MP
- Delayed intensification: Corticosteroid, VCR, PEG, anthracycline, CPM, AraC, thioguanine, intrathecal chemotherapy
- Maintenance: Oral MTX, MP, intrathecal chemotherapy, with pulses of VCR, corticosteroids

Acute Myelogenous Leukemia

- Induction I and II: Daunorubicin (DAUN), AraC, etoposide (ETOP), intrathecal AraC
- May go to hematopoietic stem cell transplant or continue with chemotherapy:
  - Intensification I: AraC, ETOP, intrathecal AraC
  - Intensification II: AraC, mitoxantrone, intrathecal AraC
  - Intensification III: High-dose AraC, *Escherichia coli* asparaginase

During induction for the standard risk patient, further risk group classification is refined by the patients' response to therapy and biology of their leukemia. This risk-adapted treatment approach has significantly increased the cure rate among patients with less favorable prognostic features while minimizing treatment-related toxicities in those with favorable features.

During induction therapy, a combination for vincristine (Vincasar), corticosteroid (prednisone or dexamethasone), and asparaginase (Elspar) (PEG-asparaginase or L-asparaginase) with or without an anthracycline (usually daunorubicin [Cerubidine]) are given to induce remission. These drugs are administered over 4 to 6 weeks. Remission is defined by a bone marrow aspirate done at the end of induction with less than 5% leukemic blasts in the setting of normal marrow elements. Approximately 98% of children with ALL reach remission at the end of induction. Patients who do not reach remission receive more intensified therapy with the goal of reaching a marrow remission or could be considered for hematopoietic stem cell transplant (HSCT).

Progress in induction is followed by a bone marrow aspirate on day 8 or day 15 or both. Early marrow response is a prognostic indicator; those patients with a rapid clearing of leukemic blasts from their marrow by day 15 fare better in terms of their EFS. Minimal residual disease (MRD) is now being measured at the end of induction by many groups. Patients with no detectable MRD have an improved EFS; patients with detectable levels of MRD (more than 0.1%) have a worse prognosis and should receive intensified therapy.

Once remission is obtained, consolidation is the second phase of treatment, during which intrathecal chemotherapy along with continued systemic therapy are given to kill lymphoblasts hiding in the meninges. Several months of intensive chemotherapy, often termed interim maintenance and intensification/reinduction therapy, follows consolidation (see Table 2). The intensification phase contributed to improved survival in pediatric ALL patients. Maintenance therapy includes daily oral mercaptopurine (Purinethol), weekly oral methotrexate (Trexall), and, often, monthly pulses of intravenous vincristine and oral prednisone or dexamethasone. Intrathecal chemotherapy is usually given every 2 to 3 months. The duration of treatment ranges between 2.5 years for girls and 3.5 years for boys in COG ALL therapy.

It is necessary to provide preventive treatment to the central nervous system (CNS) for all patients with ALL. Historically, CNS relapses occurred frequently. In current therapy, intrathecal chemotherapy is given throughout therapy to prevent a CNS recurrence. This approach is quite successful with CNS recurrences occurring in less than 5% to 10% of patients. Cranial radiation as

---

TABLE 3 Risk Classification of B-Cell and T-Cell Acute Lymphoblastic Leukemia

NIH Consensus Risk Definitions

Standard	WBC <50,000 cells/mm³ and age 1 to 10 y	
High	WBC ≥50,000 cells/mm³ or age >10 y	

Other Factors Modifying Risk

Factor Risk	Better Risk	Worse
Gender	Female	Male
DNA index	>1.16	≤1.16
Cytogenetics	Hyperdiploid	Hypodiploid
	Trisomies 4, 10, 17	t(9;22)
	T(12;21)	MLL gene (11q23) disruption
CSF status	No blasts	Blasts present
Treatment response*	Rapid	Slow

*Determined by bone marrow status at day 8 or 15 and minimal residual disease (MRD) at day 29.
Abbreviations: CSF = cerebrospinal fluid; MLL = mixed lineage leukemia; WBC = white blood cell count.

prophylaxis to prevent a CNS recurrence is still given to children with higher-risk disease (Ph+ ALL, Tcell ALL) but is now used less commonly than in earlier treatment regimens.

At diagnosis, extramedullary leukemia can be present in the CNS or in the testicles. CNS leukemia present at diagnosis is treated with cranial radiation to a dose of 1800 cGy at approximately 1 year into therapy. Boys with testicular disease at diagnosis in a current study receive additional chemotherapy with high-dose methotrexate in an attempt to delete testicular radiation therapy and spare the hormonal function of the testis.

TREATMENT OF RELAPSE

Relapse can occur as an isolated bone marrow relapse (most common), isolated CNS relapse, isolated testicular relapse, or a combination marrow with an extramedullary site. The duration of the patient's first remission is critical in treatment planning and predicting outcome. Early isolated bone marrow relapses (within 18 to 36 months of diagnosis) have a high risk of treatment failure following salvage therapy. An approach followed by many groups is to reinduce a second remission with intensive chemotherapy and try to identify a suitable stem cell donor for HSCT following reinduction therapy. For a late bone marrow relapse (more than 36 months from diagnosis or more than 6 months from the end of therapy), administration of reinduction, intensification, and maintenance chemotherapies would be a more standard approach.

The approach to isolated extramedullary relapses also depends on the timing of the relapse. An early extramedullary relapse is that which occurs within 18 months of diagnosis. An approach to treatment includes intensive reinduction chemotherapy followed by the possibility of a HSCT with a matched-related donor versus continued chemotherapy with intensification and maintenance if no donor is available. Patients with a CNS relapse also receive craniospinal radiation therapy and triple intrathecal therapy (methotrexate, cytarabine, hydrocortisone) to treat the CNS. Late isolated extramedullary relapses are treated with chemotherapy including reinduction, intensification, and maintenance for a total therapy time of 2 years. Patients with late isolated CNS relapse receive cranial radiation to a dose of 1200 cGy. Recent data have shown that the addition of high-dose methotrexate in addition to reinduction, intensification, and maintenance to a patient with testicular relapse may prevent the need to give testicular irradiation. This approach is the basis for the current COG study.

ACUTE MYELOID LEUKEMIA

Although AML accounts for only 25% of all leukemias in the pediatric/adolescent age group, it is responsible for at least a third of deaths from leukemia. Treatment for AML has evolved over the last several decades and with improvements in supportive care, the ability to provide more intensive therapy has improved the outcome for children with AML. Development of resistance to chemotherapeutic agents and treatment-related mortality continue to be reasons for treatment failure. Although congenital conditions (Diamond-Blackfan anemia, neurofibromatosis, trisomy 21, Wiskott-Aldrich, Kostmann's, and Li-Fraumeni

TABLE 4 Risk Classification of Acute Myelogenous Leukemia (AML)

Morphologic Classification (FAB)

M0	Undifferentiated leukemia
M1	Myeloblastic, no maturation
M2	Myeloblastic, with maturation
M3	Promyelocytic, hypergranular type
M3v	Promyelocytic, microgranular variant
M4	Myelomonocytic
M4Eo	Myelomonocytic, with eosinophilia
M5a	Monocytic
M5b	Monocytic, with differentiation
M6	Erythroleukemia
M7	Megakaryoblastic

Other Factors Modifying Risk

Factor	Better Risk	Worse Risk
White blood count	<100,000 cells/mm^3	>100,000 cells/mm^3
Chromosomes	t(15;17) t(8;21) Inversion 16	Deletion of 5 or 7
Other	Down syndrome	Secondary AML* Previous myelodysplasia

*Secondary leukemia occurs following chemotherapy for a prior malignancy.
Abbreviation: FAB = French-American-British.

syndromes) and acquired risk factors (ionizing radiation, cytotoxic chemotherapeutic agents, and benzenes) are associated with an increased risk of AML, the vast majority of patients have no identifiable risk factors. The improvement in outcome also somewhat relates to the improved ability to define the specific type of AML and other factors that modify risk (Table 4). Overall, the long-term survival of pediatric patients with AML is 45% to 50%.

Current AML protocols rely on the intensive administration of anthracyclines, cytarabine, etoposide,[1] mitoxantrone, and, in some protocols, dexamethasone, 6-thioguanine.[1] As with ALL, induction chemotherapy is administered after the diagnosis is made.

Remissions are successfully induced in approximately 85% of patients. Once remission is induced, therapy is continued to solidify and maintain the remission. Depending on the type of AML and the biologic features of the AML (see Table 4), two approaches are taken for continued therapy: either continued chemotherapy or HSCT. If the patient has a matched sibling donor available, HSCT is often recommended for the patient in clinical remission one (CR1).

The biologic heterogeneity of AML is becoming increasingly important therapeutically. The M3 subtype, associated with t(15;17), is currently treated with all-trans-retinoic acid (ATRA) in addition to chemotherapy with high-dose cytarabine and daunorubicin. The cure of this type of AML is good without HSCT. Another biologically distinct subtype of AML occurs in children with Down syndrome (DS), M7, or megakaryocytic AML.

---

[1]Not FDA approved for this indication.

Using less intensive treatment, remission induction rate and overall survival of these children are dramatically superior to non-DS children with AML.

RELAPSE OF AML

Marrow is the most common site of relapse for AML. Reinduction therapy following marrow relapses typically consists of a combination of high-dose cytosine arabinoside and etoposide, mitoxantrone, and/or L-asparaginase. Newer approaches include the use of an anti-CD33 monoclonal antibody (gemtuzumab ozogamicin) in combination with chemotherapy. Experimental approaches include the use of agents that block the activity of FLT3 and other targeted agents such as farnesyl-transferase inhibitors. Once remission is induced, HSCT is strongly considered, using either a matched related donor, a mismatched related donor (5/6), or a well-matched unrelated donor. The availability of cord blood stem cells allows for a greater degree of HLA disparity in the matching process with less graft-versus-host disease.

LATE EFFECTS

Late effects are an important consideration when treating children with acute leukemias. Leukemia therapy can cause significant long-term sequelae that may not manifest until years after completion of therapy. Almost any organ system can demonstrate sequelae related to previous cancer therapy. This has necessitated the creation of specialized oncology clinics whose function it is to identify and provide treatment to these patients. In addition, a recent report from the Childhood Cancer Survivor Study (CCSS) indicates that primary care physicians provide health care for most of this growing population. Late effects from leukemia therapy can include learning disabilities because of radiation, intrathecal chemotherapy, systemic chemotherapy; cardiomyopathy from anthracyclines; avascular necrosis from corticosteroids; osteoporosis from corticosteroids; growth impairment from radiation therapy; hormonal insufficiency from radiation therapy; obesity; infertility, and second malignancy from chemotherapy and radiation therapy. All of these late effects can depend on the degree of exposure to the causative treatments. As the long-term cure rate rises, one goal of future research and treatment protocols must be to lessen the late effects. Currently this is being addressed with the lower risk group of patients with ALL. Primary care providers may need to advocate for affected children and adults to ensure that they get the needed guidance and assistance in schools and with job placement. Also, it is imperative that pediatric oncologists continue to study survivors and begin to develop strategies to prevent and assist in managing these problems.

REFERENCES

http://www.survivorshipguidelines.org.
http://seer.cancer.gov/csr/1975_2000, 2003.
Alonzo TA, et al: Postremission therapy for children with acute myeloid leukemia: The children's cancer group experience in the transplant era. Leukemia 2005:19(6);965.
Friedman DL, Meadows AT: Late effects of childhood cancer therapy. Pediatr Clin North Am 2002;49:1083.
Neudorf S, Sanders J, Kobrinsky N, et al: Allogeneic bone marrow transplantation for children with acute myelocytic leukemia in first remission demonstrates a role for graft versus leukemia in the maintenance of disease-free survival. Blood 2004;103(10):3655.
Oeffinger KC, Mertens AC, Hudson MM, et al: Health care of young adult survivors of childhood cancer: A report from the childhood cancer survivor study. Ann Fam Med 2004;2:61.
Pearce JM, et al: Childhood leukemia. Pediatr Rev 2005;26(3):96.
Peters C, Schrauder A, Schrappe M, et al: Allogeneic haematopoietic stem cell transplantation in children with acute lymphoblastic leukaemia: The BFM/IBFM/EBMT concepts. Bone Marrow Transplant 2005;35:S9.
Pui CH: Treatment of Acute Leukemias, New Directions for Clinical Research. Totowa, NJ, Humana Press, 2003.
Tallman MS, Gilliland DG, Rowe JM: Drug therapy for acute myeloid leukemia. Blood 2005;106(4):1154.
Zebrack BJ, Zelter LK, Whitton J, et al: Psychological outcomes in long-term survivors of childhood leukemia, Hodgkin's disease, and non-Hodgkin's lymphoma: A report from the Childhood Cancer Survivor Study. Pediatrics 2002;110:42.

Chronic Leukemias

Method of
*Helen Enright, MD, and
Jonathan Bond, MB, MRCPI*

Chronic Lymphocytic Leukemia

Chronic lymphocytic leukemia (CLL) is the most common leukemia in the Western world with an incidence of thirty per million per year. Two thirds of patients are male. The median age at presentation is 65 to 70 years of age.

Nearly 50% of patients are asymptomatic at presentation with the diagnosis made incidentally following a routine blood count. Symptomatic presentation relates to consequences of bone marrow failure, lymphadenopathy and/or hepatosplenomegaly, constitutional symptoms, or autoimmune complications such as hemolytic anemia.

DIAGNOSIS

The presence of peripheral blood lymphocytosis of greater than 5×10^9/L is required for the diagnosis of CLL. The blood film typically shows small mature lymphocytes in addition to fragile cells damaged in the film-spreading process called smudge cells. Immunophenotyping shows a clonal population of mature B lymphocytes that aberrantly express CD5.

Diagnostic evaluation should include direct Coombs test (DCT) (positive in 35%) and serum immunoglobulin estimation.

Bone marrow aspiration and biopsy is important in delineating the extent and pattern of marrow involvement (nodular, diffuse, or interstitial) and to evaluate response to treatment. Cytogenetic analysis may reveal important prognostic information.

Two main staging systems exist (Box 1). These are based on the extent of disease and degree of bone marrow failure.

PROGNOSIS

CLL has an extremely variable clinical course. Ideally, prediction of the likely rate of progression of disease would direct therapeutic intervention.

BOX 1   The Rai and Binet Staging Systems for Chronic Lymphocytic Leukemia (CLL)

Rai System
- 0: No anemia, thrombocytopenia, or physical signs
- I: Lymphadenopathy only
- II: Splenomegaly and/or hepatomegaly but no anemia or thrombocytopenia
- III: Anemia (Hb < 11.0 g/dL)
- IV: Thrombocytopenia (platelet count <100 × 10^9/L)

Binet System
- A: 0 to 2 areas* involved—can be further subdivided into A(0), A(I), and A(II)
- B: 3 to 5 areas involved
- C: Anemia (Hb <10.0 g/dL) or thrombocytopenia (<100 × 10^9/L)

*Each general lymph node region, the liver, and the spleen constitutes an area.
Abbreviation: Hb = hemoglobin.

BOX 2   Indications for Treatment of Chronic Lymphocytic Leukemia (CLL) Suggested by the National Cancer Institute Working Group (1996)

- Progressive bone marrow failure
- Massive (>10 cm) or progressive lymphadenopathy
- Massive (>6 cm) or progressive splenomegaly
- Progressive lymphocytosis (doubling time <6 months or > 50% rise in lymphocyte count within 2 months)
- Systemic symptoms, e.g., debilitating night sweats, fevers, fatigue, weight loss
- Autoimmune cytopenias

The staging systems of Rai and Binet are the longest-standing means of assessing the prognosis of individual patients with CLL. These have inherent limitations, notably to predict if patients presenting with early stage disease would still have rapid clinical progression. Recent studies on prognostic indicators have focused on biological and molecular characteristics of leukemic cells.

Adverse cytogenetic features at diagnosis include trisomy 12 and anomalies affecting the tumor suppressor gene p53 on chromosome 17p, the latter predicting a poor response to chemotherapy.

Gene expression profiling has identified two distinct subgroups of disease based on the presence or absence of somatic mutation in the specific immunoglobulin heavy-chain variable region (IgV$_H$) genes in leukemic cells. Although technically difficult to analyze, this information has important prognostic significance, with a median survival of 25 years in *mutated* cases versus 8 years in *unmutated* cases.

Levels of expression of ZAP-70 (which normally functions as a T cell signaling molecule) by CLL cells have been shown to correlate inversely with IgV$_H$ gene mutation status. This is evaluated by flow cytometry and thus could theoretically be available as a prognostic marker in most routine hematology laboratories.

The prognostic significance of levels of CD38 expression, beta$_2$-microglobulin, lactate dehydrogenase (LDH), thymidine kinase, and soluble CD23 remains under investigation.

INDICATIONS FOR TREATMENT

CLL is a heterogeneous disease with a variable and often indolent course; a proportion of patients never require treatment for their disease. CLL is not curable by conventional treatment approaches, although reports of long-term disease-free survival (DFS) with newer treatment regimens including transplantation have led to some reconsideration of this tenet. The objective of treatment in the majority of cases, however, is disease control and palliation of symptoms.

Indications for treatment were published by the National Cancer Institute (NCI) Working Group in 1996 (Box 2). These include all Binet stages B and C and some stage A patients. Isolated lymphocytosis or hypogammaglobulinemia are not indications for treatment.

Supportive Treatment

Regular intravenous immunoglobulin (400 mg/kg every 3 to 4 weeks) should be considered in hypogammaglobulinemic patients with recurrent infections. The incidence of viral and fungal infections in CLL patients increases with the use of more intensive therapy, especially with purine analogues and alemtuzumab (Campath). Prophylaxis against *Pneumocystis carinii* is indicated in these patients. Autoimmune complications are treated in the same manner as in non-CLL associated cases, that is, usually with steroids—most patients will also require treatment of CLL in this setting. Erythropoietin may be useful in anemic patients.

Initial Treatment

The traditional first-line option for patients requiring treatment was the alkylating agent chlorambucil (Leukeran), which induces partial responses (PR) in 60% to 70% of patients. Treatment of early-stage disease does not confer a survival benefit, and there appears no difference in effect of continuous compared with intermittent dosing in patients needing treatment. There is no demonstrable therapeutic advantage to the addition of prednisone to chlorambucil, whereas combination regimens such as cyclophosphamide, hydroxydaunomycin (doxorubicin), Oncovin (vincristine), and prednisone (CHOP), despite higher overall response rates (ORR), show no relative survival benefit.

More recently, treatment with the purine analogue fludarabine (Fludara) has been shown to result in ORR of 70% to 80% in untreated disease with complete response (CR) rates of 20%, and these results have led to its increased use as a first-line agent. Intravenous treatment is given at a dose of 25 mg/m^2 for 5 days, usually for six courses at four weekly intervals. Treatment with the oral formulation of the drug (40 mg/m^2) yields comparable response rates.

Comparative studies of fludarabine and alkylator-based regimens have consistently shown increased ORR, CR, and duration of response in fludarabine-treated groups.

This has, however, not translated to an increase in overall survival, possibly because of crossover in study designs and high response rates to second-line treatment.

Fludarabine has potent immunosuppressive effects, causing increased susceptibility to serious infections. Defects in lymphocyte function may persist for months and even years after discontinuation of treatment. Transfusion should be with cytomegalovirus (CMV) seronegative and gamma-irradiated blood products. Purine analogues may also trigger autoimmune complications including refractory hemolysis and so are contraindicated in patients with a positive DCT.

Combination treatment with fludarabine with cyclophosphamide (Cytoxan) results in higher CR rates than with fludarabine alone with responses in 40% of cases previously resistant to fludarabine. The combination regimen fludarabine ($25\ mg/m^2$) and cyclophosphamide ($250\ mg/m^2$) (FCR) for 3 days with the anti-CD20 monoclonal antibody rituximab (Rituxan)[1] ($375\ mg/m^2$, day 1 only) has resulted in ORR of more than 90% and CR rates of 70% in previously untreated patients.

Second-Line Treatment

Most patients who initially respond to first-line therapy have subsequent further progression of CLL requiring retreatment. Alkylating agents may be reintroduced, but responses are usually short-lived. Patients relapsing after initial fludarabine treatment are unlikely to respond to single agent alkylator therapy.

Fludarabine produces impressive results in patients previously treated with chlorambucil with ORR of 60% to 70% in patients responsive to alkylators and 20% to 50% in those previously resistant. Retreatment with fludarabine results in approximately 85% ORR in previously sensitive patients.

Combination treatment with cyclophosphamide, vincristine, and prednisone (CVP)[1] gives ORR in 31% of previously treated patients and is commonly used in patients with bulky disease. There is little evidence that anthracycline-based regimens confer therapeutic advantage over fludarabine in patients with relapsed disease. Responses have been seen, however, in fludarabine-resistant cases, and these may be considered in this setting.

The use of alemtuzumab (Campath), a monoclonal anti-CD52 antibody that specifically targets lymphocytes, has given ORR of 33% to 40% when studied in heavily pretreated patients. The achievement of CR in this setting may be associated with long-term DFS in selected patients. Bulky lymphadenopathy is poorly responsive to this treatment. Alemtuzumab is potently immunosuppressive with a high risk of infective complications, notably CMV reactivation (seen in 10%).

Rituximab (Rituxan)[1] as a single agent has yielded disappointing results. Its use in the combination FCR, however, has shown impressive ORR of greater than 70%, with CR rates as high as 25% reported.

Patients with p53 mutations who are resistant to treatment have a particularly poor prognosis. Responses to both alemtuzumab and high-dose methylprednisolone[1] have, however, been demonstrated in this setting.

---

[1]Not FDA approved for this indication.

Stem Cell Transplantation

Peripheral blood stem cell (PBSC) and marrow transplant remain experimental in CLL. PBSC mobilization followed by high-dose therapy and stem cell rescue is feasible, although extensive pretreatment with fludarabine may compromise stem cell mobilization and harvesting.

Allogeneic transplant offers the only current potential for cure of CLL, and long-term DFS is possible, even in poor risk patients, with three-year survival rates of 46% reported, although treatment-related mortality (TRM) of 46% is also seen. The encouraging response rates seen with fludarabine-based regimens with much lower attendant morbidity means myeloablative allogeneic transplant is usually reserved for young patients with poor prognostic features.

Attempts have been made to decrease transplant toxicity while harnessing beneficial graft-versus-leukemia (GVL) effects by using nonmyeloablative conditioning regimens. These regimens have resulted in CR rates of approximately 40% with chronic graft-versus-host disease (GVHD) occurring in 75% of patients and TRM of 15% to 20%.

Richter's Syndrome

Transformation to a high-grade, usually diffuse, large-cell lymphoma occurs in 5% to 10% of CLL. Prognosis is poor with low response rates to therapy and very short survival rates (2 to 8 months).

T Cell Prolymphocytic Leukemia (T-PLL)

Typically follows an aggressive clinical course with survival usually less than 1 year. It is slightly more common in males with a median age at presentation of 65 years of age. Patients usually have hepatosplenomegaly and lymphadenopathy with skin involvement in 20% of cases. There is typically a marked lymphocytosis ($>100 \times 10^9/L$).

Treatment responses are usually disappointing. Chlorambucil, pentostatin (Nipent), or combination regimens such as CHOP are usually ineffective or give a transient short-lived PR. Recent encouraging responses have been seen with alemtuzumab with ORR of 51% to 76%, although infusion-related adverse events and infective complications are common.

T Cell Large Granular Lymphocytic (T-LGL) Leukemia

T-LGL leukemia is characterized by a persistent increase in clonal large granular lymphocytes in the peripheral blood that may infiltrate the bone marrow, liver, and spleen.

The median age at presentation is 50 to 60 years of age with males and females equally affected. The commonest clinical presentations relate to neutropenia and splenomegaly (seen in 50% of cases).

The abnormal lymphocytes usually have a mature T cell immunophenotype—expression of natural killer cell markers (e.g., CD56) is associated with a more aggressive clinical course.

Complications of neutropenia and (more rarely) red cell aplasia are believed to be cytokine-mediated. Immunologic abnormalities are common, including clinical and/or serologic evidence of rheumatoid arthritis in 30% of cases.

T-LGL leukemia usually follows an indolent clinical course, and treatment is not indicated in asymptomatic cases. Recurrent infection because of neutropenia is the commonest indication for intervention. Neutropenia may respond to corticosteroids whereas granulocyte colony-stimulating factor (G-CSF) (Neupogen)[1] may be effective in some cases.

Cyclosporine A (Neoral)[1] (5 to 10 mg/kg/day) and low-dose oral methotrexate (Rheumatrex)[1] (usually 7.5 mg/week) are used. Cyclophosphamide (Cytoxan)[1] (100 mg/day) has shown efficacy in pure red (blood) cell aplasia (PRCA).

Treatment responses in the more aggressive forms of the disease (including combination chemotherapy) have been almost universally disappointing.

Hairy Cell Leukemia

Hairy cell leukemia is characterized by malignant proliferation of mature B lymphocytes with cytoplasmic projections, giving it a characteristic morphologic appearance. Patients usually present with splenomegaly and/or pancytopenia (with monocytopenia characteristic).

Bone marrow aspiration is typically difficult because of increased fibrosis. Tartrate-resistant acid phosphatase (TRAP) stain is usually positive. The bone marrow biopsy shows an interstitial infiltrate of widely spaced lymphoid cells.

Variant cases have distinct morphology and tend to have a poorer response to treatment.

Cladribine (Leustatin) is the treatment of choice, usually given as a continuous infusion over 7 days at 0.1 mg/kg/day. CR rates of 50% to 91% with progression-free survival (PFS) and DFS at 4 years of up to 84% and 96%, respectively, are reported. Alternative dosing schedules have also been used successfully.

Pentostatin (Nipent) produces ORR of 84% with CR of 64% when given at doses of 5 mg/m[2] for 2 days every 2 weeks until maximum response.

Interferon alfa-2a (Roferon-A) (3 million IU/day by subcutaneous injection for 16 to 24 weeks initially) may be considered in cases refractory to purine analogues. Splenectomy may be considered where splenomegaly is the dominant clinical feature and other treatments have failed.

Chronic Myeloid Leukemia

Chronic myeloid leukemia (CML) is characterized by a specific chromosomal translocation resulting in the generation of an aberrant tyrosine kinase, which fuels proliferation of a malignant clone of myeloid cells.

Most patients present in chronic phase with proliferation of well-differentiated myeloid cells. Some present with more advanced disease or in blast crisis, similar to acute leukemia.

CML has an annual incidence of 1 to 2 cases per 100,000 population (accounting for 15% to 20% of all leukemia)

---

[1]Not FDA approved for this indication.

with a slight male preponderance. Typical age of presentation is 40 to 60 years of age.

CLINICAL FEATURES

Up to 20% to 50% of cases are diagnosed incidentally following blood tests performed for other reasons. Symptomatic presentation includes:

- Systemic symptoms such as sweats, fatigue and malaise
- Symptoms referable to splenomegaly, that is, abdominal discomfort or early satiety
- Rarely, may present with acute gout, priapism, or with symptoms of hyperviscosity because of very high leukocyte counts

LABORATORY FEATURES

CML usually presents with neutrophil leukocytosis. There is a "left shift" with increased myelocytes and metamyelocytes in the peripheral blood and bone marrow. The differential diagnosis includes a leukemoid reaction to infection, inflammation, or malignancy. There is typically basophilia and often eosinophilia. The platelet count is normal or elevated and mild anemia is common. Biochemical markers of increased cell turnover, such as LDH and urate, are typically elevated.

Bone marrow aspiration and biopsy show myeloid hyperplasia, but dysplastic features are not prominent.

In chronic phase, the blast count is typically less than 5%. The transition to accelerated and blast phases is defined by increasing blast percentages and other hematologic abnormalities (Box 3).

PROGNOSIS

The median survival of patients in chronic phase is 4 to 6 years. Patients with more advanced disease have much

---

BOX 3	World Health Organization Definitions of Accelerated and Blast Phases of Chronic Myeloid Leukemia (CML)

Accelerated Phase (One or more features is required for diagnosis)

- Blasts 10% to 19% (PB/BM)
- PB basophils > 20%
- Platelet count <100 × 10^9/L (unrelated to therapy)
- Platelet count > 1000 × 10^9/L
- Increasing splenic size
- Increasing WCC (all unresponsive to therapy)
- Cytogenetic evidence of clonal evolution

Blast Phase (One or more features is required for diagnosis)

- Blasts > 20% (PB/BM)
- Extramedullary blast proliferation (i.e., chloromata)
- Large foci or clusters of blasts in bone marrow biopsy

Abbreviations: BM = bone marrow; CML = chronic myeloid leukemia; PB = peripheral blood; WCC = white cell count.

shorter life expectancy with median survival of less than 1 year in accelerated phase and 3 to 6 months in blast phase.

The classic prognostic scoring system for CML is that of Sokal, devised in 1984, which includes patient age, splenic size, peripheral blood blast percentage, and platelet count at diagnosis. Other scoring systems have also been used that consider parameters such as basophil and eosinophil counts. More recently, there is increasing interest in risk assessment based on the achievement of cytogenetic and molecular responses with treatment.

MOLECULAR BIOLOGY

CML is characterized by a chromosomal translocation involving chromosomes 9 and 22, which results in the fusion of the *ABL* oncogene on chromosome 9 with the breakpoint cluster region (BCR) of chromosome 22.

In 90% to 95% of cases, this results from a t(9;22)(q34;q11) translocation resulting in the formation of the Philadelphia chromosome (Figure 1). In rare cases, variant translocations involving other chromosomes or cryptic translocations may occur. These anomalies may be detected by conventional karyotyping of metaphase cells, fluorescence in situ hybridization (FISH), or by polymerase chain reaction (PCR) techniques. Rarely, no translocation is detectable and these patients tend to have more rapid disease progression.

The abnormal *BCR/ABL* fusion gene in CML encodes an abnormal tyrosine kinase that is constitutively activated and phosphorylates proteins in signaling pathways involved in cellular proliferation and apoptosis. The resultant inhibition of apoptosis and abnormal proliferation results in the accumulation of excessive myeloid cells in the bone marrow.

TREATMENT

Nontransplant treatment options in the pre-imatinib era included hydroxyurea, busulphan, and interferon (IFN) with or without cytarabine.

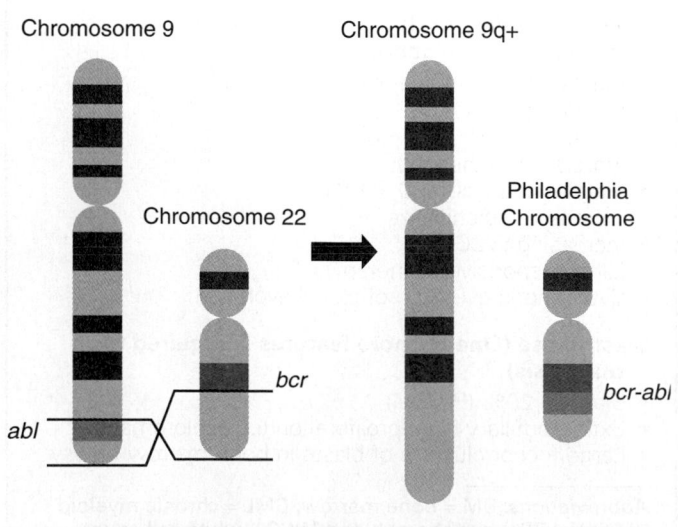

FIGURE 1. The Philadelphia chromosome.

Both hydroxyurea (Hydrea) and busulphan (Busulfex) suppress myeloid hyperplasia with reduction of the leukocyte count, although cytogenetic responses are rare, with no evidence of prolongation of overall survival.

Interferon alfa-2a (Roferon-A) (5 million U/m^2/day by subcutaneous injection) when used as a single agent produces hematologic responses in a majority of patients with complete cytogenetic remission (CCR) in 13% to 27%. IFN has well-recognized flulike adverse effects at time of injection that frequently limit dose escalation.

The combination of interferon plus cytarabine (Cytosar-U) results in increased rates of cytogenetic response compared with single agent IFN (41% versus 24% major cytogenetic response [MCR] at 12 months in one study), with improved overall survival. This combination was considered the standard of care for initial treatment of CML prior to the introduction of imatinib.

Imatinib (Gleevec) selectively inhibits the tyrosine kinase activity of *BCR/ABL* by binding its ATP-binding site, thereby inhibiting protein phosphorylation by the enzyme and blocking downstream signaling.

Following impressive preclinical and early clinical data, the International Research Information Service (IRIS) study was the first to compare the use of imatinib (400 mg/day) with conventional treatment (IFN and cytosine arabinoside [ara-C] in combination) in previously untreated patients in a randomized controlled setting. Imatinib treatment was superior in newly diagnosed chronic phase patients in several areas, notably achievement of cytogenetic responses (with MCR and CCR of 87% and 76% respectively with imatinib versus 35% and 14% in the combination group), whereas achievement of major molecular response (defined as at least a 3-log reduction in *BCR/ABL* by PCR) was seen in 39% of the imatinib group with only 2% in the combination arm achieving this response.

Significant quality of life benefits were also seen, attributable to the relative ease of administration (oral) and reduced incidence of side effects in the imatinib group. A survival benefit was not demonstrated; perhaps because of the crossover design of the study, a majority of patients in the combination group switched to imatinib treatment.

The latest data after 30 months of treatment show a still impressive MCR rate of 90% with a CCR rate of 82%.

Studies of the use of imatinib in accelerated phase disease have shown CCR in 24% of patients whereas activity has also been demonstrated in blast crisis with ORR of 55% to 70% seen. The incidence and severity of side effects seems consistent across treatment groups. These include nausea, ankle edema, skin rash, and cytopenias, all of which are usually mild to moderate in severity.

Fifteen percent to twenty percent of CML patients exhibit primary resistance to imatinib. Secondary resistance following initially successful treatment is seen in approximately 8% to 15% of chronic phase patients after 18 to 24 months.

Resistance is thought to occur by a number of mechanisms, including enhanced tyrosine kinase activity via chromosome or gene amplification, mutations within the ATP-binding site, or the development of new clonal cytogenetic abnormalities.

Ongoing studies include investigation of optimal dosage (400 mg vs. 800 mg) and the role of imatinib in combination with IFN[1] or ara-C.[1]

TREATMENT MONITORING

Response to treatment in CML has traditionally been monitored by full blood count and cytogenetic analysis. Latest data from the IRIS study suggest that CCR is associated with a decreased risk of disease progression. In addition, there is good evidence that achievement of a good molecular response as measured by quantitative PCR may result in improved PFS. Monitoring for ABL kinase domain mutations may be useful in determining likelihood of or emergence of resistance.

A broad consensus currently supports three-monthly monitoring of *BCR/ABL* mRNA levels by quantitative PCR with six-monthly assessment of cytogenetic status. A rising *BCR/ABL* level should trigger search for kinase domain mutations.

Stem cell transplantation currently provides the only proven means of achieving long-term DFS in CML. A suitable donor may not, however, be available, whereas medical co-morbidity or advanced patient age may provide unacceptable mortality risks.

Success of allogeneic transplantation is determined by several factors, notably patient age and stage of disease at time of transplant. Chronic phase patients transplanted within a year of diagnosis have significantly improved survival (70% versus 40%) than those transplanted later in the course of disease. Overall, mortality posttransplant approaches 20% in the first 100 days, mainly because of infection and GVHD.

Donor lymphocyte infusion (DLI), by inducing a GVL effect, can reestablish remission in patients relapsing following transplant, often with molecular remission and prolonged survival in responders. This maneuver may be associated with exacerbation or triggering of GVHD, and optimum dosing and scheduling remains under investigation.

Nonmyeloablative transplantation using less intensive pretransplant preparative regimens aims to harness more beneficial GVL effects with reduced transplant-related

---

[1]Not FDA approved for this indication.

CURRENT DIAGNOSIS

Chronic Myeloid Leukemia
- Neutrophil leukocytosis
- Splenomegaly
- Demonstration of t(9;22) translocation/BCR/ABL by PCR

Chronic Lymphocytic Leukemia
- Lymphocytosis (lymphocytes coexpress CD5 and CD19)
- Lymphadenopathy
- Splenomegaly
- Anemia/thrombocytopenia

Abbreviation: PCR = polymerase chain reaction.

CURRENT THERAPY

- Imatinib is the initial treatment of choice for most patients.
- Other nontransplant approaches include hydroxyurea, busulphan, and interferon (± ara-C).
- Allogeneic transplant should be considered in young patients presenting in chronic phase.
- Autologous and nonmyeloablative transplant remains experimental.

---

morbidity, and, to date, mortality has been studied in relatively small series and is currently regarded as suboptimal treatment in fit patients where a suitable donor is available. It may be used in patients medically unfit for a myeloablative procedure but remains experimental.

Transplantation using matched unrelated donor (MUD) grafts may be considered for young patients who lack a sibling donor. Improvements in transplant outcome are attributable to improved molecular typing of donors, supportive care, and GVHD prophylaxis. Data from the National Marrow Donor Program show DFS for patients younger than 35 years of age comparable to that seen with sibling donors, although rates of GVHD are higher.

The use of autologous transplant remains largely experimental. Data from UK centers show low morbidity and mortality with a suggestion of increased duration of chronic phase and prolonged survival.

TREATMENT OPTIONS IN THE IMATINIB ERA

The advent of imatinib has heralded a major change in treatment approaches to CML. This has been accompanied by increased complexity of therapeutic decisions with several ongoing areas of investigation. It is unknown if prolonged prior treatment with imatinib and consequent delayed transplant will compromise transplant outcome. Although CCR is common with imatinib, most patients do not achieve a molecular remission as measured by current techniques. It is as yet unclear if this has meaningful clinical consequences or if prolonged DFS with molecularly positive disease may prove a valid therapeutic target for many patients.

Most centers institute imatinib in all patients older than 50 years of age and most patients older than 40 years of age. Failure of or resistance to treatment may be considered an impetus to transplant in medically fit patients. The use of nonmyeloablative transplant regimens may expand the eligible patient population. The proven efficacy of transplant in younger patients (especially those younger than 30 years of age) with a suitable donor makes this still the preferred treatment option in these patients. MUD transplantation is also a valid option in this group.

Evaluation of patient wishes and expectations with regard to potential morbidity, mortality, and survival benefits is an integral part of the decision-making process. It is hoped that the evolving data on the use of imatinib and ongoing experience with transplant may aid therapeutic decisions and facilitate consistent management approaches in the years to come.

REFERENCES

Crespo M, Bosch F, Villamar N, et al: ZAP-70 expression as a surrogate for immunoglobulin-variable-region mutations in chronic lymphocytic leukemia. N Engl J Med 2003;348:1764.

Gabor EP, Mishalani S, Lee S: Rapid response to cyclosporine therapy and sustained remission in large granular lymphocyte leukemia. Blood 1996;87:1199.

Gratwohl A, Hermans J, Goldman JM et al: Risk assessment for patients with chronic myeloid leukaemia before allogeneic blood or marrow transplantation. Chronic Leukaemia Working Party of the European Group for Blood and Marrow Transplantation. Lancet 1998;352:1087.

Jaffe ES, Harris NL, Stein H, et al (eds): World Health Organization Classification of Tumours. Pathology and Genetics of Tumours of Haemopoietic and Lymphoid Tissues. Lyon, IARC Press, 2001.

Jehn U, Bortl R, Dietzfelbinger H, et al: An update: 12-year follow-up of patients with hairy cell leukemia following treatment with 2-chlorodeoxyadenosine. Leukemia 2004;18(9):1476.

Keating MJ, O'Brien S, Lerner S, et al: Long-term follow-up of patients with chronic lymphocytic leukemia (CLL) receiving fludarabine regimens as initial therapy. Blood 1998;92:1165.

Kurzrock R, Kantarjian HM, Druker BJ, et al: Philadelphia chromosome-positive leukemias: From basic mechanisms to molecular therapeutics. Ann Intern Med 2003;138:319.

O'Brien SG, Guilhot F, Larson RA, et al: Imatinib compared with interferon and low-dose cytarabine for newly-diagnosed chronic-phase chronic myeloid leukemia. N Engl J Med 2003;348:994.

Paneesha S, Milligan DW: Stem cell transplantation for chronic lymphocytic leukemia. Br J Haematol 2005;128(2):145.

Non-Hodgkin's Lymphoma

Method of
Lawrence Rice, MD, and Uday Popat, MD

Rather than representing a single disease, non-Hodgkin's lymphomas (NHLs) comprise a diverse spectrum of disorders, varying from the most rapidly growing cancer known to the most indolent of neoplasms having no impact on well-being and requiring no treatment. Together these clonal lymphocyte proliferations comprise 5% of all cancers, ranking fifth in incidence, yet their importance is far greater than their frequency. Reasons for this include that lymphomas have critically accelerated scientific understanding of neoplasia, displaying the roles of oncogenic viruses, specific genetic alterations, and the interplay of tumor with host immune factors. Lymphomas are the most common cancers in adolescents and young adults. Regarding therapy, breakthroughs in lymphomas are being applied to curing cancers more generally. The efficacy of the earliest chemotherapy drugs were established in lymphomas; the principles of combination chemotherapy and of curative radiotherapy were gleaned.

Epidemiology and Genetics

Indolent NHLs are disorders of older individuals (rare younger than age 40 years). Although large B-cell lymphomas are also most common after age 65 years, the incidence curve is much flatter such that they also represent the most common cancer in adolescents and young adults. Other lymphomas have distinctive epidemiologic patterns, such as T-cell lymphoblastic lymphoma occurring mainly in adolescent and young adult men and primary mediastinal large B-cell lymphoma in young women. Burkitt's lymphoma presents as jaw tumors in children in third-world countries related to Epstein-Barr virus (EBV) infection, but presents as abdominal masses or leukemia in young adults in developed Western countries. Hepatitis C increases the risk for several lymphomas, particularly primary splenic marginal zone B-cell lymphoma. Many lymphomas increase with HIV infection, but Burkitt's lymphoma and large B-cell lymphomas with CNS primaries are particularly common. Mucosa-associated lymphoid tissue lymphoma (MALToma) of the stomach is associated with *Helicobacter pylori*.

Lymphomas often display distinctive acquired cytogenetic abnormalities. The abnormal gene products provide clues to pathogenesis and targets for therapy. Examples include Burkitt's lymphoma where translocations involve the c-myc oncogene on chromosome 8 and immunoglobulin heavy- or light-chain genes. Follicular lymphomas have a characteristic t(14;18) affecting BCL-2 gene regulation of cellular apoptosis. In many lymphomas cytogenetic patterns provide prognostic information (e.g., small lymphocytic lymphoma) or can help establish the proper diagnosis, such as (11;14) with cyclin D overexpression in mantle cell lymphoma.

Classification of Lymphomas and Leukemias

Differentiating lymphomas from lymphoid leukemias is arbitrary and semantic, based on whether a clonal neoplasm presents mainly in lymph nodes and tissues versus prominent peripheral blood involvement. Thus, B-cell chronic lymphocytic leukemia and small lymphocytic lymphoma represent different clinical presentations of the same malignant disorder; disease behavior and treatment principles are identical. Similarly, B-cell (L3 type) acute lymphoblastic leukemia and Burkitt's lymphoma are the same disorder, as are T-cell acute lymphoblastic leukemia and lymphoblastic lymphoma.

A major advance in understanding and managing NHLs emerged 40 years ago with the Rappaport classification system. Morphologic parameters such as whether malignant cells were large or small and whether they showed a nodular (follicular) growth pattern separated disorders into clinically useful categories predicting disease behavior and responsiveness to therapies. Proliferating alternative classification schemes since have daunted students and clinicians, becoming an object for satires. Nevertheless, modern classification goes beyond morphology, bringing to bear advances in molecular biology, flow cytometry, and cytogenetics to establish homogeneous disease entities that behave more predictably. Optimizing a patient's treatment requires familiarity with up-to-date classification (Table 1).

Evaluation, Staging, and Prognosis

A thorough history specifically addresses whether the *B symptoms* of fevers, night sweats, and weight loss

TABLE 1 Proposed World Health Organization Classification Scheme for Non-Hodgkin's Lymphoma

B-Cell Neoplasms

Precursor B-cell neoplasm
Precursor B-lymphoblastic leukemia/lymphoma

Mature B-cell neoplasms
B-cell chronic lymphocytic leukemia/small lymphocytic lymphoma
B-cell prolymphocytic leukemia
Lymphoplasmacytic lymphoma
Splenic marginal zone B-cell lymphoma (± villous lymphocytes)
Hairy cell leukemia
Plasma cell myeloma/plasmacytoma
Extranodal marginal zone B-cell lymphoma of the MALT type
Nodal marginal zone B-cell lymphoma (± monocytoid B cells)
Follicular lymphoma
Mantle cell lymphoma
Diffuse large-B-cell lymphoma
    Mediastinal large-B-cell lymphoma
    Primary effusion lymphoma
Burkitt lymphoma

T-Cell and NK Cell Neoplasms

Precursor T-cell neoplasm
Precursor T-lymphoblastic lymphoma/leukemia

Mature T-cell neoplasms
T-cell prolymphocytic leukemia
T-cell granular lymphocytic leukemia
Aggressive NK cell leukemia
Adult T-cell lymphoma/leukemia (HTLV-1-positive)
Extranodal NK/T-cell lymphoma, nasal type
Enteropathy-type T-cell lymphoma
Hepatosplenic γδ T-cell lymphoma
Subcutaneous panniculitis-like T-cell lymphoma
Mycosis fungoides/Sézary syndrome
Anaplastic large-cell lymphoma, T/null cell, primary cutaneous type
Anaplastic large-cell lymphoma, T/null cell, primary systemic type
Peripheral T-cell lymphoma, not otherwise characterized
Angioimmunoblastic T-cell lymphoma

Abbreviations: HTLV-1 = human T-cell leukemia virus 1; MALT = mucosa-associated lymphoid tissue; NK = natural killer.

CURRENT DIAGNOSIS

- Precise histologic diagnosis is mandatory.
- Currently, this requires assessment of cell surface markers (e.g., by flow cytometry) and increasingly of cytogenetic and molecular markers.
- Clinical staging requires history of systemic symptoms (weight loss, fever, sweats) and careful palpation of lymph node areas, spleen, and liver.
- Evaluation requires CBC, hepatic and renal function and LD.
- Routine staging is completed by CT scans of nodal areas and bone marrow biopsy.
- Other modalities (lumbar puncture; PET scan) are for select cases or investigational.
- An international prognostic index (age, stage, number of extranodal sites, performance status, serum LD) is clinically useful.

Abbreviations: CBC = complete blood count; CT = computed tomography; LD = lactate dehydrogenase; PET = positron emission tomography.

spread such as to bone marrow, liver or pleura. *A* follows the stage if *B* symptoms are absent.

The most important factors guiding treatment and prognosis are histology and stage. Age and co-morbidities must be considered. An international prognostic index developed for large-cell lymphomas can, with some modification, also be applied to other lymphomas. Scores are generated from five parameters:

1. Age
2. Stage
3. Number of extranodal sites
4. Performance status
5. Serum LD

Another modality applicable to prognostic stratification with diffuse large-cell lymphoma is microarray gene expression profiling, able to separate good risk "germinal center like large-cell lymphoma" from poor risk "activated B-cell lymphoma."

Treatment of Some Specific Disease Entities

INDOLENT LYMPHOMAS

The common indolent lymphomas are small lymphocytic lymphoma and grade 1 follicular lymphoma, representing more than one third of NHLs. The great majority (85% to 90%) present with stage III or IV disease; in fact 90% to 100% of small lymphocytic lymphomas and 40% to 90% of follicular lymphomas have bone marrow involvement, marking them stage IV. Patients with apparent localized presentations are candidates for radiotherapy with curative intent (recognizing that two thirds will eventually relapse). Adjuvant chemotherapy is under study for such patients.

Stage III and IV patients cannot be cured with standard therapies, yet median survival for asymptomatic subgroups exceeds 10 years. So, a *watch and wait* approach with no initial therapy is appropriate for most patients, given that the disease is often asymptomatic, indolent in behavior, incurable, and associated with prolonged survival. (One cannot

are present. Physical exam pays extra attention to palpating lymph nodes and abdominal viscera. All patients require a complete blood count (CBC) with differential, blood chemistries including tests of renal function, hepatic function, calcium and lactate dehydrogenase (LD), and chest radiograph. Essential staging procedures are computed tomography (CT) scans (chest, abdomen, pelvis) and bone marrow. Bone marrow biopsy must be obtained but bilateral biopsies are not routinely indicated. Nonroutine tests for certain patients and certain disease subtypes include lumbar puncture and gallium scanning. Positron emission tomography appears promising, and its role is being investigated. The Ann Arbor staging system remains standard: Stage I is involvement of one lymph node region (or IE single extranodal site); stage II, multiple lymph node regions on the same side of the diaphragm; stage III, lymph nodes on both sides of the diaphragm; and stage IV, extralymphatic deliver palliative therapy to individuals who are asymptomatic.) Initially untreated patients average 4 years or more before disease progression mandates treatment, with no decrement in survival attributable to treatment delay. Twenty percent of patients with follicular lymphoma, and a greater number with small lymphocytic lymphoma may never require treatment even after more than 10 years of follow-up.

Factors that mandate treatment at presentation or during follow-up are mainly related to emerging cytopenias (e.g., significant anemia) or systemic symptoms. Young age and psychoemotional factors can be reasons for early therapy, but most patients readily accept no initial treatment when the rationale is fully explained. A major problem impacting survival is transformation to more histologically aggressive lymphomas (Richter-like syndrome); this may occur at 5% per year regardless of treatment.

When treatment is warranted, additions to our armamentarium have increased choices, making decisions less clear-cut. Single oral alkylating agents such as cyclophosphamide (Cytoxan) and chlorambucil (Leukeran) were mainstays and remain reasonable choices for many. Response rates are approximately 50%, few complete, but clinical problems may be dramatically reversed for years. These agents are inexpensive, convenient, and most patients experience no side-effects. Potential toxicities are myelosuppression, leukemogenesis emerging after few years (in approximately 1%), and bladder toxicity with cyclophosphamide. Cyclophosphamide (often intravenous) is the backbone of the traditional CVP regimen, with vincristine (Oncovin) and prednisone. Adding doxorubicin (Adriamycin)—the CHOP (cyclophosphamide, hydroxydaunomycin [doxorubicin], Oncovin [vincristine], and prednisone) regimen—adds toxicity without survival benefit in indolent lymphomas. Nucleoside analogues, particularly fludarabine, are active in these disorders. Response rates may exceed those of alkylating agents at the costs of toxicities and inconvenience (several days monthly of intravenous therapy). Beyond myelosuppression, long-lasting immunosuppression creates significant risks for serious opportunistic infection. Newer combinations such as FC (fludarabine, cyclophosphamide) and FND (fludarabine, mitoxantrone [Novantrone], dexamethasone) reduce the fludarabine dose, reducing toxicities. Spectacular remission rates have been observed with these regimens, making them attractive choices both for initial and salvage therapy.

The promise of monoclonal antibody therapy is realized in these disorders. Rituximab (Rituxan), an anti-CD20 monoclonal antibody, can be administered singly or in combination with any chemotherapy regimen, either initially or for salvage. It has rapidly become the world's largest selling antineoplastic agent, even though the only cancers for which it is used are B-cell lymphoproliferative disorders. It is remarkably nontoxic, with fever, chills, and manageable hypotension occurring mainly during the first infusion; infectious risks are low. Understandably, regimens such as FC-R and FND-R are becoming popular. Molecular remissions emerge with these regimens, fueling hopes that curative goals may become realistic. Other monoclonal antibodies for indolent lymphomas are more toxic and used for salvage therapy. These include anti-CD52 alemtuzumab (Campath) for small lymphocytic lymphoma, associated with high opportunistic infection risks, and anti-CD20 antibodies conjugated to radioisotopes. Recurrent or refractory disease is treated with approaches

discussed earlier, but rate and duration of response shortens with each subsequent relapse. To re-emphasize, observation without treatment is reasonable for asymptomatic relapse; more harm has resulted from overly aggressive treatment than the reverse. Patients transforming to large-cell lymphoma have a worse prognosis than de novo large-cell lymphoma, but some respond to combination chemotherapy with or without stem cell transplants. Transplants, both autologous and allogeneic, have benefited selected patients, but utility is limited by the age of patients, the anticipation of long survival, and the frequency of bone marrow involvement, which could contaminate autografts. Grade 1 and 2 follicular lymphomas are considered indolent, but grade 3 (follicular large cell) should be treated as diffuse large-cell lymphoma (in the following text), because it progresses more rapidly and because long-lasting remissions can be achieved.

DIFFUSE LARGE B-CELL LYMPHOMA

This most common lymphoma subtype comprises another one third of cases. Unlike indolent lymphomas, these are clinically aggressive with survival of few months untreated. Alkylating agents or monoclonal antibodies used alone are ineffective. Contrasting with indolent lymphomas, there is a reasonable possibility of cure with appropriate chemotherapy. Localized presentations (Stage I or II) occur in less than 30% of large-cell cases. Nonbulky localized disease is treated with three cycles of CHOP or CHOP-R (cyclophosphamide, hydroxydaunomycin [doxorubicin], Oncovin [vincristine], prednisone, and rituximab) followed by involved-field radiotherapy. A good majority of such patients are cured, as demonstrated in a randomized trial showing progression-free survival of 76% with chemoradiation compared to 67% with eight cycles of CHOP. Patients with stage III or IV disease are given six to eight cycles of CHOP or CHOP-R. Complete response to CHOP will occur in two thirds, and one third will be cured. More intensive regimens like MACOP-B (methotrexate, doxorubicin, cyclophosphamide, Oncovin, prednisone, and bleomycin), ProMACE-CytaBOM (prednisone, methotrexate [with leucovorin rescue], Adriamycin, cyclophosphamide, etoposide, cytarabine, bleomycin, Oncovin, dexamethasone), or m-BACOD (methotrexate, bleomycin, Adriamycin, cyclophosphamide, Oncovin dexamethasone) are more toxic, more difficult to administer, and no more efficacious than CHOP. The addition of rituximab improves the progression-free survival to 54% compared with 30% in patients receiving CHOP without rituximab. Hence, CHOP-R is the standard of care in patients with advanced CD20 positive diffuse large B-cell lymphomas. A baseline echocardiogram is performed because of the potential cardiotoxicity of doxorubicin. Restaging procedures are usually done after four treatment courses. Two additional courses are delivered after remission is confirmed. Prophylactic intrathecal chemotherapy should be strongly considered with involvement of the testis, ovary, breast, sinuses, bone marrow, more than one extranodal site, or a high LD. Recurrent or refractory disease carries a poor prognosis. Cure is still reasonably possible in candidates for autologous stem cell transplantation (those relatively young without serious co-morbidities). It is crucial that they have *chemotherapy-sensitive* relapse; that is, the disease is not progressing during therapy. Common salvage regimens include ICE (ifosfamide, carboplatin, etoposide),

ESHAP (etoposide, Solu-Medrol, high-dose ara-C, Platinol), and DHAP (dexamethasone, high-dose ara-C, Platinol), using ifosfamide, platinums, etoposide, cytosine arabinoside, and corticosteroids. Two thirds of patients respond, but longer outlook remains bleak unless stem cell transplant ensues (event-free survival improved from 12% to 46% in a randomized study). Patients refractory to salvage therapy may be candidates for investigational agents, allogeneic transplantation or palliative care.

Peripheral T-cell lymphoma and anaplastic large-cell lymphoma are treated similarly to diffuse large B-cell lymphoma.

LYMPHOBLASTIC AND BURKITT'S LYMPHOMAS

These represent variant presentations of T-cell and B-cell acute lymphoblastic leukemia, respectively, and they are treated with acute lymphoblastic leukemia (ALL) protocols, which employ vincristine, anthracyclines, cyclophosphamide, cytosine arabinoside, and methotrexate (e.g., Hyper-CVAD [cyclophosphamide, vincristine, Adriamycin, dexamethasone, methotrexate, cytarabine]). Prophylactic CNS therapy is mandatory. Care must be taken to avoid the tumor lysis syndrome (especially with Burkitt's lymphoma) by vigorous hydration, alkalinization of urine, allopurinol, and close monitoring. Approximately one third of patients with these disorders can be cured by chemotherapy (higher in some patient subsets).

LYMPHOMAS RELATED TO INFECTIOUS AGENTS

HIV predisposes to many lymphomas but particularly to Burkitt's lymphoma and primary CNS large-cell lymphoma. The addition of antiretroviral therapy to chemotherapy improves results. Hepatitis C also predisposes to several lymphomas, particularly primary splenic marginal zone lymphoma. Interferon therapy is highly efficacious for this lymphoma when associated with hepatitis C. (The toxicities of interferon relative to any benefit mitigate against its use in other lymphomas.) With MALToma of the stomach related to *Helicobacter pylori* infection, eradication of the organism with antibiotics results in *spontaneous* regression of the neoplasm in patients with superficial, node-negative, low-grade disease; but others often require chemotherapy or radiotherapy.

LYMPHOMAS RELATED TO IMMUNE SUPPRESSION OR DEFICIENCY

It has been known for decades that lymphomas complicate primary immunodeficiency disorders. Lymphomas with AIDS are addressed above. Post-transplant lymphoproliferative disorder is usually (but not always) a monoclonal proliferation of B-cells expressing large amounts of EBV DNA. Incidence varies from 1% in renal transplant recipients to 2% to 5% in more heavily immunosuppressed organ transplant recipients. The main therapeutic maneuver is to stop or substantially decrease immunosuppressive therapies. This leads to lymphoma resolution in half. Rituximab may be added, but antivirals have not proven beneficial. The prognosis is poor for patients who progress despite these actions, but some respond well to combination chemotherapy. Immunosuppressive drugs

CURRENT THERAPY

- Low-grade (indolent) lymphomas are usually advanced (stage III or IV) and asymptomatic—these can be followed without therapy (*watch and wait*).
- Most common indications for therapy of low-grade lymphomas are emergence of systemic systems, progressive cytopenias, or histologic transformation.
- Most effective therapies for low-grade lymphomas are alkylating agents (cyclophosphamide), nucleoside analogues (fludarabine), monoclonal antibodies (rituximab), or combinations of these.
- Corticosteroids, anthracyclines and analogues, and alkaloids are also effective.
- Large B-cell lymphomas (intermediate to high grade) require moderately aggressive chemotherapy and are potentially curable.
- The regimen of choice for large B-cell lymphomas is CHOP-R.
- High-grade lymphomas (lymphoblastic, Burkitt's) are tissue variants of acute lymphoid leukemias and should be treated with ALL-type regimens.

Abbreviations: ALL = acute lymphoblastic leukemia; CHOP-R = cyclophosphamide, hydroxydaunomycin (doxorubicin), Oncovin (vincristine), prednisone, and rituximab.

also relate to lymphomas apart from transplantation. Withdrawal of methotrexate from rheumatoid arthritis patients can produce *spontaneous* lymphoma regression.

Other Treatment Modalities

SURGICAL THERAPY

This has been advocated for isolated extranodal lymphomas, such as stomach or bowel, but its role should be relegated to obtaining biopsy material for diagnosis. Even here, it may be supplanted by needle biopsy with ancillary flow cytometry, histochemistry, and cytogenetics, sometimes allowing definitive diagnosis. (Nonsurgical therapies of gastrointestinal lymphomas do entail a small risk of bowel perforation.)

STEM CELL (BONE MARROW) TRANSPLANT

Autologous stem cell transplants, now usually collected from peripheral blood by cytapheresis, have been favored for lymphomas. This is the preferred therapy (after cytoreduction) for patients with *chemotherapy-sensitive* relapse where cure remains the goal. *Up-front* use as a form of consolidation intensification for high-risk patients is under investigation. Continuing investigations address the necessity for and means to accomplish purging of tumor cells from autografts. Allogeneic transplants, seeking the advantage of *graft versus tumor* effects, afford a chance of cure for selected patients but with increased risks of toxicity. Toxicities are being reduced by less intensive conditioning regimens.

FUTURE THERAPIES

Tumor vaccines are in clinical trials and new monoclonal antibodies loom. Molecular advances bring forth agents such as BCL-2 antisense oligonucleotides, currently in clinical trials.

REFERENCES

A predictive model for aggressive non-Hodgkin's lymphoma. The international Non-Hodgkin's Lymphoma Prognostic Factors Project. N Engl J Med 1993;329:987-994.

Ardeshna KM, Smith P, Norton A, et al: Long-term effect of a watch and wait policy versus immediate systemic treatment for asymptomatic advanced-stage non-Hodgkin lymphoma: A randomised controlled trial. Lancet 2003;362:516-522.

Coiffier B, Lepage E, Briere J, et al: CHOP chemotherapy plus rituximab compared with CHOP alone in elderly patients with diffuse large-B-cell lymphoma. N Engl J Med 2002;346:235-242.

Fisher R, Gaynor E, Dahlberg S, et al: Comparison of a standard regimen (CHOP) with three intensive chemotherapy regimens for advanced non-Hodgkin's lymphoma. N Engl J Med 1993;328:1002-1006.

Horning SJ, Rosenberg SA: The natural history of initially untreated low-grade non- Hodgkin's lymphoma. N Engl J Med 1984;311:1471-1475.

MacManus M, Hoppe RT: Is radiotherapy curative for stage I and II low-grade follicular lymphoma? Results of a long-term follow-up study of patients treated at Stanford University. J Clin Oncol 1996;14:1282-1290.

Marcus R, Imrie K, Belch A, et al: CVP chemotherapy plus rituximab compared with CVP as first-line treatment for advanced follicular lymphoma. Blood 2005;105:1417-1423.

Miller T, Dahlberg S, Cassady J, et al: Chemotherapy alone compared with chemotherapy plus radiotherapy for localized intermediate- and high-grade non-Hodgkin's lymphoma. N Engl J Med 1998;339:21-26.

Philip T, Guglielmi C, Hagenbeek A, et al: Autologous bone marrow transplantation as compared with salvage chemotherapy in relapses of chemotherapy-sensitive non-Hodgkin's lymphoma. N Engl J Med 1995;333:1540-1545.

Multiple Myeloma

Method of
Robert A. Kyle, MD, and
S. Vincent Rajkumar, MD

Multiple myeloma is characterized by the neoplastic proliferation of a single clone of plasma cells producing a monoclonal (M) protein in the serum or urine. In the United States, multiple myeloma constitutes 1% of all malignant diseases and slightly more than 10% of hematologic malignancies. The annual incidence is 4 per 100,000; the incidence in African Americans is twice that in whites. The apparent increase in rates is probably caused by increased availability and use of medical facilities and improved diagnostic techniques, particularly in the older population. The median age at diagnosis is 65 to 70 years, and only 2% of patients are younger than 40 years.

Weakness, fatigue, bone pain, recurrent infections, and symptoms of hypercalcemia or renal insufficiency should alert the physician to the possibility of multiple myeloma. Anemia is present in 70% of patients at the time of diagnosis. An M protein is found in the serum or urine in 97% of patients with multiple myeloma. Lytic lesions, osteoporosis, or fractures are present at diagnosis in 80%. Technetium bone scanning is inferior to conventional radiography and should not be used. Magnetic resonance imaging (MRI) or computed tomography (CT) is helpful in patients who have skeletal pain but no abnormality on radiographs or when spinal cord compression is suspected. Hypercalcemia is present in 25% of patients, and the serum creatinine value is 2 mg/dL or greater in almost 20% of patients at diagnosis.

CURRENT DIAGNOSIS

- Complete history and physical examination
  - Determination of values for hemoglobin, leukocytes with differential count, platelets, serum creatinine, calcium, and uric acid
  - Radiographic survey of bones, including humeri and femurs
  - Serum protein electrophoresis with immunofixation
  - Quantitation of immunoglobulins
  - Bone marrow aspirate and biopsy
  - Routine urinalysis
  - Electrophoresis and immunofixation of an adequately concentrated aliquot from a 24-hour urine specimen
- Measurement of β_2-microglobulin, C-reactive protein, lactate dehydrogenase values
- If available, cytogenetics, FISH, and plasma cell labeling index

Abbreviation: FISH = fluorescence in situ hybridization.

Diagnosis

If multiple myeloma is suspected, the patient should have, in addition to a complete history and physical examination:

- Determination of values for hemoglobin, leukocytes with differential count, platelets, serum creatinine, calcium, and uric acid
- A radiographic survey of bones, including humeri and femurs
- Serum protein electrophoresis with immunofixation
- Quantitation of immunoglobulins
- Bone marrow aspirate and biopsy
- Routine urinalysis
- Electrophoresis and immunofixation of an adequately concentrated aliquot from a 24-hour urine specimen

Measurement of β_2-microglobulin, C-reactive protein, and lactate dehydrogenase values is helpful for prognosis. Cytogenetics and measurement of the plasma cell labeling index are also important from a prognostic standpoint.

Box 1 lists the criteria for diagnosis of myeloma. Metastatic carcinoma, lymphoma, leukemia, and connective tissue disorders may resemble multiple myeloma and must be considered in the differential diagnosis. Patients with multiple myeloma must be differentiated from those with monoclonal gammopathy of undetermined significance (benign monoclonal gammopathy) and smoldering (asymptomatic) multiple myeloma because they may remain stable for long periods (Box 1). The plasma cell labeling index is helpful in differentiating monoclonal gammopathy of undetermined significance or smoldering multiple myeloma from multiple myeloma. The patient's symptoms, physical findings, and all laboratory and radiographic data must be considered in the decision to begin therapy. If there are doubts about whether to begin treatment, therapy should be withheld and the patient reevaluated in 2 to 3 months. No evidence indicates that early treatment of multiple myeloma is advantageous.

Treatment

If the patient is eligible for an autologous peripheral blood stem cell transplant, the hematopoietic stem cells should be collected before the patient is exposed to chemotherapy. Patients who are ineligible for stem cell transplantation should be treated with standard alkylating agent therapy (discussed later).

AUTOLOGOUS PERIPHERAL BLOOD STEM CELL TRANSPLANTATION

If a patient is eligible, the physician should seriously consider autologous peripheral blood stem cell transplantation. Some patients older than 70 years are physiologically younger, whereas some patients younger than 70 years may have medical problems such as heart disease, pulmonary insufficiency, or renal failure and are not suitable candidates for an autologous stem cell transplant. The patient should first be treated with an induction chemotherapy regimen that is nontoxic to the hematopoietic stem cells. Most physicians treat with the oral regimen of thalidomide (Thalomid),[1] 200 mg/day, plus dexamethasone (Decadron),[1] 40 mg/day on days 1 to 4, 9 to 12, and 17 to 20 every 28 days.

The oral regimen of thalidomide plus dexamethasone produces response rates similar to intravenous (IV) regimens such as VAD (vincristine, Adriamycin [doxorubicin], dexamethasone). Venous thrombosis, sedation, constipation, and rash constitute the most frequent side effects of thalidomide (Thalomid).[1] Patients should be anticoagulated with low molecular weight heparin or warfarin in therapeutic doses. Aspirin may reduce the risk of thromboembolic complications and is an alternative in patients unable or unwilling to take anticoagulation. Another option is the use of oral dexamethasone (Decadron)[1] as a single agent. A randomized trial comparing dexamethasone (Decadron)[1] alone to thalidomide (Thalomid)[1] plus dexamethasone (Decadron)[1] revealed a superior response rate for thalidomide (Thalomid)[1] plus dexamethasone (Decadron)[1] (63% vs. 41%) but a higher incidence of deep venous thrombosis. Although induction chemotherapy is important,

[1]Not FDA approved for this indication.

CURRENT THERAPY

Newly Diagnosed Symptomatic Myeloma

- Eligible for stem cell transplant
  - Thalidomide[1] plus dexamethasone[1]
  - Dexamethasone[1]
  - Novel agents (e.g., lenalidomide [Revlimid] plus dexamethasone, bortezomib plus dexamethasone)
- Ineligible for stem cell transplant
  - Melphalan (Alkeran) and prednisone[1]
  - Melphalan, prednisone and thalidomide (MPT)
  - Combinations of alkylating agents
  - Novel agents

Refractory or Relapsed Myeloma

- Thalidomide[1] plus dexamethasone[1]
- Dexamethasone[1]
- VAD[1]
- Bortezomib (Velcade)
- Combinations of alkylating agents
- Novel agents (e.g., lenalidomide)

[1]Not FDA approved for this indication.
Abbreviations: VAD = vincristine[1] plus doxorubicin[1] (Adriamycin)[1] plus dexamethasone.

we proceed with stem cell transplantation even if the patient has not responded to such treatment. Bortezomib (PS-341, Velcade) and lenalidomide (CC-5013, Revlimid) are currently being tested in clinical trials as initial therapy.

Most physicians use granulocyte colony-stimulating factor (G-CSF)[1] for stem cell collection. After stem cell collection, autologous stem cell transplantation can proceed as soon as the patient has recovered, or the transplantation can be delayed and the patient treated with standard alkylating agent therapy, the transplantation being reserved for relapsed disease. There is no difference in overall survival among patients who receive an autologous stem cell transplant immediately after collection and those who receive it at first relapse. We recommend autologous stem cell transplantation as soon as the patient has recovered from the stem cell collection because the patient is saved the inconvenience of prolonged chemotherapy and the potential risk of myelodysplasia from treatment with alkylating agents. Currently, more than 60% of patients receiving an autologous stem cell transplant are treated as outpatients.

Melphalan (Alkeran), 200 mg/m^2, is the most widely used preparative regimen for autologous stem cell transplantation. Melphalan (Alkeran) plus total body irradiation is rarely used because it produces more side effects, particularly mucositis, and is not more effective.

In two studies from France and the United Kingdom, peripheral stem cell transplantation was superior to combination chemotherapy. Progression-free survival was longer, and median overall survival was increased by approximately 1 year in the transplant group.

It is not known whether maintenance therapy after transplantation is advantageous. Most physicians do not give therapy after transplantation and simply follow the patient for evidence of relapse. Maintenance options are interferon alfa-2b (Intron A),[1] prednisone every 48 hours, or low-dose thalidomide (Thalomid),[1] but prospective

[1]Not FDA approved for this indication.

studies are needed to determine which, if any, prolong survival. The role of double or tandem autologous stem cell transplantation is controversial. In a randomized study from France, there was no difference in event-free or overall survival between the single and double autologous stem cell transplant groups when evaluated at 2 years, but at 7 years both event-free and overall survival were superior in the double transplant group. The investigators recommended a tandem transplant for patients who did not have a complete response or at least an excellent partial response with the first transplant. However, results of additional randomized trials are pending, and an alternative approach is to collect enough stem cells so the patient may have a second transplant at relapse.

Fortunately, the mortality rate with autologous stem cell transplantation is approximately 1% to 2%. However, the two major shortcomings are that multiple myeloma is not eradicated even with large doses of chemotherapy, and in addition, the autologous peripheral stem cells are contaminated by myeloma cells or their precursors. In an effort to improve the preparative regimen, the addition of bone-seeking radioisotopes that provide increased radiation to the bone marrow (such as holmium-166 DOTMP[2] and samarium Sm 153 EDTMP[1]) is being investigated. In an effort to reduce the contamination of hematopoietic stem cells, CD34 selection was studied. Although contaminating tumor cells were reduced by three logs, there was no prolongation of event-free or overall survival with this approach.

SYNGENEIC OR ALLOGENEIC BONE MARROW TRANSPLANTATION

Bone marrow transplantation from an identical twin donor (syngeneic) is the treatment of choice if a donor is available. Results are superior to allogeneic transplantation.

Allogeneic bone marrow transplantation is advantageous in that the graft contains no tumor cells, and there is a graft-versus-tumor effect. However, subsequent graft-versus-host disease is troublesome. Furthermore, only 5% to 10% of patients with multiple myeloma are eligible for allogeneic transplantation because an HLA-compatible donor is available in only a third of patients and 90% are 50 years or older. Allogeneic transplantation currently is associated with too high a mortality and cannot be recommended. However, efforts are under way to reduce allogeneic transplant–related mortality using T-cell depletion or nonmyeloablative regimens.

Nonmyeloablative (mini-allo) allogeneic protocols following autologous stem cell transplantation are being pursued. It is hoped that the benefits of an allograft may be realized and the toxicity associated with the procedure decreased. The mortality is 10% to 15%, and graft-versus-host disease remains troublesome. Efforts are being made to reduce the toxicity of this approach. Currently, we believe that nonmyeloablative approaches should be limited to protocol studies.

STANDARD ALKYLATING AGENT THERAPY

Alkylating agent–based chemotherapy with oral administration of melphalan (Alkeran) and prednisone produces an objective response in 50% to 60% of patients and a median survival of 2 to 3 years. We prefer to give melphalan (Alkeran) orally in a dosage of 8 to 10 mg daily for 7 days and prednisone in a dosage of 20 mg three times a day orally for the same 7 days. If the serum creatinine value is more than 2 mg/dL (177 mmol/L), the initial dose of melphalan (Alkeran) should be reduced by 25%. Melphalan (Alkeran) should be given when the patient is fasting because absorption is reduced after food is eaten. Leukocyte and platelet counts must be determined at 3-week intervals after the start of therapy and the melphalan (Alkeran) dosage altered until midcycle cytopenia occurs. The melphalan (Alkeran) and prednisone regimen should be repeated every 6 weeks. If the neutrophil count is less than 1500/mm^3 or the platelet count is less than 100,000/mm^3 at 6 weeks, chemotherapy should be delayed and the counts determined at weekly intervals until the pretreatment level is reached. If the neutrophil or platelet counts remain low or if the counts are unduly low at 3 weeks, the melphalan (Alkeran) dose in the next 7-day course must be reduced. Unless the disease progresses rapidly, at least three courses of melphalan (Alkeran) and prednisone should be given before this therapy is abandoned. An objective response may not be achieved for 6 to 12 months or longer in some patients. The natural course of multiple myeloma is one of progression, and if the patient's pain is alleviated and there is no evidence of progressive disease, the therapeutic regimen is beneficial despite the failure to reach an objective response.

Chemotherapy should be continued for at least 1 year or until the patient is in a plateau state, defined as stable serum and urine M-protein levels and no evidence of progression. Continued chemotherapy is not recommended because it may lead to the development of a myelodysplastic syndrome or acute leukemia. Patients should be followed closely during the plateau state, and the same chemotherapy should be reinstituted if relapse occurs more than 6 months later.

Because of the obvious shortcomings of melphalan (Alkeran) and prednisone, various combinations of therapeutic agents have been tried. A large meta-analysis, based on data from 6633 patients in 30 trials comparing melphalan (Alkeran) and prednisone with various combinations of chemotherapy, was performed by the Myeloma Trialists Collaborative Group. Although the response rate was higher with combination chemotherapy, there was no survival benefit over melphalan (Alkeran). This meta-analysis also failed to find any category of patients in which combination chemotherapy had a significantly different mortality rate from that with melphalan (Alkeran) and prednisone. No evidence indicated that poor-risk patients did better with combination chemotherapy than with melphalan (Alkeran) and prednisone. As a result, melphalan and prednisone has remained the standard treatment for more than 30 years. Two recent randomized trials compared melphalan and prednisone to melphalan, prednisone plus thalidomide (MPT). These trials show superior response rates and event-free survival with the latter regimen. In the French trial, there is evidence of a significant overall survival in favor of MPT. Consequently, MPT is an additional standard option for patients with newly diagnosed myeloma who are not candidates for transplantation. MPT is associated with significantly greater toxicity; therefore, care must be exercised for patient selection and during therapy.

[1]Not FDA approved for this indication.
[2]Not available in the United States.

TREATMENT FOR REFRACTORY MULTIPLE MYELOMA, INCLUDING THE USE OF NOVEL AGENTS

Almost all patients with multiple myeloma who survive eventually have relapse. If relapse occurs more than 6 months after the plateau state is reached, the initial chemotherapy regimen should be reinstituted. Most patients respond again, but the duration and quality of response are usually inferior to the initial response. Patients who are initially refractory or who become refractory to alkylating agent therapy generally have a low response rate to subsequent chemotherapy and a short survival. The highest response rates in such patients have been with VAD[1] given via IV or bolus injection. Many physicians choose single-agent dexamethasone (Decadron)[1] instead because it accounts for approximately 80% of the effect of VAD. Methylprednisolone, 2 g IV three times weekly for a minimum of 4 weeks, is helpful for patients with pancytopenia, and we find fewer side effects than from dexamethasone (Decadron).[1] Other regimens, including VBMCP (vincristine,[1] BiCNU, melphalan [Alkeran], cyclophosphamide, and prednisone[1]) or VBAP (vincristine,[1] BiCNU, Adriamycin[1] IV, and prednisone[1] orally) are useful in relapsed disease. Interferon alfa-2b (Intron A)[1] as a single agent for refractory disease has been disappointing, with objective responses of 10% to 20%.

Novel agents for the treatment of multiple myeloma include thalidomide (Thalomid)[1] and its analogue lenalidomide CC-5013 (Revlimid),[1] and the proteasome inhibitor bortezomib (Velcade, PS-341). Thalidomide (Thalomid)[1] is usually given in a dosage of 200 mg daily. Objective responses occur in approximately a third of patients and last for a median duration of approximately 12 months. The addition of dexamethasone (Decadron)[1] to thalidomide (Thalomid)[1] increases the response rate. Side effects from thalidomide (Thalomid)[1] include weakness, fatigue, constipation, and somnolence. Rashes, thrombotic events, and sensorimotor peripheral neuropathy are more troublesome side effects. Thalidomide (Thalomid)[1] alone or in combination with dexamethasone (Decadron)[1] is now a standard therapy for relapsed or refractory multiple myeloma.

The immunomodulatory thalidomide (Thalomid)[1] derivative lenalidomide (Revlimid)* CC-5013 has shown activity in previously treated patients but is not yet commercially available. Phase II studies produce response in 30% of patients, and constipation, somnolence, and neuropathy are not troublesome. Revlimid dosage for myeloma is 25 mg orally days 1 to 21, every 28 days.

Bortezomib produced objective response in 35% of patients with relapsed, refractory myeloma who had received at least two prior therapeutic regimens. It is administered as an IV bolus dose of 1.3 mg/m[2] twice weekly for 2 weeks, followed by a 10-day rest period for a maximum of eight 21-day cycles. The median duration of response is approximately 12 months. Adverse events include fatigue, anorexia, nausea, and vomiting, fever, diarrhea, constipation, anemia, asthenia, peripheral neuropathy, neutropenia, and thrombocytopenia. The agent was given accelerated approval by the Food and Drug Administration (FDA) for the treatment of relapsed, refractory myeloma in patients in whom one or more prior regimens has failed.

SUPPORTIVE THERAPY

Radiotherapy

Palliative radiation in a dose of 20 to 30 Gy should be limited to patients with disabling pain who have a well-defined focal process that has not responded to chemotherapy. Analgesics in combination with chemotherapy usually can control the pain. This approach is preferred to local radiation because pain frequently occurs at another site, and local radiation does not benefit the patient with systemic disease. In addition, the myelosuppressive effects of radiotherapy and chemotherapy are cumulative and may restrict future therapy.

Hypercalcemia

Hypercalcemia must be suspected if the patient has anorexia, nausea, vomiting, polyuria, increased constipation, weakness, confusion, stupor, or coma. If it is untreated, renal insufficiency usually develops. Hydration, preferably with isotonic saline and prednisone (25 mg orally four times daily), is effective in most patients. The dosage of prednisone must be reduced and discontinued as soon as possible. After hydration has been achieved, furosemide (Lasix) may be helpful. If these measures fail, a bisphosphonate such as zoledronic acid (Zometa) or pamidronate (Aredia) should be tried.

Renal Insufficiency

Approximately 20% of patients with multiple myeloma have a serum creatinine level of 2.0 mg/dL or more at diagnosis. Myeloma kidney and hypercalcemia are the two major causes. Myeloma kidney is characterized by the presence of large, waxy, laminated casts in the distal and collecting tubules. Some light chains are very nephrotoxic, but no specific amino acid sequence of the light chain is yet identified.

Dehydration, infection, nonsteroidal anti-inflammatory agents, and radiographic contrast media may contribute to acute renal failure. Hyperuricemia or amyloid deposition may produce renal insufficiency. Nephrotic syndrome rarely occurs in multiple myeloma unless amyloidosis is present.

Maintenance of a high fluid intake producing 3 L of urine per 24 hours is important for preventing renal failure in patients with Bence Jones proteinuria. IV pyelography or preparation for barium enema can be performed with little risk if dehydration is avoided. If hyperuricemia occurs, allopurinol (Zyloprim) in doses of 300 mg daily provides effective therapy.

Acute renal failure should be treated promptly with appropriate fluid and electrolyte replacement. Patients with acute or subacute renal failure should be treated with dexamethasone (Decadron),[1] or thalidomide (Thalomid)[1] plus dexamethasone (Decadron),[1] or VAD[1] to reduce the

---

[1]Not FDA approved for this indication.
*Available for study but not FDA approved.

---

[1]Not FDA approved for this indication.

tumor mass as quickly as possible. A trial of plasmapheresis is reasonable in an attempt to prevent chronic dialysis but is not proven. Hemodialysis and peritoneal dialysis are equally effective and are necessary for patients with symptomatic azotemia. Renal transplantation for myeloma kidney is followed by prolonged survival.

Anemia

Almost every patient with multiple myeloma eventually becomes anemic. Increase of plasma volume from the osmotic effect of the M protein may produce hypervolemia and spuriously lower the hemoglobin and hematocrit values. Erythropoietin (Epogen, Procrit) reduces the transfusion requirement and increases hemoglobin concentration in more than half of patients. Those with low serum erythropoietin values are more likely to respond. Most physicians proceed with a trial of erythropoietin (Epogen, Procrit), 150 U/kg three times weekly, or 40,000 U once a week. Darbepoetin, a long-lasting erythropoietin (Aranesp), may be given weekly or biweekly.

Skeletal Lesions

Bone lesions manifested by pain and fractures are a major problem. A skeletal radiographic survey should be repeated at 6-month intervals or sooner if pain develops. Patients should be encouraged to be as active as possible because confinement to bed increases demineralization of the skeleton. Trauma must be avoided because even mild stress may result in a fracture. Fixation of long bone fractures or impending fractures with an intramedullary rod and methyl methacrylate gives excellent results. All patients with multiple myeloma who have lytic lesions, pathologic fractures, or severe osteopenia should receive IV bisphosphonates. Zoledronic acid (Zometa), 4 mg IV over 15 minutes every 4 weeks, or pamidronate (Aredia), 90 mg IV over 2 hours every 4 weeks, are equally efficacious. The dosage of bisphosphonates should be reduced with renal insufficiency. Because renal insufficiency or nephrotic-range proteinuria may occur, serum creatinine and 24-hour urine protein monitoring is necessary. One should consider reducing the IV bisphosphonate to every 3 months after 2 years unless there is evidence of progressive skeletal disease. Osteonecrosis of the jaw is reported in patients receiving bisphosphonates. Although the relationship is unclear, it is essential to obtain a complete dental evaluation and perform preventive dental treatment prior to beginning bisphosphonates. The patient should practice good oral hygiene during therapy. Invasive procedures (especially dental extractions) should be avoided during bisphosphonate therapy. Osteonecrosis of the jaw should be managed conservatively. Vertebroplasty or kyphoplasty may be helpful for patients with compression fracture of the spine.

Infections

Bacterial infections are more common in patients with myeloma than in the general population. Pneumococcal and influenza immunization should be given to all patients despite their suboptimal antibody response. Substantial fever is an indication for appropriate cultures, chest radiography, and consideration of antibiotic therapy.

The greatest risk for infection is during the first 2 months after initiation of chemotherapy. Prophylactic trimethoprim-sulfamethoxazole (Bactrim, Septra)[1] may be useful during the first 2 months of chemotherapy. Prophylactic daily oral penicillin[1] may benefit patients with recurrent pneumococcal infections. IV-administered Ig[1] may be helpful for patients with recurrent infections, but it is too expensive for long-term therapy.

Hyperviscosity Syndrome

The symptoms of hyperviscosity may include oronasal bleeding, gastrointestinal bleeding, blurred vision, neurologic symptoms, or congestive heart failure. Most patients have symptoms when the serum viscosity measurement is more than 4 cP, but the relationship between serum viscosity and clinical manifestations is imprecise. The decision to perform plasmapheresis, which promptly relieves the symptoms of hyperviscosity, should be made on clinical grounds rather than serum viscosity levels. Hyperviscosity is more common in IgA myeloma than in IgG myeloma.

Extradural Myeloma (Cord Compression)

The possibility of cord compression must be excluded if weakness of the legs or difficulty in voiding or defecating occurs. The sudden onset of severe radicular pain or severe back pain is suggestive of compression of the spinal cord. MRI or CT is most helpful for diagnosis. Radiation therapy in a dose of approximately 30 Gy is beneficial. Dexamethasone (Decadron) should be administered during radiation therapy to reduce edema.

Emotional Support

All patients with multiple myeloma need substantial and continuing emotional support. The physician's approach must be positive in emphasizing the potential benefits of therapy. It is reassuring for patients to know that some survive for 10 years or more. It is vital that the physician caring for patients with multiple myeloma has the interest and capacity for dealing with incurable disease over the span of years with assurance, sympathy, and resourcefulness.

REFERENCES

Attal M, Harousseau JL, Facon T, et al: Single versus double autologous stem-cell transplantation for multiple myeloma. N Engl J Med 2003;349:2495-2502. (Erratum appears in N Engl J Med. 2004;350[25]:2628.)

Child JA, Morgan GJ, Davies FE, et al: High-dose chemotherapy with hematopoietic stem-cell rescue for multiple myeloma. N Engl J Med 2003;348:1875-1883.

Facon T, Mary JY, Hulin C, et al: Major superiority of melphalan prednisone (MP) plus thalidomide (THAL) over MP and autologous stem cell transplantation in the treatment of newly diagnosed elderly patients with multiple myeloma. Blood 2005;106:A780 (abstract).

Kyle RA, Rajkumar SV: Multiple myeloma: Drug therapy (review article). N Engl J Med 2004;351:1860-1873.

Myeloma Trialists' Collaborative Group: Combination chemotherapy versus melphalan plus prednisone as treatment for multiple myeloma: An overview of 6,633 patients from 27 randomized trials. J Clin Oncol 1998;16:3832-3842.

---

[1]Not FDA approved for this indication.

Palumbo A, Bringhen S, Caravita T, et al: Oral melphalan and prednisone chemotherapy plus thalidomide compared with melphalan and prednisone alone in elderly patients with multiple myeloma: Randomised controlled trial. Lancet 2006;367(9513):825-831.

Rajkumar SV, Blood E, Vesole DH, et al: Thalidomide plus dexamethasone versus dexamethasone alone in newly diagnosed multiple myeloma (E1A00): Results of a phase III trial coordinated by the Eastern Cooperative Oncology Group. J Clin Oncol 2006;24:431-436.

Rajkumar SV, Hayman S, Gertz MA, et al: Combination therapy with thalidomide plus dexamethasone for newly diagnosed myeloma. J Clin Oncol 2002;20:4319-4323.

Rajkumar SV, Hayman SR, Lacy MQ, et al: Combination therapy with lenalidomide plus dexamethasone (Rev/Dex) for newly diagnosed myeloma. Blood 2005;106(13):4050-4053.

Rajkumar SV, Kyle RA: Multiple myeloma: Diagnosis and treatment. Mayo Clin Proc 2005;80:1371-1382.

Richardson PG, Barlogie B, Berenson J, et al: A phase 2 study of bortezomib in relapsed, refractory myeloma. N Engl J Med 2003;348:2609-2617.

Richardson PG, Sonneveld P, Schuster MW, et al: Bortezomib or high-dose dexamethasone for relapsed multiple myeloma. N Engl J Med 2005; 352:2487-2498.

Singhal S, Mehta J, Desikan R, et al: Antitumor activity of thalidomide in refractory multiple myeloma. N Engl J Med 1999;341:1565-1571. (Erratum appears in N Engl J Med 2000;342[5]:364.)

Polycythemia Vera

Method of
Magda Elkabani, MD, and
Kenneth S. Zuckerman, MD

Polycythemia vera (PV) is a chronic myeloproliferative disorder in which the most prominent abnormality is a marked increase in number of red blood cells. This proliferation of red blood cells is not driven by the normal physiologic regulator of number of red blood cells, erythropoietin, which in turn is regulated by tissue oxygenation. Platelet and granulocyte numbers also are increased frequently. The cause of PV is presumed to be an undiscovered mutation or mutations in a multipotent hemopoietic progenitor cell that results in impaired programmed cell death and subsequent clonal accumulation of hemopoietic cells in the bone marrow and blood, which have acquired this selective advantage over normal bone marrow cells.

Epidemiology

PV is a disease that occurs primarily in patients older than 50 years of age, with the median age at diagnosis 60 years of age. The incidence is 1.9 per 100,000, males being slightly more commonly afflicted than females. The median survival appears to be at least 15 to 20 years, which is slightly less than that of the age-matched general population. Arterial and venous thromboses, particularly pulmonary embolism, ischemic stroke, and coronary artery thrombosis, are the most common causes of serious morbidity and mortality in PV. Progression to severe myelofibrosis occurs in approximately 15% of patients, and transformation to acute myeloid leukemia has been reported in 1.4% to 6.3% of patients with PV, but may be 10% to 15% in patients treated with alkylating agents or radioactive phosphorus. The overall death rate of patients with PV was reported to be 2.9 per 100 patient years in Polycythemia Vera Study Group (PVSG) studies, but probably has decreased with more recent therapeutic approaches.

Clinical Manifestations

Many patients are diagnosed incidentally because of plethora or elevated hematocrit and/or hemoglobin on routine blood count. Other patients present with arterial or venous thrombosis, pruritus (especially after a warm shower or bath), palpable splenomegaly, gouty arthritis, erythromelalgia (acral dysesthesia with erythema, pallor, or cyanosis of hands and feet), headaches, dizziness, or gastrointestinal symptoms (gastric erosions, increased incidence of *Helicobacter pylori,* and peptic ulcer disease).

Diagnosis

The hallmark of PV is persistently elevated red cell mass and a low erythropoietin level. The vast majority of patients with a hematocrit greater than 60 have an elevated red cell mass. A red cell mass greater than 36 mL/kg in men or greater than 32 mL/kg in females is considered elevated. However, currently there is a great deal of controversy over the necessity and value of red cell mass measurements. These studies have become very difficult to obtain in most centers, and even when available, there are many extraneous factors affecting the proper calculation and interpretation of the results. Serum erythropoietin level can be extremely helpful in making or excluding the diagnosis of PV. A low serum erythropoietin level in an untransfused polycythemic patient with a prior history of normal hemoglobin and hematocrit levels makes the diagnosis of PV highly likely. An elevated erythropoietin level makes the diagnosis of PV very unlikely. A normal serum erythropoietin level does not help to distinguish between PV and other causes of erythrocytosis. Abnormally increased leukocyte (granulocytes) and platelet counts are frequently seen and support the diagnosis of PV but are not required for diagnosis. Other commonly encountered laboratory abnormalities include microcytosis from iron deficiency, elevated vitamin B_{12} levels, and elevated leukocyte alkaline phosphatase score. These are neither sensitive nor specific enough to be of great diagnostic value.

The bone marrow of patients with PV shows hyperplasia with decreased or absent iron stores, varying degrees of reticulin fibrosis, increased erythroid lineage cells, and usually increased numbers of granulocyte lineage cells and megakaryocytes. Clustering of abnormal-appearing megakaryocytes is almost diagnostic of a myeloproliferative disorder, but it does not distinguish PV from other myeloproliferative disorders. Bone marrow examination is not essential to making the diagnosis of PV. However, it may be very useful in patients with borderline criteria for diagnosis and to establish baseline levels of marrow hyperplasia and fibrosis in all patients.

Endogenous erythroid colony (EEC) formation in vitro is determined by the generation of colonies of maturing erythroid cells derived from single erythroid precursor cells in the bone marrow, called colony-forming units-erythroid (CFUs-E), in the absence of exogenous erythropoietin. Normal erythroid precursors do not form erythroid cell colonies in the absence of erythropoietin. Increased spontaneous EEC formation has a sensitivity and specificity approaching 100% for PV when there are any other findings of a myeloproliferative disorder. However, it is a research procedure and is not widely available clinically for diagnostic testing.

Cytogenetic abnormalities associated with PV include deletion of the long arm of chromosome 20, trisomy 8, trisomy 9, and loss of heterozygosity of chromosome 9. Elevated expression of the polycythemia rubra vera-1 gene (PRV-1) in granulocytes has been described recently as a potentially useful test for distinguishing PV from secondary polycythemias, although increased PRV-1 expression also is found in patients with other myeloproliferative disorders. A majority (69% to 91%) of PV patients overexpress the PRV-1 gene. One recent report indicates that level of PRV-1 expression may be highly correlated with the leukocyte alkaline phosphatase (LAP) score, which is a simple, widely available test. Other investigational techniques that may aid in establishing the diagnosis of PV include overexpression of Bcl-xL, reduced numbers of thrombopoietin receptor on platelets, and hypersensitivity of erythroid precursors to insulin-like growth factor-1. Finally, there has been a recent breakthrough finding of a somatic mutation, V617F in the Janus Kinase 2 (JAK2) gene on chromosome 9, which results in a gain of function of this tyrosine kinase. This mutation apparently is present in at least 65% of patients with PV, and less frequently in other myeloproliferative disorders. PV patients with this mutation were found to have a longer duration of disease and a higher rate of complications. While still mainly a research tool, analysis of this mutation in patients with suspected PV may be an important diagnostic finding in the future. Other investigational techniques that may aid in establishing the diagnosis of PV include overexpression of Bcl-xL, reduced numbers of thrombopoietin receptors or platelets, and hypersensitivity of erythroid precursors to insulin-like growth factor-1.

A recent breakthrough finding has been reported by multiple groups of a somatic mutation, V617F in the Janus Kinase 2 (JAK2) gene on chromosome 9 in patients with myeloproliferative disorders. This mutation results in a gain of function of the JAK2 tyrosine kinase and is present in multiple myeloproliferative disorders, including 65% to 97% of patients with pV, approximately 50% of patients with idiopathic myelofibrosis, and approximately 30% of patients with essential thrombocythemia. PV patients with this mutation were found to have a longer duration of disease and a higher rate of complications. In the short time since the discovery of this important pathogenic mutation, it has already become a valuable diagnostic tool for patients in whom the diagnosis of PV is uncertain. Specifically, detection of this JAK2 mutation in peripheral blood or bone marrow nucleated cells by polymerase chain reaction (PCR) confirms the diagnosis of PV in patients with erythrocytosis and other findings that are not sufficient by themselves to confirm the diagnosis. In the absence of erythrocytosis, but in the presence of elevated platelet and/or myeloid cell counts in the peripheral blood, the finding of the V617F mutation in JAK2 can be important supportive data in favor of the diagnosis of other

CURRENT DIAGNOSIS

- Polycythemia is defined as Hb greater than 18.5 g/dL in men and greater than 16.5 g/dL in women on at least two measurements, and/or red blood cell mass greater than 36 mL/kg for men and greater than 32 mL/kg for women.
- Secondary polycythemia should be excluded by documenting: arterial oxygen saturation more than 92%, Pao_2 greater than 60, carboxyhemoglobin level less than 5%, no history of living at high altitude recently, no use of exogenous erythropoietin injections, no erythrocyte hypertransfusion, and no high oxygen affinity hemoglobin mutation.
- Serum erythropoietin level is low or normal.
- Increased formation of endogenous erythroid colonies (EECs) has high sensitivity and specificity.
- Bone marrow examination shows erythroid and usually granulocyte and megakaryocyte hyperplasia, iron deficiency, variable fibrosis, and clustering of abnormal megakaryocytes; cytogenetics may show abnormalities in chromosome 8, 9, and 20.
- Thrombocytosis (platelet > 400,000) and leukocytosis (white blood cells > 10,000) are variably present.
- Splenomegaly, elevated B_{12} levels, and elevated leukocyte alkaline phosphatase score may be present and are supportive of a diagnosis of PV, but are not specific for PV.
- Increased expression of PRV-1 gene may be useful in distinguishing polycythemia vera from secondary polycythemias.
- Sequencing of genomic DNA using polymerase chain reaction (PCR) techniques to identify JAK2 (V617F) mutation can be useful to identify the presence of polycythemia vera or another myeloproliferative disorder.

Abbreviations: EECs = endogenous erythroid colonies; Hb = hemoglobin; PV = polycythemia vera; PRV-1 = polycythemia rubra vera-1 gene.

myeloproliferative disorders such as essential thrombocytosis and myeloid metaplasia with myelofibrosis.

PSVG was created in 1967 to develop a set of guidelines for the optimal approach to diagnosis and treatment of PV. The diagnostic criteria have evolved over the last 35 years as certain criteria were found to be insufficiently specific and sensitive, and new tests, especially measurement of serum erythropoietin level, became available. For patients with a hemoglobin/hematocrit consistently above the reference range of normal on at least two independent measurements (Hb [hemoglobin] > 18.5 in men, Hb > 16.5 in women), the diagnostic criteria listed in the Current Diagnosis box may be used. Any patient with a history of chronic volume depletion, hypoxic pulmonary disease, sleep apnea, massive obesity (pickwickian syndrome), smoking, living at high altitude, erythropoietin-producing neoplasms, methemoglobinemia, or familial polycythemia without other signs of a myeloproliferative disorder should be evaluated for secondary or relative polycythemia. The presence of hypoxemia, elevated carboxyhemoglobin, elevated erythropoietin, or normal red cell mass indicates that secondary or relative erythrocytosis is a more likely diagnosis. One reasonable

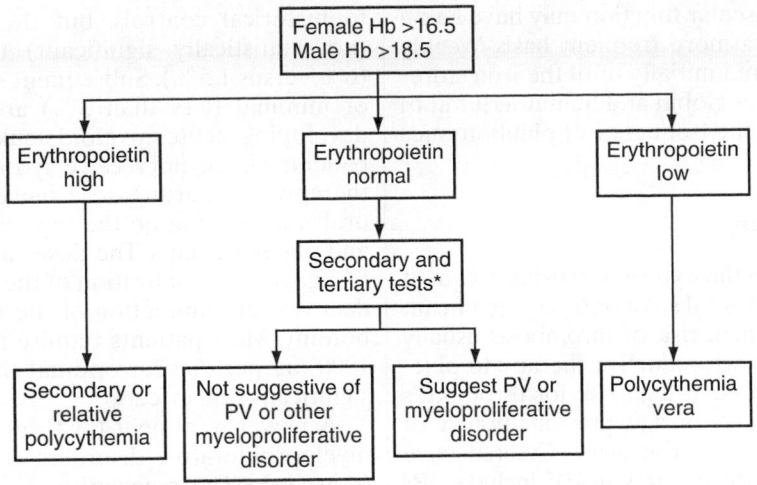

 * Secondary and tertiary tests supporting PV: bone marrow biopsy suggesting myeloproliferative disorder, increased granulocyte or platelet count, splenomegaly, elevated leukocyte alkaline phosphatase (LAP) score, elevated PRV-1 gene expression, increased endogenous erythroid colony (EEC) formation in vitro, and most importantly, presence of JAK2 (V617F) somatic mutation as detected by PCR assay.

FIGURE 1. Simplified general algorithm for diagnosis of polycythemia vera.

algorithm that may be used for patients with suspected PV is shown in Figure 1.

Treatment

More than 1600 PV patients were evaluated in the European Collaboration on Low-dose Aspirin (ECLAP) study, and 38% of those enrolled had a history of thrombosis. Therapy has been aimed at reducing thrombotic risk in these patients through the use of phlebotomy, cytoreductive therapy, and aspirin[1] at a dose of 81 to 100 mg per day. It is widely assumed that reduction of an elevated platelet count with cytoreductive therapy to the normal range or to a level less than 600,000 reduces the incidence of thromboses, although there are no firm experimental data that support that assumption. The Current Therapy box provides a summary of treatment considerations.

PHLEBOTOMY

The most commonly used therapy to treat erythrocytosis in PV patients is phlebotomy. This is not an effective treatment for thrombocytosis, which is unaffected or may even increase transiently after phlebotomy. The risk of thrombosis dramatically and progressively increases for all hematocrit levels more than 44%. Thus, the PVSG has recommended that a threshold hematocrit of 45% be used for phlebotomy therapy. A threshold hematocrit of 42% has been suggested for females, but without clear supporting data. One unit of blood (450 to 500 mL) is generally removed at a time. Elderly patients or patients

CURRENT THERAPY

- All patients should receive phlebotomy to keep Hct at less than 45% for men and less than 42% for women.
- All patients should receive low dose aspirin[1] therapy (81 to 100 mg) unless there is a contraindication to treatment.
- Cytoreductive therapy should be considered for patients at high risk of thrombosis, including patients older than 60 years of age, with a history of previous thrombosis, or with presence of cardiovascular risk factors.
- Hydroxyurea (Hydrea)[1] almost always is the cytoreductive therapy of choice, resulting in decreased morbidity and mortality associated with thrombosis, although it may be associated with a minimally increased risk of leukemic transformation.
- Anagrelide (Agrylin)[1] is an alternative cytoreductive therapy that does not alter erythropoiesis, but it lowers platelet counts and results in decreased incidence of thrombosis without risk of leukemia transformation.
- Bone marrow transplantation, imatinib,[1] and other experimental therapies are reserved for specific patient populations at this time
- Interferon-alpha may be used as cytoreductive therapy, especially as a non-teratogenic alternative in pregnant females.

[1]Not FDA approved for this indication.

[1]Not FDA approved for this indication.
Abbreviation: Hct = hematocrit.

with compromised cardiovascular function may have half a unit of blood removed on a more frequent basis. Weekly phlebotomies may be required initially until the iron stores have been depleted, and hemoglobin and hematocrit fail to rebound, but, subsequently, the frequency of phlebotomies is reduced.

CYTOREDUCTIVE THERAPY

Patients with progressive erythrocytosis requiring frequent phlebotomy, progressive or painful splenomegaly, significant thrombocytosis, or those at high risk of thrombosis usually benefit from the addition of cytoreductive therapy to phlebotomy. Those considered to be at high risk for thrombosis are patients older than 60 years of age, previous history of thrombosis, or known cardiovascular risk factors. Cytoreductive therapies that have shown effectiveness in PV include ^{32}P,[2] busulfan (Myleran),[1] chlorambucil (Leukeran),[1] pipobroman (Vercyte),[1] hydroxyurea (Hydrea),[1] interferon alfa-2a (Roferon-A),[1] interferon alfa-2b (Intron A),[1] and anagrelide (Agrylin).[1]

PSVG and European trials in the 1970s and 1980s showed that chlorambucil,[1] [32]P,[2] pipobroman,[1] and busulfan[1] were effective at reducing the incidence of thrombosis as compared to patients treated with phlebotomy alone. However, an excess mortality occurred with [32]P[2] or alkylating agents, because of the substantially increased risk of acute leukemia, gastrointestinal tumors, and skin cancers, leading to reduced survival. Because of the late increased risk of developing treatment-associated acute myeloid leukemia, these agents are generally now recommended only for patients at increased thrombotic risk, who are intolerant of or unresponsive to other treatments, and whose life expectancy is limited to less than 5 to 10 years.

Interferon-alpha (IFN-α) (Intron A, Roferon-A)[1] has been used in the treatment of PV because of its myelosuppressive effect and lack of leukemogenic potential. In a review of several small trials using IFN-α, overall response rates were 50% for hematocrit reduction and 77% for reduction in spleen size. However, IFN-α requires parenteral administration, and most patients suffer from variable severity of fatigue, sleep problems, myalgias, fever, flulike symptoms, depression, weight loss, hair loss, gastrointestinal symptoms, and cardiovascular symptoms, which results in discontinuation of interferon therapy in 25% to 35% of patients. Because it is nonteratogenic, IFN-α is a possible treatment modality for women who are pregnant. The starting dose is 3 million U subcutaneously three times per week.

Hydroxyurea (Hydrea)[1] is an antimetabolite inhibitor of DNA synthesis, which was developed in the 1970s as a noncarcinogenic drug and is the most commonly used cytoreductive drug in PV. It is usually very well tolerated, with the most common side effects being fatigue, cytopenias, and macrocytosis. Skin lesions, leg ulcers, oral ulcers, hepatotoxicity, and fever occur infrequently. The PVSG reported 51 patients with PV who were treated with hydroxyurea[1] and were compared to patients treated with phlebotomy alone (control group). The hydroxyurea group had fewer deaths and less myelofibrosis compared

to historical controls, but there was a slight tendency (not statistically significant) to more acute leukemias (6% versus 1.5%). Subsequent studies also have shown no or minimal (less than 3%) absolute increase in risk of developing acute myeloid leukemia, compared with PV patients who do not receive hydroxyurea or alkylating agent therapy. The starting dose ranges from 500 to 3000 mg/kg orally, depending on the urgency of reducing erythrocyte and platelet counts. The dose can be titrated, with an optimal goal of normalization of the platelet count and marked decrease or elimination of the need for therapeutic phlebotomy. Most patients require a long-term dose of 500 to 1000 mg per day for optimal therapeutic benefit without significant side effects.

A newer treatment for thrombocytosis associated with myeloproliferative disorders, including PV, is anagrelide (Agrylin).[1] The mechanism by which it reduces platelet counts is not completely understood, but it inhibits megakaryocyte maturation and platelet production. Approximately 85% to 90% of patients with thrombocytosis in myeloproliferative disorders achieve a platelet count less than 600,000 or 50% reduction in initial platelet count. The most common side effects include headache, fluid retention, atrial tachyarrhythmias, and diarrhea, resulting in 15% to 20% of patients discontinuing therapy. Experience with essential thrombocythemia suggests decreased risk of thrombosis and resolution of erythromelalgia with reduction of platelet counts to normal. The starting dose is 0.5 mg orally four times per day, but the dose is titrated to achieve a goal platelet count of less than 600,000, or in the normal range, if possible.

ASPIRIN

The use of aspirin[1] had been limited until recently because of the concern for gastrointestinal bleeding. A PVSG trial published in 1986 reported an increased incidence of significant gastrointestinal hemorrhage and no reduction in incidence of thrombosis with 975 mg of aspirin daily. The ECLAP trial reported in 2004 on 518 patients with PV, who had no previous history of thrombosis and were randomized to receive low dose aspirin or placebo. All patients were treated with either phlebotomy, cytoreductive therapy, or both. In patients receiving 100 mg of aspirin daily, there was a statistically significant reduction in frequency of nonfatal myocardial infarction, nonfatal stroke, pulmonary embolism, deep vein thrombosis, and death from any cardiovascular cause, and there was no increased risk of clinically significant bleeding. Unless there is a contraindication to aspirin[1] treatment, all patients with PV should receive 81 to 100 mg of aspirin[1] per day.

EXPERIMENTAL THERAPIES

Imatinib mesylate (Gleevec)[1] has been reported to treat successfully two patients with PV who were unable to tolerate hydroxyurea[1] or interferon.[1] The mechanism is unknown, although it has been proposed that inhibition of c-Kit may play a role. Allogeneic bone marrow transplantation has

---

[1]Not FDA approved for this indication.
[2]Not available in the United States.

---

[1]Not FDA approved for this indication.

been used in select patients, with some reports of cure. Given the risks associated with transplantation, this modality is generally reserved for patients who develop PV at a young age and progress rapidly.

REFERENCES

Berk P, Goldberg J, Donovan P, et al: Therapeutic recommendations in polycythemia vera based on Polycythemia Vera Study Group protocols. Semin Hematol 1986;23:132-143.

Cotes P, Dore C, Yin J, et al: Determination of serum immunoreactive erythropoietin in the investigation of erythrocytosis. N Engl J Med 1986;315:283-287.

Fruchtman S, Mack K, Kaplan M, et al: From efficacy to safety: a polycythemia vera study group report on hydroxyurea in patients with polycythemia vera. Semin Hematol 1997;34:17-23.

James C, Ugo V, Le Couedic JP, et al: A unique clonal JAK2 mutation leading to constitutive signaling causes polycythemia vera. Nature 2005:434(7037):1144-1148.

Jones C, Michael M, Dickinson T: Polycythemia vera responds to imatinib mesylate. Am J M Sci 2003;325(3):149-152.

Klippel S, Strunck E, Temerinac S, et al: Quantification of PRV-1 mRNA distinguishes polycythemia vera from secondary erythrocytosis. Blood 2004;102(10):3569-3574.

Kravolics R, Passamonti F, Buser A, et al: A gain of function mutation of Jak2 in myeloproliferative disorders. N Engl J Med 2005;352[17]:1779–1790.

Landolfi R, Marchioli R, Kutti J, et al: Efficacy and safety of low dose aspirin in polycythemia vera. N Engl J Med 2004;350(2):114-124.

Passamonti F, Rumi E, Peitra D, et al: Relation between JAK2 (V617F) mutation status, granulocyte activation, and constitutive mobilization of CD34+ cells into peripheral blood in myeloproliferative disorders

Spivak J: Polycythemia vera: myths, mechanisms, and management. Blood 2002;100:4272-4290.

Streiff M, Smith B, Spivak J: The diagnosis and management of polycythemia vera in the era since the Polycythemia Vera Study Group: A survey of American Society of Hematology member's practice patterns. Blood 2002;99(4):1144-1149.

Tartagilia A, Goldberg J, Berk P, et al: Adverse effect of antiaggregating platelet therapy in the treatment of polycythemia vera. Semin Hematol 1988;23:172-176.

Tefferi A: Polycythemia vera: A comprehensive review and clinical recommendations. Mayo Clin Proc 2003;78(2):174-194.

Vainchenker W, Constantinescu SN. A unique activating mutation in JAK2 (V617F) is at the origin of polycythemia vera and allows a new classification of myeloproliferative disease. Hematology (Am Soc Hematol Educ Program) 2005:195-200.

The Porphyrias

Method of
Claus A. Pierach, MD

The *porphyrias* present a group of mostly inherited diseases where disturbances along the heme biosynthetic pathway to heme lead to accumulations of metabolic intermediaries. Porphyria cutanea tarda can present without discernible inheritance; it can also be induced by chemicals (see the following). All steps of heme synthesis are enzymatically regulated and all porphyrias are a result of specific impasses along these transitions. Not all enzymatic defects result in clinically relevant or recognizable disease manifestations in every patient. On the one hand, the severity of the enzymatic defect plays a role. On the other, some poorly

understood revealing or unveiling cofactors are operational. The prevalence of the porphyrias is not known and fluctuates in different parts of the world.

The porphyrias can be divided between neurovisceral (acute) and cutaneous manifestations. Two types, the very rare delta-aminolevulinic acid-dehydratase deficiency porphyria and acute intermittent porphyria (AIP), have only neurological symptoms (acute attacks). Hereditary coproporphyria (HCP) and variegate porphyria (VP) may have both neurologic and dermatologic signs and symptoms. Congenital erythropoietic porphyria, porphyria cutanea tarda (PCT), and erythropoietic protoporphyria (EPP) exhibit only skin lesions but can be complicated by other problems (anemia, hepatic insufficiency).

Heme Synthesis

Succinyl coenzyme-A and glycine are the initial building blocks, subsequently transformed through eight enzymatic steps to the end product, heme, in itself essential not only for hemoglobin but also for other hemoproteins such as cytochromes, myoglobin, and other enzymes (catalase, nitric oxide synthase, and tryptophan pyrrolase). Heme synthesis happens in all cells but mostly in the liver and in the bone marrow. It is controlled by heme through feedback inhibition of the first step, delta-aminolevulinic acid synthase. Figure 1 shows the various steps, intermediaries, and resulting porphyrias. Porphyrins and their precursors, delta-aminolevulinic acid (ALA) and porphobilinogen (PBG), are only generated during heme synthesis and not during heme catabolism toward bilirubin. Specific enzymatic defects result in specific patterns of heme precursors and are of high diagnostic value when determining the

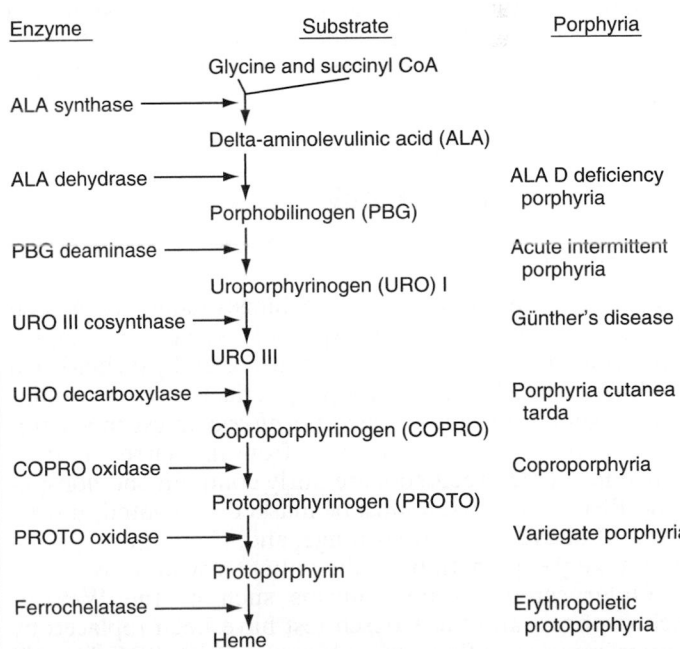

Enzyme	Substrate	Porphyria
	Glycine and succinyl CoA	
ALA synthase		
	Delta-aminolevulinic acid (ALA)	
ALA dehydrase		ALA D deficiency porphyria
	Porphobilinogen (PBG)	
PBG deaminase		Acute intermittent porphyria
	Uroporphyrinogen (URO) I	
URO III cosynthase		Günther's disease
	URO III	
URO decarboxylase		Porphyria cutanea tarda
	Coproporphyrinogen (COPRO)	
COPRO oxidase		Coproporphyria
	Protoporphyrinogen (PROTO)	
PROTO oxidase		Variegate porphyria
	Protoporphyrin	
Ferrochelatase		Erythropoietic protoporphyria
	Heme	

FIGURE 1. Heme biosynthetic pathway. Enzymes that have defects or deficiencies that cause the various porphyries are listed on the left side, heme and precursors are in the middle, and the resulting porphyrias are on the right side.

type of porphyria. Although enzyme and DNA measurements are of great interest, at present their availability is limited. The excretory pattern of heme precursors is influenced by their water solubility, which decreases toward heme; ALA and PBG are highly water soluble and measured in urine, whereas protoporphyrin is so hydrophobic that it is only excreted in stool and not in urine.

There is not just one porphyria and not just one single test revealing all porphyrias. Furthermore, the porphyric symptomatology can differ from type to type and can have considerable overlap between the various porphyrias (see previous paragraphs). Thus, highly specific and sensitive laboratory tests are necessary. All porphyrias with acute manifestations present with similar attacks, responding to similar treatment but exhibit different biochemical patterns according to their specific enzyme defect. A clinically useful grouping splits the porphyrias between acute and cutaneous.

The Acute Porphyrias

There are four types of acute porphyrias to consider:

1. The very rare ALA-dehydratase deficiency porphyria is inherited in an autosomal recessive fashion.
2. AIP, an autosomal dominant disorder, is the most common of the acute porphyrias (except for South Africa where variegate porphyria is more common).
3. HCP, again an autosomal dominant disease, is frequently misdiagnosed because coproporphyrin is often moderately and nonspecifically increased in many disorders.
4. VP is autosomal dominant and probably the mildest of the acute porphyrias.

All acute porphyrias are sensitive to a multitude of drugs and circumstances (Box 1). HCP and VP can also present with skin lesions resembling PCT. Skin lesions and acute attacks may happen at the same time or one after the other, or only one manifestation may ever be present in a given patient.

The Porphyric Attack

DIAGNOSIS

Diagnosis of the porphyric attack hinges mainly on a keen sense of suspicion. Any inexplicable symptom complex involving abdominal pain, tachycardia, and psychological findings should be suspect for porphyria. However, no clinical presentation can be called *porphyric* unless biochemically supported. Small deviations from the narrow normal range for heme precursors are fairly common and nonspecific. PBG and/or ALA must be markedly elevated, at least fivefold above the normal range, and, if not, porphyria is an unlikely explanation for the patient's symptoms.

Older screening mechanisms such as the Watson-Schwartz test and the Hoesch test have been replaced by easier, more specific tests such as the Trace PBG kit, still relying on the color reaction with Ehrlich's aldehyde. A *random* urine sample is highly sufficient for the initial diagnostic evaluation and if positive must be later followed up by more detailed tests such as quantitative measurements

---

BOX 1   Short List of Safe and Unsafe Drugs in the Acute Porphyrias

Unsafe	Safe
Alcohol	Acetaminophen
Barbiturates	Aspirin
Carbamazepine	Atropine
Carisoprodol	Bromides
Clonazepam	Cimetidine
Danazol	Erythropoietin
Diclofenac	Gabapentin
Ergotamines	Glucocorticoids
Estrogens, progesterones	Insulin
Ethchlorvynol	Narcotic analgesics
Glutethimide	Penicillins
Griseofulvin	Phenothiazine
Mephenytoin, phenytoin	Ranitidine
Meprobamate	Streptomycin
Methyprylon	Digoxin
Metoclopramide	Labetalol, propranolol
Primidone	Paraldehyde
Pyrazinamide	Bupivacaine
Pyrazolone	Chloral hydrate
Rifampin	Tetracycline
Sulfonamides	Vitamins
Valproic acid	

*Drugs not listed cannot be considered safe or unsafe.

---

of porphyrins and precursors in a 24 hour urine collection. Fecal porphyrin measurements may also be called for, but enzyme tests are only indicated if family studies can employ that test. Because the porphyrias are almost always hereditary, family studies are highly appropriate. The proper interpretation of any test result is best done with consideration for the clinical information.

CLINICAL PRESENTATION

Clinical presentations of porphyric attacks vary so much, that the term *the little imitator* has been used. No signs or symptoms are always present, but severe and poorly localized abdominal pain and unexplained tachycardia are so prevalent that their absence further complicates the diagnosis of an acute porphyric attack. The genesis of the attack is not well understood, but acutely increased demand for heme seems to be the foundation. This increased demand can be because of a wide variety of circumstances, from drugs through hormones (premenstrual phase) to stress, infection, fasting, and starvation. However, most carriers of the genetic defect for an acute porphyria remain asymptomatic for all their lives. Some have only one or two attacks, and very few suffer from many attacks.

The clinical picture with pain, fast heart rate, and neurovisceral symptoms can be complicated by, at times, severe hyponatremia, heralding seizures with therapeutic dilemmas (see Box 1) and respiratory paralysis necessitating ventilatory support. Death is rare nowadays, especially when the diagnosis is made early. The recovery is usually complete but at times prolonged, up to 1 year after a severe attack.

Superb nursing care, initially preferable in an intensive care unit, is necessary, and meticulous attention has to be paid to *all* problems. Dehydration from vomiting is common; ileus and urinary retention are not infrequent; hyponatremia occurs in approximately half of the porphyric attacks. Muscle strength must be tested frequently. Twice daily measurement of vital capacity helps to assess the necessity for tracheal intubation. High blood pressure and tachycardia deserve careful attention and, if appropriate, cautious treatment with a β-blocker. A negative caloric balance must be avoided, initially best treated with carbohydrates (if necessary intravenously with glucose), later with a balanced diet.

THERAPY

Therapy must always start with a careful look at the drugs recently taken by the patient. It is best to discontinue as many drugs as possible, especially those deemed unsafe (see Box 1). Appropriate lists of safe and unsafe drugs in porphyria are readily available via the Internet. An infection must be diligently searched for and at once be treated. Seizure precautions are especially indicated if hyponatremia is found. Analgesics should be adequately dispensed; opiates are frequently necessary in fairly large doses.

SPECIFIC THERAPY

Specific therapy was introduced a generation ago in the form of hematin* (Panhematin). This has largely replaced glucose (300 g/day), which had the main advantages of ready availability, relatively low cost, and the possibility of curbing an early or mild attack. But one must not wait for quick changes in a patient's condition and should at once take steps to obtain the definitive medication, hematin (Panhematin). This represents the equivalent to the end product, heme, and exerts its beneficial effect through repression of the deranged, and in the porphyric attack, markedly activated pathway to heme. It is still unclear whether the quick suppression of potentially toxic heme precursors (in 1 to 2 days) or a postulated replenishment of an assumed heme deficiency is the effective principle. *Early* administration of hematin (Panhematin) is strongly advocated because the course of a porphyric attack is unpredictable, and a point of no return can unfortunately be reached quickly. The infusion of hematin (Panhematin) must start as soon as possible. A daily dose of 3 to 4 mg/kg body weight is recommended for up to 4 days. Longer treatment periods are of questionable value but may be tried in severe cases for up to 2 weeks. The infusion must be strictly intravenous and with ample flushing because hematin (Panhematin) can cause thrombosis and phlebitis as it is a pro- and anticoagulant. This also makes frequent measurements of coagulation parameters advisable. Anticoagulants like coumarin should if possible be avoided. Admixture of 5% human serum albumin has been advocated to stabilize the final hematin solution and to lessen side effects. Hematin is available in many countries as heme arginate (Normosang). Its effectiveness is similar to Panhematin.

A beneficial clinical effect can be expected in 1 to 2 days, accompanied by a decrease in all heme precursors, most notably ALA and PBG. Many patients have received many treatment courses with hematin without apparent loss

*Hematin can be obtained as Panhematin from Ovation Pharmaceuticals, Inc. by calling (888) 514-5204.

of effectiveness. Prophylactic use of hematin (Panhematin) can be helpful in the treatment of women with regular premenstrual exacerbations of their porphyria. Hematin should never be given as a diagnostic test to see if unexplained symptoms lessen. The diagnosis of a porphyric attack must be as precise and as certain as possible, especially in new cases. Partial liver transplantation has been successfully undertaken and found to be curative in a patient with unrelenting porphyric attacks.

Prophylaxis of porphyric attacks is of great importance and can be accomplished to a large extent by avoidance of unsafe drugs, by stable caloric intake, and by prompt attention to intercurrent illnesses. It is a difficult decision if unsafe drugs have to be administered for a vital indication such as seizures. Here, consultation with an expert in porphyria is strongly advised.

The Cutaneous Porphyrias

The symptomatology of cutaneous porphyrias is mainly photosensitivity, often combined with skin fragility and blisters. All these findings occur because of porphyrin toxicity, resulting in cutaneous light absorption at the wavelength of 400 to 410 nm and subsequent formation of damaging reactive oxygen species. Thus, two therapeutic approaches are plausible: decrease of porphyrins and protection of the skin from light. The usual sunscreens are, however, ineffective, and reflective agents containing zinc or titanium, although better, are less popular because of their appearance.

In three porphyrias—PCT, HCP, and VP—the skin lesions are rather similar, but EPP and congenital erythropoietic porphyria can lead to very painful skin lesions, and, in the latter, even to mutilations.

PORPHYRIA CUTANEA TARDA

PCT is the most common porphyria and occurs because of uroporphyrinogen-decarboxylase deficiency and accumulation of mostly uroporphyrin. It can be inherited autosomal dominantly or may occur sporadically. It can also occur because of toxins such as halogenated aromatic hydrocarbons.

The most prominent skin manifestations are seen on the dorsa of the hands and on the face, consisting of blisters filled with mostly clear fluid, shallow, slow healing ulcers, whitish plaques, and tiny inclusion bodies, *milia*. Hypertrichosis and hyperpigmentation are frequently seen.

Unveiling factors promote the manifestation of the disease and consist mainly of liver disease, commonly because of alcohol. Hepatitis, frequently type C, and HIV infections are also common revealers. The drug list (see Box 1) is not applicable to the cutaneous porphyrias. The diagnosis is easily suspected at inspection and confirmed by measurement of urinary uroporphyrin excretion, typically manifold increased more than the normal range.

There are two treatment options with different principles but rather similar effectiveness. Repeat phlebotomies of 350 to 450 mL at 1 to 2 weeks intervals are performed and followed by hemoglobin and ferritin measurements. Overt anemia should be avoided. Ferritin usually reaches the lower end of the normal range after approximately 8 to 10 phlebotomies, and clinical remission can be expected after approximately half a year. Remission can be long lasting, especially when unveiling factors are avoided; total abstinence from alcohol is advocated. Patients should not take iron enriched vitamins because iron plays a critical role in PCT.

If phlebotomies are contraindicated (anemia, pulmonary or cardiac disease) or very inconvenient, low-dose chloroquine[1] (125 mg twice weekly) can be given orally. This flushes porphyrins from the liver and can be continued until remission is reached. In such low doses, the drug is virtually free from side effects.

Patients on chronic dialysis can develop PCT and also *pseudoporphyria*. Plasma porphyrin measurements establish the correct diagnosis. Patients with PCT and end stage renal disease respond well to erythropoietin, probably via iron (Fe) depletion through incorporation of Fe into hemoglobin. Pseudoporphyria is also seen as a side effect of many drugs, mostly nonsteroidal anti-inflammatory drugs and diuretics, but although phenotypically identical to PCT, does not respond to phlebotomies or chloroquine. Patients with PCT have a higher incidence of hepatocellular carcinoma and should be checked twice annually with hepatic imaging and measurement of alpha-fetoprotein.

CONGENITAL ERYTHROPOIETIC PORPHYRIA (GÜNTHER DISEASE)

Congenital erythropoietic porphyria (Günther disease), a rare autosomal recessive disorder, is usually apparent shortly after birth when brick-colored urine in diapers is observed because of excessive amounts of uroporphyrin (even more impressive under UV light). This porphyria and the rare homozygous PCT, hepatoerythropoietic porphyria, can be progressive and severely mutilating. Therapy is limited to sun protection and blood transfusion if hemolytic anemia is present.

ERYTHROPOIETIC PROTOPORPHYRIA

Erythropoietic protoporphyria is an autosomal dominant disorder that occurs because of deficiency of ferrochelatase, the last enzyme in heme biosynthesis. Urinary porphyrins are normal, but protoporphyrin is markedly elevated in red cells and in stool. These patients suffer from painful sun sensitivity, followed by edema and wrinkles in the

---

[1]Not FDA approved for this indication.

CURRENT DIAGNOSIS

- There is not just one porphyria, but there are at least six (and a few very rare ones because of homozygosity and dual porphyrias).
- There is not one test covering all porphyrias. For suspected acute porphyria, screening for excessive porphobilinogen is the test of choice.
- If cutaneous porphyria is in the differential diagnosis, quantitative measurements of porphyrins in urine and stool are recommended.
- Family studies are always indicated in these hereditary diseases.

CURRENT THERAPY

- Prophylaxis is mandatory and depends on the type of porphyria.
- Abstinence from alcohol is always indicated.
- The drug list should be respected in the acute porphyrias.
- Glucose therapy for the acute attack has mostly been superseded by the more effective, definitive treatment with hematin (Panhematin), to be instituted as soon as possible once the diagnosis has been made.

thickened, light-exposed skin. Approximately one fifth of these patients develop progressive liver disease secondary to hepatic accumulation of protoporphyrin. Liver transplantation can become necessary.

Therapy is often beneficial with oral β-carotene (up to 400 mg/day for adults). This leads to a harmless slight orange-yellow discoloration of the skin and often effective sun protection. Ideally, the β-carotene dose should be adjusted to a plasma level between 11 and 15 mmol/L.

REFERENCES

American Porphyria Foundation online available at: www.porphyriafoundation.com

Anderson KE, Bonkovsky HL, Bloomer JR, Shedlofsky SI: Reconstitution of hematin for intravenous infusion. Ann Intern Med 2006;144:537-538.

Anderson KE, Bloomer JR, Bonkovsky HL, et al: Recommendations for the diagnosis and treatment of the acute porphyrias. Ann Intern Med 2005;142:439-450.

Anderson KE, Sassa S, Bishop DF, et al: Disorders of heme biosynthesis: X-linked sideroblastic anemia and the porphyrias. In Scriver CR, AL Beaudet, WS Sly, et al. (eds): The Molecular and Metabolic Bases of Inherited Disease, vol 1, 8th ed. New York, McGraw-Hill, 2001, pp 2961-3062.

Badminton MN, Elder GH: Management of acute and cutaneous porphyrias. Int J Clin Pract 2002;56:272-278.

Chemmanur AT, Bonkovsky HL: Hepatic porphyrias: diagnosis and management. Clin Liver Dis 2004;8:807-838.

European Porphyria Initiative online. Available at: http://www.porphyria-europe.com

Kauppinen R: Porphyrias. Lancet 2005;365:241-252.

Therapeutic Use of Blood Components

Method of
Mahmoud Charif, MD, and
Ronald A. Sacher, MD

Blood component therapy refers to the transfusion of one or more blood components needed to treat a specific medical condition. In the United States, blood collection and processing is considered a manufacturing process performed by blood collection facilities such as independent blood centers, the American Red Cross, or hospital-based donor services. The process is regulated by the Food and Drug Administration (FDA) under the general title of Good Manufacturing Practice (GMP). Technical specifications for blood products are given in the *Circular of Information for the Use of Human Blood and Blood Components* prepared and updated by the American Association of Blood Banks (AABB), the American Red Cross, and America's Blood Centers, and it is recognized as acceptable by the FDA.

Blood component transfusion is used to treat quantitative or qualitative deficiency states resulting from blood loss, destructive or consumptive processes of cellular or acellular components, or to reverse the effects of external factors such as medications (warfarin [Coumadin] or antiplatelet drugs) (Box 1).

Loss of blood can often be managed by means other than blood component transfusion, such as fluid support with crystalloids or colloids. When making a transfusion decision, it is helpful to estimate the relative amount of blood or blood component loss, to decide whether or not transfusion is needed and to estimate the amount of replacement needed. Estimated blood volume in an adult is 70 mL/kg; in newborns, 85 mL/kg; and 100 mL/kg in low birth weight newborns.

Blood Components

WHOLE BLOOD

Fresh whole blood contains all blood elements in addition to the anticoagulant-preservative, and it is essentially red cells suspended in what is equivalent to liquid plasma (deficient in factors V and VIII) with a minimum hematocrit of 38%.

Indications

Whole blood provides oxygen-carrying capacity, blood volume expansion, and stable clotting factors (factors V and VIII decrease during storage). Whole blood is rarely available for allogeneic transfusion and is almost completely limited to autologous transfusion. Whole blood must be ABO *identical* to the recipient.

Under certain special circumstances, such as exchange transfusion in neonatal hyperbilirubinemia, when whole blood is ordered, the red cells may be suspended in AB negative fresh-frozen plasma, but this practice has a very limited indication.

One unit of whole blood is expected to raise the hemoglobin of an average adult by 1 g/dL and raise the hematocrit by approximately 3%.

RED BLOOD CELLS

Red blood cells are prepared either from whole blood with most of the plasma removed or collected by apheresis. If red blood cells are prepared from whole blood into CPD, CP2D, or CPDA-1, the final hematocrit should be less than 80%. Red cells prepared in an additive solution (AS) have a final hematocrit of 55% to 65% (Box 2).

Depending on the collection system used, a single whole blood donation typically contains either 450 mL (±10%) or 500 mL (±10%) of blood. Whole blood units are prepared at a ratio of 14 mL of anticoagulant per 100 mL whole blood collected.

After plasma is removed, the resulting component is labeled red blood cells, a component that has a hematocrit of 65% to 80% and a usual volume between 225 and 350 mL. AS may be mixed with the red cells remaining after the removal of nearly all the plasma.

The typical hematocrit of AS red blood cells is 55% to 65%, and their volume is approximately 300 to 400 mL.

Apheresis red blood cell unit contains approximately 60 g of hemoglobin compared to 50 to 80 g of hemoglobin for a whole blood collected unit, and it is comparable in all aspects. Red cells are stored at 1°C to 6°C.

Indications

The initial objective of treatment in the actively bleeding patient is restoration of oxygen-carrying capacity. Acute bleeding guidelines mandate transfusing patients who have lost 30% to 40% of their blood volume. Healthy resting adults, however, can tolerate acute isovolemic hemodilution with crystalloid or colloid replacement to a hemoglobin concentration as low as 5 g/dL. Factors to be considered when making a transfusion decision include the duration and cause of anemia, intravascular volume and perfusion criteria (e.g., urine output), the extent of the operation in patients undergoing surgery, active bleeding, the probability of massive blood loss, and the presence of other co-morbidities such as pulmonary or cardiac disease, myocardial ischemia, or cerebrovascular or peripheral vascular disease.

A hemoglobin concentration of 8 g/dL is adequate for most patients with stable cardiovascular disease.

A hemoglobin level below 6 g/dL almost always requires transfusion; however, hemoglobin above 10 g/dL rarely requires transfusion. Guidelines published by the American Society of Anesthesiologists (ASA) and the College of American Pathologists (CAP) recommend transfusing patients when hemoglobin level is 7 g/dL or hematocrit level is 21%. Objective measures that might indicate a need for transfusion are tachycardia or hypotension in the setting of normovolemia, mixed venous PO_2 less than 25, oxygen extraction ratio greater than 50%, or total oxygen consumption less than 50% of baseline.

Intensive care unit (ICU) patients who were transfused to maintain hemoglobin between 7 and 9 had a lower short-term mortality compared to patients transfused to hemoglobin between 10 and 12. A possible exception to this rule are patients with myocardial infarction and unstable angina.

Dosing

One unit of red blood cells raises the hemoglobin of an average adult by 1g/dL or the hematocrit by approximately 3%. For neonates, 10 to 15 mL/kg increases the hemoglobin by 2 to 3 g/dL.

A unit of red blood cells should be infused within 4 hours. The initial infusion rate should be slow (less than 1 mL/minute) except in urgent situations, and the patient should be observed closely for potential transfusion reactions. If the patient's condition does not allow infusion within 4 hours, smaller aliquots can be ordered for transfusion.

FROZEN RED BLOOD CELLS

Red cells can be frozen for an extended storage time, such as units of rare blood type or autologous units. The red cells can be frozen for 10 years or longer in certain circumstances. They are frozen in glycerol, a cryoprotectant that must be removed when the units are thawed. The deglycerolization process involves washing the cells with decreasing concentrations of sodium chloride. Units thawed in an open system must be used within 24 hours, whereas in an automated closed system a shelf life of up to 14 days after thawing is allowed. Thawed frozen red cells should contain at least 80% of the original red cells in the product, although units with a lower recovery rate can still be transfused, depending on the clinical circumstances, and with the approval of the transfusion facility physician.

PLATELETS

Platelets are an essential component of hemostasis and interact with von Willebrand's factor and tissue factor at the site of injury. Activated platelets aggregate and form the primary hemostatic plug, which is again stabilized by activated coagulation factors on the platelet membrane (secondary hemostasis).

Platelets normally circulate for approximately 10.5 days. Transfused platelets, however, have a life span of 4 to 5 days. Some factors can shorten the survival of platelets, such as splenomegaly, sepsis, high white cell count, hemorrhage, disseminated intravascular coagulation (DIC), auto and alloantibodies, concomitant administration of amphotericin, and cardiopulmonary bypass. Normal consumption of platelets in the body is approximately 7000 to 10,000 platelets/μL/day, and platelet function can be affected adversely by drugs, liver or kidney disease, and bone marrow disorders.

A unit of platelets is a concentrate of the platelets contained in one unit of whole blood suspended in 40 to 70 mL of plasma. Available products include *random donor pooled platelets*, which are collected from individual units of whole blood and then pooled, and *pheresis platelets*, which are collected from a single donor that usually contains an equivalent of four to eight individual single units collected by nonapheresis methods and 200 to 300 mL of plasma.

Indications

Platelet transfusion is used for treatment or prevention of bleeding related to a critical thrombocytopenia or a qualitative platelet dysfunction. An acceptable transfusion threshold for most nonbleeding patients is 5000 to 10,000/μL provided that the platelet function is normal (Box 3).

Dosing

Platelet dose depends on the clinical situation and the desired platelet count. The usual dose in an adult is 4 to 8 U or 1 U of pheresis platelets containing greater than 3×10^{11} platelets, which should increase the platelet count of an average adult by 30,000 to 60,000/μL (5000 to 10,000 per unit). In children a so-called standard dose of platelets is 1 U for each 10 to 15 kg of body weight, and in infants, 10 mL/kg of body weight.

ABO compatibility and compatibility testing are not necessary for platelet transfusion. The Rh antigen is not expressed on platelets; however, because of the small amount of red cells included with the platelets, transfusion of Rh-positive platelets to an Rh-negative woman of child-bearing age should be avoided. When it cannot be avoided, Rh immune globulin (RhoGAM, WinRho), 300 μg, which protects against 15 mL of Rh positive red cells, should be administered.

Except in unusual circumstances, the donor plasma should be ABO compatible with the recipient's red cells when this component is to be transfused to infants or when large volumes are to be transfused.

Platelet dysfunction can be caused by medications including aspirin, which irreversibly inhibits cyclooxygenase; clopidogrel (Plavix) and ticlopidine (Ticlid), which are irreversible adenosine diphosphate (ADP) antagonists; and glycoprotein IIb/IIIa antagonists such as Abciximab (ReoPro), which produces reversible (24 to 72 hours) platelet dysfunction. Eptifibatide (Integrilin) and tirofiban

---

BOX 3   Platelet Transfusion Triggers

- Prophylaxis: 5000–10,000/μL
- Planned surgical procedure: 50,000/μL; neurosurgical or retinal procedure: 100,000/μL
- Treatment: if patient bleeding, 50,000 /μL; central nervous system bleed: 100,000 /μL
- Impaired platelet function: may transfuse regardless of platelet count for prevention prior to invasive procedures and for treatment of bleeding

(Aggrastat) have a similar mechanism of action. Platelet dysfunction related to a reversible inhibition can last 5 to 7 days and often responds to platelet transfusion. Platelet dysfunction related to uremia does not respond well to platelet transfusion because the transfused platelets are affected by the uremic milieu.

Refractoriness to Platelet Transfusion

Refractoriness to platelet transfusion is defined as two consecutive 10 minutes after 1 hour posttransfusion platelet corrected count increment (CCI) less than 5000 platelets/m^2 of body surface area/μL:

$$\text{CCI} = \frac{\text{Body surface area (m}^2) \times (\text{posttransfusion platelet count/μL} - \text{pretransfusion platelet count/μL})}{\text{Number of platelets transfused } (\times 10^{11})}$$

Alloimmune platelet refractoriness is most often caused by HLA class I sensitization in the multiply transfused patient or from platelet-specific antibodies. Nonimmune causes of platelet refractoriness include massive bleeding, fever, sepsis, splenomegaly, DIC, intravenous (IV) amphotericin B, thrombotic thrombocytopenic purpura (TTP), and immune thrombocytopenic purpura (ITP). Leukoreduction of platelets reduces the risk of alloimmunization, but the use of single donor platelet transfusion does not reduce alloimmunization.

Refractoriness caused by HLA antibodies can be managed by providing HLA matched platelets that must be irradiated to prevent transfusion-associated graft-versus-host disease (TA-GVHD).

Because platelets are kept at room temperature, they are potentially more likely than other blood products to be contaminated with bacteria, usually gram positive.

Precautions and Contraindications

Platelets should not be transfused in the setting of TTP except for life-threatening hemorrhage because of the potential risk of increased thrombosis. Platelet transfusion is also not indicated in heparin-induced thrombocytopenia in the absence of clinically significant bleeding.

GRANULOCYTES

Granulocytes are collected by apheresis after stimulation of the donor with corticosteroids (prednisone, 60 mg in a single or divided doses, or 8 mg of dexamethasone) or growth factors such as granulocyte colony-stimulating factor (G-CSF), 5 to 10 μg/kg given 8 to 12 hours before collection. Granulocytes are stored at room temperature and must be infused within 24 hours after collection, which can present a logistic challenge in availability and pretransfusion testing.

Indications

Granulocytes must be Rh specific and crossmatch compatible because they contain a significant amount of red cells and should be irradiated to prevent GVHD. Alloimmunized patients should receive HLA-matched leukocytes. Leukocyte reduction filters should not be used. An adequate dose of granulocytes is 1×10^{10} granulocytes daily; higher doses are usually obtained with current donor

---

BOX 4   Granulocyte Transfusion Indications

- Neutropenia (absolute granulocyte count less than 500/μL) with positive bacterial or fungal blood cultures or progressive parenchymal infection unresponsive to appropriate antibiotic therapy.
- Myeloid hypoplasia with a reasonable chance for recovery of marrow function.
- Patients with granulocyte dysfunction during life-threatening infections.
- Neonatal sepsis.

---

stimulation regimens. The efficacy of granulocyte transfusion appears to be dose related (Box 4).

FRESH-FROZEN PLASMA

Plasma is collected either from whole blood or by the use of apheresis. Fresh-frozen plasma (FFP) is flash-frozen within 8 hours of collection and is indicated for the replacement of the coagulation factors including the labile factors V and VIII. It by definition has one international unit of each coagulation factor in each milliliter. Box 5 lists the indications.

FFP should not be used for coagulopathy that can be corrected more effectively with specific therapy such as vitamin K or factor VIII concentrate. The reversal with FFP of coagulopathy related to warfarin or liver disease is short lived (approximately 4 hours); therefore if FFP is given prophylactically before an invasive procedure, it should be given immediately prior to the procedure. FFP should not be used simply for volume expansion. A common misuse of FFP is in the setting of mild to moderate elevation in prothrombin time (PT) in patients with liver disease. Complete normalization of PT is not necessary for effective hemostasis.

Compatibility testing (crossmatch) is not necessary before plasma transfusion, but plasma must be ABO compatible with the recipient's red blood cells.

FFP should be used immediately after thawing or stored at 1° to 6°C for up to 24 hours after which it should be labeled thawed plasma. Thawed plasma can be stored for up to 5 days, and it can be used for coagulation factor replacement except for labile factors V and VIII.

There is no standard dose of plasma. The dose is determined by the clinical need, patient size, and coagulation assays. A dose of 10 to 15 mL/kg is usually sufficient for

---

BOX 5   Fresh-Frozen Plasma Indications

- Deficiency of multiple coagulation factors such as the preoperative management or bleeding in patients with liver disease; replacement in massive transfusion causing clinically significant coagulation deficiency.
- Reversal of warfarin (Coumadin)-induced coagulopathy in the setting of bleeding or surgical intervention if vitamin K use is inappropriate, when there is a need for anticoagulation shortly after the procedure.
- Plasma exchange in patients with thrombotic thrombocytopenic purpura (TTP).

temporary reversal of coagulopathy related to liver disease or warfarin.

CRYOPRECIPITATE-REDUCED PLASMA

Cryoprecipitate-reduced plasma is prepared from FFP by rapid freezing, thawing, and centrifugation, and it is deficient in factor VIII, von Willebrand's factor, fibrinogen, and factor XIII. It contains normal levels of factors II, V, VII, IX, X, XI, and albumin. Cryoprecipitation removes the high molecular weight von Willebrand's multimers.

Indications

Cryoprecipitate-reduced plasma can be used to replace deficient or defective plasma proteins except fibrinogen, factor VIII, von Willebrand's factor, and factor XIII. Because it is deficient in the large multimers of von Willebrand's factor, it is used for plasma exchange in patients with TTP refractory to FFP, although no conclusive evidence supports this practice.

CRYOPRECIPITATE

Cryoprecipitated antihemophilic factor (cryo) is produced by thawing FFP and collecting the precipitate, which is then frozen in approximately 15 mL of plasma. It contains at least 80 international units of factor VIII and 150 mg of fibrinogen (average, 200 to 250 mg) and also contains von Willebrand's factor and factor XIII. Cryoprecipitate can be pooled in a number of units according to the clinical need; a pool of 10 U is often used for adult patients. Cryo can be stored frozen for up to 1 year. Compatibility testing is not necessary for cryoprecipitate, Rh matching is not necessary, and ABO compatibility with the recipient's red cells is desired but not mandatory. Box 6 lists the indications.

BOX 6   **Cryoprecipitate Indications**

- Fibrinogen replacement:
  - Congenital or acquired fibrinogen deficiency.
  - Increased fibrinogen consumption (disseminated intravascular coagulation [DIC]) when fibrinogen level is below 80–100 mg/dL, particularly in the presence of hemorrhage.
  - Hypofibrinogenemia following massive transfusion or thrombolytic therapy.
- Dysfibrinogenemia.
- Treatment of bleeding in patients with hemophilia A (recombinant factor VIII has replaced this indication).
- Factor XIII deficiency.
- Von Willebrand's disease when factor VIII concentrates containing von Willebrand's factor (vWd) (Humate-P, Alphanate) are unavailable and desmopressin is contraindicated (type IIb vWd) or ineffective (type III vWd).
- Thrombocytopathy in some patients with renal failure for treatment of bleeding or prophylactically before invasive procedures; however, non-blood-derived factors such as desmopressin acetate (DDAVP) or erythropoietin can be used as a first-line therapy.

Dosing

Dosing of cryoprecipitate is generally based on the fibrinogen content and desired fibrinogen level.

Cryoprecipitate dose (bags) =

$$\frac{\text{Desired fibrinogen increment}^*/\text{dL} \times \text{plasma volume}^\dagger \text{ in dL}}{200 \text{ mg}}$$

*Desired fibrinogen level – current fibrinogen level.

†Plasma volume (mL) = (weight in kg × 70) × (1 – hematocrit).

The half-life of fibrinogen is 3 to 5 days; in a steady state, cryo for fibrinogen replacement may be repeated every 3 days; however, this should be based on serum fibrinogen measurements. Cryoprecipitate should be transfused within 4 hours of pooling.

Specialized Components

LEUKO-REDUCED COMPONENTS

A unit of whole blood contains 1 to 10×10^9 leukocytes. Leukocyte reduction can be achieved before storage, after storage, or at the bedside with the use of filters. The filters may remove other cellular elements; however, the leuko-reduced components have therapeutic efficacy at least equal to 85% of the regional component. Many blood centers leuko-reduce their entire inventory. Leukocyte reduction at the bedside is not subject to the same quality control as in the blood processing facilities. The use of bedside leukocyte reduction filters can result in severe hypotension in some recipients, particularly those taking angiotensin-converting enzyme (ACE) inhibitors.

Indications

Prestorage leukoreduction reduces the frequency of febrile nonhemolytic transfusion reactions and HLA alloimmunization, which can cause platelet refractoriness in the multiply transfused patient; it reduces the risk of transfusion-related cytomegalovirus (CMV) infections. Leukoreduction does not prevent GVHD and does not substitute for irradiation. Leukocyte reduction filters should not be used with granulocyte transfusion.

CMV RISK-REDUCED COMPONENTS

Transfusion-transmitted CMV is associated with cellular blood components. Acellular components such as plasma and cryoprecipitate do not require special testing to reduce this risk. CMV infection is common in healthy individuals and can be present in healthy blood donors as a latent infection. The viral genome is localized to the mononuclear cells. The presence of serologic markers for prior infection increases with age. CMV can be detected in a substantial minority of seronegative individuals when tested by polymerase chain reaction (PCR). Leukoreduction reduces the risk of transfusion-associated CMV transmission.

Indications

CMV-negative recipients who are at high risk for severe CMV infection include CMV-negative pregnant women, fetuses who may require intrauterine transfusion, low birth weight infants, CMV-seronegative bone marrow and solid organ transplant recipients, immunocompromised recipients, and seronegative HIV patients.

IRRADIATED COMPONENTS

Blood components contain viable lymphocytes and may be irradiated to prevent proliferation of T lymphocytes, which are the cause of TA-GVHD. The standard dose of gamma irradiation is 2500 cGy.

Indications

Indications are for transfusion of immunocompromised recipients, patients undergoing bone marrow transplantation, cellular components from blood relatives, intrauterine transfusion, neonates weighing less than 1200 g (some institutions irradiate cellular products for all neonates), and cellular components from donors selected for HLA compatibility. Irradiation of components transfused to all patients receiving nucleoside analogue therapy should be considered.

Irradiation causes erythrocyte membrane damage with potassium leakage, and the expiration date of irradiated red cells is shortened to 28 days postirradiation or the original expiration date, whichever is sooner. Irradiation of platelets does not change the expiration date.

SALINE WASHED COMPONENTS

Automated or manual washing with 1 to 2 L of 0.9% sodium chloride removes 99% of plasma proteins and electrolytes from cellular components including antibodies. It is associated with some loss of red blood cells and platelets. Red cells must be transfused no longer than 24 hours after washing; platelets must be transfused within 4 hours of washing. Washing results in up to 20% loss of red cells and loss of up to a third of platelets.

Indications

Indications are for recipients of cellular components who are IgA deficient and have IgA antibodies to reduce the risk of anaphylaxis and for recipients with a history of anaphylactic reactions or recurrent severe allergic reactions to transfusion. Washed platelets from the mother can be transfused to her newborn infant with neonatal immune thrombocytopenia.

VOLUME-REDUCED COMPONENTS

Platelets can be volume reduced by partial removal of the supernatant for recipients with fluid overload, renal or cardiac disease, small children requiring a large amount of platelets, or to remove supernatant substances such as ABO antibodies. Removal of the plasma can also reduce the risk of febrile nonhemolytic transfusion reaction. If an open system is used, platelets must be transfused within 4 hours, if a closed system is used and sterility is not broken, transfusion is recommended as soon as possible because the reduced amount of suspension solution has a limited capacity to support the platelets.

Special Transfusion Circumstances

MASSIVE TRANSFUSION

Massive transfusion is defined as replacement of one or more blood volumes within 24 hours, depending on the clinical circumstances and available supply. The transfusion service may change the blood provided from type identical to type compatible or from Rh-negative to Rh-positive blood. When possible this is avoided in women of childbearing age. Massive transfusion can be associated with coagulopathy from dilution or consumption. Initial empirical therapy with plasma and/or platelets may be appropriate; however, treatment should be guided by the results of coagulation parameters such as platelet count, fibrinogen level, PT, and activated partial thromboplastin time (APTT). A critical deficiency based on transfusion-related dilution alone is unlikely until 1.5 to 2 red cell volumes are transfused. Plasma or platelet transfusion should not be given after an arbitrarily determined fixed number of red cell units.

RECIPIENTS WITH ANTIBODIES

Multiply transfused individuals can develop antibodies to transfused red cell antigens. Some antibodies can cause hemolytic transfusion reactions; antibody detection and identification and finding compatible units in the transfusion service can be time consuming, particularly if the patient has multiple antibodies or an antibody to a high-frequency antigen. In patients with a known history of antibodies or multiple transfusions, it is advisable to start the process early if transfusion is anticipated to avoid delays in transfusion.

REFERENCES

Hillyer CD, Silberstein LE, Ness PM, Anderson KC (eds): Blood Banking and Transfusion Medicine: Basic Principles and Practice. November 2002.

American Association of Blood Banks: Technical manual, 15th ed.

American Association of Blood Banks: Transfusion Therapy: Clinical Principles and Practice, 2nd ed.

American Association of Blood Banks, America's Blood Centers and the American Red Cross: Circular of Information for the Use of Human Blood and Blood Components, July 2002.

Hébert PC, Wells G, Blajchman MA, et al: A multicenter randomized controlled trial of transfusion requirements in critical care. N Engl J Med 1999;340:409-417.

Heddle NM, Blajchman MA, Meyer RM, et al: A randomized controlled trial comparing the frequency of acute reactions to plasma-removed platelets and prestorage WBC-reduced platelets. Transfusion 2002;42:556-566.

Rebulla P, Finazzi G, Marangoni F, et al: The threshold for prophylactic platelet transfusions in adults with acute myeloid leukemia. N Engl J Med 1997;337:1870-1875.

TRAP Study Group: Leukocyte reduction and ultraviolet B irradiation of platelets to prevent alloimmunization and refractoriness to platelet transfusions. N Engl J Med 1997;337:1861-1869.

Vamvakas EC, Pineda AA: Determinants of the efficacy of prophylactic granulocyte transfusions: A meta-analysis. J. Clin Apheresis 1997;12:74-81.

Adverse Effects of Blood Transfusion

Method of
Phillip J. DeChristopher, MD, PhD

In the United States, an estimated 5 million recipients are transfused annually with approximately 22 million blood components, derived from approximately 5 million blood donations. These statistics position the transfusion of blood components as the most prevalent allogeneic tissue transplants practiced in medicine. Because blood components are both derived from human donors and manufactured, they are defined by the U.S. Food and Drug Administration (FDA) as both biologics and drugs. Thus it is expected that blood components have inherent, nonreducible risks of living tissues from other individuals, such as alloimmunization risks or infectious disease transmission, as well as certain limitations of drugs, such as variations in purity, potency, storage lesions, and limited shelf lives.

The safety of blood transfusion is upheld and maintained by several interlacing pillars, which include standardized blood banking operations and processes controlling transfusion administration. All U.S. blood donors are volunteers; they are currently screened by a nationally uniform Donor History Questionnaire that identifies relevant donor eligibility information, such as medical illnesses, and other disqualifying conditions, such as lifestyle and travel risks and medications. All collected blood is tested for the presence of markers for numerous transmissible infectious agents (Box 1); the application of quality management systems for the preparation, testing, storage, transportation, ordering, compatibility testing (including serologic testing, crossmatching, and serologic history checks),

and administration of blood; and the use by clinicians of practice guidelines for blood transfusion. Current Good Manufacturing Practices (cGMPs) are implemented to track and indemnify blood components from the vein of the donor to the vein of the recipient.

Overall, adverse effects of transfusion are reported in approximately 0.2% of all transfusions (albeit recognizing that clinically silent adverse effects occur much more commonly). But much higher rates for specific adverse effects are observed in chronically or heavily transfused patient cohorts. Although the risks of infectious complications of transfusion were markedly reduced in the United States over the last 25 years, a zero-risk blood supply is still not available. The constellations of clinical signs and symptoms, as well as the times to onset of symptoms (or disease), are commonly used to categorize most adverse effects of blood transfusion. The classification schemas of adverse effects are typically divided into either immune mediated or nonimmune mediated. Both categories have acute or delayed varieties, and both can have noninfectious or infectious adverse complications. The most frequent immune-mediated noninfectious transfusion hazards clearly are predicated on the fact that donor-recipient pairs in transfusion are allogeneic to one another. Such inherent genotypic/phenotypic discrepancies as well as residual or emerging infectious disease transmission risks label the practice of blood transfusion unavoidably unsafe.

The most dramatic progress over the last quarter century to improve the safety of donated blood was made in controlling viral disease transmission and other nonimmune mediated risks. These incremental improvements in the provision of a safer blood resource were made chiefly via key control steps prior to making blood available for transfusion in the clinical setting. Advances in blood preservation, storage, shipment, computerized inventory and tracking systems, regularly updated blood donor qualification schema, as well as discovery and implementation of new disease testing methods for known and emerging diseases, have all added to safeguarding donated blood. Box 1 notes the current compilation of tests applied to all blood components collected for transfusion in the United States. Table 1 gives estimates of the residual infectious disease risks of blood transfusion. (Treatment considerations for transfusion-transmitted diseases are omitted because they are the same as if the diseases were contracted outside the blood transfusion setting.) Transmission of infectious diseases—some of which can be chronic, acute, or even fatal—is not further discussed, except as noted:

- Nucleic acid test (NAT) methods for hepatitis C virus (HCV) and HIV were FDA licensed and implemented nationwide in early 2003. Application of this methodology is expected to include other analytes such as hepatitis B virus (HBV) and to continue to improve the already low levels of viral disease transmission.
- By comparison, the bacterial contamination of platelet concentrates has reemerged as a much more significant transfusion risk, with detection rates in the 1 case in the 1000 to 2000 population range. In early 2004, the American Association of Blood Banks (AABB) implemented new standards to limit and detect bacteria in platelet concentrates, which are stored at room temperature. The impact of these new standards is expected to improve the safety of platelet transfusions.

BOX 1	Required Testing of All Blood Components Collected for Transfusion in the United States

- ABO blood group and Rh type
- Antibody screening for clinically significant RBC alloantibodies
- Serologic test for syphilis
- Serologic tests, typically using an EIA technique:
- HBsAg
- Anti-HB$_c$
- Anti-HCV
- Anti-HIV-1/2
- Anti-HTLV-I/II
- Nucleic acid testing (NAT) using genomic amplification methods:
- HIV-1
- HCV
- WNV (in pilot testing under FDA IND since 2003)

Abbreviations: EIA = enzyme immunosorbent assay; FDA = Food and Drug Administration; HB$_c$ = hepatitis B$_c$ (virus); HCV = hepatitis C virus; HTLV = human T-cell lymphotrophic virus; IND = investigational new drug/device; RBC = red blood cell; WNV = West Nile Virus.

TABLE 1 Residual Infectious Disease Risks of Blood Transfusion in the United States

Infectious Agent	Estimated Frequency/Unit Transfused or Comment
Viruses	
Hepatitis B	1:220,000 to 1:488,000.
Hepatitis C	1:1,935,000.
HTLV–I/II	1:2,993,000.
HIV-1	1:2,135,000.
HIV-2	Transfusion-related cases never reported.
Hepatitis A	<1:1,000,000.
Hepatitis E	Transfusion-related cases never reported.
B19 parvovirus	1:3300 to 1:40,000 donors are viremic.
CMV	<1% of seropositive components transmit CMV; protect selected seronegative recipient populations.
EBV	Rare.
HHV-6	Seroprevalence in adults ~100%; blood transmissible, but no disease associations after transfusion.
HHV-8 (also known as KSHV)	~10% of donors are seropositive; transfusion transmission not yet documented.
GBV-C, TTV, SEN-V (putative hepatitis viruses)	Transfusion-transmissible viruses with high seroprevalence rates in asymptomatic donors; *actual clinical disease transmissions are nil*; screening not currently recommended.
Bacteria	
Gram-positive organisms (RD platelets)	1:1000 (detected by culture); 1:2500 results in clinical sepsis.
Gram-negative organisms (RD platelets)	1:2000 (detected by culture).
Platelets pheresis	1:2000 (detected by culture); 1:13,400 results in clinical sepsis.
GP or GN in RBC	1:1000 (detected by culture); 1:10,000,000 fatal sepsis.
Treponema pallidum	No transfusion transmissions reported in the last 35 years.
Borrelia burgdorferi	No transfusion-related Lyme disease case yet reported.
Parasites	
Plasmodium (all species)	0.25 per 1,000,000; 1 to 5 cases reported per year; transfusion transmission fatal in ~10% of recipients.
Babesia microti	*Rare;* ~50 cases reported, only in the United States; high seroprevalence in northeastern United States.
Trypanosoma cruzi	Transfusion-transmitted Chagas' disease *rare*; however, *T. cruzi* seroprevalence 1:9000 in Southern California.
Leishmania species	Transfusion-related cases never reported.

Abbreviations: CMV = cytomegalovirus; GBV-C = GB virus C (formerly hepatitis G virus [HGV]); GN = gram-negative; GP = gram-positive; HHV = human herpesvirus; HTLV = human T-lymphotrophic virus; KSHV = Kaposi's sarcoma–associated herpesvirus; RBC = red blood cell (unit); RD = random donor, derived from whole-blood donation; TTV and SEN-V = acronyms for patient propositi.

- In the summer of 2002, the United States experienced the largest arbovirus epidemic ever recorded in the Western Hemisphere because of the imported and emerging West Nile Virus (WNV). That year documented the first ever transmission of WNV by both blood transfusion and solid-organ transplantation. By mid-2003, NAT testing of the nation's blood supply for WNV began as an FDA investigational new drug (INV). In 2004 nearly 1000 units of donor blood contaminated with WNV were intercepted.

- Provision of cytomegalovirus (CMV)–reduced-risk cellular blood components remains a challenge because most adult donors are CMV-seropositive. In most clinical settings, reduction in CMV risk is accomplished by using either CMV-seronegative or leukoreduced components interchangeably. Both are equally safe and effective in preventing CMV transmission.

- Emerging infectious agents will certainly continue to pose threats to the blood supply. Such pressures will continue until methods are developed to sterilize donor blood. Although pathogen inactivation technologies using chemical and photochemical methods are actively being pursued in the research setting, no such methodology is licensed or available for transfusable cellular components at this time.

- Specialized blood components (such as CMV–reduced-risk, leukoreduced, and gamma irradiated) are usually reserved for specific patient populations who require reduction or removal of risk (Box 2).

Acute Adverse Effects

Table 2 shows a classification scheme for acute adverse effects of blood transfusion.

IMMUNOLOGIC

Acute (Intravascular) Hemolysis

Most acute hemolytic transfusion reactions (AHTR) are caused by the transfusion of ABO-incompatible red blood

BOX 2   Typical Major Indications for the Selective Use of Specialized Blood Components to Protect Patients at Risk

CMV-Reduced-Risk Component Support

- All intrauterine transfusions (IUT)
- Very-low-BW infants (<1200 g) born to SN mothers
- SN allograft recipients of SN solid organs or SN hematopoietic stem cells
- All SN patients with oncologic diagnoses receiving chemotherapy
- All SN candidates for any transplantation procedure
- SN pregnant women
- SN HIV-infected patients

Gamma Irradiation of Cellular Blood Components

- IUTs and exchange after IUT
- Congenital cell-mediated immunodeficiency syndromes
- Childhood solid tumors
- All BMT or PBPC recipients
- Hodgkin's lymphoma
- ALL
- Patients with leukemias, lymphomas, other malignancies requiring immunosuppressive chemoradiotherapy
- All directed blood donations
- All HLA- or crossmatch-compatible platelet components (for recipients who share a haplotype with related or unrelated HLA-homozygous donors)

Leukoreduced Cellular Blood Components

- Decreases incidence of platelet refractoriness because of HLA alloimmunization
- Prevents FNHTRs in patients
- Provides alternative supply of blood components with reduced risks for CMV transmission
- Decreases incidence of HLA alloimmunization in solid-organ transplant candidates

Abbreviations: ALL = acute lymphocytic leukemia; BMT = bone marrow transplant; BW = birth weight; CMV = cytomegalovirus; FNHTR = febrile nonhemolytic transfusion reaction; HLA = human leukocyte antigen(s); IUT = intrauterine transfusion; PBPC = peripheral blood progenitor cells; SN = (CMV–) seronegative.

cells (RBCs). The cardinal signs and symptoms include fever and chills, burning along the vein, restlessness/anxiety, and pain anywhere, as well as, ironically, being clinically silent. They can occur after the transfusion of only a small volume of blood or manifest after 1 or more units of RBCs are given. In the anesthetized patient, the only signs may be hypotension, so-called red urine, and unexpected oozing. The transfusion must be stopped immediately and the institutional policy and procedures followed for a transfusion reaction (TR) workup (see Table 2).

Although ABO-incompatible TRs occur very infrequently, improper specimen and/or patient identification all too commonly cause them. Completely enforced and documented procedures from specimen collection and labeling through to blood administration are the key preventive strategies.

The severity of an AHTR is directly proportional to the volume of incompatible blood transfused. The first essential steps in treatment include early recognition, stopping the transfusion, and preventing the transfusion of additional incompatible RBCs. Prompt and vigorous treatments for hypotension and cardiovascular support as well as maintenance of renal blood flow are the mainstays of therapy. Pressor agents may be necessary for maintenance of blood pressure, and component therapy may be necessary if the TR is complicated by disseminated intravascular coagulation (DIC).

Anaphylactic Reactions

The immediate and systemic anaphylactic reactions are mediated by an acute hypersensitivity response to proteinaceous plasmatic constituents, which trigger mast cell degranulation in multiple organ systems, including the skin, the gastrointestinal (GI) tract, the respiratory tract, and the cardiovascular system. Respiratory distress, shock, angioedema, and GI symptoms characterize this abrupt life-threatening response. The TR can occur in any clinical setting and after the administration of even vanishing small amounts of blood. Early recognition is mandatory because a combination of upper airway obstruction (laryngeal edema and bronchospasm) and severe cardiovascular collapse can occur within minutes of the first symptoms. The transfusion must be stopped immediately. Prompt administration of epinephrine (0.3 mL to 0.5 mL subcutaneously of a 1:1000 solution; injections can be repeated), volume expansion with normal saline, airway and cardiovascular support, and supplemental oxygen for patients in respiratory distress are absolutely essential. Intravenous (IV) epinephrine may be necessary for intractable hypotension. (Etiologically, the solitary identifiable protein implicated in this TR is class-specific anti-IgA in recipients who are IgA deficient; most anaphylaxis is not associated with anti-IgA in an IgA-deficient recipient.)

Fever Without Hemolysis

Febrile nonhemolytic transfusion reaction (FNHTR) is a diagnosis of exclusion that must be distinguished from AHTR and bacterial contamination. FNHTRs are characterized by fever (defined by an increase in temperature of more than 1°C above pretransfusion baseline), sometimes accompanied by chills or rigors, usually within 1 or 2 hours of transfusion. Because the differential diagnosis includes AHTR and bacterial sepsis, the transfusion is commonly suspended and discontinued. FNHTRs occur very frequently in multiply and heavily transfused recipients. Most FNHTRs are likely attributed to either cytokine showers (a storage lesion in RBC and platelets, in which proinflammatory cytokines such as IL-1, IL-6, IL-8, and tissue necrosis factor are released into the supernatant) or to preformed white blood cell (WBC) antibodies to residual WBC in the component. Treatment with antipyretic agents, either prophylactically or therapeutically, provides symptomatic relief; more severe FNHTRs can be treated more intensively with agents such as hydrocortisone (Solu-Medrol) or meperidine (Demerol). FNHTRs can be minimized in patients who experience repeated documented TRs or who are chronically or heavily transfused by using leukoreduced components (Table 3).

TABLE 2 Acute Adverse Effects of Transfusion: Classification and Frequency of Occurrence

Adverse Effect	Estimated Frequency/Unit or Comments
Immune Mediated	
Fever without hemolysis (FNHTR)	1:100 to 1:200 in adults; 6% and 12% in adult and pediatric hematologic malignancies, respectively.
Cutaneous hypersensitivity ("*allergic*")	1% to 3% of plasma transfusions.
Transfusion-related acute lung injury (TRALI) (Noncardiogenic pulmonary edema)	1:5000 to 1:7500.
Acute hemolysis, *nonfatal* (ABO incompatibility)	1:6000 to 1:33,000.
Hypotension	Incidence remains unknown; small numbers reported.
Anaphylaxis	1:20,000 to 1:47,000.
Acute hemolysis, *fatal* (ABO)	1:587,000 to 1:630,000.
Nonimmune Mediated	
Transfusional hypervolemia	Uncertain, but common, ~1:700 to 1:3000.
Bacterial contamination	1:150 to 1:2500.*
Transfusion-associated bacterial sepsis (platelets)	1:435 to 1:13,500.
Transfusion-associated bacterial sepsis (RBC)	1:1,000,000.
Fatal: transfusion-associated bacterial sepsis (RBC)	1:10,000,000.
Nonimmune hemolysis	Infrequent.
Citrate toxicity	Uncommon.[†]
Metabolic derangements (low Ca^{++}, Mg^{++}, K^+, etc.)	Uncommon.[†]
Coagulopathy, hypothermia	Uncommon

*Laboratory evidence, usually by Gram stain or culture.
[†]Typically associated with massive transfusion or therapeutic hemapheresis.
Abbreviations: FNHTR = febrile, nonhemolytic transfusion reaction; RBC = red blood cell unit.

Transfusion-Related Acute Lung Injury

Transfusion-related acute lung injury (TRALI) is a clinical diagnosis of exclusion characterized by worsening respiratory distress, dyspnea, and bilaterally symmetric pulmonary edema with hypoxemia usually developing within 2 to 8 hours after transfusion. The diagnosis of TRALI requires an interval change in the chest radiograph (demonstrating "white-out" by alveolar or interstitial infiltrates) in which cardiogenic or other causes of pulmonary edema are ruled out. Other frequent manifestations include fever and mild hypotension. Differential diagnostic considerations include anaphylactic TR, bacterial contamination, and circulatory overload. TRALI is associated with passive transfer of donor human leukocyte antibody (HLA)

TABLE 3 Delayed Adverse Effects of Blood Transfusion: Classification and Frequency of Occurrence

Adverse Effect	Estimated Frequency/Unit or Comments
Immune Mediated	
Alloimmunization to class I HLA on WBC and platelets	1:100 to 1:1000[†]; common in multiparous women.
Platelet refractoriness, clinical (can be associated with FNHTRs)	1:3300 to 1:10,000; very high in heavily transfused patients.
To RBC antigens, serologic only, with delayed hemolysis	1:1500
To RBC antigens, clinical symptoms, with delayed hemolysis	1:4000; significant in heavily transfused patients.
Graft-versus-host disease	~1:400,000.[‡]
Post-transfusion purpura	Rare; fewer than 400 cases reported worldwide; more common in multiparous women.
Immune modulation/suppression	Unknown.
Nonimmune Mediated	
Transfusional iron overload (RBCs only)	Variable, dose related; very common in chronically transfused patients with congenital hemolytic anemias.
Infectious disease transmission	Variable; see Table 2.

Abbreviations: FNHTR = febrile nonhemolytic transfusion reactions; HLA = human leukocyte antigen(s); RBC = red blood cell; WBC = white blood cell.
*Additional "relative" indications of each kind of component are matters of clinical judgment and should be individualized and clinically correlated.
[†]Incidence among selected, heavily transfused patient populations is very high (50%-100%).
[‡]Only selected patient populations are at high risk for this complication; they require prophylactic protection using gamma irradiation for cellular blood components (see Table 3).

(class I and class II) and/or granulocyte-specific antibodies. Its pathophysiology probably involves complement-mediated neutrophil lysis and pulmonary capillary leakage. Other patient-specific risk factors and component constituents also appear involved in its presentation, but its complete etiology is still under study. TRALI is associated with any blood component containing plasma. TRALI is a relatively mild form of acute respiratory distress syndrome (ARDS), and although fatal outcomes occur (usually in patients who are already sick or have co-morbidities), recovery within 48 hours is the rule. The mainstay of treatment is reversal of the progressive hypoxemia using supplemental oxygen. Aggressive treatment for respiratory failure in a critical care setting may be required. No clear preventive strategies are available.

Simple Allergic Reactions

Acute cutaneous hypersensitivity, characterized by urticaria (hives) and pruritus (itching), occur commonly after IV exposure to plasmatic components; patients requiring frequent transfusions or large amounts of plasma can experience allergic TRs in 1% to 3% of transfusion episodes. Transfused allergens in plasma cause tissue mast cell degranulation. If this TR is limited to the skin without other signs and symptoms, antihistamine administration is usually sufficient to provide symptomatic relief. The transfusion can be interrupted and if the TR does not progress, the transfusion can be restarted. These mild allergic reactions are TRs that do not need to be reported or evaluated as possible hemolytic transfusion reactions (HTRs). Transfusions can usually be safely resumed.

NONIMMUNOLOGIC

Bacterial Sepsis

Bacterial sepsis in transfusion is most commonly associated with platelet concentrates. Patients are symptomatic with very high fevers early in the transfusion episode, associated with rigors and profound hypotension, and they often experience nausea and/or diarrhea. The transfusion must be stopped and not restarted, and a TR investigation started at once (Box 3). Importantly, blood cultures must be drawn on the recipient (and later compared to blood cultures of the component). Broad-spectrum antibiotics should be administered immediately upon suspicion of bacterial sepsis because of the high likelihood of fatality. Definitive preventive measures are the current standard of practice to reduce incidence of such contaminations of platelet concentrates.

Transfusional Hypervolemia

Transfusional hypervolemia (circulatory fluid overload) is characterized by dyspnea, tachycardia, distended neck veins, hypertension, occasional cyanosis, and headache, associated with cardiogenic pulmonary edema. It is seen most frequently in patients at the age extremes and in patients who were massively transfused. Volume overload is best prevented by transfusing smaller aliquots of blood at slower rates and by close monitoring of patient's inputs/outputs and volume status. Mainstays of management include stopping the transfusion, vigorous diuresis, use of supplemental oxygen, and, less commonly, phlebotomy (in 250-mL increments).

Chemical Effects

Citrate Toxicity

Citrate is the anticoagulant used both in all blood components for transfusion and for extracorporeal manipulations involving most forms of hemapheresis. Massive transfusion or large-volume hemaphereses place patients at risk for hypocalcemia, characterized by numbness, tingling, muscular spasm, seizures, and even cardiac arrhythmias. Iatrogenic hypocalcemia is best managed by serially following

---

BOX 3   Immediate Responses to Acute Adverse Effects of Blood Transfusion

STOP (Interrupt) the Transfusion

The transfusionist performs assessment and evaluative functions

Related to patient

1. Repeat documented clerical RECHECK of ID.
2. Keep IV line open with 0.9% saline; if an HTR or other life-threatening reaction is suspected, *discontinue and disconnect* component from patient.
3. Contact treating physician for directions on patient care.
4. Administer supportive/definitive care.

Related to blood component

1. Repeat documented clerical RECHECK of label(s) on blood container(s).
2. Send administration set, blood bag, and IV fluid bag to TS.
3. Contact TS for directions for investigation.
4. Obtain blood/urine specimens from patient; send to TS with appropriate request forms and labels.

Laboratory Functions to Rule Out Acute Hemolysis

CLERICAL CHECK: Examine label on blood containers, all other records, and patient's specimen.
Check visually for hemolysis of pre- and post-transfusion serum or plasma (reliable when Hgb ≥50 mg/dL is present).
Perform DAT on post-transfusion sample.
Report findings to TS supervisor and medical director.
Report interpretation of transfusion reaction workup evaluation in the patient's medical record.
Perform additional studies per TS policies and procedures, clinically correlated to event.

Abbreviations: DAT = direct antiglobulin test; HTR = hemolytic transfusion reaction; Hgb = hemoglobin concentration; ID = identification; IV = intravenous; TS = transfusion service.

ionized serum calcium and by calcium repletion using either solutions of calcium carbonate or calcium gluconate.

Hyperkalemia or Hypokalemia

Hyperkalemia is of concern usually with very small infants (occasionally in patients with renal failure) who are exchange transfused using RBCs that are near outdating. A common strategy is to use fresher units of RBCs, which have lower absolute amounts of supernatant potassium. In patients who undergo either massive transfusion or prolonged hemapheresis procedures using citrate anticoagulant, hypokalemia is common. Citrate metabolism causes a metabolic alkalosis that causes potassium to be transported intracellularly. Electrolyte monitoring and appropriate repletion, as indicated, are recommended.

Nonimmune Hemolysis Without Symptoms

Patients may develop so-called red urine because of hemoglobinuria or because transfused RBCs were lysed by thermal extremes, mechanical means, or by chemical means (e.g., by admixture with hypo- or hypertonic drugs or parenteral solutions). All reports of red urine or findings of hemoglobinuria need to be distinguished carefully from immune hemolysis and bacterial contamination. A TR workup should aggressively seek an etiology, which usually can be traced to a remediable incident, error, or accident. Strict adherence to all standards of practice regarding the storage, transportation, and administration of blood components is the best preventive strategy.

Delayed Adverse Effects

Table 3 notes a classification list and frequency estimates of delayed adverse effects of blood transfusion.

IMMUNOLOGIC

Alloimmunization

RBC alloimmunization is possible whenever recipients are exposed to RBC antigens they lack. Because routine compatibility testing detects only the A, B, and D antigens on RBCs, transfusion recipients are at risk for alloimmunization. Risks for alloimmunization to any blood group antigen on all formed elements of blood increase in proportion to transfusion frequency. Patients can also become alloimmunized through pregnancy and transplantation. Up to 30% of heavily transfused populations, such as patients with congenital hemolytic anemias, can become alloimmunized to one or more clinically significant RBC antigens, which mandates provision of antigen-negative RBC. For patients with a history of multiple alloantibodies, the provision of appropriately antigen-negative RBCs becomes more and more problematic, ultimately requiring the finding of rare or very rare donor units to realize therapeutic benefits. An additional consideration is the disappearance of alloantibodies, which commonly happens. When this occurs, a patient transfused with an apparently compatible antigen-positive unit mounts an anamnestic humoral response and experiences a DHTR. HLA and/or other WBC alloimmunization are also frequently seen in patients who are alloimmunized to RBC antigens.

Delayed Hemolytic Transfusion Reaction

When a recently transfused patient experiences an unexplained anemia, possibly associated with hyperbilirubinemia and mild fever, within approximately 14 days of transfusion, delayed hemolysis should be suspected. DHTRs are associated with clinically significant IgG antibodies to all of the antigens of the Rh, Kell, MNSs, Duffy, and Kidd Blood Group Systems. Such hemolysis is usually antibody mediated, slow in onset, with the RBCs removed extravascularly (liver or spleen). Uncommonly, IgG-mediated hemolysis may present as an AHTR because some antibodies bind complement. RBC alloantibodies are usually demonstrable either in the patient's serum/plasma or from eluates prepared from the antigen-positive RBCs still in circulation. Except for having to transfuse again for symptomatic anemia, DHTRs generally require no specific treatment. However, an important consequence of such TRs is that all future RBC transfusions must use RBCs that lack the implicated antigen(s). When alloimmunization to multiple RBC alloantigens occurs, provision of compatible RBC becomes more difficult and can delay indicated therapy.

Platelet Refractoriness

Platelet refractoriness is suspected clinically whenever a patient's platelet count does not increase appropriately after receiving an adequate platelet transfusion dose. The refractoriness may be on an immune or nonimmune basis; nonimmune causes are the most common. If sources of platelet loss, destruction, or consumption (such as active bleeding, fever, infection, sepsis, DIC, splenomegaly, numerous drugs) can be eliminated, immune destruction may be occurring. Serial post-transfusion platelet counts, 30 to 60 minutes after transfusion, showing no platelet increment, supports immune destruction; so does a positive screen for HLA antibodies. Patients requiring chronic or heavy platelet transfusion support are at high risk for immune-mediated platelet refractoriness or may already be immunized (50% to 100% develop HLA antibodies for some period of time) because of multiparity or previous treatment. Optimally, platelet (HLA class I) alloimmunization is best prevented. In nonalloimmunized patients, immune-mediated platelet refractoriness can effectively be minimized or avoided by using leukoreduced blood components (see Table 2). In HLA alloimmunized myelosuppressed patients requiring daily platelet transfusion, obtaining suitable components could be difficult to impossible. They are at very high risk for significant bleeding complications, including death. Options to consider in the support of HLA-alloimmunized patients include use of crossmatch-compatible platelets or HLA-matched platelets if they are available.

Immunomodulation and Suppression

A growing body of literature supports transfusion-associated immunomodulation as a real biologic phenomenon associated with clinically significant deleterious effects in recipients of allogeneic blood. For example, in selected surgical

CURRENT DIAGNOSIS

The table below gives the signs and symptoms of acute transfusion reactions occurring within 24 hours or less of transfusion.

Reaction type	Component risk	Usual etiology or clinical correlate	Common signs/symptoms
Acute hemolysis, *with symptoms*	RBC; platelets; granulocyte concentrates	*ABO incompatibility,* caused by management or clerical error (specimen or patient *misidentification*); immune-mediated intravascular hemolysis because of anti-A and anti-B, from out-of-group plasma	Fever*; chills/rigors; hypotension; *pain* anywhere (chest, flank, limbs); *burning along* the vein; hemoglobinuria (*red* urine); hemolyzed serum in lab specimens; oliguria; bleeding, oozing (skin punctures)
Acute hemolysis, *usually without symptoms*	RBC	Physical disruption of RBCs because of mechanical physical forces or exposure to *nonisotonic* fluids or other parenteral drugs	Hemoglobinuria (*red* urine); might be asymptomatic
Anaphylaxis	All†	Antibody to unspecified plasma protein; anti-IgA in IgA-deficient patients; *systemic* mast cell degranulation	Hypotension; respiratory stridor/wheezing/arrest; shock and cardiovascular collapse; abdominal pain, nausea, vomiting, diarrhea; skin flushing, urticaria, pruritus
Hypotension	Plasma-containing components	Mediated by bradykinin; prekallikrein-activating factors in patients on ACE inhibitor drugs Hypovolemia	Volume resuscitation or pressor support as necessary Avoid or discontinue ACE inhibitors in patients requiring therapeutic hemapheresis procedures
Bacterial sepsis	Platelets; RBC	Bacterially contaminated components; components containing bacterial toxins	Rapidly rising, high fever; rigors; profound hypotension; nausea and/or diarrhea
Simple "allergic" reaction	All†	Antibody to unspecified plasma protein; type I hypersensitivity response	Virtually always limited to the skin; skin flushing; urticaria (hives); pruritus (itching);
Fever *without* hemolysis (*febrile, nonhemolytic*)	RBC; platelets; granulocytes	*Storage lesion* proinflammatory *cytokines;* preformed WBC antibodies in recipient	Fever* and/or chills/rigors
Transfusion-related acute lung injury	All except cryoprecipitate	*Donor* antibody to patient's WBC; acute, noncardiogenic pulmonary edema because of capillary leakage	Acute respiratory distress; shortness of breath; progressive hypoxemia; interval chest radiograph changes with symmetrical bilateral infiltrates
Transfusional hypervolemia; volume overload	All except cryoprecipitate	Circulatory overload; nonrecognition of patients at risk (age extremes)	Shortness of breath; dyspnea/cyanosis; distended neck veins; peripheral edema
Acute hypothermia	All except cryoprecipitate	Associated with massive transfusion; nonwarmed IV fluids	Chills/rigors
Citrate toxicity	All†	Often associated with massive transfusion or therapeutic apheresis procedures	Numbness, tingling (perioral, extremities); tetanic muscle cramping; seizures; cardiac arrhythmias

*Fever defined as >1°C above baseline.
†*All* includes any kind of RBC, fresh-frozen or other plasma, any platelet or granulocyte concentrates, and cryoprecipitate.
Abbreviations: ACE = angiotensin-converting enzyme; IV = intravenous; RBC = red blood cell; WBC = white blood cell.

CURRENT THERAPY

Reaction type	Usual etiology	Treatment considerations
Acute hemolysis *with symptoms*	RBC incompatibility; intravascular hemolysis, immune- or complement-mediated; circulating immune complexes	To treat renal failure: hydration, 1 L, 0.9% saline over 1-2 h; to maintain urine flow >1 mL/kg/h; administer diuretic, such as furosemide (Lasix) mg, IV; consider low-dose dopamine or other pressor support. If DIC is present: consider heparinization, 5000-U loading dose and 1500 U/h continuous infusion, to be continued for 6 to 24 h; consider component therapy, as indicated. *Under no circumstances should the transfusion be restarted.*
Anaphylaxis	Antibody to *unspecified* plasma protein(s); anti-IgA in IgA-deficient patients (less commonly)	Epinephrine (1:1000), 0.3 mL, SC; supportive measures for BP, respiratory and cardiac functions. *Under no circumstances should the transfusion be restarted.*
Hypotension	Extracorporeal volume depletion, such as in therapeutic hemapheresis; ACE inhibitor drugs	
Bacterial sepsis	Bacterially contaminated components; *sterile* components containing bacterial endo- or exotoxins	*The transfusion must be stopped and not restarted;* initiate transfusion reaction workup to include culture of component bag and IV fluids; obtain blood cultures on patient; supportive care to include antimicrobial therapy.
Fever *without* hemolysis	*Storage lesion* proinflammatory cytokines; recipient antibody to donor WBC	Acetaminophen, 650 mg, PO; rule out hemolysis and sepsis; for repeated episodes, consider prophylactic antipyretic therapy; for heavily transfused recipients, consider leukocyte reduction; for fevers with *rigors*, consider adding hydrocortisone (Hydrocortone Phosphate), injected, 50-100 mg, IVP and/or meperidine (Demerol), injected, 50 mg, IVP.
TRALI (noncardiogenic pulmonary edema)	Donor antibody (HLA or granulocyte-specific) to recipient WBC causing ARDS; possible role of patient risk factors and storage-lesion lipids in components	Reverse progressive hypoxemia, using supplemental O₂; if respiratory failure develops, intubation and mechanical ventilation, critical care support; without cardiac failure, roles for use of digoxin and diuretics unclear.
Simple allergic reactions (cutaneous hypersensitivity), urticaria and pruritus, *without* other signs and symptoms	*Type I hypersensitivity* response to plasma proteins, other allergens	Diphenhydramine (Benadryl), 25-100 mg, PO, IM, or IV; if recurrent, consider prophylactic antihistamine prior to next indicated transfusion; if urticaria is nonprogressive, may restart blood 15-30 min after antihistamine administration.
Transfusional hypervolemia (circulatory fluid overload)	Volume overload	Best prevented by transfusing smaller volumes or at slower rates (e.g., 1 mL/kg/h); consider rapid diuresis and supplemental O₂; uncommonly, therapeutic phlebotomy may be necessary.
(Nonimmune) hemolysis without symptoms	Transfusion of hemolyzed, but compatible RBC; hemolysis because of physical, chemical, drug *adulteration* of components	Cautiously rule out immune hemolysis or sepsis; perform transfusion reaction investigation to elicit etiology; watchful inaction; monitor for urine output, renal function, and evidence of DIC.
Chemical effects and derangements	Citrate toxicity; serum potassium abnormalities; hypomagnesemia; dilutional coagulopathy	Monitor for evidence of hypokalemic metabolic alkalosis; replete serum (ionized) calcium, total serum magnesium, and potassium with oral or IV preparations, as indicated; replace coagulation factors using appropriate component therapy.

Abbreviations: ARDS = acute respiratory distress syndrome; BP = blood pressure; DIC = disseminated intravascular coagulation; HLA = human leukocyte antigen; IM = intramuscular; IV = intravenous; IVP = intravenous push; O₂ = oxygen; PO = by mouth; RBC = red blood cell; SC = subcutaneous; TRALI = transfusion-related acute lung injury; WBC = white blood cell.

patients, blood transfusions are associated with earlier recurrences of malignancy after resection and/or increased rates of postoperative infections. The evaluation of such information and how to control this apparent biologic phenomenon are a matter of controversy in transfusion medicine. Although the use of leukoreduced blood components is suggested as a possible fix, currently no established preventive strategies exist.

Transfusion-Associated Graft-Versus-Host Disease

Transfusion-associated graft-versus-host disease (TA-GVHD) is an ominous and near universally fatal complication of blood transfusion. It is caused by engraftment of viable donor T lymphocytes into recipients who either cannot or do not mount a cytotoxic cellular immune response against foreign cells. Patients develop an acute syndrome within 4 to 30 days of transfusion characterized by high fever, whole body erythematous skin rash, severe GI and hepatic toxicities, and ultimately death because of bone marrow failure (bleeding and infection). Because no effective therapy is known, TA-GVHD must be prevented in susceptible populations (see Table 2). This is accomplished by gamma irradiation of cellular blood components, using at least 25 Gy (2500 rads) dose of delivered radiation, to inhibit mitotic potential of donor lymphocytes that contaminate all cellular blood components.

Post-Transfusion Purpura

The typical patient with post-transfusion purpura (PTP) is a previously transfused or multiparous middle-age woman (the female-to-male ratio is 26:1) who develops profound thrombocytopenia within 5 to 10 days of transfusion. Because of the rarity of this syndrome, the pathophysiology of PTP is only partly understood. The platelet destruction is immune mediated, caused initially by platelet-specific alloantibodies; anti-HPA-1a is a common, but not exclusive, specificity associated with this syndrome and clearance of allogeneic platelets or circulating platelet antigens. However, platelet autoantibodies also develop that destroy autologous platelets as well; the cause of thrombocytopenia in PTP remains unexplained. The duration of thrombocytopenia is typically approximately 2 weeks. Urgent treatment is necessary because the severe thrombocytopenia can last for days to weeks and has led to hemorrhagic deaths. No randomized controlled studies to optimize the treatment of PTP are available, but the optimal first-line therapy appears to be infusions of high-dose IV immunoglobulins. Plasma exchange using fresh-frozen plasma as replacement fluid is also effective. Because of its partial autoimmune nature, high-dose steroids are also used, but there is little convincing evidence for efficacy.

After recovery, prognosis of PTP is good, and it usually does not recur following subsequent transfusion.

NONIMMUNOLOGIC

Transfusional Iron Overload

Individuals who require chronic or prolonged RBC transfusion therapy, such as those with thalassemias and sickle hemoglobinopathies, inexorably accumulate excessive parenchymal iron, a complication that is ultimately life-threatening. Each unit of transfused RBC contains approximately 250 mg of iron, which saturates the monocyte-macrophage system and then deposits in the heart, liver, and endocrine system. The cardiac sequelae are the most dreadful, accounting for the majority of deaths from iron overload because of cardiac failure and conduction defects with lethal arrhythmias. Treatment with the only FDA-licensed iron chelator, deferoxamine, is currently the most effective therapy for transfusional iron overload. Its effectiveness owes to preventing cardiac toxicity, thus helping prolong survival. Compliance with chelation therapy is a real and chronic problem because deferoxamine must be administered parenterally. Oral iron chelating agents are eagerly anticipated.

REFERENCES

Brecher ME (ed): Technical Manual, 14th ed. Bethesda, Md, American Association of Blood Banks Press, 2002. (See especially Chapter 18, "Pretransfusion Testing"; Chapter 21, "Blood Transfusion Practice"; Chapter 27, "Noninfectious Complications of Blood Transfusion"; Chapter 28, "Transfusion-Transmitted Diseases.")

Brecher ME (ed): Bacterial and Parasitic Contamination of Blood Components. Bethesda, Md, American Association of Blood Banks Press, 2003.

Busch MP, Kleinman SH, Nemo GJ: Current and emerging infectious risks of blood transfusions. JAMA 2003;289(8):959-962.

DeChristopher PJ, Anderson RR: Practice parameters for transfusion medicine. Lab Med 2001;32(4):193,200-204.

Dodd RY, Notari EP, Stramer SL: Current prevalence and incidence of infectious disease markers and estimated window-period risk in American Red Cross donor population. Transfusion 2002;42(8): 975-979.

Klein HG: Pathogen inactivation technology: Cleansing the blood supply. J Intern Med 2005;257(3):224-237.

Popovsky MA (ed): Transfusion Reactions, 2nd ed. Bethesda, Md, American Association of Blood Banks Press, 2001.

Prezepiorka D, LeParc GF, Stovall MA, et al: Use of irradiated blood components. Practice parameter. Am J Clin Pathol 1996;106:6-11.

Prezepiorka D, LeParc GF, Werch J, Licthiger B: Prevention of transfusion-associated cytomegalovirus infection. Practice parameter. Am J Clin Pathol 1996;106:163-169.

Ratko TA, Cummings J, Oberman HA, et al: Evidence-based recommendations for the use of WBC-reduced cellular blood components (Conference Report). Transfusion 2001;41:1310-1319.

Silva MA (ed): Standards for Blood Banks and Transfusion Services, 23rd ed. Bethesda, Md, American Association of Blood Banks Press, 2004, pp 37-41.

The Digestive System

Cholelithiasis and Cholecystitis

Method of
Oscar Ruiz, MD

Gallstone disease is one of the most common diseases in the world. It is estimated that in the United States, more than 20 million people have gallstones. The incidence is higher in patients that are obese, diabetic, older, that have a family history of gallstones, and in certain ethnic groups (e.g., Native Americans).

Gallstone disease has always plagued humans. Gallstones were found in Chilean mummies that date back to 300 AD. The Greeks described biliary stones in the 5th century AD. Clinical jaundice related to gallstones was first described by Vesalius in the 16th century. Bile composition, physiology, and circulation were studied in the 1800s. The first cholecystectomy was performed in Berlin by Langenbach in 1882.

Most gallstones remain asymptomatic, but the gallstones that become symptomatic may cause very serious problems. Patients may develop acute cholecystitis, choledocholithiasis (with or without jaundice), gallstone ileus, gallstone pancreatitis, and/or ascending cholangitis. In these situations, prompt recognition of the problem is essential, as this leads to earlier treatment and better outcomes. For good surgical candidates, cholecystectomy remains the treatment of choice. It is estimated that more than 300,000 laparoscopic cholecystectomies are performed annually in the United States. The laparoscopic approach has become the surgical treatment of choice for gallbladder disease, leaving the open technique, cholecystostomy tubes, or endoscopic decompression, for more complicated cases.

Anatomy

The gallbladder is located between the divisions of right and left liver lobes. It is formed by the fundus (composed of smooth muscle), body (elastic tissue), infundibulum, and neck, which are connected with the cystic duct. The blood supply comes from the cystic artery that originates from the right hepatic artery. The blood return is through small vessels into the liver, and the cystic vein will drain into the portal vein. The cystic duct joins the common bile duct, where there are variations that are important to recognize for surgical approach. The lymphatic drainage goes directly into the liver and also drains into periportal lymph nodes.

Physiology

The gallbladder has a 20- to 50-mL capacity. Nearly half of the bile produced by the liver enters the duodenum directly. When the common bile duct pressure increases, the rest of the bile enters the gallbladder where water is passively absorbed over approximately 4 hours. The gallbladder then delivers the concentrated bile into the duodenum in response to cholecystokinin (CCK), secretin, and vagal stimulation from ingested food. The gallbladder relaxation is mediated by vasoactive intestinal polypeptide (VIP), pancreatic polypeptide, and somatostatin.

Gallstone Composition

The formation of gallstones is multifactorial (obstruction, inflammation, decreased solubility of bile, cholesterol crystals, etc.). The most common gallstones in the Western hemisphere are cholesterol gallstones, followed by bile pigment, the majority of which is bilirubin. The third most common are calcium, which occur predominantly as bilirubinate. There are other substances that can be found in gallstones, like carbonate, sodium, potassium, phosphate, copper, and iron, and so on.

Symptomatic and Asymptomatic Cholelithiasis

Based on numerous studies, it is generally believed that patients with asymptomatic gallstones do not require treatment. Physicians must be careful to recognize clear symptoms of gallbladder disease. The risk of observation in asymptomatic patients compared to surgical approach is definitely less. However, there are select groups of asymptomatic patients that may benefit from cholecystectomy, including patients with large gallstones (>2.5 cm), hemolytic anemia, children, and morbidly obese patients with rapid weight loss. Incidental cholecystectomies are mainly left as

573

a decision of the surgeon, depending on the individual circumstances. Identifying the different clinical presentations of symptomatic cholelithiasis, such as biliary colic, chronic cholecystitis, or acute cholecystitis, is critical for deciding the best timing of treatment.

Biliary colic, which is caused by temporary cystic duct obstruction of bile flow, is the most common manifestation of cholelithiasis. This process begins soon after meals and manifests as constant, right-upper-quadrant pain that can last for several hours. The pain often radiates to the shoulder or back. These attacks are self-limiting, and timing of recurrence is unpredictable. In addition to the previously mentioned symptoms, patients with chronic cholecystitis have more frequent attacks than in biliary colic, and are at greater risk for complications of gallstone disease. Patients with acute acalculous or calculous cholecystitis require admission to the hospital. These patients present with fever, elevated white blood count, elevated liver function tests, nausea, vomiting, and positive Murphy's sign. There is a special group of patients with the presumptive diagnosis of biliary dyskinesia that present with typical symptoms of biliary colic, but no gallstones. These individuals require a more extensive workup to rule out other etiologies for their symptoms. A paraisopropyliminodiacetic acid (PIPIDA) scan with ejection fraction (EF) will help considerably in making a diagnosis. Approximately 80% of patients with biliary dyskinesia will benefit from cholecystectomy.

Chronic Cholecystitis

Chronic attacks and inflammation of the gallbladder are most often associated with gallstones and the typical history of biliary colic. Usually, there is an obstruction in the neck of the gallbladder by a gallstone. This can produce a hydrops (mucocele), which may become secondarily infected with *Salmonella typhi*, *Streptococcus*, and *Klebsiella*. The patient usually presents with postprandial, right-upper-quadrant pain with radiation to the right shoulder, chest, or epigastrium. Significant back pain is a concern for possible choledocholithiasis. The image modality of choice is

undoubtedly an ultrasound, which shows gallstones in 90% of patients. In addition, the ultrasound may reveal thickening of the gallbladder wall, evidence of pericholecystic fluid, as well as an excellent visualization of the biliary tree, liver, pancreas, and kidney (Figure 1). Other modalities can be used to rule out additional sources of gastrointestinal pain, including computed tomography (CT) scan of the abdomen, upper endoscopy, upper or lower gastrointestinal (GI) studies, and hepatobiliary iminodiacetic acid (HIDA) scan. If the diagnosis is made with no complications, and there is resolution of the pain, the patient will be prepared for elective cholecystectomy.

TREATMENT

Cholecystectomy is one of the most common abdominal surgeries in the United States, and it is the treatment of choice for patients with symptomatic cholelithiasis. At the present time, the laparoscopic technique is the standard of care, with very low morbidity, mortality, and an incidence of clinically significant bile leaks between 1% and 3%. The decision of using the laparoscopic approach or converting to an open technique will depend on the circumstances that the surgeon encounters. The conversion rate to open cholecystectomy in elective cases of chronic cholecystitis is very low (<2%). The most common reasons for conversion are previous upper abdominal procedures, congenital ductal anomalies (5% to 7% of the general population), unexpected inflammatory processes, and Mirizzi's syndrome.

Acalculous Cholecystitis

Acute or chronic cholecystitis can occur without cholelithiasis. The incidence of chronic acalculous cholecystitis in this country is less than 5% of all cases, and occurs mainly in children. The causes are various, including anatomic anomalies, tumors that can cause obstruction, thrombosis of blood vessels, diabetes mellitus, collagen diseases, or infections (mycotic, typhoid fever, parasites). However, acute acalculous cholecystitis usually is a complication of sepsis, diabetes, multiple organ dysfunction, burns, or post–major surgical procedures. The treatment of choice is cholecystectomy, but in some cases, because of the associated disease processes, cholecystostomy tube placement (open or percutaneous) may be effective.

Acute Cholecystitis

Acute cholecystitis is usually associated with an obstruction in the infundibulum or neck of the gallbladder by stones. After direct pressure from the stones on the mucosa, the local area develops ischemia, edema, necrosis, and ulceration, which may result in a wall perforation. The etiology of acute cholecystitis may be bacterial (*Klebsiella*, *E. coli*, *Streptococcus*, *Salmonella*, *Clostridium*), sepsis from mechanical impaction of a stone, trauma, or after surgery. Less than 1% of the cases are secondary to tumors. Emphysematous cholecystitis is very rare, and is a secondary infection with gas-forming bacilli. Because of the rapid progression of this process with early perforation, the treatment of choice is early operation. Acute cholecystitis presents clinically

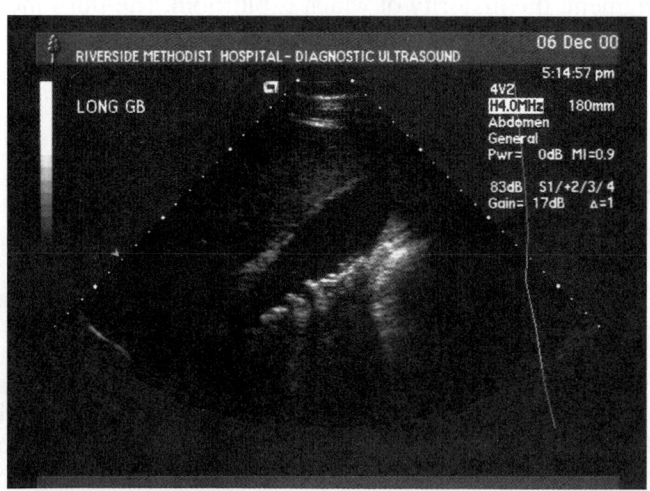

FIGURE 1. Gallbladder ultrasound demonstrates thickening of the wall, cholelithiasis.

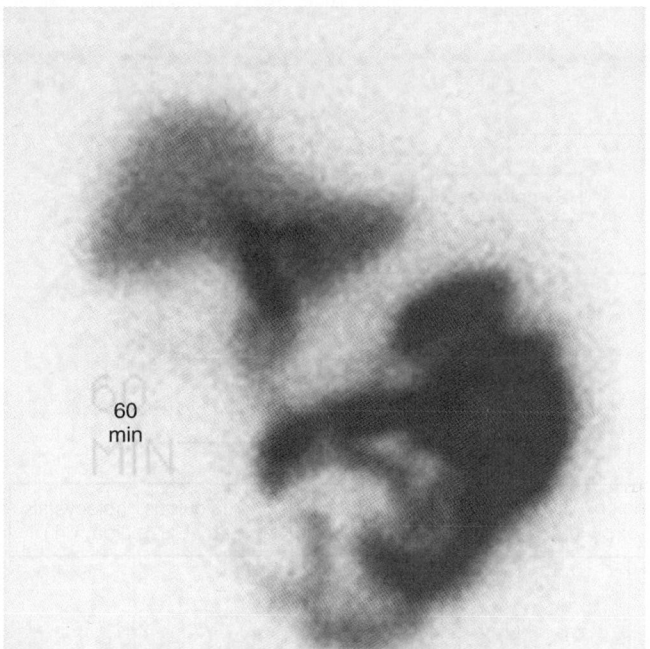

FIGURE 2. Positive HIDA scan, nonvisualization of gallbladder in 60 min.

and, by history, similarly to chronic cholecystitis and cholelithiasis. It may happen at any age, but it is most common between the 4th and 8th decades of life. The patients present with fever, elevated white blood count, positive Murphy's sign, and the gallbladder may be palpable. Mild jaundice is suggestive of extrinsic compression from the inflammatory process or choledocholithiasis. Usually leukocytosis with a shift to the left is noted. The preoperative workup includes a chest radiograph to rule out pneumonic processes, as well as a right-upper-quadrant ultrasound and HIDA scan, if needed (Figures 2 and 3).

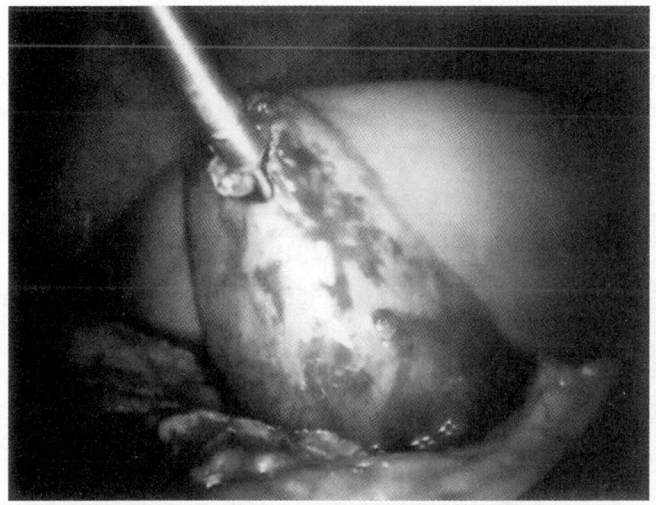

FIGURE 3. Intra-operative laparoscopic picture of acute gangrenous cholecystitis.

TREATMENT

Acute cholecystitis is the indication for laparoscopic cholecystectomy in approximately 20% of cases. There are different opinions about the optimal time for surgical intervention. Most surgeons favor early surgery (24 to 48 hours). The acute inflammation, edematous and thick gallbladder wall and sometimes gangrene of the gallbladder wall pose technical difficulties with dissection. As a result, the conversion rate to open cholecystectomy may be higher than in elective cases. The incidence of bile leak using cholescintigraphy following laparoscopic cholecystectomy for acute cholecystitis reveals a subclinical bile leak rate of 4%, similar to those for elective cases.

Choledocholithiasis

Stones in the common bile duct, single or multiple, are one of the most common and serious complications of gallstones. The incidence is difficult to determine but definitely increases with age. Common bile duct stones may be present in as many as 7% to 15% of patients that require cholecystectomy, and less than 5% may not be diagnosed before surgery. Common bile duct stones can cause acute or chronic obstruction, which may dictate the resulting clinical presentation and symptoms. The patient will typically present with right-upper-abdominal pain, jaundice, pale stools, and dark urine. The attack usually is sudden, and often precipitated by ingestion of a fatty meal. If the patient has associated ascending cholangitis, the clinical presentation is more severe. In addition to the pain and jaundice, there is also a high fever (Charcot intermittent fever). This group of patients often requires emergency removal of the common bile obstruction by endoscopic retrograde cholangiopancreatography (ERCP) and sphincterotomy, in combination with full support in the intensive care unit. If the endoscopic procedure is unsuccessful, open common bile duct exploration is necessary.

The differential diagnoses of choledocholithiasis include carcinoma of the common bile duct, viral hepatitis, drug-induced jaundice, peptic ulcer disease, myocardial infarction, pancreatitis, and pancreatic carcinoma. The main noninvasive diagnostic studies include hematology studies and evaluation of alkaline phosphatase, serum glutamic-oxaloacetic transaminase (SGOT), serum glutamic-pyruvic transaminase (SGPT), and bilirubin. The imaging studies include ultrasound, CT scan of the abdomen, magnetic resonance cholangiopancreatography (MRCP), ERCP, intraoperative cholangiogram, or transhepatic cholangiogram. For the group of surgeons that advocate routine use of intraoperative cholangiogram in cholecystectomies, the incidence of common bile duct injuries and retained bile duct stones is significantly lower. The previously mentioned radiologic studies may demonstrate a stone in the common bile duct, or dilated intra- and extrahepatic bile ducts and, importantly, exclude any tumor mass in the duct, head of the pancreas, or liver. Recently the increased use of MRCP has been a very useful noninvasive tool in the diagnosis of common bile duct stones. After the diagnosis is made, the decision is to select the best approach for each case to relieve the obstruction. This can be accomplished endoscopically with a transhepatic technique, or with a surgical approach, open or laparoscopically (Figure 4).

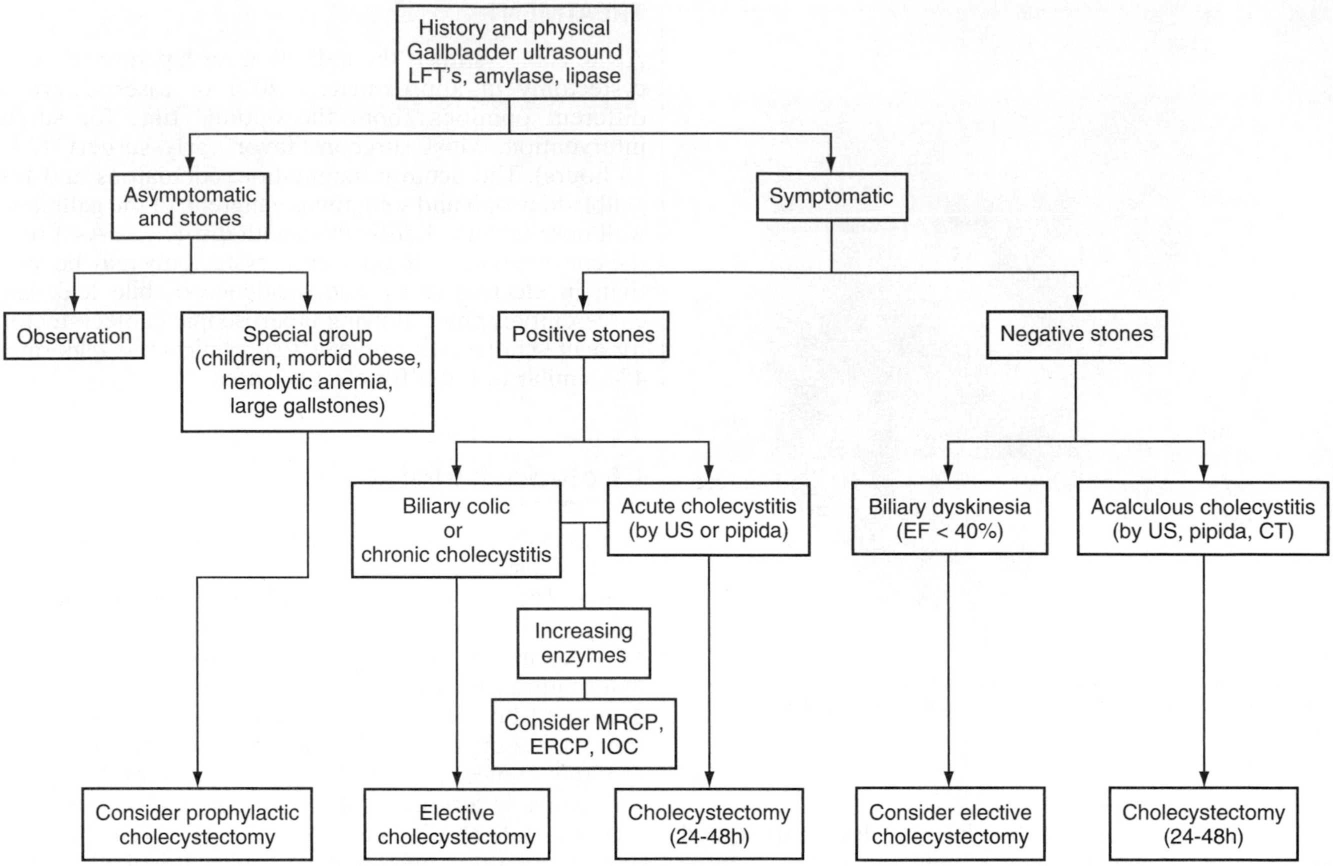

```
                        ┌─────────────────────────┐
                        │  History and physical   │
                        │  Gallbladder ultrasound │
                        │  LFT's, amylase, lipase │
                        └─────────────────────────┘
```

FIGURE 4. Protocol of management of gallbladder disease.

Flowchart boxes:

- Asymptomatic and stones
  - Observation
  - Special group (children, morbid obese, hemolytic anemia, large gallstones)
    - Consider prophylactic cholecystectomy
- Symptomatic
  - Positive stones
    - Biliary colic or chronic cholecystitis → Elective cholecystectomy
    - Acute cholecystitis (by US or pipida) → Cholecystectomy (24-48h)
      - Increasing enzymes → Consider MRCP, ERCP, IOC
  - Negative stones
    - Biliary dyskinesia (EF < 40%) → Consider elective cholecystectomy
    - Acalculous cholecystitis (by US, pipida, CT) → Cholecystectomy (24-48h)

Other Complications of Cholelithiasis

The early diagnosis of symptomatic gallstones is essential to prevent the many complications that can occur. Delay in diagnosis can lead to emphysematous cholecystitis, gallbladder perforation, gangrene, or empyema; sepsis that ensues may be difficult to counteract. Associated illnesses in this group of patients can make diagnosis difficult. Patients often need aggressive resuscitation and invasive intensive care unit (ICU) monitoring prior to abdominal exploration. Gallstone pancreatitis is a significant complication of gallstone disease. This usually occurs after one of the stones has passed into the common bile duct. Patients with gallstone pancreatitis often present with peritonitis and an acute surgical abdomen. These attacks may be transient with quick resolution of symptoms; however, 20% of these patients will need some type of surgical intervention to remove the stones. Gallstone ileus is a rare complication of cholelithiasis. This can occur when a large gallstone penetrates the wall of the gallbladder and enters the duodenum or colon forming a fistula. The stone can migrate to the terminal ileum where it becomes lodged causing a small bowel obstruction. If the patient is severely ill, the fistula between the bowel and the gallbladder may be treated in a second operation.

Another rare complication of cholelithiasis is a condition known as Mirizzi's syndrome. Mirizzi's syndrome is described as external compression of the common hepatic duct by a stone impacted in the neck of the gallbladder or in the cystic duct. This stone can erode directly through the ducts and become lodged in common bile duct causing an obstruction. In the unlikely scenario that the diagnosis is made preoperatively, the ideal management is to treat the patient conservatively. If the patient presents with an acute inflammatory process, following diagnosis with ERCP, the

---

CURRENT DIAGNOSIS

- Obtain a complete medical history (i.e., previous biliary colic attacks associated with fatty meals, history of jaundice).
- Determine pain location and type (Murphy's sign).
- Evaluate WBC, LFT, amylase, and lipase.
- Use radiologic diagnostic tools (i.e., ultrasound, HIDA scan with or without EF, CT scan).

Abbreviations: CT = computed tomography; EF = ejection fraction; HIDA = hepatobiliary iminodiacetic acid; LFT = liver function test; WBC = white blood cell count.

CURRENT THERAPY

Surgical Candidate

- Consider surgical therapy (laparoscopic cholecystectomy) for patients with diagnosis of chronic cholecystitis, acute calculous or acalculous cholecystitis, biliary dyskinesia, or gallstone pancreatitis.
- Place on low-fat diet until date of elective cholecystectomy.

Poor Surgical Candidate

- With acute cholecystitis, consider percutaneous cholecystostomy.
- With chronic cholecystitis, use conservative management.
- Prophylactic cholecystectomy should be considered in patients with gallstones, who are morbidly obese, have large gallstones, or are children with hemolytic anemia.
- If patient is pregnant, conservative management is preferred.

treatment is to proceed with cholecystectomy. This usually requires the open technique because of the challenging anatomy and the difficult dissection.

REFERENCES

Dominguez E, Ruiz O, Giammar D, et al: A prospective study of bile leaks after laparoscopic cholecystectomy in acute cholecystitis. Submitted for Publication, Riverside Methodist Hospital Department of Surgery.

Flum DR, Koepsell T, Heagerty P, et al: Common bile duct injury during laparoscopic cholecystectomy and use of intraoperative cholangiography. Arch Surg 2001;136:1287-1292.

Flum DR, Flowers C, Veenstra DL: A cost effectiveness analysis of intraoperative cholangiography in the prevention of bile duct injury during laparoscopic cholecystectomy. J Am Coll Surg 2003;196:385-393.

Friedman GD: Natural history of asymptomatic and symptomatic gallstones. Am J Surg 1993;165(4):399.

Hasl DM, Ruiz OR, Baumert J, et al: A prospective study of bile leaks after laparoscopic cholecystectomy. Surg Endosc 2001;15:1299-1300.

Phillips EH: Routine versus selective intraoperative cholangiography. Am J Surg 1993;165:505-507.

Young-Fadok TM, Smith CD, Sarr MG: Laparoscopic minimal-access surgery: Where are we now? Where are we going? Gastroenterology 2000;118:148-65.

Yu P, De Petris G, Biancani P, et al: Cholecystokinin-coupled intracellular signaling in gallbladder muscle. Gastroenterology 1994;106(3):763.

Cirrhosis

Method of
Richard K. Sterling, MD, Wissam E. Mattar, MD, and Paul Y. Kwo, MD

Cirrhosis is defined as the development of fibrosis of the liver with the formation of regenerative nodules. Typically it follows a chronic injury to hepatocytes that activate the perisinusoidal stellate cells by cytokines, which transforms them into myofibroblasts capable of proliferating and depositing collagen type 1. Progressively the normal liver histology is replaced by the fibrotic, distorted architecture. It is the resultant impairment in the synthetic, metabolic, and hemodynamic functions of the liver that defines cirrhosis clinically.

Common Clinical Manifestations

In addition to the particular expression of every etiology, most cirrhotic patients have little or no clinical features in the early stages, and many are already being followed up for abnormal liver panels before the development of cirrhosis. Patients may present with fatigue, weakness, nausea, abdominal discomfort, loss of appetite with weight loss, and pruritus. On physical examination, there may be jaundice, skin hematomas, spider angiomas, palmar erythema, gynecomastia, testicular atrophy, and caput medusae. The spleen and the liver could be palpable with tenderness in the right upper quadrant. Attention should also be given to the so-called seven hand signs of cirrhosis: palmar erythema, Dupuytren's contracture, telangiectasias, thenar wasting, leukonychia or Terry's nails, clubbing, and asterixis. As liver function decompensates, the more specific clinical manifestations of complications appear. Ascites, spontaneous bacterial peritonitis (SBP), hepatic encephalopathy (HE), esophageal varices, hepatorenal syndrome (HRS), hepatopulmonary syndrome (HPS), portopulmonary hypertension, and hepatocellular carcinoma (HCC), as well as other less apparent complications such as hematologic disturbances and hepatic osteodystrophy, are problems to address in the decompensated stage (Table 1).

CURRENT DIAGNOSIS

- Symptoms: fatigue, weakness, nausea, abdominal discomfort, loss of appetite with weight loss, pruritus
- Physical exam (general): jaundice, skin hematomas, spider angiomas, palmar erythema, gynecomastia, testicular atrophy, caput medusae, Dupuytren's contracture, thenar wasting, leukonychia or Terry's nails, clubbing, splenomegaly
- Physical exam (in decompensation): ascites, hepatic encephalopathy (asterixis)
- Complications: spontaneous bacterial peritonitis, esophageal/gastric varices, portal hypertensive gastropathy, hepatorenal syndrome, hepatopulmonary syndrome, portopulmonary hypertension, hepatocellular carcinoma

TABLE 1 Key Current Diagnoses

Ascites	Shifting dullness on physical exam, abdominal ultrasound, diagnostic paracentesis
SBP	Ascitic fluid: PMN cells count above 250/mm³, positive gram stain, positive cultures
Esophageal/ gastric varices	EGD
HE	Neuropsychiatric abnormalities; rule out other etiologies, search for precipitating factors
HRS I	Decrease of >50% in creatinine clearance or doubling of serum creatinine in less than 2 wk; rule out other etiologies of ARF
HRS II	Progressive renal failure, refractory ascites
Hepatopulmonary syndrome	Hypoxia, intrapulmonary vascular dilations, contrast-enhanced echocardiography or technetium-labeled macroaggregated albumin scanning
Portopulmonary hypertension	Pulmonary hypertension without secondary etiologies other than portal hypertension
Hepatocellular carcinoma	Lesion >2 cm with arterial enhancement or AFP >400 μg/mL, FNA in other suspicious lesions

Abbreviations: AFP = alpha-fetoprotein; ARF = acute renal failure; EGD = esophagogastroduodenoscopy; FNA = fine-needle aspiration; HE = hepatic encephalopathy; HRS = hepatorenal syndrome; PMN = polymorphonuclear neutrophil (leukocyte).

Common Laboratory and Imaging Findings

Frequently, tests confirm the clinical suspicion of cirrhosis in the presence of the characteristic physical findings of advanced liver disease. Laboratory studies could help establish the etiologic diagnosis and screen or confirm complications. In general, alanine aminotransferase (ALT) and aspartate aminotransferase (AST) are elevated but can be in the normal range. In the absence of chronic alcohol use, cirrhosis may be indicated by a higher AST than ALT. Bilirubin often increases only in advanced stages. High alkaline phosphatase pinpoints to a cholestatic component. Albumin trends to lower levels and the prothrombin time (PT) or international normalized ratio (INR) increases with the severity of the synthetic disturbance. Cytopenias, especially thrombocytopenia, are common. A low platelet count is often the only initial laboratory finding.

Imaging studies such as abdominal ultrasound (US), computed tomography (CT) scan, and magnetic resonance imaging (MRI) can suggest the diagnosis by revealing abnormalities in size, shape, and contour of the liver. However, they are not perfect, and liver biopsy remains the gold standard. Liver imaging can be helpful for the evaluation of portal hypertension and biliary tree abnormalities and to look for complications of advanced liver disease such as ascites, vascular thrombosis, and HCC.

Diagnosis

Obtaining adequate tissue from the liver confirms the diagnosis of cirrhosis. Biopsies could be obtained percutaneously except in the presence of a prolonged PT more than 3 seconds, thrombocytopenia of less than 60,000 to 80,000, or the presence of ascites. In these instances, an open biopsy or a transjugular approach can be used.

Severity of Cirrhosis

Multiple scores have been created to categorize the severity of disease. The Child-Pugh score is the most widely used (Table 2). It incorporates three laboratory values (PT, bilirubin, and albumin) and two clinical features (ascites and encephalopathy). Class A patients have an 85% 2-year survival, compared with 60% and 35% for classes B and C, respectively. The MELD (Model for End-stage Liver Disease) score has now supplanted the Child-Pugh classification for listing the patient for liver transplantation (Table 2) and is calculated by a formula that includes bilirubin, creatinine, and the INR instead of PT.

Causes

The etiologies that could lead to cirrhosis are very diverse and can be categorized into toxins and drugs, viruses, autoimmune diseases, biliary disease, metabolic, vascular and idiopathic (Table 3).

Treatment

There are limited treatments to reverse advanced fibrosis, but controlling the etiology preferably before end-stage disease ensues is highly recommended. Treatment of the complications of cirrhosis could be lifesaving or palliative.

TABLE 2 Classification of Cirrhosis

	Child-Pugh Points		
	1	**2**	**3**
Bilirubin (mg/dL)	<2.0	2.1–3.0	>3.0
Prothrombin time (seconds prolonged)	<4	4–6	>6
Albumin (g/L)	>3.5	2.8–3.5	<2.8
Ascites	None	Mild–moderate	Severe
Encephalopathy	None	Mild–moderate	Severe

Child's class A: 5–6, Child's class B: 7–9, Child's class C: 10–15.

MELD Score	**3-mo Mortality**
<10	2%–8%
10–19	6%–29%
20–29	50%–76%
30–39	62%–83%
≥40	100%

Abbreviation: INR = international normalized ratio; MELD = Model for End-stage Liver Disease. MELD Score = 11.2 ln (INR) + 3.78 ln (bilirubin) + 9.57 ln (creatinine) + 6.43

TABLE 3 Common Causes of Cirrhosis

Etiology	Diagnostic Test
Alcohol	History, AST-to-ALT ratio >2, liver biopsy
Viral hepatitis B	Surface antigen, E antigen, HBV DNA
Viral hepatitis C	HCV antibody, HCV RNA, HCV genotype
Autoimmune hepatitis	ANA, ASMA, A-LKM
Primary biliary cirrhosis	AMA
Primary sclerosing cholangitis	P-ANCA, ERCP, MRCP
Alpha 1 antitrypsin deficiency	A_1AT level, phenotype
Wilson's disease	Ceruloplasmin, serum Cu, Kayser-Fleischer rings
NASH	Liver biopsy, history of metabolic syndrome
Budd-Chiari syndrome	Duplex of the hepatic vein
Cryptogenic	Diagnosis of exclusion

Abbreviations: A-LKM = anti–liver/kidney microsome; ALT = alanine aminotransferase; AMA = antimitochondrial antibody; ANA = antinuclear antibody; ASMA = antismooth muscle antibody; AST = aspartate aminotransferase; Cu = copper; ERCP = endoscopic retrograde cholangiopancreatography; HBV = hepatitis B virus; HCV = hepatitis C virus; MRCP = magnetic retrograde cholangiopancreatography; NASH = nonalcoholic steatohepatitis; P-ANCA = perinuclear antineutrophil cytoplasmic antibody.

 CURRENT THERAPY

Procedure/Reason

- Upper endoscopy: Screen for varices.
    - If moderate or large, primary prophylaxis with nonselective β-blocker to prevent bleeding.
    - If none, then repeat q2y.
- Liver imaging (ultrasound or CT): screen/surveillance for hepatocellular carcinoma.
    - Repeat q6–12 mo.
- Alpha fetoprotein: Screen/surveillance for hepatocellular carcinoma.
    - Repeat q6–12 mo.
- Diagnostic paracentesis: Send fluid for WBC, differential, albumin, and total protein.
    - Exclude SBP (PMN <250).
    - Calculate SAAG.
- Hepatitis A and B serology: Vaccinate if negative.
- Diet: Low sodium:
    - 2 g/d if ascites.
    - 3–5 g if no ascites.
    - Avoid protein restriction unless uncontrolled encephalopathy.
- Medications: Avoid NSAIDs.
- Avoid aminoglycosides.
- Liver transplant referral/evaluation: if hepatic decompensation, variceal bleeding, or hepatocellular carcinoma.

Abbreviations: NSAIDs = nonsteroidal anti-inflammatory drugs; PMN = polymorphonuclear neutrophil (leukocyte); SAAG = serum ascites-albumin gradient; SBP = spontaneous bacterial peritonitis; WBC = white blood cell count.

Treatment of the Etiologies

CHRONIC VIRAL HEPATITIS

More information can be obtained from the article on viral hepatitis in this volume.

ALCOHOL

Alcohol abuse could lead to a spectrum of liver disease states that range from asymptomatic fatty liver to cirrhosis. The average total intake to develop cirrhosis is 80 g of ethanol per day for 20 years. Lesser doses in women, chronic viral hepatitis, and hemochromatosis could lead to higher risks of developing cirrhosis.

History, physical examination, and laboratory features can be specific for alcoholic hepatitis. An AST value more than two times the level of the ALT (related both to the deficiency in pyridoxal-6-phosphate and the direct mitochondrial toxicity of alcohol) suggests alcohol as the culprit of liver injury. If this ratio is less than 2, alcohol is unlikely to be the cause of liver injury. Aminotransferases usually do not exceed 500 UI/L. If they do, other coexisting etiologies, such as acetaminophen or acute viral hepatitis, should be excluded. Elevations in gamma glutamyl transferase (GGT) and carbohydrate-deficient transferase (CDT) could also suggest alcohol as the etiology of hepatitis. Thrombocytopenia and anemia with macrocytosis are classical findings but not specific. In acute alcoholic hepatitis (AH), alkaline phosphatase and GGT are typically and persistently elevated. Approximately 10% of the cases of AH are atypical or unclear, and in these a liver biopsy is required. A rapid bedside screening by looking for encephalopathy and ascites could evaluate the severity of alcohol-induced liver injury. If one or both are present, then calculating the MELD score and the discriminant function (DF), $4.6 \times$ (PT patient – PT control) + bilirubin in mg/dL, help assess the mortality risk and the subsequent management plan. A DF value greater than 32 predicts a 50% mortality in 1 month.

The best treatment for alcoholic liver disease is total abstinence. Progression of disease and accelerated mortality are likely in patients who continue to drink. It should be emphasized that nutritional needs are to be addressed (protein 1 to 1.5 g/kg/day with caloric needs being 1.2 to $1.4 \times$ resting energy expenditure divided as 50% from carbohydrate and 30% from fat mainly unsaturated). If dietary intake is insufficient, supplements are indicated. A nighttime snack is encouraged. The administration of 50 to 100 mg/day of thiamine along with intravenous (IV) glucose, 100 mg/day of pyridoxine (vitamin B_6), and 1 mg/day of folic acid is often required. Supplementation with phosphorus, magnesium, and potassium are necessary if serum levels are low. Colchicine[1] has no benefits and should not be prescribed. Pentoxifylline (Trental),[1] at a dose of 400 mg every 8 hours for 4 weeks, showed significant survival benefit equivalent to those reported with corticosteroids. Infliximab (Remicade)[1] with corticosteroids increased mortality from infectious complications in one study and should not be administered in acute alcoholic hepatitis.

In acute AH with a DF of 32 or with hepatic encephalopathy, it is recommended to administer 40 mg of prednisone

[1]Not FDA approved for this indication.

or 32 mg of methylprednisolone for 28 days, which can increase survival. A MELD score of 21 is suggested as a cutoff for beginning treatment with steroids. Predictors of the response to corticosteroids are decreasing DF, MELD score, and creatinine and bilirubin levels after 1 week of treatment. If these improvements are not seen, continued steroids are of little benefit. Liver transplantation is the best treatment for advanced alcoholic liver disease. Alcohol abstinence for 6 months is routinely required before transplantation in alcoholics. This time frame can be changed on an individual basis.

AUTOIMMUNE HEPATITIS

The exclusion of replicating hepatitis virus infection together with female sex, hypergammaglobulinemia, and response to immunosuppressive treatment are the hallmarks of an accurate diagnosis of autoimmune hepatitis (AIH). A score based mainly on gender, liver chemistries, immunoglobulins titers, histology, absence of viral hepatitis, and alcohol abuse was created to predict the chance of diagnosing AIH. Liver biopsy, which is essential for diagnosis, management, and prognosis, shows characteristically an increase in plasma cells with interface hepatitis.

AIH can be divided into two categories. In type 1, antibodies to nuclei (ANA) and/or to smooth muscle (SMA) are present. In type 2, anti–liver/kidney microsome-1 (ALKM-1) antibodies are most common. Untreated disease has a mortality rate of 50% at 5 years. Two fundamental goals are distinguished: induction of remission and maintenance of remission. Treatment is guided by the American Association for the Study of Liver Diseases (AASLD) guidelines, which recommend treating active disease and observing closely milder forms; severe disease is considered when aminotransferases are 10 times the normal limit, or five times the normal limit with gammaglobulins that are twice the normal, or if on histology central necrosis or bridging fibrosis is present. Some authors recommend treatment of any symptomatic patient.

The AASLD recommends treatment by corticosteroids alone or in combination with azathioprine (Imuran)[1] for its steroid-sparing effects in patients who are susceptible to the side effects of steroids. For initial induction, adults who are on prednisone alone should be on 60 mg/day and then the dose tapered by 10 mg/week to a dose of 15 to 20 mg/day by 6 months. Prednisone at 20 to 30 mg/day is sufficient if given with azathioprine[1] at a dose of 50 mg/day. Prednisone can be reduced to 15 mg/day in 5-mg decrements every 2 weeks. Once the liver panel is normalized, azathioprine[1] at 50 to 75 mg/day and prednisone at 10 to 20 mg/day are continued, and then prednisone can be decreased to 10 mg/day by 2.5 mg every 3 months. Remission is defined by a decrease by half of the aminotransferase levels and normalization of the bilirubin and the gammaglobulin levels with improvement of the histologic features. In addition to the blood work including immunoglobulins, a liver biopsy, although not required to stop therapy, is essential to confirm complete remission and is helpful in the decision process. Most patients require both drugs for a year, at which time prednisone could be tapered. Ninety percent are responders to this regimen. However, recurrence rates after stopping treatment are as high as 90% and are inversely correlated with the pathology findings. It is for this reason that many patients remain on long-term azathioprine[1] at a dose of 0.5 mg/kg/day.

PRIMARY BILIARY CIRRHOSIS

Primary biliary cirrhosis (PBC) is an autoimmune disease affecting middle-aged women. PBC results in progressive granulomatous destruction of the bile ducts. Manifestations classic of the disease are fatigue, pruritus, osteoporosis, hypercholesterolemia and skin xanthomas, sicca syndrome, vitamin deficiencies, and recurrent urinary tract infections. Most patients with PBC when discovered have no symptoms, and it is often suspected when alkaline phosphatase is elevated. Bilirubin stays in the normal range until late in the progression and is strongly correlated with prognosis. The AMA (antimitochondrial antibody) is positive in 95% of the cases. SMA and ANA can be positive in a third of the patients with PBC. Diagnosis is made by the constellation of cholestatic picture, exclusion of extrahepatic disease, positivity for AMA, and a compatible liver biopsy with granulomatous nonsuppurative cholangitis.

The first-line treatment is ursodeoxycholic acid (UDCA). It is a safe drug that lowers toxic bile acid levels and has a protective effect on the membranes of the liver cells. It is administered at a dose of 13 to 15 mg/kg/day. Cholestatic enzymes can fall to normal or near normal levels, and UDCA can delay disease progression and increase survival. It is a second-line agent for unresponsive pruritus. Although immunosuppressive therapy with methotrexate[1] at 0.25 mg/kg/week and colchicine[1] at 0.6 mg twice daily needs more verification, some authors use it in advanced stages of PBC. Their association with UDCA was additive in some reports.

Pruritus is difficult to manage; in mild cases, skin hydration (emollients and warm baths) with hydroxyzine (Atarax), 25 mg, or cyproheptadine (Periactin), 4 mg every 8 hours, can be sufficient. The first-line therapies for moderate to severe pruritus are cholestyramine (Questran) and colestipol (Colestid). Cholestyramine is taken apart from any other medication. The dose is 4 g before breakfast and dinner, with extra doses to be taken before lunch or bedtime. Second-line therapies for severe pruritus include rifampin (Rifadin),[1] at 300 to 600 mg/day twice daily, phenobarbital,[1] at 120 mg/day, opioid antagonists like naltrexone (ReVia)[1] 10 to 50 mg/day which can lead to significant decrease in the perception of pruritus. In patients who fail to respond, methotrexate,[1] colchicine,[1] sertraline (Zoloft)[1] at 75 mg/day, paroxetine (Paxil)[1] at 20 mg/day, or phototherapy (UVB) could be tried. Because plasmapheresis is inconvenient it is only used when none of the treatments just cited work because it will only give temporary relief. Liver transplantation is the only definitive treatment for severe pruritus.

Hypothyroidism and sicca syndrome associated with PBC should be addressed. Because of chronic cholestasis, fat-soluble vitamin deficiencies (A, D, and K) may occur in PBC. For osteoporosis, the only proven treatment is liver transplant, but vitamin D at 50,000 U/week can prevent

---

[1]Not FDA approved for this indication.

osteopenia and is indicated with calcium at 1 to 1.5 g/day if osteopenia is documented. If levels of 25-hydroxy vitamin D are low, supplementation at a dose of 20 µg/day is ideal. Hormone replacement therapy (HRT) is recommended in postmenopausal women. Calcitonin (Miacalcin) or alendronate (Fosamax) are considered if osteoporosis is documented. If vitamin A, which correlates to retinol-binding protein and albumin and inversely to bilirubin, is low, then 15,000 UI/day should be used; otherwise 5000 UI/day is considered as the maintenance regimen. Vitamin E at a regular dose of 400 IU/day can be supplemented. Vitamin K at 5 to 10 mg/day is only supplemented if the patient has bleeding tendencies that are obvious, which only is present if the patient is on cholestyramine and has advanced liver disease. If the patient has a steatorrhea of more than 40 g/day, then restriction of fat is indicated, with replacement by medium chain fatty acids up to a dose of 60 mL/day (medium-chain triglycerides [MCT] oil, 1 tablespoon three to four times a day).

PRIMARY SCLEROSING CHOLANGITIS (PSC)

PSC is an uncommon disease characterized by progressive diffuse inflammation of the intra- and extrahepatic bile ducts. An estimated 70% to 90% of the patients are men older than 20 years. These ducts are intermittently strictured and dilated. Up to 90% of the cases have ulcerative colitis, less commonly Crohn's disease. PSC harbors a 15% lifetime risk for developing cholangiocarcinoma. No screening for cholangiocarcinoma in patients with PSC is beneficial.

Suggestive symptoms of PSC include right upper quadrant pain, fatigue, pruritus, and jaundice; 25% are asymptomatic. Typically liver tests demonstrate a cholestatic pattern with transaminases less than 300 IU/L. Perinuclear antineutrophil cytoplasmic antibodies (P-ANCA) are associated with 70% of PSC and of inflammatory bowel disease and can be helpful in the diagnosis in difficult cases. Endoscopic retrograde cholangiopancreatography (ERCP) and magnetic resonance cholangiopancreatography (MRCP) confirm the diagnosis by showing the intra- and/or extrahepatic bile strictures, beading, and dilations and ruling out secondary causes of stenosis. Liver biopsy supports the diagnosis and determines the severity of the disease but is unnecessary to make the diagnosis. Typical findings include ductopenic and periductal fibrosis.

Treatment is limited and there are no approved therapies for PSC. Ursodiol (UDCA) at standard doses (12 to 15 mg/kg/day) is not effective and unlike in PBC, UDCA did not show survival improvement in this condition. In the presence of a dominant stricture anywhere in the biliary tree, cytologic brushing should be performed to rule out cholangiocarcinoma. Endoscopic or radiologic dilation or stent placement should be attempted while knowing that the risk of restenosis is 30% to 50% with the same failure rate for reintervention; no survival benefit is shown, but jaundice, pruritus, and liver tests improve significantly. It is recommended to administer antibiotics 1 hour before any hepatobiliary procedure for cholangitis prophylaxis. The treatment of choice for advanced PSC is liver transplantation with 70% to 80% survival at 5 years.

Treatment of pruritus, osteoporosis, steatorrhea, and fat-soluble vitamin deficiencies are the same as those for PBC. No test is recommended for cholangiocarcinoma screening; in suspicious cases, percutaneous guided-needle biopsy is the procedure of choice.

NONALCOHOLIC STEATOHEPATITIS

The majority of cryptogenic cirrhosis is caused by nonalcoholic steatohepatitis (NASH), which presents almost identically as alcoholic hepatitis, with the exception that the patient drinks less than 40 g of alcohol per week. NASH is correlated to obesity and central obesity, insulin resistance, type II diabetes, hyperlipidemia; it is now called the metabolic syndrome. Drugs like corticosteroids, estrogens, tamoxifen, and amiodarone are also associated with NASH. Total parenteral nutrition, rapid weight loss, and starvation can induce NASH. It is often suspected in patients with constantly enlarged liver, unexplained increased levels of aminotransferases, and the presence of a fatty liver on imaging studies. NASH is diagnosed on liver biopsy when steatosis and inflammation are present and after the exclusion of alcoholic, viral, metabolic, and autoimmune hepatitis by their respective laboratory tests. It is now recognized that NASH can progress to cirrhosis in a fourth of the cases. Diabetes, high body mass index (BMI), and fibrosis on diagnosis are predictors of progression. Usually ALT and AST levels are elevated, and unlike in alcoholic liver disease, ALT is the same or greater than AST.

The first-line treatment of NASH is always related to the underlying cause if present. Essentially lowering insulin resistance, which is universal in NASH, targets all components of the metabolic syndrome. Diabetes should be controlled. Weight reduction and exercise are correlated with improvement in liver enzymes. Rapid weight loss, especially after bypass surgeries, is ill advised in those with fibrosis/cirrhosis because it may precipitate liver failure by necroinflammation, portal fibrosis, and bile stasis. Although there is no proven medical therapy for NASH, some small studies encourage the use of insulin-sensitizing agents and antioxidants, either alone or in combination. However, until results from ongoing clinical trials are available, these agents cannot be recommended.

HEMOCHROMATOSIS

Hemochromatosis (HC) is defined as an excessive deposition of iron in major organs such as the liver, kidneys, heart, endocrine glands (pancreas and pituitary), and joints. The main etiology, hereditary HC, results from a genetic mutation on the short arm of chromosome 6. Most patients with clinical HC are homozygous for C282Y, whereas those with only H63D mutations are not at increased risk of liver disease. Most patients are in their 40s or 50s, and cirrhosis develops in more than 60% of the cases. Screening is recommended in persons who are symptomatic (e.g., liver disease, skin pigmentation, diabetes), who are first-degree relatives of patients with hemochromatosis, or who have abnormal iron studies. Fasting iron saturation (total iron-binding capacity [TIBC]) and ferritin levels are the first tests to be done; then genotyping is required if the iron studies are suggestive (TIBC more than 45%) or if the patient is a first-degree relative of a C282Y homozygous patient. In patients who are homozygous and older than 40 years, have signs of

---

[1]Not FDA approved for this indication.

liver disease, or have ferritin levels above 1000 μg/mL, a biopsy is recommended to exclude cirrhosis. A patient with a serum ferritin less than 1000 μg/mL without hepatomegaly and a normal AST is unlikely to have cirrhosis. Conversely, patients with a ferritin greater than 1000 μg/mL, a platelet count less than 200,000, and an elevated AST have a high probability of cirrhosis. Biopsy rules out secondary causes of iron overload (like alcohol or HCV) and assesses the fibrotic changes, which determine the prognosis.

An effective treatment of HC is serial phlebotomies. It is recommended to withdraw 1 U of blood, which contains 200 to 250 mg of iron every week and, if not tolerated, one phlebotomy every 2 to 4 weeks until the patient adapts to blood withdrawal. Once iron stores return to normal, reflected by a serum ferritin level of less than 50 μg/mL and a transferrin saturation of less than 50%, maintenance phlebotomy every 2 to 6 months is done. Hemoglobin should be monitored to avoid anemia. Levels of approximately 10 to 12 g/dL are acceptable.

HC patients must be regularly screened for hepatocellular carcinoma. Most foods are not restricted, except for iron and vitamin C supplements. Vitamin C increases iron absorption and can induce arrhythmias, but fruits and vegetables should not be limited. Daily alcohol consumption is ill advised because it will increase iron absorption, but occasional drinking is permitted in those without advanced liver disease. Liver transplantation is the definitive therapy, but cardiac involvement should be carefully evaluated. Even in acceptable candidates, survival following liver transplantation is reduced compared to most other indications.

WILSON'S DISEASE

Wilson's disease (WD), an autosomal recessive disorder, is the inability to excrete copper into bile properly and to incorporate it into ceruloplasmin (CP), leading first to inappropriate copper accumulation in the liver and later in the eyes, kidneys, and central nervous system. Liver abnormalities in WD are particular for their association with psychiatric and neurologic symptoms like dystonia, tremor, unsteady gait, slurred speech, and drooling because of the involvement of the basal ganglia. Recurrent or chronic low-grade hemolysis can be a presenting manifestation in approximately 10% of the patients.

Diagnosis of WD is confirmed when Kayser-Fleischer (KF) rings are present along with a CP level of less than 20 mg/dL. A ceruloplasmin level under 5 mg/dL or a basal 24-hour urinary copper excretion of more than 100 μg is a strong evidence of WD. If KF rings are absent or CP levels are normal, a liver biopsy should be done. Abnormal liver tests with a 24-hour urinary copper excretion of more than 40 μg with a decreased ceruloplasmin level are also an indication for liver biopsy. On quantitative copper measurement, levels greater than 250 μg/g of dry liver weight are indicative of WD. Neurologic evaluation and MR imaging are recommended prior to treatment in all patients. Screening of first-degree relatives by clinical and biologic means is indicated.

The chelating agents D-penicillamine (Cuprimine) or trientine (Syprine) are initially given at 250 to 500 mg per day, then increased to 1 to 1.5 g a day in four divided doses. Improvement appears 2 to 12 months later, and monitoring is obtained by the 24-hour urinary copper excretion, which should stay above 200 μg. Nonceruloplasmin-bound copper concentration and aminotransferases should normalize with successful treatment. The maintenance regimen is approximately 750 to 1000 mg per day. Supplementation with 25 to 50 mg of pyridoxine is required with D-penicillamine, and iron should not be administered with trientine. Many severe hypersensitivity reactions could limit their use; thus blood counts, liver function tests, creatinine, and urinalysis should be obtained regularly. Zinc gluconate, which eliminates copper from the gut, is given at 50 mg three times a day. It is the first choice for maintenance therapy and can be used in presymptomatic patients. Urinary copper excretion is required for monitoring and should be less than 75 μg in 24 hours. Maintenance therapy is lifelong. Liver and shellfish are the only banned food for patients on initiation of treatment; during maintenance therapy once a week ingestion of these foods is acceptable.

ALPHA₁-ANTITRYPSIN DEFICIENCY

Liver damage is caused by the accumulation of the mutant A_1AT in the hepatocytes. An estimated 10% to 15% of individuals with the homozygous form PiZZ (protease inhibitor phenotype ZZ) eventually develop cirrhosis with older age, Male gender and obesity are the only known predisposing factors. Most patients with liver damage are children. After excluding the most common causes of cirrhosis, diagnosis is done by phenotyping the A_1AT protein and not by measurement of the total A_1AT protein in the serum. Patients with chronic disease should be screened for hepatocellular carcinoma. An effective treatment is liver transplantation with a 5-year survival rate of 80%. Hepatocyte transplantation holds promise in this disease.

Treatment of Complications

Many patients with cirrhosis have no serious outward complications from the disease that are clinically evident. These patients are described as having compensated cirrhosis (Child's class A). For the remaining patients, several classic complications may occur, and this is described as the decompensated state. The onset of the decompensated state may herald a clinical decline with reduced survival compared to the compensated state. The major complications include ascites, bleeding from esophagogastric varices, and hepatic encephalopathy. Other common and serious complications include SBP, hepatorenal syndrome, and hepatocellular carcinoma (Table 4).

ASCITES

Ascites is the most common complication of cirrhosis. In 50% of those with compensated cirrhosis, ascites will develop within 10 years (30% in 5 years). The onset of ascites is associated with a poor prognosis, with ascites associated with a 50% mortality rate at 1 to 2 years, compared to a 10% mortality rate at 1 year in those with compensated cirrhosis. In diuretic responsive ascites, there is a 50% 2-year survival rate, but in those with diuretic-resistant ascites, there is increased mortality with a 50% 6-month survival and a 25% 1-year survival.

Portal hypertension is a prerequisite for the formation of ascites. In response to portal hypertension, there is

TABLE 4 Key Current Treatments

Ascites and peripheral edema	Sodium restriction, spironolactone and furosemide, therapeutic paracentesis with and without albumin infusion, TIPSS, OLT
SBP	Cefotaxime, ceftriaxone, ofloxacin, albumin infusion, discontinue diuretics
SBP prophylaxis	TMP-SMX, norfloxacin, ciprofloxacin
Hepatic encephalopathy	Treat precipitating etiologies, lactulose or Lactinol, metronidazole, rifaximin, or vancomycin, low-protein diet
Bleeding from esophageal/gastric varices	Hemodynamic stabilization, balloon tamponade, vasopressin, octreotide, nitroglycerin, band ligation, sclerotherapy, TIPSS
Esophageal/gastric varices prophylaxis	Propranolol or nadolol, nitrates, sclerotherapy, band ligation, TIPSS, OLT
HRS I	Treat precipitating etiologies, OLT, antibiotics, albumin, midodrine, octreotide, terlipressin, TIPSS
HRS II	Serial paracentesis, diuretics, TIPSS, OLT
Portopulmonary hypertension	Calcium channel blockers, bosentan, isoproterenol
Hepatopulmonary syndrome	OLT
Hepatocellular carcinoma	Surgical resection, OLT, chemoembolization, radiofrequency, irradiation

Abbreviations: HRS = hepatorenal syndrome; OLT = orthotopic liver transplantation; SBP = spontaneous bacterial peritonitis; TIPPS = transjugular intrahepatic portosystemic shunt; TMP-SMX = trimethoprim-sulfamethoxazole.

vasodilation of the arterioles of the splanchnic bed that is mediated by nitric oxide. In response to this vasodilation with decreased effective arterial blood volume, and as a compensatory mechanism, there is activation of the renin-angiotensin system. This leads to significant sodium retention, which, when coupled with an increase in hydrostatic pressure in the portal system and a decrease in oncotic pressure caused by hypoalbuminemia, leads to accumulation of ascitic fluid in the abdomen with ascitic fluid primarily weeping off the surface of the liver into the peritoneal cavity. The formation of ascites secondary to cirrhosis is one of the considerations for liver transplantation.

Clinical examination is unreliable in detecting small amounts of ascites (less than 2 L), especially in obese patients. Therefore US is the ideal test to detect small amounts of peritoneal fluid (as low as 100 mL) and can also be used to determine patency or thrombosis of the hepatic and portal vasculature. A paracentesis should be performed for newly diagnosed ascites and the fluid examined for total protein, cell count, cultures (inoculated at the bedside), and albumin. The serum ascites-albumin gradient (SAAG), determined by subtracting the ascitic fluid albumin from the serum albumin determined at the same time,

confirms the presence of portal hypertension as having a role in the development of ascites with more than 97% accuracy if the gradient is greater than 1.1g/dL. If the total protein in the ascitic fluid is less than 1.1 g/dL, this suggests the patient is at high risk for spontaneous bacterial peritonitis, and prophylaxis should be considered. A polymorphonuclear neutrophil (leukocyte) (PMN) count of greater than 250/mm^3 is essential for diagnosing SBP. Paracentesis carries a small risk of bowel perforation and abdominal wall hematoma (less than 1 in 1000 patients).

Ascites may be graded in severity and treatment can be tailored based on this grade. In 15% of the patients who have mild ascites, sodium restriction to 3 to 5 g/day may be sufficient if they have the ability to excrete this sodium load. For those patients with higher-grade ascites, sodium restriction to 2 g/day is recommended, as well as the initiation of diuretics. Oral spironolactone (Aldactone) is effective in 20% to 50% when used alone; additive effect is obtained when used with furosemide (Lasix). Initial doses are 100 mg and 40 mg daily, respectively, and are given once in the morning. Painful gynecomastia may result from spironolactone, and if this occurs, amiloride (Midamor), 5 to 20 mg/day, or triamterene (Dyrenium), 50 to 100 mg/day, may be substituted. Amiloride is less effective than spironolactone in reducing ascites. The dosage of furosemide and spironolactone can be increased in case of resistance every 3 to 5 days up to a maximum of 160 mg/day for furosemide and 400 mg for spironolactone or 40 mg for amiloride. Tense ascites should be treated first with therapeutic paracentesis followed by administration of diuretics and salt restriction.

A key indicator of response to diuretics is a random spot urine test to see if the ratio of sodium to potassium concentration is greater than 1. If so, then it is 90% certain that the patient is excreting a satisfactory amount of sodium (minimum 78 mmol/day). Urine sodium of less than 10 mEq/day is considered a diuretic-resistant state. A 24-hour urinary sodium more than 78 mmol is the best indicator of adequate natriuresis. The ideal weight loss should be 0.5 kg/day in patients without edema, and 1 kg/day in those with lower extremity edema. If it is observed that there is no weight loss, but patients have a good sodium clearance, then the compliance with sodium restriction must be considered and reviewed with the patient. Inpatient treatment is indicated with significant encephalopathy, bacterial infections, or gastrointestinal (GI) hemorrhage. If patients do not have these complications and are steadily losing weight, they may be followed as outpatients. Fluid restriction to 1.5 L/day may be required with development of severe (sodium less than 125 mmol/L) or symptomatic hyponatremia.

In 10% of cases of ascites, patients do not respond to diuretic therapy, reaccumulate fluid rapidly after paracentesis, or have a contraindication to the use of diuretics (encephalopathy, hyponatremia with the fluid restriction, or a creatinine more than 2 mg/dL). Then two other methods are available: serial paracentesis and transjugular intrahepatic portosystemic stent shunt (TIPSS) placement. Large-volume paracentesis is highly effective and should be followed by diuretics, which lengthen the period of reaccumulation of fluid, and should always be accompanied by cell counts to rule out SBP. Circulatory disturbance and hepatorenal syndrome are potential complications that could be prevented by the infusion of 5 to 10 g of albumin for every liter of ascites drained when removing volumes larger than 5 L.

TIPSS is a radiologically placed shunt that relieves portal hypertension by shunting blood between the portal vein and the hepatic vein. TIPSS is effective in approximately 66% of patients with refractory ascites and has the same survival benefit as serial paracentesis with a decrease in the incidence of HRS. TIPSS is recommended when it becomes necessary to draw fluid more than two times in a month or when it is impractical. The major complication of TIPSS is hepatic encephalopathy (up to 60%); thus it should be recommended with caution in those with Child-Pugh class C or in those with a MELD greater than 19. Other requirements for the successful placement of TIPSS is relatively preserved cardiac function without significant elevation of right-sided heart pressures, patency of the portal vein, and the absence of severe hepatic encephalopathy. Liver transplantation is the definitive treatment for refractory ascites and may be considered for all appropriate candidates. Another treatment for patients ineligible for transplant, TIPSS, and serial paracentesis are peritoneovenous shunts, although infection and long-term patency with these remain a problem.

SPONTANEOUS BACTERIAL PERITONITIS

SBP is the spontaneous proliferation of bacteria in the ascitic fluid in the absence of intra-abdominal source of infection. Hospitalized patients with decompensated cirrhosis have a 10% to 30% chance of having SBP. Once it occurs there is a 20% mortality rate per treated episode (90% if untreated), and SBP recurs in approximately 70% of patients at 1 year. In patients with cirrhosis and ascites, with sudden onset of fever, encephalopathy of unclear etiology, abdominal pain, renal failure, acidosis, or peripheral leukocytosis, there should be high clinical suspicion for SBP, and they should receive immediate antibiotic therapy before the data from the paracentesis and cultures are available. Cirrhotic patients with SBP may also remain clinically silent. All patients with an ascitic fluid with PMN counts above 250/mm^3 must receive empirical antibiotic therapy and be tested in their ascitic fluid for total protein, lactate dehydrogenase (LDH), glucose, and Gram stain to differentiate it from secondary peritonitis. Culture-negative neutrocytic ascites are treated as SBP. Blood and urine cultures should be done, and ascitic fluid cultures should always be in blood culture bottles at the patient's bedside. Aerobic gram-negative organisms account for 70% of the cases, with *Escherichia coli* and *Klebsiella* species predominating. Gram-positive cocci are present in 30% of the cases, with streptococci dominating. Anaerobic organisms are rare, and when isolated they should raise the suspicion of secondary peritonitis from a perforated viscus.

The treatments of choice for SBP are the third-generation cephalosporins cefotaxime (Claforan), at a dose of 2 g IV every 8 hours, and ceftriaxone (Rocephin), at 1 g every 12 hours for 5 days. Aminoglycosides should not be used because of increased nephrotoxicity. For atypical presentations a paracentesis should be considered after 48 hours and a PMN count performed again. In SBP, the PMN count should be 50% of its previous level, whereas in other sources of peritonitis, the PMN count may be higher or unchanged. Alternatively, the patient may take oral ofloxacin (Floxin) if the patient has no vomiting, shock, or hemorrhage, has a

creatinine of less than 3 mg/dL and no or mild encephalopathy. Albumin infusion at a rate of 1.5 g/kg of body weight within 6 hours after starting antibiotic treatment and readministered on the third day of treatment at 1 g/kg decreases mortality after an episode of SBP. All diuretics should be stopped during infection.

The incidence of recurrent SBP may be reduced by administration of prophylactic antibiotics. Norfloxacin (Noroxin),[1] at 400 mg/day, or trimethoprim-sulfamethoxazole (TMX) (Bactrim), at one double-strength tablet daily for 5 days a week, are indicated for prophylaxis in patients who already had an episode of SBP and those who have ascitic protein levels less than 1 g/dL on diagnostic paracentesis. Norfloxacin prophylaxis has reduced SBP occurrence by 60% and is highly cost effective. Ciprofloxacin (Cipro), at a dose of 750 mg once weekly, is also efficacious. For patients admitted to the hospital for cirrhosis and GI hemorrhage, norfloxacin,[1] at 400 mg twice a day, ofloxacin, 400 mg/day or TMX, one tablet twice a day for 7 days, decreases infection rates and prolongs survival.

ESOPHAGEAL VARICES

Patients with cirrhosis should be screened for varices when first diagnosed and then every 3 years until found. Refer to the article on esophageal varices in this volume for more information.

ENCEPHALOPATHY

HE is characterized by neuropsychiatric abnormalities that are primarily caused by nitrogenous products, endogenous ligands for benzodiazepines, and other unknown toxins released by bacteria from the colon that are incompletely metabolized by the cirrhotic liver or bypass the liver because of portal hypertension and portosystemic shunting. HE can develop in 28% of cirrhotic patients within 10 years of the diagnosis of cirrhosis and portal hypertension. Older age and severity of cirrhosis are the only known factors to predict the risk of developing HE. HE has five stages for its severity: Stage 0 is normal or only features abnormal results on psychometric tests, referred to as minimal HE, and stage 4 represents the most severe form with deep coma (Table 5).

Precipitating causes of HE include infection (usually urinary tract, pneumonia, or SBP), renal insufficiency, GI bleed, hypokalemia, excess protein in the diet, use of sedatives such as benzodiazepines and other tranquilizers and sedatives, constipation or noncompliance with lactulose, portal vein thrombosis, further hepatic parenchymal damage, hepatocellular carcinoma, and recent TIPSS placement. When assessing a mental status change in a patient with cirrhosis, other causes of motor and mental disturbance other than hepatic encephalopathy should be investigated. CT of the head must be obtained if there is any neurologic sign concerning an intracranial lesion.

Most cases of HE are preventable, and recognition of the precipitating causes just described will help prevent this complication. Lactulose (Cephulac), at 30 to 60 g/day, titrated to achieve a goal of three to four soft bowel movements a day with a pH less than 6, is effective in

---

[1]Not FDA approved for this indication.

TABLE 5 Grades and Clinical Manifestations of Hepatic Encephalopathy

Encephalopathy Grade	Level of Consciousness	Mental Status	Neurologic Signs	EEG Abnormalities
0	Normal	Normal	None	None
Subclinical	Normal	Normal	Psychometric tests may be abnormal	None
1	Day-night reversal, restlessness	Forgetful, mild confusion, Irritable	Tremor, apraxia, impaired handwriting	Triphasic waves (5 cycles/s)
2	Lethargy	Disorientation to time, inappropriate behavior	Asterixis, ataxia, dysarthria	Triphasic waves (5 cycles/s)
3	Somnolent, confused	Disorientation to time, inappropriate behavior	Asterixis, hyperreflexia, Babinski signs	Triphasic waves (5 cycles/s)
4	Coma	None	Decerebration	Delta activity

Abbreviation: EEG = electroencephalogram.

90% of the patients. Lactinol is slightly better tolerated. Excessive use leading to diarrhea is to be avoided because it can lead to prerenal azotemia and other electrolyte imbalances. In patients who have profound HE and are unable to take medications orally, Lactinol and lactulose can be administered via a nasogastric tube or as enemas at a dose of 300 mL in 700 mL of tap water two to three times a day with a response in 4 to 6 hours. Opiate analgesics, calcium, and iron supplements can all exacerbate HE and should be avoided. Also oral nonabsorbable antibiotics such as metronidazole (Flagyl),[1] at 250 mg three times a day, rifaximin (Xifaxan),[1] at 400 mg two to three times a day, and vancomycin (Vancocin),[1] at 2 g/day, can help alleviate HE in the remaining 10% of cases resistant to disaccharides. Because of renal toxicity, neomycin should be avoided. In severe HE, oral intake should be held. In milder forms, protein intake should be titrated by increasing the protein intake by 10 g/day over 3 to 5 days starting from 20 g/day to a maximum dose of 80 g/day depending on individual tolerances. Avoidance of negative nitrogen balance is crucial. An infusion of dextrose helps decrease protein catabolism. For chronic HE, lactulose and moderate protein restriction to 0.8 g/kg/day are recommended.

HEPATORENAL SYNDROME

Approximately 40% of patients with cirrhosis and ascites will develop HRS within 5 years. This complication occurs when there is avid continuous sodium retention with dilutional hyponatremia and activation of the renin-angiotensin system, in the setting of ineffective arterial blood flow because of splanchnic vasodilation. Initially, renal perfusion is maintained because of renal vasodilatation that is mediated by prostaglandins. With progressive disease, renal vasoconstriction occurs in response to arterial vasodilation, leading to reduction of renal blood flow and the glomerular filtration rates with subsequent hepatorenal syndrome.

[1]Not FDA approved for this indication.

A common precipitant of HRS is the use of nonsteroidal anti-inflammatory drugs (NSAIDs). Patients with ascites should scrupulously avoid other nephrotoxic agents such as aminoglycosides. Other precipitants are aggressive use of diuretics with volume depletion, large-volume paracentesis without albumin infusion, SBP, and sepsis. In the diagnosis of HRS, several key criteria are almost always present (Table 6).

There are two clinical types of hepatorenal syndrome, type I and type II. In type I there is a decrease of more than 50% in creatinine clearance to less than 20 mL/minute or a doubling of the creatinine level to more than 2.5 mg/dL in 2 weeks. The prognosis for type I HRS is dismal, with 80% mortality within 2 weeks after diagnosis. Type II is a more progressive form and can evolve into type I. In type II the renal deterioration does not fulfill the criteria for type I and it presents in the form of refractory ascites. Survival is 50% in type II after 6 months.

Clinical management of these patients includes an investigation for a precipitating cause, including infection such as SBP, bacteremia, or catheter-related bacteremia, and appropriate cultures should be sent. Broad-spectrum antibiotics should be started irrespective of proof of infection.

The most successful treatment for HRS is liver transplantation, with survival rates greater than 80% over 1 year. The next most effective treatment for type I HRS is albumin

TABLE 6 Diagnostic Criteria for Hepatorenal Syndrome as Proposed by the International Ascites Club

1. Serum creatinine >1.5 mg/dL indicating low glomerular filtration rate
2. Exclusion of shock, volume depletion, bacterial infection, nephrotoxic drugs
3. Failure to improve with discontinuing diuretics, volume expansion with 1.5 L normal saline
4. No evidence of proteinuria, obstruction, parenchymal renal disease

infusion (20 to 40 g/day for 20 days) with concomitant arterial vasoconstrictors. Midodrine (ProAmatine), titrated to 7.5 to 15 mg three times a day for 20 days, to achieve an increase in mean arterial blood pressure of 15 mm Hg in combination with octreotide (Sandostatin),[1] at a dose of 100 to 300 μg subcutaneously three times a day, improves renal function in selected patients with type 1 HRS in small uncontrolled trials. Similarly, terlipressin,[2] a synthetic analogue of vasopressin, infused at 0.5 to 2 mg over 4 to 6 hours for 15 days, increases the glomerular filtration rate (GFR) in up to 75% of the patients. TIPS can improve creatinine clearance and survival in well-selected patients with MELD scores less than 18. It is reasonable in patients not eligible for or awaiting liver transplantation. TIPSS in combination with midodrine, octreotide,[1] and albumin may have some benefit in HRS patients. Type II HRS is treated as refractory ascites in an outpatient setting.

HEPATOPULMONARY SYNDROME

HPS is defined in patients with cirrhosis as the increase in the alveolar-arterial gradient on room air and the documentation of intrapulmonary vascular dilations, which cause right to left shunting corrected partially by oxygen at 100%. It is associated with spider angiomata and presents as platypnea and orthodeoxia. Diagnosis is confirmed by contrast-enhanced echocardiography or technetium-labeled macroaggregated albumin scanning. The only treatment in highly selected populations is liver transplantation.

PORTOPULMONARY HYPERTENSION

Portopulmonary hypertension (PPHTN) is characterized by a mean pulmonary artery pressure measured by cardiac catheterization above 25 mm Hg on rest with a pulmonary capillary wedge pressure less than 15 mm Hg, a pulmonary vascular resistance (PVR) greater than 120 dynes/second/cm-5, and the presence of portal hypertension without any other secondary cause of pulmonary hypertension. Clinical manifestations are similar to those with primary PHTN. Treatment with calcium channel blockers is indicated if the patient has more than 20% reduction in mPAP during the trial with vasodilators on cardiac catheterization. Bosentan (Tracleer), at 62.5 mg per day for 4 weeks, increased thereafter to 125 mg daily, improves symptoms and exercise capacity. Preoperatively, Epoprostenol (Flolan) is given at 10 to 28 μg/kg/mm³ for a few months to decrease the mPAP to levels acceptable for liver transplantation. Liver transplantation may reverse minor or moderate degrees of pulmonary hypertension but is contraindicated in patients with pulmonary hypertension above 40 to 45 mm Hg because of high postoperative mortality related to cardiac failure.

HEPATOCELLULAR CARCINOMA

Patients with cirrhosis, regardless of etiology, have an increased risk for the development of HCC. An estimated 10% to 15% of patients with cirrhosis develop HCC after 10 years of diagnosis with a median survival of 6 to 20 months. Selected patients who successfully undergo orthotopic liver transplantation (OLT) for HCC have survival rates equal to those without HCC.

Screening for HCC is best accomplished by measuring serum alpha fetoprotein (AFP) and abdominal US every 6 months. Because of a sensitivity ranging between 20% and 65% (depending on the cutoff value), AFP is not proven to improve the outcome in cirrhotics from HCC. The positive predictive value for AFP levels above 20 or for a suspicious lesion on ultrasound is low; therefore imaging with triple-phase helical CT, MRI, or magnetic resonance angiography is indicated if any one of these two situations is present. These imaging modalities can reliably diagnose HCC if tumors are greater than 2 cm and there is an arterial enhancing lesion seen on two of the imaging tests just cited or seen on one test with an AFP level above 400 μg/mL. In these cases a biopsy is not required. Suspicious lesions between 1 and 2 cm should be biopsied by fine-needle aspiration (FNA), which does not worsen the outcome from tumor seeding along the needle tack, and tumors less than 1 cm should be monitored by repeat scanning every 3 months until they grow above 1 cm. Des-gamma-carboxy prothrombin (DCP) and lectin reactive AFP (AFP-L3)-to-AFP ratio are tumor markers that are measured alone or in combination with AFP and can increase the sensitivity and specificity of HCC screening.

Treatment of HCC is approached in an algorithmic fashion with surgery the ultimate goal because it is the only curative treatment. A tumor is resectable when it is confined to the liver and shows no vascular invasion and no portal hypertension. Size alone should not influence the decision. General performance of the patient, tumor stage, and assessment of liver function determine if the procedure is practical (Child's class A) or not (Child's class B/C). Prior to resection, a search for metastatic disease should be undertaken. Ninety percent of cirrhotic patients with HCC have decompensation of their cirrhosis, which contraindicates surgical resection. With earlier detection of HCC there is greater likelihood of successful outcomes with transplantation. To be a candidate for liver transplantation, the patient must have no vascular invasion, no metastatic disease, no lymphatic spread, and no more than three suspected lesions in the liver. If there are multiple lesions in the liver, all must be less than 3 cm in diameter; if only one lesion is present, it must be less than 5 cm in diameter. A major drawback of liver transplantation is long waiting times for cadaveric donor matching.

Other alternative therapies include chemoembolization, ethanol or acetic acid injection into the tumor, radiofrequency ablation, and irradiation with intra-arterial yttrium-tagged microspheres. All patients should be considered candidates for some kind of intervention. These therapies should be considered palliative, although survival for radiofrequency ablation and percutaneous ethanol injection may approach survival in surgical resection for tumors less than 3 cm. Any approach can be considered in nonresectable tumors depending on the team preferences and/or local expertise. Chemotherapy is only indicated in the context of a clinical trial.

Prevention of the development of HCC is also possible: Hepatitis B vaccine has decreased the incidence of HCC by a third in highly infected areas. Also in clinical trials for the treatment of chronic hepatitis C with interferon-based therapies, studies have suggested that patients with compensated liver cirrhosis, whether or not they

---

[1]Not FDA approved for this indication.
[2]Not available in the United States.

have a sustained response, may have reduction of their risk of HCC.

Other Considerations

VACCINATION

Hepatitis A and B vaccines should be given to all patients with chronic liver disease who are found to be nonimmune to these viruses. Pneumonia and SBP because of streptococcal pneumonia are very common in cirrhotic patients; thus all patients in this population should receive a single dose of the polyvalent pneumococcal vaccine. An annual injection of the influenza vaccine protects against influenza.

LIVER TRANSPLANTATION

Liver transplantation (LT) is the definitive treatment for a variety of irreversible problems associated with chronic liver disease. Patients with Child's class B, and those with complications from cirrhosis such as refractory ascites, variceal bleeding, and any other condition that is irreversible and progressive should be referred early for liver transplantation evaluation. HRS type 1 and HPS should expedite the referral for transplantation. The MELD score was developed to replace the Child-Pugh score as a disease severity score. A score of more than 10 is an indication for referral to a transplantation center. The MELD score (for calculation, visit www.unos.org/resources/MeldPeldCalculator.asp?index=98) is designed to improve the organ allocation system, so that available organs are directed to patients based on the severity of their liver disease rather than on the total time on the waiting list. Contraindications for liver transplantation depend on the local approach, but universal contraindications are high perioperative risk (e.g., severe cardiac failure), uncontrolled malignancies within the previous 5 years, and active alcohol or drug abuse. LT offers an overall 5-year survival rate of greater than 60% to 70%.

REFERENCES

Boyer TD, Haskal ZJ: The role of transjugular intrahepatic portosystemic shunt in the management of portal hypertension. Hepatology 2005;41:386-400.

Cardenas A, Gines P: Management of complications of cirrhosis in patients awaiting liver transplantation. J Hepatology 2005;42:S124-S133.

Czaja AJ, Freese DK: Diagnosis and treatment of autoimmune hepatitis. Hepatology 2002;36:479-497.

D'Amico G, Luca A, Morabito A, et al: Uncovered transjugular intrahepatic portosystemic shunt for refractory ascites: A meta-analysis. Gastroenterology 2005;129:1282-1293.

Levitsky J, Mailliard ME: Diagnosis and therapy of alcoholic liver disease. Semin Liver Dis 2004;24:233-247.

Moore KP, Wong F, Gines P, et al: The management of ascites in cirrhosis: Report on the consensus conference of the International Ascites Club. Hepatology 2003;38:258-266.

Murray KF, Carithers RL Jr: AASLD Practice Guidelines: Evaluation of the patient for liver transplantation. Hepatology 2005;41:1407-1432.

Runyon BA: Management of adult patients with ascites due to cirrhosis. Hepatology 2004;39:841-856.

Sanyal AJ: AGA technical review on nonalcoholic fatty liver disease. Gastroenterology 2002;123:1705-1725.

Tavill AS: Diagnosis and management of hemochromatosis. Hepatology 2001;33:1321-1328.

Bleeding Esophageal Varices

Method of
Gary C. Chen, MD, and Rome Jutabha, MD

Esophageal variceal bleeding, which is a consequence of portal hypertension, is one of the most dreadful complications of liver cirrhosis. It accounts for approximately one third of diagnoses in patients presenting with upper gastrointestinal (GI) bleeding. Despite the significant advances and improvements in the early diagnosis and treatment for esophageal variceal bleeding, the mortality rate of first episode of esophageal variceal bleeding remains very high (20% to 35%). In patients with liver cirrhosis, the prevalence of esophageal varices is approximately 60%, but newer studies with better endoscopic assessment and longer periods of follow-up suggested the prevalence could be as high as 80% to 90%. Cirrhotic patients with esophageal varices without previous variceal bleeding have a 25% to 40% chance of first variceal hemorrhage when they do not receive effective prophylactic treatment. The risk of first variceal bleeding is significantly related to the patient's Child-Pugh class, the size and wall thickness of the varices, the presence of red markings of varices observed at the time of endoscopy, and the hepatic venous pressure gradient (HVPG) or intravariceal pressure. Management of patients with esophageal varices includes prevention of the first bleeding episode (primary prophylaxis), control of actively bleeding esophageal varices, and the prevention of recurrent esophageal variceal bleeding (secondary prophylaxis).

The Child-Pugh classification system is a scoring index of liver dysfunction in cirrhotic patients (Table 1). This classification is based on the measurement of serum bilirubin level, serum albumin level, prothrombin time, and the presence of ascitic fluids and encephalopathy. For example, a patient with Child-Pugh class C cirrhosis who has red marking on large-size varices has an estimated 60% likelihood of variceal bleeding over a 2-year span. In contrast, a patient with Child-Pugh class A cirrhosis, no or small size varices, and esophageal varices without red markings would be at a much lower risk of developing variceal bleeding.

Elevated pressure within the portal venous system also increases the risk of variceal bleeding. Normal portal vein pressure is less than 10 mm Hg because the vascular

TABLE 1 Child-Pugh Classification System of Liver Disease Severity Index

Parameter	Points		
	1	*2*	*3*
Serum bilirubin, mg/dL	≤ 2	2–3	> 3
Serum albumin, g/dL	> 3.5	2.8–3.5	< 2.8
Prothrombin, sec	1–3	4–6	> 6
Ascites	Absent	Slight	Moderate
Encephalopathy	None	Grade 1–2	Grade 3–4

5–6 points = Grade A (compensated liver disease, 1-year survival is 100%).
7–9 points = Grade B (significantly functional compromised liver disease, 1-year survival is 80%).
10–15 points = Grade C (decompensated liver disease, 1-year survival is 45%).

resistance in the hepatic sinusoids is low. An elevated portal venous pressure distends the veins proximal to the site of the block and increases capillary pressure in organs drained by the obstructed veins. The HVPG is used to directly and accurately measure the portal venous pressure. This measurement is obtained by using a pressure-sensitive balloon-tipped catheter usually inserted via the transjugular route to measure pressures within the hepatic veins. The HVPG can serve as an important factor for predicting variceal bleeding. Normal HVPG is 2 to 6 mm Hg. Patients with HVPG greater than 12 mm Hg are considered having portal hypertension. A study that followed 87 patients with cirrhosis and large-size esophageal varices but without previous history of bleeding esophageal varices over a 1-year period found that 72% of the patients with HVPG greater than 16 mm Hg developed variceal bleeding. However, in patients who have presinusoidal portal hypertension such as portal or splenic vein thrombosis and schistosomiasis, HVPG can underestimate the portal venous pressure. Furthermore, measurement of the HVPG requires an invasive technique; hence, it is not commonly adopted in the clinical setting.

Nonetheless, the combination of these clinical predictors can be used to classify a patient's risk of developing bleeding esophageal varices. The mortality rate of patients with bleeding esophageal varices is 20% to 30% within 1 year after the initially hemorrhagic episode. Furthermore, there is a 70% chance of a second episode of bleeding from esophageal varices in patients who have had an episode of variceal bleeding within 1 year of the bleeding episode if left untreated. In other words, once a patient develops variceal bleeding, the risks of recurrent variceal bleeding and mortality increase. Therefore, it is logical to screen for and offer the high-risk cirrhotic patients safe and effective medical or endoscopic treatments to prevent the first episode of esophageal variceal bleeding.

Acute Bleeding From Esophageal Varices

Bleeding esophageal varices is one of the common causes of upper GI hemorrhage. It accounts for an estimated one third of diagnoses in patients presenting with upper GI bleeding. In 1985 the diagnosis of bleeding esophageal varices accounted for approximately 62,000 total hospital days in nonfederal, short-stay hospitals in the United States and was without a doubt the most expensive of all GI disorders in terms of average daily cost of hospitalization ($1091/day). Patients with bleeding esophageal varices tend to present with hematemesis and melena. Often there is evidence of large amount volume of bleeding because the high portal pressures precipitate the rupture of esophageal varices. Relevant history of chronic liver disease and thorough physical examination yielding the stigmata of liver cirrhosis can help guide clinicians toward the correct diagnosis. However, clinicians must remember that although esophageal varices are the most common cause of upper GI bleeding in cirrhotic patients requiring emergent endoscopy, peptic ulcer disease, gastric varices, Mallory-Weiss tears, and portal hypertensive gastropathy are also frequent causes of upper GI bleeding in this group of patients. In patients with active bleeding esophageal varices, only approximately half of the patients stop bleeding spontaneously, which is significantly lower than other forms of upper GI bleeding. In addition, more than 50% of the patients will have recurrent bleeding within the first week of the initial bleeding episode.

Because bleeding esophageal varices is a life-threatening medical emergency, patients with bleeding esophageal varices require immediate medical attention with admission to the hospital. All patients with hemodynamic instability (shock, orthostatic hypotension, decrease in hematocrit of at least 6%, or transfusion requirement more than 2 units of packed red blood cell (RBCs) or active bleeding (manifested by hematemesis, bright red blood per nasogastric tube, or hematochezia) should be admitted to the intensive care unit for resuscitation and close monitoring with automated blood pressure monitoring, ECG monitoring, and pulse oximetry. Because signs such as hypotension and/or tachycardia are often found in the patient, hemodynamic resuscitation is the vital first step in the treatment process. Endotracheal intubation should be considered for the severely encephalopathic, uncooperative, or unconscious patient, if the airway could be compromised, to provide adequate ventilation and prevent aspiration. Nasogastric or orogastric tube lavage should be performed to remove particulate matter, fresh blood, and clots to facilitate anticipated endoscopy examination and to decrease the risk of aspiration. Two large-bore intravenous (IV) catheters that are at least 18 gauge in size should be established. For hypotensive patients the IV catheters should be running wide open; and a central catheter should be established as well, in case pressor medications need to be initiated. It is important to remember that the initial hematocrit level poorly reflects the degree of blood loss if the bleeding is acute. Therefore, estimating the patient's volume loss could be more useful in assessing an acutely bleeding patient. Blood loss should be aggressively replaced by packed RBCs to maintain hematocrit above 30%. Patient's hemoglobin and hematocrit should be followed every 2 to 6 hours depending on the status of the patient. Platelet count should be kept above 50,000/mm^3 while the patient is actively bleeding. Desmopressin acetate (DDAVP), which is a synthetic analogue of vasopressin, can be considered in patients with concurrent renal failure in which uremia can lead to platelet dysfunction. End-stage liver disease patients often have at least some degree of coagulopathy, so transfusion of clotting factors with fresh frozen plasma should be performed if necessary. The goal is to maintain international normalized ratio (INR) less than 1.5 in these patients. Small-scale studies have suggested that recombinant human factor VIIa could assist in the treatment of coagulopathy by enhancing the normalization of serum prothrombin time. Subcutaneous (SC) administration of vitamin K can be considered if the patient is at risk for vitamin K deficiency, if the bleeding episode does not stop acutely, or if the patient has abnormal prothrombin time. It should be given at 5 to 10 mg SC/day. Three doses of vitamin K administration should adequately replenish a patient's vitamin K supply. It is also important to hold all nonsteroidal anti-inflammatory medications, anticoagulants, sucralfate, antacids, iron supplements, and food during the bleeding episode.

A synthetic and long-acting analogue of somatostatin, IV octreotide should be given if bleeding esophageal varices is suspected to assist in the reduction of portal venous pressure by indirectly causing splanchnic vasoconstriction and decreased portal flow. It can stop variceal bleeding in up to 80% of the cases. Intravenous octreotide is given as an initial 50 µg bolus followed by continuous infusion of 50 µg/hour. A higher dose of octreotide does not appear to further the lowering of portal venous pressure and perhaps could lead to elevation of systemic venous pressure. Its safety profile is generally excellent with abdominal discomfort and elevated serum glucose that can occasionally occur in patients receiving this medication. Intravenous vasopressin is an alternative medication that reduces portal pressure by directly constricting the mesenteric arterioles and decreasing portal venous inflow. It is administered by an IV bolus of 0.4 U followed by 0.4 to 0.8 U/minute infusions. Unfortunately, vasopressin is associated with potential serious side effects including myocardial, bowel, and limb ischemia because of its systemic vasoconstrictive effects. Administering nitroglycerin by IV is recommended concurrently along with vasopressin to counter the vasopressin-induced systemic vasoconstriction effect. It is administered at a rate of 10 to 40 µg/minute. We use octreotide over vasopressin in the setting of acute bleeding esophageal varices because of the lower risk of adverse events. The optimal duration of octreotide or vasopressin is unclear, but we recommend either drug to be continued for 2 to 3 days after the esophageal variceal bleeding episode is adequately controlled. Because patients with bleeding esophageal varices are at risk of having concurrent peptic ulcer disease or developing stress-induced peptic ulcers, administration of proton pump inhibitor medication is also recommended.

Another important aspect of managing this group of patients is to prevent and decrease the impact of complications associated with bleeding esophageal varices. A patient likely could achieve hemostasis but only to succumb to the associated complications such as infections including aspiration pneumonia, bacterial peritonitis, urinary tract infection, sepsis; hepatic encephalopathy; and renal failure because of acute tubular necrosis or hepatorenal syndrome. Cirrhotic patients who are hospitalized with a GI hemorrhage tend to be at high risk for developing infections. Therefore, it is reasonable to provide prophylactic antibiotic coverage in this group of patients. Most experts tend to use a fluoroquinolone class antibiotic such as ciprofloxacin or levofloxacin for 5 to 7 days total, initially administered by IV and followed by oral route. However, physicians should take the local patterns of antibiotic resistance into consideration when choosing the antibiotic regimen. Furthermore, it is important to elevate the head of the patient's bed to more than 30 degrees to decrease the risk of aspiration. Hepatic encephalopathy should be treated with lactulose to induce three loose bowel movements each day. Close monitoring of the stool output of patients with hepatic encephalopathy is important because too much watery diarrhea from lactulose can deplete these patients intravascularly, whereas too few bowel movements can worsen the encephalopathy. In terms of renal failure, it can be minimized by adequate hydration of the patient as well as avoidance of nephrotoxic drugs.

Esophagogastrodudenoscopic therapy is the definitive treatment of choice for bleeding esophageal varices; therefore, this procedure should be performed once the patient is hemodynamically stable for endoscopy exam. Endoscopy is also highly sensitive and specific for locating and identifying bleeding lesions in the upper GI tract. Modern endoscopic therapies can achieve hemostasis in up to 90% of the cases. Combining endoscopic and pharmacologic therapies has made great strides in decreasing the mortality of esophageal variceal bleeding. A complete and thorough endoscopic examination is necessary to rule out other etiologies of upper GI hemorrhage. Bleeding esophageal varices are confirmed on endoscopy if there is active bleeding from esophageal varices, a platelet plug is found on the surface of the varix, or varices are present and no other source of hemorrhage is found. Two types of endoscopic treatments can be carried out: endoscopic band ligation (Figure 1) and endoscopic sclerotherapy (Figure 2), with endoscopic band ligation as the recommended treatment option. Endoscopic band ligation is carried out by placing elastic rubber bands around the esophageal varices located in the distal portion of the esophagus. Endoscopic sclerotherapy involves the injection of a form of sclerosant into the esophageal varices. Both types of treatment measures have similar efficacy in terms of achieving hemostasis, but one study suggested band ligation has better long-term outcome. Sclerotherapy's advantages are that it is easy to use, more widely available, and a less costly procedure to perform. However, endoscopic band ligation is the preferred method mainly because it has lower risk of procedural associated complications. The potential complications of endoscopic sclerotherapy include local ulceration or bleeding, esophageal stricture formation, esophageal perforation, mediastinitis, and aspiration pneumonia. However, some endoscopists still prefer endoscopic sclerotherapy because of the ability to visualize bleeding sites, and because the application of band ligation can sometimes make the endoscopic field difficult to visualize. Endoscopists should also evaluate whether the patient has evidence of portal hypertensive gastropathy, because both treatments could potentially

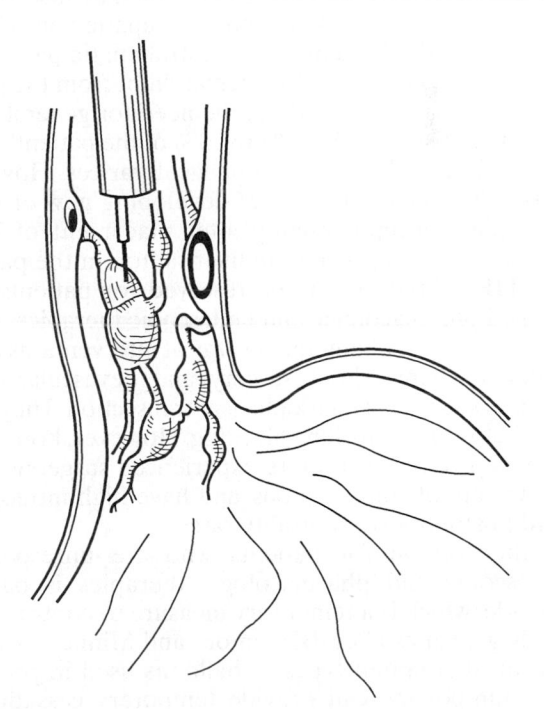

FIGURE 1. Endoscopic band ligation performed with a flexible endoscope. A varix is aspirated into the device using endoscopic suction and ensnared with an elastic band. (From Schaefer J. In GI/Liver Secrets. Philadelphia, Hanley and Belfus, 1996, p 355. Reprinted with permission.)

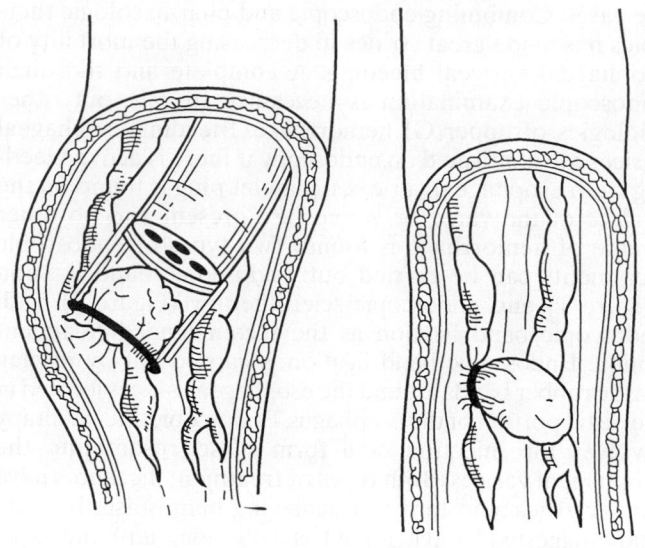

FIGURE 2. Endoscopic sclerotherapy performed with a flexible endoscope. A flexible injection needle is used to inject sclerosant into the varix. (From Schaefer J. In GI/Liver Secrets. Philadelphia, Hanley and Belfus, 1996, p 355. Reprinted with permission.)

worsen this condition and increase the risk of bleeding from the stomach.

Unfortunately, emergent endoscopic therapy fails to control acute esophageal variceal bleeding in 15% to 20% of patients. Furthermore, early rebleeding can occur after a bleeding-free period of at least 24 hours. In these circumstances the patient may require a transjugular intrahepatic portosystemic shunt (TIPS) or, in rare cases, surgical intervention to decrease portal venous pressure to control bleeding. The TIPS procedure is performed by inserting an expandable wire mesh stent into the hepatic vein via the jugular vein and advancing to the intrahepatic part of the hepatic vein, creating a portosystemic shunt from the portal vein to the hepatic vein without the need for general anesthesia or major surgery. In 80% to 90% of the patients, TIPS can control acute bleeding esophageal varices. However, there is a 30% increased risk of developing new or worsening hepatic encephalopathy after placement of TIPS. In addition it could precipitate liver failure in the patient. Hence, TIPS should solely be reserved for patients who have failed pharmacologic and endoscopic therapies. There are two main types of emergent surgical interventions available: portosystemic shunt surgery and devascularization procedures such as distal esophageal transection. They both seem effective in controlling bleeding. However, both types of surgical procedures require experienced surgeons, have a wide variety of complications, and have high intraoperative and postoperative mortality rates.

Another option for patients who are unresponsive to endoscopic and pharmacologic therapies is balloon tamponade, which is a temporary measure to control acute hemorrhage. Sengstaken-Blakemore and Minnesota tubes are the most common types of balloons used in practice. Balloon tamponade can provide temporary cessation of active bleeding in 30% to 90% of the cases, with rebleeding occurring in 50% of the cases after the balloon is deflated. The balloon typically has three parts: a gastric balloon, an esophageal balloon, and a gastric suction port. Once the tube is inserted into the patient, the gastric balloon is

inflated first, once the tube reaches the stomach, and drawn up against the gastroesophageal junction and secured in place. If this maneuver still does not control bleeding, the esophageal balloon is inflated with tension applied to the tube to directly tamponade the esophageal varices. A nasogastric tube should be placed concurrent with this procedure to prevent tracheal aspiration. This procedure requires experienced endoscopists to perform, because it is associated with significant complications including esophageal rupture, esophageal perforation, local ulceration, tracheal aspiration, and accidentally misplacing the tube into the airway. Given the high risk of complications, patients should have endotracheal intubation and mechanical ventilation support before undergoing the balloon tamponade procedure. Balloon tamponade should only be a temporary measure, and patients should have TIPS or surgical interventions performed as soon as possible (Figure 3).

Prevention of Recurrent Esophageal Variceal Bleeding

A history of bleeding esophageal varices is the best predictor of future esophageal variceal bleeding. The risk of rebleeding is 60% to 70% without further therapy after the initial bleeding episode is controlled. The risk of rebleeding is the highest in the first 6 weeks after cessation of active bleeding. The clinical predictors used to classify a patient's risk of

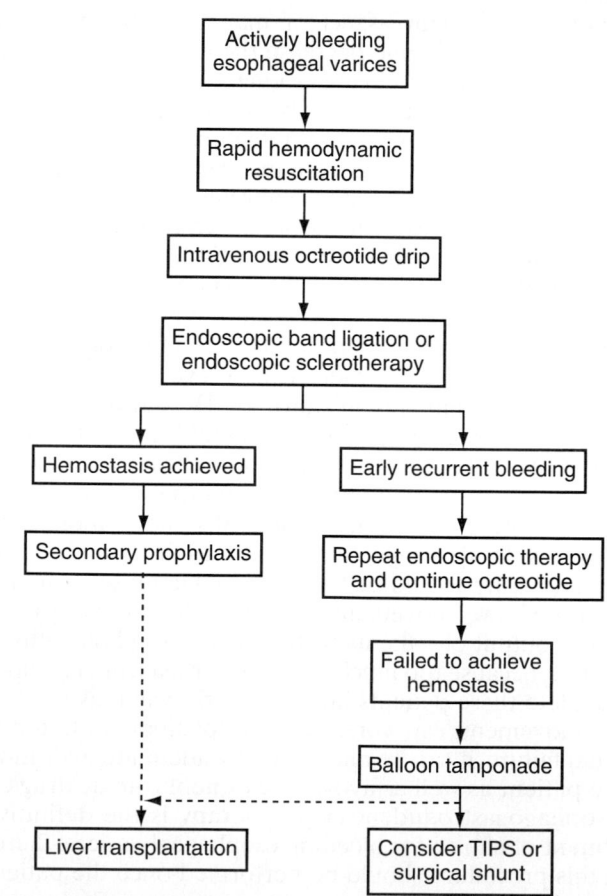

FIGURE 3. Recommended algorithm for the management of acute bleeding esophageal varices. TIPS = transjugular intrahepatic portosystemic shunt.

developing initial bleeding esophageal varices mentioned earlier can also be used to predict the risk of recurrent bleeding. Therefore, secondary prophylaxis is important to decrease the risk of rebleeding. Several treatment options are available to prevent recurrent bleeding including pharmacologic, endoscopic, surgical, TIPS, and orthotopic liver transplantation. Nonselective β-blockers such as nadolol and propranolol can decrease portal pressure and variceal blood flow. Patients who can tolerate nonselective β-blockers may start propranolol at 20 mg twice a day, or nadolol at 40 mg once a day, gradually titrating the medication dosage up until heart rate decreases by 20% to 30% or reaches 55 to 60 beats per minute. Nadolol has the advantage of being once-a-day dosing, because patient compliance can be an issue in some cirrhotic patients; however, it is a more expensive medication and less widely available. Titrating the dosage of nonselective β-blockers based on the HVPG has been evaluated by studies and appeared more effective than titration of the dosage based on heart rate alone. Unfortunately, adverse side effects and poor compliance are significant problems in achieving sustained benefit with the nonselective β-blockers. Long-acting nitrates such as isosorbide mononitrate also reduce portal pressure, but no study has demonstrated that it can decrease recurrent bleeding or mortality as a monotherapy. The mechanism of nitrates appears to be its ability to cause a decrease in outflow resistance in the portal system. Combining nonselective β-blockers and long-acting nitrates has been more effective and better tolerated than using nonselective β-blockers alone to reduce recurrent bleeding.

Endoscopic band ligation is the treatment of choice at most institutes to prevent recurrent esophageal variceal bleeding. Endoscopic band ligation appears to be at least as equally effective as sclerotherapy in preventing recurrence of bleeding and has a better complication profile. Serial endoscopic band ligation treatments are performed on an outpatient basis at 14-day intervals until varices in the distal esophagus are obliterated. Achieving complete obliteration usually requires three to four endoscopy sessions, after which follow-up endoscopy should be performed every 3 to 6 months to evaluate for any recurring varices. The main downside of band ligation is that small varices can be difficult to band and might be hard to obliterate with this technique. Patients treated with endoscopic band ligation alone have approximately 20% to 40% risk of rebleeding from the esophageal varices. However, if sclerotherapy is performed, it should be repeated 3 to 7 days after the initial session, followed by sessions at 1 to 2 weeks until all varices are completely obliterated. Treatment with sclerotherapy can reduce the risk of recurrent bleeding by 50% at 1 year, but data have not shown its ability to reduce patient mortality. Treatment combining endoscopic band ligation and nonselective β-blockers has an estimated 25% chance of rebleeding. Combination of nonselective β-blockers and sclerotherapy does not appear to be more effective than sclerotherapy alone. Whether combining nonselective β-blockers with long-acting nitrates is more effective than endoscopic therapy in decreasing the risk of rebleeding is still to be determined by future studies.

Procedures that decompress the portal system are recommended in patients who failed endoscopic and/or pharmacologic therapies. Transjugular intrahepatic portosystemic shunt is more effective at preventing recurrent esophageal variceal bleeding than endoscopic therapies. The risk of rebleeding after TIPS placement is 8% to 18% at 1 year. It also eliminates the risks of operative and postoperative complications. However, the downside of TIPS is that there is the 30% increased risk of developing new or worsening hepatic encephalopathy after placement of TIPS. Furthermore, there is no survival benefit of using TIPS over endoscopic therapies. Another problem with TIPS is that stenosis and dysfunction of the shunt are frequent. As a result, endoscopic balloon dilation or stent replacement is often needed to re-establish patency of the shunt, and frequent monitoring of stent patency is often performed using Doppler ultrasound. Unfortunately, Doppler ultrasound is neither sensitive nor specific in detecting shunt patency. All these potential problems of TIPS can lead to a significantly higher amount of overall cost. Therefore, given all these considerations, TIPS should be used as a bridge to liver transplantation.

Rebleeding occurs in 10% to 20% of patients treated with surgical shunts, which is lower in comparison to endoscopic therapies but also carries a higher risk of developing new or worsening hepatic encephalopathy. Selective shunts (e.g., distal splenorenal shunt) have lower risk of hepatic encephalopathy than nonselective shunts (e.g., portacaval interposition shunt) because it preserves better liver function. However, selective shunts are somewhat less effective in preventing rebleeding. Yet, although nonselective shunts are more effective at decompressing the portal system, it is associated with higher risk of operative and postoperative complications. Decompressive surgical shunt procedures tend to be considered in noncompliant patients, patients who are ineligible for liver transportation, Child-Pugh A and B patients, and for patients who have failed endoscopic therapies. Selective shunt is the preferred method of the two types of shunt surgeries; the nonselective shunt should only be considered in emergency situations in the hands of an experienced surgeon. Nonetheless, the choice of surgical treatment should be individualized with consideration of the surgeon's expertise, patient compliance, and severity of cirrhosis in the patient.

Of course, the best and ultimate treatment option for cirrhotic patients with history of bleeding esophageal varices is liver transplantation. Every cirrhotic patient should be evaluated for liver transplant eligibility. Nonetheless, most of the patients with Child-Pugh A and B can be managed with the treatment measures discussed earlier until liver diseases further deteriorate, whereas more severe patients should be treated adequately to control esophageal variceal bleeding in the pretransplant phase. Clinicians should follow all

CURRENT DIAGNOSIS

- Esophageal varices commonly occur in cirrhotic patients because of portal hypertension.
- A significant portion of patients with esophageal varices will develop upper GI bleeding episodes that can lead to a high mortality rate if left untreated.
- The diagnosis of esophageal varices is established by upper endoscopy but the recently developed PillCam ESO video capsule endoscope has the potential to perform rapid screening measure.

Abbreviation: GI = gastrointestinal.

patients with cirrhosis closely, and patient compliance issues should be emphasized.

Primary Prophylaxis for Bleeding Esophageal Varices

The annual risk of cirrhotic patients developing varices is approximately 6%. Because of the high mortality rate from bleeding esophageal varices, prevention of the initial bleeding episode is desirable. Therefore, endoscopy screening looking for evidence of esophageal varices is often recommended. We recommend endoscopic screening for the following subgroups of patients: all newly diagnosed cirrhotic patients and all other cirrhotic patients who are medically stable, motivated and willing to be treated prophylactically, and would benefit from medical or endoscopic therapies. Patients who are unlikely to benefit from prophylactic treatments and those with short life expectancy should be excluded from screening endoscopy. Low-risk cirrhotic patients, such as the ones that have no or small esophageal varices, may not require prophylactic treatment and a repeat screening endoscopy may be performed in 2 years. The newly developed PillCam ESO video capsule endoscope (Given Diagnostic System, Yoqneam, Israel) is equipped with miniature cameras on both ends, is approximately the size of a multivitamin, and takes approximately 20 minutes to perform with little patient discomfort; it might be a useful screening tool for monitoring esophageal varices in the near future. Study has already demonstrated PillCam ESO video capsule endoscope to be a sensitive diagnostic modality for visualization of esophageal mucosal pathology and may provide an effective method to evaluate patients for esophageal disease.

Both pharmacologic and endoscopic treatments are available for primary prophylaxis for bleeding esophageal varices. The aim in using pharmacologic therapy in this setting is, again, to reduce portal pressure and, in turn, intravariceal pressure. Nonselective β-blockers and long-acting nitrates are the main categories of medications that have been used for this purpose. In most randomized studies of prophylactic β-blocker therapy compared with control, β-blockers decreased the risk of first esophageal variceal hemorrhage and the risk of death associated with GI bleeding. In a meta-analysis of nine randomized trials comparing prophylactic β-blockers with no active treatment (i.e., placebo) to prevent first esophageal variceal bleeding, the incidence of bleeding was significantly reduced with β-blocker therapy versus control. This effect was more pronounced in patients with large- or medium-sized varices or in those with varices and an HVPG greater than 12 mm Hg. However, adverse side effects and poor compliance were significant problems in achieving sustained benefit with β-blockers. Nevertheless, prophylactic therapy with propranolol or nadolol is the standard of care for the prevention of a first esophageal variceal bleeding episode. Combination therapy with propranolol and long-acting nitrate such as isosorbide mononitrate may be superior to using β-blocker alone in the primary prevention of variceal bleeding. Unfortunately, because many patients with advanced cirrhosis often have blood pressure on the lower side, it can be difficult for them to tolerate both β-blocker and nitrate at the same time. Because of the potential to cause systemic vasodilation, nitrates should not be used as monotherapy in cirrhotic patients.

CURRENT THERAPY

- Hemodynamic resuscitation is the first step that needs to be performed in patients with actively bleeding esophageal varices.
- Combination therapy with pharmacologic and endoscopic treatments should be performed in patients with acute bleeding esophageal varices.
- Primary prophylaxis and secondary prophylaxis are important objectives in preventing initial bleeding episode and recurrent bleeding, respectively.

However, endoscopic band ligation is an effective endoscopic treatment of active variceal bleeding and secondary prevention of esophageal variceal bleeding. A recent randomized study compared endoscopic band ligation and propranolol to prevent initial variceal hemorrhage in cirrhotics with high-risk esophageal varices and concluded that prophylactic propranolol had a significantly higher treatment-failure rate than endoscopic banding. This study also concluded that propranolol was not significantly safer than banding but was associated with arithmetically more frequent severe adverse events requiring discontinuation of therapy. The direct costs of the propranolol group were not significantly less than banding. Therefore, the results of this study suggested that prophylactic banding seems to be a more promising treatment than propranolol for preventing initial variceal bleeding for compliant patients who are at high risk of initial variceal hemorrhage and who are candidates for liver transplantation. So, endoscopic band ligation perhaps should be considered as frontline for the primary prophylaxis of bleeding esophageal varices. No studies have addressed the efficacy of the effectiveness in preventing initial variceal bleeding of combining endoscopic band ligation with β-blocker treatment. Primary prophylaxis with sclerotherapy leads to a higher mortality rate than placebo or β-blocker therapy and should not be performed.

Conclusions

Bleeding esophageal varices occurs frequently in cirrhotic patients and can lead to significant mortality, disability, productivity, and costs. Because of the poor outcomes that can result once the initial bleeding episode occurs, primary prophylaxis should be carried out. It is the responsibility of clinicians to screen out the patients at risk of developing and having esophageal varices. For patients who already had a bleeding episode, secondary prophylaxis is vital in preventing future bleeds. At the present moment, combination therapies appear to be more effective for the prevention and treatment of bleeding esophageal varices. However, patient education and awareness are also important objectives that clinicians must not forget.

REFERENCES

Brown DM, Everhart JE: Cost of digestive diseases in the United States. In Everhart JE (ed.): Digestive Diseases in the United States: Epidemiology and Impact. US Department of Health and Human Services, Public Health Service, National Institutes of Health, National Institute of Diabetes and Digestive and Kidney Diseases.

(NIH Publication no. 94–1447.57–82). Washington, DC, US Government Printing Office, 1994.

Ejlersen E, Melsen T, Ingerslev J, et al: Recombinant activated factor VII (rFVIIa) acutely normalizes prothrombin time in patients with cirrhosis during bleeding from oesophageal varices. Scand J Gastroenterol 2001;36:1081.

Eliakim R, Sharma VK, Yassin K. A prospective study of the diagnostic accuracy of PillCam ESO esophageal capsule endoscopy versus conventional upper endoscopy in patients with chronic gastroesophageal reflux diseases. J Clin Gastroenterol 2005;39:572-578.

Everhart JE: Overview. In Everhart JE (ed.): Digestive diseases in the United States: Epidemiology and Impact. US Department of Health and Human Services, Public Health Service, National Institutes of Health, National Institute of Diabetes and Digestive and Kidney Diseases. (NIH Publication no. 94–1447.3–53). Washington, DC, US Government Printing Office, 1994.

Imperiale TF, McCullough AJ: Prophylactic beta-blocker therapy: Clinical implications of an aggregate analysis. Hepatology 1992;15:354-356.

Jutabha R, Jensen DM, Martin P: Randomized study comparing banding and propranolol to prevent initial variceal hemorrhage in cirrhotics with high-risk esophageal varices. Gastroenterology 2005;128:870-881.

Kovacs TOG, Jensen DM: Therapeutic endoscopy for upper gastrointestinal bleeding. In Taylor MB, Gollan J, Peppercorn MA, et al (eds.): Gastrointestinal Emergencies (2nd ed.). Baltimore: Williams & Wilkins, 1997, pp 181-198.

Nevens F, Bustami R, Scheys I, et al: Variceal pressure is a factor predicting the risk of a first variceal bleeding: A prospective cohort study in cirrhotic patients. Hepatology 1998;27:15.

Stiegman GV, Goff JS, Michaletz-Onody PA, et al: Endoscopic sclerotherapy as compared with endoscopic ligation for bleeding esophageal varices. N Engl J Med 1992;326:1527.

Thabut D, de Franchis R, Bendsten F, et al: Efficacy of activated recombinant factor VII (RFVIIA; Novoseven®) in cirrhotic patients with upper gastrointestinal bleeding: A randomized placebo-controlled double-blind multicenter trial (abstract). J Hepatol 3;38(Suppl):13.

Dysphagia and Esophageal Obstruction

Method of
*Colm O'Loughlin, MB, and
Reza Shaker, MD*

Dysphagia is the perception of an impediment to the normal passage of liquids or solids from the oral cavity to the stomach. The term *dysphagia* is derived from the Greek words *dys*, which means "with difficulty," and *phagia*, meaning "to eat." Pain with swallowing (odynophagia) may also be associated with the symptom of dysphagia in some patients. Patients may complain of difficulty initiating a swallow or a sensation of foods or fluids "sticking," "stopping," or "hanging up" while passing through the esophagus into the stomach after swallowing. The symptom of dysphagia causes concern because it may be associated with a serious underlying etiology and requires immediate investigation to determine the cause and the initiation of appropriate treatment.

Pathophysiology of Dysphagia

The transfer of an ingested food bolus through the swallowing passage depends on the size of the ingested bolus, the luminal diameter of the passage, the transport of the bolus from the oropharynx into the esophageal lumen, the peristaltic contractions of the esophagus, and deglutitive inhibition (the inhibition or relaxation that precedes the peristaltic contraction), including normal relaxation of upper and lower esophageal sphincters during swallowing. Dysphagia caused by a large bolus or luminal narrowing is termed *mechanical dysphagia*, whereas dysphagia caused by incoordination or weakness of the orderly sequence of contractions in the swallowing process is termed *motor dysphagia*. Common causes of mechanical dysphagia include peptic strictures, lower esophageal rings, and esophageal carcinoma. Dysphagia is always present when the esophagus cannot distend beyond 13 mm. Minimally obstructing lesions only induce dysphagia with large solid food boluses (meats and breads), whereas near obstructing lesions produce symptoms with both solids and liquids. Motor dysphagia may be caused by neurologic insults such as cerebrovascular accidents or disrupted orderly contractions of the esophageal body because of motility disorders. Gastroesophageal reflux disease (GERD) may cause nonobstructive dysphagia as a result of acid-induced motility disturbances with or without esophagitis. Abnormal sensory perception within the esophagus may result in dysphagia, and aberrant visceral perception could explain dysphagia in patients with no definable cause.

Classification of Dysphagia

Dysphagia can be broadly categorized into two distinct types: oropharyngeal and esophageal. Oropharyngeal dysphagia, or transfer dysphagia, arises from disease processes affecting primarily the neuromuscular apparatus of the pharynx, upper esophageal sphincter, or upper esophagus. Esophageal dysphagia arises from a variety of disease processes affecting the body of the esophagus, the lower esophageal sphincter, or the gastroesophageal junction. Table 1 reviews the primary causes of dysphagia.

TABLE 1 Common Causes of Dysphagia

Oropharyngeal	Esophageal
Neuromuscular	**Mechanical Obstruction**
Cerebrovascular accident	Benign strictures
Parkinson's disease	Webs and rings
Amyotrophic lateral sclerosis	Neoplasm
Peripheral neuropathies	Diverticula
(poliomyelitis)	Vascular anomalies
	Aberrant subclavian artery
Mechanical Obstruction	(dysphagia lusoria)
Zenker's diverticulum	Enlarged aorta (dysphagia
Cricopharyngeal bar	aortica)
Cervical osteophyte	
	Motility Disorders
Skeletal Muscle Disorders	Achalasia
Polymyositis	Spastic motility disorders
Muscular dystrophies	Scleroderma
Myotonic dystrophy	Chagas' disease
Myasthenia gravis	
Metabolic myopathies	**Miscellaneous**
(Kearns-Sayre syndrome)	Diabetes
	Alcoholism
Miscellaneous	Gastroesophageal reflux
Decreased saliva	
Medications	
Sjögren's syndrome	
Alzheimer's disease	

OROPHARYNGEAL DYSPHAGIA

Patients with oropharyngeal dysphagia have an array of complaints including an immediate awareness of "food sticking in the throat," difficulty or inability to initiate a swallow, and repeated attempts to swallow. Other complaints such as nasopharyngeal regurgitation, a choking sensation, or coughing on swallowing may occur because of a discoordinate swallowing mechanism with food material entering the trachea and nose. Similarly, oral secretions such as saliva are not swallowed and drooling may occur. Patients are aware that food has not left the oropharynx. Pain is unusual. The throat and anterior neck areas are perceived to be the focus of their complaints. The causes of oropharyngeal dysphagia relate to neuromuscular diseases affecting the striated muscles of the hypopharynx and upper esophagus and include central and peripheral neurologic lesions, such as cerebrovascular disease, Parkinson's disease, and amyotrophic lateral sclerosis; neuromuscular disease, such as myasthenia gravis; and diseases of the skeletal and muscular systems, such as dermatomyositis and polymyositis. Concomitant symptoms may include recurrent aspiration episodes, dysarthria, and unilateral extremity weakness. A crucial question in the evaluation of patients with dysphagia relates to the symptoms suggestive of oropharyngeal dysphagia because investigation of oropharyngeal dysfunction precedes testing for esophageal disorders.

ESOPHAGEAL DYSPHAGIA

Patients with esophageal dysphagia complain of material "sticking" several seconds after swallowing and relate the site of obstruction to the retrosternal or sternal notch areas. Retrosternal dysphagia usually corresponds to the location of the lesion, whereas suprasternal dysphagia is commonly referred from below. Esophageal dysphagia may be related to luminal processes: food boluses or foreign bodies; intrinsic diseases of the esophageal wall, either mucosal webs (thin mucosal folds that protrude into the lumen and are covered with squamous epithelium), peptic strictures, squamous carcinoma, and adenocarcinoma or mural processes such as leiomyomata; extrinsic lesions: malignant lymphadenopathy or pulmonary neoplasms; and smooth muscle dysfunction: achalasia, diffuse esophageal spasm, and scleroderma. Because a detailed history suggests the etiology of dysphagia and allows the physician correctly to define the cause in 80% to 85% of patients, a series of key questions must be answered (Figure 1):

1. Is dysphagia for solids, liquids, or both? Mucosal, mural, or mediastinal diseases cause dysphagia by narrowing the esophageal lumen and there is little resistance to the passage of liquids, but solids are obstructed. Hence, these diseases usually produce dysphagia for solids. Notably, high-grade mechanical obstruction of the esophagus produces dysphagia for both liquids and solids and food impaction may occur. However, diseases that disturb peristalsis by affecting the smooth muscle and its innervation (motility disorders) produce dysphagia for both liquids and solids. Patients with "achalasia" characteristically complain of regurgitation of undigested food material and may have associated weight loss. Patients with spastic esophageal dysmotility may complain of chest pain.

2. Is dysphagia progressive or intermittent? Lower esophageal mucosal rings produce intermittent and nonprogressive dysphagia. Episodes of dysphagia are

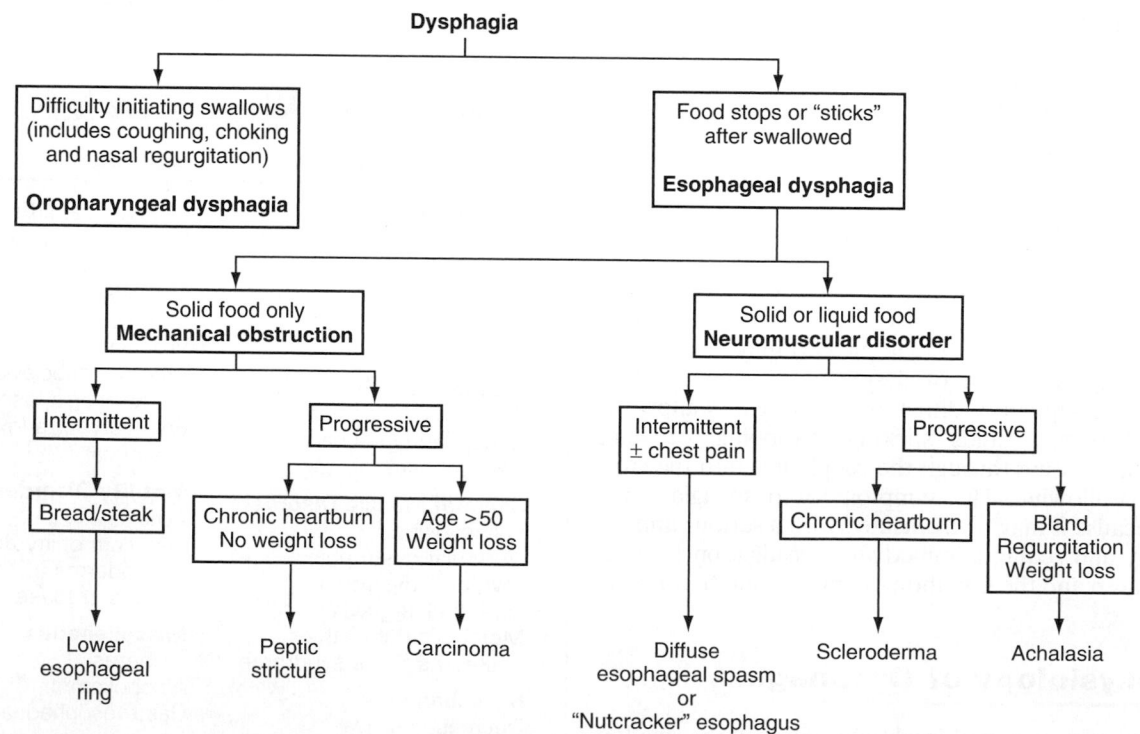

FIGURE 1. Algorithm by which patient's symptoms can be used to predict the underlying disorder and choose the initial diagnostic test. (Modified from Castell DO, Donner MW: Evaluation of dysphagia: A careful history is crucial. Dysphagia 1987;2:65; with kind permission of Springer Science and Business Media.)

typically of short duration and occur with solids, for example, "steakhouse syndrome," which is caused by a transient solid food impaction above a Schatzki ring, a thin membranous ring at the gastroesophageal junction above a hiatal hernia, which is covered by squamous mucosa on the esophageal side and columnar mucosa on the gastric side of the ring. Patients do not have dysphagia every day. Benign strictures such as those caused by peptic esophageal injury produce symptoms slowly and insidiously. Those of a malignant nature are rapidly progressive, occur in a population older than 50 years, and may be associated with weight loss.

3. Where does the food bolus stick? Patients who localize their symptoms as being below the suprasternal notch usually have dysphagia that is caused by a disorder of the distal esophagus. However, localization of symptoms above the suprasternal notch can be caused by a lesion located anywhere from the pharynx to the distal esophagus.

4. Is there a history of pill ingestion or other caustic ingestions? Medications including nonsteroidal anti-inflammatory drugs (NSAIDs), potassium chloride, antibiotics (doxycycline), and quinidine are caustic to the esophagus, and with prolonged mucosal contact they may induce ulceration (odynophagia) and stricturing with resultant dysphagia.

5. Does the patient have chronic GERD? Patients who develop peptic esophageal strictures may report a long history of heartburn. Also, many patients with dysphagia caused by adenocarcinoma in Barrett's esophagus have a history of long-standing heartburn.

6. Is there a history of underlying medical diseases such as connective tissue diseases (CTDs) or is the patient immunosuppressed? Scleroderma and other related CTDs produce vascular obliteration and fibrosis in smooth gut muscle. The subsequent effects of poor esophageal peristalsis and diminished lower esophageal sphincter pressure may result in dysphagia because of disordered esophageal motility, but they also predispose to severe gastroesophageal reflux and peptic stricture formation. Patients usually have Raynaud's phenomenon and findings of skin tightening on examination. The immunocompromised patient, whether because of medications (steroids), malignancy, HIV, or immunosuppressive medication, is at risk for viral (herpes simplex, cytomegalovirus) and fungal (*Candida*) infections of the esophagus. The primary symptoms are odynophagia and less frequently dysphagia. Late complications of infectious esophagitis may include esophageal stricturing and dysphagia.

Evaluation of Dysphagia

A barium esophagogram with videofluoroscopy is the first investigation required when oropharyngeal dysphagia is suspected. A speech pathology assessment is also essential so aspiration risk can be determined with different food consistencies and dietary modifications or alternate routes of feeding implemented.

A double-contrast barium esophagogram may be indicated prior to endoscopic evaluation as the first investigation in the evaluation of esophageal dysphagia. A 12-mm barium pill or marshmallow can also be swallowed allowing

CURRENT DIAGNOSIS

- The etiology of dysphagia can be elucidated in most cases by a careful history.
- The symptom of dysphagia is concerning for a serious underlying cause and requires immediate investigation.
- Radiographic, endoscopic, and manometric testing is performed in a directed manner depending on the clinician's suspicion of the underlying disease process.

detection of subtle narrowing or esophageal webs. Barium studies provide the clinician with valuable information, such as identifying proximal esophageal tumors or webs prior to endoscopy so that appropriate endoscopic therapies can be employed. A clinical suspicion for achalasia should be evaluated with a timed esophagogram and the diagnosis confirmed by manometry prior to esophagoscopy. This information allows the clinician to take appropriate precautions and permits timely therapeutic intervention. Upper endoscopy permits direct visualization of the oropharyngeal and esophageal mucosae, tissue to be obtained for histopathologic review, and therapeutic interventions to be undertaken. Manometric measurements of the upper and lower esophageal sphincters and esophageal body (esophageal manometry) is the gold standard in the evaluation of esophageal motility disorders such as achalasia and detection of motor disorders associated with collagen-vascular disease.

Treatment of the More Common Causes of Dysphagia

PEPTIC STRICTURES

Chronic gastroesophageal reflux may result in distal esophagitis and stricturing with subsequent dysphagia. Management of peptic strictures usually requires a combination of endoscopic dilation and acid suppressive therapy. Aggressive management of GERD is central to the

CURRENT THERAPY

- Peptic strictures require aggressive antireflux control with proton pump inhibitors that allow healing, improve dysphagia, and decrease the need for subsequent esophageal dilations.
- Malignant strictures are treated by a combination of therapies including external beam radiation, endoscopic dilation, debulking, or stenting and/or surgery.
- Achalasia may be managed pharmacologically, by endoscopic pneumatic dilation/botulinum injection, or by surgical myotomy, depending on the patient's operative candidacy.
- Eosinophilic esophagitis responds to treatment with corticosteroids (oral/topical), leukotriene inhibitors, and endoscopic dilation.

treatment of peptic esophageal strictures. Lifestyle adaptations used in the management of GERD such as dietary modification, cessation of smoking, wearing loose-fitting clothing, weight loss, and avoidance of late evening meals should be encouraged. Aggressive antireflux therapy is crucial. Pharmacologic therapy with proton pump inhibitors such as omeprazole (Prilosec), 20 mg orally daily, or pantoprazole (Protonix), 40 mg orally daily, allows healing, improves dysphagia, and decreases the need for subsequent esophageal dilations. In view of the mechanism of action, these medications should be given at least 30 minutes prior to food ingestion. Twice-daily dosing may be required in difficult cases. Prokinetic agents such as metoclopramide (Reglan), 10 mg orally four times daily, that enhance gastric emptying and improve esophageal peristaltic function and hence esophageal clearance have an adjunctive role in the treatment of GERD.

The endoscopic management of peptic strictures depends on the characteristics of the strictures in terms of length (tortuosity) and diameter. Tight or complex strictures such as those less than 10 mm in diameter or greater than 2 cm in length are best managed with wire-guided polyvinyl bougies (Savary dilators) or balloons (CRE dilation balloons) under fluoroscopic and endoscopic control. Simple strictures can be dilated with mercury-filled dilators (Maloney) that are passed orally. Esophageal dilation is performed progressively over weeks to months with a gradual increase in the diameters of the dilators. Most patients have relief of dysphagia after dilation to a diameter of 40 to 54 French or 13 to 17 mm with no requirement for maintenance dilations. Refractory strictures, those not responding to dilation and antireflux therapy, can be treated endoscopically with injection of triamcinolone acetate (Kenalog),[1] 40 mg/mL in 0.2- to 0.5-mL aliquots into the stricture in all four quadrants prior to dilation. More recently, endoscopically placed temporary nonmetallic expandable stents (Polyflex) were effective in the treatment of refractory benign strictures. Laparoscopic fundoplication may be considered in certain cases.

MALIGNANT STRICTURES

Malignant obstruction because of esophageal carcinoma is a late presentation and carries a poor prognosis. Dysphagia is rapidly progressive. Tissue diagnosis can be made by endoscopy with mucosal biopsy. Evaluation includes staging of the disease with computed tomography and endoscopic ultrasound. Endoscopic management includes dilation as performed for benign strictures that is successful in temporarily relieving symptoms in 90% of cases. Dilation can be used in conjunction with other modes of treatment such as external beam radiation therapy or endoscopic tumor ablation techniques (laser, photodynamic therapy). Per oral endoprostheses may be placed permanently for symptom control in patients with poor prognoses. Indications for esophageal stenting include advanced disease complicated by esophagotracheal fistulae and patients who are poor surgical candidates to allow for swallowing of oral secretions, prevent aspiration, and maintain a patent lumen.

RINGS AND WEBS

Other causes of dysphagia need to be excluded before embarking on a treatment regimen for esophageal mucosal rings. This may include esophageal biopsy for eosinophilic esophagitis or manometry to exclude diffuse esophageal spasm (DES). Endoscopic dilation is usually effective in the management of these patients. Dilation is performed with a large bougie or balloon (15 to 20 mm) so as to fracture the ring. Again, aggressive antireflux therapy with omeprazole (Prilosec), 20 mg orally daily, or pantoprazole (Protonix), 40 mg orally daily (as for peptic strictures described earlier), should be initiated. Persistent rings warrant another trial of dilation. Refractory rings may respond to pneumatic dilation (large balloon), electrosurgical incision, and surgical resection. Cervical webs are associated with carcinoma and warrant endoscopic evaluation and biopsy. Muscular rings (hypertrophic musculature) are rare and more frequently seen in children.

ACHALASIA

Radiographic (barium esophagogram) and manometric studies should precede endoscopy. Endoscopic evaluation is important both in the investigation and treatment of achalasia. Exclusion of pseudoachalasia such as that caused by an infiltrating carcinoma at the gastroesophageal junction is crucial prior to the implementation of invasive therapies such as pneumatic dilation (disruption of the muscle fibers of the lower esophageal sphincter) or laparoscopic myotomy. Surgery is superior to pneumatic dilation for both the short- and long-term relief of dysphagia, but it is complicated by a high frequency of GERD postoperatively. Hence, an antireflux procedure is usually performed in addition to myotomy. Failure of the first pneumatic dilation prompts repeat dilation with a larger balloon. A return of symptoms after three attempts at pneumatic dilation mandates referral for surgical myotomy. Pharmacologic therapies are used primarily in poor operative candidates. Nitrates and calcium antagonists are used with variable success. Isosorbide dinitrate (Isordil),[1] 5 to 10 mg sublingually 10 minutes before meals, produces symptomatic relief of dysphagia in up to 75% of patients. Some patients, however, cannot tolerate the side effects of these medications. Endoscopic management with botulinum toxin[1] (80 U), injected in 20-unit aliquots into each quadrant of the lower esophageal sphincter, show good short-term results with clinical remission induced for at least 6 months in 66% of patients. Therapy may need to be repeated to maintain relief of symptoms.

EOSINOPHILIC ESOPHAGITIS

Eosinophilic esophagitis is characterized by eosinophilic infiltration of the esophagus and is an increasingly recognized cause of dysphagia. It is more common in young men, and many report a history of allergic disease such as asthma or hayfever or have peripheral eosinophilia. Histopathologic review of mucosal biopsies obtained at endoscopy demonstrates the presence of more than 20 eosinophils per high-power field. Endoscopic dilation is associated with mucosal tears and perforation (often dilation in the unrecognized case), and the presence of multiple esophageal rings should

[1]Not FDA approved for this indication.

[1]Not FDA approved for this indication.

alert the clinician. The efficacy of acid-suppressive agents such as omeprazole and elimination diets is variable. Corticosteroids (Prednisolone), 1.5 mg/kg orally per day for 4 weeks, is effective; however, the unfavorable side-effect profile of steroid therapy remains of concern. Fluticasone propionate (Flovent),[1] a poorly absorbed steroid, 220 μg/puff twice daily orally (ingested rather than inhaled), provides a topical therapy that is also effective for the relief of symptoms. Montelukast, a leukotriene inhibitor (Singulair[1]), 10 mg orally daily, offers an alternate oral therapy. The dosage may need to be escalated to 100 mg[3] daily depending on response with subsequent dose reduction to a maintenance of 20 to 40[3] mg daily.

SCLERODERMA

The smooth muscle of the distal two thirds of the esophagus is very frequently involved in this diffuse disease. The most common motility abnormalities produced by atrophy and fibrosis of the smooth muscle are aperistalsis or low-amplitude contractions and low or absent lower esophageal sphincter pressure. These abnormalities alone may induce dysphagia. The resultant inadequate clearance of the esophagus also predisposes these patients to severe GERD and peptic stricture formation. Hence, treatment is directed at the prevention of GERD and its complications (as for peptic strictures described earlier).

REFERENCES

Attwood SE, Smyrk TC, Demeester TR, Jones JB: Esophageal eosinophilia with dysphagia. Dig Dis Sci 1993;38:109.

Baehr PH, McDonald GB: Esophageal infections: Risk factors, presentation, diagnosis, and treatment. Gastroenterology 1994;106:509.

Edwards DA: Discriminative information in the diagnosis of dysphagia. J R Coll Physicians Lond 1997;9:257.

Kahrilas PJ, Clouse RE, Hogan WJ: American Gastroenterological Association technical review on the clinical use of esophageal manometry. Gastroenterology 1994;107:1865.

Rose S, Young MA, Reynolds JC: Gastrointestinal manifestations of scleroderma. Gastroenterol Clin North Am 1998;27:563.

Spechler JS: AGA technical review on the treatment of patients with dysphagia caused by benign disorders of the distal esophagus. Gastroenterology 1999;117:1.

Steiner SJ, Gupta SK, Croffie JM, Fitzgerald JF: Correlation between number of eosinophils and reflux index on same day esophageal biopsy and 24 hour esophageal pH monitoring. Am J Gastroenterol 2004;99:801.

Wilcox CM, Alexander LN, Clarke WS: Localization of an obstructing esophageal lesion. Is the patient accurate? Dig Dis Sci 1995;40:2192.

Yarze JC, Varga J, Stampfl D, et al: Esophageal function in systemic sclerosis: A prospective evaluation of motility and acid reflux in 36 patients. Am J Gastroenterol 1993;88:870.

[1]Not FDA approved for this indication.
[3]Exceeds dosage recommended by the manufacturer.

Diverticula of the Alimentary Tract

Method of
Harris R. Clearfield, MD

Diverticula are often asymptomatic but may produce symptoms if they distend with food or liquid and compress the lumen (Zenker's and epiphrenic diverticula), harbor sufficient organisms to produce a bacterial overgrowth syndrome (jejunal diverticula), or become inflamed or bleed (Meckel and colonic diverticula).

Esophageal Diverticula

HYPOPHARYNGEAL DIVERTICULA

The hypopharyngeal diverticulum (Zenker's diverticulum) is found in approximately 2% of patients presenting with dysphagia, and the majority of cases occur in patients beyond the seventh decade of life. The diverticulum generally protrudes between the cricopharyngeus muscle (superior esophageal sphincter) and the inferior constrictor muscles as a result of high pressure produced by transient inadequate or uncoordinated relaxation of the superior esophageal sphincter during swallowing. Because the cervical spine prevents posterior extension, the diverticulum enlarges laterally, usually to the left side. Small diverticula are asymptomatic, but progressive enlargement can occur as a result of food-induced stretching. The opening of the diverticulum may become larger than the lumen of the esophagus, so that food and liquid can preferentially enter the diverticulum and subsequently spill over into the lumen of the esophagus. The progressively enlarging diverticulum may exert sufficient pressure on the esophagus to produce dysphagia and perhaps aspiration. Symptoms include cervical dysphagia, coughing while eating, bad breath from the fermenting food, a swelling in the neck (usually during meals or liquid ingestion) caused by the enlarging diverticulum, and nocturnal wheezing resulting from aspiration. Medications may also accumulate in the diverticulum causing erratic absorption. The symptoms may be suggestive, but barium upper gastrointestinal (GI) tract radiographic films usually establish the diagnosis. If a Zenker's diverticulum is suspected, upper endoscopy, if necessary, should be accomplished by inserting the instrument under direct vision to reduce the likelihood of perforation.

Treatment

No treatment is required for asymptomatic diverticula, but those producing symptoms often require surgery. Although external surgery such as diverticulectomy and myotomy of the superior sphincter is an effective therapy, the use of endoscopic staple diverticulotomy has become increasingly popular. It can be accomplished on an outpatient basis with a more rapid convalescence and a lower rate of complications as compared to external surgery, although there is a recurrence rate of approximately 12%.

MIDESOPHAGEAL DIVERTICULA

Midesophageal diverticula were once thought to result from a fibrotic "pull" or "traction" from an adjacent mediastinal inflammatory reaction, such as tuberculosis. This theory was largely replaced by the observation that many diverticula are associated with motility abnormalities such as achalasia or esophageal spasm. The diverticula are usually small and wide mouthed, so that food trapping rarely occurs and symptoms are unusual. If chest pain is associated with these diverticula, esophageal motility studies should be performed. No treatment is usually required for the diverticula.

EPIPHRENIC DIVERTICULA

Epiphrenic diverticula occur in the distal esophagus and are thought to result from high pressure generated by a motility disorder of the lower esophageal sphincter or distal esophagus, such as achalasia, esophageal spasm, or hypertensive lower esophageal sphincter. Most diverticula are asymptomatic, but an occasional diverticulum may progressively distend and begin to trap food and secretions, leading to dysphagia, substernal discomfort, or vomiting (often nocturnal). The diagnosis is usually established by barium upper GI studies, but upper endoscopy also reveals the lesion.

Treatment

No treatment or evaluation is required for small asymptomatic outpouchings, but detailed esophageal motility studies should be performed for larger diverticula. Symptomatic diverticula associated with a motility disorder are treated with calcium channel blockers, but medical therapy is usually ineffective. If surgery is required, myotomy of the lower esophageal sphincter down to the cardia of the stomach and proximal to the mouth of the diverticulum may suffice for relatively small diverticula, but diverticulectomy plus myotomy is best for large diverticula. The procedure is most commonly performed by an "open" approach, but increasing evidence supports a laparoscopic approach. Either type of surgery should be combined with an antireflux procedure to prevent reflux resulting from loss of the lower esophageal sphincter's competence.

Small Intestinal Diverticula

DUODENAL DIVERTICULA

Duodenal diverticula are noted in approximately 5% of patients studied with barium upper GI radiographs and in 10% to 20% of patients studied by endoscopic retrograde cholangiopancreatography (ERCP). They are the most common small bowel diverticula and are exceeded in frequency only by colonic diverticula. They usually occur within the "C loop," often adjacent to the ampulla of Vater (referred to as juxtapapillary diverticula), and are rarely found on the lateral wall of the duodenum. The diverticula increase in frequency with advancing age. They are usually composed of mucosa without muscle fibers, which suggests they are the result of duodenal pressure, but congenital diverticula may also occur. There appears to be no increased incidence of colonic diverticula in patients with duodenal diverticula, thus negating the concept of a general GI predisposition to diverticular formation.

The ERCP endoscope, which is side viewing, is best suited for the detection of juxtapapillary diverticula, but they may be observed by standard upper endoscopy and barium radiographs. Because imaging studies are usually obtained related to upper GI symptoms, it is tempting to ascribe such symptoms to the presence of the diverticula. However, it is difficult to establish a correlation between these occasionally encountered diverticula and a variety of dyspeptic or aerophagic complaints. Nevertheless, there does appear to be a correlation between the presence of juxtapapillary diverticula and infected bile, common duct stones, and gallstones. This raises the possibility that the diverticula may compromise flow in the common bile duct by exerting extrinsic pressure, thus promoting stasis and common duct calculi formation. Dysfunction of the sphincter of Oddi is ascribed to the presence of adjacent diverticula and could lead to reflux of duodenal contents and bacteria into the biliary tree. Rare cases of pancreatitis are thought to be secondary to juxtapapillary diverticula. The presence of juxtapapillary diverticula may complicate diagnostic and therapeutic ERCP procedures.

Treatment

Duodenal diverticula rarely produce symptoms and therefore usually require no therapy. Resection should be considered if studies suggest that external pressure on the common bile duct is causing obstruction or stone disease. Upper GI tract bleeding, brisk rather than occult, may rarely arise from these diverticula, but efforts should be made to define some other, more likely etiology. A causal relationship between duodenal diverticula and bleeding should be established only with convincing endoscopic or angiographic findings. The management of the bleeding is similar to that of other causes of upper GI tract hemorrhage, but emergency excision of the diverticulum could be required if supportive measures are unsuccessful. Diverticular perforation and abscess are even more uncommon and would prompt computed tomography (CT) scan, ultrasonography, or surgical exploration to establish the diagnosis. Diverticulectomy would be required for such patients.

JEJUNAL AND ILEAL DIVERTICULA

Jejunal and ileal diverticula are uncommon and are thought to be primarily of the acquired type. They tend to occur on the mesenteric border of the small bowel where blood vessels penetrate from the serosal surface, thus creating a potential weakness in the musculature. Multiple large diverticula, usually jejunal, may permit sufficient bacterial overgrowth to result in a malabsorption syndrome. This complication may be associated with a more generalized bowel motility disorder, such as scleroderma. The symptoms are those of other malabsorption syndromes and include megaloblastic anemia secondary to vitamin B_{12} or folate deficiency, steatorrhea, diarrhea, weight loss, and fat-soluble vitamin deficiency. Jejunal diverticula are also associated with intestinal pseudo-obstruction, although the retrospective nature of the published reports does not permit an estimate of the frequency of this relationship. The diverticula appear to be a manifestation of the pseudo-obstruction rather than the cause. The generalized nature of the small bowel motility disorder in these patients is illustrated by such associated findings as esophageal dysmotility, the CREST syndrome (calcinosis cutis, Raynaud phenomenon, esophageal dysfunction, sclerodactyly, and telangiectasia), and degenerated smooth muscle cells consistent with a visceral myopathy. Large small bowel diverticula have caused volvulus and are also complicated by hemorrhage and perforation (diverticulitis).

Treatment

The bacterial overgrowth of small bowel diverticulosis often responds to antibiotic therapy. Tetracycline, 250 mg four times daily, or other broad-spectrum antibiotics for 7 to 10 days may be effective. Unfortunately, relapse is common and some patients benefit from 1 week of antibiotic therapy each month. A promotility agent such as tegaserod (Zelnorm),[1] 6 mg twice daily, may be helpful. Vitamin B_{12}, folic acid, and fat-soluble vitamins should be provided, and dietary fat and milk products should be reduced. Resection of the small bowel containing the diverticula is suggested for patients with chronic symptoms, but this may prove to be ineffective if the diverticula are the result of a generalized neuropathic or myopathic process. Surgery should be reserved for acute complications such as bleeding, diverticulitis, or volvulus. It is therefore important to consider an associated motility disturbance in patients with symptomatic small bowel diverticula.

MECKEL'S DIVERTICULUM

Meckel's diverticulum, which is present in 1% to 3% of the population, represents the failure of the intestinal end of the primitive yolk duct (vitelline duct) to close completely. The diverticula usually occur on the antimesenteric surface of the ileum, approximately 60 to 80 cm from the ileocecal valve, but they may occur as far as 200 cm proximal to the valve. The diverticulum is usually several centimeters in size, but diverticula measuring up to 10 cm are described. The majority of the diverticula are asymptomatic. The major complications of bleeding, inflammation, and obstruction are seen most commonly in infants and young children (60%), with a male predominance. Adult males are also more likely to develop complications from the diverticula. The most common presenting complication in adults is bleeding, whereas the most common childhood presentation is obstruction. Bleeding generally results from the presence of ectopic gastric mucosa within the sac, a finding in approximately 50% to 70% of symptomatic patients. The acid production leads to ulceration and bleeding from within or adjacent to the diverticulum. The bleeding is more frequently maroon or red than tarry and is more likely to be brisk than occult. Obstruction, with or without a fibrous attachment to the umbilicus, can result from volvulus or intussusception and may be of the closed-loop type. Inflammation of the diverticulum (diverticulitis) is less common than appendicitis because of the diverticular wide neck that permits the fecal stream to exit easily. The motility of the ileum decreases the likelihood that the inflammation will be sealed off, increasing the possibility

---

[1]Not FDA approved for this indication.

of perforation should diverticulitis occur. The presence of painless, massive lower GI tract bleeding in an infant or child should suggest the possibility of Meckel's diverticulum. Bowel obstruction or peritonitis in this age group should also raise this suspicion. Although less common, the preceding complications can also occur in adults.

The diagnosis of Meckel's diverticulum is rarely made by barium small bowel examination, although this study (or small bowel enema) may be useful in selected patients to exclude other disorders. The ^{99m}Tc pertechnetate isotope is taken up by Meckel's diverticula containing gastric mucosa and may be helpful for establishing the diagnosis, but a negative examination does not exclude the possibility (many diverticula do not contain gastric mucosa, and even those that have the heterotopic gastric mucosa may not be visualized). Sensitivity is enhanced somewhat by pretreating patients with acid-suppressive therapy prior to isotope scanning. CT scanning has been helpful in diagnosis and should be performed if Meckel diverticulum is suspected, but false negatives also occur. The wireless videocapsule is helpful in a case report, but caution should be exercised if the process is Meckel's diverticulitis because the capsule may become lodged in an area of edema and narrowing. Mesenteric angiography may be useful during an active bleeding episode; intestinal obstruction is diagnosed on the basis of clinical and radiographic criteria; and peritonitis in an infant or child should suggest appendicitis or diverticulitis.

Treatment

The treatment of symptomatic Meckel's diverticulum requires blood replacement, localization of the bleeding point if possible by isotope scan, CT scan, angiography, or videocapsule. Diverticulectomy is advised if the symptomatic diverticulum is identified, but one study suggested that the distribution of the heterotopic gastric mucosa may be at the base of short diverticula and thus could require localized small bowel resection.

Laparoscopic resection for Meckel's diverticula in adults is reported. Occasionally patients, both young and old, may bleed intermittently posing diagnostic difficulties if the preceding localizing efforts prove unrewarding. Bowel obstruction requires immediate surgery, and Meckel's diverticulitis usually requires exploration. There is some controversy as to the management of an asymptomatic Meckel's diverticulum discovered during surgery for some other disorder. An analysis of 1476 patients at the Mayo Clinic could not support or reject the recommendation that all Meckel's diverticula found incidentally be removed. Some of the criteria that could be used for selective resection include male sex, patient younger than 50 years, and diverticular length more than 2 cm.

Diverticular Disease of the Colon

In diverticular disease of the colon, diverticula occur in two rows on either side of the colon, with a distinct clustering in the sigmoid colon. Although diverticula may also be observed in the proximal colon, it is most unusual for patients to have right-sided or transverse colonic diverticula in the absence of sigmoid involvement. The frequency of diverticula formation is almost directly related to age and increases to approximately 50% of individuals in their ninth decade. Although diverticula are uncommon before 40 years of age, complications from diverticular disease do occur in young people.

The diminished frequency of diverticula among individuals from Africa, Asia, and certain areas of South America is attributed to a high-fiber diet, which tends to decrease transit time in the gut, to increase stool frequency, and to result in softer, larger stools. This is an attractive hypothesis, but it is difficult to distinguish healthy persons from those with diverticulosis on the basis of stool weight and frequency. Another theory regarding the cause of colonic diverticula is related to the high sigmoid pressure observed in patients with the irritable bowel syndrome or those who strain during defecation. This is the basis of the supposition that increased intraluminal pressure forces the mucosa to protrude through the relatively weak areas of the colonic musculature adjacent to the blood vessels that penetrate from the serosal surface. This explanation seems reasonable, but diverticula are found in patients with no history of irritable bowel symptoms or chronic constipation. Stool weight and sigmoid pressure remain the primary explanations, but there is presently no convincing and unifying explanation for the development of colonic diverticula.

DIVERTICULOSIS

Uncomplicated diverticula do not produce symptoms, but in patients with the irritable bowel syndrome, colonic diverticula may be revealed by barium enema examination or colonoscopy. Treatment, therefore, should not be directed to the diverticula but should focus on the predominant symptoms, such as pain, diarrhea, or constipation. Consider therapy with a high-fiber diet, psyllium preparations (Metamucil, Konsyl), or methyl cellulose (Citrucel) for constipation. Crampy pain or diarrhea may respond to antispasmodic medications (Bentyl, Levbid) or antidiarrheal agents such as loperamide (Imodium) or diphenoxylate (Lomotil). Patients with diverticula and the irritable bowel syndrome should not be informed that they have diverticular disease or diverticulitis because these labels may induce added anxiety and create confusion for physicians who may subsequently evaluate the patients.

DIVERTICULAR BLEEDING

Diverticula are one of the major causes of massive colonic hemorrhage. The bleeding is usually painless and rarely accompanies clinical diverticulitis. It is thought to result from the presence of an inspissated diverticular fecalith that erodes or ulcerates into an adjacent penetrating artery. The close relationship of the diverticula to these arteries explains why bleeding is often more severe from diverticula than encountered from an arteriovenous malformation (AVM). Although right-sided diverticula are occasionally cited as the most common cause of diverticular bleeding, colonoscopy examinations suggest that the AVM is a more common etiology of right colon bleeding. The bleeding site (but not the cause) may be established by a technetium isotope bleeding study (often an initial study) or by angiography, but these studies must obviously be performed during the bleeding episode if localization is to be made with confidence. Cleansing of the colon with a lavage solution (GoLYTELY, Colyte) can be accomplished in selected patients during the bleeding episode if hemodynamic stability can be achieved, permitting a colonoscopic examination that may determine the site of bleeding and the cause (diverticula, AVM, or neoplasm). However, colonoscopy is most often performed after bleeding ceases.

Treatment

It is more important to determine which segment of the colon is the site of brisk bleeding (sigmoid, left, transverse, or right colon) than to identify the specific diverticulum or other etiology. Hemodynamic stability should be achieved before time-consuming diagnostic studies are initiated. The most common cause for death resulting from GI hemorrhage is inadequate transfusions. An isotope bleeding study may demonstrate the area of colonic bleeding but is helpful only if the patient is bleeding actively during the study window. Angiography permits the most precise localization of bleeding points if active bleeding is present. If a bleeding diverticulum is identified, angiographic embolization can be performed or vasopressin infusion may result in sufficient local vasoconstriction to permit cessation of bleeding. Colonoscopy during a colonic hemorrhage can be achieved if the patient is stable and capable of tolerating the cleansing preparation. The examination may show evidence of vascular lesions, "oozing" from a presumably culpable diverticulum, or neoplasm (benign polyps rarely bleed massively). It is useful to remember that one of the causes of lower GI bleeding is upper GI bleeding, suggesting that an upper endoscopy or enteroscopy should be considered if a colonic site is not definitely shown. If major bleeding continues and the diagnostic strategies just outlined are unrewarding, a subtotal resection with ileorectal anastomosis should be considered. A "blind" left-sided colectomy in patients with known diverticular disease may be disastrous if the bleeding originates from the right colon. If diverticular bleeding stops with conservative measures, elective surgery need not be immediately considered because there is a reasonable possibility that bleeding will not recur. Recurrent bleeding should be approached surgically if the site is identified.

DIVERTICULITIS

Diverticulitis results from a microperforation of a single diverticulum, usually into pericolic tissues. The inflammatory reaction is generally walled off by surrounding omentum or adjacent bowel loops but may progress to an abscess or phlegmon (marked cellulites without pus). If the inflammatory process is not sealed, a free perforation may rarely occur. Diverticulitis usually involves the sigmoid colon, but instances of right-sided diverticulitis are encountered.

The patient usually complains of left lower quadrant or suprapubic pain that may be accompanied by back pain, nausea, vomiting, dysuria, or fever. Gross rectal bleeding is unusual. Physical examination generally reveals tenderness over the left lower quadrant, suprapubic area, or both. Muscle guarding or rebound tenderness may be elicited.

An elevated white blood cell count has little localizing value but can be useful in distinguishing between the irritable colon (normal count) and diverticulitis (leukocytosis is common). A urinalysis may reflect the presence of cystitis secondary to an adjacent inflammatory reaction or a true colovesical fistula (ask the patient about the passage of gas during urination). An obstruction series may provide little information, but a sigmoid obstruction secondary to edema and inflammation may be noted, or a partial small bowel obstruction may result from a segment of distal jejunum or proximal ileum that becomes surrounded by the pericolonic inflammatory reaction. A CT scan provides the most useful information, such as an abscess, pericolonic inflammation, or air in the bladder if a fistula is present. The CT scan may not demonstrate these findings if obtained very early in the inflammatory process. Blood cultures should be obtained in febrile patients.

Sigmoidoscopy and colonoscopy should be avoided during the acute process so that free perforation secondary to air insufflation can be avoided. Contrast radiographic films of the colon are ordinarily deferred for the same reason, but early imaging may be required if the clinical picture is atypical, perhaps raising the possibility of ischemia, acute colitis, or perforated neoplasm. In such circumstances, meglumine diatrizoate (Gastrografin) administration given without air insufflation is usually sufficient to outline the pathology. A CT scan should be considered. This may show a fistula, partial obstruction, or evidence of an extrinsic mass effect on the colon. Colonoscopy is less useful for the diagnosis of recent diverticulitis but can be helpful in the differential diagnosis.

The differential diagnosis may include the irritable bowel syndrome, but the presence of fever, leukocytosis, and/or peritoneal signs should suggest an inflammatory reaction. Ovarian pathology, appendicitis (the appendix may extend down into the pelvis), inflammatory bowel disease, and ischemic colitis should be considered. A confined perforation of a colonic carcinoma is more difficult to exclude during the acute process. Even the surgeon may have problems making that distinction during emergency exploration because the surrounding inflammatory reaction may be intense.

Complications include fistulas to the bladder (less common in women because the uterus "protects" the bladder), small bowel, or vagina. Free perforation, which is rare but significantly increases the morbidity and mortality rate, abdominal abscess, partial or complete obstruction of the small or large bowel, and septicemia may occur. Another serious complication of diverticulitis is spread of the bacteria through the portal vein to the liver leading to pyelophlebitis (pus in the portal vein) and pyogenic liver abscess.

Treatment

Mild cases of diverticulitis with low-grade fever, tenderness without peritonitis, and modest leukocytosis may be treated on an ambulatory basis with clear liquids and a combination of oral levofloxacin (Levaquin) and metronidazole (Flagyl). If the fever subsides and clinical improvement is noted in 72 hours, the diet can be gradually increased. Immunocompromised patients should be treated earlier and more aggressively. More severe cases require hospitalization. The bowel should be kept at rest and intravenous (IV) fluids given. Nasogastric suction should be used if peritonitis or obstruction is present. Parenteral broad-spectrum antibiotic coverage against

CURRENT DIAGNOSIS

- Cervical dysphagia associated with bad breath and a swelling in the neck during eating strongly suggests Zenker's diverticulum.
- Although most duodenal diverticula are asymptomatic, those adjacent to the ampulla of Vater can cause pressure on the bile duct resulting in stasis and common duct calculi.
- The most common presenting complication of Meckel's diverticulum in adults is bleeding, whereas the most common childhood presentation is obstruction.
- Patients with the irritable bowel syndrome may present with severe left lower quadrant pain and tenderness, but diverticulitis should be suspected if there is fever, leukocytosis, or peritoneal findings.
- A negative Meckel's pertechnetate isotope scan does not exclude the diverticulum because many do not contain heterotopic gastric mucosa.
- Colonic bleeding from diverticular disease is usually more severe than that encountered from arteriovenous malformations, polyps, or neoplasms.

aerobes and anaerobes is given. Single-therapy agents include piperacillin/tazobactam (Zosyn), ticarcillin/clavulanate (Timentin), or imipenem/cilastatin (Primaxin). Combination IV therapy could include levofloxacin (Levaquin) plus metronidazole or ampicillin/sulbactam (Unasyn) plus metronidazole. Percutaneous CT-guided aspiration of a pericolonic or pelvic abscess, especially if 4 cm or larger, may hasten resolution of the process and perhaps permit a one-stage resection and anastomosis if surgery is subsequently required.

If the patient fails to improve, as judged by the white blood cell count, fever status, and abdominal findings, surgical intervention may be required. A one-stage procedure with resection of the inflamed bowel and reanastomosis is more often performed, but a staged procedure with a diverting colostomy is preferable if significant peritonitis or infection is present in the area of the planned anastomosis or if the anastomosis cannot be accomplished without tension. Laparoscopic sigmoid resection, with its attendant shorter hospital stay, is an alternative to open sigmoid resection.

If the patient responds to medical therapy, diet is gradually advanced, but the patient is instructed to avoid small hard particles such as seeds, nuts, corn, and fish bones to prevent their entrapment in diverticula (this advice seems reasonable but is not evidence based). It is also prudent to avoid constipation by increasing the fiber content of the diet, using either bran cereals, psyllium products such as Metamucil or Konsyl, or Citrucel. Elective resection of the sigmoid colon after the diverticulitis has resolved with medical therapy was once advocated, but current experience indicates that approximately 50% of patients have no further symptoms. Although some would advise surgery for a recurrent episode of diverticulitis, a prompt response to medical therapy could suggest that surgery should be deferred. Elective resection should be considered after a first attack in patients younger than 50 years (their

CURRENT THERAPY

- Symptomatic Zenker's diverticulum requires resection, most recently performed by an endoscopic staple diverticulotomy.
- Small symptomatic epiphrenic diverticula can be treated with lower esophageal myotomy, but large diverticula may also require diverticulectomy plus myotomy. Both procedures should be accompanied by an antireflux wrap procedure.
- There is controversy regarding the removal of asymptomatic Meckel's diverticula. Factors that may support excision of such diverticula include size larger than 2 cm, male sex, and patients <50 y.
- If major and continued diverticular bleeding cannot be localized by imaging studies, a subtotal colectomy is preferable to a "blind" left colectomy. If bleeding ceases, elective resection is not necessarily required.
- Moderate diverticulitis (fever, abdominal pain and tenderness, and a modest WBC elevation without other complications) may be treated on an outpatient basis with clear liquid diet and a broad-spectrum oral antibiotic plus metronidazole (Flagyl).
- Severe episodes of diverticulitis (peritoneal signs and marked WBC elevation and/or mass or abscess) require hospitalization with IV fluids and IV antibiotics.
- Elective surgery for acute diverticulitis is not necessarily required for recurrent episodes if the events are relatively mild.

Abbreviations: IV = intravenous; WBC = white blood cells.

recurrence rate appears to be higher) and in those patients who have experienced a particularly severe first attack.

REFERENCES

Chang CY, Payyapilli RJ, Scher RL: Endoscopic staple diverticulotomy for Zenker's diverticulum; Review of literature and experience in 159 consecutive patients. Laryngoscope 2003;113:957-965.

Gonzalez R, Smith CD, Mattar SG, et al: Laparoscopic vs. open resection for the treatment of diverticular disease. Surg Endosc 2004;18:276-280.

Janes S, Meagher A, Frizelle FA: Elective surgery after acute diverticulitis. Br J Surg 2005;92:133-142.

Levy AD, Hobbs CM: From the archives of the AFIP. Meckel's diverticulum: Radiologic features with pathologic correlation. Radiographics 2004;24:565-587.

Maggard MA, Chandler CF, Schmit PJ, et al: Surgical diverticulitis: Treatment options. Am Surg 2001;67:1185-1189.

Matthews BD, Nelms CD, Lohr CE, et al: Minimally invasive management of epiphrenic esophageal diverticula. Am Surg 2003;69:465-470.

Park JJ, Wolff BG, Tollefson MK, et al: Meckel diverticulum: The Mayo Clinic experience with 1476 patients (1950–2002). Ann Surg 2005;241:529-533.

Salem L, Anaya DA, Flum DR: Temporal changes in the management of diverticulitis. J Surg Res 2005;124:159.

Siewert B, Tye G, Kruskal J, et al: Impact of CT-guided drainage in the treatment of diverticular abscesses: Size matters. Am J Roentgenol 2006;186:680-686.

Zoepf T, Zoepf DS, Benz D, Riemann JF: The relationship between juxtapapillary duodenal diverticula and disorders of the biliopancreatic system, analysis of 350 patients. Gastrointest Endosc 2001;54:56-61.

Inflammatory Bowel Disease

Method of

Mark A. Peppercorn, MD, and Alan C. Moss, MD

Inflammatory bowel disease (IBD) describes the spectrum of chronic intestinal inflammation from Crohn's disease to ulcerative colitis. This condition is currently thought to occur as a consequence of a persistent and inappropriate immunologic response to gut luminal antigens. The absence of enteric parasites in developed societies and defects in mucosal innate defenses are recent additions to the many hypotheses on the pathogenesis. Irrespective of the cause, Crohn's disease (CD) and ulcerative colitis (UC) respond to a similar range of anti-inflammatory and immunomodulator therapy in inducing and maintaining remission.

Both CD and UC are characterized by mucosal ulceration, which is patchy in CD but continuous in UC. In CD the focal areas (skip lesions) of transmural inflammation and ulceration can penetrate the gut wall, leading to fistulous tracts. In 80% of patients the terminal ileum is involved, and half of these have both ileal and colonic disease. These patients typically present with crampy abdominal pain, diarrhea, and evidence of weight loss or fevers. Up to a third of patients develop perianal disease, characterized by fistulas or abscesses during their life span. Patients may also present with mouth ulcers, gastric ulceration, or skin manifestations such as erythema nodosum. These clinical patterns are dynamic, with more than 60% of patients having a change in clinical behavior over 10 years. For small intestinal disease, computed tomography (CT) with contrast is the investigation of choice, with a sensitivity of 95% in most studies. A small bowel series has advantages over CT in early disease and fistula and sinus tract delineation; magnetic resonance imaging (MRI) is superior in perianal disease. Assessment of colonic disease and tissue diagnosis is best performed with full colonoscopy and terminal ileum intubation; this allows staging of the condition and

CURRENT DIAGNOSIS

- Diagnosis should only be based on a combination of clinical, radiologic, endoscopic, and histologic features.
- Exclude tuberculosis, *Yersinia* infection, and NSAID use in suspected Crohn's disease.
- Exclude *Clostridium difficile*, *Campylobacter*, *Shigella*, and *Salmonella* infection, NSAID use, and ischemic colitis in suspected ulcerative colitis.
- Distinction between Crohn's disease and ulcerative colitis has implications for surgical interventions and prognosis.
- Nocturnal diarrhea, bloody diarrhea, weight loss, and low energy levels suggest severe disease.
- CBC, ESR, CRP, and albumin levels are useful in distinguishing disease exacerbations from functional symptoms.

Abbreviations: CBC = complete blood count; CRP = C-reactive protein, ESR = erythrocyte sedimentation rate; NSAID = nonsteroidal anti-inflammatory drug.

exclusion of other causes of terminal ileum inflammation such as tuberculosis (TB) or *Yersinia* infection. There are no diagnostic blood tests for CD per se, although erythrocyte sedimentation rate (ESR), C-reactive protein (CRP), and complete blood count (CBC) are useful markers of disease activity. CRP elevation is positively associated with clinical and endoscopic activity and severe histologic disease. Anti-*Saccharomyces cerevisiae* antibodies (ASCA) are positive in 40% to 70% of patients with CD, with a reported specificity of 95%; this may be useful in patients where the clinical pattern of colitis is nondiagnostic. In patients with a family history of CD, polymorphisms in the NOD2 gene confer an increased risk of ileal disease and fibrostenotic disease. These mutations can be found in up to 30% of patients with CD, depending on ethnic group. However, 3% of the population may also harbor such mutations, limiting their role at the diagnostic level.

UC, in contrast, is characterized by continuous inflammation proximally from the rectum; two thirds of patients have disease limited to distal to the splenic flexure at presentation, and the rest have more extensive disease. The geography of the disease is usually described in terms of its extent: proctitis (rectum), distal colitis (rectum to descending), left-sided colitis (to splenic flexure), extensive colitis (beyond splenic flexure), and pancolitis (to cecum). UC usually causes bloody diarrhea, urgency, and lower abdominal pain, progressing to fecal incontinence and nocturnal symptoms in severe disease. Up to 30% of patients progress from distal to pancolitis over 10 years. Colonoscopy remains the investigation of choice in mapping disease geography and confirming tissue diagnosis. Similar to CD, inflammatory markers such as ESR and CRP are useful to confirm clinical disease activity and predict those likely to require surgery. Antineutrophil cytoplasmic antibodies (P-ANCA) can be detected in 50% to 70% of patients with UC but in only 5% to 10% of patients with CD. These patients tend to have more aggressive disease, leading to early surgery. The main diagnoses to exclude are infective colitides, such as infection with *Clostridium difficile*, *Campylobacter*, *Shigella*, or *Salmonella*. Ischemic colitis and nonsteroidal anti-inflammatory drug (NSAID)-induced colitis can also mimic UC.

The natural history of IBD is of frequent flares of the condition in response to unknown triggers. In CD, for example, 75% of patients have a chronic intermittent course, 15% have chronically active disease, and 10% remain in remission. The management of active disease can be divided into pharmacologic therapy, surgery, and nonpharmacologic interventions. Agents are usually described in terms of obtaining remission during flare-ups and maintaining remission in the medium to long term. We describe each of these in detail and then specifically in relation to disease subtypes.

Pharmacologic Therapy

AMINOSALICYLATES

Sulfasalazine (Azulfidine), the original aminosalicylate compound, consists of sulfapyridine (an antibiotic) and 5-aminosalicylic acid (5-ASA) (an anti-inflammatory) bound with an azo bond. After ingestion, sulfasalazine reaches the colon practically unabsorbed, where the enzymatic action of colonic bacteria cleaves the azo bond to

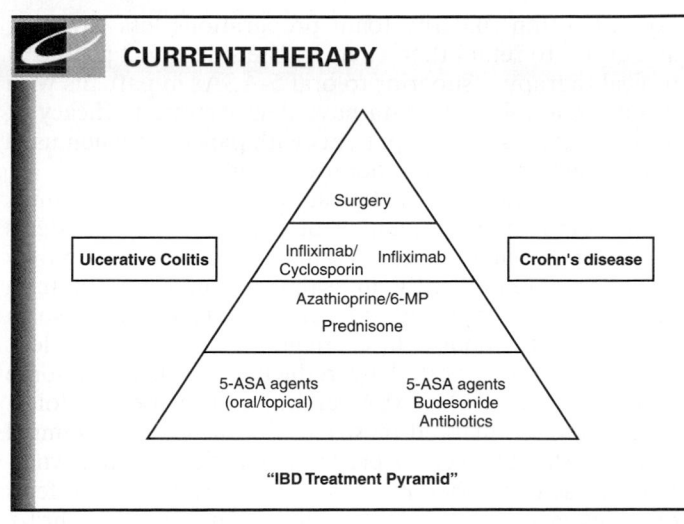

CURRENT THERAPY

"IBD Treatment Pyramid"

Ulcerative Colitis — Surgery — Infliximab/Cyclosporin — Infliximab — Azathioprine/6-MP — Prednisone — 5-ASA agents (oral/topical) — 5-ASA agents, Budesonide, Antibiotics — Crohn's disease

release the active 5-ASA from sulfapyridine. Because the sulfapyridine moiety is the cause of most of the adverse effects of sulfasalazine, most modern aminosalicylates contain 5-ASA alone or combined with an inert carrier via the azo bond. For the purposes of this discussion, we refer to the nonsulfa aminosalicylates, such as mesalamine (Asacol), balsalazide (Colazal), and olsalazine (Dipentum), as "5-ASA." The exact mechanism of action of aminosalicylates is unclear, but they appear to orchestrate a broad range of anti-inflammatory properties within the intestinal mucosa. At a molecular level they inhibit arachidonic acid metabolism and are free-radical scavengers, two pathways through which local inflammation and necrosis occurs in the intestine. They inhibit activation of peripheral and intestinal lymphocytes and their release of immunoglobulin and proinflammatory cytokines. The therapeutic effects of these alterations are dose dependent and can take up to 14 days to reach their peak clinical response. Doses of more than 2 g/day of 5-ASA are required to obtain benefit in inducing remission, occurring in 40% to 80% of patients after 4 to 8 weeks of treatment in UC. In the longer term, sulfasalazine and the 5-ASA preparations maintain remission in 60% to 80% of these patients.

A number of oral 5-ASA are preparations available. Asacol and Salofalk (in Canada) contain mesalamine coated with a pH-sensitive acrylic polymer that dissolves above pH of 6/7, typically releasing mesalamine in the terminal ileum and colon. Pentasa contains mesalamine microspheres that release 5-ASA throughout the gastrointestinal (GI) tract as these microspheres become hydrated and diffuse out of the capsule; this potentially makes it suitable for treatment of proximal small bowel disease. Olsalazine (Dipentum) contains two 5-ASA molecules joined by an azo bond that is cleaved by colonic bacteria. Balsalazide (Colazal) consists of 5-ASA bound by an azo bond to an inactive molecule, which also requires bacterial digestion to release the active 5-ASA molecules. In addition to oral therapy, topical preparations in the form of suppositories, foam, and enemas are widely used in treating distal disease. Mesalamine enemas (Rowasa) reach up to the proximal sigmoid, foam extends to the midsigmoid, whereas mesalamine suppositories (Canasa) reach the first 10 to 12 cm of the rectosigmoid region only. Patients with proctitis often find the foam preparations less irritating and easier to retain than enemas. The side-effect profile of topical therapy is superior to oral 5-ASAs in patients with distal disease. Recent data have demonstrated efficacy of topical 5-ASAs even in patients with pancolitis when used in conjunction with oral therapy.

Adverse effects from the aminosalicylate compounds are uncommon, but a number of potentially severe effects can occur. The majority of side effects occur more commonly in patients treated with sulfasalazine. The most common adverse events reported are headache, fever, and rash in up to 10% of patients. These are generally dose dependent and can be ameliorated by reducing the dose. In some patients (1% to 2%), 5-ASA can ironically cause an intolerance syndrome marked by severe diarrhea and abdominal pain; this should be considered in any patients whose symptoms worsen with therapy. Rare hypersensitivity side effects of sulfasalazine and 5-ASA include pancreatitis, nephritis, pneumonitis, pericarditis, and hepatitis. Agranulocytosis is a severe but rare side effect of sulfasalazine, which typically occurs within the first 8 weeks of therapy; it usually responds to discontinuation of sulfasalazine within 2 weeks. Infertility may also occur because of sulfasalazine in male patients by causing a reversible reduction in sperm function and number. This effect is dose dependent and can be avoided by using nonsulfa-containing 5-ASAs in these patients.

CORTICOSTEROIDS

Corticosteroids have long been used, and continue to be used, in the acute management of flares of IBD. Their exact mechanism of action is unclear, although they are a potent inhibitor of cytokine release by inducing inactivation of NFkB. This leads to a reduction in lymphocyte recruitment to inflamed areas, reduced vascular permeability, and inhibition of cytokine-mediated tissue necrosis. Although oral corticosteroids are absorbed rapidly, their biologic anti-inflammatory effects take 4 to 9 hours to take effect, regardless of mode of delivery. There appears to be no difference in the benefits of oral steroids when compared to parenteral steroids in rates of remission in IBD.

Methylprednisolone (Solu-Medrol) or hydrocortisone (Solu-Cortef) can be given parenterally in patients with severe disease or in those unable to tolerate oral intake. They are given either as bolus or continuous infusion, although no evidence indicates that either is more efficacious in obtaining remission. Intramuscular methylprednisolone induces response faster than oral prednisolone in the outpatient setting in patients with moderately active colitis. Prednisone is the most commonly used oral corticosteroid in IBD, usually at doses of 30 to 60 mg as a starting dose. The dose-response effect occurs at doses of 20 to 60 mg/day, with side effects occurring at doses greater than 40 mg. It is absorbed within 30 minutes and undergoes first-pass metabolism in the liver to produce the active drug prednisolone. In both UC and CD, steroids induce a response in approximately 80% of patients, and approximately half of these obtain remission.

These corticosteroids have little mineralocorticoid or androgenic effects, but the main risk is of suppression of the hypothalamic-pituitary-adrenal axis and Cushing's syndrome. Chronic steroid use for less than 3 weeks does not appear to suppress the hypothalamic-pituitary axis, significantly, regardless of dose. Patients receiving steroid

therapy for IBD for longer than this period should have any future reduction in steroid dose undertaken slowly (e.g., 5 mg weekly) to prevent hypoadrenalism. The main other side effect of concern is osteoporosis because up to 25% of patients with IBD have osteoporosis on bone density scans. Corticosteroid use is a major risk factor for vertebral fractures in these patients. Adequate calcium (1200 mg/day) and vitamin D (800 IU/day) are essential for patients receiving chronic steroids in IBD.

Such adverse effects with conventional synthetic steroids may be reduced with use of newer steroids such as budesonide (Entocort EC) and beclomethasone. Budesonide capsules are designed to release the active drug in the distal small bowel, where there is rapid mucosal uptake. Because of extensive hepatic metabolism, less than 10% becomes systemically available, thus reducing side effects. Beclomethasone also has high mucosal absorption with minimal systemic bioavailability.

AZATHIOPRINE/6-MERCAPTOPURINE

Azathioprine (Imuran, Azasan)[1] is a prodrug that is converted into 6-mercaptopurine[1] (6-MP, [Purinethol]) by glutathione in red blood cells. The 6-MP product is subsequently metabolized to both 6-methylmercaptopurine (6-MMP) by the TPMT enzyme, and to 6-thioguanine (6-TG) by a series of enzymatic alterations. The incorporation of 6-TG into activated lymphocytes results in activation of apoptotic pathways and inhibition of cytokine release, thus inhibiting the role of lymphocytes in IBD. These therapeutic effects take approximately 8 to 12 weeks to manifest in clinical response, which reflects the chronic inflammatory role of activated lymphocytes in IBD. Both azathioprine[1] and 6-MP (Purinethol)[1] are used in inducing and maintaining remission in both CD and UC, with efficacy rates of 60% to 70%. Azathioprine is equivalent to 6-MP in efficacy because 88% of azathioprine is metabolized to 6-MP. In practice, 6-MP is usually underdosed, whereas azathioprine is overdosed by clinicians. Full dose is 1.5 to 2.5 mg/kg for azathioprine and 1.5 mg/kg for 6-MP, although most gastroenterologists begin at a lower dose and titrate upward if no adverse effects are noted.

Side effects occur in up to 25% of patients on azathioprine[1]/6-MP,[1] but these are usually mild. Nausea and vomiting is common soon after initiation of azathioprine therapy, but in most cases this subsides or requires a trial of 6-MP instead. Bone marrow suppression and pancreatitis are two more serious adverse effects seen in patients with IBD. Leukopenia is usually dose dependent and should be prevented by monitoring CBC. We check the CBC weekly for 1 month, then every 2 weeks for 1 month, then every 3 months. Pancreatitis occurs more commonly in patients with CD and appears to be idiosyncratic. Hepatitis in the form of elevated aspartate transaminase/alanine transaminase (AST/ALT) may also occur, but this usually responds to dose reduction. There is a theoretical increased risk of infections and neoplasia in patients on immunomodulators such as azathioprine/6-MP. Meta-analysis of cohort studies reported an increased risk of lymphoma in patients with IBD treated with azathioprine/6-MP, but risk-benefit models suggest the benefits of such therapy still outweigh this risk.

---

[1]Not FDA approved for this indication.

In recent years it was recognized that an individual's level of the TPMT enzyme influences the amount of the active 6-TG metabolite they produce during azathioprine[1]/6-MP therapy.[1] Patients with low TPMT levels because of genetic polymorphisms, approximately 1 in 300 of population, produce higher levels of 6-TG and are at higher risk of leukopenia. In theory, the measurement of TPMT levels prior to commencement of therapy might identify individuals at high risk of toxicity. However, integration of TPMT testing in patients with IBD has produced mixed results in preventing toxicity; prospective data have only shown a correlation between TPMT levels and early leukopenia in patients with IBD.

METHOTREXATE

Methotrexate (MTX)[1] is a folate analogue that prevents conversion of folic acid to folinic acid, its active intracellular metabolite. This action leads to accumulation of adenosine, a potent anti-inflammatory that inhibits the production of a number of cytokines from neutrophils, macrophages, and lymphocytes. MTX also causes inhibition of proliferation and induction of apoptosis in activated T-lymphocytes. Similar to azathioprine, this effect takes up to 12 weeks to manifest clinically, and is therefore often used in patients who are steroid dependent or have failed azathioprine[1]/6-MP therapy.[1] MTX given intramuscularly shows results in 40% to 65% of patients in inducing and maintaining remission in CD. Trials using oral MTX failed to show a benefit over placebo, possibly because of variable absorption.

The main adverse effects of MTX are hepatotoxicity, myelosuppression, pneumonitis, infertility, and teratogenicity. Myelosuppression is uncommon in those receiving MTX for more than 1 year, but they should be screened for by checking the CBC every 1 to 3 months. The hepatic toxicity of MTX is well documented in other conditions where it is used at high doses, such as psoriasis. Series of IBD patients taking MTX show low prevalence of liver fibrosis with accumulated dosage greater than 2.5 g. Patients who receive MTX should have CBC and liver function tests (LFTs) frequently and further investigation if serial abnormalities appear. Folic acid supplementation is recommended in all patients who receive MTX, at least 4 hours after MTX administration.

ANTICYTOKINE THERAPY

Anticytokine therapy refers to the development of antibody therapy targeted against specific cytokines that play a role in the pathogenesis of CD, including TNF, IL-12, IL-6, and IL-8. Only anti-TNF is accepted so far into mainstream therapy based on clinical trials. Infliximab (Remicade) is a chimeric antibody (75% human, 25% mouse) against the TNF-α molecule, which leads to induction of apoptosis in activated lymphocytes. It also appears to reduce the number of inflammatory cells at the site of mucosal inflammation, possibly by inhibiting leukocyte migration. Infliximab induces and maintains remission in patients with luminal and fistulizing CD and recently induced remission in active UC. It is given as an intravenous (IV) infusion over 2 hours at 0, 2, and 6 weeks, and 8 weeks thereafter to maintain remission. In patients with CD, approximately 60% of patients respond within 2 weeks, and 30% to 50% of responders maintain response for up to 1 year. Patients who do not smoke, are also taking immunomodulators, and have nonstricturing disease achieve the best response to this therapy in CD. Recent trials in ulcerative colitis reported response rates of 70% in patients with pancolitis refractory to steroids and immunomodulators.

Adverse effects to infliximab primarily relate to immunologic reactions to the TNF antibody, which is mouse derived. Up to 60% of patients receiving infliximab develop anti-infliximab antibodies, which may cause infusion reactions and flulike illness after subsequent therapy. Thankfully these are usually mild and can be prevented by using prednisone and antihistamines prior to infusions. In the longer term up to 50% of patients may require a higher dose or shorter interval between doses to overcome loss of efficacy. More serious side effects such as reactivation of TB, cardiac events in patients with congestive cardiac failure, demyelination, and lymphoma are reported. Reactivation of latent TB occurs with an incidence of 0.46 per 1000 patient-years; therefore all patients should undergo a purified protein derivative (PPD) test and chest radiograph prior to commencement of therapy. The use of infliximab in patients with intra-abdominal collections and strictures is relatively contraindicated.

In the area of TNF inhibition, preliminary data suggest the humanized anti-TNF antibody Adalimumab (Humira)[1] and the humanized pegylated anti-TNF fragment certolizumab (Cimzia)[2] are effective in induction of response and remission in active CD. The advantage of these agents over infliximab is that they are administered subcutaneously and appear to induce fewer antibodies. Further data will be required to establish their role in CD.

CYCLOSPORINE

Cyclosporine (Neoral)[1] inhibits cytokine production primarily in activated T-helper cells by binding to calcineurin and inhibiting proinflammatory transcription factors. Its role in UC is mainly in steroid-refractory patients (no response to 72 hours of high-dose steroids) with severe colitis. It has a response rate of 80% when administered as an IV infusion for a mean of 7 days in clinical trials. However, up to 60% of responders relapse within 6 months, and by 7 years approximately 60% will have required a colectomy. The relapse rate may be reduced by immunomodulator therapy. Tacrolimus (Prograf),[1] which acts via similar pathways, shows a similar response, up to 80% in severe colitis in small studies. Cyclosporine has a number of side effects, including renal impairment, hyperkalemia, tremor, hypertension, and hirsutism. Patients with low magnesium or cholesterol are at risk of seizures. In addition there is a risk of *Pneumocystis* pneumonia, aspergillus, and cytomegalovirus (CMV) infection because of immunosuppression. Data from Europe reported mortality rates as high as 3% in patients receiving cyclosporine, although this would not be the U.S. experience.

---

[1]Not FDA approved for this indication.

[1]Not FDA approved for this indication.
[2]Not available in the United States.

ANTIBIOTICS/PROBIOTICS

Because the intestinal microflora plays a role in the pathogenesis of intestinal inflammation, manipulating the composition of this environment would be expected to ameliorate the disease process in IBD. Recent advances in the understanding of IBD suggest an impaired mucosal bacterial sensing, leading to invasion by the microflora and sustained immune response. It appears certain bacteria may be phenotype specific in the inflammatory response they elicit.

In UC, oral vancomycin (Vancocin), tobramycin (Nebcin), ciprofloxacin (Cipro), and rifaximin (Xifaxan) all improve response rates in the short term in patients with moderate to severe disease activity. IV metronidazole and tobramycin also show better response rates than placebo. These responses are not maintained in the longer term in clinical trials, however, and in the majority of trials patients were also on steroids. In practice, antibiotics are often administered to patients with severe disease requiring hospitalization as an adjunct to immunosuppressive therapy. The role of the novel nonabsorbed antibiotic rifaximin remains to be determined in active colitis and pouchitis.

The results in CD are more impressive with antibiotic therapy. Metronidazole (Flagyl) has intracellular activity against anaerobes and parasites primarily. In clinical trials it reduced colonic disease activity compared to sulfasalazine and placebo. Metronidazole is most successful in treating perianal disease, with demonstrated complete healing of chronic fistulas and symptom improvement. Finally, in patients who have undergone resection for CD, metronidazole taken for 12 weeks reduces the recurrence of endoscopic lesions at 3 months and clinical recurrence for up to 1 year. The chronicity of therapy requires close monitoring for peripheral neuropathy, the most serious adverse effect. This is unlikely to occur at daily doses less than 1 g. Patients who develop paresthesia should initially have dose reduction, followed by cessation if symptoms persist. Ciprofloxacin also produces clinical response, with 72% of patients with CD achieving complete or partial remission in recent trials. The combination of metronidazole and ciprofloxacin produces results similar to both steroids and mesalamine in patients with active disease and is a commonly used alternative to steroids. Ciprofloxacin also provides synergistic results when administered with infliximab for CD fistulas. Many gastroenterologists use antibiotic therapy in colonic and perianal CD as adjunctive therapy or as an alternative to steroids. Broad-spectrum antibiotics are also the mainstay of therapy for patients with CD who present with localized peritonitis because of a microperforation or bacterial overgrowth secondary to chronic strictures.

At the opposite end of the bacterial spectrum, probiotics have more recently been used to treat IBD. Probiotics are viable bacteria that induce beneficial therapeutic effects in intestinal mucosa. The rationale is that laboratory studies suggest that a balance between beneficial and aggressive commensal enteric microflora determines mucosal immune response in genetically susceptible individuals. Patients with IBD tend to have higher concentrations of adherent and invasive strains of bacteria such as *Bacteroides*, *Enterococci*, and *Escherichia coli*. The most studied probiotics in controlled trials to date are *Saccharomyces boulardii*, *E. coli Nissle 1917*, *Lactobacillus GG,* and a combination of eight species (*VSL#3*). In CD these randomized controlled trials produced mixed results, with some benefit demonstrated in small trials in maintenance of medically induced remission but no benefit in preventing postoperative recurrence. In ulcerative colitis, *E. coli Nissle 1917* was equal to mesalamine, and *Bifidobacteria*-fermented milk superior to placebo, in maintaining medically induced remission. No randomized controlled trials have been published in obtaining remission in patients with active disease, although a combination of bacteria showed benefit in a recent open trial. The most impressive results to date emerged in treatment of patients with pouchitis, inflammation in the ileo-anal pouch that is constructed after colectomy in patients with ulcerative colitis. *VSL#3*, a combination of eight bacterial species, is superior to placebo in preventing the development of pouchitis after pouch closure and maintaining remission after a treated episode of pouchitis. Thus, at present, the evidence suggests a definite role for probiotics as an alternative to standard therapy in prevention of pouchitis and maintenance of remission in ulcerative colitis. A number of topics in our understanding of probiotics remain to be elucidated, such as their exact anti-inflammatory mechanisms, and which probiotic strains are best suited to which conditions. A more rigorous comparison of different strains to each other and standard therapy is required. An additional approach is to stimulate the growth of an individual's commensal bacteria through dietary substances, such as oligosaccharides, inulin, and psyllium. These so-called prebiotics may tip the balance of enteric growth in favor of *Lactobacilli*, which alter luminal pH and impair invasion of disease-associated species. Some evidence indicates a potential role for this strategy in mild to moderate UC.

EXPERIMENTAL THERAPIES

As with many chronic conditions, IBD treatment still lacks a therapy that can induce high remission rates that are sustained in the long term without significant side effects. In particular, ileal CD and pancolitis that do not respond to standard therapy can prove problematic for clinicians. A high placebo response rate in CD trials (up to 50%) can make it difficult to judge the benefits of novel therapies. In response, molecular approaches targeted against specific inflammatory mediators are used with mixed effects in IBD. These include IL-11 (Oprelvekin [Neumega]),[1] thalidomide,[1] anti-IL12,* growth hormone,[1] and bone marrow transplantation. Antibodies against integrins (MLNO2, natalizumab [Tysabri]),[1] which promote translocation of lymphocytes into inflamed mucosa, improve response and remission rates in active IBD. However, the development of JC virus-related progressive multifocal leukoencephalopathy (PML) in a number of patients treated with natalizumab has raised concerns about anti-integrin therapy at present. MLNO2, which inhibits integrins specific to the gut, may avoid this rare complication. Two alternative approaches include removal of leukocytes using apheresis columns or administration of granulocyte colony-stimulating factor in patients with CD. Although many of these agents demonstrated efficacy in small trials, they are not used routinely in practice or are not licensed for treatment of IBD.

---

[1]Not FDA approved for this indication.
*Investigational drug in the United States.

NUTRITIONAL SUPPORT

Patients with IBD tend to have a high prevalence of protein-calorie malnutrition; up to 80% in some series. This tends to develop gradually in patients with small bowel CD but more rapidly in patients with UC during severe attacks. In addition to general malnutrition, specific deficits in calcium, vitamin D, vitamin B_{12}, folate, iron, zinc, and selenium are common in patients with IBD. Calcium/vitamin D depletion, in conjunction with steroid use and chronic inflammation, can lead to osteopenia in 40% to 50% of patients and to osteoporosis in up to 25%. This is associated with a 40% greater relative risk of fractures in these patients. Folate deficiency has an epidemiologic association with colorectal cancer, and supplementation may have a protective effect against dysplasia in ulcerative colitis. Zinc deficiency impairs mucosal healing, especially fistula closure, whereas selenium depletion can lead to cardiomyopathy.

Nutrition in IBD can be divided into general supportive nutrition and nutrition as primary therapy. All patients should be encouraged to maintain a balanced healthy diet without restrictions. Patients with strictures should adhere to a low-residue diet, and patients with overlap irritable bowel syndrome should avoid high-fiber foods. Calcium (1200 mg/day) and vitamin D (800 IU/day) should be taken by all patients if dietary calcium is inadequate. Folate deficiency should be sought and corrected if found. These approaches are yet to be validated in controlled trials. There is a high prevalence of lactose intolerance (40%) in patients with CD, and this should be considered and excluded if diarrhea persists despite minimal inflammatory activity. In patients with malnutrition, enteral nutrition is the preferred option as general nutritional support in most cases. Total parenteral nutrition (TPN) is associated with higher costs, greater length of stay, and more complications than enteral nutrition and should be restricted on a short term to patients with bowel obstruction or perforation, toxic megacolon, preoperatively, or for postoperative fistulas. Rarely home TPN may be required in the longer term for short-bowel syndrome after multiple resections.

Enteral nutrition as primary therapy in CD has been examined in a number of trials since the early 1980s. Systematic review of these trials concluded that enteral nutrition is superior to placebo but inferior to steroids in inducing remission in active Crohn's ileitis. Elemental diets do not appear to differ from nonelemental diets in this regard. The main problem with enteral nutrition is that it can take up to 4 weeks to demonstrate an effect, which can be difficult to comply with for these patients. Additionally, factors such as palatability, motivation, and resources can limit its use in adults. However, it remains a viable option to avoid or reduce steroids in patients with intestinal CD. There are no data to support use of enteral nutrition in ulcerative colitis, but it may be required in patients with severe colitis to supplement calorific intake.

Surgery

In the era of biologic therapy for IBD, surgery still remains an important therapeutic option for patients. In patients with UC, toxic megacolon, fulminant colitis, steroid-refractory disease, high-grade dysplasia, and cancer are all indications for colectomy. Where possible, panproctocolectomy and ileal pouch–anal anastomosis (IPAA) is the procedure of choice. This has a technical success rate of up to 95%, with the advantage of removing the diseased organ and thus cancer risk. Most patients defecate from six to eight times per day after IPAA because of the lack of colonic reservoir. Postoperative impotence in men and dyspareunia in women occurs in less than 5% of patients. In addition there is a 15% risk per year of pouchitis in the long term, which can be problematic in some patients. Hospitalized patients with severe pancolitis who do not respond to IV steroids within 72 hours should be either referred for surgery or started on cyclosporin (Neoral)[1] or infliximab (Remicade) based on current evidence. It is worthwhile for all patients with refractory UC to meet an experienced colorectal surgeon and ostomy nurse during the course of the illness to prepare them psychologically for possible surgery.

For patients with CD, indications for surgery include strictures, inflammatory collections or abscesses, fistulas, perforation, and neoplasia. Up to 70% of patients require surgery during their lifetime. Those patients who smoke or have NOD2 mutations are more likely to require surgery during the course of their disease because they are more associated with penetrating and/or stricturing disease. Local surgical therapy, such as stricturoplasty, seton placement, and limited resection, are preferred in CD because of the high rate of postoperative recurrence; approximately 50% at 5 years. Immunomodulators, such as 6-MP, and 5-ASA appear to reduce this risk and should be offered to all patients postoperatively. In those who have terminal ileum resection, bile salt diarrhea is common postoperatively and can be treated with cholestyramine. Vitamin B_{12} deficiency may occur and should be prevented with regular B_{12} injections or intranasal therapy.

Alternative Therapy

It is recognized that approximately half of all patients with IBD try nonconventional therapies during the course of their illness. The majority of these have not been assessed in randomized controlled trials or even reported in the medical literature. However, there are a number of alternative treatments we recommend to patients with mild to moderate disease who do not wish to advance to immunomodulators or biologic therapy. These are not evidence based but rather experience and anecdote based.

Aloe vera[1] has established healing properties, particularly in skin disorders. A single randomized clinical trial (RCT) in patients with mild to moderate ulcerative colitis reported that oral aloe vera gel for 4 weeks produced a significant clinical and histologic response in a small trial of 44 patients. The dose used was 100 mL of aloe vera gel taken orally per day.

Short-chain fatty acid (SCFA)[1] enemas administered daily show some promise in subsets of patients with proctitis, including those with diversion and radiation proctitis. SCFAs are an important component of mucosal nutrition, hence the rationale for their use. RCTs in ulcerative colitis reported mixed results, but they remain an option in proctitis and distal colitis that is refractory to conventional therapy.

---

[1]Not FDA approved for this indication.

Finally, dietary manipulation, in the form of the "Specific Carbohydrate Diet,"[1] has been used by a number of our patients. This involves minimizing the dietary intake of carbohydrates to monosaccharides, in an attempt to reduce the carbohydrates available for pathogenic gut bacteria. It is a restrictive diet that requires motivation. The efficacy of this dietary manipulation has not been reported in RCTs.

Management Strategies: Ulcerative Colitis

Management of UC depends on the disease geography and severity, based on prior endoscopy and symptoms. The Simple Colitis Activity Index can be used to assess disease severity in the office without laboratory results (Walmsley, 1998).

MILD TO MODERATE DISEASE

Aminosalicylates are the agents of choice for inducing remission in patients with mild to moderate UC. Patients with proctitis obtain the best response with topical therapy such as mesalamine suppositories (Canasa), 1 g once a day, whereas distal disease requires enemas (Rowasa), 4 g per day. Topical therapy is associated with a more rapid clinical response than oral 5-ASAs alone and a greater efficacy than topical steroids. Up to 80% of patients should be in remission by 6 weeks. We advise patients to insert the enema at bedtime to increase its retention. In the event of poor response or difficulty with the rectal route, oral 5-ASAs should be used. In addition, the combination of oral and topical 5-ASA agents produces better clinical results than either alone. Because the topical therapy can take up to 2 weeks to produce a clinical response, topical steroids (Cortifoam) may be used concomitantly for this period in patients who are particularly symptomatic.

In patients with left-sided extensive pancolitis, oral sulfasalazine (Azulfidine), at 2 to 4 g/day, and 5-ASA agents, at 2 to 4.8 g/day[3] should be prescribed because lower doses are not effective in inducing remission. Doses of 5-ASAs up to 4.8 g are usually well tolerated and produce clinical response in 60% of patients by 3 weeks and up to 80% in remission by 8 weeks. The dose used is probably more important than the 5-ASA agent used because there has been little comparison between the agents. Sulfasalazine has similar response rates but at a higher risk of adverse events than the other aminosalicylates, and it should be avoided in men considering fatherhood. It is significantly less expensive than the other 5-ASA agents, however, and thus more cost effective given its low absolute risk of side effects. Once remission is achieved, the same 5-ASA dose should be continued to maintain remission. As many as 90% of patients remain in remission at 1 year. Other than steroids, little evidence supports other therapies in mild to moderate disease; antibiotics, probiotics, or aloe gel may be tried in patients who cannot tolerate 5-ASAs.

SEVERE DISEASE

Approximately 9% of patients present with severely active disease, requiring supplementary therapy to 5-ASAs. It is worth excluding surreptitious NSAID use, concomitant infection by stool culture, and 5-ASA intolerance, prior to proceeding to more potent agents. In particular, *Clostridium difficile* infection in those recently hospitalized or on antibiotics, and CMV infection in those receiving steroids can cause severe colitis.

The mainstay of induction of remission in severe disease is an oral steroid. Prednisone at a dose of 40 to 60 mg/day is highly effective in inducing remission in patients with moderate to severe disease. Approximately 80% of patients respond, and 54% are in remission at 1 month. No studies have compared the efficacy of oral to IV administration. Hydrocortisone (Solu-Cortef), at 100 mg IV every 6 hours, or methylprednisolone (Solu-Medrol), 40 mg/day IV, can be used in the few patients who do not respond or have difficulty with oral absorption. Hyperglycemia occurs commonly and should be monitored for, especially in those receiving IV steroids. In those patients who respond to steroids, the aim should be to begin a steroid taper after approximately 2 weeks of high-dose therapy. The dose should be reduced by 5 mg weekly until either the steroids are withdrawn or the patient develops recurrence of symptoms. If patients are not already on 5-ASAs, they should be started during the steroid taper as maintenance therapy. If patients cannot be withdrawn from steroid therapy because of recurrence of symptoms (steroid dependent), azathioprine (Imuran, Azasan),[1] at a dose of 1.5 to 2.5 mg/kg, or 6-MP (Purinethol),[1] at a dose of 1.5 mg/kg, should be started as maintenance therapy. As discussed previously, it may take 12 weeks for full effect, and patients should have their AST, ALT, and CBC checked regularly for adverse effects. The strategy here is to remove the steroids gradually as the therapeutic effect of azathioprine/6-MP manifests. Once in remission, treatment should continue indefinitely because patients who later have their maintenance drugs stopped have a higher rate of relapse. These agents can be used for induction of remission also, but the long time to clinical effect is usually too long when patients have severe disease.

In those cases with severe colitis where steroids do not induce a clinical response, the options then are cyclosporine (Neoral),[1] infliximab (Remicade), or surgery at present. Steroids are usually given for 72 hours to determine their response before proceeding to these options, although surgery is indicated sooner for toxic megacolon, fulminant colitis, or hemorrhage. One study demonstrated that those patients with a bowel frequency of more than eight times per day or a CRP greater than 45 have an 85% chance of colectomy after 3 days of medical therapy. Cyclosporine,[1] at a dose of 2 to 4 mg/kg/day by infusion, produces a response in up to 80% of patients after 8 days of therapy. Recent data suggest the response from 2 mg/kg is similar to 4 mg/kg with less adverse events. Renal function, blood pressure, magnesium levels, cholesterol, and cyclosporine levels should be monitored during treatment. Magnesium less than 0.5 mg/dL or a cholesterol level less than 120 mg/dL increases the risk of seizures. Opportunistic infections such

---

[1]Not FDA approved for this indication.
[3]Exceeds dosage recommended by the manufacturer.

---

[1]Not FDA approved for this indication.

as *Pneumocystis* pneumonia (PCP) and *Aspergillus* should be considered if patients develop respiratory symptoms. We routinely prescribe prophylaxis against PCP with sulfamethoxazole/trimethoprim (Bactrim) because deaths from this infection are reported in patients receiving cyclosporine for ulcerative colitis. Patients usually respond within 4 days of treatment; in this case they can be switched to oral cyclosporine[1] at a dose of 5 to 7 mg/kg/day, with maintenance of serum trough levels between 150 and 250 µg/mL.

The other medical option is infliximab (Remicade) at a dose of 5 mg/kg by IV infusion. In patients with severe ulcerative colitis who are hospitalized, this halves the risk of colectomy at 90 days. For patients with moderate to severe UC, infliximab produces response in 65% and puts approximately 30% of patients into remission at 30 weeks if given at 0, 2, 6 weeks, and at 8 weeks thereafter. The precautions and side effects are similar to its use in CD. All patients should have a PPD and chest radiograph (CXR) prior to instigation of therapy, and infusion reactions can be prevented with prednisone or IV hydrocortisone. No comparison between cyclosporine and infliximab has been made in these patients to date. If these medical options do not improve individual cases, surgery will be required.

Management Strategy: Crohn's Disease

At any one time, approximately 50% of patients with CD will be in remission or have mild disease that is responsive to therapy. Of the rest, 40% will be postsurgery and 10% will have severe or treatment-refractory disease.

MILD TO MODERATE DISEASE

In patients with ileocolonic disease, there are three initial treatment options: antibiotics, 5-ASAs, or budesonide (Entocort EC). Evidence from clinical trials and clinical experience differs as to which agent to use, but all three show moderate efficacy in this setting. There is significant controversy among IBD experts about which agent should be used as first-line therapy. We generally use mesalamine (Asacol, Pentasa, Salofalk) first for ileal disease, followed by ciprofloxacin (Cipro) or metronidazole (Flagyl) in nonresponders. For ileocolonic disease we use sulfasalazine (Azulfidine) as first-line therapy, followed by the other 5-ASAs. Other experts in the field start with budesonide (Entocort EC), whereas we reserve this for nonresponders to initial therapy.

Metronidazole, at doses of 500 mg three times daily, and ciprofloxacin, at 500 mg twice daily, produce a moderate clinical response in patients with ileal and colonic disease and more marked improvements in those with perianal disease. Therapy should continue for at least 3 months to maximize the therapeutic benefit, and the development of paresthesia should warrant dose reduction or discontinuation of metronidazole. Patients on ciprofloxacin should be warned about the risk of tendon rupture. In the event of a partial response to one agent, the combination of metronidazole and ciprofloxacin is often used prior to proceeding to steroids. Antibiotic resistance does not seem to be a problem in our practice, despite prolonged therapy.

Budesonide (Entocort EC), at 3 mg three times daily, is as effective as prednisone and superior to mesalamine with fewer side effects in ileitis and ileocolonic disease. Patients who respond may be continued at a maintenance dose of 6 mg/day because this reduces relapse rates. For colonic disease, 5-ASAs are first-line therapy in CD. Mesalamine at 4 g/day or sulfasalazine (Azulfidine) at 3 g/day produces a clinical response in 50% to 60% of patients. This response takes up to 2 weeks to develop and requires adequate doses of 5-ASA. The role of 5-ASAs in maintaining remission once achieved is controversial, although probably worthwhile if patients have responded. Regardless of which agent is used to induce remission, if therapy cannot be tapered without worsening of symptoms, immunomodulator therapy should be initiated. Azathioprine (Imuran[1]), 6-MP (Purinethol[1]), and methotrexate[1] should be started in this setting.

SEVERE DISEASE

The selection of more aggressive therapy for CD should be individualized for each patient because this area is rapidly evolving. As in UC, oral steroids are highly effective first-line therapy for severe CD. Approximately 60% to 80% of cases respond to prednisone, 40 to 60 mg/day, and this should be tapered once the clinical status stabilizes. In this setting, azathioprine,[1] 1.5 to 2.5 mg/kg, or 6-MP,[1] 1.5 mg/kg, may be started during the steroid taper period or withheld until further episodes. Patients treated with immunomodulator maintenance therapy have a reduced risk of relapse in the medium term.

If patients do not respond to steroids, or they are concerned about their adverse effects, the next options are infliximab or methotrexate. Infliximab should be administered at a dose of 5 mg/kg at 0, 2 and 6 weeks initially. Patients usually notice a response within 1 to 2 weeks in the 60% of patients who respond. The development of infusion-related reactions can be prevented on subsequent doses by slowing the rate of infusion or administering prednisone, 50 mg twice daily, on the day before administration, or hydrocortisone, 200 mg IV, prior to the infusion. In those who respond to infliximab, repeated infusions every 8 weeks maintain approximately 30% to 40% in remission in the medium term. If this response wanes with time, either increase the dose to 10 mg/kg or shorten the duration between infusions. Patients with disease that requires infliximab should all be started on azathioprine[1] or 6-MP[1] as maintenance therapy because this appears to reduce antibody production against the infliximab molecule.

An alternative to infliximab in steroid-refractory disease is methotrexate.[1] Induction of remission with 25 mg IM weekly, followed by 15 mg IM weekly, induced remission in approximately 40% of patients treated and maintained 65% in remission in clinical trials at 1 year. All patients should have their AST/ALT and CBC monitored and take folic acid supplementation. This therapy is teratogenic so should be discussed prior to its use in women of child-bearing age or women intending to conceive.

Strictures that do not respond to medical therapy require surgical intervention because some of these will be "cold"

---

[1]Not FDA approved for this indication.

[1]Not FDA approved for this indication.

stenotic strictures without mucosa inflammation. Draining fistulas are primarily treated with antibiotics as above or infliximab with azathioprine[1]/6-MP[1] in more resistant cases. Deep perianal fistulas can be treated with seton placement and superficial ones with fistulotomy.

Pregnancy

Pregnancy often raises questions about both pregnancy and disease outcomes and about drug therapy for women with IBD. There is a small increased risk of low birth weight and premature delivery in women with IBD, especially those with CD. The risk of a child of an affected parent developing UC is 2% to 5% and developing CD is 5% to 10% over their lifetime. Patients in remission at the time of conception are no more likely to develop a relapse than at other times of life, although if this occurs it is most often in the first trimester. Many cases of relapse in disease activity are actually because of discontinuation of maintenance therapy once the pregnancy is confirmed. In general, patients in remission with IBD have better pregnancy outcomes than those with active disease; therefore continuation of suitable maintenance medications is important in this setting. Apart from methotrexate, most drugs used for management of IBD can safely be used during pregnancy. This includes 5-ASAs, steroids, azathioprine,[1] 6-MP,[1] cyclosporine,[1] infliximab, and metronidazole (after the first trimester). As with all drugs, the benefits need to be weighed against potential adverse effects that are unknown. Drugs that should be avoided if possible during breast-feeding include olsalazine (Dipentum), azathioprine[1]/6-MP,[1] methotrexate,[1] cyclosporine,[1] and infliximab[1] if possible. Apart from the 5-ASA agents and steroids, there is little experience documented in breast-feeding with these drugs; women in this situation should consult with their pediatrician.

Colon Cancer Surveillance

The risk of colorectal cancer (CRC) is increased in patients who have colitis for greater than 8 years; the excess risk is 19.2 for those with pancolitis and 2.8 for those with left-sided disease. At 20 years since onset of diagnosis, patients have an 8% risk of cancer. In particular, patients with primary sclerosing cholangitis and UC have a 31% risk of CRC at 20 years.

Surveillance for CRC should begin at 8 years after diagnosis for patients with disease beyond the descending colon and continue every 2 years. In patients with distal colitis and Crohn's colitis, the ideal surveillance intervals are more difficult to determine because the risk may be similar to more extensive colitis. Our personal practice is to perform surveillance on all those with UC above the rectum or extensive colonic CD after 8 years of disease. Because of the higher risk of CRC, all patients with primary sclerosing cholangitis should have surveillance regardless of their duration of UC or CD. Those patients in whom dysplasia or adenomas are detected require more intensive surveillance or consideration of colectomy. The finding of high-grade dysplasia or dysplasia-associated lesion or mass (DALM) is an indication for colectomy. However, when low-grade

dysplasia is found, the risk of neoplasia progression is controversial, varying between 5% and 50%. We most often recommend colectomy for patients with long-standing colitis and low-grade dysplasia.

In those at high risk of CRC (e.g., family history of CRC, long disease history, primary sclerosing cholangitis [PSC], extensive colitis), chemoprophylaxis should be advised. 5-ASA at doses of 1.5 to 2 g/day in some case-control studies reduced CRC risk by at least 50%. Folic acid supplements, calcium, and NSAIDs such as aspirin reduce the risk of CRC in the general population. It is not known whether a combination of these produces an additive benefit, and they have not specifically been studied in IBD.

REFERENCES

Aberra FN, Lichtenstein GR: Review article: Monitoring of immunomodulators in inflammatory bowel disease. Aliment Pharmacol Ther 2005; 21:307-319.

Banerjee S, Peppercorn MA: Inflammatory bowel disease. Medical therapy of specific clinical presentations. Gastroenterol Clin North Am 2002;31:185-202.

Campieri M: New steroids and new salicylates in inflammatory bowel disease: A critical appraisal. Gut 2002;50(Suppl 3):III43-III46.

Farrell RJ, Peppercorn MA: Ulcerative colitis. Lancet 2002;359:331-340.

Ferrero S, Ragni N: Inflammatory bowel disease: Management issues during pregnancy. Arch Gynecol Obstet 2004;270:79-85.

Hanauer SB, Korelitz BI, Rutgeerts P: Postoperative maintenance of Crohn's disease remission with 6-mercaptopurine, mesalamine, or placebo: A 2-year trial. Gastroenterology 2004;127:723-729.

Jain SK, Peppercorn MA: Inflammatory bowel disease and colon cancer: A review. Dig Dis 1997;15:243-252.

Loftus EV Jr, Schoenfeld P, Sandborn WJ: The epidemiology and natural history of Crohn's disease in population-based patient cohorts from North America: A systematic review. Aliment Pharmacol Ther 2002; 16:51-60.

Rutgeerts P, Van AG, Vermeire S: Optimizing anti-TNF treatment in inflammatory bowel disease. Gastroenterology 2004;126:1593-1610.

Thukral C, Travassos WJ, Peppercorn MA: The role of antibiotics in inflammatory bowel disease. Curr Treat Options Gastroenterol 2005;8:223-228.

Velayos FS, Terdiman JP, Walsh JM: Effect of 5-aminosalicylate use on colorectal cancer and dysplasia risk: A systematic review and metaanalysis of observational studies. Am J Gastroenterol 2005;100:1345-1353.

Walmsley RS, Ayres RC, Pounder RE, Allan RN: A simple clinical colitis activity index. Gut 1998;43:29-32.

Irritable Bowel Syndrome

Method of
Kevin W. Olden, MD, and Andrew R. Brown, MD

Irritable bowel syndrome (IBS) is a chronic disorder characterized by abdominal discomfort or pain associated with changes in stool frequency and/or stool form. IBS is considered a *functional* gastrointestinal (GI) disorder because it is characterized by abnormal gut motility, sensation, and symptom expression. The altered gut motility can be characterized by slow gut transit (constipation), fast gut transit (diarrhea), or spastic nonperistaltic colonic contractions (pain/bloating). Like other symptom-defined syndromes, such as fibromyalgia, the diagnosis is based on clinical grounds. Table 1 presents the symptom-based diagnostic criteria for IBS as defined by the Rome International Working Teams on functional GI disorders.

---

[1]Not FDA approved for this indication.

TABLE 1 Rome II Criteria for Irritable Bowel Syndrome

In the absence of structural or metabolic abnormalities to explain the symptoms: At least 12 weeks, which need not be consecutive, in the preceding 12 months the patient has experienced abdominal discomfort or pain that has at least two out of three features:

Pain or discomfort relieved with defecation; *and/or*

Onset associated with a change in stool frequency; *and/or*

Onset associated with a change in form (appearance) of stool.

Symptoms that cumulatively support the diagnosis of irritable bowel syndrome:

Abnormal stool frequency (for research purposes "abnormal" may be defined as greater than 3 bowel movements per day and less than 3 bowel movements per week).

Abnormal stool form (lumpy/hard or loose/watery stool)

Abnormal stool passage (straining, urgency, or feeling of incomplete evacuation)

Passage of mucus.

Bloating or feeling of abdominal fullness.

From Thompson WG, Longstreth G, Drossman DA, et al: Functional bowel disorders. In Drossman DA, Corazziari E, Tally NJ. et al (eds): Rome II: The Functional Gastrointestinal Disorders, 2nd ed. McLean, Va, Degnon Associates, p 355. Copyright © 2000 Degnon Associates.

It is clear that there are countless causes of diarrhea, constipation, and abdominal pain.

IBS usually presents in early adulthood, usually between 15 and 30 years of age. De novo presentation after 40 years of age is somewhat uncommon, and those patients should be worked up for other causes of abdominal pain, diarrhea, and constipation. In the absence of alarm symptoms (Table 2), the Rome criteria are very sensitive and specific for the diagnosis of IBS. The Rome criteria in patients without alarm symptoms have a sensitivity of 65%, specificity of 100%, and positive predictive value of 98% to 100%.

Epidemiology

IBS is an extremely common disorder across national and ethnic lines. Females are more likely to be affected than males (1.5–2.5:1). IBS is the most common disorder seen by gastroenterologists and accounts for 40% of all visits.

TABLE 2 Alarm Symptoms or Red Flags

Symptom onset >40 y
Short duration of symptoms
Severe, unrelenting diarrhea
Nocturnal symptoms
Unintentional weight loss
Overt or occult gastrointestinal bleeding
Family history of organic gastrointestinal diseases
Inflammatory bowel disease (IBD)
Celiac disease
Gastrointestinal malignancy
Abnormal selected laboratory evaluation

In the primary care setting, 12% of all visits are related to IBS, but only approximately 25% of IBS patients seek medical care.

Psychological Co-Morbidity

A multitude of studies show that patients with IBS are more likely to have mood and anxiety disorders. The ability to diagnose and treat these two co-morbid psychiatric disorders can lead to significant improvement in both health-related quality of life (HRQOL) and the patients' GI symptoms. Conversely, the failure to diagnose and treat concomitant psychiatric diagnoses can lead to a less than optimal response to medical management.

In addition, certain psychosocial phenomena are associated with IBS. Patients that have suffered physical or sexual abuse are much more likely to have IBS. In one study, 44% of patients with functional GI disorders reported a history of sexual or physical abuse, although only 17% had informed their physicians. Some studies even suggested that the severity of the abuse suffered correlates with the severity of the patients' IBS symptoms. Although psychological disorders and psychosocial states are associated with IBS, there is no evidence to prove causality. Screening for psychological disorders can help to treat the so-called treatment-refractory IBS patients.

Pathophysiology

No pathognomonic abnormality is identified to fully explain the symptoms of IBS. Numerous studies have documented abnormalities in gut motility. Unfortunately, commonly used agents that act on gut motility, such as prokinetics, smooth muscle relaxants (antispasmodics), and anticholinergics, show minimal benefit in lessening IBS symptoms.

Research has demonstrated increased visceral hypersensitivity in IBS patients, as shown by decreased pain thresholds with rectal balloon distention. It is known that 90% of the serotonergic neurons are found in the enteric nervous system. Abnormalities in serotonin activity are associated with IBS. Based on this information, drugs that act on serotonin receptors were developed and are beneficial in the treatment of IBS.

Diagnosis

IBS can be arbitrarily divided into three groups: diarrhea predominant, constipation predominant, and alternating. These subtypes are not well defined, and patients can migrate among groups. Recent literature suggests that patients who present with IBS and those who present with diarrhea need to be approached differently.

CURRENT DIAGNOSIS

- IBS is *not* a diagnosis of exclusion.
- Use the Rome II Criteria for diagnosis of IBS (Table 1).
- Rule out so-called alarm symptoms (Table 2),

One important form of constipation that can mimic IBS is so-called outlet constipation. It is also known as anismus and pelvic floor dyssynergia (PFD). This disorder is not a result of altered colonic motility. Rather it is a disorder of incoordination of the muscles of the pelvic floor. Patients often report inability to expel stool and often must manually disimpact themselves. The diagnosis is confirmed by anorectal manometry. As in IBS, this disorder is strongly associated with sexual or physical abuse. Treatment success rates of up to 85% are reported using anorectal biofeedback therapy.

The advocated approach to the diagnosis of IBS is a positive approach based on clinical parameters rather than as a diagnosis of exclusion. The diagnosis should be based on meeting the Rome II criteria for IBS (Table 1), the patient's presenting symptom complex (i.e., diarrhea or constipation), a thorough history and physical exam, and *selected* laboratory evaluation. Laboratory testing should include a complete blood count, routine chemistry studies, thyroid stimulating hormone (TSH) determination, stool occult blood test, and an erythrocyte sedimentation rate (ESR). Although little evidence supports the use of these tests, they are inexpensive and are part of routine evaluation. In contrast, evidence supports testing antitissue transglutaminase-IgA (TTG-IgA) levels for celiac disease, which has increased prevalence in diarrhea-predominant IBS (IBS-D).

Occult or overt bleeding, fevers, unintentional weight loss, and laboratory abnormalities such as anemia or elevated nonspecific markers of inflammation such as ESR or C-reactive protein (CRP) are inconsistent with the diagnosis of IBS. The presence of these so-called alarm symptoms (Table 2) should prompt further investigation on their own merit.

Patients with a family history of colon cancer should be screened according to current American Cancer Society (ACS) guidelines. Collagenous/microscopic colitis is common in patients older than 40 years, particularly in white females. Colonoscopy with biopsy in this patient population therefore is recommended. Findings suggestive of malabsorption should prompt the need for bacterial overgrowth testing and small bowel biopsies to rule out celiac disease. Any changes in an IBS patient's clinical picture over time may also prompt further investigation.

Treatment

The treatment of IBS (Table 3) should be aimed at improving bowel habits, abdominal discomfort, bloating/fullness, and quality of life/global well-being. Unfortunately, most of the studies regarding IBS are of poor quality and do not provide good evidence for therapy with few exceptions (noted later).

CURRENT THERAPY

- Maximize the doctor–patient relationship.
- Recognize and treat any co-morbid psychiatric diagnoses.
- Use appropriate medications based on symptoms and severity.
- Use a biopsychological approach to patient care.

TABLE 3 Irritable Bowel Syndrome Therapy

Diarrhea Predominant
Dietary measures (fiber, probiotics, etc.)
Antidiarrheals
Loperamide (Imodium)
Diphenoxylate and atropine tablet (Lomotil)
Smooth muscle relaxants (antispasmodics)
Hyoscyamine (Levsin)
Dicyclomine (Bentyl)
Serotonin antagonist
Alosetron (Lotronex)*
Antidepressants[1]
Tricyclic antidepressant (TCA)
Selective serotonin reuptake inhibitor (SSRI)
Behavior therapy

Constipation Predominant
Dietary measures (fiber, probiotics, etc.)
Serotonin agonist
Tegaserod (Zelnorm)
Laxatives
Antidepressants[1]
TCA
SSRI
Behavior therapy

---

[1]Not FDA approved for this indication.
*Alosetron (Lotronex) has monitored prescribing secondary to risk of ischemic colitis. Information regarding prescribing can be obtained at Glaxo Smith Klein (GSK) at 888-825-5249 or the FDA at http://www.fda.gov/.

PHYSICIAN–PATIENT RELATIONSHIP

An effective doctor–patient relationship is an invaluable constituent in treatment in IBS. It is important to obtain a complete history, in a nonconfrontational, nonjudgmental, patient-centered manner, along with a complete physical exam. This strengthens the patient's trust in the diagnosis. The physician should give realistic expectations regarding the prognosis and provide a thorough explanation of IBS in words the patient can understand. It is important for patients with IBS to have an ongoing relationship with their health care providers. This can greatly affect the patient's trust in the diagnosis and may prevent unnecessary tests.

TRADITIONAL THERAPY

The use of fiber, antispasmodics (smooth muscle relaxants), antidiarrheals, and laxatives were the mainstay of therapy for years with limited data supporting their use. In regard to fiber, there may be some benefit in both diarrhea and constipation, but data regarding efficacy are quite poor. Increased bloating and gas may be observed in some patients. In regard to antidiarrheals, Loperamide (Imodium) was studied and adds some modest benefit in diarrheal symptoms alone. However, it does not improve the global symptoms of IBS such as pain, bloating, and rectal urgency. Laxatives, like antidiarrheals, are a large part of the treatment of IBS and may improve constipation but do not help with the global constipation-predominant IBS (IBS-C) symptoms of bloating and abdominal pain. They also may lead to increased cramping and diarrhea. Despite the poor data regarding their effectiveness compared to placebo, traditional treatments are commonly used. The treating physician must have low expectations for their effectiveness.

ANTIDEPRESSANTS

Tricyclic antidepressants (TCA) and selective serotonin reuptake inhibitors (SSRIs) in recent high-quality trials were of reasonable benefit in IBS. TCAs decreased abdominal pain in particular. A recent study showed a statistically significant improvement in IBS symptoms with desipramine (Norpramin[1]) compared to fiber using a per protocol analysis. It is important to note that in this study, side effects caused a significant dropout rate (29%) in the desipramine (Norpramin) arm that precluded an intention to treat (ITT) analysis. This side-effect-driven reduction in patient adherence is a unique quality of the antidepressants. Clinicians must realize there may be a need to switch patients to another antidepressant that the patient can both tolerate and benefit from. Intolerance to other antidepressant drugs *does not* predict intolerance to other antidepressant drugs in the same or other classes. The dosing of TCAs (Table 4) for IBS is similar to the dosing for chronic pain, and the effects on pain are independent of the antidepressant effect.

When using a TCA for the treatment of IBS, the clinician should start off with the lowest dose possible because side effects may decrease adherence. Physicians need to realize that TCAs can be used in both IBS-C and IBS-D, but all of the TCAs have some anticholinergic effect and may therefore promote constipation. Therefore, caution needs to be exercised in IBS-C. SSRIs improve global function in IBS; however, the data in regard to pain control need more study. Paroxetine (Paxil) improves the overall well-being of depressed and nondepressed IBS patients but does not change the abdominal pain and bloating. Both TCAs and SSRIs seem to be beneficial in IBS.

SEROTONIN AGONISTS AND ANTAGONISTS

The serotonin hypothesis in regard to the brain–gut interaction is promising with the addition of drugs that have an effect on serotonin receptors. Tegaserod (Zelnorm), a

[1]Not FDA approved for this indication.

5-HT_4 partial agonist, promotes bowel motility, relieves symptoms, and should be considered first-line therapy in the management of IBS-C. In well-designed controlled studies it improved symptoms, bowel habits, pain/bloating, abdominal fullness/distention, and quality of life/global function. Alosetron hydrochloride (Lotronex) is a 5-HT_3 antagonist that is effective in relieving diarrhea, rectal urgency, and abdominal pain in female IBS-D patients. In postmarketing surveillance, an increased incidence of ischemic colitis was noted in patients using alosetron (Lotronex), and the drug was withdrawn from the market. It has since been reintroduced with a monitored prescribing program. Patients taking Alosetron (Lotronex) are counseled on the risks via *the monitoring program* and are instructed to cease therapy if they develop constipation. Any physician who "self-attests" his or her competence in the diagnosis and treatments of IBS can prescribe alosetron (Lotronex). Information regarding prescribing can be obtained from Glaxo Smith Klein (GSK) at 1-888-825-5249 or the FDA at http://www.fda.gov/.

BEHAVIORAL THERAPY

Patients often state that their symptoms completely dominate and significantly alter their lives. The preponderance of data supports the efficacy of relaxation therapy, cognitive-behavioral therapy, interpersonal psychotherapy, and hypnosis in treating IBS. Hypnosis decreases psychological distress and somatic symptoms and does so without affecting physiologic parameters. A study comparing the effectiveness of paroxetine (Paxil[1]), behavioral therapy, and placebo for severe IBS demonstrated that behavioral therapy was superior to paroxetine (Paxil), which was superior to placebo. Therefore, behavioral therapy can be a great addition to the armamentarium for patients with severe IBS.

PROBIOTICS

Probiotics may have a role in IBS as well. Interestingly, patients with IBS have abnormal IL-10 to IL-12 ratios, suggesting mild inflammation. In a recent study, *Bifidobacterium infantis* 35624* was shown in IBS patients to both improve symptoms and fix the abnormal IL-10 to IL-12 ratios.

Prognosis

The long-term prognosis of IBS is quite good. Several large-term prospective cohort studies showed no increased mortality with IBS. IBS symptoms tend to improve with time but do not often resolve. Informing patients of their positive prognosis can help calm the anxiety at the initial visit and is of vital importance. The ability to reassure patients with ongoing medical and emotional support is vital for the care of patients with this often-disabling chronic disorder.

TABLE 4 Antidepressant Gastrointestinal Dosing Guidelines

Antidepressant	Dosage (mg)	Range (mg/dL)
Amitriptyline[1] (Elavil)	10–150	50–300
Citalopram[1] (Celexa)	10–40	20–60
Desipramine[1] (Norpramin)	10–100	50–300
Escitalopram[1] (Lexapro)	5–20	5–20
Imipramine[1] (Tofranil)	10–150	50–300
Nortriptyline[1] (Pamelor)	10–150	100–210[3]
Paroxetine[1] (Paxil)	10–20	20–50

[1]Not FDA approved for this indication.
[3]Exceeds the dosage recommended by the manufacturer.

[1]Not FDA approved for this indication.
*Orphan drug in the United States.

REFERENCES

Brandt LJ, Locke R, Olden K, et al: An evidence based approach to the diagnosis of irritable bowel syndrome in North America. Am J Gastroenterol 2002;97:S1-S26.

Camilleri M, Chey WY, Mayer EA, et al: A randomized controlled clinical trial of the serotonin type 3 receptor antagonist alosetron in women with diarrhea-predominant irritable bowel syndrome. Arch Intern Med 2001;161(14):1733-1740.

Cash BD, Schoenfeld PS, Chey WD: The utility of diagnostic tests in irritable bowel syndrome patients: A systematic review. Am J Gastroenterol 2002;97:2812-2819.

Creed F, Fernandes L, Guthrie E, et al: North of England IBS Research Group. The cost-effectiveness of psychotherapy and paroxetine for severe irritable bowel syndrome. Gastroenterology 2003;124(2):303-317.

Drossman DA, Camilleri M, Mayer EA, et al: AGA technical review on irritable bowel syndrome. Gastroenterology 2002;123:2108-2131.

Drossman DA, Toner BB, Whitehead WE, et al: Cognitive-behavioral therapy versus education and desipramine versus placebo for moderate to severe functional bowel disorders. Gastroenterology 2003;125(1):19-31.

Novick J, Miner P, Krause R, et al: A randomized, double-blind, placebo-controlled trial of tegaserod in female patients suffering from irritable bowel syndrome with constipation. Aliment Pharmacol Ther 2002;16(11):1877-1888.

O'Mahony L, McCarthy J, Kelly P, et al: Lactobacillus and Bifidobacterium in irritable bowel syndrome: Symptom responses and relationship to cytokine profiles. Gastroenterology 2005;128(3):541-551.

Owens DM, Nelson DK, Talley NJ: The irritable bowel syndrome: Long-term prognosis and the physician-patient interaction. Ann Intern Med 1995;122:107-112.

Spiegel BM, DeRosa VP, Gralnek IM, et al: Testing for celiac sprue in irritable bowel syndrome with predominant diarrhea: A cost-effectiveness analysis. Gastroenterology 2004;126(7):1721-1732.

Tabas G, Beaves M, Wang J, et al: Paroxetine to treat irritable bowel syndrome not responding to high-fiber diet: A double-blind, placebo-controlled trial. Am J Gastroenterol 2004;99(5):914-920.

Thompson WG, Longstreth G, Drossman DA, et al: Functional bowel disorders. In Drossman DA, Corazziari E, Tally NJ, et al (eds): Rome II: The Functional Gastrointestinal Disorders, 2nd ed. McLean, Va, Degnon Associates, 2000, p 355.

Vanner SJ, Depew WT, Paterson WG, et al: Predictive value of the Rome criteria for diagnosing the irritable bowel syndrome. Am J Gastroenterol 1999;94(10):2803-2807.

Hemorrhoids, Anal Fissure, Perianal Abscess, and Fistula

Method of
David A. Margolin, MD, and Kerry Hammond, MD

Anorectal pathology can present a diagnostic challenge to even the most experienced clinician. An understanding of the pathophysiology and symptoms associated with common disorders of this anatomic region is essential to diagnose and treat these conditions accurately.

Hemorrhoids

ANATOMY AND PATHOPHYSIOLOGY

Hemorrhoidal disease is one of the most common disorders of the alimentary tract. Despite this prevalence, the underlying anatomy and pathophysiology that result in patient symptoms are often poorly understood.

Hemorrhoids are vascular cushions that line the inner surface of the anal canal. These submucosal vascular sinusoids lack a muscular wall. This deficiency is responsible for the amount of bleeding seen in hemorrhoid disease. Bleeding associated with hemorrhoids is arterial, originating from presinusoidal arterioles. Hemorrhoidal tissue is present at birth and thought to contribute to normal anal continence. Therefore, the presence of hemorrhoidal tissue in the absence of symptoms does not necessarily constitute a disease state.

Enlargement and prolapse of internal hemorrhoidal tissue contribute to the distressing symptoms that most patients associate with hemorrhoidal disease. Prolapse develops subsequent to the degeneration or weakening of the connective tissue structures that anchor the anal cushions to the underlying muscular layers of the internal sphincter. Constipation, excessive straining during bowel movements, and advanced age contribute to this process.

CLASSIFICATION

Hemorrhoids are classified according to their anatomic location within the anal canal. External hemorrhoids are located distal to the dentate line and covered by a layer of exquisitely sensitive anoderm (keratinized epithelium). Internal hemorrhoids are located proximal to the dentate line, where the overlying columnar mucosa lacks somatic innervation. Mixed hemorrhoids are a confluence of both internal and external hemorrhoids and encompass features of both. Columns of hemorrhoidal tissue are located in the left lateral, right anterior, and right posterior aspects of the anal canal. A four-point grading system is commonly used to further categorize internal hemorrhoids. Grade I hemorrhoids protrude into the anal canal without external prolapse. Grade II hemorrhoids spontaneously reduce after strain-induced prolapse. Grade III hemorrhoids require manual reduction when prolapse occurs. Grade IV hemorrhoids are characterized by irreducible prolapse.

CURRENT DIAGNOSIS

Differential Diagnosis of Anorectal Symptoms

SYMPTOM	POSSIBLE ETIOLOGY
Bleeding	Hemorrhoids, rectal prolapse, rectal ulcer, anal fissure, neoplasm
Itching	Hemorrhoids, pruritus ani, pinworms, dermatoses, Bowen's or Paget's disease, sexually transmitted disease
Pain	Anal fissure, thrombosed external hemorrhoid, anorectal abscess, sexually transmitted disease.
Drainage	Fistula-in-ano, anorectal abscess, anal incontinence, sexually transmitted disease
Mass	Anal or rectal tumor, hypertrophic anal papilla, abscess, hemorrhoids, anal warts

PATIENT EVALUATION

It is common for patients to attribute any anorectal discomfort or bleeding to hemorrhoidal disease. A careful history and physical examination is necessary to avoid making an incorrect diagnosis.

Typical symptoms associated with internal hemorrhoidal disease include mucus discharge, mucosal protrusion, and tenesmus. Hemorrhoidal bleeding is painless. After bowel movements, patients may notice blood in the toilet water or on the toilet tissue only. Although acute thrombosis of external hemorrhoids can cause significant pain, internal hemorrhoids are relatively painless because of their anatomic position. The evaluating physician should obtain a detailed description of bowel habits, medications, and dietary patterns from patients who present with these symptoms.

Examination of the perineum may be performed using a proctologic table or with the patient in a modified left lateral decubitus position on a standard examination table. After a careful inspection of the perianal skin, the anal canal should be visualized by gently separating the buttocks. The presence of a tender external mass with blue discoloration is characteristic of a thrombosed external hemorrhoid. The proximal anal canal can be viewed using an anoscope. Although nonenlarged internal hemorrhoids are generally not palpable, digital rectal examination remains an essential component of the physical examination. With this simple procedure, the clinician can evaluate the anal canal and lower rectum for masses while assessing the integrity of the anal sphincter.

The diagnosis of hemorrhoidal disease can usually be made on the basis of symptoms and physical findings. Further evaluation by colonoscopy or barium enema should be considered in patients over 50 or if additional symptoms are present.

TREATMENT

Several treatments for hemorrhoidal disease are available. Selection of a therapeutic regimen should be made based on the severity and acuity of the patient's symptoms.

The objective of conservative management is the alleviation of symptoms while ruling out more serious pathology. Modification of the patient's bowel habits by increasing dietary fiber is the initial therapeutic step. Dietary fiber promotes the formation of soft formed stool, which requires less straining for elimination. This can be achieved through dietary modifications, increasing insoluble fiber consumption, and/or oral fiber supplementation. Sitz baths and topical agents are also useful for symptomatic relief.

Fixation of prolapsed internal hemorrhoidal tissue in its correct anatomic position can be achieved through several nonsurgical outpatient procedures. Infrared photocoagulation, a technique by which infrared radiation is delivered directly to the hemorrhoid base, causes scarring and appropriate tissue fixation. Although this technique is extremely effective, its utility is limited by equipment expense. The most commonly employed nonsurgical procedure for grade I through III hemorrhoids is rubber band ligation. Tight bands applied anoscopically at the apex of the hemorrhoidal bundle cause vascular constriction, tissue sloughing, and scar formation that fixes the hemorrhoid tissue to the wall of the anal canal.

Surgical excision of hemorrhoidal tissue is indicated when conservative management and nonsurgical procedures fail to alleviate symptoms. It is also indicated for patients with severe mixed hemorrhoidal disease. Although grade IV hemorrhoids may respond to multiple rubber band treatments, surgical excision should be considered early in the course of therapy for this condition. The most common operation performed in the United States is the closed Ferguson hemorrhoidectomy. This technique employs sharp elliptical excision of one or multiple hemorrhoidal columns followed by suture reapproximation of the anal mucosa. Postoperative bleeding and urinary retention are the most common complications of this procedure. Stapled hemorrhoidectomy, or procedure for prolapsing hemorrhoids, has gained popularity in recent years. A circular stapling device is used to resect a circumferential strip of hemorrhoidal tissue and anal mucosa above the dentate line, reducing the mass of prolapsed tissue and disrupting the vascular supply to the remaining hemorrhoidal tissue.

 CURRENT THERAPY

Hemorrhoids

CLASSIFICATION	DESCRIPTION	THERAPEUTIC OPTIONS
Grade I (internal)	Anal canal protrusion without prolapse	■ Conservative management ■ Rubber band ligation, photocoagulation
Grade II (internal)	Prolapse with spontaneous reduction	■ Conservative management ■ Rubber band ligation, photocoagulation
Grade III (internal)	Prolapse requiring manual reduction	■ Conservative management ■ Rubber band ligation, photocoagulation ■ Excisional or stapled hemorrhoidectomy
Grade IV (internal)	Irreducible prolapse	■ Excisional hemorrhoidectomy
Acute prolapse with thrombosis (internal)	History of acute onset with physical signs of ischemia, thrombosis, or gangrene	■ Emergent excisional hemorrhoidectomy
Acute thrombosis (external)	Tender, bluish mass near the anal verge	■ Excision (acute presentation) ■ Conservative management (symptom duration >72h at time of presentation)

Although several studies have demonstrated a reduction in postoperative pain with this technique, long-term results of this procedure are yet to be determined.

Acute thrombosis of external hemorrhoids can cause considerable pain. If seen within 72 hours. complete excision of the thrombosed hemorrhoid can be performed under local anesthesia, reducing the duration of the patient's pain. However, conservative measures, including bulk agents, topical pain medications, and sitz baths, are often effective when symptoms have been present for more than 72 hours.

Anal Fissure

ANATOMY AND PATHOPHYSIOLOGY

An anal fissure is a linear ulceration or tear in the anoderm, extending from the dentate line caudally to the anal margin. The most common anatomic position of this lesion is in the posterior midline. Although rare in men, 10% to 20% of fissures in female patients occur in the anterior midline. Anal fissures located at the lateral aspects of the anal canal are less common and are associated with inflammatory bowel disease, syphilis, tuberculosis, leukemia, carcinoma, and HIV.

Although several theories pertaining to the pathogenesis of anal fissures are proposed, anal canal trauma, usually caused by the passage of a firm hard bowel movement or diarrhea, is believed to be the primary etiology of most idiopathic fissures. Internal sphincter hypertonicity is also implicated as a contributing factor by causing a relative reduction in anodermal blood flow. The resulting ischemic tissue, particularly at the poorly vascularized posterior aspect of the anal canal, is vulnerable to injury and has an impaired capacity for healing.

PATIENT EVALUATION

Patients with anal fissures usually describe an onset of severe perianal pain, a "tearing sensation," preceded by a hard firm bowel movement. Physical examination can be difficult because of the intense pain associated with anal fissure. Inspection of the perianal region and anal canal should be performed with the patient in the left lateral decubitus position or on a proctologic exam table. An acute fissure typically has distinct mucosal edges and a pink base. A fibrotic "sentinel pile" may accompany more chronic fissures. Examination under anesthesia may be necessary if patient discomfort precludes a thorough examination.

TREATMENT

Acute idiopathic anal fissures often respond to conservative therapy using bulk agents, a high-fiber diet, and warm sitz baths. Topical preparations containing nitroglycerin[1] and diltiazem (Cardizem)[1] can promote healing by reducing anal canal pressure and increasing anodermal perfusion through vasodilation. Internal sphincter tone can also be reduced with injections of botulinum toxin.

[1]Not FDA approved for this indication.

Surgical therapy is usually reserved for chronic fissures and acute fissures that do not improve with conservative treatment. The primary objective of surgical intervention for anal fissures is to disrupt the hypertonic internal sphincter and improve blood flow to the anal canal. Lateral internal sphincterotomy is the most common surgical procedure used in the United States for the treatment of anal fissures. This technique, in which sharp division of the distal third of the internal sphincter is performed, is associated with low rates of fecal incontinence and fissure recurrence. Atypically positioned anal fissures should be biopsied to rule out malignancy inflammatory bowel disease or a sexually transmitted disease (STD).

Anorectal Abscess and Fistula-in-Ano

PATHOPHYSIOLOGY

Most anorectal abscesses develop as a result of obstruction of the anal glands, a series of 4 to 10 ducts that enter the anal canal submucosa at the level of the dentate line. Fistula-in-ano is a chronic manifestation of cryptoglandular infection. Less common etiologic factors in the development of abscesses and fistulas in the anorectal region include inflammatory bowel disease, tuberculosis, trauma, radiation therapy, and malignancy.

ANATOMIC CLASSIFICATIONS OF ANORECTAL ABSCESS

To treat an anorectal abscess adequately, the clinician must be familiar with the potential anatomic spaces into which the abscess might extend. The *perianal* space is located around the anal verge and becomes continuous with the *intersphincteric* space at the level of the internal and external sphincters. The laterally located *ischiorectal* space extends from the levator ani to the perineum. The *supralevator* space lies between the levator ani and the peritoneal surface. Anorectal abscesses are classified according to the anatomic space that they inhabit. A rare fifth classification of anorectal abscess is the horseshoe abscess, which develops as suppuration extends circumferentially through the intersphincteric, supralevator, and ischiorectal spaces.

ANATOMIC CLASSIFICATIONS OF FISTULA-IN-ANO

A fistula-in-ano is an abnormal epithelialized tract extending between the rectum or anal canal and the perineum. The anatomic classification of fistula-in-ano is based on the relationship of the fistula tract to the sphincter structures. An *intersphincteric fistula* extends between the internal and external sphincters. *Transsphincteric fistulas* extend from an internal opening in the anal canal across the internal and external sphincters and terminate in the ischiorectal fossa. *Suprasphincteric fistulas* originate near the level of the dentate line, extending proximally above the puborectalis and then distally lateral to the external sphincter to a terminal point on the perineal surface. *Extrasphincteric fistulas* pass from the rectum above the levator ani and distally through the ischiorectal fossa to the perineum.

PATIENT EVALUATION

Complaints of pain, perianal swelling, and fever are common in the presence of an anorectal abscess. Patients with an abscess in the supralevator space may complain of gluteal pain. In cases of perianal and ischiorectal abscesses, physical examination typically reveals a painful, fluctuant mass. Intersphincteric abscesses are more difficult to diagnosis. On rectal exam, there may only be a slight fullness. Supralevator abscesses may not be apparent on physical examination. Computed tomography can be a useful diagnostic tool if physical examination findings do not correlate with the patient's symptoms.

Patients with fistula-in-ano often complain of bloody or purulent drainage, pain with defecation, and a decrease in swelling or pain when drainage occurs. A history of a prior abscess is common. The external fistula orifice can usually be seen on physical examination. Digital rectal examination may reveal a palpable nodule or cordlike structure at the location of the internal fistula opening. Anoscopy can be a useful adjunct for determining the extent of the fistula tract.

TREATMENT OF ANORECTAL ABSCESS

Drainage is the cornerstone of therapy for anorectal abscesses. Abscesses in the perianal and ischiorectal spaces can often be drained in the office. Under local anesthesia, an incision is made over the point of maximal fluctuance and a 10 to 14 French mushroom catheter is placed in the abscess. This provides almost instant relief. The catheter is left in place for 5 to 7 days. Antibiotics are used only in cases of immunosuppression, diabetes, or if prosthetic cardiac valves or joints are present. Treatment of anorectal abscesses with antibiotics alone is inadequate and can have devastating consequences if the infectious process progresses without surgical drainage. Abscesses that are more complex or anatomically inaccessible should be addressed in the operating room under general anesthesia.

TREATMENT OF FISTULA-IN-ANO

Obliteration of the fistula tract, preservation of sphincter function, and prevention of recurrence are the mainstays of surgical treatment. Once the internal fistula opening is identified, simple intersphincteric and low transsphincteric fistulas can be treated by fistulotomy. After inserting a probe through the tract from internal opening outward, the overlying skin is incised over the entire length of the fistula. The residual granulation tissue is then removed by curettage to promote healing from the base outward. Complex fistulas and tracts with high internal openings can be addressed with seton placement or anorectal mucosal advancement flaps. Although the rate of recurrence is higher, the use of fibrin glue injections for fistula closure does not compromise sphincter function and is a reasonable alternative for long, narrow fistula tracts.

REFERENCES

Beck DE, Wexner SD (eds): Fundamentals of Anorectal Surgery, 2nd ed. London, WB Saunders, 1998.

Billingham RP, Isler JT, Kimmins MH, et al: The diagnosis and management of common anorectal disorders. Curr Probl Surg 2004;41:586-645.

Fleshman J. Advanced technology in the management of hemorrhoids: Stapling, laser, harmonic scalpel, and ligature. J Gastrointest Surg 2002;6(3):299-301.

Hardy A, Chan CLH, Cohen CRG: The surgical management of haemorrhoids—a review. Dig Surg 2005;22:26-33.

Johanson JF: Nonsurgical treatment of hemorrhoids. J Gastrointest Surg 2002;6(2):290-294.

Lacerda-Filho A, da Silva RG: Stapled hemorrhoidectomy: Present status. Arq Gastroenterol 2005;42(3):191-194.

Metcalf AM: Anal fissure. Surg Clin North Am 2002;82:1291-1297.

Nelson R: Anorectal abscess fistula: What do we know? Surg Clin North Am 2002;82:1139-1151.

Senagore AF: Surgical management of hemorrhoids. J Gastrointest Surg 2002;6(3):295-298.

Gastritis and Peptic Ulcer Disease

Method of
Barry J. Marshall, MD

Gastritis

Gastritis literally means inflammation of the stomach. Gastritis is a nonspecific term because it can be used to describe:

- Symptoms related to the stomach.
- An endoscopic appearance of the gastric mucosa.
- Histologic change characterized by infiltration of the epithelium with inflammatory cells such as polymorphonuclear leukocytes (PMNs).

The last description is the most correct.

CLINICAL GASTRITIS

In lay terms, nausea and vomiting with epigastric pain might be called "an attack of gastritis," even though the exact pathology affecting the stomach is unknown. Use of

CURRENT DIAGNOSIS

- In the majority of cases of dyspepsia, no structural abnormality can be identified after investigation.
- Patients with dyspepsia older than 55 years or with alarm symptoms (anemia, anorexia, weight loss, early satiety, dysphagia, and gastrointestinal bleeding) should undergo upper endoscopy promptly.
- *Helicobacter pylori* infection and nonsteroidal anti-inflammatory drugs (NSAIDs) are the two most common causes of peptic ulcer disease.
- Endoscopic biopsy, urea breath test, and stool antigen testing are the most accurate ways to diagnose active *H. pylori* infection.
- Zollinger-Ellison syndrome should be suspected if there are multiple duodenal ulcers, ulcers that are refractory to treatment, or peptic ulcers associated with diarrhea.

the term *gastritis* in this situation is to be discouraged because symptoms correlate rather poorly with actual pathology present in the stomach.

ENDOSCOPIC GASTRITIS

Mucosal Redness (Erythema)

The appearance of the mucosa at endoscopy does not correlate well with the histologic diagnosis determined from a biopsy. Confusion can arise because almost every abnormality of the gastric mucosa is called gastritis by endoscopists.

The normal color of the gastric mucosa is pink, similar to the palm of your hand. An appearance of redness probably represents increased capillary blood flow in the mucosa but does not necessarily mean that inflammatory cells are present. When bile is present, the redness often appears to be diffusely present throughout the stomach.

Redness (erythema) in the gastric mucosa may be localized to the antrum or the corpus. It may be homogeneous or mottled, or present in spots from petechia size to a few millimeters. Sometimes redness is present on the top of the gastric folds of the corpus. Often, red streaks radiate upward from the pylorus. In all cases it is appropriate for the endoscopist to refer to the appearance as endoscopic gastritis, accompanied by a description of gastric mucosa. General treatment of endoscopic gastritis is to treat the patient's symptoms, usually with acid reduction therapy and avoidance of foods or medications that might aggravate the problem. Specific treatment of endoscopic gastritis depends on a histologic diagnosis. Therefore, biopsies of the gastric mucosa are necessary.

Surface Irregularity (Chicken Skin, Gooseflesh, Cobblestones)

The cause of small lumps on the antral mucosa, which are referred to as chicken skin, gooseflesh, and cobblestones, is usually *Helicobacter pylori* gastritis.

EROSIVE GASTRITIS

Erosions are breaks in the mucosa that do not extend beyond the muscularis mucosa. All lesions less than 1 mm deep are erosions. The distinction between ulcers and erosions might not have much effect on patient management because both can bleed and both are usually healed with acid-blocking therapy.

Umbilicated lumps may be a variant of erosive gastritis. As with all erosive mucosal lesions of the gastrointestinal (GI) tract, viral causes should be considered in immunosuppressed patients.

Atrophic Gastritis and Gastric Atrophy

After many years of chronic gastritis, the gastric mucosa can become atrophic (i.e., thin and translucent), with the submucosal veins easily visible. In severe cases, the folds normally present in the upper half of the stomach (the corpus) are diminished or absent (gastric atrophy). Acid secretion diminishes and the condition predisposes to adenocarcinoma of the stomach. *H. pylori* and pernicious anemia are the two main causes.

Hypertrophic Gastritis (Ménétrier's Disease)

Rarely, gastric folds are massively increased in size because of hyperplasia and hypertrophy of the specialized acid-secreting mucosa. Excessive mucus secretion leads to a syndrome of hypoalbuminemia with diarrhea, edema, or a hypercoagulable state. *H. pylori* infection is one cause; other causes are idiopathic (so far).

Portal Gastropathy and Angiodysplasia

The red lesions caused by portal gastropathy and angiodysplasia give a pattern of snakeskin and watermelon stomach, respectively, when severe. They may cause GI blood loss but are usually asymptomatic. The former is associated with portal hypertension. The latter is idiopathic and treated, when necessary, with argon plasma coagulation.

Histologic Gastritis

Histologic gastritis is present when inflammatory cells infiltrate the mucosa. Diagnostic biopsies for detection of gastritis should be taken from intact mucosa, away from any focal lesion. At least one antrum and one corpus biopsy should be examined by histology because diseases can selectively affect only the mucus-secreting mucosa of the antrum or only the parietal cell mucosa of the corpus.

If mononuclear cells are increased, chronic gastritis is present. If the PMNs are also increased, the gastritis is termed as active. In typical *H. pylori* infection, PMNs infiltrate the necks of the mucus-secreting glands of the gastric antrum causing active chronic gastritis.

Helicobacter pylori Gastritis

In the first week after infection, many PMNs and a few eosinophils infiltrate the mucosa. These are gradually replaced with the mononuclear cells. The presence of lymphoid follicles is called mucosa-associated lymphoid tissue (MALT). Rarely, MALT may become autonomous to form a low-grade, B-cell lymphoma called MALT lymphoma. When gastric tissue exists in the duodenal bulb (normally present in approximately 60% of persons), *H. pylori* may also colonize that location leading to active duodenitis.

When *H. pylori* is eradicated with antibiotics, PMNs disappear in a week or so, but reduction in the mononuclear cells is slow, often leaving mild chronic gastritis several years after *H. pylori* has disappeared.

In most countries with a high prevalence of *H. pylori*, gastric cancer is common, although diet probably also modulates the risk so that the association is not universal. Because *H. pylori* causes peptic ulcer and gastric cancer, nearly everyone with *H. pylori* chooses to be treated with antibiotics.

Non–*Helicobacter pylori* Gastritis

Because *H. pylori* is the most common cause of gastritis, and perhaps the most easily treated, non–*H. pylori* gastritis must be diagnosed with caution. Usually the *H. pylori* has been missed because of low numbers of organisms. This occurs when patients have recently taken antibiotics, or are taking proton pump inhibitors (PPIs), or have a patchy infection caused by intestinal metaplasia in the stomach (to which *H. pylori* cannot adhere). Therefore, as well as taking biopsies for urease test, histology, and culture, the physician should check serology before claiming a patient has *H. pylori*–negative histologic gastritis. Laboratory-based serologic tests are quite sensitive so can be used to confirm that *H. pylori* is not present and that the negative biopsy diagnosis is correct.

Rare causes of *H. pylori*–negative histologic gastritis are Crohn's disease, eosinophilic gastritis, gastric MALT lymphoma, as well as (very rarely) other viral and bacterial infections.

NONSTEROIDAL-INDUCED EROSIVE GASTRITIS AND ULCERS

Aspirin and nonsteroidal anti-inflammatory drugs (NSAIDs) are corrosive. Aspirin and NSAIDs inhibit prostaglandin synthesis, which is essential for maintenance of the mucus and bicarbonate barrier in the stomach. The resulting gastric erosions are often asymptomatic but sometimes lead to gastric ulcer or duodenal ulcer.

The harmful effects of NSAIDs and *H. pylori* are not synergistic because *H. pylori* boosts the prostaglandin levels, thus partially negating the deleterious effect of the NSAID.

Eradication of *H. pylori* before or at the beginning of NSAID therapy is worthwhile. Once NSAID patients have developed an ulcer, provided that treatment of the ulcer with a PPI is continued, eradication of *H. pylori* is neither urgent nor essential.

DYSPEPSIA VERSUS GASTRITIS

Dyspepsia is defined here as discomfort in the upper half of the abdomen and lower chest that is somehow related to food. Symptoms and descriptions vary widely so the patient's ethnicity needs to be taken into account when taking a history.

Regurgitation refers to reflux of gastric contents into the mouth without discomfort. Gnawing is a feeling halfway between hunger and nausea, in which case the patient tends to have small snacks to ease the symptom without vomiting. Fullness and bloating are feelings of distention that contribute to early satiety in some patients so that they are unable to finish a normal-sized meal. Burning epigastric and lower thoracic pain that is quickly relieved by antacid is likely to be caused by gastroesophageal reflux disease (GERD), although it is wise to exclude a cardiac cause.

In general, dyspepsia correlates poorly with endoscopic findings. When endoscopy is freely available at no cost to the patient, endoscopy quickly defines a management plan and gives greater patient satisfaction, according to questionnaires given to patients 12 months later. However, endoscopy-first strategies are approximately 20% more expensive.

The alternative strategy is called test and treat, where patients are selected for initial endoscopy only if they have alarm signs, are older than 50 years, or are in a high-risk category for gastric cancer. Alarm signs are dysphagia, vomiting, weight loss, blood in the stool, a family history of gastric cancer, an abdominal mass, or virtually any abnormal laboratory test.

When dyspepsia is diagnosed but there is no peptic ulcer, the condition is called nonulcer dyspepsia (NUD) or functional dyspepsia. Many NUD patients actually have GERD. If GERD is suspected, a 7-day trial of double-dose PPI therapy is worthwhile.

For patients not obviously suffering from GERD, the possibility of peptic ulcer should be considered. Because most peptic ulcers are related to *H. pylori* infection, noninvasive tests for *H. pylori* can be used to determine ulcer risk. Patients who are *H. pylori*-negative on serology are unlikely to have peptic ulcer. This means that they can be managed by trial and error until symptoms respond to therapy. Conversely, patients who are *H. pylori*-positive on serology should be regarded as possible ulcer candidates and should have the bacterium eradicated as the first step in management.

For patients who actually do have an ulcer, antibiotic therapy for *H. pylori* leads to clinical cure in approximately 70% of cases. Of the 30% who do not respond clinically, 50% have persistent *H. pylori*, and the remainder have *H. pylori*–negative dyspepsia (GERD, etc.). To differentiate these groups it is necessary to confirm cure of *H. pylori* in all patients who do not completely respond to *H. pylori* eradication. Cure is confirmed with a urea breath test. Follow-up breath test is also necessary in all patients with known peptic ulcer because these patients are at risk of ulcer relapse, with all its possible complications, if *H. pylori* persists. Because a nonendoscopic strategy does not separate ulcer from nonulcer patients at the beginning, there is a case for confirmation of *H. pylori* eradication in all patients, so that ulcer relapse never occurs.

GASTROESOPHAGEAL REFLUX DISEASE

Gastroesophageal reflux disease and symptoms related to the esophagus may be treated initially with acid reduction therapy, as needed. Antacid is used for immediate relief, and H$_2$ receptor antagonists (H$_2$RAs) or PPIs may be given at the same time to diminish acid secretion over the next few hours. Combinations of these two are available as over-the-counter (OTC) medications in the United States. If dysphagia is present (difficulty swallowing), immediate endoscopy is advised because this could be an early symptom of esophageal cancer or an acid-induced stricture.

If GERD symptoms do not completely respond, or if the patient requires the treatment just outlined on a daily basis, then endoscopy is required. Endoscopy will indicate whether the patient's symptoms correlate with the disease severity. It is important to control both clinical and endoscopic GERD because continued heartburn raises the lifetime risk of esophageal adenocarcinoma.

GERD patients should be given the following common-sense advice. Eat smaller meals, control obesity, and avoid tight clothing around the abdomen. Avoid liquids with meals, especially tea, coffee, colas, and beer. Do not eat large meals during the working day. Avoid bending or heavy work after meals. Eat the evening meal at least 3 hours before bedtime. Raise the head of the bed and sleep on the left side. Tablets that might damage the esophagus (aspirin, doxycycline, alendronate) should be taken before meals to ensure that they do not linger in the esophagus.

In spite of the management just described, many patients continue to have symptoms, and endoscopic assessment reveals acid-induced esophageal damage. In this case lifestyle measures are rarely curative, and long-term acid reduction with PPI is required. Because PPIs have long half-lives, once-daily therapy is usually sufficient. For severe GERD, start at double the usual dose and then decrease after 3 months to a single daily maintenance dose. The aim of medical therapy is complete control of acidic symptoms. Advise patients that long-term medical treatment is usually necessary.

OTHER DYSPEPSIA

Because chronic dyspeptic symptoms unrelated to GERD or ulcer do not have a specific cause or defined therapy, it is worthwhile initially to search for another, more treatable diagnosis. Be certain to exclude cardiac causes of chest pain. Intermittent pain could be esophageal spasm, which can be diagnosed with esophageal manometry. Treat with PPI to abolish any GERD component, smooth muscle relaxants for the acute episode, and calcium channel blockers (CCBs). Note that therapy for angina is quite similar, so cardiac disease needs to be ruled out before treating esophageal spasm. Some of the medical therapy causes side effects that make treatment hardly worthwhile in patients with intermittent spasm.

EPIGASTRIC DYSPEPSIA AND GASTROPARESIS

Always try to find the definitive causes of epigastric dyspepsia and gastroparesis because this allows better planning of therapy and more accurate prognosis. Endoscopy often rules out any macroscopic lesion such as an ulcer or a tumor, allowing trials of medical therapy to proceed.

If the patient has symptoms of GERD, but does not respond completely to therapy, he or she may be a rapid metabolizer of PPI. If starting with once-daily omeprazole (Prilosec), double the dose to twice daily, use a more powerful drug (esomeprazole [Nexium]), choose one with a longer half-life (pantoprazole [Protonix]), or use a drug that is less affected by metabolizer status (rabeprazole [AcipHex]). At endoscopy, avoid PPI on the day of the test and measure gastric-juice pH to see if the patient maintains a pH above 4 for the complete 24 hours after a dose. If pH is above 4.0, then the cause of the continued symptoms might not be acid reflux.

Symptoms of nausea and/or vomiting are unlikely to be caused by esophageal disease. Gastric mucosal problems or gastric outlet obstruction need to be considered. The two should be considered separately because disorders such as acute viral gastroenteritis and food poisoning cause nausea but motility is normal. Similarly, patients with chronic gastroparesis are worse off if they also have a mucosal disease such as H. pylori causing the nausea.

If H. pylori is present, it should be treated. If patients cannot take antibiotics because of nausea, try to settle them with high-dose PPI because this suppresses H. pylori in 50% of cases.

Delayed gastric emptying (gastroparesis) may be diagnosed with an isotope gastric emptying study. When present, gastroparesis is usually a chronic disorder with relapses and remissions. Eradication of H. pylori often

decreases nausea and settles the condition somewhat, but relapses still occur in most patients. Promotility agents such as metoclopramide (Reglan) and cisapride (Propulsid)* should be used (cisapride is no longer available in the United States because it has caused fatal arrhythmias). Small doses of erythromycin[1] (25 mg per day before meals) may improve gastric peristalsis because this drug is a motilin agonist. As long as obstruction is not present, a soft or liquid diet will usually empty from the stomach, even when motility is poor. Posturing the patient to stay vertical after meals, with an inclination toward the right side, should help gastric contents drain through the pylorus. Avoid uncooked vegetables because skins and salad leaves take many hours to leave the stomach. A low-residue diet is preferred whenever motility is impaired.

MANAGEMENT OF DYSPEPSIA

I usually include a test and treat strategy for H. pylori as part of any dyspepsia management plan. I also search for

---

[1]Not FDA approved for this indication.
*Investigational drug in the United States.

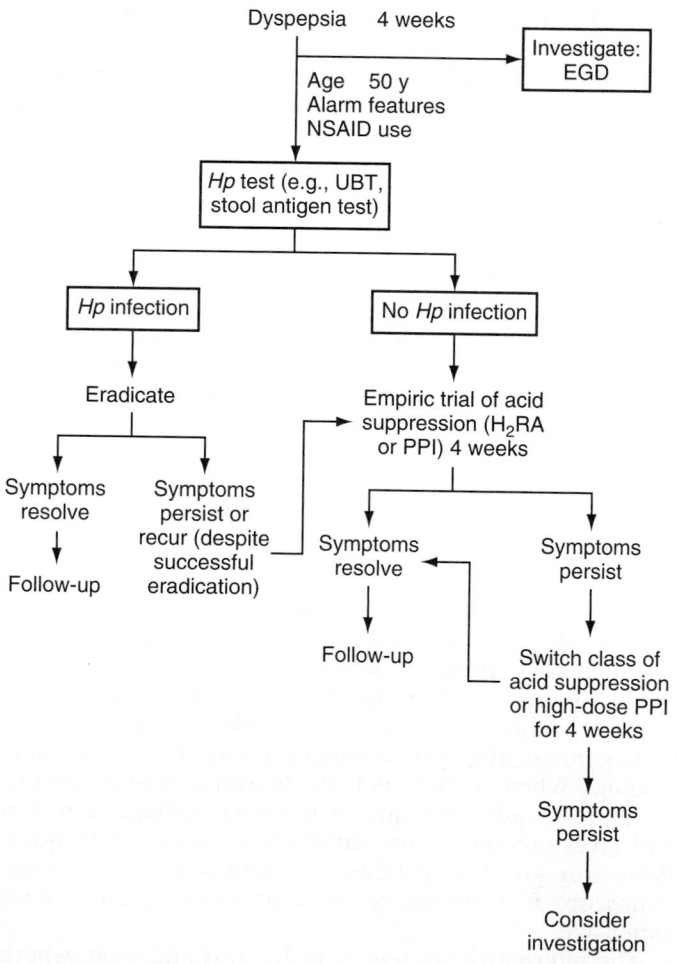

FIGURE 1. Management of uninvestigated dyspepsia. EGD = esophagogastroduodenoscopy; H₂RA = H₂ receptor antagonist; Hp = Helicobacter pylori; NSAID = nonsteroidal anti-inflammatory drug; PPI = proton pump inhibitor; UBT = urea breath test (¹³C or ¹⁴C).

and treat GERD with PPI. Lesser symptoms of GERD or vague dyspepsia may respond (if needed) to an H_2 blocker such as ranitidine (Zantac), 150 mg once or twice daily. In addition, patients can carry antacid tablets for immediate relief. Antacid-H_2RA combinations are available OTC in the United States, and these are very effective. Figure 1 shows the complete algorithm for management of dyspepsia.

Peptic Ulcer

Peptic ulcer is usually caused by *H. pylori*, NSAIDs, or a combination of the two. Rarely, hyperacidity is caused by a gastrinoma (Zollinger-Ellison syndrome) in which case a cause may not be found until serum gastrin is noted to be elevated. In any ulcer situation, resuscitate the patient and control acute bleeding endoscopically. At the first endoscopy, diagnostic biopsies should be taken for *H. pylori* (one urease test, one antrum, and one corpus for histology). If *H. pylori* is present, initiate treatment. *H. pylori* serology should be sent if the bacterium is not detected on biopsy because sometimes the acutely ill patient has taken medication that suppresses *H. pylori* in the gastric mucosa but has not eradicated the bacterium.

Ulcer patients without *H. pylori* usually have NSAIDs as the cause of the ulcer. In patients who have both *H. pylori* and NSAIDs, the sensible approach is to treat both. In most cases the NSAIDs will have been ceased and the patient given intravenous PPI, so antibiotic therapy is not the most important part of the acute therapy. Adding intravenous amoxicillin to an *H. pylori*–positive patient is an option to improve the healing rate of a dangerous ulcer. The normal oral *H. pylori* therapy can be completed a few days later when the patient tolerates a normal diet.

Peptic ulcers almost always heal once the initiating factor has been removed. However, it is usual to give H_2RA or PPI for 8 weeks to ensure a symptom-free healing period. During this time the *H. pylori* can be eradicated. At the end of 8 weeks, PPI can be changed to H_2RA, and a follow-up urea breath test (UBT) can be done to confirm eradication of the bacterium. A stool antigen test is an alternative.

◯ CURRENT THERAPY

Treatment Options for *Helicobacter pylori*

Group		Duration
A*	Bismuth	
	Ranitidine bismuth citrate (RBC),[2,‡] 400 mg bid	14 d
	Bismuth subsalicylate (Pepto-Bismol),[†] 525 mg (2 tabs) qid	14 d
	Bismuth subcitrate[1,*] (DE-NOL) 120 mg (1 tab) qid	14 d
B	Penicillin	
	Amoxicillin, 1 g bid	7, 10, or 14 d
C	Macrolide	
	Clarithromycin (Biaxin), 500 mg bid	7, 10, or 14 d
	Josamycin,[1,2,*] 1000 mg bid	7 d
D	Nitroimidazole	
	Metronidazole (Flagyl),[1] 500 mg bid or tid	7, 10, or 14 d
	Tinidazole,[1,2] 1000 mg qd	7, 10, or 14 d
E	Tetracycline	
	Tetracycline,[1] 500 mg qid	14 d
F	Quinolone	
	Ofloxacin (Floxin),[1] 1000 mg[3] qd	7–14 d
	Levofloxacin (Levaquin), 500 mg qd	7–14 d
	Ciprofloxacin (Cipro),[1] 500 mg bid	14 d
G	Nitrofuran	
	Furazolidone (Furoxone),[1] 100 mg qid	7, 10, or 14 d
H	Ansamycin	
	Rifabutin (Mycobutin),[1] 150 mg bid	14 d
I	Proton pump inhibitors (use double a normal dose)	
	Omeprazole (Prilosec), 20 mg bid	
	Esomeprazole (Nexium), 40 mg bid	
	Lansoprazole (Prevacid), 30 mg bid	
	Pantoprazole (Protonix), 40 mg bid	
	Rabeprazole (AcipHex), 20 mg bid	

[1]Not FDA approved for this indication.
[2]Not available in the United States.
[3]Exceeds dosage recommended by the manufacturer.
*Investigational drug in the United States.
†When Pepto-Bismol is not available, substitute DE-NOL, 1 tablet qid.
‡RBC is not available in all countries.
Note: Side effects are likely as doses of clarithromycin, metronidazole, and furazolidone increase. Treatment combination priorities are normally IBC, IBD, IBEG.
    For penicillin allergy, choose ICD or IAED then IFH.

In patients who are unable to cease their NSAIDs, the drug should be changed to a cyclooxygenase (COX)-2 selective agent. In addition, full-dose PPI should be continued long term. Most ulcers will then heal and not relapse. Low-dose aspirin may remove the benefit of COX-2 selective NSAIDs, so the relative benefits of aspirin should be reviewed in all patients. Prostaglandins are not a first-choice ulcer therapy because of side effects, such as cramps (in women) and diarrhea; however, they do specifically protect against erosive gastritis and peptic ulcer caused solely by NSAIDs.

TREATMENT FOR *HELICOBACTER PYLORI*

In vitro testing does not correlate with in vivo success, so treatment combinations should be used that have been proven to work in each individual country. Treatment for less than 7 days has a low cure rate, but cure rates from day 7 to day 14 are similar, and more than 14 days of treatment is usually unnecessary. The first drug to use is a PPI to render the gastric pH neutral. This enhances the cure rate for the second drug, which is usually amoxicillin (Amoxil). Clarithromycin (Biaxin) is given as the third drug. Treatment and doses vary in each country; doses in the Current Therapy box are typical for the United States and Australia.

One month after completing therapy, ensure that the patient is not taking PPI for 7 days, and then perform a UBT. Serology remains positive after treatment so it is not useful to prove eradication. If the UBT shows persistent infection, re-treat with a different regimen. As a second therapy, you may use PPI and amoxicillin again because *H. pylori* does not develop resistance to amoxicillin. The third drug should change to metronidazole (Flagyl).[1] Always repeat the UBT after therapy.

If two therapies fail, the *H. pylori* is resistant to both clarithromycin[1] and metronidazole[1]; therefore, alternatives must be chosen. In addition, the motivation of the patient and physician need to be reassessed as compliance may be an issue. A third treatment changes the PPI to a much higher dose and/or a drug less affected by the metabolizer status of the patient. Rabeprazole (AcipHex), 20 mg twice daily, might be a good choice. Amoxicillin is given as before. In addition, add ofloxacin (Floxin)[1] or levofloxacin (Levaquin)[1] plus rifabutin (Mycobutin)[1], with all four drugs being given for 14 days.

An alternative and inexpensive regimen is bismuth (Pepto-Bismol) with tetracycline,[1] metronidazole (Flagyl),[1] and a PPI. This is also called bismuth quad therapy. It is useful also when patients are allergic to penicillin. Allergic patients might also try PPI with clarithromycin (Biaxin)[1] and metronidazole[1] as the initial therapy. If patients are unable to take oral antibiotics because of nausea, start with a harmless drug such as PPI or bismuth, and then add tetracycline[1] or amoxicillin (Amoxil). After 1 week, by which time symptoms have improved, add the clarithromycin[1] or metronidazole.[1] If all else fails, high-dose PPI suppresses *H. pylori* in 30% to 50% of patients. Alternatively, because biopsy and culture with antibiotic sensitivity testing are necessary, refer patients to a gastroenterologist specializing in *H. pylori*.

---

[1]Not FDA approved for this indication.

After *H. pylori* eradication, symptoms are still present in most patients but improve gradually over 3 to 6 months. GERD symptoms may temporarily worsen, so I treat these symptoms with H_2 blockers initially because this does not interfere with the follow-up UBT. If symptoms persist, then the patient is managed as *H. pylori*–negative dyspepsia as per the algorithm in Figure 1.

REFERENCES

Chan FK, Leung WK: Peptic-ulcer disease. Lancet 2002;360:933-941.
Chan FK, Graham DY: Prevention of non-steroidal anti-inflammatory drug gastrointestinal complications—review and recommendations based on risk assessment. Aliment Pharmacol Ther 2004;1051-1061.
Stollman N, Metz DC: Pathophysiology and prophylaxis of stress ulcer in intensive care unit patients. J Crit Care 2005;20:35-45.
Suerbaum S, Michetti P: *Helicobacter pylori* infection. N Engl J Med 2002;347:1175-1186.
Talley NJ: Ameican Gastroenterological Association medical position statement: Evaluation of dyspepsia. Gastroenterology 2005:129: 1753-1755.

Acute and Chronic Viral Hepatitis

Method of
Christopher O'Brien, MD

Viral hepatitis remains a major concern to the primary care physician because it is the most common cause of liver disease worldwide and one of the most common causes in the United States. More than 20,000 to 25,000 Americans die each year as a consequence of viral liver disease. The annual cost of acute and chronic viral liver disease remains in the billions of dollars.

Disease involving the liver can be classified into acute or chronic hepatitis. Acute viral hepatitis is defined as new onset viral infection, which will resolve spontaneously within 6 months of onset. Chronic viral hepatitis is characterized by persistence of viral hepatitis (either hepatitis B, hepatitis C, or hepatitis D) for more than 6 months.

Acute Viral Hepatitis

OVERVIEW

Acute viral hepatitis is classically caused by hepatitis A, B, C, D, or E. However, the Epstein-Barr virus (EBV), the cytomegalovirus (CMV), or the herpes simplex virus (HSV) can also result in systemic infection with a hepatitis-like presentation. Other causes of acute liver disease such as medications or drug-induced hepatitis, acute alcoholic hepatitis, autoimmune liver disease, Wilson's disease, and involvement of the liver by opportunistic infections (in a patient with HIV) or lymphoma should also be considered (especially if initial serologic testing for the common hepatitis A to E viruses is negative).

Besides the specific therapy outlined for each hepatitis virus, general indications for hospitalization and/or referral for liver transplant evaluation can be found in the Treatment summary section at the end of the Acute Viral Hepatitis section.

Hepatitis A to E

HEPATITIS A

Overview

The hepatitis A virus (HAV) is a small, single-stranded ribonucleic acid (RNA) virus.

Epidemiology

This is a common virus ranging from a prevalence of 10% in patients younger than age 5 years to 74% in United States citizens older than age 50 years. The Centers for Disease Control and Prevention (CDC) estimate that almost 270,000 cases of acute HAV occur each year.

This virus is transmitted primarily by the fecal–oral route. Viral shedding in the feces, serum, and saliva occurs during the initial 4 to 6 week period before the development of symptoms and ceases within weeks after the onset of abnormal transaminases. Transmission commonly occurs either through the ingestion of contaminated water or food (particularly shellfish) or person-to-person contact (institutional, household, or sexual). Many outbreaks also occur in a community-wide fashion, with children frequently serving as reservoirs of infection.

Clinical Features

The average incubation period is approximately 30 days with a range of 15 to 50 days. The clinical presentation can vary from asymptomatic to fulminant hepatic failure. Symptoms can consist of anorexia, malaise, feeling of discomfort over the liver, dark urine, clay-colored stools, and low-grade fever. Rarely, extrahepatic manifestations can include arthritis, transverse myelitis, optic neuritis, aplastic anemia, and vasculitis.

Typically, the older the patient, the more severe the presentation and greater the case-fatality rate. Patients older than age 50 years are at the greatest risk for a fatal outcome. Duration of symptoms is most commonly for less than 2 months, but 10% to 15% can relapse with a prolonged course up to 6 months. Acute HAV resolves completely with no chronic sequelae.

CURRENT DIAGNOSIS

Acute Viral Hepatitis

- Acute liver disease is defined as the new onset of abnormal liver function tests in a patient with no prior evidence of liver disease.
- In general, hepatitis A through E are diagnosed by the presence of the IgM antibody to the virus.
- Common, ubiquitous viruses (CMV, EBV, HSV) can also have a hepatitis-like presentation.

Abbreviations: CMV = cytomegalovirus; EBV = Epstein-Barr virus; HSV = herpes simplex virus.

CURRENT THERAPY

Acute Viral Hepatitis

- Acute hepatitis in a healthy adult almost always resolves spontaneously and does not require specific treatment.
- Support therapy for acute viral hepatitis consists of normal activity, normal diet, and observation for development of complications.
- The development of confusion (encephalopathy), coagulopathy (prothrombin time greater than three seconds above control) and inability to consume adequate nutrition are all indications for hospital admission.
- Patients who develop jaundice and encephalopathy within 0 to 2 and 2 to 12 weeks of each other (fulminant and subfulminant hepatic failure, respectively) have a poor prognosis and require referral for liver transplant.

Current Diagnosis of Chronic Viral Hepatitis

- The presence of chronic viral liver disease is suspected in a patient who has abnormal liver function tests for greater than 6 months.
- Both hepatitis B and C also require direct detection by PCR.
- Other causes of chronic liver disease including medication/drug, alcohol, primary biliary cirrhosis, autoimmune hepatitis, primary sclerosing cholangitis, hemochromatosis and Wilson's disease, should also be ruled out.

Current Therapy of Chronic Viral Hepatitis

- Chronic viral hepatitis does not resolve spontaneously and requires specific treatment
- The development of a complication of chronic liver disease such as: hepatic encephalopathy, esophageal/gastric variceal bleeding, ascites, hepatorenal syndrome or the hepatopulmonary syndrome is an indication for liver transplant evaluation
- Complications of liver disease require specific therapy as outlined in the article, Cirrhosis.

Abbreviation: PCR = polymerase chain reaction.

Diagnosis

The most common finding on physical exam is hepatomegaly. Patients develop an elevation in their liver enzymes with the alanine aminotransferase (ALT) classically higher than the aspartate aminotransferase (AST). Acute hepatitis A is diagnosed by the development of an anti-HAV IgM. The anti-HAV IgM is detectable approximately when the patient presents with symptoms and persists for approximately 5 to 6 months after the initial infection. The presence of anti-HAV IgG alone represents previous infection and is evidence of recovery.

Specific Treatment

There is no specific antiviral therapy that is effective for hepatitis A infection. Treatment is supportive. Patients should be advised to practice good hygiene, especially hand washing. Indications for hospitalization and transplantation are listed in the Treatment section at the end of the Acute Viral Hepatitis section.

Prevention

Patients who have been potentially exposed to hepatitis A should receive immune globulin (BayGam) at a dose of 0.02 mL/kg by intramuscular injection. This can prevent acute HAV in 90% of cases. Immediate vaccination for hepatitis A with either HAVRIX 1 mL, 1440 ELISA Units, or VAQTA 1 mL, 50 units, should also be given followed by a second dose 6 months later.

Patients who fall in high-risk groups such as travelers to epidemic areas, men who have sex with men, as well as U.S. areas with high prevalence of hepatitis A (such as the Native American communities) should also receive preventive vaccination. Outbreaks in these communities interestingly tend to occur in a cyclical fashion every 5 to 10 years.

HEPATITIS B

Overview

The hepatitis B virus (HBV) is the smallest known, double-stranded DNA, circular virus. The virus is 100 times more infectious than HIV. It is able to survive in dried blood for up to 1 week. There are eight described genotypes (A–H) that presently are of little clinical significance.

Epidemiology

It is estimated that almost 2 billion people out of 6 billion people in the world have present or past HBV infection. The prevalence varies from regions of the world. Areas such as most of Africa, Indochina subcontinent, and northern portions of South America have a high prevalence of disease (>8%), whereas the United States has a low prevalence (<2%, except Alaska, which is >8%).

Originally, the incidence of new infections was declining with the advent of the hepatitis B vaccine. However, immigration into the United States has been originating from areas with high prevalence of hepatitis B. As a result recent estimates are that almost 78,000 cases of acute hepatitis B are now occurring each year in the United States. The incidence of new-onset hepatitis B peaks in the age group 20 to 29 years of age.

Horizontal transmission occurs via the parenteral route: through sexual activity, contaminated needles, child-to-child, and rarely as a health care worker or other percutaneous exposures. Approximately 6% infected in this fashion after age 5 years develop chronic infection.

Vertical transmission occurs by mother to infant transmission at time of childbirth. Almost 90% of infants exposed in this fashion become chronic carriers. There are no clear risk factors elicited in almost 20% to 30% of patients.

Clinical Features

The incubation period averages 2 to 3 months with a range of 1.5 to 4 months. Symptoms are nonspecific and similar to acute hepatitis A. The clinical presentation can vary from asymptomatic to fulminant hepatic failure.

Approximately 50% of patients are asymptomatic. Symptoms noted can include anorexia, malaise, a feeling of discomfort over the liver, dark urine, clay-colored stools, and low-grade fever. Extrahepatic manifestations are those of immune complex–mediated disease such as a serum sickness-like syndrome, polyarteritis nodosa, arthritis, and membranous glomerulonephritis. Typically, the older the patient, the more severe the presentation. Case fatality rates range from 0.5% to 1%.

Diagnosis

Patients develop an elevation in their serum aminotransferases. Acute hepatitis B is diagnosed by the development of an IgM antibody to the core region of the HBV (anti-HBcAb IgM). This will rise before the onset of symptoms and persist for 6 to 7 months postacute infection. The hepatitis B surface antigen (HBsAg) can be detected as soon as 1 month after initial infection and falls to nondetectable within 6 months after initial exposure signaling recovery from acute hepatitis B. The presence of an antibody to the HBV surface (anti-HBs) represents development of recovery (or a patient previously vaccinated with the HBV). Persistence of the HBsAg for more than six months indicates transition to chronic hepatitis B (see Chronic Hepatitis B section).

Specific Treatment

In general, specific antiviral therapy for acute hepatitis B is unnecessary and not recommended despite the availability of new oral antiviral medications. In theory, early antiviral therapy may actually increase the risk of developing chronic hepatitis B after the acute infection.

However, there are a number of oral agents that can be used under extremely rare situations where the patient is developing fulminant or subfulminant hepatic failure and is under consideration for a liver transplant. The rationale for the use of these treatments before liver transplant is to decrease the risk of graft loss caused by recurrent, active hepatitis B after liver transplant (Table 1). Interferon-based therapies should never be used in acute hepatitis B.

Prevention

Vaccination

The Advisory Committee on Immunization Practices recommends the routine vaccination of all infants, unvaccinated children at ages 11 to 12 years, and high-risk groups regardless of age. Three recombinant HBV vaccines are

TABLE 1 Approved Oral Agents for Hepatitis B Therapy

Generic Name	Trade Name	Dose	Route	Frequency
Lamivudine	Epivir	100 mg	PO	qd
Adefovir	Hepsera	10 mg	PO	qd
Entecavir	Baraclude	0.5/1 mg	PO	qd

TABLE 2 Hepatitis B Vaccine Dose Regimen

Vaccine	Dose	Route	Interval (mo)
Engerix-B	20 μg	IM	0, 1, and 6
Recombivax HB	10 μg	IM	0, 1, and 6
Twinrix	–	IM	0, 1, and 6

Abbreviation: IM = intramuscular.

available: Engerix-B, Recombivax HB, and Twinrix (Table 2). Surprisingly, up to 5% to 10% of healthy adults in the United States will not respond to vaccination.

HBV Immune Globulin

If previously unvaccinated, patients who have been potentially exposed to hepatitis B should receive hepatitis B immune globulin (HBIG) at a dose of 0.06 mL/kg. This provides only 3 to 6 months of temporary protection. Immediate vaccination for hepatitis B should also be given intramuscularly followed by a second dose in 1 month, and a third dose 6 months later.

HEPATITIS C

Overview

The hepatitis C virus (HCV) is a single-stranded RNA virus that was first characterized in 1989 by molecular biology techniques. There are six genotypes (see Chronic Viral Hepatitis, Hepatitis C, Overview).

Epidemiology

The rate of new infections has declined with the screening of blood products for hepatitis C. The recent estimates are now approximately 25,000 to 30,000 new infections each year. Approximately 3.9 million Americans have come into contact with the HCV, and the CDC estimates that 2.7 million chronically carry the virus.

Risk factors for acquisition of acute infection include percutaneous (occupational, injecting drug use) and perinatal exposures. Incidence of infection after an accidental needle stick from an HCV-positive patient is 1.8%. Average rate of infant infection after delivery from a HCV RNA-positive mother is 6%. There is no association with the method of delivery or breastfeeding afterwards. Sexual transmission can occur, but the rate is very low as suggested by low prevalence rates (1.5%) among long-term sex partners of patients with chronic HCV.

Clinical Features

The incubation period is short, averaging 6 weeks (range of 2 to 24 weeks). Most infections are asymptomatic. Similar to hepatitis A and B, hepatitis C can have several extrahepatic manifestations. These include vasculitis, membranoproliferative glomerulonephritis, urticaria, and erythema nodosum. Fulminant hepatitis resulting in death virtually never occurs in patients with normal immune function. However, there is a very high rate of

developing chronic infection with the HCV ranging from 75% to 85%.

Diagnosis

The diagnosis is by the detection of a positive HCV antibody (HCVAb). Although the newer assays allow earlier detection of the HCVAb, this typically is not found until 4 weeks after exposure. The presence of a positive HCVAb is confirmed by the direct detection of the virus by determination of the HCV RNA (by reverse transcriptase polymerase chain reaction [RT-PCR], or other method). This HCV RNA can be found within the first 1 to 8 weeks of infection. The serum transaminases become elevated within 6 to 12 weeks after the acute contact with HCV and normalize with resolution of the acute infection. However, up to 40% of patients who develop chronic infection can also normalize their liver function tests over the follow-up period. Therefore, it is important to monitor the HCV RNA by PCR to document resolution of the acute HCV infection. Progression to chronic infection is demonstrated by persistence of the HCV RNA for greater than 6 months from the initial detection. Approximately 15% to 25% of patients with acute hepatitis C will spontaneously clear the infection. The remainder will progress to development of chronic hepatitis C.

Specific Treatment

Unlike hepatitis B, recent studies appear to demonstrate a benefit for the treatment of acute hepatitis C because of the high rate of chronic liver disease.

Interferon-Based Regimes

Spontaneous clearance of acute HCV can occur in 20% to 30% of patients within the first 3 months of acquisition of the infection. If the patient remains positive for HCV RNA after 3 months of infection, most specialists initiate treatment with a pegylated interferon alone at full dose (see Chronic Viral Liver Disease, Hepatitis C, Specific Treatment) without simultaneous ribavirin administration for 6-month treatment duration. High, sustained virologic responses have been reported in the therapy of patients with acute HCV.

Oral Agents

There are, at present, no oral antiviral agents available for acute HCV infection. However, there are several promising candidates presently in clinical trials that may be available in the next several years.

Prevention

There is no vaccine available at the present time.

HEPATITIS D

Overview

The hepatitis D virus (HDV) is a single-stranded, defective, positive RNA virus that requires the presence of the hepatitis B virus to replicate. This virus is unable to make its own surface antigen and must acquire the HBV surface antigen for its own surface.

Epidemiology

The two major modes of transmission include percutaneous exposures (in particular with injecting drug use) and transmission during sex. Hepatitis D virus is relatively rare in the United States and occurs mainly in intravenous (IV) drug users and patients with factor VIIII deficiency.

Clinical Features

There are two general patterns: coinfection and superinfection (see Chronic Viral Hepatitis, Hepatitis D).

Diagnosis

The diagnosis of acute HDV in similar fashion to the other types of viral hepatitis is made by either the detection of the presence of the anti-HDV IgM in the blood or the HDV RNA by RT-PCR.

Specific Treatment

There is no specific treatment for acute hepatitis D.

Prevention

There is no specific vaccination against HDV. However, vaccination against HBV will also protect against either HDV coinfection or superinfection.

HEPATITIS E

Overview

Hepatitis E virus (HEV) is a small, positive, single-stranded RNA virus.

Epidemiology

Virtually all U.S. cases are linked to travel to hepatitis E endemic areas with exposure to fecally contaminated drinking water. Epidemics occur in Asia, India, and Central America, including Mexico. There is minimal person-to-person transmission. There have been reports of vertical transmission to the children born of mothers infected during the third trimester of pregnancy.

Clinical Features

Incubation period ranges for 15 to 60 days with an average of 40 days. Symptoms are similar to that of acute hepatitis A. Severity of illness, similar to hepatitis A, is more likely with increasing age of exposure. There is an overall 1% to 3% rate of fulminant liver disease and death. For reasons that are unclear, pregnant women have a particularly high fatality rate ranging from 15% to 25%. Chronic infection does not develop, and there are no chronic sequelae after the resolution of an acute infection.

Diagnosis

Similar to other forms of acute viral hepatitis, serum liver function tests become abnormal during acute infection. Serologic testing for hepatitis E is not commercially available in the United States. The CDC can test for anti-HEV IgM. The anti-HEV IgM usually is detectable before the patient becomes clinically ill and persists for only a relatively short time (less than 3 months) postexposure.

Specific Treatment

There is no specific antiviral therapy for acute hepatitis E. Treatment of acute infection is supportive only.

Prevention

The only preventive measures available are to avoid drinking water or ice, and avoid eating uncooked vegetables or fruits and shellfish when visiting regions endemic for HEV. Immune globulin from the United States does not protect against infection. No vaccine is, as yet, available.

Other Viruses with Liver Involvement

There are other viruses besides the classic hepatitis A through E that can involve the liver. Some viruses such as Epstein-Barr (EBV) commonly have liver involvement. Other widespread viruses such as cytomegalovirus (CMV) and the herpes virus (HSV) can also do so but less frequently. Presentation is influenced by other factors such as the immune status of the patient as well as the age and presence of underlying liver disease.

EPSTEIN-BARR VIRUS

Overview

The EBV is a DNA virus that most commonly is associated with the syndrome of infectious mononucleosis. Rarely, chronic EBV infections have been linked to Burkitt's lymphoma, nasopharyngeal carcinoma, and post-transplant lymphoproliferative disease (PTLD).

Epidemiology

Transmission occurs by close personal contact for infectious mononucleosis and by reactivation of latent infection in PTLD.

Clinical Features

Infectious mononucleosis can present in young adults with symptoms of fever, headache, cervical and axillary lymphadenopathy, and severe pharyngitis. Liver involvement of a variable intensity is often present in up to 90% of affected patients. Hepatosplenomegaly can be found in 17% of affected patients.

The clinical course can be variable. Serum liver function tests rise during the second to fourth weeks of involvement.

Although the hepatitis-like picture can persist for months, chronic hepatitis does not develop.

Diagnosis

The diagnosis is made by the IgM antibody to the viral capsid antigen as well as the EBV nuclear antigen. Patients who are post-transplant can have the direct detection of the EBV DNA in their blood and tissues by PCR.

Specific Therapy

Treatment of infectious mononucleosis is supportive. However, experience has shown that corticosteroids can be effective in the prompt relief of severe systemic symptoms as well as the exudative pharyngitis. The use of antivirals including acyclovir (Zovirax)[1] has not proved to be useful.

Patients after transplant, however, require the reduction of immunosuppression as well as the simultaneous administration of antivirals such as ganciclovir (Cytovene) and acyclovir.

Prevention

No vaccine is available at the present time.

CYTOMEGALOVIRUS

Overview

Cytomegalovirus is a member of the herpes viral family and, therefore, is a DNA virus. Active CMV infection can result from either primary exposure to a new infection or by reactivation of a latent viral infection.

Epidemiology

Cytomegalovirus can be found worldwide. Anywhere from 50% to 80% of the U.S. population will develop antibodies to this virus by age 30 years. The prevalence of seropositivity is more likely with increasing age. Active CMV can be intermittently present (as infectious virus) in all body fluids of any infected individual. Transmission can occur through sexual contact, contact with close family members or children, occupational contact (in particular health care workers), and finally through the receipt of infected blood products or a transplanted organ.

Clinical Features

Most CMV infections in healthy adults tend to be asymptomatic. However, primary infections can present with significant symptoms. The picture can be similar to that of infectious mononucleosis because of EBV. Patients will complain of a febrile illness with anorexia, nausea, vomiting, and malaise of 3 to 6 weeks duration with evidence of hepatitis. After resolution of the acute episode, CMV develops into a latent infection. Reactivation can occur later in life.

Similar to EBV, immunosuppressed patients can develop a much more severe liver involvement with obvious

jaundice, persistent fever, and an interstitial pneumonitis. This presentation can be caused by both new, primary infection as well as a reactivation of a latent infection.

Diagnosis

The liver enzymes are elevated during the acute episode. The diagnosis of CMV hepatitis can be suspected in the presence of more than 10% atypical lymphocytes on peripheral smear with a 50% or greater lymphocytosis. The IgM CMV antibody can be detected during the primary episode. The identification of acute CMV hepatitis can be confirmed by a fourfold rise in the IgG antibody between the initial and the convalescent blood specimens. The virus can also be cultured from urine or pharyngeal specimens.

Specific Therapy

In general, nonspecific supportive treatment is the rule for most cases of CMV infections in immunocompetent adults. In cases where the patient is immunosuppressed (such as after organ transplantation), reduction of immunosuppression in combination with an antiviral (such as ganciclovir) can be successful in treatment.

The dose and treatment duration of ganciclovir vary depending on the severity of the presentation as well as type and indication for immunosuppression. Ganciclovir is given at a dose of 10 mg/kg/day IV in two divided doses for 2 to 3 weeks. Oral ganciclovir can be used after initial treatment for suppressive therapy.

Prevention

There is no vaccine for CMV at the present time.

HERPES VIRUS INFECTIONS

Overview

Herpes simplex virus is a large DNA virus. There are two major strains of the HSV virus: HSV 1 (HSV-1) and HSV 2 (HSV-2).

Epidemiology

Herpes simplex virus is another, almost universal infection with evidence of serologic markers of infection found in 80% of humans. In general, HSV-1 causes herpes viral infections above the waist; HSV-2 causes the majority of genital herpes infections.

Clinical Features

Primary infection occurs early in life and is asymptomatic. However, generalized herpes infection can develop in pregnant women. Immunocompromised patients are especially at risk for disseminated disease with fulminant hepatitis.

Diagnosis

Diagnosis is made by detection via ELISA immunoassay to antibodies for HSV-1 or HSV-2 in the serum.

---

[1]Not FDA approved for this indication.

HSV antibodies frequently are not detectable until 2 to 3 months after the acute infections. Direct viral culture from any visible lesion is most specific.

Specific Therapy

Localized or recurrent infections will resolve spontaneously, but oral therapy with acyclovir (Zovirax) decreases the duration of infection. The treatment of choice for disseminated HSV is acyclovir at a dose of 10 mg/kg IV every 8 hours for 10 to 21 days.

Prevention

There is, as yet, no vaccine for HSV.

TREATMENT SUMMARY

Symptomatic Therapy

Patients should be advised to practice good hygiene, especially hand washing if hepatitis A or E has been diagnosed. Patients with good functional status can be observed as an outpatient.

Indications for Hospital Admission

There are three classic indications for hospital admission:

1. Intractable nausea and vomiting
2. A prothrombin time greater than 3 seconds more than control
3. Onset of confusion or other symptoms of hepatic encephalopathy

The patients with intractable nausea and vomiting require inpatient observation and IV fluid hydration. The development of any other complication is also an indication for hospital admission.

Referral for Liver Transplant

Continued elevation of the serum prothrombin time beyond 3 seconds more than the control strongly suggests that the patient should be evaluated for a liver transplant at a transplant center. The development of confusion, even if mild, implies the development of hepatic encephalopathy. This is an ominous sign because it is part of the definition of fulminant hepatic failure (FHF). The FHF syndrome is defined as the onset of hepatic encephalopathy within 2 weeks of the onset of jaundice. It has a poor prognosis with a low spontaneous recovery rate and mandates immediate referral to a transplant center.

CHRONIC VIRAL HEPATITIS

Overview

Viral liver disease that persists for greater than 6 months is termed chronic. Liver biopsy is classically recommended to determine the *grade* of inflammation present. The grade of inflammation roughly correlates with the rate of future progression. The severity of fibrosis present (stage of disease) is also graded as noted in Table 3. Chronic viral hepatitis rarely resolves spontaneously and usually requires specific therapy as outlined in the following text.

TABLE 3   Grading and Staging of Viral Liver Disease

Grade	Inflammation	Stage	Fibrosis
0	None	0	None
1	Minimal	1	Portal track only
2	Mild	2	Limited portal bridging
3	Moderate	3	Extensive portal bridging
4	Severe	4	Cirrhosis

Adapted from Batts KP, Ludwig J: Chronic hepatitis: An update on terminology and reporting. Am J Surg Path 1995;19:1409.

HEPATITIS B

Overview

There are a number of naturally occurring and treatment induced mutant varieties of HBV. Hepatitis B is now classically divided into three major phases based on the replication status of the HBV and the presence or absence of liver inflammation: the immune tolerant phase, the immune active phase, and the low replication/carrier phase.

Epidemiology

It is estimated that almost one person out of three in the world will have been infected with the hepatitis B virus sometime during the course of their lifetime. Approximately 350 to 400 million people in the world have been unable to resolve the infection and are chronic carriers of hepatitis B. This results in almost 1 million deaths/year because of chronic HBV infection.

In the United States, the CDC report that approximately 1.25 million people are chronically infected with HBV. Approximately 30% of patients with chronic HBV can progress to cirrhosis and 10% can develop hepatocellular carcinoma over the course of their lifetime. Together, it is estimated that almost 5000 deaths each year occur in the United States because of HBV.

Clinical Features

Chronic HBV infection can pursue a variable course ranging from inactive HBV characterized by low-level viral replication with normal liver enzymes and normal liver histology to active disease culminating in cirrhosis and/or the development of hepatocellular carcinoma.

The course of infection tends to fluctuate between active disease (high HBV DNA levels and either hepatitis B e antigen (HBeAg)-positive or HBeAg-negative) and the inactive or low replication state (low HBV DNA level, normal ALT, and no inflammation on liver biopsy).

Overall, it is estimated that patients with long-standing chronic HBV have approximately a 30% risk of progressing to cirrhosis; 25% of these patients with cirrhosis will progress to overt liver failure over the next 5 years. In addition, a further 10% of patients without histologic evidence of significant liver fibrosis or cirrhosis can develop hepatocellular carcinoma over the course of their lifetime. A very large recent study from Taiwan (22,707 males) has demonstrated a direct correlation between the HBV DNA level and the relative risk of the development of hepatocellular carcinoma (as well as cirrhosis) over the 12-year follow-up period of their study.

Diagnosis

The *immune tolerant phase* is characterized by the presence of a positive HBeAg and high HBV DNA levels ($>10^5$), but normal ALT levels and no or minimal liver inflammation on liver biopsy.

The *HBeAg-positive or wild type virus* has evidence of significant disease activity consisting of the presence of a high HBV DNA level ($>10^5$), abnormal ALT, and the evidence of active inflammation +/– fibrosis on liver histology. These patients can occasionally undergo spontaneous seroconversion to HBeAg-negative/HBeAb-positive state terminating active HBV replication with resolution of active disease. Two thirds of patients with spontaneous seroconversion will have sustained remission, but one third will revert to active disease. Most (80%) reactivations are because of transition to the precore mutant or HBeAb-positive virus associated with recurrence of relatively high HBV DNA level, whereas the minority will revert to the original HBeAg-positive wild type virus.

The *precore and core promoter mutant/HBeAg-negative virus* has been growing in prevalence in the population. A recent study demonstrated that 64% of patients have recurrent flares with 69% returning to normal ALT levels between flares. However, spontaneous sustained remission to the inactive or low replication state is very rare.

The *low replication/carrier phase* is characterized by low or nondetectable viral replication with normal liver function tests and essentially normal histology (Table 4).

Specific Treatment

The goals of therapy are different depending on the type of HBV virus and the patient population treated.

Patients with the HBeAg-positive (wild type) virus can seroconvert to HBeAb-positive with suppression of HBV DNA to a very low or undetectable level, normalization of serum transaminases, and resolution of liver inflammation. The present recommendation is to treat a patient who is HBeAg-positive for 6 months past the point of HBeAb-positive seroconversion and then stop. Interval monitoring to observe durability of seroconversion (approximately 82% to 92% over 1 year) should be performed on a regular basis.

HBeAg-negative patients (precore and core promoter mutants) do not have HBeAg seroconversion to HBeAb as an endpoint, and the goal is the continuous suppression of viral replication with normalization of the transaminases and improvement in liver histology.

Treatment guidelines for the selection of patients for HBV antiviral therapy have been published. In summary, patients with evidence of active inflammation by histology, or by elevated serum aminotransferases in conjunction with the presence of a detectable HBV DNA level are considered candidates for therapy.

Interferon-Based Regimes

Interferon-based therapy was the first FDA-approved therapy for patients with chronic HBV. The advantage of interferon therapy is its potential to develop a HBsAg to HBsAb seroconversion completely eliminating active hepatitis B replication. Unfortunately, that is a rare event occurring in only 2% to 3% of patients. The downside to the use of interferon is the significant number of serious side effects associated with its use.

Therefore, most physicians opt for oral antiviral therapy for treatment of chronic HBV infection. In the few situations where treatment with interferon-based therapy is used, the two interferons are available for the treatment of chronic HBV are interferon alfa-2b (Intron) and peginterferon alfa-2a (Pegasys). Interferon alfa-2b is FDA approved at the dose of 5 mIU subcutaneously (SC) on a daily basis for 4 months. Peginterferon alfa-2a is used at a fixed dose of 180 µg SC once weekly for 1 year.

In addition to the significant side effect profile of both forms of therapy, interferon treatment is usually associated with flare in the serum aminotransferases levels. This flare in ALT can be associated with a significant risk of decompensation of liver function in patients with underlying cirrhosis.

Oral Agents

There are now a number of oral agents that are effective in control of chronic HBV replication: lamivudine (Epivir), adefovir (Hepsera), and entecavir (Baraclude). These are the most common medications used for the treatment of HBV infection because of their high efficacy in controlling active viral replication. Virtually all side effects of these oral medications have been comparative to those of placebo in clinical trials reported to date.

Lamivudine was the first agent released. It is a nucleoside analogue that blocks the action of the reverse transcriptase activity of the HBV polymerase gene. Lamivudine is approved for treatment of HBV at 100 mg orally daily, but the 150-mg and 300-mg doses are commonly used in association with HIV therapy. The advantage of this particular therapy is its (relatively) low cost. The disadvantage of lamivudine therapy is the high rate of viral mutation in the region of the HBV polymerase gene resulting in loss of

TABLE 4 Classification of Chronic Hepatitis B by Replication Status

Type	HBeAg	HBeAb	HBV DNA	ALT	Histology
Immune tolerant	+	–	$> 10^6$	Normal	No activity
HBeAg (+)	+	–	$> 10^5$	Abnormal	Mild to severe
HBeAg (–)	–	+	10^4–10^6	Abnormal	Mild to severe
Healthy carrier state	–	+	$< 10^3$	Normal	No activity

Abbreviations: ALT = alanine aminotransferase; HBeAb = hepatitis B e antibody; HBeAg = hepatitis B e antigen; HBV DNA = hepatitis B viral DNA.

drug effectiveness occurring at approximately 20% per year of therapy.

Adefovir, also a nucleotide analogue, was the next agent released. The dose, 10 mg oral daily, is effective as first-line therapy as well as rescue therapy in patients who developed resistance to lamivudine. Adefovir has the advantage of a very low HBV resistance rate (1.9% at 2 years). However, patients who have underlying renal disease have to have the dose adjusted because of potential renal toxicity.

Entecavir is a guanosine nucleoside analogue that is a selective inhibitor of HBV polymerase. Entecavir does not interact with the cytochrome P450 (CYP450) system and is eliminated by renal clearance. This is the most potent agent released to date for treatment of HBV. The dose is 0.5 mg oral daily for patients who are naïve to oral therapy for HBV and 1 mg oral daily for patients who have developed lamivudine resistance. Similar to adefovir, entecavir has a very low rate of resistance reported to be 0% at year two of therapy in naïve patients and 1.6% at year one in lamivudine-resistant patients.

In general, therapy with lamivudine will result in 4 to 5 log decrease in the HBV DNA titer; adefovir a 3 to 4 log decrease, and entecavir a 5 to 7 log over the initial 48 weeks of therapy. HBeAg to HBeAb seroconversion is also greatest (21%) with entecavir in the initial one year of therapy.

A considerable advantage of all the nucleoside and nucleotide therapies for HBV is the significant improvement in histology that occurs with long-term control of HBV viral replication. In addition to the anticipated improvement in liver inflammation, many studies now document improvement in cirrhosis to appreciably lower levels of liver fibrosis in a significant percentage of patients (see Table 1).

Although it is not specifically approved by the FDA (as yet) for treatment of HBV, many coinfected patients (HBV and HIV) have been receiving tenofovir (Viread),[1] or the combination of tenofovir and emtricitabine (Truvada)[1] as part of their highly active antiretroviral therapy (HAART) for HIV. Tenofovir (Viread), alone at 300 mg oral daily or in combination with 200 mg of emtricitabine (Truvada), is highly active against the HBV viral polymerase (Table 5).

Prevention

For prevention, see section under Acute Hepatitis B.

HEPATITIS C

Overview

Hepatitis C is a small, positively stranded RNA virus with six genotypes designated 1 to 6. Each of the major genotypes

---

[1]Not FDA approved for this indication.

has several subtypes (a, b, c, etc.) The most common genotypes found in the United States are 1a, 1b, 2a, 2b, and 3a. In general 75% of the patients with chronic hepatitis C in the United States are infected with genotype 1a or 1b. Approximately 20% to 25% have either type 2 or type 3; whereas the remainders have mainly type 4. However, type 4 has been increasingly recognized because of troops returning from the Middle East, which has a high prevalence of this genotype.

Epidemiology

The worldwide seroprevalence of HCV varies by country. In some regions more than 10% of the population has a detectable HCVAb. The World Health Organization estimates that there are 170 to 200 million people with chronic hepatitis C worldwide.

The CDC National Health and Nutrition Examination Survey III study reported approximately 3.9 million people (1.8% of the population) in the United States test positive for exposure to hepatitis C. Up to 2.7 million of the U.S. population are chronically infected with the highest prevalence in the 30- to 54-year age group. However, certain groups have high prevalence, such as patients with factor VIII deficiency (85%), injecting drug users (80% to 90%), those incarcerated (16% to 41%), the homeless (22%), veterans (8%), and patients coinfected with HIV (30%).

Clinical Features

Patients are most frequently asymptomatic. However, there are many extrahepatic manifestations of chronic HCV (Table 6).

Diagnosis

The HCV Ab test is the most commonly used screening assay. If positive, and especially before considering treatment, a HCV RNA by RT-PCR should always be performed to confirm the HCVAb test and to guide treatment decisions. All patients positive by the HCV RNA assay must also have a HCV genotype performed, if treatment is to be considered.

Specific Treatment

Interferon-Based Regimes

There are, at present, two pegylated interferons available for the treatment of chronic HCV. Both pegylated interferons are combined with ribavirin treatment. The duration of therapy and the dose of ribavirin are determined by the HCV genotype. Peginterferon alfa-2a (Pegasys) is administered at a fixed dose of 180 μg, whereas peginterferon

---

TABLE 5   HAART Agents with Activity Hepatitis B in Coinfectd Patients

Generic Name	Trade Name	Dose	Route	Frequency
Tenofovir	Viread	300 mg	PO	qd
Tenofovir + emtricitabine	Truvada	300 mg + 200 mg	PO	qd

Abbreviation: HAART, highly active antiretroviral therapy.

TABLE 6 Extrahepatic Manifestations of Chronic Hepatitis C Virus

Dermatologic	**Hematologic**	**Endocrine**
Porphyria cutanea tarda	Essential mixed cryoglobulinemia	Thyroid dysfunction
Leukocytoclastic vasculitis	B-cell lymphoma	Diabetes mellitus
Lichen planus	Idiopathic thrombocytopenia	
Renal	**Neuropsychiatric**	
Membranoproliferative glomerulonephritis	Depression	

alfa-2b (PEG-Intron) is dosed at 1.5 µg/kg body weight. Both pegylated interferons are administered SC once weekly.

GENOTYPES 1 AND 4

HCV genotypes 1 and 4 are treated by the combination of a pegylated interferon with 1000 mg of ribavirin for patients weighing less than 75 kg and 1200 mg of ribavirin for patients weighing more than 75 kg for patients treated with peginterferon alfa-2a. Best evidence suggests that 10.6 mg ribavirin/kg body weight for patients treated with peginterferon alfa-2b appears to produce optimal results. Neither the dose of the pegylated interferon nor the ribavirin should be reduced in the first 3 months of therapy unless absolutely necessary. Frequently, the hemoglobin levels must be supported in the patient with weekly subcutaneous erythropoietin therapy because of the hemolytic anemia as a result of ribavirin to achieve this goal.

All genotype 1 patients should have a repeat HCV RNA drawn at month 3 of therapy. Those patients with a decrease in their HCV RNA by a 2 log or greater HCV titer from baseline should be continued on treatment. Patients who drop by 2 log titer from baseline but are not HCV RNA nondetectable should have another HCV RNA determined at month 6. Patients whose HCV RNA is nondetectable at 6 months can be continued for the full 48 weeks of treatment. Overall sustained virologic response rates have varied from 42% to 46%. Certain racial groups (African Americans) with genotype 1 have a reduced response to therapy of approximately 25%.

GENOTYPES 2 & 3

HCV genotypes 2 and 3 are treated by the combination of a pegylated interferon with 800 mg of ribavirin. Duration of therapy is 6 months for genotype 2 with a success rate of 80% to 90%. Treatment duration for genotype 3 is guided by an initial HCV PCR at month 1 of therapy. If the HCV RNA by RT-PCR is nondetectable, the treatment duration is 6 months with a success rate of 80% to 90%. If the HCV RNA by RT-PCR is detectable at month 1 of treatment, then the duration should be extended to 1 year to achieve the 80% to 90% cure rate.

Patients who are coinfected with the HIV virus have a reduced sustained virologic response to therapy varying from 29% for genotype 1 HCV to 62% for genotypes 2 and 3 HCV.

Monitoring and Side-Effect Management

Side effects of therapy occur in almost 100% of patients (Table 7). These can vary from uncomfortable to life-threatening. The pegylated interferons can cause a pancytopenia. A flulike syndrome is common at the initiation of treatment and responds to fluids, rest, and antipyretics. Depression and other mood disorders tend to improve with antidepressant

therapy. Ribavirin causes a hemolytic anemia, occasional cough and shortness of breath, rash and itching, and insomnia. Ribavirin is also considered to be teratogenic.

Contraindications to therapy include the following: the presence of hepatic decompensation, severe coronary artery disease, uncontrolled cardiac arrhythmias, significant anemia, presence of an uncontrolled autoimmune disease, poorly controlled seizure disorder, severe depression, hypersensitivity to either medication, potential pregnancy, or abnormal renal function.

Because of the side effect profile of both forms of interferon, patients have to be closely monitored for the entire duration of their treatment. A complete blood count should be monitored every 1 to 2 weeks during the initial months of therapy with follow-up monitoring monthly once the patient is stable. Usually comprehensive metabolic profiles are obtained once a month to monitor the liver tests.

Once the patient completes treatment, the HCV RNA should be checked at 6 months off therapy and again at 1 year. If the HCV RNA remains nondetectable, the patient has a sustained virologic response to therapy, and the consensus of opinion is that the patient can be considered cured of HCV.

Oral Agents

Novel treatments for chronic hepatitis C directed against various molecular targets of the hepatitis C virus may be available in the next several years. These potentially will include both polymerase as well as protease inhibitors of the HCV.

Prevention

There remains, as yet, no vaccine to prevent hepatitis C.

TABLE 7 Side Effects of Pegylated Interferon Therapy

Flulike Symptoms	**Hematologic**	**Endocrine**
Fever	Neutropenia	Thyroid dysfunction
Chills	Anemia	Diabetes mellitus
Malaise	Thrombocytopenia	
Pulmonary	**Neuropsychiatric**	**GI**
Dyspnea	Insomnia	Nausea
Cough	Depression	Vomiting
	Irritability	

Note: Pooled side effects noted in registration trials of both pegylated interferons together with those of ribavirin.
Abbreviation: GI = gastrointestinal.

HEPATITIS D

Overview

The hepatitis D virus (HDV) is a novel, positive, single-stranded defective RNA virus that requires the presence of the hepatitis B virus to replicate. This virus is unable to make its own surface antigen and must acquire the HBV surface antigen for its own surface

Epidemiology

The two major modes of transmission include injecting percutaneous exposures and transmission during sex. HDV is relatively rare in the United States and occurs mainly in the injecting drug users and patients with factor VIIII deficiency.

Clinical Features

There are two general patterns: coinfection and superinfection.

Coinfection occurs when the patient is infected with both the HBV and the HDV viruses simultaneously. The course of the infection tends to resemble that of acute HBV alone. Occasionally, this results in severe acute disease but a low risk of chronic infection. One difference, however, is the classical biphasic nature of the flare in the serum liver enzymes.

Superinfection occurs when a patient who already is already infected with HBV acquires the HDV virus at a later point in time. Because of the rapid viral spread throughout a liver already infected with HBV, up to 20% of patients can develop fulminant hepatic failure. In patients who survive the initial superinfection episode, there is a high rate of chronic persistence of the HDV virus.

Diagnosis

The diagnosis of HDV in similar fashion to the other types of viral hepatitis is made by either the detection of the presence of the anti-HDV in the blood or the HDV RNA by RT-PCR.

Specific Treatment

Clearance of the hepatitis B by specific hepatitis B therapy, if successful, eradicates the hepatitis D as a result. Surprisingly, the nucleoside analogue lamivudine has demonstrated no significant benefit in chronic HDV infection. The only medication at the present approved for the treatment of chronic HDV (and simultaneous HBV) is interferon alfa. The recommended treatment is interferon alfa-2b (Intron-A) at a dose of 9 mIU SC for 12 months. There has been little experience with the use of a pegylated interferon for chronic HDV. However, one study reported successful results with pegylated interferon alfa-2b at 1.5 µg/kg body weight SC for 1 year.

Prevention

There is no specific vaccine against HDV available. Clearly, the major means to prevent HDV infection would be vaccination against HBV with a standard HBV vaccine.

Treatment

Complications

Common complications of chronic liver disease include ascites, hepatic encephalopathy, and esophageal or gastric varices. More unusual associated problems include the development of the hepatorenal and the hepatopulmonary syndromes as well as portopulmonary hypertension.

Referral for Liver Transplant

The major indication for referral for liver transplant evaluation in the presence of chronic liver disease is the development of a complication listed previously in a patient with cirrhosis. Alternatively, many specialists would calculate the MELD score (model for end-state liver disease) as noted on the UNOS (United Network for Organ Sharing) Web site. It is now common practice to initiate a liver transplant evaluation when this score is 10 or greater. Patients can be actively listed for transplant when the MELD score reaches 15 or greater.

REFERENCES

Centers for Disease Control and Prevention on line: Available at http://www.cdc.gov/

Kim JD, Sherker AH: Antiviral therapy: Role in the management of extrahepatic diseases. Gastroenterol Clin North Am 2004;33(3): 693-708.

NIH: Consens State Sci Statements. 2002;19(3):1-46.

Polson J, Lee WM: American Association for the Study of Liver Disease. AASLD position paper: The management of acute liver failure. Hepatology 2005;41(5):1179-1197.

Schiff ER, Sorrell MK, Maddrey WC (eds.): Schiff's Diseases of the Liver (9th ed.). Philadelphia, Lippincott, Williams & Wilkins, 2003.

United Network for Organ Sharing on line: Available at: http://www.unos.org/

Zakim D, Boyer TD (eds.): Hepatology: A Textbook of Liver Disease (4th ed.). Philadelphia, Saunders, 2003.

Malabsorption

Method of
Roger L. Gebhard, MD, and
Nadeem A. Chaudhary, MD

Disorders of nutrient assimilation are collectively referred to as malabsorption or malabsorption syndrome. A diverse group of conditions produce malabsorption, including diseases of nutrient digestion, bowel motility, and enterocyte absorption and nutrient transport. The spectrum of these disorders also ranges from generalized nutrient malabsorption, as in celiac sprue, to specific nutrient malabsorption, such as lactose intolerance or pernicious anemia (vitamin B_{12}). The differential diagnosis of maldigestive or malabsorptive states requires understanding of the physiology of nutrient absorption.

Normal Absorption

Fat, protein, and most carbohydrates are eaten in polymeric form. Transport across gut epithelial cells requires that these complex nutrients first be digested to monomers. The processes are shown schematically in Figure 1. It can be seen that fat, predominantly triglycerides, requires the most complex processing. For that reason, generalized malabsorption always involves fat malabsorption (steatorrhea). Normal digestion and absorption of the primary dietary constituents are discussed in this section.

FAT

Fat assimilation begins with emulsification in the stomach, a process that allows lipase to gain access to the lipid. Although some lipase is secreted by salivary glands and stomach, most is of pancreatic origin. Entry of fat and other nutrients into the duodenum induces cholecystokinin (CCK) and secretin release from duodenal mucosa. These hormones cause secretion of bile and pancreatic juice. Appropriate timing of these secretions with the arrival of nutrients in the duodenum is important for the digestive process. In addition to lipase, the pancreas secretes colipase. Colipase facilitates the interaction between bile salts and lipase. Bile emulsifies triglycerides into micelles, consisting of the lipid plus conjugated bile salts and phospholipids. Lipase activity removes fatty acids from the end (Sn-1 and 3) positions of triglyceride, producing fatty acids and monoglyceride. Delivery of these water-insoluble products to enterocytes for absorption also requires that they be rendered water-soluble as micelles. They then diffuse through enterocyte cell membranes, bind to fatty acid binding protein, and undergo intracellular processing. The binding facilitates diffusion.

The enzymes lipase and colipase are released from pancreatic acinar zymogen granules. Lipase has 50% more activity in the presence of colipase, and its activity is present in 10-fold excess of the concentration needed for normal fat digestion. Therefore, roughly 90% of pancreatic secretory function must be lost before fat maldigestion occurs.

Liver cells secrete phospholipid and bile salts—conjugated to glycine and taurine—into bile. Conjugated bile salts are more soluble than unconjugated bile salts and are, therefore, more effective detergents. After their luminal detergent function is served, 95% of conjugated bile salts are reabsorbed via specific bile salt transporter proteins in the distal 100 cm of the ileum. They are then avidly removed from portal blood by hepatocytes and resecreted. Thus, liver cells must only synthesize approximately 30% of the total amount of bile salts secreted daily. The liver is able to increase baseline synthesis up to threefold to fivefold if needed. Inadequate bile micelles because of bile duct obstruction, deconjugation of bile salts, or dyssynchrony between release of bile and pancreatic juice and the luminal passage of fat (as seen after Billroth II gastric surgery) impairs complete fat digestion.

Fatty acids and monoglycerides entering gut mucosal cells are resynthesized into triglycerides and processed into chylomicrons with apoprotein B-48, phospholipid, and cholesterol. Chylomicrons are transported into gut villi

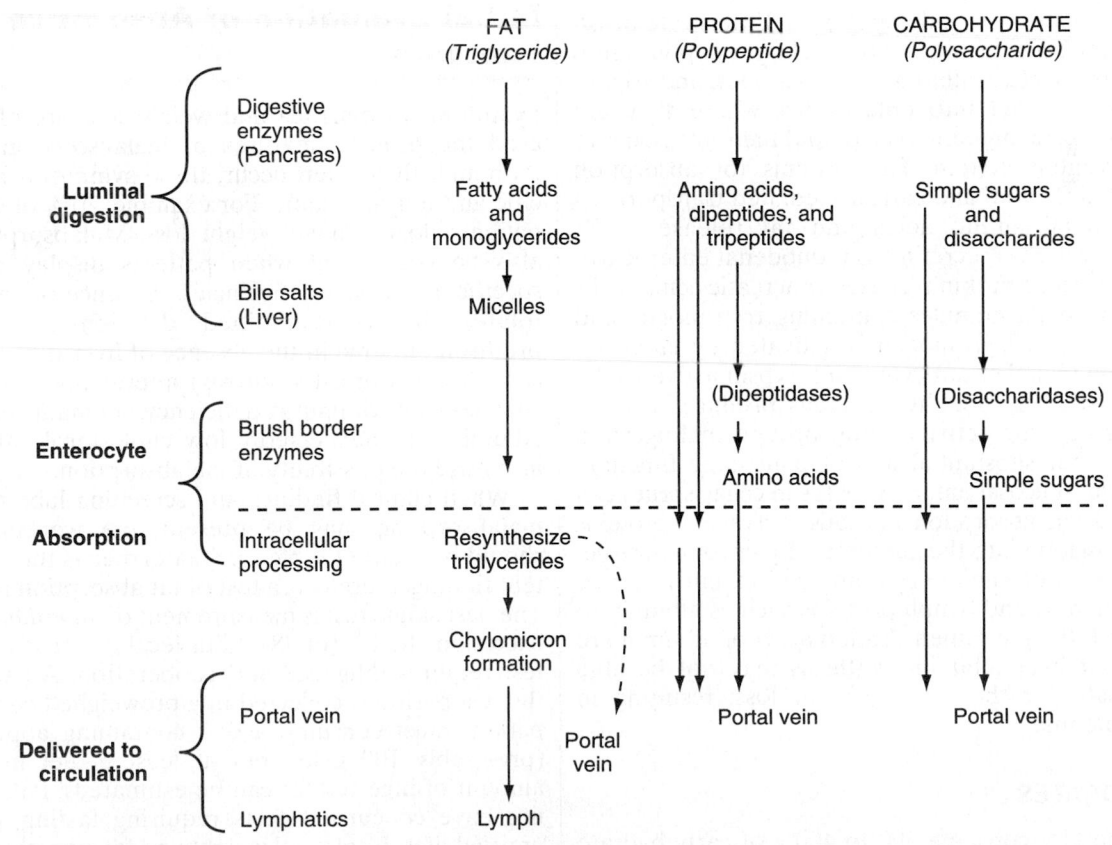

FIGURE 1. Nutrient processing.

lymphatics and enter the circulation via the thoracic duct. Some fatty acids, especially medium-chain fatty acids (C6–12), can enter the portal vein directly. The complexity of lipid transport requires healthy enterocytes and absence of lymphatic obstruction (at any level, from the gut villi to the heart) for complete fat absorption.

Undigested triglycerides, or unabsorbed fatty acids, remain as lipid particles in the gut lumen. They trap fat-soluble vitamins (D, K, A, E) within the lumen, leading to malabsorption of these vitamins. Unabsorbed fatty acids can be hydroxylated by colonic bacteria. Hydroxy fatty acids cause colonic mucosa to secrete water and electrolytes (an example is ricinoleic acid in castor oil), exaggerating the diarrhea of fatty acid steatorrhea. Patients with fatty acid malabsorption (e.g., celiac sprue) often complain of loose, watery, frothy stools, and they may not see visible oil droplets. Triglycerides (neutral fats) pass relatively inertly through the colon. Patients with triglyceride steatorrhea (e.g., pancreatic insufficiency) often complain of bulky, greasy, formed stool, and visible oil. Sudan staining of fat droplets in stool has been used as a qualitative test for steatorrhea. Triglyceride fat droplets of maldigestion stain directly with Sudan, whereas fatty acids of malabsorption must be acidified and heated to appear as fat droplets.

PROTEIN

Ingested polypeptides contact proteolytic pepsin enzymes that are acid-activated from pepsinogens secreted by gastric chief cells. Although pepsin is not required for protein digestion, proteolysis normally begins in the stomach. Pancreatic secretion of proenzymes, which are activated into trypsin, chymotrypsin, elastase, and carboxypeptidase, continues proteolysis into absorbable amino acids, dipeptides, and tripeptides. Enterocyte brush border dipeptidases further hydrolyze larger peptides into absorbable products. Amino acids, dipeptides, and tripeptides are transported into enterocytes, where they are further hydrolyzed into amino acids and then released into the portal venous system. The systems for absorption include both diffusion- and carrier-mediated transport.

Intraduodenal amino acids and fat release CCK, whereas acid releases secretin from duodenal enterochromaffin cells. Cholecystokinin causes pancreatic acinar cells to release zymogen granules containing trypsinogen and chymotrypsinogen. Trypsinogen is activated by enterokinases from duodenal enterocytes, and trypsin activates the other proteases. The healthy pancreas produces a large excess of proteolytic activity. Thus, protein maldigestion only occurs after substantial loss of pancreatic function. Damage to gut mucosal enterocytes (as in celiac sprue) can reduce amino acid absorption and cause leakage of proteins from the circulation into the gut lumen. Lymphatic obstruction does not reduce amino acid absorption, but it allows both chylomicrons and lymph proteins such as albumin to leak back into the gut lumen. Amino acids of albumin are reclaimed, but liver albumin synthesis may not be able to compensate for the rapid protein loss; resulting in hypoalbuminemia.

CARBOHYDRATES

People in the U.S. consume 300 to 400 g of carbohydrate per day, mostly as starch (50%) and sucrose (30%). Digestion of complex polysaccharides is initiated by salivary amylase. Pancreatic amylase secretion occurs concurrently with that of other pancreatic enzymes. Intraluminal starch digestion by amylase yields small two– or three–glucose-containing fragments, particularly maltose, maltriose, and limit dextrins.

Pancreatic amylase secretion has the most redundancy of all enzymes, so maldigestion of complex carbohydrates is uncommon. Ingested disaccharides, such as lactose (glucose-galactose), sucrose (glucose-fructose), and the small products of starch digestion are further digested into monosaccharides (glucose, fructose, and galactose) by enterocyte brush border enzymes. Sucrase-isomaltase and maltase enzymes are normally produced in great excess. They release glucose and fructose for active transport into enterocytes. Lactase releases glucose and galactose from lactose, but this enzyme has lower intrinsic activity and has a genetically linked propensity to be lost during aging (see the section Lactose Intolerance).

Enterocytes absorb monosaccharides by both passive and active processes or, in the case of fructose, by facilitated diffusion. Free water and electrolytes are carried passively across gut mucosa during glucose absorption. The capacity of the gut for absorption of simple sugars is remarkable—estimated at up to 22 lb/day. However, failure to digest the disaccharide lactose from milk or the trisaccharide stachyose from beans, creates an osmotic load. Excess liquid is presented to the colon, causing diarrhea. Disaccharides entering the colon are readily metabolized into hydrogen gas and short chain fatty acids by bacteria. Within limits, the colon can absorb these short chain fatty acids and prevent diarrhea. However, symptoms of intestinal gas and liquid stool may result.

Initial Evaluation of Absorptive Function

Symptoms of diarrhea and weight loss are often considered the primary features of malabsorption (Table 1). Although they often occur, these symptoms are nonspecific and not invariable. For example, 20% of celiac sprue patients do not have weight loss. Malabsorption should also be considered when patients display multiple or specific nutritional deficiencies. Presence of anemia (iron, folate, B_{12}, or combined deficiencies), prolonged prothrombin time in the absence of liver disease, hypocalcemia (tetany or osteoporosis), altered night vision or skin changes from vitamin A deficiency, edema from low serum albumin, or unexpectedly low cholesterol values should also raise the possibility of malabsorption.

When clinical findings and screening labs suggest that malabsorption may be present, the workup sequence should be logical (Table 2). Steatorrhea is the most consistent finding; therefore, a test of fat absorption is done first. The best single test is measurement of *quantitative* fecal fat excretion: the 72- (or 48-) hour fecal fat measurement. The test requires diligence and cooperation. All stool during the test period is collected in a preweighed container. The patient must consume a diet containing appreciable fat (preferably 100 g fat, but at least a diet in which the amount of ingested fat can be estimated). Patients should not have concurrent tests requiring fasting, purging, or unusual diet. Total stool weight and fat excretion are measured and expressed as g/day. In the United States, normal

TABLE 1 Malabsorption Workup
Part I: Suspecting the Diagnosis

Finding	Differential Diagnosis
Weight loss (80%)	Depression, diet, cancer, hyperthyroid
Diarrhea (80%)	Infections, irritable bowel, IBD, drugs, etc.
Nutritional abnormality (common)	
Anemia	
• Iron deficiency	• Blood loss, diet, gastric surgery
• B_{12}	• Pernicious anemia
• Folate	• Diet, drugs
• Combined	• Diet
Elevated prothrombin time	Drugs, liver disease, diet
Hypocalcemia	Hypoparathyroid, renal disease, metabolic
• Osteopenia	Aging, diet, metabolic
Hypoalbuminemia	Liver disease, nephrotic syndrome, diet
Low cholesterol	Healthy life style, cancer, metabolic, statin drugs

NOTE: For diagnosis of malabsorption first consider its possibility from the patient's history, physical exam, and basic lab tests. Diarrhea and weight loss are common symptoms, having a wide differential. Approximate symptom frequency in celiac sprue and pancreatic insufficiency are shown in parentheses.
Abbreviations: IBD = irritable bowel disease.

stool weight is less than 250 g/day, whereas normal fat output is less than 6 g/day (6% of ingested fat). Normal fat absorption is virtually complete, and stool fat is primarily of bacterial origin.

Fat excretion between 6 to 10 g/day (or percentage of intake) is suspicious for malabsorption, but not diagnostic. Most significant maldigestive or malabsorptive diseases result in values more than 10 g/day (10% of intake), with pancreatic insufficiency and celiac sprue capable of producing 40 g fat excretion per day or more. Radioactive fat absorption studies, such as measurement of serum radioactivity after [14C] triglyceride or [14C] fatty acid ingestion, are also available to evaluate steatorrhea. Tracer tests are more genteel than stool collection, but they are less reproducible and reliable because they measure small reductions in a large value (normal absorption being >95%). Quantitative fecal fat can detect a small increase in what is normally a small value (<6 g/day).

Less-expensive, qualitative tests are also used for screening. However, they have false-positive and false-negative results and are less reproducible than the quantitative test. Qualitative fecal fat (stool is placed on a slide and stained with Sudan stain for fat droplets) must include examination after heat and acidification to detect fatty acids as well as neutral fat. Serum carotene level reflects fat absorption, but there are low values in persons with poor dietary carotene intake. Three days of oral beta-carotene capsules (1 capsule per day) before testing may be advisable. Elevated serum carotene may be seen in diabetics, even in the presence of malabsorption.

If steatorrhea is found, diseases of digestion must be distinguished from diseases of absorption. Clinical clues can help to evaluate digestive dysfunction. Pancreatic insufficiency should be considered if there is a history of prior pancreatitis, alcoholism, hyperglycemia (pancreatic endocrine insufficiency) or if pancreatic calcification is seen on radiographs. Pancreatic function testing may also be used, as discussed in the section, Pancreatic Insufficiency. In the presence of impaired liver secretion of bile salt micelles, patients often have jaundice, pruritus, abnormal liver enzyme levels, or other signs of cholestasis or liver injury.

Absorption is evaluated by tests of mucosal function or structure. Absorption of the pentose D-xylose is a useful test of absorptive function. Urinary excretion and/or blood levels of D-xylose are measured after the oral ingestion of 25 g (5 g for pediatric patients). Normally, 50% of the D-xylose dose is absorbed and 50% of the absorbed dose is metabolized. Thus, at least 20% (5 g or 1 g) is excreted in urine during a 5-hour collection. Blood D-xylose level greater than 25 mg/dL (>20 mg/dL for the 5-g pediatric dose)

TABLE 2 Malabsorption Workup
Part II: Sequence of Diagnostic Workup

1. Is steatorrhea present?

   • **Yes** (**No**; then this is not generalized malabsorption)

2. Is mucosal function abnormal?
   • **Yes** (Low D-xylose absorption)
3. *Small bowel biopsy*

   • Mucosal diseases, (e.g., celiac sprue, Whipple's disease, etc.)
   • *Small bowel radiograph*
   • Bacterial overgrowth (stasis), Crohn's disease, fistula, lymphoma, etc.
4. Specific tests for bacterial overgrowth, B_{12} absorption, protein loss, etc., may be appropriate.

• *Quantitative fecal fat*
• *Qualitative fecal fat ± serum carotene*
(**No;** steatorrhea may still be isolated nutrient malabsorption, such as lactose or B_{12})
D-*xylose test*
No (Normal D-xylose absorption)
• Pancreatitis history?
• Pancreatic calcification?
• *Pancreatic function tests*
• *Therapeutic trial of pancreatic enzymes*
Consider intestinal lymphangiectasia (*biopsy*)
• Consider Crohn's disease (*radiograph*)
• Consider lymphoma (*radiograph*)

NOTE: Sequence of a logical workup involves documenting steatorrhea (generalized malabsorption) and then differentiating pancreatic insufficiency from small bowel mucosal disease or bacterial overgrowth. Differentiating lab tests are shown in italics.

1 hour after consumption is also used to indicate normal absorption. Reduced D-xylose absorption is seen in many mucosal diseases and in the presence of bacterial overgrowth. Falsely low values can be seen in persons with gastric or urinary retention, renal insufficiency, ascites, or incomplete urine collection.

When mucosal disease is suspected, gut biopsy and/or small bowel radiographs are useful. Currently, endoscopic biopsy is done more often than capsule biopsies. Endoscopy is quick and easy for patients, but the small size of endoscopic biopsy and the patchy nature of some diseases (including celiac sprue) mandates that distal duodenum or jejunum be sampled and that multiple endoscopic biopsies be taken to assure proper orientation. Small bowel barium radiographs may identify structural disease such as fistulas, Crohn's disease, small bowel stasis or diverticulosis, mass lesions, or *malabsorptive pattern* such as in celiac sprue. Absence of radiographic findings does not exclude mucosal disease.

Specific Disease Processes

PANCREATIC INSUFFICIENCY

As discussed, substantial pancreatic functional capacity (>90%) must be lost before clinical problems with nutrition are noted. History (alcohol, pancreatitis, cystic fibrosis) or concurrent hyperglycemia may be present. Patients often complain of bulky, greasy, formed stools (triglyceride steatorrhea) rather than watery diarrhea. Pain may be absent, unless ongoing chronic pancreatitis is present, and appetite may be increased. Weight loss is common. Hypoalbuminemia and anemia are not usually prominent. Iron absorption may be increased, but roughly 20% of patients have reduced B_{12} levels because of B_{12} malabsorption. Normal B_{12} absorption requires that pancreatic proteases digest a normal gastric protein, R protein, which binds to B_{12} and prevents it from linking to intrinsic factor. Deficiency of pancreatic proteases results in reduced B_{12} binding to intrinsic factor and reduced B_{12} absorption.

A history and the features described may be sufficient to justify a diagnosis of pancreatic insufficiency. However, pancreatic function testing can be required for diagnosis. A duodenal drainage tube is positioned in the second portion of the duodenum. Pancreatic secretion is stimulated using intravenous secretin and/or CCK, a Lundh test meal (protein, fat, and carbohydrate), or luminal amino acid infusion. Pancreatic secretions are collected to measure the volume, bicarbonate concentration (>70 to 80 mEq/L), or enzyme output (>400 U of amylase per 80 min). Other, less discriminating, indirect pancreatic function tests include stool chymotrypsin or elastase measurement, breath hydrogen testing after the ingestion of rice flour, and various radioactive triglyceride serum or breath tests.

The diagnosis of pancreatic insufficiency is confirmed by showing reduced fat excretion during pancreatic enzyme replacement. Usual therapy requires 30,000 U of lipase activity given orally with each meal, to reduce steatorrhea. Enzymes in nonenteric coated products are partially denatured by gastric acid; so higher dose or inhibition of acid secretion with cimetidine (Tagamet), famotidine (Pepcid), or ranitidine (Zantac) taken twice daily, or once-daily proton pump inhibitor (such as omeprazole [Prilosec]) is required

for full function. Enteric-coated products may not require acid suppression, but excessively delayed enzyme release must be considered if the clinical response is suboptimal. Doses of 2 to 6 tablets per meal are taken, based on the preparation used: Viokase 8 and Cotazym are uncoated and contain 8000 U lipase per tablet. Creon-10 and Pancrease MT10 are enteric coated and contain 10,000 U lipase per tablet, whereas Ultrase MT12 contains 12,000 U lipase per tablet. Low-fat diet may also help to reduce symptoms of steatorrhea.

DEFICIENCY OF BILE MICELLES

Reduced bile salt secretion is seen in cholestatic or severe hepatocellular disease. The bile salt pool may also be depleted in persons having resection or disease of more than 100 cm of distal ileum. The liver may not fully compensate for unresorbed bile salts by increasing synthesis. Steatorrhea is usually modest (<20 g/day), but absorption of vitamin K and other fat-soluble vitamins is particularly impaired. If large amounts of unabsorbed bile salts enter the colon, choleraic diarrhea may occur. Bile salt replacement is usually not feasible; rather, treatment is through a low-fat diet. Although cholestyramine, which binds bile acids, can reduce choleraic diarrhea, it may worsen steatorrhea.

SMALL BOWEL BACTERIAL OVERGROWTH

Factors that predispose to small bowel bacterial overgrowth include gastric achlorhydria or hypochlorhydria; hypoglobulinemia or agammaglobulinemia; small bowel bacterial contamination via enterocolic or gastrocolic fistulas; areas of stasis such as multiple jejunal diverticula, or afferent or other surgically created bowel loops; and bowel hypomotility as seen in scleroderma or diabetes. Generally, more than 10^5/mL of bacteria in the upper small intestine can impair nutrient digestion and absorption. The primary mechanism is bile salt deconjugation, resulting in impaired micelle formation. Anaerobic bacteria are particularly adept at deconjugation. Bacteria also use carbohydrates, amino acids, and nutrients such as B_{12}. Overgrowth of luminal bacteria may damage intestinal mucosa, causing villous flattening and inflammation in some cases. Thus, mucosal absorption and transport can be reduced.

Bacterial overgrowth causes steatorrhea, diarrhea, weight loss, and fat-soluble vitamin deficiencies. Vitamin K and folic acid deficiency generally do not occur, because bacteria can produce these nutrients. Useful diagnostic test abnormalities include elevated fecal fat excretion and reduced D-xylose absorption, because bacteria metabolize the pentose. Hydrogen breath tests shortly after oral sucrose (50 to 80 g) or lactulose (10 g) administration have been used, but false-negative tests occur owing to absence of hydrogen-producing bacteria in 10% to 15% of people. The measurement of $[^{14}C]$ CO_2 in the breath after oral $[^{14}C]$ D-xylose can be used. The $[^{14}C]$ bile acid breath test has lost favor. Anaerobes use B_{12}, so the Schilling test of B_{12} absorption is low but corrected with oral antibiotic therapy (so-called Part III of the Schilling test). Definitive diagnosis of bacterial overgrowth involves culturing small bowel fluid aspirated via drainage tube or endoscope. Fluid must be promptly sent for quantitative culture of aerobic and anaerobic bacteria. Greater than 10^5 organisms per mL indicates bacterial overgrowth. Small bowel followthrough or enteroclysis may demonstrate diverticula, scleroderma or other motility disorders, blind loops, or fistulas. Diagnosis is confirmed if oral antibiotics correct steatorrhea, low B_{12} or D-xylose absorption, or the abnormal breath tests described previously.

Treatment of bacterial overgrowth consists of oral antibiotics, particularly drugs such as amoxicillin-clavulanic acid (Augmentin)[1] twice daily, cephalexin (Keflex),[1] 250 mg four times daily plus metronidazole (Flagyl),[1] 250 mg three times daily; trimethoprim + sulfamethoxazole (Septra DS),[1] twice daily; ciprofloxacin (Cipro),[1] 500 mg twice daily; or rifaximin (Xifaxan),[1] 200 mg twice daily. Some patients respond to a single 2-week course, but many require repeated courses or prolonged therapy. Resistance often necessitates rotation of antibiotic type. Prokinetic drugs are not terribly effective or useful. Surgical correction of fistulas or blind loops may be curative.

CELIAC SPRUE

Also known as *gluten-sensitive enteropathy* or *celiac disease*, this is one of the most common malabsorptive diseases in the United States and Europe. Celiac sprue involves three factors:

1. Genetically determined predisposition
2. Exposure to specific grain proteins in the diet
3. Resultant immune-mediated injury to small bowel mucosa

The incidence of diagnosed celiac sprue in white North Americans is perhaps as high as 1:1000. However, celiac sprue antibody tests suggest that the prevalence of some form of the condition may be as high as 1:200 to 250, which is the prevalence of sprue in parts of Ireland. In recent years, it has become recognized that gluten sensitivity encompasses a wide spectrum of clinical features and associations beyond just malabsorption. Celiac sprue is associated with type 2 diabetes, thyroid disorders, cerebellar ataxia and other neurologic conditions, the skin disorder dermatitis herpetiformis (DH), arthritis, and a variety of other conditions. Some of these conditions (cerebellar ataxia and DH) may improve with gluten avoidance, whereas others (diabetes and thyroid disorders) do not seem to respond.

Most sprue patients possess specific, inherited histocompatibility leukocyte antigen (HLA) class cell surface immune response proteins (HLA DQ8 and DQ2). These HLA types also occur in approximately 40% of normal persons. They apparently allow the sprue patient's immune system to recognize or react to dietary wheat gluten (gliadin) or analogous proteins found in barley, rye, and perhaps oats. In the presence of gluten proteins, an immune reaction damages gut mucosa. The grain proteins involved are rich in proline and glutamine. When genetically predisposed persons consume these proteins, some will develop a cell-mediated immunologic damage to gut mucosa manifest by villous flattening, inflammation, and malabsorption. Exclusion of dietary gluten-type proteins reverses the injury and the malabsorption. Most sprue patients have serum antigliadin, antitissue transglutaminase, and antiendomysial antibodies. Whether these antibodies participate directly in mucosal injury is unclear. However, positive serum antitissue transglutaminase or antiendomysial antibody appears to be a very good, sensitive, and specific test for celiac sprue. The antigen appears to be tissue transglutaminase; interesting in that offending dietary proteins are rich in glutamine.

Although it has a genetic basis, clinical celiac disease appears at various ages, from early childhood to old age. Patients often report a history of overlooked nutrition or growth problems at the time of diagnosis. Celiac malabsorption or diarrheal symptoms in childhood may appear to abate and then return later in life. Diarrhea and weight loss is common, but many patients manifest one or several predominant nutritional deficiencies; including nutrient deficiency anemia, bleeding, or calcium deficiency. Sprue must be considered in the differential diagnosis of iron deficiency anemia. Elevated fecal fat excretion and low D-xylose absorption are seen. The most common traditional test has been intestinal biopsy. Biopsy shows substantial loss of villus height because of enterocyte destruction, deep crypts because of compensatory attempts to produce enterocytes, and a mucosal lymphocyte/plasma cell infiltrate. Increased numbers of lymphocytes in the surface epithelium of the upper small intestine is the hallmark and earliest histologic feature. The diagnosis of celiac sprue is confirmed when symptoms, absorptive tests, and/or biopsy appearance improve after rigorous exclusion of wheat, rye, barley, and (usually) oats from the diet. Although oat protein may not cross-react with gluten, most oats available in the United States are *contaminated* or commingled with wheat, so sprue patients are still advised to avoid oats. In recent years antitissue transglutaminase and antiendomysial antibody testing have become the standard screening tests for the spectrum of celiac sprue conditions. However, not all persons with positive antibody have *clinical* malabsorption. Because the required diet exclusions are difficult and lifelong, many experts prefer to confirm the diagnosis using jejunal biopsy, and even to document improvement with a repeat biopsy several months after a strict gluten-free diet. Endoscopic biopsy for celiac sprue should be performed in patients being evaluated for *iron-deficiency anemia* if they are undergoing upper gastrointestinal (GI) endoscopy to look for GI blood loss.

Villous flattening is highly suspicious for celiac sprue; but it may also be seen in other conditions: tropical sprue, viral enteritis, abdominal radiotherapy, cytotoxic chemotherapy, bacterial overgrowth, Zollinger-Ellison syndrome, thyroid and adrenal disorders, lymphoma unrelated to sprue, and other conditions. Increased numbers of intraepithelial lymphocytes is the hallmark histologic feature of sprue. It is important to follow up the clinical gluten-free diet trial with objective measures to assure improved absorptive function or biopsy histology.

A knowledgeable dietician should instruct newly diagnosed patients on the gluten-free diet. A refresher visit is advised. The food industry uses a variety of names for grain proteins, and wheat protein is found in many unexpected prepared foods (e.g., some ice creams). Educated reading of food labels is essential. If followed diligently, lifelong gluten-free diet therapy can be curative. Secondary lactase deficiency, caused by enterocyte damage, can correct itself with a gluten-free diet. The most common cause of relapse or failure to respond to diet is because of dietary mistakes—accidental or purposeful.

Complications of celiac sprue include intestinal lymphoma and other GI malignancies, *refractory sprue*,

---

[1]Not FDA approved for this indication.

the skin condition DH, pulmonary fibrosis, and neurologic disorders. Development of bowel lymphoma occurs more frequently than expected, probably more so if diagnosis of sprue has been delayed or if gluten-free diet compliance is lax. Gastrointestinal adenocarcinomas also occur more often than expected in sprue patients. Refractory and collagenous sprue are rare and not clearly related to conventional sprue, because diet response is absent by definition. However, these conditions have been seen in previously responsive patients who go off the diet. Prednisone (20 to 40 mg/day) may be needed for refractory sprue, but total parenteral nutrition is rarely necessary for the conditions. Dermatitis herpetiformis is a pruritic, vesicular eruption on extensor surfaces. Ten percent of sprue patients have DH and perhaps all DH patients have jejunal biopsy features of sprue (with or without overt malabsorption). Dermatitis herpetiformis responds to gluten exclusion, but skin improvement may take many months.

TROPICAL SPRUE

Endemic tropical areas for this condition include the West Indies (especially parts of Puerto Rico), Central America, India, Southeast Asia, the Middle East, and Africa. An uncommon diagnosis in the United States, tropical sprue is seen in visitors to these areas or expatriates. Symptoms include prolonged diarrhea and weight loss, often with steatorrhea, and macrocytic anemia. It appears to develop because of overgrowth of one or several coliform bacteria in the intestine, as a result of contaminated water and poor sanitation. Deficiency of folate and/or vitamin B_{12} is prominent. Clinical studies show steatorrhea, low D-xylose absorption, folate and/or vitamin B_{12} deficiency, villous flattening on jejunal biopsy, and a megaloblastic bone marrow. The anemia responds quickly to folate (5 mg/day orally) and B_{12} (1000 µg/wk intramuscularly [IM]) for 2 to 4 weeks. Diarrhea may also abate, but it is important to also treat with oral antibiotics to eradicate the bacteria. In addition to folate and vitamin B_{12}, oral tetracycline[1] (250 mg four times daily) or poorly absorbed sulfonamides are typically given for up to 3 to 6 months. Tetracycline therapy should be avoided in growing children.

GIARDIASIS

Poor sanitation and contaminated food or water can also result in intestinal *Giardia lamblia* infection. Although the parasite usually causes acute diarrhea, chronic infection can occur with resultant chronic diarrhea and occasional malabsorption. Malabsorption most commonly occurs in persons with IgA deficiency or hypogammaglobulinemia. Examination for ova and parasites is usually positive in acute infection but may be negative in chronic infections. Stool testing for *Giardia* antigen by enzyme-linked immunosorbent assay is a good way to detect infection, probably more reliable than ova and parasite exam. Additional tests include duodenal biopsy, parasitic exam of duodenal fluid obtained via intubation, or exam of mucus obtained by the Entero-Test string technique. *Giardia* is usually treated using oral metronidazole (Flagyl),[1] 250 mg three to four times daily for 5 to 10 days.

The drug must be avoided early in pregnancy. Tinidazole (Tindamax) has recently been approved for treatment of giardiasis, at a single oral dose of 2 g (50 mg/kg for children older than 3 years of age).

WHIPPLE'S DISEASE

This is a rare bacterial infection in which *Tropheryma whippelii* (the Whipple's bacillus) engorge macrophages in intestinal mucosa and submucosa, and often macrophages in other tissues. The clinical disease typically involves middle-aged, white males presenting with fever, migratory arthralgias, lymphadenopathy, weight loss, abdominal pain, diarrhea, and malabsorption. Central nervous system involvement, dementia, or personality change occur. Lab studies show anemia and nutritional deficiency, with steatorrhea and low D-xylose absorption. Jejunal biopsy shows mucosa infiltrated by macrophages filled with *para-aminosalicylic acid–positive bacillary bodies*. Multiple biopsies are advised, because the lesion may be spotty. The differential diagnosis includes AIDS infection complicated by mucosal *Mycobacterium avium-intracellulare* (MAI) infection, or mucosal histoplasmosis. Electron microscopy or special stains (for acid-fast bacilli or fungus) aid the diagnosis.

Polymerase chain reaction for *T. whippelii* can also confirm the diagnosis. Treatment involves long-term (1 year or longer) oral therapy with Septra DS[1] twice daily (penetrates blood brain barrier) or doxycyline[1] 100 mg twice daily. Treatment for severely ill patients includes an induction therapy with intravenous antibiotics such as penicillin,[1] with or without streptomycin,[1] or ceftriaxone (Rocephin[1]) followed by oral antibiotics. Relapse after therapy may occur.

CROHN'S DISEASE

Crohn's enteritis can cause malabsorption by a variety of mechanisms. Enterocolic fistulas may enable small bowel bacterial overgrowth. Inadequate contact of nutrients with bowel mucosa (*short bowel syndrome*) may result from fistulas, small bowel resections, or extensive areas of diseased mucosa. Small bowel radiographs, endoscopy, and tissue histology enable diagnosis. Treatment may include management of disease activity, resection of focal fistulas, or oral antibiotic therapy. Enteral nutrition with an elemental diet or parenteral nutrition may be required.

EOSINOPHILIC GASTROENTERITIS

Eosinophilic gastroenteritis refers to a diverse group of clinical entities involving eosinophilic infiltration of gastric and/or small bowel mucosa. The disease pattern may involve mucosa, muscularis, or serosa. The infiltrates may be focal and produce mass effect and obstructive symptoms (muscularis disease), or they may be diffuse. When there is diffuse involvement of small bowel, malabsorption may occur. A pediatric clinical presentation has been referred to as *allergic gastroenteritis*, manifest as diarrhea/steatorrhea, weight loss, and protein loss into the gut (mucosal disease). Peripheral eosinophilia is common. Atopy, eczema, or

---

[1]Not FDA approved for this indication.

[1]Not FDA approved for this indication.

asthma may be seen. Some children appear to respond to an elimination diet, so food allergies may be involved in some cases. In adults, eosinophilic ascites can occur (serosal disease) and true food allergy appears to be less common. Usually, no clear underlying etiology is found. Radiographs may show mucosal thickening and gut mucosal biopsy shows the eosinophilic infiltrate. Although an elimination diet may be attempted, adult patients often require steroid treatment. The clinical symptoms usually respond to low-dose prednisone therapy, 20 to 40 mg/day, for 7 to 14 days. This is often followed by dose taper. Some patients require longer treatment or repeat treatment for recurrences, which may appear years later. Before prednisone treatment, it is important to exclude parasitic infection of the GI tract—especially strongyloidiasis—by repeated, careful stool ova and parasite studies. Limited therapeutic success has been reported with oral sodium cromoglycate (Cromolyn),[1] 800 mg/day in divided doses.

HYPOGAMMAGLOBULINEMIA

Patients with hypogammaglobulinemia or agammaglobulinemia can develop malabsorption. There are probably a variety of underlying mechanisms. Chronic *Giardia* infection can produce malabsorption in IgA-deficient patients, and this can be treated with Flagyl. IgA deficiency has also been associated with celiac sprue, which is responsive to a gluten-free diet. Small bowel bacterial overgrowth can also be seen in these patients. Search for *Giardia*, small bowel biopsy and a trial of antibiotics is a reasonable approach. Some patients still have no clear mechanism found, and biopsy may show nodular lymphoid hyperplasia, villous flattening, a paucity of lymphocytes or normal mucosa.

ABETALIPOPROTEINEMIA (BASSEN-KORNZWEIG SYNDROME OR ACANTHOCYTOSIS)

This is a rare, congenital genetic defect of enterocyte apolipoprotein and chylomicron processing. Patients' enterocytes cannot transport chylomicrons; therefore, steatorrhea is prominent. Small bowel mucosal biopsy shows normal villi lined by fat-containing enterocytes. This is a systemic disorder, and extraintestinal clinical manifestations dominate and include retinopathy with blindness, cerebellar degeneration, and red blood cell acanthocytes. A deficiency of vitamin E (and other fat-soluble vitamins) seems to play a role in the neural symptoms. Low-fat diet and vitamin replacement, while monitoring fat-soluble vitamin levels in blood, are advised.

INTESTINAL LYMPHANGIECTASIA

Obstructed lymphatic drainage from gut villi results in leakage of lymph back into the gut lumen. Lymph contains chylomicron fat as well as lymphocytes, albumin, and other proteins. Hypoalbuminemia, lymphocytopenia, and steatorrhea are found. Diagnostic tests include tests for increased fecal fat, increased stool α_1-antitrypsin (for protein loss), and gut mucosal biopsy showing dilated villous lacteals. A search should be made for the level of

---

[1]Not FDA approved for this indication.

lymphatic obstruction. A congenital version, often associated with Milroy disease, is caused by embryologic failure of lymphatic channels to communicate. Acquired causes include lymphatic obstruction caused by small bowel lymphoma, retroperitoneal fibrosis or tumor, tuberculosis, lymphatic obstruction caused by surgery, thoracic duct obstruction, and even constrictive pericarditis. Underlying conditions should be treated if possible, but patients also benefit from a diet very low in long-chain fatty acids (<20 g fat/day), to reduce protein loss into the gut. Short- and medium-chain triglycerides are acceptable because they are absorbed via the portal vein.

GASTRIC SURGERY

Partial gastrectomy, especially with Billroth II anastomosis, can be associated with diarrhea (*dumping*), poor iron or B_{12} absorption, modest steatorrhea because of inadequate nutrient contact with enzymes and bile salts, low D-xylose absorption because of rapid transit, and even bacterial overgrowth.

Specific Defects in Absorption

LACTASE DEFICIENCY (LACTOSE INTOLERANCE)

Lactose is the primary disaccharide in milk and dairy products. Some processed foods contain lactose. Low activity of brush border lactase may produce osmotic diarrhea and excessive colonic gas after lactose consumption. Acquired lactase deficiency occurs in mucosal diseases such as sprue or even viral enteritis. Genetic lactase deficiency is much more common. Persons of other than Northern European heritage tend to lose lactase activity after adolescence. They may have symptoms if more than 12 g of lactose (8 oz. of milk) is consumed at once. Avoiding dairy products and lactose prevents symptoms. Lactose in yogurt may be tolerated, because yogurt bacteria possess lactase activity. Some persons benefit from using lactase-treated milk or taking lactase enzyme (LactAid) with milk. Diagnosis is by trial of dietary lactose restriction, or by measuring an excessive rise in breath hydrogen (>20 ppm) after oral consumption of 25 g of lactose (adult dosage; dose for children is 2 g/kg, up to 25 g maximum).

SUCRASE-ISOMALTASE DEFICIENCY

This uncommon genetic recessive condition presents as diarrhea and abdominal pain when sucrose-containing formula or food is introduced to the diet of infants or young adults. Starch is usually tolerated. Diagnosis is by breath hydrogen testing after oral sucrose, or mucosal biopsy for sucrase enzyme activity measurement. Treatment is by means of sucrose-restricted diet.

PERNICIOUS ANEMIA

Pernicious anemia is most commonly an autosomal dominant immune response to parietal cells and intrinsic factor (IF), which results in autoimmune metaplastic atrophic gastritis, low IF production, and B_{12} malabsorption. Rare genetic defects of ileal intrinsic factor binding, transcobalamin II deficiency, or absent intrinsic factor synthesis also produce B_{12} malabsorption. Diagnosis is by the Schilling test of B_{12} absorption. Treatment is with parenteral B_{12} (1 mg injections IM monthly). Secondary B_{12} malabsorption can be seen in pancreatic insufficiency, bacterial overgrowth, and celiac sprue.

Acute and Chronic Pancreatitis

Method of
Carmen C. Solorzano, MD, and
Richard A. Prinz, MD

Acute Pancreatitis

Acute pancreatitis is an inflammatory process of the pancreas, with variable involvement of adjacent regional tissues or remote organ systems. The clinical manifestations of acute pancreatitis are heterogeneous but usually are of rapid onset. Most patients have epigastric pain, which can range from very mild to severe with associated hemodynamic instability. Early diagnosis and staging are necessary to provide appropriate treatment.

INCIDENCE AND ETIOLOGY

The incidence of acute pancreatitis has been reported to be as high as 38 per 100,000 population per year and appears to be increasing. Around 15% to 20% of patients will develop severe life-threatening complications requiring prolonged intensive care support at considerable cost.

Gallstones and alcohol abuse are the leading causes of acute pancreatitis in the United States, accounting for up to 80% of cases. Acute alcoholic pancreatitis may occur after binge drinking, but in most cases the patient has a minimum 5- to 7-year history of regular, heavy ethanol ingestion. Controversy exists as to whether alcohol alone, without prior gland injury, can cause the condition, as only a minority of alcoholics ever develop acute pancreatitis, implying multifactorial causation. A gallstone in the common bile duct (choledocholithiasis) may incite acute pancreatitis as it passes through the sphincter of Oddi en route to the duodenum. It does so, at least in principle, by transiently obstructing pancreatic duct flow and perhaps also by promoting reflux of bile into the pancreatic duct. As with alcoholic acute pancreatitis, the exact mechanisms remain uncertain. Perhaps 10% of attacks remain "idiopathic" in spite of thorough investigation. Other infrequent causes of acute pancreatitis are listed in Table 1.

PATHOGENESIS

Although the etiologic factor is known in 85% of patients with acute pancreatitis, the pathologic basis for the condition is incompletely understood. Most patients have a mild form of acute pancreatitis, which is associated with minimal organ dysfunction and an uneventful recovery.

TABLE 1 Causes of Acute Pancreatitis

Biliary tract disease (gallstones and microlithiasis)
Alcohol abuse
Drug reaction
Pancreatic or ampullary tumors
Ampullary stenosis
Congenital anomalies of the pancreatic or biliary anatomy
Hypertriglyceridemia
Hypercalcemia
Trauma (external or iatrogenic)
Infection (mumps...)
Bites (scorpion, spiders, Gila monster)
Tropical pancreatitis
Idiopathic

These patients respond to appropriate fluid administration, with rapid normalization of physical signs and laboratory values. The predominant pathologic finding in mild acute pancreatitis is interstitial edema with occasional parenchymal necrosis. On the other hand, 10% to 15% of patients have severe acute pancreatitis, which is associated with organ failure and/or local complications, such as acute fluid collections, necrosis, abscess, and pseudocyst formation.

In most experimental models of acute pancreatitis, secretion of digestive enzymes from the acinar cell is disturbed. Inappropriate activation of the proteolytic enzyme trypsin outside the gastrointestinal tract leads to inflammation and autodigestion. Tissue destruction results in an influx of leukocytes and macrophages, which, together with the pancreas itself, elaborate numerous inflammatory mediators leading to systemic inflammatory response syndrome. This is thought to be the first step in the development of pancreatitis. Trypsinogen is activated through hydrolysis of an N-terminal peptide called *trypsinogen-activating peptide*. Several natural mechanisms prevent pancreatic autodigestion by activated trypsin. These include: production of serine protease inhibitor Kazal type 1 (SPINK1), also known as *pancreatic secretory trypsin inhibitor* (PSTI), which reversibly inhibits activated trypsin; trypsin-activated trypsin-like enzymes that degrade trypsinogen; and bicarbonate-rich secretions, which are dependent on the normal production of the cystic fibrosis transmembrane conductance receptor (CFTR). SPINK1 mutations have been identified in familial pancreatitis and in children with idiopathic chronic pancreatitis. Because SPINK1 mutations are more common than is pancreatitis, they are thought to be modifiers or promoters rather than the cause of the disease.

The cationic trypsinogen gene that causes hereditary pancreatitis was discovered in 1996. Its mutation leads to a conformational change in the structure of the trypsinogen–SPINK1 complex and may lead to an impaired SPINK1-mediated defense mechanism against activated trypsin. Hereditary pancreatitis is an autosomal dominant condition with clinical and pathologic manifestations identical to those of sporadic pancreatitis. It has an 80% penetrance and is manifested by recurrent episodes of acute pancreatitis, progression to chronic pancreatitis, and development of pancreatic cancer. Many of these mutations have also been noted in patients with idiopathic pancreatitis.

DIAGNOSIS

The predominant symptom of acute pancreatitis is severe, constant epigastric pain. The onset is rapid, although not as sudden as that of perforated duodenal ulcer. The pain frequently radiates through to the back and may be partially diminished by sitting and leaning forward, or by lying curled in a fetal position. The signs of Cullen and Grey-Turner, periumbilical and flank bruising, respectively, are rare. Nausea and vomiting are frequent. These symptoms cause most patients to seek medical attention within 6 to 12 hours of the onset of pancreatitis, although delay is often seen among inebriated patients. Patients appear acutely ill, and they are usually tachycardic. Hypotension denotes a severe attack. The abdomen is quiet, tender, and full to palpation in the epigastrium.

The simplest laboratory test that suggests the diagnosis of acute pancreatitis is an elevated serum amylase level. Acute acinar cell injury causes a rapid rise in serum amylase level. Normal kidneys efficiently clear amylase, so typically the serum amylase level returns toward normal by the third or fourth day of the attack. A number of acute abdominal surgical emergencies cause hyperamylasemia, such as perforated duodenal ulcer, but rarely to the level of elevation seen with acute pancreatitis. The severity of pancreatitis does not correlate with the degree of amylase elevation. Patients with acute biliary pancreatitis tend to have very high amylase levels, even during a mild attack, presumably because the pancreas was completely normal at the outset. A lesser elevation of serum amylase is usually observed in acute alcoholic pancreatitis, especially during a second or subsequent attack. Serum lipase concentration rises within 4 to 8 hours and returns to normal after 8 to 14 days, making it a useful method for patients presenting late.

CURRENT DIAGNOSIS

Acute Pancreatitis

CLINICAL MANIFESTATIONS

- Severe constant epigastric pain
- Pain radiates to the back
- Nausea and vomiting
- Mild pancreatitis responds to supportive treatment with no organ failure

RADIOLOGIC AND LABORATORY TESTS

- Flat and upright plain abdominal film to rule out small-bowel obstruction, perforated ulcer
- Serum amylase and lipase levels
- Ultrasound of the abdomen, with attention to the right upper quadrant (gallbladder, bile ducts, pancreas)
- Contrast-enhanced computed tomography

EVALUATE SEVERITY OF PANCREATITIS

- Ranson criteria
- Acute Physiology and Chronic Health Evaluation (APACHE) II
- Degree of pancreatic necrosis on contrast-enhanced computed tomography

TABLE 2 Ranson Criteria of Severity of Acute Pancreatitis*

On Admission	At 48 Hours
1. Age >55 years	6. Hematocrit fall >10%[†]
2. White blood cell count >16,000 cells/mm³	7. Serum calcium <8 mg/dL
3. Serum glucose >200 mg/dL	8. Base deficit >4 mEq/L
4. Serum lactate dehydrogenase >350 IU/L	9. Blood urea nitrogen increase >5 mg/dL[†]
	10. Arterial Po₂ <60 mm Hg
5. Aspartate transaminase >250 U/dL	11. Fluid sequestration >6L[‡]

*Criteria are modified slightly for gallstone pancreatitis.
[†]Compared to admission values.
[‡]Fluid volume infused minus urine and nasogastric tube output.

Lipase elevation may be more sensitive than amylase elevation in patients with alcoholic pancreatitis and is more specific as a marker of acute pancreatitis than is elevated amylase.

Plain abdominal radiographs are useful mainly to exclude other conditions, such as perforated peptic ulcer and mechanical small-bowel obstruction. Ultrasound of the abdomen may disclose edema of the pancreatic parenchyma. However, this finding is often obscured by overlying bowel gas, which acts as an acoustic barrier. Ultrasound is most useful for diagnosing gallbladder stones. It can also accurately calibrate the common bile duct diameter, suggesting choledocholithiasis if distended. A contrast-enhanced abdominal computed tomography (CT) scan (although often unnecessary) more reliably diagnoses acute pancreatitis. The severity of the attack and its outcome can be graded and correlated to the CT appearance of the pancreas and parapancreatic tissues (see next section).

QUANTIFICATION OF SEVERITY

Between 70% and 80% of all attacks of acute pancreatitis are mild, resulting in little short- or long-term morbidity and virtually no mortality. The remainder are severe attacks, involving a variable fraction of pancreatic necrosis, extensive short- and long-term morbidity, and a mortality rate between 10% and 30%. Predicting severe pancreatitis soon after hospital admission allows early triage to intensive care for supportive treatment. To this end, several systems of severity measurement have been developed and correlated with outcome. Of these systems, the best known is the scoring system devised by Ranson and associates (Table 2). They identified 11 "criteria," five of which were determined on admission and six others at 48 hours after admission, which correlated with ultimate risk of morbidity and mortality. Patients exhibiting two or fewer of the prognostic criteria are likely to survive a relatively mild attack, those with three to six criteria have progressively more severe disease and a greater probability of death, and those with seven or more criteria will almost certainly not survive. The Ranson prognostic score has the advantages of strong clinical correlation and a simple, universally available data set. Its disadvantages are that it requires 48 hours to complete, and it is not useful after 48 hours. It was originally developed to grade acute alcoholic pancreatitis. The Acute Physiology and Chronic Health Evaluation (APACHE) II evaluates 12 prognostic variables that cover all organ systems. Scores greater than 13 in acute pancreatitis have been associated with poor prognosis. An advantage of APACHE II is that it can be used at any time during the hospital course. The Balthazar Score predicts severity of acute pancreatitis based on CT appearance of the pancreas, including presence or absence of pancreatic necrosis. According to these criteria, if 30% of the pancreas is nonperfused, the chances are high that the patient will progress to complicated acute pancreatitis. The Atlanta Classification defines severe acute pancreatitis using standard clinical manifestations, three or more Ranson criteria or an APACHE II score of eight or more, evidence of organ failure, and intrapancreatic pathologic findings such as necrosis (Table 3).

MANAGEMENT OF MILD ACUTE PANCREATITIS

Although recovery without specific treatment is the rule, all patients are watched closely in a hospital setting because rapid deterioration is not always predictable. Management consists of nothing by mouth, hydration with intravenous crystalloid solution, and analgesia as needed. Prophylaxis against deep venous thrombosis with low-dose subcutaneous heparin and/or sequential calf compression should be routine. Alcoholic patients must be assessed for risk of alcohol withdrawal syndromes. Laboratory tests on admission should include either an arterial blood gas measurement or oxygen saturation measured by pulse oximetry. Oral intake of liquids is resumed when the abdomen is soft and

nontender, which usually correlates with a normalized serum amylase level. If the liquids do not exacerbate the attack, the diet can be advanced as tolerated. A right upper quadrant ultrasound is performed in all patients, even alcoholic patients, because they too may harbor gallstones. Nasogastric suction is indicated if ileus and vomiting are present because of the risk of aspiration. Likewise, gastric antisecretory agents are given only if there is concern about peptic ulcer or stress gastritis.

MANAGEMENT OF SEVERE ACUTE PANCREATITIS

Severe acute pancreatitis is usually evident on initial clinical assessment; if not, the grave situation declares itself within the subsequent 24 to 48 hours. Early mortality from severe acute pancreatitis results from cardiovascular and/or respiratory failure. Thus, patients are managed in an intensive care unit, with urinary, central venous pressure, and arterial catheters, cardiac and pulse oximetry monitoring, and close observation. Profound and ongoing intravascular volume loss results from fluid sequestration within the retroperitoneum as well as a diffuse capillary leak, which causes generalized edema. Intravascular volume is maintained by crystalloid infusion, titrated to maintain adequate tissue perfusion. Inotropic cardiac support is used as needed once intravascular volume repletion is achieved. Packed red blood cells are transfused as needed to maintain adequate oxygen-carrying capacity. Respiratory function frequently worsens precipitously in the first 24 hours, requiring endotracheal intubation and ventilatory support. Analgesia and sedation are liberally administered, as is stress ulcer prophylaxis.

At present, no pharmacologic therapy dependably ameliorates the severity of the pancreatitis or decreases the risk of systemic complications. Neither octreotide (Sandostatin),[1] a somatostatin analogue that inhibits pancreatic exocrine secretion, nor various protease inhibitors have improved mortality. Newer therapies targeting mediators of the pancreatic and systemic inflammatory response could in theory improve outcome, especially if administered very early in the attack. One such agent, a platelet-activating

---

[1]Not FDA approved for this indication.

TABLE 3 Atlanta Symposium Clinically Based Classification System for Acute Pancreatitis*

Mild Acute Pancreatitis (75%)
Clinical manifestations (abdominal tenderness, vomiting, hypoactive bowel sounds)
Lacks features of severe pancreatitis
Patients respond appropriately to fluid administration
Minimal organ dysfunction
Contrast enhancement of pancreatic parenchyma is usually normal
Intrapancreatic pathology: Interstitial edema rarely necrosis

Severe Acute Pancreatitis (25%)
Clinical manifestations (abdominal tenderness, vomiting, hypoactive bowel sounds)
Ranson ≥3, Acute Physiology and Chronic Health Evaluation (APACHE) II ≥8
Organ failure
Intrapancreatic pathology: Necrosis, less commonly interstitial edema

Pancreatic Necrosis
Nonenhanced parenchyma on contrast-enhanced computed tomography >3 cm or involving >30% of the gland
Pathology: Macroscopic focal or diffuse areas of devitalized pancreatic tissue and peripancreatic fat necrosis

*Adapted from Arch Surg 1993;128:586-990.

CURRENT THERAPY

Acute Pancreatitis

MILD ACUTE PANCREATITIS

- Supportive therapy: Intravenous fluids, pain control, diet as tolerated
- If gallstones: Cholecystectomy and cholangiogram during same hospitalization or shortly thereafter

SEVERE ACUTE PANCREATITIS

- Admission to intensive care unit
- Supportive therapy: Intravenous fluids, pain control, antibiotics, enteral or parenteral nutrition
- Surgical treatment of infected pancreatic necrosis
- Surgical or endoscopic treatment of pseudocyst

factor antagonist called *lexipafant*, showed promise in initial laboratory investigations but did not prove beneficial in clinical trials. Because retroperitoneal and peritoneal exudates contain activated digestive enzymes and a host of other vasoactive and inflammatory mediators, peritoneal dialysis might logically improve the condition of patients with severe acute pancreatitis. Indeed, several trials report amelioration of the cardiovascular collapse associated with a severe attack, although overall hospital mortality due mainly to late infectious sequela was not altered. Finally, operation has almost no role early in the course of severe acute pancreatitis (first 14 days), except to rule out another suspected cause of the acute abdomen or to resect gangrenous bowel, which has developed as a complication of the severe pancreatitis.

NECROSIS AND INFECTION

The presence of pancreatic necrosis can be detected by dynamic CT scanning or by serum markers, if available. The probability of complications and of death correlates with the amount of pancreas that is necrotic. When 20% or less of the gland undergoes necrosis, secondary pancreatic infection is rare, and survival is expected. If 50% or more of the gland is necrotic, secondary infection becomes very probable, and mortality is as high as 50%. Secondary infection of necrotic pancreatic and peripancreatic tissues is relatively common and is the principal cause of mortality from severe acute pancreatitis. Infecting organisms are usually enteric gram-negative bacilli, but infection with gram-positive organisms and fungi is now recognized as well. A trend toward reduced pancreatic infection (as well as other systemic infection) has been shown following the prolonged use of newer antibiotics, which effectively penetrate pancreatic tissue. However, infections that develop in patients treated with prophylactic antibiotics tend to involve resistant organisms. One standard prophylactic antibiotic regimen gaining acceptance uses imipenem-cilastatin (Primaxin) started soon after admission and continued for at least 2 weeks. These patients have many intravenous and invasive monitoring catheters, which are potential portals for entry of gram-positive organisms that can secondarily infect the pancreas. Rigid adherence to appropriate infection control measures is required to minimize this risk.

Infected pancreatic necrosis is the most dreaded and lethal complication of severe acute pancreatitis. The condition becomes apparent most frequently during the third and fourth weeks of hospitalization and is marked by fever, increasing pain, tenderness, and fullness in the upper abdomen. The patient usually appears septic. Contrast-enhanced CT may reveal extraluminal retroperitoneal gas, which is a radiographic hallmark of infected necrosis. Percutaneous image-guided fine-needle aspiration of the pancreas, with immediate gram stain and culture of the aspirate, can reveal the presence of organisms, which is diagnostic of infected necrosis. Infected pancreatic necrosis is almost always fatal without aggressive débridement and drainage of the retroperitoneum. The standard for wide débridement is an open laparotomy, although laparoscopic, endoscopic, and percutaneous techniques are being described and developed. Surgical strategy ranges from débridement with closed suction and irrigation of the retroperitoneum to multiple planned operative débridements every 2 to 3 days until all necrotic material is removed. All approaches are time and labor intensive, but they offer the only chance for survival of the majority of patients.

Sterile pancreatic necrosis is associated with severe acute pancreatitis but, unlike infected pancreatic necrosis, is usually managed without the need for urgent operation. Acute peripancreatic fluid collections frequently arise. They may include reactive serous effusions but likely represent secondary or even main pancreatic ductal disruption, with resultant leak of pancreatic juice into the lesser peritoneal sac or other anatomic spaces surrounding the pancreas. These acute collections often resorb spontaneously, requiring no specific treatment. If infection of the fluid is suspected or if pain and tenderness are increasing, the collections may be percutaneously aspirated or even drained. In some centers, endoscopically placed transpapillary drains are inserted into the pancreatic duct, occasionally through the disruption into the fluid collection, to accomplish drainage. Finally, if such collections do not spontaneously disappear and do not require early drainage, they may evolve into a pancreatic pseudocyst.

A few patients with sterile pancreatic necrosis fail to improve in spite of optimal, protracted conservative care. These patients deserve operative exploration and pancreatic débridement on the grounds of failed nonoperative treatment, coupled perhaps with the suspicion that a smoldering, occult infection has eluded discovery. The operation is delayed as long as is practical, to allow areas undergoing necrosis to demarcate and liquefy. This makes the débridement technically easier. The pancreas and adjacent tissues are débrided and drained, provision for enteric feeding is established, and the abdomen is closed with the expectation that the need for reoperation will be likely.

BILIARY (GALLSTONE) PANCREATITIS

Gallstone pancreatitis is caused by transient obstruction of the pancreatic duct at the ampulla of Vater. The offending gallstone need not be large; "biliary sludge" and even biliary "microlithiasis" appear to be capable of provoking acute pancreatitis. As a rule, patients with gallstone pancreatitis have multiple small gallstones within the gallbladder, a comparatively wide cystic duct (promoting passage into the common bile duct), and a distinct "common channel" of the bile and pancreatic ducts.

Nonalcoholic patients with acute pancreatitis very likely have biliary lithiasis as the underlying cause. The presence of gallstones within the gallbladder virtually makes the diagnosis. A distended common bile duct seen by ultrasound further suggests the recent passage of a stone. Serum bilirubin and/or alkaline phosphatase levels may be mildly elevated, but often both are normal. If the ultrasound fails to reveal gallbladder stones or sludge and other rare causes are excluded, an endoscopic ultrasound may identify sludge or microlithiasis in a stable patient. Endoscopic ultrasound can also complement the pancreatic anatomic findings on CT. If endoscopic ultrasound is not available or is inconclusive, the next diagnostic step includes endoscopic retrograde cholangiopancreatography (ERCP). A sample of bile can be obtained to examine for microscopic crystals (this can be achieved by duodenal drainage as well), and small stones or anatomic anomalies may be identified.

Gallstone pancreatitis is usually mild, resolving clinically within 2 to 4 days. Serum bilirubin and alkaline phosphatase levels are typically normal or return to normal within this period, suggesting a low probability of persistent stone(s) within the common bile duct. Cholecystectomy eliminates the source of further stones and thus prevents recurrent pancreatitis; it should be performed during the same hospitalization or shortly thereafter. An intraoperative cholangiogram is performed, unless it has been undertaken preoperatively. If pancreatitis resolves but liver function tests suggest a persistent stone in the bile duct, then preoperative ERCP with papillotomy and stone extraction is appropriate, followed by prompt cholecystectomy.

If the intraoperative cholangiogram shows choledocholithiasis, a laparoscopic or open common bile duct exploration or a postoperative ERCP with papillotomy with stone removal can be performed, depending on the available expertise. Severe gallstone pancreatitis is managed like severe pancreatitis of any cause. Usually, the inciting stone has passed, leaving the bile and pancreatic ducts unobstructed; therefore, routine, early ERCP is not warranted. However, if a stone is persistently obstructing the ampulla of Vater, if the patient has jaundice, or if the patient has signs of cholangitis, urgent ERCP and stone extraction may be necessary.

Chronic Pancreatitis

Chronic pancreatitis (CP) is an irreversible, progressive inflammatory disease of the pancreas characterized by pain, fibrosis, and progressive loss of exocrine and/or endocrine function. The early course of this disease may often manifest as repeated attacks of acute pancreatitis. It occurs in men more frequently than in women. Excessive alcohol consumption is usually the cause in developed countries.

INCIDENCE

In several Western industrialized countries, the estimated prevalence of CP is approximately 10 to 15 per 100,000 population, with an annual incidence of 3.5 to 4 per 100,000 population. These rates may actually underestimate the problem because the diagnosis of CP is not based on advanced diagnostic tools such as ERCP and CT scan. In a recent report from Japan using CT and ERCP, the incidence of CP is 12 per 100,000 and prevalence is 45 per 100,000 population, which are much higher than in Western countries. In southern India, the prevalence of CP has been estimated to be 125 per 100,000 with the majority being calcific pancreatitis. The cause of this tropical pancreatitis is thought to be dietary. According to estimates of the Commission on Professional and Hospital Activities, CP ranks as the 27th most common digestive disease in the United States, with a threefold higher prevalence in the black male population.

The majority of care for CP is directed toward ameliorating pain, but a substantial amount of resources is also spent on treating complications. More than half of CP patients will develop pancreatic diabetes; one third of these patients will be insulin dependent, and nearly 50% will eventually require surgical intervention for pain or other complications. Optimal care of the patient with CP relies on supportive medical management of endocrine and exocrine insufficiency and of pain. Surgical intervention is generally reserved for intractable pain and specific complications such as pseudocyst and biliary or intestinal obstruction. As many as half of all patients will die within 20 years of their diagnosis of CP, a rate much higher than their age-matched population.

ETIOLOGY AND PATHOGENESIS

CP appears to be a multifactorial process involving both a genetic predisposition and environmental factors (see Table 4). Alcohol use is by far the number one cause of CP in the Western world, accounting for an estimated 70% of the cases in the United States and Europe. About 10% of chronic alcoholics will develop CP, roughly the same percentage of alcoholics who develop hepatic cirrhosis. Average age at diagnosis of alcoholic pancreatitis is 35 to 45 years with an 11- to 18-year history of 150 to 175 g of alcohol ingestion daily.

Ingested alcohol results in direct damage to the acinar cell with increased concentration of protein secretion, decreased production of bicarbonate, and decreased fluid volume as demonstrated in experimental models and in patients with alcoholic pancreatitis. This combination appears to result in protein and calcium precipitation within the pancreatic duct system, subsequent ductal obstruction, activation of pancreatic enzymes, and autodigestion of the gland. Over time, a fibrotic response results in permanent ductal abnormalities, calcification, and stone formation.

Dietary factors, such as high-fat and high-protein intake and trace mineral insufficiency, seem to be epidemiologically associated with CP. Another theory suggests the presence of an acinar cell product, lithostatin or pancreatic stone protein, that prevents calcium precipitation. Decreased concentrations of lithostatin and decreased levels of lithostatin messenger RNA have been found in the pancreatic juice and acini of patients with chronic calcific pancreatitis, suggesting a genetic component of risk for developing the disease. Alcohol-induced derangement of lipid metabolism has also been postulated as inducing the periacinar fibrosis and changes associated with alcoholic pancreatitis. The range of experimentally identified abnormalities supports the multifactorial nature of the disease.

Another form of CP, tropical pancreatitis, may be caused by protein malnutrition and cyanogens found in cassava root. The clinical and histologic features of tropical pancreatitis are nearly identical to those of alcoholic CP. Obstructive pancreatitis results from both congenital and acquired ductal obstruction, as in pancreas divisum, congenital and acquired strictures, and neoplasia. Unlike alcoholic pancreatitis, the obstructed pancreas shows uniform inflammatory changes with preserved ductal epithelium and rare protein plugs.

TABLE 4   Causes of Chronic Pancreatitis

Alcohol	Toxic Substances
Obstruction	Tropical pancreatitis
Pancreas divisum	Hypercalcemia
Congenital strictures	Hyperlipidemia
Acquired strictures	Genetic
Acute pancreatitis	Autoimmune
Trauma	Idiopathic
Endoscopic retrograde cholangiopancreatography	
Neoplasm	
Pancreatic	
Periampullary	

The hypothesis that high intraductal pressure results in pancreatitis has been proposed based partly on the demonstration of high intraductal pressures in these patients.

Additional causes of CP include hypercalcemia, hyperlipidemia, autoimmune diseases, and genetic alterations, as seen in hereditary and idiopathic pancreatitis (see section on acute pancreatitis). The mechanism by which pancreatitis develops in these situations is unclear.

DIAGNOSIS

Patients with CP typically present with persistent midepigastric pain, often with a thoracolumbar component. The pain may be exacerbated by eating and by alcohol consumption. Nausea, vomiting, and hemodynamic instability are less frequent than with acute pancreatitis. Examination often reveals upper abdominal fullness and tenderness with frequent associated signs of malnutrition and occasionally jaundice. The classic triad of CP—pancreatic calcification, diabetes mellitus, and steatorrhea—occurs in fewer than 25% of cases, although two thirds of patients will have an abnormal glucose tolerance test at the time of presentation. Because of the difficulty of obtaining pancreatic tissue for histologic analysis, CP is usually diagnosed by pancreatic imaging with or without tests of exocrine function. Radiologic evidence of pancreatic calcification is pathognomonic and is present in only 30% to 50% of patients.

Pain is present in 75% of patients. Initially the pain is characterized by recurrent attacks but tends to become persistent with variable periods of remission. Occasionally it will "burn out" over time. The etiology of pain is uncertain. Table 5 lists some of the proposed factors. The most recent theory suggests hypoxia and damage to local sensory nerves with exposure to inflammatory irritants such as histamine, prostaglandins, and pancreatic enzymes.

Laboratory values are of limited value in evaluating CP. Pancreatic enzyme levels (amylase, lipase) may be elevated in acute exacerbations but are not a good measure of chronic disease, pancreatic function, or pancreatic reserve, nor do

TABLE 5 Proposed Factors Producing Pain in Chronic Pancreatitis
Ductal hypertension
Autodigestion
Parenchymal ischemia
Perineural inflammation

they correlate with symptoms. Functional studies are cumbersome and are rarely required to diagnose CP. However, stimulated pancreatic secretions collected from the duodenum (amylase, lipase, trypsin, chymotrypsin, and bicarbonate), urine tests (nitroblue tetrazolium–*para*-aminobenzoic acid [NBT-PABA] test, and pancreolauryl test), or serum studies (P-isoamylase and trypsin), provide reliable estimates of pancreatic functional reserve and can be useful in evaluating treatment strategies. Serum liver enzyme levels and leukocyte counts may provide important information regarding complications of the disease.

Imaging

Plain abdominal radiographs reveal pancreatic calcification in less than 50% of patients and are otherwise nonspecific in CP. Transabdominal ultrasound can determine the size and consistency of the gland, characteristics of the biliary tree, and the presence of complications. A skilled ultrasonographer may achieve 70% sensitivity in diagnosing the disease.

CT approaches 90% sensitivity and greater than 90% specificity in diagnosing CP and should be considered in all suspected patients to classify their disease and determine the presence of complications and surgically correctable lesions. CT scan is the best radiologic modality for detecting calcifications, pancreatic ductal dilation, and pseudocysts and may be the only imaging study necessary in most cases.

ERCP remains the gold standard for diagnosis and staging of CP, with a sensitivity up to 95% and specificity greater than 90%. The small but finite incidence of serious complications related to ERCP should limit its use to those patients who require anatomic definition not provided by other imaging studies and in patients suspected of ampullary or ductal obstruction amenable to ERCP treatment.

Magnetic resonance imaging (MRI), magnetic resonance cholangiopancreatography (MRCP), and CT cholangiopancreatography/angiography are rapidly evolving and can replace diagnostic ERCP in most situations. This technology provides definition of soft tissues and ductal anatomy but remains institutional and operator dependent. Likewise, endoscopic ultrasound is becoming more available and may play a role in the early diagnosis of CP.

MEDICAL TREATMENT

Medical treatment of CP consists primarily of supportive care. Pain relief, metabolic and nutritional support, as well as pancreatic endocrine and exocrine support, are the mainstays of medical therapy. Pain control is difficult, often requiring opiate analgesics. Abstinence from alcohol must be the initial goal, as alcohol consumption predicts recurrent pain even after surgical intervention. Oral pancreatic enzyme

CURRENT DIAGNOSIS

Chronic Pancreatitis

CLINICAL MANIFESTATIONS

■ Persistent midepigastric pain exacerbated by eating or alcohol consumption
■ One or more present: Malnutrition, steatorrhea, glucose intolerance

RADIOLOGIC AND LABORATORY TESTS

■ Computed tomography scan of the pancreas may show calcifications, pancreatic duct dilation, and/or pseudocyst formation
■ Endoscopic retrograde cholangiopancreatography is the gold standard diagnostic test but is used only when computed tomography is not sufficient to make the diagnosis or clarify anatomy
■ Amylase and lipase levels are not useful
■ Functional pancreatic studies are cumbersome and rarely required

CURRENT THERAPY

Chronic Pancreatitis

MEDICAL TREATMENT

- Abstinence from alcohol
- Pain control, preferably with nonopioid analgesics, pancreatic enzymes, octreotide
- Nutritional support: Low-fat foods, adequate protein and vitamins
- Management of diabetes
- Management of exocrine insufficiency with pancreatic enzymes

SURGICAL TREATMENT

- Indications: Pain refractory to medical management, inability to exclude malignancy, biliary or enteral obstruction, pseudocyst, pancreatic ascites, pancreatic fistula
- Dilated pancreatic duct: Internal drainage procedure
- Nondilated pancreatic duct: Resection
- Pseudocyst: Internal surgical drainage or endoscopic techniques

---

supplementation and octreotide[1] may provide modest pain relief, probably due to reduced pancreatic secretion. Because opiate addiction increases in proportion to duration of disease, nonsteroidal anti-inflammatory drugs should be prescribed early and chronically. Opiates should be reserved for exacerbations and intractable pain. Some authorities recommend surgical intervention prior to the chronic administration of opiates.

Malnutrition is common due to fear of pain after eating, as well as poor dietary habits and nutritional problems, in the alcoholic population. Attention should be directed at providing a low-fat diet with adequate protein and calories and vitamin supplementation. Parenteral or jejunal feedings may be required in certain situations, such as preoperative preparation and episodes of acute exacerbation.

Pancreatic exocrine insufficiency necessary to produce protein malabsorption does not occur until 90% of acinar mass has been lost. However, steatorrhea, or fat malabsorption, is a common and often troublesome problem in patents with CP. In addition to lipase from the pancreas, digestion of lipids depends on salivary and gastric hydrolysis, alkalinization in the duodenum, and adequate bile acid concentrations, all of which may be diminished in alcoholics. Pancreatic exocrine enzyme replacement is indicated to ameliorate steatorrhea. Present enzyme preparations include enteric-coated and encapsulated forms to aid delivery of active enzymes and decrease the volume of administration. Gastric acid suppression may also be necessary to provide an adequate pH environment for enzyme activity.

Endocrine insufficiency in CP is primarily manifested as pancreatic diabetes. Its treatment is similar to that for other forms of diabetes in that it may be controlled by diet, oral hypoglycemic agents, or insulin.

---

[1] Not FDA approved for this indication.

TABLE 6 Indications for Surgery in Chronic Pancreatitis

Pain refractory to medical management
Inability to exclude pancreatic malignancy
Complications
Pseudocyst
Biliary obstruction
Duodenal obstruction
Splenic vein thrombosis
Pancreatic fistula
Colonic obstruction
Pancreatic ascites
Pancreatic abscess

SURGICAL TREATMENT

The first line of therapy in CP should be noninjurious; surgical intervention should be reserved for intractable disease. Additional indications for surgical intervention are listed in Table 6. The choice of operation depends on the anatomic findings in each patient (Table 7). Pancreatic and biliary duct anatomy should be carefully evaluated preoperatively. Improvements in perioperative preparation and care have enabled routine performance of surgical procedures on the pancreas, with very low mortality and morbidity. Contemporary series of operations for CP demonstrate mortality rates less than 3% and complication rates less than 30%, comparable to the rates of other major intra-abdominal operations.

In a minority of patients, stenosis or stricture of the ampulla of Vater can be treated with simple sphincterotomy or sphincteroplasty. Initial results with this technique revealed improvement in pain, but the results were short lived and correlated with alcohol abstinence. Although these procedures have been successful in limiting recurrent acute bouts of pancreatitis in pancreas divisum, no benefit has been realized for patients with CP. This experience suggests that sphincterotomy and pancreatic duct stenting will have little effect on the long-term management of CP from other etiologies.

TABLE 7 Selection of Operation for Chronic Pancreatitis

Disease limited to tail of gland	Distal pancreatectomy
Obstruction in head of gland	
Dilated pancreatic duct	LR-LPJ
Nondilated pancreatic duct	Whipple, DPPHR
No obstruction in head of gland	
Dilated pancreatic duct	LPJ
Nondilated pancreatic duct	Distal resection (40%–95%), total pancreatectomy
Unable to tolerate major operation	Neurolysis?
Failure of primary drainage/ resection	Additional drainage/ resection, neurolysis
Inability to rule out malignancy	Resection

Abbreviations: DPPHR = duodenal preserving pancreatic head resection; LR-LPJ = local resection–longitudinal pancreaticojejunostomy.

The pancreatic duct in CP usually is either dilated diffusely or in a beaded ("chain-of-lakes") pattern. A dilated pancreatic duct is best treated with internal drainage of the pancreatic duct into a Roux-en-Y limb of jejunum. Historically, 8 mm was considered the lower limit of dilation amenable to internal drainage, but the procedure has proved tenable and successful in relieving pain in patients with duct dilation of greater than 5 mm. The Partington-Rochelle modification of the Puestow operation (lateral pancreaticojejunostomy) has resulted in good to excellent relief of pain in 70% to 80% of patients. Concomitant procedures to address complications such as pseudocyst and biliary obstruction can be incorporated into the jejunal limb. There is no evidence that surgery improves pancreatic function, as was hoped by the pioneers of ductal drainage procedures.

The Frey procedure is based on the concept that the head of the pancreas and uncinate process may not be completely drained by longitudinal pancreaticojejunostomy. This procedure entails a "coring out" or local resection of the head of the gland combined with lateral pancreaticojejunostomy. Results have been promising; only 13% of patients have reported no pain relief. Another proposed mechanism for the success of this operation is the reversal of ischemia or ductal hypertension that irritates sensory nerves in the head of the gland.

When the pancreatic duct is not dilated, decompressing procedures are not feasible. However, patients may obtain relief of pain with pancreatic resection. Debate continues on the merits and complications of partial (40%–80%) distal pancreatectomy, subtotal (95%) distal pancreatectomy (Child's procedure), pancreaticoduodenectomy (Whipple's procedure), and total pancreatectomy. Duodenum-preserving pancreatic head resection (Beger's procedure) performed in the 10% to 30% of CP patients with an inflammatory mass in the head of the gland has shown excellent pain relief, comparable to that of a Whipple procedure. Pancreatic insufficiency resulting from resection procedures is generally proportional to the extent of resection, with severe exocrine insufficiency and a particularly brittle and difficult to control form of pancreatic diabetes at the extreme. Attempts at autologous pancreatic islet cell transplantation at the time of pancreas resection were initially promising, but enthusiasm for the technique has waned because of less than satisfactory long-term results.

Several approaches to nerve ablation have been proposed based on the theory that the pain of CP is related to inflammatory involvement of the splanchnic nerves. Extraperitoneal, intraperitoneal, thoracic, and thoracoscopic splanchnicectomy as well as complete denervation procedures have been attempted to treat the pain of CP. Results have been unpredictable, often unconfirmed, and with limited follow-up. Neurotomy may be considered in patients who have not obtained relief of pain after surgical drainage or resection procedures.

PANCREATIC PSEUDOCYST

Pancreatic pseudocysts are walled-off collections of fluid and debris resulting from disruption of the pancreatic duct and are most commonly associated with acute and chronic pancreatitis. Pseudocysts will develop in up to 10% of patients after an episode of acute alcoholic pancreatitis.

They may also occur after trauma or in association with a neoplasm. The wall is vascularized inflammatory tissue without an epithelial lining and may contain pancreatic parenchyma. Pseudocysts may occur in any region of the gland and are multiple in 10% to 15% of patients. Fluid collections occurring within 3 weeks of an acute episode of pancreatitis are considered acute fluid collections, and 30% to 40% of these collections will resolve spontaneously.

The most common presentation is abdominal pain, present in 90% of patients. Physical examination often reveals a tender abdominal fullness or mass. Nonspecific complaints of nausea, vomiting, early satiety, and weight loss are common. More dramatic presentations may result from free intraperitoneal rupture, intracystic hemorrhage or infection, gastric variceal bleeding resulting from splenic or portal vein thrombosis, or intraperitoneal hemorrhage from adjacent pseudoaneurysm rupture. Laboratory findings are nonspecific, although persistent amylase elevation is common. Imaging with CT is preferable, but ultrasound is nearly as sensitive and can be recommended for follow-up to determine interval changes in size.

Sampling of a postpancreatitis fluid collection is rarely indicated. However, if there has not been a preceding episode of pancreatitis, fluid cytology and chemistry can help differentiate a pseudocyst from a more likely mucinous or serous cystic neoplasm.

The natural history of asymptomatic pseudocysts reveals that nearly half remain stable, decrease in size, or completely resolve at 1-year follow-up, irrespective of size. However, pseudocysts larger than 6 cm are more likely to require operation during follow-up. Pseudocysts present for more than 12 weeks almost never resolve spontaneously and have a high rate of complications. Therefore, current management of pancreatic pseudocysts takes into account the presence or absence of symptoms, the age and size of the pseudocyst, and the presence or absence of complications. Postpancreatitis fluid collections that are asymptomatic in a stable patient can be followed with monthly imaging to evaluate resolution, stability, and enlargement. Failure to resolve and evidence of enlargement are indications for intervention. If, on the other hand, the pseudocyst is symptomatic, early intervention should be considered. Generally, a period of 6 weeks is desired prior to surgical intervention to assure adequate maturation of the cyst wall.

The preferred operative management of a pseudocyst is internal drainage into the gastrointestinal tract. This can be accomplished by anastomosis of the opened cyst wall to the stomach (cystogastrostomy), duodenum (cystoduodenostomy), or a Roux-en-Y limb of jejunum (cystojejunostomy), depending on the location of the pseudocyst. Multiple pseudocysts can be addressed simultaneously by connecting the pseudocysts and draining them as one, separately draining each cyst into a Roux-en-Y jejunal limb, or a combination of the internal drainage procedures. A lateral pancreaticojejunostomy should be added when the pancreatic duct is dilated. The cyst wall should be biopsied on all occasions, as cystic neoplasms of the pancreas can mimic a pseudocyst. Infected pseudocysts are generally treated as pancreatic abscesses.

Simple aspiration of pseudocysts will fail to resolve the fluid collection in as many as 80% of patients. Prolonged catheter drainage has demonstrated better resolution rates but may take months of drain maintenance. New endoscopic techniques that place an endoprosthesis through the intestinal lumen into the pseudocyst and that bridge the pancreatic duct disruption with a pancreatic duct stent are currently being analyzed.

ENDOSCOPIC THERAPY

Endoscopic approaches to ductal decompression have been attempted in CP. These include endoscopic clearance of the main pancreatic duct with pancreatic sphincterotomy and basketing of stones for removal, extracorporeal shock wave lithotripsy, transpapillary drainage of pseudocysts, and dilation and stenting of ductal strictures. Various endoscopic series have reported success rates of 50% to 70% for clearing the pancreatic duct and 60% to 80% for long-term pain relief. The risk of complications is approximately 10%. The early results of endoscopic therapy are comparable with those of surgery, but all endoscopic reports have been case series, some with little long-term follow-up. Randomized controlled studies using adequate and constant methods for evaluating and reporting results and comparing endoscopic, medical, and surgical treatment modalities are now required.

REFERENCES

Balthazar EJ, Robinson DL, Megibow AJ, Ranson JH: Acute pancreatitis: Value of CT in establishing prognosis. Radiology 1990;174:331-336.

Baron TH, Morgan DE: Acute necrotizing pancreatis. N Engl J Med 1999;340:1412-1417.

Bradley EL 3rd: A clinically based classification system for acute pancreatitis. Summary of the International Symposium on Acute Pancreatitis, Atlanta, Ga, September 11 through 13, 1992. Arch Surg 1993;128: 586-590.

Howare J, Idezuki Y, Ihse I, Prinz RA: Surgical Diseases of the Pancreas, 3rd ed. Baltimore, Williams & Wilkins, 1998.

Mitchell RM, Byrne MF, Baillie J: Pancreatitis. Lancet 2003;361: 1447-1455.

Tandon RK, Sato N, Garg PK; Consensus Study Group: Chronic pancreatitis: Asia-Pacific consensus report. J Gastroenterol Hepatol 2002;17:508-518.

Triester SL, Kowdley KV: Prognostic factors in acute pancreatitis. J Clin Gastroenterol 2002;34:167-176.

Uhl W, Warshaw A, Imrie C, et al; International Association of Pancreatology: IAP guidelines for the surgical management of acute pancreatitis. Pancreatology 2002;2:565-573.

Working Party of the British Society of Gastroenterology; Association of Surgeons of Great Britain and Ireland; Pancreatic Society of Great Britain and Ireland; Association of Upper GI Surgeons of Great Britain and Ireland: UK guidelines for the management of acute pancreatitis. Gut 2005;54(Suppl. 3):iii1-iii9.

Gastroesophageal Reflux Disease

Method of
Jonathan F. Finks, MD, and John G. Hunter, MD

Epidemiology

Gastroesophageal reflux disease (GERD) is an increasingly important disease in the United States and other Western nations, with major impact on both quality of life and health care costs. In a 1988 Gallup Organization survey, 44% of U.S. adults reported monthly symptoms; 14% reported weekly symptoms and 7% reported daily symptoms. The annual cost of GERD treatment in the United States is an estimated $10 billion. Patients with GERD consistently score lower on quality-of-life surveys than patients with congestive heart failure and angina. GERD is also the most important risk factor for esophageal adenocarcinoma.

Nonerosive Reflux Disease Versus Gastroesophageal Reflux Disease

The term *GERD* applies to all individuals at risk for physical complications from gastroesophageal reflux or clinically significant impairment of health-related quality of life because of reflux-related symptoms. This definition applies equally to patients with erosive esophagitis and those with nonerosive reflux disease (NERD). This latter group accounts for approximately 70% of GERD patients. Despite the lack of endoscopic findings in patients with NERD, their symptoms are often as severe as and sometimes even more difficult to control than patients with esophagitis, and their quality of life is equally affected. Indeed, patients with NERD should be treated in a similar way to patients with erosive esophagitis.

Pathophysiology

The etiology of GERD is related to three primary mechanisms: lower esophageal sphincter (LES) incompetence, transient lower esophageal sphincter relaxation (TLESR), and hiatal hernia. Conditions such as esophageal dysmotility (achalasia, scleroderma) or impaired salivary secretion (Sjögren's syndrome) hinder esophageal clearance and can augment the injurious effect of acid reflux. Delayed gastric emptying may lead to gastric distention and distortion of the gastroesophageal (GE) junction, which may promote or intensify the symptoms of GERD.

Incompetence of the LES can result in GERD, although the LES resting pressure in most patients with reflux symptoms is normal. The most common cause of pathologic reflux disease is excessive frequency or duration of TLESRs. These events, associated with distention of the gastric fundus, are responsible for up to 70% of reflux episodes in patients with GERD.

The most important anatomic factor leading to GERD is hiatal hernia, which alters the three main components of the reflux barrier (LES, crural diaphragm, and angle of His). Hiatal hernia reduces LES pressure and leads to distension of the GE junction. Resultant stretching of the crural diaphragm impairs its ability to augment LES pressure. The herniated portion of the stomach acts as an acid reservoir, worsening the impact of reflux on the distal esophagus. Finally, upward distraction of the GE junction into the chest leads to loss of the acute cardioesophageal angle, which normally serves to prevent reflux.

Clinical Presentation

The presentation of GERD is often divided into esophageal (typical) and extraesophageal (atypical) symptoms. The most common symptoms of GERD are heartburn, a sensation of substernal burning pain, and regurgitation of swallowed food. Both symptoms typically occur in the postprandial period. Other esophageal complaints include excessive salivation (water brash) and a sensation of a foreign body in the posterior pharynx (globus hystericus).

Extraesophageal manifestations of GERD include symptoms arising from the oropharynx, airway, and respiratory tree: chronic cough, wheezing, hoarseness, choking, sinusitis, and dental caries. The presence of these atypical symptoms should prompt an evaluation for malignancy (including laryngoscopic exam) in a patient with suspected GERD. Aspiration pneumonia and asthma are also strongly associated with GERD.

So-called alarm symptoms (dysphagia, odynophagia, bleeding, anemia, and weight loss) suggest complicated disease (e.g., esophageal stricture, malignancy) and merit further evaluation.

Diagnosis

EMPIRICAL THERAPY

In patients presenting with typical reflux symptoms (heartburn or regurgitation), a trial of empirical therapy is appropriate provided the patient does not present with alarm symptoms or other indications for endoscopy (Box 1). A good response to empirical therapy is considered diagnostic of GERD, with accuracy comparable to that of 24-hour esophageal hydrogen ion concentration (pH) monitoring.

ENDOSCOPY

Box 1 lists the indications for upper gastrointestinal endoscopy upon initial presentation. Endoscopy is also

---

BOX 1   Indications for Endoscopy in Patients Presenting With Heartburn

- Presence of alarm symptoms: dysphagia, odynophagia, anemia, weight loss, gastrointestinal bleeding
- Duration of symptoms longer than 5 years
- Age more than 50 years
- Known infection with *Helicobacter pylori*
- Family history of gastroesophageal reflux disease
- Severe daily symptoms

---

indicated in patients with early or frequent relapses following an empirical trial of medical therapy. Endoscopy allows direct inspection of esophageal mucosa and is the only reliable means of diagnosing Barrett's esophagus (BE).

BARIUM ESOPHAGRAM

Although the barium esophagram has low yield in the diagnosis of GERD, it is the first test to order in a patient presenting with dysphagia. The barium swallow is the best means of detecting esophageal strictures and diverticula and can help guide the endoscopist in patients with these complications. The esophagram also serves as a road map for the surgeon preparing for an antireflux procedure.

AMBULATORY ESOPHAGEAL HYDROGEN ION CONCENTRATION TESTING

Esophageal pH testing is not necessary to diagnose GERD in all patients. The combination of typical symptoms and endoscopic changes has a specificity of 97% for GERD. Ambulatory pH testing is a useful diagnostic tool for patients with NERD or those with entirely extraesophageal symptoms. The traditional catheter-based test is limited by patient discomfort as well as somewhat variable sensitivity and specificity. The newer capsule-based system is much better tolerated and gives up to 48 hours of data, significantly improving the accuracy of the test. Another recent advance is the combined acid and impedance monitor, which allows for detection of both acid and nonacid (volume) reflux. This test may prove useful in patients with persistent symptoms despite adequate medical therapy, particularly those with extraesophageal symptoms.

MANOMETRY

An esophageal motility study allows for a functional assessment of the LES and esophageal body. Its main utility in GERD is to rule out severe motility disorders, such as achalasia or scleroderma, prior to antireflux surgery.

Treatment

The goals of therapy for most GERD patients are relief of symptoms and long-term disease control. Mucosal healing is also an important endpoint in patients with significant esophagitis or complications (stricture, BE).

LIFESTYLE MODIFICATION

Data on the efficacy of lifestyle/dietary modifications are limited, but certain recommendations may prove useful. These include smoking cessation, weight loss, avoidance of recumbency for 3 hours postprandially, and abstinence from foods known to lower LES pressure: chocolate, peppermint, coffee, and alcohol.

MEDICAL THERAPY

Over-the-counter (OTC) antacids and alginates are commonly used to treat milder forms of GERD. They offer instant relief but have a short duration of action.

Prokinetic agents, such as metoclopramide (Reglan),[1] domperidone (Motilium),[1] and cisapride (Propulsid),[*] are used to enhance foregut motility, but to date little evidence suggests they are better than placebo in controlling GERD symptoms. Baclofen (Lioresal),[1] a γ-aminobutyric acid B receptor (GABA-B) agonist, works by reducing TLESRs and decreases both acid and nonacid postprandial reflux episodes and improves symptoms in patients with GERD. Baclofen[1] is limited, however, by its side-effect profile. H_2-receptor antagonists (H_2RAs) are proving effective in numerous placebo-controlled trials, offering symptomatic relief in 60% of GERD patients, with healing of esophagitis in 50%.

Proton pump inhibitors (PPIs) remain the most effective medical therapy for GERD, providing symptom relief and esophageal healing in 80% of patients. Several large controlled trials demonstrate the superiority of PPIs over H_2RAs in terms of symptom relief, esophageal healing, and cost effectiveness. In addition, PPIs normalize the impaired quality of life associated with GERD.

Upon initial presentation with typical GERD symptoms, patients not requiring endoscopy should undergo an empirical trial of standard-dose PPIs for 4 to 8 weeks. Patients who fail therapy or relapse soon after medication withdrawal should undergo further evaluation, including endoscopy. Patients whose symptoms are relieved following an initial trial of PPIs may benefit from on-demand therapy, in which PPIs are started at the onset of symptoms and discontinued after 24 hours of symptom relief. This treatment modality may also be appropriate for patients with NERD or mild erosive esophagitis because on-demand therapy is proven cost effective in this group of patients. Patients with frequent symptom relapse, however, should be started on continuous PPI therapy. Patients with moderate to severe esophagitis and those with extraesophageal symptoms should receive continuous maintenance therapy with standard or higher doses of PPIs.

ANTIREFLUX SURGERY

Although most patients with GERD can be managed effectively with PPIs, the therapy is lifelong, and up to 50% of patients experience symptom relapses and require dose escalation. Antireflux surgery is an attractive option for patients who do not wish to take medications chronically. Surgery is also effective for patients with persistent symptoms despite maximal therapy, particularly those with volume reflux, or regurgitation. Antireflux surgery should also be considered in patients with complications of the disease such as strictures, BE, or laryngotracheal aspiration (Box 2).

Excellent results are achieved with traditional open procedures, including complete (Nissen) and partial (Toupet, Dor) fundoplications. In the last decade, however, the laparoscopic approach to antireflux surgery became the standard of care, with most surgeons favoring the so-called floppy Nissen fundoplication.

Patient selection is crucial to the success of antireflux surgery. Preoperative evaluation should include a detailed history to document reflux-associated symptoms. All patients

considered for surgery should undergo endoscopy, both to confirm the presence of GERD and to assess for strictures, BE, or malignancy. Manometry must also be performed to rule out a severe motility disorder. An ambulatory pH study should be done on patients with NERD to confirm the diagnosis of reflux disease.

Relief of heartburn and regurgitation is seen in 90% to 95% of patients following antireflux surgery, and quality-of-life scores are normalized. The most consistent preoperative predictors of successful outcome are an abnormal ambulatory pH study and a good response to PPI therapy. The response of extraesophageal symptoms to surgery is more variable, with improvement rates ranging from 60% to 80%. The response of atypical symptoms to surgery is correlated with the response to medical therapy.

Laparoscopic antireflux surgery is generally well tolerated. Side effects such as gas bloat and dysphagia are common postoperatively but typically resolve within a few months. Infrequently, patients with dysphagia may require dilation or, rarely, reoperation. Long-term outcome from surgery is excellent, with symptom relief maintained in 85% to 90% of patients in most series with at least 5 years of follow-up. Reoperative rates range from 3% to 8%. Table 1 lists the most common reasons for failure.

BOX 2 Indications for Antireflux Surgery in Patients With GERD

- Failure of medical therapy
- Patient's desire for surgery despite successful medical management (because of lifestyle considerations, including age, time, or expense of medications)
- Patients with complications of GERD (e.g., BE, grade III or IV esophagitis, esophageal stricture)
- Medical complications attributable to a large hiatal hernia (e.g., bleeding, dysphagia)
- Atypical symptoms (asthma, hoarseness, cough, chest pain, aspiration) and reflux documented on 24-hour pH monitoring

Abbreviations: BE = Barrett's esophagus; GERD = gastroesophageal reflux disease; pH = hydrogen ion concentration.
Adapted from Society of American Gastrointestinal Endoscopic Surgeons (SAGES) Guidelines: Guidelines for surgical treatment of gastroesophageal reflux disease (GERD). Surg Endosc 1998;12(2):186-188.

TABLE 1 Causes of Fundoplication Failure in 1000 Laparoscopic Antireflux Procedures

Cause of Failure	$n = 39$
Transdiaphragmatic herniation of fundoplication	29 (74%)
Twisted or slipped fundoplication	4 (10%)
Excessive tightness of fundoplication	3 (8%)
Esophageal motility disorder	2 (5%)
Disruption of fundoplication	1 (3%)

Adapted from Terry M: Outcomes of laparascopic fundoplication for gastroesophageal reflux disease and paraesophageal hernia. Surg Endosc 2001;15(7):691-699.

---

[1]Not FDA approved for this indication.
[*]Investigational drug in the United States.

TABLE 2 American College of Gastroenterology Guidelines for Surveillance of Barrett's Esophagus

Dysplasia Grade	Follow-up Endoscopy
None	3 years
Low grade	1 year
High grade	
Focal	Every 3 months
Multifocal	Intervention (resection/ablation)
Mucosal irregularity	Endoscopic mucosal resection

Adapted from Sampliner RE: Updated guidelines for the diagnosis, surveillance and therapy of Barrett's esophagus. Am J Gastroenterol 2002;97(8):1888-1895.

ENDOSCOPIC THERAPY

Several endoscopic therapies for treating GERD are available. Their use is limited to patients with esophageal symptoms, hiatal hernia smaller than 2 cm, esophagitis grade II or lower, and no evidence of BE. The Stretta procedure delivers radiofrequency energy to the distal esophagus and may act through reduction of TLESRs and alteration of neural pathways. A variety of devices work by internal plication of the stomach below the GE junction. Finally, a device approved by the Food and Drug Administration (FDA) acts to bulk up the GE junction by injection of a biocompatible polymer into the wall of the distal esophagus. Most of the data on these procedures comes from open-label trials with follow-up of a year or less. Although most series demonstrate improvement in GERD symptoms and quality-of-life scores, none of the devices normalize esophageal acid exposure. Long-term controlled trials are needed before the impact of these endoluminal therapies on GERD treatment can be assessed.

Esophageal Stricture

Excessive scar formation from erosive esophagitis can lead to stricture of the distal esophagus. The thin fibrous bands

CURRENT DIAGNOSIS

- Alarm symptoms suggest complications of GERD and include: dysphagia, odynophagia, anemia, weight loss, and gastrointestinal bleeding.
- Endoscopy at initial presentation is recommended for patients with alarm symptoms or other risk factors for Barrett's esophagus.
- Ambulatory esophageal pH testing is useful to confirm the diagnosis of GERD in patients with NERD or exclusively extraesophageal symptoms.
- Combined impedance and pH testing may be useful in patients with persistent symptoms despite adequate medical therapy, particularly those with extraesophageal symptoms.
- An empirical trial of PPI therapy has equivalent diagnostic accuracy to a 24-hour ambulatory esophageal pH study.
- Patients with Barrett's esophagus should be enrolled in a surveillance endoscopy program.

CURRENT THERAPY

- Potentially effective lifestyle modifications include weight loss, smoking cessation, avoidance of postprandial recumbency and abstinence of foods known to lower LES pressure: chocolate, peppermint, alcohol, coffee.
- Proton pump inhibitors (PPIs) are the most effective and cost-effective medical therapy available for the treatment of GERD.
- On-demand therapy with PPIs is appropriate for patients with NERD or mild esophagitis who respond to an initial trial of PPIs.
- Patients with moderate to severe esophagitis or extraesophageal symptoms should be placed on continuous PPI therapy with standard or higher doses.
- The most consistent preoperative predictors of success following laparascopic antireflux surgery are an abnormal esophageal pH study and a good response to PPIs.
- The indications for antireflux surgery include patients whose symptoms are incompletely relieved with PPIs, as well as those who do not wish to remain on lifelong medical therapy.

at the GE junction of a Schatzki's ring are usually amenable to endoscopic dilation, whereas longer fusiform strictures may prove refractory. Patients should remain on continuous PPI therapy following dilation to promote mucosal healing. Antireflux surgery is usually indicated in the presence of a benign esophageal stricture.

Barrett's Esophagus

BE represents intestinal metaplasia of the distal esophagus and is a known precursor lesion of esophageal adenocarcinoma. The yearly incidence of adenocarcinoma in patients with BE is 0.5%, nearly 40 times higher than that of patients without BE. Risk factors for BE are duration of reflux symptoms, presence of hiatal hernia, advanced age, and male gender. Patients with chronic GERD symptoms should undergo endoscopy to screen for BE, and those found to have BE should be entered into a surveillance program (Table 2). Continuous PPI therapy or antireflux surgery is recommended for patients with BE. Titration of PPIs to normalization of esophageal acid exposure may result in regression of BE, although to date no convincing evidence suggests medical or surgical therapy can prevent the development of cancer in patients with BE.

REFERENCES

Bytzer P, et al: Personal view: Rationale and proposed algorithms for symptom-based proton pump inhibitor therapy for gastro-oesophageal reflux disease. Aliment Pharmacol Ther 2004;20:389-398.

DeVault K, et al: Updated guildelines for the diagnosis and treatment of gastroesophageal reflux disease. Am J Gastro 2005;100:190-200.

Galmiche JP, et al: Treatment of gastroesophageal reflux disease in adults: An individualized approach. Dig Dis 2004;22:148-160.

Gordon C, et al: Review article: The role of the hiatus hernia in gastroesophageal reflux disease. Aliment Pharmacol Ther 2004;20:389-398.

Hunter JG, et al: A physiologic approach to laparoscopic fundoplication for gastroesophageal reflux disease. Ann Surg 1996;223(6):673-687.

Kamolz T, et al: Laparoscopic Nissen fundoplication in patients with nonerosive reflux disease: Long-term quality of life assessment and surgical outcome. Surg Endosc 2005 February.

Lind T, et al: On demand therapy with omeprazole for the long-term management of patients with heartburn without esophagitis: A placebo-controlled randomized trial. Aliment Pharmacol Ther 1999;13:907-904.

Sampliner RE: Updated guidelines for the diagnosis, surveillance, and therapy of Barrett's esophagus. Am J Gastro 2002;97(8):1888-1895.

Sharma, P: Barrett Esophagus: Will effective treatment prevent the risk of progession to esophageal adenocarcinoma? Am J Med 2004; 117(5A):79S-85S.

Terry M, et al: Outcomes of laparascopic fundoplication for gastro-esophageal reflux disease and paraesophageal hernia: Experience with 1,000 consecutive cases. Surg Endosc 2001;15:691-699.

Triadafilopoulos G, et al: GERD: The potential for endoscopic intervention. Dig Dis 2004;22:181-188.

Trus TL, et al: Improvement in quality of life measures after laparoscopic antireflux surgery. Ann Surg 1999;229(3):331-336.

Tumors of the Stomach

Method of
Scott A. Hundahl, MD

Gastric Adenocarcinoma

From earliest cancer registry activity through World War II, adenocarcinoma of the stomach ranked number one among solid organ neoplasms in the United States. Since that time, both incidence and mortality have declined. Worldwide, however, gastric adenocarcinoma remains a common neoplasm, eclipsed only by lung cancer in incidence and mortality.

Several pathology classification schemes have been proposed for gastric adenocarcinoma, including the Borrmann morphologic classification, the Broder differentiation classification, the histologic World Health Organization (WHO) classification, the Nagayo-Komagome classification, the Ming classification, and the Goseki classification. None is more widely used than the 1951 Jarvi-Lauren (aka "Lauren") classification, which divides gastric adenocarcinoma into intestinal-type (gland-forming tumors) and diffuse-type (discohesive) tumors.

The Jarvi-Lauren classification, when combined with epidemiologic information, identifies three main histoepidemiologic patterns:

1. Intestinal-type tumors arising from the distal stomach, associated with preexisting atrophic gastritis and intestinal metaplasia (*Helicobacter pylori*–associated),
2. Diffuse-type tumors involving the body of the stomach (*H. pylori*–associated) but usually not associated with significant intestinal metaplasia, and
3. Intestinal-type tumors of the gastroesophageal junction

In high-incidence regions of the world, such as Japan and Korea, up to two thirds of gastric adenocarcinomas are of the first type and are strongly associated with chronic multifocal atrophic gastritis and intestinal metaplasia from chronic *H. pylori* infection. The process usually begins at the antral-corpus junction along the lesser curvature and predisposes to cancers of the intestinal type occurring in the sixth and seventh decades of life. The second type of gastric adenocarcinoma, also associated with *H. pylori*, afflicts younger individuals in the fourth and fifth decades of life. The last type, seen in lower-incidence regions of the world, such as the United States, is associated with chronic gastroesophageal reflux and Barrett's esophagitis.

It has been estimated that 42% of gastric adenocarcinomas worldwide can be attributed to chronic *H. pylori* infection. Strains containing the cagA gene appear more dangerous. The infection usually starts by the second or third decade and, unless successfully treated, gives rise to chronic inflammation, atrophic gastritis, and eventually intestinal metaplasia, which is a premalignant histologic condition. Dietary factors, such as high-salt and high-nitrate intake, can accentuate this progression. As the condition progresses, acid-producing oxyntic mucosa is progressively eliminated, gastric pH increases, and bacterial overgrowth with non–*H. pylori* bacteria is facilitated. The original *H. pylori*, which requires an acid environment to thrive, often disappears at this point. Once intestinal metaplasia is established, dietary factors become particularly important in mitigating the risk of cancer development. Protective factors include intake of vitamin C, fresh fruits and vegetables, and antioxidants. The association of *H. pylori* infection with the development of intestinal metaplasia suggests that early detection and elimination of this infection might prevent gastric cancer. Unfortunately, in high-incidence areas, reinfection from contaminated water supplies and other sources is common, thus undermining the strategy. In addition, in prevention trials to date, any benefit is restricted to the subgroups without preexisting intestinal metaplasia.

General risk factors for gastric cancer include low socioeconomic status, smoking, a diet deficient in fresh fruits and vegetables or high in salt-preserved, nitrate-laden foods, previous gastric ulcer, ionizing radiation, family history, and previous gastric resection. Blood group A is associated with higher risk of developing a diffuse-type tumor. Predisposing genetic conditions include the Lynch syndrome (i.e., hereditary nonpolyposis colorectal cancer, a condition with microsatellite instability due to deficient DNA repair enzymes) and, for diffuse tumors, specific germline mutations in the E-cadherin gene, as first detected in certain New Zealand Maori kindreds.

In Western populations, by the time gastric cancer causes symptoms, the disease is often relatively advanced. In a large National Cancer Data Base survey of U.S. patients, presenting ascribable symptoms included weight loss (62%), abdominal/epigastric pain (52%), nausea (34%), anorexia (32%), early satiety (32%), dysphagia (26%), and melena (18%).

Mass screening combining upper GI series, endoscopy, and serum pepsinogen I/II ratio have proven beneficial in high-incidence areas, such as Japan, but cannot be justified in the United States, where incidence is low. However, for defined risk groups, such as those with established atrophic gastritis and established intestinal metaplasia, a strong family history, or hereditary nonpolyposis colorectal cancer syndrome, surveillance screening should definitely be considered.

In the United States, diagnosis is usually made by upper endoscopy. One should be aware that diffuse-type cancers presenting as linitis plastica are often associated with

CURRENT DIAGNOSIS

- Chronic *Helicobacter pylori* infection gives rise to atrophic gastritis and intestinal metaplasia, which predispose to cancer. Surveillance issue.
- Mucosal changes in diffuse-type gastric cancer presenting as linitis plastica can be minimal. Deep mucosal biopsies are required.
- Helical computed tomography, endoscopic ultrasound, and minilaparotomy or laparoscopy for pretreatment staging of gastric cancer.
- In early growth, gastrointestinal stromal tumors are rarely associated with mucosal changes.

CURRENT THERAPY

- For local-regional cancer, complete surgical resection remains the key component of curative treatment.
- Total gastrectomy and splenectomy/pancreatectomy should *not* be routine but performed only when required for negative-margin resection.
- Surgical goal with respect to node dissection for cancer is a low Maruyama index operation (see references).
- For fit patients with good postoperative caloric intake, postoperative adjuvant chemoradiation is considered standard for all but stage IA cases.
- Node dissection is not required for gastrointestinal stromal tumors.

minimal visible mucosal changes, and deep biopsies are often required for establishing the diagnosis. Furthermore, small, "early" gastric cancers ("early" defined by the Japanese as in situ and T1 cancers, with or without node involvement) can be associated with particularly subtle mucosal changes, presenting a challenge for even the most experienced endoscopist.

Extent-of-disease studies for gastric adenocarcinoma include endoscopic ultrasound, which is good for estimating depth of tumor and visualizing immediately adjacent nodes, and helical CT scanning, which is good for evaluating extraluminal extent of disease, intra-abdominal and/or mediastinal extension/spread, and liver/lung metastases. Because even high-resolution CT scanning can miss small peritoneal implants, extraregional nodal spread, and small liver metastases, staging laparoscopy and minilaparotomy are valuable adjuncts and should be considered mandatory if any preoperative treatment is considered.

Although a long-established, much-modified Japanese staging system, the "General Rules," finds widespread use in many areas of the world, the American Joint Committee on Cancer and the Union Internationale Contre le Cancer (AJCC/UICC) TNM system is by far the dominant staging system used. T stage is defined a bit differently than for colorectal cancer: muscularis propria penetration short of serosal penetration is still considered T2 disease; a serosal breach is required for T3 disease; and a T4 designation requires direct involvement of adjacent structures. Optimally accurate nodal "N" designation requires that more than 15 nodes be examined by the pathologist. N1 disease means metastases in one to six regional nodes, N2 disease means metastases in 7 to 15 regional nodes, and N3 disease means metastases in more than 15 nodes. Any N3 disease, any node-positive T4 disease, any M1 distant metastatic disease, and any involved extraregional M1 nodes translate in the staging matrix to stage IV disease. The reader is referred to the AJCC staging manual referenced at the end of this article.

Curative treatment of gastric cancer involves, as main therapy, complete negative-margin surgical resection of disease. Various experts have shown endoscopic mucosal resection and minimally invasive techniques to be appropriate for some selected in situ and T1 tumors, but most tumors in the United States are discovered at a stage where formal open surgery is required. To secure a negative intramural margin of resection, a gross margin of 2 cm is usually adequate for exophytic, noninfiltrating tumors, and a margin of at least 6 cm of grossly normal tissue is recommended for ulcerated or infiltrating tumors or diffuse histology. Closest mural margins are generally checked by frozen section at the time of surgery to confirm adequacy of resection. Total gastrectomy is not indicated as a routine procedure, except in linitis plastica, but is warranted whenever required for a negative-margin resection.

Routine splenectomy for treatment of gastric cancer, as well as routine distal pancreatectomy (performed in the past to clear splenic nodes), should be avoided unless definitely required for complete resection of visible/palpable disease.

The extent of lymph node dissection in this disease has generated—and continues to generate—international controversy. Although several prospective, randomized trials of non-Asian populations—none perfect—fail to demonstrate that routine extensive lymphadenectomy increases survival, insufficient lymphadenectomy has also been shown to definitely compromise survival. A prospectively planned analysis of a large U.S. adjuvant chemoradiation trial and a blinded reanalysis of a large Dutch surgical trial have shown that the adequacy of lymphadenectomy for a given case can be quantified using the "Maruyama index of unresected disease" (the Maruyama index), and that this measure independently correlates with survival in a "dose-response" proportional fashion. Prospectively using the Maruyama Computer Program to predict the extent of nodal spread for a given cancer case is one way to assure a low Maruyama index surgical resection.

Sentinel node biopsy, an established technique for treatment of other cancers, has failed to win support for cancer of the stomach, because of the organ's lymphatic complexity and the relatively high reported false-negative rates.

A large North American prospective, randomized trial of postoperative adjuvant 5-fluorouracil (5-FU)–based chemoradiation in completely resected gastric cancer revealed a significant increase in disease-free and overall survival with this treatment. The postoperative nature of this trial thwarted implementation of surgical guidelines, and the extent of node dissection for most patients in the trial was minimal, with survival compromise for such patients demonstrated. Practitioners in some countries, such as Japan, dismiss the necessity of adjuvant postoperative adjuvant chemoradiation with the (unproven but reasonable) argument that this is only a salvage technique for inadequate surgery.

A separate Korean chemoradiation series has shown benefit even for radically treated cases, however. For patients with good postoperative performance status, good organ function, and adequate nutrition, postoperative adjuvant chemoradiation therapy is considered standard in North America.

Recently, survival data from a U.K. study of preoperative plus postoperative epirubicin, *cis*-platinum, and continuous-infusion 5-FU (ECF) chemotherapy versus surgery alone have shown encouraging results. However, results of other preoperative chemotherapy studies have been negative. This approach, although promising, is still considered investigational in North America.

In Korea, a positive trial of adjuvant perioperative intraperitoneal chemotherapy has been reported. Considerable morbidity and mortality are associated with this adjuvant treatment, however, and this therapy likely will not be implemented without refinement and independent duplication of results.

For localized disease deemed not resectable to negative margins, chemotherapy and chemoradiotherapy have been used to convert such tumors to potentially resectable status. With successful, negative-margin resection, some of these patients survive long term. Without any surgery, administration of 5-FU–based concomitant chemoradiotherapy to patients with residual, unresected local-regional disease can also result in some degree of 5-year survival (reported in excess of 10%).

Other Gastric Tumors

Gastrointestinal stromal tumors (GISTs) present as submucosal spindle cell tumors in the sarcoma family. In contrast to leiomyosarcomas and other spindle cell sarcomas, they express the antigen CD117 and most (>80%) tumors have activating mutations of c-*kit*. Formerly considered rare, approximately 5000 of these tumors per year are now diagnosed in the United States. Owing to the pattern of growth in the gastric wall, deep to the mucosa, early symptoms are unusual, and these tumors will often grow to massive size before mucosal ulceration and hemorrhage (or other major symptoms) finally develop. GISTs are classified as sarcomas. Treatment of localized primary tumors consists of complete surgical resection, which usually can be accomplished with a 2-cm margin of grossly normal tissue. Specific lymph node dissection is not indicated for this histology. Surgical series indicate that approximately 50% of primary gastric tumors will metastasize and recur within 5 years, with risk factors including size greater than 5 cm and more than one mitosis per high-power field. For patients with widespread metastases, generally located in the peritoneal cavity or the liver, first-line therapy is now the well-tolerated oral agent imatinib mesylate (Gleevec or STI-571) at an initial dose of 400 mg daily, which generates partial responses in more than 50% of cases and stable disease in an additional 25% of cases. Side effects are minimal, and 1-year survival in treated patients is approximately 85%.

Carcinoid tumors of the stomach have a similar behavior to small-bowel carcinoids. When small (i.e., <1 cm) and unassociated with invasion of the muscularis propria, local excision to negative margins is generally deemed sufficient. For such tumors, endoscopic resection has an established role. However, even small tumors can metastasize to lymph nodes. Wider gastrectomy with lymph node dissection is generally recommended for gastric tumors larger than 1 cm. Many of these tumors are associated with serum hypergastrinemia; those without this finding tend to be more aggressive. When metastatic to the liver or other organs, surgical cytoreduction (or other means of tumor ablation) can offer considerable palliation to those with carcinoid syndrome, and this technique should always be considered. Octreotide therapy now represents a palliative mainstay in all patients with carcinoid syndrome.

Gastric lymphomas encompass most of the lymphoma subtypes, but low-grade, mucosa-associated B-cell lymphomas, so-called B-cell mucosa-associated lymphoid tissue (MALT) lymphomas, deserve special mention because they are strongly associated with *H. pylori* infection. Indeed, localized cases can be controlled simply by treating the *H. pylori* infection. In such cases, however, molecular studies indicate persistence of the offending lymphoid clone in about half of cases. In particular, if *H. pylori* infection recurs, the lymphoma in such cases returns. For further information on this and other gastrointestinal lymphomas, see the article on lymphoma.

REFERENCES

Dematteo RP, Heinrich MC, El-Rifai WM, Demetri G: Clinical management of gastrointestinal stromal tumors: Before and after STI-571. Hum Pathol 2002;33:466-477.

Greene FL, Page DL, Fleming ID, et al (eds): AJCC Cancer Staging Manual. New York, Springer, 2002.

Hartgrink HH, van de Velde CJ, Putter H, et al: Extended lymph node dissection for gastric cancer: Who may benefit? Final results of the randomized Dutch gastric cancer group trial. J Clin Oncol 2004;22:2069-2077.

Hundahl SA, Macdonald JS, Benedetti J, Fitzsimmons T: Surgical treatment variation in a prospective, randomized trial of chemoradiotherapy in gastric cancer: The effect of undertreatment. Ann Surg Oncol 2002;9:278-286.

Kim S, Lim DH, Lee J, et al: An observational study suggesting clinical benefit for adjuvant postoperative chemoradiation in a population of over 500 cases after gastric resection with D2 nodal dissection for adenocarcinoma of the stomach. Int J Radiat Oncol Biol Phys 2005;63:1279-1285.

Macdonald JS, Smalley SR, Benedetti J, et al: Chemoradiotherapy after surgery compared with surgery alone for adenocarcinoma of the stomach or gastroesophageal junction. N Engl J Med 2001;345:725-730.

Modlin IM, Lye KD, Kidd M: Carcinoid tumors of the stomach. Surg Oncol 2003;12:153-172.

Peeters KCMJ, Hundahl SA, Kranenbarg EK, et al: Low Maruyama index surgery for gastric cancer: Blinded reanalysis of the Dutch D1-D2 trial. World J Surg 2005;29:1576-1584.

Tumors of the Colon and Rectum

Method of
Alan G. Thorson, MD

The most common tumor of the colon and rectum is adenocarcinoma, which accounts for 95% of colorectal tumors. Other tumors, both benign and malignant, account for less than 5% of colorectal tumors. These tumors include carcinoid (arising from the neuroectoderm and storing 5-hydroxytryptophan), neuroendocrine carcinoma, melanoma, squamous cell and adenosquamous carcinoma, lymphoma, gastrointestinal stromal tumors (arising from the interstitial cells of Cajal), lipoma, liposarcoma, neurofibroma and other tumors of neural origin, endometriosis, colitis cystica profunda (solitary rectal ulcer syndrome), and metastatic tumors. Because most of these tumors, including adenocarcinomas, present with similar signs and symptoms, the primary importance of being familiar with the existence of these tumors lies in recognizing the need to secure a confirming histologic diagnosis, most often through biopsy, prior to initiating therapy. The remainder of this discussion is limited to adenocarcinoma.

Epidemiology

Colorectal cancer (CRC) is the third most common cancer and the second leading cause of cancer deaths in the United States. There were an estimated 148,610 new cases of CRC in the United States in 2006 and 55,170 deaths. The lifetime risk of developing CRC in the United States is about 6%. Thus, about one in 17 Americans will develop CRC at some point in their lifetime. Only lung cancer is more deadly. Although there are slight variations between the sexes with respect to CRC, overall it is considered a gender-neutral cancer.

The incidence rates for CRC declined from 66 in 100,000 in 1985 to 52 in 100,000 in 2002, the last year for which figures are available. Currently, males are affected at a rate of 65.9 per 100,000 population and females at a rate of 47.9 per 100,000 population. Since 1998, the incidence has been decreasing by 1.8% per year. The current mortality rate for males is 24.8 per 100,000 and for females is 17.4 per 100,000. This represents a decrease of 1.8% per year since 1985.

The risk of developing CRC for the average-risk individual begins to accelerate sharply at age 50 years. The risk peaks in the seventh and eighth decades. More than 90% of all CRC occurs after this age. About 5% of CRC is believed to be hereditary, another 10% to 15% familial, and 80% sporadic.

The current 5-year relative survival for all stages of CRC is 64.1%. Diagnosing CRC at an early stage has a significant impact on survival, with relative 5-year survival rates of 90.4% for local disease, 67.9% for regional disease, and 9.7% for distant disease. Only 39% of CRC is diagnosed at a local stage. Long-term survival rates have improved significantly over the last 3 decades, with an overall 5-year survival rate of 50% in 1974 to 1976 and 64% from 1995 to 2001.

African Americans experience a higher incidence of CRC compared to white Americans (72.5 versus 61.7 in males, 56.0 versus 45.3 in females) and a higher mortality (34.0 versus 24.3 in males, 24.1 versus 16.8 in females). Similarly, survival is lower for African Americans, and the difference has been increasing, from 5% lower in 1974 to 1976 to 10% lower in 1995 to 2001.

Etiology

A multifactorial process for the development of CRC is now well recognized. Both genetics and environmental influences play an important role. Of the hereditary forms of CRC, the two most prominent are familial adenomatous polyposis, which accounts for about 1% of CRC, and hereditary nonpolyposis CRC (Lynch syndrome), which accounts for about 3% to 5% of CRC. Both result in a much younger age of onset of CRC than in sporadic cases.

Patients with hereditary CRC carry a germ line genetic mutation. In a simplistic explanation, these patients are born with the first step in the multistep genetic process that occurs during the development of a mucosal polyp and its ultimate transition to a cancer. This "head start" may partially explain why patients with hereditary CRC develop cancer at an earlier age. Also, because germ line mutations affect all of the cells in the body, all tissues contain this "first step," which may partially explain the multiple cancer types often seen in these individuals. Patients with sporadic CRC harbor the necessary genetic changes for CRC only in the affected cells of the colon and must start the neoplastic process from normal cells at the molecular level.

Physicians and patients must understand the important role of family history in CRC. Patients being evaluated for newly diagnosed CRC or for CRC risk should carefully evaluate their family history not only for colon cancer but also for any of the related cancers in the known hereditary syndromes, which include, but are not limited to, endometrial, ovarian, stomach, pancreatic, and renal pelvis. Particular attention should be paid to first-degree relatives (parents, siblings, and offspring) and to age at diagnosis. A personal or family history of multiple cancers occurring before age 50 years should lead to an expanded pedigree and consideration of referral to a hereditary cancer specialist.

Numerous environmental factors have been evaluated for increased risk of CRC. Few prospective trials are available to answer these questions. However, some general statements reflect current best interpretations. Diets high in animal fat and in red and processed meats and low in fruits, fiber, and vegetables have been associated with increased risk. Calcium plays an important role in maintenance of cell membranes and signal transmission. Thus, diets low in calcium may increase risk of CRC. Obesity, lack of physical activity, smoking, and diabetes have all been associated with increased risk of CRC.

Several studies have suggested that aspirin and nonsteroidal anti-inflammatory drugs decrease the risk for CRC. The proposed mechanism of action is inhibition of cyclooxygenase (COX)-mediated prostaglandin synthesis, which could decrease polyp development. A recent study has suggested that the usual dose taken for cardiovascular effect (ASA) is not adequate to gain the desired effect on CRC. The COX-2 inhibitors have shown a 28% to 32% reduction in polyps in patients with familial adenomatous polyposis. Estrogen and progesterone hormone therapy and HMG-CoA reductase inhibitors (statin drugs) have shown contradictory epidemiologic evidence of beneficial effects on CRC. The bottom line: none of these drugs is currently recommended for prevention of CRC.

Clinical Manifestations

Symptoms associated with colon cancer are generally not specific and may include abdominal pain and bloating, change in bowel habit, rectal fullness, rectal bleeding, anemia, weakness, fatigue, anorexia, and weight loss. More often than not, these symptoms are caused by something other than CRC, for example, peptic ulcer disease, cholelithiasis, hemorrhoids, irritable bowel syndrome, inflammatory bowel disease, or even a dietary indiscretion. Generally, the greater the number symptoms, the more advanced the associated CRC. The best time to detect CRC is when no symptoms are present, which is why screening is so important. Screening can detect CRC at an early stage and provide an opportunity to remove premalignant polyps.

Rectal cancer may present with tenesmus and urgency. Both symptoms are generally associated with more advanced disease. Compared to cancers of the left colon, cancers of the right colon are less frequently associated with pain, obstruction, or change in bowel habit but are more frequently associated with anorexia, weight loss, occult bleeding, and anemia. Cancers of the left colon are more often associated with pain, overt bleeding, obstruction, and change in bowel habit. Left-sided lesions are less frequently associated with anorexia, weight loss, and anemia.

Diagnosis

Colorectal cancer is most frequently diagnosed by colonoscopy. On occasion, a barium enema demonstrates a CRC, but colonoscopy almost always will be used to confirm the diagnosis and perform a diagnostic biopsy. Similarly, if a new cancer is diagnosed by rigid proctoscopy or flexible sigmoidoscopy (FSIG), the rest of the colon must be cleared by colonoscopy because the incidence of proximal

---

 CURRENT DIAGNOSIS

Beginning at age 50 years, asymptomatic men and women of average risk* for colorectal cancer should begin screening with **one** of the following:
- Annual fecal occult blood test (FOBT) or fecal immunochemical test (FIT)
- Flexible sigmoidoscopy (FSIG) every 5 years
- Annual FOBT or FIT with FSIG every 5 years (preferred over either FOBT/FIT or FSIG alone)
- Double-contrast barium enema every 5 years
- Colonoscopy every 10 years

---

*Average-risk individuals are defined as those asymptomatic individuals age 50 years and older who have no additional risk factors for colorectal cancer.

 CURRENT THERAPY

Common chemotherapy regimens used in the management of colorectal cancer:

■ IFL	■ Irinotecan/bolus 5-FU/leucovorin
■ FOLFIRI	■ Irinotecan/infusional 5-FU/leucovorin
■ FOLFOX	■ Oxaliplatin/infusional 5-FU/leucovorin
■ CAPEOX or XELOX	■ Capecitabine/oxaliplatin
■ CAPIRI	■ Capecitabine/irinotecan

Abbreviation: 5-FU = 5-fluorouracil.

---

polyps is 30% and that of a second proximal cancer is about 2% to 3%.

Treatment

SCREENING

The most important step we can take in the treatment of CRC is to encourage screening. By identifying and removing premalignant polyps through the screening process, CRC can be prevented. By finding cancers at an early stage, curative treatment is more likely. Although technically not a treatment for CRC, screening is our best method for having the greatest impact on the disease. The components of CRC screening include fecal occult blood test (FOBT), FSIG, barium enema, and colonoscopy.

Basic Assumptions

Screening identifies individuals without signs or symptoms of disease who actually have the disease. In the case of CRC, screening identifies patients with CRC or adenomatous polyps who are without symptoms.

The concept of detecting colon and rectal cancer by testing for occult blood in the stool is based on the simple observation that cancers and polyps bleed more than normal mucosa. It is estimated that about two thirds of cancers bleed in the course of any given week. Bleeding increases as the size of a polyp or the stage of the cancer increases. Because bleeding is not continuous, blood may be distributed unevenly throughout the stool. Accordingly, it is known that the sensitivity of FOBT increases with the number of samples per stool and the number of stool samples. Therefore, the success of FOBT as a screening tool is dependent on a number of factors: samples are taken from several areas within a stool, several consecutive stools are tested (usually over 3 days), and the test is administered on an annual basis.

Most CRCs arise from preexisting adenomatous polyps. Adenomatous polyps are found in 25% to 60% of individuals by the time that they are 50 years old. It is estimated that only about 2.5 per 1000 polyps *per year* will progress to cancer. Indirect observations suggest that it takes an average of about 10 years for a polyp that is less than 1 cm in size to progress to an invasive malignancy.

This long "dwell time" is an important element in the concept of screening for CRC. Because the sensitivity of FOBT for neoplasia is relatively low, the more frequently the test is repeated, the greater the opportunity to obtain a positive result. A single test is not sufficiently accurate to be used as a screening method. FOBT is not a "hit or miss" proposition. If the process is performed appropriately, 30 stools from an individual patient will be tested over a 10-year period, which would significantly enhance the potential that even intermittent bleeding will be detected before a polyp degenerates into cancer.

Evidence for Effectiveness

Five prospective trials have conclusively shown the efficacy of FOBT in CRC screening. The first completed randomized trial was conducted in Minnesota on 46,551 patients and reported by Mandel in 1993. The 13-year cumulative mortality per 1000 patients was 5.88 for the group screened annually and 8.83 for the control group. Overall, 13-year mortality was reduced by 33% in the group screened.

A Danish study published in 1996 reported on a prospective trial of 61,993 asymptomatic patients randomized between screening every 2 years and no screening at all. Ten years after initiation of the study, an 18% reduction in CRC mortality was observed in the screened group.

An English study also published in 1996 reported on a prospective study of 150,251 asymptomatic patients randomized to undergo screening every 2 years or not at all. After a mean follow-up of 7.8 years, investigators found a 15% reduction in CRC mortality and a higher proportion of early Dukes' A cancers in the screened group.

These clinical trials used guaiac-based FOBT for detection of occult blood. Fecal immunochemical tests (FITs) are acceptable alternatives to the guaiac-based tests and contain polyclonal antihuman hemoglobin antibodies. They do not react with nonhuman hemoglobin, are specific to lower intestinal bleeding, and do not require dietary modification during testing. Currently available home test kits for use in the toilet bowl are not recommended as part of a screening program.

The other standard components of colorectal screening—FSIG, barium enema, and colonoscopy—have not been studied in well-designed prospective randomized studies. The best available evidence of their effectiveness comes from case control studies and is supportive of their use.

Colonoscopy offers several potential advantages as a screening tool. It is both diagnostic and potentially therapeutic. Ample evidence indicates that removing polyps reduces CRC incidence and that detecting CRC at an earlier stage lowers mortality. Colonoscopy will detect most polyps and most CRCs.

Cost-Effectiveness

Each of the strategies for screening as recommended by the American Cancer Society has been found to cost less than $20,000 per life-year saved, which is well within the acceptable range of cost-effectiveness established by U.S. health standards and is considerably less than the cost of screening for breast cancer. Returns on investment in terms of life-years saved are very high, ranging from 5000 to 7500 years per 100,000 persons screened.

Guidelines

The American Cancer Society recommends that, beginning at age 50 years, men and women of average risk begin screening with *one* of the following: (a) annual FOBT or FIT, (b) FSIG every 5 years, (c) annual FOBT or FIT with FSIG every 5 years [preferred over either (a) or (b) alone], (d) double-contrast barium enema every 5 years, or (e) colonoscopy every 10 years (see Current Diagnosis). People at moderate or high risk for CRC should speak with a physician about a different testing schedule (Table 1).

SURGERY

Recent advances in surgical technique include the acceptance of laparoscopic surgery as equal to open surgery in the treatment of colon cancer. The results of the Clinical Outcomes of Surgical Therapy (COST) study, a prospective randomized noninferiority trial published in the *New England Journal of Medicine* in 2004, showed rates of recurrent cancer and survival were similar after laparoscopically assisted colectomy and open colectomy. Rectal cancer has not yet been similarly studied, and laparoscopic resection is currently not recommended for rectal cancer.

Other surgical advances include the use of expandable metal stents for the management of obstructing CRC either for palliation, in the case of widespread metastatic disease, or as a bridge to surgery to allow for a single-stage resection and avoid the use of stomas. Transanal endoscopic microsurgery has expanded the role of transanal excision for selected rectal polyps and cancers that might otherwise require radical resection (Figures 1 and 2).

RADIATION

A clear dichotomy separates the treatment and follow-up of colon cancer from rectal cancer (Figures 1 and 2). This separation is most prominent in the surgical management of CRC and results largely from attempts to maintain gastrointestinal continuity without sacrificing curative intent. The use of newer surgical techniques by experienced specialists maximizes this potential to safely avoid stomas. Preoperative radiation (most commonly 4500–5040 cGy) combined with chemotherapy (neoadjuvant therapy) in the management of rectal cancer is an important part of this management. The role of radiation in colon cancer is much more limited; it is generally used only to treat localized unresectable disease in a palliative manner. Highly selected patients, especially those with localized pelvic recurrence, may benefit from the use of intraoperative radiation in specialized centers experienced with the technique.

CHEMOTHERAPY

Adjuvant therapy has become a standard of care for stage III (node positive) disease of the colon and stage II and III (full-thickness wall involvement or node-positive) disease of the rectum. In the case of rectal cancer, radiation therapy is often administered concomitantly with chemotherapy, as noted earlier. Although 5-fluorouracil (Fluorouracil) and leucovorin (folinic acid) remain the foundation of such therapy, many newer agents are finding a distinct role. These include capecitabine (Xeloda), irinotecan (Camptosar), oxaliplatin (Eloxatin), and the monoclonal antibodies

TABLE 1 American Cancer Society Guidelines on Screening and Surveillance for Early Detection of Colorectal Adenomas and Cancer: Women and Men at Increased or at High Risk

Risk Category	When to Begin	Recommendation	Comment
Increased (Moderate) Risk			
Individuals with a single, small (<1 cm) adenoma	3 to 6 yr after initial polypectomy	Colonoscopy*	If the result is normal, the individual can thereafter be screened as per average-risk guidelines.
Individuals with a large (≥1 cm) adenoma, multiple adenomas, or adenomas with high-grade dysplasia or villous elements	Within 3 yr of initial polypectomy	Colonoscopy*	If the result is normal, repeat examination in 3 yr; if normal then, the individual can thereafter be screened per average-risk guidelines.
Personal history of curative intent resection of CRC	Within 1 yr of cancer resection	Colonoscopy*	If result is normal, repeat examination in 3 yr; if normal then, repeat examination every 5 yr.
Either CRC or adenomatous polyps in any first-degree relative† before age 60 yr, or in two or more first-degree relatives at any age (if not a hereditary syndrome)	Age 40 yr or 10 yr before youngest case in the immediate family	Colonoscopy*	Every 5–10 yr. CRC in relatives more distant than first degree does not increase risk substantially above the average-risk group.
High Risk			
Family history of familial adenomatous polyposis (FAP)	Puberty	Early surveillance with endoscopy and counseling to consider genetic testing	If result of genetic test is positive, colectomy is indicated. These patients are best referred to a center with experience in the management of FAP.
Family history of hereditary nonpolyposis colon cancer (HNPCC)	Age 21 yr	Colonoscopy and counseling to consider genetic testing	If result of the genetic test is positive or if the patient has not undergone genetic testing, every 1–2 yr until age 40 yr, then annually. These patients are best referred to a center with experience in the management of HNPCC.
Inflammatory bowel disease Chronic ulcerative colitis Crohn's disease	Cancer risk begins to be significant 8 yr after onset of pancolitis or 12–15 yr after onset of left-sided colitis	Colonoscopy with biopsies for dysplasia	Every 1–2 yr. These patients are best referred to a center with experience in the surveillance and management of inflammatory bowel disease.

*If colonoscopy is unavailable, is not feasible, or is not desired by the patient, double-contrast barium enema (DCBE) alone or the combination of flexible sigmoidoscopy (FSIG) and DCBE is an acceptable alternative. Adding FSIG to DCBE may provide a more comprehensive diagnostic evaluation than DCBE alone in detecting significant lesions. A supplementary DCBE may be needed if a colonoscopic examination fails to reach the cecum, and a supplementary colonoscopy may be needed if a DCBE identifies a possible lesion or does not adequately visualize the entire colorectum.
†First-degree relative is a parent, sibling, or offspring.
Abbreviation: CRC = colorectal cancer.
From Smith RA, von Eschenbach AC, Wender R, et al: American Cancer Society guidelines for the early detection of cancer: Update of early detection guidelines for prostate, colorectal, and endometrial cancers [published erratum appears in CA Cancer J Clin 2001;51:150]. CA Cancer J Clin 2001;51:38-75.

cetuximab (Erbitux) and bevacizumab (Avastin). These drugs can be used alone or in combination. They tend to be more effective when combined into various regimens (see Current Therapy).

No single combination is best. The combination selected for any given patient is dependent upon a number of factors, including patient tolerance, side effects, and response. When used in the adjuvant setting, chemotherapy can decrease the risk of recurrence by 40% and improve survival by one third.

SURVEILLANCE

Follow-up of CRC should be tailored to the individual and his/her cancer. Approximately 30% to 50% of patients with CRC will experience a recurrence. Almost 80% of these will occur within the first 2 years and more than 95% within 5 years. Generally there is not a defensible role for the ***routine*** utilization of computed tomographic scans, blood chemistries, chest radiographs, and endoscopy on an annual basis.

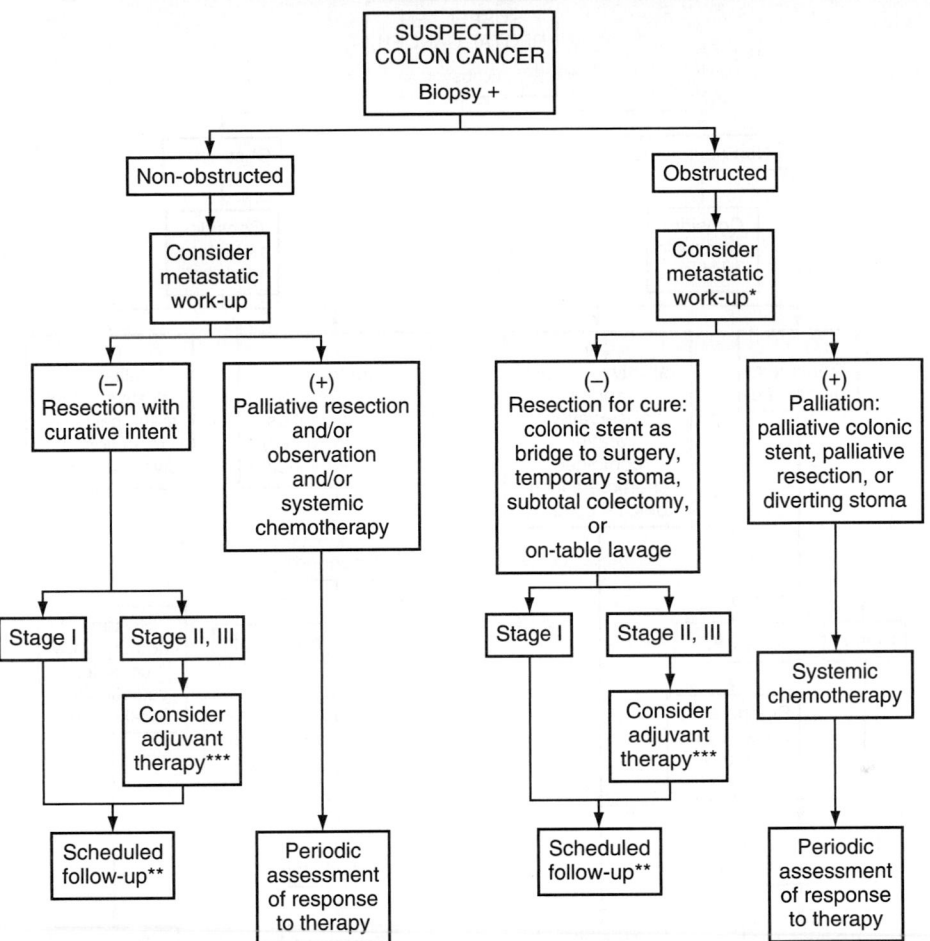

* Metastatic work-up: might include computed tomography (CT) scan of the abdomen, pelvis or chest; chest x-ray; carcinoembryonic antigen (CEA).

** Scheduled follow-up: might include periodic physical examination, CEA if it is a CEA producing tumor, CT scans for signs and symptoms suggesting recurrence including rising CEA, abnormal blood chemistries, etc. and endoscopy per American Cancer Society guidelines.

*** Adjuvant therapy is indicated in Stage III, node-positive disease; many authorities recommend therapy in Stage II disease in selected individuals.

FIGURE 1. Management of colon cancer. Resectable metastatic disease is not considered in this algorithm.

Endoscopic follow-up should adhere to the guidelines presented earlier (see Table 1). Endoscopy should focus on the detection of metachronous lesions, as most recurrences will not occur within the bowel lumen. The possible exception is the use of frequent proctoscopy in patients with a history of rectal cancer and a low anastomosis. Many centers recommend proctosigmoidoscopy every 3 months for the first 2 years in these patients and then every 6 months for another 3 years. Early detection of a local recurrence in this situation may provide an opportunity for a salvage resection. Most other tests should be based on the development of symptoms or a rising carcinoembryonic antigen (CEA) in patients who have demonstrated a CEA-producing tumor.

Summary

The best opportunity for reducing the incidence and mortality of CRC depends on the utilization of screening programs that have proven effective in prospective randomized trials. Screening for CRC provides a greater opportunity for saving lives and reducing mortality than we have with any other cancer except possibly those related to tobacco control issues. Unfortunately, only 42% of adults in the United States currently participate in such screening. The number one reason given by patients for this failure to participate is the failure of their physician or managed care organization to recommend it. This is a correctable situation that could save thousands of lives per year.

MANAGEMENT OF RECTAL CANCER
(Resectable metastatic disease not considered in this algorithm)

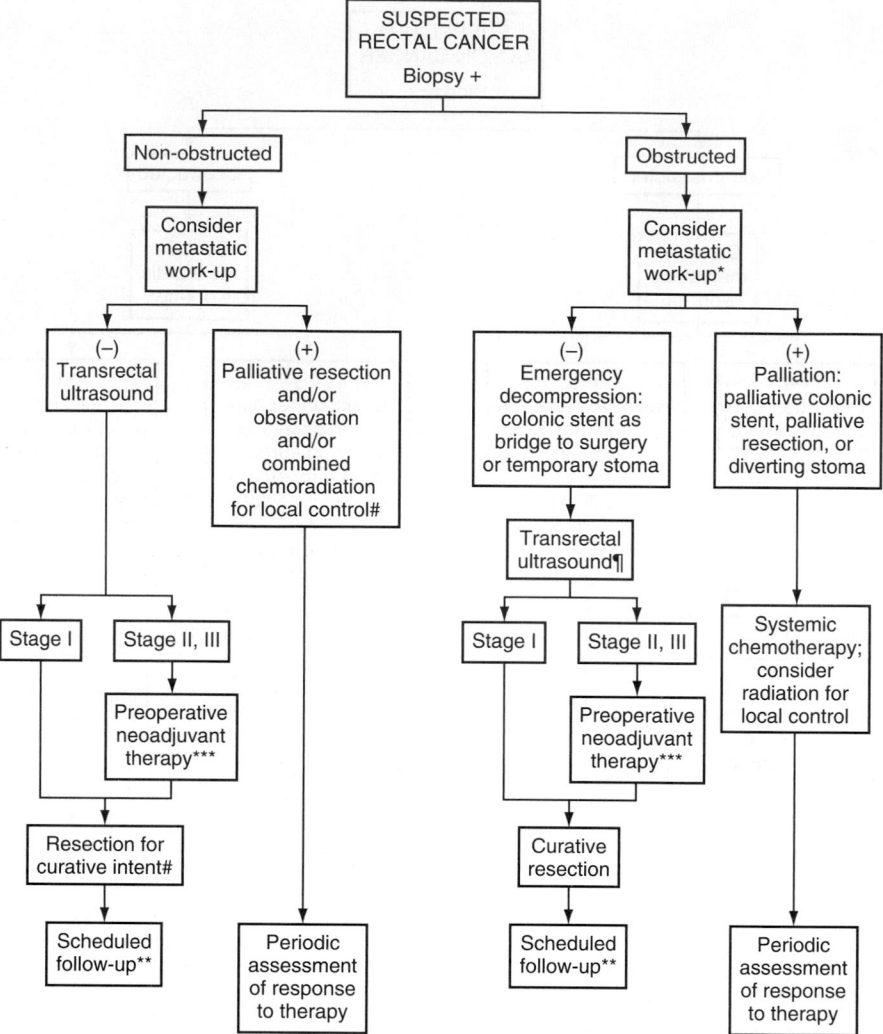

* Metastatic work-up: might include computed tomography (CT) scan of the abdomen, pelvis, chest; chest x-ray; carcinoembryonic antigen (CEA).

** Scheduled follow-up: might include periodic physical examination, CEA if it is a CEA producing tumor, CT scans for signs and symptoms suggesting recurrence including rising CEA, abnormal blood chemistries, etc. and endoscopy per American Cancer Society guidelines.

*** Adjuvant therapy is indicated in Stage II and III disease. Neoadjuvant therapy consists of combined radiation and chemotherapy.

¶ Transrectal ultrasound is performed if extent of local involvement is in doubt.

\# Transanal endoscopic microsurgery (TEM) may be utilized in selected patients with curative intent and in some patients for palliation.

FIGURE 2. Management of rectal cancer. Resectable metastatic disease is not considered in this algorithm.

REFERENCES

American Cancer Society: Cancer Facts and Figures 2006. Atlanta, GA, American Cancer Society, 2006.

Clinical Outcomes of Surgical Therapy Study Group: A comparison of laparoscopically assisted and open colectomy for colon cancer. N Engl J Med 2004;350:2050-2059.

Hardcastle JD, Chamberlain JO, Robinson MH, et al: Randomized controlled trial of faecal-occult-blood screening for colorectal cancer. Lancet 1996;348:1472-1477.

Kronborg O, Fenger C, Olsen J, et al: Randomized study of screening for colorectal cancer with faecal-occult-blood test. Lancet 1996; 348:1467-1471.

Mandel JS, Bond JH, Church TR, et al: Reducing mortality from colorectal cancer by screening for fecal occult blood: Minnesota Colon Cancer Control Study. N Engl J Med 1993;328:1365-1371.

Smith RA, von Eschenbach AC, Wender R, et al: American Cancer Society guidelines for the early detection of cancer: update of early detection guidelines for prostate, colorectal, and endometrial cancers [published erratum appears in CA Cancer J Clin 2001;51:150]. CA Cancer J Clin 2001;51:38-75.

Intestinal Parasites

Method of
Kenneth Shieh, MD, and Maria D. Mileno, MD

Parasites remain the major cause of death and disease worldwide. An understanding of intestinal parasites remains important in current medical practice. Increased global travel to regions with persistently poor sanitary conditions and the AIDS epidemic have contributed to the ongoing prevalence of parasitic infections. Protozoal infections caused by single-celled organisms, most notably giardiasis and amebiasis, often cause acute and chronic diarrhea and are especially important in travelers (Table 1). However, protozoal infections in the United States contracted through contaminated food and water, sexual contact, exposure to infants in daycare, and other means are well documented. Helminthic infections (i.e., worms) with a wide range of symptoms, depending on organ involvement, are suspected in the setting of peripheral eosinophilia and diagnosed more often in individuals residing in endemic regions.

Evaluating patients with suspected parasitic infection requires a thorough history. This includes a detailed travel history (destinations including brief airport layovers, rural vs. urban travel), dietary history (water exposure, street vendors, adventurous eaters), exposure history (blood products, fresh water, soil), sexual history, and general medical history, especially immune status. Regardless of geographic considerations, persons with AIDS are predisposed to debilitating infections with *Cryptosporidium parvum* and *Microsporidia*. Children adopted internationally are another at-risk population, and even if asymptomatic most should be screened for protozoa and for certain helminths such as *Strongyloides stercoralis* and schistosomiasis in the presence of unexplained eosinophilia. Physical findings in intestinal parasitic infections depend on the acuity and severity of the illness. Assessment should focus on general appearance and signs of severe infection, such as fever, abdominal tenderness or rebound, evidence of dehydration, and altered mental status, any of which should prompt immediate medical attention and possible hospitalization. As with any intestinal illness, consultation with a gastroenterologist should be considered for inflammatory diarrhea (characterized by fever, abdominal pain, and/or hematochezia), chronic diarrhea, or any other severe or chronic gastrointestinal complaint because endoscopic evaluation may be warranted.

This chapter focuses on the presentation, diagnosis, and therapy of the most common organisms that infect humans.

Protozoan Infections

Table 2 summarizes the drugs for the treatment of protozoal infections.

AMEBIASIS AND EXTRAINTESTINAL *ENTAMOEBA HISTOLYTICA* INFECTION

Entamoeba species infect an estimated 10% of the world's population. Amebiasis is the third most common cause of death from parasitic disease, surpassed only by schistosomiasis and malaria. Globally it affects approximately 50 million persons each year, resulting in nearly 50,000 deaths. The highest prevalence occurs in tropical regions in the developing world, particularly Mexico, India, tropical Asia and Africa, and regions of Central and South America. In developed countries, infections occur primarily among travelers to endemic regions, recent immigrants from endemic regions, homosexual men, and institutionalized

TABLE 1 Intestinal Protozoan Infections in Travelers

Infection	Parasite	Disease	Comments
Amebiasis	*Entamoeba histolytica*	Amebic dysentery, liver abscess	
Balantidiasis	*Balantidium coli*	Diarrhea, dysentery, liver abscess	Infection may be asymptomatic
Blastocystosis	*Blastocystis hominis*	Uncertain pathogenicity, diarrhea	Infections are usually asymptomatic
Giardiasis	*Giardia intestinalis*	Acute or chronic nondysenteric enteritis	
Cyclosporiasis	*Cyclospora cayetanensis*	Acute self-limited enteritis	
Dientamoebiasis	*Dientamoeba fragilis*	Diarrhea, abdominal cramps, flatulence	Most infections are asymptomatic
Cryptosporidiosis	*Cryptosporidium parvum*	Acute self-limited enteritis in the immunocompetent	Chronic enteritis and extraintestinal manifestations in the immunocompromised
Isosporiasis	*Isospora belli*	Acute or protracted nondysenteric	Chronic enteritis and malabsorption enteritis in immunocompromised patients
Microsporidiosis	*Enterocytozoon bieneusi* and other species	Disease rare in the immunocompetent	Chronic enteritis and extraintestinal manifestations in the immunocompromised
Sarcocystosis	*Sarcocystis hominis* and other species	Acute self-limited enteritis	Chronic enteritis and extraintestinal manifestations in the immunocompromised

CURRENT DIAGNOSIS

- Intestinal parasite infections should be considered in the evaluation of patients with abdominal complaints, especially diarrheal illness in the setting of travel.
- History of travel and immigration, food and water intake, exposures, sexual history, and risk factors such as HIV infection are important clues to guide the evaluation of any patient with intestinal disease.
- Physical examination should focus on features of severe illness such as fever, abdominal tenderness and rebound, dehydration, and altered mental status.
- Peripheral blood eosinophilia is an important feature of most helminthic and some protozoal infections.
- Examination of at least three stool samples for ova and parasites is an appropriate screen for most parasitic infections, and increased sampling improves yield. More sensitive and specific diagnostic tools, such as stool antigen tests and serologies, are becoming available.
- Awareness of extraintestinal manifestations of parasitic infections can assist with early diagnosis and successful management.
- Prompt referral to a gastroenterologist for possible endoscopic evaluation should be considered, especially for inflammatory diarrhea, chronic diarrhea, or any other severe or chronic gastrointestinal complaint.

individuals. Gastrointestinal infection is uncommon in travelers who have spent less than 1 month in endemic areas and is not a common cause of traveler's diarrhea. Incidence of amebiasis has increased in the southwestern United States as result of emigration from Mexico. Transmission is usually by food-borne exposure, particularly when food handlers are shedding cysts or if food is cultivated in feces-contaminated soil, fertilizer, or water. Less common routes include contaminated water, oral and anal sexual practices, and infrequently rectal inoculation through colonic irrigation devices.

After infection, approximately 90% of individuals remain asymptomatic, and the rest have clinical features ranging from dysentery to abscesses of the liver and other organs. Table 3 lists the most common signs and symptoms of amebic colitis. *E. histolytica* colonizes and penetrates colonic mucus overlying intestinal epithelium and has a remarkable ability to lyse human tissue, hence its name. In symptomatic cases, amebic colitis develops 2 to 6 weeks after the ingestion of infectious cysts and gradually develops as lower abdominal pain with mild diarrhea. This is followed by malaise, weight loss, and diffuse lower abdominal or back pain, which can mimic acute appendicitis with cecal involvement. Stool consists mainly of blood and mucus, with 10 to 12 episodes per day. Fulminant colitis is a rare complication in children and those receiving glucocorticoids. Such presentations include severe abdominal pain, an abdominal mass, high fever, profuse diarrhea, acute necrotizing colitis, toxic megacolon, or a chronic state that resembles inflammatory bowel disease. Ameboma is a localized chronic infection of the cecum or ascending colon that forms a mass of granulation tissue and presents as a right lower quadrant tender mass. Endoscopic biopsy establishes the correct diagnosis and excludes other entities such as tuberculosis, Crohn's disease, actinomycosis, or lymphoma.

The most common form of extraintestinal infection is amebic liver abscess, with 95% of such cases occurring within 5 months of infection. Liver abscess and resultant complications account for approximately 40% of deaths from amebiasis. The most frequent complication is pleuropulmonary involvement, which occurs in 20% to 30% of cases. These manifestations include sterile effusions, contiguous spread from the liver, and rupture into the pleural space. In rare cases, the skin, genitourinary tract, pericardium, spleen, and cerebrum may be involved.

Stool microscopy for detection of cysts or trophozoites is a poor test for diagnosis of intestinal amebiasis because it cannot differentiate between *E. histolytica* and the more

TABLE 2 Drugs for the Treatment of Major Protozoan Infections[1]

Infection	Drug	Adult Dosage	Pediatric Dosage
Amebiasis (*Entamoeba histolytica*) Asymptomatic			
Drug of choice	Iodoquinol (Yodoxin)	650 mg tid × 20 d	30-40 mg/kg/d (max 2 g) in 3 doses × 20 d
	or paromomycin (Humatin)	25–35 mg/kg/d in 3 doses × 7 d	25–35 mg/kg/d in 3 doses × 7 d
Alternative	Diloxanide furoate (Furamide)[2]	500 mg tid × 10 d	20 mg/kg/d in 3 doses × 10 d
Mild to moderate intestinal disease[3]			
Drug of choice[4]	Metronidazole (Flagyl)	500–750 mg tid × 7–10 d	35–50 mg/kg/d in 3 doses × 7–10 d
	or Tinidazole (Tindamax)[5]	2 g once daily × 3 d	50 mg/kg (max 2 g) in 1 dose × 3 d
Severe intestinal and extraintestinal disease[3]			
Drug of choice	Metronidazole	750 mg tid × 7–10 d	35–50 mg/kg/d in 3 doses × 7–10 d
	or Tinidazole[5]	2 g once daily × 5 d	50 mg/kg/d (max 2 g) × 5 d

TABLE 2 Drugs for the Treatment of Major Protozoan Infections[1]—cont'd

Infection	Drug	Adult Dosage	Pediatric Dosage
Balantidiasis (*Balantidium coli*)			
Drug of choice	Tetracycline[6,11]	500 mg qid × 10 d	40 mg/kg/d (max 2 g) in 4 doses × 10 d
Alternatives	Metronidazole[6]	750 mg tid × 5 d	35–50 mg/kg/d in 3 doses × 5 d
	Iodoquinol[6]	650 mg tid × 20 d	40 mg/kg/d in 3 doses × 20 d
Blastocystis hominis infection			
Drug of choice	Footnote 7		
Cryptosporidiosis (*Cryptosporidium parvum*)			
Non-HIV infected			
Drug of choice	Nitazoxanide (Alinia)[4]	500 mg bid × 3 d[6]	1–3 y: 100 mg bid × 3 d
			4–11 y: 200 mg bid × 3 d
HIV infected			
Drug of choice	Footnote 8		
Cyclosporiasis (*Cyclospora cayetanensis*)			
Drug of choice[9]	Trimethoprim-sulfamethoxazole (Bactrim)[6]	160 mg TMP, 800 mg SMX bid 7–10 d	5 mg/kg TMP, 25 mg/.kg SMX bid × 7–10 d
Dientamoeba fragilis infection[10]			
Drug of choice	Iodoquinol	650 mg tid × 20 d	30–40 mg/kg/d (max 2 g) in 3 doses × 20 d
	or Paramomycin[6]	25–35 mg/kg/d in 3 doses × 7 d	25–35 mg/kg/d in 3 doses × 7 d
	or Tetracycline[6,11]	500 mg qid × 10 d	40 mg/kg/d (max 2 g) in 4 doses × 10 d
	or Metronidazole	500–750 mg tid × 10 d	20–40 mg/kg/d in 3 doses × 10 d
Giardiasis (*Giardia lamblia*)			
Drug of choice	Metronidazole[6]	250 mg tid × 5 d	15 mg/kg/d in 3 doses × 5 d
	Nitazoxanide[4]	500 mg bid × 3 d	1–3 y: 100 mg q12h × 3 d
			4–11 y: 200 mg q12h 3 d
	Tinidazole[5]	2 g once	50 mg/kg once (max 2 g)
Alternatives[12]	Quinacrine[6]	100 mg tid × 5 d	2 mg/kg tid × 5 d (max 300 mg/d)
	Furazolidone (Furoxone)	100 mg qid × 7–10 d	6 mg/kg/d in 4 doses × 7–10 d
	Paromomycin[6,13]	25–35 mg/kg/d in 3 doses × 7 d	25–35 mg/kg/d in 3 doses × 7 d
Isosporiasis (*Isospora belli*)			
Drug of choice[14]	Trimethoprim-sulfamethoxazole[6]	160 mg TMP, 800 mg SMX bid 10 d	TMP 5 mg/kg, SMX 25 mg/kg bid × 10 d
Microsporidiosis			
Ocular (*Encephalitozoon hellem, Encephalitozoon cuniculi, Vittaforma corneae* [*Nosema corneum*])			
Drug of choice	Albendazole (Albenza) plus fumagillin[2,15]	400 mg bid	
Intestinal (*Enterocytozoon bieneusi, Encephalitozoon* [*Septata*] *intestinalis*)			
E. bieneusi[16]			
Drug of choice	Fumagillin	60 mg/d PO × 14 d	
E. intestinalis			
Drug of choice	Albendazole[6]	400 mg bid × 21 d	
Disseminated (*E. hellem, E. cuniculi, E. intestinalis, Pleistophora* species, *Trachipleistophora* species, and *Brachiola vesicularum*)			
Drug of choice[17]	Albendazole[6]	400 mg bid	

[1]Adapted from Drugs for parasitic infections. Med Lett Drug Ther, August 2004, www.medletter.com
[2]The drug is not available commercially but as a service can be compounded by Panorama Compounding Pharmacy, 6744 Balboa Blvd., Van Nuys, CA 91406 (800-247-9767) or Medical Center Pharmacy, New Haven, CT (203-688-6816).

Intestinal Parasites

663

Continued

TABLE 2 Drugs for the Treatment of Major Protozoan Infections[1]—cont'd

[3]Treatment should be followed by a course of iodoquinol or paromomycin in the dosage used to treat asymptomatic amebiasis.

[4]Nitazoxanide is FDA approved as a pediatric oral suspension for treatment of *Cryptosporidium* in immunocompetent children <12 y and for G*iardia* (Medical Letter 2003;45:29). It may also be effective for mild to moderate amebiasis (E Diaz et al: Am J Trop Med Hyg 2003;68:384). Nitazoxanide is available in 500-mg tablets and an oral suspension; it should be taken with food.

[5]A nitroimidazole similar to metronidazole, tinidazole was recently approved by the FDA and appears to be as effective and better tolerated than metronidazole. It should be taken with food to minimize gastrointestinal adverse effects. For children and patients unable to take tablets, a pharmacist may crush the tablets and mix them with cherry syrup (Humco and others). The syrup suspension is good for 7 days at room temperature and must be shaken before use. Ornidazole, a similar drug, is also used outside the United States.

[6]An approved drug, but considered investigational for this condition by the U.S. Food and Drug Administration.

[7]Clinical significance of these organisms is controversial; metronidazole 750 mg tid × 10 d, iodoquinol 650 mg tid × 20 d, or trimethoprim-sulfamethoxazole, 1 double-strength tab bid × 7 d are effective (Stenzel DJ, Borenam PFL: Clin Microbiol Rev 1996;9:563; Ok UZ, et al: Am J Gastroenterol 1999;94:3245). Metronidazole resistance may be common (Haresh K, et al: Trop Med Int Health 1999;4:274). Nitazoxanide is effective in children (Diaz E, et al: Am J Trop Med Hyg 2003;68:384).

[8]Nitazoxanide is not consistently superior to placebo in HIV-infected patients (Amadi B, et al: Lancet 2002;360:1375). A small randomized, double-blind trial in symptomatic HIV-infected patients who were not receiving HAART found paromomycin similar to placebo (Hewitt RG, et al: Clin Infect Dis 2000;31:1084).

[9]HIV-infected patients may need higher dosage and long-term maintenance (Kansouzidou A, et al: J Travel Med 2004;11:61).

[10]Norberg A, et al: Clin Microbiol Infect 2003;9:65.

[11]Use of tetracyclines is contraindicated in pregnancy and in children <8 y.

[12]Albendazole, 400 mg daily × 5 d alone or in combination with metronidazole may also be effective (Hall A, Nahar Q: Trans R Soc Trop Med Hyg 1993;87:84; Dutta AK, et al: Indian J Pediatr 1994;61:689; Cacopardo B, et al: Clin Ter 1995;146:761). Combination treatment with standard doses of metronidazole and quinacrine given for 3 wk is effective for a small number of refractory infections (Nash TE, et al: Clin Infect Dis 2001;33:22). In one study, nitazoxanide was used successfully in high doses to treat a case of *Giardia* resistant to metronidazole and albendazole (Abboud P, et al: Clin Infect Dis 2001;32:1792).

[13]Not absorbed; may be useful for the treatment of giardiasis in pregnancy.

[14]In immunocompetent patients usually a self-limited illness. Immunosuppressed patients may need higher doses, longer duration (TMP/SMX qid × 10 d, followed by bid × 3 wk) and long-term maintenance. In sulfonamide-sensitive patients, pyrimethamine, 50–75 mg daily in divided doses (plus leucovorin 10–25 mg/d) is effective.

[15]Ocular lesions caused by *E. helleum* in HIV-infected patients have responded to fumagillin eyedrops prepared from *Fumidil-B* used to control a microsporidial disease of honeybees (Diesenhouse MC, Wilson LA, Corrent GF, et al: Treatment of microsporidial keratoconjunctivitis with topical fumagillin. Am J Ophthalmol 115:293, 1993) available from Leiter's Park Avenue Pharmacy, San Jose, CA (800-292-6773; www.leiterrx.com). For lesions caused by *V. corneae*, topical therapy is generally not effective, and keratoplasty may be required (Davis RM, Font RL, Keisler MS, et al: Corneal microsporidiosis. A case report including ultrastructural observations. Ophthalmology 97:953, 1990).

[16]Oral fumagillin (Sanofi Recherche, Gentilly, France) is effective in treating *E. bieneusi* (Molina J-M, et al: N Engl J Med 2002; 346:1963) but is associated with thrombocytopenia. Highly active antiretroviral therapy (HAART) may lead to microbiologic and clinical response in HIV-infected patients with microsporidial diarrhea (USPHS/IDSA Guidelines for the Treatment of Opportunistic Infections in Adults and Adolescents with HIV, 2004; in press). Octreotide (Sandostatin) has provided symptomatic relief in some patients with large-volume diarrhea.

[17]Molina JM, Oksenhendler E, Beauvais B, et al: Disseminated microsporidiosis due to *Septata intestinalis* in patients with AIDS: Clinical features and response to albendazole therapy. J Infect Dis 171:245, 1995. There is no established treatment for *Pleistophora*. For disseminated disease caused by *Trachipleistophora* or *Brachiola*, itraconazole, 400 mg PO qd plus albendazole may also be tried (Coyle CM, et al: N Engl J Med 2004;351:42).

Abbreviations: PO = orally.

---

prevalent and noninvasive species *Entamoeba dispar*. A preferred enzyme-linked immunoabsorbent assay (ELISA) test of *E. histolytica* antigen in stools is now commercially available that is more sensitive than microscopy and can distinguish between these species. Amebic liver abscess is diagnosed based on suggestive clinical history, epidemiology, and imaging and supported by the presence of serum antibodies detectable in 92% to 97% of patients on presentation, although antibodies cannot distinguish between acute infection and past exposure. Aspiration is reserved for circumstances of diagnostic uncertainty or failure to improve with therapy. All patients with *E. histolytica* infection, even asymptomatic carriers, require therapy to diminish the risk of further invasive disease, whereas *E. dispar* requires no treatment. *Entamoeba coli* and *Entamoeba hartmanni* are also nonpathogenic. Table 2 describes treatment options for intestinal and extraintestinal amebiasis. Metronidazole (Flagyl) is a commonly used choice with response rates of approximately 90% for both intestinal disease and ameboma. Tinidazole (Tindamax) was recently approved in the United States and has a better cure rate with fewer adverse effects compared to metronidazole. Luminal agents such as iodoquinol (Yodoxin), paromomycin (Humatin), and diloxanide furoate (Formamide) are indicated as sole therapy for asymptomatic disease and as an adjunct after completion of therapy for symptomatic disease to

CURRENT THERAPY

- Effective drugs for protozoal and helminthic infections are available for most organisms in appropriate clinical situations.
- Careful attention to supportive measures, namely hydration and nutrition, is a key to the management of intestinal parasite infections.
- General principles for prevention of parasitic disease include good personal hygiene, enteric precautions, limiting exposure to untreated water, and washing and cooking food thoroughly, especially when traveling.

TABLE 3 Signs and Symptoms of Amebic Colitis

Signs and Symptoms	Percentage
Heme (+) stools	100
Diarrhea	94–100
Dysentery	94–100
Abdominal pain	12–80
Weight loss	44
Fever >38°C (100°F)	10

Modified from Petri WA Jr: Recent advances in amebiasis. Crit Rev Clin Lab Sci 1996;33:1-37 eliminate luminal cysts. For individuals residing in or traveling to areas in which the risk of amebiasis is high, prevention should include the use of bottled water and avoidance of unpeeled fruits and vegetables. Preliminary studies in the development of vaccines hold promise for minimizing the incidence and severity of the disease.

Balantidium coli

Balantidium coli is a ciliated protozoan. Pigs are its primary reservoir. It is the largest human protozoan and known to parasitize the colon. It occurs as trophozoite and cyst forms in the colon. Humans ingest infective cysts from feces-contaminated food or water that migrate to the colon and terminal ileum. Organisms dwell in the lumen, and the trophozoite form subsists on bacteria. Trophozoites can also penetrate the mucosa, cause ulcers, and rarely invade the peritoneal cavity. Most infections in humans are asymptomatic. Susceptible patients with concomitant intestinal infection, co-morbid illness, or immunosuppression are more likely to develop symptomatic disease. It has a worldwide prevalence of 1% and is reported most commonly in Latin America, Southeast Asia, and Papua New Guinea. Risk increases when persons work with pigs, handle fertilizer contaminated by excrement of infected animals, or live in areas where the water supply may be contaminated by excrement of infected animals. Patients may develop diarrhea, nausea, vomiting, abdominal pain, anorexia, weight loss, headache, mild colitis, and occasionally marked fluid loss resembling amebic dysentery.

Diagnosis can be made by wet smears of stool specimens or scrapings obtained from the periphery or invading edge of ulcers during endoscopic examination. Unstained, the trophozoite is large (50 to 100 μm long and 40 to 70 μm wide) with a short ciliary covering. It has a distinctive spiraling motility that can be seen under low power. *B. coli* does not stain well. However, on permanently stained specimens, organisms may show two characteristic nuclei: a macronucleus that is kidney shaped and a micronucleus that is spherical. Cysts may be spherical or ellipsoid, are 50 to 70 μm long and can show the nuclei, which if seen are diagnostic. Therapy with antibiotics is indicated for both asymptomatic and symptomatic disease to prevent complications such as intestinal perforation and extraintestinal spread to the liver and mesenteric lymph nodes. Tetracycline is the antibiotic of choice; metronidazole, an excellent alternative. Prevention by obtaining a clean water supply and avoiding contact with pigs or fertilizer contaminated with pig excrement is of prime importance.

Blastocystis hominis

Blastocystis hominis is a common intestinal protozoan of worldwide distribution that may cause mild, self-limited diarrhea in persons with a high burden of organisms. Four morphologic stages are vacuolar, granular, ameboid, and cystic. *B. hominis* appears to inhabit the colon but has no life cycle in humans. The transmission mode is likely fecal–oral and possibly from contaminated water or animal contact.

There is controversy whether it is truly pathogenic or simply commensal or opportunistic. Despite prevalence rates as high as 54% in Papua New Guinea, 33% in Nepal, and 23% in parts of the United States, the morbidity rate is unknown and nearly no mortality is reported with this parasitosis. Previously, many experts considered it pathogenic only with greater than five organisms per high power field (400×) and absent other infectious organisms. However, recent evidence suggests that the number of organisms correlates poorly with symptoms. Ongoing studies into the genetic diversity of blastocystis may identify disease-causing strains and thereby clarify the uncertainty surrounding its pathogenicity. Some studies have demonstrated higher rates of *B. hominis* in patients with irritable bowel syndrome, although a causal relationship is not confirmed. There is a correlation of isolation of this parasite with diarrhea in renal transplant and AIDS patients, although AIDS patients with *B. hominis* generally have spontaneous resolution of symptoms or identification of other etiologies. The most common symptoms include abdominal discomfort, diarrhea, flatulence, and occasional fever and bloating. Signs of dehydration are less common than with other intestinal protozoans.

Diagnosis is made by examination of stool by wet mount after concentration methods. Intact organisms 5 to 30 μm in size can be seen using trichrome or iron hematoxylin permanently stained smears. Metronidazole or alternatively iodoquinol or trimethoprim-sulfamethoxazole (Bactrim)[1] can reduce disease burden in symptomatic patients. Asymptomatic patients should not be treated. Adequate sanitation, hand washing, and enteric precautions can interrupt person-to-person spread.

Giardiasis

Distributed worldwide, *Giardia lamblia* (also known as *Giardia duodenalis* or *Giardia intestinalis*) is one of the most common parasitic infections in humans. Water-borne outbreaks are particularly prevalent in the mountainous regions of the United States and Canada, especially during late summer and early fall. In some developing countries, infection is nearly universal by 2 to 3 years of age. Transmission occurs by fecally contaminated water or foods and by direct fecal–oral contact. This latter mode may occur in daycare centers, custodial institutions, or with anal–oral sexual practices.

Infection results after the ingestion of as few as 10 to 25 cysts, with disease manifestations ranging from asymptomatic carriage to fulminant diarrhea, severe malabsorption, and life-threatening malnutrition. Hypochlorhydria, as from acid suppression therapy or prior gastric surgery, predisposes to infection. The majority, approximately 60%, of infections are asymptomatic, especially in children. Symptomatic cases occur after adequate cyst ingestion and an incubation period of approximately 1 to 2 weeks. Characteristically, patients complain of diarrhea with foul-smelling stools and gas, bloating, and abdominal cramps (Table 4). Acute episodes typically last 7 to 10 days, but chronic infections may emerge with or without this initial acute phase. Chronic infection may persist for many years, with symptoms occurring either continuously or episodically. Giardiasis, although a rare cause of acute traveler's diarrhea, is a frequent infectious cause of traveler's diarrhea lasting more than 2 weeks. Individuals with common variable immunodeficiency and X-linked agammaglobulinemia, who are at higher risk of a life-threatening process,

---

[1]Not FDA approved for this indication.

TABLE 4 Symptoms of Giardiasis

Symptoms	% (Range)
Diarrhea	89 (64–100)
Malaise	84 (72–97)
Flatulence	74 (35–97)
Foul-smelling, greasy stools	72 (57–79)
Abdominal cramps	70 (44–85)
Bloating	69 (42–97)
Nausea	68 (59–79)
Anorexia	64 (41–82)
Weight loss	64 (56–73)
Vomiting	27 (17–36)
Fever	13 (0–21)
Urticaria	9 (4–14)
Constipation	9 (0–17)

From Hill DR: Giardia lamblia. In Mandell GL, Bennett JE, Dolin R (eds): Mandell, Douglas, and Bennett's Principles and Practice of Infectious Diseases, 6th ed. New York, Churchill Livingstone, 2005, pp 3198-3205.

are typically more difficult to treat. *G. lamblia* can cause enteric illness in persons with AIDS, but the course of infection and the response to therapy does not appear to differ from those in persons without AIDS.

Diagnosis is made by detection of cysts or trophozoites in the stool. Because *Giardia* is excreted intermittently, submitting three samples is recommended and improves yield from 50% to 90%. Despite superior sensitivity and specificity using stool antigen testing, stool ova and parasite examination is preferred for most patients with diarrhea given the ability to reveal other pathogens. Duodenal aspiration or biopsy during endoscopy is generally reserved for cases of diagnostic uncertainty and may not be confirmatory. Metronidazole[1] is the standard of care in nonpregnant adults and pregnant women beyond the first trimester. Nitazoxanide (Alinia) and tinidazole were recently approved by the U.S. Food and Drug Administration and have comparable efficacy with fewer side effects. Children often tolerate furazolidone (Furoxone) better than metronidazole because the former is available in a more palatable elixir. Paromomycin[1] is an alternative in symptomatic pregnant women beyond the first trimester. In mild cases, in which the pregnant patient is able to maintain adequate hydration and nutrition, therapy is deferred until delivery or until progression beyond the first trimester. If treatment is required during the first trimester, metronidazole[1] or paromomycin[1] may be considered. When initial therapy fails, this is commonly the result of reemergence of the cyst form, which is unaffected by therapy. Patients should be retreated with the same agent for a longer course of 21 days, or alternatively another agent such as albendazole (Albenza)[1] or a newer agent can be administered (Table 2). Patients undergoing repeat therapy require further evaluation for a source of reinfection (family members, personal contacts, environmental sources) or possible underlying hypogammaglobulinemia. Prevention relies on good hygiene to prevent person-to-person transmission, boiling contaminated water to eliminate cysts, hand washing and care with diaper handling to prevent spread in daycare centers, and use of water treatment or water filtration devices for campers.

Cyclosporiasis

Cyclospora cayetanensis has a global distribution but is more common in developing tropical regions, especially during rainy spring and summer months. Cases reported in the United States, Central and South America, Australia, Southeast Asia, Africa, and Europe support widespread distribution. Person-to-person spread is probably limited because of a required maturation period, as seen with *Isospora belli*. Poorly defined transmission likely is water or food borne. Outbreaks occurred in 1996 and 1997 in at least 20 U.S. states and Ontario, Canada, after the ingestion of raspberries imported from Guatemala. In 1997, several outbreaks from mesclun greens and basil occurred in the United States and Canada, and an outbreak from Guatemalan snow peas occurred in Pennsylvania in 2004.

Individuals may remain asymptomatic after an incubation period of 7 days, but many develop the characteristic symptoms of watery diarrhea, abdominal cramps, nausea, anorexia, and bloating. Fatigue and malaise are also common symptoms, but fever is typically absent. The illness usually lasts 9 to 43 days, but patients may undergo periods of remission and relapse with prolonged diarrhea, anorexia, and weight loss in more severe instances. Prolonged courses are more typical in the immunocompromised host, especially individuals with AIDS presenting with protracted or fulminant diarrhea and weight loss.

The diagnosis is made by detection of acid-fast positive oocysts 8 to 10 μm in the stool. Polymerase chain reaction (PCR)-based diagnostic tests are being developed but are not yet commercially available. Cyclosporiasis responds well to trimethoprim-sulfamethoxazole (TMP-SMX[1]). Those with relapses, especially individuals with AIDS, may require retreatment, a longer course (i.e., 10 to 14 days), or longer-term maintenance therapy (TMP-SMX, 160/800 mg three times a week). Recent preliminary studies in HIV-infected patients suggest that ciprofloxacin (Cipro)[1], although less effective, may be an alternative in patients unable to take TMP-SMX.

Dientamoeba fragilis

Dientamoeba fragilis is one of the smallest parasites that can live in the human colon. It is a trichomonad nonflagellated parasite. Unlike most intestinal parasites, its life cycle has no cyst stage; thus infections are acquired via the trophozoite stage. Organisms move most actively in fresh feces but are extremely sensitive to an aerobic environment and quickly round up when left standing at room temperature. Transmission is through fecal–oral spread and possibly through ingestion of pinworm eggs (*Enterobius vermicularis*). U.S. prevalence rates are approximately 2% to 4%; however, much higher rates are associated with crowding and poor hygiene or travel to developing countries. Disease develops in 90% of colonized children compared to 15% to 25% of colonized adults. Abdominal pain and diarrhea occur during the first 2 weeks of illness with one to four episodic greenish brown stools. Stool consistency may vary and occasionally mucus is noted; however, the presence of blood in the stool is unusual. In chronic infection, abdominal pain is the predominant complaint. Other complaints include anorexia, nausea, vomiting, bloating, flatulence, weight loss, and constipation alternating with diarrhea. Nonintestinal complaints such as

[1]Not FDA approved for this indication.

[1]Not FDA approved for this indication.

headache, fever, malaise, muscle weakness, and pruritus are described.

The diagnosis is made by examination of a permanently stained smear of fresh feces preserved immediately for *D. fragilis* trophozoites. Obtaining three stool samples increases diagnostic yield by 30%. In unpreserved specimens, morphologic characteristics do not persist longer than 15 minutes. Trophozoites are 7 to 12 μm and contain one to four nuclei that have distinctive granules clumped in their center. Peripheral blood eosinophilia may be present in *D. fragilis* infection unlike most other protozoal infections, with the exception of *Isospora belli* infections. Eradication of parasites can be achieved with metronidazole for 10 days or tetracycline[1], iodoquinol, or paromomycin[1]. Spread of parasites can be limited by disinfection of surfaces used by children and diapering areas and adequate hand washing. Separation of symptomatic individuals within families is advised.

Cryptosporidiosis

Cryptosporidium parvum, widely distributed throughout developing countries, is the main species in the *Cryptosporidium* family that infects humans. In one study within the United States and Canada, oocysts were found in 87% of raw water samples. Since 1984 there have been 10 large community-based outbreaks in the United States in regions where water quality indicators either met or exceeded governmental standards. The largest such outbreak occurred in Milwaukee, Wisconsin, in 1993, affecting 403,000 people. Indirect fecal–oral transmission of highly infectious oocysts occurs in water-borne outbreaks and more directly by zoonotic and person-to-person spread.

Infection follows the ingestion of oocysts (median infectious dose of 132 oocysts in healthy volunteers) and typically results in a symptomatic course, but asymptomatic infections also occur. Diarrheal disease occurs in both immunocompetent and immunocompromised hosts. Immunocompromised patients typically have a more severe, chronic, and persistent course lasting several months, and AIDS patients may have a fulminant or even fatal course. Highly active antiretroviral therapy (HAART) in AIDS patients has resulted in a decline in the incidence of cryptosporidiosis. In the immunocompetent host, symptoms develop after an incubation period of approximately 2 to 14 days and last approximately 1 to 2 weeks. Characteristically, the diarrhea is watery, voluminous, occasionally explosive, and foul smelling. Diarrhea may result in fluid and electrolyte depletion with stools of up to 1 to 25 L per day. Symptoms such as abdominal pain, nausea, anorexia, low-grade fever, chills, sweats, myalgias, headache, fatigue, and/or weight loss occur in the majority of cases and may be severe. Rarely, extraintestinal infections are reported in the lungs, middle ear, pancreas, stomach, and especially the biliary tract. In immunocompromised hosts, the biliary tract is involved in 10% to 30% of cases, causing strictures and cholangitis.

The diagnosis is made by microscopic identification of oocysts in stool or involved tissue. Immunofluorescence microscopy and enzyme immunoassays greatly improve sensitivity and specificity. Submission of three stool specimens improves yield, which can be as low as 30% for examination of a single stool specimen. The clinical application of newer techniques in diagnosis such as stool PCR may dramatically enhance detection in the future. Organisms may also be detected in duodenal aspirates, bile secretions, and biopsy specimens from gastrointestinal tissue. Supportive care is the mainstay of therapy because the majority of cases are self-limited with resolution in 10 to 14 days in immunocompetent patients. Individuals with large-volume diarrhea and inadequate oral intake require fluid and electrolyte replacement along with antidiarrheal agents. Patients with biliary obstruction may require biliary drainage. A promising agent, nitazoxanide, has recently become available for the therapy of cryptosporidiosis in immunocompetent patients. It is the drug of choice for children 1 to 11 years of age and has also been studied in adults, although not yet approved. Chemotherapeutic agents are not proven effective in HIV-infected patients, but trials of nitazoxanide or paromomycin are reasonable. More important in HIV-infected patients is the initiation of HAART. Individuals with low CD4 counts may require maintenance therapy to prevent relapse. Prevention requires good hygiene and minimizing oral exposure to water from lakes, streams, and public swimming pools.

Isosporiasis

Isospora belli has a worldwide distribution but is more commonly found in tropical and subtropical regions with humans being the only known host. Unlike *Cryptosporidium* oocysts, excreted *Isospora* oocysts in the stool are not immediately infectious but must undergo further maturation over 24 to 48 hours. Person-to-person transmission is rare; most infections result from the ingestion of contaminated food and water with mature sporocysts from human waste.

Acute infections are typically self-limited in healthy individuals and may last several weeks or months. Symptoms begin abruptly with fever, abdominal pain, nonbloody watery diarrhea, and the unique feature of peripheral eosinophilia. Chronic cases, albeit rare, in immunocompetent hosts resemble celiac sprue with weight loss and malabsorption. Immunocompromised individuals, especially those with AIDS, often have persistent disease resembling cryptosporidiosis (i.e., chronic, profuse diarrhea).

Diagnosis of isosporiasis is made by detecting oocysts in the stool. Special stains are required because routine stool examination for ova and parasites usually cannot detect the organism. Isosporiasis responds well to chemotherapeutic agents, although relapses, especially among individuals with AIDS, may require maintenance therapy. Maintenance regimens include TMP-SMX,[1] 160/800 mg three times a week, sulfadoxine-pyrimethamine (Fansidar),[1] 500/25 mg once weekly, or pyrimethamine (Daraprim),[1] 25 mg every day if sulfonamide allergies exist.

Microsporidiosis

Microsporidiosis, recently reclassified from protozoa to fungi, causes infection in people and animals worldwide. The eight genera of *Microsporidia* implicated in human disease include *Brachiola*, *Encephalitozoon*, *Enterocytozoon*, *Microsporidia* (not otherwise specified), *Nosema*, *Pleistophora*,

---

[1]Not FDA approved for this indication.

[1]Not FDA approved for this indication.

Trachipleistophora, and *Vittaforma*. Infection occurs most commonly as an opportunistic infection in persons with AIDS, less commonly in those with other immunocompromising disorders such as post-transplant immunosuppression, and rarely among immunocompetent hosts. Although detailed risk factors for infection and routes of acquisition are not yet fully defined, transmission probably occurs by person-to-person contact, water-borne spread, or animal contacts.

Approximately 30% of AIDS patients with chronic diarrhea, particularly those with CD4 lymphocyte counts less than 100 cells per mm^3, are infected with *Microsporidia*, more commonly *Encephalitozoon intestinalis* (formerly *Septata intestinalis*) and *Enterocytozoon bieneusi*. The incidence of microsporidiosis has declined with the widespread use of HAART. Noninflammatory diarrhea, characterized by nonbloody, watery stools lacking leukocytes, has a gradual onset, frequently occurs in the morning, and is worsened by oral intake. Anorexia, weight loss, and malabsorption may result, especially when daily stools exceed 10. Fever, myositis, nephritis, prostatitis, cystitis, purulent urethritis, peritonitis, hepatitis, cholecystitis, cholangitis, pneumonitis, sinusitis, keratoconjunctivitis, bronchiolitis, and/or central nervous system involvement may follow dissemination of the organism in patients.

The diagnosis of microsporidiosis involves microscopic detection of the spores in stool or tissue specimens. Endoscopic biopsy has comparable sensitivity to stool examination. Because electron microscopy is required for speciation of the organisms, the laboratory should be alerted to the possible diagnosis. Many chemotherapeutic agents remain investigational in the treatment of microsporidiosis. Albendazole[1] is the treatment of choice for enteric infections with *E. intestinalis* but is only modestly effective against *E. bieneusi*. Fumagillin[2], not currently available in the United States for systemic use, has had some success for *E. bieneusi* infections but is limited by the risk of severe thrombocytopenia. Prevention of infection is unclear but involves good personal hygiene, consideration of boiled or bottled water, and avoidance of animals suspected of having infection, especially for immunosuppressed patients. Additional research on transmission routes and environmental sources as well as therapies and diagnostic tests using serologic and PCR-based methods are needed.

Sarcocystis hominis

Sarcocystis hominis is primarily a zoonotic infection, which can be a significant food risk for travelers to Southeast Asia. It is a protozoan parasite that requires two separate hosts for completion of its life cycle. Humans are usually accidental hosts and can have invasive disease in skeletal or cardiac muscle or enteritis after ingesting undercooked beef or pork. Humans who ingest sporocysts directly from food contaminated with animal feces can develop asymptomatic muscle cysts or myositis. Disease resulting from ingestion of tissue sarcocysts from undercooked meat leads to a gastrointestinal illness and allows for further spread of infection via feces.

S. hominis has a worldwide distribution, although most cases occur in Southeast Asia with a prevalence rate of approximately 20%. Although it can involve the heart, no deaths specifically related to myocardial involvement are

documented. The myositis form includes painful muscle swellings along with erythema, muscle tenderness, generalized muscle weakness, and fever. Bronchospasm can occur. Cardiac involvement is asymptomatic. The enteritis form of disease has been reported only in Asia and can occur within 1 day of ingesting contaminated beef or pork with occasional diaphoresis, chills, fever, vomiting, and diarrhea. Intestinal infections are usually self-limited, brief, and asymptomatic.

The workup for intestinal *S. hominis* includes identification of oocysts in freshly voided stool. They are acid fast and resemble *Isospora* cysts; however, these thin-walled oocysts usually rupture to reveal free sporocysts. Because sporocysts are not excreted in the stool for approximately 2 weeks after ingestion, serial stool examinations may be required. Complete blood count can reveal eosinophilia, and creatine kinase may be elevated in cases of myositis. Muscle biopsy can confirm the diagnosis of myositis and occasionally reveals sarcocysts, although these may be mistaken for *Toxoplasma gondii*. Toxoplasmosis of muscle can be distinguished using PCR techniques. There are currently no clinical data to guide treatment with specific antiparasitic agents. In humans the myositis form represents the terminal stage of the parasite. Corticosteroids are used to decrease inflammation associated with muscle involvement. Agents reported to be active against sarcocystis include sulfasalazine[1] and tinidazole.[1] Prevention through the avoidance of raw meat can help eliminate this parasite as well as other known pathogens present in beer or pork such as cestodes, *Trichinella*, and enterohemorrhagic *E. coli*.

Helminths

NEMATODES (ROUNDWORMS)

Ascariasis

Distributed globally, *Ascaris lumbricoides* infects approximately 25% of the world's population. Tropical and subtropical regions have the highest incidence, with more than 80% of populations infected in most countries of Asia, Africa, and South America. Approximately 4 million cases occur in the United States, especially in areas of high humidity in rural southeastern regions. The largest intestinal nematode to infect humans (reaching up to 40 cm in length), *Ascaris* is fecally to orally transmitted from contaminated soil because of poor sanitary facilities or the use of human excrement (i.e., night soil) as fertilizer and occasionally from inhalation of contaminated dust.

The majority of infected individuals maintain a low worm burden and remain asymptomatic. Symptomatic disease ranges from mild abdominal and/or pulmonary symptoms to fatal abdominal complications. Pulmonary symptoms range from a mild irritating nonproductive cough with pleurisy to more severe cases such as Löffler's syndrome including dyspnea, severe cough, and eosinophilia. Patients typically have fever greater than 38.5°C (101°F). Gastrointestinal manifestations arise with a heavy worm burden and result in abdominal discomfort, anorexia, nausea, diarrhea, and malabsorption with malnutrition in severe infections. A large mass of worms can cause intestinal obstruction, predominantly in children between 1 and 5 years of age. Migration of

---

[1]Not FDA approved for this indication.
[2]Not available in the United States.

---

[1]Not FDA approved for this indication.

worms into the biliary tree results in biliary colic, biliary strictures, cholecystitis, cholangitis, pancreatitis, intrahepatic abscesses with or without bacterial superinfection, or bile duct perforation with peritonitis.

The diagnosis of ascariasis is made by identification of characteristic eggs on stool microscopy. Unfortunately, eggs do not appear in the stool for at least 40 days after infection, hindering early diagnosis. Peripheral eosinophilia is suggestive. Imaging studies such as ultrasound and computed tomography may demonstrate collections of worms in the abdomen and biliary tree. Endoscopic retrograde cholangiopancreatography (ERCP) may establish a diagnosis of biliary ascariasis and allow for worm removal as well. Because pulmonary disease is self-limited, supportive care is the mainstay of therapy.

Effective eradication of gastrointestinal disease occurs with a single dose of drug as listed in Table 5. More complicated gastrointestinal processes such as severe intestinal, hepatobiliary, and pancreatic ascariasis require referral to a gastroenterologist. Prevention of ascariasis relies on good sanitation to prevent fecal contamination of soil, good hygiene, and drinking boiled water in high-risk communities.

Hookworm

The two organisms causing hookworm infection are *Ancylostoma duodenale* and *Necator americanus* ("American Murderer," or "New World hookworm"). The former is prevalent in southern Europe, North Africa, and northern Asia,

TABLE 5 Drugs for the Treatment of Nematode Infections[1]

Infection	Drug	Adult Dosage	Pediatric Dosage
Anisakiasis (*Anisakis*)			
Treatment of choice[3]	Surgical or endoscopic removal		
Ascariasis (*Ascaris lumbricoides*, roundworm)			
Drug of choice	Albendazole[4] (Albenza)	400 mg once	400 mg once
	or mebendazole (Vermox)	100 mg bid × 3 d[2] or 500 mg once	100 mg bid × 3 d or 500 mg once
	or ivermectin[4] (Stromectol)[7]	150–200 µg/kg once	150–200 µg/kg once
Capillariasis (*Capillaria philippinensis*)			
Drug of choice	Mebendazole[4]	200 mg bid × 20 d	200 mg bid × 20 d
Alternative	Albendazole[4]	400 mg qd × 10 d	400 mg qd × 10 d
Enterobiasis (*Enterobius vermicularis*, pinworm)			
Drug of choice[8]	Pyrantel pamoate	11 mg/kg once (max 1 g); repeat in 2 wk	11 mg/kg once (max 1 g); repeat in 2 wk
	or mebendazole	100 mg once; repeat in 2 wk	100 mg once; repeat in 2 wk
	or albendazole[4]	400 mg once; repeat in 2 wk	400 mg once; repeat in 2 wk
Hookworm (*Ancylostoma duodenale, Nector americanus*)			
Drug of choice	Albendazole[4]	400 mg once	400 mg once
	or mebendazole	100 mg bid × 3 d or 500 mg once	100 mg bid × 3 d or 500 mg once
	or pyrantel pamoate[4]	11 mg/kg (max 1 g) × 3 d	11 mg/kg (max 1 g) × 3 d
Strongyloidiasis (*Strongyloides stercoralis*)			
Drug of choice[5]	Ivermectin	200 µg/kg/d × 2 d	200 µg/kg/d × 2 d
Alternative	Albendazole[4]	400 mg bid × 7 d	400 mg bid × 7 d
	or thiabendazole (Mintezol)	50 mg/kg/d in 2 doses (max 3 g/d) × 2 d[6]	50 mg/kg/d in 2 doses (max 3 g/d) × 2 d[6]
Trichuriasis (*Trichuris trichiura*, whipworm)			
Drug of choice	Mebendazole	100 mg bid × 3 d or 500 mg once	100 mg bid × 3 d or 500 mg once
Alternative	Albendazole[4]	400 mg × 3 d	400 mg × 3 d
	Ivermectin[4]	200 µg/kg/d × 3 d	200 µg/kg/d × 3 d

[1]Adapted from Drugs for parasitic infections. Med Lett Drug Ther, August 2004, www.Medletter, com
[2]d = day.
[3]Ortega AR et al: Gastroenterol Hepatol 2003;26:341. Successful treatment of a patient with *Anisakiasis* with albendazole has been reported (Moore DA, et al, Lancet 2002;360:54).
[4]An approved drug but considered investigational for this condition by the U.S. Food and Drug Administration.
[5]In immunocompromised patients or in patients with disseminated disease, it may be necessary to prolong or repeat therapy or use other agents. Veterinary parenteral and enema formulations of ivermectin are used in severely ill patients unable to take oral medications (Chiodini PL, et al: Lancet 2000;355:43; Orem J, et al: Clin Infect Dis 2003;37:152; Tarr PE: Am J Trop Med Hyg 2003;68:453).
[6]This dose is likely to be toxic and may have to be decreased.
[7]In heavy infection, it may be necessary to extend therapy to 3 days.
[8]Because all family members are usually infected, treatment of the entire household is recommended.

and the latter is the predominant species in the Western Hemisphere and equatorial Africa. Endemic disease occurs in developing tropical and subtropical regions. Infection with either *A. duodenale* or *N. americanus* or co-infection with both species occurs in approximately a fourth of the world's population. Hookworm is transmitted when infectious filariform larvae from fecally contaminated soil come in contact with the skin. After penetration, the organism migrates to the lungs through the bloodstream and lymphatics, ascends the airways, and finally reaches the gastrointestinal tract, where the hookworm attaches to the intestinal mucosa, digests the tissue, and sucks blood from capillaries leading to loss of red blood cells and serum proteins. The oval eggs in the feces measure 40 by 60 μm, and the adults may reach 1 cm in length with a life span of 2 to 8 years.

The majority of infected individuals are asymptomatic. Symptoms occur based on repetitive insults, the worm burden, the duration of infection, and inadequate iron intake. Repeated percutaneous exposure to the larvae may cause pruritic papulovesicular dermatitis ("ground itch"), especially at the penetration site, as well as tracts because of subcutaneous migration (cutaneous larva migrans). This latter process occurs with the typical lateral epidermal migration of the dog and cat hookworm *Ancylostoma braziliense*, which does not establish intestinal infections in humans. In disease caused by human hookworms, *A. duodenale* or *N. americanus,* respiratory symptoms occur during the pulmonary phase of the worms' cycle and typically cause a mild transient pneumonitis associated with wheezing, dyspnea, and a nonproductive cough. The early intestinal phase may cause epigastric pain, diarrhea, and eosinophilia. After attachment and invasion of the organism, symptoms worsen. After the ingestion of large numbers of *A. duodenale*, symptoms of nausea, vomiting, cough, dyspnea, and eosinophilia may occur 1 to a few days after ingestion. The major concern after hookworm infection is iron deficiency anemia, especially among children and women of childbearing age. The degree of deficiency depends on the worm burden, type of hookworm (*A. duodenale* more than *N. americanus*), iron reserves of the host, and overall nutritional status of the host. Severe cases may also result in hypoproteinemia.

The diagnosis of hookworm infection is suggested by exposure history and eosinophilia and confirmed by stool examination for eggs. Eggs are not detectable until at least 2 months after initial exposure. All infections require therapy with anthelmintic drugs as listed in Table 5. Severe pulmonary symptoms may require corticosteroids. Mild cases of iron deficiency are managed by oral supplementation alone, but severe complications may require more aggressive nutritional support. Prevention is best achieved by improved sanitation in an attempt to interrupt the hookworm life cycle. Community- and school-based antihelminthic therapy in developing countries demonstrates short-term benefits, but high reinfection rates and drug resistance limit long-term effectiveness. Vaccine research holds promise for improved prevention and control.

Strongyloidiasis

Varied surveys estimate that anywhere from 3 million to 100 million people are infected worldwide by *Strongyloides stercoralis* ("threadworm"), which is distributed in hot, humid regions, particularly in Southeast Asia, Africa, and Brazil. Within the United States, *Strongyloides* is seen primarily in the rural Southeast and Appalachia, among institutionalized hosts, and among immigrants or military personnel who have resided in endemic regions. Transmission occurs with contact of fecally contaminated soil. Intestinal infection occurs after the infectious filariform larvae penetrate the skin or mucous membranes, migrate to the lungs through the venous or lymphatic systems, ascend the airways, and are swallowed to reach the intestine. The rhabditiform larvae detected in feces are typically 200 to 300 μm long, and the adult females, which remain in the small intestine, may reach 2 mm in length.

The majority of individuals with chronic disease are asymptomatic or have mild symptoms. *S. stercoralis* is unique in that it is able to replicate in the absence of a mammalian host or within the human host, and autoinfection occurs by the infective larvae penetrating the colonic wall or perianal skin, reinitiating the infectious life cycle Therefore, this organism has the ability to persist for decades without further exposure in infected individuals. Hyperinfection syndrome, usually limited to the gastrointestinal tract and pulmonary system, occurs in the setting of high-grade autoinfection with high parasite burden, often in certain immunosuppressed states and especially with chronic steroid use. Dissemination of the organism to other organs such as the central nervous system can be catastrophic. Signs and symptoms cover a wide range of patterns depending on the affected organ. These may include epigastric abdominal pain, bloating or postprandial fullness, heartburn, diarrhea alternating with constipation, bleeding (ranging from occasional occult blood to massive colonic and gastric hemorrhage), diffuse bronchopneumonia, intra-alveolar hemorrhage, gram-negative polymicrobial meningitis and sepsis related to gastrointestinal mucosal breakdown and bacterial carriage by the migrating larvae, cerebral abscess, urticarial rash, and dermatitis caused by subcutaneous larval migration (larva currens). Individuals with AIDS or congenital immunodeficiencies do not appear to be at increased risk for chronic or disseminated disease. Conversely, those with human T cell lymphotropic virus type I may be at increased risk for a higher rate of chronic carriage, an increased parasite burden, and a more severe process.

The diagnosis of strongyloidiasis is suspected in patients with unexplained eosinophilia, serpiginous skin lesions, or pulmonary and gastrointestinal symptoms. The diagnosis is confirmed by detection of rhabditiform larvae in stool specimens, although sensitivity is poor even after three stool examinations. Larvae do not appear in the stool for at least 3 weeks after initial dermal penetration. Serologies using ELISA assays are more sensitive than stool examinations but can be falsely negative in immunocompromised patients. Endoscopy, although not required for diagnosis, may also detect the organism in aspirates of duodenal fluid or biopsies of diseased mucosa. In disseminated disease, filariform larvae can be found in stool, sputum, bronchoalveolar lavage fluid, pleural fluid, peritoneal fluid, and surgical drainage fluid. Because of the catastrophic nature of disseminated disease, all individuals with proven strongyloidiasis require therapy, including those who are asymptomatic (see Table 5). Individuals on glucocorticoid therapy require tapering or discontinuation of this medication during therapy.

Trichuriasis

Trichuris trichiura ("whipworm") has a global distribution, with approximately 25% of the world's population infected. The highest prevalence occurs in tropical and subtropical regions. Individuals who live in crowded or very close conditions and who practice poor personal hygiene are at the greatest risk of infection. Children are at high risk because of their exposure risk and because partial protective immunity develops with age. Transmission occurs through the fecal–oral route, with warm, damp soil providing the best medium for transmission once fecally contaminated. The lemon-shaped eggs in the feces are typically 20 by 50 μm, and the adults may reach 3 to 5 cm in length with a life span of 1 to 3 years.

Although most infected individuals are asymptomatic, some may have mild tissue reactions and eosinophilia. More severe symptoms occur with a heavy worm burden (more than 200 adult worms). In such patients, stools may consist of mucus and frank blood with a characteristic acrid smell or may be watery and of a consistency resembling inflammatory bowel disease. Heavily infected patients may have frequent stools with nocturnal defecation. Abdominal pain, recurrent rectal prolapse, tenesmus, anorexia, iron deficiency anemia, eosinophilia, growth retardation, and clubbing of the fingers may also be present.

Diagnosis is made by stool examination for eggs, although eggs are not detectable until 3 months after initial infection. Adult worms may also be seen protruding from the bowel mucosa during endoscopic examination. The use of chemotherapeutic agents is recommended in infected nonpregnant adults (see Table 5). Prevention measures include limiting fecal exposure, appropriate hand washing, and washing of any food products grown in fecally contaminated soil. This process effectively interrupts the life cycle of these organisms and limits reinfection. Mass community therapy with albendazole is being instituted in many developing areas with variable success.

Enterobiasis

Humans are the only known host for *Enterobius vermicularis* ("pinworm" or "threadworm"). The organism is found as frequently in developed countries as in tropical regions. An estimated 40 million Americans, most commonly elementary school children, are infected. The morphologically similar *Enterobius gregorii*, a new species found to infect humans, is a significant cause of pinworm infection in Europe, Africa, and Asia. Settings of poor hygiene and overcrowding significantly increase transmission, which occurs among individuals without the requirement of a soil phase or specific arthropod vector. This person-to-person spread may occur by oral–anal sexual practices or direct skin contact, or from contaminated surfaces (i.e., bed sheets or clothing). The cycle may persist among hosts who practice poor hygiene because the remarkably gravid adult female (releasing up to 10,000 eggs during nocturnal migrations to the perianal region) enables hand-to-mouth reinfection. Microscopic demonstration of eggs and worms collected from the perianal region with cellophane tape establishes the diagnosis. Peripheral eosinophilia is uncommon because there is generally no tissue invasion. The oval-shaped eggs, with a characteristic flattening of one side, are typically 25 by 55 μm and have a double-contoured shell containing an embryo. The adults may reach 1 cm in length with a life span of 4 to 10 weeks in the female and 2 weeks in the male.

The majority of infected individuals are asymptomatic. Most commonly seen among those with symptomatic infection is nocturnal perianal pruritus (pruritus ani), which occasionally leads to eczematous perianal skin lesions and, more rarely, bacterial superinfection. A heavy worm burden may result in abdominal pain, nausea, vomiting, rectal colic, appendicitis, weight loss, and rarely eosinophilic enterocolitis and appendicitis. Pinworm migration and invasion of the female genital tract rarely causes vulvovaginitis and pelvic or peritoneal granulomas.

All individuals, including asymptomatic household members, with proven enterobiasis require therapy with chemotherapeutic agents (see Table 5) to eliminate reservoirs of potential reinfection. Improved hygiene and washing of all bedding and clothes may also interrupt the cycle of person-to-person spread.

Anisakiasis

Anisakiasis occurs more commonly in Japan, the Netherlands, and Chile because of daily consumption of raw fish. Cases in the United States are increasing because of the growing popularity of raw fish dishes. This organism has a complex life cycle involving intermediate (e.g., cephalopods, hake, sardines, tuna, cod, and mackerel) and final hosts (sea mammals such as whales, dolphins, and seals). The larvae of *Anisakis simplex* and *Anisakis physeteris* ("herring worm disease") and *Pseudoterranova decipiens* ("cod worm disease" or "sea worm disease") migrate into the musculature of a variety of fish. Infection occurs with the ingestion of the nematode larvae in raw saltwater fish, squid, and other macroinvertebrates.

Anisakid worms inhabit the stomach of their final hosts. During development, the organism buries its anterior portion into the gastrointestinal mucosa anywhere along the tract. Because humans are not definitive hosts, the parasite dies, resulting in abscess formation, inflammation, edema, and tissue eosinophilia. Occasionally, the larva enters the peritoneal cavity with the same results. Initially, individuals may describe an itching or scratchy sensation in the mouth or throat during or soon after the meal. Acutely, within hours after ingestion, patients experience severe upper abdominal and epigastric pain, nausea, vomiting (occasionally with recovery of the parasite), and symptoms mimicking an acute abdomen. Alternatively, symptoms may be delayed 1 to 2 weeks and consist of intermittent abdominal pain, diarrhea with blood and mucus followed by normal stools or constipation, nausea, and fever—a constellation of symptoms resembling Crohn's disease. Allergic reactions ranging from mild urticaria to anaphylactic shock can also occur. Extraintestinal infections are extremely rare.

The diagnosis is made by recovery of the organism if expelled or retrieved endoscopically, visualization of a threadlike defect with associated mucosal changes on barium imaging studies, or serologic testing, which is not yet widely available. Adequate chemotherapeutic agents are not available, although successful treatment with albendazole is reported. Removal of the worm surgically or endoscopically is the mainstay of therapy. Prevention can be achieved by thorough cooking or adequate freezing of fish prior to eating.

Capillariasis

Infections with *Capillaria philippinensis* occur primarily in the Philippines and Thailand, and rarely in Iran, Japan, Egypt, Indonesia, Korea, India, and Spain. Disease follows the ingestion of raw fish from fresh and brackish water infected with this organism.

Larvae released after the ingestion of the parasite subsequently mature to adults in the human intestine. Females not evacuated with the feces lay eggs that rapidly mature in the intestine. The resultant larvae enter the mucosa and develop into adults. This autoinfection explains the large number of worms found in infected hosts. Characteristically, capillariasis has an insidious onset with associated nonspecific abdominal pain and watery diarrhea because of intestinal inflammation and villous loss. Untreated hosts develop progressive autoinfection resulting in severe hypoproteinemia, malabsorption, dehydration, and, ultimately, death from cachexia, cardiac failure, or superinfection.

The diagnosis is made by detecting characteristic 45 by 20 μm eggs or larvae in fecal specimens. Table 5 lists the treatment options. Supportive measures with fluid and nutritional supplements are crucial.

Platyhelminths (Flatworms)

CESTODES (TAPEWORMS): DIPHYLLOBOTHRIASIS

Diphyllobothrium latum, found in lakes, rivers, and deltas of the Northern Hemisphere, Central Africa, China, Japan, Peru, and Chile, infects approximately 9 to 10 million people. In North America, *D. latum* is found in Canada, Alaska, Minnesota, Michigan, Florida, and California. Infection follows the ingestion of raw fish infected with the organism.

After establishing infection in the ileum and jejunum, the adult matures within 3 to 5 weeks and can survive for 10 years and reach lengths of 3 to 12 m, making it the longest known tapeworm infection in humans. Typically, infected individuals are asymptomatic. When complications arise, patients may manifest abdominal pain, bloating,

change in appetite, headache, sore gums or tongue, diarrhea, vomiting, weakness, weight loss, and sequelae of vitamin B_{12} deficiency by the tapeworm ("bothriocephalus anemia" or "tapeworm anemia"). Rarely, more severe conditions develop including acute abdominal pain, intestinal obstruction, cholangitis, and cholecystitis.

Peripheral eosinophilia is suggestive of the diagnosis, and detection in the stool of characteristic 45 by 20 μm eggs with a lidlike opening typically excreted in high numbers is confirmatory. Table 6 lists the available chemotherapeutic agents. Improved sanitation to prevent waterway contamination with the organism and adequate cooking are keys to preventing infection.

TREMATODES (FLUKES): SCHISTOSOMIASIS

Schistosoma species infect approximately 200 million people and (along with snail species that act as intermediate hosts) are distributed in tropical and subtropical regions. The three major species that infect humans include *Schistosoma haematobium*, located in Africa and the Middle East; *Schistosoma mansoni*, located in Africa, the Middle East, the Caribbean, and South America; and *Schistosoma japonicum*, located in China, Southeast Asia, and the Philippines. The other species include *Schistosoma mekongi*, located in the Mekong River area of Southeast Asia, and *Schistosoma intercalatum*, located in central and west Africa. Transmission occurs when cercarial larvae penetrate the skin of individuals who are wading or bathing in fresh water, even for brief periods.

Symptoms differ according to the stage of infection. The initial insult to the skin results in cercarial dermatitis ("swimmer's itch") within 1 day of exposure and lasting up to a week. Acute schistosomiasis ("Katayama" or "snail fever") typically occurs after heavy exposure to *S. japonicum* and *S. mansoni* infection with migration of the developing

---

TABLE 6 Drugs for the Treatment of Cestode and Trematode Infections*

Infection	Drug	Adult Dosage	Pediatric Dosage
Diphyllobothriasis (*Diphyllobothrium latum*)			
Drug of choice	Praziquantel (Biltricide)[†]	5–10 mg/kg once	5–10 mg/kg once
Alternative	Niclosamide (Yomesan)[‡]	2 g once	50 mg/kg once
Schistosomiasis (bilharziasis)			
S. haematobium			
Drug of choice	Praziquantel	40 mg/kg/d in 2 doses × 1 d	40 mg/kg/d in 2 doses × 1 d
S. japonicum			
Drug of choice	Praziquantel	60 mg/kg/d in 3 doses × 1 d	60 mg/kg/d in 3 doses × 1d
S. mansoni			
Drug of choice	Praziquantel	40 mg/kg/d in 2 doses × 1 d	40 mg/kg/d in 2 doses × 1 d
Alternative	Oxamniquine[§]	15 mg/kg once[¶]	20 mg/kg/d in 2 doses × 1 d[¶]
S. mekongi			
Drug of choice	Praziquantel	60 mg/kg/d in 3 doses × 1d	60 mg/kg/d in 3 doses × 1 d

*Adapted from Drugs for parasitic infections. Med Lett Drug Ther. August 2004, www.medletter.com
[†]An approved drug, but considered investigational for this condition by the U.S. Food and Drug Administration.
[‡]Not available in the United States.
[§]Oxamniquine is effective in some patients in whom praziquantel is less effective (Stelma FF, Sall S, Daff B, et al: Oxamniquine cures *Schistosoma mansoni* infection in a focus in which cure rates with praziquantel are unusually low. J Infect Dis 176:304, 1997). Oxamniquine is contraindicated in pregnancy.
[¶]In East Africa, the dose should be increased to 30 mg/kg, and in Egypt and South Africa, 30 mg/kg/d x 2d. Some experts recommend 40-60 mg/kg over 2-3 days in all of Africa. (Shekhar KC: *Schistosoma malalayensis*. The biologic, clinical, and pathologic features in man and experimental animals. Drugs 42:379, 1991.)

organism through the lung and hepatic circulation. *S. haematobium* rarely results in this syndrome. Symptoms develop 4 to 8 weeks after exposure, with resolution over several weeks. In severe cases, intense infection may result in death. Signs and symptoms include fever, chills, sweats, cough, headache, lymphadenopathy, hepatosplenomegaly, and eosinophilia. Acute symptoms are more common in nonimmune individuals such as travelers because of the intense immune response, whereas chronic infections involve a high burden of infection and are more common in individuals from endemic areas.

Most morbidity and mortality associated with schistosomiasis are attributed to chronic infection with resultant granuloma formation and local scarring because of repeated tissue injury and fibrosis from parasitic egg deposition in affected organs. *S. haematobium* affects the bladder, ureters, and kidneys, whereas the intestine and liver are affected by *S. mansoni, S. japonicum, S. mekongi,* and *S. intercalatum.* Depending on the organ involved, patients may have transverse myelitis, pulmonary hypertension, portal hypertension, renal failure, hydroureter and hydronephrosis, hematuria, dysuria, urinary frequency, recurrent urinary tract infections, and squamous cell bladder carcinoma.

Patients with intestinal schistosomiasis typically manifest fatigue, abdominal pain, and diarrhea. The diarrhea may progress to dysenteric bloody diarrhea and subsequent iron deficiency anemia because of granuloma and ulcer formation of the bowel wall. Granulomatous inflammation may also result in the formation of colonic pseudopolyps.

The diagnosis is usually made by demonstration of parasite eggs in stool or urine and occasionally in biopsies of affected tissues. Quantification methods can assess the intensity of the infection. Eggs are not detectable for 6 weeks after infection. Exposed individuals can also be evaluated for antigens 8 weeks after exposure by serologic testing with the Fast-ELISA assay through the Centers for Disease Control and Prevention (CDC). Chemotherapeutic agents are available as listed in Table 6. To prevent infection, persons entering endemic areas should avoid wading or bathing in fresh water. Mass chemotherapy programs in endemic areas are being implemented, and vaccines are being developed.

REFERENCES

Abramowicz M (ed): Drugs for parasitic infections. Med Lett 2004;August 1-11. Available at www.medicalletter.org

Barnett ED: Immunizations and infectious disease screening for internationally adopted children. Pediatr Clin North Am 2005;52:1287-1309.

Concha R, Harrington W Jr, Rogers AI: Intestinal strongyloidiasis: Recognition, management, and determinants of outcome. J Clin Gastroenterol 2005;39:203-211.

Dawson D: Foodborne protozoan parasites. Int J Food Microbiol 2005;103:207-227.

Didier ES: Microsporidiosis: An emerging and opportunistic infection in humans and animals. Acta Tropica 2005;94:61-76.

Fayer R: Sarcocystis spp. in human infections. Clin Microbiol Rev 2004;17:894-902.

Hlavsa MC, Watson JC, Beach MJ: Cryptosporidiosis surveillance—United States 1999–2002 and Giardiasis surveillance—United States 1998–2002. MMWR Morb Mortal Wkly Rep 2005;54/SS-1:16.

Hotez PJ, Brooker S, Bethony JM, et al: Hookworm Infection. N Engl J Med 2004;351(8):799-807.

Petri WA, Singh U: Diagnosis and management of amebiasis. Clin Infect Dis 1999;29:1117-1125.

Ramirez NE, Ward LA, Sreevatsan S: A review of the biology and epidemiology of cryptosporidiosis in humans and animals. Microbes Infect 2004;6:773-785.

Tan KSW: Blastocystis in humans and animals: New insights using modern methodologies. Vet Parasitol 2004;126:121-144.

Verdier RI, Fitzgerald DW, Johnson WD Jr, Pape JW: Trimethoprim-sulfamethoxazole compared with ciprofloxacin for treatment and prophylaxis of *Isospora belli* and *Cyclospora cayetanensis* infection in HIV-infected patients. A randomized, controlled trial. Ann Intern Med 2000;132:885.

Metabolic Disorders

Diabetes Mellitus in Adults

Method of
Shirwan A. Mirza, MD

Epidemiology

The prevalence of diabetes for all age groups worldwide was estimated to be 2.8% in 2000 and to increase to 4.4% in 2030. The total number of people with diabetes is projected to rise from 171 million in 2000 to 366 million in 2030. In the United States, the number of people with type 2 diabetes mellitus is growing to epidemic proportions. The number of people (20 years and older) in the United States who were diagnosed with diabetes in 1997 was estimated to be 10.2 million. The number of people who had undiagnosed diabetes was estimated to be 5.4 million. At diagnosis, 50% of patients have microvascular complications (diabetic neuropathy, nephropathy, or retinopathy). The risk of macrovascular complications is at least two times higher than that of the general population. Type 2 diabetes has become one of the most common chronic diseases in the United States. Recent data indicate that diabetes (diagnosed and undiagnosed combined) affects 8.7% of adults in the United States with rates reaching 18.8% at 60 years and older. This increase in prevalence portends that diabetes will continue to have a major impact on the health of the U.S. population. The risk of developing diabetes increases with age, obesity, and lack of physical activity. Type 2 diabetes is more common in individuals with a family history of the disease and in members of the minority groups in the United States. It is more common in women with a prior history of gestational diabetes and polycystic ovarian syndrome and in individuals with hypertension, dyslipidemia, impaired glucose tolerance, or impaired fasting glucose.

Diagnosis

One in five individuals in the United States has the metabolic syndrome as defined by the Adult Treatment Panel III (ATP III) criteria. Insulin resistance syndrome (IRS) is thought to be the underlying feature of the metabolic syndrome.

Prediabetes States

The American Diabetes Association (ADA) introduced the terminology of prediabetes to raise awareness of individuals who have an increased risk of developing type 2 diabetes and cardiovascular disease. Prediabetes comprises both impaired fasting glucose (IFG) and impaired glucose tolerance (IGT), and it is associated with the metabolic syndrome.

IMPAIRED FASTING GLUCOSE AND IMPAIRED GLUCOSE TOLERANCE

The Expert Committee on the Diagnosis and Classification of Diabetes Mellitus recognized an intermediate group of individuals whose glucose levels, although not meeting the criteria for diabetes, are nevertheless too high to be considered normal. This group is defined as having fasting plasma

---

 CURRENT DIAGNOSIS

ATP III Criteria for Diagnosing Metabolic Syndrome*

- Abdominal obesity:
  - Men: waist circumference >40 in
  - Women: waist circumference >35 in
- Fasting plasma glucose ≥110 mg/dL (recently changed to 100 mg/dL) and <126 mg/dL
- Blood pressure ≥130/80 mm Hg
- Triglycerides ≥150 mg/dL
- HDLC:
  - Men: <40 mg/dL
  - Women: <50 mg/dL
- The metabolic syndrome is present when three or more of these criteria are met.

Abbreviations: ATP III = Adult Treatment Panel III; HDLC = high-density lipoprotein cholesterol.

glucose (FPG) levels greater than or equal to 100 mg/dL but less than 126 mg/dL or values in the oral glucose tolerance test (OGTT) of greater than or equal to 140 mg/dL but less than 200 mg/dL. Thus,

- FPG levels less than 100 mg/dL are normal.
- FPG levels of 100 to 125 mg/dL indicate IFG.
- FPG levels greater than or equal to 126 mg/dL indicate provisional diagnosis of diabetes (must be confirmed on an alternate day).
- Symptoms of diabetes (polyuria, polydipsia, and unexplained weight loss) plus casual plasma glucose concentration of greater than or equal to 200 mg/dL indicate diabetes.

When the OGTT is used (FPG is less than 126 mg/dL and there is high suspicion for diabetes):

- FPG values remain the same as previously listed.
- Two-hour postload glucose (75 g oral glucose) less than 140 mg/dL indicates normal glucose tolerance.
- Two-hour postload glucose of 140 to 199 indicates IGT.
- Two-hour postload glucose greater than or equal to 200 mg/dL indicates provisional diagnosis of diabetes that must be confirmed on an alternate day by measurement of FPG or 2-hour postload glucose.

The use of glycosylated hemoglobin (A1C) for the diagnosis of diabetes is not recommended at this time because of lack of standardization and its insensitivity for early diagnosis. Glucometers that use capillary blood are imprecise and must not be used for diagnostic purposes.

Insulin-Resistance Syndrome

IRS is a powerful and independent predictor of developing type 2 diabetes (Box 1). Insulin-resistant individuals maintain normal or near-normal glucose levels by secreting large amounts of insulin. IRS is considered a state of enhanced vascular inflammation and endothelial dysfunction, accelerating atherosclerosis and hence causing

---

BOX 1   Other Abnormalities Associated With Insulin-Resistance Syndrome

- Hypertriglyceridemia
- Low HDLC
- Increase in small dense atherogenic LDLC particles
- Increase in inflammatory markers (e.g., C-reactive protein)
- Increase in uric acid level
- Increase in procoagulant factors (fibrinogen and plasminogen activator inhibitor-1)
- Increase in androgens (polycystic ovary syndrome)
- Sleep-disordered breathing*
- Increase in sympathetic nervous system activity*
- Increase in renal sodium retention*
- Loss of vasodilatory effects of insulin.*

---

*The last four factors comprise the underlying mechanism for increased incidence of hypertension in IRS and type 2 diabetes.
Abbreviations: HDLC = high-density lipoprotein cholesterol; IRS = insulin-resistance syndrome; LDLC = low-density lipoprotein cholesterol.

---

increased risk of cardiovascular disease. Insulin itself is not a risk factor for atherosclerosis. It is rather the elevated level of a dysfunctional insulin, an insulin unable to exert its physiologic vasodilatory and anti-inflammatory actions, which causes atherosclerosis. In insulin resistance, serum concentrations of triglycerides and free fatty acids, which are metabolic breakdown products of triglycerides, increase. These two substrates induce a state of lipotoxicity, reducing insulin production from the pancreatic β cells. Hypertriglyceridemia is also the underlying cause of nonalcoholic hepatic steatosis (fatty liver), which is now considered one of the diseases associated with IRS.

Pathophysiology

Type 2 diabetes is a multifactorial vascular disease with hyperglycemia and dyslipidemia as cardinal manifestations (Box 2). Diabetes was recently recognized as a coronary artery disease (CAD) equivalent. Type 2 diabetes is characterized by a dual defect in insulin secretion and insulin action. Insulin is essential to enhance glucose uptake at the level of muscles and adipose tissue and to reduce hepatic glucose production. Insulin resistance typically precedes the diabetes by many years, during which insulin secretion from β cells is able to increase to counter insulin resistance. In genetically predisposed individuals, however, overt diabetes occurs when β cells are overworked and exhausted and decreased insulin secretion can no longer overcome the individual's level of insulin resistance. The earliest change in insulin secretion occurs when β cells lose first-phase insulin secretion (first 5 to 6 minutes at a meal) designed to prevent postprandial hyperglycemia. At the onset of type 2 diabetes, on average 5 to 9 years have elapsed without diagnosis, chronic vascular complications are present, and 50% of β-cell mass is already lost. Most people with type 2 diabetes show a phenotype of abdominal obesity; the majority have acanthosis nigricans and skin tags commonly around the neck and axillae. Insulin exerts its anabolic action on muscles; individuals with type 2 diabetes thus have well-developed proximal muscle mass, especially the quadriceps. Individuals with diabetes who are slim and have wasted muscles, particularly the quadriceps, might have so-called type 1 diabetes, regardless of their age. Latent autoimmune diabetes of adults (LADA) is an insulin-deficient autoimmune state occurring in 10% of adult populations with diabetes, including those 60 years or older. The only difference from type 1 diabetes of childhood is that LADA has a slower onset and evolves over many years. Think of LADA in slim adults with diabetes who do not respond to oral agents. Measurement of serum C-peptide (low or low normal) and/or glutamic acid decarboxylase (GAD) antibodies (usually elevated but not in all patients) would be useful diagnostic tools.

Malnutrition-Related Diabetes

This type of diabetes, once thought to be endemic in some poor developing countries in the tropical belt, is now seen sporadically in the United States, particularly in malnourished elderly (over the age of 65) patients residing in nursing homes. These patients usually respond only to insulin therapy

BOX 2 Pertinent Laboratory Data

Blood Count

TZDs can cause or exacerbate anemia. Biguanides might cause vitamin B_{12} deficiency and red-cell macrocytosis. Anemia might raise suspicion about cancers or malnutrition. Pancreatic cancer can cause secondary diabetes; sometimes such diabetes precedes pancreatic cancer by almost a year.

Metabolic Panel

- Renal insufficiency contraindicates metformin use, and it increases risk of hypoglycemia.
- Hepatic dysfunction contraindicates TZDs, statins, and fibrates.
- Elevated transaminase might indicate liver disease (e.g., fatty liver in hypertriglyceridemic patients).
- Severe hyperkalemia contraindicates ACEI and ARB use.
- Hypercalcemia might indicate hyperparathyroidism or malignancies.
- Hyponatremia might be because of sulfonylurea-induced syndrome of inappropriate antidiuretic hormone secretion.
- A low albumin level might indicate chronic illnesses or malnutrition.
- Thyroid panel assesses:
  - Hyperthyroidism (exacerbates hyperglycemia).
  - Hypothyroidism (exacerbates hypoglycemia).
- Lipid profile assesses cardiovascular risk.
- Microalbuminuria assesses renal manifestations. Microalbuminuria is an independent risk factor for CAD through loss of vasculoprotective proteins.
- Normal iron panel and ferritin can rule out hemochromatosis.
- C-peptide and anti-GAD assess insulin deficiency and LADA.
- A1C is the single most important test to assess glycemic control.

Glycemic Control Matters

The UKPDS concluded that intensive therapy with oral agents or insulin decreased risk of microvascular complications compared to diet therapy. A 1% reduction in A1C was associated with the following:
- Microvascular endpoints: 35% reduction
- Myocardial infarction: 18% reduction
- All causes of mortality: 17% reduction

American College of Endocrinology Goals for Glycemic Control

- Target A1C is 6.5%.
- Preprandial plasma glucose target is <110 mg/dL.
- Two-hour postmeal plasma glucose target is <140 mg/dL.

Abbreviations: A1C = glycosylated hemoglobin; ACEI = angiotensin-converting enzyme inhibitor; ARB = angiotensin II receptor blocker; CAD = coronary artery disease; GAD = glutamic acid decarboxylase; LADA = late-onset autoimmune diabetes of adults; TZD = thiazolidinediones; UKPDS = United Kingdom Prospective Diabetes Study.

CURRENT THERAPY

- Any of the oral agents discussed in this chapter could be used as initial therapy.
- The current paradigm has recently shifted from a stepwise approach to a combination therapy at outset.
- Based on UKPDS, type 2 diabetes is associated with a progressive decline in β-cell function; most patients eventually need insulin when the endogenous insulin reserve is depleted.
- The natural history of type 2 diabetes is oral agent failure. The first step should be adding a bedtime long- or intermediate-acting insulin injection to the existing oral agents. Adding insulin in combination with metformin-TZD or metformin-SU is very effective in reducing A1C level.
- When insulin deficiency prevails, a full-scale insulin regimen with or without insulin sensitizers (metformin-TZDs) should be started.
- Tight lipid and blood pressure control is of utmost importance. We should also treat microalbuminuria vigorously.
- At every visit we should remind our patients of the importance of adherence to balanced nutrition and physical activity and remind them of foot care and annual dilated eye exams.

Abbreviations: A1C = glycosylated hemoglobin; SU = sulfonylurea; TZD = thiazolidinedione; UKPDS = United Kingdom Prospective Diabetes Study.

because their β cells have been destroyed by prolonged protein-calorie deficiency.

The benefit of tight blood pressure control is not less important than that of glycemic control. The goal is to achieve a blood pressure less than 130/80 mm Hg with a regimen that includes either an angiotensin-converting enzyme inhibitor (ACEI) or an angiotensin II receptor blocker (ARB).

Microalbuminuria is an independent risk factor for CAD. It should be treated rigorously with either an ACEI or an ARB. In patients with type 2 diabetes, hypertension, renal insufficiency, and macroalbuminuria, an ARB is the drug of first choice. ACEI appears to have a class effect.

Lipid Management

The American College of Physicians recommends a statin for primary and secondary prevention of cardiovascular disease for all patients with type 2 diabetes. The serum low-density lipoprotein cholesterol (LDLC) goal is less than 100 mg/dL. Updated in 2004, ADA guidelines also include a recommendation that a statin may be appropriate in adults older than 40 years with diabetes with a total cholesterol greater than or equal to 135 mg/dL, to achieve a 30% reduction in LDLC regardless of baseline level. Triglycerides should be kept less than 150 mg/dL, and high-density lipoprotein (HDL) should be greater than 40 mg/dL (more than 50 mg/dL in women). The ADA recommends aspirin therapy (75 to 162 mg daily) for secondary prevention in the presence of macrovascular disease and for primary prevention in patients older than

40 years with a family history of CAD, hypertension, smoking, dyslipidemia, and albuminuria.

Medical Nutrition Therapy

Both caloric restriction and weight loss benefit glucose metabolism. Weight loss of approximately 5% of initial body weight can significantly decrease fasting glucose and augment insulin sensitivity. There is no such thing as a diabetes diet; therefore, the terms *ADA diet, no concentrated sweets, no sugar added,* and *low sugar* should no longer be used. The goal of medical nutrition therapy (MNT) is to achieve glucose, lipid, and blood pressure control. The total amount of carbohydrates is more important than the source or type. Expert consensus suggests a diet providing 60% to 70% of energy intake from both complex carbohydrates and monounsaturated fat. Sucrose and sucrose-containing foods should be eaten in the context of a healthy diet. There is not sufficient evidence of long-term benefit of low-glycemic index diets.

Low-Carbohydrate Diets

Negative energy balance produces weight loss regardless of macronutrient composition of the diet. Popular low-carbohydrate diets are in essence high-fat diets. Although safe in the short term, their long-term effects on metabolism and cardiovascular risk are not established. A recent study compared the high-fat Atkins diet with a conventional low-fat diet. The high-fat diet produced a greater weight loss after 6 months, but at 1 year, weight loss was not significantly different between the two groups. An alternative approach to ad libitum high-fat diet is an ad libitum high-carbohydrate diet consisting of high-fiber foods with low caloric density. An example is the EatRight program employed at the University of Alabama at Birmingham. This program emphasizes the ingestion of high quantities of high-bulk, low-energy density foods (primarily vegetables, fruits, high-fiber grains, and cereals) and moderation in high-energy density foods (meats, cheeses, sugars, and fats). Participants lose on average 6.3 to 8.2 kg by the end of the 12-week program. Although nutritional counseling is usually delegated to the nutritionist, it is important for the physician to have a broad overview of the goals and problems. The dietary prescription should begin by obtaining full knowledge of the patient's dietary habits and preferences for which the patient should keep a detailed dietary log. The less flexible the dietary regimen, the less likely the patient is to comply. Choosing between a detailed exchange system, rigid meal planning, and a simpler regimen focusing on carbohydrate counting is made individually. Using dietary workshops for small groups of patients, where real food is used in educational settings, enhances patients' understanding. Giving pamphlets and theoretical information is not very effective.

Exercise

Promoting physical activity must be a core component of diabetes management. The benefit of physical activity in improving the metabolic parameters is greatest when it is used early in its progression from insulin resistance to IGT to overt diabetes. The benefits of exercise are substantial and include the following:

- Improves glycemia, lipid profile, blood pressure, and quality of life
- Prevents cardiovascular disease
- Affords modest weight loss
- Increases muscle strength and flexibility

Before starting an exercise program, CAD, peripheral vascular disease, proliferative retinopathy, nephropathy, and neuropathy should be ruled out. A single bout of exercise increases insulin sensitivity for 2 days. Regular exercise results in lower average blood glucose and A1C without a significant effect on FPG. An exercise program should consist of moderately intense aerobic exercises for 30 minutes or longer at 60% to 70% maximum heart rate (subtract age from 220) three to four times per week. In the absence of hypertension or proliferative retinopathy, resistance exercise may also be well tolerated.

Pharmacologic Therapy

Pharmacologic treatments involve the following:

- Secretagogues to enhance insulin secretion (sulfonylureas and meglitinides)
- Drugs to enhance insulin sensitivity (thiazolidinedione [TZD] and biguanide)
- Drugs that delay carbohydrate absorption (e.g., glucosidase inhibitors [α-glucosidase inhibitors, or AGIs])
- Insulin

SULFONYLUREAS

Sulfonylureas (SUs) act by stimulating insulin from pancreatic β cells (Table 1). They decrease fasting glucose by approximately 60 to 70 mg/dL and A1C by approximately 1.5% to 2%. Only 20% to 30% of newly diagnosed type 2 diabetes can be controlled on SU alone, and 75% of patients need a second agent to achieve their A1C goal. Primary failures occur in 10% to 20% of individuals. Most of these patients have insulin deficiency and may have slowly evolving type 1 diabetes. Secondary failure occurs after an initial response at a rate of 5% to 7% per year. SUs are classified as either first or second generation. The latter are more commonly used because of their increased effectiveness and fewer side effects. With half to two thirds of the maximal dose (e.g., 10 mg glyburide or glipizide; 4 mg glimepiride), 80% to 90% of their effects are seen. When target A1C is not achieved with monotherapy, either metformin, TZD, AGI, or insulin can be added. Combination therapy may result in lower A1C and better preservation of endogenous insulin.

The typical starting dose is glyburide or glipizide (2.5 mg), or glimepiride (1 to 2 mg daily), taken 30 minutes before breakfast. The dose is to be titrated over 4 weeks to 5 to 10 mg daily (glyburide or glipizide) or 4 mg daily (glimepiride). Doses above this have little further effect. Hypoglycemia risk increases with increasing age, alcohol use, poor nutrition, and renal insufficiency. Glyburide has a 19.9 episode per person-years incidence of hypoglycemia, which could last for greater than 24 hours

TABLE 1 Characteristics of Sulfonylureas

Sulfonylurea	Dose Range (mg)	Peak Level (h)	Duration of Action (h)	Half-Life (h)	Metabolites	Excretion
Tolbutamide (Orinase)	500–3000	3–4	6–10	5–7	Inactive	Renal
Chlorpropamide (Diabinese)	100–500	2–4	36–48	24–48	Active	Renal
Tolazamide (Tolinase)	100–1000	3–4	16–24	7	Weakly active	Renal
Glipizide (Glucotrol)	2.5–40	1–3	12–14	2–4	Inactive	Renal (80%) Hepatic (20%)
Glyburide (Micronase)	1.25–20	4	12–24	10	Weakly active	Renal (50%) Hepatic (50%)
Glimepiride (Amaryl)	1–8	2–3	16–24	9	Inactive	Renal (60%) Hepatic (40%)

because this medication has active metabolites. A safer SU (such as glimepiride) should preferably be used in the elderly (over the age of 65) and in patients with renal insufficiency.

MEGLITINIDES

Meglitinides are short-acting insulin secretagogues, structurally different from SUs (Box 3 and Table 2). Both repaglinide and nateglinide restore the first phase of insulin secretion. Early insulin release inhibits hepatic glucose production, which attenuates postprandial hyperglycemia.

Repaglinide

Repaglinide has a clinical efficacy similar to SUs. It can be given as monotherapy or in combination with metformin or TZDs. Risk of hypoglycemia is less than 50% of that seen with SUs.

Nateglinide

Nateglinide is indicated as monotherapy in patients who were not chronically treated with SUs or in combination with metformin or TZDs. Hypoglycemia occurs in 4.4% of nateglinide monotherapy and 2.9% of nateglinide plus metformin combination therapy.

BIGUANIDES

Metformin (Glucophage) is the only biguanide available in the United States. It enhances insulin sensitivity by inhibiting hepatic glucose output, which impacts FPG. It enhances muscle glucose uptake to a lesser degree. Metformin reduces FPG by 60 to 70 mg/dL and A1C by approximately 1.5%. An FPG of less than 140 mg/dL is achieved in 25% of patients with type 2 diabetes. A combination

with sulfonylurea lowers glucose level more than either drug alone. It reverses secondary failure to sulfonylureas in more than 50% of patients. Metformin can also be combined with meglitinides, TZDs, or insulin. Other advantages include the following:

- Lower risk of hypoglycemia
- Lipid lowering effect
- Modest weight loss

Side effects include nausea, diarrhea, and abdominal discomfort but are usually transient. The maximum effective dose is usually 2000 mg daily. Doses up to 2500 mg are approved but with little additional advantage. Lactic acidosis is extremely rare, and the risk can be reduced by avoiding use when serum creatinine is greater than 1.4 mg/dL in women and 1.5 mg/dL in men and in hypoxic states such as congestive heart failure (CHF). The long-acting formulations have reduced gastrointestinal side effects. Metformin should not be used in patients older than 80 years, unless creatinine clearance is greater than or equal to 70 mL per minute. Withhold metformin before imaging with iodinated-contrast media. Creatinine should be measured before resuming metformin.

THIAZOLIDINEDIONES

TZDs are insulin-sensitizing drugs that are selective ligands of the nuclear transcription factor peroxisomal proliferator-activated receptor (PPAR-γ) (Table 3). PPAR is abundant in adipose tissue, cells, and endothelium. It regulates the expression of several genes involved in metabolism. TZDs lower fasting and postprandial glucose concentration as well as free fatty acids. TZDs induce a "fatty acid steal" in the adipose tissue. The resulting decreased systemic availability of fatty acids, as an alternative source of fuel, improves peripheral glucose uptake by skeletal muscles and thus ameliorates insulin resistance. That is, they force glucose use as a preferred fuel rather than free fatty acids. Considerable data have recently shown that TZDs have beneficial effects on the atherogenic process; the lipid profile, especially the high-density lipoprotein cholesterol (HDLC); hemostasis; endothelial function; microalbuminuria; and inflammatory markers. Long-term trials of the effect of TZDs on cardiovascular mortality are currently in progress. Rosiglitazone and

---

BOX 3 Meglitinides

- Can be used in mild renal and hepatic insufficiency
- Have low risk of severe hypoglycemia
- Are useful in patients with an erratic lifestyle
- Should be skipped if the meal is missed

TABLE 2 Meglitinide Therapy

Drug	Dose Range	Maximum Effective Dose	Duration of Action (h)	Clearance
Repaglinide (Prandin)	0.5–4 mg tid	4 mg tid	4–6	Liver
Nateglinide (Starlix)	60–120 mg tid	120 mg tid	2–4	Liver

pioglitazone are moderately effective in achieving glycemic control. At maximum doses, A1C is reduced on average 1% to 2%. TZDs can be used as monotherapy (equal in efficacy to SUs and biguanides) or added to other antidiabetic oral agents or insulin. Rosiglitazone and pioglitazone are safe and effective for long-term therapy of type 2 diabetes. Low- and medium-dose pioglitazone and rosiglitazone (4 mg) also are indicated for use in combination with insulin but might increase the incidence of edema. These agents are contraindicated in patients with New York Heart Association (NYHA) class III or IV cardiac status. Pioglitazone should be initiated at the lowest approved dose if it is prescribed for patients with type 2 diabetes and NYHA class II CHF with an ejection fraction less than 40%.

Full effects of TZDs may take weeks to be achieved. TZDs preserve β-cell function, and they do not cause hypoglycemia when used as monotherapy or with metformin. Liver enzymes should be monitored at the start of therapy and periodically thereafter. The initial dose should be low (2 mg rosiglitazone or 15 mg pioglitazone daily). Escalate the dose slowly (over weeks), observe for signs of CHF, add diuretics judiciously as needed, reassess their usefulness, and adjust insulin doses on a regular basis.

Incretin Mimetics

EXENATIDE

Exenatide (Byetta), derived from a compound found in the saliva of the Gila monster, is an incretin mimetic agent that enhances first- and second-phase insulin secretion and reduces glucagon secretion, thus suppressing hepatic glucose output. It also regulates gastric emptying, reduces food intake, and causes sustained weight loss. The drug is indicated as an adjunctive therapy to improve glycemic control in patients with type 2 diabetes mellitus who are taking metformin, a sulfonylurea, or both but who have not achieved adequate glycemic control.

TABLE 3 Thiazolidinedione Therapy

Drug	Daily Dose Range (mg)	Usage
Rosiglitazone (Avandia)	4–8 mg	Monotherapy combination with SUs, metformin, or insulin
Pioglitazone (Actos)	15–45 mg	Monotherapy or combination with SUs, metformin, or insulin

Abbreviation: SUs = sulfonylureas.

Clinical trials have shown that exenatide, given subcutaneously twice daily, significantly reduced A1C values when maximum doses of a sulfonylurea, metformin, or both were ineffective.

Treatment is typically started with a 5-μg dose, injected subcutaneously within 60 minutes before the morning and evening meals. After the first month, the dose is increased to 10 μg, injected twice a day subcutaneously. The main side effect is nausea, occasionally associated with vomiting and diarrhea. The symptoms usually resolve after a few weeks.

PRAMLINTIDE

Pramlintide (Symlin) is a synthetic amylin analogue approved by the U.S. Food and Drug Administration (FDA) for use with mealtime insulin in patients with type 1 diabetes and patients with type 2 diabetes who are using mealtime insulin only or in the combination of insulin and metformin and/or a sulfonylurea. It produces a modest reduction in A1C. The primary adverse effects of pramlintide therapy are nausea and hypoglycemia.

α-GLUCOSIDASE INHIBITORS

Both acarbose (Precose) and miglitol (Glyset), two AGI agents, inhibit the upper gastrointestinal enzymes α-glucosidases that convert carbohydrates into monosaccharides. Although they delay digestion of carbohydrates, by shifting their absorption to distal parts of the bowel, they do not cause malabsorption. They improve postprandial blood glucose concentration. Both agents have comparable effects and are effective in monotherapy, in combination with SUs, metformin, or insulin. They decrease fasting glucose by 25 to 30 mg/dL and the A1C by 0.7% to 1%. The postprandial glucose level is reduced by 50 to 60 mg/dL. They are most useful in patients with mild fasting hyperglycemia and predominant postprandial hyperglycemia. Such patients typically present with mild fasting hyperglycemia (110 to 140 mg/dL) but with a disproportionately high A1C (more than 8%). Side effects, which include abdominal discomfort and flatulence, tend to diminish with continued use. Hypoglycemia is typically not associated with monotherapy. Acarbose is linked with elevated transaminases. AGIs are not recommended when serum creatinine exceeds 2 mg/dL. They are contraindicated in inflammatory bowel disease and in bowel obstruction. Therapy should be initiated with the lowest effective dose and titrated slowly over 2 to 4 weeks.

Combination Therapy

The availability of different classes of oral agents opened the opportunity to achieve glycemic targets in many patients but at the same time added complexity to creating a therapeutic algorithm. Any of the oral agents discussed earlier could be used as initial therapy. No one agent is considered the best for all patients. Because type 2 diabetes is a progressive disease, even patients with initial good response to monotherapy eventually require a second agent with or without insulin. Substituting one agent for another is not a good strategy. However, combining oral agents from different classes is very beneficial. The current paradigm has recently shifted from a stepwise approach to combination therapy at the outset. Fixed combinations of metformin-SU and metformin-TZD are now available and very useful and cost effective. Addition of AGIs to a combined secretagogue sensitizer has a modest supplementary effect and is costly. A combination of metformin-TZD is also effective if the patient still has a good endogenous insulin reserve. Triple oral therapy (secretagogue-metformin-TZD) is not approved, although it may work in early stages of diabetes. However, when insulin secretion is deficient, such a combination becomes inferior to a regimen of adding insulin.

Insulin Therapy

Patients who remain hyperglycemic despite adequate oral antidiabetic agents or individuals with severe hyperglycemia (glucotoxicity) may require insulin therapy. Based on the United Kingdom Prospective Diabetes Study (UKPDS), type 2 diabetes is associated with a progressive decline in β-cell function; most patients eventually need insulin when endogenous insulin reserve is depleted. The natural history of type 2 diabetes is oral agent failure. The first step should be adding a bedtime long- or intermediate-acting insulin injection to the existing oral agents. Low doses of insulin at bedtime effectively suppress nocturnal hepatic glucose production, which improves FPG. Adding insulin to a combination of metformin-TZD or metformin-SU is effective in reducing A1C level. If bedtime insulin plus daytime oral agent(s) are not sufficient, stop the secretagogues and start a full insulin regimen. Unless the patient has type 1 diabetes, continue metformin and/or TZDs with the insulin therapy. Keeping the insulin sensitizer(s) would lower insulin demand by more than 20% to 25%. The patient's attitude toward insulin reflects that of the physician's. Once insulin need is determined, we should be enthusiastic and not apologetic about insulin therapy. We should dispel the myths associated with insulin use, especially the notion that insulin is atherogenic. Many patients have had a relative who had to go on dialysis or had a limb amputation at or around the time insulin was started. We should emphasize that insulin does not cause any of these; in fact, poor glycemic control and delay in insulin therapy (when clearly needed) could lead to those complications. Once we determine that a patient needs insulin, we should start with a simple regimen using basal insulin glargine (Lantus). Neutral protamine Hagedorn (NPH), insulin zinc suspension (lente), or insulin zinc extended suspension (ultralente) could also be used once daily at bedtime. In the Treat-to-Target study, the initial glargine dose of 10 U at bedtime was adjusted on a weekly basis. The author finds a weekly adjustment regimen (by 2- to 8-U increments) not very practical in a clinical setting. Research settings have the advantage of being closely controlled and monitored. Adding 8 U to a bedtime dose of glargine could cause hypoglycemia in some patients. We advise our patients to add 1 to 2 U of glargine every third night to the 10 U at bedtime until the prebreakfast glucose reading approaches 120 mg/dL. For readings less than 70 mg/dL, we subtract 2 U. The goal is to achieve a fasting glucose of approximately 120 mg/dL. Nocturnal hypoglycemia is less frequent with glargine than with NPH.

Intensive insulin therapy is not appropriate for patients with these conditions:

- Symptomatic CAD
- Cardiac arrhythmias
- Debilitating diseases such as visual impairment and renal failure
- Advanced age (over the age of 65)

In severe diabetes (FPG more than 220 mg/dL), a full-scale insulin regimen (basal + bolus) is usually indicated. Total daily insulin requirement is between 0.5 and 1.2 U/kg daily. Insulin analogues are superior to conventional insulin. Both insulin lispro (Humalog) and aspart (NovoLog) reduce postprandial hyperglycemia and cause lower incidence of hypoglycemia. Insulin glargine has virtually no peak in contrast to NPH, lente, and ultralente. In the basal plus bolus regimen, we usually discontinue the secretagogue and maintain the insulin sensitizer(s).

Calculate the total daily insulin at 0.5 to 1.2 U/kg. The total dose is divided by two; half of this is to be given at bedtime as insulin glargine, the other half as insulin lispro or aspart (40% at breakfast, 30% at lunch, and 30% at supper). The patient checks blood glucose (sporadically) 2 hours after each meal. If 2-hour blood glucose is greater than 140 mg/dL, we fine-tune insulin lispro or aspart doses in increments of 2 U until target glucose readings are achieved. For example, a woman 50 years of age, with an A1C of 9% on a combination of metformin-TZD plus glyburide 10 mg twice daily, has a fasting glucose of more than 220 mg/dL. Her weight is 70 kg. Glyburide 10 mg daily is usually the maximum effective dose and should be given once a day. Splitting the dose is not necessary. Add 10 U of insulin glargine at bedtime. Adjust the dose by adding 2 U every night until the next morning fasting glucose is approximately 120 mg/dL. If daytime glucose readings are still high, stop glyburide and add a full-scale insulin regimen. For example:

$$70 \text{ kg} \times 1 \text{ U} = 70 \text{ U total daily dose (50\% basal,} \\ 50\% \text{ bolus)} \\ = 35 \text{ U of glargine at bedtime} \\ = 35 \text{ U of lispro or aspart:}$$

$$35 \times 40\% = 14 \text{ U at breakfast}$$

$$35 \times 30\% = \text{approximately 10 U at lunch and 10 U} \\ \text{at supper}$$

If there is concern about hypoglycemia, reduce the initial doses and adjust them later on. In the previous example, give 25 U of glargine at bedtime and 6 U of aspart or lispro right before each meal and adjust aspart or lispro based on 2-hour blood glucose level. Adjust glargine as instructed earlier. An alternative regimen would be two injections of premixed insulin (analogues) twice daily.

New Food and Drug Administration Approvals

PREGABALIN

Pregabalin (Lyrica) is an α-2 delta ligand analgesic/antiepileptic that was approved by the FDA for neuropathic pain associated with diabetic neuropathy. It is usually started at 50 mg three times a day and may increase to 100 mg three times a day within 1 week or longer. Dizziness and somnolence are the main side effects.

DULOXETINE

Duloxetine (Cymbalta) is FDA approved for the management of pain associated with diabetic neuropathy. The recommended dose is 60 mg at bedtime. Nausea is the main side effect.

INSULIN DETEMIR

Insulin detemir (Levemir) is a basal insulin analogue recently approved for use in the United States. Clinical trials demonstrated lower fasting plasma glucose levels, lower variability in plasma glucose, predictable action profile, and a reduced risk of nocturnal hypoglycemia and weight gain.

INSULIN GLULISINE

Insulin glulisine (Apidra) is an effective, safe, and well-tolerated rapid-acting insulin analogue. Insulin glulisine can be administered safely and effectively pre- and post-meal in both type 1 and type 2 diabetes. In addition, the safe administration of insulin glulisine by continuous subcutaneous insulin infusion (insulin pump therapy) is demonstrated in patients with type 1 diabetes.

REFERENCES

American Diabetes Association: Diagnosis and classification of diabetes mellitus. Diabetes Care 2004;27(Suppl 1):S5-S10.

Bell DS: Type 2 diabetes mellitus: What is the optimal treatment regimen? Am J Med 2004;8(116 Suppl 5A):23S-29S.

Calles-Escandon, Garcia-Rubi E, Mirza S, et al: Type 2 diabetes: One disease, multiple cardiovascular risk factors. Coron Artery Dis 1999;10:23-30.

DeFronzo RA: Pathogenesis of type 2 diabetes. Med Clin North Am 2004;88:787-835.

Leahy JL: What is the role for insulin therapy in type 2 diabetes? Curr Opin Endocrinol Diabetes 2003;10:99-103.

Lebovitz HE: Oral antidiabetic agents. Med Clin North Am 2004;88: 847-863.

Ritz E: Albuminuria and vascular damage: The vicious twins. N Engl J Med 2003;348:2349-2352.

Schoonjans K, Auwerx J: Thiazolidinediones: An update. Lancet 2000;355:1008-1010.

Secondary prevention of macrovascular events in patients with type 2 diabetes in the proactive study (Prospective Pioglitazone Clinical Trial in Macrovascular Events): A randomized controlled trial. Lancet 2005;366:1279-1289.

Steppel JH, Horton ES: Beta cell failure in the pathogenesis of type 2 diabetes mellitus. Curr Diab Rep 2004;4:169-175.

Diabetes Mellitus in Children and Adolescents

Method of
Lori M. B. Laffel, MD, MPH,
and Jamie R. S. Wood, MD

Diabetes mellitus is a group of metabolic disorders that have hyperglycemia as a common feature caused by inadequate insulin secretion, insulin action, or both. Chronic hyperglycemia and its numerous downstream effects lead to micro- and macrovascular complications involving the eyes, kidneys, nerves, and blood vessels. Childhood and adolescent years are periods of rapid physical growth and psychosocial change, and these two factors make the care of children and adolescents with diabetes both challenging and rewarding. The health care professional must balance the important goals of optimal glycemic control and normal growth and development along with the risks of hypoglycemia and the challenges of expected glycemic excursions during childhood. Multidisciplinary care is the hallmark of successful diabetes management for the child and adolescent with diabetes and for family members.

The American Diabetes Association (ADA) classifies diabetes mellitus into four main types: type 1 diabetes (T1D), type 2 diabetes (T2D), other specific types, and gestational diabetes mellitus (Table 1). T1D is caused by insulin deficiency, which results from the autoimmune destruction of the pancreatic β cells. There are multiple genetic loci in the major histocompatibility region of chromosome 6 that predispose (DR 3/4, DQ 0201/0302, DR 4/4, and DQ 0300/0302) or protect against (DQB1*0602, DQA1*0102) the development of T1D. T2D is caused by the combination of insulin resistance and relative insulin deficiency.

Genetic forms of diabetes include maturity-onset diabetes in the young (MODY), mitochondrial diabetes, and certain syndromes of insulin resistance. MODY is characterized by young age of onset, autosomal dominant inheritance, the lack of association with obesity, and a variable phenotype. The most common disease of the exocrine pancreas that causes diabetes in children and adolescents is cystic fibrosis. Glucocorticoids used in the treatment of systemic illnesses are also commonly associated with hyperglycemia and diabetes. Certain genetic syndromes, such as Down's syndrome, Klinefelter's syndrome, and Turner's syndrome, increase the risk for diabetes.

Diagnosis

The diagnosis of T1D in children and adolescents is typically straightforward. The classic symptoms of polyuria, polydipsia, polyphagia, and weight loss over a several-week period are common. A thorough history and physical exam may reveal perineal candidiasis or thrush. Such symptoms may be followed by nausea, abdominal pain, vomiting, lethargy, and Kussmaul respirations if diabetic ketoacidosis (DKA) and lactic acidosis develop. The presentation of T2D in children and adolescents can be more subtle and

TABLE 1 Classification of Diabetes Mellitus*

Type 1 diabetes
Type 2 diabetes
Other specific types:
- Genetic defects of β-cell function
  - MODY 1: chromosome 20, HNF-4α
  - MODY 2: chromosome 7, glucokinase
  - MODY 3: chromosome 12, HNF-1α
  - MODY 4: chromosome 13, IPF-1
  - MODY 5: chromosome 17, HNF-1β
  - MODY 6: chromosome 2, NeuroD1
  - Mitochondrial diabetes
- Genetic defects in insulin action
  - Leprechaunism
  - Rabson-Mendenhall syndrome
- Diseases of the exocrine pancreas
  - Pancreatitis
  - Cystic fibrosis
  - Pancreatectomy
- Endocrinopathies
  - Acromegaly
  - Cushing's syndrome
  - Glucagonoma
  - Pheochromocytoma
- Drug or chemical induced
  - Glucocorticoids
- Infections
  - Congenital rubella
  - Cytomegalovirus
- Other genetic syndromes associated with diabetes
  - Down's syndrome
  - Klinefelter's syndrome
  - Turner's syndrome
Gestational diabetes mellitus (GDM)

---

*Table is not all inconclusive and gives examples of each subtype of diabetes mellitus. For complete list, see American Diabetes Association: Diagnosis and classification of diabetes mellitus. Diabetes Care 2005;28 (Suppl 1):S37-S42.
Abbreviations: MODY = maturity-onset diabetes in the young.

CURRENT DIAGNOSIS

ADA Recommendations for the Diagnosis of Diabetes

- Symptoms (polyuria, polydipsia, unexplained weight loss) and a casual plasma glucose (any time of day without regard to time since last meal) ≥200 mg/dL (11.1 mmol/L) *or*
- Fasting (no caloric intake for at least 8 h) plasma glucose ≥126 mg/dL (7.0 mmol/L) *or*
- 2-hour plasma glucose ≥200 mg/dL (11.1 mmol/L) during an oral glucose tolerance test (glucose load of 75 g anhydrous glucose dissolved in water or 1.75 g/kg body weight if weight <43 kg).

Note: Criteria 2 and 3 should be confirmed on a second day if child/adolescent is asymptomatic. The OGTT is not recommended for routine clinical use and should be reserved for the asymptomatic child with incidental glucosuria/hyperglycemia or in the child with suspected diabetes but normal fasting plasma glucose.
Adapted from American Diabetes Association: Care of children and adolescents with type 1 diabetes. Diabetes Care 2005;28(1):186-212.

---

sometimes even clinically silent. However, approximately a third of adolescents with T2D have ketosis and a quarter have ketoacidosis at presentation.

The Current Diagnosis box outlines the diagnosis of diabetes mellitus. In the asymptomatic child or adolescent, diabetes is diagnosed when a fasting plasma glucose is 126 mg/dL or more, a 2-hour plasma glucose during an oral glucose tolerance test (OGTT) is 200 mg/dL or more, or a random plasma glucose is 200 mg/dL or more with confirmation on a second day. The symptomatic child or adolescent with a random plasma glucose of 200 mg/dL or more does not need repeat testing to confirm the diagnosis. Measurement of islet cell autoantibodies consistent with T1D (GAD, insulin, IA2) at diagnosis may help distinguish between type 1 and T2D. Care must be taken to avoid delay in the diagnosis and initiation of treatment because of the risk of rapid metabolic deterioration with insulin deficiency.

Initial Management

The goals of initial management of the child or adolescent newly diagnosed with diabetes mellitus are to correct fluid and electrolyte imbalances, reverse hepatic gluconeogenesis and ketogenesis by halting lipolysis with insulin replacement, and begin the process of diabetes education. The location of this initial management depends on the severity of the clinical presentation, the age of the patient, the psychosocial assessment of the child or adolescent and caregiver, and the diabetes-related resources available in the family's geographic location (availability of an outpatient education program).

Diabetic Ketoacidosis

Approximately 30% of children with newly diagnosed T1D present with diabetic ketoacidosis (DKA). Children who are younger (less than 4 years), without a first-degree relative with T1D, and from a family of lower socioeconomic status are at higher risk of DKA at onset of T1D. The majority of DKA episodes occur in patients with established diabetes, not in those newly diagnosed. Children or adolescents with established T1D are at higher risk for DKA if they are in poor metabolic control, have had a previous episode of DKA, are peripubertal/adolescent girls, have a psychiatric disorder, or are from a disadvantaged background.

Management of DKA in children and adolescents is based on the same principles used in adults and therefore is covered in a separate chapter in this book. The development of cerebral edema, however, warrants discussion because this complication is seen primarily in children and is associated with both high morbidity and mortality. Risk factors for the development of cerebral edema include lower initial partial pressure of carbon dioxide, higher initial serum urea nitrogen concentrations, treatment with bicarbonate, and an attenuated rise in measured serum sodium concentrations during therapy. In addition, children who are younger (less than 5 years), have new-onset T1D, and longer duration of symptoms may also be at an increased risk. A high index of suspicion is needed with mannitol (Osmitrol) at the bedside to allow for timely intervention.

Initiation of Insulin Replacement Therapy

Subcutaneous insulin is initiated in the patient who does not present in DKA or following intravenous insulin therapy in the child with resolved DKA who is tolerating oral intake (pH of ≥7.3, tCO$_2$ ≥18, anion gap 12 ± 2 mEq/L). The starting dose of insulin replacement therapy depends on the age, weight, and pubertal status of the patient, as well as the presence or absence of DKA. For the prepubertal child without DKA, the starting dose is usually 0.25 to 0.5 U/kg/day. For the prepubertal child with resolved DKA, the usual starting dose is 0.5 to 0.75 U/kg/day. For the pubertal child without DKA, the starting dose is 0.5 to 0.75 U/kg/day and for the pubertal child with resolved DKA, 0.75 to 1 U/kg/day. This total daily dose (TDD) of insulin is typically divided into either two or three injections per day, with the latter the preference toward implementation of intensive therapy (Figure 1). The twice-daily regimen may be selected for the younger (less than 4 years) child or if the psychosocial assessment determines that fewer injections per day would be beneficial. The use of an insulin pump at diagnosis remains within the research realm currently.

When the patient is metabolically stable, the focus turns to the psychosocial assessment of the child or adolescent and caregiver(s) and the initiation of diabetes education. A licensed social worker or other mental health professional evaluates each family and screens for circumstances that might complicate diabetes management: family composition, alternative caregiver(s), financial concerns, lack of health insurance, psychiatric or medical illness in a family member, or severe emotional distress of caregiver secondary to the diabetes diagnosis.

Diabetes education is provided by a certified diabetes nurse educator (DNE) and focuses on the set of essential skills needed to keep a child or adolescent with diabetes safe at home and school. These survival skills include techniques of blood glucose monitoring, urine or blood ketone measurement, drawing up and administration of subcutaneous insulin and glucagon, recognition and treatment of hypoglycemia and hyperglycemia, basics of sick day management, and indications for and methods of contacting the child's diabetes team. In addition to the survival skills, the child or adolescent and family should meet with a registered dietician who will assist them in developing an individualized meal plan and introduce the family to the concept of carbohydrate counting or exchanges. Once the child or adolescent (if developmentally appropriate) and caregiver(s) demonstrate the knowledge and skills needed, they are discharged with the expectation of daily phone contact with a member of their diabetes team to further titrate insulin doses and answer questions. When available and clinically indicated, a visiting nurse may assist with ongoing home-based education and support in the short term.

Outpatient Diabetes Care

The management of children and adolescents with diabetes requires a multidisciplinary team approach. Members of this team include either a pediatric endocrinologist or pediatrician with training in diabetes, a pediatric DNE, a dietician, and a mental health professional (social worker and psychologist). Members of this team need to be easily accessible to the family in times of illness or metabolic crisis. Another member of the child/adolescent's team is a pediatrician or family doctor who will continue to provide routine well child care including anticipatory guidance, immunizations, and general medical care.

In the first few months of outpatient diabetes care, patients are seen frequently by members of the diabetes team to assess the family's adaptation to the new diagnosis, reinforce skills and knowledge learned during the first few days, and expand on the skills and knowledge needed for intensive diabetes management. Patients are subsequently seen at a minimum frequency of every 3 months, alternating between their DNE and their pediatric endocrinologist. Visits with the dietician are recommended yearly or more frequently if circumstances warrant (e.g., young child or toddler, desired weight loss, initiating pump therapy, etc.).

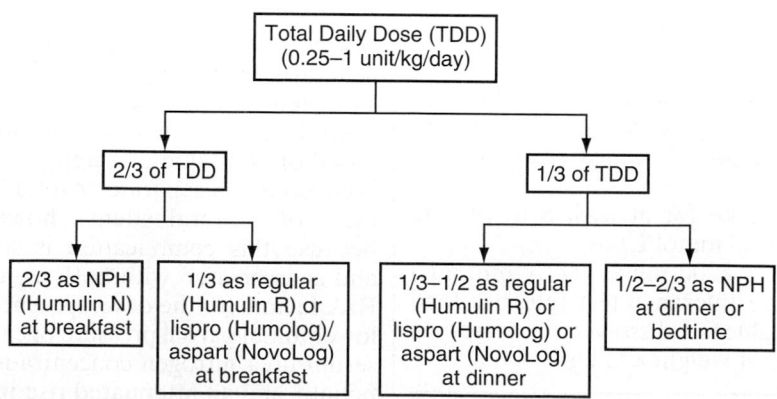

FIGURE 1. Initiation of Insulin Replacement Therapy. Two thirds of the total daily dose (TDD) is given at breakfast and further divided into NPH (two thirds) and short/rapid-acting insulin (one third). The remaining one third is either given in one injection at dinner (in a twice-daily regimen) or divided between dinner and bedtime (in a thrice-daily regimen), and should also be divided into NPH (two thirds) and short/rapid-acting insulin (one third). Short/rapid-acting insulin can be regular (Humulin R), lispro (Humalog), or aspart (NovoLog).

Diabetes Education

Diabetes education is an ongoing process with continuous need for review of previously learned material and introduction of new concepts as the family develops a more sophisticated understanding of intensive diabetes management. The educator should evaluate the patient and his or her caregiver's knowledge and skills regularly. In addition, age-appropriate issues need to be discussed as the patient matures (e.g., driving guidelines, issues related to alcohol and smoking, etc.). Diabetes education needs to be tailored to each family taking into account their educational level and cultural practices. The educator must be sensitive to the age and developmental stage of the child or adolescent, and shift his or her educational efforts from the caregiver(s) to the adolescent when it is developmentally appropriate. Continued parental involvement and supervision of the adolescent with diabetes is crucial to good metabolic control.

The health care provider should complete a focused interval history at each visit that includes recent illnesses, visits to the emergency department, hospitalizations, medications prescribed other than insulin, types of insulin and current doses, daily routine including meal plan and activity level, self-care behaviors and identifying who performs them, episodes of hypoglycemia and their precipitants, school performance, emotional health, and a review of systems focusing on symptoms of hyperglycemia (polyuria, polydipsia, polyphagia, weight loss, candidal infections) and the possible development of other autoimmune disorders. If appropriate, a history of tobacco, alcohol, recreational drugs, and sexual activity should be elicited. A focused physical examination that includes measurement of blood pressure and heart rate, weight, height, body mass index (BMI), and examination of the thyroid gland, sites of blood glucose monitoring, and insulin injections should be completed at each visit. A more thorough physical examination including Tanner staging should be performed once per year or more frequently if indicated.

The hemoglobin A1C, the fraction of hemoglobin that has glucose attached to it, is a measure of the average level of blood glucose over the preceding 2 to 3 months. It should be measured every 3 months and serves as an objective measure of blood glucose control. A discrepancy between the hemoglobin A1C and the average blood glucose levels from self-monitoring records suggests that the patient needs to monitor at different times of day, may benefit from a review of blood glucose monitoring technique and equipment, or there may be fabrication of results. Obtaining computer downloaded data helps eliminate the latter possibility.

Goals of Therapy

The Diabetes Control and Complications Trial (DCCT) demonstrated that the incidence of microvascular complications was reduced with improved blood glucose control (hemoglobin A1C approximately 7%). The reduction in complications, however, was accompanied by an increased risk of severe hypoglycemia. Because young children are more vulnerable to hypoglycemia (reduced catecholamine response to hypoglycemia, decreased ability to communicate symptoms of hypoglycemia, and risk for neuropsychologic

TABLE 2 Blood Glucose and A1C Goals for Type 1 Diabetes by Age Group

Age Group	Plasma Blood Glucose Range (mg/dL)		
	Before Meals	Bedtime/ Overnight	A1C
<6 y	100–180	110–200	7.5%–8.5%
6–12 y	90–180	100–180	<8%
13–19 y	90–130	90–150	<7.5%

Goals should be individualized; lower goals may be reasonable and achievable without hypoglycemia.
Goals should be higher in patients with frequent hypoglycemia or hypoglycemia unawareness.
Adapted from American Diabetes Association: Care of children and adolescents with type 1 diabetes. Diabetes Care 2005;28(1):186-212.

impairment from hypoglycemia), the ADA has developed age-specific glycemic targets (Table 2).

Insulin Therapy

The ideal insulin replacement therapy would be one that mirrors the basal and prandial insulin secretion in individuals without diabetes. Numerous insulin preparations are available that vary in time to onset, peak, and duration of action (Table 3). No single regimen is superior to another; thus individualization of the insulin regimen to the child or adolescent and family remains a major determinant. Important factors for consideration include blood glucose monitoring frequency, number of daily injections the family can perform, the need for flexibility in meal planning, and the unique family schedule. Regimens range in intensity from twice-a-day injections with a set dose of premixed insulin to intensive diabetes management with multiple injections per day of two or more types of insulin or use of an insulin pump (continuous subcutaneous insulin infusion [CSII]).

The typical regimen that children or adolescents begin at diagnosis was described previously (Figure 1). Some centers initiate a basal-bolus regimen in which insulin is replaced in a manner that attempts to mimic physiologic insulin release. Basal-bolus regimens include the insulin pump and glargine (Lantus) given once a day with rapid-acting insulin (lispro [Humalog] or aspart [NovoLog]) before each meal/snack and as needed for correction of hyperglycemia. The school-age child who hopes to avoid an injection at lunch often benefits from a regimen of glargine (Lantus) at dinner or bedtime, along with NPH (Humulin N) and a rapid-acting insulin at breakfast, plus a rapid-acting insulin at dinner. The peak of the NPH covers carbohydrate intake at lunch. The use of basal insulin analogue glargine (Lantus) in the evening is associated with less nocturnal hypoglycemia.

Patients on a basal-bolus regimen determine their insulin doses based on an insulin-to-carbohydrate ratio and a correction factor or sensitivity index (CF or SI). The insulin-to-carbohydrate ratio is the number of grams of carbohydrate covered by 1 U of insulin (roughly 450 divided by TDD) for each meal and snack. The CF/SI

TABLE 3 Insulin Analogues

Insulin Preparation	Onset of Action	Peak Action	Effective Duration
Rapid Acting			
Insulin lispro	5–15 min	30–90 min	2–4 h
Insulin aspart	5–10 min	60–180 min	3–5 h
Insulin glulisine*	5–15 min	30–90 min	3–5 h
Short Acting			
Regular (soluble insulin)	30–60 min	2–3 h	3–6 h
Intermediate Acting			
Lente (insulin zinc preparation)[†]	3–4 h	4–12 h	12–18 h
NPH (isophane insulin)	2–4 h	4–10 h	10–16 h
Long Acting			
Ultralente (extended insulin zinc preparation)[†]	4–6 h	8–20 h	20–24 h
Insulin glargine	1.1 h	None	24 h
Insulin detemir*	2–3 h	6–14 h	16–24 h
Insulin mixtures			
70/30 human mix[‡] (70% NPH, 30% regular)	30–60 min	dual	10–16 h
70/30 aspart analogue mix (70% intermediate, 30% aspart)[‡]	5–15 min	dual	10–16 h
75/25 lispro analog mix[‡] (75% intermediate, 25% lispro)	5–15 min	dual	10–16 h
50/50 human mix (50% NPH, 50% regular)	30–60 min	dual	10–16 h

*FDA approved for adult use only.
In many countries, including the United States, insulin preparations contain 100 U/mL and are referred to as U-100 insulin. Highly concentrated U-500 short-acting insulin is available and used primarily in adults with severe insulin resistance.
[†]Recently discontinued by manufacturer (Lilly); estimated to be available until end of 2005.
[‡]Typically used in fixed doses in twice-a-day insulin regimens.
Profiles for each insulin preparation are reasonable estimates only, based on data from adult study participants. There is variation between individuals, and time of onset, peak, and duration are also affected by size of dose, site and depth of injection, dilution, exercise, and temperature.

CURRENT THERAPY

Examples of Insulin Regimens

Injections bid:

- Insulin mixtures (70/30, 75/25) given at breakfast and dinner
- NPH and rapid- or short-acting insulin given at breakfast and dinner

Injections tid:

- NPH and rapid- or short-acting insulin given at breakfast, rapid- or short-acting insulin given at dinner, and NPH given at bedtime
- NPH and rapid- or short-acting insulin given at breakfast, rapid- or short-acting insulin given at dinner, and NPH or glargine (Lantus) given at bedtime

Injections qid:

- NPH and rapid-acting insulin given at breakfast, rapid-acting insulin given at lunch and dinner, and rapid-acting insulin and NPH given at bedtime
- NPH and rapid-acting insulin given at breakfast and lunch, rapid-acting insulin given at dinner, and NPH given at bedtime
- Rapid-acting insulin given at breakfast, lunch, and dinner, and glargine (Lantus) given at breakfast, dinner, or bedtime

Continuous subcutaneous insulin infusion (CSII)

- Rapid-acting insulin given for basal requirements and as bolus at every meal/snack and periodically to correct hyperglycemia (no more frequent than q2–3h)

is the expected decrement in glucose following 1 U of rapid-acting insulin (roughly 1650 divided by TDD). The CF/SI is applied no more than every 2 to 3 hours to lower an elevated blood glucose toward the target range to avoid so-called stacking of insulin action and subsequent hypoglycemia. For patients on a combination of intermediate-acting insulin (NPH) and rapid- or short-acting insulin, meals typically contain a certain amount of carbohydrates (e.g., 60 g or 4 carbohydrate exchanges) and require consistency in timing to avoid hypoglycemia.

The CSII, otherwise known as insulin pump therapy, comes the closest to mimicking the basal and prandial insulin secretion of an individual without diabetes. The insulin pump is steadily becoming a commonly used method to replace insulin, especially in the pediatric population. There are many advantages to the insulin pump including the elimination of multiple daily injections, increased flexibility in meal planning, ease of decreasing insulin for physical activity, fewer hypoglycemic events, and the ability to deliver very small amounts of insulin. The disadvantages are more frequent blood glucose monitoring, always being tethered to the pump, and increased risk for the development of DKA. Because only rapid-acting insulin (lispro [Humalog] or aspart [NovoLog]) is used in the insulin pump, discontinuation of insulin delivery can result in ketone production within hours. Increased vigilance, therefore, is necessary to ensure proper functioning of the insulin pump with frequent blood glucose monitoring and checking for ketones if hyperglycemia develops.

Self-Monitoring

One of the main goals of diabetes education is to teach and empower the patient and family in the self-management of diabetes. Self-management of diabetes includes measuring blood glucose and blood/urine ketone levels, recording the results along with amount of carbohydrate intake and amount of insulin administered, and the ability to make insulin dosing decisions based on the interpretation of these records. Monitoring blood glucose four or more times daily is recommended in children with T1D. Additional monitoring may be necessary postprandially, overnight, or during periods of increased physical activity to help optimize control and prevent severe hypoglycemia. Preschool or early school-age children may require more frequent monitoring because of their inability to recognize symptoms or to communicate during episodes of hypoglycemia. In addition, children and adolescents using the insulin pump typically check their blood sugar six or more times per day. Ketone measurements should be done whenever the blood glucose is greater than 250 to 300 mg/dL and/or if the patient is ill, especially with nausea, vomiting, or abdominal pain. Ketones can be measured either in the urine (acetoacetate and acetone) or blood (β-hydroxybutyric acid). Measurement of blood ketones is now available on a home meter and is the preferred method in the current era stressing blood glucose monitoring. The key to successful intensive diabetes management is frequent blood glucose monitoring, good record keeping, and communication of these results with the diabetes team at frequent intervals so that timely modifications can be made to the insulin regimen and/or meal plan.

Medical Nutrition Therapy

The meal plan remains an important component of management aimed at good glycemic control, although it is often the most difficult aspect of intensive diabetes management for families. A dietician trained in pediatric nutrition and diabetes should meet with the family at the time of T1D diagnosis and periodically thereafter. The dietician should help develop a meal plan that is individualized to the patient's daily schedule, food preferences, cultural influences, and physical activity. The meal plan is more likely to be successful if it is designed to fit into the family's already established schedule and preferences. The patient and family should also be instructed on carbohydrate counting so that either carbohydrate exchanges or insulin-to-carbohydrate ratios can be used. Like the child without diabetes, the total number of recommended calories follows the child's growth requirements along with consideration of the need for weight gain or loss. Growth velocity, weight gain, and BMI should be monitored at every visit to ensure that the meal plan is sufficient to meet the energy requirements of the patient. Unexpected weight loss or poor weight gain should prompt consideration of suboptimal metabolic control, as well as eating disorders, thyroid dysfunction, or gastrointestinal disease.

The ADA does not have pediatric specific guidelines for medical nutrition therapy, but the recommendations for adults can be extrapolated to children. The ADA recommends that carbohydrates provide 45% to 65% of total calories, with protein and fat contributing 15% and 30%, respectively. The patient and family should be educated to avoid foods high in cholesterol, saturated fat, and concentrated sweets and select foods high in complex carbohydrate and dietary fiber.

All children and adolescents are recommended to have three meals per day. If they receive intermediate-acting insulin preparations, they should also receive three snacks per day (morning, afternoon, and bedtime) to match anticipated peaks of insulin action. If the child or adolescent is on a basal-bolus regimen, snacks are optional and require insulin coverage based on insulin-to-carbohydrate ratios.

Exercise

Exercise, or periods of sustained physical activity, can be beneficial to the patient by contributing to a sense of well-being, helping achieve the recommended BMI, improving glycemic control (exercise enhances insulin sensitivity), improving the lipid panel (increasing HDL), and lowering blood pressure and improving cardiovascular fitness. All children and adolescents, especially those with diabetes, should be encouraged to participate in routine physical activity.

The child or adolescent with diabetes needs to take precautions to avoid hypoglycemia during periods of increased physical activity. The patient and family need to check blood glucose before the initiation of activity, every hour during sustained activity, and at the completion of physical activity. For the first several days of increased activity, the child should also check his or her blood sugar frequently during the 12-hour postexercise period because there is often a delayed drop in the blood glucose following exercise (i.e., the lag effect). Some children require additional carbohydrate before, during, and after activity; lower insulin doses on the days of increased physical activity; or both. It is suggested that the child take 5 to 15 g of carbohydrates, depending on age and exercise intensity, before exercise if the blood sugar is below target, and repeat the 5 to 15 g of carbohydrate for every 30 minutes of sustained activity. Rapid-acting carbohydrate should be readily available, and coaches and trainers should be aware of the diagnosis of diabetes and trained in the treatment of hypoglycemia.

Psychosocial Support

The mental health professional is an important member of the diabetes team. A thorough family assessment generally accompanies the diabetes diagnosis with appropriate referrals for additional services as needed. Thereafter, children or adolescents should be referred back to a mental health professional if social, emotional, or economic barriers to the achievement of good glycemic control are identified. Family conflict, especially conflict over diabetes care, can be associated with deterioration in glycemic control. Encouragement of ongoing family teamwork in the management of childhood diabetes promotes successful outcomes with respect to glycemic control, reducing diabetes-specific conflict, and preventing acute complications and emergency assessments.

Sick Day Management

The goals for the management of children and adolescents during sick days are never omit insulin, prevent dehydration and hypoglycemia, monitor blood glucose frequently (every 2 to 4 hours), monitor for ketosis, provide supplemental rapid- or short-acting insulin doses (5% to 20% of TDD) depending on degree of hyperglycemia and ketosis, treat underlying illness, and have frequent contact with the diabetes team. The majority of DKA among children or adolescents with established diabetes is caused by insulin omission or errors in administration of insulin. Inadequate insulin therapy in the context of an intercurrent illness accounts for the remaining small percentage. Although it is more common for children to require more insulin during illnesses, some children require a reduction of the basal and/or rapid-acting insulin dose if he or she is unable to eat and the blood glucose is less than 200 mg/dL.

Families need to be educated about symptoms that warrant immediate medical attention, including signs of dehydration (dry mouth, sunken eyes, cracked lips, weight loss, dry skin), persistent vomiting for more than 2 to 4 hours, persistence of blood glucose levels greater than 300 mg/dL or ketones for more than 12 hours, or symptoms of DKA (nausea, abdominal pain, chest pain, vomiting, ketotic breath, hyperventilation, or altered consciousness). It is helpful for the diabetes team to review sick day management annually with the family (can accompany flu immunization) to avoid metabolic decompensation during intercurrent illness.

Hypoglycemia

Fear of hypoglycemia can be a common occurrence in the management of childhood diabetes, especially among caregivers, and can be a barrier to optimal glycemic control. Recognition and treatment of hypoglycemia are important topics for diabetes education. Families are trained to treat hypoglycemia with 10 to 15 g of rapid-acting carbohydrate, recheck blood glucose in 15 minutes, repeat treatment with 10 to 15 g if blood sugar remains below target, and follow with a protein-containing snack if a meal will not follow within 1 to 2 hours. This technique avoids the natural tendency to overtreat low blood glucose levels. Caregivers should also receive glucagon training (20 to 30 μg/kg; maximum 1 mg) for severe hypoglycemia and low-dose glucagon (1 U on an insulin syringe for every year of life up to 15 years) for impending hypoglycemia, for example, in the context of a gastrointestinal illness or inadvertent insulin administration (lispro given instead of NPH). A member of the diabetes team should assess frequency, treatment, awareness, and circumstances of hypoglycemia at each visit.

Screening for Diabetes-Related Complications

Patients, families, and caregivers worry about the risk of diabetes-related complications, and therefore the diabetes team must educate families and screen for complications with sensitivity and optimism, emphasizing prevention of complications and the maintenance of health.

Screening for nephropathy, hypertension, dyslipidemia, and retinopathy are indicated.

Microalbuminuria (MA) is the first sign of diabetic nephropathy, and patients who develop persistent MA are at increased risk of progression to macroalbuminuria. Poor glycemic control, smoking, and a family history of essential hypertension are risk factors for the development of MA and nephropathy. Identification of persistent MA provides an opportunity for intervention and prevention of progressive renal disease through improvements in glycemic control and/or therapy with angiotensin-converting enzyme (ACE) inhibitors. There are currently no pediatric data on the use of angiotensin receptor blockers (ARBs). Table 4 outlines definitions, screening recommendations, and treatment.

Hypertension is an important predictor of the progression of diabetic nephropathy to end-stage renal disease. Hypertension in children and adolescents may go unrecognized because providers are not familiar with the gender-, age-, and height-specific definitions. Blood pressure should be measured every 3 months with standardized technique, using the proper size cuff. If elevated blood pressures are detected and confirmed, the first step is to exclude causes not related to diabetes. Table 4 outlines the definitions, screening recommendations, and treatment.

Dyslipidemia and diabetes are established risk factors for cardiovascular disease, and recent research suggests that a significant proportion of adolescents with diabetes already have evidence of atherosclerosis. Low-density lipoprotein (LDL) cholesterol is most closely associated with cardiovascular disease, and therefore, the ADA has developed guidelines for LDL cholesterol. Screening may be delayed until puberty if family history is negative for cardiovascular disease. A lipid profile should be performed on prepubertal children with diabetes who are older than 2 years if there is a positive family history of cardiovascular disease or if the family history is unknown. If the LDL cholesterol is less than 100 mg/dL, screening can be repeated every 5 years. The mainstay of therapy for dyslipidemia is dietary management (saturated fat less than 7% of calories and less than 200 mg/day of cholesterol). Children with levels between 130 and 159 mg/dL should be started on medication if diet and lifestyle modification are unsuccessful after 6 months or if the child has additional risk factors for cardiovascular disease, such as obesity or hypertension. Pharmacotherapy is recommended if the LDL cholesterol is more than 160 mg/dL. The LDL goal for children with diabetes is less than 100 mg/dL.

Diabetic retinopathy is a feared complication because it is the leading cause of vision loss. According to the ADA, the first ophthalmologic exam should be requested when the child is 10 years or older and has had diabetes for more than 3 to 5 years. Examinations with an eye care professional with expertise in diabetic retinopathy should occur early.

Screening for Other Autoimmune Diseases

Children and adolescents with T1D are at an increased risk for other autoimmune diseases and should be screened accordingly. Approximately 15% of patients with T1D also

TABLE 4 Screening for Diabetes-Related Complications

Complication	How to Screen	Definition	When to Screen	Therapy
Microalbuminuria	Spot urine sample timed overnight or 24-h collection	Spot urine albumin/creatinine ratio 30–299 µg/g or AER 20–199 µg/min from timed collection	Annual screening begins at 10 y or after ≥5 y duration of diabetes	Optimize glucose control, smoking cessation, normalize BP
Persistent microalbuminuria		2/3 of urine samples meet above criteria		Above, plus addition of ACE inhibitor
High-normal BP	Manual BP measurement with standard technique	Systolic or diastolic BP within the 90th–95th percentile for age, gender, and height	At every clinic visit	Dietary intervention, weight control, and exercise; if target BP not reached within 3–6 mo, then initiate pharmacologic therapy
Hypertension		Systolic or diastolic BP above the 95th percentile for age, gender, and height, or >130/80 on ≥3 occasions (whichever is lower)		Above, plus pharmacologic therapy titrated to achieve target BP

Note: Urine collection should not be performed following vigorous exercise, during an acute infection, during a female patient's menstrual cycle, or following an episode of severe hypoglycemia. Once angiotensin-converting enzyme (ACE) inhibitor is started, microalbumin excretion should be monitored q3–6 mo. Target BP is <130/80 or <90th percentile for age, gender, and height. Initial drug treatment is ACE inhibition.
Abbreviations: AER = albumin excretion rate; BP = blood pressure.

have autoimmune thyroid disease. All children and adolescents should be screened for autoimmune thyroid disease at the time of diabetes diagnosis once metabolic control is established. TSH measurement is a useful initial screen, with and without measuring the presence of thyroid autoantibodies. Screening should be repeated yearly or if there is any clinical suspicion of thyroid disease (abnormal growth rate, symptoms of hypo- or hyperthyroidism, goiter on examination, erratic blood glucose control).

Another commonly associated disorder is celiac disease. Nearly 6% of patients with T1D have elevated levels of circulating autoantibodies to tissue transglutaminase. Celiac disease can cause diarrhea, weight loss or failure to gain weight, abdominal pain, fatigue, and unexplained hypoglycemia or erratic blood glucose secondary to malabsorption. Patients with T1D should be screened with circulating IgA autoantibody to tissue transglutaminase.

A quantitative serum IgA level should be drawn at the same time to rule out IgA deficiency as a cause for falsely low IgA tissue transglutaminase levels. Positive antibodies should be confirmed with a second measurement, and if positive, a referral should be made to a gastroenterologist for small bowel biopsy. If the diagnosis is confirmed, celiac disease is treated with a gluten-free diet with recommendations and support from a registered dietician with pediatric expertise in diabetes and celiac management.

Type 2 Diabetes Mellitus in Youth

With the increasing prevalence of childhood obesity during the last two decades, there is an increased occurrence of T2D in youth. Based on National Health and Nutrition Examination survey data, the prevalence of

TABLE 5 Risk Factors and Screening for Type 2 Diabetes in Children

Criteria	Age of Initiation	Frequency	Method
Overweight (BMI >85th percentile for age and gender), weight for height >85th percentile, or weight >120% of ideal for height Plus 2 of the following risk factors: Family history of T2D in 1st- or 2nd-degree relative Race/ethnicity (American Indian, African American, Hispanic, Asian/Pacific Islander) Signs of or conditions associated with insulin resistance (acanthosis nigricans, PCOS, HTN, dyslipidemia)	10 y or at pubertal onset if puberty occurs at a younger age	q2y	Fasting plasma glucose

Note: Clinical judgment should be used to test for diabetes in high-risk patients who do not meet these criteria.
Abbreviations: BMI = body mass index; T2D = type 2 diabetes; HTN = hypertension; PCOS = polycystic ovarian syndrome.
Adapted from American Diabetes Association: Type 2 diabetes in children. Diabetes Care 2000;23(3):381-389.

TABLE 6 Medications to Treat Type 2 Diabetes

Class	Mechanism of Action	Adverse Effects
Biguanides (metformin)*	Decrease hepatic glucose production Increase peripheral glucose disposal	Gastrointestinal upset Lactic acidosis
Sulfonylureas (glimepiride, glyburide, glipizide)	Insulin secretagogues	Hypoglycemia Weight gain
Meglitinides (repaglinide, nateglinide)	Insulin secretagogues	Hypoglycemia Weight gain
α-Glucosidase inhibitors (acarbose)	Decrease gut carbohydrate absorption	Gastrointestinal upset
Thiazolidinediones (rosiglitazone and pioglitazone)	Decrease hepatic glucose production Increase peripheral glucose disposal	Weight gain Edema Increased liver enzymes Anemia

*Metformin (Glucophage) is the only medication with FDA approval for use in children.

overweight children (defined as a body mass index greater than the 95th percentile for children and youth) increased from 5% in the 1970s to more than 15% by 1999. The epidemic of obesity follows the increased consumption of fast foods, increased consumption of soft drinks, increased sedentary behavior with more television watching, and decreased physical activity. Mirroring this epidemic of childhood obesity is the occurrence of T2D in children and adolescents. Before 1990, T2D in youth was a rare occurrence. By 2000, between 8% and 45% of all newly diagnosed cases of childhood diabetes were caused by T2D. T2D occurs most commonly in those with a family history of T2D; individuals from certain racial and ethnic minority groups including Native Americans, Hispanics, African Americans, and Asian and Pacific Islanders; those with obesity falling above the 85th percentile for BMI based on age and gender; and in association with markers of insulin resistance (Table 5). Markers of insulin resistance include the occurrence of acanthosis nigricans and polycystic ovarian syndrome (PCOS). In addition, other well-known risk factors include hypertension and hyperlipidemia.

As noted earlier, the diagnosis of T2D is based on fasting plasma glucose (FPG), 2-hour glucose value during an OGTT, or a casual glucose level. Because T2D often goes without symptoms, individuals who are overweight, have a positive family history of T2D, come from one of the high-risk racial and ethnic minority groups, and/or have markers of insulin resistance warrant screening for T2D. Screening can be performed with a FPG or OGTT when clinical concerns are high and the FPG is normal.

Currently one oral medication is approved for the treatment of T2D in youth. This medication is metformin (Glucophage), which is also available in a liquid formulation. The maximum recommended daily dose of metformin (Glucophage) in youth is 2000 mg/day divided as 1000 mg twice daily. Often patients with T2D present in ketoacidosis and require initial insulin therapy. The goal of management of the child with T2D is initial stabilization often with insulin therapy, metformin (Glucophage) directed at managing the insulin resistance, and education. Once glucose levels are stabilized, insulin dosage may be lowered along with continued treatment with metformin (Glucophage) and approaches to lifestyle management. Lifestyle management involves a healthy diet, increasing exercise, and decreasing sedentary behaviors.

Other medications used to treat T2D include second-generation sulfonylureas, meglitinides, thiazolidinediones, and α-glucosidase inhibitors, none of which is currently approved for use in pediatric patients. There is ongoing studies to assess the efficacy and safety of these medications (Table 6).

REFERENCES

American Diabetes Association: Diagnosis and classification of diabetes mellitus. Diabetes Care 2005;28 (Suppl 1):S37-S42.

American Diabetes Association: Type 2 diabetes in children. Diabetes Care 2000;23(3):381-389.

Barroso I: Genetics of type 2 diabetes. Diabet Med 2005;22:517-535.

Dunger DB, Sperling MA, Acerini CL, et al: ESPE/LWPES consensus statement on diabetic ketoacidosis in children and adolescents. Arch Dis Child 2004;89:188-194.

Fox LA, Buckloh LM, Smith SD, et al: A randomized controlled trial of insulin pump therapy in young children with type 1 diabetes. Diabetes Care 2005;28:1277-1281.

Glaser N, Barnett P, McCaslin I, et al: The Pediatric Emergency Medicine Collaborative Research Committee of the American Academy of Pediatrics. N Engl J Med 2001;344(4):264-269.

Goodwin G, Volkening LK, Laffel LM: Younger age at onset of type 1 diabetes in concordant sibling pairs is associated with increased risk for autoimmune thyroid disease. Diabetes Care 2006;29(6)1397-1398.

Hannon TS, Rao G, Arslanian SA: Childhood obesity and type 2 diabetes mellitus. Pediatrics 2005;116(2):473-480.

Hirsch IB: Insulin analogues. N Engl J Med 2005;352:174-183.

Laffel LM, Vangsness L, Connell A, et al: Impact of ambulatory, family-focused teamwork intervention on glycemic control in youth with type 1 diabetes. J Pediatr 2003;142(4):409-416.

Rosenbloom AL: Cerebral edema in diabetic ketoacidosis and other acute devastating complications: Recent observations. Pediatr Diabetes 2005;6:41-49.

Silverstein J, Klingensmith G, Copeland K, et al: American Diabetes Association: Care of children and adolescents with type 1 diabetes. Diabetes Care 2005;28(1):186-212.

Wysocki T, Harris MA, Mauras N, et al: Absence of adverse effects of severe hypoglycemia on cognitive function in school-aged children with diabetes over 18 months. Diabetes Care 2003;26(4):1100-1105.

Hyperosmolar Hyperglycemic Syndrome and Diabetic Ketoacidosis

Method of
Solomon S. Solomon, MD, and
R. Dale Childress, MD

Hyperglycemic crises in patients with diabetes are generally categorized based on the presence or absence of acidosis (pH less than 7.3) as diabetic ketoacidosis (DKA) or hyperosmolar hyperglycemic syndrome (HHS), respectively. Classically, HHS is seen in type 2 diabetes, whereas DKA is more typical in type 1 diabetes. Both crises may be the presenting feature of newly diagnosed diabetes, but they most often represent a decompensation of glycemic control in patients with established diabetes receiving therapy. The leading cause of DKA in tertiary care settings is actually withdrawal of insulin therapy because of monetary and noncompliance issues. Both HHS and DKA are usually triggered by an underlying metabolic stressor such as infection or myocardial infarction.

Hallmark features shared by these two conditions include the obvious hyperglycemia and associated volume depletion. The electrolyte and pH abnormalities seen in both conditions exceed the isolated glucose disposal properties of insulin. Therapy of both conditions centers on adequate and appropriate fluid therapy, insulin therapy for hyperglycemia, treatment of electrolyte disturbances, and identification and treatment of any precipitating cause. Aggressive fluid repletion alone can significantly reverse hyperglycemia in both conditions in the absence of exogenous insulin therapy. The current standards of care recommend low doses of insulin (approximately 0.1 U/kg/hour), which reverse hyperglycemia, acidosis, and ketosis rapidly without a significant burden of hypoglycemia during treatment. Treatment of DKA in pediatric populations is associated with cerebral edema and, as such, rates of hydration and insulin delivery are often more carefully controlled in this population. Cerebral edema is virtually unknown in the treatment of hyperglycemic crises in adults, although the mechanism that limits this in adults is not yet elucidated.

Delivery of regular human insulin by intramuscular injection, subcutaneous injection, and intravenous delivery all correct hyperglycemia adequately with very similar kinetics of glucose and pH recovery. Intravenous delivery is the preferred means of therapy in most centers, primarily because of delayed clearance kinetics of ketone bodies seen with other routes of insulin delivery. Recent work, however, shows that subcutaneous short-acting insulin analogue therapy has very similar kinetics of DKA resolution to that seen with intravenous regular insulin.

It is generally accepted that the key physiologic difference between DKA and HHS is the absolute insulinopenia of DKA versus the relative insulinopenia of HHS. The presence of even suboptimal levels of insulin in HHS limits hepatic ketogenesis and adipocyte lipolysis and, as such, ketosis is not a hallmark feature of HHS. Insulin's ability to mobilize glucose transporters is diminished in both HHS and DKA. The more subtle effect of diminished insulin availability to stimulate "low km" cyclic AMP phosphodiesterase that results in elevated cyclic AMP levels sufficient to produce lipolysis, ketosis, and acidosis is only found in DKA. The underlying insulin resistance in type 2 diabetes further leads to poor glucose disposal rates in peripheral tissues and exaggerated hepatic gluconeogenesis and thus hyperglycemia (glucose more than 600 mg/dL) is frequently more pronounced in HHS than DKA. The hemodynamic consequences of this hyperosmolarity and hyperviscosity are manifested as the typical neurologic features of HHS including altered sensorium, lethargy, focal neurologic deficits, and ultimately coma.

Although this teleologic explanation of HHS and DKA is generally useful, there are well-defined cases in which patients with phenotypically evident type 2 diabetes can present with DKA. This is typically seen in certain ethnic populations including persons of African descent, referred to alternately as Flatbush syndrome or ketosis-prone type 2 diabetes. Of further interest, many patients with this presentation can subsequently be transitioned from insulin therapy to oral agents after a period of 3 to 6 months (Table 1).

Hyperglycemic Hyperosmolar Syndrome

HHS is the archetypal consequence of decompensated type 2 diabetes but is also seen in type 1 diabetes. Delayed diagnosis of HHS and the common association with an underlying physiologic stress leads to its high morbidity and mortality (above 50% in some studies). The condition usually presents with central nervous system (CNS) symptoms such as lethargy or irritability and, less commonly, with seizure or acute neurologic deficits suggestive of cardiovascular accident (CVA), which are usually reversible. Typical signs include lethargy, tachypnea, fever, and hypotension with tachycardia. Hypotension is usually attributable to volume depletion but may be because of sepsis (usually gram negative). Usual findings of dehydration (i.e., dry skin, sunken eyes, lack of sweat, hemoconcentration and elevated blood urea nitrogen [BUN]), are often present. Abdominal distention and ileus may result from osmotic effects on gastrointestinal motility. Neurologic findings, from lethargy to CVA, including both long-tract and cranial nerve findings, may be present presumably from hypoxia secondary to impaired cerebrovascular circulation. These findings frequently clear with treatment.

TABLE 1 Comparison of Diagnostic Criteria: DKA versus HHS

	DKA	HHS
Glucose (mg/dL)	>250	>600
Arterial pH	<7.3	>7.3
Serum HCO$_3$ (mEq/L)	<18	>15
Serum ketones	Present	Variable
Serum osmolality (mOsm/kg) variable	>320	
Anion gap	>12	Variable
Mental status change	Variable	Common

Abbreviations: DKA = diabetic ketoacidosis; HHS = hyperosmolar hyperglycemic syndrome.

TABLE 2 Calculation of Serum Osmolality in HHS

Plasma osmolality = 2 × [Na⁺] + [K⁺] + [glucose in mg/dL/18]
Corrected serum [Na⁺]
= [Na⁺] + 1.6 [(glucose in mg/dL) − 100]/100

Abbreviations: HHS = hyperosmolar hyperglycemic syndrome.

Laboratory findings usually demonstrate very high blood glucose (more than 600 mg/dL) in association with marked elevations of serum Na⁺, which accounts for the hyperosmolarity. Typical serum osmolarity in HHS is more than 300 mOsm/kg and may reach approximately 480 mOsm/kg. Arterial blood pH is usually only slightly low (approximately 7.30) and serum HCO₃⁻ is similarly only mildly low (15 to 20 mEq/L). (Table 2 shows how serum osmolality may be calculated.) Mild acidosis and a wide anion gap are almost always present.

The key challenge in treating HHS is identification and treatment of precipitating factors. Common triggers include: infections (gram-negative sepsis, pneumonia, urinary tract infection [UTI]); surgical abdomen, trauma, acute pancreatitis; renal failure, myocardial infarction; endocrine disorders including thyrotoxicosis, Cushing's, Addison's, acromegaly; and medications including diuretics, β-blockers, calcium channel blockers, antipsychotics. Antibiotics are routinely recommended early in HHS when fever is present. This is typically reserved for a severe hyperosmolar state (serum osmolality more than 400 mOsm/kg) even if there is no identified infectious etiology.

Treatment of HHS involves restoration of intravascular volume and hydration (up to 25% dehydration or as much as 9L of fluid loss). The usual treatment is 1 to 2 L of normal saline in the first 2 hours, followed by 5 to 9 L of hypotonic saline over 3 days. Obviously volume may be reduced in patients with left-side myocardial infarction (MI) or congestive heart failure (CHF). Because insulin is also being given (see later), D₅ NS (dextrose 5% in normal saline) or D₅ 1/2 NS are substituted when blood glucose falls below 250 mg/dL, to prevent hypoglycemia and cerebral edema. Insulin therapy causes serum glucose and K⁺ levels to fall as they enter cells as a result of insulin's action. Other ions including Ca⁺⁺, Mg⁺⁺, and PO₄²⁻ should be monitored and replaced on an individual basis. Insulin therapy in HHS may require relatively high insulin levels initially because of the peripheral insulin resistance that defines the underlying type 2 diabetes. Insulin is usually given as intravenous regular insulin with a bolus of 0.1 U/kg followed by continuous infusion of 0.1 U/kg/hour. One should err on the side of lower insulin dosing because fluid administration alone frequently reduces blood glucose significantly. Unless neurologic symptoms fail to resolve with treatment of hyperglycemia, anticoagulation is not routinely used. Continuous monitoring of the patient (both clinical and laboratory) in the hospital during treatment of HHS is essential.

Diabetic Ketoacidosis

DKA is seen primarily in patients with type 1 diabetes but is reported in certain populations with type 2 (i.e., Flatbush syndrome or ketosis-prone type 2, seen in persons of African descent). The morbidity and mortality of DKA has been improving since the isolation and use of insulin in 1922. Progress in understanding the underlying and associated abnormalities in DKA has led to improved treatment of abnormalities in electrolytes (especially potassium and phosphorus), hydration, ketosis, acidosis, and other variables independent of insulin. Current treatment guidelines emphasize so-called low-dose insulin therapy, typically with doses of approximately 0.1 U/kg/hour as a continuous infusion. This approach is associated with a lower incidence of hypoglycemia while providing adequately rapid resolution of hyperglycemia, ketosis, and acidosis. These additional therapies have lowered the morbidity and mortality independently. One confounder in the treatment success rate for DKA is the high incidence of mild DKA seen in tertiary care centers because of simple withdrawal of insulin therapy, leading to presentation of mild and otherwise uncomplicated DKA. Patients presenting in DKA with underlying metabolic triggers including sepsis and myocardial ischemia remain at elevated risk of morbidity and mortality. Despite many advances, mortality from DKA in these patients has not improved significantly since the 1970s. The most vulnerable group remains those older than 65 years.

The blood glucose in DKA is typically lower than in HHS (less than 500 mg/dL in DKA vs. more than 500 mg/dL in HHS), although severe hyperglycemia (more than 900 mg/dL) can be seen in DKA. Serum Na⁺ is usually normal in DKA and, as such, serum osmolality is usually approximately 300 mOsm/kg. Acidosis is a hallmark feature of DKA, and pH from 7.00 to 7.25 is common with ketonemia and ketonuria. Plasma HCO₃ is typically below 15 mEq/dL and often below 10 mEq/L. These changes are reflected in an anion gap, Δ[Na⁺ − (HCO₃⁻ + Cl⁻)] of greater than 10 mEq/L even in mild DKA. Severe DKA is characterized by blood glucose of more than 500 mg/dL and pH <7.00, Δ anion gap >12, and serum HCO₃⁻ <10. Total serum ketones and acetoacetate are routinely measured. Urine ketones are not routinely used anymore because they may be positive in starvation, alcohol consumption, and a number of other conditions. Unfortunately the best index of ketonemia, β-hydroxybutyrate, is not easily measured.

Patients in DKA are dehydrated, starved, with frequent nausea and vomiting. Abdominal pain, ileus, hemorrhagic gastritis, and hypotension are common. Tachypnea is a very common finding in severe DKA representing a compensatory respiratory alkalosis. Ketoacidosis may also occur in starvation and severe alcoholism absent hyperglycemia or acidosis. These must be excluded to confirm DKA. Most DKA is associated simultaneously with lactic acidosis. Many times the lactic acidosis remains when the DKA and its hyperglycemia have normalized. Although ingestion of many other agents (salicylates, ethylene glycol, and methanol) can initially present like DKA, these can usually be excluded by the medical history.

Treatment of DKA involves hydration, balancing electrolytes, and administration of insulin. As in HHS, identification of precipitating causes and appropriate specific therapy is key. Volume replacement is 1 to 2 L NS over the first 2 to 4 hours, followed by 0.45% NS, approximately 6 L, over the next 12 to 72 hours. This is titrated carefully in patients with known heart disease, CHF, or renal insufficiency. Evaluation of renal function is important before K⁺ supplement is considered. Intracellular movement of protons leads to hyperkalemia in the face of total-body depletion of potassium. The patient may initially have hyperkalemia but treatment with insulin drives potassium and glucose into peripheral tissues, resulting in hypokalemia. Hypophosphatemia must also be considered, and use of phosphate-containing fluids may be considered when hypophosphatemia is present. The routine use of HCO_3 has been abandoned in recent years. Use of HCO_3 in patients with cardiac dysfunction because of acidosis is still prudent, but the treatment of choice for acidosis in modern therapy is reversal of metabolic derangement by appropriate insulin therapy. Although hydration can largely control hyperglycemia, the absolute insulinopenia of DKA requires the use of exogenous insulin to ultimately correct ketoacidosis and other metabolic derangements. Insulin is usually given intravenously with an initial bolus of 0.1 U/kg, followed by continuous infusion at a rate starting at 0.1 U/kg per hour with a goal of producing a 50 to 100 mg/dL/hour decrease in blood glucose. The rate of insulin infusion is adjusted hourly and repeating boluses may be needed to attain the desired rate of decrease in plasma glucose. Electrolytes should be monitored frequently (basic metabolic profile at 2- to 4-hour intervals) to assess both potassium and HCO_3. When potassium falls below 4.0 mEq/L, addition of potassium to the fluids is prudent, usually with 20 mEq/L.

DKA is considered to be resolved when serum pH and HCO_3 have normalized and ketosis has resolved. After DKA has resolved, the patient can be allowed to resume oral food intake. At this point a regimen of scheduled subcutaneous insulin is instituted. Patients who were being treated with insulin prior to their hyperglycemic episode can be started on their home doses of insulin with monitoring of efficacy. During acute illness patients are insulin resistant and may require 1.5 to 2 times their usual daily insulin. In the insulin-naïve patient, a total insulin dose of 0.7 U/kg/day is a reasonable starting dose. If using twice-daily premix insulin, this is usually dosed with two thirds of the total dose before breakfast and one third before the evening meal. If the patient is treated with a basal-bolus regimen of insulin analogues, half the total dose should be given as basal (long-acting) insulin and the remaining half given in divided doses with meals (i.e., one sixth of total daily dose per meal). Any patient with DKA should be thought of as requiring insulin for life. However, a subgroup of patients with type 2 diabetes who present in DKA may be managed long term with oral agents after a period of 3 to 6 months of insulin therapy (Table 3).

Some unique complications of DKA include cerebral edema from the DKA itself or from too rapid replacement of fluid. The most likely group for this complication is young children. DKA is a condition that can usually be prevented in almost all but the most brittle diabetics. Monthly visits to the physician, coupled with diabetes and nutrition education and home monitoring, along with emergency access to the physician or his or her surrogate (i.e., preventive maintenance), remains the critical nucleus for prevention of both DKA and HHS.

REFERENCES

Fisher JN, Shahshahani MN, Kitabchi AE: Diabetic ketoacidosis: Low-dose insulin therapy by various routes. N Engl J Med 1977;297:238-247. [Clinical]

Foster DW, McGarry JD: The metabolic derangements and treatment of diabetic keto-acidosis. N Engl J Med 1983;309:159-169. [Basic science and clinical]

Majumdar G, Harrington A, Hungerford J, et al: Insulin dynamically regulates calmodulin gene expression by sequential O-glycosylation and phosphorylation of Sp1 and its subcellular compartmentalization in liver cells. J Biol Chem 2006;281(6):3642-3650. [Basic science mechanism]

Marshall SM, Alberti KGMM: Hyperosmolar non-ketotic diabetic coma. Diabetes Ann 1988;4:235-247.[Clinical]

Solomon SS, Steiner MS, Little WL, et al: Inhibitor of calmodulin and cAMP phosphodiesterase activity in BB (DIABETES1) rats. Diabetes 1987;36:210-215. [Basic science mechanism]

Turpin BP, Duckworth WC, Solomon SS: Hyperosmolarity and lipolysis: Opposing effects of sodium chloride and glucose. J Clin Invest 1979;63:403-409. [Basic science mechanism]

Umpierrez GE, Latif K, Stoever J: Efficacy of subcutaneous insulin lispro versus continuous intravenous regular insulin for the treatment of patients with diabetic keto acidosis. Am J Med 2004;117(5):291-296. [Clinical]

Hyponatremia

Method of
Biff F. Palmer, MD

Hyponatremia is a common clinical disorder. The approach to the patient with hyponatremia is outlined in Figure 1.

Is Hyponatremia Representative of a Hypo-osmolar State?

Two general causes of hyponatremia are not associated with a hypo-osmolar state. The first cause is pseudohyponatremia, which involves an abnormal measurement of the serum sodium (Na) concentration. This occurs in patients with hyperglobulinemia or hypertriglyceridemia in whom plasma water relative to plasma solids in blood is decreased, leading to less Na in a given volume of blood.

The other cause of hyponatremia in the absence of a hypo-osmolar state involves true hyponatremia but with

---

TABLE 3 Critical Issues in Current Therapy of HHS and DKA

1. Identify and treat underlying cause(s): initial laboratory chemistry, urinalysis, serum ketones, arterial blood gas, CBC, electrocardiogram.
2. Fluids (NS initially; change to 0.45% NS or D_5W after 2 L of normal saline; change to dextrose solutions when glucose <250 mg/dL).
3. Insulin (IV regular: bolus 0.1–0.15 U/kg, then continuous infusion at 0.1 U/kg/h; subcutaneous analogue 0.1 U/kg/h).
4. Monitor blood glucose hourly, ketones q2–4h, electrolytes (Chem 7) q2h.
5. Continue insulin infusion until ketones are negative (not just until pH, HCO_3, and glucose are normalized).

Abbreviations: CBC = complete blood count; DKA = diabetic ketoacidosis; D_5W = dextrose 5% in water (solution); HHS = hyperosmolar hyperglycemic syndrome; IV = intravenous; NS = normal saline.

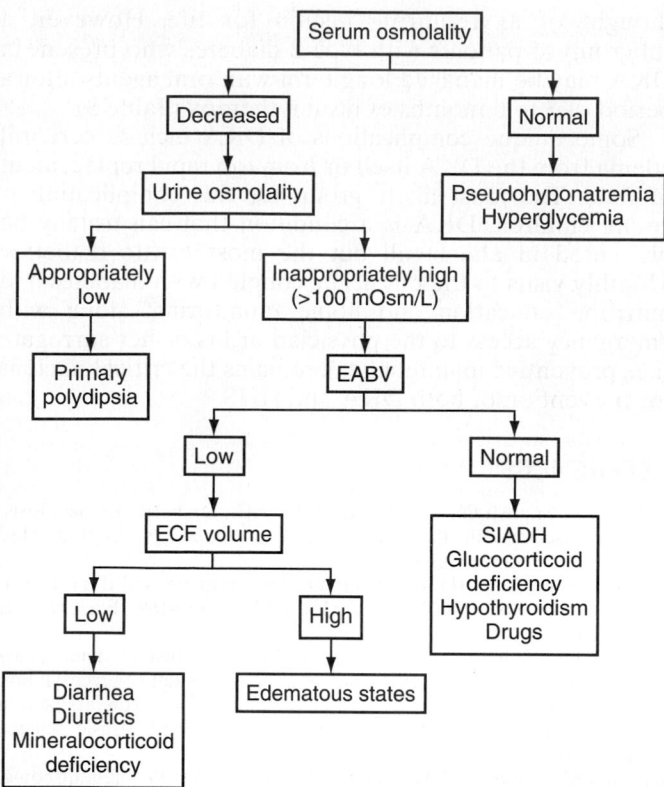

FIGURE 1. Approach to the patient with hyponatremia. *Abbreviations:* EABV = effective arterial blood volume; ECF = extracellular fluid; SIADH = syndrome of inappropriate secretion of antidiuretic hormone.

elevated concentrations of another osmole. Clinical examples include hyperglycemia, as seen in uncontrolled diabetes, and rarely hypertonic infusion of mannitol, which is used for treatment of cerebral edema. The increases in plasma glucose concentration raise serum osmolality, which pulls water out of cells and dilutes the serum Na concentration. For every 100 mg/dL rise in glucose or mannitol, the serum Na concentration quickly falls by 1.6 mEq/L. The increased tonicity stimulates thirst and arginine vasopressin (AVP) secretion, both of which contribute to further water retention. As the plasma osmolality returns toward normal, the decline in serum Na concentration will be 2.8 mEq/L for every 100 mg/dL rise in glucose.

Is the Ability of the Kidneys to Dilute the Urine Intact?

The presence of hypotonic hyponatremia implies that water intake exceeds the ability of the kidneys to excrete water. In unusual circumstances, the condition occurs even when the ability of the kidneys to excrete free water is intact. Because a normal kidney can excrete 20 to 30 L of water per day, the presence of hyponatremia with normal renal water excretion implies that the patient is drinking more than 20 to 30 L of water per day. This condition is referred to as *primary polydipsia*. These patients should have a urine osmolality less than 100 mOsm/L. Primary polydipsia is a common condition that leads to polyuria and polydipsia, but it is uncommon as a sole cause of hyponatremia.

In the absence of primary polydipsia, hyponatremia is associated with decreased renal water excretion and a urine that is inappropriately concentrated. It is important to note that in the presence of hyponatremia, urine should be maximally dilute, and a urine osmolality higher than 100 mOsm/L is inappropriate. An inappropriately concentrated urine implies a defect in renal water excretion.

Excretion of water by the kidney is dependent on three factors. First, delivery of filtrate to the tip of the loop of Henle must be adequate. Second, solute absorption in the ascending limb and the distal nephron must be normal so that the tubular fluid will be diluted. Third, AVP levels in the plasma must be low. Of these three requirements for water excretion, the failure to maximally suppress AVP levels probably is the most important factor in the genesis of hyponatremia. In many conditions, decreased delivery of filtrate to the tip of the loop of Henle also contributes.

What Is the Volume Status of the Patient?

In patients with hypotonic hyponatremia with an inappropriately concentrated urine, one needs to define whether effective arterial volume is decreased. Most causes of hyponatremia are related to a decrease in effective arterial volume, which causes baroreceptor stimulation of AVP secretion and leads to decreased distal delivery of filtrate to the tip of the loop of Henle. If effective arterial volume is low, extracellular fluid (ECF) volume can be low in the volume-depleted patient (hypovolemic hyponatremia) or high in the edematous patient (hypervolemic hyponatremia). If effective arterial volume is normal, one is dealing with the euvolemic causes of hyponatremia (isovolemic hyponatremia).

The clinical determination of effective arterial volume is usually straightforward. On physical examination, the best index of effective arterial volume is the pulse and blood pressure. Urinary electrolytes are also extremely useful in the assessment of effective arterial volume. Patients with a low effective arterial volume tend to have low urinary sodium, low urinary chloride, and low fractional excretions of sodium and chloride in the urine. Patients with euvolemic hyponatremia, however, are in balance and excrete sodium and chloride at rates that reflect dietary intake of sodium and chloride. Thus, in general they have urinary sodium and chloride concentrations greater than 20 mEq/L and fractional excretions of sodium and chloride greater than 1%.

Plasma composition can also be used to assess effective arterial volume. The blood urea nitrogen (BUN) is particularly sensitive to effective arterial volume. In patients with normal serum creatinine concentrations, a high BUN suggests a low effective arterial volume, and a low BUN suggests a high effective arterial volume. The plasma uric acid can also be used as a sensitive index of effective arterial volume. In comparing patients with the syndrome of inappropriate secretion of antidiuretic hormone (SIADH) and other causes of hyponatremia, patients with low effective arterial volume tend to have an elevated serum uric acid concentration. The serum urate concentration is low in patients with SIADH. This is due to the fact that these patients are volume expanded, although detecting the degree of volume expansion is clinically difficult.

Syndrome of Inappropriate Antidiuretic Hormone Secretion

In the setting of euvolemia, a concentrated urine and high antidiuretic hormone levels are inappropriate. The most common cause of this condition is SIADH. SIADH is generally associated with diseases of the central nervous system (CNS), usually those affecting the base of the brain, pulmonary diseases, and neoplasms (Table 1). These conditions lead to secretion of antidiuretic hormone that is inappropriate from the standpoint of both plasma osmolality and effective arterial volume. A number of other etiologic factors cause a condition of hypo-osmolality associated with euvolemia and can mimic SIADH. These include isolated glucocorticoid deficiency (normal mineralocorticoid activity), hypothyroidism, pain, nausea, acute psychosis, and a variety of drugs (Table 2).

Treatment of Hyponatremia

The principal danger of hyponatremia or hypernatremia relates to effects on CNS function due to changes in brain size. Hyponatremia initially leads to cell swelling driven by the higher intracellular osmolality. The net result is equilibration of intracellular and extracellular osmolality at the expense of increased brain volume. Cells, in general, and brain cells, in particular, then respond by decreasing the number of intracellular osmoles. As intracellular osmolality decreases, cell size returns toward normal despite the presence of hyponatremia. If the decrease in ECF osmolality is slow, no measurable cell swelling will occur. This pathophysiologic sequence correlates well with clinical observations. If hyponatremia is slow in onset, neurologic symptoms and permanent brain damage are unusual, even if the decreases in Na concentration and ECF osmolality are large. Conversely, if hyponatremia is rapid in onset, cerebral edema and significant CNS symptoms and signs can occur with lesser changes in serum Na concentration.

When treating a patient with hyponatremia, the Na concentration should be raised at the rate at which it fell (Table 3). In a patient whose serum Na concentration has fallen slowly, neurologic symptoms are generally minimal, brain size is normal, and the number of intracellular osmoles is decreased. Sudden return of ECF osmolality to normal values will lead to cell shrinkage, neurologic symptoms, and possible permanent brain damage. Specifically, rapid correction has been associated with central pontine myelinolysis. Thus, it is recommended that the serum Na concentration be corrected slowly in these patients. In a patient whose serum Na concentration has decreased rapidly, neurologic symptoms are frequently present, as is cerebral edema. In this setting, insufficient time has passed to remove osmoles from the brain, and rapid return to normal ECF osmolality merely returns brain size to normal. In general, the development of hyponatremia in the outpatient setting is more commonly chronic in duration and should be corrected slowly. By contrast, hyponatremia of short duration is more likely to be encountered in hospitalized patients receiving intravenous free water. In symptomatic patients, rapid correction may be necessary. The unusual patient with psychogenic polydipsia can also develop hyponatremia that is of short duration and, if symptomatic, may similarly require rapid correction.

Rapid Correction of Hyponatremia

In patients with acute hyponatremia and who are demonstrating CNS signs or symptoms, rapid correction is indicated. Rapid correction of hyponatremia involves intravenous administration of hypertonic saline (usually 3% NaCl). Generally, an infusion rate is used that will raise the serum Na concentration at a rate of 1 mEq/L/hr. Evidence suggests that correction at a more rapid rate may be dangerous. To calculate the amount of Na required, one should use a volume of distribution of total body water (TBW). Although Na is confined to the ECF space, in disorders of osmolality, an osmolar deficit present throughout the total body water is being replaced:

$$(\text{Desired Na} - \text{Actual Na}) \times \text{TBW} = \text{Amount of Na required.}$$

TABLE 2 Drugs Associated with Hyponatremia According to Major Mechanism of Action

Stimulate ADH Release
  Chlorpropamide
  Clofibrate
  Cyclophosphamide
  Vincristine
  Carbamazepine
  Amitriptyline
  Thiothixene, haloperidol, thioridazine
Potentiation of ADH Effect on Kidney
  Chlorpropamide
  Carbamazepine
  Nonsteroidal anti-inflammatory drugs
  Cyclophosphamide
ADH-like Action
  Oxytocin
  Deamino-D-arginine vasopressin (DDAVP)

Abbreviation: ADH = antidiuretic hormone.

TABLE 1 Disorders Associated with Syndrome of Inappropriate Secretion of Antidiuretic Hormone

Tumors
  Oat cell carcinoma
  Adenocarcinoma of the pancreas
  Hodgkin's disease
  Thymoma
Pulmonary Diseases
  Tuberculosis
  Lung abscess
  Viral and bacterial pneumonia
Central Nervous System Disorders
  Brain tumor
  Encephalitis
  Subarachnoid hemorrhage
  Acute intermittent porphyria

TABLE 3 Treatment of Hyponatremia According to Volume Status and Rapidity of Development

Correction	Low Extracellular Fluid Volume	Edematous State	Euvolemic
Acute Onset			
Slow	Normal saline	Fluid restriction	Fluid restriction
Rapid	Hypertonic saline	Hypertonic saline + furosemide	Hypertonic saline + furosemide
Chronic	Remove cause	• Remove cause	• Remove cause
		• Demeclocycline 600–1200 mg/day	• Discontinue drug
		• Vasopressin receptor antagonist (conivaptan)	• Glucocorticoid or thyroid hormone replacement
			• Treat cause of syndrome of inappropriate secretion of antidiuretic hormone

Assume a patient presents with a serum Na concentration of 110 mEq/L, has symptoms of stupor, and demonstrates seizure activity. In order to raise his serum Na concentration to 130 mEq/L, one can calculate the amount of 3% saline needed.

$$\text{Total body water (TBW)} = 70 \text{ kg} \times 60\% = 42 \text{ L}$$

$$(130 \text{ mEq/L} - 110 \text{ mEq/L}) \times 42 \text{ L} = 840 \text{ mEq Na}$$

As each liter of 3% saline contains 513 mEq of Na, one would administer 1.6 L of 3% NaCl over 20 hours in order to raise the serum Na concentration by 1 mEq/L/hr.

Use of hypertonic saline alone may be associated with volume expansion that would be dangerous in the elderly or in patients with compromised cardiac function. Patients with impaired renal function are particularly prone to volume overload with such Na loads. In this instance, a furosemide (Lasix) diuresis can be used. Hypertonic saline is infused at a rate equal to the urinary loss of Na, chloride, and potassium that is induced by furosemide.

In order to calculate the total net negative fluid balance necessary to achieve the desired Na concentration, one can use the following formulas:

$$\text{Body weight} \times 60\% = \text{Total body water (TBW)}$$
$$\text{or } 70 \text{ kg} \times 60\% = 42 \text{ L}$$

$$\text{TBW} - (\text{Actual [Na]/Desired [Na]}) \times \text{TBW} =$$
$$\text{Amount of excess water or } 42 - (110/130) \times 42 = 6.5 \text{ L}$$

When a serum Na concentration of 130 mEq/L is obtained, one can simply place the patient on fluid restriction. In this manner, neurologic sequelae resulting from rapid correction of the serum Na concentration can be avoided. It should be emphasized that these formulas are to be used as guidelines only, and that frequent monitoring of the patient and of the serum Na concentration are needed during these rapid changes in fluid balance.

In December 2005, the first AVP receptor antagonist (conivaptan [Vaprisol]) was approved for treatment of euvolemic hyponatremia. Conivaptan is initiated with a 20-mg intravenous loading dose, followed by 20 mg administered as a continuous infusion. Concurrent use of drugs metabolized by the hepatic microsomal enzyme system CYP3A4 should be avoided because of the potential for increased plasma concentrations of the coadministered drug.

REFERENCES

Adrogue HJ, Madias NE: Hyponatremia. N Engl J Med 2000;342: 1581-1589.
Palmer BF: Hyponatremia in patients with central nervous system disease: SIADH or CSW. Trends Endocrinol Metab 2003;14:182-187.
Palmer BF, Gates JR, Lader M: Causes and management of hyponatremia. Ann Pharmacother 2003;37:1694-1702.
Spital A: Diuretic–induced hyponatremia. Am J Nephrol 1999;19:447-452.

Gout and Hyperuricemia

Method of
Robert L. Wortmann, MD

Hyperuricemia is a term representing an elevated level of urate in the blood. This occurs in an absolute (or physiochemical) sense when the serum urate concentration exceeds its limit of solubility in the serum, or above approximately 6.8 mg/dL at 37°C (99°F). At values greater than this, body fluids are supersaturated with urate, a condition with the potential for urate crystal formation and deposition in body tissues. Hyperuricemia can be classified as primary or secondary (Table 1).

The term *gout* represents a heterogeneous group of disorders that includes hyperuricemia; recurrent attacks of acute, typically monoarticular arthritis, in which monosodium urate crystals are demonstrable in synovial fluid having provoked an acute inflammatory response; aggregates of sodium urate monohydrate crystals (tophi) deposited chiefly in and around joints, which can lead to deformity and crippling as a result of a chronic inflammatory reaction; renal disease involving glomerular, tubular, and interstitial tissues and blood vessels; and uric acid urolithiasis. These manifestations can occur in various combinations.

Epidemiology

Hyperuricemia is fairly common with a prevalence ranging between 2.3% and 41.4% in various populations. A variety of factors appear to be associated with higher serum urate concentrations. In adults, serum urate levels correlate

TABLE 1 Classification of Hyperuricemia

Primary
Idiopathic (molecular defects undefined)
Urate overproduction (<5%)
Uric acid underexcretion (>95%)

Secondary
Urate overproduction
Molecular defects
Hypoxanthine phosphoribosyltransferase deficiency
Phosphoribosyl pyrophosphate synthase overactivity
Glucose-6-phosphatase deficiency
Fructose-1-phosphate aldolase deficiency
Associated with accelerated ATP or nucleotide degradation
Tumor lysis syndrome
Hypoxia
Chronic alcohol use
Myeloproliferative disorder
Associated with decreased renal excretion of uric acid
Molecular defects
Familial juvenile hyperuricemic nephropathy
Familial polycystic kidney disease
Renal insufficiency
Lead intoxication
Hypothyroidism
Drugs
Diuretics
Low-dose salicylates
Pyrazinamide
Nicotinic acid
Ethambutol
Cyclosporine
Volume contraction
Acidosis
Starvation
Alcoholic ketosis
Diabetic ketoacidosis
Lactic acidosis

strongly with serum creatinine, diuretic use, body weight, age, blood pressure, and alcohol (particularly beer) intake. Hyperuricemia is present in individuals with metabolic syndrome (a cluster of abnormalities that includes resistance to insulin-stimulated glucose uptake, hyperinsulinemia, hypertension, and dyslipoproteinemia with high levels of plasma triglycerides and is associated with increased cerebrovascular disease, cardiovascular disease, and cardiovascular mortality).

The incidence of gout, which varies in populations with an overall prevalence of less than 1% to 15.3%, appears to be increasing. Gout is very rare in premenopausal women but develops in equal frequency with men after 60 years of age. The prevalence of gout seems to increase substantially with age and increasing serum urate concentrations. The annual incidence rate of gout is 0.5% for values between 7 and 8.9 mg/dL and 4.9% for urate levels greater than 9 mg/dL. For serum urate values greater than 9 mg/dL and 10 mg/dL, the cumulative incidence of gout reaches 22% and 30% after 5 years, respectively.

Clinical Features

The first attack of gouty arthritis typically follows a period of asymptomatic hyperuricemia that has been present

CURRENT DIAGNOSIS

- The only way to diagnose gout definitively is by the identification of needle-shaped, negatively birefringent monosodium urate crystals in aspirants of synovial fluid or tophaceous deposits.

for at least 15 years. The initial attack is usually intensely painful and associated with warmth, swelling, and erythema; monarticular; and associated with few constitutional symptoms. Attacks vary in duration but are time limited. The intervals between attacks are asymptomatic and are termed *intercritical* (or *interval*) *gout*. Over time, attacks recur at shorter intervals, last longer, become polyarticular, and eventually resolve incompletely. This leads to the development of chronic arthritis that progresses slowly to a crippling disease on which acute flares are superimposed.

Diagnosis of Gout

The definitive diagnosis of gout is established by aspiration of a joint or tophus and identification of intracellular needle-shaped crystals that have negative birefringence with compensated polarized light microscopy. Crystals can be identified in fluid aspirated at the time of an acute flare or after signs of inflammation have resolved.

Criteria have been proposed for the presumptive diagnosis of gout. These include, first, the triad of acute monarticular arthritis, hyperuricemia, and a dramatic response to colchicine therapy, and second, criteria proposed by the American College of Rheumatology (Table 2). Finally, some believe they can diagnose gout based on the characteristic clinical picture. Unfortunately, there are limitations to these methods. First, although the diagnosis of acute gouty arthritis can be strongly suggested by a typical presentation, not all inflammation of the great toe (podagra) in hyperuremic patients is caused by gout. Second, some

TABLE 2 Criteria for the Classification for Acute Gouty Arthritis

- The presence of characteristic urate crystals in the joint fluid, or
- A tophus proved to contain urate crystals by chemical means or polarized light microscopy, or
- The presence of 6 of the following 12 clinical, laboratory, and X-ray phenomena:
  - More than one attack of acute arthritis
  - Maximal inflammation developed within 1 day
  - Attack of monarticular arthritis
  - Joint redness observed
  - First metatarsophalangeal joint painful or swollen
  - Unilateral attack involving first metatarsophalangeal joint
  - Unilateral attack involving tarsal joint
  - Suspected tophus
  - Hyperuricemia
  - Asymmetric swelling within a joint (radiograph)
  - Subcortical cysts without erosions (radiograph)
  - Negative culture of joint fluid for microorganisms during attack of joint

patients with gout are normouricemic at the time of an acute attack, a phenomenon related to alcohol use or a consequence of IL-6 generation by the acute inflammatory process. Furthermore, diseases other than gout may improve with colchicine therapy. These include pseudogout, hydroxyapatite calcific tendinitis, sarcoid arthritis, erythema nodosum, serum sickness, rheumatoid arthritis, and familial Mediterranean fever. Finally, gout and septic arthritis can occur simultaneously, with the former masking the latter.

Treatment of Acute Gout

The therapeutic aims in gout are to terminate the acute attack as promptly and gently as possible; to prevent and reverse complications of the disease resulting from deposition of sodium urate or uric acid crystals in joints, kidneys, or other sites; and to treat associated features such as hypertension, obesity, hypertriglyceridemia, and alcoholism.

The acute gouty attack can be successfully terminated by any of several agents. For practical purposes, the choice is among colchicine, a nonsteroidal anti-inflammatory drug (NSAID), or a corticosteroid preparation. The time of initiation of therapy is more important than which agent is used. The sooner the agent is started, the more rapid the response.

Colchicine is generally preferred for patients in whom the diagnosis of gout is not confirmed because of its relative specificity against crystal-induced inflammation. NSAIDs are preferred when the diagnosis is secure. If a patient cannot take medications by mouth or has active peptic ulcer disease, the choice is among intra-articular glucocorticoid or parenteral glucocorticoids, intramuscular corticotropin,[1] or intravenous colchicine. Local application of ice packs may help control the pain of an acute attack. In some cases, analgesics, including narcotics, may be added as well. Drugs that affect serum urate concentrations, including antihyperuricemic agents, should not be

---

[1]Not FDA approved for this indication.

CURRENT THERAPY

- To terminate the acute attack as promptly and gently as possible: Initiate therapy with an NSAID, colchicine, corticosteroid or corticotropin[1] as soon after symptoms begin as possible.
- To prevent recurrences of acute gouty arthritis: Use an NSAID or colchicine in low doses to prophylax against subsequent attacks.
- To prevent or reverse complications of the disease resulting from deposition of sodium urate or uric acid crystals in joints, kidneys, or other sites: Maintain the serum urate concentration at levels below 5–6 mg/dL with xanthine oxidase inhibitors or uricosuric agents.
- To prevent or reverse associated features of the illness such as hypertension, obesity, hypertriglyceridemia, and alcoholism.

[1]Not FDA approved for this indication.
Abbreviation: NSAID = nonsteroidal anti-inflammatory drug.

---

changed (either initiated or discontinued) during an acute attack because sudden fluctuations in serum urate levels, which can precipitate acute attacks, render attacks in progress substantially worse.

COLCHICINE

Colchicine can be administered by oral or intravenous routes. Orally, a dose of 0.5 or 0.6 mg is taken hourly until one of three things occurs: signs of inflammation ease; nausea, vomiting, or diarrhea develops; or 10 doses have been taken. If 10 doses are taken without benefit, one should question the accuracy of the diagnosis. Colchicine has a low therapeutic index with steady-state plasma concentrations after acute treatment ranging between 0.5 and 3.0 μg/mL and with toxic effects occurring at approximately 3 μg/mL. Therefore, in most patients, the gastrointestinal side effects precede or coincide with improvement in joint symptoms. The drug must be stopped promptly at the first sign of gastrointestinal side effects.

Colchicine can also be given intravenously but should be done so with caution. If not used properly, intravenous colchicine is associated with significant risk of bone marrow depression and death. In addition, local extravasation during or immediately after injection causes tissue necrosis and extreme pain. The drug should not be given to patients who are neutropenic or to those with significant liver or renal disease.

When used properly, the drug abolishes the acute attack with a low incidence of gastrointestinal side effects (provided that the patient is not also taking colchicine by mouth). An initial dose of 1 or 2 mg can be followed by one or two additional 1-mg doses administered at 6-hour intervals thereafter if needed. The total dose of intravenous colchicine should not exceed 4 mg. The colchicine should be diluted with 20 mL of normal saline before administration and given slowly into an established venous access to minimize sclerosis of the vein. In addition, oral colchicine should be discontinued and no additional colchicine should be given for at least 7 days because of slow excretion of this drug.

NONSTEROIDAL ANTI-INFLAMMATORY DRUGS

In the patient with an established diagnosis of uncomplicated gout, an NSAID is the agent of choice. Indomethacin (Indocin) has been the traditional choice of agents in this class. Although this drug may be effective in doses as low as 25 mg given four times a day, an initial dose of 50 to 75 mg, followed by 50 mg every 6 to 8 hours with a maximum dose of 200 mg in the first 24 hours, is generally recommended. To prevent relapse, it is reasonable to continue this dose for an additional 24 hours, then taper to 25 to 50 mg every 8 hours for the next 2 days. Clinical trials also showed that oral naproxen (Naprosyn), fenoprofen (Nalfon), ibuprofen (Motrin), sulindac (Clinoril), piroxicam (Feldene), and ketoprofen (Orudis) as well as intramuscular ketorolac (Toradol) are effective. In fact, all members of this family of drugs can be highly effective in the treatment of acute gouty arthritis including the COX-2 selective agents. For an acute flare, the NSAID selected should generally be prescribed at the highest approved dosage.

GLUCOCORTICOIDS AND CORTICOTROPIN

Intra-articular glucocorticoids are useful in the treatment of acute gout limited to a single joint or bursa. Oral glucocorticoid usage as well as a single intramuscular or intravenous injection of a parenteral glucocorticoid can also provide relief. Anecdotally, rebound attacks have been reported as steroids were withdrawn. Intramuscular injections of corticotropin may be highly effective as well.

Prophylaxis

Unfortunately, the sudden lowering of serum urate concentrations that accompanies initiation of urate-lowering therapy often triggers acute gout attacks. This risk is reduced if the urate-lowering agent is started at a low dose and increased weekly in small increments until the appropriate urate-lowering effect is achieved (see later). In addition, giving small daily doses of colchicine as prophylaxis is 85% effective in preventing acute attacks. The use of colchicine at 0.6 mg once to three times a day is generally well tolerated, although it may produce a reversible axonal neuromyopathy. Rhabdomyolysis may also occur in these settings. In patients who are unable to tolerate even one colchicine tablet per day, indomethacin (Indocin), or another NSAID, is used prophylactically at low doses (e.g., indomethacin, 25 mg two times per day) with some success. Prophylaxis should be started 2 weeks before initiating the urate-lowering agent and usually continued until the serum urate value is maintained well within the normal range and there have been no acute attacks for 3 to 6 months. It is important to warn patients that colchicine discontinuation may be followed by an exacerbation of acute gouty arthritis and advise them what to do should an attack occur. Finally, prophylactic treatment is not recommended unless one also uses urate-lowering agents. Prophylactic colchicine may block the acute inflammatory response but does not alter the deposition of crystals in tissues. With continued deposition without the warning signs of recurrent bouts of acute arthritis, tophi and destruction to cartilage and bone can occur without notice.

Reversing the Hyperuricemia

Elimination of hyperuricemia can prevent as well as reverse urate deposition. Opinions vary as to when in the course of gout antihyperuricemic therapy should be initiated. Some regard the first gouty attack as a late event in a disorder marked by years of antecedent silent deposition of urate crystals. Others believe the patient should have had two or three attacks because it may be many years before a second attack occurs.

Regardless, once initiated, the goal is to reduce the serum urate concentration to 6.0 mg/dL or less, well below the concentration at which monosodium urate saturates extracellular fluid. Because of the physiochemistry of urate, lowering the serum urate level from 10 or 11 mg/dL to 7.5 or 8 mg/dL does not reverse the process of urate deposition; it only retards the rate at which it continues. When a level of 6 mg/dL or lower is achieved, urate deposits resolve. The lower the serum urate level achieved, the faster the reduction in tophaceous deposits. Reduction to

target levels may be achieved pharmacologically by the use of xanthine oxidase inhibitors or uricosuric agents. Xanthine oxidase inhibitors can successfully lower serum urate levels in individuals whose hyperuricemia is the result of either urate overproduction or uric acid underexcretion. Uricosuric agents are only effective in the latter situation. Whereas the uricosuric agents lose their efficacy with decreasing renal function and are contraindicated in patients with a history of urolithiasis, xanthine oxidase inhibitors can be used under those conditions. Once initiated, the antihyperuricemic agent is generally continued indefinitely.

XANTHINE OXIDASE INHIBITORS

Allopurinol (Zyloprim) is also a substrate for xanthine oxidase and is converted to oxypurinol by that enzyme activity. Oxypurinol is also an inhibitor of xanthine oxidase. Allopurinol is metabolized in the liver and has a half-life of 1 to 3 hours, but oxypurinol, which is excreted in the urine, has a half-life of 12 to 17 hours. Because of these pharmacokinetic properties, allopurinol is dosed on a daily basis, and the dosage required to achieve target serum urate levels is usually lower in patients with decreased glomerular filtration rates. The most commonly prescribed dose of allopurinol is 300 mg per day, but a maximum of 800 mg can be used.

Approximately 20% of patients who take allopurinol report side effects, with 5% of patients discontinuing the medication. More common side effects include gastrointestinal intolerance and skin rashes. The occurrence of a rash does not necessarily mean the drug should be discontinued. If the rash is not severe, the allopurinol can be held temporarily and resumed after the rash clears. Oral and intravenous protocols for desensitization to allopurinol are successful for some patients following cutaneous reactions.

Other adverse reactions include fever, toxic epidermal necrolysis, alopecia, bone marrow suppression with leukopenia or thrombocytopenia, agranulocytosis, aplastic anemia, granulomatous hepatitis, jaundice, sarcoid-like reaction, and vasculitis. The most severe reaction is the allopurinol hypersensitivity syndrome that consists of a constellation of findings and may include fever, skin rash, eosinophilia, hepatitis, progressive renal insufficiency, and death.

Allopurinol is involved in relatively few drug-drug interactions. The most important of these are azathioprine (Imuran) and 6-mercaptopurine (Purinethol). Rash may be more common in patients using allopurinol and ampicillin, and bone marrow suppression may be increased in those also taking cyclophosphamide (Cytoxan).

Phase III clinical trials have been completed with febuxostat,[4] a potent new selective inhibitor of xanthine oxidase that has a chemical structure entirely different from that of allopurinol. In phase II clinical trials, febuxostat doses of 40, 80, and 120 mg successfully lowered serum urate levels below 6.0 mg/dL in 56%, 76%, and 94% of subjects, respectively. In a phase III trial, target serum urates were reached in 53% and 62% of subjects taking febuxostat, 80 and 120 mg, respectively, compared to 21% of patients taking 300 mg of allopurinol. In a phase III trial,

---

[4]Not yet approved for use in the United States.

the side-effect profile for febuxostat and allopurinol were similar. No cases of hypersensitivity have been reported with the use of febuxostat. It appears that febuxostat is an excellent alternative for patients who cannot tolerate allopurinol. In addition, there is no need for dosage adjustment of febuxostat in patients with mild to moderate renal or hepatic dysfunction.

URICOSURIC AGENTS

A uricosuric agent increases the rate of renal uric acid excretion. Probenecid (Benemid) and sulfinpyrazone (Anturane) are the most widely used uricosuric agents available in the United States; benzbromarone is used for this purpose in other countries as well.

Probenecid is readily absorbed from the gastrointestinal tract. Its half-life in plasma is dose dependent, varying from 6 to 12 hours. The maintenance dosage of probenecid ranges from 500 mg to 3 g per day and is administered on a two or three times a day schedule. With long-term use, up to 18% of individuals develop gastrointestinal complaints and 5% develop hypersensitivity and rash. Although serious toxicity is rare, approximately a third of individuals eventually become intolerant of probenecid and discontinue its use.

Sulfinpyrazone is completely absorbed from the gastrointestinal tract and has a half-life of 1 to 3 hours. Sulfinpyrazone is usually maintained at a daily dosage of 300 to 400 mg per day given in three to four divided doses. The rates of tolerability and types of adverse reactions are similar to those with probenecid.

Benzbromarone[2] is more potent than probenecid and sulfinpyrazone. It is well tolerated and effective in cyclosporine-treated renal transplant patients. It can be used with moderate renal dysfunction (creatine clearance below 25 mL/minute). Severe hepatic toxicity is reported with its use.

Treatment Failures

Failure of urate-lowering agents to attain the target urate level is related to improper prescribing or poor compliance. At least half of the patients who use the standard dose of allopurinol, 300 mg/day, fail to attain serum urate levels below the target of 6.0 mg/dL. Higher doses clearly are required in many individuals. Compliance is often a problem when treating chronic asymptomatic conditions, and associated alcoholism can be a factor. Rarely, the tophaceous load (total body urate pool) is so large that the serum urate target can be reached only when using both a xanthine oxidase inhibitor and a uricosuric agent in combination.

Management of Gout in Patients with Organ Transplants

The management of patients with gout after organ transplantation requires careful consideration. Colchicine and NSAIDs may be inappropriate for management of acute gouty arthritis in this setting. Intra-articular glucocorticoid

---

[2]Not available in the United States.

---

or intramuscular corticotropin injections may be most helpful, and one may be forced to rely more heavily on the use of pain medications in this setting. Prophylactic colchicine can be used in patients with normal renal function, but treatment must be monitored closely. The combination of colchicine and cyclosporine has induced rhabdomyolysis.

Allopurinol can be used in patients with abnormal renal function, but the dose may need to be reduced. Allopurinol, however, has a potential severe interaction with azathioprine. If care is not taken, significant bone marrow toxicity can result. If azathioprine and allopurinol are used together, they can be started at 25 and 50 mg per day, respectively. Complete blood counts and serum urate levels are then monitored weekly, and the allopurinol dose is adjusted to bring the serum urate concentration to less than 6 mg/dL. Mycophenolate mofetil (CellCept), as an alternative to azathioprine, is used effectively with allopurinol in some transplant patients.

Ancillary Factors

In addition to anti-inflammatory agents, colchicine prophylaxis, and urate-lowering therapy, other factors may be decisive in determining whether recurrent attacks, chronic gouty arthritis, stone, or nephropathy develops. Today, dietary purine restriction solely to control serum urate levels is rarely necessary. In addition, the antihyperuricemic agents available today are so effective, if prescribed properly, that one rarely needs to resort to this kind of dietary manipulation. Nevertheless, beneficial results are reported with a diet of moderate calorie and carbohydrate restriction and increased proportional intake of protein and unsaturated fat.

In addition, diet is very important with regard to other medical problems. Many gouty patients are overweight, and restoration of ideal body weight through regulated caloric restriction is recommended. In addition, at least 75% of patients with primary gout have hypertriglyceridemia, and many patients with gout consume liberal amounts of alcohol. These issues should be addressed. Approximately a third of gouty subjects are hypertensive. The complications of hypertension are potentially more serious than those of hyperuricemia, and one should not hesitate to use whatever drugs are necessary to control the hypertension. Many hypertensive gouty patients require a thiazide diuretic. If this medication is needed to control hypertension, it should be used, with the recognition that the dosage of concomitant antihyperuricemic therapy may need to be adjusted to maintain appropriate control of serum urate levels. Because they possess mild uricosuric properties, fenofibrate (TriCor) may be a good choice for gout patients with abnormal lipids, and losartan (Cozaar) may be appropriate for those with hypertension.

Asymptomatic Hyperuricemia

The association of hyperuricemia with the manifestations of atherosclerosis has led to speculation that hyperuricemia is a risk factor for coronary artery disease. However, until that is demonstrated, it is recommended that the presence of hyperuricemia not be an indication for specific antihyperuricemic drug therapy. Rather, the finding of asymptomatic hyperuricemia should lead one to determine if an underlying and potentially reversible cause can be identified and to treat any associated conditions such as hypertension, obesity, lipid abnormalities, diabetes, and alcoholism.

REFERENCES

Becker MA, Schumacher HR, Wortmann RL, et al: Febuxostat compared with allopurinol in patients with hyperuricemia and gout. N Engl J Med 2005;353(23):2450-2461.

Choi HK, Atkinson K, Karlson EW, et al: Alcohol intake and risk of incident gout in men: A prospective study. Lancet 2004;363: 1277-1281.

Fam AG: Difficult gout and new approaches for control of hyperuricemia in the allopurinol–allergic patient. Curr Rheumatol Rep 2001;3: 29-35.

Mikuls TR, MacLean CH, Olivieri J, et al: Quality of care indicators for gout management. Arthritis Rheum 2004;50:937-943.

Perez-Ruiz F, Calabozo M, Herrero-Beites AM, et al: Improvement in renal function in patients with chronic gout after proper control of hyperuricemia and gouty bouts. Nephron 2000;86:287-291.

Perez-Ruiz F, Calabozo M, Pijoan JI, et al: Effect of urate-lowering therapy on the velocity of size reduction of tophi in chronic gout. Arthritis Rheum (Arthritis Care Res) 2002;47:356-360.

Shoji A, Yamanaka H, Kamatani N: A retrospective study of the relationship between serum urate level and recurrent attacks of gouty arthritis: Evidence for reduction of recurrent gouty arthritis with antihyperuricemic therapy. Arthritis Rheum (Arthritis Care Res) 2004;51:321-325.

Stamp L, Gow P, Sharples K, Raill B: The optimal use of allopurinol use in South Auckland. Aust N Z J Med 2000;30:567-572.

Wallace KL, Riedel AA, Joseph-Ridge N, Wortmann RL: Increased prevalence of gout and hyperuricemia over 10 years among older adults in a managed care population. J Rheumatol 2004;31:1582-1587.

Dyslipoproteinemias

Method of
Peter P. Toth, MD, PhD

The complications of atherosclerotic disease remain the number one cause of death and disability for men and women in industrialized nations. Atherosclerosis is a complex, chronic disease with a multifactorial etiology. Considerable investigation demonstrates an unequivocal relationship between disturbances in cholesterol and lipoprotein metabolism and risk for atherogenesis within the coronary, peripheral, renal, and cerebral vasculature. Dyslipoproteinemias frequently develop in response to genetic and environmental factors and are modifiable through pharmacologic intervention and lifestyle charges. As demonstrated in the Framingham Study, Multiple Risk Factor Intervention Trial and the Seven Countries Study, when serum levels of cholesterol increase, the lifetime risk for developing coronary artery disease (CAD) rises steadily. Consequently, cholesterol is one of the most important endogenous and exogenous toxins that humans are exposed to. The identification and aggressive management of dyslipidemias in both the primary and secondary prevention settings is pivotal to continued efforts to significantly reduce the prevalence of atherosclerotic disease and its clinical sequelae in populations throughout the world.

Lipoprotein Metabolism and Atherogenesis

Although it is pathogenic, cholesterol is also a critical modulator of cell membrane fluidity and is a precursor for steroid hormone biosynthesis. Consequently, a pool of cholesterol must be available for a variety of physiologic functions. Cholesterol, monoglycerides, free fatty acids, and phospholipids are absorbed from micelles in the intestinal lumen via a series of translocators located within the brush border of jejunal enterocytes. Absorbed cholesterol and lipid are assimilated with apolipoprotein (apo) B48 into chylomicrons. Chylomicrons are released into the lymph and ultimately transported to the central circulation via the thoracic duct. In serum, the triglycerides in chylomicrons are hydrolyzed by lipoprotein lipase. This lipolytic reaction produces chylomicron remnant particles that are taken up by the low-density lipoprotein (LDL) receptor-related protein and metabolized by the liver. The liver secretes very-low-density lipoprotein (VLDL), a lipoprotein enriched with triglycerides, cholesterol, and apoprotein B100. As the triglycerides in VLDL are hydrolyzed by lipoprotein lipase, the size of the lipoprotein particle decreases, eventually forming LDL. LDL particles are concentrated with cholesterol and cholesterol esters and relatively depleted of triglycerides. As the VLDL is progressively converted to LDL, it releases constituents from its surface coat (apoproteins AI, AII, and phospholipids) that are used to form high-density lipoprotein (HDL) in serum.

Patients with hypertriglyceridemia can have elevations in either serum chylomicron or VLDL levels, or both. Patients who consume very high fat diets or who are hyperabsorbers of dietary fat can be hyperchylomicronemic. In contrast, patients with excessive fat storage depots (most notably visceral adiposity) can develop elevated VLDL. Naturally occurring mutations in lipoprotein lipase and an insulin-resistant state can yield hypertriglyceridemia secondary to reduced lipolysis of chylomicrons and VLDL. Reduced lipolysis results in the formation of incompletely digested chylomicrons and VLDL, or "remnant particles" that are widely believed to be atherogenic. Patients with hypertriglyceridemia tend to have reduced serum levels of HDL because:

- There is a decreased release of surface coat constituents from chylomicrons and VLDL.
- As HDL becomes progressively more enriched with triglyceride, it becomes a better substrate for hepatic lipase, an enzyme that catabolizes HDL.

Serum VLDL remnant particles and LDL function as delivery vehicles of cholesterol to peripheral tissues, including blood vessel walls. These lipoproteins are atherogenic because they can traverse the endothelial cell barrier. Macrophages resident within the subendothelial space exposed to LDL oxidized by such enzymes as lipoxygenase or myeloperoxidase upregulate the expression of scavenger receptors (SR-A, CD-36) on their surface and actively take up excessive amounts of cholesterol. This process promotes foam cell and fatty streak development—events that precede atheromatous plaque formation.

The activation of macrophages also promotes an inflammatory response with the elaboration of cytokines, interleukins, C-reactive protein, cell mitogens, matrix metalloproteinases, and reactive oxygen species that facilitate lesion progression and instability. LDL and VLDL remnants not taken up by peripheral tissues can be cleared from the circulation by hepatic LDL receptors. Therapies targeted at the upregulation of hepatic LDL receptors are antiatherogenic by virtue of their ability to reduce circulating levels of atherogenic lipoproteins.

HDL particles appear to protect the vasculature from progressive injury and atherogenesis. With few exceptions, in prospective epidemiologic and case-control studies conducted throughout the world, high HDL levels are protective against the development of CAD. For instance, patients with familial hypoalphalipoproteinemia (low HDL) have increased risk for premature CAD, whereas patients with familial hyperalphalipoproteinemia are relatively resistant to atherosclerotic disease. In contrast to LDL, which promotes cholesterol delivery to, and uptake by, vessel wall macrophages, HDL extracts excess cellular cholesterol and delivers it back to the liver for elimination through the gastrointestinal tract in a process referred to as "reverse cholesterol transport." HDL does the following:

- Reduces endothelial cell adhesion molecule (vascular cell adhesion molecule-1, intercellular adhesion molecule-1) expression
- Augments endothelial nitric oxide and prostacyclin production
- Reduces oxidized fatty acid components of LDL
- Decreases platelet aggregability
- Inhibits endothelial cell apoptosis

Recent studies suggest that among the elderly, low HDL is a better predictor of risk for cardiovascular disease than is high LDL. An HDL greater than 60 mg/dL is a negative risk factor. The higher the level of serum HDL, the lower the risk for CAD. Therapeutic maneuvers should not be undertaken to reduce circulating levels of HDL.

Identification of Lipoprotein Targets

Dyslipoproteinemias constitute a highly prevalent and heterogeneous class of disorders. Derangements in circulating levels of specific lipoprotein classes can be the result of abnormalities in gastrointestinal absorption, enzyme activities, and/or receptor expression. A complete fasting (12 to 14 hours) lipoprotein profile should be obtained from any patient being evaluated for dyslipidemia. Because of the relationship between specific lipoprotein fractions and risk for CAD, a total cholesterol level has little practical clinical utility.

The National Cholesterol Education Program Adult Treatment Panel III (NCEP ATPIII) has systematically defined risk-stratified target levels for atherogenic serum lipoproteins based on the best available evidence to date (Table 1). Risk stratification is performed by evaluating a patient's cardiovascular risk factor burden (number of risk factors) and, if two or more risk factors are present, calculation of the Framingham risk score. Among patients being treated for primary prevention, low risk is defined as a 0-1 risk factor. Moderate and moderately high risk are defined as 2 or more risk factors and a 10-year Framingham risk of less than 10% and 10% to 20%, respectively. In the high-risk category, patients either have CAD (defined as a history of myocardial infarction [MI], stable/unstable angina, revascularization with coronary artery bypass grafting, or percutaneous angioplasty) or a CAD risk equivalent (defined as diabetes mellitus, peripheral vascular disease, significant carotid artery disease [transient ischemic attack or stroke from carotid origin or greater than 50% obstructive atheromatous plaque in a carotid artery], abdominal aortic aneurysm, and a 10-year Framingham risk that

TABLE 1 Low-density Lipoprotein Cholesterol Goals and Thresholds for Initiating Lifestyle Change and Pharmacologic Intervention

Risk Category*,†	LDLC Goal	LDLC Level at Which to Initiate TLC	LDLC Level at Which to Consider Drug Therapy
CHD or CHD risk equivalents (10-year risk >20%)	<100 mg/dL (optional goal <70 mg/dL)‡	≥100 mg/d all patients regardless of LDL	≥130 mg/dL (100-129 mg/dL: drug optional) ≥100 mg/d§ (<100 mg/dL: drug optional)
2+ risk factors (10-year risk 10%–20%)	<130 mg/dL (optional goal <100)	≥130 mg/d all patients regardless of LDL	≥130 mg/dL (<100 mg/dL: drug optional§)
2+ risk factors (10-year risk 5-10%)	<130 mg/dL	≥130 mg/dL	≥160 mg/dL
0-1 risk factor (10-year risk 0-5%)	<160 mg/dL	≥160 mg/dL	≥190 mg/dL (160-189 mg/dL: LDL-lowering drug optional)

Modified from Grundy SM, Cleeman JI, Merz CN, et al: Implications of recent clinical trials for the National Cholesterol Education Program Adult Treatment Panel III guidelines. Circulation 2004;110(2):227-239.
*CHD risk equivalents include diabetes mellitus, peripheral vascular disease, carotid artery disease, abdominal aortic aneurysm and 10 yr Framingham risk >201.
†Risk factors included in Framingham risk evaluation are age, systolic blood pressure, total cholesterol, HDLC, and smoking status.
‡The optional goal of <70 mg/dL is particularly targeted at patients who are "very high" risk, i.e., patients with a recent acute coronary syndrome, poorly controlled diabetics with multiple risk factors, etc.
§When initiating statin therapy in these patients, the goal for LDLC reduction should be 30% to 40% from baseline.
Abbreviations: CHD = coronary heart disease; HDLC = high-density lipoprotein cholesterol; LDLC = low-density lipoprotein cholesterol; TLC = therapeutic lifestyle change.

exceeds 20%). Among patients with multiple risk factors
and no history of CAD or a CAD risk equivalent, it is
important to calculate the Framingham risk score so as to
differentiate moderate, moderately high, and high risk. An
electronic version of a Framingham risk calculator for men
and women can be downloaded at www.nhlbi.nih.gov/
guidelines/cholesterol. Risk factors recognized by NCEP
are summarized in Box 1.

In ATPIII, the NCEP also instituted the following
important changes:

- An optimal low-density lipoprotein cholesterol
  (LDLC) is defined as less than 100 mg/dL for all
  patients.
- An HDL less than 40 mg/dL is now defined as a
  categorical risk factor for CAD.
- It introduced target levels for non-high-density
  lipoprotein cholesterol (HDLC). Non-HDLC (total
  cholesterol – HDLC) is a measure of the burden of
  atherogenic lipoproteins in serum (LDL + VLDL).

The risk-stratified target for non-HDLC is the LDLC
target plus 30. LDLC remains the primary target of
antilipidemic therapy. However, in patients with baseline
triglyceride levels greater than 200 mg/dL, non-HDL is the
secondary priority for therapy.

Although it is well known by the majority of health care
providers that a patient with CAD or a CAD risk equivalent
should have an LDLC less than 100 mg/dL, a number of
studies show that only 18% to 25% of these patients actually attain this target. An increasing amount of clinical trial
evidence is demonstrating that, when it comes to LDLC
reduction and CAD, "the lower, the better." In a recent
addendum to ATPIII, the NCEP has suggested that physicians consider lowering LDLC to less than 70 mg/dL and
non-HDLC to less than 100 mg/dL in very high risk patients
(e.g., recent acute coronary syndrome or a diabetic with
multiple poorly controlled cardiovascular risk factors). Other
therapeutic options recommended by the ATP III include:

- Initiation of pharmacologic intervention and therapeutic lifestyle change if baseline LDLC is greater
  than 100 mg/dL in patients with moderately high and
  high risk.

- Among patients at high risk with baseline LDLC less
  than 100 mg/dL, further reduction of LDLC by 30%
  to 40% with medication.

Such stringent criteria for LDLC and non-HDLC
reduction require the institution of intensive lifestyle
and pharmacologic interventions to ensure therapeutic
success.

Therapeutic Lifestyle Change

Therapeutic lifestyle change (TLC) constitutes front-line
therapy for all patients at risk for CAD. It is recommended
that patients who smoke achieve smoking cessation.
Smoking is associated with endothelial cell dysfunction as
well as increased levels of oxidized LDLC and reduced
serum HDLC. The amount of daily ingested cholesterol
should not exceed 200 mg. The amount of saturated fat in
the diet should be less than 7%, and the total fat intake
should not exceed 25% to 35% of calories (Table 2).
The distribution of calories from other nutrients should be
as follows: 15% protein, 50% to 60% carbohydrates, 10%
polyunsaturated fat, and 20% monounsaturated fat.
Reductions in saturated fat and increased ingestion of
mono- and polyunsaturated fats are associated with reductions in serum LDLC. The ingestion of plant stanols and
viscous fiber reduce cholesterol absorption. Patients
should be encouraged to exercise for 20 to 30 minutes five
times weekly. Exercise facilitates weight loss, which helps
to relieve visceral adiposity and insulin resistance. These
changes are associated with reduced serum triglycerides
and elevations in HDLC.

Although many types of weight loss diets were introduced in recent years, the optimal long-term approach
to weight reduction and maintenance is for patients
to continue to exercise and restrict fat consumption to
within recommended ranges (Table 3). Consultation with a
dietitian increases the likelihood of success. For patients
who are morbidly obese, bariatric surgery is emerging as
an important therapeutic alternative when aggressive
lifestyle and pharmacologic interventions fail. Bariatric
surgery facilitates significant weight reduction and relieves
insulin resistance, reduces blood pressure, and improves

**TABLE 2 NCEP ATP III Criteria for
Diagnosing the Metabolic Syndrome***

Risk Factor	Defining Level
Abdominal Obesity	
Men	Waist > 40 inches
Women	Waist > 35 inches
Triglycerides	≥150 mg/dL
HDLC	
Men	<40 mg/dL
Women	<50 mg/dL
Blood Pressure	≥130/≥85 mm Hg
Fasting Glucose	≥100 mg/dL

*Patients having any three of the five risk factors meet criteria for the
    diagnosis of the metabolic syndrome.

TABLE 3 Dietary Recommendations for Therapeutic Lifestyle Change

Dietary Component	Recommendation Allowance
Polyunsaturated fat	Up to 10% of total calories
Monounsaturated fat	Up to 20% of total calories
Total fat	25%–35% of total calories
Carbohydrate	50%–60% of total calories
Dietary fiber	20–30 g/day
Protein	Approximately 15% of total calories
Dietary cholesterol	<200 mg/day

lipoprotein profiles. In the Swedish Obese Subjects Study, gastric bypass surgery was associated with a weight loss of 20 kg (44 lb) and decreased the incidence of new-onset type 2 diabetes mellitus by 81% compared to the usual standard of care over 8 years of follow-up. Once adequate weight loss is achieved, it can only be maintained if the patient remains in an isocaloric state through sustained lifestyle modification.

Therapeutic lifestyle change is a particularly important intervention in patients with the metabolic syndrome. Metabolic syndrome develops secondary to the effects of insulin resistance and obesity and is characterized by a set of five risk factors (Table 2). The diagnosis of metabolic syndrome is made when a patient has any three or more of these defining clinical features. Although the metabolic syndrome significantly increases risk for atherosclerotic disease and diabetes mellitus, it is not defined as a CAD risk equivalent. The Framingham risk score should be calculated on all of these patients. LDL and non-HDL goals should be defined by risk stratification. If triglycerides remain elevated (200 to 499 mg/dL) after the LDL goal is reached, then consideration is given to the addition of a triglyceride lowering drug. If triglycerides are greater than 500 mg/dL, patients should be treated aggressively with triglyceride-lowering medication and a very low fat diet with less than or equal to 15% of calories derived from fat to prevent the development of pancreatitis. Although the NCEP has not defined target levels for HDL, it is recommended that an effort be made to raise low HDL (<40 mg/dL in men, <50 mg/dL in women) through lifestyle modification and drug therapy. The Expert Group on HDL suggests that HDL be raised to greater than 40 mg/dL in patients at high risk or with metabolic syndrome. The American Diabetes Association recommends that HDL be raised to more than 40 mg/dL in diabetic men and to more than 50 mg/dL in diabetic women.

Pharmacologic Interventions

STATINS

The statins are reversible, competitive 3-hydroxy-3-methylglutaryl coenzyme A (HMG-CoA) reductase inhibitors. HMG-CoA reductase is the rate-limiting step for cholesterol biosynthesis. The statins provide the most potent means currently available by which to reduce serum levels of LDLC. In addition to reducing cholesterol biosynthesis, the statins augment the clearance of atherogenic apoB100-containing lipoproteins (VLDL, VLDL remnants, and LDL) by upregulating the expression of the LDL receptor on the surface of hepatocytes. These drugs stimulate apoA-I expression and hepatic HDL secretion secondary to weak peroxisomal proliferator-activated receptor-α (PPAR-α) agonism.

The statins exert benefit distinct from their ability to alter circulating levels of lipoproteins through their "pleiotropic effects." Statins inhibit the post-translational modification and activation of small G-proteins (Rho and Ras) by blocking the production of such isoprenoids as farnesyl-pyrophosphate and geranylgeranyl-pyrophosphate. This is associated with reductions in the production of a large number of atherogenic stimuli (C-reactive protein, reactive oxygen species, tissue factor, interleukins, adhesion molecules, monocyte chemoattract protein-1, angiotensin-II receptor, and endothelin-1), decreased platelet reactivity and smooth-cell proliferation, and a reversal of endothelial dysfunction, among other effects. Consequently, statins appear to modulate inflammation, oxidative status, vasodilation, thrombotic tendency, and the capacity of a variety of cell types in vessel walls to interact and drive atherogenesis.

The statins are highly efficacious medications. In a growing number of large-scale, placebo-controlled clinical trials, these agents significantly reduced rates of myocardial infarction, stroke, and coronary and all-cause mortality in both the primary and secondary prevention settings. Statins also decrease the frequency of stable and unstable angina and reduce the rate of atheromatous plaque progression and even stimulate some degree of plaque resorption. Statins reduce event rates in men and women, diabetics, smokers, hypertensives, as well as patients older than 70 years of age. Much of the risk reduction achieved with statin therapy is attributable to LDLC reduction. Studies now show that the greater the magnitude of LDLC reduction, the greater the reduction in risk for acute coronary events. The benefits of statin therapy are widely assumed to be a class effect.

Six different statins are currently available. These drugs differ by potency and a variety of pharmacokinetic properties. The specific choice of a statin is dictated by the magnitude of LDLC reduction required (baseline versus risk-stratified NCEP target). The LDLC reducing capacity of the statins is as follows:

1. Rosuvastatin (Crestor), 45% to 63% (5 to 40 mg daily)
2. Atorvastatin (Lipitor) 26% to 60% (10 to 80 mg daily)
3. Simvastatin (Zocor) 26% to 47% (10 to 80 mg daily)
4. Lovastatin (Mevacor) 21% to 42% (10 to 80 mg daily)
5. Fluvastatin (Lescol) 22% to 36% (10 to 80 mg daily)
6. Pravastatin (Pravachol) 22% to 34% (10 to 80 mg daily).

Each doubling of the statin dose yields an additional 6% reduction, on average, in serum LDLC (the rule of 6s). The statins provide dose-dependent reductions in serum triglyceride levels (typically 10% to 25%) and elevations in serum HDLC (2% to 14%). Atorvastatin has a tendency to be less and less effective at raising HDLC as the dose is titrated to higher levels. In patients with high baseline triglycerides (>300 mg/dL), the statins increase HDLC significantly more than in patients who are normotriglyceridemic. For instance, simvastatin and rosuvastatin can raise HDLC up to 18% and 22%, respectively, in these patients.

The statins have different pharmacokinetic profiles. Because of their relatively short half-lives (1 to 4 hours), lovastatin, pravastatin, fluvastatin, and simvastatin should be taken in the evening in order to intercept the peak activity of HMG-CoA-reductase that occurs around midnight. Atorvastatin and rosuvastatin can be taken at any time during the day because of their relatively long half-lives (approximately 14 and 19 hours, respectively). The coadministration of cytochrome P450 3A4 inhibitors (azole type antifungals [ketoconazole, itraconazole], HIV protease inhibitors, macrolide antibiotics [erythromycin, clarithromycin], nefazodone [serzone], more than 1 quart of grapefruit juice daily, and cyclosporine) with simvastatin, lovastatin, and atorvastatin should be avoided as these statins are dependent on this P450 isozyme for metabolism. Concomitant dosing can lead to increased risk for toxicity. The dose of simvastatin should not exceed 20 mg daily in patients receiving verapamil or amiodarone.

The benefits of statin therapy significantly outweigh the risks. Hepatotoxicity is defined as an alanine aminotransferase elevation greater than or equal to 3 times the upper limits of normal (ULN), on two occasions at least one month apart. The average risk of this on statin therapy approximates 1%, but risk increases as a function of dose. Mild elevations in serum transaminases are relatively common, and they tend to spontaneously resolve. If transaminitis or hepatotoxicity develops, statin therapy should be discontinued until transaminase levels normalize and a different statin can be started at a lower dose. The most dreaded complication of statin therapy is rhabdomyolysis with skeletal muscle breakdown, myoglobinuria, and renal failure. The risk of this is less than 0.1%, but patients must be counseled about the possibility as well as warning signs for rhabdomyolysis (escalating muscle pain, proximal weakness, brownish-red discoloration of urine). Statins can induce myalgia. However, myalgias in general are common throughout the population. In the Heart Protection Study, among 20,536 patients randomized to either placebo or simvastatin, 40 mg daily, the incidence of myalgia was nearly identical in the two groups of patients. If a patient is experiencing significant myalgia or muscle weakness a serum creatine kinase level can be obtained. Myopathy is defined as a creatine kinase level that exceeds 10 times ULN. Statins are contraindicated in pregnant and nursing women.

EZETIMIBE

Dietary and biliary sources of cholesterol contribute substantially to circulating levels of this sterol. Although plant sterols and stanols can block cholesterol absorption, Ezetimibe (Zetia) is the first member of lipid-lowering drugs known as cholesterol absorption inhibitors. Ezetimibe inhibits a sterol transporter in the brush border of the jejunal enterocyte identified as Niemann-Pick C1 Like-1 protein that internalizes cholesterol and phytosterols from the intestinal lumen. After being glucuronidated, ezetimibe undergoes enterohepatic recirculation with negligible systemic exposure. The half-life of ezetimibe is

approximately 22 hours and is dosed at 10 mg once daily. Ezetimibe reduces serum LDLC on average by 20%, but up to 24% of patients experience a reduction of greater than or equal to 25%. Ezetimibe also decreases triglycerides by up to 8% and raises HDLC by up to 4%. Ezetimibe does not decrease the absorption of bile acids, steroid hormones (ethinyl estradiol, progesterone), or such fat-soluble vitamins as vitamins A, D, E, or α- and β-carotenes.

The risk of hepatotoxicity with ezetimibe is nearly identical to placebo (0.5% vs. 0.3%), and there is no documented evidence of increased risk for myopathy. Fixed-dose ezetimibe is also available in combination with increasing doses of simvastatin (Vytorin; 10/10; 10/20; 10/40; 10/80 mg daily). Ezetimibe can also be safely used in combination with other statins and provides additive changes in lipoprotein levels to that observed with statin therapy. The addition of ezetimibe to a statin regimen substantially reduces the likelihood of having to titrate the statin.

BILE ACID BINDING RESINS

The bile acid sequestration agents (BASAs) are orally administered anion exchange resins that bind bile acids in the gastrointestinal tract and prevent them from being reabsorbed into the enterohepatic circulation. These drugs reduce serum LDLC by two mechanisms: (1) increased catabolism of cholesterol secondary to the upregulation of 7-α-hydroxylase, the rate-limiting enzyme for the conversion of cholesterol into bile acids; and (2) increased expression of LDL receptors on the hepatocyte surface that augments the clearance of apoB100-containing lipoproteins from plasma. At maximum doses, the BASAs can reduce serum LDLC by 15% to 30% and increase HDLC by 3% to 5%. It is recommended that these drugs be used in conjunction with a statin whenever possible because BASA therapy increases HMG-CoA reductase activity in the liver, which leads to increased hepatic biosynthesis of cholesterol, thereby offsetting the effects of the BASAs over time.

There are currently three different BASAs available. These include cholestyramine (Questran; 4 to 24 g daily in two to three divided doses daily), colestipol (Colestid; 5 to 30 g in two to four divided doses daily), and colesevelam (WelChol; 1250 mg two to three times daily). The development of constipation, flatulence, and bloating are relatively frequent, though colesevelam has the most favorable side-effect profile of the three available BASAs. Increasing water and soluble fiber ingestion ameliorates some of the difficulty with constipation. The BASAs bind negatively charged molecules in a nonspecific manner. Consequently, they can decrease the absorption of warfarin (Coumadin), phenobarbital, thiazide diuretics, digitalis, β-blockers, thyroxine, statins, fibrates, and ezetimibe. These medications should be taken 1 hour before or 4 hours after the ingestion of a BASA. The BASAs can reduce the absorption of fat-soluble vitamins.

FIBRATES

The fibrates are fibric acid derivatives that exert a number of effects on lipoprotein metabolism. These agents reduce serum triglycerides by 25% to 50% and raise HDLC by 10% to 20%. Fibrates activate lipoprotein lipase by reducing levels of apoprotein CIII (an inhibitor of this enzyme) and increasing levels of apoprotein CII (an activator of lipoprotein lipase). This stimulates the hydrolysis of triglycerides in chylomicrons and VLDL. Fibrates increase HDLC by two mechanisms. First, the fibrates are PPAR-α agonists and stimulate increased hepatic expression of apoproteins AI and AII. Second, by activating lipoprotein lipase, surface coat mass derived from VLDL is ultimately used to assimilate HDL in serum. In some patients, fibrate therapy may be associated with an increase in serum LDLC (the "β" effect) secondary to increased enzymatic conversion of VLDL to LDL. This effect may diminish over time as the patient increases the expression of hepatic LDL receptors.

The fibrates are particularly valuable for treating dyslipidemia in patients with a combination of hypertriglyceridemia and low HDLC. In this patient type, posthoc evaluations of data from two studies (the Helsinki Heart Study and the Bezafibrate Infarction Prevention Study) have demonstrated substantial cardiovascular event rate reductions using fibrate therapy. In the Veterans Affairs High-Density Lipoprotein Intervention Trial (VA-HIT), men with CAD and low HDL (mean 31 mg/dL) were treated with either gemfibrozil (Lopid) 600 mg orally twice daily or placebo over a 5-year-follow-up period. With a 6% elevation in HDL, no change in LDL, and a 31% decrease in triglycerides, gemfibrozil therapy resulted in a 22% reduction in the composite endpoint of all-cause mortality and nonfatal MI compared to placebo. Gemfibrozil therapy also reduced the risk of stroke and transient ischemic attacks by 31% and 59%, respectively.

Among the diabetic patients in VA-HIT treated with gemfibrozil, there was a 32% reduction in the combined endpoint (41% in CHD death and 40% in stroke). Fibrates have been shown to exert many of the same pleiotropic effects as statins and reduce atheromatous plaque progression in native coronary vessels and in coronary venous bypass grafts.

Like the statins, fibrates are associated with a low incidence of myopathy and mild elevations in serum transaminases. Fibrate therapy can increase the risk for cholelithiasis and can raise prothrombin times by displacing warfarin from albumin binding sites. The periodic monitoring of serum transaminases (6 to 12 weeks after initiating therapy and twice annually thereafter) is recommended. The two most commonly used fibrates are gemfibrozil (Lopid; 600 mg twice daily) and fenofibrate (Tricor; 54 or 160 mg daily). Bezafibrate (Bezalip)[2] is available in Europe and is dosed at 400 mg daily. The use of therapies combining a statin and fibrate is becoming more commonplace in clinical practice, especially as the incidence of complex dyslipidemias increases. Gemfibrozil significantly reduces the glucuronidation of statins, which decreases their elimination. This increases the risk for myopathy/rhabdomyolysis and hepatotoxicity. When used in combination with gemfibrozil, the doses for simvastatin (Zocor), and rosuvastatin (Crestor), should not exceed 10 mg daily. In general, when embarking on combination therapy, fenofibrate is a safer choice, as it does not adversely impact the glucuronidation of the statins. There are no clinical trial data yet available to assess the effect of statin-fibrate combination therapy on cardiovascular morbidity and mortality.

Among patients in whom serum triglycerides do not normalize in response to a low-fat diet and fibrate therapy, consideration should be given to the addition of other agents. Patients with severe hypertriglyceridemia frequently possess mutations in lipoprotein lipase that reduce the lipolytic activity of this enzyme. In this scenario, the addition of orlistat (Xenical; 120 mg with meals) can reduce the absorption of dietary fat and hence the circulating levels of chylomicrons and triglycerides. Fish-oil capsules enriched with omega-3 (eicosapentaenoic acid) and omega-6 (docosahexaenoic acid) fatty acids can reduce serum triglyceride and VLDL levels and raise HDLC in a dose-dependent manner.

NIACIN

Niacin or nicotinic acid is a B vitamin that exerts multiple beneficial effects on lipoprotein metabolism. In contrast to statins and fibrates, niacin does not stimulate hepatic biosynthesis of HDL. Niacin appears to block HDL particle uptake and catabolism by hepatocytes without adversely impacting reverse cholesterol transport. This helps to increase circulating levels of HDL. Niacin reduces hepatic VLDL and triglyceride secretion according to two mechanisms: (1) decreasing the flux of fatty acids from adipose tissue to the liver by inhibiting lipase activity; (2) inhibiting triglyceride formation within hepatocytes by inhibiting diacylglycerol acyltransferase. Niacin also reduces serum LDLC concentrations by increasing the catabolism of apoB100. Consequently, niacin beneficially impacts all components of the lipoprotein profile.

When used as monotherapy at 3.0 g daily, crystalline niacin (Niaspan) significantly reduced the incidence of MI and stroke in patients with established CAD in the

---

CURRENT DIAGNOSIS

- Dyslipidemia is a highly heterogeneous class of metabolic disorders with an etiology that can depend on abnormalities in the gastrointestinal absorption of cholesterol and lipids and mutations in cell surface receptors and enzymes in pathways regulating lipid metabolism.
- Dyslipidemia is a widely prevalent risk factor for CAD and is associated with elevations in serum LDLC and non-HDLC and low levels of HDLC.
- When making the diagnosis of dyslipidemia, it is important to rule out and treat secondary causes of dyslipidemia, such as thyroid dysfunction, alcoholism, diabetes mellitus, and nephrotic syndrome, among others.
- A complete fasting lipoprotein profile should be performed on anyone undergoing screening for dyslipidemia.
- The diagnosis of dyslipidemia requires comprehensive, global cardiovascular risk evaluation. Target levels for LDLC and non-HDLC are risk stratified. An HDLC of less than 40 mg/dL is a categorical risk factor for CAD.

Abbreviations: CAD = coronary artery disease; HDLC = high-density lipoprotein cholesterol; LDLC = low-density lipoprotein cholesterol.

---

[2]Not available in the United States.

CURRENT THERAPY

- Dyslipidemia is a modifiable risk factor.
- Lifestyle modification is first-line therapy for all patients with dyslipidemia.
- The intensity of pharmacologic intervention depends upon risk-stratified, NCEP targets for LDLC and non-HDLC. In patients with low HDLC, therapeutic effort should be made to raise the level of this lipoprotein as much as possible.
- Dyslipidemia can be treated with statins, fibrates, niacin, and combinations thereof. These drug classes have a substantial amount of end-point driven clinical trial data supporting their use.
- In patients unable to achieve their LDLC target with lifestyle modification and statin therapy, consider adding ezetimibe.
- Patients with severe hypertriglyceridemia unable to adequately reduce serum triglycerides with a low-fat diet and a fibrate likely have a lipoprotein lipase deficiency. These patients can benefit from the addition of orlistat to their pharmacologic regimen.
- The treatment of dyslipidemia in the context of both primary and secondary prevention must be coupled with the aggressive identification and management of all risk factors patients present with, including hypertension, diabetes mellitus, obesity, cigarette smoking, as well as nephropathy and chronic kidney disease.

Abbreviations: HDLC = high-density lipoprotein cholesterol; LDLC = low-density lipoprotein cholesterol. NCEP = National Cholesterol Education Program.

Coronary Drug Project. In the HDL-Atherosclerosis Treatment Study (HATS) combinations of high-dose niacin (2 to 4 g with simvastatin) reduced cardiovascular morbidity and mortality by up to 90% compared to placebo. This combination therapy also induced atheromatous plaque stabilization over a follow-up period of 3 years. Niaspan should be started at a low dose and gradually titrated upward based on the results of follow-up lipid panels. When evaluated as a function of dose (500 to 2000 mg daily), Niaspan induces the following changes in serum lipid levels: LDLC, 3% to 16% reduction; triglycerides, 5% to 32% reduction; HDLC, 10% to 24% elevation.

Niacin therapy is associated with a number of side effects. The most common side effect with niacin is cutaneous flushing. The incidence of this can be reduced by taking a 325-mg tablet of aspirin one hour before taking niacin. The flushing is prostaglandin mediated. Limiting fat intake for 2 to 3 hours before taking niacin also helps, as fat is a source of arachidonic acid, the substrate for cyclooxygenase. Niaspan is a sustained-release preparation of niacin associated with less flushing. Other side effects include bloating, pruritus, acanthosis nigricans, transient disturbances in glycemic control, and increased serum concentrations of uric acid. Niacin appears to increase rates of proximal tubular reuptake of urate from the glomerular ultrafiltrate. Niacin is available as a combination pill with lovastatin (Advicor; 500/20 mg, 750/20 mg, 1000/20 mg, and 2000/40 mg), and the two drugs give additive changes in the levels of serum lipoproteins.

Conclusion

Dyslipidemia is a widely prevalent risk factor for CAD. Specific target levels for atherogenic lipoprotein fractions are defined by the NCEP. The treatment of dyslipidemia with lifestyle modification and pharmacologic intervention is associated with significant reductions in cardiovascular morbidity and mortality.

American Diabetes Association: Dyslipidemia management in adults with diabetes. Diabetes Care 2004;27:S68-S71.

Brown G, Albers JJ, Fisher LD, et al: Regression of coronary artery disease as a result of intensive lipid-lowering therapy in men with high levels of apolipoprotein B. N Engl J Med 1990;323: 1289-1298.

Cannon CP, Braunwald E, McCabe CH, et al., for the Pravastatin or Atorvastatin Evaluation and Infection Therapy–Thrombolysis in Myocardial Infarction 22 Investigators: Comparison of intensive and moderate lipid lowering with statins after acute coronary syndromes. N Engl J Med 2004;350:1495-1504.

Expert Panel on Detection, Evaluation, and Treatment of High Blood Cholesterol in Adults: Executive summary of the third report of the National Cholesterol Education Program (NCEP) Expert Panel on Detection, Evaluation, and Treatment of High blood Cholesterol in Adults (Adult Treatment Panel III). JAMA 2001; 285:2486-2497.

Grundy SM, Cleeman JI, Merz CN, et al: Implications of recent clinical trials for the National Cholesterol Education Program Adult Treatment Panel III guidelines. Circulation 2004;110(2):227-239.

Heart Protection Study Collaborative Group: MRC/BHF Heart Protection Study of cholesterol lowering with simvastatin in 20,536 high-risk individuals: A randomised placebo-controlled trial. Lancet 2002;360:7-22.

Mosca L, Appel LJ, Benjamin EJ, et al: Evidence-based guidelines for cardiovascular disease prevention in women. Circulation 2004; 109:672-693.

Ridker PM, Bassuk SS, Toth PP: C-reactive protein and risk of cardiovascular disease: Evidence and clinical application. Curr Atheroscler Rep 2003;5:341-349.

Robins SJ, Collins D, Wittes JF, et al. VA-HIT Study Group. Veterans Affairs High-Density Lipoprotein Intervention Trial. Relation of gemfibrozil treatment and lipid levels with major coronary events. JAMA 2001;285:1586-1589.

Sacks FM and The Expert Group on HDL Cholesterol: The role of high-density lipoprotein (HDL) cholesterol in the prevention and treatment of coronary heart disease: Expert group recommendations. Am J Cardiol 2002;90:139-143.

Sever PS, Dahlöf B, Poulter NR, et al., for the ASCOT investigators: Prevention of coronary and stroke events with atorvastatin in hypertensive patients who have average or lower-than-average cholesterol concentrations, in the Anglo-Scandinavian Cardiac Outcomes Trial—Lipid Lowering Arm (ASCOT-LLA): A multicentre randomised controlled trial. Lancet 2003:361:1149-1158.

Sjostrum CD, Peltonen M, Wedel H, et al: Differentiated long-term effects of intentional weight loss on diabetes and hypertension. Hypertension 2000;36:20-25.

Toth PP: Clinician update: HDL and cardiovascular risk. Circulation 2004;109:1809-1812.

Toth PP: Low-density lipoprotein reduction in high risk patients: How low do you go? Curr Atheroscler Rep 2004;6:348-352.

Obesity

Method of
Christopher D. Still, DO, and
Gordon L. Jensen, MD, PhD

Obesity is a heterogeneous disease that has reached epidemic proportions in the United States. For most individuals, it is chronic, relapsing, and multifactorial in origin. It encompasses genetic, environmental, socioeconomic, psychological, and behavioral factors. According to the National Health and Nutrition Examination Survey (NHANES), the prevalence of obesity in the United States has increased from approximately 25% to 33% over a single decade, and obesity now affects nearly 26 million men and 32 million women. Unfortunately, obesity does not spare children or adolescents. NHANES data indicate that approximately 30% of children are overweight (more than 10 million).

The magnitude of obesity differs widely among gender and ethnic groups. There is a marked increase in the prevalence of obesity among females of African American and Mexican American ethnic groups. Some studies estimate nearly 70% of this population is overweight.

Health care providers can no longer view obesity as simply a cosmetic issue caused by a lack of willpower. They need to have an appreciation of its complexity and the related multiple co-morbid medical problems. This chapter discusses the epidemiology, definitions, and assessment of obesity with an emphasis on its clinical consequences and the current techniques in evaluating and treating the obese patient.

Definition and Assessment

The definition of obesity has always been quite ambiguous. The once widely used determination of so-called ideal body weight based on standard height/weight tables such as the Metropolitan Life Insurance Table has fallen out of favor. Experts now recommend the routine use of the body mass index (BMI). The BMI is defined as the ratio of body weight in kilograms to the height in meters squared (kg/m^2). The BMI correlates with body fat and morbidity and mortality (Figure 1).

The BMI differentiates between overweight and obesity. Moreover, as the BMI increases, so does the risk of mortality. A so-called desirable weight individual has a BMI between 20 and 24.9 kg/m^2. The National Heart, Blood and Lung Institute defines overweight as a body mass index between 25 and 29.9 kg/m^2. Obesity, therefore,

CURRENT DIAGNOSIS

- Height, weight, and body mass index
- Waist circumference
- Exclusion of co morbid medical problems such as diabetes, obstructive sleep apnea, and hypercholesterolemia

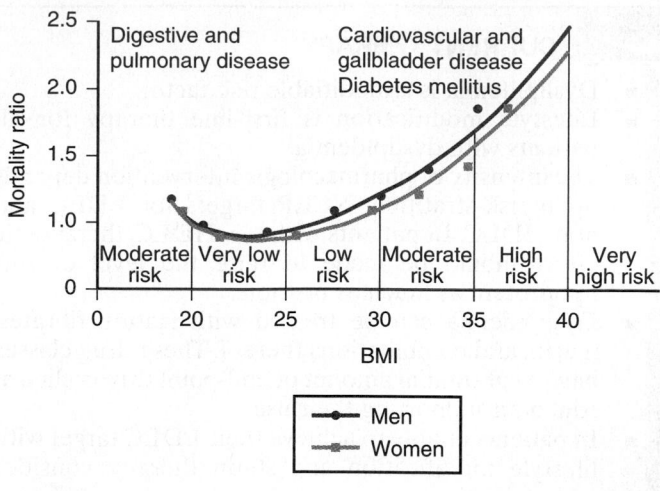

FIGURE 1. Correlation between mortality risk and increasing body mass index (BMI). As BMI increases to higher than 25, the risk for mortality from all causes increases. (Adapted with permission from Gray DS: Diagnosis and prevalence of obesity. Med Clin North Am 1989;73:1.)

is defined as a BMI more than 30. Patients with a BMI more than 27 with a co-morbid medical problem, such as diabetes mellitus, hypercholesterolemia, hypertension, or sleep apnea, are also at a higher risk of overall mortality and, therefore, more aggressive treatment options may be warranted (Table 1).

In addition to the BMI, waist circumference is another useful tool in assessing the overweight individual. A waist circumference is measured at the smallest area between the xiphoid process and the iliac crest. A waist circumference more than 35 inches in women and more than 39 inches in men reflects an android or visceral fat distribution. This visceral fat upper body distribution puts one at greater risk for developing co-morbid medical problems such as diabetes, heart disease, lipid dyscrasias, insulin resistance, and possibly cancer. In contrast, the gynoid or lower body weight obesity of the hips and buttocks is mainly subcutaneous adipose tissue that is cardioprotective and not associated with adverse sequelae.

Etiology and Pathophysiology of Obesity

Several etiologic factors classify obesity. Neuroendocrine disorder and single gene deletion syndromes include Cushing's, polycystic ovarian, gonadal failure, Prader-Willi, Cowen's, Carpenter's, and Bardet-Biedl.

TABLE 1 Clinical Use of the Body Mass Index (BMI)

BMI = ratio of weight in kilograms or weight in pounds to (height in meters)^2 or (height in inches)^2
Obesity is defined as BMI >30. If risk factors such as heart disease, hypertension, or elevated serum cholesterol levels are present, more aggressive intervention may be warranted for a BMI >27.

TABLE 2 Prescription Medications That May Promote Weight Gain

Class of Medication	Examples
Antidiabetics	Insulin, thioglitazones, sulfonylureas
Antipsychotics	Risperidone (Risperdal), clozapine (Clozaril), olanzapine (Zyprexa)
Antidepressants	Amitriptyline (Elavil), imipramine (Tofranil), doxepin (Sinequan), lithium desipramine (Norpramin), trazodone (Desyrel), tranylcypromine (Parnate)
Antiepileptics	Valproate (Depakote), carbamazepine (Tegretol)
Steroids	Glucocorticoids
Antihistamines	Astemizole[2]

[2]Not available in the United States.

Commonly prescribed medications may also promote weight gain. These include, but are not limited to, classes of drugs such as antidiabetics, antipsychotics, antidepressants, antiepileptics, steroids, hormones and adrenergic agonists (Table 2). It is always important to take a thorough medication history to ensure that no medications, either prescription or over the counter, are taken that promote weight gain.

Medical Consequences of Obesity

Obesity and its multiple medical co-morbidities are associated with a profound increase in morbidity and premature mortality. With increasing BMI there is an increased prevalence of metabolic syndrome/insulin resistance, diabetes mellitus, hypertension, coronary artery disease, lipid and cholesterol dyscrasias, gallbladder disease, respiratory compromise, degenerative joint disease, infertility, and some cancers. The major complications associated with obesity are addressed next.

INSULIN RESISTANCE/METABOLIC SYNDROME

The fundamental pathophysiologic defect that often leads to non-insulin-dependent diabetes mellitus (NIDDM) is insulin resistance. It is estimated that 25% of the population is insulin resistant, which is especially prevalent in individuals with the android type of weight distribution. Hyperinsulinemia results from compensatory pancreatic cell hypersecretion and therefore serves as a biologic and laboratory marker of insulin resistance. After prolonged hypersecretion, the insulin secretory capacity of the β cells diminishes, possibly because of the accumulation of amyloid deposits in the islet cells and eventually decompensation of insulin resistant to overt hyperglycemia. In addition, undetermined genetic factors and acquired factors such as aging, sedentary lifestyle, and obesity all contribute to insulin resistance.

Clinically, this syndrome can be associated with abdominal obesity (android adiposity), hypertension, hypertriglyceridemia, high-density lipoprotein/low-density lipoprotein (HDL/LDL) cholesterol abnormalities, hyperuricemia, fluid retention, polycystic ovarian syndrome, hypofibrinolysis, acanthosis nigricans, and skin tags. Studies revealed that treatment options in this patient population favor complex carbohydrate modification, reduced fat intake, regular exercise, and possibly the use of medications, such as metformin, that increase insulin sensitivity.

DIABETES MELLITUS

Undoubtedly, the increasing prevalence of obesity is associated with the growing prevalence of NIDDM in the United States. Some 70% to 80% of patients with NIDDM are overweight. NHANES data clearly reveal a strong correlation between the relative risk of development of NIDDM and increasing body mass index beyond 27 kg/m^2. Moreover, there exists a 10-fold increase in the prevalence of obesity in individuals with a BMI more than 40 kg/m^2. Additional individual risk factors for the development of diabetes mellitus, regardless of gender, include increasing age, family history of NIDDM, and central adipose distribution. What must be emphasized, however, is that even a modest weight loss (5% to 10% of presenting weight) can have tremendous benefit on glycemic control as well as curtailing the development and progression of the multiple co-morbidities associated with diabetes mellitus.

HYPERTENSION

Hypertension is a common, chronic disease affecting millions of individuals worldwide. A strong correlation exists between hypertension and obesity, with obesity associated with approximately 30% to 50% of the hypertension in the United States. In addition to a reduction in blood pressure, left ventricular mass, which is often associated with long-standing hypertension, has been shown to be reduced with a modest weight loss (5% to 10% of presenting weight). Moreover, a modest weight loss often leads to reduction or elimination of the need for hypertensive pharmacotherapy.

CORONARY HEART DISEASE

Until recently, obesity was considered only a minor contributor to coronary artery disease (CAD). However, in response to the emerging body of scientific, medical, and behavioral data about the link between excess adiposity and CAD, the American Heart Association reclassified obesity as a major, modifiable risk factor for CAD. In addition to obesity alone, studies suggest when other co-morbidities are present (such as hypertension, elevated LDL cholesterol, diabetes mellitus, and elevated serum triglycerides), obese individuals are at even greater risk for the development of CAD, and more aggressive treatment options may be warranted.

LIPID DYSCRASIAS

Blood lipid abnormalities are common in the obese individual. Obese individuals who possess the upper body, android, visceral adiposity often have lower HDL cholesterol leading to an increased risk of the development of CAD. On the contrary, individuals who possess the lower body, gynoid, more subcutaneous adiposity often are predisposed to an elevated HDL cholesterol concentration that is cardioprotective. Overweight and obese individuals routinely have normal or slightly elevated total or LDL cholesterol levels. Therefore, individuals with a random total cholesterol level greater than 200 mg/dL warrant a fasting lipid profile.

Unlike cholesterol, obesity predisposes individuals to higher triglyceride levels compared to normal weight individuals. Although hypertriglyceridemia alone and its association with increased morbidity and mortality have been controversial, increased portal free fatty acid availability and hyperinsulinemia increase the synthesis of very low density lipoprotein (VLDL), which is a risk factor for CAD. Pharmacologic intervention is often required when obese individuals exhibit Frederickson class IV or V hyperlipidemia.

PULMONARY ABNORMALITIES

Severe respiratory insufficiency, commonly known as pickwickian syndrome, may develop in patients with morbid obesity. Obstructive sleep apnea syndrome and obesity hypoventilation syndrome are two primary breathing disorders of the pickwickian syndrome. With obstructive sleep apnea, the tongue obstructs the glottis during sleep impeding air entry to the trachea. In moderately and morbidly obese individuals, obstructive sleep apnea is very common and often misdiagnosed. Symptoms of obstructive sleep apnea include snoring, apneic episodes, excessive daytime somnolence, memory loss, irritability, fatigue, and erectile dysfunction. Nocturnal hypoxemia, a consequence of sleep apnea, may contribute to arrhythmias, pulmonary hypertension, and right-sided heart failure. The most important and first-line intervention should be weight reduction. Moderate weight loss as a result of modified caloric intake improves oxygenation and sleep apnea in obese subjects. The most likely mechanism of improvement after a modest weight loss results from an increase in airway size or from changes in ventilatory drive, which increases upper airway muscle activity.

Treatment Options

Successful comprehensive weight management programs combine the use of nutritionally balanced, mildly hypocaloric diet regimens, modest regular activity, behavior modification techniques and, when indicated, pharmacotherapy. High rates of recidivism are seen in programs not proportionally balanced or requiring drastic dietary modification.

INITIAL EVALUATION

Individuals should undergo a comprehensive history and physical examination before initiating any diet and

CURRENT THERAPY

- Diet, exercise, and behavior modification
- Pharmacotherapy
- Bariatric surgery

exercise program. Secondary causes of obesity such as Cushing's syndrome, hypothyroidism, and diabetes mellitus should be considered in the initial evaluation. In addition, contraindications to weight reduction such as pregnancy, lactation, unstable mental illness, and medical conditions such as unstable angina or uncontrolled blood pressure should all be evaluated prior to initiation. Eating disorders such as anorexia and bulimia must also be considered. The physical examination should include both the BMI and waist circumference. These are critical to stratify patients to predict and guide various treatment options (Figure 2).

Initial blood chemistry studies including complete blood cell count, liver function studies, fasting lipid profile, determination of thyroid-stimulating hormone concentration, fasting glucose level, and renal panel should be considered as well as an electrocardiogram in appropriate individuals.

DIET

Once any secondary causes of obesity (hypothyroidism, Cushing's syndrome, etc.) are ruled out, determination of what diet regimen to best fit the overweight or obese individual is critical. The implementation of drastic, unrealistic dietary limitations makes long-term compliance difficult.

Popularized in the 1970s, very low calorie diets (VLCDs) were widely used to promote initial rapid weight loss. VLCDs are drastically limited in energy, usually between 600 and 800 calories per day, resulting in significant but usually short-term results.

VLCDs can be beneficial in the instance where rapid weight loss is needed for a specific procedure to be performed (i.e., cardiac catheterization) or life-threatening obstructive sleep apnea where rapid weight loss can significantly reduce the frequency and duration of apneic episodes. Individuals on VLCDs should be closely monitored, and additional supplementation of at least 1500 mL of water, multiple vitamins, calcium, magnesium, and

BMI category	Health risk based on BMI
<25	Minimal–low
25–<27	Low–moderate
27–<30	Moderate–low
30–<35	High–very high
35–<40	Very high–extremely high
>40	Extremely high

Health risk	Treatment options
Minimal and low	Healthful eating Increased physical activity Life style changes
Moderate	All of the above plus caloric restriction
High + very high	All of the above plus pharmacotherapy
Extremely high	All of the above plus surgical considerations

FIGURE 2. Determination of health risk based on body mass index (BMI) and various treatment options. (Adapted from the National Institute of Health: Practical Guide to the Identification, Evaluation, and Treatment of Overweight and Obesity in Adults, 1998.)

potassium are usually required. VLCDs should be used as an initial step to a less drastic conventional balance deficit meal plan.

Contraindications to VLCDs include recent myocardial infarction, unstable angina, malignant arrhythmias, type I diabetes mellitus, and pregnancy. Medications such as insulin, sulfonylurea hypoglycemics, and antihypertensives must be carefully monitored and often tapered as weight loss ensues.

Popular commercial liquid diet preparations usually contain approximately 10 to 15 g of protein, 30 to 45 g of carbohydrate, and 2 to 3 g of fat. The vastly protein-rich supplements contribute to caloric energy levels and usually range between 180 and 250 calories per serving. Rates of recidivism remain quite high with most commercial diet preparations. This is mostly because of the failure of liquid diets to provide an opportunity for the patient to alter fundamental eating and lifestyle behaviors needed for sustained weight loss.

Over the last several years, low-carbohydrate ketogenic diets such as the Atkins diet have been popular in the lay press. Although initially one may see increased satiety and rapid weight loss because of fluid loss, long-term studies on cardiovascular risk reduction and sustained weight loss over other diet options are ongoing.

What is probably most beneficial for the majority of overweight and obese individuals is a less drastic hypocaloric and balanced meal plan. These typically provide 1200 to 1800 calories per day, 20% to 30% of calories from fat, 50% to 55% from carbohydrates, and 15% to 20% from protein. These conventional diets should result in losses of approximately 1 to 2 lbs per week or 4 to 8 lbs per month. These less drastic meal plans allow individuals to make lifestyle changes, ideally long term.

To recommend a caloric concentration adequately, one must determine the caloric requirement to maintain a patient's weight upon presentation. This is crucial so unrealistic goals are not placed on individuals, setting them up for failure. For instance, in most instances it is unrealistic for a 275-lb man to adhere to 1200 calories per day. As a general rule, a 500-calorie per day deficit promotes a weight loss of 1 lb per week. A moderate degree of restriction is better tolerated, and long-term compliance should be superior to more restrictive caloric plans.

In addition to calories consumed by eating, it is also important to discern how many calories individuals are drinking. Individuals can drink thousands of calories per day and not equate them to "total calories consumed per day." Maintaining blood volume by drinking at least 64 oz of water per day and limiting or avoiding liquids with calories (i.e., regular sodas, juices, alcoholic beverages) has proven beneficial.

BEHAVIOR MODIFICATION

Behavior modification must be an integral part of any diet plan to promote the best chance of success. Several controlled trials have validated the effectiveness of behavioral techniques. However, in a busy primary care office this can be time consuming. A concise and comprehensive manual that provides specific monthly goals for the practitioner to review with patients is the Learn Program for Weight Control from the American Health Publishing Company in Dallas, Texas. This provides excellent behavior modification lessons for the patient to work through between office visits.

EXERCISE

In reviewing national weight loss registries in patients who have lost a significant amount of weight and kept it off for greater than 1 year, regular exercise is the most common denominator for weight maintenance. Unfortunately, exercise is the most difficult component of a comprehensive weight management program, partly because of unrealistic expectations placed on obese individuals. Many experts agree that 30 minutes a day, 5 days a week, of aerobic activity is the minimum exercise prescription required for weight loss and maintenance. However, it is unrealistic to expect an obese individual to sustain himself or herself, at least initially, for 30 minutes and therefore, compliance drops precipitously.

A more reasonable starting point is an occurrence type of activity program several times per day. For instance, 3 to 5 minutes of aerobic activity five to six times a day is much better tolerated by a patient, and long-term compliance is greatly enhanced. The use of a pedometer can objectively measure one's number of steps, and goals of 8000 to 10,000 steps per day should be recommended. Also, common everyday activities such as walking up stairs rather than taking the elevator or escalator, parking farther away from an entrance, or not using the television remote control add up to small but meaningful periods of increased activity, thereby increasing energy expenditure. Increased exercise, however, increases muscle mass, which weighs more than adipose tissue. Once a patient progresses to 30 minutes of occurrence exercise, 5 days per week, studies have determined a greater than 50% chance of achieving weight maintenance.

PHARMACOTHERAPY

During the 1990s, there were great ups and downs in the development of pharmacotherapy for the treatment of obesity. What must be emphasized, however, is that if pharmacotherapy is considered, it must be used as an adjunct to diet, behavior modification, and exercise to attain the best results for patients.

One of the oldest medications that is still available and used is phentermine (Ionamin). Phentermine is adrenergic medication that mildly increases norepinephrine release. This medication was popularized in the early 1990s when Weintraub studied the efficacy of phentermine used in combination with fenfluramine[1,2] or the so-called fen-phen combination. Phentermine, used alone, is not associated with cardiac valvular defects and remains available for use as a single agent for short-term use (3 months). It is available as phentermine HCl and phentermine resin. The resinate, when compared to HCl, is absorbed more slowly and blood levels reach a lower, later, and flatter peak, which is likely to result in more consistent and sustained blood levels. Potential side effects of phentermine include dry mouth, palpitations, tachycardia, hypertension, insomnia, or overstimulation.

[1]Not FDA approved for this indication.
[2]Not available in the United States.

Early in 1998, the Food and Drug Administration (FDA) approved the use of sibutramine (Meridia) for the treatment of obesity. Sibutramine is a beta-phenylethylamine that acts as a reuptake inhibitor for both norepinephrine and serotonin. Unlike fenfluramine and dexfenfluramine, sibutramine does not possess any releasing ability of serotonin. It is the potent releasing ability of dexfenfluramine and fenfluramine that has been suggested to be the cause of the valvular heart disease and pulmonary hypertension associated with these medications. To date, there have been no reports of any valvulopathies or primary pulmonary hypertension with the use of sibutramine.

Most common side effects associated with sibutramine include dry mouth, insomnia, and constipation. In addition, tachycardia and hypertension (mean blood pressure increase of 2 to 3 mm Hg and increase in pulse rate by four to five beats per minute) are reported. Therefore, pulse and blood pressure should be monitored when initiating sibutramine. Efficacy studies using sibutramine revealed an approximate 8% weight loss at the end of 12 months when used in combination with diet. Contraindications to sibutramine include use with any monoamine oxidative inhibitors or selective serotonin reuptake inhibitors or in patients with severe renal or hepatic impairment. In addition, it is contraindicated for patients with a history of CAD, congestive heart failure, arrhythmias, stroke, glaucoma, or uncontrolled hypertension.

In May 1999, the FDA approved another medication for the treatment of obesity, orlistat (Xenical). Orlistat tetrahydrolipstatin is a selective inhibitor of pancreatic lipase and thus is a novel approach to weight loss medications. Orlistat is the first nonsystemically acting medication that acts locally in the gastrointestinal tract to block gastric and pancreatic lipase and results in decreased fat absorption. Orlistat inhibits lipases for approximately 90 minutes after ingestion. Approximately a third of digested fat is excreted in the stool by patients taking orlistat.

Certain adverse events can be predicted from the mode of action of orlistat including steatorrhea, oily spotting, flatulence with discharge, and fecal urgency. Fat-soluble vitamins A, D, E, and K as well as beta carotene may be modestly decreased in individuals taking orlistat; therefore, multivitamin supplementation is recommended daily. Efficacy studies after 2 years revealed an approximate 9% weight loss when used in combination with a mildly hypocaloric meal plan.

The newest centrally active appetite suppressant medication approved in 2006 is Rimonabant* (Acomplia). Rimonabant works by blocking receptors in the brain that are part of the endocannabinoid system (EC system). These receptors, which are found throughout the body, play a critical role in the regulation of food intake and energy expenditure. Cannabinoids, chemical compounds produced by the body, latch on to specific receptors (CB 1 receptors), which are overactive in most overweight and obese individuals, sending out a signal that prompts people to eat and smoke more. This medication blocks these CB 1 receptors, which helps normalize the overactivation of the EC system, reducing hunger cravings and tobacco dependence.

The use of pharmacotherapy as an adjunct to diet, exercise, and behavior modification is indicated for individuals with a BMI more than 30 kg/m² or more than 27 kg/m² with a co-morbid medical problem relating to their obesity such as diabetes, hypercholesterolemia, or hypertension. Pharmacotherapy alone is neither indicated nor recommended. Table 3 summarizes commonly prescribed medications for the treatment of obesity.

BARIATRIC SURGERY

Bariatric surgery for the treatment of obesity, despite impressive outcomes, should be considered for patients suffering from morbid obesity. The surgical candidates who can benefit the most include patients who have failed medical management and who have a BMI more than 40 kg/m² or have a BMI 35 kg/m² and also suffer from diabetes, hypertension, obstructive sleep apnea, cardiovascular disease, gastroesophageal reflux disease, degenerative joint disease, or steatohepatitis (fatty liver). Amelioration of those common medical problems should be the prominent reason for considering bariatric surgery.

Contraindications to bariatric surgery include untreated major depression/psychosis, certain personality disorders, active alcohol or drug abuse, and noncompliance with preoperative medical, nutritional, and psychological management. Age greater than 65 years is no longer an absolute contraindication to bariatric surgery, but the risk may outweigh the benefits for patients older than 70 years.

Bariatric surgery for children and adolescents remains highly controversial. However, surgery on patients between 12 and 18 years of age who have significant medical problems relating to their obesity (diabetes mellitus, obstructive sleep apnea, reactive airway disease, steatohepatitis, and metabolic syndrome) has resolved their co-morbidities.

---

*Not yet approved in U.S. as of October 2006.

TABLE 3 Commonly Prescribed Medications for the Treatment of Obesity

Generic Name	Phentermine	Sibutramine	Orlistat
Trade Name	Ionamin	Meridia	Xenical
	Fastin		
	Adipex-P		
Mechanism of Action	Adrenergic agonist	Norepinephrine and serotonin inhibitor	Lipase inhibitor
Dose	15–30 mg	5–15 mg	120 mg
	37.5 mg		
Side Effects	CNS	CNS	GI
	CV	CV	

Abbreviations: CNS = central nervous system; CV = cardiovascular; GI = gastrointestinal.

PREOPERATIVE EVALUATION

A comprehensive team approach is supported and recommended by most physicians and insurance carriers. An ideal program would encompass a minimum of four components: medical, nutritional, psychological, and surgical. This multidisciplinary team is involved in evaluating the patient before surgery and in the education and treatment after surgery. This team ensures optimal medical, nutritional, and psychological care and ensures good insight into the lifelong lifestyle changes after bariatric surgery.

SURGICAL ASSESSMENT

Once the patient completes the preoperative medical, nutritional, and psychological evaluation and has achieved adequate metabolic control of any medical problems, he or she can be referred to the bariatric surgeon. The surgeon evaluates the patient's motivation and expectations, discusses the risks and benefits of the different surgical interventions, and chooses the most appropriate surgery for each individual patient.

Most Common Surgical Options

RESTRICTIVE PROCEDURES: GASTRIC BANDING AND THE ADJUSTABLE LAPAROSCOPIC BAND

Gastric banding has been popular in Europe, but until the 1980s did not receive much attention in the United States. Initial stapling procedures (Figure 3A) were complicated by staple-line ruptures. This has given rise to the more commonly performed vertical-banded gastroplasty (VBG) (Figure 3A). The VBG separates the stomach, forming a small pouch that joins the rest of the stomach through a small channel. This channel is banded, so to speak, with a ring of nonexpandable material that prevents the opening from enlarging. This procedure is relatively easy to perform and involves no bypass of the intestines. The VBG is not routinely performed any longer and has since been replaced by the laparoscopic adjustable band (Figure 3B).

The adjustable lap band is also a purely restrictive and relatively noninvasive procedure that requires no malabsorption. These restricted procedures are generally best suited for patients who eat large quantities of protein and carbohydrates because surgery prevents entry of a large quantity of food. Weight loss may not be adequate for patients that eat high-calorie soft foods and liquids (such as cakes, milkshakes, and ice cream) because they can rapidly pass through the channel. Expected weight loss with the adjustable lap band approximates 40% to 60% of excess body weight in properly selected individuals. However, with patients that consume soft foods and liquid calories, long-term weight loss (3 to 5 years postoperatively) may be somewhat disappointing.

COMBINED RESTRICTIVE AND MALABSORPTIVE PROCEDURES: ROUX-EN-Y GASTROPLASTY

The Roux-en-Y gastroplasty combines stomach restriction with a bypass procedure and modest malabsorption of a vast majority of the stomach and the first part of the small intestine called the duodenum. This procedure prevents entry of large amounts of food at one time while bypassing the duodenum, where calories are normally absorbed (Figure 3C).

COMMON BARIATRIC PROCEDURES

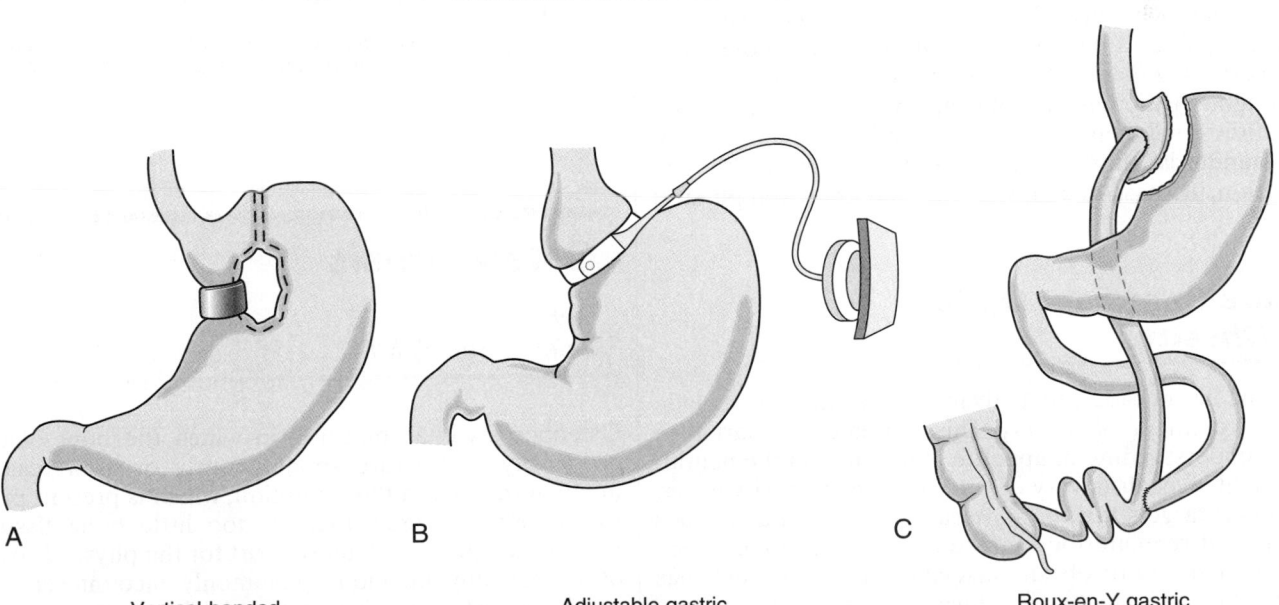

A — Vertical-banded gastroplasty

B — Adjustable gastric banding

C — Roux-en-Y gastric bypass

FIGURE 3. Techniques commonly used for the surgical treatment of obesity: vertical-banded gastroplasty (**A**), adjustable laparoscopic band (**B**), Roux-en-Y gastric bypass (**C**).

In most instances, the malabsorptive procedures are more effective than VBG and the adjustable lap band for causing and maintaining weight loss. The expected weight loss for the malabsorptive procedures are approximately 70% to 80% of a patient's excess body weight 3 years following surgery and continued maintenance 50% to 60% of excess body weight after 10 years depending on which procedure. Most importantly, co-morbid medical problems relating to obesity such as diabetes, high cholesterol, obstructive sleep apnea, fatty liver, and high blood pressure diminish or resolve after malabsorptive bariatric surgery.

All of the bariatric procedures just discussed are relatively safe, with an overall mortality of less than 2% when performed by an experienced surgeon who has performed at least 75 surgeries.

Pregnancy should be avoided for at least 12 to 18 months after undergoing malabsorptive bariatric surgery. With changes in absorption of iron/vitamins, vitamin B_{12}/folate, and protein along with rapid weight loss, women are at higher risk for spinal cord defects and other pregnancy complications. As with other medications during this period, adequate blood levels of oral birth control pills cannot be assured, and additional measures of birth control using barrier methods, patches, or injections are necessary.

Benefits of Modest Weight Loss

What is often overlooked in the obese individual with multiple co-morbid medical problems is the benefit of a modest weight loss. As health care providers, of primary importance is managing, not curing, the co-morbid medical problems of obese patients (e.g., blood sugar control, reducing cholesterol, etc.). Modest (10% to 15%) weight loss is documented in several studies to produce significant benefit in glucose control, blood pressure, and lipid management. A goal of metabolic fitness, as defined as the absence of biochemical risk factors associated with obesity, such as elevated fasting concentration of cholesterol, triglycerides, glucose, or elevated blood pressure, should be sought. Although in many instances achieving metabolic fitness still leaves patients obese by many practitioners' standards, there is tangible benefit in health risk reduction, increase in quality of life, and improved physical function.

Future Treatment Options for Obesity

Over the last decade, great advancements have been made in the treatment of obesity. This is related in part to a better understanding of appetite regulation on the neural-hormonal level, discovery of various human obesity genes, molecular targets for obesity treatment as well as various signals that regulate food intake and energy homeostasis. Characterization of obesity-associated gene products has revealed new biochemical pathways and molecular targets for potential pharmacologic intervention that will likely lead to new treatments into the millennium.

Although great strides have been made in the discovery of various hormones, genes, and gene products to develop the ideal antiobesity agent, it is likely that pharmacologic treatments will require combination therapy likely tailored to phenotype and genotype; each requiring a distinct mechanism of action. Optimism remains high for a magic bullet for the cure of obesity; however, one cannot lose sight of the fact that diet, exercise, and behavior modification will remain the cornerstone for any potential future pharmacotherapy

In conclusion, obesity in the United States has reached epidemic proportions, leading to a significant health crisis. Health care providers can no longer view obesity as a social issue but rather they must acknowledge it as a chronic medical condition, like diabetes, requiring long-term treatment. A realistic goal set at the outset to achieve metabolic fitness via a comprehensive weight management program consisting of prudent dietary changes, behavior modification, and regular aerobic exercise, with or without the adjunctive use of pharmacotherapy and/or surgery, will provide the best chance for modest weight loss and maintenance. This will be most rewarding, not only for patients, but also for health care providers managing the multiple co-morbid medical problems relating to obesity.

REFERENCES

Apovain C: The medical management of obesity and the role of pharmacotherapy: An update. Nutr Clin Pract 2000;15:5-12.

Brownell KD, Wadden TA: The Learn Program for Weight Control. Dallas, Tex, American Health Publishing Company.

Buchwald H, Avidor Y, Braunwald E, et al: Bariatric surgery: A systematic review and meta-analysis. JAMA 2004;292(14):1724-1737.

Kushner RF: Roadmaps for Clinical Practice: Case Studies in Disease Prevention and Health Promotion—Assessment and Management of Adult Obesity: A Primer for Physicians. Chicago, American Medical Association, 2003.

National Institutes of Health; National Heart, Lung and Blood Institute: North American Association for the Study of Obesity: The Practical Guide to the Identification, Evaluation, and Treatment of Overweight and Obesity in Adults. Bethesda, Md, National Institutes of Health, 2000.

National Task Force on the Prevention and Treatment of Obesity: Overweight, obesity and health risk. Arch Intern Med 2000;160: 898-904.

NIH Consensus Development Conference Panel: Gastrointestinal surgery for severe obesity. Ann Intern Med 1991;115:956-961.

Osteoporosis

Method of
Uriel S. Barzel, MD

Osteoporosis is a condition in which the bones have a propensity to fracture spontaneously or as a result of minimal trauma. In this condition, which is present primarily among the aged, there is too little bone tissue to provide adequate skeletal support for the physical stresses of normal daily life and for commonly encountered minor accidents. Osteoporosis is not clinically apparent until the patient presents with a fracture. Its most common manifestation is wrist fracture, but much more disabling are hip fractures and vertebral collapses, all without a history of severe trauma. The destructive effect of this condition is made clear by the statistics of hip fractures: 20% of patients with hip fractures (about 250,000 annually) die within 1 year of the event, 50% require nursing home care, 20% require help in the activities of daily living, and only 10% return to a normal, self-sufficient life in their own homes.

Some nonspecific radiologic findings are associated with this condition, and some patients may be suspected of having osteoporosis based upon the result of incidental observations made in radiologic procedures. Measurement of bone mineral density by dual-energy x-ray absorptiometry (DEXA) is the current gold standard for the early recognition of osteoporosis in clinical practice.

Achievement of Maximal Skeletal Growth

The achievement of maximal skeletal development requires the consumption of a normal diet with moderate amounts (4 oz per day) of animal proteins and copious amounts of fruits and vegetables, adequate intake of vitamin D and calcium, and physical exercise. Vitamin D can be endogenously synthesized through exposure of the skin to the ultraviolet rays of the sun for a few minutes per day. Vitamin D is available exogenously in cod liver oil, in deep-sea fish, and, in the United States, in non-skim milk that is fortified with vitamin D as well as some fortified fruit juices. It is also widely available singly or in therapeutic vitamin preparations. The recommended daily allowance (RDA) for vitamin D varies with age: 200 IU/day for children and adults through age 50 years, 400 IU/day for adults between 50 and 70 years, and 600 IU/day for persons older than 70 years. The RDA for pregnant and for lactating women is 200 IU/day. The RDA of calcium is also age dependent: Young children require 500 to 800 mg/day. The requirement increases at maturation, in the teens, to 1300 mg/day. For adults ages 20 to 50 years, the recommended amount is 1000 mg/day. After age 50 years, the recommended amount is 1200 mg/day. In pregnancy or lactation, the RDA is 1000 to 1300 mg/day. Both vitamin D and calcium can be obtained in adequate amounts from the ingestion of non-skim milk—one quart of milk provides 1000 mg of calcium and 400 IU of vitamin D. Calcium is also easily available in multiple over-the-counter products, as calcium carbonate, calcium citrate, and other calcium salts, and it can be taken as a supplement. Maintenance of adequate muscle strength, by the performance of weight-bearing exercises such as walking or calisthenics for 30 to 60 minutes three times weekly, is also useful. Excessive exercise may induce amenorrhea and is, therefore, counterproductive because the cessation of estrogen production in this situation results in a negative calcium balance and decreased skeletal mass.

Maintenance of Skeletal Integrity and Prevention of Osteoporosis

Maintenance of skeletal integrity, once maximal development has been achieved, requires continuation of the same regimen of normal diet, adequate intake of calcium and vitamin D, and maintenance of an exercise program. Furthermore, it is recommended that cigarette smoking and excessive alcohol consumption be avoided because these actions are associated with osteoporosis (as well as with other disabilities).

Epidemiologic studies, performed in postmenopausal white women, suggest that taking estrogen early in menopause reduces the risk of osteoporotic fractures by 50%. To eliminate the monthly bleeding associated with cyclic estrogen and progesterone therapy, a combined estrogen plus progesterone formulation, taken continuously, had been a widely accepted as an alternative hormonal treatment. *However, a recent large study—the Women's Health Initiative—found that this fixed combination has risks that outweigh its benefits. Estrogen therapy alone, given in the same study to hysterectomized women, was also found to have risks that outweigh its benefit. Both studies were stopped prematurely because of these findings.* Soy phytoestrogens have not been shown to be of value in relieving menopausal symptoms or improving bone mineral density.

Pathogenesis of Osteoporosis

The origin of this condition is multifactorial. Increased bone resorption relative to bone formation is the basic underlying mechanism. In females, an important factor is the menopausal loss of estrogen that is universally associated with an increase in bone resorption without concomitant increase in bone formation (see earlier). Decreased physical activity may be a contributory factor, as well as a diet containing excessive or insufficient amounts of animal protein, little or no fruits and vegetables, and inadequate intake of calcium. Another factor is poor intestinal absorption of calcium, which occurs frequently in the aged. In the physiologic process of bone turnover, newly laid bone matrix fails to calcify in the absence of vitamin D, leading to the development of osteomalacia in adults (and rickets in children). Bone densitometry cannot differentiate between osteomalacia and osteoporosis.

In some cases, osteoporosis is the result of an endocrinopathy or some other pathologic process. *Hyperadrenocorticism*, due to the administration of corticosteroids or to abnormal adrenal function, is commonly associated with osteoporosis. Steroid hormones block recruitment of osteoblasts (bone-forming cells) and interfere with the absorption of calcium from the gut, thus interfering with the physiologic process of bone turnover. Failure to absorb calcium in the gut results in secondary hyperparathyroidism and accelerated bone resorption (resulting in the maintenance of normal serum calcium). *Hyperparathyroidism* and excess *growth hormone* production may also result in osteoporosis. *Testosterone suppression therapy* may also cause osteoporosis.

Other, far less common causes of osteoporosis include *exercise-induced amenorrhea, anorexia nervosa, chronic heparin administration*, which stimulates resorption of bone by an unknown mechanism, *chronic anemia*, and *immobilization*, as in poliomyelitis, paraplegia, or in space flight.

Osteoporosis is most commonly seen in the elderly, especially in older women, in whom it is known as *postmenopausal osteoporosis*. Epidemiologically, it is more likely to occur in thin white female smokers of northern European extraction, but it is found in all segments of the population, including men. A large prospective follow-up study revealed that a history of hyperthyroidism, a history of a seizure disorder, poor general health, weakness of the lower extremities, and poor vision all contribute to the risk of osteoporotic fractures.

Differential Diagnosis

In the extreme, the diagnosis would be established when a patient presents clinically with an osteoporotic fracture. Wrist fracture (Colles' fracture) is the most common presenting condition of osteoporosis, followed in frequency by collapse fractures of spinal vertebrae and hip fractures. In some cases, patients sustain rib fractures as a result of leaning against a hard surface, such as the side of a bathtub. Today, however, bone "density" (mg/cm^2) is easily measurable by DEXA, which allows us to stratify subjects in terms of likelihood of fractures. People whose bone density is less than two standard deviations (T score < −2.0) from that of young, same-race, same-sex controls are classified as having osteopenia, and those with T score < −2.5 are classified as having osteoporosis.

In osteopenia and in osteoporosis, serum calcium, phosphorus, and alkaline phosphatase levels are normal, as are blood levels of parathyroid hormone and vitamin D metabolites. Urinary calcium excretion is in the normal range as well. Bones are histologically and biochemically normal. Fractures heal normally.

When a patient is found to have a low bone density, with or without fracture, she or he must be evaluated by history, physical examination, and appropriate laboratory tests for underlying conditions that may be responsible for the development of osteoporosis.

In a sample of 272 consecutive patients, mostly females with low bone density consistent with osteoporosis, we found that 17.9% had osteomalacia, 6.7% had hypercalciuria, and approximately 1% had primary hyperparathyroidism. We had one case of osteoporosis secondary to heparin therapy. Women with osteomalacia had low blood levels of 25-hydroxyvitamin D and elevated intact parathyroid hormone. In some cases of hypercalciuria (24-hour urinary calcium >250 mg), the condition was due to marked excess salt intake, but in others it was due to renal leak of calcium. Other causes of osteoporosis were not found in our patient population. We concluded that the minimum workup needed are blood calcium, 25-hydroxyvitamin D, parathyroid hormone, and a collection of 24-hour urine to

CURRENT DIAGNOSIS

- Osteomalacia
- Hypercalciuria
- Acromegaly
- Hyperparathyroidism
- Hyperthyroidism
- Hyperadrenocorticism
- Celiac disease
- Multiple myeloma
- Prolonged heparin therapy
- Lipid storage disease
- Liver disease
- Chronic anemia
- Testosterone suppression

TABLE 1 Diagnostic Evaluation

Blood calcium
25-Hydroxyvitamin D
Parathyroid hormone
Thyroid-stimulating hormone
24-Hour urinary calcium, sodium, and creatinine
N-Telopeptide (second morning urine)*
Osteocalcin*

*Used as guides to therapy.

determine total calcium and total sodium excretion. (Some physicians use the ratio of calcium to creatinine as a differential diagnostic test. A ratio >0.25 is associated with an increase in bone turnover, and a ratio <0.15 is due to malabsorption syndromes or disorders of vitamin D metabolism.) Thyroid-stimulating hormone (TSH) screening in the elderly patient may be appropriate (Table 1).

Prevention and Treatment of Osteoporosis

The major thrust today is the prevention of clinical disease. For this reason, I believe that every woman who enters the menopause should undergo determination of her bone density. If the density is normal, it can be rechecked 5 to 7 years later, after the accelerated loss of bone secondary to estrogen deficiency has run its course. If the density is still normal, it probably is reasonable not to be concerned about bone density until the patient is 65 years old.

If bone density is found to be low at either of the two earlier ages, differential diagnostic studies are imperative. If these studies reveal no abnormality, preventive treatment is undertaken leisurely, as fractures rarely occur before age 60. Thus, at this point, I stress the establishment of proper daily routines, including brisk walking for 30 minutes daily; adequate, but not excessive, animal protein intake; consumption of generous amounts of fruits and vegetables; and intake of calcium and vitamin D at the proper RDA levels. In cases of vitamin D deficiency, repletion with vitamin D (Drisdol), 50,000 U weekly or biweekly over 12 weeks, is mandatory. In cases of hypercalciuria, low sodium intake and/or hydrochlorothiazide therapy are in order. In these cases, the appropriate parameters are reexamined and dosage adjustments made as indicated.

In special situations, medical intervention can prevent the development of osteoporosis. These include patients with certain endocrine conditions, such as hyperadrenocorticism, acromegaly, and thyrotoxicosis, as well as those with ingestion of excess thyroid hormone, gastrectomy, and liver disease. To the extent possible, endocrine disease should be kept under optimal control. Patients receiving thyroxin replacement should be given this hormone in amounts that would maintain normal serum thyroxin and serum TSH levels. Suppression of the serum TSH level below the normal range should be avoided (except in cases of thyroid cancer in which this is the therapeutic goal). If patients require pharmacologic doses of corticosteroids as a long-term therapy, bisphosphonate therapy (see later) provides significant protection from osteoporosis.

CURRENT THERAPY

- Adequate intake of animal proteins
- Generous amounts of fruits and vegetables
- Calcium supplements (per recommended daily allowance)
  - Calcium carbonate
  - Calcium citrate malate
  - Calcium citrate*
- Adequate vitamin D intake (per recommended daily allowance)
- Exercise
- Teriparatide (Forteo)
- Alendronate (Fosamax)
- Risedronate (Actonel)
- Raloxifene (Evista)
- Calcitonin (Calcimar)
- Ibandronate (Boniva)
- Hydrochlorothiazide[†]
- Low sodium intake[†]

*Preferred preparation in hypochlorhydria.
[†]May be useful in controlling hypercalciuria.

Some element of protection of the skeleton can be achieved in these cases by coadministration of pharmacologic doses (50,000–100,000 U/week) of vitamin D and an adequate calcium intake. In postgastrectomy states, osteomalacia may develop unless adequate vitamin D is given regularly to overcome a degree of malabsorption that is present in this condition.

In patients with T score less than –2.5, I resort to pharmacologic therapy. The available choices include nasal calcitonin, oral antiresorptive drugs (alendronate, risedronate, ibandronate), intravenous ibandronate (see later), an oral selective estrogen receptor modulator (raloxifene), and injection therapy with teriparatide. All but teriparatide function by limiting bone resorption, thus allowing bone formation to "catch up." Teriparatide, on the other hand, achieves its effect by stimulating bone formation.

In newly diagnosed patients with markedly low bone density (T score < –4.0), teriparatide is the treatment of choice. It stimulates bone formation and increases connectivity of bone trabeculae. When used in a medically naïve case, bone density can improve by as much as 12% per year. This costly medication is available in prefilled pens and disposable needles and is administered subcutaneously at a dose of 20 µg/day. The patient who injects herself daily must be provided with instruction on use of the pen. The Food and Drug Administration (FDA) has approved the use of this drug for 18 months. It has a black box, disclosing the fact of increased osteosarcoma in rats subjected to 3 to 60 times the exposure given to humans. When given in conjunction with alendronate, the effectiveness of teriparatide is severely diminished, resulting in only 2% improvement in 1 year.

I use bisphosphonate therapy in patients with less severe osteoporosis (T score between –2.5 and –4.0). Alendronate was the first oral antiresorptive bisphosphonate approved by the FDA for treatment of osteoporosis (at a dose of 10 mg/day). Patients are instructed to take it with a large glass of water, to remain upright, and to take no food or medications for 30 minutes. Bone density improves by an average of 6% in the first year and by less in subsequent years. Some patients achieve T scores of –2.0 or better when alendronate is added to the daily regimen of calcium and vitamin D supplementation, diet, and exercise described earlier, and they are able to discontinue the medication and maintain the new bone density on this regimen. Some patients considered the requirements for daily remaining upright and avoiding food or medication for 30 minutes a hardship, and they welcomed the 70-mg alendronate formulation designed for once-per-week dosing. However, no evidence in the literature indicates improved compliance with the once-per-week regimen. A major side effect is esophageal or gastrointestinal intolerance.

I consider adherence to the regimen of *daily* taking of medication, physical activity, proper diet, and calcium and vitamin D supplements mandatory for treatment and maintenance of achieved normal bone density. I do not want my patients to assume that just taking a pill once per week will miraculously cure them. With the widespread advertising of once-per-week alendronate to the general public, I found it increasingly difficult to convince patients to maintain the daily routine that I believed was necessary for therapeutic success. When the 5-mg risedronate became available at the same time, I began using this medication with equal success. It also must be taken with a large glass of water, and the patient must remain upright and take no food or medications for 30 minutes. Its side-effect profile is similar to that of alendronate. The rates of improvement of bone density and prevention of fractures differ between risedronate and alendronate, but I consider them to be essentially equal.

It was shown recently that the residence of risedronate in the body is measured in months, whereas that of alendronate is measured in years. This fact is of potential importance in patients who do not respond to antiresorptive therapy and in whom teriparatide is the next best choice. It is theoretically likely that a drug holiday of only a few months would allow teriparatide to reach maximum effect in patients who have been taking risedronate but not alendronate.

In patients with esophageal or gastrointestinal intolerance to the bisphosphonates, raloxifene is the next choice. This selective estrogen receptor modulator, given at a dose of 60 mg daily, has been shown to be effective in improving bone density without having breast or uterine stimulating effects. It achieves about half the rate of recovery of bone density as that of bisphosphonates, but it has no gastrointestinal side effects. Its major side effects are hot flushes and thromboembolism. It is approved for treatment of reduced bone density and osteopenia but not for established osteoporosis. The recent introduction of intravenous ibandronate (see later) gives the clinician and the patient another alternative solution to the gastrointestinal/esophageal problem.

Calcitonin, a hormone with significant effect on Paget's disease, has been approved by the FDA for treatment of osteoporosis. Administered at a dose of 50 to 100 IU subcutaneously or intramuscularly every day or every other day, salmon calcitonin has a salutary effect on bone density, but the studies are too short and contain too few subjects to prove that calcitonin treatment prevents fractures. I have little experience with nasal calcitonin, which replaced the injectable formulation. Its major side effect is nasal mucosal irritation.

Ibandronate (Boniva) has been approved for daily oral administration at a dose of 2.5 mg, for monthly administration at a dose of 150 mg, and for intravenous administration of 3 mg every 3 months for treatment of osteoporosis.

A recent report identifies the rare earth mineral strontium, in the form of strontium ranelate, as another oral treatment that increases bone formation and reduces spinal fracture in osteoporotic women. It is not yet available commercially in the United States.

Denosumab, a fully human monoclonal antibody that specifically targets the receptor activator of nuclear factor kappa B ligand (RANKL), a key mediator of the resorptive phase of bone remodeling, is being studied for its possible effect in reducing bone resorption in osteoporosis. In a preliminary study of postmenopausal women with low bone mass, denosumab given intravenously every 3 months increased bone mineral density and decreased bone resorption.

Fractures

When presented with a case of apparent osteoporosis and a fracture, we treat the actual fracture and at the same time review the differential diagnosis (see Table 1) and initiate a treatment regimen for whatever underlying condition may be responsible for the development of osteoporosis. It must be remembered that patients who have experienced one osteoporotic fracture are at very high risk for a second fracture. Colles' fracture is treated by casting. Spinal collapse is treated with injection of cement into the vertebra. This method stabilizes the involved vertebra but does not protect the adjacent vertebrae from potential future collapse. Previously, the only available treatment for collapse fracture of vertebrae was complete bed rest until the acute pain had substantially diminished (72 hours to 2 weeks), followed by gradual mobilization, first to an inclined chair and later to full upright position and re-ambulation. Pain treatment in such cases should avoid narcotics, if possible, because of their tendency to produce constipation. A corset can be used for a few weeks to support the spine during recovery, followed by physiotherapy. Hip fractures generally require surgical pinning or hip replacement, followed by aggressive physiotherapy. In addition to the regimen of diet, calcium plus vitamin D, and weight-bearing physical activity, hip fracture patients and those with gait disorders or neurologic diseases that predispose them to falls may benefit from wearing a hip protector during waking hours.

REFERENCES

Barzel US, Aragaki A, Rittenbaugh C, et al: Increased risk of fractures is associated with acidogenic food intake among postmenopausal women enrolled in the observational study of the women's health initiative. Manuscript in preparation.

Cranney A, Guyatt G, Griffith I, et al: Meta-analyses of therapies for postmenopausal osteoporosis. Endocr Rev 2002:23;570-578.

Freitag A, Barzel US: Differential diagnosis of osteoporosis. Gerontology 2002;48:98-102.

Miller PD, Bilezikian JP, Deal C, et al: Clinical use of teriparatide in the real world: Initial insights. Endocr Pract 2004;10:139-148.

Paget's Disease of Bone

Method of
Paul D. Miller, MD

Diagnosis

Paget's disease is characterized by excessively high bone turnover in the involved skeletal site(s). Although the bone may appear "osteosclerotic" on radiographic evaluation, the bone strength is actually compromised and may easily fracture. Paget's disease may present with pain in the involved skeleton, or it may be asymptomatic and suspected when a patient is discovered to have either an elevated total serum alkaline phosphatase level or an unexplained elevated bone resorption marker (e.g., urine or serum collagen cross-link of type I collagen: *N*- or *C*-telopeptide). If a physician discovers an unexplained elevated total alkaline phosphatase level, then the source of this elevated enzyme must be differentiated as either hepatic or bone (assuming the patient is not pregnant because the placenta also produces alkaline phosphatase). If the alkaline phosphatase originates from bone, differential diagnosis of the possible causes of an elevated bone-specific alkaline phosphatase (BSAP) level is as follows:

1. Paget's disease
2. Metastatic cancer in bone
3. Recent large bone fracture
4. Osteomalacia
5. Hyperthyroidism
6. Hyperparathyroidism
7. Medication induced (antiseizure drugs, parathyroid hormone used for treatment of osteoporosis)
8. Immobilization/space travel
9. Vitamin D deficiency without osteomalacia

Many of these potential causes of an elevated BSAP level can be differentiated clinically and by laboratory testing. In patients who still have an elevated BSAP level of undeterminable etiology, a total body bone scan is required to locate any "hot spots" that could suggest Paget's disease. I always simultaneously order a routine radiograph of any hot spots seen on a radioisotope bone scan because Paget's disease is a radiographic, not a bone scan, diagnosis. The one radiographic finding that can be confused with Paget's disease is metastatic prostatic carcinoma. However, metastatic prostatic cancer is associated

CURRENT DIAGNOSIS

- No known cause.
- Diagnosed by radiography, not by bone scan or magnetic resonance imaging.
- Often asymptomatic.
- May be active with normal biochemical markers of bone turnover: collagen cross-links or bone-specific alkaline phosphatase.

with an elevated prostate-specific antigen level and other clinical findings of prostatic abnormalities. Given any radiographic finding that one has difficulty distinguishing between Paget's disease and prostatic cancer, a magnetic resonance image is more distinctly abnormal in metastatic cancer to bone, or, if necessary, a bone biopsy is definitive.

Painful Paget's disease requires treatment. Bisphosphonates are the treatment of choice because of their exceptional efficacy and safety when used appropriately in Paget's disease. Bisphosphonates may have the potential of "curing" Paget's disease or, at least, putting the disease into very prolonged and sustained biochemical and clinical remission.

Asymptomatic Paget's disease should also be treated. Although the proportion of patients with asymptomatic Paget's disease who progress to become symptomatic is not known, progression does occur in many patients, and who might or who might not progress cannot be predicted from the initial assessment. Because progression can lead to bony deformities, fractures, hearing loss, neurologic complications (spinal cord compression, nerve entrapment), high-output congestive heart failure, and osteogenic sarcoma, asymptomatic patients merit strong consideration for treatment. To reiterate, because the bisphosphonates are very safe, especially when required only intermittently in Paget's patients, and can be administered either by the oral or intravenous route, they should not be withheld in asymptomatic Paget's patients.

A few patients with Paget's disease may have normal BSAP but elevated bone resorption (NTX/CTX) markers. In my opinion, this combination of disassociated bone formation versus bone resorption markers may be seen in two circumstances: very early Paget's disease—classic or type 1 Paget's disease, and type 2 Paget's disease, in which the BSAP level never becomes elevated despite sustained elevation of the bone resorption markers.

Paget's disease is a disease of the osteoclasts, the cells that induce bone resorption. In pagetic bone biopsies, these osteoclasts are larger, have many more nuclei, and are increased in number compared to osteoclasts seen in normal patients or in patients with osteoporosis. The initial pathophysiologic process in Paget's disease is excessive bone resorption. Thus, the first radiologic defect seen is an osteolytic lesion (a "black" hole) in bone. Hence, early in the pagetic process, an increase in bone resorption markers is seen before the bone formation markers increase. Owing to the normal coupling process between the bone cell lines (increasing or decreasing bone resorption is followed by a directional increase or a decrease in bone formation), bone formation will, in time, also increase, and the BSAP level will ultimately rise. As the BSAP level rises, the osteolytic lesion begins to develop sclerosis and fill in with the white-appearing honeycombed pagetic features. This is the classic sequence in most pagetic patients.

Type 2 Paget's disease looks just like type 1 on radiography: the initial osteolytic lesion is present. The difference between the two forms of Paget's disease is that the osteolytic lesion persists: the bone resorption markers remain elevated without a rise in BSAP or filling in of the osteolytic lesion. There is something different about this very uncommon form of Paget's disease that both I and my colleagues, who see many Paget's patients, have observed in clinical practice. The normal coupling between bone cell lines seems to be absent. It is possible that these patients started out with a low BSAP level, and that it did increase but never above the upper limits of the normal reference range. It may also be true that type 2 Paget's disease is a different disease from a pathophysiologic point of view than type 1 Paget's disease. It is important, however, to stress that even if the BSAP level never becomes elevated, the high NTX/CTX ratio confers enough evidence of high bone turnover of a sufficient magnitude to warrant treatment because these persistent osteolytic pagetic lesions are highly prone to fracture. Multiple myeloma is another clinical condition characterized by high bone resorption and elevated bone resorption markers without an increase in either bone formation or in the bone formation markers BSAP. Despite the presence of many osteolytic lesions in patients with advanced multiple myeloma, the BSAP level never becomes elevated. Hence, myeloma represents another situation in which there is uncoupling between bone resorption and bone formation, as may be seen in type 2 Paget's disease.

Do the two different forms of Paget's disease respond differently to treatment? Probably not, although the proportion of patients with type 2 Paget's disease is small and insufficient for a head-to-head study with type 1 disease to determine any differences in treatment response.

Treatment

The Food and Drug Administration (FDA)–approved therapies for treatment of Paget's disease are calcitonin and bisphosphonates. Off-label use of gallium nitrate (Ganite)[1] or pliamycin[2] is available for the very rare

---

[1]Not FDA approved for this indication.
[2]Not available in the United States.

 CURRENT THERAPY

- Bisphosphonates are the treatment of choice.
- Bisphosphonates should be used in asymptomatic patients who have elevated bone turnover markers.
- May be mono-ostotic (single bone involvement) or polyostotic (more than one bone involved). Once the patient is diagnosed with either mono-ostotic or polyostotic Paget's disease, those bones will be the only ones ever involved. Paget's disease does not spread from one bone to another.
- Recent data suggest that the greater the magnitude of normalization of the total or bone-specific alkaline phosphatase level achieved with treatment, the longer the duration of remission.
- Prevalence is highly variable throughout the world: estimated to be 2% of the white population of North America, declining in northern England, and very rare in China. However, the accuracy of prevalence data must be interpreted in the context that many asymptomatic patients are radiographed, and population radiographic studies that assessed prevalence radiographed only specific skeletal sites, so some involved areas could have been missed.

recalcitrant patient. I have not needed to use either gallium nitrate or pliamycin for more than 20 years because of the exceptional response rate to bisphosphonates. In addition, the response rate seems far greater with bisphosphonates than with calcitonin, which for Paget's disease must be given parenterally and has a high nausea side-effect profile.

Injectable calcitonin has been used for more than 25 years as therapy for Paget's disease and may be considered an option in patients who might not be able to tolerate or to be given a bisphosphonate. Subcutaneous administration of 100 IU/day[3] often leads to an average 50% reduction in bone turnover markers 3 to 6 months after therapy. The nasal spray formulation of calcitonin (Miacalcin) is not FDA approved for Paget's disease.

The bisphosphonates available for treatment of Paget's disease are: etidronate (Didronel), alendronate (Fosamax), risedronate (Actonel, oral formulations), and pamidronate (Aredia). Zolendronic acid[4] is currently under review by the FDA for registration for Paget's disease.

The bisphosphonates alendronate and risedronate have the most robust data showing an exceptional positive effect in the treatment of Paget's disease. Alendronate (Fosamax) at a dose of 40 mg/day for 6 months or risedronate (Actonel) at a dose of 30 mg/day for 2 months can rapidly normalize the NTX/CTX ratio or BSAP level in the majority of patients. No head-to-head clinical trials have compared the efficacy of these two bisphosphonates in Paget's disease, although a head-to-head study did compare etidronate to risedronate in active Paget's disease. Risedronate was clearly more effective in reducing the BSAP level and inducing a longer remission than was etidronate. Selection between the two aminobisphosphonates (alendronate and risedronate) probably is based on physician preference, tolerability, and costs. With either bisphosphonate, bone turnover marker should be measured at the end of the treatment period. If the BSAP level has not normalized, either a second course of the oral bisphosphonate or a change to an intravenous bisphosphonate should be considered. As previously stated, normalization of the BSAP level is the goal of treatment, and the lower the BSAP level, the greater the probability of a longer duration of remission.

Recently, clinical trial data on the efficacy of intravenous zolendronic acid[4] in the treatment of Paget's disease were published. The study showed that 5 mg of intravenous zolendronic acid given over 15 minutes induced a more rapid therapeutic response along with a larger proportion of patients who responded with normalization of BSAP level than was seen with risedronate. In addition, in the 6-month posttreatment follow-up, a greater proportion of patients who received zolendronic acid were still in remission than those who had received risedronate. This finding is consistent with the observations suggesting that the duration of remission is related to the magnitude of suppression of BSAP.

Zolendronic acid[4] has also been shown to have a greater effect on alkaline phosphatase than pamidronate, the other available intravenous nitrogen-containing bisphosphonate.

Hence, with highly effective oral and intravenous bisphosphonates available for treatment of Paget's disease, the clinician must choose which one to use. In my practice, all Paget's disease patients who have pain receive an intravenous bisphosphonate because the pain reduction or elimination is very fast. On the other hand, for asymptomatic Paget's patients, I often use an oral bisphosphonate, saving the intravenous formulations for recalcitrant patients or for patients with relapses. This approach may change as the data evolve, confirming that the duration of remission is prolonged with greater suppression of BSAP. Certainly, costs may become a consideration in the choice, as will upper gastrointestinal conditions that could make an oral bisphosphonate risky. On the other hand, in the zolendronic acid versus risedronate clinical trial, more patients receiving zolendronic acid experienced the acute-phase reaction (fever, muscle pain), which was transient and without sequelae. Nevertheless, intravenous formulations may not be preferred in some patients.

Resistance to bisphosphonates may develop in Paget's disease. After repeated doses of a particular bisphosphonate, some patients stop responding to that particular bisphosphonate but do respond to a different bisphosphonate. The reason for resistance development is unknown because it has not been described in patients treated with bisphosphonates for osteoporosis. Another unexplained phenomenon in Paget's patients who develop resistance to a particular bisphosphonate is that often they again become responsive to the bisphosphonate to which they had become unresponsive after a period of not receiving that specific bisphosphonate.

Finally, there are a few instances in the treatment of Paget's disease in which the clinician must use extra diligence. One is the patient with a painful osteolytic lesion in the proximal femur. Bisphosphonate administration will often relieve the pain promptly, which may encourage the patient to increase activity and weight bearing, and then the hip may fracture. In these circumstances, the patient should be cautioned about this potential and provided with a cane to support the leg until the osteolytic lesion fills in (several months). Another area of caution is the patient who does not respond to any treatment, who relapses quickly and has a rapidly progressive radiographic pagetic change, or develops more pain, swelling, and redness over the pagetic bone. Osteogenic sarcoma could be a distinct possibility, and the lesion may require biopsy. Finally, a third area of caution is the patient in whom neurologic impairment may be related to pagetic bone encroachment, spinal cord compression with long-tract signs, spinal stenosis, or basilar skull invagination with neural compromise. Close consultation with a neurosurgeon is needed to help decide on a possible surgical intervention through a highly vascular pagetic bone. Administration of intravenous bisphosphonate 1 to 2 days before surgery might mitigate bleeding because bisphosphonates reduce blood flow in highly vascular areas for a period of time.

Paget's disease is manageable and may be put into very long-term remission by normalization of the biochemical markers of bone turnover. Asymptomatic patients with high bone turnover should be treated to prevent potential long-term complications. Treatment in these patients is very reasonable given the evidence that the newer aminobisphosphonates are highly effective and very safe when used appropriately.

---

[3]Exceeds dosage recommended by the manufacturer.
[4]Not yet approved for use in the United States.

REFERENCES

Altman RD, Bloch DA, Hochberg MC, Murphy WA: Prevalence of pelvic Paget's disease of bone in the United States. J Bone Miner Res 2000;15:461-465.

Miller PD, Brown JP, Siris ES, et al: A randomized, double-blind comparison of risedronate and etidronate in the treatment of Paget's disease of bone. Am J Med 1999;106:513-520.

Reid IR, Miller PD, Lyles K, et al: Comparison of a single infusion of zolendronic acid with risedronate for Paget's disease. N Engl J Med 2005;353:22-32.

Reid IR, Nicholson GC, Weinstein RS, et al: Biochemical and radiologic improvement in Paget's disease of bone treated with alendronate: A randomized, placebo-controlled trial. Am J Med 1996;101:341-348.

Total Parenteral Nutrition in Adults

Method of
Gail Cresci, MS, RD, and
Robert Martindale, MD, PhD

The era of parenteral nutrition (PN) began in the 1960s when a technique to access the central venous circulation was demonstrated. Placement of a central venous catheter allows for the delivery of large volumes of hypertonic PN formulations, which are rapidly diluted in the high-flow central vein. Previously, the provision of PN was limited to isotonic or slightly hypertonic solutions infused through a peripheral vein. Limitations of peripheral PN are the need for large fluid volumes to meet the patient's nutritional needs leading to potential fluid overload and frequent loss of peripheral venous access. Extensive knowledge about the provision of total parenteral nutrition (TPN) has evolved over the past 45 years. There is now a multitude of commercial products available for inclusion in TPN formulations such as amino acids, carbohydrates, lipid emulsions, electrolytes, vitamins, minerals, and trace elements.

Indications

Like any invasive therapy, TPN has inherent risks (Table 1). TPN is indicated when nutrient provision via the enteral route is inadequate or not tolerated for periods greater than 7 days, the enteral route should be avoided, or when the enteral route may be detrimental to the disease process. A number of meta-analyses of the use of PN in different patient populations including intensive care, oncology, and surgery have not shown benefit and have generally reported increased complications. Therefore, careful patient selection for TPN is necessary and should only be considered when the enteral route is not an option.

TPN offers the obvious advantage that a functional gastrointestinal (GI) tract is not required. The parenteral route provides considerable ease in nutrient delivery, and as shown in several recent large series, the nutritional requirements are met more consistently. These *ease of delivery* advantages may be overshadowed by TPN's alleged disadvantages. The adverse effect of TPN on the mucosal barrier and gut-associated lymphoid tissue (GALT) has been extensively investigated. Other adverse effects often associated with TPN are hepatic impairment including steatosis, cholestasis and cholelithiasis, systemic immunosuppression, venous thrombosis, and local complications at the venous access site.

The proposed advantages of enteral nutrition (EN) over parenteral in surgical and critically ill patients are now well described. They include attenuation of the metabolic response to stress, improved nitrogen balance, better glycemic control, increased visceral protein synthesis, increased GI anastomotic strength, and increased

TABLE 1 Indications for Total Parenteral Nutrition

Clinical Condition	TPN Indicated	Comments
Critical illness	EN preferred; TPN may be necessary during low flow states to supplement enteral feeding; prolonged ileus	PN glutamine shown benefit PN lipids containing n-3 FA, MCT, MUFA beneficial
Acute pancreatitis	EN preferred; TPN as alternative in those without jejunal enteral access, severe ileus; combined with EN when it's not fully tolerated, hemodynamic instability	PN lipids do not exacerbate disease; n-3 FAs, MCT lipids preferred
Hepatic failure	EN preferred; TPN if active GI bleeding, bowel obstruction, hemodynamic instability, supplement to enteral	High BCAA formulations for refractory HE
Renal failure	EN preferred; TPN if enteral contraindicated or needs supplementing	Use of standard amino acid solutions preferred more than those containing low amounts of nonessential amino acids
SBS	TPN initially until patient stable, fluid/electrolyte balance maintained; introduce enteral feeding slowly, monitor for tolerance, wean TPN accordingly	Additional vitamins and trace elements may be required for stool outputs >1 L/d
Enterocutaneous fistula	TPN initially until patient stable, fluid/electrolyte balance maintained; introduce enteral feeding slowly, monitor for tolerance, wean TPN accordingly	Additional vitamins, trace elements, protein, and fluid outputs >500 mL/d

Abbreviations: BCAA = branched-chain amino acid; EN = enteral nutrition; FA = fatty acid; GI = gastrointestinal; HE = hepatic encephalopathy; MCT = medium-chain triglyceride; MUFA = monounsaturated fatty acid; PN = parenteral nutrition; SBS = short bowel syndrome; TPN = total parenteral nutrition.

collagen deposition. Other benefits of EN include decreased nosocomial infections, enhanced visceral blood flow, increased variety of nutrients available for delivery, and decreased risk of GI bleeding. Many of the proposed physiologic benefits of EN are based on animal studies with limited corroborating human data.

Recommendations for the use and specific indications for TPN are provided by several nutrition societies, including the American Society of Parenteral and Enteral Nutrition. When specialized nutrition support is indicated, TPN should only be used when the GI tract is not functional, cannot be safely accessed, or when adequate nutrients (approximately 60% nutritional needs) are not tolerated by oral diets and/or EN in which a combination of TPN and enteral feeding may be provided. TPN should be initiated in the aforementioned patients in whom inadequate oral intake is expected over a 7- to 14-day period.

There are several disease states and clinical situations where TPN is preferred over EN because of hemodynamic instability and low visceral blood flow states, inadequate nutrient absorption, or enteral feeding intolerance.

Guidelines for Diseases

CRITICAL ILLNESS

Most critically ill patients exhibit one or more organ system dysfunctions necessitating active medical intervention. The systemic inflammatory response syndrome (SIRS) or sepsis is frequently present in critically ill patients. Metabolic alterations caused by cytokine, neuroendocrine, and hormone changes in response to the metabolic insult result in hypermetabolism, hyperglycemia and insulin resistance, and proteolysis with increased nitrogen losses. Nutrition intervention in these patients is supportive because it can slow the rate of net protein catabolism. Enteral feeding is the preferred route of nutrient delivery in critically ill patients. However, even with best efforts, adequate nutrient provision with enteral feeding is not always tolerated in the critically ill. Also, in early stages of critical care admissions, patients may often be hemodynamically unstable and require vasopressor support for stability, which results in decreased visceral blood flow. Therefore, TPN may be necessary to solely provide nutrient needs or supplement the patient's enteral intake if nutritional goals cannot be safely met after 7 to 10 days of attempts.

Supplementation with a variety of nutrients at pharmacologic doses has been investigated, primarily in trauma and surgical patients. Various TPN amino acid solutions have been reviewed in critically ill patients. Studies of branched-chain amino acid (BCAA)-enriched TPN solutions have not demonstrated a decreased catabolic rate or a reduction in morbidity or mortality. Although there are theoretical reasons for the use of BCAA-enriched solutions in the critical care population, they are not consistently superior to standard amino acid solution. Glutamine is a nonessential amino acid but may be essential in certain clinical settings (i.e., critical illness) because the body is unable to synthesize sufficient amounts. Glutamine[1] is not currently included in parenteral amino

---

[1]Not FDA approved for this indication.

acid solutions because of limited solubility (3.5 g/dL) and stability (degradation with heat sterilization and prolonged storage). In the critically ill, decreased complications and hospital length of stay as well as improved survival have been associated with PN glutamine supplementation at doses from 0.26 to 0.57 g/kg per day. Intravenous (IV) lipids should be provided to critically ill patients to prevent essential fatty acid (FA) deficiency. However, because the solutions in the United States are very rich in n-6 FAs, provisions greater than 25% of total calories are associated with inflammation and immunosuppression. Outside the United States various parenteral lipid emulsions are available. Those containing omega-3 FAs, medium-chain triglycerides (MCT), and monounsaturated FAs (MUFAs) have shown beneficial effects such as decreased inflammatory responses and immune function.

ACUTE PANCREATITIS

Most patients with acute pancreatitis have a mild or self-limiting illness that resolves within 5 to 7 days. These patients can usually start with an oral diet within the first 3 days of onset if their pain is diminished, and the pancreatic enzymes have a tendency to return to normal. The patients who should be targeted for aggressive nutrition support are those at risk for developing severe necrotizing pancreatitis or infected pancreatic necrosis. Specific nutritional support depends on the severity of the disease. It is therefore essential to define the patients at risk and assess their nutritional needs throughout the course of the disease. Traditionally TPN was used to avoid stimulation of the exocrine pancreatic secretory response, or *pancreatic rest*. However, recent studies have shown that enteral feeding is superior to TPN in mild to severe necrotizing pancreatitis. EN when compared to TPN was found to attenuate the acute phase response in acute pancreatitis and attenuate disease severity and improve clinical outcome.

TPN is indicated in patients in whom a jejunal feeding tube near or distal to the ligament of Treitz cannot be placed, those with a severe ileus, as a supplement to enteral feeding, or in those who are hemodynamically labile. IV lipids have not been shown to exacerbate the disease and can be provided in the majority of patients with pancreatitis.

HEPATIC FAILURE

The liver plays a central role in metabolism, storage, and distribution of nutrients leading to protein calorie malnutrition and nutritional deficiencies in patients with hepatic failure. The pathophysiology of malnutrition is multifactorial and complex. Dietary restrictions and GI symptoms may limit nutrient intake, fat malabsorption may occur because of altered bile acid production, and total nutrient malabsorption may occur because of medication therapy (lactulose, neomycin). Therefore, the provision of nutritional support to patients with hepatic failure can be a life-saving treatment modality.

Altered amino acid metabolism is the hallmark of liver disease, characterized by low levels of circulating BCAA and elevated levels of aromatic amino acids (AAAs). This altered amino acid profile is thought to be responsible for the production of *false neurotransmitters,* resulting in ineffective neurotransmission and the induction of hepatic encephalopathy (HE). Historically, the general recommendation for patients with HE has been to restrict protein intake to avoid excessive ammonia production. However, severe restriction of protein can worsen nutritional deficits and liver function. Trials have demonstrated that patients with hepatic failure can tolerate normal or increased protein intake of up to 70 g per day without exacerbating HE. Special amino acid formulations that are high in BCAA but low in AAA have been considered the alternative for protein intolerance in HE. They were initially administered to correct the abnormal serum amino acid profile and prevent the changes in blood brain barrier transport abnormalities and formation of *false neurotransmitters*. However, several randomized controlled trials of BCAA have not shown major beneficial effects on morbidity and mortality. A recent trial of 174 patients, comparing outcomes after 1 year of dietary supplements of BCAA versus lactalbumin or maltodextrin, showed significantly lower mortality, decreased hospital admission, and shorter hospital stay in the BCAA arm of the study.

PN is generally reserved for patients who cannot receive EN, as in cases of active GI hemorrhage or small bowel obstruction. The use of central PN is preferred over peripheral because less fluid volume is required to provide calories and protein because these patients are often fluid restricted. Parenteral BCAA solutions should be reserved for patients who have refractory HE.

RENAL FAILURE

Renal failure causes a variety of metabolic and clinical abnormalities that can affect a patient's nutritional status. The degree of actual nutritional impairment or risk of its development is dependent on the metabolic stress, the degree and duration of renal failure (acute versus chronic), and the medical intervention for its treatment. The type of medical intervention for treatment of renal failure greatly impacts nutrient delivery and its tolerance. Renal failure patients undergoing dialysis have elevated protein needs compared to those who do not. Often dialysis patients are malnourished because of nutrient restrictions and resultant inadequate consumption of allowed unpalatable foods.

Nutritional support is for those unable to consume adequate nutrients orally. Enteral feeding is preferred over parenteral. TPN is for patients unable to tolerate adequate enteral nutrients or where EN is contraindicated. There are several commercially available parenteral amino acid solutions designed for patients with renal compromise. These products contain predominantly essential amino acids as well as histidine. One product also contains arginine, which is important in the urea cycle, and another contains lower amounts of nonessential amino acids. The essential amino acid solutions for renal failure were based on the principles established for treating patients with chronic renal failure (CRF) with a low-protein diet and an essential amino acid supplement using the concept that the patient can endogenously produce the nonessential amino acids via transamination. Because of underlying differences in the metabolic response between chronic and acute renal failure, essential-only amino acid solutions may not meet protein needs. The benefits of modified amino acid solutions for renal failure over standard amino acids in acute renal failure remain controversial. For most patients with acute renal failure, a standard amino acid solution that contains both essential and nonessential amino acids should be used. In the event where dialysis is not used, protein should be restricted for a short period. Intradialytic TPN has been used as a supplement to protein and calorie intake for malnourished patients receiving maintenance hemodialysis. This therapy has several disadvantages and should be reserved for situations such as gut failure or when access problems exist inhibiting the ability to provide enteral feeding or TPN.

Intestinal Diseases

SHORT BOWEL SYNDROME

Short bowel syndrome (SBS) is secondary to either an anatomic or functional loss of mucosal absorptive surface resulting in malabsorption, and/or maldigestion, diarrhea, and steatorrhea. Although intestinal resection accounts for the majority of SBS cases, mucosal diseases such as Crohn's disease can result in functional SBS. With a normal small bowel length of 300 to 500 cm, symptoms of SBS typically begin when more than 50% of the small intestine is lost. Determinants of disease severity depend on the length of bowel resected or diseased, anatomic location of bowel affected (jejunum, ileum), and the presence or absence of the ileocecal valve.

Following resection, fluid, electrolyte, and nutrient absorption are compromised, and patients frequently become dehydrated. Most patients require TPN for a specific length of time; patients with less than 100 cm of small bowel distal to the ligament of Treitz and without a colon often require TPN indefinitely. Once the patient is stabilized and fluids and electrolytes are balanced, enteral feeding may be introduced. The goal is to maintain stool losses at less than 1 L per day. Often a combination of EN and TPN can be tolerated; early attempts at enteral feeding are crucial because enteral feeding is trophic to gut mucosa. TPN is reduced gradually as enteral intake is tolerated, diarrhea decreases, and nutritional status is maintained. For patients with distal resections, fat-soluble vitamin supplementation and vitamin B_{12} injections may be required.

ENTEROCUTANEOUS FISTULA

Abdominal operations account for the majority of enterocutaneous fistulas (EF); other predisposing conditions include Crohn's disease, neoplasia, infection, and radiation. Fistulas are classified by their location in the GI tract and by their output (>500 mL per day is high output; <500 mL per day is low output). Early management of extracellular fluid (ECF) is similar to SBS with control of sepsis, drainage of abscesses, aggressive resuscitation by restoring intravascular volume and electrolyte abnormalities. Skin protection and aggressive nutrition support are the next main priorities because these patients are typically malnourished.

Although enteral feeding is the preferred method of nutrient provision, TPN is often provided in the early stages of ECF to promote bowel rest and control fistula output and potential spontaneous fistula closure. The spontaneous closure rate ranges from 30% to 70%

depending on EC location, co-morbid factors, and nutritional state. Location of the fistula largely dictates the route of feeding. If at least 100 cm of bowel exists between the ligament of Treitz and the fistula, then enteral feeding should be attempted. Often a combination of TPN and enteral feeding is provided. Patients require additional vitamins, minerals, trace elements, fluids, protein, and electrolytes with high output fistulas.

Administration

ROUTE OF TOTAL PARENTERAL NUTRITION DELIVERY

Central venous access is the preferred route for infusion of TPN because it allows for maximizing nutrient delivery while minimizing volume. Peripherally inserted central catheters (PICCs) are inserted into a peripheral vein and advanced into a central vein. They also are useful for administering long-term home TPN or antibiotics. Peripheral lines are limited to parenteral solutions containing 900 mOsm/L or less, whereas central venous lines are for solutions greater than 900 mOsm/L. Incidence of phlebitis, pain, inflammation, and vessel thrombosis increases dramatically in peripheral veins once solution osmolality exceeds 900 mOsm/L. Other factors that can contribute to phlebitis besides osmolality include insertion site, vein size, duration of insertion, cannular size, material, and colonization. Peripheral lines should be rotated every 48 to 72 hours to prevent thrombosis and phlebitis.

ENERGY REQUIREMENTS

Provision of calories equal to energy expenditure is usually the goal, but under some circumstances hypocaloric feeding is acceptable or even desirable. Indirect calorimetry remains the *gold standard* method for determining a patient's energy needs. However because of many factors (including expense), most facilities do not employ this technology and therefore rely on predictive equations. There are multiple predictive equations for determining energy requirements for patients, many of which have not been validated. Common practice for predicting resting metabolic rate in patients is to calculate healthy resting metabolic rate (often using the Harris-Benedict equations) and then to multiply this rate by a stress factor (Table 2). Total energy needs are then provided to the TPN patient with dextrose, protein, and lipids; the ratios of each depend on the medical situation.

PROTEIN REQUIREMENTS

Protein requirements will vary depending on the patient's metabolic state, wound-healing needs, and organ function (e.g., kidney, liver). In general most TPN patients will require more than the recommended daily allowance (RDA) (0.8 g/kg per day) for protein with limits up to 2.0 g/kg per day at which no further improvement in use occurs (Table 3). Providing amounts greater than this only increases the rate of ureagenesis or accumulates eventually producing additional clinical problems. However, this upper limit may not apply for those with protein-losing conditions such as open wounds, major thermal burns, or high-output EC fistulas. In those with organ dysfunction, the medical therapy dictates how much protein can be provided. Protein calories should be considered into the total energy provision.

NONPROTEIN CALORIES

The remaining energy needs, once protein calories are subtracted, are divided between dextrose and lipids. Box 1 shows a sample TPN calculation. Excessive amounts of IV lipid are not only proinflammatory but also immunosuppressive as the solutions in the United States are rich in omega-6 FAs. Lipid infusion should comprise

---

TABLE 2 Commonly Used Predictive Energy Equations

Name of Equation	Equation	Explanation of Abbreviations
Harris-Benedict equation $BEE = kcal/d$	$BEE(male) = 13.7(W) + 5(H) - 6.8(A) + 66$ $BEE(female) = 9.6(W) + 1.7(H) - 4.7(A) + 655$ Add injury/activity factor to BEE for total energy expenditure (10% to 40% above BEE)	W = weight in kg H = height in cm A = age in years
Penn State equation (for ventilated patients) $RMR = kcal/d$	$RMR = RMR(healthy)(0.85) + V_E(33) + T_{max}(175) - 6433$	RMR = BEE via Harris Benedict equation (actual body weight used), V_E = minute ventilation in L/min, T_{max} = maximum body temperature in the previous 24 hours (degrees centigrade)
Ireton-Jones equation $EEE = kcal/d$	Spontaneous breathing patients: $EEE(s) = 629 - 11(A) + 25(W) - 609(O)$ Ventilator-dependent patients: $EEE(v) = 1784 - 11(A) + 5(W) + 244(G) + 239(T) + 804(B)$	A = age in years W = weight (kg) O = presence of obesity; >30% above ideal body weight or BMI >27 (0 = absent, 1 = present) G = Gender (0 = female, 1 = male) T = Trauma diagnosis (0 = absent, 1 = present) B = Burn diagnosis (0 = absent, 1 = present)
General equation	20-35 kcal/kg	

Abbreviations: BEE = basal energy expenditure; EEE = estimated energy expenditure; RMR = resting metabolic rate.

TABLE 3 Protein Requirements

Metabolic State	Recommended Amounts
Normal condition, no stress	0.8 g/kg/d
Mild stress	1.0-1.2 g/kg/d
Moderate stress	1.2-1.5 g/kg/d
Severe stress	1.5-2.0 g/kg/d
Renal failure, predialysis	0.6-0.8 g/kg/d
Renal failure, dialysis	1.2-1.5 g/kg/d
Hepatic failure	0.8-1.2* g/kg/d

*If high branched-chain amino acid formulation used.

TABLE 4 Laboratory Values and Recommended Monitoring

	Baseline	Daily	Biweekly
CBC	X	X	
Basic metabolic panel (Na, K, Cl, CO_2, Ca, BUN, Cr)	X	X	
PO_4, Mg^{2+}	X	X	
Liver function tests (AST, ALT, ALK PHOS, T bili, D bili)			X
Visceral proteins (albumin, prealbumin)			X
Serum triglycerides			X

Abbreviations: ALK PHOS = alkaline phosphatase; ALT = alanine aminotransferase; AST = aspartate aminotransferase; BUN = blood urea nitrogen; Ca = calcium; CBC = complete blood count; Cl = chloride; CO_2 = carbon dioxide; Cr = chromium; D bili = direct bilirubin; K = potassium; Na = sodium; T bili = total bilirubin.

10% to 30% of total calories and is better tolerated when infused over longer time periods (18 to 24 hours). Lipids should be withheld in those with serum triglyceride levels >400 mg/dL. Most patients can tolerate up to 10 days without lipids before concern for essential FA deficiency arises.

Carbohydrate, provided as dextrose, administered in excess can result in hyperglycemia, increased CO_2 production leading to increased ventilatory requirements, and hepatic steatosis. In addition to hyperglycemia, critically ill patients are commonly hyperinsulinemic and exhibit peripheral insulin resistance. Alterations in nutrient metabolism associated with critical illness often result in mobilization of FAs and therefore elevated triglyceride levels. The maximal total glucose oxidation rate in a human is 5 mg/kg per minute, or in a 70-kg human it is 500 g per day. Critical illness and resultant hypermetabolism can account for up to 3 mg/kg per minute endogenous glucose production; providing excessive exogenous glucose during hypermetabolism exacerbates hyperglycemia.

BOX 1 Sample Total Parenteral Nutrition Macronutrient Calculation

- Energy needs: 2000 kcal/d.
- Protein needs: 120 g/d.
- Fluid needs: 2400 mL/d.
- TPN:
  Protein contains 4 kcal/g, so 120 g protein = 480 kcal.
  2000 total kcal − 480 protein kcal = 1520 kcal (to provide as nonprotein kcal).
- Lipid: 1520 kcal × 0.25 = 380 kcal.
  Provided as 20% Intralipid: has 2 kcal/mL (380 kcal ÷ 2 kcal/mL) = 190 mL Intralipid.
- Dextrose: 1520 kcal × 0.75 = 1140 kcal.
  Dextrose has 3.4 kcal/g (1140 kcal ÷ 3.4 kcal/g) = 335 g dextrose.
  Volume (using 10% amino acid, and 70% dextrose solutions).
- Protein: 120 g ÷ 0.1 = 1200 mL.
- Dextrose: 335 g ÷ 0.7 = 478 mL.
- Lipid: 190 mL.
- Electrolytes and other additives: approximately 100 mL.
- Total volume = 1968 mL.
- Fluid needs: 430 mL sterile water.

Abbreviation: TPN = total parenteral nutrition.

INITIATION OF TOTAL PARENTERAL NUTRITION

Prior to initiating TPN patients should be adequately resuscitated and serum electrolytes should be normalized. Baseline laboratory values should be obtained (Table 4). Once the macronutrient composition goals have been determined (see Box 1), a formulation may either be provided via a nonstandard prescription, or many institutions may carry a standard TPN solution in which the dextrose and amino acid concentrations are preformulated, and the amount the patient will receive is dependent on the TPN volume provided; lipids can then be provided separately. A standard solution is often adequate for nonstressed patients and may be convenient and cost effective for community-based facilities where the number of TPN patients does not justify maintaining the necessary compounding equipment and staff.

The dextrose concentration in PN should be increased gradually to avoid hyperglycemia and electrolyte abnormalities with initial amounts of 100 to 150 g dextrose per day. It is imperative to take all dextrose-containing solutions into account when calculating daily carbohydrate intake. When serum glucose levels are controlled, preferably between 80 to 150 mg/dL, the dextrose concentration may be increased toward the goal. Calculated protein and lipid requirements can be provided at goal amounts initially. Electrolytes should be provided daily based on individual requirements (Table 5) and adjusted according to laboratory values. Vitamins and trace elements should be provided daily unless contraindicated based on medical condition.

METABOLIC COMPLICATIONS

Metabolic complications related to macronutrient and micronutrient composition of PN can be minimized by following published guidelines as well as fastidious monitoring.

HYPERVOLEMIA

Hypervolemia is more common in critically ill patients than hypovolemia because of fluid overload from

TABLE 5   Electrolyte Requirements for Adults

Substrate	Usual Dose	Range
Sodium	2 mEq/kg/d	0.5-5 mEq/kg/d
Potassium	1 mEq/kg/d	0.5-2 mEq/kg/d
Chloride*	2 mEq/kg/d	0.5-4 mEq/kg/d
Acetate*	1 mEq/kg/d	0.5-2 mEq/kg/d
Calcium	10 mEq/d	5-15 mEq/d
Magnesium	16 mEq/d	8-32 mEq/d
Phosphorus	15 mmol/d	5-30 mmol/d

*Chloride and acetate to maintain acid-base balance.

increased vascular permeability associated with the SIRS. Hence, TPN volume restriction to as low as 1 L per day is sometimes necessary. Other patients at risk of hypervolemia include the elderly, and those with cardiac, renal, pulmonary, and hepatic failure. Using concentrated macronutrient substrates (15% amino acids, 70% dextrose, 30% lipid) with no additional sterile water allows for maximizing nutrient delivery while minimizing volume.

HYPERGLYCEMIA

Hyperglycemia is extremely common in the critical care setting. Causes include overly rapid advancement of dextrose delivery in the face of underlying metabolic stress, infection, sepsis, and diabetes mellitus. These high-risk patients should have capillary glucose measurements taken three to four times daily with a sliding scale insulin regimen provided with a goal of maintaining blood glucose at 80 to 150 mg/dL. Critically ill patients may require a continuous insulin infusion to maintain optimal blood glucose levels; for those on an insulin infusion, capillary glucose measurements should be hourly with adjustments made in the insulin delivery accordingly. In a large prospective intensive care unit (ICU) study, practising meticulous maintenance of blood glucose levels between 80 and 110 mg/dL resulted in significantly reduced mortality and morbidity. Dextrose concentrations should only be advanced to goal amounts when blood glucose levels are well maintained within desired ranges.

REFEEDING SYNDROME (HYPOKALEMIA, HYPOPHOSPHATEMIA, HYPERMAGNESEMIA)

Refeeding syndrome may result in malnourished patients with the initiation of aggressive specialized nutrition support as a result of the body's shifting from using stored body fat for energy to carbohydrates; it is a potentially lethal condition. As blood glucose levels rise, serum insulin levels also increase causing the intracellular movement of electrolytes from the systemic circulation. Circulating levels of potassium, phosphorus, and magnesium subsequently are reduced. Refeeding is associated with sodium retention and expansion of the extracellular space resulting in weight gain, thereby leading to an increase in cardiovascular demands. Fluid shifts can result in cardiac failure, dehydration or fluid overload, hypotension, prerenal failure, and sudden death. Patients at risk for developing

refeeding syndrome include malnourished individuals, especially patients with an unexplained weight loss of more than 10% in <6 months, and critically ill patients who haven't been fed for 7 to 10 days. Overzealous feeding with specialized nutrition support should be avoided. Prior to initiating specialized nutrition support, electrolyte and mineral abnormalities should be corrected and fluid status adequately resuscitated. TPN dextrose should also be advanced slowly with patients monitored closely for signs of heart failure. Serum electrolytes, mineral, and glucose levels (e.g., potassium, magnesium, phosphorus) in addition to fluid status should be monitored closely for several days to allow for repletion of suboptimal levels, control of blood glucose should hyperglycemia occur, and restoration of fluid balance as needed.

LIVER DYSFUNCTION

Hepatic complications can occur if the patient is being overfed or receiving more carbohydrate than the liver can oxidize. Alterations in hepatic enzymes may not be seen for two to three weeks, but liver enzymes should be monitored on a weekly basis. Elevation of the serum transaminases and alkaline phosphatase can be seen within 1 week, whereas an increase in bilirubin usually occurs later. If elevations do occur, all etiologies of hepatic inflammation/dysfunction should be investigated before assuming PN is the culprit. PN administration has been associated with cholestasis, fatty changes, portal inflammation or triaditis, bile duct proliferation, and fibrosis. In the case of biliary sludge formation, providing some enteral feeding, particularly long-chain FAs, in combination with TPN may be beneficial to stimulate bile flow.

INFECTIOUS COMPLICATIONS

Many infections are related to the central venous catheter (CVC) with the incidence ranging from 3% to 20% in hospitalized patients. Rates are 2 to 5 times higher in the critically ill patient. Bacterial systemic infections related to the catheter occur in 3% to 7% of CVCs. Risk factors influencing sepsis include patient characteristics, therapy, catheter properties, and maintenance procedures. Because the glucose content in central PN is a good medium for bacterial growth, it is recommended that whenever possible, TPN be administered through a dedicated port of a central line that has not been used for any other therapy. The maximum hang time for IV fat emulsions

CURRENT DIAGNOSIS

- Obtain medical and surgical history.
- Obtain nutrition history, daily intake and output.
- Obtain pertinent laboratory parameters.
- Obtain current medications and fluids.
- Obtain height, actual body weight, and usual body weight.
- Obtain current interventions (e.g., mechanical ventilation, dialysis).
- Evaluate current access sites (e.g., central versus peripheral venous access).

- Evaluate need for PN:
  Enteral feeding not indicated.
  Enteral nutrient provision inadequate (e.g., <60% nutritional needs tolerated for >7 days).
- Perform nutrition assessment:
  Calculate or measure energy requirements.
  Estimate protein requirements.
  Estimate fluid requirements.
- Calculate PN formulation:
  Protein: 1 to 2 g/kg per day (dependent on disease state and medical intervention).
  Dextrose: 40% to 60% kcal per day (2 to 5 mg/kg/min per day).
  Lipid: 10% to 30% kcal per day.
  Electrolytes per needs reflected in laboratory measurements and medical interventions.
  Vitamins, minerals based upon disease state.
  Extra fluid if need to meet fluid needs solely via parenteral feeding.
- Monitor daily clinical status, laboratory values, fluid status, and adjust parenteral formulation as needed.

Abbreviations: PN = parenteral nutrition.

recommended by the Centers for Disease Control and Prevention (CDC) is 12 hours. This recommendation was subsequent to reports of increased microbial growth in contaminated IV fat emulsions hung for greater than 12 hours as well as reports of gram-negative sepsis associated with the administration of IV fat emulsion. TPN is associated with an increase in non–catheter-related infections that may be related to overfeeding, hyperglycemia, immunosuppression by n-6 fatty rich IV lipid, missing nutrients (e.g., taurine, choline, glutamine, vitamins, minerals), and nonluminal delivery of nutrients. Therefore to minimize these infections, changes in TPN therapy have been made over the years. Recommended calorie intake is less, more aggressive blood glucose control is becoming standard of therapy, EN is encouraged when possible, new lipid products are being evaluated, and a variety of missing nutrients are being studied for their usefulness in specialized nutrition support.

REFERENCES

ASPEN Board of Directors: Guidelines for the use of parenteral and EN in adult and pediatric patients. JPEN J Parenter Enteral Nutr 2002;26(Suppl):1SA-137SA.

Christensen M: Parenteral nutrition formulations. In Cresci G (ed): Nutrition Support for the Critically Ill: A guide to practice. Boca Raton, Fla, CRC Press, 2005.

Forbes A: Parenteral nutrition: New advances and observations. Curr Opin Gastroenterol 2004;20:114-118.

Pipkin W, Gadacz T: Nutritional considerations for dealing with intestinal disease in the intensive care unit. In Shikora S, Martindale R, Swaitzberg S (eds): Nutritional Considerations in the Intensive Care Unit. Dubuque, Iowa, Kendall/Hunt, 2002, pp 281-283.

Szesezski E, Benjamin S: Complications of total parenteral nutrition. In Cresci G (ed): Nutrition Support for the Critically Ill: A Guide to Practice. Boca Raton, Fla, CRC Press, 2005.

Parenteral Fluid Therapy for Infants and Children

Method of
Thomas R. Welch, MD

The background behind our contemporary approach to parenteral fluid therapy in children is inextricably intertwined with the history of American pediatrics. The formulae and methods that have been used to calculate fluid requirements developed hand in hand with the evolution of our understanding of the physiology of dehydration.

The most common indication for parenteral fluid therapy originally was overwhelmingly diarrheal dehydration. Although this is still important, many children requiring such therapy today have complex disorders, multiorgan system failure, parenteral nutrition requirements, and other complicating factors. Nonetheless, the principles underlying our approach today are largely unchanged. In fact, a solid grounding in these principles actually allows a more simplified approach than has classically been taught.

Normal Maintenance Fluid Requirements

The concept of *maintenance fluid therapy* quite simply implies that patients are to be maintained in a net fluid balance of zero: Fluid intake from all sources equals fluid output from all sources. The vast majority of healthy individuals manage to keep themselves in a net zero fluid balance every day, providing their own maintenance fluid therapy.

Parenteral maintenance fluid therapy is necessary when a child is unable to meet these needs orally. This could only occur today in limited situations such as children for whom oral feedings are being withheld awaiting a diagnostic or surgical procedure, children recuperating from surgery whose gastrointestinal tract is unable to tolerate oral feedings, or children unable to feed because of a recent change in neurologic status. Note that *by definition* maintenance fluid therapy does not apply to a child who is dehydrated or otherwise has a deficit, real or functional, in intravascular volume.

COMPONENTS OF NORMAL MAINTENANCE FLUID REQUIREMENTS

Understanding the usual requirements for maintenance fluid *input* requires knowledge of the usual sources of *output*, which generally are only *insensible* water loss from the skin and lung and urinary losses. Although a few additional sources of output exist (and at least one source of metabolic input), these are usually so trivial in magnitude that they may be ignored for purposes of calculating fluid therapy.

Insensible water loss and urine loss are calculated on caloric expenditure. Thus the first step in writing a prescription for maintenance fluid is estimating caloric expenditure. Other systems for calculating fluid

TABLE 1 Estimation of Caloric Expenditure From Body Weight*

Body Weight	Caloric Expenditure
0 to 10 kg	100 kcal/kg/d
10 to 20 kg	1000 kcal plus 50 kcal/kg/d for weight >10 kg
>20 kg	1500 kcal plus 20 kcal/kg/d for weight >20 kg

*Note that for children with normal renal function who are euvolemic and who have no additional ongoing losses, the daily kcal expenditure translates into an approximation of mL fluid requirement.
Modified from Holiday MA, Segar WE: The maintenance need for water in parenteral fluid therapy. Pediatrics 1957;19:823-832.

therapy may be based on body surface area; surface area, which must be estimated from a nomogram, is only a surrogate for caloric expenditure.

Classic studies in hospitalized children have shown that caloric expenditure can be estimated closely by weight, using the calculation in Table 1. Thus, a 30-kg child is predicted to have a resting caloric expenditure of 1700 kcal per day.

Some factors operating in hospitalized children may raise the actual caloric expenditure above that estimated from body weight. The most obvious of these is the hypermetabolic state associated with fever; a 12% increase in basal caloric expenditure should be allowed for each degree centigrade above 37°C (98.6°F). Thus, if a 30-kg child has a temperature of 40°C (104°F), the estimated caloric expenditure will increase to approximately 2300 kcal per day.

Insensible Water Loss

The usual allowance for insensible water loss is 45 mL per 100 kcal, of which approximately one-third (15 mL/100 kcal) represents loss of water through expired air and two-thirds (30 mL/100 kcal) through the skin. It should be stressed that both of these represent *electrolyte-free* water; there is no appreciable sodium in insensible water loss. Insensible water loss from the skin is not to be confused with *sweat*. Insensible skin losses are constant evaporative losses of free water. Sweat is an adaptive process by which electrolyte-containing water is actively secreted by glands in the skin. Sweat losses are rarely encountered in hospitalized children today.

Urinary Water Loss

The allowance for urinary water losses is considerably less fixed than that provided for insensible water loss. Within a wide range of physiologic tolerance, the kidney is able to maintain a net zero fluid balance by excreting water taken in excess of daily need. To calculate a safe allowance for urine output, however, it is crucial to appreciate the role of the kidney in excreting solute. Two factors determine the required urine output: the *solute load* requiring excretion and the *urine concentration* at which these solutes are excreted.

Solute load consists of most of the daily intake of the electrolytes, sodium, potassium, and chloride, in addition

to urea. The latter, as the ultimate breakdown product of protein metabolism, is more difficult to quantitate precisely, being determined by protein intake, the child's metabolic state, and the intake of nonprotein calories.

Using reasonably conservative assumptions regarding solute load and renal concentrating ability, 55 mL/100 kcal per day is suitable for the component of maintenance fluids related to obligatory urine output. Add to this amount 45 mL/100 kcal per day for insensible water loss, one derives a useful allowance for normal maintenance fluid of 100 mL/100 kcal per day. Because this formula fortuitously equates to 1 kcal/1 mL, the 100-50-20 rule (see Table 1) used to estimate caloric expenditure in kilocalorie per day can also be used to calculate the normal maintenance fluid requirement in milliliters per day.

MODIFICATIONS TO NORMAL MAINTENANCE FLUID REQUIREMENTS

By definition, maintenance fluids are provided for children who are euvolemic. The fluid therapy of dehydration, therefore, is *not* maintenance therapy and will be addressed separately in this article.

There are a variety of situations in which the *normal* requirements for maintenance fluid therapy may need to be adjusted. By understanding the physiologic principles on which the normal requirements are derived, it is relatively straightforward to make such adjustments. Note that this approach avoids such shorthand imprecisions as placing a child on *half maintenance* or *twice maintenance* fluid therapy.

Increased Metabolic Rate

Adjustments for the increased metabolic rate of fever were discussed previously. In this situation the estimated daily caloric expenditure is adjusted upward by 12% per degree centigrade. The usual allowance of 100 mL fluid per 100 kcal per day is still employed.

Altered Insensible Water Loss

Several factors may impact the allowance for insensible water loss. Children breathing humidified air, such as in a *croup tent* or on a ventilator, will have a lower volume of lung water loss than the 15 mL/100 kcal usually estimated. Reducing the normal maintenance allowance by this amount (i.e., from 100 to 85 mL/100 kcal/day) is rational in such settings, but the overall impact on fluid balance would be trivial.

Children with burns or other extensive denuding skin lesions have significant evaporative water losses from loss of the skin barrier, contributing to a substantial increase in cutaneous insensible water loss. The fluid therapy of severe burns, especially in the first few days, is complex and beyond the scope of this article. During recuperation, once intravascular volume has been returned and tissue edema reduced, an increase in the allowance for insensible loss beyond the 30 mL/kcal per day is required; the precise amount is directly related to the extent of the burns.

Altered Requirement for Urinary Loss

The allowance for urinary output may also require modification under specific circumstances. The major reason for such modification is a limitation on the kidney's ability to concentrate or dilute the urine. The 55 mL/kcal per day estimated urine allowance is based on the assumption of a normal dietary solute load and that urine concentration is in the range of 280 mOsm/L—easily achievable in virtually any child. Some intrinsic renal disorders (e.g., renal dysplasia, nephrogenic diabetes insipidus), however, may make even that degree of concentration impossible. A child with dysplastic kidneys and a maximal urine osmolality of 140 mOsm/L, for example, would probably become significantly dehydrated if provided normal maintenance fluids at 100 mL/kcal per day. Given that the child's urinary concentration is half that on which the 55 mL/kcal per day estimate is predicated, a more appropriate allowance would be 110 mL/100 kcal per day for urine loss. Adding in the (unchanged) 45 mL/100 kcal per day allowance for insensible water loss, the appropriate total maintenance fluid for this child would be 155 mL/100 kcal per day.

An opposite problem to a concentrating deficit occurs when a child is unable to dilute urine. Assuming that volume contraction has been excluded (in which case the fluid therapy would not be maintenance and isotonic volume resuscitation would be necessary), the most common cause of this would be the syndrome of inappropriate secretion of antidiuretic hormone (SIADH). This is a scenario that must be considered in children receiving parenteral fluids postoperatively and is likely consequent to pain, stress, and neurohormonal factors. Here again measurement of urine osmolality allows appropriate calculation of the allowance for urine output. A child with urine concentration of 540 mOsm/L, for example, would require *half* the usual allowance, which is based on a urine osmolality of approximately 270 mOsm/L. Thus the urine allowance for the child would be 27 mL/100 kcal per day, for a total daily maintenance fluid allowance of 72 mL/100 kcal per day.

Allowance for Other Continuing Losses

In most children requiring maintenance fluid therapy, only urinary and insensible losses need to be replaced. Occasionally, however, a child will have an additional, substantive loss, which needs to be replaced on an ongoing basis. Again, it must be stressed that ongoing replacement of continuing losses should not be confused with restoring accumulated loss; the latter is not maintenance therapy.

One of the most common sources of additional ongoing losses is gastric fluid loss from continuous nasogastric (NG) suction. Failure to replace NG losses can quickly result in metabolic alkalosis from chloride depletion. Ongoing losses such as this can be replaced milliliter for milliliter separate from the rest of the maintenance fluid. Typically, this is recalculated on a per shift basis, with total losses over the past shift replaced during the duration of the next. In very small infants with particularly voluminous losses, the interval for recalculation may need to be shorter than the usual 8- or 12-hour shift.

The content of these replacement fluids is driven by the measured electrolyte content of the fluid being lost. For gastric fluid this is usually approximately 50% isotonic saline. Some losses (chest tube drainage, for example) may contain substantial amounts of protein that, if the losses are substantial, may also need to be replaced.

Normal Maintenance Requirements for Electrolytes

SODIUM

The concept of a fixed daily maintenance requirement for sodium and its accompanying anions is frequently misunderstood. Although growing infants have a slightly positive sodium balance, reflecting net accretion, the fate of virtually all ingested sodium is to be excreted in the urine. Daily dietary intake of sodium virtually always matches urinary losses. Rather than being an essential nutrient, sodium is a ubiquitous accompaniment of most other nutrients, which must then be excreted. Thus, the concept of estimating a daily *requirement* for sodium by calculating the concentration of the element in foodstuffs such as milk is fundamentally flawed.

The frequently quoted daily sodium requirement of 2 to 4 mEq/kg per day actually derived from calculation of the average sodium intake of infants consuming equal caloric volumes of various milks. The relevance of such figures to the provision of brief courses of parenteral fluids to children of varying ages is questionable.

The danger of providing a fixed daily sodium allowance to a child receiving parenteral fluids is that the sodium intake may be considered in isolation from water intake. Consequently, a child whose total daily fluid intake has been restricted but who continues to receive a fixed sodium allowance could actually develop a free water deficit and be unable to excrete the solute load. Although this scenario would be unlikely in providing a brief course of normal maintenance fluid to a child with normal kidneys, it is a real concern in this provision of long-term total parenteral nutrition.

A more rational approach to the provision of sodium in maintenance fluid therapy is to index it to total fluid requirements rather than body weight. Providing parenteral fluid in the form of D_5 ¼ isotonic saline (0.2% NaCl), ensures the provision of adequate sodium to address the trivial ongoing losses in a healthy child, while providing adequate free water to permit excretion of solute and replace insensible water losses.

POTASSIUM

As is the situation with sodium, there is no true fixed daily requirement for potassium. Children with no pre-existing reason to have a potassium deficit (e.g., diarrheal dehydration, diuretic use) require no potassium during brief courses of parenteral maintenance fluid therapy. Children who have risk factors for potassium deficiency may have potassium chloride added to their parenteral fluids to achieve a concentration of 20 mEq/L.

CALCIUM, PHOSPHATE, AND OTHER ELECTROLYTES

Although provision of calcium and phosphate is essential for growing children and is a critical component of total parenteral nutrition, they are generally not provided during the course of normal maintenance fluid therapy. The same applies to trace minerals such as magnesium.

GLUCOSE

Although not an electrolyte, glucose is an important additive in intravenous fluids. It is impossible to provide sufficient calories to meet total daily needs solely by providing glucose in conventional maintenance fluids. Thus, children unable to take sufficient calories orally for more than a few days will require parenteral nutrition—a procedure outside the scope of this article.

Glucose serves two roles when used in normal maintenance fluid therapy. Solutions that are less than isotonic (e.g., ¼ isotonic saline [0.2%] and ½ isotonic saline [0.45%]) can be provided in 5% glucose (D_5). In theory this will minimize the hypotonic lysis of erythrocytes in the immediate vicinity of the infusion if these dilute solutions did not contain glucose; the clinical importance of this is probably minimal. More importantly, the absorbed glucose from this fluid will provide some calorie intake (approximately 20 kcal for each 100 kcal expended, if the foregoing maintenance calculations are used) and may moderate ketosis.

Fluid Therapy for Children With Preexisting Deficits

The foregoing discussion applies to a child who is euvolemic at the time of beginning parenteral fluid therapy. In most hospitalized children requiring parenteral fluids, however, a deficit will be present. This may result from preexisting losses (e.g., diarrhea and vomiting from gastroenteritis), decreased intake (e.g., a febrile infant with an acute respiratory infection that has impaired feedings), or *third space* losses (e.g., movement of fluid out of the vasculature into the interstitial space following surgery). Using the maintenance scheme presented previously in such children would be inappropriate for two reasons. First of all, the rate of fluid administration would be inadequate to replace the deficit and restore circulation. Additionally, the free water provided in normal maintenance fluid is not excreted in states of volume contraction consequent to antidiuretic hormone (ADH) release and increased urinary concentration. This could result in the abrupt development of hyponatremia, which could have devastating neurologic consequences.

Some schemes for the parenteral fluid therapy of children with deficits are predicated on an estimation of the volume of the deficit, and provision of this volume over a fixed period of time; typically 8, 12, or more hours.

There are two problems with this approach. First, none of the systems for estimating the volume of a deficit from physical findings has ever been validated (but a uniform system for grading the *severity* of dehydration has been developed recently—Table 2). Second, if a fluid deficit compromising or potentially compromising circulation is present, there is no physiologic rationale for delaying its repair for several hours. It is for these reasons that the classical *deficit* approach to fluid therapy has recently been questioned.

The initial priority in managing a child with a fluid deficit is securing vascular access. If this cannot be accomplished expeditiously, the intraosseous route can be lifesaving. As this is being done, an objective assessment of the clinical signs of dehydration (see Table 2) should be obtained and recorded, to provide a baseline to assess response to therapy. A blood specimen for electrolyte determination should also be obtained, although initiation of therapy should never be delayed awaiting the results of this.

Once vascular access has been secured, restoration of the circulation with an isotonic solution is the next priority. Either isotonic (normal, 0.9%) saline or lactated Ringer's solution is appropriate. The latter has the advantage of providing some of its anion in the form of lactate. This may attenuate the transient worsening of acidosis that predictably accompanies volume expansion when chloride is the only anion. The usual dose of isotonic fluid is 20 mL/kg, given as rapidly as possible. Both of these solutions are also available with added dextrose, which may be important in small infants at risk for hypoglycemia.

After this initial dose of isotonic fluid, the child's response is assessed by such clinical measures as heart rate, capillary refill, urine output, state of consciousness, and the other measures of dehydration severity outlined in Table 2. Up to three additional such doses of isotonic fluid, to a total of 80 mL/kg, may be given. In most children with diarrheal dehydration, objective measures of circulatory restoration will be evident after this isotonic expansion. If not, careful assessment for confounding issues such as hypoglycemia, sepsis, or cardiac dysfunction may be required, and additional support such as pressors may be necessary.

If the child shows objective improvement after isotonic expansion, the next phase of therapy may be planned. Ideally this therapy can be provided orally. The likelihood of inducing dangerous osmotic shifts is much less when oral rehydration is employed. An oral electrolyte solution is one such option; formula or human milk is another.

TABLE 2 A Scale for the Quantitation of Dehydration Severity*

Characteristic	0	1	2
General appearance	Normal	Thirsty, restless, lethargic, but irritable when touched	Drowsy, limp, cold, sweaty, ± comatose
Eyes	Normal	Slightly sunken	Very sunken
Mucous membranes (tongue)	Moist	Sticky	Dry
Tears	Tears present	Tears decreased	Tears absent

*This scale results in total points ranging from 0 for no clinical evidence of dehydration to 8 for severe dehydration.
Modified from Friedman JN, Goldman RD, Srivastava R, Parkin PC: Development of a clinical dehydration scale for use in children between 1 and 36 months of age. J Pediatr 2004;145:201-207.

TABLE 3 Typical Correlations Between Urinary Specific Gravity and Urinary Osmolality*

Urine Specific Gravity	Urine Osmolality
1.010	300 mOsm/L
1.020	600 mOsm/L
1.030	900 mOsm/L

*These approximations are appropriate in the absence of glycosuria and/or proteinuria.

In the event that oral therapy is not an option, further parenteral fluids will be required, which will be designed to provide for normal maintenance requirements and to address any ongoing losses (e.g., persistent diarrhea). The volume of the maintenance component of therapy can be calculated as outlined above. Keep in mind that the allowance for urinary losses in these calculations was based on fairly dilute urine. In the event that urine is more concentrated than 280 mOsm/L, some of the 55 mL/100 kcal per day allowance for urinary losses will be retained. Thus, any remaining small deficit after the isotonic expansion will be restored with this maintenance fluid. In fact, occasional assessment of urine osmolality provides a measure of the adequacy of therapy. Once an intravascular fluid deficit has been repaired, the osmolality of urine in a child receiving normal maintenance fluids should be <300 mOsm/L. If timely urine osmolality measurements are not available, specific gravity is a useful surrogate, as long as glycosuria or proteinuria are not present (Table 3). Instead of providing maintenance therapy as D_5 ¼ isotonic saline, it is prudent to provide D_5 ½ isotonic saline (0.45% NaCl) as long as urine concentration is >300 mOsm/L to avoid retention of free water and hyponatremia.

The only other modification to provide in this phase of therapy for dehydration is to provide potassium, typically by adding KCl to a final concentration of 20 mEq/L of fluid. This will begin replenishment of potassium lost during the acute phase of the illness.

Modification of Therapy in the Presence of Electrolyte Disturbances

ACID-BASE

Some degree of metabolic acidosis is very typical in diarrheal dehydration. Most often, this is a normal anion gap acidosis, resulting from stool bicarbonate losses. In severe dehydration, however, an elevated anion gap may reflect circulatory compromise and lactic acidosis.

Either type of acidosis will be corrected by the kidney once circulation has been restored. If the initial expansion is performed with isotonic saline, however, there may actually be a transient worsening of acidosis before correction occurs. This can usually be avoided if the initial expansion is with lactated Ringer's solution.

Persistence of serious acidosis after circulation and urine output have been restored for over 24 hours is

CURRENT DIAGNOSIS

- Assess the child clinically for evidence of fluid deficit.
- Assess the child for coexisting metabolic abnormality: hypernatremia/hyponatremia, acidosis, and so on.
- Determine the extent and composition of any ongoing losses.
- Estimate the child's caloric expenditure.

unusual and should prompt further investigation for a complicating factor such as renal dysfunction or sepsis.

SODIUM DISORDERS

Most diarrheal dehydration today is *isotonic*, much as if the serum sodium is normal. Some children with diarrheal dehydration, however, may be *hyponatremic* at presentation. Typically, this results from consumption of low osmolality fluids in the face of the avid renal water retention, which characterizes dehydration. This situation should be viewed as a relative excess of free water rather than a relative deficit of sodium. Typically, once volume has been restored, the stimulus for urine concentration and renal water retention (ADH) is lost and the relative free water excess is excreted. With appropriate volume expansion, urine concentration should then fall and serum sodium rise. The correction of serum sodium is made by the coordinated activity of hypothalamic osmoreceptors, the pituitary, and the kidney. Thus, once the circulation has been restored, the process of correcting hyponatremia is not driven by the fluid therapy prescription but by the child's normal physiologic processes. The thought that the rate of correction of hyponatremia is under the control of the prescriber of the fluid therapy reflects hubris rather than physiologic reality.

There have been reports of some individuals with severe hyponatremia developing demyelinating central nervous system (CNS) lesions during the course of repair. The bulk of these reports have been in adults, often in the perioperative setting, and usually with rapid movement of serum sodium concentrations to levels above normal. This should not be a concern in children with hyponatremic dehydration treated in the fashion described.

CURRENT THERAPY

- Secure venous access. In urgent situations, if venous access is not easily obtained, immediately secure intraosseous access.
- Provide rapid volume expansion with an isotonic solution in 20 mL/kg increments if the child is assessed as volume depleted.
- Begin maintenance fluid therapy based on the child's estimated caloric needs, as well as any additional ongoing losses when volume depletion is repaired and if oral intake is not feasible.
- Monitor and adjust therapy based on objective changes in clinical status, urine output and concentration, and changes in measured serum chemistries.

Some children with diarrheal dehydration may be *hypernatremic*. This is a much less common disorder and is unusual. It was more common in an era when the treatment of diarrhea included hyperosmolar liquids such as scalded skimmed milk. Today hypernatremic dehydration is most commonly seen in the context of breast-feeding insufficiency in infants.

The rapid correction of hypernatremia can result in significant osmotic shifts in the CNS and may precipitate cerebral edema. Treatment of hypernatremic dehydration with the protocol outlined above, in which rapid expansion of the circulation with an isotonic solution is the initial step, will avoid this complication. If the child is unable to tolerate oral feedings after isotonic volume expansion, the subsequent maintenance fluid should initially be more concentrated than usual, at least D_5 $1/2$ isotonic saline (0.45% NaCl). More frequent reassessments of the serum sodium concentration may be needed to ensure that adequate free water is being provided to allow a correction of the hypernatremia.

REFERENCES

Finberg L: Hypernatremic (hypertonic) dehydration in infants. N Engl J Med 1973;289:196-198.

Friedman JN, Goldman RD, Srivastava R, Parkin PC: Development of a clinical dehydration scale for use in children between 1 and 36 months of age. J Pediatr 2004;145:201-207.

Holliday MA, Segar WE: The maintenance need for water in parenteral fluid therapy. Pediatrics 1957;19:823-832.

Holliday M: The evolution of therapy for dehydration: Should deficit therapy still be taught? Pediatrics 1996;98:171-177.

Winters RW: Maintenance fluid therapy. In Winters RW (ed): The Body Fluids in Pediatrics. Boston, Little, Brown, 1973, pp 113-133.

The Endocrine System

Acromegaly

Method of
Mark E. Molitch, MD

Pretreatment Evaluation

Acromegaly is an insidious disorder, usually present for years before the diagnosis is made. The prevalence is approximately 50 cases per million population with an annual incidence of new diagnoses of approximately 3 to 4 per million. The excess growth hormone (GH) secretion may cause considerable morbidity, including hypertension, diabetes, heart disease, progressive arthritis, sleep apnea, muscle weakness, overgrowth of facial features and appendages, and colonic neoplasia. Colonoscopy is indicated routinely for the evaluation for neoplasia. When the GH excess starts before epiphysial closure at puberty, gigantism may result. Mortality is also increased two- to threefold over the general population. Morbidity and mortality are related to the amount of hormone as well as the duration of disease and can be greatly ameliorated by early diagnosis and treatment that normalizes GH and insulin-like growth factor-1 (IGF-1) levels. The diagnosis must be made biochemically by demonstrating failure of normal suppression of GH levels by hyperglycemia and increased IGF-1 levels.

The definition of an abnormal basal serum GH level was difficult to ascertain in the past because of the poor sensitivity of GH assays and episodic secretion. Some patients with active acromegaly may have basal GH levels less than 2 µg/mL using conventional radioimmunoassays (RIAs). However, normal GH levels are even lower, using immunoradiometric (IRMA) and enzyme-linked immunosorbent assays (ELISA). Except for the episodic secretory surges, a level of 2 µg/mL may well be the upper limit of normal for basal GH levels. For establishing the diagnosis and clinical activity of acromegaly, it is necessary to document the failure to suppress GH levels with an oral glucose load (75 to 100 g) to less than 1.0 µg/mL using an RIA and less than 0.40 µg/mL using the IRMA or ELISA assays. Elevation of levels of IGF-1, using age-adjusted normal

CURRENT DIAGNOSIS

Acromegaly is diagnosed using the following criteria:
- GH not suppressed <1 µg/mL (conventional RIA) or >0.4 µg/mL (2-site assays) during a glucose tolerance test
- IGF-I levels elevated (age corrected)
- Tumor size and extension assessed by MRI
- Visual fields performed if tumor found to be abutting optic chiasm on MRI
- Colonoscopy performed to rule out polyps/cancer
- Other pituitary function assessed in patients with macroadenomas
- Prolactin measured to determine if the tumor co-secretes this hormone

Abbreviations: MRI = magnetic resonance imaging; RIA = radioimmunoassay.

values, has also become accepted as a criterion for the diagnosis of active acromegaly. IGF-1 levels correlate with indexes of disease activity better than GH levels in most but not all studies.

Approximately 30% to 40% of patients with acromegaly have elevated prolactin (PRL) levels. Uncommonly, patients will present with symptoms caused by the hyperprolactinemia, such as decreased libido, impotence, galactorrhea, or amenorrhea, rather than the normal presenting symptoms of acromegaly.

Almost all patients with acromegaly have GH-secreting pituitary adenomas. The size and degree of any extrasellar extension of the adenoma are best assessed by magnetic resonance imaging (MRI). Compression of the optic chiasm by the adenoma can be determined with Goldmann visual field testing when MRI shows that the tumor abuts the optic chiasm. Approximately three quarters of patients have macroadenomas (more than 10 mm in diameter), and 15% to 20% have suprasellar extension of the adenoma. Large adenomas may cause hypopituitarism by directly compressing the normal pituitary or interfering with stalk function; a detailed evaluation of anterior and posterior pituitary function determines whether hormone replacement is necessary.

Rarely, no evidence of pituitary adenoma is found or, if surgery is performed, hyperplasia of the somatotropes may

733

be found. Such patients may have a syndrome in which growth hormone-releasing hormone (GHRH) is being secreted by a pancreatic, carcinoid, hypothalamic, or other tumor. If one of these GHRH-secreting tumors is suspected, then GHRH blood levels can be measured.

Goals of therapy include elimination of effects because of the mass of the tumor (hypopituitarism, visual field defects, etc.); reduction of elevated GH levels and IGF-I levels to normal; amelioration of the end-organ effects of the elevated GH levels; avoidance of damage to remaining normal hypothalamic or pituitary function; and minimizing other potential adverse effects of therapy.

Treatment

TRANSSPHENOIDAL ADENOMECTOMY

Transsphenoidal surgery offers the patient a chance for cure. The newer technique of endoscopic, endonasal transsphenoidal surgery is associated with fewer local symptoms postoperatively and a faster recovery time, but cure rates are no better than with the standard approach. Even when cure is not achieved, surgery may effect a significant

 CURRENT THERAPY

- Transsphenoidal surgery is generally the initial treatment for most patients.
- Cure is defined as suppression of GH to <1 µg/mL (RIA) or <0.4 µg/mL (2-site assay) during an oral glucose tolerance test and normalization of IGF-I.
- Adjunctive therapy is indicated for random GH levels >2 µg/mL and elevated IGF-I levels postoperatively.
- Gamma-knife stereotactic radiotherapy is reserved for patients not cured by surgery and often is used only when medical therapy also fails.
- Medical therapy is usually used in patients not cured by surgery.
- Cabergoline (Dostinex)[1] results in normalization of GH/IGF-I levels in 10%–20% of patients but often is tried as initial therapy. It may also provide further benefit in patients whose levels are not normalized by somatostatin analogues.
- Somatostatin analogues are the mainstay of medical therapy and result in normalization of GH/IGF-I levels in approximately 60% of patients.
- Tumor size reduction of 10%–50% occurs in up to 75% of patients when octreotide is used primarily and approximately 50% when used adjunctively following surgery.
- Pegvisomant (Somavert) results in normalization of IGF-I levels in >90% of patients but has no effect in decreasing tumor size.
- Octreotide LAR (Sandostatin LAR) may also be used primarily in patients whose tumors appear to be nonresectable.
- Patients must be carefully monitored with GH and IGF-I levels and MRI scans.

[1]Not FDA approved for this indication.

Abbreviations: GH = growth hormone; IGF-1 = insulin-like growth factor-1; MRI = magnetic resonance imaging; RIA = radioimmunoassay.

reduction in GH levels and considerable amelioration of clinical symptoms. As would be expected, the smaller the tumor and the lower the basal GH levels, the better the surgical result. The actual cure rates depend on the criteria used. Using the criteria of postoperative, glucose-suppressed GH levels less than 1 µg/mL with a conventional RIA or 0.4 µg/mL with the newer two-site assays and normal IGF-I levels (age adjusted), so-called cure rates of 60% to 80% can be expected for intrasellar lesions and 25% to 50% for larger tumors when the operation is performed by experienced neurosurgeons. However, studies show that the increased mortality can be reduced to normal and much of the morbidity reversed when GH levels are maintained below 2 µg/mL (RIA). Relapses occur in approximately 5% of patients who initially achieve glucose-suppressed GH levels of less than 2 µg/mL but less than 2% when 1 µg/mL is used. Approximately a quarter of patients have discordant IGF-I and glucose-suppressed GH levels, and these patients appear to have a higher risk for relapse.

With microadenomas, the risks of surgery are very small. The mortality from surgery approaches that of anesthesia alone. Transient diabetes insipidus (DI) may occur in 10% to 20% of patients, but it is rare for the patient to need treatment following discharge from the hospital. Hypopituitarism occurs in less than 1%, and other complications such as meningitis and cerebrospinal fluid leak also occur in less than 1% of patients. The total complication rate for this surgery by an experienced pituitary neurosurgeon, except for transient DI, is less than 3%. The complication rate is higher for larger tumors, with risks for CSF leak, meningitis, and permanent DI reaching 2% each. Loss of one or more anterior pituitary hormones occurs in 5% to 10% of patients.

Rarely, patients with very large tumors may need craniotomy and a subfrontal lobe approach. This may be necessary if the tumor has a large suprasellar extension with a dumbbell configuration. Risks are much higher with craniotomy, and mortality reaches 5% in some series.

Another approach for patients whose tumors are so large or invasive that they obviously cannot be cured by surgery and if there is no visual field defect is to use medical therapy with somatostatin analogues primarily (see later). Whether debulking tumors before medical therapy is better than primary medical therapy without surgery is controversial.

Pituitary function tested 6 to 8 weeks postoperatively determines whether the patient is cured or whether there is persistent GH hypersecretion. Testing involves obtaining basal GH and IGF-I levels and showing suppression of GH with glucose. Those patients who appear to be cured need to be followed to detect potential relapse. Testing of other pituitary function detects other hormonal deficiencies that may need treatment. We routinely place patients with macroadenomas on maintenance glucocorticoids (5 mg daily of prednisone or 20 to 30 mg of hydrocortisone) until this time of postoperative testing, in case loss of adrenocorticotropic hormone (ACTH) function has occurred. Because loss of ACTH is very unlikely following surgery for microadenomas, we usually do not prescribe maintenance glucocorticoids unless the patient is symptomatic or is found to be deficient on the formal testing carried out at 6 to 8 weeks.

IRRADIATION

Irradiation is sometimes used in patients following surgery when a cure is not obtained. Many experienced clinicians also restrict this treatment modality to patients whose GH and IGF-I levels cannot be normalized with medical therapy. Irradiation is used as primary therapy generally only in those patients who are believed to be unable to tolerate surgery and who do not respond to medical therapy.

Conventional irradiation, given at a dose of 4500 cGy through two or three fields over 5 weeks, lowers GH levels substantially in more than 80% of patients. The destructive effects of the irradiation are cumulative over time; levels of GH continue to decrease for up to 20 years of follow-up. GH levels decrease to less than 5 µg/ml in 15% to 20% of treated cases by 2 years, in approximately 40% by 5 years, and in approximately 70% by 10 years.

At the same time that irradiation affects tumor function, it also affects the normal pituitary. By 10 years after irradiation, approximately 20% of patients are hypothyroid, 35% to 40% are hypoadrenal, and approximately 50% are hypogonadal. During irradiation therapy some patients complain of fatigue. If a patient is deficient in ACTH and on glucocorticoid replacement therapy, a doubling of the glucocorticoid dose is sometimes needed during radiation therapy. In rare patients, irradiation may cause subtle but permanent cognitive and short-term memory deficits. Patients may complain of difficulty concentrating, a poor memory, and lack of initiative.

Tumor infarction may occur following irradiation and usually presents with the sudden onset of severe headache and often coma and vascular collapse, a syndrome referred to as "pituitary apoplexy." Computed tomography (CT) or MRI usually shows evidence of hemorrhage. Such patients must be supported with glucocorticoids in stress doses, and consideration should be given to emergency transsphenoidal decompression. Lesser degrees of tumor infarction may also occur, and the patient may have either no symptoms or a mild headache with evidence of infarction being found only later on scan or at surgery. With conventional radiotherapy, there is also a twofold increased risk of stroke and approximately a fourfold increased risk of brain tumors.

Stereotactic radiotherapy using the gamma-knife apparatus or linear accelerator (LINAC) has become the most common way to administer radiotherapy because it can be given over a single day and may have a somewhat better therapeutic benefit-to-risk ratio. The irradiation is given through multiple ports and is shaped to correspond with the tumor visible on MRI. Achievement of GH levels less than 5 µg/mL occurs a little more quickly than with conventional irradiation, with some centers finding that 50% of patients achieve this level by 3 to 4 years. Complications of this type of radiotherapy appear to be much less than with conventional radiotherapy, although the experience is much less and the follow-up periods are much shorter thus far. However, hypopituitarism appears to occur in a proportion of patients similar to that found with conventional irradiation. The cranial nerves that pass through the cavernous sinus (i.e., III, IV, V_1, V_2, and VI) are relatively resistant to this form of irradiation, and thus this technique is particularly useful for residual tumor in the cavernous sinus. The optic nerves, tracts, and chiasm are more radiosensitive, and therefore this form of radiotherapy is less useful for tumors with considerable suprasellar extension.

MEDICAL THERAPY

Medical therapy is generally reserved for patients who fail to achieve GH levels less than 2 ng/mL (RIA) and normal IGF-I levels with surgery. In that population, it may be used alone or may be given following irradiation while awaiting the effects of the irradiation. A select group of patients may also be considered for primary medical therapy: those who are medically unable to undergo surgery and those who have tumors that extend into the cavernous sinus and thus are not curable by surgery and who do not have a visual field deficit. In this second group, somatostatin analogues often cause a 10% to 50% shrinkage of the tumor, and growth during such treatment occurs in less than 2% of patients.

Medical Therapy with Dopamine Agonists

Approximately 10% to 20% of patients respond to cabergoline (Dostinex)[1] with a normalization of GH and IGF-I levels, although this drug is not approved by the U.S. Food and Drug Administration for this indication and published experience is limited. Patients with concomitant secretion of PRL may have a better chance of responding. Thus, although the chance of successful therapy is relatively low, I generally give a therapeutic trial with cabergoline because it is generally well tolerated, given orally, and less expensive than other medical options. If there is no response, I switch to another medical agent. Side effects are uncommon but may include nausea and constipation.

Medical Therapy with Somatostatin Agonists

The somatostatin analogue octreotide (Sandostatin) results in substantial reductions of GH and IGF-I in 90% of patients, and in approximately 60% IGF-I levels can be brought into the normal range. Two long-acting preparations of somatostatin agonists are available and are the ones currently used in most patients. Octreotide LAR (Sandostatin LAR) is given monthly intramuscularly in 10-, 20-, or 30-mg doses, depending on the GH and IGF-1 responses. Rarely, higher doses are necessary. Prior to starting the intramuscular preparations, octreotide should be given subcutaneously for 2 weeks to be sure there are no unacceptable side effects (mainly gastrointestinal). In patients who achieve normalization of GH and IGF-I with 10 mg per month, the interval between doses can sometimes be lengthened to 5 to 8 weeks. Lanreotide Autogel[4] is given every 2 weeks subcutaneously, the timing depending on the GH and IGF-1 responses. MRI scans show 10% to 50% tumor size reduction as a result of therapy with somatostatin analogues in approximately 30% to 50% of patients when used adjunctively following surgery and in up to 75% of patients when used primarily. Tumor size reduction with octreotide LAR appears to be better than that seen with lanreotide. In patients who respond but do

---

[1]Not FDA approved for this indication.
[4]Not yet approved for use in the United States.

not normalize GH and IGF-1 levels with these drugs, the addition of cabergoline is often helpful.

Side effects include mild abdominal bloating, nausea, moderate diarrhea, steatorrhea, and gastritis. Cholelithiasis and gallbladder sludge because of poor gallbladder contractility occur in up to 25% of patients. Cholecystitis occurs in less than 1% of patients and is treated by laparoscopic cholecystectomy rather than stopping the drug if the patient is having a good GH/IGF-1 response. The glucose intolerance of acromegaly usually improves with treatment, but occasionally some patients worsen with octreotide use and glucose levels should be monitored.

Medical Therapy with Pegvisomant

Pegvisomant (Somavert) is a biosynthetic GH analogue that is a GH receptor blocker. It functions as a competitive inhibitor to GH, blocking its action in all tissues and decreasing the generation of IGF-I. It normalizes IGF-I levels in more than 95% of patients when given by daily subcutaneous injection. It does not directly work on the tumor, so GH levels do not fall and actually rise because of loss of negative feedback by IGF-I. In a few patients treated with pegvisomant, tumor size increased, but it is uncertain whether this is because of the pegvisomant or just because of the natural history of tumor growth in those patients. Two patients also had reversible liver function test abnormalities. Glucose intolerance usually improves with pegvisomant. It is controversial whether pegvisomant should be used as first-line medical therapy or just in those patients who do not have adequate responses to octreotide. At present, most clinicians reserve its use for patients who do not normalize GH and IGF-I levels with octreotide. During treatment, only IGF-I levels are monitored and used for dose adjustment because the drug cross-reacts with GH in the standard assays for GH. Liver function tests must also be monitored. Because of the risk of tumor size enlargement, MRI scans of the pituitary must be monitored. There is very limited experience in using pegvisomant together with octreotide.

Conclusion

In conclusion, in patients with microadenomas and intrasellar macroadenomas, transsphenoidal surgery offers a 60% to 80% chance of cure, depending on the experience of the neurosurgeon. The recurrence rate after apparent cure is less than 5%. Thus, this would appear to be the best choice as primary therapy for such patients. In patients with larger tumors, surgery can cause a considerable debulking of the tumor with a concomitant reduction in GH levels, but the cure rate decreases as tumor size and invasiveness increase.

Because radiotherapy may take several years to bring GH levels to normal, I believe it should be regarded as second- or even third-line therapy to be used if an operation has not resulted in cure or is contraindicated. Stereotactic radiotherapy appears to cause a moderately faster reduction of GH levels with less adverse effects, especially when the residual tumor is in the cavernous sinus, and it is now the preferred mode of irradiation. Hypopituitarism is the primary complication.

Medical therapy is generally reserved for patients not cured by surgery and/or radiotherapy or in whom ablative therapy is contraindicated. When the parasellar extent of a tumor indicates that it cannot be cured surgically and there is no visual field deficit, primary medical therapy with somatostatin analogues may be appropriate. Additionally, these drugs may be useful while awaiting the eventual destructive effects of irradiation.

Because of ease of use and lower cost, I often try cabergoline first, realizing that the success rates for dopamine agonists are relatively low. In those patients in whom dopamine agonists are ineffective, a long-acting somatostatin agonist such as octreotide LAR can be given with good expectations of success at normalizing GH and IGF-1 levels. However, cabergoline may also help to bring GH and IGF-1 levels into the normal range when added to octreotide. Pegvisomant has a very high rate of success in normalizing IGF-I levels and if tumor size is not an issue can be considered for early medical therapy or in patients who do not respond to octreotide.

In all cases, patients need to be followed carefully following surgery and/or radiotherapy and during medical treatment. GH and IGF-I levels need to be monitored as well as tumor size by MRI. Other pituitary function may also need to be monitored and treated if there is hypopituitarism.

REFERENCES

Ayuk J, Stewart SE, Stewart PM, Sheppard MC and the European Sandostatin LAR Group: Efficacy of Sandostatin LAR (long-acting somatostatin analogue) is similar in patients with untreated acromegaly and in those previously treated with surgery and/or radiotherapy. Clin Endocrinol 2004;60:375-381.

Beauregard C, Truong U, Hardy J, Serri O: Long-term outcome and mortality after transsphenoidal adenomectomy for acromegaly. Clin Endocrinol 2003;58:86-91.

Caron P, Bex M, Cullen DR, et al: One-year follow-up of patients with acromegaly treated with fixed or titrated doses of lanreotide Autogel. Clin Endocrinol 2004;60:734-740.

Castinetti F, Taieb D, Kuhn J-M, et al: Outcome of gamma knife radiosurgery in 82 patients with acromegaly: Correlation with initial hypersecretion. J Clin Endocrinol Metab 2005;90:4483-4488.

Clemmons DR, Chihara K, Freda PU, et al: Optimizing control of acromegaly: Integrating a growth hormone receptor antagonist into the treatment algorithm. J Clin Endocrinol Metab 2004;88:4759-4767.

Cozzi R, Attanasio R, Lodrini S, Lasio G: Cabergoline addition to depot somatostatin analogues in resistant acromegalic patients: Efficacy and lack of predictive value of prolactin status. Clin Endocrinol 2004;61:209-215.

Freda PU: Somatostatin analogs in acromegaly. J Clin Endocrinol Metab 2002;87:3013-3018.

Growth Hormone Research Society and the Pituitary Society Consensus Conference: Biochemical assessment and long-term monitoring in patients with acromegaly. J Clin Endocrinol Metab 2004;89:3099-3102.

Holdaway IM, Rajasoorya RC, Gamble GD: Factors influencing mortality in acromegaly. J Clin Endocrinol Metab 2004;89:667-674.

Puder JJ, Nilavar S, Post KD, Freda PU: Relationship between disease-related morbidity and biochemical markers of activity in patients with acromegaly. J Clin Endocrinol Metab 2005;90:1972-1978.

Terzolo M, Reimondo G, Gasperi M, et al: Colonoscopic screening and follow-up in patients with acromegaly: A multicenter study in Italy. J Clin Endocrinol Metab 2005;90:84-90.

Van der Lely AJ, Hutson KR, Trainer PJ, et al: Long-term treatment with pegvisomant, a growth hormone receptor antagonist. Lancet 2001;358:1754-1759.

Adrenocortical Insufficiency

Method of
Andjela Drincic, MD, and Robert J. Anderson, MD

Adrenal insufficiency encompasses endocrine disorders of high morbidity that are fatal if the patent is undiagnosed and untreated. Patients' dramatic responses to treatment underscore the necessity for accurate and timely diagnosis and treatment. Adrenal insufficiency is divided into two categories on the basis of the anatomic location of the deficit in the hypothalamic-pituitary-adrenal axis. Primary adrenal insufficiency refers to the loss of cortisol and mineralocorticoid because of destruction or drug-induced dysfunction of the adrenal gland. Secondary adrenal insufficiency refers to lack of adrenocorticotropic hormone (ACTH) because of pituitary damage or destruction. Hypothalamic etiologies that lead to loss of corticotropin-releasing hormone (CRH) (so-called tertiary insufficiency) are included in the secondary group for convenience because the differentiation is often difficult and the treatment is the same.

Primary Adrenocortical Insufficiency

ETIOLOGY

Primary adrenocortical insufficiency (Addison's disease) is an uncommon but urgent clinical problem that has multiple causes (Table 1). The most common cause (approximately 80% of cases) is autoimmune destruction of the adrenal glands. The autoimmune disease can occur as an isolated disorder, or it can be associated with other autoimmune deficiencies in polyglandular failure syndrome type I (primary adrenal insufficiency, hypoparathyroidism, chronic mucocutaneous candidiasis, and pernicious anemia) and polyglandular failure syndrome type II (primary adrenal insufficiency, primary hypothyroidism, type I diabetes mellitus, and vitiligo). The second most common etiology is infection (approximately 20% of cases). Within this group tuberculosis and histoplasmosis are the most frequent. Fungal infections—blastomycosis, cryptococcosis and coccidioidomycosis—are also reported as causes. The adrenal necrosis commonly seen in patients with HIV is usually caused by associated opportunistic infections, especially cytomegalovirus and

CURRENT DIAGNOSIS

- Adrenal insufficiency (AI) is characterized by low cortisol level and lack of cortisol response to ACTH stimulation.
- Primary and secondary AI differ according to ACTH level: In primary AI, ACTH is elevated; in secondary AI, ACTH level is normal or low.
- In primary AI, both glucocorticoid and mineralocorticoid secretion are diminished. In secondary AI, only glucocorticoid hormone is deficient.

TABLE 1 Causes of Primary Adrenal Insufficiency

Autoimmune adrenalitis: up to 80% of cases
Infectious: up to 20% of cases
- Tuberculosis
- Histoplasmosis
- Blastomycosis
- Cryptococcosis
- Coccidioidomycosis
- Bacterial
- HIV and associated opportunistic infections

All other causes:
- Bilateral adrenal hemorrhage: postoperatively, trauma, heparin
- Surgical: bilateral adrenalectomy
- Metastatic disease: lung, breast, gastric
- Congenital adrenal hyperplasia
- Adrenoleukodystrophy (X-linked)
- Drugs
  - *Decreased cortisol biosynthesis:* Mitotane (Lysodren), ketoconazole (Nizoral), aminoglutethimide (Cytadren), metyrapone (Metopirone)
  - *Accelerated cortisol metabolic clearance:* rifampin (Rifadin), phenytoin (Dilantin), phenobarbital (Luminal)

tuberculosis. Increased awareness and better imaging techniques have led to more frequent reports of bilateral adrenal hemorrhage in patients after abdominal surgery or trauma. Table 1 includes drugs that may lead to partial or complete cortical dysfunction and adrenal insufficiency either by decreasing cortisol biosynthesis (metyrapone [Metopirone], mitotane [Lysodren], aminoglutethimide [Cytadren], and ketoconazole [Nizoral]) or by enhancing cortisol catabolism via induction of hepatic microsomal enzymes (rifampin [Rifadin], phenytoin [Dilantin], phenobarbital [Luminal]). Patients taking corticosteroid replacement have increased corticosteroid requirements when treated with rifampin or similar agents.

CLINICAL PRESENTATION

Acute and chronic courses are the major modes of presentation of adrenal insufficiency. A patient with a rapid onset of primary adrenal insufficiency is usually ill enough with the underlying disease to present in adrenal crisis. Major manifestations are dehydration, fever, hypotension with cardiovascular collapse associated with hyponatremia, hyperkalemia, and hypoglycemia. The patient responds to fluid resuscitation, glucose, and blood pressure maintenance initially but often expires if the cortisol lack is unrecognized. If acute primary adrenal insufficiency is suspected, it should be treated first, and the diagnostic testing completed when the patient is stable (see later).

Chronic primary adrenal insufficiency, the second major mode of presentation, may include more clues to the diagnosis. The patients decline in health over months with gradual weakness, fatigue, anorexia, weight loss, and postural hypotension. They develop hyperpigmentation of the skin (described by Addison as "a dingy or smoky appearance of various tints or shades of deep amber or chestnut brown"), especially at the palmar creases, extensor surfaces (particularly the knuckles, elbows, and knees), buccal mucosa, recent scars, and sun-exposed areas. Vitiligo that is either stippled or expansive in confluent areas may be present. These findings, together with hyperkalemia, hyponatremia, fasting hypoglycemia, possible hypothyroidism, pernicious anemia, and other deficiencies, assist in diagnosis. Patients may have difficulties with minor illnesses. They are always at risk for the third major mode of presentation—catastrophic acute adrenal crisis concomitant with the underlying chronic insufficiency—if the stress is severe enough. Vigilance, early diagnosis, and timely treatment are lifesaving for these patients.

Secondary Adrenocortical Insufficiency

ETIOLOGY

Causes of secondary adrenal insufficiency commonly involve hypothalamic-pituitary tumors and accompanying anatomic and therapeutic sequelae (Table 2). Other causes include trauma, infarction, infiltrative and infectious diseases, and autoimmune disease. The most common cause of secondary adrenal insufficiency is iatrogenic: the use and withdrawal of exogenous glucocorticoid preparations. Patients who have received a course of high-dose glucocorticoids for a month or more within the previous year can have variable degrees of suppression and recovery of the hypothalamic-pituitary-adrenal axis. The possibility of secondary adrenal insufficiency must be considered in these individuals.

CLINICAL PRESENTATION

General malaise, fatigue, weakness, hypotension, and lack of skin hyperpigmentation are suggestive findings. Hyponatremia can occur and some patients may present with symptomatic hypoglycemia as the main finding. Female patients may have loss of pubic and axillary hair

TABLE 2 Causes of Secondary Adrenal Insufficiency

Iatrogenic:
- Discontinuation of exogenous glucocorticoid treatment or inadequate coverage during stress in patients on long-term or intermittent glucocorticoids by any route

Tumors:
- Pituitary adenomas: functioning or nonfunctioning
- Craniopharyngioma

Isolated ACTH deficiency

Trauma

Infarction/vascular:
- Ischemic necrosis
- Sheehan's syndrome (postpartum pituitary necrosis), diabetes mellitus, sickle cell disease
- Pituitary apoplexy: necrosis of tumor

Radiation of pituitary:
- Usually gradual and progressive decline in function

Infiltrative and infectious disease:
- Sarcoidosis
- Hemochromatosis
- Meningitis
- Tuberculosis

Autoimmune
- Lymphocytic hypophysitis

Idiopathic

because of the lack of adrenal androgens. Patients also may present with other manifestations of pituitary disease, such as mass effect of the lesion with headache and cranial nerve paralysis. The combined effects of one or more overproduced hormones may occur with variable pituitary hormone losses because of tumor compression or destruction of normal pituitary cells. Patients given exogenous glucocorticoids may be cushingoid but may present in the interesting situation of having secondary adrenal insufficiency with clinical Cushing's syndrome if the glucocorticoid therapy is withheld or withdrawn. Careful review of the patient's history and drug records should help avoid secondary adrenal insufficiency.

Diagnosis

CLINICAL

Typical skin hyperpigmentation and vitiligo help with the diagnosis of primary adrenocortical insufficiency. Because isolated ACTH deficiency is rare, the diagnosis of chronic secondary adrenal insufficiency can be assisted by the finding of accompanying pituitary hormone hypofunction and/or hyperfunction. Skin hyperpigmentation is not present. A careful history is useful to detect exogenous glucocorticoid administration and subsequent interruption of treatment. Diagnosis of acute adrenal crisis depends on laboratory results.

LABORATORY

Clinical evaluation of an ambulatory patient with suspected adrenal insufficiency should start with a morning measurement of serum cortisol and plasma ACTH. In primary adrenal insufficiency, the serum cortisol value is low and the ACTH is high (more than 200 pg/mL). The usual findings in secondary hypoadrenalism are a low or "normal" ACTH level (0 to 50 pg/mL) in association with a low serum cortisol. However, there is significant overlap in cortisol values between normal and hypoadrenal patients. Therefore, the morning cortisol is useful only if it is very low (≤ 3 µg/dL), thus confirming the diagnosis of adrenal insufficiency, or elevated (≥ 19 µg/dL), thereby excluding this diagnosis. Most patients need dynamic testing with synthetic $a_{1,24}$-ACTH (cosyntropin [Cortrosyn]). A baseline plasma cortisol is obtained, 250 µg of ACTH is given intravenously (or intramuscularly), and cortisol levels are drawn at 30 and 60 minutes. A normal response is a cortisol level of at least 18 µg/dL at any time during the test. Simultaneous aldosterone levels should rise to 16 µg/dL at 30 minutes. In secondary adrenal insufficiency, lack of endogenous ACTH leads to adrenal atrophy, and the response of cortisol to cosyntropin is usually also less than 18 µg/dL at 30 and 60 minutes. However, if the ACTH deficiency is partial, or of recent onset, one may see a normal response to stimulation using 250 µg of cosyntropin. A low-dose cosyntropin test using 1 µg of ACTH is proposed as a more sensitive test for diagnosis of secondary adrenal insufficiency, but it is limited by the cumbersome, and potentially inaccurate, need to dilute a standard vial containing 250 µg of ACTH. The metyrapone test or insulin-induced hypoglycemia test may be needed to confirm secondary adrenal insufficiency by demonstrating a lack of cortisol response associated with low ACTH. Both tests entail risks and can precipitate an adrenal crisis. The reader is referred to standard endocrinology texts for detailed protocols of these tests. In patients with other autoimmune diseases, level of adrenal autoantibodies correlates with the degree of adrenal dysfunction and may help identify subclinical disease.

Computed tomography (CT) or magnetic resonance imaging (MRI) of the adrenals can be helpful in the differential diagnosis of primary adrenal insufficiency. In autoimmune adrenalitis, the glands are small, atrophied, and difficult to visualize, whereas chronic granulomatous adrenal diseases are associated with enlargement, and calcifications are present in approximately 50% of the patients with adrenal insufficiency because of tuberculosis. Bilateral enlarged adrenals are present in hemorrhage, metastases, and granulomatous diseases. MRI scanning is equally informative in hemorrhage and may be superior in differentiating inflammatory from metastatic disease.

The diagnosis of adrenal insufficiency in a critically ill patient poses a special dilemma. On one hand, patients with hypoproteinemia (albumin concentration of 2.5 g/dL or less) can have a spuriously low cortisol level because of a decrease in binding proteins. In such patients, serum free cortisol concentration should be measured. On the other hand, there are recent concerns that patients in refractory septic shock may have relative adrenal insufficiency despite high basal cortisol levels. If a patient presents in an acute crisis with cardiovascular collapse, a serum cortisol level of less than 20 to 25 μg/dL is highly suggestive of adrenal dysfunction.

Treatment

ACUTE ADRENAL CRISIS

The treatment for acute adrenal insufficiency is the same whether it is primary or secondary. Hydrocortisone sodium succinate (Solu-Cortef), 100 mg intravenously every 6 hours, should be given for the first 24 hours with full fluid resuscitation with dextrose and normal saline. Mineralocorticoid replacement is not needed because of the adequate mineralocorticoid effect with a glucocorticoid dose of 100 mg/day or greater. The dose of hydrocortisone can be reduced by half each day as the patient improves. Oral treatment can be resumed rapidly once the patient recovers. An aggressive review is required to define and to treat the precipitating event and associated illnesses. If adrenal insufficiency is suspected in an unstable patient who cannot wait for diagnostic studies, instead of hydrocortisone, dexamethasone (4 mg) should be given intravenously. Baseline ACTH and cortisol levels are useful if obtainable. Cosyntropin stimulation testing can be performed immediately after dexamethasone is given because it does not interfere with subsequent measurement of serum cortisol levels. Hydrocortisone is then initiated after the stimulation test.

CHRONIC PRIMARY AND SECONDARY ADRENAL INSUFFICIENCY

Glucocorticoid replacement in both chronic disorders is the same. The major goal of treatment is to restore normalcy by attempting to reproduce the diurnal rhythm of cortisol production with a glucocorticoid preparation. Determining the best way to achieve this goal is still controversial. Glucocorticoid preparations differ according to their half-life and mineralocorticoid potency, which should be kept in mind when choosing therapy for a particular patient. The optimal dose of medication chosen is lower than what was recommended in the past. The previous typical hydrocortisone dose of 30 mg daily often led to chronic overreplacement with increased risks of bone loss and cardiovascular disease. We prefer to use hydrocortisone (Cortef) at a dose of 10 to 15 mg in the morning, 5 mg at noon, and 5 mg in the late afternoon titrated to

	CURRENT THERAPY	
	Treatment	**Items to Monitor**
Acute: Primary and Secondary	Hydrocortisone sodium succinate (Solu-Cortef), 100 mg IV q6h; dextrose 5% in normal saline; treat underlying illness, precipitating event	Blood pressure, electrolytes, glucose
Chronic: Primary	Hydrocortisone (Cortef), 10–15 mg PO, AM, 5 mg PO noon, 5 mg PO, PM *or* Prednisone (Deltasone), 5.0 mg PO, AM *or* Cortisone acetate (Cortone), 15 mg PO, AM, 10 mg PO, PM *and* Fludrocortisone (Florinef), 0.05–0.2 mg PO/d (usual dose: 0.1 mg/d)	Sense of well-being, strength, blood pressure, electrolytes; avoid cushingoid changes; skin pigmentation
Secondary	Same as Primary except no fludrocortisone	Same as Primary except skin changes do not occur and potassium is usually normal

Abbreviations: IV = intravenous; PO = orally.

the patient's needs. Cortisone acetate (Cortone), 25 mg daily (divided in two doses), or prednisone (Deltasone), 5 mg in the morning, can also be used, but both preparations rely on hepatic metabolism for bioactivity. We avoid longer acting preparations, such as dexamethasone (Decadron, Hexadrol) because of the higher occurrence of exogenous Cushing's syndrome. Occasionally, short-acting hydrocortisone allows for continuous stimulation of ACTH secretion overnight. This may lead to persistent hyperpigmentation and sometimes even pituitary hyperplasia. Such a patient may do better on dexamethasone therapy at bedtime (or in the morning, if insomnia is a problem). Conversely, short-acting hydrocortisone is the ideal choice for a patient with glucocorticoid-induced secondary adrenal insufficiency because it facilitates recovery of pituitary adrenal axis.

In primary adrenal insufficiency, the mineralocorticoid preparation fludrocortisone (Florinef) is used at a dose of 0.05 to 0.2 mg/day (usual dose, 0.1 mg/day). Too little Florinef leads to hyperkalemia, hyponatremia, and dehydration. Too much causes upright and supine hypertension and hypokalemia. Rarely, a patient does not require the mineralocorticoid because of an adequate effect from the glucocorticoid or residual adrenal mineralocorticoid production. In most cases of secondary adrenal insufficiency, a mineralocorticoid preparation is not required because the renin-angiotensin system is intact.

Androgen replacement therapy using DHEA (25 to 50 mg daily) has been studied in women with primary and secondary adrenal insufficiency. A positive impact on well-being and mood were noted. The addition of DHEA can be considered for some women with adrenal insufficiency. One caveat is that DHEA is considered a food supplement in the United States and its quality is not monitored by the Food and Drug Administration.

How do we know how much glucocorticoid replacement is enough? Unfortunately, we do not have precise means for exact laboratory assessment of therapy of either primary or secondary adrenal insufficiency. A 24-hour urine free cortisol may be helpful to determine significant over- or undersupplementation. It is limited in value because of the marked individual variability in urine cortisol achieved after different doses of hydrocortisone. The use of plasma hydrocortisone patterns (by obtaining cortisol levels after the morning dose, before lunch, and before the afternoon dose) is proposed, but this method has practical limitations. The ACTH level is not a good measure of adequate replacement because it may not be suppressed into the normal range in some patients with primary adrenal insufficiency. In both primary and secondary adrenal insufficiency, the best approach is to follow the clinical examination and history for a sense of well-being and good appetite and to monitor blood pressure and serum electrolyte levels. In primary adrenal insufficiency, progressive increases in the skin hyperpigmentation may serve as an indication of inadequate replacement. An occasional patient may become cushingoid and require a smaller replacement dose. In secondary adrenal insufficiency the corticosteroids may unmask underlying mild diabetes insipidus in some patients. Mineralocorticoid therapy is monitored with assessment of blood pressure, presence of edema, electrolyte imbalance, and, if needed, a plasma renin activity, which should be normal to slightly elevated, not suppressed. If DHEA therapy is started, DHEA sulfate and testosterone levels should be assessed periodically.

GLUCOCORTICOID COVERAGE FOR MEDICAL AND SURGICAL STRESS

The patient must understand the need to increase the glucocorticoid dose during sick days. Each patient should receive a detailed sheet that lists how to adjust the medicine. Various recommendations for adrenal supplementation therapy exist, but they are the result of expert opinions rather than a product of systematic research. We recommend that the patient double the dose during the 1 to 3 days of a moderate illness such as the "flu" with a low-grade fever (100°F [38°C] or less) and triple the dose if a higher fever (more than 100°F [38°C] is present. Patients are given 1.0-mL vials with injectable dexamethasone (Decadron Phosphate, 4 mg/mL in 1.0-mL vials) to use if they are vomiting and cannot get to medical care quickly. Patients administer the dose intramuscularly (4 mg) and repeat if necessary every 12 hours before arriving at the hospital. They frequently keep one vial at work and one in the car, taking care to renew them as needed. Patients must get medical information bracelets or necklaces that detail their need for cortisol.

Glucocorticoid coverage for surgery and stressful procedures is the same for primary and secondary adrenal insufficiency. We give a depot of 100 mg hydrocortisone sodium succinate intramuscularly on call to surgery and then 50 to 100 mg hydrocortisone intravenously every 6 hours (starting in surgery) the first 24 hours. The intramuscular dose is given to ensure a depot in case the intravenous access is interrupted. The dose is decreased by 50% each postoperative day as indicated by patient progress until the oral glucocorticoid (and mineralocorticoid for primary adrenal insufficiency) can be resumed.

REFERENCES

Arlt W, Allolio B: Adrenal insufficiency. Lancet 2003;361(9372):1881-1893.

Arlt W, Callies F, van Vlijmen JC, et al: Dehydroepiandrosterone replacement in women with adrenal insufficiency. N Engl J Med 1999;341(14):1013-1020.

Cooper MS, Stewart PM: Corticosteroid insufficiency in acutely ill patients. N Engl J Med 2003;348(8):727-734.

Coursin DB, Wood KE: Corticosteroid supplementation for adrenal insufficiency. JAMA 2002;287(2):236-240.

Crown A, Lightman S: Why is the management of glucocorticoid deficiency still controversial: A review of the literature. Clin Endocrinol (Oxf) 2005;63(5):483-492.

Dorin RI, Qualls CR, Crapo LM: Diagnosis of adrenal insufficiency. Ann Intern Med 2003;139(3):194-204.

Hamrahian AH, Oseni TS, Arafah BM: Measurements of serum free cortisol in critically ill patients. N Engl J Med 2004;350(16):1629-1638.

Howlett TA: An assessment of optimal hydrocortisone replacement therapy. Clin Endocrinol (Oxf) 1997;46(3):263-268.

Krasner AS: Glucocorticoid-induced adrenal insufficiency. JAMA 1999;282(7):671-676.

Salvatori R: Adrenal insufficiency. JAMA 2005;294(19):2481-2488.

Ten S, New M, Maclaren N: Clinical review 130: Addison's disease 2001. J Clin Endocrinol Metab 2001;86(7):2909-2922.

Cushing's Syndrome

Method of
Kathryn G. Schuff, MD

The diagnosis of Cushing's syndrome is one of the most difficult but potentially most important that can be made in a patient. The consequences of pathologic hypercortisolism are significant, and excess mortality and morbidity improve with cure of the disease. Although the evaluation and management often involve specialty referral, the primary care provider plays a pivotal role in suspecting the diagnosis and initiating the workup.

Clinical Presentation

Although traditionally considered a rare disease with an incidence of 1 to 2 per 100,000, more recently Cushing's syndrome has been reported to occur in up to 3% to 4% of the obese, uncontrolled diabetic population. The classic presentation (moon facies, purple striae, central obesity) is uncommonly seen, and the presentation more commonly overlaps that of polycystic ovary syndrome, the metabolic syndrome, and depression. Given the nonspecific presentation, health care providers should have a low threshold for screening patients for the disease. More specific features (Table 1) that should prompt evaluation include difficult-to-control diabetes mellitus or hypertension, unexplained osteoporosis, and menstrual irregularities. In addition, physical signs that are disquieting include facial rounding, plethora, supraclavicular fat pad filling, central obesity, thin skin (including spontaneous ecchymoses), and proximal muscle weakness, particularly if a change in appearance can be demonstrated. Children exhibit poor linear growth, generalized obesity, and menstrual irregularities. The etiologies of hypercortisolism are varied (Box 1)

TABLE 1 Clinical Features of Cushing's Syndrome (In Order of Decreasing Specificity)

Feature	Sensitivity (%)	Specificity (%)
Hypokalemia (K+ <3.6)	25	96
Ecchymoses	53	94
Osteoporosis	26	94
Weakness	65	93
Diastolic blood pressure ≥105 mm Hg	39	83
Red or violaceous striae	46	78
Acne	52	76
Central obesity	90	71
Hirsutism	50	71
Plethora	82	69
Oligomenorrhea	72	49
Generalized obesity	60	38
Abnormal glucose tolerance	88	23

BOX 1 Etiologies of Hypercortisolism

- Pseudo-Cushing's syndrome (nonpathologic hypercortisolism)
  Acute/chronic medical illness
  Psychiatric illness
  Alcoholism
- Subclinical Cushing's syndrome (subtle hypercortisolism without features of overt Cushing's syndrome)
  Adrenal adenoma (incidentaloma)
  Adrenal macronodular hyperplasia (rare)
  Pituitary corticotroph adenoma (rare)
  Aberrant receptor expression (rare)
- Cushing's syndrome (pathologic hypercortisolism)
  Exogenous glucocorticoid use
  Oral glucocorticoids (prednisone, dexamethasone [Decadron], hydrocortisone [Cortef])
  Topical glucocorticoids (inhaled, intranasal, dermal)
  Injected glucocorticoids (articular, periarticular, intramuscular)
  Naturopathic preparations
  Endogenous glucocorticoid production
    ACTH-dependent
      Pituitary corticotroph adenoma
        MEN1 (rare, also includes hyperparathyroidism and pancreatic islet cell tumors)
      Pituitary corticotroph hyperplasia (some because of ectopic CRH)
      Ectopic ACTH syndrome
        Oat-cell lung carcinoma
        Foregut carcinoid tumors (bronchial, thymic, splenic)
        Pheochromocytoma
        Medullary thyroid carcinoma
        Islet cell tumors
    ACTH-independent
      Adrenal adenoma
      Adrenocortical carcinoma
      Rare: micronodular hyperplasia
      Macronodular hyperplasia
        Aberrant receptor expression (gastric inhibitory peptide–food responsive, 5-hydroxytryptamine, angiotensin II, interleukin-1, luteinizing hormone and human chorionic gonadotropin, vasopressin, β-adrenergic)
      Pigmented micronodular hyperplasia (Carney's triad)
      Adrenal rests
      McCune-Albright (activating mutations)

Abbreviations: ACTH = adrenocorticotropic hormone; CRH = corticotrophin-releasing hormone; MEN1 = multiple endocrine neoplasia, type 1.

and include both pathologic etiologies causing subclinical and overt Cushing's syndrome as well as pseudo-Cushing's syndrome, which is temporary, nonpathologic hypercortisolemia caused by concurrent medical or psychiatric illness.

SUBCLINICAL CUSHING'S SYNDROME

Subtle hypothalamic-pituitary-adrenal (HPA) axis abnormalities and autonomy have been demonstrated in 5% to 20% of patients with incidentally discovered adrenal masses. These patients do not exhibit frank signs, symptoms, or biochemical abnormalities of Cushing's syndrome, and thus this entity is termed subclinical Cushing's syndrome. However, there are higher rates of hypertension, impaired glucose tolerance, and diabetes in these patients, which often improve with removal of the lesion, and a higher prevalence of cardiovascular dysfunction. Although this syndrome is considered a very mild form of Cushing's syndrome, there appears to be a low rate of progression to overt Cushing's syndrome, and therapeutic decisions must be individualized.

Diagnostic Evaluation

EXOGENOUS GLUCOCORTICOIDS

Cushing's syndrome caused by exogenous glucocorticoid use can be obvious, but careful investigation for unsuspected or surreptitious use must be undertaken in all patients. Infrequently recognized culprits are intraarticular, epidural, topical (inhaled, intranasal, and dermal), and naturopathic preparations. Variations in the metabolic clearance of synthetic glucocorticoids can lead to markedly prolonged glucocorticoid exposure and development of Cushing's syndrome. Detection of the synthetic glucocorticoid may require tandem mass spectrometry evaluation.

ENDOGENOUS HYPERCORTISOLISM

Evaluation of suspected endogenous hypercortisolemia must follow a stepwise approach (Figure 1). The first step is to make the diagnosis of Cushing's syndrome. The second step is to determine if the abnormal cortisol secretion is adrenocorticotropic hormone (ACTH)-dependent (from either a pituitary adenoma (Cushing's disease) or the ectopic ACTH syndrome) or ACTH-independent (primary adrenal disease). Finally, in ACTH-dependent Cushing's syndrome, the health care provider must distinguish pituitary sources of ACTH from the ectopic ACTH syndrome. Proceeding in the evaluation in a stepwise approach is critical for correct interpretation of test results because the premise of many of the tests is that preliminary biochemical diagnoses have been confirmed. For example, Cushing's syndrome must be confirmed before the ACTH level can be interpreted. In addition, because of the high prevalence of incidental pituitary and adrenal lesions and the finding of nodular adrenal disease in some cases of Cushing's disease caused by pituitary adenomas, imaging should not be performed until the biochemical diagnoses have been established. Finally, as many as 15% of patients with Cushing's syndrome will have intermittent hypercortisolemia, and care must be taken that the evaluation is performed when the patient is symptomatic or has documented hypercortisolism.

STEP ONE: DIAGNOSE CUSHING'S SYNDROME

The first step in the evaluation is to establish the diagnosis of Cushing's syndrome by demonstrating pathologic hypercortisolism, either by measuring cortisol overproduction, abnormal HPA regulation, or absent diurnal variation. We recommend four tests for this purpose: the 1 mg overnight dexamethasone suppression (1 mg ON dex) test, measurement of 24-hour urine-free cortisol (24-hour UFC) excretion, assessment of diurnal variation with a midnight serum or salivary cortisol level, and the dexamethasone-suppressed corticotrophin-releasing hormone stimulation (dex-CRH) test.

One Milligram Overnight Dexamethasone Suppression Test

The 1 mg ON dex test has sensitivity sufficiently high to exclude the diagnosis of Cushing's syndrome; however, it lacks sufficient specificity to confirm the diagnosis, with false-positive rates from 5% to 30%. The test is simple to perform and involves administering 1 mg of dexamethasone (Decadron) by mouth at 11 PM. The serum cortisol at 8 AM the next morning should be less than 5 µg/dL; more strict criteria require suppression to less than 2.5 or 3 µg/dL. A simultaneous dexamethasone (Decadron) level can detect false positives that occur in patients taking medications that accelerate dexamethasone (Decadron) metabolism (phenytoin [Dilantin], phenobarbital [Luminal], rifampin [Rifadin], and primidone [Mysoline]). False positives may also be seen with estrogen therapy and tamoxifen (Nolvadex).

Measurement of 24-Hour Urine-Free Cortisol Excretion

Because of the high false-positive rate, an abnormal 1 mg ON dex test must be confirmed, usually by measurement of 24-hour UFC excretion. Alternatively, a 24-hour UFC measurement may be the initial step in the evaluation. As shown in Figure 1, marked elevations in 24-hour UFC (>300 µg/day) confirm the diagnosis, but intermediate levels require additional evaluation. Because of potential problems with incomplete collections and intermittent hypercortisolemia, creatinine should be measured in the specimen, and normal 24-hour UFC excretion should be demonstrated on 2 or 3 occasions before the diagnosis of Cushing's syndrome is excluded. Acute medical illness can cause marked elevations in 24-hour UFC, false positives can occur with high urine volumes, and carbamazepine (Tegretol) can cross-react in the high-pressure liquid chromatography (HPLC) assay.

Midnight Serum or Salivary Cortisol Levels

Loss of the diurnal rhythm in cortisol secretion is a characteristic feature in Cushing's syndrome (Figure 2). Demonstration of a midnight serum cortisol greater than 7.5 µg/dL distinguishes patients with Cushing's syndrome from normal and pseudo-Cushing's patients with high sensitivity and specificity. More recent improvements in the salivary cortisol assay allow collection of a saliva sample at home, avoiding the logistic difficulties in arranging a blood draw at night. Cut-off values for salivary cortisol measurements vary by assay, but normal suppression is generally between less than 0.2 and 0.55 µg/dL.

Dexamethasone-Suppressed Corticotropin-Releasing Hormone Stimulation Test

The dex-CRH test detects the relative resistance to dexamethasone (Decadron) suppression and over-responsiveness to ovine corticotropin-releasing factor (oCRH [Acthrel]) in various tumors. It improves on the poor specificity of the 1 mg ON dex test with a higher dose of dexamethasone (Decadron), 0.5 mg by mouth every 6 hours starting at 12 PM and ending at 6 AM on the second day. Because this

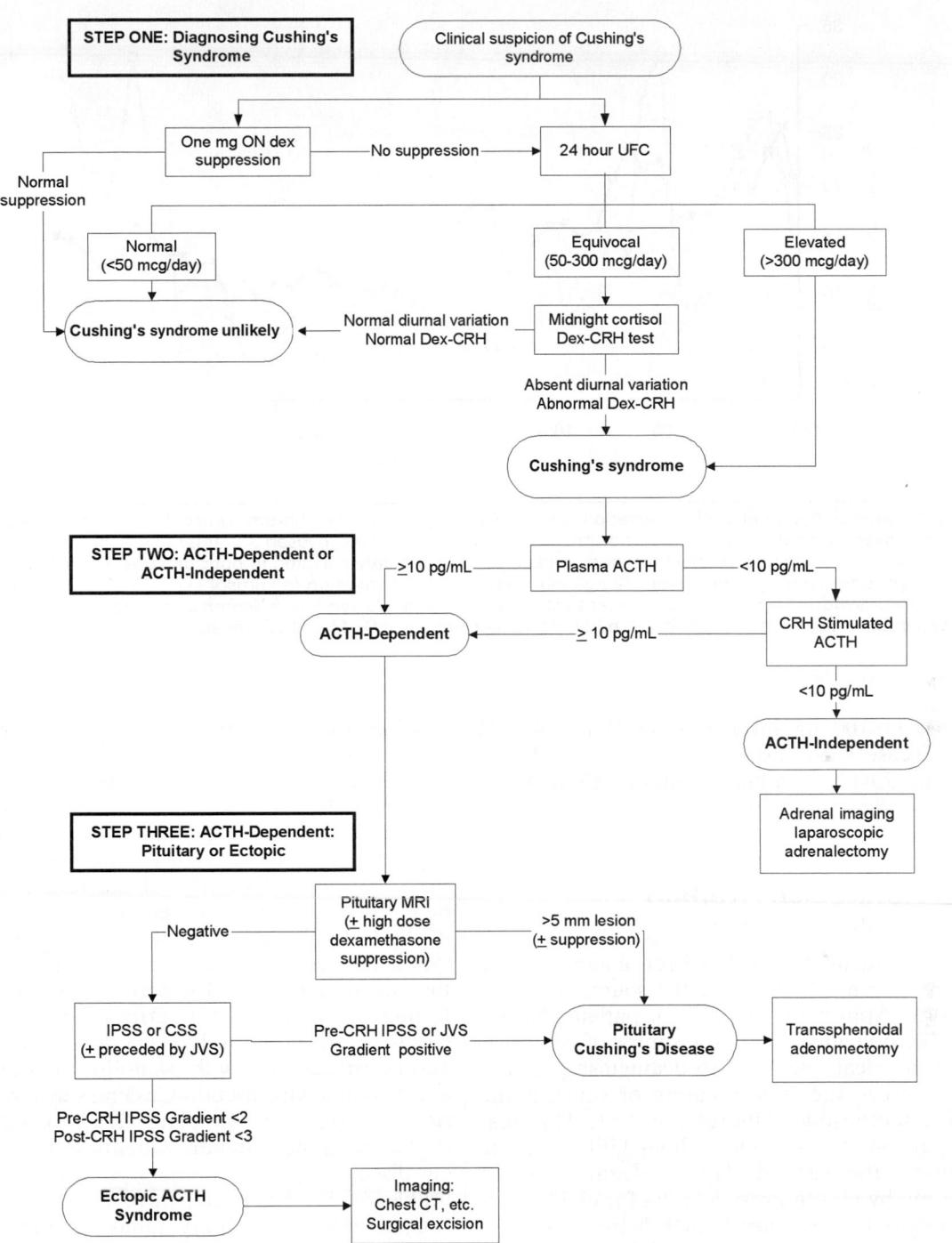

FIGURE 1. Stepwise approach to the diagnosis and differential diagnosis of Cushing's syndrome. ACTH = adrenocorticotropin; CRH = corticotrophin-releasing hormone; CSS = cavernous sinus sampling; CT = computed tomography; dex = dexamethasone; IPSS = inferior petrosal sinus sampling; JVS = jugular venous sampling; MRI = magnetic resonance imaging; ON = overnight; UFC = urine-free cortisol.

dose of dexamethasone (Decadron) will suppress many pituitary adenomas, sensitivity of the test is retained by administration of oCRH (Acthrel)[1] 100 μg intravenously at 8 AM on the final day followed by cortisol and ACTH levels every 15 minutes for 1 hour. A plasma cortisol greater than 1.4 μg/dL distinguishes patients with Cushing's syndrome from those with pseudo-Cushing's with high accuracy.

---

[1]Not FDA approved for this indication.

STEP TWO: ACTH-DEPENDENT OR ACTH-INDEPENDENT DISEASE

Once the diagnosis of Cushing's syndrome has been established, the next step is to determine if the abnormal cortisol secretion is dependent on ACTH. A random ACTH level greater than 10 pg/mL confirms ACTH-dependent disease. However, because ACTH is secreted in a pulsatile, episodic fashion and is rapidly degraded, a low ACTH level must be confirmed by lack of stimulation to more than 10 pg/mL by

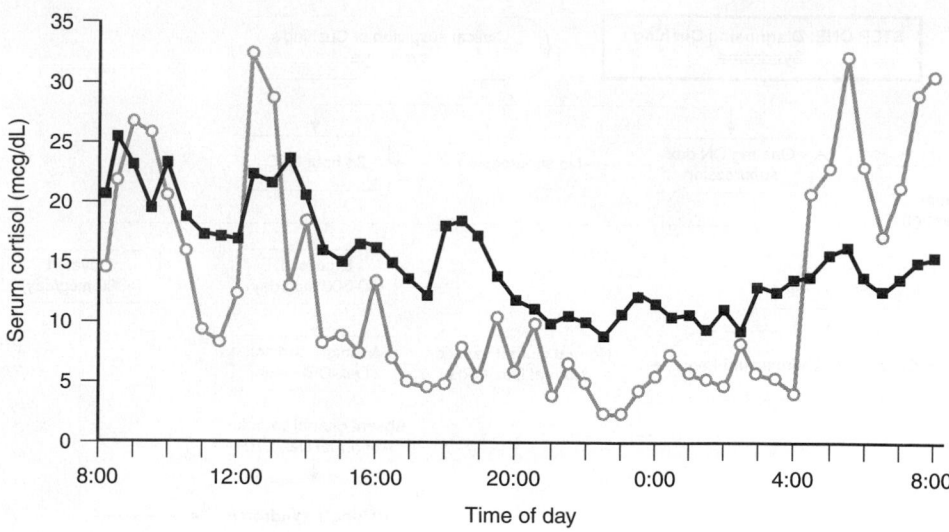

FIGURE 2. Diurnal rhythm of cortisol secretion is lost in Cushing's syndrome. Serum cortisol levels were measured every 30 minutes over 24 hours in a patient with proven Cushing's syndrome *(closed squares)* and a patient with pseudo-Cushing's syndrome *(open circles)*. Urine free cortisol (UFC) was mildly elevated in both patients (Cushing's syndrome, 75 μg/day; pseudo-Cushing's syndrome, 76 μg/day). Loss of diurnal variation in cortisol secretion is seen in the patient with Cushing's syndrome, whereas the patient with pseudo-Cushing's syndrome demonstrated normal diurnal variation with low serum cortisol levels (2.2 μg/dL) at midnight. (Data courtesy of Dr. Mary H. Samuels.)

oCRH (Acthrel),[1] 100 μg intravenously. When ACTH independent disease is confirmed, we then proceed with adrenal imaging, usually with high-resolution (3- to 5-mm sections), computed tomography (CT) to evaluate primary adrenal disease.

STEP THREE: DISTINGUISH PITUITARY FROM ECTOPIC SOURCES OF ACTH

Once ACTH-dependent disease has been confirmed, the health care provider must determine the source of excess ACTH secretion. Approximately 90% of patients have a pituitary corticotroph adenoma as the source of ACTH. A number of biochemical tests exist to distinguish pituitary from ectopic sources, the most accurate of which is the high-dose dexamethasone suppression test. This test involves comparison of a baseline 24-hour UFC with one collected during the second day of dexamethasone (Decadron) 2 mg by mouth every 6 hours for eight doses. Although failure to suppress more than 90% from the baseline UFC has been reported to have 100% specificity for identifying ectopic tumors, the sensitivity of this test is poor, and there have been subsequent reports of lower specificity. Because of this, we do not rely on biochemical testing. Rather, once ACTH-dependent disease is confirmed, we perform magnetic resonance imaging (MRI) of the pituitary gland. In approximately one half of patients, a definite tumor is identified, and we then proceed with transsphenoidal adenomectomy. However, another reasonable strategy is to proceed with pituitary surgery only if both MRI and high-dose dexamethasone testing suggests a pituitary tumor.

If a tumor is not definitely identified, inferior petrosal or cavernous sinus sampling with oCRH stimulation is required to localize the ACTH source. Finding a central (cavernous sinus or petrosal sinus) to peripheral ratio of more than 2.0 before oCRH or greater than 3.0 after oCRH is highly accurate for identifying a pituitary source of ACTH. In addition, a pre-oCRH lateralization (right to left or left to right) ratio more than 1.4 suggests the intrapituitary location of the tumor. Sampling must be performed by experienced personnel, and the accuracy of the test is highly dependent on oCRH administration, symmetric catheter placement, symmetric flow through the venous sinuses, and hypercortisolemia at the time of testing. In addition, it is critical that the diagnosis of Cushing's syndrome and ACTH-dependence be confirmed before proceeding with sampling. Normal individuals and patients with pseudo-Cushing's syndrome have inferior petrosal sinus sampling (IPSS) results that falsely suggest a pituitary tumor. Patients with ACTH-independent disease (primary adrenal disease) with low but measurable ACTH levels can have IPSS results that falsely suggest either a pituitary tumor or the ectopic ACTH syndrome.

Recently, internal jugular venous sampling has been evaluated as a less invasive alternative to petrosal sinus sampling. A jugular to peripheral ratio of greater than 1.7 before oCRH or more than 2.5 after oCRH indicate a pituitary source with high accuracy. Nondiagnostic ratios are unreliable and should be further evaluated with inferior petrosal or cavernous sinus sampling.

If sampling suggests an ectopic source of ACTH, imaging is then performed to locate the tumor, starting with high resolution CT or MRI of the chest. If those areas are unrevealing, neck, abdomen, and pelvis CT are performed. Octreotide scanning may be helpful but only rarely identifies an abnormality not already seen on anatomic imaging. Often, the culprit lesion is not seen at initial imaging, but becomes apparent on serial studies performed every 6 to 12 months.

[1]Not FDA approved for this indication.

Although IPSS is highly accurate, occasional false-negative and rare false-positive results have been reported. In situations where IPSS ratios indicate the ectopic ACTH syndrome but no ectopic tumor can be found, distinguishing a truly occult ectopic ACTH-producing tumor from a false-negative IPSS is extremely difficult. Review of the response of peripheral ACTH levels to oCRH stimulation should be done, because pituitary adenomas have significantly more robust responses than ectopic tumors. Repeat IPSS and consideration of pituitary exploration are appropriate, particularly if the ACTH response to oCRH, biochemical testing, and/or MRI are consistent with a pituitary adenoma.

Therapeutic Interventions

EXOGENOUS GLUCOCORTICOID USE

Once identified, the treatment for iatrogenic Cushing's syndrome is straightforward but often difficult because of the therapeutic benefit of pharmacologic glucocorticoids. Tapering the steroid needs to occur gradually, with close monitoring of the underlying disease process and optimization of nonsteroid therapeutics. Alternate-day dosing regimens may assist in HPA axis recovery but may be limited by the underlying disease process. Patients should wear Medic Alert identification until the taper is completed and normal HPA function is demonstrated.

ENDOGENOUS CUSHING'S SYNDROME

The therapeutic intervention in essentially all etiologies of endogenous Cushing's syndrome is surgical resection of the autonomous tumor or tissue, except for the case of lung carcinomas causing the ectopic ACTH syndrome, where therapy is tailored to the stage of the cancer. Postoperatively, all patients are treated with stress doses of glucocorticoids, tapering quickly to doses approximately twice physiologic replacement, usually hydrocortisone (Cortef)[1] 20 mg by mouth twice or three times daily. Further slow taper is done over the next several months as tolerated by cortisol withdrawal symptoms and recovery of the HPA axis. A morning serum cortisol level less than 2 μg/dL on the second postoperative day is highly predictive of surgical cure; patients with low but detectable serum cortisol levels, such as less than 5 μg/dL, have varying

[1]Not FDA approved for this indication.

TABLE 2 Drugs Used in the Medical Therapy of Cushing's Syndrome

Medication	Mechanism of Action	Typical Dosage	Reported Efficacy	Common Toxicities
Steroid Biosynthesis Inhibitors				
Ketoconazole (Nizoral)[1]	Blocks multiple steps in cortisol synthesis	200-1200 mg/d	70%	Hepatotoxicity, gynecomastia, nausea, edema, rash
Metyrapone (Metopirone)[1]	Blocks 11β-hydroxylase	500-6000 mg/d	85%	Hirsutism, acne, lethargy, dizziness, ataxia, edema, nausea, rash
Aminoglutethimide (Cytadren)	Blocks cholesterol to pregnenelone conversion	750-2000 mg/d	>60% Useful additive to metyrapone	Lethargy, somnolence, dizziness, rash, fever, nausea, anorexia, hyopthyroidism
Mitotane (o,p′-DDD, Lysodren)[1]*	Blocks side-chain cleavage Adrenolytic	500-12,000 mg/d	83%	Gastrointestinal, impaired mentation, dizziness, hyperlipidemia, gynecomastia, transient rash, hepatotoxicity
ACTH Release Inhibitors				
Cyproheptadine (Periactin)[1]	Impairs ACTH secretion	24 mg/d	30%-50%	Somnolence, hyperphagia, weight gain
Bromocriptine (Parlodel)[1]	Impairs ACTH secretion	3.75-30 mg/d	25%-42%	Nausea, dry mouth, postural hypotension
Octreotide (Sandostatin)[1]	Inhibits ACTH release	100-600 μg/d	Limited experience, additive to ketoconazole	Diarrhea, gallstones
Valproic acid (Depakene)[1]	Potentiates GABA inhibition of CRH and ACTH release	1-2 g/d	Limited experience, additive to metyrapone	Sedation, nausea, hepatotoxicity, pancreatitis
Glucocorticoid Receptor Antagonist				
Mifepristone (RU-486, Mifeprex)[1]	Glucocorticoid receptor antagonist	10-25 mg/kg/d	Limited experience	Nausea, vomiting, irregular menses

[1]Not FDA approved for this indication.
*FDA approved for treatment of adrenocortical carcinoma.
Abbreviations: ACTH = adrenocorticotropic hormone; CRH = corticotropin-releasing hormone; GABA = gamma-aminobutyric acid.

cure rates. Periodic morning cortisol levels and cosyntropin (Cortrosyn)[1] stimulation testing assess recovery of the HPA axis during and after the glucocorticoid taper.

Cushing's Disease

Transsphenoidal adenomectomy is recommended for the vast majority of patients with pituitary tumors, except where extensive cavernous sinus involvement indicates a transfrontal approach. Intraoperative ultrasound or MRI can assist in the localization of tumors. If a tumor is not identified at surgery, hemihypophysectomy based on preoperative MRI and/or IPSS or CSS lateralization ratios may result in cure. Often, tumors are not identified on pathology, because they are semiliquid and "lost" during suctioning.

Mortality and morbidity are generally low in experienced centers, but complications can include cerebrospinal fluid leaks, meningitis, visual impairment, hypopituitarism, hemorrhage, venous thromboembolism, and death. Careful monitoring for abnormalities in vasopressin secretion postoperatively is required, both for diabetes insipidus and the syndrome of inappropriate antidiuretic-hormone secretion. Testing of pituitary function including free T4, IGF-1 with possible growth hormone stimulation testing and testosterone levels or menstrual history is performed at 6 weeks postoperatively.

Even in experienced hands, long-term cure of hypercortisolemia is difficult, with initial success rates reported from 68.5% to 91% and relapse rates of up to 15% over a 10-year period. Cure rates are worse for macroadenomas or invasive tumors and second surgeries, reported at 40% to 55%. Even with biochemical cure and improvement in symptoms, studies show persistent compromise in quality of life.

Primary Adrenal Disease

The laparoscopic approach has essentially replaced open surgery with similar mortality, morbidity, and operative times; and shorter postoperative recovery, hospital stays, and decreased acute and chronic pain. The laparoscopic approach is not used in cases of adrenocortical carcinoma or patients with coagulopathy, previous surgery or trauma. Lesion size was previously a limitation, but with increasing experience appears to no longer be a significant factor. Unilateral adrenalectomy is indicated for adrenal adenomas and adrenocortical carcinomas; the rare nodular hyperplasias are treated with bilateral surgery. Adrenalectomy is curative for adrenal adenomas and hyperplasia, but carcinomas are often advanced at presentation and generally have a poor prognosis. Adrenolytic therapy with mitotane (Lysodren) may be necessary to control hypercortisolemia and tumor growth in carcinomas postoperatively.

Secondary Therapy for Failed Pituitary Surgery or Occult Ectopic Tumors

If transsphenoidal surgery fails to resolve the hypercortisolemia, patients can be offered pituitary irradiation. If a lesion can be targeted, stereotactic radiosurgery with a linear accelerator (LINAC) system, gamma-knife system,

CURRENT DIAGNOSIS

- The clinical presentation of Cushing's syndrome is nonspecific and overlaps that of other more common diseases such as polycystic ovary syndrome, the metabolic syndrome, and depression.
- Signs and symptoms more specific for Cushing's syndrome include unexplained osteoporosis, muscle weakness, spontaneous ecchymoses, hypokalemia, central obesity, and plethora. Children present with growth failure, generalized obesity, and menstrual irregularities.
- A stepwise approach to the diagnosis helps avoid pitfalls in the interpretation of diagnostic tests. The first step is to confirm the diagnosis of Cushing's syndrome. The second step is to determine if the patient has ACTH-dependent or ACTH-independent disease. The final step is to determine if the ACTH source is eutopic (from the pituitary gland) or ectopic (the ectopic ACTH syndrome).
- The 1 mg ON dex test is easy to perform and has good sensitivity for diagnosing Cushing's syndrome. However, because of its poor specificity, confirmatory testing with measurement of urine free cortisol, midnight serum or salivary cortisol or the dex-CRH test is required.
- Random or CRH-stimulated ACTH levels greater than 10 pg/mL indicate ACTH-dependent disease.
- Biochemical testing is inadequate for distinguishing pituitary tumors from the ectopic ACTH syndrome. Jugular venous sampling has a high positive predictive value, but if negative, inferior petrosal or cavernous sinus sampling with CRH stimulation is required.
- Pituitary MRI is positive in only approximately one half of patients with corticotroph adenomas.

Abbreviations: ACTH = adrenocorticotropic hormone; CRH = corticotrophin-releasing hormone; dex = dexamethasone; MRI = magnetic resonance imaging; 1 mg ON dex test = 1 mg overnight dexamethasone suppression test.

or proton beam system offers lower radiation exposure to surrounding normal tissue and theoretically more effective higher doses to the residual tumor than conventional fractionated radiation therapy. Time to control of hypercortisolemia is variable, reported from 6 to 36 months, requiring interim control of hypercortisolemia by either medical therapy or adrenalectomy. Complications of radiation therapy include hypopituitarism, rare optic neuropathy, and rare (and debated) induction of second tumors and brain necrosis. The risk of Nelson's syndrome (rapid and aggressive growth of corticotroph tumors after adrenalectomy) may be lessened with radiation therapy.

Alternatively, and in the cases of ectopic tumors remaining occult, bilateral adrenalectomy can be performed offering immediate control of hypercortisolemia. Both glucocorticoid and mineralocorticoid (fludrocortisone [Florinef] 0.1 mg by mouth once or twice daily) replacement are generally required. Glucocorticoids are tapered as described above to physiologic doses of hydrocortisone (Cortef)[1] 20 to 30 mg by mouth daily in single or divided doses. Continued surveillance with imaging is

---

[1]Not FDA approved for this indication.

[1]Not FDA approved for this indication.

CURRENT THERAPY

- Treatment for Cushing's syndrome is primarily surgical and targeted to the pathologic lesion.
- Transsphenoidal adenomectomy is recommended for pituitary-dependent Cushing's disease, but has a long-term success rate of only 60% to 80%.
- Laparoscopic adrenalectomy has replaced open approaches in the management of primary adrenal lesions except for adrenocortical carcinoma, and for second-line treatment after failed pituitary surgery or failure to localize an occult ectopic tumor.
- Definitive secondary treatments for failed pituitary surgery include pituitary irradiation and bilateral adrenalectomy.
- Medical therapy for Cushing's syndrome is difficult, and reserved for surgical failures awaiting benefit from radiation therapy or in preparation for surgical therapy.

required, because of the risk of development of Nelson's syndrome and the occasional, locally invasive, and rarely metastatic potential of ectopic tumors.

Medical Management of Hypercortisolemia

Medical management of hypercortisolemia has an inadequate efficacy and side-effect profile for primary or long-term use. However, it has a very important role in temporizing the pathologic effects of long-standing Cushing's syndrome in preparation for surgical treatment and while awaiting definitive cure from radiation therapy. Strategies include medications (Table 2) that block glucocorticoid synthesis, inhibit pituitary ACTH secretion, or block glucocorticoid action. None of the agents that inhibit ACTH release is very effective but might be useful in combination therapy. The most effective medications are those that block glucocorticoid synthesis including ketoconazole[1] (Nizoral), metyrapone[1] (Metopirone), and mitotane[1*] (o,p'DDD, Lysodren). These are usually dosed to partially block cortisol production, suppressing it into the normal range. Alternatively, complete adrenal blockade with replacement hydrocortisone can be attempted. Finally, very limited experience with blockade of the glucocorticoid receptor with mifepristone (Mifeprex)[1] has shown clinical efficacy. Because glucocorticoid levels are unaffected, titration of this medication must be done on clinical grounds.

REFERENCES

Bochicchio D, Losa M, Buchfelder M: Factors influencing the immediate and late outcome of Cushing's disease treated by transsphenoidal surgery: A retrospective study by the European Cushing's disease survey group. J Clin Endocrinol Metab 1995;80:3114-3120.

Hammer GD, Tyrrell JB, Lamborn KR, et al: Transsphenoidal microsurgery for Cushing's disease: Initial outcome and long-term results. J Clin Endocrinol Metab 2004;89:6348-6357.

Ilias I, Chang R, Pacak K, et al: Jugular venous sampling: An alternative to petrosal sinus sampling for the diagnostic evaluation of adrenocorti-

---

cotropic hormone-dependent Cushing's syndrome. J Clin Endocrinol Metab 2004;89:3795-3800.

Leinung MC, Zimmerman D: Cushing's disease in children. Endocrinol Metab Clin North Am 1994;23:629-39.

Mahmoud-Ahmed AS, Suh JH: Radiation therapy for Cushing's disease: A review. Pituitary 2002;5:175-180.

Nieman LK: Medical therapy of Cushing's disease. Pituitary 2002; 5:77-82.

Oldfield E, Doppman J, Nieman L, et al: Petrosal sinus sampling with and without corticotropin-releasing hormone for the differential diagnosis of Cushing's syndrome. N Engl J Med 1991;325:897-905.

Papanicolaou DA, Mullen N, Kyrou I, Nieman LK: Nighttime salivary cortisol: A useful test for the diagnosis of Cushing's syndrome. J Clin Endocrinol Metab 2002;87:4515-4521

Reincke M: Subclinical Cushing's syndrome. Endocrinol Metab Clin North Am 2000;29:43-56.

Yanovski J, Cutler G, Chrousos G, Nieman L: Corticotropin-releasing hormone stimulation following low-dose dexamethasone (Decadron) administration. JAMA 1993;269:2232-2238.

Diabetes Insipidus

Method of
Jennifer Kelly, DO, and Arnold M. Moses, MD

General Principles of Treating Central (Neurogenic) Diabetes Insipidus

The hormonal treatment of diabetes insipidus is accomplished using the synthetic nanopeptide desmopressin (1-deamino [8-D-arginine] vasopressin; DDAVP). Arginine vasopressin (AVP) is the natural hormone of humans.

CURRENT DIAGNOSIS

Central diabetes insipidus (DI) can be diagnosed as follows:

1. Ensure urine volume is increased to ≥3 L/day in adults.
2. Rule out glycosuria (dipstick will suffice).
3. Measure serum sodium concentration during ad libitum fluid intake.
4. If the serum sodium concentration is *above* normal while urine osmolality is *less than* 300 mOsm per kilogram of water, injection of desmopressin (DDAVP) at least doubles the urine osmolality in patients with central DI. If the urine osmolality response is less, the patient may have nephrogenic DI.
5. If the serum sodium concentration is *normal* while urine osmolality is *less than* 300 mOsm per kilogram of water, additional procedures, including a water deprivation or saline infusion test, may be required. Refer to an experienced specialist.
6. Magnetic resonance imaging to detect the presence or absence of the pituitary hyperintense signal may be helpful in differentiating central DI from primary polydipsia. Plasma arginine vasopressin levels do *not* differentiate these two polyuric conditions.

---

[1]Not FDA approved for this indication.
*FDA approved only for adrenocortical carcinoma.

Trade Name	Chemical Composition	Concentration	Size	Pharmaceutical Company
Intranasal Preparations				
Desmopressin Rhinal Tube	Desmopressin acetate	100 µg/mL	2.5-mL bottle with rhinal tube delivering sprays of 10–20 µg	Ferring
DDAVP Rhinal Tube	Desmopressin acetate	100 µg/mL	2.5-mL bottle with rhinal tube delivering sprays of 10–20 µg	Aventis
DDAVP Nasal Spray	Desmopressin acetate	100 µg/mL	5.0-mL bottle with spray pump delivering 50 sprays of 10 µg each	Aventis
Oral Preparation				
DDAVP Tablets	Desmopressin acetate	Not applicable	0.1-mg, 0.2-mg tablets	Aventis
Injectable Preparations (Subcutaneous, Intravenous)				
DDAVP Injection	Desmopressin acetate	4 µg/mL	1.0, 10.0 mL/vials	Aventis
Pitressin Injection	Arginine vasopressin	20 U/mL	1 mL/vial	Monarch
Arginine Vasopressin Injection	Arginine vasopressin	20 U/mL	0.5, 1, and 10 mL/vials	American Regent

Caution: Stimate Nasal Spray (desmopressin acetate) is marketed by Aventis Pharmaceuticals in a 2.5-mL nasal spray bottle. It is designed for treating bleeding disorders and contains 1.5 mg/mL desmopressin. Stimate can be confused easily with the less concentrated preparations of desmopressin acetate that are used for treating diabetes insipidus.

Desmopressin is a synthetic analogue of AVP that does not constrict smooth muscle and has a longer antidiuretic action than does the natural hormone. Because of its lack of vasoactivity, desmopressin can be used without precipitating angina, abdominal cramps, or headaches. It can also be used to treat diabetes insipidus during pregnancy because it resists inactivation by placental vasopressinase. The available preparations of vasopressin are listed in the table above. The durations of antidiuretic responses to the different preparations are listed in Table 1.

For most patients with diabetes insipidus, the treatment of choice is intranasal desmopressin (100 µg/mL). Two delivery systems are available: a nasal (rhinal) tube, which the patient uses to blow measured amounts (0.05–0.2 mL) into the nose, and a compression pump system, which delivers 0.1 mL (see Current Therapy). Treatment is usually initiated with 10 µg of intranasal desmopressin. Patients are instructed to repeat this dose when polyuria recurs. Some patients respond better if the hormone is administered on a more defined schedule. The dose administered can be increased or decreased in accordance with the patient's response. Patients should be told to drink only when they are thirsty.

Some patients prefer to start therapy with oral desmopressin; others can be switched to the oral preparation when absorption of the intranasal form is decreased in the presence of nasal congestion. The starting dose of the tablet is usually 0.05 mg (half of a 0.1-mg tablet) twice per day. The maintenance dose is gradually adjusted to provide an adequate limitation of water turnover. The daily oral dose may range from 0.1 to 1.2 mg in divided doses. We do not currently recommend the use of nonhormonal agents such as chlorpropamide (Diabinese),[1] clofibrate,[1,2] or carbamazepine.[1]

In the uncooperative or unconscious patient with diabetes insipidus, desmopressin should be injected subcutaneously, usually starting with 0.5 or 1.0 µg (see Table 1 for duration of action). Subcutaneous AVP is sometimes used in patients with acute onset of diabetes insipidus after head trauma or neurosurgical procedures. Its short duration of action might help prevent water intoxication in patients receiving poorly monitored intravenous fluids. As with

---

[1]Not FDA approved for this indication.
[2]Not available in the United States.

TABLE 1 Mean Time That Urine Remains Hypertonic in Adults with Diabetes Insipidus*

Route of Administration	Amount Administered	Mean Duration of Action (hr)
Intranasal desmopressin	10 µg (0.1 mL)	12
	15 µg (0.15 mL)	16
	20 µg (0.2 mL)	20
Subcutaneous or intravenous desmopressin	0.5 µg	10
	1.0 µg	14
	2.0 µg	18
	4.0 µg	22
Oral desmopressin	0.1 mg	6–8
	0.2 mg	8–12
	0.4 mg	16–20
Subcutaneous arginine vasopressin	5 U	4

*Note: Onset of antidiuretic action of subcutaneous or intravenous preparation is 30–45 minutes. Onset of antidiuretic effect of tablets is about 60 minutes.

desmopressin, it is safest to administer subsequent doses of AVP when polyuria reappears.

As long as untreated patients with diabetes insipidus are conscious, retain normal thirst, and have enough fluid to drink, they seldom become dehydrated. However, severe dehydration with extremely high serum sodium concentrations may occur acutely when patients with untreated diabetes insipidus do not receive adequate fluids (orally or intravenously).

The most common and important problem in the hospitalized patient with diabetes insipidus is iatrogenic hyponatremia. Particularly when it occurs rapidly, hyponatremia may cause severe neurologic problems. Hyponatremia in this setting is caused by overhydration (only rarely does sodium loss contribute) in patients receiving vasopressin and can be prevented by allowing patients to self-regulate their oral intake of fluids whenever possible. When such self-regulation is not feasible because the patient is obtunded, has a defective thirst mechanism, or cannot drink, extreme care must be taken in ordering intravenous fluids to prevent hyponatremia. The patient can be maintained in an antidiuretic state by giving vasopressin when the urine becomes dilute. The intravenous fluid should consist largely of 5% dextrose in water with amounts of normal saline gauged to replace daily urinary sodium losses. The volume of intravenous fluid for every 8-hour period should replace 8-hour urine volumes plus estimated 8-hour insensible losses and fluid losses through perspiration and other routes. The amount of intravenous fluid should be adjusted according to plasma sodium, blood urea nitrogen, and creatinine levels. If hypernatremia occurs, the amount of intravenous fluids should be increased accordingly.

If a major decrease in serum sodium concentration occurs, intravenous fluids should be temporarily discontinued, and, if necessitated by clinical manifestations, the patient should be given 200 to 300 mL of 3% saline, perhaps with 40 mg of furosemide (Lasix) intravenously. Temporary discontinuation of vasopressin should also be considered.

To emphasize, the patient with central diabetes insipidus whose fluid intake is maintained intravenously presents a major medical problem and must be followed up carefully to maintain normonatremia.

Pregnancy is associated with significant alterations in water metabolism. The osmotic threshold for secretion of vasopressin is lowered and the threshold for thirst reduced, with a resulting decrease in plasma osmolality by about 10 mOsm per kilogram of water. A deficiency of plasma vasopressin can also result from increased degradation of the hormone by placental vasopressinase. This disorder is referred to as *gestational diabetes insipidus* because the symptoms of diabetes insipidus occur only during pregnancy and remit soon after delivery. An underlying subclinical deficiency in vasopressin secretion may also be involved. Gestational diabetes insipidus is treated successfully with desmopressin, which is not degraded by vasopressinase. The dose of desmopressin should be about the same as that used in the nonpregnant state, but the normal range for serum sodium is about 5 mEq/L lower.

Principles of Treating Specific Problems

THE ALERT PATIENT WITH INTACT THIRST

When antidiuretic therapy is initiated in the alert patient with diabetes insipidus, the patient must consciously avoid excessive drinking for at least several days. By that time, the thirst mechanism usually adapts to the more normal urine volume. However, some patients must be reminded to avoid excessive drinking, which causes the syndrome of inappropriate antidiuresis. Thirst may be perceived with normal or low serum sodium concentration because of a dry mouth, as might occur with mouth breathing, anticholinergic drugs, β-adrenergic blockers, or cigarette smoking. An occasional patient is hyperdipsic because of increased circulating angiotensin II levels or from hypothalamic involvement, as may occur with sarcoidosis involving the hypothalamus. Use of ice may help limit fluid intake.

THE ALERT PATIENT WITH ADIPSIA

The alert patient with adipsia presents a difficult management problem in the hospital and particularly after the patient is discharged from the hospital. Because of the loss of thirst perception, normal serum sodium concentration is maintained only with great difficulty. The patient and family must closely and continuously monitor the patient's intake and output of fluids, body weight, and vital signs. Serum sodium concentration and blood urea nitrogen, uric acid, and creatinine levels should be checked often. Such a patient must always relate fluid intake to volume of urine plus fluid losses through perspiration and the gastrointestinal tract. Failure to properly monitor these patients may allow their condition to go unrecognized until they develop severe dehydration. This may require the infusion of normal saline to restore pulse and blood pressure and then water orally or dextrose in water intravenously. Appropriate antidiuretic therapy should be instituted along with the fluids.

THE CONFUSED, OBTUNDED, OR UNCONSCIOUS PATIENT

When confused, obtunded, or unconscious, such as postoperatively or after head trauma, the patient with diabetes insipidus is monitored in the same ways described for the alert patient with adipsia. The only major difference is that vasopressin must be given by injection or infusion and the fluids given intravenously. In the presence of hypernatremia and associated hypovolemia, normal saline is required to help restore pulse and blood pressure to normal. Otherwise, patients with hypernatremia should be treated with dextrose in water (see later) while antidiuretic therapy is instituted and maintained.

Postoperative hypernatremia should be prevented by the early recognition of diabetes insipidus before, during, and after surgery and by avoidance of osmotic diuretic use during surgery. The patient should be switched to oral fluids as soon as possible, and the adequacy of the patient's thirst mechanism to control fluid intake appropriately should be evaluated. Diabetes insipidus that occurs postoperatively or after head trauma may be variable (biphasic or triphasic), and frequently the diabetes insipidus is transient. Therefore, hormonal treatment should be withheld periodically to determine whether the symptoms of diabetes insipidus recur. After 6 months of diabetes insipidus, remission is very unlikely.

Special Problems of Fluid Balance

THE HYPERNATREMIC PATIENT

Hypernatremia in patients with diabetes insipidus is usually associated with normal total body sodium. The hypernatremia is due to loss of free water by way of the kidneys, but losses from the skin and lungs can aggravate the problem. Alterations in the composition of water and solutes in the brain cells may contribute to the symptoms of hypernatremia. An abrupt increase in plasma sodium concentration causes more severe symptoms than does a gradual rise to the same sodium level.

The goal of treating hypernatremia in patients with diabetes insipidus is restoration of normal plasma volume and tonicity. Desmopressin should be injected to maintain concentrated urine. If the patient has circulatory disturbances due to hypovolemia, isotonic saline should be given until systemic hemodynamics are stabilized. In fact, isotonic saline is relatively hypotonic to plasma in patients with severe hypernatremia and simultaneously corrects both volume and water deficits. After volume deficits are corrected, the hypernatremia can be treated intravenously with 5% dextrose in water, or water can be given by mouth if the patient is able to drink.

The water deficit in these patients can be calculated on the basis of the serum sodium concentration and on the assumption that 60% of body weight is water. For example, if the patient's usual weight is 75 kg, total body water would normally be 75 kg × 0.6 = 45 L. If the serum sodium value is 154 mEq/L, the patient has a 10% deficit of water (154 − 140) ÷ 140 and theoretically requires 4.5 L of water to correct the deficit. Continuing losses of water must also be replaced. Despite inaccuracies, including the assumption

that body water is always 60% of the body weight and the postulate that water is lost uniformly throughout all body cells, this approach provides an approximate value that can be used in planning therapy. The major problem is determining the appropriate rate at which to lower serum sodium concentration to normal. Because seizures or even fatal cerebral edema may occur when serum sodium concentration is lowered rapidly, the best recommendation is to correct the hypernatremia over 48 to 72 hours and at a rate not exceeding 0.5 to 2.0 mEq/L/hr. As total body water expands, the serum sodium concentration may fall proportionately. Serum electrolyte values should be monitored frequently to ensure an appropriate response.

Treatment of the hypernatremia due to water loss, as occurs in untreated patients with diabetes insipidus, must also address associated electrolyte abnormalities and underlying medical and surgical conditions. An example is the patient with diabetes insipidus with coexisting hyperglycemia. In this case, the "corrected" serum sodium concentration should be used to calculate the water deficit. Slightly low or abnormal serum sodium concentrations in the presence of high serum glucose often result, when corrected, in hypernatremic values. The corrected serum sodium concentrations can be calculated by increasing the sodium concentration by 1.5 mEq/L for every 100 mg/dL increment in the serum glucose concentration above 100 mg/dL. For example, in a patient with a sodium level of 138 mEq/L and a glucose level of 700 mg/dL, the corrected serum sodium concentration is 138 + (1.5 × 6), or 147 mEq/L.

THE HYPONATREMIC PATIENT

Hyponatremia in diabetes insipidus occurs almost exclusively in patients who are overhydrated orally or parenterally while they are being treated with desmopressin. The severity of hyponatremia correlates closely with the magnitude of fluid overload. The amount of excessive body water can be calculated using the same approach as described for hypernatremia. Rarely, the hyponatremia is aggravated by large amounts of sodium in the urine, probably related to increased levels of atrial natriuretic peptide and glomerular filtration rate and inhibition of aldosterone. The hyponatremia due to natriuresis in the water-overloaded patient can be corrected only partially with saline infusions, because the natriuresis continues until the hypervolemic state is corrected. Hyponatremia can be caused or aggravated by adrenal or thyroid insufficiency.

A large body of literature on the appropriate rate at which to correct hyponatremia is available. Rapidly occurring (acute) and marked hyponatremia can be lethal and should be treated urgently. Under these conditions, and when neurologic symptoms are severe, initial therapy should raise the serum sodium concentration by 1 to 2 mEq/L/hr regardless of the duration of the electrolyte abnormality. Most authorities agree that the rate of change in serum sodium concentrations should not exceed 12 to 20 mEq/L/day. However, in patients with chronic hyponatremia, correction of serum sodium concentration approximating this rate occasionally causes serious, even fatal complications by inducing central pontine myelinolysis.

Fluid restriction is adequate for treatment of the asymptomatic mildly hyponatremic patient. Urine should be analyzed every 4 to 8 hours for volume and osmolality, and fluid replacement should be ordered in relation to *urine volume*. Remember that insensible fluid losses of about 600 mL of free water per day occur in the usual adult. *It is **NOT** appropriate to write for a fixed amount of fluid replacement*. Plasma sodium concentration should be checked frequently and fluid replacement adjusted according. The complaint of thirst by a water-restricted patient should not be ignored. Long-term management is usually less disrupted by adjusting fluid intake than by discontinuing hormonal therapy and allowing the patient to "break through." Alternatively, when the patient has symptomatic or severe hyponatremia (serum sodium concentration <115 mEq/L in chronic hyponatremia or 125 mEq/L in acute hyponatremia), intravenous furosemide (Lasix), may help by causing the excretion of urine that is lightly hypotonic or isotonic. After injection of 40 mg or more of furosemide, 100 mL of 3% saline should be infused in the first hour. This rate should be decreased or discontinued subsequently if symptoms have ameliorated or if the plasma sodium concentration has increased by more than 2 mEq/L in that hour. Infusion of more than a total of 250 mL of 3% saline is rarely necessary.

PREPARATION FOR DIAGNOSTIC TESTS OR TREATMENT

Special care must be taken when patients with treated diabetes insipidus are subjected to certain "standard protocols" associated with many diagnostic and therapeutic procedures. These protocols require the patient to be either fluid restricted, as for preparation for intravenous pyelography, or hydrated, as for intravenous administration of chemotherapy. Tests requiring that a patient receiving no oral fluids should be performed with adequate intravenous hydration matched to the patient's urine output. Intravenous fluids should be started from the time the patient is no longer able to take oral fluids and can be discontinued when oral fluids are again allowed. In contrast, patients receiving antidiuretic therapy for diabetes insipidus should not be made to "force fluids" beyond the amounts determined by thirst or be subject to hydration orders at rates not related to urine output. If high urine flow rates are needed, the patient's antidiuretic therapy must be discontinued. Oral or intravenous fluids can then be given to match the large urine volumes. Sometimes, it may be appropriate (to obtain more precise timing of a diuresis) to continue antidiuretic therapy and administer intravenous furosemide. Close monitoring of serum sodium levels will greatly assist in determining the status of fluid balance in these situations.

Nephrogenic Diabetes Insipidus

Nephrogenic diabetes insipidus is characterized by resistance of the kidney to the antidiuretic action of vasopressin. This disorder is often hereditary, caused by inactivating mutations of the V2 receptor or of the vasopressin-regulated water channel protein aquaporin 2. Standard doses of desmopressin or AVP do not decrease the polyuria. The urine volume can be decreased by 25%

to 40% by severe solute restriction and by further inducing hypovolemia with thiazide diuretics. Rarely, very high doses of desmopressin may be effective in females. Occasionally, acquired nephrogenic diabetes insipidus resolves by eliminating the underlying cause (i.e., treating the hypercalcemia or hypokalemia or discontinuing lithium therapy). Nephrogenic diabetes insipidus due to long-term lithium therapy may persist after discontinuation of lithium. Treatment of lithium-induced nephrogenic diabetes insipidus is limited to a low-sodium diet and possibly diuretics. Treatment may reduce urine volume by up to 30% or 40%. Caution must be taken because solute restriction, especially with a diuretic, may lead to lithium toxicity.

REFERENCES

Adrogue HJ, Madias NE: Hypernatremia. N Engl J Med 2000;342: 1493-1499.

Gross P: Treatment of severe hyponatremia. Kidney Int 2001;60: 2417-2427.

Moses AM, Clayton B, Hochhauser L: Use of T1-weighted MR imaging to differentiate between primary polydipsia and central diabetes insipidus. AJNR Am J Neuroradiol 1992;13:1273-1277.

Moses AM, Moses LK, Notman D, Springer J: Antidiuretic responses to injected desmopressin, alone and with indomethacin. J Clin Endocrinol Metab 1981;52:910-913.

Moses AM, Scheinman SJ, Oppenheim A: Marked hypotonic polyuria resulting from nephrogenic diabetes insipidus with partial sensitivity to vasopressin. J Clin Endocrinol 1984;59:1044-1049.

Rose BD, Post TW: Clinical Physiology of Acid-Base and Electrolyte Disorders, 5th ed. New York, McGraw-Hill, 2001, pp 716-719, 764-775.

Primary Hyperparathyroidism and Hypoparathyroidism

Method of
John P. Bilezikian, MD

Primary Hyperparathyroidism

INCIDENCE AND GENERAL CHARACTERISTICS

Primary hyperparathyroidism (PHPT) is a relatively common endocrine disease with an incidence as high as 1 in 500 to 1 in 1000. The high visibility of PHPT today marks a dramatic change from several generations ago when it was considered rare. The increased incidence is undoubtedly due to widespread use of the multichannel autoanalyzer. PHPT occurs in individuals of all ages but occurs most frequently in the sixth decade of life. Women are affected more often than men by a ratio of 3:1. PHPT in children is an unusual event. It might be a component of one of several endocrinopathies with a genetic basis, such as multiple endocrine neoplasia (MEN), type I or II. PHPT is caused by excessive secretion of parathyroid hormone (PTH) from one or more parathyroid glands. A benign,

TABLE 1 Differential Diagnosis of Hypercalcemia

Primary hyperparathyroidism
Malignancy
Other endocrinopathies
    Hyperthyroidism
    Pheochromocytoma
    Adrenal insufficiency
    VIPoma
Medications
    Lithium
    Thiazides
    Thyroid hormone
    Vitamin D
    Vitamin A
Granulomatous diseases
Familial hypocalciuric hypercalcemia
Immobilization

solitary adenoma is found in 80% of patients. Less commonly, in 15% to 20% of subjects, all four glands are hyperplastic. Four-gland parathyroid disease may occur sporadically or in association with the MEN syndromes. The most uncommon presentation of PHPT is parathyroid cancer, occurring in less than 0.5% of patients with PHPT.

DIFFERENTIAL DIAGNOSIS

The major diagnostic distinction to be made is between PHPT and malignancy, the other most common cause of hypercalcemia. These two etiologies account for more than 90% of all patients with hypercalcemia (Table 1). A much longer, complete list of potential causes of hypercalcemia is considered after these two etiologies are ruled out or if there is reason to believe that a different cause is likely. Today, PHPT presents most often as an asymptomatic disorder. In contrast, malignancy-associated hypercalcemia is usually found at a later stage of the malignant process and is associated with symptoms. Besides a major difference in clinical presentation between these two most common causes of hypercalcemia, the PTH immunoassay is a helpful distinguishing point. In patients with PHPT, the PTH level will be elevated or in the upper range of normal, whereas in malignancy, the PTH level is invariably suppressed.

PATHOPHYSIOLOGY, MOLECULAR GENETICS, AND PATHOLOGY

The pathophysiology of PHPT relates to the loss of normal feedback control of PTH by extracellular calcium. Why the parathyroid cell loses its normal sensitivity to calcium is not known. Genetic abnormalities that could be linked to sporadic parathyroid tumors have been described. A rearrangement of the cyclin D1/(PRAD1) proto-oncogene has been seen in some patients with PHPT. The rearrangement associates the PTH gene with the growth promoter cyclin D1. Only a small number of parathyroid tumors have been demonstrated to harbor this defect. Tumor suppressors, such as the gene associated with MEN-I, have generated interest, as have potential abnormalities in the gene for the calcium-sensing receptor. Although the gene for the calcium receptor has been implicated in familial hypocalciuric hypercalcemia and neonatal severe hyperparathyroidism, there is little evidence for this genetic abnormality in the sporadic form of PHPT. Even the vitamin D receptor has been implicated in pathogenetic abnormalities associated with parathyroid neoplasia.

The typical parathyroid adenoma is an enlarged, oval-shaped, smooth, red-brown gland. A visible rim of normal yellow-brown parathyroid tissue is sometimes seen. The typical parathyroid adenoma is between 300 and 500 mg, much larger than a normal gland that generally weighs 35 to 50 mg. Microscopically, the parathyroid adenoma consists of a network of cells arranged alongside a capillary network, resembling classic endocrine microanatomy. Fat cells are reduced or absent. The form of PHPT characterized by four-gland hyperplasia is seen grossly as enlarged glands that may be of equal size. Microscopically, solid masses of chief cells are seen in the absence of fat cells. In contrast to the adenoma, in which a rim of normal tissue can sometimes be seen, normal tissue is absent in hyperplastic disease.

SIGNS AND SYMPTOMS

PHPT is associated classically with skeletal and renal complications. In severe cases, the skeleton can be involved in a process called *osteitis fibrosa cystica.* Subperiosteal resorption of the distal phalanges, tapering of the distal clavicles, a "salt and pepper" appearance of the skull, bone cysts, and brown tumors of the long bones are all overt manifestations of hyperparathyroid bone disease. This form of hyperparathyroid bone disease is now most unusual, occurring in fewer than 5% of patients with PHPT. Much less severe, but nevertheless significant, skeletal involvement in PHPT is detected by dual energy x-ray absorptiometry (see later). Similar to the reduced incidence of gross skeletal disease, the kidney is also involved in PHPT much less commonly than before. From an incidence of approximately 33% in the 1960s, most series place the incidence of nephrolithiasis now to be no more than 15% to 20%. Nephrolithiasis, nevertheless, is still the most common complication of PHPT. Other renal features of PHPT include diffuse deposition of calcium–phosphate complexes in the parenchyma (nephrocalcinosis). The frequency of this complication is unknown. Hypercalciuria (daily calcium excretion of >250 mg in women or >300 mg in men) is seen in 30% to 40% of patients. PHPT may be associated with a reduction in creatinine clearance, in the absence of any other cause. Classic associations exist between PHPT and other organs, such as the neuromuscular system, the gastrointestinal tract, and the cardiovascular and articular systems, but such panopleistic features of PHPT are rarely seen today. More vexing are nonspecific elements associated with PHPT, such as easy fatigability, a sense of weakness, and a feeling that the aging process is advancing faster than it should be. This is sometimes accompanied by an intellectual weariness and a sense that cognitive faculties are less sharp. Whether these nonspecific features of PHPT are truly part of the disease process, reversible upon successful parathyroid surgery, remains under active investigation.

CLINICAL FORMS OF PRIMARY HYPERPARATHYROIDISM

Asymptomatic PHPT with serum calcium levels within 1 mg/dL above the upper limits of normal is the most common clinical presentation. Most patients do not have specific complaints and do not show evidence of any target organ complications. In parts of the world where severe vitamin D deficiency is common, more symptomatic PHPT is seen. Unusual clinical presentations of PHPT include MEN-I and MEN-II, familial PHPT not associated with any other endocrine disorder, familial cystic parathyroid adenomatosis, jaw tumor syndrome, and neonatal PHPT. A new presentation of PHPT is being described, namely, in individuals with normal serum calcium concentrations but elevated PTH levels. Potential secondary causes of elevated PTH levels are considered but have not been found. It is considered likely that these patients represent the earliest stage of PHPT, when there is glandular over-production of hormone, before hypercalcemia becomes evident.

DIAGNOSIS AND EVALUATION

Hypercalcemia and elevated levels of PTH establish the diagnosis. The serum phosphorus concentration tends to be in the lower range of normal. Serum alkaline phosphatase activity may be elevated. More specific markers of bone formation (bone-specific alkaline phosphatase, osteocalcin) and bone resorption (urinary deoxypyridinoline, N-telopeptide of collagen) tend to be in the upper range of normal. In some patients, the actions of PTH in altering renal acid-base handling leads to a small increase in the serum chloride concentration and a concomitant small decrease in the serum bicarbonate concentration. Urinary calcium excretion, when elevated, is not generally excessively high. The circulating 25-hydroxyvitamin D concentration is low, and the 1,25-dihydroxyvitamin D concentration is high in some patients.

ROLE OF BONE MASS MEASUREMENT

Dual-energy x-ray absorptiometry shows a pattern of skeletal involvement that is consistent with the physiologic actions of PTH, that of eroding cortical bone while sparing cancellous sites. The typical patient with PHPT shows reductions in bone density that are most marked in the distal third of the forearm, a cortical site, with much less

CURRENT DIAGNOSIS

Primary Hyperparathyroidism

- Most common cause of hypercalcemia.
- Diagnosis established by elevated serum calcium concentration and parathyroid hormone level that is frankly elevated or is in the upper range of normal.
- In some patients, the parathyroid hormone level is elevated but the serum calcium concentration is normal.

Hypoparathyroidism

- Much less common than primary hyperparathyroidism.
- Most often due to destruction or removal of the parathyroid glands.
- Diagnosis is established by hypocalcemia and low parathyroid hormone levels.

CURRENT THERAPY

Primary Hyperparathyroidism

- When symptoms are present, parathyroid surgery is indicated.
- In the absence of symptoms, surgery is recommended if any one of five criteria are met (see Table 2).
- Preoperative localization testing prior to surgery has become routine.
- Medical management is reserved generally for those who do not meet surgical criteria.
- Prudent use of calcium, hydration, and ambulation is encouraged.
- Pharmacologic agents, such as bisphosphonates and calcimimetics, show promise.

Hypoparathyroidism

- Acute management of hypocalcemia is a medical emergency and requires intravenous administration of calcium.
- Chronic treatment is based upon adequate calcium, vitamin D, and, in some cases, the active vitamin D metabolite 1,25-dihydroxyvitamin D.

involvement of the lumbar spine, a cancellous site. The hip region, a mixture of cortical and cancellous bone, shows changes that are intermediate between changes in the forearm and the lumbar spine.

TREATMENT

Localization Tests Prior to Surgery

Imaging of abnormal parathyroid tissue is accomplished most accurately with technetium-99m sestamibi. Sestamibi is taken up by both thyroid and parathyroid tissue, but it persists in the parathyroid glands. Various approaches to the use of technetium-99m sestamibi include using the imaging agent alone, and thereby depending upon a difference in uptake kinetics between thyroid and parathyroid tissue, or in combination with iodine 123 (^{123}I). Some believe that use of dual isotopic methods provides better definition of the thyroid from which the image obtained with sestamibi can be subtracted. Even more sophisticated approaches have been developed using sestamibi imaging with single-photon emission computed tomography. Ultrasound, computed tomography, and magnetic resonance imaging are also used to localize abnormal parathyroid tissue. Invasive localization tests with arteriography and selective venous sampling for PTH are used when noninvasive studies have not been successful. In the past, parathyroid imaging was reserved for patients who had undergone neck surgery. With greater success in parathyroid imaging and the increasing popularity of minimally invasive parathyroid surgery, preoperative imaging is becoming routine in all patients.

SURGERY

PHPT is cured when abnormal parathyroid tissue is removed. Asymptomatic patients are advised to have

TABLE 2 Guidelines for Surgical Management of Asymptomatic Primary Hyperparathyroidism*

Serum calcium >1 mg/dL above normal
Hypercalciuria >400 mg/day
Reduced creatinine clearance by >30%
Reduced bone density below T score of −2.5 at any site
Age <50 years

*These guidelines are meant only for asymptomatic patients with primary hyperparathyroidism. For patients who are symptomatic (i.e., kidney stones, fractures), surgery is recommended unless there are extenuating medical circumstances.

surgery if they meet current guidelines (Table 2). Symptomatic patients are always advised to undergo parathyroid surgery. At the present time, a number of different surgical procedures can be performed. The standard four-gland parathyroid gland exploration is performed under general or local anesthesia. The single adenoma is removed, and the other glands are ascertained to be normal but not removed. In the case of multiglandular disease, the approach is to remove all tissue except for a remnant that is left in situ or autotransplanted in the nondominant forearm. A popular recent advance in parathyroid surgery is the minimally invasive parathyroidectomy. This procedure depends upon preoperative localization by an imaging technology and confirmation of the success of parathyroid surgery with intraoperative PTH measurements. The circulating PTH level should fall to less than 50% of the preoperative value within minutes after removal of the parathyroid adenoma.

MEDICAL MANAGEMENT

In patients who do not meet surgical guidelines or who, for other reasons, will not undergo parathyroid surgery, the following medical principles apply. Adequate hydration and ambulation are always encouraged. Thiazide diuretics are to be avoided because they may lead to worsening hypercalcemia. Dietary intake of calcium should be moderate, avoiding both high- and low-calcium diets. Low-calcium diets theoretically could fuel abnormal parathyroid tissue to secrete more PTH. High-calcium diets could be detrimental by worsening hypercalcemia, especially if the 1,25-dihydroxyvitamin D level is elevated. Monitoring with biannual measurements of the serum calcium and annual measurement of bone mass by dual-energy x-ray absorptiometry are recommended. In patients whose 25-hydroxyvitamin D level is low, careful replacement seems reasonable. The serum calcium concentration must be monitored to guard against the potential for worsening hypercalcemia in some patients.

Oral phosphate will lower the serum calcium concentration in PHPT by approximately 0.5 to 1 mg/dL, but concerns about ectopic calcium–phosphate deposition limit its utility. Prior to the results of the Women's Health Initiative, estrogen was an option in postmenopausal women. The serum calcium concentration would fall by about 0.5 mg/dL; estrogens are no longer advised for this specific reason. Preliminary observations suggest that raloxifene, a selective estrogen receptor modulator, may have calcium-lowering effects similar to those of estrogen in postmenopausal women with PHPT.

The bisphosphonate alendronate (Fosamax) has shown promise in patients with PHPT. Lumbar spine bone density improves by as much as 5% in the first year of therapy. Neither the serum calcium concentration nor the PTH level falls significantly. Patients who will not undergo parathyroid surgery but in whom lumbar spine bone density is reduced may benefit from bisphosphonate therapy.

An early clinical experience with hyperparathyroid postmenopausal women has shown that, in principle, a calcimimetic can significantly reduce PTH and serum calcium levels in patients with the disease. By binding to a site on the calcium-sensing receptor, the calcimimetic increases the affinity of the calcium receptor for extracellular calcium. The result is an increase in intracellular calcium and thus reductions in PTH synthesis and secretion. Even though the drug has not yet been approved for use for PHPT in the United States, early data are promising. The serum calcium concentration typically becomes normal and remains within normal limits for as long as the drug is used. Interestingly, the serum PTH level falls only modestly and continues to be elevated despite correction of the hypercalcemia by the drug.

Hypoparathyroidism

Hypoparathyroidism is much more uncommon than is PHPT. It results from the destruction, removal, or dysfunction of all parathyroid tissue.

ETIOLOGY

The most common causes of hypoparathyroidism are neck surgery and an autoimmune process (Table 3). Surgical hypoparathyroidism can follow the operation by many years and can occur after any neck surgery. Autoimmune destruction of the parathyroid glands can occur in an isolated fashion or in connection with a variety of polyglandular syndromes. The two major forms are type I (multiple endocrine gland failure along with candidiasis,

TABLE 3 Causes of Hypoparathyroidism

Parathyroid gland destruction
Postsurgical
Autoimmune
Sporadic
Polyglandular syndromes
Activating antibodies against the calcium-sensing receptor
Infiltration
Iron, copper
Malignancy
Granulomatous
Genetic
Activating mutations of the calcium-sensing receptor
Inactivating mutations in the PTH gene
DiGeorge syndrome
Impaired secretion and/or action of PTH
Hypomagnesemia
Pseudohypoparathyroidism

Abbreviation: PTH = parathyroid hormone.

pernicious anemia, and/or alopecia) and type II (with adrenal or thyroid failure and/or diabetes mellitus). Activating mutations of the calcium-sensing receptor or of the parathyroid gene itself can be associated with hypoparathyroidism. Parathyroid gland destruction is rarely due to infiltration of the glands by iron, copper, granulomas, or malignancy. In severe magnesium deficiency, parathyroid secretion is impaired along with a peripheral resistance to the actions of PTH. Mild hypoparathyroidism can become symptomatic in the presence of a potent bisphosphonate such as alendronate.

CLINICAL FEATURES

Increased neuromuscular irritability is the clinical hallmark of hypoparathyroidism. Features of hypoparathyroidism can range from mild paresthesias around the mouth, fingers, and toes to muscle cramping, and, at their worst, carpal, pedal, or laryngospasm. Central nervous system seizure activity is also seen as a severe manifestation of hypocalcemia. These symptoms are due, in part, to the actual serum calcium level but also to the rate at which the serum calcium level falls. Rapid declines in the serum calcium concentrations are more likely to be associated with symptoms than to situations in which the serum calcium concentration has fallen gradually. If respiratory or metabolic alkalosis is present, symptoms can worsen because the partition between bound and free calcium is shifted to the bound state when the blood pH rises. Signs of hypocalcemia include the Chvostek sign (evoked facial nerve irritability), the Trousseau sign (carpal spasm when the blood pressure cuff is inflated to pressures above systolic), and a prolonged QT interval on the electrocardiogram. When severe hypocalcemia is present, impaired cardiac contractility, unresponsive to inotropic agents until the hypocalcemia is corrected, has been reported. Pseudopapilledema and subcapsular cataracts can be seen. In some individuals, hypoparathyroidism is detected only by an asymptomatic reduction in the serum calcium concentration. Pseudohypoparathyroidism is a group of genetic disorders of the PTH receptor/G-protein transduction system responsible for PTH action. In the type I variant, subjects have a classic phenotype (Albright's hereditary osteodystrophy) with short stature, brachydactyly, subcutaneous and basal ganglia calcifications, rounded facies, shortened neck, seizures, and below-average intelligence. Other endocrine glands, such as the thyroid and gonads, can also be dysfunctional. In the type II form of pseudohypoparathyroidism, PHT resistance is present in the absence of the clinical phenotype.

DIAGNOSIS

Hypocalcemia and an elevated serum phosphorus concentration in association with absent PTH levels confirm the diagnosis of hypoparathyroidism. In pseudohypoparathyroidism, PTH levels are elevated, reflecting the PTH-resistant state, but otherwise the biochemical findings of hypocalcemia and hyperphosphatemia are similar to those of hypoparathyroidism. The urinary calcium concentration is usually not elevated because the filtered load of calcium is low, but actually renal handling of calcium is impaired in this setting because of the lack of PTH. Such individuals have an increase in urinary calcium for the given filtered calcium load, even though the actual amount of urinary calcium excretion might not be excessive.

TREATMENT

The goals of treatment are to establish a serum calcium concentration that is not associated with symptoms or signs and to prevent long-term complications of hypocalcemia. Acute, symptomatic hypocalcemia is a medical emergency and must be treated urgently. The management of chronic hypocalcemia follows a different set of guidelines.

Acute Management

The initial approach is to infuse intravenously 1 to 2 ampules of calcium gluconate (90–180 mg of elemental calcium), diluted in 50 to 100 mL of 5% dextrose over a 10- to 15-minute period. If the acute symptoms are not quickly ameliorated, another 1 to 2 ampules can be administered. To raise the serum calcium concentration further, but more gradually, an infusion of 15 mg/kg of calcium gluconate in 1 L of 5% dextrose over 8 to 10 hours will raise the serum calcium concentration by 2 to 3 mg/dL. Because 1 ampule of calcium gluconate contains 90 mg of elemental calcium, 9 to 11 ampules of calcium gluconate are required for an average-size adult (60–70 kg). The serum calcium concentration should be monitored frequently. If the hypocalcemia is due to magnesium deficiency, these measures are also appropriate while magnesium is being replaced. Acute administration of magnesium without calcium will not immediately correct hypocalcemia because peripheral resistance to PTH, one component of hypocalcemia induced by magnesium deficiency, is not corrected for several days. Intravenous replacement of magnesium is 2.4 mg/kg, up to 180 mg, over a 10-minute period or a continuous infusion of 576 mg of magnesium over 24 hours.

Chronic Management

Oral calcium supplementation is required in virtually all patients. The amount varies but is generally in the range of 1 to 3 g in divided doses. The carbonate or citrated form of calcium is most commonly used. Calcium carbonate is generally preferred because it contains the highest amount of elemental calcium. When calcium preparations are given with meals, both the carbonate and the citrated form of calcium are equally bioavailable. The presence of food obviates the need for gastric acid when calcium carbonate is used.

Most patients also require vitamin D. The amount of ergocalciferol (vitamin D_2) or cholecalciferol (vitamin D_3) ranges from 25,000 to 200,000 IU daily (1.25–10 mg). These large amounts are required because the absence of PTH and hyperphosphatemia both limit the amount of vitamin D that ultimately is converted to 1,25-dihydroxyvitamin D, the active metabolite in the kidney. Because activation of vitamin D is impaired, much more vitamin D is required. There is no impairment of the first activation step in the liver, namely, from vitamin D to 25-hydroxyvitamin D, the storage form. Because there is no impairment in this step, large amounts of 25-hydroxyvitamin D can accumulate in fat tissues. At times and unpredictably, these stores can be mobilized and lead to hypercalcemia. Sometimes, the hypercalcemia is severe, requiring emergent treatment.

Other times, a simple adjustment in the amount of calcium and/or vitamin D is sufficient. In any event, patients receiving large doses of vitamin D should always be regularly monitored for serum calcium concentrations approximately every 3 to 6 months.

Although many patients with hypoparathyroidism can be adequately managed with oral calcium and vitamin D, other patients also require therapy with 1,25-dihydroxyvitamin D, the active metabolite of vitamin D. 1,25-Dihydroxyvitamin D is used in addition to, but not in place of, vitamin D because 1,25-dihydroxyvitamin D alone does not provide for smooth control. Perhaps this is because 1,25-dihydroxyvitamin D is not stored to any appreciable extent in fat tissue. The half-life of 1,25-dihydroxyvitamin D is as short as 6 hours. Therefore, patients managed without parent vitamin D but with 1,25-dihydroxyvitamin D as the only source of vitamin D are more likely to have unpredictable fluctuations in serum calcium concentration. The amount of 1,25-dihydroxyvitamin D ranges from 0.5 to 1.0 µg/day. Some patients require more. Enhanced gastrointestinal absorption of calcium with 1,25-dihydroxyvitamin D can lead to hypercalciuria because in hypoparathyroidism there is no PTH to facilitate calcium reabsorption in the renal tubule. Urinary calcium should be checked on a regular basis. If hypercalciuria occurs, the dose of 1,25-dihydroxyvitamin D and/or vitamin D should be adjusted downward. In this situation, a thiazide diuretic such as hydrochlorthiazide[1] can be used to reduce urinary calcium excretion. In pseudohypoparathyroidism, hypercalciuria is less likely to occur because PTH is present and does have some renal effects in reabsorbing filtered calcium.

Another reason for variability in the control of serum calcium concentration in hypoparathyroidism is a change in medications. For example, if a thiazide or loop diuretic is started for hypertension, the serum calcium concentration may increase or decrease, respectively. Glucocorticoids can lead to a reduction in the serum calcium concentration because glucocorticoids interfere with vitamin D action in the gastrointestinal tract. Bile-sequestering resins can interfere with vitamin D absorption. Midcycle changes in estrogen levels in premenopausal women can lead to altered control.

Hypoparathyroidism is one of the few endocrine disorders for which the replacement hormone, namely, PTH, is not yet available, but it is being studied in some clinical trials.

REFERENCES

Arnold A, Shattuck TM, Mallya SM, et al: Molecular pathogenesis of primary hyperparathyroidism. J Bone Miner Res 2002;17(Suppl. 2): N30-N36.

Bilezikian JP, Silverberg SJ: Management of asymptomatic primary hyperparathyroidism. N Engl J Med 2004;350:1746-1751.

Bilezikian JP, Silverberg SJ: Primary hyperparathyroidism. In Favus M (ed): Primer on the Metabolic Bone Diseases and Disorders of Calcium Metabolism, 5th ed. Washington DC, American Society for Bone and Mineral Research, 2003, pp 230-235.

Bilezikian JP, Brandi ML, Rubin M, Silverberg SJ: Primary hyperparathyroidism: new concepts in clinical, densitometric, and biochemical features. J Int Med 2005;257:6-17.

Bilezikian JP, Potts JT, El-Hajj Fuleihan G, et al: Summary statement from a workshop on asymptomatic primary hyperparathyroidism: A perspective for the 21st century. J Bone Miner Res 2003; 17(Suppl. 2):N2-N11.

Khan AA, Bilezikian JP, Kung AWC, et al: Alendronate in primary hyperparathyroidism: a double-blind, randomized, placebo-controlled trial. J Clin Endocrinol Metab 2004;89:3319-3325.

Marx SJ: Hyperparathyroid and hypoparathyroid disorders. N Engl J Med 2000;343:1863-1875.

Miller PD, Bilezikian JP: Bone densitometry in asymptomatic primary hyperparathyroidism. J Bone Miner Res 2002;17(Suppl. 2):N98-N102.

Peacock M, Bilezikian JP, Klassen PS, et al: Cinacalcet hydrochloride maintains long-term normocalcemia in patients with primary hyperparathyroidism. J Clin Endocrinol Metab 2005;90:135-141.

Silverberg SJ, Bilezikian JP: Clinical presentation of primary hyperparathyroidism in the United States. In Bilezikian JP, Marcus R, Levine MA (eds): The Parathyroids, 2nd ed. San Diego, CA, Academic Press, 2001, pp 349-360.

Silverberg SJ, Bilezikian JP: "Incipient" primary hyperparathyroidism: A "forme fruste" of an old disease. J Clin Endocrinol Metab 2003;88:5348-5352.

Stock JL, Marcus R: Medical management of primary hyperparathyroidism. In Bilezikian JP, Marcus R, Levine MA (eds): The Parathyroids, 2nd ed. San Diego, CA, Academic Press, 2001, pp 459-474.

Primary Aldosteronism

Method of
Raymond R. Townsend, MD

Aldosterone is an important regulatory component in human physiology. Excess of aldosterone as a mechanism of hypertension was first noted in 1955. Primary aldosterone overproduction has several causes. Certain clinical presentations and interpretations of laboratory testing assist clinicians with diagnosis. Today, clinically important dysregulation of aldosterone metabolism in disorders of electrolyte or blood pressure control may be detected by the ability to easily assay aldosterone in the urine and plasma and the concurrent ability to measure renin activity. Diagnosis leads to the evaluation of effective surgical and medical approaches to aldosterone regulation management

History

In prior years, primary aldosterone excess was recognized by unprovoked (i.e., not due to diuretic therapy or diarrhea) hypokalemia in a patient with hypertension. A measurement of the failure of increased salt intake and exogenous mineralocorticoid administration defined the aldosterone production as relatively autonomous. An assay of plasma renin activity was incorporated into the workup of this kind of patient due to occasionally increased aldosterone production resulting from an activated renin system (through angiotensin II). This is driven by renal ischemia from renal artery disease and termed "secondary" aldosterone excess. These aldosterone excess workups tended to be tedious because a proper assay of aldosterone production was generally undertaken in a drug-free state (discontinuing most, if not all, antihypertensive medications for at least 2, if not 4, weeks), with potassium repletion (often requiring considerable supplemental potassium chloride) and ensured sodium excess (potentially driving blood pressure higher) with sodium chloride tablets. Questionable cases also involved infusion of 2 L of normal saline over 4 hours with aldosterone and renin activity determinations taken at baseline, 2 hours, and 4 hours. This allowed the known suppressing activity of sodium chloride to maximally curtail that portion of the renin-angiotensin-aldosterone axis still susceptible to regulation. When the workup ended in an imaging procedure showing an adrenal tumor, surgery (when feasible) was usually recommended and was generally effective in curing or improving the hypertension.

Such complex physiologic endeavors were often relegated to an endocrine specialist because of the attention to detail needed to produce results that would be used to support an operative indication. Two events have relegated such investigations to a more historical category. The first is the observation that many patients do not have hypokalemia or a tumor when aldosterone excess is present, yet they benefit by blood pressure reduction from procedures that specifically interrupt aldosterone action. The second is the finding that about 3% of individuals have a computed tomography (CT) scan showing a detectable adrenal mass. Thus, false-positive associations of an increase in aldosterone to an incidentally discovered adrenal mass are possible because of the relative rarity of a true adrenal aldosterone-producing tumor.

Physiology

Like many regulatory systems, the aldosterone axis defends against a lack, rather than an abundance, of its target substrate—sodium chloride. When a diet relatively high in potassium and relatively low in sodium is consumed, aldosterone secretion from the adrenal cortex (zona glomerulosa) facilitates sodium conservation and potassium loss through specific effects on transport epithelia in the kidney, colon, salivary glands, and skin. The primary target tissue for sodium regulation is the kidney, which possesses the unique ability to adjust total body electrolyte balance. The following are principal stimuli to aldosterone production and release:

- The renin axis is activated by detection of reduced sodium in the kidney with the ultimate production of angiotensin II, which in turn stimulates aldosterone production and release.
- Potassium intake increases, which also stimulates aldosterone production and release by poorly understood mechanisms.
- Pituitary adrenocorticotropic hormone (ACTH) is released, causing a modest stimulatory effect on aldosterone, which assumes importance when testing aldosterone concentrations at different times of the day (circadian aspects) or when pursuing one of the rare forms of aldosterone excess (glucocorticoid-remediable aldosteronism, described later).

Aldosterone acts by binding to the mineralocorticoid receptor in a target cell, stimulating production of proteins that results in:

- Insertion of sodium channels in the portion of the cell oriented to a lumen (e.g., the luminal side of the distal convoluted tubule in the nephron)

TABLE 1 Aldosterone Effects—Beyond Blood Pressure

Action	Organ	Result
Collagen synthesis and fibrosis	Heart	Cardiomyopathy, heart failure
	Vessels	Stiff noncompliant vessels
	Kidney	Interstitial fibrosis, loss of renal function

- Exchange of potassium (or hydrogen ion) for sodium recovered from the lumen and finally increased activity of the sodium/potassium adenosine triphosphatase (Na^+,K^+-ATPase) pump. This pump handles the increase in incoming sodium by promoting its transit through the cell to the basolateral (blood) side, where extruded sodium is exchanged for potassium and returned to the circulation. Said potassium is now available for exchange on the lumen side, so the cycle continues until the stimulus is remitted.

Conversely, when the diet is relatively enriched in sodium chloride and depleted in potassium, the high-salt intake should suppress the entire renin-angiotensin-aldosterone system. Aldosterone action is not needed during this process and becomes, if anything, unwelcome because retention of sodium chloride only fuels the blood pressure level, contributes further to poor overall potassium balance, and mitigates renal natriuresis systems. This process labors to diminish, rather than preserve, overall body salt balance.

Aldosterone does play a role in heart failure and as an inflammatory mediator. These roles are not discussed here, although these actions are important and deserve consideration in their appropriate clinical circumstances. The other effects of aldosterone are listed in Table 1.

The clinician should be aware of expected drug effects on the renin-angiotensin-aldosterone system. In their discussions on testing for aldosterone excess, endocrinology textbooks usually categorize drugs based on their effects of increasing the activity in either part or all of the renin-angiotensin-aldosterone system. Diuretics increase renin and aldosterone activity. Angiotensin-converting enzyme inhibitors (ACEIs) and angiotensin receptor blockers (ARBs) increase renin activity, but ACEI suppresses aldosterone activity and ARB has a relatively neutral effect on aldosterone. β-Blockers suppress renin activity. Calcium channel blockers tend to increase renin activity. Vasodilators and mineralocorticoid antagonists tend to increase renin and aldosterone activity. Testing of aldosterone status (see later) must be interpreted in light of these drug effects, especially when determining aldosterone activity is important but discontinuing antihypertensive agents is unwise.

Clinical Presentations

In the past, patients with primary aldosterone excess presented with low serum potassium concentration, elevated blood pressure, and a metabolic alkalosis (from

TABLE 2   Clinical Presentation of Primary Aldosterone Excess

Age	Usually 30–50 yr
Potassium	Low:<3.5 mEq/L
Acid-base	Metabolic alkalosis: HCO$_3$ >30 mEq/L
Adrenal adenoma	Almost always unilateral
Serum sodium	Sometimes in upper range of normal: 140–145 mEq/L
Arrhythmia	Associated with low potassium levels
Magnesium	Low levels in some patients

CURRENT DIAGNOSIS

- Establish aldosterone excess relative to plasma renin activity.
- Consider a localizing study (adrenal imaging procedure; computed tomography/magnetic resonance imaging) to detect the presence of an adrenal cortex adenoma.
- If the result of the first localizing study is positive, consider a second localizing study (e.g., selective adrenal vein sampling) that can link the anatomy (adenoma) to excess aldosterone production.

stimulation of hydrogen ion excretion in exchange for sodium, especially as body potassium stores become depleted). When assays of renin activity became available in the early 1960s, a suppressed renin activity completed the biochemical evaluation. These patients do not generally have edema. Their serum sodium concentration tends to be in the higher range of normal, and the reduced potassium concentration often leads to impaired urinary concentration and complaints of nocturia. These signs form the classic Conn's syndrome of unilateral aldosteronoma patients. A significant number of patients with aldosterone excess have bilateral hyperplasia (idiopathic hyperaldosteronism). The relative occurrence of Conn's syndrome compared with idiopathic hyperaldosteronism (which together account for almost all the cases of aldosterone excess) is a moving target (60:40). Table 2 summarizes common and less common clinical aspects of primary aldosteronism.

Other forms of unprovoked hypokalemia include syndromes of apparent mineralocorticoid excess. These are mostly disorders of the sodium channel that allow the unregulated reabsorption of sodium at the expense of the loss of potassium. This process results in a form of hypertension with hypokalemia clinically indistinguishable from primary aldosteronism except that aldosterone is usually suppressed when measured.

A rare patient has a family or personal history of stroke at a young age (often before age 50 years). In such patients who have low or low–normal potassium values, the clinician may consider the syndrome of glucocorticoid-remediable aldosteronism. These patients have a splice variant gene that links aldosterone production to cortisol regulation and results in much more aldosterone production. These patients are identified by elevated aldosterone concentrations that decline dramatically when they are treated with dexamethasone for a few days.

In current practice, aldosterone excess is now most often pursued in patients presenting with drug-resistant hypertension. Drug-resistant hypertension is usually defined as a blood pressure greater than 140/90 mm Hg (usually the systolic blood pressure is uncontrolled) in patients given adequate dosages of a three-drug regimen that should include a diuretic.

Diagnosis

The workup is designed to show the autonomous production of aldosterone and identify a functioning adrenal cortex adenoma (if one is present). Autonomous production of aldosterone is usually shown by suppressed renin activity. Many now use the aldosterone-to-renin ratio. When the Sealey assay of plasma renin activity is used (which has normal values of about 1.5–4 ng of angiotensin I per milliliter of plasma per hour) in conjunction with a standard serum assay of aldosterone (which has normal values of 5–30 ng/dL), an aldosterone-to-renin ratio greater than 25 to 30 is considered evidence of aldosterone excess. Evaluation of such patients may include measurements of plasma renin activity and serum aldosterone concentration when other remediable causes of drug refractoriness are not found. When the aldosterone returns at values of 15 to 20 ng/dL and higher, the presence of suppressed renin activity (or a low direct renin assay) is evidence of aldosterone excess. An attractive feature of such simple office testing is that it does not require holding or discontinuing blood pressure medication but is predicated on subjects being up and around for at least 2 hours to yield the most representative aldosterone concentration. These patients usually have normal potassium concentrations. Two caveats to keep in mind: β-blockers may suppress renin activity independently of autonomous aldosterone production, and treatment with spironolactone will increase both renin and aldosterone concentrations.

Other measures are sometimes undertaken, including a 4-hour infusion of 2 L of normal saline during which aldosterone concentrations are assayed at time 0 minutes and repeated at 2 and 4 hours (Table 3). Aldosterone normally is suppressed to less than 5 ng/dL with this maneuver. Aldosterone values that remain higher than 10 ng/dL are relatively diagnostic of autonomous aldosterone production. Alternatively, patients may be placed on a high-salt diet with sodium chloride supplements to raise their salt intake up to more than 200 mEq of sodium per day (equal to 10–12 g of sodium chloride daily). Aldosterone concentrations are measured after 3 days of such a regimen. It is important to keep potassium normal during salt loading because low serum potassium will reduce the release of aldosterone, even in aldosterone excess states, and cloud the diagnosis.

Once confirmatory biochemical findings of aldosterone excess are found, the adrenal gland is usually imaged. If no tumor is seen, the patient likely has bilateral adrenal hyperplasia, although a small (<6 mm) adenoma may be missed with a conventional CT scan. When a tumor is found, it is strongly recommended that an effort be made to link the tumor to aldosterone excess. This is recommended because of the frequency of incidentally discovered adrenal masses (3%) in the population at large. Either adrenal vein

TABLE 3 Tests and Interpretations for Aldosterone Excess

Test Name	Procedure	Test	Normal Response	Primary Aldosterone Excess
Saline suppression test	2 L of saline IV over 4 hr	Aldosterone time 0 min Aldosterone 120 min Aldosterone 240 min	Serum: <10 ng/dL (some use <5 ng/dL)	Aldosterone usually >15–17 ng/dL supine and remains above 10 ng/dL throughout the study
Salt load	10–12 g NaCl daily for 3 days	Serum aldosterone, and 24-hr urine collection	Urine aldosterone <14 μg/day in presence of large amount of sodium (>200 mmol)	Daily aldosterone secretion >14 μg/day, often >20 μg/day
Captopril suppression test	Administer 50 mg captopril at 9:00 AM	Serum aldosterone at baseline and 90 min after captopril	Reduction of 20% from baseline and usually to <15 ng/dL	Aldosterone does not suppress
Position test	Measure hormones supine and after 2–4 hr upright posture	Plasma renin activity and serum aldosterone	50% increase in aldosterone upright compared with supine	Renin remains suppressed and aldosterone does not increase
Aldosterone-to-renin ratio	Measure hormones after patient has been up and around for 2 hr	Plasma renin activity and serum aldosterone	Aldosterone usually <15 ng/dL; renin variable	Renin usually <1.0 ng of angiotensin I/mL/hr and aldosterone >15–17 ng/dL
Dexamethasone suppression test	Administer 0.5 mg dexamethasone every 6 hr for 48 hr	Serum aldosterone on third day at 8 AM	<4 ng/dL	
Genetic screen	Perform analysis for gene associated with GRA	Send sample with DNA to address per *www.brighamand womens.org/gra*	Negative	

Abbreviations: GRA = glucocorticoid-remediable aldosteronism; NaCl = sodium chloride.

sampling (for aldosterone and cortisol) or adrenal scintigraphy with radioactive iodinated cholesterol after 3 days of dexamethasone suppression is useful. Adrenal vein sampling with samples obtained after ACTH (Cortrosyn) infusion is preferred. Examples of a positive and a negative adrenal vein sampling in two patients, each with biochemical evidence of aldosterone excess, are shown in Figure 1. Lateralization of aldosterone secretion is said to be present when the ratio of the concentration of aldosterone from one side to the other is greater than 10:1. Normally the ratio of aldosterone (in ng/dL) to cortisol (in μg/dL) is less than 6:1. The right adrenal vein is often very short (6–7 mm), difficult to catheterize, and prone to dilution.

Treatment

Two modes of treatment are available to hypertensive patients with aldosterone excess: surgery and medication. Most surgical procedures are laparoscopic, as the tumors are

CURRENT THERAPY

- Blockade with a mineralocorticoid receptor antagonist or amiloride will address both the hypertension and the electrolyte abnormalities in patients with aldosterone excess.
- Patients without a clear adrenal adenoma can be managed for many years with the drugs mentioned in text. In some cases, the adenoma may have been too small to detect when the aldosterone excess was first noted. A subsequent computed tomography scan (i.e., 1–2 years later) during follow-up is reasonable to consider.
- Adrenalectomy surgery may be curative. However, patients with a family history of hypertension and a personal history of hypertension for at least 3 to 5 years are less likely to be cured, although they may benefit from less medication needed to control their hypertension.

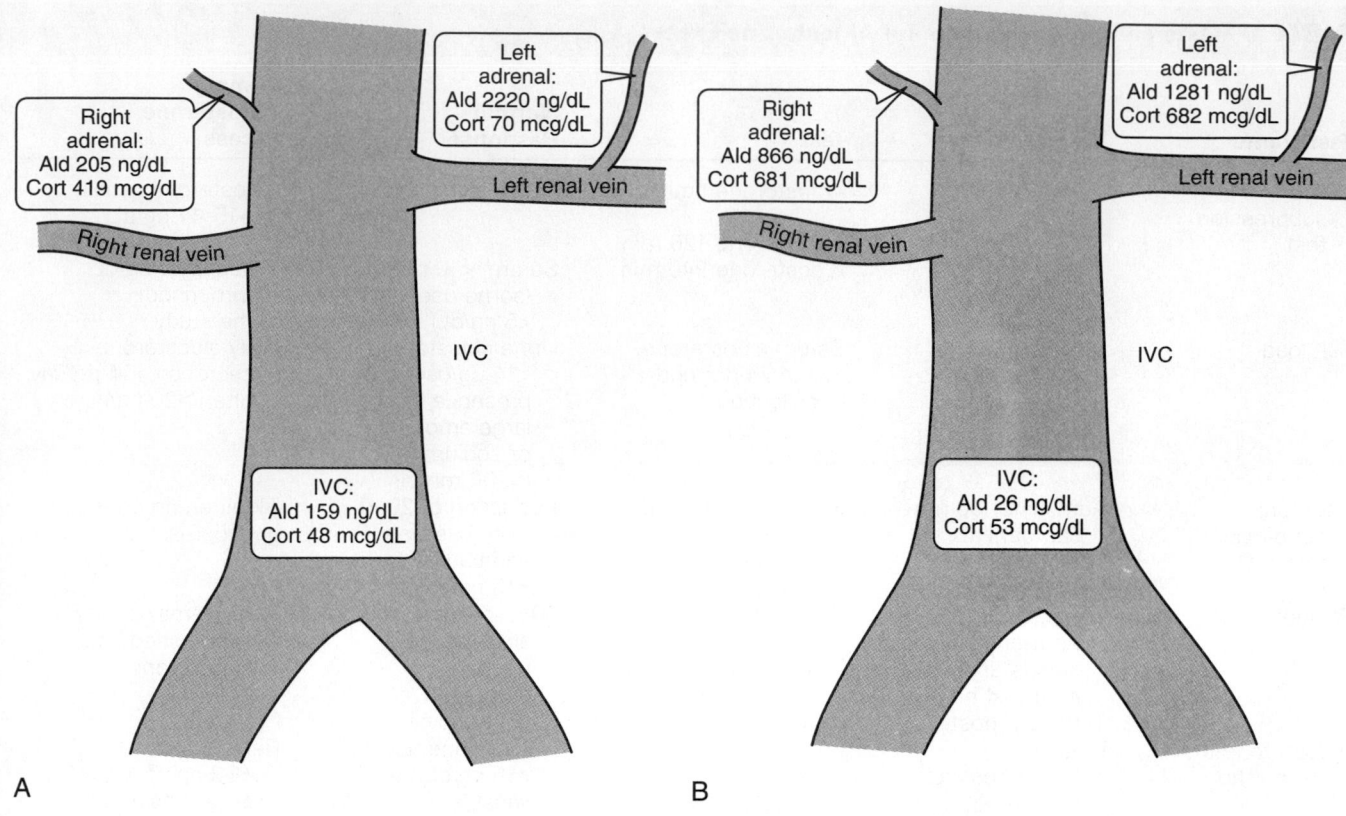

FIGURE 1. **A,** Adrenal vein sampling results in a patient with a left adenoma on computed tomography scan. The ratio of left-to-right aldosterone is greater than 10:1. This lateralization is consistent with Conn's syndrome (aldosteronoma). **B,** Adrenal vein sampling results in a different patient with biochemical signs of aldosterone excess and a "nodular" appearance in the left adrenal gland. Lateralization did not occur in this patient. In both patients, the results are seen after adrenocorticotropic hormone (Cortrosyn) infusion. *Abbreviations:* Ald = aldosterone; Cort = cortisol; IVC = inferior vena cava.

rarely larger than 4 to 5 cm and almost always unilateral. Surgery is more effective in subjects who have a relatively recent onset of hypertension (<5 years), a negative family history of hypertension, and clear unilateral secretion. Such patients have a good chance of cure of their hypertension after surgery, although some patients who undergo surgery may have, or someday may develop, primary hypertension (note that the incidence of primary hypertension in 30- to 50-year-olds is about 20%).

Medication treatment involves blockade of aldosterone effect. Antihypertensive treatment, which does not address the sodium retentive effects of aldosterone, is often ineffective at controlling blood pressure. This is accomplished by either direct mineralocorticoid antagonism with spironolactone (Aldactone) or eplerenone (Inspra), or with blockade of the kidney's luminal channels, which recover filtered sodium, by the use of amiloride (Midamor) or triamterene (Dyrenium). Often 4 weeks or longer is needed to achieve an improvement in blood pressure. A conventional diuretic (e.g., a thiazide) is a frequent adjunct to the use of either a mineralocorticoid receptor antagonist or amiloride. Triamterene, the weakest agent among these choices, is infrequently used.

When medication is used, drugs that block the mineralocorticoid receptor may be advantageous in long-term management because they are true antagonists of mineralocorticoid activity. Amiloride does not block the mineralocorticoid receptor; it only antagonizes the downstream effects of receptor activation. Although no comparative long-term trials of a mineralocorticoid antagonist compared with a luminal sodium channel blocker such as amiloride have been performed, specialists typically reserve amiloride for patients intolerant of mineralocorticoid antagonists.

The choice of surgery versus long-term medical management is easy when clear-cut signs of aldosterone excess are present in a relatively young person with unilateral secretion of aldosterone from the adrenal gland noted to have a tumor. Successful long-term (>25 years) management with medication is achievable without obvious detriment (other than long-term medication administration itself) in those with glucocorticoid-remediable aldosteronism or when no lateralization (idiopathic hyperaldosteronism) has occurred. This is a reasonable option for patients who are not surgical candidates.

REFERENCES

Conn JW: Primary aldosteronism, a new clinical syndrome. J Lab Clin Med 1955;45:3-17.

Dunnick NR, Doppman JL, Mills SR, Gill JR Jr: Preoperative diagnosis and localization of aldosteronomas by measurement of corticosteroids in adrenal venous blood. Radiology 1979;133:331-333.

Gallay BJ, Ahmad S, Xu L, et al: Screening for primary aldosteronism without discontinuing hypertensive medications: Plasma aldosterone-renin ratio. Am J Kidney Dis 2001;37:699-705.

Townsend RR: Aldosterone redux. J Clin Hypertens 2003;5:300.

Young WF Jr: Minireview: Primary aldosteronism-changing concepts in diagnosis and treatment. Endocrinology 2033;144:2208-2213.

Hypopituitarism

Method of
Mary Lee Vance, MD

Definition

Hypopituitarism is target endocrine gland failure because of insufficient hypothalamic or pituitary hormone stimulation of the target gland or tissue. Loss of hypothalamic or pituitary hormone production may cause secondary adrenal insufficiency, secondary hypothyroidism, secondary gonadal failure, growth hormone (GH) deficiency, and/or diabetes insipidus (DI), alone or in combination. Regardless of the etiology, replacement of glucocorticoid and thyroid hormone is necessary to sustain life; replacement of gonadal steroids, GH, and antidiuretic hormone is necessary for normal function and for prevention of morbidity. Loss of all pituitary function is termed *panhypopituitarism;* loss of one or more pituitary hormones is termed *partial hypopituitarism.*

Etiology

The most common cause of hypopituitarism is a pituitary lesion (pituitary adenoma, craniopharyngioma, Rathke's cleft cyst) or infiltrative disease (lymphocytic hypophysitis, sarcoidosis, metastatic tumor) (Table 1). In general, the larger the pituitary lesion, the greater the likelihood of loss of pituitary function. Infiltrative disease often causes permanent loss of pituitary function. Selective removal of a pituitary adenoma, taking care to avoid damage to remaining normal pituitary tissue, may result in recovery of pituitary function.

Hypopituitarism also occurs as a result of any type of pituitary radiation for a pituitary lesion, total brain radiation for a brain lesion, or head and neck radiation for carcinoma (the radiation field often involves the pituitary gland). Head trauma may cause loss of pituitary function, occurring in up to 36% of patients studied. Less commonly, developmental defects of the hypothalamus or pituitary cause loss of pituitary function.

Diagnosis

The diagnosis of pituitary deficiency is often straightforward but sometimes requires a definitive stimulation test to assess hypothalamic-pituitary-adrenal function and GH reserve. In a patient who presents with a large pituitary lesion, the most critical determination is the need for glucocorticoid and thyroid hormone replacement before recommending surgical resection or medical treatment (macroprolactinoma). A subnormal morning serum cortisol or subnormal free thyroxine (FT$_4$) concentration indicates the need for immediate replacement. In a patient who has undergone pituitary surgery, it is important to review the operative note to assess the amount of resection and to make an estimate of remaining pituitary gland (unfortunately, this estimate is not always mentioned in the operative report).

CURRENT DIAGNOSIS

- Diagnosis is biochemical in association with clinical features. Diagnosis may require a stimulation test to determine the need for replacement of glucocorticoid, growth hormone, or both.
- Initial patient evaluation should include measurement of concentrations of early-morning serum cortisol, adrenocorticotropic hormone (ACTH), FT$_4$, gonadotropins (luteinizing hormone [LH], follicle-stimulating hormone [FSH]), insulin-like growth factor-1 (IGF-1), and testosterone (in men); menstrual history should be obtained from premenopausal women.

A history of frequent nocturia, polyuria, and excessive thirst is indicative of DI. Diabetes insipidus most commonly occurs in patients with a craniopharyngioma, Rathke's cleft cyst, or infiltrative disease such as lymphocytic hypophysitis or sarcoidosis. An extensive surgical resection in a patient with one of the aforementioned lesions involving the pituitary stalk indicates a high probability of permanent DI. Extensive surgical resection may also damage the pituitary stalk and cause DI. Serum sodium concentration is usually normal in these DI patients who have normal thirst sensation. Serum osmolality usually is normal; urine osmolality usually is low. The diagnosis of DI is made

TABLE 1 Causes of Hypopituitarism

Hypothalamic Disease
- Histocytosis
- Eosinophilic granuloma
- Sarcoidosis
- Hypothalamic tumor (gangliocytoma, hamartoma, optic nerve glioma, third-ventricle tumor)
- Metastatic tumor
- Congenital midline defects

Pituitary Disease
- Pituitary adenoma
- Craniopharyngioma
- Rathke's cleft cyst
- Pilocytic astrocytoma
- Infiltrative disease (giant cell granuloma, sarcoidosis, lymphocytic hypophysitis, lymphoma, plasmacytoma, metastatic tumor)
- Chordoma with pituitary involvement
- Parasellar/suprasellar meningioma
- Pituitary apoplexy (hemorrhage into pituitary adenoma, postpartum hemorrhage)
- Congenital pituitary hypoplasia

Radiation
- Cranial
- Pituitary
- Head/neck

Infection
- Tuberculosis
- Mycoses

Miscellaneous
- Head trauma
- Empty sella
- Carotid-cavernous aneurysm

clinically for a patient with a pituitary lesion and does not usually require a formal water deprivation test. A subnormal morning serum cortisol or FT_4 level concentration requires prompt glucocorticoid or thyroxine replacement.

A patient who has a large pituitary lesion commonly has loss of some or all anterior pituitary hormone production. This loss is less common in a patient with a small pituitary lesion but requires evaluation and replacement as indicated. In general, a stimulation test to assess for hypothalamic-pituitary-adrenal function to determine the need for cortisol replacement and for GH deficiency should be conducted after surgical removal of the lesion. Recovery of pituitary function after surgical removal of the lesion may occur but is not common; approximately 6% of patients have recovery of some pituitary function after surgery. Postoperative or postradiation assessment should include clinical history (menses in premenopausal women, sexual function in men, symptoms of hypothyroidism, adrenal insufficiency, DI) and basal and dynamic endocrine testing.

A subnormal morning serum cortisol concentration (without administration of steroid for 2–3 days) is usually adequate to diagnose secondary adrenal insufficiency; the serum ACTH concentration may be low or in the normal range. A normal morning serum cortisol concentration does not provide information regarding the ACTH-cortisol response to stress; the definitive study is an insulin hypoglycemia test in which the serum glucose concentration decreases to 40 mg/dL or less and the serum cortisol concentration increases to 18 µg/dL or greater to exclude secondary impaired hypothalamic-pituitary-adrenal reserve. This test is also the most rigorous test of GH reserve to determine the need for GH replacement (stimulated serum GH concentration <5 ng/mL indicates GH deficiency). Cortisol stimulation with ACTH (Cortrosyn stimulation test) may be misleading in patients with recent ACTH deficiency in whom the cortisol response is normal but the ACTH response to stress is impaired. For this reason, an ACTH stimulation test should not be performed in the immediate postoperative period. It is prudent to wait 4 to 6 weeks after surgery before performing this test.

A subnormal serum FT_4 concentration, often in the setting of a "normal" serum thyroid-stimulating hormone (TSH) concentration (not normal for a low FT_4), indicates the need for thyroid hormone replacement.

SECONDARY GONADAL FAILURE

The diagnosis of secondary gonadal failure is straightforward. Chronic amenorrhea in a premenopausal woman indicates gonadotropin insufficiency. In premenopausal women, serum LH and FSH concentrations are typically either low or "normal"; the estradiol level is usually low or in the follicular phase range. In men, a low serum testosterone concentration indicates gonadal insufficiency; a low serum testosterone concentration but LH and FSH concentrations within the "normal" range indicate secondary gonadal failure.

GROWTH HORMONE DEFICIENCY

The diagnosis of GH deficiency is more complicated, usually requiring a stimulation test. In a patient with three or four other pituitary hormone deficiencies, the probability of GH deficiency is 96% and 99%, respectively. Three or four pituitary hormone deficiencies and a serum IGF-1 concentration less than 84 µg/L reliably predicted GH deficiency in more than 95% of patients. Despite this finding, many third-party payers (insurance companies) require the results of a stimulation test confirming GH deficiency because of the cost and misuse of GH. The most rigorous test for determining GH deficiency is the insulin hypoglycemia test; the next "best" test is the arginine–growth hormone-releasing hormone test. Other tests of GH reserve, such as arginine or clonidine, are less reliable.

Treatment

Treatment of hypopituitarism requires replacement of all hormone deficiencies with adjustment of hormone doses based on both hormone levels and clinical response. Optimal hormone replacement is the goal. Optimal hormone replacement often requires a great deal of time and effort; "one dose" is not suitable for all patients.

Glucocorticoid replacement exemplifies the "art of medicine": no blood test accurately assesses the adequacy or insufficiency of a glucocorticoid dose. In general, a daily dose of hydrocortisone (Cortef) 15 mg on awakening and 5 mg at 6 PM or prednisone 5 mg on awakening and 2.5 mg at 6 PM should be adequate replacement. However, patients who gain weight on this regimen may feel well with a lower dose of hydrocortisone 10 mg on awakening and 5 mg at 6 PM or only 5 mg of prednisone on awakening. Rarely, a patient receiving hydrocortisone replacement requires dosing three times daily. Glucocorticoid replacement with dexamethasone is discouraged because of the long biologic half-life and cumulative effect causing symptoms of Cushing's syndrome and bone loss. Mineralocorticoid therapy (fludrocortisone [Florinef]) is not required in a patient with secondary adrenal insufficiency because mineralocorticoid (aldosterone) secretion is not regulated chronically by pituitary ACTH secretion. Patients should be instructed to double the glucocorticoid dose during intercurrent illness (such as flu, urinary tract infection) and to always wear a medical alert necklace or bracelet.

THYROID HORMONE REPLACEMENT

Thyroid hormone replacement with L-thyroxine (Synthroid, Levoxyl) should be monitored by measuring FT_4, not TSH. Because the TSH level in patients with hypopituitarism is often low, basing hormone replacement therapy on TSH level could result in an inappropriate reduction of the thyroid hormone dose. In healthy patients with no history of coronary artery disease or angina,

CURRENT THERAPY

- All hormone deficiencies require replacement. Optimal replacement often requires dose adjustments.
- Dose adjustments should be made at appropriate intervals (e.g., after 6 weeks of thyroid hormone or GH replacement).
- Dose adjustments may be necessary in pregnancy (thyroid hormone) or with addition of estrogen (growth hormone).
- Growth hormone replacement is not approved during pregnancy.

a beginning dose of 0.088 or 0.1 mg daily is reasonable, with dose adjustment after 1 month of therapy according to the serum free T$_4$ concentration and clinical response. Thyroid hormone replacement in the elderly or in patients with coronary artery disease should be initiated with a small dose (e.g., 0.025 mg/day) and gradually increased to achieve a normal serum FT$_4$ concentration.

GONADAL STEROID REPLACEMENT

Gonadal steroid replacement in men is most often accomplished physiologically with either a testosterone gel (AndroGel) or a testosterone patch (Androderm) that delivers a physiologic dose over 24 hours. Intramuscular testosterone, testosterone enanthate (Delatestryl), and testosterone cypionate are not physiologic and often result in supraphysiologic levels soon after injection and subphysiologic levels before the next injection. Depending on the interval after injection, intramuscular testosterone may cause mood swings, including irritability and depression. This formulation may cause erythrocytosis and elevated hemoglobin and hematocrit levels. If the patient must use the intramuscular formulation, hemoglobin and hematocrit levels should be monitored periodically. A buccal formulation of testosterone (Striant) is available and requires multiple daily doses; irritation of the gums may occur. Men should undergo a prostate examination and determination of serum prostate-specific antigen concentration yearly. Testosterone replacement does not cause prostate cancer but may promote growth of an undiagnosed carcinoma. Premenopausal women should receive cyclic estrogen and progesterone replacement for its beneficial effect on bone physiology and libido and for prevention of hot flashes. This can be accomplished with an oral contraceptive or cyclic estradiol and progesterone treatment. Annual gynecologic and breast examinations are necessary.

HORMONE REPLACEMENT FOR DIABETES INSIPIDUS

Hormone replacement for DI with desmopressin acetate (DDAVP) can be administered as an oral formulation or as a nasal spray. Because the duration of biologic activity varies among patients, the beginning dose should be low (0.1-mg tablet at bedtime), and dose frequency should be changed according to the duration of activity. Some patients are controlled with a single bedtime dose, whereas others require dosing two or three times daily. The patient can sense when the effect of desmopressin wears off because of frequent urination and return of increased thirst.

GROWTH HORMONE REPLACEMENT

Growth hormone (Genotropin, Humatrope, Norditropin, Nutropin) replacement is indicated in GH-deficient adults. The recommendation is to begin with a small dose (0.3 mg/day by subcutaneous injection) and then titrate the dose every 4 to 6 weeks according to the serum IGF-1 level and symptoms. An optimal serum IGF-1 level is at the middle or a little above the middle of the age-adjusted normal range. Women usually require a higher final dose than do men, and women receiving oral estrogen replacement usually require a higher final dose to achieve an optimal serum IGF-1 level than do women not receiving oral estrogen. Patients should be informed that a beneficial effect on energy, endurance, body composition, and serum lipid levels may not be noted for several months (6 months or more). Patients receiving GH replacement should be monitored every 6 months with a serum IGF-1 measurement, to determine the adequacy of the dose, and yearly serum lipid measurements.

Summary and Conclusions

Loss of pituitary function is common in patients with a hypothalamic or pituitary lesion, resulting either from the lesion or the treatment; these patients require regular monitoring and treatment as indicated. Patients who have undergone pituitary or cranial radiation therapy are always at risk for developing a new pituitary deficiency. Knowing if, or when, a new pituitary deficiency will occur is not possible, thus emphasizing the need for regular endocrine assessment. Optimal hormone replacement is similar to the best possible management of a patient with diabetes mellitus—frequent monitoring and adjustment of hormone doses based on hormone measurements and clinical response. The goal is accurate diagnosis and optimal replacement to prevent risk of premature mortality. With hormone replacement, a patient can lead a normal and productive life.

REFERENCES

Cook DM, Ludlam WH, Cook MB: Route of estrogen administration helps to determine growth hormone (GH) replacement dose in GH-deficient adults. J Clin Endocrinol Metab 1999;84:3956-3960.

Hartman ML, Crowe BJ, Biller BM, et al: Which patients do not require a GH stimulation test for the diagnosis of adult GH deficiency? J Clin Endocrinol Metab 2002;87:477-485.

Kelly KF, Gonzalo IT, Cohan P, et al: Hypopituitarism following traumatic brain injury and aneurysmal subarachnoid hemorrhage: A preliminary report. J Neurosurg 2000;93:743-752.

Lieberman SA, Oberoi AL, Gilkison CR, et al: Prevalence of neuroendocrine dysfunction in patients recovering from traumatic brain injury. J Clin Endocrinol Metab 2001;86:2752-2756.

Vance ML: Hypopituitarism. N Engl J Med 1994;330:1651-1662.

Hyperprolactinemia

Method of
Anthony A. Luciano, MD, and
Danielle E. Luciano, MD

Hyperprolactinemia is estimated to affect approximately 0.4% of an unselected female population. However, approximately one third of women with amenorrhea, and three quarters of women with galactorrhea and oligomenorrhea are found to have elevated prolactin levels. Prolactinomas are the most common cause of hyperprolactinemia, and they represent approximately 80% of all pituitary adenomas.

Prolactin is a polypeptide with 198 amino acids synthesized by the anterior pituitary lactotrophs. Its half-life is approximately 20 minutes; it is excreted by both the liver and the kidneys. Prolactin is similar in structure to growth hormone and has three biological forms, all of which are immunoreactive and detected by assay. The most biologically active form is the *small form*, which is secreted along with the less biologically active *big form* and *big-big form*. Prolactin, unlike any other pituitary hormone, is under tonic inhibition by the hypothalamus via dopamine secreted through the pituitary portal system. Therefore, hyperprolactinemia results from interference with this inhibition through blockage of the pituitary portal system and the hypothalamic release of dopamine.

Clinical Manifestations

The main symptoms of hyperprolactinemia in women include galactorrhea, menstrual disturbances, and symptoms from the mass effect of the adenoma, if present. Galactorrhea is the nonphysiologic mammary secretion of milky fluid that can be either unilateral or bilateral or occurs in parous women more than 12 months after delivery or weaning.

Menstrual disturbances caused by hyperprolactinemia can result in amenorrhea and infertility. Elevated prolactin levels inhibit pulsatile gonadotropin-releasing hormone in a dose-dependent manner. Prolactin levels of 20 to 50 ng/mL can cause oligomenorrhea or amenorrhea, and levels greater than 100 ng/mL can cause hypogonadism and hypoestrogenemia. Hyperprolactinemia can cause hirsutism, acne, and osteoporosis and has also been associated with hyperinsulinemia, polycystic ovary syndrome, and an increased risk for metabolic syndrome.

Mass effect symptoms from prolactinoma include headaches, visual disturbances (specifically bitemporal hemianopsia), cranial neuropathies, and seizures. Other pituitary functions can also be affected, and symptoms of panhypopituitarism can be seen.

Diagnosis and Evaluation

Diagnosis of hyperprolactinemia is usually made on the basis of blood results from symptomatic women. The upper limit for normal prolactin levels is 20 to 25 ng/mL. However, prolactin levels are affected by sleep, exercise, stress, food intake, recent breast exam, and diurnal variation with peak levels occurring during sleep. Therefore, confirmatory testing of elevated levels should be done with a fasting early morning sample.

A thorough examination of a patient with hyperprolactinemia should include a detailed diagnostic history

CURRENT DIAGNOSIS

Reconfirm hyperprolactinemia:
- Retest fasting in the early morning

Exclude other causes:
- Get detailed history (especially medications) and physical exam; obtain hCG and TSH levels; obtain LFTs, BUN/Cr levels

Head imaging:
- MRI (preferable) or CT scan
- Obtain imaging with persistent elevated prolactin levels; perform visual field testing if mass is >1 cm

Abbreviations: BUN = blood urea nitrogen; Cr = creatinine; CT = computed tomography; hCG = human chorionic gonadotropin; LFT = liver function test; MRI = magnetic resonance imaging; TSH = thyroid-stimulating hormone.

TABLE 1 Differential Diagnoses of Hyperprolactinemia

Hypothalamic conditions	• Craniopharyngioma • Meningioma • Sarcoidosis • Other cancers • Vascular accidents
Pituitary conditions	• Prolactinoma (<1-cm microadenoma, ≥1-cm macroadenoma) • Empty sella syndrome • Other adenomas • Acromegaly • Cushing's syndrome • Transection of pituitary stalk
Medications	• Phenothiazines • MAOIs • Tricyclic antidepressants • Butyrophenones • Methyldopa (Aldomet) • Metoclopramide (Reglan) • Verapamil (Calan) • SSRIs • Narcotics
Other	• Hypothyroidism • Pregnancy • Renal failure • Cirrhosis • Neurogenic (spinal cord or chest wall lesions) • Idiopathic

Abbreviations: MAOI = monoamine oxidase inhibitor; SSRI = selective serotonin reuptake inhibitor.

and evaluation of clinical signs and symptoms to exclude or include all physiologic, pathologic, and pharmacologic causes. The differential diagnoses of hyperprolactinemia can be subgrouped into hypothalamic conditions, pituitary conditions, medications, and other (Table 1). Prolactin levels between 20 to 60 ng/mL should be confirmed; if still elevated, computed tomography (CT) or magnetic resonance imaging (MRI) of the head is necessary to rule out a pituitary adenoma. Levels of human chorionic gonadotropin (hCG) and thyroid-stimulating hormone (TSH) should be drawn and liver and kidney function tests should be administered. If a mass *more than* 1 cm (macroadenoma) is seen on MRI or CT, visual field testing should be performed. Once the cause of hyperprolactinemia is ascertained, a treatment plan can be determined.

Treatment

PROLACTINOMA

Some patients with micro- or macroadenomas and no symptoms may be followed expectantly. In some patients, no change in size or clinical symptoms occurs; these patients can avoid treatment. However, most patients require therapy; and indications include significant symptoms of infertility, galactorrhea, ovulatory dysfunction, visual field defects, cranial nerve palsies, osteopenia, or increased prolactinoma size after observation.

The first-line treatment for both micro- and macroadenomas is dopamine agonist therapy. The principal goals of this treatment are normalization of the prolactin levels and improvement in symptoms. Hopefully, treatment also results in a reduction or stabilization in size of the tumor and prevents recurrence or progression. Bromocriptine (Parlodel) is the most commonly used medication and has been found to normalize prolactin levels and reduce tumor size in greater than 80% of patients. Menses will usually normalize in approximately 6 weeks with galactorrhea improving in approximately 12 weeks. Visual disturbances will often improve before noticeable changes in tumor size occur. Bromocriptine is available in 2.5-mg tablets, and the usual starting dose is 1 tab by mouth at bedtime with weekly increases as needed up to 7.5 to 10 mg daily. The normal dose is 2.5 mg by mouth two times daily. Side effects include nausea or vomiting, headache, faintness, dizziness, fatigue, nasal congestion, and abdominal cramps. These side effects can be relieved by taking the medication at night and with food, or by taking it per vagina to avoid liver first pass. Vaginal administration often requires a reduced dosage because it is better absorbed. Approximately 12% of patients find this medication intolerable, and some prolactinomas are not responsive, necessitating trial of another medication.

Cabergoline (Dostinex) is a long-acting dopamine receptor agonist useful in patients resistant to or intolerant of bromocriptine. It is more effective with fewer side effects in normalizing prolactin levels and reducing symptoms. Cabergoline is a long-acting drug that can be dosed twice weekly starting with 0.25 mg by mouth two times a week and increasing every 4 weeks by 0.25 mg until normalized prolactin levels are observed. Maximum dosing is 1.5 mg by mouth twice weekly.

Pergolide (Permax)[1] is a more potent, longer-lasting dopamine agonist used primarily in the treatment of Parkinson's disease and has been found to be comparable to bromocriptine in efficacy. It is given in 0.05 mg by mouth once daily but is currently not approved for treatment of prolactinomas.

Surgery for a prolactinoma is generally reserved for large lesions unresponsive to medications. Trans-sphenoidal surgery is the procedure of choice with an acceptable short-term cure rate of approximately 80% with microadenomas and 40% with macroadenomas. However, there is a high recurrence rate of 30% in microadenomas and 70% to 80% in macroadenomas, even in experienced hands. Although patients complain of hyperprolactinemia symptoms, some recurrences are not visualized radiographically. Surgery has a low mortality rate (<0.5%), and side effects include panhypopituitarism (10% to 30%), cerebral spinal fluid leaks, meningitis, and diabetes insipidus (temporary 10% to 40%, long-term <2%).

Radiotherapy is reserved for adjunctive therapy in patients with large infiltrative macroadenomas. Side effects include panhypopituitarism (up to 50%) and optic nerve damage.

IDIOPATHIC, MEDICATION-INDUCED, AND OTHER CAUSES

A key to managing patients with hyperprolactinemia but no prolactinoma is treating any underlying condition they may have. For example, patients taking medications that affect dopamine action may respond to medication changes or alterations to minimize their prolactin effects. Hypothyroidism is responsible for approximately 3% to 5% of the cases of hyperprolactinemia; the mechanism is through elevated TRH levels stimulating pituitary lactotrophs. Thyroid replacement should normalize both thyroid and prolactin levels. Cushing's disease as well as other systemic disorders should be treated. Once these underlying conditions are addressed, if symptoms persist or prolactin levels do not normalize, dopamine agonist therapy is the treatment of choice. In women desiring pregnancy, bromocriptine is the agonist of choice because it has the most long-term safety data during pregnancy.

PREGNANCY

As a general rule, bromocriptine should be used as little as possible during pregnancy. Bromocriptine therapy should be stopped once the presence of fetal heart tones has been established. Long-term data have not shown any increase in spontaneous abortions, ectopics, or pregnancy complications. There has also been no data that indicated fetal effects when bromocriptine was used in this fashion. Symptoms exhibit slow progression during pregnancy with less than 2% growth in microadenomas and a 15% to 30% growth in macroadenomas. Prolactin levels increase in pregnancy so periodic checking is not useful. Visual field testing and MRIs are also not useful for screening during pregnancy and should only be used in patients complaining of headache or other tumor mass symptoms, such as visual disturbances.

If a patient complains of tumor enlargement symptoms, she should be treated with bromocriptine. Women prescribed bromocriptine have been shown to have a quick response with no adverse fetal effects. Although bromocriptine is a dopamine agonist, it does not affect amniotic fluid prolactin or electrolyte balance. Amniotic fluid prolactin is made by the decidual tissue and is regulated by estrogen and progesterone, not dopamine. Other dopamine agonists such as cabergoline and pergolide have not been tested in pregnancy.

Surgical resection is rarely indicated during pregnancy because bromocriptine is usually highly effective. However, up to 25% of patients with large macroadenomas (>3 cm) do not respond to bromocriptine during pregnancy; these patients may best be treated with trans-sphenoidal resection prior to conception. Surgery is also indicated if the tumors continue to grow despite dopamine agonist therapy.

Breastfeeding is not contraindicated in patients with prolactinomas because it does not affect tumor growth. Dopamine agonist therapy should be avoided, and prolactin levels should be checked 2 to 3 months postpartum. MRIs should be performed as indicated by symptoms, and patients should be treated accordingly.

Hyperprolactinemia should be treated based on its cause. Once any underlying conditions or medications have been identified and resolved, first-line therapy should be dopamine agonist medication. If the patient desires pregnancy, bromocriptine is the first line of treatment. Surgery should be reserved for prolactinomas unresponsive to medication therapy.

---

[1]Not FDA approved for this indication.
[3]Exceeds dosage recommended by the manufacturer.

CURRENT THERAPY

Treat underlying condition:

- Hypothyroidism-thyroid replacement, change medications

Prolactinoma first line therapy: dopamine agonists

- Bromocriptine (Parlodel), especially if patient desires pregnancy, start at 2.5 mg qhs with food; usual dose 2.5 mg bid; max dose 5 mg bid cabergoline (Dostinex); start 0.25 mg 2×/wk, max dose 1.5 mg[3] 2×/wk pergolide (Permax)[1]

Surgery only when indicated:

- Adenoma unresponsive to medical therapy with neurologic symptoms

Pregnancy:

- Bromocriptine until positive fetal heart tones; and then if symptoms recur, no contraindication to breastfeeding

[1]Not FDA approved for this indication.
[3]Exceeds dosage recommended by the manufacturer.

REFERENCES

Biller BMK, Luciano AA, Crosignanai PG, et al: Guidelines for the diagnosis and treatment of hyperprolactinemia. J Reprod Med 1999; 44(12):1075-1084.

Di Sarano A, Landi ML, Cappabianca P, et al: Resistance to cabergoline as compared with bromocriptine in hyperprolactinemia: Prevalence, clinical definition, and therapeutic strategy. J Clin Endocrinol Metab 2001;86:5256-5261.

Luciano AA: Clinical presentation of hyperprolactinemia. J Reprod Med 1999;44(12):1085-1090.

Moltich ME: Management of prolactinomas in pregnancy. J Reprod Med 1999;44(12):1121-1126.

Olive D: Indications for hyperprolactinemia therapy. J Reprod Med 1999;44(12):1091-1094.

Schlechte JA, Dolan K, Sherman B, Luciano AA: The natural history of untreated hyperprolactinemia: A prospective analysis. J Clin Endocrinol Metab 1989;68:412-418.

Webster J, Piscitell G, Polli A, et al: A comparison of cabergoline and bromocriptine in the treatment of hyperprolactinemic amenorrhea. N Engl J Med 1994;331:904-909.

Hypothyroidism

Method of
John T. Nicoloff, MD, and
Jonathan S. LoPresti, MD, PhD

Diagnosis and treatment of hypothyroidism is an extremely rewarding experience both for the patient and clinician because lifelong restoration of a euthyroid state can be safely and economically achieved with the appropriate use of oral L-thyroxine (T_4) replacement therapy. Although there are many potential causes for hypothyroidism (Table 1), autoimmune thyroiditis (chronic thyroiditis, lymphocytic thyroiditis, Hashimoto's thyroiditis) represents most spontaneously occurring cases of primary hypothyroidism. The initial phases of the disease often start in early adolescence; the incidence of hypothyroidism

TABLE 1 Etiology of Hypothyroidism

Primary Hypothyroidism
- Chronic autoimmune thyroiditis (Hashimoto's, lymphocytic)
- Iatrogenic: [131]I therapy, thyroidectomy, external radiation
- Drugs: methimazole (Tapazole), PTU, perchlorate, lithium, amiodarone
- Immune modulators: interferon-α, interleukins, postpartum period
- Congenital: complete or partial thyroid gland absence, peroxidase deficiency
- Severe dietary iodine deficiency
- Thyroid infiltrative diseases (rare): lymphoma, Riedel's struma, amyloidosis, hemochromatosis

Central Hypothyroidism
- Pituitary TSH deficiency (secondary hypothyroidism): Sheehan's syndrome, pituitary tumors, hypophysitis, trauma (surgery, radiation, head injury), empty sella syndrome
- Hypothalamic TRH deficiency (tertiary hypothyroidism): tumor, craniopharyngioma, Sheehan's syndrome, infiltrative diseases (sarcoidosis, tuberculosis, histiocytosis, lymphoma, eosinophilic granuloma)

Transient Hypothyroidism
- Subacute thyroiditis
- Postpartum thyroiditis

Congenital Thyroid Hormone Resistance (Genetic)
- Peripheral variant
- Central variant

Abbreviations: [131]I = iodine-131; PTU = propylthiouracil; TRH = thyrotropin releasing hormone; TSH = thyroid-stimulating hormone.

often reaches its peak in older patient populations in which some degree of biochemical hypothyroidism becomes demonstrable in approximately 8% of males and 20% of females by the age of 70 years. This pattern is the result of the inherently slow, progressive, and unremitting nature of the underlying destructive autoimmune process. Unfortunately, establishing a clinical diagnosis of hypothyroidism generally is a difficult task, especially during the early stages of the disease. The insidious character of thyroid destruction and the lack of specific symptoms that raise suspicion in either the patient or physician make the diagnosis of hypothyroidism problematic. However, this diagnostic limitation can be overcome by establishing the presence of what is most often termed *biochemical* or *subclinical* or *mild* hypothyroidism as defined by consistent elevations in serum thyroid-stimulating hormone (TSH) concentrations when serum free thyroxine (FT_4) levels still remain within the normal range. This diagnosis may be further bolstered by the additional findings of detectable serum antithyroperoxidase (anti-TPO) antibodies and the presence of a small, firm goiter. Therefore, the diagnosis of hypothyroidism secondary to chronic autoimmune thyroiditis can definitively be diagnosed at the earliest stages of the disease before the development of significant morbidity occurs. Furthermore, advances in technology have both reduced the cost and improved the accuracy of serum TSH measurements, thereby making it possible to perform cost-effective serum TSH screening on large *at-risk* populations. Therefore, the challenge for the clinician is to identify populations that are likely to be *at risk* for developing hypothyroidism, establish a diagnosis of subclinical disease, and initiate oral T_4 therapy before overt signs and symptoms of hypothyroidism become clinically apparent.

Etiology

PRIMARY HYPOTHYROIDISM

Chronic autoimmune thyroiditis is responsible for most spontaneously occurring cases of thyroid gland failure. As its name implies, chronic autoimmune thyroiditis results from an immunologic process characterized by the insidious, cell-mediated destruction of the thyroid gland. Lymphocytic thyroiditis and Hashimoto's thyroiditis represent specific pathologic terms that describe histologic variants of this autoimmune thyroid gland destruction. The disorder is characterized by progressive infiltration of the thyroid by lymphocytes, lymphoid follicles, and other inflammatory cells over many years, ultimately producing a remnant scar where the gland was located. The onset of the disease commonly occurs in early adolescence and primarily in females (5:1 female-to-male ratio) who display a small, irregular, firm, nontender goiter (so-called adolescent goiter) in an otherwise healthy young adult. Even in this initial phase of the disease, serum TSH concentrations can become persistently elevated; and serum anti-TPO antibodies are frequently detectable. The former is responsible for the compensatory goiter formation, and the latter serving as a nonspecific marker of the underlying thyroid autoimmunity. With advancing age, the cumulative incidence of hypothyroidism gradually rises in both females and males with the female-to-male ratio declining from an initial value of 5:1 to a 2:1 ratio by age 70 years. This latter finding is consistent with the concept of a genetic predisposition for developing autoimmune thyroiditis with thyroid dysfunction displayed earlier in the female population. It is noteworthy that this same age/sex pattern is commonly observed with other autoimmune diseases as well. Exposure to iodine-containing drugs such as intravenous (IV) contrast dyes and to immune modulating agents such as interferon can precipitate or exacerbate this underlying autoimmune process in susceptible individuals, occasionally producing an abrupt onset of thyroid gland failure and development of hypothyroidism. However, on withdrawal of these agents, thyroid function usually returns to the pretreatment status. In a similar context, postpartum thyroiditis represents a transient autoimmune exacerbation of thyroid dysfunction occurring during early postpartum in women with either preexisting or the genetic tendency for autoimmune thyroid disease. Although most of these women subsequently experience a spontaneous resolution of this mild and transient form of biochemical hypothyroidism within a few weeks, they should be considered to be an at-risk population for developing spontaneous hypothyroidism in the future.

UNCOMMON CAUSES OF PRIMARY HYPOTHYROIDISM

Severe dietary iodine deficiency, surgical thyroidectomy, iodine-131 (^{131}I) ablation, and excessive antithyroid drug administration represent obvious and anticipated causes of primary hypothyroidism and therefore should not represent either a diagnostic or therapeutic problem for the clinician. Approximately one third of patients with subacute thyroiditis will experience a mild to moderate primary hypothyroidism from 6 weeks to 6 months following the onset of this virally mediated destruction of the thyroid. However, in contrast to chronic autoimmune thyroiditis, this form of hypothyroidism is transient in character; eventual full recovery of thyroid gland function and histology is the norm. Neonatal hypothyroidism, or cretinism, represents a rare but important treatable cause of infant mental retardation. Although clinically difficult to recognize at birth, the widespread use of neonatal thyroid screening testing and early T_4 replacement therapy has essentially abolished this form of hypothyroidism in medically advanced countries. Fortunately, thyroid neonatal screening programs are also rapidly spreading to the underdeveloped regions of the world to address this treatable form of hypothyroidism.

CENTRAL HYPOTHYROIDISM

Central hypothyroidism is a rarely encountered entity representing less than 1% of all cases of hypothyroidism. It results from a wide variety of pathologic conditions that impair pituitary TSH, secondary hypothyroidism, and/or hypothalamic thyrotropin-releasing hormone (TRH), tertiary hypothyroidism production, or secretion resulting in a decline in function of the thyroid gland. Common causes of central hypothyroidism include pituitary tumors, empty sella syndrome, trauma, postpartum pituitary necrosis (Sheehan's syndrome), hypophysitis, whole-brain radiation, and a variety of infiltrative diseases (see Table 1). Of considerable diagnostic importance is that the biologic properties of the TSH secreted in secondary hypothyroidism are often altered (because of impaired TRH action on TSH formation) resulting in forms of TSH that have markedly reduced bioactivity while retaining normal immunoactivity. This phenomenon often results in falsely normal TSH values reported in patients who are otherwise biochemically and clinically hypothyroid. Therefore, the utility of serum TSH measurements by immunoassay in accurately assessing thyroid status is essentially lost either for establishing the initial diagnosis or monitoring the adequacy of T_4 replacement therapy in patients with secondary hypothyroidism.

Diagnosis

The clinical diagnosis of hypothyroidism is inherently difficult to establish because the classic features of this condition only become fully evident in the latest stages of the disease. Furthermore, the classic signs and symptoms of hypothyroidism such as weight gain, hypertension, dry skin, hair loss, cold intolerance, chronic fatigue, constipation, and fluid retention are nonspecific in character and commonly occur in populations without hypothyroidism. Only the presence of an asymptomatic, small, firm goiter and delayed deep tendon reflexes provide findings of some diagnostic utility and specificity. However, these signs are usually not routinely assessed unless a suspicion that the patient is at risk for developing hypothyroidism is present. Common risk factors include a positive family history of thyroid or other autoimmune diseases and the

CURRENT DIAGNOSIS

- Hypothyroidism presents with nonspecific signs and symptoms. Therefore, hypothyroidism requires biochemical diagnosis.
- Screening of all adults older than 35 years of age should be considered.
- Definitive indications for screening include a positive family history and/or the presence of a goiter on exam.
- Routine screening tests include a serum TSH level and anti-TPO titer.
- Primary hypothyroidism is confirmed by elevated serum TSH levels and low T_4 values.
- Secondary hypothyroidism is diagnosed by low serum T_4 levels.
- Subclinical hypothyroidism is defined as a normal T_4 and a minimally elevated TSH level.

Abbreviations: anti-TPO = antithyroperoxidase; T_4 = L-thyroxine; TSH = thyroid-stimulating hormone.

detection of an elevated serum TSH value with routine blood tests.

AT-RISK POPULATIONS FOR PRIMARY HYPOTHYROIDISM

Because the propensity for the development of autoimmune diseases is strongly influenced by genetic factors, it is not surprising to find that hypothyroidism secondary to chronic thyroiditis is a familial disorder. Therefore, eliciting a family history either of an *underactive* or *overactive* thyroid condition, the use of thyroid medications, or the presence of a goiter all point toward the possibility of the patient harboring an occult thyroid disorder. If any of these conditions are present in the family, undertaking of a more careful neck examination palpating for a goiter, eliciting deep tendon reflexes evaluating for a slow relaxation phase, and measuring serum TSH and anti-TPO levels can be justified. A positive family history for other autoimmune disorders such as vitiligo, pernicious anemia, myasthenia gravis, Addison's disease, and type 1 diabetes mellitus increases the risk of developing autoimmune hypothyroidism. The discovery of such a history of familial autoimmunity is considerably useful because it raises the probability of detecting subclinical hypothyroidism.

LABORATORY DETECTION OF SUBCLINICAL HYPOTHYROIDISM

Measurement of serum TSH levels occupies a central role in establishing the laboratory diagnosis of primary hypothyroidism, especially in its earliest subclinical stage. Because thyroxine secretion declines as a result of the progressive destruction of the thyroid gland from chronic thyroiditis, even a small decrease in serum FT_4 concentration within the normal range promptly produces a reciprocal increase in the serum TSH value. Importantly, the relative magnitude of this serum TSH rise far exceeds the fall in FT_4 resulting from an *amplified* hypothalamic–pituitary negative feedback response, for example, a two-fold change in FT_4 produces a 100-fold change in TSH. Therefore, this isolated elevation in serum TSH not only serves as an early

marker for impending thyroid gland failure but also acts to stimulate the preferential secretion of more biologically active triiodothyronine (T_3) by the thyroid gland, thereby masking the onset of the signs and symptoms of hypothyroidism. This latter phenomenon helps, in part, to explain the subclinical character of this syndrome. When such an isolated elevation in serum TSH is detected, the serum TSH determination should be repeated along with a serum anti-TPO measurement for diagnostic verification and as an indicator of the underlying autoimmune nature of the process. If not already performed, complete a careful family history, as characterized earlier; a careful neck examination for the presence of a goiter; and an assessment of deep tendon reflexes.

WHEN ARE SERUM THYROID-STIMULATING HORMONE ELEVATIONS SIGNIFICANT?

In ambulatory, clinically well individuals, any persistent serum TSH elevation should be considered as strong evidence for the presence of primary hypothyroidism, even when the serum FT_4 values remain within the normal range. With a normal reference range of serum TSH concentration of 0.5 to 3.5 mU/L, individuals displaying TSH increases from 3.5 to 10 mU/L or even higher are often remarkably free of hypothyroid symptoms, particularly in younger patients. However, bolstered by the additional findings of detectable anti-TPO antibodies, a positive family history for thyroid or other autoimmune diseases as well as the presence of a small firm goiter, this suspicion evolves into the realm of diagnostic certainty, even with modest rises in serum TSH levels. If, however, these additional confirmatory findings are absent but serum TSH elevations persist, some clinicians may choose to defer making a diagnosis of primary hypothyroidism, especially if the rise in serum TSH is minimal (less than 10 mU/L). In this case, the physician should continue to monitor serum TSH concentrations at 6- to 12-month intervals to ascertain the persistence and progression of hypothyroidism rather than to initiate lifelong oral T_4 therapy. Keep in mind, however, that many patients with mild subclinical hypothyroidism may experience unexpected symptomatic benefit as well as lowering of serum lipid levels following the initiation of T_4 replacement therapy. In this sense, *subclinical* hypothyroidism may represent a misnomer.

TRANSIENT SERUM THYROID-STIMULATING HORMONE ELEVATIONS ASSOCIATED WITH SYSTEMIC ILLNESSES

In contrast to the relatively stable serum TSH values encountered in healthy ambulatory populations, serum TSH values can become quite labile with acute illnesses where serum TSH values are commonly in the range characteristic of both hyper- and hypothyroidism. Generally, as the illness worsens, serum TSH concentrations become suppressed whereas during recovery they can rebound to elevated values. Obviously, these transient changes in serum TSH levels greatly impair the utility of serum TSH determination as a diagnostic tool. Therefore, greater reliance must be placed on serum FT_4 measurements in sick patients. Interestingly, the therapeutic use of both glucocorticoids and dopamine will also cause dramatic transient reductions in serum TSH levels during their acute administration, followed by rebound elevations when these agents are withdrawn. It is believed that this results from direct inhibitory action on the release of TSH from the pituitary. Presumably, a similar inhibitory action from the endogenous cortisol increase on TSH secretion in response to major stress is responsible for the spontaneous decline in serum TSH in acute illness. When such transient changes in serum TSH occur in ambulatory patient populations, acute therapeutic glucocorticoid administration most often proves to be the culprit, such as asthma therapy. However, when chronic glucocorticoid therapy is employed, serum TSH concentrations generally remain in the normal range in the euthyroid patient.

THYROID-STIMULATING HORMONE SCREENING OF ADULT POPULATIONS

Serum TSH screening of adult populations is cost effectively performed because of technological advances made in the automation of TSH assay methods. This fact has led the American Thyroid Association to recommend screening of the entire population for thyroid disease starting at age 35 years and at 5-year intervals thereafter if initial screening results are normal. Other more restrictive population screening recommendations include testing the entire prenatal population and all the adult population starting at age 60 years. Certainly, all individuals providing a familial history of thyroid or other autoimmune diseases also make up a logical group deserving of TSH screening, as well. In the final analysis, it comes down to what is perceived to be the cost-to-benefit ratio of such an undertaking. Presently, a broad consensus in the medical community on this subject has not yet been formed regarding screening for thyroid disease in the population.

Treatment

ORAL L-THYROXINE ALONE AS THE SOLE FORM OF THYROID HORMONE REPLACEMENT THERAPY

The advantages of employing oral LT_4 (Synthroid) as the sole thyroid replacement therapy are many and include the following:

- The availability of several well-standardized, competitively priced brands of synthetic oral LT_4 (Table 2)
- A long biological half-life approximating 7 days, thereby making day to day compliance less critical

TABLE 2 Thyroid Hormone Preparations

Generic Name	Brand Name
Levothyroxine sodium (LT_4)	• Levothroid • Levoxyl • Unithroid
Liothyronine sodium (LT_3)	Cytomel
Liotrix (LT_4 and LT_3 combination)	Thyrolar
Thyroid USP (LT_3 and LT_4 extract)	Armour Thyroid

Abbreviations: LT_4 = levothyroxine; LT_3 = liothyronine.

CURRENT THERAPY

- Treatment of choice for hypothyroidism should be a nongeneric levothyroxine preparation.
- Interchanging of brands is contraindicated because each levothyroxine preparation has a unique absorption profile.
- Levothyroxine sodium (Synthroid) dosing should start at 25 μg daily and be increased slowly until the ideal dose is reached as determined by a serum TSH level.
- Goal of levothyroxine therapy in primary hypothyroidism is a serum TSH value between 0.5 mU/L and 2.0 mU/L.
- Goal of therapy in secondary hypothyroidism is a normal T_4 level.
- Treatment of subclinical hypothyroidism should be determined on a case-by-case basis.

Abbreviations: T_4 = L-thyroxine; TSH = thyroid-stimulating hormone.

- Production of remarkably stable circulating levels of FT_4, which can be easily and accurately measured by routine laboratory testing methods
- Production of stable physiologic circulating levels of triiodothyronine (T_3), the active form of thyroid hormone, derived from the peripheral tissue conversion from T_4
- Allows the physiologically adaptive regulation of T_4 to T_3 conversion to occur in response to alterations in nutrition and stresses associated with illness and injury

In contrast, the use of oral LT_3 (Cytomel) alone or in combination with LT_4 possesses none of these important advantages and therefore is not recommended for use as standard hormone replacement therapy.

INITIATION AND MAINTENANCE OF OPTIMAL LT_4 REPLACEMENT THERAPY IN PRIMARY HYPOTHYROIDISM

It is important to initiate oral LT_4 replacement therapy slowly, starting with a LT_4 dose of 25 μg daily and subsequently increasing the dose by 25 μg every 6 weeks until the serum FT_4 levels reach the midnormal range. A total daily LT_4 dose ranging between 50 and 125 μg usually is required to achieve this goal of a normal FT_4 value (a daily dose of 125 μg of LT_4 is needed for full replacement in an adult with no residual thyroid function). This deliberate treatment approach is essential to allow sufficient time for the myriad of metabolic alterations produced by T_4 therapy to take place. After achieving this initial goal of normal serum FT_4 levels, serial serum TSH levels can be measured to achieve an optimal individualized TSH target value ranging between 0.5 to 2.0 mU/L. However, with each LT_4 dosage adjustment, it is important to allow a period of at least 6 weeks for a new metabolic equilibrium to be achieved before serum TSH is remeasured. As noted, this LT_4 titration process requires that considerable time and patience be practiced by both by the clinician and patient. Once the final optimal serum TSH level is achieved, this daily oral LT_4 dose requirement rarely changes as long as the patient remains compliant and the brand of T_4 medication is not altered. One possible exception to this rule is that a slight reduction in LT_4 dose requirement often occurs after the age of 60 years presumably in association with a general slowing of overall metabolism.

TREATMENT OF CENTRAL HYPOTHYROIDISM

The initiation of oral LT_4 therapy in patients with central hypothyroidism is essentially the same as detailed previously for primary hypothyroidism. However, before starting LT_4 therapy, special care must be exercised to ensure adequate glucocorticoid replacement as thyroid hormone may accelerate glucocorticoid disposal and thereby may precipitate an Addisonian crisis. Additionally, because the measurement of serum TSH concentrations cannot serve as a useful therapeutic end-point in patients with central hypothyroidism, the adequacy of LT_4 replacement therapy must then rely on normalizing serum FT_4 values.

COMMON PITFALLS IN OPTIMAL ORAL L-THYROXINE THERAPY

The clinician should become suspicious that a problem likely exists in the management of LT_4 therapy when marked variability in serum TSH values occurs on a fixed LT_4 maintenance dose. The three most likely causes for this phenomenon are as follows:

1. Noncompliance: Poor compliance represents the most commonly encountered problem causing suboptimal LT_4 maintenance therapy. The principal reason for noncompliance usually relates to the fact that patients do not experience any immediate change in their state of health when stopping LT_4 therapy. This often results in patients missing their daily LT_4 dose or when they run out of their T_4 supply, not promptly replacing it. To compound the problem, when the patients are asked, "Are you taking your thyroid medication?" they can honestly say, "Yes," because they may have recently restarted therapy in anticipation of the next physician visit. Therefore, one might ask, "How often do you forget to take your thyroid medication?" to remove the stigma from noncompliance. Patients often look puzzled when queried in such a manner but they then rapidly understand when their physician reassures them, "We all forget to take our medication at some time—I certainly do." Experience indicates that such misinformation is the most common cause for physicians inadvertently prescribing excessive dosages of oral LT_4 therapy

2. Drugs and other factors altering T_4 absorption and metabolism: Table 3 lists some of the most common causes leading to a need for an increase in oral LT_4 dose requirements. Drugs or conditions that reduce gastric acidity also decrease T_4 absorption because the hormone is more readily absorbed in its acidic form. Because T_4 is highly lipophilic, drugs that interfere with fat absorption also will impair thyroxine absorption, as well. Still other drugs act to accelerate hepatic T_4 disposal by the so-called hepatic "first pass effect." Administering oral LT_4 separately in the morning before taking drugs that interfere with GI absorption can mitigate this problem. Otherwise, compensatory increases in the oral LT_4 dosing schedule will be required.

TABLE 3 Common Causes Requiring Oral Levothyroxine Dosage Adjustment

Increased LT_4 Administration Required
- Poor compliance
- Decreased gastrointestinal absorption: oral iron, lipid-binding drugs, sucralfate, calcium carbonate, achlorhydria, proton-blocking drugs
- Altered T_4 metabolism: phenobarbital, phenytoin, carbamazepine, rifampin, HAART
- Pregnancy
- Nephrotic syndrome

Decreased LT_4 Administration Required
- Aging

Abbreviations: HAART = highly active antiretroviral therapy; LT_4 = levothyroxine; T_4 = L-thyroxine.

3. Switching oral LT_4 brands: The T_4 content of oral thyroxine preparations is well standardized and carefully monitored by the FDA. However, variations in tablet dissolution characteristics and other features of the tablet structure appear to influence the efficiency of T_4 gastrointestinal absorption. These facts make it desirable not to switch the brand of an oral LT_4 preparation once the optimal dose has been ascertained for any given patient. For the same reason, generic T_4 brands should be avoided because the source of the T_4 tablets may vary over time.

Special Situations

PREGNANCY

Women with hypothyroidism who become pregnant usually require substantial increases in their oral LT_4 maintenance dose. Such upward dose adjustments must be performed very early in pregnancy because normal fetal brain development in the first 12 weeks of gestation depends on maternal thyroxine as its source of thyroid hormone. Furthermore, there is strong circumstantial evidence that a deficiency in maternal T_4 at this stage of pregnancy is associated with a subsequent reduction in intelligence quotient in the offspring. It is noteworthy that one possible cause for this increased oral LT_4 requirement results from the concurrent use of oral iron supplements, which interfere with T_4 absorption (Table 3). To reduce this effect of iron on T_4 absorption, it is advisable to take the oral LT_4 dose and the iron at separate times.

SURGICAL PROCEDURES

Surgery usually does not present a special problem for hypothyroid patients who have received adequate preoperative oral LT_4 replacement therapy. The failure to receive oral medications for a few days postoperatively also is not a therapeutically important problem by virtue of the long 7-day half-life of thyroxine. However, in rare cases of prolonged restriction of oral intake, LT_4 can then be administered as a 500 μg IV bolus every 5 days until oral intake can be restarted. In the untreated or inadequately treated hypothyroid patient requiring elective surgery, surgery should be deferred until a euthyroid state is restored with LT$_4$ therapy to significantly reduce operative and postoperative morbidity. In those instances of surgical emergencies or in patients with severe coronary artery disease, surgery should proceed because such surgery is reasonably well tolerated if IV LT$_4$ therapy is administered in the immediate postoperative period.

MYXEDEMA COMA

Myxedema coma is a somewhat imprecise term in that this syndrome should be more appropriately termed *decompensated* hypothyroidism. Myxedema coma does not simply represent the natural progression of severe hypothyroidism but signifies an instance where intervening illness or events are responsible for precipitating a significant deterioration in mental status (i.e., acute psychosis, confusion, stupor, and coma) and producing cardiovascular collapse in the patient. The key to therapy is determining the precipitating cause and promptly initiating appropriate therapy. Occult infection and sepsis represent the most common etiologies of decompensation, but a long list of primary and contributing causes includes blood loss, excessive use of diuretics, carbon dioxide retention, oversedation with medications, overuse of tranquilizers and narcotics, and so forth. The use of IV LT$_4$ at an initial dose of 500 µg undoubtedly plays a positive role in marshalling an improved host response but is only useful in conjunction with the identification and reversal of the precipitating event(s).

REFERENCES

Foley TP Jr.: Hypothyroidism. Pediatr Rev 2004;25: 94-100.
Green WL: New questions regarding bioequivalence of levothyroxine preparations: A clinician's response. AAPS J 2005;7:54-58.
LoPresti JS: Thyroid function tests. In Shindo M, Singer P (eds.): *Clinics in Otolaryngology*. WB Saunders, Philadelphia, pp 557-576, 1996.
LoPresti JS, Nicoloff JT: Myxedema coma: A form of decompensated hypothyroidism. In Ober KP (ed.): Endocrinology and Metabolism Clinics of North America. WB Saunders, Philadelphia, 1993, pp 279-290.
Roberts CG, Ladenson PW: Hypothyroidism. Lancet 2004;363:1558-1594.
Surks MI, Goswami G, Daniels GH: The thyrotropin reference range should remain unchanged. J Clin Endocrinol Metab 2005;90: 5489-5496.
Wartofsky L, Dickey RA: The evidence for a narrower thyrotropin reference range is compelling. J Clin Endocrinol Metab 2005;90:5483-5488.

Hyperthyroidism

Method of
Kenneth D. Burman, MD

Hyperthyroidism is a condition resulting from overproduction of L-thyroxine (T$_4$) and/or L-triiodothyronine (T$_3$) (Box 1). The clinical diagnosis should always be confirmed with thyroid function tests and sometimes by radioisotope studies. Treatment of hyperthyroidism should preferably be conducted in consultation with an endocrinologist.

BOX 1   Causes of Endogenous Hyperthyroidism

Common
- Graves' disease
- Toxic adenoma
- Multinodular goiter
- Thyroiditis (subacute, postpartum)
- Amiodarone

Uncommon
- TSH-secreting pituitary adenoma
- Metastatic differentiated thyroid cancer
- Struma ovarii

Abbreviations: TSH = thyroid-stimulating hormone.

Diagnosis

HISTORY AND PHYSICAL EXAMINATION

Classically, by history and/or examination, the patient usually has one or more of the following: nervousness; weight loss; increased appetite; palpitations; tachycardia; generalized pruritus; hand tremor; hyperdefecation; diaphoresis; irritability; insomnia and muscle weakness; widened pulse pressure with systolic hypertension; hyperreflexia; lid lag; warm, moist skin; irritability; and inability to concentrate. However, a given patient may exhibit these findings to a varying extent. Elderly patients in particular may present in a more subtle fashion, perhaps demonstrating only weight loss, weakness, depression, or atrial fibrillation. Commonly, patients have an enlarged thyroid gland. In Graves' disease the thyroid gland is enlarged and smooth possibly with an overlying bruit. Patients with Graves' disease may demonstrate extrathyroidal findings such as diplopia, burning or itching eyes, lid lag or retraction, extraocular muscle involvement, proptosis, or even, on rare occasions, decreased vision. Pretibial myxedema, onycholysis, and acropachy may occur. The thyroid gland is nodular in patients with a multinodular goiter or solitary autonomous nodule. Patients with granulomatous (de Quervain's thyroiditis) subacute thyroiditis may have a history of recent viral infection, neck pain that can radiate to the jaw or chest, and a tender goiter. Patients with postpartum thyroiditis present within 6 to 12 months of gestation. Subacute, postpartum, and silent thyroiditis tend to evolve through various stages of hyperthyroidism and hypothyroidism before usually returning to the euthyroid state. Patients with exogenous thyrotoxicosis may have no goiter. Those with iodine-induced thyrotoxicosis have a history of recent exposure to iodinated contrast agents (e.g., computed tomography [CT] scan, angiogram). Rarer causes of hyperthyroidism are a thyroid-stimulating hormone (TSH)-secreting pituitary tumor and human chorionic gonadotropin (hCG)-mediated disease. Metastatic follicular cancer and struma ovarii are usually evident by history and physical examination.

LABORATORY EVALUATION

The diagnosis is established by having an undetectable TSH (<0.01 mU/L) and elevated T$_4$ and/or T$_3$. TSH assays vary in their sensitivity, and in some assays a TSH less than 0.05 mU/L is also consistent with the diagnosis. Free T_4 (FT_4) hormone determinations are preferable to total T_4. Total T_3 is still more easily obtained than Free T_3 (FT_3). Binding protein abnormalities such as elevated thyroxine-binding globulin (TBG) induced by pregnancy and estrogen administration interfere with total hormone assays. However, a variety of circumstances such as systemic illness and medications may interfere with TSH and FT_4 and FT_3 assays. Secondary hypothyroidism, nonthyroidal illness, Amiodarone (Cordarone),[1] glucocorticoid therapy, and excess exogenous thyroid hormone administration may cause discordant thyroid hormone tests results, usually with relatively decreased T_3 concentrations. It is always prudent to interpret the thyroid function tests carefully with consideration of the clinical condition.

A radioactive iodine uptake (RAIU) and scan may be helpful (Box 2). Patients can be divided into high uptake hyperthyroidism (Graves' disease, multinodular goiter, toxic adenoma) and low uptake hyperthyroidism (subacute, silent, postpartum thyroiditis, Amiodarone (Cordarone)[1]-induced disease, and exogenous thyroid hormone administration). Patients taking thyroid hormones for replacement therapy may have subclinical or overt hyperthyroidism because of overtreatment. Thyrotoxicosis may also occur when patients unwittingly take over-the-counter *nutraceuticals* containing thyroid hormone extracts or analogues or when they surreptitiously take thyroid hormone for weight loss or other purposes. In both cases, patients usually do not have a goiter and the thyroid uptake is low (<3%; normal 24-hour 131-I uptake is 8% to 30%). Measurement of a serum thyroglobulin level (not antibody) may be helpful in discriminating different causes of low uptake hyperthyroidism. If a patient is taking exogenous L-thyroxine, the serum thyroglobulin level is low (e.g., <5 ng/mL) because there is no intrathyroidal synthesis and secretion of iodothyronines. If the patient has destructive thyroiditis (e.g., subacute, silent, postpartum), however, the serum thyroglobulin level is elevated (usually greater than 20 ng/mL) because there is release of hormones into the circulation.

Except for over-replacement with exogenous L-thyroxine administration, in all age groups, Graves' disease is the most common cause of hyperthyroidism. Graves' disease is an autoimmune disease in which thyrotropin receptor-stimulating antibodies stimulate thyroid gland growth, thyroid hormone synthesis, and release. The most important differential diagnosis is with thyroiditis (through disruption of the thyroid follicles and release of preformed thyroid hormones) and toxic nodular disease (multinodular goiter or toxic adenoma). Graves' disease is associated with increased thyroid hormone production and is associated with high-normal (in spite of suppressed TSH levels) or more typically increased 131-I uptake. Although TSH receptor antibodies are present in almost all patients with Graves' disease, I measure them only in specific circumstances (e.g., diagnosis in doubt, pregnancy with hyperthyroidism).

Thyroiditis may be indistinguishable from Graves' disease in the absence of extrathyroidal manifestations of the latter. In contrast to Graves' disease, thyroiditis is associated with low 131-I uptake (<3%). Additionally, patients with granulomatous (subacute) thyroiditis may have anterior neck pain, elevated sedimentation rate, and elevated white blood count. Patients with transient lymphocytic thyroiditis may have a painless goiter, family history of autoimmune disease, and antithyroperoxidase (anti-TPO) antibodies. Postpartum thyroiditis occurs within approximately 6 months of delivery and also occurs more frequently in patients with thyroid antibodies.

Toxic multinodular goiters (Plummer's disease) are more frequent in the elderly and may be difficult to diagnose. Patients usually present with large multinodular glands, but in some patients the goiter could be substernal and, therefore, not palpable in the neck. Elderly patients may present with cardiac arrhythmias, weight loss, and fatigue. Patients with multinodular goiter are especially prone to developing thyrotoxicosis after iodine exposure (e.g., following radiocontrast injection). A patient with a toxic solitary adenoma has a *hot* nodule on thyroid isotope scan.

Therapy

GRAVES' DISEASE WITH HYPERTHYROIDISM

The first goal of therapy is to render the patient euthyroid with an antithyroid agent and to treat hyperadrenergic activity with a β-blocker. Thionamides are antithyroid drugs that inhibit the synthesis of thyroid hormones with gradual decreases in the concentrations of T_3 and T_4 over several weeks of treatment. I start propylthiouracil (PTU) at doses of 50 to 100 mg orally every 8 hours for mild or moderate disease and 200 mg every 8 hours for more severe disease. Alternatively, methimazole (Tapazole) at doses of 10 to 20 mg (once daily) are used for mild to moderate disease and 20 to 40 mg (once daily) for more severe disease. In men and postmenopausal women I prefer methimazole (Tapazole), rather than PTU, because it can be administered once daily. The frequency of possible complications (skin rash, arthralgias, liver toxicity, and bone marrow suppression) is probably comparable with these two medications. Methimazole (Tapazole) has been associated with a congenital defect called *aplasia cutis*. It is preferable to use PTU in child bearing aged women who may become pregnant or breast-feed as PTU binds more strongly to serum proteins (as compared with methimazole [Tapazole]), and only a small amount of PTU crosses the

---

[1]Not FDA approved for this indication.

placenta or gets into breast milk. PTU inhibits T_4 to T_3 conversion, but this effect probably is of minimal clinical effect. It generally takes approximately 2 to 8 weeks of antithyroid drug (ATD) treatment for the thyroid function tests to normalize. At this point, the conversations regarding definitive therapy should become more intense. Occasionally, the serum TSH concentration remains suppressed for a long time, regardless of the serum T_4 and T_3 levels. Accordingly, serum T_4 and T_3 levels and the clinical condition must be interpreted in the context of the serum TSH level to assess when a patient is euthyroid. In some instances, I administer definitive therapy initially when the patient originally presents with hyperthyroidism. This approach is also reasonable but in the majority of cases I prefer to render the patient euthyroid first. The reasons for this approach include the observation that occasionally 131-I therapy may exacerbate hyperthyroidism but, most importantly, hyperthyroid patients may have difficulty concentrating and making rational, well-considered decisions. Treatment with ATDs for several weeks prior to definitive therapy allows the patient (and family) to carefully consider the options and make the best individual decision.

Definitive treatment options include ATDs, 131-I therapy, or surgery (Box 3). ATDs may be used for an arbitrary time period (usually a year) in an effort to induce a *permanent* remission. The likelihood that a persistent remission will occur is relatively unusual and appears to correlate with multiple factors. Favorable factors at initial presentation include mild hyperthyroidism, small goiter, and negligible or undetectable titers of thyrotrophin receptor stimulating antibodies. The ATD dose is modulated on a frequent basis for the year of treatment to maintain a normal FT_4 and T_3. TSH should not be used as the sole indicator of thyroid function. To monitor for possible adverse effects of ATD, I suggest measuring CBC with differential, liver function tests and thyroid function tests every 4 to 6 weeks while taking an ATD. The long-term remission rate after ATD is discontinued is probably in the 10% to 20% range. Relevant articles in the literature are difficult to apply to a given patient population because of varying degree of initial hyperthyroidism and varying follow-up intervals after putative remission. If someone has or is suspected of having a major side effect, the patient is asked to immediately discontinue the offending agent and to contact their primary care doctor or the emergency room if they develop a sore throat or any significant febrile illness. It is appropriate to see these patients expeditiously and obtain appropriate laboratory studies. Patients receiving ATDs require close monitoring of thyroid function during initiation, maintenance, and discontinuation to ascertain recurrence of hyperthyroidism. In my practice, few patients opt for this approach and often prefer other forms of therapy.

In some instances as initial therapy and also in a patient who has a recurrence (usually 3 to 6 months after ATD discontinuation), radioactive iodine (RAI) or surgery is then recommended. RAI therapy has been used for more than 60 years and is very effective and safe. The goal of 131-I therapy is permanent hypothyroid. Hypothyroidism typically develops approximately 2 to 3 months after 131-I administration. Patients require close follow-up during this time period and frequently require ATD for 1 to 2 months after 131-I therapy. As the FT_4 and total T_3 (TT_3) return to the normal range, the dose of ATD is gradually decreased and then discontinued. When the FT_4 decreases to the lower portion of the normal range or to below it, I start L-thyroxine therapy. Frequently the TSH rises to above the normal range, but some patients have persistent suppression of this axis even despite the development of hypothyroidism. Few patients require a second dose of 131-I, which would not be given until at least 6 months after the initial dose.

The 131-I dose is estimated from goiter size and RAI uptake using the following formula:

$$\frac{100 - 200\ \mu Ci \times thyroid\ gland\ weight\ [g]}{24\ RAIU\ [\%]}$$

The usual dose is 10 to 20 mCi. In adult women of childbearing potential a negative pregnancy (and appropriate clinical history) is required within 2 to 3 days of the 131-I therapy. Patients are informed of the recommended radiation precautions. Some patients may experience a short-lived exacerbation of thyroid symptoms or anterior neck pain following 131-I treatment. Serum FT_4/FT_3 and TSH are checked roughly every 4 weeks after treatment. When the TSH rises above the normal range and/or the FT_4 starts to fall into the lower portion of the normal range or below the normal range, I start levothyroxine (Synthroid) (1.7 μg/kg per day) with the goal to achieve a TSH between 0.5 to 3.0 mU/L (and FT_4/T_3 within the upper part of the normal range). This therapy is continued for life with yearly monitoring. Patients with significant ophthalmopathy may have an exacerbation of their eye problems following 131-I treatment. Smoking is also considered a risk factor for ophthalmopathy. Patients with significant ophthalmopathy are given prednisone 0.5 mg/kg per day starting several days prior to 131-I therapy and continued for approximately 2 weeks with tapering over the following 1 to 2 weeks.

Near-total or bilateral subtotal thyroidectomy represents an effective treatment that resolves the thyrotoxic symptoms, usually resulting in postoperative hypothyroidism requiring lifelong levothyroxine (Synthroid) replacement. Thyroidectomy is an effective option for patients who require immediate relief of their thyrotoxic symptoms, with large goiters (especially with compressive symptoms), with suspicious or malignant nodules,

---

BOX 3   Treatment Options

- Short term
  Thionamide (PTU or methimazole [Tapazole])
  β-blocker
- Rare
  SSKI or Lugol's[1] solution
  Lithium
  Potassium perchlorate[1]
- Definitive therapy
  Thionamide
  131-I
  Thyroidectomy

---

[1]Not FDA approved for this indication.
Abbreviations: PTU = propylthiouracil; 131-I = radioactive iodine; SSKI = saturated solution of potassium iodide.

with contraindications to 131-I (pregnancy) or ATDs, and preferring definitive treatment without radiation. Surgical morbidity is lower in centers with more surgical experience. As a result, permanent hypoparathyroidism, vocal cord dysfunction because of recurrent laryngeal nerve injury, infection, and hematoma are rare complications.

When any thyrotoxic patient requires control of β-adrenergic symptoms, I tend to use either once daily long-acting propranolol (Inderal LA)[1] 80 mg per day, or atenolol (Tenormin),[1] 50 mg per day. Occasionally, propranolol (Inderal)[1] 20 mg twice a day may be used. β-blockers[1] provide faster relief than ATDs and are particularly useful in the preoperative period. The goal is to maintain a pulse rate below 100 beats per minute (bpm). β-Blockers[1] do not directly affect thyroid gland secretion. Stable iodine (see Box 3) decreases the release of glandular hormones and is effective for approximately 7 to 14 days. Lugol's solution (8 mg iodide per drop) given as 5 drops three times per day or saturated solution of potassium iodide (SSKI, 40 mg iodide per drop) given as 1 to 2 drops three times per day can be beneficial as adjunctive therapy in the preparation of patients for surgery (in combination with β-blockers and ATD). In atypical additional circumstances Lugol's solution or SSKI can be used as adjunctive therapy to lower thyroid hormone levels in patients who require rapid restoration of thyroid hormone levels to normal. However, stable iodine should be given cautiously because iodine-containing preparations may actually exacerbate hyperthyroidism when given to unblocked patients, especially when used for more than 10 to 14 days. Stable iodine preparations abrogate the ability of the thyroid gland to concentrate 131-I probably for at least several weeks or longer.

SPECIAL SITUATIONS

Toxic Multinodular Goiter (Plummer's Disease)

131-I therapy or thyroidectomy represent effective treatment choices for patients with a toxic multinodular goiter. If the RAIU is sufficiently elevated, a relatively high dose (30 mCi) of 131-I can be administered with follow-up measurements of TSH, FT_4 and TT_3 levels. 131-I can also be considered in patients who are poor surgical candidates, assuming the RAIU is sufficiently elevated. 131-I therapy is associated with approximately a 20% chance of recurrence, in which case patients can receive a second dose of 131-I or opt for thyroidectomy.

Toxic Adenoma

For young patients and patients with a small (less than 4 cm) toxic nodule, either radioactive iodine therapy or surgery can be used. A single dose of 20 to 30 mCi 131-I results in resolution of the hyperthyroidism with hypothyroidism occurring in approximately 28% of patients at 5 years of age and in approximately 60% at 20 years of age. The thyroid nodule may decrease its function but remain as a structural entity in approximately 50% of cases. Patients with larger nodules are generally recommended to have surgery. Although there is a scant likelihood of malignancy, I frequently recommend a fine-needle aspiration.

Subacute Thyroiditis

For patients with subacute thyroiditis, treatment is supportive with β-blockers and analgesics. Patients with moderate to severe pain, usually who also have an elevated white blood count and sedimentation rate, prednisone therapy (40 mg per day for 7 to 10 days with tapering over 1 to 2 weeks) may provide immediate relief of the neck pain but is not believed to affect the natural evolution of the thyroid hormones.

Amiodarone (Cordarone)[1]

Amiodarone (Cordarone)[1]-associated hyperthyroidism may be related to iodine excess (type 1) or to a toxic effect of the molecule on the thyroid gland, resulting in thyroiditis (type 2). Type 1 disease is treated with ATD and rarely with potassium perchlorate,[1] which inhibits the ability of the thyroid gland to trap iodine, but this medication may be associated with agranulocytosis in rare circumstances. When use of potassium perchlorate[1] is necessary, it should be only for a short time. Type 2 disease can be treated with prednisone (40 mg per day for 7 to 10 days with tapering over 1 to 2 weeks). In patients with mild to moderate amiodarone (Cordarone)[1]-associated hyperthyroidism, I use β-blockers[1] and ATD. If this does not control the disease or if the original presentation is severe, the additional use of prednisone and/or perchlorate may be indicated. Most patients do not have a pure presentation of either type 1 or type 2 disease. Because 131-I therapy can not be used because of the iodine contained in amiodarone (Cordarone),[1] thyroidectomy must be considered in some patients when the medical modalities fail. Thyroidectomy in these patients is inherently fraught with difficulty: The patients may not be euthyroid and they obviously have underlying cardiac disease. The adverse thyroid effects can persist or become manifest as long as 6 to 12 months after amiodarone (Cordarone)[1] is discontinued. Amiodarone (Cordarone)[1] associated thyrotoxicosis may be very complex, and it is preferable an experienced team treats these patients.

Subclinical Hyperthyroidism

Subclinical hyperthyroidism is defined as subnormal TSH in the context of normal T_4 and T_3. Subclinical hyperthyroidism represents part a continuum of disease, and in general the signs and symptoms are less pronounced than in patients with overt hyperthyroidism (elevated T_4 and T_3 with decreased TSH). Patients with subclinical hyperthyroidism are at increased risk for atrial fibrillation and enhanced bone loss, especially if they are older than 60 years of age. Thyroid function tests should be repeated several times over several weeks or months to ensure the persistence of disease. The intervals of assessing repeat thyroid function tests depend on the severity of clinical disease. Because patients may even be asymptomatic, they are less willing, perhaps appropriately, to accept definitive

---

[1]Not FDA approved for this indication.

[1]Not FDA approved for this indication.

therapy such as 131-I therapy or surgery. I prefer to offer this group of patients ATD for 6 to 12 months in an effort to induce a remission. In contrast to overt symptomatic Graves' disease, patients with subclinical hyperthyroidism may have a higher chance of persistent remission following discontinuation of ATD. Nonetheless, the pathophysiology of the subclinical hyperthyroidism is not well studied, and the likelihood of inducing a remission is also unclear. TSH values that apply to this patient group are less than 0.1 mU/L and most frequently less than 0.01 mU/L. Patients who have a TSH of 0.1 to 0.45 mU/mL may not require therapy and could be monitored, although this is a case-by-case decision.

Pregnancy

Thyrotoxicosis during pregnancy is almost always caused by Graves' disease and tends to improve as the pregnancy proceeds. PTU is the ATD of choice with the goal of keeping serum FT_4 levels in the upper part of the normal range. FT_3 is preferable to follow as compared with total T_3. FT_3 levels should be maintained in the middle portion of the normal range. TSH receptor antibodies should be measured in the second or third trimester because this helps predict the development of neonatal hyperthyroidism. Close cooperation is required with the obstetrician. Maternal thyroid function tests should be monitored frequently, and it may be helpful for the obstetrician to monitor fetal thyroid gland size. Mothers may experience an exacerbation of thyrotoxicosis after delivery. All infants of mothers with Graves' disease should have thyroid function tests within the first few days of life and should be seen by a neonatologist.

A separate cause of hyperthyroidism in pregnancy is because of hCG elevations. During the first trimester, in some women hCG elevations bind to the thyroidal TSH receptor and induce thyroid gland secretion with an elevation of T_4/T_3 and resultant TSH inhibition. This cause of hyperthyroidism is usually mild and may be associated with hCG-induced hyperemesis. This type of hCG-induced hyperthyroidism is usually temporary and does not typically require treatment, except in extremely unusual

CURRENT DIAGNOSIS

- Use the history and physical examination, in conjunction with the thyroid function tests, to assess the degree and severity of hyperthyroidism.
- Graves' disease may be associated with extrathyroidal manifestations.
- Assessment of RAIU (low versus high) may help determine the etiology.
- TSH should be undetectable for patients with hyperthyroidism.
- Be alert for unusual or unexpected complications or special circumstances, such as thyroid nodules that may harbor malignancy, adverse effects of medications, worsening disease, or pregnancy.
- Discuss therapeutic options with the patient.

Abbreviations: RAIU = radioactive iodine uptake; TSH = thyroid-stimulating hormone.

CURRENT THERAPY

- All patients should have thorough history and physical examinations as well as complete laboratory evaluations.
- Assess clinical status; more severely ill patients should be monitored closely and treated more aggressively.
- Close monitoring with frequent analysis of clinical status and laboratory studies are important.
- In most circumstances restore moderate or severely hyperthyroid patients to the euthyroid state prior to giving definitive therapy.

circumstances. In contrast to Graves' disease patients, patients with hCG-induced elevations of thyroid secretion do not have a significantly enlarged thyroid gland, TSH receptor antibodies are negative, there is no ophthalmopathy, and in general the degree of elevations of FT_4 and T_3 is minimal.

REFERENCES

Burman KD, Cooper DS: The diagnostic evaluation and management of hyperthyroidism due to Graves' disease, toxic nodules and toxic multinodular goiter. In Cooper DS (ed): Medical Management of Thyroid Disease. New York, Marcel Dekker, 2001, pp 33-92.

Burman KD, Wartofsky L: Iodine effects on the thyroid gland: Biochemical and clinical aspects. Rev Endocr Metab Disord 2000; 1:19-25.

Burman KD: Graves' disease in women: Proper therapy depends on an accurate diagnosis. Women's Health in Primary Care. 2001;4:306-308

Ceccarelli C, Bencivelli W, Vitti P, et al: Outcome of radioiodine-131 therapy in hyperfunctioning thyroid nodules: A 20 years' retrospective study. Clin Endocrinol (Oxf) 2005;62:331.

Cooper DS: Antithyroid drugs in the management of patients with Graves' disease: An evidence-based approach to therapeutic controversies. J Clin Endocrinol Metab 2003;88:3474.

Cooper DS: Antithyroid drugs. N Engl J Med 2005;352:905.

Kazlauskaite R, Weintraub BD, Burman KD: Evaluation of thyroid function tests. In Humes HD (ed): Kelley's Textbook of Internal Medicine, Fourth Edition. New York, Lippincott Williams & Wilkins, 2000, pp 2821-2829.

Martino E, Bartalena L, Bogazzi F, Braverman LE: Amiodarone and the thyroid. Endocr Rev 2001;22:240.

Reinwein D, Benker G, Lazarus JH, Alexander WD: A prospective randomized trial of antithyroid drug dose in Graves' disease therapy: European multicenter study group on antithyroid drug treatment. J Clin Endocrinol Metab 1993;76:1516.

Surks MI, Ortiz E, Daniels GH, et al: Subclinical thyroid disease: Scientific review and guidelines for diagnosis and management. JAMA 2004;291:228.

Torring O, Tallstedt L, Wallin G, et al: Graves' hyperthyroidism: Treatment with antithyroid drugs, surgery, or radioiodine. A prospective, randomized study. Thyroid study group. J Clin Endocrinol Metab 1996;81:2986.

Weetman AP: Graves' disease. N Engl J Med 2000;343:1236.

Thyroid Cancer

Method of
Debra G. Koivunen, MD

A discussion about thyroid cancer necessarily entails an overview of thyroid nodules. As much as 8% of the population will harbor a nodule in their thyroid, but only 5% of these will prove to be malignant. Therefore, the diagnostic approach to a patient presenting with a mass in his or her thyroid must be able to differentiate the few patients with a malignant process from the greater majority with benign disease. Of note, over the last several years, the workup of thyroid nodules has changed, allowing a nonoperative approach and thus sparing many patients diagnostic surgery. With the increased use of ultrasonic and radiological visualization of the neck for other nonendocrinologic diseases, more patients with occult lesions in the thyroid are being brought to our attention, thus making our understanding of the precise diagnostic approach and decision for surgery even more important. From the patients' perspective, the good news remains that the majority of thyroid malignancies are slow growing and associated with a long survival.

Diagnosis

Although the history and physical examination may lead one to suspect a malignancy, the majority of patients do not have suggestive complaints or findings. Certainly, a history of a rapidly growing mass, new onset of hoarseness, low-dose head or neck irradiation, or family history of medullary carcinoma will all raise suspicion of malignancy, as would a hard irregular or fixed mass in the thyroid or cervical lymphadenopathy on physical examination. However, many patients with benign disease can also present with some of these findings, and most patients with malignancy will have none. The risk of thyroid cancer is considered equally as high for incidentally discovered nodules less than 10 mm as for larger nodules detected on palpation or by symptomatology. The fact that the thyroid is located relatively deep in the neck behind muscles and fat makes the physical detection of nodules as large as 2 cm difficult in some patients and subsequently insensitive for differentiating malignancy. Nearly all patients presenting with a thyroid nodule will be clinically and chemically euthyroid, but a suppressed serum thyroid-stimulating hormone (TSH; thyrotropin) level indicates a possible benign hyperfunctioning nodule. These particular patients should then undergo a radionuclide thyroid scan to confirm this entity. Chemically euthyroid patients need not undergo a thyroid scan because 90% of their nodules will be nonfunctioning (or "cold") and only 5% of these nodules will be malignant, rendering the radionuclide scan of little help.

Ultrasonography can give an accurate measurement of the thyroid nodule and detect nonpalpable lesions. It can distinguish solid nodules from simple cysts and mixed (cystic and solid) lesions, and it reveals characteristics suggestive of malignancy, such as hypoechogeneity, microcalcifications, irregular margins, nodular dimensions that are taller than wide, and increased blood flow within the nodule. Ultrasonography is also used to guide needle aspiration biopsy of thyroid nodules, adding an element of accuracy during this procedure for both palpable and nonpalpable lesions of interest.

Ultimately, the only way to prove malignancy is to obtain tissue for microscopic evaluation. Fine-needle aspiration is an inexpensive, safe, and uncomplicated modality that is performed in the clinical setting with or without ultrasonic guidance. It has a false-positive rate of only 1% to 2%, and a low false-negative rate of 2% to 5%. Cytologists can accurately diagnose papillary, medullary, and anaplastic carcinomas from the aspirated cells, and they can usually differentiate lymphoma and metastatic lesions. However, follicular neoplasms and Hürthle cell lesions cannot be judged benign or malignant based on fine-needle aspiration cytology; patients with these lesions must be directed to a surgeon for diagnostic unilateral thyroid lobectomy. Obviously, any aspiration attempts that fail to produce a diagnosis ("insufficient" or "nondiagnostic") must be repeated or the patient sent for surgical biopsy (lobectomy). Nodules proven to be cytologically benign may be observed, managed medically, or surgically removed based on the patient's symptoms, change in nodule size over time, or the patient's level of concern.

A special mention is needed concerning solitary cervical lymph nodes that yield "thyroid cells" on needle aspiration biopsy. These patients should be considered to have a thyroid malignancy that has manifested initially as a metastasis to a node, and they require no further workup other than referral to a surgeon.

Histologic Classification and Pathophysiology

Although only 5% of thyroid nodules are malignant, thyroid cancer is the most common endocrine malignancy, accounting for more than 22,000 new cases each year. Of these cases, papillary cancer is the most common, constituting

---

CURRENT DIAGNOSIS

- History
  - New-onset hoarseness
  - Rapid growth
  - Head or neck low-dose irradiation
  - Family history
- Physical Examination
  - Hard or fixed mass in thyroid lobe
  - Cervical lymphadenopathy
- Laboratory Test: Serum Thyroid-Stimulating Hormone Level
  - If suppressed, obtain radionuclide thyroid scan
- Consider Ultrasound to Characterize Nodule
- Fine-Needle Aspiration Biopsy (Possible Outcomes)
  - Papillary, medullary, anaplastic, lymphoma
  - Follicular neoplasms, Hürthle cell neoplasms
  - Benign nodular hyperplasia or colloid nodule
  - Insufficient or nondiagnostic

75% to 80% of all thyroid malignancies and 90% of radiation-induced thyroid tumors. Papillary cancers arise from follicular cells and include multiple variants: papillary, papillary–follicular mixed, tall cell, columnar cell, oxyphilic, encapsulated, and occult microcarcinomas. The latter are most often incidental microscopic findings from a thyroid lobe surgically removed for another unrelated lesion. Papillary cancers are characterized microscopically by psammoma bodies, intranuclear grooves, and cytoplasmic inclusions. They are multifocal in 30% to 50% of cases and bilateral in 33%. They tend to metastasize initially to cervical lymph nodes, with 30% to 50% of patients having cervical node involvement at the time of diagnosis. Only 2% of patients will present initially with systemic metastases. Papillary cancer is familial in 3% of patients. Because of the follicular origin of papillary cancer, the cells concentrate radioiodine, which can be used for adjuvant therapy and follow-up. The 20-year survival rate for patients with papillary cancer is excellent at 90%.

Follicular cancers also arise from follicular cells and account for 10% of all thyroid cancers. They tend to be solitary lesions, and because the diagnosis is based on invasion of the tumor capsule, neither fine-needle aspiration biopsy nor frozen section pathologic evaluation at the time of surgery can distinguish between this cancer and its benign counterpart, the follicular adenoma. Follicular cancers tend to spread hematogenously to lungs and bone, with only 10% of patients developing cervical lymph node metastases. Similar to papillary cancer, follicular cancer cells concentrate radioiodine. The overall 10-year survival rate for patients with follicular carcinoma is 86%.

Hürthle cell carcinomas are similar to follicular cancers but display greater involvement of cervical lymph nodes. They have a benign counterpart, the Hürthle cell adenoma. The malignant version accounts for only 5% of all thyroid cancers. Unlike the more common follicular thyroid cancer, 90% of Hürthle cell carcinomas do not concentrate radioiodine, and they have higher recurrence and mortality rates. The 10-year survival rate for patients with these tumors is 70%.

Anaplastic cancers are markedly more lethal malignancies, constituting 2% to 4% of thyroid cancers. They occur in patients older than 60 years and tend to arise within well-differentiated cancers of follicular origin or occasionally within long-standing goiters. These tumors are fast growing, locally invasive, and respond poorly to most therapies. Anaplastic cancer cells do not have the ability to concentrate iodine. The overall 5-year survival rate is only 3%.

Medullary thyroid cancers are different from the preceding malignancies in that their cell of origin is the "C cell" or parafollicular cell, which produces calcitonin. Medullary cancers account for only 5% of all thyroid malignancies, and 75% of these will be sporadic. Most of the nonfamilial cases will be unilateral. The familial cancers tend to be bilateral and associated with C-cell hyperplasia. They are autosomal dominant disorders that occur as a result of one of several germ line mutations in the RET proto-oncogene (which codes for a tyrosine kinase receptor) and can be a component of the multiple endocrine neoplasia (MEN) type 2 syndromes (Table 1). Because of this situation, patients diagnosed with medullary carcinomas must undergo screening for pheochromocytomas before undergoing thyroidectomy in order to avoid severe intraoperative blood pressure fluctuations.

TABLE 1 Familial Medullary Thyroid Carcinoma

Familial Non-MEN Medullary Thyroid Carcinoma

Multiple Endocrine Neoplasia Type 2A (Sipple's Syndrome)

Medullary thyroid carcinoma	100%
Pheochromocytoma	30%–40%
Hyperparathyroidism	25%–35%

Multiple Endocrine Neoplasia Type 2B

Medullary thyroid carcinoma	100%
Pheochromocytoma	50%–90%
Mucosal neuromas	100%
Marfanoid body habitus	100%

Familial medullary carcinoma as a single entity and as part of the multiple endocrine neoplasia (MEN) type 2 syndromes. Percentages indicate the frequency of the different components of the syndrome types.

Patients who are diagnosed as having MEN type 2A or 2B syndrome with associated pheochromocytomas will require localization, biochemical block, and surgical removal of their adrenal/extra-adrenal tumors prior to undergoing thyroid surgery. Conversely, asymptomatic members of families known to carry a RET proto-oncogene mutation should be screened for the mutation at an early age. It has been recommended that children carrying this mutation undergo total thyroidectomy any time between the ages of 6 months to 10 years (depending on the specific mutation detected) to avoid the 100% certainty of medullary cancer later in life along with its associated 10-year mortality rate of 25% to 40%.

Lymphomas of the thyroid account for less than 1% of all thyroid malignancies and are often associated with Hashimoto's thyroiditis. They are usually non-Hodgkin's, B-cell type and of intermediate or high grade. They are more common in women and present as a rapidly enlarging goiter. After tissue diagnosis has been established, patients with a thyroid lymphoma should undergo the appropriate workup and medical management of their disease. Surgery for debulking is rarely indicated and is helpful for prognosis only if the disease is confined to the thyroid.

Rarely, other malignancies manifest by metastasizing to the thyroid. The most common primary lesions that can present in this manner include melanoma, breast cancer, renal cell, and lung carcinomas.

Treatment

The universally accepted therapy for most thyroid cancers is surgical resection; the controversy arises when discussing how extensive the excision should be and whether adjuvant therapy is necessary. This argument applies only to thyroid cancers of follicular cell origin (papillary and follicular cancers). Medullary carcinomas must be subjected to total thyroidectomy because parafollicular cells do not take up radioiodine, negating the ability to use this modality postoperatively for treatment or follow-up of patients. Central neck node dissection is also usually performed and supplemented by a modified lateral neck node dissection for larger tumors or evidence of

CURRENT THERAPY

- Follicular and Hürthle Cell Neoplasms
  - Unilateral lobectomy until pathology is determined
  - Return to operating room for contralateral procedure if pathology malignant
- Papillary Cancers
  - If diagnosis is known preoperatively, perform bilateral resection
  - If malignancy is determined after unilateral procedure, consider contralateral resection based on risk-group prognosis and ease of follow-up
- Postoperative Management of Papillary and Follicular Cancers
  - If only unilateral resection was performed, lifelong suppression of thyroid-stimulating hormone, followed by physical examination and possibly ultrasonography
  - If bilateral resection was performed and based on risk-group prognosis and stage, consider radioiodine ablation, then follow long term with thyroid scans and possibly thyroglobulin assays
- Medullary Thyroid Cancer
  - Bilateral total thyroidectomy with node dissection
  - Follow long term with calcitonin and carcinoembryonic antigen assays

involved nodes. Occasionally, performance of bilateral neck node dissections is necessary, particularly in patients with familial disease. As mentioned earlier, it is imperative to rule out the presence of a pheochromocytoma in patients with medullary carcinoma before subjecting them to a thyroidectomy.

No prospective randomized studies have evaluated the extent of thyroidectomy, management of cervical node metastases, or the added value of postoperative radioiodine ablative therapy for patients with differentiated thyroid cancer of follicular cell origin. Many of these patients will be diagnosed with papillary or follicular cancer only after they have undergone unilateral lobectomy for a solitary nodule. The question then arises as to whether they would benefit from a second surgical procedure without incurring more risk of complications. These risks include injury to the recurrent and/or superior laryngeal nerves (bilateral injury to the recurrent laryngeal nerves can compromise the patient's airway, necessitating a tracheostomy) as well as hypoparathyroidism if more than two glands are compromised during surgery. Additionally, postoperative radioactive iodine ablation and scans for long-term follow-up cannot be used unless a bilateral thyroid resection has been performed. In an attempt to provide a better understanding of long-term prognosis for these patients and to aid in determining extent of therapy, several scoring systems have been developed over the years. Most notable are the **AMES** (Lahey Clinic; **A**ge, distant **M**etastases, **E**xtent of primary, **S**ize) and the **MACIS** (Mayo Clinic; distant **M**etastases, **A**ge, **C**ompleteness of resection, local **I**nvasion, tumor **S**ize) prognostic scales, both of which sort patients into low- and high-risk groups for both recurrence and mortality. In any

prognostic or staging system (Tables 2 and 3), age is the most important variable, with younger patients faring noticeably better. Tumor size is also important, but the presence of cervical lymph node metastases does not necessarily portend a worse survival for most patients.

Most experts agree that patients with papillary cancers smaller than 1 cm and minimally invasive follicular cancers

---

TABLE 2 Low- and High-Risk Groups for Recurrence and Mortality from Papillary and Follicular Thyroid Cancer

Low Risk
- Women <50 yr
- Men <40 yr
- Well- or moderately well-differentiated tumors
- Tumors <4 cm in diameter
- Tumor confined to the thyroid gland
- No distant metastases

High Risk
- Women ≥50 yr
- Men ≥40 yr
- Poorly differentiated tumors, tall cell, columnar cell, or oxyphilic variants of papillary carcinoma
- Tumor >4 cm in diameter
- Local invasion
- Distant metastases

TABLE 3 Staging of Thyroid Cancer

A. Definitions
- Primary tumor (T)
  - T0 = No evidence of primary tumor
  - T1 = Tumor ≤1 cm
  - T2 = Tumor >1 cm but ≤4 cm
  - T3 = Tumor >4 cm
  - T4 = Tumor extending beyond the thyroid capsule
- Nodal disease (N)
  - N0 = No regional lymph node metastases
  - N1 = Regional lymph node metastases
- Systemic metastases (M)
  - M0 = No distant metastases
  - M1 = Distant metastases

B. American Joint Committee on Cancer Stage Grouping

Papillary, follicular, and Hürthle cell cancer

	Age <45 yr	Age ≥45 yr
Stage I	Any T, any N, M0	T1N0M0
Stage II	Any T, any N, M1	T2 or T3, N0M0
Stage III	T4 or N1M0	
Stage IV	Any T, any N, M1	

Medullary thyroid cancer

Stage I	T1N0M0
Stage II	T2 or T3 or T4, N0, M0
Stage III	Any T, N1, M0
Stage IV	Any T, any N, M1

Anaplastic thyroid cancer (all cases are classified as stage IV)

Stage IV	Any T, any N, any M

can appropriately undergo thyroid lobectomy and isthmusectomy followed by lifetime suppression of TSH secretion with L-thyroxine. Patients who fall into a high-risk group (see Table 2) should undergo either a total or near-total thyroidectomy followed by radioiodine scanning and ablation of any remaining tissue. Patients who fall in the low-risk category will cause the most consternation regarding therapy; most endocrinologists favor completion contralateral resections if the patient is willing to undergo additional surgery. This then allows the ability to follow patients with postoperative scans and thyroglobulin assays. My personal preference is to perform a bilateral procedure initially if the diagnosis of papillary cancer has already been established, because by definition the tumor in question is no longer an "occult" cancer. However, if a papillary cancer (<1 cm) is found "incidentally" in a lobectomy specimen removed for another separate focus of pathology, I am comfortable placing the patient on L-thyroxine suppression, assuming he or she falls into the low-risk category for prognosis. Most endocrinologists prefer a bilateral procedure if the initial lobectomy yields a follicular cancer, because the long-term survival statistics are not as impressive as seen with papillary cancer and they want to be able to reliably screen the patient for recurrent disease.

The other controversy involves the use of radioiodine ablation. Two relatively sensitive means are available to follow papillary and follicular thyroid cancer patients for recurrence: radioactive iodine total body scans and thyroglobulin assays. Both are based on the premise that no functioning thyroid tissue remains in the patient's body. In order to use either technique, the patient must have most or all of his or her thyroid surgically removed, followed by radioiodine ablation of any microscopic residue during a hypothyroid (high TSH) state. Subsequent scans may then be performed at 6- to 12-month intervals, again in a high-TSH state. An alternative mode of screening for recurrent disease is to assay thyroglobulin levels in patients following the ablation of thyroid tissue described. Patients need not be hypothyroid for this periodic measurement because thyroglobulin is not present in any thyroid hormone replacement preparations. If at any time thyroglobulin is detected, the patient then undergoes radioiodine total body scanning in a hypothyroid state to localize (and potentially treat) the site of tumor.

The most pressing concern in patients with anaplastic thyroid cancer is assurance of a patent airway while they undergo external beam radiation and/or chemotherapy. This most often requires the placement of a tracheostomy. Rarely, these patients present with a surgically resectable tumor.

Long-Term Follow-up

Regardless of whether a unilateral or bilateral resection has been performed, patients with follicular or papillary thyroid cancer must be placed on L-thyroxine suppression, keeping the serum TSH level less than 0.3 μIU/mL. Differentiated thyroid cancers of follicular cell origin have TSH receptors in the cell walls and respond to TSH stimulation. For patients who have undergone total ablation of their thyroid glands through a combination of bilateral resection and radioiodine ablation, it is now possible to use recombinant human thyrotropin (rhTSH) in preparation for a subsequent total body follow-up scan instead of rendering patients uncomfortably hypothyroid. Another alternative is to stop their L-thyroxine therapy and place them on liothyronine (Cytomel) for approximately 3 weeks while their circulating T_4 levels disappear. They then can stop taking liothyronine and develop the needed high TSH levels over the course of 7 to 10 days, greatly diminishing the length of time needed to develop the necessary clinical hypothyroidism to facilitate the scan. As mentioned earlier, an alternative or complementary method for detecting recurrent or metastatic disease is measurement of the serum thyroglobulin level. This can usually be done with the patient in the euthyroid state (on thyroid replacement therapy), but occasionally patients develop disease without detectable circulating levels of thyroglobulin. It is recommended that a TSH-stimulated thyroglobulin level (using rhTSH) be checked periodically to rule out the possibility in patients who are at high risk for recurrent disease. Patients who underwent only unilateral surgical resections can be followed by only physical examination of their necks supplemented by ultrasonography, searching for enlarged lymph nodes or unexplained masses in either the operative site or the contralateral lobe.

Patients with medullary thyroid cancer are followed postoperatively with serum calcitonin and carcinoembryonic antigen levels every 3 to 6 months for the first 2 years, then yearly thereafter if no elevations are detected. Because medullary thyroid cancer cells are not affected by TSH stimulation, it is only necessary to maintain patients on replacement (instead of suppressive) doses of L-thyroxine postoperatively. There is no role for thyroid scans or thyroglobulin measurements in these patients. All patients with thyroid cancer should also be followed with thorough routine physical examinations of their necks, looking specifically for evidence of local recurrence or new lymphadenopathy.

REFERENCES

Hay ID, Thompson GB, Grant CS, et al: Papillary thyroid cancer managed at the Mayo Clinic during six decades (1940-1999): Temporal trends in initial therapy and long-term outcome in 2444 consecutively treated patients. World J Surg 2002;26:879-885.

Hegedus L: The thyroid nodule. N Engl J Med 2004;351:1764-1771.

Hundahl SA, Cady B, Cunningham MP, et al: Initial results from a prospective cohort study of 5583 cases of thyroid carcinoma treated in the United States during 1986: An American College of Surgeons Commission on cancer patient care evaluation study. Cancer 2000;89:202-217.

Mazzaferri EL, Robyn J: Postsurgical management of differentiated thyroid carcinoma. Otolaryngol Clin North Am 1996;29:637-662.

Quayle FJ, Moley JF: Medullary thyroid carcinoma: including MEN 2A and MEN 2B syndromes. J Surg Oncol 2005;89:122-129.

Sanders LE, Cady B: Differentiated thyroid cancer: Reexamination of risk groups and outcome of treatment. Arch Surg 1998;133:419-425.

Schlumberger MJ: Medical progress: papillary and follicular thyroid carcinoma. N Engl J Med 1998;338:297-306.

Pheochromocytoma

Method of
Massimo Mannelli, MD, and
Jacques W. M. Lenders, MD, PhD

Pheochromocytoma is a tumor arising from the chromaffin cells of the adrenal medulla. These cells derive from the embryonic neural crest and are sympathetic in origin. When the tumor occurs in chromaffin cells located in the abdomen and thorax, it is called paraganglioma.

Both pheochromocytomas and thoracic and abdominal paragangliomas secrete catecholamines (CAs) with both metabolites and variable amounts and types of peptides. Paragangliomas can arise also in the head and neck region. These tumors are parasympathetic in origin and do not secrete CAs. The most frequent localization is in the carotid body; but the vagal, jugular, and tympanic ganglions can also be affected.

Pheochromocytomas are rare tumors causing hypertension in approximately 0.1% of all hypertensive patients. Pheochromocytoma is clinically relevant as a cause of cardiovascular damage and as a potentially life-threatening condition in cases of massive and abrupt, spontaneous, or provoked secretion.

Clinical Presentation

Pheochromocytoma and paraganglioma secretions are characterized by high variability; this accounts for the large variation in their clinical picture. No signs, symptoms, or associations are specific enough to permit diagnosis on a clinical basis. The most frequent signs and symptoms are reported in Table 1. These are mainly caused by the activation of adrenergic receptors caused by CAs released by the tumor.

The possibility of a pheochromocytoma should be considered in the event of a hypertensive crisis, but not every hypertensive spell is caused by a pheochromocytoma. Approximately one third of patients with pheochromocytoma have no symptoms, and one fifth does not even have hypertension. Sometimes the clinical picture is so

TABLE 1 Most Frequent Signs and Symptoms in Patients with Pheochromocytoma and Paraganglioma

Signs or Symptoms	Frequency (%)
Headache	90-50
Sweating	75-50
Palpitations	70-60
Paroxysmal hypertension	60-30
Anxiety	40-35
Nausea	40-20
Dyspnea	20
Dizziness	20
Postural hypotension	15
Diarrhea or constipation	10
Fever	2

insignificant (or absent) that the first sign of the condition is the discovery of an adrenal incidentaloma, and many pheochromocytomas are first discovered at autopsy.

Hypertension can be continuous or intermittent, and hypertensive crises can supervene a condition of hypertension or normotension. Because of the ambiguous characterization of the disease, pheochromocytoma has been nicknamed *the great mimic*, and clinicians need a high degree of clinical alertness to diagnose pheochromocytoma. The primary symptoms that may suggest pheochromocytoma are the presence of a hypertensive crisis, intermittent or resistant hypertension, especially in young patients, or the finding of an adrenal incidentaloma.

Head and neck paragangliomas do not generally secrete CAs and are diagnosed by the discovery of a neck mass or compression symptoms such as dysphagia, dysphonia, or neurologic deafness. They may also be discovered during radiologic examination of the neck, such as a thyroid sonography.

Genetics

Recent advances in genetics have clearly shown that the familial forms of pheochromocytoma and paraganglioma occur more frequently than previously thought, accounting for at least 25% of all cases. The susceptibility genes known to predispose to pheochromocytoma and paraganglioma formation are the von Hippel-Lindau (VHL), RET and neurofibromatosis type I (NF1) genes, and the more recently discovered genes encoding for three (SDHD, SDHB, and SDHC) of the four subunits of the mitochondrial complex 2, succinate-dehydrogenase (SDH). The characteristics of these genes are reported in Table 2.

There are families affected by pheochromocytomas where no germline mutations of these susceptibility genes have been found. This suggests that other, still unknown genes might be involved in the pathogenesis of these tumors. As one out of four patients with a pheochromocytoma or paraganglioma is a carrier of a germline mutation, genetic screening might be suggested for every affected patient. Genetic testing is mandatory in young patients, patients with multiple or recurrent pheochromocytomas and paragangliomas, or in those showing an association with clinical features suggesting one of the previously mentioned syndromes (Table 3). Detection of a germline mutation is clinically relevant for patients and their relatives. Each mutation carrier is at risk for developing additional pheochromocytomas, paragangliomas, and other syndrome-related diseases whose prognosis is ameliorated by an early diagnosis.

Diagnosis

Pheochromocytomas and paragangliomas that are sympathetic in origin are diagnosed based on the measurement of secreted CAs or their metabolites in plasma or urine. Diagnosis of head and neck paragangliomas starts from the discovery of a mass or from mass-induced neurologic complications, such as deafness, dysphagia, or dysphonia. The sensitivity and specificity of the different assays for the diagnosis of pheochromocytoma or paraganglioma is reported in Table 4. In cases of suspected

TABLE 2 Characteristics of Genes Responsible for Familial Forms of Pheochromocytoma

Gene	Syndrome	Chromosome	Exons	Protein
VHL	von Hippel-Lindau	3p25-26	3	pVHL19 pVHL30
RET	MEN2	10q11.2	21	Tyrosine-kinase receptor
NF1	NFI	17q11.2	59	Neurofibromin
SDHB	PGL4	1p36.13	8	Catalytic iron-sulfur protein
SDHC	PGL3	1q21.23	6	CybL (membrane-spanning subunit)
SDHD	PGL1	11q23	4	CybS (membrane-spanning subunit)

Abbreviations: MEN2 = multiple endocrine neoplasia, type 2; NF1 = neurofibromatosis type 1; PGL = paraganglioma; SDH = succinate dehydrogenase; VHL = von Hippel-Lindau.

pheochromocytoma and paraganglioma, it is important to avoid false negative results. The best tests are those with a higher sensitivity, such as measurement of plasma and urinary metanephrines (MNs). Metanephrines should be measured differentially because in some patients the tumor, especially if small, might secrete only mild amounts of a single compound. For example, in patients affected by a small pheochromocytoma caused by a RET mutation, MN might be the only increased compound.

The higher sensitivity of MNs in comparison to CAs is because pheochromocytomas and paragangliomas possess high metabolic intratumoral activity and secrete MNs continuously, whereas CA secretion is often periodic. In a minority of affected patients showing a mild increase in plasma or urinary MNs, the diagnosis may need a confirmatory test, such as the clonidine suppression test. Oral administration of 300 µg of clonidine can normalize plasma CAs in cases of an increased release by sympathetic activation, but it does not decrease plasma CAs secreted by the tumor.

Localization

Once diagnosed, the tumor must be localized. Approximately 90% of all tumors are in the adrenal glands, and most extra-adrenal tumors are in the abdomen. The first recommended radiologic exams are an abdominal

TABLE 3 Clinical Pictures of Syndromes Associated with Pheochromocytoma and Paraganglioma

Multiple Endocrine Neoplasia	Von Hippel-Lindau Disease	Neurofibromatosis Type 1	Paraganglioma Syndromes (PGL1, PGL3, PGL4)
Type 2A: Medullary thyroid carcinoma • Pheochromocytoma • Hyperparathyroidism • Lichen cutaneous	**Type 1:** Without pheochromocytoma • Hemangioblastomas (retinal and CNS) • Renal cysts and carcinomas • Pancreatic cysts and tumors • Endolymphatic sac tumors • Epididymal cystoadenomas	Multiple neurofibromas on skin and mucosae	Head and neck paragangliomas (carotid body, vagal, jugular, tympanic)
FMTC: Isolated familial thyroid carcinoma	**Type 2:** With pheochromocytoma **2A:** • Hemangioblastomas (retinal and CNS) • Pheochromocytomas • Endolymphatic sac tumors • Epididymal cystoadenomas	*Café au lait* spots on skin	Abdominal or/and thoracic paragangliomas
Type 2B: Medullary thyroid carcinoma • Pheochromocytoma • Marfanoid habitus • Multiple mucosal neuromas	**2B:** • Hemangioblastomas (retinal and CNS) • Renal cysts and carcinomas • Pheochromocytomas • Pancreatic cysts and tumors • Endolymphatic sac tumors • Epididymal cystoadenomas **2C:** Pheochromocytoma (only)	Pheochromocytoma	Pheochromocytomas

Abbreviations: CNS = central nervous system; FMTC = familial medullary thyroid carcinoma; PGL = paraganglioma.

CURRENT DIAGNOSIS

- Because of the high variability of the signs and symptoms, the suspicion of pheochromocytoma requires high clinical alertness by the physician. Hypertensive spells are the clinical hallmark. Pheochromocytoma should be suspected in the presence of hypertension, especially if labile, resistant, or in young patients; or in the presence of an adrenal incidentaloma or of a genetic syndrome characterized by the presence of a tumor.

- Diagnosis stems from laboratory tests demonstrating excessive or abnormal levels of catecholamines or metabolites in plasma or urine. The most sensitive and most recommended assays are plasma or urinary metanephrines.

- Approximately 90% of pheochromocytomas are in the adrenals. The first step to localize the tumor is a CT or NMR scan of the abdomen. Total body scintigraphy with ^{123}I-MIBG is a complementary test that permits the diagnosis of multiple or metastatic lesions. The PET scan with fluorodopa or fluorodopamine is a new and promising scintigraphic tool.

- Genetic screening for mutations in one susceptibility gene (VHL, RET, NF1, SDHD, SDHB, SDHC) is recommended, especially in young patients, in the case of multiple tumors, or a clinical picture suggesting familial syndromes.

- Malignancy is diagnosed only by the presence of metastases.

Abbreviations: CT = computed tomography; ^{123}I-MIBG = ^{123}I-meta-iodobenzylguanidine; NF1 = neurofibromatosis type I; NMR = nuclear magnetic resonance; PET = positron emission tomography; VHL = von Hippel-Lindau.

computed tomography (CT) or nuclear magnetic resonance imaging (NMRI). Both offer high sensitivity, especially for adrenal pheochromocytomas, but lack specificity because they can only suggest and not assure the chromaffin origin of the tumor. Chromaffin origin can be suspected at NMRI by finding high T2-weighted signal intensity.

Conversely, total body scintigraphy using ^{123}I-meta-iodobenzylguanidine (^{123}I-MIBG) offers high specificity, but sensitivity is less than 90%. It also permits detection of multiple chromaffin tumors and metastatic lesions. Similar specificity and higher sensitivity seem to be offered by the positron emission tomography (PET) scan using fluorodopa

TABLE 4 Sensitivity and Specificity of Different Biochemical Tests for Diagnosis of Pheochromocytoma

Assay	Sensitivity (%)	Specificity (%)
Plasma-free MNs	99	89
Urinary fractionated MNs	97	69
Urinary catecholamines	86	88
Plasma catecholamines	84	81
Urinary total MNs	77	93
Vanillylmandelic acid	64	95

Abbreviation: MNs = metanephrines.

or fluorodopamine as a tracer. In very limited cases, when both radiology and nuclear medicine do not permit tumor localization, CA measurement in specimens sampled along the main venous tree may indicate the tumor site showing a concentration gradient.

Therapy

The therapy for pheochromocytomas and paragangliomas is surgical. Medical therapy is pivotal before and during surgery. Medical therapy with α-adrenoceptor blockers, introduced after 1950, substantially changed the intraoperative and postoperative mortality rates of patients with pheochromocytoma.

PREOPERATIVE MEDICAL TREATMENT

Before and during surgery, risk is constituted by a massive spontaneous or provoked release of CAs by the tumor, causing generalized vasoconstriction by the activation of α-adrenoceptors, thus eliciting a sharp increase in blood

CURRENT THERAPY

- Surgery is the only curative therapy. The laparoscopic technique is the first choice.

- In cases of bilateral pheochromocytoma, adrenal sparing surgery is recommended to avoid chronic hypocortisolism.

- Presurgical medical preparation of the patient stems from therapy with α-antagonists. The most widely used drugs are phenoxybenzamine and doxazosin.

- β-Blockers can be used to reduce tachycardia but only after an adequate α-blockade.

- Volume expansion with saline or plasma expanders is recommended in the days before surgery.

- Anesthesia should be performed using inhalation or IV agents that do not cause catecholamine release.

- Continuous monitoring of the patient's cardiovascular parameters should be performed during and after surgery.

- Supervening hypertensive spells can be treated with IV phentolamine (Regitine), magnesium sulphate, or nitroprusside (Nitropress).

- Supervening arrhythmias can be treated with IV lidocaine or short-acting β-blockers.

- Therapy of malignant pheochromocytoma is palliative. It is based on primary tumor debulking, α-methyl-*p*-L-tyrosine (Demser) (to reduce catecholamine synthesis), α-antagonists (to reduce catecholamine adverse effects), chemotherapy, and/or radiopharmaceutical administration of ^{131}I-MIBG.

- Strict clinical control of the patient is recommended in the first 24 to 48 hours after surgery to prevent complications such as hypoglycemia or hypotension.

- Recurrences, including subsequent development of metastases, remain possible after successful resection of a pheochromocytoma; thus, each patient should be advised to undergo periodic biochemical testing for detecting recurrent disease.

Abbreviations: ^{131}I-MIBG = ^{131}I-meta-iodobenzylguanidine; IV = intravenous.

pressure (BP). These adverse cardiovascular effects are reduced by α-blockers.

After surgery, risk for patient is constituted by a deep and long-lasting decrease in BP caused by a general vasodilatation once the surgeon has clamped the venous pole of the tumor, thus reducing the plasma CA concentration abruptly. The fall in BP is made more profound by the reduction in plasma volume, caused by the previous general vasoconstriction and by the reduced vascular sensitivity to endogenous or exogenous amines caused by receptor down-regulation.

When given before surgery, α-antagonist administration decreases BP, increases plasma volume, and limits receptor down-regulation, reducing postoperative risk of severe hypotension. Therefore, α-blocking therapy before surgery is highly recommended. The most used α-antagonists are phenoxybenzamine (Dibenzyline) and doxazosin (Cardura).[1] Phenoxybenzamine is a noncompetitive, nonselective α-antagonist. It binds covalently with both α_1- and α_2-adrenoceptors, offering a stable receptor blockade whose duration depends on receptor recycling. Phenoxybenzamine is administered orally in capsules of 10 mg. Recommended doses range from 10 to 80 mg/day. Binding to presynaptic α_2-adrenoceptors causes an increase in norepinephrine release from the sympathetic nerve endings. As a consequence, tachycardia ensues and needs to be controlled by β-blockers, such as propranolol (Inderal) or bisoprolol (Zebeta). The long-lasting effect of phenoxybenzamine is desirable before and during surgery, but it can be negative once the tumor is removed. Therefore, some authors suggest administering the last dose at least 12 hours before surgery. Additional, less-important side effects of phenoxybenzamine are postural hypotension, nasal stiffness, and anejaculation.

Doxazosin[1] is a competitive, selective α_1-antagonist available for oral use in tablets of 1, 2, 4, or 8 mg. It can be displaced from adrenoceptors by endogenous amines. The higher the plasma CA level, the higher the dose of doxazosin to be administered. Daily doses range from 6 to 30 mg,[3] administered in one or more doses. Being a selective α_1-antagonist, doxazosin does not cause tachycardia, and β-blocker administration is seldom required. Side effects are limited to postural hypotension. Other less used α_1-antagonists are terazosin (Hytrin)[1] or prazosin (Minipress).[1] Their shorter half-life necessitates more frequent dosing.

It is important to remember that β-blockers must never be used before an appropriate α-blockade has been established. By antagonizing vasodilator β-receptors, β-blockers can worsen a hypertensive crisis. Labetalol (Normodyne, Trandate)[1] is a mixed α- and β-antagonist with higher β- than α-blocking activity, and some authors do not recommend its use in patients with pheochromocytoma. Calcium antagonists, such as Nifedipine (Adalat)[1] or other dihydropyridines, can be administered as alternative or in addition to α-antagonists to improve vasodilatation. Medical preparation for surgery also requires volume expansion, which can be obtained by saline infusion (1.5 to 2.0 L daily, 2 to 3 days before surgery).

There are no established clinical parameters to assure the clinician of a good presurgical preparation, but 24-hour BP monitoring showing a permanent decrease in BP values less than 160/90 mm Hg should be accepted as a favorable index.

Some patients with pheochromocytoma and paraganglioma are normotensive, and treating them with α-antagonists is still debated. Many authors recommend to treat normotensive patients, especially those who, in spite of their normal BP, show elevated plasma or urinary CAs.

Pheochromocytoma occurring during pregnancy is exceptionally rare and extremely dangerous. Mother's and fetal's survival are greatly improved by predelivery diagnosis and treatment. The tumor should be suspected in any pregnant women affected by hypertension, especially if in the first trimester or paroxysmal. Differential diagnosis with preeclampsia is difficult. Phenoxybenzamine has been widely used without adverse consequences to the fetus and the mother. After appropriate medical preparation, laparoscopic removal can be performed, preferably during the second trimester. If pheochromocytoma is diagnosed later, surgery is delayed until delivery.

INTRAOPERATIVE MEDICAL TREATMENT

Good medical preparation should eliminate or limit hypertensive spells before or during surgery. These are still possible depending on the tumor's tendency to release large amounts of CAs or with surgical manipulation of the tumor. Hypertensive crises should be promptly treated with intravenous (IV) phentolamine (Regitine) administration. Phentolamine is available in ampules of 10 mg and should never be administered as a bolus but infused slowly, monitoring the decrease of BP. Alternative drugs are magnesium sulphate or nitroprusside (Nitropress).

Cardiac arrhythmias ensuing during surgery can be treated with lidocaine or β-blockers, such as esmolol (Brevibloc), propranolol (Inderal), or metoprolol (Lopressor).

Medical presurgical treatment should eliminate consistent fall in BP once the tumor is removed. Should this happen, hypotension can be corrected by volume expansion or, in severe cases, by phenylephrine, vasopressin, or hydrocortisone infusion. Hypoglycemia, which may occur after tumor excision, should be treated by infusion of 5% dextrose.

ANESTHESIA

General anesthesia is generally preceded by the patient's sedation with benzodiazepines or barbiturates. Induction can be achieved using thiopental, propofol (Diprivan), or etomidate (Amidate). Agents that can cause direct or indirect release of CAs, such as ketamine (Ketalar), ephedrine, morphine, and droperidol (Inapsine) should be avoided. Muscle relaxation is obtained using pancuronium (Pavulon), Cisatracurium (Nimbex), or vecuronium (Norcuron). Other muscular blockers such as succinylcholine (Quelicin), atracurium (Tracrium), tubocurarine,[2] gallamine (Flaxedil), and curare[1] are not recommended. Inhalation agents, sevoflurane (Ultane), isoflurane (Forane), and enflurane (Ethrane) are the most widely used. Halothane and desflurane (Suprane) are not recommended.

---

[1]Not FDA approved for this indication.
[3]Exceeds dosage recommended by the manufacturer.

[1]Not FDA approved for this indication.
[2]Not available in the United States.

MEDICAL TREATMENT OF METASTATIC PHEOCHROMOCYTOMA

Malignant pheochromocytomas and paragangliomas are characterized by the presence of metastasis and cannot be effectively cured. Malignancy is present in approximately 10% of all cases but is higher in large paragangliomas, especially in SDHB-mutated tumors where it is higher than 35%. Metastatic tissue determines high levels of circulating CAs, and palliative therapy is directed to limiting hypertension and the toxic effects of CAs, especially on the heart. Debulking surgery is indicated for large primary tumors, followed by medical therapy with α-methyl-*p*-L-tyrosine, associated or not to α- and β-blockers.

α-Methyl-*p*-L-tyrosine (Demser) reduces the synthesis of CAs by inhibiting tyrosine hydroxylase, the rate-limiting enzyme in the synthesis of CAs. Although sometimes used before surgery, it is generally administered to patients with metastatic pheochromocytomas presenting high levels of CAs and poorly controlled BP. Recommended doses range from 250 to 500 mg three to four times a day.

Malignant pheochromocytomas are resistant to chemotherapy, but partial remission has been reached in approximately 50% of patients after combined administration of vincristine (Oncovin), dacarbazine (DTIC-Dome), and cyclophosphamide (Cytoxan).

An additional option is radiopharmaceutical therapy with high doses of ^{131}I-MIBG. This therapy is able to improve symptoms in approximately 70% of patients and reduce plasma CAs in approximately 50%; complete remissions are very rare. Additional palliative options can be external beam radiation, radiofrequency, cryoablation, or arterial embolization. Malignant pheochromocytoma is a progressive disease, but combined palliative treatment is able to improve quality of life and life expectancy significantly. Although the course of the disease can be very variable, some patients are still alive 15 or more years after identification of metastases.

SURGICAL TREATMENT

Surgery is the only way to cure pheochromocytomas and paragangliomas. Laparoscopic removal of the tumor is the best option. Although abdominal insufflation can cause CAs release, tumor manipulation is highly reduced using this technique. Reduced surgical invasiveness and cosmetic damage, shorter hospitalization period, and faster recovery are major additional advantages. Several laparoscopic approaches have been performed, including the anterior or lateral transabdominal approaches and the posterior or lateral retroperitoneal approaches.

In the case of bilateral pheochromocytomas, despite a higher risk of recurrency, sparing adrenalectomy on at least one gland is often recommended to avoid chronic hypocortisolism, which requires lifelong treatment with glucocorticoid and mineralocorticoid replacement therapy. After the successful removal of a pheochromocytoma, approximately 60% of hypertensive patients become normotensive.

Laparoscopic surgery can also be performed to remove abdominal paragangliomas. Head and neck paragangliomas should be removed by an experienced head and neck surgeon. In the absence of other chromaffin tumors in the abdomen or the thorax, patients can undergo surgery without α-antagonist pretreatment. Surgical risk is mainly represented by local hemorrhage and permanent lesions of the head and neck nerves.

Follow-up

A patient with a sporadic tumor is considered disease free if laboratory test results are normal 4 to 6 weeks after surgery. Control of plasma or urinary MNs is recommended annually because in some cases, benign pheochromocytomas turn out to be malignant with metastatic spread many years after surgery. In patients receiving surgery for a familial pheochromocytoma, clinical, laboratory, and radiologic control is recommended approximately twice a year throughout the life of the patient.

Pheochromocytomas and paragangliomas are rare tumors, difficult to diagnose, and dangerous because of their potential cardiovascular complications. Correct management of these patients can be achieved only through close collaboration between experienced endocrinologists, anesthesiologists, and surgeons.

REFERENCES

Baysal BE, Willett-Brozick JE, Lawrence EC, et al: Prevalence of SDHB, SDHC and SDHD germline mutations in clinic patients with head and neck paragangliomas. J Med Genet 2002;39:178-183.

Bravo EL, Tagle R: Pheochromocytoma: State-of-the-art and future prospects. Endocr Rev 2003;24:539-553.

Eisenhofer G, Bornstein SR, Brouwers FM, et al: Malignant pheochromocytoma: Current status and initiatives for future progress. Endocr Relat Cancer 2004;11:423-436.

Gimenez-Requeplo AP, Favier J, Rustin P, et al: Mutations in the SDHB gene are associated with extra-adrenal and/or malignant phaeochromocytomas. Cancer Res 2003;63:5615-5621.

Kinney MA, Narr BJ, Warner MA: Perioperative management of pheochromocytoma. J Cardiothorac Vasc Anesth 2002;16:359-369.

Lenders JW, Pacak K, Walther MM, et al: Biochemical diagnosis of pheochromocytoma: Which test is best? JAMA 2002;287:1427-1434.

Lenders JWM, Eisenhofer G, Mannelli M, Pacak K: Pheochromocytoma Lancet 2005;366:665-675.

Maher ER, Eng C: The pressure rises: update on the genetics of pheochromocytoma. Hum Mol Genet 2002;11:2347-2354.

Neumann HP, Bausch B, McWhinney SR, et al: Germ-line mutations in nonsyndromic pheochromocytoma. N Engl J Med 2002;346:1486-1488.

Pacak K, Eisenhofer G, Goldstein DS: Functional imaging of endocrine tumors: Role of positron emission tomography. Endocr Rev 2004;25:268-280.

Plouin PF, Duclos JM, Soppelsa F, et al: Factors associated with perioperative morbidity and mortality in patients with pheochromocytoma: Analysis of 165 operations at a single center. J Clin Endocrinol Metab 2001;86:1480-1486.

Pry-Roberts C, Farndon JR: Efficacy and safety of doxazosin for perioperative management of patients with pheochromocytoma. World J Surg 2002;26:1037-1042.

Thyroiditis

Method of
Petros Perros, BSc, MBBS, MD

To pathologists the term *thyroiditis* applies to conditions associated with acute or chronic inflammatory infiltration of the thyroid gland. The list of pathologies is long and includes rarities that most clinical practitioners are unlikely to encounter (Table 1). From the clinical perspective, thyroiditis is a distinct syndrome that typically consists of an initial phase of thyrotoxicosis followed by hypothyroidism and finally by spontaneous restoration of the euthyroid state over a period of weeks or months (Figure 1). The pathophysiologic basis of this triphasic natural history is that thyroid epithelial cells are traumatized by one of a variety of insults; thus, preformed thyroid hormones stored in colloid are released to the systemic circulation causing thyrotoxicosis. The serum thyroxine concentration tends to be more raised in relation to the triiodothyronine (T_3) concentration compared to other causes of thyrotoxicosis, such as toxic multinodular goiter or Graves' disease. The damaged thyroid epithelium then is unable to synthesise thyroid hormones for a period of time thus leading to hypothyroidism. In due course thyrocytes recover and euthyroidism ensues.

Subacute Thyroiditis (de Quervain's Thyroiditis)

The typical presentation is that of a viral illness usually with a sore throat associated with pain and tenderness in the thyroid bed. Painful dysphagia may also be a feature, and in some cases patients are aware of a tender goiter. The thyrotoxic phase occurs a few weeks after the viral illness. It is unclear whether there is direct invasion of thyrocytes by viruses or whether the immune response to the virus causes the thyroiditis. Histologically, giant cells are seen infiltrating the thyroid. Common respiratory

TABLE 1 Causes of Thyroiditis

Common
- Viral (de Quervain's) thyroiditis
- Postpartum thyroiditis
- Silent thyroiditis
- Amiodarone-induced thyroiditis
- Cytokine-induced thyroiditis
- Radiation-induced thyroiditis

Rare
- Acute suppurative thyroiditis
- Riedel's thyroiditis
- Lithium-induced thyroiditis

viruses are implicated. The diagnosis can be confirmed by raised inflammatory markers (elevated erythrocyte sedimentation rate [ESR], C-reactive protein [CRP]) and reduced or absent iodide uptake on thyroid scanning during the thyrotoxic phase (Figure 2). Management of this condition is symptomatic with analgesics (paracetamol [acetaminophen], 1 g four times a day) if required and β-blockers (propranolol [Inderal][1] slow release, 80 to 160 mg once daily) during the initial phase. Antithyroid drugs are ineffective because the problem lies in release of preformed thyroid hormones rather than new synthesis. In severe cases where the thyrotoxicosis is marked and/or the pain severe, a short course of steroids (prednisolone 40 mg once daily for 7 to 10 days) is effective. The hypothyroid phase is usually mild; but in some cases when patients are symptomatic, thyroxine may be justified for a few weeks or months (levothyroxine sodium [Synthroid], 50 to 100 μg daily). Permanent hypothyroidism follows in approximately 5% of cases. Occasionally subacute thyroiditis can recur.

Postpartum Thyroiditis

Postpartum thyroiditis (PPT) occurs in approximately 5% of women within 12 months of childbirth or after a miscarriage. The presence of antithyroid peroxidase antibodies

---

[1]Not FDA approved for this indication.

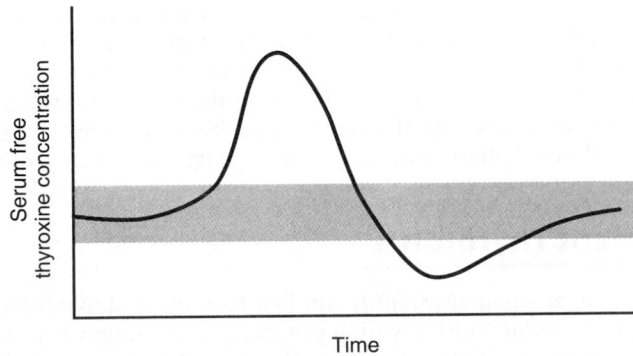

FIGURE 1. Natural history of thyroiditis, illustrating the transient phases of thyrotoxicosis, hypothyroidism, and euthyroidism. The hatched area represents the normal range for serum FT_4 concentration. *Abbreviation:* FT_4 = free thyroxine.

CURRENT DIAGNOSIS

- Patients presenting with thyrotoxicosis should be investigated to make an accurate diagnosis
- A tender goiter in association with thyrotoxicosis is highly suggestive of subacute thyroiditis
- A high serum FT_4 to FT_3 ratio is a clue that the underlying cause of thyrotoxicosis is thyroiditis
- A thyroid scan showing low or absent iodide uptake during the thyrotoxic phase is diagnostic of thyroiditis
- Serum anti-TPOAbs are raised in the vast majority of cases of postpartum, silent, and lymphocytic thyroiditis
- Inflammatory markers (ESR, CRP) are typically raised in subacute thyroiditis

Abbreviations: anti-TPOAb = antithyroid peroxidase antibody; CRP = C-reactive protein; ESR = elevated erythrocyte sedimentation rate; FT_3 = free triiodothyronine; FT_4 = free thyroxine.

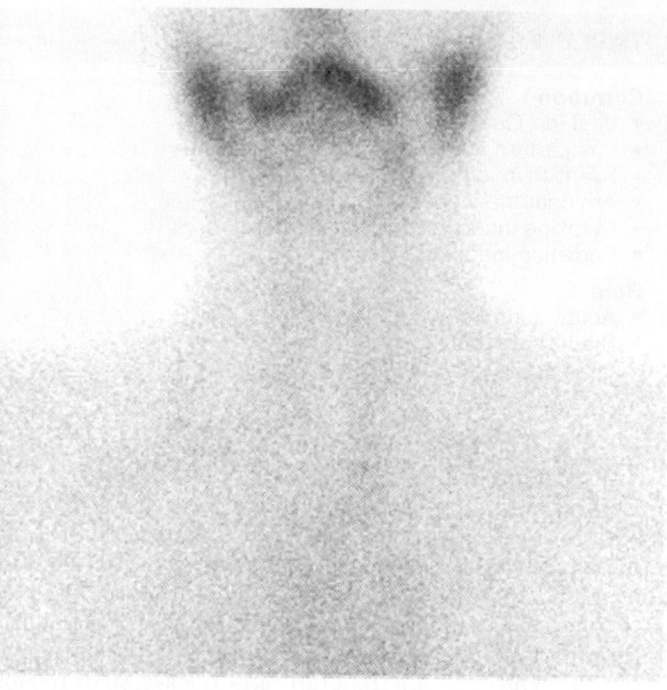

FIGURE 2. ^{123}I scan of the thyroid in a patient with viral thyroiditis demonstrating absence of isotope uptake in the thyroid bed, a typical feature of thyroiditis. *Abbreviation:* ^{123}I = iodine-123.

(anti-TPOAbs) prepartum increases the risk of PPT to 50%, but in most cases it is subclinical. Pain is not a feature of PPT. Different variants exist in addition to the classical thyrotoxic–hypothyroid–euthyroid scenario and include a thyrotoxic phase alone, a hypothyroid phase alone, and occasionally hypothyroidism followed by thyrotoxicosis. The underlying cause is autoimmune, and the thyroid gland shows typical features of lymphocytic thyroiditis. One hypothesis about the pathogenesis of PPT proposes that fetal cells settle in the maternal thyroid during pregnancy and subsequently provide the stimulus to the maternal immune system. A previous episode of PPT and smoking are risk factors for PPT. The diagnosis is confirmed by usually strongly positive anti-TPOAb and reduced or absent uptake on iodide scanning during the thyrotoxic phase. It is important to recognise PPT because the symptoms may be vague and mistakenly attributed to the upheaval of having and caring for a new infant. Furthermore, a previous episode of PPT is a significant risk factor for subsequent development of permanent hypothyroidism in up to 70% of women. Treatment may be required for symptomatic relief with blockers during the thyrotoxic phase. A course of thyroxine may be considered if the hypothyroid phase is accompanied by significant symptoms.

Silent Thyroiditis

The term *silent thyroiditis* applies to a clinical syndrome rather similar to PPT, which is unrelated to pregnancy and can occur in either sex. The pathophysiology is essentially the same as PPT. There is lymphocytic infiltration of the thyroid; strongly positive anti-TPOAb, low or reduced uptake on iodide scanning; and usually a triphasic clinical course. Management is similar to that of PPT.

Amiodarone-Induced Thyroiditis

Amiodarone has several complex effects on the thyroid, including direct toxicity on thyroid epithelial cells. Thyrotoxicosis in a patient receiving amiodarone (Cordarone) therapy is thought to result from two etiologies, but this is an oversimplification and an overlap probably exists. Patients with thyroid autonomy (usually caused by undiagnosed toxic nodular goiter or Graves' disease) can become frankly thyrotoxic because of the increased iodide availability provided by amiodarone. In such cases there is increased synthesis of thyroid hormones, and the treatment of choice is thionamide antithyroid drugs. Amiodarone-induced thyroiditis occurs because of release of preformed thyroid hormones. The clinical features of thyrotoxicosis may be masked because of the β-blocking effects of amiodarone and partly because the serum concentration of the biologically active thyroid hormone (T_3) is usually not markedly elevated. This effect is caused by blockade of the peripheral conversion of T_4 to T_3 by amiodarone. The thyrotoxic phase of amiodarone-induced thyroiditis may be prolonged and not followed by hypothyroidism. Amiodarone-induced thyroiditis may be effectively treated with steroids (prednisolone 30 to 40 mg daily for several weeks) or iopanoic acid[1] (500 mg twice daily for several weeks), but in some cases additional measures are required; and management can be difficult, particularly if the patient's cardiovascular status is compromised. In extreme cases plasma exchange and thyroidectomy may be necessary. Withdrawal of amiodarone should be considered particularly if other cardiac medications can be employed to treat the underlying arrhythmia effectively, or when the initial indication for amiodarone was not life-threatening. The effect of amiodarone withdrawal on the thyroid, however, is not immediate because significant amounts of drug are stored in fat.

Cytokine-Induced Thyroiditis

The introduction of interferon-α and interleukin-2 (Proleukin) in clinical practice for treatment of viral, autoimmune, and neoplastic diseases was followed by episodes of thyroiditis in a significant proportion of patients (up to 15% in interferon-α–treated patients). The clinical picture and management are similar to silent thyroiditis. Whether withdrawal of cytokine therapy is necessary is unclear at present. The underlying etiology is thought to be autoimmune in at least some cases and anti-TPOAbs are usually raised. Patients with positive anti-TPOAb before the introduction of these drugs have a higher risk of thyroiditis.

Radiation-Induced Thyroiditis

Thyroiditis can occur following external beam irradiation to the neck for malignant disease or after large doses of iodine-131 (^{131}I). The treatment is symptomatic as for other types of thyroiditis.

---

[1]Not FDA approved for this indication.

Chronic Lymphocytic Thyroiditis

Chronic lymphocytic thyroiditis is the most common cause of permanent hypothyroidism. The thyroid is often atrophic and shows evidence of lymphocytic infiltration. Lymphocytic thyroiditis may also be associated with a firm nodular goiter, and this clinical presentation is usually referred to as Hashimoto's thyroiditis. The goiter consists of infiltrating lymphocytes forming germinal centers. Hashimoto's thyroiditis may be associated with normal thyroid function or subclinical or clinical hypothyroidism. Occasionally Hashimoto's thyroiditis can cause alternating episodes of hyper- and hypothyroidism (also known as hashitoxicosis) caused by changes in the dominant autoantibodies to the TSH receptor from stimulatory to blocking types. The thyrotoxic phase of hashitoxicosis is caused by increased synthesis of thyroid hormones, and antithyroid drugs or radioiodine are effective. The underlying pathogenesis is autoimmune, and anti-TPOAbs are raised in most patients. Hashimoto's thyroiditis is closely related to postpartum and silent thyroiditis.

Other Rare Causes of Thyroiditis

Suppurative thyroiditis may be caused by bacteria or other microorganisms such as fungi and parasites. It usually occurs in immunocompromised patients and is accompanied by fever, pain, and obstructive symptoms. Treatment consists of antibiotics and surgical drainage.

Riedel's thyroiditis usually presents with a hard painless goiter. Thyroid autoantibodies are elevated in most cases, and many patients become eventually hypothyroid. The fibrotic process may spread to adjacent tissues and cause symptoms. Surgery may be required, although steroids and other drugs (methotrexate [Trexall] and tamoxifen [Nolvadex][1]) are also beneficial.

Lithium-treated patients have a greater-than-expected risk of both hypo- and hyperthyroidism.

REFERENCES

Ando T, Davies TF: Clinical Review 160: Postpartum autoimmune thyroid disease: The potential role of fetal microchimerism. J Clin Endocrinol Metab 2003;88:2965-2971.

Bogazzi F, Bartalena L, Cosci C, et al: Treatment of type II amiodarone-induced thyrotoxicosis by either iopanoic acid or glucocorticoids: A prospective, randomized study. J Clin Endocrinol Metab 2003;88:1999-2002.

Fatourechi V, Aniszewski JP, Fatourechi et al: Clinical features and outcome of subacute thyroiditis in an incidence cohort: Olmsted County, Minnesota, study. J Clin Endocrinol Metab 2003;88:2100-2105.

Lazarus JH, Ammari F, Oretti R, et al: Clinical aspects of recurrent postpartum thyroiditis. Br J Gen Pract 1997;47:305-308.

Monzani F, Caraccio N, Dardano A, Ferrannini E. Thyroid autoimmunity and dysfunction associated with type I interferon therapy. Clin Exp Med 2004;3:199-210.

Muller AF, Drexhage HA, Berghout A: Postpartum thyroiditis and autoimmune thyroiditis in women of childbearing age: Recent insights and consequences for antenatal and postnatal care. Endocr Rev 2001;22:605-630.

Oppenheim Y, Ban Y, Tomer Y: Interferon induced Autoimmune Thyroid Disease (AITD): A model for human autoimmunity. Autoimmun Rev 2004;3:388-393.

Pearce EN, Farwell AP, Braverman LE: Thyroiditis. N Engl J Med 2003;348:2646-2655.

Vestergaard P: Smoking and thyroid disorders—A meta-analysis. Eur J Endocrinol 2002;146:153-161.

Weetman AP: Autoimmune thyroid disease. Autoimmunity 2004;37:337-340.

[1]Not FDA approved for this indication.

CURRENT THERAPY

- In most patients with thyroiditis presenting with thyrotoxicosis, no treatment is required because symptoms are mild or absent and spontaneous recovery is expected.
- If the thyrotoxic symptoms are troublesome, β-blockers (propranolol[1] slow release, 80 to 160 mg once daily) are the treatment of choice. Thionamide drugs (carbimazole[2]/propylthiouracil) are ineffective and inappropriate because thyroid hormone synthesis is not increased in thyroiditis.
- Severe hypothyroid symptoms may merit thyroxine therapy (levothyroxine 50 to 100 μg once daily); but because the hypothyroidism is unlikely to be permanent, this treatment should be withdrawn after a few months.
- Women with a history of postpartum thyroiditis are at high risk of developing permanent hypothyroidism after several years.
- The management of amiodarone-induced thyroiditis is difficult and such patients should be managed by a specialist.

[1]Not FDA approved for this indication.
[2]Not available in the United States.

The Urogenital Tract

Bacterial Infections of the Urinary Tract in Males

Method of
*Brian A. VanderBrink, MD, and
Robert M. Moldwin, MD*

Epidemiology

The incidence of urinary tract infections (UTIs) in males follows a bimodal distribution with peaks in infancy and after 50 years of age likely secondary to the presence of foreskin and the effects of prostatic enlargement, respectively. Urinary tract infections in males of all ages are traditionally classified as *complicated* because of the high incidence of associated urologic abnormalities, including incomplete emptying, urolithiasis, and obstruction.

Infant Evaluation

Early diagnosis and treatment of a febrile UTI in the male infant is critical to preserve renal function of the growing kidney and to prevent progression to life-threatening septicemia. A history of vesicoureteral reflux (VUR) in a sibling suggests up to a 34% risk of VUR in the patient. When a UTI is suspected, obtaining a reliable urine culture, preferably by sterile urethral catheterization, is crucial to confirm the diagnosis. Once therapy is completed, a course of prophylactic antibiotics should begin to prevent further infections while evaluation continues. Further evaluation entails both ultrasound and voiding cystourethrogram to assess if obstruction or reflux exists, respectively.

Although epidemiology suggests the presence of foreskin is associated with a higher risk of neonatal UTI, recommending circumcision for prevention of recurring UTIs remains controversial. The benefits of circumcision may be more profound later in life because recent observational studies have demonstrated a protective effect of circumcision against HIV infection in high-prevalence regions.

Epididymitis

Bacterial infection of the epididymis is typically the result of sexual activity or bladder outlet obstruction, and the causative agent may differ dependent on the mechanism of inoculation. In males younger than 35 years of age with acute epididymitis, the most common isolated organisms include *Neisseria gonorrhoeae*, *Chlamydia trachomatis*, and *Ureaplasma urealyticum*, which are transmitted during unprotected sexual intercourse. Homosexual men who practice unprotected anal intercourse have a higher incidence of coliforms as the causative agent.

In males older than 35 years of age, *Escherichia coli* is the most frequent cause of epididymitis. Epididymitis is also potentiated by elevated intravesical pressures generated in patients with bladder outlet obstruction, thereby resulting in urethral-vasal reflux of enteric organisms. Tuberculosis is a rare but important cause of epididymitis that assumes a greater relative importance in high-prevalence regions.

Scrotal pain is present in all cases of epididymitis but is not pathognomonic, and the clinician must remember that the pain may be referred in origin. The significant findings on physical exam include preservation of cremasteric reflexes, a normal vertical lie of the testicle without foreshortening of the spermatic cord, and tender scrotal contents with particular tenderness and induration of the epididymis. A *reactive* hydrocele may be present, which precludes a complete physical examination of the scrotal contents. Doppler ultrasound is a useful adjunct to the history and physical examination, helping to differentiate acute epididymitis from surgical emergencies such as acute testicular torsion or an incarcerated inguinal hernia. Ultrasound may also be useful to diagnose scrotal abscess or guide scrotal drainage.

Prostatitis

Most forms of prostatitis are associated with pelvic, perineal, penile, and/or scrotal pain, but frequently no overt microbial etiology can be identified; hence, in 1995 the National Institutes of Health workshop on prostatitis classified prostatitis into four main categories:

1. Acute bacterial
2. Chronic bacterial
3. Chronic pelvic pain syndrome
4. Asymptomatic inflammatory prostatitis, collectively termed *chronic prostatitis/chronic pelvic pain syndrome* (CP/CPPS).

The hallmark features of category 1 prostatitis usually include those of acute bacterial cystitis and constitutional symptoms such as fever and chills. Acute urinary retention, progression to prostatic abscess, and frank sepsis is more common in diabetic and other immunocompromised patients. Category 2 prostatitis is typified by recurring urinary tract infections yet constitutes a small percentage of chronic prostatitis patients. In one study only 7% of 656 patients seen in a urology clinic for evaluation of prostatitis symptoms had bacteriologically proven category 2 disease.

Historically, categorization of prostatitis has been based on leukocyte and bacterial localization studies (from urine and expressed prostatic secretions) originally described in 1968 and simplified in 1997. However, even these *gold-standard* localization studies have been called into question with recent studies showing comparable rates of uropathogenic bacteria in both expressed prostatic secretions and postmassage urine cultures from men with chronic prostatitis/chronic pelvic pain syndrome and asymptomatic controls (8.0% versus 8.3%, respectively).

Key Treatment

Clinical presentation dictates medical care of the male presenting with UTI. For example, category 1 prostatitis may be associated with urinary retention for which Foley catheter or suprapubic drainage is required. Radiographic imaging to exclude abscess should be contemplated in the category 1 prostatitis or epididymitis patient with unremitting infection despite *adequate* antibiotic therapy.

Patients who appear nontoxic and are able to tolerate oral medications can be safely treated as outpatients. Empirical selection of the antibiotic and its duration is influenced by a number of variables including site of infection, antibiotic tissue penetration, patient allergy profile, patient current medications, and co-morbidities. Trimethoprim-sulfamethoxazole (TMP-SMZ) (Bactrim) is effective against most uropathogens with the notable exception of *Enterococcus* and *Pseudomonas* species; however, resistance to community-acquired organisms continues to grow. Because of their broad spectrum of activity and excellent tissue penetration, such as prostate and kidney, fluoroquinolones are an attractive class of antibiotics for outpatient therapy, especially in areas where TMP-SMZ resistance is high. Patients requiring hospitalization may require intravenous antibiotics to provide broad spectrum coverage while awaiting urine and blood culture and sensitivities.

Urinary tract infections in males are almost always characterized as complicated and therefore require 7 or more days of antibiotic therapy. With reference to duration of antibiotic therapy, no standard of care has been developed for genitourinary infections that are not associated with bacteremia. Common practice has been 10 to 14 days of antimicrobial therapy for epididymitis and 4 to 6 weeks of therapy for category 2 prostatitis (chronic bacterial prostatitis). Prophylactic antibiotic therapy should be considered for patients who frequently relapse. In male patients who have a chronic indwelling catheter, bacteriuria should only be treated if acute symptoms referable to urinary tract are present (i.e., flank, suprapubic, or scrotal pain) or before genitourinary tract procedures.

REFERENCES

Berger RE, Alexander ER, Harnisch JP, Paulsen CA: Etiology, manifestations and therapy of acute epididymitis: Prospective study of 50 cases. J Urol 1979;121:750-754.

Craig JC, Knight JF, Sureshkumar P, et al: Lack of circumcision increases the risk of urinary tract infection in young men. J Pediatr 1996;128:23-27.

Griebling TL: Urologic diseases in America project: Trends in resource use for urinary tract infections in men. J Urol 2005;173:1288-1294.

Kass EJ, Kernen KM, Carey JM: Pediatric urinary tract infection and the necessity of complete urological imaging. BJU Int 2000;86:94-96.

Krieger JN, Nyberg L Jr, Nickel JC: NIH consensus definition and classification of prostatitis. JAMA 1999;282:236.

Meares EM, Stamey TA: Bacteriologic localization patterns in bacterial prostatitis and urethritis. Invest Urol 1968;5:492-518

Nickel JC, Alexander RB, Schaeffer AJ, et al: Leukocytes and bacteria in men with chronic prostatitis/chronic pelvic pain syndrome compared to asymptomatic controls. J Urol 2003;170:818-822.

Nickel JC: The Pre and Post massage Test (PPMT): A simple screen for prostatitis. Tech Urol 1997;3:38-43.

Noe HN: The long-term results of prospective sibling reflux screening. J Urol 1992;148:1739-1742.

Reynolds SJ, Shepherd ME, Risbud AR, et al: Male circumcision and risk of HIV-1 and other sexually transmitted infections in India. Lancet 2004;363:1039-1040.

Ulleryd P, Zackrisson B, Aus G, et al: Selective urological evaluation in men with febrile urinary tract infection. BJU Int 2001;88:15-20.

Weidner W, Schiefer H-G: Inflammatory disease of the prostate: Frequency and pathogenesis. In Garraway M (ed.): Epidemiology of Prostate Disease. New York, Springer, 1995, pp 85-93.

Urinary Tract Infections in Women

Method of
Burke A. Cunha, MD

General Concepts

Urinary tract infections (UTIs) are common in adult women. The two major clinical manifestations of UTIs in adult women are cystitis or pyelonephritis. Young adult women may also present with so-called dysuria pyuria syndrome (abacteriuric cystitis), previously known as acute urethral syndrome, as outpatients. Hospitalized compromised female hosts with cystitis may be complicated by bacteremia or ascending infection. Renal abscess may complicate pyelonephritis in normal or compromised female hosts.

Cystitis Versus Pneumonias

The therapeutic approach to UTIs in adult women depends on accurate localization of the site of infection in the urinary tract. The most common clinical problem is differentiating cystitis from pyelonephritis. Patients with acute bacterial cystitis present with dysuria and frequency, which may or may not be accompanied by suprapubic discomfort or lower back pain. The fever accompanying cystitis is $\leq$ to 38.9°C (102°F) and is not usually associated with chills. The clinical manifestation of cystitis is confirmed by finding pyuria and significant bacteriuria, (i.e., $\geq 10^6$ CFU/mL) in such patients. The urinalysis in acute cystitis is not usually accompanied by microscopic hematuria.

Staphylococcus saprophyticus is the only uropathogen in the ambulatory setting that is responsible for the majority of cases of UTIs accompanied by microscopic hematuria. Microscopic hematuria in a urinalysis in a patient with an apparent UTI should be carefully observed and should disappear after therapy of the UTI. If the microscopic hematuria disappears, then the physician can safely assume it was related to the UTI. Particularly in elderly patients, if the microscopic hematuria persists after eradication of the UTI, then the patient should be investigated for a bladder or renal source of the microscopic hematuria.

Dysuria-Pyuria Syndrome

There are three other types of UTIs that mimic or resemble cystitis. In sexually active young women, the dysuria-pyuria syndrome manifests with the symptoms of cystitis but with negative urine cultures, or if organisms are cultured, they are present in low numbers ($\leq 10^3$ CFU/mL). Most cases of dysuria-pyuria syndrome are caused by *Chlamydia trachomatis*. In patients with dysuria-pyuria syndrome, if the urine is cultured for *Chlamydia*, cultures are frequently positive.

Catheter-Associated Bacteriuria (CAB)

Hospitalized patients with indwelling Foley catheters often acquire bacteriuria as a function of time that the Foley catheter is in place. Pyuria is often in the urine of patients with indwelling Foleys because the catheter elicits inflammation of the urinary tract. The presence of pyuria and bacteriuria in a patient with an indwelling Foley suggests either UTI or CAB. The majority of such patients are asymptomatic and afebrile. More than 95% of the time these patients have colonization of the urinary tract without infection. The urinalysis in patients with indwelling Foley catheters is helpful if either bacteria without pyuria or pyuria without bacteria is demonstrated. Bacteriuria without pyuria signifies colonization of the urinary tract, whereas pyuria without bacteriuria indicates inflammation of the urinary tract. In non–Foley catheter patients, the presence of pyuria plus significant bacteriuria is diagnostic of a UTI. This is not the case with CAB. As mentioned in the setting of the Foley catheter, bacteriuria plus pyuria almost always represents colonization and not a UTI.

Benign Bacteriuria of the Elderly

In elderly female patients, varying degrees of relaxation of the pelvic musculature are common. Patients often have varying degrees of cystocele of rectocele, which changes anatomic relationship and the angularity of the urethra as it enters the bladder and predisposes to colonization of the bladder urine by the introital flora, such as coliform flora derived from the colon. For this reason, elderly female patients often have bacteriuria with few or no symptoms of a UTI. The presence of bacteriuria/pyuria is often discovered on a routine urinalysis obtained as part of either admission laboratory work or an outpatient workup/screening test battery. The presence of bacteriuria/pyuria in an elderly female patient without underlying genitourinary (GU) disease or impaired host defenses has been appropriately termed *benign bacteriuria of the elderly*; it has been shown that these patients do not go on to have symptomatic UTIs, ascending infection (e.g., pyelonephritis/renal abscess), or bacteremia from the urinary tract.

Recurrent Urinary Tract Infections: Reinfection Versus Relapse

Most UTIs in women are acute. CAB is often incorrectly considered a chronic UTI because in most cases it represents colonization rather than infection. Recurrent UTIs are chronic in the sense that they persist over a long period of time, but are really episodic infections. However, the approach to recurrent UTIs is based on determining whether the recurrence is on the basis of reinfection or relapse. The reinfection variety of recurrent UTIs is defined as a recurrent UTI because of different organisms being cultured during each UTI episode. The relapse form of recurrent UTIs is defined as demonstrating the same organism during repeated bouts of UTIs. The reinfection form of recurrent UTIs is usually because of rapid colonization of the vaginal introitus/entry into the urethra, usually following sexual intercourse. The relapse variety of recurrent UTI by the same organism recovered during each episode suggests an underlying structural abnormality of the GU tract. The correct diagnostic approach to recurrent UTIs because of relapse is a thorough investigation of the GU tract from the urethra to the kidneys, which determines a possible source for the focus for the organisms to periodically reappear as a relapsing UTI. Relapse UTIs cannot be successfully approached therapeutically without correcting the underlying condition predisposing to relapse (i.e., bladder calculi, kinked ureters, renal stones, renal abscesses).

Acute Pyelonephritis

Acute pyelonephritis is most common in pregnancy and as a complication of an ascending infection from cystitis/GU instrumentation. An acute episode of pyelonephritis may occur in patients who have chronic pyelonephritis; the acute episode is superimposed on the chronic condition. Renal abscess may complicate acute and chronic pyelonephritis. Renal cortical abscesses are often caused by gram-positive cocci (e.g., staphylococci acquired hematogenously), whereas medullary abscesses are usually caused by aerobic gram-negative bacilli (e.g., coliforms or enterococci).

Acute pyelonephritis may be differentiated from cystitis by the presence of unilateral costovertebral angle (CVA) tenderness (otherwise unexplainable) and a temperature of ≥ 38.9°C (102°F). Bilateral pyelonephritis is unusual, and the presence of bilateral CVA tenderness should suggest an alternative diagnosis. Pyelonephritis is often bilateral pathologically, but clinically it is almost always unilateral in its presentation with CVA tenderness. The urinalysis in pyelonephritis is the same as in cystitis, for example with significant pyuria/bacteriuria in addition to the findings suggestive of pyelonephritis. The clinical presentation of renal abscess may resemble pyelonephritis if CVA tenderness is present, but this is not an invariable finding. The urinalysis in renal abscess may reveal pyuria and bacteria if the abscess is medullary but only pyuria if the renal abscess is cortical. Renal imaging studies are usually unnecessary in cystitis or pyelonephritis. If there is confusion regarding the presence or absence of chronic pyelonephritis, then a computed tomography/magnetic resonance imaging (CT/MRI) scan of the abdomen or renal ultrasound is appropriate.

Chronic Pyelonephritis

Chronic pyelonephritis results in shrunken and distorted kidneys with a distorted collecting system. If the patient presents with *chronic pyelonephritis* and has kidneys of normal or large size, then an alternate explanation should be sought. The only way to diagnose a renal abscess with certainty is with renal imaging studies. For this purpose, the CT/MRI of the kidneys is vastly superior in picking up small lesions than is the renal ultrasound. For the purposes of excluding a renal abscess, a negative renal ultrasound should never be used to rule out the diagnosis. A negative renal ultrasound should always be followed with a renal CT/MRI of the kidneys if a renal abscess is in the differential diagnosis.

Therapeutic Considerations

ACUTE CYSTITIS

The initial episode of acute complicated cystitis in a normal host without GU abnormalities/preexisting renal disease need not be treated with antimicrobial therapy. Usually treatment with phenazopyridine (Pyridium), which has no antibacterial effect, is sufficient to relieve bladder spasm and the relative urine obstruction because of the bladder spasm, and the bacteria will spontaneously clear itself without antimicrobial therapy. Repeated episodes of acute cystitis should have appropriate diagnostic studies, for example a urinalysis and urinary culture with sensitivities with each episode to differentiate reinfection from relapse. If cystitis occurs in a nonleukopenic compromised host (e.g., with diabetes mellitus, systemic lupus erythematosus, multiple myeloma, cirrhosis, etc.), then a seven-day course of therapy is recommended with an oral agent such as nitrofurantoin (Macrodantin), trimethoprim-sulfamethoxazole (TMP-SMX) (Bactrim), or amoxicillin (Amoxil). Ampicillin

should be avoided because of its resistance potential with coliform bacteria.

DYSURIA-PYURIA SYNDROME

The dysuria-pyuria syndrome because of *Chlamydia* should be treated with a two-week course of doxycycline (Vibramycin). Patients unable to tolerate doxycycline (Vibramycin) may be treated with a macrolide for the same period of time. A grossly hemorrhagic cystitis suggests a viral etiology for which no specific therapy is available. Patients with cystitis and microscopic hematuria are often infected with *S. saprophyticus*.

Fortunately, *S. saprophyticus* is susceptible to a wide range of antibiotics and virtually any agent selected to treat a UTI will be effective. Antimicrobial resistance has not been a problem in *S. saprophyticus* UTIs. Chronic interstitial cystitis is not an infectious disorder and therefore antimicrobial therapy is unnecessary.

CATHETER-ASSOCIATED BACTERIURIA

CAB in hospitalized patients who are normal hosts without structural abnormalities need not be treated, because virtually all of these patients are colonized and not infected. CAB in nonleukopenic compromised hosts (with diabetes mellitus, systemic lupus erythematosus, multiple myeloma, cirrhosis, and so forth), should be treated to prevent ascending infection/bacteremia from the lower urinary tract. Such individuals should be treated with an oral agent such as amoxicillin (Amoxil), nitrofurantoin (Macrodantin), or TMP-SMX (Bactrim) for 1 to 2 weeks.

Nonleukopenic compromised hosts with enterococci CAB are best treated with oral nitrofurantoin (Macrodantin), which is effective against enterococcal strains such as *E. faecalis* (non-vancomycin-resistant *Enterococcus* [non-VRE]) as well as *E. faecium* [VRE]). *Enterococcus faecalis* strains may also be treated with oral amoxicillin (Amoxil). These instances represent prophylaxis/early therapy because the majority of patients who are nonleukopenic-compromised hosts will have colonization of the urinary tract prior to catheterization or rapidly develop it soon thereafter. Therefore, prevention of ascending infection/bacteremia is the primary aim of therapy in patients with CAB who are compromised on the basis of their host defenses or GU tract abnormalities (e.g., ureteral stents).

ACUTE PYELONEPHRITIS

Acute pyelonephritis may be caused by aerobic gram-negative bacilli, such as coliforms or enterococci (almost always *E. faecalis*). The empirical treatment of pyelonephritis is based on a Gram stain of the urine, which, if the diagnosis is pyelonephritis, will show significant pyuria and a single predominant organism. In a patient with presumed pyelonephritis, the absence of bacteria in the Gram stain of the urine in an acutely ill patient essentially eliminates the diagnosis of pyelonephritis from further consideration, and an alternate explanation for the patient's fever and CVA tenderness should be sought (e.g., renal imaging studies).

Because acute pyelonephritis is often accompanied by bacteremia (urosepsis), parenteral agents may be used initially followed by oral agents; or in mild-to-moderate

CURRENT DIAGNOSIS

- Acute uncomplicated cystitis is the most common type of UTI in adult women.
- The initial peak incidence of cystitis occurs with sexual intercourse and gradually increases through adulthood.
- Cystitis may occur as a single event or may be recurrent because of reinfection or relapse.
- Cystitis is usually caused by coliform or enterococci from the fecal flora or by *Staphylococcus saprophyticus* from the skin flora.
- Clinically, cystitis is marked by low-grade fever (≤38.9°C [102°F]) with lower abdominal/ suprapubic discomfort, and/or dysuria.
- *Staphylococcus aureus*, *Streptococcus pneumoniae*, groups A, C, G streptococci, and *Bacteroides fragilis* are not uropathogens in cystitis.
- In elderly women, *cystitis* manifests as pyuria and bacterluria without fever or dysuria, which is termed *benign bacteriuria of the elderly*.
- A variant of cystitis, the so-called *dysuria/pyuria syndrome*, is also known as *abacteriuric cystitis*.
- Dysuria/pyuria syndrome, most common in young adult women, manifests as cystitis, but urine cultures are negative for bacteria or uropathogens such as *Escherichia coli* are present in low numbers. *Chlamydia trachomatis* is frequently isolated if the urine is cultured for *Chlamydia*.
- Pyelonephritis in women may occur as an uncommon complication of cystitis or during pregnancy.
- It is not possible to predict the uropathogen of cystitis from clinical features except for *S. saprophyticus*.
- *S. saprophyticus* cystitis is characterized by a fishy urine odor, microscopic hematuria, and an alkaline urinary pH.
- Cystitis with alkaline urine suggests infection secondary to *S. saprophyticus*, *Ureaplasma urealyticum*, or a struvite stone with associated infection caused by a urea-splitting organism such as *Proteus*.
- Microscopic hematuria is common with *S. saprophyticus* cystitis but is uncommon with other uropathogens. If a patient with cystitis and microscopic hematuria fails to promptly resolve with antimicrobial therapy, work up the patient for a bladder/renal neoplasm or renal TB.
- The diagnosis of cystitis in women is made by demonstrating pyuria and significant bacteriuria (≥ 10^6 col/mL) in the setting of cystitis symptoms.
- Cystitis symptoms with gross hematuria should suggest a viral hemorrhagic cystitis or a renal lesion.
- Pyuria without bacteriuria indicates urinary tract inflammation. Persistent pyuria without bacteriuria should suggest interstitial cystitis or renal TB.
- With cystitis, the specific gravity of the urine is not decreased in contrast to pyelonephritis where the specific gravity is decreased.
- Urinary concentration returns to normal with treatment in pyelonephritis.
- Pyelonephritis may be differentiated from cystitis by the presence of fever ≥38.9°C (102°F) and otherwise unexplained unilateral CVA tenderness.
- The urine analysis/culture findings in pyelonephritis and cystitis are the same. Bacteremia frequently occurs with pyelonephritis but is not a feature of cystitis in normal hosts.
- Nonleukopenic compromised hosts, such as diabetes mellitus, systemic lupus erythematosus, multiple myeloma, cirrhosis, and so on, with cystitis may be complicated by pyelonephritis or bacteremia.
- Pyelonephritis is caused by the same uropathogens that cause cystitis; however, *S. saprophyticus* occurs only in cystitis.
- Acute pyelonephritis clinically improves unless complicated by renal abscess.
- Clinically, pyelonephritis is almost always unilateral, but pathophysical findings may be bilateral.
- Bilateral CVA tenderness should suggest an alternate diagnosis.
- In pyelonephritis, radiologic studies typically show unilateral renal involvement characterized by cortical scarring, medullary abnormalities, and renal shrinkage.
- Bilateral, normal-sized, or enlarged kidneys should suggest an alternate diagnosis to pyelonephritis.

Abbreviations: CVA = costovertebral angle; TB = tuberculosis; UTI = urinary tract infection.

cases, oral agents may be used for the entire course of therapy. The parenteral agents useful in the treatment of acute pyelonephritis because of aerobic gram-negative bacilli include aminoglycosides, aztreonam (Azactam), antipseudomonal penicillin (e.g., ticarcillin [Ticar]), piperacillin (Pipracil), or a renally excreted respiratory quinolone. Patients presenting with acute pyelonephritis, who have streptococci in the Gram stain of the urine indicating enterococci, may be treated empirically with ampicillin and antipseudomonal penicillin, ticarcillin (Ticar), piperacillin (Pipracil), or meropenem (Merrem). In the rare instance where there is enterococcal urosepsis complicating acute pyelonephritis because of VRE, then linezolid (Zyvox), quinupristin-dalfopristin (Synercid), or daptomycin (Cubicin) may be used. In patients presenting with acute pyelonephritis where a Gram stain is unobtainable or unavailable, then empirical coverage for both aerobic gram-negative bacilli and enterococci (*E. faecalis*), may be achieved with antipseudomonal penicillins, nonrenally eliminated respiratory quinolones, or meropenem (Merrem). After the organism responsible for the pyelonephritis is subsequently identified by urine/blood culture, then the patient may be switched to one of the agents mentioned. Similarly, if the patient is shown to have enterococci as the cause of the urosepsis, it may be treated initially as non-VRE, as indicated previously in the article. Patients with pyelonephritis are usually treated for 1 to 2 weeks.

- Virtually all cases of initial uncomplicated cystitis will resolve spontaneously with or without treatment. No urine analysis/culture is needed with the initial episode of cystitis.
- For the dysuria of cystitis, phenazopyridine (Pyridium), which has no antibacterial properties but relieves pain and relative urinary obstruction from muscle spasm, may be used. Relief of spasm promptly clears the bacteriuria.
- Recurrent cystitis of the reinfection variety is because of different uropathogens with each episode that the urine is cultured. Reinfection is related to vaginal introital colonization following sexual intercourse and may be treated with a postcoital/HS of an appropriate antibiotic.
- Although the initial attack of cystitis resolves in virtually all patients without treatment, those who prefer to treat may use single-dose therapy with nitrofurantoin (Macrodantin), TMP-SMX (Bactrim), or amoxicillin (Amoxil).
- Cystitis in a nonleukopenic compromised host (discussed previously) should be treated for 1 to 2 weeks to prevent bacteremia/ascending infection, such as pyelonephritis/renal abscess.
- Ampicillin should be avoided because of its high resistance potential. Amoxicillin should be used instead, which has not been associated with resistance and is effective against the common coliforms and enterococci (*Enterococcus faecalis*).
- Nitrofurantoin has no resistance potential, is effective against all common uropathogens and all enterococci, such as *E. faecalis* (non-VRE) and

Enterococcus faecium (VRE). Nitrofurantoin (Macrodantin) is useful in cystitis or catheter-associated bacteremia but is not to be used in pyelonephritis/bacteremia.

- Recurrent UTI of the relapse variety is caused by the same uropathogen with each occurrence. The problem in relapse UTIs is not therapeutic but diagnostic. Relapsing UTIs have an underlying structural abnormality or ureteral shunts that do not permit antimicrobial therapy to be effective.
- The treatment of pyelonephritis is with IV or PO antibiotics, depending on the severity of the clinical manifestation. Treatment is for 2 to 4 weeks with an effective antibiotic.
- For pyelonephritis, parenteral agents useful against coliforms are cephalosporins, aztreonam (Azactam), aminoglycosides, TMP-SMZ (Bactrim), or renally eliminated quinolones. Against enterococci (most of which are non-VRE), parenteral ampicillin, antipseudomonal penicillins, and meropenem (Merrem) are useful.
- Oral antibiotics useful against coliform causes of pyelonephritis include renally eliminated quinolones, amoxicillin (Amoxil), antipseudomonal penicillins, or TMP-SMZ (Bactrim).
- Linezolid (Zyvox) may be used for pyelonephritis caused by enterococci (non-VRE), amoxicillin (Amoxil), or for VRE.
- Patients with acute pyelonephritis become afebrile/nearly afebrile within 72 hours with or without treatment. Persistence of high fevers for greater than 72 hours should be considered as representing a renal abscess until proved otherwise.

Abbreviations: HD = half dose; IM = intramuscular; IV = intravenous; TMP-SMZ = trimethoprim-sulfamethoxazole; UTI = urinary tract infection; VRE = vancomycin-resistant *Enterococcus.*

Particularly in critically ill patients, initial therapy is often started parenterally. Patients may be switched to an oral agent as soon as the patient clinically defervesces or treated entirely by an oral agent for the duration of therapy. The ideal oral antibiotic has the same spectrum as its parenteral counterpart and has excellent bioavailability; blood/tissue levels are approximately the same after intravenous/oral (IV/PO) administration. For example, by giving 1 g of amoxicillin (Amoxil) every 8 hours, the same blood/tissue levels are achieved as by giving ampicillin by intramuscular injection (IM). Nonrenally eliminated respiratory quinolones, such as levofloxacin (Levaquin) and gatifloxacin (Tequin), achieve the same blood and tissue levels when given either by the IV or PO route. This permits completion of therapy at home and does not require 2 to 4 weeks of inpatient hospitalization for intravenous drug therapy. There is some rationale for treating acute pyelonephritis for an extended period, such as 2 to 4 weeks, to prevent chronic pyelonephritis.

CHRONIC PYELONEPHRITIS

Patients with chronic pyelonephritis are a therapeutic challenge because of the distorted intrarenal architecture

and decreased blood supply to the kidney, which limits access of white blood cells (WBCs), impairs host defenses, and limits penetration of the antibiotic into the infected/diseased areas of the kidney. Treatment of chronic pyelonephritis should be based on susceptibility testing of the isolates that are present in the urine. In chronic pyelonephritis, bacteriuria is intermittent but is present over a long period of time and will persist after short or inadequate treatment. The antibiotic selected should be effective against the isolate recovered from the urine in patients with chronic pyelonephritis and possess the ability to penetrate into diseased kidneys. The ideal oral agents for therapy are TMP-SMX (Bactrim), doxycycline (Vibramycin), or a nonrenally eliminated respiratory quinolone.

RENAL ABSCESS

Acute pyelonephritis treated appropriately results in a rapid defervescence of temperature and decrease in CVA tenderness within 72 hours. If the temperature does not decrease after 72 hours of appropriate therapy, suggest a renal abscess until proved otherwise. Renal abscesses should be treated for the presumed organism based on the location of the abscess by renal imaging studies. If sensitivities from an isolate available from the urine or percutaneous aspiration of the abscess are unavailable, then empirical treatment directed against aerobic gram-negative bacilli for medullary abscesses is indicated. Treatment is the same as for pyelonephritis except is more prolonged and should be given until the abscess is drained or it resolves. For cortical abscesses in the absence of culture and sensitivity data, antibiotic therapy should be directed against *Staphylococcus aureus* and *E. faecalis*, and treated in the same manner as pyelonephritis but for an extended period of time. Acute pyelonephritis with or without acteremia is usually treated for 7 days.

RECURRENT UTIs

Reinfection may be treated with nitrofurantoin (Macrodantin), TMP-SMX (Bactrim), or amoxicillin (Amoxil) as a single postcoital dose. Therapeutic approach to relapse is to remove the underlying condition responsible for perpetuating the bacteriuria. Antimicrobial therapy may be selected based on the susceptibility of the organism, but antimicrobial therapy alone will not eradicate the relapsing form of recurrent UTI.

REFERENCES

Cunha BA: Clinical concepts in the treatment of urinary tract infections. Antibiotics for the Clinician 1999;3:88-93.
Cunha BA: Nosocomial catheter-associated urinary tract infections. Hosp Physician 1986;22:13-16.
Cunha BA: *Staphylococcus saprophyticus* urinary tract infections. Intern Med 1985;6:82-89.
Cunha BA: Single-dose therapy of urinary tract infections. Hosp Physician 1983;19:35-37.
Cunha BA. Urinary tract infections: Pathophysiology/diagnosis. Postgrad Med 1981;70:141-145.
Cunha BA: Urinary tract infections: Therapy. Postgrad Med 1981;70: 149-157.
Cunha BA, Comer JB: Pharmacokinetic considerations in the treatment of urinary tract infections. Conn Med 1979;43:347-353.
Gupta K, Hooton TM, Roberts PL, Stamm WE: Patient-initiated treatment of uncomplicated recurrent urinary tract infections in young women. Ann Intern Med 2001;135:9.
Hooton TM: The current management strategies for community-acquired urinary tract infection. Infect Dis Clin North Am 2003;17:303-332.
Kahan E, Kahan NR, Chinitz DP: Urinary tract infection in women—Physician's preferences for treatment and adherence to guidelines: A national drug utilization study in a managed care setting. Eur J Clin Pharmacol 2003;59:663-668.
Kraft JK, Stamey TA: The natural history of symptomatic recurrent bacteriuria in women. Medicine (Baltimore) 1977;56:55.
Meiland R, Geerlings SE, Hoepelman LI: Management of bacterial urinary tract infections in adult patients with diabetes mellitus. Drugs 2002;62:1859-1868.
Miller LG, Tang AW: Treatment of uncomplicated urinary tract infections in an era of increasing antimicrobial resistance. Mayo Clin Proc 2004;79:1048-1053.
Nicolle LE: Urinary tract infection: Traditional pharmacologic therapies. Am J Med 2002;113(Suppl 1A):35S-44S.
Nicolle LE, Ronald AR: Recurrent urinary tract infection in adult women: Diagnosis and treatment. Infect Dis Clin North Am 1987;1:793.
Ronald AR, Conway B: An approach to urinary tract infection in women. Infection 1992;20(Suppl 3):S203.
Schaeffer AJ, Stuppy BA: Efficacy and safety of self-start therapy in women with recurrent urinary tract infections. J Urol 1999;161:207.
Wong ES, McKevitt M, Running K, et al: Management of recurrent urinary tract infections with patient administered single-dose therapy. Ann Intern Med 1985;102:302.

Bacterial Infections of the Urinary Tract in Girls

Method of
Candice E. Johnson, MD, PhD

Urinary tract infections (UTIs) are bacterial infections of any mucosal surface of the urinary tract including the urethra, the bladder, the ureters, and the renal calyces, as well as the renal parenchyma (Box 1). The best indicator for differentiating clinical pyelonephritis from cystitis is fever higher than 38.5°C (101.3°F). The classification of UTIs by anatomic location is complicated by the ascending nature of virtually all these infections. Thus, a girl with pyelonephritis usually has cystitis and urethritis simultaneously. Box 2 gives the colony count criteria generally accepted for clinical use, although research studies are usually more stringent.

Epidemiology and Pathogenesis

Approximately 2.2% of girls will have a UTI in the first 24 months of life. In the first year of life, most UTIs in females are febrile and may be hard to diagnose. Because of this difficulty, girls younger than 36 months with no source of fever should have a urine culture and urinalysis obtained. Unfortunately, the sensitivity of a standard urinalysis is only 82%, although it is 92% specific. For unknown reasons, the prevalence of UTI is much higher in white compared with African American girls, with Hispanics having a rate between the two groups.

Risk factors for UTI include:

- A history of recurrent UTI in the mother
- Family history of vesicoureteral reflux (VUR)
- Dysfunctional voiding patterns
- Constipation

BOX 1   Classification of Urinary Tract Infections

- **Urethritis:** Dysuria, frequency or enuresis, accompanied by pyuria, but colony count of 10^3/mL of urine or less.
- **Cystitis:** Afebrile UTI. Dysuria, frequency or enuresis with colony count of at least 10^4/mL of urine. Hematuria may be present, but casts, flank pain, temperature more than 38.5°C (101.3°F) and systemic toxicity are absent.
- **Clinical pyelonephritis:** Febrile UTI (≥38°C [100.4°F]), usually accompanied by flank and abdominal pain. The colony count is usually greater than or equal to 10^5/mL of urine except with *Staphylococcus saprophyticus* or enterococci. Cystitis symptoms may also be present.
- **Proved pyelonephritis:** Shows evidence of acute inflammation on radiologic evaluation by CT, ultrasound, or radionuclide scan.

Abbreviations: CT = computed tomography; UTI = urinary tract infection.

BOX 2   Colony Count Criteria for Urinary Tract Infection in Children

- If suprapubic aspiration is performed any growth is significant for UTI
- If catheterization of female is performed, greater than 1000 CFU/mL is significant for UTI
- If clean-void urine is performed, greater than 10,000 CFU/mL in pure culture is suggestive; >100,000 CFU/mL is highly likely.
- Growth of two or more species suggests contamination, but does not exclude true infection. Repeat the culture.

Cleanliness and methods of wiping with toilet paper are not risk factors. In girls, an "unstable bladder" is the main cause of dysfunctional voiding. An unstable bladder has strong contractions at volumes 50% to 75% of capacity. These contractions cause both frequency and incontinence, and girls may sit on their feet to attempt to prevent voiding (Vincent's curtsy). In the most severe cases the girl tightens the external sphincter during bladder contraction, and this leads to high bladder pressure. A thickened and trabeculated bladder often occurs as well as VUR.

Diagnosis

A high index of suspicion is needed to diagnose all UTIs, especially those in infants and toddlers. In addition to fever, manifesting symptoms include anorexia and emesis, abdominal pain, fussiness, neonatal jaundice, poor weight gain, enuresis, and hematuria.

Urine should be collected only by catheter or suprapubic aspiration until the child is toilet trained, because urine bags have contamination rates of up to 50%. Box 2 shows the colony counts that best differentiate real UTIs from contamination.

Urinalysis continues to be performed in most laboratories by a dipstick combined with spun urine sediment. This continues despite studies since 1983 showing that unspun urine counted in a hemocytometer is more sensitive and specific. In a private office, the dipstick results for leukocyte esterase, nitrites, and hematuria are sufficient to decide on empirical treatment of girls. Urine cultures should still be sent, even with a negative dipstick, because, unlike adult women, radiologic workups may be needed for confirmed UTIs in girls.

Treatment of Afebrile Urinary Tract Infection

Treatment of a girl with an afebrile UTI (cystitis or lower tract) is straightforward, requiring only a knowledge of national and local antibiotic resistance rates. *Escherichia coli* causes more than 90% of cystitis in girls, with other Enterobacteriaceae and *Staphylococcus saprophyticus* comprising the remainder. *E. coli* is resistant to amoxicillin

---

BOX 3   Antibiotic Choices for the Treatment of Urinary Tract Infections

Oral

- Trimethoprim (Primsol oral solution)—8-12 mg/kg/day divided every 12 hours (max dose 320 mg).
- Trimethoprim-sulfamethoxazole (TMP/SMX) (Bactrim, Septra)—8-12 mg of TMP component divided every 12 hours (max dose 320 mg).
- Amoxicillin (Amoxil)—children <40 kg: 40 mg/kg/day divided every 12 hours; children >40 kg: 875 mg every 12 hours.
- Cephalosporins:
  Cefprozil (Cefzil)[1]—30 mg/kg/day divided every 12 hours (max dose 1 g/day).
  Cefixime (generic only)—infants and children: 8 mg/kg/day divided every 12 hours; adolescents and adults: 400 mg/day divided every 12-24 hours.
  Cefdinir (Omnicef)[1]—Infants and children (older than 6 months to 12 years): 14 mg/kg/day divided every 12 hours (max dose 600 mg/day).
  Cephalexin (Keflex)—25-50 mg/kg/day divided every 6 to 8 hours (max dose 4 g/day).
- Nitrofurantoin (Macrodantin) for afebrile infections only— 5-7 mg/kg/day divided every 6 hours; children older than 12 years and adults, 300 mg every 12 hours or 600 mg every 24 hours.

Parenteral

- Gentamicin (Garamycin)—5-6 mg/kg/day divided every 8 hours or 5 mg/kg as a single dose every 24 hours (with measured levels after third dose).
- Trimethoprim-sulfamethoxazole (Bactrim, Septra) at 8 mg/kg/day of the TMP component, divided every 12 hours.
- Cephalosporins:
  Ceftriaxone (Rocephin)—50 mg/kg/day once every 24 hours.
  Ceftazidime (Fortaz)—100-150 mg/kg/day divided every 8 hours; (max dose 600 mg)
  Cefotaxime (Claforan)—50-150 mg/kg/day divided every 6-8 hours. (max dose 12 grams/day)
- Fluoroquinolones are not approved for under age 18 years, but may be required for resistant organisms.

---

[1]Not FDA approved for this indication.

(Amoxil) more than 50% of the time, so this is not appropriate initial therapy. Rates of resistance to trimethoprim (Proloprim) and sulfonamides are highest in the Pacific Coast states, and rates of first-generation cephalosporin resistance vary widely. Drugs that retain high sensitivity rates are the second- and third-generation cephalosporins and nitrofurantoin (Macrodantin). Box 3 provides doses of commonly used drugs, and amoxicillin is preferred if the organism is sensitive.

Treatment of Febrile Urinary Tract Infection

Unlike the majority of viral and bacterial infections, a single kidney infection may cause permanent damage

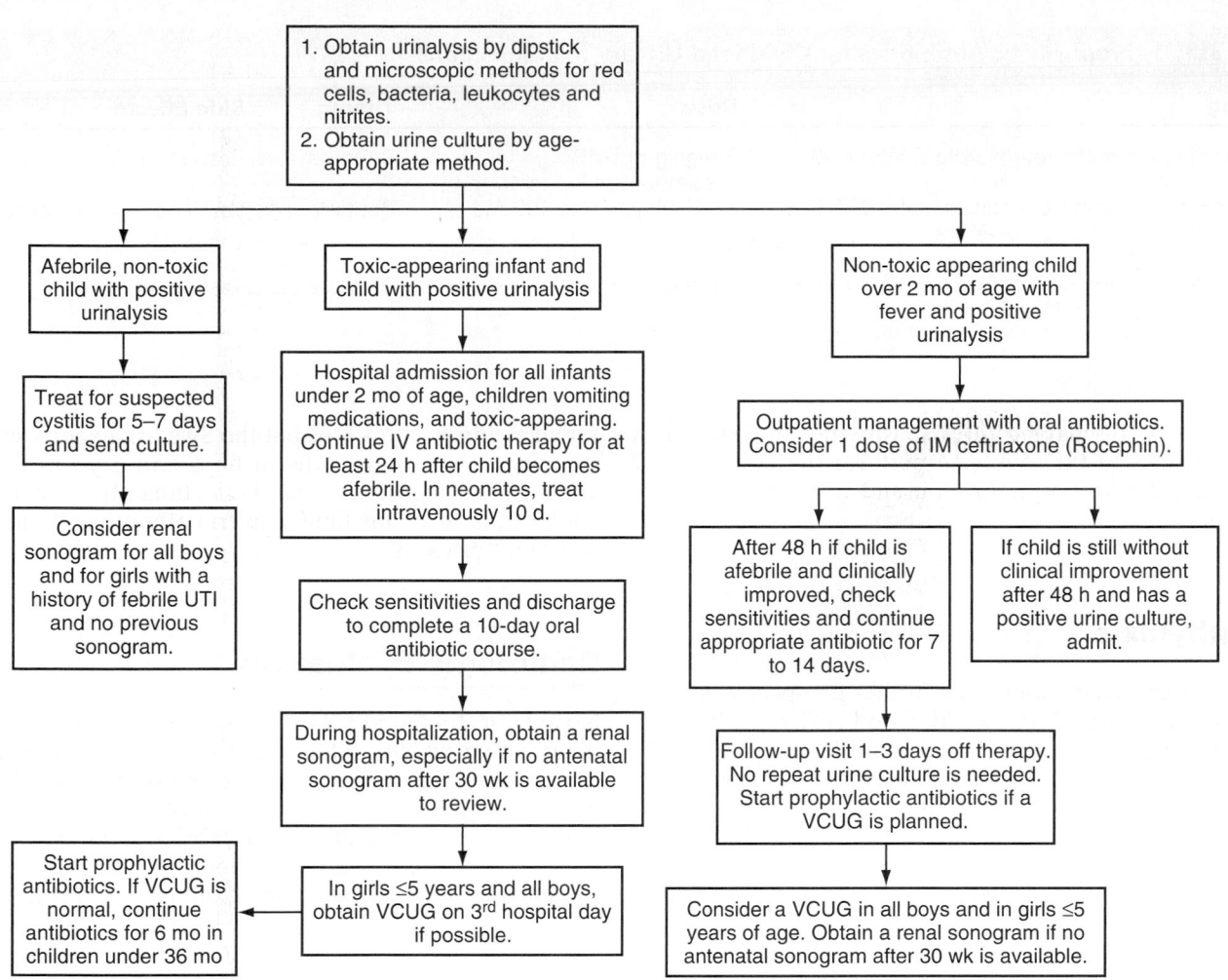

FIGURE 1. Treatment of suspected urinary tract infection in children younger than 13 years old.

(i.e., renal scarring) if not treated rapidly and with effective antibiotics. In 1999, outpatient management of febrile UTIs was demonstrated to be effective in a study of 306 children under 24 months of age. A 2004 study in Montreal of 291 patients who were 3 months to 5 years of age showed that at least 75% of febrile children with UTI could be managed in a day treatment center (DTC). These children had a mean of 3.5 visits to the DTC for intravenous gentamicin (Garamycin), followed by an oral antibiotic to complete 10 days of treatment. Successful treatment was seen in 97% of the UTI episodes, and all first UTIs were evaluated by renal sonography and cystography at the DTC.

Because the DTC concept is not widely available for children in the United States, Figure 1 shows a suggested decision tree that does not use a DTC. Inpatient management is recommended for infants younger than 8 weeks as they do not absorb oral antibiotics predictably. Box 4 lists other variables to consider in deciding on inpatient versus outpatient treatment. Antibiotic choices are given in Box 3. Duration of symptoms before presentation is very important, because renal scarring was seen in British studies after as few as 5 days of delayed diagnosis.

Once on antibiotic therapy, defervescence may be expected in approximately 68% of children younger than 2 years by 24 hours and in 89% by 48 hours. The 11% who remain febrile at 48 hours were no more likely to have renal abscesses or hydronephrosis than the others, and

---

BOX 4   Proposed Criteria for Hospitalization of Children With Febrile Urinary Tract Infection

- Sufficient emesis is present to prevent oral therapy.
- Family is judged likely to be noncompliant with antibiotics or follow-up appointments.
- Toxic or ill-appearing child which is suggestive of sepsis.
- Age is younger than 2 months.
- Prolonged duration of symptoms exists (>5 days).
- Renal scarring or impaired renal function is known to be present.
- Diabetes, AIDS, sickle cell, or other serious chronic disease is present.

TABLE 1 Prophylactic Antibiotics for Childhood Urinary Tract Infections

Drug	Dose	Timing	Side Effects
Trimethoprim-sulfamethoxazole (TMP-SMX) (Bactrim)	2 mg/kg of TMP component (up to 40 mg)	Bedtime	Rash in ~6%
Nitrofurantoin (Macrodantin capsules 25, 50, or 100 mg preferred over oral suspension)	1-2 mg/kg/d up to 100 mg	Bedtime	Vomiting, abdominal pain
Trimethoprim (Primsol oral solution 50 mg/mL or 100 mg tablets)	2 mg/kg up to 40 mg	Bedtime	Rash in ~1%

they may be discharged after sensitivities are known. It is convenient to the family to perform the cystogram, if indicated, during hospitalization and it greatly improves compliance.

Prophylaxis

There is expert agreement that further prospective studies of antibiotic prophylaxis for childhood UTI are needed. In adult women, the cost-to-benefit ratio favors prophylaxis with three or more UTIs per year. In children, because young age is the major risk for renal scarring, studies are lacking, but expert opinion favors 6 months of prophylaxis after a febrile UTI, with or without VUR. Guidelines from the American Urological Association also suggest prophylaxis

for all children with VUR, but the Swedish experts suggest stopping at age 24 months in boys and 5 years in girls. Table 1 lists suggested agents. Unfortunately, the choice of antibiotic is becoming limited as trimethoprim (Proloprim) resistance rates rise.

Radiologic Evaluation

No area of childhood UTI evaluation is as controversial as determining which children merit sonography, radionuclide scans, and cystograms. Two recent studies have helped clarify these issues, and several professional academies have agreed on guidelines for febrile children younger than 2 years of age (Pediatrics, Family Practice, Emergency Physicians, Urological, and College of Radiology).

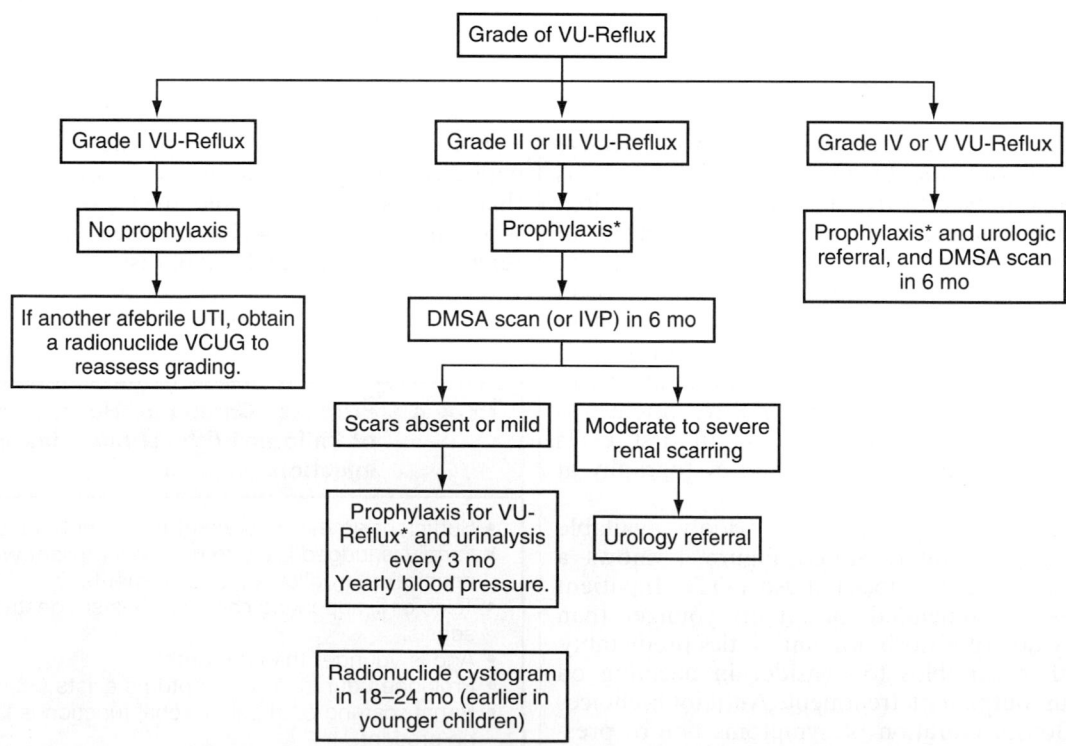

*Trimethoprim (Primsol) (1–2 mg/kg/d at bedtime) or nitrofurantoin (Macrodantin) (same dosage)

FIGURE 2. Radiologic management of a child with vesicoureteral reflux.

CURRENT DIAGNOSIS

- A high level of suspicion is required in all febrile infants.
- Boys outnumber girls 10:1 in the neonatal period.
- Girls are at highest risk for UTI when younger than 12 months of age and again at 3 to 5 years of age.
- Urine for culture should not be obtained with a bag, but requires a catheterization or suprapubic aspiration, if the child is not toilet trained.
- The colony count cutoff to define a UTI differs with the method used for collection.
- With a negative urinalysis, febrile UTI becomes much less likely, but an afebrile UTI cannot be ruled out.

Abbreviations: UTI = urinary tract infection.

These associations recommend a renal sonogram and a voiding cystogram soon after the first febrile UTI. Figure 2 indicates that the initial cystogram should be a standard fluoroscopic examination to permit accurate grading of VUR. Follow-up cystograms may be radionuclide studies, which carry less risk of gonadal radiation.

Hoberman and colleagues also question the value of the initial renal sonogram. In a cohort of 309 febrile children who had paired dimercaptosuccinic acid (DMSA) radionuclide renal scans and sonography performed within 48 hours of diagnosis, neither study changed management. All had had an antenatal sonogram after 30 weeks of gestation, and anomalies were presumably corrected before UTI could occur. The argument in favor of doing this painless and medically safe study is that children with "dilating reflux" (i.e., grades III-V) would be identified, and the doctor could track down these children if they fail to keep an appointment for a cystogram. In other words, in the absence of a cystogram, a sonogram with hydronephrosis or pelvic caliectasis *will* change management. In the patient with no health insurance who cannot afford both studies, the more important study is the voiding cystogram, not the sonogram.

CURRENT THERAPY

- Outpatient therapy of febrile UTIs is usually appropriate in infants older than 2 months of age.
- A single dose of intramuscular ceftriaxone (Rocephin) will cover the first 24 hours after diagnosis when emesis is most likely to occur and antibiotic sensitivities are unknown.
- Febrile girls should be seen between 36 and 48 hours after diagnosis to assess clinical improvements and check urine culture results.
- A voiding cystogram remains essential for febrile girls younger than 5 years of age and all boys.

Abbreviations: UTI = urinary tract infection.

REFERENCES

Abelson Storby K, Osterlund A, Kahlmeter G: Antimicrobial resistance in *Escherichia coli* in urine samples from children and adults: A 12 year analysis. Acta Paediatr 2004;93:487-491.

Bollgren I: Antibacterial prophylaxis in children with urinary tract infection. Acta Paediatr 1999;(Suppl 431):48-52.

Gauthier M, Chevalie I, Sterescu A, et al: Treatment of urinary tract infections among febrile young children with daily intravenous antibiotic therapy at a day treatment center. Pediatrics 2004;114: 469-476.

Hellerstein S: Urinary tract infections in children. Infections in Medicine 2002;19:554-560.

Hoberman A, Charros M, Hickey RW, et al: Imaging studies after a first febrile urinary tract infection in young children. N Engl J Med 2003;348(3):195-202.

Hoberman A, Wald ER, Hickey RW, et al: Oral versus initial intravenous therapy for urinary tract infections in young febrile children. Pediatrics 1999;104(1)79-86.

Jakobsson B, Esbjorner E, Hansson S: Minimum incidence and diagnostic rate of first urinary tract infection. Pediatrics 1999; 104(2 Pt):222-226.

Johnson CE: Dysuria. In: Kliegman RM, Greebaum LA, Lye PS, (eds): Practical Strategies in Pediatric Diagnosis and Therapy, 2nd ed. Philadelphia, WB Saunders, 2004, pp 397-411.

Lin D-S, Huang F-Y, Chiu N-C, et al: Comparison of hemocytometer leukocyte counts and standard urinalysis for predicting urinary tract infections in febrile infants. Pediatr Infect Dis J 2000;19:223-227.

Lowe LH, Patel MN, Gatti JM, Alon US: Utility of follow-up renal sonography in children with vesicoureteral reflux and normal initial sonogram. Pediatrics 2004;113:548-550.

Roberts KB: A synopsis of the American Academy of Pediatrics' practice parameter on the diagnosis, treatment, and evaluation of the initial urinary tract infection in febrile infants and young children. Pediatr Rev 1999;20(10):1-4.

Rushton HG: Urinary tract infections in children: Epidemiology, evaluation, and management. Pediatr Clin North Am 1997;44(5): 1133-1169.

Childhood Enuresis

Method of
Frank R. Cerniglia, Jr., MD

In general, *enuresis* is associated with purely nighttime wetting. The term, however, means involuntary wetting (day or night) beyond the age of anticipated control. Childhood enuresis includes both day (diurnal) and night (nocturnal) wetting. The latter is further subdivided into primary and secondary nocturnal enuresis. Enuresis is one of the most common problems seen by the pediatric primary care physician and is referred to the pediatric urologist.

The problem, which dates back to as early as 1500 BC, has been the subject of many dissertations on diagnosis, causes, and remedies. Childhood wetting problems, or voiding dysfunctions, affect 5% to 10% of school-aged children and can be a profound source of distress for the child and family as a whole. The number of potential causes for abnormal voiding include anatomic, neuropathic, and functional disorders. Most children who present with day and/or nighttime wetting have a non-neurologic functional voiding abnormality requiring no complex evaluation or invasive study.

Development of Bladder Control

Urinary continence develops in an ordered process of sequenced maturation that requires no teaching. To attain continence, one needs a low-pressure storage vessel surrounded by smooth muscle to "squeeze" out the urine from the bladder, an "involuntary" internal sphincter, and a complex external sphincteric mechanism with intertwined smooth and skeletal muscle that is under voluntary control. These three mechanisms work in accord to accomplish bladder emptying. The neonate voids by reflex through the sacral spinal cord. The bladder reaches a functional capacity stretch point, and afferent signals are sent to the spinal cord to activate sympathetic outflow to the bladder and urethra. The result is relaxation of the external sphincter and contraction of the detrusor; bladder emptying ensues.

Urinary frequency, incontinence, and nocturnal enuresis are all normal occurrences in the very young child. Infants are asleep approximately 60% of the time with 40% of their voiding episodes occurring during sleep. In year 1 of life, the child voids approximately 20 times per day. During the next 2 years, voiding frequency decreases by as much as 50% while the voided volumes (and bladder capacity) increase by as much as three to four times. Beginning at age 2 years, conscious sensation of bladder fullness develops, although control is not yet mastered. By 4 years, most children have achieved an adult pattern of voiding in which micturition can occur at less than total bladder capacity or be postponed until absolute functional bladder capacity is reached. For the transition to this pattern, three separate events must occur:

1. Capacity of bladder must increase so it can function as a reservoir.
2. The child must gain control over the external sphincter so urination can be allowed or terminated at will.
3. Direct voluntary control over the voiding reflex must develop to allow the child to initiate or inhibit bladder contraction voluntarily.

Simply put, urinary control is obtained when the bladder fills under low pressure to an adequate capacity and then can be emptied, with a detrusor contraction coordinated with complete relaxation of the external sphincter. However, one needs to understand this happens on a continuum. Nocturnal bowel control occurs first, followed by daytime bowel control, daytime urine control, and finally nighttime dryness. Most, but not all, children achieve these functions by the 4th year.

Evaluation

Pure voiding dysfunction is urinary incontinence without any underlying structural or obvious neurologic abnormality. On the whole, patients with an anatomic abnormality usually have leaked their entire lives, unable to gain continence at any point. The incontinence, instead of being diurnal or nocturnal only, is a combination of both. Children with suspected anatomic defects should be evaluated with imaging of both the kidneys and bladder by ultrasound and voiding cystogram with or without a fluoroscopic urodynamics study. Children with voiding dysfunction are able to gain continence for a varying period of time followed by incontinence.

It is important during history taking to ask the child's primary caregiver for valuable insight into the general aspects of the child's voiding habits. One should ask precise questions, understandable to the child, in order to get accurate answers. This information can be augmented with a voiding diary because many parents may not be totally aware of the specifics and finer points of the child's voiding habits.

ONSET

At what age was the child toilet trained? If the child was trained, at what point did he or she start wetting? Were there any occurrences in the child's life coinciding with the onset of wetting? Has the child ever been able to be toilet trained? Is the wetting new over the last few days, weeks, or months?

FREQUENCY

Voiding diaries can be very helpful in diagnosing and treating voiding abnormalities. They can be kept over a 3- to 4-day period and include voiding times, volumes, wet versus dry, and any associated symptoms. Appropriate volumes can be calculated as age (in years) plus 2 oz. One should determine if the volumes are less than expected. Does the child void infrequently with larger-than-anticipated amounts? How many voids per day? How many accidents per week? Does the child wet multiple times during the day or only at night?

CHARACTER OF VOIDING

Does the male child compress his urethra while or after voiding? Does he sit or stand to void? Can the parent hear him voiding (good forceful stream) or does he dribble? Does the little girl void with her legs tightly closed? Does she sit back on the toilet or perch on the edge of the seat to help maintain balance (causing pelvic contraction)? Is the child in a rush? Does he or she delay voiding? Is there posturing (squatting, crossing legs)?

DEGREE

Does the child wet enough to require clothes to be changed, or does the wetting consist of only spotting in the underwear? Is the wetting before voiding (unstable bladder) or after voiding (vaginal pooling)?

Two other important aspects of the history are bowel habits and family history of wetting. Any bowel dysfunction must be corrected before one can treat any wetting abnormality successfully. One should obtain a family history because it is now evident that a genetic component is linked to conditions such as primary nocturnal enuresis. One should also ask about other associated urologic, neurologic, or nephrologic conditions (valves, reflux, renal insufficiency) or any previous surgeries.

Physical Examination

Once the history is taken, the physical examination should be performed, taking into account not only vitals (height, weight, blood pressure), as a basic starting point, but the general appearance of the child. Uncleanliness, poor hygiene, or poor dentition may suggest neglect or abuse. An abdominal examination should seek to identify masses, a palpable bladder, or stool in the colon. Careful inspection of the child's back for occult spinal dysraphisms includes looking for lipomas, scoliosis, hair patches, cutaneous lesions, sacral or coccygeal defects, or gluteal asymmetry. A basic neurologic examination is essential and should include such points as gait, reflexes, and brief examination room maneuvers to substantiate that no nerve deficits are contributing to the incontinence. Examination of the rectal area is important, but often passed over, and should incorporate assessing sphincter tone, ruling out pelvic masses, and looking for signs of fecal soiling. Additionally, one should inspect the external genitalia to diagnose labial adhesions in young girls, female epispadias (causing total incontinence), and signs of vaginal pooling (butterfly "rash" and irritation of the labia and perineal and perianal areas). In boys, one should look for narrowing or inflammation of the meatus, unretractable foreskin, hypospadias, or epispadias. If the physician can observe the child void, valuable information can be gained about the quality and pattern of the urinary stream.

Laboratory/Radiograph Examination

A urinalysis should be performed to check for infection, glucosuria, and proteinuria. A specific gravity test can exclude polyuria as a cause for incontinence and indicates if the kidneys concentrate properly. If indicated, a urine culture should be done. If all of the tests just mentioned are normal, no further testing is needed at this initial stage. After the history, physical examination, and urinalysis, the abnormality is classified as anatomic, functional, or neurogenic. When an anatomic problem is suspected, imaging of the upper tract as well as the bladder is needed. Usually a renal ultrasound and voiding cystourethrogram is performed. The same is required if the urine is infected, a neurologic disorder is diagnosed, or there is history of either. More complex testing (magnetic resonance imaging [MRI] or computed tomography [CT] scan) may need to be done if abnormal physical findings of the lower spine or sacrum are found. Although urodynamics testing may be invasive and is not done routinely as a screen, it may be valuable in those select patients with severe symptoms refractory to standard treatment or in the child with a neurologic lesion.

Diurnal Enuresis

Daytime wetting, or diurnal enuresis, is much more troubling to the school-aged child and adolescent because it is often obvious to family, friends, and peers as well as being socially unacceptable and a source of embarrassment and ridicule. Children who are wet during the day generally experience urge and urge incontinence and may be wet at night as well. They may posture, and when the urine volume is measured, a small bladder capacity may be found. Children generally outgrow daytime wetting as they mature, but until that time treatment can be offered, which parents generally expect. Initial treatment measures are usually directed toward placing the child on a timed voiding schedule (every 2 to 3 hours to empty the bladder before the child has an uninhibited bladder contraction), practicing good hygiene, and, of utmost importance, correcting constipation with stool softeners and a high-fiber diet.

The next step commonly is pharmacologic treatment of the voiding dysfunction. This must be tailored to the type of abnormality and whether there is associated infection or vesicoureteral reflux. For many years, the drug of choice has been oxybutynin (Ditropan) because the mainstay of treatment has been long-term anticholinergic use. Once the underlying bladder overactivity or instability is quashed and the overactivity of the external sphincter lessened, the result is diminished or eliminated elevated intravesical pressure. Another preparation used recently is tolterodine (Detrol).[1] Both of these drugs are now available in once-a-day long-acting formulations (Ditropan XL, Detrol LA). Both have been reported to have side effects in varying degrees such as facial flushing, dry mouth, diminished sweating, occasional blurred vision, and constipation. Other drugs, which have been used with varying levels of success, include hyoscyamine sulfate (Levsin),[1] propantheline (Pro-Banthine),[1] and dicyclomine hydrochloride (Bentyl).[1]

The child who fails initial treatment may need a further workup with fluoroscopic urodynamics studies to assess bladder function, filling pressure, and sphincter coordination with voiding.

Nocturnal Enuresis

Nocturnal enuresis (NE) has been described in early literature dating back to the Ebers papyrus with various documented causes and remedies across the centuries. It continues to be a very common problem affecting 15% to 20% of school-aged children. The prevalence falls to 5% at 10 years old and affects 1% of 15-year-old teenagers. Fifteen percent of children with monosymptomatic primary nocturnal enuresis experience spontaneous resolution each year. NE can have a serious impact on the child, leading to shame, guilt, and diminished self-esteem. Only about one third of parents seek medical attention; about the same number punish the child for wetting, mistakenly thinking laziness or purposeful behavior has caused the problem. It is therefore incumbent on anyone who treats young children to screen for bed-wetting, educate the parents, and offer treatment if appropriate.

There is no one isolated cause for bed-wetting. It has been attributed to a multifactorial maturational delay in arousal to a full bladder, a delay in maturation of the bladder resulting in a diminished nocturnal bladder capacity, and a diminished circadian rhythm of antidiuretic hormone production. Even a genetic component is implicated because bed-wetting has been shown to run in families.

Although bed-wetting is considered benign from a physical standpoint, because of the previously described negative impact, treatment options should be offered to the child age 6 years and older. The focus of the physician

---

[1]Not FDA approved for this indication.

treating NE should be to ensure the child has no physical abnormality causing the bed-wetting. The child who has pure monosymptomatic nocturnal enuresis needs no further evaluation than a good history and physical examination and a urinalysis.

Treatment should be first directed at treating constipation or any daytime frequency or wetting component, which can be a benign association in 15% to 25% of cases. Treatment measures should include patient education because once the child (and parents) have an understanding of the mechanisms behind bed-wetting, compliance and success of treatment often improve. Initial therapy should also center on evening fluid restriction, avoidance of caffeine and artificial dyes (particularly red number 40), and motivational therapy with rewards and praise for dry nights. The child has no control over wet nights and should never be punished for a wet bed.

If the parents decide treatment is desirable, they can choose between pharmacologic and nonpharmacologic options. For those wishing to avoid medication, conditioning therapy with a moisture-sensitive alarm is an option. Several enuresis alarms are available on the market, all with the goal of awakening the child at or shortly after the time of micturition. The first drops of urine complete a circuit, activating a buzzer designed to awaken the child. It is important for a family member to be involved in the process to ensure the child wakes up and completes the voiding process in the toilet. Over time a conditioned response develops, and the child awakens voluntarily to a full bladder without help from the alarm. This process can take weeks to months, therefore requiring a patient and dedicated family and child to achieve success. The overall success rate has been stated as 50%, but with family involvement and proper use it can be as high as 70% to 90%.

Additional nonpharmacologic treatments offered include motivational therapy, bladder training exercises, hypnotherapy, bladder training, night wakening, and fluid restriction and diet therapy. All except motivational therapy have shown disappointing results.

The alternative to the alarm is pharmacologic treatment. The most commonly used drug now is desmopressin acetate (DDAVP) in tablet form and less commonly nasal spray. Desmopressin acetate is a synthetic analogue of vasopressin, a potent antidiuretic hormone produced by the pituitary gland. Desmopressin acetate tablets are dosed starting at 0.2 mg 1 hour before bed (food and drink should be withheld 1 hour before dosing) and increased by one tablet per week up to 0.6 mg or until dryness is achieved at a lower dose. Success rates increase with higher doses and can be as high as 60% to 70%. Side effects are rare even at

CURRENT DIAGNOSIS

- Obtain a good voiding history, including family history of wetting, history of all elimination habits, and dietary history.
- Do a thorough physical examination, including neurologic and rectal if appropriate and indicated.
- Educate the family and debunk any myths about wetting.
- Give the family multiple treatment options, both pharmacologic and nonpharmacologic, including observation.

the higher doses. If a child responds, that dose is continued for 3 to 6 months before structured weaning by one less tablet a night per week. The drug can also be used long term without reservation. Another advantage is its ability to be used intermittently in situations like nightly or weekend sleepovers at a friend's house or overnight trips.

Another acceptable alternative is imipramine (Tofranil), a tricyclic antidepressant that has generalized effects on the bladder including weak α-adrenergic and anticholinergic effects. It weakly increases arousal and additionally may have some antidiuretic properties. Dosage begins at 25 mg at bedtime and is increased if necessary to 50 mg at bedtime in preadolescents and 75 mg per night in adolescents. There has been some hesitancy recently using imipramine because of certain profound side effects that have been observed. These include insomnia, weight loss, extrapyramidal symptoms, anxiety, and personality changes. Fatal cardiac dysrhythmias have been reported with overdosage. If dosed properly, imipramine can be an effective and safe drug. If effective, medicine is dosed for 6 months before attempts to wean.

REFERENCES

Cendron M: Primary nocturnal enuresis: Current concepts. Am Fam Physician 1999;59(5):1205-1214, 1219-1220.
Hinsl KK, Hurwitz RS: Urol Clin North Am 1991;18(2):283-293.
Roth DR: Enuresis. In Rakel RE, Bope ET (eds): Conn's Current Therapy 2003, 55th ed. Philadelphia, Elsevier Science, 2003.
Rushton HG: Wetting and functional voiding disorders. Urol Clin North Am 1995;22(1):75-93.
Rushton HG, Belman AB: Enuresis and voiding dysfunction: A national kidney foundation guide to the child who wets. Washington, DC, Children's National Medical Center, 1999.

CURRENT THERAPY

- Treatment of constipation is the initial measure.
- Children should not be punished for wet nights.
- For the bed-wetting alarms to be effective, family involvement is critical.
- Patience and understanding of the process are important for compliance with therapy and attaining success.

Urinary Incontinence

Method of
E. Ann Gormley, MD

Urinary incontinence is a significant problem that affects millions of Americans. Patients may not report incontinence to their primary care providers because of embarrassment or misconceptions regarding treatment.

TABLE 1 Etiology of Incontinence

Bladder Dysfunction
1. Urge incontinence
   - Detrusor overactivity
     - Idiopathic
     - Neurogenic origin
   - Poor compliance
2. Overflow incontinence

Urethral Dysfunction
3. Stress incontinence
   - Anatomic
   - Intrinsic sphincter deficiency

Because incontinence is often treatable, it behooves the health care professional to identify patients who might benefit from treatment. Given that the treatment of incontinence varies depending on the etiology, the aim of evaluation is to identify the etiology.

Etiology

Urinary incontinence is generally the result of either bladder or urethral dysfunction (Table 1). Incontinence also may result from a nonurologic cause and is usually reversible when the underlying problem is treated (Table 2). More uncommon causes of incontinence are urinary fistulae and ectopic ureteral orifices.

BLADDER DYSFUNCTION

Bladder dysfunction causes urge or overflow incontinence. *Urge incontinence* occurs when the bladder pressure is sufficient to overcome the sphincter mechanism. Elevated bladder or detrusor pressure tends to open the bladder neck and urethra. An elevation in detrusor pressure may occur from intermittent bladder contractions (detrusor overactivity) or because of an incremental rise in pressure with increased bladder volume (poor compliance). Detrusor overactivity may be idiopathic, or it may be associated with a neurologic disease (detrusor overactivity of neurogenic origin). Detrusor overactivity is common in the elderly and may be associated with bladder outlet obstruction. Poor bladder compliance results from loss of the viscoelastic features of the bladder or because of a change in neuroregulatory activity. The patient with urge incontinence may appreciate a sudden sensation to void but then is unable to suppress the urge fully. In severe cases, the patient may not be aware of the sensation of needing to void until he or she is actually leaking. The amount of leakage in patients with urge incontinence is variable, depending on the patient's ability to suppress the contraction. Patients with urge incontinence will often have frequency and nocturia in addition to urgency and urge incontinence. They may also have nocturnal enuresis.

Overactive bladder is a newer term that describes patients with frequency and urgency with or without urge incontinence.

Overflow incontinence occurs at extreme bladder volumes or when the bladder volume reaches the limit of the bladder's viscoelastic properties. The loss of urine is driven by an elevation in detrusor pressure. Overflow incontinence is seen in the case of incomplete bladder

TABLE 2 Transient Causes of Incontinence (*DIAPPERS*)

Cause	Comment
Delirium	Incontinence may be secondary to delirium and will often stop when acute delirium resolves.
Infection	Symptomatic infection may prevent a patient from reaching the toilet in time.
Atrophic vaginitis	Vaginitis may cause the same symptoms as an infection.
Pharmacologic	
• Sedatives	Alcohol and long-acting benzodiazepines may cause confusion and secondary incontinence.
• Diuretics	A brisk diuresis may overwhelm the bladder's capacity and cause uninhibited detrusor contractions, resulting in urge incontinence.
• Anticholinergics	Many nonprescription and prescription medications have anticholinergic properties. Side effects of anticholinergics include urinary retention with associated frequency and overflow incontinence.
• α Adrenergics	Tone in the bladder neck and proximal sphincter is increased by α-adrenergic agonists and can cause urinary retention, particularly in men with prostatism.
• α Antagonists	Tone in the smooth muscles of the bladder neck and proximal sphincter is decreased with α-adrenergic antagonists. Women treated with these drugs for hypertension may develop or have an exacerbation of stress incontinence.
Psychological	Depression may be occasionally associated with incontinence.
Excessive urine production	Excessive intake, diabetes, hypercalcemia, congestive heart failure, and peripheral edema can all lead to polyuria, which can lead to incontinence.
Restricted mobility	Incontinence may be precipitated or aggravated if the patient cannot get to the toilet quickly enough.
Stool impaction	Patients with impacted stool can have urge or overflow urinary incontinence and may also have fecal incontinence.

From Resnick NM: Urinary incontinence in the elderly. Med Grand Rounds 1984;3:281-290.

CURRENT DIAGNOSIS

Urge Incontinence

Symptoms
- Urgency
- Frequency
- Nocturia
- Unable to reach the toilet with urge

Stress Incontinence

Symptoms
- Leakage with physical activity

Signs
- Bladder neck mobility
- Positive stress test

Mixed Incontinence

Symptoms
- Urgency
- Frequency
- Nocturia
- Unable to reach the toilet with urge
- Leakage with physical activity

Signs
- Bladder neck mobility
- Positive stress test

Overflow Incontinence

Symptoms
- Frequency
- Nocturia
- Urgency
- Leakage with physical activity

Signs
- High postvoid residual

emptying caused by either obstruction or poor bladder contractility. Obstruction is rare in women but can result from severe pelvic prolapse or following surgery for stress incontinence. Patients with overflow incontinence complain of constant dribbling, and they may also describe extreme frequency.

URETHRAL-RELATED INCONTINENCE

Urethral-related incontinence, or *stress incontinence*, occurs because of either urethral hypermobility or intrinsic sphincter deficiency (ISD). Incontinence associated with urethral hypermobility has been called *anatomic incontinence* because the incontinence is due to malposition of the sphincter unit. Displacement of the proximal urethra below the level of the pelvic floor does not allow for transmission of abdominal pressure that normally aids in closing the urethra. Some women with mobility of the bladder neck or urethra do not experience incontinence. ISD was initially believed to occur after failure of one or more operations for stress incontinence. Other causes of ISD include myelodysplasia, trauma, and radiation. Some authors have theorized that all incontinent patients must have an element of ISD in order to actually leak. The patient with stress incontinence leaks urine with any sudden increase in abdominal pressure. In patients with severe ISD, the increase in abdominal pressure required to cause leakage is small, so patients may leak urine with minimal activity.

Evaluation of the Incontinent Patient

The evaluation of the incontinent patient includes a history, physical examination, laboratory tests, and possibly urodynamic testing. The onset, frequency, severity, and pattern of incontinence should be sought, as well as any associated symptoms such as frequency, dysuria, urgency, and nocturia. Incontinence may be quantified by asking the patient if he or she wears a pad and how often the pad is changed. Obstructive symptoms, such as a feeling of incomplete emptying, hesitancy, straining, or weak stream, may coexist with incontinence, particularly in males and in female patients with previous incontinence procedure, cystoceles, or poor detrusor contractility. Female patients should be asked about symptoms of pelvic prolapse, such as recurrent urinary tract infection, a sensation of vaginal fullness or pressure, or the observation of a bulge in the vagina. All incontinent patients should be asked about bowel function and neurologic symptoms. Response to previous treatments, including drugs, should be noted. Important features of the history include previous gynecologic and urologic procedures, neurologic problems, and past medical problems. A list of the patient's current medications, including over-the-counter medications, should be obtained.

Although the history may define the patient's problem, it may be misleading. Urge incontinence may be triggered by activities such as coughing, so according to the patient's history, he or she seems to have stress incontinence. A patient who complains only of urge incontinence may also have stress incontinence. Mixed incontinence is very common; at least 65% of patients with stress incontinence have associated urgency or urge incontinence.

A complete physical examination is performed, with emphasis on the neurologic assessment and on the abdominal, pelvic, and rectal examinations. In females, the condition of the vaginal mucosa and the degree of urethral mobility are determined. Simple pelvic examination with the patient supine is sufficient to determine if the urethra moves with straining or coughing. The degree of movement is not as important as the determination of whether movement occurs. The presence of associated pelvic organ prolapse should be noted because it can contribute to the patient's voiding problems and may have an impact on diagnosis and treatment. A rectal examination in both males and females includes the evaluation of sphincter tone and perineal sensation.

A urinalysis is performed to determine if there is any evidence of hematuria, pyuria, glucosuria, or proteinuria. A urine specimen is sent for cytologic examination if there is hematuria and/or irritative voiding symptoms. The urine is cultured if there is pyuria or bacteriuria. Infection should be treated prior to further investigations or interventions. Hematuria consisting of more than three red cells per high-power field warrants further investigation.

A postvoid residual (PVR) should be measured either with pelvic ultrasound or directly with a catheter.

CURRENT THERAPY

Urge Incontinence

Behavioral Changes
- Avoidance of bladder irritants
- Timed voiding
- Pelvic muscle exercises

Anticholinergics—Antimuscarinics—Nonselective for M3 Receptor
- Propantheline (Pro-Banthine)[1] 7.5 to 30 mg orally, three to five times daily
- Tolterodine (Detrol LA) 4 mg orally, daily
- Trospium (Sanctura) 20 mg orally, two times daily
- Solifenacin (Vesicare) 5–10 mg orally, daily

Anticholinergics—Antimuscarinics—Selective for M3 Receptor
- Darifenacin (Enablex) 7.5–15 mg orally, daily

Anticholinergics—Antimuscarinics/Smooth Muscle Relaxants
- Oxybutynin
- Regular (Ditropan) 2.5–5 mg orally, one to three times daily
- Extended-release (Ditropan XL) 5–30 mg orally, daily
- Transdermal (Oxytrol) 3.9-mg patch, twice per week
- Hyoscyamine (Levsin) 0.125–0.375 mg orally, two to four times daily

Anticholinergics/α Agonist—For Urge or Mixed Incontinence
- Imipramine (Tofranil)[1] 10–25 mg, once to three times daily

Stress Incontinence

Behavioral Changes
- Weight loss
- Quitting smoking
- Pelvic muscle exercises

α Agonists
- Pseudoephedrine (Sudafed)[1] 30–60 mg, up to four times daily

Surgery
- Anatomic
  - Retropubic suspensions
    - Burch
    - Marshall-Marchetti-Krantz
  - Slings
  - Pubovaginal
  - Midurethral
  - Obturator
- Intrinsic Sphincter Deficiency
  - Slings
    - Pubovaginal
    - Midurethral
    - Obturator
  - Artificial sphincter
- Submucosal Injections with Bulking Agents
  - Collagen (Contigen)
  - Carbon-coated zirconium oxide beads (Durasphere)
  - Ethylene vinyl alcohol copolymer (Tegress)

[1]Not FDA approved for this indication.

A normal PVR is less than 50 mL, and a PVR greater than 200 mL is abnormal. A significant PVR urine may reflect either bladder outlet obstruction or poor bladder contractility. The only way to distinguish outlet obstruction from poor contractility is with urodynamic testing.

Urodynamic testing is used to accurately diagnose the etiology of a patient's incontinence; however, many patients can be successfully treated without urodynamic testing. The purpose of urodynamic testing is to examine compliance, diagnose stress incontinence, and rule out obstruction as a cause of either overflow or urge incontinence. Urodynamic testing should ideally be performed prior to invasive therapies and certainly in patients who are undergoing repeat procedures following failed procedures.

Treatment of Urinary Incontinence

URGE INCONTINENCE

Patients with urge incontinence need to understand that they leak urine because their bladder contracts with little or no warning. The first line of treatment is timed voiding. Often, reminding patients to void every 1 to 2 hours during the day, before they get an urge to void, will result in them staying dry. Other behavioral interventions, such as modification of fluid intake, avoidance of bladder irritants, and bladder retraining, where the patient attempts to consciously delay voiding and to increase the interval between voids, may also have a role in the treatment of urge incontinence.

Anticholinergics are the mainstay of medical therapy in achieving continence. The side effects of anticholinergics include urinary retention, dry mouth, constipation, nausea, blurred vision, tachycardia, drowsiness, and confusion. They are contraindicated in patients with narrow-angle glaucoma. Anticholinergics are also used to decrease bladder pressure in patients with poor compliance. Anticholinergics are combined with clean intermittent catheterization in patients who have a significant PVR prior to treatment and in patients who develop retention while taking anticholinergics.

Patients with intractable detrusor overactivity may require surgical intervention, consisting of neuromodulation with a sacral nerve stimulator or various forms of bladder augmentation.

The primary goal in caring for the patient with poor compliance is treating the high bladder pressure. Complete bladder emptying with clean intermittent catheterization combined with anticholinergics will often lower bladder pressure to a safe range. Some patients may require a combination of anticholinergics and α agonists. Bladder augmentation is required when medical management fails.

OVERFLOW INCONTINENCE

Overflow incontinence is treated by emptying the bladder. If the cause of overflow is obstruction, then relieving the obstruction should lead to improved emptying. Anatomic obstruction in males derives from either urethral stricture disease or prostatic obstruction. Depending on the severity of urethral stricture disease, the patient may require urethral dilation, internal urethrotomy, or urethroplasty. Prostatic obstruction may be treated in a variety of ways, but transurethral resection remains the gold standard. If a woman is obstructed from previous surgery or from pelvic prolapse, she may benefit from urethrolysis or surgical correction of the prolapse. Clean intermittent catheterization is an option in the obstructed patient who does not want or could not tolerate further surgery.

The patient with overflow incontinence secondary to poor detrusor contractility is best treated with clean intermittent catheterization.

Indwelling catheters are not an optimum treatment modality for treatment of incontinence. All patients with indwelling catheters will have infected urine, which predisposes them to bladder calculi and ultimately to squamous cell carcinoma of the bladder. Any foreign object in the bladder can cause or exacerbate elevated bladder pressure that is associated with hydronephrosis, ureteral obstruction, renal stones, and eventually renal failure.

STRESS INCONTINENCE

The amount of incontinence and how it affects the patient often determines the aggressiveness of treatment. The patient who is severely restricted because of severe leakage with minimal movement may not want to try medical therapy but may opt for surgical treatment, whereas the patient who leaks small amounts infrequently may choose conservative treatment. Pelvic floor exercises can improve anatomic stress urinary incontinence by augmenting closure of the external urethral sphincter and by preventing descent and rotation of the bladder neck and urethra. To benefit from the exercises, women must be taught to do the exercises properly, and they must do them. Adjuncts to learning pelvic floor exercises include weighted vaginal cones, a perineometer, and electrical stimulation.

α Agonists such as phenylpropanolamine[1] and pseudoephedrine (Sudafed)[1] can be used for treatment of stress incontinence. The bladder neck and proximal urethra have abundant α receptors. Activation of these receptors by α agonists leads to an increase in smooth muscle tone. The usual dose is twice daily, but some women who are incontinent with exercise may benefit from taking an α agonist 1 hour before exercise. Tricyclic antidepressants, such as imipramine (Tofranil),[1] have both α-agonist and anticholinergic properties.

Surgical therapy for stress incontinence is indicated when a patient does not wish to pursue nonsurgical therapy, or if such therapy has failed. The type of surgical therapy depends on the diagnosis. Patients who have anatomic stress incontinence can benefit from a variety of surgical repairs that restore the bladder neck to its normal retropubic position or improve urethral support. Patients with ISD usually have a well-supported bladder neck. These patients require a procedure that will close or coapt the proximal urethra. Coaptation may be achieved with a variety of bulking agents that are injected into the bladder neck or proximal urethra. A pubovaginal sling is the ideal procedure for the patient with both ISD and anatomic stress incontinence, as a sling will coapt the proximal urethra and restore the bladder neck to its normal location.

---

[1]Not FDA approved for this indication.
[2]Not available in the United States.

BOX 1	Overview of Treatments

Behavioral Changes
- Avoidance of bladder irritants
- Weight loss
- Quitting smoking
- Pelvic muscle exercises

Medical Therapy
- α Agonists
  - Stress incontinent patients
  - Mixed incontinent patients
- Anticholinergics
  - Urge incontinent patients
- Anticholinergics/α agonists
  - Mixed incontinent patients

Surgical Therapy
- Stress incontinent patients
- Rare patients with urge incontinence

Synthetic midurethral slings are ideal for the patient with anatomic stress incontinence who wishes surgery with minimal recovery time. In one of the rare randomized surgical trials for stress incontinence, the result with tension-free vaginal tape has been shown to be comparable to that of a Burch colposuspension at 6, 12, and 24 months. The newest sling is a transobturator sling that is placed transversely underneath the urethra from one obturator foramina to the other. The advantage of this sling is that the retropubic space is avoided, with low risk of bladder, bowel, and major vessel injury.

Randomized trials comparing midurethral or transobturator slings to pubovaginal slings have not been performed.

MIXED INCONTINENCE

Stress and urge incontinence often coexist. Burgio et al. advocate pelvic muscle exercises with biofeedback for treatment of stress and urge incontinence. Behavioral therapy can result in a reduction in incontinence episodes and patient-perceived improvement.

Imipramine (Tofranil)[1] is beneficial in patients with mixed (stress and urge) incontinence. The recommended dose is 10 to 25 mg, three times daily.

Seventy percent of patients with combined incontinence (stress and urge) will be relieved of urge incontinence following a procedure for stress incontinence. Patients whose urge incontinence does not respond to anticholinergics preoperatively may have a good response to anticholinergics once their stress incontinence is treated. Box 1 provides an overview of treatments.

REFERENCES

Blaivas JG, Groutz A: Urinary incontinence: Pathophysiology, evaluation, and management overview. In Walsh PC, Retik AB, Vaughan ED Jr, Wein AJ (eds): Campbell's Urology, vol 2, 8th ed. Philadelphia, WB Saunders, 2002, p 1027.

---

[1]Not FDA approved for this indication.

Burgio KL, Locher JL, Goode PS, et al: Behavioral vs drug treatment for urge urinary incontinence in older women: A randomized controlled trial. JAMA 1998;280:1995-2000.

Leach GE, Dmochowski RR, Appell RA, et al: Female Stress Urinary Incontinence Clinical Guidelines Panel summary report on surgical management of female stress urinary incontinence. The American Urological Association. J Urol 1997;158:875.

Ward KL, Hilton P: A randomized trial of colposuspension and tension-free vaginal tape (TVT) for primary genuine stress incontinence: 2 year follow-up. Int Urogynecol J Pelvic Floor Dysfunct 2001; 12[Suppl. 2]:S7-S8.

Epididymitis

Method of
Michael Thomas Gambla, MD,
and Darren Chapman, MD

Epididymitis refers to inflammation or infection of the epididymis. *Acute epididymitis* is defined by a duration of symptoms of less than 6 weeks, typically with pain and swelling. *Chronic epididymitis* refers to a longer duration of pain, usually not accompanied by swelling.

Epidemiology

Acute epididymitis is a major cause of urologic morbidity. In a survey published by Collins and colleagues of almost 60,000 ambulatory office visits of all medical specialties, epididymitis accounted for 1 in 345 (0.29%), making it the fifth most common urologic cause of an office visit, behind prostatitis, urinary tract infection (UTI), kidney stones, and sexually transmitted diseases (STDs) in men ages 18 to 50 years. In a review of 121 patients, Kaver and Matzkin found it most commonly occurs in patients ages 16 to 30 and 51 to 70 years. Mittemeyer and colleagues' data on 610 U.S. Army soldiers also demonstrated a peak incidence in the 20- to 29-year-old age range. There is no predilection for laterality, and up to 9% of cases can be bilateral. There is no racial bias.

Pathophysiology

Before Berger published his landmark paper in 1979, reflux of urine into the vas deferens was considered the cause of epididymitis. Using cultures and epididymal aspirates, however, Berger proved that most cases of epididymitis are caused by bacterial infection. The causative organisms vary according to the age of the patient. *Neisseria gonorrhoeae* and *Chlamydia trachomatis* are the common isolates in men younger than 35 years; *Escherichia coli* is usually found in men older than 35 years. Thus in younger, sexually active men, it is the common causes of sexually transmitted urethritis that cause epididymitis, whereas in the older age groups, it is the common urinary pathogens. Note that in men who practice anal intercourse, coliform bacteria are the common causative organisms. Less common pathogens include the sexually transmitted *Ureaplasma*

urealyticum, as well as the common urinary pathogens *Proteus* species, *Klebsiella pneumoniae, Pseudomonas aeruginosa,* and *Haemophilus influenzae. Mycobacterium tuberculosis* is a rare cause of epididymitis but must be considered in patients at risk for this disease. One fifth of men with mumps develop acute epididymo-orchitis because of the virus. Cytomegalovirus (CMV) is another viral cause of epididymitis, but it is associated with HIV-positive patients. Noninfectious causes are the vasculitides as well as the antiarrhythmic amiodarone (Cordarone).

Presentation and Evaluation

The most comprehensive review of the presentation of epididymitis was published by Kaver and Matzkin. In their evaluation, 90% of patients presented with a duration of symptoms of 1 week or less. Dysuria was present in one third, and 75% had a temperature higher than 37.5°C (99.5°F), but only 20% reported chills. Orchitis, an infection of the testicle, was present in 58%. Scrotal skin erythema was present in 62%. Peripheral leukocytosis occurred in 64%. Hematuria was present in 53%, and pyuria in 79%.

The Centers for Disease Control and Prevention (CDC) has made recommendations for the evaluation of patients with epididymitis. An intraurethral swab or Gram stain as well as a culture of the urethral exudate should be obtained. Patients with a gonoccocal infection should be identified. If the urethral Gram stain is negative, a urinalysis, urine Gram stain, and urine culture should be obtained. Syphilis serology and HIV testing should also be performed.

Differential Diagnosis

The most important differentiation that must be made is between acute epididymitis and torsion of the testicle. Physical findings can be helpful in that torsion manifests with a high transversely oriented testicle, whereas the testicle is in its normal anatomic position in epididymitis. A swollen, tender epididymis often can be palpated in the patient with acute epididymitis. Prehn's sign, or relief of pain with elevation of the testicle, may be present in epididymitis, whereas elevating a torsed testicle generally induces more pain. The physical examination may be difficult in a patient with an inflamed hemiscrotum and

CURRENT DIAGNOSIS

- Onset greater than or equal to 1 week
- Pain on palpation of epididymis
- Scrotal skin erythema
- Leukocytosis
- Elevated temperature
- Pyuria
- Association with gonorrhea, chlamydia, or *Escherichia coli* infection
- Scrotal ultrasound to differentiate epididymitis, testicular torsion, and tumor

a reactive hydrocele. Testicular ultrasound is a reliable noninvasive test that can distinguish between epididymitis and testicular torsion. If the diagnosis is in question, immediate surgical exploration is warranted because time is critical in the treatment of torsion. Testicular cancer, although less commonly misdiagnosed as epididymitis, should also be considered. An ultrasound is helpful in making this distinction as well. If this diagnosis is considered, tumor markers (α-fetoprotein, β-human chorionic gonadotropin [β-hCG], and lactic dehydrogenase [LDH]) should be sent.

Management

Patients should be treated with empirical antibiotic therapy. For patients with presumptive gonococcal or chlamydial infections, a single dose of ceftriaxone (Rocephin) 250 mg intramuscularly and doxycycline (Vibramycin) 100 mg orally twice a day for 10 days is the regimen recommended by the CDC. An oral dose of 1 g of azithromycin (Zithromax) may be substituted for doxycyline if compliance is an issue. In patients whose epididymitis is caused by coliform bacteria, or in those who are allergic to cephalosporins and/or tetracyclines, a 10-day course of ofloxacin (Floxin), 300 mg orally twice a day, should be prescribed. For symptomatic improvement, a 2-week course of anti-inflammatories begun at the time of antibiotics has proved very effective in reducing both pain and swelling. Patients should adhere to a regimen of decreased activity and scrotal elevation. Those who do not improve within 3 to 5 days should be reevaluated. Patients who are systemically ill, or those with a scrotal abscess or pyocele, should be hospitalized and treated with intravenous antibiotics. Surgical therapy is usually reserved for the most severe cases.

Prognosis

Acute epididymitis caused by a sexually transmitted infection usually resolves quickly with appropriate therapy. Complications are more common in cases caused by coliforms and include testicular abscess, testicular infarction, and testicular atrophy. Reduced spermatogenesis and subfertility may also occur. Chronic pain is uncommon but is a clinical and therapeutic dilemma.

CURRENT THERAPY

Age Younger Than 35 Years
- Ceftriaxone (Rocephin) 250 mg IM × 1 *and either*
- Doxycycline (Vibramycin) 100 mg PO bid × 10 days *or*
- Azithromycin (Zithromax) 1 g PO × 1

Age Older Than 35 Years
- Ofloxacin (Floxin) 300 mg PO bid × 10 days

All Patients
- Anti-inflammatories
- Decreased activity
- Scrotal elevation
- Pain control

Abbreviations: bid = twice a day; IM = intramuscular; PO = by mouth.

REFERENCES

Berger RE, Alexander ER, Harnisch JP, et al: Etiology, manifestations and therapy of acute epididymitis: Prospective study of 50 cases. J Urol 1979;121:750-754.

Berger RE, Lee JC. Sexually transmitted diseases: The classic diseases. In Walsh PC, Retik AB, Vaughan ED, et al. (eds): Campbell's Urology, 8th ed. Philadelphia, WB Saunders, 2002, pp 671-691.

Centers for Disease Control and Prevention. Sexually transmitted diseases treatment guidelines. MMWR 1998;47:1-118.

Collins MM, Stafford RS, O'Leary MP, et al: How common is prostatitis? A national survey of physician visits. J Urol 1998;159:1224-1228.

Kaver I, Matzkin H: Epididymo-orchitis: A retrospective study of 121 patients. J Fam Pract 1990;30:548-552.

Luzzi GA, O'Brien TS: Acute epididymitis. BJU Int 2001;87:747-755.

Mittemeyer BT, Lennox KW, Borski AA: Epididymitis: A review of 610 cases. J Urol 1966;95:390-392.

Primary Glomerular Disease

Method of
Daniel Cattran, MD,
and Penny Turner, MD

Primary, or idiopathic, glomerular diseases encompass a wide variety of clinical scenarios and management. They vary from the treatment of asymptomatic urinary abnormalities to the complexity of renal replacement therapy. This article focuses on their clinicopathologic correlations and management.

Clinical Presentation

The most common presentations and their histologies are described in the following text and summarized in Table 1.

- Acute nephritic syndrome (ANS): This is defined by the presence of hypertension, active urine sediment, and usually some degree of renal insufficiency. Active sediment implies that dysmorphic (misshapen) red blood cells (RBCs) and RBC casts are in the urine. Rapidly progressive glomerulonephritis (RPGN) is the most extreme example of this syndrome. Renal function declines rapidly over weeks or months, often to the point of requiring dialysis.
- Nephrotic syndrome: This is defined by the presence of edema, hypoalbuminemia, hypercholesterolemia, and proteinuria greater than 3.5 g per day (>50 mg/m^2 in children). Renal function is usually normal.
- Asymptomatic microhematuria and/or proteinuria: This state is defined by the results of a positive urine dipstick test for blood and/or protein in a completely asymptomatic individual.
- Gross hematuria: This is characterized by redness in the urine that can be seen by the naked eye.
- Uremic syndrome: This state is accompanied by symptoms of chronic renal failure, including decreased appetite, weight loss, pruritus, decreased energy, and other symptoms of chronic kidney failure.

TABLE 1 Primary Glomerular Diseases and Their Common Presentations

Primary Glomerular Disease	Presentation
Minimal Change Disease	Nephrotic syndrome
FSGS	Nephrotic syndrome, +/– reduced renal function, +/– hypertension in up to 50%
Membranous Glomerulopathy	Nephrotic syndrome, usually normal renal function
MPGN	Nephritic (10-30%), nephrotic syndrome (40-50%), asymptomatic proteinuria (20-40%)
Diffuse Proliferative GN	Acute nephritic syndrome
IgA Nephropathy	Asymptomatic hematuria +/– proteinuria (40-70%), nephrotic syndrome (2-30%), acute nephritic syndrome (10-20%)
Crescentic GN	Acute nephritic syndrome

TABLE 2 Secondary Glomerular Diseases Pathology and Their Common Causes

Pathology Type	Causative Factor
Minimal Change Disease	Medications
	Malignancy
Focal Segmental	HIV
Glomerulosclerosis	Obesity
	Reflux nephropathy
Membranous	Hepatitis B
Nephropathy	Systemic lupus erythematosus
	Malignancy
	Medications
MPGN Type 1	Hepatitis C
	Systemic lupus erythematosus
Diffuse Proliferative GN	Bacterial infection
IgA Nephropathy	Liver disease
Type 1 Crescentic GN	Antiglomerular basement Membrane antibodies
Type 2 Crescentic GN	Systemic lupus erythematosus Bacterial infection
Type 3 Crescentic GN	Systemic vasculitis

Approach to Diagnosis

All patients with suspected primary glomerular disease should have serum creatinine, urinalysis, and a quantitative estimate (24-hour urine collection or aliquot for protein-to-creatinine ratio) of proteinuria if positive on dipstick. The urine dipstick is a sensitive test for microhematuria and proteinuria, often the two earliest signs of glomerular disease. If the dipstick results are positive, perform a urine microscopic examination to identify other signs of glomerular disease such as dysmorphic RBCs, RBC casts, granular casts, and oval fat bodies.

Patients with signs or symptoms suggesting glomerular disease, such as persistent proteinuria and/or impaired renal function, should be considered for renal biopsy. This is the best way to classify the primary glomerular diseases for prognosis and treatment. The risk of biopsy is low. The only major hazard is significant bleeding, and in expert hands it occurs in fewer than 1% of procedures.

Secondary glomerular renal disease can occur as a consequence of a systemic process, often closely mimics primary glomerular disease, and can only be excluded after close clinical and laboratory evaluations (Table 2). Treatment is targeted at the underlying causative factor and is often different from primary glomerular disease.

Treatment

TARGETS OF THERAPY

The therapy goals are to:

- Slow or prevent loss of renal function
- Complete reversal of proteinuria
- Reduce proteinuria

The management of primary glomerular diseases can be divided into conservative and specific therapies.

CONSERVATIVE THERAPY

Conservative therapy is aimed at slowing the progression of the underlying glomerular disease. Blood pressure (BP) targets are substantially lower than in the past; 130/80 mm Hg or lower (e.g., 125/75 mm Hg in patients with ≥1 g/day of proteinuria) is recommended. The initial agent should be an angiotensin-converting enzyme inhibitor (ACEI) because it not only lowers BP but also has an independent renal protective benefit. The latter is reflected in greater reductions in proteinuria compared with other classes of antihypertensive agents per mm Hg BP decrease. Angiotensin receptor blockers (ARBs) also have a similar additive benefit. ACEIs used in combination with ARBs are synergistic in regard to their benefit in proteinuria and renal function preservation. The serum creatinine may initially rise 5% to 10% with the initiation of an ACEI or ARB, but this is hemodynamic rather than nephrotoxic and will stabilize after 2 to 3 months. An important caveat with single or combined ACEI/ARB therapy is the careful monitoring of the serum potassium level because hyperkalemia is a risk, especially if renal function is 50% of normal or less.

Diuretics like furosemide (Lasix) are used as necessary to control symptoms secondary to volume overload and work well if used in conjunction with a low-sodium diet. Spironolactone (Aldactone) is often a useful addition, especially if the nephrotic syndrome is severe. Again, watch for hyperkalemia if ACEI/ARB plus spironolactone (Aldactone) is used.

Metolazone (Zaroxolyn), a powerful thiazide diuretic, may need to be added in cases of refractory edema and/or if renal insufficiency is severe. Care must be taken to maintain euvolemia. Excessive intravascular volume depletion not only increases the risk of decreased renal perfusion and acute renal failure, but it may also increase the thrombotic tendency in the severely nephrotic patient and accentuate muscle cramping.

Cholesterol is usually elevated with either nephrotic range proteinuria and/or chronic kidney impairment. The hyperlipidemia is an independent cardiovascular risk factor and lipid-lowering therapy, most commonly with beta-hydroxy-β-methylglutaryl-coenzyme A (HMG-CoA) reductase inhibitors such as atorvastatin (Lipitor) 20 to 40 mg daily to achieve a low-density lipoprotein (LDL) cholesterol of less than 100 mg/dL is recommended. Ezetimibe (Ezetrol), a new lipid-lowering agent that inhibits intestinal absorption of cholesterol, is a useful addition in resistant cases or when statins are not tolerated.

SPECIFIC THERAPY

The *specific* therapy of primary glomerular diseases, based on their underlying renal pathology, is discussed in the following text; and Table 3 summarizes it as well.

MINIMAL CHANGE DISEASE

Pathology

Minimal change disease (MCD) is named for the absence of any abnormalities on light and immunofluorescence microscopy. The identifying characteristic of this disease is diffuse effacement of the epithelial foot processes with loss of slit diaphragms on electron microscopy.

Treatment

MCD remains the most common cause of the idiopathic nephrotic syndrome in children. Treatment for children is prednisone at 60 mg/m^2 per day (up to 80 mg/day) for

4 weeks, and then 40 mg/m^2 on alternate days for 4 to 8 weeks, slowly tapering off over 4 to 6 weeks. Remission is achieved in more than 90% of cases within 8 weeks. Up to 75% of children will have at least one relapse, and 50% will have a frequently relapsing course, defined by two or more relapses within a 6-month period. Initially, most relapses are retreated with prednisone alone. Renal biopsy in this age group is usually only performed after at least 4 weeks of therapy, if the patient is unresponsive, or if the response is incomplete. Approximately 10% of children will have steroid-resistant disease and most will subsequently have focal and segmental glomerulosclerosis on biopsy.

MCD is an uncommon cause of the nephrotic syndrome in adults, but its presentation is similar. In contrast to children, however, there may be age-related renal insufficiency and/or hypertension. Treatment with prednisone in doses of 1 mg/kg per day up to a maximum of 80 mg per day is often required, but for a longer period (12 to 16 weeks) before a complete remission is induced. In addition, there is a lower rate (approximately 75%) of success than in children.

Steroid-resistant and steroid-dependent patients (especially if maintenance is >10 mg/day and/or drug toxicities are accumulating with prednisone) will require treatment with an immunosuppressive agent such as cyclophosphamide (Cytoxan)[1] or cyclosporine (Neoral).[1] Cyclophosphamide (Cytoxan)[1] in doses of 1.5 to 2 mg/kg per day for 12 weeks in combination with low-dose prednisone is an effective regimen. Careful monitoring for cytopenias and infections is essential. If cyclosporine (Neoral)[1] is selected, it is initiated at 3 to 4 mg/kg in two divided doses and adjusted to maintain a 12-hour trough level of 100 to 175 ng/mL. This drug is also often used in combination with low-dose prednisone. Therapy with cyclosporine (Neoral),[1] if the patient responds, should be continued for up to 12 months before tapering, always with careful monitoring of renal function to minimize nephrotoxicity. If one of these routines is unsuccessful, consider using the other, often after a drug-free holiday (off all immunosuppressive agents for 2 to 4 months). Any patient on prolonged high-dose steroids and/or an immunosuppressive agent should be on *Pneumocystis carinii* pneumonia (PCP) prophylaxis with trimethoprim-sulfamethoxazole (Bactrim or Septra) 80 mg/400 mg daily, barring sulfa drug allergy. In addition, bisphosphonate therapy should be considered if prolonged oral corticosteroids are used to minimize osteoporosis.

FOCAL AND SEGMENTAL GLOMERULOSCLEROSIS

Pathology

In focal and segmental glomerulosclerosis (FSGS), focal (some glomeruli) and segmental (parts of individual glomeruli) scarring of the glomerular tuft at the vascular pole, with or without adhesions to Bowman's capsule, and mesangial collapse in these areas are the classic lesions on light microscopy. Immunofluorescence may show nonspecific IgM and C1 trapping in these areas, and

TABLE 3 Immunosuppressive Treatment of Primary Glomerular Disease

Primary Glomerular Disease	Specific Therapy
Minimal Change Disease	First Line: prednisone Second Line: cyclosporine[1] (Neoral) or cytotoxics
FSGS	First Line: prednisone Second Line: cyclosporine[1]
Membranous Glomerulopathy	First Line: cyclosporine[1] or cytotoxics/corticosteroids Second Line: mycophenolate mofetil[1] (CellCept)
MPGN	Alternate day low dose prednisone for children
Diffuse Proliferative GN	Supportive therapy only, unless crescents
IgA Nephropathy	ACE inhibitors and/or ARBs, fish oil supplements,[1] corticosteroids[1] +/– cyclophosphamide[1] (Cytoxan)
Crescentic GN	Corticosteroids, cyclophosphamide[1] +/– azathioprine[1] (Imuran) +/– plasmapheresis, mycophenolate mofetil,[1] rituximab[1]

[1]Not FDA approved for this indication.

[1]Not FDA approved for this indication.

electron microscopy demonstrates diffuse epithelial foot process effacement.

Treatment

Treatment of primary FSGS should begin with prednisone in a dose of 1 mg/kg per day up to 80 mg maximum per day for up to 16 weeks before steroid resistance can be declared. If a patient is at risk of steroid toxicity (e.g., the patient is older than age 60 years, obese, or has a family history of diabetes) and/or if a 50% reduction in proteinuria is not seen by 8 weeks, the addition of a second agent is recommended with an associated taper of steroids to more acceptable levels (10 to 20 mg/day) to minimize complications.

Cyclosporine (Neoral)[1] therapy is effective in the treatment of steroid-resistant or steroid-dependent FSGS. The initial dose and management are the same as in steroid-resistant MCD. If there is no significant change in proteinuria (a minimum 50% decrease) by 6 months, and/or there is a sustained rise in serum creatinine (30% or more) unimproved by a reduction in cyclosporine (Neoral)[1] dosage, it should be discontinued. If the patient is responsive to cyclosporine (Neoral),[1] it should be continued at the lowest possible dose for at least 1 year before slowly tapering it off.

There is insufficient evidence from retrospective reviews to support prolonged cytotoxic therapy with an agent such as cyclophosphamide (Cytoxan)[1] in steroid-resistant FSGS.

MEMBRANOUS NEPHROPATHY

Pathology

Glomeruli look normal on light microscopy at the earliest phase of disease, but as the immune complexes continue to be deposited, there is glomerular basement membrane (GBM) matrix increase and the capillary loops begin to look rigid and diffusely thickened. On silver stain, spikes of matrix may be visible on the epithelial side of the capillary wall, representing new GBM enclosing the immune complex deposits. Subepithelial immune complexes are confirmed by electron microscopy, positive granular staining along the GBM for IgG, and complement on immunofluorescence.

TREATMENT

The prognosis in idiopathic membranous glomerulonephritis (MGN) follows the rule of thirds: one third will progress slowly to end-stage renal disease (ESRD), one third will have persistent low- to medium-grade proteinuria with preserved renal function over many years, and one third will have a spontaneous remission. Demographic markers of a poor outcome at onset include male gender, older age, hypertension, interstitial fibrosis and tubular atrophy on renal pathology, and reduced renal function and high-grade proteinuria (>8 g/day) on laboratory examination. These factors should all be considered before deciding how to manage the patient. Conservative therapy should be initiated immediately, but an observation period of up to 6 months is recommended before deciding if immunosuppressive treatment is warranted. A semiquantitative assessment that can categorize the patients in terms of their risk of progression has been constructed and validated. Its application can substantially help in assessing the risk benefit of immunosuppressive therapy for both the physician and the patient. If proteinuria remains less than 4 g per day for 6 months, continued conservative treatment is recommended; seriously consider immunosuppressives if proteinuria remains between 4 and 8 g per day; and if more than 8 g per day and/or progressive deterioration in renal function ensues, immunosuppressive therapy should be initiated even prior to the completion of 6 months of observation. Options include corticosteroids with cytotoxics or cyclosporine (Neoral).[1] Prednisone as monotherapy is not sufficient treatment. A 6-month course of alternating monthly prednisone, 0.5 mg/kg per day, with a month of either chlorambucil (Leukeran),[1] 0.2 mg/kg per day, or cyclophosphamide (Cytoxan),[1] 2.5 mg/kg per day orally, is effective. Cyclosporine (Neoral)[1] therapy initiated at 3 to 4 mg/kg in two divided doses targeting a 12-hour trough level of 100 to 175 ng/mL for a minimum of 6 months has also been proved to be effective in a randomized controlled trial.

Mycophenolate mofetil (CellCept),[1] 500 to 2000 mg daily, in an open-label pilot study significantly reduced and stabilized renal function in approximately 30% of a group of MGN patients resistant to other forms of therapy and can be considered if all else fails. Rituximab (Rituxan),[1] a monoclonal antibody against B-cell marker CD20, has also had positive results in a pilot study.

MEMBRANOPROLIFERATIVE GLOMERULONEPHRITIS

Pathology

There is mesangial hypercellularity, increased mesangial matrix, and capillary-wall thickening on light microscopy in both subtypes of membranoproliferative glomerulonephritis (MPGN). Immunofluorescence is varied and nondiagnostic. On electron microscopy there are subendothelial immune complex deposits in type I MPGN, and ribbon-like, dense deposits within the GBM in MPGN type II.

Treatment

C3 complement levels are reduced in both types I and II MPGN, and the C4 complement component is low in type I, but usually normal in type II. Treatment of idiopathic MPGN is challenging, and few treatments have demonstrated a significant benefit over conservative therapy alone. Alternate day, prolonged (>2 years), low-dose prednisone in children has the best evidence, but even it is limited to retrospective albeit long-term analyses. Cyclophosphamide (Cytoxan)[1] has been reported to be of benefit in a small study, but was associated with significant toxicity, and based on current evidence cannot be recommended. Initially, aspirin[1] and dipyridamole (Persantine)[1] were felt to have a favorable effect on proteinuria, but later results from these studies have suggested no long-term benefits on either proteinuria or renal survival.

---

[1]Not FDA approved for this indication.

[1]Not FDA approved for this indication.

DIFFUSE PROLIFERATIVE GLOMERULONEPHRITIS

Pathology

In diffuse proliferative glomerulonephritis (DPGN), light microscopy shows proliferative glomerular lesions with increases in both mesangial and endothelial cells, often with an associated intracapillary inflammatory infiltrate of polymorphs. Immunofluorescence shows varying amounts of complement and Ig deposition, and on electron microscopy the characteristic subepithelial *humps* or deposits along the GBM are evident. In severe cases epithelial crescent formation may be found.

Treatment

The most common known causal factor in DPGN is infection. Poststreptococcal glomerulonephritis (PSGN) is less prevalent in the developed world with antibiotic use, but it can still occur. Other bacteria commonly associated with subtle chronic infections such as endocarditis, infected atrioventricular shunts, skin infections, and visceral abscesses can also be associated with proliferative glomerulonephritis (PGN).

Hypocomplementemia is often found in the acute phase. The symptoms and signs of DPGN usually spontaneously resolve within 4 to 8 weeks. Conservative therapy includes BP control, diuretics, and sodium restriction. Dialysis support may be necessary during the acute phase. The underlying infection should be treated if it has not resolved spontaneously. In children the prognosis is excellent with little long-term sequelae, and more than 80% of adults will have no residual renal dysfunction. If crescent formation is present, these patients should be treated as outlined in the idiopathic crescentic GN section later in this article.

IMMUNOGLOBULIN A NEPHROPATHY

Pathology

IgA nephropathy has mesangial hypercellularity and matrix expansion on light microscopy. Crescents are rarely present and are usually segmental in nature. Immunofluorescence shows mesangial IgA (± IgG) and complement deposits and their location is confirmed on electron microscopy.

Treatment

Management depends on the clinical features, the degree of proteinuria, and the severity of renal insufficiency. Patients with only microhematuria, no proteinuria, and normal renal function with no hypertension need only be followed at regular intervals. If proteinuria is less than 1 g per day and the patient has a normal serum creatinine, treatment should include ACEI and/or ARBs therapy, even in the absence of hypertension, to reduce proteinuria to the lowest level possible. If proteinuria is greater than 1 g per day with normal renal function, ACEI and/or ARBs should be instituted and proteinuria and BP normalization targeted. Fish oil supplements[1] at a dose of 1.8 g per day of eicosapentaenoic acid (EPA) and 1.2-g per day doses of docosahexaenoic acid (DHA) daily should be considered.

Although results from trials have been varied, the risk of this treatment is negligible. If renal function is deteriorating or proteinuria persists at doses of ≥1 g per day despite maximum conservative therapy after 6 months, immunosuppressive therapy should be considered. In the group with persistent proteinuria but stable, well-preserved renal function, pulse methylprednisolone (Solu-Medrol) doses of 1 g per day for 3 days in the beginning of months 1, 3, and 5 with low-dose prednisone (0.5 mg/kg/day) on alternate days for 6 months has been shown to be effective. In the group with persistent proteinuria and rising serum creatinine, cytotoxic therapy should be considered in addition to prednisone. Prednisone doses of 40 mg per day, tapering to 10 mg per day within 2 years, combined with cyclophosphamide (Cytoxan)[1] orally for 3 months followed by azathioprine (Imuran)[1] for a minimum of 2 years, both at 1.5 mg/kg per day, has been studied in this type of patient in a RCT with good results. A recent RCT using mycophenolate mofetil (CellCept)[1] as a single agent showed no benefit on either proteinuria or renal survival if initial serum creatinine was 3 mg/dL or more. This would support the futility of using immunosuppressive therapy once severe chronic renal insufficiency (creatinine clearance ≤35 mL/minute) has been reached.

CRESCENTIC GLOMERULONEPHRITIS

Pathology

Light microscopy will show varying degrees of cellular or fibrocellular crescent formation in Bowman's space, surrounding, and in some cases obliterating, the glomerular tuft. Immunofluorescence staining helps distinguish between the three main types: Type 1, or anti-GBM disease, has linear IgG staining of the GBM; type 2, or immune complex disease, has diffuse granular staining along the GBM; and type 3, or pauci-immune, has little or no staining in the glomeruli.

Treatment

Rapid institution of treatment is critically important to reverse or stabilize renal function. The overall renal survival rate in crescentic GN is 75% to 85% and patient survival rate is 85% to 90%. Therapy should be focused first on induction and then on maintenance treatment. Induction should be with methylprednisolone (Solu-Medrol) at 5 to 15 mg/kg per day for 3 days, then prednisone at 1 mg/kg per day. Additional immunosuppressive therapy includes

---

[1]Not FDA approved for this indication.

CURRENT DIAGNOSIS

- All persistent hematuria and proteinuria above 150 mg per day need to be investigated.
- Secondary causes of glomerular disease must be excluded.
- Renal biopsy is often necessary for proper classification, prognosis, and therapy.

---

[1]Not FDA approved for this indication.

CURRENT THERAPY

- Blood pressure (BP) should be controlled below 130/80 mm Hg or less than 125/75 mm Hg if significant proteinuria is present (>0.5 g/d).
- Angiotensin-converting enzyme inhibitors and angiotensin receptor blockers provide renal protection independent of their effect on BP control.
- Specific immunosuppressive therapy in primary glomerular disease depends on careful assessment of the likelihood of progression/complication of the disease and the risks of therapy.
- Treatment is directed at the underlying cause in secondary glomerular diseases.

cyclophosphamide (Cytoxan),[1] 1.5 to 2.5 mg/kg per day orally. The dose of cyclophosphamide (Cytoxan)[1] should be reduced in elderly patients in proportion to their degree of renal failure aiming to maintain a neutrophil count above 2.5 cu[3]. Cyclophosphamide (Cytoxan)[1] is not always required in the induction phase. It is not recommended, for instance, in idiopathic type-2 crescentic GN of postinfectious origin. When pulmonary hemorrhage is present in anti-GBM disease (and also associated with vasculitis), plasma exchange is added for up to 10 exchanges, or until anti-GBM antibodies are negative, using 4-L exchanges with albumin (or fresh-frozen plasma if bleeding risk is high). Rituximab has been shown in pilot studies to be very effective and less toxic. In the vasculitis type, maintenance consists of cyclophosphamide (Cytoxan)[1] for 3 months, then azathioprine (Imuran) maintenance therapy is substituted at 1 to 2 mg/kg per day if the disease is quiescent. Mycophenolate mofetil is an effective alternate. Long-term maintenance therapy is unnecessary in anti-GBM crescentic GN, and all therapy can usually be discontinued after 6 to 9 months.

REFERENCES

Bakris GL, Weir MR: Angiotensin-converting enzyme inhibitor-associated elevations in serum creatinine: Is this a cause for concern? Arch Intern Med 2000;160:685-693.

Ballardie FW, Roberts ISD: Controlled prospective trial of prednisolone with cytotoxics in progressive IgA nephropathy. J Am Soc Nephrol 2002;13:142-148.

Cattran DC, Appel GB, Hebert LA, et al: A randomized trial of cyclosporine in patients with steroid-resistant focal segmental glomerulosclerosis. Kidney Int 1999;56:2220-2226.

Cattran DC, Appel GB, Hebert LA, et al: Cyclosporine in patients with steroid-resistant membranous nephropathy: A randomized trial. Kidney Int 2001;59:1484-1490.

Cattran DC, Pei Y, Greenwood CM, et al: Validation of a predictive model of idiopathic membranous nephropathy: Its clinical and research implications. Kidney Int 1997;51:901-907.

ISEN Group (Gruppo Italiano di Studi Epidemiologici in Nefrologia): Randomised placebo-controlled trial of effect of ramipril on decline in glomerular filtration rate and risk of terminal renal failure in proteinuric, non-diabetic nephropathy. Lancet 1997;349: 1857-1863.

Jayne D, Rasmussen N, Andrassy K, et al: A randomized trial of maintenance therapy for vasculitis associated with antineutrophil cytoplasmic autoantibodies. N Engl J Med 2003;349:36-44.

Klahr S, Levey AS, Beck GJ, et al: The effects of dietary protein restriction and blood-pressure control on the progression of chronic renal disease. N Engl J Med 1994;330:877-884.

Miller G, Zimmerman R, Radhakrishnan J, Appel G: Use of mycophenolate mofetil in resistant membranous nephropathy. Am J Kidney Dis 2000;36:250-256.

Nakao N, Yoshimura A, Morita H, at el: Combination treatment of angiotensin-II receptor blocker and angiotensin-converting-enzyme inhibitor in non-diabetic renal disease (COOPERATE): A randomised controlled trial. Lancet 2003;361:117-124.

Pei Y, Cattran D, Delmore T, et al: Evidence suggesting under-treatment in adults with idiopathic focal segmental glomerulosclerosis. Am J Med 1987;82:938-944.

Ponticelli C, Altieri P, Scolari F, et al: A randomized study comparing methylprednisolone plus chlorambucil versus methylprednisolone plus cyclophosphamide (Cytoxan) in idiopathic membranous nephropathy. J Am Soc Nephrol 1998;9:444-450.

Praga M, Gutierrez E, Gonzalez E, et al: Treatment of IgA nephropathy with ACE inhibitors: A randomized and controlled trial. J Am Soc Nephrol 2003;14:1578-1583.

Acute Pyelonephritis

Method of
Kurt A. McCammon, MD,
and Carol F. McCammon, MD

Acute pyelonephritis results from infection and inflammation of the renal parenchyma and renal pelvis. Most infections ascend to the kidney from the lower urinary tract (LUT), and many patients relate a history of recent dysuria, frequency, or urgency. Patients in general present ill-appearing, febrile, and complain typically of unilateral flank pain often associated with nausea and vomiting.

Physical findings include fever, costovertebral angle (CVA) tenderness, and sometimes mild abdominal discomfort on examination. Although the majority of patients may be treated as outpatients successfully, remember that inadequate or delayed eradication of infection can result in serious sequelae including hypertension, renal scarring, and end-stage renal disease (ESRD). Fortunately, timely diagnosis and appropriate treatment can greatly reduce the risk of these complications.

Etiology

The most common pathogens causing acute pyelonephritis are aerobic gram-negative bacteria. Most cases result from ascending lower urinary tract infections (LUTIs); therefore, the etiologic agents parallel. Nearly 85% of community-acquired cases of acute pyelonephritis result from *Escherichia coli.* Other less-common pathogens include *Proteus, Klebsiella, Enterococcus,* and *Staphylococcus saprophyticus.* Nosocomial infections are predominantly caused by *E. coli* (approximately 50%); other pathogens include (in order of frequency) *Enterococcus, Klebsiella, Enterobacter, Citrobacter, Serratia, Pseudomonas aeruginosa,* and *Staphylococcus epidermidis.* Urine cultures usually produce single bacterium because pyelonephritis is rarely polymicrobial.

---

[1]Not FDA approved for this indication.

Pathology

The susceptible host frequently develops acute pyelonephritis from the LUT. Colonization of the perineum by the intruding organism may be the initial event. If untreated at the LUT level, the organism may further ascend the urinary tract (UT) via the ureters to the renal pelvis and renal parenchyma, resulting in the clinical manifestations of acute pyelonephritis. This retrograde progression may result from the presence of fimbriae on the surface of many bacteria that invade the UT. Culture-proved fimbriated organisms occur in 8% of cases of acute pyelonephritis.

Hematogenous seeding of the renal parenchyma from a remote site of infection causes pyelonephritis in approximately 5% of cases. Patients will more frequently exhibit bilateral flank pain, and CVA tenderness and sources other than the UT must be sought and appropriately treated. Individuals at risk include patients on immunosuppressive therapy or a history of intravenous (IV) drug use. A gram-positive bacterial urine culture is nearly always a result of blood-borne, distant infection.

Epidemiology

There are 250,000 cases of acute pyelonephritis each year in the United States. Women are most frequently affected by acute pyelonephritis with a 50% chance of developing a LUTI. Only 2% of these LUTIs are found to ascend. Pregnancy adds a significant risk, particularly in the second and third trimesters when ureteral compression and urinary stasis from the enlarging uterus play anatomic roles in establishing urinary infection. Thus, treatment of asymptomatic bacteriuria is recommended in pregnant women. In children, vesicoureteral reflux and anatomic anomalies are most often associated with the development of pyelonephritis.

Differential Diagnosis

Any disease process that causes fever and flank or abdominal pain must be considered in the differential diagnosis of acute pyelonephritis. Generally, diverticular disease, appendicitis, cholecystitis, hepatitis, and pancreatitis should be considered. Renal colic from calculi or other obstructing lesions may manifest similarly. In women, consider pelvic inflammatory disease, Fitz-Hugh-Curtis syndrome, and when pregnant, hemolysis, elevated liver enzymes, and low platelet (HELLP) syndrome. Men should also be evaluated for prostatitis, epididymitis, and orchitis as well, and their presence may be a preceding factor in the cause of acute pyelonephritis. Overall, the patient's history, physical examination, and appropriate ancillary testing will help distinguish between these numerous possibilities in differential diagnosis.

Ancillary Testing

Urinalysis and urine culture are indicated preferably before institution of antibiotic therapy when appropriate because pyelonephritis, by definition, is a complicated UTI. Urinalysis and urine culture require adequate clean urine; in females, a catheterized specimen is recommended. The urinalysis frequently shows pyuria, bacteria, esterase, and nitrites. It should not contain epithelial cells, which indicate contamination and renders the specimen inadequate for culture.

White blood cell (WBC) casts are often seen in the setting of acute pyelonephritis. Taking blood for complete blood cell count and culture should also be considered because the WBC count can be followed for signs of response to treatment along with clinical progress. The blood culture is useful in the treatment of particularly ill-appearing patients, and 20% to 30% of patients will have a positive blood culture. Renal function should also be ascertained because acute pyelonephritis may cause renal dysfunction in severely affected patients, those with co-morbid conditions, or those with a single kidney. Antibiotic choice and further radiographic evaluation may be altered in the patient with a disturbance in renal function. Empirical treatment should promptly begin while awaiting culture results.

Patients with significant co-morbid conditions and those who do not respond well to initial antimicrobial therapy, prepubescents, and the elderly should be considered for radiographic evaluation. Indications include pyelonephritis in pregnancy, history of urolithiasis, prior genitourinary surgery, recurrent pyelonephritis, and fever for more than 5 to 7 days without appropriate medical evaluation.

Intravenous pyelogram (IVP) is the initial study of choice in nonpregnant patients with adequate renal function. IVP will demonstrate segmental or global renal enlargement, delay in nephrograms, anatomic anomalies, and/or UT obstruction. However, 75% of studies prove normal.

Alternatively, computed tomography (CT) may be useful (without contrast) to quickly evaluate for obstructing stones. Other abnormalities may also be suggested by the CT, which could help in patient management. Ultrasound (US) is less invasive, safe in pregnancy, and will not disturb renal function; however, it may not provide as much information as IVP. It is sensitive in identifying the presence of perinephric or intrarenal abscess, segmental renal abnormalities, and hydronephrosis and may detect larger renal calculi.

Management

First, it must be determined whether the patient has a complicated or uncomplicated case of acute pyelonephritis. Patients with uncomplicated cases of acute pyelonephritis are generally treated as outpatients (Figure 1). After an adequate urinalysis and culture are obtained, the patient can be started on oral antibiotics, most often a fluoroquinolone or other antibiotic with similar coverage (Box 1). Antipyretics, analgesia, and fluids are recommended. The patient should be re-evaluated in 72 hours and, if the patient is appropriately improving, may continue outpatient treatment for 14 to 21 days. At the end of treatment, the patient should return for repeat urinalysis and culture to prove complete adequate treatment. If this culture is positive, retreatment with an appropriately targeted antibiotic should be started and radiographic evaluation of the

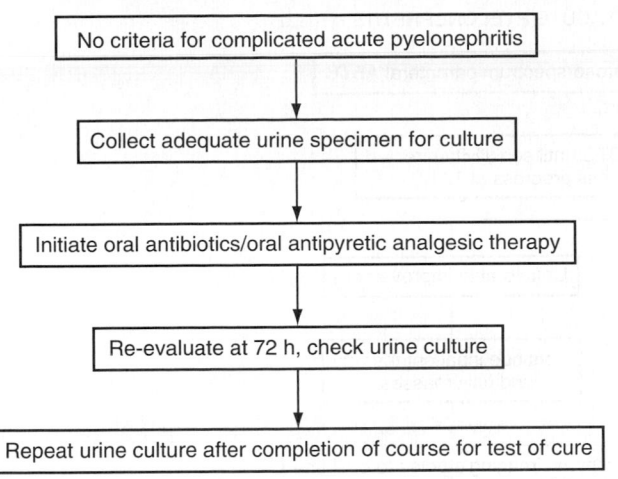

FIGURE 1. Treatment algorithm for uncomplicated acute pyelonephritis.

UT considered. Nonsteroidal anti-inflammatory drugs[1] and vitamins A[1] and E may potentially decrease renal scarring even if there is a delay in initial antibiotic treatment.

Patients with complicated cases of acute pyelonephritis should be strongly considered for inpatient treatment with at least 3 days of IV antibiotics (Box 2 and Figure 2). These patients are at risk for serious sequelae in the face of treatment failure and should be monitored closely. After adequate urinalysis and culture, the patient should promptly be started on an IV broad-spectrum antibiotic regimen (Box 3). The patient should have a complete blood cell count, blood culture, and creatinine level drawn. Supportive measures of IV fluids, antipyretics, analgesia, and antiemetics should be administered. Radiographic evaluation in

[1]Not FDA approved for this indication.

BOX 1   Oral Antibiotic Regimens for Outpatient Treatment*

Primary

Ciprofloxacin (Cipro)[1] 500 mg bid
Ofloxacin (Floxin)[1] 200-400 mg PO q12h
Levofloxacin (Levaquin) 250-500 mg qd

Alternative

Amoxicillin/clavulanate (Augmentin)[1] 875 mg bid
Cephalexin (Keflex)[1] 500 mg tid-qid
Cefadroxil (Duricef)[1] 1-2 g divided bid
Cefaclor (Ceclor)[1] 250-500 mg tid
Cefprozil (Cefzil)[1] 250-500 mg bid
Cefdinir (Omnicef)[1] 600 mg qd
Cefpodoxime (Vantin)[1] 100-400 mg bid
Ceftibuten (Cedax)[1] 400 mg qd
Trimethoprim/sulfamethoxazole DS PO bid

---

*Check antibiotic resistance patterns in your region to guide empirical therapy.
[1]Not FDA approved for this indication.
Abbreviations: bid = twice daily; PO = orally; qd = every day; qid = four times daily; tid = three times daily.

BOX 2   Criteria for Complicated Pyelonephritis[1]

- Anatomic or functional urinary tract abnormalities
- Immunocompromised host
- Prepubertal age
- Male gender
- Sepsis
- Nausea and vomiting
- Significant co-morbid conditions

---

[1]Consider admission.

---

the hemodynamically stable patient should be considered early in the course of treatment. If fever abates and there is clinical improvement within 72 hours, the patient may be switched to a tailored oral regimen. Another day of observation is recommended to make certain the patient remains afebrile. If the patient does not improve within 72 hours, review cultures and sensitivity and perform studies to rule out renal abscess, perinephric abscess, UT obstruction, or other abnormality. If any are present, appropriate management by an urologist is indicated.

Management in Pregnancy

Obstetric/gynecologic (OB/GYN) consultation in these patients is appropriate in management of acute pyelonephritis. Antibiotic regimens that are category B or C are acceptable under most circumstances, provided the patient has no allergies. Nearly all of these patients should have IV antibiotics and initial inpatient management because preterm labor and miscarriage are risks of persistent infection. Avoid sulfa during the third trimester because newborns may develop kernicterus. Tetracycline discolors teeth in the fetus and therefore is also contraindicated in all trimesters. Fluoroquinolones have been shown to cause cartilaginous disorders in fetal animals and are not recommended.

Special Pediatric Considerations

Pediatric patients with acute pyelonephritis are likely to have UT anomalies. These patients must have radiographic evaluation to include renal US and voiding cystourethrography to further evaluate the anatomy of the UT. Once initial infection is eradicated, the patient with an anatomic abnormality should be maintained on daily antibiotic suppressive therapy until it is deemed unnecessary by the urologist or the abnormality is appropriately corrected.

Neurologic Impairment

Patients with spinal cord injury above the level of renal innervation (T11 or higher) can have a delayed presentation and much more vague symptomatology. Similarly, patients with multiple sclerosis (MS) and other neurologic diseases can have an atypical presentation because of sensory loss.

CRITERIA FOR COMPLICATED ACUTE PYELONEPHRITIS

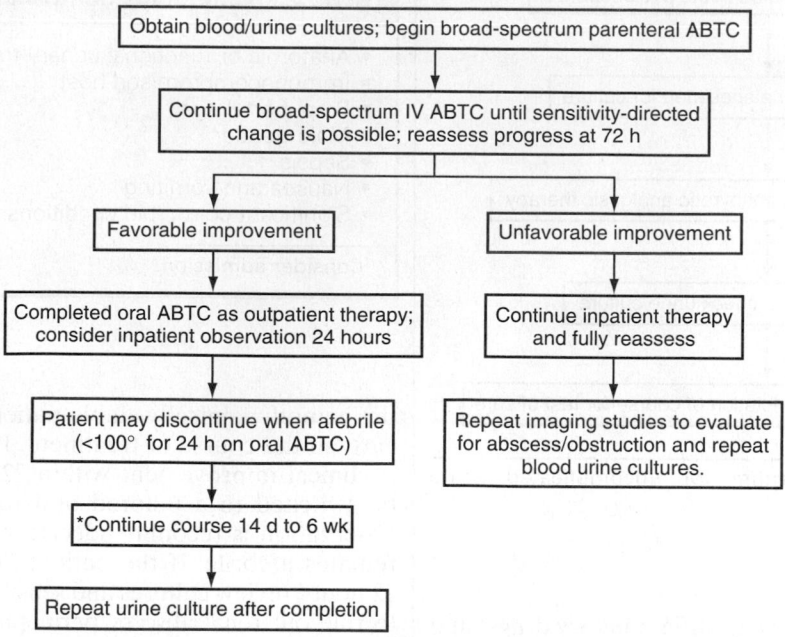

FIGURE 2. Treatment algorithm for complicated acute pyelonephritis. ABTC = antibiotic; IV = intravenous.

They may be unable to identify dysuria, flank pain, and other classic symptoms of pyelonephritis; additionally, many of these patients have indwelling or intermittent catheterization, which can interfere with interpretation of urinalysis. The presence of fever and pyuria/bacteriuria with absence of other foci of infection may be the only clinical indicators of the presence of pyelonephritis. These patients should undergo radiographic imaging to rule out upper-urinary obstruction in addition to management in the complicated pyelonephritis pathway.

Complications

Aggressive early treatment of acute pyelonephritis prevents most complications of the disease. However, patients who are inadequately treated or who present late in a fulminant process can suffer significant complications, including sepsis and death. Emphysematous pyelonephritis is a rare form and occurs primarily in diabetics. It is a fulminant, necrotizing infection, commonly caused by *E. coli.* An examination of the kidney, ureter, and bladder may show air in the nephric shadow. The involved kidney functions poorly; therefore, an IVP is not helpful in confirming the diagnosis. Emphysematous pyelonephritis is an indication for emergency nephrectomy. Percutaneous drainage helps in the appropriate clinical setting. Renal and perinephric abscess should be evaluated by a urologist and may respond to antibiotics alone. Some may require percutaneous or surgical drainage or possibly nephrectomy. Chronic renal scarring may lead to hypertension. Recurrent episodes can cause enough scar formation to contribute to chronic renal failure.

BOX 3 **Intravenous Antibiotic Regimens for Inpatient Treatment* of Adults with Normal Renal Function**

Primary

Ciprofloxacin[1][†] 400 mg q12h
Levofloxacin (Levaquin) 250-500 mg q24h
Ofloxacin (Floxin)[1][†] 200-400 mg q12h
Ampicillin 1-2 g q4-6h plus gentamicin 3-5 mg/kg/day divided q8h[2]
Ceftriaxone (Rocephin)[1][†] 1 g q24h
Ceftizoxime (Cefizox)[1][†] 1-2 g q8-12h
Ceftazidime (Fortaz)[1][†] 1-2 g q8-12h
Cefotaxime (Claforan)[1][†] 1-2 g q6-8h

Alternative

Ticarcillin/clavulanate (Timentin)[1][†] 3.1 g q4-6h
Ampicillin/sulbactam (Unasyn)[1][†] 1.5-3 g q6h
Piperacillin/tazobactam (Zosyn)[1] 3.375-4.5 g q6h
Ertapenem (Invanz)[1] 1.0 g IV qd

---

*Check antibiotic resistance patterns in your region to guide empirical therapy.
[1]Not FDA approved for this indication.
[2]Follow peak/trough levels during treatment.
[†]For gram-positive organisms, consider adding vancomycin 1 g q12h.

Trauma to the Genitourinary Tract

Method of
Noel A. Armenakas, MD, and
J. James Bruno II, MD

Injuries to the genitourinary tract often occur in conjunction with injuries to other organs in a polytraumatized patient. Only after the assessment of the "ABCs" (*A*irway, *B*reathing, *C*irculation) should attention be directed to specific organ injuries. Priorities include treatment of life-threatening injuries, control of major hemorrhage and their sequelae (e.g., coagulopathy, hypothermia, metabolic disturbances), and management of intra-abdominal contamination. The urologic consultation is frequently requested after the initial emergency or operating room resuscitation. Overall, genitourinary injuries occur in 10% to 15% of abdominal and pelvic traumas. Of all civilian genitourinary traumas, the kidneys have the highest incidence of involvement, followed by the bladder, urethra, genitals, and ureters (Figure 1).

Renal Trauma

ETIOLOGY

Kidney trauma in the civilian population accounts for 60% to 70% of all genitourinary organ injuries. The majority of renal injuries (85%–90%) result from blunt abdominal trauma, including motor vehicle accidents, falls, and assaults. Most blunt renal injuries are low grade. Occasionally, blunt abdominal injuries result in renovascular injuries, usually from rapid deceleration. The most frequently associated injuries occur to the head and central nervous system and less frequently to the abdomen, with splenic and liver injuries prevailing. Penetrating renal injuries most frequently result from gunshot wounds. These are associated with multisystem injuries, most commonly involving the liver, bowel, and spleen.

DIAGNOSIS

A renal injury is diagnosed by combining a carefully performed history and physical examination with the appropriate laboratory and radiologic evaluations. This comprehensive evaluation allows for accurate staging and appropriate treatment selection. The historical details of the injury can provide significant information regarding potential renal involvement. For example, deceleration injuries from high-speed motor vehicle accidents and falls from heights may be associated with major vascular and/or parenchymal renal damage. On the physical examination, flank contusions, seatbelt marks, lower rib or lumbar vertebral fractures, and upper abdominal or flank tenderness are all clinical indicators of a potential renal injury. Initial blood pressure should be noted because patients with renovascular injuries often present in shock. Any penetrating injury to the flank or upper abdomen suggests the possibility of renal trauma, although the site of injury (i.e., abdomen, flank, back) does not reliably predict its extent. Weapon and ballistics information (e.g., gun type and caliber, knife length) can be helpful in assessing the depth of penetration and potential débridement requirements.

SITES OF GENITOURINARY TRAUMA

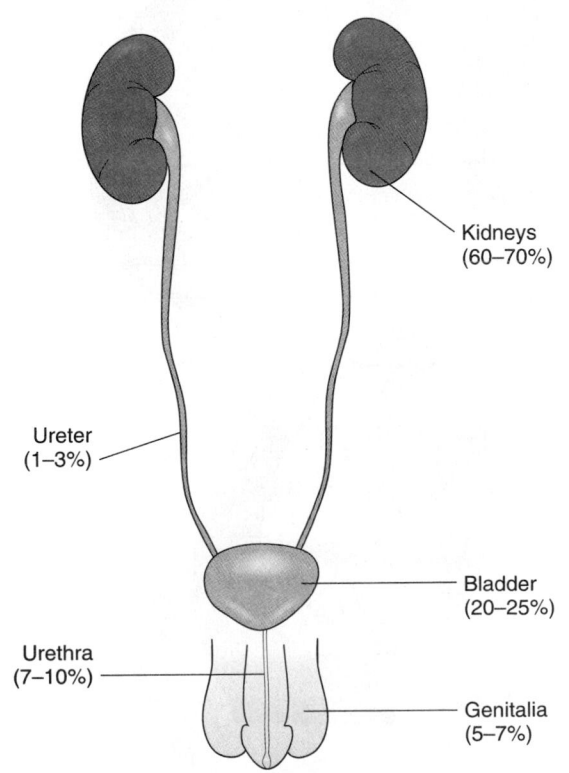

Kidneys (60–70%)

Ureter (1–3%)

Urethra (7–10%)

Bladder (20–25%)

Genitalia (5–7%)

FIGURE 1. Genitourinary injuries.

 CURRENT DIAGNOSIS

- Renal Trauma
  - History and physical examination
  - Laboratory evaluation (urinalysis, hematocrit)
  - Radiographic assessment
- Ureteral Trauma
  - Radiographic evaluation
  - Intraoperative inspection
- Bladder Trauma
  - History and physical examination (including pelvic and rectal examinations)
  - Urinalysis
  - Cystogram
- Genital Trauma in Males
  - History and physical examination
  - Scrotal sonogram
  - Retrograde urethrogram
- Urethral Trauma
  - History and physical examination (inability to void, pelvic fracture, blood at the meatus, or vaginal introitus)
  - Urinalysis
  - Retrograde urethrogram

Urine should be obtained and evaluated for hematuria by either dipstick or microscopic analysis. It is important to collect the first voided or catheterized specimen to avoid false-negative results from dilution after intravenous hydration. The presence of hematuria, defined as more than five erythrocytes per high-power field in adults, is the primary laboratory indicator of a renal injury. However, the amount of hematuria does not correlate with the degree of renal trauma, and its absence cannot exclude a major parenchymal or vascular injury. Other important laboratory tests include a complete blood count and chemistry profile.

Radiographic imaging enables the extent of injury to be defined and should be considered once the patient has been stabilized. The need for radiographic renal imaging is determined by the presence of any of the following criteria:

1. Any *penetrating* injury to the abdomen, flanks, back, or lower chest
2. Any *blunt* injury presenting with either (a) gross hematuria, (b) microscopic hematuria and an initial blood pressure less than 90 mm Hg, or (c) any clinical indicator of renal injury

In adult patients who sustain blunt trauma and are hemodynamically stable with only microscopic hematuria, a clinical diagnosis of a low-grade renal injury can be accurately made without the need for radiographic renal assessment. This recommendation is based on results from several large series that have documented the rarity of an isolated high-grade renal injury in this subgroup. Historically, pediatric patients sustaining blunt abdominal trauma who present with any degree of hematuria, irrespective of hemodynamic stability, have been evaluated radiographically. Newer data confirm that children can be evaluated with the same guidelines as used for adult patients providing the urinalysis shows *fewer than 50* erythrocytes per high-power field. Children who present with blunt abdominal trauma and more than 50 erythrocytes per high-power field should be evaluated radiographically.

Radiographic imaging is undertaken to define the extent and type of renal injury and to complete the staging process accurately. The appropriate imaging study should determine the presence and function of the contralateral kidney and delineate the renal parenchyma and collecting system on the involved side. Currently, computed tomography (CT) is the preferred imaging modality to evaluate renal injuries. If CT is unavailable, a complete excretory urogram (intravenous pyelogram [IVP]) can be obtained. Ultrasonography has a limited role in the acute evaluation of renal trauma because of its inability to differentiate blood from urine, but it can be used for follow-up. Angiography is rarely necessary simply for diagnostic purposes but can have an important therapeutic role in vascular embolization. Magnetic resonance imaging is comparable to CT in identifying renal injuries, but it is more expensive and less readily available, which limits its use.

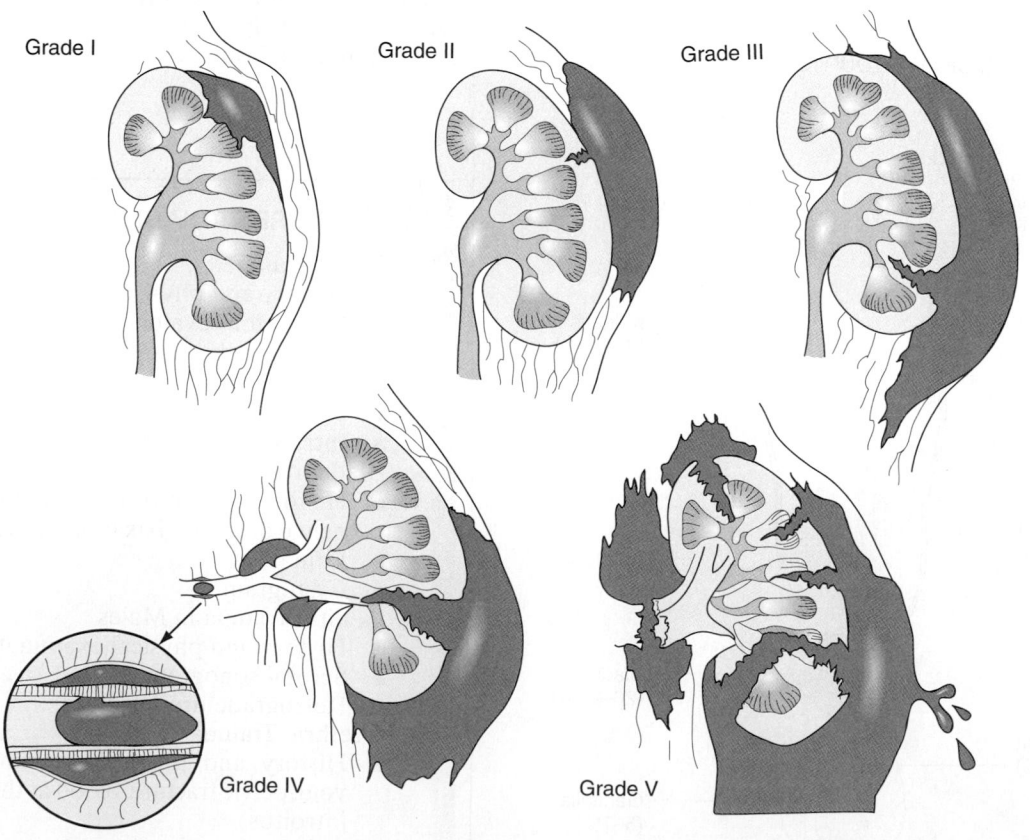

FIGURE 2. Classification of renal injuries by grade. (Modified from Organ Injury Scaling Committee of the American Association for the Surgery of Trauma. Copyright © 2003, Elsevier Science (USA). All rights reserved.)

On the basis of the information obtained radiographically or clinically, renal injuries are classified according to severity into five grades (Figure 2):

Grade I: Renal contusion or subcapsular hematoma
Grade II: Less than 1-cm parenchymal (cortex) laceration
Grade III: Greater than 1-cm parenchymal (cortex and medulla) laceration *without* urinary extravasation
Grade IV: Parenchymal laceration through renal cortex, medulla, and collecting system *with* urinary extravasation or a contained vascular injury
Grade V: Shattered kidney or avulsion of renal hilum

In cases in which the patient's instability precludes a complete abdominal radiographic assessment, prior to renal exploration, a "one-shot" IVP should be performed in the operating room. This limited imaging study provides information primarily about the presence and function of both kidneys, but it lacks accuracy in defining anatomic details of the injury (Figure 3).

MANAGEMENT

Low-grade renal injuries (I and II), whether blunt or penetrating, can be managed safely nonoperatively. If they present only with microscopic hematuria, hospitalization is usually not required. Patients with gross hematuria should be hospitalized and maintained on bed rest until the hematuria visibly clears. Overall, more than 95% of blunt renal injuries can be managed nonoperatively.

High-grade renal injuries (III through V) with associated intra-abdominal organ injuries requiring laparotomy and most renovascular injuries are best explored and reconstructed. Nonoperative management can be chosen for *select accurately staged* high-grade renal injuries, providing the patient is stable and does not have any other injuries requiring abdominal exploration. By following these recommendations, approximately 55% of renal stab wounds and 25% of renal gunshot wounds can be managed nonoperatively.

Absolute indications for renal exploration include an expanding or pulsatile retroperitoneal hematoma and hemodynamic instability from renal hemorrhage. Relative indications include urinary extravasation, nonviable renal parenchyma with a major laceration, a renovascular injury

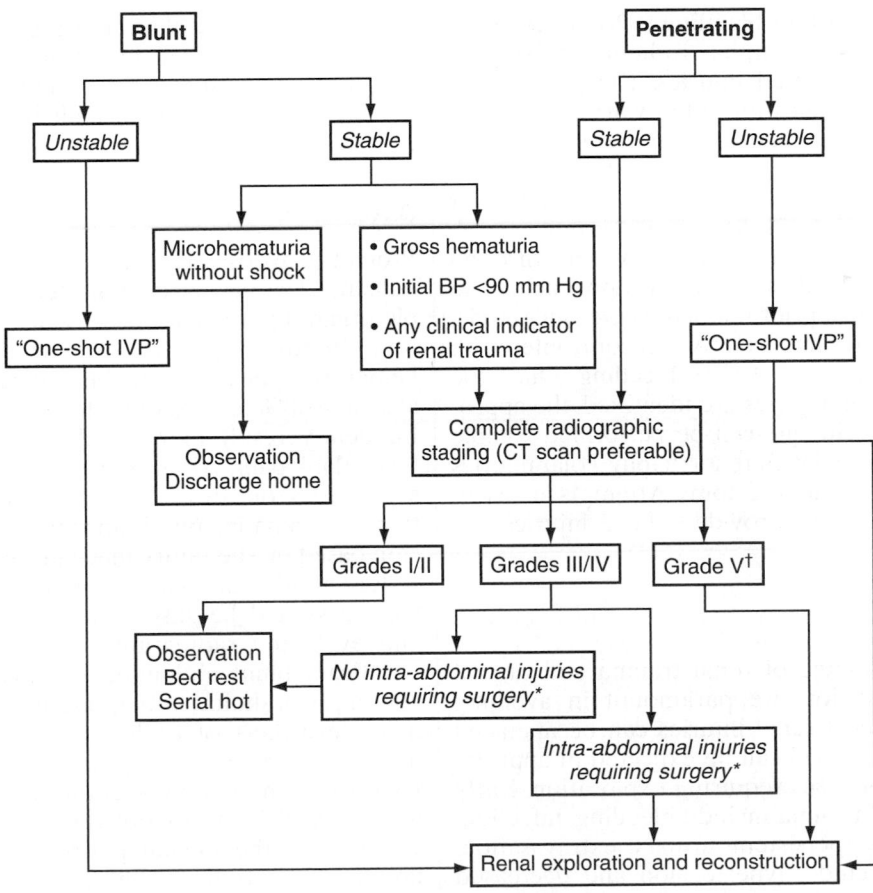

* Select injuries with large devitalized segments or with significant extravasation may require renal exploration and reconstruction.

† Select injuries may be managed by observation.

FIGURE 3. Algorithm for the diagnosis and management of renal trauma (abdominal, flank, back, or chest injury). *Abbreviations:* BP = blood pressure; CT = computed tomography; IVP = intravenous pyelogram; Hct = hematocrit.

CURRENT THERAPY

- Renal Trauma
  - Observation with close monitoring of vital signs and hematocrit
  - Renal exploration and attempted reconstruction
- Ureteral Trauma
  - Urinary diversion (via a ureteral stent or percutaneous nephrostomy tube)
  - Ureteral exploration and repair (immediate or delayed)
- Bladder Trauma
  - Catheter drainage
  - Bladder exploration and repair
- Genital Trauma in Males
  - Surgical exploration and repair
- Urethral Trauma
  - Transurethral catheterization
  - Suprapubic urinary diversion
  - Endoscopic realignment
  - Urethral suturing

in a solitary kidney, persistent bleeding (>2 U packed red blood cells per 24 hours), incomplete radiographic staging, and laparotomy for associated injuries. The presence of more than one relative indication often warrants surgical treatment. The selective embolization of hemorrhage via interventional radiology, used more commonly in splenic and hepatic injuries, is a promising new modality for nonoperative management of select renal injuries.

Operative renal exploration is performed through a midline transperitoneal abdominal approach. The renal vessels are identified prior to opening Gerota's fascia. Vascular control becomes important when confronted with deep renal parenchymal or vascular bleeding. Once the kidney is exposed and all injuries are identified, the appropriate reconstructive technique can be performed. Simple lacerations can be managed with renorrhaphy. Polar injuries are best treated by partial nephrectomy. Attempts at vascular repair should be made provided these injuries are discovered promptly.

OUTCOME

Aggressive accurate staging of renal trauma and careful attention to reconstruction are paramount in avoiding renal loss. Although most renal injuries can be managed nonoperatively, renal salvage can be expected in approximately 70% to 90% of cases requiring exploration. Early complications of renal trauma include bleeding, infection, abscess formation and persistent urinary extravasation. Late complications include hypertension and decreased renal function. Hypertension occurs in approximately 5% of cases and is believed to be caused by mechanisms that activate the renin-angiotensin system. It usually manifests within the first few months of injury, but further delayed onset has been documented. Blood pressure should be measured regularly for the first year and annually thereafter.

Ureteral Trauma

ETIOLOGY

Ureteral injuries from external trauma constitute approximately 1% to 3% of all genitourinary injuries. The ureter's mobility and anatomic characteristics protect it from trauma; its narrow diameter and retroperitoneal location between the spine, major muscle groups, and the peritoneal contents make it an unlikely target. Most external ureteral injuries occur from gunshot wounds. The bullet need not physically transect the ureter to cause significant damage. If the bullet's path is simply near the ureter, the temporary cavitation created by the missile can cause significant tissue destruction and delayed necrosis. Such injuries can be difficult to identify initially and often present with delayed sequelae. Penetrating ureteral injuries are almost always associated with multiple organ injuries. The most common sites, in order of decreasing frequency, are the small bowel, colon, liver, and iliac vessels. Ureteral injuries from blunt trauma are rare. They usually occur in children during rapid deceleration, causing excessive hyperextension of their flexible vertebral column with disruption at the ureteropelvic junction. Blunt ureteral injuries also are associated with multiple organ injuries, most commonly to the liver, spleen, and skeletal system.

Iatrogenic ureteral injuries are the most common. They most frequently occur during ureteroscopy, hysterectomy, low anterior colon resection, vaginal surgery, and abdominal aneurysm repair and usually involve the lower ureteral segment.

DIAGNOSIS

Prompt diagnosis is the first step toward a successful outcome. This may be complicated by the presence of multiple organ injuries and the absence of clinical and laboratory findings specific for ureteral trauma. Indeed, hematuria, which is a reliable indicator of renal trauma, is absent in 30% to 45% of ureteral injuries. These limitations frequently result in delayed recognition manifested by fever, flank pain, urinoma, fistula formation, and eventually sepsis. To avoid this additional morbidity, it is imperative that the evaluating physician maintain a high index of suspicion based on the injury mechanism and location.

Essentially any patient with penetrating abdominal trauma should be suspected of having a ureteral injury and evaluated radiographically. Similarly, children with significant blunt abdominal trauma and multiple associated injuries should undergo radiographic ureteral assessment regardless of findings on urinalysis. Urinary tract imaging can be obtained using either a CT scan or an IVP. Extravasation of contrast is the sine qua non of a ureteral injury. On CT, the extravasated contrast usually will be confined to the medial perirenal space. With complete ureteral disruption, no contrast material will be seen in the distal ureter on delayed images. Extravasation may be seen on an IVP, but frequently the findings are more subtle, such as delayed renal function or mild ureteral dilation or deviation. If the results of the CT or IVP are inconclusive, a retrograde ureterogram can be performed. Although this is the most accurate ureteral imaging test, it is often impractical in the acute trauma setting.

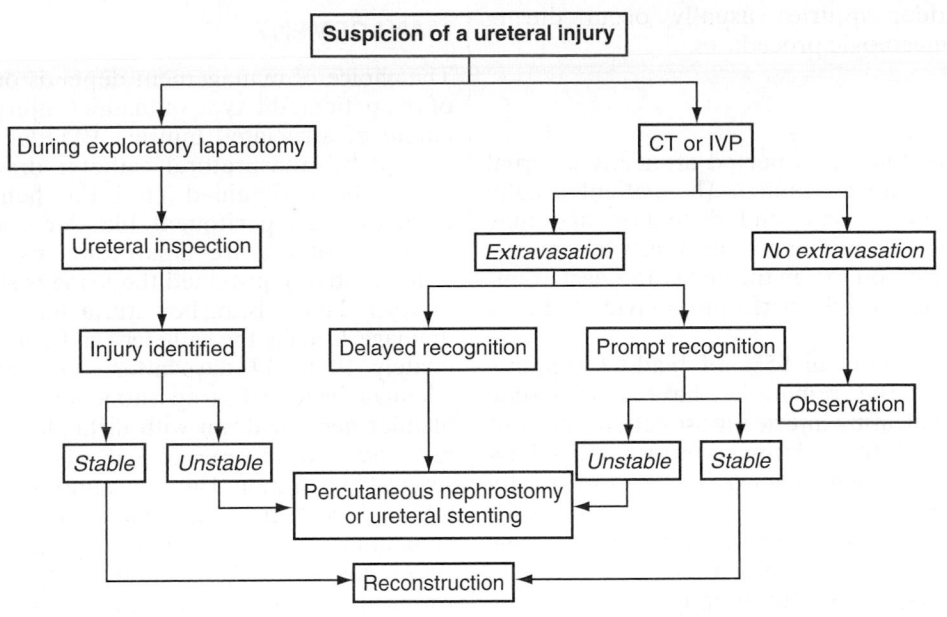

FIGURE 4. Algorithm for the diagnosis and management of ureteral trauma (abdominal or rapid deceleration injury). *Abbreviations:* CT = computed tomography; IVP = intravenous pyelogram.

Most penetrating ureteral injuries are diagnosed intraoperatively during the initial exploratory laparotomy performed for management of the associated abdominal injuries. In this setting, direct visual inspection is the most reliable method for assessing ureteral integrity. Intravenous or intraureteral injection of indigo carmine or methylene blue may aid in injury recognition (Figure 4).

Iatrogenic ureteral injuries are usually discovered more than 24 hours after the insult. Often they present with signs of acute infection from prolonged urinary extravasation or with incisional urinary leakage.

MANAGEMENT

Selection of the appropriate management of a ureteral injury depends on the patient's condition, the site and extent of injury, and the time of diagnosis. Most patients with ureteral injuries from external trauma require prompt operative exploration for management of the associated abdominal injuries. Concomitant intra-abdominal organ or vascular injuries should not preclude ureteral reconstruction in a stable patient. Ureteral repair can be performed using a variety of reconstructive techniques, depending on the level and length of the injured segment. Regardless of the location, successful surgical repair includes the use of healthy ureteral segments (taking thermal effect into consideration) and a watertight, tension-free anastomosis. Injuries to the distal lower third of the ureter are best managed by bladder reimplantation. For injuries involving the entire lower third of the ureter, a psoas hitch can be used. However, in patients with insufficient bladder capacity or with severe pelvic scarring, a transureteroureterostomy can be fashioned. Injuries encompassing the lower half of the ureter are best managed with an anterior bladder wall (Boari-Ockerblad) flap. Short mid or upper ureteral defects can be bridged with a primary ureteroureterostomy. Complete ureteral avulsions are managed with an ileal interposition or renal autotransplantation.

Ureteral injuries in a patient in whom diagnosis was significantly delayed or in an unstable patient are best managed initially by percutaneous nephrostomy drainage or endoscopic ureteral stenting. Definitive repair can be scheduled electively, if necessary. Approximately 50% of iatrogenic ureteral injuries heal simply with temporary urinary diversion.

OUTCOME

Early diagnosis and careful reconstruction of ureteral injuries are important in minimizing complications and preserving renal function. Complications are rare but include prolonged extravasation, infection, fistula formation, and stricture.

Bladder Trauma

ETIOLOGY

The bladder is second to the kidneys in frequency of injury, accounting for 20% to 25% of all genitourinary injuries. Bladder injuries are caused by either blunt or penetrating trauma to the lower abdomen, pelvis, or perineum. Blunt trauma is the more common mechanism, usually by a severe external force such as a motor vehicle accident, fall, or crush injury. Associated injuries include pelvic and long bone fractures as well as central nervous system and chest injuries. Factors that contribute to bladder rupture include pelvic fracture, bladder distention, and any previous pelvic surgery. The location of the bladder deep within the bony pelvis protects it from most penetrating trauma; however, the possibility of bladder trauma should be considered with any lower abdominal gunshot or stab wound.

Iatrogenic bladder injuries usually occur during transurethral or gynecologic procedures.

DIAGNOSIS

A bladder injury should be suspected after any external lower abdominal or pelvic trauma. The patient usually complains of abdominal pain and distention and may be unable to urinate. Hemodynamic instability is common because of extensive blood loss in the pelvis. Physical examination should include carefully performed pelvic and rectal examinations.

Gross hematuria occurs in 95% of bladder ruptures from blunt injuries; the remainder have microscopic hematuria. With penetrating injuries, most patients present with microscopic hematuria. Urine is best obtained by urethral catheterization, which must be performed only after inspection of the urethral meatus. *Blood at the meatus is a contraindication to urethral catheterization* because this finding strongly suggests a urethral injury and requires confirmation by retrograde urethrography.

Cystography is the most accurate imaging test to diagnose a bladder injury. With conventional cystography, a plain film of the pelvis is first obtained and then 350 mL of water-soluble contrast material is infused through a catheter by gravity to distend the bladder; anteroposterior and drainage films should be taken. Alternatively, CT cystography can be used, provided the bladder is filled in a retrograde manner (via a transurethral catheter). In most cases, extravasation of contrast is not seen, and the injury is classified as a contusion. Such injuries result in damage to the mucosa or muscularis without loss of bladder wall continuity. With extravasation of contrast material, the distinction between an extraperitoneal and intraperitoneal bladder rupture must be made. Extraperitoneal bladder ruptures are more common. On cystography, these injuries are characterized by extravasation confined to the perivesical soft tissues. With intraperitoneal bladder ruptures, the contrast extravasates in the peritoneal cavity, outlining the bowel loops. Although cystography can accurately diagnose bladder injuries, the amount of contrast extravasated does not correlate with the extent of injury (Figure 5).

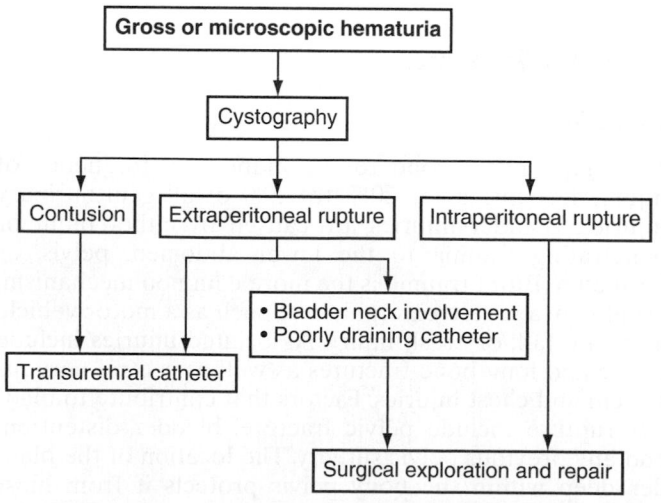

FIGURE 5. Algorithm for the diagnosis and management of bladder trauma (lower abdominal or pelvic injury).

MANAGEMENT

The choice of management depends on the overall status of the patient, the type of bladder injury sustained, and the extent of associated injuries. Bladder contusions can be treated by transurethral catheter drainage alone, which should be maintained until the hematuria completely resolves. Extraperitoneal bladder ruptures in patients who do not require laparotomy can also be managed nonoperatively, provided the urine is sterile at the time of injury and the existing hematuria does not obstruct catheter drainage. Usually the catheter can be removed after approximately 10 to 14 days after a repeat cystogram shows adequate healing. Extraperitoneal ruptures that involve the bladder neck or drain with difficulty should be surgically repaired. All intraperitoneal bladder ruptures require surgical exploration. This is accomplished through a midline infraumbilical incision, avoiding dissection of the pelvic hematoma. The peritoneum is opened and the abdominal viscera inspected; the bladder injury is then repaired from within the bladder lumen, and a transurethral catheter is maintained for 7 to 10 days.

OUTCOME

Mortality in patients with bladder trauma approaches 20% and is due to the associated injuries rather than the bladder rupture. Short-term complications of the bladder injury include persistent bleeding, urinary extravasation, and infection. Long-term complications are rare but can include fistula formation, urinary incontinence, and bladder instability.

Genital Trauma in Males

ETIOLOGY

Injuries to the male genitalia constitute 5% to 7% of all civilian genitourinary injuries. However, in some wartime series, they were the most common genitourinary injuries (60%). This high incidence was the result of the widespread use of ground-level explosives during combat.

Genital injuries include those occurring to the testes, scrotum, and penis. Most testicular injuries result from blunt trauma and are usually unilateral; penetrating testicular injuries from gunshot and stab wounds are less common. Similarly, scrotal trauma from gunshot or stab wounds occurs infrequently; most scrotal injuries occur as a consequence of burns or avulsions. Penile injuries have diverse mechanisms, including ruptures (usually occurring during sexual intercourse), amputations (usually self-inflicted or from entrapment of clothes by heavy machinery), and strangulations (usually from constricting penile rings used to enhance erections). Penetrating injuries (mostly gunshot wounds) can occur, although they usually cause little tissue destruction apart from the entrance and exit wounds.

DIAGNOSIS

Accurate determination of the extent of a testicular injury by clinical means alone may be difficult; the diagnosis is enhanced by scrotal ultrasonography. A heterogeneous intratesticular echo pattern is the most common

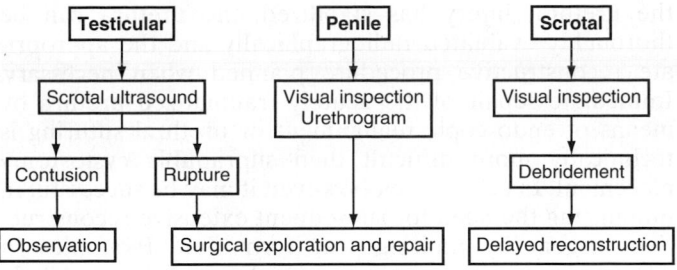

FIGURE 6. Algorithm for the diagnosis and management of genital trauma.

ultrasonographic finding of a testicular rupture. In addition, extruded testicular tissue or disruption of the tunica albuginea can be seen occasionally but is not a required sonographic criterion to confirm a rupture. Penile and scrotal injuries can be accurately diagnosed by visual inspection in conjunction with a thorough history. Any patient with trauma to the penis should undergo a retrograde urethrogram because the incidence of a concomitant urethral injury approaches 80%, depending on the mechanism of injury (Figure 6).

MANAGEMENT

All penetrating testicular injuries and any blunt testicular injury suggestive of a rupture should be surgically explored. Attempts at testicular repair should be made, with orchiectomy limited to extensive unreconstructable injuries. Similarly, penile ruptures and penetrating injuries should be explored promptly and the defect repaired, sparing unnecessary débridement, which could further compromise valuable erectile tissue. Penile amputations should be managed by microsurgical reimplantation, provided the amputated segment is viable. The management of scrotal burns or avulsions requires surgical excision of all nonviable tissue and meticulous wound care. Techniques for delayed scrotal closure include split-thickness skin grafts, rotational thigh flaps, and tissue expanders.

OUTCOME

Genital injuries usually can be diagnosed easily and should be managed promptly. The goal is preservation of genital function and maintenance of cosmesis. Untoward sequelae can be minimized by limiting excessive débridement of penile and testicular tissues and instituting prompt aggressive local wound care with scrotal trauma. Complications of penile and testicular injuries include erectile and reproductive dysfunction, infection, tissue necrosis, and urethral stricture.

Urethral Trauma

ETIOLOGY

Urethral injuries compose approximately 7% to 10% of all genitourinary injuries. These injuries are anatomically subdivided into posterior and anterior injuries. In males, the posterior urethra is proximal and the anterior urethra is distal to the external (striated) sphincter. Only the posterior urethra exists in females.

Injuries to the posterior urethra occur almost exclusively with pelvic fractures. Specifically, with a crush or deceleration-impact injury, the severe shearing forces necessary to fracture the pelvis are transmitted to the prostatomembranous junction, the weakest portion of the urethra. Overall, the male posterior urethra is injured in up to 10% of all pelvic fractures and the female urethra in up to 4% of all pelvic fractures.

In contrast to posterior urethral trauma, injuries to the anterior urethra are not associated with pelvic fractures. External anterior urethral injuries result from blunt or penetrating trauma. Blunt injuries are more common and are caused by vehicular accidents (often bicycles), falls (straddle-type injuries), and direct blows to the perineum or penis. Penetrating anterior urethral injuries, usually from gunshot wounds, are less frequent but often occur in conjunction with penetrating penile or testicular trauma.

Iatrogenic urethral injuries are by far the most frequent cause of urethral trauma. Examples include inadvertent Foley catheter balloon inflation in the urethra and traumatic lower urinary tract endoscopy (cystoscopy, transurethral surgery). These injuries are often minor and tend to be underreported.

DIAGNOSIS

The diagnosis of urethral trauma should be suspected from the history. A pelvic fracture or any external penile or perineal injury can be suggestive of urethral trauma. In a conscious patient, a thorough voiding history should be obtained to establish the time and characteristics of the last urination. A urinalysis is an important laboratory adjunct.

The following clinical indicators of urethral trauma warrant a complete urethral evaluation:

1. *Blood at the urethral meatus.* This is the most consistent and accurate clinical indicator of urethral trauma. Its presence should preclude any attempts at urethral instrumentation until the entire urethra is adequately imaged.
2. *Blood at the vaginal introitus.* In female patients following pelvic fracture, this finding is highly suggestive of a urethral injury.
3. *Hematuria.* Although this finding is nonspecific, it is a reliable indicator of urethral trauma. All patients who are able to urinate after a urethral injury will have some degree of hematuria on a first-voided specimen.
4. *Pain on urination or inability to void.* Painful urination occurs after urethral trauma from edema or urinary extravasation. The inability to void suggests urethral disruption.
5. *High-riding prostate.* This may be palpated after a posterior urethral injury because of superior displacement of the prostate, but it is not a very reliable finding.

Assessment of concomitant rectal and genital injuries is mandatory in every case of external urethral trauma. All patients should have a rectal examination with stool Hemoccult testing. In addition, a complete pelvic examination should be performed on female patients.

Retrograde urethrography is the cardinal diagnostic procedure in male patients suspected of having sustained urethral trauma. This must be performed prior to any attempt at transurethral catheterization. Urethroscopy should not be used in the initial diagnosis of urethral trauma in males. In females, however, the short urethra precludes adequate imaging with retrograde urethrography, making urethroscopy the diagnostic modality for identification and staging of these injuries.

Urethral injuries are simplistically classified as follows:

1. *Contusion*, whereby the urethral mucosa remains intact
2. *Partial disruption*, with segmental maintenance of mucosal continuity
3. *Complete disruption* with separation of both urethral ends

The distinction is made by retrograde urethrography. Although any degree of urethral disruption will result in contrast extravasation, the absence of contrast material in the bladder suggests a complete disruption (Figure 7).

MANAGEMENT

The goal of initial treatment of any urethral trauma is avoidance of any maneuver that can potentiate the injury. Only urethral contusions can be managed safely with transurethral catheterization. With a urethral disruption, the blind passage of a transurethral catheter should be avoided because this can extend the urethral tear, introduce infection, and disrupt a pelvic hematoma. Urinary diversion by means of a suprapubic cystostomy is the easiest and safest option for the initial management of any urethral disruption (partial or complete). After the patient has adequately recovered from the associated injuries and the urethral injury has stabilized, the urethra can be thoroughly evaluated radiographically and the appropriate reconstructive procedure planned when necessary. Immediate repair of the acutely traumatized urethra by means of endoscopic realignment or urethral suturing is technically more difficult than suprapubic cystostomy placement. In select cases, however, it may be successful in minimizing the need for subsequent extensive reconstructive surgery by limiting scar formation. Examples in which primary urethral repair may be considered include most penetrating urethral injuries (by suturing), urethral injuries associated with penile fractures (by suturing), and select partial posterior urethral disruptions (by realignment).

A urethral disruption in a female requires immediate surgical repair because any tear involving the short female urethra likely will extend to the bladder neck and disrupt the sphincteric mechanism. Prompt urethral and bladder neck reconstruction is necessary in order to limit posttraumatic incontinence.

OUTCOME

Urethral injuries from external trauma are some of the most devastating and difficult genitourinary injuries. Major long-term complications, which include urinary incontinence, erectile dysfunction, stricture formation, and recurring infections, are often a result of the initial injury. Adhering to the principles outlined earlier can minimize additional complications.

REFERENCES

Brandes S, Coburn M, Armenakas NA, McAninch JW: Diagnosis and management of ureteric injury: an evidence-based analysis. BJU Int 2004;94:277-289.

Chapple C, Barbagli G, Jordan, G, et al: Consensus statement on urethral trauma. BJU Int 2004;93:1135-1202.

Gomez RG, Ceballos L, Coburn M, et al: Consensus statement on bladder injuries. BJU Int 2004;94:27-32.

Morey AF, Metro MJ, Carney KJ, et al: Consensus on genitourinary trauma: External genitalia. BJU Int 2004;94:507-515.

Santucci RA, Wessells H, Bartsch G, et al: Evaluation and management of renal injuries: Consensus statement of the renal trauma subcommittee. BJU Int 2004;93:937-954.

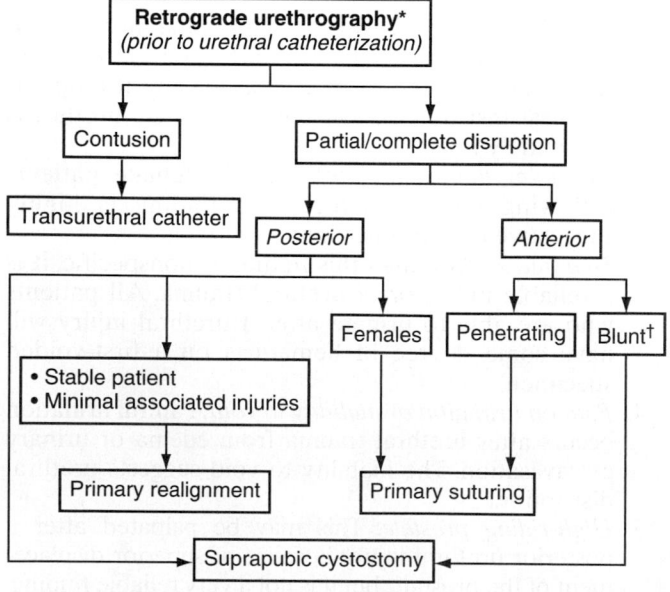

* In females only, proceed to urethroscopy.
† Except in association with penile fractures.

FIGURE 7. Algorithm for the diagnosis and management of urethral trauma (penile or perineal injury, pelvic fracture).

Prostatitis

Method of
Ira W. Klimberg, MD

Prostatitis is one of the most common urologic problems. Nearly 50% of men will experience the symptom complex of "prostatitis" at some time. Prostatitis has been traditionally classified as acute or chronic bacterial prostatitis, nonbacterial prostatitis, or prostatodynia (pelviperineal pain). In 1995, the U.S. National Institutes of Health (NIH) developed a new classification system that emphasized the differences between bacterial prostatitis and the myriad of other clinical conditions that can produce similar

TABLE 1 National Institutes of Health Classification of Prostatitis

Category I	Acute bacterial prostatitis
Category II	Chronic bacterial prostatitis
Category III	CPPS
Category IIIA	Inflammatory CPPS
Category IIIB	Noninflammatory CPPS
Category IV	Asymptomatic inflammatory prostatitis

Abbreviation: CPPS = chronic pelvic pain syndrome.

symptoms and categorized all of these other idiopathic conditions as the chronic pelvic pain syndrome (CPPS; Table 1). This new classification system has provided a clearer conceptual framework for prostatitis; however, we remain ignorant of the pathophysiology underlying chronic pelvic pain (category III prostatitis).

Bacterial prostatitis, either acute or chronic, accounts for no more than 10% of cases in clinical practice and is readily diagnosed from the presence of pyuria and a positive urine culture. Ninety percent of men will have category III prostatitis, which is more accurately defined as CPPS. Nonbacterial prostatitis, an inflammatory process that mimics the symptoms of chronic bacterial prostatitis, is now classified as category IIIA, or inflammatory prostatitis.

Prostatodynia is a term that causes urologists to shudder and has produced much of the confusion about prostatitis. Prostatodynia defines symptoms that fit the clinical picture of prostatitis but are unaccompanied by any objective evidence of infection or inflammation localizable to the urinary tract or prostate. The term has been used to describe any unexplained pelviperineal complaints in men. The NIH designation of "chronic pelvic pain syndrome, noninflammatory" (category IIIB) is appropriate and more correct! Stamey referred to this spectrum of real or putative prostatic diseases as a "wastebasket of clinical ignorance."

I find it useful to try to differentiate men whose symptoms can reasonably be attributed to the prostate from those who have other sources of pelviperineal pain and/or voiding symptoms. Patients with a prostatic nexus for their symptoms would be expected to have evidence of significant inflammation in their prostatic fluid. This is clinically defined as the presence of 10 or more white blood cells per high-power field of their expressed prostatic secretions (EPS). The diagnosis of prostatitis cannot be rationally entertained in the absence of inflammatory cells in the EPS; it is the sine qua non of prostatitis. Meares and Stamey described segmented urine cultures to aid in the diagnosis of prostatitis and localize urinary tract infections. The patient collects the first 10 mL of voided urine (VB1), which represents the urethra, and a midstream urine specimen (VB2), which represents the bladder. Prostatic massage is then performed, and the EPS are collected. The first 10 mL of voided urine after the prostatic massage (VB3) is also collected. Each sample is subjected to microscopic examination and quantitative cultures.

Physicians (and patients) have found this technique to be cumbersome and uncomfortable. It has largely been replaced by the two-glass test; urine samples obtained before and after prostatic massage. Performing prostatic massage vigorously enough to recover EPS in all suspected cases of prostatitis is frequently painful to patients. A valuable surrogate for the EPS specimen is the VB3 specimen, which can be obtained easily and painlessly after digital rectal examination. Virtually all cases of bacterial prostatitis manifest with concomitant urinary tract infection and are readily identifiable by the presence of pyuria in the initial urine collection and a positive urine culture. If the initial urine specimen is clear, 10 white blood cells per high-power field in the EPS is diagnostic of prostatitis; if EPS are unobtainable, pyuria in VB3 is highly suggestive of prostatic inflammation. If inflammatory cells are absent from all of the specimens, then the diagnosis of prostatitis cannot be made.

Acute Bacterial Prostatitis

Acute bacterial prostatitis is usually manifested by the sudden onset of fever, urinary frequency, urgency, and dysuria. Low back pain, suprapubic or perineal pain, and varying degrees of bladder outlet obstruction often accompany these symptoms of bacteriuria. An extremely tender, enlarged, sometimes swollen and "boggy"-feeling prostate are characteristic. Vigorous prostatic massage should be avoided because of the risk of bacteremia and patient discomfort. Obtaining EPS is not necessary because the bacterial pathogen can be easily identified from the voided urine. *Escherichia coli* and other members of the Enterobacteriaceae predominate; *Pseudomonas* and *Enterococcus* organisms are less common.

Many men with acute bacterial prostatitis will require hospitalization. Signs of bacteremia and sepsis are frequent. Hydration, analgesics, antipyretics, and stool softeners are helpful supportive measures. Acute urinary retention is common, and Foley catheter placement may be required. For toxic patients, I obtain blood and urine cultures and initiate therapy with ceftriaxone (Rocephin),[1] 1 g intravenously every 24 hours, and a fluoroquinolone such as

---

[1]Not FDA approved for this indication.

CURRENT DIAGNOSIS

- Acute bacterial prostatitis is readily diagnosed by pyuria and positive urine cultures. Vigorous prostatic massage should be avoided.
- Chronic bacterial prostatitis frequently demonstrates pyuria and positive urine cultures; however, some patients require prostatic massage and expression of prostatic secretions or a postmassage urine specimen to identify pyuria or infection limited to the prostate.
- Inflammatory chronic pelvic pain syndrome is diagnosed when white blood cells are present in the expressed prostatic secretions or in postmassage urine.
- The majority of men have noninflammatory chronic pelvic pain syndrome and demonstrate normal-appearing urine and prostatic secretions.

CURRENT THERAPY

- Acute bacterial prostatitis patients may have a toxic condition and require hospitalization, with administration of intravenous ceftriaxone (Rocephin)[1] 1 g/day or gentamicin (Garamycin)[1] 5 mg/kg/day in addition to fluoroquinolone therapy with ciprofloxacin (Cipro) 500 mg bid, levofloxacin (Levaquin) 400 mg qd, or ofloxacin (Floxin) 500 mg qd.
- For patients who are not seriously ill, oral quinolones alone are usually effective. A single dose of gentamicin 5 mg/kg and antipyretics may be indicated for febrile patients who wish to be managed as outpatients.
- Oral fluoroquinolones, which have excellent tissue penetration into the prostate, are the mainstays for treatment of chronic prostatitis.
- Long-term antibacterial therapy (4–8 weeks) appears to be more effective than shorter-duration regimens in achieving bacteriologic cure in patients with chronic prostatitis.
- α_1-Adrenergic blockers, such as tamsulosin (Flomax)[1] 0.4 to 0.8 mg daily or alfuzosin (Uroxatral)[1] 10 mg daily, are useful adjuncts in men with significant obstructive voiding symptoms.

[1]Not FDA approved for this indication.

ciprofloxacin (Cipro) 500 mg intravenously or orally every 12 hours, ofloxacin (Floxin) 500 mg, or levofloxacin (Levaquin) 400 mg, both intravenously or orally once daily. Intravenous gentamicin (Garamycin)[1] at 5 mg/kg/day in a single dose can be substituted for the ceftriaxone.

These patients usually respond dramatically to antibiotic therapy. By the time the urine culture and sensitivity results are available, patients can usually be treated with oral fluoroquinolone therapy alone. If the patient does not rapidly improve, prostatic abscess must be excluded by computed tomographic imaging of the prostate. If the patient is not acutely ill and does not require hospitalization, oral fluoroquinolone therapy alone is usually effective. I frequently add a single intravenous dose of gentamicin at 5 mg/kg and antipyretics for febrile patients managed as outpatients. Oral antimicrobial therapy is continued for a minimum of 14 days.

Chronic Bacterial Prostatitis

The hallmark of chronic bacterial prostatitis is recurrent urinary tract infections caused by the same pathogen. Pathogenic bacteria may persist unaltered in the prostatic fluid during therapy with some older antimicrobial agents because these agents accumulate poorly in prostatic secretions. This entity has all but disappeared in recent years as a result of the fluoroquinolone antibiotics that exhibit excellent penetration into prostatic tissue and secretions.

Patients complain of irritative voiding symptoms such as urgency, frequency, and dysuria during episodes of bacteriuria. Ill-defined pelvic or perineal pain, symptoms

of bladder outlet obstruction, ejaculatory pain, and hematospermia, may accompany these symptoms.

Long-term antibiotic therapy (4–8 weeks) appears to be more effective than short-term therapy in achieving permanent bacteriologic cure. Oral fluoroquinolones, such as ciprofloxacin, ofloxacin, or levofloxacin (at the doses previously indicated) are the mainstays of treatment. Trimethoprim-sulfamethoxazole (TMP-SMZ; Septra, Bactrim)[1] one double-strength tablet (160 mg TMP and 800 mg SMZ) orally bid for 12 weeks can be used alternatively or in cases of bacterial resistance to the quinolones. Antibiotic therapy should be tailored to microbiologic sensitivity results.

Chronic Pelvic Pain Syndrome (Nonbacterial Prostatitis)

A paucity of clinical trial results or evidence-based medicine is available for reference when confronted with men having CPPS. Fortunately, the majority of patients show symptomatic improvement with a course of antimicrobial therapy, and antibiotics should be considered first-line empirical therapy. I prefer quinolone antimicrobials because of their broad clinical spectrum and excellent tissue penetration into the prostate. I generally prescribe 10 to 14 days of therapy, with several refills if the patient clinically responds while undergoing therapy and then relapses. I frequently coadminister naproxen (Aleve) 400 mg orally twice daily for its anti-inflammatory effect.

The uroselective α_1-adrenergic blocker tamsulosin (Flomax)[1] 0.4 to 0.8 mg daily or alfuzosin (Uroxatral)[1] 10 mg daily is a useful adjunct in men who experience significant obstructive voiding symptoms. I have obtained sporadic results with amitriptyline (Elavil)[1] 50 to 100 mg daily in patients whose predominant symptoms are pain unaltered by antibiotic treatment. Prednisone in short courses has been effective at times.

In the majority of men, prostatitis is a self-limited process, with symptoms resolving spontaneously within several weeks. The repetitive administration of antimicrobial drugs is unwarranted and uniformly ineffective in the treatment of recalcitrant prostatitis symptoms. Patient education and symptomatic treatment with anti-inflammatory drugs, α_1-adrenergic-blockers, and hot sitz baths are advised. Avoidance of caffeine, alcoholic beverages, and dietary triggers is recommended. Men with unrelenting symptoms should be referred for more complete urologic evaluation to rule out undiagnosed pelvic pathology.

REFERENCES

Karlovsky ME, Pontari MA: Theories of prostatitis etiology. Curr Urol Rep 2002;3:307-312.

Krieger JN, Nyberg L Jr, Nickel JC: NIH consensus definition and classification of prostatitis. JAMA 1999;282:236.

Litwin MS, McNaughton-Collins M, Fowler FJ Jr, et al: The National Institutes of Health chronic prostatitis index: Development and validation of a new outcome measure. Chronic Prostatitis Collaborative Research Network. J Urol 1999;162:369-375.

Nickel JC: Prostatitis syndromes: Update for urologic practice. Can J Urol 2000;7:1091-1098.

True LD, Shoskes D, Alexander R, et al: Special report on prostatitis: State of the art. Rev Urol 2001;3:[KMcC1]

[1]Not FDA approved for this indication.

[1]Not FDA approved for this indication.

Benign Prostatic Hyperplasia

Method of
Gopal H. Badlani, MD,
and Matthew E. Karlovsky, MD

Epidemiology

Bladder outlet obstruction (BOO) secondary to benign prostatic hyperplasia (BPH) is one of the most common medical conditions in older men and represents up to a 40% clinical risk for urinary retention in a man's lifetime. It is the most prevalent condition in the aging male, affecting 14 million men in the United States, with an annual cost of $4 billion to treat. Age and normal androgenic function are two of the better established risk factors. Whereas BPH is rare before the age of 40, the prevalence of histologic BPH at autopsy is 50% by 60 years of age and 90% by 85 years of age. Approximately 40% of males 70 years of age or older have lower urinary tract symptoms (LUTS) secondary to BPH, and with age, the prevalence increases. Symptomatically, approximately 25% of 55-year-old men experience decreased urinary flow rate and other symptoms of BPH. By 75 years of age, the appearance of this symptom increases to 50%. Age, however, is not a causative factor of BOO. Although the risk for developing symptoms from BPH doubles for each decade of life between 60 and 90 years of age, clinical symptoms of the individual patient do not necessarily progress with age. BPH is more commonly diagnosed because of increased life expectancy and a greater tendency today to seek medical advice at an earlier disease stage.

Normal androgenic function is required for development of BPH. Both androgenic and estrogenic hormonal stimulation can induce prostatic hypertrophy. Other factors, such as race, sexual activity, smoking, socioeconomic status, vasectomy, alcohol intake, and diet, have been implicated in BPH development. Identifying men at clinical risk for BPH and its progression has clinical usefulness in selecting the appropriate intervention when necessary.

Pathophysiology

The pathophysiology of BPH is poorly understood because no direct correlation can be made between prostatic glandular enlargement and the symptomatology of BPH. Because the condition is rare in those younger than 40 years of age and does not develop in castrated men, it is accepted that BPH development requires aging and functional testes for androgen production. BPH is believed to originate in the transitional zone of the prostate, which surrounds the prostatic urethra between the bladder neck and the verumontanum, and is progressive.

Both a static and a dynamic component are involved in BPH development. The static component relates to epithelial and stromal cell proliferation in the prostatic transitional zone (TZ); enlargement is evident as median or lateral lobe hypertrophy. Proliferation is induced by testosterone and its biologically active conversion product, dihydrotestosterone. Conversion of testosterone to dihydrotestosterone occurs via the enzyme 5α-reductase. Two forms of this enzyme have been described, type 1 and type 2. Type 1 is present in liver, skin, and other organs. Type 2 is present in urogenital tissues. Individuals lacking 5α-reductase type 2 do not develop genitalia and prostates.

Conversely, the dynamic component relates to prostatic smooth muscle. High concentrations of α_1-adrenergic receptors occur in the prostatic capsule and bladder neck. An increase in smooth muscle tone is responsible for increased urethral resistance and pressure. Pharmacologic blockade with α_1 antagonists blocks prostatic smooth muscle contraction and decreases urethral resistance and pressure, subsequently relaxing the dynamic component of BPH.

Symptoms

The diagnosis of BPH is presumptive, based on symptoms. These symptoms, commonly referred to as lower urinary tract symptoms (LUTS), are not specific for BPH. LUTS include frequency, retention, intermittency, decreased force of stream (FOS), straining, urgency, and nocturia. Individuals with LUTS should be carefully assessed to determine the cause, to confirm diagnosis of BPH, and to exclude other bladder and prostate processes. Normal prostate size on digital rectal examination (DRE) does not rule out a diagnosis of BPH because palpable prostate size does not correlate with degree of obstruction or severity of LUTS. However, the odds of having moderate to severe symptoms are five times higher for men with enlarged prostates compared with those with normal prostates. Symptoms of BPH are difficult to assess and quantify, yet they are the keys to proper diagnosis and treatment. Because the vast majority of procedures performed for BPH are to provide symptomatic relief, it is necessary to quantify the level of interference in the quality of life of the patient. Assessment of interference on quality of life can be reliably accomplished using the well-validated International Prostate Symptom Score (IPSS) (Figure 1). Symptoms based on overall score are classified as mild (0 to 7), moderate (8 to 19), and severe (20 to 35). The subjective impact of these symptoms on overall quality of life must also be taken into account. The patient with a severe-range IPSS may feel the symptoms are less bothersome than a patient with a lower IPSS, and this subjective impact on quality of life can direct therapeutic options.

Diagnosis

Diagnosis of BPH relies on an accurate medical history eliciting the specific voiding complaints, as well as quantification of these symptoms using the IPSS. Other possible causes of LUTS also must be ruled out, including urinary tract infection (UTI), urolithiasis, diabetes, urethral stricture, overactive or neurogenic bladder, prostate/bladder cancer, or congestive heart failure. Medications that can exacerbate obstructive symptoms include tricyclic antidepressants, anticholinergic agents, diuretics, narcotics, and first-generation antihistamines and decongestants. Physical examination should include DRE for prostatic abnormalities, such as palpable nodules, induration or irregularities of malignancy, or infection. On DRE, the posterior lobes,

Name: _____   Date: _____

	Not at all	Less than 1 time in 5	Less than half the time	About half the time	More than half the time	Almost always	Your score
Incomplete emptying Over the past month, how often have you had a sensation of not emptying your bladder completely after you finish urinating?	0	1	2	3	4	5	
Frequency Over the past month, how often have you had to urinate again less than two hours after you finished urinating?	0	1	2	3	4	5	
Intermittency Over the past month, how often have you found you stopped and started again several times when you urinated?	0	1	2	3	4	5	
Urgency Over the past month, how difficult have you found it to postpone urination?	0	1	2	3	4	5	
Weak stream Over the past month, how often have you had a weak urinary stream?	0	1	2	3	4	5	
Straining Over the past month, how often have you had to push or strain to begin urination?	0	1	2	3	4	5	

	None	1 time	2 times	3 times	4 times	5 times or more	Your score
Nocturia Over the past month, how many times did you most typically get up to urinate from the time you went to bed until the time you got up in the morning?	0	1	2	3	4	5	

Total IPSS score	

Quality of life due to urinary symptoms	Delighted	Pleased	Mostly satisfied	Mixed—about equally satisfied and dissatisfied	Mostly dissatisfied	Unhappy	Terrible
If you were to spend the rest of your life with your urinary condition the way it is now, how would you feel about that?	0	1	2	3	4	5	6

FIGURE 1. International prostate symptom score (IPSS).

not the transition zone, are palpable. Abdominal examination may detect a suprapubic or low abdominal mass in a patient with BPH-induced retention. The American Urological Association and the American Cancer Society recommend all men older than age 50 receive an annual prostate-specific antigen (PSA) serum level to screen for prostate cancer. In black men or men with a family history of prostate cancer in a first-degree relative, PSA screening should begin at 40 years of age or younger. The normal range for PSA is up to 4.0 µg/mL. Other valuable laboratory data include urinalysis to rule out infection or hematuria, a serum creatinine level to determine renal function, and urine cytologic studies if irritative voiding symptoms are present. More sophisticated studies, such as urinary flow rate, postvoid residual, and pressure flow urodynamic studies, are appropriate for evaluation of men with more severe symptoms (IPSS >8) or with more complex comorbidities. These tests are often used to determine baseline function prior to initiation of therapy or to determine subsequent response to therapy. In patients who fail medical therapy, urodynamic pressure-flow studies and cystoscopy may be appropriate to evaluate the need for operative intervention and to rule out other urologic pathologies. Cystoscopy is also reserved for situations in which invasive treatment is strongly considered. If watchful waiting or noninvasive therapies are appropriate,

TABLE 1 Common Medications for Benign Prostatic Hyperplasia

Medication	Class	Dose	Schedule
Alfuzosin (Uroxatral)	α-1 Blocker	10 mg	Once daily
Doxazosin (Cardura)	α-1 Blocker	1-8 mg, titrated	Once daily at bedtime
Tamsulosin (Flomax)	α-1a Blocker	0.4 mg	Once daily
Terazosin (Hytrin)	α-1 Blocker	1-10 mg, titrated	Once daily at bedtime
Dutasteride (Avodart)	5-α Reductase inhibitor	0.5 mg	Once daily
Finasteride (Proscar)	5-α Reductase inhibitor	5 mg	Once daily

invasive diagnostic tests are usually not necessary. The variables of importance of disease progression in an artificial neural network analysis were PSA, obstructive symptom score, and transitional zone volume. The Olmsted County study showed risk progression of acute urinary retention (AUR) with age. Overall, a 60-year-old man has a 23% chance of AUR if he survives the next 20 years. The average annual change in prostate volume was 1.6% for all ages. The annual increase was not significantly related to baseline age but was significantly related to baseline prostate volume.

Treatment

WATCHFUL WAITING

Indications for treatment of BPH rely, in large part, on the subjective nature of the symptoms. For the majority of patients with BPH, symptoms are not severe or bothersome enough to warrant long-term medical or surgical intervention. Men with an IPSS of less than 8 are usually treated with expectant management. Advising the patient toward lifestyle modifications, such as minimizing evening fluid intake, avoiding caffeine, and avoiding decongestants, anticholinergics, and other medications that impair voiding, often provides an effective resolution of symptoms. In a study of 556 men with moderate symptoms of BPH comparing outcomes following transurethral resection of the prostate (TURP) with watchful waiting for more than 3 years, 8% of men randomized to TURP and 17% of men with watchful waiting failed treatment. Treatment failure with watchful waiting was mostly because of high postvoid residuals and significant increases in IPSS symptoms. Patients who respond poorly to watchful waiting have multiple medical and surgical options for treatment of BPH.

α₁-ADRENERGIC BLOCKING AGENTS

The α_1-adrenergic antagonists have been shown in numerous randomized placebo-controlled trials to be safe and effective in the treatment of BPH. The most commonly prescribed α_1-adrenergic blockers appear to have similar safety profiles and clinical efficacy and are the common first approach for urologists. Terazosin (Hytrin) and doxazosin (Cardura) were the first α antagonists available for treatment of BPH; however, orthostatic hypotension was a significant concern, requiring careful dose titration. Tamsulosin (Flomax), a highly selective α-blocker, does not induce orthostatic hypotension and so does not require dose titration. Overall, the most common side effects include

headaches, dizziness, asthenia, and drowsiness. Sexual side effects are limited to retrograde ejaculation. Alfuzosin (Uroxatral), a newer nonspecific α-blocker, has minimal vasoactive or retrograde ejaculation side effects. Table 1 provides a list for medication dosing and schedules.

5α-REDUCTASE INHIBITION

Finasteride (Proscar) and dutasteride (Avodart) are 5α-reductase inhibitors (type 1 and type 1/2, respectively) that block conversion of testosterone to dihydrotestosterone, the androgen involved in development of BPH. These medications represent the paradigm for androgen suppression of BPH. They have their greatest therapeutic effect in men with prostates greater than 40 g, and treatment for 6 months or more is usually required for a clinical response. The first randomized, multicenter, double-blind, placebo-controlled trial investigating the efficacy of finasteride demonstrated significant improvements in maximum flow rate and decreased prostatic volume. Since then, further studies have confirmed a reduced risk of acute urinary retention and surgical intervention with finasteride use. Finasteride can reduce BPH-associated hematuria. It is effective as adjuvant therapy, following other treatments, and as neoadjuvant therapy prior to minimally invasive therapy. Adverse effects include decreased libido, ejaculatory dysfunction, and gynecomastia. In the patient being monitored for prostate cancer with PSA testing, finasteride therapy must be taken into account when interpreting PSA values; finasteride decreases PSA values by 50%, leading to a false-negative result.≠

Efficacy of Medical Therapy

The Medical Therapy of Prostate Symptoms (MTOPS) study evaluated the efficacy of doxazosin and finasteride to determine if medical therapy delays or prevents disease progression. At 4 years, combination therapy was most effective for reducing risk of clinical progression (AUR) and improving symptom score and urinary flow rate. Finasteride and combination therapy significantly reduced the risk of AUR and invasive therapy over 4 years. Monotherapy with either medication reduced symptom score and improved flow significantly, but to a lesser degree than combination therapy. Doxazosin delayed time to progression of AUR and invasive therapy but not the risk. Without treatment, the risk of BPH progression was 20% more during the trial. Risk factors for progression include baseline prostate volume (>40 g) and higher serum PSA value (>2 μg/mL).

Phytotherapy

Saw palmetto (*Serenoa repens*)[1,2] extract is the most popular phytotherapeutic agent. Its likely mechanism is inhibition of 5α-reductase. A recent meta-analysis of numerous randomized trials using saw palmetto described a mild to moderate improvement in flow and LUTS; however, because of small study sample, varying products, short treatment times, and varying outcomes, these study conclusions are difficult to interpret. Other popular preparations are African plum (*Pygeum africanum*)[1,2] and South African star grass (*Cynodon nlemfuënsis*).[1,2] The former has been shown to have several in vitro effects, such as antiestrogen effects, leukotriene blockade, and inhibition of fibroblast growth factors. The latter has been shown in vitro to increase plasminogen activators, as well as to stimulate release of transforming growth factor-β, an inducer of apoptosis, yet these in vitro effects have not been shown to occur in vivo. A meta-analysis of four clinical trials of South African star grass extract, β-sitosterol, concluded that β-sitosterol improved urologic symptoms and flow rates in men.

There is no standard of care for management of patients using phytotherapy. Nor have the long-term safety effects been established. Patients should be cautioned that doses, efficacy, side effects, and drug interactions with phytotherapy are unknown. For the patient refusing medical therapy of α-blockers and 5α-reductase inhibitors, phytotherapy may be attempted as long as the patient understands the limitations of these agents. If retention, UTI, calculi, or decreased renal function occurs, phytotherapy should be discouraged and more aggressive medical and surgical management undertaken.

Minimally Invasive Therapies

The most commonly employed surgical procedure, and the gold standard for BPH, is transurethral resection of the prostate (TURP), involving endoscopic resection of the obstructive component of the prostate. TURP is highly effective, improving symptoms in up to 95% of patients. Common complications include inability to void postoperatively, clot retention, incontinence, impotence, and retrograde ejaculation. A number of new minimally invasive therapies have been developed to reduce the complications associated with TURP, as well as provide alternatives for the unfavorable surgical candidate. Most minimally invasive therapies use energy, such as radio waves, laser, ultrasound, microwaves, or electrical current.

Transurethral incision of the prostate (TUIP) involves endoscopic placement of one to two incisions into the prostate and capsule to reduce urethral constriction. This procedure is highly effective on prostate glands less than 30 g and is well documented and safe, with efficacy comparable with TURP. TUIP is associated with a 78% to 83% improvement of symptoms. Because TUIP is associated with fewer retrograde ejaculations, less morbidity, and a reoperation rate of less than 1% in 10 years, this procedure is the treatment of choice for small gland BPH in men concerned with fertility and ejaculation.

[1]Not FDA approved for this indication.
[2]Available as a dietary supplement.

In transurethral needle ablation (TUNA), low-level energy is transferred by radiofrequency to the prostate, creating a well-defined necrotic lesion within the prostatic parenchyma while preserving the urethral mucosa. A cystoscope-like instrument with two needles set at 90 degrees from each other ablates tissue in 3 to 5 minutes when needles reach temperatures of 27° to 38°C (80° to 100°F). Urethral and rectal temperatures are also vigorously monitored as the device adjusts. Preliminary studies show an increase in peak flow and a decrease in symptom score following TUNA, with no major complications. Transient urinary retention is reported in 10% to 40% of patients. In a prospective study, TURP was superior to TUNA in increasing flow rates but demonstrated comparable improved symptoms at 1 year postoperatively. Transurethral microwave thermotherapy (TUMT) heats prostatic transitional zone tissue to between 60° and 80°C (140° to 176°F), inducing tissue damage. Thermotherapy preferentially destroys smooth muscle by coagulative necrosis while water-conductive cooling of the urethral mucosa preserves periurethral tissues. Although prospective studies indicate that TURP produces more pronounced urinary improvements versus TUMT, thermotherapy consistently improves symptom scores by 75% and increases peak flow rates by 75%. Furthermore, TUMT is a procedure done under local anesthesia. Retrograde ejaculation and urinary retention with prolonged catheterization occurs in greater than one third of patients.

Ultimately, therapeutic decisions depend in large part on symptom scores. Men with low symptom scores without bother are appropriately managed through watchful waiting. As scores increase, or if progression with clinical morbidity develops, more aggressive management is appropriate.

REFERENCES

Bhargava S, Canda AE, Chapple CR: A rational approach to benign hyperplasia evaluation: Recent advances. Curr Opin Urol 2004;14:1-6.

Djavan B, Waldert M, Ghawidel C, Marberger M: Benign prostatic hyperplasia progression and its impact on treatment. Curr Opin Urol 2004;14:45-50.

Fong YK, Milani S, Djavan B: Role of phytotherapy in men with lower urinary tract symptoms. Curr Opin Urol 2005;15:45-48.

Hoffman RM, MacDonald R, Monga M, Wilt TJ: Transurethral microwave thermotherapy vs. transurethral resection for treating benign prostatic hyperplasia: A systematic review. BJU Int 2004;94:1031-1036.

Walsh PC, Retik A, Vaughan D (eds): Campbell's Urology, 8th ed. Philadelphia, Saunders Elsevier Science, 2002.

Erectile Dysfunction

Method of
Luciano Kolodny, MD

The term *erectile dysfunction* (ED) is relatively new, having replaced *impotence* approximately a decade ago. ED is defined as the "inability of the male to attain or maintain an erection sufficient for satisfactory sexual intercourse." ED affects millions of men worldwide with implications that go far beyond sexual activity alone. ED is now recognized as a sentinel event in cardiovascular disease, diabetes mellitus (DM), and depression. It can also be damaging to interpersonal relationships and self-esteem.

Epidemiology

The Massachusetts Male Aging Study is one of the pivotal studies on the prevalence of ED. Between 1987 and 1989, men between the ages of 40 and 70 years received questionnaires inquiring about several aspects of their sexual health. Of the 1790 men who received the questionnaires, 1290 responded. They revealed that 52% of them had some degree of dysfunction, 17% with minimal, 25% with moderate, and almost 10% with complete absence of erectile function. It also showed the extremely detrimental link between coronary artery disease (CAD), DM, and ED. A few years later another group used the same patient database and followed up on these subjects. The risk of ED was 26 cases per 1000 men annually, which increased with age, lower education, DM, heart disease, and hypertension.

Physiology of Erection

The penile erection requires intact vascular, neuronal, and hormonal systems. The intricate details of this process are beyond the scope of this article, but in summary, after any sensorial stimulation, which can be visual, tactile, auditory, or olfactory, nitric oxide (NO) and other neurotransmitters are released at the cavernous nerve terminals. The endothelial cells then release vasoactive relaxing factors, which lead to vasodilatation of the penile blood vessels and increased blood flow. As blood flow increases, compression of the subtunical venular plexuses will substantially decrease venous outflow and finally cause the penis to change from flaccid to erect (Figure 1).

NO is the principal neurotransmitter involved in penile erection, but other vasoactive substances such as vasoactive intestinal peptide, neuropeptide Y, calcitonin gene-related peptide (CGRP), substance P, and serotonin also play roles. High levels of intrapenile NO facilitate the relaxation of intracavernosal trabeculae, thereby maximizing blood flow and penile erection. Nonadrenergic, noncholinergic neurons have been found to release NO, leading to increased production of cyclic guanosine monophosphate (cGMP). Through a series of reactions, cGMP will lead to relaxation of the smooth muscle, directly impacting the ability to go from a flaccid to an erect penile state. The return from erect to flaccid requires the hydrolysis of cGMP to guanosine monophosphate (GMP) by phosphodiesterase 5 (PDE5) (see Figure 1).

Testosterone and Erectile Function

Testosterone provides intrapenile nitrous oxide synthase (NOS), which has an important role in enhancing the production of NO, subsequent local vasodilatation, and penile erection. There is no correlation between serum testosterone levels and the degree of ED. However, hypogonadal men may experience significantly reduced libido. Hypogonadism is associated with decreased self-esteem, depression, osteoporosis, insulin resistance, increased fat mass, decreased lean body mass, and cognitive dysfunction.

Pathophysiology of Erectile Dysfunction

ED can be classified as psychogenic, organic (hormonal, vascular, drug-induced, or neurogenic), or mixed psychogenic and organic. Up to 80% of ED cases have an

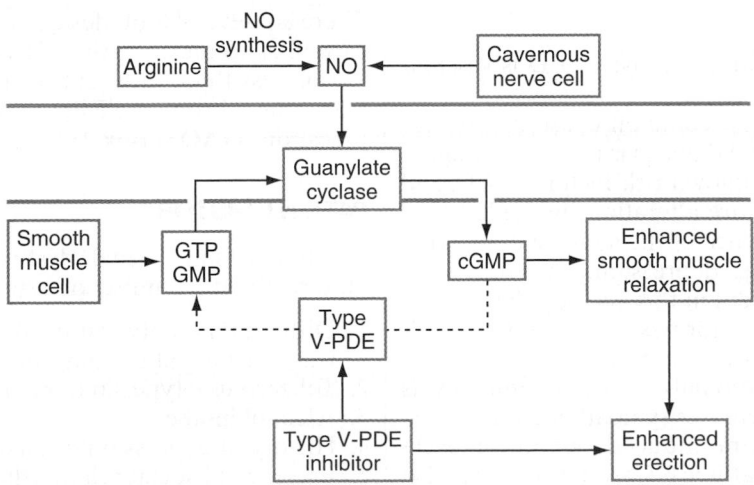

FIGURE 1. The biochemical process involved in erections and the mechanism of action of sildenafil citrate (Viagra). The cavernous nerves (S2-S4) innervate the penis and release NO. NO stimulates the production of cGMP in the smooth muscle cells of the penis. cGMP is directly responsible for increasing smooth muscle relaxation, which leads to increased arterial inflow and an erection. When cGMP is metabolized by PDE5, the penis undergoes detumescence. Sildenafil citrate (Viagra) inhibits PDE5 and increases the available cGMP, thereby leading to an enhanced erection. cGMP = cyclic guanosine monophosphate; NO = nitric oxide; PDE5 = phosphodiesterase 5.

BOX 1   Classification of Erectile Dysfunction

Endocrine
- Hypogonadism
- Hyperprolactinemia

Drug Induced
- β-Blockers
- Calcium channel blockers
- Alcohol
- Nicotine
- Antiandrogens
- Cocaine
- Heroin
- Marijuana
- Cimetidine
- Metoclopramide
- Antidepressant medications
- Antipsychotic medications

Vascular
- Coronary artery disease
- Peripheral vascular disease
- Hypertension
- Diabetes mellitus

Psychogenic
- Depression
- Performance anxiety

Neurogenic
- Spinal cord injury
- Neuropathy (diabetic, hypertensive)
- Cerebrovascular disease
- Radical prostatectomy
- Pelvic surgery

Multifactorial
- Aging
- End-stage renal disease
- Pelvic trauma (neurogenic and vasculogenic)
- Diabetes mellitus (neurogenic, vasculogenic, drug induced)

organic origin. The most common cause of ED is vascular disease (Box 1).

Atherosclerosis is the most common cause of vasculogenic ED, whereas endothelial damage is the most common mechanism. Aging is a well-known risk factor for ED, and it is hypothesized that there are alterations in the levels of NO that occur as a consequence of the aging endothelium. Additionally, chronic illness, depression, and lack of a sexual partner are all prevalent in this age population.

Chronic tobacco use is a major risk factor for the development of vasculogenic ED because of its effects on the vascular endothelium. Additionally, blood nicotine levels rise after smoking, which increases sympathetic tone in the penis and leads to nicotine-induced, smooth-muscle contraction in the cavernosal body. Chronic smoking also leads to decreased penile NOS activity and neuronal NOS content.

DM is a major risk factor for ED. In the Massachusetts Male Aging Study, the diabetic subset had a threefold increased prevalence of ED compared with nondiabetic subjects (28% versus 9.6%). In the same study, the overall incidence rate of ED was 26 cases per 1000 man-years in nondiabetics and 50 cases per 1000 man-years in the diabetic population. The pathogenesis of ED in the diabetic patient is related to accelerated atherosclerosis, alterations in the corporal erectile tissue, and neuropathy.

Hypertension is another major risk factor for ED. Whether ED in patients with hypertension is related to the disease itself or to the use of antihypertensive medications has been debated for years. In a study looking at 104 subjects, the differences in incidence or severity of ED were minor between distinct types of antihypertensive medications or the number of agents being used simultaneously. This favors the concept that antihypertensive agents as well as the disease itself contribute to the appearance of ED. There are, however, classes of antihypertensive medications that are notorious for their negative impact on erectile function such as thiazides and β-blockers. The only β-blocker not associated with significant incidence of ED is carvedilol (Coreg).

Hyperlipidemia is another etiologic factor for ED. It is believed to contribute to ED by its relationship to endothelial dysfunction. One study showed that decreasing total cholesterol to less than 200 mg/dL by using atorvastatin (Lipitor) led to significant improvement of ED as measured by the International Index of Erectile Function (IIEF).

ED may be a sentinel manifestation of vascular disorders. In a study of 980 subjects seeking ED advice, 18% were suffering from undiagnosed hypertension, 16% had DM, 5% had ischemic heart disease, 15% had benign prostatic hyperplasia, 4% had prostate cancer, and 1% had depression. ED can itself be an independent marker for CAD. In addition, the extent of CAD correlates with the prevalence of ED.

Quantification of the Severity of Erectile Dysfunction and Improvement

There are several tools designed to assess the severity of ED, as well as to measure the efficacy of different treatments. We discuss three different measures, the IIEF, the Sexual Encounter Profile (SEP), and the Global Assessment Question (GAQ) (Box 2).

PATIENT HISTORY

When assessing sexual dysfunction, it is important to inquire about a number of issues:

1. Differentiate between decreased libido and ED: assess whether the patient has one or both
2. Tobacco use: type, amount, duration
3. Alcohol intake
4. History of depression or anxiety disorder
5. Presence of social/relationship stressors
6. Ability to have erections while masturbating versus when with partner
7. List of all prescription, over-the-counter, and herbal medications
8. Knowledge of whether nocturnal erections are present

Tools used in the quantification of the severity of erectile dysfunction (ED) include the International Index of Erectile Function (IIEF), the Sexual Encounter Profile (SEP), and the Global Assessment Question (GAQ).

International Index of Erectile Function

The IIEF is a standardized questionnaire designed to measure ED and detect treatment-related changes. It is a 15-item questionnaire addressing five different domains: erectile function, orgasmic function, sexual desire, intercourse satisfaction, and overall satisfaction. The IIEF is the most frequently used efficacy measurement employed in ED drug trials. Using a scale from 1 (never/almost never) to 5 (almost always/always), men grade each domain. It is very sensitive and specific, and has been validated in 20 languages to assess treatment-related changes in sexual function. The questions 1-5 and 15 are used to quantify erectile dysfunction severity and are as follows:

1. How often were you able to get an erection during sexual activity?
2. When you had erections with sexual stimulation, how often were your erections hard enough for penetration?
3. When you attempted sexual intercourse, how often were you able to penetrate (enter) your partner?
4. During sexual intercourse, how often were you able to maintain your erection after you had penetrated (entered) your partner?
5. During sexual intercourse, how difficult was it to maintain your erection to completion of intercourse?
15. How do you rate your confidence that you could get and keep an erection?

And it is scored as follows:

26-30	Normal ED
22-25	Mild ED
17-21	Mild to moderate ED
11-16	Moderate ED
≤10	Severe ED

Sexual Encounter Profile

SEP is a five-question survey provided to patients with ED in clinical studies of oral therapies. The survey is completed after each sexual attempt. The questions are as follows:

1. Were you able to achieve at least some erection?
2. Were you able to insert your penis into your partner's vagina?
3. Did your erection last long enough to have successful intercourse?
4. Were you satisfied with the hardness of your erection?
5. Were you satisfied with the overall sexual experience?

Answers to questions 2 and 3 are the ones most often used in the literature.

Global Assessment Questions

GAQ is usually administered at the end of the treatment period during efficacy studies.
Question 1: Has the treatment taken during the study improved your erections?
Question 2: If yes, has the treatment improved your ability to engage in sexual activity?
This is very subjective, and its responses tend to be valued less than SEP and IIEF.

9. History of drug use: marijuana, cocaine, other recreational drugs
10. History of genitourinary trauma
11. History of prostatic disease, or possible related symptoms
12. History of hypertension, hyperlipidemia, CAD, peripheral vascular disease, cerebrovascular disease
13. History of DM
14. History of spinal cord injury
15. History of penile plaques: possible Peyronie's disease
16. Frequency of intercourse or attempted intercourse
17. Ability to ejaculate

PHYSICAL EXAMINATION

The physical examination should include a careful testicular examination to assess testicular size, asymmetries, presence of hernias, or varicoceles. Additionally, a digital rectal examination to assess the prostatic size, consistency, and presence of nodules is warranted. Penile inspection and palpation should be performed, with special attention to possible fibrotic plaques. Palpation and auscultation of femoral arteries for possible bruits is another important part of the examination.

LABORATORY STUDIES

Laboratory workup on a patient with ED should include total and bioavailable testosterone levels drawn in the morning, prolactin, prostate-specific antigen, fasting glucose, and fasting lipid panel. Further studies may be warranted depending on the results of the aforementioned.

Management of Erectile Dysfunction

The landscape of ED was revolutionized with the introduction of sildenafil citrate (Viagra), the first oral medication for the treatment of this condition. Since then, oral agents have become the preferred mode of treatments by patients in surveys worldwide. There are three oral agents that inhibit PDE5 currently on the market:

1. Sildenafil citrate (Viagra)
2. Vardenafil (Levitra)
3. Tadalafil (Cialis)

All three drugs work by inhibiting PDE5, which maintains intracavernosal levels of cGMP, subsequently producing vasodilatation and penile erection (see Figure 1).

SILDENAFIL CITRATE (VIAGRA)

Sildenafil citrate (Viagra) is an orally active, potent, and selective inhibitor of cGMP-specific PDE5. The predominant phosphodiesterase isoform in the penile tissue is type 5. The selectivity of sildenafil citrate (Viagra) for PDE5 is approximately 4000-fold greater than its selectivity for phosphodiesterase 3 (PDE3), the isoform involved in the control of cardiac contractility. Sildenafil citrate (Viagra) is absorbed rapidly after oral administration, with an absolute bioavailability of 40%. The time of maximal (T-max) plasma after oral dosing in the fasting state is between 30 and 120 minutes. A high-fat meal increases the time to peak plasma concentration by 60 minutes and reduces the peak plasma concentration by 29%. The half-life of the drug is from 3 to 5 hours. Sildenafil citrate (Viagra) is metabolized by hepatic microsomal cytochrome P450 isoenzyme 3A4 for the most part. Cytochrome P450 3A4 inhibitors, cimetidine (Tagamet), erythromycin, ketoconazole (Nizoral), and protease inhibitors may retard the metabolism of sildenafil citrate (Viagra).

The recommended dose is from 25 to 100 mg as needed approximately 1 hour before sexual activity. In some individuals, the onset of activity may be seen as early as 11 to 19 minutes, but this is not the norm. The usual starting dose is 50 mg.

The maximum recommended dose is 100 mg, and the maximum dosing frequency is once daily. A starting dose of 25 mg can be considered for patients older than age 65 years as well as for patients with severe hepatic cirrhosis or severe renal impairment.

There are more than two dozen, randomized, double-blind, placebo-controlled studies involving this agent. It produces positive results regardless of the etiology of ED. It has been studied in patients with DM, CAD, postcoronary artery bypass graft (post-CABG), spinal cord injury, depression, hypertension, prostate cancer post-prostatectomy, benign prostate enlargement post-transurethral resection of the prostate (TURP), patients on hemodialysis, as well as recipients of renal transplants. Results vary according to the underlying condition causing ED in the first place, ranging from 50% to 85%.

The most common side effects of sildenafil citrate (Viagra) include vasodilatory effects such as headaches, flushing, and nasal congestion caused by hyperemia of the nasal mucosa, as well as dyspepsia. Up to 30% of patients may get at least one side effect. Another side effect that presents on occasion is blurred or blue-green vision because of inhibition of phosphodiesterase 6 (PDE6) in the retina. It is absolutely contraindicated in men taking long-acting or short-acting nitrate drugs, and men taking any form of nitrates should be informed about the dangerous interaction.

Do not prescribe sildenafil citrate (Viagra) to patients with unstable CAD who need nitrates. Assess the need for ordering treadmill testing in select patients. Initial monitoring of blood pressure (BP) after the administration of sildenafil citrate (Viagra) may be indicated in men with complicated congestive heart failure (CHF). α-Blockers should not be used in combination with sildenafil citrate (Viagra) because of possible orthostatic hypotension.

VARDENAFIL (LEVITRA)

Vardenafil (Levitra) is a highly potent inhibitor of PDE5. It was approved for use in the United States in late 2003. It is a more selective PDE5 inhibitor than sildenafil citrate (Viagra). The absorption of vardenafil (Levitra) is delayed by a fatty content of more than 30% in a meal. However, that does not seem to affect its effectiveness in different trials. The half-life of vardenafil (Levitra) is 4.4 to 4.8 hours, and the clinical effectiveness may be as long as 12 hours. The time for maximum plasma concentration is between 42 and 54 minutes. The first trial using the agent included 580 patients, excluding patients with spinal cord injury, radical prostatectomy, hypogonadism, thyrotoxicosis, or DM.

The successful rates of intercourse were 71% to 75% on patients taking 5 or 10 mg at a time. Those taking 20 mg had a success rate of 80%. The placebo groups had an average success rate of 30%.

Vardenafil (Levitra) has been tested in patients with type 2 DM; 452 patients were enrolled in a double-blind, placebo-controlled trial. The success rate in the vardenafil (Levitra) group ranged from 57% to 72%.

In a different study involving 736 subjects including men with DM and stable CAD, the success rates were 28% for the placebo group, 65% for those taking 5 mg, 80% for those taking 10 mg, and 85% for the 20-mg group.

Patients who were unresponsive to sildenafil citrate (Viagra) at a dose of 100 mg on several attempts were given vardenafil (Levitra) in doses of 10 and 20 mg (proved in trial). Vardenafil (Levitra) produced statistically and clinically significant results compared with placebo in men who were historically unresponsive to sildenafil citrate (Viagra). The dose that offers the best clinical results is 20 mg. It should not be taken more than once every 24 hours. Safety studies have shown no deleterious effects with long-term daily use of this drug for up to 12 months.

The most common side effects include headaches (10% to 21%), flushing (5% to 13%), rhinitis (9% to 17%), and dyspepsia (1% to 6%) because vardenafil (Levitra) does not inhibit PDE6. Unlike sildenafil citrate (Viagra), it does not produce problems of blurred vision or blue-green visual disturbances. The same warning regarding the use of nitrates as sildenafil citrate (Viagra) applies to vardenafil (Levitra). Patients taking vardenafil (Levitra) may use α-blocking agents with caution.

TADALAFIL (CIALIS)

The third oral agent of this class is tadalafil (Cialis). It has a half-life of 17.5 hours, with two thirds of patients experiencing clinical benefits of this drug up to 36 hours after its use. The clinical onset of action occurs in less than 1 hour. There is no interaction between food and alcohol on the absorption of the drug.

There have been numerous phase II and III studies in Europe, Canada, and the United States using doses of 2, 5, 10, and 25 mg of the drug in comparison with placebo. The average success rates on these studies averaged 17% for placebo, 51% for the 2-mg dose, and 80% for the other doses, as well as up to 88% on the 25-mg dose in one study. In one study looking at 216 subjects with type 2 DM, improved erections were reported in 56% to 64% of the patients.

A recent article looking at all the previously published patient data showed that among 2102 men studied in 11 randomized placebo-controlled trials lasting 12 weeks, each mean improvement in IIEF at 20 mg of tadalafil (Cialis) was 8.6. Mean positive Sexual Encounter Profile Diary Question 3 (SEP3) response was 68% versus 31% in placebo groups. Mean GAQ was 84% versus 33% in placebo group.

In a multicenter, randomized, double-blind, crossover study looking at 181 men who received either sildenafil citrate (Viagra) or tadalafil (Cialis), 73% (132) preferred tadalafil (Cialis) at 20 mg instead of sildenafil citrate (Viagra) at 50 or 100 mg.

The most clinically effective dose of tadalafil (Cialis) is 20 mg. It should be taken at least 30 minutes before intercourse. It may be used with caution in patients using α-blocking agents. Nitrates are absolutely contraindicated for use in patients taking tadalafil (Cialis). The most common side effects include headaches, dyspepsia, back pain, rhinitis, and flushing. There are no visual side effects reported.

APOMORPHINE (UPRIMA)[1]

Apomorphine (Uprima)[1] is a potent emetic that acts on central dopaminergic receptors. The stimulation of central dopaminergic receptors transmits excitatory signals down the spinal cord to the sacral parasympathetic nucleus, stimulating activity of the sacral nerves supplying the penis. It has been used successfully in up to 67% of patients when administered through a sublingual preparation. Subcutaneous injections[2] of apomorphine (Uprima)[1] produce almost a 100% erectile response, but nausea and vomiting are limiting factors to this mode of administration.

The most common side effects are headache, nausea, and dizziness. Rare syncopal episodes have been reported.

PHENTOLAMINE (REGITINE)

Phentolamine (Regitine) is an α$_1$- and α$_2$-adrenergic receptor antagonist.

The sympathetic system via the release of noradrenaline (NA) is the primary determinant of cavernosal smooth muscle contraction and detumescence. A relative predominance of NA-induced contraction over NO-induced smooth muscle relaxation may contribute to ED.

In large phase III studies, 55% to 59% of patients receiving 40 and 80 mg were able to achieve vaginal penetration. Adverse effects include nasal congestion (10%), headaches (3% to 5%), dizziness (3% to 5%), tachycardia (3%), and nausea.

TRAZODONE (DESYREL)[1]

Trazodone (Desyrel)[1] is a serotonin reuptake inhibiting agent. Its action in ED is believed to be the result of central serotonergic and peripheral α-adrenolytic activity. The efficacy of trazodone is poorly demonstrated; however, it may have a place in those with performance anxiety. Side effects include drowsiness, insomnia, headaches, and weight loss.

DIETARY SUPPLEMENTS AND ERECTILE DYSFUNCTION

Yohimbine[1] is an α$_2$-adrenoreceptor antagonist with short duration of action. It is administered orally, and it is believed to have a central effect at adrenergic receptors in brain centers associated with libido and penile erection. A meta-analysis of seven studies established that it is superior to placebo, although results can be very erratic. Side effects include palpitations, tremors, and anxiety. Yohimbine should *not* be recommended as part of the management of ED.

A study with 60 patients who had failed papaverine[1] injections (50 mg or less) were treated with an extract of *Ginkgo biloba*, 60 mg for 12 to 18 months. After 6 months, 50% of the patients reported improvement in erectile function. A placebo-controlled randomized trial using 240 mg of *Ginkgo biloba* extract daily for 24 weeks in patients with vasculogenic ED did not demonstrate significant differences between the groups.

L-Arginine[1] is an amino acid that is the precursor to NO. Three small studies are looking at this drug. There are encouraging results in one study.

Zinc is found in high concentrations in seminal fluid. Anecdotal reports of improvement in ED.

ALPROSTADIL (PROSTAGLANDIN E1, CAVERJECT, MEDICATED URETHRAL SYSTEM FOR ERECTION)

Prostaglandin E1 (PGE$_1$) exerts a number of pharmacologic effects including systemic vasodilatation, inhibitory actions on platelet aggregation, and relaxation of smooth muscle. PGE$_1$ binds to PGE receptors and causes a relaxation response mediated by cyclic adenosine monophosphate (cAMP). It can be administered intracavernosally or intraurethrally.

It has been used in combination with papaverine,[1] and the combination was superior to PGE$_1$ alone. The intracavernosal administration seems to be more effective than transurethral (medicated urethral system for erection [MUSE]). MUSE should be administered in 1-mg doses, applied intraurethrally. Responses to intracavernosal injections (Caverject) as high as 80% may be expected in patients with organic ED with a dose of 20 μg, and much lower to MUSE (35% to 43%). Injections are given with 27- to 30-gauge needles. The administration of PGE$_1$ is usually relegated as an alternative in patients who have contraindications to the use of phosphodiesterase 5 (PDE5) inhibitors. The possible side effects include penile fibrosis, priapism, urethral bleeding, hypotension, or syncopal episodes.

Papaverine[1] is a nonspecific phosphodiesterase inhibitor that increases cAMP and cGMP levels in penile erectile tissue. It produces smooth muscle relaxation and vasodilatation. It decreases the resistance to arterial inflow and increases the resistance to venous outflow. It is highly effective in psychogenic and neurogenic ED but not vasculogenic. It has been commonly used in combination with phentolamine (Regitine). Major side effects include priapism, corporeal fibrosis, and possible elevation of liver transaminases.

Moxisylyte chlorohydrate[2] is an α-blocking agent. In a study where 156 subjects received either alprostadil or moxisylyte in a dose-escalating fashion, alprostadil had much better success rates (46% versus 81%).

Chlorpromazine (Thorazine)[1] is useful when given in combination with alprostadil or papaverine. It has α-blocking properties, and it is cheaper than phentolamine (Regitine).

Decreased concentration of vasoactive intestinal polypeptide (VIP)* has been reported in the penile tissue of men with ED. VIP is believed to play a role in the

---

[1]Not FDA approved for this indication.
[2]Not available in the United States

---

[1]Not FDA approved for this indication.
[2]Not available in the United States
*Investigational drug in the United States.

erectile process. It is ineffective when administered alone but can be quite effective in combination with phentolamine (Regitine). In a small study of 52 subjects with organic ED, 100% of them achieved an erection sufficient for intercourse. Further studies into the effectiveness of VIP may be needed.

PENILE PROSTHESES

This surgical approach used to be quite common before the advent of oral agents. The use of prostheses is still a suitable alternative for those who are unresponsive to less invasive treatments. Prostheses can be classified as rod, one-piece inflatable, two-piece inflatable, and three-piece inflatable. Postsurgical infections and malfunctions are the most common complications. Patients are usually satisfied with the results of prosthetic placement.

Vacuum Constrictive Device

Vacuum constrictive device is a plastic cylinder that is placed over the penis and connected to a pump that creates a partial vacuum. After achieving penile rigidity, a band is placed around the base of the penis to maintain the erection. This is a safe, noninvasive, and effective method of treating ED. It requires an understanding partner and the quality of the erection is not ideal; but patients are usually satisfied.

Testosterone

Patients who have low testosterone levels may benefit substantially from replacement. Men may expect significant improvements in libido, self-esteem, and overall energy levels. Additionally, testosterone is necessary for NO generation in the penile tissue.

The different testosterone preparations include injections such as testosterone enanthate (Delatestryl), cypionate (Depo-Testosterone) given as an intramuscular (IM) injection in doses of 100 to 200 mg, every 2 weeks on average. They also include transdermal testosterone patches (Androderm and Testoderm, 5 mg/d) or transdermal gel (AndroGel 5-g packets, one daily; or Testim 1% testosterone gel, one packet daily). Testosterone gel

---

CURRENT DIAGNOSIS

- The risk factors for ED include tobacco, alcohol, and drug use, as well as DM, hypertension, hyperlipidemia, and prostate disease.
- ED is widely prevalent, and incidence sharply increases with age.
- ED is a cardiovascular sentinel event, and its occurrence warrants a cardiac workup.
- The workup of ED should include checking testosterone levels, prolactin, glucose, and lipid levels.
- First-line therapies include the use of PDE5 inhibitors such as sildenafil citrate (Viagra), vardenafil (Levitra), and tadalafil (Cialis).

Abbreviations: DM = diabetes mellitus; ED = erectile dysfunction; PDE5 = phosphodiesterase 5.

CURRENT THERAPY

- PDE5 Inhibitors
  Sildenafil citrate (Viagra) 25-100 mg
  Vardenafil (Levitra) 10-20 mg
  Tadalafil (Cialis) 10-20 mg
- Alprostadil (PGE₁)
  Intracavernosal injections (Caverject) 20 µg
  Intraurethral application (MUSE) 1-mg pellet
- Papaverine injections[1] 30-60 mg
- Agents not yet approved for use by the FDA:
  Apomorphine (Uprima)[1] 3, 4, 6 mg
  Phentolamine (oral)[1] 40, 60, 80 mg

[1]Not FDA approved for this indication.
Abbreviations: MUSE = medicated urethral system for erection; PDE5 = phosphodiesterase 5; PGE₁ = prostaglandin E1.

---

preparations provide physiologic replacement of testosterone and are preferred more than depot IM injections.

Future Trends

In the next few years we will see a sharp rise in the use of combination drugs, such as PDE5 inhibitors and apomorphine (Uprima),[1] PDE5 inhibitors and phentolamine (Regitine), and combinations of PDE5 inhibitors and intraurethral and intracavernosal agents. ED will be recognized universally as a cardiovascular sentinel event and also as a risk factor for vascular disease in general.

REFERENCES

Archer SL: Potassium channels and erectile dysfunction. Vascul Pharmacol 2002;38:61-71.
Burchardt M, Burchardt T, Baer L, et al: Hypertension is associated with severe erectile dysfunction. J Urol 2000;164(10):1188-1191.
Carson CC, Rajfer J, Eardley I, et al: The efficacy and safety of tadalafil: An update. BJU Int 2004;93:1276-1281.
Crowe SM, Streetman DS: Vardenafil treatment for erectile dysfunction. Ann Pharmacother 2004;38:77-85.
Feldman HA, Goldstein I, Hatzichristou DG, et al: Impotence and its medical and psychosocial correlates: Results of the Massachusetts Male Aging Study. J Urol 1994;151(1):54-61.
Jackson G, Betteridge J, Dean J, et al: A systematic approach to erectile dysfunction in the cardiovascular patient: A consensus statement—Update 2002. Int J Clin Pract 2002;56(9):663-671.
Jaynat D, Shepherd MD: Evaluation and treatment of erectile dysfunction in men with diabetes mellitus. Mayo Clin Proc 2002;77(3):276-282.
Johannes CB, Araujo AB, Feldman HA, et al: Incidence of erectile dysfunction in men ages 40 to 69 years old: Longitudinal results from the Massachusetts Male Aging Study. J Urol 2000;163(2): 460-463.
Kirby M, Jackson G, Betteridge J, et al: Is erectile dysfunction a marker for cardiovascular disease? Int J Clin Pract 2002;55(9): 614-618.
Lue TF: Drug therapy: Erectile dysfunction. N Engl J Med 2000; 342(24):1802-1813.
Michelakis E, Tymchak W, Archer S: Sildenafil: From the bench to the bedside. CMAJ 2000;163(9):1171-1175.
NIH Consensus Development Panel on Impotence: Impotence (NIH Consensus Conference). JAMA 1993;270(1):83-90.
Padma-Nathan H: Intra-urethral and topical agents in the management of erectile dysfunction. In Carson CC III, Kirby RS, Goldstein I (eds): Textbook of Erectile Dysfunction. Oxford, Isis Medical Media, 1999, pp 323-326.

[1]Not FDA approved for this indication.

Rhoden EL, Teloken C, Mafessoni R, et al: Is there any relation between serum levels of testosterone and the severity of erectile dysfunction? Int J Impot Res 2002;14:167-171.

Shokeir AA, Alserafi MA, Mutabagani H: Intracavernosal versus intraurethral alprostadil: A prospective randomized study. BJU Int 1999;83:812-815.

Spahn M, Manning M, Juenemann KP: Intracavernosal therapy. In Carson CC III, Kirby RS, Goldstein I (eds): Textbook of Erectile Dysfunction. Oxford, Isis Medical Media, 1999, pp 345-353.

Sullivan ME, Thompson CS, Dashwood MR, et al: Nitric oxide and penile erection: Is erectile dysfunction another manifestation of vascular disease? Cardiovasc Res 1999;43:658-665.

Acute Renal Failure

Method of
Steven D. Weisbord, MD, MSc,
and Paul M. Palevsky, MD

Definition, Epidemiology, and Outcomes of Acute Renal Failure

Acute renal failure (ARF) is a clinical syndrome broadly defined as an abrupt decline in renal function over a period of hours to days. Its clinical characteristics relate to the retention of nitrogenous and metabolic waste products and of extracellular fluid resulting from a reduction in the glomerular filtration rate (GFR). Although the initial manifestation of ARF may be decreased urine output, urine volume may remain normal or even increase, with the decline in renal function manifested by increases in blood urea nitrogen and serum creatinine concentrations. Despite a clear conceptual understanding of the syndrome, a universally accepted, operational definition of ARF does not exist, leading to the use of a variety of definitions in clinical studies and confounding efforts to characterize its epidemiology. Definitions have been based on absolute or proportional changes in the serum creatinine concentration, as direct measurement of GFR in the clinical setting is technically difficult. Commonly used definitions have included absolute increases in serum creatinine concentration of 0.5 to 1.0 mg/dL and relative increases of 25% to 100% over 1 to several days. Although expert panels have been convened to develop consensus definitions, the lack of sensitive and easily measured biomarkers of early renal damage has limited such efforts.

The reported incidence of ARF is dependent on both the patient population studied and the definition of renal failure used. ARF develops in as many as 7% of hospitalized patients and complicates up to 30% to 50% of admissions to intensive care units. Its incidence among ambulatory patients is substantially lower. Unfortunately, outcomes associated with ARF have changed little over the past several decades. In-hospital mortality rates in excess of 50% continue to be reported in critically ill patients with ARF despite technologic advances in renal replacement therapies and other supportive care. Multiple studies have identified demographic and clinical factors that portend adverse outcomes from ARF. Older age, male gender, and respiratory, liver, and hematologic failure have all been directly correlated with in-hospital mortality, whereas serum creatinine and urea nitrogen concentrations (presumably reflecting nutritional factors) as well as urine output have inverse relationships with in-hospital mortality. Whereas associated comorbidities contribute to the high mortality associated with ARF, multiple studies have demonstrated that the development of ARF, in and of itself, is a strong predictor of mortality independent of concomitant comorbid conditions. The impact of a change in renal function on hospital outcomes is underscored by a recent study that found that even very small elevations in serum creatinine concentration (0.1–0.2 mg/dL) following cardiac or thoracic aortic surgery were associated with increased 30-day postoperative mortality.

Classification of Acute Renal Failure

ARF can be broadly classified into prerenal, postrenal, and intrinsic renal etiologies (Table 1). Prerenal ARF is the most common cause of acute renal dysfunction, resulting from hemodynamically mediated reductions in renal blood flow. The hallmarks of prerenal azotemia are the absence of demonstrable pathologic damage to the renal parenchyma and the prompt restoration of renal function following correction of the hemodynamic abnormality.

The second broad category of ARF is postrenal, which is characterized by obstruction of the urinary collecting system. ARF may develop with obstruction of either the lower urinary tract (bladder or urethra) or the upper urinary tract (ureters and kidneys). Upper tract obstruction must, however, be bilateral or affect a solitary functioning kidney in order to cause ARF.

Intrinsic ARF involves renal parenchymal injury. The most common form of intrinsic ARF is acute tubular necrosis (ATN), which develops as the result of nephrotoxic, ischemic, or septic injury to the kidney. With ATN there is renal tubular epithelial cell injury, apoptosis and necrosis of the tubular epithelium, denuding of the epithelial basement membrane, and obstruction of tubular lumens by sloughed epithelial cells and debris. Glomerular histology is preserved, and the decline in renal function is mediated by a combination of intrarenal vasoconstriction, back-leak of glomerular ultrafiltrate across the denuded epithelium, and tubular obstruction. Acute interstitial nephritis, acute glomerulonephritis, rapidly progressive GN, and macrovascular- and microvascular-mediated injury are less common forms of intrinsic ARF.

ARF can also be categorized based on urine volume as nonoliguric, oliguric, or anuric. Oliguria is defined as daily urine output less than 400 mL and anuria as daily urine output less than 50 mL, the latter most commonly encountered in the setting of bilateral urinary tract obstruction or severe ATN associated with shock. In general, nonoliguric ARF is associated with a better prognosis than is oliguric or anuric disease, reflecting lesser degrees of renal injury.

TABLE 1 Classification of Etiologies of Acute Renal Failure

Prerenal Acute Renal Failure
- Decreased Absolute Blood Volume
  - Blood loss: Hemorrhage
  - Cutaneous losses: Burns, sweating
  - Gastrointestinal losses: Diarrhea, vomiting, drainage from intestinal, pancreatic or biliary fistulas
  - Renal losses: Diuretics, osmotic diuresis
- Decreased Effective Blood Volume
  - Heart failure
  - Cirrhosis
  - Nephrotic syndrome
- Intrarenal Hemodynamic Effect
  - Nonsteroidal anti-inflammatory drugs

Postrenal Acute Renal Failure
- Upper Tract Obstruction: Bilateral obstruction or unilateral obstruction with single functioning kidney
  - Intrinsic: Nephrolithiasis, papillary necrosis, blood clot, transitional cell carcinoma
  - Extrinsic: Retroperitoneal or pelvic malignancy, retroperitoneal adenopathy, retroperitoneal fibrosis, endometriosis, abdominal aortic aneurysm
- Lower Tract Obstruction
  - Transitional cell carcinoma of the bladder, prostate cancer, benign prostatic hypertrophy, urethral stricture, neurogenic bladder, bladder stones

Intrinsic Acute Renal Failure
- Acute Tubular Necrosis
  - Ischemic
  - Nephrotoxic
    - Exogenous: Radiocontrast media, aminoglycosides, amphotericin B (Fungizone), cis-platinum (Platinol), acetaminophen (Tylenol)
    - Endogenous: Rhabdomyolysis, hemolysis
  - Sepsis
- Acute Interstitial Nephritis
  - Medications: Penicillins, cephalosporins, sulfonamides, rifampin (Rifadin), phenytoin (Dilantin), furosemide (Lasix), nonsteroidal anti-inflammatory drugs
  - Infections: Bacterial, viral, rickettsial, mycobacterial
  - Autoimmune disorders: Systemic lupus erythematosus, Sjögren's syndrome, sarcoidosis
- Acute Glomerulonephritis
  - Poststreptococcal glomerulonephritis
  - Postinfectious glomerulonephritis
  - Endocarditis-associated glomerulonephritis
  - Vasculitis/autoimmune disease
  - Thrombotic microangiopathy (hemolytic uremic syndrome, thrombotic thrombocytopenic purpura)
  - Rapidly progressive glomerulonephritis
- Acute Vascular Syndromes
  - Large-vessel disease: Bilateral renal artery thromboembolism or dissection, bilateral renal vein thrombosis
  - Small-vessel disease: Atheroembolic disease
- Intratubular Obstruction
  - Crystals: Calcium oxalate, uric acid, acyclovir (Zovirax), indinavir (Crixivan)
  - Protein: Light-chain nephropathy

Diagnostic Features of Specific Syndromes of Acute Renal Failure

PRERENAL ACUTE RENAL FAILURE

Prerenal ARF results when hemodynamic factors lead to renal hypoperfusion. Prerenal ARF may occur in the setting of true hypovolemia, as may result from diarrhea, vomiting, decreased oral intake, and overly aggressive use of diuretics, or it may occur in relation to clinical conditions associated with decreased effective circulating volume, such as congestive heart failure and chronic liver disease. Clinical findings of volume depletion may include absolute or relative hypotension, orthostatic changes in pulse and/or blood pressure, decreased jugular venous pressure, dry mucous membranes, and tenting of the skin. However, many of these physical findings are nonspecific, especially in the elderly and in chronically ill patients. The utility of these physical findings may be diminished in patients with cardiac or liver disease, in whom effective circulating volume may be decreased despite extracellular volume overload with edema.

Assessment of urine chemistry may be helpful in the diagnosis of prerenal azotemia. The urine sodium concentration is usually low (<20 mEq/L), with a fractional excretion of sodium [FE_{Na} (excreted sodium divided by filtered sodium) calculated as $(U_{Na}/P_{Na}) \div (U_{Cr}/P_{Cr})$, where U_{Na} and P_{Na} are the urine and plasma concentrations of sodium, respectively, and U_{Cr} and P_{Cr} are the urine and plasma concentrations of creatinine, respectively] of less than 1% as the result of avid tubular reabsorption of filtered sodium. However, in patients taking diuretics or having underlying chronic kidney disease with impaired sodium conservation, the urinary sodium and fractional excretion of sodium may be elevated. In such cases, a low fractional excretion of urea (<35%) supports the diagnosis of prerenal ARF. Other possible urinary findings are evidence of urinary concentration (urine osmolality >300 or specific gravity >1.015) and a bland urine sediment without casts. In prerenal states, the ratio of blood urea nitrogen to serum creatinine may be increased to greater than 20:1 as a result of increased tubular reabsorption of urea. Table 2 provides a summary of diagnostic findings associated with various etiologies of ARF.

Nonsteroidal anti-inflammatory drugs (NSAIDs) are commonly used medications that can precipitate or exacerbate prerenal ARF. In settings of decreased absolute or effective circulatory volume, local synthesis of vasodilatory prostaglandins opposes the vasoconstrictive effects of angiotensin II on the afferent (preglomerular) arteriole in order to maintain GFR. In settings in which the renin-angiotensin axis is activated, inhibition of prostaglandin synthesis by the kidney results in unopposed vasoconstriction, markedly diminishing GFR. NSAID use, particularly in the setting of chronic kidney disease, older age, concomitant use of angiotensin-converting enzyme inhibitors, use of angiotensin receptor blockers or diuretics, and clinical conditions associated with decreased effective circulating volume (e.g., heart failure and advanced liver failure), is associated with a markedly increased risk of prerenal ARF and an increased risk of developing ATN.

TABLE 2 Diagnostic Findings in Acute Renal Failure

	BUN/Cr Ratio	U$_{Na}$ (mEq/L)	FE$_{Na}$	Urinalysis	Other Findings
Prerenal Acute Renal Failure	>20:1	<20	<1%	Normal or hyaline casts Specific gravity >1.015	FE$_{Urea}$ <35%
Intrinsic Acute Renal Failure					
Acute tubular necrosis	10:1	>40	>2%*	Muddy-brown casts, tubular epithelial cells Specific gravity ~1.010	FE$_{Urea}$ >50%
Acute interstitial nephritis		>20	>1%	Hematuria, WBCs, WBC casts, eosinophils	Eosinophilia
Acute glomerulo-nephritis		<20	<1%	Dysmorphic RBCs, RBC casts	—
Intratubular obstruction		Variable	Variable	Crystalluria or Bence-Jones proteinuria[†]	Monoclonal paraprotein on electrophoresis
Acute vascular syndromes		>20	Variable	Hematuria	Elevated lactate dehydrogenase with renal infarction
Postrenal Acute Renal Failure	>20:1	>20	Variable	Variable	Fluctuating urine output

*Fractional excretion of sodium (FE$_{Na}$) can be low in cases of radiocontrast nephropathy and pigment nephropathy.
[†]Calcium oxalate crystals with ethylene glycol intoxication; uric acid crystals with uric acid nephropathy; Bence-Jones proteins, associated with multiple myeloma, can be detected using the sulfosalicylic acid test of urine.
Abbreviations: BUN = blood urea nitrogen; Cr = creatinine; FE$_{Urea}$ = fractional excretion of urea; U$_{Na}$ = urine concentration of sodium; RBC = red blood cell; WBC = white blood cell.

POSTRENAL ACUTE RENAL FAILURE

The second broad category of ARF is postrenal or obstructive disease, which is characterized by obstruction of the urinary collecting system. ARF develops only when obstruction affects both kidneys or with unilateral upper urinary tract obstruction in the setting of a solitary functioning kidney. The disorders that cause postrenal ARF are usually categorized by the level of urinary tract obstruction. Obstruction to the lower urinary tract (bladder outlet and urethra) commonly results from benign or malignant prostate disease, bladder cancer, or urethral stricture. Obstruction to the upper urinary tract commonly stems from pelvic and retroperitoneal malignancy, retroperitoneal lymphadenopathy, transitional cell carcinoma of the renal pelvis and ureters, bilateral kidney stones, or retroperitoneal fibrosis.

The clinical findings depend on the degree and level of obstruction to urinary flow. Anuria can be seen with complete obstruction, whereas normal urine volume, polyuria, or fluctuating urine output may occur with partial obstruction. Gender-related anatomic differences, notably a longer urethra and periurethral prostatic tissue, make postrenal ARF more common in men. Careful abdominal examination may reveal a tender, distended bladder, suggesting the presence of bladder outlet obstruction. The gold standard diagnostic test is the renal ultrasound, which demonstrates dilation of the renal collecting system (hydronephrosis and/or hydroureter). However, in up to 20% of cases, particularly early in the clinical course or in cases associated with intravascular volume contraction or retroperitoneal fibrosis, ultrasound may fail to demonstrate hydronephrosis despite the underlying presence of obstructive ARF. Documentation of a postvoid bladder urine volume of at least 100 mL by bedside ultrasound or catheterization suggests lower urinary tract obstruction. Outcomes with postrenal ARF depend greatly on the duration and degree of obstruction. With complete obstruction, the likelihood of recovery of renal function decreases after approximately 1 week. Recovery from partial obstruction is more difficult to predict and depends on the severity and duration of obstruction along with other complicating factors.

INTRINSIC RENAL DISEASE

Acute Tubular Necrosis

Most cases of ATN can be linked to renal ischemia, use of nephrotoxic agents, or sepsis. Unlike prerenal azotemia, ATN is characterized by tubular epithelial cell injury leading to impaired reabsorption of sodium with a urine sodium concentration greater than 40 mEq/L and a fractional excretion of sodium greater than 2%. Urine in patients with ATN is typically isosthenuric (isotonic with plasma), with a specific gravity of approximately 1.010. The urine sediment typically demonstrates "muddy brown" coarse granular casts on microscopic analysis. The blood urea nitrogen concentration usually rises in proportion to the serum creatinine concentration, leading to maintenance of the normal ratio of approximately 10:1.

Radiocontrast-Associated Acute Tubular Necrosis

The administration of intravascular radiocontrast media results in one of the most common forms of ATN, accounting for approximately 10% of hospital-acquired ARF. The administration of intravascular radiocontrast often results in a transient and clinically insignificant (0.1–0.2 mg/dL) rise in the serum creatinine concentration. Radiocontrast nephropathy (RCN) develops when more pronounced reductions in kidney function follow radiocontrast administration. The pathogenesis of RCN is multifactorial and is mediated by both renal vasoconstriction, particularly affecting the renal medulla, and direct epithelial cell toxicity. Clinically, RCN manifests as an abrupt decline in kidney function 24 to 72 hours after radiocontrast administration. The serum creatinine concentration typically peaks within 3 to 5 days and returns to baseline by 7 to 10 days. Several clinical factors increase the risk for RCN, including preexisting chronic kidney disease, diabetes mellitus with or without diabetic nephropathy, congestive heart failure, volume depletion, and increasing dose of radiocontrast media. In contradistinction to other forms of ATN, the fractional excretion of sodium may be low in RCN.

Aminoglycoside-Associated Acute Tubular Necrosis

Aminoglycoside antibiotics are associated with nephrotoxicity in 10% to 15% of patients. Aminoglycosides are actively taken up and accumulate in proximal tubular cells, leading to toxicity as intracellular concentrations rise. ARF usually develops 7 to 10 days after the initiation of therapy. Because aminoglycosides are renally excreted, dosing of these agents is central to their nephrotoxicity. Aminoglycoside-induced ATN is typically nonoliguric, and near-complete or full recovery of renal function is common, although the course of ARF may be protracted.

Myoglobinuric Acute Tubular Necrosis

Rhabdomyolysis develops from injury to skeletal muscle and results in the release of cellular constituents, such as creatine phosphokinase and myoglobin, into the systemic circulation. When myoglobin is filtered in large quantities by the kidney, tubular damage and ATN can ensue. Although the classic description of rhabdomyolysis involves severe trauma with crush injuries, an increasing number of cases are linked to nontraumatic etiologies, including use of medications, such as statins, and use of illicit drugs, primarily cocaine. Typical symptoms include muscle soreness and weakness. A dramatically elevated creatine phosphokinase level is the sine qua non of this condition. Commonly, hyperphosphatemia, hyperuricemia, and hyperkalemia complicate rhabdomyolysis due to release of the respective components from damaged muscle. Additionally, hypocalcemia may occur, resulting primarily from calcium deposition in the injured muscle. Subsequent release of deposited calcium during the recovery phase may result in hypercalcemia. Urine findings include heme-pigmented casts and a positive dipstick for heme pigment in the absence of red blood cells on microscopic examination.

Postoperative Acute Renal Failure

ARF is a relatively common complication following vascular, cardiac, and major abdominal surgical procedures and is associated with particularly high mortality rates. Its development can usually be linked to perioperative episodes of hypotension and/or sepsis. Depending on the definition of ARF and the risk profile of the patient population, ARF develops in 1% to 40% of patients undergoing cardiac surgery, with 1% to 7% of these patients requiring dialysis. Specific clinical factors that increase the risk for ARF following cardiac surgery include cardiogenic shock, decreased baseline renal function, emergent surgery, left ventricular dysfunction, age greater than 70 years, peripheral vascular disease, and left main coronary artery disease. Additionally, valve surgery, particularly of the aortic valve, is associated with greater risk than is coronary artery bypass surgery, with the greatest risk in patients undergoing combined procedures.

Acute Interstitial Nephritis

Acute interstitial nephritis (AIN) results from inflammatory damage to the renal interstitium. Antibiotics and NSAIDs are the most common etiologic agents, although the list of drugs that can precipitate AIN is extensive. Less commonly, infections and autoimmune diseases lead to AIN. Eosinophilia, fever, and rash classically accompany AIN, although the presence of this complete triad is seen in only approximately one third of patients. Examination of the urine reveals hematuria and sterile pyuria with or without white blood cell casts. Although eosinophiluria is associated with AIN, the sensitivity and positive predictive value of this finding are poor. In contrast, the negative predictive value of this finding is high, making the absence of eosinophiluria a useful test for ruling out AIN. The clinical features of AIN typically develop several days to weeks after exposure to the offending agent, and recovery is common following discontinuation of the agent.

Acute Glomerulonephritis

Acute GN and rapidly progressive GN are uncommon causes of ARF that can result from myriad conditions and are characterized by primary injury to the glomerulus. The hallmark findings of GN-associated ARF are dysmorphic red blood cells and red blood cell casts on microscopic examination of the urine sediment. The prototypic form of acute GN is poststreptococcal GN; however, acute GN may also develop in the setting of endocarditis and other infections, systemic vasculitis, and autoimmune disease, or it may present as an idiopathic renal-limited disease. Serologic assays for complement levels (C3 and C4), hepatitis markers, antistreptococcal antibodies (ASO), antinuclear antibodies (ANA), antiglomerular basement membrane antibodies (anti-GBM), and antineutrophil cytoplasmic antibodies (ANCA) may be helpful in making a diagnosis; however, renal biopsy is commonly required to determine the specific etiology.

Intratubular Obstruction

Intratubular obstruction to the flow of urinary filtrate can occur in certain clinical settings and result in an acute decline in renal function. The obstruction may result from precipitation of either crystals or protein within the tubular lumen. Ethylene glycol ingestion is associated with intratubular precipitation of calcium oxalate crystals. This diagnosis should be suspected when ARF develops in the setting of acute intoxication and high anion-gap metabolic acidosis and is usually accompanied by a preponderance of calcium oxalate crystals on examination of the urine sediment. *Tumor lysis syndrome* is a term applied to a constellation of metabolic and clinical findings that may occur after treatment of rapidly proliferative neoplastic disorders, usually of hematologic origin. Marked hyperuricemia leads to intratubular precipitation of uric acid crystals in the distal nephron. Other associated findings include hyperphosphatemia, hyperkalemia, and hypocalcemia. This form of ARF is typically oliguric or anuric. The urine sediment usually demonstrates abundant uric acid crystals or amorphous urates in the setting of an acidic urine. Characteristically, the ratio of urine uric acid to creatinine is greater than 1 in acute uric acid nephropathy, compared to values of less than 0.6 to 0.75 in ARF of other etiologies. Intratubular precipitation of acyclovir and indinavir is the major mechanism of ARF with use of these drugs. Tubular obstruction is also one of the well-recognized complications of multiple myeloma. Monoclonal immunoglobulins and/or light chains precipitate in distal tubules, leading to intratubular obstruction and ARF.

Acute Vascular Syndromes

Acute vascular syndromes that cause ARF can be broadly divided into large-vessel disease and small-vessel disease. Although uncommon, etiologies for large-vessel disease include bilateral thromboembolism, renal vein thrombosis, and large vessel vasculitis leading to renal infarction. More common is small-vessel disease resulting from atheroemboli that involve the distal renal vasculature. Cholesterol crystals released from atheromatous plaques deposit in small arteries and arterioles. Although nonobstructive, these emboli induce an inflammatory reaction that ultimately leads to fibrosis and obliteration of vessels. Acute and/or subacute renal failure are common sequelae. Along with renal involvement, cutaneous manifestations such as livedo reticularis, abdominal pain from intestinal ischemia and pancreatitis, myositis, and neurologic involvement from emboli to the central nervous system and spinal cord can complicate the clinical picture. Renal atheroemboli should be suspected in any case of ARF that occurs subsequent to instrumentation of the vasculature. Laboratory clues to the diagnosis include eosinophilia, eosinophiluria, and hypocomplementemia, although these findings are not universally present.

Prevention and Treatment of Acute Renal Failure

PRERENAL ACUTE RENAL FAILURE

Treatment of prerenal azotemia is directed at augmenting renal perfusion. With true hypovolemia, administration of intravascular isotonic fluid is the primary therapy. Treatment directed at the cause of volume loss, such as diarrhea or vomiting, should also be implemented. In cases of overdiuresis, diuretics should be discontinued and judicious intravascular volume expansion provided. With severely decompensated heart failure, renal perfusion can be optimized using intravenous inotropic agents, although this is usually only a temporizing measure. Cautious intravascular volume expansion can be beneficial in prerenal azotemia in advanced liver disease; however, this must be balanced against the risk of total body volume overload. No data support the routine use of intravenous albumin for expansion of the intravascular space in the majority of patients with advanced liver disease. However, use of intravenous albumin has proved beneficial in preventing renal dysfunction in the treatment of spontaneous bacterial peritonitis and in patients undergoing large volume paracentesis. Prevention of NSAID-related prerenal azotemia hinges on avoiding these agents in patients with chronic kidney disease or other factors that predispose to renal underperfusion. To prevent the evolution of NSAID-associated prerenal ARF into ischemic ATN, prompt discontinuation of the offending NSAID, along with other potentially nephrotoxic agents, is essential.

POSTRENAL ACUTE RENAL FAILURE

Treatment of postrenal ARF hinges on the prompt relief of obstruction. Placement of a bladder catheter provides relief of functional or anatomic bladder outlet obstruction. Upper tract obstruction requires the placement of ureteral stents or percutaneous nephrostomy tubes.

INTRINSIC ACUTE RENAL FAILURE

Acute Tubular Necrosis

General Therapeutic Considerations

In the majority of patients, the development of ARF is unpredictable. For this reason, with the exception of specific clinical settings discussed later, preventive measures are limited to broad recommendations for avoidance of nephrotoxic agents when possible, for cautious dosing of such agents when they must be used, particularly in the elderly and in patients with underlying chronic renal insufficiency, and for avoidance of hypovolemia and hypotension. Similarly, the pharmacologic management of established ATN is ineffective. Although multiple agents, including diuretics, renal vasodilators, natriuretic peptides, and growth factors, have shown promise in animal models and preliminary clinical trials, none has proved to be clinically effective when rigorously evaluated.

The role of loop diuretics in the management of ATN has been controversial. It was hypothesized that decreased oxygen demand resulting from inhibition of sodium transport might reduce the extent of renal injury; however, this benefit has not been substantiated in clinical trials. In addition, diuretics have been used to convert oliguric to nonoliguric ARF in the hope that this will improve prognosis. Although the increased urine volume simplifies fluid management, there is no evidence that the conversion to a nonoliguric state actually impacts outcomes. Rather, the response to diuretics merely identifies patients with less severe renal injury. A recent observational study suggested that diuretic use was associated with an increased risk of death and with nonrecovery of renal function, although these findings were not confirmed in a subsequent trial. Nevertheless, these findings highlight the concern that diuretic therapy may result in delays in initiation of renal replacement therapy. Therefore, we believe that a trial of high-dose furosemide (Lasix; 160–200 mg intravenously) or an equivalent dose of other loop diuretics is reasonable in oliguric patients who are not intravascularly volume depleted, but that diuretic therapy should not be used to delay the initiation of otherwise indicated renal replacement therapy. Repeated dosing of diuretics is not warranted in patients who do not respond.

Dopamine (Intropin) increases renal plasma flow, GFR, and sodium excretion when administered at doses of 0.5 to 2 µg/kg/min. Although such "renal-dose" dopamine has been widely used in the management of ARF, clinical trials have not established any benefit with regard to survival or need for renal replacement therapy with this agent. Given the risk of complications, especially cardiac tachyarrhythmias, there is no role for low-dose dopamine in the management of ARF. Similarly, there is no established role for fenoldopam mesylate[1] (Corlopam), a selective dopamine-1 receptor agonist, in the management of ARF.

Renal Replacement Therapy

In the absence of effective pharmacologic therapy, renal replacement therapy remains the primary treatment of severe ARF, providing an effective means for managing hyperkalemia, metabolic acidosis, volume overload, and uremic manifestations. Multiple forms of renal replacement therapy, including intermittent hemodialysis, continuous renal replacement therapy, newer hybrid forms of slow hemodialysis such as sustained low-efficiency dialysis, and peritoneal dialysis, can be used in patients with ARF. Only limited data are available to guide selection of modality of renal replacement therapy. Specifically, no data support improved outcomes associated with continuous renal replacement therapy compared to intermittent hemodialysis, although continuous renal replacement therapy and sustained low-efficiency dialysis both are associated with less hemodynamic instability and more effective volume removal than is intermittent hemodialysis. Therefore, selection of modality should be based on local capabilities and expertise.

Generally accepted indications for initiation of renal replacement therapy in patients with ARF include volume overload, hyperkalemia, metabolic acidosis, and overt uremic manifestations such as encephalopathy and pericarditis. An optimal threshold for initiation of therapy based on level of azotemia is not established, although preemptive initiation of therapy prior to the development of uremic symptoms is well recognized to be associated with improved outcomes. Therefore, it is generally accepted that, in the absence of other indications, renal replacement therapy should be initiated when the blood urea nitrogen concentration reaches approximately 90 to 100 mg/dL, although some data suggest that earlier initiation of therapy may be associated with improved outcomes.

Despite substantial technologic advancements in the dialysis apparatus, the optimal dose of renal replacement therapy in ARF remains uncertain. Although daily intermittent hemodialysis was associated with improved survival compared to alternate-day dialysis in a prospective study, several methodologic issues related primarily to the relatively low dose of dialysis provided with each treatment raise questions regarding the applicability of the results of this study to general practice. Similarly, although a single-center randomized controlled trial demonstrated improved survival with increased intensity of therapy, these results have not been confirmed in subsequent published studies. It is hoped that ongoing clinical trials will resolve this issue in the near future.

Therapeutic Considerations for Specific Etiologies of Acute Tubular Necrosis

RADIOCONTRAST NEPHROPATHY. Most radiographic procedures that utilize intravascular radiocontrast are planned in advance, making RCN one of the forms of ARF most amenable to preventive measures. Three strategies have been conclusively shown to decrease the risk for RCN in high-risk patients. First is intravascular volume expansion with intravenous fluids. Volume expansion with isotonic saline (1 mL/kg/hr for 12 hours before and 12 hours after the administration of radiocontrast) is more effective than the same volume of hypotonic saline. Recently, a single-center study found that administration of isotonic sodium bicarbonate at 3 mL/kg/hr starting 1 hour before the procedure followed by 1 ml/kg/hr for 6 hours after the administration of radiocontrast was superior to similar doses of isotonic saline. Whether this regimen is superior to the more prolonged administration of isotonic saline is not established. Second, low-osmolar radiocontrast agents are associated with less nephrotoxicity than are older high-osmolar agents. In a small study of high-risk diabetic patients with chronic kidney disease, iodixanol (Visipaque), an iso-osmolar agent, was less nephrotoxic than iohexol (Omnipaque), a low-osmolar agent. Whether this benefit is seen in other high-risk populations is not established. Third, minimizing the dose of radiocontrast decreases renal damage.

Along with these measures, the administration of N-acetylcysteine[1] (Mucomyst), an antioxidant agent, may be associated with protection from RCN. Although clinical trials have yielded conflicting results and meta-analyses have failed to conclusively demonstrate a beneficial effect, this agent is inexpensive and free of deleterious side effects. Therefore, use of N-acetylcysteine (600-1200 mg orally twice daily on the day before and on the day of the procedure) is not inappropriate, albeit not in lieu of proven preventive strategies. Similarly, with the well-recognized relationship between intravascular volume depletion/renal underperfusion and risk for RCN, discontinuation of diuretics and NSAIDs prior to radiocontrast administration is advisable. Mannitol,[1] dopamine[1] (Intropin), fenoldopam[1] (Corlopam), calcium channel blockers, and human β-type natriuretic peptide[1] (Natrecor) are not effective and have no role in the prophylaxis of RCN. Likewise, prophylactic intermittent or continuous hemodialysis has no role in the prevention of RCN. An algorithm for the prevention of RCN is shown in Figure 1.

AMINOGLYCOSIDE-ASSOCIATED ACUTE TUBULAR NECROSIS. Based on the observation that proximal tubule uptake of aminoglycosides is saturable, use of once-daily dosing of these

---

[1]Not FDA approved for this indication.

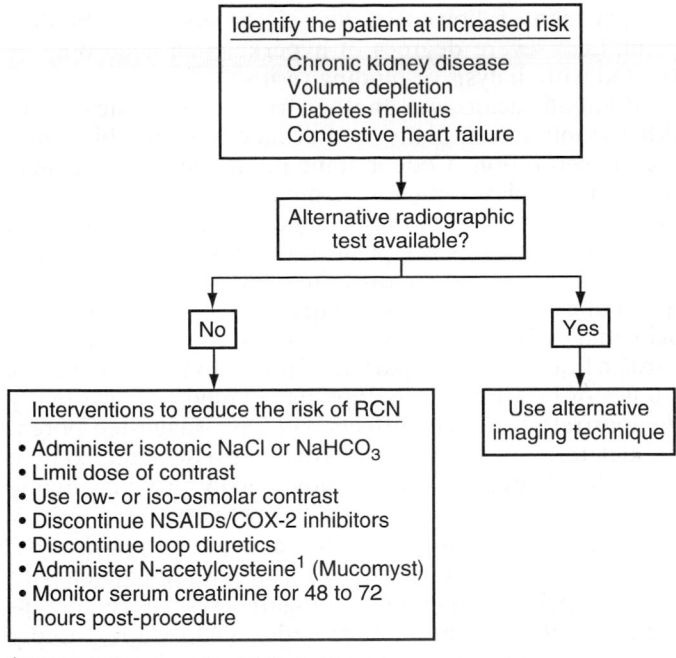

FIGURE 1. Management algorithm for the prevention of radiocontrast nephropathy (RCN). [1]Not FDA approved for this indication. *Abbreviations:* COX-2 = cyclooxygenase-2; NaCl = sodium chloride; NaHCO$_2$ = sodium bicarbonate; NSAIDs = nonsteroidal anti-inflammatory drugs.

antimicrobial agents may be less nephrotoxic than multiple-daily dosing schemes. Although conclusive data are lacking, a series of studies and meta-analyses support the use of once-daily dosing. Therefore, it is not unreasonable to consider once-daily dosing in clinically appropriate circumstances to reduce the risk of ARF. Additional preventive strategies that should be implemented include monitoring of drug levels, discontinuing concomitant nephrotoxic agents, limiting the duration and total dose of therapy, and switching to non-nephrotoxic agents guided by antibiotic sensitivities.

MYOGLOBINURIC ACUTE RENAL FAILURE. Rhabdomyolysis is associated with sequestration of large volumes of fluid in the injured muscle. Because the risk of ARF in rhabdomyolysis is associated with intravascular volume depletion, patients with rhabdomyolysis should be aggressively administered large volumes of isotonic electrolyte solutions to maintain intravascular volume. In patients with crush injuries, the use of aggressive fluid resuscitation with administration of normal saline at 1 L/hr has been shown to minimize the risk of ARF. Optimally, this strategy should be initiated in the field, prior to extraction of the patient. Although use of mannitol as an osmotic diuretic and urinary alkalinization with bicarbonate have been recommended, data supporting the superiority of these agents over isotonic saline alone are inconclusive. Hypocalcemia should not be treated unless the patient is symptomatic because calcium administration increases the risk of hypercalcemia during the recovery phase of rhabdomyolysis.

POSTOPERATIVE ACUTE RENAL FAILURE. No specific therapies have been demonstrated to be effective for the prevention or treatment of postoperative ATN.

Acute Interstitial Nephritis

The primary treatment of AIN is discontinuation of the offending agent. In most patients, renal function recovers, although this can take several weeks. Use of glucocorticoids for treatment of AIN remains controversial. Although case series have suggested a potential benefit of glucocorticoids, their use has not been evaluated in prospective randomized trials. Nonetheless, a trial of glucocorticoids is a reasonable therapeutic option in patients with biopsy-proven AIN in whom renal function fails to improve after discontinuation of the offending drug.

ACUTE GLOMERULONEPHRITIS

Therapy for acute GN is dependent upon the specific diagnosis. The treatment of poststreptococcal GN is supportive. In patients with endocarditis-associated GN and other forms of infection-associated GN, treatment is directed at the underlying infection. Plasma exchange should be initiated in patients with hemolytic uremic syndrome and thrombotic thrombocytopenic purpura. High-dose glucocorticoids and cytotoxic or immunosuppressive therapy are usually required in patients with vasculitis-associated GN and rapidly progressive GN. In patients with anti-GBM disease, plasmapheresis is often required in addition to high-dose glucocorticoids and cytotoxic therapy.

INTRATUBULAR OBSTRUCTION

Oxalate Nephropathy

Fomepizole (Antizol), a competitive inhibitor of alcohol dehydrogenase, and intravenous ethanol[1] are the primary therapies for ethylene glycol intoxication. By inhibiting formation of oxalate, these therapies can prevent the development or arrest the progression of acute oxalate nephropathy. Maintenance of high urinary flow rates with intravenous fluids may help minimize calcium oxalate precipitation. Mannitol can be used as an osmotic diuretic to maintain urine flow rates. Intravenous sodium bicarbonate may be necessary to treat the metabolic acidosis that commonly complicates this form of ARF. Dialysis may be beneficial for rapidly lowering plasma ethylene glycol levels and acutely decreasing the concentrations of plasma oxalate and other metabolites.

Acute Uric Acid Nephropathy

Tumor lysis syndrome and acute uric acid nephropathy characteristically develop after the initiation of chemotherapy, allowing initiation of treatment to prevent this form of ARF. Volume expansion with intravenous saline to maintain high urine flow rates minimizes the intratubular precipitation of uric acid crystals and is the mainstay of therapy. The role of urinary alkalinization with intravenous sodium bicarbonate is less certain. Although the solubility of uric acid is increased in alkaline urine, the benefit of alkalinization compared to saline alone has not been demonstrated, and it may promote the deposition of calcium phosphate in patients with concomitant hyperphosphatemia. Allopurinol (Zyloprim; 600–900 mg/day) should be initiated in advance of chemotherapy to inhibit xanthine oxidase and block the

---

[1]Not FDA approved for this indication.

generation of uric acid. In patients unable to take oral medications, an intravenous form of allopurinol ($200–400$ mg/m^2/day) is available. Alternatively, rasburicase (Elitek; $0.15–0.2$ mg/kg/day), a recombinant form of uricase, rapidly metabolizes uric acid to the more soluble allantoin and is approved for use in children. Rasburicase is contraindicated in patients with glucose-6-phosphate dehydrogenase deficiency. In patients who develop ARF, hemodialysis may rapidly lower uric acid concentrations and facilitate recovery of renal function.

Multiple Myeloma

Acute light-chain nephropathy should be treated with aggressive intravascular volume expansion. Concomitant hypercalcemia, which increases the risk of acute nephropathy, should be treated. Chemotherapy should be initiated to decrease the light-chain burden. Plasmapheresis may be of benefit in some patients by rapidly lowering the filtered light-chain burden.

Atheroembolic Disease

No specific therapy for atheroembolic disease exists. Treatment with antiplatelet agents, steroids, and iloprost[1] (Ventavis), a prostacylin analogue, have all been investigated, with no definitive benefit seen. Supportive care, including the withdrawal of anticoagulants, avoidance of additional intravascular manipulation, and therapy to lower serum cholesterol concentrations with statins, may improve outcomes. Overall mortality from renal atheroembolic disease remains greater than 60% to 80% in some series, underscoring the importance of primary prevention.

Complications and Additional Therapeutic Considerations

Electrolyte and Acid-Base Complications

Hyperkalemia is a common complication of ARF, developing as a result of decreased renal excretion, particularly in patients with oliguric ARF. If severe, hyperkalemia can lead to life-threatening arrhythmias. Therapy depends on the degree of elevation of the serum potassium concentration, with severe hyperkalemia requiring urgent therapy. In patients with electrocardiographic changes of hyperkalemia, the initial therapy is intravenous calcium ($10–20$ mL of 10% calcium gluconate or 10 mL of 10% calcium chloride). This should be followed by intravenous insulin ($10–20$ U regular insulin), combined with an infusion of dextrose (250 mL of 20% dextrose in water over 1 hour) to prevent hypoglycemia and inhaled albuterol[1] (Proventil) ($10–20$ mg by nebulizer) to translocate potassium from the extracellular to intracellular compartments. Potassium removal from the body can be achieved by administration of oral or rectal polystyrene sulfonate (Kayexalate) or by initiation of dialysis. In patients with serum potassium concentrations greater than 6 mEq/L but without electrocardiographic changes, intravenous calcium is not required, and treatment should begin with insulin/glucose and/or albuterol to translocate potassium into the intracellular

compartment, followed by dialysis or potassium-binding resin. Less severe degrees of hyperkalemia need only be treated with dialysis or binding resins.

Metabolic acidosis is another frequent complication of ARF, manifested initially by a decline in serum bicarbonate concentration. Concomitant pulmonary disease may result in the development of mixed acid-base disorders; hence, confirmation of the presence of acidemia by blood gas analysis is necessary prior to initiation of therapy. The role of bicarbonate therapy in patients with anion-gap metabolic acidosis remains controversial. Although severe acidemia (pH <7.1) may be associated with decreased cardiac function and impaired response to catecholamines, studies of bicarbonate therapy have failed to consistently demonstrate beneficial effects and have suggested potential deleterious consequences from the associated sodium load. Renal replacement therapy usually provides highly effective correction of metabolic acidosis.

Hyperphosphatemia is common in patients with ARF and, if severe, warrants the use of oral binding agents. In severe hyperphosphatemia (>7 mg/dL), short-term administration of aluminum hydroxide[1] (Alu-Cap) rapidly lowers the serum phosphate concentration. Once the serum phosphate concentration is less than 7 mg/dL, calcium-based binders should be used (calcium acetate [PhosLo] $667–1364$ mg or calcium carbonate[1] [Tums] $0.5–1.0$ g administered with meals). Sevelamer (Renagel), a newer non–calcium-containing polymer that binds intraintestinal phosphate, can be used in patients with hypercalcemia or an elevated calcium-phosphate product. Hemodialysis and renal replacement therapy are highly effective in lowering the plasma phosphate concentration and may lead to hypophosphatemia.

Hypermagnesemia can occur with ARF and is usually due to exogenous magnesium administration in the setting of impaired renal excretory capacity. Extreme caution should be used when administering magnesium to patients with severely decreased GFR. Hemodialysis can be used in severe cases to lower the serum magnesium level.

Hematologic Complications

ARF can result in platelet dysfunction, predisposing to bleeding complications. The uremic platelet defect is manifested by prolongation of the bleeding time in the setting of a normal platelet count, normal prothrombin time (PT), and normal activated partial thromboplastin time (aPTT). This defect is usually corrected, at least in part, by dialysis. If the platelet dysfunction is severe and is complicated by active bleeding, administration of 1-deamino (8-D-arginine) vasopressin (DDAVP[1]; 0.3 µg/kg intravenously) may be of benefit; however, tachyphylaxis usually develops after two to three doses. Intravenous estrogens (conjugated estrogen[1] [Premarin] 0.6 mg/kg) administered daily for 5 days has been shown to correct the platelet defect for up to 14 days. Pooled cryoprecipitate is of benefit but is associated with risk of transmission of viral diseases. Anemia is a common occurrence with ARF; however, the role of recombinant human erythropoietin[1] (Procrit) and other erythropoietic agents in the management of this complication is not well characterized.

---

[1]Not FDA approved for this indication.

[1]Not FDA approved for this indication.

Infectious Complications

Infection is a common comorbidity in patients with ARF. Intravascular and bladder catheters frequently serve as routes of infection. Whenever possible, bladder catheters should be removed and intermittent bladder catheterization used. Temporary dialysis catheters are a frequent source of bacteremia. To reduce the risk of infection, femoral dialysis catheters should be avoided whenever possible and should remain in place for as brief a duration as possible. In patients with prolonged ARF, the use of tunneled dialysis catheters will decrease the risk of infection. In a single small clinical trial, use of antibiotic-impregnated dialysis catheters was associated with a reduced risk of catheter-associated bacteremia. Additional studies confirming these results are needed before this approach can be recommended.

Early recognition and initiation of systemic antimicrobial therapy for blood-borne infections related to central venous catheters are essential, as is the appropriate dosing of antibiotics in the setting of reduced GFR. Removal of central venous catheters in the setting of bacteremia is highly dependent on the clinical status of the patient, the pathogenic organism, and the need for short-term vascular access.

Cardiopulmonary Complications

Cardiac and pulmonary problems are protean in patients with ARF. Arrhythmias, hypertension, pericarditis, and pericardial effusion can be seen with ARF. Pericarditis, which can be life-threatening, should be treated with intensification of renal replacement therapy. Pulmonary vascular congestion or overt pulmonary edema resulting from impaired diuresis and natriuresis may precipitate the need for renal replacement therapy. In patients with acute lung injury or the acute respiratory distress syndrome who are mechanically ventilated using low-tidal volumes as a lung-protective strategy, the dialysis prescription may require adjustment to provide adequate control of the acidemia resulting from hypercapnia.

Nutritional Management

The optimal approach to nutritional therapy in the setting of ARF remains a matter of debate. ARF is usually a catabolic state. Although caloric and protein requirements should be individualized based on the overall clinical condition of the patient, protein intake should not be restricted and generally should range from 1.2 to 1.6 g/kg/day, with a minimum daily caloric intake of 30 kcal/kg. Enteral routes of nutritional supplementation are greatly preferred. Renal replacement therapy can be associated with loss of proteins and amino acids, necessitating adjustments in the nutritional prescription. Among nondialysis patients, close attention should be paid to limit intake of potassium (<60 mEq/day) and phosphate (<1.0 g/day).

REFERENCES

Chertow GM, Levy EM, Hammermeister KE, et al: Independent association between acute renal failure and mortality following cardiac surgery. Am J Med 1998;104:343-348.

Friedrich JO, Adhikari N, Herridge MS, Beyene J: Meta-analysis: Low-dose dopamine increases urine output but does not prevent renal dysfunction or death. Ann Intern Med 2005;142:510-524.

Lassnigg A, Schmidlin D, Mouhieddine M, et al: Minimal changes of serum creatinine predict prognosis in patients after cardiothoracic surgery: A prospective cohort study. J Am Soc Nephrol 2004;15:1597-1605.

Mehta RL, Pascual MT, Soroko S, Chertow GM: Diuretics, mortality, and nonrecovery of renal function in acute renal failure. JAMA 2002;288:2547-2553.

Merten GJ, Burgess WP, Gray LV, et al: Prevention of contrast-induced nephropathy with sodium bicarbonate: A randomized controlled trial. JAMA 2004;291:2328-2334.

Mueller C, Buerkle G, Buettner HJ, et al: Prevention of contrast media-associated nephropathy: Randomized comparison of 2 hydration regimens in 1620 patients undergoing coronary angioplasty. Arch Intern Med 2002;162:329-336.

Nash K, Hafeez A, Hou S: Hospital-acquired renal insufficiency. Am J Kidney Dis 2002;39:930-936.

Pannu N, Manns B, Lee H, Tonelli M: Systematic review of the impact of N-acetylcysteine on contrast nephropathy. Kidney Int 2004;65:1366-1374.

Ronco C, Bellomo R, Homel P, et al: Effects of different doses in continuous veno-venous haemofiltration on outcomes of acute renal failure: A prospective randomised trial. Lancet 2000;356:26-30.

Schiffl H, Lang SM, Fischer R: Daily hemodialysis and the outcome of acute renal failure. N Engl J Med 2002;346:305-310.

Stone GW, McCullough PA, Tumlin JA, et al: Fenoldopam mesylate for the prevention of contrast-induced nephropathy: A randomized controlled trial. JAMA 2003;290:2284-2291.

Tepel M, van der Giet M, Schwarzfeld C, et al: Prevention of radiographic-contrast-agent-induced reductions in renal function by acetylcysteine. N Engl J Med 2000;343:180-184.

Uchino S, Doig GS, Bellomo R, et al: Diuretics and mortality in acute renal failure. Crit Care Med 2004;32:1669-1677.

Chronic Renal Failure

Method of
Jeffrey A. Kraut, MD

Chronic renal failure is defined as a reduction in glomerular filtration rate (GFR) below the normal values of approximately 120 to 130 mL/minute developing over months to years. Its incidence has increased significantly over the last several years, but this probably reflects more accurate estimations of GFR. However, there is an increased prevalence of type II diabetes mellitus, a frequent cause of renal disease, in Western societies that could contribute to a higher incidence of chronic renal failure. When renal failure is severe (GFR <10 mL/minute), renal replacement therapy, either dialysis or renal transplantation, is required to preserve life. However, even before several renal failure ensues, the presence of chronic renal failure has an important impact on organ function and can contribute to the development of significant electrolyte derangements, important hormonal abnormalities, and anemia. Also, its presence can alter the metabolism and therefore the blood concentrations and tissue concentrations of drugs administered for the treatment of various diseases. Moreover, a reduced GFR is associated with an increased risk of death, increased incidence of cardiovascular events, and hospitalizations independent of known risk factors or a history of cardiovascular diseases. Finally, the mortality of several surgical procedures is substantially increased by the presence of chronic renal failure. Therefore, detecting and treating patients with chronic renal failure is extremely important.

Causes of Chronic Renal Failure

Many disorders can cause chronic renal failure. However, epidemiologic studies indicate that diabetes mellitus and hypertension account for the majority of cases (>60%). Chronic glomerulonephritis, polycystic kidney disease, obstructive uropathy, and ischemic nephropathy caused by atherosclerotic renal artery stenosis are less common, but important causes of renal impairment. The latter disorder is postulated to be more frequent than previously believed and is an important undiagnosed cause of chronic renal impairment.

Recent studies have indicated that a reduction in GFR occurs with aging in the absence of factors known to produce renal injury such as hypertension or diabetes. Indeed, the average GFR of subjects in the 8th decade of life in one large study was 40 to 50 mL/minute. Pathologic examination of these individuals, when available, may reveal only benign nephrosclerosis.

Importantly, because a majority of individuals older than 60 years of age have lower muscle mass, the reduced GFR is not accompanied by a rise in serum creatinine concentration. Therefore, renal failure is not detected unless the physician considers other variables such as the patient's age and muscle mass in assessing GFR (see the following section).

Approach to the Diagnosis of Chronic Renal Failure

The first step in the diagnosis of chronic renal failure is, of course, to detect a reduction in GFR. In the past, estimations of GFR were based on the measurement of serum creatinine concentration alone. In adults, the normal serum creatinine ranges between 0.6 and 1.3 mg/dL. Individuals with values greater than this are said to have renal failure. However, there is a wide range of normal values. Also, creatinine production, which is dependent on muscle mass, is a critical variable affecting serum creatinine concentration. Thus, a large group of individuals with reduced muscle mass can have serum creatinine values within the normal range, but a decreased GFR. The most common situation in which this paradox is encountered is in the elderly and in individuals with malignancy or chronic liver disease.

Precise measurement of GFR is accomplished by calculating the clearance of creatinine in a timed urine collection, generally 24 hours in duration:

Creatinine clearance (mL/minute) = Ucr (mg/dL) × volume (mL)/Scr(mg/dL)/1440.

where Ucr = urine creatinine concentration,
Scr = plasma creatinine concentration

However, timed urine collections are often inaccurate because of errors in collection. Moreover, as renal function progresses and serum creatinine rises, or in the presence of nephrotic range proteinuria, GFR tends to be overestimated by creatinine clearance. Most recently, formulas derived from studies of large groups of patients—such as those by Cockroft and Gault and the Modification of Diet in Renal Disease (MDRD) in which GFR was correlated with other factors (e.g., body weight, age, and serum albumin)—are sufficiently accurate to use for clinical purposes:

Cockroft-Gault: CrCl (mL/minute) = {(140 − age) × wt × [1 − (0.15 × gender)]}/(0.814 × Scr)

MDRD: $GFR = 170 \times [PCr]^{-0.999} \times [Age]^{-0.176} \times [0.762\ female] \times [1.180\ if\ patient\ is\ black] \times [SUN]^{-0.170} \times [Alb]^{+0.318}$

Once renal function is depressed, the physician determines whether this represents acute or chronic renal failure, When previous measurements of GFR are available, it is relatively easy to determine if the renal failure is chronic in nature. However, if these studies are not available, demonstration that the kidneys are small in size (less than 8 to 9 cm when they are normally approximately 10 to 12 cm) by renal ultrasound will confirm the chronicity of the disease. Evidence of increased echogenicity reflecting augmented fibrous deposits is also suggestive of chronic disease. However, several disorders associated with chronic renal failure have normal kidney size such as diabetes mellitus, polycystic kidney disease, and amyloidosis. Therefore, normal kidney size does not exclude chronic renal failure. If individuals have normal kidney size, the presence of anemia and/or certain abnormalities of divalent ion metabolism can also suggest the disease is chronic in nature.

Once impaired renal function is recognized, measurements of blood urea nitrogen (BUN), sodium, potassium, chloride, bicarbonate, hemoglobin and hematocrit, and calcium and phosphorus are obtained. A urinalysis is obtained looking for increased excretion of protein, presence of blood in the urine, and abnormal cellular elements. In patients with diabetes, studies to find microalbuminuria (albumin urine concentrations less than 300 mg per day) are important to detect the early stages of renal disease. A 24-hour or spot urine protein and creatinine determination

---

CURRENT DIAGNOSIS

The following lists the optimal care of patients with chronic kidney disease:

- Test for albuminuria and estimate glomerular filtration rate using MDRD formula yearly for early diagnosis and stratification of CKD.
- If possible, determine cause of kidney disease.
- Initiate treatment to delay or prevent progression of disease including use of converting enzyme inhibitors and/or angiotensin receptor blockers to reduce BP to less than 138/80 and urine protein excretion to less than 1 g/24 hours.
- Control or prevent biochemical or clinical abnormalities including those of serum potassium, serum bicarbonate, serum phosphorus, parathyroid hormone, and hemoglobin.
- Evaluate patients for presence of and treat important co-morbid conditions, particularly heart disease.
- If the GFR is less than 30 mL/min, consider referral to a nephrologist.

Abbreviations: BP = blood pressure; CKD = care of patients with chronic kidney disease; GFR = glomerular filtration rate; MDRD = modification of diet in renal disease.

to assess the urine's protein-to-creatinine ratio is obtained to quantitate the amount of protein being excreted. Urine protein excretion in excess of 3.5 g daily indicates the presence of glomerular pathology, whereas interstitial disease is characterized by values below 2 g. However, urine protein excretion can vary with glomerular disease so values below 3.5 g are still consistent with this diagnosis. Assessment of urine protein excretion is important for diagnostic purposes, but also because urine protein excretion is often followed to assess effectiveness of therapy.

Obstruction uropathy, an important cause of chronic renal failure and exacerbation of renal failure, can be excluded in the majority of cases by ultrasound of the kidneys. Doppler ultrasound of the renal arteries performed at the same time is helpful in excluding obstruction of the renal arteries. The necessity of obtaining other diagnostic studies such as measurement of serum complement, blood and urine eosinophils, serum and urine and protein electrophoresis, antiglomerular basement membrane antibodies, anti–double-stranded DNA (dsDNA) antibodies, hepatitis B and C antibodies, sedimentation rate, and HIV studies depends on the context of the renal failure.

Finally, a renal biopsy may be required in certain situations to make a definitive diagnosis. Because treatment of specific diseases can vary, making a precise pathologic diagnosis can be extremely important for proper management. Unfortunately, once the renal failure is moderate to severe in nature, renal pathologic examination may not always be helpful in determining the cause.

Clinical and Laboratory Abnormalities in Chronic Renal Failure

Because the kidney plays a critical role in the regulation of the serum concentrations of sodium, potassium, bicarbonate, chloride, calcium, and phosphorus as well as the levels of hemoglobin and hematocrit, blood pressure and extracellular volume, chronic renal injury can lead to derangements in these parameters as summarized in Table 1.

TABLE 1 Clinical and Electrolyte Abnormalities Noted With Chronic Renal Failure

Clinical or Laboratory Disorder	GFR or Stage of Renal Failure*
Hypertension	GFR <60 mL/min (stage 3)
Hyponatremia or hypernatremia	GFR <30 mL/min (stage 4)
Hyperkalemia*	GFR <30 mL/min (stage 4)
Hyperphosphatemia*	GFR <30 mL/min (stage 4)
Metabolic acidosis	GFR <30 mL/min (stage 4)
Anemia	GFR <60 mL/min (stage 3)
Uremic symptoms Nausea, vomiting, disturbances in sleep	GFR <15 mL/min (stage 5)

*Descriptions of the various stages are presented in the text. These electrolyte abnormalities can be seen at higher levels of GFR.
Abbreviations: GFR = glomerular filtration rate.

HYPONATREMIA AND HYPERNATREMIA

The kidney plays an essential role in excreting water by producing a dilute urine (less than 1/6 plasma osmolality) or retaining water by producing a concentrated urine (three to four times plasma osmolality). The ability to concentrate or dilute the urine in the majority of cases is usually retained until GFR falls to less than 30% of normal, and therefore hyponatremia or hypernatremia are uncommon until that time. If the disease is primarily interstitial in nature, alterations in urine concentrating ability can appear prior to significant reductions in GFR. However, even with higher levels of GFR the patient can be at risk for either of these electrolyte abnormalities should they ingest large quantities of fluid or be deprived of appropriate fluid intake.

HYPERKALEMIA

The kidney plays the most critical role in the regulation of potassium balance. Adaptive changes in renal tubular function and possible colonic function enable the kidney to maintain serum potassium within the normal range until GFR falls below 20% to 25% of normal (serum creatinine of 4 mg/dL or greater). Recent studies indicate a tendency for elevations in serum potassium to appear at even modest reductions in GFR (<60 mL/min). When disease of the kidney involves the medullary portion or hormonal derangements such as hyporeninemic hypoaldosterinism are present, hyperkalemia can be observed prior to significant declines in GFR. In addition, patients with even moderate renal failure have a reduced reserve to eliminated potassium and therefore can develop hyperkalemia if potassium load is increased dramatically.

METABOLIC ACIDOSIS

A fall in plasma bicarbonate concentration in association with a reduced blood pH (metabolic acidosis) is frequently observed when GFR falls below 20% to 25% of normal. The acidosis results from acid excretion falling below acid production leading to positive proton balance. Recent studies have documented that a tendency to the development of metabolic acidosis can be seen with mild reductions in GFR (<60 mL/min).

The electrolyte pattern seen with the metabolic acidosis of renal failure is often of the high anion gap variety, but frequently a hyperchloremic (normal anion gap) or combined anion gap and hyperchloremic pattern can be observed. The degree of acidosis is usually mild to moderate with plasma bicarbonate concentration ranging from 12 to 22 mEq/L. Of interest, at any given level of GFR, the acidosis is often not progressive, but plasma bicarbonate concentration remains stable unless renal function declines further or there is an increment in acid production.

ABNORMAL DIVALENT IN METABOLISM

Serum phosphorus is regulated by the kidney but in most cases remains within the normal range until GFR falls below 20% to 25% of normal. This stabilization of serum phosphorus is attributed to increased tubular excretion of phosphorus as a result of increased parathyroid hormone secretion. As with potassium and bicarbonate, recent studies demonstrate a tendency for elevation in serum phosphorus can be observed with mild renal failure (<50 to 60 mL/min). Serum calcium is usually in the normal range, but varies receiprocally with serum phosphorus. Because of derangements in divalent ion metabolism bone disease with increased tendency to fractures and disordered soft tissue structures can be observed.

Hyperparathyoridism is a common occurrence in patients with renal failure, the values usually being higher with a greater degree of renal impairment. The elevated PTH values are usually induced by hypocalcemia, although increased serum phosphorus concentrations independent of serum calcium values can also play a role. The increased parathyroid hormone levels can induce damage to bone and soft tissue structures, but also may affect other functions such as cardiac function and the production of red blood cells.

ANEMIA

The kidney is the source of erythropoietin, the hormone that regulates bone marrow production of red blood cells. Thus, with the development of renal impairment, there is a fall in red blood cell production. A fall in red cell survival also contributes to development of anemia. Anemia generally appears when GFR falls below 60 mL/minute. There is a rough correlation between the severity of renal failure and the degree of anemia: the more severe the renal failure the greater the degree of anemia. However, this relationship is not invariable, and many patients have only mild reductions in hemoglobin and hematocrit.

Anemia initially was believed to contribute only to changes in oxygen delivery. However, recent studies show that anemia can contribute to the genesis of left ventricular hypertrophy and other cardiomyopathies noted with chronic renal failure and can raise mortality in patients with chronic renal failure.

HYPERTENSION

Recent studies emphasize the importance of the kidneys in the regulation of blood pressure, and the bulk of patients with diabetes or other glomerular disease will develop hypertension in the course of their renal failure. In many instances, hypertension does not develop until GFR is below 40% to 50% of normal. The type of renal disease underlying chronic renal failure appears to be important, as hypertension is less common with pyelonephritis. Hypertension might be observed earlier in the course of renal failure, however, in patients with polycystic kidney disease or ischemic nephropathy. Because hypertension is one of the most critical factors in the genesis of cardiovascular disease and can accelerate the progression of renal failure, careful attention of control of hypertension is important.

VOLUME OVERLOAD

Salt retention often accompanies chronic renal failure even when GFR is not severely compromised. The degree of salt retention can be profound if significant albuminuria with resultant hypoalbuminemia is seen and is more severe as GFR falls below 20% to 25% of normal. Salt retention is a critical factor in the development of hypertension and can promote congestive heart failure.

Symptoms and Signs of Renal Failure

Patients with chronic renal failure are often asymptomatic with little evidence of disease other than laboratory abnormalities until late in the course of renal failure. If anemia is present, patients may complain of fatigue; and if significant elevations in parathyroid hormone levels are noted, bone pain, ruptured tendons or other disorders of soft tissue structures can be noted. Once moderate to severe renal failure appears, symptoms of the electrolyte abnormalities can be observed. Hyperkalemia, if severe, can lead to arrhythmias or heart block and muscle weakness. Metabolic acidosis can contribute to fatigue. Anemia can contribute to fatigue and changes in mentation and physical stamina. Weight loss related to metabolic acidosis and or retention of various uremic toxins may occur. Sexual dysfunction characterized by reduced libido and reduced fertility are common with moderate to severe renal failure.

Once severe renal failure develops (stage 4 or 5), the uremic syndrome can be observed characterized by a decreased appetite, nausea, vomiting, and subtle changes in mental status including changes in sleep patterns. However, even with severe renal failure many patients feel surprisingly well.

Management of Chronic Renal Failure

STAGING OF CHRONIC RENAL FAILURE

As noted earlier, within the last several years, a great deal of effort has been expended into developing guidelines for the evaluation, monitoring, and treatment of patients with chronic renal failure. To this end, experts working with the National Kidney Foundation have divided chronic renal failure into different states based on measurements or estimations of GFR. The value of staging to the physician is that the studies necessary to monitor patients and the complications of chronic renal failure are often different depending on the stage of renal failure.

Stage 0 (GFR Greater Than 90 mL/minute With Risk Factors for Renal Disease)

Patients at stage 0 have increased risk for development of chronic renal failure, such as those with diabetes or hypertension but who have GFR greater than 90 mL/minute in the absence of proteinuria or urinary sedimentary abnormalities. These patients should have their blood pressure and diabetes controlled. Estimates of GFR should be obtained approximately every 6 months from measurement of serum creatinine, and qualitative tests for urine protein excretion should be obtained. In diabetics measurement of microablumin should also be obtained. Because control of disease may forestall progression glycosylated hemoglobin (HbA1C) values should also be obtained.

Stage 1 (GFR Greater Than 90 mL/minute With Albuminuria)

Once evidence of renal damage is obtained, as reflected by microalbuminuria or proteinuria, but GFR is either normal or increased, patients are said to be in stage 1. These individuals should be monitored more closely and strict attention must be given to maintain blood pressure below 130/80. Furthermore, angiotensin converting enzyme inhibitor (ACEI) or angiotensin receptor blocker (ARB) should be given to prevent evolution of microalbuminuria to full-blown proteinuria (see the following). No clinical or laboratory abnormalities are observed at this stage.

Stage 2: Mild Renal Failure (GFR 60 to 90 mL/minute)

When GFR is mildly reduced to values from 60 to 90 mL/minute, patients are in stage 2. These patients should also be carefully monitored and blood pressure tightly controlled. If diabetes is present, strict attention to maintaining HbA1C within recommended guidelines should be given. Again, it is rare at this stage for any significant clinical abnormalities other than hypertension to be present.

Stage 3: Moderate Renal Failure (GFR 30 to 59 mL/minute)

When GFR ranges between 30 to 59 mL/minute, patients are in stage 3. At this point hypertension may appear, mild abnormalities in serum phosphorus might be observed, and anemia can be seen. Also in some patients an elevation in serum potassium can be noted, particularly if they are ingesting a relatively high potassium diet. These patients need to be followed more closely, and it is recommended that patients at this stage be monitored by a nephrologist.

Stage 4: Moderate to Severe (GFR from 15 to 29 mL/minute)

Once GFR falls to values from 15 to 29 mL/minute, patients have severe renal failure, or stage 4 disease. At this level of GFR, significant electrolyte abnormalities such as metabolic acidosis, hyperkalemia, and hyperphosphatemia are frequent. Anemia is common and the patient may begin to note reductions in appetite and have a fall in muscle mass. However, there is great variability in the appearance of symptoms or laboratory derangements.

Stage 5: Severe (GFR Less Than 15 to 29 mL/minute)

When GFR falls below 15 mL/minute, severe electrolyte abnormalities are often present, anemia is common. Clinical symptoms can develop. Renal replacement therapy, either dislysis or transplantation, is usually required at this stage.

Recommendations for treatment of patients are summarized below. The frequency of patient visits, of course, largely depends on the complications of renal disease present and co-morbid conditions. Therefore, these are only general recommendations for frequency of examination.

When patients are in stage 0, they should be seen once per year for renal evaluation. When GFR remains normal or elevated, but proteinuria is present, renal evaluation should be performed every 6 months. When stage 3 develops, we usually repeat renal evaluation every 3 months. Patients in stage 4 are seen more frequently, usually at the minimum of once per month. Patients with end-stage disease require renal replacement therapy.

GENERAL APPROACH TO TREATMENT OF CHRONIC RENAL FAILURE

Treatment of chronic renal failure can be divided into the modalities that are specific to the underlying disorder and those that are used to treat all patients with chronic renal failure. Thus, patients with systemic lupus erythematosus or other immune-mediated or inflammatory disease may benefit from treatment with steroids and immunosuppressive agents. Treatments specific for individual disorders are beyond the scope of this article.

The physician treating the patient with renal failure has two goals: preventing or delaying progression of renal failure, and alleviating the electrolyte and hormonal abnormalities that can lead to symptoms or complications of the disease. Understanding the methods to accomplish the former requires knowledge of those factors that are integral to progression of the disease.

FACTORS CAUSING PROGRESSION OF CHRONIC RENAL FAILURE

It has been recognized for several years that once renal failure has developed, renal function can decline at a predictable rate in the absence of further insults to the kidney. Essential to the optimal approach used to treat chronic renal failure, therefore, is an understanding of those factors that can cause progression of renal failure, including:

- Systemic and intraglomerular hypertension
- Glomerular hypertrophy
- Intrarenal precipitation of calcium and phosphorus
- Hyperlipidemia
- Altered metabolism of prostanoids
- Metabolic acidosis
- Anemia
- Tubulointerstitial disease
- Proteinuria

Intraglomerular Hypertension and Glomerular Hypertrophy

As nephrons are lost, changes are induced in the kidney to preserve GFR such as renal vasodilatation, an increase in glomerular capillary pressure, and an increment in size of individual glomeruli raising wall stress. These adaptive mechanisms probably induce damage by causing endothelial cell damage with detachment of epithelial cells allowing enhanced flux of water and solutes that might cause narrowing of capillary lumens. Also, strain on mesangial cells causes them to produce cytokines and extracellular matrix with resultant expansion of the mesangium and glomerular sclerosis.

Proteinuria

Although proteinuria has traditionally been a marker of glomerular injury, with greater amounts of urinary protein excretion being associated with more severe injury, recent studies indicate that proteinuria, can induce mesangial and tubular damage. Therefore, treatments to reduce proteinuria, may be beneficial in limiting further renal damage.

Tubulointerstitial Disease

Some component of tubulointerstitial disease is generally found in individuals with chronic renal failure even when the primary process affects the glomerulus. It has been postulated that the tubulointerstitial disease can produce atrophy of tubules or obstruction destroying individual nephrons. Even when tubular inflammation is treated, progressive scarring can continue unabated. Thus, treatments designed to reduce interstitial fibrosis may be important for preventing progression of disease. At present, only experimental drugs not available for human use have been examined for this purpose.

Hyperlipidemia

Hyperlipidemia is frequently observed in disorders associated with nephrotic range proteinuria, but is also noted in a large percentage of the general population without renal disease. Experimental evidence obtained from animal studies shows hyperlipidemia can promote progression of renal failure. Thus, loading with cholesterol augments renal injury and treatment with cholesterol-lowering drugs slows the rate of progression. This effect is synergistic to that achieved by lowering blood pressure.

The mechanisms underlying the effects of lipids are not well understood, but possible explanations include mesangial lipid deposition leading to glomerular injury or tubular injury. A few studies performed in human subjects have demonstrated benefit from lipid lowering on the progression of renal injury, although they are not conclusive. Because patients with chronic renal failure have a high prevalence of cardiovascular disease, it is reasonable to initiate therapy with statin drugs to lower serum cholesterol and lipid levels.

Calcium-Phosphate Deposition

A rise in serum phosphorus, usually seen at the later stages of renal failure, can lead to precipitation of calcium phosphate in the renal interstitium. The deposits can then induce an inflammatory response producing interstitial fibrosis and tubular atrophy. Some have indicated that the deposits may form prior to detectable elevations in serum phosphorus concentrations.

Increased Glomerular Prostaglandin Production

An increment in glomerular prostaglandin production has been found in several studies of chronic renal failure. The increased prostanoids produce renal vasodilatation and a rise in intraglomerular pressure, factors that augment progression of disease.

METABOLIC ACIDOSIS

Metabolic acidosis commonly develops in the course of chronic renal failure. In response to the acidosis, ammonia production per residual functioning nephron is augmented. It has been postulated that the increased local production of ammonia in some way induces tubulointerstitial damage. This issue remains controversial, as some studies do not support this possibility.

SPECIFIC TREATMENT MEASURES

Treatment of patients with chronic renal failure should be designed to ameliorate those factors that can cause progression of renal injury, treat or prevent important complications, and normalize important laboratory abnormalities that contribute to symptoms of the disease.

Measures Designed to Reduce the Rate of Progression of Renal Failure

CONTROL OF SYSTEMIC AND INTRAGLOMERULAR HYPERTENSION

Experimental and human studies demonstrate that control of systemic hypertension can slow the rate of progression of renal disease substantially. Recent evidence indicates that target blood pressure levels should be lower than recommended for the general population (<130/80). Control of hypertension with the use of myriad agents can benefit the patient with renal failure. However, as indicated previously, reduction in intraglomerular hypertension may be the most important factor underlying the benefits from blood pressure control. Therefore, when possible, treatment with ACEIs, ARBs, or the combination of these agents should be first-line antihypertensive therapy in these patients. Patients who do not tolerate these drugs might benefit from administration of non-dihydropyridine calcium channel blockers. In patients with proteinuria, even if blood pressure is controlled or they are normotensive, the doses of ACEIs or ARBs should be raised to levels even greater than recommended to reduce urine protein excretion to levels less than 500 mg. This reduction in proteinuria is the most optimal in protecting the kidney.

Potentially serious complications with ACEIs or ARBs include acute reduction in GFR and hyperkalemia. If these complications occur, a reduction in dose or even discontinuation of these agents might be required. It is recommended that these agents be continued less than 20 mL/minute. Given the potential severity of these complications, patients should be monitored closely.

PROTEIN RESTRICTION

The benefits of protein restriction in preventing progression are unclear, but it has suggested that reducing protein intake to 0.8 to 1.0 g/kg body weight of high biologic value is beneficial. Others have indicated that 0.6 g/kg body weight should be used. In patients with substantial proteinuria,

CURRENT THERAPY

The recommendations for the treatment of patients with renal failure is as follows:

Recommendation	Goal
Control BP	130/80
Reduce proteinuria by administering angiotensin converting enzyme inhibitors or angiotensin receptor blockers. In some cases both agents may have to be given concomitantly.	Decrease urine protein excretion to less than 1 g per day by gradual titration of dose.
Control phosphate concentrations with phosphate binders with noncalcium containing binders when possible.	Serum phosphate <4.5 mg/dL
Prevent hyperparathyroidism with vitamin D or calcimimetics.	Maintain PTH <150 pg/mL
Correct anemia with erythropoietin and iron replacement as needed.	Maintain Hg between 11 and 12 mg/dL
Administer diuretics to control hypertension and volume overload.	Maintain euvolemia when possible
Control serum potassium with dietary restriction, diuretics, and/or potassium exchange resin as necessary.	Maintain serum potassium <5.0 mEq/L
Keep protein intake at 0.6 to 0.8 g/kg body weight per day.	Slow progression of renal disease while preventing protein depletion
Control metabolic acidosis with administration of sodium citrate (Citra pH).	Maintain serum HCO₃ >20 mEq/L

Abbreviations: BP = blood pressure; HCO₃ = bicarbonate; Hg = mercury; PTH = parathyroid hormone.

the quantity of protein recommended will have to be adjusted to prevent hypoalbuminemia. Once patients reached later stage 4, protein restriction may be useful to prevent expression of uremic symptoms. Reducing protein intake will have the added benefit of decreasing acid, potassium, and phosphate production.

CONTROL OF LIPIDS

Control of cholesterol with statins may help prevent progression and should reduce the burden of cardiovascular disease, which remains the most lethal disorder for patients with chronic renal failure. Adherence to the newly proposed aggressive recommendation appears reasonable.

Measures Designed to Treat Significant Laboratory Abnormalities

ANEMIA

Patients with renal anemia should be treated with erythropoietin (Procrit). Although this requires subcutaneous injection once per week, newer, long-lasting forms (darbepoetin [Aranesp]) enable patients to be treated every 3 weeks. Because iron stores need to be repleted for anemia to be successfully treated, these should be monitored and iron given. Because of the vagaries of ferritin measurements, we use serum iron and iron binding capacity with the goal of maintaining saturation above 20% and near 30%. At present, the target hemoglobin and hematocrit varies between 11 mg/dL and 12 mg/dL 33 and 36, respectively.

METABOLIC ACIDOSIS

Controversy exists as to the target value of bicarbonate for patients with chronic renal failure. Some experts recommend raising plasma bicarbonate to levels above 20 mEq/L, whereas others recommend complete normalization of plasma bicarbonate. To properly raise plasma bicarbonate concentration, the deficit should be calculated from the formula:

Desired – prevailing level of plasma bicarbonate
× 50% body weight = Total bicarbonate deficit.

The deficit should be corrected slowly over several days.

Because patients experience gas when the base is given as bicarbonate, the base is usually administered as Shohl's solution sodium citrate,* the citrate being metabolized to bicarbonate in the liver. Each milliliter of Shohl's solution represents 1 mEq of the base.

DIVALENT ION METABOLISM

Serum phosphorus is controlled by administration of phosphate binders usually starting with calcium citrate (Citracal) or acetate (PhosLo). If these are not successful or if patients have elevated calcium levels, then sevelamer (Renagel) can be used either alone or in combination with calcium binders. Physicians should aim to maintain serum phosphorus levels below 5 mg/dL and keep serum calcium phosphorus product below 60.

Parathyroid hormone (PTH) levels should be maintained below 150 pg/mL, or less depending on stage; levels associated with proper bone remodeling but not to values observed in patients without kidney disease. Suppression of

---

*May be compounded by pharmacists.

parathyroid hormone secretion can be achieved by administration of various vitamin D analogues. The recent recognition of the calcium-sensing receptor and development of calcimimetic drugs that are extremely effective in lowering PTH secretion may make using vitamin D compounds obsolete in the future.

HYPERKALEMIA

As this is the most serious electrolyte disorder encountered, patients should be monitored closely. Serum potassium concentrations should be maintained below 5 mEq/L. If hyperkalemia develops during treatment with ACEIs or ARBs, the doses of these agents should be reduced or discontinued. Diuretic administration, often given for control of hypertension, can help control hyperkalemia, but if it should develop, particularly when GFR falls below 20% of normal, it can be treated with the potassium exchange resin, sodium polystyrene sulfonate (Kayexalate).

ELEVATED BLOOD UREA NITROGEN CONCENTRATION

The precise solutes that are retained, which are important for the pathogenesis of the uremic syndrome, are not clear. However, BUN is a marker for other retained solutes and is roughly correlated with development of uremic symptoms. When the BUN is greater than 100 mg/dL and serum creatinine concentration is greater than 8 mg/dL uremic symptoms may develop. These symptoms will often abate merely with protein restriction and reduced production of these compounds. Protein restriction is usually not instituted until GFR is less than 15% to 20% of normal. Prior to that time, it is important to maintain protein intake to keep serum albumin within the normal range.

VOLUME OVERLOAD

Because salt retention is an essential component of the development of hypertension and underlies volume overload, diuretic administration is usually necessary in the treatment of chronic renal failure. Thiazides frequently used in the treatment of hypertension or volume overload in subjects with normal renal function may not be efficacious once GFR is less than or equal to 33% of normal. Therefore, loop diuretics, such as furosemide (Lasix) or a combined loop and proximal tubule diuretic such as metolozone (Zaroxolyn), are generally indicated. Because the effectiveness of both agents requires access to the tubule lumen, the effective dose is often higher than in those with normal renal function. Once patients are in stage 4 renal failure, use of diuretics is hampered by worsening of renal failure and often must be used cautiously.

REFERENCES

Beco JA, Bansal VK: Medical nutrition therapy in chronic kidney failure: Integrating clinical practice guidelines. J Am Diet Assoc 2004; 104:404-409.

Clase CM, Garg AX, Kiberd BA: Prevalence of low glomerular filtration rate in nondiabetic Americans: Third National Health and Nutrition Examination Survey (NHANES III). J Am Soc Nephrol 2002;13.

Cleveland DR, Jindal KK, Hirsch DJ, et al: Quality of pre-referral care in patients with chronic renal insufficiency. Am J Kidney Dis 2002;40:30-36.

Curtin RB, Becker B, Kimmel PL, Schatell D: An integrated approach to care for patients with chronic kidney disease. Semin Dial 2003; 16:399-402.

Djamali A, Kendziorski C, Brazy PC, Becker BN: Disease progression and outcomes in chronic kidney disease and renal transplantation. Kidney Int 2003;64:1800-1807.

Kopple JD: National Kidney Foundation K/DOQI clinical practice guidelines for nutrition in chronic renal failure. Am J Kidney Dis 2001;37:S66-S70.

Maschio G, Alberti D, Janin G, et al: Effect of the angiotensin-converting-enzyme inhibitor benazepril on the progression of chronic renal insufficiency. N Engl J Med 1996;334:939-945

Tonelli M, Gill J, Pandeya S, et al: Slowing the progression of chronic renal insufficiency. Can Med Assoc J 2002;166:906-907.

Malignant Tumors of the Urogenital Tract

Method of
Michael S. Cookson, MD,
and Sam S. Chang, MD

CARCINOMA OF THE PROSTATE

Carcinoma of the prostate is the most common solid malignancy in men and the second leading cause of male cancer mortality in the United States. In 2005, it was estimated there would be 232,090 new cases and 30,350 deaths from prostatic cancer alone. The incidence of prostatic carcinoma increases with age, and this is anticipated to continue to increase for the next 25 years in direct relationship to the aging U.S. population. A familial pattern is identified, and prostatic carcinoma is more common in African Americans than in the white population. A high-fat diet is implicated as a contributing factor in some studies. Hereditary prostatic carcinoma has been identified in approximately 9% of patients and may account for as much as 40% of the early age of onset cancers. In fact, the hereditary prostate cancer gene (HPC1) was identified on the long arm of chromosome 1 and is thought to be intimately related to the development of carcinoma of the prostate.

Diagnosis

More than 95% of prostatic cancers are adenocarcinomas. Prostatic carcinoma can be identified at autopsy in more than 75% of individuals older than 80 years, yet clinically the risk of being diagnosed is estimated at one in six men. Thus, there is a large discrepancy between the microscopic presence of the disease and clinically significant disease. Most men with early-stage prostatic cancer have no disease-related symptoms. Prostatic cancer and benign prostatic hypertrophy (BPH) may occur simultaneously, but there is no apparent causal relationship. Obstructive voiding symptoms or hematuria may be present. Patients with advanced disease may present with pelvic pain, ureteral obstruction, or bone pain from distant metastasis.

Early detection has allowed more patients to be identified with lower stage clinical disease, and as a result,

Carcinoma of the Prostate

- Average-risk patient offered screening with PSA and DRE at 50 years of age
- High-risk patients with strong family history or African Americans at age 45 years
- Patients with an elevated PSA or abnormal DRE referred for discussion regarding risks, benefits, and alternatives to biopsy of the prostate
- Diagnosis made with transrectal ultrasound-guided biopsy of the prostate
- Staging with bone scan for patients with high-grade tumors (Gleason grade 4 or 5), PSA levels >20 µg/mL, elevated alkaline phosphatase levels, or bone pain

Abbreviations: DRE = digital rectal examination; PSA = prostate-specific antigen.

such men have had higher recurrence-free survival rates after treatment. Recommendations from groups such as the American Urologic Association and American Cancer Society generally include annual screening with serum prostate-specific antigen (PSA) determination and a digital rectal examination (DRE) for all men older than 50 years and for all African American men and men with a family history of prostatic cancer starting at 40 years of age. These recommendations are not uniformly accepted; the U.S. Public Health Service Task Force does not endorse screening for prostatic cancer because of a lack of convincing prospective data that screening has an impact on the prostatic cancer death rate. The goal of screening is to detect clinically significant prostatic cancer in individuals with at least 10 years of life expectancy.

Serum PSA is specific for the prostate but is secreted by both benign and malignant prostatic epithelial cells. PSA may be elevated in men with prostatitis, BPH, or prostatic cancer. PSA values differ somewhat depending on the assay used. In general, a level of less than 4.0 µg/mL is considered normal, and in younger men, a value of greater than 2.5 ng/mL may be considered abnormal. Approximately 25% of prostatic carcinoma may occur despite what is considered a normal PSA level, and in some studies, the incidence of prostatic carcinoma is 15% even when the PSA is less than 2 µg/mL.

Serum PSA occurs in several forms, with the majority bound to a alpha-1-antichymotrypsin and another portion that is unconjugated or free in serum. The relative proportion of the two forms can be used to improve the specificity of PSA testing. A greater proportion of free PSA is seen in men with BPH compared to those with prostatic cancer. In general, the lower the percentage of free fraction, the more likely it is to reflect a diagnosis of cancer, with a percentage of less than 25% most commonly associated with prostatic cancer as compared to higher percentages. Newer tests such as complexed PSA are being used to improve the specificity of PSA testing.

Most often, transrectal ultrasonography (TRUS) is used for imaging and as a guide for biopsy of the prostate. TRUS can distinguish the zonal anatomy of the prostate and is an accurate measure of the size of the prostate.

Prostatic cancers typically are located in the peripheral zone and may have a hypoechoic pattern. Because of its lack of sensitivity and specificity, TRUS is not used as a screening test.

The grading of prostatic carcinoma is based on the degree of differentiation of the tumor. This provides important prognostic information. Most often, the Gleason grading system is used. Tumors with a Gleason score of 2 to 4 are usually considered to be well differentiated; 5 to 7, moderately differentiated; and 8 to 10, poorly differentiated. Prognosis is strongly linked to grade and Gleason score. Most cancers found through early detection or screening programs are of an intermediate grade (Gleason score 5 to 7).

Staging of prostatic cancer defines the local, regional, and distant extent of disease. The TNM staging system is used to allow categorization of nonpalpable tumors detected because of PSA or ultrasound abnormalities (stage T1c). The primary staging modality for local disease is DRE. Serum PSA levels correlate only roughly with disease extent. However, bone metastasis is quite uncommon in patients with a PSA of less than 20 µg/mL. Radionucleotide bone scanning is the most sensitive method for detection of bone metastases. Bone scan in the absence of symptoms is not required routinely if the PSA value is less than 10 µg/mL and a Gleason sum of less than or equal to 7. Computed tomography (CT) scanning is not routinely used because grossly positive nodes are detected rarely with clinically localized tumor.

Lymph node staging is important in selecting patients for therapy. CT scanning may show enlarged lymph nodes in patients with high-volume or high-grade primary tumors. Laparoscopic pelvic lymphadenectomy is feasible and can provide adequate sampling of the pelvic lymph nodes among those patients not selecting surgery. More commonly, lymph node dissection is performed through an open incision immediately prior to radical prostatectomy.

Treatment

The optimal therapy for localized prostatic cancer is controversial and must be individualized. For men with a life expectancy of less than 10 years, observation alone may be appropriate. Also, some men choose active surveillance rather than initial treatment but later opt for treatment when clinical evidence indicates worsening disease. Surgery and radiation therapy are the most commonly used treatments. For organ-confined tumors, the 15-year disease-free survival rates are greater than 90% for patients treated with surgery. Moreover, the survival outcome is similar after radiation therapy or surgery; however, randomized comparisons among similarly staged patients are lacking. Brachytherapy involves the use of radioactive seeds (iodine 125 or palladium 103) placed into the prostate. This is also a valid option, with similar long-term disease-free survival in low- and intermediate-risk patients. High-dose radiation (HDR) therapy is also an emerging treatment option that allows high doses of radiation therapy to be administered in a relatively short period of time. Cryotherapy (i.e., freezing of the prostate) is also approved in the treatment of men with prostatic carcinoma, but long-term outcomes are not available.

Radical prostatectomy (RP) may be performed via an open surgical approach or by a laparoscopic technique. Most commonly, it is performed via open surgery through a retropubic approach, although some are performed through a perineal incision. Laparoscopic and robot-assisted RPs are being performed with a reduction in blood loss and seemingly comparable oncologic results as compared to open surgery. These minimally invasive techniques may have the potential for improved functional outcomes. In patients who were sexually active before therapy, potency can be retained in nearly 40% to 70% by preservation of the neurovascular bundles. In patients with organ-confined disease, there is an excellent prognosis, with a life expectancy similar to men without prostatic cancer. In patients with positive surgical margins or positive lymph nodes, adjuvant radiation and hormonal therapy may be used, respectively.

Serum PSA should be undetectable after radical prostatectomy because all PSA-producing cells are removed. After radiation therapy, superior results are achieved in patients in whom the PSA level decreases to less than 1 µg/mL. An increasing serum PSA is evidence of tumor recurrence. There is controversy about when to initiate hormonal therapy in men with a rising PSA level after treatment, although several studies suggest early hormonal therapy may be of benefit among those with more aggressive tumors.

Prostatic cancer is a partially androgen-dependent disease. Therefore, the primary treatment for metastatic carcinoma of the prostate is androgen deprivation. Suppression of serum testosterone can be achieved by orchiectomy. Alternatively, medical therapy may be considered. Luteinizing hormone-releasing hormone (LHRH) analogues effectively suppress testosterone to the castrate range within 1 month of administration. LHRH analogues are associated with few serious side effects but do cause vasomotor hot flashes in approximately two thirds of patients. Loss of libido and impotence are also a consequence of treatment.

The median response to hormonal therapy in patients with metastatic disease is approximately 18 to 24 months. After that time, disease progression often occurs and ultimately progresses to death. Once the cancer fails to respond to hormonal therapy, the patient usually dies of the disease, although survival rates of greater than 40 months are reported. Recently, published trials have documented improved survival with docetaxel (Taxotere) chemotherapy among patients with androgen-independent prostatic cancer (AIPC) treatments. In addition, mitoxantrone (Novantrone) is now approved for palliative relief for symptomatic bone pain from AIPC. Radiation can also be effective palliation for isolated sites of bone metastasis. The mechanisms through which prostatic carcinoma escapes hormonal control and achieves androgen independence is an area of intense research.

TUMORS OF THE RENAL PARENCHYMA

Malignant tumors of the renal parenchyma are either primary or metastatic. Among the primary renal lesions, the tumors may be either malignant or benign. The most common malignant tumor is renal cell carcinoma (RCC), whereas other tumor types such as papillary, collecting duct carcinoma, medullary carcinoma, and sarcomas occur infrequently. The most common benign renal tumors are angiomyolipomas and oncocytomas, the latter of which is often indistinguishable from malignant lesions on radiographic imaging. Metastatic lesions such as lung, breast, and ovary may occur, and lymphoma may be present in the kidney.

RENAL CELL CARCINOMA

RCC is the most common primary neoplasm of the kidney and accounts for greater than 85% of all primary renal cancers. In the United States, an estimated 36,160 new cases are diagnosed, and approximately 12,660 patients die of the disease each year. Renal cell carcinoma represents approximately 3% of all adult malignancies. It is a tumor that usually occurs in adults between 40 and 60 years of age, although it is reported in younger age groups. It has a 2:1 male-to-female preponderance and a well-documented association with von Hippel-Lindau disease.

RCCs arise from the proximal convoluted tubules. The most consistent chromosomal changes in RCC are deletions and translocations of the short arm of chromosome 3. No specific agent is implicated as the cause of RCC. Tobacco smoking poses an approximately twofold relative risk for developing kidney cancer. Patients with end-stage renal disease (ESRD) with acquired cystic disease of the kidney (ACDK) have an increased risk of RCC as well. Of these patients, RCC develops in 1% to 2%, with younger dialysis patients having the greatest risk. Renal ultrasound is recommended in these patients annually, with CT scans for more complex cysts.

Diagnosis

Hematuria is the single most common sign associated with renal cell carcinoma; it occurs in 29% to 60% of cases. Flank pain and a palpable mass occur next most frequently, but the classic triad of hematuria, flank pain, and a palpable abdominal mass is reported in only 10% of cases. Other common signs and symptoms are fever, anemia, and elevated sedimentation rate. Although serum lactate dehydrogenase and alkaline phosphatase may be elevated, there are no reliable tumor markers for RCC. RCCs can present only with nonspecific symptoms such as weight loss, fever, or weakness. Most, however, are asymptomatic and are detected incidentally on radiographic imaging.

TNM staging is currently the most commonly used system to determine the extent of the primary lesion, involvement of contiguous structures, vascular involvement, and whether the tumor has metastasized. It allows for a distinction between venous involvement and nodal invasion and stratifies the extent of each stage. RCCs often involve the renal vein and vena cava and may even extend into the right atrium. Five-year survival rates for stages T1N0M0 (less than 7 cm) and T2N0M0 (more than 7 cm) are 80% to 90%, for stages T3N0M0 40% to 60%, and N1–3 and M1 are 10% to 20%.

Treatment

Radical nephrectomy is the primary treatment of RCC. This classic procedure removes the kidney en bloc within Gerota's fascia along with the ipsilateral adrenal gland and lymph nodes. Radical nephrectomy traditionally is performed as an open procedure (flank, transabdominal, or thoracoabdominal incision). Radical nephrectomy has evolved, with adrenalectomy performed for upper pole tumors, very large tumors, or lesions that directly extend into the adrenal gland. If the RCC extends into the inferior vena cava, open as compared to laparoscopic nephrectomy is usually the preferred approach. Rarely, cardiopulmonary bypass is needed to remove the entire tumor thrombus, which is particularly important for those thrombi that extend above the level of the diaphragm. Laparoscopic radical nephrectomy, both hand assisted and pure laparoscopic, is equally efficacious as compared to open surgery and is potentially less morbid, allowing patients a faster recovery.

A partial nephrectomy is performed in patients with solitary kidneys, in those with bilateral RCC, and in patients with compromised renal function. It is also generally agreed that partial nephrectomy or tumor enucleation may be used in patients with lesions 4 cm or less and a normal contralateral kidney, with local recurrence rates less than 5%. Like radical nephrectomy, laparoscopic techniques are emerging as viable alternatives to open surgical removal. In addition, there is an emergence of minimally invasive approaches that will likely compete with partial nephrectomy in the near future. These include radiofrequency ablation and cryotherapy, which may effectively treat smaller lesions under radiologic guidance, thus reducing or eliminating the need for surgery.

Up to 25% of patients initially seen with symptoms have metastatic disease. Sites of metastasis in decreasing frequency include the lungs, lymph nodes, liver, bone, and adrenal gland. Chemotherapy and radiation have little to no survival benefit, with radiation only palliating painful metastasis. The mainstay of treatment is immunotherapy, with 5-year survival rates of 10% to 20%. Emerging evidence suggests an improved survival in those undergoing nephrectomy prior to immunotherapy.

BENIGN RENAL TUMORS

Benign solid tumors of the kidney are encountered occasionally. An angiomyolipoma can usually be diagnosed by the characteristic appearance of fat within the lesion on CT scan. An angiomyolipoma may occur as an isolated

CURRENT DIAGNOSIS

Benign Renal Tumors

- Angiomyolipomas are diagnosed by the characteristic appearance of fat within the lesion on computed tomography (CT) scan.
- Angiomyolipomas may occur as an isolated phenomenon or in association with tuberous sclerosis.
- Tuberous sclerosis is characterized by mental retardation, epilepsy, and adenoma sebaceum. Approximately 50% of patients with tuberous sclerosis develop angiomyolipomas, and many are bilateral and multifocal.
- Oncocytomas are benign renal tumors that account for between 5% and 10% of solid renal lesions.
- Oncocytomas are more difficult to differentiate from RCC but usually are round and of uniform density; they may have a central scar or spoke-wheel appearance on CT scan.
- Oncocytomas are a pathologic diagnosis characterized by eosinophilic granular cells. These masses should be considered malignant until proven otherwise.

phenomenon or in association with tuberous sclerosis. Tuberous sclerosis is a disease characterized by mental retardation, epilepsy, and adenoma sebaceum. Approximately 50% of patients with tuberous sclerosis develop angiomyolipomas, and many are bilateral and multifocal. The management of angiomyolipomas is controversial. In asymptomatic lesions smaller than 4 cm, observation with annual imaging is reasonable. In patients with an acute bleeding episode, angioinfarction may be used to stabilize the patient. In symptomatic lesions or lesions greater than 4 cm, surgical excision is considered the standard therapy.

Oncocytomas are benign renal tumors that account for between 5% and 10% of solid renal lesions. Renal oncocytomas are more difficult to differentiate from RCCs but usually are round, of uniform density, and may have a central scar or spoke-wheel appearance on CT scan. From a practical standpoint, renal oncocytomas are a pathologic diagnosis, and characteristic masses should be considered to be malignant until proven otherwise. Histologically, they are characterized by eosinophilic granular cells. The cell of origin is thought to be that of distal renal tubules.

CURRENT THERAPY

Benign Renal Tumors

- The management is controversial. In asymptomatic lesions <4 cm, observation with annual imaging is reasonable.
- In patients with acute bleeding, angioinfarction may stabilize the patient. In symptomatic lesions or lesions >4 cm, surgical excision is considered standard therapy.

Metastatic Renal Lesions

Lung cancer is the most common solid tumor to metastasize to the kidney, although lymphoma and ovarian, bowel, and breast tumors are also seen. Lymphoma of the kidney is almost always a metastatic manifestation of a systemic disease, and therefore surgical treatment is rarely indicated in the absence of symptoms. However, approximately 15% of renal lymphomas present as solitary masses. It is a challenge to differentiate these tumors from renal cell carcinoma preoperatively.

TUMORS OF THE RENAL PELVIS/URETER

Tumors of the renal pelvis account for approximately 10% of all renal tumors and approximately 5% of all urothelial tumors. Ureteral tumors are even less common, representing approximately 25% of upper tract urothelial tumors. Ureteral tumors are three times more common in men than in women and twice as common in whites as in blacks. Cigarette smoking is strongly associated with an increased risk of developing upper tract transitional cell carcinomas. Additionally, analgesic abuse and cyclophosphamide are associated with an increased risk.

The risk of upper tract tumors is approximately 4% among patients with bladder cancer. However, in patients with carcinoma in situ and high-grade urothelial lesions, the risk may approach 20% with long-term follow-up. Conversely, patients with upper tract tumors have a 40% to 70% risk of developing bladder cancer. Therefore, patients with upper tract tumors should undergo periodic surveillance cystoscopy. The incidence of bilateral upper tract tumors is 2% to 5%. In addition to transitional cell carcinomas, squamous cell carcinomas and adenocarcinomas are included in the differential diagnosis; particularly in a patient with a history of recurrent urinary tract infections or staghorn calculi.

Diagnosis

As with renal cell carcinomas, the most common presenting symptom of tumors of the renal pelvis/ureter is hematuria. In patients with normal renal function, the diagnostic workup usually includes an intravenous pyelogram (IVP) and urine cytologic examination followed by cystoscopy. However, it must be kept in mind that a voided urine cytologic examination may be falsely negative in up to 85% of patients with a low-grade lesion. Approximately 50% to 75% of patients have a filling defect on IVP. The differential diagnosis includes a tumor, blood clot, fungal ball, sloughed papilla, and radiolucent stone. A retrograde ureteropyelogram may be helpful in documenting the persistence of the filling defect; however, ureteroscopy with biopsy or brushings may be diagnostic. In renal pelvic defects, a noncontrast CT scan with 3-mm cuts through the kidney is usually able to differentiate a stone from a soft-tissue mass because even radiolucent stones on standard urography are opaque on CT scan. The TNM system is recommended for staging.

CURRENT DIAGNOSIS

Tumors of the Renal Pelvis/Ureter

- Renal pelvic tumors account for 10% of all renal tumors and approximately 5% of all urothelial tumors.
- Ureteral tumors are even less common, occurring approximately 25% of the incidence of renal pelvic tumors.
- These tumors are three times more common in men than in women.
- Cigarette smoking is strongly associated with an increased risk. Additionally, analgesic abuse and cyclophosphamide are implicated.
- Most common presenting symptom is hematuria.
- Diagnostic workup usually includes an IVP and cytologic examination of the urine followed by cystoscopy.
- Cytologic examination of the urine may give a false-negative result in up to 85% of patients with a low-grade lesion.
- 50%–75% of patients have a filling defect on IVP. The differential diagnosis includes a tumor, blood clot, fungal ball, sloughed papilla, and radiolucent stone.
- The risk of upper tract tumors is approximately 4% among those patients with bladder cancer. In patients with CIS and high-grade lesions, the risk may approach 20%.
- Patients with upper tract tumors have a 40%–70% risk of developing bladder cancer.

Abbreviations: CIS = carcinoma in situ; IVP = intravenous pyelogram.

Treatment

Patients with low-grade, low-stage lesions do well with conservative or radical treatment. Patients with intermediate- or high-grade tumors are best managed with aggressive surgical resection. Solitary low-grade and low-stage

CURRENT THERAPY

Tumors of the Renal Pelvis/Ureter

- Low-grade, low-stage lesions do well with conservative or radical treatment.
- Intermediate- or high-grade tumors are best managed with aggressive surgical resection.
- Solitary low-grade and low-stage upper ureteral tumors may be managed with segmental resection. Similar distal ureteral tumors can be managed with distal ureterectomy and ureteroneocystostomy.
- High-grade and high-stage tumors are treated by nephroureterectomy with removal of a cuff of bladder at the ureteral orifice.
- Hand-assisted laparoscopic nephroureterectomy is the preferred surgical approach, allowing for complete tumor removal through a single incision and often quicker convalescence.

upper ureteral tumors may be managed with segmental resection. Similar distal ureteral tumors can be managed with distal ureterectomy and ureteroneocystostomy. Treatment of high-grade and high-stage tumors is nephroureterectomy with removal of a cuff of the bladder at the ureteral orifice because of the high incidence of ipsilateral ureteral orifice and bladder involvement. This can be accomplished through a single extended flank or midline incision but is often performed through two incisions. Currently, hand-assisted laparoscopic nephroureterectomy is the preferred surgical approach, allowing for complete tumor removal through a single incision and offers the advantage of quicker convalescence. Successful endoscopic management including percutaneous and retrograde approaches is reported in selected cases.

CARCINOMA OF THE BLADDER

Transitional Cell Carcinoma of the Bladder

Bladder carcinoma is the fifth most common malignancy in the United States with more than 63,210 new cases annually. It is almost three times more common among men than women, in whom it is the fourth most common cancer. Because of frequent recurrences, particularly among patients with superficial tumors, bladder cancer is the second most prevalent cancer. Bladder cancer is the fifth most common cause of cancer deaths among men. It is approximately four times more prevalent among cigarette smokers and is associated with known carcinogens including occupational exposures such as those of rubber and oil refinery workers. In addition, patients treated with cyclophosphamide (Cytoxan) have up to a ninefold increased risk of developing bladder cancer. This is believed to be secondary to acrolein, a urinary metabolite of cyclophosphamide.

Approximately 90% of bladder malignancies are transitional cell carcinomas. Of these, 70% of tumors are papillary, 10% are sessile, and 20% are mixed. Approximately 20% to 25% of noninvasive tumors progress to muscle invasion during follow-up. However, of patients with muscular invasive bladder cancer, approximately 80% to 90% have invasion at the time of initial presentation. A strong correlation exists between tumor grade and stage; most well-differentiated tumors are superficial and most poorly differentiated tumors are invasive. Carcinoma in situ (CIS) is a poorly differentiated transitional cell carcinoma that is confined to the urothelium. CIS may be found as a solitary or multifocal process and is found in association with invasive carcinoma in approximately 25% of cases. It is associated with a poor prognosis. Between 10% and 20% of patients treated with cystectomy for diffuse CIS are found to have microscopic muscle-invasive disease.

Diagnosis

Gross painless hematuria is a common presenting sign of bladder cancer. However, approximately 20% of patients may present with only microscopic hematuria. Irritative voiding symptoms such as frequency and urgency may also

CURRENT DIAGNOSIS

Carcinoma of the Bladder

- Painless, gross hematuria is the most common presenting symptom.
- 20% may present with only microscopic hematuria.
- Irritative voiding symptoms such as frequency and urgency may also suggest a malignancy, particularly CIS.
- Patients suspected of bladder cancer should undergo an evaluation of their upper tracts (IVP or CT scan), cystoscopy, and cytologic examination of the urine.
- Transurethral biopsy or resection confirms the diagnosis.
- 90% of bladder cancers are transitional cell carcinoma, and 80% are nonmuscle invasive (superficial) at presentation.

Abbreviations: CIS = carcinoma in situ; CT = computed tomography; IVP = intravenous pyelogram.

suggest a malignancy, particularly CIS. Patients suspected of bladder cancer should undergo an evaluation of their upper tracts (IVP or CT scan), cystoscopy, and cytologic examination of the urine. Transurethral biopsy or resection confirms the diagnosis.

Treatment

Management of bladder carcinoma depends on tumor stage. The TNM system is recommended for staging. For most superficial bladder carcinomas, transurethral resection of the tumor is often the only treatment required. However, for CIS or high-grade superficial tumors, tumors that involve the lamina propria (stage T1), and rapidly recurrent tumors, treatment with intravesical agents such as thiotepa (Thioplex), doxorubicin (Adriamycin), and mitomycin C (Mutamycin)[1] or intravesical bacillus Calmette-Guérin (BCG, Tice) may be indicated.

Bladder surveillance is mandatory because the recurrence rate in the bladder may be as high as 50% at 5 years. Surveillance protocols include cystoscopy and urinary cytologies every 3 months for the first year, every 4 months for the second year, semiannually in year 3, and annually thereafter. Periodic evaluation of the upper tract should be performed to rule out the presence of carcinoma of the bladder in that area.

The risk of progression to muscle invasive disease is relatively low (less than 10%) for stage Ta tumors but increases as tumor stage advances (stage T1) or with high-grade lesions. For superficial tumors that progress in stage or fail conservative therapy, and in those that invade the bladder muscle (stage T2 to T3), a radical cystectomy is the treatment of choice. In addition, a thorough lymphadenectomy is performed at the time of surgery; there have been reports of improved survival based on the completeness of the dissection.

[1]Not FDA approved for this indication.

CURRENT THERAPY

Carcinoma of the Bladder

- Treatment depends on tumor stage.
- Superficial bladder (Ta) cancers are managed with transurethral resection.
- CIS or high-grade stage Ta, tumors that involve the lamina propria (stage T1), and recurrent tumors are managed with transurethral resection and intravesical therapy such as thiotepa (Thioplex), doxorubicin (Adriamycin), and mitomycin C (Mutamycin)[1] or intravesical bacillus Calmette-Guérin (BCG, Tice).
- Bladder surveillance is mandatory because the recurrence rate in the bladder may be as high as 50% at 5 years.
- Surveillance protocols include cystoscopy and urinary cytologic examinations every 3 months for the first year, every 4 months for the second year, semiannually in year 3, and annually thereafter.
- Periodic evaluation of the upper tracts should be performed as well.
- In superficial tumors that progress in stage or fail conservative therapy and in those that invade the bladder muscle (stages T2–3), a radical cystectomy and urinary diversion is the treatment of choice.
- Urinary diversion may be either incontinent (conduit) or continent (orthotopic or continent cutaneous).
- Five-year survival rates are 85%–60% after cystectomy for stages T2a and T2b, respectively. For stage T3a and T3b tumors, the 5-year survival decreases to 60% and 40%, respectively, whereas patients with node-positive disease have a 5-year survival of <30%.
- Patients with T2–T4 disease may be offered either neoadjuvant or adjuvant chemotherapy. There have been reports of modest survival advantages (<10%) using MVAC in the neoadjuvant setting.
- Patients with M1 disease are generally treated with chemotherapy as well.
- The standard regimen over the past decade has been methotrexate (Trexall),[1] vinblastine (Velban),[1] doxorubicin (Adriamycin), and cisplatin (Platinol) (MVAC); however, durable complete response rates are <15%.
- Newer agents such as gemcitabine (Gemzar) along with cisplatin appear to offer similar response rates and reduced toxicity.

[1]Not FDA approved for this indication.
Abbreviations: CIS = carcinoma in situ.

Each year there are an estimated 13,180 deaths in the United States from bladder cancer. Five-year survival rates are approximately 85% to 60% after cystectomy for stages T2a and T2b, respectively. For stage T3a and T3b tumors, the 5-year survival decreases to 60% and 40%, whereas patients with node-positive disease have a 5-year survival of less than 30%. Adjuvant chemotherapy is generally offered to patients at high risk for failure (pathologic stages T3b, T4, and N1/2 disease). The standard regimen over the past decade has been methotrexate (Trexall),[1] vinblastine (Velban),[1] doxorubicin (Adriamycin), and cisplatin (Platinol) (MVAC); however, durable complete response rates have been less than 15%. There have been recent reports of modest survival advantages (less than 10%) using MVAC in the neoadjuvant setting. Newer agents such as gemcitabine (Gemzar)[1] along with cisplatin appear to offer similar response rates and reduced toxicity.

Urinary diversion may be accomplished with an ileal or colon conduit, which requires wearing a collection appliance. A continent cutaneous diversion may be created; most often using the right colon with a tapered and a catheterizable efferent limb of ileum (Indiana pouch) or with creation of a nipple valve (Koch pouch). Approximately 50% of cystectomy patients undergo continent diversion. An orthotopic neobladder allows creation of a reservoir using detubularized ileum or colon with direct anastomosis to the urethra. With the development of orthotopic urinary diversion, functional status and quality of life among patients following cystectomy has improved significantly.

Adenocarcinoma of the Bladder

Adenocarcinomas account for less than 2% of bladder cancers. They are classified into three groups: primary bladder, urachal, and metastatic. Most adenocarcinomas are poorly differentiated and invasive. They are commonly associated with cystitis glandularis rather than CIS. Adenocarcinomas also are found in association with bladder augmentations. Adenocarcinoma is the most common type of cancer in patients with bladder exstrophy. Radical cystectomy with pelvic lymphadectomy is the treatment of choice.

Squamous Cell Carcinoma of the Bladder

Squamous cell carcinoma accounts for approximately 6% of bladder cancers in the United States but more than 75% of bladder cancers in Egypt. Chronic bladder inflammation, as occurs with chronic indwelling Foley catheters, recurrent bladder infections, or bladder diverticula, is associated with an increase risk of squamous cell carcinoma. Approximately 80% of squamous cell carcinomas in Egypt are associated with *Schistosoma haematobium* infestation. These cancers are known as bilharzial bladder cancers and occur in patients 10 to 20 years younger than those affected with transitional cell carcinoma. The prognosis for squamous cell carcinoma is generally poor, and radical cystectomy is the standard treatment for patients who are surgical candidates. Chemotherapy, particularly regimens used in transitional cell carcinoma, is not effective in squamous cell carcinoma. The benefit of neoadjuvant radiation therapy prior to radical cystectomy is unproved in patients with squamous cell carcinoma with the possible exception of bilharzial cancers.

---

[1]Not FDA approved for this indication.

CURRENT DIAGNOSIS

Urethral Carcinoma

- Urethral carcinoma is the only urologic malignancy that is more common in females than males.
- 50% of cases are associated with urethral stricture.
- May present as hematuria, obstructive voiding, or a palpable mass.
- Transurethral biopsy is usually required for diagnosis.

URETHRAL CARCINOMA

Diagnosis

Urethral carcinoma is the only urologic malignancy that is more common in women than men. It usually occurs after 60 years of age. Although the etiology remains undetermined, approximately 50% of cases are associated with urethral stricture. A patient should be evaluated for urethral carcinoma when a urethral mass is palpable, obstruction does not respond to conventional stricture management, a urethral abscess and/or fistula occurs, hematuria is present, or inguinal adenopathy becomes evident. The treatment of the primary tumor is surgical excision. Urethrectomy is performed via a perineal incision. Proximal tumors of the bulbar urethra are managed with cystoprostatectomy and en bloc urethrectomy.

Although the etiology of female urethral carcinoma remains obscure, there is an association with urethral malakoplakia and urethral caruncles. Most patients are white and older than 50 years. The usual presenting symptom is a papillary or fungating urethral mass and hematuria.

Treatment

For tumors of the proximal urethra or in cases of extension into adjacent structures, cystectomy with en bloc urethrectomy and anterior vaginectomy along with pelvic

CURRENT THERAPY

Urethral Carcinoma

- Treatment of the primary tumor is surgical excision and varies based on location and stage of tumor.
- In men, urethrectomy is performed via a perineal incision.
- Proximal tumors of the bulbar urethra are managed with cystoprostatectomy and en bloc urethrectomy.
- Among women, tumors of the proximal urethra or, in cases of extension, into adjacent structures, cystectomy with en bloc urethrectomy and anterior vaginectomy along with pelvic lymphadenectomy are usually required.
- Radiation therapy is also reported to provide local control in selective cases.

lymphadectomy are usually required. Radiation therapy also provides local control in selected cases. In advanced cases, multimodality treatment with chemotherapy and either surgical excision or radiation therapy provides the best chance for cure, although to date no specific regimen has emerged as standard treatment.

PENILE CANCER

Diagnosis

Penile cancer is relatively rare in the United States. Poor personal hygiene and retained phimotic foreskin are implicated in the etiology of penile carcinoma. Penile cancer is extremely rare in men circumcised at birth. Squamous cell carcinoma of the penis occurs most commonly in the sixth decade. The symptoms are related to ulceration, necrosis, suppuration, and hemorrhage of the penile lesion. The clinical evaluation of patients with penile cancer includes physical examination with palpation of the inguinal region, liver function tests, chest radiograph, CT of the abdomen and pelvis, and bone scan.

Treatment

The TNM stage is based primarily on depth of invasion and usually dictates treatment. Small penile cancers limited to the prepuce can be treated by circumcision alone. Partial penectomy with at least a 1-cm margin of normal tissue is used to treat smaller (2 to 5 cm) distal penile tumors. The remaining penis should be long enough to permit voiding in the standing position. The 5-year cure rate for patients treated with partial penectomy is 70% to 80%. Larger distal penile lesions or proximal tumors require total penectomy and perineal urethrostomy. If the scrotum, pubis, or abdominal wall is involved, radical en bloc excision may be necessary.

Many patients have inguinal lymphadenopathy at presentation. However, inguinal lymph node enlargement before excision of the primary tumor may be the result of infection and not metastatic disease. Clinical assessment of the inguinal region thus should be delayed 4 to 6 weeks during which time the patient is treated with antibiotics. If inguinal lymphadenopathy persists or develops, there is a high likelihood of metastatic disease, and ilioinguinal

lymphadenectomy should be performed. However, if inguinal lymphadenopathy resolves, prophylactic lymph node dissection may not be necessary. Radiation of the primary tumor and regional lymph nodes is an alternative to surgery in patients with small (2 cm or less) low-stage tumors.

TESTICULAR CANCER

Malignant disease of the testes can be divided into germinal neoplasms, which includes seminomatous and nonseminomatous germ cell tumors (NSGCTs) and secondary neoplasms. Ninety-five percent of tumors originating in the testis are germ cell tumors. Fewer than 10% of all germ cell tumors arise from extragonadal primary sites. The mediastinum and retroperitoneum are the most common extragonadal sites. Testicular cancer, although relatively rare, represents the most common malignancy in men in the 15- to 35-year-old age group, with 8010 new cases occurring annually.

Testicular cancer has become one of the most curable solid neoplasms and serves as a paradigm for the multimodal treatment of malignancies. The dramatic improvement in survival resulting from the combination of effective diagnostic techniques, improved tumor markers, effective multidrug chemotherapeutic regimens, and modifications of surgical technique has led to a decrease in patient mortality from greater than 50% before 1970 to less than 10% currently.

Germ cell tumors are seen principally in the white population. Recent data show a ratio of approximately 5:1 in white versus black individuals, and a report from the U.S. military showed a relative incidence of 40:1. The cause of germ cell tumors is unknown. Familial clustering is observed, particularly among siblings. Cryptorchidism and Klinefelter's syndrome are predisposing factors in the development of germ cell tumors arising from the testis and mediastinum, respectively. Orchidopexy performed before puberty may not reduce the risk of germ cell tumors but improves the ability to observe the testis.

Diagnosis

A painless testicular mass is pathognomonic of a primary testicular tumor. This occurs in a minority of patients. The majority of testicular tumors present with diffuse testicular pain, swelling, hardness, or some combination of these findings. Because infectious epididymo-orchitis is more common than a testicular tumor, a trial of antibiotics is often undertaken. If testicular discomfort does not abate or the findings do not revert to normal within 2 to 4 weeks, testicular sonography is indicated. A radical inguinal orchiectomy with ligation of the spermatic cord at the internal ring is required for all patients with suspected testicular tumors.

Regional metastasis first appears in the retroperitoneal lymph nodes below the renal vessels. Right testicular tumors usually metastasize to nodes between the aorta and inferior vena cava (interaortocaval nodes), and left testicular tumors to nodes lateral to the aorta (para-aortic). Left supraclavicular adenopathy and pulmonary nodules may occur with or without retroperitoneal disease. CT scan of the abdomen and pelvis and chest radiography are required. Lymph nodes in the primary lymphatic drainage areas (landing zones) of their respective affected testicle

that measure between 1 and 2 cm are involved by germ cell tumors in approximately 70% of cases. CT imaging of the chest is required if mediastinal, hilar, or lung parenchymal disease is suspected.

Treatment

Testicular cancer is one of the few neoplasms associated with accurate serum markers, human β-chorionic gonadotropin (β-hCG), and α-fetoprotein (AFP). These accurate tumor markers allow careful follow-up and intervention earlier in the course of disease. AFP production is restricted to NSGCTs, specifically embryonal carcinoma

CURRENT THERAPY

Testicular Cancer

- A radical inguinal orchiectomy with ligation of spermatic cord at the internal ring is required for all patients with suspected testicular tumors.
- Once a diagnosis is made, serum tumor markers are determined before, during, and after treatment.
- Radiographic staging is performed with a CT scan of the chest/abdomen/pelvis.
- Histologically, seminoma is the most common germ cell tumor, and is initially considered good risk because of its generally favorable response to treatment. Therapy for low-stage (stage 1, 2a, or 2b) seminomas following radical inguinal orchiectomy is irradiation to the retroperitoneal and ipsilateral pelvic lymph nodes. Relapse occurs in approximately 4% of patients with stage 1 seminomas and 10% of patients with stage 2a or 2b seminomas. Chemotherapy cures >90% of patients who have a relapse after radiation therapy. Thus, approximately 99% of patients with low-stage seminomas are cured.
- NSGCTs include embryonal cell carcinoma, choriocarcinoma, yolk sac carcinoma, teratoma, and mixed germ cell tumors. The rate of cure for patients with NSGCTs in clinical stage 1 exceeds 95%.
- Surveillance and RPLND are both standard treatment options for this group of patients. Twenty percent of clinical stage 1 NSGCT patients have lymph node involvement, and those with vascular invasion or predominance of embryonal cell carcinoma are at increased risk (50%).
- RPLND is a major abdominal operation in which lymph nodes from the retroperitoneum are removed from the renal hilum down to the level of the common iliac artery, with lateral margins being confined by the ureters.
- Patients found to have node-positive disease are generally recommended for chemotherapy with usually two cycles.
- Patients with persistently increased concentrations of AFP, β-hCG, or both but without other clinical evidence of disease following orchiectomy usually have systemic disease and are treated with chemotherapy.

CURRENT DIAGNOSIS

Testicular Cancer

- Testicular cancer, although relatively rare, represents the most common malignancy in males in the 15- to 35-year-old age group, with 8010 new cases annually.
- Usually presents as a painless enlarging testicular mass.
- Malignant disease of the testes can be divided into germinal neoplasms, which includes seminomatous and nonseminomatous germ cell tumors, and secondary neoplasms.
- 95% of tumors originating in the testis are germ cell tumors. Fewer than 10% of all germ cell tumors arise from extragonadal primary sites. The mediastinum and retroperitoneum are the most common extragonadal sites.
- Testicular cancer is one of the few neoplasms associated with accurate serum markers, β-hCG, and AFP.

Continued

CURRENT THERAPY—cont'd

Testicular Cancer

- Initial chemotherapy is required in approximately one third of patients with germ cell tumors. Because relapse is frequent in patients with clinical stage 2c disease or in patients with primary retroperitoneal or mediastinal seminomas who receive radiation alone, these patients are treated initially with chemotherapy. Patients also receive initial chemotherapy if they have stage 3 NSGCTs or multifocal retroperitoneal lymph node involvement, lymph nodes >3 cm in diameter, or tumor-related back pain.
- Postchemotherapy RPLND is usually reserved for residual masses (>3 cm) in patients after treatment for seminoma. In NSGCT, the need for postchemotherapy RPLND is controversial. Some advocate surgery in all patients with initial bulky retroperitoneal disease, whereas others advocate observation rather than surgery in patients with >90% shrinkage of retroperitoneal nodes, no residual nodes >1.5 cm, and no teratomatous elements in the primary tumor.
- Owing in part to the multimodality approach to these tumors, 90%–95% of patients are ultimately cured of their disease.

Abbreviations: AFP = α-fetoprotein; β-hCG = β-chorionic gonadotropin; CT = computed tomography; NSGCT = nonseminomatous germ cell tumor; RPLND = retroperitoneal lymph node dissection.

and yolk sac tumor. Patients with an increased AFP and the finding of pure seminoma on pathologic examination of the orchiectomy specimen should be treated as a NSGCT. Increased serum concentrations of β-hCG may be observed in both seminomatous and nonseminomatous tumors. Increased concentrations of β-hCG are seen in 40% to 60% of patients with metastatic NSGCT and 15% to 20% of patients with metastatic seminomas. A third serum marker, lactate dehydrogenase, is less specific but has independent prognostic value in patients with advanced germ cell tumors. Serum lactate dehydrogenase concentrations are also increased in approximately 60% of patients with NSGCT and 80% of those with seminomatous germ cell tumors.

Increased concentrations of α-fetoprotein, β-hCG, or both without radiographic or clinical findings imply active disease and are sufficient reason to initiate treatment if likely causes of false-positive results are ruled out. The serum half-lives of α-fetoprotein and β-hCG are 5 to 7 days and 30 hours, respectively. Slow clearance suggests residual active disease.

Histologically, seminoma is the most common germ cell tumor, and it is initially considered to be good risk because of its favorable response to treatment. Therapy for low-stage (stages 1, 2a, or 2b) seminomas following radical inguinal orchiectomy is irradiation to the retroperitoneal and ipsilateral pelvic lymph nodes. Relapse recurs in approximately 4% of patients with stage 1 seminomas and 10% of patients with stage 2a or 2b seminomas. Chemotherapy cures more than 90% of patients who have a relapse after radiation therapy. Thus, approximately 99% of patients with low-stage seminomas are cured.

NSGCTs include embryonal cell carcinoma, choriocarcinoma, yolk sac carcinoma, teratoma, and mixed germ cell tumors. The rate of cure for patients with NSGCTs in clinical stage 1 exceeds 95%. Twenty percent of patients with stage 1 tumors with no lymphatic or vascular invasion or invasion into the tunica albuginea, spermatic cord, or scrotum are discovered to have regional lymph node or distant metastasis. Surveillance and nerve-sparing retroperitoneal lymph node dissection (RPLND) are both standard treatment options for this group of patients. If patients have stage 1 disease confined to the testes, attention must be paid to the surgical pathology. In any patient with embryonal histology or the presence of lymphovascular invasion or extension beyond the tunica albuginea, RPLND is recommended. The rationale for this treatment stems from a 30% relapse rate in stage 1 patients with these findings.

RPLND is a major abdominal operation in which lymph nodes from the retroperitoneum are removed from the renal hilum down to the level of the common iliac artery, with lateral margins confined by the ureters. In the past, this procedure resulted in lack of ejaculation and infertility in 100% of patients. By performing a modified-template RPLND, the contralateral area of aorta below the inferior mesenteric artery is not manipulated. This maneuver serves to preserve the confluence of sympathetic fibers along the aorta that are responsible for ejaculation, with a 60% to 88% rate of preservation of ejaculation and no reports of recurrence for stage 1 disease. Patients with persistently increased concentrations of α-fetoprotein, β-hCG, or both but without other clinical evidence of disease following orchiectomy usually have systemic disease. These patients should undergo three or four cycles of standard chemotherapy rather than surgery.

Patients with stage 2 NSGCTs are treated initially with either RPLND or chemotherapy depending on the extent of the disease, serum tumor marker concentrations, and the presence or absence of tumor-related symptoms. Asymptomatic patients with solitary retroperitoneal lymph nodes less than 3 cm in diameter as assessed by CT imaging generally undergo retroperitoneal lymph node dissection, whereas bulky stage 2 disease (more than 5 cm) undergo initial chemotherapy. Recurrences within the retroperitoneum are rare after a properly performed operation.

Adjuvant chemotherapy is an important consideration when any lymph node is more than 2 cm in diameter, at least six nodes are involved, or there is extranodal invasion. The majority of patients in this group who relapsed did not receive adjuvant chemotherapy. Although the rate of cure is the same when chemotherapy is withheld until relapse, patients who received adjuvant therapy require fewer cycles of chemotherapy and avoid additional surgery.

Initial chemotherapy is required in approximately one third of patients with germ cell tumors. Because relapse is frequent in patients with clinical stage 2c disease or in patients with primary retroperitoneal or mediastinal seminomas who receive radiation alone, these patients are treated initially with chemotherapy. Patients also receive initial chemotherapy if they have stage 3 NSGCTs or multifocal retroperitoneal lymph node involvement, lymph nodes more than 2 cm in diameter, or tumor-related back pain.

Postchemotherapy RPLND is usually reserved for residual masses (more than 3 cm) in patients after treatment for seminoma. In NSGCT, the need for postchemotherapy RPLND is controversial. Some groups advocate surgery in all patients with initial bulky retroperitoneal disease, whereas others advocate observation rather than surgery in patients with greater than 90% shrinkage of retroperitoneal nodes, with no residual nodes greater than 1.5 cm, and with no teratomatous elements in the primary tumor. There is no debate, however, concerning the need for removal of any significant postchemotherapy residual mass.

The first combination chemotherapy regimens containing cisplatin (Platinol), vinblastine (Velban), and bleomycin (Blenoxane) resulted in complete remission in 70% to 80% of patients with metastatic germ cell tumors. Subsequent studies show that prolonged maintenance chemotherapy was unnecessary, and vinblastine was replaced by etoposide (Vepesid), which is less toxic and probably more efficacious. Serious adverse effects of combination chemotherapy include neuromuscular toxic affects, death from myelosuppression for bleomycin-induced pulmonary fibrosis, and Raynaud's phenomenon.

Leydig cell tumors make up between 1% and 3% of all testicular tumors. Although the majority of cases are recognized in men between 20 and 60 years of age, approximately a fourth are reported before puberty. The prognosis for Leydig cell tumors following radical inguinal orchiectomy is good because of their generally benign nature.

Gonadoblastoma is a rare tumor occurring almost exclusively in patients with some form of gonadal dysgenesis. Gonadoblastomas constitute approximately 0.5% of all testicular neoplasms and occur in all age groups from infancy to beyond 70 years, although the majority occur in individuals younger than 30 years. Radical orchiectomy is the first step in therapy. The high incidence of bilaterality (50%) mandates a contralateral gonadectomy when gonadal dysgenesis is present. The prognosis is excellent for patients with gonadoblastoma.

The most common secondary neoplasm of the testis and the most frequent of all testicular tumors in patients older than 50 years is lymphoma. The median age is approximately 60 years of age. As with lymphomas elsewhere, patients with poorly differentiated lymphocytic types tend to survive longer than those with the histocytic type. Survival is poor with bilateral disease and among patients presenting with lymphoma at other sites who later experience a testicular tumor relapse. However, among those patients with disease apparently confined to the testis, survival appears to be good.

REFERENCES

Carver BS, Sheinfeld J: Germ cell tumors of the testis. Ann Surg Oncol 2005;12:871.

Cohen HT, McGovern FJ: Renal-cell carcinoma. N Engl J Med 2005;353:2477.

Cooperberg MR, Moul JW, Carroll PR: The changing face of prostate cancer. J Clin Oncol 2005;23:8146.

Jemal A, Murray T, Ward E, et al: Cancer statistics, 2005. CA Cancer J Clin 2005;55:10.

Stein JP, Lieskovsky G, Cote R, et al: Radical cystectomy in the treatment of invasive bladder cancer: Long-term results in 1,054 patients. J Clin Oncol 2001;19:666.

Management of Urethral Stricture Disease*

Method of
Andrew C. Peterson, MD

Urethral strictures are defined as an area of narrowing in the urethra, usually occurring from scar tissue formation. The strictures may occur anywhere in the urethra from the bladder to the meatus of the penis. They are well documented in ancient literature dating from the Greek and Egyptian period. Urethral stricture disease is relatively common today, mostly acquired from injury or infection. Recently, iatrogenic causes, including urologic instrumentation and placement of indwelling catheters, that cause strictures anywhere in the urethra are the most common cause.

The urethra is commonly described as having two sections: the posterior urethra (starting at the bladder neck, including the prostatic urethra and membranous urethra) and the anterior urethra (starting at the bulbar urethra, including the pendulous urethra and the fossa navicularis and meatus). Posterior urethral strictures are commonly caused by trauma with pelvic fractures and concomitant urethral injuries. Anterior urethral injuries commonly result from direct, blunt penile or perineal trauma, instrumentation, catheterization, and infections.

Diagnosis and Preoperative Evaluation

Obstructive voiding symptoms are the most common complaints causing patients to seek medical attention, including decreased force of stream, hesitancy, urgency, nocturia, and sometimes acute urinary retention. Urinary tract infections, urethral bleeding, and, rarely, urethrocutaneous fistula and periurethral abscess may develop. Young men diagnosed with recurrent epididymitis and so-called prostatitis should be completely evaluated for urethral strictures because this is often a missed diagnosis in these cases.

---

*The views expressed in this article are those of the author and do not reflect the official policy or position of the United States Army, Department of Defense, or the U.S. government.

CURRENT DIAGNOSIS

- Young men with recurrent so-called prostatitis and epididymitis should be considered for workup of urethral stricture disease.
- Obstructive voiding symptoms are the most common complaints causing patients to seek medical attention for urethral stricture disease.
- The retrograde urethrogram is the key diagnostic study for evaluation of urethral stricture disease.

Retrograde urethrography (RUG) is the study of choice for diagnosis. An antegrade voiding study through a previously placed suprapubic tube combined with a RUG often helps define the length and complexity of the stricture. Penile ultrasound may also help define the extent of spongiofibrosis and aid in planning for a surgical reconstruction.

Cystourethroscopy allows for identification of the true caliber of a urethral stricture, and a small flexible ureteroscope may be used to determine the length of the stricture and the quality of the proximal urethra. It may be important to examine the bladder through a suprapubic tract as well for concomitant injury and bladder calculi.

Magnetic resonance imaging (MRI) studies can be invaluable in some cases of posterior urethral strictures after pelvic fracture. This is an important study to define the post-traumatic anatomy, allowing the surgeon to plan the reconstructive approach. MRI should always be used in conjunction with RUG and cystogram and not as a sole technique for evaluation.

Management

After the final diagnosis and staging of the urethral stricture are completed, the choice of treatment depends heavily on location, etiology, and length. Treatment options for urethral strictures continue to include simple dilation, incision of the urethral stricture using endoscopes (urethrotomy), the UroLume stent, and a wide spectrum of reconstructive surgical techniques that include possible use of skin flaps, skin grafts, and more complex reconstructive techniques. Although no single procedure is appropriate for all strictures, dilation and urethrotomy continue to be most commonly employed. However, these interventions have high recurrence rates, and many patients eventually progress to surgical repair.

DILATION AND URETHROTOMY

Office/clinic dilation of urethral stricture continues to be the most common initial treatment and is often the first treatment attempted. Techniques used in the office include filiforms and followers, serial dilators, and balloon dilation under endoscopic control. Afterward, patients can be taught self-calibration with a soft catheter for ongoing management. Few patients, however, accept this option in the long term.

Visual internal urethrotomy is performed using local, spinal, or general anesthesia and is ideally aided by a guidewire placed through the stricture under direct vision. The incision is made at either the 12 o'clock or at the 3 and 9 o'clock positions with a cold knife, laser, or cautery. Urethrotomy is especially suited for short strictures in the bulbar urethra and has high failure rates for long strictures associated with significant spongiofibrosis and those located in the pendulous urethra.

Although both of these procedures may be curative, most often the patient requires retreatment. Both dilation and internal urethrotomy have equivalent long-term outcomes for the treatment of short urethral strictures. In those who ultimately require formal operative repair, there is not a higher failure rate if that patient first underwent a prior endoscopic treatment. Therefore, this practice of initial treatment of short urethral strictures with repeat dilations or internal urethrotomies may be reasonable.

UROLUME STENTS

The UroLume stent (American Medical Systems, Minnetonka, MN) is a permanent, self-expanding metal stent that is FDA approved for the treatment of bulbar urethral strictures. Enthusiastically introduced in 1988, postplacement problems, including postvoid dribbling, perineal pain, erectile pain, and recurrent stricture, significantly limited the use of this device. It is helpful to manage recalcitrant anastomotic bladder neck contracture following radical prostatectomy and in the very elderly who may not be able to tolerate an open operative repair of a urethral stricture.

SURGICAL INTERVENTION

Surgical options for urethral stricture disease are based primarily on the location and length of the stricture. Tissue, including local grafts or flaps from the penis or scrotum and grafts from remote sources such as mouth, thigh, and preauricular areas, often are needed to reconstruct the urethra. Buccal graft harvested from the mouth currently has the most support.

Management of Strictures in the Pendulous Urethra

Optimal management of strictures of the pendulous urethra consists of onlay flap repairs using penile skin as described by Orandi, Quartey, McAninch, Turner-Warwick, and Mundy. Strictures from lichen sclerosis, however, require significantly different treatment (see later). The stricture is opened on the ventral side of the penis and the incision carried into healthy urethra on either side. It is then patched with an island of skin carried on a vascular pedicle. Although the ideal skin consists of hairless penile skin, island flaps can be made in the longitudinal or a transverse orientation and may reach up to 15 cm in length and 2 cm in width. Even circumcised men invariably have ample penile skin for these flaps.

CURRENT THERAPY

- Office/clinic dilation of urethral stricture continues to be the most common initial treatment and is often the first treatment attempted.
- Both dilation and internal urethrotomy have equivalent long-term outcomes for the treatment of short urethral strictures.
- Surgical options for urethral stricture disease are based primarily on the location and length of the stricture.
- In treatment of lichen sclerosis, all of the native surrounding genital skin is subject to this disease so the entire affected urethra must often be excised and replaced with extragenital tissue for reconstruction

Bulbar Strictures

Historically, flap-based repairs and tubularized single-staged graft urethroplasties were often performed for these strictures. However, these had a failure rate up to 56%, and currently the interest has shifted to excision of tight segments of the stricture and use of grafts (ideally buccal) to augment the anastomosis or to address the stricture in its entirety.

For strictures less than 2 cm long, stricture excision and primary reanastomosis remains the ideal procedure with excellent reported long-term results exceeding 90% success rates (Figure 1). For strictures measuring 2 to 4 cm, the latest evolution is the excisional augmented anastomotic urethroplasty. In this procedure, the worst section of the stricture is excised and the repair is augmented with a buccal graft or other onlay (Figure 2). Long strictures where segmental excision is not feasible are best managed with a dorsal onlay alone without excision (Figure 3). Occasionally, very long and dense strictures require a staged repair. Depending on the clinical situation, the entire urethra may need to be excised, replacing with a flat grafted area of buccal mucosa tissue, split-thickness skin graft from the thigh or other areas such as preauricular skin, and rarely bladder or rectal mucosa. The graft is allowed to heal for 6 to 12 months after which the patient is brought back to the operating room for tubularization.

Strictures from Lichen Sclerosis (Balanitis Xerotica Obliterans)

Balanitis xerotica obliterans, first described in 1928, is a form of lichen sclerosis (LS) and occurs in up to 1 in 300 men. The cause is unclear, and changes from LS most commonly occur in the glans penis and prepuce, causing phimosis

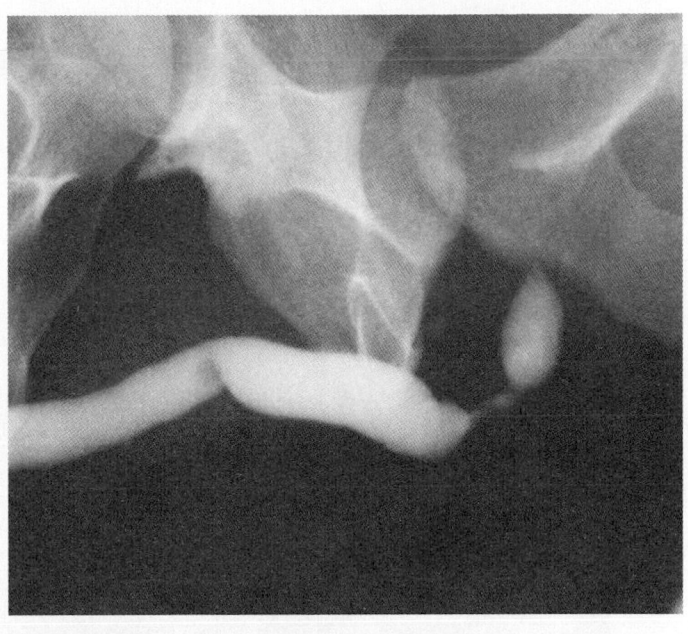

FIGURE 2. Retrograde urethrogram showing a longer, more complex, bulbar urethral stricture needing excision of the most significant area of stricture and onlay of the remaining stricture: the excisional, augmented anastomotic urethroplasty.

with more extensive disease affecting the urethra as far back as the midbulb (Figure 4).

Management includes medications and surgery. Topical steroids, such as clobetasol (Temovate),[1] 0.05% cream applied two to four times daily, may cause significant regression of the scarring process. Surgical therapy ranges

---

[1]Not FDA approved for this indication.

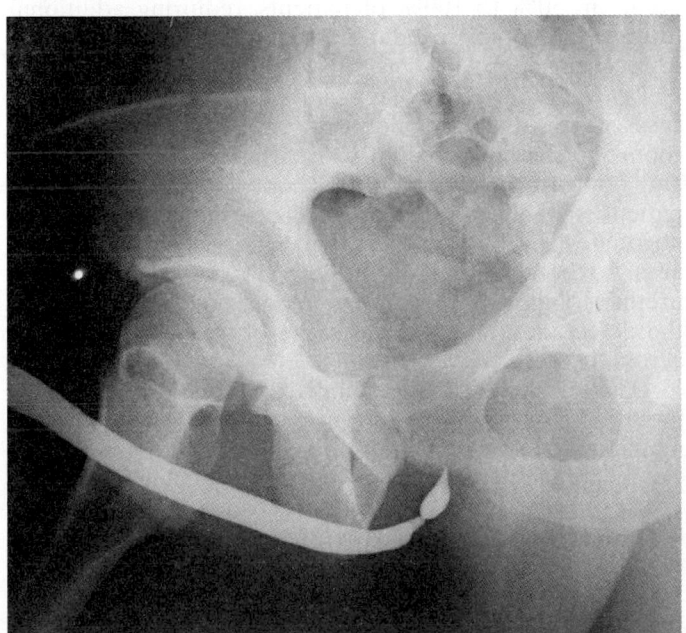

FIGURE 1. Retrograde urethrogram showing a short bulbar urethral stricture amenable to excision with primary anastomosis.

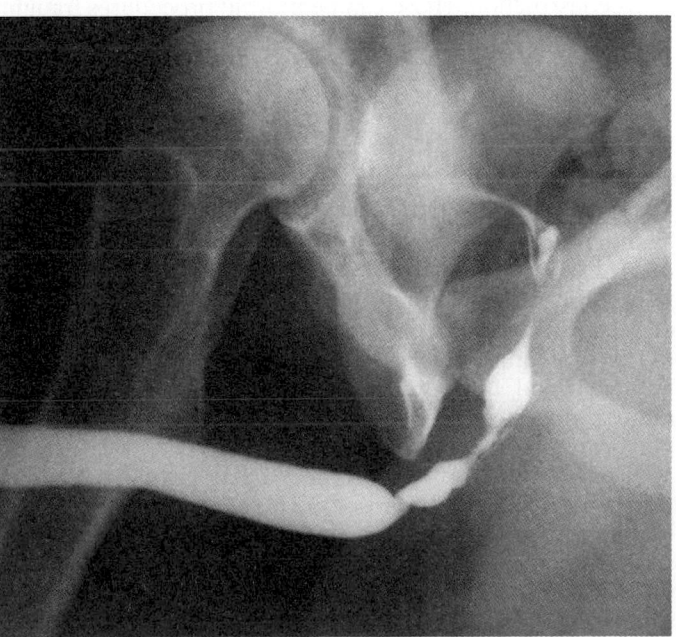

FIGURE 3. Retrograde urethrogram showing a very long and complex stricture needing repair with dorsal onlay.

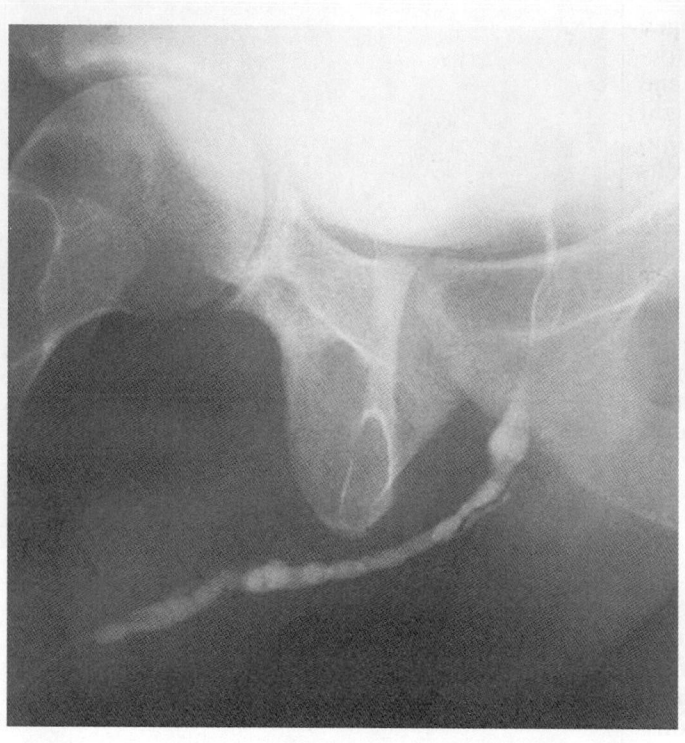

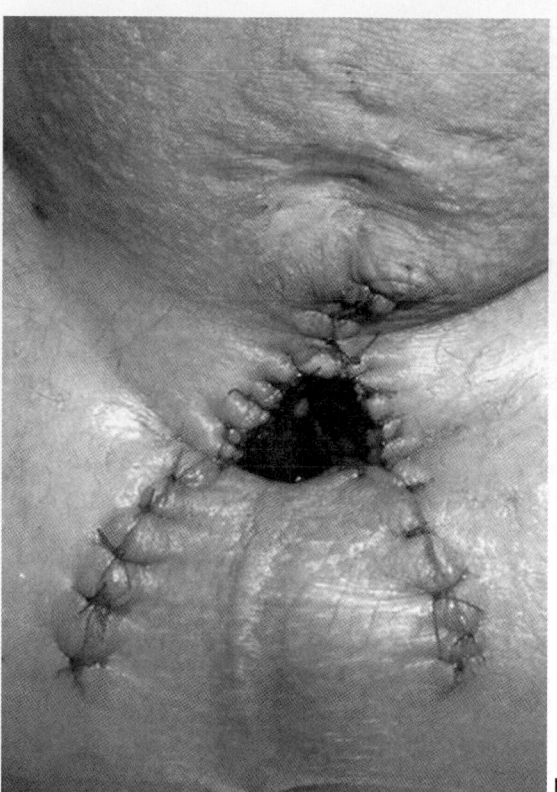

FIGURE 4. Retrograde urethrogram (**A**) showing a pan-pendulous urethral stricture from lichen sclerosis. These may be repaired with complex staged reconstruction. However, a simple perineal urethrostomy (**B**) may be appropriate for some patient populations.

from extended simple meatotomy for distal strictures to complex staged repairs for more extensive disease. Because all of the native surrounding genital skin is subject to progression of LS, the entire affected urethra must often be excised and replaced with extragenital tissue for reconstruction. These can be morbid procedures fraught with complications and high failure rates up to 71%. Placement of a perineal urethrostomy may provide a good alternative to complex staged repair (Figure 4).

Posterior Urethral Strictures

Traumatic injury to the prostatomembranous urethra occurs in approximately 10% of pelvic fractures. This injury may range from urethral elongation without tearing of the urethra to complete transection. With any suspicion of urethral injury in a pelvic trauma patient, a RUG should be performed. If no extravasation is seen, a Foley catheter may be inserted and a cystogram or upper tract study performed as indicated.

When a catheter cannot be placed into the bladder through the urethra because of a posterior urethral injury, bladder drainage should be managed acutely with a suprapubic (SP) catheter. Definitive treatment after 3 to 6 months of recovery allows resolution of hematoma and shortening of the defect. Acute surgical intervention is indicated only in the uncommon situations where there is an associated rectal, bladder, or bladder neck injury or when there is another indication for laparotomy.

Immediate (primary) realignment is performed without the preceding indications using a variety of techniques. All involve the acute placement of a catheter across the urethral defect with magnetic guides, interlocking guides, or an open surgical procedure. Long-term restricturing occurs in 50% to 100% of patients, requiring additional future endoscopic procedures, intermittent catheterization, or reconstruction.

Delayed (primary) management is an alternative in cases whose recovery allows for return to the operating room 5 to 10 days after injury. An SP tube is placed acutely and realignment accomplished endoscopically when the patient is stable. An antegrade placed flexible endoscope negotiates the bladder neck and emerges in the injured area. A second retrograde endoscope is placed through the urethra to allow for hematoma irrigation, visualization of the defect, and antegrade passage of a stenting catheter across the defect.

Delayed (secondary) repair is delayed for 3 or more months following the injury; in the interim the patient is managed by SP catheter drainage. Most of these defects can be repaired with a one-stage perineal anastomotic urethroplasty. This remarkably versatile procedure manages long obliterative strictures well in more than 95% of cases.

The progressive perineal anastomotic repair involves the mobilization of the urethra with transection at the point of obliteration. The bulbar urethra is then reconnected to the prostatomembranous urethra proximal to the obliteration. Depending on the length of the repair needed, one to four of the following well-described sequential steps are used to accomplish a tension free anastomosis:

1. Circumferential mobilization of the distal urethra provides 2 to 3 cm of length sufficient for anastomosis in 8% of cases.
2. Separation of the proximal corporal bodies shortens the distance by 1 to 2 cm and is sufficient for anastomosis in another 41% of cases.
3. Inferior pubectomy with resection of a wedge of bone from the inferior surface of the pubis further shortens the defect by 1 to 2 cm, facilitating anastomosis in another 28% of cases.
4. Rerouting the urethra around the lateral surface of a corporal body provides another 1 to 2 cm of length and is needed for the remaining 23% of cases.

Future Trends

The current evolution is pointing toward development and acceptance of artificial tissue replacements, allografts, and xenografts for the urethra, obviating the need for graft harvesting. These include Apligraf, a bioengineered product composed of a bovine-collagen fibroblast-containing matrix integrated with a sheet of stratified human epithelium that is similar to human skin. Also, many are currently developing a promising off-the-shelf collagen matrix based on cultured human cadaveric bladder mucosa.

REFERENCES

Attwater HL: History of urethral stricture. BJU Int 1943;15:39.
Barbagli G, Palminteri E, Lazzeri M, et al: Long-term outcome of urethroplasty after failed urethrotomy versus primary repair. J Urol 2001;165(6 Pt 1):1918-1919.
Barbagli G, Selli C, Tosto A, Palminteri E: Dorsal free graft urethroplasty. J Urol 1996;155(1):123-126.
Depasquale I, Park AJ, Bracka A: The treatment of balanitis xerotica obliterans. BJU Int 2000;86(4):459-465.
El Kassaby AW, Retik AB, Yoo JJ, Atala A: Urethral stricture repair with an off-the-shelf collagen matrix. J Urol 2003;169(1):170-173.
Flynn BJ, Delvecchio FC, Webster GD: Perineal repair of pelvic fracture urethral distraction defects: Experience in 120 patients during the last 10 years. J Urol 2003;170:1877-1880.
Glass RE, Flynn JT, King JB, Blandy JP: Urethral injury and fractured pelvis. Br J Urol 1978;50(7):578-582.
Guralnick ML, Webster GD: The augmented anastomotic urethroplasty: Indications and outcome in 29 patients. J Urol 2001;165(5):1496-1501.
Iselin CE, Webster GD: Dorsal onlay graft urethroplasty for repair of bulbar urethral stricture. J Urol 1999;161(3):815-818.
Kane CJ, Tarman GJ, Summerton DJ, et al: Multi-institutional experience with buccal mucosa onlay urethroplasty for bulbar urethral reconstruction. J Urol 2002;167(3):1314-1317.
McAninch JW: Reconstruction of extensive urethral strictures: circular fasciocutaneous penile flap. J Urol 1993;149(3):488-491.
Orandi A: One-stage urethroplasty. Br J Urol 1968;40(6):717-719.
Quartey JK: One-stage penile/preputial island flap urethroplasty for urethral stricture. J Urol 1985;134(3):474-475.
Santucci RA, Mario LA, McAninch JW: Anastomotic urethroplasty for bulbar urethral stricture: Analysis of 168 patients. J Urol 2002;167(4):1715-1719.
Steenkamp JW, Heyns CF, de Kock ML: Internal urethrotomy versus dilation as treatment for male urethral strictures: A prospective, randomized comparison. J Urol 1997;157(1):98-101.
Venn SN, Mundy AR: Urethroplasty for balanitis xerotica obliterans. Br J Urol 1998;81(5):735-737.
Webster GD, Ramon J: Repair of pelvic fracture posterior urethral defects using an elaborated perineal approach: Experience with 74 cases. J Urol 1991;145(4):744-748.
Webster GD, Sihelnik S: The management of strictures of the membranous urethra. J Urol 1985;134(3):469-473.

Renal Calculi

Method of
Nicholas J. Hegarty, MD, FRCS,
and Stevan B. Streem, MD

Urolithiasis affects 5% to 15% of adults and the incidence of stone disease appears to be increasing. Calcium stones are the most frequent, and they present most often between the 3rd and 5th decades of life. They are two to three times more common in males than females. Incidence is threefold higher in whites than African Americans with people of Asian or Hispanic background having an intermediate incidence. More than one half of those presenting with their first stone episode will suffer a second stone event within 10 years. Thus, there are two important considerations in approaching patients with stone disease: the management of the initial stone episode and the prevention of further stone formation.

Presentation and Initial Management

The most common presenting symptom is acute onset flank pain. This is generally described as severe and colicky in nature, but may be mild. Pain may radiate anteriorly, to the groin and ipsilateral testis or labia. Associated symptoms may include nausea and diaphoresis. Patients are often restless, moving about in an attempt to obtain relief. Other than indicating the side of the stone, pain location does not correlate well with the position of the stone in the ureter. The onset of irritative bladder symptoms, however, suggests progression of the stone to the ureterovesical junction. The presence of fever or systemic symptoms is worrisome as they suggest the coexistence of a urinary tract infection and the need for urgent treatment (Figure 1). Physical examination may reveal upper quadrant or renal angle tenderness, but no guarding nor rebound, which indicates peritonitis. Basic investigations include urinalysis and microscopy, which usually, but not invariably, show the presence of red blood cells. A pregnancy test is performed in women of childbearing age prior to abdominal imaging, and blood urea nitrogen (BUN) creatinine, and electrolytes are performed prior to the administration of contrast, in order to give an indication of renal function. Pain relief should not be delayed and requires a nonsteroidal anti-inflammatory drug (NSAID) such as ketorolac (Toradol), 30 mg every 6 hours, or opiates such as morphine sulfate or meperidine (Demerol), 1mg/kg every 8 hours, or a combination of these.

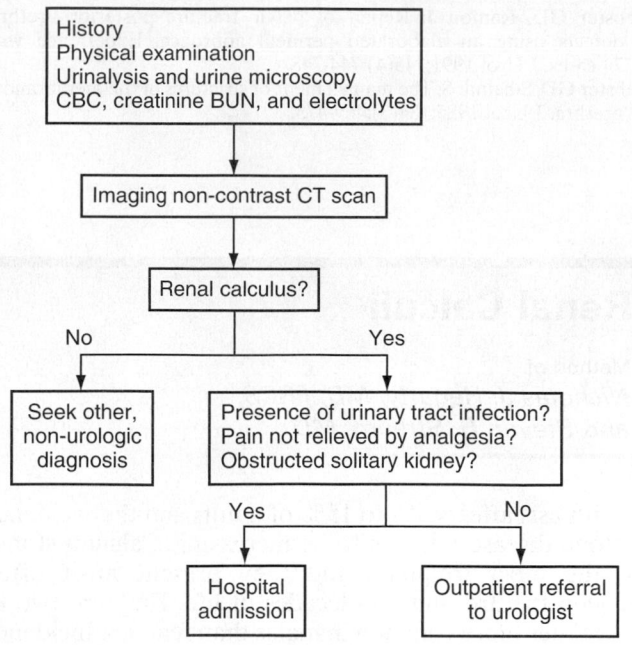

History
Physical examination
Urinalysis and urine microscopy
CBC, creatinine BUN, and electrolytes

↓

Imaging non-contrast CT scan

↓

Renal calculus?

No ← → Yes

Seek other, non-urologic diagnosis

Presence of urinary tract infection?
Pain not relieved by analgesia?
Obstructed solitary kidney?

Yes ← → No

Hospital admission

Outpatient referral to urologist

FIGURE 1. Acute stone episode algorithm.

Imaging

Radiologic imaging is performed to confirm the diagnosis and determine stone size, location, and degree of obstruction. Other findings that may influence treatment are urinary tract anatomy and ipsilateral and overall renal function. Local availability and the clinical setting influence the choice and combination of imaging technique(s). Abdominal plain radiograph will reveal more than 90% of calcium-containing stones, but small stones or those composed of uric acid or cystine are difficult to visualize. Renal ultrasound can demonstrate shadowing of renal stones and hydronephrosis, but is limited in showing ureteral calculi. Intravenous pyelogram (IVP) is the traditional urologic investigation of choice, as it identifies the location of stones in the collecting system. It offers some functional detail and demonstrates the presence or absence of obstruction and any renal or ureteral anomalies. However, it does require exposure to radiographs and intravenous iodine-based contrast. It can also be quite time-consuming, particularly if there is delayed excretion secondary to obstruction. In most centers, noncontrast computed tomography (CT) has superseded IVP. It has greater sensitivity and specificity comparable with that of IVP. All stones, other than certain drug-related crystals, are visualized by this method. Thin-cut spiral CT can be performed in one breath hold and can also provide details of nonurologic causes of abdominal pain. Magnetic resonance urography has little role in stone disease, but may be considered in pregnancy or a patient who has a complex genitourinary anatomy. In some chronic and complicated cases, radionuclide studies are performed to assess remaining function in a compromised kidney, prior to deciding between stone removal and nephrectomy.

Indications for Intervention

The presence of ureteral calculus and urinary tract infection constitutes a surgical emergency that requires prompt intervention. Impaired function in the obstructed kidney mandates an increase in antimicrobial dosage (intravenous administration is usually required). Drainage, either by percutaneous nephrostomy or retrograde stent placement, further assists the resolution of infection prior to considering definitive management. Similarly, an obstructing calculus in an anatomically or functionally solitary kidney may result in anuria and acute renal failure. In general, there is less urgency associated with the treatment of stones and many can be treated expectantly if pain control is sufficient. Stone size is the single most important determinant of the likelihood of spontaneous stone passage. The majority of stones less than 5 mm can be expected to pass, whereas almost all stones greater than 8 mm will require intervention. Along with analgesia, hydration and activity are recommended (although there is, in fact, little evidence to suggest these measures result in an improved outcome). Studies of ureteral physiology have proposed a number of strategies including calcium channel blockers,[1] steroids,[1] and phosphodiesterase inhibitors.[1] Perhaps the most promising of these are the α-adrenergic blocking agents.[1] The vesicoureteral junction is rich in α-adrenergic receptors. Oral administration of α_1-blockers in the acute stone episode reduces analgesic requirements and results in more rapid and higher overall rates of spontaneous stone passage. Experience with their use in benign prostatic hyperplasia has shown their safety, tolerability, and freedom from interaction with other drug groups (other than phosphodiesterase inhibitors). How long to wait is a question that remains unanswered. With complete obstruction, renal damage is evident at 2 weeks and irreversible damage at 6 weeks, although truly "complete" obstruction rarely develops from ureteral calculi. Longer periods of partial or intermittent obstruction can be tolerated, and many studies show few untoward effects in the follow-up of nonobstructing distal ureteral calculi after 1 year. Nevertheless, we feel that failure to progress at 4 to 6 weeks probably corresponds to a high probability that the stone is unlikely to progress with further observation. We generally recommend intervention at this stage if there has been no caudal stone movement.

Interventional Options

SHOCK WAVE LITHOTRIPSY

Shock wave lithotripsy (SWL) is a noninvasive technique whereby shock waves from an external source bring about stone fragmentation. Radiograph fluoroscopy, ultrasound, or dual imaging is used to bring the stone to the focal point of the shock wave generator. Typical treatments are comprised of 3000 shock waves, and, in most cases, the procedure is performed as an outpatient. It is an option for patients with relatively small renal and ureteral

---

[1]Not FDA approved for this indication.

stones—although the need for re-treatment is higher than some other minimally invasive alternatives. SWL is less invasive than ureteroscopy or percutaneous management, and its side-effect profile is less. Cystine and calcium oxalate monohydrate stones are resistant to fragmentation by SWL, and radiolucent uric acid stones may pose difficulty with focusing. Obesity may also give rise to difficulty with stone visualization, and dissipation of shock wave energy by excessive interposed adipose tissue can reduce treatment efficacy. Reduced power settings are recommended in children to protect the growing kidney. Use can be extended to stones larger than 1 cm in children, but ureteral stenting is often required to prevent obstruction as fragments are passing. The presence of distal ureteral obstruction is a contraindication to SWL, and certain abnormalities of collecting system anatomy, particularly in dependent lower poles, may preclude drainage of stone debris, despite successful fragmentation.

URETEROSCOPY

Ureteroscopy or ureterorenoscopy can be performed with rigid, semirigid, or flexible scopes. It provides direct visualization of stones during manipulation and extraction. Early series reported a 2% to 6% rate of ureteral injury or perforation. We recommend the use of a floppy-tipped safety wire in all cases, as this allows placement of a ureteral stent if injury occurs, or in the rare instance that an impacted stone cannot be removed. Two wires are required for flexible ureteroscopy—a working wire, for introducing a ureteral access sheath or guiding the flexible scope into the ureter, and a safety wire. Large stones require fragmentation prior to extraction. A number of modalities are available, the most frequently used being holmium laser lithotripsy. Laser fibers allow stone break-up with little propulsion of fragments. The holmium laser is capable of fragmenting all stone types, but care must be taken to avoid ureteral damage. Laser fibers are suitable for use in rigid, semirigid, and flexible ureteroscopes, and most centers now use a holmium laser almost exclusively as the fragmentation modality of choice.

PERCUTANEOUS EXTRACTION

This is recommended for renal stones greater than 1 to 1.5 cm and stones refractory to SWL. Fragmentation can be accomplished with an ultrasound wand or, more recently, a single device combining both ultrasound and pneumatic lithotripsy. Laser fragmentation is considerably slower but can be used with a flexible scope to access difficult calyces or the ureter in an antegrade manner. Fragments inaccessible to percutaneous management can be treated by SWL to achieve greater stone clearance rates. Percutaneous surgery also allows correction of coexisting infundibular stenosis or ureteropelvic junction (UPJ) obstruction. The indications for open or laparoscopic surgery are progressively fewer, and today such management is applied to less than 1% of stone patients requiring intervention. Nephrectomy is an option for a stone-bearing kidney with irreversible loss of function (with a differential function less than 10% to 15% on radionuclide scanning).

<table>
<tr><td colspan="2">BOX 1   General Recommendations for All Calcium Stone Formers</td></tr>
<tr><td colspan="2">

General dietary measures include the following:
- Fluid intake >2 liters per day
- Low sodium (<4 g NaCl per day)
- Normal calcium intake
- Oxalate restriction
- Moderate protein restriction
- Low fat, high fiber diet
- Avoidance of vitamin C and D supplements

</td></tr>
</table>

Stone Prevention

General recommendations can be given to reduce the incidence of further stones. These include maintaining adequate hydration and reducing intake of dietary purines, oxalates, and vitamin supplements (Box 1). Opinions differ on which patients should undergo metabolic evaluation, when they should be tested, and how extensive testing should be. A comparable incidence of finding a treatable abnormality is found in those presenting with their first stone as compared with subsequent stones. However, full investigation of all stone formers would incur considerable expense and inconvenience for such a large patient group. This has prompted some units to propose an abbreviated investigation for the majority of patients, with full investigation for a small minority. In our unit, we recommend complete investigation for those who are likely to require medical treatment (Box 2). Serum studies include electrolytes, creatinine, BUN, calcium, phosphorus, and uric acid. The need for more detailed investigations with further tests such as parathyroid studies should be assessed based on initial results. A single, 24-hour urinary collection is taken, with the patient on a normal diet. Urinary volume, creatinine, calcium, citrate, oxalate, uric acid, and sodium are all measured. A creatinine value of 1 to 2 g per day is an important indicator of a properly collected specimen. The most frequently detected abnormalities are hypercalciuria, hyperuricosuria, hypocitraturia, hyperoxaluria, and a combination of these.

HYPERCALCIURIA

In the absence of hypercalcemia, hypercalciuria is termed idiopathic. It may be considered absorptive or "renal leak," but we do not differentiate between them as both represent an increased sensitivity to vitamin D and respond to thiazide diuretics (hydrochlorothiazide, 25 to 50 mg per day).[1] Thiazides reduce the urine calcium load by increasing its tubular absorption and increasing calcium availability to the bones. Calcium supplements are restricted to 600 mg daily, but we do not restrict dietary calcium because longitudinal studies show that dietary calcium restriction may promote stone formation, and because creating a negative calcium balance promotes bone resorption and

---

[1]Not FDA approved for this indication.

BOX 2 Metabolic Evaluation

Serum
- Blood urea nitrogen
- Creatinine
- Sodium
- Potassium
- Chloride
- Calcium
- Phosphorus
- Uric acid
- Parathormone*

24-Hour Urine
- Volume
- Creatinine
- Calcium
- Citrate
- Oxalate
- Uric acid
- Sodium
- Cystine†

Stone Analysis
- Calcium oxalate
- Calcium phosphate
- Uric acid
- Struvite
- Cystine

---

*Parathormone levels performed if calcium elevated or phosphorus low.
†Test for urinary cystine if cystine stone on stone analysis or family history of cystine stones.

 CURRENT DIAGNOSIS

- **General**
  Consider and rule out life-threatening causes of acute abdominal pain (e.g., abdominal aortic aneurysm rupture).
  Rule out concurrent urinary tract infection.
- **Imaging**
  Computed tomography stone protocol provides greatest sensitivity and specificity.
- **Metabolic**
  Full metabolic workup is indicated in those likely to require medical treatment.
  Serum studies, stone analysis, and a single 24-hour urine usually provide sufficient information to guide treatment.

---

osteoporosis. We routinely recommend dietary sodium restriction, as a high sodium intake increases urinary calcium, especially in hypercalciuric patients.

HYPERURICOSURIA

Hyperuricosuria may be primary or secondary to high dietary purine intake. If it persists with dietary restriction, allopurinol (Zyloprim), 300 mg daily, should be commenced. Persistent acid urine and elevated serum uric acid suggest gout. Treatment is aimed at alkalinization of the urine with potassium citrate (Urocit K), 10 to 20 mEq three or four times per day, or sodium bicarbonate.

HYPOCITRATURIA

Acidosis inhibits citrate production causing hypocitraturia. Most often, it is associated with alkaline loss from inflammatory bowel disease (IBD) or hypokalemia connected with thiazide use. IBD may also cause malabsorption of citrate. Treatment is aimed at correcting the underlying condition and citrate replacement (typically Urocit K, 30 to 60 mEq per day). Marked hypocitraturia may suggest the presence of renal tubular acidosis. Usually, there will be an associated hyperchloremic, hypokalemic acidosis. Where electrolytes are normal, an acid load test may be considered to confirm the diagnosis.

HYPEROXALURIA

Hyperoxaluria may result from endogenous, or, more frequently, exogenous sources. Endogenous causes include congenital deficiencies of glyoxylate transamination or oxidation, excess vitamin C ingestion, or pyridoxine deficiency. Hydration, vitamin C restriction, and dietary oxalate restriction are recommended initially. In those with persistent hyperoxaluria, vitamin B_6 (pyridoxine),[1] starting at 200 mg daily, may be effective. Exogenous causes include malabsorption from previous gastrointestinal surgery or inflammatory bowel disease. Malabsorption promotes saponification of calcium. There is less calcium available to bind oxalate in the gut, which is then absorbed in greater quantities. Treatment is the same as for endogenous causes, along with treatment of the underlying condition. Calcium citrate may reverse metabolic acidosis and increase oxalate binding in the gut. In those with stones from jejunoileal bypass, bypass reversal may be required if stones cannot otherwise be controlled.

Cystine Stones

Cystinuria is an autosomal recessive condition characterized by abnormal intestinal and renal absorption of dibasic amino acids (cystine, ornithine, lysine, and arginine). Excess urinary cystine leads to stone formation in a minority of patients. Initial treatment is aimed at increasing the solubility of cystine by increasing fluid intake to 2 to 3 L per day and alkalinization with citrate or bicarbonate. If this fails, D-penicillamine (Cuprimine) 1.5 to 2 mg per day or α-mercaptopropionyl-glycine (Thiola), 800 to 1200 mg per day, should be commenced.

Staghorn Calculi

Typically these are infective (struvite) in nature, but may also be composed of uric acid, cystine, or calcium oxalate. Infection-related stones form only in the setting of

---

[1]Not FDA approved for this indication.

CURRENT THERAPY

Acute Stone Event

- Pain relief to be instituted and diagnosis established.
- Choice of treatment influenced by position and size of stone, patient comorbidity and preference, and available treatment modalities.
- α-Adrenergic blockade[1] may facilitate spontaneous stone passage.
- Presence of urinary tract infection, persistent pain, obstruction in a solitary kidney, and patient social circumstances may mandate prompt intervention.

Intervention

- Minimally invasive techniques have all but replaced open stone surgery.
- Shock wave lithotripsy is suitable first-line treatment for small ureteral and renal calculi.
- Ureteroscopy has higher treatment success rates, but is more invasive than SWL.
- In an otherwise healthy patient, staghorn calculi, even when asymptomatic, should be treated.
- Percutaneous extraction is the first-line treatment for most patients with large stones, and certainly for staghorn calculi.

Stone Prevention

- Hydration and general stone preventive measures should be recommended to all stone formers.
- Medical treatment is tailored to the individual patient, based on lifestyle and metabolic findings.
- Metabolic abnormalities frequently coexist.

[1]Not FDA approved for this indication.

urease-producing organisms, and patients typically have a high urinary pH. Untreated, these tend to result in chronic pyelonephritis with atrophy of the kidney or life-threatening pyonephrosis. Unless the patient's condition precludes treatment, it is generally recommended that staghorn calculi be treated, that is, removed. Infection remains within the stone matrix and is probably impossible to completely eradicate in the presence of the stone. Percutaneous extraction is the treatment of choice for most staghorn calculi. The position and number of access tracts will be determined by the stone morphology and anatomy of the collecting system. Repeat procedures may be required or SWL may be used to treat remaining or inaccessible fragments. Entire stone clearance is usually required for eradication of infection and to prevent further stone formation. Where there is little useful function remaining in a kidney with a staghorn calculus, nephrectomy is a reasonable option.

REFERENCES

Dellabella M, Milanese G, Muzzonigro G: Efficacy of tamsulosin in the medical management of juxtavesical ureteral stones. J Urol 2003;170(6):2202-2205.

Fielding JR, Steele G, Fox LA, et al: Spiral computerized tomography in the evaluation of acute flank pain: A replacement for excretory urography. J Urol 1997;157(6):2071-2073.

Klein LT, Frager D, Subramanium A, Lowe FC: Use of magnetic resonance urography. Urology 1998;52(4):602-608.

Pak CY, Peterson R, Poindextrer JR: Adequacy of a single stone risk analysis in the medical evaluation of urolithiasis. J Urol 2001;165(2):378-391.

Segura JW, Preminger GM, Assimos DG, et al: Ureteral Stones Clinical Guidelines Panel summary report on the management of ureteral calculi: The American Urological Association. J Urol 1997;158(5):1915-1921.

Segura JW, Preminger GM, Assimos DG, et al: Nephrolithiasis Clinical Guidelines Panel summary report on the management of staghorn calculi: The American Urological Association Clinical Guidelines Panel. J Urol 1994;151(6):1648-1651.

Stamatelou KK, Francis ME, Jones CA, et al: Time trends in reported prevalence of kidney stones in the United States: 1976-1994. Kidney Int 2003;63(5):1817-1823.

The Sexually Transmitted Diseases

Chancroid

Method of
Stanley M. Spinola, MD

Chancroid is caused by the gram-negative bacillus *Haemophilus ducreyi*. Chancroid is endemic in resource-poor countries in Africa, Asia, South America, and the Caribbean and occurs in sporadic outbreaks in industrialized nations. The annual global prevalence of chancroid is estimated to be 6 million cases, but diagnostic tests for *H. ducreyi* are not routinely performed and its epidemiology is poorly defined. The male-to-female ratio ranges from 3:1 to 25:1. Lack of circumcision is associated with infection in men. Like other agents of genital ulcer disease (GUD), *H. ducreyi* facilitates both acquisition and transmission of HIV-1, and chancroid contributes substantially to the HIV-1 pandemic in Asia and sub-Saharan Africa.

H. ducreyi has a short duration of infection, and chancroid can be perpetuated only by highly sexually active populations such as commercial sex workers (CSWs). Infected men usually report intercourse with CSWs. In the United States, chancroid is now rare; less than 100 cases were reported annually from 2000 to 2004. However, outbreaks occurred as recently as 1995 in New Orleans and Jackson, Mississippi. In these outbreaks, additional risk factors for infection included crack cocaine use, exchange of drugs for sex, or sex with a partner who used crack. Elimination of chancroid from CSWs controls outbreaks and reduces endemic disease.

Diagnosis

H. ducreyi enters the skin through breaks in the epithelium that occur during sex, and erythematous papules form at each entry site within hours to days. Papules evolve into pustules in 2 to 3 days. After several weeks, the pustules ulcerate, and patients usually develop one to four soft painful ulcers with ragged edges. The ulcer may be covered by a yellow or gray purulent exudate and frequently bleeds when scraped. The most frequent sites of the ulcer are the foreskin and the entrance of the vagina. Internal vaginal and cervical ulcers may be painless and go unnoticed by infected women. Suppurative inguinal lymphadenopathy occurs in up to 50% of patients with ulcers. The classic presentation of chancroid occurs in a minority of patients, and chancroid cannot be reliably distinguished from syphilis or herpes on clinical grounds. Mixed infections with *H. ducreyi*, *Treponema pallidum*, and herpes simplex virus (HSV) are common, occurring in approximately 17% of proven chancroid cases. Mixed infection may account for the variable clinical presentations of chancroid and treatment failures.

Confirmation of chancroid is difficult because culture is at best 80% sensitive. A highly sensitive multiplex polymerase chain reaction assay for GUD was developed but not marketed. Culture is the only reliable diagnostic test available for most settings. In practice, the diagnosis of chancroid is typically made by exclusion of HSV and syphilis. If patients with GUD and inguinal lymphadenitis or treatment failures for presumed primary syphilis appear in a community, public health authorities should be notified and diagnostic testing initiated.

Treatment

H. ducreyi is usually resistant to ampicillin, chloramphenicol (Chloromycetin), tetracyclines, trimethoprim (Proloprim), and sulfonamides and is susceptible to macrolides,

---

CURRENT DIAGNOSIS

- Patients usually develop 1–4 soft painful ulcers with ragged edges on the foreskin or at the entrance of the vagina. Infected women may also have painless internal vaginal and cervical ulcers. Regional lymphadenitis occurs in 10%–50% of cases.
- Infected men have usually had contact with CSWs.
- Diagnosis is typically made by culture after exclusion of HSV and syphilis.

Abbreviations: CSWs = commercial sex workers; HSV = herpes simplex virus.

873

CURRENT THERAPY

- CDC recommends single-dose azithromycin (Zithromax), 1 g orally, or ceftriaxone (Rocephin[1]), 250 mg IM, ciprofloxacin (Cipro[1]), 500 mg PO bid for 3 days, or erythromycin base,[1] 500 mg PO tid for 7 d.
- Low dose erythromycin (250 mg tid for 7 d) may be as effective as the standard 500 mg regimen.
- Single-dose oral ciprofloxacin, 500 mg, may be as effective as single-dose azithromycin and multiple-dose ciprofloxacin regimens.
- Even if *H. ducreyi* is successfully treated, ulcers may persist if HSV or syphilis is present and not treated.
- Recommend HIV testing at time of presentation and 3 mo later if initial test is negative.

[1]Not FDA approved for this indication.

Abbreviations: IM = intramuscularly; HSV = herpes simplex virus; PO = orally.

quinolones, and third-generation cephalosporins. The Centers for Disease Control and Prevention (CDC) recommends single-dose azithromycin (Zithromax), 1 g orally, or ceftriaxone (Rocephin[1]), 250 mg intramuscularly (IM), ciprofloxacin (Cipro[1]), 500 mg orally twice a day for 3 days, or erythromycin base,[1] 500 mg orally three times a day for 7 days. Low-dose erythromycin (250 mg three times a day for 7 days) may be as effective as the standard 500 mg regimen. Single-dose oral ciprofloxacin, 500 mg, may be as effective as the single-dose azithromycin and multiple-dose ciprofloxacin regimens.

Within 1 week of treatment, there should be no purulence and the ulcers should be less tender. Most ulcers heal in 2 weeks, but large ulcers may take 4 weeks to heal. Patients co-infected with HIV and *H. ducreyi* may have a greater number of ulcers that do not heal as quickly as patients infected with *H. ducreyi* alone. However, the antibiotic treatment efficacy of single-dose azithromycin or ciprofloxacin for chancroid in HIV seropositive and seronegative patients is similar. When evaluating the response to treatment, one must distinguish between bacteriologic and clinical cure. Even if *H. ducreyi* is successfully treated, ulcers may persist if HSV or syphilis is present and not treated. Fluctuant buboes may be treated by incision and drainage or needle aspiration; the former lessens the need for repeated procedures. All patients with chancroid should undergo testing for HIV at the time of presentation and 3 months later if the initial test is negative. All sexual contacts should be examined and treated even if GUD is not present.

REFERENCES

Ballard RC, Ye H, Matta A, et al: Treatment of chancroid with azithromycin. Int J STD AIDS 1996;7(Suppl 1):9-12.

Bong CTH, Bauer ME, Spinola SM: Haemophilus ducreyi: Clinical features, epidemiology, and prospects for disease control. Microbes Infect 2002;4:1141-1148.

Ernst A, Marvez-Valls E, Martin D: Incision and drainage versus aspiration of fluctuant buboes in the emergency department during an epidemic of chancroid. Sex Transm Dis 1995;22(4):217-220.

Kimani J, Bwayo JJ, Anzala AO, et al: Low dose erythromycin regimen for the treatment of chancroid. East Afr Med J 1995;72:645-648.

Lewis DA: Diagnostic tests for chancroid. Sex Transm Infect 2000;76: 137-141.

[1]Not FDA approved for this indication.

Malonza IM, Tyndall MW, Ndinya-Achola JO, et al: A randomized, double-blind, placebo-controlled trial of single-dose ciprofloxacin versus erythromycin for the treatment of chancroid in Nairobi, Kenya. J Infect Dis 1999;180:1886-1893.

Martin DH, Sargent SJ, Wendel GD, Jr., et al: Comparison of azithromycin and ceftriaxone for the treatment of chancroid. Clin Infect Dis 1995;21:409-414.

Moodley P, Sturm PDJ, Vanmali T, et al: Association between HIV-1 infection, the etiology of genital ulcer disease, and response to syndromic management. Sex Transm Dis 2003;30:241-245.

Trees DL, Morse SA: Chancroid and *Haemophilus ducreyi*: An update. Clin Microbiol Rev 1995;8:357-375.

Tyndall MW, Agoki E, Plummer FA, et al: Single dose azithromycin for the treatment of chancroid: A randomized comparison with erythromycin. Sex Transm Dis 1994;21:231-234.

Gonorrhea

Method of
David M. Bamberger, MD

Gonorrhea is a common sexually transmitted disease of epithelial tissue that usually causes urethral infection in men and cervical infections in women. Conjunctival infections, proctitis, and pharyngeal infections are also observed. *Neisseria gonorrhoeae* is a gram-negative, aerobic, piliated but nonmotile coccus that grows in pairs with adjacent, flattened sides.

Epidemiology

In 2004, 330,132 cases of gonorrhea were reported in the United States. The rate of 113.5 per 100,000 people was the lowest ever reported, and it reflects a large decrease in incidence from 1976 to 1996 but only a small decrease from 1996 to 2004. Infection rates are much higher in the southeastern states. Rates among women and men are almost equal. The highest rates are observed among women 15 to 19 years of age and men 20 to 24 years of age. Rates among blacks are higher than in whites, Hispanics, Asian/Pacific Islanders, or American Indians/Alaskan natives. Although rates are highest among blacks and those living in the South, the rates have been declining over the past 5 years in these populations and have been increasing among whites and those living in the West. Rates in developing countries are estimated to be substantially higher than in the United States. An estimated 60 million cases of gonorrhea occur worldwide every year.

Cases reported to state and local health departments are underreported. On the basis of a population-based study performed in 2001–2002 in adults 18 to 26 years of age, the prevalence of gonococcal infections was 0.43%. This rate was approximately 10-fold less than for chlamydial infections, the other common cause of urethritis and cervicitis. The population-based study confirmed the substantially higher rate among blacks than whites and a lower rate in the West compared to the South. Most men and women with gonococcal infections in the survey were asymptomatic.

Rates of gonococcal infection are also high among men who have sex with men, lower socioeconomic and educational attainment, users of illicit drugs, and commercial sex workers. Among men having sex with men, the rate of infection increased between 1999 and 2003, particularly from western U.S. cities. Acquisition of infection is more related to differences in sex partner networks, societal factors, and access to health care than the number of sexual partners. Transmission usually occurs among those with no or minimal symptoms. The risk of transmission from a single sexual encounter from an infected woman to her male partner is approximately 20% and is approximately 50% from an infected man to his female partner. The U.S. Preventive Services Task Force recommends that clinicians screen all sexually active women under the age of 25, including those who are pregnant, for gonorrhea infection if they have a history of sexually transmitted infections, new or multiple sex partners, inconsistent condom use, sex work, or drug use.

Clinical Manifestations

In men, the usual incubation is 2 to 5 days, followed by a urethral discharge that is typically purulent, as opposed to the clear or whitish discharge of chlamydial urethritis. Extragenital infections, such as proctitis or pharyngitis, are more likely to be asymptomatic. Symptoms of proctitis may include tenesmus, rectal discharge, and pain. Acute epididymitis is the most common complication of urethral infection.

In women, the usual symptoms are vaginal discharge or pruritus and dysuria. Pelvic pain is often because of ascending infection. On cervical exam, a mucopurulent discharge is often observed. Vaginal involvement, including periurethral (Skene's) glands and involvement of the Bartholin ducts, is more common in postmenopausal women and prepubertal girls. Rectal involvement is often asymptomatic and caused by contamination with cervicovaginal secretions. Pelvic inflammatory disease (PID) (see the appropriate article) is estimated to occur in 10% to 20% of women with cervical infections. Perihepatitis (Fitz-Hugh-Curtis syndrome) is caused by involvement of the liver capsule. Pharyngeal involvement in both men and women may be a source of transmission and is usually asymptomatic. Autoinoculation of the eye is the usual cause of adult gonococcal conjunctivitis.

Bacteremic dissemination is estimated to occur in 0.5% to 3% of patients, but these estimates may be high because of declining prevalence in strains associated with dissemination (serotype IA, auxotype AHU, failure to express outer membrane protein II). It occurs more often in women or in men who have sex with men; in women it is associated with menstruation or pregnancy, and it may be associated with deficiencies in the terminal components of complement. During the initial phase of illness, patients usually develop fever and polytenosynovitis of the knees, elbows, wrists, and joints of the hands and feet. Discrete papulopustular skin lesions on an erythematous base occur. As the illness continues, septic arthritis manifests in one or two joints, typically the knees, elbows, ankles, or wrists.

Microbiology and Diagnosis

In men with symptomatic purulent urethritis, a Gram stain of the purulent discharge revealing intracellular gram-negative diplococci is both sensitive and specific. The use of a Gram stain in the diagnosis of cervical infection has lower sensitivity and specificity. Cultures of urethral specimens from men and cervical specimens from women should be plated

CURRENT DIAGNOSIS

- Urethral discharge in men and vaginal discharge and dysuria in women are the common symptoms of gonococcal infections, but many women and some men have asymptomatic or minimally symptomatic infections.
- Urethral Gram stain is an inexpensive sensitive and specific test in men but not women.
- Newer generation nucleic acid amplification tests are highly sensitive and specific in cervical specimens in women and in urethral and urine specimens in men, but some lack sensitivity in urine specimens from women. Nucleic acid amplification tests should not be used in testing specimens from pharyngeal or rectal sources.

directly onto media to improve yield and transported promptly to the microbiology laboratory. A special medium such as Thayer-Martin, which inhibits the growth of contaminating organisms, is used for nonsterile sites such as the urethra, cervix, rectum, or pharynx. Plates are incubated at 35°C to 36°C (95°F to 97°F) in 3% to 5% carbon dioxide (CO_2).

Nonculture methods are increasingly replacing cultures in the diagnosis of gonococcal infections. Three commercially available nucleic acid amplification tests are currently marketed: the polymerase chain reaction (PCR) assay (Amplicor, Roche), a transcription mediated amplification assay (Aptima, Gen-Probe), and the DNA strand displacement assay (Probe-Tec, Becton Dickinson). These assays are highly sensitive and specific in testing male urethral, female cervical, and male urine specimens. An important advantage of the assays is their utility in testing urine specimens from both men and women and self-collected vaginal specimens from women. The PCR assay was only 55% to 65% sensitive when testing urine samples from women. The strand displacement and transcription mediated amplification assay are moderately more sensitive in testing female urine specimens but sensitivity remains less than 95%. Although most of the current nonculture assays have a specificity of approximately 99%, there is a suboptimal positive predication if testing a population with very low prevalence. Cultures are still considered the gold standard test in forensic settings and offer the advantage of preserving the specimen for antimicrobial testing. Cultures remain the only approved diagnostic testing methodology for pharyngeal and rectal specimens.

Treatment

Treatment for gonococcal infections is best provided at the time of initial presentation with a regimen that is highly effective with single-dose therapy. Adherence with therapy wanes with prolonged outpatient treatment courses. Antimicrobial resistance rates are increasing, and susceptibility testing results are generally not available at the time treatment is provided. In the U.S. Gonococcal Isolate Surveillance Project (GISP) report in 2004, 15.9% of isolates were resistant to penicillin, tetracycline, or both, and 6.8% of isolates demonstrated resistance to ciprofloxacin (Cipro).

CURRENT THERAPY

- Uncomplicated urethritis, cervicitis, or rectal infections should be treated with a single dose of:
- Ceftriaxone (Rocephin), 125 mg IM
- Cefixime (Suprax), 400 mg PO
- Ciprofloxacin (Cipro), 500 mg PO
- Levofloxacin (Levaquin[1]), 250 mg PO
- Ofloxacin (Floxin), 400 mg PO
- Fluoroquinolone resistance is increasing, and fluoroquinolones should not be used in:
  - Locales with 3%–5% rates of resistance (see text)
  - Men who have sex with men
  - Patients with sexual partners from locales with high rates of resistance
- Alternative therapies include:
  - Azithromycin (Zithromax), 2 g PO
  - Cefpodoxime (Vantin), 200–400 mg PO
- Patients should be treated for concomitant chlamydial infection with
  - Azithromycin (Zithromax), 1 g PO *or*
  - Doxycycline (Vibramycin), 100 mg PO bid for 7 d
- Sexual partners of infected patients should be evaluated and treated for gonorrhea and chlamydia and evaluated and counseled for other sexually transmitted diseases.

[1]Not FDA approved for this indication.

Chlamydial infection is detected in approximately 20% of men and 42% of women with laboratory-documented gonococcal infections, necessitating the need for co-treatment of *Chlamydia trachomatis* (see Obstetrics and Gynecology section) in patients with gonococcal infections, unless a nucleic acid amplification test is negative for the presence of chlamydia at the time of treatment. Patients with gonococcal infections should also be screened and counseled regarding other sexually transmitted diseases, including HIV and syphilis, and offered hepatitis B vaccination.

An ideal treatment regimen for gonococcal infections of the urethra, cervix, or rectum is inexpensive, well-tolerated, and a single dose. Ceftriaxone (Rocephin), 125 mg given intramuscularly (IM) as a single dose, is highly efficacious for urogenital and rectal infections. It may be reconstituted in 1% lidocaine (Xylocaine) to reduce injection site pain. The 2006 *STD Treatment Guidelines* from the Centers for Disease Control and Prevention (CDC) included four oral choices: cefixime (Suprax) at 400 mg, ciprofloxacin (Cipro) at 500 mg, ofloxacin (Floxin) at 400 mg, and levofloxacin (Levaquin[1]) at 250 mg. Manufacture of cefixime (Suprax) as an oral tablet ceased in 2002 but may be reintroduced. An oral suspension (100 mg/5 mL) is marketed. Since 2002 quinolone resistance has increased. Several countries in Southeast Asia have rates of fluoroquinolone resistance that exceed 50%. Within the United States, data from the GISP in 2004 indicated a rate of greater than 5% resistance in most West Coast U.S. cities, Denver, Miami, Minneapolis, and Phoenix. Rates varied among U.S. cities. Albuquerque, Birmingham, Detroit, and St. Louis did not identify any resistant strains. Outside of the GISP, high rates of

fluoroquinolone resistance (approximately 3%) are also reported in Hawaii, Massachusetts, Michigan, New York, and New Hampshire. The rate of fluoroquinolone resistance in men who have sex with men is 23.8% compared to 2.9% in heterosexuals. Fluoroquinolones are not recommended when local public health officials report rates of resistance of greater than 3% to 5%, among men who have sex with men, and in people with sexual contacts from areas with resistance rates greater than 3% to 5%. Fluoroquinolones should also not be used during pregnancy.

Oral cefpodoxime (Vantin) is an alternative to cefixime but is slightly less active in vitro. At a dose of 200 mg, the efficacy is 96.5% (95% confidence interval [CI], 94.8 to 98.9) and is approved for urethritis in males and females and rectal infections in females by the FDA, but not recommended by the CDC because the lower limit of the 95% CI was less than 95%. Use of a 400 mg oral dose is recommended by some state health departments as an alternative, but published efficacy data are limited. A 2 g single oral dose of azithromycin (Zithromax) is highly efficacious but associated with more gastrointestinal intolerance, and azithromycin resistance has occurred. Spectinomycin (Trobicin), given as a single 2 g IM dose, is an alternative to ceftriaxone (Rocephin) in patients with a history of allergy to cephalosporins or anaphylaxis to penicillin, but it may not be available in the United States as of May 2006.

Pharyngeal infections are generally less responsive to treatment. Treatment options include 125 mg IM ceftriaxone (Rocephin), a 2 g dose of oral azithromycin (Zithromax), or 500 mg of oral ciprofloxacin (Cipro) in areas and populations in which quinolone resistance is known to be less than 3% to 5%. Conjunctival infections in adults are treated with a single dose of 1 g IM ceftriaxone (Rocephin); ophthalmia neonatorum is treated with 25 to 50 mg/kg, not to exceed 125 mg, of intravenous (IV) or IM ceftriaxone. All neonates should receive ocular prophylaxis against gonococcal ophthalmia with 0.5% erythromycin (Ramycin), or 1% tetracycline.

Sexual partners of infected patients should be evaluated and treated for gonorrhea and chlamydia and evaluated and counseled for other sexually transmitted diseases. Expedited partner therapy involves a strategy in which patients deliver treatment and counseling information with medication or a prescription to their partner. This strategy reduces recurrent infections. Operational issues regarding the patient–physician relationship with uncertain current legal status in some states are a barrier in the use of this strategy.

Patients who have uncomplicated gonorrhea and are treated with any of the CDC-recommended regimens do not need to return for a confirmation of cure testing. Patients who have symptoms that persist after treatment should be evaluated by culture for *N. gonorrhoeae,* and any gonococci isolated should be tested for antimicrobial susceptibility.

Disseminated gonococcal infection is treated with 1 g of ceftriaxone (Rocephin) daily, and once a response has occurred may be switched to oral therapy with cefixime (Suprax) or a fluoroquinolone (in populations in which fluoroquinolone resistance is low) to finish 1 week of therapy. Gonococcal endocarditis is treated with 4 weeks of ceftriaxone (Rocephin), and meningitis with 10 to 14 days of ceftriaxone (Rocephin). Treatment of PID is described in the appropriate article.

[1]Not FDA approved for this indication.

REFERENCES

Centers for Disease Control and Prevention. Sexually transmitted diseases treatment guidelines 2006. MMWR Recomm Rep 2006;55(No. RR-11): 42-49.

Centers for Disease Control and Prevention: Increases in fluoroquinolone-resistant *Neisseria gonorrhoeae* among men who have sex with men—United States, 2003, and revised recommendations for gonorrhea treatment, 2004. MMWR Wkly Rep 2004;53:335-338.

Centers for Disease Control and Prevention: Sexually transmitted disease surveillance 2003 Supplement: Gonococcal Isolate Surveillance Project (GISP) annual report—2003. Atlanta, Ga, U.S. Department of Health and Human Services, November 2004.

Centers for Disease Control and Prevention: STD Surveillance 2004: Accessed December 2, 2004, at http://www.cdc.gov/std/stats/04pdf/NatProfileAll.pdf

Cook RL, Hutchison SL, Ostergaard L, et al: Systematic review: Noninvasive testing for *Chlamydia trachomatis* and *Neisseria gonorrhoeae*. Ann Intern Med 2005;142:914-925.

Golden MR, Wrightington WLH, Handsfield HH, et al: Effect of expedited treatment of sex partners on recurrent or persistent gonorrhea or chlamydial infection. N Engl J Med 2005;352:676-685.

Miller WC, Ford CA, Morris M, et al: Prevalence of chlamydia and gonococcal infections among young adults in the United States. JAMA 2004;291:2229-2236.

Nongonococcal Urethritis

Method of
Heidi M. Bauer, MD, MS, MPH, and
Kimberly Workowski, MD

Nongonococcal urethritis (NGU) is estimated to affect more than 4 million men in the United States every year. This syndrome is characterized by urethral inflammation that may be asymptomatic in 30% to 50% of cases. Symptoms of urethritis include urethral discharge, dysuria, or meatal pruritus. The majority of infectious cases are sexually transmitted. Because of its well-defined role in the development of upper tract disease and infertility in women, *Chlamydia trachomatis* remains the most important pathogen, accounting for 15% to 40% of cases of NGU. Other etiologies include *Mycoplasma genitalium, Trichomonas vaginalis*, and herpes simplex virus. Diagnostic and treatment procedures for these organisms are reserved for situations in which these infections are suspected (e.g., contact with trichomoniasis and genital lesions or severe dysuria and meatitis, which might suggest genital herpes) or when NGU is not responsive to therapy. Enteric bacteria have been identified as an uncommon cause of NGU and might be associated with insertive anal sex. The role of *Ureaplasma urealyticum*, enteric bacteria, anaerobes, and *Candida* species is less well defined. Complications of untreated NGU include epididymitis in less than 3% of cases and, rarely, Reiter syndrome. Although NGU can be caused by chemical, allergic, or autoimmune processes, the syndrome should be presumed infectious. Evaluation and treatment for both gonorrhea and chlamydia is warranted. Furthermore, clinical evaluation and treatment of sex partners is critical for preventing complications and interrupting sexual transmission. Pathogens responsible for NGU are associated with cervicitis, pelvic inflammatory disease (PID), and tubal infertility.

Diagnosis

Although the clinical presentation varies, the incubation of NGU averages 7 to 14 days with gradual onset of mild dysuria and mucoid discharge. In some high-risk populations, up to 50% of infections are asymptomatic.

Because of its high sensitivity and specificity, the Gram stain is the preferred rapid diagnostic test for evaluating urethritis. Gonococcal infection can be established by documenting the presence of white blood cells (WBCs) containing intracellular gram-negative diplococci. The presence of gram-negative rods should raise the suspicion for enteric bacteria. Confirmatory tests are important for identifying a specific etiology, which may improve compliance and facilitate partner management. *Neisseria gonorrhoeae* and *C. trachomatis* can be detected using culture, DNA hybridization tests on a urethral specimen, or nucleic acid amplification tests (NAATs) on a urethral or urine specimen. Because of their increased sensitivity, NAATs are recommended for chlamydia testing. For urine-based NAATs, 10 to 15 mL of first-catch urine is collected.

Diagnostic tests for mycoplasmas are available in research settings; however, these are not available for routine clinical use. Although culture is available for *T. vaginalis*, specific medium is necessary for isolation; both urethral and urine specimens are recommended.

Treatment

If gonorrhea cannot be ruled out with a stat test (i.e., Gram stain of urethral exudate), patients should be treated for both gonorrhea and chlamydia. Both azithromycin (Zithromax) and doxycycline (Vibramycin) are highly effective in treating chlamydial NGU. Azithromycin provides convenient dosing and the opportunity for directly observed therapy. Doxycycline is inexpensive but requires a twice-daily dosing for a full week. Alternatives include erythromycin (E-Mycin) and fluoroquinolones.

Among patients with erratic health care seeking behavior in whom poor compliance is anticipated, azithromycin offers the easiest administration. Further, *M. genitalium* appears to respond better to macrolides compared with tetracyclines. Patients should be advised to abstain from sex until seven days after treatment, symptoms have resolved, and until seven days after sex partners have been treated. Patients should return for evaluation and treatment if their symptoms persist or recur after completion of therapy.

 CURRENT DIAGNOSIS

The diagnosis of urethritis is confirmed by documenting evidence of inflammation on a urethral smear or in the urine:

- Urethral discharge that is mucoid or purulent
- Gram stain of urethral exudate demonstrating five or more white blood cells (WBCs) per oil immersion field (×1000)
- Positive leukocyte esterase test on first-void urine or microscopic examination of first-void urine sediment demonstrating 10 or more WBCs per high power field (×400)

CURRENT THERAPY

Recommended Regimens

- Azithromycin (Zithromax), 1 g PO in a single dose
- Doxycycline (Vibramycin), 100 mg PO bid × 7 days

Alternative Regimens

- Erythromycin base (E-Mycin, ERYC, E-Base), 500 mg PO qid × 7 days
- Erythromycin ethylsuccinate (EES), 800 mg PO qid × 7 days
- Ofloxacin (Floxin), 300 mg PO bid × 7 days
- Levofloxacin (Levaquin), 500 mg PO qd × 7 days

Abbreviations: bid = two times a day; PO = by mouth; qd = once daily; qid = four times a day.

Patients should refer all sex partners in the past 60 days for evaluation and treatment. Sexual contacts of patients with NGU should be offered evaluation and treatment.

Persistent or Recurrent Urethritis

Chronic urethritis is defined as persistent or recurrent urethritis within 6 weeks following treatment. An estimated 20% to 40% of NGU cases do not respond to first-line therapy. Although up to 20% of men with chlamydial NGU have recurrence, up to 50% of men with nonchlamydial NGU have recurrence. Noncompliance and reinfection are important considerations. Other causes include organisms that do not respond to the standard treatment regimens, such as trichomoniasis, tetracycline-resistant *Ureaplasma*, viral etiologies, and other bacteria. Up to 30% of NGU has no identifiable infectious etiology. These cases may involve allergy and postinfectious immunologic response. Before administering therapy, the presence of urethral inflammation should be documented. Patients with persistent or recurrent urethritis who did not comply with therapy or who had exposure to an untreated sex partner should be retreated with the initial drug regimen. Otherwise, recommended treatment regimens include metronidazole (Flagyl) 2 g orally in a single dose or tinidazole (Tindamax) 2 g orally in a single dose, plus azithromycin (Zithromax) 1 g orally in a single dose (if not used for the initial episode).

REFERENCES

Bradshaw CS, Tabrizi SN, Read TRH, et al. Etiologies of nongonococcal urethritis: bacteria, viruses, and the association with orogenital exposure. J Infect Dis 2006;193:336-345.

Centers for Disease Control and Prevention. Sexually transmitted diseases treatment guidelines—2006. MMWR 2006 (in press).

Centers for Disease Control and Prevention: Screening tests to detect *Chlamydia trachomatis* and *Neisseria gonorrhoeae* infections—2002. Morb Mortal Wkly Rep 2002;51(RR-15):3-19.

Jensen JS: *Mycoplasma genitalium:* The aetiological agent of urethritis and other sexually transmitted diseases. J Eur Acad Dermatol Venereol 2004;18(1):1-11.

Kodner C: Sexually transmitted infections in men. Prim Care 2003; 30:173-191.

Granuloma Inguinale (Donovanosis) and Lymphogranuloma Venereum

Method of
A. A. Hoosen, MSc, MB, ChB, MMed, FC Path

The initial clinical presentation of granuloma inguinale (GI) (or donovanosis) and lymphogranuloma venereum (LGV) is genital ulceration, and these conditions are considered in the differential diagnosis of genital ulcer disease (GUD) or genital ulcer syndrome (GUS).

In view of the difficulty in making an accurate clinical diagnosis of the exact etiology of GUD and also because more than one sexually transmitted pathogen may cause an infection concurrently in high-risk populations, syndromic management of sexually transmitted infections (STIs) is promoted. The World Health Organization (WHO) has published guidelines for syndromic management, which are being followed in many countries; however, other countries have modified these according to the local prevalence of STIs. Antimicrobial agents shown to be efficacious for the eradication of GI (donovanosis) and LGV are always included in the protocols for the management of genital ulcer disease.

Management is important with these diseases not only, for public health reasons, to curtail their spread among the population but also because these diseases enhance the spread of HIV.

Granuloma Inguinale

Granuloma inguinale (GI)/donovanosis is a chronic, progressive ulcerative condition of the genitalia caused by an encapsulated bacterium called *Calymmatobacterium granulomatis*. A recent proposal is that this organism be reclassified as *Klebsiella granulomatis*. The infection occurs in selected foci worldwide including southeast India, Papua New Guinea, the Caribbean, Brazil, eastern South Africa, Zimbabwe, Zambia, and Australia.

The primary lesion begins as a small, painless papule that ulcerates to form an exuberant, beefy red granulomatous ulcer with rolled edges. The lesions are painless and bleed easily on contact. Healing may be accompanied by scar formation and, in severe cases, lymphedema with resultant elephantiasis and deformities. In men, the lesions usually appear on the penile shaft, coronal sulcus, and prepuce; in women they occur commonly on the labia and fourchette. Intravaginal and cervical lesions mimic carcinoma of the cervix clinically and may result in complications such as hydronephrosis.

In large characteristic beefy lesions, the diagnosis is usually made clinically. However, for smaller lesions and where mixed infections are suspected, tests to exclude other causes of GUD need to be undertaken. The mainstay of laboratory diagnosis for GI is visualization of characteristic intracellular Donovan bodies in monocytes in tissue smears stained by Giemsa and Wright stains. Donovan bodies are encapsulated, short rods showing a characteristic bipolar staining. Specimens are collected by taking scrapings or swab specimens from the edge of lesions. Tissue biopsy lesions taken from the edge of the lesions assist in excluding malignancy, and these are stained with Giemsa and silver stains for ease of diagnosis. The causative organism has been successfully cultured in monocytes and in HEp-2 cells, but this requires elaborate laboratory facilities and expertise, which are not readily available in many routine diagnostic laboratories. Molecular diagnostic assays are not available commercially and have only been used in a few research studies.

A number of antimicrobial agents provide successful therapy for GI. The recommended duration of therapy is until lesions re-epithelize. Our recommendation for patients with severe lesions is hospitalization and administration of an aminoglycoside (e.g., gentamicin at 4.5 to 5 mg/kg per day or amikacin 15 mg/kg per day intravenously in a single daily dose for 10 to 14 days) together with a macrolide agent (e.g., erythromycin at 500 mg four times per day until resolution of lesions). Tetracycline, 500 mg four times per day; doxycycline, 100 mg twice daily; and trimethoprim/sulfamethoxazole, 80/400 mg twice daily, are also reported to be effective by various centers. There is no difference in clinical outcome for HIV co-infected individuals.

Lymphogranuloma Inguinale

Lymphogranuloma venereum (LGV) is caused by serovars L1, L2, and L3 of *Chlamydia trachomatis*. The initial clinical presentation is a small transient papular lesion; the characteristic regional lymphadenopathy occurs later. The disease is endemic in Africa, India, Southeast Asia, South America, and the Caribbean.

Classic LGV disease has three distinct stages. The first stage is the formation of the primary lesion, usually on the genitalia, which is a papular ulcer and is usually asymptomatic. The lesion appears approximately 3 days to 3 weeks after acquisition of infection and heals without scar formation. The secondary stage is characterized by regional lymphadenopathy and manifestation of systemic symptoms. In men, the inguinal area is usually affected, and in the majority of cases it is a unilateral lymphadenopathy. In women vulval lesions lead to inguinal and femoral lymphadenopathy, and for upper vaginal or cervical lesions the iliac nodes are affected. The simultaneous enlargement of the femoral and inguinal lymph nodes gives an appearance of a groove and this "groove sign" is said to be characteristic of LGV. The lymph nodes coalesce and form a bubo that may rupture spontaneously and lead to fistulae and sinus tracts. In the third stage, there is chronic granulomatous enlargement with ulceration of the external genitalia. These changes may lead to lymphatic obstruction resulting in elephantiasis.

Diagnosis of a chlamydial infection is usually made either by demonstrating the causative agent in stained smears, by antigen detection, by culture, by serologic tests, or by molecular tests such as the polymerase chain reaction (PCR). For the diagnosis of LGV, Giemsa-stained smears of ulcerative lesions are not helpful because of the presence of competing genital flora. Antigen detection by monoclonal immununofluoresence assays has been used; culture in HEp-2, HeLa, and McCoy cell lines have shown yields of up to 30%; and molecular tests are not currently commercially available. Diagnosis is usually made by serologic assays. The classic complement fixation test is rarely used nowadays; the current test of choice is the microimmunofluorescence test (MIF or micro IF) as it allows for discrimination between the serovars of *C. trachomatis*.

A number of antibacterial agents such as tetracycline, doxycycline, minocycline, chloramphenicol, and erythromycin have been used for successful therapy. The recommended duration of therapy is at least 14 days in view of the unique intracellular life cycle of this pathogen. The Centers for Disease Control and Prevention (CDC) recommends the use of doxycycline, 100 mg twice daily for 21 days, with erythromycin and sulfisoxazole as alternative agents. The use of the azalide azithromycin (1 g orally) allows for a single-dose regimen for the

---

CURRENT DIAGNOSIS

Clinical

GRANULOMA INGUINALE

- Characteristic, large beefy, exuberant, painless lesions which bleed easily on contact
- Mainstay of diagnosis is demonstration of characteristic bipolar staining of "Donovan bodies" in monocytes in Giemsa-stained tissue smears
- Biopsied tissue stained with Giemsa and silver stains

Laboratory

LYMPHOGRANULOMA VENEREUM

- Transient papular ulcer followed by regional lymphadenopathy which develops into bubo and may suppurate
- Serology is most widely used
- Current test of choice is the micro IF or MIF test

CURRENT THERAPY

GRANULOMA INGUINALE

- For large lesions – combination therapy with intravenous aminoglycoside plus oral erythromycin followed by oral erythromycin till re-epithelialization of lesions.
- Antimicrobials such as tetracycline, ceftriaxone, azithromycin, chloramphenicol, and co-trimoxazole have been used with good success.

LYMPHOGRANULOMA VENEREUM

- Widely used agent is doxycline 100 mg bid for 2-3 weeks
- Alternative agents include erythromycin, sulfisoxazole
- Fluctuant buboes must be aspirated before they rupture

management of chlamydial infections, and this may allow for better compliance of therapy.

It is extremely important to aspirate fluctuant buboes to prevent complications of rupture and sinus tract formation.

REFERENCES

Carter J, Hutton S, Sriprakash KS, et al: Culture of the causative organism of donovanosis (*Calymmatobacterium granulomatis*) in Hep-2 cells. J Clin Microbiol 1997;35:2915-2917.

Carter JS, Bowden FJ, Bastian I, et al : Phylogenetic evidence for reclassification of *Calymmatobacterium granulomatis* as *Klebsiella granulomatis* comb. Nov. Int J Syst Bacteriol 1999;49:1695-1700.

Centers for Disease Control and Prevention: Sexually transmitted diseases: Treatment guidelines, 2002. MMWR Morb Mortal Wkly Rep 2002;51(RR6):1-80.

Hoosen AA, Draper G, Moodley J, Cooper K: Granuloma inguinale of the cervix: A carcinoma look-alike. Genitourin Med 1990;66: 380-382.

Hoosen AA, Mphatsoe M, Kharsany ABM, et al: Granuloma inguinale in association with pregnancy and HIV infection. Int J Gynaecol Obstet 1996;53:133-138.

Kharsany ABM, Hoosen AA, Kiepiela P, et al: Growth and cultural characteristics of *Calymmatobacterium granulomatis*—the aetiological agent of granuloma inguinale (donovanosis). J Med Microbiol 1997;46:579-585.

Mahony JB, Coombes BK, Chernesky MA: *Chlamydia* and Chlamydophila. In: Murphy PR, et al (eds): Manual of Clinical Microbiology. Washington, DC, American Society of Microbiology, 2003, pp 991-1004.

O'Farrell N, Hoosen AA, Coetzee K, van der Ende J: A rapid stain for the diagnosis of granuloma inguinale. Genitourin Med 1990;66: 200-201.

Richens J: The diagnosis and treatment of donovanosis (granuloma inguinale). Genitourin Med 1991;67:441-452.

Stamm WE, Jones RB, Balteiger BE: *Chlamydia trachomatis*. In: Mandell GL, Bennett JE, Dolin R (eds):. Principles and Practice of Infectious Diseases. New York, Churchill Livingstone, 2005, pp 2239-2255.

Wasserheit JN: Effect of changes in human ecology and behaviour on patterns of sexually transmitted diseases, including human immunodeficiency virus infection. Proc Natl Acad Sci U S A 1994;91:2430-2435.

World Health Organization. Guidelines for the management of sexually transmitted infections. World Health Organization, 2003, pp 1-91.

Syphilis

Method of
Mrunal Shah, MD

One of the oldest infections known, syphilis dates back more than 500 years. It was known as "The Great Pox" because of its skin manifestations; in contrast to the "small pox" seen around the same time. Studies were done before the use of antibiotics, which is where most of our natural history information comes from. The most recent epidemic occurred in 1990 (20.3 cases per 100,000 population) and has fallen steadily each year since. In the year 2000, the rate was at an all time low of 2.2 cases per 100,000 population. This was a 9.6% drop since 1999. The Centers for Disease Control and Prevention (CDC) hopes to eradicate the disease completely by 2005, but this may be difficult.

Peak ages are 30 to 39 years of age in men and 20 to 24 years of age in women. African Americans have always had higher incidences than whites. In the 1990s, it was 60:1, but the incidence has since declined to 30:1.

Microbiology

Treponema pallidum is the bacterium responsible for causing syphilis. It is very small and cannot be detected by ordinary microscopy, a feature that complicates diagnosis. The organism can be seen with darkfield microscopy, a technique that uses a special condenser to cast an oblique light. This allows visualization of a corkscrew-shaped organism with tightly wound spirals. This organism is extremely sensitive to penicillin, as is discussed later in the article. It has a very slow doubling rate, therefore requiring longer courses of treatment.

Pathophysiology

T. pallidum initiates infection when it gains access to subcutaneous tissues through microabrasions that can occur during sexual intercourse. Even though it has a slow doubling time (30 hours), it escapes host immune defenses and leads to the initial ulcerative lesion, the chancre. These can be seen anywhere around the genitalia including the cervix, perianal and rectal areas, and the oral mucosa. Regional lymphadenopathy also can be seen. As the host immune system fights the initial infection, *T. pallidum* is disseminated throughout the host. This is known as latency, as the patient will have no symptoms. There is also vertical spread in utero or during delivery, which is why prenatal panels include screening tests for syphilis.

Clinical Manifestations

The initial clinical manifestation is also called *primary* syphilis. This usually consists of a painless chancre at the site of inoculation. Primary syphilis represents a local infection, but it quickly becomes systemic with widespread dissemination of the spirochete. Because it is painless, most people do not seek medical attention. Even without treatment, the chancre will resolve in 4 to 6 weeks. It is this painlessness that helps separate it from herpes simplex virus (genital herpes) and *Haemophilus ducrey*i (chancroid).

In approximately weeks to months after the resolution of the chancre, patients will develop *secondary* syphilis, which includes systemic symptoms of rash, fever, headache, malaise, anorexia, and diffuse lymphadenopathy. The rash typically involves the palms and soles but can also include mucosal surfaces. Many patients do not realize that they had these lesions. These symptoms usually resolve spontaneously but can relapse for up to 5 years.

After symptoms resolve, and for up to many years later, the disease goes into *latent* syphilis, which is characterized by a lack of symptoms but seropositive test results. This can be separated into early and late latent phases based on being potentially infectious in the early phase. This is defined by the United States Public Health Service (USPHS) as infection of 1 year's duration or less. Anything longer is late latent.

TABLE 1 Clinical Manifestations and Treatment of Syphilis

Stage	Clinical Manifestation	Treatment
Primary	Painless ulcer (chancre), adenopathy	Benzathine penicillin G (Bicillin LA), 2.4 million U IM × 1
Secondary (weeks to months)	Rash, mucocutaneous lesions, adenopathy, hepatitis, arthritis, glomerulonephritis, condyloma lata	Benzathine penicillin G, 2.4 million U IM × 1
Latent	Asymptomatic	
Early (<1 year)		Benzathine penicillin G, 2.4 million U IM × 1
Late		Benzathine penicillin G, 2.4 million U IM weekly × 3
Tertiary (late) 1-30 years		
Cutaneous	Gummatous lesions	Benzathine penicillin G, 2.4 million U IM weekly × 3
Cardiovascular	Aortic aneurysm, aortic insufficiency	Benzathine penicillin G, 2.4 million U IM weekly × 3
CNS	Neurosyphilis, tabes dorsalis, Argyll-Robertson pupils, paresis, seizures, subtle psychiatric manifestations, dementia; may be asymptomatic	Aqueous crystalline penicillin G, 18-24 million U/d given as 3-4 million units IV q4h for 10-14 days or Procaine penicillin (Wycillin), 2.4 million U qd with probenecid 500 mg PO qid for 10-14 days

Abbreviations: CNS = central nervous system; IM = intramuscularly; IV = intravenously; PO = orally; qd = daily; qid = 4 times per day.
Adapted from the CDC: Guidelines for the treatment of STDs. MMWR Morb Mortal Wkly Rep 2002;51(RR-06):1-80.

Finally, for the next 1 to 30 years, untreated patients have a 25% to 40% risk of developing *late* or *tertiary* syphilis. It may involve many tissue types, so the spectrum of disease can be very confusing. Moreover, patients need not have had symptoms of primary or secondary syphilis prior to developing late syphilis. Tissues involved include cutaneous (gumma formation), cardiovascular (aortic disease), and central nervous system (CNS) (tabes dorsalis, meningitis, neurosyphilis) diseases (Table 1).

Diagnosis

The quickest, most direct method of diagnosing primary and secondary syphilis is direct visualization of the spirochete of moist lesions by means of darkfield microscopy. This is difficult and requires using laboratories that perform a high volume of sexually transmitted disease analyses. In general, a moist lesion should be cleaned with saline (not iodine because of bacteriocidal effect). Then, using gauze, the lesion should be unroofed. Any serosanguineous material should be collected on a dry slide for examination.

More common is serologic testing that can be done in most laboratories. The two most common screening tests are rapid plasma reagin (RPR) and the Venereal Disease Research Laboratory (VDRL) test. These tests are designed to test for IgM and IgG antibodies against a cardiolipin-cholesterol-lecithin antigen. Positive tests are reported as a dilutional titer. False positives are less than 1:4, whereas higher titers (1:16 to 1:128) are found in secondary and early latent syphilis. This titer is important as a benchmark to follow treatment. Lack of expected decreases in titer indicate inadequate treatment, false-positive result, re-infection, or late-stage therapy.

Before treatment, a positive screening test needs to be confirmed with specific *T. pallidum* antigen testing, such as the fluorescent treponemal antibody absorption test (FTA-ABS). These tests are expensive and have a high false-positive rate, making them unsuitable as screening tests. They also remain positive for life in most people.

Newer molecular tests include the use of polymerase chain reaction (PCR), which can be used to detect multiple organisms. It has high sensitivity and specificity and can distinguish among *H. ducreyi*, herpes simplex virus, and *T. pallidum*. This test is very expensive and is likely to be available only in specialized laboratories, for now.

The most significant morbidity of syphilis occurs during the tertiary phase and includes neurosyphilis. *T. pallidum* can be found in the cerebrospinal fluid (CSF) during primary and secondary phases, but it usually resolves on its own. Those patients who have an abnormal CSF during the latent phase are at higher risk for symptomatic neurosyphilis, making it helpful to distinguish asymptomatic neurosyphilis. The CDC recommends that CSF testing be done whenever there is clinical evidence of neurosyphilis or vision changes, active tertiary syphilis, treatment failure, or HIV infection. CSF-VDRL is highly specific, but, unfortunately, very insensitive (as low as 30%) and therefore can rule in but cannot exclude neurosyphilis.

Although the HIV epidemic showed a resurgence of syphilis, it is controversial as to what diagnostic changes occurred in testing. Several studies show contradictory information; one shows that there was an increase in the false-positive rates, whereas a second study showed a decrease in true-positive rates, and a third study showed higher false negatives. In any case, testing should still be performed as in non-HIV patients and followed accordingly.

Pregnancy poses only increased risk, including perinatal death, premature delivery, low birth weight, congenital anomalies, and active congenital syphilis of the neonate. Physical examination and serologic testing should be performed in any female considering pregnancy or during initial antepartum testing at least. Treatment, discussed below, should be given as if the patient is not pregnant.

Treatment

In all stages, the main reason for treatment is to prevent progression and spread of the disease. Historic treatments included mercury, salvarsan (an arsenic derivative), fever therapy, and malarial injection. Today's treatment has been in use since 1943, since the introduction of penicillin. Because there has been no reported resistance, penicillin remains the treatment of choice, so much so that penicillin-allergic patients have undergone desensitization therapy in order to receive it. Although penicillin G, given parenterally, is the preferred drug, the preparation used (benzathine, procaine, crystalline), dosage, and duration of therapy depend on stage and clinical manifestations (see Table 1). Oral penicillin is not considered appropriate for treatment. Alternative treatments could include doxycycline (Vibramycin), tetracycline, erythromycin, or ceftriaxone (Rocephin).[1]

Once treatment is started, physicians should be aware of a potential complication called the Jarisch-Herxheimer reaction. It is an acute, febrile reaction accompanied by headache and myalgias, which represents treponemal cell death and release of toxins. It peaks within 2 hours and subsides within 24 hours, and is most common in primary and secondary disease.

Follow-up of Treated Patients

Any patient with syphilis diagnosed at any stage should get testing for HIV and should be retested in 3 to 6 months if a member of a high-risk population. After treatment, repeat serologic testing should be done at 6 and 12 months and titers at 24 months. If there is not at least a fourfold decrease in 6 months, there is likely treatment failure. A lumbar puncture should be done to rule out neurosyphilis, and retreatment with three weekly injections of 2.4 million units of benzathine penicillin (Bicillin LA) is recommended unless there is evidence of neurosyphilis.

Partners of patients with syphilis should also be notified and treated. In primary disease, any partner within the previous 3 months should be identified. Empiric treatment is recommended unless there is good follow-up and serologic surveillance.

---

[1] Not FDA approved for this indication.

Contraceptive Methods

Method of
Lama L. Tolaymat, MD, MPH, and
Andrew M. Kaunitz, MD

Each year, nearly 2% of U.S. women of reproductive age have an induced abortion. This sobering statistic underscores the importance of women and couples having access to the effective hormonal, intrauterine, and surgical methods of contraception described here.

 CURRENT THERAPY

- Two percent of U.S. women of reproductive age have an induced abortion annually.
- Noncontraceptive benefits of oral contraceptive include decreasing the risk of endometrial cancer, ovarian cancer, ectopic pregnancy, and pelvic inflammatory disease as well as treatment of dysmenorrhea, menorrhagia, and acne.
- Combination estrogen-progestin birth control methods (pills, patch, and ring) are contraindicated in women who are smokers >35 y and those with a history of DVT, with cardiovascular disease, or with active liver disease.
- Progestin-only birth control methods (pills, injections, or the progestin-releasing IUD) represent appropriate contraceptive options for women who have medical problems contraindicating combination birth control methods.
- Women with menorrhagia or dysmenorrhea may benefit from extended-cycle oral contraceptive pills (Seasonale).
- Plan B, a progestin-only formulation, is the only oral formulation currently marketed for emergency contraception. Although package labeling indicates it should be taken within 72 hours, effective postcoital contraception is provided if Plan B is taken up to 5 d following unprotected intercourse.
- Copper and progestin-releasing IUDs offer users convenient birth control as effective as sterilization yet completely reversible.
- The copper IUD (ParaGard) may increase menstrual flow and thus may not be a good method for women with menorrhagia.
- Use of the progestin (levonorgestrel)-releasing IUD (Mirena) is associated with noncontraceptive benefits including reduction in heavy menstrual flow because of fibroids or adenomyosis and decreased pain in women with endometriosis.
- Surgical tubal sterilization is associated with a 10-y cumulative failure rate of 1.8%–3%.
- A device for occlusion of the fallopian tubes using hysteroscopy (Essure) was approved for use in the United States in 2002.
- The failure rate associated with vasectomy is 0.94% at 1 y and 1.1% at 5 y, representing pregnancy rates higher than previously reported.

Abbreviations: DVT = deep vein thrombosis; IUD = intrauterine device.

Estrogen/Progestin Combination Oral Contraceptive Pills

Oral contraceptive (OC) use is safe for the majority of users with many noncontraceptive benefits, such as decreasing the risk of endometrial cancer, ovarian cancer, ectopic pregnancy, and pelvic inflammatory disease and treating dysmenorrhea, menorrhagia, and acne. Although OCs represent a highly effective birth control method for correct consistent users, inconsistent or incorrect use accounts for the annual failure rate of 8% experienced overall by OC users.

OCs are usually initiated on the first day of menses or the first Sunday after menses starts. In these cases, a backup method of contraception is not needed. It is helpful to associate pill taking with a daily routine such as tooth brushing to improve compliance.

Conventional combination OC formulations include 21 active and 7 inactive tablets. The progestin component of the OCs suppresses the pituitary secretion of luteinizing hormone (LH), preventing ovulation. The estrogen component (ethinyl estradiol) suppresses secretion of follicle-stimulating hormone (FSH) and enhances cycle control (regular withdrawal bleeding with minimal unscheduled or so-called breakthrough bleeding). If 1 or 2 tablets are missed, the patient should take 1 tablet as soon as possible. Then 1 tablet should be taken twice a day until all the missed tablets are taken. Breast tenderness and nausea, common OC side effects, are related to the estrogen dose. Accordingly, if these side effects persist for more than several cycles, changing to a lower estrogen dose (e.g., switching from a 30- to 35-μg to a 20- to 25-μg) formulation may be useful.

Breakthrough (unscheduled) bleeding and spotting occurs more often in women taking 20-μg estrogen OCs than in those taking 30- to 35-μg formulations. Box 1 lists medical contraindications to all estrogen-progestin contraceptives.

Combination Oral Contraceptives with Reduced Pill-Free Intervals and/or Extended Cycles

OC formulations with reduced pill-free intervals appear to achieve superior cycle control (less unscheduled or breakthrough bleeding/spotting) despite use of very low doses of estrogen and may achieve higher contraceptive efficacy than conventional 21/7 OC formulations. Three 28-day OC formulations are formulated with 20 μg ethinyl estradiol and have fewer than 7 hormone-free days. One (Mircette), formulated with the progestin desogestrel, includes 2 days of inactive tablets and 5 ethinyl estradiol tablets in place of the 7 inactive tablets. Two recently approved formulations contain 24 active tablets followed by 4 days of inactive pills. One (Yaz) is formulated with the progestin drospirenone and improves symptoms associated with premenstrual dysphoric disorder. The other (Loestrin 24) is formulated with the progestin norethindrone acetate and has a shorter duration of withdrawal bleeding than other OCs.

The first extended-cycle OC (Seasonale) to be marketed in the United States includes 84 (12 weeks) of active pills followed by 7 placebo pills, rather than the conventional 21 active tablets followed by 7 placebos. Each active pill contains 150 μg of levonorgestrel and 30 μg of ethinyl estradiol. Over time, this extended approach to OC leads to 4 rather than 13 withdrawal bleeding episodes each year. Women considering extended OC use should be counseled to expect an initially higher rate of breakthrough bleeding and spotting, which declines over time. Women with a history of menorrhagia or dysmenorrhea may be candidates for extended-cycle OC use. In the future, extended-cycle OC formulations with no hormone-free days may become available. A recently approved OC (Seasonique) is identical to Seasonale but substitutes 10 μg of estrogen in place of the 7 placebo tablets that follow the 12 weeks of active tablets in each pack.

Progestin-Only Oral Contraceptives

Also known as minipills, the progestin-only OC formulation (Micronor) contains even lower doses than combination OCs. The documented rates of failure for progestin-only pills are comparable to those of combination OCs in women who are meticulous about taking the pill at the same time every day. If one pill is taken 3 or more hours late, backup contraception is needed for 48 hours. Most commonly in the United States, minipills are used by lactating women who intrinsically have low fecundability; in this subgroup of women, contraceptive failures with progestin-only OC use are not common.

Emergency Contraception

With the manufacturer no longer making a dedicated combination emergency contraception (EC) formulation (Preven) as of summer 2004, the only dedicated EC formulation currently available is the progestin-only formulation (Plan B), which consists of two levonorgestrel 750 μg tablets.

Progestin-only EC is more effective and causes less nausea and emesis than combination EC. Package labeling for Plan B indicates that 1 tablet should be taken within 72 hours of unprotected intercourse, followed 12 hours later by a second tablet. Taking the 2 tablets together, however, may be as effective in preventing pregnancy as dividing the dose. Furthermore, Plan B may retain its efficacy in pregnancy prevention when taken up to 5 days after unprotected intercourse. Although EC is currently only available by prescription, it may become available over the counter in the future.

BOX 1 Contraindications to Combination Hormonal Methods

- Smokers: ≥35 y
- Hypertension: Uncontrolled or ≥35 y
- Diabetes: Vascular disease or ≥35 y
- Migraines: Focal neurologic symptoms or ≥35 y
- Vascular disease: Associated with systemic lupus erythematosus
- Personal history of breast cancer or thromboembolism
- Coronary artery or cerebrovascular disease
- Acute or chronic hepatocellular disease with abnormal liver function
- Cholestatic jaundice with prior pregnancy or contraceptive use

Adapted from http://www.arhp.org/healthcareproviders/cme/onlinecme/wellwoman/TOC.cfm?ID=336

Injectable Contraception

PROGESTIN ONLY

Depomedroxyprogesterone acetate (DMPA) (Depo-Provera) is an injectable contraceptive that provides long-acting reversible birth control, as effective as sterilization. The standard dose is 150 mg (1 mL) of DMPA intramuscularly every 3 months (or every 12 to 13 weeks). As with combination OC use, DMPA suppresses ovulation and ovarian estradiol production. In contrast with combination OC use, DMPA includes no estrogen component. Therefore, bone mineral density (BMD) declines during prolonged use of DMPA. On November 2004, the FDA placed a black box in DMPA package labeling warning of the risk of significant loss of bone density during DMPA use. Fortunately, in adolescents as well as adult users, BMD rapidly recovers after discontinuation of DMPA, and no evidence indicates that DMPA use causes postmenopausal osteoporosis or fractures. The short-term impact that DMPA has on BMD appears analogous to that of lactation (which also lowers background estrogen levels). Lactation is not a risk factor for osteoporosis later in life. Skeletal health concerns should not restrict use of DMPA in adults or teens, nor should use of DMPA be considered by itself an indication for testing BMD.

Although concerns regarding weight gain may discourage some women, small randomized clinical trial data found that DMPA did not cause weight gain or increased appetite in short-term users. A subcutaneous DMPA formulation that should facilitate self-administration became available in 2005.

Combination Patch

Ortho Evra is a once-a-week transdermal contraceptive patch applied for 3 consecutive weeks, followed by a patch-free week during which withdrawal bleeding is anticipated. The patch can be applied to the lower abdomen, upper outer arm, buttock, or upper torso (except for the breast). The patch delivers a daily systemic dose of 150 μg of norelgestromin and 20 μg of ethinyl estradiol. In a randomized clinical trial, the contraceptive efficacy of the patch was comparable to that of oral contraception. If the patch is detached for greater than 24 hours, the user should start a new patch cycle and use a backup contraceptive method (such as condoms) for 1 week. A recent randomized pharmacokinetic trial found that serum ethinyl estradiol exposure was lower in the users of the vaginal contraceptive ring compared to oral contraceptives and the transdermal patch. This led to the concern that the risk of venous thromboembolus may be higher in women using the transdermal patch. A recent clinical trial, however, observed that the risk of nonfatal venous thromboembolus for the contraceptive patch is similar to the risk for OCs containing 35 μg of ethinyl estradiol.

Combination Vaginal Ring

NuvaRing is worn for 3 weeks, then removed for 1 week, during which withdrawal bleeding is anticipated. The ring is composed of a flexible ethylene vinyl acetate copolymer, which releases approximately 120 μg of etonogestrel and 15 μg of ethinyl estradiol per day. The ring is self-inserted and removed. In comparative clinical trials, rates of breakthrough bleeding and spotting were lower with the ring than with OCs. As with the patch, contraceptive efficacy of the ring is similar to that of combination OCs in clinical trials. Backup contraception is needed for 7 days if the ring remains outside of the vagina for more than 3 hours.

Intrauterine Devices

Intrauterine devices (IUDs) offer users convenient birth control as effective as sterilization yet completely reversible. In women in the United States, use of IUDs has declined from approximately 10% in the mid-1970s to 1% today. Concerns among clinicians and women that IUDs cause salpingitis and tubal infertility account for much of this decline. A systematic review found that if any increased risk in salpingitis is associated with IUD use, it is small and appears confined to the first month postinsertion. Likewise, use of an IUD is not associated with a subsequent increased risk of tubal infertility.

The copper IUD (ParaGard) is approved for up to 10 years of use. It is appropriate for women who prefer regular cycles. Because use of the copper IUD can increase flow and cramps, it is appropriate for women who have no excess menstrual flow or cramps at baseline. The Food and Drug Administration (FDA) approved liberalized safety labeling revisions for the copper IUD in September 2005. The revised labeling states that although the IUD may now be used in women with a history of pelvic inflammatory disease (PID) or sexually transmitted disease, it is contraindicated in those with acute PID or current behavior suggesting a high risk thereof. The prior language discouraging use of the IUD in nulliparous women was likewise removed.

The levonorgestrel-releasing IUD (Mirena) is approved for up to 5 years of use. It releases 20 μg of levonorgestrel a day. This progestin-releasing IUD reduces menstrual flow and is therefore appropriate for women who would like their birth control method to reduce flow. Women interested in using the levonorgestrel-releasing IUD should be aware, however, that initial irregular spotting or bleeding is common after insertion of this device. Hormonal side effects, including acne and ovarian cysts, also occur in some users. Box 2 details the important noncontraceptive benefits associated with use of the levonorgestrel IUD.

Progestin-Releasing Implants

Progestin-releasing contraceptive implants provide highly effective, convenient birth control. Although Norplant and Jadelle are approved by the FDA, neither is currently marketed in the United States.

Norplant levonorgestrel consists of six capsules and provides contraception up to 5 years. The difficulty with insertion and, in particular, removal of the six capsules, along with frequent complaints of irregular bleeding among users, explains why U.S. clinicians, women, and the manufacturer lost interest in this contraceptive system, which initially was in great demand when introduced in 1991.

> **BOX 2 Noncontraceptive Health Benefits of the Levonorgestrel-Releasing Intrauterine Device**
>
> - Reduces menorrhagia, including when caused by uterine fibroids or adenomyosis and as an alternative to endometrial ablation or hysterectomy
> - Relieves pain caused by endometriosis
> - Prevention of endometrial hyperplasia in menopausal women using estrogen therapy; also, treatment of endometrial hyperplasia/cancer
> - Prevention of endometrial proliferation and polyps in patients taking tamoxifen (Nolvadex)

Jadelle consists of an implant of two rods each containing 150 mg of levonorgestrel. A single-rod progestin (Etonogestrel) implant (Implanon)* is easier and quicker to insert and remove than Norplant, and its use is associated with less bleeding. This highly effective single-rod implant system received FDA approval in 2006.

Female Sterilization

Tubal sterilization involves using rings (Falope), clips (Filshie or Hulka), electrocautery, or ligature/segmental excision (Pomeroy) to interrupt the patency of the fallopian tubes surgically. In the United States, approximately 700,000 tubal sterilizations are performed annually. Approximately half of them follow delivery, and half of these are performed as outpatient interval procedures. Sterilization is associated with a 10-year cumulative failure rate of 1.8% to 3%. The failure rate is higher in women younger than 28 years. Although sterilization can be reversed in some women and assisted reproductive technology can also be used to achieve pregnancy in many women following sterilization, this procedure should nonetheless be considered permanent.

Hysteroscopic tubal occlusion (Essure) is a device developed and approved for use in the United States in 2002. This device (2 mm in diameter and 4 cm long) is made of titanium, stainless steel, and nickel, and it contains Dacron fibers that induce an inflammatory reaction and fibrosis in the tubal lumen. A hysterosalpingogram is recommended following placement of the Essure device to confirm bilateral tubal occlusion.

Male Sterilization

Vasectomy involves interruption of the vas deferens, preventing passage of sperm into seminal fluid. This office-based surgical procedure does not interfere with male sexual performance. After vasectomy, couples should use backup contraception until the sperm count reaches zero. According to Jamieson, recent data indicate the failure rate following vasectomy is 9.4 per 1000 procedures at 1 year and 11.3 at 5 years, higher than the previously estimated failure rate.

REFERENCES

Anderson FD, Gibbons W, Portman D: Safety and efficacy of an extended-regimen oral contraceptive utilizing continuous low-dose ethinyl estradiol. Contraception 2006;73(3):229-234.

Anderson FD, Hait H: A multicenter, randomized study of an extended cycle oral contraceptive. Contraception 2003;68:89-96.

Audet MC, Moreau M, Koltun WD, et al: Evaluation of contraceptive efficacy and cycle control of a transdermal contraceptive patch vs. an oral contraceptive: A randomized controlled trial. JAMA 2001; 285:2347-2354.

Bjarnadottir RI, Tuppurainen M, Killick SR: Comparison of cycle control with a combined contraceptive vaginal ring and oral levonorgestrel/ ethinyl estradiol. Am J Obstet Gynecol 2002;186:389-395.

Edelman AB, Koontz SL, Nichols MD, Jensen JT: Continuous oral contraceptives: Are bleeding patterns dependent on the hormones given? Obstet Gynecol 2006;107(3):657-665.

Hubacher D, Lara-Ricalde R, Taylor DJ, et al: Use of copper intrauterine devices and the risk of infertility among nulligravid women. N Engl J Med 2001;345:561-567.

Jain J, Jakimiuk AJ, Bode FR, et al: Contraceptive efficacy and safety of DMPA-SC. Contraception 2004;70:269-275.

Jamieson DJ, Costello C, Trussell J, et al: US Collaborative Review of Sterilization Working Group: The risk of pregnancy after vasectomy. Obstet Gynecol 2004;103:848-850.

Jick SS, Kaye JA, Russmann S, Jick H: Risk of nonfatal venous thromboembolism in women using a contraceptive transdermal patch and oral contraceptives containing norgestimate and 35 micrograms of ethinyl estradiol. Contraception 2006;73(3):223-228.

Jones RK, Darroch JE, Henshaw SK: Contraceptive use among U.S. women having abortions in 2000–2001. Perspect Sex Reprod Health 2002;34:294-303.

Kaunitz AM: Revisiting progestin-only OCs. Contemp OB/GYN 1997;42:91-108.

Kaunitz AM: Beyond the pill: New data and options in hormonal and intrauterine contraception. Am J Obstet Gynecol 2005;192:998-1004.

Kaunitz AM: Depo-Provera's black box: Time to reconsider? Contraception 2005;72:165-167.

Ubeda A, Labastida RM, Dexeus S: Essure: A new device for hysteroscopic tubal sterilization in an outpatient setting. Fertil Steril 2004;82:196-199.

Van den Heuvel MW, Van Bragt AJ, Alnabawy AK, Kaptein MC: Comparison of ethinyl estradiol pharmacokinetics in three hormonal contraceptive formulations: The vaginal ring, the transdermal patch and an oral contraceptive. Contraception 2005;72(3):168-174.

Westhoff C: Depot-medroxyprogesterone acetate injection (Depo-Provera): A highly effective contraceptive option with proven long-term safety. Contraception 2003;68(2):75-87.

Westhoff C: Emergency contraception. N Engl J Med 2003;349:1830-1835.

Westhoff C, Davis A: Tubal sterilization: Focus on the U.S. experience. Fertil Steril 2000;73:913-922.

Yonkers KA, Brown C, Pearlstein TB, et al: Efficacy of a new low-dose oral contraceptive with drospirenone in premenstrual dysphoric disorder. Obstet Gynecol 2005;106(3):492-501.

---

*Investigational drug in the United States.

Diseases of Allergy

Anaphylaxis and Serum Sickness

Method of
Stephen F. Kemp, MD

Anaphylaxis

Anaphylaxis has no universally accepted definition and both its morbidity and mortality are probably underestimated. A variety of statistics on the epidemiology of anaphylaxis are published, but the lifetime risk per person in the United States is presumed to be 1% to 3%, with a mortality rate of 1%. In this discussion, anaphylaxis is an acute life-threatening reaction, usually but not always mediated by an immunologic mechanism that results from the sudden systemic release of mast cell and basophil mediators. It has varied clinical presentations, but respiratory compromise and cardiovascular collapse cause the most concern because they are the most frequent causes of fatalities. Urticaria and angioedema are the most common manifestations (more than 90% in retrospective series) but may be delayed or absent in rapidly progressive anaphylaxis. The more rapidly anaphylaxis occurs after exposure to an offending stimulus, the more likely the reaction is to be severe and potentially life threatening. Anaphylaxis often produces signs and symptoms within 5 to 30 minutes, but reactions sometimes may not develop for several hours.

PATHOPHYSIOLOGY

The chemical mediators that cause anaphylaxis are preformed and released from granules (histamine, tryptase, and others) or are generated from membrane lipids (prostaglandin D_2, leukotrienes, and platelet-activating factor) by the activated mast cell or basophil.

Tryptase is concentrated selectively in the secretory granules of all human mast cells. Its plasma levels during mast cell degranulation correlate with the clinical severity of anaphylaxis but need not be elevated in all forms of anaphylaxis (e.g., food-associated anaphylaxis).

Histamine exerts its pathophysiologic effects via both H_1 and H_2 receptors. Erythema (flushing), hypotension, and headache are mediated by both H_1 and H_2 receptors, whereas tachycardia, pruritus, bronchospasm, and rhinorrhea are associated with H_1 receptors alone.

Increased vascular permeability during anaphylaxis can produce a shift of 50% of intravascular fluid to the extravascular space within 10 minutes. This shift of effective blood volume causes compensatory catecholamine release, activates the renin-angiotensin-aldosterone system, and stimulates production of endothelin-1.

Mast cells accumulate at sites of coronary plaque erosion and rupture and they may contribute to coronary artery thrombosis. Because antibodies attached to mast cells can trigger mast cell degranulation, some investigators suggest that anaphylaxis may promote plaque rupture.

AGENTS THAT CAUSE ANAPHYLAXIS

Cause and effect often is confirmed historically in subjects who experience recurrent, objective findings of anaphylaxis upon inadvertent reexposure to the offending agent. Diagnostic testing, where appropriate, may confirm the presence of specific IgE and/or the degranulation of mast cells and basophils.

Virtually any agent capable of activating mast cells or basophils may potentially precipitate anaphylactic or anaphylactoid reactions. Table 1 lists common causes of anaphylaxis classified by pathophysiologic mechanism.

 CURRENT DIAGNOSIS

- Cutaneous: urticaria, angioedema, diffuse erythema, generalized pruritus
- Respiratory: tachypnea, bronchospasm, laryngeal or tongue edema, dysphonia
- Cardiovascular: tachycardia, bradycardia, hypotension, angina, cardiac arrhythmias
- Gastrointestinal: nausea, emesis, diarrhea, abdominal cramps, dysphagia
- Other: rhinitis, conjunctivitis, uterine cramps, headache, dizziness, syncope, blurred vision, seizure

TABLE 1 Representative Agents That Cause Anaphylaxis

IgE dependent:
- Foods (such as peanuts, tree nuts, and crustaceans)
- Medications (such as antibiotics)
- Venoms (fire ants, yellow jackets, others)
- Allergen extracts
- Latex
- Exercise (where food or medication dependent)
- Hormones

IgE independent:
- Nonspecific degranulation of mast cells and basophils
  - Opioids
  - Muscle relaxants
  - Idiopathic
  - Physical factors
    - Exercise
    - Cold, heat
- Disturbance of arachidonic acid metabolism
  - Aspirin and other nonsteroidal anti-inflammatory drugs (NSAIDs)
- Immune aggregates
  - Intravenous immunoglobulin
- Cytotoxic
  - Transfusion reactions to cellular elements (IgM, IgG)
- Multimediator complement activation/activation of contact system
  - Radiocontrast media
  - Angiotensin-converting enzyme (ACE) inhibitor administered during renal dialysis with selected dialysis membranes
  - Protamine (possibly)

Psychogenic

Modified and abridged from Kemp SF, Lockey RF: Anaphylaxis: A review of causes and mechanisms. J Allergy Clin Immunol 2002;110:341-348.

Idiopathic anaphylaxis, anaphylaxis with no identifiable cause, has accounted for approximately a third of cases in most retrospective studies of anaphylaxis. However, of 593 patients evaluated more than two decades in a university-affiliated practice (the largest retrospective series), 77% of subjects were deemed to have idiopathic anaphylaxis.

Idiopathic anaphylaxis remains a diagnosis of exclusion, however. Serial histories and diagnostic tests for foods, spices, and vegetable gums occasionally identify a specific culprit in subjects previously presumed to have idiopathic anaphylaxis. The most common identifiable causes of anaphylaxis are foods, medications, insect stings, and immunotherapy injections. Anaphylaxis to peanuts and/or tree nuts causes the greatest concern because of its life-threatening severity, especially in subjects with asthma, and the tendency for subjects to develop lifelong allergic responsiveness to these foods.

RECURRENT ANAPHYLAXIS

Depending on the report, recurrent (biphasic) anaphylaxis occurs in up to 20% of subjects who experience anaphylaxis. Signs and symptoms experienced during the recurrent phase of anaphylaxis may be equivalent to or worse than those observed in the initial reaction and may occur up to 28 hours after apparent remission. Thus, it may be necessary to monitor subjects up to 24 hours after apparent recovery from the initial phase.

DIFFERENTIAL DIAGNOSIS

Several systemic disorders share clinical features with anaphylaxis. The vasodepressor (vasovagal) reaction probably is the condition most commonly confused with anaphylactic reactions. In vasodepressor reactions, however, urticaria is absent, dyspnea is generally absent, the blood pressure is usually normal or elevated, and the skin is typically cool and pale. Tachycardia is the rule in anaphylaxis. Bradycardia may be underrecognized in anaphylaxis, however. Brown and others conducted sting challenges in 19 subjects known to be allergic to jack jumper ants (*Myrmecia*). All eight subjects who became hypotensive developed bradycardia after an initial tachycardia.

Systemic mastocytosis, a disease characterized by mast cell proliferation in multiple organs, usually features urticaria pigmentosa (brownish macules that transform into wheals upon stroking them) and recurrent episodes of pruritus, flushing, tachycardia, abdominal pain, diarrhea, syncope, or headache. Other diagnostic considerations include myocardial dysfunction, pulmonary embolism, foreign body aspiration, acute poisoning, and seizure disorder.

MANAGEMENT OF ANAPHYLAXIS

Table 2 outlines a sequential approach to management. Assessment and maintenance of airway, breathing, circulation, and mentation are necessary before proceeding to other management steps. Subjects are monitored continuously to facilitate prompt detection of any treatment complications. The recumbent position is strongly recommended. In a retrospective review of prehospital anaphylactic fatalities in the United Kingdom, the postural history was known for 10 individuals. Four of the 10 were associated with assumption of an upright or sitting posture and postmortem findings consistent with "empty heart" and pulseless electrical activity.

Epinephrine is the treatment of choice for acute anaphylaxis. Aqueous epinephrine 1:1000 dilution, 0.2 to 0.5 mL (0.01 mg/kg in children; maximum dose, 0.3 mg) administered intramuscularly every 5 minutes, as necessary, should be used to control symptoms and sustain or increase blood pressure. Comparisons of intramuscular injections to subcutaneous injections during acute anaphylaxis are not available. However, absorption is more rapid and plasma levels are higher in asymptomatic individuals who receive epinephrine intramuscularly in the anterolateral thigh.

All subsequent therapeutic interventions depend on the initial response to epinephrine and the severity of the reaction. Development of toxicity or inadequate response to epinephrine injections indicates that additional therapeutic modalities are necessary.

The α-adrenergic effect of epinephrine reverses peripheral vasodilation, which alleviates hypotension and also reduces angioedema and urticaria. It may also minimize further absorption of antigen from a sting or injection. The β-adrenergic properties of epinephrine increase myocardial output and contractility, cause bronchodilation, and suppress further mediator release from mast cells and basophils.

Fatalities during witnessed anaphylaxis usually result from delayed administration of epinephrine and from severe respiratory and/or cardiovascular complications.

TABLE 2 Management of Anaphylaxis

Immediate intervention:
- Assessment of airway, breathing, circulation, and adequacy of mentation.
- Administer aqueous epinephrine 1:1000 dilution, 0.2–0.5 mL (0.01 mg/kg in children; maximum dose, 0.3 mg) *intramuscularly* q5min, as necessary, to control symptoms and blood pressure.

Possibly appropriate, subsequent measures depending on response to epinephrine:
- Place subject in recumbent position and elevate lower extremities.
- Establish and maintain airway.
- Administer oxygen.
- Establish venous access.
- Use normal saline IV for fluid replacement.

Specific measures to consider after epinephrine injections, where appropriate:
- An epinephrine infusion might be prepared. Continuous hemodynamic monitoring is essential (see reference for specific details).
- Diphenhydramine (Benadryl). Note: In the management of anaphylaxis, a combination of diphenhydramine and ranitidine (Zantac)[1] is superior to diphenhydramine alone.
- For bronchospasm resistant to epinephrine, use nebulized albuterol (Proventil).
- For refractory hypotension, consider dopamine (Intropin), 400 mg in 500 mL D_5W, administered IV at 2–20 µg/kg/min titrated to maintain adequate blood pressure. Continuous hemodynamic monitoring is essential.
- Where use of β-blockers complicates therapy, consider glucagon,[1] 1–5 mg (20–30 µg/kg; maximum: 1 mg in children), administered IV over 5 min followed by an infusion, 5–15 µg/min. Aspiration precautions should be observed.
- For patients with a history of asthma and for those who experience severe or prolonged anaphylaxis, consider methylprednisolone (Solu-Medrol) (1.0–2.0 mg/kg/d).
- Consider transportation to the emergency department or an intensive care facility.

Interventions for cardiopulmonary arrest occurring during anaphylaxis:
- High-dose epinephrine and prolonged resuscitation efforts are encouraged, if necessary, because efforts are more likely to be successful in anaphylaxis where the subject (often young) has a healthy cardiovascular system (see reference for specific details).

Observation and subsequent outpatient follow-up:
- Observation periods after apparent resolution must be individualized and based on such factors as the clinical scenario, co-morbid conditions, and distance from the patient's home to the closest emergency department. After recovery from the acute episode, patients should receive epinephrine syringes (EpiPen or TwinJect) and be instructed in proper technique. Everyone postanaphylaxis requires a careful diagnostic evaluation in consultation with an allergist-immunologist.

[1]Not FDA approved for this indication.
Abbreviation: IV = intravenous.
Modified from Lieberman P, Kemp SF, Oppenheimer J, et al (chief eds). Joint Task Force on Practice Parameters. The diagnosis and management of anaphylaxis: An updated practice parameter. J Allergy Clin Immunol 2005;115:S483-S523.

There is no absolute contraindication to epinephrine administration in anaphylaxis.

Oxygen should be administered to subjects with anaphylaxis who require multiple doses of epinephrine, receive inhaled β_2 agonists, have protracted anaphylaxis, or have preexisting hypoxemia or myocardial dysfunction.

Antihistamines (H_1 and H_2 antagonists) support the treatment of anaphylaxis. However, these agents act much slower than epinephrine and should never be administered alone as treatment for anaphylaxis. Antihistamines thus should be considered as *second-line* treatment.

Systemic corticosteroids have no role in the acute management of anaphylaxis because even intravenous administration of these agents may have no effect for 4 to 6 hours after administration. Although corticosteroids traditionally are used in the management of anaphylaxis, their effect has never been evaluated in placebo-controlled trials. Corticosteroids administered during anaphylaxis might provide additional benefit for patients with asthma or other conditions recently treated with corticosteroids.

Numerous cases of unusually severe or refractory anaphylaxis are reported in subjects receiving β-blocking agents. Greater severity of anaphylaxis observed in usual doses of epinephrine administered during anaphylaxis to subjects taking β-blockers may not produce the desired clinical response. In such situations, both isotonic volume expansion and glucagon[1] administration are recommended. Glucagon may potentially reverse refractory hypotension and bronchospasm because it bypasses the β-adrenergic receptor and directly activates adenyl cyclase.

Persistent hypotension despite epinephrine injections should first be treated with intravenous crystalloid solutions. Saline is generally preferred. One to 2 L of normal saline might need to be administered to adults at a rate of 5 to 10 mL/kg in the first 5 minutes. Children should receive up to 30 mL/kg in the first hour. Large volumes (e.g., 7 L) are often required.

Vasopressors should be administered if epinephrine injections and volume expansion fail to alleviate hypotension. Dopamine (Intropin) frequently increases blood pressure while maintaining or enhancing renal and splanchnic perfusion. These agents would not be expected to work as well in patients already maximally vasoconstricted by their internal compensatory response to anaphylaxis.

PREVENTION OF ANAPHYLAXIS

Table 3 outlines the basic principles for the prevention of future anaphylactic episodes in high-risk individuals. An allergist-immunologist can provide comprehensive professional advice on these matters.

All subjects at high risk for recurrent anaphylaxis should carry epinephrine syringes and know how to administer them. An EpiPen (Dey Laboratories) is a spring-loaded, pressure-activated syringe with a single 0.3 mg dose (1:1000 dilution) of epinephrine. It is easy to use and injects through clothing. An EpiPen Jr, which delivers 0.15 mg (1:2000 dilution) epinephrine, is appropriate for children weighing less than 30 kg. The TwinJect (Verus Pharmaceuticals) is a prefilled, pen-sized, epinephrine auto-injector with two doses of either 0.3 or 0.15 mg.

[1]Not FDA approved for this indication.

TABLE 3 Preventive Measures for Subjects with Anaphylaxis

General measures:
- Obtain thorough history to diagnose life-threatening food or drug allergy.
- Identify cause of anaphylaxis and those individuals at risk for future attacks.
- Provide instruction on proper reading of food and medication labels, where appropriate.
- Patient should avoid exposure to antigens and cross-reactive substances.
- Manage asthma and coronary artery disease optimally.

Specific measures for high-risk subjects:
- Individuals at high risk for anaphylaxis should carry self-injectable syringes of epinephrine (EpiPen or TwinJect) at all times and receive instruction in proper use with placebo trainer.
- Individuals should wear a Medic Alert bracelet or chain.
- Other agents for β-adrenergic antagonists, angiotensin-converting enzyme (ACE) inhibitors, tricyclic antidepressants, and monoamine oxidase inhibitors should be substituted whenever possible.
- Agents suspected of causing anaphylaxis should be administered slowly, supervised, and orally if possible
- Where appropriate, use specific preventive strategies, including pharmacologic prophylaxis, short-term challenge and desensitization, and long-term desensitization.

Modified from Kemp SF: Anaphylaxis: Current concepts in pathophysiology, diagnosis, and management. Immunol Allergy Clin N Am 2001;21:611-634.

TABLE 4 Representative Agents That Cause Serum Sickness

Medications: β-lactam antibiotics, sulfonamides, ciprofloxacin (Cipro), metronidazole (Flagyl), rifampin (Rifadin), allopurinol (Zyloprim), carbamazepine (Tegretol), phenytoin (Dilantin), fluoxetine (Prozac), bupropion (Wellbutrin), methimazole (Tapazole), propylthiouracil, thiazide diuretics, captopril (Capoten), propranolol (Inderal), verapamil (Calan), streptokinase (Streptase), others
Heterologous (animal-derived) antisera:
- Horse: snake and spider venom, tetanus, botulism, diphtheria
- Horse or rabbit: anti-lymphocyte globulin
Mouse: monoclonal antibodies (muromonab-CD3 [Orthoclone OKT3], rituximab [Rituxan], infliximab [Remicade])
Homologous (human-derived) antisera: cytomegalovirus, hepatitis B, rabies, tetanus, perinatal $RH_0(D)$

Serum Sickness

Serum sickness is a clinical syndrome of fever, malaise, and urticarial and/or morbilliform cutaneous eruption that is often preceded by generalized erythema and pruritus. Arthralgias or arthritis (mainly large joints), neuropathy, lymphadenopathy, nephritis, abdominal pain (emesis or melena are possible), or vasculitis (cutaneous or systemic) may occur in some cases. Cutaneous vasculitis, also known as hypersensitivity vasculitis, is often manifested by palpable purpura, which most commonly are found on the lower extremities of ambulatory individuals or on the sacral or gluteal region of patients with restricted mobility. These purpura reflect vascular leakage from inflamed postcapillary venules. Systemic vasculitis may occur in association with autoimmune diseases, infection, or malignancy.

Many agents may produce serum sickness or serum sickness–like reactions (Table 4). *Serum sickness* classically refers to the immune complex syndrome caused by immunization with heterologous serum proteins (often equine or murine). The most frequent cause is immune complex-mediated drug hypersensitivity. A serum sickness–like drug reaction generally develops 6 to 21 days after the culprit medication is started, but it can occur within 12 to 48 hours in previously sensitized individuals.

PATHOGENESIS AND LABORATORY ABNORMALITIES

Healthy individuals regularly generate low levels of circulating immune complexes, which are either excreted by the kidneys or extracted in the liver and spleen by monocytes and macrophages. It is hypothesized that serum sickness results when a drug (hapten) binds to plasma protein and antibodies are generated in response to the drug-protein complex. Complement activation occurs when large quantities of soluble antigen-antibody (immune) complexes fix to vascular endothelial receptors. Complement fragments attract and activate neutrophils, which release proteases that induce tissue injury. The urticaria in serum sickness probably results from immune complex necrotizing vasculitis and complement activation that induces mast cell degranulation. IgE-dependent mechanisms likely are also contributory in some individuals. Laboratory abnormalities include elevated erythrocyte sedimentation rate, leukopenia (acute phase), occasional plasmacytosis, and decreased total hemolytic complement (CH50), C3, and C4. Slight albuminuria, hyaline casts, and microscopic hematuria may also occur.

TREATMENT

Stoppage of the culprit agent, when identified, is recommended. Serum sickness is usually self-limited and rarely life threatening when the offending drug or protein is stopped or removed. Symptoms generally improve over 2 to 4 weeks as patients clear their immune complexes. Evidence-based treatment recommendations for serum sickness are very limited. Long-acting, less-sedating H_1 antihistamines such as cetirizine (Zyrtec), desloratadine (Clarinex), fexofenadine (Allegra), or loratadine (Claritin) generally control urticaria. Systemic corticosteroids (e.g., prednisone, 0.5 to 1.0 mg/kg/day) may help severe symptoms. Fever and arthralgias typically resolve within 48 to 72 hours of treatment, and the formation of new cutaneous eruptions usually ceases within the same time frame. Antihistamine therapy is continued for 1 week after apparent resolution of symptoms and then slowly discontinued. Skin testing with heterologous antisera is performed routinely to avoid anaphylaxis to future administration of heterologous serum.

REFERENCES

American Heart Association in collaboration with International Liaison Committee on Resuscitation: 2005 American Heart Association guidelines for cardiopulmonary resuscitation and emergency cardiovascular care. Anaphylaxis. Circulation 2005;112(Suppl 4):143-145.

Brown SGA, Blackman KE, Stenlake V, Heddle RJ: Insect sting anaphylaxis: Prospective evaluation of treatment with intravenous adrenaline and volume resuscitation. Emerg Med J 2004;21:149-154.

Kemp SF, Lockey RF: Anaphylaxis: A review of causes and mechanisms. J Allergy Clin Immunol 2002;110:341-348.

Lieberman P, Kemp SF, Oppenheimer J, et al. (cheif eds). Joint Task Force on Practice Parameters. The diagnosis and management of anaphylaxis: An updated practice parameter. J Allergy Clin Immunol 2005;115:S483-S523.

Project Team of the Resuscitation Council (UK): Emergency medical treatment of anaphylactic reactions. J Accid Emerg Med 1999;16:243-247.

Pumphrey RSH: Fatal posture in anaphylactic shock. J Allergy Clin Immunol 2003;112:451-452.

Pumphrey RSH: Fatal anaphylaxis in the UK, 1992–2001. Novartis Found Symp 2004;257:116-128.

Simons FER, Gu X, Simons KJ: Epinephrine absorption in adults: Intramuscular versus subcutaneous injection. J Allergy Clin Immunol 2001;108:871-873.

Simons FER, Roberts JR, Gu X, Simons KJ: Epinephrine absorption in children with a history of anaphylaxis. J Allergy Clin Immunol 1998;101:33-37.

Wener M: Serum sickness and serum sickness-like reactions. In: Rose BD (ed): UpToDate, www.uptodateonline.com, Version 14.2 (current through April 2006), Wellesley, Ma.

Asthma in Adolescents and Adults

Method of
Louis-Philippe Boulet, MD

Asthma is one of the most common respiratory diseases in adults and children, and its prevalence has been increasing worldwide. This rise is mostly attributed to an increase in allergic diseases, probably of multifactorial origin. With the recent improvements in our understanding of the disease and the availability of various therapeutic options, it should have a minimal impact in most asthma sufferers, but the human and socioeconomic burden of asthma is unfortunately still high.

Definition and Pathophysiology: Targets for Therapy

Asthma is defined as a condition characterized by paroxysmal or persistent symptoms such as wheezing, chest tightness, phlegm production, and cough, associated with variable airway obstruction and hyperresponsiveness to various stimuli. These changes are mostly caused by underlying airway inflammation and structural changes (remodeling). The asthmatic airway inflammatory process, in which eosinophils, mast cells, and lymphocytes are abundant compared to normal subjects, is caused by the influence of TH_2 cells, producing mediators such as interleukin (IL)-3, IL-4, IL-5, IL-13, and granulocyte-macrophage colony-stimulating factor (GM-CSF). Some of these mediators (IL-4) activate B lymphocytes to produce immunoglobulin E (IgE) or perpetuate eosinophilic airway inflammation

(IL-3, IL-5, GM-CSF). Changes in airway structure in asthma include epithelial damage, subepithelial fibrosis, increased airway vasculature, changes in proteoglycans, and increased smooth muscle mass, among many others.

The etiology of asthma is unknown, but its development likely results from environmental exposures in individuals genetically predisposed to develop this condition. Many genes determine the susceptibility to develop asthma, and the number of polymorphisms associated with asthma is still increasing. In regard to environmental exposures, allergen sensitization plays a major role. According to the hygiene hypothesis, the increase in allergic diseases observed in the last two decades may be related to a change in the immune system in favor of a TH_2-type lymphocyte response, mostly programmed at producing antibodies against environmental allergens, to the detriment of the mostly anti-infectious TH_1-type response; this may be the result of reduced exposure to infectious agents and therefore endotoxins, in the context of an expanding so-called Western lifestyle. In regard to ambient or outdoor pollutants, their influence on asthma is complex, but they may contribute to its development. The increasing prevalence of various sensitizers at the workplace may also be involved.

Diagnosis

Although typical symptoms of asthma may suggest its diagnosis, the disease should be confirmed by objective measures that demonstrate either variable airway obstruction or hyperresponsiveness because various conditions may mimic asthma. Box 1 lists the diagnostic criteria. Ideally, spirometry should be done to measure expiratory flows; otherwise, a peak expiratory flow (PEF) may be measured with a portable device. A bronchoprovocation test may reveal airway hyperresponsiveness, a classic hallmark of symptomatic asthma. Physical examination is often normal unless the patient is seen during an asthma exacerbation. Chest radiograph is usually normal except in the presence of an associated condition or complication.

Triggers and Inducers

Box 2 categorizes exposures causing or increasing airway inflammation (inducers) and noninflammatory stimuli that provoke symptoms (triggers). Indoor allergens such as

CURRENT DIAGNOSIS

- The diagnosis of asthma should be confirmed by the objective measures of variable airflow limitation or airway hyperresponsiveness.
- Control of asthma is the main parameter to adjust the treatment and should be assessed regularly according to current guideline criteria, including symptoms and expiratory flows.
- Triggers (particularly relevant allergen exposure, workplace sensitizers, smoking) and co-morbidities (e.g., rhinitis, gastroesophageal reflux) of asthma should be identified.

BOX 1 Diagnostic Criteria of Asthma

Variable Airway Obstruction

- Improvement of FEV_1
  >12% postbronchodilator, ideally 15% (minimum 180 mL for adults)
  >20% over time or after corticosteroid treatment (minimum 250 mL for adults)
- Improvement in PEF
  >20% postbronchodilator or over time

Airway Hyperresponsiveness

- Positive bronchial provocation test (e.g., with methacholine)

Abbreviations: FEV_1 = forced expiratory volume in 1 second; PEF = peak expiratory flow.
Adapted from Boulet LP, Becker A, Bérubé D, et al., on behalf of the Canadian Asthma Consensus Group: Canadian asthma consensus report. Can Med Assoc J 1999;30; 161(11 Suppl):S1-S61.

---

animal danders and house dust mites are recognized as more "asthmogenic" than outdoor ones. Various sensitizers may be present at the workplace, divided into high (e.g., flour) or low molecular weight (e.g., isocyanates) substances. Potential environmental exposures and their relationship to symptoms should be documented. Allergy skin prick

BOX 2 Triggers and Inducers of Asthma

Inducers of Airway Inflammation

- Allergens (indoors): domestic animals, house dust mites, cockroaches, molds, etc.
- Allergens (outdoors): pollen, molds, foods (more rarely)
- Workplace sensitizers:
  Animal origin: laboratory animals, seafood processing, etc.
  Vegetable origin: flour, wood dust, etc.
  Chemical: isocyanates, phthalic anhydrides, etc.
  Biologic agents: *Bacillus subtilis*
  Metals: nickel, platinum salts
- Viral respiratory infections

Factors That Can Increase or Modify the Type of Airway Inflammation

  Environmental pollutants (sulfur dioxide [SO_2], nitrogen dioxide [NO_2], ozone)
  Tobacco smoke

Other Potential Triggers of Asthma in Most Asthmatic Patients

- Exercise, cold air, temperature changes, humidity
- Strong odors, respiratory irritants
- β-Blockers
- Emotional stress

Other Potential Triggers of Asthma in Selected Subgroups of Patients with Asthma

- Aspirin and nonsteroidal anti-inflammatory agents
- Food additives (sulfites, benzoates, monosodium glutamate)
- Premenstrual increase in asthma
- Gastroesophageal reflux

tests help determine if IgE antibodies are produced against the common airborne allergens. Upper and lower respiratory tract infections, particularly of viral origin, may lead to asthma exacerbations and could be involved in the development of asthma in predisposed individuals. Finally, exposure to respiratory irritants, cold air, or emotional stress can result in bronchoconstriction, depending on the degree of airway responsiveness. Tobacco smoke can trigger asthma, and when tobacco is used regularly it may reduce the efficacy of treatment. Gastroesophageal reflux is common in asthma, and its contribution to asthma symptomatology should be assessed. Exercise may induce asthma symptoms that could be prevented by taking a fast-acting bronchodilator beforehand. Increasing bronchoconstrictive response to exertion suggests a loss of control of the asthma.

Management and Treatment

Table 1 summarizes the global management of asthma, and Figure 1 shows the therapeutic scheme of asthma treatment. According to the international guidelines "Global Initiative on Asthma: (GINA) (http://www.ginasthma.com), asthma management includes the following:

- Educate patient to develop a partnership in asthma management.
- Assess and monitor asthma severity with symptom reports and, when possible, measurement of lung function.
- Avoid exposure to risk factors.
- Establish an individual medication plan for long-term management.

TABLE 1 General Management of Asthma

Confirm the diagnosis and assess initial severity.	Evaluate symptoms and measure expiratory flows ± airway responsiveness.
Determine possible triggers and inducers.	Questionnaire, allergy tests, other tests (assess environment, workplace, etc.)
Initiate treatment.	Prescribe medication required and treat associated triggers to achieve asthma control conditions.
Initiate education.	Provide basic elements and refer to an asthma educator.
Determine the achievable best results.	Check asthma control criteria (symptoms, activities, rescue medication needs, expiratory flows).*
Determine the medication needed.	Once asthma is well controlled, reduce medication while keeping control.
Devise an action plan.	Write and discuss with the patient a plan for management of exacerbations.
Ensure regular follow-up.	Check control criteria, including expiratory flows.*

*And maybe in the near future from noninvasive measures of airway inflammation.
Adapted from Boulet et al: What is new since the last (1999) Canadian Asthma Consensus guidelines? Can Respir J 2001.

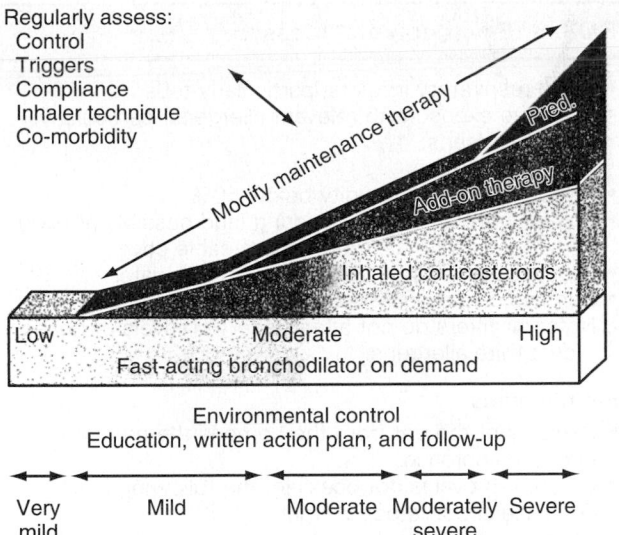

Regularly assess:
Control
Triggers
Compliance
Inhaler technique
Co-morbidity

FIGURE 1. Therapeutic Scheme of Asthma. The Canadian Guidelines suggest that asthma management be considered as a continuum: Inhaled corticosteroids (ICSs) are introduced as initial maintenance treatment, even with symptoms less than three times a week. LTRAs (leukotriene receptor antagonists) are a second-choice alternative, particularly for patients who cannot or will not use ICS agents. If control is inadequate on low-dose inhaled corticosteroids, the reasons for poor control are researched, and, if needed, additional therapy with long-acting β_2-agonists, LTRAs, or theophylline, as a third therapeutic option, is offered. The dose of inhaled corticosteroid is adapted to the severity of asthma. Severe asthma may require additional systemic steroids. Asthma control, compliance, and maintenance therapy must be regularly reassessed. (See Stepwise Approach for Managing Asthma in Adults and Children Older Than 5 Years of Age [p. 132]. Available online at http://www.nhlbi.nih.gov/guidelines/asthma/execsumm.pdf)

- Establish an individual plan for managing exacerbations.
- Provide regular follow-up care.

GOALS OF TREATMENT

The goals of asthma treatment are to promote a normal active life, including adequate exercise tolerance, no or minimal asthma symptoms, optimal pulmonary function; to prevent exacerbations; to reduce asthma severity or the potential for irreversible airflow limitation; and to minimize asthma-related morbidity and mortality while experiencing no significant side effects from treatment.

These goals could be achieved by obtaining rapid and long-term optimal control of asthma, including optimal pulmonary function, from avoidance of triggers, particularly those inducing airway inflammation. The minimal medication allowing optimal control of symptoms should be determined and reevaluated regularly (Table 2). The patient with asthma must fully understand the disease and its treatment and know how to avoid triggers and exposures that could induce symptoms but, more importantly, those that could increase airway inflammation.

Assessment of Control and Severity

Treatment needs are based on achievement of control criteria, which means minimal symptoms and rescue medication needs and optimal pulmonary function. Additional measures of control have been suggested, such

 CURRENT THERAPY

- Asthma education, environmental control, and smoking cessation are mandatory for optimal treatment.
- A fast-acting bronchodilator should be available for occasional symptoms and used at the minimal frequency and dosing.
- If asthma symptoms become regular (e.g., every week or more), an anti-inflammatory agent (first choice: inhaled corticosteroid) should be introduced.
- If an inhaled corticosteroid at low doses is not sufficient to control asthma, after compliance, environmental, inhaler technique, and co-morbidities are checked, an add-on therapy such as an inhaled long-acting β_2-agonist or a leukotriene antagonist should be introduced.
- If asthma is severe or difficult to control, it should be reassessed by an asthma specialist.
- Compliance with therapy and environmental measures, as well as inhaler techniques, should be verified regularly.
- Regular medical and educational follow-up should be ensured.

as airway responsiveness, airway eosinophilia from induced sputum analysis, and nitric oxide (NO) measurement in expired air, but they are not currently recommended in most guidelines. Severity is best defined by the minimum medication needed to achieve asthma control (Table 3).

Asthma Education

Education of asthmatic patients and their families is mandatory to achieve adequate asthma control and optimize treatment compliance and self-management, particularly at the onset of asthma exacerbations. A written individualized action plan should indicate how to manage these exacerbations. Various programs and networks offer asthma education. The educational intervention initiated

TABLE 2 Asthma Control Criteria

Parameters	Frequency or Value
Daytime symptoms	<4 d/wk
Nighttime symptoms	<1 night/wk
Physical activity	Normal
Exacerbations	Mild, infrequent
Absenteeism from work or school because of asthma	None
Need for β_2-agonist as needed	<4 doses/wk*
FEV1 or PEF	≥90% of personal best
PEF diurnal variation	<15%

*May use one dose per day before exercise.
Abbreviations: FEV$_1$ = forced expiratory flow in 1 second; PEF = peak expiratory flow.
Adapted from Boulet LP, Becker A, Bérubé D, et al, on behalf of the Canadian Asthma Consensus Group: Canadian asthma consensus report. Can Med Assoc J 1999;30;161(11 Suppl):S1-S61; and Lemiere C, Bai T, Balter M, et al: Adult Asthma Consensus Guidelines Update 2003. Can Respir J 2004;11(Suppl A):9A-18A.

TABLE 3 Asthma Severity According to Long-Term Treatment Needs

Severity*	Symptoms	Treatment Required
Very mild	Mild/infrequent	None, or inhaled β_2 agonist, rarely
Mild	Well controlled	β_2 agonist occasionally + low-dose ICS
Moderate	Well controlled	β_2 agonist low/moderate doses ICS ± additional therapy
Severe	Well controlled	β_2 agonist + high doses ICS + additional therapy
Very severe glucocorti-costeroid	Not well controlled	β_2 agonist + high doses ICS + well-controlled additional therapy + oral

*The primary measure of asthma severity in the treated patient should be the minimum therapy required to achieve acceptable control.
Abbreviation: ICS = inhaled corticosteroid.
Reproduced from Boulet LP, Becker A, Bérubé D, et al., on behalf of the Canadian Asthma Consensus Group: Canadian asthma consensus report. Can Med Assoc J 1999;30;161(11 Suppl):S1-S61.

in the physician's office is ideally completed by an asthma educator. Education should result in an improvement in the patient's health behaviors and self-management abilities. Asthma-control criteria must be explained and instructions provided on preventive measures and ways to adjust the treatment rapidly in case of exacerbation. Meta-analyses show that asthma education, including a written action plan and regular review, could lead to a reduction of asthma-related morbidity. Asthma education should especially be offered to patients with high asthma-related morbidity or severe asthma. Good communication between the patient and the physician/educator is essential, and the patient's feedback should be obtained to address any barrier to an adequate control of the disease.

ENVIRONMENTAL CONTROL AND AVOIDANCE OF TRIGGERS

Environmental control is another important aspect of asthma management. Contacts with respiratory irritants, particularly with allergens to which patients are sensitized, should be avoided. Although preventive measures are usually implemented for house dust mites, they are more rarely done for domestic animal avoidance. However, control of indoor exposures in sensitized subjects is key to asthma control (Box 3). The best measure for an allergy to domestic animals is to stop exposure to the animal, although secondary measures may be applied if the patient is unwilling in this regard. Asthmatic patients who smoke have an accelerated decline in lung function, respond less to treatment, and suffer an increased asthma-related morbidity. All of these patients should be offered participation in a smoking cessation program when available.

Asthmatic patients with nasal polyps are often intolerant of aspirin and nonsteroidal anti-inflammatory agents (e.g., for arthritis) and should avoid them. β-Blockers are contraindicated in asthma because they can trigger severe bronchospasm. Regular exercise is recommended and

---

BOX 3 Environmental Measures

- Avoid respiratory irritants, particularly tobacco smoke.
- Minimize exposure to relevant allergens, particularly indoor allergens:
  House dust mites
- Maintain relative humidity below 50%.
- Encase mattress and box spring (and possibly pillows) in mite- and mite allergen-impermeable covers.
- Launder bed linen in hot (55°C [131°F]) water.
- Remove carpeting whenever possible.
  Note: Air filters do not affect reservoir levels of house dust mite allergens.

Pet Allergens

- Removal of the pet from the home is the most effective approach.
- Where removal is not possible, the following may decrease airborne pet allergens:
  Pet exclusion from the bedroom
  HEPA (high-efficiency particulate air [filter]) room air cleaner
  Mattress and pillow covers
  Removal of carpeting
  Frequent vacuuming of upholstered furniture with a HEPA-filtered vacuum
  Washing the pet may temporarily reduce allergen load, but the allergic individual must not do the washing

Adapted from Boulet et al: What is new since the last (1999) Canadian Asthma Consensus guidelines? Can Respir J 2001.

---

associated with improved asthma control. Finally, weight loss should be promoted in obese patients because it reduces asthma severity.

Pharmacotherapy

Asthma medications are usually categorized as relievers for acute intermittent symptoms and as controllers for long-term maintenance treatment and prevention of the manifestations of asthma (Box 4). Therapeutic plans are

---

BOX 4 Categories of Asthma Medications

Relievers

- Short-acting β_2-agonists
- Formoterol (if already used with an inhaled corticosteroid)
- Anticholinergics (if intolerance to β_2-agonists)*

Controllers

- Anti-inflammatory medications
  Corticosteroids: inhaled and systemic
  Nonsteroidal agents: Leukotriene receptor antagonists:
    Omalizumab (Anti-IgE)*
  Cromoglycate and nedocromil (antiallergics)
  Methotrexate, ketotifen*
- Bronchodilators
  Long-acting β_2-agonists
  Theophyllines*

*More rarely prescribed.

suggested by current guidelines, either in the form of a continuum of treatment or using a stepwise approach (Figure 1). Basically, that medication should be adapted to the severity of the disease, and the minimum amount of drugs and dosage required to keep asthma controlled is a good index of its severity.

RELIEVERS

Fast-acting β_2-agonists, such as the short-acting agents salbutamol, fenoterol, and terbutaline or the long-acting formoterol (in certain patients already using this medication and an inhaled corticosteroid), are used for treating intermittent asthma symptoms. For this purpose, however, they should be used on demand at the least frequent dose possible. A frequent or increasing need for these drugs reveals a loss of asthma control and/or abuse of the medication and is associated with increased incidence of severe asthma events.

CONTROLLERS

Inhaled Corticosteroids

Inhaled corticosteroids (ICSs) are the mainstay of long-term asthma treatment and act at numerous sites of the inflammatory cascade. They should be prescribed for all patients with more than very mild asthma. They help obtain and maintain asthma control by reducing symptoms and improving lung function, decreasing airway responsiveness, preventing asthma exacerbations, and reducing the morbidity and mortality associated with asthma. Most of the benefit is obtained at low to moderate doses. Depending on asthma severity, the dose response of the therapeutic effect of ICS agents plateaus at moderate to high doses. Table 4 shows the comparative potency of the available agents.

Too much phobia still exists about using inhaled corticosteroids. The side effects of low to moderate doses in adolescents and adults are minimal, mostly in the form of occasional dysphonia or oropharyngeal candidiasis, reduced by rinsing the mouth after intake or the use of a spacer. At high doses, they may slightly increase bone loss and produce ecchymosis and, possibly, in predisposed groups of patients, promote the development of glaucoma or cataracts. Osteoporosis prophylaxis is not recommended for patients on ICS agents unless they regularly use high doses, particularly with intermittent or regular oral corticosteroids.

Recent studies suggest that introducing an ICS early in the course of the disease may be beneficial because it may reduce asthma-related events; whether this could influence the course of the disease remains to be documented. An ICS cannot be stopped in most asthmatic patients without recurrence of symptoms and reduction in pulmonary function, indicating that the ICS may control the disease but does not induce a long-term remission. A reduction of doses to the minimum that keeps asthma under control is warranted, and if doses higher than low (to sometimes moderate) are needed, there are benefits to adding another controller.

Long-Acting β_2-Agonists

The long-acting β_2-agonists (LABAs) salmeterol (Serevent) and formoterol (Oxeze) are now introduced earlier in the asthma treatment plan than before and are an excellent choice as add-on treatment when low to moderate doses of an ICS alone are insufficient to control asthma. Because LABAs have little or no effect on airway inflammation, they should always be taken with a corticosteroid. As monotherapy, they are associated with an increased incidence of severe asthma events and even, although very rarely, to fatal asthma, particularly with overuse of the medication. Unlike with short-acting β_2-agonists, their regular use with an ICS leads to improved asthma control in a large number of patients. LABAs improve airway caliber for 12 hours or more and therefore are usually prescribed twice daily. Although they seem to add little to an ICS in mild corticosteroid-naive patients compared to an ICS alone, in patients already on this last type of medication, even on low doses, they provide an added benefit, compared to doubling the dose of ICS. A possible synergy with ICS is suggested at the molecular level, but its clinical relevance is not confirmed. Formoterol has a rapid onset of action and could also act as a reliever in patients on ICS already using this medication. The prescription of a combination of ICS and LABA in the same inhaler (combination therapy) may simplify the treatment, improve compliance, and prevent the use of LABA as monotherapy. Such formulations include budesonide and formoterol (Symbicort) or fluticasone and salmeterol (Advair).

Leukotriene Receptor Antagonists

Leukotriene receptor antagonists (LTRAs), such as montelukast (Singulair) and zafirlukast (Accolate), block the effects of leukotrienes, acting as receptor antagonists. Most guidelines consider LTRAs the second-best choice for anti-inflammatory treatment of asthma, and they may be useful in those who cannot or will not use inhaled corticosteroids. They may possibly act even better at earlier stages of asthma, and their proposed role in the treatment of rhinitis may improve asthma as well and possibly

TABLE 4 Inhaled Corticosteroid Equivalences

Product	Dose (μg/d)		
	Low	Medium	High
BDP pMDI and spacer (CFC)	≤500	501–1000	>1000
BUD Turbuhaler*	≤400	401–800	>800
FP pMDI and spacer	≤250	251–500	>500
FP Diskus[†]	≤250	251–500	>500
BDP pMDI (HFA)[‡]	≤250	251–500	>500
BUD wet nebulization[§]	≤1000	1001–2000	>2000

Note: For children, the consensus group defines low dose as <400 μg of BDP delivered via a pMDI attached to a spacer.
*Budesonide Turbuhaler.
[†]Fluticasone propionate Diskus.
[‡]In solution with alcohol (QVAR); other HFA inhalers may provide dose equivalencies similar to BDP delivered with a traditional pMDI.
[§]Budesonide solution for wet nebulization.
Abbreviations: BDP = beclomethasone dipropionate; BUD = budesonide; FP = fluticasone propionate; HFA = hydrofluoroalkane (propellant); pMDI = pressurized metered-dose inhaler.
Adapted from Boulet LP, Becker A, Bérubé D, et al., on behalf of the Canadian Asthma Consensus Group: Canadian asthma consensus report. Can Med Assoc J 1999;30;161(11 Suppl):S1-S61.

influence its natural history, although we need more studies to determine if that is the case.

LTRAs may also be prescribed as an add-on therapy to corticosteroids when asthma is not sufficiently controlled. Some patients may like the fact that they are used in an oral form. They are considered very safe. Most of their therapeutic effect is usually seen within the first 2 weeks of treatment. Zafirlukast is given twice daily, should not be taken with food, and interacts with warfarin. Montelukast does not have these limitations and is taken once daily. In regard to lipoxygenase inhibitors, Zileuton is available in the United States. Its effects are similar to LTRAs. It may be associated with an increase in liver enzymes.

OTHER MEDICATIONS

So-called antiallergic drugs, such as cromolyn (Intal) and nedocromil (Tilade), are now infrequently prescribed because low doses of ICS agents or LTRAs have replaced them. Furthermore, they have to be taken four times a day. They may still have an adjunct role in the prevention of exercise-induced asthma.

Theophylline has immunomodulatory properties and is suggested as a third choice add-on treatment because it is less effective than LABAs and has a narrow therapeutic window. Ipratropium (Atrovent) and tiotropium (Spiriva) are rarely used for the long-term treatment of asthma unless there is an associated component of chronic obstructive pulmonary disease (COPD). Ipratropium is used in acute asthma and as a reliever in patients intolerant to β_2-agonists.

Omalizumab (Xolair) is a monoclonal antibody that is now available. Although asthma guidelines have not yet evaluated its role in asthma treatment, it could be particularly useful for the treatment of severe allergic asthma. Its cost and the need to be administered subcutaneously may be considered limitations, however.

Oral corticosteroids are required in very few patients today for long-term treatment of severe asthma. Their need should be carefully assessed, dosage kept at the minimum required, and compliance to the other treatments and environmental measures checked. Prophylaxis for osteoporosis is required in these patients. Some immunosuppressive drugs, such as methotrexate, gold salts, and cyclosporine, may reduce oral steroid needs, but their benefits are sometimes small compared to their potential side effects. If considered, they should be used only in specialized centers after extensive evaluation.

Immunotherapy is used variably from one country to another. It is generally reserved for patients in whom environmental measures and medication are insufficient to control the disease adequately. It is more beneficial in allergic rhinitis. Its benefits should be weighed against the possible occurrence of complications (transient increase in asthma, local allergic responses, etc.), its cost, time involvement, and the possibility of achieving control by other means.

Other Measures

An increased prevalence of asthma or asthma-like symptoms is described in the obese patient. Weight loss is associated with an improvement of asthma.

Vaccination for influenza is recommended in asthmatic subjects.

Although some studies suggest the asthmatic's diet should include sufficient antioxidants to help reduce inflammatory responses and that omega 3 (e.g., in fish oil) may have some beneficial effects, no specific dietary measures, other than those dictated by general health principles, are currently recommended, in the absence of a food allergy, which is rare.

Yoga and stress reduction techniques may sometimes improve asthma, but their effect is small.

Controlling Asthma

Asthma control should be assessed regularly and the treatment adjusted accordingly. Box 5 summarizes some of the reasons asthma control may not be achieved. If the cause of this lack of adequate control is uncertain or if asthma is severe, the patient benefits from a referral to an asthma specialist.

FOLLOW-UP

Asthma is a chronic condition and remissions are rare. Regular medical and educational follow-up should be ensured to adjust treatment and repeat the essential information needed to obtain an effective self-management of the disease. Box 6 outlines the ideal elements for follow-up visits.

MANAGEMENT OF EXACERBATIONS

Asthma exacerbations are an important cause of morbidity and health care costs. Patients should be educated about how to modify their medication according to control criteria, and these guidelines should be summarized in a written action plan. Basically, corticosteroid treatment should be rapidly stepped up (dose more than doubled) until symptoms and expiratory flows improve. If exacerbation is severe, systemic (usually oral) corticosteroids should be prescribed.

THE FUTURE OF ASTHMA MANAGEMENT

Asthma in most patients can be well controlled with the available therapies, and most often, insufficient asthma control is because of inadequate treatment and insufficient self-management skills. We should nevertheless improve

---

BOX 5 Possible Causes of Uncontrolled Asthma

- Wrong diagnosis
- Current smoking
- Noncompliance with medication
- Environmental exposures
- Untreated co-morbidities
- Chronic obstructive pulmonary disease (COPD) component
- Inadequate inhaler technique
- Steroid resistance
- Severe asthma

BOX 6 Follow-up Visits

When asthmatic patients are seen at follow-up or unscheduled visits, the following elements should be checked:
- Control criteria (symptoms, expiratory flows)
- Current treatment: understanding and compliance
- Untoward reactions to the medication
- Exacerbations, emergency department visits, or hospital admissions
- Current exposure to triggers (particularly cigarette smoke, relevant allergens, workplace exposures)
- Inhaler technique
- Co-morbidities (e.g., rhinitis, gastroesophageal reflux disease [GERD]) (additional investigation required?)
- Possible reassessment of treatment and educational needs
- Understanding and use of an action plan to manage exacerbations
- New prescriptions; follow-up visit scheduled

modes of delivery of asthma care and better integrate evidence-based asthma guidelines into current practice. Asthma education is still not integrated into care enough, and self-management skills should be acquired by those suffering from asthma, including adequate assessment of asthma control from symptoms and ideally occasional measurement of expiratory flows. Goals of treatment should be understood by the patient, and information and advice provided by caregivers should be consistent and their interventions well articulated.

Current Diagnosis and Assessment

New medications and procedures are being developed and could be useful in the future treatment of asthma. New corticosteroids such as mometasone and ciclesonide should be available soon. Phosphodiesterase 4 (PDE4) inhibitors are proposed as a means to reduce airway inflammation. Cytokine inhibitors, such as anti-IL-5 and anti-IL-4, are being tested, but results are not conclusive. Other potential therapies include inhaled modulation of the TH_1/TH_2 balance through vaccines or oligonucleotides, as well as more targeted immunotherapy and inhibition of various adhesion molecules, chemokines, and mediators. Bronchothermoplasty is an intriguing new procedure for the treatment of asthma currently in the experimental stage. Finally, progress is being made in the field of gene therapy that may lead to the identification of individuals at risk of developing asthma or better targeting of treatments.

REFERENCES

Abramson MJ, Puy RM, Weiner JM: Allergen immunotherapy for asthma. Cochrane Database Syst Rev 2000;(2):CD001186.
Boulet LP: Asthma guidelines and outcomes. In Adkinson NF, Adkinson Jr NF, Yunginger JW, Busse WW, et al: (eds): Middleton's Allergy Principles and Practice, 6th ed. St. Louis, Mo, Mosby, 2003, pp 1283-1301.
Boulet LP, Becker A, Bérubé D, et al., on behalf of the Canadian Asthma Consensus Group: Canadian asthma consensus report. Can Med Assoc J 1999;30;161(11 Suppl):S1-S61.
Gibson PG, Powell H, Coughlan J, et al: Self-management education and regular practitioner review for adults with asthma (Cochrane Review). Cochrane Database Syst Rev 2003;(1):CD001117.
Global Initiative on Asthma: Available online at http://www.ginasthma.com
Lemiere C, Bai T, Balter M, et al: Adult Asthma Consensus Guidelines Update 2003. Can Respir J 2004;11(Suppl A):9A-18A.
Masoli M, Fabian D, Holt S, Beasley R: Global Initiative for Asthma (GINA) Program. The global burden of asthma: Executive summary of the GINA Dissemination Committee report. Allergy 2004;59:469-478.
National Expert Report Guidelines for the Diagnosis and Management of Asthma: Update on selected topics 2002. National Asthma Education and Prevention Program (NAEPP). Available online at http://www.nhlbi.nih.gov/guidelines/asthma/execsumm.pdf
Partridge MR, Hill SR: Enhancing care for people with asthma: The role of communication, education, training and self-management. 1998 World Asthma Meeting Education and Delivery of Care Working Group. Eur Respir J 2000;16:333-348.
Tattersfield AE, Knox AJ, Britton JR, Hall IP: Asthma. Lancet 2002;360:1313-1322.

Asthma in Children

Method of
Gerald B. Kolski, MD, PhD, FAAAAI, FAAP

Asthma is the most common cause of significant childhood morbidity. This includes school absenteeism, hospitalizations, emergency department visits, and acute care visits. Its prevalence has been increasing throughout the 1990s and into this century. An estimated 5 million children younger than 15 years have asthma as identified by the National Health Interview Survey of 2003. According to this survey, the prevalence of asthma in the general population is somewhere between 6% and 10%. Prevalence in inner-city populations and especially in African Americans is closer to 14% to 15%. Pediatricians and family practitioners are often reluctant to make the diagnosis because of difficulty with giving prognostic information to parents. Wheezing during the first few years of life can often be associated with acute viral infections, especially respiratory syncytial virus (RSV). Longitudinal studies suggest there are three patterns to wheezing in children. There are a group of children who wheeze during infancy associated with viral infections, a second group that wheeze during infancy and also as they get older, and a third group that only develops wheezing later after sensitization with allergens. Because of these groups it is oftentimes difficult to give prognostic information to parents until you have seen the pattern that a child will follow.

Despite tremendous improvement in medications and treatments for asthma, deaths from asthma continue to occur. Most recently, however, the mortality rates seem to have leveled off or decreased slightly.

One theory for the high prevalence of asthma is the "hygiene hypothesis." Studies done in homogeneous populations in Europe and Scandinavian countries have noted less asthma and allergies in rural populations versus those that live in urban environments. Attempts have been made to correlate this with endotoxin exposure during infancy and/or infections during this period of time that turn on immune responses that do not promote allergies. This concept favors an immune response, which postulates that certain infections and endotoxin exposure promote a T_H1 T cell response in which interferon gamma and interleukin(IL)-2 predominate, whereas a lack of these infections promotes a T_H2 response where there is an IL-4, IL-13, and IL-5 predominance with increased IgE production.

Pathophysiology

Over the last several decades the idea that reversible bronchoconstriction is the main element in asthma has changed. It has become apparent that in addition to bronchoconstriction there is considerable inflammation involving increased mucus production, inflammatory cell infiltrates, and airway thickening. With longitudinal studies it has become apparent that there may in fact be some fibrosis that leads to "airway remodeling." The increased inflammatory infiltrates lead to increasing airway reactivity characterized by hyperresponsiveness to various stimuli. The inflammatory cell infiltrates can include eosinophils, lymphocytes, basophils, neutrophils, and macrophages depending on the stimulus. Unchecked inflammation is believed to be the cause of the fibrosis. Clearly it is important to try and identify the triggers in an individual patient that are causing the inflammation as well as treating the inflammation.

Differential Diagnosis

Determining the cause of wheezing in infancy can often be difficult. During the first year of life if the wheezing is associated with a viral infection, a diagnosis of bronchiolitis is often made. A clinical response to bronchodilators might be helpful in assessing whether this is going to be a child with asthma. Recurrent wheezing in an atopic child with a strong family history of asthma would strongly suggest that the child has underlying asthma. An association with eczema and/or other allergic manifestations might also be suggestive of asthma. Because of the difficulty in doing pulmonary functions during the first few years of life, clinical assessment is the key. In addition to asthma, Table 1 lists the other diagnoses that have to be considered. Cystic fibrosis, gastroesophageal reflux disease, and foreign body aspiration probably are the most common diagnoses that have to be entertained. Recurrent infiltrates should make you worry about immune deficiencies including hypogammaglobulinemia and ciliary defects such as immotile cilia syndrome.

Diagnostic tests such as a sweat test, immunoglobulins, skin or radioallergosorbent assay test (RAST), barium swallow, bronchoscopy, or chest radiograph may be indicated.

In older children asthma may be diagnosed by doing pulmonary functions. Spirometry can often be done in the office and can be a reproducible way to measure the extent of airway disease in known asthmatics as well as diagnostic by looking at pre- and postbronchodilator responses. The forced expiratory volume at 1 second (FEV_1) is often thought to be a measure of large airway obstruction. The FEF_{25-75} or expiratory flow between the

TABLE 1   Differential Diagnosis of Wheezing

Infants	Older Children
Laryngomalacia	Asthma
Tracheomalacia	Cystic fibrosis
Vascular rings	Gastroesophageal reflux disease
Subglottic stenosis	Foreign body aspiration
Airway congenital masses	Airway tumors
Gastroesophageal reflux	Viral infections (RSV, adenovirus)
Bronchiolitis	Tuberculosis
Pneumonia	

Abbreviations: RSV = respiratory syncytial virus.

25th and 75th percentile of the forced vital capacity (FVC) is often thought to be a measure of small airway disease. A 15% increase in FEV_1 pre- and postbronchodilator or 25% increase in FEF_{25-75} is thought to be diagnostic of asthma. Inhalation challenges with methacholine (Provocholine) or histamine are often used to measure airway reactivity in experimental studies. Bronchoconstriction with these inhalation challenges can determine the degree of airway hyperreactivity. Similar results can also be obtained with exercise challenges or cold air challenges. These tests are often used to diagnose asthma in children whose pulmonary functions at baseline are not significantly depressed. In children with asthma, peak expiratory flow rates (PEFRs) are often used to monitor the asthma as well as the management. This test is effort dependent.

Key Diagnostic Points Consistent with Asthma

- Recurrent wheezing responding to bronchodilators
- Coughing or wheezing shortly after exercise
- Pulmonary functions that show obstruction responding to bronchodilators
- Strong family history of asthma
- Associated allergic symptoms including seasonal rhinitis, eczema, or urticaria

 CURRENT DIAGNOSIS

- Always focus on the ABCs (airway, breathing, and circulation).
- Start prescription early and aggressively (titrate β-agonist to effect).
- Reevaluate frequently (try to avoid intubation at all cost).
- Lack of wheezing is not always a good thing.
- Plan ahead in case things go bad.
- Ensure adequate hydration.

BOX 1 Asthma Triggers

- Allergies: perennial or seasonal
- Viral infections
- Irritants, especially cigarette smoke and air pollution
- Exercise
- Weather changes
- Gastroesophageal reflux
- Medications including aspirin and nonsteroidal anti-inflammatory drugs (NSAIDs)
- Sinusitis

History

Once a diagnosis of asthma is made, it is important to determine the trigger for this individual's asthma symptoms or exacerbations. The history is very important in determining treatment. Box 1 lists the most common causes for asthma exacerbations.

The most common perennial allergens are dust mites, cockroaches, mold, and pets. In the inner cities, cockroaches and dust mites are very common causes for allergic sensitization. They are extremely common and very difficult to control. Dust mites need moisture and thus are much more common in humid areas. With increased humidity, molds also can play a significant role. Children are often treated with humidifiers or vaporizers for upper respiratory infections, which may exacerbate dust mite and mold exposure. In drier climates, pets, especially indoor animals, are often exacerbating causes. Recent studies have indicated that more than two or three pets decreased the likelihood of sensitization, whereas an isolated pet is more likely to be associated with the development of allergy. This may have to do with endotoxin and the previously discussed hygiene hypothesis.

Children who only have difficulty with their asthma in the spring and fall may have sensitization to the pollens. This is very regional and often associated with being outdoors. Pollination and dissemination is most problematic with dry windy days. Keeping the windows closed at night as well as air conditioning may benefit individuals with seasonal allergies. These children may need medications at particular times of the year but not throughout the year. Airway reactivity often continues even 4 to 6 weeks after the allergen is no longer present.

Children who have trouble with viral infections may also have increased reactivity from perennial or seasonal exposures that exacerbate the asthma with infection. It is often helpful to reduce allergy exposure in these individuals so as to reduce their response to viral infections. Parents may be alerted to signs of upper respiratory infection so that they can increase asthma treatment at those times.

At all times cigarette smoke causes increased mucus production as well as decreases mucociliary clearance. Children with asthma thus are especially prone to having difficulty around cigarette smoke. During infancy, cigarette smoke exposure is associated with a two- to threefold increase in risk of asthma as well as upper respiratory infections, ear infections, and pneumonia. Smoking during pregnancy is also associated with a sustained decrease in infant pulmonary functions. Smoke is a form of indoor air pollution. Outdoor air pollution, especially small particles, ozone, nitrogen dioxide, and sulfur dioxide, all can be exacerbating factors in asthma.

Exercise is associated with asthma exacerbations because of the inhalation of cold dry air. Exercise is often associated with mouth breathing. The nose normally moisturizes, filters, and warms the air. Nasal congestion secondary to allergies, viral infections, or nasal obstruction can all lead to more difficulty with exercise as well as with breathing cold dry air at any time.

Weather changes are often a problem secondary to what is in the air or the changes in temperature of the air. Children who have trouble with weather changes are often responding to changes in pollen distribution or other allergens or irritants.

Children who have reflux as the exacerbating cause of their asthma often have difficulty at night when they lie down, shortly after meals, or when ingesting very acidic substances. Often there will be considerable coughing and if the child is old enough to talk some significant heartburn. Reflux is often worse when the asthma is a problem because the lower esophageal sphincter tone decreases with hyperinflation at that time.

Children with sensitivity to aspirin or nonsteroidal anti-inflammatory drugs (NSAIDs) often have associated sinusitis, nasal polyps, and profuse rhinorrhea with aspirin exposure. It often goes undiagnosed until adulthood. Nasal polyps should always raise this possibility in addition to a diagnosis of cystic fibrosis.

Sinusitis can be associated with significant exacerbations of asthma. Often treating the sinusitis treats the asthma exacerbation. Purulent nasal discharge for 5 to 7 days associated with significant coughing and maxillary tenderness may be suggestive of underlying sinusitis. In children with allergic rhinitis, complications of sinusitis often occur.

In all children with asthma it is very important that you try and assess severity of disease. There should be questions asked about whether the patient has ever been intubated or had an intensive care unit admission. In addition questions about recent use of oral corticosteroids should be asked to determine the recent course of asthma. Children with underlying seizure disorders are also important to identify because they are at greater risk for mortality. Signs of mental illness or depression should also be noted because this predisposes children to significant morbidity and mortality.

Physical Examination

In examining a patient with asthma, the complete physical is extremely helpful. Children with skin findings of eczema or hives associated with an exacerbation of asthma may often lead to a search for an allergy exposure that is responsible for symptoms. Nasal examination may show boggy turbinates suggestive of allergy or erythematous turbinates suggestive of infection. Purulent discharge associated with sinus tenderness may suggest sinusitis. Nasal polyps should also be looked for to ascertain whether the patient may have underlying cystic fibrosis or aspirin-sensitive asthma. Enlarged tonsils and adenoids may predispose to mouth breathing and exacerbate underlying asthma. Examination of the chest may show whether there is a pectus suggesting chronic disease or whether there is hyperinflation with a barrel chest. Supraclavicular, intercostal, and subcostal muscular activity give information as to the work of breathing. The cardiac examination should focus on heart rate as well as any sign that might indicate this is cardiac wheezing instead of asthma. Abdominal examination is important to evaluate any signs of liver or spleen enlargement that might indicate evidence of pulmonary hypertension or cardiac disease. Examination of the extremities is important to look for clubbing and/or cyanosis. The neurologic exam is especially important acutely to ascertain whether the patient is having any change in mental status secondary to hypoxia.

Treatment

Treatment for asthma has changed considerably since the mid 90's. The chronic management of asthma has focused on assuring that the patient functions as normally as possible with the following goals of asthma management:

- No nocturnal asthma
- Full exercise activity
- No emergency department visits or hospitalizations
- No lost time from school or work
- No or minimal side effects from medication

Asthma treatment has focused on the anti-inflammatory nature of the disease to eliminate long-term damage to the lungs. Asthma treatment has followed the National Heart, Lung, and Blood Institute (NHLBI) guidelines with assessment of asthma severity and management based on the classifications (Table 2). We developed a color-coded questionnaire that gives an indication of asthma control.

 CURRENT THERAPY

- **Severe:** ABCs, oxygen, monitors, POX, IV, isotonic fluids to maintain volume.

Start with (consider SC epinephrine if really tight):

- Albuterol, 0.5% inhalation solution, 0.5 mL (<20 kg), 0.75 mL (>20 kg) q20min × 3 (may give as mini-Nebs or start continuous at 2–3 mL/h). After initial stabilization patient will likely need q2h Nebs or continuous albuterol.
- Methylprednisolone (Solu-Medrol), 2 mg/kg IV (maximum, 125 mg) then start 1 mg/kg q6h (maximum, 80 mg/dose).
- Ipratropium bromide (Atrovent), 250 µg (<5 y), 500 µg (>5 y) × 2, then q4h.

If minimal improvement:

- Magnesium sulfate,[1] 45 mg/kg IV over 20 min (maximum, 2 g).

If still severe, consider terbutaline drip:

- Terbutaline (Brethine), 2–10 µg/kg loading dose, then start infusion at 0.1–0.4 µg/kg/min (maximum, 6 µg/kg/min). **Needs pediatric intensive care unit (PICU).**

At any time if minimal air entry, use:

- Epinephrine (1:1000), 0.01 mL/kg SC (maximum, 0.3 mL)
  or
- Terbutaline, 0.01 mg/kg SC (maximum, 0.25 mg)

Note: Adequate volume can be critical in maintaining circulatory volume (preload), so use volume freely. Also buffering with THAM for severe acidosis can be useful. These two strategies may help you avoid intubation.

If you really need to intubate (impending respiratory failure), use atropine, 0.02 mg/kg IV (minimum), 0.1 mg (maximum, 1 mg); ketamine (Ketalar), 1–2 mg/kg IV; or vecuronium (Norcuron), 0.1–0.2 mg/kg IV.

- **Moderate:** ABCs, POX, oxygen, monitors. ± IV

Start with

- Albuterol, 0.5 mL (<20 kg), 0.75 mL (>20 kg) q20min × 3 (may start with mini Nebs or continuous). Then patient will likely need q2h Nebs or continuous albuterol (2 mL/h <10 kg, 3 mL/hr >10 kg)
- Ipratropium bromide, 250 µg (<5 y), 500 µg (>5 y) × 2, then q4h
- Prednisone, 2 mg/kg (maximum, 80 mg) if tolerating PO
  or
- Methylprednisolone, 2 mg/kg (maximum, 80 mg) (continue steroids for 5 d, 2 mg/kg/d)

If minimal improvement:

Consider magnesium sulfate as above.
- **Mild:** ABCs, POX

Start with

- Albuterol Nebs or MDI with spacer q2–4h
- Prednisolone, 2 mg/kg loading dose (maximum, 80 mg), then 2 mg/kg/d divided bid × 5 d

For mild to moderate exacerbation, discharge home may be considered if patient shows good improvement, is no longer dyspneic or hypoxic, tolerates Nebs q4h, and has good supervision at home.

CXR: Consider for a first-time wheezer; a condition other than asthma (i.e., FB); a febrile child with clinical signs of pneumonia; or no clinical improvement or worsening condition (pneumothorax, pneumomediastinum).

Continuous albuterol: To calculate the total amount of albuterol and normal saline, remember that the total amount of solution per hour must equal 30 mL.

Example: For a child >10 kg, the albuterol dose for continuous Nebs is 3 mL/h so you need to add 27 mL of NSS to run for 1 h (to set it up for 4 h, total mL = 120 with 12 mL albuterol + 108 mL NSS).

---

[1]Not FDA approved for this indication.
Abbreviations: ABCs = airway, breathing, and circulation; CXR = chest radiograph; FB = foreign body; IV = intravenous; Nebs = nebulized; NSS = normal saline solution; POX = pulse oximeter; SC = subcutaneous; THAM = tromethamine.

TABLE 2 Stepwise Approach for Managing Asthma in Children

Classify Severity: Clinical Features Before Treatment or Adequate Control			Medications Required to Maintain Long-Term Control
	Symptoms/Day	*PEF or FEV₁*	
	Symptoms/Night	*PEF Variability*	*Daily Medications*
Step 4 Severe persistent	Continual Frequent	<60% >30%	**Preferred treatment:** • High-dose inhaled corticosteroids, *and* • Long-acting inhaled β₂-agonists (combination preferred) *and*, if needed, • Corticosteroid tablets or syrup long term (2 mg/kg/d, generally do not exceed 60 mg/d). (Make repeat attempts to reduce systemic corticosteroids and maintain control with high-dose inhaled corticosteroids.)

Step 3:
Moderate
persistent
	Daily
	>1 night/wk
		>60%–<80%
		>30%
			• **Preferred treatment:**
			  • Low- to medium-dose inhaled corticosteroids.
			• **Alternative treatment** (listed alphabetically):
			  • Increase inhaled corticosteroids within medium-dose range
			  or
			  • Low to medium–dose inhaled corticosteroids and either leukotriene modifier or theophylline.
			
			If needed (particularly in patients with recurring severe exacerbations):
			• **Preferred treatment:**
			  • Increased inhaled corticosteroids within medium-dose range and add long-acting inhaled β₂-agonists (combination inhaler preferred).
			• **Alternative treatment** (listed alphabetically):
			  • Increase inhaled corticosteroids within medium-dose range, and add either leukotriene modifier or theophylline.

Step 2
Mild persistent
	>2/wk but <1/d
	>2 nights/mo
		>80%
		20%–30%
			• **Preferred treatment:**
			  • Low-dose inhaled corticosteroids.
			• **Alternative treatment** (listed alphabetically):
			  • Cromolyn (Intal).
			  • Leukotriene modifier.
			  • Nedocromil (Tilade) *or* sustained-release theophylline (Slo-bid Gyrocaps) to serum concentration of 5–15 µg/mL.

Step 1 Mild intermittent	<2 d/wk <2 nights/mo	>80% <20%	• **No daily medication needed.** • Severe exacerbations may occur, separated by long periods of normal lung function and no symptoms. A course of systemic corticosteroids is recommended.

Note: Children <5 y cannot do adequate peak flows.

Quick relief All patients	• Short-acting bronchodilator: 2–4 puffs short-acting inhaled β₂-agonists as needed for symptoms. • Intensity of treatment depends on severity of exacerbation; up to 3 treatments at 20-min intervals or a single nebulizer treatment as needed. Course of systemic corticosteroids may be needed. • Use of short-acting β₂-agonists >2 times/wk in intermittent asthma (daily, or increasing use in persistent asthma) may indicate the need to initiate (increase) long-term-control therapy.
↓ Step down Review treatment q1–6mo; a gradual stepwise reduction in treatment may be possible.	**↑ Step up** If control is not maintained, consider step up. First, review patient medication technique, adverse effects from medications.

Notes:

The stepwise approach is meant to assist, not replace, the clinical decision-making required to meet individual patient needs.

Classify severity: Assign patient to most severe step in which any feature occurs (PEF is percentage of personal best; FEV₁ is percentage predicted).

Gain control as quickly as possible (consider a short course of systemic corticosteroids); then step down to the least medication necessary to maintain control.

Minimize use of short-acting inhaled β₂-agonists. Overreliance on short-acting inhaled β₂-agonists (e.g., use of approximately 1 canister/mo even if not using it every day) indicates inadequate control of asthma and the need to initiate or intensify long-term control therapy.

Provide education on self-management and controlling environmental factors that make asthma worse (e.g., allergens and irritants).

Refer to an asthma specialist if there are difficulties controlling asthma or if step 4 care is required. Referral may be considered if care at level step 3 is required.

Continued

TABLE 2 Stepwise Approach for Managing Asthma in Children—cont'd

Usual Dosages for Long-Term-Control Medications

Medication	Dosage Form	Child Dose
Systemic Corticosteroids		
Methylprednisolone (Medrol)	2-, 4-, 8-, 16-, 32-mg tablets	0.25–2 mg/kg daily in single dose in AM or qod as needed for control
Prednisolone (Prelone) (Orapred)	5-mg tablets 5 mg/5 mL, 15 mg/5 mL	Short-course "burst": 1–2 mg/kg/d, maximum
Prednisone (Orasone)	1-, 2.5-, 5-, 10-, 20-, 50-mg tablets: 5 mg/5 mL, 5 mg/mL	60 mg/d for 3–10 d
Long-Acting β2-agonists		
(Do not use for symptom relief or for exacerbations.)		
Salmeterol (Serevent)	DPI 50 μg/blister	1 blister q12h
Formoterol (Foradil)	DPI 12 μg/single-use capsule	1 capsule q12h
Combine Medication		
Fluticasone/salmeterol (Advair)	DPI 100, 250, or 500 μg/50 μg	1 inhalation bid; dose depends on severity of asthma
Mast Cell Stabilizer		
Cromolyn (Intal)	MDI 800 μg/puff Nebulizer 20 mg/ampule	1–2 puffs tid–qid 1 ampule tid–qid
Nedocromil (Tilade)	MDI 1.75 mg/puff	1–2 puffs bid–qid
Leukotriene Modifiers		
Montelukast (Singulair)	4- or 5-mg chewable tablet 10-mg tablet	4 mg qhs (2–5 y) 5 mg qhs (6–14 y) 10 mg qhs (>14 y)
Zafirlukast (Accolate)	10- or 20-mg tablet	20 mg daily (5–11 y) (10-mg tablet bid)
Methylxanthines		
(Serum monitoring is important.)		
Theophylline (Slo-Phyllin)	Liquids, sustained-release tablets and capsules	Starting dose 10 mg/kg/d; usual maximum: <1 y: 0.2 (age in wks) + 5 = mg/kg/d >1 y: 16 mg/kg/d

Estimated Comparative Daily Dosages for Inhaled Corticosteroids

Drug	Low Daily Dose	Medium Daily Dose	High Daily Dose
Beclomethasone HFA (QVAR) 40 or 80 μg/puff	80–160 μg	160–320 mcg	>320 μg
Budesonide DPI (Pulmicort) 200 μg/inhalation	200–400 μg	400–800 mcg	>800 μg
Budesonide inhalation suspension for nebulization (Pulmicort Respules)	0.5 mg	1.0 mg	2.0 mg
Flunisolide (AeroBid) 250 μg/puff	500–750 μg	1000–1250 μcg	1250 μg
Fluticasone (Flovent) MDI: 44, 110, or 220 μg/puff DPI: 50, 100, or 250 μg/inhalation	88–176 μg 100–200 μg	176–440 μg 200–400 μg	>440 μg >400 μg
Triamcinolone acetonide (Azmacort) 100 μg/puff	400–800 μg	800–1200 μg	>1200 μg
Mometasone fumarate (Asmanex) 220 mg	220 μg	440 μg	880 μg

Abbreviations: DPI = daily permissible intake; FEV$_1$ = forced expiratory volume at 1 second; MDI = metered-dose inhaler; PEF = peak expiratory flow (rate).

Medications

Asthma medications are classified according to medications that are used for acute relief of symptoms called *relievers* and those that are used for chronic control of symptoms characterized as *controllers*. This classification was established to give patients a better understanding of the role of their individual medications. It is also a better way to educate patients as to why they have to continue to take medications even when they are not having symptoms. It is important to discuss these individual classifications and medications for both acute and chronic management.

TABLE 3 Medications for the Acute Relief of Symptoms

Generic β-agonist	Brand Name*
Albuterol	Ventolin, Ventolin HFA, Proventil HFA, Proventil
Pirbuterol	Maxair, Maxair Autohaler
Terbutaline	Brethaire, Brethine, Bricanyl
Metaproterenol	Alupent
Levalbuterol	Xopenex

*Many of these drugs are available in liquid, tablet, inhalation aerosol, as well as metered-dose inhalers.
Albuterol is also available in an inhaler in combination with ipratropium bromide (Combivent).

RELIEVERS

Various bronchodilators are used for acute management of asthma. These bronchodilators are predominantly β-agonists such as albuterol (Proventil) and terbutaline (Brethine) that are selective for $β_2$-receptors. Table 3 gives the generic as well as trade names for these medications. The short-acting β-agonists are used for acute relief in most circumstances. In children anticholinergics such as ipratropium bromide (Atrovent) are often used in the emergency department and hospital setting acutely but are rarely given chronically. Chronic use of β-agonists is avoided because of a decrease in effectiveness as well as an increase in airway reactivity with their chronic use. With chronic use there is also a decrease in both the number and affinity of β-receptors for these bronchodilators. The affinity as well as number of β-receptors is increased with the use of corticosteroids.

In the management of acute episodes of asthma, an algorithm is used (see Current Therapy box). β-agonists are given either by nebulizer or inhaler. In addition to albuterol, a selective stereoisomer levalbuterol (Xopenex) is also available but is more expensive. This isomer may cause fewer side effects and have a slightly longer duration of action. In the acute setting, treatments are often given every 20 minutes times three and then are continued every 2 to 3 hours for hospitalized patients. In critical situations, albuterol may also be given continuously. It is during the acute situation where ipratropium bromide is beneficial for the first 24 to 48 hours of treatment. It can be given by nebulizer every 4 to 6 hours.

Injectable epinephrine is still recommended especially in the acute attack if it is thought to be secondary to allergies or anaphylaxis. It also can be used in the acute situation to make sure that inhaled drugs can reach the lower airway.

Magnesium sulfate[1] is used intravenously in severe asthmatics for its bronchodilator properties to prevent intubation or respiratory failure. This is outlined again in the acute management algorithm (Current Therapy box).

Theophylline (Theolair) was often the mainstay of asthma management in the 1980s, but its toxicity and the difficulty in having to monitor levels has reduced its use.

[1]Not FDA approved for this indication.

Nausea, vomiting, abdominal pain, and an increase in hyperactivity often lead to noncompliance. With the selective β-agonists their use has been minimal. They can be used for chronic management in patients to decrease corticosteroid need.

Oral or systemic corticosteroids are always indicated in acute management of episodes of asthma exacerbation. The usual recommended starting dose is 2 mg/kg and should be continued during the episode. Prolonged use of corticosteroids may require a taper, but a short course of 4 to 5 days does not usually require a taper. Any patient who was admitted for an acute exacerbation of asthma should go home on a controller with an action plan for future attacks.

In the chronic management of asthma, albuterol is still the mainstay of acute attacks, pre-exercise, and for any reduction in peak flow or pulmonary functions. Albuterol (Proventil) is usually given by metered-dose inhaler and for most patients it is recommended that it be given with a spacer. Spacers increase the deposition in the lower airway and increase the effectiveness of inhaled drugs. In the chronic management of asthma, the NHLBI guidelines recommend that if albuterol is being used more than two or three times a week a step up in controller medications is suggested (Table 2).

CONTROLLERS

Inhaled corticosteroids are established as the mainstay of chronic management of asthma. Various preparations are available either by dry powder inhaler or metered-dose inhaler. Table 2 outlines the doses and route. Side effects of growth suppression and decreases in bone mineralization are dose related as well as preparation dependent. Individuals on any of the corticosteroids need to have their growth monitored and also to have instructions on mouth rinsing after inhalation to reduce fungal colonization in the oropharynx.

Leukotriene antagonists are available in oral preparations. These offer some advantage in pediatric patients in that they do not require good inhalation technique and can be given once a day. This may improve compliance and offer benefit in asthma as well as allergic rhinitis. They are not as effective as inhaled corticosteroids but offer some benefit in mild disease or as an adjunct to inhaled corticosteroids.

Cromolyn (Intal) and nedocromil (Tilade) are available as inhaled medications. Both of these drugs are mast cell stabilizers and appear to be most effective in allergic patients. These drugs should be taken three to four times a day, which makes their compliance more difficult. There are no significant side effects to these medications, however, and they are used in children because of their safety profile. They are used primarily in the mildest of patients and as pretreatment before allergy exposure.

Long-acting β-agonists are characterized as controllers, but these medications cannot be taken as anti-inflammatory agents. They have an increased risk of mortality when taken alone. For this reason only the preparations that are in combination with inhaled corticosteroids should be used in children. The drug preparations contain varying doses of inhaled corticosteroid with one standard dose of long-acting β-agonist.

Oral corticosteroids have been used for asthma since they were developed. They were used for patients with severe or chronic asthma before inhaled steroids were available. Because oral corticosteroids have significant side effects they should be used with caution. Prolonged use of systemic steroids leads to adrenal suppression, osteoporosis, and growth suppression. With prolonged use the dose should be reduced gradually. Inhaled corticosteroid effects can be similar to the systemic corticosteroids, especially if they are used at doses higher than recommended.

OMALIZUMAB

Omalizumab (Xolair) is a monoclonal antibody that is humanized and was developed against IgE. It is expensive and requires monthly injections. It is most effective when allergies are the main trigger for asthma. It is also used in patients with severe anaphylaxis.[1] It is indicated for children with moderate to severe persistent asthma that is exacerbated by significant documented allergies. Because it is nonspecific it does not reduce specific allergies and cannot be used in patients who have no significant atopy.

IMMUNOSUPPRESSIVE AGENTS

Various experimental studies in patients with chronic steroid-dependent asthma have used immunosuppressive agents such as methotrexate[1] (Trexall), IV gammaglobulin[1] (Gamimune N), and anti-inflammatory monoclonal antibodies against cytokines. None of these produced dramatic results and none is available or can be recommended at this time.

IMMUNOTHERAPY

Specific injections of extracts of allergens to which the patient is allergic is effective for allergic rhinitis that is secondary to certain allergens. Therapy with allergy extracts is effective for pollens, and by reducing allergic rhinitis symptoms it can affect nasal breathing and therefore benefit asthma. Because of the risk of reactions to immunotherapy it should be used cautiously when the patient is having significant asthma symptoms at the time of injection. Studies in Europe suggest that in the future sublingual immunotherapy may be effective. Well-documented studies in this country have not been done and it is not approved as an FDA procedure.

Education and Environmental Control

Education of the individual asthmatic is important. Action plans in which treatment of acute episodes is outlined is recommended. Parents and patients should be taught about the patient's triggers as well as steps they should take to increase or decrease their medications depending on symptoms. Environmental precautions such as dust mite avoidance have had some success. Pet avoidance has not worked unless the pet is totally eliminated.

[1]Not FDA approved for this indication.

REFERENCES

Castro-Rodriguez JA, Holberg CJ, Wright AL, Martinez FD: A clinical index to define risk of asthma in young children with recurrent wheezing. Am J Respir Crit Care Med 2000;162:1403-1406.

National Institutes of Health/National Heart, Lung, and Blood Institute: NAEPP expert panel report 2: Guidelines for the diagnosis and management of asthma. Publication no. 97-4051. Bethesda, Md, The Institutes, 1997.

O'Connor GT: Allergen avoidance in asthma: What do we do now? J Allergy Clin Immunol 2005;116:26-30.

Romagnani S: Immunologic influences on allergy and the TH1/TH2 balance. J Allergy Clin Immunol 2004;113:395-400.

Spahn JD, Szefler SJ: Childhood asthma: New insights into management. J Allergy Clin Immunol 2002;109:3-13.

Allergic Rhinitis Caused by Inhalant Factors

Method of
Richard W. Weber, MD

Atopy is an inherited disposition manifested by any or all of allergic rhinitis, asthma, or atopic eczema. It is closely, but not invariably, linked to the ability to generate specific allergic antibody, IgE, in greater than normal amounts. Allergic rhinitis is the most prevalent of the atopic diseases, affecting 25% to 35% of persons, depending on the population studied. The atopic disorders have become steadily more prevalent over the past century, although the exact reason for this increase is not clear.

Although allergic rhinitis is considered by nonsufferers to be a trivial disease, it delivers a significant personal impact on quality of life. It is responsible for an enormous economic burden in terms of direct medical costs for physician visits and medication and indirect costs of missed work and school and lost productivity. This cost in the United States was recently estimated at more than $2 billion annually and is now presumably even greater.

Pathogenesis

IgE, like IgA, is a mucosal antibody, produced by plasma cells beneath the mucosal surfaces of the eyes, upper and lower airways, and the gut. IgE is a homocytotropic antibody, binding to specific high-affinity receptors on basophils in the circulation and mast cells in various tissues. Bridging by allergen of two specific IgE molecules on the cell surface is sufficient to cause activation of the basophils or mast cells. This is followed by the release of vasoactive mediators such as histamine, tryptase, leukotrienes, and prostaglandins, as well as several chemokines and cytokines. The former mediators are responsible for the immediate allergic (early-phase) reaction, manifested by sneezing, itching, rhinorrhea, and nasal congestion. Chemotactic factors result in the recruitment of inflammatory cells such as basophils, eosinophils, and polymorphonuclear leukocytes. The influx of these cells is accompanied by fresh release of vasoactive substances, culminating in the delayed (late-phase) reaction with a recrudescence of symptoms.

With a single allergen exposure, the early and late phases are easily discernible, the latter occurring 4 to 6 hours after the initial reaction. With persistent exposure, such as with indoor allergens such as dust mite or animal dander, the late-phase inflammatory process is ongoing, resulting in chronic symptoms. With outdoor allergens such as pollens, the persistence of inflammation from prior exposure results in greater sensitivity to further exposures, with lesser pollen amounts resulting in greater symptoms. This is called the priming effect.

The proclivity to produce IgE is caused by a shift of helper T-cells cytokine release to a T_H2 profile. Two central cytokines to this allergic phenotype are IL-4 and IL-5. The former causes isotype switch in B-cells to IgE production. The latter cytokine is crucial for eosinophil activation and longevity. Once this shift to a T_H2 profile occurs, it tends to self-perpetuate. Atopic persons are presumably genetically predisposed to the T_H2 phenotype.

In the great majority of instances, allergic rhinitis sensitization is to an airborne, inhalant factor. These aeroallergens may emanate from indoor or outdoor sources and be perennial, relatively constant, or with seasonal peaks. Outdoor sources are usually of plant or fungal origin, namely, pollen grains or spores. These frequently have seasonal peaks whose timing frequently aids in diagnosing the airborne culprit. Depending on the region, tree pollens pollinate in the winter into the early spring, although certain trees shed pollen in the fall. Grasses generally pollinate from May into July, with longer seasons in the southern states, and year round in Hawaii and southern Florida. Although some weeds overlap with the grasses, most pollinate from July into the fall. Aeroallergens indoors are more likely animal in origin: dust mite or cockroach emanations or animal dander. Mold spores are possible, especially with water damage or high humidity, but less likely. The exposures are usually perennial, but there are seasonal peaks in these as well: dust mite in late summer to early fall, cat and dog dander in late winter, and cockroach in summer. A recent study showed that the allergens from dog and cat dander can be found in the dust of essentially all homes, whether pets are present or not.

Differential Diagnosis and Co-Morbid Conditions

Irritant rhinitis was previously referred to as vasomotor rhinitis, with nasal symptoms driven by perturbations in the environment, and is as frequent as allergic rhinitis. The cause of the increased susceptibility to irritants is not fully understood, although the resultant release of mediators is similar to that seen with allergic rhinitis. A variant of irritant rhinitis is "gustatory rhinitis," where the act of eating triggers rhinorrhea. Viral infection (upper respiratory infection [URI]) is perhaps the most common cause of nasal symptoms; other infectious agents are distinctly less common. Hormonal factors such as hypothyroidism and pregnancy can lead to increased nasal congestion. Medication-induced nasal congestion was commonly seen with older hypotensive agents and is certainly seen with topical α-adrenergic agonist abuse. Intolerance to aspirin and nonsteroidal anti-inflammatory drugs (NSAIDs) may manifest as asthma, chronic sinusitis, or both. Vasculitides such as Wegener's can present with chronic sinusitis.

An expert panel convened by the World Health Organization developed a position statement, "Allergic Rhinitis and Its Impact on Asthma (ARIA)." This document emphasized several important issues. Its scope is not just industrialized countries, but developing countries as well, and it discusses resources with a global perspective. One of the major messages is the frequent concordance of allergic rhinitis and asthma. It is crucial to suspect rhinitis and inflammation of the upper airway as an aggravant in asthma, just as the lower airway should be evaluated in patients with rhinitis. The position statement also suggests that the terms *seasonal* and *perennial* be replaced by *intermittent* and *persistent* in keeping with the phraseology recommended by the National Asthma Education and Prevention Program (NAEPP) and the Global Initiative for Asthma (GINA) guidelines for management of asthma.

Evaluation

Evaluation of rhinitis is greatly aided by a careful history: presence of itching and sneezing, severity, seasonality, and progression of symptoms, identifiable triggers, occupational exposures, alleviating factors, and medication usage. A positive family history of atopic disease is helpful. The impact of disease and medication on daily activity is likewise important. The presence of co-morbid conditions is suggested by a history of headache, loss of smell and taste, purulent discharge, cough, chest tightness or wheezing, snoring, and sleep disturbance.

Physical examination of the head may reveal characteristic findings. Dennie's lines are folds under the eyes caused by edema. Dark discoloration under the eyes, or so-called allergic shiners, is caused by venous engorgement. A transverse crease across the nose may be seen in children who chronically push their palm upward under the nose because of rhinorrhea or itching. The turbinates appearing edematous with a bluish mother-of-pearl hue is believed to be pathognomonic but may be seen in non-allergic rhinitis also. Likewise, turbinates may be engorged and erythematous. Lymphoid hyperplasia, or cobblestoning, may be seen on the posterior pharynx. Chronic mouth breathing in children caused by nasal obstruction can cause the allergic facies in the developing facial features. These include open mouth with receding chin and overbite, elongation of the face, and arching of the hard palate.

Diagnosis is frequently determined by the appropriate history and findings and supported by demonstration of specific IgE antibodies against a variety of airborne agents. Percutaneous (prick or puncture) skin testing remains the most specific and cost-effective diagnostic modality, although newer CAP-RAST (radioallergosorbent assay) testing is approaching similar sensitivity. Intradermal skin testing is more sensitive but introduces a higher false-positive rate and is not believed to add any diagnostic value to prick testing of potent pollen extracts. There may, however, be a role for intradermal testing with less potent extracts.

Pharmacotherapy

Pharmacotherapy for allergic rhinitis is the most used mode of treatment, although perhaps not the most effective. H_1 antihistamines have the largest market share of

CURRENT DIAGNOSIS

Appropriate history of exacerbants:

- Perennial or seasonal symptoms, with timing to identify pollens or spores
- Symptom triggering with identifiable agents such as animals

Familial history of asthma, allergic rhinitis, or atopic eczema

Medication and medical history:

- Oral aggravants such as ASA, NSAIDs, hypotensive agents
- Topical aggravants such as α-agonists
- Hypothyroidism
- Pregnancy

Physical findings:

- Rhinorrhea
- Nasal congestion
- So-called allergic facies

Corroborative findings:

- Immediate hypersensitivity skin testing
- Serum-specific IgE

Co-morbid conditions:

- Sinusitis
- Nasal polyposis
- Asthma
- Eustachian tube dysfunction and serous otitis media

Abbreviations: ASA = acetylsalicylic acid (aspirin); NSAIDs = nonsteroidal anti-inflammatory drugs.

rhinitis remedies, although, again, they are not the most effective. Oral first-generation H_1 receptor antagonists have been available for more than a half century, and many are obtainable as over-the counter (OTC) preparations. Typical benefits are inhibition of sneezing, itching, and rhinorrhea; oral antihistamines are notoriously ineffective for nasal congestion. Drawbacks are sedation and anticholinergic effects of overdrying. Second-generation antihistamines have the advantage of less anticholinergic effects and little to no sedation. Loratadine (Claritin) is available as an OTC formulation, whereas others such as fexofenadine (Allegra) are still prescription items. Cetirizine (Zyrtec), the active metabolite of hydroxyzine (Atarax), possesses potential for sedation. Topical azelastine (Astelin) is a twice-daily nasal spray as well as an ophthalmic preparation (Optivar). In addition to typical antihistaminic effects, it is modestly anti-inflammatory, improving nasal congestion, presumably through inhibition of ICAM-1, lipoxygenase, and leukotriene C4 synthase. It can cause sedation. Several topical ophthalmic antihistamine preparations are available for associated allergic conjunctivitis.

Leukotriene receptor antagonists were initially approved by the Food and Drug Administration (FDA) for use in asthma, but montelukast (Singulair) was more recently approved for allergic rhinitis therapy as well. However, a recent systematic review and meta-analysis showed these agents to be modestly better than placebo, as effective as antihistamines, and inferior to nasal corticosteroids in improving symptoms and quality of life in patients with seasonal allergic rhinitis. There seems little reason to use leukotriene modifier for treatment of uncomplicated allergic rhinitis. There may be some rationale for using montelukast or zafirlukast[1] (Accolate) with zileuton[1] (Zyflo) in the treatment of rhinitis complicated by sinusitis with polyposis, although evidence-based data are still missing.

Topical glucocorticoids are the most effective pharmacotherapy for allergic rhinitis. Topical corticosteroids decrease nasal T_H2 cytokines, IgE, and eosinophils. A meta-analysis showed superiority over antihistamines in 15 of 16 controlled trials, evaluating symptoms such as rhinorrhea, congestion, and sneezing. Another meta-analysis of nine studies again showed superiority of intranasal corticosteroids over topical antihistamines for nasal symptoms and no difference for ocular symptoms. Even if used on an as-needed basis only, nasal corticosteroids are superior for symptom relief to oral antihistamines. In a short-term 2-week study, the combination of montelukast with cetirizine each once daily was shown to be as effective as once-daily intranasal mometasone in improvement of nasal peak flow and total nasal symptoms.

Although steroid potency based on receptor affinity is very important in the management of asthma, the dose-response curves for most topical nasal corticosteroids are such that all preparations appear to be equally effective. Choice is therefore predicated on patient preference, which is usually affected by effects of expedients. The most common side effect is epistaxis. Septal perforation is reported, presumably caused by topical vasoconstriction, but is exceedingly uncommon and appears to be adverted by proper administration technique. Concern over systemic side effects is generally not warranted. Fluticasone (Flonase) and mometasone (Nasonex) have very low levels of systemic bioavailability via the nasal route; the levels of budesonide (Rhinocort), triamcinolone (Nasacort), beclomethasone (Vancenase AQ), and flunisolide (Nasalide) are higher. Even so, reports of adverse effects are not common with nasal preparations. For severe symptoms, oral steroids such as prednisone are sometimes used for very short periods to achieve quick improvement. The well-known complications of long-term therapy are not justifiable in the management of rhinitis. In some parts of the United States, intramuscular corticosteroids are considered standard of care for severe symptoms induced by large exposures such as seen with mountain cedar fever. The wisdom of this practice is debatable.

An anticholinergic topical preparation, ipratropium bromide (Atrovent 0.06% Nasal Spray), is useful for rhinitis associated with more profuse rhinorrhea. It may be beneficial in allergic rhinitis but has a larger role in nonallergic irritant rhinitis such as cold air–induced, gustatory rhinitis, and the profuse rhinorrhea associated with viral URIs. Ipratropium has no effect on nasal congestion. Methscopolamine (Pamine) is an oral quaternary ammonium anticholinergic used as a drying agent and found primarily in combination with antihistamines such as chlorpheniramine and decongestants such as phenylephrine (Dura-vent/DA). Cromolyn (NasalCrom), a mast cell stabilizer, can be used as a topical nasal spray for allergic rhinitis but needs to be used every 4 hours for optimal efficacy.

The use of decongestants is problematic: data on oral efficacy are wanting, and benefit may be overridden by

---

[1]Not FDA approved for this indication.

side effects. Potential for significant adverse reactions with overuse resulted in removal of phenylpropanolamine from the U.S. market. Similar problems are arising with pseudoephedrine. Phenylephrine is most often found in combination products. Overuse of topical decongestants like phenylephrine (Neo-Synephrine) and oxymetazoline (Otrivin) results in well-described rebound nasal congestion.

The use of saline nasal washes is highly recommended. A commercially available clear squeeze bottle with packets of sodium chloride and baking soda (Neilmed) is effective. This modality is especially useful in patients with complicating chronic sinusitis but is helpful for perennial allergic rhinitis as well.

Avoidance and Environmental Controls

Although avoidance of outdoor aeroallergens can be frequently only achieved by remaining indoors, avoidance of indoor allergens is more amenable to intervention. Pets can be removed from the home, although levels of allergenic proteins may take months to subside. And many pet owners choose not to remove an allergenic animal. The value of allergen-impermeable bedding linens is either supported or disavowed by contradictory studies. Control of indoor humidity may provide the best avenue for dust mite and mold abatement. Cockroach control is very difficult to achieve, and sublethal boric acid treatment may actually increase the release of cockroach allergen.

Allergen Immunotherapy

Allergen vaccine immunotherapy, administered via subcutaneous route, was shown by double-blind placebo-controlled studies to be effective in the treatment of allergic rhinoconjunctivitis. Extracts used include pollens such as short ragweed, timothy grass, other northern grasses, mountain cedar, and pellitory, fungi such as *Alternaria* and *Cladosporium*, house dust mites, and cat and dog dander. Immunologic changes include induction of specific IgG, blunting of specific IgE, decreased end-organ responsiveness, decreased recruitment of effector cells, shift from T_H2 to T_H1 cytokine profile, and induction of T regulatory cells. Sublingual/oral route of administration was studied extensively in Europe, requires high dose of allergen, and appears to have an excellent safety profile but is less effective than subcutaneous immunotherapy and is slower in onset of benefit.

Biologic Modifiers

Omalizumab[1] (Xolair), the chimeric monoclonal antibody directed against IgE, is effective for allergic rhinitis, although presently approved only for use in steroid-requiring perennial allergic asthmatics. It would be an exceedingly costly way of treating hayfever, but those patients using it

---

[1]Not FDA approved for this indication.

CURRENT THERAPY

Allergen avoidance
Pharmacotherapy
- Topical corticosteroids as first-line monotherapy:
    - Mometasone (Nasonex)
    - Fluticasone (Flonase)
    - Budesonide (Rhinocort Agua)
    - Triamcinolone (Nasocort AQ)
    - Flunisolide (Nasalide)
- Oral antihistamines used as add-on therapy or alone for mild symptoms:
    - Fexofenadine (second generation) (Allegra)
    - Cetirizine (second generation) (Zyrtec)
    - Loratadine(second generation) (Claritin)
    - Hydroxyzine (Atarax)
    - Chlorpheniramine (Chlor-Trimeton)
    - Diphenhydramine (Astelin)
- Topical antihistamine (azelastine)
- Oral leukotriene modifiers (montelukast [Singulair]) as add-on only
- Oral decongestants:
    - Pseudoephedrine (Sudafed)
    - Phenylephrine (Ah-Chew D)
- Topical cromolyn (NasalCrom)
- Nasal saline irrigation (Ocean)
- Allergen immunotherapy

for asthma control could expect benefit in concomitant allergic rhinitis symptoms.

Considerations in Pregnancy

Older antihistamines like chlorpheniramine (Chlor-Trimeton), hydroxyzine (Atarax), and tripelennamine (Pyribenzamine, PBZ) are safe in pregnancy, and data are likewise reassuring for loratadine (Claritin) and cetirizine (Zyrtec). Topical corticosteroids, especially after the first trimester, appear safe; budesonide (Rhinocort) is category B.

Cromolyn (NasalCrom) is category B also and can be used for mild disease. Pseudoephedrine (Sudafed) carries a category C, and oral decongestants are best avoided if possible. Allergen immunotherapy with stable maintenance dosing is safe.

In conclusion, pharmacotherapy is the most used therapeutic modality in allergic rhinitis because of inhalant factors. Second-generation antihistamines are preferable because of decreased sedation and anticholinergic effects. Topical corticosteroids remain the best and preferred method of treatment, both for seasonal and perennial allergic rhinitis. Addition of antihistamines and antileukotrienes to topical steroids may be beneficial because of a more rapid onset of effect, and they may be withdrawn as control is achieved. Allergen avoidance is recommended but may be difficult depending on the incriminated agent. Allergen vaccine immunotherapy is effective and should be strongly considered in the face of poor response to pharmacotherapy and avoidance.

REFERENCES

Benson M, Strannegård I-L, Strannegård Ö, Wennergren G: Topical steroid treatment of allergic rhinitis decreases nasal fluid T_h2 cytokines, eosinophils, eosinophil cationic protein, and IgE but has no significant effect on IFN-γ, IL-1β, TNF-α, or neutrophils. J Allergy Clin Immunol 2000;106:307-312.

Bousquet J, Van Cauwenberge P, Khaltaev N: Allergic rhinitis and its impact on asthma, J Allergy Clin Immunol 2001;108:S147-S334.

Frew AJ: Immunotherapy of allergic disease. J Allergy Clin Immunol 2003;111:S712-S719.

Incaudo GA, Takach P: The diagnosis and treatment of allergic rhinitis during pregnancy and lactation. Immunol Allergy Clin N Am 2006;26:137-154.

Kaszuba SM, Baroody FM, deTineo M, et al: Superiority of an intranasal corticosteroid compared with an oral antihistamine in the as-needed treatment of seasonal allergic rhinitis. Arch Intern Med 2001; 161:2581-2587.

Pedersen S: Assessing the effect of intranasal steroids on growth. J Allergy Clin Immunol 2001;108:S40-S44.

Weber RW: Immunotherapy with allergens. JAMA 1997;278:1881-1887.

Weiner JM, Abramson MJ, Puy RM: Intranasal corticosteroids versus oral H1 receptor antagonists in allergic rhinitis: Systematic review of randomized controlled trials. BMJ 1998;317:1624-1629.

Wilson AM, O'Byrne PM, Parameswaran K: Leukotriene receptor antagonists for allergic rhinitis: A systematic review and meta-analysis. Am J Med 2004;116:338-344.

Wilson AM, Orr LO, Sims EJ, Lipworth BJ: Effects of monotherapy with intra-nasal corticosteroid or combined oral histamine and leukotrienes receptor antagonists in seasonal allergic rhinitis. Clin Exp Allergy 2001;31:61-68.

Yanez A, Rodrigo GJ: Intranasal corticosteroids versus topical H1 receptor antagonists for the treatment of allergic rhinitis: A systematic review with meta-analysis. Ann Allergy Asthma Immunol 2002;89:479-484.

Allergic Reactions to Drugs

Method of
Donald McNeil, MD

Drug allergic reactions fall under the broader category of adverse drug reactions (ADRs), which also include toxic drug effects, drug interactions, drug intolerance, and, finally, allergic (or immunologic) drug reactions. Adverse drug reactions are common and often result in only trivial consequences. Some may be severe and life-threatening, and may result from both allergic and nonallergic causes.

The incidence of adverse drug effects is unknown but estimates of 20% of hospital admissions are not unreasonable. A skin rash is the most common manifestation; more importantly, however, severe life-threatening reactions occur, of which only a small portion have an allergic etiology. Most drug reactions are the result of unknown mechanisms. Drug intolerance, drug overdose, and side effects of drugs, as well as drug interactions, all play a significant role. These reactions should be considered both common and predictable.

Although allergic drug reactions are potentially severe, they are also the least common and least predictable. Allergic drug reactions are given particular attention because of the unpredictable, costly, and severe consequences that occasionally arise.

Several mechanisms may play a role in the underlying etiology of immunologic drug reactions. Immediate IgE-mediated reactions represent the classic allergic reaction.

This is well characterized and the best understood, but other mechanisms also exist, for example, a cytotoxic reaction in which drug-induced antibodies result in hemolytic anemia. Another example is immune complex formation resulting in organ damage. This is commonly referred to as a "serum sickness" reaction and is characterized by fever, rash, and arthralgia beginning 2 to 4 weeks after initiation of drug. Finally, a delayed-type hypersensitivity reaction occurs when drug-specific T-lymphocytes react. This completes the picture of the four types of immunologic-mediated drug reactions according to the original Gell and Coombs classification. These are referred to as Type I, II, III, or IV reactions, respectively.

Cutaneous reactions comprise the most frequent type of allergic drug reaction. Approximately 94% cause a morbilliform rash and only 5% cause an urticarial reaction. Idiosyncratic reactions are still the most likely cause for a rash and occur much more frequently than a true drug-induced allergic reaction. Ampicillins in conjunction with a viral hepatitis or sulfa drugs taken in the AIDS population are common examples.

Both allergic and nonallergic reactions are known to be associated with severe reactions, including fatalities. Contrast media agents, allergic extracts, anesthetics, and antibiotics are the most commonly implicated drugs. Penicillin remains the most common cause of fatal drug reactions and accounts for up to 75% of these severe drug reactions in the United States.

An allergy to penicillin is the most frequently reported, but as many as 90% of patients labeled "penicillin allergic" are able to tolerate penicillin. This allergy is often mislabeled because of underlying illness or interaction between antibiotic and illness. Unfortunately one third to half of vancomycin (Vancocin) prescriptions in hospitals are given because of a history of "penicillin allergy." This raises the incidence of drug-resistant bacteria because of broad-spectrum antibiotic overuse. The economic impact of treating antibiotic-resistant infections is roughly $4 billion annually.

Pathophysiology

Some drugs are capable of reacting in the body without further alteration in chemical structure, whereas others must first be metabolized to become immunogenic. Many drugs are too small to be immunogenic alone and are incapable of eliciting an immune allergic response. These drugs require binding to a high-molecular-weight protein followed by antigen processing and presentation by the macrophage in the presence of major histocompatibility complex (MHC)-specific antigen to appropriate T-cell receptors.

Penicillin is capable of inducing an allergic reaction in more than one manner. Benzylpenicilloyl, the major penicillin determinant, is able to produce a strong antigenic response. A commercially available product, benzylpenicilloyl-polylysine (PPL) (Pre-Pen), provides the means to reproduce the same allergic response by simple skin testing. Minor determinants are metabolic derivatives of penicillin that may also produce an immune response. The diagnostic capabilities of a penicillin allergy are strengthened by including some measure of the allergic response to the minor determinants when skin testing is conducted for penicillin (Figure 1).

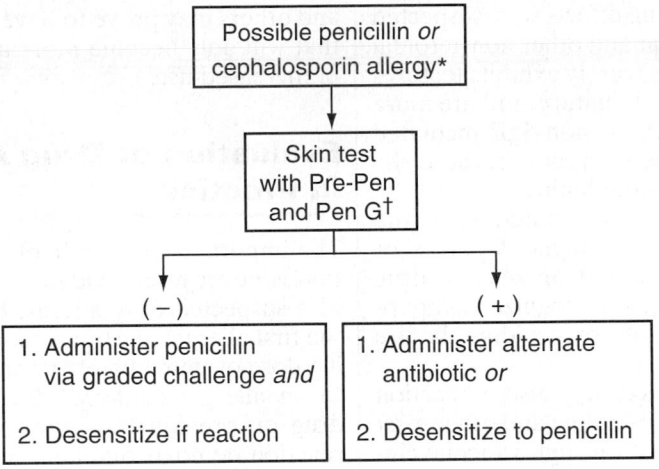

```
          ┌─────────────────────────┐
          │    Possible penicillin or  │
          │   cephalosporin allergy*   │
          └─────────────────────────┘
                       │
                       ▼
          ┌─────────────────────────┐
          │        Skin test          │
          │     with Pre-Pen          │
          │      and Pen G†            │
          └─────────────────────────┘
              │                    │
           ( − )                ( + )
     ┌──────────────────┐  ┌──────────────────┐
     │ 1. Administer     │  │ 1. Administer     │
     │    penicillin     │  │    alternate      │
     │    via graded     │  │    antibiotic or  │
     │    challenge and  │  │                   │
     │                   │  │                   │
     │ 2. Desensitize if │  │ 2. Desensitize to │
     │    reaction       │  │    penicillin     │
     └──────────────────┘  └──────────────────┘
```

*Only 10%–20% of patients who report a penicillin allergy are actually allergic.
†Benzylpenicilloyl-polylysine (Pre-Pen) and penicillin G (Pen G) will not include all potential penicillin derivatives. The additional benefit of testing with the minor determinant mixture is impractical and usually not available.

FIGURE 1. Penicillin allergy evaluation.

Patients with a history of penicillin allergy but negative skin testing to PPL and the minor determinants rarely experience allergic reactions on re-exposure. If they should occur, these are not fatal, but rather mild and self-limited.

PPL alone will potentially miss a significant percentage of allergic reactions to penicillin. Allergy testing with fresh benzylpenicillin G, aged penicillin (reconstituted more than 24 hours) as well as skin testing with the specific penicillin in question will greatly enhance the likelihood of uncovering of penicillin allergy in a patient with a positive history.

Cephalosporins do not provide the same degree of certainty with respect to an allergic evaluation. Cross-reactivity with penicillin allergy patients is known to exist, and although uncommon, it is also unpredictable. To err on the side of safety, a patient with a known penicillin allergy should not be treated with a cephalosporin. A patient with a previous cephalosporin reaction with a negative penicillin skin test cannot safely receive penicillin or another cephalosporin unless further diagnostic measures are taken. This patient may be allergic to a side chain on the cephalosporin that has not been identified by penicillin skin testing. Others recommend a graded oral challenge using a cephalosporin with a different side chain. The latter should be done realizing that standardized procedures have not been developed for this and therefore false negative results may occur.

Successful desensitization to penicillin has permitted a similar approach with other drugs. If the drug in question is required, either intravenous or oral drug administration is possible by incremental doses given usually every 15 minutes. A 10,000-fold dilution of the initial dose is usually sufficient to begin, followed by higher doses, 2-fold or greater. The vital signs are monitored throughout the procedure with timely medical intervention if problems arise.

Sulfonamides typically cause cutaneous reactions, infrequently in healthy individuals but extremely common in AIDS patients. Reactions may be relatively benign in nature such as urticaria or fixed-drug eruption, but may also cause more serious reactions (Stevens-Johnson syndrome, toxic epidermal necrolysis). A variety of mechanisms may exist, alone or in combination, using IgE antibody response, T-lymphocytes, and inflammatory cytokines. Because of our inadequate understanding of these mechanisms, there are no universally acceptable means of evaluating sulfonamide hypersensitivity. Unless there has been previously severe reaction, a graded challenge with the drug in question is considered a reasonable alternative (Box 1). Although a theoretical risk exists between sulfonamides and drugs with sulfonamide derivatives (diuretics, COX-2 inhibitors), little data show this is actually true.

Radiographic contrast media (RCM) produce an anaphylactoid reaction by an unknown mechanism. Conventional RCM is hypertonic. The newer nonionic RCM with lower osmolarity are associated with fewer anaphylactoid or allergic-like reactions. Complement system activation, which is capable of causing histamine release, is thought to be the method by which this reaction occurs.

BOX 1 Graded Challenge

1. Cautious administration of medications to patient not likely allergic to drug.
2. Not to be considered equivalent to desensitization.
3. Used when insufficient evidence available to exclude drug allergy.
4. Medication administered in incremental doses beginning at 1:100 dilution of final dose.
5. Adequate medical resources exist to treat allergic reaction.

In the continuum of adverse drug effects with suspected hypersensitivity, exposure to *aspirin* and other nonsteroidal anti-inflammatory drugs (NSAIDs) rarely exhibits features that are IgE mediated and allergic in nature, and are more often nonimmunologic mediated. A non–IgE-mediated event must still be approached with caution because the consequences are potentially life-threatening.

More commonly, NSAIDs are associated with the asthma triad syndrome associated with nasal polyps or rhinitis, and severe asthma. This is not an allergic drug reaction, but it represents a largely unrecognized subpopulation of asthmatics who will benefit by avoiding the use of NSAIDs.

The antibiotic *vancomycin* (Vancocin) causes a reaction referred to as *red man syndrome*. Histamine and other mast cell mediators are released, but not through vancomycin-induced IgE antibody (rare cases have been reported). Most, but not all, cases of the red man syndrome are related to the rate of the infusion, and most will subside once the medication is stopped. A graded challenge with the drug or a full course of desensitization usually permits resumption of treatment.

Angiotensin-converting enzyme (ACE) inhibitors are well known to be associated with cough and angioedema, but like NSAIDs, the mechanism is unknown. Newer ACE inhibitors have been described to cause similar reactions but at a much lower incidence. The symptoms of cough and angioedema may continue to recur for several months and up to a year after the discontinuation of the drug.

As seen from the discussion above, IgE-mediated allergic drug reactions represent only a portion of immune-mediated drug reactions. To assist in the diagnosis, a 7- to 10-day delay in the appearance of the drug reaction after initial treatment or immediate reactivation on re-exposure suggests an immunologic etiology. Oftentimes, only the history will provide this index of suspicion. Confirmation by positive skin testing with the drug in question is highly predictive of IgE-mediated hypersensitivity.

Attempts to label reactions as either IgE- or non–IgE-mediated may prove to be costly, time-consuming, and of no immediate benefit. Non-IgE reactions are capable of eliciting changes in vital signs, pulmonary function, and cutaneous effects similar to anaphylaxis and are referred to as anaphylactoid. These need to be regarded with the same degree of caution as IgE-mediated reactions. Narcotics, radiographic contrast media, and chemotherapeutic agents may directly affect mast cell mediator release with the consequences listed above. Antihistamines and corticosteroids given prior to administration of these drugs are usually sufficient to prevent a reoccurrence, or at least to minimize these reactions.

Drug desensitization is indicated for those patients with positive skin tests who must receive the drug, but should not be assumed to be universally safe or protective. Some chemotherapeutic agents, such as etoposide (VePesid) and teniposide (Vumon), have a much higher incidence of anaphylactoid reactions. Readministration of these drugs in the face of a previous reaction and in spite of prophylactic measures often leads to disappointing results.

Current biologic response modifier agents, as well as others soon to arrive, are associated with adverse reactions. Monoclonal antibodies, T- and B-cell inactivators, and others may prove to have adverse immunologic effects that will only become more apparent with the experience of increased use.

Evaluation of Drug Allergy in Practice

The importance of a reliable history in a medical evaluation is never more evident than during the initial workup of a suspected drug allergy. The timing of exposure, with the first allergic reaction occurring within days of the priming dose or immediately upon re-exposure, strongly points to an allergic etiology. Multiple exposures to the same drug on previous occasions do not preclude an allergic reaction de novo. Similarly, a previous history of an allergic drug reaction does not by itself predict a reoccurrence on re-exposure. The allergic diathesis may wane over time for drugs just as it may occur for other allergens.

Armed with this suggestive drug history and clinical findings such as a rash, fever, bronchospasm, or anaphylaxis, the evaluation becomes more straightforward. In the appropriate clinical setting, eosinophilia will also support a drug-allergic reaction.

Avoiding the implicated drug may be the simplest approach because confirmation of the diagnosis with appropriate skin testing is often unavailable. (Standardized skin testing exists only for penicillin, but even this does not provide 100% reliability.) Skin testing with the drug is questionable, but using both a positive and negative control of histamine and saline may still provide useful information. A positive skin test would certainly discourage use of this drug unless adequate precautions were taken.

If a non–life-threatening history of a reaction exists and the drug cannot be appropriately substituted, the option exists for a graded oral challenge to confirm the diagnosis. This should not be considered to be the same as desensitization because it involves higher doses and exposure over a shorter period of time than would be considered safe in a truly allergic individual. A challenge such as this should be conducted in suitable medical facilities under close medical supervision.

If the drug in question has been shown to cause an allergic reaction but still must be used, then a carefully monitored drug desensitization program should be considered. Under medical supervision, the drug should be administered orally or intravenously beginning with doses that are tenfold more dilute than the final strength. Incrementally higher doses of the drug should be administered every 15 minutes, increasing the dose twofold each time.

Drug-induced skin reactions are common and warrant particular attention. Early recognition is necessary to avoid an incorrect diagnosis and to institute appropriate interventional measures as soon as possible.

The following points will assist the physician in arriving at a correct diagnosis. The *timing of the onset* of the reaction in relation to the time the drug was given provides an important clue. Often signs and symptoms develop 1 to 2 weeks after time of initial drug exposure. Symptoms may develop rapidly on repeat exposure. *Pruritic urticarial lesions* strongly suggest an adverse drug reaction. A *symmetrical or truncal distribution* or a rash that occurs only in sun-exposed areas (polymorphous light eruption) also supports an ADR finding. The morphology

TABLE 1 Drugs Used to Treat AIDS/HIV

Drug	Reaction
Zidovudine, AZT (Retrovir)	Hyperpigmentation
Zalcitabine, ddC (Hivid)	Oral ulcers
Abacavir (Ziagen)	Severe rash/anaphylaxis
Nevirapine (Viramune)	Toxic epidermal necrolysis
Foscarnet	Urethral ulceration
Trimethoprim-sulfamethoxazole (TMP-SMX) (Bactrim)	Morbilliform rash or erythema multiforme

of the reaction is helpful, although many types occur (lichenoid, morbilliform, eczematous). The histopathology of the lesion on skin biopsy may reveal eosinophils, which may also be detected in the peripheral blood.

Drugs that commonly cause ADRs tend to be antibiotics. The most common is the morbilliform rash when ampicillin is given in the presence of a viral infection such as infectious mononucleosis or cytomegalovirus. Rarely is this IgE mediated and it should not be regarded as a basis for a history of penicillin allergy. It should also be noted that not all ADRs are caused by prescription medications. A patient may fail to disclose over-the-counter medications that might be responsible (e.g., St. John's wort).

The *response to treatment* may aid in the recognition of an ADR. An incomplete response to topical steroids is typical of an ADR and systemic steroids may turn out to be the therapy of choice. Finally, the *response to withdrawal* of drug may range from a rapid recovery to slow clearing over many weeks, but a favorable response nonetheless.

Table 1 lists several drugs used to treat AIDS/HIV that are worthy of mention. Not all should be considered to be an allergic cause of ADR.

A careful and systematic approach to the patient with a suspected drug allergy will provide valuable information for both the immediate and the long-term management of the patient. A suspected drug allergy that is disproved will facilitate good medical care because unnecessary expense and the risk of further sensitizing the patient to a new medication will be spared if the patient is not allergic. On the other hand, a positive screen for a suspected drug allergy will result in a safe alternative. It should be emphasized, however, that neither a family history of a drug allergy nor a patient requesting a "test" for a possible drug allergy without other reason is an indication for further drug allergy evaluation because of the risk of false-negative results.

Allergic Reactions to Insect Stings*

Method of
David B. K. Golden, MD

Insect bites and stings normally cause temporary localized swelling, redness, pain, and itching. Allergic swelling can also result from insect bites or stings, but stinging insects of the order Hymenoptera can cause anaphylaxis. Allergic reactions to stings from honeybees, vespids (yellow jackets, hornets, wasps), and fire ants are caused by IgE antibodies directed against the protein allergens in the venoms (but not in the bodies or saliva) of these insects. Yellow jacket and hornet venoms are almost identical and are partially cross reactive with wasp venoms, but honeybee venom and fire ant venom are each unique. Commercial venom vaccines are available for honeybee, yellow jacket, yellow hornet, white-faced hornet, and *Polistes* wasps (ALK Laboratories; Hollister-Stier Laboratories). For fire ant sting allergy, imported fire ant whole body extract is the only commercial available material. Although it contains sufficient venom allergens for diagnostic use and for immunotherapy, evidence indicates that venom is superior.

Allergic reactions may be localized or systemic. Large local reactions have a late-phase inflammatory mechanism that progresses for 24 to 48 hours after the sting, causing a painful induration that is often larger than 6 inches in diameter and lasts for 5 to 10 days. A large local reaction to a sting can mimic laryngeal edema (from a sting in the mouth or throat) or cellulitis (lymphangitic drainage from the reaction on an extremity). Systemic reactions are immediate hypersensitivity reactions with manifestations distant from the site of the sting, which can include any one or more of the signs or symptoms of anaphylaxis including urticaria, angioedema, flushing, throat or chest tightness, dyspnea, dizziness, or hypotensive shock. The reported frequency of 50 to 100 fatal reactions per year in the United States is certainly an underestimate. Elevated serum tryptase and venom-specific IgE antibodies are reported in postmortem blood samples in cases of unexpected death in young individuals. Half of fatal reactions occurred in persons with no prior history of reactions to stings, and most occur in individuals older than 45 years. The population at risk is greater than generally appreciated: 3% of adults in the United States have a history of a systemic allergic reaction to insect stings, and more than 20% have IgE antibodies to venom allergens detectable in the skin or blood.

Diagnosis

A detailed history provides the most important diagnostic information. The exact features and time course of the reaction can distinguish large local, systemic, and

*This work was supported by National Institutes of Health (NIH) grant AI08270.

CURRENT DIAGNOSIS

- History of systemic allergic reactions to sting
- Positive venom skin tests or radioallergosorbent assay test (RAST)
- Degree of test reaction not correlated with severity of sting reaction
- Low risk if previous large local sting reactions
- Low risk in children with mild systemic reactions
- Quality of life and frequency of exposure a consideration

nonallergic reactions. Objective signs and documented clinical observations are more reliable than subjective descriptions. Venom-specific IgE antibodies can be demonstrated by skin testing or serologic methods (radioallergosorbent assay test [RAST]) but must be interpreted in the context of the clinical history. Skin testing with the five Hymenoptera venoms (or fire ant whole body extract) is recommended for patients who have had systemic allergic reactions to a sting but is not required for large local reactions. Skin tests are performed with superficial intradermal injection of 0.02 mL of each venom at concentrations starting at 0.001 μg/mL and increasing incrementally up to 1.0 μg/mL, if needed, until a positive wheal and flare reaction is elicited. Diagnostic laboratory measurement of venom-specific IgE antibodies (RAST) may be useful when skin testing is inconclusive or cannot be performed but is less sensitive than skin testing. The venom RAST is positive in 10% of affected patients with negative skin tests, and conversely, the RAST is negative in 20% of patients with positive skin tests. A positive venom skin test in an individual with no history of sting reaction is associated with a 17% frequency of systemic reaction to a subsequent sting. The level of sensitivity on skin test or RAST is not correlated consistently with the severity of the sting reaction.

Assessing the risk of a systemic reaction to a future sting is based on the detailed history of previous reactions, the presence of venom-specific IgE antibodies, and the known natural history of the condition (Table 1). In adults with positive venom skin tests and a prior history of systemic reactions, the risk of systemic reaction is 30% to 60%, with the higher risk in patients with the most severe reactions (airway obstruction, unconsciousness) and the lower frequency in patients who had cutaneous systemic signs (urticaria, angioedema) and/or mild dizziness or throat tightness. The risk declines with time, but remains at 15% to 20% even after 20 to 30 years. The risk of systemic reaction is known to be low in the general population and in some subgroups of sensitized individuals (Table 2). The majority of affected children (16 years and younger) have had systemic reactions limited to skin manifestations, including generalized hives and angioedema of the face or lips but with no tongue or throat swelling and no dyspnea or hypotension. In these children, subsequent stings cause no systemic reaction in 90%, mild cutaneous systemic reactions in 5%, and more severe systemic reaction in less than 5% of cases. Patients with large local reactions generally have strongly positive venom skin tests but have only a 5% risk of systemic reaction to future stings.

Treatment and Avoidance of Sting Reactions

Local sting reactions can be treated symptomatically with ice and oral antihistamines. Large local reactions may require a burst of oral prednisone (e.g., 40 to 60 mg the first day, tapering over 4 to 7 days) but almost never require antibiotic treatment. Systemic reactions generally require the intramuscular administration of epinephrine (1:1000), 0.3 mg in an adult (0.01 mg/kg in children), with the availability of oxygen, intravenous fluids, or airway support if needed. Corticosteroids have no benefit in the acute stage, but despite a lack of supporting evidence are often administered in the hope of preventing late-phase manifestations. The patient should be monitored for 3 to 6 hours because more than 20% of severe cases develop biphasic or protracted anaphylaxis. Any patient judged to have a risk for anaphylaxis to future stings should have a prescription for an epinephrine injection kit and detailed instructions on when to use or not use it. Commercial kits include the EpiPen (0.3 mg epinephrine) and EpiPen Jr (0.15 mg epinephrine) (Dey Laboratories) and the Twinject (two doses of either 0.15 or 0.3 mg epinephrine) (Verus Pharmaceuticals). Such individuals should also be referred to a specialist for evaluation and discussion of risks and treatment options. Sting-allergic patients should avoid nesting areas, trash receptacles, eating or drinking outdoors, lawn mowing, or going barefoot.

TABLE 1 Clinical Recommendations Based on History of Sting Reactions, Age, and Results of Venom Skin Test (or RAST)

Reaction to Previous Sting	Skin Test (or RAST)	Risk of Systemic Reaction	Clinical Recommendation
No reaction	Positive	10%–15%	Avoidance
Large local	Positive	5%–10%	Avoidance
Cutaneous systemic	Positive: child	5%–10%	Avoidance
	Positive: adult	15%–20%	Venom immunotherapy
Anaphylaxis	Positive	30%–60%	Venom immunotherapy
	Negative	5%–10%	Repeat skin test/RAST

Abbreviations: RAST = radioallergosorbent assay test.

CURRENT THERAPY

- Epinephrine Autoinjector (EpiPen or Twinject) and avoidance strategies for low-risk patients is suggested.
- Venom immunotherapy is for high-risk patients.
- Venom immunotherapy is up to 98% effective.
- Most patients can discontinue venom immunotherapy after 5 years.
- Highest risk patients may need indefinite venom immunotherapy.

Prevention of Sting Reactions (Venom Immunotherapy)

Systemic reactions to insect stings can be prevented with up to 98% efficacy with venom immunotherapy. The indications for therapy are simply a positive history (of systemic reaction to stings) and positive venom skin tests (or RAST), although the severity of previous reactions and the patient's age at the time are also important variables (Table 3). Venom immunotherapy, and therefore skin testing, is not considered necessary for low-risk patients because more than 90% will never have a systemic reaction, such as in patients with large local reactions and in children with cutaneous systemic reactions.

Venom immunotherapy should begin with all of the venoms giving a positive skin test and follows a dose schedule described in the product package insert (ALK Laboratories; Hollister-Stier Laboratories). Injections are generally administered weekly for 8 to 26 weeks to achieve the full maintenance dose of 100 µg of each venom. More rapid treatment is not associated with more frequent adverse reactions. This dose is then repeated every 4 weeks for at least 1 year, then every 6 weeks for 1 to 2 years, and every 6 to 8 weeks thereafter. During immunotherapy, systemic reactions occur in 5% to 15% of cases, with variable degrees of urticaria, airway obstruction, or hypotension. The majority of such reactions are mild, but some require aggressive treatment for anaphylaxis. Venom injections also cause large local reactions in many patients during the first few months of therapy, but they are not predictive of systemic reactions and should not interfere with attaining the full recommended dose. All adverse reactions are much less common during maintenance treatment.

TABLE 2 Considerations in Stopping Venom Immunotherapy

Severity/pattern of systemic reaction
Age (child/teen, adult, senior)
Skin tests/RAST (persistent strong)
Time/duration of venom immunotherapy
Systemic reaction during venom immunotherapy
 (to injection or sting)
Quality of life/exposure

Abbreviation: RAST = radioallergosorbent assay test.

TABLE 3 Patients with Low Risk for Anaphylaxis

Minimal (<5%)	General adult population
	Patients on venom immunotherapy
	Children with cutaneous systemic reactions
Low (5%–10%)	Large local reactors
	Discontinued venom immunotherapy after 5 y

The frequency of systemic reactions is similar with venom immunotherapy and immunotherapy with inhalant allergens. Periodic monitoring of venom skin test or RAST sensitivity is recommended every 2 to 5 years to determine possible early discontinuation of therapy. The level of venom-specific IgG antibodies is correlated with clinical protection and may be measured during the first 3 years of venom immunotherapy, especially to determine whether protection is adequate with single-venom therapy and when maintenance intervals are extended. Some patients require higher doses for full protection.

The duration of venom immunotherapy remains a matter of judgment. The product package insert advises that venom immunotherapy should be continued indefinitely. Some experts advocate stopping treatment if skin tests (or RAST) become negative, but this occurs in only 25% of patients treated for 5 years and in 60% of those treated for 7 to 10 years. When venom immunotherapy is stopped after at least 5 years of maintenance treatment, the chance of reaction to a sting is 10% for each sting that occurs, even 10 to 15 years after stopping even if there are uneventful intervening stings and even if skin tests become negative. The cumulative risk of reaction is 15% to 20% more than 10 years after discontinuing treatment. The risk of a very severe reaction exists primarily in patients who had such a reaction prior to treatment, and they should therefore consider remaining on therapy indefinitely. Other high-risk patients who should consider continuing treatment beyond 5 years include those who had a systemic reaction during treatment whether to an injection or a sting. The relapse rate is also higher in honeybee allergic patients, as is the frequency of systemic reactions to venom injections and the failure rate for reaction to stings during therapy. Both the relapse rate and the level of venom-specific IgE (or skin test) are higher in patients who stop therapy after only 3 years compared to 5 years. Some investigators have suggested that lower risk patients (e.g., children with reactions of any severity and adult patients with mild reactions) might be able safely to stop after 3 years of treatment, but there are limited data published about this.

REFERENCES

Bernstein JA, Kagan SL, Bernstein DI, Bernstein IL: Rapid venom immunotherapy is safe for routine use in the treatment of patients with Hymenoptera anaphylaxis. Ann Allergy 1994;73:423-428.

Freeman TM: Hypersensitivity to Hymenoptera stings. N Engl J Med 2004;351:1978-1984.

Freeman TM, Highlander R, Ortiz A, Martin ME: Imported fire ant immunotherapy: Effectiveness of whole body extracts. J Allergy Clin Immunol 1992;90:210-215.

Golden DBK: Insect sting allergy and venom immunotherapy: A model and a mystery. J Allergy Clin Immunol 2005;115:439-447.

Golden DBK, Kagey-Sobotka A, Norman PS, et al: Outcomes of allergy to insect stings in children with and without venom immunotherapy. N Engl J Med 2004;351:668-674.

Golden DBK, Kwiterovich KA, Kagey-Sobotka A, et al: Discontinuing venom immunotherapy: Outcome after five years. J Allergy Clin Immunol 1996;97:579-587.

Golden DBK, Marsh DG, Kagey-Sobotka A, et al: Epidemiology of insect venom sensitivity. JAMA 1989;262:240-244.

Hamilton RG: Diagnostic methods for insect sting allergy. Curr Opin Allergy Clin Immunol 2004;4:297-306.

Hoffman DR: Fatal reactions to Hymenoptera stings. Asthma Allergy Proc 2003;24:1-5.

Hunt KJ, Valentine MD, Sobotka AK, et al: A controlled trial of immunotherapy in insect hypersensitivity. N Engl J Med 1978;299:157-161.

Moffitt JE, Golden DBK, Reisman RE, et al: Stinging insect hypersensitivity: A practice parameter update. J Allergy Clin Immunol 2004;114:869-886.

Stafford CT: Hypersensitivity to fire ant venom. Ann Allergy Asthma Immunol 1996;77:87-95.

Diseases of the Skin

Acne and Rosacea

Method of
Guy F. Webster, MD, PhD

Acne

Acne vulgaris is an extremely common disease. To some degree, signs of the disease can be found in nearly all adolescents, and regardless of severity, acne is often of greater psychological effect than cutaneous. Most patients overestimate the severity of their disease, whereas most doctors underestimate the impact of acne on their patients. Studies show that those with severe acne as teens are less employable as adults, and self-esteem in acne patients is low. These facts, combined with routine adolescent tensions, make acne a difficult disease to treat.

PATHOGENESIS

The pathogenesis of acne is multifactorial with disturbances of keratinization, hormonal secretion, and immunity. The central defect involves the formation of the comedo, a plug in the follicle that results from aberrant desquamation of the follicular wall. Comedones are described clinically as *open* if the pore is visible and *closed* if it is not. The black tip of an open comedo results from the oxidation of sebaceous lipid and melanin, and it is not dirt (contrary to worldwide maternal advice). The cause of comedo formation is not known but may relate to bacterial stimulation of aberrant keratinization within the sebaceous duct. Comedones do not result from poor hygiene or diet or use of name-brand cosmetics (big companies have a reputation to lose and test for acnegenicity).

The acne of many patients remains in this first noninflamed stage, but it may progress to inflammatory lesions of varying severity. The target of inflammation is *Propionibacterium acnes*, an aerotolerant anaerobic member of the normal flora in sebaceous regions of the skin. *P. acnes* lives in the follicle and metabolizes sebaceous triglycerides into fatty acids and glycerol. It consumes the glycerol and casts off the fatty acids. In years past it was believed the fatty acids in sebum were the cause of acne

inflammation, but it is now clear the organism itself is the target.

P. acnes is a highly inflammatory, activating complement, secreting neutrophil and monocyte chemotactic factors, activating toll-like receptors and lymphocytes, and inducing lysosomal enzyme release. In addition, the organism is degraded only very slowly, resulting in a persistent follicular inflammatory response.

Because all individuals have significant levels of *P. acnes* and some degree of follicular plugging, it is curious that everyone does not have active acne. The explanation lies in the level of the immune response to the organism. Patients with excessive humoral and cellular immunity to *P. acnes* mount a more destructive inflammatory response that produces clinical lesions. This response represents a true hypersensitivity to *P. acnes*, in that the organism is a beneficial commensal and of minimal infectious potential.

A minority of women have an endocrine aspect to their acne. Although not necessarily severe, their acne may become very refractory. Such patients may give a history of irregular menses, be overweight, or have increased facial hair or androgenetic alopecia. Measurement of serum androgen levels and subsequent corrective therapy usually improves their acne as well. Although only two contraceptives are currently approved for marketing as acne therapy, probably all oral contraceptives are of some benefit.

There are many acne grading systems. Those that involve pimple counting are useful for clinical trials but too cumbersome for office use. A gestalt system is more useful, in which the physician and patient reach some consensus on the degree of the acne by combining severity of actual lesions with the impact of the disease on the patient. Inflammatory acne lesions range from superficial pustules to deep scarring nodules. Patients generally have a mixture of lesion types, and their acne should be graded based on the most severe lesions present (i.e., a patient with 3 scarring nodules has more severe acne than one with 50 superficial pustules). The presence of acne on the chest or back also connotes more severe and hard-to-treat disease.

The terms *inverse acne, triad acne,* and *hidradenitis suppurativa* all describe a follicular process that results in comedo formation and inflammation in the scalp, axilla, and groin. In the past, this was believed to be an apocrine disease, but recent work describes it as a disease of the hair follicle, like acne. Unlike acne, *P. acnes* plays little or no role in this acne of nonsebaceous regions. Various bacteria, enterics, pseudomonads, and streptococci colonize these lesions and provoke inflammation and scarring. Sinus tract formation is common and results in disease that is often best treated surgically.

TREATMENT

The first step in treatment of patients with acne is to be certain they (and their parents) have not fallen prey to the numerous myths about the disease. Acne is not caused by dirt, diet, or impure thoughts. Patients commonly believe one particular food, usually a greasy or sweet one (never asparagus), worsens their acne. Trying to correct this misconception is fruitless; it is better to focus on the proper use of medicine. Hair on the forehead does not make pimples, and the disease cannot be treated effectively with soap and water. Although satisfying, popping pimples is bad; it promotes scarring and prolongs the life of many lesions. Stress may play a role in acne, but it is a small one, and most patients' acne does not benefit from tranquilizers.

Patients and doctors need to communicate particularly well during the treatment of acne. During the first visit, patients should be given realistic expectations and disabused (if possible) of incorrect ideas. Teens, in particular, expect quick results. They must understand that 3 to 6 weeks (although an eternity) is the quickest that acne can be expected to improve. Bigger lesions may take longer, as do open comedones. To most patients, so-called scarring is any mark on the face after a pimple is gone; they need to learn to distinguish between true scars and transient postinflammatory pigment changes.

Acne regimens vary widely among dermatologists. Some use one or two drugs in each patient; others use five or six. In general, one or two properly chosen drugs do better and are easier to comply with than a more complex regimen.

The central lesion in acne is the microcomedo in both comedonal and inflammatory acne types. Thus most effective regimens include a retinoid such as adapalene, tretinoin or tazarotene. Indeed, with sufficient patience, topical retinoids are excellent monotherapy for all but the most severe acne. But because topical retinoid monotherapy takes several months to really clear inflammatory acne, it is sensible to add a drug that reduces inflammation by reducing *P. acnes* populations. Purely noninflammatory (comedonal) acne is the mildest form of disease but can be the hardest to treat. Comedones are usually firmly ensconced in the follicle and, untreated, they cannot be easily expressed. Tretinoin (vitamin A acid) cream is the standard against which all other anticomedonal agents are compared. It inhibits comedo formation and eliminates comedonal acne in a few months. The only significant side effect is the irritation that is greatest after a few weeks. It usually does not require intervention, but if desired, a moisturizing lotion may be prescribed. Because their skin is inherently irritable, patients with atopic diseases may not tolerate topical retinoids even with moisturization. Other drugs are also useful for noninflammatory acne. Adapalene is a naphthoic acid derivative that binds to nuclear retinoid receptors and has retinoid effects. It is effective for comedonal acne and also has a measure of anti-inflammatory activity. Adapalene is roughly equivalent to topical tretinoin but with somewhat less irritation.

Tazarotene is a potent anticomedonal retinoid cream that is only slightly more irritating than tretinoin.

In the past 15 years, most dermatologists have observed a reduced efficacy of topical erythromycin and clindamycin. When first introduced the drugs were quite effective, but they have become of little use because of a dramatic increase in the resistance of *P. acnes* to the drugs. Fortunately, this resistance does not translate into hard-to-treat infections, just in hard-to-treat acne. The solution to the problem is to use the two drugs along with benzoyl peroxide, which effectively prevents the acquisition of resistance.

Oral antibiotics that are effective in acne include erythromycins, tetracyclines, trimethoprim-sulfamethoxazole, and ciprofloxacin. Because of concerns about generating resistant gastrointestinal (GI) flora, the latter two drugs should be reserved for problematic patients. Tetracyclines have the significant advantage of additional anti-inflammatory activity in acne and are the most widely prescribed. Doxycycline and minocycline have the greatest effect on acne and are well tolerated and generally safe.

Because of the clear link to androgens, acne is often perceived as a hormonal disease, but it is unusual for a hormonal drug to be effective as monotherapy. Adding a hormonal therapy to acne regimens in women is occasionally helpful. Two types of drug may be used: oral contraceptives and spironolactone. As stated earlier, although only two oral contraceptives are currently approved for marketing as an acne treatment, it is likely that most are helpful in acne to a degree.

In treating acne during pregnancy, tetracyclines may cause staining of teeth and bones and are contraindicated. Although commonly thought to be a teratogen, topical tretinoin does not raise circulating vitamin A levels or result in fetal deformity when used. Nevertheless, many patients and doctors are concerned and do not use the drug during pregnancy. Benzoyl peroxide, azelaic acid, and oral erythromycin are generally agreed to be safe for use during pregnancy; however, because nausea and heartburn often accompany pregnancy, avoiding erythromycin and treating acne topically is recommended.

Although occasionally helpful, topical steroids actually cause acne and invariably cause atrophy of facial skin if used for any length of time. They should be avoided. Intralesional triamcinolone acetonide is useful to calm big nodules but can cause pitting and hypopigmentation, both of which eventually resolve (0.05 mL of a 2 mg per mL dosage is commonly used).

Nodular scarring acne that resists oral antibiotics and topical retinoids is usually treated with oral isotretinoin, a potent and effective therapy for severe acne. After 4 to 6 months, most patients have little or no disease. Eighty percent have a complete long-term remission (possible cure) of their acne if treated with 1 mg/kg per day for 4 to 6 months. The duration of benefit after therapy is linked to dosage; lower dosages minimize side effects but increase the relapse rate.

Unfortunately, isotretinoin has significant side effects. There is an initial flare of acne in many patients that can be blunted by beginning at a low dose (e.g., 20 mg) and then increasing to around 1 mg/kg after 1 month. Patients with truncal acne may have a particularly severe flare of disease known as acne fulminans. This is a vicious scarring process that must be avoided. These patients are usually started on 20 mg of isotretinoin along with 20 mg of prednisone for the first month. The drug also produces dry skin and mucosae, elevated triglycerides in approximately 30% of patients, and occasional muscle or joint aches. Transaminases are occasionally elevated, but investigation usually determines they are muscle derived rather than of hepatic origin. Patients who exercise vigorously are at greater risk for muscle enzyme leakage.

Much public concern focuses on depression caused by isotretinoin, but both personal experience and large studies fail to show a correlation between the drug and mental illness. Unfortunately, disproving a negative can be nearly impossible. Discussing the issue with patients and parents and agreeing to bring up any problems that arise is beneficial.

The major issue with isotretinoin is teratogenicity. The drug produces a tremendous rate of miscarriage and deformed babies, and pregnancy must be rigorously prevented while patients are undergoing treatment. Fortunately, isotretinoin is rapidly eliminated, and patients may conceive safely one full menstrual period after stopping the drug. Perhaps surprisingly, the patient most likely to become pregnant while taking isotretinoin is in her 20s or 30s. All female patients taking the drug must be either surgically sterile or use two means of contraception; one hormonal and one barrier method. A negative pregnancy test must be obtained monthly.

Rosacea

Although usually considered along with acne, rosacea is a distinct disease. Comedo formation, the hallmark of acne, is absent. Rather, the predisposing factor seems to be vascular hyperreactivity. Patients who blush, especially the fair skinned, often develop some degree of rosacea, although the condition is not limited to the very pale and can be seen in all races if closely observed.

The mildest form of disease is the permanent malar blush. Telangiectasia may follow as may inflammatory papules and nodules. Some patients develop sebaceous overgrowth, particularly on the nose. Termed *rhinophyma*, this process is disfiguring and stigmatizing because people believe it is a sign of alcoholism.

Approximately 50% of rosacea patients also have ocular involvement. Styes, blepharitis, and corneal surface disease may result. The severity of ocular rosacea bears no relation to the severity of facial disease, and all patients should be questioned about symptoms and have their conjunctivae examined.

The pathogenesis of rosacea is a matter of great debate, and few hard facts are available. Vasodilation clearly plays a role, but what it does to promote the process is unclear. The resulting edema fluid is suggested as the cause of

CURRENT THERAPY

- Topical retinoids are the cornerstone of acne therapy.
- Mild disease is well treated with topical therapy (e.g., retinoid plus benzoyl peroxide or clindamycin).
- More severe inflammatory acne usually requires oral doxycycline or minocycline.
- Resistant nodular acne may be treated with isotretinoin.
- Ocular rosacea is best treated with doxycycline.

inflammation. Any food or medication that induces blushing worsens rosacea, but probably no one's rosacea has ever been treated effectively by diet alone. *P. acnes* probably plays a role in some patients' inflammatory disease, but drugs that reduce the organism without anti-inflammatory activity are not very effective. *Demodex* mites and gastrointestinal *Helicobacter* were suggested for years as having a role in rosacea, but no convincing studies exist.

No medication adequately treats the vascular phase of rosacea. The temptation to use topical corticosteroids must be avoided; it always makes the condition worse in the long run.

Inflammatory rosacea may be treated topically with azelaic acid or metronidazole creams. Benzoyl peroxide is sometimes helpful. Because vasodilation worsens disease, creams should be used that are not irritating to the patient. Oral therapy with tetracyclines, especially doxycycline and minocycline, is best for refractory, severe, or ocular rosacea. In extreme cases, isotretinoin is an appropriate last resort.

REFERENCES

Webster GF: Acne vulgaris. BMJ 2002;325:475-479.
Leyden JJ: A review of the use of combination therapy for the treatment of acne vulgaris. J Am Acad Dermatol 2003;49:S200-S210.

Diseases of the Hair

Method of
Kimberly May Eickhorst, MD,
and Eyal Levit, MD

The chief complaint of hair loss or disease is ubiquitous throughout all medical practices. Therefore it is important to have a general understanding of the normal physiologic hair growth cycle and how alterations in this cycle manifest as different hair diseases. Diagnosis and treatment of hair disease can at times be frustrating for both the physician and the patient because of a lack of unequivocal diagnostics and effective treatments. However, a thorough and appropriately directed history armed with a few key diagnostic techniques can help direct care to maximize treatment and patient satisfaction.

CURRENT DIAGNOSIS

- Determine severity of acne: comedonal, papular, nodular.
- Evaluate possibility of endocrinopathy.
- Evaluate rosacea patients for ocular involvement.

A hair cycles through three stages: anagen, catagen, and telogen. The duration of each cycle varies from one body area to the other. Within each body area, each follicle cycles at a different periodicity but maintains the same growth control characteristics. However, in this chapter we concentrate on the scalp. During the first stage (anagen), the bulb or hair root is located in the subcutaneous or dermal portion of the skin and actively grows for a period of approximately 2 to 5 years. As the cycle continues and the hair matures, the hair bulb begins to progress toward the scalp surface. After transiently passing through the catagen or resting phase (2 to 4 weeks), the hair enters telogen (3 to 4 months). It is in this final stage that the hair is ultimately dislodged from the follicle and shed. At any given moment, the telogen-to-anagen ratio is 85% to 15% in females and 90% to 10% in males. Hair grows at a rate of approximately 1 cm per month. An average scalp contains approximately 100,000 hairs, with no known racial or sexual differences; this translates into a completely normal hair loss of approximately 100 to 150 hairs per day, in any given individual. Alterations in this physiologic cycle often result in different types of hair loss; inherent metabolic insults or abnormalities can result in other hair disorders.

History is critical to guiding the physician toward a correct diagnosis. Table 1 lists several questions to pose to your patient when formulating a differential diagnosis. Box 1 lists some specific diagnostic techniques.

Additionally, examine all hair-bearing areas, making note of hair quality (fine, terminal, or vellus; brittle, dry,

---

TABLE 1 Key Questions to the Patient

Timing
When did you first notice changes in your hair?

Quality
Is the hair thinning or shedding?
Is the hair falling out from the root or breaking off?
Associated itching, pain, or burning of scalp?

Quantity
How much hair is lost daily? *(100–150 daily is normal)*
When did you last wash your hair? *(affects hair-pull test)*

Associated Factors
Have you *ever* used permanents, relaxers, hair dyes, hair picks, curlers, braiding, hot comb or curlers, hairpins, rubber bands, or worn tight hairstyles (repeat chronic use can lead to CCCA)?
Family members with similar patterns of hair loss?
Changes in medications (prescribed/OTC/herbals)?
Any recent changes in your health:
• Autoimmune disorders?
• High fever, severe illness, or surgery?
• High stress (emotional/physical)?
• Psychiatric history (depression/anxiety)?
• Pregnant (abortion, miscarriage, delivery) in the last 6 mo?
• Endocrine disorders (hirsutism, acne, irregular periods, change in voice)?
• Nutrition and significant weight loss/gain?
• Chemotherapy/radiation?
What treatments have been tried for your hair loss?

Abbreviations: CCCA = central centrifugal cicatricial alopecia; OTC = over the counter.

BOX 1 Hair: Specific Diagnostic Techniques

• **Hair-pull test:** Gather approximately 40 hairs between the fingers, and then while holding the hairs up away from the scalp under tension, slowly pull along the hair shafts until the distal ends are reached. This technique should be repeated approximately seven times in different areas of the scalp. If more than 4–6 hairs are shed during any one of the eight pulls, the test is considered positive and indicative of an effluvium.
• **Hair parting:** Make a coronal part at the vertex. Measure the width of the part. Proceed to part other areas of the scalp and compare widths among different scalp locations. A widened coronal part with retention of the frontal hairline is seen in female androgenetic alopecia.
• **Laboratory data** and **scalp biopsy** (Table 3):
  • **Light microscope examination of hair bulb:** aids in determining stage of hair cycle during which alopecia is occurring (Figures 1A and B).

---

frayed, or sharp distal ends), density, distribution, and associated skin changes (erythema/inflammation/scale/scar/follicular plugging). Remember, with the exception of the palms, soles, glans, and prepuce, hair grows on all skin surfaces. A magnifying glass and side lighting can be of great assistance. Additionally, the nails, oral mucosa, and thyroid should be closely evaluated. Certain types of hair loss are associated with distinct nail findings (i.e., alopecia areata), lichen planus and lupus can have oral lesions, and thyromegaly can indicate a thyroid disorder.

If hair loss is the complaint, a hair-pull test can be extremely instrumental. This maneuver serves to estimate the number of hairs in telogen. The test is performed by gathering approximately 40 hairs between the fingers, and then while holding the hairs up away from the scalp under tension, slowly pulling along the hair shafts until the distal ends are reached. This technique should be repeated approximately seven times in different areas of the scalp and should be mildly uncomfortable to the patient if done correctly. More than six to eight hairs dislodged on any one pull indicates an increased percentage of hairs in the telogen phase and a positive test. The classic telogen hair has a clublike root. A *caveat*: The hair-pull test is highly subjective and strongly influenced by its relation to the last shampoo/combing.

If a patient has vigorously brushed or shampooed the hair prior to the visit, a large amount of telogen hairs may have already been dislodged, thus confounding the hair-pull test with increased false-negative results. If factors exist that prohibit a valid hair-pull test, the patient can also be instructed to collect *all* hairs lost over a 1-day period and store them in a small sealable plastic bag. Over the course of 7 full days, each day's worth of lost hair should be counted by the patient, stored in an individual bag labeled with the date and hair number, and brought to the physician's office. This collection should include hair lost on the pillow, in the shower, and on combs/brushes.

The hairs harvested from the hair-pull test can also be examined under the light microscope. The proximal ends of the hairs can be placed under a coverslip with potassium hydroxide (KOH) as background media or simply sandwiched between two glass slides and viewed under low power. The hairs can then be evaluated simultaneously for stage of cycling (anagen/telogen) and the presence of fungus. An anagen has retention of pigment at its proximal "root" as well as some remnants of root sheath, creating an irregularly shaped and glistening bulb. In contrast, a telogen hair has a more swollen, white, rounded, and cornified bulb likened to a cotton applicator tip (Figure 1). Fungus presents as hyphae or spores within or lining the hair shaft and may clinically be associated with cervical lymphadenopathy or "black dot alopecia," in which stubbles of darker hair are seen at the follicular orifices.

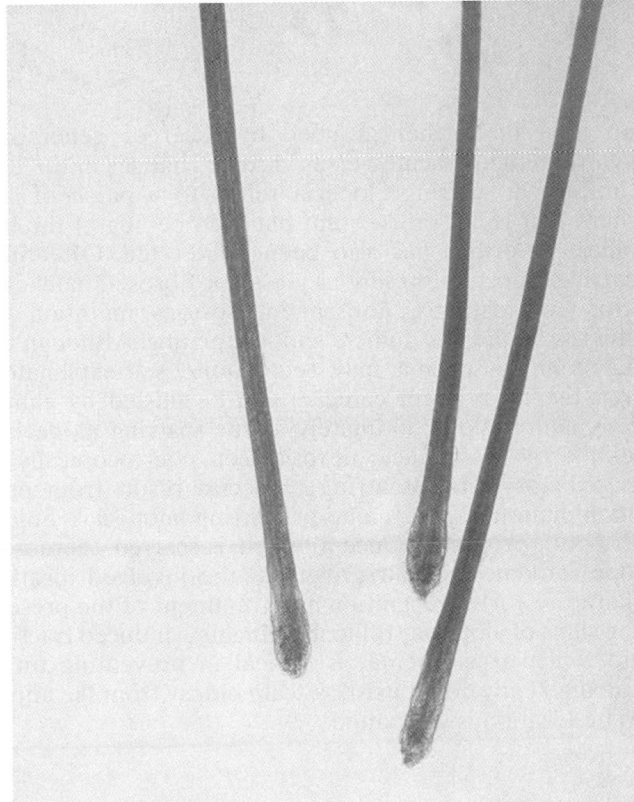

A

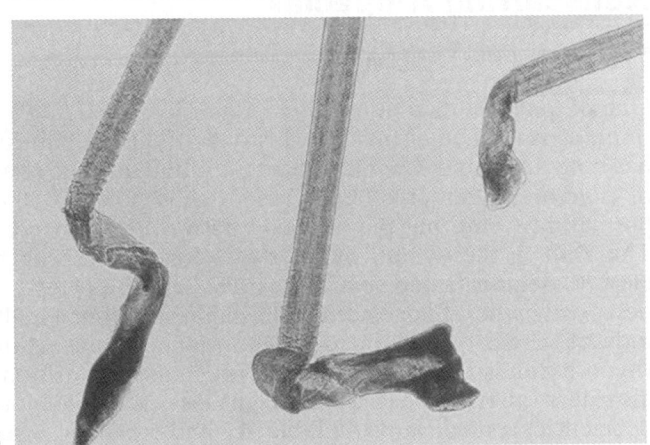

B

FIGURE 1. What to expect when examining a hair-pull test hair under the light microscope: telogen hair (**A**); anagen hair (**B**). (From Bolognia JL, Jorizzo JL, Papini RP: Dermatology, vol 1, 1st ed. Alopecias. New York, Mosby, 2003, p. 1035.)

The scalp should also be parted in several different locations to compare the width of the parts. Parting not only helps define and compare hair density throughout the scalp but can also be a diagnostic tool. A midline widened coronal vertex part that resembles a "Christmas tree" pattern and displays central thinning while maintaining the frontal hairline is characteristic of female androgenetic alopecia.

Scalp biopsy is usually reserved as a later step in the hair disease workup when alopecia is refractory, when suspicion is high for a scarring component, or when the patient simply desires a definitive reason, specifically proof, for his or her hair disease. Scalp biopsy entails infiltrating an area of the scalp with local anesthesia and then using a 4- to 6-mm punch biopsy to obtain a full-thickness skin specimen down to the fat, where many of the hair bulbs reside. A 6-mm biopsy or two 4-mm punches are recommended over a single smaller diameter punch biopsy. It is also suggested that two biopsies from different involved scalp sites be harvested. The specimen is then sent for both vertical and horizontal sectioning. If scarring is suspected, direct immunofluorescence testing should also be considered (Table 2). Overall, a scalp biopsy is extremely useful in definitively identifying scarring versus nonscarring alopecia and the presence and type of inflammation.

Certain laboratory data (see Table 2) can also help unravel the mystery of troubling hair disease. Equipped with a thorough history and exam, one can begin to narrow the differential diagnosis of hair disease and to test and treat the suspected malady. Following is a brief discussion of some of the more commonly encountered hair disorders, as well as suggested diagnostics and treatment.

Alopecia

Hair loss, or alopecia, is commonly divided into scarring and nonscarring alopecia (Table 3). Variants of hair loss

 CURRENT DIAGNOSIS

- Detailed history (Table 1)
- All hair-bearing sites should be examined using specific techniques:
    - Hair quality (dry, brittle, fine, short/long, sharp or frayed distal ends)
    - Scarring versus nonscarring; diffuse versus focal involvement description
    - Hair-pull test
    - Part width measurements and comparisons
- Appropriate laboratory data collected (Table 2)
- Two 4-mm or a single 6-mm punch biopsy of the scalp helps distinguish scarring from nonscarring alopecias:
    - The specimen should be harvested from the involved edge of the scalp where some hair is still present. The specimen should then be sent for *horizontal* and *transverse* sectioning by an experienced dermatopathologist.
    - If connective tissue disease is suspected, another 3-mm biopsy should be sent for direct immunofluorescence (DIF).

CURRENT THERAPY

- Start aggressive treatment early. True scarring alopecias are permanent. However, if diagnosed and treated early, scarring can be prevented.
- Regarding topical Minoxidil 5% (Rogaine):
  - Once started, it must be continued indefinitely; if stopped, all the hair gained will shed, usually within the next 4–6 mo.
  - Patients should always wash their hands after scalp treatment application to prevent accidental unwanted hair growth on the face.
  - Warn patients that they may first experience a small increase in hair loss at the very beginning of treatment as the growth of new anagen hairs replaces old telogen hairs out of the hair follicle.
- Physicians should be prepared to refer patients to reputable stylists and shops that can provide alternative natural hair styling and accoutrements.

TABLE 2 Suggested Laboratory Testing for Alopecia

Rule out anemia:
- CBC
- Iron
- TIBC
- Ferritin
- MCV, RDW

Rule out autoimmune disorders:
- ANA, SSA, SSB
- Scalp biopsy for direct immunofluorescence

Rule out syphilis:
- RPR, FTA-Abs

Rule out thyroid disorder:
- TSH
- Anti-thyroglobulin Abs
- Thyroid peroxidase Abs

Rule out hormonal aberrations:
- DHEA, DHEAS (adrenal)
- LH, FSH (polycystic ovary disease)
- Free and total testosterone (ovarian/testicular)
- Antihormone binding globulin
- Morning cortisol levels
- Scalp biopsies (Bx): usually taken from involved edge; should be sent for transverse and horizontal sectioning to an experienced dermatopathologist who is familiar with transverse section reading; now considered the standard of care for proper diagnosis of alopecias
- Scalp Bx for DIF should be sent if lupus is suspected.

Abbreviations: ANA = antinuclear antibody (test); CBC = complete blood count; DHEA = dehydroepiandrosterone; DHEAS = dehydroepiandrosterone sulfate; FSH = follicle-stimulating hormone; FTA-Abs = fluorescence treponemal antibody absorption; LH = luteinizing hormone; MCV = mean corpuscular volume; RDW = red (blood cell) diameter width; RPR = rapid plasma reagent (test); TIBC = total iron-binding capacity; SSA = anti-Ro/single stranded DNA strand A; SSB = anti-La/single stranded DNA strand B; TSH = thyroid-stimulating hormone.

TABLE 3 Scarring versus Nonscarring Classification of Alopecia*

Scarring	Nonscarring
Lichen planopilaris	Androgenetic alopecia
Discoid lupus erythematosus	Telogen effluvium
Central centrifugal cicatricial alopecia (CCCA)	Alopecia areata
Trichotillomania/traction (chronic)	Trichotillomania/traction (acute)
Folliculitis decalvans	Anagen effluvium
	Syphilitic alopecia

*Arranged from most to least common.

can then be further grouped by focal or generalized involvement and acute versus chronic changes in the hair. Clinically, a scarring alopecia refers to a patch of skin where hair is not only absent but the opening of the hair follicle or orifice has also been obliterated. Oftentimes scarring alopecias present as glossy or fibrosed patches of skin. Contrastingly, nonscarring lesions maintain the integrity of the hair follicle and its opening. Although this dichotomous schema may seem quite self-explanatory, even the most adept clinician can be misled by clinical examination alone; ultimately a true scarring alopecia is defined by hair follicle fibrosis seen microscopically on scalp biopsy. Most scarring alopecias result from prior inflammation. Unfortunately, scarring alopecias hold a very poor prognosis. Once a follicle is scarred, there is no hope for renewed hair growth at the involved location. Therefore early recognition and treatment of the prescarring signs of alopecia (follicular plugging, induced traction, and follicular erythema) is critical in preventing future scarring. If any doubt exists, a scalp biopsy from the appropriate location is warranted.

Nonscarring Alopecias

TELOGEN EFFLUVIUM

One of the most common causes of hair loss/shedding and thinning is telogen effluvium. This type of diffuse hair loss has both acute and chronic variants, but both are the result of a greater number of hairs (more than 10% to 20%) prematurely entering the telogen phase of the hair cycle. This shift in the overall number of telogen hairs can be clearly demonstrated by a positive hair-pull test, as described earlier. Telogen effluvium can result from a multitude of medical states including hormonal abnormalities (hypothyroidism, hyperthyroidism, pregnancy), nutritional disorders (anorexia, excessive weight loss, iron/zinc/biotin deficiencies), medications (Table 4) and systemic stress (high fever, surgery, systemic lupus erythematosus, dermatomyositis). In approximately 33% of cases of acute telogen effluvium, no trigger can be identified. Anxiety, depression, and other types of emotional stress are commonly blamed for causing telogen effluvium. However, little scientific

TABLE 4 Drugs Associated with Telogen Effluvium*

Angiotensin-converting enzyme (ACE) inhibitors
Anticoagulants
β-Blockers
Interferon
Lithium
Oral contraceptives
Oral retinoids (isotretinoin, acitretin)
Valproic acid
Vitamin A excess

*Greater than 1% incidence.

evidence exists to support the belief that everyday life stress is sufficient to induce diffuse hair loss.

Telogen effluvium is usually self-limited but can become chronic if the triggering factors are not removed. Clinically, at least 15% to 25% of scalp hairs must be lost before telogen effluvium can be objectively observed. It is important to reassure patients that although they may suffer temporarily from decreased hair density, they will *not* go completely bald, despite what might appear to be continued hair loss. The diagnosis of telogen effluvium is usually clinched with a positive hair-pull test and a history describing some recent (within the past 6 weeks to 4 months) physiologic/emotional stress, followed by diffuse scalp hair loss/shedding. In addition to removing any persistent causative factors, topical 2% or 5% minoxidil (Rogaine) applied twice daily to the scalp can encourage new hair growth until the distribution of hairs throughout the hair cycle returns to baseline.

ANAGEN EFFLUVIUM

Anagen effluvium results from acute and direct insult to the nearly 90% of hairs in the initial hair growth phase. Chemotherapy, followed by radiation and poisoning (e.g., arsenic), are the more common culprits. During this toxic event, the follicle and stem cells are neither harmed nor converted to a different stage in the hair cycle. However, mitosis is inhibited. The result is a hair that is proximally weakened and narrowed. As a consequence of this proximal hair shaft weakness, the affected hairs usually break off as they approach the scalp. Anagen hair shedding may begin approximately 1 to 2 weeks following the inciting event. But hair loss may be most evident after approximately 1 to 2 months and can be clinically profound. Patients should be assured that this condition is completely reversible and once the insult to the metabolic function of the hair follicle is removed, normal hair production and growth should resume. If chemotherapy is anticipated, a prophylactic approach to anagen effluvium involves applying a pressure cuff around the scalp during chemotherapy.

ALOPECIA AREATA

An autoimmune, cell-mediated disorder, alopecia areata may be found in association with vitiligo, thyroid disorders, lupus, atopic dermatitis, or Down's syndrome. There may also be a strong familial predominance. However, it most commonly presents without any other disease associations. Clinically, asymptomatic or mildly pruritic ovoid patches of hair loss are seen. These patches can be small and focal (Figure 2A) or extend over large areas of skin (Figure 2B). At times there can be such diffuse focal involvement that the scalp begins to look almost "moth eaten." In this instance a rapid plasma reagent (RPR) test may be warranted to rule out syphilitic alopecia, which can take on a similar appearance.

When complete loss of scalp hair is seen as a result of alopecia areata, the condition is called *alopecia totalis*. When hair is absent on *all* hair-bearing areas of the body, the term *alopecia universalis* is used. *Ophiasis* describes alopecia areata in a bandlike distribution over the periphery of the temporal and occipital scalp, whereas the term *sisaipho* describes the inverse, with balding of the superior scalp. At the periphery of many of these balding patches, hair may seem loose. Forcefully dislodging these hairs can

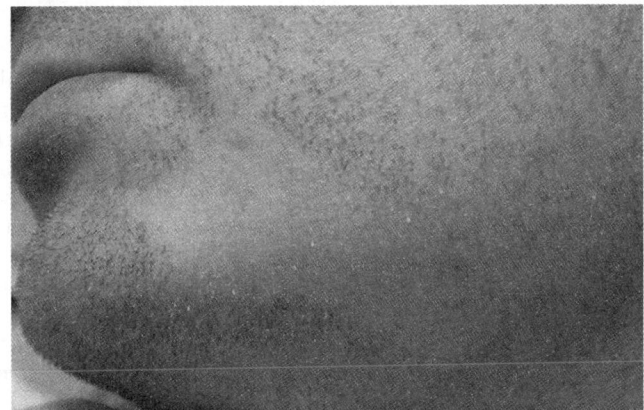
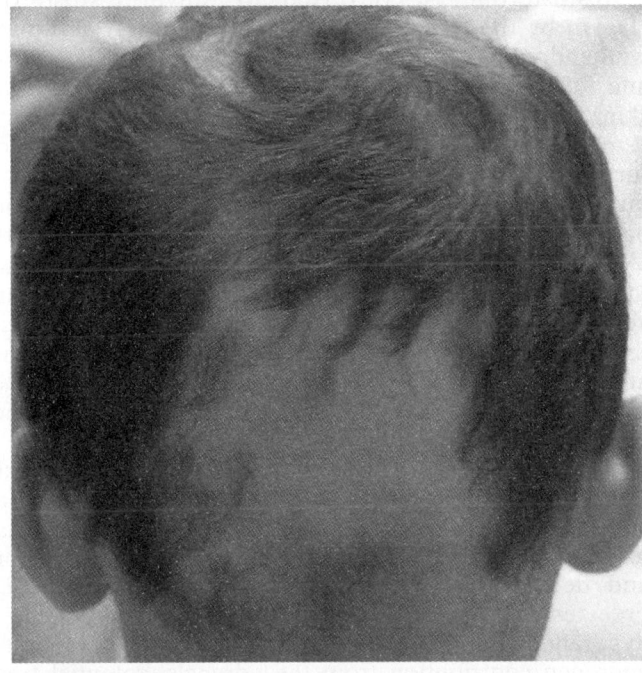

FIGURE 2. A, Small patches of hair loss on the chin and neck. White hairs are seen in some areas and represent signs of early hair regrowth. **B,** Large patch of alopecia areata on the occipital scalp with patches of regrowth at the edges.

reveal a more tapered proximal end of the hair shaft. Thus, these hairs are called *exclamation hairs*. Gridlike nail pitting is another hint to the presence of alopecia areata.

Although alopecia areata may spontaneously remit, treatment is encouraged and decreases disease duration. Intralesional triamcinolone (Kenalog) is used for localized disease, but more diffuse scalp involvement usually lends itself to topical application of high potency class I topical steroids and calcineurin inhibitors like topical pimecrolimus (Elidel) or tacrolimus (Protopic). Steroid treatment demands close follow-up to avoid hypothalamic-pituitary axis (HPA) suppression or skin atrophy signs such as hypopigmentation, thinning, and telangiectasias. If these treatments fail, the use of anthralin or squaric acid dibutyl ester can be cautiously attempted with gradual increase in contact exposure time. Refractory cases may even require PUVA (oral psoralen plus UVA light treatment) or a short course of oral steroids for response. Atopic dermatitis, childhood onset, widespread involvement, ophiasis, duration longer than 5 years, and onychodystrophy tend to predict a poor prognosis.

ANDROGENETIC ALOPECIA

Androgenetic alopecia can occur in both males and females and is by and large linked to the presence of excess androgens that subsequently cause follicular miniaturization and loss of hair. The reduction in the size of the follicle is accompanied by shortening of the anagen phase and increased telogen shedding. In males there is clinical regression of the frontal-temporal hairline, whereas in women there is retention of the frontal hairline but widening of the coronal part and decreased hair density over the vertex. In both sexes, a similar family history of patterned hair loss is often present. Interestingly, a higher risk of coronary heart disease is associated with male-patterned baldness.

Testosterone is converted to dihydrotestosterone (DHT) by the enzyme 5-α reductase (type II). In males with androgenetic alopecia, 5-α reductase (type II) activity and DHT are increased as opposed to nonbalding scalp skin. Therefore, finasteride (Propecia), a 5-α reductase (type II) inhibitor, at 1 mg orally daily, can halt or slow further hair loss in men. Pregnant women should not so much as touch this drug because pregnant women handling of finasteride (Propecia) risks feminization of the fetus. Female-patterned baldness is most commonly seen in the perimenopausal stages of life, although younger and younger patients of both sexes seem to be presenting with this complaint. Although this process may begin at any age after puberty, it usually becomes clinically apparent in men by 17 years of age and in androgenetically normal women by 25 to 30 years of age.

When younger patients, especially in the face of coexistent hirsutism, present with this classic patterned hair loss, and/or females present with a male-patterned hair loss, laboratories should be drawn to assess testosterone and dehydroepiandrosterone sulfate (DHEAS) levels. Free testosterone represents the ovarian component of hyperandrogenism, whereas DHEAS levels represent androgen contribution from the adrenals. Potential treatments for female-patterned hair loss include oral contraception with relatively higher estrogen levels or antiandrogens like spironolactone (Aldactone) at 50 to 200 mg orally daily. Although many of my female patients have had success

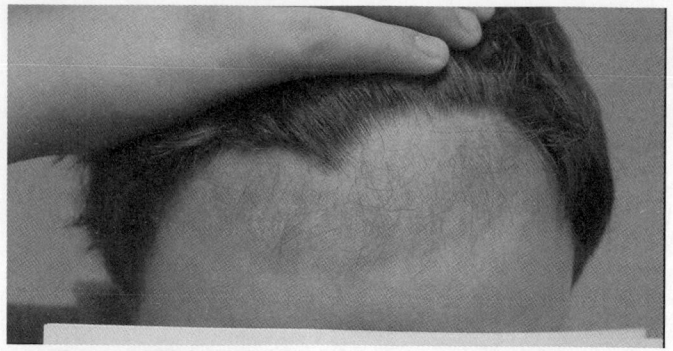

FIGURE 3. Traction alopecia. Hairs of varying lengths with a well-defined border.

using Finasteride (Propecia), 1 mg orally every day, a single small study by Merck failed to show statistical benefits. Topical Minoxidil 5% (Rogaine) may also be helpful, but like finasteride, it must be continued indefinitely to maintain its effect.

TRICHOTILLOMANIA

Trichotillomania refers to the act of forcibly pulling/plucking out one's hair, resulting in patchy or full alopecia of the scalp. The scalp is the most frequent hair-pulling site, followed by the eyebrows, eyelashes, pubic area, trunk, and extremities. This type of chronic alopecia forms with more linear, well-defined borders, which include hairs of varied lengths (Figure 3). The occiput generally tends to be spared. Although patients with obsessive-compulsive disorders and neurotic personality traits are suspect for this variant of alopecia, a scalp biopsy can confirm the diagnosis with evidence of abundant catagen hairs, retained follicular pigment, and hemorrhage. Observed or reported hair-pulling behavior from family and friends may help avoid a biopsy. Such pulling can also be caused from tightly styled hair as with ponytails or braiding. Additionally, if trichotillomania is high on the differential, as a last resort, shaving a 3 × 3 cm area of the scalp may help clinch the diagnosis. Subsequent normal hair growth would support the diagnosis; these new hairs will be too short for the patient to pull out.

Treatment is difficult, and just breaking the hair-pulling habit is key. Sometimes instructing the patient to apply any salve (e.g., olive oil) to the scalp area each night under a shower cap and wearing it to bed may break the habit. Even if treatment fails, patients are often relieved to find that others pull out hair. Organizations offering educational materials and support contacts can help. Although clomipramine is the only drug that was effective in controlled trials, other selective serotonin reuptake inhibitors (SSRIs) have anecdotally led to improvement. Additionally, behavior therapy, hypnosis, insight-oriented psychotherapy, habit modification, and close, lengthy follow-up should also be treatment considerations.

Scarring (Cicatricial) Alopecia

Scarring alopecia represents fibrosis of the hair follicle, most commonly secondary to previous inflammation.

Discoid lupus erythematosus, lichen planopilaris, and central, centrifugal scarring alopecia are the most common forms of scarring hair loss. The most helpful methods to differentiate these subtypes are scalp biopsy, early in the process, and bacterial and/or fungal culture if active signs of superficial inflammation such as pustules or crusts are present. Early diagnosis is key. If the insulting inflammatory process can be halted before complete follicle fibrosis, there is still hope for improvement. However, if complete fibrosis occurs, the result is a burnt-out, noninflammatory, end-stage scarring alopecia termed pseudopelade of Brocq that has no recourse.

Discoid Lupus Erythematosus

Discoid lupus erythematosus (DLE), a cutaneous form of lupus, manifests as sharply demarcated atrophic plaques with adherent scale and follicular plugging. Plaques are often circumscribed by a fine outline of hyperpigmentation (Figure 4). Key areas of involvement, in addition to the scalp, include the ear, perioral, and perinasal regions. Despite the often classic clinical appearance, a scalp biopsy for direct immunofluorescence (DIF) and H&E (hematoxylin & eosin) should be sent (Current Diagnosis box). Although DLE can progress to systemic lupus in approximately 5% of individuals, it is predominantly stable and can be most effectively treated with sun protection and topical and intralesional steroids. Refractory cases may also respond well to antimalarials, systemic retinoids, and dapsone.

LICHEN PLANOPILARIS

Four more times common in women, this entity is a follicular-based variant of lichen planus. The scalp, as well as other hair-bearing areas, can be involved (Graham Little syndrome). The hair-pull test is positive for anagen hairs. Clinically this condition begins as perifollicular erythema that then leads to hyperkeratotic and spiny follicles and eventual permanent scarring. If early in the disease process, successful treatment can include potent topical and intralesional steroids as well as antimalarials.

CENTRAL CENTRIFUGAL CICATRICIAL ALOPECIA

Largely an umbrella term for "hot comb alopecia," the "follicular degeneration syndrome," and central centrifugal scarring alopecia. Central centrifugal cicatricial alopecia (CCCA) is defined as premature desquamation of the inner root sheath eventually leading to loss of the follicular epithelium and replacement with fibrosis. Patients may be asymptomatic or complain of sensations of pruritus, pain, or pins and needles. Most commonly found in a subset of African American women, this insidious, noninflammatory primary scarring alopecia starts in the central midline scalp and spreads centrifugally over the vertex. At times polytrichia, multiple hairs exiting one hair follicle ostia, can be observed. There is little scalp bogginess or tautness, but this type of alopecia has long been associated with the hair care regimens of certain ethnic backgrounds. However, this anecdotal association remains to be scientifically validated. If treated in the early stages, the condition can be improved with both high potency topical steroids and tetracycline (500 mg orally twice a day) and cessation of any traumatic or chemical hair care practices.

FOLLICULITIS DECALVANS

Folliculitis decalvans, a recurrent, inflammatory process, is defined by well-circumscribed patches, along which follicular papules and pustules line the advancing margins (Figures 5A and B). If progressive, these often boggy

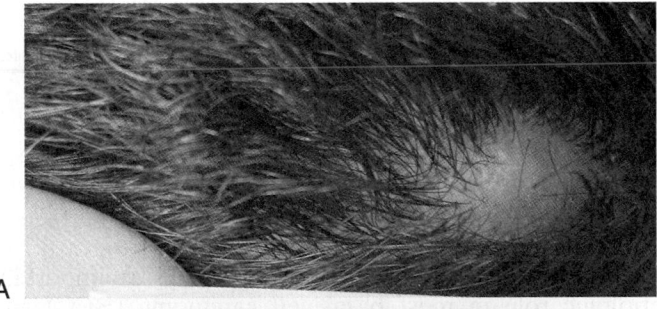

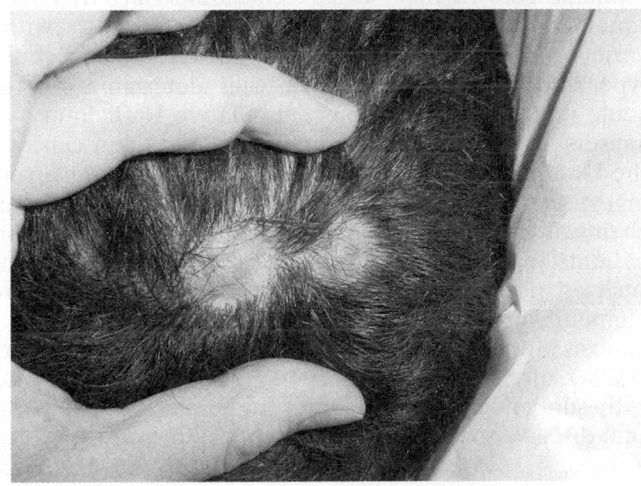

FIGURE 5. A, Folliculitis decalvans. Well-defined carbuncle on the scalp with overlying hair loss. **B,** Folliculitis decalvans. Well-circumscribed patches of boggy scarred scalp with few areas showing "tufted" folliculitis.

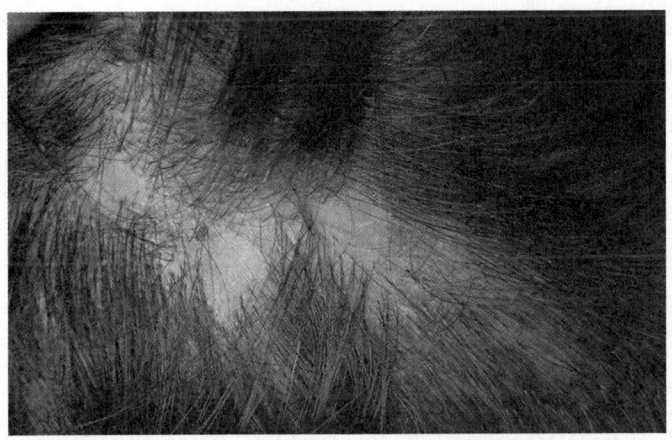

FIGURE 4. Discoid lupus erythematosus (DLE). Scalp showing whitish old burned-out areas and newly inflamed erythematic patches with perifollicular scale, crust, and erosions.

scalp areas eventually become scarred. Variants include so-called tufted folliculitis in which multiple hairs emerge from erythematous and crusted follicles resembling doll-like hair. During active disease, there is an abundance of gram-positive organisms. Hypotheses exist affirming *Staphylococcus aureus* to be the causative agent. However, the true etiology is unknown. Fungal and bacterial cultures are warranted as well as screening for potential immune deficiency. Long-term oral and topical antibiotics and/or retinoids are the mainstay of therapy.

REFERENCES

Freedberg IM, et al: Fitzpatrick's Dermatology in General Medicine, vol 1, 6th ed. Disorders of epidermal appendages and related disorders. New York, McGraw-Hill, 2003, pp 633-655.

Odom RB, et al: Andrews' Diseases of the Skin: Clinical Dermatology, 9th ed. Philadelphia, WB Saunders, 2000, pp 943-952.

Ross EK, Tan E, Shapiro J: Update on primary cicatricial alopecias. J Am Acad Dermatol 2005;53(1):1-37.

Sinclair R, Jolley D, Mallari R, Magee J: The reliability of horizontally sectioned scalp biopsies in the diagnosis of chronic diffuse telogen hair loss in women. J Am Acad Dermatol 2004;51(2):189-199.

Berger RS, Fu JL, Smiles KA, et al: The effects of minoxidil, 1% pyrithione zinc and a combination of both on hair density: A randomized controlled trial. Br J Dermatol 2003;149(2):354-362.

Hautmann G, Hercogova J, Lotti T: Trichotillomania. J Am Acad Dermatol 2002;46(6): 807-821.

Harrison S. Sinclair R: Telogen effluvium. Clin Exp Dermatol 2002;27(5):389-385.

Sperling LC, Solomon AR, Whiting DA: A new look at scarring alopecia. Arch Dermatol 2000;136:235-242.

Dawber R, Van Neste D, Dunitz M: Hair and Scalp Disorders. Common Presenting Signs, Differential Diagnosis and Treatment, 2nd ed. Philadelphia, Lippincott, 1995.

Cancer of the Skin

Method of
Richard F. Wagner, Jr., MD

Ultraviolet light (UVL) skin damage plays an important etiologic role in most basal cell carcinoma (BCC) and squamous cell carcinoma (SCC). UVL interacts with a variety of factors, including host genotype, Fitzpatrick skin type, and immunocompetence, that determine whether acute (sunburn) and chronic cumulative UVL injury will cause skin cancer. Less frequent causes of skin cancer in the United States are ionizing radiation exposure, arsenic ingestion, traumatic skin injury, tobacco (SCC of lip), and chemical carcinogen. Many genetic disorders predispose patients to skin cancer through a variety of mechanisms, such as albinism, basal cell nevus syndrome, xeroderma pigmentosum, and epidermolysis bullosa. Genital SCC is almost always associated with human papilloma virus (HPV), often identified as HPV-16 or -18. HPV interacts with sunlight to result in life-threatening SCC in a rare skin disease, epidermodysplasia verruciformis.

Clinical Features

Nodular BCC is the most common subtype of BCC (80%), and it classically manifests as a shiny papule with visible telangiectasia. Nodular BCC may be pigmented and can be confused with nodular melanoma. Superficial BCC (15%) usually appears as an erythematous thin plaque on the trunk, with a subtle threadlike raised border. The most difficult type of primary BCC to recognize clinically is the morpheaform or sclerotic type, appearing much like a scar. Neglected BCC, although usually painless, may ulcerate ("rodent ulcer") and bleed, have a foul odor, and reach enormous size.

SCC may be difficult to distinguish clinically from BCC. The presence of keratotic scale and the absence of classic BCC morphology are the best clinical indicators for SCC. Organ transplant patients on immunosuppressive therapy are more likely to have SCC than BCC. SCC remains the most common malignancy of the mucosal lip. Bowen's disease, or SCC in situ (SCCIS), may resemble superficial BCC. When SCCIS arises on the uncircumcised mucosal penis (erythroplasia of Queyrat), it is typically moist and bright red with sharp clinical margins. SCCIS may develop into invasive SCC, and invasive SCC may also arise from actinic keratoses. Invasive SCC classically manifests as a red papule or nodule with scale. The keratoacanthoma is regarded by many dermatopathologists as a subtype of well-differentiated invasive SCC, often having a history of sudden rapid growth and a central keratotic crater. Large (2-cm diameter or greater) invasive SCCs are more likely to have perineural invasion, especially if the tumor is recurrent.

Regional lymph nodes should be examined for patients with BCC and SCCs, and a bimanual examination of the mouth is recommended for patients with SCC of the mucosal lip. Pathologic lymph nodes should be referred to a specialist for fine-needle aspiration (FNA) and imaging studies to exclude metastatic skin cancer to lymph nodes, the most frequent site of metastasis.

Treatment Cryosurgery

Cryosurgery with liquid nitrogen, an effective treatment for BCC and SCC, relies on the destructive effect of the freeze-thaw cycle on living cells. It should be performed under the guidance of a thermocouple to ensure an adequate depth of freeze. Cold sensitivity disorders such as cryoglobulinemia are contraindications.

Electrodesiccation and Curettage

Electrodesiccation and curettage (EDC) remains the most frequently used treatment modality for BCC and SCC in the United States. It is highly effective in selected tumors, and although variability is reported among physicians using the technique, 95% cure rates are cited for small primary BCC and SCC. It is often the fastest and least expensive treatment, and it is very effective for small BCC and SCC (5 mm or less) that arise on areas of skin that are not high tumor recurrence zones, such as on the arms, legs, and trunk. It can also be effective for superficial BCC and SCCIS, as long as the tumor does not extend down the hair follicle. EDC treatment sites heal by second intention and are usually flat and hypopigmented. In one private dermatology practice setting, there was no statistical difference in recurrence rates for primary BCC and SCC treated with either EDC or excision, although previous studies from academic centers favored excision.

Other Destructive Options

Surgical lasers such as the carbon dioxide and the erbium:yttrium-aluminum-garnet (Er:YAG) are also used to ablate small or superficial BCC and SCCIS.

Standard Surgical Excision

For primary BCC less than 2 cm in diameter, excision with a 4-mm margin yields a 95% cure rate. Margins for primary SCC of the same size should be 4 to 6 mm, adjusted for specific tumor characteristics. If excision is initially attempted and the surgical margin is subsequently reported positive, Mohs' micrographic surgery (MMS) or adjuvant radiation therapy should be considered.

Mohs' Micrographic Surgery

Mohs' micrographic surgery fully integrates the roles of dermasurgeon and dermatopathologist, and it achieves the highest statistical cure rates for BCC and SCC with maximal conservation of uninvolved tissue. MMS has a wide range of indications, including BCC and SCC arising in areas of high recurrence (nose, lip, eyelid, ear, etc.) or areas where maximal tissue sparing is needed and for tumors that are recurrent, have specific histologic subtypes, show perineural invasion, have poorly defined clinical margins, or have a diameter greater than 1 cm on the face or 2 cm elsewhere.

Photodynamic Therapy

The basis of photodynamic therapy (PDT) is the activation of selectively absorbed photosensitizers by skin cancer and subsequent destruction of these cells by visible light. Superficial BCC and SCCIS are successfully treated with topically applied photosensitizers, but currently this method is not widely available in the United States.

Radiation Therapy

Fractionated radiation therapy (typical total of 4000 to 6000 cGy) is an effective but costly treatment for primary and recurrent BCC and SCC, with reported 90% cure rates. It is especially useful for treating tumors in patients with co-morbid medical conditions that put them at high risk for surgical complications or when surgical treatment would result in extensive morbidity. Because of the lower statistical cure rate than MMS and the risk for late local cutaneous complications, including the rare risk of another primary tumor in the radiation portal (SCC is most common), primary radiation therapy for BCC and SCC is not widely employed in healthy patients younger than 50 years in the United States. For surgically treated SCC with perineural invasion and unusually aggressive BCC and SCC, adjuvant radiation therapy is offered at many medical centers to decrease the risk of tumor recurrence.

It is relatively contraindicated for patients with basal cell nevus syndrome, xeroderma pigmentosum, and epidermodysplasia verruciformis.

Topical Medicines

Topical 5-fluorouracil (Efudex) is used successfully to treat superficial BCC, but patients frequently cannot complete the recommended treatment course because of brisk local inflammation (pregnancy category X). Imiquimod (Aldara) cream, a biologic response modifier, recently gained FDA approval for nonfacial superficial BCC that are less than 2.0 cm in diameter in immunocompetent adults and are not located in the hands, feet, or anogenital skin, when surgery is less appropriate and patient follow-up is likely (pregnancy category C).

Systemic and Topical Chemoprophylaxis

No FDA-approved prescription medications for skin cancer prevention are currently available.

Patient Follow-up and Aftercare

Scheduled follow-up visits every 6 months in the case of primary BCC and every 3 months for recurrent BCC and primary or recurrent SCC are recommended to check for tumor recurrence. Patients presenting with a BCC skin cancer have approximately a 36% risk for additional primary BCC.

Patients with a history of nonmelanoma skin cancer should be advised to reduce their UVL exposure. It is reasonable to advise these patients to take daily oral supplemental vitamin D every day (200 IU to age 50, 400 IU from age 51 to 70, and 1000 IU at age 71 and older) to compensate for decreased sunlight exposure. People of color and burn patients may also require supplemental dietary vitamin D because of decreased skin synthesis of cholecalciferol to natural sunlight. Immunosuppressed patients may be vitamin D deficient because of sun avoidance and other factors, and they may require specialized protocols and monitoring to normalize and maintain their vitamin D levels.

REFERENCES

Brodland DG, Zitelli JA: Surgical margins for excision of primary cutaneous squamous cell carcinoma. J Am Acad Dermatol 1992; 27(2 Pt 1):241-248.

Robinson JK: Risk of developing another basal cell carcinoma. A 5-year prospective study. Cancer 1987;60(1):118-120.

Shriner D, McCoy DK, Goldberg DJ, Wagner RF Jr: Mohs micrographic surgery. J Am Acad Dermatol 1998;39(1):79-97.

Taub AF: Photodynamic therapy in dermatology: History and horizons. J Drugs Dermatol 2004;3(1 Suppl):S8-S25.

Werlinger KD, Upton G, Moore AY: Recurrence rates of primary nonmelanoma skin cancers treated by surgical excision compared to electrodesiccation-curettage in private dermatological practice. Dermatol Surg 2002;28(12):1138-1142.

Wolf DJ, Zitelli JA: Surgical margins for basal cell carcinoma. J Am Acad Dermatol 1987;123(3):340-344.

Cutaneous T Cell Lymphoma

Method of
Marie-France Demierre, MD

Cutaneous T cell lymphomas (CTCLs) are primary lymphomas of the skin belonging to the category of extranodal non-Hodgkin lymphomas. The most common type of CTCL is mycosis fungoides (MF), a malignancy of thymus-derived helper lymphocytes, usually CD4+ in phenotype, that present as patches, plaques, or tumors. Sézary syndrome (SS) is a more aggressive form of CTCL with peripheral blood involvement. Mycosis fungoides and SS account for 70% to 80% of all CTCLs diagnosed in North America. Primary cutaneous CD30+ lymphoproliferative disorders, lymphomatoid papulosis (self-healing, recurrent papules), and primary cutaneous CD30+ anaplastic large cell lymphoma (CD30+ tumors) represent 15% of CTCLs in North America. Epidemiologic data for MF only is known. Males are affected twice as often as females, and although all races appear to be affected, African Americans have a higher incidence than whites. The average age at onset is approximately 55 years. Young adults less than 20 years of age and even children can be affected.

The appropriate medical management and selection of therapeutic modalities varies with the subtype of CTCL and staging. Diagnosis, staging, and a summary of current therapies used for MF and SS patients are presented.

Diagnosis of Mycosis Fungoides

MF often begins with subtle lesions that may be mistaken for eczema (ill-defined erythematous patches or plaques) or psoriasis (well-defined erythematous plaques). The lesions often present in sun-protected areas, the bathing trunk distribution (breast, abdomen, belt line, buttocks). Patient may have pruritus. Other presentations include hypopigmented patches, poikiloderma atrophicans vasculare with patches of telangiectasia, atrophy, pigmentation resembling radiation dermatitis, and folliculotropic mycosis fungoides with grouped follicular papules or indurated plaques devoid of hair. In large-plaque parapsoriasis, scaly, pink to dusky, sometimes slightly infiltrated patches are suggestive of MF, but full criteria for its diagnosis are lacking. Patches of MF can evolve to plaques that can be thickened, annular, serpiginous, and finally to tumors. Characteristic skin histology of MF shows numerous atypical lymphocytes with convoluted nuclei near and within the epidermis as well as clusters within the epidermis (Pautrier's microabscess).

CURRENT DIAGNOSIS

- Mycosis fungoides is the most common type of cutaneous T cell lymphoma.
- Lesions can present as patches, plaques, or tumors.
- Erythroderma is the hallmark of Sézary syndrome.
- Staging is relevant to manage patients appropriately.

TABLE 1 Frequency and Disease-Specific 5-Year Survival for Primary Cutaneous Lymphomas

WHO-EORTC Classification	Disease-Specific 5-Year Survival (%)
Indolent Clinical Behavior	
Mycosis fungoides (MF)	88
Folliculotropic MF	80
Pagetoid reticulosis	100
Granulomatous slack skin	100
Primary cutaneous anaplastic large cell lymphoma	95
Lymphomatoid papulosis	100
Subcutaneous panniculitis-like T cell lymphoma	82
Primary cutaneous CD4+ small/medium pleomorphic T cell lymphoma[†]	75
Aggressive Clinical Behavior	
Sézary syndrome	24
Primary cutaneous NK/T cell lymphoma, nasal type	NR
Primary cutaneous aggressive CD8+ T cell lymphoma[†]	18
Primary cutaneous γ/δ T cell lymphoma[†]	NR
Primary cutaneous peripheral T cell lymphoma, unspecified[‡]	16

Data are based on 1905 patients with a primary cutaneous lymphoma registered at the Dutch and Austrian Cutaneous Lymphoma Group between 1986 and 2002.
[‡]Primary cutaneous peripheral T cell lymphoma, unspecified excluding the three provisional entities indicated with a single dagger (†).
Abbreviations: MF = mycosis fungoides; NR = not reached; WHO-EORTC = World Health Organization-European Organization of Research and Cancer Treatment.
Data obtained from Willemze, R, Jaffe ES, Burg G, et al: WHO-EORTC classification for cutaneous lymphomas. Blood 2005;105(10):3768-3785.

In SS, itching is severe, and erythroderma is the hallmark. SS is accompanied by ectropion, hair loss, keratoderma, fissures, cutaneous pain, enlarged lymph nodes, and large numbers of circulating atypical lymphocytes in the peripheral blood. Molecular techniques and immunophenotyping are helpful to confirm diagnosis. In the context of clinically suspicious lesions, demonstration of dominant clonality in the skin, lymph nodes, and blood, particularly of the T cell receptor gene, represents strong evidence of malignancy, even in early-stage lesions.

Staging of Mycosis Fungoides

Staging classification is helpful in the management of patients. The World Health Organization-European Organization for Research and Treatment of Cancer (WHO-EORTC) classification pertains to prognostic categories, indolent versus aggressive (Table 1); the TNM nomenclature permits more precise clinical staging for MF and SS (Tables 2 and 3). The extent of skin (T of TNM) and peripheral lymph node enlargement (N of TNM) involvement are significantly associated with survival in patients with CTCL. Generally, a lymph node biopsy is not obtained in patients with early patch/plaque disease because

CURRENT THERAPY

- Optimal treatment depends on stage of disease.
- Skin-directed therapies are for early-stage patients.
- Systemic therapy is used for more advanced disease.
- Treatment of pruritus is relevant for all patients.

TABLE 2 TNM Classification for Cutaneous T Cell Lymphoma (Mycosis Fungoides and Sézary Syndrome)*

Skin (T)

T0	Clinically and/or histologically suspicious lesions
T1	Limited plaques, papules, or eczematous patches covering <10% of skin surface
T2	Limited plaques, papules, or eczematous patches covering ≥10% of skin surface
T3	Tumors (≥1)
T4	Generalized erythroderma

Lymph Nodes (N)

N0	No clinically abnormal peripheral lymph nodes; pathologic findings not CTCL
N1	Clinically abnormal peripheral lymph nodes; pathologic findings not CTCL
N2	No clinically abnormal peripheral lymph nodes; pathologic findings positive for CTCL
N3	Clinically abnormal peripheral lymph nodes; pathologic findings positive for CTCL

Peripheral Blood (B)

B0	Atypical circulating cells not present (<5%)
B1	Atypical circulating cells present (≥5%)

Visceral Organ (M)

M0	No visceral organ involvement
M1	Visceral involvement (must have pathologic confirmation)

*Peripheral blood involvement (B) is not incorporated into the staging classification for this disorder.
Abbreviation: CTCL = cutaneous T cell lymphoma
Modified from Bunn PA Jr, Lamberg SI: Report of the Committee on Staging and Classification of Cutaneous T-Cell Lymphomas. Cancer Treat Rep 1979;63:725-728.

TABLE 3 Staging Classifications for Cutaneous T-Cell Lymphoma

Stage	Skin	Lymph Nodes	Visceral Involvement
IA	T1	N0	M0
IB	T2	N0	M0
IIA	T1, T2	N1	M0
IIB	T3	N0, N1	M0
III	T4	N0, N1	M0
IVA	T1–T4	N2, N3	M0
IVB	T1–T4	N0–N3	M1

Modified from Lamberg SI, Bunn PA Jr: Cutaneous T cell lymphomas: Summary of the Mycosis Fungoides Cooperative Group-National Cancer Institute Workshop. Arch Dermatol 1979;115:1103-1105.

lymph nodes are rarely positive or show only dermatopathic lymphadenitis by light microscopy. In the setting of histologically proven lymph node involvement or extracutaneous lymphoma in blood (B) or viscera (M of TNM), prognosis is impacted.

Table 4 lists the tests recommended for the evaluation and staging of patients with MF or SS. Computed tomography (CT) scans are obtained in advanced disease but are not justifiable as a routine evaluation procedure in patients with early-stage disease.

Treatment

Optimal therapy for MF and SS depends on the stage of disease, patients' co-morbidities, insurance coverage (where applicable), and accessibility (Table 5). Long remissions and possible cures are possible in patients with early disease, but current treatments are not curative in patients with more advanced disease. A National Cancer Institute (NCI) study confirmed that late-stage patients with extensive plaques, tumors, or erythroderma did more poorly when treated aggressively, usually because of increased susceptibility to superinfection.

The optimal schedules of current treatments and investigation of new therapies only occur if patients with MF and SS are entered into ongoing treatment protocols. Information regarding finding studies in progress can be obtained in the references list.

GENERAL MEASURES

Pruritus is a common, sometimes overwhelming problem for patients with MF or SS. Moderate relief may be gained by the use of systemic antihistamines such as hydroxyzine (Atarax) at 25 mg orally every 4 hours as needed, topical emollients such as Aquaphor, or topical corticosteroids such as betamethasone, fluocinonide (Lidex), or triamcinolone (Aristocort) in ointment form applied as needed or overnight under plastic wrap occlusion. For severe itch, gabapentin (Neurontin), mirtazapine, or drugs that treat neuropathic pain are indicated.

In most cases, skin-directed therapies are used for patients with disease considered to be confined to the skin, and systemic therapy is used for more advanced disease.

SPECIFIC MEASURES

Skin-Directed Therapies

Phototherapy

Phototherapy with ultraviolet B (UVB) treats limited patch or plaque T1 disease, resulting in up to 74% complete response rate. Psoralen ultraviolet A-range (PUVA) long-wavelength light penetrates the skin more deeply: 90% of stage IA and 76% of stage IB patients may achieve complete remission. Recently, narrowband UVB showed similar response rates to PUVA without the adverse events of nausea from psoralen. However, patients with thicker plaques need frequent maintenance light treatments to maintain control along with other modalities.

TABLE 4 Recommended Evaluation Procedures

	Routine	Investigational
History and physical examination	X	
Skin biopsy	X	
Complete blood count and differential, renal function tests, uric acid, serum calcium, lactate dehydrogenase (LDH)	X	
Peripheral smear to determine the absolute lymphocyte count and percentage of Sézary cells	X	
Chest radiograph	X	
Scans and/or biopsies of organs when history or physical examination suggests abnormalities	X	
Lymph node biopsy*	See text	
Bone marrow biopsy†		X
Abdominal ultrasound/computed tomography	X	
Positron emission tomography scans		X

*Lymph node biopsy would be justifiable in patients with enlarged lymph nodes (>1.5 cm in diameter) and in those with tumor stage.
†Bone marrow biopsy is indicated in those patients with peripheral blood involvement and tumor stage.

TABLE 5 Comparison of Treatment Options

	Advantages	Disadvantages
Topical steroids	Symptomatic relief Defer more definitive Rx to observe the course	Alter skin pathology Questionable long-term benefit No effect on infiltrated plaques
Phototherapy	Skin clearing in early disease Side effects minimal	High relapse rate without maintenance No effect on thick plaques or tumors Associated with other late skin cancers (PUVA) "Cure" rate low
Mechlorethamine (HN2, Mustargen)	Ease of use at home 10% long-term remission of early MF	High rate of allergic reactions No effect on thick plaques or tumors
Carmustine (BCNU, BiCNU)	Ease of use at home Response rate like that of topical HN2 Low rate of allergic contact dermatitis	Potential bone marrow suppression Telangiectasia, pigmentation, skin tenderness
Bexarotene gel (Targretin)	Ease of use at home Not carcinogenic	May irritate skin Expensive
Total skin electron beam therapy	High long-term disease-free rates One course of therapy	Significant cutaneous side effects Expensive
Bexarotene (Targretin)	Benefits 30% of patients who failed prior treatments Single oral dosage Can be adjuvant to other treatment	Limited availability Increases triglycerides and decreases TSH and T_4 Expensive
Interferons	May salvage late-stage disease Adjuvant with other modalities	Significant side effects Expensive Intramuscular dosage required
Photopheresis	Effective in Sézary syndrome Minimal side effects	Limited availability Slow response to treatment Expensive
Denileuken diftitox (Ontak)	Can treat late-stage disease (10%–35%)	Need expertise to administer Possible serious side effects Expensive
Systemic chemotherapy	May maintain remissions Sometimes induces remissions Palliation of late stage	Significant side effects Complete response unlikely Increases susceptibility to infection

Abbreviations: HN2 = nitrogen mustard; MF = mycosis fungoides; PUVA = psoralen plus ultraviolet light of A wavelength; Rx = prescription; T_4 = thyroxine; TSH = thyroid-stimulating hormone.

Topical Mechlorethamine

Topical application of mechlorethamine (nitrogen mustard [HN2], Mustargen) is a proven regimen for the control of early stage MF with 94% complete response rates in stage IA and 59% in stage IB. Limitations of this treatment modality include a high rate of hypersensitivity reactions (up to 20%), and the need for continuous daily application.

A liquid preparation or ointment form is used. Although there are no studies comparing the preparations, the ointment form is helpful for patients who experience significant dryness from the liquid preparation. Treatment should be carried out daily to the total body, neck down, until complete clearing, which may take several months to a year or longer. Once clear, therapy should be continued for 6 to 24 months, perhaps at a decreased frequency, and then discontinued. Many patients clear except for one or a few patches. These patients often require continuous therapy to maintain control or an alternative topical therapy. For those patients who become allergic, half can be desensitized by graded increases of diluted HN2, managed by experienced dermatologists.

Topical Carmustine

Although less frequently used than HN2, topical carmustine (BiCNU) is an effective alternative for early-stage disease, especially in patients who became allergic to HN2. Local irritation and persistent telangiectasias usually develop. Because the drug is absorbed, patients have a risk of reversible bone marrow depression with decreased leukocytes and platelets, usually delayed for 6 weeks after use. The patient can be supplied with a stock solution by prescribing a 100-mg vial of BiCNU dissolved in 50 mL of absolute or 95% ethanol to be stored at home in the refrigerator. Once each day, the patient should add 5 mL of the stock to approximately 60 mL of water and paint the solution onto affected areas. Because of the potential for bone marrow suppression, treatment should only continue for 6 to 8 weeks. If the response is incomplete, this course can be followed immediately by treating individual lesions with the undiluted alcoholic stock solution up to twice daily (up to 70 mg or 35 mL/week). Alternatively, after a 6-week rest period, the patient can be retreated with twice the concentration (10 mL stock per 60 mL water) for another 6 to 8 weeks. The cycle of treatment may be repeated as necessary to suppress visible lesions.

Complete blood counts, including platelet counts, should be obtained every 2 to 4 weeks during and for 6 weeks after total body and intensive local applications.

Topical Bexarotene Gel

Bexarotene (Targretin) gel is the topical form of the retinoid X receptor (RXR), approved by the Food and Drug Administration (FDA) for the skin manifestations of MF. Bexarotene gel is initially applied once every other day for the first week, with application frequency increased at weekly intervals to once, twice, three times, and up to four times daily, depending on individual lesion tolerance. Irritation is common. Most patients require several weeks of treatment before a response is evident. The medication is expensive; its use is reserved for resistant lesions or lesions on palms and soles.

Radiotherapy

Mycosis fungoides is radiosensitive, and conventional orthovoltage radiation therapy has been used for decades. It can be appropriate for a single plaque or tumor. For patients with extensive skin disease or tumors, total skin electron beam (TSEB) therapy is a better consideration. The penetration of electrons can be controlled to reach depths as shallow as a few millimeters, whereas orthovoltage radiation passes deeply into tissues. A large surface dose can be given with electron beam radiotherapy without deep tissue injury or bone marrow suppression.

With TSEB therapy, most patients in early stages achieve a complete remission, and up to a third remain clear and, perhaps, cured. Therapy is usually fractionated over a period of 6 to 10 weeks to a total of approximately 3000 to 3600 cGy. All portions of the body must be treated; a higher recurrence rate was found in patients who elect scalp shielding to prevent loss of scalp hair. Acute side effects include skin edema, erythema, and fissuring. Hair, nails, and sweat gland function usually return in 3 to 6 months. Limitations of TSEB therapy include its high cost and its availability, although most large cities have medical centers capable of TSEB therapy.

Biologic Disease Modifying Agents

Interferons

Interferons, especially recombinant interferon alpha-2a (Roferon-A[1]), interferon alpha-2b (Intron A[1]), and gamma-1b (Actimmune[1]), are helpful as primary treatment in early-stage CTCL and in combination with retinoids, phototherapy, or extracorporeal photopheresis in later stages. Response rates of approximately 50% are shown with 20% of patients undergoing full remission. Although low doses, 3 million U three times a week, can be offered, doses as high as 12 million U three times a week, given intramuscularly or subcutaneously, may be needed for maximal response. Toxicity depends on dose and includes fever, chills, myalgia, anorexia, and bone marrow suppression.

The degree of leukopenia is the dose-limiting side effect, but recovery is rapid.

Retinoids

Bexarotene (Targretin) for oral use is approved by the FDA for the treatment of CTCL refractory to at least one previous course of systemic therapy. The recommended oral dose is 300 mg/m^2/day, a level at which approximately a third of patients achieve at least a partial response. For a 70-kg, 6-foot person, the surface area is approximately 2m^2. Therefore, eight 75-mg capsules per day are required. Side effects at the recommended dosage can be significant. They often include high lipid levels that require systemic agents for control, central hypothyroidism, and signs and symptoms of retinoid therapy that may be seen with etretinate and isotretinoin, including headache, dry skin, leucopenia, pruritus, and nausea.

With antilipemic agents and thyroid replacement, side effects can be minimized. Liver function tests should be performed at baseline; after weeks 1, 2, 4; and once stable, at 8-week intervals. Thyroid function tests should be obtained at baseline and then monitored to watch for decreases in thyroid-stimulating hormone and thyroxine levels. Blood lipid levels, especially triglycerides, should be determined at baseline, weekly until the lipid response is established, and then at 8-week intervals. Alterations, especially if triglyceride levels are greater than 400 mg/dL, should be controlled with antilipemic therapy (not gemfibrozil) and dose reduction. White blood cell counts and differential should be obtained at baseline and at regular intervals.

Extracorporeal Photopheresis

Extracorporeal photopheresis has been approved by the FDA for the treatment of CTCL since 1988. It is principally used for erythrodermic MF or SS. Complete clinical responses are 15% to 25%. In this procedure, the patient's centrifugally separated white blood cells are exposed to UVA in the presence of psoralen and then infused back into the patient. Whether because of a direct cytotoxic effect on the lymphocytes or because of an additional anti-idiotype antibody reaction induced by lymphocyte damage, a substantial reduction in the number of circulating atypical cells is seen in most patients. Skin lesions also often improve, presumably because of movement of atypical cells from the skin into the circulation, where they can be targeted. Side effects are minimal, but expertise in a hospital setting is necessary.

Interleukin-2 Fusion Toxin

Denileukin diftitox (Ontak) is the product of the fusion of sequences of interleukin-2 (IL-2) with amino acid sequences of diphtheria toxin fragments that targets the malignant cell, the activated T-helper lymphocyte. The combination directs the cytocidal action of diphtheria toxin to cells that express the IL-2 receptor. Response rates are based on patients with at least 20% of the cells in skin lesions positive for CD25, the α-chain of the IL-2 receptor. Initial reported response rates were 30% with 10% complete response in patients who had been refractory to at least two prior therapies. Administer the drug

---

[1]Not FDA approved for this indication.

at 9 to 18 μg/kg/day intravenously for 5 consecutive days and repeat every 3 weeks. The major side effects are a flulike syndrome, which occurs in most patients, and capillary leak syndrome, seen in 10%. Excluding patients who have a low albumin can minimize side effects.

Systemic Chemotherapy

In resistant or progressive disease, systemic chemotherapy may be necessary. Single-agent chemotherapy, particularly low-dose methotrexate (Rheumatrex), 5 to 50 mg per week, is used for resistant plaque disease and erythrodermic MF or SS.

Chemotherapeutic agents that are effective in some cases include liposomal doxorubicin (Doxil), fludarabine (Fludara[1]), deoxycoformycin (pentostatin), gemcitabine (Gemzar[1]), CHOP (cyclophosphamide [Cytoxan], hydroxydaunomycin [Adriamycin], Oncovin [vincristine], and prednisone), and EPOCH (etoposide, prednisone, Oncovin, cyclophosphamide, and hydroxydaunomycin [doxorubicin]).

TREATMENT BY STAGE

Early Mycosis Fungoides Apparently Confined to the Skin

Ninety percent of patients with limited patch stage disease do not progress beyond this stage (T1 and N [any] or T2 and N0–N1 [M0]). Because most patients receive some form of therapy, it is unclear whether it is the treatment or the natural history of the disease that confers the good prognosis in patients in this group. Data from the Mycosis Fungoides Cooperative Group (MFCG) show 5-year survival rates decreased to 83% in comparison to insurance data for what was expected for persons without MF of the same age and sex. Therapies are generally skin directed and include phototherapy, topical chemotherapy (nitrogen mustard, carmustine), or, more aggressively, TSEB.

Later Stage Mycosis Fungoides Confined to the Skin

In patients with T2 and N2 or T3 (M0) (B0), although curative therapy is not likely in most instances, sustained remissions are possible. Combination of skin-directed therapies with a biologic disease modifying agent (bexarotene (Targretin), interferon,[1] extracorporeal photopheresis, denileukin diftitox [Ontak]) helps achieve remission. Maintenance therapy is necessary. Treatment of pruritus and prevention of infections are relevant. Five-year survival rates are reduced in this group of patients to 64% and for tumor stage 50% (MFCG data).

Late Stage with Visceral Involvement, Failure of Previous Therapy, or Sézary Syndrome

Treatment in the late stage is palliative. Because aggressive systemic chemotherapy may shorten the survival of patients with late-stage disease by increasing the chance of sepsis, biologic disease modifying agents that are immunomodulators rather than immunosuppressors are better treatment options. These agents are often combined to achieve higher

response rates. Examples of combination of agents include oral bexarotene with interferon[1] and extracorporeal photopheresis with interferon or with oral bexarotene. Oral bexarotene increases response rates to denileukin diftitox. Pruritus can be severe in advanced stages, and a multidisciplinary approach may be needed to treat all dimensions of the disease. Five-year survival drops to 35% in SS (stage T4) patients (MFCG data), and, if extracutaneous involvement is present (stage M1), to less than 20% (2001 Stanford data).

REFERENCES

Foss F: Mycosis fungoides and the Sézary syndrome. Curr Opin Oncol 2004;16(5):421-428.
Girardi M, Heald PW, Wilson LD: The pathogenesis of mycosis fungoides. N Engl J Med 2004;350(19):1978-1988.
Lundin J, Osterborg A: Therapy for mycosis fungoides. Curr Treat Options Oncol 2004;5(3):203-214.
Willemze R, Jaffe ES, Burg G, et al: WHO-EORTC classification for cutaneous lymphomas. Blood 2005;105(10):3768-3785.
Information on mycosis fungoides and Sézary syndrome studies in progress can be obtained by calling the Cancer Information Service, NCI, Bethesda, MD, at 1-800-4CANCER or from the NCI Web site, http://www.cancer.gov/search/clinical_trials/

[1]Not FDA approved for this indication.

Papulosquamous Disorders

Method of
Chai Sue Lee, MD, and John Koo, MD

Psoriasis

Psoriasis is a genetically influenced, immune-mediated chronic disorder. It is one of the most commonly encountered conditions in dermatologic practice and is regularly seen in primary care practice. Psoriasis affects approximately 2.6% of U.S. population, or approximately 7 million people. Between 150,000 and 260,000 new cases of psoriasis are diagnosed annually. Although slightly more prevalent in women than men, psoriasis affects all ages, races, and ethnicities.

Psoriasis is characterized by sharply demarcated, erythematous, scaly plaques. The most common sites of involvement are the scalp, elbows, and knees followed by the nails, hands, feet, and trunk, including the intergluteal fold.

One of the most important decisions that physicians must make is whether the patient's psoriasis can be adequately treated with topical medications alone or whether it requires phototherapy and/or systemic therapies. This critical decision should take into account the severity of psoriasis, the disease's impact on the patient's quality of life, responsiveness or lack of response to topical therapies, and the presence of or absence of psoriatic arthritis.

Psoriasis can range from mild to severe. In clinical practice, the severity of psoriasis is usually defined by the percentage of body surface area (BSA) involved. The palm

[1]Not FDA approved for this indication.

CURRENT DIAGNOSIS

- Sharply demarcated, scaly, erythematous plaques.
- The most common sites of involvement are scalp, elbows, and knees followed by the nails, hands, feet, and trunk (including the intergluteal fold).
- Psoriatic arthritis is the major associated systemic manifestation; the most common presentation is asymmetric oligoarthritis of the small joints of the hands and feet.

CURRENT THERAPY

Topical therapies
- Corticosteroids
- Calcipotriene (Dovonex)
- Tazarotene (Tazorac)
- Anthralin
- Tar
- Salicylic acid

Phototherapy
- Broadband UVB
- NBUVB
- PUVA

Oral therapies
- Acitretin (Soriatane)
- Methotrexate
- Cyclosporine (Neoral)

Biologic agents
- Etanercept (Enbrel)
- Efalizumab (Raptiva)
- Alefacept (Amevive)

Abbreviations: NBUVB = narrowband ultraviolet light B; PUVA = psoralen plus ultraviolet light of A wavelength.

of the patient's hand, including the fingers and the thumb (i.e., from the wrist to the top of the fingers), constitutes approximately 1% of the BSA. In clinical trials, severe psoriasis is defined as the presence of lesions over more than 10% of the BSA. In general, if 10% or more BSA is involved, it becomes impractical, if not unrealistic, for most patients to treat their psoriasis with topical medications. Not only does it become tedious and time consuming, it also becomes difficult to obtain sufficient quantities of topical medications. Furthermore, some of the more frequently used and effective topical treatments for psoriasis, such as superpotent topical steroids and calcipotriene (Dovonex), have limitations on the amount of medication that is allowed to be used per unit time for safety reasons. Therefore, patients with more than 10% BSA involvement should probably be managed by a dermatologist so that phototherapy and/or systemic therapy can be used. It is estimated that approximately 30% of psoriasis patients, or approximately 1.5 million U.S. adults, have moderate to severe psoriasis.

When determining severity the impact of psoriasis on the patient's quality of life, including both psychologic and emotional well-being, should also be taken into consideration. Psoriasis may also be deemed severe even when the BSA involved is less than 10%, and phototherapy or systemic therapy should be considered if the psoriasis proves unresponsive to optimized topical treatments. This is especially true if the psoriasis is physically debilitating or emotionally, occupationally, or socially devastating to the patient. For example, a person may only have the palms and/or soles (i.e., 2% BSA) affected by psoriasis, but the impact on quality of life may be profound if the psoriasis impairs the use of the hands or feet; aggressive therapy may be warranted.

Approximately 10% to 40% of patients with psoriasis, or approximately 1 million or more people, have psoriatic arthritis. A major clinical difference between psoriasis and psoriatic arthritis is that psoriasis does not leave behind a permanent scar as long as the patient does not excoriate or damage the skin in other ways once the psoriasis is adequately treated, whereas psoriatic arthritis, if it is severe enough, can cause irreversible bony destruction. No topical medications are known to help psoriatic arthritis, and systemic therapies such as methotrexate and etanercept (Enbrel) are FDA approved for both psoriasis and psoriatic arthritis.

There are also many different forms of psoriasis. Plaque-type psoriasis is the most common form and comprises 80% to 90% of those with psoriasis. Other less-common forms of psoriasis include pustular psoriasis, erythrodermic psoriasis, guttate psoriasis, and inverse psoriasis. When determining treatment, the form of psoriasis should also be taken into consideration because certain forms of psoriasis are more responsive to certain therapies. Trigger factors for psoriatic flares are listed in Table 1.

TREATMENT

There are many topical and systemic medications to choose from to treat psoriasis. Our recommendation is to learn a few of these agents well, with a good understanding of appropriate patient selection, expected results, and side effects, because mastering all available agents for psoriasis is probably beyond the scope of a general practitioner.

Topical Therapies

Topical steroids and calcipotriene (Dovonex) are two of the most useful topical agents, especially in a primary care setting, and will be discussed in some detail. Other perhaps more complicated topical agents, such as tazarotene, anthralin, and tar preparations, will be briefly described.

TABLE 1 Triggers for Psoriatic Flare

- Traumatic injury to the skin
- Streptococcal infection
- Stress
- Cold weather
- Drugs: systemic corticosteroid withdrawal, β-blockers, ACE inhibitors, lithium, antimalarials, interferons
- Excessive alcohol

Abbreviation: ACE = angiotensin-converting enzyme.

Topical Steroids

Topical steroids are best suited for a *quick fix* or rapid improvement when the patient first presents. To obtain an adequate response in psoriasis, however, the physician usually must use a stronger topical steroid than what is typically used when treating other common, chronic inflammatory conditions such as eczema or seborrheic dermatitis. Topical steroids weaker than medium potency generally are ineffective for plaque-type psoriasis, especially in nonsensitive areas such as the elbows and knees, where often a high-strength or even superpotent topical steroid is necessary to control the psoriasis adequately.

The most distressing adverse effects associated with topical steroids are skin atrophy, including striae or stretch marks because of their unsightliness and irreversibility, and the risk of adrenal suppression. Steroid-sensitive areas that need special consideration include face, axillae, inframammary folds, abdominal pannus, inner thighs, and groin. If steroids must be used in high-risk areas, physicians should first try those from classes 5, 6, or 7. Topical steroids from class 4 are usually the highest potency acceptable for use in steroid-sensitive areas.

Adrenal suppression can occur with any of the medium-potent to superpotent topical steroids. The amount of superpotent topical steroid applied each week should be limited to no more than 50 to 60 g/week for an adult to avoid risk of adrenal suppression. The FDA recommends that class I, or superpotent, topical steroids such as clobetasol (Temovate) or halobetasol (Ultravate) be used for no more than 2 weeks at a time.

Topical steroid use in psoriasis is also well known to be associated with tachyphylaxis, a phenomenon in which the drugs initially work well, but efficacy gradually diminishes with continuous use. To regain efficacy, the physician needs to increase steroid potency or give the patient a *steroid holiday* lasting several months.

Whenever topical steroids are discontinued, they should be tapered off rather than abruptly stopped, because abrupt discontinuation may lead to a rebound phenomenon. In this rare phenomenon, psoriasis suddenly becomes worse than pretreatment after the medication is discontinued.

Calcipotriene

A topical vitamin D analogue, known as calcipotriene (Dovonex) in the United States and calcipotriol (Daivonex) in other countries, is not only the first elegant nonsteroidal alternative for the treatment of psoriasis but is also the most prescribed single agent for psoriasis worldwide. Twice daily application of calcipotriene ointment has been shown in two randomized, double-blind, multicenter studies to be more effective than a high-potency topical steroid ointment, fluocinonide (Lidex), twice daily.

One of the most important features of calcipotriene that makes it an excellent agent for primary care physicians as well as dermatologists is its safety profile. It is steroid free, and thus free from steroidal side effects such as skin thinning, striae formation, and adrenal suppression. The main side effect of calcipotriene is lesional and perilesional (around the lesion) irritation. Irritation from calcipotriene usually presents with a red ring of inflamed skin surrounding the treated lesions. Patients may report a mild stinging or burning sensation. This is usually transient and patients quickly become accustomed to it. In clinical trials of calcipotriene, only 1 in 25 research subjects had to discontinue treatment because of skin irritation. Skin irritation from calcipotriene is usually more pronounced on the face and occluded parts of the body such as the axillae and groin. This is because skin irritation appears to depend largely on the penetration of calcipotriene through the skin; the intertriginous areas are occlusive by nature and, therefore, enhance the penetration of calcipotriene through the skin. Furthermore, calcipotriene is lipophilic and more readily absorbed by skin containing oily sebaceous glands, such as the face, which also helps to explain why it tends to be more irritating on the face.

Calcipotriene irritation does not necessarily preclude its use. This can often be prevented by decreasing the penetration of calcipotriene through the skin. One way is to use the cream formulation instead of the ointment formulation. Using smaller amounts and reducing the frequency of application to once a day or every other day instead of twice a day is another method of reducing penetration and irritation. Once this regimen is tolerated, the frequency of application can be increased carefully. Another strategy used by many dermatologists at the initiation of therapy is combining calcipotriene with a topical steroid. Calcipotriene has been proven to be chemically compatible with the topical steroid halobetasol propionate (Ultravate) when mixed and applied together for up to 48 hours. Rarely, calcipotriene may cause excessive peeling and apparent expansion of erythema beyond the original border of the psoriatic lesion. If this peculiar perilesional peeling occurs, and if the patient is asymptomatic, it is best to reassure the patient that this reaction is self-limited and to encourage continued use of calcipotriene.

The systemic side effect to be aware of when prescribing calcipotriene is hypercalcemia. Hypercalcemia has been reported only in rare instances when a patient has used large amounts of this medication on the body. A good guideline to follow is to limit total weekly use of calcipotriene to no more than 100 to 120 g/week. One can instruct the patient to use no more than one large tube per week, because 120 g is the largest tube size available.

For those who wish for at least 75% or better improvement, which is what most patients would consider satisfactory response, it is good to know that the efficacy of once-daily calcipotriene is approximately half that of twice-daily use. Because many patients find time to apply topical medications only once a day, which may lead to slow onset of action and relative dissatisfaction, most dermatologists in the United States use calcipotriene not as monotherapy but rather in combination with other treatments. Combination of calcipotriene with other treatments not only increases the rate of improvement and offers greater improvement but, in the case of topical steroids, also a reduction of side effects. The topical steroid decreases the risk of skin irritation by calcipotriene, and calcipotriene prevents skin atrophy by the topical steroid.

One of the authors' favorite topical combination therapy for psoriasis is sequential therapy (Table 2).

Other Topical Agents

Other topical agents that are either less effective, have more side effects, or involve special instructions are described in the following text.

TABLE 2 Topical Sequential Therapy

Step I (clearing phase): 2 weeks to 1 month
- Halobetasol (Ultravate)* + calcipotriene (Dovonex) bid (mixed immediately prior to application)

Step II (transitional phase): 1 month to indefinitely for some patients
- Calcipotriene (Dovonex) bid on weekdays
- Calcipotriene (Dovonex) + halobetasol (Ultravate) bid on weekends

Step III (maintenance phase): indefinitely or until clearance
- Calcipotriene (Dovonex) bid

*Generic halobetasol or clobetasol can be substituted if necessary, but chemical compatibility with calcipotriene (Dovonex) is unknown.

Tazarotene (Tazorac) is the only topical retinoid approved in the United States for plaque-type psoriasis. It is available in two strengths, 0.05% and 0.1%, and two formulations, cream and gel. It is applied once daily in the evening. Tazarotene offers a somewhat longer duration of remission than other topical agents for psoriasis but tends to be significantly much more irritating. Tazarotene should be applied sparingly only to the psoriatic plaques, avoiding the surrounding normal skin. Concurrent use of a topical steroid every morning increases efficacy and reduces tazarotene irritation. Mometasone furoate (Elocon) has demonstrated a synergistic effect when used in combination with tazarotene. Tazarotene is a category X medication, which is contraindicated during pregnancy.

Anthralin has been used to treat psoriasis for more than 100 years. However, it is one of the less commonly used agents in the United States because of its tendency to stain skin, clothing, and linens; risk of irritation; and moderate efficacy. Anthralin is applied once daily to affected areas for 30 minutes to 1 hour and then washed off.

Coal tar is a mixture of at least 10,000 components, most of which have not been identified. Tar products are available in many different formulations and strengths. Crude coal tar in combination with phototherapy in a specialized daycare setting is still the most effective and safe treatment available for moderate to severe psoriasis since it was first described by Goeckerman in 1925. Messiness is the main drawback. Compared to other treatments, tar remains one of the safest. In response to a California lawsuit, the FDA has ruled that there is no convincing evidence of carcinogenic risk with human therapeutic use of coal tar in concentrations up to 5%.

Salicylic acid is a keratolytic agent that acts to remove excess scale and hyperkeratosis associated with psoriasis. It does not affect erythema or induration. Salicylic acid is commercially available over the counter as 6% Keralyt gel. Salicylic acid can produce local irritation and erythema. It is probably best to avoid salicylic acid in patients with diabetes, because systemic absorption of salicylic acid can inhibit gluconeogenesis and lead to hypoglycemia in diabetics.

Systemic Therapies

For moderate to severe psoriasis, phototherapy or systemic therapy is usually required. Phototherapy options include ultraviolet B (UVB) light and psoralen plus ultraviolet light of A wavelength (PUVA). There are two types of UVB phototherapy: broadband and narrowband. Narrowband UVB (NBUVB) is more effective for psoriasis than broadband UVB therapy. Oral agents approved by the FDA for psoriasis include acitretin (Soriatane), methotrexate, and cyclosporine (Neoral) (Table 3). There are now three FDA-approved biologic agents for psoriasis: etanercept (Enbrel), efalizumab (Raptiva), and alefacept (Amevive) (Table 4). Specialized centers can also provide Ingram therapy (anthralin and UVB combination therapy) and Goeckerman therapy (tar and UVB combination therapy).

Seborrheic Dermatitis

Seborrheic dermatitis is a common, chronic inflammatory scaling condition of unknown cause typically confined to the sebaceous gland-rich skin of the head and trunk. It is seen in early infancy and in adulthood and is more common in men than women. Seborrheic dermatitis affects

TABLE 3 Summary of Oral Agents

Drug	Dose	Laboratory Monitoring	Main Adverse Effects
Acitretin (Soriatane)	10–50 mg qd	• CBC • LFT • Fasting lipid profile • Pregnancy test	• Mucocutaneous changes • Teratogenicity • Hyperlipidemia • Hepatotoxicity
Methotrexate	15–30 mg/wk	• CBC • LFT • BUN and creatinine • Liver biopsy • Pregnancy test	• Bone marrow suppression • Teratogenicity
Cyclosporine (Neoral)	3–5 mg/kg/d divided bid	• CBC • LFT • BUN and creatinine • Fasting lipid profile • Urinalysis • Potassium and magnesium • Blood pressure	• Nephrotoxicity • Hypertension • Paresthesias • Hyperlipidemia

Abbreviations: BUN = blood urea nitrogen; CBC = complete blood count; LFT = liver function test.

TABLE 4 Summary of Biologic Agents

Drug	Dose	Laboratories	Adverse Events
Etanercept (Enbrel)	50 mg biweekly for 3 months, then either 50 mg once weekly or 25 mg biweekly		• Reactivation of TB* • Multiple sclerosis* • Congestive heart failure* • Lupus* • Bone marrow suppression*
Efalizumab (Raptiva)	1 mg/kg SC weekly	CBC with platelet counts recommended but not required	• Flulike symptoms • Psoriasis worsening • Arthritis worsening* • Thrombocytopenia* • Hemolytic anemia*
Alefacept (Amevive)	15 mg IM weekly for 12 weeks	CD4 counts weekly during treatment	• Decreased CD4 count if the count becomes less than 250

*Causal relationship with the drug has not been established because of the rarity of these cases.
Abbreviations: CBD = complete blood count; IM = intramuscularly; SC = subcutaneously; TB = tuberculosis.

approximately 3% to 5% of adults. Patients infected by HIV have a higher prevalence of seborrheic dermatitis.

Infantile seborrheic dermatitis typically involves the scalp, the flexural creases, and the diaper area. Thick, yellowish-white plates of scales often develop on the scalp, and this has been colloquially termed *cradle cap*. Erythematous plaques with sharply defined borders and a glazed or shiny surface are characteristic. Small erythematous papules with fine scales may be scattered around and between larger plaques. Scales may be absent in flexural areas.

Adults with seborrheic dermatitis usually have diffuse erythema and scaling of the hair-bearing portions of the scalp. Typical lesions are well-defined pink plaques with powdery scale that form in the eyebrows, glabella, nasolabial folds, and the postauricular sulci. Occasionally, the presternal, interscapular, or genital skin is affected. Pruritus may or may not be present.

Mild seborrheic dermatitis can be treated with shampoos containing tar, selenium sulfide (Selsun), or zinc pyrithione (Head & Shoulders). These may be used daily on the affected areas including scalp, face, and other involved sites until the condition is under control, then once or twice weekly for maintenance. Moderate cases often respond to shampoos or creams containing 2% ketoconazole (Nizoral), used daily until it is under control, then once or twice weekly for maintenance. Low-potency topical steroids such as 1.0% to 2.5% hydrocortisone cream (for recalcitrant cases, stronger topical steroids such as desonide [DesOwen] cream) once or twice daily may be used initially but ideally not for maintenance therapy. Topical pimecrolimus (Elidel)[1] or topical tacrolimus (Protopic)[1] can be used as steroid-sparing agents. Thick scalp scales may be loosened with overnight application of salicylic acid 6% gel under occlusion or with Derma-Smoothe/FS oil.

Pityriasis Rosea

Pityriasis rosea is a common, acute, inflammatory dermatosis that affects mainly older children and young adults. It is characterized by a self-limited course that often starts with a primary isolated scaly plaque followed by a secondary, generalized, symmetrical, papulosquamous eruption typically distributed on the trunk and proximal extremities. The disease is more prevalent in the cooler months of the year in temperate zones. The exact cause is unknown, but a viral etiology has been speculated.

Typically, most patients will initially develop a lesion referred to as the *herald patch*, which is an asymptomatic, solitary papule that enlarges rapidly in 1 to 2 days to form an oval patch 2 to 10 cm in diameter with an erythematous, salmon-colored border with fine scaling. The trunk, primarily the anterior chest, is the most common location for the herald patch. Several days later, numerous smaller patches will appear, mainly on the trunk and proximal parts of the extremities. They are typically oval, faint pink, with a collarette of delicate scales well inside the border of the lesion. On the back, longitudinal axes of the lesions run down and out relative to the orientation of the spine in a pattern that, with imagination, has been likened to a Christmas tree. The patient may have associated itching, but pruritus is often absent. The eruption usually lasts between 2 and 10 weeks and then resolves spontaneously. There are usually no complications except for occasional postinflammatory hypopigmentation or hyperpigmentation, which resolves slowly over time, often months. Recurrence of pityriasis rosea is infrequent; occurring in less than 3% of cases.

Because secondary syphilis can mimic pityriasis rosea closely, a serologic test for syphilis should be ordered in all cases of *atypical* pityriasis rosea; for example, if there is no herald patch, if the distal extremities (especially the palms and soles) are involved or if the patient is systemically ill.

Offering the patient reassurance is usually all that is necessary for this self-limited disease. Antipruritics such as calamine lotion, a mild-potency topical steroid, or oral antihistamines may be prescribed if necessary. For severe cases, UVB phototherapy has been shown to be effective in controlling the symptoms as well as in inducing a faster remission.

REFERENCES

Feldman S, Koo J, Lebwohl M, et al: The Psoriasis and Psoriatic Arthritis Pocket Guide. Portland, OR, National Psoriasis Foundation, 2005.

[1]Not FDA approved for this indication.

Koo J, Cheung L, Lee CS: Contemporary Diagnosis and Management in Primary Care Dermatology. Newtown, PA, Handbooks in Health Care, 2002.

Koo J, Kochavi G, Kwan J: Contemporary Diagnosis and Management of Psoriasis. Newtown, PA, Handbooks in Health Care, 2004.

Koo J, Lebwohl M, Lee CS: Therapy of Mild-to-Moderate Psoriasis. New York, Taylor & Francis, 2006.

Connective Tissue Disorders

Method of

John Varga, MD, Susan M. Manzi, MD, MPH, and Gabriella Lakos, MD, PhD

Systemic lupus erythematosus (SLE), scleroderma (or systemic sclerosis), and the inflammatory myopathies are distinct but related idiopathic autoimmune connective tissue diseases. Each of these diseases is associated with significant morbidity and mortality. Each is characterized by considerable clinical heterogeneity and a chronic and unpredictable clinical course, often with remissions and relapses. Each is more common in women than men and associated with progressive damage to multiple organs. Prominent target organs include the skin, the cardiovascular system, the lungs, and the musculoskeletal system; in SLE, the brain and the kidneys are also affected. At the tissue level, inflammation and progressive scarring are prominent. Furthermore, each of these diseases is associated with high levels of autoantibodies in the circulation. Autoimmunity, a hallmark of connective tissue diseases, reflects a fundamental breakdown in immunologic self-tolerance. Although the connective tissue diseases have no cure, many effective treatment options are currently available. Because of their clinical heterogeneity, protean multiorgan systemic manifestations, and chronic and unpredictable course, the evaluation and management of patients with connective tissue diseases present unique challenges.

Systemic Lupus Erythematosus

Chronic inflammation and immune dysregulation characterize SLE. The precise etiology is unknown but likely results from a combination of genetic, hormonal, and environmental factors. The spectrum of manifestations in SLE is quite broad and the time course extremely variable. Some patients develop life-threatening irreversible organ damage, whereas the most incapacitating condition in others may be fatigue. Therapy should be tailored to the individual patient and designed not only to suppress disease activity but also to alleviate symptoms as well. Patients with SLE are optimally managed by a team of specialists that may include, in addition to the rheumatologist, a dermatologist, nephrologist, cardiologist, psychiatrist, psychologist, pulmonologist, gastroenterologist, orthopedic surgeon, and physical therapist.

Although a definitive cure for SLE remains elusive, recent advances, both nonpharmacologic and pharmacologic, have significantly improved survival and quality of life. According to Manzi, established treatments fall into four main categories: nonsteroidal anti-inflammatory drugs, antimalarial agents, corticosteroids, and cytotoxic and immunosuppressive agents. Choosing an appropriate treatment regimen requires careful thought in light of the complexity and marked clinical heterogeneity of the disease and the potential long-term side effects of the drugs used. Consultation with a rheumatologist or other subspecialist with expertise in lupus is recommended.

GENERAL PRINCIPLES OF THERAPY

As patients become more information savvy, the role of health professionals in patient education becomes crucial. Physicians and their staff should assist patients in evaluating the flow of information available through modern technology such as the Internet. A patient may be alarmed by hearing or reading about worst-case scenarios. Reassurance that the manifestations and course of disease vary considerably may ease this anxiety. Providing information about support groups may also be helpful. Moreover, physicians should recognize and address the psychological impact that a diagnosis of a chronic, potentially serious disease may have on a previously healthy individual.

Although not life-threatening, fatigue is a challenge for many SLE patients. Physicians should search for contributing factors such as hypothyroidism, fibromyalgia, or depression and must emphasize the importance of adequate rest. Overexposure to ultraviolet (UV) radiation may cause systemic disease flares in addition to skin rashes. Photosensitive patients should avoid excessive exposure to sunlight and wear protective clothing and sunscreen (SPF [sun protection factor] of 35) routinely. Certain prescription drugs, including sulfa drugs and other antibiotics, can exacerbate photosensitivity as well as other lupus disease activity.

Unexplained fever should not be ignored because lupus patients are susceptible to infections. To minimize this risk, physicians should exercise caution when prescribing immunosuppressive agents and corticosteroids and consider influenza and pneumococcal immunizations. Because a disease flare during pregnancy poses risk to the fetus, pregnancies in women with lupus are considered high risk. High-dose estrogen contraceptives should generally be avoided, particularly in patients with increased risk of blood clots; low-dose estrogen, progesterone-only pills, or other effective means of contraception should be considered. Planning pregnancies during periods of disease remission and careful monitoring of both the mother and fetus can improve the chances for healthy outcomes.

Other considerations in the general management of patients with SLE include their increased risk of cardiovascular disease and osteoporosis. Patients should be screened for these conditions and be advised to adopt a cardioprotective lifestyle and take measures to ensure their bone health. These actions include smoking cessation, moderate intake of alcohol, heart-healthy diet, adequate intake of dietary calcium and vitamin D, and regular weight-bearing exercise. Although no definitive link is established between SLE and malignancy, routine gynecologic testing and breast examinations should be performed.

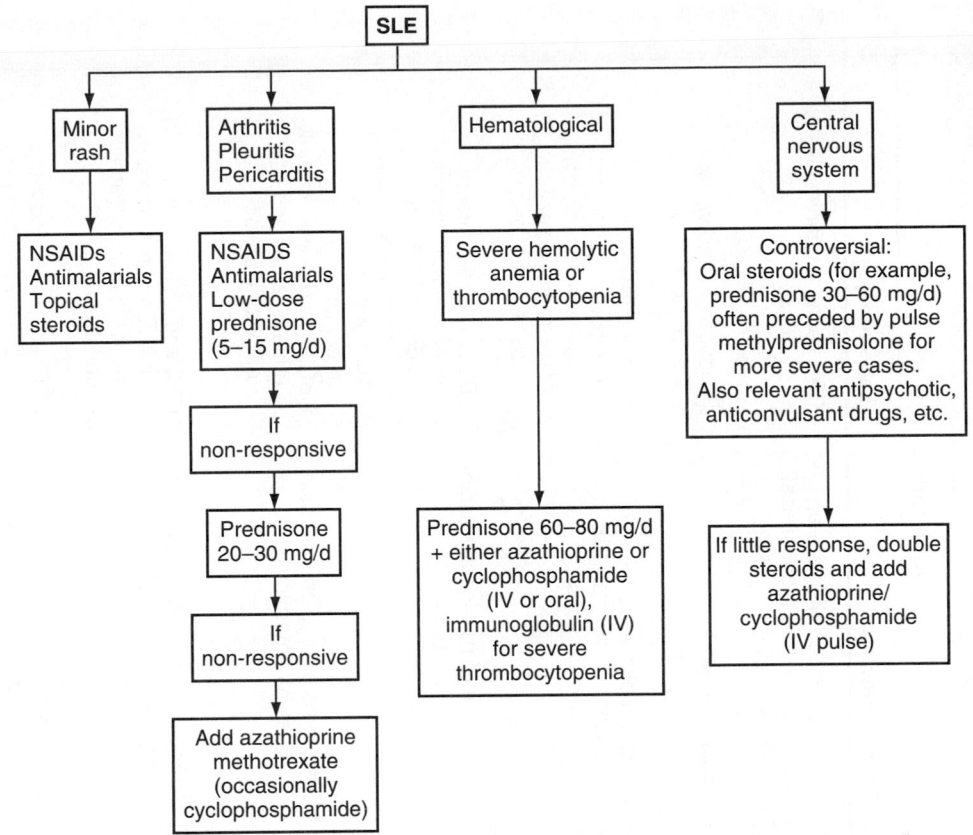

FIGURE 1. Management of nonrenal lupus. (Adapted from Ioannou Y, Isenberg DA: Current concepts for the management of systemic lupus erythematosus in adults: A therapeutic challenge. Postgrad Med J 2002;78:599-606.)

NONSTEROIDAL ANTI-INFLAMMATORY DRUGS

Although nonsteroidal anti-inflammatory drugs (NSAIDs) do not have disease-modifying properties in SLE, they are used to treat fever, pleuritis, pericarditis, and musculoskeletal complaints (Figure 1). Because SLE patients may take NSAIDs for long periods of time, consideration should be given to gastroprotective agents. Furthermore, the potential adverse effects of these drugs on the kidney, liver, and central nervous system may be confused with worsening disease activity. Table 1 lists the general recommendations for monitoring NSAIDs and other commonly used agents in SLE.

ANTIMALARIAL AGENTS

Antimalarial agents are frequently prescribed in the treatment of SLE. The most commonly used are hydroxychloroquine (Plaquenil)[1] and chloroquine (Aralen).[1] Antimalarials are regularly used in the management of cutaneous and musculoskeletal manifestations, constitutional symptoms, and in some cases serositis. Antimalarials may be used in combination when one agent by itself is ineffective because their actions can be synergistic. A particular benefit of antimalarial agents is their steroid-sparing effect. Hydroxychloroquine[1] (200 to 400 mg daily) is generally

[1]Not FDA approved for this indication.

well tolerated, but it may take 6 to 8 weeks for the benefit to become apparent. Because of potential ophthalmologic toxicity, patients should have an ophthalmologic examination when they begin treatment and every 6 to 12 months thereafter. Although it is unclear whether antimalarials prevent major organ disease, they do have lipid-lowering and possible antiplatelet activities.

CORTICOSTEROIDS

Corticosteroids are used to treat a broad spectrum of lupus manifestations. Oral administration of 5 to 30 mg of prednisone daily in single or divided doses is effective in treating constitutional symptoms, cutaneous disease, arthritis, and serositis. Once immediate relief is achieved, their dose is often tapered while slower-acting agents such as antimalarials or immunomodulatory therapy are added. For more serious organ involvement, such as nephritis, central nervous system or hematologic abnormalities, or systemic vasculitis, prednisone at higher doses (1 to 2 mg/kg) daily or parenteral corticosteroid preparations in equivalent doses are given. Pulses of methylprednisolone (1000 mg) can be given for 3 consecutive days in severe situations. According to Ionnaou and Isenberg, the infusion should be given over several hours to minimize the risk of reactions such as joint pain, flushing, headache, or tachycardia. Although high-dose corticosteroids may be required to preserve major organ function, patients who require such aggressive treatment over extended periods are subjected to

TABLE 1 Standard Drug Therapies in Systemic Lupus Erythematosus and Recommended Monitoring Strategies

Drug	Toxicities Requiring Monitoring	Baseline Evaluation	Monitoring	
			System Review	Laboratory
Salicylates, nonsteroidal anti-inflammatory drugs	Gastrointestinal bleeding, hepatic toxicity, hypertension	CBC, creatinine, urinalysis, AST, ALT	Dark/black stool, dyspepsia, nausea/vomiting, abdominal pain, shortness of breath, edema	CBC yearly, creatinine yearly
Hydroxychloroquine	Macular damage	None unless patient is over 40 y of age or has previous eye disease	Visual changes	Funduscopic and visual fields q 6-12 mo
Glucocorticoids	Hypertension, hyperglycemia, hyperlipidemia, hypokalemia, osteoporosis, avascular necrosis, cataract, weight gain, infections, fluid retention	BP, bone densitometry, glucose, potassium, cholesterol, triglycerides (HDL, LDL)	Polyuria, polydipsia, edema, shortness of breath, BP at each visit, visual changes, bone pain	Urinary dipstick for glucose q 3-6 mo, total cholesterol yearly, bone densitometry yearly to assess osteoporosis
Azathioprine	Myelosuppression, hepatotoxicity, lymphoproliferative disorders	CBC, platelet count, creatinine, AST or ALT	Symptoms of myelosuppression	CBC and platelet count q 1-2 wk with changes in dose (q 1-3 mo thereafter), AST yearly, PAP test at regular intervals
Cyclophosphamide	Myelosuppression, myeloproliferative disorders, malignancy, immunosuppression, hemorrhagic cystitis, secondary infertility	CBC and differential and platelet count, urinalysis	Symptoms of myelosuppression, hematuria, infertility	CBC and urinalysis monthly; urine cytology and PAP test yearly for life
Methotrexate	Myelosuppression, hepatic fibrosis, cirrhosis, pulmonary infiltrates, fibrosis	CBC, chest radiograph within past year, hepatitis B, C serology in high-risk patients, AST, albumin, bilirubin, creatinine	Symptoms of myelosuppression, shortness of breath, nausea/vomiting, oral ulcer	CBC and platelet count, AST or ALT, and albumin q 4-8 wk, serum creatinine, urinalysis
Mycophenolate mofetil	Myelosuppression, gastrointestinal	CBC and differential and platelet count, creatinine, AST, ALT	Symptoms of myelosuppression, nausea, diarrhea	CBC and platelet count q1-2 wk with changes in dose (q 1-3 mo thereafter), AST, ALT, creatinine q 1-3 mo.

Abbreviations: ALT = alanine transaminase; AST = aspartate transaminase; BP = blood pressure; CBC = complete blood count; HDL = high-density lipoprotein; LDL = low-density lipoprotein.
Adapted from Manzi S: Treatment of systemic lupus erythematosus. In Klippel JH, Stone J, Weyand C, Crofford LJ (eds): Primer on the Rheumatic Diseases. Atlanta, Arthritis Foundation, 2001, pp 346-352.

highly unfavorable side effects, including emotional lability, weight gain, hypertension, hyperlipidemia, diabetes, glaucoma, risk of infection, avascular necrosis of bone, and osteoporosis. It is recommended that treating physicians attempt to taper corticosteroids to discontinuation or to a minimal dose administered daily or on alternate days once disease activity is controlled.

CYTOTOXIC AGENTS

Aggressive therapy with cytotoxic agents is required for patients with severe disease involving major organs. In general, such therapy should be administered by specialists aware of the potential dangers involved. Cyclophosphamide (Cytoxan)[1] and azathioprine (Imuran),[1] are the agents most commonly prescribed. Methotrexate (Rheumatrex),[1] mycophenolate mofetil (CellCept),[1] and intravenous immunoglobulin (IVIG)[1] also show promising results.

Cyclophosphamide

According to Ortmann and Klippel, cyclophosphamide[1] is the drug of choice for treating most forms of lupus nephritis (Figure 2). Glucocorticoids in combination with intravenous bolus regimens of cyclophosphamide (0.5 to 1.0 g/m^2) is more effective than glucocorticoids alone in preserving renal function. Cyclophosphamide[1] appears to be most effective in diffuse proliferative lupus nephritis, although it may also be useful in membranous nephropathy. Less severe forms of lupus nephritis are commonly treated with corticosteroids alone; however, physicians should be prepared to administer immunosuppressive agents if more severe nephritis develops or if patients develop unacceptable side effects from corticosteroids. Renal biopsy is helpful in determining the therapy of choice. Regardless of the type of immunosuppressant used, it is necessary to control blood pressure effectively to prevent irreversible organ damage. Cyclophosphamide[1] is also effective in nonrenal manifestations of SLE, such as cytopenia, central nervous system disease, pulmonary hemorrhage, and vasculitis.

Cyclophosphamide[1] has numerous undesirable side effects. Nausea, vomiting, hair loss, infertility, and bone marrow suppression are the most common. Gastrointestinal toxicity can be minimized with the administration of antiemetics, and hair loss is normally reversible when treatment is discontinued. Older age and cumulative dose appear to be the major risk factors for infertility. Adjusting the dose of cyclophosphamide[1] can often regulate leukopenia, which typically peaks 8 to 12 days after intravenous administration. Patients on cyclophosphamide[1] are also at increased risk for infections, particularly herpes zoster. Bladder carcinoma can develop even years after cyclophosphamide[1] therapy has stopped; thus urinalysis, urine cytology, and cystoscopy are indicated in patients with hematuria.

Azathioprine (Imuran)

Azathioprine[1] can be used for lupus nephritis, as a steroid-sparing agent in patients with nonrenal manifestations, and

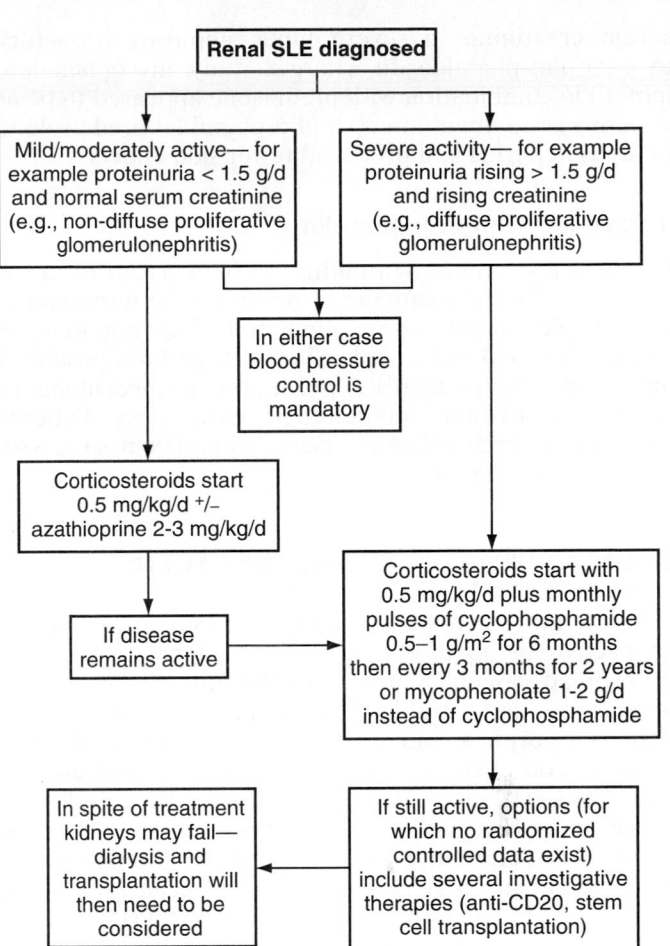

FIGURE 2. Management of renal lupus. (Adapted from Ioannou Y, Isenberg DA: Current concepts for the management of systemic lupus erythematosus in adults: A therapeutic challenge. Postgrad Med J 2002;78:599-606.)

in patients at low risk for progressive renal failure. Azathioprine[1] is generally started at 50 mg daily and increased by 25 mg per week to a maintenance dose of 2 to 3 mg/kg daily. Azathioprine[1] is generally better tolerated than cyclophosphamide[1]; however, bone marrow, hepatic, and gastrointestinal toxicity are common.

Methotrexate (Rheumatrex)

Much evidence supports the effectiveness of methotrexate in rheumatoid arthritis, but very few controlled studies have been conducted in SLE. Evidence suggests that methotrexate at 15 to 20 mg per week is effective in controlling cutaneous and articular manifestations. Because side effects are common at high doses, methotrexate[1] is currently used primarily as a steroid-sparing agent in milder SLE.

Mycophenolate Mofetil (CellCept)

Mycophenolate mofetil[1] (500 to 1000 mg twice daily) appears to be effective for lupus nephritis. In one small study, it is effective in reducing proteinuria and improving

---

[1]Not FDA approved for this indication.

[1]Not FDA approved for this indication.

serum creatinine in severe lupus nephritis refractory to cyclophosphamide. In a larger study, mycophenolate mofetil in combination with prednisone appeared to be as effective as combination cyclophosphamide[1]/prednisolone in lupus nephritis and produced fewer side effects.

Intravenous Immunoglobulin

Intravenous immunoglobulin (IVIG)[1] is used most commonly for the treatment of refractory thrombocytopenia. Platelet counts rise rapidly following initiation of treatment at 400 mg/kg daily. Similar doses have produced improvements in arthritis, nephritis, fever, mucocutaneous manifestations, and immunologic parameters. Patients with SLE-associated IgA deficiency should be treated with alternative therapies.

Scleroderma/Systemic Sclerosis

Scleroderma, or systemic sclerosis (SSc), is a chronic connective tissue disease characterized by evidence of widespread vascular injury, autoimmunity, fibroproliferative process, and variable clinical course. Localized sclerodermas (morphea and linear scleroderma) are distinct from SSc, occur more frequently in children, and are not associated with internal organ involvement. According to Mayes and colleagues, median survival in SSc is 11 years. Survival is determined by the extent of internal organ involvement. Prominent target organs include the skin, lungs, heart, kidneys, and gastrointestinal tract (Box 1). SSc has substantial clinical heterogeneity. Based on the constellation of clinical and laboratory findings present, patients are subclassified as "limited cutaneous SSc" or "diffuse cutaneous SSc" (Box 2). These two subtypes predict distinct patterns of organ involvement, clinical course, and survival. Some patients with SSc show features of overlap with other autoimmune diseases and manifest sicca syndrome, arthritis, myositis, or thyroiditis.

GENERAL PRINCIPLES OF THERAPY

In light of the clinical heterogeneity of SSc and its variable course, treatment must be individualized according to the

---

[1]Not FDA approved for this indication.

> **BOX 1 Prominent Organ Involvement in Systemic Sclerosis (SSc)**
>
> - Skin (inflammation, induration and tethering; hyper- and hypopigmentation, calcinosis)
> - Lungs (alveolitis and pulmonary fibrosis; pulmonary arterial hypertension)
> - Heart (restrictive cardiomyopathy, pericarditis)
> - Peripheral vascular (mucocutaneous telangiectasia, Raynaud's phenomenon, digital ulcers and infarction, watermelon stomach, male erectile dysfunction)
> - Gastrointestinal tract (see Box 4)
> - Muscle (myositis)
> - Joints (contractures, arthralgia, tendon friction rubs)

> **BOX 2 Clinical Features of Systemic Sclerosis (SSc) Subsets**
>
> - Limited cutaneous SSc
>   - Limited extent of skin induration (distal extremities and face); no truncal skin involvement; slowly progressive
>   - Prominent vascular involvement (cutaneous telangiectasia, Raynaud's phenomenon, digital ulcers; pulmonary hypertension)
>   - Calcinosis cutis
>   - Antibodies to centromere
> - Diffuse cutaneous SSc
>   - Progressive and diffuse skin induration; truncal involvement frequent
>   - Pulmonary fibrosis
>   - Scleroderma renal crisis
>   - Antibodies to topoisomerase-I

unique needs of each patient; some need early aggressive intervention, whereas others need a conservative symptom-based approach with close monitoring. According to Bryan and colleagues, predictors of poor outcome include older age onset (>60 years of age), anemia, evidence of significant cardiac or pulmonary involvement, tendon friction rubs, and the presence of antitopoisomerase antibodies. In general, therapies fall into two groups: those that target the underlying pathophysiologic process, and those that alleviate or reverse target organ complications. Because major internal organ involvement develops early, disease-modifying interventions should be considered before tissue damage becomes established. Because SSc is invariably a multisystem disease, a coordinated approach to evaluation and management by an integrated multidisciplinary team including a rheumatologist, pulmonologist, cardiologist, gastroenterologist, vascular or orthopedic surgeon, and physical therapist is desirable. Patients should also be given the opportunity to participate in controlled clinical trials on novel therapeutic agents.

DISEASE-MODIFYING THERAPIES

To date, no therapy is shown conclusively to be disease modifying in SSc. Nonetheless, based on historical or anecdotal evidence or empirical considerations, many agents are used widely in an attempt to reverse or halt the progression of the immunologic, vascular, and fibrotic damage (Box 3). In light of the potential toxicities associated with these therapies and their lack of proven benefit, decisions regarding their use must be considered carefully. In patients with limited SSc and stable disease, organ-based treatments directed toward specific complications of the disease (see later) are generally more appropriate than these generalized disease-modifying treatment strategies.

ORGAN-BASED TREATMENT APPROACHES

Therapy for Skin Involvement

Skin induration can be progressive and widespread in diffuse cutaneous SSc, whereas it is generally not prominent in limited cutaneous form. Extensive skin involvement often, but not invariably, predicts severe internal

BOX 3 Potentially Disease-Modifying Interventions for Systemic Sclerosis (SSc)

- Immunomodulatory
  - Methotrexate*
  - Cyclophosphamide*
  - Mycophenolate mofetil*
  - Antithymocyte globulin
  - Autologous stem cell therapy (with or without immune oblation)
- Antifibrotic
  - D-Penicillamine*
  - Interferon γ

*Although commonly used, to date these interventions have not been demonstrated in controlled clinical trials to be of unequivocal benefit in the treatment of SSc.

TABLE 2 Oral Vasodilator Therapy for Raynaud's Phenomenon in Systemic Sclerosis

Agent	Dose
Calcium Channel Blockers	
Nifedipine (Procardia)	10-30 mg three times daily
Diltiazem (Cardizem)	30-120 mg three times daily
Amlodipine (Norvasc)	5-20 mg daily
Felodipine (Plendil)	2.5-10 mg daily
Angiotensin II Receptor Antagonists	
Losartan (Cozaar)	25-100 mg daily
Valsartan (Diovan)	80-320 mg daily
Sympatholytic Agents	
Prazosin (Minipress)	1-5 mg daily
Doxazosin (Cardura)	1-16 mg daily
Nitroglycerin	2% ointment topically once daily

Adapted from Wigley FM: Raynaud's phenomenon. N Engl J Med 2002;347(13):1001-1008.

organ involvement. In diffuse SSc, skin induration generally peaks in the first 2 to 4 years of SSc, after which it regresses with spontaneous softening. In early disease, inflammation of the skin dominates, with edema, erythema, and pruritus. Patients at this stage benefit form antihistamines such as hydroxyzine (Atarax),[1] 25 mg at bedtime. Low-dose glucocorticoids such as prednisone,[1] 5 mg daily, provide substantial symptomatic relief for inflammation in early SSc but should be used with caution in light of the increased risk of scleroderma renal crisis (see later); patients taking low-dose prednisone[1] should be instructed to monitor their blood pressure daily. Digital ulcers can be managed using Duoderm[1] application to promote healing and topical povidone-iodine (Betadine)[1] solution for cleansing.

Therapy for Vascular Involvement

Raynaud's Phenomenon and Its Complications

Widespread damage of small and medium-sized peripheral blood vessels is virtually universal in SSc. Endothelial cell injury is associated with release of vasoconstrictors such as thromboxane and endothelin 1 (ET1), impaired production of vasodilators such as nitric oxide and prostacyclin, and platelet aggregation and thrombosis. What starts out as a reversible dysfunction of vascular smooth muscle often progresses to irreversible structural alterations characterized by intimal layer proliferation, medial hypertrophy, and adventitial fibrosis. Reduced blood flow and repeated episodes of ischemic reperfusion in the digits, kidneys, lungs, heart, and other involved organs cause tissue ischemia, progressive vascular damage, and fibrosis.

Cold-induced Raynaud's phenomenon is the most common presenting problem in SSc and may precede other manifestations of the disease by years. Repeated and increasingly severe Raynaud's episodes lead to digital ischemia, resulting in painful ulcers and nonhealing pitting scars and, in extreme cases, digital infarction and gangrene. Patients should be counseled to stop smoking and to avoid cold exposure, which triggers vasoconstriction; not only

the hands but the whole body should also be kept warm. Mild Raynaud's phenomenon can be effectively treated with orally active vasodilators (Table 2) and treatment is most commonly started with calcium channel blockers. Infection complicating digital ulcers should be treated aggressively with antibiotics; such ulcers may take months to heal and may progress to osteomyelitis. The ET1 receptor blocker bosentan (Tracleer),[1] 125 mg twice daily, is effective in preventing digital ulcers. Patients with impending digital infarction may respond to intravenous epoprostenol (Flolan),[1] 0.5 to 6 μg/kg body weight per minute for 6 to 24 hours, or nonpharmacologic interventions such as sympathetic ganglion blockade and surgical digital sympathectomy. The role of statin drugs, antioxidants such as tocopherol (vitamin E)[1] (400 IU daily), and diets rich in fish oils in preventing vascular damage in Raynaud's phenomenon are not yet adequately studied.

Pulmonary Arterial Hypertension

Pulmonary arterial hypertension (PAH), which occurs in at least 15% of SSc patients, has a major impact on survival. PAH may complicate interstitial pulmonary fibrosis or may occur in the absence of parenchymal lung disease; the latter is indistinguishable from primary (idiopathic) and familial pulmonary hypertension. Because PAH may be asymptomatic until advanced, it was historically underdiagnosed in SSc. Moderately severe PAH is associated with exertional dyspnea, chest pain, and syncope; right-sided heart failure is seen in late-stage disease. Emphasis must be placed on early preclinical recognition of PAH. A combination of pulmonary function testing and Doppler echocardiography is appropriate for screening and should be performed yearly. Right heart catheterization is the gold standard for determining pulmonary arterial pressures and cardiac index and for excluding pulmonary embolism.

[1]Not FDA approved for this indication.

[1]Not FDA approved for this indication.

Several new classes of agents provide at least short-term symptomatic and hemodynamic improvement in PAH. Patients with New York Heart Association functional class III or IV symptoms (ordinary activity causing dyspnea, chest pain, or near syncope) should start an orally active ET1 receptor blocker such as bosentan (Tracleer). In addition, warfarin anticoagulation (to achieve an INR [international normalized ratio] of 1.5 to 2.0), low-flow oxygen therapy, diuretics, and digitalization are generally indicated. Patients who fail to respond to ET1 antagonists may benefit from parenteral prostacyclin analogues such as inhaled iloprost (Ventavis), every 2 hours up to 45 μg daily, or continuous infusions of subcutaneous treprostinil (Remodulin) 1.25 μg/kg per minute, or intravenous epoprostenol (Flolan), 2 to 10 μg/kg per minute. A major limitation of these therapies is their cost, now exceeding $30,000 per year. Furthermore, because of their short half-lives, prostacyclin analogues must be administered by continuous infusion or frequent inhalations. Epoprostenol requires long-term ambulatory central venous catheterization, which may be complicated by line sepsis and pump failure with potentially catastrophic consequences. Combinations of a prostacyclin analogue together with an ET1 antagonist or a phosphodiesterase type 5 inhibitor such as sildenafil (Viagra),[1] up to 50 mg three times daily, appear to be well tolerated and provide added benefit. Surgical options for patients unresponsive to pharmacologic therapies include atrial septostomy and lung transplantation. In light of the complexity involved, the evaluation and management of PAH in SSc patients should be coordinated by specialized centers having appropriate expertise.

Therapy for Interstitial Lung Disease

Some degree of interstitial lung disease is present in most patients with SSc and is a leading cause of death. The extent and progression of pulmonary fibrosis are major determinants of outcome. Combined with pulmonary function testing, high-resolution computed tomography (HRCT) scan of the chest is more sensitive for interstitial lung disease screening than chest radiography. A ground-glass appearance generally correlates with active inflammation (alveolitis). Patients with alveolitis may benefit from cyclophosphamide (Cytoxan)[1] (orally up to 50 mg daily, or intravenously as pulse therapy up to 1000 mg/m² monthly) to stabilize lung function. Low-dose prednisone[1] (up to 20 mg daily) is often used in combination with cyclophosphamide. The optimal duration of cyclophosphamide[1] treatment is uncertain, but some experts recommend at least a year. General supportive measures include pneumococcal vaccination and yearly influenza immunization, avoidance of smoking, prevention of gastroesophageal reflux, nasal oxygen supplementation, and bronchodilators. Respiratory tract infections should be treated with empirical antibiotics. For selected patients with progressive respiratory decline, lung transplantation remains an option.

Therapy for Gastrointestinal Tract Involvement

Gastrointestinal involvement is common, can be extensive, and significantly contributes to the morbidity of SSc.

> **BOX 4 Gastrointestinal Tract Complications of Systemic Sclerosis (SSc)**
>
> - Esophageal dysmotility leading to dysphagia and chronic gastroesophageal reflux; dyspepsia, esophagitis, strictures, ulcers, pulmonary aspiration; Barrett's esophagus and esophageal adenocarcinoma
> - Watermelon stomach with upper gastrointestinal bleeding
> - Gastroparesis and small bowel hypomotility
> - Blind loop syndrome with malabsorption, weight loss, diarrhea
> - Large bowel pseudo-obstruction
> - Colonic perforation
> - Pneumatosis cystoides intestinalis

Gastroesophageal reflux may be associated with dyspepsia, dysphagia, and regurgitation and can lead to chronic esophagitis and its complications (Box 4). Reflux should be managed by elevating the head of the bed, eliminating triggers such as chocolates, alcohol, and tobacco, and restricting food intake before going to sleep. Most patients require long-term treatment with proton pump inhibitors such as omeprazole (Prilosec)[1] in doses sufficient to suppress reflux symptoms (up to 160 mg daily). Prokinetic agents such as metoclopramide (Reglan)[1] (10 mg four times daily) or erythromycin[1] (250 mg three times daily) may be effective for gastroparesis. Chronic diarrhea and malabsorption caused by small bowel bacterial overgrowth can be treated with periodic courses of tetracycline[1] (500 mg four times daily) or metronidazole (Flagyl)[1] (500 mg three times daily). Some patients benefit from subcutaneous octreotide injections (Sandostatin,)[1] (50 μg one to four times daily). Nutritional assessment and support are important aspects of management. Gastric vascular ectasia (watermelon stomach) is frequent in SSc and causes recurrent occult gastrointestinal bleeding. It can be effectively treated with laser argon ablation.

Therapy for Renal Involvement

Scleroderma renal crisis, which develops in up to 15% of patients with SSc, was uniformly fatal in the pre–angiotensin-converting enzyme (ACE)[1] inhibitor era. Risk factors include progressive skin induration, male sex, and glucocorticoid use. Renal crisis characteristically manifests with an abrupt rise in blood pressure, frequently associated with retinal hemorrhages, and occasionally with seizures and pulmonary hemorrhage, microangiopathic hemolysis, and rapidly progressive oliguric renal insufficiency. The key to controlling this dreaded complication of SSc is early recognition. Accordingly, high-risk patients should monitor their blood pressure daily, and if there is a rise in blood pressure, a new onset of proteinuria, or a rise in creatinine, patients should be hospitalized for close monitoring and aggressive management. Some patients (<10%) develop scleroderma renal crisis in the absence of hypertension. Treatment with increasing doses of ACE inhibitors such as captopril (Capoten)[1] (up to 200 mg daily) should be

---

TABLE 3 Clinical Characteristics of Idiopathic Inflammatory Myopathies

Dermatomyositis	Polymyositis	Inclusion	Body Myositis
Female to male	2:1	1:1	1:3
Age (y)	10-80	30-60	50-70
Muscle atrophy	Frequent	Rare	Frequent
Skin rash	Yes	No	No
Lung disease	Frequent	Frequent	
Dysphagia	Frequent	Rare	Rare
Arthralgia	Frequent	Rare	No
Malignancy	5%-17%	Rare	No

started immediately. The creatinine may continue to rise even on ACE inhibitor therapy[1] and with adequate blood pressure control. Despite aggressive treatment, progressive renal insufficiency may ensue, necessitating dialysis. Nevertheless, up to 40% of patients may ultimately recover adequate renal function to discontinue dialysis. There is insufficient evidence to support prophylactic use of ACE inhibitors[1] in SSc.

Polymyositis/Dermatomyositis

Idiopathic inflammatory myopathies (IIM) include adult and childhood dermatomyositis (DM), polymyositis (PM), myositis associated with malignancy or other connective tissue diseases, and inclusion body myositis (IBM) (Table 3). Although the etiology of IIM is unknown, the presence of cellular infiltrates in the muscle provides strong evidence for an immune mechanism of muscle damage. In DM, the main immune effector response appears to be humoral and directed against the microvasculature, whereas in both PM and IBM, cytotoxic CD8+ T cells and macrophages invade and destroy muscle fibers. Inflammatory myopathies are characterized by progressive symmetric weakness of the proximal muscles, causing difficulty walking, standing, and lifting objects. In DM, a characteristic erythematous rash on the face, eyelids, neck, upper chest, and back is seen. Muscle biopsy is helpful in differentiating PM/DM from drug-induced myopathies and from endocrine and metabolic myopathies. Myositis-specific antibodies may be of prognostic value; patients with Jo-1 or other anti–aminoacyl-tRNA autoantibodies are at high risk for

[1]Not FDA approved for this indication.

interstitial lung disease (ILD) and show poor response to therapy. The levels of serum creatine kinase (CK) are useful in assessing disease activity. Involvement of the gastrointestinal muscles can lead to dysphagia. Patients with new myositis and especially adults with dermatomyositis, should be carefully screened for malignancy.

GENERAL PRINCIPLES OF THERAPY

Immunosuppressive therapies are the primary treatment for the IIM. Early intervention is crucial to prevent irreversible muscle damage. Because long-term administration of high doses of corticosteroids is associated with significant morbidity, a second-line agent such as methotrexate[1] or azathioprine[1] should be introduced early. Intravenous Ig therapy,[1] cyclophosphamide (Cytoxan),[1] and cyclosporine (Neoral)[1] are also used with some benefit. Rehabilitative and physical therapeutic interventions are essential to complement pharmacologic therapy. Although PM and DM can usually be controlled by immunosuppressive agents, the treatment of IBM remains unsatisfactory.

Corticosteroids

Prednisone[1] (1 mg/kg daily) is effective as initial therapy in the majority of the cases. In patients with rapidly progressive myositis or extramuscular manifestation such as ILD, intravenous pulse methylprednisolone[1] (1 g daily for 3 days) may be used. Both muscle strength and functional status and serum levels of CK should be checked regularly. Clinical improvement usually follows a fall in CK levels. Prednisone at 10 mg daily may be needed for 6 to 12 months.

[1]Not FDA approved for this indication.

BOX 5 Rationale for Using a Second-Line Immunosuppressive Agent in Idiopathic Inflammatory Myopathy (IIM)

- Increased risk of corticosteroid-related side effects (diabetes mellitus, osteoporosis)
- Disease relapse after corticosteroid tapering attempts jeopardy
- Corticosteroid complications (myopathy)
- Severe or progressive myositis
- Serious extramuscular manifestations
- Lack of efficiency of corticosteroid as a single agent

CURRENT DIAGNOSIS

- Protean manifestations in multiple organs
- Marked clinical heterogeneity
- Unpredictable, often remitting-relapsing clinical course
- Diagnosis based on characteristic constellations of clinical and laboratory features (criteria)
- Accurate diagnosis, specific subset, and stage of disease must be established

Progressive weakness in the face of declining CK levels suggests steroid myopathy.

Other Immunosuppressive Agents

In patients who fail to respond to corticosteroids, azathioprine[1] (2 mg/kg daily) or methotrexate[1] (20 mg weekly) may be used. Box 5 shows the indications for using second-line agents. Blood cell counts and liver functions should be closely monitored. Intermittent bolus IVIG (up to 2 g/kg infused every 4 to 8 weeks) may also be effective in some steroid-resistant DM patients and for severe esophageal involvement.

Treatment of Extramuscular Manifestations

Alveolitis and ILD are frequent complications. Some experts recommend high-dose daily corticosteroids in combination with a second-line immunosuppressive agent (cyclophosphamide,[1] azathioprine,[1] or cyclosporine[1]) early in the treatment. Skin rash can be effectively treated with hydroxychloroquine (Plaquenil)[1] (200 to 400 mg daily). Patients with severe proximal dysphagia may need a feeding tube to prevent aspiration and malnutrition.

Rehabilitative Measures

The goal of physical therapy is to preserve existing muscle function and to prevent muscle atrophy and joint contractures. Bedridden patients should receive passive exercise, stretching, and massage. As muscle strength improves, resistive exercise followed by an active aerobic conditioning regimen can be introduced. Proximal oropharyngeal dysphagia should be managed by speech therapy.

REFERENCES

Bryan C, Knight C, Black CM, Silman AJ: Prediction of five-year survival following presentation with scleroderma: Development of a simple model using three disease factors at first visit. Arthritis Rheum 1999;42(12):2660-2665.

Dalakas MC: High-dose intravenous immunoglobulin in inflammatory myopathies: Experience based on controlled clinical trials. Neurol Sci 2003;24(Suppl 4):S256-S259.

Ionnaou Y, Isenberg DA: Current concepts for the management of systemic lupus erythematosus in adults: A therapeutic approach. Postgrad Med J 2002;78:599-606.

Isenberg DA, Allen E, Farewell V, et al: International consensus outcome measures for patients with idiopathic inflammatory myopathies. Development and initial validation of myositis activity and damage indices in patients with adult onset disease. Rheumatology (Oxford) 2004;43(1):49-54.

Manzi S: Treatment of systemic lupus erythematosus. In Klippel JH, Stone J, Weyand C, Crofford LJ (eds): Primer on the Rheumatic Diseases. Atlanta, Arthritis Foundation, 2001, pp 346-352.

Mayes MD, Lacey JV Jr, Beebe-Dimmer J, et al: Prevalence, incidence, survival, and disease characteristics of systemic sclerosis in a large US population. Arthritis Rheum 2003;48(8):2246-2255.

Oddis CV: Idiopathic inflammatory myopathies: A treatment update. Curr Rheumatol Rep 2003;5(6):431-436.

Ortmann RA, Klippel JH: Update on cyclophosphamide for systemic lupus erythematosus. Rheum Dis Clin North Am 2000;26:363-375.

Ramirez A, Varga J: Pulmonary arterial hypertension in systemic sclerosis: Clinical manifestations, pathophysiology, evaluation, and management. Treat Respir Med 2004;3(6):339-352.

Wigley FM: Raynaud's phenomenon. N Engl J Med 2002;347(13): 1001-1008.

---

[1]Not FDA approved for this indication.

Cutaneous Vasculitis

Method of
Manisha J. Patel, MD, and
Joseph L. Jorizzo, MD

Vasculitis refers to inflammation and necrosis of blood vessels. It can be local or systemic and may be primary or secondary to another disease process. In patients with systemic involvement, the kidneys, gastrointestinal (GI) tract, or peripheral nerves may be involved. The classic cutaneous manifestation of small-vessel vasculitis is palpable purpura; the clinical manifestation greatly depends on the size and type of the vessel affected.

Clinical Presentation

The typical primary skin lesion of small-vessel cutaneous vasculitis (CV) is palpable purpura with lesions ranging in size from 1 mm to several centimeters (Figure 1). The lesions arise as a simultaneous *crop* and result from the exposure to an inciting stimulus. Usually macular in the early stages, lesions may progress to wide array of lesions including, papules, nodules, vesicles, plaques, bullae, or pustules. Secondary findings include ulceration, necrosis, and postinflammatory hyperpigmentation. Other cutaneous findings include livedo reticularis, edema,, and urticarial lesions. Lesions most commonly occur on dependent areas, such as ankles and lower legs or other areas prone to stasis.

Although normally asymptomatic, local symptoms may include pruritus, pain, or burning. Systemic symptoms including fever, arthralgias, myalgias, anorexia, or GI pain should raise the suspicion that the CV may be associated with a systemic vasculitis.

Typically 50% of all patients with CV experience an acute or transient course, 30% develop chronic disease, and 20% experience relapsing disease. The percentage of patients with CV who have systemic involvement of one or more systems depends on the subspecialty of the series authors and the definition of systemic involvement. Most patients

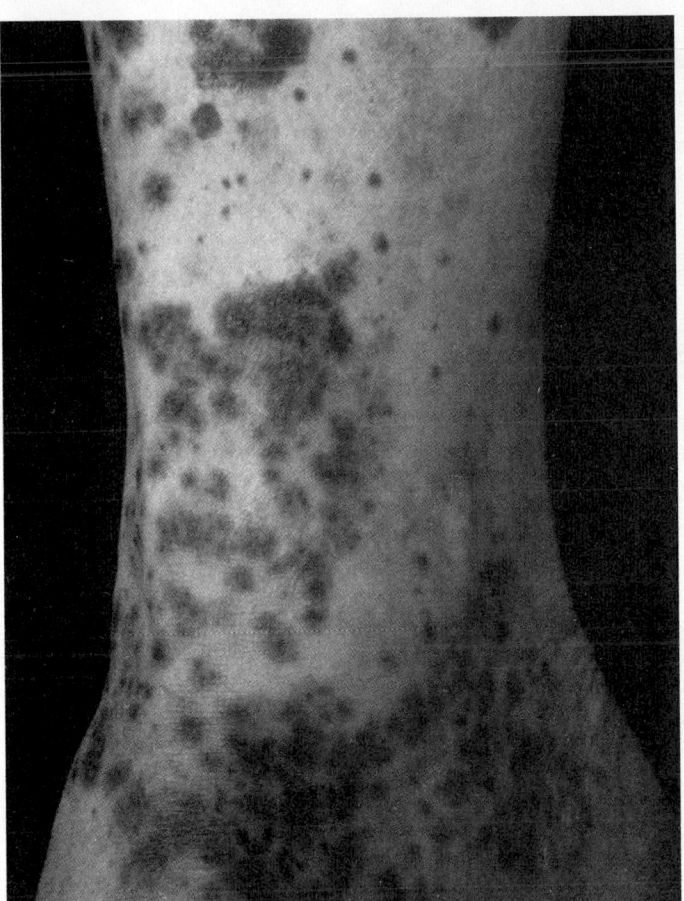

FIGURE 1. Small-vessel cutaneous vasculitis. Palpable purpura and early central necrosis are seen on the distal lower extremity. (Courtesy of Dr. Kelly Barham, Wake Forest University School of Medicine, Winston-Salem, NC.)

of IgM or activated third component of complement (C3) in the superficial dermal papillary vessels. One exception is the deposition of IgA in patients with Henoch-Schönlein purpura. Documenting leukocytoclastic vasculitis in biopsy specimens is essential to confirming the diagnosis.

Etiology

Small-vessel CV is considered to be an aberrant immune complex response that is usually triggered by an infection, exposure to a drug, or association with an autoimmune disease; most etiologic factors identified have been incriminated by association rather than by direct demonstration. Between 50% and 60% of patients have no identifiable cause. Of the approximately 50% of patients in whom a cause is identifiable, 20% are associated with infections; and another 20% are thought to be triggered by an exposure to a drug. Bacterial infections associated with CV include streptococcus, staphylococcus, and gram-negative organisms. Several viral agents include HIV, hepatitis B and C, herpes simplex virus (HSV), and influenza. Suspected medications include antibiotics (penicillins, sulfonamides), anticonvulsants, isoniazid (Laniazid), oral contraceptives, and thiazides. Less than 5% of patients have underlying connective tissue disease. There have been patients with small-vessel CV reported rarely in patients with malignancies, especially Hodgkin's disease, mycosis fungoides, and adult T-cell lymphoma.

Differential Diagnosis

Not all dermatoses associated with purpura are a result of vasculitis. In the differential diagnosis of vasculitis, be aware of disorders that may present with livedo or infarcted lesions secondary to vascular occlusion disorders. Some examples of vaso-occlusive disorders include cryoglobulinemia, cholesterol emboli, Sneddon's syndrome, septic emboli, and malignant atrophic papulosis (Degos' disease). The histopathology in these disorders results from either initially occlusive or mediation by antiphospholipid antibodies, and therefore, falls into the category of microvascular occlusion. The differential diagnosis also includes trauma, coagulopathies, and thrombocytopenia. Purpuras secondary to coagulopathies and thrombocytopenia are noninflammatory and often nonpalpable; they can be distinguished promptly on histologic and laboratory testing.

Given the wide array of systemic diseases that can be associated with small-vessel CV, it is important to carefully

presenting to dermatologists do not have significant systemic involvement, excluding arthralgias, myalgias, fever, and serum sickness-like symptoms. It is best to consider that every patient with small-vessel CV may have systemic disease; this mandates a careful history, physical examination, and laboratory evaluation. Table 1 summarizes the key steps in evaluating suspected small-vessel CV and highlights the assessment for possible systemic involvement.

Histopathology

The hallmark histopathologic pattern of small-vessel CV is leukocytoclastic vasculitis. The histologic specimen shows an infiltration of neutrophils within and around blood vessel walls; leukocytoclasia (degranulation and fragmentation of neutrophils leading to the production of nuclear dust); fibrinoid necrosis of the damaged vessel walls; and necrosis, swelling, and proliferation of the endothelial cells. New clinical lesions should be selected for biopsy because specimens taken too late (i.e., older than 48 hours) may show the pathology of repair more than of the initial injury. Direct immunofluorescence microscopic studies on fresh lesions frequently demonstrate perivascular deposits

---

CURRENT DIAGNOSIS

- Clinical spectrum of lesions ranging from purpura to palpable purpura, urticarial lesions, or ulcers: concentrated on dependent areas
- Small-vessel CV involves postcapillary venules only
- Histologic finding: leukocytoclastic vasculitis
- Pathogenesis: circulating immune complexes, neutrophils, cytokines, and adhesion molecules

Abbreviation: CV = cutaneous vasculitis.

TABLE 1 Evaluation of Suspected Small Vessel Cutaneous Vasculitis

Confirming Histopathologic Correlation	Assessing the Extent of the Disease	Establishing Etiology
Punch biopsy early lesion	General • Myalgia • Arthralgia • Fever	Infection (bacterial, viral, fungal, acid-fast bacilli, other)
Incisional biopsy for suspected larger vessel vasculitis	Renal involvement (acute and chronic renal failure) • Proteinuria • Hematuria Nervous system • Central or peripheral • Diffuse or local findings	Drugs Diseases associated with immune complexes • Connective tissue/autoimmune diseases • Malignancy (especially myelodysplastic) • Inflammatory bowel disease Idiopathic (50%)
	Musculoskeletal involvement • Nonerosive polyarthritis Gastrointestinal system • Abdominal pain (colicky, nausea, vomiting, diarrhea) • Gastrointestinal bleeding (melena or hematemesis) Pulmonary involvement • Pleural effusion • Pleuritis • Hemoptysis Pericardial involvement (myocardial angiitis or pericarditis) • Pericardial effusion Ocular involvement (retinal vasculitis) • Conjunctivitis • Keratitis Other	

Modified from Barham KL et al: Rook's Textbook of Dermatology, 7th ed. Oxford, Blackwell Publishing, 2004.

evaluate each patient for coexistent disease; the first manifestation of large-vessel vasculitis is often small-vessel disease.

HENOCH-SCHÖNLEIN PURPURA

Henoch-Schönlein purpura (HSP) deserves specific mention given its history and frequent occurrence. Heberden first described a single patient with HSP in 1801. Johann Schönlein and Eduard Henoch elucidated features in the mid-19th century as a tetrad of palpable purpura, arthritis, and GI and renal involvement. Henoch-Schönlein purpura is defined by the Chapel Hill Consensus Conference as a vasculitis affecting small vessels, involving deposition of IgA immune complexes that characteristically involves the skin, GI system, and glomeruli with or without arthralgia or arthritis. Approximately 30% of cases follow an upper respiratory infection. The clinical outcome is excellent with fewer than 10% of patients developing chronic disease. A small percent of patients will develop persistent renal or GI disease requiring systemic immunosuppressive therapy.

URTICARIAL VASCULITIS

Another important subtype of small-vessel CV is urticarial vasculitis. Urticarial vasculitis is a chronic disorder consisting of episodic urticarial and/or angioedematous lesions lasting longer than 24 hours that histologically manifest features of leukocytoclastic vasculitis. Urticarial vasculitis may range from patients with only urticarial skin lesions to those with urticarial vasculitis associated with hypocomplementemia with some systemic features; this meets criteria for systemic lupus erythematosus. Patients with urticarial vasculitis may also have underlying autoimmune connective tissue diseases, infections (hepatitis B and C), neoplastic processes, or medications as underlying etiologic factors. Treatment is directed at underlying etiologies and/or follows the same therapeutic ladder as for small-vessel CV (Table 2).

Treatment

Because small-vessel CV is generally self-limited, treatment is often unnecessary except for symptomatic relief. When possible, identification and removal of a causative agent (e.g., infection, drug, chemicals, food) should be accomplished. Removal of an inciting agent is occasionally followed by rapid resolution of the lesions and no other treatment is indicated; otherwise, local and systemic therapies are recommended. Symptomatic improvement may be achieved with leg elevation, gradient support stockings, nonsteroidal anti-inflammatory drugs, and antihistamines.

TABLE 2 Therapeutic Ladder for Small-Vessel Cutaneous Vasculitis

	Double-Blind Studies	Case Series	Case Reports
Skin lesions alone	Colchicine[1]	Nonsteroidal anti-inflammatory drugs Dapsone[1]	Supportive therapy • Antihistamines • Pentoxifylline (Trental)[1] • Hydroxychloroquine (Plaquenil)[1] • Thalidomide (Thalomid)[1] • Low-dose weekly methotrexate (Rheumatrex)[1]
Ulcerative skin lesions alone		Prednisone[1]	
Systemic disease	Interferon-α and ribavirin (Rebetron) (if associated with hepatitis C) 3 million units 3/wk and 1000 mg/d, respectively	Prednisone[1] Azathioprine (Imuran)[1] 1–2.5 mg/kg/d PO as single dose or divided in half Cyclophosphamide (Cytoxan)[1] pulsed dosing regimen, 40–50 mg/kg IV in divided doses over 2–5 d or 10–15 mg/kg IV q 7–10 d or 3–5 mg/kg IV 2/wk	Mycophenolate mofetil (CellCept)[1] 500–2000 mg PO bid Cyclosporine (Neoral, Sandimmune)[1] 2.5 mg/kg/d PO divided in half qd; after 4 wk, dose may be increased 0.5 mg/kg/d at 2-wk intervals; maximum of 4 mg/kg/d • IV gammaglobulin (Gammagard)[1] • Extracorporeal immunomodulation • Biologic agents: infliximab (Remicade),[1] etanercept (Enbrel)[1] (TNF-α inhibitors)
	Methotrexate (Trexall)[1] 7.5–15 mg once a week*		

*There is no study associated with this drug.
[1]Not FDA approved for this indication.
Abbreviations: IV = intravenously, TNF-α = tumor necrosis factor-α.
Modified from Barham KL et al: Rook's Textbook of Dermatology, 7th ed. Oxford, Blackwell Publishing, 2004.

Cutaneous Vasculitis

Small-vessel CV with persistent palpable purpura without significant internal organ complications may respond to treatment with oral colchicine[1] in doses of 0.6 mg two to three times daily. Dosing is limited by GI symptoms. This therapy is supported by anecdotal reports, but a statistically significant difference was not confirmed in a randomized controlled trial. Dapsone[1] (50 to 200 mg per day) has also been used in patients only having skin involvement.

Systemic treatment is advised for patients with small-vessel CV who have significant systemic manifestations or significant cutaneous ulceration. However, almost no double-blind, placebo-controlled prospective trials exist. Table 2 describes a therapeutic ladder for small-vessel CV. The medications discussed in Table 2 have not been FDA approved for this indication. Oral corticosteroids (Prednisone[1] 0.5 to 1 mg/kg per day) are indicated for progressive, symptomatic nodular, vesicular, or ulcerating purpura as well as systemic involvement. Once the patient's symptoms have stabilized, prednisone should be tapered gradually over 3 to 6 weeks because a rapid taper can lead to clinical disease rebound.

Small-vessel CV can manifest clinically with a spectrum of cutaneous lesions; palpable purpura is the classic presentation. The hallmark histologic appearance is a leukocytoclastic vasculitis. There is a presumed immune complex mediated pathogenesis. The therapeutic approach requires elimination of the cause (drugs, chemicals, infection) when possible. In most patients, only the skin is involved and can be treated with supportive measures. The most important step in evaluation is the full workup to find etiology and extent (systemic involvement) of the disease process. Skin manifestations alone may be managed with nonsteroidal anti-inflammatory drugs, gradient support stockings, colchicine, and dapsone. Systemic treatment is advised in small-vessel CV with significant systemic manifestations or those with significant cutaneous ulceration.

---

[1]Not FDA approved for this indication.

 CURRENT THERAPY

- Small-vessel CV is generally self-limited; treatment is often unnecessary except for symptomatic relief, which may be achieved with leg elevation, gradient support stockings, nonsteroidal anti-inflammatory drugs, and antihistamines.
- Skin manifestations alone may be managed with agents such as colchicine and dapsone.
- Systemic treatment is advised for patients with significant systemic manifestations or those with significant cutaneous ulceration.

Abbreviation: CV = cutaneous vasculitis.

[1]Not FDA approved for this indication.

REFERENCES

Fiorentino DF: Cutaneous vasculitis. J Am Acad Dermatol 2003;48(3): 311-340.

Gonzalez-Gay MA, Garcia-Porrua C, Pujol RM: Clinical approach to cutaneous vasculitis. Curr Opin Rheumatol 2005;17(1):56-61.

Lamprecht P: TNF-alpha inhibitors in systemic vasculitides and connective tissue diseases. Autoimmun Rev 2005;4(1):28-34.

Lotti T, Ghersetich I, Comacchi C, Jorizzo JL: Cutaneous small-vessel vasculitis. J Am Acad Dermatol 1998;39(5 Pt 1):667-687.

Diseases of the Nails

Method of
Bianca Maria Piraccini, MD, PhD,
and Matilde Iorizzo, MD

Nail abnormalities are frequent and their etiology extremely variable, including physiologic, inflammatory, traumatic, infective, and neoplastic causes. The diagnosis of nail diseases requires a good knowledge of nail anatomy and physiology because nail symptoms are strictly related to the portion of the nail apparatus that is affected (Table 1). The nail plate is continuously produced throughout life (at a rate of 2 to 4 mm/month for fingernails and 1 to 2 mm/month for toenails) by the matrix, which lies under the proximal nail fold. The nail plate emerges from the proximal nail fold in correspondence to the cuticle and moves distally, strictly adhering to the epithelium of the underlying nail bed. The strong nail plate nail bed adhesion is essential for the tactile, grasping, and defensive functions of the nail. The nail detaches from the nail bed at the end of the digit, in the area of the hyponychium, where the distal nail plate appears white.

The healthy nail plate is transparent and appears pink because it permits visualization of the color of the highly vascularized nail bed. The proximal part of the nail plate covers the distal matrix, which appears as a distally convex whitish crescent, the lunula.

The clinical examination of a patient with nail dystrophy includes a careful examination of all 20 nails, the skin, hair, and all the mucosae and a detailed clinical history. Optional diagnostic tools include microbiologic examinations, radiography, magnetic resonance imaging, and histopathology.

When treating nail diseases, keep in mind the following:

- Topical drugs do not reach the nail matrix, which lies beneath the nail plate and proximal nail fold.
- Because drugs do not easily penetrate the nail plate, removal of the nail plate may be indicated to treat nail bed diseases.
- Owing to the slow growth rate, complete replacement of a fingernail takes approximately 6 months and that of a toenail 1 year. For this reason improvement of nail symptoms is slow, and treatment should last longer than treatment for skin conditions. This should be clearly explained to patients to avoid unrealistic expectations and poor treatment compliance.

- Duration of systemic treatment is best chosen according to the improvement of the nail condition because nail growth rates and treatment responses vary between patients. Follow-up of once a month or once every 2 months is the best way to achieve correct management of patients.

Table 2 lists all systemic/intralesional treatments mentioned in this article, summarizing dosages, modalities of administration, and special care measures.

Acute Paronychia

Acute inflammation of the proximal nail fold is a common consequence of biting or chewing the periungual tissues and usually affects children. It can also be a consequence of an excessively aggressive manicure. Gram-positive bacteria, usually *Staphylococcus aureus*, invade and proliferate in the space under the fold, giving rise to the acute inflammation that may lead to abscess formation.

Differential diagnosis includes herpes simplex infection: In this case, acute paronychia occurs most commonly in adults, especially health workers; the flare is recurrent; and vesicles are often observed on the periungual skin or under the nail plate. Swabs for microbiologic study should be taken for a correct diagnosis.

Trachyonychia

Trachyonychia, also known as 20-nail dystrophy, is a chronic disease characterized by a mild inflammation of the proximal nail matrix that results in the production of a brittle, rough, opaque nail plate. The damage is limited to the superficial layer of the nail plate because this is the portion produced by the proximal nail matrix. More common in children, it usually affects patients with severe alopecia areata, in which it is considered a nail localization of the disease. The course of trachyonychia does not parallel that of alopecia areata.

Even if several studies have shown that the pathology of patients with trachyonychia may lead to a diagnosis of psoriasis or lichen planus, the clinical features and the outcome of the disease are always the same: Nail lesions last for a long time and tend to improve slowly and spontaneously.

Ingrowing Toenails

Ingrowing toenails are the most common nail disease of teenagers, who usually seek advice when the problem has been present for a long time and conservative treatment is no longer possible. Nail ingrowing is the final results of several factors:

- Lateral deviation of the nail plate in respect to the longitudinal axis of the digit (congenital malalignment), which predisposes to penetration of the lateral edge of the nail into the fold
- Improper cutting or manual removal of the distal edge of the nail, a frequent habit of children and teenagers, which produces a sharp nail plate edge

Nail Portion	Function	Symptoms When Damaged
Nail matrix	Nail plate production	• Nail plate abnormalities • Nail plate absence
Nail bed/hyponychium	Nail plate attachment to underlying tissues	• Nail detachment (onycholysis) • Subungual hyperkeratosis • Nail uplifting
Proximal nail fold	Protection of the matrix through sealing the skin of the digit to the nail plate by the cuticle	• Absence of the cuticle • Erythema and swelling • Nail matrix damage
Nail matrix	Nail plate production	• Nail plate abnormalities • Nail plate absence • Nail detachment (onycholysis)
Nail bed/hyponychium	Nail plate attachment to underlying tissues	• Subungual hyperkeratosis • Nail uplifting • Absence of the cuticle
Proximal nail fold	Protection of the matrix through sealing the skin of the digit to the nail plate by the cuticle	• Erythema and swelling • Nail matrix damage

• Hyperhydrosis of the feet, which facilitates nail plate breaking with formation of sharp edges.

All these factors contribute to the formation of a sharp spicule on the distolateral edge of the nail plate that with walking penetrates and damages the soft tissues of the lateral fold. This produces pain and periungual inflammation (stage 1, according to Zaias' classification); with time, the injured dermis of the nail fold gives rise to a granulation tissue (pyogenic granuloma), which emerges from the lateral fold and appears as a painful bleeding nodule (stage 2). If the condition lasts longer, the granulation tissue induces the growth of a newly formed skin epithelium that partially covers the nail plate, fixing it in place (stage 3).

Chronic Paronychia

Chronic paronychia is a common condition that typically affects predisposed persons whose hands are in frequent contact with water, humidity, detergents, and irritants, such as housewives and food handlers. Irritation and maceration of the proximal nail fold lead to inflammation and swelling of the fold with arrested production of the cuticle. Because the role of the cuticle is to protect the nail matrix from the environment by sealing the skin of the dorsal digit to the nail plate, its disappearance causes penetration of water, dirt, food particles, and microorganisms under the nail fold. This results in nail matrix damage with production of a nail plate with an irregular surface where dirt and microorganisms (*Pseudomonas aeruginosa*) easily accumulate, causing a greenish-black irregular discoloration. *Candida albicans* is frequently isolated from nails with paronychia, but the yeast is only a secondary colonizer and not the primary cause of the disease.

Nail Fragility

Nail brittleness is a common problem for women, who complain of cosmetic and functional problems associated with the condition. Overall, it is similar to skin dryness, and results from excessive dehydration of the nail plate caused by environmental and intrinsic factors. The nail is fragile and tends to split in horizontal layers in its distal portion, causing irregularities and breakages of the free edge. Nail fragility is very difficult to cure, and predisposed individuals tend to have frequent recurrences.

Onychomycosis

Onychomycosis is one of the most frequent nail disorders, usually affecting the toenails of adults. The most common form (up to 70% of the cases, according to our experience) is distal subungual onychomycosis caused by dermatophytes, where fungi invade the nail bed causing onycholysis and subungual hyperkeratosis with typical yellow-brown scales accumulated under the nail plate. White superficial onychomycosis is frequently seen in elderly people, in whom it involves several toenails and appears as white opaque patches on the superficial nail. Invasion of the nail by nondermatophytic molds is not rare in Italy, where it accounts for 15% of onychomycosis, but different figures have been reported in other countries. What characterizes mold onychomycosis (caused by *Fusarium* species, *Aspergillus* species, and *Scopulariopsis brevicaulis*) is the particular clinical feature, consisting of acute periungual inflammation associated with the findings of a severe distal subungual onychomycosis or of a proximal subungual onychomycosis. In proximal subungual onychomycosis, the nail shows a patch of subungual yellow-white discoloration that starts from under the cuticle. White superficial onychomycosis may be also caused by nondermatophytic molds: in this case, the nail plate is invaded more deeply and diffusely, and the periungual tissues are mildly erythematous.

Onychomycosis caused by *Candida* species is rare and only seen in patients with immunodeficiencies, such as HIV infection, iatrogenic immunodepression, or chronic mucocutaneous candidiasis. *Candida* invades all nail epithelia, causing a total onychomycosis characterized by paronychia, nail plate opacity and friability, and nail bed hyperkeratosis.

TABLE 2 Systemic/Intralesional Treatments with Dosages, Modalities of Administration, and Special Care Measures

Type of Treatment	Modality of Administration	Dosage	Duration	Notes
Systemic Steroids				
Triamcinolone acetonide (Kenalog)	IM 1/mo	0.5 mg/kg	4–6 mo	
Methylprednisolone (Medrol)	PO	32 mg/d	2 wk	Add gastric antacids
Intralesional Steroids				
Triamcinolone acetonide (Kenalog)	Injections into matrix or nail bed	2–3 mL per digit of 10 mg/mL solution	1–2 mo	• Some skills necessary • Local anesthesia required
Systemic Antifungals				
Terbinafine (Lamisil)	PO	250 mg/d	• 2 mo fingernails • 4 mo toenails	• Not effective in *Candida* • Not if hepatic problems
Itraconazole (Sporanox)	PO	200 mg bid × 1 wk/mo	• 2 mo fingernails • 4 mo toenails	• Not if hepatic problems • Possible drug interactions
Systemic Retinoids				
Acitretin (Soriatane)	PO	0.3–0.5 mg/kg/d	4–6 mo	• Monitor hepatic and renal functions • Contraception needed in women
Systemic Steroids				
Triamcinolone acetonide (Kenalog)	IM	0.5 mg/kg	4–6 mo	
Methylprednisolone (Medrol)	PO	1/mo 32 mg/d	2 wk	Add gastric antacids
Intralesional Steroids				
Triamcinolone acetonide (Kenalog)	Injections into matrix or nail bed	2–3 mL per digit of 10 mg/mL solution	Once every 1–2 mo	• Some skills necessary • Local anesthesia required
Systemic Antifungals				
Terbinafine (Lamisil)	PO	250 mg/d	• 2 mo fingernails • 4 mo toenails	• Ineffective in *Candida* • Not if hepatic problems
Itraconazole (Sporanox)	PO	200 mg bid × 1 wk/mo	• 2 mo fingernails • 4 mo toenails	• Not if hepatic problems • Possible drug interactions
Systemic Retinoids				
Acitretin (Soriatane)	PO	0.3-0.5 mg/kg/d	4–6 mo	• Monitor hepatic and renal functions • Contraception needed in women

Abbreviation: IM = intramuscularly.

Psoriasis

Nail psoriasis is not rare, even in patients without skin or scalp involvement. The nail lesions may vary considerably in different patients, and diagnosis is not always easy. Onychomycosis is the most important differential diagnosis, especially in the toenails, where psoriasis causes nondiagnostic signs such as onycholysis and subungual hyperkeratosis.

Pustular psoriasis of the nails (Hallopeau's acrodermatitis continua) is also not an infrequent occurrence:

It usually involves one digit, with recurrent episodes of painful acute pustular eruptions of the nail bed and periungual tissues, leading to partial or total onycholysis.

Idiopathic Onycholysis

Onycholysis, which is detachment of the nail plate from the nail bed, is a frequent sign of different nail diseases. The term *idiopathic onycholysis* identifies a condition common

CURRENT DIAGNOSIS

Acute Paronychia

- Acute onset
- One digit
- Pulsating pain, swelling, and erythema of the periungual skin, usually more marked on one side

Trachyonychia

- Usually young patients
- One to several to all twenty nails may be affected
- Nail plate surface totally rough and scaly, as if sandpapered
- Family personal history of alopecia areata frequent

Ingrowing Toenails

- Great toenail(s)
- Painful periungual inflammation with/without pyogenic granulomas
- Nail plate distal margin irregular or not visible

Chronic Paronychia

- Fingernails
- Middle-aged women
- Swelling of the nail fold, absence of cuticle, nail plate surface abnormalities, and discoloration

Nail Fragility

- Fingernails
- Adult women
- Distal nail plate horizontally split and broken

Onychomycosis

- Toenails
- Adults and elderly people
- Onycholysis and nail bed hyperkeratosis (in distal subungual onychomycosis)
- Superficial opaque white patches (in white superficial onychomycosis)
- Tinea pedis plantaris or interdigitale often associated
- Periungual inflammation associated if a nondermatophytic mold is responsible

Psoriasis

- Onycholysis with erythematous border in one or more fingernails
- Salmon patches of the nail bed in one or more fingernails
- Nail plate thickening and crumbling

Idiopathic Onycholysis

- Fingernails
- Women
- White or greenish-black subungual space

---

in women, possibly caused by the same environmental traumas that produce chronic paronychia. In predisposed individuals, the frequent contact with water and irritants damages the distal portion of the nail bed (the so-called onychocorneal band), where nail plate–nail bed adhesion is stronger, and causes nail plate detachment. The newly formed space under the nail plate is penetrated by water and dirt and colonized by different microorganisms that may cause discoloration.

 CURRENT THERAPY

Acute Paronychia

- Mechanical drainage is necessary if pus is present.
- Treatment involves topical application of creams containing antibiotics, such as mupirocin (Bactroban) for 5 to 7 days.
- When swelling and pain are severe, the association of a topical steroid, such as betamethasone cream (Diprolene), for 4 to 5 days induces a more rapid regression of symptoms.
- Systemic antibiotics (amoxicillin/clavulanate potassium tablets (Augmentin) 2 g/day for 5 days) are required in severe cases.

Trachyonychia

- Trachyonychia affects the nail matrix, and topical drugs are therefore ineffective. Moreover, trachyonychia is a benign condition, so medical treatment is not advisable in children and when only one or a few nails are affected. In these patients, topical application of emollients containing urea several times a day may produce cosmetic benefit, as does the use of nail lacquers.
- In adults with trachyonychia of several nails, the cosmetic discomfort may be severe, and systemic steroids may be useful in these cases (see Table 2). Trachyonychia responds well and rapidly to systemic steroids, and recurrences are rare.
- Intralesional injection of steroids (see Table 2) into the nail matrix is an option in adults when only one or two nails are involved.

Ingrowing Toenails

- The final goals of treatment of ingrowing toenails are to remove the spicule that penetrates and damages the lateral nail fold and to help the nail plate to grow over the distal edge of the fold. This can be easily done in stage 1, but it requires the previous removal of the pyogenic granuloma in stage 2. In our experience two modalities of treatment are effective, both needing good patient compliance and 30 to 40 days of time:
  - Uplifting the nail plate by insertion under its edge of a small cylinder of cotton gauze soaked in antiseptic, such as povidone-iodine (Betadine). The patient should then be instructed to keep the gauze in place or reinsert it if necessary until the lateral nail reaches and grows over the distolateral fold.

Continued

- Pushing down the lateral and distal folds with a tape sealed on the skin of the distal digit and rolled all along the digit to increase traction. The tape should be applied by the patient every night and kept on for 12 hours. This should be done until the nail has grown completely over the distal border.
- When inflammation and pyogenic granuloma are present, they can be treated by topical application of high-potency topical steroids, such as clobetasone propionate ointment (Temovate) in occlusion at bedtime followed by topical mupirocin (Bactroban) in the morning until remission.
- Severe pyogenic granuloma may also be removed by electrodesiccation or by intralesional injection of steroids (see Table 2).
- Stage 3 ingrowing toenails always require an invasive approach with chemical (phenolization) or surgical removal of the lateral portion of the matrix to obtain production of a narrower nail plate that will not ingrow any more.

Chronic Paronychia

- Cure of chronic paronychia cannot be achieved until the patient avoids hand contact with the humid environmental condition by wearing cotton gloves under rubber gloves during manual activities.
- Topically apply medium- or high-potency steroids, such as fluocinolone (Synalar), betamethasone (Diprolene), and clobetasone propionate (Temovate) creams at bedtime followed by morning application of an antimicrobial cream, such as econazole (Spectazole).
- In severe cases, topical treatment can be preceded by a 15-day course of oral steroids (see Table 2).
- Treatment of chronic paronychia should be continued until the disease is cured, which is achieved when the cuticle has completely regrown.

Nail Fragility

- Avoid environmental factors known to dehydrate the nail plate, including water and irritants, and nail polish and nail lacquers.
- Trim the nails short because the longer the plate, the more it tends to lose water.
- Topical moisturizers containing urea or α-hydroxy acids to be applied on the nail plate several times a day and after each hand washing.
- Oral biotin (D-Biotin) at a dose of 5 mg/day for at least 6 months.

Onychomycosis

- Mycologic examination (KOH and cultures) is mandatory before starting therapy because treatment varies depending on type and etiology of onychomycosis.
- Onychomycoses caused by nondermatophytic molds (except for those caused by *Aspergillus* species) are difficult to treat because they usually do not respond to systemic antifungals.
- Topical treatment alone is indicated in white superficial onychomycosis caused by dermatophytes, distal subungual onychomycosis limited to the distal

one third of one digit, and onychomycosis caused by *Scopulariopsis brevicaulis* and *Fusarium* species. Suggested options include the following:
  - Nail lacquers containing antifungals may be effective, such as amorolfine (Loceryl) applied once a week or ciclopirox (Penlac) applied daily.
  - Another option is periodic mechanical or chemical removal of the affected portion of the nail associated with the daily application of antifungal creams. For chemical nail avulsion, we use 40% urea in petrolatum kept on the nail in occlusion for 7 days, after covering the periungual soft tissues with tape to avoid their maceration. After removal of the medication, the affected nail is soft and easy to clip away.
- Systemic treatment (see Table 2) is, in our experience, more effective when associated with topical therapy.
- Complete cure of onychomycosis (clinical and mycologic) may require a duration of systemic treatment longer than what is suggested by the manufacturer. For this reason we use a modality of treatment *à la carte*: After an initial treatment of 2 or 4 months (for fingernail and toenail onychomycosis, respectively), we perform a mycologic examination and continue therapy until its results are negative.
- Clinical cure may take more time than mycologic cure, so we continue to follow mycologically negative patients for a further 4 to 6 months.
- An annual follow-up of cured patients is advisable to check for recurrences that occur in up to 20% of patients.

Psoriasis

- Explain to patients that psoriasis is a chronic disease with improvements and relapses that are often induced by trauma (Koebner phenomenon).
- Topical treatment is suitable only for signs of nail bed psoriasis, such as onycholysis and hyperkeratosis. After clipping away the detached nail plate, different topicals can be applied on the nail bed epithelium. Topical steroids, such as betamethasone (Diprolene) and clobetasone propionate (Temovate) creams, or the association of steroids with keratolytics (Diprosalic ointment) are effective but can be applied only for short periods of time to avoid skin atrophy. However, tazarotene cream (Tazorac) and calcipotriene cream or ointment (Dovonex) can be used for a long time. A possible treatment modality can be the alternate use of vitamin D–derived topicals from Monday to Friday with steroid creams on Saturday and Sunday.
- Intralesional steroids (see Table 2) are effective in nail matrix psoriasis and are the treatment of choice when a few fingernails are involved. Injections of steroids into the nail bed via the lateral folds can be used to treat nail bed disease.
- Severe nail matrix psoriasis and pustular psoriasis of the nails greatly improve with systemic retinoids (see Table 2). Other effective systemic treatments are methotrexate and biologicals, but they are only suitable in patients with associated severe cutaneous or arthropathic psoriasis.

Idiopathic Onycholysis

- The detached nail plate should be clipped away to expose the nail bed to keep it clean and dry. This is not easily accepted by patients but should be done periodically until regrowth of a totally attached plate.
- Cotton gloves inside rubber gloves should be worn when handling water and irritants.
- The nail bed should be dried carefully after each hand washing.
- Daily soaking of the affected finger in a mild antiseptic solution, such as sodium hypochlorite (Dakin's solution) for 2 to 3 minutes.
- Application of a topical steroid, such as betamethasone cream (Diprolene), at bedtime for the first 10 to 15 days, and then of a topical antiseptic in an evaporating vehicle, such as 4% thymol in chloroform.

Abbreviation: KOH = potassium hydroxide.

REFERENCES

Baran R, Kaoukhov A: Topical antifungal drugs for the treatment of onychomycosis: An overview of current strategies for monotherapy and combination therapy. J Eur Acad Dermatol Venereol 2005; 19:21-29.

de Berker DA, Lawrence CM: A simplified protocol of steroid injection for psoriatic nail dystrophy. Br J Dermatol 1998;128:90-95.

Haneke E: Nail surgery. Eur J Dermatol 2000;10:227-241.

Piraccini BM, Tosti A: White superficial onychomycosis: Epidemiological, clinical, and pathological study of 79 patients. Arch Dermatol 2004;140:696-701.

Tosti A, Piraccini BM: Twenty-nail dystrophy. Curr Opin Dermatol 1997;2:82-86.

Tosti A, Piraccini BM, Ghetti E, Colombo MD: Topical steroids versus systemic antifungals in the treatment of chronic paronychia: An open, randomized double-blind and double dummy study. J Am Acad Dermatol 2002;47:72-76.

Tosti A, Piraccini BM, Lorenzi S, Iorizzo M: Treatment of nondermatophyte mold and Candida onychomycosis. Dermatol Clin 2002;2: 491-497.

Uyttendaele H, Geyer A, Scher RK: Brittle nails: Pathogenesis and treatment. J Drugs Dermatol 2002;2:48-49.

Keloids

Method of
Woraphong Manuskiatti, MD

Keloids are a frequent reason for dermatologic consultation requests. Clinically, keloids appear as firm, bulbous nodules or markedly elevated plaques following the healing process of a skin injury that extends beyond the confines of the original wound. They do not regress spontaneously and tend to recur after excision. Histologically, keloids are characterized by foci of markedly thickened, brightly eosinophilic-staining collagen bundles arranged randomly that appear within the mass of fibrillary collagen. The presence of a keloid is often cosmetically unacceptable to the affected individuals. In addition, it may be painful or pruritic, and it may restrict range of motion. Keloids represent abnormal wound healing in response to cutaneous surgery, physical trauma, or inflammatory responses. Keloids occur in all races, with a preponderance in individuals with darker pigmentation.

Pathogenesis

The exact mechanisms of keloid pathogenesis are yet to be determined and may be multifactorial. Studies have demonstrated both overproduction of collagen and increased procollagen levels, as well as decreased levels of collagenase in keloidal tissue. Proposed mechanisms for the cause of keloid formation include tension and vessel occlusion, as well as genetic, hormonal, and immune-mediated mechanisms. Much of the current research is concentrated on the immunoregulation of collagen production and deposition.

Treatment

Prevention should be the first rule of keloid therapy. Nonessential surgical and cosmetic procedures should not be performed on patients with histories of forming keloids or in anatomical regions prone to keloid formation, including the midchest, shoulder, back, and posterior neck. All postoperative and cutaneous trauma sites should be treated with appropriate antibiotics to prevent infection. All surgical wounds should be closed with normal tension. If possible, incision should not cross joint spaces, and skin excisions should be horizontal ellipses in the same direction as the skin tension lines.

Several forms of treatment are used with varying degrees of success. No single therapy is superior. Use of multiple modalities is often necessary to treat the lesions successfully. The selection of therapeutic techniques typically depends on size, location, depth, patient age, past responses to treatment, and the economic status of individuals (Table 1).

Medical Therapies

CORTICOSTEROID INJECTIONS

Intralesional corticosteroid injections are the mainstay therapy for treatment of keloids. Corticosteroids decrease excessive scarring by reducing synthesis of collagen and glycosaminoglycans and by reducing inflammatory mediators and fibroblast proliferation during the wound healing process. The most commonly used corticosteroid is triamcinolone acetonide (Kenalog-10),[1] 10 to 40 mg/mL, administrated intralesionally at 2- to 4-week intervals over the course of months to years. Response rates vary from 50% to 100%, with a recurrence of 9% to 50%. Results are improved when corticosteroids are combined with other

---
[1]Not FDA approved for this indication.

TABLE 1   Common Therapeutic Regimens for Keloids

Treatment Modality	Regimen	Treatment Interval
IL corticosteroids	TAC (10-40 mg/mL)	q 2-4 wk
IL 5-FU plus TAC	5-FU (45 mg/mL) mixed with TAC (1 mg/mL)	q 1-2 wk
Excision	Scalpel or CO_2 laser excision	Should be followed by another treatment modality
Cryosurgery	Two to three freeze-thaw cycles of 10 to 30 sec	q 3-4 wk
Pressure therapy	Pressure maintained between 24 and 30 mm Hg, 18 to 24 hr per day	At least 6-12 mo
Pulsed-dye laser	7-mm spot, 5-7 J/cm²	q 2-4 wk
Silicone gel sheeting	Apply for at least 12 h per day	At least 3 mo

Abbreviations: CO_2 = carbon dioxide; 5-FU = 5-fluorouracil; IL = intralesional; q = every; TAC = triamcinolone acetonide.

therapies such as excision and cryosurgery. Complications of repeated corticosteroid injections include atrophy, telangiectasia, and hypopigmentation at and around the injection sites (Figure 1).

INTERFERON

Interferon (IFN)[1] causes a decrease in collagen I and III synthesis by reducing cellular messenger ribonucleic acid. Intralesional IFN-γ injection administered twice weekly for 4 weeks shows improved to complete resolution of keloids. But injections tend to be exceedingly painful and complicated by flulike symptoms.

5-FLUOROURACIL[1]

Treatment of keloids with intralesional 5-fluorouracil (5-FU) (Adrucil)[1] injection combined with corticosteroids

is as effective as intralesional corticosteroids alone, but the latter is much more likely to cause adverse effects. 5-FU[1] appears to work by decreasing keloid fibroblast proliferation. Injections are given once a week at the beginning and then adjusted up or down according to the therapeutic response. Side effects of intralesional 5-FU include spots of purpura, pain during injection, and localized superficial tissue slough.

IMIQUIMOD[1]

A study on the effect of postoperative application of imiquimod (Aldara)[1] 5% cream on the surgically excised keloids for a period of 8 weeks noted a lower recurrence rate than that of excision alone. Theoretically, imiquimod induces production of IFN, thus down-regulating collagen synthesis. Reported side effects include local skin irritation and mild hyperpigmentation.

[1]Not FDA approved for this indication.

[1]Not FDA approved for this indication.

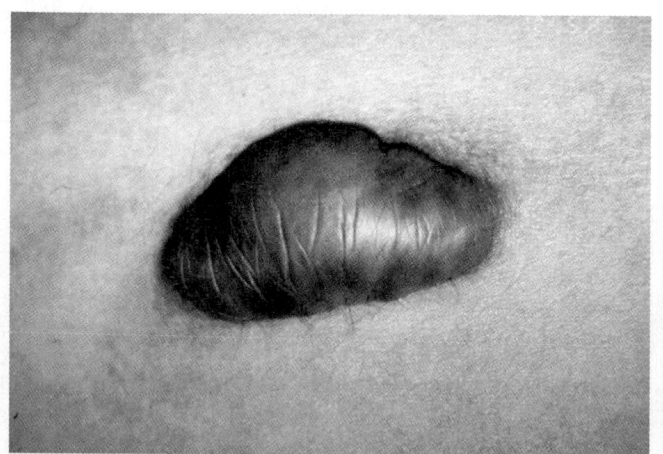
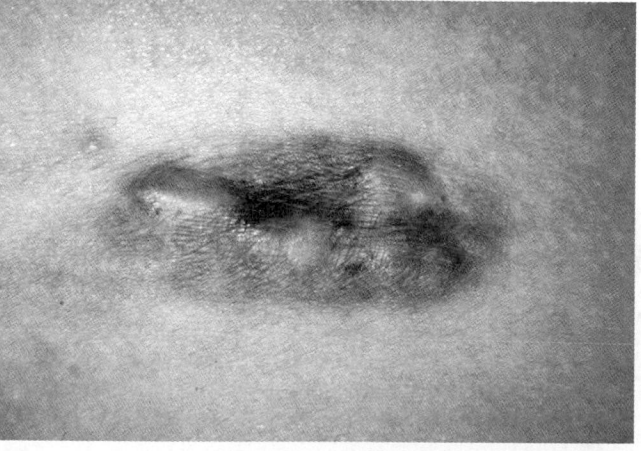

A   B

FIGURE 1. A keloid on the back before (**A**) and after (**B**) four intralesional corticosteroid (10 mg/mL) injections. Note side effects of skin atrophy, telangiectasia, and hypopigmentation. (Adapted from Manuskiatti W: Guidelines for the treatment and management of keloids and hypertrophic scars. Siriraj Hosp Gazette 2003;55:251.)

Surgical Therapies

EXCISION

Surgical excision of keloids without adjunctive therapy yields a high rate of recurrence (45% to 100%). Decreased recurrence rates are consistently reported with excision in combination with other postoperative treatment modalities, such as intralesional corticosteroids, radiation, pressure therapy, silicone gel sheeting (SGS), or imiquimod cream. Surgical techniques to minimize tissue trauma, closing with minimal tension and using buried sutures when necessary for layered closure, are recommended to decrease the possibility of recurrence.

CRYOSURGERY

Freezing keloids with cryogen such as liquid nitrogen affects the microvasculature and causes cell damage. This occurs via intracellular crystallization leading to tissue anoxia with subsequent tissue necrosis and sloughing, followed by tissue flattening. Cryosurgery alone causes complete flattening in more than half of patients after two or more sessions performed at 3- to 4-week intervals. Limitations to this treatment include postoperative pain, slow healing, and hypopigmentation (especially in patients with darker skin).

Radiation Therapy

Radiation may be used as a monotherapy or combined with surgery to prevent recurrence of keloids following excision. Radiation therapy theoretically works by inhibiting fibroblast proliferation and neoangiogenesis in wound healing. When used as a monotherapy, radiation is not very effective, with a high recurrence rate of 50% to 100%. The risks of carcinogenicity associated with radiotherapy are controversial. Caution is advised when treating young children or when treating areas around the breasts and thyroid because of the increased radiosensitivities of these tissues.

Physical Modalities

PRESSURE THERAPY

The mechanism involved in how pressure therapy reduces keloid formation is unknown, but it is hypothesized that pressure induces tissue hypoxia, resulting in fibroblast degeneration and subsequent collagen degradation. It is generally recommended that the pressure be maintained between 24 and 30 mm Hg, 18 to 24 hours a day for at least 6 to 12 months, for this therapy to be effective. Pressure therapy is commonly used in combination with other modalities such as SGS and postsurgical excision. Patient compliance is the limiting factor, given the need for long-term pressure application for therapeutic success.

LASER THERAPY

At present, the common use of lasers to treat keloids is based on two different approaches. One technique is an application of a carbon dioxide (CO_2) laser for nonspecific destruction of keloids. Keloid vaporization or excision by CO_2 laser alone results in high (40% to 90%) recurrence rate and provides no distinct advantage over scalpel excision. The CO_2 laser is now reserved for debulking large keloids, prior to the initiation of other treatment modalities. Another method used is 585-nm pulsed-dye laser (PDL) for selectively damaging the microvasculature of the keloids (Figure 2). Multiple (more than two) PDL treatment sessions decrease scar height and erythema and improve scar texture and dysesthesia.

 CURRENT DIAGNOSIS

- Clinical characteristic: A raised, firm scar, possibly painful or pruritic, extending beyond wound borders
- Histologic characteristics: Thick bundles of hyalinized collagen arranged in dense swirls or nodules

---

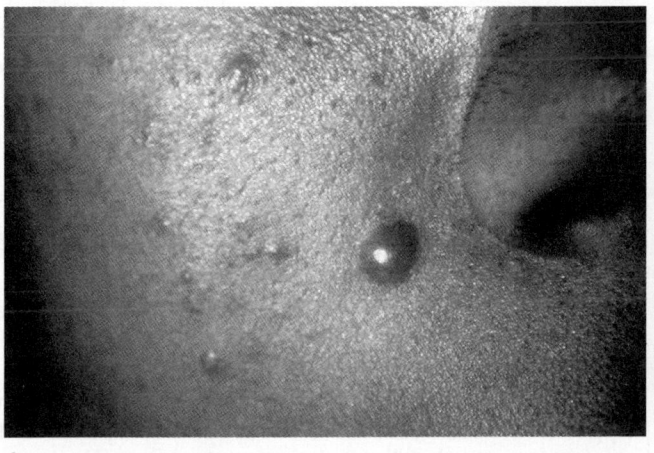

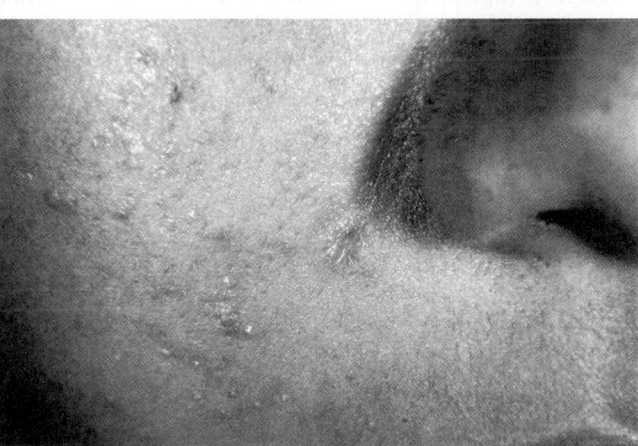

A

B

FIGURE 2. A keloid developing after acne on the cheek before (**A**) and after (**B**) two pulsed-dye laser treatments, combined with two intralesional corticosteroids plus 5-fluorouracil injections.

CURRENT THERAPY

Medical Therapies

- Corticosteroid injections[1] (Kenalog-10)
- Interferon (IFN)[1]
- 5-Fluorouracil (5-FU) (Adrucil)[1]
- Imiquimod (Aldara)[1]

Surgical Therapies

- Primary excision
- Cryosurgery

Radiation Therapy

Physical Modalities

- Pressure therapy
- Laser therapy
- Silicone gel sheeting (SGS)

Miscellaneous Therapies

- Topical vitamin E,[1] onion extract cream (Mederma),[1] topical retinoic acid (Retin-A),[1] IL verapamil,[1] colchicines,[1] ultraviolet A1 phototherapy

[1]Not FDA approved for this indication.

SILICONE GEL SHEETING

The mode of action of SGS is unknown but thought to occur through an increased scar hydration effect provided by the sheet, leading to anti-keloidal effects. To be effective, the sheets must be applied for at least 12 hours daily. SGS may be especially useful in children and others who cannot tolerate the pain associated with other treatment modalities.

Miscellaneous Therapies

Although additional novel therapies are available, many treatments are anecdotal and require confirmation of efficacy and safety through formal studies. Some of these therapies include topical vitamin E,[1] onion extract cream (Mederma),[1] topical retinoic acid (Retin-A),[1] intralesional verapamil,[1] colchicines,[1] and ultraviolet A1 phototherapy.

In conclusion, therapeutic management of keloids remains a challenge because of their high rate of recurrence and lack of curative treatment. Treatment approaches to keloids depend not only on the size of the lesion but also on the age and location. Use of several approaches in combination or sequentially, based on the patient's individual requirements and responses, is recommended to maximize the therapeutic outcome.

REFERENCES

Alster TS, Handrick C: Laser treatment of hypertrophic scars, keloids, and striae. Semin Cutan Med Surg 2000;19:287-292.

Berman B, Flores F: The treatment of hypertrophic scars and keloids. Eur J Dermatol 1998;8:591-596.

Manuskiatti W, Fitzpatrick RE: Treatment response of keloidal and hypertrophic sternotomy scars: Comparison among intralesional corticosteroid, 5-fluorouracil, and 585-nm flashlamp-pumped pulsed-dye laser treatments. Arch Dermatol 2002;138:1149-1155.

[1]Not FDA approved for this indication.

Murray JC: Keloids and hypertrophic scars. Clin Dermatol 1994;12:27-37.

Mustoe TA, Cooter RD, Gold MH, et al: International clinical recommendations on scar management. Plast Reconstr Surg 2002;110:560-571.

Niessen FB, Spauwen PH, Schalkwijk J, Kon M: On the nature of hypertrophic scars and keloids: A review. Plast Reconstr Surg 1999;104:1435-1458.

Urioste SS, Arndt KA, Dover JS: Keloids and hypertrophic scars: Review and treatment strategies. Semin Cutan Med Surg 1999;18:159-171.

Warts (Verrucae)

Method of
Tamara Salam Housman, MD, and
Phillip M. Williford, MD

Viral warts afflict approximately 10% of the population and are caused by human papillomavirus (HPV). HPV, a nonenveloped, double-stranded DNA virus, is of the papovavirus class and invades both mucous and squamous epithelium. At least 130 known types of HPV have been identified. HPV causes both clinical and subclinical infection and plays a role in certain cutaneous carcinomas, including squamous cell carcinoma (SCCa) of the anogenital area and nail unit. HPV is found in the basal layer of the epidermis but replicates only in the superficial, well-differentiated layer. The subsequent cellular proliferation gives rise to thick, hyperkeratotic lesions generally known as warts.

Cutaneous warts are mainly divided into common warts, plantar warts, flat warts, and genital warts. Common warts account for 70% of all cutaneous warts and are probably associated with HPV types 1, 2, and 4. Two thirds of untreated common warts spontaneously regress within 2 years, but these previously infected individuals have a higher rate of developing new warts than those who were never infected. Treatment of warts with salicylic acid and/or cryotherapy has demonstrated a 60% to 80% cure rate.

Transmission is via skin-to-skin contact, including sexual, and is seen with greater frequency where groups of people are in close contact, including in school-age children, with a frequency of 20% for common warts. Extent of infection is determined by the immune response, and immunocompromised hosts are at increased risk. Symptoms may include pain and bleeding, and warts may interfere with daily functioning, especially if located on the palms, soles, or digits. Warts can be professionally and socially stigmatizing, especially if located on the hands or fingers of patients who must touch others on a daily basis.

Types of Warts

Verrucae vulgares (common warts) are flesh-colored, hyperkeratotic, verrucous, fissured, firm papules that disrupt normal skin lines on fingers and toes. They may be distinguished from calluses and corns by paring down of the stratum corneum (the uppermost horny layer of skin) to reveal thrombosed/bleeding capillaries seen as brown/black dots. A subtype is a butcher's wart, which is

TABLE 1 Treatment of Verrucae

	Available Preparations	Mechanism of Action	Application	Dosage	Disadvantages/Adverse Effects
Salicylic acid (keratolytic) (Compound W)	Solution Gel/lotion/cream Plaster Pad 10%-60%	Destruction of infected epidermis; irritation leads to stimulation of immune response.	Patient applied. Adjunct to other treatment modalities. May pare down/shave wart then apply keratolytic to increase penetration.	qhs until clear, usually weeks to months.	Irritation
Cryosurgery	Liquid nitrogen (−196°C [−320.8°F]): cryospray or cotton-tipped applicator	Destruction of infected epidermis; induces inflammation leading to stimulation of immune response.	Physician applied. Paring of thick lesions; liquid nitrogen freeze for 30-60 sec to include a 1-2 mm rim around wart → let thaw → repeat × 2 cycles total.	May repeat q 3-4 wk.	Pain Erythema Vesicle/bullae Crusting Possible infection Hypopigmentation Scarring (if freeze too deep) Onychodystrophy (if not careful with periungual warts)
Cantharidin[1,2]	Colloidal solution, 0.7%	Destruction of epidermis and leads to blister formation; extract of blister beetle.	Adjunct to other treatment modalities. Careful with periungual warts, overlying tendons, and on lower extremities. Physician applied. Paring of thick lesions. Apply using very fine applicator only to wart then patient is to wash off in 6-8 h. Painless—good for children.	May repeat q 2-4 wk.	Vesicle/bullae Crusting Avoid face or near eyes
Surgical excision Curettage Electrocautery	N/A	Destruction by surgical removal of wart.	Physician applied. Surgical excision of wart or surgical removal by curetting wart then cauterizing the base.	Usually only performed once but may repeat if wart recurs.	Painful (minimal if use local anesthesia but some postoperative pain) Scarring
Trichloroacetic acid (Tri-Chlor) Bichloroacetic acid	Solution, up to 50% concentration	Destruction of infected epidermis.	Physician applied.	Most useful for mucosal warts.	Painful reactions
Lasers: Carbon dioxide Pulsed-dye Erbium:YAG	N/A	Destruction of infected epidermis.	Physician applied.	May repeat q 4-6 wk.	Expensive Risk of viral spread via laser plume Not superior to conventional therapy
Imiquimod	Cream, 5%	Immunomodulator: indirect in vivo antitumor and antiviral effects mediated by induction of cytokines—IFN-α, TNF-α, IL-1, -6, -8, and others.	Patient applied. On nonmucosal skin, including plantar/palmar warts, apply keratolytic, followed by occlusion in PM, followed by imiquimod in AM; may also occlude imiquimod if not getting any erythema. If irritation is severe, stop regimen for few days then resume, if possible. May initiate therapy with cryosurgery followed by keratolytic-imiquimod combination therapy for 6 wks then repeat if necessary.	3 times/wk on mucosal skin; 5-7 times/wk on keratinized skin.	Irritation Erythema Pruritus Burning Crusting Infection Scarring

Continued

TABLE 1   Treatment of Verrucae—cont'd

	Available Preparations	Mechanism of Action	Application	Dosage	Disadvantages/ Adverse Effects
Cimetidine (Tagamet)[1]	Tablets: 200 mg, 300 mg, 400 mg, 800 mg; liquid: 300 mg/5 mL	Immunomodulator: at high doses may enhance immune response.	Patient initiated.	25 to 40 mg/kg daily, divided bid to qid.	True efficacy unclear
DPC[1] SADBE[1] DNCB[1]	Acetone solution, 0.001-2% Acetone solution, 0.01-1%	Immunomodulator: inducing a delayed hypersensitivity reaction thus leading to stimulation of immune response.	Physician applied. Sensitize patient by applying 2%-3% solution of SADBE/DPC to 1 cm area on inner arm → may need to resensitize every 10-14 d until get local reaction (erythema/vesicle).	After sensitization, apply to wart using 0.03%-2% solution once per wk until clear.	DNCB—possibly mutagenic May be unable to sensitize some patients Irritation Erythema Vesicle/bullae
Retinoids	Acitretin (Soriatane),[1] 10 mg or 25 mg tabs Isotretinoin (Accutane),[1] 10 mg, 20 mg, 40 mg tabs Topical tretinoin (Retin-A),[1] cream/microgel	Antimitotic: interferes with epidermal differentiation and proliferation.	Patient applied/initiated. Good prevention for immunosuppressed/ immunocompromised patients with multiple warts or EDV. Topical retinoids for flat warts.	Systemic: least effective qd or qod dose. Topical: apply qhs to warts only.	Topical: local irritation, erythema, and dryness Systemic: mucocutaneous dryness, abnormal liver function tests, elevated triglycerides,
Bleomycin (Blenoxane)[1]	Aqueous solution, 0.1% (1 mg/mL)	Antimitotic.	Physician applied. Intralesional.	Single dose of 0.1 mL of 1 unit/mL in 0.1% solution with normal saline (unclear if repeat q 2-3 wk).	Pain (use with local anesthesia) Tissue necrosis Scarring Loss of nail Raynaud's at local site Possible significant systemic absorption
5-Fluorouracil (Adrucil)	Cream, 5%	Antimitotic: inhibition of DNA and RNA synthesis leading to keratinocyte death.	Patient applied. May be combined with topical tretinoin therapy	Once per wk.	Irritation Erythema Edema

[1]Not FDA approved for this indication.
[2]Not available in the United States.
Abbreviations: bid = twice daily; DNCB = dinitrochlorobenzene; DPC = diphencycloproprenone; EDV = epidermodysplasia verruciformis; q = every; qd = every day; qhs = at bedtime; qid = four times daily; qod = every other day; SADBE = squaric acid dibutylester; YAG = yttrium-aluminum-garnet.

seen on the hands of butchers and fish and meat handlers/packers, and appears as large, cauliflower plaques. Differential diagnoses (DDx) include seborrheic keratosis, molluscum contagiosum, keratoacanthoma, amelanotic melanoma, SCCa in situ, and invasive SCCa. Verrucae vulgares warts are associated with HPV subtypes 1, 2, 4.

Verrucae plantares (plantar warts) are flesh-colored, hyperkeratotic, endophytic papules or plaques located on the soles of the feet that also disrupt normal skin lines and may have thrombosed capillaries manifested as brown/black dots. These can be quite painful and interfere with mobility and daily functioning, especially if located on sites of pressure. A mosaic wart occurs if multiple plantar warts coalesce into a plaque. DDx include callus, corns, exostosis, and acral melanoma. Verrucae plantares warts are associated with HPV subtypes 1, 2, 4, 27, 57.

Verrucae planae (flat warts) are tan- to flesh-colored, flat, sharply demarcated papules located on the dorsum of hands, distal lower extremities, and face; and are often in a linear arrangement after trauma. DDx include molluscum contagiosum, epidermodysplasia verruciformis, and benign syringomas on the face. Verrucae planae warts are associated with HPV subtypes 3, 10.

Epidermodysplasia verruciformis (EDV) is a rare, autosomal recessive, hereditary disorder manifesting with extensive, flesh-colored to pink to tan, round, flat papules on the trunk, hands, upper and lower extremities, and face. These do have malignant potential, especially on the face on sun-exposed areas. Patients with EDV are usually infected with multiple types of HPV. DDx include seborrheic keratosis, actinic keratosis, basal cell carcinoma, SCCa in situ, or invasive SCCa. EDV warts are classified into more than 30 associated HPV subtypes, including types 3, 5, 8, 9, 12, 14, 15, 17, 19-25, 36-38, 47, 49, 50.

Verrucous carcinoma is a slow-growing variant of SCCa arising in three sites:

1. Oral mucosa (oral florid papillomatosis)
2. Anogenital region (giant condyloma of Buschke and Löwenstein)
3. Plantar foot (epithelioma cuniculatum)

Verrucous carcinoma warts are associated with HPV subtypes 6, 11.

Diagnosis

Diagnosis is mainly based on clinical findings. In immunocompromised or immunosuppressed patients, biopsy should be performed in large or suspicious lesions to rule out SCCa.

Therapy

It is well accepted that the treatment of warts must be individualized and that usually more than one therapeutic modality is required to achieve complete resolution (Table 1). Conventional destructive treatments include repeated application of topical chemotherapy (i.e., salicylic acid [Compound W], cantharidin,[2] podophyllin [Podofin], 5-fluorouracil [Adrucil], etc.), cryosurgery, surgical excision,

[2]Not available in the United States.

curettage and/or electrosurgery, and laser therapy. Other approaches include immunotherapy (i.e., intralesional interferon [IFN] [Alferon N], diphencyprone[2]), tape occlusion, and observation. In 20% of immunocompetent individuals, the warts will spontaneously resolve within 3 months. Cure rates for common and plantar verrucae with salicylic acid vary from 60% to 80%. Also, overall cure rates with cryosurgery range from 60% to 80%; and with carbon dioxide and pulsed-dye laser, they range from 45% to 90%. However, these methods are usually painful and expensive. Nonetheless, with most methods, recurrence is common, and repeat visits to the physician are costly.

Intralesional IFN-α, although promising with a 36% to 62% clearance rate of anogenital warts, requires multiple injections in the physician's office, is expensive, and may cause systemic adverse effects. Imiquimod (Aldara),[1] a self-applied topical agent that induces interferon production at the site of application, is reported to have a 50% eradication rate in the treatment of genital warts. Other treatments include:

- Hyperthermia with hot water (113°F [45°C]) immersion
- Intralesional injection of *Candida*[1]/mumps[1] antigen
- Photodynamic therapy with aminolevulinic acid (Levulan Kerastick)[1] followed by red light irradiation
- Hypnosis
- Duct tape occlusion

Special attention should be paid to immunosuppressed or immunocompromised patients in whom there is a higher rate of malignant transformation of warts and in whom warts tend to be more resistant and more numerous and thus may require systemic retinoids as a maintenance regimen.

[1]Not FDA approved for this indication.
[2]Not available in the United States.

Condyloma Acuminatum (Genital Warts)

Method of
*Karl R. Beutner, MD, PhD,
and Alice N. Do, DO*

Genital warts are the most common manifestation of infection of the genital area with the human papilloma virus (HPV). Genital HPV infection is the most common viral sexually transmitted disease. Approximately 1% of the general population has genital warts at any time.

Proliferation of HIV-infected keratinocytes results in a genital wart. More than 100 genotypes of HPV exist. Low-risk HPV types 6 and 11 cause genital warts. High-risk HPV, most often types 16 and 18, are commonly associated with squamous cell carcinoma (SCC) in situ, also known as bowenoid papulosis or vulvar intraepithelial neoplasia of the external genital area, as well as abnormal Papanicoulau

(Pap) smears including in situ and invasive SCC of the cervix. In immunocompetent hosts, in situ SCC of the skin rarely, if ever, evolves into invasive SCC. Genital skin appears not to be as susceptible to the oncogenic potential of HPV as are the transformation zones of the uterine cervix and the anal canal.

Diagnosis is clinical, so identification of various presentations of genital warts involves understanding the different genital skin types that influence wart morphology. Three types of genital skin are fully keratinized hair-bearing, fully keratinized non–hair-bearing, and partially keratinized non–hair-bearing. The later appears moist and is often mistakenly referred to as mucous membranes. However, there are no mucus glands, and it appears moist because it is partially keratinized.

Treatment can be directed by skin type and wart morphology. The four morphologic types of genital warts are:

1. Cauliflower-type, or condyloma acuminatum
2. Smooth papular type, which are skin-colored, dome-shaped, 1 to 4 mm papules
3. Keratotic type, which may mimic seborrheic keratoses or common warts
4. Flat type, which are slightly raised.

Condyloma acuminatum occurs most commonly on moist, partially keratinized skin, whereas the smooth papular and keratotic types are seen most frequently on fully keratinized areas; the flat type is seen on all types of genital skin.

Genital warts may appear on the penile shaft, scrotum, perineum or perianal areas, labia, vulva, or pubic area, or in the crural folds. They can also be found in the urethra or bladder or in the oral cavity. The oral cavity should also be examined in patients being evaluated for genital warts.

Biopsy is usually unnecessary to confirm a clinical diagnosis of external genital warts. However, a biopsy should be considered when lesions are atypical, pigmented, ulcerated, indurated, or fixed to underlying tissue; fail to respond to treatment or worsen during treatment; frequently recur; exhibit individual (noncoalescent) warts larger than 1 cm in diameter; or are suspicious for malignancy. Biopsy should also be considered when diagnosis is unclear.

Acetowhitening to aid in diagnosis of external genital warts is no longer recommended because it lacks adequate specificity and sensitivity.

Differential diagnosis includes lichen planus, skin tags, seborrheic keratoses, molluscum contagiosum, condyloma latum, pearly penile papules, sebaceous glands, lichen nitidus, Crohn's disease, and SCC in situ.

Treatment

Genital warts may spontaneously resolve or persist. Discuss expectations of therapy with patients. The goal is to eliminate symptoms, namely visible wart lesions, rather than to address HPV infection. Rather than a treatment, a course of therapy is required to achieve a wart-free state. It is unknown whether wart elimination will decrease or eliminate the patient's infectivity to current or future sexual partners. Even after proper treatment, recurrence is due to latent HPV in the surrounding normal tissue, and not necessarily due to reinfection. Once two individuals are infected with the same HPV type, they will not continue

to reinfect one another. Any given treatment carries a 40% to 75% change of clearing and a 25% to 50% chance of recurrence. Recurrence is responsible for a prolonged course for the patient. Treatment failure is commonly caused by improper selection or use of a therapeutic modality. At the present time, all treatments are comparable in effectiveness.

Choice of Treatment

Selection of treatment is influenced by wart morphology, anatomic site, total wart area, wart count, clinician's experience, and patient preference. Not all patients respond equally well to all modalities. Proper matching of patient with modality will usually shorten treatment duration. Pregnancy and immunosuppression are associated with larger and more numerous genital wart lesions. Certain treatment modalities are more appropriate in pregnancy. Immunosuppressed patients do not respond as well to therapy and have a high recurrence rate. These patients have a higher incidence of SCC. Have a plan or set protocol, particularly when a limited number of modalities are available. In general, if after three to four treatments with a given therapy a clinically significant response is not seen, or if after six treatments no clearance is achieved, the treatment modality should be changed and the diagnosis should be re-evaluated.

TREATMENT MODALITIES

Current treatments are divided into provider-administered and patient-applied therapies. Provider-administered therapies include cryotherapy, podophyllin resin (Podocon-25), trichloroacetic acid (Tri-Chlor)[1], and surgery. Patient-applied therapies allow the patient greater control and include podofilox (Condylox) and imiquimod (Aldara). However, these require good compliance and that the patient be able to view and reach the warts.

PROVIDER-ADMINISTERED THERAPIES

Cryotherapy

Cryotherapy works well for small, flat, few warts in dry or moist areas. It can be used on the penile shaft and vulva with little scarring. It can be used during pregnancy. It is not recommended for large wart areas, which can be quite painful and cause wound-care issues. A small, tightly wound cotton swab (Q-tip) that holds inadequate amounts of liquid nitrogen cannot effectively freeze a wart. Apply liquid nitrogen with a large, loosely wound piece of cotton on a wooden stick or with a cryoprobe.

A few small warts can be frozen without an anesthetic. Patients with more warts should be offered local anesthesia, with either injection of 1% lidocaine[1] or topical application of a eutectic mixture of 2.5% lidocaine and 2.5% prilocaine (EMLA cream).[1] Freeze the wart and 1- to 2-mm surrounding border. For larger warts, two freeze-thaw cycles are effective. How *hard* to freeze the warts can be learned with experience.

Cryotherapy requires proper training. Complications are rare but inexperienced clinicians often underfreeze

---

[1]Not FDA approved for this indication.

areas, reducing efficacy. Overfreezing increases pain and the probability of scarring and other complications. Warn patients about post-treatment pain and blistering.

Podophyllin Resin

Podophyllin resin (Podofin, Podocon-25, Podofilm) is from the plant species *Podophyllum peltatum* or *Podophyllum emodii*. This resin contains podofilox (podophyllotoxin), 4-dimethylpodophyllotoxin, α-peltatum, and β-peltatum, which cause cellular mitotic arrest and lead to tissue necrosis. It is a good choice for moist warts and up to a 10 cm² surface area. It is ineffective in dry areas, such as the scrotum, penile shaft, and labia majora.

Podophyllin resin lacks a standardized preparation, but it is commonly used as a 10% to 25% solution in tincture of benzoin. Use a cotton tip and apply a thin layer directly to the wart and allow to air dry before the patient assumes a normal anatomic position. Traditionally, patients were advised to wash off podophyllin 2 to 4 hours after application, but benzoin is water insoluble and cannot be removed simply with soap and water. Another ill-advised but not uncommon practice is to create a *barrier* around the wart with Vaseline or K-Y jelly, and apply podophyllin resin to the central wart. Body temperature thins the barrier, which mixes with the podophyllin resin, and spreads over the entire area, creating an impressive irritant reaction. I advise patients to leave the podophyllin resin on overnight and avoid washing, bathing, or sexual contact until the next day. Local side effects include erythema, pain, and irritation. Systemic side effects are caused by increased toxic absorption and are associated with large treatment area (>10 cm²) or allowing the resin to absorb for an extended time. Avoid podophyllin resin in pregnancy.

Trichloroacetic Acid (Tri-Chlor)[1]

Trichloroacetic acid ([TCA] Tri-Chlor)[1] chemically coagulates warts and adjacent skin. Use for small, few, moist warts. TCA[1] can be used during pregnancy. Although 30% to 70% solutions are employed, the optimal concentration is undetermined. Use extreme caution with the higher concentrations, which can be highly caustic. Apply sparingly to lesions, being careful not to let the solution run onto normal skin. Treatment can be repeated weekly, or every other week, as needed. TCA[1] can be neutralized, if needed, with soap and sodium bicarbonate.

Surgery

Surgery renders the patient wart free with a single visit. It is a good choice for limited or large treatment areas. There is no clearly superior surgical modality. Selection of a surgical approach depends on clinician experience and availability of equipment. Good results can be achieved with superficial tangential scissors, electrodesiccation, hot cautery, curettage, or CO_2 laser.

PATIENT-APPLIED THERAPIES

Podofilox

The major active lignin in podophyllin resin is podofilox, available as a 0.5% solution or gel (Condylox). Apply to warts twice daily for 3 days followed by a treatment-free period of 4 days. Repeat this cycle four to six times to achieve wart clearance. A maximum of 10 cm² should be treated, and podofilox should be avoided in pregnancy.

Imiquimod

Imiquimod (Aldara) is a 5% cream, applied three times weekly at bedtime to moist wart areas. Dry and nonintertriginous areas may respond better to daily application. It can be used for up to 16 weeks. As imiquimod stimulates an inflammatory response, however, local irritation, burning, and ulceration are expected side effects and are similar to those seen with other modalities.

5-Fluorouracil

5-Fluorouracil creams (Carac, Effudex),[1] used previously for genital warts, are no longer recommended because of side effects, unproven efficacy, and the availability of other treatments.

Transmission and Prevention

HPV is a sexually transmitted disease (STD). Educate patients to tell sexual partners that they have this infection.

---

[1]Not FDA approved for this indication.

[1]Not FDA approved for this indication.

 CURRENT DIAGNOSIS

Diagnosis of genital warts requires their identification on physical exam. The clinician should become adept at recognizing the various morphologies of genital warts, which are influenced by the overlying genital skin type.

External Wart Morphology	Description	Skin Type
Condyloma acuminatum	Coalescent cauliflower-like plaques	Moist/partially keratinized
Smooth papular	Skin-colored, dome-shaped, 1 to 4 mm papules	Fully keratinized
Keratotic		Fully keratinized
Flat type	Discrete, warty papules Slightly raised, flat-topped papules	Moist/partially keratinized or fully keratinized

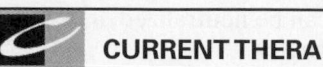

CURRENT THERAPY

Treatment modalities can be divided into either provider-administered or patient-applied therapies. The choice of therapy will depend on skin type, wart quantity, and location.

Treatment	Mechanism	Good Choice for	Poor Choice for	Procedure
Provider administered				
Cryotherapy	Direct tissue destruction	• Small, flat, few warts • Dry or moist warts • Pregnancy OK	• Large wart areas (> 10 cm^2)	• Liquid nitrogen applied on a large, loosely wound piece of cotton on a wooden stick; or with a cryoprobe, by the spray technique • Freeze the wart and 1- to 2-mm surrounding border
Podophyllin resin	Arrest in mitosis leading to tissue necrosis	• Moist warts	• Dry wart areas • Do not exceed 10 cm^2 treatment area • Not for pregnancy	• Use a cotton tip and apply a thin layer to wart and allow to air-dry before the patient assumes a normal anatomic position • Leave on overnight and avoid washing, bathing, and sexual contact • Repeat treatment 1 week later, as needed
TCA (Tri-Chlor)[1]	Chemical coagulation of wart proteins	• Small, moist, few warts • Pregnancy OK	• Large wart areas (> 10 cm^2) • Dry warts	• Apply sparingly to the lesion, being careful not to let the solution run onto normal skin • Repeat weekly or every other week, as needed
Surgery	Direct removal of lesions	• Large or small treatment areas • Rectal lesions OK • Pregnancy OK	• Bleeding disorders	• Superficial tangential scissor excision, electrodesiccation, hot cautery, curettage, or CO$_2$ laser may be used
Patient applied				
Podofilox (Condylox)	Arrest in mitosis → tissue necrosis	• Moist warts	• Do not exceed 10 cm^2 treatment area • Not for pregnancy • Poor compliance	• Apply bid for 3 days following by a 4-day treatment-free period • Repeat weekly cycles four to six times, as needed
Imiquimod (Aldara)	Immunomodulator	• Moist warts	• Large wart areas (> 10 cm^2) • Dry warts • Poor compliance	• Apply every other night on moist warts or intertriginous areas, or every night on dry warts • May be used for up to 16 weeks, as tolerated

[1]Not FDA approved for this indication.
Abbreviations: TCA = trichloroacetic acid.

Condoms may decrease transmission but do not completely prevent infection. Asymptomatic partners can harbor a subclinical infection, and examination for genital warts is appropriate if lesions are suspected. It is unknown whether treatment of genital wart lesions eliminates infectivity. Discuss the oncogenic potential of HPV types associated with bowenoid papulosis. Women with external genital warts or whose male partners have lesions should have a Pap smear and remain in the system for monitoring for cervical cancer. Investigations for other STDs should be done if suspected.

Acquiring an STD carries a negative social stigma and emotional trauma. Patients often fear discovery and rejection and feel guilty and victimized. They view themselves as less sexually desirable, enjoy sex less, and have concerns about transmission. Teaching and educational materials are available from the American Social Health Association (1-919-361-8422).

REFERENCES

Beutner KR, Richwald GA, Wiley DJ, et al: External genital warts: Report of the American Medical Association consensus conference. Clin Infect Dis 1998;27:796-806.

Beutner KR, Wiley DJ, Douglas JM, et al: Genital warts and their treatment. Clin Infect Dis 1999;28(Suppl 1):S37-S56.

Habif TP: Sexually transmitted viral infections. In Hodgson S, Cook L (eds): Clinial Dermatology, A Color Guide to Diagnosis and Therapy, 4th ed. Philadelphia, Mosby 2004, pp 336-342.

Odom RB, James WD, Berger TG: Viral diseases. In Fathman EM, Geisel EB, Salmo A (eds): Andrews' Diseases of the Skin, Clinical Dermatology, 9th ed. Philadelphia, WB Saunders, 2000; pp 541-519.

Nevi

Method of
Scott C. Wickless, DO,
and Joan Guitart, MD

Nevi (singular, nevus) are considered benign proliferations of normal skin constituents. Although the term *nevi* describes an assortment of nonmelanocytic and melanocytic entities of the skin, the scope of this discussion is limited to congenital and common acquired types of melanocytic nevi, also known as nevocellular nevi or moles.

Epidemiology

Melanocytic nevi commonly appear in childhood and adolescence (acquired). Less commonly, nevi may also be present at birth (congenital). The incidence of melanocytic nevi increases during the first 3 decades of life. The prevalence of nevi is related to race and age. Genetic factors and sun exposure may encourage their development as well. Individuals with a fair complexion (Fitzpatrick types I and II) are more likely to have higher counts of acquired nevi, especially if they have extensive sun exposure. Furthermore, an increased risk of melanoma is associated with high counts of nevi with or without dysplastic features. Broad-spectrum sunscreens may decrease the development of melanocytic nevi when used in children. The highest counts of melanocytic nevi are seen in the fourth and fifth decades of life, and the incidence with each successive decade decreases. In contrast, congenital melanocytic nevi are best regarded as an error in the development and migration of neuroectodermal elements. They present at birth or soon thereafter, but some small congenital nevi remain inconspicuous until years later.

Clinical Presentations

Nevi may appear as macules (flat), papules (raised), or even nodules with varying degrees of pigmentation. Common acquired nevi are usually symmetrical and smaller than 0.5 cm. Infrequently, they may be grouped. Nevi are characterized histologically by their nested collections of cells present in the dermis and/or epidermis capable of producing melanin pigment in the early stages of the lesions and under certain circumstances, such as sun exposure or hormonal influence. Melanocytes present only in the dermoepidermal junction are referred to as junctional nevi, often occurring on the acral surfaces as pigmented macules. Melanocytes present in the dermoepidermal junction and the dermis are referred to as compound nevi. These are often raised and may be papillomatous. Melanocytes present exclusively in the dermis are referred to as dermal nevi. These are typically flesh colored. Each has a typical clinical presentation, but considerable overlap of features is seen (Table 1). Lesions larger than 0.5 cm are often dysplastic nevi or congenital nevi.

Congenital nevi are present at birth and have the specific histologic characteristics of nevus cells occurring deep around skin structures. They are divided into small (<1.5 cm), medium (1.5 to 20 cm), and large (>20 cm) (Table 2). Small congenital nevi have a low risk for melanoma development, whereas large congenital melanocytic nevi have a substantially higher risk of cutaneous or even leptomeningeal melanoma. Because the melanocytes occur deep in the subcutaneous fat and even fascia, excision can be quite disfiguring.

Many variants of melanocytic nevi exist. Halo nevi (Sutton's nevi) are pigmented nevi surrounded by a well-circumscribed white halo caused by the cytotoxic effect of

CURRENT DIAGNOSIS

- The diagnosis of a nevus is based on the clinical presentation. If the clinician suspects a possible melanoma, the diagnosis is confirmed by histologic examination.
- A thorough physical examination of patients with lesions should be performed in adequate lighting that involves careful inspection of the lesion in question, as well as a recommended total skin examination. This includes the scalp, palms, soles, genitalia, buttocks, axillae, and between digits.
- Nevi must be distinguished from melanoma.
- Suspicious lesions are usually larger than 0.6 cm.
- Irregular borders, asymmetry, and variable pigmentation also suggest melanoma (see Box 1).
- Patient education regarding clinical signs of melanoma is imperative, and sun protection should be encouraged.
- Any patient history with persistent change in a long-lasting pigmented lesion or the development of a new pigmented lesion warrants careful inspection.
- Appropriate documentation of the lesion should include the location, color, and size of the lesion. A simple drawing or chart may be beneficial. A magnifying lens may also be useful to visualize lesions.
- Dermoscopy (epiluminescence microscopy, dermatoscopy) in the hands of an experienced clinician may provide further diagnostic accuracy by using a handheld magnifier (×10) with or without polarization and oil interface.
- Photographic documentation of lesions is helpful for people with multiple lesions who require comparative examinations in the future.

TABLE 1 Clinical and Histologic Features of Common Acquired Melanocytic Nevi

Feature	Junctional	Compound	Dermal
Size	<5 mm	<5 mm	<10 mm
Color	Tan to brown	Brown	Flesh colored to tan or pink
Primary lesion	Macule (flat)	Papule (raised)	Papule (raised)
Clinical location	Head, neck, trunk, upper extremities	Head, neck, trunk	Face, head, neck, trunk, upper/lower extremities
Histologic location	Dermoepidermal junction	Dermoepidermal junction and dermis	Dermis

infiltrating T lymphocytes. Halo nevi are more common in adolescents than in adults. Patients older than age 40 years with halo nevi, especially if multiple lesions are present, should be evaluated for the presence of melanoma elsewhere on the body or in the lesion.

Blue nevi are typically heavily pigmented lesions and usually located on the dorsal hands and feet, as well as the scalp and sacral region. They are believed to arise from dermal melanocytes that failed to complete migration to the epidermis during gestation. It is important to note that not all blue nevi appear blue, and the color varies depending on the light source and the depth of pigment deposition in the skin. Dark brown, black, or even gray hues are often noted. Although color variation exists, blue nevi have a hard consistency and are typically small and symmetric.

Nevus spilus (speckled lentiginous nevus) most commonly affects the trunk and extremities. It is characterized by a tan patch (flat) ranging from 1 to 4 cm with a tan background and a dark brown speckled pattern. Microscopically, the epidermis contains increased single melanocytes at the dermoepidermal junction. Meanwhile, the 1- to 6-mm smaller interspersed multiple speckles of dark brown macules or papules may demonstrate increased single melanocytes or melanocytic nesting with or without dermal involvement (compound or junctional nevus).

Spitz nevi or epithelioid and spindle cell nevus were formerly known as benign juvenile melanoma. Although benign, these single flesh-colored or slightly pigmented papules or nodules commonly seen on children and young adults can occasionally mimic melanoma histologically.

Rarely, they occur with multiple lesions grouped together. This form is known as agminated Spitz nevus. The head and neck region is the most common site, but they may be present on the trunk or extremities. Clinically, Spitz nevi are often difficult to distinguish from conventional nevi. Some Spitz nevi can be heavily pigmented and demonstrate hemangioma-like features, but in general they are less pigmented than common nevi, appearing as tan-colored dome-shaped papules.

Dysplastic or atypical melanocytic nevi (Clark's nevus, nevus with architectural disorder) are pigmented lesions with irregular borders in a haphazard variety of colors ranging from pink, brown, and dark brown to black. Erythema may be present around the nevus as a perilesional halo or within the lesion. These may be flat or raised and in general are larger than common acquired nevi. Lesions most commonly involve the trunk but can be identified in any skin location, and the number can range from one to hundreds of lesions. Atypical isolated lesions have a low risk of melanoma, whereas patients with a strong family history of melanoma and patients with multiple larger lesions are at an increased risk for the development of melanoma.

Recurrent nevi (pseudomelanoma) result from incompletely removed nevi, especially after shave removal. The lesion is usually macular and demonstrates irregular borders and coloration within or adjacent to the previous surgical scar (Box 1). Loss of pigment and stippling and mottling may be present. More than half of recurrent nevi are noted to occur within 6 months after the procedure.

Treatment

Although most melanocytic nevi require no treatment because of their static and benign appearance and nature, occasionally, some may require a biopsy with complete histologic examination to exclude the possibility of

TABLE 2 Clinical Features of Small, Medium, and Large Congenital Nevi

Feature	Small and Medium	Large
Size	<1.5 cm (small) 1.5–20 cm (medium)	<20 cm
Color	Tan to brown with follicular accentuation	Brown to black
Primary lesion	Plaquelike, pebbled	Plaquelike, furrowed
Clinical location	Anywhere, especially head, neck	Anywhere, including involvement of major anatomic region

---

BOX 1 The ABCD Approach to the Clinical Evaluation of Suspicious-Appearing Lesions

- Asymmetry in shape
- Border irregularities
- Color variation
- Diameter more than 6 mm

CURRENT THERAPY

- Although most melanocytic nevi are static and benign in appearance, some require a biopsy with complete histologic examination to exclude the possibility of melanoma.
- Indications for biopsy and treatment include typical clinical appearance suspicious for melanoma (see Box 1); changing lesion; repeated irritation including bleeding, ulceration, pruritus, pain; incomplete removal or recurrence of an old lesion; presence of a new lesion; or cosmetic reasons (see Box 2).
- Patients should be informed of the potential for scarring if the indication is purely cosmetic.
- Although multiple biopsy/treatment methods for nevi are available, certain variables may help to determine which procedure is most appropriate: convenience, amount of healing time, adequacy of specimen for histologic examination, and cosmetic result.
- Pigmented melanocytic lesions should never be destroyed by cryosurgery because it impairs the ability to diagnose the lesion properly. Treatment may include biopsy and/or excision.

melanoma. Indications for biopsy and treatment include typical clinical appearance suspicious for melanoma (see Box 1); changing lesion; repeated irritation (including bleeding, ulceration, pruritus, pain); incomplete removal or recurrence of an old lesion; presence of a new lesion; or cosmetic reasons (Box 2).

SHAVE BIOPSY/EXCISION

The shave biopsy is a quick method performed with a scalpel (usually a number 15 blade). A straight razor blade allows for easily controlling depth by increasing or decreasing the convexity of the blade. Shave biopsy/excision is not generally used for pigmented lesions, because an unanticipated melanoma cannot be properly staged if only the superficial portion is removed. Shave biopsies are preferred for lesions with less suspicious pathology confined to the epidermis, such as actinic keratoses, skin tags, and superficial basal cell carcinomas (see Box 2).

The saucerization technique involves deeper removal of the lesion by taking 1- to 2-mm margins of normal skin surrounding the lesion. This technique provides significantly more tissue for histologic evaluation of depth.

BOX 2   Indications for Biopsy/Excision

- Atypical clinical appearance suspicious for melanoma
- Changing lesion
- Repeated irritation (including bleeding, ulceration, pruritus, pain)
- Recurrence of old lesion
- Presence of new lesion
- Cosmetic reasons

PUNCH BIOPSY/EXCISION

The punch biopsy uses a round cutting instrument ranging in diameter from 2 to 10 mm. The punch is an ideal procedure for diagnostic skin biopsy because it provides full-thickness evaluation while providing a better cosmetic result than a shave biopsy. Punch biopsies are quick and easily performed, with a low incidence of significant scarring. Ideally, the entire lesion should be removed for proper evaluation.

ELLIPTICAL EXCISION

Elliptical excision removes the pigmented lesion with a variable amount of clinically normal skin. It is indicated for any lesion that is suspicious for malignancy, especially when lesions cannot be removed with a punch because of depth, location, or size. This type of excision provides plentiful tissue for histologic interpretation and provides a good cosmetic result with rapid healing.

REFERENCES

Barnhill RL: Textbook of Dermatopathology, 2nd ed. New York, McGraw-Hill, 2004.
Bolognia JL, Jorizzo JL, Rapini RP, et al: Dermatology. St Louis, Mosby, 2003.
Freedburg IM, Eisen AZ, Wolff K, et al: Fitzpatrick's Dermatology in General Medicine. New York, McGraw-Hill, 2003.
James WD, Berger TG, Elston DM: Andrews' Diseases of the Skin Clinical Dermatology. New York, Elsevier, 2006.
Massi G, LeBoit PE, Pasquini P, et al: Histological Diagnosis of Nevi and Melanoma. Darmstadt, Germany, Steinkopff-Verlag, 2004.
Weedon D: Skin Pathology. New York, Churchill Livingstone, 2002.

Melanoma

Method of
Frank G. Haluska, MD, PhD

Melanoma is the most lethal of all solid cancers: prognostically, no other tumor carries the severe implication that its diagnosis does. An early-stage, solitary 3-cm lesion for lung cancer, responsible for most cancer deaths, may confer 5-year mortality of 20% to 30% on discovery. In contrast, a primary melanoma only 1 mm in depth confers a similar prognosis spread over 10 years. Melanoma offers a constant challenge to improve prevention, detection, diagnosis, and treatment.

Epidemiology

The incidence of melanoma is rapidly increasing with approximately 62,190 new cases projected in the United States in 2006 and 7910 deaths as a consequence. Risk factors include a changing mole, dysplastic nevi either arising in the setting of family history or sporadically, or a personal history of melanoma or congenital nevi. Sensitivity to sun and a history of sunburns and freckling are also associated with risks for melanoma. Prevention and

CURRENT DIAGNOSIS

- Pigmented or unusual nonpigmented skin lesions should be carefully evaluated for ABCD:
  - *A*symmetry or unusual contours
  - *B*order irregularity
  - *C*olor that is blue, black, red, or white (regressed); is variegated or changing
  - *D*iameter that is larger than 6 mm (a pencil eraser's diameter) or is enlarging
- Elevated, ulcerated or bleeding lesions require evaluation.
- Diagnosis by biopsy must be excisional or incisional.

CURRENT THERAPY

- Proper surgery is the mainstay of treatment.
- The primary tumor should be completely excised with recommended margins.
- A sentinel lymph node biopsy is recommended for lesions 1 mm and deeper.
- Palpable regional lymph nodes should be biopsied and resected if involved.
- There is no adjuvant medical therapy for stage I and II, but interferon alpha-2B is recommended for stage III.
- Stage IV DTIC chemotherapy and interleukin-2 cytokine therapy are FDA approved, but clinical trial entry is an important option.

early detection depend on taking a careful history from patients in such risk categories.

Clinical Features and Diagnosis

Melanomas can arise on any cutaneous surface, on any mucous membrane, in structures of the eye, or as a metastasis lacking a primary site, but they typically arise on sun-exposed skin surfaces. The most common sites of occurrence in males are the trunk and back, and in females the lower legs and back.

The clinician should have a high index of suspicion for any lesion that is new, has changed, or is out of the ordinary. The visible features requiring further investigation include irregularity of surface texture, border contour, or coloration. Growth, manifested as an increase in diameter, nodularity or elevation, is worrisome. Surface ulceration and overt hemorrhage are also hallmarks of melanoma. The clinician should have a low threshold for biopsy for lesions with any of these characteristics. Patients should be taught the features (ABCD) as well: lesion asymmetry (A), an irregular border (B), changing or variegated color (C), and a diameter (D) larger than a pencil eraser.

An expert dermatologist can augment diagnostic accuracy at the bedside using epiluminescence microscopy or by using dermoscopy with sophisticated digital photography and image analysis. The standard for diagnosis is histopathologic evaluation by excisional biopsy of the lesion with a narrow margin. An incisional biopsy may be used when lesions are large or in a difficult anatomical site. In both instances the objective should be to allow for full-thickness histopathologic assessment of the lesion. Other biopsy techniques (e.g., shave or curettage) and local ablative therapies such as liquid nitrogen are contraindicated if melanoma is considered in the differential diagnosis. Correctly performing biopsy is critical in arriving at an accurate tissue diagnosis and providing subsequent treatment.

Treatment

SURGICAL THERAPY OF PRIMARY MELANOMA

Melanoma, detected early, is a curable disease; but most cases cured are by surgical, not medical, means.

Surgical care encompasses primary excision integrated with regional lymph node assessment and removal.

Planning the Primary Excision

The goals of primary surgical excision of melanoma are threefold. First, the procedure must account for the potential need for assessment of regional lymph node involvement. Second, the lesion must be completely excised with curative intent. Third, the margin of excision should be planned to minimize the risk of local recurrence.

The assessment of the regional lymph nodes is controversial. No randomized clinical trial has demonstrated that elective lymph node dissection of the draining lymph node basin influences the median survival of a population of melanoma. Regional lymph node mapping, or sentinel lymph node (SLN) biopsy, has the same findings; but technical accessibility, reliability, proven prognostic value, relative lack of morbidity, and the potential for therapeutic value have led to its widespread use. SLN biopsy involves injection of a blue dye and radioactive tracer, which migrate to the lymph node providing drainage of the primary site; intraoperative identification of the node with a small radiation counter; and excision for histopathologic examination. Approximately 17% of patients referred for SLN biopsy ultimately have involved sentinel lymph nodes. Patients with involved (positive) sentinel nodes should then be taken to complete lymph node dissection of the involved basin. Sentinel lymph node biopsy, at the time of excision with an intermediate thickness (1 mm or greater) melanoma and in selected cases of high-risk thinner melanomas, is now the standard of surgical care for the melanoma patient.

Initial wide local excision of a primary tumor may interfere with the normal pattern of lymphatic drainage; consequently, lymphatic mapping may be impaired or precluded. Therefore, it is important to perform SLN biopsy concurrent with wide excision. Excision of the lesion is designed to remove all melanoma at the local site. Typically, the incision used is elliptical, and the tumor should be removed en bloc with the underlying tissues to the level of the muscular fascia.

Local metastases, or satellites, can spread to the skin immediately surrounding the primary tumor, and a margin

TABLE 1 Surgical Treatment of Primary Melanoma

Breslow Depth	Margin	Sentinel Node Biopsy
<1.00 mm	1 cm	Only if adverse prognostic feature*
1.00–2.00 mm	2 cm	Yes
>2.00 mm	At least 2 cm	Yes

*For example, ulceration.

of normal tissue should be excised to minimize the risk that these metastases will manifest later as local recurrences. The most recent of five randomized clinical trials assessing adequacy of margins suggests that thicker tumors require wider margins, but none show that margins affect survival. Recommendations for excisional margins vary from center to center. Table 1 lists the surgical care guidelines used in the Massachusetts General Hospital Melanoma Center.

If local lymph nodes are palpable at the time of diagnosis, therapeutic lymph node dissection is required.

ADJUVANT MEDICAL THERAPY OF HIGH-RISK DISEASE

The most important prognostic features obtainable at the time of diagnosis, incorporated into the American Joint Committee on Cancer (AJCC) staging system, are Breslow depth, the presence of ulceration of the primary tumor, and lymph node involvement (Table 2). The 10-year survival rate for patients with stage I melanoma (localized and 2 mm or thinner) is approximately 85%; for stage II (localized but thicker than 2 mm) survival is 55%; and for stage III (metastatic to the local skin or lymph nodes), it is 35%. Biologically, at the time of diagnosis, occult metastases are present in a subset of patients who will eventually succumb to recurrence. This provides an opportunity for early therapy in an at-risk population or adjuvant therapy.

There are no adjuvant therapies at present for stage I and stage II melanoma, providing an active area for research. The United States Food and Drug Administration (FDA) has approved interferon alpha-2b (Intron A) for patients with a high risk of systemic recurrence (T4 lesions 4 mm deep or greater, or stage III melanoma).

TABLE 2 Survival by Stage and Sentinel Node Status

Stage	10-yr Survival	Median Survival
I	85%	-
II	55%	-
III	35%	-
IV	8%	8 months

Sentinel Node Status	3-yr Disease-Free Survival	3-yr Overall Survival
Negative	88.5%	96.8%
Positive	55.8%	69.9%

This yearlong course of adjuvant therapy is expensive with a significant side-effect profile, primarily a severe flu-like syndrome, with hepato- and myelotoxicity. Yet, interferon alpha-2b is the only therapy proven in the randomized controlled setting to alter the natural history of this disease. Interferon alpha-2b prolongs relapse-free survival reproducibly; two trials suggested improvement in overall survival of approximately 10% as well, though a recent meta-analysis demonstrates this is not statistically significant.

MEDICAL THERAPY OF ADVANCED DISEASE

The median survival of stage IV melanoma patients is approximately 8 months. Melanoma can spread to any site, but metastases most commonly involve skin, lymph nodes, brain, lung, and liver. No treatment for metastatic melanoma has ever been proven to effectively prolong survival in a randomized clinical trial; thus, for many patients, entry into a clinical study is an important option for stage IV therapy.

CYTOTOXIC THERAPY

Like many other solid tumors, such as metastatic pancreatic or renal cell cancer, melanoma is relatively refractory to the systemic administration of cytotoxic chemotherapy. Response rates to most single agents, including alkylating agents, platinum compounds, and taxanes, range from 5% to 20%. Dacarbazine (DTIC) is the only chemotherapy agent approved for use in melanoma. Temozolomide (Temodar),[2] an oral drug metabolized to the same active agent (MTIC) as DTIC, is often used in its place. In recent randomized clinical trials using modern RECIST response-evaluation criteria, response rates for DTIC were approximately 7%. Complete response rates were low: approximately 1%. A recent European randomized trial suggested fotemustine might improve response rate compared to DTIC, but no single drug has improved the survival of treated patient populations.

Combination chemotherapy has been studied extensively. Two common regimens are as follows:

1. The Dartmouth regimen: DTIC, carmustine (BCNU), cisplatin (Platinol), and tamoxifen (Nolvadex)
2. Cisplatin, DTIC, and vinblastine (CVD)

Although single-institution studies suggest improved response rates with these regimens, in randomized trials survival rates are no better with these regimens than with single agent treatment.

IMMUNOTHERAPY

Interleukin-2 (IL-2), recombinant (Proleukin), is a second drug approved by the FDA and available for use in patients with stage IV disease. The major toxicity of IL-2 is a systemic inflammatory state, which manifests as capillary-leak syndrome and hypotension. Most patients require pressors or intensive care during treatment. Clinicians should restrict IL-2 use to a select subset of patients with excellent performance status and features predictive of response to therapy.

[2]Not available in the United States.

Melanoma

967

Initial dramatic responses were reported with systemic IL-2 therapy, but the response rate is now approximately 15%. Patients with metastases confined to the skin demonstrate a response rate of 54%, but for patients with disease other than that confined to skin and lymph nodes, the response rate is approximately 11%. At the National Cancer Institute (NCI) approximately 3% of patients experience durable complete responses. But overall, IL-2 therapy is of limited benefit to most patients with visceral metastatic melanoma.

BIOCHEMOTHERAPY

The hypothesis that combining chemotherapy and immunotherapy might join therapies having different mechanisms of action and drug resistance led to the development of biochemotherapy. Most biochemotherapy regimens include combination chemotherapy, interleukin-2, and interferon, but a variety of regimens have been tested. A randomized study of biochemotherapy compared with chemotherapy conducted at the NIH was stopped early because the outcome favored chemotherapy alone; a second single-institutional randomized study suggested an improved response rate and a marginal survival improvement from biochemotherapy but with severe toxicity (90% of patients requiring pressors). Recently, several large multi-institutional randomized studies demonstrated that biochemotherapy is more toxic but no more effective than chemotherapy alone.

Clinical Trial Directions: Targeted Therapies, Vaccines, and New Approaches

The potential for progress in treating melanoma depends on the development of new approaches tested in clinical trials. The first area of promise is the use of small molecule inhibitors of biochemical pathways important in the pathogenesis of melanoma. The most frequent somatic mutations in melanoma involve the RAS signal transduction cascades: the BRAF protein is mutated in 60% to 70% of cutaneous melanomas. Inhibitors of this protein, including the new agent sorafenib,[1] are in clinical trials alone and in combination with other small molecules and cytotoxic agents. The BCL-2 protein has also been targeted in this disease, and continued study of antisense inhibitors of BCL-2 expression is ongoing.

The second important avenue of research is active immunotherapy, using approaches designed to augment host antitumor immunity. Approaches include the use of surgically resected autologous melanoma as vaccine (in GM-CSF-gene transduced preparations, or in conjunction with autologous heat shock proteins), allogeneic vaccines (e.g., Canvaxin and Melacine), melanoma antigen-derived peptide vaccines, lymphodepletion protocols, and antibodies to immunoregulatory molecules (anti-CTLA4). Although none of these approaches has yielded positive results in randomized trials, single-institution reports often suggest potential efficacy. A focus on immunotherapy will likely remain an important component of investigational therapy for melanoma.

REFERENCES

Atkins MB, Lee S, Flaherty LE, et al: A prospective randomized phase III trial concurrent biochemotherapy with cisplatin, vinblastine, dacarbazine (CVD), IL-2 and interferon alpha-2b versus CVD alone in patients with metastatic melanoma (E3695): An ECOG-coordinated intergroup trial. Proc ASCO 2003;22:708.

Avril MF, Aamdal S, Grob JJ, et al: Fotemustine compared with dacarbazine in patients with disseminated malignant melanoma: A phase III study. J Clin Oncol 2004;22:1118-1125.

Balch CM, Buzaid AC, Soong SJ, et al: Final version of the American Joint Committee on Cancer staging system for cutaneous melanoma. J Clin Oncol 2001;19:3635-3648.

Chapman PB, Einhorn LH, Meyers ML, et al: Phase III multicenter randomized trial of the Dartmouth regimen versus dacarbazine in patients with metastatic melanoma. J Clin Oncol 1999;17:2745-2751.

Gershenwald JE, Thompson W, Mansfield PF, et al: Multi-institutional melanoma lymphatic mapping experience: The prognostic value of sentinel lymph node status in 612 stage I or II melanoma patients. J Clin Oncol 1999;17:976-983.

Kirkwood JM, Manola J, Ibrahim J, et al: A pooled analysis of Eastern Cooperative Oncology Group and intergroup trials of adjuvant high-dose interferon for melanoma. Clin Cancer Res 2004;10:1670-1677.

Krown SE, Chapman PB: Defining adequate surgery for primary melanoma. N Engl J Med 2004;350:823-825.

McMasters KM, Reintgen DS, Ross MI, et al: Sentinel lymph node biopsy for melanoma: controversy despite widespread agreement. J Clin Oncol 2001;19:2851-2855.

Middleton MR, Grob JJ, Aaronson N, et al: Randomized phase III study of temozolomide versus dacarbazine in the treatment of patients with advanced metastatic malignant melanoma. J Clin Oncol 2000;18:158-166.

Phan GQ, Attia P, Steinberg SM, et al: Factors associated with response to high-dose interleukin-2 in patients with metastatic melanoma. J Clin Oncol 2001;19:3477-3482.

Premalignant Lesions

Method of
Donald Clemons, MD

Premalignant Lesions

Premalignant lesions of the skin are those that, if left untreated, can evolve into malignant invasive and potentially metastasizing tumors. With early treatment, these lesions can be managed and the threat of malignancy averted. These premalignant diseases include actinic keratosis (AK), actinic cheilitis, Bowen's disease, bowenoid papulosis, porokeratosis, and nevus sebaceus.

Nonmelanoma skin cancer's worldwide economic and health implications are enormous, because it is the most prevalent form of cancer. However, it is also one of the most preventable cancers and, in early stages, relatively easy to diagnose and treat. We must educate our patient population to not only recognize and seek treatment for these early manifestations but to also act as public health advocates regarding modification of behavioral patterns of our at-risk population.

---

[1]Not FDA approved for this indication.

CURRENT DIAGNOSIS

Actinic keratosis
- Tender, rough adherent scale on erythematous base
- Background of photo-damaged skin
- Suspect SCC if indurated or hyperkeratotic

Actinic cheilitis
- Protuberant lower lip mucosa, fair skin, photo damage
- Often history of pipe or chewing tobacco use
- Up to 25% metastatic incidence with invasion

Bowen's disease
- Erythematous sharply demarcated plaque with variable scale
- Involves hair follicles
- Frequently recurs if inadequately treated
- May affect genital mucosal skin

Bowenoid papulosis
- Clinically indistinguishable from warts
- Genital skin
- Histologically indistinguishable from Bowen's disease
- Associated with HPV-16

Porokeratosis
- Papules or annular plaques with thin peripheral collarette of scale
- Discrete or linear
- Sun damaged skin or palms or soles
- Coronoid lamella seen histologically

Nevus sebaceus
- Perpetual elevated often inapparent plaques usually on head or neck
- Postpubertal evolve into yellow-orange papillomatous plaques devoid of hair
- Malignancies are usually low grade

Abbreviations: HPV-16 = human papilloma virus type 16; SCC = squamous cell carcinoma.

CURRENT THERAPY

Actinic keratosis
- Cryotherapy, light curettage, dermabrasion, or chemical peels
- Topical or systemic tretinoin (Retin-A), fluorouracil (Efudex), diclofenac (Solaraze), imiquimod (Aldara), or PDT

Actinic cheilitis
- Cryotherapy, fluorouracil, imiquimod
- Vermilionectomy, laser, PDT

Bowen's disease
- All methods used for actinic keratosis
- Excision to include Mohs' surgery

Bowenoid papulosis
- Same as Bowen's
- Imiquimod may be treatment of choice

Porokeratosis
- Cryosurgery, salicylic plaster and fluorouracil, topical tretinoin[1]
- Imiquimod

Nevus sebaceus
- Watchful waiting with appropriate biopsies
- Excision

[1]Not FDA approved for this indication.
Abbreviations: PDT = photodynamic therapy

Premalignant lesions are most commonly located on chronic sun-exposed and sun-damaged skin in lighter-skinned individuals who easily burn, have light hair color, have blue or green eyes, and freckle. Both genetic and extrinsic factors are responsible for the development and progression of these lesions. Chronically damaged skin, such as burn scars and long-standing ulcers, infections, and areas having received ionizing radiation are also more likely to develop malignant transformation. Other factors placing patients at increased risk include chronic arsenic exposure and immunosuppression as seen in the elderly, organ transplant recipients, HIV-infected individuals, and patients receiving systemic steroid therapy. This large subset of patients is more likely to rapidly develop malignant transformation and show aggressive behavior in their lesions. They should be closely monitored and considered for long-term prophylactic care.

Actinic Keratosis

Actinic keratosis, a form of squamous cell carcinoma (SCC) in situ, is usually found on photo-damaged skin and is characterized clinically by rough adherent scale on an erythematous nonindurated occasionally friable and tender base. The background is usually telangiectatic with areas of dyspigmentation. Hyperpigmented and atrophic variations can be seen. They may be palpated easier than visualized but can progress to thickened hyperkeratotic plaques. Rapidly enlarging lesions or those that are excessively hyperkeratotic or indurated should be biopsied to rule out malignant progression to SCC. Histologically, AKs are characterized by a partial thickness disordered wind-blown maturation of atypical epidermal keratinocytes and a thickened compact stratum corneum. The hair acrotrichium and sweat duct acrosyringium are spared involvement and no invasion is seen. The epidermis can be thickened or atrophic.

TREATMENT OF ACTINIC KERATOSIS

Treatment can be by physical disruptions or chemically applied methods. Among the physical methods, liquid nitrogen cryosurgery is most commonly used. Care must be taken to adequately freeze and destroy the lesion yet minimize significant pigment alteration or scarring. The length of the freeze time will vary by size, thickness, and location of the tumor, ethnic skin color, and concomitant systemic illness such as lupus erythematosus or cryoglobulinemia.

Light curettage, medium-depth chemical peels, and dermabrasion can be used for more extensive lesions. Carbon dioxide (CO_2) and Er:YAG (erbium:yttrium-aluminum-garnet) lasers, although more expensive and having more potential complications, are effective methods of treatment. Surgical excision is usually reserved for clinically suspicious discrete lesions or treatment recalcitrant lesions.

The topically applied chemical methods include topical tretinoin (Retin-A, Differin, Tazorac[1]), fluorouracil cream or solution (Efudex, Fluoroplex, Carac), diclofenac sodium gel (Solaraze), imiquimod cream (Aldara), or 20% aminolevulinic acid (ALA) (Levulan) with photodynamic therapy. Tretinoin[1] cream or gel is applied daily to photo-damaged skin indefinitely. Results are usually not clinically evident for 4 to 6 months of therapy. Side effects of dryness and scaling can be improved by judicious use of medication; moisturizers; and initially alternate- or every-third-day therapy, gradually increasing as tolerated. Ultraviolet A (UVA) and ultraviolet B (UVB) blocking sunscreens are critical to retard further skin damage.

Fluorouracil can be found in a 0.5%, 1%, or 5% cream or 1% solution and is applied once or twice daily for up to 8 weeks as tolerated. It is highly effective; but side effects of redness, pain, erosion, and allergic reaction may limit its usefulness. Side effects often persist for weeks after therapy has ceased. Diclofenac gel is applied twice daily for 2 to 3 months; although better tolerated clinically, it is expensive, requires compliance, and can have side effects similar to fluorouracil as well as photosensitive and anticoagulative effects. Imiquimod cream 0.5% is a new class of immunomodulator drug that is applied once daily 2 to 5 times per week for 4 to 6 weeks.[2] It can cause erythema, scaling, and erosion but is usually relatively painless and resolves as the lesions clear. It is expensive but may offer more long-term clearing and may be effective against concomitant superficially invasive cancers.

Topical photodynamic therapy (PDT) is the most recent addition to the treatment arm. After acetone pretreatment, 20% ALA (Levulan) is applied and allowed to incubate for 1 to 3 hours. It is activated by a light source such as a blue light, an intense pulsed light, or a long pulse dye laser causing destruction of individual lesions and cosmetic improvement of photo-damaged skin. One to three treatments at 3-week intervals are needed. The therapy is expensive, requires equipment, causes 24- to 36-hour photosensitivity, and is variably uncomfortable. This therapy is also highly effective, and cosmetic downtime is lessened. Lack of scarring or dyspigmentation and less noncompliance issues combined with superior cosmetic photodamage repair make this a useful alternative treatment. Hypertropic extremity lesions can be pretreated for 5 days with fluorouracil before PDT.

Oral tretinoin (acitretin)[1] 25 mg or 0.4 mg/kg/day as tolerated can be an effective treatment for chronic AKs in immunosuppressed individuals minimizing the progression to invasive SCC. Benefits cease with disruption of therapy.

Actinic Cheilitis

Actinic cheilitis (leukokeratosis or leukoplakia of the lip) usually occurs on the lower lip mucosa. Predisposing factors include chronic photodamage, fair skin, protuberant lower lip, and pipe or chewing tobacco use. This disease is essentially AK, and much of what was previously discussed about AK applies here. Unfortunately, the incidence of invasion is higher and the subsequent chance of metastatic spread may approach 25%. Clinically, actinic cheilitis can appear as a tender whitish plaque adherent to the mucosa. Erosion, induration, and erythema should be evaluated further because these are often signs of invasion; a biopsy of the most clinically affected area may be necessary to rule invasion out.

TREATMENT OF ACTINIC CHELITIS

Treatment is often accompanied by pain, discomfort, erosion, and slow healing. The most commonly used method of treatment is liquid nitrogen spray. If fluorouracil or imiquimod (Aldara) are used, only 2 to 3 weekly applications may be tolerated; treatment may be necessary for 6 to 8 weeks with erosion persisting for many weeks afterward.

Surgical advancement of normal mucosa (vermilionectomy) with removal of affected tissue or CO_2 laser ablation can be performed, but these procedures are technically difficult and potentially scarring. Recently, another form of photodynamic therapy using 20% ALA incubated for 2 to 3 hours followed by activation with a pulse dye laser 595 nm long pulsed has been reported very effective with minimal discomfort and erosive side effects. This therapy might be an alternative treatment, if this laser is available.

Bowen's Disease

Bowen's disease is a form of SCC in situ that differs histologically from AK by involving the full thickness of the epidermis to include involvement of the hair follicle acrotrichium. Because of hair follicle involvement, superficial treatments that are effective on actinic keratosis often fail when treating Bowen's disease. Recurrence as well as development of invasive squamous cell carcinoma may occur. Bowen's disease occurring on non–sun-exposed hair-bearing skin is suggestive of arsenic exposure; concomitant lymphoreticular or gastrointestinal malignancies may develop. Bowen's disease on mucosal surfaces of the penis or labia (erythroplasia of Queyrat) has a higher incidence of invasion and metastasis (20% to 30%) and, therefore, should be managed more aggressively and closely monitored. Clinically, these lesions appear as an erythematous sharply demarcated plaque with light to moderate scale on sun-damaged skin. It can often be mistaken for eczema or psoriasis. On mucosal surfaces, it may be more indurated and velvety. Care must be taken to ensure that there is no involvement of the urethral meatus.

TREATMENT OF BOWEN'S DISEASE

Treatment modalities include aggressive liquid nitrogen therapy, topical fluorouracil (Efudex) two times a day for 6 to 8 weeks[2], and curettage; but there is a significant risk of recurrence on hair-bearing skin. Topical imiquimod (Aldara) 3 to 5 times weekly for 6 to 8 weeks may be more effective, especially on mucosal skin, but long-term cure rates are uncertain. Simple excision, or Mohs' surgery, probably affords the most effective and curative method

---

[1]Not FDA approved for this indication.

[2]Exceeds dosage recommended by the manufacturer.

available; but there is significant potential for scarring and may result in a mutilating procedure on genital skin.

Bowenoid Papulosis

Bowenoid papulosis represents SCC in situ on genital skin associated primarily with human papilloma virus type 16 (HPV-16) that can progress to invasive SCC. Clinically, these lesions are indistinguishable from common warts, or condyloma acuminatum, and present as tan or reddish-brown papules or plaques. Histologically, viral changes are absent and show classic features of Bowen's disease.

TREATMENT OF BOWENOID PAPULOSIS

The same treatment modalities used in Bowen's disease are effective; although imiquimod may be the treatment of choice to cure additional clinically inapparent or distal lesions on cervix or vaginal mucosa. Daily application 3 times weekly[2] for 8 weeks has shown cure. In addition, PDT activated by a Diode laser and topical cidofovir (Vistide)[1] may also have use in recalcitrant lesions.

Porokeratosis

Porokeratosis presents as papules or annular plaques, which may be discrete or linear and occur on photo-damaged skin or on palms or soles. Clinically, they show central flattening and a peripheral fine thin collarette of scale and may show centrifugal spread. These lesions may be congenital or acquired and are represented by five distinct variants with several types sometimes present in one patient. They may evolve into invasive SCC. Histologically, they are all characterized by having a thin angled parakeratotic column over a focus of dyskeratotic cells without a granular cell layer (coronoid lamella), which represents the advancing margin.

TREATMENT OF POROKERATOSIS

Successful treatment of these lesions is often difficult. Hard cryosurgery is effective but may scar. Topical tretinoin[1] 0.1% gel daily for 4 months or a combination of salicylic acid plaster pads (Mediplast)[1] in the morning and fluorouracil in the afternoon or evening has been successful. Topical 5% imiquimod 3 times weekly for at least 3 weeks may be used as well as topical or systemic fluorouracil, as tolerated.

Nevus Sebaceus

Nevus sebaceus is a congenital hamartoma of infancy comprised of immature sebaceous, follicular, and apocrine elements. Following puberty, benign pilosebaceous and apocrine tumors may develop as well as low-grade malignant neoplasms. Rarely, aggressive malignant sebaceous and apocrine carcinomas have been reported. Clinically, they are slightly elevated often inapparent linear plaques

---

[1]Not FDA approved for this indication.
[2]Exceeds dosage recommended by the manufacturer.

---

most often present on the head or neck. At puberty, they evolve into yellow-orange plaques devoid of hair with a velvety or papillomatous surface.

TREATMENT OF NEVUS SEBACEUS

Treatment is by surgical excision or watchful waiting. Large lesions can be removed by staged excisions. Development of nodules or ulcerations should be biopsied to rule out tumor development.

REFERENCES

Dereli T, Ozyurt S, Ozturk G: Porokeratosis of Mibelli: Successful treatment with cryosurgery. J Dermatol 2004;31(3):223-227.

Jones E, Korzenko A, Kriegel D: Oral isotretinoin in the treatment and prevention of cutaneous squamous cell carcinoma. J Drugs Dermatol 2004;3(5):498-502

Jorrizo J, Carney P, Ko W, et al: Treatment options in the management of actinic keratosis. Cutis 2004;74(6s):9-15.

Villa A, Berman B: Immunomodulators for skin cancer. J Drugs Dermatol 2004;3(5): 533-539.

Bacterial Diseases of the Skin

Method of
Ronald Lee Nichols, MD

The spectrum of bacterial diseases of the skin ranges from superficial, localized, easily recognized, and treated skin eruptions to deep, aggressive, gangrenous, or necrotizing infections that might appear innocuous at first but quickly become life threatening. The prompt recognition and treatment of these infections is paramount in limiting morbidity and mortality. A healthy respect for the aggressiveness of gangrenous and necrotizing infections of the skin and soft tissues is developed by first harboring a high index of suspicion to provide early recognition and appropriate treatment before overwhelming clinical infection occurs.

COMMON INFECTIONS

Impetigo

Impetigo is the most common bacterial infection of the skin. It is highly contagious and can occur at any age from infancy to adulthood, but it is most common in preschool-aged children. There are two classic forms of impetigo: nonbullous and bullous. Both forms have a predominantly staphylococcal etiology, but they present with different morphologic characteristics.

Nonbullous (crusted) impetigo can be recognized by the development of a serous, yellow-brown exudate, which dries into a golden crust. Lesions rarely elicit pain but can be associated with erythema and pruritus. They are most common on exposed areas such as the hands, feet, and legs

CURRENT DIAGNOSIS

- Most infections are superficial and local and not associated with systemic toxicity.
- Deeper infections may involve many layers of the soft tissues including fascia and muscle.
- Systemic toxicity is always present in the deeper infections.
- Rapid advancement of the local infection with areas of necrosis indicates more serious infections including necrotizing and gangrenous processes.
- Streptococci and clostridial microorganisms are the cause of most gangrenous infections.
- Mixed aerobic and anaerobic microflora cause most necrotizing infections.

and are often associated with a traumatic event such as an insect bite or laceration. Crusted impetigo is usually associated with a heavy mixed flora of both staphylococci and streptococci.

The bullous variety usually presents as a rapidly spreading papule, which may progress to a thin-walled vesicle if the lesion is infected with *Staphylococcus aureus*, an organism that produces an exfoliative toxin. These lesions occur most often in warm, moist areas of the body. Predisposing factors include warm ambient temperatures, humidity, poor hygiene, and crowded living conditions.

Treatment of impetigo begins with eradication or with the environmental factors thought to be influential in its development. Aggressive lesion débridement with mesh gauze sponges or brushes and antibacterial soap is encouraged. Special attention to hygiene and disinfection of towels and bedding is also necessary. Topical antibiotic treatment with mupirocin (Bactroban) has been effective in mild to moderate cases. In more extensive cases, oral antibiotic therapy with a penicillinase-resistant synthetic penicillin (oxacillin) is the treatment of choice (Table 1). However, it should be remembered that a high percentage of methicillin-resistant strains of *S. aureus* are now isolated in both institutional and community settings. Patients should be treated for at least 5 to 7 days. If no improvement is seen,

CURRENT THERAPY

- Local care and oral antibiotics chosen for the suspected or culture proven pathogens are the usual treatment of most limited skin infections.
- Infections that show evidence of rapid advancement associated with bullae, blebs, crepitus, or necrosis require parenterally administered antibiotics and prompt surgical débridement.
- Morbidity and mortality rates associated with the deeper infections increase with delays in antibiotic therapy and surgical débridement.
- Antibiotic therapy should be guided by clinical presentation and changed if necessary when culture and sensitivity studies are available.

lesions should be cultured and antibiotics adjusted appropriately.

Systemic complications from impetigo are very uncommon. Cellulitis has occurred but is usually susceptible to systemic antibiotic therapy. Septicemia and staphylococcal scaled skin syndrome are exceedingly rare complications of impetigo; when they occur systemic therapy is indicated.

FOLLICULITIS

Folliculitis is a pyoderma that arises within a hair follicle. The process is known as a furuncle (boil) when the infection extends beyond the hair follicle. These lesions occur most frequently in the moist areas of the body and in areas subject to friction and perspiration. Host factors known to predispose one to folliculitis include obesity, blood dyscrasias, defects in neutrophil function, immune deficiency states (such as diabetes, transplant-related immunosuppression, and AIDS), and treatment with corticosteroids or cytotoxic agents. The offending organism in most immunocompetent patients is *S. aureus*; however, when immunosuppression impairs host defenses, gram-negative organisms (*Klebsiella*, *Enterobacter*, and *Proteus* species) can be involved. *Pseudomonas* species such as *aeruginosa* or *cepacia* are associated with hot-tub folliculitis, which is usually self-limited, resolving in 7 to 10 days.

Successful treatment of folliculitis depends on correcting the predisposing factors that promote the development of this condition. For patients with localized disease, topical wound care including antibiotics such as mupirocin (Bactroban) is effective. Patients with furunculosis or multiple lesions should be treated with orally administered systemic antibiotics that are effective against *S. aureus*. Any fluctuant nodules or masses should be incised and drained, and recurrent disease should receive extended treatment.

CELLULITIS

Cellulitis is an acute infection of the skin and underlying soft tissues. It commonly begins as a hot, red, edematous, sharply defined eruption and may progress to lymphangitis, lymphadenitis, or in severe cases, necrotizing fasciitis and gangrene. Cellulitis usually occurs in local skin trauma caused by insect bites, abrasions, surgical wounds, contusions, or other cutaneous lacerations. Immunosuppressed patients are particularly susceptible to the progression of cellulitis to regional or systemic infections, and these patients should be treated aggressively with systemic antibiotics, drainage, and débridement where indicated.

Initial presentation is that of a rapidly expanding, tender, erythematous, firm area of skin. An ascending lymphangitis may be present, especially in cellulitis involving an extremity often associated with regional lymphadenopathy. Systemic signs and symptoms can eventually evolve and when present, mandate hospitalization and treatment with systemic antibiotics. Offending organisms are most commonly group A β-hemolytic *Streptococcus* (GABHS) species and *S. aureus*.

Treatment of localized processes is with oral antibiotics (see Table 1). If fever, septicemia, or other signs of advancement to deeper tissues are present, the patient should be admitted to the hospital for blood and wound

TABLE 1 Suggested Antibiotic Therapy for Gram-Positive Bacterial Isolates

| | Drugs of Choice | |
Isolate	Oral	Parenteral
GABHS	• Penicillin G or V • Erythromycin • First-generation cephalosporin	• Penicillin G • Ampicillin/sulbactam (Unasyn) • First-generation cephalosporin
Staphylococcus aureus (methicillin sensitive)	Penicillinase-resistant synthetic penicillin (Oxacillin)	• First-generation cephalosporin • Clindamycin (Cleocin) • Oxacillin
Staphylococcus aureus (methicillin resistant)	Linezolid (Zyvox)	• Vancomycin • Daptomycin (Cubicin) • Linezolid (Zyvox)
Clostridial species	• Penicillin G or V • Clindamycin (Cleocin) • Metronidazole (Flagyl)	• Penicillin G • Clindamycin • Metronidazole

Abbreviation: GABHS = group A β-hemolytic *Streptococcus.*

cultures, parenteral antibiotics (see Table 1), and observation. If a prompt response is not noted after parenteral antibiotic treatment, surgical exploration of the involved area may be indicated to rule out the presence of necrotic or gangrenous tissue. Immunosuppressed patients or patients with recurrent cellulitis should be extensively examined to exclude chronic sources of infection; and these patients should be treated with parenteral antibiotics until the cellulitis resolves, followed by 5 to 7 days of oral antibiotics.

ABSCESS

Local skin signs and symptoms such as pain (dolor), redness (rubor), warmth (calor) and swelling (tumor) often denote an abscess. Loss of function associated with fluctuation may also indicate abscess formation. Localization of purulent fluid necessitates surgical drainage and local wound care. The administration of oral or parenteral antibiotic therapy should not be used routinely after incision and drainage of localized abscesses. They should be administered only when clinically indicated, and antibiotic therapy should be based on culture and sensitivity testing.

Life-Threatening Infections

GROUP A β-HEMOLYTIC STREPTOCOCCAL GANGRENE

Group A β-hemolytic streptococcal gangrene is an extremely rapid progressing skin and soft tissue infection commonly caused by *Streptococcus pyogenes*. These organisms secrete hemolysins and streptolysins O and S, which are cardiotoxic, leukocytic, and responsible for the characteristic hemolysis. Gangrene results when the cutaneous blood vessels thrombose, a finding that is often associated with intense local pain. The involved skin is initially erythematous and indurated and quickly evolves to hemorrhagic blebs with focal necrotic zones. The potential for extensive tissue loss and mortality exists, especially if treatment is delayed. Prompt, aggressive tissue débridement and antibiotic therapy are necessary for a favorable outcome (see Table 1).

SYNERGISTIC NECROTIZING CELLULITIS

Synergistic necrotizing cellulitis (SNC) is an extremely aggressive, often lethal, polymicrobial infection of the skin and soft tissues, which exhibits progressive invasion superficial to fascial planes. This condition may initially begin as a benign process with scant indication of its impending severity. The initial lesion is typically an erythematous, tender pustule or abscess with a small area of necrosis. The benign appearance of this lesion belies the widespread and aggressive tissue destruction that has occurred beneath it.

Direct inspection through skin incisions reveals extensive gangrene of the superficial tissues and fat that very rarely involves the underlying fascia and muscles. These lesions characteristically exude a thin, brown, malodorous discharge, which presents mixed flora with abundant polymorphonuclear leukocytes on a Gram stain. Crepitus, which is caused by the accumulation of gas in the tissue produced by facultative and/or obligate anaerobes, can be palpated in 25% of patients and mandates immediate surgical attention.

The most common site of involvement is the perineum, which is involved in 50% of patients with SNC. Predisposing factors include perirectal abscess and ischiorectal abscess, both of which may track to the deeper structures of the pelvis, leading to abscess formation and subsequent septicemia. The thigh and leg are involved in approximately 40% of patients. This infection can occur after amputation and is usually associated with diabetes mellitus (75% of cases) and/or peripheral vascular disease (50% of cases). The relative immunosuppression and poor circulation that accompany these significant causes of morbidity are also responsible for upper extremity and neck SNC, which account for the remaining 10% of cases.

Synergistic necrotizing cellulitis is commonly caused by mixed flora originating in the gastrointestinal (GI) tract.

TABLE 2 Suggested Parenteral Antibiotic Therapy for Mixed Infections

Organisms	Primary Choice
Aerobic: Must include an agent effective against anaerobic organisms	• Amikacin (Amikin) • Aztreonam (Azactam) • Ceftriaxone (Rocephin) • Ciprofloxacin (Cipro) • Gentamicin (Garamycin) • Levofloxacin (Levaquin) • Tobramycin (Nebcin)
Anaerobic: Must include an agent effective against aerobic organisms	• Chloramphenicol (Chloromycetin) • Clindamycin (Cleocin) • Metronidazole (Flagyl)
Aerobic and anaerobic coverage	• Ampicillin/sulbactam (Unasyn) • Imipenem/cilastatin (Primaxin) • Meropenem (Merrem) • Piperacillin/tazobactam (Zosyn) • Tigecycline (Tygacil)

Coliforms are the most prevalent aerobes (*Escherichia coli*, *Klebsiella*, *Proteus*), and anaerobic flora include *Bacteroides*, *Peptostreptococcus*, *Clostridium*, and *Fusobacterium*. The primary treatment modality is aggressive débridement of nonviable skin and subcutaneous tissues. This may involve several operations and dressing changes under general anesthesia, which should be performed until all necrotic tissue is removed. Rotation or free myocutaneous flaps and split-thickness skin grafting may cover areas of tissue loss when necessary. If the perineum is involved, fecal diversion by colostomy may be necessary to facilitate healing. Empiric parenteral antibiotics effective against polymicrobial gram-positive and gram-negative aerobic and anaerobic flora are also a mainstay of therapy. However, antibiotic coverage must be modified as soon as culture and susceptibility testing reveal specific offending organisms (Table 2) to reduce the emergence of resistant organisms.

CLOSTRIDIAL MYONECROSIS (GAS GANGRENE)

Clostridial myonecrosis is a destructive infectious process of muscle associated with infections of the skin and soft tissues. It is often associated with local crepitus and systemic signs of toxemia, which are caused by the anaerobic, gas-forming bacilli of the *Clostridium* species. This infection most often occurs after abdominal operations on the GI tract; penetrating trauma, such as gunshot wounds, and frostbite can also expose muscle, fascia, and subcutaneous tissues to these organisms. Common to all these conditions is an environment-containing tissue necrosis, low oxygen tension, and sufficient nutrients of amino acids and calcium to allow germination of clostridial spores and production of the lethal α toxin.

Clostridia are gram-positive, spore-forming, obligate anaerobes that are widely found in soil contaminated with animal excreta. They have also been isolated in the human GI tract and skin, most importantly in the perineum and oropharynx. *Clostridium perfringens* is the most common isolate (present in 80% of cases) and is among the fastest growing clostridial species, having a generation time, under ideal conditions, of approximately 8 minutes. This organism produces collagenases and proteases that cause widespread tissue destruction as well as α toxin, which is associated with the high mortality of clostridial myonecrosis. The α toxin causes extensive capillary destruction and hemolysis, leading to necrosis of the muscle and overlying fascia, skin, and subcutaneous tissues.

Historically, clostridial myonecrosis was a disease associated with battle injuries, but presently, 60% of cases now occur after trauma: 50% after automobile accidents and the remainder after crush injuries, industrial accidents, and gunshot wounds. Mortality can be the result of a failure to recognize that clostridial infection is under way, which leads to a delay in the débridement of devitalized tissues. Patients often complain of a sudden onset of pain at the site of trauma or surgical wound, which increases rapidly in severity and extends beyond the original borders of the wound. The skin initially exhibits tense edema, its pale appearance progresses to a magenta hue. Hemorrhagic bullae and a thin, watery, foul-smelling discharge are common. A Gram stain examination of wound discharge reveals abundant gram-positive rods with a paucity of leukocytes.

The diagnosis of gas gangrene is based on the appearance of the muscle on direct visualization by surgical exposure, because many changes are not apparent when inspected through a small traumatic wound. Initially, the muscle is pale, edematous, and unresponsive to stimulation. As the disease process continues, the muscle becomes frankly gangrenous, black, and extremely friable. This occurs as a late event and is often accompanied by septicemia and shock. Despite profound hypotension and impending organ failure, these patients may be remarkably alert and extremely sensitive to their surroundings. They feel their impending doom and often panic just before slipping into toxic delirium and eventually coma.

The clinical features should arouse suspicion early in the course, so the disease can be recognized and treated with aggressive surgical débridement. Gas in the wound is a relatively late finding, and by the time crepitation is observed, the patient may be near death. Approximately 15% of blood cultures are positive, but this too is a late finding. Serum creatinine kinase levels, although relatively nonspecific, are always elevated in cases with muscle involvement.

The mortality rate of gas gangrene is as high as 60%. It is highest in cases involving the abdominal wall and lowest in those affecting the extremities. Among the signs that prognosticate a poor outcome are leukopenia, thrombocytopenia, hemolysis, and severe renal failure. Myoglobinuria is common and can contribute significantly to worsening renal function. Frank hemorrhage may also be present and indicates disseminated intravascular coagulation.

Successful treatment of this life-threatening infection depends on early recognition and débridement of devitalized and infected tissues. Hyperbaric oxygen and systemic antibiotics are also important adjuncts. Surgical intervention should include wide débridement of all necrotic tissue and amputation if extremities are involved. Hyperbaric oxygen (100% O_2 at 3 atm) has been reported to reduce associated tissue loss and mortality; however, core treatment is surgical débridement and should never be delayed to arrange for hyperbaric oxygen treatments. A parenteral antibiotic is directed toward the offending organism (see Table 1). Cardiovascular collapse mandates careful monitoring of intravenous fluid resuscitation, which may require large volumes. Failure to adequately resuscitate these patients compromises therapy by limiting oxygen delivery and antibiotic distribution to the affected tissues and may promote progression to multisystem organ failure.

A less life-threatening form of this disease is known as clostridial cellulitis. In this process the bacterial tissue invasion is primarily superficial to the fascial layer without muscle involvement. Prompt recognition and treatment, as described earlier, can reduce morbidity and mortality.

NECROTIZING FASCIITIS

Necrotizing fasciitis is an aggressive soft tissue infection involving the fascia with extensive undermining and tracking along anatomic planes. This process usually occurs in patients with significant co-morbidity such as diabetes mellitus or peripheral vascular disease but is also seen in obese or malnourished patients and intravenous drug abusers. Cellulitis is a frequent occurrence, and progressive necrosis to subcutaneous tissue results from thrombosis of the perforating vessels. Classically associated with GABHS and staphylococci, the disease is usually caused by a variety of organisms, including aerobic streptococci, staphylococci, and coliforms, as well as anaerobic *Peptostreptococcus* and *Bacteroides*. Ninety percent of these infections are polymicrobial in etiology, and it is common to culture up to 5 organisms from the fascial planes involved with this infection.

Necrotizing fasciitis most commonly evolves from a benign-appearing skin lesion (80% of cases). Minor abrasions, insect bites, injection sites, and perirectal abscesses have all been implicated. Rare cases have been reported in women with Bartholin's gland abscess, from which the infection has spread to fascial planes of the perineum and thigh. The remaining 20% of patients have no visible skin lesion. Surgical procedures, especially bowel resections and penetrating trauma, can be complicated by superficial wound infections that evolve into necrotizing fasciitis. The infection commonly involves the buttocks and perineum, which result from untreated perirectal abscesses or decubitus ulcers; intravenous drug abusers commonly participate in *skin popping*, which leads to infections of the upper extremities. The idiopathic form, commonly known as spontaneous necrotizing fasciitis, is particularly dangerous because of the frequent delay in diagnosis.

The initial presentation is a slowly advancing cellulitis that progresses to a firm, tense, woody feel of the subcutaneous tissues. This entity may be distinguished from other aggressive anaerobic soft tissue infections (i.e., SNC) by the brawny, pale, erythematous appearance of the skin overlying subcutaneous tissues that are unyielding, making fascial planes and muscle groups indistinguishable during palpation. Often a broad erythematous tract along the route of the underlying fascial plane can be discerned through the skin. If an open wound exists, probing the edges with a blunt instrument permits ready dissection of the superficial fascia well beyond the wound margins, and this is the most important diagnostic feature of necrotizing fasciitis. On direct inspection, the fascia is swollen and dully gray in appearance with stringy areas of fat necrosis. A thin, brown exudate can be expressed from the wound, and frank purulent drainage is rare. These wounds are remarkably insensate when found and mandate immediate débridement.

As with other gangrenous soft tissue infections, the most important component of the treatment plan is aggressive, total débridement of all devitalized and necrotic tissue. This may often necessitate frequent operations and dressing changes. Wide débridement and parenteral antibiotics have a profound effect on survival, and limited or staged débridement has no place in the treatment of this very aggressive, life-threatening infection. Parenteral antibiotics (see Table 2) should be directed against the polymicrobial aerobic and anaerobic microorganisms isolated from these infections. Every effort should be made to quickly identify the offending organisms, and antibiotic therapy should be changed accordingly.

There is a rarely reported monomicrobial form of this disease known as *idiopathic necrotizing fasciitis*. When erythema, induration, and warmth occur without trauma or other obvious cause of the infection, consider this entity, which often arises without any obvious portal of entry. Misdiagnosis and delay in diagnosis are common and associated with significant morbidity and mortality. Surgical exploration with débridement of infected and necrotic tissue, in addition to systemic antibiotic therapy, directed toward the aerobic *Streptococcus* can result in decreased morbidity and mortality (see Table 1).

Special Circumstances

FOURNIER'S GANGRENE

Fournier's gangrene is a necrotizing fasciitis that originates as a necrotic black area on the scrotum of male patients or the labia in females and most often has a cryptogenic origin. In the author's experience, Fournier's gangrene occurs more commonly without a predisposing event or after routine, uncomplicated hemorrhoidectomy. Less commonly, this condition has occurred after urologic manipulation or as a late complication of deep anorectal suppuration. Fournier's gangrene is characterized by necrosis of the skin and soft tissues of the scrotum and/or perineum associated with a fulminant, painful, and severely toxic infection. Definitive diagnosis is made by identification of a necrotic black area on the scrotum associated with local and systemic signs of infection. Left untreated, death ensues from uncontrolled, severe systemic sepsis and multiple organ failure. Prompt recognition and treatment can minimize tissue loss, specifically the skin and soft tissues of the scrotum, labia, and perineum, and may prevent complete loss of genitalia.

The infection is often polymicrobial, as with necrotizing fasciitis, with several species of aerobic and anaerobic bacteria predominating. Successful treatment is, again, based on early recognition and vigorous surgical débridement, occasionally including diversion of the fecal stream. Empirical treatment is appropriate until results of culture and susceptibility testing are available (see Table 2). The therapeutic benefit of hyperbaric oxygen treatments remains to be proved and should only be used as an adjunct to surgical débridement at this time.

ECTHYMA GANGRENOSUM

Occasionally, hospitalized patients with overwhelming pseudomonal septicemia develop a patchy dermal and subcutaneous necrosis. Although sepsis caused by *Pseudomonas aeruginosa* is often indistinguishable from other types of gram-negative sepsis, a characteristic skin lesion may develop with erythematous macular eruptions that quickly become bullous with central ulceration and necrosis. This lesion may resemble a decubitus ulcer with the characteristic black eschar. There are usually multiple lesions occurring in different stages of development. They may concentrate on the extremities or the gluteal region. These lesions may be distinguished from the lesions of pyoderma gangrenosum (a noninfectious dermatosis) by their association with clinical signs of infection (i.e., fever and leukocytosis) in addition to the isolation of *P. aeruginosa* from culture of the lesion. Treatment is primarily by administration of antimicrobial therapy effective against the *Pseudomonas* organism and by débridement of the multiple lesions, which may lessen the bacterial burden, perhaps allowing greater antibiotic efficacy.

SEA WATER INFECTIONS

Infections caused by *Vibrio vulnificus* and *Aeromonas hydrophilia* can be extremely aggressive, with necrosis often occurring within hours and necessitating rapid, wide débridement. Although infections caused by these organisms cannot be differentiated from those caused by mixed infections, a history of exposure to sea water and the rapidity with which the infection spreads often suggest the true etiology of the infection. The antibiotics of choice for *V. vulnificus* infection are doxycycline (Vibramycin) or tetracycline and an aminoglycoside. In cases with impaired renal function, chloramphenicol may be used.

Conclusion

The wide range of soft tissue infections caused by bacteria may be distinguished by their wide variety of presenting signs, symptoms, and body location and by the time course of the pathologic processes unique to each. Early recognition is of paramount importance to the effective treatment plan, which most often includes aggressive surgical débridement and specific antimicrobial therapy. This approach can often minimize tissue damage and promote recovery.

REFERENCES

Adinolfi MF, Voros DC, Moustoukas NM, et al: Severe systemic sepsis resulting from neglected perineal infections. South Med J 1983;76:746-749.

Craig ML, Hardin WD Jr, Fox LS, et al: Ecthyma gangrenosum: A deadly complication. Hosp Physician 1987;23:65-71.

Moustoukas NM, Nichols RL, Voros D: Clostridial sepsis: Usual clinical presentations. South Med J 1985;78:440-445.

Nichols RL: Postoperative infection in the age of drug-resistant gram-positive bacteria [review]. Am J Med 1998;104 (Suppl. 5A):11S-16S.

Nichols RL, Florman S: Clinical presentations of soft-tissue infections and surgical site infections. Clin Infect Dis 2001;33(Suppl. 2):84-93.

Viral Diseases of the Skin

Method of
Jacqueline M. Losi-Sasaki, MD,
and Angela Yen Moore, MD

Human Herpesviruses

HERPES SIMPLEX VIRUS TYPES 1 AND 2

Etiology and Epidemiology

Herpes simplex virus types 1 (HSV-1/human herpesvirus [HHV-1]) and 2 (HSV-2/HHV-2) belong to the family Herpesviridae and the subfamily Alphaherpesvirinae. The two viruses cause clinically indistinguishable mucocutaneous findings. Classic clinical manifestations are grouped or clustered vesicles and erosions on an erythematous base, often with secondary crusting. Predilection for the mucocutaneous surfaces is the rule, with perioral and anogenital surfaces most commonly affected. Herpes simplex virus type 1 is the most common culprit of orofacial HSV, which typically presents at and around the oral surfaces. The etiology of most genital herpes infections is HSV-2 (70% to 90%), but recent reports demonstrate an increasing incidence associated with HSV-1 (10% to 30%).

Herpes simplex virus type 1 seropositivity is approximately 90% worldwide in adults 20 to 40 years old, with an estimated one third of the world's population able to transmit the virus during periods of viral shedding. Despite the high worldwide seropositivity, only 20% to 40% of infected individuals have a history of lesions, translating to a high number of infected individuals unaware of their ability to transmit disease. In the past two decades, there has been an alarming increase in the seroprevalence of HSV-2 in the United States, with approximately 1.6 million individuals acquiring primary genital HSV annually. An estimated 25% to 30% of women and 20% of men in the United States is infected with HSV-2. Factors associated with the transmission of genital herpes include the number of lifetime partners, the age of greatest sexual activity, black or Hispanic race, lower socioeconomic status, female gender, homosexuality, and HIV infection.

Pathogenesis

Herpes simplex virus types 1 and 2 are transmitted primarily through direct contact with active lesions, contaminated saliva, semen, or cervical secretions. More commonly, transmission occurs in patients without active disease, in whom subclinical or asymptomatic viral shedding occurs. Following viral replication at the mucocutaneous site of contact, viral nucleocapsids travel by retrograde axonal flow to the dorsal root ganglia and establish latency until reactivation. Latent virus has been recovered from trigeminal, sacral, and vaginal ganglia both ipsilateral and contralateral to the clinical lesion. Reactivation accounts for repeated episodes of viral shedding that result in further transmission or dissemination of disease. Many instances of reactivation are spontaneous, but others are caused by physical or emotional stress, fever, exposure to ultraviolet light, compromised skin barrier function (abrasion or other trauma), immune suppression, menses, or fatigue.

Clinical Features

Herpes simplex virus infections are variable in clinical expression, and most cases are, in fact, subclinical. In primary infections, a prodrome of fever, malaise, and lymphadenopathy as well as tingling, burning, or localized pain may be present. These symptoms are followed days later by the development of characteristic painful and grouped papules, vesicles, ulcers, or erosions on an erythematous base with secondary crusting and re-epithelialization. Lesions typically heal in 7 to 10 days without scarring. Recurrent outbreaks may be preceded by prodromal symptoms and are characterized by subsequent lesions that are decreased in number, severity, and duration.

Orofacial labialis, also known as herpes labialis, is the most common manifestation of HSV infection. Worldwide, 20% to 30% of children older than age 5 years are seropositive for HSV-1. In the United States 68% of children older than age of 12 years are seropositive for HSV-1, and 22% are seropositive for HSV-2. Primary infection with HSV-1 typically presents as herpetic gingivostomatitis in children and young adults. Sore throat and fever develop, as well as painful vesicles and erosions on the tongue, palate, gingiva, buccal mucosa, and lips. Edema, pain, and ulceration may cause associated dysphagia, anorexia, and drooling. Young adults may have an associated pharyngitis and mononucleosis-like syndrome. In men herpetic folliculitis of the beard area may occur and is often mistaken for a bacterial etiology because of its pustular appearance. Prodromal symptoms and recurrent episodes are historical clues to the diagnosis.

Primary genital herpes infection, usually caused by HSV-2 infection, produces an exquisitely painful erosive balanitis, vulvitis, or vaginitis. Involvement of the cervix, buttocks, and perineum with associated lymphadenopathy may be seen in women. Associated fever, dysuria, urinary retention, or aseptic meningitis may occur in decreasing order of frequency in 10% to 20% of affected females. The glans penis or shaft is typically involved in men. Recurrent disease may be subclinical or less severe in nature. Resolution occurs within 1 week in recurrences versus 2 to 3 weeks in primary infection. The severity of the primary infection correlates with the frequency of recurrences. Prodromal symptoms of tingling or burning may precede episodes of reactivation, with lesions typically occurring at the site of initial manifestation.

Eczema herpeticum, also known as Kaposi's varicelliform eruption, is a widespread dissemination of HSV that occurs in patients with atopic dermatitis, burns, or other underlying skin conditions. Painful, monomorphous, and crusted papules or vesicles develop over mucocutaneous surfaces including the face, extremities, or trunk. Secondary bacterial infection may be present and often hinders diagnosis. The presence of pain and grouped lesions are clues to the diagnosis.

Herpetic whitlow is HSV infection of a digit, most commonly observed in children and medical professionals, caused by direct contact or autoinoculation of HSV-1 or HSV-2.

Herpes gladiatorum occurs in contact-sport athletes such as wrestlers. Direct contact with active lesions or areas of asymptomatic shedding in an infected individual underlies this condition that is most commonly seen on the head, neck, or proximal trunk.

Herpes simplex virus keratitis is a major cause of blindness worldwide, most often caused by infection with HSV-1. Clinical manifestations are unilateral or bilateral keratoconjunctivitis with eyelid edema, photophobia, and preauricular lymphadenopathy. Fundic exam reveals branching dendritic lesions. Complications include corneal ulceration, scarring, globe rupture, and blindness.

Herpes simplex virus encephalitis most often affects the temporal lobe and presents with bizarre behavior changes and altered mental status. Fever and focal neurologic deficits may be present. Mortality is significant at 70% and long-term sequelae are often observed.

Herpes simplex virus in HIV patients is often severe and may be chronic. Bone marrow and solid organ transplant patients as well as chemotherapy patients are also vulnerable. Atypical clinical manifestations include large verrucous papules or plaques, pustules, ulcers, widespread distribution, and visceral organ involvement.

Neonatal HSV continues to be an important public health concern, with most instances transmitted by mothers unaware of their HSV-2 infection. The risk of transmission is highest in women with first-episode genital herpes at or near the time of delivery. Associated neonatal morbidity and mortality is high. Disseminated disease with liver, adrenal, or encephalopathic involvement is a poor prognostic indicator.

VARICELLA-ZOSTER VIRUS

Varicella-zoster virus (VZV/HHV-3) is the cause of varicella (chickenpox), and herpes zoster (shingles). A widespread, pruritic vesicular eruption is highly characteristic of VZV. Following transmission via airborne droplets or direct contact with vesicular fluid, replication and viremia ensue. Epidermal invasion results from virus transmigration from the endothelial cells. Varicella-zoster virus eventually establishes latency in the dorsal root ganglia via mechanisms similar to HSV.

Before the introduction of live attenuated varicella vaccine, more than 90% of children in the United States contracted the primary infection before the age of 10 years. Since the advent of the vaccine, an overall decrease in incidence approaching 87% has been observed between 1995 and 2000. The greatest decline in varicella incidence has been observed in preschool children. This decline correlates with the reduction in the number of hospitalizations for varicella. Reports of outbreaks of varicella in highly immunized groups have shown a milder disease course with fewer lesions and fewer complications than the disease among previously unvaccinated children. These results provide support for ongoing efforts aimed at universal immunization in children in the United States.

Herpes zoster occurs in up to 20% of people infected with VZV and may present at any time after the primary varicella infection. Zoster is, in its classic form, recognized by a dermatomal distribution of blisters. This eruption is caused by reactivation of VZV from latently infected sensory ganglia and is most commonly observed in immunocompetent individuals older than 50 years old with a known prior history of varicella. Younger adults or children with herpes zoster typically experience a primary varicella infection relatively early, typically within the first year of life.

A prodrome of pain, pruritus, tingling, tenderness, or hyperesthesia often precedes the classic sensory dermatomal vesicular eruption. Pain that persists for more than 1 month after resolution of the herpes zoster rash is known as postherpetic neuralgia, a complication that is often chronic and refractory to treatments. The effect of the varicella vaccine on the incidence of postherpetic neuralgia appears to be unclear, with different studies showing both an increase and a decrease in the incidence of this complication. Other complications include secondary bacterial infection, ophthalmic zoster, meningoencephalitis, pneumonitis, and hepatitis.

Ophthalmic zoster is a serious complication that occurs in 5% to 10% of cases with an associated significant risk of blindness. Vesicles or crusted papules along the nasal tip, sidewall, or base is known as Hutchinson's sign and signifies involvement of the nasociliary branch of the trigeminal nerve. This clinical presentation is an indication for immediate empiric antiviral therapy and ophthalmology referral.

Severe or disseminated herpes zoster (>20 vesicles outside the primarily involved dermatome) is most frequently observed in the immunosuppressed population. Atypical clinical manifestations such as crusted, verrucous papules and plaques may also be noted.

DIAGNOSIS

Herpes Simplex Virus

Viral culture, serology, direct immunofluorescence, and molecular techniques are available laboratory tests for the diagnosis of HSV infection. Viral culture is a useful method of diagnosis in first-time genital outbreaks or few mucocutaneous lesions. The cell culture technique is most reliable at the onset of symptoms, before healing or crusting of the vesicular lesions. False negative results may occur, especially in lesions that are already healing.

Direct fluorescent antibody staining of vesicle base scrapings is 95% diagnostic and can be used to distinguish VZV from HSV. In one study direct immunofluorescence and culture were shown to be equally sensitive at 88% in detection of HSV, whereas direct immunofluorescence was four times more sensitive (100% versus 18%) than culture in the case of VZV.

The gold standard of serologic diagnosis is the Western blot test, which is 99% sensitive and 99% specific for HSV antibodies. To distinguish between HSV-1 and HSV-2, type-specific serologic assays based on type-specific glycoproteins from HSV-1 and HSV-2 are available and approved by the Food and Drug Administration (FDA).

The Tzanck smear offers a rapid and useful bedside test of HSV infection and relies on the identification of multinucleated giant cells in vesicular scrapings. However, this test does not differentiate among HSV-1, HSV-2, or VZV.

On histopathologic examination, characteristic ballooning degeneration of keratinocytes, spongiosis or frank vesiculation, and nuclear molding may be observed. Intranuclear inclusion bodies may also be present.

Polymerase chain reaction (PCR) of the cerebrospinal fluid is the test of choice for HSV infections of the central nervous system.

Varicella-Zoster Virus

A thorough history and physical examination are critical in diagnosis and often prompt initial antiviral therapy. The Tzanck smear (see previous mention) may aid in prompt diagnosis but will not distinguish between HSV and VZV. Similar limited information may be provided by histopathologic specimens of lesional skin.

Direct fluorescent antibody, viral culture, serology, and PCR may all distinguish between HSV and VZV. Viral culture is the most specific, albeit a less-sensitive test.

Polymerase chain reaction is the test of choice for detection of VZV in the cerebrospinal fluid. Serologic tests have limited utility, because most of the population is seropositive.

TREATMENT

Both topical and systemic antiviral treatments are useful in the management of orolabial herpes in immunocompetent people. Oral valacyclovir (Valtrex), 2 grams orally taken twice in one 24-hour period,[3] and topical 1% penciclovir result in decreased duration of pain, clinical lesions, and duration of viral shedding.

Systemic antiviral agents are the agents of choice for the treatment of primary and recurrent genital herpes (see Table 1). Three highly effective and well-tolerated antivirals are acyclovir (Zovirax), valacyclovir (Valtrex), and famciclovir (Famvir). All have been shown to shorten the duration, severity, pain, and period of viral shedding for initial and recurrent genital herpes infections. Because they inhibit only actively replicating viral DNA, these

CURRENT DIAGNOSIS

- Grouped or clustered vesicles and erosions on an erythematous base should prompt consideration of herpetic etiology.
- The presence of painful crusted, eroded, or vesicular lesions on the nose should prompt immediate ophthalmologic evaluation and empiric antiviral therapy (the so-called Hutchinson's sign, a diagnostic urgency implicating possible herpes keratitis).
- A high suspicion for herpetic etiology in an immunosuppressed patient is critical.
- Laboratory tests:
  - Viral culture is useful in first-time outbreaks, however time sensitive.
  - Serology
    - Western blot
    - Type-specific serologic assays based on glycoproteins
  - Direct immunofluorescence: rapid and specific
  - Tzanck smear:* rapid, but nonspecific
  - Polymerase chain reaction of cerebrospinal fluid

*This test does not differentiate between HSV-1, HSV-2, or VZV.
Abbreviations: HSV-1 = herpes simplex virus type 1; HSV-2 = herpes simplex virus type 2; VZV = varicella-zoster virus.

---

[3]Exceeds dosage recommended by the manufacturer.

CURRENT THERAPY

- Both topical and systemic antiviral treatments may be used to manage orolabial herpes in immunocompetent people.
- Systemic agents offer the best treatment for primary and recurrent genital herpes.
- Immunosuppressed individuals need more aggressive management with oral or IV antivirals.
- Early treatment and empirical therapy are critical for herpes zoster.
- Prompt ophthalmologic evaluation and empirical therapy is critical for nasal herpetic presentations.

Abbreviation: IV = intravenous.

---

medications are not useful for the treatment of latent infection.

Intravenous (IV) acyclovir is reserved for neonatal HSV infection, severe HSV infections in immunocompromised hosts, and HSV patients with systemic complications. Immunosuppressed individuals require more aggressive management with oral or IV antivirals until complete mucocutaneous clearing is observed. For patients with greater than six outbreaks per year, chronic suppressive therapy is indicated and is associated with a 95% reduction of asymptomatic viral shedding (see Table 1).

Acyclovir-resistant HSV and VZV are increasing in frequency, especially in those who are immunosuppressed. Most commonly, a mutation in thymidine kinase is responsible. Antivirals that are thymidine kinase dependent are ineffective in such cases. Alternative antivirals include foscarnet (Foscavir) and cidofovir (Vistide).

Early treatment with antiviral agents is critical for herpes zoster, and empiric therapy is warranted (see Table 1). Acyclovir, valacyclovir, and famciclovir are FDA approved for herpes zoster and result in decreased VZV duration and pain. Adequate pain control with narcotics or other appropriate agents are required. Intravenous acyclovir is the treatment of choice for herpes zoster in patients with complications or immunosuppression.

Postherpetic neuralgia (PHN) correlates with active viral replication at the dorsal root ganglion and poses a difficult therapeutic challenge. Both famciclovir and valacyclovir are effective at reducing the duration and pain of PHN. Low-dose tricyclic antidepressants and gabapentin (Neurontin) are also shown to be effective in reducing pain and sleep disturbances. Narcotics, analgesics, capsaicin, biofeedback, and nerve blocks are other options.

Human Parvovirus B19

A small, single-stranded DNA virus and member of the family Parvoviridae, human parvovirus B19 is transmitted through respiratory droplets with peak infection rates noted in patients between ages 4 and 15 years. Human parvovirus B19 is responsible for several clinical syndromes including the benign childhood exanthem known as erythema infectiosum, or fifth disease. Less commonly, purpuric eruptions or severe complications including aplastic anemia and hydrops fetalis may occur.

TABLE 1 Systemic Antiviral Therapy for Herpes Simplex Virus and Varicella Zoster Virus

Herpes Simplex Virus Infection

First episode of genital herpes

Acyclovir (Zovirax)	400 mg PO tid for 7–10 d
Acyclovir	200 mg PO 5 times/d for 7–10 d
Famciclovir (Famvir)	250 mg PO tid for 7–10 d
Valacyclovir (Valtrex)	1 g PO bid for 7–10 d

Recurrent episode of genital herpes

Acyclovir	400 mg PO tid for 5 d
Acyclovir	200 mg PO 5 times/d for 5 d
Acyclovir	800 mg PO bid for 5 d
Famciclovir	125 mg PO bid for 5 d
Valacyclovir	500 mg PO bid for 3–5 d
Valacyclovir	1.0 g PO bid for 5 d
Valacyclovir	2.0 g PO bid for 1 d[3]

Chronic suppressive therapy

Acyclovir	400 mg PO bid
Famciclovir	250 mg PO bid
Valacyclovir	500 mg PO qd (<10 outbreaks/y)
Valacyclovir	1.0 g PO qd (≥10 outbreaks/y)

Recurrent orolabial or genital HSV in immunosuppressed patients

Acyclovir	400 mg PO tid for 5–10 d
Acyclovir	200 mg 5 times/d for 5–10 d
Acyclovir	5 mg/kg intravenously q8h for 7–10 d
Famciclovir	500 mg PO bid for 5–10 d
Valacyclovir	1.0 g PO bid for 5–10 d

Chronic suppressive HSV therapy in immunosuppressed patients

Acyclovir	400–800 mg PO bid to tid
Famciclovir	500 mg PO bid
Valacyclovir	500 mg PO bid

Varicella-Zoster Virus Infection

Varicella

Acyclovir	20 mg/kg (800 mg maximum dose) PO qid for 5 d

Zoster

Acyclovir	800 mg PO 5 times/d for 7–10 d
Famciclovir	500 mg PO tid for 7 d
Valacyclovir	1 g PO tid for 7 d
Adult immunosuppressed patients: Acyclovir	10 mg/kg IV q8h for 7–10 d
Pediatric immunosuppressed patients: Acyclovir	10 mg/kg IV q8h for 7–10 d

[3]Exceeds dosage recommended by the manufacturer.
Abbreviations: IV = intravenous; PO = orally.

Classic clinical manifestations of erythema infectiosum include low-grade fever and mild upper respiratory symptoms that occur 2 to 3 days prior to the onset of the easily recognized *slapped cheeks* erythema over the bilateral malar cheeks with circumoral pallor. A pink lacy or reticular eruption over the trunk and extremities shortly follows. Duration is 7 to 14 days and occurs without scarring or long-term sequelae. Adolescents and other susceptible individuals may present with arthralgias or arthritis; severe disease is only seen in immunosuppressed patients, including pregnant women.

Papular purpuric gloves and socks syndrome is also associated with acute B19 infection and is most common in young adults in the spring. Burning and pruritus are associated. Fetal B19 infection may result in fetal hydrops, anemia, spontaneous miscarriage, or stillbirth.

Diagnostic confirmation of B19 infection may be confirmed by detection of serum anti-B19 IgM antibody. Polymerase chain reaction assays may also be used.

Symptomatic management of most B19 infections is adequate. Affected fetuses may require in utero blood transfusions. Intravenous immunoglobulin has been used in select cases of B19 infection in the immunosuppressed.

Hand-Foot-and-Mouth Disease

Hand-foot-and-mouth disease is a common benign exanthem of childhood, characterized by a palmoplantar vesicular eruption and stomatitis. The causative agent is an enterovirus, most often coxsackievirus serotype A16. Transmission is via the oral–oral or fecal–oral route. A prodrome of malaise, low-grade fever, anorexia, abdominal pain, or upper respiratory symptoms may occur. Oval-shaped erythematous macules progress to small vesicles on the palms, soles, tongue, buccal mucosa, palate, and tonsillar pillars. Buttocks and perineal surfaces are rarely involved. The vesicles evolve into yellow-gray ulcerations with peripheral erythema in the same distribution. Self-limited resolution occurs without scarring. Treatment is symptomatic.

Poxviruses

MOLLUSCUM CONTAGIOSUM

Molluscum contagiosum is caused by the molluscipoxvirus genus of Poxviridae, a family of large, brick-shaped, double-stranded DNA viruses. Children, sexually active adults, and immunosuppressed individuals are the most frequent hosts, and transmission is via direct contact or fomites. In children molluscum contagiosum is a common, benign, self-limited eruption characterized by numerous, scattered dome-shaped pearly papules with central umbilication that show predilection for the face, trunk, and skin folds. The presence of Henderson-Patterson bodies (intracytoplasmic inclusion bodies) may be demonstrated by lesional scrapings and aid in the diagnosis.

Treatment is not required, but numerous modalities including topical cantharidin, curettage, electrodesiccation, cimetidine, topical tretinoin, and chemical peels are available. Similar cutaneous findings are observed in sexually active adults, but the distribution favors the perineal areas, lower abdomen, and thighs in this population. Immunosuppressed individuals exhibit atypical, larger eroded papules or plaques that are often widespread and deforming.

ORF AND MILKER'S NODULES

Orf, or ecthyma contagiosum, is caused by a parapoxvirus endemic in sheep and goats. Direct contact with infected animals or fomites results in transmission to humans. The clinical presentation is typically on the dorsal digits or hands with single or multiple 1.5- to 5.0-cm discrete plaques or nodules. Initial lesions typically progress through several stages, including maculopapular, targetoid, nodular, regenerative, papillomatous, and regressive lesions prior to eventual healing 35 to 40 days later. Diagnosis is by history and physical examination. Treatment is symptomatic.

Milker's nodule (bovine papular stomatitis) is a similar clinical entity to orf and arises from a closely related parapoxvirus transmitted from infected cattle. Physical manifestations are indistinguishable from orf. Milker's condition is benign and self-limited. Treatment is supportive.

REFERENCES

Armstrong GL, Schillinger J, Markowitz L: Incidence of herpes simplex virus type 2 infection in the United States. Am J Epidemiol 2001; 153:91-99.

Centers for Disease Control and Prevention: Sexually transmitted diseases treatment guidelines 2002. MMWR Morb Mortal Wkly Rep 2002;51(RR-6):1-80.

Corey L, Adams H, Brown A, Holmes KK: Genital herpes simplex virus infections: Clinical manifestations, course and complications. Ann Intern Med 1983;98:958-972.

Douglas MW, Johnson RW, Cunningham, AL: Tolerability of treatments for postherpetic neuralgia. Drug Saf 2004;27(15):1217-1233.

Johnson LS, Nahmias AJ, Magder RE, et al: A seroepidemiological survey of the prevalence of herpes simplex virus type 2 infection in the United States. N Engl J Med 1989;321:7-12.

Langtry LAA, Ostlere AS, Hawkins DA, Staughton RCD: The difficulty in diagnosis of cutaneous herpes simplex virus infection in patients with AIDS. Clin Exp Dermatol 1994;19:224-226.

Miron D, Lavi I, Kitov R, Hendler A: Vaccine effectiveness and severity of varicella among previously vaccinated children during outbreaks in day-care centers with low vaccination coverage. Pediatr Infect Dis J 2005;24(3):233-236.

Nahmias AJ, Lee FK, Bechman-Nahmia S: Sero-epidemiological and sociological patterns of herpes simplex virus infection in the world. Scand J Infect Dis 1990;69:19-36.

Stalkup JR, Yeung-Yue K, Brotjens M, Tyring SK: Human herpesviruses. In JL Bolognia (ed): Dermatology. Spain, Mosby, 2003, pp 1245-1253.

Takahashi M: Effectiveness of live varicella vaccine. Expert Opin Biol Ther 2004;4(2):199-216.

Vázquez M: Varicella zoster virus infections in children after the introduction of live attenuated varicella vaccine. Curr Opin Pediatr 2004;16:80-84.

Zirn JR, Tompkins SD, Huie C, Shea CR: Rapid detection, and distinction of cutaneous herpesvirus infections by direct immunofluorescence. J Am Acad Dermatol 1995;33:724-728.

Parasitic Diseases of the Skin

Method of
Andreas Katsambas, MD, PhD, and
Electra Nicolaidou, MD, PhD

A parasite is an organism that obtains food and shelter from another organism and derives all benefits from this association. Parasites responsible for diseases with skin manifestations include protozoa, helminths, and arthropoda. Most parasitic diseases are more common in tropical and subtropical regions, but, mostly because of traveling and immigration, they are also encountered in temperate climates. Updated treatment guidelines for these diseases are available at the Centers for Disease Control (CDC) Web site, www.cdc.gov/travel/diseases.htm.

Diseases Caused by Protozoa

AMEBIASIS

Amebiasis is caused by *Entamoeba histolytica*. Infection occurs by ingestion of mature cysts in fecally contaminated food and water and through fecal exposure during sexual contact. Clinical presentation includes asymptomatic infection, invasive intestinal amebiasis, and invasive extra intestinal amebiasis. Cutaneous findings include purulent nodules, cysts, and sinuses. *Entamoeba histolytica* can be identified microscopically in the stool as well as in aspirates or biopsy samples obtained during colonoscopy or surgery. Treatment of choice for extraintestinal disease is metronidazole (Flagyl), 750 mg by mouth (PO) three times daily for 7 to 10 days or tinidazole (Tindamax), 2 g once daily for 5 days. Tinidazole was recently approved by the Food and Drug Administration (FDA) and appears to be as effective

CURRENT DIAGNOSIS

Diseases Caused by Protozoa

AMEBIASIS

- Purulent nodules, cysts, and sinuses
- Microscopic identification of *Entamoeba histolytica* in stool or biopsy samples

LEISHMANIASIS

- Well-demarcated ulcer with encrusted center
- Isolation of *Leishmania* by direct examination or culture

TRYPANOSOMIASIS

CHAGAS' DISEASE

- Erythematous induration with a subcutaneous nodule (chagoma)
- Cardiomyopathy, megaesophagus, and megacolon
- Microscopic identification of *Trypanosoma cruzi* in fresh anticoagulated blood or blood smears
- Isolation of the parasite by culture

AFRICAN SLEEPING SICKNESS

- Painful chancre surrounded by a white halo
- Fever, lymphadenopathy, and generalized pruritic eruptions with erythematous annular plaques
- Headaches, somnolence, abnormal behavior, loss of consciousness, and coma
- Identification of trypanosomes by microscopic examination

Diseases Caused by Helminths

CUTANEOUS LARVA MIGRANS

- Intense pruritus, papular lesions, and linear, minimally elevated, serpiginous tracts

DRACUNCULIASIS

- Erythematous papule or blister that ulcerates and may become secondarily infected
- Identification of the worm in the ulcer

Filariasis

LYMPHATIC FILARIASIS

- Fever with lymphangitis and lymphadenitis, chronic pulmonary infection, and progressive lymphedema leading to massive tissue thickening, especially of the legs and scrotum (elephantiasis)

- Identification of microfilariae microscopically in blood

ONCHOCERCIASIS

- Subcutaneous nodules, dermatitis, depigmentation, skin atrophy, lymphadenopathy, lymphedema, and blindness
- Identification of microfilariae in skin snips

LOIASIS

- Pruritus, subcutaneous swelling containing the worm, serpiginous lesion on the sclera conjunctiva
- Microfilariae identified in the blood by microscopic examination

SCHISTOSOMIASIS

- Pruritic papular dermatitis
- Verrucous papules and nodules, secondary infection, ulceration, and development of squamous cell carcinoma
- Identification of eggs in urine or stool, enzyme-linked immunoabsorbent assay (ELISA) tests

Diseases Caused by Arthropoda

SCABIES

- Intense pruritus, especially at night
- Burrows
- Scaly papules on the nipples and the male genitals
- Identification of the mite, its eggs, or its feces in skin samples

PEDICULOSIS

PEDICULOSIS CAPITIS

- Intense pruritus of the scalp
- Nape dermatitis
- Identification of lice and nits on the hair

PEDICULOSIS CORPORIS

- Intense pruritus, erythema, urticarial lesions, papules, nodules, and excoriations
- Identification of lice and nits on clothing

PEDICULOSIS PUBIS

- Pruritus
- Blue macules
- Identification of lice and nits on pubic hair

CURRENT THERAPY

Diseases Caused by Protozoa

AMEBIASIS

- Metronidazole (Flagyl), 750 mg PO tid for 7–10 d *or*
- Tinidazole (Tindamax), 2 g once daily for 5 d.
- Treatment with either metronidazole or tinidazole should be followed by iodoquinol (Yodoxin), 650 mg PO tid for 20 d.

LEISHMANIASIS

- Sodium stibogluconate (Pentostam),[2] 20 mg/kg/d IV or IM for 20 d.

TRYPANOSOMIASIS

CHAGAS' DISEASE

- Nifurtimox (Lampit),[2] 8–10 mg/kg/d PO in 3–4 doses for 90–120 d.

EAST AFRICAN SLEEPING SICKNESS

- Suramin (Germanin),[2] 100–200 mg (test dose) IV, then 1 g IV on days 1, 3, 7, 14, and 21.
- For late disease with involvement of the central nervous system (CNS), melarsoprol (Mel-B)[2] is used in the following dosage scheme: 2–3.6 mg/kg/d PO for 3 days; after 7 d, 3.6 mg/kg/d for 3 d; and the latter repeated after 7 d.

WEST AFRICAN SLEEPING SICKNESS

- Pentamidine isethionate (Pentam 300, NebuPent),[1] 4 mg/kg/d IM for 10 d.
- In cases of late disease with CNS involvement, either melarsoprol (Mel-B),[2] 2.2 mg/kg/d PO for 10 d, or eflornithine (Ornidyl), 400 mg/kg/d PO in 4 doses for 14 d.

Diseases Caused by Helminths

CUTANEOUS LARVA MIGRANS

- Albendazole (Albenza), 400 mg daily PO for 3 d, or ivermectin (Stromectol),[1] 200 µg/kg/d for 1–2 d.

DRACUNCULIASIS

- Slow extraction of the worm, which is facilitated by metronidazole (Flagyl), 250 mg PO tid for 10 d.

FILARIASIS

LYMPHATIC FILARIASIS

- Diethylcarbamazine (Hetrazan), as follows: d 1: 50 mg, d 2: 50 mg tid, d 3: 100 mg tid, d 4–14: 6 mg/kg in 3 doses.

ONCHOCERCIASIS

- Ivermectin (Stromectol), 150 µg/kg PO q6–12mo until asymptomatic.

LOIASIS

- Diethylcarbamazine (Hetrazan), as follows: d 1: 50 mg, d 2: 50 mg tid, d 3: 100 mg tid, d 4–14: 9 mg/kg in 3 doses.

SCHISTOSOMIASIS

- Praziquantel (Biltricide), 40 mg/kg/d[3] in 2 doses for 1 day (*S. haematobium* and *S. mansoni)* and 60 mg/kg/d[3] in 3 doses for 1 day (*S. japonicum).*

Diseases Caused by Arthropoda

SCABIES

- 5% permethrin (Nix, Elimite), applied for 10 h; application can be repeated after 10–14 d.

PEDICULOSIS

PEDICULOSIS CAPITIS

- Malathion (Ovide) 0.5% lotion, applied for 8–12 h before being washed off, or permethrin (Nix, Elimite) 1% cream rinse, applied to shampooed hair and washed off after 10 min; a second application 1 wk later is recommended.

PEDICULOSIS CORPORIS

- Disinfection of clothes.

PEDICULOSIS PUBIS

- Same treatment as pediculosis capitis.

---

[1]Not FDA approved for this indication.
[2]Not available in the United States.
[3]Exceeds dosage recommended by the manufacturer.

---

as and better tolerated than metronidazole. Treatment with either metronidazole or tinidazole should be followed by iodoquinol (Yodoxin), 650 mg PO three times daily for 20 days.

LEISHMANIASIS

Leishmaniasis is caused by *Leishmania* species, which are transmitted by sandflies. In the cutaneous form of the disease, an initial solitary red papule develops into a well-demarcated ulcer with encrusted center that, if untreated, heals spontaneously with a scar. Diagnosis is based on a history of exposure to sandflies, symptoms and isolation of

the organisms from the lesion aspirate, or biopsy by direct examination or culture. Treatment includes sodium stibogluconate (Pentostam),[2] 20 mg/kg/day intravenously (IV) or intramuscularly (IM) for 20 days.

TRYPANOSOMIASIS

There are three different types of trypanosomiasis:

- American trypanosomiasis or Chagas' disease, caused by *Trypanosoma cruzi*

---

[2]Not available in the United States.

- East African sleeping sickness, caused by *Trypanosoma brucei rhodesiense*
- West African sleeping sickness, caused by *Trypanosoma brucei gambiense*

Chagas' disease can be transmitted to humans by blood-sucking triatomae bugs as well as by blood transfusions, organ transplantation, and transplacentally. The acute reaction at the bite site may include an erythematous induration with a subcutaneous nodule, known as chagoma. The chronic stage of the disease is characterized by cardiomyopathy, megaesophagus, and megacolon. Microscopic identification of the parasite in fresh anticoagulated blood and in blood smears or its isolation by culture confirms the diagnosis. Drug of choice for the treatment of Chagas' disease is nifurtimox (Lampit),[2] 8 to 10 mg/kg/day PO in three to four doses for 90 to 120 days.

African sleeping sickness, East and West, is transmitted through an infected tsetse fly bite. A painful chancre surrounded by a white halo can develop at the site of inoculation. This is followed by a hemolymphatic stage with fever, lymphadenopathy, and generalized pruritic eruptions with erythematous annular plaques. In the meningoencephalitic stage, invasion of the central nervous system (CNS) can cause headaches, somnolence, abnormal behavior, and lead to loss of consciousness and coma. Diagnosis is confirmed by identification of trypanosomes by microscopic examination in chancre fluid, lymph node aspirates, blood, bone marrow, or, in the late stages of infection, cerebrospinal fluid. East African sleeping sickness is treated with suramin (Metaret) (Germanin),[2] 100 to 200 mg (test dose) IV, then 1 g IV on days 1, 3, 7, 14, and 21. For late disease with involvement of the CNS, melarsoprol (Mel-B)[2] is used in the following dosage scheme: 2 to 3.6 mg/kg/day PO for 3 days; after 7 days, 3.6 mg/kg/day for 3 days, the latter repeated after 7 days. For West African sleeping sickness, the drug of choice is pentamidine isethionate (Pentam 300, NebuPent),[1] 4 mg/kg/day IM for 10 days. In cases of late disease with CNS involvement, either melarsoprol (Mel-B)[2] 2.2 mg/kg/day PO for 10 days, or eflornithine (Ornidyl), 400 mg/kg/day PO in four doses for 14 days can be used.

Diseases Caused by Helminths

CUTANEOUS LARVA MIGRANS

Cutaneous larva migrans, or creeping eruption, is caused when various nematode larvae penetrate the skin and migrate through it. These larvae are unable to complete their life cycle or reach internal organs. Larvae of *Ancylostoma braziliense, Ancylostoma caninum, Ascaris suum, Bunostomum phlebotomus*, and others can cause creeping eruptions. Infection is acquired by exposure to contaminated soil. Initially, there is intense pruritus and papular lesions, but, as the larvae begin to migrate, the classic linear, minimally elevated, serpiginous tract becomes apparent. Excoriations and secondary infections are common. The diagnosis is usually clinical; sometimes the larva can be found within a tunnel. Treatment of choice is

either albendazole (Albenza), 400 mg daily PO for 3 days, or ivermectin ((Stromectol),[1] 200 µg/kg/day for 1 to 2 days.

DRACUNCULIASIS

Dracunculiasis, one of the oldest infections on record, is caused by *Dracunculus medinensis*. Infection occurs by drinking water that contains crustaceans of the *Cyclops* family infected with the larvae of *D. medinensis*. Crustaceans release the mature larvae in the intestine. From the intestine they migrate to the subcutaneous tissue and, finally, the female worm moves into the skin, producing an erythematous papule or blister. The blister ulcerates and may become secondarily infected. The female worm can often be seen in the ulcer. Treatment of choice is slow extraction of the worm combined with wound care. Metronidazole (Flagyl), 250 mg PO three times daily for 10 days, decreases inflammation and facilitates removal of the worm.

FILARIASIS

Filariasis is caused by nematodes (roundworms) that inhabit the lymphatics and subcutaneous tissues. The most common filarial infections include lymphatic filariasis, onchocerciasis, and loiasis.

Lymphatic Filariasis

Lymphatic filariasis is caused by *Wuchereria bancrofti, Brugia malayi*, and *Brugia timori*. It is transmitted by mosquitoes. Adult worms block lymphatics and produce microfilariae. Many patients are asymptomatic, but some may develop fever with lymphangitis and lymphadenitis, chronic pulmonary infection, and progressive lymphedema leading to massive tissue thickening, especially of the legs and scrotum (elephantiasis). The overlying skin is thickened. Diagnosis is made by identifying the microfilariae microscopically in blood. Antigen detection using an immunoassay for circulating filarial antigens may also be used. Treatment is with diethylcarbamazine (Hetrazan), as follows: day 1: 50 mg; day 2: 50 mg three times daily; day 3: 100 mg three times daily; days 4 through 14: 6 mg/kg in three doses.

Onchocerciasis

Onchocerca volvulus is the causative organism of onchocerciasis and transmitted by the blackflies *Simulium*. Onchocerciasis is manifested with subcutaneous nodules, dermatitis, depigmentation, and skin atrophy and, in later stages, with lymphadenopathy and lymphedema. The eyes are another favorite site for the microfilariae, and the infection can lead to blindness (river blindness). Diagnosis is based on identification of microfilariae in skin snips. The drug of choice for onchocerciasis is ivermectin (Stromectol), 150 µg/kg PO every 6 to 12 months until asymptomatic.

Loiasis

Loiasis is caused after the transmission of the filarial parasite *Loa loa* by deerflies *(Chrysops)*. It is usually manifested by pruritus and a subcutaneous swelling containing the worm. In some cases, there is subconjunctival migration of the adult worm producing a migrating serpiginous lesion on the sclera conjunctiva. Microfilariae can be identified in the blood by microscopic examination. Diethylcarbamazine (Hetrazan) is used for the treatment of loiasis, according to the following scheme: day 1: 50 mg; day 2: 50 mg three times daily; day 3: 100 mg three times daily; days 4 through 14: 9 mg/kg in three doses.

SCHISTOSOMIASIS

Schistosoma haematobium, Schistosoma japonicum, and *Schistosoma mansoni* are the main trematodes that cause schistosomiasis in humans. All trematodes have a life cycle that involves the snail as an intermediate host. The infective cercariae leave the snail, swim, and penetrate the human skin, causing a pruritic papular dermatitis. *S. mansoni* primarily causes hepatosplenomegaly, colonic pseudopolyps, and pulmonary lesions, whereas *S. haematobium* mostly affects the bladder. *S. japonicum* primarily involves the liver, but its eggs are more likely to be found in ectopic sites, such as the spinal cord and brain. In the skin, the eggs elicit an inflammatory response with verrucous papules and nodules. Secondary infection, ulceration, and development of squamous cell carcinoma may follow. Diagnosis is established by identification of the eggs in the urine or stool. Enzyme-linked immunoabsorbent assay (ELISA) tests are also available. The infection is treated with praziquantel (Biltricide), 40 mg/kg/day[3] in two doses for 1 day (*S. haematobium* and *S. mansoni*) or 60 mg/kg/day[3] in three doses for 1 day (*S. japonicum).*

Infection of the skin by cercariae of nonhuman schistosomes leads to *cercarial dermatitis* or *swimmers' itch*, manifested by intensely pruritic macules and papules that may coalesce and produce diffuse erythema and swelling. The rash usually disappears within a week because the cercariae only live for 2 to 3 days. Symptomatic treatment with topical steroids and oral antihistamines may be needed.

Diseases Caused by Arthropoda

SCABIES

Scabies is caused by the mite *Sarcoptes scabiei var humanus*, an obligate parasite to humans. Transmission requires close personal contact, such as sexual intercourse, contact between family members, sharing a bed, or holding hands. Live mites can be found in the environment of patients, where they survive for 2 to 3 days.

The fertilized female crawls through the stratum corneum creating tiny tunnels (burrows), where she lays her eggs. The eggs hatch in approximately 1 week.

Initial infestation is usually asymptomatic for approximately 6 weeks, after which an immune response develops to the mites or their feces. Reinfestation provokes symptoms within only 1 to 3 days.

The classic symptom of scabies is intense pruritus, especially at night. Papules, pustules, excoriations, and crusting can appear, especially at the interdigital spaces, the wrists, the axillary folds, the nipples, and the genitals.

Pathognomonic signs of scabies include the burrows made by the female mite and the appearance of scaly papules on the nipples and the male genitals. In adults, the head is usually spared, whereas in infants involvement of the scalp, palms, and soles is common.

Crusted scabies (Norwegian scabies) is an aggressive infestation that usually occurs in immunodeficient, debilitated, or malnourished persons. The skin is inhabited by thousands of mites per square millimeter, and clinically there is a proliferative, hyperkeratotic response.

Diagnosis of scabies is confirmed by finding either an intact burrow or the mite, its eggs, and its feces in skin samples from the infected area.

Adults should be treated from the neck down; in infants the scalp should also be treated. Topical therapy of choice is with 5% permethrin (Nix, Elimite), applied for 10 hours. Application can be repeated after 10 to 14 days. Alternatively, crotamiton 10% topical (Eurax), applied once daily for 2 days, or ivermectin (Stromectol),[1] 200 µg/kg once (the dose can be repeated in 10 to 14 days), can be used. Ivermectin, either alone or in combination with a topical scabicide, is the drug of choice for crusted scabies in immunocompromised patients. All sexual and close personal and household contacts within the preceding 6 weeks should be treated at the same time, regardless of whether they have symptoms or not. Bedding and clothing should be decontaminated (i.e., either machine washed and dried using the hot cycle or dry cleaned) or removed from body contact for at least 3 days.

PEDICULOSIS

Lice are blood-sucking insects and are obligate parasites of humans. There are three major types of lice: *Pediculus humanus capitis* (head louse), which lives on the scalp, *Pediculus humanus corporis* (body louse), which lives in a person's clothes, and *Phthirus pubis* (pubic louse), which lives mostly on pubic hair.

Pediculosis Capitis

Pediculosis capitis is caused by *Pediculus humanus capitis*. The louse attaches its eggs or nits firmly to the hair shaft. Children and individuals with long hair are mostly affected. Transmission is accomplished either directly from human to human or through sharing combs and brushes. Clinically, there is intense pruritus of the scalp, which is sometimes accompanied with nape dermatitis, secondary bacterial infection, and lymphadenopathy. Diagnosis is established by identification of lice and nits on the hair.

Treatment of choice for pediculosis capitis is either malathion (Ovide) 0.5% lotion, applied for 8 to 12 hours before being washed off, or permethrin (Nix, Elimite) 1% cream rinse, applied to shampooed hair and washed off after 10 minutes. A second application is recommended with permethrin 1 week later to kill hatching progeny. Alternatively, pyrethrins with piperidyl butoxide (RID) can be applied to the affected area and washed off after 10 minutes. Ivermectin (Stromectol)[1] can also be used at a dose of 200 µg/kg on days 1, 2, and 10. In combination with insecticide treatment, combing of wet hair with a fine-toothed comb every 3 to 4 days for 2 weeks, to remove all

---

[3]Exceeds dosage recommended by the manufacturer.

[1]Not FDA approved for this indication.

lice as they hatch, can be very helpful. Bedding and clothing should be decontaminated (as for scabies) or removed from body contact for at least 2 weeks.

Pediculosis Corporis

Pediculosis corporis is associated with poor hygiene and unsanitary living conditions (vagabond's itch). *Pediculus humanus corporis*, the body louse, lives and lays its eggs on clothes, especially on seams. Transmission occurs mainly through contact with contaminated clothing or bedding. *P. humanus corporis* is capable of transferring several infectious diseases, especially epidemic typhus.

The infestation is manifested with intense pruritus, erythema, urticarial lesions, papules, and nodules. Excoriations, secondary infections, and lymphadenopathy may also be seen. The lice and nits usually can be found in the clothing.

For treatment, disinfection of clothes is enough. They should be washed and rinsed in hot water following by ironing. Items that cannot be washed should be removed from body contact for 2 weeks. Skin lesions can be managed with topical antipruritics or corticosteroids.

Pediculosis Pubis

Phthirus pubis is usually transmitted during sexual intercourse, although any intimate personal contact suffices. Lice and nits are found mostly on pubic hair, but other body parts and, especially in children, eyelashes and the periphery of the scalp can be involved. Patients present with pruritus. Blue macules, or *maculae caeruleae*, are often found and result from intracutaneous hemorrhages whose hemoglobin has been altered by the saliva of the lice.

Pediculosis pubis can be treated in the same way as pediculosis capitis. Some recommend treatment with permethrin (Nix, Elimite) 5% or ivermectin (Stromectol),[1] as for scabies (see earlier). Infestation of eyelashes should be treated by applying occlusive ophthalmic ointment to the eyelid margins twice a day for 10 days. Bedding and clothing should be decontaminated (as for scabies) or removed from body contact for at least 2 weeks. Sexual partners within the last month should also be treated.

REFERENCES

Braun-Falco O, Plewig G, Wolff HH, Burgdorf WHC: Diseases caused by worms. In: Dermatology, 2nd ed. Springer, Berlin Heidelberg, 2000, pp 383-402.

Ectoparasitic infections. In: Centers for Disease Control and Prevention: Sexually transmitted diseases treatment guidelines-2006. MMWR Morb Mortal Wkly Rep 2006;55(RR11):1-94.

Orion E, Matz H, Wolf R: Ectoparasitic sexually transmitted diseases: Scabies and pediculosis. Clin Dermatol 2004;22:513-519.

Braun-Falco O, Plewig G, Wolff HH, Burgdorf WHC: Protozoan diseases. In: Dermatology, 2nd ed. Springer, Berlin Heidelberg, 2000, pp 299-312.

Drugs for Parasitic Infections. The Medical Letter on Drugs and Therapeutics. The Medical Letter Inc, New Rochelle, NY, August, 2004;1-12.

Tsoureli-Nikita E, Campanile G, Hautmann G, Hercogova J: Pediculosis. In: Katsambas AD, Lotti TM (eds): European Handbook of Dermatologic Treatments, 2nd ed. Springer, Berlin Heidelberg, 2003, pp 377-381.

---

[1]Not FDA approved for this indication.

Fungal Diseases of the Skin

Method of
Adelaide A. Hebert, MD

Fungal infections are caused by organisms that infect keratin-containing tissues such as skin, nails, and hair shafts. The most common organism involved in these processes is a group known as the dermatophytes (*Trichophyton, Microsporum, Epidermophyton*), often referred to as tinea infections, but fungal infections can also be caused by nondermatophytes such as yeast (*Candida*) or *Malassezia* species.

The spores and hyphae of dermatophytes rarely invade growing tissues, confining themselves to the soft keratin composing the skin of the trunk, arms, and ventral feet and hands. For this reason, topical therapeutics can penetrate and cure these cutaneous infections, which include tinea corporis, tinea manuum, tinea faciei, and tinea cruris.

Hair and nails are composed of hard keratin, which topical medications cannot penetrate. Oral therapy must be used for hair and nail involvement, as well as for more chronic or extensive skin involvement.

Diagnosis

Diagnosis is often clinically based, but 20% potassium hydroxide (KOH) preparations for microscopic visualization of hyphae can confirm the diagnosis. In skin and scalp infections, a sample can be obtained by lightly scraping the scaly area with a #15 blade. Nail samples must be acquired by curetting the affected surface of the nail plate, scraping under the nail bed, or taking nail clippings, depending on the region of the nail involved. Fungal cultures are still useful to verify the causative organism, particularly in scalp or nail infections where oral therapy will be required for successful infection control.

TINEA PEDIS

Tinea pedis is the most common fungal infection of the skin in the United States, popularly known as athlete's foot. Most commonly caused by *Trichophyton rubrum*, this infection commonly appears as maceration between the toes with fissuring. Tinea pedis can also involve more diffuse erythema and scaling favoring the plantar surface of the foot (moccasin-type). Differential diagnosis includes contact dermatitis, dyshidrotic eczema, and cellulitis.

TINEA CRURIS

Tinea cruris, or jock itch, affects men more than women, occurring in the groin where there is increased sweating and friction. This condition more often occurs in warm, humid environments or in the summer months; causal organisms include *T. rubrum, Trichophyton mentagrophytes*, or *Epidermophyton floccosum*. The pruritic plaques are well demarcated in the inner thighs, usually sparing the scrotum. This sparing is in contrast to a candidal infection in the groin, which can involve the scrotum. The differential

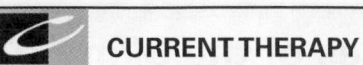
Section 13 Diseases of the Skin

986

	Preferred Treatment	Alternatives	Comments or Considerations
Dermatophytes			
Tinea pedis	**Systemic:** terbinafine (Lamisil) 250 mg/day for 2 wk; itraconazole (Sporanox) 200 mg bid for 2 wk **Topical:** butenafine (Mentax) 1-2 times daily for 2-4 wk	**Systemic:** fluconazole (Diflucan) 150 mg/wk for 4 wk	Topicals can be used concurrently with oral therapy. Prevent recurrence with moisture-absorbing foot powder, wide-toe shoes, and frequent changes of socks and shoes.
Tinea cruris	**Topical:** miconazole, bid, 4 wk clotrimazole, bid, 4 wk econazole, bid, 4 wk	Systemic therapy for resistant cases: **Oral:** griseofulvin ultramicrosized 333 to 500 mg/day for 2 wk; terbinafine 250 mg/day for 2 wk; fluconazole 150 mg once a week for 2-4 wk	Inflamed lesions: butenafine (Mentax) qd for 4 wk.
Tinea corporis	**Topical:** clotrimazole or terbinafine bid for 2 wk **Systemic** (for extensive involvement): itraconazole 200 mg/d 2 wk	**Topical:** miconazole bid, 2 wk **Oral:** terbinafine 250 mg/d 2 wk **Oral:** fluconazole 150 mg once a week for 4 wk	Watch for secondary bacterial infections in these cases.
Tinea capitis	**Systemic:** griseofulvin liquid microsized 20-25 mg/kg/d for 8 wk; griseofulvin pill ultramicrosized 15-20 mg/kg/d for 8 wk	**Systemic:** terbinafine 5 mg/kg/d for 4-8 wk	Concurrent topical use of 2% ketoconazole or 1% selenium sulfide shampoo helps kill spores on the hair, decreasing transmission. Topicals should not be used as monotherapy, as systemic therapy is required.
Tinea barbae	**Systemic:** griseofulvin ultramicrosized 500 mg or 330 mg 1-2/d	**Systemic:** itraconazole 200 mg/d for 2-4 wk terbinafine 250 mg/d for 2-4 wk	
Tinea unguium *(Onychomycosis)*	**Systemic:** terbinafine 250 mg/d for 6 wk (fingernails), 12 wk (toenails)	**Systemic:** itraconazole 400 mg bid for 1 wk, repeat in next 1 to 2 mo fluconazole 300 mg once a week for 6-9 mo	Nails will not look clear after 12 wk; patients must be reassured. Onychomycosis can be caused by *Candida* alone or in combination with dermatophytes; treat accordingly
Nondermatophytes			
Tinea versicolor	**Topical:** miconazole, clotrimazole, econazole bid for up to 4 wk Selenium sulfide 2.5% lotion; use an antiseborrheic shampoo 2/wk **Systemic:** itraconazole 200 mg/d for 1 wk or ketoconazole (Nizoral) 400 mg once	ketoconazole (Nizoral) can be used for 3 d Salicylic acid soap, terbinafine spray	Oral therapy reserved for nonresponsive, extensive involvement Recurrence rates are high Pityrosporum folliculitis, also caused by same *Pityrosporum orbiculare* is treated with similar drugs and dosing

Treatment of Cutaneous Fungal Infections

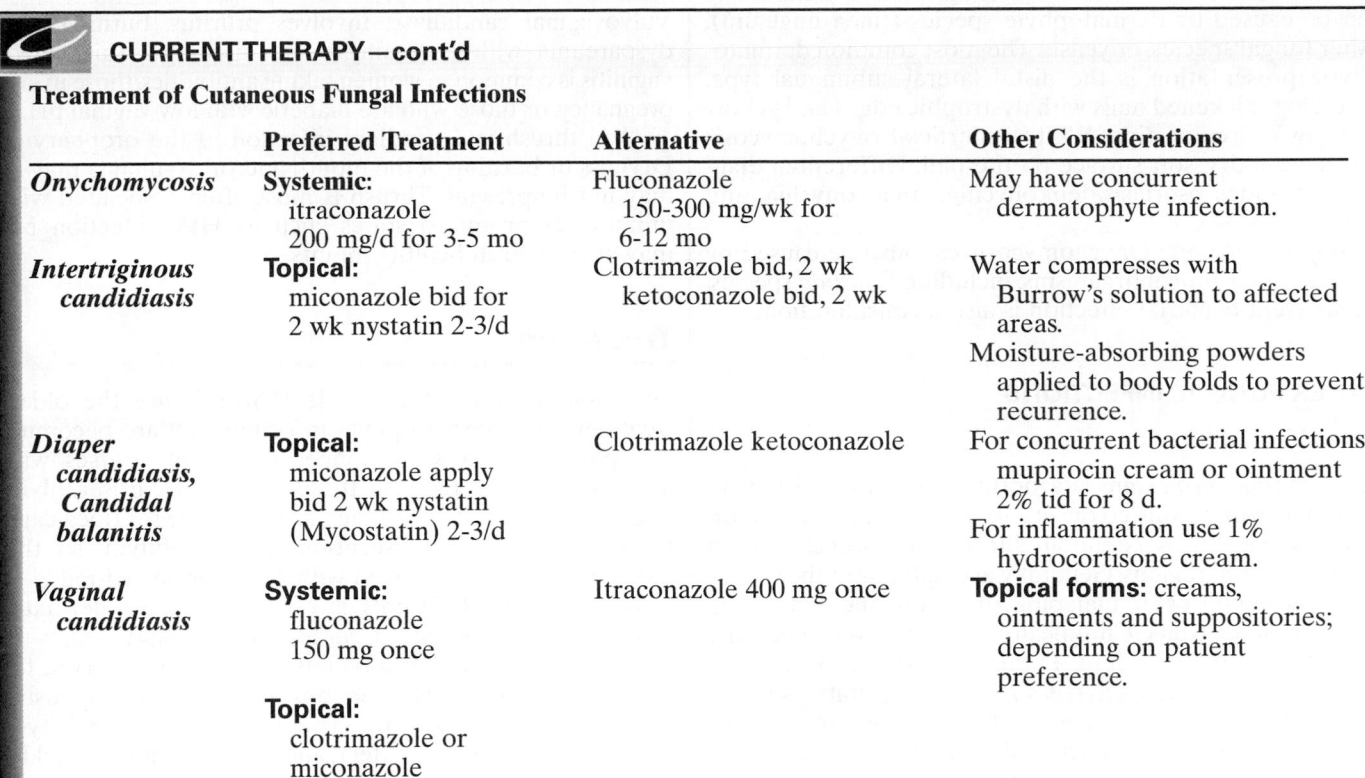

	Preferred Treatment	Alternative	Other Considerations
Onychomycosis	**Systemic:** itraconazole 200 mg/d for 3-5 mo	Fluconazole 150-300 mg/wk for 6-12 mo	May have concurrent dermatophyte infection.
Intertriginous candidiasis	**Topical:** miconazole bid for 2 wk nystatin 2-3/d	Clotrimazole bid, 2 wk ketoconazole bid, 2 wk	Water compresses with Burrow's solution to affected areas. Moisture-absorbing powders applied to body folds to prevent recurrence.
Diaper candidiasis, Candidal balanitis	**Topical:** miconazole apply bid 2 wk nystatin (Mycostatin) 2-3/d	Clotrimazole ketoconazole	For concurrent bacterial infections: mupirocin cream or ointment 2% tid for 8 d. For inflammation use 1% hydrocortisone cream.
Vaginal candidiasis	**Systemic:** fluconazole 150 mg once **Topical:** clotrimazole or miconazole	Itraconazole 400 mg once	**Topical forms:** creams, ointments and suppositories; depending on patient preference.
Mucocutaneous candidiasis	**Systemic:** fluconazole 150 mg/wk for 4 wk	Clotrimazole lozenges nystatin suspension swish and swallow	

must include psoriasis, seborrheic dermatitis, erythrasma, and candidiasis.

TINEA CORPORIS

Fungal infections can occur on the trunk or extremities and are commonly caused by *T. rubrum*. Characteristic findings include circular lesions with central clearing, but follicular pustules can also be seen. Differential diagnosis includes nummular eczema and pityriasis rosea. Watch for secondary bacterial infections in these cases.

Important note: Cutaneous fungal infections that have been misdiagnosed and treated with topical steroids can have unusual features caused by the reduced inflammation with a loss of defined borders and scale. This condition is known as tinea incognito. In such cases discontinue the use of topical steroids and treat with topical antifungals or appropriate oral therapy if progression is extensive.

TINEA MANUUM

Some patients with tinea pedis may also have involvement of the hands with a diffuse erythema along with fairly well-demarcated scaling. Dry, peeling skin can be slowly progressive and mildly pruritic. Tinea manuum is most often unilateral, and in more acute presentations it may be related to animal or soil contacts. Hand involvement can also mimic eczema, dyshidrosis, keratolysis exfoliativa, or the palmoplantar pustulosis type of psoriasis.

TINEA CAPITIS

Trichophyton tonsurans is the common culprit in scalp fungal infections in the majority of the United States. Tinea capitis is most often seen in children, causing patchy hair loss with scaling and possibly a boggy scalp with tender plaques (kerion). Cervical lymphadenopathy is common in this condition. The differential includes alopecia areata, which has no scale, and seborrheic dermatitis, which may have scaling with minimal to no hair loss. In black-dot tinea capitis, the hair shaft is brittle and breaks off at the level of the scalp. Differential diagnosis includes seborrheic dermatitis, psoriasis, eczema, poor hygiene, or adherent scalp products such as styling gels.

TINEA BARBAE

In men's beard and mustache areas, a fungal infection is typically unilateral and spares the upper lip. In contrast to the other main differential diagnosis, bacterial folliculitis, tinea barbae is more insidious. The causal organisms include *T. mentagrophytes* and, more rarely, *Trichophyton verrucosum*. Secondary bacterial infection is common and can cause regional lymphadenopathy.

TINEA UNGUIUM (ONYCHOMYCOSIS)

Fungal infections of the nail are more common in adults (affecting approximately 2% of the U.S. population) and can be caused by dermatophyte species (tinea unguium), other fungal species, or yeasts. The most common dermatophytic presentation is the distal lateral subungual type, involving thickened nails with dystrophic edges and yellow to brown discoloration. White superficial onychomycosis produces a dry, soft surface on the nail. Differential diagnosis includes psoriasis, leukonychia, trachyonychia, and onycholysis.

Important note: Onychomycosis can also be caused by various other fungal organisms, including *Candida* species. Concurrent bacterial infection is also a consideration.

OTHER FUNGAL INFECTIONS

Tinea Versicolor

Pityrosporum orbiculare is a normal inhabitant of human skin, but overzealous colonization defines tinea versicolor. Tinea versicolor is common during adolescence and in humid, tropical regions. Generally asymptomatic, the lesions manifest acutely as circular, pink, or hypopigmented scaling macules on the trunk. Chronically, these lesions can become greyish-tan and confluent. Differential diagnosis includes vitiligo, pityriasis alba, pityriasis rosea, and guttate psoriasis. Diagnosis is confirmed with a KOH examination of the scale, which will reveal a characteristic *spaghetti and meatballs* appearance of the hyphae and spores.

Pityrosporum Folliculitis

This is an infection of the hair follicle caused by the yeast *Pityrosporum orbiculare*. The condition causes an itchy, diffuse papulopustular eruption of the upper trunk and shoulders. Differential diagnosis includes acne, bacterial folliculitis, and scabies.

CANDIDIASIS

Most cutaneous candidiasis is caused by the yeast *Candida albicans* infecting skin and mucous membranes. This species is part of normal human flora, growing best in moist, warm areas or where skin touches skin. Pregnancy, diabetes, immunosuppression, and the use of birth control pills, topical steroids, and antibiotics can all predispose to these skin infections. The presentation usually includes pustules with a red, glistening border. A KOH preparation is helpful but not always diagnostic in differentiating these pseudohyphae from dermatophytes.

Intertriginous candidiasis involves skin folds such as the axillae, submammary folds, groin, and perineum areas. Obese and diabetic patients are at particular risk, with moisture, heat, and friction predisposing the skin to these infections.

Diaper dermatitis, diaper rash, appears as erythematous small pustules with similar satellite lesions involving the genitalia, buttocks, and perineum, but characteristically sparing the genitocrural folds. Bacterial superinfection and/or concurrent contact diaper dermatitis can occur. Pseudohyphae can be seen on KOH prep. *Candida*-induced diaper dermatitis must be differentiated from staphylococcus impetigo, atopic dermatitis, or contact diaper dermatitis.

Candidal balanitis involves erythema and vesiculopustules on the glans penis and is especially prevalent in the uncircumcised penis or in cases of poor hygiene. Vulvovaginal candidiasis involves pruritus, burning, and dyspareunia with a creamy white discharge. This vulvovaginitis is common in women taking antibiotics, those in late pregnancy, or those who are diabetic with low vaginal pH.

Oral thrush is a candidal infection in the oropharynx. Dryness or burning of the mouth and/or dysphagia may or may not be present. Thrush is most often associated with immunocompromised states such as HIV infection but may also occur in healthy infants.

Treatment

Griseofulvin and ketoconazole (Nizoral) are the oldest treatments for dermatophyte infections but are becoming less popular because of longer treatment courses with lower cure rates. Despite these drawbacks, griseofulvin, which is fungistatic, is still the drug of choice for tinea capitis. Fat aids in the absorption of griseofulvin, so this medication should be taken with meals or dairy foods.

Ketoconazole (Nizoral) is effective against dermatophyte, *Malassezia,* and *Candida* species and comes in cream, shampoo, and oral tablets. This drug is reserved for recalcitrant cutaneous infections and those unresponsive to topical therapies or oral griseofulvin. Hepatotoxicity is a rare but possible side effect, and liver function should be monitored regularly.

The development of imidazole derivatives has ushered in broad-spectrum efficacy. The triazole antifungal itraconazole (Sporanox) is active against dermatophytes, *Candida,* and even some molds. Reversible hepatitis is a risk, and liver function should be monitored in patients with liver problems. Other problems include cardiac side effects (such as congestive heart failure) and multiple drug interactions. Fluconazole (Diflucan) has high oral absorbability and may become a favored alternative for infections previously treated with griseofulvin. Side effects are usually mild and include nausea and headaches.

Allylamines make up another newer class of antifungals and include naftifine (Naftin) and terbinafine (Lamisil). Some patients taking these medications report taste changes that persist for a period after therapy is concluded. The benzylamine drug butenafine (Mentax) is another option with the added benefit of an anti-inflammatory effect. Mentax is useful for dermatophyte infections with marked inflammatory reactions in the infected tissue.

Ciclopiroxolamine (Loprox) comes in a lotion, cream, or shampoo form for *Candida* and dermatophyte infections of the skin. Ciclopirox 8% (Penlac Nail Lacquer) is the only topical nail treatment approved for infections not involving the lunula, but it must be applied daily for up to a year with only limited cure rates being reported.

Nystatin (Mycostatin) is a polyene available in both oral and topical versions and is only effective for *Candida* infections. *Candida* can also be treated with both topical and oral imidazole derivatives, such as ketoconazole (Nizoral). Ciclopiroxolamine and allylamines such as terbinafine are also effective options.

The key to successful management of dermatophyte, tinea versicolor, and *Candida* infections is to correctly identify the diagnosis prior to initiating therapy. Simple techniques such as KOH examinations and cultures can support clinical findings and validate a diagnosis in most cases. Therapy should be directed at the causative agent with consideration given to the patient's other medical conditions, treatments, and ability to comply with the outlined regimen.

REFERENCES

Aly R, Forney R, Bayles C: Treatments for common superficial fungal infections. Dermatol Nurs 2001;12(2):91-94.

Boucher HW, Groll AH, Chiou C, Walsh T: Newer systemic antifungal agents: Pharmacokinetics, safety and efficacy. Drugs 2004;64(18): 1997-2000.

Chan YC, Freidlander SF: New treatments for tinea capitis. Curr Opin Infect Dis 2004;17:97-103.

Cribier BJ, Bakshi R: Terbinafine in the treatment of onychomycosis: A review of its efficacy in high-risk populations and in patients with nondermatophyte infections. Br J Dermatol 2004;150:414-420.

Foster KW, Ghannoum M, Elewski B: Epidemiologic surveillance of cutaneous fungal infection in the United States from 1999 to 2002. J Am Acad Dermatol 2004;50(5):748-752.

Greenburg HL, Shwayder TA, Bieszk N, Fivenson DP: Clotrimazole/betamethasone dipropionate: A review of costs and complications in the treatment of common cutaneous fungal infections. Pediatr Dermatol 2002;19(1):78-81.

Grin C: Tinea: Diagnostic clues, treatment keys. Consultant 2004; 44(2):14.

Gupta AK: Systemic antifungal agents. In Wolverton SE (ed): Comprehensive Dermatologic Drug Therapy. Philadelphia, WB Saunders, 2001, pp 55-70.

Gupta AK, Bluhm R: Ciclopirox (Loprox) gel for superficial fungal infections. Skin Therapy Lett 2004;9(7):4-5.

Gupta AK, Chaudhry M, Elewski B: Tinea corporis, tinea cruris, tinea nigra, and piedra. Dermatol Clin 2003;21(3):395-400.

Gupta AK, Ryder J, Summerbell RC: Comparison of efficacy criteria across onychomycosis trials: need for standardization. Int J Dermatol 2003;42;312-315.

Habif et al: Skin disease: Diagnosis and treatment, St. Louis, Mosby, 2001, pp 206-209.

Loeffler J, Stevens DA: Antifungal drug resistance. Clin Infect Dis 2003;36(2):S31.

Piraccini BM, Tosti A: White superficial onychomycosis: Epidemiological, clinical and pathological study of 79 patients. Arch Dermatol 2004; 140:696-701.

Vander Straten MR, Hossain MA, Ghannoum MA: Cutaneous infections dermatophytosis, onychomycosis, and tinea versicolor. Infect Dis Clin North Am 2003;17(1):87-112.

Weinstein A, Berman B: Topical treatment of common superficial tinea infections. Am Fam Physician 2002;65(10):2095-2102.

Diseases of the Mouth

Method of
Carl M. Allen, DDS, MSD

A wide variety of disease processes other than dental caries and periodontal disease affect the oral region. These diseases may be classified based on the etiopathogenesis of the disease (e.g., viral, neoplastic); the clinical form of the lesions (e.g., plaque, vesicle, ulcer); or the anatomic region affected (e.g., lips, buccal mucosa). The clinical form and anatomic region are particularly useful for the clinician confronted by an unknown lesion. An accurate diagnosis is the most important aspect of patient management because treatment is predicated on diagnosis. The lesions that tend to affect certain oral mucosal sites preferentially are listed here according to their frequency; space limitations prohibit discussion of rare entities.

Generalized Oral Involvement

Xerostomia is the subjective feeling of a dry mouth. In most instances, it is caused by any of a variety of medications (antihypertensives, antihistamines, psychoactive drugs), and withdrawal or substitution of the medication may be helpful. A smaller number of patients may have xerostomia secondary to autoimmune destruction of the salivary gland tissue (Sjögren's syndrome) or caused by radiation therapy of the head and neck region. Such patients may develop a number of problems. The mucosa is not as well lubricated and becomes susceptible to traumatic ulceration. The dry environment predisposes the individual to the erythematous or angular cheilitis forms of oral candidiasis. If the patient has natural teeth, a marked increase in dental caries is noted.

A number of over-the-counter artificial saliva substitutes, in both liquid and gel form, are available to help manage the symptoms of dryness. Oral ulcerations should be managed conservatively using a protective hydroxypropylcellulose medication (Zilactin),[1] applied as often as necessary. Oral candidiasis can be treated with any of several antifungal medications, although those with high sucrose content, such as nystatin pastilles (Mycostatin Oral Pastilles), should probably be avoided in dentulous patients because these agents could contribute to caries activity. A prescription-strength topical fluoride preparation, such as 1.1% neutral sodium fluoride gel (PreviDent), should be used daily by patients who have natural teeth to prevent dental decay. Application of the topical fluoride is best performed at night after brushing the teeth and before retiring. Several drops of the fluoride gel should be placed on the toothbrush and gently massaged onto the surfaces of the teeth next to the gum tissue.

Lips

COMMON CONDITIONS

Fordyce's Granules

Fordyce's granules, a variation of normal anatomy, are heterotopic sebaceous glands seen in more than 80% of adults. They occur as 1-mm yellow-white submucosal dots distributed on the lateral upper lip and the buccal mucosa. No treatment is indicated because of the completely benign nature of the condition.

Angular Cheilitis

Angular cheilitis is characterized by inflammation of the corners of the mouth, accompanied by fissuring and sometimes scaling. This condition was thought to be caused by B vitamin deficiency, but the vast majority of these lesions are now thought to be caused by a low-grade infection of *Candida albicans*, with or without *Staphylococcus aureus*.

These lesions can be easily treated with a topical antifungal agent such as nystatin-triamcinolone cream (Mycolog-II Cream). Another alternative is iodoquinol-hydrocortisone cream (Vytone Cream),[1] which is both antifungal and antibacterial but must be used externally. Either medication should be applied three to four times daily for at

---

[1]Not FDA approved for this indication.

least 1 week. With recurrence, a careful search for an intra-oral source of infection may be indicated, and the possibility of HIV infection may need to be ruled out. Angular cheilitis with associated intraoral candidiasis requires treatment. Topical agents include clotrimazole troches (Mycelex Oral Troches) and nystatin pastilles, each dissolved in the mouth four to five times daily for 7 to 10 days. Systemic therapy with fluconazole (Diflucan) may be more convenient for some patients because it is given orally, 200 mg the first day, followed by 100 mg daily for the next 6 days.

Herpes Labialis

Recurrent herpes labialis affects approximately 25% of the population. Reactivation of the virus is usually triggered by sun (ultraviolet light) exposure, with many patients experiencing an itching or tingling sensation in the prodromal phase. A cluster of vesicles then develops on the vermilion zone of the lip or on perioral skin, rupturing within 1 to 3 days and leaving a crusted area that resolves after a few more days.

No curative therapy exists for this condition, and treatment results may be difficult to interpret because of the strong placebo effect in some instances. High sun protection factor (SPF) sun-blocking agents significantly reduce the frequency of episodes triggered by exposure to ultraviolet light. Low-dose acyclovir (Zovirax)[1] or valacyclovir (Valtrex)[1] may prevent attacks if it is taken continuously (400 mg twice daily; 1 g per day, respectively), but attacks resume as usual once the medication is stopped. Systemic valacyclovir, 2-g doses 12 hours apart given during the prodromal phase, reduces lesion formation in a subset of individuals affected by this condition. Topical acyclovir ointment shows no benefit in double-blind, placebo-controlled trials in immunocompetent patients, whereas topical penciclovir cream (Denavir) has only a modest effect on the course of the lesions.

Melanotic Macule

Melanotic macule, a solitary lesion, usually develops on the vermilion zone of the lips, but it may be seen intra-orally. The lesion occurs as a 1- to 5-mm macule that exhibits a uniform, well-demarcated brown to black color.

If the patient indicates the lesion has been present for several years and has not observed any change in size or color, no treatment is indicated unless the patient is concerned about cosmetic appearance. If changes in the lesion are recent, excisional biopsy is indicated to rule out the possibility of an early melanoma.

Actinic Keratosis (Cheilitis)

Actinic keratosis is a premalignant process affecting the lower vermilion zone of the lip of fair-skinned adults with a history of chronic sun exposure. The lesions have a scaly texture and ill-defined margins.

Excision, by either scalpel or laser, or cryosurgery is indicated for treatment. Excision is often accomplished by vermilionectomy, in which the entire vermilion zone is removed as a strip for histopathologic examination. The labial mucosa is then advanced over the resulting defect.

[1]Not FDA approved for this indication.

When topical chemotherapy with fluorouracil (Efudex) is used, dysplastic epithelial cells persist histologically. All patients with sun-damaged lips should be advised to use a sunscreen with high SPF, applied particularly to the lower lip when sun exposure is anticipated.

UNCOMMON CONDITIONS

Squamous Cell Carcinoma

The malignancy of squamous cell carcinoma affects the lower vermilion zone, typically arising in a preexisting actinic keratosis. Such lesions usually have a relatively slow, steady growth, with a roughened or ulcerated surface. The diagnosis should be established by biopsy. Wide surgical excision, obtaining at least a 1-cm margin of normal tissue, is usually adequate treatment because these lesions are rather indolent and do not metastasize until relatively late in their course.

Reactive Cheilitis

Patients may present occasionally with a complaint of fissured, painful lips. Evaluation of the problem should include a history of onset, duration, and use of medications and cosmetics. Lipstick and artificially flavored cinnamon products may produce a contact cheilitis. Isotretinoin (Accutane) often causes exfoliative cheilitis. Solitary chronic lip fissures, which usually occur in the winter months, may respond to topical antibiotic preparations, with surgical excision reserved for resistant lesions. Many cases of reactive cheilitis appear to be factitial, although patients may be reluctant to admit their habit of licking and nibbling at the vermilion zone. Constant moistening of the lips also predisposes the individual to a superimposed candidal infection, which exacerbates the inflammatory symptoms, and petrolatum-based lip balms may contribute to the problem by trapping moisture and thereby promoting the growth of yeast.

Telangiectasias

Superficial dilated blood vessels may occur on the vermilion zone of the lips as an isolated finding or, if multiple, as a component of either hereditary hemorrhagic telangiectasia or CREST (calcinosis, Raynaud's phenomenon, esophageal dysfunction, sclerodactyly, and telangiectasias) syndrome. Patients should be evaluated to distinguish between these two entities because their prognoses are different. Treatment of the telangiectatic lesions can be performed by laser excision, cryotherapy, or electrodesiccation.

Labial Mucosa

COMMON CONDITIONS

Mucocele

The mucocele represents a collection of extravasated mucin within the submucosal connective tissue caused by the disruption of a minor salivary gland duct by minor trauma. Most mucoceles develop on the lower labial mucosa, appearing suddenly as a painless, soft, bluish, circumscribed swelling. A cycle of swelling, breaking, and swelling again is typical.

Surgical excision of the mucous deposit and the associated gland usually is necessary for resolution of the problem.

Varix

The varix, similar to varicose veins of the leg, is seen on the labial mucosa, lips, buccal mucosa, and tongue of patients older than 50 years. Patients usually describe the gradual onset of a painless purplish or bluish nodule.

Generally, no treatment is indicated. If the lesion is a cosmetic problem or if it occurs in areas likely to be traumatized, the varix may be treated by surgical excision or cryotherapy.

Aphthous Ulcer (Canker Sore)

The aphthous ulcer is perhaps one of the most misdiagnosed, mismanaged, and misunderstood of all oral diseases. Most authorities believe that aphthous ulcers are immunologically induced. No convincing scientific data link the process to viral infection. Furthermore, studies suggesting the lesions are associated with certain foods or vitamin deficiencies have not been duplicated. Several mechanisms may initiate the abnormal immune response leading to focal destruction of the oral mucosa. The lesions are typically recurrent, ranging from 1 to 24 episodes per year. The most common form of aphthous ulcer is the minor aphthous ulcer, manifesting as a 1- to 10-mm ulceration with an erythematous periphery and smooth borders. From one to five ulcers may develop simultaneously. Aphthous ulcers are located on movable mucosa, not mucosa bound to periosteum, a situation directly opposite to recurrent intraoral herpes. The patient typically reports pain that seems out of proportion to the size of the lesion. With no treatment, minor aphthae heal within 5 to 10 days. Patients with frequent attacks should be questioned regarding ocular complaints or genital ulcerations to rule out Behçet's syndrome. Infrequently, aphthous-like oral ulcerations may be a manifestation of Crohn's disease as well.

Topical application of a relatively strong corticosteroid, such as fluocinonide (Lidex Gel),[1] betamethasone dipropionate (Diprolene Gel),[1] or clobetasol (Temovate Gel),[1] is most effective in controlling the lesions. For optimum response, small amounts of the medication should be applied as a thin film often (four to five times daily) and as early in the course of the lesion as possible.

UNCOMMON CONDITIONS

Major Aphthous Ulcers

Major aphthae are debilitating oral lesions that resemble minor aphthae, except they are much larger (ranging up to 3 cm), and they persist for periods of up to 6 weeks before healing. Topical application of fluocinonide,[1] betamethasone dipropionate,[1] or clobetasol[1] usually controls this process. If the lesions are in the posterior segments of the mouth, betamethasone syrup (Celestone Syrup),[1] used as a mouth rinse and swallowed (10 mL after meals and at bedtime for 7 to 10 days), often provides relief.

---

[1]Not FDA approved for this indication.

Herpetiform Aphthous Ulcers

Herpetiform aphthous ulcers resemble primary herpetic gingivostomatitis, and they can be distinguished from that condition by their history of recurrence. Herpetiform aphthae are most effectively treated with one of the topical corticosteroid preparations or rinses described earlier.

Angioedema

Angioedema is thought to occur because of localized release of histamine from mast cells. Most cases are sporadic and harmless. The lips are most frequently affected, followed by the tongue. A tingling sensation usually precedes the sudden onset of rather dramatic, nontender swelling. The overlying skin appears normal, and the patient is otherwise asymptomatic; these features should help distinguish this condition from cellulitis associated with a dentoalveolar abscess. With no treatment, the condition resolves in 24 to 48 hours; however, oral antihistamine therapy seems to speed resolution. Attacks are commonly recurrent, and the precipitating factor is often difficult to identify. A rare hereditary form, caused by a deficiency of C1 esterase inhibitor, can be life-threatening if the laryngeal tissues are involved. With persistent swelling, biopsy may be indicated to rule out relatively rare conditions such as orofacial granulomatosis (cheilitis granulomatosa, Melkersson-Rosenthal syndrome).

Buccal Mucosa

COMMON CONDITIONS

Linea Alba

The oral linea alba merely represents a mild thickening of the epithelium along the plane of occlusion in dentate patients. The extent to which it is evident varies tremendously from patient to patient. No treatment is indicated for this completely benign condition.

Leukoedema

Leukoedema is considered a variation of normal. Clinically, it has a whitish, filmy, almost opalescent appearance, usually affecting the buccal mucosa. Stretching the mucosa causes the white appearance to diminish greatly or disappear completely. The surface epithelial cells histologically are edematous but otherwise normal, and no treatment is necessary for this benign condition.

Cheek-Chewing

Cheek-chewing is a harmless chronic habit. Although the anterior buccal mucosa is the most common site, the labial mucosa and lateral tongue may also be affected. A white, ragged alteration of the mucosa is seen clinically. Actual ulceration is uncommon because only the outer layers of the epithelium (which have no nerve fibers) are nibbled. The patient usually admits to the habit if questioned. This habit is completely benign and requires no further management once it is identified.

Fibroma (Irritation Fibroma, Focal Fibrous Hyperplasia)

The fibroma represents an accumulation of dense collagenous connective tissue at a site of irritation. For this reason, most of these lesions are found on the buccal mucosa. The lesion appears clinically as a sessile, dome-shaped, smooth-surfaced nodule. Patients may complain because they bite the lesion inadvertently.

Because this lesion cannot be definitively differentiated clinically from a wide array of other neoplasms, excisional biopsy is generally indicated. Recurrence is uncommon.

Lichen Planus

Lichen planus is an immunologically mediated condition of unknown cause that affects adults. The oral lesions manifest in two patterns: reticular and erosive. The reticular pattern is more common and usually seen bilaterally on the posterior buccal mucosa, occurring as white fine interlacing lines or papules. The gingivae and the tongue may also be affected. The erosive form of the condition is symptomatic because of the presence of ulcerations. These ulcerations usually have a central yellow-white area of fibrin surrounded by an erythematous halo and radiating white striae.

Reticular lichen planus requires no treatment. In 20% of cases, candidiasis is present, which should be treated with an antifungal agent. Erosive lichen planus can usually be managed effectively with the more potent topical corticosteroids such as fluocinonide,[1] betamethasone dipropionate,[1] or clobetasol.[1] Application of a thin film of medicationto the lesional areas, four to five times daily, often resolves the ulcers within a few days. Other conditions, such as epithelial dysplasia, lichenoid amalgam reactions, contact stomatitis, lichenoid drug reactions, and systemic lupus erythematosus, may mimic lichen planus clinically; biopsy is thus warranted if classic clinical features are not present. Malignant transformation of reticular lichen planus is not thought likely, although erosive lichen planus could possibly be premalignant. Affected patients should be reevaluated periodically for evidence of significant mucosal change, with rebiopsy performed if necessary.

UNCOMMON CONDITIONS

Verrucous Carcinoma

Verrucous carcinoma is a relatively low-grade malignancy of surface epithelial origin. It appears as a diffuse, white, rough-surfaced, spreading plaquelike lesion affecting the buccal mucosa, palate, or alveolar process in patients over 65 years of age.

Treatment is complete surgical excision, via scalpel or laser, with evaluation of the lesional tissue histopathologically because 25% of verrucous carcinomas may contain foci of routine squamous cell carcinoma. The prognosis is generally good because this lesion does not metastasize.

Oral Mucosal Cinnamon Reaction

The oral mucosal cinnamon reaction affects the buccal mucosa, the lateral tongue, and gingivae. The lesions appear

[1]Not FDA approved for this indication.

as diffuse areas of mucosal erythema with varying degrees of superimposed white plaques and, less commonly, ulceration. Such lesions may be mistaken clinically for lichen planus, candidiasis, leukoplakia, or erythroplakia. Discontinuing the artificially flavored cinnamon product (usually chewing gum) resolves the lesions within 1 week. The diagnosis can be confirmed by challenging the oral mucosa with the offending agent, although patients are often reluctant to do so after their lesions clear.

Hard Palate

COMMON CONDITIONS

Torus

Palatal tori are common developmental lesions representing a benign accumulation of dense bone in the midline posterior hard palate region. The diagnosis can be made clinically because no other condition manifests as a bony hard midline palatal mass. No treatment is necessary for this benign process, although denture construction may be hampered. Removal of the torus by an oral surgeon is recommended in that situation.

Denture Stomatitis

Denture stomatitis is almost invariably associated with a maxillary removable denture worn 24 hours per day. The palatal mucosa directly beneath the denture appears red, although it is asymptomatic. The redness is confined to the denture-bearing mucosa.

In many cases, simply having the patient remove the denture at night may resolve the palatal erythema. If the patient has a complete upper denture, it can be soaked in a mild sodium hypochlorite solution (Clorox) (1 teaspoon in 8 ounces of water) each night for a week to disinfect it. (Note: Chrome-cobalt metal denture frameworks should not be soaked in Clorox; severe corrosion will result and ruin the denture.) Because denture stomatitis is a benign and asymptomatic condition, treatment need not be a top priority.

Inflammatory Papillary Hyperplasia

Inflammatory papillary hyperplasia (IPH) (denture papillomatosis) is seen almost exclusively in patients who wear ill-fitting complete upper dentures. The lesions appear as multiple, erythematous 1- to 2-mm papules typically confined to the palatal vault area. These papules are composed of dense fibrous connective tissue that has accumulated secondary to chronic irritation in the superficial mucosa.

Treatment of this benign process is somewhat controversial. Some prosthodontists prefer to have these lesions surgically removed prior to constructing a new denture, although this procedure may not be necessary in every case.

UNCOMMON CONDITIONS

Recurrent Intraoral Herpes

Recurrent intraoral herpes is much less common than aphthous ulcerations, a condition with which it is frequently confused. Recurrent intraoral herpes affects only the hard palate and the attached gingiva (the paler firm gum tissue directly adjacent to the teeth). Most patients experience mild symptoms and may give a history of recurrent episodes. Lesions appear as a cluster of 1- to 2-mm shallow ulcerations that heal within 1 week. Generally no treatment is necessary, although the patient should be cautioned that virus is being shed from the lesion.

Salivary Gland Tumors

The posterior hard palate/anterior soft palate region is the most common site for the development of intraoral salivary gland neoplasia. This type of lesion presents as a slowly growing, rubbery firm, nontender mass that may or may not be ulcerated. The clinical appearance does not distinguish benign form malignant tumors, so a biopsy should be obtained that includes a margin of normal adjacent tissue. Approximately 50% of these tumors are pleomorphic adenomas, whereas the remainder represent mucoepidermoid carcinoma, polymorphous low-grade adenocarcinoma, adenoid cystic carcinoma, or acinic cell carcinoma. Complete excision is recommended for the pleomorphic adenoma, including overlying mucosa and underlying periosteum. The malignancies should be treated with a much more aggressive surgical approach, depending on the histologic type, the extent of bone involvement, and the size of the lesion. Adjunctive radiation therapy may be indicated for adenoid cystic carcinoma and high-grade mucoepidermoid carcinoma.

Soft Palate/Tonsillar Pillars

COMMON CONDITIONS

Papilloma

The squamous papilloma is the most common benign epithelial neoplasm that affects the oral mucosa, typically occurring as a solitary exophytic growth with numerous finger-like or frondlike projections on its surface. The soft palate/tonsillar pillar region is the most common site for the papilloma, and its color may range from pink to white.

Excisional biopsy, including the base of the lesion, should be performed. For those lesions of the posterior soft palate, periodic observation may be appropriate, particularly if the patient is experiencing no symptoms and the lesion is clinically characteristic.

UNCOMMON CONDITIONS

Pemphigus Vulgaris

Pemphigus vulgaris is an immunologically mediated condition characterized by the formation of vesicles and bullae secondary to attack of desmosomal complexes of the surface epithelium by autoantibodies. The condition usually is first seen intraorally, with painful, erosive lesions distributed diffusely on the oral mucosa. The soft palate is a primary site of involvement. Diagnosis should be established by light microscopy with direct and indirect immunofluorescence studies. Systemic immunosuppressive therapy is necessary to control this condition addressed in other areas of the text.

Tongue

COMMON CONDITIONS

Coated and Hairy Tongue

Coated and hairy tongue represents the accumulation of excess keratin on the filiform papillae of the dorsal tongue, resulting in the formation of elongated filamentous strands that superficially resemble hairs. Contrary to the description in numerous textbooks, this condition is not caused by an overgrowth of yeast.

No treatment is required, but if the patient is concerned about the appearance of the tongue, gentle daily débridement with a tongue scraper or the edge of a spoon assists in removing the accumulations of dead keratinized cells.

Fissured Tongue

Fissured tongue is essentially a variation of normal that usually develops sometime after the first decade of life. The patient may be concerned about the appearance of the tongue, but no symptoms are associated with the condition. The extent and pattern of fissuring can vary, and no treatment is indicated.

Benign Migratory Glossitis (Erythema Migrans, Geographic Tongue)

Benign migratory glossitis, a condition of unknown etiology, is seen in approximately 2% of the population. Most patients are asymptomatic, with lesions detected on routine examination. The dorsal tongue exhibits one or more well-demarcated zones of papillary atrophy that are surrounded, at least partially, by yellow-white slightly raised linear serpentine borders. The lesions typically resolve in one area and move to another, appearing in various stages of resolution and activity concurrently.

Because this is a benign condition, treatment is usually unnecessary. Approximately 5% of patients complain of sensitivity to hot or spicy foods when their lesions are active, but usually they do not require treatment. With severe symptoms, topical fluocinonide (Lidex Gel)[1] or one of the other stronger topical corticosteroids, applied as a thin film to the lesions several times daily, seems to reduce the discomfort.

Traumatic Ulcer

The traumatic ulcer occurs most frequently on the lateral tongue, buccal mucosa, and overlying bony prominences such as tori and exostoses. Most of these lesions are associated with relatively little pain. The traumatic ulcer manifests clinically as a defect covered by creamy white fibrin. Although most of these lesions heal within a week or so, some tend to persist, developing a rolled margin and peripheral induration.

Often no treatment is required because of the minimal degree of discomfort and the rapid healing time. If the patient complains of tenderness when eating salty or acidic foods, a protective medication (Zilactin) can be applied as needed. Topical corticosteroids should probably not be used because they may delay healing in this situation. If an

---

[1]Not FDA approved for this indication.

ulcer is present for longer than 2 weeks, with or without previous treatment, a biopsy is mandatory to rule out malignancy. A possible exception to this rule might be those ulcers overlying tori because they are notoriously difficult to resolve.

Burning Tongue Syndrome (Idiopathic Glossopyrosis)

The burning tongue syndrome seems to affect post-menopausal women predominantly. The patient often reports the rather sudden onset of a sensation that feels like the tongue was scalded. Symptoms are usually localized to the anterior tongue, although the labial mucosa and anterior hard palate may also be affected. Clinically, the mucosa appears normal. If mucosal erythema is identified, a variety of conditions should be ruled out, including candidiasis, anemia, local trauma, and erythema migrans. A culture for *Candida albicans* should be performed. If the workup shows no evidence of these conditions, a diagnosis of burning tongue syndrome can be made. Because there is no medically proven therapy, no specific treatment exists. The numerous suggested treatments in the literature have generally not been examined in controlled trials, and their efficacy is typically no more than that of the placebo effect. Reassuring patients this is a harmless condition, nothing more than a nuisance, and that the condition often resolves spontaneously after a period of months or years is usually sufficient.

UNCOMMON CONDITIONS

Squamous Cell Carcinoma

The lateral/ventral tongue is one of the most common sites for squamous cell carcinoma. In the early stages, the lesion is relatively asymptomatic, which underscores the importance of a regular and thorough oral mucosal examination. Slight thickening or nodularity within a white or red plaque frequently heralds the onset of invasion. As the lesion grows, the surface becomes ulcerated and symptoms of pain and tenderness develop. On palpation, squamous cell carcinomas are usually firm and show infiltrative borders. Biopsy is mandatory because other chronic ulcerative processes, such as chronic traumatic ulcer, deep fungal infections, mycobacterial infections, Wegener's granulomatosis, and other malignancies, may have a similar clinical presentation.

Treatment consists of wide surgical resection or radical radiation therapy, or both, depending on a number of factors. Prognosis is directly related to the tumor stage, although, in general, these patients do poorly because their lesions are not diagnosed until the later stages.

Hairy Leukoplakia

Hairy leukoplakia is an HIV-related lesion, significant because it often heralds a rapid decline in the patient's immune status. The lesion affects the lateral borders of the tongue, usually bilaterally, appearing as white plaques with vertical streaks. Sometimes the degree of keratinization may be great enough to produce hairlike projections, hence the name. Because this is otherwise a benign condition, no treatment is necessary. Hairy leukoplakia is caused by Epstein-Barr virus, thus medications used against other herpes viruses, such as acyclovir (Zovirax),[1] valacyclovir (Valtrex),[1] and dihydroxypropoxymethyl guanine (DHPG) (ganciclovir [Cytovene]),[1] may produce transient resolution.

Herpes in the Immunocompromised Host

With an immunocompromised host, the normal rules governing the location of the lesions of recurrent herpes are not applicable. The virus is not contained by the host, as in the normal individual, and the result is the formation of large, shallow, painful ulcerations with slightly elevated serpentine or scalloped margins. The diagnosis should be established by exfoliative cytology or viral culture, and treatment should be instituted immediately with systemic acyclovir, orally or intravenously, depending on the severity of the clinical infection.

Macroglossia

Macroglossia is the term used to describe enlargement of the tongue. Among the more frequent causes of macroglossia are hemangiomas and lymphangiomas. Hemangiomas are usually present at birth or develop shortly thereafter, with the tongue the most common site. These lesions are typically red or purple in color. If no compromise in function of the involved tissue is seen, treatment should be delayed until the child is older than 6 years of age because many of these lesions regress spontaneously. For those lesions that do not regress, argon laser excision is the optimal therapy. Other methods of management include cryotherapy and sclerosing agents.

Lymphangiomas affecting the oral tissues often exhibit a characteristic so-called frog-egg or tapioca-pudding surface morphology because of the dilated lymphatic vessels that are close to the surface. Treatment is surgical excision, although the decision to treat may depend on the size and site of the lesion. Recurrence rates as high as 40% are reported in some series of cases.

Other causes of macroglossia are much less common and include amyloidosis as well as benign and malignant tumors. Biopsy would be indicated to establish a diagnosis prior to treatment planning.

Floor of the Mouth

COMMON CONDITIONS

Leukoplakia

Leukoplakia is a clinical term that should be applied only to those white patches of the oral mucosa that cannot be wiped off and cannot be diagnosed as any other condition clinically. Leukoplakia is considered a premalignant condition and usually diagnosed in the sixth and seventh decades of life. Clinically, the condition appears as a well-defined white plaque that may show varying degrees of redness. The most worrisome sites of involvement include areas prone to cancer development, such as the lateral tongue, floor of the mouth, and the tonsillar pillar region.

---

[1]Not FDA approved for this indication.

Ideally, treatment is complete removal with microscopic evaluation of the excised specimen. Cryotherapy and laser excision may be used, but tissue may be rendered unsuitable for histopathologic examination. More concern should be given to leukoplakias found in nonsmokers, in high-risk areas for oral cancer, in lesions with a red component, in multifocal lesions, or those found in patients 20 to 50 years of age. If complete excision is accomplished, 30% of leukoplakias still recur, so careful follow-up with rebiopsy is indicated.

Sialolithiasis

Sialolithiasis (salivary duct stones) may appear with symptoms or be discovered on routine examination. The classic presentation is sudden painful unilateral swelling of the involved salivary gland occurring at mealtime. Most stones involve the submandibular gland, and these can be palpated as a hard submucosal mass in the floor of the mouth. Treatment usually involves surgical removal of the stone with repositioning of the salivary duct opening proximally. Sialography should then be performed to assess the function of the gland, and if it appears abnormal, it should probably be removed to prevent subsequent episodes of chronic recurrent sialadenitis.

UNCOMMON CONDITIONS

Erythroplakia

The premalignant lesion of erythroplakia represents the nonkeratinized version of leukoplakia. Erythroplakia appears as a well-demarcated, velvety red plaque that is typically asymptomatic. Dysplastic changes are likely, and treatment should consist of complete removal by the most expedient means.

Squamous Cell Carcinoma

The clinical appearance of squamous cell carcinoma at this site is similar to that of the lateral tongue, as is the treatment.

Alveolar Process/Gingiva

COMMON CONDITIONS

Mandibular Tori/Exostoses

Mandibular tori/exostoses are benign developmental lesions that consist of dense, viable bone. Mandibular tori are located on the lingual surface of the mandible in the premolar region, whereas exostoses occur on the alveolar process in other sites. Radiographic evaluation of any asymmetric bony swelling is indicated, and the exostosis should appear as a well-defined radiopacity. Generally, no treatment is necessary unless the bony outgrowths interfere with denture construction, in which case surgical removal is indicated.

Amalgam Tattoo

The amalgam tattoo is produced by the iatrogenic implantation of dental amalgam into the oral soft tissues.

Amalgam tattoos are usually macular and range in color from gray to blue to black or brown. Periapical radiographs often show the fine radiopaque metallic particles.

No treatment is necessary if the diagnosis can be made definitively from the radiograph. If no radiopacity is seen, biopsy is generally indicated to rule out a relatively rare oral melanocytic process such as a nevus or melanoma.

Dental Sinus Tract (Parulis)

The lesion of the dental sinus tract (parulis) represents a proliferation of granulation tissue at the drainage site of a sinus tract originating form the apical root portion of a nonvital tooth. Clinically, the parulis appears as an erythematous papule on the alveolar mucosa. Symptoms of pain may wax and wane. Treatment consists of either extraction or endodontic therapy for the offending tooth, and the prognosis is good.

Acute Necrotizing Ulcerative Gingivitis (Trench Mouth, Vincent's Infection)

Acute necrotizing ulcerative gingivitis is a disease produced by bacteria that are normal inhabitants of the oral microflora. The condition, which occurs in the third or fourth decade of life, is associated with poor oral hygiene, poor diet, and stress. College students are especially vulnerable during final examinations, and the condition may be seen in HIV-positive patients as well. Patients invariably present with a complaint of painful, foul-smelling gingivae. Examination shows punched-out ulceration of the interdental papillae. Acute necrotizing ulcerative gingivitis is frequently confused with primary herpes, which also is associated with pain and ulceration, but the punched-out interdental papillae are not seen in herpes infection.

Débridement, often requiring topical or local anesthesia, or both, is very important. This should be combined with systemic antibiotic therapy, such as tetracycline,[1] 250 mg every 6 hours, or potassium penicillin V, 500 mg every 6 hours. HIV-infected patients should also use chlorhexidine (Peridex) mouth rinse twice daily to prevent recurrence of acute necrotizing ulcerative gingivitis. For non-HIV patients, the prognosis is reasonably good, assuming they improve their diet and oral hygiene status.

Primary Herpetic Gingivostomatitis

Primary herpetic gingivostomatitis is caused by the initial exposure of the patient to herpes simplex virus, usually type I. Most of these infections occur during childhood, but occasionally an individual escapes contact with the virus until adulthood. Patients present with fever, cervical lymphadenopathy, malaise, and oropharyngeal pain. Examination of the oral mucosa reveals multiple shallow ulcerations distributed diffusely throughout the mouth, although the gingivae are often markedly affected. The gingival involvement is different from that of acute necrotizing ulcerative gingivitis, in that the interdental papillae do not show the punched-out ulcerations with the herpetic infection.

Patients should be managed symptomatically with analgesics, antipyretics, and topical anesthetics as indicated. Dehydration is sometimes a problem if oral pain prevents intake of fluids. Having the patient rinse with 5 mL of viscous lidocaine (Xylocaine Viscous) or dyclonine HCl (Dyclone) prior to meals provides temporary relief. Systemic acyclovir (Zovirax)[1] or valacyclovir (Valtrex)[1] may have a significant impact on the course of this disease if given during the first few days of the infection.

Inflammatory Fibrous Hyperplasia (Denture Epulis, Epulis Fissuratum, Denture Fibroma)

Inflammatory fibrous hyperplasia is caused by low-grade irritation from an ill-fitting denture. Clinically, the lesions are seen as smooth-surfaced sessile masses that appear to arise from the mucosa of the alveolar process or vestibule. Sometimes a groove or fissure runs lengthwise across the lesion, corresponding to the denture flange. Ulceration of the surface may be seen.

Surgical excision of the lesion is indicated prior to construction of new dentures. If the lesion is removed and the patient continues to wear the old denture, inflammatory fibrous hyperplasia recurs, but it is a completely benign process that does not undergo malignant transformation.

UNCOMMON CONDITIONS

Pyogenic Granuloma, Peripheral Giant Cell Granuloma, and Peripheral Ossifying Fibroma

Pyogenic granuloma, peripheral giant cell granuloma, and peripheral ossifying fibroma are benign gingival lesions probably initiated by chronic irritation in most instances. Although they are histologically distinctive, their clinical appearance and biologic behavior are similar. All of these lesions appear as sessile, dome-shaped masses that develop mainly on the gingiva (although pyogenic granuloma may be seen on any surface). They range from pink to reddish purple in color and are often ulcerated. Excisional biopsy is recommended to rule out the less likely possibility of metastatic neoplasm, which may clinically appear very similar. A recurrence rate of 15% can be expected for each of these lesions.

Generalized Gingival Hyperplasia

Generalized gingival hyperplasia usually develops as a side effect of medication: phenytoin (Dilantin), calcium channel blocking agents, or cyclosporine (Sandimmune). Only 30% to 50% of patients receiving one of these drugs show the diffuse gingival enlargement, which is usually related to the level of oral hygiene of the patient. If the drug cannot be discontinued or substituted, periodic periodontal surgery with reinforcement of oral hygiene instruction can usually control the problem. Rarely such enlargement may be associated with any of several genetic syndromes. These patients typically require periodic surgical reduction of the gingival tissues by a periodontist. Generalized gingival hyperplasia may also be a manifestation of myelomonocytic leukemia, although these patients usually complain of other signs and symptoms related to

their leukemic state. Biopsy and appropriate hematologic evaluation are necessary to establish a diagnosis.

Desquamative Gingivitis

Desquamative gingivitis is a descriptive term for a reaction pattern that affects the gingival tissues of adults. Patients complain of red, tender gingival mucosa that has a tendency to slough with minor manipulation. Vesicles may sometimes be reported. This condition must be biopsied for light microscopic evaluation as well as direct immunofluorescence studies because it invariably represents one of several distinct entities: erosive lichen planus, cicatricial pemphigoid, linear IgA disease, pemphigus vulgaris, or chronic ulcerative stomatitis. Once the definitive diagnosis is established, the patient can be managed appropriately.

REFERENCES

Neville BW, Damm DD, Allen CM, Bouquot JE: Oral and Maxillofacial Pathology, 2nd ed. Philadelphia, Elsevier Science, 2002.

Neville BW, Day TA: Oral cancer and precancerous lesions. CA Cancer J Clin 2002;52:195-215.

Regezi JA, Sciubba JJ, Jordan RCK: Oral Pathology. Clinical Pathologic Correlations, 4th ed. Philadelphia, Elsevier Science, 2003.

Sapp JP, Eversole LR, Wysocki GP: Contemporary Oral and Maxillofacial Pathology, 2nd ed. Philadelphia, Elsevier Science, 2004.

Scully C, Gorsky M, Lozada-Nur F: The diagnosis and management of recurrent aphthous stomatitis: A consensus approach. J Am Dent Assoc 2003;134:200-207.

Venous Stasis Ulcers

Method of
Tania J. Phillips, MD, and
Chukwuemeka N. Etufugh, MD

Epidemiology

Chronic venous ulceration is an increasingly important disease because of its impact on health care costs and effect on the quality of life. The estimated annual cost of ulcer treatment in the United States is reported to be $1 billion per year, with the average cost of one patient over a lifetime exceeding $40,000. An estimated 5% to 8% of the world population suffers from venous disease, and 1% of the world's population develops venous ulcers. In the United States alone, 5 million individuals have venous disease and approximately 500,000 individuals have chronic venous ulcers. Of the three main varieties of ulcer disease, arterial, venous, and neuropathic, venous ulcers account for 80% to 90% of all ulcers.

Pathogenesis

The venous system of the lower extremity is made up of the deep, superficial, and communicating veins. During ambulation, the calf muscles contract and act as a pump that promotes the return of venous blood to the heart with

---

[1]Not FDA approved for this indication.

one-way venous valves preventing retrograde flow. When the calf muscles contract, deep venous pressure decreases, thus moving blood from superficial veins through communicating veins into the deep venous system. The deep veins of the leg are emptied and the total volume of blood in the lower extremities is diminished. Individuals with venous disease because of incompetent valves, immobility, abnormality of calf muscle pump, or a combination of all three factors have a less than normal decrease in venous pressure during calf pump action. These individuals have elevated ambulatory venous pressure (so-called venous hypertension).

How this leads to ulcer formation is unclear. Hypotheses include the theory of pericapillary fibrin cuffs with leukocyte and growth factor trapping and cytokine release, which leads to capillary dysfunction and eventual ischemia, ulceration, and impaired healing of surrounding tissue.

Clinical Features

Patients with chronic venous ulcers report having a feeling of heaviness of the affected limb and leg swelling and aching, which improves with elevation and is worse at the end of the day. These patients may also have a history of deep venous thrombosis (DVT) and are prone to allergic contact dermatitis to several topical medications.

Venous ulcers are generally found in the gaiter area, the area from the midcalf to the ankle. They are shallow with irregular borders and can vary in size and shape. Other clinical findings include periulcer hyperpigmentation caused by hemosiderin deposits, lipodermatosclerosis, which is a chronic fibrosing process of the dermis, and subcutaneous tissue because of venous insufficiency that makes the skin feel firm and indurated. Varicose veins, lower extremity edema, and eczema caused by either venous or stasis dermatitis also occur. With advanced venous disease, the patient may develop a so-called champagne bottle leg, where because of chronic venous obstruction, the proximal leg swells and the distal leg constricts as a result of loss of subcutaneous fat and fibrosis.

Diagnosis and Treatment

A complete history and physical examination should be performed in all patients. Although most venous ulcer cases are diagnosed clinically, noninvasive techniques can aid in the diagnosis and evaluate the anatomy of the venous vasculature. Color duplex ultrasound scanning is the gold standard for evaluation of the anatomy of the venous system because of its accuracy and reproducibility. It can provide an analysis of venous anatomy and physiology and provide additional information about other anatomic structures in the leg, which might produce signs and symptoms that mimic venous disease such as arterial aneurysms and masses. Continuous-wave Doppler, photoplethysmography, and air plethysmography also can be used. In patients with a history of DVT, screening for coagulation defects may reveal activated protein C resistance caused by a point mutation in the gene for factor V Leiden. Other mutations in the prothrombin gene, proteins C and S, and antithrombin III can also cause venous thrombosis.

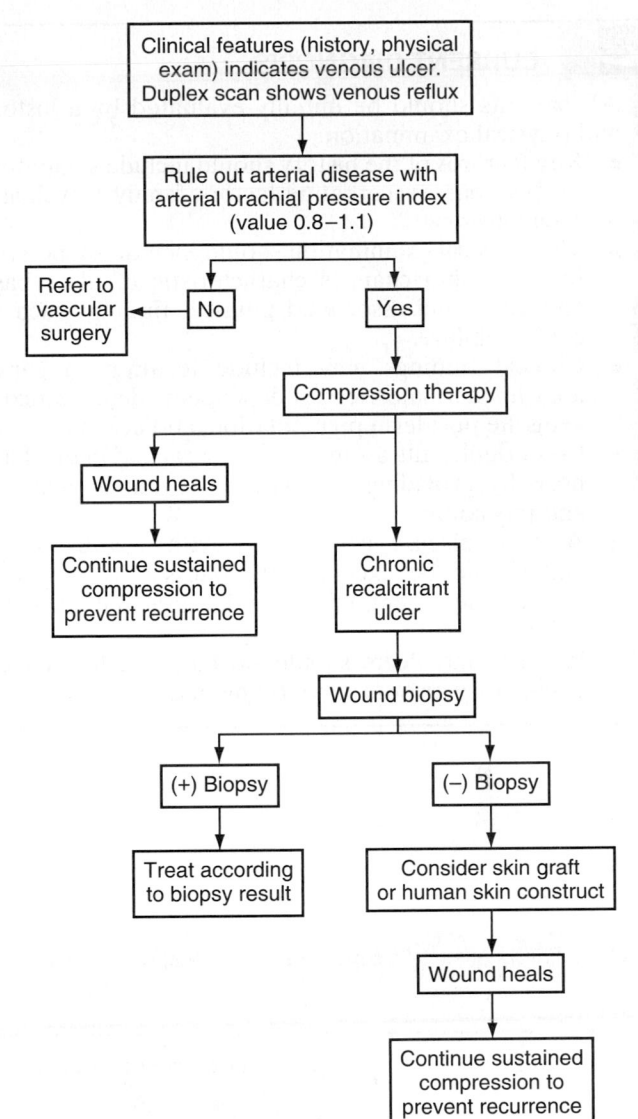

FIGURE 1. Scheme for treatment of venous ulcer.

Arterial disease, which can coexist with venous ulcers, should be excluded by the use of the ankle-brachial index (ABI) because palpation of the pedal pulses alone is not always reliable. The ABI is the ratio of systolic pressure between the ankle and the arm. An ABI in the range of 0.8 to 1.1 is considered normal, whereas a value less than 0.8 is abnormal, and the patient should be evaluated by a vascular surgeon. An ABI value of more than 1.1 suggests less compressible vasculature that is typically seen in diabetics or the elderly over 70 years of age because of vessel calcification. In these patients, the toe-brachial pressure index can be calculated by measuring the arterial pressure in the toe.

In the management of venous ulcers, compression is the mainstay of therapy. The goal of compression therapy is to counteract venous hypertension by facilitating venous return toward the heart. Several different compression devices are available, including compression pumps, elastic and nonelastic bandages, orthotic devices, and compression stockings (Table 1). Sustained graduated pressure of 30 to 40 mm Hg at the ankle is optimal. However, it is

CURRENT DIAGNOSIS

All patients should be initially evaluated by a history and physical examination.

- Key features of the history should include symptoms, medications, exacerbating factors, family, travel, and social history.
- The physical examination should include shape, size, location, skin changes characteristic of ulcer base and edge, and associated physical findings such as cardiac failure.
- Clinical findings may include location in gaiter area, lipodermatosclerosis, dependent edema, varicose veins, hemosiderin pigmentation, and eczema.
- Color duplex ultrasound scanning can aid in the diagnosis by providing an analysis of venous anatomy and physiology.
- Arterial disease can coexist with venous ulcers and should be excluded by assessment of pulses and measurement of the ankle-brachial pressure index.
- Recalcitrant ulcers should be biopsied to exclude malignancy or other underlying disease.

CURRENT THERAPY

- Treatment should involve optimum wound care, leg elevation, and compression therapy.
- Sustained graduated pressure of 30 to 40 mg Hg at the ankle is optimal for compression therapy.
- A variety of dressings are available that can promote wound granulation and débridement.
- Wound débridement at regular intervals can accelerate venous ulcer healing.
- Skin grafting or human skin constructs can be used to treat large slow to heal ulcers.
- Venous ulcers frequently recur.
- Compression therapy should be maintained when an ulcer is healed to prevent recurrence.

unclear which of these compression systems is the most effective.

A variety of dressings are also used along with compression therapy in the management of venous ulcers. These dressings help promote wound granulation, promote débridement, and absorb exudate (Table 2). Some dressings that contain cadexomer iodine or silver can have antimicrobial activity without adversely affecting wound healing. Sharp débridement on a regular basis can accelerate venous

TABLE 1   Types of Compression Therapy

Bandage	Advantage	Disadvantage
Elastic wraps	Inexpensive; can be reused.	Often applied incorrectly by patient. Tend to unravel. Do not maintain sustained compression. Lose elasticity after washing.
Self-adherent wraps	Self-adherent; maintain compression.	Expensive. Cannot be reused.
Unna boot	Comfortable. Protects against trauma. Full maintenance of ambulatory outpatient status. Minimal interference with regular activities. Substitute for failing pump.	Pressure changes over time. Needs to be applied by well-trained physicians and nurses. Does not accommodate highly exudative wounds.
Four-layered bandage	Comfortable. Can be left in place for 7 d. Protects against trauma. Maintains a constant pressure for 7 d because of the overlap and elasticity of bandages. Used for highly exudative wounds.	Needs to be applied by well-trained physicians and nurses. Expensive.
Graduated compression stockings	Reduces the ambulatory venous pressure. Increases the venous refilling time. Improves calf pump function. Different types of stockings accommodate different types of legs. Dressing underneath can be changed frequently.	Often cannot monitor patient compliance. Difficult to put on.
Orthotic device	Adjustable compression. Sustained pressure. Easily put on and removed. Comfortable.	Expensive. Bulky appearance.
Compression pump	Augments venous return. Improves hemodynamics and microvascular functions. Enhances fibrinolytic activity Prevents postoperative thromboembolic complications in high-risk patients.	Expensive. Requires immobility for a few hours per day.

From Choucair M, Phillips T: Compression therapy. Dermatol Surg 1998;24:141-148.

TABLE 2 Dressing Recommendations Based on Ulcer Type

Type of Ulcer	Dressing Recommended
Heavy exudate	Foam, alginate, hydrofiber
Moderate exudate	Hydrocolloid, foam
Mild exudate	Hydrocolloid, hydrogel
Malodorous	Foam, alginate, hydrocolloid, charcoal
Recalcitrant	Collagen

From Bello Y, Phillips T: Therapeutic dressings. Adv Dermatol 2000; 16:253-270.

ulcer healing. Drugs such as pentoxifylline, at doses of 800 mg three times a day, can accelerate healing of chronic venous ulcers.

Venous ulcers tend to heal slowly, but the majority of ulcers respond well to management with compression therapy. Large ulcer size, ABI less than 0.8, ulcer of long duration, history of venous ligation, and the presence of fibrin on more than 50% of wound surface are poor prognostic factors for healing of venous ulcers.

Large slow to heal ulcers may be treated with autologous split-thickness or pinch grafting. Another approach includes use of an allogeneic human skin construct made of keratinocytes and fibroblasts cultured in bovine type 1 collagen. Up to 40% of patients with venous ulcera have superficial venous insufficiency. In this group, ulcer recurrence can be prevented by stripping or sclerotherapy of affected veins. If the ulcer does not heal, it should be biopsied to exclude malignancy or other causes of ulceration. Once the ulcer heals, sustained compression is recommended to prevent recurrence.

REFERENCES

Araujo T, Federman D, Kirsner R, Valencia I: Managing the patient with venous ulcers. Ann Intern Med 2003;138:326-334.

Bello Y, Phillips T: Chronic leg ulcers: Types and treatment. Hosp Pract 2000;35:101-108.

Bos J, Loots A, Mekkes J, Van der wal A: Causes, investigation and treatment of leg ulceration. Br J Dermatol 2003;148:388-401.

Callam M, Ruckley C, Harper D, Dale J: Chronic ulceration of the leg: Extent of the problem and provision of care. BMJ 1985;290: 1855-1856.

Cullum N, Fletcher A, Nelson E, Sheldon T: Compression for venous leg ulcers. Cochrane Database Syst 2004, volume (1).

Dix F, Simon D, McCollum C: Management of venous leg ulcers. BMJ 2004;328:1358-1362.

Eaglstein W, Falabella A, Kirsner R, Trent J: Venous ulcers: Pathophysiology and treatment options. Ostomy Wound Manage 2005;51:38-54.

Eaglstein W, Falabella A, Kirsner R, Valencia I: Chronic venous insufficiency and venous leg ulceration. J Am Acad Dermatol 2001;44:401-421.

Goldman M, Fronek A: The Alexander House Group: Consensus paper on venous leg ulcer. J Dermatol Surg Oncol 1992;18:592-602.

Ruckley C: Socioeconomic impact of chronic venous insufficiency and leg ulcers. Angiology 1997;46:67-69.

Vanhoutte P, Corcaud S, De Montrion C: The demographics of venous disease of the lower limbs. Angiology 1997;48:557-558.

Pressure Ulcers

Method of
David R. Thomas, MD

A pressure ulcer is the visible evidence of pathologic changes in blood supply to the dermal and underlying tissues, usually because of compression of the tissue over a bony prominence.

A differential diagnosis of ulcer type is critical to treatment. Chronic ulcers of the skin include arterial ulcers, venous stasis ulcers, diabetic ulcers, and pressure ulcers. Pressure ulcers generally appear in soft tissue over a bony prominence. A classic presentation aids the diagnosis. For example, arterial ulcers occur in the distal digits or over a bony prominence, diabetic ulcers occur in regions of callus formation, and venous stasis ulcers occur on the lateral aspect of the lower leg. However, atypical presentations may occasionally obscure the etiology. The treatment of these various etiologies differs considerably. This discussion is limited to the treatment of pressure ulcers and should not be used to treat other types of ulcers.

Seven principles of management guide treatment of pressure ulcers. The chief cause of these ulcers is pressure applied to the tissues that compromises blood flow. Therefore, the first treatment principle is to relieve pressure. Pressure relief can be obtained by positioning the patient frequently at a fixed interval to relieve pressure over the compromised area. Turning and positioning may be difficult to achieve because of a patient's self-positioning or medical treatments that interfere with the ability to position the patient. Because of this difficulty, a number of medical devices are designed in an attempt to relieve pressure. These devices can be classified as static or dynamic. Static devices include air-, gel-, or water-filled containers that reduce the tissue–surface interface. Dynamic devices use a power source to fill compartments with air that support the patient's weight or alternate the pressure on different areas of the body. Choose a static device when the patient has good bed mobility. Choose a dynamic device when the patient cannot self-position in bed.

At the present time, results of reported clinical trials do not favor one device over another. The choice should be based on durability, ease of use, and patient comfort. A simple check for so-called bottoming out should be done for all devices. Your hand should be inserted palm upward under the patient's sacrum between the device and the bed surface. If there is not an air column between the patient and the bed surface, the device is ineffective and should be changed. No device is effective in reducing heel pressure, the second most common site for pressure ulcers. Bridging with pillows is effective in reducing heel pressure in immobile patients; patients with high bed mobility may require boot devices to elevate the heel off the bed surface.

CURRENT DIAGNOSIS

- Differentiate among pressure, diabetic, venous stasis, and arterial ulcers.

CURRENT THERAPY

Seven Principles of Pressure Ulcer Therapy

- Relieve pressure.
- Assess pain.
- Assess nutrition and hydration.
- Remove necrotic debris.
- Maintain a moist wound environment.
- Encourage granulation and epithelial tissue formation.
- Control infection.

Patients who fail to improve or who have multiple pressure ulcers should be considered for a dynamic-type device, such as a low-air-loss bed or air-fluidized bed.

The second principle of pressure ulcer therapy is to assess pain. Pressure ulcers do not always result in pain, particularly in insensate patients. However, some pressure ulcers do result in pain and should be treated aggressively. Oral or parenteral pain medications should be used to control symptoms.

The third principle of ulcer therapy is to assess nutrition and hydration. Pressure ulcers occur in sicker individuals in whom nutrient intake may be reduced by coexisting illness. Increased intake of protein (1.2 to 1.5 g/kg/day) is associated with higher healing rates. Achievement of high protein intake may be difficult because of anorexia of aging or anorexia associated with coexisting diseases. Adequate calories, adjusted for stress (30 to 35 kcal/kg/day), should be prescribed. Adequate dietary intake should provide adequate vitamins and minerals. No difference in healing rates is associated with supertherapeutic doses of vitamin C or zinc. If adequate dietary intake is compromised, a supplemental vitamin/mineral prescription at RDA (recommended daily allowance) doses should be considered. Adequate hydration can be maintained by 30 mL/kg/day of water. The decision to institute enteral feeding in patients with pressure ulcers who are unable to maintain adequate oral intake should not be undertaken lightly. The decision to use enteral feeding must consider the patient's wishes, overall goal of care, and the complications of enteral feeding. In several studies, the long-term result of enteral feeding was associated with poorer outcomes in patients with pressure ulcers.

The fourth principle of pressure ulcer management requires removing necrotic debris. Phagocytosis removes necrotic debris naturally. Accelerating the rate of removal may shorten healing time. Options include sharp surgical débridement, mechanical débridement with gauze dressings, application of exogenous enzymes, or autolytic débridement under occlusive dressings. Choose surgical débridement if the ulcer is infected. Surgical débridement is the fastest method but may remove some viable tissue, cause discomfort, and is the most expensive method, especially if done in an operating room. Applying moist gauze that is allowed to adhere to the ulcer bed by drying is a form of débridement. When the dry dressing is removed, nonselective tissue removal occurs. This method can be associated with discomfort, may delay healing while débridement is in progress, and is often defeated when the dressing is remoistened before removal. Enzymatic débridement can digest necrotic material. Three enzymatic preparations are available in the United States: collagenase, papain/urea, and papain/urea combined with chlorophyll. Enzyme preparations are nonselective, possibly resulting in some damage to fibroblasts, epithelial cells, or granulation tissue. Enzymatic débridement is slower, can be associated with discomfort, and should be limited in duration until a clean wound bed is obtained. Autolytic débridement is achieved by allowing autolysis under an occlusive dressing. Both enzymatic and autolytic débridement may require 2 to 6 weeks to achieve a clean wound bed. A total of five clinical trials did not show that enzymatic agents increased the rate of complete healing in chronic wounds compared to control treatment. Unless clinically infected, heel ulcers are better left undébrided because they occur in poorly vascularized tissues.

The fifth principle of pressure ulcer management is to maintain a moist wound environment. Maintaining a moist wound environment is associated with more rapid healing rates compared to dressings that are allowed to dry. Continuously moist saline gauze is the historical standard dressing for stage II through IV pressure ulcers. Care must be taken to change the gauze frequently to prevent drying because this may delay healing. Newer wound dressings provide a low moisture vapor transmission rate (MVTR), a measure of how quickly the dressing allows drying. A MVTR of less than 35 g of water vapor per square meter per hour is required to maintain a moist wound environment. Woven gauze has a MVTR of 68 $g/m^2/hour$, and impregnated gauze has a MVTR of 57 $g/m^2/hour$. By comparison, hydrocolloid dressings have a MVTR of 8 $g/m^2/hour$. Dressings with low MVTR provide a healing environment that encourages granulation tissue formation and epithelialization.

The use of occlusive-type dressings is more cost effective than gauze dressings primarily because of a decrease in nursing time for dressing changes. A meta-analysis of five clinical trials comparing a hydrocolloid dressing with a dry dressing demonstrated that treatment with a hydrocolloid dressing resulted in a statistically significant improvement in the rate of pressure ulcer healing (odds ratio: 2.6).

Occlusive dressings can be divided into broad categories of polymer films, polymer foams, hydrogels, hydrocolloids, alginates, and biomembranes. Each has advantages and disadvantages. No single agent is perfect. The choice of a particular agent depends on the clinical circumstances. Nonpermeable polymers can be macerating to normal skin. Polymer films are not absorptive and may leak, particularly when the wound is highly exudative. Most films have an adhesive backing that may remove epithelial cells when the dressing is changed. Hydrogels are hydrophilic polymers that are insoluble in water but absorb aqueous solutions and are available in amorphous gels or sheet dressings. They are poor bacterial barriers and are nonadherent to the wound. Because of their high specific heat, these dressings are cooling to the skin, aiding in pain control and reducing inflammation. Most of these dressings require a secondary dressing to secure them to the wound. Hydrocolloid dressings are complex dressings similar to ostomy barrier products. They are impermeable to moisture and bacteria and highly adherent to the skin. Hydrocolloid dressings have an accelerated healing of 40% compared to moist gauze dressings. Hydrocolloid dressings are particularly suited for areas subject to urinary and fecal incontinence. Their adhesiveness to surrounding skin is higher than some surgical tapes, but they are nonadherent to wound tissue and do not damage epithelial tissue in the wound. The adhesive barrier is frequently overcome in highly exudative wounds. Hydrocolloid dressings cannot be used over tendons or on wounds with eschar formation. Alginates are complex polysaccharide dressings that are highly absorbent in exudative wounds. This high absorbency is particularly suited to exudative wounds. Alginates are nonadherent to the wound, but if the wound is allowed to dry, damage to the epithelial tissue may occur with removal. Alginates may be used under other dressings to absorb exudate. The biomembranes are very expensive and not readily available.

Stages I and II pressure ulcers can be managed with a polymer film or hydrocolloid dressing. Stages III and IV dressings may require a wound filler, such as a calcium alginate or an amorphous hydrogel, to obliterate dead space and decrease anaerobic colonization.

Vacuum-assisted closure is used in both acute and chronic wounds. Only two randomized, controlled trials in pressure ulcers are reported. In both trials, vacuum-assisted closure was equivalent to treatment with a hydrogel or moistened gauze.

Electrotherapy is used for stages III and IV pressure ulcers unresponsive to conventional therapy. Several clinical trials suggest that electrotherapy is likely to be marginally effective. Hyperbaric oxygen, ultrasound, infrared, ultraviolet, and low-energy laser irradiation have insufficient data to recommend their use currently. No data support the use of a systemic vasodilator, hemorheologics, serotonin inhibitors, or fibrolytic agents in the treatment of pressure ulcers. Topical agents such as zinc, phenytoin,[1] aluminum hydroxide,[1] honey, sugar, yeast, aloe vera gel, or gold[1] were not effective in clinical trials.

Because the theory of augmenting ulcer healing under the newer dressings suggests that wound fluid contains favorable healing factors, it is important not to change the dressings too frequently. Unless the wound fluid seeps from under the dressing, it should not be changed more often than every 3 to 7 days.

The sixth principle of pressure ulcer treatment is to encourage granulation tissue formation and promote reepithelialization. Growth factors show promising early results, but the data do not suggest accelerated healing of pressure ulcers. It is important not to affect granulation and epithelial tissue negatively. A number of wound cleaners and antiseptics are toxic to fibroblasts and epithelial tissues, including benzalkonium chloride, povidone-iodine solution (Betadine), Dakin's solution, hydrogen peroxide, Granulex, Hibiclens, and pHisoHex. The use of these agents in a pressure ulcer should be limited to use in infected ulcers and strictly limited in duration.

The seventh principle of pressure ulcer management is to control infection. Quantitative microbiology alone is a poor predictor of clinical infection in chronic wounds. All pressure ulcers are colonized with bacteria, usually from skin or fecal flora. The presence of microorganisms alone (colonization) does not indicate an infection in pressure ulcers. The diagnosis of infection in chronic wounds must be based on clinical signs: erythema, warmth, pain, edema,

---

[1]Not FDA approved for this indication.

---

odor, fever, or purulent exudate. In the presence of clinical signs of infection, enteral or parenteral antibiotics should be used. In ulcers that are not progressing toward healing, an empirical trial of topical antimicrobials may be considered, although the data are inconclusive.

REFERENCES

Thomas DR: The role of nutrition in prevention and healing of pressure ulcers. Geriatr Clin North Am 1997;13:497-512.
Thomas DR: Are all pressure ulcers avoidable? J Am Med Dir Assoc 2001;2:297-301.
Thomas DR: Improving the outcome of pressure ulcers with nutritional intervention: A review of the evidence. Nutrition 2001;17:121-125.
Thomas DR: Issues and dilemmas in managing pressure ulcers. J Gerontol Med Sci 2001;56:M238-M340.
Thomas DR: Prevention and management of pressure ulcers. Rev Clin Gerontol 2001;11:115-130.
Thomas DR: The promise of topical nerve growth factors in the healing of pressure ulcers. Ann Intern Med 2003;139:694-695.
Thomas DR: Management of pressure ulcers. J Am Med Dir Assoc 2006;7:46-59.

Atopic Dermatitis

Method of
Sarah L. Chamlin, MD

Atopic dermatitis (AD) is a prevalent chronic inflammatory skin condition occurring in 7% to 17% of school-age children with most children developing the disease before they are 5 years of age. The pathophysiology of atopic dermatitis includes a complex interrelationship of genetic, environmental, skin barrier, psychological, and immunologic factors. The goals of management of AD in children include skin hydration, decreasing skin inflammation and itch, identifying and treating skin infection, and assessing the psychosocial impact of disease on the child and family.

Diagnosis

AD is characterized by pruritus, a chronic relapsing course, an atopic history (personal or family), and a dermatitis in the typical morphology and distribution for age (facial and extensor surface in infants; flexural surfaces and lichenification in older children and adults). In addition,

---

CURRENT DIAGNOSIS

Atopic dermatitis is characterized by:
- Pruritus
- Chronic relapsing course
- Atopic history both personal or family
- Dermatitis in the typical morphology and distribution for age, including facial and extensor surface in infants and flexural surfaces and lichenification in older children and adults

CURRENT THERAPY

- Treatment of dryness should focus on hydration and lubrication to repair skin and reduce water loss. Both emollients and topical anti-inflammatory medications are recommended. Showers and baths should be no longer than 10 min using fragrance-less soap.
- Topical steroids are the first-line of therapy for treatment of the dermatitis. Ointments are often preferred to creams. Consider body location and severity of dermatitis.
- Topical therapies often relieve pruritus, but additional use of sedating antihistamines may be indicated. If nighttime sleep disruption occurs, sedating antihistamines such as diphenhydramine (Benadryl, 1 mg/kg) or hydroxyzine (Atarax, 1 mg/kg) can be given before bedtime.
- Flaring of disease caused by bacterial superinfection may improve with topical corticosteroids alone, but systemic antibiotics should be considered. A 10–14 d course is most often prescribed.

Table 1 lists other cutaneous features and findings present in affected patients.

Treatment

DRY SKIN

Treatment of dryness is one of the most critical aspects of management. Patients with atopic dermatitis have an abnormal skin barrier that leads to increased transepidermal water loss and dryness. Treatment of dryness focuses on hydration and lubrication of the skin to repair the skin and reduce water loss. Both emollients and topical anti-inflammatory medications are most often needed for

TABLE 1 Cutaneous Findings and Associated Features in Atopic Dermatitis

Xerosis
Ichthyosis vulgaris
Hyperlinear palms
Keratosis pilaris
Cutaneous infections
Hand and/or foot dermatitis
Nipple eczema
Cheilitis
Recurrent conjunctivitis
Dennie-Morgan infraorbital folds
Periorbital darkening
Midfacial pallor
Pityriasis alba
Itch when sweating
Intolerance to wool/soaps
White dermatographism
Elevated serum IgE

TABLE 2 Bathing and Emollient Recommendations

Daily lukewarm baths or showers for 5–10 min
Sparing use of gentle shampoo for hair
Mild fragrance-free soap or soap substitute (e.g., Dove, Cetaphil)
Avoidance of harsh soaps and bubble baths
Applying emollient while still damp (e.g., petrolatum, Cetaphil Cream, Eucerin Cream)
Reapplying emollient once or twice daily
If topical corticosteroids or topical immunomodulators (TIMs) used, applying them first followed by emollient

this repair. Baths or showers are recommended daily or every other day and should last no longer than 10 minutes. Recommended soaps lack fragrance and often contain a moisturizer, a humectant, and a mild synthetic surfactant (Table 2). Dryness worsens with excessive bathing or showering, exposure to detergents, and low humidity. Although ointments and creams are preferred to lotions because of increased oil content, widespread use of thick creams and ointments may not be tolerated in hot climates.

INFLAMMATION

Topical steroids are the first line of therapy for treatment of the dermatitis and are effective and safe when used appropriately. Many parents are fearful of using of topical corticosteroids because of potential side effects and need reassurance that low- to mid-potency corticosteroids applied for limited periods of time are safe. Ointments are often preferred to creams because they are more moisturizing and less irritating. Consider body location and severity of dermatitis when choosing a topical corticosteroid. Low-potency corticosteroids can be safely used on the face and intertriginous areas, whereas higher potency topical corticosteroids are needed for effective treatment of dermatitis on the trunk and extremities. Liquid or foam preparations are recommended for scalp dermatitis.

Topical immunomodulators (TIMs) should be considered as second-line therapy for atopic dermatitis. Tacrolimus ointment (Protopic) 0.03% ointment is approved for use in children 2 to 15 years of age and 0.1% for use in children and adults older than 15 years. Pimecrolimus 1% cream (Elidel) is approved for patients 2 years and older. Both act via inhibition of T cell cytokine production and may have the side effects of stinging and burning with application. Short-term safety profiles remain reassuring, but long-term safety remains unknown. Sun protection is recommended while using TIMs.

Topical mid-potency corticosteroids are very effective for initial treatment of an acute flare of atopic dermatitis. When the flare is improving (5 to 7 days), treatment alternatives include low-potency topical corticosteroids or TIMs. TIMs are effective for facial dermatitis, particularly in the periocular region (Tables 3 and 4).

PRURITUS

Controlling itch is an important step in breaking the disease-propagating itch-scratch cycle. Topical therapies

TABLE 3 How to Apply Topical Steroids and Topical Immunomodulators (TIMs)

Apply to area affected by dermatitis (rough, red, and scaly plaques).
Coat area with thin greasy layer (it should look shiny).
Use twice daily until skin feels smooth (ignore changes in pigment).
Switch to emollients alone after treated area smooth.
If used for 2 weeks and the dermatitis not clearing:
- Medication may not be strong enough.
- Medicine is being used too sparingly.
- Skin infection may be present.

often relieve pruritus, but additional use of sedating antihistamines may be indicated. If nighttime sleep disruption occurs because of pruritus, sedating antihistamines such as diphenhydramine (Benadryl, 1 mg/kg) or hydroxyzine (Atarax, 1 mg/kg) can be given prior to bedtime. The doses can be titrated to minimize daytime sleepiness. Long-standing sleep disruption because of pruritus can lead to learned behaviors and associations including nighttime awakening even when the dermatitis is in remission. To prevent these behaviors from forming, therapy with sedating antihistamines is warranted. Nonsedating antihistamines are effective for symptoms associated with allergic rhinitis and other allergic diseases, but they are less effective for relief from the itch of atopic dermatitis.

INFECTION

The most common complication of atopic dermatitis is infection with *Staphylococcus aureus*. Bacterial infection of the skin in atopic dermatitis not only causes the clinical signs of erosion, crusting, and weeping but may also trigger a flare of the disease. The presence of infection may not be obvious or generalized and may be as subtle as a few pustules. Although flaring of disease because of bacterial superinfection may improve with topical corticosteroids alone, systemic antibiotics should be considered. Most often a 10- to 14-day course is prescribed, but a longer course may be needed for children with frequent recurrent infections. Although use of antibiotics is often required, they should be prescribed judiciously because of the increase in community-acquired methicillin-resistant *S. aureus* in the United States. Localized infection can be treated with mupirocin 2% ointment (Bactroban). A skin culture may be helpful in identifying the antibiotic sensitivity of the bacterial organism. Recommended systemic antibiotics include cephalexin (Keflex), dicloxacillin (Dynapen), and clindamycin (Cleocin).

If eczema herpeticum, herpes simplex virus superinfection, is suspected, therapy with systemic acyclovir (Zovirax) is warranted. If the patient is febrile, dehydrated, or ill appearing, hospitalization with intravenous acyclovir and fluids is indicated.

Recalcitrant Atopic Dermatitis

A small proportion of patients with atopic dermatitis are not controlled with topical therapy. Although oral corticosteroid treatment is an effective therapy, its use is limited by its systemic toxicities and the flare of disease that often occurs after discontinuation. The use of phototherapy (UVB [ultraviolet B] and PUVA [psoralen plus ultraviolet light of A wavelength], narrow-band UVB) is often reserved for older children with recalcitrant disease. Excessive phototherapy increases risk for skin malignancies later in life, and children often miss school several times weekly for treatment, limiting its use. Systemic immunosuppressants such as cyclosporine A (Neoral[1]) may be useful in the treatment of recalcitrant atopic dermatitis. These should only be used with careful monitoring and after a thorough discussion of the short- and long-term risks and benefits.

Psychosocial Impact

Atopic dermatitis affects the quality of life of afflicted children and their families. Childhood behavior abnormalities, parent stress and anxiety, and sleep disturbance for both the child and their parents are well documented in this population. When severity of the disease decreases, quality of life for the child improves. Physicians caring for children with atopic dermatitis should ask children and their parents about sleep quality and about the life changes that have occurred because of atopic dermatitis.

TABLE 4 Site-Specific Recommended Treatment

Body Location	Topical Medication
Face/groin/axillae	Pimecrolimus 1% cream (Elidel)
	Tacrolimus 0.03% or 0.1% ointment (Protopic)
	Hydrocortisone 1% or 2.5%
	Desonide 0.05% (DesOwen)
	Alclometasone 0.05% (Aclovate)
Scalp (oil, solution, foam, or lotion)	Fluocinolone 0.01% (Synalar)
	Hydrocortisone butyrate 0.1% (Locoid)
	Fluocinolone 0.01% oil (Derma-Smoothe FS)
	Betamethasone 0.12% foam (Luxiq)
Trunk/extremities	Triamcinolone 0.1% (Kenalog)
	Fluocinolone 0.025% (Synalar)
	Pimecrolimus 1% cream (Elidel)
	Tacrolimus 0.03% or 0.1% ointment (Protopic)
Thickened nonfacial areas (monitored closely and used for short periods of time)	Betamethasone 0.05% (Diprosone)
	Mometasone 0.1% (Elocon)
	Fluocinonide 0.05% (Lidex)

REFERENCES

Balkrishnan R, Housman TS, Grummer S, et al: The family impact of atopic dermatitis in children: The role of the parent caregiver. Pediatr Dermatol 2003;20(1):5-10.

[1]Not FDA approved for this indication.

Chamlin SL, Frieden IJ, Williams ML, Chren MM: The effects of atopic dermatitis on young American children and their families. Pediatrics 2004;114:607-611.

Chamlin SL, Mattson CL, Frieden IJ, et al: The price of pruritus: Sleep disturbance and cosleeping in atopic dermatitis. Arch Pediatr Adolesc Med 2005;159(8):745-750.

Charman CR, Morris AD, Williams HC: Topical corticosteroid phobia in patients with atopic eczema. Br J Dermatol 2000;142:931-936.

Drake L, Prendergast M, Maher R, et al: The impact of tacrolimus ointment on health-related quality of life of adult and pediatric patients with atopic dermatitis. J Amer Acad Dermatol 2001;44: S65-S72.

Hanifin JM, Rajka G: Diagnostic features of atopic dermatitis. Acta Derm Venereol Suppl (Stockh) 1980;92:44-47.

Laughter D, Istvan JA, Tofte SJ, Hanifin JM: The prevalence of atopic dermatitis in Oregon schoolchildren. J Amer Acad Dermatol 2000;43:649-655.

Stalder JF, Fleury M, Sourusse M, et al: Local steroid therapy and bacterial skin flora in atopic dermatitis. Br J Dermatol 1994;131: 536-540.

Whalley D, Huels J, McKenna SP, Van Assche D: The benefit of pimecrolimus (Elidel, SDZ ASM 981) on parents' quality of life in the treatment of pediatric atopic dermatitis. Pediatrics 2002;110: 1133-1136.

Erythema Multiforme, Stevens-Johnson Syndrome, and Toxic Epidermal Necrolysis

Method of
Marcia G. Tonnesen, MD

Historically, erythema multiforme (EM), Stevens-Johnson syndrome (SJS), and toxic epidermal necrolysis (TEN) were considered a disease spectrum, and therefore they are addressed together here. Current evidence, however, supports a clear distinction between EM, with characteristic acrally distributed target lesions and an etiologic link to herpes simplex virus (HSV) infection, and SJS/TEN, with focal to widespread skin and mucous membrane involvement, characterized by epidermal destruction, and an etiologic link to adverse drug reactions. EM is typically mild and self-limited and requires only symptomatic care. In contrast, because of the degree and extent of epidermal and mucosal involvement that occurs in SJS and TEN, careful monitoring is critical and hospitalization for supportive care often required. Thus early diagnosis is critical. Elimination of any identified or presumed precipitating factors is of prime importance. Therapy should combine symptomatic and supportive measures with observation for and treatment of associated complications, depending on the clinical characteristics and severity of the episode. Optimal therapeutic intervention is hindered because specific pathogenic mechanisms of tissue injury are not yet completely defined. In addition, few controlled studies have evaluated the effectiveness of proposed therapeutic agents. Nevertheless, recent advances elucidating unique morphologic features and novel mechanisms of epidermal necrosis enhance the likelihood of successful therapeutic intervention.

Erythema Multiforme

EM is an acute, self-limited, but frequently recurrent, inflammatory cutaneous disorder, characterized by the sudden onset of a symmetric erythematous eruption with primarily an acral distribution. Skin lesions begin as fixed (lasting longer than 24 hours) erythematous flat macules, rapidly progress to erythematous raised papules, and then develop a pale or dusky central zone because of edema or bulla formation. This characteristic morphology is now termed *raised atypical target.* Some further evolve to form distinctive raised target lesions with at least three zones of color (dusky/bullous center, pale edematous halo, erythematous border), termed *typical target.* Individual lesions occasionally sting or itch, appear in successive crops for 24 to 72 hours, and spontaneously resolve within 1 to 4 weeks. Mucosal involvement, when present, is usually limited to the lips, buccal mucosa, and tongue.

Most recurrent EM cases are associated with herpes simplex virus (HSV) type I or II infection and typically occur 3 to 14 days after the appearance of a recurrent HSV lesion (oral, genital, or other location). Subclinical episodes of herpes can also induce EM. HSV DNA is detected in EM lesions. Herpes-associated erythema multiforme is currently believed to result from the HSV-specific host immune response.

THERAPEUTIC APPROACH

Elimination of Etiologic Factor

In recurrent herpes-associated EM, a course of acyclovir (Zovirax), 200 mg orally five times daily for 5 days, should be initiated at the first symptom of HSV infection. Acyclovir therapy is not effective if initiated after the development of HSV or EM lesions.

Symptomatic Measures

For pruritic or painful skin lesions, systemic antihistamines or analgesics may provide symptomatic relief. Topical acyclovir and topical corticosteroids are not beneficial. Care for skin and mouth erosions is addressed in the following section.

Preventive Measures

Because of the common etiologic association between recurrent HSV infections and EM, measures that attempt to prevent recurrences of HSV may lessen the frequency of subsequent episodes. Avoidance of sun exposure by using sunscreens (SPF [sun protection factor] 15 or higher), sun sticks (sunscreen-containing lip balm), and UV (ultraviolet)-protective clothing and by minimizing sun exposure from 10 AM to 3 PM (the peak period for ultraviolet B [UVB]) may reduce ultraviolet light–induced HSV recurrences. Attempts should be made to minimize stress, a well-known precipitating factor of HSV. Topical antiviral preparations do not prevent or abort recurrent HSV infections.

Prophylactic administration of acyclovir abolishes recurrent HSV infections and ensuing episodes of EM. In patients with frequently recurring, debilitating, herpes-associated EM, the treatment of choice is daily oral acyclovir for a period of 6 months or longer. The recommended adult starting dose is 400 mg orally twice daily, with tapering of the dose after the disease is brought under control. Because asymptomatic subclinical HSV episodes can also trigger EM, patients with so-called idiopathic recurrent EM often benefit from prophylactic antiviral therapy. If acyclovir fails to prevent recurrences of HSV, newer antiviral agents with enhanced bioavailability, such as valacyclovir (Valtrex) or famciclovir (Famvir), should be tried. Because of the known occurrence of acyclovir resistance and the unknown long-term side effects of chronic acyclovir therapy, the drug should be stopped periodically and the need for its continuance reassessed.

Patient Education

Patients should be reassured regarding the usual benign, self-limited course, educated regarding the frequent association of EM with recurrent HSV infections, and advised regarding preventive measures.

Stevens-Johnson Syndrome and Toxic Epidermal Necrolysis

SJS is a severe mucocutaneous illness characterized by an extensive blistering eruption with a primarily facial and truncal distribution and extensive mucosal erosions, typically involving the mouth and conjunctivae. A prodrome with constitutional symptoms and fever usually heralds the onset of the eruption. Skin lesions begin as erythematous flat macules, frequently develop dusky central vesiculation, and may progress to bullae formation with epidermal necrosis. The current morphologic terms for these characteristic lesions are *macule with or without blister* if only one color and *flat atypical target* if two concentric zones of color are present. Epidermal detachment may involve up to 10% body surface area (BSA). Painful mucosal erosions result in characteristic hemorrhagic-crusted lips, foul-smelling mouth, and decreased oral intake. Ocular involvement with photophobia and painful conjunctival erosions may lead to residual scarring, lacrimal abnormalities, and permanent visual impairment. Disease duration is 4 to 6 weeks. Recurrences are infrequent. SJS is now recognized as strongly related to adverse drug reactions and linked to some infections, particularly *Mycoplasma pneumoniae*, but never to herpes virus infection.

TEN is characterized by widespread sheetlike necrosis and sloughing of the epidermis, involving greater than 30% of the BSA. (Epidermal detachment between 10% and 30% of the BSA is classified as SJS/TEN overlap.) Following a 1- to 3-day prodrome of fever and flulike symptoms, the cutaneous eruption characteristically begins symmetrically on the face and upper body. Initial painful erythema rapidly progresses within hours to days to widespread bulla formation. Sheetlike areas of epidermal necrosis with extensive denudation involve significant or total BSA. Alternatively, TEN may begin as erythematous or violaceous macules that then develop bullae and coalesce. Involvement of multiple mucosal surfaces is present in nearly all patients. The order of frequency is oropharynx (in severe cases extending to larynx and tracheobronchial tree), eyes, genitalia, and anus. TEN is considered a manifestation of "acute skin failure" with abnormal barrier function resulting in fluid, electrolyte, and protein loss, increased

BOX 1 Drugs With Highest Risk of Stevens-Johnson Syndrome/ Toxic Epidermal Necrolysis

Antibiotics
- Sulfonamides
- Cephalosporins
- Quinolones
- Tetracycline
- Aminopenicillins
- Imidazole antifungals

Anticonvulsants/Antianxiety
- Carbamazepine
- Chlormezanone[2]
- Phenytoin
- Phenobarbital
- Valproic acid
- Lamotrigine
- Nonsteroidal anti-inflammatory drugs, particularly oxicams
- Allopurinol
- Antiretroviral agents

[2]Not available in the United States.

susceptibility to infection, impaired thermoregulation, altered immune status, and increased energy expenditure. Morbidity is significant, and the mortality rate is 25% to 40%. The leading cause of death is sepsis.

Adverse drug reactions are the only well-documented cause of TEN. The most common offenders (Box 1) include antibiotics, particularly sulfonamides, anticonvulsants, nonsteroidal anti-inflammatory agents (NSAIDs), and more recently antiretroviral agents, although more than 100 drugs are implicated. The greatest risk for antibiotics occurs during the initial weeks of use; for most anticonvulsants, the risk is highest during the first 2 months. Although the specific pathogenic mechanism is not fully elucidated for SJS/TEN, the characteristic epidermal necrosis is now believed to be a result of keratinocyte apoptosis. Current evidence supports important roles in the induction of keratinocyte death for Fas/Fas ligand–mediated apoptosis, cytokines such as tumor necrosis factor-α (TNF-α), and cytotoxic T lymphocytes, as well as specific genetic defects in detoxification of reactive drug metabolites. Recent novel attempts at therapeutic intervention are based on these proposed mechanisms of epidermal necrosis.

THERAPEUTIC APPROACH

Elimination of Etiologic Factors

Immediate withdrawal of any suspected or potential causative drug(s) is critical because cessation of the offending agent no later than the stage of early blister formation may decrease mortality. For SJS, *Mycoplasma pneumoniae* and other infections, if diagnosed, should be appropriately treated.

Intervention with Systemic Therapy to Stop Progression

Indication for the use of systemic therapy in SJS/TEN is highly controversial because no randomized, controlled trials document efficacy of any systemic intervention. Because widespread epidermal necrosis is associated with a high mortality rate, however, early administration of systemic therapy in the progressive phase of the disease process is advocated to attempt to limit the extent of tissue damage. Use of systemic glucocorticosteroids has proved particularly controversial. There is no evidence-based documentation of their efficacy, and some retrospective studies indicate that patients treated with systemic steroids have an increased incidence of morbidity, prolonged hospitalization, and mortality. Thus other agents are currently being assessed and advocated. Case studies or uncontrolled trials involving small numbers of patients report benefit from a variety of systemic agents. Immunosuppressive therapy with oral cyclosporine (Sandimmune)[1] or high-dose intravenous cyclophosphamide (Cytoxan)[1] is claimed to help several patients. Plasmapheresis may be of some benefit. Innovative treatment is not without risk, however. For example, a double-blind, placebo-controlled trial of thalidomide, which suppresses production of TNF-α, had to be aborted because of a dramatic increase in thalidomide-related mortality.

---

[1]Not FDA approved for this indication.

Currently the most promising and widely advocated systemic therapy is the early administration of high-dose intravenous immunoglobulin (IVIG)[1] to inhibit epidermal apoptosis mediated by the Fas/Fas ligand death receptor. An initial landmark pilot study by Viand and colleagues of 10 TEN patients treated with IVIG demonstrates rapid cessation of disease progression and 100% survival. Subsequently, numerous case reports, retrospective analyses, and uncontrolled prospective studies support the overall safety as well as the efficacy of IVIG to decrease mortality, with only a few dissenting. Improved survival appears to depend on use of high-dose IVIG (1 g/kg/day given more than 3 to 4 days for a total dose of 3 to 4 g/kg) because increased risk of mortality occurs at lower total doses (2 g/kg/day or less). A randomized placebo-controlled trial of IVIG for TEN has not yet been done and will be challenging to accomplish, given the rarity of the disease and the high mortality rate.

In the absence of documented efficacy, use of systemic therapy to limit disease progression in a specific patient remains at the discretion of the physician. However, it is now clear that if systemic intervention is administered, once disease progression ceases and the wound healing

---

[1]Not FDA approved for this indication.

 CURRENT DIAGNOSIS

Erythema Multiforme

- Symmetric erythematous acral eruption with target lesions
- Acute: Onset over 24 to 72 hours
- Unique clinical morphology: key to diagnosis
   Raised atypical target lesions
- Palpable round red with central edema/bulla
- Two concentric zones of color
   Typical target lesions
- Palpable round red with pale halo and dusky center
- Three concentric zones of color
- Mucosal involvement variable, oral only
- Self-limited: Spontaneous resolution within 1 to 4 weeks
- Recurrent EM
   Associated with HSV type I or II
   Occurs 3 to 14 days after HSV lesion

Stevens-Johnson Syndrome

- Severe mucocutaneous disease
   Extensive symmetrical blistering eruption
   Mucosal erosions: mouth, conjunctivae, then oropharynx, genitalia
- Characteristic erosions with hemorrhagic crust on lips
- Initial prodrome with fever and flulike symptoms
- Skin lesions: Erythematous/violaceous macules
   Often with central vesicles/bullae
   May progress to epidermal necrosis (<10% BSA)
- Unique clinical morphology: key to diagnosis
   Macules with or without blisters
- Flat nonpalpable (except central blister)

- Red or dusky
- May become confluent face/trunk
   Flat atypical target lesions
- Flat nonpalpable (except central blister)
- Round red/dusky or pale central blister
- Two concentric zones of color
- Duration 4 to 6 weeks; infrequent to no recurrences
- Severe adverse reaction to drug
   Or if infection: *Mycoplasma pneumoniae,* never HSV

Toxic Epidermal Necrolysis

- Severe adverse drug reaction
- Initial 1- to 3-day prodrome of fever, flulike symptoms
- Initial painful erythema of the face and upper trunk
- Rapid progression of skin involvement:
   Central, then acral
      Dusky red flat macules to flaccid blisters to large sheets of epidermal necrosis
- Unique clinical morphology: key to diagnosis
   Macules with or without blisters
- Flat nonpalpable (except central blister)
- Red or dusky
- Become confluent
   Flat atypical target lesions
- Flat nonpalpable (except central blister)
- Round red/dusky or pale central blister
- Two concentric zones of color
   Extensive areas of confluent epidermal denudation
- >30% BSA (may involve >90% BSA)
- Involvement of multiple mucosal surfaces usual
- High morbidity; mortality rate: 25% to 40%

Abbreviations: BSA = body surface area; EM = erythema multiforme; HSV = herpes simplex virus.

process begins, or if no response is noted within 3 to 6 days, treatment should be abruptly discontinued to minimize risk of associated complications.

Supportive Care

Because of the extensive epidermal and mucosal necrosis and detachment that can occur in SJS and TEN, careful monitoring is critical and hospitalization is often required. Early referral of severe cases to an intensive care or burn unit decreases mortality. Poor outcome can be predicted by a TEN-specific severity of illness score and correlates with the number of specific independent risk factors for mortality present within the first 24 hours after admission to an intensive care unit (Box 2).

BOX 2 SCORTEN: A Severity-of-Illness Score Predictive of Mortality in Toxic Epidermal Necrolysis

- Age >40 y
- Presence of malignancy
- Initial epidermal detachment >10% BSA
- BUN >28 mg/dL
- Glucose >252 mg/dL
- HCO_3 slightly <20 mEq/L
- Heart rate >120 beats/min

Abbreviations: BSA = body surface area; BUN = blood urea nitrogen; HCO_3 = bicarbonate.

 CURRENT THERAPY

Erythema Multiforme

- Eliminate/prevent etiologic factor by initiating acyclovir (Zovirax), 200 mg orally five times daily, for 5 days at the first symptom of HSV recurrence but not after HSV or EM lesions appear.
- Reduce UV-induced HSV recurrences.
    Apply sunscreens (SPF 15 or higher).
    Use sunscreen-containing lip balm.
    Wear UV-protective clothing and minimize sun exposure from 10 AM to 3 PM.
- Consider prophylactic acyclovir if frequent severe recurrences.
    Prescribe 400 mg orally twice daily for at least 6 months.
    Taper dose after disease under control.
    Stop periodically to reassess need.

Stevens-Johnson Syndrome/Toxic Epidermal Necrolysis

- Eliminate/prevent etiologic factor:
    Immediately stop suspected drug(s).
    Avoid exposure to causative drug and chemically related agents.
    Treat *Mycoplasma pneumoniae* if present.
- Stop progression of epidermal necrosis:
    Administer high-dose IVIG[1]
    Give total dose of 3 to 4 g/kg over 3 to 4 consecutive days, 1g/kg/day for 3 to 4 days; if renal insufficiency: lower daily dose, and lengthen the duration.
    Initiate as early as possible.
    Discontinue once disease progression ceases, or if no response in 3 to 6 days, to minimize complications.

Supportive Care

SKIN CARE

For crusted, erosive discrete skin lesions:
- Apply open wet-to-damp compresses of sterile water for 20 minutes three to four times per day to cleanse and soothe.

- Observe for secondary infection; culture and treat with appropriate systemic antibiotic.
- Use systemic antihistamines or analgesics for discomfort.

For extensive epidermal detachment (10% to 20% BSA):
- Transfer immediately to intensive care or burn unit.
- Guard against iatrogenic infection:
    Stop all systemic steroids.
    Avoid indwelling lines and catheters.
    Limit antibiotic use to specific culture-proven infections.
    Perform daily surveillance cultures of denuded skin, eyes, mouth, sputum, and urine.
    Treat sepsis aggressively if it occurs.
- Provide supportive care:
    Try an air-fluidized bed.
    Give intravenous fluid therapy.
    Provide tube feedings.
    Provide pain relief.
    Give respiratory and physical therapy.
    Provide eye care by an ophthalmologist.
    Avoid all unnecessary medications.
    Apply wound dressings—synthetic, biologic, or silver nitrate, or use allografts/porcine xenografts.

MOUTH CARE

- Use hygienic mouthwash such as hydrogen peroxide (1.5%) or sterile normal saline every 2 hours.
- Use a pain-relief mouthwash such as viscous lidocaine or a 1:1 mixture of Kaopectate[1] and elixir of diphenhydramine (Benadryl).
- Provide a liquid/soft diet or tube feedings.

EYE CARE

- Provide daily continuing care by an ophthalmologist:
    Use sterile irrigation and compresses.
    Perform lysis of adhesions.
    Provide instillation of topical antibiotics.

---

[1]Not FDA approved for this indication.
Abbreviations: BSA = body surface area; EM = erythema multiforme; HSV = herpes simplex virus; IVIG = intravenous immunoglobulin; SPF = sun protection factor; UV = ultraviolet.

Skin Care

For crusted erosive discrete skin lesions, mild drying, gentle débridement, and cleansing as well as a soothing antipruritic effect is achieved with open wet to damp compresses of tepid water applied for 20 minutes three or four times per day. Lesions should be observed for signs of secondary infection, cultured when indicated, and treatment initiated with the appropriate systemic antibiotic. Topical corticosteroids are not beneficial. For pruritic or painful skin lesions, systemic antihistamines or analgesics provide symptomatic relief.

If extensive, advanced tissue necrosis occurs or is already evident (10% to 20% total BSA involvement), immediate transfer of the patient to an intensive care or burn unit under the care of an experienced dermatologist and skilled nurses is strongly advocated. Therapeutic protocols consist of the following:

- Measures to guard against iatrogenic infection, including withdrawal from systemic steroids; avoidance of indwelling lines and catheters whenever possible; limitation of antibiotic use to specific culture-proven infections; daily cultures of denuded skin, eyes, mouth, sputum, and urine; and aggressive treatment of sepsis if it occurs.
- Supportive care consisting of use of an air-fluidized bed, intravenous fluid therapy to restore fluid and electrolyte balance, tube feedings to ensure adequate caloric intake, adequate pain relief, respiratory and physical therapy as needed and tolerated, and continuing eye care by an ophthalmologist.
- Avoidance of all unnecessary medications, particularly those that are known etiologic factors of SJS/TEN, such as sulfonamides (including sulfa-containing eye preparations and topical dressings).
- Skin care with emphasis on wound dressings to protect the denuded dermis from desiccation and secondary infection and to facilitate rapid re-epithelialization. Reduced mortality and faster healing result from the use of synthetic dressings, biologic dressings, silver nitrate dressings, allografts, or porcine xenografts.

Mouth Care

When extensive painful mouth lesions are present, good oral hygiene is critical to minimize infection and discomfort. Hydrogen peroxide (1.5%) or sterile normal saline mouthwash every 2 hours provides cleansing and gentle débridement. Topical anesthetics, such as dyclonine, viscous lidocaine, or a 1:1 mixture of Kaopectate[1] and elixir of diphenhydramine (Benadryl), used as a mouthwash, often provides pain relief. A liquid or soft diet, usually better tolerated, contributes to the maintenance of hydration and nutrition. More aggressive nutritional support is usually required for severe oral involvement.

Eye Care

Because of the potential for long-term sequelae resulting in loss of vision, careful monitoring of eye involvement is mandatory, and early consultation and daily continuing care by an ophthalmologist is strongly recommended. Suggested therapeutic measures might include sterile irrigation and compresses to cleanse the eye, lysis of adhesions, and instillation of topical antibiotics.

Preventive Measures

In drug-associated SJS or TEN, future avoidance of the causative drug or chemically related agents is mandatory.

Patient Education

For SJS and TEN, patients should be advised the course is self-limited but potentially severe and life-threatening, educated regarding the association with adverse drug reactions, and warned to avoid future use of the implicated medication(s).

REFERENCES

Bachot N, Revuz J, Roujeau J-C: Intravenous immunoglobulin treatment for Stevens-Johnson syndrome and toxic epidermal necrolysis: A prospective noncomparative study showing no benefit on mortality or progression. Arch Dermatol 2003;139:33-36.

Bastuji-Garin S, Rzany B, Stern RS, et al: Clinical classification of cases of toxic epidermal necrolysis, Stevens-Johnson syndrome, and erythema multiforme. Arch Dermatol 1993;129:92-96.

Green JA, Spruance SL, Wenerstrom G, Piepkorn MW: Post-herpetic erythema multiforme prevented with prophylactic oral acyclovir. Ann Int Med 1985;102:632-633.

Halebian PH, Madden MR, Finklestein JL, et al: Improved burn center survival of patients with toxic epidermal necrolysis managed without corticosteroids. Ann Surg 1986;204:503-512.

Kelemen JJ, Cioffi WG, McManus WF, et al: Burn center care for patients with toxic epidermal necrolysis. J Am Coll Surg 1995; 180:273-278.

Lehrer-Bell KA, Kirsner RS, Tallman PG, Kerdel FA: Treatment of the cutaneous involvement in Stevens-Johnson syndrome and toxic epidermal necrolysis with silver nitrate–impregnated dressings. Arch Dermatol 1998;134:877-879.

Prins C, Kerdel FA, Padilla S, et al: Treatment of toxic epidermal necrolysis with high-dose intravenous immunoglobulins: Multicenter retrospective analysis of 48 consecutive cases. Arch Dermatol 2003;139:26-32.

Roujeau J-C, Kelly JP, Naldi L, et al: Medication use and the risk of Stevens-Johnson syndrome or toxic epidermal necrolysis. N Engl J Med 1995;333:1600-1607.

Tatnall FM, Schofield JK, Leigh IM. A double-blind, placebo-controlled trial of continuous acyclovir therapy in recurrent erythema multiforme. Br J Dermatol 1995;132:267-270.

Trent JT, Kirsner RS, Romanelli P, Kerdel FA: Analysis of intravenous immunoglobulin for the treatment of toxic epidermal necrolysis using SCORTEN. Arch Dermatol 2003;139:39-43.

Viard I, Wehrli P, Bullani R, et al: Inhibition of toxic epidermal necrolysis by blockade of CD95 with human intravenous immunoglobulin. Science 1998;282:490-493.

Wolkenstein P, Latarjet J, Roujeau J-C, et al: Randomized comparison of thalidomide versus placebo in toxic epidermal necrolysis. Lancet 1998;352:1586-1589.

[1]Not FDA approved for this indication.

Bullous Diseases

Method of
Sarah E. Dick, MD, and Victoria Werth, MD

The autoimmune bullous diseases are a group of rare disorders with potential significant morbidity and mortality. Although our scientific knowledge of these conditions is advancing and our armamentarium of therapies is growing, evidence-based practice guidelines are still lacking. Given the rarity of these diseases and the absence of common terms and endpoints for assessing disease extent, activity, and therapeutic response, the paucity of randomized controlled studies of the bullous diseases is not surprising. Thus, the true effectiveness of the available therapies remains unclear. The following treatment recommendations are based on published data and on the authors' personal experiences with patients with bullous disease.

Pemphigus Vulgaris

Pemphigus vulgaris (PV) is characterized by nonscarring, fragile vesicles and bullae of the mucous membranes with or without cutaneous involvement. Systemic corticosteroid use and other advances in management have dramatically decreased the mortality rate for PV from 75% in untreated cases to 5% to 10% in treated cases. At present, the primary causes of morbidity and mortality in PV are complications resulting from treatment. Thus, the goal of PV management is to induce and maintain remission with the lowest medication doses possible. Therapies can be divided into those with a rapid effect and those with a delayed effect. Treatments that act rapidly, such as systemic corticosteroids, pulse corticosteroid therapy, intravenous immunoglobulin (IVIg), and plasmapheresis, are usually used to induce remission. Therapies with a delayed effect, such as immunosuppressive medications, dapsone,[1] and antibiotics, are generally used to decrease the need for systemic steroids.

The management of PV can be divided into three therapeutic phases: control, consolidation, maintenance. During the *control phase*, the medication doses should be rapidly increased to a level at which no new lesions form and established lesions start to heal. Without this initial successful disease suppression, tapering of treatment can be difficult. In the *consolidation phase*, the current therapy should be maintained until about 80% of the established lesions are healed. During the *maintenance phase*, medications are gradually decreased to the lowest doses needed to prevent the appearance of new lesions. If multiple medications are being given, they should be tapered one at a time, with tapering of corticosteroids usually occurring first because of the significant toxicity associated with prolonged systemic corticosteroid use.

Systemic corticosteroids are the most effective and rapidly acting treatment for PV. Low to moderate doses of oral prednisone (Deltasone; 0.5 mg/kg/day) can be started for mild disease. Higher doses of prednisone (1 mg/kg/day) should be used for more severe disease. These starting doses can be increased every 1 to 2 weeks by 50% increments until disease activity is controlled. Different and/or adjuvant therapies should be considered if patients do not respond to an oral prednisone dose of 1.5 to 2 mg/kg/day. Often adjuvant immunosuppressive therapy is started concurrently with systemic corticosteroids in order to maximize disease control and minimize the steroid dose. Pulse corticosteroid therapy with intravenous methylprednisolone (Solu-Medrol) has been shown to have long-lasting benefits and should be considered in patients who are not responsive to prednisone. It is used at a dose of 1 g/day over 1 to 3 hours for 3 consecutive days. The advantage of pulse steroid therapy is that remission can be quickly achieved and long-term side effects of chronic steroid use minimized.

Once remission is achieved and maintained, prednisone doses can be tapered cautiously, with a decrease of 5 to 10 mg every 1 to 2 weeks. If a few new lesions appear during the taper, they can be treated with intralesional corticosteroids, such as triamcinolone (Kenalog), or with high-potency topical corticosteroids, such as clobetasol (Temovate), while the current dose of systemic medications is unchanged. If many new lesions appear, the dose of prednisone should be increased in increments of 25% to 50% until control is re-established.

Other rapidly acting agents for PV include IVIg (Gamimune, Gammagard) and plasmapheresis. IVIg appears to be most effective when used with immunosuppressive therapies or when used as a steroid-sparing agent. However, IVIg has also been shown to be effective as monotherapy. The usual dose is 2 g/kg over 3 to 5 days. Multiple cycles given every 4 weeks are generally needed. The effectiveness of plasmapheresis for PV is controversial. In a controlled study, plasmapheresis used in combination with prednisone was found to have no advantage over the use of prednisone alone. However, plasmapheresis in combination with immunosuppressive therapy may be a valuable treatment for severe and/or unresponsive PV. Plasmapheresis is normally performed three times per week, with approximately 2 L of plasma removed at each treatment. Concurrent use of immunosuppressive medications helps prevent a rebound in the antibody concentrations that usually occurs. With both plasmapheresis and IVIg, serum antibody concentrations can be monitored to determine a response to therapy.

Immunosuppressive medications used for treatment of PV include azathioprine[1] (Imuran) at doses of 3 to 5 mg/kg/day, cyclophosphamide[1] (Cytoxan) at doses of 2 to 3 mg/kg/day or as pulse therapy of 0.5 to 1 g/m² monthly combined with low-dose oral cyclophosphamide,[1] mycophenolate mofetil[1] (MMF; CellCept) at doses of 2 to 3 g per day, methotrexate[1] (Rheumatrex) at doses up to 20 mg/week, chlorambucil[1] (Leukeran) at doses of 4 to 10 mg/day, and cyclosporine[1] (Neoral, Sandimmune) at doses of 3 to 6 mg/kg/day. These therapies are thought to have a lag phase of 4 to 6 weeks before they become effective. They are generally used as adjuvant therapy. In a randomized trial, cyclosporine[1] was shown to be ineffective as adjuvant therapy to corticosteroids in the treatment of PV. Nevertheless, based on case reports, some experts still believe that it may be beneficial as adjuvant therapy to corticosteroids in long-term maintenance.

---

[1]Not FDA approved for this indication.

[1]Not FDA approved for this indication.

Dapsone[1] (Avlosulfon) has been shown to reduce steroid dependence in PV patients. It is used at doses of 50 to 300 mg/day. It is usually started at a dose of 50 mg daily and increased by 25 mg weekly until a response is obtained.

Other treatments for PV that can be considered as alternatives to the adjuvant therapies mentioned include gold,[1] tetracycline[1] (Sumycin) with or without niacinamide,[1] and hydroxychloroquine[1] (Plaquenil).

For severe and refractory PV that has failed conventional therapies, extracorporeal photopheresis can be considered. This procedure requires collaboration with specialists.

New potential treatments for PV include rituximab (Rituxan),[1] infliximab (Remicade),[1] etanercept (Enbrel),[1] and pyridostigmine bromide (Mestinon).[1] Rituximab (Rituxan)[1] is a chimeric murine-human monoclonal antibody against CD20. It has been shown to be effective in refractory PV at a dose of 375 mg/m[2]/week for 4 weeks. Infliximab (Remicade)[1] is a chimeric murine-human monoclonal antibody against tumor necrosis factor-α (TNF-α). Recent reports suggest that TNF-α blockade might be a short-term therapeutic option for immediate control of refractory PV. Etanercept (Enbrel)[1] is a fusion protein of TNF-α receptor that acts as a competitive inhibitor of TNF-α. It may have a beneficial role in the treatment of PV. Pyridostigmine bromide[1] is an acetylcholinesterase inhibitor that is being investigated for treatment of PV.

Pemphigus Foliaceus

Pemphigus foliaceus (PF) typically presents with nonscarring superficial, cutaneous erosions and crusts with a similar distribution as PV. In contrast to PV, there is no mucosal involvement. The principles and practice of managing PF are similar to those for PV. However, monotherapy with dapsone[1] can be effective. In addition, because PF may remain localized for several years, topical steroids such as triamcinolone (Kenalog) and clobetasol (Temovate) may suffice for many years before systemic treatment in needed.

Paraneoplastic Pemphigus

Paraneoplastic pemphigus (PNP) is frequently associated with an underlying lymphoproliferative neoplasm (most commonly non-Hodgkin's lymphoma, chronic lymphocytic leukemia, and Castleman disease). Clinically, there are polymorphous mucocutaneous lesions. The oral lesions are typically severe and refractory to treatment. Other organs, especially the lungs, can be affected.

Management of PNP involves treatment of the underlying neoplasm as well as immunosuppression. Excision of associated benign neoplasms may result in remission, whereas excision of malignant neoplasm often does not. High-dose systemic corticosteroids, such as prednisone at doses of 1 to 2 mg/kg/day, are usually the first-line therapy. Patients rarely have a complete response to systemic corticosteroids alone. The addition of immunosuppressive therapies, such as cyclosporine, azathioprine, MMF, and cyclophosphamide, have all been used with variable success. Although there may be a concern about treatment with immunosuppression in a patient with a known malignancy, the extremely high morbidity and mortality associated with PNP warrants MMF use. Other therapies to consider for treatment of recalcitrant PNP include IVIg, plasmapheresis, immunophoresis, and photopheresis. Both rituximab and alemtuzumab (Campath)[1] are new therapies that have been shown to be beneficial in the treatment of PNP. Alemtuzumab is a humanized monoclonal antibody against CD52.

Bullous Pemphigoid

Bullous pemphigoid (BP) usually presents as nonscarring tense blisters with a predilection for the flexural aspects of the limbs. Mucosal lesions occur in 10% to 35% of patients. Even without treatment, BP is usually a self-limited disease. Remission is likely to occur within 5 years. Despite this limited course of BP, its mortality rate appears to be between 20% and 40% with or without therapy. The aim of treatment should be to heal established lesions, halt the development of new lesions, and minimize side effects from medications.

Localized or limited disease should be treated with potent topical corticosteroids, such as clobetasol ointment twice daily. Moderate and even severe BP can also be treated with potent topical steroids. In a randomized trial, potent topical steroids used for extensive BP had a lower 1-year mortality rate compared to prednisone at a dose of 1 mg/kg/day. Nevertheless, most patients with generalized disease require systemic therapy. Systemic corticosteroids are currently the best-established treatment. They have a rapid effect (within days) and well-documented effectiveness. Prednisone alone is often sufficient as monotherapy at doses of 0.5 to 0.75 mg/kg/day. Once remission is achieved, prednisone doses can be tapered in a manner similar to that described for PV.

Immunosuppressive medications can be considered in the treatment of BP, especially for patients who cannot tolerate corticosteroids or who have severe, difficult to control disease. In randomized trials, azathioprine[1] has been shown to have a steroid-sparing effect, but it has also been associated with more side effects when used with prednisolone in comparison to prednisolone alone. It is used at doses of 2 to 3 mg/kg/day. MMF has been shown to be effective both as monotherapy and in combination with corticosteroids. It is used at doses of 2 to 3 g/day. An ongoing randomized trial is comparing azathioprine[1] and MMF.[1] Other immunosuppressive medications to consider include cyclophosphamide,[1] methotrexate,[1] chlorambucil,[1] and cyclosporine.[1]

Antibiotics have been shown to have a beneficial effect in the treatment of BP and should be considered for treatment of mild disease or as a steroid-sparing agent. In a randomized trial, the combination of tetracycline[1] and niacinamide[1] was equally as effective as prednisone alone. Tetracycline[1] is given at a dose of 500 mg four times daily with or without niacinamide[1] at a dose of 500 mg three times daily. Doxycycline[1] (Vibramycin) or minocycline[1] (Minocin) 100 mg twice daily can be given rather than tetracycline.

---

[1]Not FDA approved for this indication.

[1]Not FDA approved for this indication.

Dapsone[1] (50–300 mg/day) can be used as a steroid-sparing agent in the treatment of BP. It is usually started at a dose of 50 mg daily and increased by 25 mg weekly until a response is obtained.

For recalcitrant disease, IVIg and plasmapheresis can be used. Both are very costly. Randomized trials studying plasmapheresis suggest it has a steroid-sparing effect.

Mucous Membrane Pemphigoid

Mucous membrane pemphigoid (MMP) is also known as cicatricial pemphigoid and mucosal pemphigoid. Lesions of MMP can be scarring and predominantly involve the oral cavity and conjunctiva. Limited cutaneous disease with fragile vesicles, bullae, and erosions is present in approximately one third of patients. Mucosal involvement of the nasopharynx, pharynx, esophagus, larynx, trachea, genitals, and anus can occur.

Treatment of MMP is dictated by the site, extent, and severity of disease as well as by the rapidity of progression. Patients with ocular, nasopharyngeal, laryngeal, esophageal, and/or genital lesions are considered high risk because involvement of these sites can lead to blindness, airway obstruction, esophageal stricture, and urinary and sexual dysfunction. For high-risk patients with severe or rapidly progressing disease, initial treatment should consist of cyclophosphamide[1] (1-2 mg/kg/day) and prednisone (1-1.5 mg/kg/day). A small randomized controlled trial found the combination of cyclophosphamide[1] and prednisone to be more effective than prednisone alone. Azathioprine[1] or MMF[1] (at doses similar to those used for BP) given with prednisone can also be considered if cyclophosphamide[1] is ineffective or not tolerated. IVIg has been shown to have a beneficial effect and can be used for refractory MMP. Subconjunctival mitomycin can be used to help reduce mucosal fibrosis and prevent scarring. For milder disease in high-risk patients, dapsone[1] (50-300 mg daily) may be given. A small randomized controlled trial showed that cyclophosphamide[1] was superior to dapsone[1] in the treatment of severe MMP with ocular involvement. However, the study concluded that dapsone can be beneficial for mild to moderate disease. Other treatments to consider in recalcitrant cases include methotrexate,[1] thalidomide (Thalomid),[1] etanercept,[1] and plasmapheresis. All MMP patients should be evaluated and managed in conjunction with the appropriate subspecialist (e.g., ocular involvement requires ophthalmologic monitoring) with surgical intervention as needed.

MMP patients with only oral mucosal involvement, with or without cutaneous lesions, are considered low risk. Because these patients are less likely to have mucosal scarring, a more conservative therapeutic approach can be taken. In addition to good oral hygiene, moderate- to high-potency topical corticosteroids, such as triamcinolone or clobetasol (two to four times daily), can be used for the initial treatment. An insertable prosthetic device/retainer is useful for the oral topical application of corticosteroids. Intralesional corticosteroids, such as triamcinolone, may also be beneficial for refractory oral mucosal lesions. Tetracycline[1] with or without niacinamide[1] (at doses similar to those used for BP) can be effective in managing low-risk patients. If disease control is not achieved with topical corticosteroids or oral antibiotics, other treatments to consider include dapsone[1] (50-200 mg/day) or low-dose prednisone (0.5 mg/kg/day) with or without low-dose azathioprine[1] (100-150 mg/day). For MMP with severe oral disease, the treatments recommended for high-risk patients may be needed.

Epidermolysis Bullosa Acquisita

Epidermolysis bullosa acquisita (EBA) has heterogeneous clinical features. Classically, patients have skin fragility and present with bullae and/or erosions at areas of friction and trauma. However, EBA patients can also present with lesions resembling BP, linear immunoglobulin A (IgA) bullous dermatosis, or MMP. Lesions heal with scarring and milia formation. Complications similar to those with MMP, such as blindness and esophageal stricture, can occur. EBA may be associated with various systemic diseases, most commonly inflammatory bowel disease.

EBA is very difficult to treat. It appears that the classic presentation is the most resistant to therapy. Any measures that decrease friction and trauma to the skin will help. Systemic corticosteroids such as prednisone (0.5-2 mg/kg/day) can be beneficial, especially with inflammatory EBA. Dapsone[1] or colchicine[1] used as adjuvant agents or monotherapies should also be considered. Dapsone[1] (50-300 mg/day) is believed to be particularly appropriate with inflammatory EBA that has a neutrophilic predominance in histology. Colchicine[1] (0.5-2 mg/day) may not be tolerated because of gastrointestinal side effects, especially in patients with associated inflammatory bowel disease.

Cyclosporine[1], with or without systemic corticosteroids, can result in a rapid response and should be considered for the initial treatment of EBA. Doses of 3 to 9 mg/kg/day can be started and then increased or decreased as needed. Long-term toxicity of the medication limits its use.

Immunosuppressive agents, such as azathioprine,[1] cyclophosphamide,[1] methotrexate,[1] and MMF,[1] may be considered for treatment of EBA. They can be used in regimens and at doses similar to those used for PV.

IVIg can be effective when given as monotherapy or in combination with immunosuppressive agents and/or systemic corticosteroids. This treatment is expensive and is best reserved for recalcitrant cases. Extracorporeal photopheresis and plasmapheresis can also be considered for treatment of recalcitrant EBA. Plasmapheresis has been shown to be beneficial when given in combination with IVIg, systemic corticosteroids, or cyclophosphamide.[1]

As with MMP, patients with EBA should be followed by the appropriate subspecialists, such as ophthalmologists and gastroenterologists, if mucosal membranes are involved.

Linear Immunoglobulin A Bullous Dermatosis

Linear IgA bullous dermatosis (LABD) has heterogeneous clinical features. It typically presents with annular or grouped pruritic papules, vesicles, and bullae on the

---

[1]Not FDA approved for this indication.

elbows, knees, and buttocks. These lesions can be indistinguishable from those of dermatitis herpetiformis. However, the lesions can also resemble those of BP and EBA. Mucosal lesions resembling MMP may occur.

LABD can have an unpredictable course with occasional spontaneous remissions. Treatment with dapsone[1] usually results in a rapid dramatic response and is considered the first-line treatment of LABD. Doses as described for PV are used. Sulfapyridine[1] can also be used with similar results. The initial dose for sulfapyridine[1] is 500 mg twice daily. This can be increased by 1 g every 1 to 2 weeks until disease control, or a maximum dose of 4 g, is reached. Tetracycline[1] in combination with niacinamide[1] (at doses similar to those used for BP) has been shown to have a beneficial effect in the treatment of LABD. Prednisone can be added to these therapies when clinical responses

___

[1]Not FDA approved for this indication.

are incomplete. Several other medications, such as MMF,[1] azathioprine,[1] cyclosporine,[1] and methotrexate,[1] have also been shown to be helpful in the management of patients with difficult to control disease. For recalcitrant cases, cyclosporine[1] (3-6 mg/kg/day) or IVIg can be used. Oral mucosal lesions may be more resistant to treatment and require therapy with topical steroids.

As with MMP and EBA, patients with LABD should be followed by the appropriate subspecialists if mucosal membranes are involved.

Dermatitis Herpetiformis

Dermatitis herpetiformis (DH) presents as intense pruritus with grouped papules and vesicles distributed on the

___

[1]Not FDA approved for this indication.

 CURRENT DIAGNOSIS

Pemphigus Vulgaris

- Flaccid blisters: Mucocutaneous.
- Suprabasilar intraepidermal blisters.
- DIF is positive for epidermal intercellular IgG deposition.
- IIF on monkey esophagus is positive for circulating autoantibodies.
- ELISA identifies antibodies to desmoglein-3 with/without desmoglein-1.

Pemphigus Foliaceus

- Flaccid blisters: Cutaneous only.
- Subcorneal intraepidermal blisters.
- DIF is positive for epidermal intercellular IgG deposition.
- IIF on guinea pig esophagus is positive for circulating autoantibodies.
- ELISA identifies antibodies to desmoglein-1 only.

Paraneoplastic Pemphigus

- Polymorphous lesions: Mucocutaneous.
- Intraepidermal blisters, keratinocyte necrosis, and interface dermatitis.
- DIF is positive for IgG and C3 deposition at epidermal intercellular sites and at the dermal-epidermal junction.
- IIF on rodent bladder is positive for circulating autoantibodies. Immunoblotting and immunoprecipitation identify antibodies to desmoglein and multiple plakin antigens (at a minimum, periplakin and/or envoplakin).

Bullous Pemphigoid

- Tense blisters: Mostly cutaneous, can be mucocutaneous.
- Subepidermal blisters with eosinophils.
- DIF is positive for IgG and C3 deposition at the dermal–epidermal junction.

- IIF on salt-split skin is positive for autoantibodies on the epidermal side (roof) of the blister. BPAg2 is the target antigen.

Mucous Membrane Pemphigoid

- Scarring blisters: Mucosal.
- Subepidermal blister.
- DIF is positive for IgG and C3 deposition at the dermal-epidermal junction.
- IIF on salt-split skin can be positive for autoantibodies on the epidermal side (roof) of the blister, dermal side (floor) of the blister, or both. Target antigens are BPAg2, integrin subunit β_4, and laminin-5.

Epidermolysis Bullosa Acquisita

- Skin fragility at sites of trauma with scarring and milia: Mostly cutaneous, can be mucosal.
- Subepidermal blister.
- DIF is positive for IgG deposition at the dermal-epidermal junction.
- IIF on salt-split skin is positive for autoantibodies on the dermal side (floor) of the blister.
- ELISA identifies antibodies to type VII collagen.

Linear IgA Disease

- Pruritic grouped papules: Mucocutaneous.
- Subepidermal blisters with neutrophils.
- DIF positive for linear deposition of IgA at the dermal-epidermal junction.
- IIF can be negative or detect low levels of circulating IgA autoantibodies.

Dermatitis Herpetiformis

- Pruritic grouped papules associated with a gluten sensitive enteropathy: Cutaneous.
- Subepidermal blisters with neutrophils.
- DIF positive for granular deposition of IgA in the dermal papillary tips.

Abbreviations: BPAg2 = bullous pemphigoid antigen–2; C3 = complement 3; DIF = direct immunofluorescence; ELISA = enzyme–linked immunosorbent assay; IgA = immunoglobulin A; IgG = immunoglobulin G; IIF = indirect immunofluorescence.

CURRENT THERAPY

Pemphigus Vulgaris

- Rapid effect: systemic corticosteroids.
- Delayed effect: Immunosuppressive agents, dapsone,[1] and antibiotics.
- Resistant disease: Intravenous immunoglobulin, rituximab[1] (Rituxan).
- Bone prophylaxis for systemic corticosteroid use.

Pemphigus Foliaceus

- Similar management as pemphigus vulgaris.

Paraneoplastic Pemphigus

- Treat underlying neoplasm.
- High-dose systemic corticosteroids plus immunosuppressive agents.

Bullous Pemphigoid

- Generalized or severe disease: Systemic corticosteroids, immunosuppressive agents, dapsone.[1]
- Limited or mild disease: Topical corticosteroids, tetracycline[1] with niacinamide.[1]

Mucous Membrane Pemphigoid

- High-risk patients: Cyclophosphamide[1] (Cytoxan) plus prednisone.
- Low-risk patients: Topical corticosteroids, tetracycline[1] plus niacinamide,[1] dapsone.[1]

Epidermolysis Bullosa Acquisita

- Difficult to treat.
- Decrease friction and trauma to skin.
- Systemic corticosteroids, dapsone,[1] colchicine.[1]

Linear IgA Disease

- Dapsone.[1]

Dermatitis Herpetiformis

- Dapsone and gluten-free diet.

---

[1]Not FDA approved for this indication.
Abbreviations: IgA = immunoglobulin A.

---

extensor surfaces of the elbows, knees, buttocks, and back. It can be indistinguishable from LABD. DH appears to be caused by an immune response to gluten, and it is associated with a gluten-sensitive enteropathy.

Dapsone is considered the first-line therapy for DH. It usually causes a rapid and dramatic response at doses described for PV. Sulfapyridine[1] can also be used when dapsone cannot be tolerated. The initial dose of sulfapyridine is 500 mg three times daily. This can be increased by 1 g every 1 to 2 weeks until disease control, or a maximum dose of 4-6 g, is reached. Other medications have been used with variable success, including tetracycline[1] with niacinamide,[1] heparin,[1] colchicine,[1] azathioprine,[1] prednisone, and cholestyramine,[1] and can be considered for patients who are intolerant or allergic to dapsone and sulfapyridine.[1]

---

[1]Not FDA approved for this indication.

A gluten-free diet is important for the long-term management of DH for several reasons. First, DH symptoms improve and can allow for reduction or even discontinuation of medications. Second, associated gastrointestinal symptoms improve and can resolve. Third, the associated risk of gastrointestinal lymphoma significantly decreases and disappears after 5 to 10 years.

REFERENCES

Ahmed AR, Dahl MV: Consensus statement on the use of intravenous immunoglobulin therapy in the treatment of autoimmune mucocutaneous blistering diseases. Arch Dermatol 2003;139:1051-1059.
Bystryn JC, Steinman NM: The adjuvant therapy of pemphigus. An update. Arch Dermatol 1996;132:203-212.
Chaffins ML, Collison D, Fivenson DP: Treatment of pemphigus and linear IgA dermatosis with nicotinamide and tetracycline: A review of 13 cases. J Am Acad Dermatol 1993;28:998-1000.
Chan LS, Ahmed AR, Anhalt GJ, et al: The first international consensus on mucous membrane pemphigoid: Definition, diagnostic criteria, pathogenic factors, medical treatment, and prognostic indicators. Arch Dermatol 2002;138:370-379.
Engineer L, Ahmed AR: Emerging treatment for epidermolysis bullosa acquisita. J Am Acad Dermatol 2001;44:818-828.
Fleischli ME, Valek RH, Pandya AG: Pulse intravenous cyclophosphamide therapy in pemphigus. Arch Dermatol 1999;135:57-61.
Garioch JJ, Lewis HM, Sargent SA, et al: 25 years' experience of a gluten–free diet in the treatment of dermatitis herpetiformis. Br J Dermatol 1994;131:541-545.
Heaphy MR, Albrecht J, Werth VP: Dapsone as a glucocorticoid-sparing agent in maintenance-phase pemphigus vulgaris. Arch Dermatol 2005;141:699-702.
Ioannides D, Chrysomallis F, Bystryn JC: Ineffectiveness of cyclosporine as an adjuvant to corticosteroids in the treatment of pemphigus. Arch Dermatol 2000;136:868-872.
Khumalo N, Kirtschig G, Middleton P, et al: Interventions for bullous pemphigoid. Cochrane Database Syst Rev 2005 (3):CD002292.
Mimouni D, Anhalt GJ, Cummins DL, et al: Treatment of pemphigus vulgaris and pemphigus foliaceus with mycophenolate mofetil. Arch Dermatol 2003;139:739-742
Werth VP: Treatment of pemphigus vulgaris with brief, high-dose intravenous glucocorticoids. Arch Dermatol 1996;132:1435-1439.

Contact Dermatitis

Method of
Peter C. Schalock, MD, and
Kathryn A. Zug, MD

Eczema is well described by the word's Greek roots, with "ek" meaning "out or over" and "zein" meaning "to boil." Thus, this boiling over pattern of superficial inflammatory skin diseases of the skin is one of the most common reaction pattern seen by dermatologists. Pruritus is the most characteristic skin sensation associated with eczema.

Irritant Contact Dermatitis

Contact dermatitis (CD) is caused by exogenous substances coming into contact with the skin. Irritant contact dermatitis (ICD) is the most common form of CD, caused by frequent or chronic exposure to an irritating substance. ICD will eventually occur in any person exposed to these irritating substances in sufficient concentration. This type of reaction is the most common form of occupational skin disease and is a problem for many individuals worldwide. The most common location for ICD is the hands. Other locations commonly involved are the palms, fingers, and dorsal web spaces. As opposed to allergic contact dermatitis, the dorsal hands are most often spared from dermatitis.

Allergic Contact Dermatitis

Two types of immune reactions are seen in allergic contact dermatitis (ACD): type I immediate-type hypersensitivity and type IV delayed-type hypersensitivity. Immediate-type reactions are most commonly caused by animal or plant proteins that are able to bind to mast cells and cause mast cell degranulation, leading to an urticarial or anaphylactic reaction. The most commonly recognized cause of this type of immediate hypersensitivity is natural rubber latex proteins. Allergy to these proteins is caused by exposure to products containing natural rubber latex, especially rubber gloves. Type IV allergy is caused by substances that are taken up by Langerhans cells in the epidermis and processed and presented to T cells in the regional lymph node, thus creating memory T cells that are capable of reacting the next time the individual is exposed to the substance. The delayed reaction is due to the time needed to mount the immune response. Frequent culprits are urushiol (poison ivy/oak), topical antibiotics, nickel, and formaldehyde/formaldehyde-releasing preservatives.

Diagnosis

Evaluation for the etiology of CD reactions depends upon the type of allergy sought. Evaluation for type I immediate-type allergy is different than for type IV delayed-type reactions. Testing for type I allergy can be achieved by in vivo and in vitro methods. Prick testing can be performed for panels of suspected allergens. For the prick test, the skin on the flexor forearm or other area is cleaned, and a small amount of a pure dilution of the suspect protein is placed on the skin. The skin is pricked using a sterile lancet, and the patient is observed for a wheal and flare reaction. Histamine should also be used as a positive control. This type of testing can elicit an anaphylactic type of reaction and should be performed with caution. Many allergens that elicit a type I reaction can also be tested by the allergen-specific immunoglobulin E antibody test or radioallergosorbent assay test (RAST).

Type IV allergy is best evaluated by patch testing. A patch test is made with hypoallergenic tape to which Finn chambers (small metal chambers) or IQ Ultra chambers (Chemotechnique Diagnostics, Vellinge, Sweden) are placed with a purified potential allergen. The patches are placed most often on the patient's upper back and left for 48 hours. The patches are then removed, the locations of the allergens marked, and the initial reading performed. The patient is seen again in another 48 hours for the final reading. Two readings are preferable to allow assessment of some reactions that appear after the patch has been removed and of some reactions initially thought to be positive that may actually have been irritant reactions. Patch testing technique has been described in detail by Corey.

Once the patient's sensitivities are determined, the information is useful to help educate the patient regarding avoidance of the offending allergen. There is no "cure" for ACD. The Contact Allergen Replacement Database available through the American Contact Dermatitis Society is a useful tool for helping patients avoid their allergens (available at: www.contactderm.org). The patient can enter each allergen into the database, and a list of products free of the allergens is generated.

In the United States, only the 23 thin-layer rapid-use epicutaneous (TRUE) test allergens are Food and Drug Administration (FDA) approved for use. A multitude of other allergens for patch testing are available in Europe. Chemotechnique AB (Malmo, Sweden) and Hermal (Reinbek, Germany) both manufacture many standard and specialty series of allergens. Patch testing with an expanded series of allergens can be useful in identifying relevant allergens. TRUE test allergens encompass 1.4% of the more than 3700 known allergens, although 28% of patients are fully evaluated with this panel. By expanding the series to the 65 standard allergens used by the North American Contact Dermatitis Group (NACDG), 50.2% of relevant allergies are identified. Although use of the TRUE test may be a good starting point for evaluation of ACD, an expanded panel of allergens with additional testing for suspected agents to which the patient may have contact gives a much greater return on testing.

Treatment

Treatment of CD hinges upon four premises: education of the patient regarding skin care and the etiology of the dermatitis, postexposure skin care, strict avoidance of the offending allergen(s), and pharmacologic therapy of active dermatitis. Patients educated on the basics of good skin care and on the cause of their ICD and ACD had less dermatitis than did those without intervention. For patient with ICD and ACD, postexposure skin care plays an important role in treatment. ICD can play a role in the development and perpetuation of ACD by allowing greater penetration of allergens. Good skin care, such as the use of appropriate barrier creams, bland emollients, and avoidance of wet work or macerating gloves, can decrease skin irritation and transepidermal water loss. Good skin care and prevention of irritation should be an integral part of preventing and treating ACD.

 CURRENT DIAGNOSIS

Type I Allergy

- Prick test
- Use test (perform with caution)
- Radioallergosorbent assay test (RAST) for specific allergens

Type IV Allergy

- Patch test using a broad panel of allergens and patient's personal care products most helpful
- Repeated open application test (ROAT)/use test

In cases of mild to moderate dermatitis, a medium- or high-potency topical steroid, such as triamcinolone acetonide (Aristocort A) 0.1% or desoximetasone (Topicort) 0.25%, can be used two to three times daily for monotherapy. For widespread cases, a 1-lb (454 g) jar of generic triamcinolone acetonide 0.1% is preferable. Ointments are preferable to creams because the water and preservatives present in creams may worsen the irritant reaction. Simple, greasy lubricants, such as Aquaphor or Vaseline, should be used every time the body or hands are washed or appear dry. Widespread dermatitis will often improve rapidly with open wet dressings preceded and followed by a topical corticosteroid cream. For hand dermatitis, use of the steroid or of Vaseline under cotton gloves can be helpful, either for short periods or overnight. For sensitive areas such as the face and genitalia, topical calcineurin inhibitors can be useful. Either tacrolimus (Protopic) 0.1% ointment or pimecrolimus (Elidel) 1% cream twice daily can be used. For more severe cases of dermatitis, topical therapy and a corticosteroid taper can be helpful in alleviating the patient's symptoms as well as calming the dermatitis. Short prednisone tapers (i.e., "dose packs") will not always be adequate, with the patient flaring after the short taper is finished. Using prednisone in a 4-week course with 7-day tapering steps, such as 60-40-20-10 mg, can be helpful in breaking the cycle of chronic inflammation and excoriation/pruritus. Open wet dressings with application of topical corticosteroid before and after can diminish dermatitis quickly. For patients with severe pruritus, especially at night, hydroxyzine (Atarax) 10 to 50 mg orally or doxepin[1] (Sinequan) 10 to 20 mg orally at bedtime can be helpful.

---

[1]Not FDA approved for this indication.

CURRENT THERAPY

- Strict avoidance of the offending allergen(s) and pharmacologic therapy for active dermatitis.
- Patient education on good skin care and prevention of irritation.
- Simple, greasy lubricants, such as Aquaphor or Vaseline, should be used every time the body or hands are washed or appear dry.
- Groin or face dermatitis: Tacrolimus (Protopic) 0.1% ointment or pimecrolimus (Elidel) 1% cream twice daily
- Mild to moderate dermatitis: Medium- or high-potency topical steroid such as triamcinolone acetonide (Aristocort A) 0.1% or desoximetasone (Topicort) 0.25% bid-tid for monotherapy.
  - Widespread dermatitis: Generic triamcinolone 0.1% cream (454-g jar) bid-tid
  - Pruritus: Hydroxyzine (Atarax) 10-50 mg PO bid–tid PRN
- Severe Dermatitis
  - Prednisone in a 4-week course with 7-day tapering steps, such as 60-40-20-10 mg
  - Open wet dressings with topical steroid application

Conclusion

Contact dermatitis is a broad diagnosis encompassing both immediate- and delayed-type hypersensitivities. Testing can be helpful in characterizing specific allergens and in guiding the patients as to which substances to avoid to prevent dermatitis. The RAST or prick test is useful for determining immediate-type hypersensitivity and patch testing for delayed-type allergy. TRUE tests will fully evaluate 28% of patients. Broadening the screen with other allergens, such as the NACDG panel, can be useful for defining ACD in patients with dermatitis. Treatment of CD consists of topical steroids, open wet dressings, moisturization, topical calcineurin inhibitors, and infrequently oral corticosteroids.

REFERENCES

Bauer A, Kelterer D, Stadeler M, et al: The prevention of occupational hand dermatitis in bakers, confectioners and employees in the catering trades. Preliminary results of a skin prevention program. Contact Dermatitis 2001;44:85-88.

Corey G: Applying patch tests from a technician's or nurse's point of view. Am J Contact Dermat 1993;4:175-181.

Kalimo K, Kautiainen H, Niskanen T, Niemi L: "Eczema school" to improve compliance in an occupational dermatology clinic. Contact Dermatitis 1999;41:315-319.

Saripalli YV, Achen F, Belsito DV: The detection of clinically relevant contact allergens using a standard screening tray of twenty–three allergens. J Am Acad Dermatol 2003;49:65-69.

Pruritus Ani and Vulvae

Method of
Libby Edwards, MD

Anogenital pruritus, or itching, is a symptom, not a diagnosis. The word *itching* encompasses a number of sensations, including irritation, prickling, and crawling sensations as well as a sensation of needing to scratch. Specifically excluded are burning, soreness, and other pain adjectives.

Unlike medication for pain, no nonspecific anti-itch medications are available. Thus the management of anogenital pruritus begins with an evaluation to diagnose the underlying cause, followed by specific therapy for that etiology (Box 1). The usual causes of itching are infection, dermatosis, neuropathy, or anxiety/depression. Several factors may play a role.

Acute itching is most often related to infection, especially *Candida albicans*. Herpes simplex virus infection, trichomoniasis, *Staphylococcus aureus,* and scabies are less common causes of itching. The most common dermatosis to produce sudden-onset itching is allergic or irritant contact dermatitis, in which something touching the skin (overcleaning, stool retained in skin folds, topical medications, etc.) causes itching.

Chronic itching is most often caused by skin disease, often with exacerbating factors such as secondary infection or irritation from topical medications. The most common dermatoses to cause chronic itching are

---

BOX 1 Causes of Anogenital Itching

Acute Itching
Infection
- *Candida albicans*
- Pinworms
- Trichomoniasis
- Herpes simplex virus infection
- Mollusca contagiosa
- Genital warts, bacterial vaginosis, group B streptococcus

Dermatoses
- Irritant or allergic contact dermatoses
- Eczema, lichen sclerosus, psoriasis, lichen planus

Chronic Itching (Often Multifactorial)
- Dermatoses: Lichen simplex chronicus/eczema, lichen sclerosus, psoriasis, lichen planus
- Neuropathy
- Anxiety/depression
- Infection: Usually only a complicating factor in the face of underlying dermatosis

---

BOX 2 Treatment of Anogenital Itching

Nonspecific Measures
- Patient education and reassurance
- Careful evaluation for infection and dermatoses
- Elimination of irritants: Overwashing, infection, nighttime scratching, unnecessary topical medications and lubricants, infections
- Topical anesthetics: Topical lidocaine (Xylocaine) jelly 2%/ointment 5%, as needed; pramoxine (Summer's Eve Anti-itch Gel) as needed; topical benzocaine (Vagisil) and diphenhydramine (Benadryl) should be avoided
- Nighttime sedation
- Cool soaks/ice (frostbite avoided by wrapping ice in a towel)

Specific Measures
- Itching because of infection
  Acute itching: Treatment with standard therapy.
  Chronic itching: Evaluation for concomitant dermatosis; infection treated and suppressed long enough for skin to heal and itching to respond to therapy for concomitant process.
- Itching because of dermatoses
  Lichen sclerosus: Clobetasol propionate (Temovate) ointment two times per day until skin texture is normal, then three times per week for life (prepubertal girls occasionally experience remission at puberty; boys remit after circumcision). Or (less effective and concern regarding squamous cell carcinoma) chronic tacrolimus (Protopic) 0.1%, two times per day.
  Eczema/lichen simplex chronicus (LSC): Clobetasol propionate ointment two times per day until skin is normal and itching controlled, then frequency tapered to three times weekly, twice weekly, once weekly, then discontinued; restarted when flares occur. Or (less effective) tacrolimus (Protopic) or pimecrolimus (Elidel), two times per day.
- Itching without objective abnormalities
  Treated as for eczema/lichen simplex chronicus with clobetasol propionate for presumed subtle eczema/LSC.
  Amitriptyline (Elavil) (tapered up as high as 150 mg at bedtime), venlafaxine (Effexor) (tapered up as high as 150 mg extended release per day), gabapentin (Neurontin) (up to 3600 mg per day) for neuropathic pain
  Anxiety/depression addressed

---

eczema/lichen simplex chronicus (LSC) and lichen sclerosus (LS). Less common pruritic dermatoses that can affect anogenital skin include psoriasis and nonerosive lichen planus (LP). Although infection is almost never the primary cause of chronic anogenital itching, infection can complicate and perpetuate itching from dermatoses. Some patients exhibit chronic itching despite a normal physical examination and negative cultures. Most often these patients have subtle eczema, but itching on the basis of neuropathy or anxiety/depression can occur. These diagnoses are made by excluding infection and skin disease and by response to therapy.

Management

The first step in management is a very careful examination of the anogenital area, including vulvar and perianal skin folds and the vaginal epithelium (Box 2). Severe symptoms sometimes are produced by subtle signs. Cultures of vaginal secretions and scrapings of scaling skin to evaluate for infection are indicated.

Acute itching on the basis of an infection can generally be cleared rapidly and definitively by treatment of the infection. All dermatoses, whether producing acute or chronic itching, can be treated with an ultrapotent topical corticosteroid ointment (e.g., clobetasol propionate [Temovate]). Ointments are less irritating than creams or gels. Although potent corticosteroids can produce atrophy, striae, and steroid dermatitis when used chronically without supervision, short-term twice-daily use produces safe and rapid control of symptoms. The frequency of application can be tapered when itching is controlled, or a lower potency medication can be substituted. Some dermatoses (LS, psoriasis) require long-term or lifetime thrice-weekly dosing of a corticosteroid to maintain control, whereas others (LSC) usually achieve remission, and medication can be discontinued, at least for prolonged times. Tacrolimus and Pimecrolimus can be beneficial for LSC, LS, and LP, but less so than Clobetasol, and current concerns for secondary squamous cell carcinoma also limit their use for LS and LP.

In addition, they are slow in onset and produce burning with application. Itchy anogenital skin without evidence of an infection or a visible dermatosis should be treated with a potent topical corticosteroid. If unresponsive to a steroid, the addition of medication for neuropathy (amitriptyline [Elavil], gabapentin [Neurontin], venlafaxine [Effexor]) or attention to anxiety/depression should be considered.

 CURRENT DIAGNOSIS

- Examination for skin disease
- Microscopic examinations and cultures for infection
- History of contactants and irritants

CURRENT THERAPY

- Careful evaluation for underlying etiologies
- Specific therapies for all appropriate underlying etiologies
- Specific therapy continued long enough for the skin to heal and the itch-scratch cycle to cease
- Patient education regarding the chronic/recurrent nature of itching and the role of irritants
- Consideration of neuropathy and anxiety/depression in patients without observable disease who are resistant to topical corticosteroid therapy

Whatever the cause, certain nonspecific measures can improve itching and contribute to a more rapid response to specific therapy, including the following:

- Avoidance of irritants, such as overwashing and unnecessary topical medications.
- Topical anesthetics (lidocaine [Xylocaine] jelly 2% or ointment 5%) that can temporarily improve itching and minimize ongoing irritation from scratching (but topical benzocaine [Vagisil] and diphenhydramine [Benadryl], which can be irritating and allergenic, should be avoided).
- Nighttime sedation, which can both provide well-needed respite from sleepless itchy nights and protect the skin from irritating scratching during nighttime hours. Tricyclic medications such as amitriptyline and doxepin (Sinequan) produce deeper sleep and less scratching than diphenhydramine and hydroxyzine (Atarax).

Although many clinicians use antihistamines for all itching, this class of medication has no intrinsic anti-itch properties and is generally useful only for the histamine-mediated itch of urticaria, usually a generalized rather than anogenital process.

Other, less potent measures that can be used in patients with recalcitrant symptoms include topical doxepin (Zonalon), tacrolimus (Protopic 0.1%), or pimecrolimus (Elidel). These medications are beneficial primarily in patients with mild to moderate eczema/LSC.

Patients should be advised that all causes of itching can be chronic or recurrent. Thus recurrence of itching does not necessarily reflect a failure of diagnosis or therapy but rather a need for recurrent or chronic therapy that is sufficiently prolonged for the skin to heal completely and for the itch-scratch cycle to be broken.

REFERENCES

Bohm M, Frieling U, Luger TA, et al: Successful treatment of anogenital lichen sclerosus with topical tacrolimus. Arch Dermatol 2003; 48:444-448.
Bornstein J, Heifetz S, Kellner Y, et al: Clobetasol dipropionate 0.05% versus testosterone propionate 2% topical application for severe vulvar lichen sclerosus. Am J Obstet Gynecol 1998;178(1, Pt 1): 80-84.
Cohen AD, Masalha R, Medvedovsky E, Vardy DA: Brachioradial pruritus: A symptom of neuropathy. J Am Acad Dermatol 2003; 48(6):825-828.
Farage MA: Vulvar susceptibility to contact irritants and allergens: a review. Arch Gyneol Obstet 2005;272:167-172.
Koca R, Altin R, Konuk N, et al: Sleep distubance in patients with lichen simplex chronicus and its relationship to noctunal scratching: A case control study. South Med J. 2006;99:482-485.
Margesson LJ: Contact dermatitis of the vulva. Dermatol Ther 2004;17:20-27.
Stellon A: Neurogenic pruritus: An unrecognized problem? A retrospective case series of treatment by acupuncture. Acupunct Med 2002;20(4):186-190.
Weichert GE: An approch to the treatment of anogenital pruritus. Dermatol Ther 2004;17:129-133.

Urticaria and Angioedema

Method of
Eugene W. Monroe, MD

Urticaria (hives) is a skin reaction pattern characterized by transient, pruritic, edematous, lightly erythematous papules or wheals, frequently with central clearing. *Angioedema* describes swellings of the deep dermis or subcutaneous tissue involving mucous membranes and loose tissues around the eyes, lips, or genitalia. Urticaria is extremely common. Approximately 15% to 20% of the general population have at least one episode of urticaria, angioedema, or both during their lives. The potential causes of urticaria are numerous, including drugs, food, infections, internal diseases, inhalants, bites/stings, contactants, immunologic processes, psychogenic factors, genetic abnormalities, and physical agents (dermographism and pressure, cholinergic, cold, solar, and heat urticaria).

Classification

Urticaria is classified as acute or chronic, depending on the duration of the condition. Most cases of urticaria are classified as acute because they persist for only a few days to a few weeks. The incidence of acute urticaria is between 10% and 20% of the population. The etiology is usually detected, often an allergic reaction to a food or medication, or related to an acute infection. Many cases of urticaria are never seen by a physician. The initial aspect of therapy is the elimination of any suspected cause. Drug therapy should begin with the use of a so-called nonsedating H_1 antihistamine. In severe urticarial reactions or in cases associated with asthma or laryngeal edema, stronger medical management is required, including the use of subcutaneous injection of epinephrine or systemic corticosteroids.

When urticaria persists longer than 6 weeks, it is classified as chronic urticaria. The incidence of this form is between 0.1% and 3% of the population. The course is variable, from months to years, with 20% lasting longer than 20 years. Approximately 40% of the cases are associated with angioedema. Unfortunately, the etiology is not found in 60% to 95% of these cases, with most either idiopathic or autoimmune in nature. Treatment programs for chronic urticaria focus on measures that provide symptomatic relief.

TABLE 1 Comparison of Second-Generation H₁ Antihistamines

Drug	Recommended Dosage	Efficacy in Urticaria	Side Effects at Recommended Dosage	Side Effects at Higher than Recommended Dosage
Loratadine (Claritin)	10 mg qd	+++	None	Mild sedation
Cetirizine (Zyrtec)	10 mg qd	+++	Mild sedation	Dose-related increases in sedation
Fexofenadine (Allegra)	60 mg bid or 180 mg qd	+++	None	None
Desloratadine (Clarinex)	5 mg qd	+++	None	Mild sedation

Abbreviations: bid = twice per day; qd = every day.

Diagnosis

The clinical diagnosis of urticaria is reasonably easy. Finding an underlying cause, especially for chronic urticaria, however, is usually extremely frustrating for the patient and the physician.

The most important diagnostic test in the evaluation of a patient with urticaria is a detailed history, which should include the location of lesions, morphology of lesions, pattern of attacks, precipitating factors, review of medical systems, and review of potential etiologies of urticaria. Diagnostic tests are selected on the basis of suspicions elicited by a meticulous history and physical examination. Potential minimal baseline tests might include a complete blood count with differential, a chemistry panel, and a sedimentation rate. Other possible tests based on the history might include thyroid autoantibodies, physical urticaria challenge tests, autologous serum skin testing, and so on.

Treatment

The ideal treatment for urticaria is identification and removal of its cause. If that is not possible, the reduction of various triggering factors should be attempted, especially in cases of physical urticaria. The drug management of urticaria centers around four theoretical treatment approaches: blocking the effects of already released histamine on the receptor sites of cutaneous blood vessels; blocking the release of histamine and other mediators from mast cells; blocking mediators other than histamine that can cause hives; and modulating the inflammatory, cellular, and immunologic components of the urticarial process.

H₁ antihistamines remain the first line of therapy for urticaria. First-generation antihistamines such as hydroxyzine (Atarax), diphenhydramine (Benadryl), and chlorpheniramine (Chlor-Trimeton) are moderately effective in treating urticaria. The usefulness of these agents is sometimes limited by undesirable side effects, however, especially central nervous system (CNS) effects such as daytime sedation and anticholinergic effects. Because of these problems, a new class of peripherally acting second-generation antihistamines, most of which are labeled "nonsedating," are now available.

Four second-generation antihistamines are currently available on the market in the United States. In order of their FDA approval, these are loratadine (Claritin), cetirizine (Zyrtec), fexofenadine (Allegra), and desloratadine (Clarinex). Table 1 compares these agents in terms of dosing, potency, and side effects.

In clinical studies of chronic urticaria, the efficacy of the second-generation antihistamines is statistically superior to placebo and clinically comparable to the strongest of the first-generation agents such as hydroxyzine. The few clinical studies comparing the second-generation agents with each other in chronic urticaria show no statistically significant differences in efficacy.

The second-generation H₁ antihistamines are a heterogeneous group of compounds with lesser sedation than the first generation. Loratadine, desloratadine, and fexofenadine are nonsedating at the recommended dosage. Cetirizine is sedating at recommended dosage, but less than the first-generation agents. Only fexofenadine is totally nonsedating at any dosage above recommended levels.

What if monotherapy with a second-generation H₁ antihistamine does not adequately control the signs and symptoms of urticaria? Figure 1 summarizes a practical treatment algorithm for patients with chronic urticaria. The next step is to add another H₁ antihistamine to the original second-generation antihistamine, either an additional second-generation agent or a first-generation agent at night. The next option is to add an agent that blocks the H₂ receptors, either a tricyclic antidepressant such as doxepin (Sinequan) or an H₂ receptor antagonist.

The use of H₂ receptor antagonists is supported by the evidence that the cutaneous blood vessels possess H₂ receptors as well as the commonly recognized H₁ receptors, and these receptors are involved in the mediation of cutaneous vasodilatation and vascular permeability. Tricyclic antidepressants such as doxepin are potent H₁ and H₂ antihistaminic antagonists. Studies show doxepin to have comparable efficacy and side effects to hydroxyzine in the treatment of chronic urticaria. The usual initial dosage is 10 to 25 mg at night, which can be increased to two or three times daily if necessary. Several clinical studies show that the combination of an H₁ antihistamine and an H₂ antihistamine in both chronic urticaria and dermographism has added benefit compared to the use of an H₁ antihistamine alone. The dosage of the H₂ antihistamine is similar to that

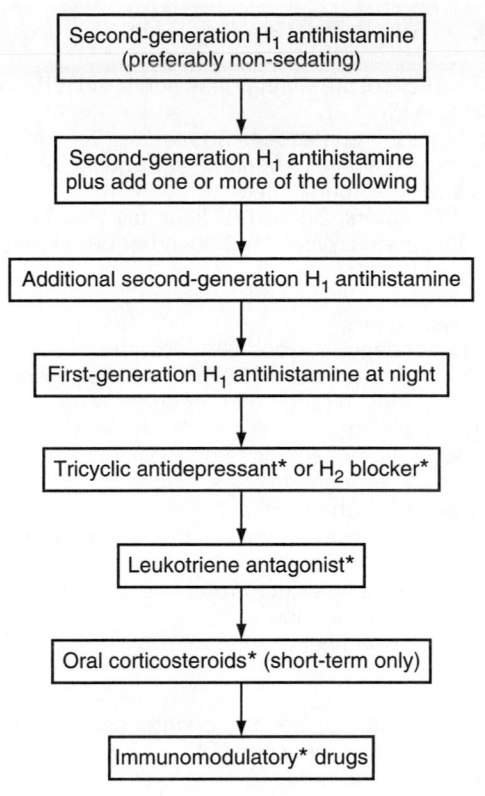

 CURRENT THERAPY

- H_1 antihistamines remain the first choice of therapy for urticaria, both acute and chronic.
- The second-generation, so-called nonsedating antihistamines, are the treatment of choice for many patients, with urticaria because of their comparable efficacy and better safety profile compared to the first-generation antihistamines.
- Several other agents demonstrate additive value when monotherapy with H_1 antihistamines is not sufficient to control the refractory cases of chronic urticaria.

Second-generation H_1 antihistamine (preferably non-sedating)

Second-generation H_1 antihistamine plus add one or more of the following

Additional second-generation H_1 antihistamine

First-generation H_1 antihistamine at night

Tricyclic antidepressant* or H_2 blocker*

Leukotriene antagonist*

Oral corticosteroids* (short-term only)

Immunomodulatory* drugs

* Not FDA approved in this indication.

FIGURE 1. Treatment algorithm for patients with chronic urticaria.

used for gastrointestinal disease—cimetidine (Tagamet), 300 mg four times daily, or ranitidine (Zantac), 150 mg twice daily.

Several mediators other than histamine can increase vascular permeability and thus cause hives. A few recent studies show that leukotriene receptor antagonists, such as montelukast (Singulair, 10 mg once daily) and zafirlukast (Accolate, 20 mg twice daily), may be beneficial in some cases of chronic urticaria.

Systemic corticosteroids are sometimes indicated for the management of moderate to severe acute urticaria, pressure urticaria, or urticarial vasculitis. They have no place in extended therapy of chronic urticaria, although they may occasionally be used as a short course of therapy to break the cycle of a resistant case. A common routine is the use of prednisone beginning at 30 to 40 mg daily, tapered over 2 to 4 weeks. Systemic corticosteroids should

be discontinued as soon as possible or at most maintained on an alternate-day basis.

In refractory cases of severe chronic urticaria or cases of "steroid-dependent" urticaria, other medications might be considered. Cyclosporine (Neoral, Sandimmune) in doses of 4 mg/kg per day is shown in some controlled studies to be effective in severe refractory cases of chronic urticaria or autoimmune urticaria.

In urticarial vasculitis, patients present clinically with urticaria that by skin biopsy is shown to be leukocytoclastic vasculitis. Treatment of this condition is often unsatisfactory. In addition to the use of antihistamines, other occasionally beneficial agents include nonsteroidal anti-inflammatory drugs such as indomethacin (Indocin), 25 to 50 mg three times daily; colchicine, 0.6 mg twice daily; dapsone, 50 to 300 mg daily; or hydroxychloroquine (Plaquenil), 200 to 400 mg per day. Systemic corticosteroids are also sometimes effective.

REFERENCES

Finn AF, Kaplan AP, Fretwell R, et al: A double-blind, placebo-controlled trial of fexofenadine HCl in the treatment of chronic idiopathic urticaria. J Allergy Clin Immunol 1999;103:1071-1078.

Grattan CEH, Sabroe RA, Greaves MW: Chronic urticaria. J Am Acad Dermatol 2002;46:645-657.

Greaves M: Chronic urticaria. J Allergy Clin Immunol 2000;105:664-672.

Kaplan AP: Chronic urticaria and angioedema. N Engl J Med 2002;346:175-179.

Kaplan AP: Chronic urticaria: Pathogenesis and treatment. J Allergy Clin Immunol 2004;114:465-474.

Lee EE, Maibach HI: Treatment of urticaria. An evidence-based evaluation of antihistamines. Am J Clin Dermatol 2001;2:151-158.

Monroe EW: Urticaria. Curr Probl Dermatol 1993;V:113-140.

Monroe E, Finn A, Patel P, et al: Efficacy and safety of desloratadine 5 mg once daily in the treatment of chronic idiopathic urticaria: A double-blind, randomized, placebo controlled trial. J Am Acad Dermatol 2003;48:535-541.

Zuberbier T: Urticaria. Allergy 2003;58:1224-1234.

 CURRENT DIAGNOSIS

The key clinical features of urticaria are the following:

- Erythematous, edematous papules or wheals, often with central clearing
- Pruritus (usually without signs of excoriation) and transient nature of individual lesions, which last 1 to 12 hours but definitely less than 24 to 48 hours.

Pigmentary Disorders

Method of
Norman Levine, MD

Skin pigmentation is the body's best defense against ultraviolet light radiation and is an important cultural and social characteristic. Almost all of the skin's characteristic hue comes from melanin, a complex protein produced in epidermal melanocytes. Disorders of pigmentation occur if an abnormal number of melanocytes is present, if the melanocytes produce an inappropriate amount of melanin, or if the pigment is deposited in anomalous sites.

Hyperpigmentary Disorders

MELASMA

Clinical Findings

Melasma is a reticulated hyperpigmentation of the face, neck, and forearms that occurs most commonly in women taking oral contraceptives or in women who are pregnant ("the mask of pregnancy"). Men and nonpregnant women may also be affected. Hormonal and genetic factors are operative, but the exact cause of this malady is unknown. Sunlight exacerbates the condition.

Treatment

If the extra pigment is located primarily in the epidermis, the patches are tan. These lesions respond well to bleaching agents. Pigment that is situated deeper in the dermis is blue or gray and does not lighten well even after prolonged treatment. A combination of hydroquinone, tretinoin, and fluocinolone (Tri-Luma) applied daily for at least 8 weeks and for as long as 1 year[3] can produce substantial lightening, particularly in those with predominantly epidermal hyperpigmentation. Avoidance of sun exposure and use of potent sunscreens and other forms of sun protection (Table 1) are mandatory because sun-induced pigmentation can reverse the positive effects of the medication. Some hydroquinone products, such as Viquin Forte and Solaquin Forte, contain sunscreens. Patients should avoid using hydroquinone-containing agents on skin that is sunburned, windburned, dry, chapped, or irritated or on open wounds. Azelaic acid 20% cream (Azelex)[1] applied twice daily with or without tretinoin 0.025% cream for 6 months may also bleach the patches.

Physical means of removing the excess pigment may be helpful in those with fair skin and mainly epidermal melanin deposition. Mid-depth trichloroacetic acid[1] (Tri-Chlor) or glycolic acid chemical peels, nonablative laser resurfacing, or intense pulse light therapy will lighten the skin, but the results are incomplete and recurrences are common. Use of hydroquinone after these procedures may provide long-term improvement.

---

[1]Not FDA approved for this indication.
[3]Exceeds dosage recommended by the manufacturer.

TABLE 1 Sun Protection Strategies

- Avoid sun exposure during peak hours of UVB and UVA (9 AM to 4 PM)
- Apply high-SPF sunscreens 30 minutes before exposure and again 15 minutes after going into the sun
  - Organic Absorbers/Filters
    - PABA esters: Good UVB filter; fair UVA filter
    - Cinnamates: Weak UVB absorber but stabilizes other agents
    - Salicylates: Weak UVB absorber but stabilizes other agents
    - Benzophenone: Good UVA absorber
    - Avobenzone (Parsol 1789): Good UVA absorber, particularly in range that produces drug phototoxicity
    - Mexoryl (Capital Soleil Sun Block Cream and others): Very good UVA absorber
  - Inorganic Absorbers/Filters
    - Titanium dioxide: Protects over wide UV range but may leave white film
    - Microfine zinc oxide: Protects over wide UV range
- Wear protective clothing
  - Tightly woven fibers
  - Thick fabrics
  - Dark fabrics
  - Fabrics cleansed in optical brighteners or UV absorbers (e.g., Tinosorb FD)
  - Hats with wide brims

Abbreviations: PABA = *para*-aminobenzoic acid; SPF = skin-protection factor; UV = ultraviolet; UVA = ultraviolet A; UVB = ultraviolet B.

SOLAR LENTIGO

Clinical Findings

Solar lentigines are present in many fair-skinned white individuals older than 50 years. They are strongly related to cumulative and intermittent intense sun exposure, are considered a sign of photodamage, and are largely confined to sites of chronic sun exposure.

Lentigines presumably arise as a protective mechanism against ultraviolet light injury. The lesions are stellate brown macules that occur mostly on the dorsa of the hands, on the face, and over the shoulders.

Treatment

Because solar lentigines have no malignant potential, the purpose of treatment is cosmetic only. Bleaching creams containing hydroquinone (Tri-Luma) or azelaic acid (Azelex) work slowly and incompletely in most cases. The addition of tretinoin (Retin-A) cream may improve the results. A combination of mequinol 2% and tretinoin 0.01% (Solage) may be more effective. Light liquid nitrogen cryotherapy or destruction by electrodesiccation and curettage is effective for localized lesions; there is a risk for posttherapy hypopigmentation, particularly with cryotherapy. Mid-depth trichloroacetic acid or glycolic acid chemical peels can eradicate multiple lesions in a single sitting. The Nd-YAG laser, the Q-switched ruby laser, and the nonablative resurfacing laser are very effective at removing lentigines, but the treatments are costly.

DRUG-INDUCED HYPERPIGMENTATION

Clinical Findings

Several medications can produce abnormal skin or nail pigmentation because of either deposition of the drug or its metabolite in the skin or drug-induced increased melanin production by melanocytes. Compounds such as 5-fluorouracil (Efudex), gold, and amiodarone (Cordarone) produce preferential darkening in sun-exposed sites. Other medications, such as bleomycin (Blenoxane) and cyclophosphamide (Cytoxan), cause pigmented bands in the nails. Minocycline (Minocin) may produce brown-gray discoloration in old scars. The color changes seen with medication reactions range from tan to slate gray to blue-black (Table 2).

Treatment

In most instances, the dyspigmentation associated with drugs slowly fades after the drug is discontinued. Certain medications, such as gold and topical hydroquinone (Solaquin), produce color changes that may be irreversible. Use of sunscreens is encouraged in patients with drug-induced hyperpigmentation to minimize additional pigment production from the sun.

POSTINFLAMMATORY HYPERPIGMENTATION

Clinical Findings

After an epidermal injury, such as occurs with a superficial burn, melanin either is carried into or falls into the dermis, where it is engulfed by macrophages. This pigment may remain indefinitely and results in hyperpigmentation. If the melanin is close to the surface, the lesions are tan or brown. If the pigment is deposited deeper in the dermis, the skin becomes gray or blue-gray.

Treatment

If the pigment is superficial, the areas can be lightened somewhat with the regimens previously noted for melasma. This process will not work well for deep dermal melanosis. Q-switched lasers may accelerate pigment removal. Sunscreens are helpful for minimizing increased tanning at sites that are already dark.

Hypopigmentary Disorders

VITILIGO

Clinical Findings

Vitiligo is a common condition of uncertain etiology characterized by loss of skin pigment. The typical lesion is a milk-white macule or patch. The hair in the affected sites may also be white. The lesions often have a remarkably symmetrical distribution. There is also a variety in which the depigmentation occurs in a segmental pattern along the path of a peripheral nerve.

Treatment

Treatment can be tailored to suit the extent of the disease, the location of the depigmented patches, the degree of psychosocial disruption that the condition causes, and the amount of time that the patient has to treat this chronic problem. For limited lesions, a trial of high-potency topical corticosteroids, such as clobetasol (Temovate), applied twice daily for at least 3 months[3] is indicated. For facial lesions, less potent corticosteroids, such as fluocinonide (Lidex) 0.05% cream, are safer but still can produce cutaneous atrophy and steroid-induced rosacea if used for a prolonged period. Topical immune modulators, such as

---

[3]Exceeds dosage recommended by the manufacturer.

TABLE 2 Medication-Induced Hyperpigmentation

Medication	Clinical Findings
Amiodarone (Cordarone)	Gray discoloration, particularly in sun-exposed skin
Bleomycin (Blenoxane)	Hyperpigmentation over joints and nails
	Linear pigmented bands after trauma
Busulfan (Myleran)	Addison disease-like generalized hyperpigmentation
5-Fluorouracil (Adrucil)	Increased pigmentation in sun-exposed areas of skin
Dactinomycin (Cosmegen)	Generalized hyperpigmentation with accentuation on the face
Daunorubicin (Cerubidine)	Transverse nail bands and sun-induced hyperpigmentation
Doxorubicin (Adriamycin)	Nail pigmentation and increased pigment on palms, soles, and oral mucosa
Gold	Blue-gray discoloration in sun-exposed areas, particularly around the eyes
Hydroxychloroquine (Plaquenil)	Brown to gray dyspigmentation over anterior legs and face
Hydroxyurea (Hydrea)	Hyperpigmentation over pressure points and in the nails
L-Dopa (Sinemet)	Diffuse hyperpigmentation
Methotrexate (Rheumatrex)	Sun-induced hyperpigmentation
Minocycline (Minocin)	Blue-black discoloration in old scars, on the lower extremities, and on the oral mucosa
Oral contraceptives	Melasma, darkening of nipples and nevi
Silver (Silvadene)	Generalized gray discoloration, including nails and sclerae

tacrolimus[1] 0.1% ointment (Protopic), are often very effective for lesions on the head and neck regions when used twice daily for many months.

The most effective therapy for widespread vitiligo is phototherapy, most often given as narrowband ultraviolet B phototherapy. Photochemotherapy (psoralen plus ultraviolet A [PUVA]) also works well, but the skin cancer risks and the expense and side effects associated with ingestion of methoxsalen before each ultraviolet A treatment makes this form of phototherapy less desirable. A minimum of 50 treatments is usually needed for repigmentation to occur. Localized areas of depigmentation can be treated with the excimer laser, which is a means for delivering high-intensity narrowband ultraviolet B light to small areas of involved skin.

For dark-skinned patients with depigmentation involving more than 50% of the body, bleaching of the uninvolved skin may make the skin tones uniform by causing complete depigmentation of the integument. Monobenzyl ether of hydroquinone (Benoquin) 20% cream applied twice daily for 3 to 6[3] months to the normal skin can cause permanent loss of pigment. Before embarking on this treatment, the patient must understand that he or she will never have his or her normal skin color again. Vitiliginous skin contains no protective melanin. Thus, the patient is highly susceptible to sunburn and the chronic effects of sun exposure, such as actinic keratoses and skin cancer. Daily sunscreen use and protective clothing will aid in retarding the development of sun-damaged skin (see Table 1).

The extent of psychological devastation that may accompany the progression of vitiligo should not be underestimated. Support and reassurance can be very therapeutic. Referral to a trained cosmetologist who can teach the patient the proper use of cover-up cosmetics is helpful. Self-tanning products containing dihydroxyacetone, such as Self Tanning Lotion by Almay or Sunless Tanning Lotion by Vaseline Intensive Care, can help to cover the white spots.

IDIOPATHIC GUTTATE HYPOMELANOSIS

Clinical Findings

Idiopathic guttate hypomelanosis is an extremely common condition in which patients develop asymptomatic confetti-like white macules on the extremities. The spots rarely are larger than 1 cm in diameter and have no tendency to involute spontaneously. Thus, over many years, hundreds of hypopigmented macules may be acquired. The cause of this condition is unknown, but it may be related in some way to sun exposure.

Treatment

Careful destruction with trichloroacetic acid[1] (Tri-Chlor) 25% occasionally causes isolated lesions to gain pigment. For the individual with hundreds of lesions, a full-extremity trichloroacetic acid chemical peel may result in more uniform pigmentation. This is particularly true for the person with concomitant sun-damaged skin who has widespread cutaneous mottling.

[1]Not FDA approved for this indication.
[3]Exceeds dosage recommended by the manufacturer.

CURRENT DIAGNOSIS

- Melasma is exacerbated by sunlight exposure.
- Lentigo occurs on chronically sun-exposed areas in individuals with fair skin.
- Drug-induced hyperpigmentation may involve the nails and mucosal surfaces.
- Superficial postinflammatory hyperpigmentation is tan in color, whereas deeper pigmentation has a bluer hue.
- Depigmented patches of vitiligo often show bilateral symmetry.
- Idiopathic guttate hypomelanosis presents with a confetti-like hypopigmentation of the extremities.
- Pityriasis alba typically appears in children with atopic dermatitis.

PITYRIASIS ALBA

Clinical Findings

Pityriasis alba is a common form of hypomelanosis that occurs mainly in children and young adults with atopic dermatitis, often with darker skin types. The process begins as poorly defined pink, scaly papules, which evolve into hypopigmented plaques with a fine, powdery scale. The lesions are found on the face, upper extremities, and upper trunk. In most instances, this condition represents postinflammatory hypopigmentation after a flare of eczema.

Treatment

Mild- or moderate-strength topical corticosteroids, such as hydrocortisone 1% cream or triamcinolone (Kenalog) 0.1% cream, applied twice daily help to reduce residual inflammation and thus to delimit the process. Emollient creams will mask the scale and improve the appearance and texture of the skin. Judicious sun exposure will stimulate epidermal melanocytes to produce more melanin and will darken the affected sites.

CURRENT THERAPY

- Melasma: Tri-Luma applied daily for at least 8 weeks.
- Lentigo: Nd-YAG laser or Q-switched ruby laser for multiple lesions.
- Drug-induced dyspigmentation: Stop the offending medication if possible.
- Postinflammatory hyperpigmentation: Tri-Luma cream applied daily for at least 8 weeks.
- Vitiligo: Clobetasol 0.05% cream applied twice daily for months[3] or tacrolimus[1] (Protopic) 0.1% ointment applied twice daily for months.
- Idiopathic guttate hypomelanosis: Trichloroacetic acid 25% solution used as chemical peel.
- Pityriasis alba: Hydrocortisone 1% cream applied twice daily.

[1]Not FDA approved for this indication.
[3]Exceeds dosage recommended by the manufacturer.

REFERENCES

Bastiaens M, Hoefnagel J, Westendorp R, et al: Solar lentigines are strongly related to sun exposure in contrast to ephelides. Pigment Cell Res 2004;17:225-229.

Grimes P: New insights and new therapies in vitiligo. JAMA 2005;293:730-735.

Jarratt M: Mequinol 2%/tretinoin 0.01% solution: An effective and safe alternative to hydroquinone 3% in the treatment of solar lentigines. Cutis 2004;74:319-322.

Kanwar AJ, Dogra S, Parsad D, Kumar B: Narrow-band UVB for the treatment of vitiligo: An emerging effective and well-tolerated therapy. Eur J Dermatol 2005;44:57-60.

Kullavanijaya P, Lim H: Photoprotection. J Am Acad Dermatol 2005;52:937-958.

Nanda S, Grover C, Reddy BS: Efficacy of hydroquinone (2%) versus tretinoin (0.025%) as adjunct topical agents for chemical peeling in patients with melasma. Dermatol Surg 2004;30:385-388.

Torok HM, Jones T, Rich P, et al: Hydroquinone 4%, tretinoin 0.05%, fluocinolone acetonide 0.01%: a safe and efficacious 12-month treatment for melasma. Cutis 2005;75:57-62.

Sunburn

Method of
Henry W. Lim, MD, and Camile Hexsel, MD

Ultraviolet (UV) radiation is subdivided into UVC (wavelengths ranging from 270–290 nm), UVB (290–320 nm), and UVA (320–400 nm). UVA is further subdivided into UVA2 (320–340 nm) and UVA1 (340–400 nm). The stratosphere blocks most of the UVC and large amounts of the UVB rays before they reach the earth's surface; however, little or no UVA is filtered.

Sunlight at noon consists of 95% UVA and only 5% UVB. Because UVB is 1000-fold more erythemogenic compared to UVA, sunburn is predominantly a reflection of the biologic effect of UVB. UVB-induced erythema becomes visible 2 to 6 hours after irradiation, reaches a maximum in 8 to 24 hours, and fades after about 72 hours, depending on the individual's skin phototype. The erythema, which fades rapidly, is followed by delayed tanning at 72 hours.

Because UVA has long wavelengths, it penetrates deeper into the dermis compared to UVB. Approximately 10% of solar erythema is caused by UVA. UVA-induced erythema is biphasic. It becomes visible immediately after exposure, subsides by 4 hours, and reaches a second peak in 6 to 15 hours, fading within 24 to 120 hours. The predominant effect of UVA is cutaneous pigmentary alterations (pigment darkening and delayed tanning).

Various mediators of inflammation, including histamine, eicosanoids, interleukins, tumor necrosis factor, and adhesion molecules play a role in sunburn reaction.

Clinical Manifestations

Following excessive sun exposure, erythema, edema, warmth, and tenderness are present in the exposed areas. Pruritus may also be present. Vesicle and bullae formation

CURRENT DIAGNOSIS

- Erythema, edema, and tenderness develop on sun-exposed areas 2 to 24 hours after irradiation, followed by desquamation and tanning.
- Relatively sun-protected areas, such as nasolabial folds, submental and postauricular areas, and inner aspect of arms and forearms, are spared.

with occasional erosions and ulcerations can develop within 24 to 48 hours in more severe cases. Massive UV exposure is accompanied by constitutional symptoms of headache, weakness, fever, and chills, with or without tachycardia and hypotension. The distribution of the eruption is diagnostic. It is seen exclusively in sun-exposed areas, with sharp cutoffs at areas protected by clothing. Therefore, there is accentuated involvement of the forehead, nose, chin, V area of the neck, extensor forearm, and dorsum of the hand. Areas that are naturally protected from sun exposure, such as the nasolabial folds and other skin folds, submental and postauricular areas, and the inner aspects of the arms and forearms, are spared. Resolution of the erythema is followed by desquamation and tanning, which occurs in about 1 week.

Treatment

Because eicosanoids are a known mediator of sunburn, topical corticosteroids and nonsteroidal anti-inflammatory drugs (NSAIDs), usually used in combination, is the treatment of choice. Topical corticosteroids and NSAIDs must be started within 24 hours after the exposure and ideally within the first 4 to 6 hours. In severe cases, a 7- to 10-day course of oral prednisone at a dose of 1 mg/kg, with a maximum of 80 mg, is indicated.

Oral antihistamines for treatment of sunburn have not been extensively studied, and their benefit is not completely known. A few studies reported lack of efficacy. However, they are commonly used as an antipruritic measure. Topical antihistamines should not be used because of the possibility of induction of allergic contact dermatitis.

Topical and oral antioxidants, such as polyphenols from tea, vitamin C, vitamin E, and fish oil, have been shown to decrease UV-induced inflammation in animal models and in studies involving a few human subjects. Further investigation using a larger number of subjects is needed before the benefit of antioxidants can be confirmed.

Supportive treatments, which include cool compresses, emollients, oral hydration, rest, and sun avoidance for a few days, are usually necessary. The presentation of acute sunburn is an excellent opportunity for patient education on photoprotection (see next section).

Prevention

Preventive measures for sunburn are summarized in Table 1.

Sunscreen is an integral part of photoprotection. In the United States, UV filters are regulated as over-the-counter

CURRENT THERAPY

- Treatment is based on symptoms and includes cool compresses, emollients, oral hydration, and rest as appropriate.
- In severe cases, topical and systemic corticosteroids and nonsteroidal anti-inflammatory drugs (NSAIDs), alone or in combination, are appropriate.
- Prevention is key to the management of sunburn (see Table 1).
- Sunscreens are regulated by the Food and Drug Administration as over-the-counter substances. They are usually a combination of more than one organic or inorganic filters that provide ultraviolet A and ultraviolet B protection.
- Cutaneous effects of excessive ultraviolet radiation are classified into acute and chronic effects. Acute effects are sunburn, vitamin D synthesis, photodermatoses, and acute photoimmunosuppression. Chronic effects are development of photoaging changes, solar lentigines, actinic keratoses, and, most importantly, skin cancers.

---

medications by the Food and Drug Administration (FDA). In 1999, the FDA issued a monograph listing 16 UV filters; these are the only filters that can be marketed in sunscreen products. UV filters are divided into *inorganic* (previously termed physical or nonchemical) filters and *organic* (previously termed chemical) filters. Commercially available sunscreens are often a combination of more than one agent. These agents are discussed later.

Only two inorganic filters are listed in the FDA monograph: titanium dioxide and zinc dioxide. These filters are broad-spectrum filters. The organic filters can be divided into UVA and UVB filters. The UVA filters available in the United States are the benzophenones (oxybenzone, sulisobenzone, dioxybenzone), butyl methoxydibenzoyl (avobenzone [Parsol 1789]), and meradimate (methyl anthranilate). Mexoryl and Tinosorb are UVA photostable sunscreens used in most parts of the world but are not listed in the FDA monograph. Mexoryl SX (ecamsule) was recently approved by the FDA for marketing in the United States.

TABLE 1 Preventive Measures for Sunburn

- Avoid sun exposure between 10 AM and 4 PM. If avoidance is not possible or practical, protect the skin with photoprotection measures.
- Apply broad-spectrum sunscreen with a skin-protection factor (SPF) of 15 or above.
- If possible, sunscreens should be applied at least every 2 hours and after swimming, sweating, and towel drying.
- Use of physical barriers, such as shades, wide-brimmed hats, tightly woven protective clothing, and sunglasses, is recommended.
- For individuals at risk of vitamin D insufficiency, oral vitamin D supplements are recommended.
- Photoprotection should be applied to children.
- Children younger than 6 months should be protected mainly by physical measures. Application of sunscreen to exposed areas only is probably safe.

UVB filters include *para*-aminobenzoic acid (PABA) derivates (PABA and padimate O or octyl dimethyl PABA), cinnamates (octinoxate and cinoxate), salicylates (octisalate or octyl salicylate, homosalate or homomenthyl salicylate, trolamine salicylate), octocrylene, and ensulizole.

REFERENCES

Benvenuto-Andrade C, Cestari TF, Mota A, et al: Photoprotection in adolescence. Skinmed 2005;4:229-233.

Cavallo J, DeLeo VA: Sunburn. Dermatol Clin 1986;4:181-187.

Driscoll MS, Wagner RF Jr: Clinical management of the acute sunburn reaction. Cutis 2000;66:53-58.

Han A, Maibach HI: Management of acute sunburn. Am J Clin Dermatol 2004;5:39-47.

Hönigsman H: Erythema and pigmentation. Photodermatol Photoimmunol Photomed 2002;18:75-81.

Kullavanijaya P, Lim HW: Photoprotection. J Am Acad Dermatol 2005;52:937-958.

Lovato CY, Shoveller JA, Peters L, Rivers JK: Canadian National Survey on Sun Exposure & Protective Behaviours: Youth at leisure. Cancer Prev Control 1998;2:117-122.

Maier T, Korting HC: Sunscreens—Which and what for? Skin Pharmacol Physiol 2005;18:253-262.

Thompson L: Trying to look SUNsational? Complexity persists in using sunscreens. FDA Consum 2000;34:15-21.

The Nervous System

Alzheimer's Disease

Method of
Monica Peterson Gordon, MD,
and L. Jaime Fitten, MD

Definition and Clinical Presentation

Alzheimer's disease (AD) is a progressive, neurodegenerative disorder characterized by a gradual decline of cognitive processes, such as memory, language, judgment, behavior, and global functioning. According to the *Diagnostic and Statistical Manual of Mental Disorders, Fourth Edition (DSM-IV, 2000)*, dementia of the Alzheimer's type is the development of multiple cognitive deficits manifested by both memory impairment and one or more cognitive disturbances, such as aphasia, apraxia, agnosia, and disturbance in executive functioning. The deficits must cause significant impairment in social or occupational functioning and represent a decline from previous levels of functioning and cannot be due to psychiatric, systemic, substance-induced states, or delirium that cause cognitive impairment or produce the dementia syndrome. Other more detailed, research-oriented criteria also have been developed by the National Institute of Neurological and Communicative Disorders and Stroke and the Alzheimer's Disease and Related Disorders Association (NINCDS-ADRDA, 1984).

Alzheimer's disease has a gradual onset often beginning after age 60 years but most commonly after age 70 years. The rarer familial forms can have an onset as early as the fourth decade of life. Recent studies suggest that an isolated, mild but progressive forgetfulness, in the absence of functional or other cognitive impairment, signals a preclinical stage of the disease in a high percentage of cases and has been referred to as *mild cognitive impairment* of the amnestic type. Typically, AD has a 10- to 12-year progressive course. In its early stage, the disease is characterized by a declarative memory deficit that makes it difficult for patients to learn new information or recall recently experienced events. During this stage, language

deficits are not always immediately apparent; however, a degree of word finding difficulty may exist. In addition, minor difficulties with visuospatial and drawing skills may be found. Mild executive dysfunction or subtle personality changes, such as reduction in spontaneity and initiative, may be present. Variations in mood may occur. As the disease progresses, memory deficits become more profound, and most of the patient's capacity for new memory formation is lost. Access to old memories becomes increasingly impaired. Language and other cognitive deficits become more pronounced, with clear evidence of aphasia, apraxia and agnosia. The ability to manipulate concepts is lost, and thought becomes increasingly simple and concrete. During this phase, patients usually begin to exhibit behavioral and psychiatric symptoms, such as agitation, wandering, and irritability. They may experience circadian abnormalities, such as sleep cycle reversal. They may also develop psychotic symptoms such as persecutory delusions, and auditory or visual hallucinations. In the advanced stages, patients have more profound cognitive and memory deficits such that meaningful communication even at its basic level may be difficult. The loss of autonomy and the emergence of difficult to manage behavioral and psychiatric symptoms during this stage frequently lead to institutionalization. Patients invariably need full assistance for their activities of daily living and may be incontinent. Motor disturbances and difficulty walking emerge, and the patient becomes bed or chair bound in the end stages of the illness (Table 1).

Although AD accounts for more than 50% of dementias in the United States and Europe, other dementing conditions must be included in the differential diagnosis. The second and third most commonly occurring dementias are dementia with Lewy bodies and vascular dementia. Dementia with Lewy bodies can be characterized by symptoms of global cognitive impairment, including memory, and earlier neuropsychiatric disturbance than occurs in AD, with the appearance of visual hallucinations and parkinsonism. In vascular dementia, executive dysfunction is more prominent than in AD, and memory difficulties may be minimal early in the course of the illness. In contrast to AD, in which behavioral and psychiatric symptoms appear later in the progression of the illness, in vascular dementia these symptoms may appear earlier in the course. However, more than one etiologic factor may exist in

CURRENT DIAGNOSIS

Criteria	Description
Intellectual functioning	Development of multiple cognitive deficits, including memory impairment plus one or more of the following attributes: ■ Aphasia (language disturbance) ■ Agnosia (impaired recognition) ■ Apraxia (impaired motor activity) ■ Executive dysfunction (difficulties in planning and organization)
Functional capacity	Cognitive deficits cause significant impairment in social, occupational, or usual activities of daily living and represent a significant decline from a previous level of functioning.
Course of symptoms	Symptoms have a gradual or insidious onset, and patient experiences a continuous cognitive decline.
Absence of delirium	Cognitive deficits do not occur solely during the course of delirium.
Other neurologic and medical conditions excluded	Cognitive defects described are not caused by other central nervous system disorders that cause progressive deficits in memory and cognition (e.g., cerebrovascular disease, Huntington's or Parkinson's disease, subdural hematoma, normal-pressure hydrocephalus, brain tumor) or by systemic conditions known to cause the dementia syndrome (e.g., hypothyroidism, vitamin B_{12} or folic acid deficiency, hypercalcemia, neurosyphilis, HIV infection)
Psychiatric conditions excluded	Disturbance is not caused by another major psychiatric disorder (e.g., schizophrenia, major depression, substance abuse)

patients with dementia. At autopsy, neuropathologic findings of concomitant AD and cerebrovascular disease have been reported in the brain tissue of 7% to 25% of patients who received a diagnosis of probable AD. Comorbid AD and dementia with Lewy bodies could account for as many as 20% of patients diagnosed with dementia. The frontotemporal group of dementias has a much lower incidence. These dementias occur earlier in life by a decade or two from the typical appearance of AD and often present initially with behavioral disturbances such as disinhibition, inappropriateness, apathy, and executive dysfunction. Other cognitive functions and memory become clearly impaired later in the disease process. Depression may, at times, be accompanied by cognitive impairment, producing a dementia-like clinical impression (Table 2). Elements of a diagnostic evaluation for AD are given in Table 3.

Epidemiology

An estimated eighteen million people worldwide currently suffer from AD. This number is expected to double within the next 25 years. The current prevalence of AD in the United States has been estimated between 1.1 and

---

TABLE 1 Stages of Alzheimer's Disease

Stage	Mild	Moderate	Severe
Folstein Mini Mental State Examination (MMSE) Score	20–29	10–19	0–9
Symptoms	Memory impairment evident Early language problems (e.g., word-finding difficulty) Decreased insight and scope of judgment Early mood and personality changes Withdrawal from more demanding activities May need assistance with some instrumental ADLs	Unable to learn or recall new information Worsening long-term memory and recall Language, orientation, executive and other cognitive functions impaired Development of behavioral and psychiatric disturbances Sleep disturbance common Requires help with most all instrumental ADLs	Major, broad cognitive deterioration Loss of language; mutism Motor disturbances and unstable gait Dysphagia, frequent weight loss Poor basic ADLs to complete dependence Progresses to bedridden state Institutionalization common

Abbreviation: ADL = activity of daily living.

TABLE 2 Causes of Dementia Syndrome

Causal Condition	Approximate Incidence*
Common	
• Alzheimer's disease	50%–70%
• Dementia with Lewy bodies	15%
• Vascular dementia	10%
• Alzheimer's disease and vascular dementia (mixed dementia)	10%
• Depression	5%–10%
Less Common	
• Toxic-metabolic disorders	<5%
• Parkinson's disease	<5%
• Frontotemporal dementias	<5%
• Infections	<3%
• Space-occupying lesions	<3%
• Other neurodegenerations	<2%
• Immune inflammatory	<1%
• Prion diseases	<1%

*Considerable geographic variation has been reported.

4.8 million cases. Although symptoms of the disease usually appear after age 60 years, the incidence of AD increases sharply and steadily after age 70 years. It has been estimated that nearly half of all people 85 years and older have some form of dementia. The National Institutes of Health estimates that, if the current trend continues, 8.5 million Americans will have AD by the year 2030.

Research has shown that the major risk factor for AD is age. Other risk factors include genetics (presenilin-1 and presenilin-2, apolipoprotein E4 status, Down syndrome), female gender, lack of education, head trauma, and myocardial infarction. The influences of presenilin on AD are based on the autosomal dominant forms of the disease, which account for 1% to 2% of all cases and result from missense mutations of genes that encode the amyloid precursor protein APP (chromosome 21) or proteolytic enzymes that cleave APP (chromosomes 1 and 14). Such mutations are associated with an increased production of β-amyloid peptide (Aβ) and result in early-onset AD. Apolipoprotein E (ApoE) status has been suggested as a risk factor for typical AD (chromosome 19). ApoE is a protein involved in cholesterol transport and has three alleles: e2, e3, and e4. Homozygous individuals who carry two ApoE e4 alleles have an increased probability of developing AD by age 85 years and do so about 10 years earlier than individuals carrying the other allelic variants. Possible mechanisms are ApoE e4 enhancement of β-amyloid deposition and amyloids reduced clearance from extracellular space.

Pathology

The brains of AD patients are atrophic with ventricular and sulcal enlargement. Histologic specimens are significant for progressive neuronal loss, β-amyloid deposition with formation of senile and neuritic plaques, and intraneuronal neurofibrillary tangles. Early changes are most abundant in the mesial temporal lobe (entorhinal cortex, hippocampus). With disease progression, parietal and frontal association areas become involved. Primary sensorimotor cortex involvement is last. The current prevailing hypothesis of AD pathogenesis contends that the initial pathogenic event is extraneuronal and intraneuronal accumulation of a misfolded protein, amyloid β-peptide, which initiates a pathogenic cascade that results in neurotoxicity, neural dysfunction, and neuronal death and culminates in the clinical syndrome of AD.

TABLE 3 Elements of a Dementia Evaluation

Historical Information
- Symptoms (onset, duration of cognitive, psychiatric, behavioral, and personality changes).
- Functional status (driving, cooking, finances, social contacts, other basic and instrumental activities of daily living).
- Past history (medical, neurologic, psychiatric, social functioning, family history of major medical and neuropsychiatric disorders).
- Medications.

Mental Status Examination
- Evaluation of behavior at interaction, mood, thought content and process, psychosis, insight, and judgment, as well as cognitive evaluation that includes orientation, attention, memory, language, calculations, visuospatial abilities, executive functions.
- Folstein Mini Mental State Examination and the Clock Drawing Test are useful brief instruments.
- Neuropsychologic testing is occasionally indicated in some cases for diagnostic clarity.

Review of Symptoms
- Falls, constipation, urinary incontinence, sensorial deficits, dentition, pain, sleep difficulties.

Physical and Neurologic Examination
Laboratory evaluation
- Complete blood cell count, standard chemistry panel, vitamin B$_{12}$, folate, thyroid-stimulating hormone, neurosyphilis treponemal screen (e.g., *Treponema pallidum* hemagglutination assay), urinalysis.
- Additional tests may be indicated under specific circumstances.

Neuroimaging
- Magnetic resonance imaging frequently used for exclusion of other conditions and for diagnostic clarity
- Positron emission tomography may be indicated when frontotemporal dementia is in the differential diagnosis.

Treatment and Management of Cognitive Symptoms

More than 30 years ago, researchers first showed decreased cholinergic markers, such as choline acetyltransferase, in the cortex of AD patients. Others subsequently demonstrated loss of basal forebrain cholinergic neurons innervating neocortex and hippocampus in AD patients. These collective findings were the basis of a cholinergic hypothesis of AD that resulted in efforts to treat AD through a variety of cholinergic interventions. Cholinesterase inhibitor (ChE-I) therapy in use today evolved from those early efforts and received FDA approval based on its good tolerability and modest efficacy. ChE-Is are believed to increase acetylcholine signaling in damaged cortical areas where neurodegeneration has occurred. Three ChE-Is are in use today: donepezil (Aricept), rivastigmine (Exelon), and galantamine (Razadyne). Tacrine (Cognex), the ChE-I first approved in 1993, is rarely used today because of its hepatoxicity. In blinded controlled studies, donepezil treatment resulted in cognitive and global functioning benefits for up to 1 year in patients with mild to moderate AD. Patients treated with rivastigmine for 6 months also showed improvement in cognitive and global functioning. Well-controlled trials of galantamine in AD have shown comparable cognitive gains for patients treated for 5 to 6 months. More recent work has indicated that ChE-Is appear to reduce the rate of cognitive decline for periods of 6 months to 1 year or possibly longer, rather than producing a significant cognitive improvement after the start of therapy.

All three agents have comparable efficacy, although their side-effect profiles and dosing schedules vary (Table 4).

Donepezil (Aricept) has an elimination half-life of about 70 hours, needing only once-daily dosing. A starting dose of 5 mg/day is given orally for 4 to 6 weeks. The dose is then increased to a maximum of 10 mg/day as tolerated. Donepezil is taken with or without food but preferably in the morning because vivid dreams may disturb sleep in some patients. Rivastigmine (Exelon) is given twice daily because of its shorter elimination half-life. Dosing starts at 1.5 mg twice daily and is titrated upward slowly, every 2 weeks, to a maximum of 6 to 12 mg/day. If rivastigmine is taken with food and titration occurs in 1.5-mg twice daily increments over 4-week intervals, cholinergic side effects are reduced. Dose reduction is suggested in patients with renal or hepatic impairment. Galantamine (Razadyne) also requires twice-daily dosing. Starting dose is 4 mg twice daily. After 4 weeks, the dose is slowly augmented over several weeks to a maximum of 12 mg twice daily if tolerated. Dose reduction is advised in patients with moderate renal or hepatic impairment. The total dose should not exceed 16 mg/day. Galantamine is contraindicated in patients with severe hepatic or renal impairment.

The side effects of all ChE-Is are similar. However, some agents may be better tolerated than others. The most common side effects are nausea, vomiting, diarrhea, anorexia, weight loss, vivid dreams, insomnia, and muscle cramps. Donepezil appears to have a lesser frequency of gastrointestinal side effects than do galantamine or rivastigmine. In all three agents, these side effects tend to be dose related and transient. The vagotonic effects of

TABLE 4 Pharmacologic Treatment of Cognitive Impairment

Medication	Disease Stage	Recommended Dose	Half-Life	Main Side Effects	Hepatic Cytochrome P-450 Metabolism
Donepezil (Aricept)	Mild to moderate	Start 5 mg qd for 4–6 wk then increase to 10 mg as tolerated	70 hr	Nausea, diarrhea, insomnia, hypertension/hypotension, bradycardia, urinary obstruction	Partial inhibition by ketoconazole, quinidine Induction by carbamazepine
Galantamine (Razadyne, previously Reminyl)	Mild to moderate	Start 4 mg bid for 4 wk and taper slowly to a maximum of 12 mg bid	7 hr	Nausea, vomiting, diarrhea, bradycardia, syncope Contraindicated in severe hepatic or renal disease	Partial inhibition by ketoconazole, paroxetine Clearance reduced by fluoxetine, quinidine, amitriptyline
Rivastigmine (Exelon)	Mild to moderate	Start 1.5 mg bid and increase slowly every 2 wk to a final dose of 6–12 mg/day	1.5 hr	Dizziness, vomiting, headache, diarrhea, anorexia, abdominal pain; titrate slowly with hepatic or renal disease	Not affected by a wide variety of commonly used medications
Memantine (Namenda)	Moderate to severe	Start 5 mg qd and after 1 wk can be increased in 5-mg increments to a maximum of 20 mg daily	60–80 hr	Hypertension, constipation, dizziness, hallucinations, headache, Stevens-Johnson syndrome	Predominantly renal metabolism and clearance

ChE-I therapy can cause bradycardia. Therefore, patients with a history of sick sinus syndrome, supraventricular tachycardia, congestive heart failure, and acute coronary artery disease should be monitored. The patient's ability to tolerate side effects is a major factor affecting medication adherence. However, an optimal ChE-I medication trial should consist of at least 3 to 4 months of treatment at the maximally tolerated dose prior to discontinuation of therapy for inadequate response, because that period of time is needed to establish that the patient has continued to deteriorate at the expected nontreated rate. If the patient does not respond to one ChE-I, another can be tried.

In 2003, memantine (Namenda), a noncholinergic-related *N*-methyl-D-aspartate (NMDA) receptor antagonist, was approved by the FDA for treatment of moderate to severe AD based on the results of two controlled studies involving more than 600 moderately to severely demented AD patients. The first 28-week study involved memantine alone versus placebo. Results demonstrated that memantine treatment was of moderate benefit to patients in terms of both cognitive and functional measures. For 12 weeks, cognition remained stable in the memantine group then declined afterward; however, significantly less impairment was noted at endpoint in the memantine group than in the placebo group. The second study evaluated memantine in AD patients already receiving donepezil. The patients treated with donepezil plus memantine showed a modest but better therapeutic effect in cognition sustained from baseline than did the donepezil with placebo group. Treatment of mildly demented AD patients with memantine has produced less robust results, and memantine is not currently FDA approved for this use (see Table 4).

Memantine should be started at 5 mg once daily for 1 week. It can be increased in 5-mg increments per week to a maximum dose of 20 mg/day. It is then best given 10 mg twice daily. Memantine is generally well tolerated and can be taken with or without food. Because of its partial renal clearance, dosage reduction is recommended for patients with significant renal insufficiency. Potential side effects include headache, agitation, confusion, constipation, dizziness, hallucinations, and insomnia. Memantine can be used as monotherapy in patients with moderate to severe AD who do not respond to or tolerate ChE-Is. A decreased rate of cognitive decline for a period of time, as with ChE-Is, appears to be the main therapeutic effect. Best use of memantine may be in combination with a ChE-I, as benefits of the combination appear to be superior to that of either drug used alone.

Treatment of Behavioral and Psychiatric Symptoms

Patients with AD frequently develop behavioral and psychiatric symptoms in addition to cognitive impairments. These symptoms become more prominent as the disease progresses and often lead to institutionalization. When dementia is well established, patients commonly develop some form of agitation (excessive purposeless activity), either motoric or verbal, during the day or evening hours. They may become intermittently irritable and aggressive with family members. Nearly half will develop psychosis, either as hallucinations (auditory or visual) or simple delusions of infidelity or persecution, such as believing someone is stealing from them. They may manifest apathy (loss of motivation) and disordered mood with symptoms of depression, anxiety, and irritability. Optimal management is both nonpharmacologic and pharmacologic.

NONPHARMACOLOGIC MANAGEMENT

Often patients are confused and agitated as a consequence of temporal-spatial disorientation and need to be reassured and redirected with regularity. Environmental cues, such as the posted date and visible familiar objects and pictures of loved ones, may help. Agitated and/or aggressive behavior may be exacerbated by environmental triggers, such as insufficient (e.g., poor daytime lighting) or excessive (too much activity) sensorial stimulation. These elements can and should be adjusted. It is important to educate the patient, family, and staff (if the patient is institutionalized) regarding target behavioral symptoms and the environmental and behavioral techniques useful in their management. Implementation of a management plan can then proceed with better consistency and effectiveness wherever the patient resides. Managing AD patients is a large burden for caregivers. According to studies, caregivers have a 52% prevalence of psychiatric symptoms compared with 15% to 20% in the general population. As part of an overall management plan, caregivers will need support through reassurance, education, and referral to important community resources, such as the Alzheimer Association, caregiver support groups, day care centers, and social or legal services.

PHARMACOLOGIC TREATMENT

Pharmacologic management of behavioral and mood symptoms depends on accurate analysis of problem moods and behaviors and should be individualized. Broadly speaking, depression and anxiety are managed with newer antidepressants (selective serotonin reuptake inhibitors [SSRIs], mirtazapine [Remeron], trazodone [Desyrel]). Dementia-related psychotic symptoms and aggression are treated with atypical antipsychotics. Pure agitation without aggression can be treated with trazodone,[1] buspirone[1] (BuSpar), SSRIs,[1] or anticonvulsants.[1] Newer studies also suggest that cholinesterase inhibitors and memantine (Namenda) may be helpful in the management of this condition. Certain benzodiazepines are occasionally a useful adjunct for short-term treatment of anxiety-driven agitation or anxiety with depression (Table 5).

Depressive symptoms requiring treatment (e.g., withdrawal, appetite loss, worsening sleep, negativism, irritability, somatization) are more common than the classic major depressive syndrome in demented AD patients. Because of their safety profile, tolerability, and efficacy, newer antidepressants, such as the SSRIs or venlafaxine (Effexor; 50–300 mg/day) and mirtazapine (15–45 mg/day), are the mainstay of treatment. The SSRIs have comparable efficacy, but agents with low drug–drug interactions and low side-effect profiles, such as citalopram (Celexa; 10–60 mg/day) and sertraline (Zoloft; 50–200 mg/day), are preferred. Onset of action of the antidepressants may require 1 to several weeks. Patience and dose adjustments are needed. Treatment of the first episode of depression should last 1 year at the therapeutic dose before the

---

[1]Not FDA approved for this indication.

TABLE 5 Pharmacologic Treatment of Behavioral and Mood Symptoms

Medication	Indication	Recommended Dose	Main Side Effects	Caution
Antidepressants				
Citalopram (Celexa)	Depression, agitation,[1] irritability,[1] anxiety[1]	10–60 mg/day	Headache, nausea, hyponatremia, insomnia, diarrhea, somnolence	
Sertraline (Zoloft)	Depression, agitation,[1] irritability,[1] anxiety[1]	50–200[3] mg/day	Headache, nausea, hyponatremia, insomnia, diarrhea, somnolence	Adjust dose in hepatic impairment
Mirtazapine (Remeron)	Depression, agitation,[1] irritability,[1] anxiety[1]	15–45[3] mg/day	Somnolence, increased appetite, arrhythmia, hypercholesterolemia agranulocytosis	
Venlafaxine (Effexor)	Depression, agitation,[1] irritability,[1] anxiety[1]	50–300 mg/day	Hypertension, hyponatremia, nausea, headache, nervousness, dizziness	
Trazodone (Desyrel)	Agitation alone,[1] mild anxiety,[1] insomnia[1]	25–200 mg/day	Somnolence, dizziness, headache, nausea, priapism, orthostasis	
Antipsychotics				
Haloperidol (Haldol)	Acute psychosis with agitation or aggression[1]	0.25–3 mg/day, IM, if oral dosing not possible	Hypertension, hypotension, tachycardia, movement disorders	Parkinsonism, tardive dyskinesia, neuroleptic malignant syndrome
Quetiapine (Seroquel)	Subacute or chronic psychosis without or with agitation or aggression[1]	25–200 mg/day PO	Weight gain, dizziness, headache, agitation, sedation	QT_c prolongation possible, glucose intolerance, increased stroke risk? Monitor
Risperidone (Risperdal)	Subacute or chronic psychosis without or with agitation or aggression[1]	0.25–2 mg/day PO	Hypotension, hyperglycemia, insomnia, agitation, headache, weight gain, extrapyramidal symptoms	QT_c prolongation possible, glucose intolerance, increased stroke risk? Monitor
Olanzapine (Zyprexa)	Subacute chronic psychosis without or with agitation or aggression[1]	Start 2.5–5 mg/day PO, increase by 2.5 mg/wk to a maximum of 10–15 mg/day	Hyperglycemia, headache, agitation, dizziness, dyspepsia, hypotension, weight gain, somnolence	QT_c prolongation possible, glucose intolerance, type 2 diabetes mellitus?, increased stroke risk? Monitor
Anticonvulsants				
Divalproex (Depakote)	Aggression with or without agitation or irritability[1]	Start 125 mg/day and may increase slowly to a maximum of 1500 mg/day	Liver toxicity, pancreatitis, thrombocytopenia, somnolence, dizziness, diarrhea, tremors, nausea, vomiting	Adjust dose for hepatic and renal impairment

[1]Not FDA approved for this indication.
[3]Exceeds dosage recommended by the manufacturer.

TABLE 5 Pharmacologic Treatment of Behavioral and Mood Symptoms—cont'd

Medication	Indication	Recommended Dose	Main Side Effects	Caution
Benzodiazepines and Other Anxiolytics				
Lorazepam (Ativan)	Anxiety	1–2 mg/day	Memory impairment, sedation, dizziness, falls	For short-term use only while concomitant antidepressants are titrated to effectiveness
Oxazepam (Serax)	Anxiety	15 mg/day	Hepatic dysfunction, leukopenia, dizziness	For short-term use only while concomitant antidepressants are titrated to effectiveness
Buspirone (BuSpar)	Anxiety, agitation only[1]	30–60 mg/day	Dizziness, sedation	

antidepressant is tapered off. In a patient with a history of episodes of depression, therapy should be maintained indefinitely. It is useful to match the side-effect profile of the antidepressant with the patient's main symptoms. For example, for an inactive, withdrawn patient, an activating antidepressant such as venlafaxine or sertraline may be useful. On the other hand, for an anxious patient who is not sleeping or eating well, a calming agent that enhances appetite and can increase evening sedation, such as mirtazapine, may be a preferable initial choice.

The newer antidepressants are also effective in treating anxiety and irritability, both of which commonly occur in AD, although the onset of action of these agents may not be immediate. When relief of anxiety is needed more quickly, a benzodiazepine of moderately short duration of action, such as oxazepam (Serax; 15 mg/day) or lorazepam (Ativan; 1–2 mg/day), can be initiated at the same time an antidepressant at low dose is started. Over a period of 2 to 3 weeks, as the antidepressant dose is titrated upward, the benzodiazepine is tapered off to reduce exposure to possible benzodiazepine side effects, such as memory loss, falls, confusion, and behavioral disinhibition. The antidepressant should now exert a greater anxiolytic effect. For patients with mild anxiety, trazodone[1] (25–200 mg/day) or buspirone (BuSpar) can be tried.

The newer, atypical antipsychotics are helpful in treating psychosis alone and psychosis associated with aggression/agitation. These medications have demonstrated some utility in treating irritability and aggression but not agitation alone. Patients with acute psychosis who are unable to take oral medication may respond to haloperidol (Haldol) intramuscularly 0.25 to 3 mg/day, although side effects are more prominent with this conventional antipsychotic. Patients with subacute and chronic psychotic symptoms can be treated with oral risperidone[1] (Risperdal; 0.25–2 mg/day), quetiapine[1] (Seroquel; 25–200 mg/day), or olanzapine[1] (Zyprexa; 2.5–15 mg/day). Movement disorders, such as

parkinsonism and tardive dyskinesia, are less frequent with atypical antipsychotics than with conventional ones. In addition to the use of atypical antipsychotics for aggression with psychosis, aggression alone or with irritability can be treated with SSRIs having low drug–drug interactions, such as citalopram[1] (Celexa; 10–60 mg/day) or sertraline[1] (Zoloft; 50–200 mg/day), with mirtazapine[1] (Remeron; 7.5–45 mg/day), or with anticonvulsants, such as divalproex[1] (Depakote; 125–1500 mg/day). Persistent male sexual aggression may benefit from treatment with medroxyprogesterone[1] (Depo-Provera) intramuscularly 150 mg biweekly or monthly. Agitation alone without psychosis or aggression may respond to environmental adjustments in combination with trazodone[1] (25–200 mg/day), buspirone[1] (30–60 mg/day), or a ChE-I. Apathy may improve in some patients with standard doses of ChE-Is.

Caution is necessary when prescribing most medications to the elderly because of their sensitivity to adverse reactions. Specifically, newer antipsychotic medications can cause QT_c prolongation, weight gain, hyperlipidemia, increased glucose resistance, and type 2 diabetes mellitus. They have even been associated with a possible small increase in stroke or death risk in exposed demented populations, although additional prospective studies are needed to reach more definitive conclusions. When prescribing atypical antipsychotics to patients with a vulnerable cardiac or metabolic status, a baseline and treatment electrocardiogram, lipid panel, chemistry panel, and weight measurement should be performed, with subsequent monitoring as indicated.

In refractory patients, combination therapies may be necessary, and in such cases pharmacologic agents belonging to different classes should be combined. However, certain cautions should be observed. Only one change should be introduced at a time, and lower initial doses should be used. Avoid olanzapine (Zyprexa) and clozapine (Clozaril) in patients with diabetes. The following combinations are

---

[1]Not FDA approved for this indication.

[1]Not FDA approved for this indication.

CURRENT THERAPY

- If delirium, acute psychosis, depression, or major aggression/agitation is present initially, treat this condition first and then re-evaluate.
- If no acute psychosis, depression, or major behavioral perturbation is evident, treat cognitive symptoms with a memory enhancer such as a ChE-I or memantine (Namenda; an *N*-methyl-D-aspartate receptor antagonist) as appropriate for disease stage.
- Mild Alzheimer's disease: ChE-I—donepezil (Aricept), galantamine (Razadyne), or rivastigmine (Exelon).
- Moderate Alzheimer's disease: ChE-I and/or memantine (Namenda).
- Severe Alzheimer's disease: ChE-I and/or memantine.
- Consider nonpharmacologic interventions for behavioral and mood problems.
- Treat persistent psychiatric and behavioral symptoms as follows:
  - Acute psychosis with agitation/aggression: Haloperidol[1] (Haldol)
  - Subacute, chronic psychosis with or without aggression/agitation: Atypical antipsychotic
  - Depression, irritability: Second generation non-TCA antidepressant
  - Agitation alone: Trazodone[1] (Desyrel), second generation non-TCA antidepressant, nonpharmacologic intervention
  - Anxiety: Atypical antidepressant with or without short-term benzodiazepine, trazodone,[1] or buspirone[1] (BuSpar)
  - Insomnia: Trazodone,[1] short-term only benzodiazepine, or similar hypnotic

[1]Not FDA approved for this indication.
Abbreviation: ChE-I = cholinesterase inhibitor.

---

best avoided: clozapine (Clozaril) and carbamazepine (Tegretol); ziprasidone (Geodon) and tricyclic antidepressants; conventional antipsychotics and fluoxetine (Prozac); and conventional antipsychotics and lithium, divalproex (Depakote), or lamotrigine (Lamictal). However, divalproex and risperidone (or haloperidol) is an acceptable combination. Key therapeutic points are summarized in Current Therapy.

Sleep Disorders

Method of
David N. Neubauer, MD

In recent years there has been increasing recognition of the high prevalence and significant consequences of sleep disorders and the effects of insufficient sleep. The National Sleep Foundation estimates that about 70 million Americans have problems with their sleep. Research has documented various medical and psychiatric comorbidities with sleep disorders and how sleep disturbances can increase the risk of other disorders. While the number of sleep specialists and sleep disorder centers continue to grow, primary care medicine remains the frontline in the clinical evaluation and treatment of sleep disorders. This chapter provides a broad overview of the common sleep disorders encountered in clinical practice. Sleep-disordered breathing is covered in greater detail in the article on Sleep Apnea.

The foundation of understanding sleep disorders is an appreciation of the two primary processes normally regulating the sleep-wake cycle. A *homeostatic* sleep drive determines the amount of sleep we need for alertness and vigilance during our waking hours. For most individuals, a daily sleep total of approximately 8 hours is ideal. Insufficient sleep, whether acute or chronic, leads to increased sleepiness. The ability to achieve sufficient sleep at night and subsequent wakefulness throughout the daytime and evening is optimized by the *circadian* process, which is coordinated through the suprachiasmatic nucleus in the anterior hypothalamus with input from the photoperiod. The circadian process generates maximum arousal in the evening to offset the homeostatic sleepiness that evolves throughout the day. These two processes together promote sustained wakefulness for about 16 hours and sleep for about 8 hours in synchrony with the day-night cycle.

The homeostatic and circadian processes describe the normal pattern of alertness and sleepiness, but they also may help explain clinical problems associated with insufficient sleepiness (insomnia) and excessive sleepiness. Daytime or evening napping reduces the homeostatic sleep drive available to promote sleep onset and maintenance during a desired nighttime sleep period. This may lead a patient to complain of insomnia. Difficulty falling asleep and remaining asleep also may result from attempts to sleep outside the normal photoperiod-reinforced circadian zone of increased sleep propensity. Sleep difficulty associated with shift work is a typical example.

Symptoms of Sleep Disorders

The evaluation of patients with sleep difficulties should begin with a thorough history of their sleep-related symptoms. How long has it been a problem? Is it intermittent, or a daily or nightly problem? What time of the day or night do the symptoms occur? Are there obvious precipitants or consequences? Is there impairment in normal functioning? What have been the typical sleep-wake hours for the individual. and what is the current pattern? Are there medical or psychiatric disorders or medications that might be influencing the sleep-related symptoms? Input from a bed partner or other informant can be invaluable. Having patients maintain sleep logs can offer a concise view of the patterns of their sleep disturbances and help demonstrate the effects of treatment strategies. Questionnaires and scales (e.g., Epworth Sleepiness Scale, Pittsburgh Sleep Quality Index) can be useful for screening patients for possible sleep disturbances.

Symptoms of sleep disorders may include an inability to sleep at desired times (insomnia), an inability to remain fully awake and attentive at desired times (excessive sleepiness), snoring and fluctuations in breathing patterns during sleep, uncomfortable sensations prior to sleep onset, abnormal movements before and during sleep, and abnormal behaviors emanating from sleep (parasomnias). Although insomnia, excessive daytime sleepiness, and parasomnias are the primary symptom clusters, individual patients may experience overlapping symptoms. For instance, sleep-disordered breathing can be associated with disrupted nighttime sleep and excessive daytime sleepiness.

Insomnia

Insomnia is difficulty falling asleep or remaining asleep when people expect to be able to sleep and when there is an opportunity for them to be in bed sleeping. An insomnia disorder persists for at least 1 month and is associated with daytime impairment. Insomnia affects about 30% of the general adult population intermittently and about 10% on a chronic basis. Insomnia is a problem for more than half of patients with chronic medical conditions. Insomnia may occur idiopathically or may result from distressing circumstances; psychological conditioning; environmental factors; jet lag and shift work schedules; medication effects; and medical, psychiatric, and sleep disorders.

Treatment of insomnia may require multiple strategies that involve correction of sleep hygiene problems, bedtime routine and schedule modifications, cognitive and other psychotherapeutic techniques, strategically timed exposure to bright light, and use of medications. Additionally, optimizing the management of comorbid conditions (e.g., major depression, chronic pain, sleep-disordered breathing, and congestive heart failure) may be necessary for sleep quality improvements. General sleep hygiene recommendations are listed in Table 1. Delaying bedtime may help patients spending excessive frustrating wakeful time in bed. Cognitive therapy techniques may be especially helpful for the patients who catastrophize about their sleep problems.

Significant advances in the pharmacologic treatment of insomnia have been made in recent years. Patients may experience improved sleep with sedating medications prescribed for comorbid conditions (e.g., antidepressants). The medications indicated for treatment of insomnia (Table 2) include both traditional benzodiazepines and newer nonbenzodiazepine hypnotics. All of these hypnotics function through enhancing the inhibitory responses of γ-aminobutyric acid (GABA)-A receptors. The newer medications have pharmacokinetic and pharmacodynamic characteristics that improve their safety profile. Ramelteon (Rozerem), a nonsedating, selective melatonin receptor agonist that targets activity of the circadian system, also is approved for treatment of insomnia.

The duration of action of the newer generation hypnotics ranges from the very short-acting zaleplon (Sonata) to the progressively longer-acting zolpidem (Ambien), modified-release zolpidem (Ambien CR), and eszopiclone (Lunesta). Food and Drug Administration (FDA) approval is anticipated for immediate-release indiplon,* which will join this class of relatively short-acting hypnotics. The pattern of patients' sleep disturbances influences the selection of hypnotics. Exclusive sleep-onset difficulty may be treated

---

*Investigational drug in the United States.

TABLE 1 Sleep Hygiene Recommendations

- Try to maintain a regular sleep-wake schedule.
- Avoid afternoon or evening napping.
- Allow yourself enough time in bed for adequate sleep duration (e.g., 11 PM to 7 AM).
- Develop a relaxing evening routine for the hours approaching bedtime.
- Spend some idle time reflecting on the day's events before going to bed. Make a list of concerns and how some might be resolved.
- Reserve the bed for sleep and sex. Do not do homework, pay bills, or engage in serious domestic discussions in bed.
- Avoid evening alcohol.
- Avoid caffeine in the afternoon and evening.
- Minimize annoying noise, light, or temperature extremes.
- Consider a light snack before bedtime.
- Exercise regularly, but not late in the evening.
- Do not try harder and harder to fall asleep. If you are unable to sleep, do something else out of bed and in another room, if possible.
- Avoid smoking.

adequately with a very short-acting medication; however, most insomnia patients have combined difficulty falling asleep and maintaining sleep. Accordingly, moderately short-acting medications that do not cause residual morning sedation generally are optimal.

Until recently, all prescription sleep-promoting medications were approved for short-term treatment of insomnia; however, beginning in 2005 the FDA began approving sleep-promoting agents simply for treatment of insomnia without the implied short-term restriction. Whereas the majority of patients taking hypnotic medications require

TABLE 2 Medications Indicated for Treatment of Insomnia

Medication	Available Doses (mg)	Duration of Action
Hypnotic		
Benzodiazepines:		
Estazolam (ProSom)	1, 2	Intermediate-long
Flurazepam (Dalmane)	15, 30	Long
Quazepam (Doral)	7.5, 15	Long
Temazepam (Restoril)	7.5, 15, 22.5, 30	Intermediate
Triazolam (Halcion)	0.125, 0.25	Short-intermediate
Nonbenzodiazepines:		
Eszopiclone (Lunesta)	1, 2, 3	Intermediate
Zaleplon (Sonata)	5, 10	Very short
Zolpidem (Ambien)	5, 10	Short
Zolpidem (Ambien CR) extended-release	6.25, 12.5	Short-intermediate
Melatonin Receptor Agonist		
Ramelteon (Rozerem)	8	Short

help with their sleep only for limited periods of time, others with chronic insomnia have experienced continued improvement in nighttime sleep and daytime functioning with longer-term nightly or intermittent hypnotic use. All of the currently approved benzodiazepine receptor agonist hypnotics remain Schedule IV controlled substances. In contrast, ramelteon (Rozerem) is not classified as a controlled substance.

Circadian Rhythm Disorders

Although the circadian system typically promotes night-time sleep from approximately 10 to 11 PM until about 6 to 7 AM, many individuals have long-standing tendencies to experience either earlier or later sleep propensity zones. An individual's circadian phase can contribute to complaints of insomnia or excessive sleepiness, although this influence often is not recognized. Adolescents and young adults are more likely to have later sleep propensities, whereas elderly individuals tend to have an earlier onset and offset of sleepiness. People with an *advanced sleep phase* are early birds; they become sleepy earlier in the evening and then are unable to sleep later in the morning. They may complain of persistent early morning awakening as well as daytime fatigue and sleepiness. Night owls with a *delayed circadian phase* have difficulty falling asleep early and tend to sleep later in the morning. This can represent a significant clinical problem. Patients may report sleep-onset insomnia or excessive daytime sleepiness, particularly during the morning hours. Melatonin receptor agonists given prior to bedtime also may help advance and stabilize the sleep onset and morning awakening times for delayed sleep phase patients. Evening bright light exposure may help patients with a long-term predisposition for early evening sleepiness and bother-some early morning awakening. Conversely, bright light exposure upon awakening may help those with a night-owl pattern.

Excessive Daytime Sleepiness

Excessive sleepiness during waking hours is a major public health problem most evident in associated workplace and vehicular accidents, injuries, and fatalities. Excessively sleepy patients typically complain of sleepiness for major portions of the day and report a high propensity for falling asleep during sedentary activities. In severe cases, patients may fall asleep while driving, conversing, or attending important meetings. Chronic sleepiness may lead to educational, occupational, and social difficulties. The most common cause of excessive sleepiness is insufficient sleep, whether due to work schedules or lifestyle choices. Sedating medications and other substances can lead to excessive sleepiness. Emerging evidence suggests that sleep deprivation may contribute to metabolic and immune impairment, even in healthy young individuals.

Patients complaining of difficulty remaining awake during the daytime should be evaluated at a sleep center unless there is an obvious and reversible cause. Sleep laboratory testing includes the standard nighttime polysomnography and possibly a series of daytime nap opportunities that objectively assess sleep onset latency and sleep stages.

The key sleep disorders associated with excessive daytime sleepiness are narcolepsy, hypersomnolence disorders, and sleep-disordered breathing. To a limited extent, insomnia and other disorders causing frequent arousals and awakenings, or awakenings with difficulty returning to sleep, may contribute to daytime sleepiness. The latter might include restless legs syndrome, periodic limb movement disorder, and parasomnias.

Narcolepsy

Although *narcolepsy* is the classic disorder of excessive sleepiness, it affects only about 0.05% of the population. It is characterized by persistent sleepiness and difficulty maintaining attention. Symptoms typically begin to evolve by the late teens and continue through life. In addition to disturbed daytime wakefulness and nighttime sleep, narcolepsy patients have symptoms reflecting dysregulation of the characteristics of rapid eye movement (REM) sleep. *Cataplexy* is the loss of postural muscle tone that occurs during waking and is precipitated by heightened emotion, such as anxiety or laughter. The effects may range from a barely noticeable jaw drop to the patient lying on the ground awake but unable to move for up to several minutes. *Sleep paralysis* occurs at the transition to sleep when a person becomes aware of a complete inability to move any muscles voluntarily. It resolves spontaneously within minutes. Cataplexy and sleep paralysis both involve the intrusion of the normal paralysis that accompanies REM sleep; however, it occurs at an abnormal time. Narcolepsy patients also are more likely to experience *hypnagogic hallucinations*, which are dreamlike experiences occurring at sleep onset. Sleep laboratory testing confirms the diagnosis.

Treatment of narcolepsy begins with the establishment of therapeutic goals, typically including maximizing attention and alertness during certain hours of the day, along with the elimination of cataplexy. Narcolepsy patients should be careful to allow sufficient hours for nighttime sleep, as sleep deprivation will exacerbate their symptoms. Scheduled brief naps and periods of increased physical activity during the daytime may be very helpful. Most narcolepsy patients will require pharmacotherapy to enhance daytime alertness. Modafinil (Provigil) may be adequate for some patients; however, many will respond best to amphetamine medications. Antidepressants (e.g., venlafaxine[1] [Effexor]) may reduce cataplexy. Sodium oxybate (Xyrem), which is taken in two nighttime doses, has been shown to improve nighttime sleep, reduce cataplexy, and increase daytime alertness in narcolepsy patients.

Hypersomnolence Disorders

In addition to narcolepsy, various central nervous system processes can cause persistent sleepiness that interferes with daytime functioning. Patients with hypersomnolence may sleep for extended periods and nap during the day, but they still never feel fully alert and refreshed. This condition may be idiopathic, or it may be related to head trauma, viral infections, encephalitis, tumors, and

---

[1]Not FDA approved for this indication.

neurodegenerative disorders. As with narcolepsy, stimulants represent the primary treatment approach but often are less reliable in providing significant benefit for these patients.

Sleep-Disordered Breathing

This topic is covered in greater detail in the article on Sleep Apnea. *Sleep-disordered breathing* involves fluctuations in airflow during sleep. Most commonly it is due to an obstructive process involving an abnormal collapsibility of the upper airway, which may result in recurrent episodes of hypopneas and apneas. Alternately, it may involve a decreased respiratory drive associated with central mechanisms, as can occur with congestive heart failure with a prolonged circulation time. Sleep apnea can cause frequent arousals that undermine sleep quality and lead to excessive sleepiness during the daytime.

Restless Legs Syndrome and Periodic Limb Movements

Although the primary discomfort of restless legs syndrome (RLS) occurs prior to sleep, it is considered a sleep disorder because it is associated with delayed and disrupted sleep and because the irresistible urge to move the legs follows a circadian pattern with increasing symptoms as bedtime approaches. As the condition worsens over time, the sense of restlessness may begin earlier in the afternoon or morning. The discomfort is most bothersome when patients are at rest. Moving the legs offers only very brief relief. In severe cases, patients often experience such intense restlessness that they are unable to sleep for long periods and often will pace until exhaustion finally allows sleep. During sleep, about 80% of RLS patients exhibit periodic limb movements. In some patients, these involuntary jerking movements occur frequently and cause arousals that further undermine sleep quality. Occasionally patients have periodic limb movements during sleep without the pre-sleep restlessness.

Although RLS often occurs idiopathically, there also is a significant familial component. Other risk factors are iron deficiency, peripheral neuropathies, renal failure, and use of certain medications, including most antidepressants, sedating antihistamines, and centrally acting dopamine antagonists. Pregnancy may be associated with a temporary worsening of symptoms.

Iron supplementation may be beneficial for RLS patients with low ferritin levels (<50 ng/mL). Otherwise, the first-line approach consists of dopamine agonists, such as ropinirole (Requip). Selected patients may benefit from opiates (e.g., propoxyphene[1] [Darvon] and methadone[1] [Dolophine]), benzodiazepines (e.g., clonazepam[1] [Klonopin]), or gabapentin[1] (Neurontin).

Parasomnias

Behaviors and other symptoms emanating from sleep are considered *parasomnias*. Although most parasomnias are

[1]Not FDA approved for this indication.

CURRENT DIAGNOSIS

- Patient should be screened routinely for problems associated with sleep and wakefulness.
- Ask patients and bed partners about difficulty falling and staying asleep, movements and behaviors during sleep, and snoring and breathing irregularities during sleep.
- The most common sleep disorders encountered in primary care settings are insomnia, sleep-disordered breathing, and restless legs syndrome. Parasomnia, narcolepsy, and other hypersomnolence disorders are relatively uncommon.
- Excessive sleepiness is a potentially dangerous condition that should be evaluated aggressively. Sleep laboratory testing is appropriate for cases not easily explained by sleep deprivation.

relatively benign, occasionally injuries to patients or bed partners result from these behaviors. Evaluation of patients with parasomnias should include a consideration of sleep-disordered breathing as a possible precipitant to the abnormal behaviors. Most parasomnias can be categorized according to their association with non-REM or REM sleep.

Slow-wave sleep, classified as non-REM stages 3 and 4, generally occurs during the first few hours of sleep. Children have the most slow-wave sleep, and the amount declines with age. Compared with other sleep stages, it is most difficult to awaken from these stages. *Sleep terrors, sleepwalking, sleep-related eating disorder,* and *confusional arousals* all represent incomplete awakenings. Often people experiencing these parasomnias have no recollection of them the following morning. These parasomnias may be exacerbated by sleep insufficiency when there is an increase in slow-wave sleep intensity during recovery sleep. Sleep terrors may be especially dramatic. When they

CURRENT THERAPY

- Patients with persistent insomnia may benefit from improved sleep hygiene measures, cognitive-behavioral therapy, and pharmacologic agents.
- Sleep-promoting medications approved by the Food and Drug Administration include benzodiazepine and nonbenzodiazepine hypnotics, and a selective melatonin receptor agonist.
- Iron supplementation may benefit patients with restless legs syndrome and low ferritin levels. Otherwise, dopamine agonists are the first-line treatment.
- Narcolepsy can be treated with central nervous system stimulants, rapid eye movement suppressants, and sodium oxybate (Xyrem).
- Parasomnia behaviors should be treated when they frequently disrupt sleep or represent a danger to the patient or bed partners.

are frequent or involve dangerous behaviors, then treatment with a benzodiazepine receptor agonist may be appropriate.

REM sleep is associated with the most intense dreaming experiences and markedly decreased skeletal muscle tone. It occurs intermittently throughout the night but for the longest periods during the last few hours of the night. *Nightmares* are distressing awakenings from REM sleep with the awareness of frightening dream content. *REM sleep behavior disorder*, which is more common among elderly individuals, involves an incomplete muscle paralysis during REM sleep leading patients to move during REM sleep. Patients seem to be acting out intense dream experiences. The results can be dangerous because patients may thrash about in bed, fall out of bed, or even attack bed partners before awakening. Bedtime clonazepam[1] (Klonopin) has been the standard treatment; however, recent studies suggest melatonin[1] also may be beneficial.

Summary

Sleep disorders can have a significant impact on a patient's quality of life and on comorbid conditions. Initial screening for sleep-wake cycle disturbances is as simple as asking patients how they are sleeping and whether they feel awake and alert throughout the daytime. Most sleep disorders can be identified with a thorough history in a primary care setting; however, consultation with a sleep specialist and sleep laboratory testing may be helpful in the evaluation and management of complex insomnia, hypersomnia, and parasomnia patients.

REFERENCES

The International Classification of Sleep Disorders: Diagnostic & Coding Manual, ICSD-2, 2nd ed. Westchester, IL, American Academy of Sleep Medicine, 2005.

Chokroverty S: Sleep Disorders Medicine: Basic Science, Technical Considerations, and Clinical Aspects. Boston, Butterworth-Heinemann, 1994.

Earley CJ: Clinical practice: Restless legs syndrome. N Engl J Med 2003;348:2103-2109.

Kryger MH, Roth T, Dement WC: Principles and Practice of Sleep Medicine, 4th ed. Philadelphia, Elsevier/Saunders, 2005.

Mahowald MW, Bornemann MC, Schenck CH. Parasomnias. Semin Neurol 2004;24:283-292.

Neubauer DN: Understanding Sleeplessness: Perspectives on Insomnia. Baltimore, Johns Hopkins University Press, 2003.

Reid KJ, Zee PC: Circadian rhythm disorders. Semin Neurol 2004;24: 315-325.

Thorpy M: Current concepts in the etiology, diagnosis and treatment of narcolepsy. Sleep Med 2001;2:5-17.

---

[1]Not FDA approved for this indication.

Intracerebral Hemorrhage

Method of
James M. Gebel, Jr., MD

Parenchymal intracerebral hemorrhage (ICH) represents approximately 10% of all strokes and two thirds of hemorrhagic strokes in the United States. Despite advances in ICH diagnosis and improved understanding of its natural history and prognosis, mortality is unchanged over the past 30 years.

Epidemiology

The incidence of ICH is more than twice that of subarachnoid hemorrhage and kills more than 20,000 Americans annually. An estimated 67,000 cases of ICH occurred in the United States in 2002. The incidence of ICH fell in the 1960s and 1970s with the increasing prevalence of antihypertensive therapy but then has leveled off over the past 30 years.

The risk of ICH increases dramatically with age. Ethnicity is a second important nonmodifiable ICH risk factor. A recent population-based study estimates the annual incidence of ICH at 18 per 100,000 for whites and 37 per 100,000 per year for blacks. Rates of ICH in blacks ages 55 or younger are especially disproportionately higher as compared to whites, with up to a fivefold relative risk. Persons of Asian and, to a lesser extent, Hispanic ethnicity are also at increased risk of ICH.

Risk Factors and Causes

HYPERTENSION

Hypertension is the single most significant and prevalent modifiable risk factor for so-called spontaneous, primary, or hypertensive ICH, and it accounts for the vast majority of preventable attributable risks for ICH. Merely treating hypertension in those in whom it is suboptimally controlled would eliminate an estimated 17% to 28% of all ICHs. As expected, a dose-response curve exists between hypertension severity and subsequent ICH risk. Table 1 reviews this dramatic risk relationship.

CEREBRAL AMYLOID ANGIOPATHY

Cerebral amyloid angiopathy is a common cause of lobar ICH in the elderly (age 65 years or older). Distinct from generalized amyloidosis, the amyloid protein is selectively deposited in the subcortical arterioles of the brain. Dementia and recurrent lobar ICH are its primary clinical manifestations. Its prevalence dramatically increases with age, observed in approximately 5% to 8% of persons in their 60s versus 55% to 60% of those 90 years of age or older. Magnetic resonance imaging (MRI), specifically with gradient echo sequencing that detects previous microscopic hemorrhages, should be employed in anyone with suspected cerebral amyloid angiopathy.

TABLE 1 Annual Incidence of Intracerebral Hemorrhage as Related to Initial Systolic Blood Pressure in Hiroshima and Nagasaki, Japan

Initial Systolic Blood Pressure (mm Hg)	Subsequent Annual Incidence Per 100,000 Persons
Less than 110	0
110-139	30
140-179	113
180 or greater	252

COAGULOPATHY

Coagulopathy is implicated in up to 7.8% of cases with ICH and is most often caused by warfarin therapy, which increases relative ICH risk by 6- to 11-fold overall, with risk paralleling the degree of anticoagulation. Absolute risk of ICH from warfarin therapy ranges from 0.3% to 1.7% per year, depending on the reason for anticoagulation.

STRUCTURAL LESIONS

Vascular malformations, which are often treatable, account for a progressively larger fraction of ICH etiologies with decreasing age. They should be strongly considered in any patient with ICH under age 45 years, including those with hypertension, and represent a significant ICH fraction (4% to 5%) in some series. Up to 10% of aneurysmal ruptures result in parenchymal ICH. Angiography and brain MRI are recommended in all patients with ICH under age 45 years, and in older patients who lack traditional risk factors for ICH.

DRUG-RELATED CASES

Drug abuse is a final important consideration in nontraumatic ICH, representing approximately 0.5% of overall ICH, but a much higher percentage in adolescents and young adults. Cocaine and amphetamine abuse, in particular, represent important identifiable and potentially modifiable etiologies for ICH. A toxicology screen should generally be performed in any young patient with ICH. Finally, alcohol, the most commonly abused drug in American society, is associated with increased ICH risk.

Diagnosis

With the advent of computed tomography (CT) scanning, ICH diagnosis is greatly facilitated. Patients classically present with headache, depressed or diminishing level of consciousness, and gradually evolving, rather than sudden maximal-at-onset, focal neurologic deficits, which often fail to conform to a specific vascular territory. Many patients with ICH fail to conform to this classic presentation, however, so CT scanning is mandatory to differentiate ischemic from hemorrhagic stroke.

Special mention should be given to the presenting signs of cerebellar hemorrhage, namely headache, nausea and vomiting, nystagmus, and dysmetria or ataxia. Unless thin 3-mm or 5-mm posterior fossa cuts are ordered, it is possible to miss a cerebellar hematoma by routine 10-mm-thickness CT scanning. Because cerebellar hemorrhage is readily treatable by surgical decompression, which is often both life and disability saving, it is important to maintain a high level of suspicion for patients with the appropriate clinical presentation, as well as to walk the patient to detect truncal ataxia, which is often the only clinically apparent examination finding (if any).

Treatment

INITIAL MEDICAL THERAPY

Medical therapy begins with the ABCs (airway, breathing, circulation). Airway protection in patients whose level of consciousness or gag reflex is markedly diminished is mandatory. Extremes of blood pressure should be promptly treated.

BLOOD PRESSURE MANAGEMENT

Controversy exists over how aggressively and quickly blood pressure should be lowered. A large clinical trial funded by the National Institutes of Health (NIH) is investigating whether or not aggressive lowering of blood pressure in patients with acute ICH reduces the frequency of hematoma growth during the first 24 hours post-ICH, which is as high as 38%. Studies of perihematomal cerebral blood flow by both MRI and xenon CT suggest that in the vast majority of patients, unlike ischemic stroke, little or no penumbra is present. Overly aggressive use of potent vasodilating antihypertensive medications, however, can precipitate herniation in those with large hematomas by increasing intravascular volume. Current American Heart Association practice guidelines recommend lowering mean arterial pressure (MAP) to below 130 mm Hg in those with a prior history of hypertension. In patients with elevated increased intracranial pressure (ICP), cerebral perfusion pressure should be kept above 70 mm Hg. Pressors are recommended in those patients whose *systolic* blood pressure drops below 90 mm Hg.

TREATMENT OF INCREASED INTRACRANIAL PRESSURE

Intubation and hyperventilation are often the fastest way to lower ICP. Osmotic diuretics such as intravenous mannitol or glycerin are also used. Neither is shown to improve overall mortality or functional outcome in patients, although clinical trials employ arbitrary, regularly scheduled, fixed dosing of such agents, which does not mirror their use in clinical practice. Corticosteroids are *not* shown to benefit overall outcome of these patients. In fact, infection and hyperglycemic complication rates are much higher in dexamethasone-treated patients in clinical trials employing steroid use.

SURGICAL TREATMENT

Data are available from eight randomized controlled trials of surgical versus conservative therapy for ICH (Table 2).

TABLE 2 Summary of All Prospective, Randomized Placebo-Controlled Trials for the Treatment of Intracerebral Hemorrhage in the Post–Computed Tomography Era

Study/year	Number of Patients	Intervention	Benefit
ISTICH/2003	1024	Early (<24 h) surgery	None
Yu/1992	216	Glycerol	None
Batjer/1990	21	Surgery	None
Auer/1989	100	Endoscopic surgery	Yes*
Juvela/1989	52	Surgery	None
Italian/1988	164	Hemodilution	None
Poungvarin/1987	93	Dexamethasone	None
Tellez/1973	40	Dexamethasone	None

*Decreased mortality in surgically treated (30%) versus medically treated (70%) patients ($P < .05$); increased proportion of neurologically intact patients in surgically treated arm ($P < .01$).

Early trials were greatly limited by no imaging confirmation and/or small size. Auer and colleagues demonstrated a lower mortality rate for endoscopically surgically treated patients with deep ICHs with a trend toward better survival in patients whose ICH volume was less than 50 mL, despite not demonstrating an overall statistically significant benefit.

The most significant clinical trial of surgical therapy for ICH is the 1024-patient International Surgical Trial of ICH (ISTICH), which evaluated the efficacy of early craniotomy (within 24 hours of admission) versus a conservative therapy group, which underwent craniotomy only when signs of impending herniation were evident, in patients presenting within 72 hours of ICH onset. No difference was discerned in the rate of favorable outcome in the early surgery group (26.1%) and the conservative management group (23.8%), nor in mortality rates. A trend did favor early surgery for lobar ICH.

TREATMENT OF COAGULOPATHY-RELATED INTRACEREBRAL HEMORRHAGE

Warfarin-related ICH should be treated immediately with recombinant factor VIIa where available, which is now FDA-indicated for life-threatening warfarin-related bleeding. It can reverse warfarin in 5 minutes or less. Fresh-frozen plasma and vitamin K should also be administered because factor VIIa has only a 3-hour half-life.

MEDICAL COMPLICATIONS

Much of ICH mortality is caused ultimately by medical complications such as aspiration pneumonia. As with any patient with an impaired level of consciousness or stroke, swallowing function should be carefully assessed and aspiration risk-monitored and treated as necessary with aspiration-reducing strategies including early tracheostomy and gastrostomy in patients who are likely to have sustained aspiration risk. Deep venous thrombosis prophylaxis with pneumatic air stockings in paretic or paraplegic legs can begin immediately. Decubitus prophylaxis should be tailored to individual patient risk as ascertained by Braden score or other comparable risk assessment tool. Fall risk assessment should be performed in potentially ambulatory patients. Adequate hydration and nutrition, especially protein, should be maintained while considering aspiration risk.

Secondary Prevention

Only one large clinical trial indirectly addresses the issue of pharmacologic means of recurrent ICH prevention above and beyond reduction of modifiable risk factors. The perindopril protection against recurrent stroke study (PROGRESS) trial reported a 75% relative risk reduction in recurrent hemorrhagic stroke in patients treated with a combination of perindopril and indapamide as compared to placebo. The effect of these medications appears not to be explained simply by their blood pressure reduction effect, suggesting that additional effects (such as on the endothelium of cerebral arterioles) may be responsible for part or all of the treatment effect.

Outcome

Overall outcome in ICH is poor. Mortality rates for so-called spontaneous ICH generally remain in the 30% to 50% range. A simple bedside prognostic scale, the ICH score, is used in clinical practice to determine mortality risk in patients with ICH, and incorporates factors most strongly correlated to ICH mortality risk, such as age,

---

 CURRENT DIAGNOSIS

- Obtain an emergency noncontrast CT scan of the brain upon arrival.
- Determine whether the patient is on anticoagulant therapy.
- Ascertain antecedent hypertension history and control.
- Order MRI/MRA and/or angiography for underlying cause in patients younger than 45 years of age or for lobar ICH.

Abbreviations: CT = computed tomography; ICH = intracerebral hemorrhage; MRI/MRA = magnetic resonance imaging/magnetic resonance arteriography.

TABLE 3 The Intracerebral Hemorrhage (ICH) Score

Variable	ICH Score Points
Glasgow Coma Score 3-4	2
Glasgow Coma Score 5-12	1
Glasgow Coma Score 13-16	0
ICH volume 30 mL or greater	1
ICH volume < 30 mL	0
Intraventricular extension present	1
Intraventricular extension absent	0
Infratentorial ICH	1
Supratentorial ICH	0
Age ≥ 60 y: check	1
Age < 60 y	0

Note: Mortality rate for score of 0 = 0%; 1 = 13%; 2 = 26%; 3 = 72%; 4 = 97%; 5 or 6 = 100%.

hematoma volume, hydrocephalus, and intraventricular extension (Table 3).

Emerging Therapies

Recently completed and ongoing studies are evaluating the efficacy of ultra-early hemostatic medications such as recombinant factor VIIa, neuroprotective drugs such as NXY-059, aggressive versus conservative blood pressure reduction, and aggressive versus conventional management of hyperglycemia.

ICH represents a significant fraction of all strokes and causes a disproportionate amount of stroke-related morbidity and mortality, especially in blacks age 55 years or younger. Treatment of hypertension is the single most important means of preventing ICH. Although diagnosis is greatly improved in the CT/MRI era, morbidity and mortality remain essentially unchanged. A high level of suspicion for cerebellar hemorrhage must be maintained. A toxicology screen, MRI, and angiography should be strongly considered in all patients with ICH under age 45 years. Patients presenting with hyperacute ICH need to be closely monitored because there is a 38% risk of rebleeding within the first 24 hours post-ICH onset. Patients with warfarin-related ICH should be immediately treated with recombinant factor VII infusion. Corticosteroids are of no value in ICH treatment and may increase risk of

CURRENT THERAPY

- Remember the ABCs (airway/breathing/circulation).
- Reverse warfarin coagulopathy immediately with recombinant factor VII, vitamin K, and fresh-frozen plasma.
- Lower extreme hypertension aggressively upon presentation.
- Monitor for rebleeding within the first 24 hours.
- Do not use corticosteroids.

hyperglycemia and infection. Mortality risk can be predicted by the ICH score, a useful bedside prognostic scale.

REFERENCES

Broderick JP, Adams HP Jr, Barsan W, et al: Guidelines for the management of spontaneous intracerebral hemorrhage. Stroke 1999;30:905-915.

Broderick JP, Brott T, Tomsick T, et al: ICH is more than twice as common as subarachnoid hemorrhage. J Neurosurg 1993;78:188-191.

Brott TG, Broderick JP, Kothari R, et al: Early hemorrhage growth in patients with ICH. Stroke 1997;28:1-5.

DelZoppo GJ, Mori E: Hematologic causes of ICH and their treatment. Neurosurg Clin North Am 1992;3:637-658.

Hemphill JC, Bonovich DC, Besmertis L, et al: The ICH Score: A simple, reliable grading scale for ICH. Stroke 2001;32:891-897.

Kissela B, Schneider A, Kleindorfer D, et al: Stroke in a biracial population: The excess burden of stroke among blacks. Stroke 2004;35:426-431.

Mendelow AD, Gregson BA, Fernandes HM, et al: Early surgery versus initial conservative treatment in patients with spontaneous supratentorial intracerebral haematomas in the International Surgical Trial in Intracerebral Haemorrhage (STICH): a randomised trial. Lancet 2005;365(9457):387-397.

Poungvarin N, Bhoopat W, Viriyavejakul A, et al: Effects of dexamethasone in primary supratentorial ICH. N Engl J Med 1987;316: 1229-1233.

PROGRESS Collaborative Group. Randomised trial of a perindopril-based blood-pressure lowering-regimen among 6,105 individuals with previous stroke or transient ischaemic attack. Lancet 2001; 358(9287):1033-1041.

Woo D, Haverbusch M, Sekar P, et al: The effect of untreated hypertension on hemorrhagic stroke. Stroke 2004; 35:1703-1708.

Zhu XL, Chan MSY, Poon WS: Spontaneous ICH: Which patients need diagnostic cerebral angiography? A prospective study of 206 cases and a review of the literature. Stroke 1997;28:1406-1409.

Ischemic Cerebrovascular Disease

Method of
Elzbieta Wirkowski, MD

A rupture of a blood vessel causes a hemorrhagic stroke. A hemorrhagic stroke can be either intracerebral or subarachnoid, and together it makes up 25% of all strokes.

An ischemic stroke is caused by an acute blood vessel occlusion and can be divided into three categories: lacunar, embolic, and atherothrombotic. A rapid distinction between hemorrhagic and ischemic strokes is crucial because each requires a different therapeutic approach.

Stroke is the third leading cause of death in the United States behind cancer and heart disease. It is the second leading cause of death worldwide, surpassed only by heart disease. An estimated 730,000 new or recurrent strokes occur every year in the United States.

Cerebral ischemia is caused by diminished blood flow. This interrupts the oxidative metabolic pathways in the brain ultimately leading to the destruction of neurons and glial cells. The extent of the tissue damage depends on the size of the occluded vessel, the patency of collaterals, and the speed of occlusion. When the cerebral blood flow falls below 10 mL/100 g/minute even for a few minutes, it results in permanent brain tissue damage. This area is called the core of the infarct. The surrounding tissue, with cerebral blood flow in the range of 10 to 20 mL/100 g/minute, is still potentially salvageable and called the ischemic penumbra. An understanding of the ischemic penumbra is extremely important in the development of new diagnostic techniques and therapeutic approaches.

Computed tomography (CT) is based on image reconstruction from a set of quantitative X-ray measurements through the brain. CT is especially useful for identifying an acute hemorrhage. An ischemic stroke may not be detectable for several hours. Early radiographic signs of stroke include a loss of gray–white matter differentiation, a loss of insular ribbon, and a dense vessel sign. After several days from the time of onset, one can find a hypodensity that ultimately obtains a well-defined dark appearance of CSF (cerebrospinal fluid).

A newer technique, CTA (CT angiography) and CTP (CT perfusion), can be very helpful in an early diagnosis of stroke. CTA can image the vascular anatomy of the neck and brain vessels. It requires intravenous (IV) contrast but is not as invasive as a formal angiogram. The CT perfusion scan when performed at stroke onset detects perfusion failure and therefore ischemia immediately.

Using a combination of noncontrast CT to exclude hemorrhage, followed by CTA to check for vascular occlusion and finally CTP to confirm ischemia, is particularly useful before the administration of tissue plasminogen activator (t-PA) in patients who have defibrillators or pacemakers.

MRI (magnetic resonance imaging) uses magnetic properties of the tissue that are displayed as maps of signal intensity. It provides a better definition of anatomic structures, especially the posterior fossa and the brainstem. MRI has several disadvantages: need for the patient's cooperation, inability to use in patients with pacemakers, defibrillators, and foreign metallic bodies. In spite of that, MRI is the modality of choice for the diagnosis of acute ischemic stroke. The ability to acquire diffusion-weighted imaging (DWI) and perfusion-weighted imaging (PWI) can identify salvageable ischemic penumbra within minutes of the stroke. In the future this may help extend the therapeutic window for acute thrombolysis.

MRA (magnetic resonance angiography) can determine the patency of the main vessels of the neck and brain without the need to administer potentially nephrotoxic contrast. Neurosonology plays yet another very important role in the diagnosis of acute stroke. MRA and duplex sonography of the carotid arteries are the most common methods used for an evaluation of carotid stenosis. The formal cerebral angiogram carries a significant number of risks for stroke (0.3% to 5.7%). In older patients with atherosclerotic disease, this number can increase two- to threefold.

Main indications for TCD (transcranial Doppler) use are sickle cell disease, right to left shunt, patent foramen ovale (PFO), intracranial stenosis, monitoring during acute thrombolysis, and detection of vasospasm.

TCD is particularly useful in the detection of PFO with sensitivity and specificity above 95% for paradoxical emboli detection. TCD can test autoregulation and vasomotor reactivity, which can help select patients for extracranial-intracranial (EC-IC) bypass surgery or endarterectomy. The main drawback of the technique is an inadequate acoustic window that limits insonation in 5% to 20% of patients.

ATHEROTHROMBOTIC STROKE AND CAROTID DISEASE

Carotid occlusive disease is responsible for 25% of ischemic strokes. The main risk factors are hypercholesterolemia, smoking, hypertension, and diabetes. Clinical presentation may be preceded by the brief loss of vision in one eye on the side of stenosis. Carotid bruit may suggest a presence of carotid stenosis, but there is no correlation between the degree of stenosis and the presence or absence of the bruit.

Carotid endarterectomy is currently the accepted standard of treatment for carotid occlusive disease. The North American Symptomatic Carotid Endarterectomy Trial (NASCET) reported an unequivocal benefit of surgery over the best medical management in symptomatic patients with carotid stenosis of 70% or more. The surgical intervention reduced the 2-year risk of any ipsilateral stroke from 26% to 9%. The overall rate of perioperative stroke was 6.5%. The results of the European Carotid Surgery Trial (ECST) were in accordance with NASCET.

The results of carotid stenting vary. In the Stenting and Angioplasty with Protection in Patients at High Risk for Endarterectomy (SAPPHIRE) trial, perioperative stroke and death rates were 7.3% for surgery and 4.4% for stenting. SAPPHIRE data analysis showed long-lasting effectiveness of the stent. The Carotid Revascularization Endarterectomy versus Stent Trial (CREST) is ongoing. Stenting therapy may need to pass the learning curve in the same way that carotid endarterectomy did.

For the intracranial stenosis of the large vessels of the circle of Willis, aspirin appears to be adequate and safe.

CARDIOEMBOLIC STROKE

Cardioembolic stroke accounts for 20% to 57% of all ischemic strokes. The main risk factors for cardioembolic stroke are mechanical prosthetic valve, mitral stenosis with atrial fibrillation (AF), AF (other than lone AF) left atrial thrombus, sick sinus syndrome, recent myocardial infarction (MI), left ventricular thrombus, dilated cardiomyopathy, akinetic left ventricular segment, atrial myxoma, and infective endocarditis.

Anticoagulation is recommended in AF with the exception of patients younger than 75 years old with lone AF, when aspirin can be acceptable. Warfarin (Coumadin) is otherwise recommended with an international normalized ratio (INR) between 2.0 and 3.0. In patients with MI and mural thrombus, anticoagulation with INR 2, 0 to 3.0 is recommended for 3 months to 1 year. To prevent a secondary ischemic coronary event, aspirin is frequently added. Adding aspirin to the warfarin can double the risk of bleeding complications. The Combination Hemotherapy and Mortality Prevention (CHAMP) trial compared aspirin 162 mg to warfarin (mean INR: 1.8) plus aspirin 81 mg after MI. The combination has not been better in the prevention of death, recurrent MI, or stroke. The possibility of a major hemorrhage was significantly increased in the combination therapy group. For patients with mechanical

TABLE 1 Clinical Syndromes of Lacunar Stroke

Silent (asymptomatic)
Pure motor hemiparesis
Ataxic hemiparesis
Sensory hemiparesis
Sensory motor
Clumsy hand dysarthria

prosthetic heart valves, oral anticoagulation with INR 2.5 to 3.5 is recommended.

PFO and atrial sepal aneurysm (ASA) are common, occurring in 25% of the general population. They are associated with unexplained ischemic strokes in younger patients less than 55 years. An evaluation for the presence of sepal defects with TCD or transesophageal echocardiography (TEE) should be a part of the standard workup of stroke in the younger population. If the hypercoagulable state is not an issue, antiplatelet therapy should be the initial treatment for secondary stroke prevention in younger patients with cryptogenic stroke and isolated PFO. In patients older than 55 years, even in the presence of PFO, other risk factors play more important roles in the occurrence of the stroke.

LACUNAR STROKES

Lacunar strokes occur because of the occlusion of small so-called end vessels in the brain (Table 1). Antiplatelet therapy is the treatment of choice for this type of ischemic stroke. The best treatment, however, is primary prevention by controlling the most prevalent risk factors: hypertension, diabetes, smoking, excessive drinking, and a sedentary lifestyle.

Secondary prevention includes aspirin, the combination of aspirin with extended-release dipyridamole (Aggrenox), and clopidogrel (Plavix) (Table 2). Positive statistically significant effects of aspirin therapy in stroke, MI, or vascular death prevention are documented in many trials.

TABLE 2 Current ACCP Guidelines for Noncardioembolic Stroke Prevention

Every patient who has experienced a noncardioembolic stroke or transient ischemic attack (TIA)
should receive treatment with an antiplatelet agent (grade 1A)
Acceptable options for initial therapy:
- Aspirin (50–325 mg)
- Combination of aspirin and ER-dipyridamole (Aggrenox) (25/200 mg bid)
- Clopidogrel (Plavix), 75 mg/d
Recommend antiplatelet agents over oral anticoagulation (grade 1A)
Suggest the use of the combination of aspirin and ER-dipyridamole over aspirin (grade 2A) and clopidogrel over aspirin (grade 2B)

Abbreviations: ACCP = American College of Chest Physicians.

The Warfarin Aspirin Recurrent Stroke Study (WARSS) did not show statistical benefits of warfarin compared to aspirin in noncardioembolic stroke, including antiphospholipid antibodies syndrome, PFO, or aspirin failure. Warfarin posed a slightly higher hazard in patients with hypertension, moderate stroke, and brainstem infarcts.

The European Stroke Prevention Study (ESPS2) trial compared aspirin 50 mg daily to a combination of 50 mg of aspirin and dipyridamole 400 mg (ER-DP). The aspirin/ER-DP combination showed a 23% relative risk reduction (RRR) compared to aspirin for stroke prevention. The main concern with this low dose of aspirin is the potential lack of protection against concomitant coronary artery disease. Fortunately, in this subgroup of patients, aspirin/ER-DP achieved a relative risk reduction for MI comparable to aspirin.

The Clopidogrel versus Aspirin in Patients at Risk for Ischemic Event (CAPRIE) study compared the effectiveness of aspirin versus clopidogrel in patients with stroke, MI, and PVD (peripheral vascular disorder). Clopidogrel showed an 8.7% overall risk reduction for cluster but did not reach statistical significance in stroke prevention.

The Management of Atherothrombosis with Clopidogrel in High-Risk Patients with Recent Transient Ischemic Attack (MATCH) trial showed that adding aspirin to clopidogrel did not provide any additional protective value compared with clopidogrel monotherapy. There was a significant increase in major bleeding complications in the clopidogrel plus aspirin group.

For patients with acute ischemic stroke, the use of full-dose anticoagulation is not recommended. The exceptions are: a high degree of carotid stenosis, a dissection of the cerebral arteries, and sinus vein thrombosis.

Regardless of the etiology of the ischemic stroke, thrombolysis with IV t-PA is currently the Food and Drug Administration (FDA)-approved way of the acute stroke treatment (Table 3). Only a small fraction of stroke victims

TABLE 3 Use of t-PA in Ischemic Stroke

Indication for t-PA	Contraindications for t-PA
Ischemic stroke Onset of symptoms <3 h	Time of onset >3 h Evidence of intracranial hemorrhage, mass effect, or edema on CT scan Clinical presentation that suggests subarachnoid hemorrhage Known bleeding diathesis Coumadin with INR >1.5; PTT >1.5 control Platelets <100,000 mm^3 Major surgery, trauma, GI and GU hemorrhage in the previous 2 wk History of previous stroke in the last 3 mo Intracranial or intraspinal surgery in the last 2 mo Glucose <50 and >400 mg/dL

Abbreviations: CT = computed tomography; GI = gastrointestinal; GU = genitourinary; INR = international normalized ratio; PTT = partial thromboplastin time; t-PA = tissue plasminogen activator.

CURRENT DIAGNOSIS

- Neurologic exam consistent with stroke is reliable.
- Presence or absence of bleeding on the head CT guides therapy.
- Hyperintensity on DWI (diffusion-weighted images) MRI is diagnostic.
- Presence of flow in the major neck or brain vessels determines the therapy.

Abbreviations: CT = computed tomography; MRI = magnetic resonance imaging.

receive t-PA. Treatment is demanding and requires an organized, team approach. The crucial information that needs to be obtained before the administration of t-PA is the last time the patient was seen well, a head CT to rule out a bleed, blood pressure control, and the size of the stroke. There are many misconceptions about t-PA. It is thought to be a very risky drug, yet 11 more patients out of 100 who received t-PA had a resolution of symptoms. Patients who receive t-PA have a higher risk of bleeding complications (6%); however, they still have better survival and recovery rates.

The intra-arterial (IA) use of thrombolytics has not been universally approved and is still considered experimental. The combined IA and IV use showed no difference in clinical outcomes in spite of better recanalization in the IV/IA group.

The Merci Retriever device offers acute intervention beyond 3 hours. Unfortunately the Mechanical Embolus Removal in Cerebral Ischemia (MERCI) trial showed that the rates of nonhemorrhagic complications (primarily embolization and dissection) were 5.7%. The hemorrhage rates were 9%.

The Neurocritical Care of Stroke

Close to 70% of patients with acute stroke have an elevation of blood pressure (BP) more than 170/100 with spontaneous decline by day 4. BP control in acute brain ischemia is controversial, and some studies favor lowering the BP by 20%, whereas others favor aggressive pressor therapy. Current American Stoke Association (ASA) guidelines recommend treatment if systolic BP is more than 220 and diastolic BP is more than 120. Patients who undergo thrombolysis require better BP control with systolic BP less than 180. Normothermia as well as glucose control and admission to a dedicated stroke unit improves outcomes.

CURRENT THERAPY

- Maintain proper perfusion using isotonic fluids.
- Involve a stroke team for best recovery results.
- Initiate t-PA if symptoms are <3 h and no hemorrhage is seen.
- Start antiplatelet agent in every nonhemorrhagic stroke unless t-PA is given or the patient has atrial fibrillation.

Abbreviation: t-PA = tissue plasminogen activator.

REFERENCES

AHA 2002 Heart and Stroke Statistical Update.

Antithrombotic Trialists Collaboration: Collaborative meta-analysis of randomised trials of antiplatelet therapy for prevention of death, myocardial infarction, and stroke in high risk patients. BMJ 2002;324:71-86.

Adams HP Jr, Adams RJ, Brott T, et al: Guidelines for the early management of patients with ischemic stroke: a scientific statement from the Stroke Council of the American Stroke Association. Stroke 2003;34:1056-1083.

Diener HC, Cunha L, Forbes C, et al: European Stroke Prevention Study. 2. Dipyridamole and acetylsalicylic acid in the secondary prevention of stroke. J Neurol Sci 1996;143:1-13.

Dyken M: Stroke risk factors in presentation of stroke. In Norris JW, et al (eds): New York, Springer-Verlag, 1991, pp 83-102.

Foulkes MA, Wolf PA, Price TR, et al: The NINDS Stroke Data Bank: Design, methods, and baseline characteristics. Stroke 1988;19:547-554.

Merritt's Neurology, 11th ed. Philadelphia, Lippincott Williams and Wilkins, 2005.

Mohr JP, Thompson JL, Lazar RM, et al: A comparison of warfarin and aspirin for the prevention of ischemic stroke. N Engl J Med 2001;345:1444-1451.

Risk factors for stroke and efficacy of antithrombotic therapy in atrial fibrillation. Analysis of pooled data from 5 randomized control trials. Arch Intern Med 1994;154:1449-1457.

Rehabilitation of the Stroke Patient

Method of
Karl J. Sandin, MD

Of the approximately 700,000 Americans who will have a stroke this year, an estimated half of them will need some sort of rehabilitation effort to maximize function. Whether because of thromboembolic disease, subarachnoid hemorrhage, or intracerebral hemorrhage, stroke is the third leading cause of disability in the United States. Although typically ineffective or unnecessary for either the minimally affected or tremendously impaired stroke survivor, for the large middle cohort of individuals with mild, moderate, or severe disability after stroke, rehabilitation programs provide improvements in outcome over natural recovery alone.

Rehabilitation is a coordinated program that provides reliable, conscientious, patient-centered restorative care to minimize impairment, disability, and handicap caused by a particular set of medical conditions. *Impairment* is any loss or abnormality of psychological, physical, or anatomic structure or function. *Disability* is any restriction to perform an activity in the manner within the range considered normal for a human being. *Handicap* is a social disadvantage that results from impairment or disability that limits fulfillment of a normal role. After stroke, a patient may have hemiparesis (impairment) that limits ambulation (disability), subsequently affecting ability to work (handicap). Some authors prefer to emphasize functions that remain after stroke, so they speak of ability and participation instead of disability and handicap. When rehabilitation is delivered by a well-functioning team, it provides a level of service excellence greater than the sum of its parts.

Rehabilitation settings include acute-care hospitals, acute rehabilitation hospitals and units, skilled nursing facilities, outpatient facilities and departments, the community (including the home, licensed residential care facilities, and assisted living centers), and transitional living facilities. Typically a patient with stroke is admitted through the emergency department to the hospital, preferably to a dedicated stroke unit. Use of these specialized service areas decreases morbidity and mortality after stroke and sets the stage for maximal recovery. From there patients with a substantial level of disability, yet good endurance for rehabilitation efforts and a reasonable prognosis to achieve a functional level that will allow them to live in a community setting, are referred to acute comprehensive stroke rehabilitation. Patients with less endurance or community discharge uncertainty are often referred to skilled nursing facilities for a less intensive program of rehabilitation. Some patients with less disability are referred directly from hospital care to outpatient or home health programs. Patients move from setting to setting as their medical condition and rehabilitation needs demand; services should continue in the least restrictive setting possible until the patient reaches a plateau. Younger stroke survivors, for whom community and vocational reentry is paramount, benefit greatly from transitional living center care. Gresham and colleagues in *Post-Stroke Rehabilitation* (in Chapter 5) effectively summarize decision trees to help choose a rehabilitation setting.

Apart from the patient and family, rehabilitation team clinical members include physicians (especially physiatrists—medical doctors specializing in physical medicine and rehabilitation—internists, and neurologists), nursing personnel of all levels, therapists (physical, occupational, recreational), speech/language pathologists, counselors (vocational, psychological), case/program managers, and others (dietitians, pharmacists, chaplains, etc.). The degree of involvement of each team member depends primarily on the setting and the stroke survivor's rehabilitation needs. In general, doctors are very involved in stroke rehabilitation as primary physician and team captain in acute rehabilitation settings but less so in community-based programs. Therapists are often more peripheral in intensive care unit settings but integral in home- and community-based treatment.

The antiquated term *cerebral vascular accident* (CVA) should never be used to describe a stroke. Accidents happen without warning or foreknowledge, whereas definable, manageable risk factors for stroke include homocystinemia, cardiac rhythm disturbances such as atrial fibrillation, obesity, dyslipidemia, nicotine dependence/tobacco use, stress, cocaine use, hypertension, diabetes, and autoimmune disease. Although nonmodifiable risk factors for stroke exist such as age (the older the person the higher the risk), gender (women die more of stroke than men, but men have more strokes), ethnicity (even controlled for other risk factors, people of color have more strokes than whites), and family history, primary and secondary stroke risk can be managed. Using the best medical care, family counseling, and education, stroke rehabilitation efforts should always seek to prevent future stroke. Secondary prevention of stroke through diet, exercise, cessation of smoking, and compliance with medical regimens remains a primary rehabilitation concern.

Prevention and early recognition of medical complications of stroke maximize neurologic and functional recovery. Thromboembolic disease, respiratory complications, cardiac problems, neurologic change, bowel and bladder dysfunction, skin breakdown, and pain can particularly affect stroke rehabilitation. All rehabilitation providers have the opportunity to recognize the signs and symptoms of these obstacles to improvement. Prompt recognition and diagnosis of medical problems improve patient care and outcome.

After stroke, deep venous thrombosis (DVT) and pulmonary embolism (PE) occur 40% to 50% and 9% to 15% of the time, respectively. These phenomena are the fourth most common cause of death in the first 30 days after stroke. Risk factors for their development include venous stasis, hypercoagulability, and endothelial injury. The first two are typically present in the stroke survivor because of immobility and acute-phase reaction. Primary prevention of these complications is critical. Stroke survivors not on systemic anticoagulation need either heparin or inferior vena caval filter placement. Because of lower morbidity compared with standard heparin, most stroke patients (including those with CNS [central nervous system] hemorrhage not requiring neurosurgical evacuation) receive low-molecular-weight fractionated heparin (enoxaparin sodium [Lovenox], 40 mg every day). Heparin prophylaxis continues until thromboembolic risk is minimized, typically defined as walking without physical assistance for 200 feet at a time. Pragmatically, prophylaxis is often stopped at institutional discharge but should be continued for at least 3 weeks after stroke. Intermittent pneumatic compression has little relevance in rehabilitation programs because patients are spending considerable time out of bed; elastic stockings provide no DVT/PE prevention. Recognition of failure of prevention requires clinical vigilance and forethought because 50% of DVT cases are clinically silent. A low threshold to check for DVT using Doppler ultrasound or other noninvasive testing or for PE using spiral chest computed tomography (CT) should inform the physician caring for the stroke survivor.

Pneumonia is the third major cause of death in the first 30 days after stroke. An estimated 32% of all stroke survivors develop pneumonia, especially after subarachnoid hemorrhage and in patients with coma because of stroke. Common risk factors include aspiration of oral contents, including saliva, liquids, and food, decreased chest wall compliance, poor expiratory muscle strength, decreased immune response after stroke, and general debility. Although pneumonia classically presents with shaking chills, hemoptysis, and pleuritic pain, in the stroke survivor the only symptom(s) may be low-grade fever, lethargy, loss of neurologic or functional status, or malaise. Prevention of pneumonia requires early assessment for and treatment of dysphagia, strict oral hygiene, such as sterilizing the mouth with an oral antiseptic (chlorhexidine gluconate [Peridex] on a foam-tipped mouth brush every 8 hours, preventive respiratory care including frequent incentive spirometry and inspiratory muscle training, and supervised posturally appropriate eating. Treatment of pneumonia includes rest, antibiotics, and tracheobronchial hygiene and may interrupt the stroke rehabilitation program.

At least 75% of patients with stroke have cardiac disease, which may have caused the stroke (e.g., atrial fibrillation) and may affect stroke recovery (e.g., cardiomyopathy). Cardiac disease is the second leading cause of early mortality and the leading cause of late mortality after stroke. Of stroke patients, 66% have coronary artery disease, 50% have dysrhythmias, and 20% have congestive heart failure (CHF). Effective management of CHF improves function after stroke. Cardiovascular and neurovascular disease commonly exist together, so stroke rehabilitation providers should assume all stroke survivors younger than 70 years have at least latent heart disease. Regardless of rehabilitation setting, patients should be monitored for vital signs and for signs and symptoms of well-being at the inception of the exercise components of stroke rehabilitation (and to some degree throughout).

Neurologic conditions may change or appear after stroke. Seizures complicate less than 10% of strokes; half occur in the first few days after stroke. Patients who seize after stroke typically have more brain damage and therefore a worse prognosis. Many patients with large bland infarcts or intracerebral and subarachnoid hemorrhage are placed on antiseizure agents as a prophylaxis against seizures. This controversial practice may impair the function of surviving normal brain and is discouraged in rehabilitation settings. A short (1-week) course of seizure prophylaxis is warranted after craniotomy. Bland infarcts may hemorrhagically transform, often presenting with changes in neurologic or functional status. A low threshold for repeat neurologic imaging (especially brain CT) should uncover this phenomenon and enable transfer, as is typically required, to a higher level of medical care. Change in neurologic status because of new stroke or intolerance of medications is not unusual during rehabilitation.

Neuromuscular conditions aggravate and facilitate stroke rehabilitation. After stroke, many survivors are initially hypotonic. As a result, their joints are poorly protected, so normal assistance moving in bed can result, for example, in shoulder trauma and pain. In the first few months after stroke, flaccidity is typically replaced with spasticity, a symptom complex of resistance to passive stretch, brisk reflexes, and hypertonicity because of loss of descending inhibition of spinal interneurons. Although spasticity can have its benefits, such as causing lower extremity rigidity that provides knee and ankle stiffness and allows a stable circumducted gait, it also can cause pain, contracture, and loss of function. Physical exercises, medications (dantrolene sodium [Dantrium], up to 100 mg four times daily), chemodenervation (botulinum toxin A [Botox]), and neuro destructive techniques seek to preserve some level of tone, thereby allowing maximal motor control. Yet much of the disability after stroke is caused by underlying weakness or sensory disturbances, losses not impacted by spasticity control.

Most stroke survivors have bowel and bladder dysfunction. Bladder problems include infection, incontinence, retention, and preexisting genitourinary disease, and they are often complicated by impairments in cognition, language, and mobility in the stroke patient. Continence, a complex feat of awareness, control, mobility, and dexterity, is vulnerable at many points to the direct and indirect effects of stroke. Cortical lesions can cause symptoms of urinary urgency at low urine volumes because of an unstable detrusor, the most common finding on urodynamic testing of stroke survivors with persistent incontinence. Brainstem strokes can cause detrusor sphincter dyssynergia. Patients with large strokes that cause aphasia, alteration in consciousness, or high levels of physical disability are typically bladder incontinent during initial stroke care. Patients with postvoid urinary retention (demonstrated by ultrasound postvoid measurement of bladder volume) have higher rates of incontinence and infection.

Urinary tract infection occurs in almost all stroke survivors and responds well to targeted antibiotic therapy. Incontinence rates drop in the first 3 months after stroke. Stroke survivors often require bladder retraining with timed voiding every 2 to 3 hours around the clock, elimination of medications with anticholinergic side effects that cause increased sphincter tone, and voiding trials in upright rather than recumbent positions to regain continence. Bowel dysfunction is common after stroke because of physical inactivity, inadequate fluid and/or dietary fiber, direct effect of a neurologic lesion of central defecation centers, side effects of medication, or impaction because of prolonged constipation. Conversely, some patients have diarrhea after stroke because of antibiotic side effects including *Clostridium difficile* infection, overstimulation of the colon with laxative, or obstipation. To normalize bowel function, stroke survivors require proper fluid, nutrition, fiber, and opportunity to eliminate in an upright position on their normal schedule. Often patients require a stimulant laxative (senna [Senokot], 2 to 4 tablets) followed 8 hours later by a postprandial rectal suppository (bisacodyl [Dulcolax]). Excessive use of bulk-forming agents does not help restore bowel regularity in the stroke survivor with altered mobility.

Neuropathic and nociceptive pain are common after stroke. Most worrisome is shoulder-hand syndrome (reflex sympathetic dystrophy, CPRS [Complex Regional Pain Syndrome, type 1]) that presents with pain in the eponymous parts, edema, dystrophic skin, and vasomotor instability. Triple-phase radionuclide bone scanning complemented by diagnostic and therapeutic blockade confirm the diagnosis. Additional therapies include transdermal clonidine, contrast baths, and axial loading extremity exercises. Most shoulder pain after stroke is caused by contracture, glenohumeral subluxation, rotator cuff disease, or bicipital tendonitis. Many stroke survivors have co-morbid conditions, such as osteoarthritis, which flare symptomatically with restorative efforts. True neuropathic pain because of stroke (central poststroke pain) is rare and difficult to treat.

Impairments after stroke include weakness (hemiparesis), loss of coordination (ataxia), hemisensory loss, visual deficits, agnosia, apraxia, disorders of language, and cognitive losses. After stroke, weak extremities often swell, usually because of flaccidity, loss of muscle control, or clot. If a thrombus is ruled out, extremity swelling requires elevation, such as for the upper extremity on a hemilap tray, or an external pressure gradient such as a 25 to 35 mm Hg below-knee compression stocking. Stroke survivors may have loss of light touch, pinprick, temperature, proprioception, kinesthetic, or vibratory sense, singularly or in combination. Even with normal strength, the patient with sensory loss may be very disabled. Visual deficits after stroke include field cuts, disregard, and disorders of perception. Anecdotal reports of improvement in visual functioning through behavioral optometry are not supported by well-designed studies. Agnosia (a deficit in afferent processing or inability to interpret or recognize information in one sensory modality when the end-organ is intact) particularly involves vision, touch, and hearing. Apraxia (a deficit in efferent processing or the inability to perform purposefully despite normal coordination and motor function) can involve language, dressing, or construction. Language problems include aphasia (impairment of the capacity to interpret and formulate multimodal language symbols), dysarthria (imprecise or poorly coordinated speech production with decreased articulation and intelligibility without problems in word retrieval or comprehension), and speech apraxia (a verbal or oral impairment of voluntary execution of complex speech-motor activities). Cognitive sequelae of stroke are inattention, memory loss, and loss of insight and judgment, which in combination may result in inability to initiate, plan, and complete (executive functioning) daily tasks. Various rehabilitation techniques such as transfer of training, neurodevelopmental technique (NDT) of Bobath, cutaneous stimulation of Rood, proprioceptive neuromuscular facilitation (PNF) of Voss and Knott, and motor relearning have particular disciples and adherents, although most rehabilitation therapists use a combination of various theories to improve function.

Strict attention to patient safety vis-à-vis falls and swallowing limits morbidity after stroke. Stroke survivors, regardless of location, have high fall rates. Falls can be prevented by placing the patient near the nurse's station, using bed movement alarms and mobility monitors, eliminating wet or uneven surfaces, providing one-to-one supervision, and avoiding polypharmacy, especially with cognitively impairing medications. Approximately 50% of stroke survivors have dysphagia because of deficits in oral, pharyngeal, or esophageal stages of swallowing. Of those, one third aspirate (some silently), defined as entrance of material into the airway below the level of the true vocal folds. Although the history and physical offer some tools to identify and treat swallowing problems, most rehabilitation therapists use functional endoscopic or videofluoroscopic swallowing studies to determine swallowing ability and guide management of dysphagia. Stroke survivors with dysphagia should eat only in highly structured, distraction-free environments using techniques such as double swallow and chin tuck to mitigate risk of aspiration. At time of advancement to more difficult diet textures or consistencies, strokes survivors should receive special attention to ensure a safe transition.

In the past, stroke rehabilitation paradigms focused almost exclusively on disability limitation. Today, changes in medical and societal perspective and improved neuroscience understanding are leading to newer techniques of care that seek to first improve physical function, automatically lessening disability. Examples of such efforts in stroke rehabilitation include partial weight-bearing treadmill training, constraint-induced movement therapy, and residential aphasia training. Although there is some overlap with disability treatment, a primary goal of these interventions is to avoid or eliminate learned nonuse, demanding maximal performance of the CNS for the physical or cognitive task at hand. At a cellular level, stroke rehabilitation improves outcome in two major ways: synaptogenesis and uncovering of dormant or vestigial CNS pathways.

Neuropharmacology augments the stroke rehabilitation process. Deficits in attention can be decreased by stimulants (methylphenidate [Ritalin], up to 10 mg twice daily). The addition of dextroamphetamine (Dextrostat) biweekly to speech/language pathologist language retraining improves aphasia and verbal apraxia compared to therapy alone. Although no controlled studies exist, many practitioners use acetylcholinesterase inhibitors designed to treat dementia (donepezil [Aricept], 5 to 10 mg every day) for cognitive disorders after stroke. Selective serotonin reuptake inhibitor (SSRI) and serotonin-norepinephrine reuptake inhibitor (SNRI) antidepressants effectively treat poststroke depression and may directly improve neural recovery after stroke.

Regardless of setting, stroke rehabilitation affects outcome beneficially. Major outcome measurement tools include the National Institutes of Health (NIH) stroke scale, a 14-item assessment scoring various impairments. Functional (disability) scales are the bedrock of analysis of stroke rehabilitation success and include, most prominently, the Barthel index and the Functional Independence Measure (FIM). Few scales assess participation, although arguably ability to return to active community living best reflects stroke rehabilitation success. Using diagnostic and demographic data and FIM scores, stroke survivors undergoing acute comprehensive rehabilitation paid by Medicare are assigned to a case-mix group (CMG) from which prospective payment derives. Payment for stroke rehabilitation is a controversial topic because rehabilitation hospitals, skilled nursing facilities, outpatient departments, and home health agencies all believe current funding schemes under-reimburse their services.

Perhaps the biggest burden after stroke is psychosocial. Depression and anxiety are common after stroke, with an incidence of approximately 40% each at 6 months. Many standard tests for these psychological conditions require normal cognitive and language function, so they have limited usefulness in the stroke survivor. Emotionalism (emotional lability) is present up to 1 year after stroke in 21% of patients. Social problems after stroke include economic strain (46%), social isolation (53%), decreased community involvement (43%), disruption of family function (52%), poor motivation, dependency, and loss of control. Social isolation is more common in women and those with higher educational achievement. Families are often called on to provide care for stroke survivors, but they may have neither the emotional nor physical ability to do so. As a result, caregivers burn out, culminating in severe situations with neglect or abuse. The incidence of depression in spouses of stroke patients is three times that of controls. To maximize the chances of a satisfying life for stroke survivors and their families, liberal use of community services within the entire first year after stroke should be encouraged. If the challenges of resuming a meaningful life are not met, patients and their families may respond with illness and maladaptive behaviors (Current Therapy Box).

 CURRENT THERAPY

- Stroke rehabilitation improves outcome over natural recovery alone.
- Stroke rehabilitation is most effective when team members work together on shared functional goals.
- Reduction of future stroke risk is a primary stroke rehabilitation concern.
- Most common medical problems after stroke include DVT/PE, pneumonia, UTI, and CHF, conditions that can usually be prevented, and if they occur must be managed well to secure stroke rehabilitation success.

Abbreviations: CHF = congestive heart failure; DVT/PE = deep venous thrombosis/pulmonary embolism; UTI = urinary tract infection.

REFERENCES

Bode RK, Heinemann AW, Semik P, Mallinson T: Patterns of therapy activities across length of stay and impairment levels: Peering inside the "black box" of inpatient stroke rehabilitation. Arch Phys Med Rehabil 2004;85(12):1901-1908

Bogey RA, Geis CC, Phillip R, et al: Stroke and neurodegenerative disorders: III. Stroke: Rehabilitation management. Arch Phys Med Rehabil 2004;(Suppl 1)85(3):15-20

Da Cunha IT Jr, Lim PA, Qureshy H, et al: Gait outcomes after acute stroke rehabilitation with supported treadmill ambulation training: A randomized controlled pilot study. Arch Phys Med Rehabil 2002;83:1258-1265.

Dettmers C, Teske U, Hamzei F, et al: Distributed form of constraint-induced movement therapy improves functional outcome and quality of life after stroke. Arch Phys Med Rehabil 2005;86(2): 204-209.

Gresham GE, Duncan PW, Stason WB, et al: Post-Stroke Rehabilitation. Clinical Practice Guideline, No. 16. Rockville, Md, U.S. Department of Health and Human Services. Public Health Service, Agency for Health Care Policy and Research. AHCPR Pub. No. 95-0662. May 1995.

McLean DE: Medical complications experienced by a cohort of stroke survivors during inpatient, tertiary-level stroke rehabilitation. Arch Phys Med Rehabil 2004;85:466-469.

Sandin KJ, Mason KD: Manual of Stroke Rehabilitation. Boston, Butterworth-Heinemann, 1996.

Seizures and Epilepsy in Adolescents and Adults

Method of
Erik K. St. Louis, MD,
and Mark A. Granner, MD

Epilepsy is a common public health problem afflicting approximately 2.5 million Americans and 30 million persons worldwide. Epilepsy is equally prevalent between the sexes until older age, where the increased incidence of epilepsy in elderly men mirrors that of cerebrovascular disease.

Epilepsy was recognized in antiquity, described by Hippocrates as "the falling sickness." The etymology of epilepsy stems from the Greek *epilepsia*, "to be seized or taken hold of," derived from the erroneous belief and unfortunately persistent stigma that epileptic seizures result from supernatural or spiritual, rather than medical, causes. Such historical misunderstandings, coupled with limited availability of effective treatments, have instilled fear of epilepsy for centuries in patients, their families and caregivers, and society. Fortunately, an evolving medical understanding of epilepsy and its many causes and imitators has enabled improved diagnostic testing and an ever-expanding palette of effective, tolerable antiepileptic drug and surgical therapies over the last three decades. All clinicians should be familiar with epilepsy not only because of its prevalence, but because its treatments are increasingly adopted for a wide variety of neurologic and psychiatric conditions including migraine, pain, and mood disorders.

Seizures and Epilepsy Defined

An epileptic seizure is a sudden, transient alteration in behavior caused by an abnormal, excessive neuronal discharge in the cerebral cortex. Everyone has a seizure threshold and holds the potential to have a seizure. Only a small subset of the population, however, experiences spontaneous seizures or develops epilepsy. The lifetime prevalence of experiencing a single seizure is approximately 10%, but only approximately 30% of incipient seizures recur and become epilepsy.

Seizures are most often provoked by an extrinsic (systemic) or intrinsic (brain) factor. Table 1 lists the causes of provoked seizures. An individual may have recurrent provoked seizures without developing epilepsy. In most cases, a provoked seizure does not recur when the provoking factor is successfully corrected, avoided, or removed. The tendency toward recurrent provoked seizures speaks either to the root cause (e.g., recurrent episodes of alcohol withdrawal seizures) or to a heightened sensitivity to seizures in the individual (e.g., a lower than average seizure threshold).

Epilepsy is characterized by recurrent, unprovoked seizures. The prevalence of epilepsy in the general population is approximately 1%. The principal clinical symptoms and signs of epilepsy include ictal (during a seizure), postictal (immediately following seizure termination), and interictal (between seizure episodes) manifestations. Behavioral alterations accompanying epileptic seizures are diverse, ranging from subjective feelings reported by the patient, to objectively witnessed behavioral arrest, unresponsiveness, or involuntary movements. The nature of the ictal behavioral disturbance depends on the location of seizure onset in the brain and its pattern of propagation.

Diagnosis of Seizure Type and Epilepsy Syndrome

A seizure is only a symptom of brain dysfunction, and the seizure type is not in itself an etiologic diagnosis. A diversity of underlying causative pathologies may result in identical phenotypes of clinical seizure behavior and electroencephalographic (EEG) manifestations. The patient's prognosis and treatment are directed by a diagnosis of the underlying epilepsy syndrome, which incorporates an understanding of the cause of the seizures as well as the clinical and EEG characteristics. Epilepsy syndromes are regarded as idiopathic, symptomatic, or cryptogenic.

The International League Against Epilepsy (ILAE) has created consensus terminology defining different seizure types and, in parallel, descriptions of epilepsy syndromes. Diagnosis of ILAE seizure type and epilepsy syndrome is based on electroclinical criteria, including the description of seizure behavior and EEG manifestations. Most experts now also use neuroimaging to diagnose the most likely seizure type and epilepsy syndrome. The seizure type and epilepsy syndrome diagnoses are crucial steps in the approach to the patient with epilepsy because this information determines the patient's prognosis, which type of antiepileptic drug (AED) therapy is indicated, and whether surgical therapies can potentially be offered if AEDs are ineffective.

The two principal varieties of epileptic seizures are partial (also known as focal or localization-related) and generalized seizures. Partial seizures begin in one brain region, whereas generalized seizures have their onset simultaneously in both cerebral hemispheres. Differentiating epileptic seizure type and syndrome is often difficult in

TABLE 1 Common Causes of Provoked Seizures

Drugs of Abuse
Alcohol
- Severe acute alcohol intoxication
- Alcohol withdrawal

Amphetamine and methamphetamine
Cocaine
Lysergic acid diethylamide (LSD)
Phencyclidine

Iatrogenic (Prescription Drugs)
Antibiotics
- High-dose intravenous penicillin
- Imipenem

Antiarrhythmic agents
- Lidocaine (Xylocaine)
- Procainamide (Pronestyl)
- Propafenone (Rythmol)

Insulin overdose
Pain medications
- Opiate analgesics, especially meperidine (Demerol)
- Tramadol (Ultram)

Psychotropic drugs
- Antidepressants
  - Clomipramine (Anafranil)
  - Bupropion (Wellbutrin)
- Antipsychotics
  - Clozapine (Clozaril)

Stimulants
- Amphetamines mixed (Adderall), methylphenidate (Ritalin)

Infection
Brain abscess
Cerebritis
- Lyme disease
- Neurosyphilis

Encephalitis
- Cytomegalovirus
- Herpes simplex virus type 1
- Varicella-zoster virus
- West Nile virus

Acute meningitis
- Bacterial
- Fungal
- Viral

Metabolic Disorders
Hypocalcemia
Hypoglycemia
Hyperglycemia
- Nonketotic hyperosmolar state
- Diabetic ketoacidosis

Hypomagnesemia
Hyponatremia
Hypernatremia
Hypophosphatemia

Herbal Products
Guarana
Ma Huang

---

new-onset epilepsy. Many partial seizures present clinically as a secondarily generalized tonic–clonic seizure without focal features, and patients usually present for evaluation after only one or a few seizures have occurred, so the full spectrum of their epilepsy is not yet apparent.

Partial seizures are subclassified as simplex, complex, and secondarily generalized seizures. A simple partial seizure is restricted at onset to one focal cortical region and does not impair consciousness. Simple partial seizures are synonymous with the term *aura* and involve autonomic, gustatory, cognitive, somatosensory, or involuntary motor activity depending on where they begin in the brain. When a simple partial seizure propagates beyond the initial seizure focus, it may evolve into a complex partial or secondarily generalized seizure. A complex partial seizure is defined by the feature of altered consciousness (although often not full loss of consciousness) and may involve behavioral arrest, blank staring, oral automatisms such as chewing or swallowing, limb automatisms including aimless fumbling movements of the hands, and amnesia. A complex partial seizure may or may not be preceded by an aura, and it may propagate to the whole brain to become a generalized tonic–clonic seizure. There may be considerable variability of behavioral characteristics between different patients with partial seizures or even within a given patient (although a patient's personal seizures tend to be rather monomorphic). Table 2 provides a summary of characteristic auras and behavioral manifestations of partial seizures according to the region of seizure onset. An EEG during a partial seizure usually demonstrates focal rhythmic activity overlying the region of seizure onset.

Generalized seizures involve simultaneous seizure onset in both cerebral hemispheres. By definition, consciousness is impaired from seizure onset, although myoclonic seizures may be too brief to detect an alteration in consciousness. Absence seizures, frequently confused with complex partial seizures because both were previously (and unfortunately) referred to as petit mal seizures, are brief episodes (typically less than 10 seconds) of behavioral arrest, staring with unresponsiveness, and oral or limb automatisms. Absence seizures lack an aura or postictal state. Tonic seizures involve symmetric tonic posturing of the extremities and, if prolonged, may have prominent autonomic instability. Atonic (also known as astatic) seizures involve loss of tone and may lead to falls. Generalized tonic–clonic seizures involve an initial phase of tonic posturing, generally lasting less than 20 seconds, followed by symmetric clonic movements of the limbs for 1 to 3 minutes. Ictal EEG during generalized seizures demonstrates generalized epileptiform patterns of repetitive spike-wave discharges, polyspikes, or background attenuation.

The accurate diagnosis of an epilepsy syndrome in each patient is an important tenet in epilepsy care; whereas diagnosis of the habitual seizure type describes the ictal seizure characteristics, an epilepsy syndrome diagnosis reaches further, inferring knowledge of the underlying etiology and therefore determining the prognosis and most appropriate therapy. Despite rigorous diagnostic testing, many times the epilepsy syndrome remains ambiguous in new-onset epilepsy cases.

Partial seizures and their associated epilepsy syndromes are most common in adolescents and adults, representing approximately 70% of all epilepsy in these age groups. Most partial epilepsy is related to known acquired etiologies such as head injury, cerebrovascular disease, or tumors. Conversely, idiopathic or cryptogenic partial epilepsies and idiopathic generalized epilepsies are often inherited. The basis of inherited epilepsies is a rapidly evolving field. Many of the known gene effects relate to ion channelopathies.

TABLE 2 Typical Partial Seizure Characteristics According to Region of Seizure Onset

	Simple Partial	Complex Partial	Secondary Generalized
Frontal	Focal clonic motor or none	Amnestic Automatisms Hypermotor common	Frequent

Temporal	Mesial (none possible)
	 • Autonomic
	 • Dysmnesic
	   • Déjà vu
	   • Jamais vu
	 • Gustatory
	Lateral/posterior neocortical
	Auditory
	Complex visual
		Amnestic
		Automatisms
		
		Amnestic
		Automatisms
			Less frequent

Parietal	Somatosensory or none	Amnestic Automatisms	Frequent
Occipital	Simple visual or none	Amnestic Automatisms	Frequent

The Differential Diagnosis of Paroxysmal Spells

The differential diagnosis of epilepsy is wide. Numerous paroxysmal non-neurologic and neurologic disorders may closely mimic the behavioral alterations of an epileptic seizure. Table 3 differentiates commonly confused seizure types and nonepileptic paroxysmal spells by behavioral characteristics, duration, and usual ictal EEG findings. Although most of these conditions are reviewed elsewhere in this text, psychological mimicry of epilepsy is particularly common. Psychogenic nonepileptic spells (also known as pseudoseizures) are most often an expression of a conversion disorder with subconsciously motivated spells of behavioral unresponsiveness or unusual movements that may closely resemble epileptic seizures. Psychogenic spells, however, frequently involve behavioral characteristics of eye closure, nonphysiologic patterns of movements, prominent pelvic thrusting, prolonged duration (often over 5 to 10 minutes), lack of stereotypy between episodes, and failure to respond to antiepileptic drugs. Because true epileptic seizures may also share all of these characteristics, the diagnosis of psychogenic nonepileptic spells is necessarily a diagnosis of exclusion and requires diagnostic ictal video-EEG monitoring for confirmation.

Clinical Approach to the Patient with Seizures

The fundamental goals in epilepsy care are both diagnostic and therapeutic: to understand the underlying cause of epilepsy and determine the epilepsy syndrome when possible; and to strive for seizure freedom without adverse side effects of treatment whenever feasible (or, at the very least, to minimize disabling, injurious seizures and limit adverse effects). The approach to new-onset seizures and chronic care of the patient with established epilepsy is now considered.

THE SINGLE SEIZURE AND NEW-ONSET EPILEPSY

The focus during the approach to new-onset seizures is different than in chronic epilepsy. The emphasis for new-onset seizures is prompt diagnosis of the underlying cause because it is imperative to ensure there is no symptomatic etiology requiring further diagnosis or therapy (e.g., brain mass or vascular malformation). Diagnostic tests also help determine the epilepsy syndrome diagnosis and judge the prognosis for future seizure recurrence.

After an apparent single seizure, the physician should take a detailed history from the patient and any available collateral historians about the presenting event. Although serum laboratory values are frequently obtained after a first seizure, these tests actually have little value in the diagnosis of most uncomplicated first seizures in adolescents and adults. Electrolytes and complete blood count may assure overall general health and serve as a baseline prior to contemplation of antiepileptic drug therapy. A serum or urine drug screen is often appropriate to exclude drug abuse or intoxication as a cause of provoked seizures in adolescents and adults.

The two most important diagnostic tests in the initial evaluation of new-onset seizures are a magnetic resonance image (MRI) of the brain and an EEG; the former provides a measure of structure and the latter a complementary measure of function. A computed tomography (CT) of the head is insufficient to disclose subtle epileptogenic pathology in the brain. The only reason to obtain a head CT after a new-onset seizure is for emergency exclusion of acute neurologic catastrophes requiring urgent attention, such as cerebral hemorrhage or infarction. If a patient has recovered to baseline and neurologic examination is normal, head CT can often be deferred if a definitive brain MRI and neurologic consultation may be obtained promptly (i.e., within 1 week following the seizure). If there is a question of head or neck trauma, head CT should be performed emergently, and cervical radiographs may be necessary. EEG is particularly valuable when brain MRI is normal because it may disclose

TABLE 3 Differentiating Epileptic Seizures from Nonepileptic Spells

	Premonitory Symptoms	Behavioral Characteristics	Duration	Postictus Symptoms	Ictal EEG Findings
Absence seizure	None	Staring, automatisms	<10 sec	None	Generally 3-Hz spike wave
Partial complex seizure	Aura variable; if sensory march, brief over 10–30 sec	Staring, automatisms, posture often preserved	30–180 sec	Common; amnesia, aphasia, sleepiness, ± incontinence	Focal rhythmic activity
Generalized tonic–clonic seizures	Aura variable	Sequence of tonic limb posturing for 10 sec, then clonic movements	1–3 min	Invariable; frequently amnesia, sleep, incontinence, tongue biting	Repetitive spikes (tonic phase); spike wave (clonic phase)
Psychogenic nonepileptic spells (pseudoseizures)	Variable	Variable; behavioral unresponsiveness Nonstereotypy, and unusual movements common	Variable; may be prolonged (>10 min)	Variable; often none	None, other than movement artifact
Syncope	Common; lightheadedness	Falling, eye closure, variable convulsive movements, incontinence	Minutes	None to brief confusion; no postical amnesia	Suppression
Migraine	Prolonged; sensory march over minutes	"Positive" symptoms (e.g., tingling paresthesias)	20–30 min	None	Slowing/suppression
Transient ischemic attack (TIA)	Sensory march rapid (<10 sec)	More often "negative" (e.g., anesthetic numbness, weakness)	Variable; <1 h	None	Slowing/suppression
Sleep disorders: Cataplexy	Emotional provocation	Behavioral sleep	Minutes	None	REM stage sleep
Parasomnias	None	Sleep-onset only	Minutes	Brief confusion	Onset in REM/NREM sleep

Abbreviations: EEG = electroencephalogram; NREM = nonrapid eye movement (sleep); REM = rapid eye movement (sleep).

functional evidence for a heightened epileptogenic potential by demonstrating interictal epileptiform discharges that help determine risk of seizure recurrence after a single seizure or diagnose the epilepsy syndrome when there have been recurrent spells.

Additional diagnostic studies such as ictal video-controlled EEG (V-EEG) monitoring, positron emission tomography (PET) of the brain, magnetoencephalography (MEG), and neuropsychological testing may be used later in the course of a patient's evaluation if empirical medical therapy is unsuccessful and if surgical candidacy is questioned, but they are of generally limited value in new-onset seizure disorders. V-EEG is appropriate when psychogenic nonepileptic spells are the suspected diagnosis to exclude epilepsy and to allow prompt triage to appropriate psychological care, thereby sparing the patient

from an errant diagnosis and the potential risks of unnecessary antiepileptic drug therapy.

The risk of seizure recurrence following a single seizure is approximately 30% when both MRI and EEG are normal. Multiple seizures occurring over a single day should still be considered as a single seizure episode. The risk of recurrence following a second remote seizure is variable, ranging from roughly 50-80%. Evidence is conflicting on the precise prognostic value of an abnormal EEG following a first seizure, but most experts consider EEG abnormalities to raise the risk of seizure recurrence substantially, especially when the EEG shows generalized epileptiform discharges.

Following a second unprovoked seizure, most experts diagnose epilepsy and recommend treatment. Treatment may be considered even following a first seizure if a structural cortical lesion is found because the risk of seizure recurrence is more than 50% in such instances, or if the patient leads a lifestyle where a second seizure would be highly undesirable (such as dependency on driving or a risky occupation).

All patients with new-onset epilepsy must be counseled regarding safety and driving. All patients with consciousness-impairing seizures should be instructed to avoid work, hobbies, or sports activities exposing them to heightened risk of personal injury until seizures are controlled for at least 3 to 6 months. Driving is a critical personal and public safety concern with legal implications to both patient and physician. Because laws vary between states, clinicians must ensure intimate familiarity with the law governing epilepsy in their own jurisdiction and counsel patients appropriately, then document their discussion in the medical record. A few states require physicians to report epilepsy patients.

CHRONIC EPILEPSY CARE AND DETERMINATION OF REFRACTORY EPILEPSY

The approach to the patient with chronic epilepsy is to determine whether the epilepsy is benign or refractory (also known as medically intractable, pharmacoresistant). Following from the tenet in new-onset epilepsy evaluation, determination of the patient's epilepsy syndrome directs the choice of AED therapy most likely to control seizures successfully and allows prognosis for future remission or commitment to long-term AED therapy. Symptomatic or cryptogenic partial or generalized epilepsies and juvenile myoclonic epilepsy rarely remit and usually require long-term AED treatment. Idiopathic partial epilepsy or unclassified epilepsy syndromes more frequently remit after 2 to 5 years of treatment, suggesting future AED withdrawal is worth considering. Drug withdrawal is a complicated decision that is best made in consultation with a neurologist.

Determination of the epilepsy syndrome is more readily achieved during longitudinal continuity of care, given information derived from observations of seizure episodes and further opportunities to obtain interictal or ictal EEG recordings. With repeated or prolonged interictal EEG recording, the yield of identifying interictal epileptiform discharges increases. However, even after repeated outpatient EEGs, or with intensive inpatient V-EEG recording, approximately 20% of those with eventually proven epilepsy lack definite interictal EEG abnormalities. It is important to realize that the diagnosis of epilepsy remains at heart a clinical determination. The absence of abnormalities on MRI or interictal laboratory EEGs does not exclude an epilepsy diagnosis. If MRI or EEG has not been performed prior to evaluation, it is helpful to begin with these investigations to determine the patient's epilepsy syndrome and to exclude symptomatic pathology. Inpatient V-EEG is the gold standard for establishing a diagnosis of epilepsy and should be considered when patients are refractory to one to two empirical AED treatment trials. Even if a patient has infrequent seizures while maintained on AED therapy, admitting patients to an epilepsy monitoring unit allows an opportunity for withdrawal of medication in a safe, carefully supervised environment with a goal of increasing seizure frequency so that one or more habitual clinical seizures may be recorded. Ambulatory EEG or outpatient V-EEG are also available at many centers but have lower yield, given limitations of the inability to withdraw AEDs safely, to conduct behavioral testing or capture video, and to accomplish a technically adequate recording.

Patients continuing to experience breakthrough seizures may have refractory epilepsy. Just more than 10% of patients who have an efficacy failure on their first AED ever become seizure free during future AED trials, suggesting the need for vigilance toward achieving the clinical goals of seizure freedom without AED side effects. If a patient fails to achieve seizure freedom following one to two AED monotherapy trials, referral to a comprehensive epilepsy center should be strongly considered to permit appropriate seizure classification and consideration of surgical options.

Approximately one-third of those with epilepsy, approximately 750,000 in the United States, have medically refractory epilepsy (i.e., epilepsy that is resistant to AEDs with continued breakthrough seizures and intolerable AED adverse effects). Those afflicted with refractory epilepsy consistently report lower quality of life for multiple reasons, including lost productivity at work or school, inability to drive, self-injury, and the fear of living with the constant uncertainty of when their next seizure may occur. Even more alarming, growing evidence indicates that patients with refractory epilepsy are at a heightened risk for mortality from sudden unexplained death in epilepsy (SUDEP). Even in patients who are well controlled on their drug treatment, approximately half of those surveyed are not satisfied with their current regimen of AEDs, in most instances because of unpleasant or disabling drug-related side effects. A determination of refractory epilepsy from breakthrough seizures or intolerable AED adverse effects should be made relatively early in the course of treatment to permit other potentially more effective care options to be considered. Because of the limitations of current AEDs, both patients and their physicians may be lulled into a dangerous complacency by the desperation of chronic refractory epilepsy, perhaps figuring that any further efforts toward improvement of the situation will prove futile. However, given the severe morbidity and potential mortality of refractory epilepsy, clinicians must aspire beyond the status quo of a so-called acceptable seizure burden and educate their patients that intensive evaluation may lead to more effective treatment for their seizures. Patients who may benefit from referral to a comprehensive epilepsy center include those with these situations:

- An uncertain diagnosis of spells (i.e., the diagnosis of epilepsy is still in question)
- Failure to achieve complete seizure control
- Adverse effects on current AED therapy
- Injury from their seizures
- Lost productivity at work or school because of seizures or adverse effects
- A complicated regimen of concurrent medications and/or other confounding medical, psychiatric, or psychosocial conditions

Epilepsy Therapies

The goals of all epilepsy therapies are to achieve seizure freedom without adverse effects of treatment.

Choosing between the numerous options available for epilepsy treatment can be daunting for physicians and patients alike. The last two decades have seen the release of a number of newer AEDs into clinical use, many of which offer improved tolerability and safety profiles. Another advent is vagus nerve stimulation (VNS), the first device using the novel approach of electrical stimulation in epilepsy approved by the Food and Drug Administration (FDA). Centers offering expert evaluation for epilepsy surgery have also become more widely available.

Guidelines for choosing among epilepsy therapies are currently lacking. Until evidence-based guidelines are developed, optimal therapeutic triage must be highly individualized by synthesizing available data, clinical wisdom, and the patient's preference.

All AEDs have the potential to cause dose-related neurotoxic adverse effects. Fortunately, these may be obviated in most patients by dose reduction or substituting for a better tolerated AED.

ANTIEPILEPTIC DRUG THERAPY

Table 4 itemizes specific AEDs with accompanying information on clinical spectrum of uses, pharmacokinetics, typical dosing and blood levels, and cardinal adverse effects. There are currently no clear evidence-based algorithms to guide the temporal sequencing of different AED trials. Nonetheless, common treatment principles underlie the choosing, dosing, sequencing, and monitoring of AED therapy in epilepsy care. Here are several basic principles:

- Choose AED therapy appropriate for the epilepsy syndrome.
- Consider patient characteristics and co-morbidities when choosing AEDs.
- Employ AED monotherapy at the lowest effective dosage to achieve seizure freedom.
- Reserve AED polytherapy (combining two or more AEDs) for refractory patients and minimize total drug load to limit adverse effects.
- Treat according to the patient's clinical response, not the AED level.
- Monitor for long-term complications of older AED therapy and consider withdrawal of therapy when appropriate.
- Choose affordable AED therapy.

Choosing an AED appropriate for the patient's epilepsy syndrome is an important tenet of epilepsy care. AEDs have different spectrums of efficacy for various seizure types within epilepsy syndromes. Some AEDs are narrow in their spectrum of efficacy, whereas others are broader, treating a variety of different seizure types well. Broad-spectrum AEDs may be favored when the epilepsy syndrome diagnosis is ambiguous because they offer potential efficacy against most seizure types and have less potential to aggravate some epilepsy syndromes. To some degree, the spectrum of efficacy of an AED is related to its postulated mechanism of action. AEDs that chiefly antagonize sodium channel ionophores or promote γ-aminobutyric acid (GABAergic) neurotransmission are generally most effective in partial-onset seizures, whereas drugs that combine these and other mechanisms of action may have broader efficacy in primary generalized seizure types.

Evidence from prospective, blinded, randomized clinical trials is only available for certain AEDs for monotherapy use. Gabapentin (Neurontin), oxcarbazepine (Trileptal), and lamotrigine (Lamictal) possess randomized controlled trial evidence for monotherapy treatment of partial-onset seizures, and topiramate (Topamax) has evidence for monotherapy use in new-onset epilepsy. All older AEDs and other newer AEDs have either comparator trial or anecdotal monotherapy evidence. All marketed newer AEDs have randomized controlled trial evidence for use as adjunctive treatment in partial-onset seizures, whereas older AEDs have comparator trial evidence.

Patient characteristics and co-morbidities may affect the choice of an AED. For example, weight is an important consideration. Valproate (Depakene), pregabalin (Lyrica), and carbamazepine (Tegretol) may contribute to weight gain, whereas topiramate (Topamax) and zonisamide (Zonegran) may include weight loss among their adverse effect profile. The patient with both epilepsy and migraine might favor topiramate or valproate, drugs that are efficacious for both conditions.

In general, AED monotherapy is just as effective—or more effective—than polytherapy. Monotherapy limits the potential for adverse effects and drug interactions. AED dosing must be individualized to achieve optimal results. Our strategy is to titrate the AED toward a target dose that has proven effective for most individuals in clinical studies and in our experience. Dose adjustment can then be made in the event of adverse drug reactions or recurrent seizures. If the endpoint of seizure freedom is preserved, maintaining a lower but clinically therapeutic AED dosage is entirely acceptable. If a patient continues to experience breakthrough seizures, raising the AED dose to the maximal dose tolerated is sometimes necessary, although recent evidence demonstrates that only a minority of patients become seizure free when dosed above the usual therapeutic range, so a practical viewpoint of treatment futility should be realized when patients experience frequent breakthrough seizures despite adequate AED dosages. Therapeutic change should be made when seizure freedom is not maintained at AED doses effective for most patients. Overlapping AEDs in transitional polytherapy (where the baseline AED is maintained at the current dose to limit breakthrough seizures, the newly added AED is titrated to a protective dose, then the original drug is tapered and discontinued) is the preferred method when introducing a new AED monotherapy. Abruptly stopping the existing AED increases the risk of seizures (and perhaps status epilepticus), whereas introducing the new AED too rapidly may induce adverse effects that taint the patient's perception of what could be an effective therapy.

Many medically refractory epilepsy patients require chronic polytherapy. Overall, only a small minority of refractory patients can be rendered seizure free with AED polytherapy, but they may benefit substantially by reduction of seizure burden. Although no good evidence for specific AED polytherapy combinations exists, augmenting monotherapy with an AED offering a different or complementary mechanism of action may be considered. Great care must be taken to avoid excessive drug dosing and drug–drug interactions. Initiating and maintaining AED polytherapy is difficult and requires oversight by a neurologist with extensive knowledge of clinical pharmacology.

TABLE 4 Properties of the AEDs

	Spectrum of Effect	Daily Adult Dosage/Interval	Usual Level (µg/mL)	Severe Adverse Effects	Toxicities	Idiosyncratic Interactions
Older AEDs						
Carbamazepine (Tegretol)	Partial	400–1600+ mg (bid–qid)	4–12+	Diplopia, dizziness, ataxia, hyponatremia	Yes	Bidirectional (AEDs, OC, AC, many)
Ethosuximide (Zarontin)	Absence	500–1500+ mg (bid)	40–100+	Nausea, sedation	Yes	Unidirectional
Phenobarbital	Partial	90–180+ mg (qd)	15–40	Sedation, psychomotor slowing	Yes	Bidirectional (AEDs, OC, AC, many)
Phenytoin (Dilantin)	Partial	200–400+ mg (qd–bid)	8–20+	Sedation, dizziness, ataxia, gingival hyperplasia	Yes	Bidirectional (AEDs, OC, AC, many)
Primidone (Mysoline)	Partial	500–1500+ mg (bid–tid)	5–12 (measure phenobarbital)	Sedation, psychomotor slowing	Yes	Bidirectional (AEDs, OC, AC, many)
Valproate (Depakene)	Broad	750–2500+ mg (qd–tid)	50–100+	Nausea, tremor, hair loss, weight gain	Yes	Bidirectional (AEDs)
Newer AEDs						
Felbamate (Felbatol)	Broad	1800–4800+ mg (bid–tid)	30–100+	Irritability, insomnia, weight loss	Yes	Bidirectional (AEDs, OC, AC)
Gabapentin (Neurontin)	Partial	900–3600+ mg (tid–qid)	4–20++	Sedation, dizziness, weight gain	No	None
Lamotrigine (Lamictal)	Broad	300–600+ mg (qd–bid)	1–20+	Dizziness, rash	Yes	Bidirectional (AEDs, OC)
Levetiracetam (Keppra)	Broad	1000–3000++ mg (bid)	5–40++	Sedation, dizziness	No	None
Oxcarbazepine (Trileptal)	Partial	600–3600+ mg (bid)	10–40+ (MHD)	Sedation, dizziness	Yes	Bidirectional (AEDs, OC)
Tiagabine (Gabitril)	Partial	16–64 mg (bid–tid)	100–300 µg/mL	Sedation, weight gain	No	Unidirectional
Topiramate (Topamax)	Broad	100–600+ mg (qd–bid)	10–20+	Sedation, cognitive complaints, paresthesias, weight loss, rare nephrolithiasis	No	Bidirectional (AEDs, OC at high doses)
Zonisamide (Zonegran)	Broad	100–600+ mg (qd–bid)	10–40+	Sedation, paresthesias, weight loss, rare nephrolithiasis	Yes	Unidirectional

Notes: AED = antiepileptic drug; + = higher doses/levels often additionally effective, as tolerated; ++ = considerably higher doses/levels sometimes additionally effective in intractable patients, as tolerated; MHD = 10, 11 Monohydroxy derivative active metabolite of oxcarbazepine. Interactions: Unidirectional indicates that other AEDs or drugs may affect this AED; bidirectional indicates that other drugs may affect this AED, and this AED affects other drugs; OC = oral contraceptives, AC = anticoagulants; many = many other non-AEDs.

AED dosing should be adjusted to achieve the clinical goals of seizure freedom without adverse effects. This may indeed be a delicate balancing act for some patients because all AEDs have the potential to cause dose-related so-called neurotoxic adverse effects. Fortunately, adverse effects may be obviated in most patients by dose reduction or substituting for a better tolerated AED.

Philosophies on the use of AED blood level monitoring differ, but most agree that blood levels should in most cases be considered only a guideline to treatment. AED levels should not be perceived as an absolute indication for altering AED dosing, divorced from clinical judgment of the patient's seizure control or adverse effects. Blood-level monitoring can help guide therapy, but so-called therapeutic levels are derived from treatment of populations. An individual patient may require a lower or higher intensity of AED therapy to achieve optimal results. For example, some patients develop breakthrough seizures even at supratherapeutic or toxic levels, others may experience adverse effects within the usual therapeutic range, whereas some patients become seizure-free on levels in a subtherapeutic range. The danger of overreliance on AED blood levels is twofold: levels may lead both physicians and patients to a false sense of therapeutic adequacy or may lead to errant manipulation of AEDs in patients who require no adjustments. Typical clinical scenarios where clinicians should obtain AED levels include the following:

1. After reaching steady-state administration of an AED, to establish a patient's individual personal baseline against which future comparisons can be made in event of breakthrough seizures.
2. While titrating individual AEDs in complex polypharmacy regimens, when drug interactions may influence either the new adjunctive AED or baseline antiepileptic and other medications.
3. Adjusting for alterations in AED metabolism during aging, disease states, and during each trimester of pregnancy when AED levels can fluctuate substantially based on altered drug absorption, metabolism, protein binding, and clearance. With some heavily protein-bound drugs, especially phenytoin (Dilantin), obtaining free drug levels is necessary to discern the biologically active fraction of the drug, especially in chronically or critically ill patients.
4. When trying to determine the AED responsible for adverse effects in a patient receiving polytherapy.

In summary, AED levels are most useful when testing a clinical hypothesis. We discourage the use of routine or scheduled levels, an exception being chronic phenytoin therapy in institutionalized patients (where zero-order kinetics from nonlinear hepatic metabolism may lead to drug accumulation and toxicity).

With chronic AED therapy, intermittent blood testing for monitoring of liver function tests and hematologic functions is reasonable although not of proven value. The highest risk of idiosyncratic reactions associated with AEDs such as serious rash, hepatotoxicity, and hematologic dyscrasias is during the first 6 to 12 months of therapy and extremely rare thereafter. There is, however, mounting concern that patients on chronic maintenance therapy with older AEDs are at risk for osteopenia and osteoporosis. Any enzyme-inducing AED (carbamazepine [Tegretol], phenytoin [Dilantin], phenobarbital, primidone [Mysoline], and oxcarbazepine [Trileptal]) has the potential to decrease bone density. Valproate (Depakote) may also lead to decreased bone density. Chronic phenytoin exposure is of particular concern, given its rare association with cosmetic adverse effects including gingival hyperplasia (which may be severe enough to warrant repeated gingivectomies), peripheral neuropathy, and irreversible cerebellar ataxia. Considering AED withdrawal in appropriate candidates or transition to another newer AED therapy without such untoward effects is often reasonable.

AED cost is a crucial social issue that may trump all other medical principles in selection and maintenance of AED therapy in patients who lack adequate medical insurance. Choosing expensive AEDs that a patient cannot afford may erode the patient's adherence to treatment and trust in the physician. Insurance and financial status must therefore be considered, so that available resources (i.e., indigent federal- or state-sponsored insurance or corporate pharmaceutical assistance programs) can be summoned if a prohibitively expensive newer AED is the best therapeutic choice. Some of the patents of newer AEDs will expire by publication of this book, leading to increased availability of generic drug formulations that could reduce the impact of medication cost, but the pharmacokinetic reliability of these generic formulations must also be established before their widespread use is recommended.

Withdrawal from chronic AEDs is a difficult consideration in the older adolescent or adult with epilepsy because seizure recurrence may impact driving and work abilities. In general, it is worthwhile to consider an attempt at withdrawing AED therapy when the patient has been seizure free for an arbitrary period between 2 and 5 years. Available data suggest that approximately 25% to 70% of patients experience seizure recurrence with AED withdrawal. The decision to withdraw AED therapy must be discussed in the context of the patient's lifestyle and responsibilities because driving and work considerations may be paramount and trump the medical prognosis. Neurologic consultation should be strongly considered when AED withdrawal is contemplated.

EPILEPSY SURGERY

Evaluation for epilepsy surgery should be strongly considered in patients with refractory partial epilepsy. A syndrome particularly amenable to surgical intervention is mesial temporal-lobe epilepsy (MTLE), characterized by medically refractory complex partial seizures, often a history of complex febrile seizures in infancy, and hippocampal sclerosis on brain MRI.

Resective surgery for epilepsy has been performed for over a century, and advances in EEG and neuroimaging have increased the widespread application of epilepsy surgery. A pivotal clinical trial established the clear superiority of anterior temporal lobectomy over medical therapy for chronically refractory MTLE in carefully selected patients.

Identification of potential candidates for epilepsy surgery remains the biggest challenge for tertiary care epilepsy centers. Some have estimated that nearly 75,000 potential surgical candidates in the United States remain under care in primary care settings with ongoing seizures, yet only 3000 or fewer surgical procedures for epilepsy are performed annually.

Potential candidates for resective epilepsy surgery have refractory epilepsy with ongoing seizures that have been resistant to at least two to three appropriately administered AEDs. The precise seizure burden meriting an aggressive, invasive approach remains a subject of conjecture, but even one to two consciousness-impairing seizures annually may be highly disabling in patients who aspire to work and drive.

The basic approach in epilepsy surgery involves identification and precise localization of the epileptogenic zone, the region of the brain that is necessary and sufficient to cause clinical seizures; determining whether the patient possesses appropriate functional reserve for safe removal of that seizure focus; and subsequent operative resection of this area.

A variety of investigations must be performed at specialized comprehensive epilepsy centers to determine if epilepsy surgery would be effective and safe for an individual patient. The most useful and important initial investigations are a high-resolution volumetric brain MRI (with thin cut coronal plane acquisition perpendicular to the hippocampal long axis) and inpatient prolonged ictal V-EEG monitoring that permits intimate correlation and offline, post hoc detailed analysis of the ictal behavior and

EEG to localize the patient's habitual clinical seizures. Additional techniques that help localize the epileptic focus preoperatively include functional imaging techniques such as single photon emission computed tomography (SPECT) and PET, magnetoencephalography, and neuropsychological testing. An intracarotid sodium amytal test is necessary in all patients to lateralize memory functions accurately and estimate functional reserve prior to surgery. In some cases, invasive EEG recording with surgically implanted subdural or parenchymal strips or grids of electrodes is necessary to confirm the seizure focus precisely and allow mapping of eloquent functional cerebral cortex to reduce operative morbidity.

When a structural epileptogenic mesial temporal brain lesion evident on MRI is concordant with well-localized habitual clinical seizures by ictal V-EEG, there is a 60% to 90% chance that surgery will produce seizure freedom. Resection in neocortical epilepsies offers a 30% to 80% chance of achieving a seizure-free outcome, depending largely on whether a MRI lesion concordant with the seizure focus is present. Surgical efficacy contrasts with a 5% or less chance that additional AED therapy will render the refractory patient seizure free. Favorable seizure outcome must be balanced with a 3% or less risk of major morbidity (i.e., hemorrhage, infection, stroke, memory, language, or hemianopic visual field deficit) incurred by surgery. Risk may be higher in extratemporal epilepsy surgery for postoperative motor, sensory, and visual deficits, depending on the location of the seizure focus. Memory or language deficits may occur in temporal lobe operations.

OTHER ALTERNATIVE THERAPIES

Some patients with refractory partial epilepsy are not suitable epilepsy surgical candidates because of diffuse or unlocalizable epileptic foci, whereas others may choose not to undergo brain surgery despite suitable candidacy. In these cases, other options may still exist.

The vagus nerve stimulator (VNS) is the only electrical device currently approved as an adjunctive treatment for partial-onset seizures. A battery-operated generator and programmable computerized stimulator are placed surgically in a subcutaneous pocket on the left anterior chest. The device looks much like a cardiac pacemaker and has electrical leads connected to the left vagus nerve in the neck. Once implanted, the device is programmed by means of a radiofrequency wand in the physician's office and provides a small electrical current to the nerve at preset intervals and amounts. The patient also has the opportunity to trigger a stronger current to attempt to abort or lessen an oncoming seizure by means of a magnet that is passed externally over the device.

The efficacy of VNS for seizure reduction is roughly comparable to that of AEDs; approximately 40% of patients experience a 50% or greater reduction in their seizures, and up to 15% of patients become seizure free. Although there are no current evidence-based guidelines for the best timing of VNS placement, we reserve VNS for patients who are not resective surgery candidates or who refuse surgery and those who have failed most older and newer AEDs. In addition to reducing seizure burden, VNS may improve a patient's quality of life by improving alertness, mood, and memory. Predictors of which patients are most likely to benefit from VNS, and the optimal dosing of the device once it is implanted, are yet to be defined in prospective clinical trials.

Specialized diets may be a useful adjunctive treatment for epilepsy. The best studied of these is the ketogenic diet, a high-fat, low-protein, low-carbohydrate diet that induces systemic ketosis, which has an antiepileptogenic effect on the brain. The ketogenic diet is most often successfully used in children, but it may also be tried in adolescents and adults. Unfortunately, unless rigid compliance is assured, the ketogenic diet produces little benefit and, in general, most adolescents and adults have limited tolerance of the diet. However, highly motivated and desperately refractory epilepsy patients may benefit from the ketogenic diet. An alternative that is often more tolerable, but not yet robustly studied, is the modified Atkins diet, a high-fat, moderate-protein, low-carbohydrate diet that induces mild ketosis.

Identifying and treating seizure aggravators is an important consideration. Recent studies have suggested that obstructive sleep apnea syndrome (OSAS) is a frequent comorbidity in refractory epilepsy, and nasal central positive airway pressure in patients with refractory epilepsy and comorbid OSAS may lead to seizure reduction. Primary sleep disorders such as restless legs syndrome and periodic limb movements of sleep may fragment sleep and worsen seizure burden in patients with refractory epilepsy. If a primary sleep disorder is suspected, a diagnostic polysomnogram should be ordered, and aggressive treatment for the sleep disorder should be initiated.

STATUS EPILEPTICUS: IDENTIFICATION AND MANAGEMENT

Status epilepticus is a prolonged, unremitting epileptic seizure that constitutes a medical emergency. Until the last decade, status epilepticus was defined as a seizure lasting 30 minutes or longer (from onset through the end of the ictal period, exclusive of the postictal recovery phase that may in itself last well over 30 minutes). However, more recent data suggest that most seizures that self-terminate do so by 3 minutes after onset, indicating that longer lasting seizures are unlikely to stop without intervention.

Status epilepticus may be convulsive or nonconvulsive. Status epilepticus frequently begins with a prolonged generalized tonic–clonic or partial motor seizure, followed by a minimally convulsive or nonconvulsive phase with or without subtle motor features such as facial or eyelid twitching, or nystagmus. Status epilepticus thus evolves in a manner analogous to a lethal cardiac dysrhythmia, proceeding from clinically overt convulsive movements toward an eventual electromechanical dissociative state where the epileptic seizure continues as a subclinical electrographic discharge evident only during EEG monitoring.

Management of status epilepticus begins with securing the airway, respiration, and circulation and placement of two large-bore intravenous catheters for drug administration and fluid resuscitation. Obtaining a stat glucose is appropriate before rapid administration of thiamine, followed by intravenous dextrose (to avoid Wernicke encephalopathy in malnourished patients). If intravenous access is not readily available, rectal diazepam (Diastat) or intramuscular fosphenytoin (Cerebyx) can be used. Rectal diazepam is also useful in the out-of-hospital treatment of prolonged seizures or seizure clusters in adolescents and adults, potentially obviating escalation into status epilepticus and preventing an emergency department visit.

Initial pharmacotherapy of status epilepticus begins with intravenous lorazepam (Ativan) given at 2 mg/minute to a goal of 0.1 mg/kg (or 8 mg total) with cautious respiratory monitoring, then loading with phenytoin (Dilantin) at 20 mg/kg, given no faster than 50 mg/minute to avoid hypotension, with ECG and hemodynamic monitoring. Phenytoin should be given through a dedicated peripheral intravenous line because of potential for cardiotoxicity and to avoid precipitation by other drugs. Intravenous phenytoin, a highly insoluble alkaline solution, may lead to substantial soft-tissue toxicity (including the much feared purple-glove phenomenon). An alternative is fosphenytoin, which may be administered at up to 150 mg/min, and is not associated with tissue injury if extravasation occurs.

The success of treatment of status epilepticus can be measured clinically, but if the patient remains unresponsive after the convulsive movements stop, an urgent EEG may be needed to exclude nonconvulsive status epilepticus. Refractory status epilepticus can be treated with midazolam (Versed),[1] propofol (Diprivan),[1] pentobarbital (Nembutal), sodium pentothal (Thiopental), or phenobarbital.[1] An advantage of short-acting agents such as midazolam and propofol is the rapidity with which pharmacologically induced coma can be reversed to examine the patient.

Conclusion

Epilepsy is characterized by recurrent, spontaneous seizures. Epilepsy has many causes and represents a collection of syndromes that have varying natural histories and responses to therapy. Diagnosis is based on the history and may be supported by physical examination. The two most important investigations in initial evaluation of the patient with new-onset seizures or epilepsy are high-resolution brain MRI and EEG. There are many mimickers of epilepsy requiring careful differential diagnosis. When confronted with spells of an uncertain type, evaluation with VEEG may secure the correct diagnosis.

The past decade has seen tremendous expansion in available AED therapies, many of which are more tolerable and safer for long-term use. Choice of AED in an individual patient depends on the epilepsy syndrome, consideration of available efficacy evidence, patient characteristics and co-morbidities, and cost. AED monitoring should reinforce, and not replace, clinical judgment. Chronic complications of certain older AEDs may include osteopenia, adverse cosmetic effects, weight gain, and neuropathy. Withdrawal of AEDs in selected seizure-free patients or transition to AEDs without chronic toxicities should be considered in such instances.

Unfortunately, despite advances in available AEDs, more than a third of patients with epilepsy are refractory. Early determination of refractory epilepsy and triage to intensive diagnostic and therapeutic resources at a comprehensive epilepsy care center is critical. Epilepsy surgery may render carefully selected patients seizure free, and VNS is a viable alternative when surgery is not possible, leading to reduced seizure burden and improved quality of life. Physicians should approach their patients with epilepsy with enthusiasm and hope for effecting an improvement in their condition.

REFERENCES

French JA, Kanner AM, Bautista J, et al: Efficacy and tolerability of the new antiepileptic drugs: I. Treatment of new-onset epilepsy: Report of the Therapeutics and Technology Assessment Subcommittee and Quality Standards Subcommittee of the American Academy of Neurology and the American Epilepsy Society. Neurology 2004;62(8):1252-1260.

French JA, Kanner AM, Bautista J, et al: Therapeutics and Technology Assessment Subcommittee of the American Academy of Neurology; Quality Standards Subcommittee of the American Academy of Neurology; American Epilepsy Society. Efficacy and tolerability of the new antiepileptic drugs: II. Treatment of refractory epilepsy: Report of the Therapeutics and Technology Assessment Subcommittee and Quality Standards Subcommittee of the American Academy of Neurology and the American Epilepsy Society. Neurology 2004;62(8):1261-1273.

Kwan P, Brodie MJ: Early identification of refractory epilepsy. N Engl J Med 2000;342(5):314-319.

Wiebe S, Blume WT, Girvin JP, Eliasziw M: A randomized, controlled trial of surgery for temporal-lobe epilepsy. N Engl J Med 2001; 345:311-318.

Epilepsy in Infancy and Childhood

Method of
Raj D. Sheth, MD

Definition

Seizures are a sudden self-limited clinical event that results from abnormal and excessive firing of cortical neurons. Paroxysmal events that are not cerebral in origin may mimic seizures, and in infants these commonly include breath-holding spells, vasovagal syncope, or cardiac arrhythmias.

Classification

Seizures can be classified based on their onset as either *partial* (starting in a focal area of the brain), *partial with secondary generalization* (starting as a partial seizure but then secondarily spreading to other areas of the brain, usually involving both cerebral hemispheres), or *primary generalized* (involving all of the brain from the onset of the seizure) (Box 1). Partial seizures may be either simple partial, if consciousness is preserved during the seizures, or complex partial, if impairment of consciousness or confusion occurs during the seizure. Partial seizures typically present with brief motor movement, sensation, or autonomic symptoms.

Such a classification scheme, which works well in a child older than 7 years, may be difficult to apply to a younger child or infant. This feature adds considerable difficulty in determining if an event is an epileptic seizure or simply a

BOX 1 Seizure Classification

Partial (or focal)
- Simple partial
  - Motor
  - Sensory
  - Autonomic
- Complex partial
  - Focal or generalized secondarily

Generalized
- Absence
  - Typical or atypical absence
- Myoclonic
- Tonic/clonic or tonic–clonic
  - Atonic

behavioral phenomenon. For example, a young child with staring spells might simply be daydreaming or might be having an epileptic seizure such as an absence seizure or a complex partial seizure. Useful features to distinguish these events are that seizures may occur in both active and passive modes, whereas behavioral staring events are typically only seen in a passive mode (e.g., while watching television).

Generalized seizures include absence seizures, myoclonic seizures, or primary generalized tonic-clonic seizures.

Provoking Factors

Seizures may be acutely provoked by a fever (febrile seizures) or be symptomatic of an underlying acute cerebral insult such as a severe head injury, central nervous system infection, electrolyte imbalance, or metabolic derangement. In these patients, treatment is directed at the underlying cause of the seizure. Patients with acute symptomatic seizures may require temporary seizure medication to control seizures but may not need long-term treatment with seizure medication.

Idiopathic and Symptomatic Epilepsy

Epilepsy is the occurrence of two or more unprovoked seizures and indicates an underlying tendency toward seizures. Epilepsy that does not appear to be caused by an underlying cerebral abnormality (normal neurologic examination and cognitive function and a normal cranial magnetic resonance imaging [MRI] scan) is referred to as idiopathic epilepsy. Approximately 50% of childhood cases are idiopathic. The prognosis for idiopathic epilepsy is usually good for either spontaneous remittance of seizures or for their control. Idiopathic epilepsy is frequently related to a genetic multifactorial tendency toward the disorder. When it is a symptom of underlying remote cranial trauma, congenital cerebral malformations, tumors, or vascular anomalies, it is referred to as symptomatic epilepsy. Approximately two thirds of these patients have difficult to control seizures. When a cause cannot be identified but cognitive impairment is present, epilepsy is called cryptogenic. Patients with cryptogenic epilepsy have a similar prognosis as those with symptomatic epilepsy.

Epidemiology

Approximately 3% to 5% of all children experience a single seizure, with febrile seizures the most frequent. The incidence of seizures is highest in the first year of life, particularly in the neonatal period (first 4 weeks of life). Approximately 1% of these children have unprovoked seizures, and half of those have two or more seizures and are said to have epilepsy. Of those with epilepsy, approximately half have generalized seizures. Half of all children have epilepsy that is symptomatic of an underlying brain lesion, with the remainder having idiopathic epilepsy indicative of a genetic tendency.

Diagnosis

The first priority is to determine if the event the patient experienced was a seizure or a nonepileptic paroxysmal event. Nonepileptic events in children include breath-holding spells, temper tantrums, vasovagal syncope, night terrors, hyperventilation, and panic attacks. The history is often sufficient to differentiate these events from seizures.

Evaluation of seizures requires a careful history, with particular attention given to the onset of the seizure (eye deviation, fear) and any focal weakness following the seizure to determine if the seizure was partial. The neurologic examination is very useful. When a child exhibits neurologic deficits, it strongly suggests the seizure resulted from a focal brain lesion and warrants a cranial MRI.

ELECTROENCEPHALOGRAM

The electroencephalogram (EEG) is central to the evaluation of seizures and should be obtained in all patients who had a seizure other than those with a simple febrile seizure. The EEG can help diagnosis and guide treatment by helping classify seizures, and it also offers some indication about prognosis. Generally, two features on the EEG are helpful in the evaluation: the background EEG activity and the epileptiform discharges. Background activity may be in either the normal or slow range. Normal background activity typically suggests idiopathic epilepsy, whereas background slowing is more indicative of seizures that are symptomatic of an underlying cerebral abnormality. Epileptiform discharges can occur even when the patient is not acutely seizing and are seen in approximately two thirds of patients known to have epilepsy. They are also seen in approximately 1% of children who have never experienced a seizure. Importantly, epileptiform discharges can help differentiate between partial and generalized seizures, thereby guiding treatment. Focal epileptiform discharges are present in one part of the brain and indicate partial epilepsy. Generalized epileptiform discharges occur throughout the brain. Specific generalized seizures can be diagnosed: 3-Hz generalized spike-and-wave activity (indicative of absence seizures) or polyspike-and-wave activity (indicative of myoclonic or tonic–clonic seizures) are suggestive of generalized epilepsy. Severe forms of epilepsy, including infantile spasms, are associated with hypsarrhythmia, and the Lennox-Gastaut syndrome, associated with slow spike-and-wave activity, can be diagnosed with the EEG.

CRANIAL IMAGING

In an acute situation, a cranial computed tomography (CT) can help evaluate urgently for intracranial blood or trauma, although a comprehensive evaluation requires an MRI scan in most patients. New-onset seizures may require evaluation with gadolinium enhancement to exclude a brain tumor. Patients with temporal lobe epilepsy require specific studies, which include a temporal lobe protocol to determine if there is mesial temporal sclerosis.

DIFFERENTIAL DIAGNOSIS

Movement in the neonatal period can be difficult to differentiate from seizures. In an intensive care unit (ICU) setting, approximately 90% of events thought to be epileptic seizures turn out to be nonepileptic. Jitteriness can be separated from seizures because seizures can be stopped by changing the position of the limb. Clonic movements are the most specific for epileptic seizures. An EEG is very helpful at this point. A consistent precipitant suggests nonepileptic events. Breath holding can be associated with brief nonepileptic convulsive activity. Importantly, seizures are stereotypic. Parental home videos of the events can be helpful in better characterization.

In children older than age 5 years and adolescents, complicated migraine, sleep disorders, and syncope may be difficult to separate from seizures. Hyperventilation and panic events should also be considered. When there is doubt about the diagnosis, an EEG may be very helpful, with approximately 70% of patients showing epileptiform discharges between seizures.

Epilepsy Syndromes

FEBRILE SEIZURES

Febrile seizures occur between ages 6 months and 5 years, with the majority presenting by age 3 years. Simple febrile seizures last less than 15 minutes, with a single seizure within a 24-hour period, and they are not associated with Todd's paralysis. All other seizures are complex and may require further evaluation. Antipyretic measures and therapy are often recommended, although no evidence indicates this strategy prevents recurrence. Approximately one third of patients experience a recurrence. Rectally administered diazepam (Diastat) may help reduce the length of a seizure and is typically recommended for seizures that last longer than 5 minutes. Phenobarbital and valproate (Depakene) are effective in preventing recurrence of febrile seizures, although given the adverse effect of chronic therapy they are rarely indicated. Patients with prior febrile seizures who subsequently experience a seizure without fever should be evaluated for epilepsy.

INFANTILE SPASMS AND LENNOX-GASTAUT SYNDROME

Infantile spasms and Lennox-Gastaut syndrome, although uncommon, are severe epilepsies and should be evaluated promptly. Infantile spasms occur between ages 3 and 18 months, and Lennox-Gastaut syndrome is typically diagnosed after that. Untreated infantile spasms often transition into Lennox-Gastaut syndrome.

Spasms are typically brief, lasting 1 to 5 seconds, with symmetric contraction of the trunk, extension of the arms, and tonic extension of the legs. Spasms, which occur in clusters, are associated with irritability and often seen as the child awakens or transitions to sleep. The EEG is hypsarrhythmic, showing a markedly abnormal and chaotic background with multifocal epileptiform discharges. The triad of infantile spasms, hypsarrhythmia, and developmental regression is referred to as West's syndrome. An underlying etiology is present in 80% of infants and usually associated with a poorer outcome than those in whom an etiology is not found. Corticotropin (ACTH)[1] treatment frequently results in control of spasm, improvement in EEG background, and an improvement in development. Vigabatrin (Sabril)* is an oral agent that can control infantile spasms, particularly those associated with tuberous sclerosis.

Lennox-Gastaut syndrome develops in 50% of children with infantile spasms. The EEG shows a diffuse slow spike-and-wave pattern. Patients have a combination of tonic, myoclonic, and atypical absence seizures. Seizures are intractable to medical treatment and the outcome is poor, with mental retardation seen in up to 90% of patients.

ABSENCE EPILEPSY

Absence seizures resemble staring spells, although they may occur in both an active or passive state. Fifty seizures a day are typical, with subtle behavioral arrest that may be associated with eyelid twitching. The EEG shows 3-Hz generalized spike and waves. Absence seizures occur in childhood absence, juvenile absence, and juvenile myoclonic epilepsy.

Childhood absence epilepsy develops between 4 and 10 years of age and remits in most patients by 10 years of age. Seizures are easily treated with ethosuximide (Zarontin), although valproate (Depakote) and lamotrigine (Lamictal) can also be used.

Juvenile absence epilepsy develops between ages 6 and 10 years and usually does not remit. Unlike the childhood form, seizures do not remit and may be associated with tonic–clonic seizures. Ethosuximide is usually not effective for the tonic–clonic seizures, and valproate or lamotrigine are usually considered.

Juvenile myoclonic epilepsy, the most common epilepsy syndrome seen in children of normal intellect, has a similar age of onset as juvenile absence epilepsy and does not remit. The EEG shows generalized polyspike-and-wave discharges. Valproate is an effective medication for

---

[1]Not FDA approved for this indication.
*Investigational drug in the United States.

this epilepsy, although lamotrigine can also be considered. The latter is not as effective as valproate in controlling myoclonic seizures, although it has a better side-effect profile compared to valproate.

BENIGN PARTIAL EPILEPSY WITH CENTROTEMPORAL SPIKE

Benign partial epilepsy with centrotemporal spike (BECTS) accounts for approximately 15% of epilepsy in childhood. Seizures are partial, with face twitching, of which the child is usually aware. Generalized tonic–clonic seizures may occur at night. The EEG shows a normal background with epileptiform spikes in the centrotemporal regions. If the child is only experiencing simple partial seizures, treatment may be withheld. Seizures remit in the vast majority of children. Control of seizures is seen with low-dose medication, and carbamazepine (Tegretol) or oxcarbazepine (Trileptal) are both effective treatment options.

Treatment

After a careful diagnosis of epileptic seizures, treatment decisions are made to reduce the risk of seizure-associated injury, prevent the risk of prolonged seizures (status epilepticus), reduce the adverse cognitive effects of frequent seizures, and deal with social factors, such as driving. Decisions should be discussed with the child and family, weighing the benefits with the risks of treatment. Factors that help guide treatment include seizure type, etiology, frequency, duration, and impact on the patient's life, along with age and level of activity.

The goal of treatment is prevention of seizures; therefore, assessment of the recurrence risk should be made. Following a first unprovoked seizure, there is a 50% risk of a second seizure. With the second seizure, the risk of the third increases to 80%. A normal neurologic examination, MRI, and EEG are all factors that lower the risk to 25% to 33%, whereas abnormalities found in these tests and a family history of epilepsy increase the recurrence risk to 75%. An EEG that shows 3-Hz generalized spike wave discharges seen in absence of seizures, however, increases that risk to virtually 100%. Treatment is often suggested after a patient has a second unprovoked seizure.

The underlying principles guiding treatment are that the patient should be free from both seizures and the adverse effects of medications (Table 1). Choosing among the different medications requires an understanding of adverse effects and efficacy. Seizures that respond well to treatment include the benign syndromes discussed earlier. In these patients, the lowest dose of recommended medication should be tried and gradually titrated depending on response (Table 2).

Medications should be titrated slowly to minimize adverse effects. Medication serum levels can help guide treatment, but medications should be titrated to response. Serum levels can be helpful in deciding if breakthrough seizures are a result of noncompliance or lack of efficacy. Some patients require more than one medication to control seizures. Unfortunately, many patients, despite multiple medications, continue to have seizures.

TABLE 1 Commonly Used Antiepileptic Medications

Agent	Pediatric Dose (mg/kg/d)	Half-life (h)*	Dosing Schedule	Side Effects
Carbamazepine (Tegretol)	10-35	25-65 (initial) 12-17 (chronic)	bid-qid	r, hep, bd, s, n dip, hypn, ost
Clonazepam (Klonopin)	0.01-0.2	18-50	bid-tid	s, a, h, b
Ethosuximide (Zarontin)	10-15 (initial) 15-40 (maint)	30-40	qd-tid	gi, n, an, s, d, b, r, bd
Gabapentin (Neurontin)	30-60	5-7	tid-qid	s, d, a, ny, wg
Lamotrigine (Lamictal)				
Off valproate	0.6 (initial) 5-15 (maint)	7	bid	r, hep, d, a, s, n
On valproate	0.15 (initial) 1-5 (maint)	45	qd-bid	
Levetiracetam (Keppra)†	20-60	6-8	bid	s, d, ha, b
Oxcarbazepine (Trileptal)	8-10 (initial) 20-50 (maint)	8-10	bid	r, hep, s, diz, n dip, a, ha, hypn
Topiramate (Topamax)	1-3 (initial) 5-9 (maint)	18-30	bid	s, an, ks, ps, wl
Valproic acid (Depakote)	15-60	9-20	bid-qid	hep, bd, n, s, d, wg, hl, r, gi
Zonisamid (Zonegran)†	2-4 (initial) 4-8 (maint)	50-70	qd-bid	r, bd, hep, s, diz, an, n, ha, wl, ks

*Half-life is based on monotherapy and assumes normal renal function.
†Not FDA approved for this indication in children.
Abbreviations: a, ataxia; an, anorexia; b, behavioral difficulties; bd, blood dyscrasia; d, dizziness; dip, diplopia; gi, gastrointestinal distress; h, hyperactivity; ha, headache; hep, hepatotoxicity; hl, hair loss; hypn, hyponatremia; ks, kidney stones; maint, maintenance; n, nausea; ny, nystagmus; ost, osteomalacia; ps, psychomotor slowing; r, rash; s, sedation; wg, weight gain; wl, weight loss.

TABLE 2 Which Medications for Which Seizure Types?

Seizure Type	First-Line Therapy	Second-Line Therapy	Third-Line Therapy
Partial (all types)	CBZ, OXC	LTG, VPA, GBP, TPM, PHT	TGB, LEV,[A] ZNS,[A] PB
Generalized			
Tonic-clonic	VPA	LTG, TPM, PHT	PB, ZNS[A]
Myoclonic	VPA	LTG, CZP	PB, ZNS[A]
Tonic	VPA	LTG	CZP, TPM, ZNS[A]
Absence (before age 10)	ESM*	VPA, LTG	ZNS, TPM
(after age 10)	VPA	LTG	ESM, TPM, ZNS[A]
Epilepsy Syndromes			
CAE	ESM	VPA, LTG	ZNS, TPM
JAE	VPA	LTG	ESM, TPM, ZNS[A]
JME	VPA, LTG	TPM, ZNS[A]	CZP, PHT
Lennox-Gastaut	VPA	LTG, TPM	CZP, ZNS,[A] FBM
Infantile spasms	ACTH, VGB[†]	VPA, TPM, TGB, CZP	FBM, ZNS[A]
BECTS	CBZ, OXC	VPA, PHT, CBZ	LTG, TPM

*Assuming no convulsive seizures.
Abbreviations: ACTH, adrenocorticotropic hormone; BECTS, benign epilepsy of childhood with centrotemporal spikes; CAE, childhood absence epilepsy; CBZ, carbamazepine (Tegretol); CZP, clonazepam (Klonopin); ESM, ethosuximide (Zarontin); FBM, felbamate (Felbatol); GBP, gabapentin (Neurontin); JAE, juvenile absence epilepsy; JME, juvenile myoclonic epilepsy; LEV, levetiracetam (Keppra); LTG, lamotrigine (Lamictal); OXC, oxcarbazepine (Trileptal); PB, phenobarbital; PHT, phenytoin (Dilantin); TGB, tiagabine (Gabitril); VGB, vigabatrin (Sabril); ZNS, zonisamide (Zonegran).
[A]Not FDA approved for this indication in children.
[†]Investigational drug in the United States.

WHEN MEDICATIONS FAIL TO CONTROL SEIZURES

Approximately 33% of patients' seizures are not controlled by medication, and alternative approaches can be considered. Options include the vagus nerve stimulator, the ketogenic diet, and epilepsy surgery. The first two measures typically reduce but do not abolish seizures. These decisions are best made using a multidisciplinary approach and require referral to a comprehensive epilepsy center. Patients who do not respond to a first medication choice should be referred for consultation.

STOPPING MEDICATIONS

Discontinuing medications depends on the type of seizures and epilepsy. Generally, when a patient is seizure free for 2 years, discontinuing medication can be considered. With this strategy, 60% to 75% of patients remain seizure free. However, a higher relapse rate is seen in remote symptomatic epilepsy, epileptiform discharges on EEG, and structural cerebral lesions on MRI. Recurrences usually occur in the first year, but late recurrence is also seen. Discontinuing medications should be considered before adolescents start driving because once patients are driving the decision to stop medication becomes much more complicated.

Attention Deficit Hyperactivity Disorder

Method of
Timothy Wilens, MD, Thomas Spencer, MD, and Joseph Biederman, MD

Attention deficit hyperactivity disorder (ADHD; the term used in this article refers to previously used definitions including hyperkinesis and ADD with or without hyperactivity) is the most common emotional, cognitive, and behavioral disorder that pediatricians, family physicians, neurologists, and psychiatrists treat in children. It is a major clinical and public health problem because of its associated morbidity and disability. Epidemiologic studies indicate that ADHD is prevalent throughout the world, with a general consensus that from 6% to 9% of youth and 4% of adults have the disorder. Follow-up studies of ADHD children into adolescence and early adulthood indicate that ADHD is associated with significant psychopathology, school and occupational failure, and peer and emotional difficulties throughout the life span. Although previously thought to remit in early adolescence, ADHD is now seen as a chronic condition continuing into adolescence in approximately three quarters of cases and into adulthood in approximately half of childhood cases. These higher persistence findings are related to more recent information indicating that whereas many of the overt hyperactive-impulsive symptoms diminish over time, the bulk of attentional problems continue and are correlated with later difficulties. For example, in one study, 90% of ADHD adults presenting for treatment endorsed functionally impairing inattentive symptomatology. Predictors of ADHD

CURRENT DIAGNOSIS

Cognitive Disturbance(s)

- Inattention (focus, vigilance, arousal)*
- Distraction (shifting, modulating, filtering)*
- Working memory (manipulation, problem solving)
- Executive function deficits (organization, time management, sequential work)

Behavioral Difficulties

- Impulsivity (rash decisions, interrupting, poor judgment)*
- Hyperactivity (fidgety, overactive, restlessness)*
- Talkativeness*
- Easily frustrated*
- Oppositionality/rigidity
- Immaturity
- Moodiness

*Denotes *Diagnostic and Statistical Manual of Mental Disorders, Fourth Edition (DSM-IV)* core symptom criterion.

persistence include prominent hyperactivity or impulsivity, aggression, co-occurring psychiatric and learning disorders, and a family history of ADHD.

Diagnosis

The diagnosis of ADHD is made by careful clinical history applying *Diagnostic and Statistical Manual of Mental Disorders, Fourth Edition (DSM IV)* criteria available in a user-friendly primary care version. Youth with ADHD are characterized by a considerable degree of inattentiveness, distractibility, impulsivity, and often hyperactivity that is inappropriate for the developmental stage of the child. Other common symptoms include low frustration tolerance, shifting activities frequently, difficulty organizing, and daydreaming. These symptoms are usually pervasive; however, they may not all occur in all settings. Children with predominantly inattention may have more difficulties in school and in completing homework but not manifest difficulties with peers or family. Conversely, children with excessive hyperactive or impulsive symptoms may perform acceptably academically but have difficulties at home or in situations of less guidance and structure. Adults tend to present with prominent attentional difficulties affecting work, schooling, and relationships. ADHD adults frequently also manifest residua of impulsivity (intrusiveness, impatience) and hyperactivity (fidgetiness, restlessness).

Children, adolescents, and adults who have the cognitive features of the disorder (i.e., inattention, distractibility, shifting activities, etc.) but lack hyperactive or impulsive features are considered to have ADHD. Previously anchored by overactivity and impulsivity, connected to brain dysfunction and damage, the disorder has been reconceptualized based on *impaired cognition* as a core feature. Hence, depending on what symptoms predominate, *DSM-IV* recognizes three subtypes of ADHD (percentage occurrence): a combined subtype (50% to 75% of cases), a predominantly inattentive subtype (20% to 30%), and a predominantly hyperactive-impulsive subtype (less than 15%).

Although not diagnostic, rating scales, checklists, and neuropsychiatric batteries may be helpful in providing evidence for the disorder and accompanying co-morbid conditions. Rating scales such as the Vanderbilt (downloadable from www.AAP.org) can be useful in assessing and monitoring ADHD. Although neuropsychological testing is not relied on to diagnose ADHD, testing may serve to identify particular weaknesses within ADHD or specific learning disabilities along with ADHD.

More than half of youth with ADHD are at risk for the development of co-occurring psychiatric disorders. Common co-occurring disorders include oppositional (40% to 60% of ADHD cases), conduct (10% to 20%), anxiety (30% to 40%), depression (20% to 30%), and bipolar disorder (less than 20%). For example, whereas only a minority of ADHD individuals develop mood disorders, an excess of ADHD is noted in depressed (20% to 30%) and bipolar youth (50% to 90%). ADHD and its associated co-morbid conditions also are a significant risk for higher rates and earlier ages of onset of cigarette smoking and alcohol and drug abuse. Not surprisingly, recent data suggest that these adolescents and young adults may be self-medicating mood and sleep issues with substances of abuse.

Males are more commonly affected with ADHD than females; although underidentification in girls remains a major concern. ADHD females share with their male counterparts the prototypical features of the disorder such as inattention, impulsivity and hyperactivity, high rates of school failure, and high levels of familial connection. Compared to boys, girls with ADHD have lower rates of disruptive behavior including conduct and oppositional disorders—common flags to ADHD in youth.

Although its precise neural and pathophysiologic substrate remains unknown, a large literature suggests the presence of abnormalities in (pre)-frontal networks or frontal-striatal dysfunction. Studies generally show reduced corpus callosum, cerebellum, and caudate volumes and reduced prefrontal cortex and anterior cingulate activity, with recent imaging studies demonstrating reversal in baseline abnormalities in ADHD adults with stimulant administration. Both dopaminergic and noradrenergic dysfunction appear to be important in the underlying neurochemistry of ADHD. Data from family—genetic, twin, and adoption studies as well as segregation analysis—suggest a genetic origin for some forms of the disorder. Molecular genetic studies have implicated the dopamine D2, D4, and the dopamine transporter, as well as a serotonin receptor and storage protein (SNAP) as candidate genes. Studies evaluating the relationship between genetic subtypes or vulnerabilities and the expression of the ADHD and response to treatment are currently under way.

Treatment

The management of ADHD includes consideration of two major areas: nonpharmacologic (educational remediation, individual and family psychotherapy) and pharmacotherapy. Support groups for ADHD are invaluable and an inexpensive way for families to learn about ADHD and resources available for their children or themselves. Support groups can be accessed by calling an ADHD hot line, large support group organization, or on the Internet (e.g., www.CHADD.org).

Specialized educational planning based on the child's difficulties is necessary in a majority of cases. Identification of co-morbid learning disorders, found in approximately a third of ADHD youth, should translate into the development of appropriate remediation plans. Parents should be encouraged to work closely with the child's school guidance counselor, who can provide direct contact with the child as well as a valuable liaison with teachers and school administration. The school's psychologist can be helpful in providing cognitive testing as well as assisting in the development and implementation of the individualized education plan. Educational adjustments should be considered in ADHD youth with difficulties in behavioral or academic performance. Increased structure, predictable routine, learning aids, resource room time, and checked homework are among typical educational considerations in these youth. Similar modifications in the home environment should be undertaken to optimize the child's ability to complete homework. Frequent parental communication with the school about the child's progress is essential.

Focused therapies incorporating cognitive-behavioral features are reportedly effective in children, adolescents, and adults with ADHD; however, the long-term benefit of these treatments independent of pharmacotherapy is yet to be determined. Behavioral modification with the child and parents is useful in cases of co-occurring disruptive behaviors, inflexibility, anxiety, or outbursts. More traditional insight-oriented psychotherapy should be considered in ADHD cases with evidence of self-esteem issues, adjustment problems, or depression. Social skills remediation for improving interpersonal interactions and coaching for improving organization and study skills are useful adjuncts to treatment.

Pharmacotherapy

Medications remain a mainstay of treatment for ADHD. In fact, large multisite studies support that medication management of ADHD is the most important variable in outcome in context to multimodal treatment. Stimulants, adrenergic agents, arousal agents, antihypertensives, and antidepressants comprise the available agents for ADHD).

STIMULANTS

The stimulants are considered among the first-line agents for ADHD based in part on their extensive efficacy and safety data. Stimulants are sympathomimetic drugs that increase intrasynaptic catecholamines (dopamine and norepinephrine) by inhibiting the presynaptic reuptake mechanism and releasing presynaptic catecholamines. The most commonly used compounds in this class include d,1-methylphenidate (Ritalin [LA], Concerta, Metadate, methylphenidate transdermal patch [MTS, Daytrana]), d-methylphenidate (Focalin [XR]), amphetamine compounds (Adderall [XR]), and d-amphetamine (Dexedrine). The stimulants are available in immediate-release short-acting preparations that last 2 to 4 hours and extended-release forms that last from 8 to 12 hours. Differences among the

constellation of the stimulants exist (e.g., racemic and single isomer, different release mechanisms, different "early" and "late" day concentrations with extended release).

Despite the findings on efficacy of the stimulants, studies also report consistently that typically a third of ADHD individuals do not respond or cannot tolerate this class of agents. Although methylphenidate is the best studied stimulant, the literature suggests more similarities than differences in response to the various available stimulants. However, based on marginally different mechanisms of action, some patients who lack a satisfactory response or manifest adverse effects to one stimulant may respond favorably to another. Stimulants should be initiated at the lowest available dosing once daily and increased every 3 to 7 days until a response is noted or adverse effects emerge. Parameters for upward daily dosing of the stimulants typically are 1 mg/kg/day for the amphetamines and 2 mg/kg/day for methylphenidate (1 mg/kg/day for transdermal or d-methylphenidate).

Predictable short-term adverse effects include reduced appetite, insomnia, edginess, and gastrointestinal (GI) upset. A number of controversial issues are related to chronic stimulant use. Although stimulants may produce anorexia and weight loss, their effect on ultimate height is less certain. Although initial reports suggested a persistent stimulant-associated decrease in growth in height in children, other reports failed to substantiate this finding, and still others questioned the possibility that growth deficits may represent maturational delays related to ADHD itself rather than to stimulant treatment. Stimulants may precipitate or exacerbate tic symptoms in ADHD children. Recent work suggests that up to a third of children with tics may have worsening of their tics with stimulant exposure. Long-term exposure to stimulant treatment of ADHD appears to decrease the risk of subsequent substance abuse; however, diversion and misuse of immediate-release stimulants in older adolescents and young adults remains a concern.

NORADRENERGIC AGENTS

Antidepressants

The antidepressants are not approved by the Food and Drug Administration (FDA) for ADHD and are considered second-line agents. Bupropion (Wellbutrin, Zyban[1]) is an antidepressant with indirect dopamine and noradrenergic effects that was effective for ADHD in controlled trials of children and adults. Given its usefulness in reducing cigarette smoking, improving mood, lack of monitoring requirements, and tolerability, bupropion is often used for complex ADHD patients with substance abuse or an unstable mood disorder. Adverse events include activation, irritability, insomnia, and rarely seizures. The serotonin reuptake inhibitors (e.g., fluoxetine [Prozac][1]) are not useful for core symptoms of ADHD. The tricyclic antidepressants[1] are also effective in treating ADHD but require electrocardiogram (ECG) and blood monitoring and have substantial adverse effects (dry mouth, constipation, cardiac). Both bupropion and tricyclics may require up to 6 weeks to see a full therapeutic effect.

---

[1]Not FDA approved for this indication.

CURRENT THERAPY

Medications Used in Attention Deficit Hyperactivity Disorder

Generic Medication	Brand Name	Daily Dose (mg/kg)[3]	Common Adverse Effects
Stimulants			All age groups:
Methylphenidate	Ritalin (LA*)	1.0–2.0	■ Insomnia, decreased appetite, weight loss, dysphoria
	Concerta*	0.5–1.0	
	Metadate (CD*)	0.3–1.5	
	MTS (patch)*[4]	(1 mg/kg/day)	
D-methylphenidate	Focalin (XR*)	(1 mg/kg/day)	■ Possible reduction in growth velocity with chronic use
Amphetamines			
Dextroamphetamine	Dexedrine	(1 mg/kg/day)	■ Rebound phenomena with immediate release
Amphetamine compound	Adderall (XR*)	(1 mg/kg/day)	
Noradrenergic Agents			
Atomoxetine	Strattera	0.5–1.8	■ GI upset
			■ Hypersomnia and insomnia
			■ Irritability/activation
Arousal Agents			
Modafinil[1]	Provigil	200–400 (mg/d)	■ Insomnia
			■ Appetite suppression
			■ Headache
Antidepressants			All age groups:
Bupropion[1]	Wellbutrin (SR, XL)	3–6 (mg/kg/day)	■ Irritability, insomnia, seizure risk
			■ Contraindicated in bulimics
Tricyclics (TCA)[1]			■ Dry mouth, constipation
Imipramine, Desipramine;	Tofranil, Norpramin,	2.0–5.0	■ Weight loss
Nortriptyline	Pamelor	1.0–3.0	■ Vital sign and ECG changes
			■ Nausea
			■ Sedation
Antihypertensives			Juveniles only:
Clonidine[1]	Catapres	3–10 µg/kg	■ Sedation, depression, confusion
			■ Rebound hypertension
			■ Dermatitis with patch
Guanfacine[1]	Tenex	30–100 µg/kg	Similar to clonidine but less sedation

[1]Not FDA approved for this indication.
[3]Exceeds dosage recommended by the manufacturer.
[4]Not yet approved for use in the United States.
*Denotes extended-release preparation of stimulant.

Atomoxetine

Atomoxetine (Strattera) is a potent norepinephrine-specific reuptake inhibitor that was studied in more than 1800 youths with ADHD. In contrast to stimulants, atomoxetine does not increase dopamine availability in the nucleus accumbens or striatum, which may explain why it is not associated with euphoria. Although useful in uncomplicated ADHD, atomoxetine is particularly useful in ADHD co-morbid with oppositional, tic, anxiety, and substance use disorders. Dosing of atomoxetine is up to 1.8 mg/kg/day and should be reduced if patients are on concomitant medications that interfere with its metabolism (e.g., fluoxetine). Adverse effects associated with atomoxetine include GI upset, change in sleep pattern, nausea, irritability, and rare hepatitis and suicidal ideation (0.37%). Atomoxetine also had no long-term effect (less than 3 years) on growth in height and weight. Recent data show continued effectiveness and good tolerability in children and adolescents up to to 2 years.

AROUSAL AGENTS

Modafinil (Sparlon)[1] is a nonstimulant recently tested FDA approved for pediatric ADHD. Recently published trials have shown efficacy in both the cognitive and hyperactive-impulsive symptoms in ADHD children. Despite efficacy, the precise mechanism or areas of action of modafinil in relation to the treatment of ADHD is not fully understood. Modafinil seems to exert effects on the hypothalamus and attenuates cholinergic, cathecolaminergic and monoaminergic components of the ascending reticular activating system. Activation of the frontal cortex and anterior cingulate may be directly related to the positive effect on ADHD symptoms. Modafinil may be particularly useful in addressing the various aspects of attentional dysfunction in ADHD such as impaired vigilance, arousal,

[1]Not FDA approved for this indication.

motivation, and executive functioning. There may be a delayed onset to full effect, and adverse effects include reduced appetite, insomnia, and headaches. Long-term studies indicate similar tolerability to that described with stimulants. Although relatively free of drug interactions, modafinil reduces the effectiveness of some oral birth control pills.

ANTIHYPERTENSIVES

The antihypertensives clonidine (Catapres)[1] and guanfacine (Tenex)[1] are used to treat the hyperactive-impulsive symptoms of ADHD. Clonidine is a relatively short-acting compound with usual daily dose ranges from 0.05 mg to 0.4 mg. Guanfacine is longer acting and less potent than clonidine with usual daily dose ranges from 0.5 mg to 3 mg. The antihypertensives are used for the treatment of ADHD as well as associated tics, aggression, and sleep disturbances, particularly in younger children. Two multisite studies suggest that α-agonists may be useful in ADHD plus tics, alone and in combination with stimulants. Although sedation is more commonly seen with clonidine, both agents may cause depression and rebound hypertension. Older reports have implicated the combination of clonidine plus methylphenidate in the deaths of four children; however, many mitigating and extenuating circumstances were operative, making these cases uninterpretable. Cardiovascular monitoring (vital signs, ECG) remains optional.

Combined pharmacologic approaches can be used for the treatment of co-morbid ADHD, as augmentation strategies for patients with insufficient response to a single agent, pharmacokinetic synergism, and for the management of treatment-emergent adverse effects. Examples include the use of atomoxetine plus methylphenidate to enhance treatment responsivity, an antidepressant plus a stimulant for ADHD and co-morbid depression (fluoxetine [Prozac] plus methylphenidate), the use of clonidine to ameliorate stimulant-induced insomnia, and the use of a mood stabilizer or atypical antipsychotic plus an anti-ADHD agent to treat ADHD co-morbid with bipolar disorder (e.g., divalproex [Depakote] plus amphetamine compounds).

Unfortunately, a number of individuals either do not respond to or are intolerant of the adverse effects of medications used to treat their ADHD. Youth who are nonresponders to one stimulant should be considered for another stimulant trial or for a nonstimulant. If two stimulant trials are unsuccessful, a nonstimulant should be considered starting with atomoxetine (Strattera), and later considering modafinil (Sparlon)[1] or bupropion (Wellbutrin)[1] and the tricyclic antidepressants.[1] Antihypertensives may be useful for younger children or those with prominent hyperactivity, impulsivity, aggressiveness, or tics/Tourette's disorder. Cognitive activators such as donepezil may be considered for refractory youth.

In summary, there is increasing recognition that ADHD is a heterogeneous disorder that persists in a number of cases through adolescence into adult years. The scope of co-morbidity has expanded to include not only disruptive disorders but also mood, anxiety, and substance use disorders as well. Emerging findings support a genetic and neurobiologic basis for ADHD with catecholaminergic dysfunction as a central finding. An extensive literature supports the effectiveness of pharmacotherapy not only for the core behavioral symptoms of ADHD but also improvement in linked impairments including cognition, social skills, and family function. Similarities between juveniles and adults in the characteristics, biology, and pharmacologic responsivity of ADHD supports the continuity of the disorder across the life span.

REFERENCES

A 14-month randomized clinical trial of treatment strategies for attention-deficit/hyperactivity disorder. The MTA Cooperative Group. Multimodal Treatment Study of Children with ADHD [see comments]. Arch Gen Psychiatry 1999;56(12):1073-1086.

Barkley R: Attention-Deficit/Hyperactivity Disorder: A Handbook for Diagnosis and Treatment, 2nd ed. New York, Guilford Press, 1998.

Biederman J, Newcorn J, Sprich S: Comorbidity of attention deficit hyperactivity disorder with conduct, depressive, anxiety, and other disorders. Am J Psychiatry 1991;148:564-577.

Biederman J, Spencer T, Wilens T: Evidence based pharmacotherapy for attention deficit hyperactivity disorder. Int J Neuropsychopharmacol 2004;7(1):77-97.

Castellanos FX, Lee PP, Sharp W, et al: Developmental trajectories of brain volume abnormalities in children and adolescents with attention-deficit/hyperactivity disorder. JAMA 2002;288(14):1740-1748.

Faraone SV, Biederman J: Neurobiology of attention deficit hyperactivity disorder. In Charney DS, Nestler EJ (eds): Neurobiology of Mental Illness, 2nd ed. New York, Oxford University Press, 2004.

Hinshaw SP: Preadolescent girls with attention-deficit/hyperactivity disorder: I. Background characteristics, comorbidity, cognitive, and social functioning, and parenting practices. J Consult Clin Psychol 2002;70(5):1086-1098.

Kurlan R: Treatment of ADHD in children with tics: A randomized controlled trial. Neurology 2002;58:527-536.

Michelson D, Faries D, Wernicke J, et al: Atomoxetine in the treatment of children and adolescents with attention-deficit/hyperactivity disorder: A randomized, placebo-controlled, dose-response study. Pediatrics 2001;108(5):E83.

Spencer T, Biederman J, Wilens T: Growth deficits in ADHD children. Pediatrics 1998;102(Suppl 2):501-506.

Wilens T, Faraone S, Biederman J, Gunawardene S: Does stimulant therapy of ADHD beget later substance abuse: A metanalytic review of the literature. Pediatrics 2003;11(1):179-185.

Gilles de la Tourette Syndrome

Method of
Roger D. Freeman, MD

Tourette's syndrome (TS), otherwise known as Gilles de la Tourette syndrome or Tourette's disorder, is characterized by waxing and waning motor and vocal tics over a period of at least 1 year. For historic and arbitrary reasons, at least one vocal tic is required to fulfill all criteria, although lists of tics often confuse the issue by incorrectly including sniffing as "vocal." (There seems to be no valid reason to privilege a vocal tic in the definition.) A child with multiple changing tics (not necessarily simultaneous) almost certainly fulfills criteria for TS later, even if only a few weeks have passed; the 12-month rule is again arbitrary. The media loves to portray coprolalia, the involuntary

---

[1]Not FDA approved for this indication.

emission of expletives or unacceptable words, noises, or phrases, but it occurs in only approximately 5% to 15% of cases as a significant problem and may be transient. Tics, like other neurodevelopmental disorders, are highly familial and probably influenced by multiple genetic and environmental factors.

Clinical Features and Course

Tics are very common, occurring in up to 20% of boys in any one school year. Most of these are single tics that may resolve with further development and never come to a physician's attention. It is now generally accepted that the current criteria for TS is satisfied by approximately 0.5% to 1% of the child population, with boys outnumbering girls by approximately four to one and a mean age at onset of 6 to 7 years. These two stable findings around the world indicate that the underlying process is neurodevelopmental and may be influenced by gender-specific factors, but it is unlikely that diet, environmental toxins, allergies, or infections is a major cause. Psychological factors are not sufficient to cause tics but may sometimes influence their severity or form. "Automatic suppression" of tics in the presence of strangers may mean the physician sees many fewer symptoms than the parents do, and the teacher sees less than at home. The experience of having obvious tics is the result of a complex mixture of biologic, psychological (learning, meanings), family, and sociocultural factors in which information, attitudes, talent, time, and support have important roles to play. Tics are at their most severe and unstable prior to puberty (approximately 10 to 12 years of age) and usually diminish gradually and become more stable in or after adolescence. Follow-up studies and clinical experience agree that no matter how severe the tics in childhood, substantial improvement is likely. The quality of life is then determined not by the cross-sectional severity or impairment, but by how childhood is endured with the tics and the kind of individual who emerges into adulthood. Home medical encyclopedias and medical dictionaries (and their equivalent on the Web) rarely provide more than a bleak view of TS and its future. If this were one's sole source of information, one would never guess that having TS can (eventually) fall into place as a small or even insignificant part of life. This is a distortion that renders a real disservice to parents and receives too little emphasis.

Co-occurring Conditions and Problems

Depending on whether subsyndromal obsessive-compulsive symptoms are included as a disorder, approximately 12% to 20% of clinical cases simply have tics (TS-Only); the remainder, varying by clinic from almost all to approximately 60%, have (on average) two co-occurring disorders (TS+) by our current classification system and may therefore present with (or develop) a wide variety of problems; often the tics are the least of these. Attention deficit hyperactivity disorder (ADHD) and obsessive-compulsive disorder (OCD) are the most common co-occurring conditions, and the trio is well known by all clinicians in the field, typically starting with ADHD, tics developing around

6 to 8 years of age, and OCD often somewhat later. Those patients with this complex picture are also at risk for learning disabilities; anxiety disorders, oppositional-defiant disorder, and mood disorders. Families need to understand that the evolution of a complex clinical picture with multiple diagnoses does not mean separate diseases are acquired, but that the complexity of the underlying problem and its adaptive manifestations has changed and will likely evolve further. All disorders or problem behaviors cannot be treated simultaneously or rigidly; assessment of all areas of functioning, strengths as well as weaknesses, is required to determine the need for treatment. Patients with TS-Only that persists for a few years without the development of co-morbid disorders are unlikely to have problem behaviors, self-injurious behavior (SIB), sleep disorders, or a learning disability.

Assuming the diagnosis is made correctly, the goals in the management of TS are these:

- The development of tolerance for tics, which minimizes the need for long-term medication and the burden of suffering.
- The development of ways of thinking conducive to a balanced view of the child.
- Suppression of tics in some cases at some times.
- Treatment of co-occurring disorders or problems.

The Development of Tic Tolerance

Parents do not like to see their child acting strangely or others looking askance at them. They may hesitate to take their child to the movies or to church where their tics will be noticeable or hear their child complaining of sore muscles or teasing. Many actions can be taken to reduce the impact for most children:

- Ensure that both parents have a basic understanding of key information. Other important family members may need the same information, especially absent fathers and involved grandparents.
- Seek school support with understanding by staff and schoolmates, advocacy where necessary, and monitoring of teasing and bullying. Teachers may need explanations tailored to the individual child if tics are prominent, causing misunderstanding/rejection or interfering with attention, writing, or peer relationships.
- Offer the child explanations at his or her level and the opportunity to develop brief, simple explanations of symptoms for peers and others.
- Find ways to work around certain tics like eye rolling, which results in a loss of focus on the line while reading.
- Manage muscle soreness conservatively (heat, massage, analgesics), especially with a frequent new tic.
- Optimize family functioning and activities to promote positive experiences.
- Ensure the continued accessibility of the clinician for questions about new symptoms and for reassessment as needed. This works best in the context of a continuing relationship.
- Learn not to attribute all problems to tics. Ask, "Could the same or a similar problem occur without tics?" Often the answer is "yes." Resist trying obsessively to find causes for new symptoms or distinguish a tic from compulsions and all other behaviors.

- Find support groups after the situation is stabilized that share tips and reduce a sense of negative uniqueness. Note: Support groups may create problems if attended primarily by persons with worse difficulties or with an idiosyncratic agenda.

A Balanced View

At first, many parents react as if the tics and associated symptoms override all other characteristics of their child. In cases in which the child has good social skills, interests, and talents, these important qualities need to be gradually restored to their rightful place in the parental repertoire of reactions and meanings. An exploration of the individual significance of that child and his or her success in life or apparent suffering for being different may be helpful and is sometimes necessary when a balanced view cannot be restored. The continuing influence of spouses and relatives must also be taken into account, and sometimes it is necessary to help them with their understanding.

Tic Suppression

Except in extreme instances, the need for a tic suppressant is not determined by the tics themselves but by their specific effects and meanings at a particular stage of development of the child and family and in an individual context. If a rapid response is needed, a neuroleptic is the first choice (pimozide, haloperidol, or risperidone), followed by tetrabenazine (available in Canada and probably soon in the United States). The general principle is to start very low and increase dosages slowly. If that rule is followed, concurrent usage of antiparkinsonian agents is usually unnecessary, and acute extrapyramidal (dystonic) reactions are very rare. The dosage-related onset of school or work avoidance as a new problem is reason to suspect the "neuroleptic separation anxiety syndrome" and to test its relationship to neuroleptic dosage. Tardive dyskinesia is fortunately a very rare occurrence but may not always be reversible, so the need for medication must be very clear.

CURRENT DIAGNOSIS

- *DSM-IV-TR* diagnosis requires multiple waxing and waning tics (at least 2 motor and 1 vocal) over ≥12 mo. An additional questionable criterion is no period of ≥3 mo without tics.
- Tics do not have to be present simultaneously and there is no impairment criterion; coprolalia phenomena are not required.
- All repetitive behaviors are not tics.
- There is a wide variety of severity, manifestations, and degree of impairment.
- Common eyelid muscle twitches are usually not tics; they are benign ocular myokymia (sometimes also termed fasciculations).
- Most (about 85%) clinical cases are co-morbid.

Abbreviation: DSM-IV-TR = Diagnostic and Statistical Manual of Mental Disorders, Fourth Edition, Text Revision.

Information about the long-range side effects of the atypical neuroleptics is still emerging (prolactin effects, weight gain, increased risk of diabetes or cardiovascular disease), so their advantage over the typical neuroleptics may not be great. If a slower response is tolerable, clonidine or guanfacine may be tried. Refractory cases should be treated by (or in consultation with) a TS expert. Finally, there are three important rules:

1. Complete tic suppression is undesirable. It leads to excessive drug dosages and obscures the continuing need for medication.
2. Because tics wax and wane spontaneously, there should be a delay in responding to an upsurge, and because of confusion caused by rebound, medication dosage should be tapered rather than suddenly stopped.
3. A baseline electrocardiogram and close monitoring are essential to minimize complications, especially when a new drug is initiated and dosages are changed.

Co-occurring Disorders or Problems

Co-occurring ADHD, with all of its ramifications, is diagnosed in approximately 60% of clinical TS cases. Because ADHD is itself highly familial, other family members with such problems may need consideration in comprehensive management. The use of stimulant medications is usually quite successful without causing tic exacerbations beyond that which could occur by chance with any medication. Experience with the nonstimulant atomoxetine (Strattera) is just beginning but looks promising.

In approximately 25% of TS cases, OCD is diagnosed. Subthreshold but significant symptoms appear in another 35%. Treatment with selective serotonin reuptake inhibitors (SSRIs) or clomipramine is the usual approach, with low-dosage pimozide augmentation for some refractory cases with tics. Cognitive behavior therapy (with or without medication) is also useful for fixed symptom patterns in cooperative patients and may have longer lasting effects than medication.

Sleep disorders (25%) are highly associated with ADHD, not tics, although new or complex tics may make it difficult to fall asleep. When sleep initiation difficulty fails to respond to modifications in sleep hygiene, timing of stimulant medication, or treatment of obsessive-compulsive symptoms, 0.1 mg of clonidine[1] or 3 to 9 mg of melatonin* are effective for many children.

Anger control problems, sometimes referred to as "rage," are uncommon in TS-Only but common in TS+ cases (40% or more). Co-occurring obsessive-compulsive features or mood lability may serve as triggers, but problems occurring in school may also have a learning problem (often unrecognized) as a factor. It is important to try to identify target symptoms that may be contributing to these problems.

SIB is reported in 15%. SIB is not uncommon in the general population and in many of the childhood neuropsychiatric disorders. It is much more common in

---

[1]Not FDA approved for this medication.

*Weiss M, Wasdell M, Bomben M, et al: Sleep hygiene and melatonin treatment for children and adolescents with ADHD and initial insomnia. J Am Acad Child Adolesc Psychiatry 2006;45:1-8

TS+OCD than in TS-Only, and it may take bizarre forms. It may or may not respond to neuroleptic and/or anti-obsessional treatment.

Anxiety disorders are diagnosed in 15% to 20%. Many of the same measures used in childhood anxiety without tics can be equally useful, but SSRI medications have more unpredictable effects than in adults and may have paradoxical effects.

Mood disorders are diagnosed in 20%. In practice, formal mood disorders seem less common than complaints about "moodiness," high reactivity, or a negative approach to problems and frustrations. The distinction between juvenile bipolar disorder and ADHD may be difficult in some cases.

Pervasive developmental disorders (PDDs) are diagnosed in approximately 5%. Several epidemiologic studies show a high rate of tics and TS in children with Asperger's syndrome and autism; as those children age, obsessive-compulsive symptoms and severe sleep disorders may become very troublesome. These cases typically require consultation or management by a specialist.

Management of the Typical Case of Tourette's Syndrome-Only

Children with TS are now brought to physicians significantly earlier than in the past. The child is usually not the one worried about the tics. The parents may already have done research, perhaps with resulting confusion and likely with considerable anxiety. Almost certainly they have heard something about TS and require remedial learning. They often fear social rejection (especially because of coprolalia, a dire prognosis from cases shown on television) and the use of potentially dangerous drugs. They may have guilt over blaming the child for deliberate behavior rather than involuntary symptoms, disagreeing with each other over the nature of the tics and fruitless attempts at

diagnosis and treatment. If the child has friends, reasonable intelligence, hobbies and interests, and at least average school achievement, reassurance and education are usually all that is needed. Parents can learn that these positive features are the most important. Even with competent diagnosis and information, however, the next few upsurges often require support before tolerance of tics develops. The school may need confirmation of the diagnosis or explanation of its significance. As development proceeds, monitoring school progress, social development, and any new symptoms that may indicate the presence of a co-morbid disorder is important, and parents need to know whom to contact in that event. If parental anxiety does not diminish, more work to uncover its current or remote sources may be necessary.

Management of the More Complex Case (TS+)

Complexity in management is not always correlated with the number of co-morbid disorders. Some TS-Only cases can be more difficult to manage than cases with three or more diagnostic labels, but ongoing management of difficult cases is really the province of the specialist with extensive experience. Additional consultation with colleagues may be indicated. Psychological testing is often helpful, especially when there are school problems, either academic or behavioral. When medications are needed for tics, they need to be started at very low dosages and raised and lowered slowly (Table 1).

Management of Adults

Many of the same considerations as previously outlined apply to adults with TS. The original assessment may be inadequate by current standards, however, and a fresh look

TABLE 1 Medications for Tics

Drug	Starting Dose	Maintenance Dose	Side Effects	Comments
Haloperidol (Haldol)	0.25 mg every morning	0.5–3 mg/d	Cognitive blunting at higher dosages; extrapyramidal symptoms	Drops available
Pimozide (Orap)	0.5 mg every morning or evening	2–6 mg/d	Tremor, akinesia, extrapyramidal symptoms	May be used bid
Risperidone (Risperdal)	0.25 mg/d	0.5–4 mg/d	Extrapyramidal symptoms, weight gain, diabetes	Oral solution available; off label
Clonidine (Catapres)	0.025 bid–tid	0.1 mg tid	Somnolence, dry mouth	(Off-label use)
Guanfacine (Tenex)	1 mg every morning	1–2 mg/d	Somnolence, dry mouth	(Off-label use)
Olanzapine (Zyprexa)	2.5 mg	5–10 mg/d	Extrapyramidal symptoms, weight gain, diabetes	(Off-label use)
Quetiapine (Seroquel)	25 mg bid	100–300 mg/d	Diabetes, extrapyramidal symptoms	Not well established yet for TS
Ziprasidone (Geodon)	20 mg/d	40–120 mg/d	Increased QTc interval, possibly less weight gain	Not yet well evaluated for tics

Abbreviations: QTc = corrected for heart rate; TS = Tourette's syndrome.

CURRENT THERAPY

- Keep a high threshold for prescribing medication for tic suppression until the situation and the patient and family's tolerance are well explored. Most patients do not require medication for tics.
- Co-morbidity is common and always needs to be explored, especially ADHD, OCD, anxiety, and learning disabilities. Co-morbid disorders are more likely to require treatment than tics.
- In questionable cases, obtain a videotape of the tics.
- School-related problems need timely and sometimes comprehensive attention.
- Psychological testing may be advisable.

Abbreviation: ADHD = attention deficient disorder with hyperactivity; OCD = obsessive-compulsive disorder.

therefore needs to be taken. The delay between onset of tics and the diagnosis may be quite long. Discussion of etiology years ago may have centered on psychogenic factors. The consequences of misunderstanding the nature of the condition and the effects on family relationships may be severe and enduring. Education or reeducation of the patient and important family members must be considered.

A knowledgeable and interested clinician can manage many cases of TS-Only, and—with the advice of a specialist—some co-morbid TS+ cases. In spite of tics and other symptoms, patients and families who can develop a well-balanced perspective may experience a good quality of life.

REFERENCES

Bloch MH, Peterson BS, Scahill L, et al: Adulthood outcome of tic and obsessive-compulsive symptom severity in children with Tourette syndrome. Arch Pediatr Adolesc Med 2006;16:65-69.

Chowdhury U, Heyman I: Tourette's syndrome in children. BMJ 2004;329:1357-1358.

Cohen AJ, Leckman JF: Sensory phenomena associated with Gilles de la Tourette's syndrome. J Clin Psychiatry 1992;53:319-323.

Como PG, LaMarsh J, O'Brien KA: Obsessive-compulsive disorder in Tourette's syndrome. Adv Neurol 2005;96:249-261.

Freeman RD, Fast DK, Burl L, et al: An international perspective on Tourette syndrome: Selected findings from 3,500 individuals in 22 countries. Dev Med Child Neurol 2000;42:436-447.

Gadow KD, Nolan EE, Sprakin J, et al: Tics and psychiatric comorbidity in children and adolescents. Dev Med Child Neurol 2002;44:330-338.

Goetz CG, Leurgans S, Chmura TA: Home alone: Methods to maximize tic expression for objective videotape assessments in Gilles de la Tourette syndrome. Mov Disord 2001;16:693-697.

Grados MA, Riddle MA, Samuels JF, et al: The familial phenotype of obsessive-compulsive disorder in relation to tic disorders: The Hopkins OCD family study. Biol Psychiatry 2001;50:559-565.

Hoekstra PJ, Minderaa RB: Tic disorders and obsessive-compulsive disorder: Is autoimmunity involved? Int Rev Psychiatry 2005;17:497-502.

Hoekstra PJ, Steenhuis MP, Kallenberg CG: Association of small life events with self reports of tic severity in pediatric and adult tic disorder patients: A prospective longitudinal study. J Clin Psychiatry 2004;65:426-431.

Hoekstra PJ, Steenhuis MP, Troost PW, et al: Relative contribution of attention-deficit hyperactivity disorder, obsessive-compulsive disorder, and tic severity to social and behavioral problems in tic disorders. J Dev Behav Pediatr 2004;25:272-279.

Kadesjö B, Gillberg C: Tourette's disorder: Epidemiology and comorbidity in primary school children. J Am Acad Child Adolesc Psychiatry 2000;39:548-555.

Kurlan R: Tourette's syndrome: Are stimulants safe? Curr Neurol Neurosci Rep 2003;3:285-288.

Kurlan R, Como PG, Miller B, et al: The behavioral spectrum of tic disorders: A community-based study. Neurology 2002;59:414-420.

Kushner HI: A Cursing Brain? The Histories of Tourette Syndrome. Cambridge, Mass, Harvard University Press, 1999.

Leckman JF: Tourette's syndrome. Lancet 2002;360:1577-1586.

Leckman JF, Cohen DJ (eds): Tourette's Syndrome—Tics, Obsessions, Compulsions: Developmental Psychopathology and Clinical Care. New York, John Wiley, 1999.

Leckman JF, Zhang H, Vitale A, et al: Course of tic severity in Tourette syndrome: The first two decades. Pediatrics 1998;102:14-19.

Mantel BJ, Meyers A, Tran QY: Nutritional supplements and complementary/alternative medicine in Tourette syndrome. J Child Adolesc Psychopharmacol 2004;14:582-589.

Scahill L, Sukhodolsky DG, Williams SK, et al: Public health significance of tic disorders in children and adolescents. Adv Neurol 2005;96:240-248.

Singer HS, Giuliano JD, Zimmerman AM, et al: Infection: A stimulus for tic disorders. Pediatr Neurol 2000;22:380-383.

Snider LA, Seligman LD, Ketchen BR, et al: Tics and problem behaviors in schoolchildren: Prevalence, characterization, and associations. Pediatrics 2002;110:331-336.

Headache

Method of
R. Michael Gallagher, DO

Headache is a disturbing and sometimes fearsome affliction that has plagued humankind throughout recorded history. It often is debilitating and particularly disturbing to the sufferer because the pain is located in the head, the very center of the body's cognitive and control functions. With its accompanying pain and debilitating symptoms, stress can mount and the headache can become all consuming.

Headache is experienced by all age groups from young children to the elderly. It is more common than asthma, diabetes, mental illness, and rheumatoid arthritis. In fact, the World Health Organization identifies severe migraine, along with psychosis and quadriplegia, as "one of the most debilitating chronic conditions." Although the majority of Americans experience tension-type headaches at some time in their lives, approximately 30 million experience migraine headache: 13% of women and 6% of men, predominantly in their most productive years between the ages of 13 and 55 years. Prepubescent boys and girls suffer equally; however, boys often outgrow their migraine attacks as they mature, and they are less subjected to hormonal influences. Smaller percentages of people, by comparison, suffer with other chronic headaches, such as cluster headache and chronic daily headache.

No sure diagnostic tests are available to differentiate headache types. The headache condition can progress over time in frequency, severity, and debilitation. Each sufferer can be different and may require a detailed evaluation and individualized treatment plan; more frequent or prolonged attacks often necessitate a more comprehensive treatment plan. Thus, the headache problem can be a challenge for both the sufferer and the clinician.

During the 20th century, dramatic advancements were made in medicine. Longevity and quality of life improved for many individuals. Unfortunately, for headache sufferers, most of these advances were for maladies that killed or maimed rather than for non–life-threatening conditions. It was not until the 1960s that even a reasonable preventive medication, propranolol (Inderal), was introduced, and by the 1980s only a handful of medications were available for wide use. Physicians had to improvise with medications and treatments that were originally designated for other medical conditions.

In the late 1980s and 1990s, epidemiologic, psychosocial, and pharmacologic research resulted in an increase in available headache information and treatment possibilities. The development of the triptans, serotonin agonists, brought a new awareness to both physicians and sufferers. Today, seven triptans and two relatively new preventive medications are available. In spite of this, a minority of migraine sufferers use these options, and more than 50% continue to self-treat without benefit of professional care.

In the past, patients wanted the physician to believe their headache problem was real. They hoped that they would be taken seriously and that the physician would make a sincere attempt to help them. The headache patient has changed. The headache sufferer who seeks treatment today is more knowledgeable and interested in rapid relief and tolerability of medication.

Evaluation and Diagnosis

An accurate diagnosis is essential for effective management of patients with the more commonly encountered headaches. Because no biologic markers or diagnostic tests exist to determine headache type, the history is the single most important element in the evaluation of the headache patient. Various headache types sometimes have similar initial presentations, or patients may suffer with more than one type of headache (e.g., migraine and tension-type headache), which can be confusing at first, but the careful history usually differentiates the headache type. In general, little in the way of diagnostic testing is needed unless a physical cause is suspected. Some physicians prefer to perform simple laboratory tests to establish a baseline for medication toleration and monitoring as necessary (Table 1).

The headache complaint on occasion can be a sign of a more serious medical condition, such as a tumor, infection, or aneurysm. For this reason, the clinician always must be cautious and diligent in establishing an accurate and timely diagnosis. Certain so-called red flags in the history require immediate attention. These include any complex of symptoms or history that does not fit a typical headache type; report of a significant neurologic deficit; late-onset migraine (patient older than 30 years); sudden onset of a new head pain without history of similar headaches; changes in headache character; headache associated with elevated temperature; or completely unresponsive attacks in the absence of analgesic or caffeine overuse. When any of these symptoms are present or physical examination reveals significant findings, further diagnostic evaluation with imaging studies and consultation is imperative.

The appropriate headache patient evaluation includes a thorough history, physical examination with special attention to the head and the neurologic, cardiovascular, and musculoskeletal systems, and diagnostic tests when appropriate. The history should include headache onset, location, pain character (e.g., pressure, throb), frequency, duration, associated symptoms, aura or prodrome, triggers, previous treatment, and family history. Certain clues in the history may lean toward the diagnosis of migraine, such as motion sickness, absence of headache during pregnancy, and headache relationship to menses, sun glare, oversleep, fatigue, fasting, foods, or alcohol.

Various diagnostic screening questionnaires and tools have been developed over the years to assist busy clinicians in establishing the diagnosis of migraine. Most are long and cumbersome and do not easily become a part of routine patient evaluation. A simple three-question screener for migraine is helpful for generalist clinicians. A "yes" answer to all three questions indicates a strong possibility of the migraine diagnosis:

1. Do you experience headaches severe enough to see a physician?
2. Are your headaches accompanied by other symptoms?
3. Are your headaches intermittent (i.e., nondaily)?

Note: This screener should not be substituted for a complete history; it should be used only for screening purposes.

TENSION-TYPE HEADACHE

Tension-type headache (TTHA) is the most common of headaches and first was believed to be caused by sustained muscle contraction of the neck, jaw, scalp, or facial muscles. However, it is now thought that the sustained muscle contraction can, in fact, be an epiphenomenon to possible central disturbances rather than a primary process. Evidence suggests that altered levels of serotonin, substance P, and neuropeptide Y in the serum or platelets of patients with TTHA are responsible.

TTHA is characterized by intermittent or persisting bilateral pain, usually described as a squeezing pressure or a bandlike sensation around the head. Most patients experience their symptoms in the frontal, temporal, or occipital areas of the head. Location frequently varies with the attack, and tightness of the neck and shoulders is common. Intensity varies greatly. The attacks can last from hours to days, and in some extreme cases they may last for months. Aura, nausea, photophobia and phonophobia, and incapacitation are not typically associated with TTHA.

CURRENT DIAGNOSIS

- Seizures may be partial (focal or localization-related) or generalized in onset. Clinical history, EEG, and imaging data assist the clinician in determining the seizure type and epilepsy syndrome.
- The most important initial diagnostic tests for evaluating new-onset epilepsy in adolescents and adults are high-resolution brain magnetic resonance imaging and EEG.
- In refractory epilepsy or spells of an uncertain type, the patient should be referred for video-EEG monitoring to document and localize the seizure type.

TABLE 1 Current Diagnosis

Symptoms	Frequency	Duration
Tension-Type Headache		
Bilateral variable pain	Variable	Hours to days
Squeezing or bandlike	Often related to known precipitant	
Tightness of head and shoulders		
Migraine Headache		
Unilateral mostly	1–6 mo	Hours to days
Throbbing or constant pain	Sometimes cyclic	
Nausea, vomiting		
Photophobia/phonophobia		
Fluid disturbances		
Mood changes		
Can be associated with aura		
Cluster Headache		
Unilateral severe boring pain	Multiple daily	45–90 min
Ipsilateral lacrimation, scleral injection, rhinorrhea	Near-daily	Cycles of attacks
Eyelid droop		
Restlessness		

Many TTHA sufferers easily recognize the origin of their attacks. TTHA typically results from emotional upset, periods of stress, and major life changes. Anxiousness, poor adaptation skills, and anxiety and depression often are present. Physical causes, such as degenerative joint disease, trauma to the head or neck, poor posture, or temporomandibular joint dysfunction, also can precipitate attacks. Persons older than 50 years are prone to excessive muscle contraction because of arthritis of the neck and jaw, poor posture, or stress. TTHA that is consistently precipitated by tension or pathology of the neck frequently is referred to as a *cervicogenic headache*. In contrast to migraine headache, TTHA is more likely to begin in later life.

MIGRAINE HEADACHE

Migraine headache is a familial disease characterized by unilateral or bilateral paroxysmal headache lasting hours to days. Adult women experience attacks more than men by a ratio of 3:1. Children and the elderly experience migraine equally. Attacks occur from as infrequently as one or two per year to several times weekly. Associated symptoms usually occur and frequently include throbbing, nausea, vomiting, photophobia, phonophobia, fluid retention, and mood changes.

The two basic types of migraine headache are *migraine with aura* (previously called classic migraine) and *migraine without aura* (previously called common migraine). Migraine with aura is preceded by an aura, a transient neurologic symptom that usually is visual, such as scotoma, teichopsia, tunnel vision, or visual field deficit, lasting 10 to 30 minutes. Migraine without aura is more commonly experienced and comes on gradually or is present on awakening from sleep. In some patients, these headaches are associated with a nonspecific prolonged prodrome, such as mood changes, food cravings, or fluid retention hours before the pain.

The underlying cause of migraine headache is not clearly established, and various theories are proposed.

Migraine appears to be of genetic origin and to be an inflammatory disease that causes disturbances in serotonin use and activity. Strong evidence indicates the migrainous attack originates in the central nervous system by stimulation of the locus ceruleus and dorsal raphe nuclei. Resultant changes alter cerebral and extracranial blood flow, activate the trigeminovascular system, and cause vascular dilation, neurogenic inflammation, and pain. Various precipitants are known, and many sufferers report that migraine attacks frequently are associated with menstruation or are triggered by foods containing vasoactive amines, strong odors, too much or too little sleep, sun glare, stress, altitude, weather changes, exertion, or fasting (Boxes 1 and 2, Table 2).

Some physicians classify migraine according to its precipitant or description (e.g., menstrual migraine, exertional migraine, coital migraine, cervicogenic migraine, cyclic migraine, acephalic migraine). Regardless, the fundamentals of evaluation and treatment are the same.

BOX 1 Migraine Dietary Triggers

- Dairy: Ripened cheese (cheddar, brie, camembert, half-cup of sour cream)
- Meats: Processed lunch meats, hot dogs, sausage, bologna, salami, chicken liver
- Fish: Pickled or dried herring
- Grains: Sourdough bread
- Fruits: Bananas, raisins, figs, avocado, half-cup limit of citrus
- Vegetables: Broad and fava beans, onions, snow peas
- Other: Chocolate, nuts, peanut butter, pickled foods, Chinese food with monosodium glutamate (MSG)
- Beverages: Most wines and alcohol, 200-mg daily limit of caffeine
- Additives: MSG, soy sauce, meat tenderizers, aspartame, sulfites, garlic

BOX 2   Migraine Triggers

- Altitude
- Alcohol
- Caffeine withdrawal
- Fluorescent or flickering lights
- Sun glare
- Weather changes
- Stress, stress letdown
- Foods
- Skipping meals
- Smoky environment
- Noisy environment
- Strong odors
- Lack of sleep, oversleep
- Exertion
- Hormonal changes

CLUSTER HEADACHE

The cause of cluster headache is unknown, and little credible research is available. Various possibilities or theories are suggested and include, but are not limited to, disturbances in histamine production or use; hypothalamic biorhythm dysfunction; or serotonin and neurotransmitter mechanisms similar to those of migraine. Some authorities consider cluster headache one of the most severe pain conditions known to humankind.

Cluster headache predominantly affects men, with a male-to-female ratio of 6:1. It occurs in well under 0.5% of the population. Onset later in life (after age 30 years) is common, and patients sometimes report head injury or a traumatic event occurring months before onset. Attacks occur on a daily or near-daily basis for weeks or months at a time and mysteriously disappear for months to years regardless of treatment, only to recur and cycle again. Although nonspecialist physicians only occasionally encounter the patient with cluster headaches, it is important to consider cluster headaches in the differential diagnosis.

The typical patient with a cluster headache experiences relatively brief attacks (45–90 minutes) of horrible unilateral head pain associated with ipsilateral lacrimation, scleral injection, rhinorrhea, or eyelid droop. The hallmark of the syndrome is its associated symptoms and its severe and intense pain. During attacks, most cluster patients move about, trying unsuccessfully to get more comfortable, similar to renal colic, in contrast to migraine sufferers, who prefer to lie quietly in a dark quiet room. Few triggers are identified, and alcohol almost always precipitates an attack during a cluster "on" cycle. A rare form of cluster headache does not cycle and continues on a daily or near-daily basis without cessation.

Treatment

The doctor–patient relationship frequently is the key to successful treatment in the headache patient. Although to some this statement seems an obvious truism, its importance cannot be overemphasized. Patients who experience frequent, near-daily, or daily headaches invariably require a comprehensive treatment program that necessitates good communication. Anxious patients sometimes do not comprehend medical explanations or instructions; busy doctors sometimes do not have or take the time to ensure that the patient understands.

The two elements of headache treatment are *abortive treatment*, directed at attacks once they have begun, and *prophylactic treatment*, directed at preventing or reducing the frequency of attacks. In general, the abortive approach is used for patients who suffer infrequent attacks and for those who experience breakthrough attacks while undergoing prophylactic therapy. Prophylactic therapy should be instituted when headaches are frequent, when headaches are unresponsive to abortive medication, or when there are contraindications to abortives (Table 2).

Headache treatment can include nonpharmacologic measures, such as physical exercise, stretching, stress avoidance, relaxation exercises, biofeedback, manipulation, massage, or cold/warm packs. Pharmacologic therapies can include a vast array of medicaments from over-the-counter (OTC) drugs to prescription drugs such as triptans, other vasoconstrictors, β-blockers, antiepileptic agents, antidepressants, nonsteroidal anti-inflammatory drugs (NSAIDs), analgesics, muscle relaxants, anxiolytics, and others.

Treatment, whether prophylactic or abortive, should follow a definite plan incorporating the clinician and patient into a team focused on reducing the headache frequency, severity, and disability. As mentioned earlier, impressions and physical findings should be explained to the patient in as much detail as necessary to ensure the patient's complete understanding. The complexity of the headache condition needs to be explained, emphasizing its chronicity, rather than its curability, and that the goal of treatment is disease control.

The comprehensiveness of the treatment plan depends on the frequency of the patient's attacks. The more frequent and severe the attacks, the more detailed plan may be necessary. Patients experiencing infrequent attacks

TABLE 2 Current Therapy

Headache Type	PRN	Prophylaxis
Tension	OTC*	Stress/precipitant avoidance
	NSAIDs	Stretching
	Muscle relaxants	Warm packs
	Combination analgesics	Relaxation techniques
	NSAIDs	
	Muscle relaxants	
	Antidepressants	
Migraine	NSAIDs*	Biofeedback
	Triptans*	β-Blockers*
	Ergotamine*	Divalproex sodium*
	Dihydroergotamine*	Topiramate*
	Isometheptene*	TCA antidepressants
	Combination analgesics	Calcium channel blockers
Cluster	Oxygen	No alcohol
	Triptans	Calcium channel blockers
	Dihydroergotamine	
	Ergotamine	Divalproex sodium
	Lithium	NSAIDs
	Steroids	

*FDA indication.
Abbreviations: NSAID = nonsteroidal anti-inflammatory drug; OTC = over-the-counter; TCA = tricyclic antidepressant.

(e.g., once or twice monthly) may require only an abortive medication and little else. Patients with more frequent attacks may benefit from dietary restrictions, psychosocial intervention, biofeedback relaxation training, manipulation, and physical modality intervention, in addition to medication.

TENSION-TYPE HEADACHE TREATMENT

TTHA often is associated with emotional stress and muscle strain or tension of the shoulders and neck. Simple self-administered measures, such as stress avoidance, stretching, warm packs, or relaxation techniques, can be helpful in reducing or relieving attacks. More comprehensive professional intervention, such as manipulation, physical therapy, local injections, or biofeedback training, are considerations for more frequent or severe cases.

Prophylactically, the use of OTC or prescription medications can be considered in addition to nonmedicinal measures for reducing the frequency and duration of attacks. NSAIDs, muscle relaxants, or antidepressants (tricyclic antidepressant [TCA], selective serotonin reuptake inhibitor [SSRI]), at the lowest effective doses, are more commonly used.

Daily use of the longer-acting NSAIDs, such as naproxen[1] (Naprosyn) or celecoxib[1] (Celebrex), in the appropriately screened patient over a 2- to 3-week period, can be an effective preventative. TCAs, such as nortriptyline[1] (Pamelor)

or amitriptyline[1] (Elavil), in low doses at night over 1 to 3 months, are frequently effective, especially in patients with anxiety or mild depression. The SSRI drugs, such as fluoxetine[1] (Prozac) or sertraline[1] (Zoloft), similarly can be useful. The muscle relaxant cyclobenzaprine[1] (Flexeril), at low doses, with a similar mechanism to the TCAs, can be administered at night for limited periods. Other muscle relaxants occasionally can be effective. Potential side effects can limit the use of NSAIDs (gastrointestinal irritation) and the TCAs (fatigue and weight gain).

Abortive or symptomatic treatment of TTHA can include simple OTC medications (e.g., aspirin or acetaminophen), NSAIDs (short-acting), muscle relaxants, combination analgesics, and, in some cases, opioid or opioidlike drugs. Caution should be exercised in prescribing potentially habituating drugs. Daily or near-daily use of analgesics can lead to analgesic rebound headache, which can compound the patient's headache problem.

Botulism toxin[1] (Botox) reportedly is helpful in the treatment of tension-type and migraine headache, but controlled studies are limited. In this treatment, a diluted solution of botulism toxin is injected into various muscles of the face, scalp, neck, or shoulders. Because this treatment frequently is used in headache specialty and pain centers, simultaneous comprehensive measures and medication may contribute to positive results. Side effects from botulism toxin are low when injected properly.

MIGRAINE TREATMENT

Migraineurs are unique individuals, and the effectiveness and tolerance of medications can vary from patient to patient. Medication changes, combinations of medications, and trial and error may be necessary in the early stages of treatment.

Nonmedicinal measures for migraine sufferers include biofeedback stress reduction, caffeine and dietary restrictions, regimentation of meals and sleep, rest, exercise, stretching, and avoidance of work or activity overload. Limiting caffeine to less than 200 mg/day is important to prevent the caffeine headache (rebound headache). Elimination of vasoactive foods, such as chocolate, aged cheese, and processed meats, and avoidance of fasting for more than 4 hours can be helpful for patients with more frequent attacks (Table 3). Regular exercise and stretching, planned relaxation, regular sleep schedules, and following a healthy lifestyle are frequently included in a comprehensive treatment regimen. In some patients, especially children and adolescents, biofeedback stress reduction or psychotherapeutic intervention may be necessary.

The more commonly used medications for prophylaxis are β-blockers, calcium channel blockers, antiepileptics (neurostabilizers), and the antidepressants. Treatment should be continued for a 4- to 8-week trial before discontinuation for ineffectiveness. Determination of which medication to use depends on comorbidities, interactions with concomitant medications, and tolerability.

β-Blockers such as propranolol (Inderal) and timolol (Blocadren) are nonselective and are approved by the Food and Drug Administration (FDA) for migraine prevention. Other β-blockers, such as nadolol[1] (Corgard),

---

[1]Not FDA approved for this indication.

[1]Not FDA approved for this indication.

TABLE 3 Triptans

Medication	Brand Name	Half-life	Form/Strength
Sumatriptan	Imitrex	1.5 hr	Oral: 25, 50, 100 mg; NS: 20 mg; injection: 6 mg
Naratriptan	Amerge	6 hr	Oral: 2.5 mg
Zolmitriptan	Zomig	3 hr	Oral: 2.5, 5 mg; Melt: 2.5, 5 mg; NS: 5 mg
Rizatriptan	Maxalt	2–3 hr	Oral: 5, 10 mg; Melt: 10 mg
Almotriptan	Axert	3–4 hr	Oral: 6.25, 12.5 mg
Frovatriptan	Frova	25 hr	Oral: 5 mg
Eletriptan	Relpax	4 hr	Oral: 20, 40 mg

[1]Not FDA approved for this indication.
Abbreviations: Melt = oral disintegrating; NS = nasal steroid.

metoprolol[1] (Lopressor), and atenolol[1] (Tenormin), also can be effective. The mechanism of action in migraine is not wholly understood, but it is thought to involve anxiolytic effects as well as vascular changes and stabilization. The usual dosage is recommended (e.g., timolol 10–30 mg/day, propranolol 120–160 mg/day), and many consider the nighttime dose the more significant.

Calcium channel antagonists are well tolerated in general and can be as effective as the β-blockers. They are believed to alter serotonin release and inhibit platelet serotonin uptake and release within the brain. Verapamil[1] (Calan) is considered the more effective and is commonly recommended to patients. Dosage can vary from 120 to 480 mg/day. Nimodipine[1] (Nimotop) is equally effective, but it is rarely used in the United States because of its high cost.

Antiepileptic medications such as phenytoin[1] (Dilantin) and carbamazepine[1] (Tegretol) have been prescribed for migraine prevention over the years, with mixed results. Their use is now limited with the advent of newer, more easily tolerated agents, such as divalproex sodium (Depakote) and topiramate (Topamax).

Divalproex sodium is effective in reducing migraine attacks and is particularly useful in patients with coexisting head injury, seizure disorders, and bipolar disorders. It is thought to improve inhibitory and excitatory amino acid imbalance in the brain. It is best to start with a lower dose and to gradually increase as needed and tolerated. The dosage of 500 to 1000 mg/day is more frequently prescribed. A commonly experienced side effect is sedation, which can sometimes be used to the patient's advantage when anxiolytic effects are needed.

Topiramate is the most recent preventive medication approved by the FDA for migraine prophylaxis. It has multiple mechanisms of action, but its exact mechanism in migraine headache is unknown. Its effectiveness is believed to involve sodium ion channel stabilization, calcium ion channels, GABA (γ-aminobutyric acid) receptors, and neuronal membrane stabilization. The average daily dose is variable and ranges from 30 to 100 mg/day. A most unusual side effect of weight loss or appetite suppression can be used to the patient's advantage in preventing weight gain, which frequently accompanies migraine prophylactic medications.

The TCAs can be useful in patients who experience frequent attacks and in those who experience anxiety and depression. The TCAs inhibit synaptic reuptake of serotonin, thereby reducing neuron firing and release of neurotransmitters. Starting with a low dose in the evening and titrating up to efficacy and tolerability is recommended. Significant anticholinergic and sedation effects sometimes limit their use. The SSRIs[1] are reported helpful in some patients, but their use in migraine prevention is limited.

In general, prophylactic medications should be taken for 6 to 8 weeks to determine efficacy. If effective, a course of 4 to 6 months is recommended before an attempt is made to discontinue medication.

A variety of abortive treatment options are available for migraine sufferers. Although the triptans (Table 3) have generated much interest and are frequently prescribed, other medications continue to be used, including ergotamine and its derivatives, isometheptene, and NSAIDs. Many of the abortive medications carry significant prescribing limitations that must be taken into consideration. Vasoconstrictor medications are contraindicated in patients with cardiovascular or peripheral vascular disease. NSAIDs should not be used in those with gastrointestinal or bleeding disorders. As with all medications, the clinician must consider appropriate prescribing, contraindications, and side-effect information.

The vasoconstrictor ergotamine is available in oral, rectal (Ergocaf PB), and sublingual forms (Ergomar). Ergotamine has a relatively long half-life and duration of action (up to 3 days) and should be used no more frequently than every 4 to 5 days to avoid ergotamine rebound headache. The ergot derivative dihydroergotamine (DHE-45, Migranal NS) is available for intramuscular (IM), subcutaneous (SC), intravenous (IV), and intranasal use. IV dihydroergotamine (DHE-45) sometimes is used for intractable migraine (status migrainosus) in emergency departments and inpatient settings. The intranasal form (Migranal) is an effective treatment when administered correctly by the patient. Unfortunately, dihydroergotamine is not absorbed by the gastrointestinal tract, and, unlike other abortive nasal sprays, any swallowed medication will be wasted. Dihydroergotamine has a low headache recurrence rate of approximately 12%. All forms of ergotamine and dihydroergotamine are more effective when taken early in attacks.

Isometheptene is used in combination with dichloralphenazone and acetaminophen (Midrin, Duradrin). It is slow acting and more effective when taken early in attacks and when used for attacks preceded or accompanied by stress and muscle tension of the neck. Although isometheptene is considered less potent than ergotamine and triptans, it is preferred by many patients whose headaches have features of both migraine and TTHA.

At the present time, seven serotonin agonists (triptans) are approved for abortive migraine treatment in the

[1]Not FDA approved for this indication.

[1]Not FDA approved for this indication.

United States (see Table 3). As a category, the triptans are approximately 65% to 70% effective in published clinical trials. Their similarities are greater than their differences, but each triptan is not necessarily effective for all patients, and familiarity with their differences can be helpful to the treating physician. Half-life, onset and duration of action, adverse events, tolerability, recurrence of headache, and routes of administration may vary and allow the physician to match the medication to the individual patient. For example, a slower onset of action and longer-lasting triptan may be appropriate for slow-onset, longer-lasting migraine attacks.

Like other treatments, oral triptan tablets are more effective in the early phases of migraines. It is thought that peripheral sensitization—allodynia—is a sign of later phase migraine, and treating the attack before this phenomenon occurs is important. When treatment is delayed or the patient awakens with severe migraine, the injection, nasal spray, or rapidly acting triptans may be more beneficial. Although triptans as a group are very effective, recurrence of headache, after initial relief, requiring retreatment is common and can be as high as 40%. The recurrence rate tends to be less with triptans having a longer half-life.

The ergots and triptans are contraindicated in patients with ischemic heart disease, uncontrolled hypertension, and cerebrovascular disease. Physicians initially were extremely cautious about recommending triptans to their patients when the triptans were first introduced in the United States. However, significant human exposure to the triptans has revealed that catastrophic myocardial infarction or serious ischemia is rare. Chest pain following triptan use affects a small percentage of patients, and because the significance of this finding is not clear, refraining from future triptan use in these patients is recommended.

Sumatriptan (Imitrex), the first triptan approved in the United States, is available in nasal spray (20 mg), SC (6 mg), and oral formulations (25, 50, 100 mg). Its half-life is approximately 1.5 hours, and its duration of action is less than 4 hours. The injectable form produces rapid relief in 70% to 80% of patients, and it appears to be the most effective of all the available triptan forms. Conversely, it appears to cause the most side effects, and, for this reason, it should be used only for the more severe attacks. The oral forms are more favorable with regard to adverse effects, and their effectiveness is similar to that of other triptans (approximately 65%). Because of sumatriptan's short half-life and duration of action, recurrence of headache is common, necessitating repeat dosing.

Zolmitriptan (Zomig) is available in 2.5- and 5-mg oral and oral disintegrating tablets (ZMT) and as a 5-mg nasal spray. The efficacy of oral zolmitriptan is approximately 65% and that of the nasal form is 70%. The half-life of oral zolmitriptan is 3 hours, and its duration of action is longer than the nasal form, which improves on the need to re-medicate. The nasal spray has a biphasic absorption curve, which accounts for its favorable adverse effect profile over the 5-mg oral tablet.

Naratriptan (Amerge) was the first to be approved of the gradual-onset, longer-acting triptans. It is available as oral 2.5-mg tablets and has a half-life of 6 hours. Naratriptan is well tolerated by patients and often is used by patients with slow-onset migraine. Some specialists prescribe daily naratriptan for limited periods for treatment of menstrual or intractable migraine attacks.

Rizatriptan (Maxalt) is available as oral 5- and 10-mg tablets and as an oral disintegrating form (MLT). It has a relatively rapid onset of action and a favorable one-dose 2-hour response rate. Patients who are undergoing concomitant treatment with propranolol should take the lesser 5-mg rizatriptan dose because of higher resultant rizatriptan plasma levels.

Almotriptan (Axert) is available in 6.25- and 12.5-mg tablets. It has a half-life of 3.5 hours and, because of a broad T_{max} (time of maximal concentration) range of 1.4 to 3.8 hours, a relatively rapid onset of action. Almotriptan has favorable adverse effect and headache recurrence profile. Chest pain symptoms after almotriptan use are similar to placebo in clinical trials.

Frovatriptan (Frova) is a long-acting triptan available in 2.5-mg oral tablets. It has the longest half-life of 25 hours and a favorable recurrence rate. Frovatriptan is frequently used for treatment of menstrual migraine and for attacks of longer duration. Some specialists prescribe daily frovatriptan for a limited period for menstrual and prolonged migraine attacks.

Eletriptan (Relpax) is the most recently approved triptan. It is available in 20- and 40-mg oral tablets and has a half-life of nearly 5 hours. Eletriptan has a relatively rapid onset but a longer duration of action and a favorable recurrence rate. In studies, some patients who were unresponsive to other triptans responded to eletriptan.

Various attempts have been made to compare triptans. Head-to-head trials mostly have compared one triptan to sumatriptan. A meta-analysis of 53 clinical trials published in 2001 compared the efficacy, recurrence, duration of action, and tolerability of all available triptans. Almotriptan and eletriptan were rated favorably across the major parameters of onset of action, efficacy, adverse events, and recurrence. In spite of efforts to adjust for variations in protocols and placebo response, specialists reached no clear consensus as to the validity or value of the meta-analysis or the preferability of one triptan over another.

NSAIDs frequently are recommended for treatment of acute migraine and can be effective when taken early. Their effects on the physiology of pain, inflammation, and platelets are believed to be the mechanisms responsible. Various agents are used, but none of the rapid-acting NSAIDs appears to have significant efficacy superiority. OTC ibuprofen (Motrin) and aspirin, in combination with caffeine and acetaminophen (Excedrin Migraine), is approved by the FDA for treatment of migraine.

Symptomatic treatment of pain may be necessary in patients who do not respond to recommended abortive treatment. Any effective analgesic can be appropriate, provided it is used infrequently and not on a daily or near-daily basis. In general, the more effective analgesics have anti-inflammatory and sedative properties.

CLUSTER HEADACHE TREATMENT

Cluster headache is one of the more unusual pain conditions occasionally encountered by physicians. Pain onset is rapid, and the duration of the attack is brief. For this reason, prophylactic treatment usually is the most practical. Abortive prescriptions frequently are given, but, for the most part, the cluster attack is resolving by the time medication is absorbed.

Nonmedicinal prophylactic measures are extremely limited. The reduction of cigarette smoking, the addressing

TABLE 4 Cluster Headache Prophylactic Medications

Medication	Brand	Average Daily Dose
Verapamil[1]	Calan, Isoptin, Verelan	240–420 mg
Divalproex[1]	Depakote	500–1500 mg
Topiramate[1]	Topamax	50–200 mg
Indomethacin[1]	Indocin	100–150 mg
Naproxen[1]	Naprosyn	1000–1500 mg
Lithium[1]	Lithobid	600–1200 mg*
Ergotamine[1]	Bellergal[1]	1 tablet bid[†]
Prednisone[1]	—	100 mg, decrease to 0

[1]Not FDA approved for this indication.
*With serum level monitoring.
[†]Ergotamine 0.6 mg with phenobarbital 40 mg and 0.2 mg L-alkaloids of belladonna.

of individual stress and hostility issues when appropriate, and the complete cessation of alcohol consumption during cluster periods should be part of any treatment program. Prophylactic medications include the calcium channel blockers verapamil[1] (Calan) and nimodipine[1] (Nimotop), the neurostabilizers valproate[1] (Depakote) and topiramate[1] (Topamax), various NSAIDs, ergotamine,[1] lithium[1] (Eskalith), and, in extreme cases, steroids.[1] These medications are used in average therapeutic doses, and combinations of medications are commonly needed (Table 4). The preventatives should be used during the cluster cycle and discontinued during off-cycle periods.

Abortive treatment is less preferred for cluster headache, as noted previously. However, inhalation oxygen via facial mask at 6 L terminates cluster attacks in 75% to 80% of sufferers within 12 minutes. Other possibilities include sumatriptans (Imitrex) SC or nasal spray,[1] zolmitriptan (Zomig ZMT) nasal spray,[1] ergotamine (Ergomar) sublingual, or dihydroergotamine injection (DHE-45) or nasal spray[1] (Migranal). The occasional patient reports relief with the oral triptans or analgesics. When triptans, ergotamine, or analgesics are used, appropriate prescribing and frequency guidelines should be followed. In general, with the exception of oxygen, daily as-needed medications should be avoided.

Headache continues to present a challenging problem for clinicians as well as for suffering patients. In spite of recent treatment advances and more public awareness, millions continue to needlessly endure pain and debilitation. At first glance, the headache problem appears complex and difficult when, in actuality, most sufferers experience straightforward, easily diagnosed headaches. The interested generalist or specialist who takes the time to elicit a careful history can establish the headache diagnosis and direct a simple treatment plan that can make a tremendous difference in the headache sufferer's life.

REFERENCES

Astin JA, Ernst E: The effectiveness of spinal manipulation for the treatment of headache disorders: A systematic review of randomized clinical trials. Cephalalgia 2002;22:617-623.

[1]Not FDA approved for this indication.

Diamond ML, Dalessio DJ (eds): Diamond and Dalessio's The Practicing Physician's Approach to Headache, 5th ed. Philadelphia, WB Saunders, 1999.
Ferrari MD, Roon KI, Lipton RB, et al: Oral triptans (serotonin 5HT-IB/ID-agonists) in acute migraine treatment: A meta-analysis of 53 trials. Lancet 2001;358:1668-1675.
Gallagher RM, Kunkel R: Migraine medication attributes important for patient compliance: Concerns about side effects may delay treatment. Headache: J Head Face Pain 2003;43:36-43.
Goadsby PJ, Lipton RB, Ferreri MD: Migraine current understanding and treatment. N Engl J Med 2002;346:257-270.
Silberstein SD, Lipton EB, Dalessio DJ: Wolff's Headache and Other Head Pain, 7th ed. New York, Oxford University Press, 2001.
Vernon H, McDermaid C, Hagino C: Systematic review of randomized clinical trials of complementary/alternative therapies in the treatment of tension-type and cervicogenic headache. Complement Ther Med 1999;7:142-155.

Viral Meningitis and Encephalitis

Method of
Mark J. Abzug, MD

Viral meningitis is the most common cause of aseptic meningitis, an inflammatory process involving the meninges in which usual bacterial etiologies cannot be identified. Encephalitis is an inflammatory process that affects the brain parenchyma, typically producing more severe illness. Many viral infections of the central nervous system produce inflammation of both the meninges and brain tissue (meningoencephalitis). Encephalitis may result from acute viral invasion of the brain and a concomitant inflammatory response or from a postinfectious, autoimmune process characterized by demyelination following a viral illness or vaccination (acute disseminated encephalomyelitis). The majority of the approximately 8000 to 13,000 cases of aseptic meningitis and approximately 20,000 cases of encephalitis reported annually in the United States are caused by viral infections.

Clinical Features

Regardless of etiology, most cases of viral meningitis present similarly. Infants and young children display nonspecific symptoms, such as fever, irritability, lethargy, anorexia, and emesis. More specific findings suggestive of meningeal inflammation, such as nuchal rigidity, bulging fontanelle, and photophobia, are often absent. In older children and adults, these signs, along with fever, headache, and emesis, are more frequent. Focal neurologic findings and seizures are uncommon presenting findings in viral meningitis, although approximately 10% of children hospitalized with viral meningitis may develop acute complications such as obtundation, seizures, increased intracranial pressure, and inappropriate antidiuretic hormone secretion. Illness can last up to 1 to 2 weeks, with protracted headache not uncommon in adults.

Encephalitis is distinguished from meningitis by a change in sensorium and/or by focal neurologic findings.

In younger children, encephalitis typically presents with irritability and/or lethargy, often after a febrile illness. Older children may manifest headache, disorientation, unusual behavior, abnormal speech, bizarre movements, and disorientation in addition to fever, nausea, emesis, myalgias, and photophobia. Generalized or, less commonly, focal neurologic abnormalities, including seizures and motor deficits, may be present. Progression to extreme lethargy, stupor, or coma may ensue.

Etiology

In recent studies, a specific etiologic agent was identified in 55% to 70% of presumed cases of viral meningitis and in only 25% to 65% of cases of encephalitis despite thorough investigation. The list of implicated viruses is extensive (Table 1). Enteroviruses (EVs) are the most common cause of both viral meningitis and encephalitis of proven etiology. Other important agents include arboviruses (transmitted by arthropod vectors such as mosquitoes or ticks), herpes simplex virus (HSV), influenza virus, Epstein-Barr virus, varicella-zoster virus, adenovirus, and rabies virus.

Diagnosis

Important diagnostic clues may come from history (respiratory or gastrointestinal symptoms, family exposures, seasonality, prevalent diseases, travel, animal and insect exposure, and recreational activities) and physical examination (see Table 1). The presence of a rash may suggest specific agents, such as varicella-zoster virus or EVs. Whereas identification of a mucocutaneous vesicle in a neonate may be key to the diagnosis of HSV infection, cold sores in older children and adults are *not* predictive of HSV encephalitis. The combination of findings of

CURRENT DIAGNOSIS

Differential diagnosis of meningitis and encephalitis is broad and includes:

- Bacteria: *Streptococcus pneumoniae, Neisseria meningitidis, Haemophilus influenzae, Listeria monocytogenes, Mycobacterium tuberculosis, Borrelia burgdorferi, Mycoplasma pneumoniae, Mycoplasma hominis, Bartonella henselae,* syphilis, leptospirosis, brucellosis, rickettsial and ehrlichial infections
- Parasites: Neurocysticercosis, toxoplasmosis, amebic encephalitis
- Fungi: *Cryptococcus neoformans, Coccidioides immitis*
- Parameningeal focus: Brain abscess or subdural or epidural empyema
- Kawasaki disease
- Sarcoidosis
- Connective tissue disease: Systemic lupus erythematosus, cerebral vasculitis, Wegener's granulomatosis, Hashimoto's disease
- Medication-induced meningitis: Nonsteroidal anti-inflammatory drugs, sulfa antibiotics, immune globulin, cytosine arabinoside (Cytarabine), muromonab-CD3 (Orthoclone OKT3), carbamazepine (Tegretol)
- Metabolic derangements: Inborn errors of metabolism, leukodystrophy, uremia, hepatic encephalopathy, Reye's syndrome
- Cerebrovascular hemorrhage and/or infarct
- Malignancy
- Drug toxicity (e.g., neuroleptic malignant syndrome)
- Toxins

Historical information may suggest specific etiologic viruses:

- Respiratory symptoms: Influenza virus, adenovirus, other respiratory viruses
- Gastrointestinal symptoms: Rotavirus
- Family exposure: Influenza virus, EV
- Seasonality and prevalent diseases in the community: EV, West Nile virus, other arboviruses, influenza virus, other respiratory viruses
- Travel to areas with endemic or epidemic disease: West Nile virus, EV 71, Japanese encephalitis virus, other arboviruses
- Animal exposure: Rabies virus, lymphocytic choriomeningitis virus
- Mosquito exposure: West Nile virus, other arboviruses
- Tick exposure: Colorado tick fever virus, Powassan virus
- Recreational activities: Spelunking-associated bat exposure and rabies infection, hiking-associated mosquito and tick exposure and arbovirus infection

Useful laboratory evaluations for viral meningitis and encephalitis include CSF examination, imaging (especially magnetic resonance imaging), and electroencephalography. Imaging abnormalities may suggest certain pathogens (see Table 1). CSF PCR, serum IgM assays, and viral culture/antigen detection/PCR of mucosal specimens are especially useful specific diagnostic tests.

- CSF PCR is a more sensitive technique than viral culture for detection of viruses such as EVs; HSV; varicella-zoster virus, cytomegalovirus, human herpesvirus 6, Epstein-Barr virus, and JC virus in immune-compromised patients; measles virus; parvovirus B19; and human immunodeficiency virus. CSF PCR for other viruses, such as adenovirus, influenza virus, and arboviruses (including West Nile virus), have low or variable sensitivity. PCR of saliva has high sensitivity for rabies virus (other testing includes immunostain of a nape of neck biopsy, corneal impression, buccal mucosa, or brain tissue).
- The etiology of encephalitis is elusive in many cases. Extensive investigations ultimately are able to identify a specific etiologic agent in only 25% to 65% of cases.

Abbreviations: CSF = cerebrospinal fluid; EV = enterovirus; PCR = polymerase chain reaction.

TABLE 1   Epidemiology and Clinical Features of Viral Meningitis and Encephalitis

Enteroviruses
Epidemiology
- Most common proven cause of viral meningitis and encephalitis (up to 85%–95% of viral meningitis and 80% of viral encephalitis).
- Majority of meningitis and encephalitis occurs in children <1 year old; incidence of meningitis exceeds that of encephalitis.
- Epidemic in warm seasons in temperate climates.
- Poliovirus infection decreased with widespread immunization.
- Enterovirus 71 frequently occurs in regional outbreaks, e.g., Asia since the late 1990s. Severe disease occurs primarily in children <5 years old.

Clinical Features
- Meningitis and severe encephalitis more common in younger children, especially neonates. Encephalitis may be part of systemic illness in newborns.
- Encephalitis typically generalized, although focal seizures and other abnormalities may occur, especially in neonates.
- May have biphasic febrile course; meningeal and encephalitic symptoms occur during second phase.
- Rash (macular, maculopapular, petechial, vesicular), enanthem, conjunctivitis, respiratory symptoms, pleurodynia, pericarditis, myocarditis, diarrhea, myalgias may accompany.
- Chronic meningoencephalitis with waxing and waning neurologic symptoms and high fatality rate occur in hypogammaglobulinemic patients.
- Enterovirus 71 associated with hand-foot-and-mouth disease, herpangina, and neurologic disease (meningitis, brainstem encephalitis, myelitis/acute flaccid paralysis, Guillain-Barré syndrome).
  - Signs of brainstem encephalitis include myoclonic jerks, tremors, ataxia, cranial nerve palsy, limb weakness, altered consciousness, seizures, increased intracranial pressure.
  - Imaging reveals high-intensity lesions in the midbrain, brainstem, and spinal cord anterior horn cells and ventral roots.
  - Pulmonary edema/hemorrhage, cardiac failure, shock may develop rapidly.

Herpes Simplex Virus
Epidemiology
- ~1%–3% of viral meningitis.
  - Predominantly associated with primary type 2 HSV genital infection and less frequently with primary type 1 HSV genital infection, nonprimary HSV genital infection (either type), or without recent genital disease.
  - Mollaret's meningitis (recurrent, benign aseptic meningitis) mostly associated with type 2 infection without signs of genital infection and occasionally with type 1 HSV or with Epstein-Barr virus.
- ~10%–20% of encephalitis in the United States.
  - Encephalitis primarily due to type 2 HSV in neonates and type 1 HSV in older age groups.
  - Encephalitis occurs in ~50% of neonatal HSV infections.
  - ~33%–50% of non-neonatal HSV encephalitis is caused by primary HSV infection and ~50%-67% is caused by HSV reactivation.
  - Most common focal viral encephalitis in nonepidemic settings; most common sporadic fatal encephalitis.

Clinical Features
- Neonatal encephalitis characterized by seizures (focal and generalized), lethargy, irritability, tremors, anorexia, temperature instability, bulging fontanelle.
  - Central nervous system–only disease frequently begins in temporal lobe and then becomes bitemporal.
  - Encephalitis with disseminated disease more commonly is diffuse.
- Non-neonatal encephalitis characterized by fever and focal encephalitis with necrosis and hemorrhage.
  - Tropism for temporal lobe: Aphasia, anosmia, temporal lobe seizures, other focal findings.
  - Findings include headache, emesis, altered consciousness, bizarre behavior, personality changes, disorientation, ataxia, hallucinations, hemiparesis.
  - Focal findings are not always present; bilateral disease, widespread disease, or brainstem encephalitis may occur.
  - Elevated red blood cell count may be present in CSF; CSF protein levels may be normal early and increase over time.
  - Focal abnormalities on imaging studies, especially involving one or both temporal lobes, are suggestive of HSV disease. However, focal disease may occur with other viruses, other regions of the brain may be affected by HSV, and imaging may be normal in early HSV.
  - Temporal lobe focality on electroencephalography, especially with periodic lateralizing epileptiform discharges, is characteristic of HSV but is not specific.
  - Rapid progression is common; however, atypical and mild, slowly progressive cases are increasingly being reported.

Arboviruses
Epidemiology
- ~5% of viral meningitis and important cause of encephalitis.
- Prevalent during warm and/or wet seasons; incidence related to mosquito or tick exposure.
- Leading agents in the United States.
  - West Nile virus: U.S. outbreaks since late 1990s; July to December predominance. Lower incidence and severity in children. Risk factors for severe neurologic disease include older age and immune compromise.
  - La Crosse virus: Central, eastern United States. Incidence of encephalitis approximately equal to that of meningitis; affects children more than adults.

- St. Louis encephalitis virus: Central, western, southern United States. Incidence of encephalitis less than that of meningitis; lower incidence and severity of encephalitis in children.
- Japanese encephalitis virus: Most common cause of epidemic encephalitis worldwide; causes encephalitis more than meningitis. Prevalent in Asia and Australia; affects children more than adults.
- Other important viruses
  - Eastern equine encephalomyelitis virus: Causes encephalitis more than meningitis.
  - Western equine encephalomyelitis virus: Causes encephalitis more than meningitis.
  - Venezuelan equine encephalomyelitis: Causes encephalitis more than meningitis.
  - Colorado Tick Fever virus: Rocky Mountains; tickborne. Meningitis in up to 18% of cases; encephalitis uncommon.
  - Powassan, Rocio, Murray Valley, Kyasuma Forest, Jamestown Canyon, California encephalitis, tickborne encephalitis, Ilheus, Snowshoe Hare, Rift Valley viruses.

Clinical Features
- West Nile virus
  - ~20% of infections are symptomatic; West Nile fever in majority of these infections.
  - Neurologic illness in ~1/150 infected; of these, meningitis in ~30% and encephalitis in ~65%. Neurologic manifestations also include acute asymmetrical flaccid paralysis, polyradiculitis, transverse myelitis, Guillain-Barré syndrome, optic neuritis, and chorioretinitis.
  - Encephalitis is characterized by altered consciousness, cranial nerve palsies (brainstem involvement), generalized or focal motor deficits (weakness, tremor, myoclonus), movement disorders, sensory deficits, and ataxia. Focal temporal lobe disease may mimic HSV. Case fatality rate ~10%.
  - Fever, emesis, maculopapular rash (especially in children) frequently accompany neurologic disease.
- Japanese and Eastern equine encephalitides
  - Thalamic, midbrain, basal ganglia, brainstem lesions characteristic.

Influenza Virus
Epidemiology
- Rare cause of meningitis.
- Cause of 8%–10% of encephalitis.
  - More commonly associated with influenza A than with influenza B.
  - Encephalitis may be acute or postinfectious.
  - Acute necrotizing encephalopathy reported primarily in 1- to 5-year-old children in Asia since the late 1990s.
- Neurologic spectrum includes Reye's syndrome (influenza B), myelitis, Guillain-Barré syndrome.

Clinical Features
- Acute necrotizing encephalopathy
  - Fever, altered consciousness, prolonged seizures; rapid progression to coma.
  - Elevated CSF protein, usually without pleocytosis.
  - Magnetic resonance imaging: Bilateral thalamic lesions and multifocal symmetrical lesions (brainstem, putamina, medulla, periventricular white matter, cerebellum).
  - Mortality ~30%; severe sequelae among survivors.

Varicella-Zoster Virus
Epidemiology and Clinical Features
- Chickenpox associated with cerebellar ataxia, meningitis, encephalitis, postinfectious encephalitis/ADEM, transverse myelitis, Guillain-Barré syndrome.
- Zoster associated with encephalitis, granulomatous hemiparesis, myelitis, cranial neuritis (including Bell's palsy). Neurologic complications may occur with rash, weeks to months after rash or without rash (especially in immune-compromised patients).

Epstein-Barr Virus
Epidemiology and Clinical Features
- Neurologic complications occur in 1%–5% of primary infections.
- Etiology of 2%–5% of acute viral encephalitis.
- Spectrum includes meningitis, encephalitis, ADEM, cranial nerve palsy (including Bell's palsy), transverse myelitis, and Guillain-Barré syndrome. Alice in Wonderland syndrome, consisting of visual seizures with metamorphopsia, may accompany encephalitis.
- Neurologic disease more frequent in immune compromised hosts.
- Typical features of infectious mononucleosis, atypical lymphocytosis, and heterophile antibody often absent in Epstein-Barr virus neurologic syndromes.

Cytomegalovirus
Epidemiology and Clinical Features
- Encephalitis primarily in congenitally infected neonates and immune-compromised hosts.
- Insidious progression.

Human Herpesvirus 6
Epidemiology and Clinical Features
- Meningoencephalitis occasionally occurs with primary infection.
- Increased incidence of encephalitis in immune-compromised hosts.
- Confusion, headache, seizures may accompany encephalitis; disease may be focal and mimic HSV encephalitis.

Continued

TABLE 1   Epidemiology and Clinical Features of Viral Meningitis and Encephalitis—cont'd

Adenovirus
Epidemiology and Clinical Features
- Neurologic spectrum includes acute encephalitis, postinfectious encephalitis, Reye's syndrome-like encephalopathy, and transient encephalopathy.
  - Acute encephalitis is characterized by seizures, CSF pleocytosis, and severe disease.
  - Transient encephalopathy is characterized by obtundation, normal CSF, and complete recovery within several days.

Lymphocytic Choriomeningitis Virus
Epidemiology and Clinical Features
- Transmission by rodent secretions.
- Meningitis and encephalitis more commonly occur in developing countries.
- Spectrum includes encephalitis, hydrocephalus, transverse myelitis.

Human Immunodeficiency Virus
Epidemiology and Clinical Features
- Transient meningitis and, more rarely, encephalitis may accompany primary infection (acute retroviral syndrome).
- Chronic infection may be associated with subacute encephalopathy (loss of developmental milestones in young children, dementia).
- Acute encephalitis may accompany treatment failure during chronic infection (uncommon).

Rabies Virus
Epidemiology and Clinical Features
- Relatively uncommon in United States; major sources are bats, raccoons, foxes, skunks.
- Important cause of encephalitis in developing countries; important sources are dogs and cats.
- Incubation period can vary from weeks to months to years. Pain, pruritus, or paresthesias at bite wound is followed by prodromal fever and anxiety and then by encephalitis.

Measles, Mumps, Rubella Viruses
Epidemiology and Clinical Features
- Meningitis occurs in ~30% of measles infections; measles also causes acute encephalitis, postinfectious encephalitis, and delayed subacute sclerosing panencephalitis.
- Mumps was the leading cause of meningitis in the prevaccine era.
- Meningitis and encephalitis due to each virus dramatically decreased with widespread immunization in developed countries.

Other Viral Agents
- Parainfluenza virus, respiratory syncytial virus, human metapneumovirus, rhinovirus, coronavirus, parvovirus B19, rotavirus, encephalomyocarditis virus, hepatitis C virus, simian herpes B virus, human T-lymphotropic virus, JC virus, Lassa fever virus, yellow fever virus, Hendra virus, Nipah virus, Australian bat Lyssavirus.

Acute Disseminated Encephalomyelitis
Epidemiology
- Implicated in 10%–15% of cases of encephalitis in the United States.
- Increased incidence in infants and children.
- Onset days to weeks after respiratory tract infection (influenza, enteroviruses, measles, mumps, rubella, *Mycoplasma pneumoniae*, and others), gastroenteritis (rotavirus), and other infections (HSV, Epstein-Barr virus, varicella-zoster virus, human herpesvirus 6, cytomegalovirus).
- History of preceding infection or vaccination elicited in up to two thirds of cases.
- Winter–spring predominance in some series.

Clinical Features
- Diffuse, often multifocal symptoms reflecting regions of brain affected. Spectrum includes motor deficits, cranial nerve palsies, optic neuritis, cerebellar ataxia, altered consciousness, psychosis, seizures, transverse myelitis, peripheral neuritis.
- Multifocal, asymmetrical demyelinating lesions in imaging studies, with predilection for white matter.
- CSF cytology may be normal or show pleocytosis; CSF protein elevated in 50%–70%.
- Typically monophasic; occasionally relapses occur.
- Acute hemorrhagic leukoencephalitis is a rare entity representing the fulminant end of the spectrum. It primarily affects young adults and is characterized by seizures, coma, cerebral edema, and a rapid, often fatal course.

Abbreviations: ADEM = acute disseminated encephalomyelitis; CSF = cerebrospinal fluid; HSV = herpes simplex virus.

encephalitis and myelitis in the same patient is suggestive of infection with an EV (especially EV 71), West Nile virus, or Japanese encephalitis virus. Although focal signs are present in the majority of older children and adults with HSV encephalitis, the positive predictive value of focal findings for HSV is low.

Examination of the cerebrospinal fluid (CSF) is indicated in suspected meningitis or encephalitis unless contraindicated by concern for a space-occupying lesion or increased intracranial pressure. CSF in viral meningitis typically has a low-grade pleocytosis (100–1000 white blood cells [WBCs]/mm^3, range <100 to ≥2000 WBC/mm^3).

Polymorphonuclear leukocytes may predominate early then become mononuclear within 8 to 48 hours. In general, CSF protein is normal or slightly increased, and the glucose concentration is normal or slightly decreased, although exceptions occur. The CSF in encephalitis typically has a predominantly mononuclear pleocytosis, increased protein, and normal glucose, although CSF may be normal in 3% to 5% or more of cases, especially early in the course. Certain viruses, including influenza and parvovirus B19, typically cause encephalopathies characterized by the absence of pleocytosis.

Imaging and electroencephalography (EEG) are useful adjuncts, particularly for encephalitis. Magnetic resonance imaging generally has better sensitivity than does computed tomography, especially early in disease. Characteristic imaging findings may suggest specific pathogens (see Table 1), and imaging can exclude alternative diagnoses; for example, a parameningeal focus or tumor. EEG is the most sensitive tool for confirming encephalitis and can distinguish infection from metabolic encephalopathy.

Viral culture, polymerase chain reaction (PCR), and serology are the major techniques for specific virologic diagnosis. Sensitivity of CSF viral culture is better for meningitis than for encephalitis. Sensitivity reaches 65% to 75% for EVs, and CSF culture may be positive in young infants lacking pleocytosis. CSF culture is positive in 25% to 40% of neonates with HSV encephalitis but in less than 2% of older children and adults. CSF PCR is generally more sensitive than culture in both meningitis and encephalitis. CSF PCR for EVs has greater than 95% sensitivity and specificity. Sensitivity and specificity of CSF PCR for HSV are between 75% and 100% in neonatal HSV encephalitis and 91% and 98% in older children and adults with HSV encephalitis. Importantly, HSV PCR may be falsely negative within the first 3 to 4 days of illness in up to 25% of cases; repeat testing 4 to 7 days later is generally positive. In many viral encephalitides, viral cultures, antigen detection tests, and PCR of non-CSF specimens have better yields than do CSF culture and PCR (e.g., throat and stool/rectum for EV 71, for which CSF culture and PCR are more often negative, and respiratory specimens for influenza, adenovirus, and other respiratory viruses). Detection of serum and CSF antibodies can be performed for many viruses (e.g., most arboviruses and lymphocytic choriomeningitis virus), frequently requiring acute and convalescent specimens. Serum and CSF IgM assays can be diagnostic for West Nile virus, Japanese encephalitis virus, Epstein-Barr virus, and EV 71. A brain biopsy should be considered in a patient with symptoms that are progressive or do not improve, with an uncertain diagnosis, and with a focal, accessible lesion.

Treatment

The mainstay of therapy for viral meningitis and encephalitis is supportive care. In patients in whom there is difficulty distinguishing between bacterial and viral meningitis (e.g., young children, especially those younger than 1 year), hospitalization and parenteral antibiotics (vancomycin [Vancocin] plus a third-generation cephalosporin such as cefotaxime [Claforan] or ceftriaxone [Rocephin]) are administered until bacterial cultures are negative and/or

 CURRENT THERAPY

- General supportive measures for patients with severe meningitis or encephalitis include:
  - Analgesics for headache, antiemetics, intravenous fluids and medications for patients with depressed consciousness, anticonvulsants for seizures, provision of a quiet environment
  - Intensive care for severely ill patients, including tracheal intubation for airway protection and respiratory support, cardiorespiratory monitoring
  - Mild fluid restriction for cerebral edema or inappropriate antidiuretic hormone secretion
  - Head of bed elevation, hyperventilation, osmotic (mannitol) and loop diuretics, and control of temperature, pain, and seizures for increased intracranial pressure
- Specific antiviral agents available for meningoencephalitis include acyclovir (Zovirax) for HSV and varicella-zoster virus, ganciclovir (Cytovene) for cytomegalovirus and human herpesvirus 6, foscarnet (Foscavir) for cytomegalovirus and human herpesvirus 6, amantadine (Symmetrel) for influenza A, rimantadine (Flumadine) for influenza A, and oseltamivir (Tamiflu) for influenza A and B.
- Rehabilitative therapy and neurodevelopmental follow-up are frequently necessary after the acute phase of encephalitis regardless of the etiologic agent.
- Prognosis for viral meningitis is generally favorable without long-term sequelae, although fatigue, decreased concentration, and irritability may last for several weeks.
- Prognosis for viral encephalitis is variable and may be difficult to predict, especially early in the course of illness. In general, a worse prognosis is associated with extremes of age (infants <1 year and older adults), specific etiologies (HSV, enterovirus 71, West Nile virus, Japanese encephalitis virus, rabies), more severe illness (lower Glasgow Coma Scale) and extensive brain involvement, and, in the case of HSV, longer duration prior to initiation of treatment.

Abbreviation: HSV = herpes simplex virus.

an alternative diagnosis is made. Additionally, newborns or other immune-compromised patients with EV meningitis may require supportive therapy for severe disseminated disease (e.g., hepatitis, coagulopathy, or myocarditis). A presumptive diagnosis of viral meningitis can often be made in older children and adults who are not very ill based on clinical and CSF examination (low-grade pleocytosis with mononuclear predominance initially or 8–24 hours later, normal to slightly depressed glucose concentration, normal to slightly increased protein level). Lumbar puncture may alleviate symptoms such as headache, irritability, and emesis. Therefore, in older children and adults, hospitalization and empirical antibiotic treatment are indicated for patients who appear ill, including those requiring parenteral hydration and/or analgesics, those in whom viral and bacterial infection cannot be readily distinguished, and those who manifest findings of encephalitis. Presumptive therapy for *Mycobacterium tuberculosis* may be indicated if the exposure history, clinical presentation, CSF examination, and imaging findings are suggestive of this agent.

There are few proven specific antiviral therapies for meningitis and encephalitis. Acyclovir[1] (Zovirax) can hasten recovery from HSV meningitis, although HSV meningitis without encephalitis generally has an excellent outcome without antiviral treatment. Valacyclovir[1] (Valtrex) and famciclovir[1] (Famvir) are also available for oral therapy of HSV meningitis associated with genital HSV in immune-competent patients.

For children and adults with encephalitis, empirical therapy with acyclovir (30 mg/kg/day up to 45–60 mg/kg/day intravenously divided every 8 hours) should generally be initiated pending diagnostic studies, particularly in the presence of fever and any evidence of focal neurologic abnormality (clinical examination, imaging, or electroencephalography). Treatment for 14 to 21 days* is indicated if HSV infection is confirmed or if clinical and diagnostic findings are strongly suggestive in the absence of other proven etiologies; a 21-day course is generally favored for more severe disease. Acyclovir (60 mg/kg/day intravenously divided every 8 hours) should be presumptively administered to newborns with encephalitis with focal or generalized findings. Treatment of proven or highly suspect neonatal HSV encephalitis is generally continued for 21 days and until an end-of-therapy CSF PCR is negative, although proof that extending therapy until the PCR is negative is beneficial is lacking. Whether higher doses (60 mg/kg/day) or longer courses (21 days) confer additional benefit outside the neonatal period is not established. Relapse within the first 1 to 3 months after therapy of neonatal and childhood/adult HSV encephalitis has been reported with variable incidence, in some cases correlated with lower daily dose and treatment duration. Whether relapses reflect active viral replication or an immune-mediated phenomenon is controversial, although CSF PCR positivity in some cases suggests the former.

Whether encephalitis associated with varicella-zoster virus is due more often to direct viral infection or an immune-mediated parainfectious process is not established. Thus, although acyclovir is frequently used for varicella-zoster virus encephalitis, including cerebellar ataxia, the role of antiviral therapy is unproven. Ganciclovir (Cytovene) and foscarnet (Foscavir) are used for meningoencephalitis in immune-compromised hosts caused by cytomegalovirus and human herpesvirus 6.

Pleconaril (Picovir) is an experimental agent that has been studied for treatment of EV meningitis and encephalitis, including chronic meningoencephalitis in hypogammaglobulinemic patients, with some evidence of benefit; however, the agent is not currently available. Intraventricular, intrathecal, and intravenous administration of immune globulin[1] have been used to suppress or stabilize chronic EV meningoencephalitis in immune-compromised patients.

The mainstays of management of severe EV 71 neurologic disease are close monitoring, fluid restriction, osmotic diuretics, and cardiorespiratory support. Various agents, including pleconaril, interferon α,[1] intravenous immune globulin, and corticosteroids have been tried, but none has been proven to be effective.

Influenzal encephalitis is frequently treated with oral antivirals, including amantadine (Symmetrel) for influenza A, rimantadine (Flumadine) for influenza A, and oseltamivir (Tamiflu) for influenza A and B; corticosteroids and immune globulin[1] have also been tried. However, none of these agents has been proven to be effective for influenzal encephalitis. A combination of antiviral treatment, corticosteroids, and intravenous immune globulin has been suggested to reduce mortality due to influenzal acute necrotizing encephalopathy. There currently are no established therapies for West Nile virus encephalitis. Ribavirin (Rebetol),[1] interferon, high-titer immune globulin, and corticosteroids have been used, and therapeutic trials are currently ongoing. No specific therapies have been proven to be effective for encephalitis due to other arboviruses or for rabies. Corticosteroids, intravenous immune globulin, and plasmapheresis have been used for acute disseminated encephalomyelitis, but efficacy trials have not been performed.

REFERENCES

Beaman MH, Wesselingh SL: Acute community-acquired meningitis and encephalitis. Med J Aust 2002;176:389-396.

Chang L, Hsia S, Wu C, et al: Outcome of enterovirus 71 infections with or without stage-based management: 1998-2002. Pediatr Infect Dis J 2004;23:327-331.

Glaser CA, Gilliam S, Schnurr D, et al: In search of encephalitis etiologies: Diagnostic challenges in the California encephalitis project, 1998-2000. Clin Infect Dis 2003;36:731-742.

Huang C, Morse D, Slater B, et al: Multiple-year experience in the diagnosis of viral central nervous system infections with a panel of polymerase chain reaction assays for detection of 11 viruses. Clin Infect Dis 2004;39:630-635.

Kennedy PGE: Viral encephalitis: causes, differential diagnosis, and management. J Neurol Neurosurg Psychiatry 2004;75(Suppl 1):i10-i15.

Kimberlin DW: Herpes simplex virus infections of the central nervous system. Semin Pediatr Infect Dis 2003;14:83-89.

Rotbart HA: Viral meningitis. Semin Neurol 2000;20:277-292.

Watson JT, Gerber SI: West Nile virus: A brief review. Pediatr Infect Dis J 2004;23:355-358.

Weitkamp J, Spring MD, Brogan T, et al: Influenza A virus-associated acute necrotizing encephalopathy in the United States. Pediatr Infect Dis J 2004;23:259-263.

Whitley RJ, Gnann JW: Viral encephalitis: Familiar infections and emerging pathogens. Lancet 2002;359:507-514.

---

[1]Not FDA approved for this indication.
*Exceeds duration recommended by the manufacturer.

---

[1]Not FDA approved for this indication.

Multiple Sclerosis

Method of
Randall T. Schapiro, MD

Multiple sclerosis (MS) has been called a primary demyelinating disease of the central nervous system, but that is somewhat inaccurate. Charcot's description of MS included damage to the axon, which has been especially emphasized in the past decade. Today MS is described not only as a disease of myelin, but also of the cell that makes myelin (oligodendrocyte) and also the axon. All these are primary targets in the destructive process that appears to be directed by the immune system, and thus MS is more properly called an immune-mediated disorder. The immune system can cause direct destruction and inflammation. It also can program the targets (cells, axons) to self-destruct over time (apoptosis).

The pathology of MS has been elucidated more thoroughly in the past several years thanks to international projects that began with descriptions of biopsied specimens from brain lesions of patients with the disease. Some individuals had a high involvement of the immune system; a minority had less. Four different varieties are separable. These types (I through IV) provide a way to separate the disease potentially into different categories. This combination of possibilities puts MS into both the inflammatory and degenerative categories. Much work is left to do in this area, but in the next decade treatments may be dictated by the variety of pathologic processes occurring as the disease changes over time.

While describing MS at a microscopic level, it is easy to lose sight of the fact that, at a global level, it is a disease of people with all of their complexities. The person with MS is typically diagnosed early in the third decade of life and has a family, work, and responsibilities in the community, making this potentially disabling disease one of the most important acquired, nontraumatic neurologic diseases in the world.

Relative to the past, MS today is a disease with very active treatment strategies aimed in three general directions. The ideal goal is to slow or stop the disease itself. Disease management is now routine, with five Federal Drug Administration (FDA)-approved medications available to slow MS. Symptom management remains one of the principal directions of treatment in MS. Superimposed on these two very obvious directions is the psychological support necessary to keep people with neurologic dysfunction performing at their highest level. The psychological area is often ignored in the office but is of equal importance in offering a quality of life for those with the disease.

Etiology

The cause of multiple sclerosis remains unknown. Despite numerous advances, the discussion of MS causation has changed little in the past decade. No simple explanation is available for why MS occurs. For more than 40 years, a population gradient to MS has been understood. As one moves away from the equator north and south, the number of MS cases increases. Much of that may be because of the ethnic origin of the people in those areas. They tend to be northern European and Scandinavian, but migration studies demonstrate that the disease spreads beyond ethnic backgrounds when generations remain in the targeted geographic regions. Studies in the Faeroe and Shetland/Orkney islands off the coast of Scotland and other regions give credence to the possibility of a viral or other infectious influence. Despite decades of modern viral isolation techniques, no virus has stood the test of time in MS. Each decade has produced its own target virus. In the 1970s, it was the measles virus, in the 1980s, the herpesvirus, and in the 1990s, the retroviruses of tropical spastic paraparesis. Then, one after another, the human herpesvirus type 6 and the chlamydia bacteria were implicated. None appeared conclusive, although many continue under investigation.

What does seem clear is the involvement of the immune system in MS. The understanding of the influence of the immune system continues to evolve as newer and better techniques to explore this complex area develop. MS is now described as an immune-mediated disease to distinguish it from a classic autoimmune disease. The immune system clearly is more active toward a central nervous system antigen. Just what that antigen is remains mysterious, but several candidates have emerged, including myelin and it components, the oligodendrocyte, the axon, and other surrounding tissues and cells. For the immune system to attack the nervous system, something must trigger it. That is likely the environmental influence, and after it is programmed to attack a nervous system element, it must make its way through the blood–brain barrier to find the target. It is the very complexity of the process that may make it susceptible to intervention. Strategies are being or have been developed to interfere with the initial reaction of the antigen-presenting cell (macrophage) to the antigen, the passage through the blood-brain barrier, and the reaction once in the central nervous system.

The immune system appears to be the genetic link in MS. Although MS is said to be nonhereditary, it clearly has a genetic component. The likelihood of getting MS with no one in the family having it is approximately 0.2%. If a parent has the disease and the child is a girl, the risk jumps to 3% to 4%. If the child is a boy, the risk is 2%. If an identical twin has MS, the risk to the sibling is 30%. But if MS were wholly a hereditary disease, it would be 100%.

Thus the cause of MS is unknown, but it must be a multifactorial process. It takes a susceptible individual who has an immune system capable of being genetically stimulated by an exogenous factor, and all these factors must be at the right time in the right place.

Course of the Disease

The disease has numerous presentations. Virtually any symptom that can result from an irritated central nervous system may be present in MS. Fatigue is the single most common symptom, but numbness, tingling, dizziness, visual distortion, weakness, clumsiness, pain, urinary, bowel, sexual, and psychological effects are often present as well. The course of MS is also very unpredictable and variable. Today MS is divided into four broad categories. Approximately 80% of MS begins with a fluctuating course with relapses of neurologic deficit followed by periods of relative quiet, termed *relapsing-remitting MS.*

Over time, half of those untreated with relapsing-remitting MS stop fluctuating and slowly get worse. This is called *secondary progressive MS*. If the course of secondary progressive MS fluctuates, it is called *secondary progressive with relapses*. The common feature of the progressive variety is that it progresses between relapses if relapses are present.

Approximately 10% of MS gets worse from the beginning, which is called *primary progressive*, and approximately 5% begins progressive and then has a relapse or two and is labeled *progressive-relapsing*.

Even though MS is divided into categories, it remains MS, which is especially true of the relapsing-remitting and secondary progressive types that are almost certainly the same process. Primary progressive and progressive-relapsing may be variants, but the two of them are also almost certainly the same process.

Approximately 20% of people with MS do fairly well, with their disease accumulating little disability over time, even untreated. The exact number is controversial, but even autopsy studies demonstrate repeatedly that MS appears without clinical evidence much more than would be expected. Those autopsied died from other causes and did not even recognize they had MS.

Many experts believe MS is a spectrum of diseases that appear clinically similar. Little actual data support the theory, but in the past few years when researchers at the Mayo Clinic, together with many others around the world, looked at biopsied specimens of lesions that turned out to be MS, they saw great variability among them. This discovery has prompted a new classification based on the pathology that divides MS into four broad categories. At one end is a very immunologically based pathology, at the other end is a very degenerative pathology, and in between are two that blend between the extremes. Thus MS is highly diverse, both clinically and pathologically, and yet there is also much similarity.

Diagnosis

Under normal circumstances, MS typically is not difficult to diagnose when following simple clinical dictums. There are three criteria in the clinical diagnosis of MS:

1. The person should be relatively young, between the ages of 15 and 55 years.
2. She or he should have neurologic symptoms that fluctuate.
3. The neurologic examination should demonstrate multiple abnormalities within the central nervous system, hence the name *multiple* sclerosis.

Other obvious reasons for the clinical picture should be ruled out, and then the diagnosis of MS can be made very accurately. Schumacher codified these criteria in the 1970s before the days of elaborate testing. When evoked potentials and spinal fluid tests became more accurate, Poser and his committee added the use of those modalities to allow for a diagnosis when a clinical piece is missing. Magnetic resonance imaging (MRI) advanced the cause rapidly, allowing for more precision in diagnosis, and recently the McDonald committee added its use to speed the diagnostic process. The MRI scan has to show significant specific abnormalities to be substituted for a clinical

loss, and to be effective, all these criteria still depend on the initial clinical presentation.

Despite the emphasis on the clinical picture in diagnosing MS, laboratory testing continues to play a role in confirming the diagnosis. Evoked potentials are electrical potentials stimulated within the brain by a stimulus (visual, auditory, or somatosensory). They can be measured via electrodes placed on the scalp. With the aid of computerized signal averaging, normal transmission can be separated from abnormal, thus extending the neurologic examination to find more subtle abnormalities of the sensory system. The spinal fluid can be analyzed in a very sophisticated way for immune abnormalities. Detection of unique oligoclonal banding in the IgG spectrum is characteristic of MS. Increased production of IgG and the presence of myelin basic protein are also common.

Blood (and sometimes cerebrospinal fluid) should be analyzed to eliminate mimicking diseases such as lupus, Sjögren's, sarcoid, B_{12} deficiency, Lyme disease, vasculitis, and other autoimmune processes.

Management

The complexity and variability of multiple sclerosis make it a classic example of a disease best managed by a team approach. The team may require participation from physicians, nurses, rehabilitation professionals, psychologists, and social workers. The extent of participation should be determined by the complexity of the individual situation. It is not necessary or appropriate for all professionals to be involved with all patients, but an educated team makes the management of complicated patients much more effective.

With the advent of immune-modulating medication, treatment has expanded greatly. These medications have revolutionized the medical approach toward the disease, but their expense and their lack of total efficacy must be taken into consideration when determining their use.

It is abundantly clear that patients cannot get back what is lost in the destruction of the central nervous system. Thus the goal of management is to prevent loss and maintain function. In MS the immune system becomes programmed to attack the myelin, oligodendrocyte, or other nerve component. Whether that programming antigen is a virus or other stimulus does not change the fact that an antigen-presenting cell (usually a macrophage) engulfs the antigen and presents it. This causes a stimulation of T-helper cells, which separate into the highly inflammatory Th1 and the anti-inflammatory Th2 cells. In MS there is a shift of the balance, with increased Th1 allowing for increased destruction. The programmed cells then cross the blood–brain barrier looking for the part of the nervous system that resembles their programming. Stopping this from occurring has become the principal treatment strategy. The interferons appear to keep the flow of Th1 cells from crossing the blood–brain barrier, thus decreasing their likelihood of destruction. Glatiramer acetate appears to cross the barrier and stimulate increased Th2 production, changing the balance of immune regulation toward a more modulating course. Another agent awaiting approval (Natalizumab, Antegren) works to shore up the blood–brain barrier by preventing it transport across via inhibition of adhesion molecule movement.

Keeping an activated immune system from getting to the myelinated central fibers appears to slow the process of demyelination in MS. Therefore the principle of treatment in MS today revolves around immune modulation. Over the past dozen years more scientifically proven treatments for MS have evolved than in all other years combined. Today five FDA-approved medications are available.

Interferons are proteins that the body makes in response to a foreign stimulation. Thus with a viral infection the body makes interferons that modulate the immune system. The three main categories of interferon are alfa (α), beta (β), and gamma (γ). Interferon γ stimulates the immune system and makes MS worse, whereas interferon β calms the system down and decreases attack rates, increases the time between attacks, and decreases the damage seen on MRI scans.

Studies done in various ways show approximately one third of the attacks in an actively affected MS population can be diminished during the first 2 years. The preponderance of information leads to the conclusion that the higher the dose of interferon, the more potent the response. Many studies show that in the appropriate person, with the appropriate dose, interferons change the course of the disease. The potent anti-inflammatory effects of interferons have a dramatic effect on the MRI, with a decrease in T2 and T1 contrast-enhancing lesions. These human gene interferons come in two formulations: interferon beta-1a (Avonex, Rebif) made in a hamster and interferon beta-1b (Betaseron) made in bacteria. The recommended doses of Rebif and Betaseron appear to be equivalent (three to four times per week); that of Avonex is significantly lower (once per week).

Glatiramer acetate is a polypeptide that appears to fool the immune system. As noted earlier, it shifts the Th1-Th2 balance toward the Th2. Appearing to mimic myelin, it may also decrease the attack by blocking the cells headed toward myelin and preventing damage. It, too, appears to decrease attack rates by approximately a third in the first 2 years of use.

All of these medications are administered parentally. They all have side effects and are all costly. The β-interferons may be toxic to the blood and liver and can exaggerate depression in a susceptible individual that is generally mild but should be monitored. Glatiramer acetate has less toxicity but can cause a systemic reaction that mimics a heart attack, although it is not, and clears in 20 minutes. Although rare, this reaction can be frightening. All of the drugs can produce skin reactions except for the intermuscular interferon beta-1a (Avonex).

All of these agents were studied in the relapsing forms of MS. Although this does not preclude effectiveness in more progressive forms, there is a paucity of data for that use. Clinical experience, together with evidence-based data, gives a picture of the high-dose interferons having the most potent effect, followed by glatiramer acetate, and then low-dose interferon.

Based on the aggressiveness of the MS and the lifestyle of the patient, the physician should select the agent. The goal must include maintaining the person on the medication and preventing noncompliance. Although patients must be included in the decision making, they should not be given the choice without a recommendation from the health professional. Many neurologists tend to abdicate the decision making to patients, who are not prepared to make such a decision.

Knowing that approximately 20% of patients do well without treatment and many more do well for a significant period of time without treatment begs the question of how early to treat. As stated earlier, it is impossible to retrieve damaged neurons consistently. The issue is whether to treat 100% of patients with MS immediately at the time of diagnosis if only 80% will need to be treated eventually. If the drugs were curative, time limited, or inexpensive, all would agree on treating all patients. Given the fact they are not, who should be treated and when is an issue.

All experts agree that early treatment is necessary, but the question is how to define "early." Much controversy surrounds the question of whether it is advisable to wait and see into what group an individual falls. Studies on so-called pre-MS, what is called the "clinically isolated syndrome," do not answer the question. The clinically isolated syndrome is a first attack, usually accompanied by an abnormal MRI. Two attacks are required for diagnosis. Studies clearly show that the second attack, leading to the diagnostic label, can be delayed by treatment, but that says nothing about long-term disability. This dilemma is especially pertinent because often the disease quiets after diagnosis and can go decades or more before reactivating. Attempts to look at that issue scientifically have come up short. The CHAMPS (Controlled High Risk Avonex Multiple Sclerosis) study looked at people with a first attack who did not meet the criteria for clinically definite MS. The study showed that the immune treatment (interferon beta-1a [Avonex]) did delay the second attack, but it says nothing about whether such early treatment changes disability later in life, a very important question that remains unanswered. A European study (ETOMS [Early Treatment of MS] with interferon beta-1a [Rebif]) leaves the same question.

Prognostic indicators can help predict whether a more aggressive course is impending. A large burden of disease on initial MRI scanning and the presence of weakness, ataxia, cognitive problems, frequent attacks, and spinal cord symptoms all point to a worse prognosis and should lead to earlier treatment. Numbness, tingling, blurred vision, dizziness, pain, and fatigue do not usually evolve into the more aggressive forms of MS, and immediate treatment may not be as necessary. All experts agree with the National Multiple Sclerosis Society's practice guideline, which states that if the disease is *active*, treatment should be instituted with one of the four agents.

Thus prevention is the key, but despite best efforts, breakthrough attacks do occur. People, treated or untreated, may develop new symptomatology, which is deemed a relapse. The use of the potent anti-inflammatory cortisone agents has been used to settle attacks for many decades. There are many regimens that individual experts use depending on the severity of the attack. If the attack is relatively minor and not encroaching on function, a hand-holding approach with no steroids is recommended. If the attack is slightly more severe, two dose packs of methylprednisolone may be given simultaneously. If the attack is even more severe with increased disability, 1000 mg of methylprednisolone may be administered each day for 3 to 5 days. If the attack is such that aggressive inpatient rehabilitation is warranted, a dose of dexamethasone beginning at 64 mg with a taper over 1 week is given. After either the outpatient high-dose or the inpatient high-dose steroid plan, a 1-month taper of oral methylprednisolone is included. All of these are based on experience rather than evidence-based data.

Once the decision is made that the person has active disease, requiring ongoing immunomodulation, a decision about which agent to use becomes paramount. If the disease is highly inflammatory with aggressive relapses and/or MRI evidence of blood–brain barrier breakdown (contrast-enhancing lesions), a high-dose β-interferon is used. If the person's lifestyle cannot tolerate that, an adjustment of medication to a less anti-inflammatory agent (glatiramer acetate or interferon beta-1a, at a lower dose) is suggested. If the disease is less aggressive but the patient is experiencing much depression, glatiramer is preferred. The use of medication is not random but represents the best fit of the drug to the situation. This is with the understanding that high-dose interferon β (Betaseron, Rebif) is the most potent, with glatiramer acetate (Copaxone) following and low-dose interferon beta-1a (Avonex) next.

If the disease cannot be controlled with the four immunomodulating medications, as seen by ongoing progression of disability with continued relapses, immunosuppression with mitoxantrone (Novantrone) is administered. The MRI scan can be of some help in the decision making but correlates poorly with the clinical picture. Thus it should not be the most important factor in decision making. Mitoxantrone is administered intravenously in a regimen of 12 mg/m². There is a total lifetime dose of 140 mg/m² before heart damage becomes a major concern. Examination of the heart at appropriate levels for ejection fraction and function is necessary. A typical course is 1 year of therapy and then continued evaluations without further mitoxantrone until (or if) progression resumes.

The use of oral immune suppressants including azathioprine (Imuron) and methotrexate (Rheumotrex) were more popular before the newer agents became available. They are still used as adjunct therapy in difficult cases of progressive disease.

Natalizumab (Tysabri, previously called Antegren) is a monoclonal antibody that prevents immune cells from moving from the blood to the central nervous system by blocking integrin, the adhesion molecule. It was originally approved by the FDA on the basis of impressive data obtained in the first year of a 2-year study. There is a dramatic lowering of relapse rate and a significant decrease in MRI activity. This treatment is a once-monthly intravenous infusion. Two large studies were conducted. One was Tysabri versus placebo and the second was Tysabri plus Avonex versus placebo plus Avonex. Unfortunately, shortly after release of the treatment by the FDA, two cases of progressive multifocal leukoencephalopathy (PML) were found in the Avonex and Tysabri group and one died and the other became much more disabled. A third case of PML was discovered in a Tysabri-treated patient with Crohn's disease. As a result, the distribution of Tysabri was halted pending further evaluation.

Studies on intense immunosuppression with bone marrow transplantation (autologous and stem cell) continue but are not positive enough to recommend its use.

Despite the time, effort, and success given to slow the disease, the bulk of a clinician's time with multiple sclerosis is devoted to symptomatic management. The tools available include pharmacologic, rehabilitative, and psychological approaches. Fatigue is the single most common and most disabling symptom seen in MS. Five different "fatigues" are apparent in MS: normal, neuromuscular, deconditioning, fatigue of depression, and lassitude (MS-related fatigue). Normal fatigue is the same that occurs in everyone who tires after working hard. Neuromuscular fatigue is the tiring of muscles when they are required for activities such as walking. The fatigue of deconditioning is the result of a lack of sufficient activity to maintain endurance. Depression can result in poor sleep and ongoing fatigue. The most common fatigue is a tiredness that occurs without significant activity. It comes on spontaneously and is likely the result of a neurochemical imbalance in the brain. Neurochemically active drugs including amantadine and modafinil are helpful in its management. Occupational therapy can teach energy conservation and improve activities of daily living to increase efficiency and decrease fatigue. In managing fatigue the health professional must rule out a sleep disturbance or other contributing confounding problem and then develop a plan based on the specific fatigue present.

Spasticity is managed with a multicentered approach. Noxious stimuli are minimized initially because they can increase muscle tone. An exercise program emphasizing stretching and range of motion is instituted. If more management is necessary, baclofen, tizanidine, benzodiazepines, and gabapentin may be added to appropriate doses. Failing all of the preceding, intrathecal administration of baclofen via a pump or selected muscle weakening with botulinum toxin is effective.

The bladder and bowel are often involved with MS. Bladders may become hypertonic, small, and fail to store or they may become hypotonic, large, and fail to empty. Sometimes the bladder and the sphincter become dyssynergic. Anticholinergic medication often helps the small bladder and controls the bladder spasms. Catheterization techniques may help the large bladder (self, intermittent, and indwelling). Combinations of therapy can aid the dyssynergic bladder including α-adrenergic blocking agents. A bowel program can lead to improved independence by scheduling the bowel movement rather than allowing it to be entirely spontaneous. Taking advantage of the gastrocolic reflex, attempting evacuation following a meal with the judicious use of bulking agents, stool softeners, and suppositories is the start to taking charge.

Sexual function may require attention. Erectile dysfunction in men is managed with Viagra, Levitra, or Cialis. Injection of prostaglandin (Caverject) is clearly more potent than the oral agents but requires the ability to directly inject the penis. Prostaglandin suppository (Muse) places the medication within the urethral orifice but is less potent than the injection. Women often experience decreased libido, decreased sensation, decreased lubrication, or sometimes pain. The use of various vibrators along with external water-soluble lubricants with the gentle application of cold can be helpful. Many of the commonly used antidepressant medications can decrease sexual desire and may need adjustment.

Neuropathic type pain is surprisingly common in MS (50%). The newer anticonvulsants, including gabapentin, Trileptal, Topamax, and Lamictal, are commonly dosed sufficiently to decrease the pain. Amitriptyline can be helpful, especially at night.

Cognitive problems likewise occur in approximately 50% of those with MS. Watching for depression and the contribution of other medications to the problem is essential. Keeping people in society and not allowing them to withdraw may decrease the secondary exaggeration of the symptom.

Ataxia, tremor, and balance problems often go together and are very difficult to manage. Although a number of medications can help any one person, none are consistent. Bracing across a joint can be helpful. Compensatory training for balance sometimes helps that symptom.

A number of paroxysmal symptoms relatively unique to MS are managed with anticonvulsant medications. These include spasms of an extremity. Sensory aberrations rapidly coming and going may include the pain of trigeminal neuralgia or fluctuating pain in an extremity. Paroxysmal visual blurring or speech slurring can be seen. These fluctuations may occur many times a minute, only to settle down for hours.

Ambulation can be affected through many mechanisms including weakness and ataxia. Ambulatory support through the appropriate use of devices (canes, crutches, walkers, and ankle-foot orthoses) is recommended to enhance mobility. If ambulation becomes too difficult, other mobility devices should be used freely. One of the major answers to disability is maintaining mobility.

Progressive resistive exercises must take into account the strength of innervation of the specific muscle. Fatigue results from the overzealous use of strengthening exercises. If a muscle is not used, however, atrophy results. Thus an intelligent strengthening program can be helpful if not overdone.

The role of aerobic exercise has evolved significantly over the past 2 decades, and an appropriate training program can benefit an individual if tailored to his or her deficits. The program must emphasize the slow buildup of intensity of the exercise over as much time as it takes to prevent fatigue from becoming overwhelming with each session.

Because of the individuality of the disease for each person, generalizations are hard to make. What is clear is that simply having the diagnosis causes a ripple effect even in the patients with the mildest symptoms. The family experiences the problems of their loved ones and thus this

CURRENT THERAPY

- Education and psychological support
- Symptomatic management of appropriate symptoms
- Immune modulation with interferon beta-1a, interferon beta-1b, or glatiramer acetate early in the active disease course and ongoing
- Regular follow-up with clinical examination and magnetic resonance imaging if additional information is needed

becomes a family disease like few others. The age of the patient influences vocational planning. It also influences family roles and child rearing. Thus counseling may be a very necessary component of a well-rounded approach. The complexity of all of this has made MS centers a popular choice for many who have issues surrounding the MS. These allow for experienced therapists to communicate with the medical professionals and the patients to develop a comprehensive management strategy.

The diagnosis and management of MS has drastically evolved over the past 2 decades. It has gone from a disease characterized by the late Labe Scheinberg, MD, as "diagnose and adios" to one in which physicians are arguing about how early and how aggressively treatment strategies should be applied. We have come a long way but still have far to go to find the cause and eventual cure to this very difficult problem.

REFERENCES

Jacobs LD, Cookfair DL, Rudick RA, et al: Intramuscular interferon beta-1a for disease progression in relapsing multiple sclerosis. Ann Neurol 1996, 39(3):285-294.

Johnson KP, Brooks BR, Cohen JA, et al: Copolymer 1 reduces relapse and improves disability in relapsing-remitting multiple sclerosis: Results of a phase III multi-center, double-blind, placebo-controlled trial. Neurology 1995;45:1268-1276.

Petajan JH, White AT: Recommendations for physical activity in multiple sclerosis. Sports Med 1999;27(3):179-191.

PRISMS Study Group and University of British Columbia MS MRI Analysis Group: PRISMS-4: Long-term efficacy of interferon-beta 1a in relapsing MS. Neurology 2001;56:1628-1636.

Rao S, Leo GT, Bernardin L, Unverzagt F: Cognitive dysfunction in multiple sclerosis: I. Frequency, pattern and predictors. Neurology 1991;41(5):685-691.

Sadovnik AD, Remick RA, Allen J, et al: Depression and multiple sclerosis. Neurology 1996;46:628-632.

Schapiro RT: The Management of MS Symptoms. New York, Demos Medical Publishing, 2003.

The IFNB Multiple Sclerosis Group, University of British Columbia MS/MRI Analysis Group: Interferon beta-1b in the treatment of multiple sclerosis: Final outcome of the randomized controlled trial. Neurology 1995;45:1277-1285.

CURRENT DIAGNOSIS

- Clinical history of fluctuating neurologic symptoms (exacerbations and remissions)
- Multiple abnormalities seen on neurologic examination
- Absence of other systemic disorder (e.g., lupus, Lyme, other autoimmune processes)
- Confirmatory laboratory studies of benefit: MRI (using McDonald criteria); CSF, looking for increased immune activity including oligoclonal IgG banding, increased IgG synthesis, and index; abnormal evoked potentials indicating multiple abnormalities potentially not found on routine neurologic examination

Abbreviations: CSF = cerebrospinal fluid; MRI = magnetic resonance imaging.

Myasthenia Gravis and Related Disorders

Method of
Jenice Robinson, MD,
and Milind J. Kothari, DO

Myasthenia gravis (MG) is a relatively uncommon disease of the postsynaptic neuromuscular junction (NMJ). Most patients with myasthenia have an acquired immunologic abnormality, but other uncommon inherited forms of myasthenia may result from structural abnormalities of the NMJ. The following discussion focuses on acquired (autoimmune) MG.

The physiologic abnormality in autoimmune MG results from the reduction in concentration of the nicotinic acetylcholine receptor (AChR) on the endplates of somatic muscles at the NMJ. Although the cause of the disorder is unknown, the pathogenesis of autoimmune MG is now well understood. Two antigens have been described: AChR and muscle-specific receptor tyrosine kinase (MuSK). Antibodies against AChR are found in 80% to 90% of patients with MG. Antibodies against MuSK are found in 40% of the remaining patients. Strong evidence supports the role of antibodies in the pathogenesis of MG. Anti-AChR antibodies cause disruption of myotubes in culture and cause myasthenic symptoms when transferred to experimental animals. Removal of anti-AChR antibodies results in clinical improvement. The thymus plays an important but incompletely understood role in MG.

Clinical Features

The hallmark of MG is fluctuating or fatigable weakness. MG presents with ocular symptoms of ptosis or diplopia in 60% of patients. Diplopia may not fluctuate, and an ocular misalignment may appear fixed. This presentation may mimic a neuropathy of the third, fourth, or sixth cranial nerves, or an internuclear ophthalmoplegia. Abnormalities of pupillary function should not be present in MG. Patients may present initially to an optometrist or ophthalmologist for these problems. Ocular symptoms eventually develop in almost all patients with MG. Presenting symptoms are bulbar (dysarthria, dysphagia, or facial weakness) in 10%, leg weakness in 10% to 20%, and generalized weakness in 10%. Symptoms often worsen with exercise and improve with rest. Symptoms are often most prominent late in the day. Weakness in MG arises from fluctuating strength of the voluntary muscles and always causes a functional deficit, such as an inability to hold the arms above the head when washing the hair or leg weakness resulting in sudden falls. If a patient has only generalized fatigue or tiredness, MG is unlikely. Chronic pain and sensory complaints are not features of MG. Respiratory dysfunction is the initial presenting symptom in only 1% of patients but, if present, requires admission to the hospital for monitoring and treatment because respiratory failure may occur rapidly. Weakness in MG can be worsened by infection, physical stress such as surgery, emotional stress, and medications.

TABLE 1 Medications Reported to Exacerbate Myasthenia Gravis

Antibiotics
Aminoglycosides, ampicillin sodium, ciprofloxacin hydrochloride (Cipro), erythromycin, imipenem (Primaxin), kanamycin sulfate (Kantrex), pyrantel (Antiminth), chloroquine (Aralen)

Cardiovascular Agents
β-Blocking agents (propranolol hydrochloride [Inderal], oxprenolol hydrochloride[2] [Trasicor], timolol maleate [Blocadren]), procainamide (Procanbid), verapamil hydrochloride (Calan), propafenone hydrochloride (Rythmol), quinidine
Penicillamine (Cuprimine)
Corticosteroids (transiently when initiating therapy)
Magnesium salts and lithium carbonate (Eskalith)
Phenothiazine antipsychotics
Phenytoin sodium (Dilantin)

Neuromuscular Blocking Agents
Vecuronium bromide (Norcuron), succinylcholine chloride (Anectine)

Ocular Drugs
Timolol maleate (Timoptic), proparacaine hydrochloride (Alcaine), tropicamide (Mydriacyl)

Anticholinergic Agents
Trihexyphenidyl hydrochloride (Artane)
Acetazolamide (Diamox)

[2]Not available in the United States.

Medications that reportedly worsen strength in MG are listed in Table 1.

The prevalence of MG is estimated to be 14 per 100,000 people. MG may present at any age, but the most common ages of onset are in the second and third decades in women and in the seventh and eighth decades in men. In the past MG was more common in women than men, but with aging of the population, MG now is more common in men. Associated autoimmune diseases, such as thyroid disease, rheumatoid arthritis, lupus, and pernicious anemia, are present in 5% to 10% of patients. Approximately 10% of MG patients have an associated thymoma, and 50% to 70% of patients have thymic hyperplasia. Familial occurrence of autoimmune MG is rare, although the incidence of autoimmune diseases in first-degree relatives of patients with MG may be increased.

Diagnosis

An accurate diagnosis prior to initiating treatment for MG is crucial. A critical assessment of the patient's symptoms is the most important initial step in evaluation. The differential diagnosis of MG is quite limited in most patients. Disorders that may mimic MG are listed in Table 2.

All patients suspected of having MG should undergo testing consisting of a complete blood count (CBC), erythrocyte sedimentation rate, thyroid-stimulating hormone and thyroxine levels, rheumatoid factor concentration, and liver and renal profiles. Autoimmune thyroid disease may mimic or accompany MG. In addition to excluding other

CURRENT DIAGNOSIS

- Hallmark of MG is fluctuating or fatigable weakness.
- Initial symptom is ptosis or diplopia in 60% of patients.
- Generalized fatigue or tiredness alone is not a symptom of MG.
- Diagnostic evaluation includes:
  - Laboratory evaluation: Thyroid-stimulating hormone level, complete blood count, erythrocyte sedimentation rate, rheumatoid factor, liver and renal function studies
  - Edrophonium chloride (Tensilon) test: >90% sensitivity, but be certain to choose a defined clinical endpoint (e.g., improvement in ptosis)
  - Antibody testing: Send AChR binding antibodies first. Binding antibodies are found in ~90% of patients with generalized MG, and 50% with ocular MG. If negative, send AChR modulating antibodies. If both are negative, send muscle-specific receptor tyrosine kinase antibody.
  - All patients with suspected MG should undergo chest computed tomography with contrast for thymoma
  - If antibodies are negative or if searching for evidence of generalized MG in a patient with pure ocular symptoms, obtain electromyography with repetitive nerve stimulation. This test result is abnormal in >70% of patients with generalized MG but is less sensitive in patients with pure ocular symptoms
- If diagnosis remains unclear, refer to neuromuscular specialist.

Abbreviations: AChR = acetylcholine receptor; MG = myasthenia gravis.

TABLE 2 Clinical Presentations and Diagnostic Considerations in Myasthenia Gravis

Site of Predominant Weakness	Alternative Diagnoses
Ocular	Brainstem and cranial nerve disorders due to processes such as neoplasm, stroke, and multiple sclerosis
	Horner syndrome
	Oculopharyngeal muscular dystrophy
	Kearns-Sayre syndrome
	Graves' disease
	Congenital myasthenia
	Botulism (if symptom onset is acute)
	Miller-Fischer variant of GBS
Bulbar	Brainstem and multiple cranial nerve dysfunction due to processes such as neoplasm, stroke, and multiple sclerosis
	Bulbar-onset ALS
	Obstructive lesion of the oropharynx or laryngeal lesion
	Botulism (if symptom onset is acute)
Proximal extremity weakness	Inflammatory myopathies (e.g., polymyositis, dermatomyositis)
	LEMS
	GBS
	Periodic paralysis
	Acid maltase deficiency
Isolated respiratory weakness	ALS
	Polymyositis
	LEMS
	Myotonic dystrophy
Isolated neck weakness	ALS
	Inflammatory myopathies
	Paraspinous myopathy

Abbreviations: ALS = amyotrophic lateral sclerosis; GBS = Guillain-Barré syndrome; LEMS, Lambert-Eaton myasthenic syndrome.

diagnoses, these tests are important because treatments of MG may have adverse effects on the bone marrow, liver, and kidneys.

The role of specific testing for MG is to confirm the clinical diagnosis. For a patient with ptosis, the ice test is easy and convenient. A small amount of ice is placed over the ptotic lid for a few minutes. Improvement of the ptosis with cooling is suggestive of a defect of neuromuscular transmission. Further testing should then be pursued.

EDROPHONIUM CHLORIDE (TENSILON) TEST

The edrophonium (Tensilon) test is readily available, but the result may be invalid if the test is not properly performed. A defined clinical endpoint is needed, and vague patient reports of improvement in strength are not acceptable. Cranial nerve deficits, such as ptosis, dysconjugate gaze, and limitation of extraocular movements, provide the most reliable endpoints. The test should be performed in a location where syncope, hypotension, or respiratory failure can be managed, as these complications can rarely occur in supersensitive individuals. Atropine sulfate 0.4 mg should be available in case of symptomatic bradycardia. An intravenous line is often started for the test, although some practitioners use a butterfly needle for administration. Edrophonium 10 mg (1 mL) is drawn up in a syringe. The strength or maximum excursion of the target muscles is assessed immediately prior to administration of the edrophonium. A 2-mg (0.2-mL) test dose is given to ensure that the patient is not supersensitive to the drug. If no respiratory or cardiac side effects occur, 3 mg (0.3 mL) of edrophonium is given. Re-examination of the target muscle is performed. If no definite improvement is observed at 60 seconds, the remaining 5 mg (0.5 mL) of edrophonium is given. If unequivocal improvement in the strength of the target muscle occurs within 60 seconds of administration of a dose of edrophonium, the test is considered positive. Edrophonium 10 mg will not weaken normal muscles, but the full dose may induce weakness in a patient with a defect in neuromuscular transmission. For this reason, the medication should be given in the manner described so that any improvement in muscle strength is not missed.

The edrophonium (Tensilon) test is positive in more than 90% of patients with MG, but a positive result is not specific for MG. Positive edrophonium tests have been reported in patients with the Lambert-Eaton myasthenic syndrome, motor neuron disease, lesions of the oculomotor nerves, and conditions affecting the extraocular muscles.

ANTIBODY TESTING

Acetylcholine receptor antibodies (AChR-Ab) are present in 90% of patients with generalized MG and in approximately 50% to 60% of patients with ocular myasthenia. They are the most specific test for MG. False-positive results can occur but are rare. Antibody levels are not predictive of the severity of MG in an individual patient.

Three different tests for AChR-Ab are available commercially: binding, modulating, and blocking antibodies. The binding antibody is the antibody most commonly found in MG and should be tested first. If the test result is negative, a modulating antibody test should be performed because this may be positive in a small number of patients who do not have binding antibodies. The blocking antibody titer adds little additional diagnostic value and is not generally indicated.

Recently, antibodies against muscle-specific receptor tyrosine kinase (MuSK-Ab) have been described in approximately 40% of patients with "seronegative" MG. Evidence indicates that MuSK is involved in the proper distribution of AChR at the muscle endplate, and some evidence indicates that MuSK-Abs are pathogenic in these patients. The MuSK-Ab test is commercially available. Patients with MuSK-Ab are almost always seronegative for AChR-Ab. For this reason, the MuSK-Ab test should be sent only if the patient has already been tested for AChR-Ab and is seronegative. MG in patients with MuSK-Ab may have a different natural history and response to treatment, and this is an area of active investigation. Patients with MuSK-Ab more likely are young women and present with bulbar, neck, or respiratory symptoms. Edrophonium (Tensilon) testing is less likely to yield a positive result. Whether thymectomy should be performed in patients with MuSK-Ab is unclear.

Striational antibodies are a marker for thymoma, although false-positive and false-negative results are common. Chest computed tomography (CT) with contrast to evaluate for possible thymoma is indicated for all patients diagnosed with MG. The added value of performing striational antibodies has not been definitely demonstrated.

ELECTROPHYSIOLOGIC TESTING

Electrophysiologic testing is indicated for evaluation of possible MG if the AChR-Ab test is negative. In antibody-positive patients, electrophysiologic testing is often not necessary unless the test is being performed to evaluate for evidence of generalized disease in those with purely ocular symptoms. Typically, routine nerve conduction studies and needle electromyography (EMG) are normal. These tests are performed to ensure that other disorders of the peripheral nerves or muscles are not present. Repetitive nerve stimulation (RNS) is then performed if the study was ordered to evaluate for an NMJ disorder. RNS has a sensitivity of approximately 50% to 60% in all patients with MG, with a higher yield in patients with generalized MG and a lower yield in patients with pure ocular MG. RNS of the spinal accessory and facial nerves may increase the yield of testing. It should be emphasized that abnormal RNS is not specific for MG, and routine nerve conduction studies and needle EMG must be performed to exclude other conditions. Single-fiber EMG (SFEMG) is a highly specialized and demanding technique with a sensitivity of approximately 90% to 95% in patients with MG. SFEMG is abnormal in many neuromuscular diseases and therefore should be performed only in the correct clinical context and after a routine EMG with RNS has been performed. Because of the demanding nature of the study, SFEMG is usually performed by a neuromuscular specialist.

OTHER INVESTIGATIONS

Currently all patients diagnosed with MG should undergo a CT scan of the chest with contrast to evaluate for an associated thymoma. Routine chest radiography or determination of antistriational antibodies is not an adequate substitute.

Prognosis

The natural history of MG is highly variable. Ocular symptoms are the presenting symptoms in approximately 50% to 60% of MG patients. Weakness subsequently develops in other muscles in most patients. Weakness remains restricted to the extraocular muscles for the entire course of MG in 15% to 20% of patients (pure ocular myasthenia). Patients with initial ocular involvement typically develop weakness in other muscles within the first year of having the disease. If no generalized symptoms develop after 2 years, subsequent generalization is unlikely. The maximal weakness from MG occurs within the initial 3 years of symptoms in 70% of patients. Mortality from MG is now low because of advances in critical care; however, quality of life is often affected by MG. Long-lasting remission occurs spontaneously in approximately 10% to 15% of patients if no immunosuppressive agents are used. Spontaneous remissions may be more frequent in patients with pure ocular myasthenia.

Treatment

CHOLINESTERASE INHIBITORS AS FIRST-LINE THERAPY

Cholinesterase inhibitors (ChEIs) are first-line therapy in all patients with MG. The commonly available ChEIs are listed in Table 3. Acetylcholinesterase (AChE) is anchored in the synaptic cleft on the postsynaptic membrane. AChE normally cleaves acetylcholine (ACh) released from the presynaptic nerve terminal, which normally prevents repeat binding of ACh to the AChR. ChEIs reduce the hydrolysis of ACh and increase the amount of ACh available at the postsynaptic membrane. ChEIs used for treatment of MG are reversible inhibitors of AChE and cause few central nervous system side effects because they do

CURRENT THERAPY

Be certain of the diagnosis
- Ocular symptoms only or mild weakness: Cholinesterase inhibitors
- Moderate to severe weakness:
  - Cholinesterase inhibitors, and
  - Thymectomy for patients younger than 60 years (with complete removal of the gland)
- If symptoms are uncontrolled with cholinesterase inhibitors, use immunosuppression:
  - Prednisone if urgent or severe
  - Azathioprine[1] (Imuran) or mycophenolate mofetil[1] (CellCept)
    - As a steroid-sparing agent to facilitate prednisone taper
    - Prednisone fails to elicit patient response
    - Prednisone contraindicated
    - Excessive prednisone side effects
- Plasma exchange or intravenous immune globulin[1]
  - Myasthenic crisis
  - Preoperative (i.e., before thymectomy)
- If the above measures fail:
  - Refer to neuromuscular specialist

[1]Not FDA approved for this indication.

not cross the blood–brain barrier efficiently. Absorption from the gastrointestinal tract is inefficient, and oral bioavailability is low.

Pyridostigmine bromide (Mestinon) is the most widely used ChEI. Onset of action is within 15 to 30 minutes of an oral dose, with peak action at 1 to 2 hours and gradual wearing off at 3 to 4 hours. All ChEI medications have muscarinic side effects, including cramping, diarrhea, salivation, lacrimation, and bradycardia. For this reason, the medication should always be introduced in low dose, preferably on the weekend. Pyridostigmine tablets are double scored and can be easily split. Start the patient with a half tablet (30 mg) of pyridostigmine once daily in the morning. The dose is then increased by a half tablet each day to a dose of a half tablet (30 mg) four times daily. Subsequently, the dose can be increased further to a full tablet (60 mg) four times daily. If necessary for symptom relief, pyridostigmine can be increased to a maximum dose of 120 mg every 3 to 4 hours, but 60 mg every 4 hours usually provides optimum benefit. If a patient has weakness while eating, pyridostigmine doses can be timed to be taken 1 hour before meals. If a patient has significant weakness upon awakening, the extended-release formulation of pyridostigmine (Mestinon Timespan) can be given at bedtime; however, absorption is too unpredictable for daytime use. If a patient requires parenteral dosing of medications, intravenous pyridostigmine is given at $\frac{1}{30}$ the oral dose (usually 1–2 mg intravenously) every 3 to 4 hours.

When symptoms are not controlled with 60 to 120 mg of pyridostigmine every 4 hours, possible initiation of an immunosuppressive agent must be discussed fully with the patient. Most patients with generalized MG will require immunosuppressive treatment in order to induce a remission of symptoms. Pyridostigmine is often initially very effective, but therapeutic efficacy usually gradually diminishes. The immunosuppressive agents used in MG are corticosteroids, azathioprine[1] (Imuran), mycophenolate mofetil[1] (CellCept), cyclosporin A[1] (Neoral), and cyclophosphamide[1] (Cytoxan). Each of these agents is discussed separately in Table 4. Important considerations are the clinical severity of the MG, the patient's perception of his or her disability, any coexisting medical conditions, as well as the patient's age, gender, and overall lifestyle. For example, a physically active patient will be less tolerant of weakness than a patient with a sedentary lifestyle.

TREATMENT OF PURE OCULAR MYASTHENIA GRAVIS

From 15% to 20% of patients with MG have only visual symptoms for the entire course of their disease. Visual symptoms in patients with MG result from ptosis or

[1]Not FDA approved for this indication.

TABLE 3 Commonly Available Cholinesterase Inhibitors

Medication	Route of Administration	Unit Dose	Average Dose (Adult)	Children's Dose
Pyridostigmine bromide tablet (Mestinon)	Oral	60-mg tablets, double-scored for splitting	30–60 mg every 4–6 hours, maximum 120 mg every 3 hours	1 mg/kg every 4–6 hours
Pyridostigmine bromide syrup	Oral	12 mg/mL	30–60 mg every 4–6 hours	1 mg/kg every 4–6 hours
Pyridostigmine bromide sustained-release (Mestinon Timespan)	Oral	180-mg tablet (not crushable)	1 tablet at bedtime	—
Pyridostigmine bromide	Intravenous	5 mg/mL ampules	$\frac{1}{30}$ of usual oral dose, i.e., 1–2 mg every 3–4 hours	—
Neostigmine bromide (Prostigmin)	Oral	15-mg tablets	7.5–15 mg every 3–4 hours	
Edrophonium (Tensilon)	Intravenous		Used for diagnosis	Used for diagnosis

TABLE 4 Oral Immunosuppressive Agents Used on Myasthenia Gravis

Medication	Starting Dose	Therapeutic Dose	Time to Clinical Effect	Laboratory Monitoring	Side Effects	Advantages
Prednisone[1]	60–80 mg daily (see text)	60–80 mg daily (or 120 mg every other day)	Days to weeks	May need to follow blood glucose level; follow bone density every 6 mo	Many serious long-term side effects (see text); always start with calcium 1500 mg/day and vitamin D 400 IU/day; may also require bisphosphonate	Short time to clinical effect; long clinical experience in MG; not teratogenic; relatively safe in pregnancy; no increase in malignancy
Azathioprine[1] (Imuran)	50 mg daily	2–3 mg/kg/day in divided doses	4–12 mo	CBC, LFT weekly as dose increased; may then check once per month; if WBC <2500, stop azathioprine	~10% fever, nausea, abdominal pain during first weeks of treatment; increased risk of malignancy with long-term use; teratogenic	Long clinical experience; predictable; fewer long-term side effects than prednisone
Mycophenolate mofetil[1] (CellCept)	500 mg twice daily	1000–1500 mg twice daily	2–6 mo	CBC monthly, but significant myelosuppression is uncommon	Diarrhea; risk of malignancy with long-term use is currently unclear; should not be used in pregnancy because safety is unknown; clinical experience in MG is limited—randomized study is ongoing	Usually well tolerated; few serious side effects; faster onset of clinical effect than azathioprine
Cyclosporine[1] (Sandimmune, Neoral)	3–5 mg/kg/day in divided doses	3–5 mg/kg/day in divided doses	2–6 mo	Renal function, trough cyclosporine levels, electrolytes monthly; follow blood pressure	Significant renal toxicity is common and is a frequent reason to stop the drug; hypertension; should not be used in pregnancy; many drug interactions; use only under guidance of neuromuscular specialist	Faster onset of clinical effect than azathioprine
Cyclophosphamide[1] (Cytoxan)	25 mg/day orally; parenteral administration may be used in severe, refractory MG	2–5 mg daily		CBC monthly	Significant myelosuppression, hemorrhagic cystitis, risk of opportunistic infections; increased risk of malignancy; absolutely contraindicated during pregnancy; use only under guidance of neuromuscular specialist	May be effective in patients refractory to other treatments

[1]Not FDA approved for this indication.
Abbreviations: CBC = complete blood count; LFT = liver function test; MG = myasthenia gravis; WBC = white blood cell count.

ocular misalignment. Approximately 50% of patients will experience significant relief of visual symptoms with ChEIs alone and will be satisfied with their treatment. The effect on symptoms should be clear within 1 month of beginning pyridostigmine (Mestinon) therapy. In general, pyridostigmine provides significant relief of ptosis and is less helpful for ocular misalignment.

Among the 50% of patients who achieve significant control of ocular symptoms using pyridostigmine, this may be the only treatment necessary. If symptoms are not controlled, the patient's perception of his or her disability and lifestyle are very important to treatment. A patient who is unable to work because of visual misalignment will require further treatment. Nonpharmacologic options for symptom management include eyelid taping or eyelid crutches for ptosis and eye patching for ocular misalignment.

If the patient requests further treatment, prednisone[1] can be started at 10 mg/day, with an increase of 5 mg every other day until a dose of 40 to 60 mg/day is reached. This dose should be continued for approximately 1 month. The vast majority of patients will improve. At 1 month, a taper at 5 mg/wk can be started; at 20 mg the taper should be slowed to improve the chances of maintaining remission.

The role of corticosteroids in the treatment of pure ocular MG is controversial. Some data suggest that corticosteroids decrease the chance of developing generalized MG. However, corticosteroids have many undesired effects. In general, corticosteroids are used for ocular myasthenia only when the symptoms are significant to the patient and are uncontrolled by ChEIs.

CORTICOSTEROIDS

Corticosteroids are usually the first-line immunosuppressive agent. After 6 weeks of treatment with a corticosteroid, approximately 90% of patients have improvement in symptoms. Approximately 30% of patients treated with prednisone obtain remission, and 50% experience marked improvement. Paradoxically, 50% of patients have an initial increase in weakness during the first weeks of treatment with corticosteroids. The reasons for this effect are not well understood. Some practitioners begin treatment at the full therapeutic dose of prednisone 60 to 80 mg/day, with careful monitoring for increased weakness. If weakness worsens, the patient may require hospitalization and treatment with plasma exchange or intravenous immune globulin[1] (IVIG; Gamimune N). Others begin treatment at a lower dose with a gradual increase to the target dose over 1 month with the goal of avoiding the initial worsening of strength. An example of this method begins with a dose of prednisone 20 mg once daily. The dose is increased by 5 mg every third day until the target dose of 60 to 80 mg/day is reached. Alternate-day dosing with a target dose of 100 to 120 mg every other day can also be used. When beginning prednisone, calcium, vitamin D, and a bisphosphonate medication should be started at the same time unless a contraindication is present. This is appropriate because most patients will require long-term therapy with prednisone.

A clinical effect is typically seen within 6 weeks. If a remission is achieved, the full dose should be maintained for 6 weeks, followed by a slow taper. Initially the daily prednisone dose can be decreased by 5 mg/month. When the daily dose reaches 30 mg/day. the taper should be slowed, with further decreases in dose of 2.5 mg/month. Clinical exacerbations are frequent when the daily dose of prednisone reaches 20 to 30 mg/day, and a slower taper may prevent this problem. If an exacerbation occurs, the daily prednisone dose should be increased by 5 to 10 mg. The new dose can be maintained for 6 weeks, followed by a slower taper. Some practitioners use alternate-day dosing, with tapering from an initial dose of 100 to 120 mg every other day.

Long-term use of corticosteroids is associated with serious complications, including osteoporosis, fractures, medication-induced diabetes mellitus, obesity, glaucoma, cataracts, gastric and duodenal ulcers, anxiety or depression, myopathy, opportunistic infections, and avascular necrosis of the large joints. Most patients are not able to completely discontinue prednisone and require a minimum dose to maintain improvement of their MG. The decision to start a steroid-sparing agent is often not clear-cut. In general, if a patient has more than one relapse when tapering off steroids, therapy with a steroid-sparing agent should be considered. If a patient does not have a remission with steroids, combined therapy with a steroid-sparing agent should be considered. In the older patient population, treatment with a steroid-sparing agent should be considered early in the course. In a young patient, particularly a woman in her childbearing years, steroid-sparing drugs should be avoided when possible because of teratogenicity and the increased risk of lymphoma with long-term use of these agents.

OTHER IMMUNOSUPPRESSIVE AGENTS

Azathioprine[1] (Imuran) has been extensively used in MG, usually as a steroid-sparing medication. Azathioprine is an inhibitor of purine synthesis and therefore affects rapidly dividing cell populations, such as lymphocytes. A large double-blind, randomized study demonstrated improvement in steroid tapering with the use of azathioprine. The major drawback of azathioprine is that a clinical effect may not be seen until 12 months. Side effects are less common than with steroids. Approximately 10% of patients have an idiosyncratic reaction in the first weeks of therapy, with fever, nausea, vomiting, and abdominal pain. Symptoms resolve with cessation of the drug but usually recur if azathioprine is restarted. Azathioprine may cause leukopenia or thrombocytopenia, vomiting, or hepatic dysfunction. Mild leukopenia occurs in 25% of patients but is usually not significant. Elevation of hepatic enzyme levels occurs in 5% of patients but is usually reversible with cessation of the drug. The risk of lymphoma increases slightly after 10 years of use. Azathioprine is potentially teratogenic and should be avoided in women of childbearing age. The initial dose is 50 mg/day (or 1 mg/kg/day). The dose is increased over a few months until the therapeutic dose of 2 mg/kg/day in divided doses is reached. CBC with differential and liver function tests initially should be tested weekly and monthly after the target dose has been reached. Leukopenia may develop even after several years of treatment. If the white blood cell count drops below 2500 cells/mm^3 or the absolute neutrophil count

---

[1]Not FDA approved for this indication.

[1]Not FDA approved for this indication.

below 1000 cells/mm³, the drug should be stopped. Overall, approximately 50% of patients improve with azathioprine therapy. Relapse after discontinuation of azathioprine occurs in more than 50% of patients.

Mycophenolate mofetil[1] (CellCept) is a newer immunosuppressant that inhibits proliferation of T and B lymphocytes by blocking de novo purine synthesis. Lymphocytes are selectively affected because they are unable to use the purine salvage pathway. The major advantages of mycophenolate are its relatively fast onset of clinical effect and its favorable side-effect profile. Side effects are usually mild and include diarrhea, abdominal pain, nausea, peripheral edema, and mild leukopenia. The long-term risk of malignancy with use of mycophenolate is unclear; however, an elderly MG patient who developed primary central nervous system lymphoma in association with mycophenolate use has been recently reported. Treatment trials of patients with MG are ongoing. Some practitioners use mycophenolate to induce remission without the concomitant use of steroids. Others use mycophenolate only as a steroid-sparing agent in steroid-dependent patients. The standard starting dose is 500 mg twice daily. The therapeutic dose for treatment of MG is 1000 to 1500 mg twice daily. Significant myelosuppression is uncommon; however, a monthly check of CBC with differential is standard practice.

Cyclosporine[1] (Sandimmune, Neoral) is an inhibitor of T-helper cell function through blockade of calcineurin-mediated cytokine signaling. Cyclosporine is of limited use for treatment of MG because of renal toxicity. Cyclosporine is used for cases of severe MG when steroids and azathioprine are not tolerated or are ineffective. The standard dosage for treatment of MG is 3 to 5 mg/kg/day in divided doses. Anecdotally, a lower target dose of 2 mg/kg/day may decrease the incidence of renal insufficiency while still achieving clinical improvement. A clinical effect is usually seen within the first 6 months of treatment. Renal function and trough cyclosporine levels should be followed monthly. Creatinine levels greater than 50% of the pretreatment levels are an indication to stop the drug. A rise in creatinine level typically occurs after several years of use. Hypertension is a frequent side effect, and blood pressure must be monitored regularly. In general, this medication should be used for treatment of MG under the guidance of a neuromuscular specialist.

Cyclophosphamide[1] (Cytoxan) is an alkylating agent that acts on DNA, inhibiting cell proliferation. Cyclophosphamide has limited use in MG because of multiple serious toxicities. Cyclophosphamide is used in patients with severe MG when steroids and azathioprine are ineffective or not tolerated. It appears effective at inducing remission when used in this manner. Cyclophosphamide has been used in combination with steroids for patients with severe disease who have not responded to steroids alone. The risk of side effects from cyclophosphamide is high. Cyclophosphamide may cause severe bone marrow suppression, severe opportunistic infections, bladder toxicity, and increased risk of neoplasm. Cyclophosphamide is a chemotherapeutic agent at higher doses, and parenteral high-dose administration has occasionally been used for patients with refractory, severe MG. In general, this medication should be used for treatment of MG only under the guidance of a neuromuscular specialist.

SHORT-TERM IMMUNOTHERAPY: PLASMA EXCHANGE AND INTRAVENOUS IMMUNE GLOBULIN

Plasma exchange (i.e., plasmapheresis) is a well-established intervention that produces short-term clinical improvement in patients with MG. Plasmapheresis is typically used in a MG patient with rapid worsening of weakness or myasthenic crisis. Plasma exchange treatments may be performed prior to an elective surgical procedure, such as thymectomy, to decrease the likelihood of a myasthenic exacerbation. Rarely a patient is refractory or intolerant of all long-term therapies and requires periodic plasma exchange on an ongoing basis. Typical treatment of a myasthenic exacerbation consists of five exchanges of 3 to 4 L each over a period of approximately 2 weeks. The effect is rapid and improvement is seen within days of starting therapy, but the effect is short lived. Typically the beneficial effects of plasma exchange last only a few weeks. Central venous access, typically with a large-bore catheter, is required. Complications of plasma exchange are usually related to the vascular access. Patients are at risk for significant iatrogenic infections, particularly because many of these patients are undergoing long-term therapy with immunosuppressive agents. Hematoma at the site of line placement, pulmonary embolism from venous thrombosis, electrolyte imbalance, pneumothorax, and hypotension during plasma exchange treatments can occur.

IVIG[1] is used for identical indications as plasma exchange. The standard dose is 400 mg/kg/day for 5 days. The only large, randomized study of IVIG in MG found IVIG equivalent to plasmapheresis for treatment of myasthenic crisis. Some practitioners anecdotally believe plasma exchange produces more rapid improvement in strength. The advantages of IVIG are that it is generally more widely available than is plasmapheresis, and it does not require central venous access. The most common side effects are headache and transient flulike symptoms. However, IVIG may cause volume overload, vascular events such as ischemic stroke, and venous thrombosis. IVIG should be used with caution in patients with risk factors for these conditions. IVIG cannot be used in patients with IgA deficiency, a relatively frequent condition. An IgA level must be determined prior to the first IVIG treatment to avoid a potentially serious allergic reaction. Anecdotally, some patients refractory to IVIG will have a good response to plasma exchange.

THYMECTOMY

Thymectomy has been standard therapy for treatment of MG for more than 50 years, but it has never been evaluated in a large, prospective, randomized controlled trial. Thymectomy appears to be effective in improving the course of MG in patients without thymoma. If a thymoma is present, thymectomy is mandatory. The procedure is not a cure for MG, but it appears to increase the likelihood of clinical remission, particularly if performed within the first year of symptom onset. Approximately 75% of patients

---

[1]Not FDA approved for this indication.

[1]Not FDA approved for this indication.

appear to receive some benefit from the procedure, but the effect may be apparent only after several years. Thymectomy appears to be more effective in younger patients, which may reflect the involution of the thymus with aging. Patients younger than 60 years with moderate to severe MG are candidates for thymectomy. Patients with pure ocular myasthenia do not usually undergo thymectomy unless a thymoma is suspected. Thymic tissue may be present throughout the neck and the mediastinum. The majority of surgical centers perform a combined transsternal–transcervical exposure with en bloc removal of the thymus to ensure complete removal of the gland. Incomplete resections have been followed by persistent symptoms that were later relieved by removal of residual thymus at reoperation. Referrals for thymectomy should be made to an experienced surgeon willing to perform a maximal resection. In the days preceding thymectomy, patients often undergo plasma exchange to decrease the likelihood of an exacerbation due to the surgery. The surgery involves sternotomy and a 4- to 6-week convalescence. Serious complications are uncommon when the surgery is performed at an experienced center by anesthesiologists and neurologists familiar with the perioperative management of MG.

TREATMENT OF MYASTHENIC CRISIS

A myasthenic crisis is an exacerbation of MG producing respiratory weakness or profound muscle weakness. Myasthenic crisis is a neurologic emergency. Patients with worsening weakness should undergo tests including chest radiograph, blood and urine cultures, CBC with differential, and serum chemistries to screen for concurrent infections. The patient's medication list should be scrutinized and any recent additions or changes noted. Patients occasionally increase their ChEI dose to toxic levels without consulting their physician, resulting in increased muscle weakness and a "cholinergic crisis." This event is relatively uncommon, but recent consumption of ChEI must be determined in all myasthenic patients with increasing weakness. Signs of cholinergic crisis include abdominal cramps, diarrhea, nausea and vomiting, excessive secretions, and miotic pupils; these are not characteristics of myasthenic crisis. If cholinergic crisis is a consideration, the ChEI must be stopped. A patient in myasthenic crisis should be admitted to an intensive care unit if any signs of respiratory failure are present because respiratory deterioration may occur quickly. The vital capacity and peak negative inspiratory force should be followed as measures of respiratory strength. As a rule, elective intubation should be performed when the vital capacity falls below 15 mL/kg and peak negative inspiratory force below −20 cm H_2O. Arterial blood gas measurements do not accurately reflect the degree of respiratory muscle weakness in MG. PCO_2 and pO_2 measurements may be normal until just prior to respiratory collapse. While a patient is ventilated, it is reasonable to discontinue pyridostigmine (Mestinon) because this medication may increase respiratory secretions. Any immunosuppressive agents should be continued. If the patient is a new-onset myasthenic, it is appropriate to begin prednisone therapy 60 to 80 mg/day while the patient is ventilated. Options for improving strength during crisis are plasma exchange treatments and IVIG (discussed earlier). Readiness for weaning from the ventilator can be assessed using the vital capacity and peak negative inspiratory force measurements. Weaning from the ventilator may otherwise be performed according to standard protocols. Once the patient is successfully extubated, treatment with ChEIs can be resumed. A treatment plan to prevent future myasthenic crises should be developed.

Other Issues

TRANSIENT NEONATAL MYASTHENIA

Transient neonatal myasthenia occurs in 10% of infants of mothers with autoimmune MG. Following delivery, the infant has a weak cry or suck, appears floppy, and may require mechanical ventilation. The symptoms result from maternal antibodies transferred across the placenta to the infant in utero and resolve within a few weeks. Infants with severe weakness can be treated with oral pyridostigmine 1 to 2 mg/kg every 2 hours.

LAMBERT-EATON MYASTHENIC SYNDROME

Lambert-Eaton myasthenic syndrome (LEMS) is an uncommon autoimmune disorder of the presynaptic NMJ. LEMS is characterized by fluctuating proximal extremity weakness. Symptoms typically include difficulty walking, standing up from a chair, and climbing stairs. Patients may complain of autonomic symptoms, such as dry mouth, blurry vision, anhidrosis, or constipation. Unlike MG, in LEMS ptosis, diplopia, dysphagia, and dysarthria are usually not prominent. Respiratory failure may occur but is uncommon. Patients may report improvement in muscle strength after sustained activity. Other frequent symptoms include myalgias, muscle stiffness, paresthesias, and a metallic taste in the mouth.

On examination, patients typically have proximal muscle weakness, more prominent in the lower extremities. The objective weakness may be less than expected given the patient's symptoms. Characteristically, muscle stretch reflexes are absent. Sustained muscle grip strength often increases over the first several seconds (Lambert's sign).

LEMS is a paraneoplastic syndrome in 60% of patients, most often due to a small cell carcinoma of the lung. In patients without malignancy, LEMS is often associated with other autoimmune conditions. Male patients older than 40 years are more likely to have an associated malignancy, whereas patients without malignancy are more often young women. All patients with suspected LEMS should undergo a thorough evaluation for malignancy, however. If no malignancy is found, the evaluation should be repeated at regular intervals. Presentation of LEMS may antedate the discovery of a malignancy by up to 2 years.

LEMS is believed to result from autoantibodies against the presynaptic voltage-gated calcium channels of cholinergic nerve terminals. At the NMJ, decreased release of acetylcholine from the presynaptic nerve terminal results in muscle weakness. The cholinergic nerve terminals of the autonomic nervous system are also affected. Seventy-five percent of patients with LEMS have detectable serum IgG antibodies against voltage-gated P/Q calcium channels. The diagnosis of LEMS should always be confirmed by electrophysiologic studies. Nerve conduction studies reveal diffusely low compound motor action potential (CMAP) amplitudes with normal sensory responses. RNS shows a CMAP decrement with slow rates of stimulation but marked increment of the CMAP response after brief exercise. A similar increment is seen with fast rates of RNS.

In LEMS with an associated malignancy, treatment of the malignancy may lead to improvement of LEMS symptoms. For symptomatic treatment, some patients achieve improvement with use of ChEIs such as pyridostigmine (Mestinon). 3,4-Diaminopyridine (DAP) increases release of ACh from the presynaptic nerve terminal by decreasing potassium conductance. 3,4-DAP is not approved by the Food and Drug Administration (FDA) for use in the United States. In countries where 3,4-DAP is approved, it represents the first-line symptomatic therapy for LEMS. The typical starting dose is 10 mg every 4 to 6 hours. In patients with disabling symptoms, immunosuppressive therapies such as long-term corticosteroids, plasma exchange treatments, and IVIG[1] can be used.

REFERENCES

Chaudry V, Cornblath DR, Griffin JW, et al: Mycophenolate mofetil: a safe and promising immunosuppressant in neuromuscular diseases. Neurology 2001;56:94-96.

Drachman DB: Myasthenia gravis. N Engl J Med 1994;330:1797-1810.

Gajdos PH, Chevret S, Clair B, et al: Clinical trial of plasma exchange and high-dose intravenous immunoglobulin in myasthenia gravis. Ann Neurol 1997;41:789-796.

Jaretzki A, Steinglass KM, Sonett JR: Thymectomy in the management of myasthenia gravis. Semin Neurol 2004;24:49-62.

Kaminski HJ (ed): Current Clinical Neurology: Myasthenia Gravis and Related Disorders. Totowa, NJ, Humana Press, 2002.

Katirji B, Kaminski HJ: Electrodiagnostic approach to the patient with suspected neuromuscular junction disorder. Neurol Clin 2002; 20:557-586.

Palace J, Newsom-Davis J, Lecky B: A randomized double-blind trial of prednisolone alone or with azathioprine in myasthenia gravis. Neurology 1998;50:1778-1783.

Pascuzzi RM, Coslett HB, Johns TR: Long-term corticosteroid treatment of myasthenia gravis: Report of 116 patients. Ann Neurol 1984;15: 291-298.

Richman DP, Agius MA: Treatment of autoimmune myasthenia gravis. Neurology 2003;61:1652-1661.

Saperstein DS, Barohn RJ: Management of myasthenia gravis. Semin Neurol 2004;24:41-48..

Seybold ME, Drachman DB: Gradually increasing doses of prednisone in MG. N Engl J Med 1974;290:81-84.

Vincent A, Leite MI: Neuromuscular junction autoimmune disease: Muscle specific kinase antibodies and treatments for myasthenia gravis. Curr Opinion Neurol 2005;18:519-525.

[1]Not FDA approved for this indication.

Trigeminal Neuralgia

Method of
Ronald F. Young, MD

Trigeminal neuralgia (TN) is one of the most devastating pain conditions that people endure. The pain is frequently misdiagnosed as being of dental or paranasal sinus origin. Unnecessary dental procedures, such as root canals and extractions or sinus surgery, are often performed in misguided attempts to treat the pain. The condition is also referred to as *tic douloureux* because of the sudden facial grimacing that may be seen as a reaction to the pain. The illness is estimated to affect about 1 in 20,000 people and becomes more frequent with advancing age. TN may be of primary (idiopathic) origin or secondary origin due to a variety of structural conditions, such as tumors (meningiomas and vestibular schwannomas in particular), multiple sclerosis (MS), vascular malformations, and cysts of the posterior cranial fossa. The exact etiology of TN is still debated, but it is generally accepted that most cases of idiopathic TN are due to compression of the trigeminal nerve root near its entry into the brainstem at the pons by adjacent blood vessels, most commonly arteries. Such compression is thought to result in segmental demyelination due to the constant pulsatile forces directed against the nerve root. The underlying pathology is thought to be related to the aging process wherein arteries (particularly the superior cerebellar artery) that normally course superior to, but not in contact with, the nerve root gradually come into contact and then compress and distort the nerve root as a result of constant pulsatile pressure. Such pressure causes localized demyelination and loss of the normal insulating function of the myelin. Ephaptic or nonsynaptic transmission and abnormal local depolarization are then postulated to result in ectopic impulse generation. Such impulses are thought to activate nerve fibers in the trigeminal nerve root that generate the pain of TN. Ephaptic transmission is also thought to account for the "triggering" of pain by usually innocuous stimuli, such as lightly touching the face or brushing the teeth.

Diagnosis

In spite of modern technology, TN is a diagnosis based almost exclusively on the medical history. Neither laboratory nor imaging studies establish the diagnosis conclusively,

CURRENT DIAGNOSIS

- Sudden, sharp, severe pain on one side of the face
- Confined to the cutaneous or intraoral distribution of the trigeminal nerve
- Triggered by otherwise innocuous stimulation of the face or mouth
- Usually due to arterial compression of the trigeminal nerve root but may be due to multiple sclerosis, tumors, or vascular malformations

although properly formatted magnetic resonance imaging (MRI) scans recently have been thought to contribute to the correct diagnosis if they demonstrate arterial compression of the trigeminal nerve root. Three aspects of the history are critical to the diagnosis: (1) the type of pain, (2) the location of the pain, and (3) the factors that trigger or activate the pain. The pain of TN is sharp, sudden, severe, and brief in character, usually lasting only a few seconds but often occurring in repeated bursts. The pain is often described as feeling like an electric shock or ice pick jabbing into the face. Pains that are of longer duration and described as burning, aching, boring, or like pressure are not typical of TN; when such symptoms are described, an alternative diagnosis should be considered. The pain of TN is confined within one or more of the major three peripheral divisions of the trigeminal nerve: the first division encompassing the anterior two thirds of the scalp, the forehead, the eye, and the upper portion of the nose; the second division encompassing the edges of the nares, the upper lip and cheek, the upper teeth, gums, and mucosal lining of the mouth; and the third division encompassing the skin over the mandible, including the lower lip as well as the lower teeth, gums, and anterior two thirds of the tongue. Pain that is located in the mastoid or occipital region, deep within the ear canal, extending below the edge of the mandible onto the neck or traversing the midline is not trigeminal in origin. TN is almost exclusively a unilateral condition. Bilateral pain is estimated to occur in less than 1% of cases; when bilateral, the pain on the two sides is often different with regard to the age of the patient at onset and the location of the pain. Most cases of bilateral TN occur in patients with MS wherein the pain is due to demyelination in the trigeminal nerve root secondary to an MS plaque. One of the most characteristic historical features of TN is the triggering of jabs or jolts of pain by stimuli that usually are innocuous. Such triggers include a variety of light mechanical stimuli, such as touching the face lightly, brushing the teeth, talking, attempting to eat and drink, and even a light breeze blowing against the face. Light, gentle stimuli are often more effective in eliciting the pain than are more forceful ones. Facial pain, even severe pain, probably is not TN if trigger phenomena are not described. The time course of TN is marked by unexplained, erratic exacerbations and remissions that may last days, weeks, months, or even years. The exacerbations tend to be less severe and shorter in duration at the onset of the illness and tend to become more severe and longer in duration and marked by shorter interval remissions as the illness persists over time. Patients who complain of persistent, unremitting facial pain, often with durations of weeks, months, or even years, probably do not suffer from TN. TN is often misdiagnosed as being of dental or paranasal sinus origin, but conversely other forms of facial pain are often misdiagnosed as TN. Most commonly misdiagnosed is so-called atypical facial pain. Such pain, often seen in young or middle-aged women but seen in men as well, usually is described as a strong, unremitting pressure or burning sensation that encompasses an area of the head and/or neck outside of the distribution of the trigeminal nerve, unassociated with trigger phenomena, often of prolonged durations (years), and usually unresponsive to a variety of medical interventions. Patients with atypical facial pain often express feelings of depression and hopelessness. Such pain is unresponsive to surgical intervention, and ill-advised surgical procedures often aggravate the pain and may leave the patient with new medical problems due to complications of the surgical procedures.

Physical Examination

In classic, or idiopathic, TN due to vascular compression of the trigeminal nerve root, the physical examination is usually completely unremarkable. Specifically, at least by the usual clinical examination techniques, facial sensation including the corneal reflex is normal. When loss of facial sensation to innocuous or painful stimuli is detected, a structural cause of TN should be sought. Tumors, vascular malformations, and MS are usually accompanied by other abnormal neurologic examination findings, including double vision, unilateral hearing loss, and facial weakness. MRI scanning is recommended in all patients with a suspected diagnosis of TN because even in some cases of TN caused by structural lesions, the examination may be normal, and the diagnosis of TN may be strengthened if an MRI scan demonstrates arterial compression of the trigeminal nerve root. Occasionally, an MRI scan discloses a completely unexpected cause of TN, such as a tortuous vertebrobasilar artery complex compressing the nerve root or even a large contralateral tumor or cyst displacing the brainstem. Such findings may radically alter any surgical recommendations made for treatment of TN. Patients who are unable to undergo MRI scanning because they have a cardiac pacemaker, for instance, should undergo thin-section computed tomography scanning, which cannot detect arterial vascular compression and small tumors but can detect larger tumors, vascular malformations, and vertebrobasilar artery compression.

Treatment

MEDICAL TREATMENT

The anticonvulsant family of drugs is the mainstay of medical treatment of TN. Carbamazepine (Tegretol) and oxcarbazepine (Trileptal)[1] are the best drugs for initial medical treatment of TN. Both should be started in relatively low doses, for example, 100 to 200 mg once or twice daily and then increased gradually and slowly until either satisfactory control of the pain or intolerable side effects occur. Such side effects include drowsiness, weakness, difficulty with recent memory, and unsteadiness of gait.

---

[1]Not FDA approved for this indication.

 CURRENT THERAPY

- Usually responds to oral anticonvulsant medications, such as carbamazepine (Tegretol) or oxcarbazepine (Trileptal).[1]
- Early radiosurgical treatment offers a good chance of curing the illness with minimal side effects.
- Microvascular decompression is the most effective surgical treatment of TN, but it is associated with the greatest risk of serious complications.

[1]Not FDA approved for this indication.

Older patients are particularly sensitive to such side effects, and the initial dose and maximum tolerable dose are usually lower in older patients, particularly those in their 70s and older. From 5 to 7 days should elapse between dosing increments in order to allow development of a stable blood level of medication. Additional increments of 100 to 200 mg/day are recommended. Laboratory tests of serum levels of the medications are of little or no help in the treatment of TN. In order to establish a consistent blood level of these medications and to provide the best chance for achieving lasting pain relief with minimum side effects, counseling of the patient by the physician regarding the correct dosing regimen is essential. Patients often regard these medications as analgesics and vary the dosage on an as-needed basis, some days taking little or no medication and other days taking large amounts. Because of their pharmacokinetics, these medications must be taken in a consistent dosage on a daily basis in order to maximize the chance of success. It is surprising how hard it may be for patients to understand and adhere to such a regimen, but maintaining the regimen is essential for successful pain relief. Gabapentin (Neurontin)[1] has become popular for the treatment of TN, but experience indicates it is a secondary medication only. It may be useful when pain control cannot be achieved with carbamazepine (Tegretol) or oxcarbazepine (Trileptal) or when those medications cannot be tolerated because of side effects. Other potential second-line medications include a variety of other anticonvulsants (e.g., lamotrigine [Lamictal],[1] phenytoin [Dilantin][1]) as well as baclofen (Lioresal). A variety of toxicities, including liver dysfunction, bone marrow suppression, and allergic reactions, may accompany use of these medications, so appropriate laboratory surveillance should be performed per manufacturers' recommendations.

SURGICAL TREATMENT

In the past, surgery was reserved for patients who did not respond to medical management of TN because the medication was ineffective or the side effects or toxicities were intolerable. However, some studies suggest that the longer the illness persists, the smaller the chance for lasting successful surgical relief of the pain. Many patients considered the potential side effects and complications of the surgical procedures unacceptable, and neurologists often referred patients for surgical procedures only as a last resort. With the advent of radiosurgery as a viable, successful, and safe surgical treatment of TN, consideration of surgical intervention earlier rather than later in the disease course may be better. Microvascular decompression (MVD) is the most effective, yet most dangerous, of the surgical procedures for TN. About 90% of patients will achieve immediate relief of TN after MVD, but this success rate drops to about 75% in long-term follow-up. MVD is the only surgical procedure that treats the putative cause of TN, namely, vascular compression of the trigeminal nerve root. In the MVD procedure, a small posterior fossa craniotomy is performed. The trigeminal nerve root is visualized using the operating microscope, any compressing vessels are dissected free of the nerve, and future contact is prevented by placing a shock-absorbing material, usually

shredded Teflon felt, between the vessel and the nerve. Fatal complications may occur in up to 1% of patients undergoing the MVD procedures. From 15% to 20% of patients who undergo MVD experience some complication of the procedure, such as cerebellar edema, brainstem infarction, subdural and epidural hematomas, facial paralysis, unilateral hearing loss, cerebrospinal fluid leakage, meningitis, and infection. Percutaneous procedures (e.g., radiofrequency electrocoagulation, glycerol rhizolysis, balloon compression) are considerably safer than MVD, but loss of facial sensation usually accompanies such procedures. Loss of facial sensation should be avoided in order to prevent secondary complications such as anesthesia dolorosa and loss of the corneal reflex with subsequent corneal ulceration or loss of vision. The initial success rate is about 90% with the percutaneous procedures, but recurrences are frequent. Serious side effects, such as meningitis, brain abscess or hematoma, and carotid artery to cavernous sinus fistulas, occasionally occur. One of the attractive features of percutaneous procedures is that they can be repeated fairly easily if pain recurs. Radiosurgery is gaining increased acceptance as a surgical method for treating TN. Although considered a form of surgery, the procedure is accomplished without an incision, instead using either gamma rays (Gamma Knife, Elekta, Inc.) or high-energy x-rays (linear accelerator [LINAC]) that are focused on the trigeminal nerve root adjacent to the brainstem. The treatment is planned using MRI or computed tomography scanning, and the radiation is guided to the target at the trigeminal nerve root in such a way as to avoid injury to adjacent structures. The procedure provides pain relief in about 60% of patients with TN without the need for medication; another 15% to 20% of patients experience pain relief with small tolerable doses of medication. Radiosurgery is attractive to patients and referring physicians because of the ease of performing the procedure and the minimum risk of side effects. Radiosurgery is a destructive form of treatment of TN, but the degree of damage to the nerve root is usually minimal enough that normal facial sensation is maintained. Permanent losses of facial sensation may occur in as few as 5% of patients treated with radiosurgery, depending on the dose of radiation used for the treatment. Drawbacks of radiosurgery include delayed onset of pain relief after treatment (usually a few months) and recurrences. Radiosurgery can be repeated in the event of initial failure of the treatment or in case of recurrence after an initially successful treatment. The reasonable success rate, the ease of performance of the procedure, and the minimal risk of side effects make radiosurgery a treatment that can be recommended early in the treatment of TN, once the diagnosis has been well established, because it may provide permanent cure of the disease with minimal risk.

REFERENCES

Bagheri SC, Fairhdvash F, Perciaccante VJ: Diagnosis and treatment of patients with trigeminal neuralgia. Am Dent Assoc 2004;135:1713-1717.

Kres B, Schindler M, Rasche D, et al: MRI volumetry for the preoperative diagnosis of trigeminal neuralgia. Eur Radiol 2005;15:1344-1348.

Liu JK, Apfelbaum RI: Treatment of trigeminal neuralgia. Neurosurg Clin North Am 2004;15:319-334.

---

[1]Not FDA approved for this indication.

Shetter AG, Aabramisk JM, Speiser BL: Microvascular decompression after gamma knife surgery for trigeminal neuralgia: intraoperative findings and treatment outcomes. J Neurosurg 2000;102(Suppl.):259-261.

Young RF: Stereotactic procedures for facial pain. In Apuzzo M (ed): Brain Surgery: Complication Avoidance and Management. New York, Churchill Livingstone, 1993, pp 2097-2114.

Young RF: Radiosurgery versus microsurgery for trigeminal neurlagia: current techniques in neurosurgery. In Salcman M (ed): Current Medicine. New York, Springer, 1998, pp 35-43.

Young RF, Vermeulen SS, Grimm P, et al: Gamma knife radiosurgery for treatment of trigeminal neuralgia: Idiopathic and tumor related. Neurology 1997;48:608-614.

Young RF, Vermeulen SS, Posewitz A: Gamma knife radiosurgery for treatment of trigeminal neuralgia. Stereotact Funct Neurosurg 1998;70:192-199.

Acute Facial Paralysis (Bell's Palsy)

Method of
Bruce J. Gantz, MD, Ted A. Meyer, MD, PhD, and Peter C. Weber, MD

Bell's palsy and *idiopathic facial paralysis* are synonymous terms for acute facial paralysis of unknown etiology. McCormick first postulated that Bell's palsy was caused by herpesvirus in 1972. More recently, Murakami and coworkers (1996) further substantiated this claim when they identified DNA fragments of herpes simplex virus type 1 (HSV-1) in the perineurial fluid of 11 of 14 subjects undergoing facial nerve decompression during the acute phase of the illness. Burgess and colleagues (1994) found HSV-1 DNA in a temporal bone section in the region of the geniculate ganglion in a patient who had died of other causes 6 days after the onset of Bell's palsy. These two independent pieces of evidence strongly support the concept that the facial paralysis known as Bell's palsy is caused by a viral infection that induces inflammatory edema within the facial nerve. The nerve lies within the bony fallopian canal as it traverses the temporal bone. The labyrinthine segment, which has a diameter of approximately 0.6 mm, lies just medial to the geniculate ganglion. As the facial nerve swells, it is constricted to the greatest extent in the labyrinthine segment, and the ensuing neural conduction block causes paralysis of the voluntary facial musculature seen in Bell's palsy. An animal model of Bell's palsy has also been developed by inoculating the auricles and tongues of mice with herpes simplex virus, providing further evidence that a viral infection is an important cause in this disease. Together, this information provides more than circumstantial support for a herpes simplex viral etiology of Bell's palsy. This article highlights the epidemiology, clinical manifestations, evaluation, and treatment of Bell's palsy, taking into account the new information regarding etiology.

Epidemiology

The incidence of Bell's palsy is approximately 30 cases per 100,000 individuals per year, thus making it the most common cause of unilateral facial paralysis. Approximately 40,000 cases occur in the United States each year. There appears to be no gender predilection, and the ages range from infancy to elderly, with manifestation in the fifth and sixth decades of life most common. Right- and left-sided facial palsies occur equally. Recurrence may be unilateral or contralateral in up to 10% of patients, but the physician should be alerted to perform a rigorous examination to rule out other causes. Pregnancy triples the risk, whereas hypertension and diabetes mellitus are associated with only a small increase in incidence. Roughly 10% have a familial orientation, and 70% of patients relate an upper respiratory tract infection preceding the onset.

Recovery begins within 3 weeks for 85% of the patients, with full recovery occurring in 6 months. Approximately 10% to 15% of patients are troubled with asymmetric movement, mass movement of all branches, or movement of the mouth when closing the eye (synkinesis). Only 4% to 6% of patients, however, experience severe deformity with minimal return of facial movement. Some of these patients are completely unable to close the eye. Identification of this poor recovery group using electrophysiologic testing must be accomplished within 2 weeks of the onset of complete paralysis. Delay beyond 2 weeks renders approximately 50% of this group with residual facial dysfunction for the rest of their lives.

Evaluation

A detailed history is mandatory for any patient with facial paralysis. Date of onset, duration of associated symptoms, and other precipitating factors are important to document. Many patients report an antecedent viral illness 7 to 10 days before the onset of paralysis. A description of otalgia associated with skin and auricular blebs or blisters is not Bell's palsy but rather herpes zoster oticus (Ramsay Hunt syndrome), which is best treated with antiviral agents (valacyclovir [Valtrex][1]). The facial paralysis in Bell's palsy may be abrupt or worsen over 2 to 3 days. It is not slowly progressive over weeks to months. Patients with Bell's palsy do not complain of facial twitching, decreased hearing, otorrhea, severe otalgia, or balance dysfunction. It is equally important to rule out recent trauma, tick bites (Lyme disease), or current ear infections.

Physical examination should confirm a facial paralysis of all branches. If the forehead is intact, a central etiology is of concern, whereas involvement of a single branch indicates a parotid tumor or trauma. The middle ear, tympanic membrane, and external canal should be normal. No aural or oral vesicular lesions should be seen. The parotid gland is palpated bimanually to ensure against a deep lobe tumor. All other cranial nerves should function normally, including cranial nerve V, even though patients may complain of vague facial numbness.

Audiometric evaluation is necessary for every patient. Unilateral hearing loss or acoustic reflex decay is suggestive of a cerebellopontine angle tumor and an indication for further retrocochlear evaluation. If vestibular complaints are present, an electronystagmogram (ENG) is obtained.

Although radiographic studies are important in patients with facial paralysis, it is not necessary to image all patients with acute facial paralysis immediately, especially

[1]Not FDA approved for this indication.

patients with classic symptoms of Bell's palsy. Imaging studies are obtained immediately if the signs and symptoms are not compatible with Bell's palsy or if no return of facial motion is observed at 6 months. Both high-resolution computed tomography (HRCT) and magnetic resonance imaging (MRI) with gadolinium are useful. Computed tomography (CT) allows better visualization of the fallopian canal and associated temporal bone structures. Magnetic resonance imaging can demonstrate inflammatory changes associated with Bell's palsy as well as tumors.

Electrodiagnosis

Electroneurography (ENog) and voluntary electromyography (EMG) are the two electrical diagnostic tests used most often to assess facial paralysis. ENog can estimate the amount of severe nerve fiber degeneration from an injury or conduction block, such as neurapraxia. It takes approximately 3 days for wallerian degeneration to occur after severe injury; therefore, ENog is not performed until more than 3 days after total paralysis. Electrical testing is not employed if a patient exhibits paresis, because the presence of even minimal voluntary motion after 3 days indicates minor injury, with full recovery to be expected.

ENog uses an electrical stimulus to activate the facial nerve as it exits the temporal bone at the stylomastoid foramen. Resulting facial movement generates a compound muscle action potential (CMAP) that is measured with surface electrodes. The amplitude of the CMAP biphasic response correlates with the number of remaining stimulatable fibers. The CMAP from the paralyzed side can be compared with the CMAP of the normal side. The percentage of functioning or degenerated nerve fibers can then be calculated. Degeneration of 90% or more of the fibers indicates poor recovery in more than 50% of patients. Conversely, if 90% of degeneration is not obtained by 2 weeks, a good prognosis is indicated. In addition to the percentage of degeneration, the time course of the degeneration is important. Patients reaching 90% degeneration within 5 days have a far worse prognosis than those who exhibit 90% degeneration in 2 to 3 weeks.

If the ENog demonstrates 100% degeneration and no CMAP is discernible, then voluntary EMG testing is performed, which measures voluntary motor activity: The patient is asked to make forceful facial muscle contractions, and the single motor unit action potentials are recorded. Because all nerve fibers must synchronously depolarize to generate a CMAP, no response may be seen on ENog, even when polyphasic potentials (a sign of regenerating nerve fibers) are noted on EMG. ENog is also not of benefit in long-standing facial paralysis (>3 weeks) because of polyphasic potentials when degeneration and regeneration are occurring. For similar reasons, ENog is not a useful diagnostic test for facial paralysis caused by tumors.

Treatment Protocols

The management of patients with idiopathic facial paralysis depends on a number of variables. An overview of our

treatment protocol is shown in the flow chart in Figure 1. This chart is a general guide. Alterations may be made on an individual basis depending on specific circumstances.

Patients with paresis (partial paralysis) seen within the initial 2 days of onset are treated with oral corticosteroids and antiviral medication. Electrodiagnostic evaluation is not performed until at least 3 days of total paralysis. Prednisone[1] is usually prescribed at 60 to 80 mg per day for 7 days without tapering, and the recommended dosage of valacyclovir (Valtrex)[1] is 500 mg three times per day for 7 days. Patients are re-evaluated within 5 days to assess the progress of the disease. If during the course of treatment complete flaccid paralysis ensues, the patient is managed according to the acute paralysis protocol (see Figure 1). Patients coming to medical attention more than 14 days after onset are followed with only intermittent examinations.

Patients with complete paralysis seen within the first 14 days are started on oral prednisone,[1] 60 to 80 mg per day, and valacyclovir (Valtrex),[1] 500 mg three times a day. ENog is performed no sooner than the third day after the onset of paralysis. If degeneration is less than 90%, medical management is continued for a full 7 days. ENog testing is repeated based on the percentage of degeneration until 2 weeks have elapsed from the date of onset of total paralysis. If more than 90% neural degeneration occurs within the 2-week period after complete paralysis, then surgical decompression of the internal auditory canal, labyrinthine segment, and tympanic portion of the facial nerve through a middle cranial fossa approach is recommended.

Surgical decompression of the facial nerve in Bell's palsy has been controversial since it was reported in 1932. Decompression of the mastoid segment of the nerve provides no benefit to severely degenerated facial nerves compared with the natural history of the disease. Decompression of the nerve medial to the geniculate ganglion, including the meatal foramen, through a middle cranial fossa craniotomy, improves facial nerve return in cases of severe degeneration. We have reported a series of patients with severely degenerated facial nerves that were decompressed through the middle fossa approach (Gantz and colleagues, 1999). Ninety-one percent of decompressed patients exhibited normal or near-normal return of facial function 6 months after the onset of their paralysis. A group of control patients electing not to undergo decompression exhibited normal or near-normal facial function in only 42% of the cases. This study demonstrates that surgical decompression of the meatal foramen and labyrinthine segment of the facial nerve in severely degenerated cases of Bell's palsy provides significantly improved return of facial function compared to those with similar neural degeneration not decompressed ($P = .0002$). Surgical decompression through the middle fossa more than 2 weeks after the onset of paralysis provided results similar to the control group and did not result in improved facial function. If ENog demonstrates 100% degeneration, voluntary EMG is performed to confirm that complete wallerian degeneration has occurred. EMG testing is also performed if patients come to medical attention more than 3 weeks after the onset of paralysis. EMG testing

---

[1]Not FDA approved for this indication.

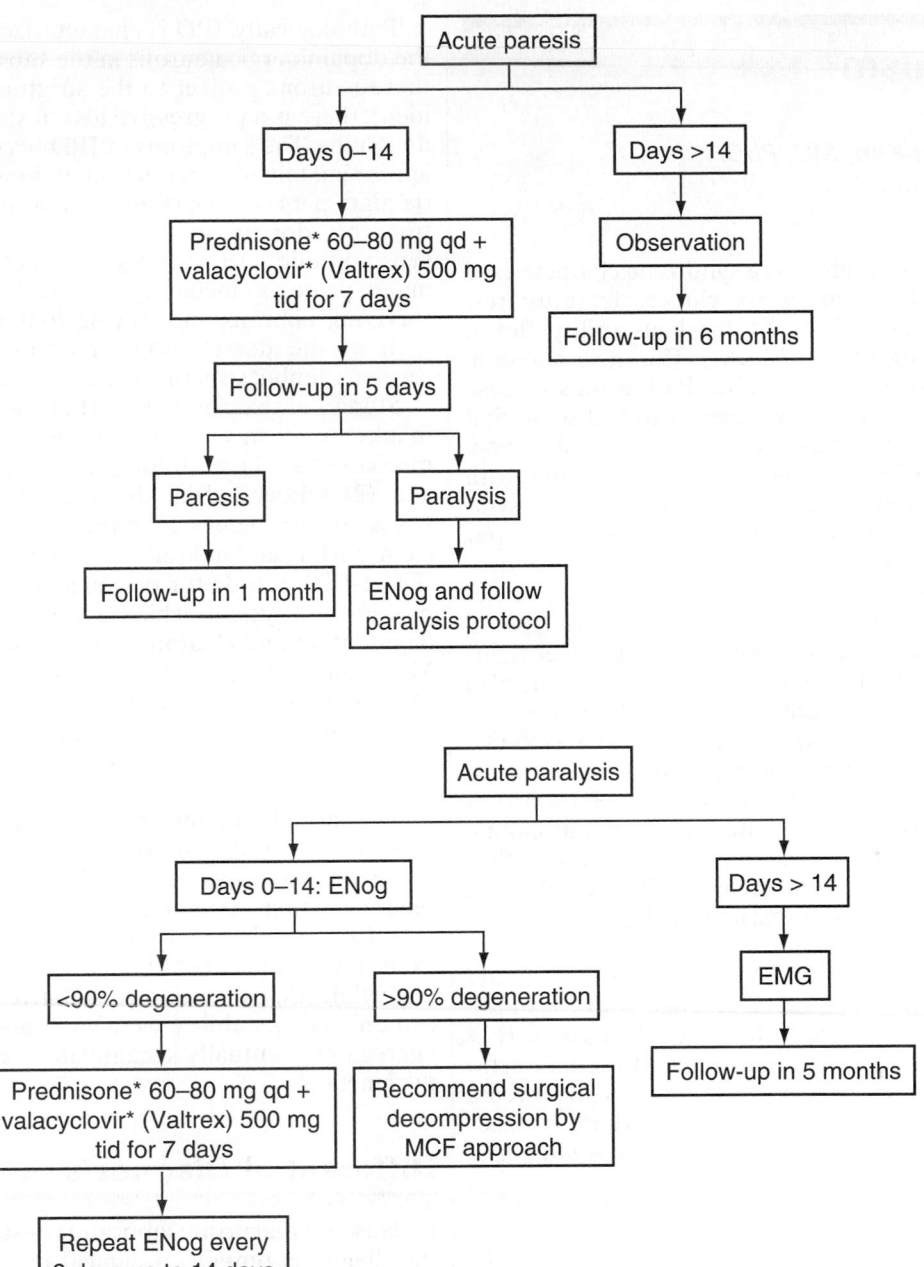

FIGURE 1. Acute facial paralysis flow chart. *Abbreviations*: EMG = electromyography; ENog = electroneurography; MCF = middle cranial fossa.

will demonstrate nerve regeneration with polyphasic potentials.

Preventive eye care is mandatory for all patients with Bell's palsy. Failure to keep the eye moist (with drops during the day and ointment/moisture chamber at night) may result in corneal abrasions and ulcers. Any problems that develop with the eye should be managed by an ophthalmologist. Bell's palsy invariably demonstrates some improvement by 6 months. If no movement is identified 6 months after the onset of paralysis, the original diagnosis of Bell's palsy should be questioned and imaging studies, to rule out a neoplastic process, must be performed.

Parkinsonism

Method of
*Julie Leegwater-Kim, MD, PhD,
and Cheryl Waters, MD*

The term *parkinsonism* refers to a syndrome characterized by any of a combination of six clinical features: rest tremor, bradykinesia, rigidity, postural instability, flexed posture, and freezing (motor blocks). The most common cause of parkinsonism is idiopathic Parkinson's disease (primary parkinsonism), a neurodegenerative disease first described by Dr. James Parkinson, an English physician, in 1817. The onset of Parkinson's disease is insidious, with approximately 70% of patients presenting with an asymmetrical 3- to 5-Hz resting tremor, usually of the upper extremity. Other signs are bradykinesia, slowing of movement, which manifests as difficulties with fine finger movements (e.g., tying shoelaces, buttoning buttons), decreased arm swing, hypophonia, and hypomimia. Cogwheel rigidity, a ratchet-like resistance to passive movement, also develops. Over time, the disease progresses to involve the contralateral side of the body, and postural instability, flexed posture, and freezing of gait eventually develop. In addition to the motor symptoms of idiopathic Parkinson's disease (IPD), patients frequently develop autonomic symptoms, such as constipation, urinary urgency, and orthostatic hypotension. Depression occurs in 50% of patients, and dementia can develop, especially in individuals with older age at onset.

The mean age at onset of IPD is 60 years. Both the prevalence and incidence increase with age, with 1% of the population older than 60 years affected by the disease. IPD affects men more than women, with a male-to-female ratio of 3:2. Onset of primary parkinsonism before age 20 years is referred to as *juvenile parkinsonism*, whereas onset between ages 20 and 40 years is known as *young-onset parkinsonism*.

Pathogenesis

The etiology is unknown in the vast majority of cases of IPD (sporadic Parkinson's disease), but epidemiologic data and the identification of novel genes in familial forms of the disease implicate a combination of environmental and genetic factors. The finding that l-methyl-4-phenyl-1,2,3,6-tetrahydropyridine (MPTP) intoxication can cause levodopa-responsive parkinsonism has suggested that similar environmental toxins play a role in the pathogenesis of IPD. Exposure to pesticides and herbicides, living in a rural environment, and drinking well water have been associated with an elevated risk of IPD. Cigarette smoking and consumption of caffeine appear to reduce the risk of developing IPD.

From 5% to 10% of cases of IPD are familial, and a number of genes have been identified in the pedigrees studied: α-synuclein (autosomal dominant), LRRK2 (autosomal dominant), parkin (autosomal recessive), DJ-1 (autosomal recessive), and PINK1 (autosomal recessive). Several of these genes encode proteins that appear to play roles in protein degradation (see following).

Pathologically, IPD is characterized by degeneration of the dopaminergic neurons in the substantia nigra. Because these neurons project to the striatum (caudate and putamen), there is a progressive loss of striatal as well as nigral dopamine. The symptoms of IPD become evident upon an approximately 60% reduction of dopamine in the substantia nigra pars compacta and an approximately 80% reduction of dopamine in the striatum. Lewy bodies (eosinophilic intracytoplasmic inclusions that contain many proteins, including α-synuclein) are seen in the surviving neurons and can be found in other structures, such as the dorsal motor nucleus of the vagus, locus ceruleus, limbic structures, and cortex.

Studies of toxic models of IPD and the genes implicated in inherited forms of IPD point to two major pathogenetic mechanisms: (1) misfolding and aggregation of proteins and (2) mitochondrial dysfunction leading to oxidative stress. Several genes identified in familial IPD (α-synuclein, parkin, and ubiquitin carboxy-terminal hydrolase L1 [UCH-L1]) encode for proteins involved in the ubiquitin-proteosome system, which is responsible for the normal degradation and clearance of proteins in eukaryotic cells. Mutations in these genes appear to be linked to mishandling and accumulation of proteins, which in turn lead to cell death. The potential role of mitochondrial dysfunction and subsequent oxidative stress in the pathogenesis of IPD was first suggested by the discovery that MPTP blocks the mitochondrial electron transport chain. Inhibition of this pathway can produce toxic products, including harmful reactive oxygen species that can cause cellular damage by reacting with proteins, lipids, and nucleic acids. It is important to recognize that these theories are not mutually exclusive, and they could be involved sequentially in causing cell death. For example, oxidative stress to α-synuclein can enhance its ability to misfold and aggregate, and the aggregates eventually accumulate because of proteosomal dysfunction.

Differential Diagnosis

Because no diagnostic laboratory test for IPD is available, the diagnosis remains a clinical one. Distinguishing IPD from other causes of parkinsonism is paramount because prognosis and treatment options vary according to disease. The most helpful clinical signs supporting a diagnosis of IPD are asymmetry of presentation, presence of resting tremor, absence of atypical clinical features (i.e., cerebellar dysfunction, pyramidal signs), and clear improvement with levodopa/carbidopa (Sinemet) therapy. A number of neurologic diseases can often mimic IPD and therefore deserve mention (Table 1).

Drug-induced parkinsonism (DIP) can occur with exposure to dopamine receptor-blocking agents, such as antipsychotic medications (e.g., haloperidol [Haldol]) and antiemetic agents (e.g., metoclopramide [Reglan]). Because DIP can be reversed with discontinuation of the offending drug, it is important to carefully review the patient's current medications when investigating possible causes of parkinsonism. Symptoms of DIP tend to be symmetrical. When DIP is suspected, the dopamine receptor-blocking agent should be stopped, if possible, or substituted with an atypical neuroleptic with a low incidence of extrapyramidal side effects (e.g., quetiapine [Seroquel]). The symptoms

- *Parkinsonism* refers to a syndrome characterized by any or a combination of six clinical features: resting tremor, bradykinesia, rigidity, postural instability, flexed posture, and freezing (motor blocks).
- Idiopathic Parkinson's disease (IPD) is the most common cause of parkinsonism.
- The vast majority of cases of IPD are sporadic. The etiology of IPD is hypothesized to involve a complex interaction between environmental and genetic factors.
- The pathologic hallmarks of IPD are loss of dopaminergic neurons in the substantia nigra pars compacta and the presence of Lewy bodies (intracytoplasmic eosinophilic inclusions).
- Asymmetry of presentation, presence of resting tremor, absence of atypical signs (i.e., ataxia, pyramidal signs), and clear response to levodopa/carbidopa (Sinemet) are important features in distinguishing IPD from other forms of parkinsonism.

of DIP usually resolve within weeks to months after discontinuation of the drug.

Essential tremor (ET) is a disorder characterized by a 4- to 12-Hz tremor usually beginning in the arms. Unlike Parkinson's disease, the tremor of ET is a kinetic tremor (brought on by an action such as finger-to-nose testing). There is often a postural tremor as well, which is usually bilateral at onset. Common presenting complaints include difficulty drinking from a cup or spoon or spilling while pouring. The handwriting of patients with ET is large and tremulous, not micrographic. In 30% to 50% of patients, tremor may spread to involve the neck (head); in rare cases

TABLE 1 Classification of Parkinsonism

Primary Parkinsonism (Idiopathic Parkinson's Disease)
- Sporadic
- Familial

Secondary Parkinsonism
- Drug-induced (i.e., dopamine receptor–blocking agents)
- Vascular
- Normal pressure hydrocephalus
- Toxin-induced (i.e., manganese)
- Infectious
- Postencephalitic
- Structural lesion (i.e., tumor)

Parkinson-Plus Syndromes/Atypical Parkinsonism
- Progressive supranuclear palsy
- Multiple system atrophy
- Corticobasal ganglionic degeneration
- Dementia with Lewy bodies

Heredodegenerative Disorders
- Frontotemporal dementia
- Wilson's disease
- Huntington's disease

there is isolated head tremor. A family history of tremor in an autosomal dominant pattern is common. Another distinguishing feature of ET is that the tremor can often be temporarily improved by alcohol. Bradykinesia, rigidity, and loss of postural reflexes are absent.

The Parkinson-plus syndromes—progressive supranuclear palsy, multiple system atrophy, corticobasal ganglionic degeneration, and dementia with Lewy body disease—are rare neurodegenerative diseases that are often confused with IPD, especially in their early stages. The presence of atypical clinical features and the lack of response to levodopa therapy are key in helping to distinguish between these diseases and IPD. Progressive supranuclear palsy typically presents with postural instability and recurrent falls. A supranuclear gaze palsy, usually affecting downgaze first, develops, and truncal rigidity with nuchal extensor rigidity predominates. Patients often have an "astonished" facial expression and deepened nasolabial folds. Multiple system atrophy is a sporadically occurring neurodegenerative disease characterized by a variable combination of parkinsonism, cerebellar dysfunction, pyramidal signs, and autonomic dysfunction. Unlike IPD, autonomic dysfunction occurs early in the clinical course and tends to be severe. Stridor can develop, and some patients exhibit the "cold hands sign": dusky violaceous fingers with delayed capillary refill after blanching. Corticobasal ganglionic degeneration typically presents asymmetrically with gradual development of stiffness, jerking, and cortical sensory loss in a limb, usually the arm. Cortical reflex myoclonus and apraxia develop in the affected limb. Over time, other limbs become involved. Dementia with Lewy body disease is characterized by parkinsonism and dementia. Although dementia can also be seen in IPD, the dementia of dementia with Lewy body disease occurs early on in the course and is associated with prominent hallucinations and delusions and fluctuations in mental status.

Normal pressure hydrocephalus and vascular parkinsonism typically present with a predominantly lower body type of parkinsonism. Normal pressure hydrocephalus is classically defined by a clinical triad of gait disturbance, urinary incontinence, and dementia, although many cases can present with isolated gait disturbance. The gait is usually wide based and shuffling, with features of gait apraxia and prominent retropulsion. Gait dysfunction can improve after a large-volume lumbar puncture or lumbar drain trial. Vascular parkinsonism results from multiple lacunar infarcts of the basal ganglia. Patients often have a wide-based apraxic gait with frequent freezing. Neither normal pressure hydrocephalus nor vascular parkinsonism demonstrates a significant clinical response to levodopa therapy. When these diseases are suspected, brain magnetic resonance imaging (MRI) should be obtained as part of the workup.

Other rarer causes of parkinsonism should be considered if indicated by history. Toxin exposure (i.e., carbon monoxide poisoning, manganese intoxication), head trauma, structural brain lesions, and infection can produce parkinsonism. Brain imaging is important in ruling out these etiologies.

The differential diagnosis of parkinsonism in pediatric patients and young adults should include heredodegenerative and metabolic diseases. Wilson's disease, an autosomal recessive disorder characterized by abnormal copper metabolism, should be considered in all young-onset cases of parkinsonism because the disease is treatable. Dysarthria, dystonia, and ataxia are common accompanying symptoms. Ophthalmologic examination with slit lamp to rule out Kayser-Fleischer rings (present in 100% of Wilson's disease patients with neurologic symptoms), serum ceruloplasmin, and 24-hour urine copper should be obtained to rule out this disorder. Brain MRI can reveal evidence of copper deposition within the basal ganglia. Pantothenate kinase-associated neurodegeneration (formerly called Hallervorden-Spatz disease), a genetic disorder involving a disturbance of iron metabolism, can present with parkinsonism. Dystonia is also a prominent feature. Brain MRI should be obtained to look for evidence of iron deposition in the basal ganglia. Genetic testing for PANK2, a gene implicated in pantothenate kinase-associated neurodegeneration, is now available. Juvenile Huntington's disease, unlike the adult-onset form, often presents with parkinsonism and should be considered in any patient with a family history suggestive of this disorder. Genetic testing is diagnostic.

CURRENT THERAPY

- Treatment of idiopathic Parkinson's disease (IPD) consists of improving motor symptoms and treating nonmotor symptoms, such as autonomic dysfunction, depression, psychosis, dementia, and sleep disturbance.
- Pharmacologic therapy for early IPD should begin when motor symptoms become disabling or sufficiently bothersome.
- Treatment of motor symptoms in early IPD usually begins with either carbidopa/levodopa (Sinemet) or dopamine agonist (e.g., pramipexole [Mirapex]) monotherapy because these drugs provide the greatest symptomatic benefit. In general, dopamine agonist monotherapy is preferred in younger patients, whereas levodopa/carbidopa (Sinemet) monotherapy is preferred in elderly patients (>70 years).
- As IPD progresses, motor complications develop, including wearing-off, on–off phenomena, and dyskinesias. A variety of approaches can be used to smooth out motor fluctuations. Wearing-off can be treated with more frequent levodopa dosing, use of extended-release levodopa/carbidopa (Sinemet CR), addition of a catechol-*O*-methyltransferase inhibitor, or addition of a dopamine agonist. On–off phenomena can be treated with liquefied levodopa/carbidopa (Sinemet). Dyskinesias can be reduced by lowering the levodopa dose or by adding amantadine (Symmetrel) or clozapine (Clozaril).[1]
- Surgical therapy for IPD includes deep brain stimulation and ablative techniques. Appropriate selection of patients for these procedures is crucial. Clinical features that have been associated with successful outcomes include clinically definite IPD, good clinical response to levodopa, persistent disabling medically intractable motor fluctuations, intact cognitive status, and younger age.

[1]Not FDA approved for this indication.

Treatment

Treatment of IPD includes both nonpharmacologic and pharmacologic therapies (Table 2). A regular exercise regimen is important for both medical and psychologic well-being, and physical therapy is helpful in maintaining range of motion and flexibility and in gait and balance training. Speech therapy can improve dysarthria and hypophonia. Psychologic support to patients and families is critical and support groups are important resources. Pharmacologic treatment of IPD comprises neuroprotective strategies and symptomatic treatment of both motor and nonmotor symptoms.

TABLE 2   Treatment Strategies in Idiopathic Parkinson's Disease

Nonpharmacologic
- Regular exercise
- Physical therapy
- Speech therapy
- Psychosocial support

Pharmacologic
Motor symptoms
- Levodopa/carbidopa (Sinemet)
- Dopamine agonists
- Anticholinergics
- Selegiline (Eldepryl)
- Amantadine (Symmetrel)

Motor fluctuations
- Wearing-off
  - More frequent levodopa/carbidopa (Sinemet) dosing
  - Extended-release levodopa/carbidopa (Sinemet CR)
  - Add dopamine agonist
  - Add catechol-*O*-methyltransferase inhibitor
  - Selegiline (Eldepryl), rasagiline[*]
- On–off phenomena
  - Liquefied levodopa/carbidopa (Sinemet)
  - Intraduodenal infusion of levodopa[1]
  - Apomorphine (Apokyn)
- Dyskinesias
  - Reduce levodopa/carbidopa (Sinemet) dose
  - Amantadine (Symmetrel)
  - Clozapine (Clozaril)[1]

Nonmotor symptoms
- Orthostatic hypotension
  - Increase salt and fluid intake
  - Midodrine (ProAmatine)
  - Fludrocortisone (Florinef)[1]
- Urinary urgency/frequency
  - Oxybutynin (Ditropan)
- Constipation
  - High-fiber diet
  - Stool softeners, laxatives
- Depression
  - Selective serotonin reuptake inhibitor antidepressants
  - Tricyclic antidepressants
- Psychosis
  - Quetiapine (Seroquel), clozapine (Clozaril)[1]
- Dementia
  - Cholinesterase inhibitors

[1]Not FDA approved for this indication.
[*]Investigational drug in the United States.

NEUROPROTECTION

To date, no drug has been categorically proven to retard the progression of or reverse the course of IPD. Selegiline (Eldepryl),[1] a monoamine oxidase type B inhibitor, and vitamin E were evaluated in the Deprenyl and Tocopherol Antioxidative Therapy of Parkinsonism (DATATOP) study, a placebo-controlled trial that studied the potential neuroprotective effects of each drug separately and in combination in patients with early IPD. Vitamin E conferred no neuroprotective benefit in IPD. Selegiline delayed the onset of disability and levodopa therapy, but this finding was confounded by the fact that selegiline has mild symptomatic effects. Coenzyme Q10[1,*] was studied in a small, double-blind, placebo-controlled trial, which showed a trend toward slowed symptom progression in early IPD at a dose of 1200 mg/day. However, larger and longer-term studies are needed to confirm this finding.

SYMPTOMATIC TREATMENT OF MOTOR SYMPTOMS

Pharmacologic treatment of IPD should be initiated when motor symptoms are sufficiently bothersome or cause functional disability. In general, tremor, bradykinesia, and rigidity are responsive to treatments, whereas postural instability, flexed posture, and freezing of gait are more intractable to treatment. The two mainstays of therapy are levodopa/carbidopa (Sinemet) and the dopamine agonist (DA) drugs, as these medications have the greatest symptomatic benefit. Selegiline (Eldepryl) monotherapy[1] has mild symptomatic benefit. Amantadine (Symmetrel), an N-methyl-D-aspartate (NMDA) antagonist, provides modest symptom relief in approximately two thirds of patients with early IPD. Selegiline (Eldepryl) can be started as a 5-mg dose at breakfast for 1 week and increased to two 5-mg doses taken in the morning and at noon. Amantadine (Symmetrel) can be given at a dose of 100 mg up to four times per day. Anticholinergic drugs such as trihexyphenidyl (Artane) can be especially effective for tremor but should be used with caution in the elderly because of the tendency of anticholinergic drugs to cause confusion and cognitive disturbance. Trihexyphenidyl (Artane) can be started at 2 mg/day and increased to 2 to 5 mg three times per day.

The choice of whether to start levodopa/carbidopa (Sinemet) or a DA in patients with early IPD is controversial. Important consideration should be given to the patient's age, cognitive status, lifestyle, and degree of impairment. Because DAs are less likely to induce dyskinesia and they have good symptomatic efficacy in mild disease, DA monotherapy is preferred in younger patients with early IPD, as this population is more prone to the development of levodopa-induced motor fluctuations and dyskinesias. In addition, the side effects of DAs (hallucinations, somnolence, obsessive-compulsive behaviors) are usually better tolerated by younger patients. Conversely, levodopa monotherapy is the preferred first-line treatment in elderly patients (older than 70 years) because levodopa-induced motor complications are less likely to develop in this population, and the potential side effects, especially hallucinations, are better tolerated than those associated with the DAs.

DAs directly stimulate dopamine receptors and do not require metabolic conversion to active metabolites. The available DAs—pramipexole (Mirapex), ropinirole (Requip), pergolide (Permax), cabergoline (Dostinex),* bromocriptine (Parlodel), and apomorphine (Apokyn)—all activate the D2 receptors. Bromocriptine, pergolide, and cabergoline are ergot derivatives and carry the rare but serious risk of retroperitoneal, pulmonary, and cardiac valve fibrosis. A yearly transthoracic echocardiogram is advised to monitor for valvular disease. Among the nonergot DAs, pramipexole and ropinirole are used most commonly. Pramipexole (Mirapex) is started at 0.125 mg three times per day and increased slowly over 4 to 5 weeks to 3 mg/day. Ropinirole (Requip) is started at 0.25 mg three times per day and is usually titrated to 12 mg/day over a 7-week period. Cabergoline (Dostinex) has the longest half-life of the DAs; it is used in Europe but is not approved for IPD in the United States. Apomorphine (Apokyn), a potent D1/D2 agonist, is not available in oral form and must be injected or given sublingually. Recently, it has been developed as a "rescue" therapy in IPD patients with predictable "off" periods. Rotigotine,[†] a nonergot DA, is currently being studied as the first transdermally delivered DA.

The DAs have similar side-effect profiles, including nausea, sleepiness, orthostatic hypotension, leg edema, hallucinations, and obsessive-compulsive behaviors. Both pramipexole (Mirapex) and ropinirole (Requip) carry the rare risk of sleep attacks. Obsessive-compulsive behaviors include compulsive eating, spending, hypersexuality, hoarding, and gambling. Because these behaviors are not often volunteered by the patient and can be harmful to both the patient and his or her family, the physician should always ask the patient and the caregiver or spouse about these potential side effects. The side-effect spectrum of DAs varies among patients, so if one DA is not tolerated, another should be tried.

Levodopa/carbidopa (Sinemet) remains the most potent drug used for treatment of the symptoms of IPD. Levodopa, the precursor of dopamine, is administered with carbidopa, a peripheral decarboxylase inhibitor that inhibits the conversion of levodopa to dopamine. Side effects of levodopa/carbidopa (Sinemet) include nausea, vomiting, orthostasis, somnolence, and hallucinations. Long-term levodopa use has been linked to the development of motor fluctuations and dyskinesias. Levodopa/carbidopa (Sinemet) is available in standard-release (Sinemet 10/100, 25/100, 25/250) and extended-release forms (Sinemet CR 25/100, 50/200) as well as a disintegrating tablet form (Parcopa 10/100, 25/100, 25/250). The extended-release form provides a longer plasma half-life and lower peak plasma levels by slowly releasing the drug from a matrix. Standard-release levodopa/carbidopa (Sinemet) is started at half to one tablet 25/100 three times daily and increased gradually to a dose that gives optimal symptomatic benefit. Alternatively, extended-release levodopa/carbidopa (Sinemet CR) can be started at 25/100 three times daily and titrated to benefit. Despite the longer half-life, extended-release levodopa/carbidopa

---

[1]Not FDA approved for this indication.
*Available as a dietary supplement.

*Not available in this form.
[†]Investigational drug in the United States.

(Sinemet CR) has not been shown to delay the development of levodopa-induced motor complications. In elderly patients, extended-release levodopa/carbidopa (Sinemet CR) may be preferred because the lower rate of absorption and lower peak plasma level decrease the likelihood of peak-dose confusion or somnolence. The side effects of levodopa/carbidopa (Sinemet) include nausea, vomiting, somnolence, orthostasis, and hallucinations. Nausea and vomiting can often be relieved by administration of levodopa/carbidopa (Sinemet) with meals. If this is unsuccessful, addition of carbidopa (Lodosyn) can be helpful. Carbidopa (Lodosyn) is available in 25-mg tablets and can be given with each levodopa/carbidopa (Sinemet) dose. At doses of 150 mg/day, carbidopa (Lodosyn) may enter the brain and block central conversion of levodopa to dopamine, so care should be taken not to exceed this value. Domperidone (Motilium),[2] a peripheral dopamine antagonist, can also be given with levodopa/carbidopa (Sinemet) to relieve nausea and vomiting. Hallucinations and delusions can be troublesome side effects of both levodopa/carbidopa (Sinemet) and the DAs, and they can be effectively treated with the atypical neuroleptics quetiapine (Seroquel)[1] and clozapine (Clozaril).[1]

The development of motor fluctuations in IPD is well known, and management of these complications can be challenging. Approximately 25% to 50% of patients taking levodopa will develop motor fluctuations after 5 years of therapy, and this risk increases substantially with younger age of onset. Although the exact mechanism underlying the development of motor complications is unclear, findings suggest that both the progression of disease and levodopa therapy play a role. Early on, motor complications occur in a predictable pattern. The earliest symptom is end-of-dose "wearing-off," in which the same dose of levodopa lasts for a shorter period, and the antiparkinson effect wears off before the next dose is taken. Patients become slower, stiffer, and more tremulous. In addition, they may have nonmotor wearing-off symptoms, including cognitive changes, depression, and autonomic and sensory disturbances. Over time, patients may develop "on–off" phenomena, consisting of sudden, unpredictable shifts between mobility and immobility. Dyskinesias are involuntary movements that can occur after years of levodopa therapy. Peak-dose dyskinesia, the most common type, consists of choreiform movements of the head, trunk, and limbs. Diphasic dyskinesias occur in 15% to 20% of patients receiving chronic levodopa therapy and consist of dyskinetic movements that occur at the beginning and end of each dose.

A number of different strategies reduce motor fluctuations and "smooth out" the patient's clinical course. Wearing-off can be treated in a variety of ways. Perhaps the simplest approach is to give levodopa more frequently. Another option is to substitute extended-release levodopa/carbidopa (Sinemet CR) for regular levodopa/carbidopa (Sinemet). The major disadvantage to this approach is that absorption of the extended-release form is often unpredictable. Catechol-O-methyltransferase (COMT) inhibitors function to lengthen the half-life of levodopa by inhibiting its catabolism. The available COMT inhibitors

are entacapone (Comtan) and tolcapone (Tasmar). Tolcapone (Tasmar) is the more potent inhibitor with a half-life of 2 hours (versus 1 hour for entacapone [Comtan]), but rare cases of acute hepatotoxicity have limited its use. Liver function tests must be monitored closely, every 2 weeks in the first year of use. Explosive diarrhea has been associated with tolcapone (Tasmar). Entacapone (Comtan) can cause a benign orange discoloration of the urine. Tolcapone (Tasmar) can be administered 100 to 200 mg three times per day. Entacapone (Comtan) is available in 200-mg tablets and can be given up to eight times per day. Recently, a combination tablet of levodopa/carbidopa/entacapone (Stalevo) was approved and is available in 12.5/50/200 (Stalevo 50), 25/100/200 mg (Stalevo 100), and 37.5/150/200 mg (Stalevo 150). DAs can also be added to smooth out motor complications. They should be used with caution in the elderly. Because DAs enhance the effects of levodopa, levodopa doses may need to be decreased gradually with titration of DA. Rasagiline, a second-generation irreversible monoamine oxidase type B inhibitor, has been shown to reduce levodopa-induced motor complications as well. Two recent phase III trials (Lasting Effect in Adjunct Therapy with Rasagiline Given Once Daily [LARGO] and Parkinson's Rasagiline: Efficacy and Safety in the Treatment of "Off" [PRESTO]) have found that adjunctive rasagiline therapy in patients with levodopa-induced motor fluctuations reduced the off state by at least 1 hour per day. In a recent double-blind randomized trial of Zydis selegiline,[‡] a dissolvable form of selegiline that undergoes pregastric absorption, patients taking the drug were found to have significant reduction in daily off time when compared with placebo. Currently, investigation of the adenosine A_{2A} receptor antagonist istradefylline* (KW-6002) is being studied as a potential agent in reducing wearing-off periods.

Treatment of on–off phenomena and "yo-yoing" (a combination of fluctuations and dyskinesias) can be challenging and relies on smooth activation of dopamine receptors throughout the day. One approach involves use of liquefied levodopa/carbidopa (Sinemet). The patient makes a solution of levodopa/carbidopa (Sinemet) and takes small sips of the solution throughout the day. Levodopa/carbidopa (Sinemet) is not stable at room temperature unless it is in an acidified solution. Patients can dissolve tablets in ascorbic acid solution or dietetic soda. Liquefied levodopa/carbidopa (Sinemet) should be prepared fresh daily in a 1 mg/1 mL concentration (four tablets of 25/250 levodopa/carbidopa in 1 L of liquid). A more invasive strategy for treating on–off phenomena involves infusion of levodopa through an intraduodenal pump.[1]

Sudden off periods and dose failures can be treated with liquefied levodopa/carbidopa (Sinemet) or subcutaneous apomorphine (Apokyn). Administration of apomorphine (Apokyn) requires treatment with an antiemetic for 3 days before injection. Onset of action is relatively rapid (<20 minutes) and lasts up to 40 minutes. Side effects include hypotension, chest discomfort, dyskinesias, and yawning.

Effective therapies for dyskinesias include reduction of the levodopa dose and addition of amantadine or clozapine.

---

[1]Not FDA approved for this indication.
[2]Not available in the United States.

*Investigational drug in the United States.
[1]Not FDA approved for this indication.

Amantadine (Symmetrel) has been shown to reduce dyskinesias in patients with advanced IPD by 60% when compared with placebo. Its antidyskinetic effect has been attributed to inhibition of the NMDA receptor. Clozapine (Clozaril)[1] has also been shown to suppress levodopa-induced dyskinesias. In a recent double-blind, placebo-controlled trial of 50 patients, there was a significant reduction in "on" levodopa-induced dyskinesias at a mean dosage of 39.4 mg/day. The main drawback to clozapine (Clozaril) administration is the 1% to 2% risk of agranulocytosis, which warrants frequent blood monitoring.

SYMPTOMATIC TREATMENT OF NONMOTOR SYMPTOMS

In addition to motor symptoms, patients with IPD experience nonmotor complications, such as autonomic disturbances, sleep disorders, depression, psychosis, and dementia. Autonomic symptoms include orthostatic hypotension, urinary frequency and urgency, constipation, and sexual dysfunction. Orthostatic hypotension can occur as a result of the IPD itself or as a complication of levodopa and DA therapies. Increased salt and fluid intake should be tried first. If these conservative measures are unsuccessful, medications such as fludrocortisone (Florinef)[1] 0.1 to 0.5 mg/day or midodrine (ProAmatine) 2.5 to 10 mg three times per day can be tried. Urinary symptoms are usually a result of detrusor hyperreflexia and can be helped by a peripheral anticholinergic medication such as oxybutynin (Ditropan) 5 to 10 mg/day. Low-dose amitriptyline (Elavil) 25 mg at bedtime can also be considered in a patient with concomitant depression or insomnia.[1] Both drugs should be avoided in the elderly population because anticholinergic effects can lead to cognitive disturbance. Constipation is a frequent complaint in patients with IPD. Regular exercise and adequate fluid and fiber intake should be encouraged. Stool softeners, such as docusate sodium (Colace) 100 mg two to three times per day and polyethylene glycol (MiraLax) 17 g per day, are also effective. Sexual dysfunction is not uncommon in patients with IPD, but its occurrence is frequently not volunteered by the patient. Oral medications, such as sildenafil (Viagra), can be helpful but may exacerbate hypotension.

Sleep difficulties in patients with IPD are common and can be due to rapid eye movement (REM) sleep behavior disorder, periodic leg movements of sleep, restless legs syndrome, motor symptoms (e.g., difficulty turning in bed), and daytime somnolence. A nighttime dose of clonazepam (Klonopin)[1] 0.5 mg is helpful in treating REM behavior disorder. Propoxyphene (Darvon)[1] has been effective in treating restless legs syndrome. A dose of extended-release levodopa/carbidopa (Sinemet CR) 25/100 or 50/200 can help relieve nighttime motor symptoms. Daytime somnolence is a common complaint and can be a result of the IPD itself or of certain medications; I prefer to prescribe levodopa/carbidopa (Sinemet) and DAs. The activating agent modafinil (Provigil)[1] can be useful in combating daytime sleepiness. As mentioned previously, sleep attacks have been reported as a rare side effect of pramipexole (Mirapex) and ropinirole (Requip). If sleep attacks occur, driving should be curtailed, and the medication should be changed.

Depression is common in individuals with IPD, affecting nearly half of all patients. The causes are likely twofold: reactive depression and depression secondary to disease pathology. The selective serotonin reuptake inhibitors (SSRIs) fluoxetine (Prozac) and citalopram (Celexa) have been used safely and successfully in many IPD patients. Tricyclic antidepressants are less commonly used because their anticholinergic and antiadrenergic effects can cause confusion and hypotension, respectively. In the patient refractory to medication treatment, electroconvulsive shock therapy may be necessary.

Psychosis in IPD is usually due to antiparkinsonian medications, but intercurrent illness should always be considered as a cause. DAs, levodopa/carbidopa (Sinemet), anticholinergic drugs, and amantadine (Symmetrel) can all cause hallucinations. Management of psychosis should include discontinuing anticholinergic drugs, amantadine (Symmetrel), and DAs and using the lowest effective levodopa dose possible. If an antipsychotic medication is needed, the atypical neuroleptic medications quetiapine (Seroquel)[1] or clozapine (Clozaril)[1] should be started, as these agents have a low risk of exacerbating parkinsonism. Because clozapine (Clozaril) requires regular blood monitoring to prevent the serious risk of agranulocytosis, quetiapine (Seroquel) is the antipsychotic prescribed by most practitioners. Quetiapine (Seroquel) is started at 12.5 to 25 mg and should be given at night because of its potential to cause drowsiness. The dose can be titrated until symptomatic benefit is achieved. If quetiapine (Seroquel) is ineffective or cannot be tolerated, clozapine (Clozaril) should be tried next, starting with 12.5 mg at bedtime and titrating to effect. Baseline white blood cell (WBC) and differential counts must be obtained before clozapine (Clozaril) treatment. During treatment, WBC counts should be monitored every week for the first 6 months, every 2 weeks for the next 6 months, and monthly thereafter. Recent studies comparing the atypical neuroleptics and placebo in the treatment of elderly demented patients with behavioral disorders found a 1.6- to 1.7-fold increase in mortality in patients taking the atypical antipsychotics. Patients should be warned about this possible side effect, and both quetiapine (Seroquel) and clozapine (Clozaril) should be used at the minimum effective dose.

Dementia is encountered frequently in patients with IPD, with an average prevalence of 40%. Risk factors include advanced age, longer duration of disease, and older age at onset of disease. Recent data suggest that cholinesterase inhibitors can improve cognitive function in IPD patients with dementia without significantly worsening IPD symptoms. The available cholinesterase inhibitors are donepezil (Aricept),[1] rivastigmine (Exelon),[1] and galantamine (Razadyne).[1] The main side effects (nausea, vomiting, and diarrhea) are related to the cholinergic action of these agents. Memantine (Namenda),[1] an NMDA receptor antagonist, has recently been approved for moderate to severe Alzheimer's dementia. It has yet to be studied in patients with IPD, but anecdotal reports suggest a benefit in IPD patients with dementia.

---

[1]Not FDA approved for this indication.

[1]Not FDA approved for this indication.

SURGICAL THERAPY

Advances in the understanding of both the pathophysiology of IPD and the circuitry of the basal ganglia have led to the development of surgical treatments of IPD. Current surgical approaches include ablative techniques and deep brain stimulation (DBS). Ablative surgery involves stereotactic lesioning of specific areas of the basal ganglia. Unilateral pallidotomy has been shown to alleviate tremor and levodopa-induced dyskinesias. Bilateral pallidotomies, however, have been associated with significant morbidity (hypophonia, dysarthria, and cognitive deterioration) and are rarely performed. Subthalamotomy has not been studied widely because of concerns about inducement of hemiballism, but preliminary data suggest motor improvement comparable to that with pallidotomy. Unilateral lesioning of the ventral intermediate nucleus of the thalamus is highly effective in improving parkinsonian tremor but does not improve bradykinesia or rigidity.

Ablative procedures are gradually being replaced by DBS, as the latter is a reversible procedure and can be performed bilaterally. Moreover, the stimulation parameters are adjustable. In DBS, high-frequency stimulation is delivered to a precise target in the basal ganglia, effectively mimicking a lesion. The exact mechanism by which DBS exerts its effects is unclear. Thalamic DBS, like thalamotomy, has been shown to be very effective in the relief of tremor, with no significant benefit with regard to other symptoms of IPD. The main side effect of stimulation of the ventral intermediate nucleus of the thalamus is dysarthria, which occurs in 20% of patients. DBS of the internal globus pallidus improves all of the cardinal motor symptoms of IPD and suppresses levodopa-induced dyskinesias. Complications associated with DBS of the internal globus pallidus include rare reports of mood disorder and cognitive decline. DBS of the subthalamic nucleus, like stimulation of the internal globus pallidus, is effective in alleviating all the motor symptoms of IPD. Moreover, stimulation of the subthalamic nucleus has been associated with reduced levodopa requirements after surgery. However, stimulation of the subthalamic nucleus has been associated with more reports of adverse effects on mood and cognition. Although no prospective randomized double-blind trials have compared stimulation of the internal globus pallidus with stimulation of the subthalamic nucleus, stimulation of the subthalamic nucleus has become the preferred choice because it appears to be the best target for controlling bradykinesia and allows for subsequent reduction of the levodopa dosage.

The efficacy of surgical therapy for Parkinson's disease is critically dependent on the appropriate selection of patients. Patients with a clear response to levodopa therapy and clinically definite IPD have better outcomes with surgical therapy. Patients with medically intractable motor fluctuations, drug-induced dyskinesias, and on–off phenomena may have good response to surgery. The cognitive status of all patients should be assessed by neuropsychologic testing prior to surgery, because patients with significant cognitive impairment tend to have worse outcomes. Any premorbid psychiatric disturbances (depression, anxiety) should be adequately treated before surgery. In general, younger patients tend to do better after surgery because of fewer comorbid illnesses, but there is no absolute age cutoff. Finally, because DBS requires close clinical follow-up for parameter adjustment, a history of good patient compliance and adequate family support are critical.

REFERENCES

Fahn S: Description of Parkinson's disease as a clinical syndrome. Ann NY Acad Sci 2003;991:1-14.
Jankovic JJ, Tolosa E (eds): Parkinson's Disease and Movement Disorders, 4th ed. Philadelphia, Lippincott, Williams & Wilkins, 2002.
Pahwa R, Lyons KE, Koller WC (eds): Handbook of Parkinson's disease, 3rd ed. New York, Marcel Dekker, 2003.
Walter BL, Vitek J: Surgical treatment for Parkinson's disease. Lancet Neurol 2004;3:719-728.
Waters CH: Diagnosis and Management of Parkinson's Disease. New York, Professional Communications, 2005.

Peripheral Neuropathies

Method of
Marina Grandis, MD, and
Michael E. Shy, MD

Peripheral neuropathy is the common term for disorders affecting the peripheral nervous system (PNS). The PNS consists of motor, sensory, and autonomic neurons that extend outside the central nervous system (CNS) and are associated with Schwann cells or ganglionic satellite cells. The PNS includes the dorsal and ventral spinal roots, spinal and cranial nerves, sensory and motor terminals, and the bulk of the autonomic nervous system. Motor neurons extend from their cell body in the ventral horn of the spinal cord to the neuromuscular junctions at the muscle they innervate. The cell bodies of primary sensory neurons lie outside the spinal cord in the dorsal root ganglia (DRG) where they extend peripherally to specialized sensory end-organs including nociceptors, thermoreceptors, and mechanoreceptors. Central projections from the DRG enter the spinal cord through the dorsal roots. At each spinal segment the ventral roots, carrying motor axons, and the dorsal roots, carrying sensory axons, join to form mixed sensorimotor nerves. In the cervical, brachial, and lumbosacral areas, the mixed spinal nerves form plexuses from which the major anatomically defined limb nerves emanate. Each mixed nerve is composed of large numbers of myelinated and nonmyelinated nerves of varying diameters. The large myelinated axons include motor neurons and large fiber sensory nerves that subserve position and vibration senses. Small thinly myelinated or nonmyelinated axons primarily subserve nociception and autonomic modalities. Preganglionic sympathetic autonomic fibers begin in the intermediolateral column of the spinal cord and synapse in the sympathetic trunk with sympathetic ganglia. Preganglionic parasympathetic fibers travel long distances from their cell bodies in the brainstem or sacral spinal cord to reach terminal ganglia that are near the organs the parasympathetic fibers innervate. The sympathetic and parasympathetic divisions work synergistically to mediate motivational and emotional states as well to monitor the body's basic physiology.

An Approach to the Patient With Peripheral Neuropathy

The use of a systematic approach is essential to evaluate a patient with peripheral nerve disease. A multitude of laboratory abnormalities, toxins, and hereditary and acquired disorders can cause peripheral neuropathy. A so-called shotgun approach in which every conceivable cause of neuropathy is excluded is expensive, may not identify the cause of the neuropathy, and is therefore not in the patient's best interests. It is better to use the history and physical examination to demonstrate peripheral nerve disease, use neurophysiologic testing to characterize the demyelinating or axonal nature of the process, and then order the relevant tests to diagnose the neuropathy.

SYMPTOMATOLOGY

Peripheral neuropathies are characterized by negative symptoms, caused by a loss of function of motor, sensory, or autonomic nerve fibers, and positive symptoms, mainly caused by abnormal electrical activities in damaged peripheral nerves.

Motor Symptoms

Weakness and loss of muscle bulk are the main motor symptoms associated with peripheral neuropathies. Weakness is usually length dependent, so the lower extremities are more involved than upper extremities. Furthermore weakness is often most accentuated in muscles providing foot dorsiflexion and eversion (anterior tibialis, peroneus brevis, and longus) and in intrinsic hand muscles (first dorsal interosseus, adductor digiti minimi, and abductor pollicis brevis). Loss of muscle bulk (atrophy) can occur with either demyelinating or axonal neuropathies (see later) because even demyelinating neuropathies develop axonal loss and denervation secondary to the demyelination.

Positive motor symptoms include cramps, fasciculations, and myokymia. Cramps are painful spontaneous contractions of a muscle and frequently occur with chronic denervation. Fasciculations, defined as the spontaneous electric discharge of a motor unit (motor neuron, its axon, and the muscle fibers it innervates), appear as irregular twitches of a muscle. Although fasciculations are most characteristic of motor neuron disorders, they can occur in peripheral neuropathies, particularly in the case of conduction blocks. Finally, myokymia is a continuous rippling contraction of the muscles and can be localized or generalized in a disorder such as Isaacs' syndrome.

Sensory Symptoms

Sensory symptoms are separable into those involving small thinly myelinated or unmyelinated fibers and those affecting large myelinated fibers. Small-fiber symptoms involve pain and temperature; large-fiber symptoms involve proprioception, or position sense. Common complaints in small-fiber neuropathy include feeling like one's feet are "walking on pebbles" or difficulties determining bath water temperature with one's feet. Large-fiber symptoms usually involve an unsteady gait, particularly at night or in crowds where it is more difficult to use vision as a way to compensate for the neuropathy.

Positive sensory symptoms can either occur spontaneously or in response to stimulation; they include *paresthesias*, such as tingling and prickling feelings, and painful *dysesthesias,* such as burning, cutting pain, or the feeling of being stuck with pins. Paresthesias and dysesthesias are associated with small-fiber abnormalities, and, like weakness and sensory loss, they tend to be length dependent.

Autonomic Symptoms

Autonomic symptoms are particularly frequent in certain neuropathies such as those associated with diabetes and amyloidosis. They include urinary retention or incontinence, abnormalities of sweating, constipation alternating with diarrhea, and lightheadedness when changing position. Impotence is a frequent component of autonomic neuropathies.

FINDINGS ON NEUROLOGIC EXAMINATION

Muscle Weakness

Muscle weakness is usually distal and expressed as an abnormality of gait or clumsiness in running. Some increased instability at the ankle, a tendency to varus deformity of the foot, and steppage gait are typically observed. In steppage gait, the knees have to be raised higher than normal to lift the feet off the ground. Muscle weakness and atrophy typically begin insidiously in the foot and leg muscles and especially affect intrinsic foot and peroneal muscles. Calf and intrinsic hand muscles are affected later. Occasionally, in more severe cases, proximal thigh muscles become affected. The atrophy tends to affect the distal part of the gastrocnemius, soleus, and distal quadriceps muscles, leaving only a small mass of muscle at the proximal end. Muscle tendon reflex loss, particularly at the Achilles tendon is frequent, *although not invariable.*

Sensory Findings

Sensory loss is usually found in a stocking-glove distribution for both large- and small-fiber neuropathy. Cold, erythematous, or bluish discolored feet suggest a loss of small-fiber function, although other factors may also contribute. Large-fiber sensory loss, or "sensory ataxia," in the upper extremities is often detected by the inability of the patient to localize the thumb with the opposite index finger accurately while eyes are closed or by the presence of a characteristic irregular tremor (pseudoathetosis) of the fingers. The sensory examination should include vibration, position, and light touch as well as pain and temperature. A determination of the degree and the extent of sensory loss as well as the pattern of the deficits (symmetric or asymmetric; distal or generalized; focal, multifocal, or diffuse) in both upper and lower extremities is important.

Most peripheral neuropathies involve motor and sensory abnormalities. Occasional forms involve primarily motor or sensory findings (Tables 1 and 2). In addition, autonomic abnormalities are particularly frequent in neuropathies (Table 3).

TABLE 1 Predominantly Motor Neuropathies

Immune Mediated
- Guillain-Barré syndrome
- Chronic inflammatory demyelinating polyneuropathy (CIDP)
- Multifocal motor neuropathy (MMN) (often with conduction block)

Toxic
- Lead
- Dapsone

Paraneoplastic
- Motor neuropathy associated with lymphoma

Hereditary
- Distal hereditary motor neuropathies (HMNs)
- Porphyria
- Hexosaminidase A deficiency

LABORATORY EVALUATION

Determining when to order particular tests is one of the major challenges in caring for patients with neuropathy. There are literally hundreds of different causes of neuropathy, tests can be expensive, and neuropathies with different etiologies can present similarly. Certain laboratory tests are routinely ordered on most patients when they are first evaluated. For example, it is usually necessary to obtain a blood sugar, as well as a set of electrolytes, to evaluate renal function and a complete blood count (CBC) to evaluate hemoglobin levels and red blood cell morphology (for macrocytosis). In the absence of an obvious cause of neuropathy, many also order vitamin B_{12} levels, HIV, rapid plasma reagent (RPR), and serum immunofixation electrophoresis (IFE) early in the evaluation of a patient. This test for monoclonal gammopathy is more sensitive and specific than serum protein electrophoresis (SPEP) or routine immunoelectrophoresis (IPEP). It is at this point that neurophysiologic testing should be obtained.

Specifically, testing is not advisable at this time for the presence of specific antibodies or for genetic causes of neuropathy without an electromyelogram (EMG), even if there is a family history of neuropathy. Interpreting the significance of antibodies reacting with ganglioside G_{M1} or myelin-associated glycoprotein (MAG) should be done in the context of the patient's clinical presentation and physiology. Similarly, genetic testing is most effective when candidate genes are selected based on the patient's nerve conduction studies, inheritance pattern, and clinical presentation. Testing for the presence of specific antibodies or genes is expensive, not always useful, and is most helpful when ordered based on characteristic presentations with characteristic neurophysiology.

Unless the history suggests specific toxin ingestion or deficiency states, testing for these substances without an EMG should not be considered because different toxins or deficiency states present with different nerve conduction abnormalities. Finally, diabetic neuropathies, acquired demyelinating neuropathies, infectious neuropathies, and vasculitic neuropathies all have characteristic patterns of EMG abnormalities.

TABLE 2 Predominantly Sensory Neuropathies

Large-Fiber Neuropathies
Immune mediated
- Sensory neuropathy associated with Sjögren's syndrome

Toxic/metabolic
- Cisplatin

Vitamin E deficiency
Vitamin B_{12} deficiency
Excess vitamin B_6
Paraneoplastic
- Sensory neuropathy with "anti-Hu" antibodies

Hereditary
- Hereditary sensory neuropathy
- Abetalipoproteinemia

Small-Fiber Neuropathies
Associated with systemic disease
- Diabetes mellitus
- Amyloidosis
- HIV

Toxic metabolic
- Alcoholic neuropathy
- Nucleoside reverse transcriptase inhibitors (NRTIs)
- Vincristine

Hereditary
- Hereditary sensory neuropathy
- Fabry's disease
- Tangier disease

TABLE 3 Neuropathies With Autonomic Features

Associated With Systemic Disease
- Diabetes mellitus
- Amyloidosis

Toxins
- Vacor

Hereditary
- Riley-Day syndrome
- Shy-Drager syndrome
- Hereditary sensory and autonomic neuropathies (HSANs)

NEUROPHYSIOLOGY

The use of EMG, including nerve conduction studies (NCS), suggests whether a neuropathy is primarily demyelinating or axonal and whether the process is symmetrical or asymmetrical. If the neuropathy is demyelinating, NCS can determine whether the disorder is purely motor (as seen in multifocal motor neuropathy), distally accentuated (as seen in anti-MAG neuropathies), or uniformly slow (as seen in many genetic neuropathies). If the neuropathy is axonal, the EMG can help distinguish between symmetric axonal neuropathies or the asymmetric mononeuritis multiplex. It can also help identify whether the neuropathy is chronic. These distinctions are important because they identify potentially treatable neuropathies. Acquired demyelinating neuropathies or mononeuritis multiplex may respond to specific treatments. But interpretation of EMG findings works best when the study is used as an extension of the neurologic examination. When EMG studies are performed in the absence of quality clinical information, the testing is much less useful. The Current Diagnosis box lists common laboratory tests useful in evaluating neuropathies.

Classification and Approach to Peripheral Neuropathies

ACQUIRED NEUROPATHIES

Neuropathies Associated With Metabolic Disorders

Diabetes mellitus (DM) is the most frequent cause of neuropathy in the Western world. The estimated prevalence of peripheral nervous system impairment in diabetic patients varies in different studies from 30% to 60% as a result of differences in the measures used for assessment. Although diabetes is associated with a broad spectrum of peripheral nervous system complications, the most typical is the diabetic polyneuropathy (DPN).

Clinical features of DPN include a length-dependent, distal, symmetric, predominantly sensory nerve disorder that may occur in both type I and type II DM patients. DPN tends to develop after several years of metabolic impairment and is associated with other diabetic complications such as nephropathy and retinopathy.

The pathogenesis of diabetic neuropathy is probably multifactorial, involving both microvascular and metabolic abnormalities. The Diabetes Control and Complication Trial (DCCT), performed in 1983, confirmed a definitive causal link between increased blood glucose level and the development and progression of diabetic neuropathy. In particular, the study evaluated conventional therapy versus intensive treatment and demonstrated a 60% reduction in the intensively treated patients compared with conventionally treated ones. A strict control of diabetes remains the only established therapy for diabetic neuropathy. The mechanisms by which hyperglycemia causes nerve dysfunction are probably multiple and still not completely elucidated.

Current pathogenic mechanisms thought to cause DPN include activation of the polyol pathway, extensive glycation, altered diacylglycerol (DAG)/protein kinase activity (PKC), and oxidative stress. All these factors are targeted by new therapeutic approaches, and many clinical trials are under way. Additionally, a large body of evidence, mainly derived from animal model studies, suggests a role for neurotrophic factors, in particular nerve growth factor (NGF), which selectively supports small fiber sensory and sympathetic neurons, in future treatments of DPN. Specific treatments for diabetic neuropathy are still not available, however, and the current therapy is based on the control of hyperglycemia, the management of symptoms, and foot care. Nonetheless, an increasing understanding of the pathogenic mechanisms may lead to truly effective treatment.

Diabetic patients may also develop acute mononeuropathies, including mononeuropathy multiplex, although the incidence is much less than with the symmetrical sensory neuropathy. The basis for these mononeuropathies is probably nerve infarction. Typical clinical presentations of these focal neuropathies are ophthalmoplegia (third, fourth, or sixth nerve palsies), proximal leg weakness (femoral neuropathy or "diabetic amyotrophy"), and thoracic pseudoradiculopathy (intercostal neuropathies). The mononeuropathies usually present with pain followed by loss of function of the nerve involved. Thus symptoms may be motor or sensory depending on the nerve. Gradual recovery of function may occur over a period of months. Finally, patients with diabetes also are more likely to develop compression neuropathies such as carpal tunnel syndrome, tarsal tunnel syndrome, or ulnar neuropathy.

Polyneuropathies Associated With Other Metabolic Disorders

A peripheral neuropathy may complicate severe renal failure, but these are now less common, in part because of better care for renal disease such as dialysis. Hypothyroidism may be associated with PNS impairment, particularly in the form of entrapment syndromes such as carpal tunnel syndrome. In both cases, therapy should address the underlying metabolic disease.

Toxic and Deficiency Neuropathies

In Western countries, toxic neuropathies are more frequently side effects of medications rather than a result of environmental exposures. In most cases iatrogenic neuropathy presents as length-dependent or dying-back axonal neuropathies. The treatment involves a correct diagnosis and the discontinuation of the drug, but improvement is often slow and may take several months.

Neuropathies Associated With Antineoplastic Agents

Vincristine is a vinca alkaloid, used for solid tumors, lymphoma, and leukemia, which acts by blocking tubulin polymerization into microtubules, thus arresting the cell cycle. The neuropathy manifests as a distal, painful, sensory-predominant axonal polyneuropathy. Occasionally vincristine is administered to patients with subclinical hereditary neuropathy, causing an acute and severe PNS impairment.

Paclitaxel (Taxol) is a taxoid mainly administered for ovarian and breast cancers. Similar to vincristine, paclitaxel blocks the polymerization of tubulin and causes a painful axonal polyneuropathy. A recent randomized trial with vitamin E demonstrated promising results in preventing the neuropathy.

Cisplatin is a platinum-derived compound, generally used for ovarian and small cell lung tumors. Cisplatin treatment is limited by a dose-dependent sensory neuronopathy because of toxicity on DRG. Many studies address the role of possible neuroprotectant agents, including NGF, acetyl-L-carnitine, BNP7787, and its derived molecule mesna, to prevent the neuropathy, but data are not conclusive.

Suramin is an old medication that recently demonstrated anticancer properties. It may be associated with both a dose-dependent axonal neuropathy and a more severe, acute, demyelinating neuropathy, similar to Guillain-Barré syndrome.

Thalidomide recently demonstrated anticancer properties and is used against brain tumors and multiple myeloma. Similarly to cisplatin, it causes a sensory neuronopathy by inducing DRG degeneration.

Neuropathies Associated With Antimicrobials

A peripheral neuropathy is described in association with several antibiotic molecules, including chloramphenicol, chloroquine, dapsone, isoniazid, metronidazole, and nitrofurantoin. In most cases the peripheral neuropathy is a prevalent sensory polyneuropathy, with the exception of dapsone, a basic drug for leprosy, which produces a predominantly motor neuropathy.

Isoniazid-induced neuropathy is caused by a vitamin B_6 deficiency and may be prevented by pyridoxine administration (100 mg per day).

Nucleoside reverse transcriptase inhibitors (NRTIs), including zidovudine, zalcitabine, didanosine, stavudine, and lamivudine, are associated with a distal painful sensory axonopathy that is difficult to distinguish from a sensory neuropathy caused by HIV. If the neuropathy is caused by the medications, it usually begins near the onset of the therapy and may ameliorate after its suspension.

Neuropathies Associated With Cardiac Medications

Different medications commonly used for cardiac disease may determine a peripheral neuropathy. Amiodarone, an antiarrhythmic drug, and perhexiline, commonly used for angina pectoris, may bind to Schwann cell lysosomes and cause a demyelinating sensorimotor neuropathy. *Hydralazine* is an antihypertensive drug that, similarly to isoniazid, may cause a polyneuropathy related to a vitamin B_6 deficiency.

Neuropathies Associated With Other Medications

Colchicine, used for gout, may, like vincristine and paclitaxel, prevent tubulin polymerization into microtubules.

FK 506 (tacrolimus) is an immunosuppressant associated with a CIDP (chronic inflammatory demyelinating polyneuropathy)-like neuropathy, usually responding to plasma exchange (PE) or intravenous immunoglobulin (IVIG). *Gold salts,* used for rheumatoid arthritis, can cause both a subacute, mainly demyelinating polyneuropathy and a chronic axonal disease with myokymia. *Phenytoin,* an anticonvulsant drug, may be rarely responsible for a mild polyneuropathy. *Disulfiram* (Antabuse), employed in alcohol abuse discontinuation, may cause peripheral nerve damage. *Pyridoxine* (vitamin B_6) in doses greater than 200 mg per day causes a degeneration of DRG, leading to a severe sensory polyneuropathy.

Neuropathies Associated With Heavy Metals

Several heavy metals are associated with peripheral neurotoxicity, but the observation of related neuropathies is becoming less frequent because of better public control on health hazards. The treatment remains the removal of the source of contamination, eventually associated with chelating agents in case of severe poisoning.

Lead, no longer used in water containers and pipes, is still used as a component for solder and batteries and may cause a prevalent motor neuropathy typically affecting the wrist extensors and the dorsal tibialis.

Today the intoxication of *arsenic* mainly derives from homicide or suicide attempts, but, rarely, intoxication may derive from by-products of copper and lead smelting or from pesticides that may contaminate the soil and water. In case of severe intoxication, systemic symptoms prevail; if the dosage is not life-threatening, however, a painful sensory neuropathy may occur.

Organic *mercury* may be concentrated in fish and shellfish, whereas inorganic mercury is widely used in scientific instruments such as thermometers and barometers, potentially causing a poisoning in subjects working in the production of such instruments, but also in research institutions where such instruments are used extensively. Concerns regarding the safety of silver-mercury amalgam fillings continue to be raised but are unfounded.

Thallium is used in pesticides and rodenticides. A sensory painful neuropathy may accompany hair loss, which is the main clinical manifestation.

Neuropathies Associated With Chemical Compounds

The monomeric form of *acrylamide,* used in plastic and grouting industries, may cause a sensory ataxic neuropathy, particularly through skin contact.

Carbon disulfide is employed in the manufacture of rayon and cellophane and may be responsible for a sensory neuropathy. The intoxication is rare, however, because of the continuous monitoring of workers exposed to this substance.

Ethylene glycol is the main compound in automobile antifreeze and may be ingested accidentally or following a suicide or homicide attempt. It causes a prevalent renal failure associated with a polyradiculopathy with cranial nerve involvement.

The *hex carbons* n-hexane and methyl-n-butyl ketone are proven neurotoxic agents. They enter the composition of glue and solvents, and the inhalation may occur in workers exposed to those products or may be intentional (glue sniffing). The chronic exposure causes a slowly progressive sensory neuropathy characterized by giant axonal swellings observed on pathologic examination, whereas acute exposure may cause a subacute, prevalently motor neuropathy, mimicking Guillain-Barré syndrome (GBS).

Organophosphate esters, molecules used in the plastic industry and as insecticides in agriculture, are acetylcholinesterase inhibitors, which may give rise to an acute intoxication because of a direct anticholinesterase effect. As a result of a chronic low-dose exposure, particularly to triorthocresyl phosphate, a slowly progressive predominantly motor neuropathy, associated with pyramidal signs, may occur, secondary to the inhibition of a specific neuropathy target esterase.

Vacor, a rodenticide usually ingested for suicidal purposes, results in diabetes and severe autonomic neuropathy. Early niacinamide may be successful in preventing these episodes.

Deficiency Neuropathies

In Western countries a severe *vitamin B₁ deficiency* is usually secondary to severe ethanol consumption, even if an additive direct toxic effect of ethanol is likely.

Vitamin B₁₂ deficiency may cause a mild chronic sensorimotor polyneuropathy, but the prominent signs are caused by the spinal cord impairment.

Vitamin E deficiency may be genetically determined and is associated with ataxia (AVED [ataxia with vitamin E deficiency]) or, more frequently, occurs secondary to disorders affecting vitamin E absorption such as liver disease or disorders of fat metabolism (abetalipoproteinemia).

Infectious Neuropathies

The peripheral nervous system may be involved in all phases of HIV infection. The most common peripheral neuropathy is a distal, painful, sensory polyneuropathy, which is very similar to the toxic neuropathy caused by NRTIs; as already mentioned, a temporal criteria may help in the differential diagnosis, but in several cases both factors overlap. When a mainly iatrogenic neuropathy is suspected, the removal of NRTIs may improve the symptoms, whereas a direct HIV-related neuropathy may stabilize or ameliorate with a specific antiretroviral scheme. In the initial phases of HIV infection, inflammatory neuropathies prevail and may present as either acute or chronic inflammatory demyelinating neuropathies. Differently from idiopathic inflammatory neuropathies, the cytoalbuminemic dissociation usually present in the cerebrospinal fluid (CSF) is less evident in HIV patients because of a mild mononuclear pleocytosis. The response of those neuropathies to plasma exchange or IVIG is generally good. In the late stages, cytomegalovirus (CMV) may cause both an acute lumbosacral polyradiculopathy because of the direct invasion of nerve roots or a mononeuritis multiplex through a vasculitic mechanism. CMV complications are usually treated with ganciclovir.

Varicella-zoster virus (VZV) tends to remain latent in cranial or spinal ganglia after the resolution of a systemic infection. Reactivation tends to occur in elderly persons or immunocompromised patients and determines a vesicular skin eruption, associated with pruritus and dysesthesias. Herpes zoster normally undergoes a spontaneous resolution but is frequently followed by a severe postherpetic neuralgia, which is defined as a pain persisting for more than 6 weeks after the rash appearance. Early treatment with oral acyclovir (800 mg, five times daily for 7 days) may reduce both the duration of the acute phase and the chances of developing a postherpetic neuralgia, which is usually treated with symptomatic drugs for neuropathic pain (see later).

Neuropathy Associated With Lyme Disease

Borrelia burgdorferi causes a disease in which three stages may be recognized. Shortly after a tick bite, in the same area, a nonpruritic rash develops (erythema migrans) and spontaneously disappears after a few weeks. The second phase is frequently associated with neurologic complications such as lymphocytic meningitis, focal and multifocal peripheral and cranial neuropathies, in particular unilateral or bilateral facial palsy, and radiculitis. The third stage is associated with severe neurologic complications, including encephalopathy, encephalomyelitis, and mainly sensory axonal polyneuropathy. A lymphocytic pleocytosis on the CSF analysis associated with a serologic demonstration of *B. burgdorferi* infection on serum or CSF are the main laboratory findings. Whereas early stages are treated with a 3-week course of oral antibiotics (doxycycline, 100 mg twice daily, or amoxicillin, 500 mg three times daily), intravenous penicillin or cephalosporins should be given in late stages.

Neuropathy Associated With Leprosy

Leprosy is the main cause of peripheral neuropathy in developing countries, although it is infrequent in the Western world. Leprosy may manifest in different forms, depending on the host's immune system. Patients with a normal cell-mediated immunity are more likely to have a tuberculoid form characterized by hypopigmented skin lesions associated with hypoesthesia, whereas patients with inefficient immune responses may develop a lepromatous form, which is a more severe disease leading to large disfiguring lesions. A multineuropathic pattern with a prominent superficial sensory loss is the more typical clinical presentation of leprosy. A long-term multiple-drug regimen (daily dose of dapsone, 100 mg, associated with rifampicin, 600 mg, and clofazimine, 50 mg) is normally applied.

Neuropathy Associated With Diphtheria

Although infrequent in the Western world because of intensive vaccination, diphtheria is still an important cause of subacute neuropathy in developing countries. Some strains of *Corynebacterium diphtheriae* produce a potent neurotoxin that causes a palatal weakness, accommodation deficit, and extraocular palsies, followed by an ascending paralysis because of a demyelinating neuropathy that shares many clinical features with GBS. The treatment is based on horse serum antitoxin, as early as possible, and erythromycin or penicillin to eradicate the infection and stop the toxin production.

Immune-Inflammatory Neuropathies

Immune-mediated neuropathies are frequent disorders and potentially treatable conditions. Because many therapies are described in literature, we will focus on the most frequently used schedules.

Guillain-Barré Syndrome

Also defined as acute inflammatory demyelinating polyneuropathy (AIDN), GBS is a rapidly evolving sensorimotor polyneuropathy characterized by prevalent motor deficits, usually with an ascending pattern involving initially the distal parts of the limbs and gradually spreading to the proximal segments. Typically, a progressive phase develops in a few days or weeks (up to 4) followed by stabilization and finally by a slow spontaneous recovery lasting weeks or months. Most of the patients undergo either a complete recovery or are left with minor problems; approximately 20% report a persistent significant disability, and 5% to 8% die from complications of the disease.

GBS frequently is preceded by a respiratory tract infection (cytomegalovirus, Epstein-Barr virus) or gastroenteritis (*Campylobacter jejuni*) that is thought to trigger an autoimmune response directed against myelin antigens of the PNS, probably because of a molecular similarity (molecular mimicry) between a viral or bacterial antigen and myelin proteins epitopes.

Examination of the CSF reveals an increase of protein content with a normal or only moderately elevated (less than 10) cell count (myoalbumin dissociation). Electrodiagnostic studies are characterized by slow nerve conductions and partial or complete conduction blocks.

Recent evidence suggests the clinical presentation of GBS may be more heterogeneous than previously thought. Acute motor axonal neuropathy (AMAN) and acute motor sensory axonal neuropathy (AMSAN) define two variants of GBS characterized by a prominent axonal damage, frequently preceded by *C. jejuni* gastroenteritis.

Miller Fisher syndrome is another variant of GBS with specific clinical features, including ophthalmoplegia, ataxia, and areflexia, and associated with distinct antibodies recognizing the GQ1b ganglioside that appears to be particularly expressed in the paranodal region of oculomotor nerves.

A main point in the management of GBS, particularly for nonambulant patients, is careful medical and nursing care, including proper positioning and frequent turning to avoid cutaneous pressure sores, urinary catheterization to prevent urinary infections, and subcutaneous heparin and support stockings to avoid venous thromboembolism. Patients should be strictly monitored to select those who will require intensive care measures. In the presence of a rapid disease progression, bulbar dysfunction, bilateral facial weakness, dysautonomic signs, and rapid decrease in vital capacity, patients should be admitted to intensive care units and eventually intubated to start mechanical ventilation.

Therapies directed at nonspecifically modulating the immune system are proving effective in many of these disorders. PE was the first treatment to prove superior to supportive measures alone and is therefore considered the gold standard therapy. The usual PE regimen involves four exchanges of 1.5 L of plasma, each spread over a 10-day period. Two PE are sufficient in mild cases, whereas six exchanges are not superior to four in severely affected patients. The therapy should be administered preferentially within the first 2 weeks and not later than 4 weeks from clinical onset.

IVIG therapy, given at a dose of 2 g per kg divided over 2 to 5 days, is equally effective as PE. The shorter scheme acts more rapidly but is associated with higher rates of adverse effects. The effects of IVIG are ascertained if the therapy is administered within the first 2 weeks. Because both PE and IVIG are equally effective, at least in the first 2 weeks, IVIG is often preferred because of the technical convenience of this treatment compared with PE, unless there are contraindications such as low serum immunoglobulin A (IgA) levels, renal failure, severe hypertension, or hyperosmolar state.

Ten percent of GBS patients experience a secondary worsening of their neurologic condition after successful PE or IVIG, but they usually respond to a second cycle of the previously effective treatment. A combined treatment of PE followed by IVIG does not significantly change the prognosis and is therefore not recommended.

A recent examination of the use of corticosteroids in different forms (intravenous methylprednisolone, oral prednisolone or prednisone, intramuscular ACTH [adrenocorticotropic hormone]) by a Cochrane systematic review did not find them beneficial. A recent Dutch trial examined the effects of intravenous methylprednisolone (500 mg per day for 5 days) in association with IVIG compared with IVIG alone, showing a slight initial advantage for the combination regimen, without significant differences in disability at long-term evaluation.

Chronic Inflammatory Demyelinating Polyneuropathy

Considered a closely related disorder to GBS, CIDP shares an autoimmune pathogenesis and a demyelinating damage of motor and sensory peripheral nerves. The clinical course develops insidiously over weeks to months (minimum 8 weeks) or years, however, and may be slowly progressive or relapsing-remitting. Unlike GBS, an antecedent infection is rare, and although considered treatable, the prognosis of CIDP overall is less favorable compared to monophasic GBS. Laboratory features include an increase of CSF protein levels, with a normal or only mildly elevated cell count, and slow conduction velocities. Laboratory tests to evaluate diabetes and monoclonal gammopathy should always be performed because those conditions may be associated with CIDP and influence the clinical course of the disease; in particular, the association of CIDP with IgM monoclonal gammopathy of unknown significance predicts a worse prognosis.

Corticosteroids are the traditional therapy for CIDP and are proven effective. A standard approach is to use oral prednisone (1 mg/kg/day) for 6 to 8 weeks, followed by very slow tapering over several months. To prevent serious side effects, H_2-receptor antagonists; osteoporosis prophylaxis; and sodium-restricted, low-carbohydrate, and a protein-rich diet should be prescribed. Long-term corticosteroid therapy leads always to weight gain, however, and it frequently causes diabetes and hypertension. Particularly because improvement with prednisone may take several months to occur, PE and IVIG are at the moment the usually preferred initial therapies.

Different immunosuppressive drugs (azathioprine, cyclosporine A, cyclophosphamide, methotrexate, mycophenolate mofetil, rituximab, and interferons α and β) are administered to patients who are refractory to conventional therapies, but no definitive evidence proves the efficacy of these drugs.

Multifocal Motor Neuropathy

Multifocal motor neuropathy (MMN), originally considered related to CIDP, is now described as a distinct neuropathy characterized by progressive, predominantly distal, asymmetric limb weakness, mainly affecting the upper limbs. Mild sensory symptoms may be present, but a definitive sensory deficit is usually absent. Electrophysiologic features include the presence of conduction blocks in motor nerves outside the normal sites of nerve compression, prolonged distal motor and F wave latencies, and normal sensory conduction parameters. The CSF examination is often normal, but in some cases a mild increase of protein content may be observed. Anti-G_{M1} IgM antibodies are reported by ELISA (enzyme-linked immunosorbent assay) in 30% to 80% of MMN patients and, even if their pathogenetic role has never been proven, they may be helpful in differentiating MMN from other lower motor neuron syndromes.

Unlike in CIDP, MMN patients usually do not respond to corticosteroids and PE and may even experience a clinical worsening of neurologic deficits following both kinds of treatments. The large majority of patients rapidly improve after an IVIG cycle (2 g/kg over 2 to 5 days), but in most cases the effect is short lasting and the treatment must be repeated every 3 to 4 weeks to prevent neurologic deterioration. Because of the high costs of this therapy, immunosuppressive drugs have been tried to reduce or eliminate the dependency of MMN patients on IVIG. Cyclophosphamide, azathioprine, mycophenolate mofetil, and interferon beta-1a have been used, but controlled studies are not available for these therapies. Table 4 lists some of the more common immune-inflammatory neuropathies.

Neuropathy Associated With Vasculitis

Vasculitic neuropathy may be associated with primary or secondary systemic vasculitides or, less frequently, may be restricted to the PNS. Primary systemic vasculitides include polyarteritis nodosa, Wegener's granulomatosis, Churg-Strauss syndrome, and microscopic polyangiitis. In secondary systemic vasculitides, blood vessel inflammation occurs in the context of the following conditions:

- Connective tissue diseases: rheumatoid vasculitis, Sjögren's syndrome, systemic lupus erythematosus, sarcoidosis, systemic scleroderma
- Systemic infections: HIV, hepatitis B and C viruses (HBV and HCV), with or without mixed cryoglobulinemia, cytomegalovirus, human T cell leukemia/lymphoma virus, Epstein-Barr virus, tuberculosis, Lyme disease
- Vaccinations
- Tumors: paraneoplastic vasculitis (described in the paraneoplastic neuropathies)
- Drug reactions: carbimazole, amiodarone, naproxen, allopurinol, hydralazine, sulfasalazine

The clinical appearance reflects multifocal ischemic nerve damage, presenting as mononeuritis multiplex or asymmetric polyneuropathy with subacute evolving burning pain and sensory loss, whereas motor deficits are less frequent and appear later. If the neurologic evaluation is made late in the disorder, mononeuritis multiplex may be mistaken for a symmetric process because of multiple nerve involvement.

If a vasculitic neuropathy is suspected, beyond a complete blood count and a metabolic panel, serum should be checked for:

- ESR (erythrocyte sedimentation rate)
- ANA (antinuclear antibody)
- ENA (extractable nuclear antigen)
- Rheumatoid factor
- p-ANCA (perinuclear antineutrophil cytoplasmic antibody)
- c-ANCA (cytoplasmic antineutrophil cytoplasmic antibody)
- Complement and circulating immunocomplex levels
- Cryoglobulins
- HBV, HCV, and HIV
- Angiotensin-converting enzyme level

In case of a PNS-restricted vasculitis, these examinations are usually normal. Nerve conduction studies may confirm a multifocal axonal neuropathy. Protein content of CSF is usually normal or mildly elevated, except in paraneoplastic neuropathy, in which proteins may be markedly increased. A sural nerve biopsy may show fibrinoid necrosis, obstruction of epineural arteries lumen, perivascular inflammation, and hemosiderin deposits.

In the case of systemic vasculitides, treatment usually requires a high dosage of glucocorticosteroids (prednisone, 1 mg/kg/day, or intravenous methylprednisolone, 1000 mg/day for 3 to 5 days followed by oral prednisone), eventually associated with an immunosuppressant drug like cyclophosphamide, for very acute multisystemic diseases, or methotrexate and azathioprine, for milder forms. In the case of a PNS-restricted vasculitis, a less aggressive approach is applied, including oral prednisone, azathioprine, or weekly methotrexate.

TABLE 4 Immune-Inflammatory Neuropathies

Guillain-Barré syndrome: rapid onset
CIDP: subacute to chronic onset
Associated with plasma cell dyscrasia: chronic onset
IgM anti-MAG: subacute to chronic onset
IgG with POEMS: subacute to chronic onset
MMN with conduction block: subacute to chronic onset

Abbreviations: CIDP = chronic inflammatory demyelinating polyneuropathy; IgG anti-MAG= immunoglobulin G anti-myelin-associated glycoprotein; IgM = immunoglobulin M; MMN = multifocal motor neuropathy; POEMS = polyneuropathy, organomegaly, endocrinopathy, monoclonal protein, and skin changes.

Neuropathy Associated With Paraproteinemia

Paraproteinemia includes different disorders such as monoclonal gammopathy of undetermined significance (MGUS), multiple myeloma, solitary plasmocytoma, osteosclerotic myeloma, Waldenström's macroglobuline-mia, primary amyloidosis, and cryoglobulinemia, all characterized by a monoclonal antibody produced by a single clone of abnormally proliferating plasma cells. A monoclonal protein may be found in approximately 5% of all patients with polyneuropathy, in approximately 10% of patients with idiopathic neuropathies, but also in 3% of the general population over the age of 50 years. The presence of a monoclonal antibody therefore does not necessarily mean it is causing a neuropathy. The neuropathy frequently is the main clinical manifestation of an underlying hematologic disorder. Even if in some cases the monoclonal protein may react against nerve antigens, in most cases the causal link between the monoclonal protein and the neuropathy is not clear.

Neuropathy Associated With Monoclonal Gammopathy of Undetermined Significance

MGUS refers to an asymptomatic and often benign condition that may rarely evolve into a malignant form (1% per year). The neuropathy, frequently the only sign of the disease, is more common with IgM-MGUS compared with IgG- or IgA-MGUS. In approximately half of the patients with neuropathy associated with IgM-MGUS, the monoclonal protein reacts against the MAG, a protein mainly localized in the paranodal region of myelinated fibers, suggesting a direct role of anti-MAG monoclonal protein.

The clinical features of this neuropathy, affecting mainly the elderly, are well defined and include predominant sensory impairment presenting with hypoesthesia, paresthesia, dysesthesia, and unsteadiness of gait. Distal weakness tends to develop in the course of the disease, whereas a postural tremor in the upper limbs may occur in the early phases. The clinical evolution tends to be slowly progressive, but approximately 50% of the patients report a significant disability after 15 years.

Electrophysiologic studies show demyelinating features with extremely prolonged distal latencies. Sural nerve biopsy demonstrates a demyelinating neuropathy with a typical enlargement of myelin lamellae at the electron microscopy and, in most cases, deposits of IgM and complement can be seen around myelin sheaths.

Different forms of neuropathies are also associated with IgG- or IgA-MGUS, but the causal link between the hematologic disorder and the neuropathy is not at all definite.

Based on the likely hypothesis that anti-MAG involves pathogenetic factors, patients are treated with both immunomodulatory and immunosuppressive therapies, including steroids, plasma exchange, cyclophosphamide, chlorambucil, IVIG, fludarabine, interferon alfa with partial responses in open studies, although the effects were never confirmed by randomized trials. Because those patients are usually elderly and all the cited treatments may have important chronic side effects, some caution should be used before starting an aggressive regimen. The anti-B lymphocyte (CD20) humanized monoclonal antibody (rituximab) is being studied in open pilot trials with promising results, and a randomized controlled trial is currently under way.

Neuropathy Associated With Multiple Myeloma

Neuropathy, although not very frequent, may be the presenting sign or may be found along with fatigue, bone pain, anemia, hypocalcemia, and increased erythrocyte sedimentation rate. The clinical presentation of the neuropathy is heterogeneous, probably reflecting different pathogenetic mechanisms, including nerve root compression because of lytic bone lesions, metabolic and toxic effects of both myeloma and the chemotherapeutic drugs, and rarely amyloidosis deriving from light chain deposition. Treatment of the myeloma is only rarely associated with the improvement of the neuropathy.

Neuropathy Associated With Osteosclerotic Myeloma

Although osteosclerotic myeloma is a rare disease, peripheral neuropathy may occur in approximately 50% of the patients and is often the presenting sign. Osteosclerotic myeloma is frequently associated with a complex syndrome called POEMS (polyneuropathy, organomegaly, endocrinopathy, monoclonal protein, and skin changes). The neuropathy is a mainly distal sensorimotor polyneuropathy associated with electrophysiologic demyelinating features and increased CSF protein content. Local radiation or surgical excision of the sclerotic lesions may improve the PNS impairment, especially in the case of a single lesion. Patients with multiple bone lesions are treated with alkylates, prednisone, PE, and tamoxifen.

Neuropathy Associated With Waldenström's Macroglobulinemia

Waldenström's macroglobulinemia (WM) is a monoclonal IgM gammopathy (with κ light chain in most cases), clinically characterized by fatigue, weight loss, bleeding, organomegaly, and hyperviscosity syndrome (dizziness, numbness, visual disturbances, hearing problems, epistaxis, and congestive heart failure). A peripheral neuropathy may occur in more than 10% of cases, and in 30% to 40% of the patients it is associated with an anti-MAG immunoreactivity of the monoclonal protein, sharing the same pathogenetic and clinical features of the neuropathy described in association with IgM-MGUS. In most patients, neuropathy presents as a sensorimotor polyneuropathy that may derive from different mechanisms, including cryoglobulinemia or amyloidosis. Plasma exchange, prednisone, melphalan, chlorambucil, the nucleoside analogues fludarabine or cladribine, rituximab, and allogeneic bone marrow transplantation have been tried, but definitive conclusions cannot be drawn.

Neuropathy Associated With Primary Amyloidosis

Primary systemic amyloidosis includes rare hereditary forms caused by mutations in the transthyretin gene and acquired lymphoproliferative disorders associated with a monoclonal paraprotein, usually IgG or IgM. Congo red–stained deposits of amyloid are found in different organs and consist in the majority of cases of fragments from the variable region of the immunoglobulin light chains or the light chains themselves and misfolded transthyretin in the hereditary ones. The neuropathy is a painful, distal, sensory polyneuropathy with prominent autonomic involvement (orthostatic hypotension and impotence), frequently associated with bilateral carpal tunnel syndrome. Liver transplantation is the only therapy for familial amyloidosis, whereas hematologic disorders may be treated with prednisone and melphalan to slow the progression of renal and cardiac involvement and prolong survival. It is rare, however, to see improvement in the neuropathy.

Neuropathy Associated With Cryoglobulinemia

Cryoglobulins are immunoglobulins that undergo reversible precipitation at low temperatures and may damage peripheral nerves through immune complex deposition and consequent vasculitis. Cryoglobulins are usually divided into three groups:

1. Type I (monoclonal) associated with lymphoproliferative disorders and mixed cryoglobulinemia
2. Type II (monoclonal and polyclonal)
3. Type III (polyclonal) associated with autoimmune disorders or chronic infections, particularly HCV infection

Peripheral nerve involvement is a common complication and may manifest as a multiple mononeuropathy or, more frequently, as a distal sensorimotor polyneuropathy. The therapy is based on corticosteroids, cyclophosphamide, and plasma exchange. In case of HCV infection, the treatment is based on interferon-alfa, alone or associated with ribavirin.

Paraneoplastic Neuropathies

The peripheral nervous system is frequently involved in paraneoplastic neurologic syndromes. The pathogenetic link between the tumor and the neurologic impairment is probably represented by a host immune response to cancer antigens cross-reacting with neural epitopes. The tumors more likely related to paraneoplastic peripheral neuropathies include small cell carcinoma of the lung (SCLC) followed by carcinoma of the stomach, breast, colon, rectum, ovary and prostate, lymphoma and Hodgkin's disease.

Subacute Sensory Neuronopathy

The best clinically characterized paraneoplastic neuropathy is the subacute sensory neuronopathy (Denny-Brown syndrome), presenting with neuropathic pain and progressive sensory loss leading to numbness and ataxic gait. The clinical course is generally rapidly evolving, but a slowly progressive evolution may be possible. In most cases it is associated with SCLC, and frequently the neuropathy is the first clinical sign of the underlying disease. Laboratory findings include the demonstration of serum anti-Hu (ANNA-1 [anti-neuronal nuclear antibody) antibodies by immunohistochemical reaction against the Purkinje cells on rat cerebellar section, a normal or mildly elevated CSF protein content, and a marked decrease or absence of sensory nerve action potential (SNAPs).

The detection and treatment of the tumor may stabilize the neuropathy, although a remission is infrequent, whereas immunomodulant treatments (corticosteroids, PE, and IVIG) are usually unhelpful.

Other Paraneoplastic Neuropathies

A sensorimotor polyneuropathy may occur in a variable percentage of neoplastic patients (5% to 50%), without a specific association to a particular histotype, but the causal association between the neoplasm and the neuropathy is always very difficult to prove and therefore the best treatment remains undetermined.

A prevalent motor neuropathy may be associated with non-Hodgkin's lymphoma. A few cases of paraneoplastic neuropathies presenting with prominent dysautonomic features also have been described recently. Finally, different types of neoplasms (SCLC, lymphoma, renal, stomach, and prostate cancers) are associated with a paraneoplastic vasculitis of peripheral nerves presenting as an asymmetric painful neuropathy with increased protein content. This neuropathy usually responds to the treatment of the cancer associated with steroids and cyclophosphamide.

Because many of the neuropathies described in the preceding few sections can present as mononeuritis multiplex, Table 5 presents a brief list of neuropathies presenting in this manner.

Inherited Neuropathies

Charcot-Marie-Tooth (CMT) disease, a class of heritable peripheral neuropathies, is among the most frequent of the genetic neuromuscular disorders with a prevalence of approximately 1:2500. In recent years, more than 30 different genes causing CMT have been identified, and loci are known for at least another 10 causes (http://www.molgen.ua.ac.be/CMTMutations/default.cfm). Despite a marked genetic heterogeneity, some prevalent clinical features may provide clues to the etiology. Patients with CMT tend to be slow runners in childhood, develop

TABLE 5 Axonal Causes of Mononeuritis Multiplex

Diabetes mellitus
Vasculitis
- Polyneuritis nodosa (PAN)
- Wegener's granulomatosis
- Allergic granulomatous angiitis (Churg-Strauss syndrome)
- Rheumatoid arthritis

Chronic inflammatory diseases
- Sarcoidosis

Infectious
- HIV (cytomegalovirus)
- Leprosy
- Cryoglobulinemia

Amphetamine abuse
Tumors (myeloma, neurofibromatosis)

foot problems in their teenage years because of high arches and hammertoes, and often require orthotics for ankle support as adults. Sensory loss is variable and affects both large- and small-fiber modalities. Although the combination of weak ankles and decreased proprioception often leads to problems with balance, the vast majority of patients remain ambulatory throughout their life, which is not shortened by their disease. The most frequent form, CMT1A, is caused by a duplication on chromosome 17, containing the gene-encoding peripheral myelin protein 22 (PMP22), leading to an overexpression of PMP22 and producing a demyelinating polyneuropathy. Although no cures are available for CMT, rehabilitation and orthopedic surgery may improve the quality of life and help preserve independence.

NEUROPATHIC PAIN

Pain is a major problem in many peripheral neuropathies, significantly affecting the quality of life of patients. This section reviews the main medications used to control neuropathic pain.

Topical Agents

Topical anesthetic creams may provide a local relief without systemic toxicity and are therefore indicated in case of localized neuropathic pain. *Capsaicin cream* acts by depleting P substance from unmyelinated fibers and may be beneficial for some patients. When the treatment is started it may cause a temporary worsening of the burning sensation, which then decreases with repeated use. *Lidocaine* and *prilocaine emulsion* are also used topically for the treatment of postherpetic neuralgia.

The tricyclic antidepressants *amitriptyline, nortriptyline,* and *desipramine* are low-cost efficacious medications. Amitriptyline is the most frequently administered drug in this category. The dosage required for pain control may be significantly lower compared with the doses normally used for antidepressive purpose. Patients should begin at 10 mg,

CURRENT THERAPY

Neuropathic Pain

TOPICAL AGENTS

- Capsaicin cream
- Lidocaine emulsion
- Prilocaine emulsion

TRICYCLIC ANTIDEPRESSANTS

- Amitriptyline
- Nortriptyline
- Desipramine

ANTIEPILEPTIC DRUGS

- Gabapentin
- Pregabalin
- Lamotrigine
- Carbomazepine
- Oxcarbazepine

2 hours before bedtime, and slowly increase in increments of 5 to 10 mg every 3 to 5 days until reaching a significant improvement. The usual dosage is included between 50 and 200 mg daily, but some patients respond to lower ranges. The main side effects include orthostatic hypotension, dry mouth, urinary retention, confusion, and somnolence. They may also increase the risk of cardiac arrhythmias.

Antiepileptic Drugs

The anticonvulsant *gabapentin* is widely used for the treatment of neuropathic pain. The mechanism of action of this molecule is not completely clear, but it was designed as a precursor of GABA and shown to increase the GABA content in brain synapses. It is also supposed to decrease the influx of calcium ions into neurons. The standard dosage for neuropathic pain is between 1200 to 3600 mg per day, divided in three doses. The initial dose is 300 mg, taken 2 hours before bedtime, with a gradual increase of 300 mg per day every 3 days. A slow increase is associated with a reduced risk of dizziness and gait problems, thus improving the compliance, especially in elderly patients. The main side effects—dizziness, gait problems, and somnolence—usually disappear after 10 days of treatment and may be minimized by slow increases in dosage. The only contraindication is renal failure.

Pregabalin, a GABA analogue with similar structure and actions to Gabapentin, was recently approved by the FDA for neuropathic pain. The usual dosage is from 150 to 600 mg, divided into two or three doses. It is a well tolerated treatment which may be associated to mild to moderate somnolence and dizziness.

Lamotrigine acts through the inhibition of voltage-gated sodium-channels and is efficacious in the painful neuropathy associated with HIV. The usual dose is 200 to 500 mg per day divided in two doses. The starting dose is 50 mg, which should be incremented by 50 mg every 2 weeks. The reason for slow increments is to prevent hypersensitivity. Side effects include dizziness, ataxia, and nausea. If a skin rash appears, the drug should be discontinued because more serious allergic reactions may develop. Multiorgan failure or blood dyscrasias rarely occur.

Carbamazepine is mainly used for trigeminal neuralgia but also is proposed for other painful neuropathies. The dosage is 200 to 1200 mg, divided in two doses daily. The most common side effects, dizziness, ataxia, and dyspepsia, may be prevented by advancing the dose by slow increments. A complete blood count should be carefully monitored to detect blood dyscrasias, including agranulocytosis and aplastic anemia, which may occur as a result of idiosyncrasy.

Oxcarbazepine, a second-generation antiepileptic drug, has proven to be as efficacious as carbamazepine in reducing neuropathic pain, but with significantly fewer side effects. The usual starting dose is 300 mg, twice daily. Most patients respond to a daily dose ranging from 600 to 1200 mg, but occasionally it may require 2400 mg/day.

REFERENCES

Dyck PJ, Davies JL, Wilson DM, et al: Risk factors for severity of diabetic polyneuropathy: intensive longitudinal assessment of the Rochester Diabetic Neuropathy Study cohort. Diabetes Care. 1999 Sep;22(9): 1479-86.

Hughes RA: Systematic reviews of treatment for chronic inflammatory demyelinating neuropathy. Rev Neurol (Paris). 2002 Dec;158 (12 Pt 2):S32-36.

Shy ME, Lewis RA: An approach to patients with peripheral neuropathy. In Miller AE (ed): Continuum, Lifelong Learning in Neurology. Lippincott, Williams & Wilkins, 2003, vol 9, pp 11-18.

Sommer C: Painful neuropathies. Curr Opin Neurol 2003;165(5):623-628.

Vincent AM, Feldman EL: New insights into the mechanisms of diabetic neuropathy. Rev Endocr Metabol Disord 2004; 5:227-236.

Wicklund MP, Kissel JT: Paraproteinemic neuropathy. Curr Treat Options Neurol 2001 Mar;3(2):147-156.

Management of Head Injuries

Method of
Todd W. Vitaz, MD

Traumatic brain injury (TBI) most commonly results from motor vehicle crashes (MVC) and typically affects males in the 2nd through 4th decades of life. These sudden random acts can have long-lasting effects on the patient and family, but these events also impact society as a whole when a young, viable working-age individual becomes suddenly disabled and dependent on the care of others. TBI has no regard for age or gender, however, and can be seen in infants as a result of nonaccidental trauma as well as in geriatric patients following falls. The management of these patients can become extremely complicated and often requires the close interaction of numerous different health care providers ranging from trauma, orthopedic, and neurologic surgeons to nurses, social workers, speech, occupational, and physical therapists. Unfortunately, current interventions are still limited to the avoidance or minimization of secondary injury and rehabilitative intervention. However, when these patients are managed with aggressive, comprehensive, multidisciplinary approaches, the outcomes at times can be rewarding.

TBI can be categorized based on numerous factors. Most commonly it is differentiated based on mechanism and injury type (closed versus penetrating), whether it has occurred with or without systemic injuries (isolated versus multisystem), and the severity (mild, moderate, severe). The Glasgow Coma Scale (GCS) (Table 1), which was initially developed as a prognostic indicator following closed head injury, has become the principal triage tool for evaluating these patients. Patients are scored based on their best response in each of the three categories (eye opening, verbal responses, and motor score) and then subdivided into mild (13 to 15), moderate (9 to 12), and severe (3 to 8). One caveat to this assessment tool is that it can be affected by numerous alterations: hypoxia, hypotension, hypothermia, intoxication, infection, and other metabolic derangements, which are commonly seen in the trauma population.

Pathology

Another common classification system following TBI is based on pathophysiologic findings. Concussion commonly occurs following mild or moderate TBI as the result of transient (typically seconds to minutes) neurologic dysfunction in the setting of a normal computed tomography (CT) scan. Brief loss of consciousness, commonly with amnesia regarding the event, is not uncommon and is often associated with nausea, vomiting, headache, dizziness, and transient visual obscuration. These symptoms may persist for several hours to weeks as part of the *postconcussive syndrome* and, in rare instances, especially following repetitive injury, these alterations may become long-lasting. As a result of these persistent problems, in addition to a better understanding of the neurocognitive effects following this type of injury, there has been an enormous emphasis placed on their prevention (see text following).

Skull fractures may occur in isolation or be associated with other types of brain injuries. They are commonly classified based on whether they are open (overlying laceration) or closed, linear or comminuted, nondepressed or depressed. Skull fractures occur either as the result of a large force directed to a small area (i.e., depressed skull fracture following a blow to the head with a golf club) or when larger forces are dissipated throughout the skull resulting in fracture through the weakest area (linear fractures through frontal skull base, petrous, or squamous temporal bone). Linear fractures are commonly associated with raccoon eyes (frontal skull base fractures), Battle's sign (posterior skull base fracture), cerebrospinal fluid leak (otorrhea or rhinorrhea) or olfactory, facial or acoustic nerve injury (amnesia, facial palsy, sensorineuronal deafness).

In addition, temporal bone fractures may also be associated with epidural hematomas (EDHs). These extraaxial blood clots are most commonly caused by laceration of the middle meningeal artery and result in accumulation of *high-pressure arterial bleeding* in the potential space between the dura and skull. EDHs are more commonly seen in younger individuals probably because of the

TABLE 1 Glasgow Coma Scale

Best Motor Score	Best Verbal Response	Best Eye Opening
6 Obeys commands	5 Normal speech	4 Spontaneous
5 Localizes to pain	4 Confused	3 To voice
4 Withdraws to pain	3 Inappropriate words	2 To pain
3 Flexor posturing	2 Incomprehensible sounds	1 No eye opening
2 Extensor posturing	1 No verbal response	
1 No motor reponse	Intubated patients receive a 1 with the suffix T added to score	

decreased skull thickness and lack of adhesions between the skull and dura mater in this population. Commonly, these lesions appear on CT scan as lens-shaped, extra-axial hematomas most often in the temporal region and can be rapidly expansive secondary to the high-pressure arterial bleeding. The clinical course in these patients is classically described by a brief loss of consciousness from the initial concussion, followed by a "lucid interval" in which the patient may be awake and alert, which then gives way to another episode of decreased mental status that may be rapidly progressive and associated with signs of brain stem compression (flexor or extensor posturing, dilated nonreactive pupil). EDHs are usually treated surgically unless they are extremely small and constitute one of the few true neurosurgical emergencies where mere minutes may make an enormous difference in the patient's outcome.

Unlike EDHs, subdural hematomas (SDHs) are often associated with other types of brain injury and thus typically involve an altered level of consciousness (LOC) from the onset. SDHs are typically caused by bleeding from bridging veins that get torn when the brain moves within its cerebrospinal fluid (CSF) buffer while the veins remain tethered at their dural insertions; however, other causes such as venous or arterial hemorrhage from a brain laceration also exist. CT scanning reveals that these lesions commonly appear more crescent-shaped but never cross the dural boundaries (falx or tentorium). Unlike the high-pressure EDHs, SDHs typically expand at a slower rate but still cause devastating neurologic dysfunction from compression of the underlying brain. In addition mortality rates tend to be higher with worse outcome for SDH as a result of the common underlying brain injury. Once again these extra-axial clots frequently require surgical evacuation unless they are small and fail to have substantial compression on the underlying brain, where they are managed with serial imaging and close neurologic observation. In patients for whom a small SDH is not treated surgically, the physician must remain cognizant of the fact that a small proportion of these will increase in size between 1 and 4 weeks following the trauma and can be a cause of delayed deterioration or increased headache and new neurologic findings.

Intraparenchymal hematomas occur quite commonly following TBI and can be either hemorrhagic or nonhemorrhagic. These lesions range in size from 1 to 2 mm, up to several centimeters, and can cause a full range of symptoms and neurologic findings based on their location, size, and degree of compression on surrounding structures. Just like extra-axial hematomas, these lesions may increase in size and commonly coalesce or mature and *blossom* during the first 12 to 24 hours following the trauma. In addition, larger hematomas incite an inflammatory reaction in the surrounding brain resulting in increased edema around the lesion, which may result in increases in the intracranial pressure (ICP) (commonly seen on postinjury days [PIDs] 3 to 7). Management of these lesions depends on their size, location, and associated findings and ranges from serial observation and repeat imaging, surgical evacuation of the hematoma, or decompressive craniectomy with or without lobectomy.

The final category of pathologic abnormalities following TBI occurs as the result of shear injury to the axons themselves, called diffuse axonal injury (DAI). This is caused by either acceleration and deceleration or rotational forces to the axons resulting in micro- or macroscopic areas of injury and axonal transection. Most commonly this is encountered in the setting where a patient clinically has signs of a severe TBI, often with a GCS score less than 6; however, the CT scan is either unimpressive or shows only small areas of petechial hemorrhage. In addition ICP recording typically shows normal or only slightly elevated values. Magnetic resonance imaging (MRI) is commonly used in this subset of patients and can be used as a predictive indicator for determining the severity of injury, especially if CT is negative. MRI commonly shows areas of increased intensity on fluid attenuation inversion recovery (FLAIR) and T2-weighted sequences in the brainstem, diencephalon, deep white matter tracts, or corpus callosum. Recovery following this type of injury is variable and depends more on the injury location (reticular activating system of brainstem versus supratentorial white matter tracts) rather than the injury volume.

In addition to these abnormalities, patients with TBI are also at risk for damage to the spinal cord and vertebral and carotid arteries. Thus, patients with altered LOC should be assumed to have spinal instability and possible spinal cord injury (SCI); they should remain immobilized until the absence of these can be confirmed. The incidence of carotid and vertebral artery injury associated with severe TBI is unknown, but patients with facial or cervical fractures and those with soft tissue neck or chest injury (seat belt sign) have been found to be at higher risk. The appropriate screening for and treatment of these injuries have become a topic of intense debate in recent years but should be suspected in a patient with focal neurologic findings without identifiable cause on other imaging.

INTRACRANIAL PRESSURE AND THE MONROE-KELLIE DOCTRINE

Regardless of the pathophysiologic type of injury, the end result commonly is the generation of increases in the ICP, which can then lead to secondary brain injury. ICP dynamics are easily understood if one considers the principles of the volume pressure relationships outlined by the Monroe-Kellie doctrine. The basis of this principle resides on the fact that the skull is a fixed and rigid volume; because of this any changes to the volume of its contents will directly affect the pressure within this rigid space. In simplest terms the intracranial cavity contains blood, water, and tissue. Blood may be intravascular (IV) or extravascular (EV) in the case of extra-axial blood clots; water includes not only cerebrospinal fluid, which may build up in cases of hydrocephalus, but also edema following traumatic injuries; brain parenchyma typically compromises the tissue component but in select instances tumors or cysts may also fall into this category.

As increases in any or all three of these categories occur, the pressure inside the cranial cavity increases proportionally. At first compensatory changes occur, which accommodate for these increases, resulting in only mild pressure changes; however, eventually a critical volume is reached where the compensatory mechanisms are saturated, resulting in rapid and dramatic pressure changes. The following scenario illustrates these principles. A patient is involved in a motor vehicle crash and suffers a head injury with a small epidural hematoma. Initially he is awake and alert without any focal neurologic findings.

The epidural hematoma creates an increase in the EV blood component of the Monroe-Kellie doctrine; however, compensatory changes in intracranial CSF volume result in decreases in the water component, thus preventing significant changes in ICP. However, the hematoma continues to enlarge, causing increases in ICP exhibited clinically by slow deterioration in the patient's level of consciousness. The patient is now intubated and mildly hyperventilated causing vasoconstriction, therefore decreasing the intravascular blood component and reducing ICP with an improvement in the patient's neurologic condition. Unfortunately, as the operating room (OR) is being prepared, the patient suffers a rapid decrease in his level of conscious, becoming unresponsive with flexor posturing and a nonreactive pupil. Although the hematoma has expanded at a constant rate over time, the rapid change in the patient's condition is the result of him reaching the critical point where all compensatory mechanisms have been exhausted, thus causing profound rapid changes in the patient's ICP.

Treatment of Elevated Intracranial Pressure

Acute changes in ICP result in altered LOC, and at times other localizing neurologic findings such as *blown* (dilated, nonreactive) pupils and flexor or extensor posturing, and such findings may be the sign of impending herniation and death without immediate intervention. In a patient without a ventricular drain already in place, hyperventilation is the most rapid mechanism for acutely lowering elevated ICP. Currently, aggressive hyperventilation ($PCO_2 < 30$) is recommended only for short durations in cases of impending cerebral herniation while patients are being stabilized. As stated previously, hyperventilation causes vasoconstriction, which reduces intravascular blood within the cranial vault and almost instantaneously lowering ICP. However, several studies have now shown that the routine use of aggressive hyperventilation in the management of patients with severe closed head injury (CHI) results in decreased outcomes because of hypoxic injury and possible stroke caused by the sustained hyperventilation. Our current practice is to maintain PCO_2 values between 35 and 38 with controlled ventilation in all patients with severe CHI; because of this we leave all these patients intubated and mechanically ventilated until their ICPs normalize and all other therapies are withdrawn.

Adequate sedation and pain control are also important elements of ICP control. Patients who are restless and agitated will have higher ICPs than similar patients who are resting quietly in bed. Another important point is the prevention of venous congestion. This occasionally is evident in cervical collars, which are fastened too tight or with the use of trach ties that are wrapped too tightly around the neck to hold the endotracheal tube in place.

Several medications are available for the treatment of elevated ICP with the most common one being mannitol. Although this agent acts as an osmotic diuretic and helps pull excess interstitial fluid into the vascular space and thus lower ICP, there are several other hypothetical mechanisms that probably also increase its efficacy such as increasing RBC flexibility, decreasing RBC and platelet clumping in small arterioles and capillaries, and increasing

intravascular volume, thus improving cardiac function. Other diuretics such as furosemide (Lasix)[1] or urea (Ureaphil) may also be used but have less dramatic effects on ICP. Hypertonic saline (NaCl 3% to 5%)[1] has also been used more recently by some physicians and has been shown to have many of the same effects as mannitol.

CSF diversion is one of the simplest, quickest acting methods for decreasing ICP especially if a ventricular drain is already in place. The emergent surgical evacuation of mass lesions such as large epidural, subdural, or intraparenchymal hematomas is also extremely effective for controlling ICP, and in many instances it is also life-saving. However, in some instances, underlying brain injury or stroke from prolonged brain compression may be exhibited as massive intraoperative brain swelling and in these instances may necessitate that the bone flap be left off (craniectomy).

Management of Severe Closed Head Injury

The current recommendations of the Brain Trauma Foundation Guidelines for the management of closed head injuries call for the placement of ICP monitors in all patients who fall into the severe category (GCS score < 9). At our institution we routinely place combination intraventricular monitors and drains in all patients with a postresuscitation GCS score of less than 7. Monitors are inserted into patients with a GCS score of 7 to 9 on an individual basis depending on whether there are distracting reasons, such as intoxication, to cause the altered LOC. If patients are intubated and not following commands but are purposeful in their movements, we will sometimes elect not to place a ventriculostomy and follow the patient's clinical course over several hours. Other factors include CT findings and the need to go to the operating room during the acute period for the treatment of other life-threatening injuries, age, or for heavy sedation secondary to other injuries or pulmonary problems. At times patients in this GCS range will be given 6 to 12 hours and treated medically to see whether or not they improve prior to placement of an ICP monitor.

Once an ICP monitor and drain have been placed elevations in ICP are treated in a systematic order. Target values include attempts to keep ICP less than 15 to 20 and cerebral perfusion pressure (CPP) greater than 60. Low CPP (CPP = mean arterial blood pressure [MAP] – ICP) is caused by either elevated ICP or low MAP. For patients with low MAP or uncontrolled ICP, vasopressors may be used to increase blood pressure (BP) and central venous pressure. At the University of Louisville, dopamine (Intropin) is used as a first line agent, followed by phenylephrine (Neo-Synephrine) and norepinephrine (Levophed) in refractory cases. ICP elevations are initially treated with adequate sedation and pain control, such as midazolam (Versed),[1] propofol (Diprivan), and/or morphine (Lioresal),[1] to prevent agitation and elevated airway pressures, which can further increase ICP and intermittent CSF diversion. In cases where this fails to control ICP, mannitol is then added to the treatment protocol along with more continuous CSF diversion and finally chemical paralysis.

[1]Not FDA approved for this indication.

Mannitol is administered as a bolus infusion in doses ranging from 0.25 to 1.0 mg/kg body weight every 4 to 8 hours with the endpoints being either ICP control or measured serum osmolarity greater than 315 mOsmL.

Patients who continue to have sustained increases in their ICP despite these interventions are considered to have refractory ICP and at our facility are considered for one of two potential salvage treatments. Pentobarbital (Nembutal)[1] coma has been used successfully on occasion in young patients without mass lesions to decrease the metabolic demands of the brain during these periods of sustained ICP. Patients need to be chosen wisely for this therapy because it carries enormous risks in addition to the possibility of preserving the patient in a long-term, nonfunctional, persistent vegetative state. Initiation of pentobarbital (Nembutal)[1] coma causes severe hypotension, and patients almost always require the use of pressors in addition to volume expansion. At our facility we also place all of these patients on a Rotorest bed in an attempt to minimize the pulmonary complications that frequently occur with the use of this technique.

The second salvage therapy is decompressive craniectomy. This procedure involves the removal of a significant area of skull, typically almost an entire hemisphere or both frontal regions with opening of the dura. This permits the injured swollen brain to herniate through the opening and is the only intervention that increases the volume of the intracranial compartment, thereby reducing pressure. In addition this technique allows for the evacuation of large hemorrhagic contusions, or in cases of extreme ICP elevations it can be coupled with either frontal or temporal lobectomy. Once again, patients must be selected carefully for this intervention. Decompressive craniectomy is used much more frequently than pentobarbital (Nembutal)[1] coma at our institution. We use this strategy for patients with elevated ICP—more than 30 to 40 for more than 30 minutes—or a significant change in neurologic condition that is nonresponsive to all other interventions. In order for either of these two salvage approaches to be effective, they must be used at the first signs of refractory ICP prior to the occurrence of complications such as ischemic infarcts or brainstem compression or hemorrhage.

Patients treated with decompressive craniectomies are at risk for significant alterations in CSF dynamics that may result in delayed deterioration. Signs of hydrocephalus either in the form of ventriculomegaly or extra-axial or interhemispheric CSF fluid collections will be evident in 50% to 80% of these patients. When necessary these patients will be treated with external ventricular or subdural drains followed by early cranioplasty (replacement of the bone plate). In many instances these changes will resolve following cranioplasty and therefore avoid the need for ventriculoperitoneal shunting, with its associated risks and complications.

All patients with abnormal head CT scans (regardless of GCS score) are treated with close neurologic observation most commonly in an intensive care unit (ICU) setting, serial CT scans (4 to 6 hours later and on PID 1), and placed on 7 days of phenytoin (Dilantin). Temkin and colleagues showed that patients with post-traumatic intracranial hemorrhage were at increased risk of suffering seizures in the acute period; treatment with antiepileptics beyond 7 days did not decrease the risk of these patients from developing epilepsy or delayed seizures but there were increased risks associated with side effects from medication administration. Patients who experience a seizure following CHI (with the exception of acute post-traumatic seizures) should be maintained on antiepileptics for at least 3 to 6 months and possible indefinitely depending on their clinical condition and EEG results. Patients with acute post-traumatic seizures (within the first several minutes following the event) are not felt to be at increased risk for developing further seizures and receive the routine 7-day treatment. At the University of Louisville we have found that changing phenytoin dosing to a weight-based schedule (15 mg/kg load, 2 mg/kg every 8 hours unless elderly [≥70 years old], then 2 mg/kg every 12 hours) increases the chance of achieving a therapeutic dose earlier in the treatment course and lowers the costs of monitoring these agents.

Finally, the treatment of these patients requires a tight-knit group of specialists and ancillary service providers with open communication channels. We have found that the use of a time-independent phased outcome clinical pathway helps maximize the level of patient care and maintain cost-effectiveness. By using such an approach all routine interactions are initiated at the time of admission and each care provider has a clear role and responsibility; one of the most important aspects of this system is the creation of a clinical coordinator whose responsibility includes ensuring that all aspects of patient care and family education are completed at the appropriate intervals. We believe another key component of this is our philosophy toward early feeding (prior to PID 3) and early tracheotomy and percutaneous endoscopic gastrostomy (PEG) feeding tube placement in a majority of these individuals (PID 4). We have shown that such an aggressive approach to these issues helps reduce infectious complications and minimizes length of ICU stay.

Treatment of Mild and Moderate Traumatic Brain Injury

In many circumstances patients with moderate TBI are treated almost as though they had severe TBI, with the exception of invasive ICP monitoring. Many patients will be intubated at the time of admission and require sedation and adequate pain management. This can be difficult because it is of utmost importance to maintain the ability to perform serial neurologic examinations. Therefore, we commonly use a combination of propofol (Diprivan) infusions and intermittent morphine (Lioresal)[1] injections in these patients, thereby allowing hourly assessment of neurologic function. We have found that a subset of patients (older than age 45 years, multisystem trauma, presence of early pneumonia) with moderate TBI requires more aggressive treatment with early tracheostomy and PEG tube placement and at times ICP monitors.

The subset of patients with moderate TBI who are not intubated at the time of admission are also watched closely

---

[1]Not FDA approved for this indication.

[1]Not FDA approved for this indication.

in the ICU. Once again, close monitoring of neurologic function and vigorous pulmonary toilet is of key importance because some patients may be lethargic and are at risk of pulmonary decompensation. We have found ipratropium (Atrovent)[1] and albuterol (Proventil)[1] nebulizers and early mobilization minimize pulmonary problems. Patients with progressive lethargy, worsening neurologic function, hypoxia, hypercapnia, or the inability to protect their airways are intubated and placed on mechanical ventilation. Once again, patients unable to tolerate a diet by PID 3 have a nasogastric feeding tube placed to allow for early enteral nutritional support; however, PEG tubes are not placed until later in the hospital course in the predischarge phase because many patients in this category will improve throughout their hospitalization and be able to tolerate an oral diet by the time of discharge.

Patients with mild TBI are treated over a much wider continuum, ranging from discharge from the emergency room (ER) with appropriate adult supervision to observation in the ICU to immediate surgical treatment of surgical mass lesions. The two most important factors in determining treatment algorithms for these patients are presence or absence of abnormal CT findings and neurologic function, with associated symptoms such as nausea, vomiting, dizziness, or visual problems. Headache is a common complaint in all of these patients and must be taken in context with other complaints and imaging results. Patients with severe headaches, dizziness, and vomiting (postconcussive syndrome) may commonly require a brief hospital stay to allow for delayed imaging and at least partial resolution of some of the complaints.

Early and Delayed Neurologic Changes

Any patient suffering a significant neurologic injury requires close neurologic monitoring. Although most patients remain unchanged or show gradual improvement in the early phases, a small percentage will show signs of neurologic deterioration. At first these signs may be subtle (agitation, mild increase in lethargy, protracted vomiting); but eventually they may become more profound and can be precursors to impending neurologic demise and death. When these changes are the result of either expanding mass lesions or increases in ICP, treatment instituted in the early phases is more likely to be more successful compared to instances when interventions are performed under conditions associated with cerebral herniation syndromes. Thus any patient showing persistent signs of neurologic decline should be promptly evaluated by a physician and many may also require repeat CT scanning.

However, not all neurologic changes are the result of changes in ICP or expansion of mass lesions, and such irregularities may be caused by a long list of other metabolic or neurologic conditions. Some of the more common causes are seizures, strokes (especially from carotid or vertebral dissections), electrolyte imbalances, hypoxia, hypercarbia, fever, excess sedation, or drug and/or alcohol withdrawal.

Concussions and Sports-Related Injuries: Return to Play Guidelines

Over the past 2 decades, the knowledge regarding the detrimental effects of repetitive mild head injuries has led to intense public debate concerning whether athletes should be allowed to return to play following such injuries. Concussions are not uncommon among participants of competitive sports including football, hockey, baseball, and soccer. Concerns regarding the full negative impact of repetitive, almost innocuous injury have led many youth soccer leagues to ban or modify rules regarding *heading* of the ball. In addition, other concerns exist following more severe concussions such as development of other life-threatening neurologic injuries such as subdural or epidural hematomas, development of the double-impact syndrome (rapid uncontrolled increases in ICP following sequential minor traumas), and the long-term neuropsychological impact of these injuries. As a result of these concerns, the guidelines concerning when and if an athlete should be allowed to return to play have undergone modification since development of the earlier criteria. Because of these frequent changes, readers are encouraged to check with their local medical agencies or recent publications and Internet sources if faced with these issues. In short, if a player loses consciousness or has persistent symptoms (>15 to 20 minutes), they should not be allowed to return to play on that day or even not for 1 to 2 weeks following the complete resolution of all symptoms. It should also be stressed that an individual may have a concussion without loss of consciousness and that concussion is defined as any transient change in mental status. To this end many organizations including the National Football League have developed a sideline neuropsychological screening test that can often help illustrate these deficits even when the athlete appears normal.

 CURRENT DIAGNOSIS

Classification of Head Injuries

- Closed versus penetrating
- Isolated versus multisystem injuries
- Severity
  - Mild (GCS 13-15)
  - Moderate (GCS 9-12)
  - Severe (GCS 3-8)

Pathologic Findings with Closed Head Injuries

- Skull fractures
- Epidural hematomas
- Subdural hematomas
- Parenchymal contusions
- Intraparenchymal hematomas
- Diffuse axonal injury

---

[1]Not FDA approved for this indication.

Restorative Therapies

Patients suffering any type of TBI can have long-lasting cognitive, psychological, and emotional dysfunction in addition to their functional and neurologic deficits. Although most people assume that the resolution of decreased alertness and consciousness symbolizes resolution of the overall neurologic injury, this is not the case in most patients. In our series of patients with moderate TBI, we found that almost 50% of patients at median follow-up of 27 months complained of persistent emotional or cognitive problems that interfered with their lifestyle despite the fact that they all were discharged from the hospital with a GCS score of 14 to 15. Long-term speech and cognitive therapies as well as individual, group, and family counseling will be helpful for many of these patients.

In the late hospital and early rehabilitative stages, numerous pharmacologic agents may be helpful to overcome some of the neurologic side effects following TBI. Patients with autonomic storms (intermittent episodes of diaphoresis, tachycardia, fever, agitation) may respond to adrenergic antagonists such as clonidine (Catapres)[1] or propanolol (Inderal),[1] in addition to volume resuscitation, morphine (Lioresal),[1] baclofen,[1] and bromocriptine (Parlodel).[1] Patients with hypoarousal are treated with amantadine[1] (Symmetrel), 100 mg at 8 AM and 12 PM, and bromocriptine,[1] 5 to 15 mg every day. Trazodone (Desyrel), 50 to 100 mg at bedtime, may be helpful in restoring sleep-wake cycles, whereas risperidone (Risperdal),[1] olanzapine (Zyprexa),[1] and quetiapine (Seroquel)[1] may be helpful to control agitation and combativeness during the subacute recovery phases.

Future Considerations

The previously mentioned treatment strategies include what is considered common practice at the University of Louisville; however, newer, more aggressive treatments and monitoring capabilities are always being developed. Some of the newer monitoring systems under development include cerebral oximetry measurements (frequently through invasive indwelling catheters) or cerebral microdialysis systems, in which continuous assessments are performed

---

[1]Not FDA approved for this indication.

CURRENT THERAPY

Management of Elevated Intracranial Pressure

- Prevention of venous engorgement
- CO_2 control (mild hyperventilation)
- Sedation and pain control
- Cerebrospinal fluid drainage
- Mannitol
- Lasix
- Hypertonic saline
- Decompressive craniectomy
- Pentobarbital coma

---

to determine the concentrations of critical markers such as lactate in the brain or CSF. Both of these methods provide physiologic feedback for the metabolic environment of the brain, are sensitive enough to predict changes in regional oxygenation, and have been found to be correlated with outcomes in small nonrandomized studies.

REFERENCES

Brain Trauma Foundation: Management and Prognosis of Severe Traumatic Brain Injury. New York, Brain Trauma Foundation, 2000.

Mcilvoy L, Spain DA, Raque G, et al: Successful incorporation of the Severe Head Injury Guidelines into a phased-outcome clinical pathway. J Neurosci Nurs 2001;33(2):72-78, 82.

Miller PR, Fabian TC, Bee TK, et al: Blunt cerebrovascular injuries: Diagnosis and treatment. J Trauma 2001;51(2):279-286.

Temkin NR, Dikmen SS, Wilensky AJ, et al: A randomized, double-blind study of phenytoin for the prevention of post-traumatic seizures. N Engl J Med 1990;323:497-502.

Vitaz TW, McIlvoy L, Raque GH, et al: Development and implementation of a clinical pathway for severe traumatic brain injury. J Trauma 2001;51(2):369-375.

Vitaz TW, McIlvoy L, Raque GH, et al: Development and implementation of a clinical pathway for spinal cord injuries. J Spinal Disord 2001;14(3):271-276.

Vitaz TW, Jenks J, Raque GH, Shields CB: Outcome following moderate traumatic brain injury. Surg Neurol 2003;60(4):285-291.

Traumatic Brain Injury in Children

Method of
Stephen R. Deputy, MD

Traumatic brain injury (TBI) is one of the leading causes of death and disability among children, adolescents, and young adults. An estimated 185 per 100,000 children (ages 0 to 14 years) and 550 per 100,000 adolescents (ages 15 to 19 years) are hospitalized each year for TBI. The etiology of TBI varies depending on the age of the patient, with younger children more likely to be injured from falls and pedestrian injuries, and adolescents more often injured in motor vehicle accidents and assaults. Inflicted TBI (shaking-impact syndrome of infancy) is the leading cause of injury-related deaths in children younger than 4 years of age and accounts for 80% of deaths from head trauma in children younger than 2 years of age.

Types and Severity of Head Injury

Closed head injury is the most common type of TBI seen in children. Forces from rapid deceleration are applied diffusely throughout the brain and consciousness is frequently impaired. *Open head injuries*, in which the dura is breached, are caused by focal penetrating forces, and the risk of post-traumatic epilepsy is relatively high.

Primary brain injury is caused by the mechanical forces of the trauma itself. Diffuse axonal injury is an example of primary brain injury. During rapid deceleration, angular forces applied to the head cause the brain to rotate about its center of gravity. Shifting regions of differing densities within the brain itself result in shearing along planes such as the gray-white junction, corpus callosum, and brainstem. The shearing of axons effectively serves to "disconnect" the cortex from the brainstem and consciousness becomes impaired. Translational (straight-line) forces applied to the head produce impact-loading contact phenomena, resulting in focal injuries to the scalp, skull, and brain, such as lacerations, skull fractures, cerebral contusions, and epidural hematomas. *Subdural hematomas* may occur because of tearing of fragile dural bridging veins during rapid decelerations.

Secondary brain injury follows and is the consequence of primary injury. Examples include hypoxic-ischemic injury (secondary to low cerebral perfusion pressure or anoxia), disrupted cerebral autoregulation, seizures or status epilepticus, diffuse cerebral edema, hydrocephalus, and raised intracranial pressure. The goal of treatment for TBI is to reduce or prevent secondary brain injury from occurring because the primary brain injury has already happened at the time of trauma and cannot be altered.

The severity of TBI can be broken down into mild, moderate, and severe. *Mild* TBI is defined as head trauma with an initial Glasgow Coma Scale (GCS) score of 13 to 15. *Moderate* TBI occurs with an initial GCS score of 9 to 12. *Severe* TBI occurs with an initial GCS score of 8 or less. The GCS is modified for use in infants under the age of 36 months (Table 1).

Special attention should be given to those infants with TBI who do not show evidence of external facial or head trauma and who may not be presented by their caregivers as having a history of head injury. The *shaking-impact syndrome* is usually found in infants younger than 3 years of age with a peak incidence in infants younger than 1 year of age. Presenting symptoms include irritability, lethargy, or coma, apnea or breathing irregularities, and seizures. Retinal hemorrhages may be found in from 65% to 95% of these patients and should be actively looked for with a dilated funduscopic examination in any case where head trauma is suspected. Computed tomography (CT) imaging most commonly shows evidence of acute or remote subdural hematomas with or without evidence of cerebral infarction. Workup should include a skeletal survey to look for evidence of skull, posterior rib, or long bone fractures of different healing stages. Infants may be more susceptible to shaking-impact syndrome given their relatively large head size compared to their underdeveloped neck musculature. Infants also have thinner skulls, and translational forces may cause more severe contusions. Relatively longer subdural veins that bridge the infant's enlarged subarachnoid spaces can be easily lacerated from angular forces, resulting in subdural hematomas.

Management of Traumatic Brain Injury in Children

MILD TRAUMATIC BRAIN INJURY

Mild TBI accounts for more than 90% of all pediatric admissions for TBI. Children in this category should have a GCS score of 15 upon arrival to the emergency room, no focal neurologic deficits, and no signs of increased intracranial pressure (ICP). These children may have had a brief loss of consciousness (less than 1 minute), amnesia for the event, an immediate impact seizure, vomiting, or lethargy (as long as the GCS score is 15 during the evaluation). Children without loss of consciousness or amnesia may be observed or sent home with competent caregivers without performing neuroimaging studies. Vigilance for any change in the child's neurologic status should be maintained for up to 72 hours after the injury. If there has been a brief loss of consciousness or amnesia for the event, the risk of intracranial hemorrhage is still relatively low, and it is up to the discretion of the treating physician whether CT imaging is warranted.

Clinical predictors of intracranial hemorrhage are less reliable for children under the age of 2 years, and nonaccidental trauma also comes into consideration in this age group. Therefore, most children under the age of 2 years with TBI should undergo CT imaging followed by careful observation.

MODERATE TRAUMATIC BRAIN INJURY

Patients who fall within the moderate category generally need more intensive monitoring and medical management to avoid secondary brain injuries. As with all critical illness, attention should first be paid to following the ABCs (airway, breathing, circulation).

TABLE 1 Glasgow Coma Scale for Children

Score	Eyes Open	Best Verbal Response	Best Verbal Response	Best Motor Response (<36 mo)	Best Motor Response (<36 mo)
6	—	—	—	Follows commands	Normal spontaneous movements
5	—	Oriented and converses	Coos and babbles	Localizes pain	Withdraws to touch
4	Spontaneously	Confused	Irritable to pain	Withdraws to pain	Withdraws to pain
3	To verbal commands	Inappropriate words	Cries to pain	Flexor posturing	Flexor posturing
2	To painful stimuli	Nonspecific sounds	Moans to pain	Extensor posturing	Extensor posturing
1	None	None	None	No response	No response

Airway

Patients with a GCS score of 9 or greater usually do not require endotracheal intubation for airway protection, although they should be kept NPO (nothing by mouth) in case of clinical deterioration.

Breathing

Hypoxemia and hypoventilation may increase ICP, so supplemental oxygen by nasal cannula may be helpful.

Circulation

It is important to avoid hypotension to maintain adequate cerebral perfusion pressure (CPP). Isotonic intravenous fluids should be provided with care to avoid fluid overload, hypoglycemia, or hyperglycemia. Careful attention should be paid to fluid and sodium balance because these patients may be at risk for developing diabetes insipidus. Likewise, the head of the bed should be raised to 30 degrees and the patient's head kept midline to optimize venous return from the cranium to the right side of the heart. Sedation with short-acting sedatives (propofol [Diprivan] or midazolam [Versed]) or opioids may be necessary to avoid agitation, which can also reduce venous return to the heart.

Early post-traumatic seizures are fairly rare in children with moderate TBI. The need for empirical anticonvulsant therapy in this group remains controversial and should be reserved for those patients in whom raised intracranial pressure is of concern. Likewise, empirical use of mannitol has little clinical support for this group.

SEVERE TRAUMATIC BRAIN INJURY

Patients in the severe group are at the highest risk for secondary brain injuries. The following additional interventions are recommended.

Airway

By definition, these patients have a GCS score of 8 or lower and require endotracheal intubation for airway protection.

Breathing

Hyperventilation with a goal Pco_2 of 26 to 30 mm Hg should be performed only if there is impending brainstem herniation or to bridge the gap until more definitive neurosurgical intervention can be performed to lower intracranial pressure. The benefit of hyperventilation is generally short lived (1 to 24 hours) and may worsen local ischemia following trauma or acute stroke.

Circulation

In the setting of suspected raised intracranial pressure, the goal of fluid and blood pressure management should be to maintain the cerebral perfusion pressure greater than 50 to 70 mm Hg. Recall that CPP equals MAP (mean arterial blood pressure) minus ICP. Because children generally have a lower MAP than adults, it is not always necessary to provide vasopressor therapy to keep the CPP above 70 mm Hg unless there is evidence of raised ICP. Invasive intracranial pressure monitoring should be considered if the GCS score is lower than 8 or in the setting of elevated ICP to optimize CPP.

Other Techniques to Lower Intracranial Pressure

NEUROSURGICAL

Obvious mass lesions, such as hydrocephalus, subdural and epidural hematomas, and contused cortical tissue should be surgically evacuated whenever feasible. CT scanning is able to identify most of these surgical lesions. Decompressive craniectomy is now used more frequently to relieve pressure when multifocal contusions or diffuse cerebral edema is present. As mentioned earlier, ICP monitoring is usually warranted for all severe TBI patients.

OSMOTHERAPY

Mannitol (20% solution) may be given as an initial bolus of 0.5 to 1 g/kg. Repeat doses of 0.25 to 0.5 g/kg are given every 6 to 8 hours as needed to maintain the serum osmolality and sodium levels to less than or equal to 320 mOsmL and 150 mEq, respectively. Osmotic diuretics should be used with caution in patients with renal insufficiency. The beneficial effects occur within minutes, peak at 1 hour, and last 4 to 24 hours. Potential disadvantages include worsening of focal cerebral edema in areas where the blood-brain barrier is disrupted.

BARBITURATES

Sedating agents may lower ICP by reducing pain as well as by making the brain metabolically less active. Pentobarbital is given as a loading dose of 5 to 20 mg/kg, followed by a continuous infusion of 1 to 4 mg/kg per hour. Continuous EEG monitoring to maintain a burst suppression pattern is warranted with this therapy. Potential disadvantages include systemic hypotension and a long half-life that may interfere with the declaration of brain death.

ANTICONVULSANT THERAPY

Children with severe TBI are at a high risk for early post-traumatic seizures, which can further elevate the ICP.

 CURRENT DIAGNOSIS

- Children under the age of 2 years with traumatic brain injury (TBI) may require neuroimaging because clinical predictors of intracranial hemorrhage are less reliable in this age group.
- Children under the age of 1 year presenting with lethargy, irritability, apnea, or seizures should be evaluated with computed tomography (CT) imaging and a dilated funduscopic examination to rule out shaking-impact syndrome.

CURRENT THERAPY

- Children with mild TBI and a GCS score of 15 at presentation can usually be observed clinically without the need for neuroimaging.
- The goal of treatment for TBI is to minimize *secondary* brain injury.
- In the setting of raised ICP, it is important to maintain CPP above 50 to 70 mm Hg.
- Early post-traumatic seizures are relatively frequent in open head injury and in severe TBI. They should be empirically treated in any patient in whom raised ICP is a concern.
- Direct intracranial pressure monitoring should be considered in any TBI patient with a GCS score of 8 or less.

Abbreviations: CPP = cerebral perfusion pressure; ICP = intracranial pressure; GCS = Glasgow Coma Scale; TBI = traumatic brain injury.

It is generally recommended empirically to load these children with 20 mg/kg of intravenous phenytoin (Cerebyx). Maintenance therapy can be achieved with 5 mg/kg per day divided every 8 hours with target blood levels of 10 to 20 mg/dL.

HYPOTHERMIA

More centers are including hypothermia as an option for patients with elevated ICP not responsive to medical or surgical management. The best method of cooling (i.e., whole body versus head only) and the optimal core temperature are not established for children.

Of note, apart from neurosurgical interventions, none of the techniques just described are shown definitively to reduce morbidity or mortality in children with severe TBI.

REFERENCES

Annegers JF, Grabow JD, Grover RV, et al: Seizures after head trauma: A population study. Neurology1980;30:683-689.
Bruce DA, Zimmerman RA: Shaken impact syndrome. Pediatr Ann 1989; 18:482-494.
Committee on Quality Improvement, American Academy of Pediatrics: The management of minor closed head injury in children. Pediatrics 1999;104(6):1407-1415.
Deputy SR: Shaking-impact syndrome of infancy. Semin Pediatr Neurol 2003;10(2):112-119.
Kraus JF, Nourjah P: The epidemiology of uncomplicated brain injury. J Trauma 1988;28:1637-1643.
Schutzman SA, Barnes P, et al: Evaluation and management of children younger than two years old with apparently minor head trauma: Proposed guidelines. Pediatrics 2001;107:983-993.

Brain Tumors

Method of
*Ashwatha Narayana, MD, and
Eve S. Ferdman, BA*

Primary brain tumors accounted for an estimated 18,400 new cases diagnosed and 12,690 deaths in the year 2004 in the United States. Several histopathologically different tumors arise in the brain, reflecting the diversity of phenotypically distinct cells within the central nervous system (CNS) that have a capacity for neoplastic transformation. Gliomas, the most common tumors, are considered first in this article, followed by a description of many of the principles of brain tumor management. Then less common tumors are briefly presented, and the article closes with a discussion about managing metastatic brain tumors.

Gliomas

INCIDENCE

Malignant gliomas make up 35% to 45% of primary brain tumors, and of these, nearly 85% are glioblastoma multiforme. The incidence of anaplastic astrocytoma peaks in children younger than 10 years of age and then remains constant in each subsequent decade of life. In contrast, the incidence of glioblastoma multiforme increases dramatically after the age of 40 years. Low-grade astrocytomas make up 5% to 15% of primary brain tumors and 67% of low-grade gliomas. The remainder of low-grade gliomas are mixed oligoastrocytomas (19%) and oligodendrogliomas (13%). Unlike their malignant counterparts, low-grade gliomas are most common between the ages of 20 and 40 years and rarely occur after the age of 50 years.

GENETICS AND ETIOLOGY

Genetic abnormalities are demonstrated for 50% to 75% of adult astrocytomas. It is hypothesized that p53 gene mutations are associated with the transition to grade II tumors. Malignant progression to anaplastic astrocytoma is associated with loss of heterozygosity (LOH) for chromosomes 9p, 13q, or 19q and CDK4 gene amplification. Subsequent LOH on chromosome 10 and amplification of the epidermal growth factor receptor genes characterize further progression to glioblastoma multiforme. A second, p53-independent, pathway that leads more directly to glioblastoma multiforme development is also described.

Losses of genetic information from chromosomes 1p and 19q are commonly seen in oligodendroglioma specimens, whereas losses on 17p and p53 gene mutations are notably less frequent, suggesting that early events in their oncogenesis are distinct from those associated with astrocytic tumors.

Although some environmental factors are linked with brain tumor development, they do not appear responsible for most brain tumors. Radiation-induced gliomas are reported, mainly in children with acute leukemia who received prophylactic cranial irradiation and chemotherapy.

The hereditary syndromes associated with an increased risk of brain tumors include neurofibromatosis type 1 and neurofibromatosis type 2, tuberous sclerosis, Li-Fraumeni syndrome, familial polyposis, Turcot's syndrome, Gardner's syndrome, and von Hippel-Lindau disease.

PATHOLOGY

CNS tumors are generally classified as follows (Table 1):

- Gliomas
- Neuronal/glioneuronal neoplasms

TABLE 1 Histopathology of Brain Tumors

Major Classification	Variants	WHO Grade
Gliomas		
Astrocytic: circumscribed	Pilocytic astrocytoma	I
	Subependymal giant cell astrocytoma (SEGA)	I
	Pleomorphic xanthoastrocytoma (PXA)	II
Astrocytic: diffuse	Astrocytoma	II
	Anaplastic astrocytoma	III
	Glioblastoma multiforme	IV
Oligodendroglial	Oligodendroglioma	II
	Anaplastic oligodendroglioma	III
Mixed gliomas	Oligoastrocytoma	II
	Anaplastic oligoastrocytoma	III
Ependymal	Subependymoma	I
	Myxopapillary ependymoma	I
	Ependymoma	II
	Anaplastic ependymoma*	III
Choroid plexus	Choroid plexus papilloma	I
	Choroid plexus carcinoma*	III
Cranial and Peripheral Nerve Tumors	Schwannoma	I
Neuronal and Glioneuronal Tumors	Gangliocytoma/ganglioglioma	I–III
	Desmoplastic infantile ganglioma (DIG)	I
	Dysplastic cerebellar gangliocytoma	I
	Central neurocytoma	I
	Dysembryoplastic neuroepithelial tumor	I
	Paraganglioma	I
Pineal Parenchymal Tumors (PPTs)	Pineocytoma	II
	PPT with intermediate differentiation	III
	Pineoblastoma	IV
Embryonal Tumors	Medulloepithelioma*	IV
	Primitive neuroectodermal tumor (PNET),* including medulloblastoma and variants*	IV
	Atypical teratoid/rhabdoid tumor (AT/RT)	IV
	Cerebral neuroblastoma/ganglioneuroblastoma	IV
	Ependymoblastoma*	IV
	Olfactory neuroblastoma (esthesioneuroblastoma)	IV
Meningeal Tumors	Meningioma	I
	Atypical meningioma	II
	Anaplastic (malignant) meningioma	III
Germ Cell Tumors	Hemangiopericytoma†	II–III
	Germinoma	NA
	Mature teratoma	NA
	Nongerminomatous germ cell tumors	NA
Tumors of the Sellar Region	Craniopharyngioma: adamantinomatous	I
	Craniopharyngioma: papillary	I
Hemopoietic Neoplasms	Primary central nervous system lymphoma (PCNSL)	NA
	Secondary lymphoma/leukemia	NA
	Histiocytic tumors and histiocytoses	NA
Secondary Tumors/Metastases	Carcinomas and sarcomas	NA

*Indicates those tumors with a tendency to disseminate throughout the central nervous system (CNS).
†The origin of hemangiopericytoma is uncertain.
Abbreviations: WHO = World Health Organization; NA = not applicable.

- Embryonal neoplasms
- Meningeal neoplasms
- Miscellaneous nonglial neoplasms

Reliance on a pathologic classification of brain tumors is a requisite for treatment. Indeed, histopathology is more important than anatomic staging in determining the clinical behavior and prognosis of these tumors. Neuropathologists do not all agree on a uniform classification system for astrocytic gliomas. The World Health Organization system, which divides astrocytic tumors into four grades—from grade I, corresponding to pilocytic astrocytomas, to grade IV, corresponding to the glioblastoma multiforme—is used more often.

Low-grade astrocytomas are well-differentiated tumors that display increased cellularity compared with normal brain tissue and have mild to moderate nuclear pleomorphism (Figure 1). The cytoplasmic processes that extend from the astrocytes contain a characteristic filamentous protein, glial fibrillary acidic protein (GFAP), which provides an immunohistochemical marker for these tumors. Over time, at least 50% of these tumors transform into more anaplastic lesions. The characteristic histopathologic features of anaplastic astrocytomas include moderate hypercellularity, moderate cellular and nuclear pleomorphism, variable mitotic activity, and microvascular proliferation. The presence of tumor necrosis is the hallmark that distinguishes anaplastic astrocytoma from glioblastoma multiforme (Figure 2).

Oligodendrogliomas, in contrast, are composed of small uniform cells with round central nuclei and distinct cytoplasmic borders. Formalin fixation causes a perinuclear halo that produces a "fried egg" or "honeycomb" appearance. The cells lack fibrillary cytoplasmic processes. Calcification is a frequent feature.

CLINICAL PRESENTATION

The presenting symptoms and signs of brain tumors include those associated with a mass effect and increased intracranial pressure and those that are focal. The most common presenting symptom with gliomas is headache. Approximately two thirds of adult patients with low-grade astrocytomas and 20% of patients with malignant

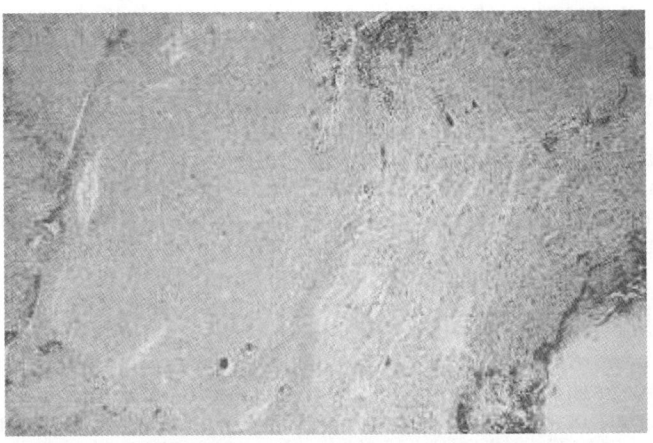

FIGURE 1. Low-grade astrocytoma showing mildly increased cellularity with uniform cells and nuclei.

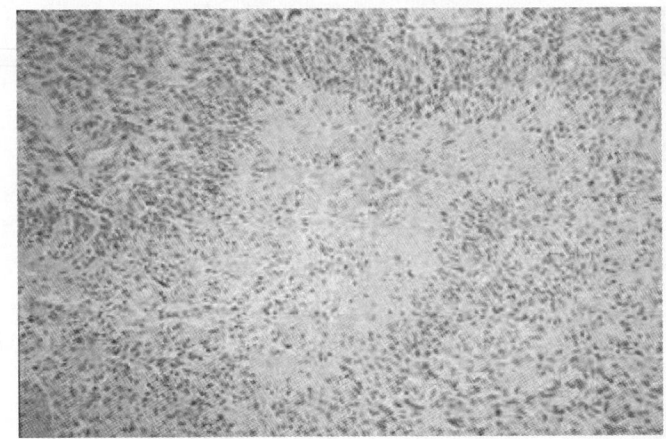

FIGURE 2. Glioblastoma multiforme with the hallmark features of necrosis with peripheral pseudopalisading of neoplastic nuclei.

tumors present with seizures but are otherwise neurologically intact. Others exhibit a slowly progressive neurologic syndrome consisting of headache, vomiting, motor deficit, visual or sensory loss, language disturbance, or personality change. Symptoms may be present for months or years before the diagnosis is made.

ROUTES OF SPREAD

The most common route of spread for gliomas is through local extension. As they enlarge, malignant gliomas extend directly into adjacent lobes and disseminate along anatomically defined nerve fiber pathways. Multicentric gliomas are found in less than 5% of patients. Dissemination by seeding through the CPF pathways occurs in approximately 10% of cases but is usually a late event. Metastases rarely arise outside the CNS.

DIAGNOSTIC STUDIES

Computed tomography (CT) and magnetic resonance imaging (MRI) play indispensable roles in the management of brain tumors. CT is a reliable screening and diagnostic method for suspected supratentorial brain tumor lesions. MRI, now more frequently used in patients with malignant brain tumors, is the screening procedure of choice for diagnosing and localizing tumors in the brainstem, posterior fossa, and spinal cord. Ordinary astrocytomas appear as diffuse, poorly defined, low-density, nonenhancing lesions. Approximately 40% of ordinary astrocytomas enhance, and calcification is found in 10% of cases. Although the majority of malignant gliomas enhance with contrast media, as many as 30% of anaplastic astrocytomas present as nonenhancing lesions. In both low-grade and malignant gliomas, parenchymal infiltration by isolated tumor cells may be present in regions of T2-weighted abnormality that appear normal on CT (Figures 3 and 4). Positron emission tomography (PET), single-photon emission computed tomography (SPECT) with thallium-201 (^{201}Tl), and magnetic resonance spectroscopy (MRS) are other imaging approaches used in brain tumor management.

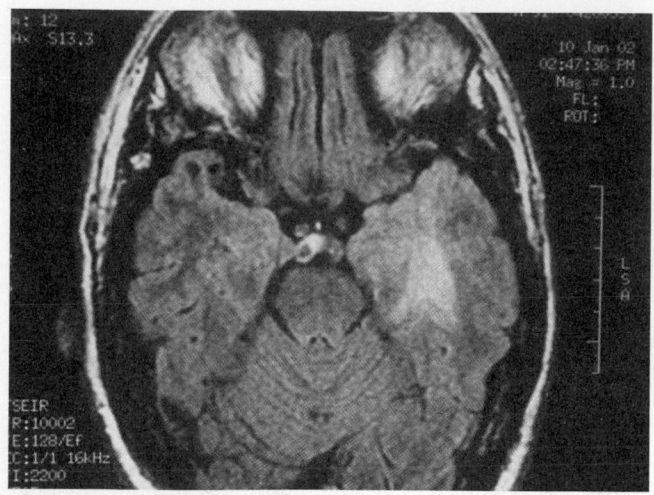

FIGURE 3. Axial magnetic resonance imaging scan of low-grade astrocytoma of left temporal lobe.

STAGING

No accepted staging system exists for primary brain tumors. The American Joint Committee on Cancer proposed a staging scheme for primary brain tumors based on tumor size and metastases as well as tumor grade. Because this system was not generally adapted to clinical use, it was subsequently removed.

PROGNOSTIC FACTORS

Age, histologic appearance, Karnofsky performance score (KPS), mental status, duration of symptoms, neurologic functional class, extent of surgery, and radiation dose are identified as significant partitioning covariates in clinical trials.

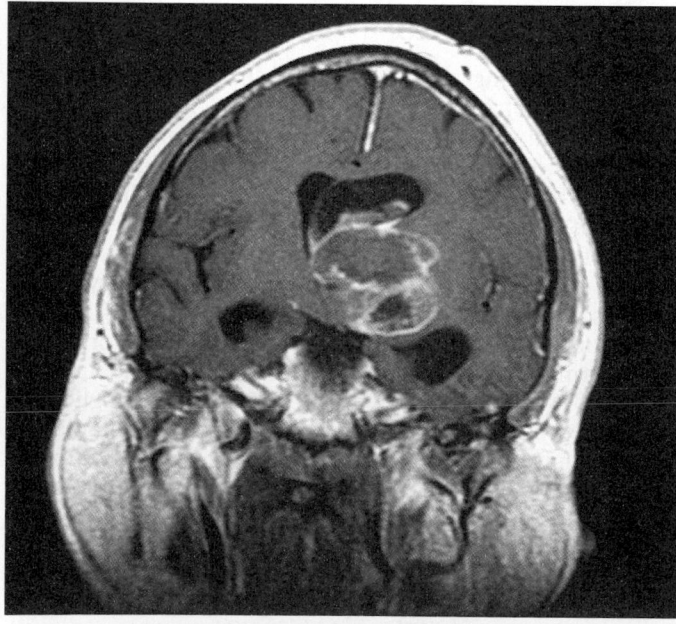

FIGURE 4. Coronal magnetic resonance imaging scan of high-grade astrocytoma of left internal capsule and brainstem region.

This information is important for correctly interpreting the results of studies comparing different treatment regimens and for assessing the potential of new therapeutic methodologies.

STANDARD THERAPEUTIC APPROACHES FOR GLIOMAS

Surgery

The combination of surgery, radiation therapy, and chemotherapy represents the standard approach to the treatment of gliomas. The goals of surgery are to provide a histologic diagnosis, to alleviate intracranial hypertension and focal neurologic deficits because of a mass effect, and to permit rapid corticosteroid dose tapering. Pilocytic astrocytomas are relatively well circumscribed, and 60% to 80% are amenable to total removal. Resection of the more common diffuse astrocytomas is limited by the lack of clear demarcation between the infiltrating tumor and normal brain tissue. Evidence suggests that patients with more complete resections live longer and have an improved functional status compared with those who undergo a biopsy or partial resection only. Advances in neurosurgery, including diagnostic ultrasound, lasers, ultrasonic tissue aspirators, cortical mapping, functional imaging, and computer-assisted stereotactic laser techniques, have improved the ability of neurosurgeons to radically remove intracranial tumors.

Radiation Therapy

Limited radiation fields are used for the treatment of gliomas. Three-dimensionally designed complex treatment plans with multiple fields are used whenever appropriate to limit the high-dose volume and to minimize the risk of long-term radiation sequelae. Doses of 50.4 to 54 Gy are usually recommended for low-grade gliomas and 59.4 to 60 Gy for high-grade gliomas. Rapid fractionation schemes (such as 30 to 36 Gy) may be appropriate for some elderly or poor performance status patients with glioblastoma multiforme who have relatively short survival expectancies.

In low-grade gliomas, the role of radiation therapy is debatable. Although it improves disease-free survival, overall survival is not altered, indicating that deferring postoperative therapy is an option for selected group of patients. Evidence also indicates that lower doses of radiation therapy are probably as effective as higher doses of radiation for low-grade gliomas.

Randomized trials provide seminal evidence that external beam irradiation favorably affects the outcome of malignant gliomas. These trials demonstrate both a significant survival advantage and ability to maintain a full or partial working capacity for irradiated patients.

Chemotherapy

Chemotherapy has little established role in adult low-grade astrocytomas, but adjuvant chemotherapy is part of the standard therapeutic regimen for malignant gliomas. The addition of chemotherapy to radiation therapy improves the 1-year survival by 10% and the 2-year survival by 8.6%. The nitrosoureas, especially BCNU

(*N,N′*-bis(2-chloroethyl)-*N*-nitrosourea, carmustine), are the most active single agents. No benefit of chemotherapeutical agents such as tirapazamine, topotecan (Hycamtin), paclitaxel (Taxol), B-IFN (Avonex), and thalidomide (Thalomid) is noted when used with standard radiation in clinical trials. Temozolomide (Temodar) is an alkylating agent that demonstrates an improvement in survival by an additional 2 to 3 months when given concurrently with radiation in high-grade gliomas. Anaplastic oligodendrogliomas are chemosensitive tumors. PCV (procarbazine, lomustine [CCNU], and vincristine) chemotherapy regimens produce response rates of 50% to 75% in both recurrent and newly diagnosed anaplastic oligodendrogliomas. Unfortunately, improved response to chemotherapy does not translate into improved survival for these tumors.

Some of the newer biologic agents explored today in gliomas include tyrosine kinase inhibitors, matrix metalloproteinase inhibitors, and antitenascin antibodies.

Outcome

The 5-year recurrence-free survival rates of patients with low-grade astrocytomas or mixed oligoastrocytomas who undergo total or radical subtotal tumor resection range from 52% to 95%. The median survival times for high-grade gliomas using conventional radiation therapy alone or with chemotherapy consistently range from 9 to 14 months. The median survival for patients with glioblastoma multiforme is 10 to 12 months, whereas the 3-year survival rate is only 6% to 8%. The median survival for patients with anaplastic astrocytoma is 36 months, and the 3-year survival rate is approximately 50%.

Uncommon Primary Brain Tumors

PRIMARY CENTRAL NERVOUS SYSTEM LYMPHOMA

Primary CNS lymphomas (PCNSLs) represent approximately 2% to 5% of all intracranial neoplasms. During the last 2 decades, the incidence has increased in both the AIDS and immunocompetent general population. PCNSLs most frequently arise in the supratentorial paraventricular region of the brain. Multifocal tumors are present at diagnosis in 25% to 50% of immunocompetent patients and in 60% to 80% of AIDS patients. Cytologic examination of CPF reveals malignant cells in up to two thirds of immunocompetent patients and in nearly all AIDS patients. The neoplastic cells are similar to those of non-Hodgkin's lymphoma arising in extranodal sites. Single or multiple uniformly contrast-enhancing lesions in the paraventricular regions, basal ganglia, thalamus, or corpus callosum on MRI are characteristic findings.

The role of surgery is to establish a tissue diagnosis only. Primary CNS lymphomas respond dramatically to corticosteroid therapy. At least 90% of patients improve clinically, whereas 40% of lesions shrink considerably. Whole-brain irradiation with corticosteroids is the standard treatment for PCNSL. Recommended doses range from 36 to 45 Gy. Several reports document improved survival when chemotherapy is added to radiation therapy. The outcome is better with high-dose methotrexate-based regimens, often combined with intrathecal chemotherapy.

Survival times for primary CNS lymphoma with no treatment or steroids alone are approximately 1 to 4 months. The median survival for radiotherapy alone varies from 12 to 20 months. Median survival times for treatment programs that include high-dose methotrexate-based chemotherapy range from 33 to 42 months.

EPENDYMOMA

Ependymomas represent approximately 5% of all intracranial gliomas. The incidence peaks at 5 years and again at 34 years of age. Approximately 60% to 70% of ependymomas arise in the infratentorial brain. Ependymomas are separated into low-grade and high-grade lesions. The 5-year survival for low-grade tumors ranges from 60% to 80%, whereas it varies from 10% to 47% for high-grade tumors. Supratentorial ependymomas generally have a poorer prognosis than their infratentorial counterparts.

Most ependymomas cannot be completely excised because of their location and growth characteristics. Postoperative irradiation improves local tumor control and survival and is an accepted part of the standard treatment for these tumors. Although most ependymomas are slow growing, others are more aggressive and may disseminate throughout the CSF pathways. Current therapy for high-grade ependymomas after surgical debulking is with local fields to a dose of 59.4 Gy. The value of chemotherapy in adults with ependymomas and anaplastic ependymomas is not well defined.

BRAINSTEM GLIOMA

Brainstem gliomas account for less than 2% of brain tumors. Children constitute approximately two thirds of the reported cases. Diagnostic imaging is sufficient for the majority of the cases. The role of surgery is minimal and limited to biopsy only if there are questions about the diagnosis. Radiation therapy alone by conventional fractionation to 54 Gy in symptomatic or large brainstem lesions is recommended. Chemotherapy does not show any benefit in the management of brainstem gliomas. The median survival time is 9 to 12 months.

MEDULLOBLASTOMA

Medulloblastoma accounts for a third of pediatric brain tumors and is the most common tumor arising in the posterior fossa in children. It arises from the roof of the fourth ventricle or from the vermis. The presenting symptoms include headache, vomiting, and imbalance. On microscopic examination, small blue undifferentiated cells are noted consistent with primitive neuroectodermal tumor. CSF involvement is noted in 25% to 40% of the patients. Five-year survival rates range from 50% to 80%, and 10-year rates vary from 40% to 55%.

Surgery involves maximal resection of the tumor. Radiation therapy to the entire craniospinal axis is essential. The dose to the craniospinal axis is 23.4 to 36 Gy. A boost of 18 to 31.4 Gy is given to the posterior fossa to bring the total to 54 Gy. The role of chemotherapy is to decrease the craniospinal radiation dose and to improve the survival in poor-risk patients. Combinations of vincristine, CCNU, and *cis*-platinum are used.

Brain Metastases

EPIDEMIOLOGY

Metastases to the brain occur in as many as 30% of patients with systemic cancer and represent the most common type of intracranial tumor. Brain metastases exert a profound effect on the quality and length of survival, and despite the best current management, they represent the direct cause of death in 25% to 30% of affected patients. Melanoma and carcinomas of the lung, breast, and colorectum have a higher propensity to metastasize to the brain. Approximately 50% of patients present with a solitary lesion. Most brain metastases, particularly those that arise from primary sites other than the lung, occur at a late stage when metastatic dissemination is present elsewhere in the body.

STANDARD TREATMENT APPROACHES

Because the majority of patients with metastatic brain lesions have or will soon develop widely disseminated disease, treatment is dictated by the need to achieve immediate short-term palliation and the desire for durable symptom-free remission. The median survival of patients with symptomatic brain metastases is approximately 1 month without treatment and 2 months with corticosteroid administration. Survival is longer and the quality of life better if brain metastases are treated.

Corticosteroids

Corticosteroids rapidly ameliorate many symptoms of brain metastasis and should be used at the onset for all symptomatic patients. Symptomatic but stable patients can begin with approximately 16 mg of dexamethasone daily in two to four divided doses. Patients who are receiving whole-brain irradiation should receive steroids for at least 48 hours before treatment. Steroid tapering may begin during week 2 of radiotherapy. For patients receiving 16 mg of dexamethasone, the drug should be tapered by 2 to 4 mg every fifth day.

Surgery

Surgery establishes the diagnosis of metastatic brain disease when it is uncertain and serves as a treatment for single metastases. Surgery can provide better local control and immediate relief of neurologic signs and symptoms because of a mass effect. Surgically treated patients also live longer, have fewer recurrences of cancer in the brain, and enjoy a better quality of life compared with those treated by radiotherapy alone. Only 10% of patients are ideal candidates for surgical extirpation, however.

Whole-Brain Radiation Therapy

Radiotherapy is the appropriate treatment for most patients with brain metastases, including those with multiple lesions and those with single metastases who are not candidates for surgery. The standard approach is to treat the whole brain to 30 Gy in 10 daily fractions over 2 weeks. Depending on the symptom, the response rate varies from 70% to 90%. Neurologic function is improved overall in 50% of patients. The median survival with radiation therapy is 4 to 6 months. Overall, 75 to 80% of remaining life is spent in an improved or stable neurologic state.

Stereotactic Radiosurgery

Stereotactic radiosurgery (SRS) is an excellent alternative to surgical extirpation of solitary and multiple brain metastases. The procedure involves the delivery of a single large dose of radiation to a small volume of the brain region under stereotactic frame guidance. Recently, data from a large randomized trial show that addition of SRS to whole-brain radiation therapy improves both the survival and the quality of life in patients with limited brain metastases. Although surgery and SRS have never been compared directly in a clinical trial, local control, survival, and quality of life in selected patients seem comparable in retrospective trials.

Chemotherapy

Chemotherapy can be considered in selected patients who progress locally after whole-brain irradiation. Systemic chemotherapy shows a response rate of 25% to 50%. Temozolomide shows promise both as an adjuvant to whole-brain radiation therapy and in patients who fail radiation therapy.

REFERENCES

Andrews DW, Scott CB, Sperduto PW, et al: Whole brain radiation therapy with or without stereotactic radiosurgery boost for patients with one to three brain metastases: Phase III results of the RTOG 9508 randomised trial. Lancet 2004;363:1665-1672.

Deangelis LM, Hormigo A: Treatment of primary central nervous system lymphoma. Semin Oncol 2004;31:684-692.

Henson JW, Gaviani P, Gonzalez RG: MRI in treatment of adult gliomas. Lancet Oncol 2005;6:167-175.

Jemal A, Tiwari RC, Murray T, et al: Cancer statistics, 2004. CA Cancer J Clin 2004;54:8-29.

Kleihues P, Cavenee WK: Pathology and Genetics: Tumours of the Nervous System, 2nd ed. Lyon, France, IARC Press, 2000, pp 6-7.

Narayana A, Leibel SA: Primary and metastatic brain tumors in adults. In Leibel SA, Philips TL (eds): Textbook of Radiation Oncology, 2nd ed. Philadelphia, WB Saunders, 2004, pp 463-496.

Patchell RA, Tibbs PA, Regine WF, et al: Postoperative radiotherapy in the treatment of single metastases to the brain: A randomized trial. JAMA 1998;280:1485-1490.

Reifenberger G, Collins VP: Pathology and molecular genetics of astrocytic gliomas. J Mol Med 2004;82:656-670.

The Locomotor System

Rheumatoid Arthritis

Method of
Joseph C. Shanahan, MD,
and E. William St. Clair, MD

Rheumatoid arthritis (RA) is a chronic disease characterized mainly by a polyarthritis, with frequent progression to articular cartilage and bone damage, physical dysfunction, and work disability. Most patients with RA have circulating autoantibodies such as rheumatoid factor (RF) and anticyclic citrullinated peptide (anti-CCP) reflecting the autoimmune features of this disease. RA is a common illness, with an estimated worldwide prevalence of 1% to 2%. It typically develops in the fourth to sixth decades, with predominance among women of approximately 2.5:1. RA may be associated with extra-articular inflammatory features, including fatigue, subcutaneous nodules, pleuritis and pericarditis, interstitial lung disease, vasculitis, and Sjögren's syndrome. Patients with RA have excess mortality, but the most frequent cause of death appears to be complications of atherosclerotic cardiovascular disease. The increased risk of cardiovascular disease in this population occurs independently of traditional cardiovascular risk factors and corticosteroid therapy and may be related to the systemic inflammatory process.

The natural history of RA is a steady decline in joint function caused by progressive cartilage damage, bone erosions, and tendon rupture. As a result, work disability rates among patients with RA are more than 50% within 10 years of disease onset. Early rheumatoid arthritis is characterized by bone erosions detectable within 2 years of disease onset in as many as 70% of patients. In some patients RA progresses rapidly, leading to early work disability if effective therapy is not started to control the inflammatory response and joint damage.

Most patients with RA are initially treated with a combination of nonsteroidal anti-inflammatory agents and corticosteroids to provide sufficient time to confirm the persistence of joint inflammation and complete the diagnostic workup. Shortly thereafter, disease-modifying antirheumatic drugs (DMARDs) are added because they can afford long-term protection from joint damage and disability. DMARDs (Box 1) are defined by the ability to reduce the signs and symptoms as well as slow the progression of joint damage, as measured by radiographic changes in the amount of bone erosions and joint space narrowing.

Over the past 20 years there has been an evolution in the treatment paradigm for RA. These advances derive from early initiation of DMARD therapy and the expanded availability of effective DMARDs. Moreover, clinical trials examining the effect of multi-DMARD treatment for early RA have shown a long-lasting and improved benefit in terms of both disease control and improved health-associated quality of life compared with single DMARD therapy. As a result, the present treatment paradigm for RA incorporates the following three goals:

1. Early diagnosis and intervention
2. First-line therapy with DMARDs that reduces progressive joint damage followed by adding more DMARDs if disease activity persists
3. Management of co-morbidities such as disease- and treatment-related osteoporosis

Traditional DMARDs notable for their excessive toxicity, such as gold and penicillamine, are no longer in widespread use. However, the availability of safer DMARDs that can be used effectively in combination has expanded RA treatment options. In particular, a major advance has been the development of tumor necrosis factor-α (TNF-α) blocking agents that include etanercept (Enbrel), infliximab (Remicade), and adalimumab (Humira). Encouraging results from phase II clinical trials involving B-cell–directed therapies and other novel biologic immune response modifiers suggest that better RA control and possibly remission-inducing treatments are on the horizon. For now, RA remains a chronic illness usually managed with lifelong, anti-inflammatory, and immunomodulating treatment aimed at abrogating joint damage and minimizing disability.

Diagnosis

In the absence of a definitive diagnostic test, the diagnosis of RA is based on clinical features and supportive laboratory tests. Established in 1987, the American College of Rheumatology (ACR) criteria require at least four of seven features be present for longer than 6 weeks to make

BOX 1   Drugs Used for Treatment of Rheumatoid Arthritis

Traditional DMARDs
- MTX
- Leflunomide (Arava)
- Sulfasalazine (Azulfidine)
- Gold (intramuscular or oral) (Myochrysine, Solganal, Auranofin)
- Azathioprine (Imuran)
- Cyclosporine (Neoral)
- Corticosteroids

Biologic Agents
- Anti-TNF monoclonal antibodies
- Infliximab (Remicade)
- Adalimumab (Humira)
- Soluble TNF receptor
- Etanercept (Enbrel)
- IL-1ra
- Anakinra (Kineret)

Abbreviations: DMARD = disease-modifying antirheumatic drug; IL-1ra = interleukin-1 receptor antagonist; MTX = methotrexate; TNF = tumor necrosis factor.

TABLE 1   American College of Rheumatology Criteria for Rheumatoid Arthritis Diagnosis*

Criterion	Definition
Morning stiffness	In and around joints lasting at least 1 h before maximal improvement
Arthritis in at least three joint areas[†]	Simultaneously involved by soft tissue swelling or fluid observed by a physician
Arthritis of hand joints	At least one area swollen: wrist, MCP, PIP
Symmetric arthritis	Simultaneous involvement of the same joint areas on both sides of the body (bilateral involvement of PIPs, MCPs, or MTPs acceptable without absolute symmetry)
Rheumatoid nodules	Subcutaneous nodules over bony prominences, extensor surfaces, or in extra-articular regions observed by a physician
Serum rheumatoid factor	Abnormal amounts by any method for which the result has been positive in <5% of normal control subjects
Radiographic changes	Typical of RA on posteroanterior hand and wrist radiographs, which must include erosions or unequivocal bony decalcification localized or most obvious adjacent to involved joints (osteoarthritis changes alone do not qualify)

*Patient must satisfy four of the seven criteria listed. Criteria 1 through 4 must be present at least 6 weeks.
[†]Joint areas (14 total) include: right or left PIP, MCP, wrist, elbow, knee, ankle, and MTP joints.
Abbreviations: MTP = medial tibial plateau; MCP = metacarpophalangeal; PIP = proximal interphalangeal; RA = rheumatoid arthritis.

the diagnosis (Table 1). These criteria were not originally designed for use in the clinic; they were to classify subjects diagnosed with RA for the purpose of clinical research. As a result, the ACR criteria are highly sensitive (95%) but only modestly specific (75% to 89%) for making the clinical diagnosis of RA in patients with established disease. In studies of early inflammatory arthritis, the ACR criteria are poorly sensitive in the first 2 years following disease onset, but improve thereafter. Although characteristic radiographic lesions, particularly marginal joint erosions, strongly support the diagnosis of RA, such lesions are only present in up to 70% of patients within the first 2 years of disease. Recently, both musculoskeletal ultrasound (US) and magnetic resonance imaging (MRI) have been shown to detect erosive lesions early in the disease course, and in many cases, before they are evident on plain radiographs. However, the impact of these imaging techniques on diagnostic accuracy in early RA remains uncertain. Another recent diagnostic advance is the measurement of anti-CCP antibodies. In studies of stored sera, these autoantibodies are detectable as long as 10 years before the clinical diagnosis of RA. Anti-CCP antibodies are more specific, but less sensitive, for the diagnosis of RA than serum RF. RF such as IgM or IgG antibodies with binding specificity for the Fc portion of γ-globulin are detectable in approximately 70% of patients with RA. The presence of either RF or anti-CCP increases the diagnostic sensitivity for RA to more than 80%.

Primary care providers play an important role in the diagnosis of RA. Recognition of inflammatory arthritis and rapid referral to rheumatologists leads to early initiation of effective, joint protective therapies. Early inflammatory polyarthritis may not always meet diagnostic criteria for RA; however, approximately 30% of these cases of undifferentiated arthritis will ultimately evolve into RA.

The importance of early, accurate diagnosis of RA has grown with evidence that early, intensive therapy, using multiple DMARDs, can alter the natural history of the disease. In one study subjects with early RA (less than 2 years of disease duration) were randomized to intensive, multidrug therapy consisting of high-dose corticosteroids, methotrexate (MTX), and sulfasalazine or monotherapy with sulfasalazine alone. The combination therapy was gradually withdrawn over 6 months until all subjects were taking sulfasalazine alone. At 1 year, no differences in disease activity were noted between the groups; however, long-term radiographic follow-up showed at 5 years that progression of joint damage was slower in the group originally treated with multiple DMARDs, even after controlling for DMARD treatment after the initial year of the study. Several other studies supporting the outcomes of the Combinatietherapie Bij Reumatoide Artritis (COBRA) trial have shown that early introduction of combination therapy using a variety of different DMARDs with and without corticosteroids benefits long-term radiographic outcomes. Whether this translates into corresponding reductions in work disability is still under investigation.

Therapeutic Goals

Successful treatment of RA is predicated on reduction in symptomatic joint pain and swelling, relief of joint stiffness, return of lost function, and prevention of joint damage (Figure 1). Clinically, response to therapy may be determined by examining joints for tenderness and swelling, obtaining laboratory measures of inflammation (erythrocyte sedimentation rate [ESR] and C-reactive protein [CRP]), and assessing patient-reported outcomes using questionnaires, such as the Health Assessment Questionnaire (HAQ), or visual analogue scales. Long-term therapy goals include reducing missed work days, delaying disability, and decreasing early mortality. Frequent surrogates for long-term outcomes are radiographic changes indicative of joint damage (e.g., joint erosions and joint space narrowing). In clinical trials radiographic outcomes are quantified using the van der Heijde modification of the Sharp score, a validated scoring system in which the extent of joint space narrowing and erosions are quantified on standard radiographs of the hands, wrists, and feet.

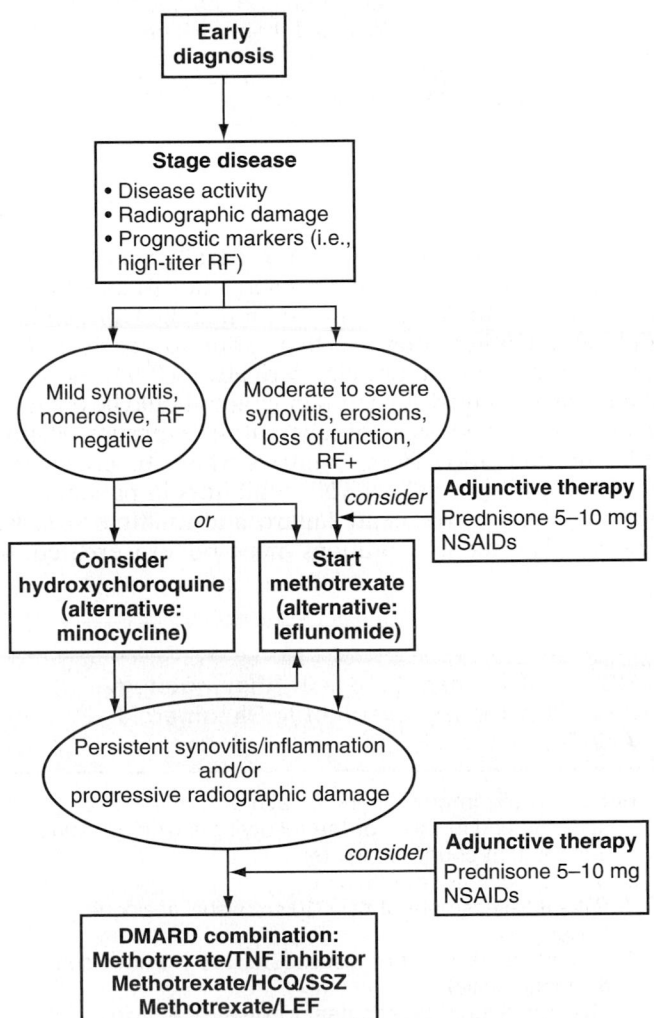

FIGURE 1. This flow diagram illustrates key decision points for RA therapy, based on the recommendations of the ACR. RA = rheumatoid arthritis. (American College of Rheumatology Subcommittee on Rheumatoid Arthritis Guidelines: Guidelines for the management of rheumatoid arthritis: 2002 update. Arthritis Rheum 2002;46:328-323.)

Both short- and long-term goals may be reached using DMARDs that reduce joint inflammation as well as retard the development of radiographic joint damage. The most commonly used DMARD, MTX, has a long track record of efficacy and acceptable toxicity and is often the treatment against which other agents or regimens are compared. Other DMARDs used previously for the treatment of RA, such as gold salts, penicillamine, azathioprine, and cyclophosphamide, are rarely used today because of either relatively poor efficacy or excessive toxicity, or both. A generation of novel DMARDs that inhibit inflammatory cytokines, termed *biologic response modifiers*, have essentially taken their place.

Methotrexate

A purine antimetabolite, MTX reduces symptoms of joint inflammation and decreases radiographic joint damage in patients with RA. Evidence of clinical efficacy has been shown in many studies. MTX is generally well tolerated; the majority of patients still use the drug after 5 years of treatment. Side effects may be divided into so-called nuisance toxicities, including nausea, diarrhea, mucosal ulcerations, and alopecia, and serious complications such as hepatotoxicity, bone marrow suppression, and pneumonitis (Table 2). Nuisance toxicities are an infrequent cause of MTX discontinuance and can often be managed with folic acid supplementation or by switching from oral to parenteral administration. Hepatotoxicity is typically characterized by fibrosis and cirrhosis, which occur rarely with frequent monitoring for possible toxicity. The ACR guidelines recommend monitoring hepatic transaminases and serum albumin at 4- to 8-week intervals and reserving liver biopsy for an otherwise unexplained decrease in albumin or persistent or recurrent elevation of transaminases. A rare complication, MTX-induced pneumonitis typically develops early after initiation and is characterized by cough, dyspnea, and fever. Chest radiographs reveal diffuse interstitial changes. The development of pneumonitis after MTX initiation should be managed with immediate drug discontinuation, and consideration of corticosteroid treatment in severe cases. Pneumonitis recurs frequently with rechallenge; therefore, patients experiencing this complication should be treated with an alternative DMARD. MTX is contraindicated in patients with impaired renal function because delayed clearance increases drug levels, and hence, the risk of side effects.

MTX is administered in once-weekly doses. It is important to maximize the beneficial effects of MTX by titrating to 20 to 25 mg per week because lower doses are often less effective. There has been little additional benefit observed in patients treated with doses greater than 25 mg per week; however, toxicities become more common at these higher doses.

Inhibitors of Tumor Necrosis Factor-α

TNF-α is a pleiotropic cytokine expressed by activated T lymphocytes and macrophages and acts in an autocrine and paracrine fashion to upregulate production of other proinflammatory cytokines, including interleukin (IL)-1

TABLE 2   Disease-Modifying Antirheumatic Drug Monitoring

DMARD	Tests	Interval
Methotrexate (MTX)	Hepatic transaminases, serum creatinine, CBC, albumin	Baseline and q 4-8 wk
	CXR, HBV and HCV serology, β-HCG	Baseline
Leflunomide (Arava)	Hepatic transaminases, serum creatinine, CBC, albumin, HBV and HCC serology, β-HCG	Baseline
	ALT	q mo for 6 mo, then q 6-8 wk
	Hepatic transaminases, serum creatinine, CBC, albumin	q 6-8 wk
TNF inhibitors (etanercept, infliximab, adalimumab [Humira])	PPD, CXR (if positive PPD, emigration from TB endemic country, or TB exposure history), CBC	Baseline
	CBC	q 6-8 wk
Sulfasalazine (Azulfidine)	CBC, hepatic transaminases, creatinine	Baseline and q 2 wk for 3 mo, then q 4 wk for 3 mo, then q 12 wk
	G6PD screen	Baseline
Hydroxychloroquine	Serum creatinine and G6PD deficiency screen	Baseline
	Ophthalmologic evaluation: visual acuity and retinal function tests	Baseline and q 6 mo
Cyclosporine (Neoral)	Serum creatinine, hepatic transaminases, CBC, potassium, blood pressure	Baseline and q 2 wk until dosage is stable, then q mo
Azathioprine (Imuran)	CBC, hepatic transaminases, creatinine	Baseline and then q 2 wk for 3 mo, then q mo for 3 mo, then q 2-3 mo
Anakinra (Kineret)	CBC	Baseline and then q 4-8 wk

Abbreviations: ALT = alanine aminotransferase; CBC = complete blood count; CXR = chest radiograph; DMARD = disease-modifying antirheumatic drug; G6PD = glucose-6-phosphatase deficiency; HBV = hepatitis B virus; HCC = hepatitis contagiosa canis; HCV = hepatitis C virus; q = every; TB = tuberculin.

and IL-6, matrix metalloproteinases, and reactive oxygen intermediates that provoke inflammation and injure articular cartilage and bone. In addition, TNF-α promotes receptor activation of nuclear factor-κB ligand (RANK ligand) expression that leads to differentiation and activation of osteoclasts. In RA, osteoclasts are responsible for articular bone loss characterized by erosions and osteopenia. In addition, TNF-α drives the differentiation of synoviocytes into a fibroblastic phenotype that confers invasive, tumor-like qualities on these cells. Fibroblast-like synoviocytes form the synovial pannus, a tumor-like mass unique to rheumatoid joints that invades and damages cartilage.

Clinical studies of several TNF-inhibiting agents have demonstrated the therapeutic benefits of TNF blockade on RA disease activity and joint damage. The three TNF-inhibiting drugs approved for the treatment of RA—etanercept (Enbrel), infliximab (Remicade), and adalimumab (Humira)—appear similarly efficacious for the treatment of this disease, but they have not been directly compared in clinical trials. Many clinical trials have compared treatment using TNF inhibitors with placebo controls in patients with active RA despite taking MTX. In these studies, 40% to 60% of patients met American College of Rheumatology (ACR) criteria for improvement at week 20 (Box 2). Approximately 10% to 20% of patients improved even more, reaching ACR 70 criteria. The add-on design of these trials simulates current practice patterns in which a second DMARD is added to MTX in patients with persistent synovitis. Long-term follow-up of subjects enrolled in these trials has shown clinically important improvement in quality-of-life measures and reduction of disability.

The TNF-blocking agents are generally well tolerated. However, an increased risk for reactivation of latent tuberculosis has led to the recommendation in the United States and certain other countries that, prior to use of a TNF inhibitor, a purified protein derivative (PPD) skin test should be performed. A chest radiograph should be obtained in patients with a history of tuberculosis exposure, positive PPD, or emigration from countries where tuberculosis is endemic. Clinical trials of TNF inhibitors in patients with advanced congestive heart failure and multiple sclerosis suggest that these conditions may be exacerbated by

---

BOX 2   American College of Rheumatology 20 Criteria for Improvement in Rheumatoid Arthritis

Requires 20% improvement in each of the first two domains and in three of the following seven domains:
1. Tender joint count (68 joints)
2. Swollen joint count (66 joints)
3. Patient assessment of pain (10 cm visual analogue scale)
4. Patient assessment of disease activity (10 cm visual analogue scale)
5. Physician global assessment of disease activity (10 cm visual analogue scale)
6. Patient assessment of physical function (HAQ score)
7. Serum CRP or erythrocyte sedimentation rate

Abbreviations: CRP = C-reactive protein; HAQ = Health Assessment Questionnaire.

these drugs. Demyelinating syndromes have been reported rarely in association with therapeutic TNF blockade. TNF inhibitors have been associated in trials with a slight increase in minor infections (primarily upper respiratory). Postmarketing surveillance suggests that infections with organisms that promote granulomatous inflammatory responses, such as histoplasmosis, coccidioidomycosis, and listeriosis may occur more frequently in patients treated with TNF inhibitors. There have been rare reports of lupus-like syndromes characterized by rash, serositis, and antinuclear and anti–double-stranded DNA autoantibodies.

A total of three TNF-inhibiting agents are commercially available. Etanercept (Enbrel) is a soluble TNF-receptor type II (p75)-to-Fc fusion protein. Infliximab (Remicade) is a chimeric human-to-mouse monoclonal anti-TNF antibody, whereas adalimumab (Humira) is a fully human anti-TNF monoclonal antibody. Etanercept (Enbrel) is administered by subcutaneous injection at a dose of 25 mg twice weekly or 50 mg once weekly. Adalimumab (Humira) is administered subcutaneously at a dose of 40 mg every 1 or 2 weeks. Infliximab (Remicade) is given as an intravenous infusion. Standard initial dosing for infliximab (Remicade) calls for 3 mg/kg to be given at 0, 2, and 6 weeks followed by regular infusions at 8-week intervals. The dosage may vary among patients from 3 to 10 mg/kg, and the interval may be adjusted between 4 and 8 weeks, depending on the individual's clinical response. Although TNF inhibitors may be used as monotherapy, more commonly they are added to MTX or other DMARD therapy to improve disease control. However, clinical trials in early RA suggest that combining MTX with a TNF inhibitor may be more effective than either therapy alone.

Other DMARDs

Other DMARDs may be used alone or in combination to treat RA. Some traditional DMARDs such as gold and D-penicillamine are now rarely used because of toxicity concerns. In some cases of mild RA, agents such as hydroxychloroquine or minocycline may be useful, particularly in early disease. Hydroxychloroquine is an antimalarial drug that may be used by itself in early and mild RA, or as part of a combination regimen. It is typically prescribed at doses of 5 to 7.5 mg/kg per day. The primary serious side effect is retinal toxicity, so routine ophthalmologic evaluation is suggested. Gastrointestinal side effects and skin rashes may also occur with hydroxychloroquine use.

Leflunomide is a pyrimidine antimetabolite that has been shown in clinical trials to be as efficacious as MTX. The recommended starting dose is 20 mg per day. The dose may be reduced to 10 mg per day when used in combination with MTX or if the starting dose is not tolerated. Leflunomide side effects are typically observed 2 to 4 weeks after starting treatment. The most important serious toxicities are hepatotoxicity and cytopenias. Therefore, laboratory monitoring of hepatic transaminases and a complete blood count should be performed at 4- to 8-week intervals. Leflunomide is an alternative to MTX as a first-line DMARD in patients intolerant of MTX or with renal insufficiency. Leflunomide may be used in combination with MTX. Because both drugs cause hepatotoxicity, however, hepatic transaminases and serum albumin should be monitored carefully. The safety data for combining leflunomide

with TNF-α blockers are limited to open-label studies with infliximab (Remicade), but suggest that leflunomide may be used safely in combination with TNF inhibition.

Other DMARDs include sulfasalazine and cyclosporine. With respect to efficacy, these agents compare similarly with MTX as monotherapy, and also improve control of synovitis when combined with MTX. Sulfasalazine treatment is started at 500 mg twice daily and may be titrated gradually to 4.5 g per day, given in two or three divided doses. Gastrointestinal toxicity may limit the dose. Interval monitoring for hepatotoxicity and cytopenias is also required. Cyclosporin is started at 2.0 to 2.5 mg/kg per day in two divided doses. It may be titrated to 4.5-5 mg/kg per day, but the dose may be limited by hypertension or renal toxicity. Long-term side effects such as nephrotoxicity and hirsutism make it difficult for most patients to maintain therapy with cyclosporin for long periods. Gold salts administered parenterally provide significant clinical improvement in up to 30% of patients with RA and prolonged complete remissions have been observed. Unfortunately, many patients are forced to discontinue gold because of side effects that include cytopenia, nephropathy, and cutaneous hypersensitivity.

Anakinra (Kineret), a recombinant IL-1 receptor antagonist (IL-1ra), is a biologic agent that blocks the proinflammatory activities of IL-1. IL-1 shares many of the proinflammatory abilities of TNF-α in promoting the symptoms of arthritis and joint damage in RA. IL-1ra is a naturally occurring anti-inflammatory molecule that competes with soluble IL-1β for binding to cells expressing the IL-1 receptor type I. IL-1ra binding does not induce signaling through the IL-1 receptor, resulting in IL-1 inhibition. Anakinra modestly reduces joint pain and swelling when administered in combination with MTX to patients with RA that is refractory to MTX monotherapy. Anakinra use has been limited by cost and aversion to daily subcutaneous administration (100 mg/day). Many patients develop local injection site reactions, but these are self-limited and usually subside over time.

Azathioprine and cyclophosphamide, traditional cytotoxic agents, have shown efficacy in RA, but their use is limited by toxicity. These drugs are usually reserved for use in life-threatening extra-articular manifestations of RA such as interstitial lung disease or vasculitis.

Corticosteroids

Corticosteroids are potent anti-inflammatory agents used for controlling signs and symptoms of synovitis. The use of corticosteroids in RA is limited by the side effects associated with long-term therapy. For short periods, high doses (0.25 to 0.5 mg/kg/day) may be used to control severe flare-ups of arthritis. However, corticosteroids are most commonly used in low daily doses (5 to 10 mg/day) as bridge treatment while a DMARD takes effect or as adjuvant therapy to control persistent symptoms in patients with DMARD-refractory disease. In clinical studies, low-dose corticosteroids can reduce the number of radiographic erosions that develop early after disease onset. These doses are rarely sufficient to completely control synovitis, and are therefore most commonly used in conjunction with traditional DMARDs or biologic agents. Low-dose corticosteroids are generally well-tolerated, but careful monitoring for complications, particularly osteoporosis, should be performed.

An alternative to systemic corticosteroids is intra-articular injection of triamcinolone (Kenalog, Aristocort), betamethasone (Celestone), or methylprednisolone (Depo-Medrol), particularly for disproportionately inflamed joints or joints responding slowly to systemic therapies. Clinicians should be careful not to assume a disproportionately swollen joint is because of RA. In such cases, synovial fluid aspiration is performed first to exclude infection because RA is a leading risk factor for joint sepsis.

Combination Therapy

Although many patients' disease appears to be well controlled using a single DMARD, persistent synovitis or progressive radiographic joint damage is common with such an approach. The current treatment paradigm favors a rapid *step-up* strategy, which calls for the addition of a second or third DMARD if synovitis persists despite adequate dosing with a single DMARD. There are several possible approaches. One approach is that inadequate responders to MTX can add a TNF inhibitor. Another approach is to convert to *triple therapy,* which consists of sulfasalazine and hydroxychloroquine in addition to MTX. Triple therapy reduces disease activity in patients with an inadequate response to MTX. An alternative combination regimen, adding leflunomide to MTX, reduces joint inflammation in otherwise refractory disease states. Available data suggest that combination therapy improves radiographic and functional outcomes for patients with RA inadequately controlled with a single DMARD. In subjects with RA refractory to combination therapy, alternative DMARDs may be used, either singly or in combination; but such patients, albeit in the minority, represent a small group that may be difficult to treat with currently approved agents.

Nonsteroidal Anti-Inflammatory Drugs

Nonsteroidal anti-inflammatory drugs (NSAIDs) are used widely to reduce pain, swelling, and stiffness in joints affected by RA. Although NSAIDs are useful adjunctive agents, they are not considered disease-modifying drugs. Traditional NSAIDs inhibit cyclooxygenase (COX) enzymes and therefore block the conversion of arachidonic acid into prostaglandins, molecules that may stimulate inflammation. Two forms of COX enzymes exist, COX-1 and COX-2. COX-1 is expressed constitutively in the gastric mucosa, where it functions to protect the stomach from luminal acid secretion, and in the kidney, where it serves to maintain renal perfusion. COX-2 is expressed at sites of inflammation and is also expressed constitutively in the kidney. Traditional NSAIDs, which block the function of both COX-1 and COX-2, have anti-inflammatory effects, but they also produce gastrointestinal toxicity that may manifest as gastritis, peptic ulcers and hemorrhage, or enteritis. NSAIDs that specifically antagonize COX-2 activity, termed *coxibs* (celecoxib [Celebrex]), have similar anti-inflammatory efficacy as the nonselective NSAIDs; but they cause significantly less gastrointestinal toxicity. Some evidence suggests that the gastrointestinal benefits of coxibs may be reduced by the concurrent use of aspirin. In addition, rofecoxib (Vioxx) and valdecoxib (Bextra) have been associated with an increased risk of cardiovascular and cerebrovascular events and have been withdrawn from the market.

Emerging Biologic Therapies

Novel biologic agents are being developed that target various inflammatory pathways or mediators deemed to be important in the pathogenesis of RA. T-cell activation, for example, is believed to be a central mechanism that initially triggers RA. The activation of T cells requires two interactions between cell surface receptor-ligand pairs. The first interaction occurs between the T-cell receptor (TCR) and an antigen complexed with an HLA molecule on the surface of an antigen-presenting cell (APC). On their surface, T cells also express CD28, which provides a second activating signal to the T cell when it associates with its ligands B7-1 or B7-2 (CD80/86), which are expressed on the APC. Failure of inducing a second signal through CD28 may result in anergy, which is a process that silences T cells. Cytotoxic T-lymphocyte antigen-4 (CTLA4, CD152) is also expressed on T-cell surfaces and competes with CD28 for binding to B7-1 and B7-2. CTLA-4 does not send an activating signal after binding to B7 molecules; however, it appears to downregulate T-cell activation. Abatacept, a fusion protein consisting of CTLA4 and the Fc portion of IgG, is presently under development for treatment of RA. It binds to B7-1 and B7-2 (CD80/86) and thereby blocks the costimulatory signal for T cells and inhibits T-cell activation. Studies show that abatacept can reduce disease activity in RA.

Recently, B cells have emerged to play an important role in the pathogenesis of RA. This belief is supported by the recognition that rituximab, an anti-CD20 monoclonal antibody that depletes B cells, can improve the signs and symptoms of RA. Rituximab is currently approved for the treatment of certain types of lymphoma and is under development as a possible treatment for RA.

 CURRENT DIAGNOSIS

- Synovitis—palpable swelling or effusions are present.
- Symmetry—similar joints are involved on both sides of the body.
- RA-specific joints—MCP and wrist involvement is present with DIP sparing.
- Persistence—synovitis lasting longer than 6 weeks excludes most reactive arthritis.
- Synovial fluid—joint aspiration is favored to exclude crystal-induced polyarthritis.
- Imaging—erosions in the hands or feet are commonly found early in disease; periarticular osteopenia reflects intra-articular inflammation.
- Laboratory features include:
  Inflammation—elevated ESR or CRP
  Autoimmunity—rheumatoid factor and/or anti-CCP antibodies

Abbreviations: CRP = C-reactive protein; DIP = distal interphalangeal; ESR = erythrocyte sedimentation rate; MCP = metacarpophalangeal; RA = rheumatoid arthritis.

CURRENT THERAPY

- Early initiation of DMARD
- Regular reassessment of disease progression
- MTX (or leflunomide if MTX contraindicated or poorly tolerated) as first-line DMARD
- Step up to combination therapy
- NSAIDs as tolerated for improved symptom control
- Low-dose corticosteroids to reduce synovitis and damage early after diagnosis
- Regular monitoring for associated diseases that contribute to morbidity
- Regular BP monitoring
- Annual fasting lipid profile
- Annual assessment of glucose tolerance (HbA$_{1c}$ or fasting glucose)
- DEXA scan

Abbreviations: BP = blood pressure; DEXA = dual-energy radiograph absorptiometry; DMARD = disease-modifying antirheumatic drug; HbA$_{1c}$ = glycosylated hemoglobin; MTX = methotrexate; NSAID = nonsteroidal anti-inflammatory drug.

Other biologic therapies that block the function of proinflammatory cytokines include anti–IL-6 receptor antibody, anti–IL-12, and anti–IL-15 have also shown efficacy for treating RA. These agents are at earlier stages of clinical development.

Overview of RA Treatment Strategies

The effectiveness of RA treatment has improved dramatically with recent advances in early diagnosis, the development of less toxic and more effective disease-modifying treatments, and more intensive DMARD regimens that control persistent synovitis and progressive radiographic damage. Furthermore, recognition of the impact of associated disorders including osteoporosis and atherosclerotic disease, in addition to appropriate therapeutic intervention for these disorders, will likely result in improved morbidity and mortality among patients with RA. Figure 1 depicts the most commonly employed strategy in use today, and the strategy favored by the authors. Effective treatment begins with early initiation of effective DMARDs before substantial joint damage has occurred. Careful follow-up, particularly using objective measures that account for physical findings, patient disease assessment, and laboratory measures of systemic inflammation, should guide clinicians about the need for combination therapy, in which new DMARDs are added to existing ones, with special attention to suppressing joint inflammation as much as possible. Most patients today are able to live productively with RA because of the advent of new drugs and more intensive early treatment. The future likely holds an expanded therapeutic armamentarium, which promises to afford even better disease control and less disability.

REFERENCES

Arnett FC, Edworthy SM, Bloch DA, et al: The American Rheumatism Association 1987 revised criteria for the classification of rheumatoid arthritis. Arthritis Rheum 1988;31:315-324.

Hansen KE, Cush J, Singhal A, et al: The safety and efficacy of leflunomide in combination with infliximab in rheumatoid arthritis. Arthritis Rheum 2004;51:228-232.

Kirwan JR: Effects of glucocorticoids on joint destruction in rheumatoid arthritis. N Engl J Med 1995;333:142-146.

Kremer JM, Alarcon GS, Lightfoot RW Jr, et al: Methotrexate for rheumatoid arthritis. Suggested guidelines for monitoring liver toxicity. American College of Rheumatology. Arthritis Rheum 1994;37:316-328.

Kremer JM, Genovese MC, Cannon GW, et al: Concomitant leflunomide therapy in patients with active rheumatoid arthritis despite stable doses of methotrexate. A randomized, double-blind, placebo-controlled trial. Ann Intern Med 2002;137:726-733.

Landewe RB, Boers M, Verhoeven AC, et al: COBRA combination therapy in patients with early rheumatoid arthritis: Long-term structural benefits of a brief intervention. Arthritis Rheum 2002;46:347-356.

Lee DM, Schur PH: Clinical utility of the anti-CCP assay in patients with rheumatic diseases. Ann Rheum Dis 2003;62:870-874.

O'Dell JR, Haire CE, Erikson N, et al: Treatment of rheumatoid arthritis with methotrexate alone, sulfasalazine and hydroxychloroquine, or a combination of all three medications. N Engl J Med 1996;334:1287-1291.

St. Clair EW, Wagner CL, Fasanmade AA, et al: The relationship of serum infliximab concentrations to clinical improvement in rheumatoid arthritis: Results from ATTRACT, a multicenter, randomized, double-blind, placebo-controlled trial. Arthritis Rheum 2002;46:1451-1459.

van der Heijde DM: Plain x-rays in rheumatoid arthritis: Overview of scoring methods, their reliability and applicability. Baillieres Clin Rheumatol 1996;10:435-453.

van Everdingen AA, Jacobs JW, Siewertsz Van Reesema DR, Bijlsma JW: Low-dose prednisone therapy for patients with early active rheumatoid arthritis: Clinical efficacy, disease-modifying properties, and side effects: A randomized, double-blind, placebo-controlled clinical trial. Ann Intern Med 2002;136:1-12.

Juvenile Idiopathic Arthritis

Method of
Terry L. Moore, MD

Juvenile rheumatoid arthritis (JRA), now mainly known by the International League of Associations of Rheumatologists (ILAR) classification as juvenile idiopathic arthritis (JIA), is a protean disorder whose variable modes of onset and patterns of disease course are accompanied by a myriad of diverse signs, symptoms, and manifestations. JIA affects approximately 250,000 children in the United States. No distinct race predilection is noted at this time. It is the most common disease cause of children missing school in the United States. It is also the second leading cause of eye pathology in children. JIA presents a difficult diagnostic problem because of its lack of specific serologic abnormalities. This represents a dual problem to a clinician in that it makes it difficult to establish an early diagnosis of JIA when the clinical picture is not clear, and even after the diagnosis is established, it is difficult to know when the disease has remitted or an exacerbation is beginning. The diagnosis of JIA is usually made clinically. Serologic studies can be informative, but in the past no routine laboratory tests have been diagnostic.

Diagnostic criteria for JIA include children younger than 16 years with persistent arthritis of one or more joints for at least 6 weeks. Arthritis is defined as swelling of a joint or limitation of motion with heat, pain, and tenderness.

JIA Subtypes

These are the seven basic subgroups or categories of JIA:

1. *Polyarthritis (RF positive)*: 19S IgM rheumatoid factors (RF) are present in the peripheral blood on testing and usually anticyclic citrullinated peptide antibodies (αCCP Ab). This group is manifested by arthritis in five or more joints in the first 6 months of disease. The joints most commonly affected are peripheral joints, including the knees, ankles, wrists, and fingers, but all synovial joints can become involved. There may also be an associated tendonitis. The classical joints involved are predominantly the metacarpophalangeal (MCP) and proximal phalangeal (PIP) joints producing fusiform-shaped swelling of the fingers. The knees are usually the first joints to limit function. They may exhibit deformity and flexion contractures. Polyarthritis (RF positive) is seen in approximately 5% to 10% of the children with JIA. The incidence of this type increases with age with the highest incidence found in adolescent females. The disease course in these children is generally believed to be one of a lifelong constantly active, or recurrent, relapsing pattern. It is associated with subcutaneous nodules and a higher incidence of vasculitis than the other forms of JIA. Radiograph films may show erosions with greater frequency than other forms of arthritis in children and may be helpful in diagnosis. Antinuclear antibodies (ANA) are present in approximately 80%.

2. *Polyarthritis (RF negative)*: This group by definition also has arthritis in five or more joints involved during the first 6 months; however, RF testing is negative, but αCCP Ab may be present. The disease pattern is similar to that of the RF-positive polyarthritis group. The course of these patients may be long term; however, most improve over a period of time. This type of onset occurs in approximately 20% to 30% of children with JIA. This type also shows female predominance.

3. *a. Oligoarthritis (pauciarthritis) with iridocyclitis* (inflammation of the iris and ciliary body in the posterior uveal tract of the eye): Oligoarthritis is manifested by arthritis of one or more joints involved in the first 6 months, but less than five joints. This type of onset is seen in approximately 50% of children with JIA and again shows female predominance. The most common children presenting are younger than 4 years at onset and have ANA present on testing. The ANA positivity is found in approximately 90% of the children developing chronic iridocyclitis. This group has a very good prognosis with little residual joint damage. There may be occasional asymmetric growth and leg length differences that develop; however, the process usually produces no long-term abnormalities. Approximately 50% of these children develop some type of iridocyclitis. Most children with iridocyclitis are easily controlled with anti-inflammatories such as naproxen, local steroid drops, or mydriatics (dilators). Therefore, any child being considered for a diagnosis of JIA requires frequent slit-lamp examinations by an ophthalmologist. *b. Extended oligoarthritis*: This type has an oligoarticular onset and then becomes more widespread, developing polyarthritis with five or more joints involved after the first 6 months of disease.

4. *Enthesitis related*: This category is predominantly seen in males who may later develop sacroiliitis and ankylosing spondylitis. This type of onset is associated with an enthesitis such as Achilles tendonitis or arthritis of the lower extremities again involving fewer than five joints in the first 6 months. The large joints, such as knees, ankles, hips, and sacroiliac joints, are usually involved. Anterior uveitis may be associated. The onset type is predominantly male, usually from 8 to 14 years of age, and may progress on to true ankylosing spondylitis. It is seen in approximately 10% to 15% of children with JIA. There is a high incidence of familial predisposition in these patients with an 80% to 95% occurrence of the HLA-B27 antigen found. Sacroiliitis is often present on radiographs before symptoms develop and precedes the development of real limitation of motion of the spine.

5. *Systemic arthritis*: Initially seen with daily temperatures rises usually late afternoon from normal to exceeding 39°C (103°F) in an intermittent, spiking pattern. This usually occurs for more than 2 weeks. The onset of this type may include a salmon-colored, transient skin rash, lymphadenopathy, splenomegaly, hepatomegaly, pleuritis, pericarditis, or abdominal pain. It is seen in approximately 20% of children with JIA. RF, αCCP Ab, and ANA are usually negative, but white blood cell counts may exceed 30 to 40,000/mm³. Erythrocyte sedimentation rate (ESR) and C-reactive protein (CRP) are elevated and anemia may rapidly develop. This group also shows a male predominance. Approximately 50% of children develop an oligoarticular pattern and remit quickly, but many of the children go on to develop a long-term symmetric polyarthritis. This type of onset causes the most consternation in the diagnosis because it may mimic severe localized infections, sepsis, or neoplasms, such as lymphomas or leukemias.

6. *Psoriatic arthritis*: Arthritis and psoriasis or dactylitis with nail pitting and onycholysis. Usually there is a first-degree relative with a psoriasis. RF is negative.

7. *Other arthritis*: Children with arthritis of unknown cause that persists for at least 6 weeks and does not fulfill criteria for any of the other categories or fulfills criteria for more than one of the other categories.

JIA Evaluation

The workup on a JIA patient includes a complete blood count (CBC) that may show an anemia, leukocytosis, and thrombocytosis in systemic onset. ESR and CRP are quite high in systemic and polyarticular disease but may be minimally elevated or normal in oligoarticular disease. RF is only positive in the late-onset polyarticular patients and αCCP Ab also mainly appears in this group but may be seen in a small number of RF-negative polyarticular and oligoarticular patients. ANA are found in the polyarticular group and also in the oligoarticular group, associated with the presence of iridocyclitis. Other immunologic testing and liver, muscle, and kidney function tests should be in the normal range. Radiographs should be performed of involved joints looking for periarticular demineralization, joint space narrowing, and/or erosions.

JIA Prognosis

The course and outcome of JIA is generally good, however, the disease needs to be treated early and aggressively to prevent asymmetrical skeletal development, osteopenia, chronic eye disease, or systemic manifestations. Approximately 75% of the children do well long term, with the oligoarticular group rarely having any residual damage. Approximately 25%, usually found in the polyarthritis and systemic groups, develop continuous arthritis with some long-term disability.

JIA Therapy

The therapy of JIA begins with the use of physical and occupational therapy (PT/OT). The object of PT is to strengthen muscles, improve range of motion, and decrease the impact loading on the joints. The object of OT is to improve body mechanics, posture, and other modalities to decrease any kind of impact loading on the joints. Medical therapy begins with the judicious use of nonsteroidal anti-inflammatory drugs (NSAIDs). Oligoarthritis patients are usually placed on a NSAID, usually naproxen (Naprosyn), at a dosage of 10 to 20 mg/kg in two divided doses. Naproxen has an advantage over other NSAIDs in that it comes in both a tablet and a liquid form at 125 mg/5 mL and has a long half-life so it can be given in two doses, which is more amenable to taking before and after school for compliance. The other nonsteroidal in tablet form generally used is tolmetin sodium (Tolectin) at a dosage of 20 to 30 mg/kg in three to four divided doses. One other medication, meloxicam (Mobic), which comes in a tablet and a liquid form, was recently approved by the Food and Drug Administration (FDA). It has an advantage of a long half-life and can be given once daily at dosages of 0.125 to 0.25 mg/kg. The liquid form is 7.5 mg/5 mL. Two other medications are approved for the use of children with JIA including aspirin (dosages of 80 to 120 mg/kg in four divided doses) and ibuprofen at 30 to 40 mg in three or four divided doses. A liquid preparation comes at 100 mg/5 mL. Other NSAIDs recently used in trials in JIA but not FDA approved include nabumetone (Relafen),[1] at 30 mg/kg. This medication has an advantage in that it is only once a day and also can be used in a liquid form by crushing the tablet and dissolving in warm water. Other agents are occasionally used such as oxaprozin (Daypro), at 10 to 20 mg/kg in one to two doses; fenoprofen (Nalfon), at 40 to 50 mg/kg[3] three to four times per day; diclofenac sodium (Voltaren), 20 to 40 mg/kg[3] twice to three times per day; sulindac (Clinoril), 4 to 6 mg/kg in a twice daily dosage; or celecoxib (Celebrex), a cyclooxygenase-2 (COX-2) inhibitor, at 4 to 6 mg/kg in two doses. Laboratory studies including CBC, urinalysis, and comprehensive metabolic panel should be drawn every 4 months to monitor medication toxicity.

Children who have erosions on radiograph or show more aggressive disease at time of onset, usually those with polyarthritis, with systemic disease with polyarthritis, or with very aggressive oligoarticular disease, benefit greatly by combination therapy to reduce long-term disability. This means being aggressive with therapy in the first 2 years of disease. The first 2 years of disease are the period in which the most erosions and joint damage occurs. Combination therapy has become the standard of care of patients with JIA. The most common combination is the use of two or more of the disease-modifying antirheumatic agents (DMARDs), which include methotrexate (MTX), hydroxychloroquine (Plaquenil) [HCQ], or some of the new biologic preparations. MTX, a purine inhibitor, in dosages of 10 to 20 mg/m² once weekly along with folic acid at 400 µg to 1 mg daily is a very efficacious DMARD with little toxicity. MTX can be given orally or by intramuscular (IM) or subcutaneous (SC) injection. Dosages more than 20 mg should always be administered IM or SC. These children, however, do need to be monitored monthly to every 6 weeks with CBC, urinalysis, and liver and kidney function tests to monitor the medication toxicity. The combination of MTX and HCQ is the most common with the addition of HCQ in dosages of 6 mg/kg as an excellent adjunct along with the NSAID. Eye exams every 6 months to monitor HCQ toxicity are indicated. MTX is also monitored once a year with a chest radiograph and also if any cough is present. The toxicities of these medications are relatively minimal in patients with JIA. Other DMARDs, although not approved in children, are cyclosporine (Neoral)[1] at 2.5 to 3 mg/kg, intramuscular gold[1] at a dosage of 1 mg/kg weekly for 20 weeks, and sulfasalazine (Azulfidine) (SSZ) at doses of 50 mg/kg beginning at 500 mg per day and up to 2 g twice a day.[3] These are used with efficacy in JIA patients. Also, leflunomide (Arava)[1], a pyrimidine synthetase inhibitor, is effective in children. It also has liver toxicity, so it should be monitored like MTX. Abdominal complaints such as diarrhea are the most common side effects. The drug has a long half-life and potential teratogenicity, so it should be used with caution in females of childbearing age. Recently, the use of biologics

---

CURRENT THERAPY

- Anti-inflammatory agents (NSAIDs: naproxen [Naprosyn], ibuprofen [Advil], tolmetin [Tolectin], meloxicam [Mobic]) and intra-articular steroids for oligoarticular disease
- NSAIDs, disease-modifying agents (methotrexate [Rheumatrex], hydroxychloroquine [Plaquenil], sulfasalazine [Azulfidine], etc.) and/or biologics (etanercept) for polyarticular and systemic disease

Abbreviation: NSAIDs = nonsteroidal anti-inflammatory drugs.

[1]Not FDA approved for this indication.
[3]Exceeds dosage recommended by the manufacturer.

or anticytokines in JIA has brought about a great deal of improvement in some of the patients. One medication is etanercept (Enbrel) at 0.4 mg/kg SC two times per week or 0.8 mg/kg SQ once per week. It has brought about marked improvement in many patients with long-standing polyarthritis. Efficacy has been sustained for up to 4 years now. This medication has caused marked decrease in joint swelling, tenderness, decreased sedimentation rate, and marked improvement in fatigue. The mechanism of action is that of blocking tumor necrosis factor (TNF), a cytokine that increases the inflammatory response in joints. Etanercept is produced to function like the p75 receptor for TNF. It binds to TNF and keeps it from binding to its own receptor and increasing the inflammatory response. It is the only biologic approved for JIA by the FDA. It is well tolerated with the main side effect injection site reactions. TNF blockers can exacerbate an underlying tuberculosis infection, so before starting the medication a chest radiograph and purified protein derivative (PPD) skin test should be performed and then yearly while on the medication. Its counterpart, infliximab (Remicade), a chimeric monoclonal antibody to TNF, also is very efficacious in JIA. It is used as an intravenous (IV) preparation at 3 mg/kg given at baseline, 2 weeks, 6 weeks, and 8 eight weeks thereafter in an IV infusion over a 2-hour period. This agent markedly decreases the inflammatory response. It has mainly been used in older children with polyarticular disease. A fully humanized monoclonal antibody to TNF, adalimumab (Humira), is still in trials in children at 20 to 40 mg SC every 2 weeks. Also, studies are being run on the interleukin (IL)-1 receptor antagonist, Anakinra (Kineret), in children. It is given daily at 50 to 100 mg SC. This medication shows a more favorable response in children with systemic-onset than with polyarticular or oligoarticular disease. A high number of children experience injection site reactions. Other biologic medications are in trials, including an IL-6 receptor antagonist (tocilizumab)[2] in systemic onset JIA, anti-B cell therapy (rituximab) (Rituxan), or T-cell therapy (abatacept) (Orencia).

Prednisone still may be used in severe systemic disease to control fever, rash, and/or other systemic manifestations in dosages of 1 to 2 mg/kg. The possibility of long-term side effects such as growth retardation, avascular necrosis, osteoporosis, weight gain, and acneiform lesions from steroids make their long-term use tentative in children. If disease is controlled, steroids should be tapered. Steroid eye drops may be used at times for severe iridocyclitis or orally in those patients with severe eye disease. Intraarticular (IA) steroids may be used in all onset-types if one or more joints are severely involved at one point in time. Local injections of 10 to 40 mg of triamcinolone hexacetonide may provide symptomatic relief in one specific joint. In the long course of the disease, other immunosuppressives such as cyclophosphamide (Cytoxan), azathioprine (Imuran), and chlorambucil (Leukeran)[1] are used in certain cases of severe systemic or polyarthritis, but the use of these has waned with the new biologic medication.

The use of PT and OT is indicated at the first onset of disease. The child, after being evaluated, is sent to PT for instructions in the use of moist heat to the joints such as hot packs, the judicial use of rest, and two to three periods each day of passive or active assisted exercises performed by the patient or aided by the parent. Splints that protect joints may be prescribed to decrease the development of deformities. Splints can be made out of lightweight plastic that is molded while warm to fit the child in the desired position. The wrists and knees are the most amenable to splinting, but finger splints may hold the entire hand in slight dorsiflexion to decrease ulnar drift. If flexion contractures occur, splints can be used to hold the joint in maximum extension. The use of OT begins with the instructions for the patient in posture, body mechanics, improvement in activities of daily living, and instructions in joint protection. These instructions help the patient learn to protect and not increase the impact loading on the joints. Exercises are important in all stages of the care of the child with arthritis. During appearance of disease activity, excessive exercises exacerbate the inflammation. In these stages, passive range of motion exercise should maintain range of motion along with active assistive exercise. As joints improve and the inflammation is reduced, the exercise should be increased to a more active form. Resistive and strengthening exercises should be introduced along with isometric exercises to help provide muscle tone. Swimming or hydrotherapy or water aerobics for exercise may greatly aid in improving muscle strength. The use of regular cycling exercises may also be helpful. If the child has a lot of morning stiffness in the hands, the use of paraffin baths may be of great help, and the use of Theraputty to squeeze and improve muscle strength in the hands is indicated.

In conclusion, children with JIA should be diagnosed as soon as possible and treated aggressively. It is not a benign condition if left partially treated or untreated. Early treatment prevents further disease progression, maintains range of motion of the joints, and promotes normal growth and development. Combination therapy of NSAIDs, DMARDs, and/or biologics should be used early in those patients identified with aggressive disease. The team approach of the pediatric rheumatologist, ophthalmologist, and physical and occupational therapists will best benefit the JIA patient for a good long-term outcome.

REFERENCES

Cassidy JT, Petty RE: Juvenile rheumatoid arthritis. In Cassidy JT, Petty RE (eds): Textbook of Pediatric Rheumatology. Philadelphia, WB Saunders, 2001, pp 218-322.

Kietz DA, Pepmueller PH, Moore TL: Therapeutic use of etanercept in polyarticular course juvenile rheumatoid arthritis over a two-year period. Ann Rheum Dis 2002;61:171-173.

Lovell D, Giannini EH, Reiff A, et al: Etanercept in children with polyarticular juvenile rheumatoid arthritis. N Engl J Med 2000;342:763-769.

Low JM, Chauhan AK, Kietz DA, et al: Determination of anti-cyclic citrullinated peptide antibodies in sera of patients with juvenile idiopathic arthritis. J Rheumatol 2004;31:1829-1833.

Moore TL: Immunopathogenesis of juvenile rheumatoid arthritis. Curr Opin Rheumatol 1999;11:377-383.

Petty JE, Southwood TR, Manners P, et al: International League of Associations for Rheumatology classification of juvenile idiopathic arthritis: Second revision, Edmonton, 2001. J Rheumatol 2004;31:390-392.

Wallace CA, Huang B, Bandeira M, et al: Patterns of clinical remission in select categories of juvenile idiopathic arthritis. Arthritis Rheum 2005;52:3554-3562.

---

[1]Not FDA approved for this indication.
[2]Not available in the United States.

Ankylosing Spondylitis

Method of
Maxime Breban, MD, PhD

Ankylosing spondylitis (AS) is the prototypical form of a group of inflammatory rheumatic disorders, referred to as the spondyloarthropathies (SpAs). The prevalence and burden of SpA are very similar to those of rheumatoid arthritis (RA). Until recently, however, few therapeutic options were available to treat SpA. This situation changed dramatically with the arrival of the very efficacious anti–tumor necrosis factor-α (TNF-α) biologic therapies. The clinical manifestations of SpA usually begin early in adulthood (average age at onset is 22 to 23 years). The evolution tends to be chronic, with fluctuations, including the possibility of remissions and relapses. Male predominance is well established, albeit this characteristic was overrated in the past, and female cases are frequent and sometimes serious. Genetic predisposition is strong, with a trend to familial aggregation, which is partially accounted for by the striking association with the human leukocyte antigen (HLA)-B27.

Birth and Rise of the Spondyloarthropathy Concept

Recognition and even definition of SpA bear some difficulties, which relate to the nature of the disease:

- Presentation of SpA is variable from patient to patient.
- Some of the key manifestations tend to remit.
- Clinical manifestations lack specificity.
- Morphologic and biologic investigations are poorly contributive.
- Pathophysiology remains largely unexplained.

The different entities that make up the SpAs were originally identified on the basis of their most striking presentation features. Accordingly, AS refers to the following: an axial disorder predominantly affecting the spinal and the pelvic skeleton; psoriatic arthritis as defined by the concomitance of arthritis and psoriasis; arthritis of inflammatory bowel disease (IBD), by the combination of arthritis with Crohn's disease or ulcerative colitis; reactive arthritis, as the onset of sterile arthritis following an infection of the gastrointestinal or the urethral mucosa by invasive bacteria.

Frequent overlap of manifestations between these different entities in the same patient (simultaneously, or consecutively) and within multicase families is indicative of shared genetic background. Part of this genetic predisposition was explained by the identification of HLA-B27 as a genetic factor shared by the different entities. Classification criteria were then developed to distinguish SpAs from other unrelated rheumatic disease conditions. However, only recently was it shown in the context of familial disease that different SpA subtypes correspond to variations of the same disease, rather than to distinct entities. This assumption is consistent with the description of enthesitis (i.e., inflammation at the sites of attachment of tendons, ligaments, and capsules to bone) as a unifying target lesion shared by all SpA subtypes, as opposed to RA.

Key Manifestations of Spondyloarthropathies

AXIAL SKELETON

The most frequent manifestation of the spondyloarthropathies is back pain, which is typically persistent (i.e., 3 months) and inflammatory (responsible for nocturnal awakening and morning stiffness, improved by exercise). Symptoms usually begin in the lumbar region and diffuse upward, affecting the thoracic and less frequently the cervical spine. The sacroiliac joint is also an early affected site, manifesting as buttock pain, irradiating posteriorly to the thigh. Another frequent symptom is pain in the anterior chest wall, impairing breathing. When such symptoms occur in a young adult, 15 to 35 years of age, without alternative explanation, such as disk herniation or another mechanical spinal condition, a diagnosis of SpA must be seriously considered, even if physical examination is poor. Clear-cut improvement of the pain by nonsteroidal anti-inflammatory drugs (NSAIDs) is also indicative of the inflammatory nature of the disease. Other symptoms must then be carefully retrieved from past medical history because they are frequently absent at the time of examination.

PERIPHERAL SKELETON

Peripheral arthritis typically presents as an asymmetric oligoarthritis predominating in the large joints of lower limbs, as opposed to arthritis because of RA or other connective tissue diseases. It frequently runs an acute remitting course. It may be destructive, however, particularly in the hip and shoulder. Enthesitis most typically affects insertions of the Achilles tendon or the plantar fascia, on the calcaneus, revealing as posterior or subtalar pain, but it may affect a variety of sites, such as knee, elbow, hip, and shoulder. The physical examination is frequently poorly contributive. Dactylitis (sausage-like digit or toe) is less frequent but most typical of SpA.

EXTRA-ARTICULAR MANIFESTATIONS

The most frequent extra-articular manifestation is acute anterior uveitis, which happens at least once in 40% of the patients over 20 years of disease duration. Psoriatic skin or nail lesions are very common (15% to 20% in SpA versus 2% in the general population). Overt inflammatory bowel disease (IBD) occurs in 5% of the patients, but occult IBD could be detected more frequently by performing systematic ileocolonic investigations, including biopsies and microscopic examination. Other less frequent extra-articular manifestations are valvular insufficiency and heart conduction block.

Diagnosis

Validated classification criteria require the presence of advanced radiographic sacroiliitis for the diagnosis of AS. A major issue with this criteria is its dependency on evolution time and its inadequacy for an early diagnosis.

Biologic alterations such as raised erythrocyte sedimentation rate (ESR) or C-reactive protein (CRP) level in the serum are inconstant and not specific. The HLA-B27 allele confers a 100-fold increase in the risk of developing SpA. Thus the detection of this antigen is helpful in case of doubt. However, HLA-B27 positivity is neither mandatory nor sufficient for the diagnosis (i.e., 10% of SpA patients lack this antigen and less than 3% of HLA-B27–positive individuals ever develop SpA).

Amor and colleagues' (1990) classification criteria recapitulate all major findings typical of SpA and attribute to each of them a weight proportional to their specificity (Table 1). Although not developed for this purpose, they are frequently used as a diagnostic tool because their specificity and sensitivity are quite good, even in early disease.

To face the need for more reliable early diagnosis instrument, the most recent imaging modalities, such as magnetic resonance imaging (MRI) and ultrasonography (US), coupled with pulsed-wave Doppler (PwD), bear some hope. Both techniques may demonstrate early inflammatory changes adjacent to the affected sites (i.e., the spine, the sacroiliac or the peripheral joints, and the enthesis). Their diagnostic performance has yet to be studied systematically. However, the sensitivity of sacroiliac or spinal MRI changes seems rather poor in early SpA. In contrast, US PwD could offer greater sensitivity by showing vascularized peripheral enthesitis in most SpA patients, a very specific finding as it appears.

Treatment

NONSTEROIDAL ANTI-INFLAMMATORY DRUGS

NSAIDs remain the cornerstone of the pharmacologic treatment of SpA. Molecules of this class can be efficacious on all osteoarticular manifestations. Selection of the molecule must be adapted to individual cases because of the high variability of response and tolerance from patient to patient. The half-life of the molecule must be considered and time of intake (bedtime is the most useful) must be adapted to obtain the greatest relief of inflammation during the second half of the night. A great proportion of patients can be satisfactorily treated with NSAIDs alone, but high dosages are required to control the most severe cases and may even be inefficacious in some cases.

CORTICOSTEROIDS

Oral or even parenteral corticosteroids are usually ineffective for skeletal manifestations. In contrast, local injections of slow-acting corticosteroids at the site of inflammation are very efficacious. Most extra-articular manifestations, such as psoriatic lesions and acute anterior uveitis, also benefit from corticosteroids.

DISEASE-MODIFYING ANTIRHEUMATIC DRUGS

Efficacy of the classic disease-modifying antirheumatic drugs (DMARDs) used to treat RA, such as gold salts or methotrexate (Rheumatrex),[1] is rarely achieved in SpA and not supported by any convincing study. Trials show some efficacy of sulfasalazine (Azulfidine),[1] 1 g two or three times daily, on peripheral manifestations but not on axial disease. These drugs were used routinely in the past to treat the most severe patients, with limited success.

In contrast, the anti–TNF-α biologic therapies in several controlled study are very efficacious in treating even the most seriously affected patients. Both the anti–TNF-α antibody infliximab (Remicade)[1] and the TNF p75-soluble receptor etanercept (Enbrel)[1] are approved to treat NSAID-resistant AS. As many as 50% of the patients enrolled in a controlled study experienced a sustained decrease of disease activity, including normalization of ESR and CRP. Patients receiving anti–TNF-α for SpA can usually decrease and frequently discontinue NSAIDs. Remicade is administered intravenously, starting with a loading regimen of three infusions (5 mg/kg per infusion) within a 6-week interval (weeks 0, 2, and 6), followed by retreatment every other 6 to 8 weeks. Enbrel is administered subcutaneously, twice weekly (25 mg per injection). Both treatments must be given permanently because relapse predictably happens upon discontinuation. The most serious adverse effects are infections, which should be minimized by a careful investigation for latent tuberculosis before treatment initiation, including a chest radiograph and a purified

TABLE 1   Classification Criteria for Spondyloarthropathy*

Clinical Symptoms or Past History	Scoring
Lumbar or dorsal pain at night or morning stiffness of lumbar or dorsal pain	1
Asymmetric oligoarthritis	2
Buttock pain	1
or	
If alternate buttock pain	2
Sausage-like toe or digit	2
Heel pain or other well-defined enthesitis	2
Iritis	1
Nongonococcal ureteritis or cervicitis within 1 mo before the onset of arthritis	1
Acute diarrhea within 1 mo before the onset of arthritis	1
Psoriasis, balanitis, or IBD (i.e., ulcerative colitis or Crohn's disease)	2
Radiologic findings	
Sacroiliitis (bilateral grade 2 or unilateral grade 3)	3
Genetic background	
Presence of HLA-B27 and/or family history of ankylosing spondylitis, reactive arthritis, uveitis, psoriasis or IBD	2
Response to treatment	
Clear-cut improvement within 48 hours after NSAIDs intake or rapid relapse of the pain after their discontinuation	2

*A patient is considered suffering from a spondyloarthropathy if the score is greater than or equal to 6.
Abbreviations: HLA = human leukocyte antigen; IBD = inflammatory bowel disease, NSAIDs = nonsteroidal anti-inflammatory drugs.
From Amor et al. (1990).

[1]Not FDA approved for this indication.

CURRENT DIAGNOSIS

- Retrieve relevant skeletal (axial/peripheral) and extra-articular symptoms from medical history (personal and familial).
- Search evidence for inflammation, both clinically and biologically.
- Search for clinical spinal stiffness, joint alterations, and psoriasis.
- Screen for human leukocyte antigen (HLA)-B27 positivity in case of doubt.
- Use imaging modalities as needed: pelvic radiography, tomodensitometry, magnetic resonance imaging, bone scan.

protein derivative (PPD) test. A 9-month prophylactic course of isoniazid should be undertaken in patients having a suspicion of untreated latent tuberculosis.

PHYSICAL THERAPY

Whenever possible, physical exercises are recommended, and physical readaptation is an important aspect of AS treatment. One to three physical therapy sessions per week are recommended, especially in patients with severe stiffness and deformities. The aim of exercises is to relax muscle stiffness, to avoid posture deformities, and to maintain muscle strength.

Follow-Up and Evaluation

Adjustment of the treatment may require a number of visits. Clinical variables to be monitored systematically are a disease activity self-assessment index, such as the Bath Ankylosing Spondylitis Disease Activity Index (BASDAI), a functional self-assessment index, such as the Bath Ankylosing Spondylitis Functional Index (BASFI), and several metrologic parameters, reflecting spinal deformity (height, occiput to wall distance, C7 spinous process to wall distance, Schober index). Other variables such as synovitis and enthesitis counts are appropriate for patients with peripheral manifestations.

The course of disease is variable during a lifetime for all patients, who must be taught how to adapt their medications. For instance, intake of NSAIDs may need to be increased during a flare, whereas discontinuation of the

CURRENT THERAPY

- Use nonsteroidal anti-inflammatory drugs (NSAIDs) as first-line therapy.
- Add physical therapy.
- Consider local corticosteroid injections.
- Consider second-line therapy for patients with a Bath Ankylosing Spondylitis Disease Activity Index (BASDAI) of 4 out of 10 despite NSAIDs.

drug can be achieved in the case of complete remission. In the absence of clinical manifestation, including pain, swelling, stiffness, and fatigue, there is no absolute need for active treatment. Only periodic examination will then be required to check for the lack of evolution. There is no need to treat isolated biologic findings, such as elevated ESR or CRP.

REFERENCES

Amor B, Dougados M, Mijiyawa M: Critère diagnostique des spondylarthropathies. Rev Rhum Mal Ostéoartic 1990;57:85-89.
Braun J, Sieper J: Biological therapies in the spondyloarthritides—the current state. Rheumatology (Oxford) 2004;43(9):1072-1084.
Breban M, Said-Nahal R, Hugot JP, Miceli-Richard C: Familial and genetic aspects of spondyloarthropathy. Rheum Dis Clin North Am 2003;29(3):575-594.
Collantes E, Veroz R, Escudero A, et al: Can some cases of 'possible' spondyloarthropathy be classified as 'definite' or 'undifferentiated' spondyloarthropathy? Value of criteria for spondyloarthropathies. Spanish Spondyloarthropathy Study Group. Joint Bone Spine 2000;67(6):516-520.
D'Agostino MA, Said-Nahal R, Hacquard-Bouder C, et al: Assessment of peripheral enthesitis in the spondylarthropathies by ultrasonography combined with power Doppler: A cross-sectional study. Arthritis Rheum 2003;48:523-533.
Dougados M, van der Heijde D: Ankylosing spondylitis: How should the disease be assessed? Best Pract Res Clin Rheumatol 2002; 16(4):605-618.
Dougados M, Van der Linden S, Juhlin R, et al: The European Spondylarthropathy Study Group preliminary criteria for the classification of spondylarthropathy. Arthritis Rheum 1991;34:1218-1227.
Maksymowych WP, Breban M, Braun J: Ankylosing spondylitis and current disease-controlling agents: Do they work? Best Pract Res Clin Rheumatol 2002;16(4):619-630.
McGonagle D: Diagnosis and treatment of enthesitis. Rheum Dis Clin North Am 2003;29(3):549-560.
van der Linden S, Valkenburg HA, Cats A: Evaluation of diagnostic criteria for ankylosing spondylitis. A proposal for modification of the New York criteria. Arthritis Rheum 1984;27:361-368.

Cervico-Cranio-Mandibular Disorders

Method of
Per-Olof Eriksson, DDS, PhD,
and Hamayun Zafar, PT, PhD

Anatomic structures are more diverse in the orofacial region than in any other region. No other location expresses so many systemic and local diseases as does the oral cavity. It serves as a focal point of interest to more medical and dental specialties than any other single part of the body. Intraoral and dental diseases are the most common cause of jaw–face pain, but a number of possible etiologic factors have to be considered in patients seeking care for pain and functional impairment in the jaw–face–head region. Jaw–face pain and dysfunction may originate from dental, neurologic, otolaryngologic, vascular, cervical spine, metaplastic, infectious, or systematic diseases. Outside the dental profession, it is less known that long-standing pain and disturbed function in the jaw–face are often caused by musculoskeletal disorders, which in fact are as prevalent as the two other major dental diseases, caries and periodontitis, and therefore constitute a significant health problem. Thus the dental profession is responsible for three major so-called dental diseases that can explain jaw–face pain and dysfunction. The human jaw–face muscles show unique fiber types and contractile proteins, both for the extrafusal and the intrafusal (muscle spindles) fibers, and changes with aging in fiber type and myosin composition are opposite those of limb muscles.

Development and Maturation of Structure and Function of the Jaw–Face Region

It is generally agreed that there is an orderly development and maturation of motor control, including postural control, in a cephalocaudal direction. First comes the ability to stabilize the head, followed by stabilization of the shoulder, trunk, and hips, to allow control of the lower limbs. Similarly, development is directed proximal-distal, which means the child first learns to control proximal body segments, such as the trunk, shoulders, and hips, and hand movements after that.

The orofacial muscles are the first to develop in the body, in keeping with the cephalocaudal sequence of fetal development, and facial premuscle masses are formed between the gestational ages of 8 and 9 weeks. Muscular response to a stimulus first develops in the perioral region and is elicited at 7.5 weeks' gestational age, as a result of tactile cutaneous stimuli applied to the lips, indicating that the trigeminal nerve is the first cranial nerve to become active. Stroking the face of the 7.5-week-old embryo produces a reflex bending of the head and upper trunk away from the stimulus, an avoiding reaction, as a total neuromuscular response. Stimulation of the lips at 8.5 weeks' gestational age results in incomplete but active reflex opening of the mouth. Swallowing begins at 12 weeks' gestational age in association with extension reflexes and occurs when the fetus drinks the amniotic fluid in which it is bathed. Tongue movements may begin at 12.5 weeks' gestational age and lip movements at 14.5 weeks' gestational age. The earliest functional movements include oral actions, such as suckling and swallowing, and full swallowing and suckling permitting survival occur at only 32 to 36 weeks of fetal age. Head movements remain strongly associated with mouth movements even into the postnatal period, whereby perioral stimulation leads to ipsilateral head rotation, which in the infant is associated with suckling. Respiratory movements may be elicited by stimulation as early as 13 weeks, but spontaneous rhythmic respiration necessary for survival does not occur until much later. Increasingly complex muscle movements, producing mastication and speech, depend on development of the appropriate reflex proprioceptive mechanisms. All of the complex interrelated orofacial movements of suckling, swallowing, and breathing are reflex in origin, rather than learned, and they constitute unconditioned congenital reflexes necessary for survival. Conditioned acquired reflexes develop with maturation of the neuromuscular system and are generally learned habits. The conversion of infantile swallowing, using predominantly facial nerve muscles, into mature swallowing when molar teeth have

erupted and the trigeminal nerve muscles come into action, infantile suckling into mastication, and infantile crying into speech are all examples of the substitution of conditioned reflexes acquired with maturation for the unconditioned congenital reflexes of the neonate. Superimposed on these reflex movements are voluntary activities under conscious control that are acquired by learning and experience.

Pain and Dysfunction in the Jaw–Face Region

A number of diseases may give rise to similar symptoms and signs of pain and dysfunction in the jaw–face region. Assessment, management, and treatment outcome are therefore related to the profession of the care provider. Thus pain experienced in the ear may be of muscular origin, referred to the ear region from adjacent painful jaw muscles. If such pain is interpreted as caused by infection instead of dysfunction, treatment will fail instead of being beneficial and cost-effective for the patient and society.

Symptoms and signs of musculoskeletal disorders in the jaw–face region originate preferentially in the temporomandibular joint (TMJ) and the jaw–face–head muscles. They typically include feelings of fatigue and stiffness in the jaw and face; pain in the jaw, face, ear, head, and neck regions; sounds in the TMJ; limitation of mandibular movements; and tenderness to palpation above the TMJ and jaw muscles. Pain is aggravated during jaw movements. These joint and muscle problems hamper unrestrained motor control with regard to amplitude, speed, force, coordination, direction, and endurance of movement, and they may result in difficulties in gaping, biting, chewing, and swallowing (i.e., eating behavior, yawning, and speech).

Terminology, Epidemiology, and Sex Differences

Musculoskeletal disorders in the jaw–face region are generally termed a *craniomandibular disorder* (CMD) or a *temporomandibular disorder* (TMD). Epidemiologic studies report a high prevalence of signs and symptoms of CMDs, although prevalence rates vary. Recent data, including mild symptoms and signs, reveal average values for perceived and clinically assessed CMDs to be 30% and 44%, respectively. Severe pain and dysfunction, which need treatment, are estimated to occur in about 5% to 10% of the adult population. A strong female preponderance among patients seeking care for CMDs is observed, and symptoms and signs of CMDs are more frequent, severe, and long-lasting in women than in men. No conclusive explanation for gender differences in CMD is as yet reported, in accordance with what is known for musculoskeletal disorders in other body regions.

Etiology and Treatment of Craniomandibular Disorders

Knowledge about mechanisms behind musculoskeletal disorders is in general limited. Consequently, treatment and preventive care are hampered. This is the case also for musculoskeletal disorders in the jaw–face region. Generally, it is a matter of load and capacity, and both central and peripheral factors seem important. Central factors include lifestyle-related psychogenic muscular tension and stress-induced clenching of the jaws. Peripheral factors include the stability of the bite (i.e., the relation between the lower jaw, mandibular teeth and the upper jaw, skull, or "head–neck" teeth at rest and during jaw movements). Psychogenic tension and jaw clenching in a bite that lacks stability may to various degrees give rise to an overload of dental and musculoskeletal components and accordingly result in pain and dysfunction.

Studies on treatment outcome involve both dental and nondental therapies, and between 65% and 95% of CMD patients who seek care for the first time are reported to improve. Treatment usually includes the following:

- Counseling
- Jaw exercises for tension relief and to regain movement skills
- A decrease of load on dental, muscle, and joint tissues by improving bite stability, which can be fulfilled by using reversible methods (e.g., intraoral appliances, bite splints) and irreversible methods (e.g., dental fillings and selective grinding of teeth)
- Drugs for relief of pain and tension
- TMJ surgery when pain and dysfunction are caused by internal derangement

Functional Coupling Between the Jaw and the Neck Regions

Evidence from neuroanatomic and neurophysiologic studies in animals demonstrates close connections between the trigeminal and the neck neuromuscular systems. In humans, a functional coupling between the craniomandibular and the cervical spine regions is suggested by intimate anatomic and biomechanical relationships, by findings of reflex activities in the neck muscles following electrical stimulation of trigeminal nerve branches, and from observations of simultaneous activation of jaw and neck–shoulder muscles during mandibular movements. The earliest reflex found in the human embryo is the trigeminal neck reflex, which consists of contraction of neck muscles elicited by light touch of the perioral region. Thus previous studies in animals and humans indicate a close functional linkage between the jaw and the neck regions. Systematic studies of integrated mandibular and head–neck behavior during natural jaw function, however, are lacking.

A series of studies in humans, using optoelectronic wireless technique for three-dimensional movement recording and electromyography, showed concomitant and well-coordinated mandibular and head–neck movements during both single and rhythmic jaw opening-and-closing tasks (Figure 1). Such movements are invariant in nature. The findings led to a new concept for natural jaw function. In this concept, functional jaw movements are the result of jointly activated jaw as well as neck muscles, leading to simultaneous movements in the temporomandibular, atlanto-occipital, and cervical spine joints. These jaw and head–neck movements have neural commands in common

and are preprogrammed. Furthermore, when combined with observations in ultrasonographic studies on human fetal yawning, findings indicate that mouth opening and closing are accompanied by head extension-flexion movements, respectively, and the functional connection between the jaw and the neck in natural jaw function is innate. Thus, based on results from studies in animals and people, "natural jaw function," by definition, includes integrative jaw–neck behavior.

Significance of Functional Coupling Between the Jaw and the Neck

Connections between the trigeminal system and neck motoneurons are important for head withdrawal reactions in all species. Any sudden or unexpected stimulus in the orofacial region leads to fast head aversion, hence paralleling the flexor reflex of the limbs. Such connections are also likely critical for coordinating jaw and head–neck motions and in timing of jaw opening and closing with head–neck movements during daily activities such as eating and communication.

Free neck movements are a prerequisite for natural maximal gaping. A reduced head extension ability may limit the three-dimensional space for the mandibular movement because of impingement of the mandible with suprahyoid and airway structures. A connection between the jaw and the neck motor systems is probably of importance to allow simultaneous mandibular and head–neck movements, aimed at optimizing both the magnitude of the gape and the positioning of the gape in space. From an evolutionary perspective, such a mechanism, to optimally direct the jaw motor system (i.e., the mouth or the gape) in basic actions such as feeding, attack, and defense behavior, is probably of great survival value (e.g., during catching of prey).

Craniomandibular Disorders and Pain and Dysfunction in the Neck

Clinical trials demonstrate an association between CMDs and neck symptoms; pain and dysfunction in the neck are often present in patients with CMD. It is also known that patients with neck problems may have signs and symptoms of CMD. In fact, randomized controlled trials show that treatment of CMD in patients who were on sick leave for neck–shoulder pain and dysfunction, but who also had CMD, provided relief of both CMD and neck–shoulder symptoms. Notably, treatment outcome was measured in terms of reduced number of days on sick leave and use of medical services. The treatment consisted of improvement of bite stability by selective grinding of the lower and upper teeth. Such adjustment of peripheral input probably influences the relation between the mandible and the head–neck biomechanically, by changing the functional load on jaw and neck components, and with regard to integrative sensorimotor control of the jaw and neck.

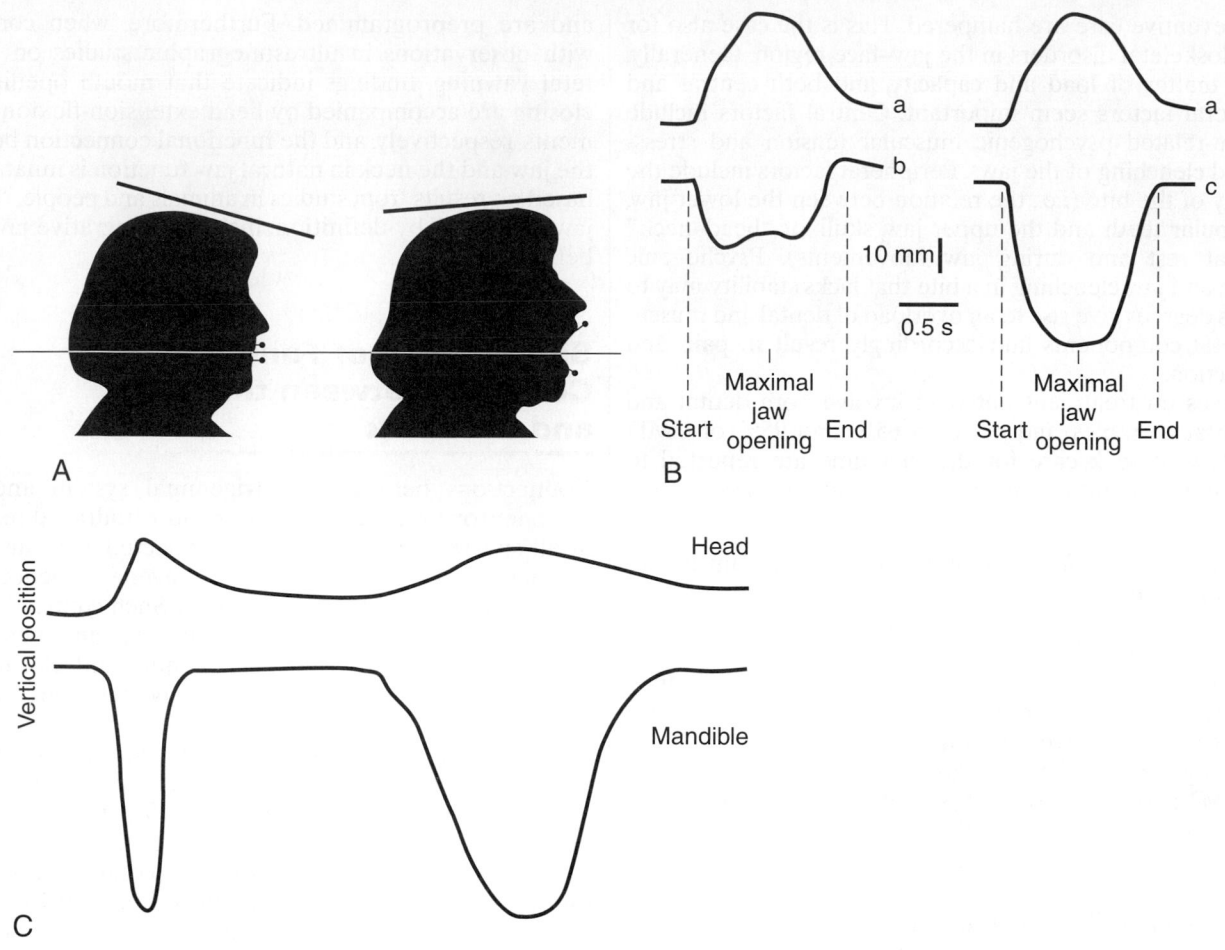

FIGURE 1. **A,** Head position at rest (*left*) and at maximal jaw opening (*right*). Note change in head position indicated by reference line above the head and recording markers attached to the upper and lower frontal teeth. Note also the relatively unchanged midposition of the gape at maximal jaw opening, indicated by the horizontal reference line. **B,** Movement trajectories in vertical dimension over time of the mandible (*b, c*) and the head (*a*) for a maximal jaw opening–closing movement. Start and end of movement are labeled. The *left* panel (*b*) illustrates the mandibular movement "in space," i.e., the trajectory is the result of the combined mandibular and head–neck movements. The *right* panel (*c*) shows the magnitude of the mandibular movement after mathematical compensation for head movement, i.e., in relation to the head. **C,** Movement trajectories in vertical dimension over time of head–neck and mandibular movements at fast (*left*) and slow (*right*) jaw opening–closing tasks, and after mathematical compensation for head movements. Note simultaneous start of mandibular and head movements.

Craniomandibular Disorders in Whiplash-Associated Disorders

Trauma to the neck from a motor vehicle accident or some other type of head–neck trauma, generally called whiplash trauma or injury, may lead to a condition comprising a number of symptoms and signs in the neck and head termed whiplash-associated disorders (WADs). Studies indicate that such head–neck trauma can result in pain and dysfunction in the jaw–face region (i.e., CMD), although the matter is under debate.

Studies on integrated jaw–neck motor control in healthy subjects and in WAD patients led to an explanatory model for the development of CMD in subjects who met with whiplash injury. Given that natural jaw actions require a healthy state with unrestricted motion of both the TMJ and the atlanto-occipital and cervical spine joints,

it can be assumed that an injury to or disease of any of these three joint systems might derange natural jaw motor control. Furthermore, such a functional impairment would be reflected by disturbed jaw–neck behavior, which could be detected by recording and analyzing concomitant mandibular and head–neck movements during natural jaw actions. We recently tested this hypothesis by studying integrative jaw–neck function in patients suffering from WADs and pain and dysfunction in the jaw–face. The results show an association between neck trauma and disturbed jaw–neck function, indicating that coordinated jaw–neck motor control during both single and rhythmic jaw opening-closing movements indeed can be disturbed following neck injury. Thus *cervico-cranio-mandibular disorder* (CCMD) is an appropriate term for the clinical condition comprising both jaw–face and head–neck pain and dysfunction.

Treatment Model for Improvement of Mandibular and Head–Neck Mobility

Studies on integrative jaw–neck function include measurement of magnitude, temporal coordination, speed, and spatiotemporal consistency of concomitant mandibular and head–neck movements. By applying the methods we developed for analysis of healthy jaw–neck behavior in investigations of patients, we found signs of disturbed jaw–neck function in individuals suffering from WADs. Based on the findings in healthy subjects and in patients, we developed a new model for treatment of pain and dysfunction in the jaw–face and WADs. This treatment approach is aimed at improving both mandibular and head–neck mobility, thereby regaining natural jaw function. The model is based on the fact that motor control starts to develop and mature in the jaw-orofacial region (as described earlier). Data from numerous studies in animals and people suggest a close linkage between the jaw and the neck sensorimotor systems in natural jaw function. Consequently, treatment for improving jaw function should include the neck. Our studies to test this treatment model in patients with jaw–face pain and dysfunction and WADs show improvement of both jaw and neck function, results that merit further studies in randomized clinical trials.

Figure 2 shows a typical example. It is based on data from a female patient, 30 years of age, who had a car accident and developed WAD 4 years before she was referred to the department of Clinical Oral Physiology, Umeå University Hospital, Umeå, Sweden, for assessment and management of pain and dysfunction in the jaw and face. The patient had received all the care and treatment for WAD available according to routines used by the health care system. Our examination revealed severely impaired jaw and neck function and widespread pain in all body regions. The initial, pretreatment, investigation of concomitant mandibular and head–neck movements during jaw opening-and-closing tasks, using our routine protocol and optoelectronic wireless three-dimensional movement recording technique, verified the functional impairment of jaw–neck behavior. As Figure 2 illustrates, the follow-up recordings after 4 and 7 months show an increase in magnitude of movement amplitudes of both the mandibular and the head–neck movement. In addition, the speed of movement increased. The figure also shows that functional impairment, as well as change in behavior in response to treatment, can be measured and documented qualitatively and quantitatively by objective recording methods.

Treatment Regimen for Craniomandibular Disorders and Whiplash-Associated Disorders

The general aim of the treatment regimen is to regain natural jaw function by reprogramming faulty jaw–neck sensorimotor behavior. In short, this is performed in three ways:

1. Education, advice, and instructions with regard to anatomy, physiology, pathophysiology, and treatment
2. Specific jaw–neck exercises, including mandibular and head–neck movements to gain successive increase in movement amplitude and speed in very minor steps (i.e., to slowly reteach the neuromuscular system to

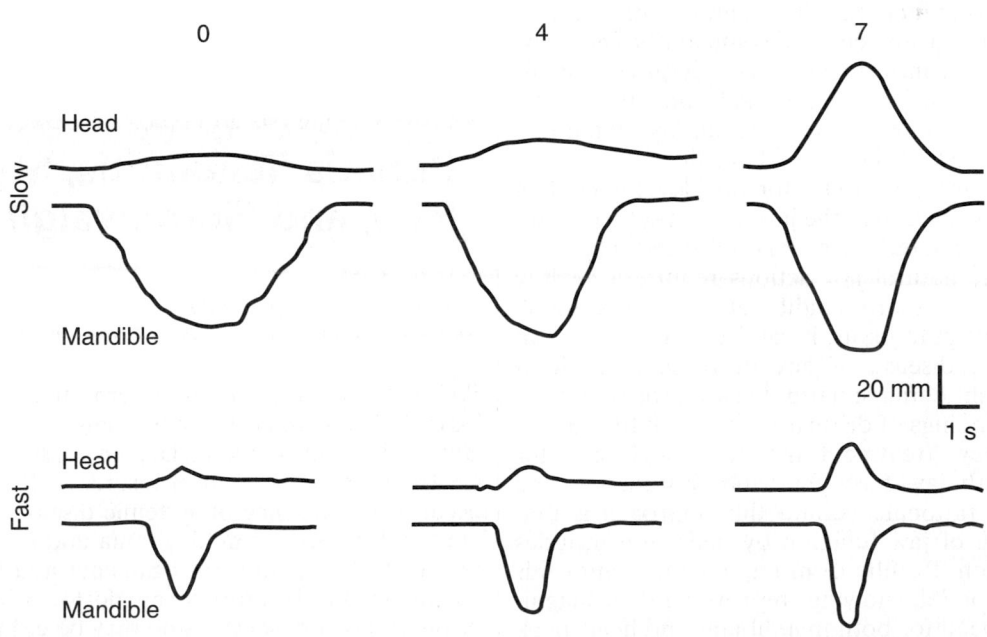

FIGURE 2. Repeated movement recordings in a female patient, 30 years old, suffering from whiplash-associated disorders and pain and dysfunction in the jaw–face. Trajectories for the vertical dimension over time of mandibular and head–neck movements at slow (*upper panel*) and fast (*lower panel*) maximal jaw opening-and-closing tasks: initial, pretreatment, recording (0), and recordings after 4 and 7 months of treatment. Note post-treatment increase in amplitude and speed for both mandibular and head–neck movements, and for both slow and fast jaw opening and closing tasks.

CURRENT DIAGNOSIS

- Because different diseases in the jaw–orofacial region may give rise to similar symptoms, proper examination and diagnosis must precede treatment.
- Musculoskeletal disorders in the jaw–face region, generally termed *craniomandibular disorders* (CMDs), are as prevalent as the two major dental diseases, caries and periodontitis, and constitute a significant health problem.
- There is a strong female preponderance among patients seeking care for CMD, and symptoms and signs are more frequent, severe, and longer lasting in women than in men.
- Between 65% and 95% of CMD patients who seek care for the first time are reported to improve.

execute coordinated mandibular and head–neck movements in a cost-effective way)
3. A custom-made intraoral appliance (bite splint) attached to the upper teeth for day and night use, to change biomechanical relations (reducing detrimental load on sensitized components of the jaw–neck motor system and give pain relief) and to modulate sensorimotor settings for control of jaw–neck behavior and

CURRENT THERAPY

- A new concept for natural jaw function suggests that "functional jaw movements" are the result of jointly activated jaw and neck muscles, leading to simultaneous movements in the temporomandibular, atlanto-occipital, and cervical spine joints. These jaw and head–neck movements have neural commands in common, are preprogrammed, and are innate. Accordingly, natural jaw function, by definition, includes integrative jaw–neck behavior.
- A new explanatory model for the development of pain and dysfunction in the jaw–face in subjects with whiplash-associated disorders (WADs) proposes that because natural jaw actions require a healthy state of the temporomandibular, atlanto-occipital, and cervical spine joints, it can be assumed that an injury to or disease of any of these three joint systems might derange natural jaw motor control.
- Based on findings of disturbed jaw–neck function in WAD, a new treatment model is suggested for patients with jaw–face pain and dysfunction and WAD. The rationale behind this approach is that intervention of jaw function by definition includes neck function. Results from implementation of this treatment model, showing improvement of magnitude and speed for both mandibular and head–neck movements, are reported.
- Finally, an appropriate term for the clinical condition comprising both jaw–face and head–neck pain and dysfunction is *cervico-cranio-mandibular disorders* (CCMDs).

disturb jaw-clenching habits. In fact, ongoing studies in our laboratory indicate that this device is associated with significant changes in control mechanisms of posture and movement.

REFERENCES

Carlsson GE: Epidemiology and treatment need for temporomandibular disorders. J Orofac Pain 1999;13:232-237.

Eriksson P-O, Zafar H, Nordh E: Concomitant mandibular and head-neck movements during jaw opening-closing in man. J Oral Rehabil 1998;25:859-870.

Eriksson P-O, Häggman-Henrikson B, Nordh E, Zafar H: Coordinated mandibular and head-neck movements during rhythmic jaw activities in man. J Dent Res 2000;79:1378-1384.

Eriksson P-O, Zafar H, Häggman-Henrikson B: Deranged jaw-neck motor control in whiplash-associated disorders. Eur J Oral Sci 2004;112:25-32.

Häggman-Henrikson B, Zafar H, Eriksson P-O: Disturbed jaw behavior in whiplash-associated disorders during rhythmic jaw movements. J Dent Res 2002;81:747-751.

Häggman-Henrikson B: Neck function in rhythmic jaw activities. [Doctoral Dissertation] Umeå University, Sweden 2004; pp 1-53.

Johansson H, Windhorst U, Djupsjöbacka M, Passatore M [Eds]: Chronic work-related myalgia. Neuromuscular mechanisms behind work-related chronic muscle pain syndromes. Gävle University Press Gävle, Sweden 2003; pp 1-310.

Kirveskari P, Alanen P: Effect of occlusal treatment on sick leaves in TMJ dysfunction patients with head and neck symptoms. Community Dent Oral Epidemiol 1984;12:78-81.

Monemi M, Kadi F, Liu JX, et al: Adverse changes in fibre type and myosin heavy chain compositions of human jaw muscle vs. limb muscle during ageing. Acta Physiol Scand 1999;167:339-345.

Sperry GH: Craniofacial embryology. 4th ed. Wright. 1989.

Zafar H: Integrated jaw and neck function in man. Studies of mandibular and head-neck movements during jaw opening-closing tasks. [Doctoral Dissertation] Swed Dent J Suppl 2000;(143):1-41.

Zafar H, Nordh E, Eriksson P-O: Spatiotemporal consistency of human mandibular and head-neck movement trajectories during jaw opening-closing tasks. Exp Brain Res 2002;146:70-76.

Zafar H, Nordh E, Eriksson P-O: Impaired positioning of the gape in whiplash-associated disorders. Swed Dent J 2006;30:9-15.

Bursitis, Tendonitis, Myofascial Pain, and Fibromyalgia

Method of
Keith K. Colburn, MD

Soft tissue rheumatism is a term that describes musculoskeletal pain and other symptoms not caused by arthritis. Bursitis, tendonitis, myofascial pain syndrome, and fibromyalgia belong to this group of disorders. These maladies may occur in the absence of systemic disease. They are associated with persistent mild trauma and overuse of muscles, bursae, tendons, entheses, ligaments, and fascia, conditions commonly seen by primary care doctors. Localized tendonitis or bursitis is very specific and may be either self-limiting or relieved by topical or oral anti-inflammatory medications or treated with a well-placed injection. Fibromyalgia is more diffuse and may be very difficult to treat. There are no abnormal laboratory tests consistently associated with soft tissue rheumatism. Radiologic tests and scans may show abnormalities of soft tissue; it is only occasionally necessary, however, to do expensive tests to get an accurate diagnosis of these conditions. Diagnosis requires a good history and a careful physical examination of the musculoskeletal system.

Bursitis and Tendonitis

Bursitis and tendonitis may occur in any one of hundreds of locations throughout the body. A bursa is a synovial membrane-lined sac containing synovial fluid. Bursae are found in areas of potential friction, such as where tendons, ligaments, and bone rub against each other. Bursitis may occur alone or in conjunction with inflammation of a tendon in close proximity. Tendons and ligaments are fibrous cords or bands that attach muscle to other structures, usually bone. Bursitis and tendonitis are considered together here by regions of the body because diagnosis and treatment share some common principles. Treatments specific to unique locations are mentioned in the text. Otherwise, general treatment principles are listed in the Current Therapy box.

SHOULDER REGION

Shoulder pain is a common problem that increases with age. Because the shoulder has an extensive range of motion, it one of the most unstable joints in the body. Numerous ligaments, tendons, and bursae surround the shoulder joints. *Rotator cuff tendonitis*, or the *impingement syndrome,* is the most common cause of shoulder pain. *Subacromial bursitis* may be secondarily present with the impingement syndrome. Pain on active abduction and internal rotation of the glenohumeral joint and aching over the deltoid area are the main symptoms of this condition. The impingement syndrome may be acute from a recent injury or chronic with calcific tendonitis sometimes seen on radiographs. *Rotator cuff tears* may be partial or complete, acute or chronic, exquisitely painful or hardly felt. Weakness and pain on abduction, night pain, and tenderness on palpation may indicate the presence of a torn rotator cuff. The diagnosis may be established by a shoulder arthrogram, ultrasonogram, or magnetic resonance imaging (MRI) scan. Although incomplete tears often are best treated by conservative means, over time they often become complete tears. Complete tears can often be surgically repaired, especially if they are acute and occur in younger patients. *Bicipital tendonitis* often presents as anterior shoulder pain. Sometimes the pain is diffuse, but rolling the long head of the biceps tendon under the examiner's thumb elicits localized tenderness if the tendon is inflamed. Rupture of the long head of the biceps tendon presents as an enlargement of the distal end of the biceps muscle. This complication is usually not repaired because it results in only a minor loss of strength in the biceps muscle. *Adhesive capsulitis,* or *frozen shoulder,* presents as generalized pain and tenderness of the shoulder area with a marked loss of active and passive range of motion and with muscle atrophy. Inflammatory arthritis, diabetes, immobility, low pain threshold, depression, or improper treatment of a painful shoulder can result in a frozen shoulder. Arthrography demonstrates a contracted joint capsule space. Less common painful conditions associated with the shoulder region include the *thoracic outlet syndrome, brachial plexopathy,* and *neuropathies.*

ANTERIOR CHEST WALL

Pain in the anterior chest wall is common and often needs to be differentiated from cardiac, pulmonary, or gastrointestinal pain. Point tenderness helps delineate actual chest wall pain from pain generated from an internal organ. *Costochondritis (Tietze's syndrome)* is manifested by tenderness at the costochondral junction of the anterior ribs. There is usually one distinct tender spot, although more can occur simultaneously. *Xiphodynia* is characterized by tenderness and pain over the xiphoid area.

ELBOW REGION

Olecranon bursitis occurs with repetitive mild trauma and abrasion over the elbow or with an inflammatory condition including gout, pseudogout, rheumatoid arthritis, and infection. Range of motion of the elbow is usually relatively normal and pain minimal except when infection is present. Aspiration of an uninfected bursa alone or combined with an injection of a corticosteroid is the usual treatment. Crystal identification with a polarized microscope is helpful to differentiate gout or pseudogout from infection. Antibiotic treatment, after a Gram stain and culture of purulent fluid, is indicated in a suspected infected bursa. *Lateral epicondylitis,* or tennis elbow, is a common finding in repetitive use of one's arms. Tenderness is elicited by pressing the extensor tendons 1 to 2 cm distal to the lateral epicondyle. Shaking hands or lifting a bag causes pain in the same location. *Medial epicondylitis,* or golfer's elbow, is less common but diagnosed by palpating the flexor tendons attached to the medial epicondyle. A soft forearm brace may be helpful if patients would prefer not to have an injection of the tender spot. *Ulnar nerve entrapment* and *tendonitis of the musculotendinous insertion of the biceps* are conditions also found in the elbow region.

HAND AND WRIST REGION

A *ganglion* is a cyst arising from a tendon sheath or a joint, commonly located on the dorsum of the wrist. It is lined with synovium and contains a thick jelly-like liquid. *De Quervain's tenosynovitis* is inflammation and tenderness of the sheath of the abductor pollicis longus and extensor polices brevis tendons located over the radial styloid. Repetitive trauma, pregnancy, and systemic rheumatoid diseases are causes for this disorder. *Carpal tunnel syndrome* caused by the compression of the median nerve by the surrounding structures in the wrist is the most common cause of numbness and tingling in the hands. A positive Tinel or Phalen sign with a confirming nerve conduction test makes the diagnosis fairly simple. Trauma, pregnancy, and a host of metabolic or inflammatory diseases are often responsible for this condition. Treatment starts with wrist splinting at night. The use of 200 mg of vitamin B_6 daily[1] until the symptoms subside may be controversial, but in my opinion is often very helpful. If these measures are unsuccessful, a corticosteroid injection on the ulnar side of the carpal tunnel, a few millimeters away from the median nerve, usually relieves the numbness and tingling, often for months. In many patients, surgery is eventually required to release the median nerve. Other less frequent

---

[1]Not FDA approved for this indication.

hand and wrist soft tissue problems include *pronator teres syndrome, anterior interosseous nerve syndrome, radial nerve palsy, ulnar nerve entrapment at the wrist, volar flexor tenosynovitis,* and *Dupuytren's contractures.*

HIP REGION

The trochanteric bursa lies on the posterior portion of the greater trochanter. Pain from *trochanteric bursitis* is felt in the trochanteric area and lateral thigh, and it is often thought inaccurately to be hip joint pain, which is usually felt in the groin and high in the buttock. Excessive trauma to the bursal area, such as a long hike, can precipitate trochanteric bursitis. Osteoarthritis of the lumbar spine or hip, scoliosis or leg length discrepancies, and age can contribute to trochanteric bursitis. *Iliopsoas (iliopectineal) bursitis* causes groin and anterior thigh pain, made worse on passive hyperextension and sometimes flexion of the hip with resistance. *Ischial (ischiogluteal) bursitis,* or *weaver's bottom,* is caused by trauma or sitting for a long time on hard surfaces. Pain from ischial bursitis is felt down the back of the thigh with point tenderness over the ischial tuberosity. Soft seat cushions and a corticosteroid injection of the bursa usually help relieve the pain. *Piriformis syndrome* is not well understood. The predominant symptom is pain over the buttocks sometimes radiating down the back of the thigh and leg. Trauma is usually involved in the etiology. The diagnosis is often made on rectal or vaginal examination by detecting tenderness in the piriformis muscle. *Meralgia paresthetica* is caused by the compression of the lateral femoral cutaneous nerve (L2-L3). It causes intermittent burning pain, hyperesthesia, and numbness of the anterolateral thigh. This syndrome is seen most often in patients with obesity or diabetes, or who are pregnant.

KNEE REGION

Popliteal cysts, or Baker cysts, are associated with knee joint effusions, causing a synovial herniation into the popliteal fossa. The cyst may rupture and dissect down the calf, often to the ankle, where it may leave a purpuric "crescent sign" beneath the malleolus. A ruptured Baker cyst is acutely painful and must be differentiated from thrombophlebitis. An arthrogram or ultrasound examination of the knee may be used to diagnose a Baker cyst with or without a rupture. A venogram can exclude concomitant thrombophlebitis if necessary. An injection of a corticosteroid[1] into the cyst or the knee joint often shrinks the cyst. Surgical removal of the cyst may be necessary if the injection is ineffective. *Anserine bursitis* is diagnosed by tenderness over the medial aspect of the knee an inch or two below the joint line and occurs in predominantly obese middle-age to elderly women (35 to 80 years of age) with osteoarthritis of the knee. *Prepatellar bursitis,* or *housemaid's knee,* presents as a mildly tender swelling over the patella. It is usually caused by trauma from frequent kneeling. Aspiration of the bursa is important because occasionally septic prepatellar bursitis is present. Because the bursa does not communicate with the knee joint, treatment with oral antibiotics appropriate for the organism cultured is adequate. For sterile bursitis, an injection of a

[1]Not FDA approved for this indication.

corticosteroid is helpful, as is protection of the knee from trauma. Less common painful soft tissue conditions of the knee include *patellar tendonitis, popliteal tendonitis, medial plica syndrome, rupture of the quadriceps tendon,* and *infrapatellar tendon* and *patellofemoral pain syndrome (chondromalacia patellae).*

ANKLE AND FOOT REGION

Achilles tendonitis has two predominant causes. One is trauma. The other is a group of inflammatory conditions including rheumatoid arthritis, the spondyloarthropathies, and pseudogout. Tenderness, pain, and swelling occur proximal to or at the Achilles tendon attachment to the calcaneus. Shoe corrections, heel lifts, a splint with plantar flexion, and careful stretching of the tendon constitute the safest treatment. The inflamed Achilles tendon is vulnerable to rupture, especially if a corticosteroid is injected around it. The differential diagnosis of Achilles tendonitis includes *retrocalcaneal bursitis* and *subcutaneous Achilles bursitis. Plantar fasciitis* is characterized by burning, lancing or aching pain, and tenderness over the plantar surface of the heel from a variety of kinds of trauma or overuse. *Tarsal tunnel syndrome* is caused by compression of the posterior tibial nerve, posterior and inferior to the medial malleolus. A positive Tinel sign may be elicited by percussion over the entrapment site. Numbness, paresthesias, and burning pain are felt from the toes to the medial malleolus. Changing shoes and conservative therapy may help in the treatment of this condition, but surgery is often needed to decompress the nerve and provide relief. *Morton's neuroma*

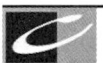

CURRENT DIAGNOSIS

Bursitis and Tendonitis

- Localized tenderness is usually palpated directly over an affected bursa or tendon.
- Most often, *active* range of motion in the affected tendon or bursa is painful, but unlike with arthritis, *passive* range of motion is frequently painless.
- With a few exceptions, blood tests and radiographs are usually normal.

Fibromyalgia

- A longer than 3-month history of chronic, widespread pain both above and below the waist and on both sides of the body in the absence of another condition to explain the pain.
- The presence of at least 11 of 18 tender points by digital palpation at previously published locations.
- Tender point sites include bilateral locations on the following locations:
  Occiput
  Anterior lower neck (C5-C7)
  Trapezius
  Supraspinatus
  Second anterior costochondral junction
  Lateral epicondyle
  Buttocks in the upper outer quadrant
  Greater trochanters
  Medial fat pad of the knees

is an entrapment neuropathy of the interdigital nerve most commonly found between the third and fourth toes. This condition is often detected in middle-age women (35 to 60 years old) wearing high heels or tight shoes. Pain is often felt in the fourth toe as a burning, aching pain with paresthesias. Treatment consists of a metatarsal bar or a corticosteroid[1] injection in the web space of the toe where the tenderness is palpated. If these are unsuccessful, surgery to remove the neuroma may be necessary. Less common causes of nonarthritic foot pain include *posterior tibial tendonitis, hallux valgus, bunionette (tailor's bunion)*

---

[1]Not FDA approved for this indication.

of the fifth toe, hammertoes, metatarsalgia, pes planus (flat foot), pes cavus (claw foot), and a variety of *tendon ruptures* or *displacements* including the Achilles, posterior tibialis, and the peroneal tendons.

Myofascial Pain Syndrome

Myofascial pain syndromes are often referred to as localized or regional fibromyalgia. They include regional pain disorders like chronic whiplash, repetitive strain syndrome, and temporomandibular joint syndrome. Myofascial pain is characterized by the presence of trigger points, defined as localized areas of deep muscle tenderness located in a

---

 CURRENT THERAPY

Bursitis and Tendonitis

- Use conservative measures first in treating bursitis and tendonitis. These include rest, modifying wear-and-tear activities, heat and/or ice, physical therapy, weight loss, splinting, topical analgesics, nonsteroidal anti-inflammatory drugs (NSAIDs), and well-placed lidocaine injections with or without corticosteroids.
- There are numerous NSAID preparations, including naproxen (Naprosyn), 500 mg twice a day, ibuprofen (Motrin),[1] 400 to 800 mg every 6 to 8 hours, and the newer COX-2 selective agents, including celecoxib (Celebrex),[1] 100 to 200 mg one to two times daily. (If the patient is taking aspirin, even a baby aspirin, the COX-2 effect is eliminated. A proton pump inhibitor such as lansoprazole (Prevacid), 15 to 30 mg daily, with a traditional NSAID, gives the equivalent gastrointestinal protection of the COX-2 agents.)
- Corticosteroid injections using 0.5 to 1.0 mL of methylprednisolone acetate (Depo-Medrol) or triamcinolone acetonide (Kenalog-40) are best administered after 1 to 10 mL of lidocaine (Xylocaine) is injected with a separate syringe, leaving the needle in place while changing the syringe. This avoids the possibility of subcutaneous fat atrophy at the injection site from the corticosteroid.
- Inject around, not into, a tendon to avoid tendon rupture. For patient comfort, a number 25 or 27 needle of appropriate length should be used. (Ethyl chloride spray on the skin obscures the pain of the needle stick. Adding bicarbonate to the syringe neutralizes the stinging sensation of lidocaine.)
- Surgical solutions for bursitis and tendonitis are reserved for unresponsiveness to conservative measures.

Fibromyalgia

INITIAL THERAPY

- See Other Tested and Possibly Helpful Therapies later in this box.
- Daily aerobic exercise, starting with as little as 5 minutes at first, progressing to between 30 to

60 minutes, is ideal. Emphasize to patients that without the progressive aerobic exercise part of treatment (i.e., walking, swimming in warm water, bicycling, jogging, etc.), they are unlikely to improve very much no matter what medications they take. It usually takes 6 to 12 months of exercise by unusually motivated patients to attain the level of fitness that is likely to diminish most or all the pain. Even some exercise is still beneficial.
- Tramadol (Ultram),[3] 50 mg, progressively up to 8 tablets daily in divided doses, for pain.
- Zolpidem (Ambien), 10 mg at bedtime (this drug is less habit forming and gives the deepest—that is, stage 3 or 4—sleep of any other sleeping medications).

SECOND-LINE THERAPY

- May be added onto or substituted for one of the first-line medications depending on drug interactions and efficacy.
- Gabapentin (Neurontin),[1] 1800 to 3600 mg daily, in progressive, divided doses, for pain.
- Amitriptyline (Elavil),[1] 10 to 200 mg, or trazodone (Desyrel),[1] 25 to 250 mg at bedtime, for sleep, depression, and mild pain relief.
- A selective serotonin reuptake inhibitor agent such as sertraline (Zoloft),[1] 50 mg daily, for depression and mild pain relief.

OTHER TESTED AND POSSIBLY HELPFUL THERAPIES

- Muscle relaxants, such as tizanidine (Zanaflex), 4 to 8 mg three times per day, or cyclobenzaprine (Flexeril), 10 mg at bedtime, for pain and rest.
- Newer antidepressants, such as duloxetine (Cymbalta), 60 mg two times per day, for pain and, secondarily, for depression.
- Magnesium, 500 mg, combined with malic acid, 1200 to 2400 mg daily, for fatigue.
- Narcotics should be avoided.
- NSAIDs are rarely helpful.
- Prolonged bed rest and inactivity and expensive and/or dangerous alternative therapies should be avoided.

---

[1]Not FDA approved for this indication.
[3]Exceeds dosage recommended by the manufacturer.
Abbreviations: NSAID = nonsteroidal anti-inflammatory drug.

taut band in the muscle that when palpated are referred to distant zones of perceived pain. In addition to the referred pain, a local "twitch response," or muscle contraction, is seen with pressing on a trigger point. Tender points of fibromyalgia are not characterized by referred pain. Treatment includes injecting the trigger points and often adding the treatment modalities outlined in the fibromyalgia section (Current Therapy box).

Fibromyalgia Syndrome

Fibromyalgia is a chronic, diffuse pain syndrome of unknown etiology. It is characterized by widespread musculoskeletal pain of variable intensity and specific "tender points" to palpation (Current Diagnosis box). Fibromyalgia is associated with a lack of deep sleep and a relative intolerance of physical activities because of pain. Box 1 outlines the signs and symptoms associated with fibromyalgia. Many patients also complain of a history of either an emotional or physical traumatic event prior to the onset of symptoms of fibromyalgia. The incidence of fibromyalgia is estimated at 2% of the population; 90% of these cases are found in women. Primary fibromyalgia is remarkable for the lack of abnormal laboratory and radiologic tests routinely done for rheumatologic diseases. Secondary fibromyalgia, fibromyalgia linked to another disease (Box 2), may improve when the primary disease is treated. Concurrent fibromyalgia or fibromyalgia coexisting together with other conditions (see Box 2) may not respond to treatment of the other disease. The American College of Rheumatology has published diagnostic criteria for fibromyalgia (see Current Diagnosis box). Digital palpation of the tender points is done at approximately 4 kg of force, which is roughly enough pressure to blanch the thumbnail. It is extremely important that patients are made aware by the treating physician that they own this diagnosis and it requires effort on their part to get better. It then becomes the patient's responsibility to take charge of their own problem and carry out the treatment recommendations by their physicians and appropriately trained staff. Treatment with narcotics,[1] because of potential dependency problems, should be avoided if at all possible. Because there is no reliable program that eliminates all of the patient's pain, there are many treatment protocols for fibromyalgia. Self-motivated patients may find relief for a significant portion of their discomfort. My preferred method of treatment is outlined in the Current Therapy box. A compassionate, experienced physician is essential

---

[1]Not FDA approved for this indication.

BOX 2 Conditions Associated or Concurrent with Fibromyalgia

Secondary Fibromyalgia	Concurrent Fibromyalgia
Hypothyroidism	Chronic fatigue syndrome
Polymyalgia rheumatica	Autoimmune diseases
Tapering off corticosteroids	(systemic lupus
Drugs (lipid-lowering	erythematosus,
and antiviral agents)	rheumatoid arthritis)
Cervical stenosis?	Myofascial pain syndrome
Malignancy	Irritable bowel syndrome
	Gulf War syndrome
	Migraine headaches
	Interstitial cystitis
	Viral infections
	(e.g., parvovirus,
	Lyme disease,
	hepatitis C)

---

for the successful treatment of fibromyalgia. Psychological counseling may be helpful if it is presented to the patient as a modality in helping to cope with pain and not a suggestion that the patient's problems are "just" psychological. Encouraging the patient to expect small increments of improvement and not to anticipate a cure helps expectations remain realistic. Patients may be referred to support groups backed by organizations like the Arthritis Foundation. Online Web sites for fibromyalgia associated with universities or reputable foundations may be very helpful to patients by providing accurate information about their condition and its treatment.

REFERENCES

Biundo JJ, Jr: Regional rheumatic pain syndromes. In: Klippel JH, Crofford LJ, Stone JH, Weyand CM (eds): Primer on the Rheumatic Diseases, 12th ed. Atlanta, Arthritis Foundation, 2001, pp 174-187.

Clauw DJ: Fibromyalgia and diffuse pain syndromes. In: Klippel JH, Crofford LJ, Stone JH, Weyand CM (eds): Primer on the Rheumatic Diseases, 12th ed. Atlanta, Arthritis Foundation, 2001, pp 188-193.

Fransen J, Russell IJ: Medical management of fibromyalgia. In Fransen J, Russell IJ (eds): The Fibromyalgia Help Book. St. Paul, Minn, Smith House Press, 1996, pp 35-58.

Goldenberg DL: Fibromyalgia and related syndromes. In: Hochberg MC, Silman AL, Smolen JS, et al (eds): Rheumatology, 3rd ed. St. Louis, Mo, Mosby, 2003, pp 701-712.

Sheon RP: Overview of soft tissue rheumatic disorders. UpToDate, online 12.3, 2004. Available online at http://www.uptodate.com.

BOX 1 Signs and Symptoms of Fibromyalgia

- Sleep disturbance
- Fatigue
- Paresthesias
- Stiffness
- Depression
- Dry eyes and mouth
- Raynaud's syndrome
- Headaches

Osteoarthritis

Method of
George E. Ehrlich, MD

In some respects, the term *osteoarthritis* is a misnomer because it refers only to a subset of joint changes—those accompanied by inflammation. An older, and still popular name in some parts of the world, is osteoarthrosis, which implies a condition of the joints without inflammation, and perhaps this should be revived for a majority of cases, in which pain is minimal at worst. A former synonym, degenerative joint disease, has been largely discarded, as it implies a specificity that cannot be supported. The confusion arises from the fact that no adequate definition of the term exists, and osteoarthritis occurs in almost all individuals past middle life, as well as in many individuals who are younger, but symptomatic osteoarthritis afflicts only a minority of these. Part of the reason no adequate definition exists derives from the roentgenographic criteria; a narrowing of "joint space" implies loss of cartilage (there is no real space in a joint, only the distance between the bones, composed of cartilage, which is radiolucent unless it contains crystals or metabolic derivatives), but other attributes, such as marginal osteophytes, are part of the repair process, and geodes (cysts in the subchondral bone) may even be part of the pathogenesis. The pathologist's definition includes diminished cartilage, fibrillation of cartilage, cartilaginous debris, the osteophytes and geodes, eburnation (smoothing of exposed bone denuded of its cartilage), and, in many instances, angiogenesis and increased vascularity. The clinician is confronted chiefly by symptomatic osteoarthritis, although roentgenograms taken for any purpose that include diarthrodial joints may disclose joint changes that can delude one into attributing symptoms to these; this is particularly true of spinal changes at the discs and intervertebral neural foramina.

From the standpoint of therapy, only symptomatic osteoarthritis requires treatment, and even much of that remains under dispute. Prevention would obviously be best, if it could be achieved, but in such a slowly developing process as osteoarthritis, it would require a lifetime of effort and may still not be attainable. Osteoarthritis, then, is not a disease but a final common pathway for all insults, overuse, and abuse of a joint, begun by trauma, diseases of metabolism, heritable and genetic predisposition, hormonal influences, and inflammatory diseases of the joints. The initial insult may well have occurred in childhood, but the expression as osteoarthritis takes years to develop (faster when the insult is severe, as in athletic injury, slower if because of repetitive minor trauma, and slower yet if the inception was minimal). When it becomes symptomatic, however, osteoarthritis fits the definition of disease and challenges treatment paradigms.

Osteoarthritis must be viewed as a reparative process, as confirmed by its antiquity: it is found in skeletons of prehistoric animals and early hominids and afflicted all vertebrates that lived long enough. At that, it is not a manifestation of aging, only a slowly developing process that requires time and is, therefore, more common in elderly individuals. Weather changes influence symptoms but not the process itself. There is no particular geographic predilection. Although some patterns are more common in some populations (e.g., interphalangeal osteoarthritis, which, except as a consequence of trauma, is rarely found in Africans and East Asians), that applies chiefly to interphalangeal osteoarthritis in which rows of joints are involved, and not to single large joints. Obesity has been cited as a precursor, a reasonable contention for affliction of weight-bearing joints, but equally true for interphalangeal osteoarthritis, where it should theoretically play no role. Increased bone density seems to parallel osteoarthritis, but whether causal or consequential needs to be determined (similarly, osteoporosis and osteoarthritis tend to be mutually exclusive, but again cause and effect are problematic). Some investigators have looked for causes in the bone. Subchondral microfractures and bone marrow edema have been cited, but again the relationship to expression remains controversial. Box 1 lists some of the known precursors, and Box 2 lists some of the resumed risk factors. Ultimately, osteoarthritis is thought to be a disease of chondrocyte fatigue, accelerated when the weakened chondrocytes can no longer replace proteoglycans, leading to structural alterations. Chondrocalcinosis, with deposition of hydroxy apatite or calcium pyrophosphate dihydrate, commonly accompanies symptomatic osteoarthritis, but may play more of a role in causing symptoms than contributing to pathogenesis. Although some would classify osteoarthritis as primary or secondary, it probably is always secondary, even if the inception is remote in the past and long forgotten. Remember that osteoarthritis is not an acute disease, even if punctuated by

---

BOX 1 Precursors of Osteoarthritis

- Congenital
  Slipped femoral epiphysis
  Legg-Calvé-Perthes disease
- Bone dysplasias
  ? Kashin-Beck disease
  ? Mseleni joint disease
  ? Familial
  Mediterranean fever
- Metabolic
  Ochronosis
  Hemochromatosis
  Calcium pyrophosphate deposition disease
  Gout
- Traumatic
  Acute (e.g., athletic injury)
  Chronic (repetitive trauma)
- Endocrine
  Diabetes mellitus
  Acromegaly
  ? Obesity (cofactor?)
- Idiopathic
  Rheumatoid arthritis
  Septic arthritis disease
  Joint disease
- Vascular
  Avascular necrosis
- Neurologic
  Charcot joint
  Charcot-Marie-Tooth disease
- Bone disease
  Paget's disease (osteitis deformans)

BOX 2   Risk Factors

Aging	Time duration; weak muscle control (lower extremities)
Sex	Women: interphalangeal osteoarthritis, predilection knees in valgus
Obesity	May be cofactor (interphalangeal, knees in women)
Genetics	Symmetric Heberden's nodes, Ehlers-Danlos syndrome, genetic collagen abnormalities
Endocrine	Elevated growth hormone concentrations (postmenopause?)
Diet?	
Bone density	Increased bone density; osteoporosis
Race	Site predilections that may be racially related
Occupation	Jackhammers and similar tools, habitual usage (e.g., specific finger joints in knitting shop workers, elbows in foundry workers, knees in professional football running backs, shoulders in baseball pitchers)
Avocation	Knees and hips in joggers and runners on hard surfaces (not those who continue but those who drop out)
Inflammation	Calcium pyrophosphate dihydrate, hydroxy apatite, other crystal depositions
Trauma	Acute and severe, repetitive but mild to moderate

acute painful episodes in approximately 15% to 20% of those in whom roentgenographic evidence of osteoarthritis exists.

Regional Issues

Patterns differ and give clues to pathogenesis. The knees are more frequently afflicted in women, perhaps because the broader pelvis leads to genu valgum and predisposes to knee afflictions. However, although cartilage loss on the gliding surface of the patella generally results in symptoms, even major cartilage loss in the opposing surfaces of the femur and tibia may not, and the anatomic features fail to correlate with symptomatic expression. Although proprioceptive changes were thought to play a role in the pathogenesis of knee osteoarthritis, recent studies refute this contention.

The hips tend to be more often afflicted in men. The classic FABERE maneuver (flexion, abduction, external rotation, and extension) reveals limitations of motion and elicits pain. However, in time, knee and hip osteoarthritis are nearly gender equal.

Osteoarthritis of the distal interphalangeal (DIP) joints (Heberden's nodes) and proximal interphalangeal joints (PIP), usually symmetric, occurs in white women at about the time of menopause (earlier after total hysterectomies) and implies genetic predisposition; nonsymmetric involvement of these joints is often a consequence of specific traumas or work exposure. The symmetric variety often bares erosive changes at the joint margins, and is accompanied by the traditional signs of inflammation at presentation: redness, heat, swelling, pain, and functional deficits. The joints at the bases of the thumbs (first carpometacarpal, or trapeziometacarpal joints) tend also to be involved, and even the metacarpophalangeal joints, which rarely develop osteoarthritis in other circumstances. In these women, accompanying osteoarthritis at other joints is unrelated to the hereditary familial variety, bearing a casual, not causal, relationship.

The encroachment of osteophytes on the intervertebral foramina in the movable sections of the spine (cervical and lumbar) leads to referred pain in the areas served by the appropriate nerves. The shoulders are rarely a site of osteoarthritis, but sometimes severe destructive changes (the Milwaukee shoulder) do occur. Elbows are generally spared, but "cystic" protrusions through the joint capsules of distended fluid-filled joints lead to antecubital "cysts," the corollaries of the popliteal cysts at the knees; the latter can rupture, simulating thrombophlebitis in the calves. Wrists and ankles are almost always spared, because the mosaic distribution of the small bones diffuses forces. The first metatarsophalangeal joint is subject to osteoarthritis (the bunion) but rarely other joints of the toes (thought to be spared because shoes act as splints).

Although several studies claim that jogging and running do not predispose to osteoarthritis, these studies dealt with individuals who habitually exercised and not with those who gave up exercising, so they may well not conclusively prove the advantages of exercise for the majority of patients.

I have left out the molecular biology, the catalytic enzymes and debris, and even the synovial fluid changes, as these are of greater interest to the investigator than to the clinician responsible for counseling and treating patients. They are giving us some clues to better treatments in the future, however, and a later version of this article might well give them more prominence. Of greatest importance is not necessarily to ascribe symptoms to osteoarthritis detected on imaging; false attributions can delay correct diagnoses and appropriate treatment.

Management

PREVENTION

As osteoarthritis is the culmination of all life events at the joints, it cannot really be prevented. Attempts to use bovine cartilage extracts and other substances failed to retard progression and have been largely abandoned. However, as osteoarthritis is consequent to trauma or inflammation, aggressive treatment of this initial insult might delay its onset years later, but this remains unproven. Attention must be paid to the risk factors (see Box 2), minimizing them as much as possible; weight reduction obviously decreases the load on knee and hip joints in overweight individuals. Keeping joints supple through exercising and not exposing them to shear factors (particularly in sports), jogging on soft surfaces rather than on unyielding pavement, wearing supportive footwear (spike heels may not lead to osteoarthritis per se but can lead to accidents that do, and flat heels put excessive strain on the calf muscles and later the knees), and in general maintaining physical fitness are all helpful. Despite recently published studies that isometric exercises, especially of the quadriceps, probably cannot prevent osteoarthritis of the knees, these apply chiefly to radiographic changes and not to symptoms; it is still wise to recommend exercises that strengthen the muscles that move a joint, because function will be retained even if the anatomic changes continue. Osteoarthritis found on radiographs taken for another purpose, if asymptomatic, requires no treatment; the old dictum, "treat the patient, not the radiograph," applies. Architectural barriers should be avoided; ramps are particularly troublesome for knee and hip osteoarthritis, especially descending (that applies to stairs as well, as descent requires knee extension, which increases joint discomfort).

Symptomatic osteoarthritis occasions discomfort at times of weather changes, but the symptoms are often mild and tolerated. Many people treat themselves for these, before seeing a physician. It is important to know what they may be taking, as they often do not consider these as medicines, and potential drug interactions can occur.

COMPLEMENTARY AND ALTERNATIVE TREATMENTS

Analgesics, such as acetaminophen (Tylenol and other unbranded generics) and aspirin, and several nonsteroidal anti-inflammatory drugs are readily available on supermarket shelves and pharmacies. In these days of global travel and ethnic migrations, other approaches also are common. Ayurvedic medicine is another system, popular in Southeast Asia and spreading from there; its medicines are based on plant extracts. Ayurvedic schools are found in India and the medicines themselves are carefully prepared and tested. The most popular treatment for osteoarthritis is composed of winter cherry, Indian frankincense, turmeric, and ginger (Artrex).

Herbal medicines available chiefly in health food stores have become popular throughout the United States. These are exempted by law from testing and approval by the FDA, and their safety and efficacy remain problematic. Potential interactions with prescribed drugs have not been studied. Ginger is especially popular, but among the other preparations are boron,[1] borage oil,[1] evening primrose oil,[1] and avocado soybean saponifiables,[1] all of which are claimed to be anti-inflammatory.

Yoga is currently being studied as a potential treatment for knee osteoarthritis, and acupuncture is said to provide considerable pain relief. Chiropractic adjustment is popular, especially for back pain attributed to osteoarthritis. However, the placebo effect is very striking in most osteoarthritis; even follow-up telephone calls from the doctor's office inquiring about the health of the patient lead to improvement. Do not slight the placebo effect, though—it is, after all, an effect.

GENERAL PRINCIPLES

A recent symposium on osteoarthritis concluded that osteoarthritis is all about biomechanics, and normalization thereof yields better results than drug therapy (that means splints, braces, canes, shoe corrections, abolition of unsound architectural and style features). Joint damage is not the main determinant of pain, but psychosocial factors,

compensation systems, and inaccurate labeling play a major role. Also, people who have osteoarthritis, because of the long duration of its inception, tend to be elderly and therefore more likely to tolerate drug therapy and surgery poorly, and because many have concurrent problems under treatment, are prone to untoward drug interactions.

As stated, only approximately 15% to 20% of individuals have sufficient pain to seek medical attention. This pain waxes and wanes, and considerable controversy addresses the best approaches to treatment. A much cited study compared acetaminophen 4 g per day with ibuprofen 1200 and 2400 μg a day during a span of 4 weeks, and concluded that there was no difference in results. However, the span is short, and proves only that analgesics are analgesic. Most patients prefer a nonsteroidal anti-inflammatory drug (NSAID), especially in anti-inflammatory dosage, as confirmed in epidemiologic and observational studies. Physical and occupational therapy can help joint-sparing mobility, ergonomic principles help at the work site, and sexual counseling, for those afflicted with hip involvement in particular, should be part of the treatment program.

For inflammatory erosive osteoarthritis of the fingers, the overnight wearing of nylon and spandex stretch gloves can inhibit nodose deformities if started early enough, before these excrescences become bony and function is compromised.

DRUG THERAPY

The severe pain of osteoarthritic joints—knees, hips, and fingers, chiefly—may be the result of secondary inflammation, caused by cartilaginous debris inciting cytokine response. A whole array of nonsteroidal anti-inflammatory drugs is available by prescription (from indomethacin [Indocin] and ibuprofen [Motrin, Advil, generics] through naproxen [Naprosyn] and diclofenac [Voltaren], with doses usually lower than those for rheumatoid arthritis), and others, not available in the United States, may be taken by patients who purchased them abroad (e.g., tiaprofenic acid[2]). These inhibit cyclooxygenase, an enzyme necessary for prostaglandin synthesis that has been found to have at least two components, COX-1, which helps protect against gastric erosion and other consequences, and COX-2, which is evoked by inflammatory mediators and may lead to adverse gastric mucosal effects (a COX-3 has been proposed as well). To avoid the latter complication, misoprostol (Cytotec) may be prescribed or incorporated into a combination formulation with diclofenac (Arthrotec), but that is not without its own complications, namely, diarrhea and cramps. To avoid the adverse effects, a series of selective (at least in recommended dosage) COX-2 inhibitors were developed (e.g., celecoxib [Celebrex, 200 μg per day]). Lumiracoxib (Prexige),[2] 100 to 200 μg per day, was recently approved for short-term relief in osteoarthritis outside the United States. As of this writing, recommended doses may vary, so the package insert should always be consulted to determine the current appropriate dose. Gastric mucosal protection appears to be better, but there are renal consequences associated with its use and other problems are imputed. It must be stated that compounds considered safer are usually given to the patients most at risk, so the profiles do not address

---

[1]Not FDA approved for this indication.

[2]Not available in the United States.

comparable populations. Moreover, the coxib NSAIDs are currently more expensive and not approved by all medical payment plans. Other NSAIDs, such as sulindac (Clinoril) and nabumetone (Relafen), are prodrugs, converted after absorption and hepatic biotransformation. Etodolac (Lodine) seems to work by a different mechanism; nimesulide is popular in Europe under a variety of trade names, but not available in the United States, is more COX-2 selective but less expensive, and may be brought back by travelers. Licofelone (as below) is awaiting approval in Europe. The choice of NSAIDs is relatively arbitrary; patients may respond well to one and not to another. In most instances, the most severe symptoms can be brought to a level patients will tolerate within a few days to weeks, and long-term therapy may not be necessary.

Aspirin, once the mainstay of treatment, has largely been superseded. Gastrointestinal intolerance, irreversible inhibition of platelet aggregation, and animal studies that show it to be deleterious to cartilage may be the reasons, but nonacetylated salicylates, such as salsalate (Disalcid) and choline magnesium trisalicylate (Trilisate), and simple analgesics, such as propoxyphene (Darvon)[1] and tramadol (Ultram), alone or in combination, are given alone or with NSAIDs. Narcotics are best avoided because of the potential for addiction.

Gastric mucosal erosions are found by endoscopy but usually do not translate into clinical problems. Similarly, elevation of hepatic enzymes is noncongruent with hepatotoxicity. Adverse effects on gastric mucosa are the most common; however, liver, kidney, and bone marrow complications, although uncommon, need also to be guarded against.

In most parts of the world, NSAIDs are available in creams and ointments for topical administration. The FDA is not convinced that this is more than a placebo effect so these formulations are not currently available in the United States. However, topical capsaicin, the spice in pepper plants, has been approved for use in osteoarthritis and is available under a number of trade names over the counter (a prescription no longer is necessary). During the initial period of administration, localized burning is usual. Capsaicin is also available on a patch, which is especially popular in Asia.

INTRA-ARTICULAR THERAPY

For nearly 50 years, cortisol derivatives have been injected into joints, usually after removal of the excess synovial fluid through arthrocentesis. When even symptomatic osteoarthritis was deemed not to be inflammatory, many clinicians cautioned that the resultant lack of pain indicated an insensitivity that could lead to further joint destruction, similar to the neuropathic Charcot joint. This fear has not been borne out and now arthrocentesis and corticosteroid instillation, preferably of a depot compound, in appropriately calibrated dosage, depending on the size of the joint, can effect long-lasting relief. However, patients should be admonished not to overuse the joint, at least for the first 3 days, as the lesions have not healed, even if the symptoms have abated. A general rule for counseling: do no more than when it hurt.

On the assumption that lubrication of the joint is impaired and corticosteroids are strictly palliative, preparations of hyaluronate have been approved for intra-articular instillation. While this procedure is called viscosupplementation, there is as yet little evidence that the instilled material is long retained in the joint or that it improves lubrication. Nevertheless, the results usually are as good as those with corticosteroids, and the duration of effect often long-lasting. The two preparations currently available are sodium hyaluronate (Hyalgan) and hylan G-F 20 (Synvisc), administered as a short series of three to five weekly injections; why they should work is problematic, and some controlled trials concluded that they were no more effective than placebo. This has been claimed for many preparations, however, because the placebo effect on pain is quite potent. Functional impairment remains, in most instances, especially at the hip, but often also at the knee. Hyaluronic acid is not indicated for interphalangeal injection, although small doses of corticosteroid into these tiny joints can sometimes lead to dramatic relief.

GLUCOSAMINE AND CHONDROITIN SULFATE

Oral glucosamine[1] is said to be as analgesic as NSAIDs and acetaminophen. Multicenter controlled trials seem to agree, but there is still much skepticism about this treatment. There is no rationale to explain why it should be analgesic, but all studies show glucosamine to be superior to placebo or reference compounds, even if not statistically in all cases. It appears to be harmless, with no untoward interactions, and the hypothesis that it might aggravate diabetes mellitus has not been borne out. Most preparations are available over the counter. The likelihood exists that any patient with symptomatic osteoarthritis is taking glucosamine, and so are many rheumatologists, empirically trusting that it has a salutary effect. Chondroitin sulfate[1] has not been shown to add anything, except in some poorly designed studies. However, the combination of glucosamine and chondroitin sulfate is marketed more frequently than either compound alone, and whole shelves in markets and pharmacies are devoted to these.

DISEASE MODIFICATION

By the time osteoarthritis becomes symptomatic and fulfills roentgenographic criteria, it is already well established. Thus, it is too late to think of "disease modification," as is now possible in rheumatoid arthritis. Nevertheless, the search for disease-modifying osteoarthritis drugs (DMOADs) goes on. All the compounds cited as possible DMOADs have been tested in animals only; no satisfactory assessment exists for studies in humans. Tetracycline derivatives, such as doxycycline,[1] seem to have merit. Drugs that work on the inner mechanisms of cells, such as chloroquine (Aralen),[1] are also under study on theoretical grounds, but have not yet proved themselves. Antioxidant vitamins, tamoxifen (Nolvadex),[1] nitric oxide inhibitors, metalloproteases, and the aforementioned nutraceuticals have all been mentioned, but no reliable protocol exists that can measure their effect on cartilage and the joint. Specialized radiography that requires positioning is too crude for the purpose; magnetic resonance imaging

---

[1]Not FDA approved for this indication.

[1]Not FDA approved for this indication.

and ultrasound have yet to be validated and standardized for this condition.

Studies are currently underway in Europe of diacerein (Diadar)[2] and growth factors, including insulin-like growth factor β, somatomedins, fibroblast growth factor, chondrocyte growth factor, and cartilage-derived and transforming growth factors. The problem of what to study and what outcome measures to use, and the duration of the trial, also bedevil these studies. While it is true that these are experimental treatments, not currently in use, and may never come to pass, they are mentioned here to counter the argument that the neurologist diagnoses untreatable disease and the rheumatologist treats untreatable disease. If not these, other treatments deriving from our better understanding of arthritis and its pathogenesis surely are in the offing. Included among these are mesenchymal stem cells that can produce site-specific tissue, thus restoring lost cartilage and bone, but how can that be done while mechanical impediments remain? The same is true for gene manipulation, and if new cartilage and bone are created, even with no counterpressures, how will the new attach to the older remnants and what will determine that? Cartilage transplants and chondrocyte transfer and stimulation are also being investigated. A polymer of glucosamine is also available (POLY-Nag).

SURGERY

Surgery is the consequence of failure of medicine. Our inability to effect healing and repair leads to treatments that would be forestalled if we could anticipate who, and under what circumstances, develops symptomatic disease and offer appropriate medical treatments. Barring that, the surgical treatment of osteoarthritis has made remarkable progress during the past 40 years. By and large, the osteotomies that were formerly performed have faded into well-deserved oblivion. Arthroscopy was hailed as a less invasive way to deal with motion-impeding osteophytes and derangements and meniscal tears, especially if combined with lavage, but the results do not materially differ from those achieved with placebos. Indeed, removal of the meniscus seems to hasten the development of the ultimate osteoarthritic lesion. The major advance was the total joint replacement, first for hips, then knees and even fingers and other small joints of the hands. These have given back life content and quality of life to myriad recipients, more than 100,000 people annually in the United States alone! While surgery is clearly not a last resort, it has successfully addressed the functional deficits and pains and permitted recipients to resume their life styles. Shut-ins are liberated. Despite the trepidation of orthopedists, travel, skiing, tennis, and golf become achievable, even with bilateral surgery. Newer materials and methods of bonding have improved the longevity of these interventions.

Osteoarthritis remains an enigma, despite the major scientific advances of the past few years. Paradoxically, we have become more effective in treating advanced osteoarthritis and symptomatic disease (because of our better understanding of inflammation and the recognition that it plays a major role in evoking symptoms) than in addressing the variety of presentations. Symptomatic relief

---

[2]Not available in the United States.

is achievable, and restoration of function; roentgenographic and pathologic changes may fulfill the definition but do not necessarily demand treatment. The removal of infectious and other killer diseases that curtailed life expectancy in the past has paradoxically resulted in the emergence of more chronic disorders. As stated in the World Health Organization's catalogue of disabilities, the killer diseases remove the consumer shortly after the consumer ceases to be a producer; the crippling diseases leave the consumer long after the consumer ceases to be a producer. The expense and increased suffering require a humane and scientifically sound understanding.

Giant Cell Arteritis and Polymyalgia Rheumatica

Method of
John H. Stone, MD, MPH

Giant cell arteritis (GCA), the most common form of primary systemic vasculitis in adults, preferentially affects the extracranial branches of the carotid artery and also often involves the aorta and its primary branches. Polymyalgia rheumatica (PMR), an aching and stiffness of the shoulders, neck, and hip-girdle area, occurs in up to 50% of GCA cases but usually occurs alone. Age is the greatest risk factor for either GCA or PMR; essentially all patients with these conditions are older than 50 years of age. The mean age at disease onset is 72 years. PMR occurs two to four times more often than GCA. Both GCA and PMR have a predilection for individuals of northern European ancestry and occur three to four times more frequently in women than in men.

Diagnosis

The classic presenting manifestations of GCA are PMR symptoms, headache, jaw claudication, and visual disturbances (Table 1). The onset may be gradual or sudden. PMR symptoms are characterized by pain and stiffness in the neck, shoulders, and hip-girdle area that is usually much worse in the morning. Patients with PMR may report great difficulty getting out of bed, raising their arms over their heads, or rising from the commode. The most striking feature of the headache is that it is new or different from other headache patterns. Many patients describe tenderness of the scalp when brushing their hair. Some localize the tenderness to the temporal arteries, but these are enlarged or nodular in only a minority of patients. Jaw claudication—pain in the master muscles that occurs with chewing—has the highest specificity of any GCA symptom.

Approximately one third of patients present with visual symptoms, chiefly amaurosis fugax or diplopia. Blindness, which can develop abruptly, is usually preceded by episodes of blurred vision or amaurosis fugax. Visual loss results most often from infarction of the posterior ciliary artery, which supplies blood to the optic nerve head. Both eyes

TABLE 1 Likelihood Ratios for Symptoms and Signs Among Patients with Suspected GCA

Symptom/Sign	Likelihood Ratio*
Symptoms	
Anorexia	1.2
Weight loss	1.3
Arthralgia	1.1
Diplopia	3.4
Fatigue	1.2
Fever	1.2
Temporal headache	1.5
Any headache	1.2
Jaw claudication	4.2
Myalgia	0.9
Polymyalgia rheumatica	1.0
Unilateral visual loss	0.9
Any visual symptoms	1.1
Vertigo	0.7
Signs	
Optic atrophy or ischemic optic neuropathy	1.6
Scalp tenderness	1.6
Synovitis	0.4
Beaded temporal artery	4.6
Prominent/enlarged temporal artery	4.3
Tender temporal artery	2.6
Absent temporal artery pulse	2.7

*Likelihood ratio is the probability of a positive temporal artery biopsy in a patient with a certain symptom or sign, compared to the probability of a positive biopsy in a patient without that same finding.
From Seo P, Stone JH: Large-vessel vasculitis. Arthritis Rheum 2004;51(1): 128-139.

may be affected, sometimes in close temporal succession. Almost all patients with classic GCA features also have nonspecific manifestations such as malaise, fatigue, and anorexia. Weight loss of 2 to 10 kg is common.

Clinically overt involvement of large arteries—the aorta and its major branches—develops in at least 15% of the patients. The most commonly affected vessels include the aorta (often involving the proximal aorta, leading to valvular incompetence) and the vertebral, carotid, subclavian, and axillary arteries. Aortic involvement may lead to thoracic aortic aneurysm, the risk of which is increased 17-fold in GCA patients. Aortic aneurysm is usually a late complication of GCA, developing on average 7 years after diagnosis of the vasculitis. Abdominal aortic aneurysms, while less common, also occur in GCA.

The most common physical finding is an abnormal temporal artery, found in up to two thirds of patients. The temporal artery may be enlarged, tender, nodular, or found to have decreased pulsation. Normal temporal arteries do not exclude the diagnosis, however. Approximately 10% to 15% of patients will have axillary or subclavian disease revealed by diminished pulses, unequal arm blood pressures, or by bruits heard above or below the clavicle or along the upper arm.

The laboratory hallmarks of GCA and PMR are marked elevations of the acute phase reactants, the erythrocyte sedimentation rate (ESR), and C-reactive protein. Nearly 90% of patients with GCA present with an ESR greater than 50 mm/hour. Normochromic, normocytic anemia and thrombocytosis are also common. Approximately 20% of patients with GCA demonstrate a mildly elevated alkaline phosphatase (of liver origin). Radiologic studies such as magnetic resonance imaging (MRI) and ultrasound (US) may reveal abnormalities compatible with PMR or GCA, but the clinical uses of these tests are unclear. Neither replaces temporal artery biopsy as the gold standard for the diagnosis of GCA. Guidelines for making the diagnosis of PMR and classifying patients with GCA have been developed. The diagnosis of PMR rests almost entirely on clinical grounds, namely symptoms of proximal limb stiffness associated with an elevated ESR and a dramatic response to prednisone.[1] Classification criteria for GCA are designed for use in the research setting, not for use as diagnostic criteria per se.

Treatment

Any patient strongly suspected of having GCA should be started on 40 to 60 mg of prednisone[1] per day and referred for temporal artery biopsy. Temporal artery biopsy, the only test that can secure the diagnosis of GCA, is recommended in all cases. Although it is traditional to obtain the temporal artery biopsy quickly, evidence suggests that the pathology remains intact for at least 2 weeks after the start of corticosteroid treatment. Unilateral and bilateral temporal artery biopsies are approximately 90% and 95% sensitive, respectively, at least when performed by experts in the procedure. In any setting, some patients whose histories are compelling for the diagnosis of GCA will have negative biopsies.

Patients suspected of having GCA who have experienced transient visual loss should receive high-dose intravenous methylprednisolone[1] (e.g., 1000 mg/day) for 3 days. Low-dose aspirin[1] (81 or 325 mg/day) is also prudent in patients with GCA. Patients with PMR alone are treated usually with prednisone,[1] 10 to 20 mg per day. Patients with PMR or GCA usually respond dramatically to corticosteroid treatment within 2 days or earlier. Approximately 10% of patients, however, require a week of therapy before feeling better.

Prednisone[1] tapers usually begin after 1 month. The overall goal of the prednisone taper is to discontinue the medication within 9 to 12 months. Because of the substantial toxicities of corticosteroids, one reasonable approach is to taper prednisone[1] more quickly at higher doses than at lower doses, aiming to reach 20 mg per day by 2 or 3 months after the start of treatment. Once patients with GCA reach 15 mg of prednisone[1] or PMR patients reach 10 mg, decrements of 1 mg about every 2 weeks may reduce the chance of flare. Mild to moderate ESR elevations, common during corticosteroid tapers, should not necessarily trigger increases in the prednisone[1] dose. Rather, increases in prednisone[1] should be dictated by the recurrence of clinical symptoms.

Unfortunately, 50% to 80% of patients with PMR or GCA relapse during or after the prednisone[1] taper. (Relapses at prednisone[1] doses higher than 15 mg/day

[1]Not FDA approved for this indication.

CURRENT DIAGNOSIS

Simple Diagnostic Criteria for Polymyalgia Rheumatica

- Age at onset is older than 50 years of age
- Symmetric ache/pain for at least 1 month in two of three muscle groups below, associated with morning stiffness lasting longer than 30 minutes:
  Neck or torso
  Shoulders or proximal arms
  Hips or proximal thighs
  ESR more than 40 mm per hour (Westergren method)
  Prompt, dramatic response to glucocorticoids (equivalent to prednisone[1] 20 mg once per day or less)

Criteria for the Diagnosis of Giant Cell Arteritis

- Age older than 50 years at disease onset
- New headache
- Temporal artery abnormality
- Temporal artery tenderness to palpation or decreased pulsation unrelated to arteriosclerosis of cervical arteries
- Elevated erythrocyte sedimentation rate more than 50 mm per hour
- Abnormal temporal artery biopsy
- Biopsy specimen with vasculitis characterized by a predominance of mononuclear cell infiltration or granulomatous inflammation, usually with multinucleated giant cells
- For classification purposes, a patient with vasculitis shall be said to have GCA if at least three of these seven criteria are present. The presence of any three or more criteria yields a sensitivity of 93.5% and a specificity of 91.2%.

[1]Not FDA approved for this indication.
Abbreviations: GCA = giant cell arteritis; ESR = erythrocyte sedimentation rate.
From Hunder GG, Bloch DA, Michel BA, et al: The American College of Rheumatology 1990 criteria for the classification of giant cell arteritis. Arthritis Rheum 1990;33:1122-1128.

CURRENT THERAPY

- No treatment other than glucocorticoids has been shown convincingly to be effective in either GCA or PMR.
- A majority of patients flare within 1 year as glucocorticoid doses are tapered.
- An appropriate strategy is to taper patients to low doses (<10 mg of prednisone/day) within several months and then to maintain 5 mg of prednisone/day for approximately 1 year. Ultimately prednisone should be tapered at the rate of only 1 mg/month.
- The usual starting dose of prednisone in GCA is 60 mg per day. The usual starting dose in PMR is 15 mg per day.

Abbreviations: GCA = giant cell arteritis; PMR = polymyalgia rheumatica.

are rare.) Patients who experience recurrent symptoms usually respond to increasing the prednisone[1] dose 5 to 10 mg above the last dose at which the patient was asymptomatic. A substantial minority of patients require some prednisone[1]—usually in the range of 5 to 10 mg per day—for longer than 2 years. No corticosteroid-sparing agent has been proven consistently effective. Reports of the efficacy of methotrexate[1] in both PMR and GCA have been conflicting. Controlled studies of tumor necrosis factor-α inhibitors[1] are not yet available.

To prevent osteoporosis, patients starting on prednisone[1] should take 1500 to 1800 mg of calcium daily with 400 to 800 units of vitamin D. If bone density measurements indicate osteopenia or osteoporosis, bisphosphonates are usually the first-line agents for treatment.

REFERENCES

Caporali R, Cimmino MA, Ferraccioli G, et al: Methotrexate plus prednisone combined therapy in polymyalgia rheumatica. Ann Intern Med 2004;141(7):493-500.

Hoffman GS, Cid MC, Hellmann DB, et al: A multicenter, randomized, double-blind, placebo-controlled trial of adjuvant methotrexate treatment for giant cell arteritis. Arthritis Rheum 2002;46(5):1309-1318.

Hoffman GS, Stone JH. Disparate results in studies of methotrexate plus corticosteroids in the treatment of giant cell arteritis. Arthritis Rheum 2003;48(4):1160-1161.

Jover JA, Hernandez-Garcia C, Morado IC, et al: Combined treatment of giant cell arteritis with methotrexate and prednisone. A randomized, double-blind, placebo-controlled trial. Ann Intern Med 2001;134:106-14.

Salvarani C, Cantini F, Boiardi L, et al: Medical progress: Polymyalgia rheumatica and giant-cell arteritis. N Engl J Med 2002;347:261-271.

Seo P, Stone JH: Large-vessel vasculitis. Arthritis Rheum 2004;51(1):128-139.

Smetana GW, Shmerling RH: Does this patient have temporal arteritis? JAMA 2002;287:92-101.

Stone JH: Methotrexate in polymyalgia rheumatica: Kernel of truth or curse of Tantalus? Ann Intern Med 2004;141(7):568-569.

[1]Not FDA approved for this indication.

Osteomyelitis

Method of
Luca Lazzarini, MD

Osteomyelitis is a complex disease often associated with high morbidity and considerable health care costs. This condition can be classified by duration (acute or chronic), pathogenesis (hematogenous or contiguous spread), site, extent, and by the type of patient (infant, child, adult, or compromised host). The Waldvogel classification system subdivides osteomyelitis as being either hematogenous or secondary to a contiguous focus of infection. Contiguous focus osteomyelitis has been further subdivided into osteomyelitis with or without vascular insufficiency. An alternative to the Waldvogel classification system has been developed by Cierny and Mader. The Cierny-Mader staging system is based on the anatomy of the bone infection and the physiology of the host (Box 1). The anatomic types

TABLE 1 Principal Antibiotics Used in the Initial Intravenous Treatment of Osteomyelitis

Staphylococci, methicillin sensitive	Nafcillin (Unipen) 2 g q4-6h (+ rifampin[Rifadin][1] 600 mg qd PO)
Staphylococci, methicillin resistant	Vancomycin (Vancocin) 1 g q12h (+ rifampin [Rifadin][1] 600 mg qd PO)
Streptococci	Penicillin[1] 2 MU q4h
Anaerobes, gram-positive	Clindamycin[1] (Cleocin) 900 mg q8h
Anaerobes, gram-negative	Metronidazole[1] (Flagyl) 500 mg q8h
Enterobacteriaceae, *Pseudomonas*	Ciprofloxacin (Cipro) 400 mg q12h

[1]Not FDA approved for this indication.
Abbreviations: PO = orally; q = every; qd = every day.

Staphylococcus aureus, *Streptococcus agalactiae*, and *Escherichia coli* are most frequently isolated from blood or bones. However, in children more than 1 year of age, *S. aureus*, *Streptococcus pyogenes*, and *Haemophilus influenzae* are most commonly isolated. The incidence of *H. influenzae* infection decreases after age 4 years. However, the overall incidence of *H. influenzae* as a cause of osteomyelitis is decreasing because of the new *H. influenzae* vaccine now given to children. In adults, *S. aureus* is the most common organism isolated. Multiple organisms are usually isolated from the infected bone in contiguous focus osteomyelitis. *S. aureus* remains the most commonly isolated pathogen. However, gram-negative bacilli and anaerobic organisms are also frequently isolated. Other microorganisms, such as mycobacteria and fungi, can be involved as well.

Clinical Manifestations

SIGNS AND SYMPTOMS

Hematogenous osteomyelitis in children may present with acute signs of infection including abrupt fever, irritability, lethargy, and local signs of inflammation. However, 50% of children present with vague complaints, including pain of the involved limb of 1 to 3 months in duration and minimal, if any, temperature elevation.

Adults with hematogenous osteomyelitis usually present with vague complaints consisting of nonspecific pain and few constitutional symptoms lasting 1 to 3 months. However, acute clinical presentations with fever, chills, swelling, and erythema over the involved bone(s) are occasionally seen. The source of bacteremia may be from a trivial skin infection or from a more serious infection such as acute or subacute bacterial endocarditis. Hematogenous osteomyelitis that involves either long bones or vertebrae is an important complication of injection drug abuse.

Patients with contiguous focus osteomyelitis often present with localized bone and joint pain, erythema, swelling, and drainage around the area of trauma, surgery,

of osteomyelitis are medullary (stage 1), superficial (stage 2), localized (stage 3), and diffuse (stage 4). Stage 1 infection is confined to the medullary surface of the bone. Hematogenous osteomyelitis and infected intramedullary rods are examples of this anatomic type. Stage 2 is a contiguous focus infection occurring when an exposed infected necrotic surface of bone lies at the base of a soft tissue wound. Stage 3 is usually characterized by a full-thickness, cortical sequestration that can be removed surgically without compromising bony stability. Stage 4 is a through-and-through process that usually requires an intercalary resection of the bone to arrest the disease process. Further, the patient is classified as an A, B, or C host. An A host represents a patient with normal physiologic, metabolic, and immunologic capabilities. The B host is either systemically compromised, locally compromised, or both. When the morbidity of treatment is worse than that imposed by the disease itself, the patient is given the C host classification. This classification system aids in the understanding, diagnosis, and treatment of bone infections in children and adults (Table 1).

Etiology

In hematogenous osteomyelitis, a single pathogenic organism is almost always recovered from the bone. In infants or wound infection. Signs of bacteremia such as fever, chills, and night sweats may be present in the acute phase of osteomyelitis, but not in the chronic phase.

The sedimentation rate is usually elevated, reflecting chronic inflammation, but the leukocyte count is usually normal. The chronic disease is usually either not progressive or slowly progressive. If a sinus tract becomes obstructed, the patient may present with a localized abscess and or an acute soft tissue infection. A sedimentation rate that returns to normal during the course of therapy is a favorable prognostic sign.

MICROBIOLOGY

The diagnosis and determination of the etiology of long bone osteomyelitis rests on the isolation of the pathogen(s) from the bone lesion or blood or joint culture. Except in hematogenous osteomyelitis, where positive blood or joint fluid cultures may suffice, antibiotic treatment of osteomyelitis should be based on meticulous cultures of bone taken at débridement surgery or from deep bone biopsies. If possible, cultures should be obtained before antibiotics are initiated. Sinus tract cultures are unreliable for predicting which organisms will be isolated from infected bone; however, those growing *S. aureus* show a positive correlation with bone cultures.

RADIOLOGY

In hematogenous osteomyelitis, radiographic changes usually correlate with the destructive process and are usually seen when at least 50% to 75% of the bone matrix is destroyed. This happens at least 2 weeks after the infection was initiated. The earliest radiologic changes are swelling of the soft tissue, periosteal thickening and/or elevation, and focal osteopenia. Radiographic improvement may lag behind clinical recovery, even when the patient is receiving appropriate antimicrobial therapy. In contiguous focus osteomyelitis, the radiographic changes are subtle, often found in association with other nonspecific radiographic findings, and require a careful clinical correlation to achieve diagnostic significance. Computed tomography (CT) may play a role in the diagnosis of osteomyelitis. Increased marrow density occurs early in the infection, and intramedullary gas has been reported in patients with hematogenous osteomyelitis. The CT scan can also help identify areas of necrotic bone and assess the involvement of the surrounding soft tissues. One disadvantage of this study is the scatter phenomenon, which occurs when metal is present in or near the area of bone infection. Magnetic resonance imaging (MRI) has been recognized as a useful modality for diagnosing the presence and scope of musculoskeletal infection. The resolution of MRI makes it useful in differentiating between bone and soft tissue infection, often a problem with radionuclide studies. Radionuclide scans may be obtained when the diagnosis of osteomyelitis is ambiguous or to help gauge the extent of bone and soft tissue inflammation.

Treatment

Therapy of osteomyelitis is both surgical and medical and includes adequate drainage and débridement, obliteration of dead space, soft tissue coverage, and specific antimicrobial treatment. If the patient is a compromised host, an effort is made to correct or improve the host defect.

ANTIBIOTIC TREATMENT

According to the results of animal studies, the optimal duration of antibiotic treatment is 4 to 6 weeks. The time needed for bone revascularization after débridement surgery is approximately 3 weeks. Shorter durations are probably successful when the infection is superficial (stage 2) and a complete débridement is performed and when ablative surgery (amputation above the infected region) is performed.

Antibiotic treatment for osteomyelitis is traditionally administered by the intravenous (IV) route. To reduce hospitalization and health care costs, outpatient IV therapy is currently used. This modality of administration reduces treatment cost and improves patient quality of life.

Antistaphylococcal penicillins (nafcillin [Unipen],[1] oxacillin [Prostaphlin][1]) are used for the treatment of methicillin-sensitive staphylococcal osteomyelitis. A first-generation cephalosporin, cefazolin (Ancef), is effective in the treatment of staphylococcal osteomyelitis. The glycopeptides vancomycin (Vancocin)[1] and the oxazolidinone antibiotic linezolid (Zyvox)[1] are used to treat methicillin-resistant staphylococcal osteomyelitis. Several third- and forth-generation cephalosporins, such as cefotaxime (Claforan)[1] or cefepime (Maxipime)[1] can be used to treat osteomyelitis because of gram-negative bacilli.

Oral antibiotics have also been successfully used to treat osteomyelitis. Several oral drugs, such as clindamycin (Cleocin),[1] rifampin (Rifadin),[1] cotrimoxazole (Bactrim),[1] and fluoroquinolones (e.g., ciprofloxacin [Cipro] and levofloxacin [Levaquin][1]) are currently used in the treatment of osteomyelitis. Clindamycin (Cleocin), a lincosamide antibiotic active against most gram-positive bacteria, possesses an excellent bioavailability and is currently used orally, after an initial IV treatment of 2 weeks. Oral therapy using quinolones for gram-negative organisms is used in adult patients with osteomyelitis. The current quinolones have variable *S. aureus* and *Staphylococcus epidermidis* coverage. Pediatric patients should not be given the quinolone class of antibiotics because of possible damage to cartilage.

The initial treatment of most cases of osteomyelitis usually starts on an empirical basis. After cultures are obtained, a parenteral antimicrobial regimen is begun, covering the clinically suspected pathogens. Once the organism is identified, different antibiotics can be selected by appropriate sensitivity methods. If possible, antibiotics should not be initiated until the results of the bone bacterial culture and sensitivities are known.

ANTIBIOTIC TREATMENT BY CIERNY-MADER STAGE

Stage 1 osteomyelitis in children usually responds to antibiotics alone. Stage 1 osteomyelitis in adults is more refractory to therapy and is usually treated with antibiotics and surgery. The patient is treated for 4 to 6 weeks with appropriate antimicrobial therapy, dated from the initiation of

---

[1]Not FDA approved for this indication.

therapy or after the last major débridement surgery. If after 48 hours there is no clinical improvement, surgical treatment may be needed in conjunction with another 4-week course of antibiotics.

In stage 2 osteomyelitis shorter courses of antibiotics, such as 2 weeks, are usually given. In stages 3 and 4 osteomyelitis the patient is treated with 4 to 6 weeks of antimicrobial therapy dated from the last major débridement surgery. This long treatment is needed because even when all necrotic tissue has been adequately débrided, the remaining bed of tissue must be considered contaminated with the responsible pathogen(s).

SUPPRESSIVE ANTIBIOTIC THERAPY

When surgical treatment of osteomyelitis is not feasible, a long-term antibiotic therapy is usually given to control the disease and to prevent flare-ups. Oral antibiotics are usually used. Suppressive therapy has been studied extensively in the setting of infected orthopedic implants. The efficacy of suppressive treatment in osteomyelitis without implants has not been determined. Suppressive therapy is usually administered for 6 months. If recurrence of the infection occurs after discontinuation, a new, culture-directed suppressive regimen is begun and administered indefinitely.

SURGICAL TREATMENT

Surgical treatment of osteomyelitis includes adequate drainage, extensive débridement of all necrotic tissue, obliteration of dead spaces, adequate soft tissue coverage, and restoration of an effective blood supply.

Adequate débridement may leave a large bony defect termed *dead space*. The goal of dead space management is to replace dead bone and scar tissue with vascularized tissue. Local tissue flaps or free flaps may be used to fill dead space. An alternative technique is to place cancellous bone grafts beneath local or transferred tissues where structural augmentation is necessary. Antibiotic-impregnated acrylic beads may be used to sterilize and temporarily maintain dead space. The beads are usually removed within 2 to 4 weeks and replaced with a cancellous bone graft. The most commonly used antibiotics in beads are vancomycin (Vancocin),[1] tobramycin,[1] and gentamicin.[1] Because beads act as a biomaterial surface to which bacteria adhere, infection associated with the use of beads has been described.

---

[1]Not FDA approved for this indication.

CURRENT DIAGNOSIS

- Clinical signs
- Plain radiographs
- CT, NMR, and bone scans obtained in selected cases
- Cultures from sinus tract are unreliable
- Perform bone biopsy for culture and histology whenever possible

Abbreviations: CT = computed tomography; NMR = nuclear magnetic resonance.

CURRENT THERAPY

- Stabilization (if needed) and surgical débridement
- Antibiotic treatment of 4 to 6 weeks after surgical débridement
- Select antimicrobial according to in vitro sensitivity tests; consider toxicity, allergy, costs
- Antibiotic suppressive therapy in selected cases

If movement is present at the site of infection, measures must be taken to achieve permanent stability of the skeletal unit. Stability may be achieved with plates, screws, rods, and/or an external fixator. External fixation is preferred more than internal fixation because of the tendency of medullary rods to become secondarily infected and to spread the extent of the infection. The Ilizarov fixator is a type of external fixator that allows reconstruction of segmental bone defects and difficult infected nonunions. The technique is used for difficult cases of osteomyelitis when stabilization and bone lengthening is necessary.

Adequate soft tissue coverage of the bone is often necessary to arrest osteomyelitis. Small soft tissue defects may be covered with a split thickness skin graft. In the presence of a large soft tissue defect or with an inadequate soft tissue envelope, local muscle flaps and free vascularized muscle flaps may be placed in a one- or two-stage procedure. Local muscle flaps and free vascularized muscle transfers improve the local biologic environment by bringing in a blood supply important in host defense mechanisms, antibiotic delivery, and osseous and soft tissue healing.

REFERENCES

Cierny G, Mader JT, Pennick JJ: A clinical staging system for adult osteomyelitis. Contemp Orthop 1985;10:17-37.

Lew DP, Waldvogel FA: Osteomyelitis. Lancet 2004;364:369-379.

Shuford JA, Steckelberg JM: Role of oral antimicrobial therapy in the management of osteomyelitis. Curr Opin Infect Dis 2003;16:515-519.

Simpson AH, Deakin M, Latham JM: Chronic osteomyelitis. The effect of the extent of surgical resection on infection-free survival. J Bone Joint Surg Br 2001;83:403-407.

Common Sports Injuries

Method of
Julie J. Chuan, MD,
and Kenneth S. Taylor, MD

Sports-related injuries are commonly evaluated and treated in a physician's office. Injuries can be from acute trauma, such as a fracture or burner/stinger (see definition later), or repetitive stress, such as patellofemoral syndrome. To manage all of these injuries, the provider needs to do a focused evaluation to make the diagnosis and decide on a plan for treatment. Treatment should include rehabilitation, injury prevention, and safe return to play.

Evaluation, Diagnosis, and Treatment

When evaluating any patient with a sports injury, the date of injury and chronicity of symptoms should be determined. The mechanism of injury for all acute injuries, including when, how, and what happened after the injury, should be established. A head injury with persistent headache sustained a week ago is much more concerning for a serious concussion than one sustained an hour ago. If the patient says he or she sustained a twisting knee injury and recalls a pop followed by immediate swelling and was able to walk, an anterior cruciate ligament (ACL) injury is likely. Finally, knowing what happens after the injury can be useful. For example, weight bearing after an ankle injury makes a significant fracture much less likely.

If the injury is more chronic, a history of the sport must be obtained, including change in level or type of activity. The level of activity is important to gauge overuse injuries, including frequency, duration, and intensity. Distance runners with shin pain after increasing their distance is concerning for a stress reaction or fracture. Learning about the type of activity and evaluating for proper biomechanics can often help lead to the diagnosis. Any swimmer who complains of shoulder pain with overhead activity who recently changed from breaststroke to a freestyle stroke likely has some subacromial impingement. This is also important in rehabilitation, which should focus on correcting the biomechanics to prevent reinjury.

After the history, a focused examination of the injury, including palpation, range of motion, and neurovascular status, should be documented. Plain radiographs are useful to assess for fractures and bony alignment. Magnetic resonance imaging (MRI) is helpful to visualize soft tissues and often performed if a diagnosis is in question.

Treatment should include acute injury management, rehabilitation, and return to play. Acute injuries often respond well to rest, ice, compression, elevation, and protection/immobilization, as indicated. If pain cannot be controlled with this alone, non-narcotic analgesics can be used acutely for comfort. Rehabilitation should start as soon as the injury is stable and pain is controlled. It can range from a home exercise program to formal physical therapy. Home exercise programs can be more convenient for the patient and are most appropriate for motivated people who understand how to do the exercises properly. Physical therapists incorporate modalities such as ultrasound (phonophoresis) and electrical stimulation (iontophoresis), and they provide controlled, supervised stretching and strengthening programs that can be individualized for each patient. Finally, the decision to return to play should be addressed and be made when the injury has had adequate time to heal and rehabilitate and the patient understands how to prevent reinjury.

Specific Injuries

HEAD AND NECK INJURIES

Concussions

Concussions are traumatic brain injuries that can occur with any sport and they range in severity. Initial evaluation should include neurologic and physical examinations. Obtaining a history from the patient to assess for post-traumatic amnesia, level of awareness, concentration, and confusion, as well as history of prior concussions, can help determine the severity of injury. Friends and witnesses can be helpful to confirm the history and verify if any loss of consciousness occurred. Concussion symptoms can include but are not limited to headache, dizziness, mood lability, loss of concentration, fatigue, nausea, and vision changes. The physical examination should include pupillary response, coordination, gait, balance, and cranial nerve and strength testing. If there was minimal or no loss of consciousness and the patient is asymptomatic with a normal examination within 15 minutes after injury, the injury is mild. In the patient with prolonged loss of consciousness (more than 1 minute), prolonged or progressive symptoms (hours to days), abnormal physical examination, or severe amnesia, imaging should be strongly considered to look for more severe injury such as an intracranial bleed. Return to play should be determined based on the extent of injury and duration of symptom-free days from injury.

Burners and Stingers

Burners and stingers are neck injuries caused by brachial plexus traction or compression. They are common in contact sports, up to 38% in one study of 190 sports injuries. They are acute injuries usually sustained by one of three mechanisms:

1. Lateral flexion force distracting the head and neck away from the shoulder of the affected side
2. Compression injury with neck and head flexion toward the affected side
3. Direct blow to the supraclavicular region

This results in numbness, tingling, or burning down the arm into the hand, usually in the C5 or C6 distribution. Minor injuries resolve within minutes, but more severe injuries involving weakness can last hours to weeks. Athletes often do not seek treatment because symptoms resolve within a few minutes in more than 90% of injuries. If patients do complain of symptoms, evaluation should include a neck examination with palpation and range of motion, shoulder examination, and upper extremity neurologic examination. If more than one extremity is involved, the patient should be immobilized and radiographs obtained to exclude cervical spine injury. Electromyelograms (EMGs) are useful for evaluating severe injuries but may take up to 3 weeks after injury to become abnormal. Burners or stingers involving weakness for more than 72 hours have an abnormal EMG at 4 weeks. Prolonged injury can be treated with physical therapy for range of motion and strengthening. Natural history is not been well studied because permanent neurologic symptoms are rare. Return to play should not be considered until the athlete is asymptomatic with neck and shoulder range of motion and has a normal neurologic examination, including symmetric strength testing.

SHOULDER INJURIES

Acromioclavicular Separation

Shoulder pain can be from injury to the acromioclavicular (AC) joint or the glenohumeral joint. Acromioclavicular joint separations occur from a direct blow to the shoulder, an axial load from the elbow, or an axial load with an extended arm. The trauma is acute and results in swelling, bruising, pain at the AC joint, and occasionally deformity. A focused neurovascular examination should be performed because the brachial plexus is at risk of injury. Shoulder radiographs should be obtained including a true anterior-posterior, 10- to 15-degree cephalic anterior-posterior, and axillary lateral views. If the diagnosis is in question, comparison views of the contralateral side can be useful, but weighted views are not recommended because they rarely change the diagnosis and may exacerbate the injury. Separations are classified by the extent of ligamentous disruption, which is determined by examination and radiographs. Types I and II separations can be treated conservatively with a sling and early range-of-motion exercises. Type III separation treatment is not clearly defined and should be managed individually. Any type IV, V, or VI injury is unstable and usually needs surgical fixation. Treatment should be immobilization with a sling for comfort for all AC separations and referral if warranted (Table 1). Return to play in nonsurgical cases can be considered when there is no pain on palpation of the AC joint.

Shoulder Impingement

Glenohumeral joint pain in active patients without history of acute trauma is often from overuse. Repetitive overhead or throwing activities can lead to impingement or subacromial bursitis symptoms. Examination elicits pain at 70 to 120 degrees of abduction, often with positive provocative tests, such as Hawkins (passive forward flexion of the shoulder and elbow to 90 degrees with internal rotation eliciting pain) and Neer (passive forward flexion

with elbow extended eliciting pain). These tests impinge the greater tuberosity against the acromion and have 75% to 90% sensitivity for bursitis and 88% sensitivity for rotator cuff pathology. Rotator cuff strength should be carefully tested for deficits suggestive of muscle or tendon tears. Radiographs are useful to assess for fractures, calcium deposits for calcific tendonitis, acromial shape for bony spurs, and alignment of the glenohumeral joint for rotator cuff or degenerative pathology. If soft tissue injury is suspected, MRI can be a useful diagnostic tool. Treatment should consist of relative rest with limited overhead activity, ice, and analgesics as needed. Strengthening the rotator cuff and focusing on kinetic chain function can help restore biomechanical motion. Subacromial injections can be used for diagnostic and therapeutic purposes. If the examination is limited by pain, a subacromial anesthetic injection usually offers significant if not complete pain relief if the source is impingement. Physical therapy is important for restoration of function, but it can be difficult for the patient to tolerate secondary to pain. A subacromial steroid injection may offer temporary pain relief that can facilitate physical therapy. If the injection does not provide any relief, consider referral for surgical decompression and débridement. This is an option for more definitive treatment and can often be performed arthroscopically to provide significant symptom relief. Return to play is contingent on the patient's level of pain. Sometimes patients can return to activity if they minimize the overhead activity that reproduces the symptoms.

KNEE INJURIES

Patellofemoral Pain

Knee injuries are a common complaint in athletes, both from overuse and acute trauma. The most common overuse injury seen in the athlete under 40 years old is patellofemoral joint pain. The pathophysiology, however, is not clear, but most accepted theories involve a combination of stress-induced cartilage defects and abnormal extensor mechanism biomechanics. The patient usually complains of anterior knee pain as well as pain after long periods with the knee held in flexion, which closes the

---

TABLE 1   Acromioclavicular Separation

Acromioclavicular Separation	Ligamentous Disruption	Radiographs	Treatment
Type I	AC ligament sprain	Normal	Nonsurgical
Type II	AC ligament and capsule disruption	<50% AC subluxation	Nonsurgical
Type III	AC and CC ligaments disrupted; unstable joint	>25% CC separation, >50% AC separation	Nonsurgical versus surgical; controversial
Type IV	AC and CC ligaments disrupted; unstable joint	Type III with *posterior* displacement of the clavicle	Surgical
Type V	AC and CC ligaments disrupted; unstable joint	Type III with *superior* displacement of the clavicle	Surgical
Type VI	AC and CC ligaments disrupted; unstable joint	Type III with inferior displacement of the clavicle	Surgical

Abbreviations: AC = acromioclavicular; CC = coracoclavicular.

patellofemoral joint (movie theater sign). There may be an inciting incident such as blunt trauma to the patella or simply a change in activity. Examination and treatment should focus on correction of the biomechanics of the patellofemoral joint. Femoral and tibial torsion, patellar tilt, foot hyperpronation, and varus or valgus knee malalignment can put uneven forces on the knee extensor mechanism. This is often evident by vastus medialis oblique muscle weakness or decreased muscle bulk and tightness of the lateral patellar retinaculum, rectus femoris, and/or hamstring on examination. The biomechanics can usually be improved with hamstring stretching, vastus medialis oblique strengthening, activity modification, and orthotics as needed. If symptoms are refractory to therapy, surgical intervention is an option to correct the malalignment. Return to play is contingent on the patient's level of pain and ideally should be close to pain-free prior to returning to play.

Anterior Cruciate Ligament Injury

Acute knee injuries in sports commonly result in injury to the anterior cruciate ligament (ACL). The mechanism is usually a twisting injury and/or a valgus force on the knee. The patient often reports hearing or feeling a pop followed by a significant effusion. With the high-energy force causing ACL tears, there is often associated meniscal, collateral ligament, chondral injury, or fracture. If there is an isolated ACL tear, patients are usually able to ambulate and the pain is mild. They may present chronically with complaints of instability with twisting or cutting activity because the ACL functions to provide stability for torsional forces. On examination, a Lachman test, anterior drawer, and/or pivot shift test may be positive. The Lachman test is performed with the patient lying supine and relaxed with the knee in 20 to 30 degrees of flexion. Stabilizing the femur, the examiner gently pulls the tibia forward to assess for an endpoint and anterior translation relative to the normal knee. The anterior drawer is performed in a similar fashion, except with the knee at 90 degrees of flexion; however, studies do not show it to be as sensitive as the Lachman test. The pivot shift is performed with the knee in extension, and the examiner passively internally rotates and flexes the knee while applying a valgus stress to the knee. The tibia shifts into place around 20 to 30 degrees of flexion when the ACL is torn but can only be done when the patient is completely relaxed. For the experienced clinician, the Lachman test has a high negative predictive value and the pivot shift a high positive predictive value. In acute injuries, the range of motion of the knee should be examined to ensure there is no soft tissue or bony block that may require earlier surgical intervention. If the patient is guarding or has a large knee effusion acutely and no fracture is suspected, range-of-motion bracing and/or crutches for comfort should be considered and repeat the examination a few days later when pain has decreased. Knee range of motion and strength should be optimized prior to surgery and initiated as soon as the patient's pain is controlled. Partial ACL tears can be managed conservatively with therapy and strengthening if there is no instability. Partial or complete ACL tears with clinical instability should be referred for surgical evaluation. Return to play in nonsurgical cases depends on the degree of instability and may require modification of activities.

Meniscal Injury

Meniscal injuries are a common cause of knee pain seen with acute and chronic degenerative trauma. Patients often complain of symptoms of locking, catching, giving way, and localized areas of pain. Examination of any meniscal injury should include inspecting for effusion, palpating for joint line tenderness, testing passive range of motion, and performing McMurray and Apley provocative tests. Joint line tenderness helps localize the area of injury and is a sensitive but not very specific test. The McMurray test is performed by palpating the joint line with one hand and internally and externally rotating while flexing and extending the knee. A positive test elicits a click or catch with pain at the joint line. The Apley test is performed with the patient prone and the knees flexed to 90 degrees. An axial load is placed on the knee while internally and externally rotating the tibia to load each of the menisci with a positive test reproducing the symptoms. In evaluating acute meniscal injuries, range of motion should be documented, specifically extension, to ensure there is no evidence of an extension lag suggestive of a bucket-handle meniscal tear that needs earlier surgical intervention. Because the medial and lateral menisci are much more vascular in the margins, or peripheral third areas, there is a higher chance of healing of tears in those areas. Degenerative tears occur from repetitive knee-loading activities, ranging from running to squatting (baseball catchers) or kneeling (gardening). Patients usually present with more insidious symptoms of pain in certain positions, and they rarely have locking, catching, or giving-way symptoms as in acute meniscal injuries. If meniscal symptoms are persistent, surgical intervention can repair or remove the area of damaged meniscus, depending on the area and extent of the damage. Return to play in nonsurgical cases is appropriate when the patient is symptom free, suggestive of meniscal healing, and there are no signs of meniscal injury on examination.

ANKLE INJURIES

Ankle Sprain

Ankle sprains, specifically lateral ankle sprains, are the most common sports injuries and usually occur with an inversion and plantar flexion mechanism. This usually disrupts the anterior talofibular ligament (ATFL), followed by the calcaneofibular ligament and posterior talofibular ligament. In the acute setting, swelling and pain may limit the examination and should be treated symptomatically and reevaluated to get a better examination a few days later. The examination should look for swelling, ecchymosis, areas of tenderness, and instability. Swelling, ecchymosis, and tenderness over the ATFL are suggestive of a ligament disruption. The anterior drawer test may be difficult to perform in the acute setting and should be repeated for a more accurate result approximately 5 to 7 days after injury when pain and swelling have subsided. The ankle anterior drawer test is performed with the patient seated with the foot hanging over the table. The examiner stabilizes the leg with one hand and uses the other to hold the heel and pull forward to look for anterior translation. The anterior drawer test is 73% sensitive and 97% specific. Tenderness over the ATFL with a positive anterior drawer increases sensitivity to 100% and specificity to 77%. Finally, bony tenderness suggestive of any fractures that

If any of the following are positive, films are
  recommended:
- Unable to walk four steps immediately after injury and
  in the office
- Tenderness over the distal 6 cm of the tibia or fibula,
  including the malleoli
- Midfoot or navicular tenderness
- Tenderness over the proximal fifth metatarsal

require imaging should be checked. Box 1 lists the criteria for the Ottawa ankle rules, a useful guide to determine whether an ankle sprain requires imaging.

Swelling and pain can be treated with relative rest, ice, compression, elevation, and support (RICES). Rest may involve the use of crutches for a few days if it is difficult to bear weight, but early mobilization should be encouraged. Icing is recommended for 15- to 20-minute periods to stimulate vasoconstriction and decrease swelling. Compression acutely can be managed by an Ace wrap or pneumatic splint placing pressure on the areas of swelling to promote

CURRENT DIAGNOSIS

- Concussions
  History of head trauma
  Loss of consciousness determined
  Neurologic examination
- Burner/stingers
  History of flexion or direct blow to the head
    or neck
  Duration of symptoms
  Neurologic deficits
- AC separations
  History of direct fall on or blow to the shoulder
  Palpation of the AC joint
  Deformity at the AC joint
- Impingement
  History of pain with overhead activity
  Neer impingement test
  Hawkins impingement test
- Patellofemoral syndrome
  History of possible increased level of activity
  Pain with prolonged sitting
- ACL injury
  History of twisting injury, instability
  Lachman test
  Pivot shift test
  Anterior drawer test
- Meniscal injury
  History of pain, clicking, locking, giving way
  McMurray test
  Apley test
- Ankle sprain
  History of injury, pain, swelling
  Anterior drawer
  Pain over the ATFL

Abbreviations: AC = acromioclavicular; ACL = accessory collateral ligament;
  ATFL = anterior talofibular ligament.

CURRENT THERAPY

- Concussions
  Monitor for resolution of symptoms
  Image for persistent symptoms, prolonged loss of
    consciousness, or neurologic deficit.
  Return to play when asymptomatic. If symptoms
    severe, may need to be asymptomatic for days to
    weeks prior to return to play.
- Burner/stingers
  Monitor for resolution of symptoms.
  Consider EMG if symptoms persist.
  Return to play when asymptomatic.
- AC separations
  Provide sling for comfort.
  Refer for grade III and above injuries.
  Return to play when asymptomatic.
- Impingement
  Order physical therapy for strengthening and
    biomechanical retraining.
  Prescribe NSAIDs and steroid injections to improve
    symptoms temporarily.
  Consider referral for surgical débridement if
    symptoms persist.
- Patellofemoral syndrome
  Order physical therapy for strengthening.
  Correct any malalignment.
- ACL injury
  Order physical therapy for strengthening and
    range of motion.
  Make surgical referral for reconstruction.
- Meniscal injury
  If symptoms persist, make surgical referral for
    repair or débridement.
- Ankle sprain
  Prescribe RICES.
  Order physical therapy for range of motion,
    strengthening, and proprioception training.

Abbreviations: AC = acromioclavicular; ACL = accessory collateral ligament;
  EMG = electromyelogram; NSAIDs = nonsteroidal anti-inflammatory drugs;
  RICES = rest, ice, compression, elevation, and support.

fluid resorption. Elevation decreases swelling because it increases venous and lymphatic drainage to the heart. Finally, supportive devices are useful in improving swelling and stability in the acute phase. Analgesics such as acetaminophen or mild narcotics can be used acutely, but a nonsteroidal anti-inflammatory drug (NSAID) should be reserved until 48 hours after injury when bruising and swelling have stabilized because it may exacerbate bleeding and swelling acutely. Finally, rehabilitation should be started when the patient is pain-free and should include range-of-motion exercises (writing the alphabet in the air), balance/proprioception exercises (balancing on the injured ankle on the floor, balance board, or trampoline), and strengthening exercises (controlled elastic band exercises). Return to play can be considered when the athlete gradually progresses to his or her previous level of activity, has near to full range of motion, swelling has resolved, has the ability to hop and perform sport-specific tasks without pain or instability, and has regained at least 90% of the strength of the noninjured side.

Discussion

Sports injuries are common in the active population of all ages. When evaluating any injury, understanding the patient's level of activity and goals for return to play are important in treatment. Graded return to play should be emphasized to the patient because full return to play after any injury makes reinjury likely. Physical therapists and athletic trainers are important in treating the injury, and if they are used, the clinician should monitor progress and determine the appropriate time to return to play. Finally, if the patient is not improving appropriately or the diagnosis is unclear, further imaging or referral to a specialist for evaluation should be considered.

REFERENCES

Adams WB: Treatment options in overuse injuries of the knee: Patellofemoral syndrome, iliotibial band syndrome, and degenerative meniscal tears. Curr Sports Med Rep 2004;3(5):256-260.

Bossart PJ, Joyce SM, Manaster BJ, Packer SM: Lack of efficacy of 'weighted' radiographs in diagnosing acute acromioclavicular separation. Ann Emerg Med 1988;17(1):20-24.

Cohen RS, Balcom TA: Current treatment options for ankle injuries: Lateral ankle sprain, Achilles tendonitis, and Achilles rupture. Curr Sports Med Rep 2003;2(5):251-254.

Dugan S, Weber K: Selected topics in sports medicine. Disease-A-Month. September 2002;48(9)572-616.

Ferrante MA: Brachial plexopathies: Classification, causes, and consequences. Muscle Nerve 2004;30(5):547-568.

Fithian DC: Fate of the anterior cruciate ligament-injured knee. Orthop Clin North Am 2002;33(4):621-636.

Guskiewicz KM, Bruce SL, Cantu RC, et al: National Athletic Trainers' Association Position Statement: Management of Sport-Related Concussion. J Athletic Training 2004;39(3):280-297.

Pyne SW: Diagnosis and current treatment options of shoulder impingement. Curr Sports Med Rep 2004;3(5):251-255.

Safran MR: Nerve injury about the shoulder in athletes: II. Long thoracic nerve, spinal accessory nerve, burners/stingers, thoracic outlet syndrome. Am J Sports Med 2004;32(4):1063-1076.

Tennet TD, Beach WR, Meyers JF: A review of the special tests associated with shoulder examination: I. The rotator cuff test. Am J Sports Med 2003;31(1):154-160.

Van Dijk CN: Management of the sprained ankle. Br J Sports Med 2002;36(2):83-84.

Zanda P: Shoulder pain: Involvement of the acromioclavicular joint. Am J Roentgenol Radium Ther Nucl Med 1971;112(3):493-506.

Obstetrics and Gynecology

Antepartum Care

Method of
Faith Joy Frieden, MD, and Ying Chan, MD

Pregnancy offers the health care provider a window of opportunity to influence the health of today's women and tomorrow's children. Although the cornerstone of treatment during this unique time period is antepartum care, the ideal time to begin is prior to conception.

Preconception Care

At a preconception visit, a basic history and physical examination should be performed, along with a risk assessment. Special areas of concern include preexisting maternal medical conditions, medication use, family history of birth defects, carrier screening for inherited diseases, occupational hazards, and recreational drug use, including cigarettes and alcohol. This visit provides an opportunity to determine susceptibility to infectious diseases, such as toxoplasmosis, cytomegalovirus, varicella, rubella, and HIV, and to vaccinate as appropriate. When risk factors are identified, the patient can be advised of the potential consequences. In some situations (such as uncontrolled diabetes, recent vaccination, recent viral infection, or potentially teratogenic exposure), pregnancy can be postponed until the risk factor is managed and the risk reduced.

Routine Care

INITIAL PRENATAL VISIT

At the initial prenatal visit, a thorough history is obtained, including age, menstrual history, prior obstetrical history, past medical and surgical history, family history, genetic screening, medication or drug use, and history of exposure to infections (tuberculosis, hepatitis B, genital herpes, HIV, and other sexually transmitted diseases, etc.). Any risk factors identified should be addressed and incorporated

into the plan of care for the pregnancy. Certain obstetrical conditions, such as prior preterm birth, recurrent pregnancy loss, or preeclampsia remote from term, are associated with a relatively high recurrence risk, compared with women with no such history. Medical conditions, such as diabetes, hypertension, lupus, asthma, or a seizure disorder, must be stabilized as quickly as possible. In counseling the pregnant woman with underlying medical disorders, we must consider the effects of the medical condition on a pregnancy and the effects of pregnancy on the woman's health. We also must weigh the risk of medication compared with the risks of not treating the condition. The general rule of thumb is that the best predictor of a healthy infant is a healthy mother. Many medications are available that are not known to incur any increased risk of birth defects above the background risk in the general population.

The initial physical examination should include a general physical exam as well as a pelvic exam. The prepregnancy height and weight are recorded, along with the initial vital signs. It is important to perform a thorough exam at this time because many women have not had a physical exam prior to becoming pregnant. Also, at subsequent prenatal visits, less emphasis will be placed on nonobstetric areas in the absence of complaints. The pelvic exam should include assessment of the cervix, uterine size, and adnexa, as well as a clinical impression of the adequacy of the pelvis. Table 1 lists the recommended initial and subsequent laboratory tests.

FOLLOW-UP PRENATAL VISITS

In general, prenatal visits are repeated every 4 weeks until 28 weeks, then every 2 to 3 weeks until 36 weeks, then weekly until delivery. Of course, this schedule should be individualized to the patient, and more frequent visits may be appropriate. The purpose of each prenatal visit is to assess maternal and fetal well-being. Therefore, in a systematic fashion at each visit, the patient's weight and blood pressure are recorded, along with the presence or absence of edema. A urine dipstick is performed to check for protein and glucose. The height of the uterine fundus is measured and fetal heart tones are recorded. The fetal heart rate usually can be auscultated using a Doppler device by 12 weeks. The patient is also asked about the

TABLE 1 Recommended Prenatal Laboratory Screening

Preconception or First Visit	15-20 Weeks	26-28 Weeks	35-37 Weeks
Hemoglobin and hematocrit	Maternal serum screening	Diabetic screening	GBS culture
Blood type/RH factor/antibody screen			
Rubella titer		Hemoglobin and hematocrit	
Hepatitis B test		Antibody screen if indicated	
Syphilis test			
Tests for chlamydia and gonorrhea			
HIV test (offered)			
Urine analysis and culture			
Pap smear			

GBS, Group B streptococcus; HIV, human immunodeficiency virus.
Modified from Gabbe SG, Niebyl JR, Simpson JL: Obstetrics: Normal and Problem Pregnancies, 4th ed, 2002.

perception of fetal movement, which is usually apparent by 20 weeks.

NUTRITION IN PREGNANCY

Pregnant women should increase their daily caloric intake by approximately 300 kcal. The American College of Obstetricians and Gynecologists (ACOG) recommends total weight gain for healthy women with singleton gestation to be 25 to 35 pounds. Underweight women may gain 28 to 40 pounds and overweight women 15 to 25 lb. Women carrying twins may gain 35 to 45 pounds. Pregnant women should receive 30 mg of ferrous iron supplements daily. Folic acid supplementation is advised, both on a hematologic basis and to decrease certain birth defects. The Centers for Disease Control and Prevention (CDC) recommends folic acid, 0.4 mg per day, while attempting pregnancy and during the first trimester of pregnancy for prevention of neural tube defects (NTDs). A woman with a history of a prior NTD-affected pregnancy can reduce the 3% recurrence risk of NTDs by more than 70% if she supplements her daily diet with 4 mg of folic acid for the month before conception and for the first trimester of pregnancy.

VACCINATION OF PREGNANT WOMEN

The benefits of immunization to pregnant women usually outweigh the theoretical risks to the fetus. In general, live-virus vaccines are contraindicated because of the theoretical risks of transmitting vaccine virus to the fetus. Vaccinating pregnant women with inactivated virus, bacterial vaccines, or toxoids is not contraindicated. Although the MMR (measles-mumps-rubella) vaccine is contraindicated in pregnancy, no cases of congenital mumps, measles, or rubella syndromes are identified among infants born to women who were vaccinated within 3 months prior to conception or early in pregnancy. Similarly, no adverse fetal outcomes are reported in pregnant mothers who received varicella vaccine inadvertently. In October 2001, the CDC changed the recommendations concerning the pregnancy interval after receiving rubella vaccine, reducing it from 3 months to 1 month. Influenza vaccine, tetanus-diphtheria booster, hepatitis A vaccine, hepatitis B vaccine, rabies vaccine, and pneumococcal vaccine are safe in pregnancy and should be administered if appropriate.

HERBAL MEDICINES

Herbal medicines are increasing in popularity nowadays. Herbs were traditionally used to deal with a wide range of pregnancy complications, including morning sickness, threatened miscarriage, labor problems, and poor milk production. Some of the most commonly used herbal medicines are ginger,[1] St. John's wort,[1] and ginseng.[1] Because they originate from plants, most pregnant women perceive them as safe. But herbal medicines can potentially alter maternal hemodynamic parameters and increase bleeding complications associated with regional anesthesia and childbirth. Ginger is a potent inhibitor of thromboxane synthetase, and ginseng has an antiplatelet component. Drug-herb interactions are also described. Therefore, it is imperative that health care providers routinely ask about their use in pregnant women.

COMMON COMPLAINTS

Nausea and vomiting frequently complicate early pregnancy. Nonpharmacologic remedies include frequent small feedings and avoiding spicy foods. Several medications are used as well, including diphenhydramine (Benadryl),[1] metoclopramide (Reglan),[1] prochlorperazine (Compazine), promethazine (Phenergan), and trimethobenzamide (Tigan). One of the newer considerably successful treatment modalities is a continuous infusion of metoclopramide via subcutaneous infusion pump.

Heartburn is a frequent problem, which occurs because of relaxation of the esophageal sphincter with reflux of gastric contents into the lower esophagus. Patients should avoid spicy foods and lying completely flat. Antacids may be helpful, especially in liquid form that coats the lining of the esophagus.

Constipation occurs as a result of smooth muscle relaxation and delayed bowel transit time. It can usually be treated successfully with dietary modification, incorporating

---

[1]Not FDA approved for this indication.

increased fruits, vegetables, and water. Stool softeners may also be helpful.

Environmental Hazards and Exposures

Whenever considering the teratogenic potential of an exposure, it is imperative to keep in mind the 3% background risk of major birth defects in the general obstetric population. Only a small percentage of birth defects can actually be linked to a known agent. Examples include such infectious agents as rubella virus and *Toxoplasma gondii,* drugs such as alcohol, thalidomide, and isotretinoin, physical agents such as ionizing radiation and hyperthermia, and chemicals such as lead, organic solvents, and methylmercury.

METHYLMERCURY EXPOSURE IN PREGNANCY

Fish and shellfish are an important part of a balanced diet for pregnant women. Almost all fish and shellfish contain traces of methylmercury. However, some fish contain higher levels of methylmercury that may be harmful to susceptible populations. High levels of methylmercury can impair an unborn fetus's nervous system. In April 2004, the Food and Drug Administration and Environmental Protection Agency issued a joint advisory regarding this issue. Pregnant women and women who might become pregnant should not eat shark, swordfish, tilefish, and king mackerel. They may eat up to 12 ounces, two average meals per week, of fish and shellfish that are lower in mercury: shrimp, canned light tuna, salmon, pollock, catfish.

Prenatal Diagnosis

The purpose of prenatal diagnosis is to provide information that optimizes medical care and enables the patient to make informed reproductive decisions. As health care providers, our responsibility is to assess the risks unique to each pregnancy, convey that information to the patient, and guide her through the testing process while allowing her to choose a course of action that is right for her. This nondirective approach, based on the principle of patient autonomy, is critical to the process of genetic counseling and prenatal diagnosis.

CARRIER SCREENING

Several autosomal recessive disorders occur with increased frequency in certain ethnic groups. Carrier detection should be offered whenever one or both expectant parents belong to the group at increased risk. The most frequently encountered of these conditions are Tay-Sachs disease in the Ashkenazi Jewish population, sickle cell disease in the African American population, and the thalassemias in people of Mediterranean, African, and Asian descent. Cystic fibrosis (CF) is the most common serious autosomal recessive disorder in the Caucasian population. In 2001 the American College of Obstetricians and Gynecologists and American College of Medical Genetics published clinical guidelines for CF screening. It is recommended that CF screening be offered to couples in ethnic or racial groups considered at higher risk for carrying the CF gene: Caucasians, particularly those of Ashkenazi Jewish or European descent. It is also recommended that CF testing be available to those of Hispanic, African, and Asian descents, although screening in these populations is less conclusive. Screening for other genetic disorders on the basis of family history may also be indicated (e.g., fragile X syndrome for family history of mental retardation). It is important to counsel patients that a negative test result does not guarantee an unaffected pregnancy, but rather it decreases the risk.

NUCHAL TRANSLUCENCY AND BIOCHEMICAL MARKERS SCREENING

First-trimester screening, consisting of nuchal translucency, free β-human chorionic gonadotropin (hCG), and pregnancy-associated plasma protein A (PAPP-A), may be available in some centers. First-trimester screening is typically performed at 11 to 14 weeks. This allows for earlier detection and diagnosis of some fetal chromosomal and structural abnormalities. Median level of free β-hCG is higher in affected Down syndrome pregnancies. Conversely, median level of PAPP-A is lowered in affected Down syndrome pregnancies. Increased nuchal translucency is associated with chromosomal abnormalities such as trisomy 21, 18, and 13, 45, X, and triploidy. It is also associated with congenital anomalies such as cardiac defects, skeletal abnormalities, and some genetic disorders. The prevalence of major cardiac defects increases with increasing nuchal translucency thickness. In fetuses with increased nuchal translucency measurement and normal chromosomes, detailed anatomic survey and fetal echocardiography are recommended.

Second-trimester maternal serum screening is offered at approximately 16 weeks' gestation. This test generally evaluates three markers, namely α-fetoprotein (AFP), hCG, and unconjugated estriol. AFP is produced by the fetus and is present in high concentrations in the amniotic fluid and, to a lesser extent, in maternal serum. Elevated levels of maternal serum AFP are associated with open neural tube defects, ventral wall defects, some renal abnormalities, multiple gestation, certain skin disorders, maternal tumors, fetal demise, placental abnormality, and otherwise unexplained adverse perinatal outcome. Low levels of maternal serum AFP are associated with Down syndrome. The addition of the other two markers enhances the detection rate, from 25% using AFP alone to approximately 60% using all three. This test is especially useful for younger women, who might not otherwise pursue prenatal diagnosis. In the event of an abnormal result, patients are offered ultrasound for confirmation of gestational age and for anatomic survey. They also have the option of amniocentesis for direct assessment of the fetal chromosomes and AFP level.

In general, first-trimester screening has comparable detection rates and positive screening rates for Down syndrome as second-trimester screening. However, integrated screening (i.e., combined first- and second-trimester screening) is believed to be the most sensitive and cost-effective test. Detection rate for fetal Down syndrome with this approach can be as high as 92%.

AMNIOCENTESIS AND CHORIONIC VILLUS SAMPLING

Genetic amniocentesis is the most commonly performed invasive prenatal diagnostic procedure. It is generally performed at 15 to 20 weeks. Although it is performed under ultrasound guidance, using sterile technique, it still carries a pregnancy loss rate attributable to the procedure of approximately 0.5%. The amniotic fluid is sent for fetal karyotyping and AFP determination, although other specific genetic testing can also be performed.

An alternative to traditional amniocentesis is chorionic villus sampling (CVS), which allows a first-trimester diagnosis. CVS can be performed at 10 to 12 weeks, using the transabdominal or transcervical approach. The pregnancy loss rate is approximately 1.3% with CVS, which is somewhat higher than with traditional amniocentesis, according to a large multicenter trial conducted by the National Institute of Child Health and Human Development. Another drawback is that AFP cannot be measured in villi. It is conceivable, therefore, that an amniocentesis might be necessary later to evaluate an elevated maternal serum AFP. Subsequent amniocentesis could also be indicated to clarify an ambiguous CVS finding, which occurs in approximately 1% of cases.

FETAL BLOOD SAMPLING

Sometimes it becomes necessary to sample fetal blood directly for rapid karyotyping, evaluating for fetal infection, or diagnosing platelet disorders prenatally. This technique, of accessing fetal blood via the umbilical cord, is known as percutaneous umbilical blood sampling (PUBS) and has an estimated fetal loss rate of 1% to 2%.

Antepartum Testing

ULTRASOUND

A variety of noninvasive techniques are available for evaluating fetal health. The most powerful tool, and perhaps the most controversial, is diagnostic ultrasound. Ultrasound technology has fundamentally altered the practice of obstetrics and refined the art of prenatal diagnosis. Its clinical utility is under constant scrutiny, analysis, and expansion. Although academics disagree about whether routine ultrasound screening is useful or cost effective in low-risk pregnancies, this tool is almost universal in the United States.

NONSTRESS TEST

The nonstress test (NST) is a simple, noninvasive method of monitoring fetal well-being by recording fetal heart rate patterns along with the maternal perception of fetal movement. It is based on the premise that the heart rate of a nonacidotic or non–neurologically depressed fetus accelerates in response to fetal movement. If two or more accelerations of 15 beats per minute, lasting for 15 seconds, are present in a 20-minute period, the test is considered "reactive," or normal. The major pitfall of this test is the high false-positive rate because "nonreactivity" is more likely associated with a fetal sleep cycle than with actual central nervous system depression.

BIOPHYSICAL PROFILE

Biophysical profile testing combines multiple biophysical parameters to assess fetal well-being, in an attempt to identify the compromised fetus more accurately. It is composed of the NST and four parameters evaluated by ultrasound, namely fetal breathing movement, fetal body movement, fetal tone, and assessment of amniotic fluid volume.

Medical Complications

DIABETES MELLITUS

Diabetes in pregnancy encompasses two very different groups of women—diabetic women who become pregnant and pregnant women who become diabetic. The former group, although smaller in number, is greater in terms of the impact on a pregnancy. Preconception counseling is most important for this group. With a two- to fourfold increase in the risk of major malformations in infants of diabetic mothers, congenital malformations are the most important cause of perinatal loss in these pregnancies. The organ systems most frequently affected are the cardiovascular, skeletal, and central nervous systems. It has been demonstrated repeatedly that excellent glycemic control at the time of conception and organogenesis can dramatically reduce this risk. Fetal overgrowth because of maternal hyperglycemia can be another complication because delivery of excessively large infants occurs up to 10 times more often in diabetic women than in the nondiabetic population. If maternal blood glucose levels are not controlled adequately, these newborns are also subject to metabolic derangements, including hypoglycemia, magnesium deficiency, and hyperbilirubinemia, as well as respiratory distress and polycythemia. When the diabetes is associated with vasculopathy, such as nephropathy or retinopathy, the fetus is at risk for intrauterine growth restriction. Therefore, it is essential that diabetic women maintain meticulous glycemic control, adhering to an appropriate diet and monitoring blood glucose levels from four to seven times daily. Target values are fasting capillary blood glucose of 60 to 90 mg/dL and 1-hour postprandial values less than 120 mg/dL. In addition, it is useful to monitor glycosylated hemoglobin levels in these women, which indicate the overall level of control for the preceding 6 weeks. Fetal well-being is assessed with ultrasound and echocardiography in the second trimester and with nonstress tests and biophysical profile exams in the third trimester. Because of the increased risk of adverse perinatal outcome in these pregnancies, delivery is usually recommended at term, as soon as fetal lung maturity is assured.

Approximately 3% of pregnant women develop carbohydrate intolerance, or gestational diabetes, during the latter part of pregnancy. Because roughly half of these women have no identifiable risk factors, it is good practice to screen all pregnant women for this condition at 28 weeks with the 1-hour 50-g oral glucose challenge test (GCT). If this result is elevated, the 3-hour 100-g OGTT is

TABLE 2 Recommended Cutoff Values by Carpenter and Coustan to Diagnose Gestational Diabetes Mellitus With a 100-g Oral Glucose Tolerance Test (OGTT)

100-g OGTT	Plasma (mg/dl)
Fasting	95
1 hour	180
2 hours	155
3 hours	140

performed. In contrast to GCT, which can be performed at any time of the day, OGTT should be performed in the morning after an overnight fast of at least 8 hours and after at least 3 days of unrestricted diet (150 g carbohydrate or more per day) and physical activity. Table 2 shows the recommended cutoff values by Carpenter and Coustan. A woman who meets or exceeds two or more values is diagnosed with gestational diabetes. Approximately 15% of women with a positive GCT have a positive OGTT. The mainstay of management is diet with self-monitoring of blood glucose, in most cases four times daily (fasting and 1 hour after meals). If the target glucose values cannot be reached and maintained with this regimen, insulin therapy may be necessary. Although carbohydrate intolerance should resolve following delivery, gestational diabetic patients should know that they have a 50% chance of becoming diabetic later in life.

Surgery in Pregnancy

Whenever the physician is faced with the decision of whether to take a pregnant woman to the operating room, the risks of surgery must be weighed against the risks of conservative management, keeping in mind that the sequelae of nonintervention could actually be more severe in a pregnant patient. If surgery is performed, a general rule of thumb is to minimize uterine manipulation to minimize the risk for preterm labor. Cesarean section should be reserved for obstetric indications.

Appendicitis is the most common nonobstetric emergency during pregnancy. The diagnosis is complicated by the overlap of the symptoms of appendicitis with some common symptoms in pregnancy. In addition, the position of the appendix becomes higher as pregnancy advances, making it more difficult to pinpoint the source of the pain. Maternal and fetal complications are directly associated with advanced disease and delay in treatment. Therefore, once acute appendicitis is suspected in pregnancy, emergency surgery should be performed. To lower maternal and fetal morbidity, we accept a higher negative exploration rate than in the nonpregnant population.

Gallbladder disease is the second most common nonobstetric surgical condition in pregnancy, usually presenting with right upper quadrant pain, nausea, and vomiting. Medical management includes bed rest, no oral feedings, intravenous fluids for hydration, and antibiotics. When attacks are recurrent or if the patient develops an acute abdomen, cholecystectomy should be performed.

Trauma in Pregnancy

Trauma and violence are the leading causes of death in women of reproductive age. The first priority when encountering a pregnant trauma victim is treatment and stabilization of the woman. Only then should attention be directed to the fetus. Pregnancy should not alter the necessary evaluation and treatment. It cannot be overstated that necessary radiographic studies should be performed without delay, with efforts made to minimize the dose to the lower abdomen. A systematic approach to evaluation should be used, consisting of the ABCs (airway, breathing, and circulation). There are some considerations unique to pregnancy. The patient should be tilted or wedged in the left lateral position, thus deflecting the uterus off the inferior vena cava and aorta. The pregnant trauma victim requires a greater volume of blood replacement to maintain her cardiovascular integrity than a nonpregnant patient. In gestations beyond 20 weeks, electronic monitoring for uterine contractions, as well as fetal heart rate, is helpful in evaluation for placental abruption and other injury.

Motor vehicle accidents are a significant source of trauma and death, especially when the victim is ejected from the car. The three-point lap belt/shoulder harness restraint is superior to the lap belt alone in preventing maternal and fetal injury.

Perhaps the most insidious form of trauma in pregnancy is domestic violence. The actual incidence is not known, but an estimated 25% of women in the United States are abused by a current or former partner sometime in their lives. Because obstetricians are the primary care providers for many women, they are in a unique position to identify women who are victims of abuse and offer them help. If an abusive relationship is identified, the woman should be encouraged to leave the violent situation and be referred to appropriate agencies, to protect both herself and her children.

Obstetrical Complications

PRETERM BIRTH

Preterm birth, occurring prior to the completion of 37 weeks of gestation, complicates 9% of all births in the United States and accounts for 75% of the neonatal deaths that are not caused by congenital malformations. Despite the advent of new diagnostic and therapeutic modalities, the preterm birth rate has remained unchanged over the past 40 years. This may be largely because of the multifaceted nature of this problem. Approximately one third of such births are iatrogenic, in that they are indicated because of medical or obstetric disorders that place the mother or fetus at increased risk, such as hypertension, diabetes, hemorrhage, or intrauterine growth restriction. The remaining two thirds are attributed to preterm labor, preterm premature rupture of membranes, and cervical incompetence. Some current therapies directed at early diagnosis and treatment include home uterine activity monitoring, tocolytic therapy, ultrasonographic measurements of cervical length, and assays of fetal fibronectin levels in cervicovaginal secretions. When preterm birth is imminent, delivery in a setting with appropriate neonatal intensive care optimizes perinatal outcome.

PROLONGED PREGNANCY

A postdate or post-term pregnancy is defined as one that reaches 42 weeks after the last menstrual period. Perinatal morbidity and mortality increase dramatically after 40 weeks and especially after 42 weeks. Possible maternal complications include an increased incidence of cesarean section, hemorrhage, and trauma because of fetal macrosomia. Potential problems of these neonates include birth trauma from macrosomia and meconium aspiration. Good outcomes can be expected with accurate dating, careful fetal surveillance, and intervention when indicated.

MULTIPLE GESTATIONS

The incidence of twinning in the United States is approximately 1.2% of all pregnancies. With the increased use of assisted reproductive technologies, the incidence of higher-order multiple gestations (triplets and higher) is approximately 0.3%. These pregnancies pose special concerns for management of the mother as well as the fetuses. Increased maternal risks include an increased strain on the cardiovascular system, pulmonary edema, preeclampsia, anemia, complications related to tocolysis, and delivery complications. The greatest fetal risk is that of prematurity. In addition, when identical twin fetuses have a single placenta and a shared placental circulation, there is a significant risk for twin-twin transfusion syndrome, a potentially fatal complication of twinning. Early diagnosis of multiple gestations, frequent checkups to monitor maternal health, serial ultrasound exams to assess fetal growth and well-being, reduced maternal activity level, prompt treatment of preterm labor, close intrapartum surveillance, and appropriate neonatal personnel in the delivery room all contribute to optimizing the outcome of these pregnancies.

Infections

Certain perinatal infections, such as toxoplasmosis, cytomegalovirus, human parvovirus B19, rubella, varicella, and syphilis, have the potential for teratogenicity or fetal loss. Some infections have the potential for other adverse perinatal sequelae. For example, vertical transmission of hepatitis B has been demonstrated. Group B β-hemolytic streptococcus, although a frequent component of vaginal flora, is one of the most common and dangerous perinatal pathogens in susceptible newborns, requiring intrapartum prophylaxis. Genital herpes can colonize newborns during passage through an infected birth canal. Chorioamnionitis, or bacterial infection of the amniotic cavity and membranes, is an important cause of perinatal morbidity and mortality, best treated with intrapartum antibiotics and delivery. Increasing evidence indicates that exposure to such intrauterine infection may be associated with an increased risk of cerebral palsy.

Special attention must be paid to HIV, which is estimated to complicate 7000 pregnancies per year in the United States. HIV testing should be offered to all pregnant women, in light of the findings of the landmark study, Pediatric AIDS Clinical Trials Group 076. This study demonstrated a significant reduction in mother-to-infant transmission of the virus, from 26% in the placebo group to 8% in the group using zidovudine (ZDV, Retrovir). According to this protocol, prophylactic ZDV therapy is given to HIV-positive women starting at 14 weeks and continued throughout pregnancy, in an oral dose of 100 mg five times daily. During labor, it is given intravenously in a 1-hour loading dose of 2 mg/kg body weight, followed by a continuous infusion of 1 mg/kg body weight every hour until delivery. The neonate is then given zidovudine syrup at a dose of 2 mg/kg body weight every 6 hours for the first 6 weeks of life.

Other risk factors may affect perinatal transmission. Prolonged fetal exposure to ruptured membranes, fetal scalp sampling, fetal scalp electrodes, and any other fetal abrasions should be avoided. Breast-feeding is contraindicated in HIV-positive women because it also increases transmission.

New multiple antiretroviral regimens are available for the treatment of HIV and AIDS. Although data are limited on their use in pregnancy, they should be administered as necessary for the life and well-being of the mother and certainly should not be avoided,

---

 CURRENT DIAGNOSIS

- Preconceptual and initial pregnancy evaluation should include complete blood count (CBC), type and screen, rubella, syphilis, and hepatitis testing. HIV testing should also be offered.
- The following genetic disorders based on racial and ethnic background should be screened for:
  Sickle hemoglobinopathies (African American).
  B-thalassemia (Mediterranean, Southeast Asian, and African American).
  Tay-Sachs disease (Ashkenazi Jews, French Canadians, Cajuns).
  Canavan disease and familial dysautonomia (Ashkenazi Jews). Carrier screening is also available for Gaucher's disease, Niemann-Pick disease, mucolipidosis IV, Fanconi anemia, maple syrup urine disease, Bloom syndrome, glycogen-storage disease type 1a, and so on.
  Cystic fibrosis (Caucasians of European and Ashkenazi Jewish descent).
- Both first-trimester nuchal translucency/ PAPP-A/free ß-hCG and second-trimester maternal serum screening may detect women at increased risk for chromosomal abnormalities.
- Total weight gain should be 25 to 35 pounds for women of normal prepregnancy weight with a singleton gestation. Underweight women may gain 28 to 40 pounds, and overweight women 15 to 25 pounds.
- All pregnant women should be screened for gestational diabetes mellitus at 26 to 28 weeks with the 1-hour 50-g oral glucose challenge test. If it is elevated, then the 3-hour 100-g oral glucose tolerance test is performed (fasting, <95 mg/dL; 1 hr, <180 mg/dL; 2 hr, <155 mg/dL; 3 hr, <140 mg/dL). A woman who meets or exceeds two or more values is diagnosed with gestational diabetes.

Abbreviations: hCG = human chorionic gonadotropin; PAPP-A = pregnancy-associated plasma protein A.

CURRENT THERAPY

- Although some vaccines are safe to receive during pregnancy, it is best to have all needed immunizations before becoming pregnant. Susceptible women should have MMR (measles-mumps-rubella) and varicella vaccines at least 1 month before conception. Influenza vaccine, tetanus-diphtheria booster, hepatitis A vaccine, hepatitis B vaccine, rabies, and pneumococcal vaccines are safe in pregnancy.
- The amount of folic acid found in prenatal vitamins (1 mg) is sufficient for most women. For women at increased risk for neural tube defects, the recommended dose is 4 mg of folate starting before conception and continuing through week 12 of gestation.
- Pregnant women and women who might become pregnant should not eat shark, swordfish, tilefish, and king mackerel. They may eat up to 12 ounces per week of fish and shellfish that are lower in mercury.
- In pregnant women who are HIV-positive, antepartum, intrapartum, and neonatal treatment with zidovudine (ZDV) are recommended.

especially after the first trimester when organogenesis is completed.

Fetal Therapy

With improved prenatal diagnosis and the resultant opportunity for antenatal therapy, the concept of the fetus as a patient is emerging. This therapy has taken two main forms: pharmacologic manipulation of the fetal environment via maternal medication that crosses the placenta and the exciting and challenging new frontier of fetal surgery. Perhaps the most frequently used form of in utero therapy is maternal administration of betamethasone (Celestone),[1] a corticosteroid, for the purpose of accelerating fetal lung maturity when delivery is anticipated prior to 34 weeks. The recommended dosage is 12 mg given by intramuscular injection for two doses, 24 hours apart. Maternally administered antiarrhythmics, such as digoxin, are useful in treating certain fetal cardiac arrhythmias, which, if left untreated, may lead to fetal congestive heart failure. Another striking example of in utero drug therapy is the use of dexamethasone (Decadron)[1] in pregnancies at risk for congenital adrenal hyperplasia to prevent the external genital masculinization of affected female fetuses.

When fetal anemia is suspected as a cause of fetal hydrops, such as in cases of certain congenital infections or hemolytic disease because of Rh or other maternal blood group antibodies, the fetal circulation can be accessed through percutaneous umbilical blood sampling. This allows for measurement of the fetal hematocrit as well as direct intravascular fetal transfusion. A handful of fetal treatment centers in the country use fetal surgery to treat such conditions as obstructive uropathy, congenital diaphragmatic hernia, and spina bifida.

---

[1]Not FDA approved for this indication.

Ethical Issues

As medical technology advances, it inevitably raises new questions regarding when and how to apply it in clinical practice. Ethical principles require full disclosure of the diagnosis, prognosis, and management alternatives. The wishes of the pregnant woman, who still retains autonomy, must always be respected. An even more perplexing ethical question is how to handle feto-fetal conflicts, such as in the case of twins with competing interests, when surgery or delivery of the affected twin will jeopardize the unaffected one. Such cases are optimally managed by carefully balancing these concerns and striving for the safety of both fetuses.

Considering all the facets of antepartum care just described, it is clear why physicians who care for pregnant women play a pivotal role in guiding them through this most important time.

REFERENCES

American College of Obstetricians and Gynecologists and American College of Medical Genetics: Preconception and prenatal carrier screening for cystic fibrosis: Clinical and laboratory guidelines. Washington, DC, ACOG, October 2001.

Braun L: Herb-drug interaction guide. Aust Fam Physician 2001; 30(4):357-358.

Carpenter MW, Coustan DR: Criteria for screening tests for gestational diabetes. Am J Obstet Gynecol 1982;144(7):763-773.

Connor EM, Sperling RS, Gelber R, et al: Reduction of maternal-infant transmission of human immunodeficiency virus type 1 with zidovudine treatment. Pediatric AIDS Clinical Trials Group Protocol 076 Study Group. N Engl J Med 1994;331(18):1173-1180.

Hyett J, Perdu M, Sharland G, et al: Using fetal nuchal translucency to screen for major congenital cardiac defects at 10-14 weeks of gestation: Population based cohort study. BMJ 1999;318: 81-85.

Revised ACIP recommendation for avoiding pregnancy after receiving rubella-containing vaccine. MMWR Morb Mortal Wkly Rep 2001; 50:1117.

Wald NJ, Rodeck C, Hackshaw AK, et al: First and second trimester antenatal screening for Down's syndrome: The results of the Serum, Urine, and Ultrasound Screening Study (SURUSS). J Med Screen 2003;10(2):56-104.

Ectopic Pregnancy

Method of
Gary H. Lipscomb, MD

In the United States, the incidence of ectopic pregnancies has increased dramatically during the last several decades. Commonly cited risks include prior pelvic inflammatory disease (PID), previous tubal surgery, intrauterine device (IUD) use, previous ectopic pregnancy, ovulation induction and in vitro fertilization, progestin-containing contraceptives, smoking, previous abdominal surgery, in utero diethylstilbestrol (DES) exposure, and previous induced abortion.

A high degree of suspicion is necessary for the early diagnosis of an ectopic pregnancy. Almost all ectopic pregnancies have episodes of vaginal bleeding or lower abdominal pain prior to rupture. Such patients are appropriate candidates to evaluate for ectopic pregnancy. Figure 1 illustrates

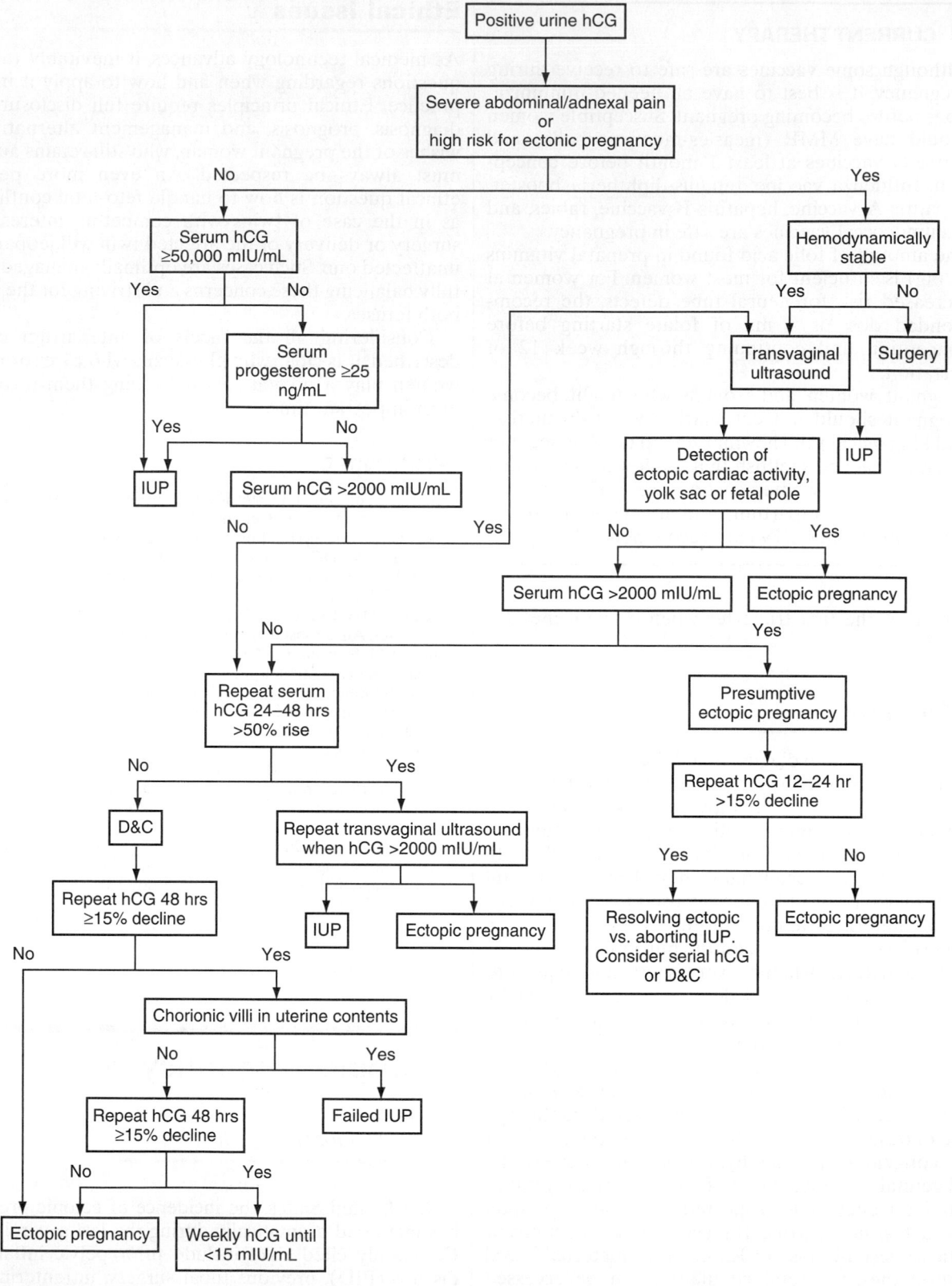

FIGURE 1. University of Tennessee Diagnostic Algorithm. D&C = dilation and curettage; hCG = human chorionic gonadotropin.

CURRENT DIAGNOSIS

- Screening for symptomatic patients or those with risk factors
- Diagnostic algorithm to coordinate testing
- hCG titers every 48 hours
- Ultrasound at hCG level of 2000 mIU/mL
- D&C for inappropriate hCG rise (<50% in 48 hours) below 2000 mIU/mL

Abbreviations: D&C = dilation and curettage; hCG = human chorionic gonadotropin.

a diagnostic algorithm that is useful in efficiently coordinating and interpreting the tests used in the diagnosis of ectopic pregnancy.

Diagnosis

Serum progesterone levels are helpful as an initial screening test for ectopic pregnancy. Levels higher than 25 ng/mL are associated with ectopic pregnancy in only 1% to 2% of cases; levels less than 5 ng/mL are associated with a nonviable pregnancy (either intrauterine or ectopic) more than 99% of the time. If progesterone levels are not readily available in a timely manner, however, human chorionic gonadotropin (hCG) levels alone may be used.

Levels of hCG rise in an essentially linear fashion until after 41 days of gestation. By this gestational age, an intrauterine pregnancy (IUP) should be seen on ultrasound. In 85% of normal pregnancies, hCG doubles approximately every 2 days, rising at least 66% in 48 hours. However, 15% of normal IUPs rise less than this in 48 hours. Conversely, 15% of ectopic pregnancies rise more than 66%. But a rise of less than 50% is associated with an abnormal pregnancy 99.9% of the time.

Because the interassay variability of hCG is 15%, a change of less than this amount is considered a plateau. Plateaued levels are the most predictive of ectopic pregnancy. The use of a urine pregnancy test to rule out the possibility of phantom hCG is strongly recommended prior to surgical or medical treatment. This phenomenon, caused by heterophilic serum antibodies, produces false-positive hCG levels usually less than 1000 IU/L.

The sonographic identification of an intrauterine gestational sac essentially excludes an ectopic pregnancy. A viable IUP should always be visualized at an hCG titer of 2000 IU/L by transvaginal scan and by 6500 IU/L with transabdominal ultrasound. An adnexal mass, in a patient with a presumed ectopic pregnancy and hCG levels less than 2000 IU/L, should not automatically be assumed to be an ectopic without the presence of a yolk sac, fetal pole, or cardiac activity. Such masses are frequently corpus luteum cysts associated with an early IUP.

Except in the rare case of heterotopic pregnancy, the identification of chorionic villi in uterine contents essentially eliminates the diagnosis of ectopic pregnancy. The use of dilation and curettage (D&C) also eliminates giving methotrexate unnecessarily to a patient with a failed IUP.

A D&C is particularly important in patients with hCG titers below the discriminatory zone of ultrasound. In these patients, the appropriate use of hCG doubling times and

serum progesterone levels is necessary to avoid interrupting a viable IUP. Patients with hCG titers that plateau (less than 15% change) or an hCG rise of less than 50% in 48 hours should undergo D&C to differentiate between a failed IUP and an ectopic pregnancy. Villi is absent on final histology in up to 50% of these cases. Because only the presence of villi is diagnostic, those without villi require serial hCG titers. While awaiting final histologic pathology, hCG titers are also followed. As noted in the ectopic algorithm, a serum hCG drawn after D&C is followed by a repeat level in 12 to 24 hours. Rising or inappropriately falling levels after D&C are considered diagnostic of an ectopic pregnancy.

Laparoscopy remains the gold standard for the diagnosis of ectopic pregnancy. It should be employed in any patient with suspected ectopic rupture, unreliable patients, or any others suspected of ectopic pregnancy for which the diagnostic algorithms are inappropriate.

Treatment

Surgery is the classic treatment for ectopic pregnancy and remains the treatment of choice in hemodynamic unstable patients, those desiring no further pregnancies, or those who are unsuitable or unwilling to risk medical therapy.

Medical therapy with methotrexate[1] is an acceptable option to surgical therapy. Reported success rates range from 75% to 96%, with an average of approximately 90%. Whether a multidose or single-dose methotrexate protocol is most effective remains debatable, but single-dose methotrexate is the most popular because of its ease of use and low incidence of side effects.

Contraindications to medical therapy remain ill defined, but Boxes 1 and 2 note frequently used contraindications.

---

[1]Not FDA approved for this indication.

CURRENT THERAPY

- Surgery: treatment of choice for unstable patients
- Methotrexate success: correlation with hCG levels
- Multidose methotrexate: 1 mg/kg body weight IM alternate days with leucovorin 0.1 mg/kg IM until hCG declines 15%
- Multidose treatment follow-up: daily hCG until decline, then weekly
- Single-dose methotrexate: 50 mg /m² based on actual body weight
- Single-dose treatment follow-up: hCG on days 1, 4, 7, then weekly if 15% decline between days 4 and 7

Abbreviations: hCG = human chorionic gonadotropin; IM = intramuscularly.

The hCG level is the single factor most predictive of failure. With hCG levels of 5000 to 9999, success rates fall to approximately 87%, further dropping to 82% for levels 10,000 to 14,999 and 68% if more than 15,000. These levels can be used to counsel patients about the risk of failure.

MULTIDOSE METHOTREXATE

Intramuscular methotrexate, 1 mg/kg of actual body weight, alternating with citrovorum rescue factor (Leucovorin), 0.1 mg/kg, is given daily and continued until a 15% decline in two consecutive daily hCG titers. Human chorionic gonadotropin levels are then followed weekly. A repeat course of methotrexate/citrovorum is given if levels fall to less than 15% or rise between two consecutive hCG titers.

SINGLE-DOSE METHOTREXATE PROTOCOL

Methotrexate, 50 mg/m² based on actual body weight, is given intramuscularly. The day methotrexate is given is considered day 1. A repeat hCG is performed on days 4 and 7. If there is an appropriate decline, hCG levels are followed weekly. If the hCG level declines less than 15% between days 4 and 7, a second dose of methotrexate is given and the protocol restarted at a new day 1. Although this protocol is referred to as "single-dose methotrexate," approximately 20% of patients require more than one treatment cycle.

In conclusion, the incidence of ectopic pregnancy has reached epidemic proportions in the United States. Nevertheless, the mortality associated with this disease is steadily declining. This decline is primarily because of earlier diagnosis that allows treatment prior to rupture This earlier diagnosis is the result of improved assays for progesterone, hCG, transvaginal ultrasound, and the use of diagnostic algorithms that do not require the use of laparoscopy. Once diagnosed, numerous treatment options are now available, including the option of medical therapy. Future developments ideally will provide for an even earlier diagnosis as well as data on the optimum candidates for each form of treatment.

REFERENCES

Brenaschek G, Rudelstorfer R, Csaicsich P: Vaginal sonography versus serum human chorionic gonadotropin in early detection of pregnancy. Am J Obstet Gynecol 1988;158:608-612.

Kadar N, Freedman M, Zacher M: Further observation on the doubling time of human chorionic gonadotropin in early asymptomatic pregnancy. Fertil Steril 1980;54:783-787.
Lipscomb GH, McCord ML, Huff G, et al: Predictors of success of methotrexate treatment in women with tubal ectopic pregnancies. N Engl J Med 1999;341:1874-1878.
Lipscomb GH, Stovall TS, Ling FW: Nonsurgical treatment of ectopic pregnancy. N Engl J Med 2000;343:1325-1329.
Stovall TS, Ling FW, Buster JE: Nonsurgical diagnosis and treatment of tubal pregnancy. Fertil Steril 1990;54:537-538.
Stovall TG, Ling FW, Gray LA, et al: Methotrexate treatment of unruptured ectopic pregnancy: A report of 100 cases. Obstet Gynecol 1991;77: 749-753.

Vaginal Bleeding in Late Pregnancy

Method of
Jami Star Zeltzer, MD

Vaginal bleeding in late pregnancy complicates approximately 6% of pregnancies and is associated with increased maternal and fetal morbidity and mortality. Excluding labor, the most likely causes are placenta previa and placental abruption, followed by uterine rupture and vasa previa; less common etiologies include trauma, cervical lesions, and coagulopathy. The primary focus in obstetric hemorrhage, regardless of cause, is maternal hemodynamic assessment and stabilization. Given the extraordinary blood flow to the uterus at term (600 to 800 mL/min), exsanguination can occur rapidly. Additionally, redistribution of maternal blood flow may lead to fetal hypoxia.

Early maternal signs of hemodynamic compromise include tachycardia and tachypnea; later, hypotension, weakened pulses, and oliguria ensue, along with evidence of fetal compromise. Further decompensation can ultimately result in the death of both mother and fetus. Guidelines for restoration of maternal circulating volume are approximately 3 mL of intravenous crystalloid, (i.e., normal saline or Ringer's solution) per 1 mL of blood lost (often underestimated). Laboratory evaluation includes a complete blood count, blood type, and crossmatch; in the setting of thrombocytopenia (less than 100,000 platelets), coagulation studies (prothrombin time [PT], partial thromboplastin time [PTT], fibrinogen, fibrin degradation products [FDPs]) are recommended. Packed red blood cells, fresh-frozen plasma, platelets, and/or cryoprecipitate are given to maintain maternal hemoglobin near 10 g/dL and correct coagulopathy (unlikely if whole blood is observed to clot in less than 8 minutes). Additional measures include administration of oxygen, lateral displacement of the uterus and, rarely, vasopressors. Fetal evaluation and treatment, including consideration of delivery, follow stabilization of the mother.

Placenta Previa

Placenta previa, or the implantation of the placenta adjacent to or covering the internal os, complicates approximately 0.5% of all deliveries. The degree of placenta previa may be:

- Complete (internal os covered entirely)
- Partial (portion of internal os covered)
- Marginal (placental edge at cervix or less than 2 cm away)
- Low lying (not a true previa, where the placental edge implants in the lower uterine segment but doesn't reach the cervix)

Box 1 lists the risk factors. The pathophysiology appears to involve endometrial damage, with resulting limitation of healthy uterine tissue for implantation.

The hallmark symptom is painless vaginal bleeding, presumably initiated by development of the lower uterine segment. Usually, this occurs by 29 to 30 weeks of gestation, although in approximately 33% of cases, there is no bleeding until labor. The first bleed may be self-limited, but rebleeding complicates approximately 60% of cases. The diagnosis is often made in the absence of symptoms on routine ultrasound. The incidence of placenta previa is 5% to 10% in mid-gestation; this resolves in most cases with development of the lower uterine segment (*placental migration*). When asymptomatic, expectant management is appropriate, although vaginal precautions after 28 weeks' gestation may be advised.

When a patient presents with third-trimester bleeding, speculum exams are contraindicated until placenta previa is ruled out. The most accurate method of diagnosis is transvaginal ultrasound, which is safe in experienced hands; transperineal or transabdominal ultrasound carry greater risks of false-positive and false-negative results.

Observation in the hospital is recommended following a bleed, during which time approximately 50% of patients will deliver. Steroids are indicated for enhancement of fetal lung maturation. Tocolysis can be administered if the mother and fetus are stable, preferably with magnesium sulfate to minimize cardiovascular effects. Outpatient management is acceptable if bleeding ceases, as long as the patient is compliant and has ready access to a hospital. Serial ultrasound assessment is recommended because there is an increased risk of intrauterine growth restriction. Transfusion should be offered to maintain hemoglobin greater than 10 mg/dL.

Urgent delivery by cesarean section is indicated when there is ongoing maternal hemorrhage or evidence of fetal compromise. In the stable patient, a planned cesarean section can be performed at 35 to 36 weeks, generally after an amniocentesis is performed to confirm fetal lung maturity. Vaginal delivery is preferable in the setting of fetal demise; it may be attempted if delivery is imminent, or

with marginal previa, although a *double setup* for emergent cesarean section is advised.

Placenta previa predisposes to postpartum hemorrhage, either from atony of the lower uterine segment or inability to remove the placenta because of absence of the decidua basalis. The most common form of this latter condition is placenta accreta, where the trophoblast adheres to the myometrium. Less common forms include placenta increta (the trophoblast invades the myometrium) and placenta percreta (trophoblast invades uterine serosa and/or adjacent organs). The primary risk factor for placenta accreta is the number of previous cesarean sections, with an incidence approaching 40% in patients with two prior cesarean sections and a placenta previa. Other risk factors include age, parity, and history of curettage. Color Doppler ultrasound and magnetic resonance imaging (MRI) are helpful but not always definitive for diagnosis. If placenta accreta is suspected, preparations can be made for scheduled delivery with trained personnel and blood products available. At delivery, the placenta should be left in place if a cleavage plane cannot be developed easily. Cesarean–hysterectomy is often required for hemostasis, although conservative management, including preoperative and intraoperative selective embolization and/or use of methotrexate, has been reported. With placenta percreta, bladder invasion may require cystoscopy and urologic repair.

Vasa Previa

Vasa previa is a rare condition (estimated 1 in 2500 deliveries) in which fetal blood vessels cross over the membranes in advance of the presenting part. This is most often associated with velamentous insertion of the umbilical cord (vessels reach the placenta after coursing through the membranes rather than by direct insertion); Box 2 lists the risk factors. Vasa previa carries a profound risk of fetal mortality from exsanguination, particularly at the time of membrane rupture (fetal blood volume at term is approximately 250 mL). Even in the absence of bleeding, vessel compression may result in compromise of the fetal circulation.

Signs include hemorrhage, as well as fetal heart rate abnormalities. A high index of suspicion is required, and advances in imaging techniques (color Doppler, transvaginal ultrasound) make prenatal diagnosis possible. If there is unexplained bleeding, an Apt test or Kleihauer-Betke test can identify fetal red blood cells. If the diagnosis of vasa previa is strongly suspected at term, or if hemorrhage is significant, prompt cesarean delivery is recommended, followed by neonatal resuscitation.

Uterine Rupture

Most often reported following prior cesarean section, uterine rupture can also occur in an unscarred uterus (1 in 8000 to 1 in 15,000 deliveries). This phenomenon implies complete separation of the uterine wall (as compared to uterine dehiscence), with or without expulsion of the fetus. Box 3 lists risk factors and differential diagnoses.

Common signs and symptoms include abdominal pain/tenderness and vaginal bleeding; additional complaints include epigastric or shoulder pain, abdominal distention, and constipation. The fetal tracing may show sudden variable decelerations or abrupt and prolonged bradycardia, often accompanied by recession of the presenting part. Maternal and fetal morbidity and mortality are high, particularly with delayed diagnosis. Treatment is urgent cesarean delivery, with repair of the uterus and/or hysterectomy as needed. Repeat cesarean section is advised in the future because of the risk for recurrence.

Placental Abruption

Abruption of the placenta, or separation of the normally implanted placenta before birth, complicates 1% to 2% of pregnancies. Bleeding into the decidua basalis, with subsequent separation of varying amounts of placental tissue from the endometrium, may result in fetal compromise and/or demise. The exact pathophysiology is unclear. Box 4 lists the risk factors.

Vaginal bleeding in the second half of pregnancy is assumed to be caused by placental abruption, once placenta previa and other rare causes are ruled out. Concealed hemorrhage, present in 10% to 20% of cases, can complicate the diagnosis. Abdominal pain, back pain, uterine contractions (often described as low amplitude, high frequency), hypertonus, uterine tenderness, and/or idiopathic premature labor may be present. While ultrasound can identify placenta previa, it cannot be relied upon to definitively diagnose abruption, as clot is sonographically visible in less than 50% of cases. The differential diagnoses include uterine rupture, appendicitis, and chorioamnionitis, as well as other causes of abdominal pain.

Most commonly, bleeding is not profuse and, if the episode is self-limited, expectant management of a preterm gestation includes observation, serial fetal growth assessment, fetal well-being testing, and steroid therapy to accelerate fetal lung maturation. With ongoing significant blood loss, stabilization of the mother, fetal assessment, and laboratory evaluation are indicated. Coagulopathy is rare in the absence of fetal demise. If tocolysis is required, magnesium sulfate is preferred, as β-sympathomimetics may mask maternal cardiovascular decompensation.

Vaginal delivery is appropriate if mother and fetus are stable. Amniotomy may decrease extravasation of blood into the myometrium by head compression. Not uncommonly, effacement will precede dilatation; oxytocin (Pitocin) is acceptable for labor dysfunction. In the event of an intrauterine demise, vaginal delivery is preferred. Acute hemorrhage requires immediate cesarean delivery, with blood and coagulation factor replacement as needed.

Potential complications of abruption include hemorrhagic shock, disseminated intravascular coagulation (unlikely unless there is greater than 2000 mL blood loss and/or fetal demise), ischemic necrosis of maternal organs (especially kidney), and Couvelaire uterus (extravasation of blood into uterine muscle). Recurrence is approximately 5% to 15%, increasing with each subsequent event. There are no known preventive measures other than correcting modifiable risk factors.

Hypertensive Disorders of Pregnancy

Method of
David G. Weismiller, MD

Hypertension is the most common medical disorder during pregnancy. It occurs in 6% to 8% of pregnancies and contributes significantly to stillbirths and to neonatal morbidity and mortality. Hypertensive disorders during pregnancy are the second leading cause of maternal mortality in the United States after thromboembolism, accounting for almost 15% of such deaths. For this reason, strategies to diagnose, prevent, treat, and reduce the risk for hypertensive disorders of pregnancy receive considerable attention.

Classification of the Hypertensive Disorders of Pregnancy

The most important factor to consider in classifying disease in which blood pressure rises abnormally in pregnancy is whether the hypertensive disorder antedates the pregnancy or whether it is a potentially more ominous disease peculiar to pregnancy: preeclampsia. Elevated blood pressure is the cardinal pathophysiologic feature in chronic hypertension, whereas in preeclampsia, increased blood pressure is important primarily because it signals the underlying disorder and is a potential cause of maternal morbidity.

According to the National High Blood Pressure Education Program, increased blood pressure in pregnancy is divided into four main categories:

- Preeclampsia-eclampsia
- Chronic hypertension
- Preeclampsia superimposed on chronic hypertension
- Gestational hypertension (transient or chronic)

PREECLAMPSIA-ECLAMPSIA

Preeclampsia-eclampsia usually occurs after 20 weeks of gestation. The rate of preeclampsia ranges from 2% to 7% in healthy nulliparous women and is substantially higher in women with twin gestation (14%) and those with previous preeclampsia (18%). The disorder may occur earlier with trophoblastic diseases such as hydatidiform mole or hydrops. Preeclampsia is determined by increased blood pressure accompanied by proteinuria in a woman who is normotensive before 20 weeks (Box 1). The finding of proteinuria usually correlates with 30 mg/dL (1+ dipstick) or greater in a random urine determination with no evidence of urinary tract infection. Because of the discrepancy between random protein determinations and 24-hour urine protein in preeclampsia (which may be either higher or lower), it is recommended that the diagnosis be based on a 24-hour urine, if at all possible, or a timed collection corrected for creatinine excretion, if a 24-hour urine is not feasible.

In the absence of proteinuria, preeclampsia is highly suspect when increased blood pressure is accompanied by the symptoms of headache, blurred vision, and abdominal pain or when it is accompanied by abnormal laboratory tests, specifically low platelet counts and abnormal liver enzymes. Diastolic blood pressure is determined by the disappearance of sound (Korotkoff 5). Gestational blood pressure elevation should be defined on the basis of at least two determinations. No randomized controlled trial evidence supports the use of ambulatory blood pressure monitoring during pregnancy.

In the past, an increase of 30 mm Hg systolic or 15 mm Hg diastolic blood pressure was used as a diagnostic criterion in preeclampsia, even when absolute values were below 140/90 mm Hg. But this diagnostic criterion is not included in the classification criteria set forth by the National High Blood Pressure Education Program. The only available evidence demonstrates that women in this group are not likely to suffer increased adverse outcomes. Still, some experts believe that women who have a rise of 30 mm Hg systolic or 15 mm Hg diastolic blood pressure warrant close observation, especially if proteinuria and hyperuricemia of 6 mg/dL or more are also present. Edema is also removed as a marker in hypertension schemes because it occurs in too many normal pregnant women to be discriminant.

Eclampsia is the occurrence of seizures that cannot be attributed to other causes in a woman with preeclampsia. Up to 40% of eclamptic seizures occur before delivery. Approximately 16% occur more than 48 hours after delivery.

Preeclampsia always presents potential danger to the mother and the fetus. As the certainty of the diagnosis of preeclampsia increases, the requirements for careful assessment and consideration for delivery also increase (Table 1).

CHRONIC HYPERTENSION

Chronic hypertension is defined as hypertension that is present and observable before week 20 of gestation, with hypertension defined as a blood pressure of 140 mm Hg systolic or 90 mm Hg diastolic or greater. Hypertension diagnosed for the first time during pregnancy that does not resolve postpartum is also classified as chronic hypertension.

BOX 1 Criteria for Diagnosis of Preeclampsia

- Blood pressure of 140 mm Hg systolic or higher or 90 mm Hg diastolic or higher that occurs after 20 weeks of gestation in a woman with previously normal blood pressure.
- Proteinuria, defined as urinary excretion of 0.3 g protein or higher in a 24-hour urine specimen.

TABLE 1 Findings That Increase Certainty of Diagnosis of Preeclampsia Syndrome

Findings	Value
Blood pressure	160 mm Hg or more systolic or 110 mm Hg or more diastolic.
Proteinuria	2.0 g or more in a 24-hour urine collection (2^+ or 3^+ g on qualitative examination). The proteinuria should occur for the first time in pregnancy and regress after delivery.
Serum creatinine	Greater than 1.2 mg/dL unless known to be previously elevated.
Platelet count	Less than 100,000 cells/mm^3 and/or evidence of microangiopathic hemolytic anemia (with increased lactic acid dehydrogenase).
Hepatic enzymes	Elevated ALT or AST.
Central nervous system	Persistent headache or other cerebral or visual disturbances.
Abdomen	Persistent epigastric pain.

Abbreviations: ALT = alanine aminotransferase; AST = aspartate aminotransferase.

TABLE 2   Findings That Increase Certainty of Diagnosis of Preeclampsia Superimposed Upon Chronic Hypertension

Finding	Value
Proteinuria	New-onset proteinuria (in women with hypertension and no proteinuria prior to 20 weeks' gestation) defined as the urinary excretion of 300 mg protein or greater in a 24-hour specimen or in women with hypertension and proteinuria before 20 weeks' gestation or sudden increase in proteinuria
Blood pressure	Sudden increase in blood pressure in a woman whose hypertension has been previously well controlled
Platelet count	Thrombocytopenia with a platelet count of less than 100,000 cells/mm^3
Hepatic enzymes	Increase in ALT or AST to abnormal levels

Abbreviations: ALT = alanine aminotransferase; AST = aspartate aminotransferase.

BOX 2   Risk Factors for Preeclampsia

Pregnancy-Associated Factors
- Chromosomal abnormalities
- Hydatidiform mole
- Hydrops fetalis
- Multifetal pregnancy
- Oocyte denotation or donor insemination
- Structural congenital abnormalities
- Urinary tract infection

Maternal-Specific Factors
- Age greater than 35 years
- Age less than 20 years
- Black race
- Family history of preeclampsia
- Nulliparity
- Preeclampsia in a previous pregnancy
- Specific medical conditions: gestational diabetes mellitus, type I diabetes, obesity, chronic hypertension, renal disease, thrombophilias
- Stress

Paternal-Specific Factors
- First-time father
- Previously fathered a preeclamptic pregnancy in another woman

SUPERIMPOSED PREECLAMPSIA

Superimposed preeclampsia complicates almost 25% of pregnancies in women with chronic hypertension. The prognosis for mother and fetus is worse than with either condition alone. The incidence of superimposed preeclampsia is even higher in women who have underlying renal insufficiency, chronic hypertension that has been present 4 or more years, or who have had a hypertensive disorder complicate a previous pregnancy. Distinguishing superimposed preeclampsia from worsening chronic hypertension is a challenge (Table 2).

GESTATIONAL HYPERTENSION

Gestational hypertension refers to blood pressure elevation without proteinuria that is detected for the first time after midpregnancy. The hypertension may be accompanied by other signs of the preeclampsia syndrome, which impacts management. The final determination that the woman does not have the preeclampsia syndrome is made retrospectively postpartum. Gestational hypertension is subdivided into two types. If preeclampsia has not developed and blood pressure has returned to normal by 12 weeks postpartum, the diagnosis of transient hypertension of pregnancy is assigned. If the blood pressure elevation persists, the woman is diagnosed as having chronic hypertension.

Pathophysiology of Preeclampsia

Preeclampsia is a syndrome with well-defined maternal and fetal manifestations. The maternal disease is characterized by vasospasm, activation of the coagulation system, and derangement in many humoral and autacoid systems that are associated with volume and blood pressure control. Oxidative stress and inflammatory-like responses may also be important in the pathophysiology of this syndrome.

The pathologic changes are primarily ischemic in nature and affect the placenta, brain, liver, and kidney. Several of the so-called nonhypertensive complications can be life-threatening, even in the face of otherwise mild blood pressure elevations. Risk factors for preeclampsia are related to medical conditions, such as antiphospholipid antibody syndrome and nephropathy, or they may be related to the pregnancy itself or may be specific to the mother or father of the fetus (Box 2).

The etiology of most cases of hypertension during pregnancy, particularly preeclampsia, remains unknown. Many consider the placenta the pathogenic focus for all manifestations of preeclampsia because delivery is the only definitive cure of the disease. Much research centers on the changes in the maternal blood vessels that supply blood to the placenta. Discoveries on how alterations in the immune response at the maternal interface might lead to preeclampsia address the link between placental and maternal disease. A nonclassical human leukocyte antigen (HLA), HLA G is expressed in normal placental tissue and may play a role in modulating the maternal immune response to the immunologically foreign placenta. Additional evidence for alterations in immunity in pathogenesis includes the disease's prominence in nulliparous gestations with subsequent normal pregnancies, a decreased prevalence after heterologous blood transfusions, long cohabitation before successful conception, and observed pathologic changes in the placental vasculature in preeclampsia that resemble allograft rejection.

BLOOD PRESSURE CHANGES

Women with preeclampsia typically do not develop frank hypertension until the second half of gestation, but vasoconstrictor influences may be present earlier. Alterations in vascular reactivity may be detected by gestational week 20, and numerous surveys suggest that women destined to develop preeclampsia have slightly higher "normal" blood pressure (e.g., diastolic levels more than 70 mm Hg) as early as the second trimester, confirmed by ambulatory blood pressure monitoring techniques. Blood pressure normalizes postpartum, usually within the first few days of the puerperium, but may take as long as 2 to 4 weeks, especially in severe cases.

CARDIAC CHANGES

Typically the heart is not affected in preeclampsia. The decrements in cardiac performance represent a normally contracting ventricle against a markedly increased afterload.

RENAL CHANGES

The renal lesion characteristic of preeclampsia is termed *glomerular endotheliosis*. The glomeruli become enlarged and swollen. Both glomerular filtration rate and renal blood flow decrease in preeclampsia, leading to a decrease in filtration fraction. Because renal function normally rises 35% to 50% during pregnancy, creatinine levels in women with preeclampsia may still be below the upper limits of normal for pregnancy (0.8 mg/dL). Fractional urate clearance decreases, producing hyperuricemia. Although an elevated serum uric acid level (6.0 mg/dL) represents a useful confirmatory test for the diagnosis of preeclampsia, it has very poor predictive value among patients without preexisting hypertension. But when the patient has chronic hypertension, the serum uric acid level may be of some value. One investigator has reported that a serum uric acid level of 5.5 mg/dL or greater could identify women with an increased likelihood of having superimposed preeclampsia, which is an important marker of preeclampsia. Proteinuria may appear late in the clinical course and tends to be nonselective. Preeclampsia is associated with hypocalciuria, in contrast with the increased urinary calcium excretion observed during normal pregnancy. Even when edema is marked, plasma volume is lower than that of normal gestation, and there is evidence of hemoconcentration, believed to be caused, in part, by extravasation of albumin into the interstitium. Oliguria, commonly defined as less than 500 mL in 24 hours, also may occur, secondary to the hemoconcentration and decreased renal blood flow.

COAGULATION SYSTEM CHANGES

Thrombocytopenia is the most common hematologic abnormality in preeclampsia. Circulating fibrin degradation products occasionally may be elevated, and unless the disease is accompanied by placental abruption, plasma fibrinogen levels are unaffected. Platelet counts below 100,000 cells/mm³ signal serious disease, and if delivery is delayed, levels may continue to fall precipitously. The cause of thrombocytopenia is unclear.

HEPATIC CHANGES

Liver damage accompanying preeclampsia may range from mild hepatocellular necrosis with serum enzyme abnormalities (aminotransferase and lactate dehydrogenase) to the ominous hemolysis, elevated liver enzymes, and low platelet count (HELLP) syndrome, with markedly elevated enzyme levels and even subcapsular bleeding or hepatic rupture. HELLP represents serious disease and is associated with significant maternal morbidity. A disproportionate elevation of lactate dehydrogenase (LDH) levels in serum may be a sign of hemolysis.

CENTRAL NERVOUS SYSTEM CHANGES

Eclampsia is the convulsive phase of preeclampsia and remains a significant cause of maternal mortality. Other central nervous system manifestations are headache and visual disturbances, including blurred vision, scotomata, and, rarely, cortical blindness. Focal neurologic signs occasionally develop, which should prompt radiologic investigation.

Clinical Considerations

Expectant mothers with hypertension are predisposed to the development of potentially lethal complications, notably abruptio placentae, disseminated intravascular coagulation, cerebral hemorrhage, hepatic failure, and acute renal failure. The clinical spectrum of preeclampsia ranges from mild to severe forms. In most women, progression through this spectrum is slow, and the disorder may never proceed beyond mild preeclampsia. In others, the disease progresses more rapidly, changing from mild to severe in days or weeks. In the most serious cases, progression may be rapid and fulminant, with mild disease progressing to severe preeclampsia or eclampsia.

DIAGNOSIS

Decisions regarding hospitalization and delivery that have significant impact on maternal and fetal health are often based on whether the patient is believed to have preeclampsia or a more benign hypertensive disorder of pregnancy, such as chronic or gestational hypertension.

The period in gestation when hypertension is first documented is helpful to consider in determining the correct diagnosis. Documentation of hypertension before conception, or before gestational week 20, favors a diagnosis of chronic hypertension (either essential or secondary). High blood pressure presenting at midpregnancy (weeks 20 to 28) may be caused by early preeclampsia (rare before 24 weeks), transient hypertension, or unrecognized chronic hypertension. Blood pressure normally falls in the initial trimesters, and this physiologic decrement may even be exaggerated in patients with essential hypertension, masking the diagnosis in pregnancy. Hypertension may be noted later in pregnancy, however, as part of the normal third trimester rise in blood pressure or when superimposed preeclampsia occurs.

LABORATORY EVALUATION

Laboratory tests recommended to diagnose or manage hypertension in pregnancy serve primarily to distinguish preeclampsia from either chronic or transient hypertension. They are also useful in assessing the severity of disease, particularly in the case of preeclampsia, which is usually associated with laboratory abnormalities that deviate significantly from those of normal pregnant women.

The same measurements are usually normal in women with uncomplicated chronic or transient hypertension. Efforts to identify an ideal screening or predictive test for preeclampsia are not successful to date. At present, no single screening test is considered reliable and cost effective for predicting preeclampsia. Numerous clinical, biophysical, and biochemical tests are proposed for the prediction or early detection of preeclampsia. Most of these tests suffer from poor sensitivity and poor predictive values, although this situation may be changing. Low levels of placental growth factor (PGF) predict subsequent development of preeclampsia. Decreased urinary PGF at mid-gestation is strongly associated with subsequent early development of preeclampsia.

The laboratory evaluation of hypertensive disorders can be approached by classifying women into one of three categories:

1. High-risk patients presenting with normal blood pressure
2. Patients presenting with hypertension before gestation week 20
3. Patients presenting with hypertension after midpregnancy

High-Risk Patients Presenting With Normal Blood Pressure

Pregnant women whose gestations are considered high risk for preeclampsia benefit from a database of laboratory tests performed in early gestation. Those who are at high risk for preeclampsia include women who have a history of high blood pressure before conception or in a previous gestation (especially before week 34); women with diabetes, collagen vascular disease, underlying renal vascular disease, or renal parenchymal disease; and women with a multifetal pregnancy.

Tests that by later comparison assist in establishing an early diagnosis of preeclampsia (pure or superimposed) include hematocrit and platelet count as well as serum creatinine and uric acid levels. Observation of 1+ protein by routine urine analysis, documented by a clean-catch specimen, should be followed by a 24-hour collection for measurement of protein, as well as creatinine content, to determine accuracy of collection and to permit calculation of the creatinine clearance. High-risk patients require accurate dating and assessment of fetal growth. If circumstances are not optimal for clinical dating, sonographic dates should be established as early in the pregnancy as possible. A baseline sonogram for evaluating fetal growth should be considered at 25 to 28 weeks in these circumstances.

Patients Presenting With Hypertension Before Gestation Week 20

Most women presenting with hypertension before gestation week 20 have (or will develop) essential hypertension. Women with hypertension should be evaluated before pregnancy to define the severity of their hypertension and to plan for potential lifestyle changes that a pregnancy may require. As recommended by the Joint National Committee on Prevention, Detection, Evaluation, and Treatment of High Blood Pressure (JNC VII Report), the diagnosis should be confirmed by multiple measurements and may

TABLE 3 Laboratory Evaluation and Rationale for Women Who Develop Hypertension After Midpregnancy

Test	Rationale
Hemoglobin or hematocrit	Hemoconcentration supports the diagnosis of preeclampsia, and it is an indicator of severity. Note that values may be decreased if hemolysis accompanies the syndrome.
Platelet count	Thrombocytopenia suggests severe preeclampsia.
Quantification of protein excretion	Gestational hypertension with proteinuria should be considered preeclampsia (pure or superimposed), until it is proved otherwise.
Serum creatinine level	Abnormal or rising serum creatinine levels, especially in association with oliguria, suggest severe preeclampsia.
Serum uric acid level	Increased serum uric acid levels suggest the diagnosis of preeclampsia (>6.0 mg/dL).
Serum transaminase levels	Rising serum transaminase values suggest severe preeclampsia with hepatic involvement.
Serum albumin, lactic acid dehydrogenase, blood smear, and coagulation profile	For women with severe disease, these values indicate the extent of endothelial leak (hypoalbuminemia), presence of hemolysis (lactic acid-dehydrogenase level increase, schizocytosis, spherocytosis), and possible coagulopathy, including thrombocytopenia.

incorporate home or other out-of-office blood pressure readings. If hypertension is confirmed, and particularly if it is severe (stage 3, systolic pressure of 180 mm Hg or more and diastolic pressure of 110 mm Hg or more), a woman should be evaluated for potentially reversible causes.

Patients Presenting With Hypertension After Midpregnancy

Table 3 summarizes the recommended laboratory tests in the evaluation of women with hypertension after midpregnancy and the rationale for testing them biweekly or more often, if clinical circumstances lead to hospitalization of the patient. Such tests help distinguish preeclampsia from chronic and transient hypertension and are useful in assessing disease progression and severity. Note that in women with preeclampsia, one or more laboratory abnormalities may be present, even when blood pressure elevation is minimal.

Prevention of Preeclampsia

Preventing preeclampsia is a challenge because of the limited knowledge of its etiology. During the past two decades, numerous clinical reports and randomized trials

TABLE 4 Effectiveness of Agents in Prevention of Preeclampsia

Agent	Prevention
Low-dose aspirin prophylaxis	Minimal to no reduction in the incidence of preeclampsia. The prevailing opinion is that women without risk factors do not benefit from treatment. Overall, administration of low-dose aspirin to women at risk leads to a 19% reduction in the risk of developing preeclampsia. On average, for every 69 women treated, 1 case is prevented. Starting aspirin before 12 weeks and/or using higher doses cannot be recommended for clinical practice until more information is available about safety. As the reductions in risk are small to moderate, relatively large numbers of women need to be treated to prevent a single adverse outcome.
Calcium supplementation	No data indicate that dietary supplementation with calcium prevents preeclampsia in low-risk women in the United States. Randomized trials of calcium supplementation in women considered at high risk of gestational hypertension (teenagers, previous preeclampsia, women with increased sensitivity to angiotensin II, preexisting hypertension) and in communities with low dietary calcium intake (mean intake equals 900 mg per day) demonstrate significant reductions in incidence of preeclampsia.
Magnesium supplementation	Prophylactic magnesium is not beneficial in preventing preeclampsia.
Zinc supplementation	No benefit in preventing preeclampsia.
Fish oil supplementation	No reduction in the incidence of preeclampsia.
Antioxidant therapy (vitamin C[1] and vitamin E[1])	Limited data show some promise in preventing preeclampsia.
Salt restriction	No benefit in preventing preeclampsia.
Diuretic therapy[1]	No benefit in preventing preeclampsia.

[1]Not FDA approved for the indication.

described the use of various methods to reduce the rate and/or severity of preeclampsia. Table 4 summarizes current opinion and data on the prevention of preeclampsia. Prevention focuses on identifying women at higher risk and conducting close clinical and laboratory monitoring, to recognize the disease process in its early stages. Although these measures do not prevent preeclampsia, they may be helpful for preventing some adverse maternal and fetal sequelae.

Management of Hypertensive Disorders of Pregnancy

Three factors underlie any management scheme in hypertension and pregnancy. First, delivery is always appropriate therapy for the mother but may not be for the fetus. Second, the pathophysiologic changes of severe preeclampsia indicate that poor perfusion is the major factor leading to maternal physiologic derangement and increased perinatal morbidity and mortality. Third, the pathogenic changes of preeclampsia are present long before clinical diagnostic criteria are manifest.

For maternal health, the goal of therapy is to prevent eclampsia as well as other severe complications of preeclampsia. If there is a rationale for management other than delivery, it is to palliate the maternal condition to allow fetal maturation and cervical ripening.

ANTICONVULSIVE THERAPY

Anticonvulsive therapy is usually indicated either to prevent recurrent convulsions in women with eclampsia or to prevent convulsions in women with preeclampsia. There is universal consensus that women with eclampsia should receive anticonvulsive therapy. Several randomized studies indicate that parenteral magnesium sulfate reduces the frequency of eclampsia more effectively than phenytoin (Dilantin). Parenteral magnesium sulfate is given during labor and delivery and for variable durations postpartum. There is no clear agreement concerning the use of prophylactic magnesium for women with preeclampsia. Although parenteral magnesium sulfate should be given peripartum to women with severe preeclampsia, its benefits with mild gestational hypertension or preeclampsia remain unclear.

Women with eclampsia require prompt intervention. When an eclamptic seizure occurs, the woman should be medically stabilized. First, it is important to control convulsions and prevent their recurrence with intravenous or intramuscular magnesium sulfate. One protocol is a 4- to 6-g loading dose diluted in 100 mL fluid and administered intravenously for 15 to 20 minutes, followed by 2 g per hour as a continuous intravenous infusion.

ANTIHYPERTENSIVE THERAPY

Therapy in Acute Hypertension

Antihypertensive therapy is indicated when blood pressure is dangerously high or rises suddenly in women with preeclampsia, especially intrapartum. Pharmacologic treatment with antihypertensives can be withheld as long as maternal pressure is only mildly elevated. Some experts treat persistent diastolic blood pressure of 105 mm Hg

TABLE 5 Medications to Treat Acute Severe Hypertensive Crises in Pregnancy

	Route of Dose	Pharmacologic Agent	Administration Notes
Arterial vasodilator (hydralazine: e.g., Apresoline)	IV or IM	5 mg over 1-2 min	After 20 min, subsequent doses are dictated by initial response; once desired response, repeat as necessary (usually 3 h)
β-Blockers (labetalol: e.g., Normodyne or Trandate)	IV	20-40 mg bolus or 1 mg/kg infusion (max 220 mg)	If effect is suboptimal to initial 20 mg IV, give 40 mg 10 min later and 80 mg every 10 min for additional two doses. Avoid in women with asthma and in those with congestive heart failure (CHF).
Calcium antagonists (nifedipine: e.g., Adalat, Procardia)	PO	10 mg PO and repeat in 30 min, if necessary	The JNC VII recommends rapidly acting nifedipine not be used for treating hypertension or hypertensive emergencies.
Sodium nitroprusside (Nipride)	IV	0.25 µg/kg/min to a maximum of 5 µg/kg/min	After failure of hydralazine, nifedipine, and labetalol. Fetal cyanide poisoning may occur if used more than 4 h.

Abbreviations: IM = intramuscularly; IV = intravenously; JNC VII = Joint National Committee on Prevention, Detection, Evaluation, and Treatment of High Blood Pressure; PO = by mouth.

or above. Others withhold treatment until the diastolic blood pressure reaches 110 mm Hg. Table 5 summarizes the medications used to treat acute elevations in blood pressure. The goal of blood pressure reduction in emergency situations should be a gradual reduction to the normal range.

Therapy in Chronic Hypertension

The role of antihypertensive therapy for pregnant women with mild to moderate chronic hypertension (stage 1 or 2 hypertension, defined as systolic blood pressure of 140 to 179 mm Hg or diastolic blood pressure of 90 to 109) is unclear. Among women with stage 1 to 2 preexisting essential hypertension and normal renal function, most pregnancies have good maternal and neonatal outcomes. Because there is no immediate need to lower blood pressure, the rationale for treatment is that it will prevent or delay progression to more severe disease, thereby benefiting the woman and/or her infant and reducing consumption of health service resources. In addition to reducing blood pressure, these drugs are believed to reduce the risk of preterm delivery and placental abruption and improve fetal growth. A wide variety of drugs are advocated, and each group has different potential side affects and adverse effects (Table 6). More importantly, these women are candidates for nonpharmacologic therapy because to date no evidence indicates that pharmacologic treatment results in improved neonatal outcomes. Because blood pressure usually falls during the first half of pregnancy, hypertension may be easier to control with less or no medication.

The value of continued administration of antihypertensive medications to pregnant women with chronic hypertension continues to be debatable. Although it may be beneficial for the mother with hypertension to reduce her blood pressure, lower pressure may impair uteroplacental perfusion and thereby interfere with fetal development. On the basis of available data, some centers currently manage women with chronic hypertension by stopping antihypertensive medications under close observation. In patients who have had hypertension for several years, show evidence of target organ damage, or take multiple antihypertensive agents, medications may be tapered on the basis of blood pressure readings, but medications should be continued if they are needed to control blood pressure. The end point for reinstituting treatment includes exceeding threshold blood pressure levels of 150 to 160 mm Hg systolic or 100 to 110 mm Hg diastolic or the presence of target organ damage. Methyldopa (Aldomet) is preferred by most practitioners. Women who are well controlled on antihypertensive therapy before pregnancy may be kept on the same agents during pregnancy, with the exception of angiotensin-converting enzyme inhibitors and angiotensin II receptor antagonists.

For women with severe hypertension (stage 3 hypertension, usually defined as 160 to 170 mm Hg or more systolic blood pressure or 110 mm Hg or more diastolic blood pressure), there is a risk of direct arterial damage, so antihypertensive medications are indicated to lower blood pressure (see Table 6). The most effective antihypertensive drug is unclear.

Fetal Assessment

FETAL ASSESSMENT IN PREECLAMPSIA

Nonstress testing (NST), ultrasound assessment of fetal activity and amniotic fluid volume (biophysical profile [BPP]), and fetal movement counts constitute the most common fetal surveillance techniques. Although weekly to biweekly assessment usually suffices, daily testing is appropriate for women with severe preeclampsia who are being managed expectantly. If fetal surveillance (nonreactive NST, oligohydramnios, nonreassuring BPP) indicates possible fetal compromise, the decision to deliver must be significantly weighted by fetal age (Box 3).

FETAL ASSESSMENT IN CHRONIC HYPERTENSION

Much of the increased perinatal morbidity and mortality associated with chronic hypertension can be attributed to superimposed preeclampsia and/or fetal growth restriction.

TABLE 6 Antihypertensive Drug Selection

Drug	Example	Usual Dose Range in mg/day (Daily Frequency)	Notes
Central α_2-agonists	Methyldopa (e.g., Aldomet)	250-1000 (2)	First-line therapy on the basis of reports of stable uteroplacental blood flow and fetal hemodynamics.
β-Blockers	Labetalol (e.g., Normodyne, Trandate)	200-800 (2)	There is a suggestion that β-blockers prescribed early in pregnancy, specifically atenolol (Tenormin), may be associated with growth restriction. None of these agents are associated to date with any consistent ill effect.
Calcium antagonists	Nifedipine long-acting (e.g., Adalat CC, Procardia XL)	30-60 (1)	Experience is limited, with most reported uses late in pregnancy.
Diuretic	Hydrochlorothiazide (e.g., HydroDIURIL)	12.5-50 mg (1)	Use is controversial; however, if their use is indicated, they are safe and efficacious agents; they can markedly potentiate the response to other antihypertensive agents, and they are not contraindicated, except in settings where uteroplacental perfusion is already reduced (preeclampsia and IUGR).
ACE inhibitors	Captopril (e.g., Capoten)	Contraindicated	Contraindicated because of association with fetal growth restriction, oligohydramnios, neonatal renal failure, and neonatal death. Fetal risks with ACE inhibitors depend on timing and dose.
Angiotensin II receptor antagonists	Losartan (e.g., Cozaar)	Contraindicated	Data are limited. Adverse effects likely to be similar to those reported with ACE inhibitors, and these agents should be avoided.

Abbreviations: ACE = angiotensin-converting enzyme; IUGR = intrauterine growth retardation.

1187

A plan of antepartum fetal assessment is directed by these findings. Thus efforts should be directed toward the early detection of superimposed preeclampsia and fetal growth restriction. If these conditions are excluded, extensive fetal antepartum testing is less essential.

Most authorities recommend an initial sonographic assessment of fetal size and dating at week 18 to 20 of gestation. Fetal growth should be carefully assessed thereafter. If this assessment is not possible with usual clinical estimation of fundal height, sonographic assessment should be performed at 28 to 32 weeks and every 4 weeks until term. If growth restriction is evident, fetal well-being should be assessed by nonstress tests or biophysical profiles as usual for the growth-restricted fetus. Similarly, if preeclampsia cannot be excluded, fetal assessment as appropriate for the fetus of a woman with preeclampsia is mandatory. If the infant is normally grown and preeclampsia can be excluded, however, these studies are not indicated.

Maternal Assessment

MATERNAL ASSESSMENT IN PREECLAMPSIA

Antepartum monitoring has two goals. The first goal is to recognize preeclampsia early; the second is to observe progression of the condition, both to prevent maternal complications by delivery and to determine whether fetal well-being can be safely monitored with the usual intermittent observations. Current clinical management of preeclampsia is directed by overt clinical signs and symptoms. Although rapid weight increase and facial edema may indicate the fluid and sodium retention of preeclampsia, they are neither universally present nor uniquely characteristic of preeclampsia. These signs are, at best, a reason to monitor blood pressure and urinary protein more closely. Early recognition of impending preeclampsia is based primarily on blood pressure increases in the late second and third trimesters. Once blood pressure starts to rise, a repeat examination within 1 to 3 days is recommended. The woman should be evaluated for symptoms suggestive of preeclampsia and undergo laboratory testing for platelet count, renal function, and liver enzymes. Quantification of a 12- to 24-hour urine sample for proteinuria is recommended. The frequency of subsequent observations is determined by the initial observations and the ensuing clinical progression. If the condition appears stable, weekly observations may be appropriate.

MATERNAL ASSESSMENT IN CHRONIC HYPERTENSION

No consensus exists as to the most appropriate fetal surveillance test(s) or interval and timing of testing in women with chronic hypertension. Testing should be individualized, based on clinical judgment and on the severity of disease. There are no conclusive data to address either the benefits or the harms of various monitoring strategies for pregnant women with chronic hypertension. Box 3 lists the current proposed recommendations for

BOX 3 Fetal Monitoring in Hypertensive Disorders

- Gestational hypertension—Hypertension only without proteinuria, with normal laboratory test results, and without symptoms.
  1. Perform estimation of fetal growth and amniotic fluid status at diagnosis. If results are normal, repeat testing only if a significant change occurs in maternal condition.
  2. Perform NST at diagnosis. If NST is nonreactive, perform BPP. If BPP value is 8 or if NST is reactive, repeat testing only if a significant change occurs in maternal condition.
- Mild preeclampsia—Mild hypertension plus proteinuria (300 mg or more per 24-hour period), normal platelet count, normal liver enzymes values, and no maternal symptoms.
  1. Perform estimation of fetal growth and amniotic fluid status at diagnosis. If results are normal, repeat testing every 3 weeks.
  2. Perform NST, BPP, or both at diagnosis. If NST is reactive or if BPP value is 8, repeat weekly. Repeat testing immediately if abrupt change in maternal condition occurs.
  3. If estimated fetal weight by ultrasound is less than 10th percentile for gestational age, or if there is oligohydramnios (amniotic fluid index equals or is less than 5 cm), perform testing at least twice weekly.
- Severe preeclampsia—Severe hypertension in association with abnormal proteinuria; hypertension in association with severe proteinuria (at least 5 g per 24-hour period); presence of multiorgan involvement such as pulmonary edema, seizures, oliguria (less than 500 mL per 24-hour period), thrombocytopenia (platelet count less than 100,000/mm^3), abnormal liver enzymes in association with persistent epigastric or right upper quadrant pain; persistent severe central nervous system symptoms (altered mental status, headaches, blurred vision, or blindness).
  1. Term
     Hospitalize, prevent seizures, control hypertension, and proceed with delivery.
  2. Remote from term
     Provide care in a tertiary-care setting.
     Perform laboratory evaluation and fetal surveillance (as outlined for mild preeclampsia earlier) daily depending on the severity and progression of the disorder.[1]
- Chronic hypertension—Mild hypertension (BP more than 140/90 mm Hg) or severe hypertension (BP equal or more than 180/110 mm Hg) present before the 20th week of pregnancy or hypertension present before pregnancy.
  1. Perform baseline ultrasonography at 18 to 20 weeks and repeat at 28 to 32 weeks of gestation and monthly thereafter until delivery, to monitor fetal growth.
  2. If growth restriction is detected or suspected, monitor fetal status frequently with NST or BPP.[1]
  3. If growth restriction is not present and superimposed preeclampsia is excluded, these tests are not indicated.[1]

[1]Not FDA approved for this indication.
Abbreviations: BPP = biophysical profile; NST = nonstress test.

antepartum monitoring. When chronic hypertension is complicated by intrauterine growth retardation (IUGR) or preeclampsia, fetal surveillance is warranted.

Indications for Delivery

INDICATIONS FOR DELIVERY IN PREECLAMPSIA-ECLAMPSIA

Delivery is the only definitive treatment for preeclampsia; Box 4 lists some suggested indications for delivery. All women with the diagnosis of preeclampsia should be considered for delivery at 40 weeks' gestation. Delivery may be indicated for women with mild disease and a favorable cervix at 38 weeks' gestation and should be considered in women who have severe preeclampsia beyond 32 to 34 weeks' gestation. Prolonged antepartum management with severe preeclampsia is possible in a select group of women with fetal gestational age between 23 and 32 weeks but should be attempted only at centers equipped to provide close maternal and fetal surveillance. Vaginal delivery is preferable to cesarean delivery, thus avoiding the added stress of surgery to multiple physiologic aberrations. Labor induction should be carried out aggressively once the decision for delivery is made. In a gestation that is remote from term in which delivery is indicated and fetal and maternal conditions are stable enough to permit pregnancy to be prolonged 48 hours, glucocorticoids can be safely administered to accelerate fetal pulmonary maturity.

The patient with eclampsia should be delivered in a timely fashion. Once the patient is stabilized, the method of delivery should depend, in part, on gestational age, fetal presentation, and cervical examination findings.

INDICATIONS FOR DELIVERY IN CHRONIC HYPERTENSION

Pregnant women with uncomplicated chronic hypertension of a mild degree generally can be delivered vaginally at term; most have good maternal and neonatal outcomes. Cesarean delivery should be reserved for other obstetric indications. Women with mild hypertension during pregnancy and a prior adverse pregnancy outcome (e.g., stillbirth) may be candidates for earlier delivery after documentation of fetal lung maturity (as long as fetal status is reassuring). Women with severe chronic

BOX 4 Indications for Delivery in Preeclampsia

Maternal
- Gestational age ≥38 wk
- Platelet count <100,000 cells/mm^3
- Progressive deterioration in hepatic and/or renal function
- Suspected abruption placentae
- Persistent central nervous system (CNS) manifestations: headaches or visual changes
- Persistent severe gastric pain, nausea, or vomiting

Fetal
- Severe fetal growth restriction
- Nonreassuring fetal testing results
- Oligohydramnios

hypertension during pregnancy most often either deliver prematurely or have to be delivered prematurely for fetal or maternal indications. Delivery should be considered in all women with superimposed severe preeclampsia at or beyond 28 weeks of gestation and in women with mild superimposed preeclampsia at or beyond 37 weeks of gestation. Magnesium sulfate should be used for women with superimposed preeclampsia to prevent seizures.

Postpartum Management

Acute hypertensive changes induced by pregnancy usually dissipate rapidly, within the first several days after delivery. Resolution of hypertension is more rapid in patients with gestational hypertension and may lag in those with preeclampsia, especially those with longer duration of preeclampsia and greater extent of renal impairment. Oral antihypertensive agents may be needed after delivery (see Table 6) to help control maternal blood pressure, particularly for women who were hypertensive before pregnancy. If prepregnancy blood pressures were normal or unknown, it is reasonable to stop oral medication after 3 to 4 weeks and observe the blood pressure at 1- to 2-week intervals for 1 month, then at 3- to 6-month intervals for 1 year. If hypertension recurs, it should be treated. If the abnormalities persist, the pathology will probably be chronic.

Limited data are available on which to base our knowledge of the natural history and pathogenesis of postpartum hypertension. The women who appear to be at greatest risk for postpartum hypertension are those with antenatal preeclampsia, particularly those with higher urinary protein, serum uric acid, and blood urea nitrogen. For previously normotensive women, the risk of postpartum hypertension appears lower. Beyond the postnatal period, it is not known whether women with isolated

CURRENT DIAGNOSIS

- The most important factor to consider in classifying disease in which blood pressure rises abnormally in pregnancy is whether the hypertensive disorder antedates the pregnancy or arises during the pregnancy.
- Preeclampsia–eclampsia usually occurs after 20 weeks of gestation. Chronic hypertension is defined as hypertension that is present and observable before the 20th week of gestation.
- Gestational blood pressure elevation is defined as a blood pressure greater than 140 mm Hg systolic or 90 mm Hg diastolic in a woman normotensive before 20 weeks.
- Proteinuria in pregnancy is defined as the urinary excretion of 300 mg protein or greater in a 24-hour specimen.
- Laboratory tests recommended to diagnose or manage hypertension in pregnancy serve primarily to distinguish preeclampsia from either chronic or transient hypertension.
- No single screening test is considered reliable and cost effective for predicting preeclampsia.

CURRENT THERAPY

- Prevention focuses on identifying women at higher risk and conducting close clinical and laboratory monitoring to recognize the disease process in its early stages.
- Delivery is always appropriate therapy for the mother but may not be for the fetus.
- For maternal health, the goal of therapy is to prevent eclampsia as well as severe complications of preeclampsia. Parenteral magnesium sulfate is given during labor and delivery and for variable durations postpartum to women with eclampsia and severe preeclampsia. Its benefits in mild gestational hypertension or preeclampsia remain unclear.
- Antihypertensive medications are indicated to lower blood pressure for women with severe hypertension, usually defined as 160 to 170 mm Hg or more systolic blood pressure or 110 mm Hg or more diastolic blood pressure.
- Antihypertensive therapy is indicated intrapartum when diastolic blood pressure is persistently 105 to 110 mm Hg or above.
- The goal of blood pressure reduction in emergency situations should be a gradual reduction of blood pressure to the normal range.

postpartum hypertension are at increased risk of chronic hypertension.

Risk of Recurrence

Women who have had preeclampsia are more prone to hypertensive complications in subsequent pregnancies. Risk is best established for multiparas with a history of preeclampsia; the magnitude of the recurrence rate increases the earlier the disease manifested during the index pregnancy. The recurrence rate for women with one episode of HELLP is 5%. Recurrence rates are higher for those experiencing preeclampsia as multiparas compared with nulliparous women. Risk is also increased in multiparas who conceive with a new father, even when their first pregnancy was normotensive, the incidence being intermediate between that of primiparous women and monogamous multiparous women who have not had a preeclamptic pregnancy.

REFERENCES

Abalos E, Duley L, Steyn DW, Henderson-Smart DJ: Antihypertensive drug therapy for mild to moderate hypertension during pregnancy (Cochrane Review). In The Cochrane Library, Issue 4. Chichester, UK, John Wiley, 2004.

Agency for Healthcare Research and Quality: Management of chronic hypertension during pregnancy. Evidence Report/Technology assessment no. 14. AHRQ Publication No. 00-E011. Rockville, Md, Author, 2000.

American College of Obstetricians and Gynecologists: ACOG Practice Bulletin No. 29. Chronic hypertension pregnancy. Obstet Gynecol 2001;98:177-185.

Atallah AN, Hofmeyr GJ, Duley L: Calcium supplementation during pregnancy for preventing hypertensive disorders and related problems (Cochrane Review). In The Cochrane Library, Issue 4. Chichester, UK.: John Wiley, 2004.

Bergel E, Carroli G, Althabe F: Ambulatory versus conventional methods for monitoring blood pressure during pregnancy (Cochrane Review). In The Cochrane Library, Issue 4. Chichester, UK, John Wiley, 2004.

Cunningham FG, Gant NF, Leveno KJ, et al: Hypertensive disorders in pregnancy. In Cunningham FG (ed): Williams Obstetrics, 21st ed. New York, McGraw-Hill, 2001, pp 567-618.

Duley L, Henderson-Smart DJ: Drugs for treatment of very high blood pressure during pregnancy (Cochrane Review). In The Cochrane Library, Issue 4. Chichester, UK, John Wiley, 2004.

Joint National Committee: The Seventh Report of the Joint National Committee on Prevention, Detection, Evaluation, and Treatment of High Blood Pressure (JNC VII). JAMA 2003;289:2560-2571.

Levine RJ, Thadhani RT, Qian C, et al: Urinary placental growth factor and risk of preeclampsia. JAMA 2005;293:77-85.

Lim KH, Friedman SA, Ecker JL, et al: The clinical utility of serum uric acid measurements in hypertensive diseases of pregnancy. Am J Obstet Gynecol 1998;178:1067-1071.

Lucas JL, Leveno KJ, Cunningham FG: A comparison of magnesium sulfate with phenytoin for the prevention of eclampsia. N Engl J Med 1995;333:201-205.

Magee L, Sadeghi S: Prevention and treatment of postpartum hypertension (Cochrane Review). In The Cochrane Library, Issue 4. Chichester, UK, John Wiley, 2004.

Report of the National High Blood Pressure Education Program: Working group report on high blood pressure in pregnancy. Am J Obstet Gynecol 2000;183:S1-S22.

Sibai BM: Prevention of preeclampsia: A big disappointment. Am J Obstet Gynecol 1998;179:1275-1278.

Postpartum Care

Method of
Lisa R. Nash, DO

The postpartum period, or puerperium, is defined as the time needed for the anatomic and physiologic changes of pregnancy to revert to the normal state, lasting from immediately after delivery of the placenta to 6 to 8 weeks following birth.

The First 4 to 6 Hours

During the first few hours after delivery, blood pressure (BP), pulse, respiratory rate, temperature, vaginal bleeding, urination, and pain should be monitored every 15 minutes until the patient is stable. Complications that can occur during this time include hypotension, hemorrhage, dyspnea, fever, hypertensive disorders of pregnancy, and urinary retention. Table 1 describes the differential diagnosis and management of these disorders. Table 2 lists oxytocics used to control uterine atony.

Early skin-to-skin contact between the mother and her healthy infant should be ensured to facilitate bonding. Early breast-feeding should be encouraged. The first breast-feeding should occur prior to transfer of the healthy newborn to the nursery in facilities where rooming-in is unavailable.

The First 24 to 72 Hours

Hospitalization generally lasts 24 to 48 hours after an uncomplicated vaginal delivery and up to 72 hours after a typical cesarean delivery. During this time, the following should be addressed:

- Signs and symptoms of potential complications described in Table 1
- Transition of lochia to diminishing reddish-brown discharge
- Fundal height below umbilicus by 24 hours postpartum
- Perineal inflammation or edema and proper perineal hygiene
- Signs and symptoms suggesting deep venous thrombosis
- Resumption of normal ambulation
- Return of bowel/bladder function
- Lactation establishment
- Pain management
- Maternal mood, bonding, and family adjustment
- Contraceptive planning
- Any special requirements such as administration of $Rh_0(D)$ immune globulin (RhoGAM) or rubella vaccine

Symptoms of breast engorgement for mothers who will not breast-feed may be relieved by breast support, ice packs, and nonsteroidal anti-inflammatory medications.

Routine hospital discharge instructions should include direction to contact the physician for any of the following: heavy uterine bleeding; purulent lochia; worsening perineal pain; abdominal or breast pain; redness, warmth, tenderness, or swelling of the lower legs/calves; dysuria; fever (temperature >38°C [100°F]) and/or chills; presence of depression or problems with family adjustment. The patient should be instructed to maintain pelvic rest (nothing in the vagina) for 4 to 6 weeks, and encouraged to resume normal activities and diet.

The 2-Week Newborn Check

The 2-week newborn check provides a good opportunity to reassess the maternal condition. Persistence of any depressive symptoms should be explored. Postpartum *blues* generally resolve by the 10th postpartum day. Although rare, postpartum psychosis generally manifests in this same time period and requires emergent intervention because of the risks of suicide and infanticide. Additional areas to assess include family adjustment, breast-feeding progress or problems, urinary incontinence, anticipated time of return to sexual intimacy, and contraceptive plans. If early postpartum complications were experienced, a repeat complete blood count or urinalysis may be indicated.

The Traditional Postpartum Assessment

This assessment is generally scheduled at 6 weeks after delivery. Assessment should include vital signs and physical examination of the thyroid gland, breasts, heart, lungs, abdomen, perineum, pelvis (uterus and ovaries), and lower extremities. Papanicolaou smear should be obtained. Items listed previously for the 2-week assessment should be readdressed.

TABLE 1 Potential Complications of the Immediate Postpartum Period : Key Diagnostic and Treatment Considerations

Condition	Differential Diagnosis	Management
Hypotension	Vagal response Hypovolemia Reaction to anesthesia Blood loss	For All: Supportive – Trendelenburg position, 500 – 1000 mL IV crystalloid (normal) saline or lactated Ringer's solution For blood loss: packed RBCs
Immediate hemorrhage	Uterine atony (most common)	See Table 2 for oxytocics
	Retained placental tissue or blood clots	Evaculation, oxytocics, surgical assistance as appropriate
	Laceration or hematoma	Repair
	Bleeding disorders	Blood products
Delayed hemorrhage (>24 hours after delivery)		IV crystalloids and blood products for all etiologies, as appropriate
	Subinvolution of former placental site	Oxytocics, as needed
	Retained placental tissue or blood clots	Evacuation, oxytocics, surgical assistance as appropriate
Dyspnea	Amniotic fluid embolism	Respiratory and cardiovascular support, treatment of disseminated intravascular coagulation
	Pulmonary embolus	Antithrombolytics, anticoagulation
	Exacerbation of asthma	Nebulized albuterol
Temperature >38 degrees Centigrade (100 degrees Fahrenheit) on any 2 days beyond first 24 hours OR temparature >39 degrees Centigrade (102.2 degrees Fahrenheit) at any time	Endometritis	Clindamycin (Cleocin) 900 mg IV q8h + gentamicin (Garamycin) 100 mg (2 mg/kg) IVPB then 80 mg (1.0-1.5 mg/kg) IVPB q8h OR 2nd/3rd generation cephalosporin ± metronidazole (Flagyl)
	Breast engorgement (<48 hours after delivery)	Ice packs to relieve vascular congestion (note: if >48 hrs after delivery, increase breastfeeding and/or pumping)
	Septic pelvic thrombophlebitis	Anticoagulation with heparin
	Other: abdominal wound or perineal infection, UTI, DVT, pneumonia	Antibiotic as appropriate for source
Hypertensive disorders: postpartum preeclampsia, postpartum eclampsia		Magnesium sulfate 4 g slowly IV over 15 – 30 min, followed by 1 to 3 g/h to keep serum magnesium levels between 4 and 7 mEq/L IV hydralazine (Apresoline) titrated to maintain blood pressure about 130/80
Urinary retention	Trauma of delivery Anesthesia	In-and-out bladder catheterization if spontaneous voiding does not occur within 6 h of delivery

TABLE 2 Oxytocics Used for Control of Uterine Atony

Drug	Dose	Maintenance	Contraindications
Oxytocin (Pitocin)	10 U IM or infuse 10 to 40 U in 1 L of IV fluid	IV infusion maintained 1-4 h	None
Methylergonovine (Methergine)	0.2 mg IM	Repeat q 2-4 h	Hypertension, toxemia
$PGF_{2\text{-}alpha}$ carboprost; (Hemabate)	0.25 mg IM	Repeat q 15-90 min	Cardiac or pulmonary disease
PGE_2 (Prostin E_2)	20 mg suppository inserted into rectum	Repeat q 2-4 h	Hypotension (use $PGF_{2\text{-}alpha}$ instead)

Abbreviations: IM = intramuscular; IV = intravenous; PG = prostaglandin.

Postpartum Depression

Postpartum depression is common, occurring in approximately 20% of parturients. Postpartum thyroid dysfunction may present with similar or overlapping symptoms and should be investigated when postpartum depression is suspected. Management may be supportive and could include individual or group psychotherapy or medication. Antidepressant medications acceptable for breast-feeding mothers include sertraline (Zoloft), paroxetine (Paxil), amitriptyline (Elavil), and desipramine (Norpramin).

Family Adjustment

Many women experience transient feelings of vulnerability, inadequacy, and anxiety during the family adjustment that occurs following the addition of a new infant. Feelings of attachment may vary initially but usually increase over time. Conflicting emotions elicited by increased responsibility for meeting the demands of the expanded family are common. Significant changes in lifestyle, relationships, and careers often must be made. Assessment of emotional, tangible (financial, household, childcare, etc.), and informational support can identify families who may benefit from referral to additional resources. Men typically have concerns about infant care skills, decreased personal time, changes in the marital relationship, financial security, and the health of their partner and the newborn. Common sibling responses to arrival of the new infant include behaviors that are imitating, aggressive, solicitous, or anxious. Siblings may also withdraw or become more independent. Many authorities recommend that siblings have contact with the mother during the postpartum hospitalization. Allowing siblings to assist (as age permits) in infant care and maintaining separate time for siblings to interact with parents (such as the newborn's nap time) may reduce adjustment problems. Reading children's books about new babies and discussing feelings with siblings are additional options.

CURRENT DIAGNOSIS

- Hypo- or hypertension, tachypnea, fever, excessive vaginal bleeding, inability to void, and excessive abdominal or perineal pain are potential indicators of postpartum complications.
- Return to normal ambulation, bowel and bladder function, establishing lactation, and family adjustment and bonding are tasks for the first 24 to 72 hours postpartum.
- Persistence of depressive symptoms, family adjustment, breast-feeding progress or problems, urinary incontinence, return to sexual intimacy, and contraceptive plans should be addressed at the 2- and 6-week postpartum visits.
- Single parents, adopting parents, and parents experiencing a perinatal loss or the birth of a child with a serious illness or congenital anomaly will likely require additional/special information, services, and resources.

Return to Sexual Activity and Contraception

The return to sexual activity and contraception should be discussed. Most couples will resume sexual activity between 6 weeks and 3 months postpartum, although some will do so sooner if perineal discomfort has resolved. The most common barriers to resumption of sexual activity include perineal pain (25%), lack of interest (more common in breast-feeding than bottle-feeding mothers), and fatigue. Anticipatory guidance is helpful for negotiating this time of transition. Breast-feeding mothers should be advised they may require a vaginal lubricant because of the hormonal changes related to breast-feeding.

Postpartum anovulatory infertility persists for 5 weeks in nonlactating women and 8 weeks or more in lactating women. The anticipated time to resume sexual activity and infant feeding plans should be considered in determining the best time to initiate contraceptive measures postpartum.

Contraceptive effects of lactational amenorrhea provide approximately 98% protection in the first 6 months if there is little or no supplemental feeding. Other options for postpartum contraception include natural family planning, barrier methods, oral contraceptives, contraceptive patch (Ortho Evra) and ring (NuvaRing), the injectable contraceptive medroxyprogesterone acetate (Depo-Provera), intrauterine device, and sterilization (Table 3).

The usual amount of time off work allowed for employed mothers is 6 weeks.

Special Circumstances

THE SINGLE PARENT

The single parent often experiences financial and time pressures exceeding those of two-parent families. Enlisting an extended support network of family and friends in addition to a supportive and empathic physician will be helpful.

ADOPTING PARENT(S)

Adopting parent(s) usually have experienced stressful approval and unpredictable placement processes. They may have as little as a few hours' notice to make plans for the arrival of their newborn. Loss issues related to infertility may exist at various stages of resolution. Other issues may include decisions about timing and telling the adoption story to the child(ren) as well as ethnic and cultural considerations when parents and child(ren) have different backgrounds.

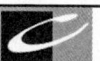

CURRENT THERAPY

- Specific interventions for potential complications of the immediate postpartum period are outlined in Tables 1 and 2.
- The anticipated time to resume sexual activity and infant feeding plans should be considered in the choices of contraceptive method and when to initiate contraceptive measures postpartum.

TABLE 3 Postpartum Contraception

Method	Earliest Initiation	Special Considerations
Lactational amenorrhea	Immediately postpartum	Additional measures required for any of the following: >6 mo postpartum, supplemental infant feeding initiation or resumption of menses
Natural family planning	Depends on return of normal menstrual cycle	
Barrier methods: condom diaphragm	3 w postpartum (coincident with earliest recommended time to resume sexual activity) 6 w postpartum	Requires full uterine involution AND refitting for patients who previously used this method
Medroxyprogesterone acetate (Depo-Provera)	Prior to hospital discharge	Does not diminish lactation Many physicians delay to 2 wk postpartum because of the potential risk for prolonged bleeding
Progesterone-only pills (Micronor)	Prior to hospital discharge	Same as medroxyprogesterone acetate (Depo-Provera)
Combination oral contraceptives	Non–breast-feeding women: 3 wk postpartum Breast-feeding women: 1 mo after lactation becomes well established	May diminish lactation
Contraceptive patch (Ortho Evra), ring (NuvaRing)	Same as combination oral contraceptives	Same as combination oral contraceptives
Intrauterine device (Mirena, ParaGard)	Within 20 min of delivery of placenta OR 6 wk postpartum	Full uterine involution must be achieved
Sterilization	After delivery/prior to hospital discharge OR 6 wk postpartum	Full uterine involution must be achieved

PERINATAL GRIEVING

Perinatal grieving occurs both for parents experiencing the death of an infant and parents of a child with a serious illness or congenital anomaly. Physicians can be helpful in this process by providing information and acknowledging when an answer is unknown. The medical team should recognize the infant as a person by using his or her name, encouraging the family's involvement in care of the infant as much as possible and providing opportunities for family members to express and discuss emotions. Parents experiencing a perinatal death should be encouraged to touch and hold their infant and photographs should be offered. Physicians should assist parents with plans for notifying siblings, friends, and relatives. Identifying available community and medical resources such as parent support groups can also be very helpful.

REFERENCES

Anderson GC, Moore E, Hepworth J, Bergman N: Early skin-to-skin contact for mothers and their healthy newborn infants. Cochrane Database Syst Rev 2003(2);CD003519.

Anonymous: Postpartum care of the mother and newborn: A practical guide. Technical Working Group, World Health Organization. Birth 1999;26(4):255-258.

Baxley E: Postpartum biomedical concerns. In Ratcliffe SD, Byrd JE, Sakornbut EL (eds): Handbook of Pregnancy and Perinatal Care in Family Practice: Science and Practice, Philadelphia, Hanley & Belfus, 1996, pp 430-446.

Driscoll CE: Postpartum Care. In Rakel RE, Bope ET (eds): Conn's Current Therapy 2004, Philadelphia, WB Saunders, 2003, pp 1076-1078.

Gabbe SG, Niebyl JR, Simpson JL (eds): Obstetrics: Normal & Problem Pregnancies, 4th ed. New York, Churchill Livingstone, 2002, pp 753-779.

Hatcher RA, Nelson AL, Zieman M, et al: A pocket guide to managing contraception. Tiger, Georgia, Bridging the Gap Foundation, 2003, p 27.

Killeen I, Osborn C: Postpartum care: Psychosocial concerns. In Ratcliffe SD, Byrd JE, Sakornbut EL (eds): Handbook of Pregnancy and Perinatal Care in Family Practice: Science and Practice. Philadelphia, Hanley & Belfus, 1996, pp 447-458.

Levitt C, Shaw E, Wong S, et al: Systematic review of the literature on postpartum care: Selected contraception methods, postpartum Papanicolaou test, and rubella immunization. Birth 2004;31(3):203-212.

Montgomery, AM: Breast-feeding and postpartum maternal care. In Larimore WL (ed): Primary Care: Clinics in Office Practice. Update in Maternity Care, Vol. 27, No. 1. Philadelphia, WB Saunders, 2000, pp 237-250.

Resuscitation of the Newborn

Method of
Derek S. Wheeler, MD,
and Martin J. McCaffrey, MD

Numerous and dramatic changes must occur more or less in sequential order around the time of birth, at which time the fetal cardiovascular and respiratory systems must undergo an instantaneous transition to life outside the liquid-filled uterine environment. Several events occurring prior to or at the time of delivery may interrupt this transition and lead to problems ranging from mild respiratory distress to shock, organ dysfunction, and death. Fortunately the vast majority of term newborns require no resuscitation beyond routine warming, drying, suctioning of the airway, and mild stimulation. However, rapid identification and resuscitation of those newborns experiencing a difficult transition to extrauterine life may dramatically improve outcome. Neonatal resuscitation is a team effort and requires the coordinated execution of several, simultaneous psychomotor and procedural skills. Adequate knowledge of the normal fetal, transitional, and neonatal physiology, as well as prior planning and preparation is essential to achieving the most favorable outcomes following neonatal resuscitation.

Fetal, Transitional, and Neonatal Circulations

The fetal circulation is characterized by parallel circulations, the presence of intracardiac and extracardiac shunts, a high pulmonary vascular resistance, and a relatively low systemic vascular resistance (attributed to the low-resistance placental circulation). Conversely, on delivery the right and left ventricles are in series, shunts functionally close, pulmonary vascular resistance decreases, and systemic vascular resistance increases. During intrauterine life, gas exchange occurs in the placenta; but during extrauterine life, gas exchange occurs in the lungs. An understanding and appreciation for these differences is essential to the optimal care and resuscitation of the newborn infant.

The fetal cardiovascular anatomy differs from that of the normal newborn infant. The fetal circulation contains the two atria, two ventricles, and two great arteries but is further complemented by a foramen ovale, ductus arteriosus, and ductus venosus. In utero there exist two large anatomic shunts. One occurs between the right and left atria (the foramen ovale). The second exists between the pulmonary artery and aorta (the ductus arteriosus). The origin of blood flowing through these shunts is crucial. A streaming pattern of fetal blood flow is observed at the level of the right atrium. Less oxygenated blood from the lower body streams along the lateral wall of the inferior vena cava (IVC) crosses the tricuspid valve, and enters the right ventricle. The right ventricle also receives poorly oxygenated blood from the superior vena cava (SVC) (from the brain and upper body) and coronary sinus (from the heart). Because of the high pulmonary vascular resistance (PVR) during intrauterine life, little of the blood pumped from the right ventricle enters the pulmonary circulation. Rather, the right ventricle ejects this poorly oxygenated blood (approximately two thirds of total cardiac output) into the main pulmonary artery and into the descending aorta via the ductus arteriosus, thereby reaching the placenta (via the paired umbilical arteries) where the blood is reoxygenated. In contrast, oxygenated blood from the umbilical-placental circulation (via the single umbilical vein) bypasses the liver via the ductus venosus and travels along the medial wall of the IVC. The majority of this relatively oxygenated stream is directed across the foramen ovale into the left atrium, crosses the mitral valve, and enters the left ventricle. Although the left ventricle also receives a small percentage of poorly

oxygenated blood from the lungs, the majority is relatively well oxygenated. In sum, blood in the fetal left ventricle is 20% more saturated than the blood in the right ventricle. The left ventricle ejects this blood (approximately one-third of total cardiac output) into the ascending aorta to supply the heart, brain, and upper fetal body with relatively well-oxygenated blood. A smaller percentage of left ventricular output crosses the aortic arch to the descending aorta. Therefore, the fetal right and left ventricles are functionally arranged in parallel, such that the right ventricle supplies the lower portion of the body, including the placenta, and the left ventricle supplies the upper portion of the body, including the brain. This arrangement assures that the brain receives blood with relatively higher oxygen content than does the placenta.

During birth, a number of complex events occur simultaneously. Clamping of the umbilical cord removes the low-resistance placental capillary bed from the systemic circulation, and blood flow to the placenta ceases abruptly, resulting in an increase in systemic vascular resistance (SVR). The fluid-filled lungs rapidly expand and fill with air with the first few breaths. Initiation of respirations is followed by a marked fall in PVR, and blood flow to the lungs dramatically increases. The increase in SVR results in an increase in left-sided heart pressures. The further increase in left atrial pressure resulting from increased pulmonary venous return results in closure of the foramen ovale, because left atrial pressure exceeds the right atrial pressure. Functional closure of the ductus arteriosus occurs and shunting of blood from the pulmonary artery to the aorta ceases. The fall in PVR and functional closure of the ductus arteriosus depend on several factors, the most important of which are initiation of respirations with subsequent lung inflation and increased oxygen saturation. In the majority of cases, the transition from intrauterine to extrauterine life occurs smoothly and uneventfully. However, up to 10% of all newborn infants will require some degree of intervention (e.g., positioning, suctioning, and/or stimulation to breathe) to assist with this transition. A smaller percentage will require more intensive resuscitative efforts. Certain high-risk conditions (Box 1) may preclude a smooth transition, and further resuscitation may be required to restore and support cardiopulmonary function. For example, several studies suggest that approximately 1% of newborns in the delivery room setting will require assisted ventilation.

Perinatal Asphyxia

Perinatal asphyxia occurs when oxygen delivery is insufficient to meet metabolic demands, resulting in hypoxia, hypercarbia, and metabolic acidosis. Initial compensatory mechanisms, including tachycardia and vasoconstriction, may allow adequate oxygen delivery to the vital organs for a time. However, without resolution or treatment, these compensatory mechanisms will eventually fail, leading to a fall in heart rate and blood pressure (BP) with eventual cardiopulmonary arrest. World Health Organization (WHO) estimates from 1995 conclude that birth asphyxia is responsible for 19% of the 5 million neonatal deaths that occur annually. Intrauterine asphyxia manifests as alterations in fetal heart rate (late decelerations, bradycardia), passage of meconium (see text following), fetal gasping, and eventual apnea, termed *primary apnea*. This initial

BOX 1 Risk Factors for Neonatal Resuscitation

Maternal Factors	Intrapartum Factors
Chronic or pregnancy-induced hypertension	Size for date discrepancy
Diabetes mellitus	Polyhydramnios or oligohydramnios
Previous fetal or neonatal death	Breech presentation
Maternal age >35 y or <18 y	Decreased fetal movement
Anemia	Prolonged labor (>24 h)
Rh isoimmunization	Prolonged rupture of membranes (>12 h)
Prematurity (<37 wk gestation)	Meconium-stained amniotic fluid
Postmaturity (>42 wk gestation)	Placental abruption
Premature rupture of the membranes	Prolapsed cord
Malnutrition or poor weight gain	Fetal distress (fetal heart rate abnormalities, fetal acidosis)
Lack of prenatal care	Emergent operative delivery
Substance abuse (including alcohol)	
Antepartum hemorrhage	
Multiple gestation	
Chronic disease (cardiovascular, rheumatologic, neurologic, etc.)	

period of apnea is followed by further gasping, which gradually weakens in intensity, eventually terminating in what is termed *secondary apnea*. In the delivery room spontaneous respirations can be elicited in newborns with primary apnea by stimulation (vigorous warming and drying) or a brief trial of positive-pressure ventilation (PPV). Newborns with secondary apnea, on the other hand, have suffered a prolonged period of inadequate oxygen delivery and require aggressive resuscitation to prevent further decompensation, cardiac arrest, and death. The longer the delay in initiating resuscitation for primary apnea, the longer the time required to establish spontaneous respirations following PPV. Because there is no definitive method of differentiating between primary and secondary apnea following delivery, the neonatal resuscitation team must promptly recognize and institute proper treatment for all newborn infants with apnea and suspected perinatal asphyxia.

Neonatal Resuscitation

Neonatal resuscitation is directed toward assuring a smooth transition to extrauterine life by achieving the following goals:

- Maintaining or restoring normal body temperature
- Maintaining or establishing effective ventilation and oxygenation
- Maintaining or restoring adequate cardiac output and tissue perfusion
- Avoiding hypoglycemia

Neonatal resuscitation follows an orderly sequence known as the ABCs (airway, breathing, circulation) of resuscitation. Concurrently, the overall physiologic status of the newborn is continuously monitored via a cycle of repeated assessment and intervention (assess-intervene-assess).

Unique to newborn infants is an increased ratio of body surface area to volume; and they are at risk for significant heat loss and temperature. Temperature instability and cold stress will increase oxygen consumption and may impede an effective resuscitation. Therefore, initial efforts should be directed toward minimizing heat loss. On delivery the infant should be placed on a radiant warmer. Other heat sources such as a heating lamp may be used if a radiant warmer is not available. Heated bags of intravenous (IV) fluid should be avoided because they may cause burns. The infant is then dried vigorously with a warm, sterile towel. To minimize conductive heat losses, wet linens should be removed as soon as possible. If the newborn is otherwise stable, he or she may be placed naked against the mother's skin and covered with a clean blanket or towel.

Initial resuscitative efforts are directed toward maintaining the airway. Properly positioning the infant on his or her back, with the head and neck in a neutral, midline position will assist in opening the airway. A towel roll may be placed beneath the shoulders to assist in opening the airway. Hyperextension, which may lead to airway obstruction, should be avoided. The mouth and nose should be suctioned with a bulb syringe to remove any secretions that may contribute to airway compromise.

Drying, positioning, and suctioning usually provide sufficient stimulation to help the newborn initiate effective breathing. If respirations are adequate and cyanosis is present, supplemental oxygen should be administered, and an appropriately sized face mask should be available. Acrocyanosis (bluish discoloration of the hands and feet), on the other hand, is a normal physical finding that is often present in the first few minutes of life and does not require oxygen supplementation. Using a bag-valve-mask PPV is indicated for those infants with either absent (apnea) or slow, gasping respiratory movements. In addition, because one of the most common causes of bradycardia is lack of sufficient oxygen, PPV is indicated when the heart rate is below 100 beats per minute (bpm).

Both neonatal-sized self-inflating bags and anesthesia bags (Figure 1) are acceptable for administering PPV in the delivery room. The main advantages to using an anesthesia bag are that these devices are capable of either delivering 100% blow-by oxygen or continuous positive airway pressure (CPAP). Inspiratory pressures can be controlled and titrated with the use of an in-line manometer when using an anesthesia bag. The use of an anesthesia bag requires more expertise, however, and some centers preferentially use a self-inflating bag because of its simplicity. The main disadvantages to the self-inflating bag are that these devices require an additional oxygen reservoir attachment and inspiratory pressures cannot be closely titrated. Both devices are acceptable for use in neonatal resuscitation provided that staff is familiar with the requirements of each device.

Proper placement and sizing of the face mask is required to produce an effective seal around the mouth and nose (Figure 2). Adequate ventilation is assured using a rate of 40 to 60 breaths per minute, with a tidal volume sufficient enough to produce adequate, symmetric expansion of

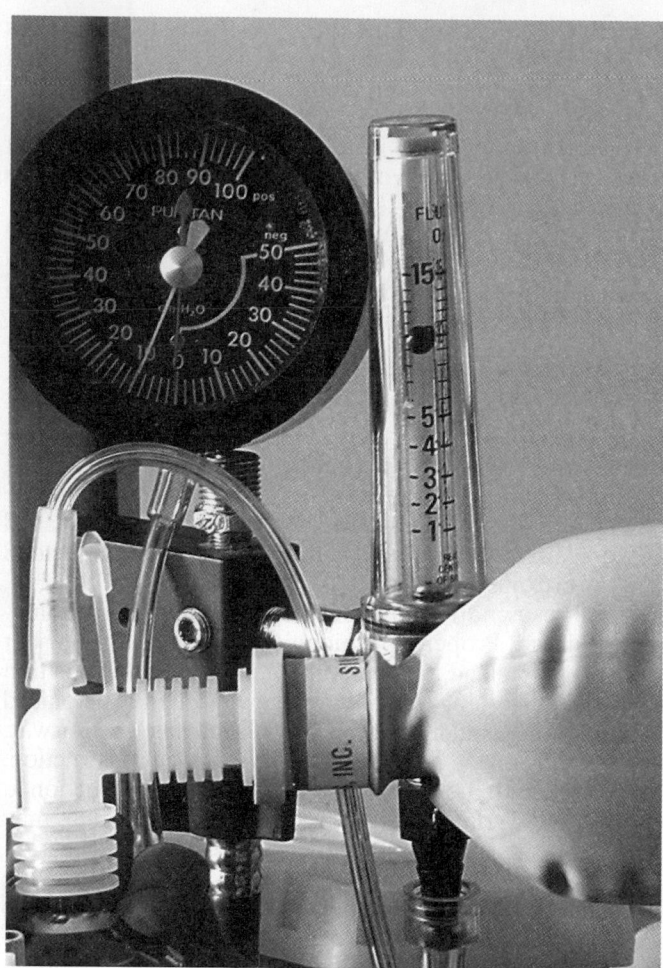

FIGURE 1. Anesthesia bag preparation. Setting the initial flow rate to 8 to 10 L/minute and the end-respiratory pressure to 8 to 10 cm H$_2$O allows for effective bag filling while providing positive-pressure ventilation.

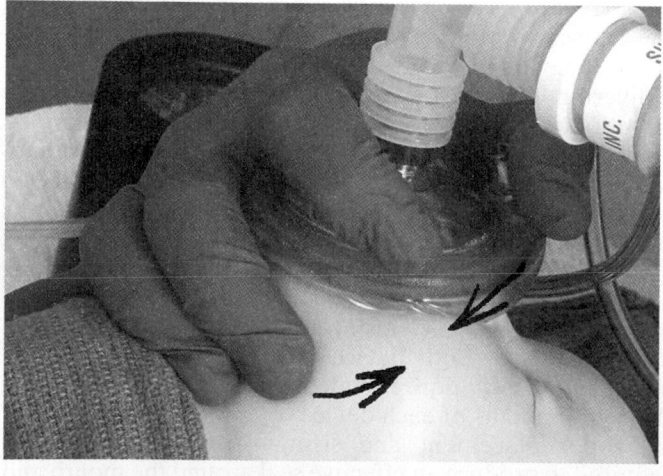

FIGURE 2. Proper placement and seal of face mask. The thumb and third finger (which is on the mandible or ramus of the mandible) are being squeezed toward each other in a *C hold.*

the chest. Initially, inspiratory pressures as high as 30 cm H$_2$O or more may be required for adequate lung inflation. Smaller pressures (generally 20 cm H$_2$O or less) are generally sufficient for subsequent breaths. An 8 or 10 F orogastric tube may be placed to decompress the stomach and improve ventilation. Ventilation via the bag-valve-mask is relatively simple to perform and can be life sustaining. Endotracheal intubation should be considered if bag-valve-mask ventilation is ineffective after attempts to optimize, if it appears that prolonged ventilation will be required or if an intravascular route for epinephrine administration is unattainable. However, intubation should only be attempted by providers experienced with the management of the neonatal airway. Intubation of a newborn requires careful assessment to determine that the tube has been properly placed. In addition, careful ongoing assessment is required to determine that the tube remains properly positioned. Use of a disposable CO$_2$ indicator should be considered to confirm proper endotracheal tube placement initially and during the course of the resuscitation.

Once adequate ventilation and oxygenation are assured, attention is directed toward the circulatory system. Heart rate is assessed by palpating the brachial pulse, palpating the pulse at the base of the umbilical cord, or by auscultation of cardiac sounds with a stethoscope. The heart rate in a newborn normally ranges from 100 to 170 bpm. As mentioned previously, PPV should be initiated for infants whose heart rates are less than 100 bpm. However, chest compressions should be performed immediately if the heart rate is less than 60 bpm after 30 seconds of effective PPV with 100% oxygen (Box 2). Chest compressions are performed using either the two-thumb technique (Figure 3) or two-finger technique (Figure 4), but the two-thumb technique is thought to provide a more controlled depth of compression and better cardiac output. Team members should coordinate ventilations with chest compressions. After three compressions, a positive pressure breath with 100% oxygen should be administered (for a compression to breath ratio of 3:1). Chest compressions should be continued until the heart rate is greater than 60 bpm.

Resuscitation medications (Table 1) should be administered if the heart rate remains less than 60 bpm despite 30 seconds of chest compressions and adequate PPV. Vascular access should be established at this time, as drug, fluid and dextrose administration may be necessary, but endotracheal administration of drugs may be the most accessible route. The medication is either flushed through the endotracheal tube with 0.5 to 1 mL normal saline or pushed through a 5 F feeding tube passed to the tip of the endotracheal tube. Both methods of drug administration should be followed by several positive-pressure breaths.

Vascular access may be achieved most readily via umbilical vein cannulation. The umbilical vein is easily identified and cannulated and is therefore the preferred site of vascular access in the newborn. The umbilical vein is identified as a single, thin-walled, larger vessel compared to the small, thick-walled pair of umbilical arteries (Figure 5). A 3.5 or 5.0 F catheter is inserted until the tip of the catheter is below the skin or until blood can readily be aspirated. This should be done sterilely if possible. If not placed sterilely, however, after stabilization the catheter must be replaced to avoid potential infections. A peripheral IV line is also perfectly acceptable but may be difficult to establish by inexperienced providers.

BOX 2 Newborn Resuscitation Equipment for the Emergency Department

Airway
- Bulb syringe
- DeLee suction catheter
- Meconium aspirator
- Laryngoscope and straight blades (sizes 0, 1)
- Endotracheal tubes, uncuffed (sizes 2.5, 3.0, 3.5, and 4.0 mm)
- Stylet
- Suction catheters (5 F, 8 F, 10 F)
- Suction source with manometer
- Nasogastric tube
- Feeding tubes (8 F, 10 F)

Breathing
- Face masks (premature, newborn, and infant sizes)
- Self-inflating ventilation bag (450 to 750 mL), with oxygen reservoir and manometer
- Oxygen source
- Chest tubes (8 and 10 F)

Circulation
- Sterile umbilical vessel catheterization tray
- Umbilical catheters (3.5 F, 5.0 F)
- Three-way stopcocks
- Syringes (tuberculin, 1, 3, 10, and 20 mL)
- Medication and fluids:
  - Epinephrine 1:10,000 concentration
  - Naloxone hydrochloride
  - Sodium bicarbonate (0.5 mEq/mL or 4.2% solution)
  - Normal saline
  - Lactated Ringer's
  - 10% Dextrose
  - 5% Albumin

Miscellaneous Equipment
- Radiant warmer or heat lamps
- Sterile towels
- Pulse oximeter
- Cardiorespiratory monitor with small electrocardiographic leads
- Sterile gowns, gloves
- Resuscitation chart

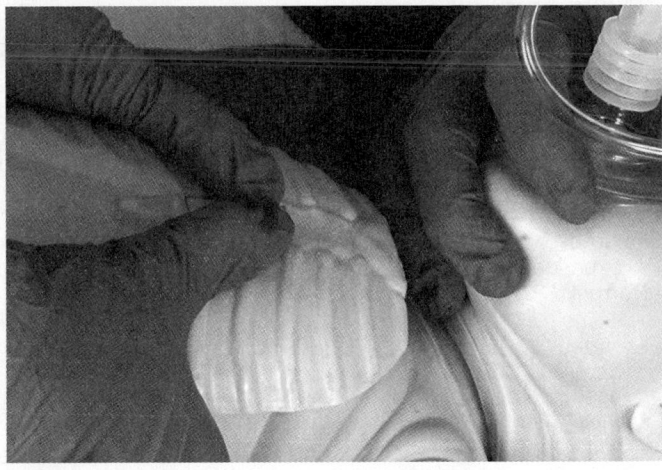

FIGURE 3. Two-thumb chest-encircling external cardiac massage technique. This is the preferred technique. Note that the thumbs are above the xyphoid process in the midsternum region.

and in whom heart rate and color are normal, but severe respiratory depression persists. However, naloxone (Narcan) will precipitate acute narcotic withdrawal and seizures if administered to newborns born to women with known or suspected drug abuse. IV glucose (2 mL/kg $D_{10}W$) is administered for suspected or documented hypoglycemia. Sodium bicarbonate should only be given in cases of documented severe acidosis or in prolonged resuscitations with no response to other described interventions. Finally, surfactant preparations (Survanta, Infasurf) may be administered in the delivery room to preterm newborns with respiratory distress.

It should be emphasized that resuscitation proceeds according to the above protocols, and not according to the result of the Apgar score. The Apgar score is based on five objective signs (Table 2) and was designed to provide an easily reproducible measure of the status of a

Epinephrine is the drug used most frequently during resuscitation of the newborn. It may be administered via the IV or endotracheal routes for either asystole or heart rate less than 60 bpm despite effective ventilations and chest compressions. Generally, the dose is 0.01 to 0.03 mg/kg (0.1 to 0.3 mL/kg of the 1:10,000 solution) administered as needed every 3 to 5 minutes. Volume expanders are also used frequently and are indicated for the treatment of hypovolemia. Generally, 10 mL/kg of either normal saline or lactated Ringer's are administered through an IV or intraosseous catheter over 5 to 10 minutes. If there is concern for significant anemia in the fetus or newborn, O-negative blood, crossmatched with the mother if possible, should be considered as a volume expander. If time does not allow, emergent-release O-negative blood should be used to initially resuscitate the severely anemic infant. Naloxone (Narcan) is administered to newborns whose mothers had narcotics within 4 hours of delivery

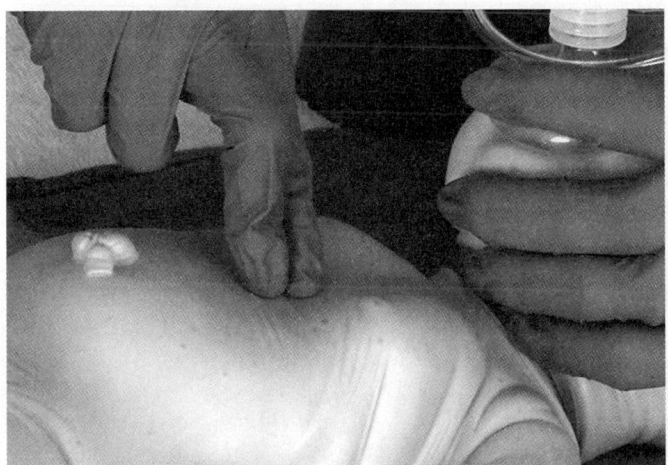

FIGURE 4. Two-finger external cardiac massage technique. Fingers are above xyphoid process; approximately one finger width beneath the nipple line.

TABLE 1 Drugs for Resuscitation/Stabilization

Medication	Concentration	Dosage/Route	Indications	Comment
Epinephrine	1:10,000	0.1-0.3 mL/kg/ dose IV or via ETT	Asystole Bradycardia that is unresponsive to PPV and chest compressions	Dilute dose with 1-3 mL normal saline for ETT. May repeat dose q 3-5 min.
Volume expanders Normal saline Lactated Ringer's		10 mL/kg IV	Hypovolemia Shock	
Glucose	10%	2 mL/kg IV	Hypoglycemia	May need to repeat.
Naloxone (Narcan)		0.1 mg/kg IV, IM, or ETT	Respiratory depression secondary to maternal narcotics	May precipitate acute life-threatening withdrawal in neonates born to drug-abusing mothers.
Sodium bicarbonate	0.5 mEq/mL	2 mL/kg IV	Documented severe metabolic acidosis or prolonged resuscitation with no response to other interventions	Administer slowly (≈2 mL/min).

Abbreviations: ETT = endotracheal tube; IM, intramuscularly; IV = intravenously; PPV = positive-pressure ventilation; q = every.

newborn shortly after birth. Scores are usually determined at 1 and 5 minutes of life. Resuscitation should *not* be delayed while awaiting the results of the 1-minute Apgar score.

Meconium Staining of the Amniotic Fluid

Meconium is a viscous, greenish-black substance consisting of gastrointestinal (GI) secretions, blood, bile acids, amniotic fluid, and cellular debris present in the fetal GI tract. In the majority of cases, meconium is cleared from the GI tract with the first few bowel movements. However, in approximately 10% to 15% of all deliveries, meconium is passed prior to birth, leading to meconium staining of the amniotic fluid, which increases an infant's risk of developing the meconium aspiration syndrome (MAS), a disease with serious morbidity and mortality. Current recommendations for management of meconium-stained amniotic fluid advise that as soon as the infant's head is delivered, and before the shoulders are delivered, that the mouth, nose, and pharynx should be vigorously suctioned with a specialized apparatus called a DeLee suction catheter, regardless of whether the meconium staining is thin or thick. After the infant is delivered, if the amniotic fluid contains meconium and the infant has absent or depressed respirations, decreased muscle tone, or heart rate less than 100 bpm, the infant is tracheally intubated and the trachea is suctioned using a meconium aspirator attached directly to the endotracheal tube. Resuscitation is then performed in the usual sequence, if required. Recent studies have called into question several of the aforementioned practices, including suctioning of the mouth, nose, and pharynx prior to delivery of the shoulders and routine endotracheal intubation and suctioning of the otherwise vigorous newborn. However, until further research is available, current recommendations continue to suggest the use of the previously discussed protocol.

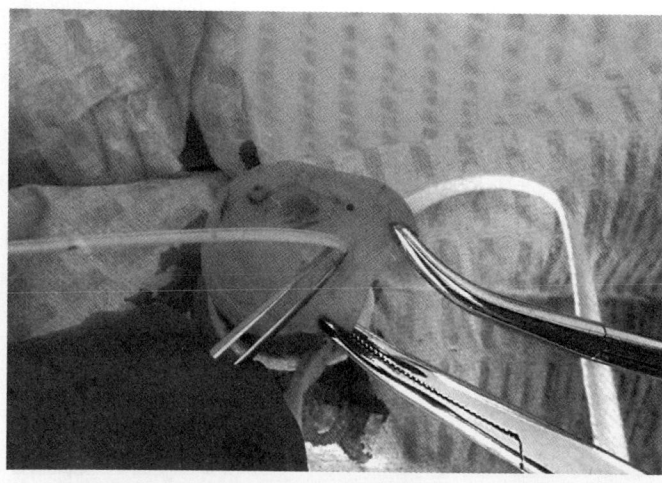

FIGURE 5. Umbilical vein catheterization. The umbilical vein is the preferred route for immediate venous access for drug medication and volume administration.

Newborn Resuscitation Outside the Delivery Room

Ideally, newborn resuscitation should take place in the delivery room setting. Unfortunately, many newborns are born outside the delivery room setting, such as in the home, en route to the hospital, or in the emergency department. Many mothers who deliver either outside the hospital setting or in the emergency department are more likely to represent high-risk groups (multiparous births, trauma-induced labor, lack of prenatal care, adolescent pregnancy,

TABLE 2 The Apgar Score*

Sign	0	1	2
Heart rate	Absent	Slow (less than 100 bpm)	Greater than 100 bpm
Respirations	Absent	Slow, irregular	Good, crying
Muscle tone	Limp	Some flexion	Active motion
Reflex irritability (catheter in nares)	No response	Grimace	Cough or sneeze
Color	Blue or pale	Acrocyanosis	Pink

*A score of 0, 1, or 2 is assigned in each category at 1 and 5 minutes of life.
Abbreviations: bpm = beats per minute.

placental abruption, etc.). Therefore, all emergency providers should be familiar with the resuscitation of the newborn. Resuscitation of the newborn infant presents several unique challenges to emergency care providers that are infrequently found during resuscitation of either the adult or child.

In many cases, deliveries in the emergency department will occur with little prior notice. Therefore, advanced preparation and an organized approach to resuscitation are essential. In addition to a standard obstetrical tray, airway, vascular access, and other equipment unique to newborn resuscitation should be readily available (see Box 2). There is often insufficient time to obtain a complete prenatal history from the mother; however, three key pieces of information are often helpful in determining the initial priorities of resuscitation. First, if labor is premature (i.e., fewer than 37 weeks' gestation), a lengthy resuscitation with a possible need for prolonged PPV can be anticipated. Second, if twins are expected, two resuscitation teams and two sets of equipment should be available. Finally, if the membranes have ruptured, the presence of meconium will indicate the need for an additional, more specialized resuscitation sequence (see previous discussion).

Ongoing Assessment

Neonatal resuscitation consists of a cycle of repeated assessment and therapeutic intervention (assess-intervene-assess) until cardiorespiratory and hemodynamic stability are achieved. The cycle of assess-intervene-assess should continue once the critically ill newborn has stabilized. During stabilization a complete blood cell count (CBC), serum electrolytes, blood urea nitrogen (BUN), creatinine, blood glucose, and an arterial blood gas to assess acid-base status should be obtained. A chest radiograph should be obtained to confirm proper placement of the endotracheal and orogastric tubes. Additional vascular access should be obtained. In the intubated patient, further deterioration should prompt rapid, close assessment for potential endotracheal tube complications. These complications can be easily recalled at the bedside by the mnemonic *DOPE*:

Dislodged: Has the endotracheal tube moved distally into the right or left main bronchus?
Obstructed: Is the endotracheal tube obstructed with inspissated secretions or blood?
Pneumothorax: Is there a pneumothorax?
Esophagus: Is the endotracheal tube in the esophagus?

In conclusion, the dramatic changes in cardiovascular and respiratory physiology that occur around the time of birth pose several potential problems that could lead to an unfavorable outcome. Proper education and training in neonatal resuscitation is imperative for all health care providers working in the deliver room and nursery setting. Health care providers in these settings, as well as those physicians working in the emergency department who may

CURRENT DIAGNOSIS

- Intrauterine asphyxia manifests as alterations in fetal heart rate (late decelerations, bradycardia), passage of meconium, fetal gasping, and eventual apnea, termed *primary apnea*. This initial period of apnea is followed by further gasping, which gradually weakens in intensity, eventually terminating in what is termed *secondary apnea*.

- Spontaneous respirations can be elicited in newborns with primary apnea by stimulation (vigorous warming and drying) or a brief trial of PPV. Newborns with secondary apnea, onthe other hand, have suffered a prolonged period of inadequate oxygen delivery and require aggressive resuscitation to prevent further decompensation, cardiac arrest, and death.

- The longer the delay in initiating resuscitation for primary apnea, the longer the time required to establish spontaneous respirations following PPV. Because there is no definitive method of differentiating between primary and secondary apnea following delivery, the neonatal resuscitation team must promptly recognize and institute proper treatment for all newborn infants with apnea and suspected perinatal asphyxia.

- Neonatal resuscitation is directed toward assuring a smooth transition to extrauterine life by achieving the following goals:
  Maintaining or restoring normal body temperature
  Maintaining or establishing effective ventilation and oxygenation
  Maintaining or restoring adequate cardiac output and tissue perfusion
  Avoiding hypoglycemia

- Neonatal resuscitation consists of a cycle of repeated assessment and therapeutic intervention (assess-intervene-assess) until cardiorespiratory and hemodynamic stability are achieved.

Abbreviation: PPV = positive-pressure ventilation.

- Initial efforts should be directed toward minimizing heat loss. On delivery, the infant should be placed on a radiant warmer. The infant is then dried vigorously with a warm, sterile towel.

- Properly positioning the infant on his or her back, with the head and neck in a neutral, midline position will assist in opening the airway. The mouth and nose should be suctioned with a bulb syringe to remove any secretions that may contribute to airway compromise.

- If respirations are adequate and cyanosis is present, supplemental oxygen should be administered.

- PPV, using a bag-valve-mask is indicated for those infants with either absent (apnea) or slow, gasping respiratory movements, and when the heart rate is below 100 bpm.

- Chest compressions should be performed immediately if the heart rate is less than 60 bpm after 30 seconds of effective PPV with 100% oxygen using either the two-thumb technique (preferred) or two-finger technique.

- Resuscitation medications should be administered if the heart rate remains less than 60 bpm despite 30 seconds of chest compressions and adequate PPV.

Abbreviations: bpm = beats per minute; PPV = positive-pressure ventilation.

also be called on to resuscitate newborn infants should have advanced knowledge and understanding of normal fetal, transitional, and neonatal physiology so that potential problems can be recognized and treated early. Only through the early recognition, resuscitation, and stabilization of the critically ill newborn will the best possible outcome be realized.

REFERENCES

Saugstad OD: Practical aspects of resuscitating newborn infants. Eur J Pediatr 1998;157(Suppl 1):S11-S15.

Palme-Kilander C: Methods of resuscitation in low-Apgar-score newborn infants: A national survey. Acta Pediatr 1992;81:739-744.

Apgar V: A proposal for a new method of evaluation of the newborn infant. Anesth Analg 1953;32:260-267.

Gelfand SL, Fanaroff JM, Walsh MC: Meconium stained fluid: Approach to the mother and the baby. Pediatr Clin North Am 2004;51:655-667.

Vain NE, Szyld EG, Prudent LM, et al: Oropharyngeal and nasopharyngeal suctioning of meconium-stained neonates before delivery of their shoulders: multicentre, randomised controlled trial. Lancet 2004;364:597-602.

Wiswell TE, Gannon CM, Jacob J, et al: Delivery room management of the apparently vigorous meconium-stained neonate: Results of the multicenter, international collaborative trial. Pediatrics 2000;105:1-7.

Niermeyer S, Kattwinkel J, Van Reempts P, et al: International guidelines for neonatal resuscitation: An excerpt from the Guidelines 2000 for Cardiopulmonary Resuscitation and Emergency Cardiovascular Care: International Consensus on Science. Contributors and Reviewers for the Neonatal Resuscitation Guidelines. Pediatrics 2000;106:E29.

The views presented are those of the author and do not necessarily represent the views of the Department of Defense or its components.

Care of the High-Risk Neonate

Method of
Dilcia McLenan, MD

Despite advances in prenatal care and diagnosis, the overall prematurity rate has not changed in the last two decades. The rate remains at 10% to 12% of all births in the United States. Although the overall mortality rate and the short-term morbidity rate have improved with the advances in neonatal care, premature births are still responsible for 75% to 85% of neonatal deaths. Congenital anomalies are associated with 20% to 30% of perinatal deaths. The early identification of the high-risk neonate is essential to improve outcome. The goal is to prevent the development or progression of more serious illnesses and to minimize the risk of both morbidity and mortality.

The definition of the high-risk neonate can be applied in the prenatal, perinatal or postnatal period. Approximately 75% of risk factors affecting the fetus are identified in the prenatal period. Maternal high-risk factors include age, race, socioeconomic status, nutrition and past obstetric history, current pregnancy problems, and maternal drug use. Maternal acute and chronic illness can also adversely affect the fetus. The placenta is considered fetal tissue; all conditions that affect the placenta will also affect the fetus, and vice versa. Fetal factors are limited to genetic conditions (chromosomal and nonchromosomal), and metabolic.

The prenatal diagnosis of the high-risk neonate uses many tools, such as chorionic villus sampling (CVS), amniocentesis, maternal serum screening, and cordocentesis. With the use of cytogenetics, molecular biology, and the fluorescence in situ hybridization, many genetic disorders and infectious conditions can be diagnosed. Fetal ultrasonography is another valuable tool in diagnosing high-risk conditions, including fetal growth abnormalities, which are associated with increased perinatal morbidity and mortality. The Doppler can assess blood velocity in the umbilical and fetal vessels. There is increased morbidity and mortality in fetuses with absent umbilical artery flow or with reverse end diastolic flow. The measurement of the nuchal translucency, done between 10 and 14 weeks of gestation by fetal ultrasound (US) in conjunction with the maternal serum markers, increases the detection rate of Down syndrome and other chromosomal and genetic syndromes, fetal structural malformations, and adverse pregnancy outcome.

Prenatal care facilitates the diagnosis and care of the high-risk neonate through a multidisciplinary approach. This multidisciplinary approach sets the stage for counseling, referrals, and the plan of care pre- and postnatally. When counseling the family, consider the gestational age at diagnosis, effect on maternal outcome and neonatal prognosis with or without therapy, plans for delivery, intrapartum management, and surgical intervention when applicable. General discussion with the parents during the intrapartum period regarding the preterm or high-risk neonate will include such things as anticipated birth weight and gestational age, the need for respiratory support, procedures to be expected, the need for transfusion of blood products, short- and long-term complications of each problem or condition, the need for other specialists, and morbidity and mortality. Involving the neonatologist in the counseling can aid families in making difficult decisions. One should also explain the need for transport, if delivered at a nontertiary care center, and the role the parents will have while their infant is in the neonatal intensive care unit (NICU).

The delivery management of the high-risk neonate is influenced by the factors identified in the antepartum and intrapartum period. In the intrapartum period, neonatal resuscitation facilitates the transition from the intrauterine to the extrauterine life. Approximately 5% to 10% of all newborns need help making this transition; 1% of all newborns need a more extensive intervention. The fetus is dependent on its mother and the placenta for the delivery of oxygen and nutrients as well as removal of carbon dioxide. After the umbilical cord is clamped and cut, the newborn needs to expand its lungs, establishing respirations and convert from a fetal (parallel) to an adult (in series) circulation for a successful transition, and avoid the development of asphyxia.

Resuscitation aims at facilitating the transition and reversing the process of asphyxia by clearing the airway, providing adequate oxygenation and ventilation, ensuring adequate cardiac output, and keeping oxygen consumption to the minimum. These objectives can be achieved by adhering to the four principles of neonatal resuscitation.

Principles of Neonatal Resuscitation

The American Heart Association (AHA) and the American Academy of Pediatrics (AAP) Neonatal Resuscitation Program (NRP) have defined the following principles of neonatal resuscitation:

- **Anticipation.** Risk factors in the antepartum and intrapartum history help identify instances that may potentially require intervention (Box 1).
- **Preparation.** In preparing the area, equipment should be assembled and checked, and drugs should be readied.
- **Availability of qualified personnel.** At every delivery there should be at least one person skilled in neonatal resuscitation whose only responsibility is the newborn; skills include the proper use of the bag and mask. In cases of emergency or if further intervention is needed, additional competent personnel should be immediately available.
- **Organized response to the emergencies—evaluation, decision, and action.** The ABCs (airway, breathing, and circulation) of resuscitation is the order in which assessment and needed intervention will be evaluated. The evaluation assesses the breathing, heart rate, and color, then the decision or diagnosis is made followed by the action or treatment .

The initial steps of resuscitation provide the support needed to make the transition from the intrauterine to the extrauterine life (Table 1).

BOX 1 Antepartum/Intrapartum Factors Associated with Potential Asphyxia

Antepartum Factors

Age >35 years	Post-term gestation
Maternal diabetes	Multiple gestation
Pregnancy-induced hypertension	Size-dates discrepancy
	Drug therapy, e.g.:
Chronic hypertension	Lithium carbonate
Anemia or isoimmunization	Magnesium
Previous fetal or neonatal death	Adrenergic blocking drugs
Bleeding in 2nd or 3rd trimester	Maternal substance abuse
Maternal infection	Fetal malformation
Hydramnios	Diminished fetal activity
Oligohydramnios	No prenatal care
Premature rupture of membranes	

Intrapartum Factors

Emergency cesarean section	Nonreassuring fetal heart rate pattern
Breech or other abnormal presentation	Use of general anesthesia
Premature labor	Uterine tetany
Prolonged rupture of membranes >24 h before delivery	Narcotics administered to mother within 4 h of delivery
Precipitous labor	Meconium-stained amniotic fluid
Prolonged labor (>24 h)	
Prolonged second stage of labor (>2 h)	Prolapsed cord
	Abruptio placentae; Placenta previa

Note: Keep these factors in mind because they will alert you that depression and possibly asphyxia are potential problems.

From Bloom RS, Cropley C: The AHNAAP Neonatal Resuscitation Program Steering Committee. Textbook of Neonatal Resuscitation. Dallas, TX, 1994, Copyright American Heart Association.

Shortcutting these steps prolongs the resuscitation process, increases the risk for asphyxia, and increases the likelihood of morbidity and mortality. In cases where further intervention is needed beyond the initial steps of resuscitation, a thorough evaluation should be done to diagnose conditions that might have contributed to the

TABLE 1 At Birth

Initial Step	Objective
Provide warmth.	Prevent heat loss, maintain oxygen consumption at a minimum, and prevent hypoglycemia.
Position, clear the airway (as necessary).	Establish an airway.
Dry stimulate and reposition.	Initiate breathing and open the airway.

need for further resuscitation, such as congenital abnormalities of the airway, heart, gastrointestinal (GI) tract, genitourinary (GU) system, or secondary cardiopulmonary disorders. Infants with Apgar scores below 7 at 10 minutes should be admitted to the NICU for further observation and management.

Asphyxia

Asphyxia is the result of prolonged decrease of oxygen delivery to the tissues. During the event, there is redistribution of blood flow to the heart, brain, and adrenals. The continuation of the insult results in bradycardia, impaired gas exchange, and reduced tissue perfusion. These series of events can occur prenatally, intrapartum, or postnatally. In severe cases of asphyxia almost every organ of the body is affected:

- Central nervous system (CNS): hypoxic ischemic encephalopathy
- Cardiovascular: myocardial dysfunction
- Renal: renal dysfunction and or acute renal failure
- GI: liver dysfunction and increased risk of necrotizing enterocolitis
- Hematologic: coagulopathy
- Pulmonary: activation of the mechanisms that cause persistent pulmonary hypertension of the newborn, surfactant (Survanta) deficiency, and meconium aspiration syndrome (MAS)
- Metabolic: acidosis, hypoglycemia, and hypocalcemia

After birth the normal newborn goes through a period of transition that lasts for several hours. During this period the cardiovascular, pulmonary, and sympathetic systems regulate themselves to adjust to extrauterine life. During the transition, abnormalities in color, respirations, heart rate, sleep state, motor activity, GI function, and temperature stability can be identified and will require care in the NICU. Clinical manifestations of abnormal transition include persistent tachypnea, nasal flaring, grunting, retractions, persistent cyanosis, apnea and bradycardia, pallor, temperature instability, blood pressure (BP) instability, lethargy, and other neurologic symptoms.

Postnatal Care

The postnatal care of the high-risk neonate is extremely important. There are interventions and supportive care that are common to the high-risk neonates to ensure the best possible outcome. These include thermoregulation, nutrition, developmental care, and parental involvement. Notwithstanding, individualized care that will address specific needs of each infant should always be kept in mind.

THERMOREGULATION

Thermoregulation is the balance between heat production and heat loss. It is closely linked to morbidity and mortality. In the neonate, heat loss can exceed heat production because of larger surface area to body mass ratio, decreased subcutaneous (SC) tissue or fat, increased permeability to water and small radius of curvature of exchange surfaces.

The newborn generates heat by nonshivering mechanisms—brown fat, increased muscular activity, flexion, and increased metabolic rate with increased oxygen consumption. The newborn loses heat through conduction, convection, evaporation, and radiation (Table 2).

In the neonate there is always a combination of types and mechanism of heat loss. The prevention of cold stress and hypothermia is critical for intact survival of the neonate (Figure 1).

Heat production is a result of metabolic processes that generate energy by oxidative metabolism of glucose (most efficient in the premature infant), fat, and protein. In the newborn, heat or energy production is low relative to heat or energy losses. Brown adipose tissue generates more energy than any other tissue in the body. The brown adipose tissue cells begin to differentiate by 26 to 30 weeks of gestation and continue to develop until 3 to 5 weeks after birth; they constitute 10% of the adipose tissue in term infants.

Thermoregulation is achieved by providing the appropriate thermal environment to prevent heat loss, hypothermia, and cold stress. The neutral thermal environment (NTE) is an idealized range of ambient temperature at which the body temperature is normal, metabolic rate or

---

TABLE 2   Thermoregulation: Types, Mechanisms, and Management

Type/Definition	Mechanism	Prevention
Conduction, transfer of heat from the body core to surface, and object in contact with body.	Cold surfaces, cold objects in contact with the body	Use rubber mattresses, warm blankets, and warm mattresses.
Convection, heat transfer from the body surface to the surrounding air.	Cool rapid air flow, cold oxygen flow	Swaddle using a cap, warm oxygen, and placing infant away from draft. Servo control air or skin incubators, warm room temperature.
Evaporation, moisture on the body surface or respiratory tract evaporates. Major source of heat loss after delivery or during bath. Inversely related to gestational age.	Wet skin, increase of activity, tachypnea, under radiant warmer and phototherapy	Dry infant immediately after birth and bath; increase humidity; use warm soaks and solutions; use polyethylene wraps, warm and humidified oxygen.
Radiation, transfer of heat from the body to surrounding cooler surfaces not in contact with the infant.	Dependent on ambient temperature, air speed and other heat loss mechanisms	Double-wall incubators, radiant warmer, and heat shield.

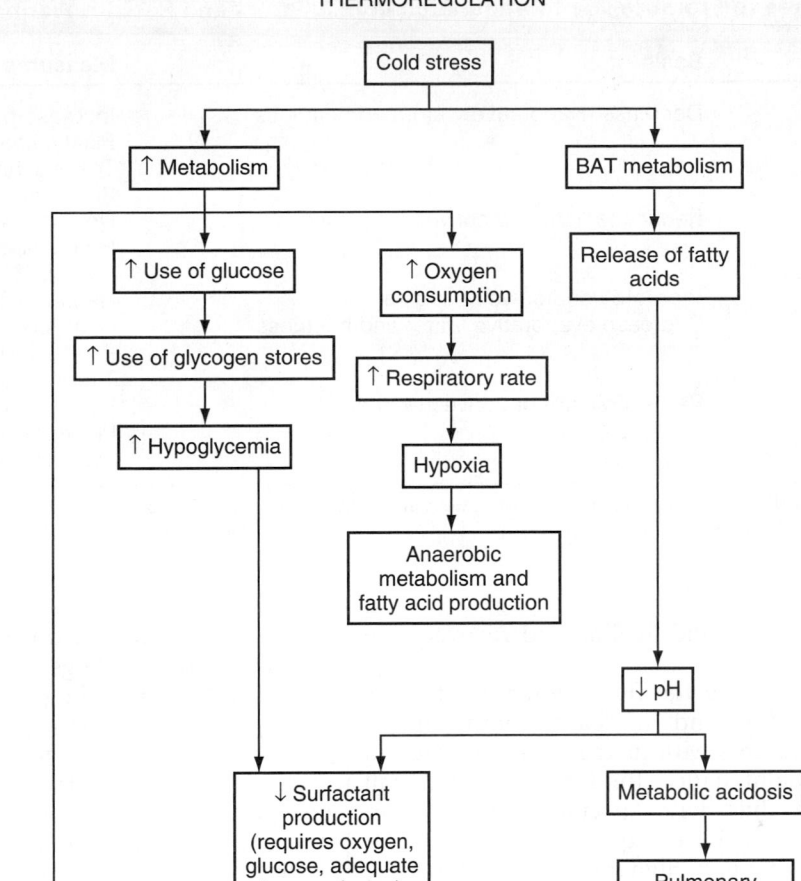

FIGURE 1. Physiologic consequences of cold stress. BAT = Brown adipose tissue.

oxygen consumption is minimal, and thermoregulation is achieved by basal nonevaporative physical processes. It promotes growth and stability and minimizes heat (energy) and water loss. Newborns have a narrow control range that make them vulnerable to alterations in the thermal environment. The NTE is achieved for the:

- Term infant at 32°C (89.6°F) to 33.5°C (92.3°F)
- Preterm infant greater than 1500 g at 34°C (93.2°F) to 35°C (95°F)
- Preterm infant less than 1500 g at 36.7°C (98.1°F) to 37.3°C (99.1°F)

The two common methods of supporting thermoregulation are the radiant warmer and the incubator (Table 3).

NUTRITION

Proper nutrition is essential for adequate growth, development, and healing. Protein and lipid stores are decreased in the neonate, who has a higher baseline energy requirement compared to children and adults. The low-birth-weight (LBW) infant and the premature infant have even higher baseline requirements. The premature infant has minimal stores of fat and carbohydrates and rapidly develops nutritional deficiencies in calcium, phosphorus, iron trace elements, and vitamins. Nutritional requirements of calories and protein increase even further in the critically ill neonate with overwhelming infections, severe lung disease, and major surgical conditions. These conditions obviate the enteral route of delivering adequate nutrition as well as the immature digestive pathways of the GI tract. In these cases parenteral nutrition is the only option. In premature infants nutritional support is aimed at achieving an intrauterine growth pattern of 15 to 30 g per day. To achieve comparable weight at term-corrected age, compared to a term infant, the daily growth rate would have to be higher to achieve catch-up growth. When there is early positive nitrogen balance, weight loss is less, there

TABLE 3 Measures to Promote Thermoregulation in Incubators and Radiant Warmers

Bed	Basis	Measures
Incubator	Decrease evaporative water and heat loss	Increase humidity
		Plastic heat shield
		Thermal blanket
		Semiocclusive dressings or emollients
	Reduce radiant and convective losses	Double-walled incubator
		Heat shield
		Thermal blanket
Radiant warmer	Promote conductive heat gain	Heated mattress
	Decrease evaporative water and heat loss	Heat shield
		Plastic wrap
		Thermal blanket
	Reduce radiant or convective losses	Heat shield
		Plastic wrap
		Thermal blanket

Modified from Sinclair, J. (1992). Management of the thermal environment. In J.C. Sinclair and M.B. Brocker (eds). Effective care of the newborn infant. Oxford: Oxford University Press.

is a better rate of growth, and healing and recovery are faster.

With parenteral nutrition the fluid requirement starts at 80 mL/kg per day and increases daily up to 150 mL/kg per day. Infants with increased fluid losses, in addition to their maintenance fluid requirement, will require replacement fluid with specific electrolytes to offset their losses. The caloric requirement varies from 80 kcal to 120 kcal/kg per day. Higher caloric needs of 20% to 30% more are required in the extremely premature infants and in the critically ill neonate. To achieve the expected postnatal growth pattern, the total nonprotein calories requirement should be at least 70 to 105 kcal/kg per day; and the protein intake should be 2.7 to 3.5 g/kg per day of protein for positive nitrogen balance, adequate nitrogen accretion, and good neurodevelopmental outcome. Protein is given in the form of an amino acid solution. These amino acids are the building blocks required for growth, preservation of skeletal muscle protein mass, tissue repair, and appropriate inflammatory response. Protein intake starts at the recommended daily intake of 3 to 4 g/kg per day. Critically ill neonates will also require an increase in protein intake by 10% to 20%.

Calories or energy is given through carbohydrates and fat. Glucose is the carbohydrate used in parenteral nutrition and is the preferred substrate for the brain. It provides 3.4 cal/g of glucose. Fat is given as a 20% lipid emulsion solution, and it provides 2 cal/mL. The use of the lipid emulsion will prevent essential fatty acid deficiency, improve protein use and will not increase significantly CO_2 production or metabolic rate compared to glucose. This is an important factor in infants with chronic lung disease and retention of carbon dioxide. The infusion rate of fat begins at 0.5 g/kg per day and is advanced by 0.5 g daily up to 2 to 4 g/kg per day. Close monitoring of triglycerides is required. A level above 250 mg/dL is considered high, so the rate of infusion should then be cut back. Adequate energy intake will promote or facilitate positive nitrogen balance and nitrogen accretion. Other components of parenteral nutrition are calcium, phosphorus, vitamins, and trace minerals. Sodium and potassium are added based on the serum electrolyte results. Carnitine is added when premature infants are on prolonged parenteral nutrition with no enteral feedings.

The task of providing adequate nutrition is multidisciplinary; the neonatologist, pharmacist, and nutritionist form part of the team. Close metabolic monitoring for glucose, electrolytes, urea, lipids, and acid–base balance is an integral part of the nutritional management of the high-risk neonates. This will help assess and meet nutritional needs as well as monitor for complications such as metabolic acidosis, electrolyte imbalance, cholestatic jaundice, increased triglyceride levels, and infection. When enteral feeding is possible, human milk should be considered. Although it may not provide adequate caloric and protein intake, it has many other assets that are important in promoting healing, neurodevelopment, and protection against infection.

DEVELOPMENTAL CARE

The NICU environment plays a major role in the growth and development of the high-risk neonate and may contribute to the morbidity of these fragile infants. The amount of abnormal sensory stimulus that these fragile beings are exposed to is the source of overwhelming stress at sensitive periods of their development, and in turn will modify their brain development. The cortex of the brain is part of the sensory system, and both deprivation and over-stimulation can modify its development. The sensitive period when this occurs is between 28 and 40 weeks of gestation. Therefore the NICU environment is crucial as part of the care of the sick newborn infant. These infants are subject to numerous stress factors, unpleasant procedures, continuously disrupted sleep, frequent noxious oral stimulus, noise, and bright lights. Stress causes autonomic instability, with secretion of cortisol and catecholamines. These hormones in turn interfere with tissue healing and growth.

When considering the NICU environment and the input or stimuli that could be beneficial to these high-risk neonates, one has to take into consideration the in utero environment and how the sensory stimulus would have been perceived in that environment, and the normal development of the sensory system for planned interventions. The hierarchical organization, maturation, and integration of the sensory system is as follows:

- Tactile
- Vestibular
- Gustatory
- Olfactory
- Auditory
- Visual

The visual sensory system is the least mature at term and maturation continues after birth. There is overlapping regarding when a sensory system maturation begins and ends, but there is clear evidence that disruption of one sensory system will affect the maturation of the system that has not yet developed. The same is true when a later sensory system is stimulated earlier than expected.

The interventions that support the development of the sensory system are as follows:

- Minimal handling
- Clustering of care
- Soft swaddling
- Stroking, rocking, and holding when appropriate
- Non-nutritive sucking
- Positioning prone or on the side
- Nesting
- Placing the infant in an infant seat; then swaddle and nest
- Soothing, soft, simple repetitive, and harmonic sounds with limited dynamic range
- Limit ambient light
- Shield eyes and chest from bright lights
- Limit the initial visual stimulus to the human face
- Massage therapy

These suggested interventions should take into consideration the gestational age and the clinical acuity of the high-risk patient. The goal is to improve growth and neurodevelopmental outcome of the high-risk neonate.

PARENTAL INVOLVEMENT

When looking at specific high-risk situations, one can appreciate the scope of support needed by these high-risk neonates from various subspecialists and ancillary health care professionals. One of the things often forgotten is the major role the parents play in the healing and development of their sick infant. Parents have a sense of loss from the time their sick newborn has to be resuscitated and/or is admitted to the NICU. They have a sense of loss for delivering prematurely, for not having a healthy full-term infant, loss of self-esteem, and social status as parents. Involving the parents in the care of their infant will provide some emotional, psychosocial, and spiritual support to the parents. The literature continues to support the need for and the benefits of parental involvement in the NICU as part of the care of the high-risk neonate.

Kangaroo care, or skin-to-skin contact between the parent and the infant, provides sustained multimodal stimulation of tactile, vestibular, proprioceptive, olfactory, and auditory sensory systems. Physiologic benefits such as stable temperature; stable oxygen consumption; higher saturation levels; increased quiet sleep, which lowers cortisol levels resulting in fewer infections; and better growth have been described. It promotes non-nutritive sucking, and there is a better letdown in breast-feeding mothers. Kangaroo care acts as a behavioral organizer or facilitator, decreases motor activity, increases the quiet state in stable preterm infants, and reduces the effect of painful stimuli. These infants are also discharged sooner.

Parents can also participate in massage therapy. It has a calming effect on infants; they express fewer stress behaviors, are more alert, actively respond to face and voice, and show more organized limb movements on the Brazelton behavioral scale. Better weight gain and early discharge have been reported. At 8 months these infants continue to show better weight gain and higher scores on the Bayley Scales of Infant Development.

Conditions Associated With Abnormal Transition

A few conditions associated with abnormal transition are described in the following text.

HYALINE MEMBRANE DISEASE

Hyaline membrane disease (HMD) is the result of surfactant deficiency. Surfactant reduces the surface tension of the alveoli and prevents them from collapsing. This disorder is common to preterm infants. The clinical presentation of HMD is that of respiratory distress characterized by grunting, retractions, and flaring. Grunting is used to maintain the intra-alveoli pressure and prevent it from collapsing. The blood gas typically has hypoxemia and to a lesser degree respiratory acidosis. Radiographically the lungs have a ground glass appearance (this represents microatelectasis) and air bronchograms (the contrast of the air-filled bronchi against the collapse parenchyma). These infants are managed with ventilator support and/or continuous positive airway pressure (CPAP), and surfactant (Survanta) replacement therapy. The use of antenatal steroids has decreased the incidence of HMD and the need for exogenous surfactant in the premature newborn, especially in infants who are 28 weeks' gestation or more.

TRANSIENT TACHYPNEA OF THE NEWBORN

Transient tachypnea of the newborn (TTN) is described as the retention of lung fluid or transient pulmonary edema. During labor the increased level of prostaglandins causes dilation of the lymphatic vessels in the lungs promoting the absorption of the pulmonary interstitial fluid. After birth, this process is further accelerated by the expansion of the lungs with air-filled alveoli and increased pulmonary circulation. Any delay in this process will result in tachypnea and occasional grunting and flaring. This is common after elective cesarean section. The arterial blood gas shows various degrees of respiratory acidosis and some hypoxemia. The typical chest radiographic findings reveal increased interstitial marking with fluid in the fissure and on occasion pleural effusion. This condition is self-limited, resolving in 1 to 2 days. These infants are managed with oxygen support by hood and rarely require ventilator support.

MECONIUM ASPIRATION SYNDROME

Meconium staining of the amniotic fluid occurs in 10% to 25% of all deliveries. It is seen in fetuses beyond 35 weeks of gestation. Passage of meconium in utero is often the result of a hypoxemic event. Meconium can be aspirated before, during, or after delivery. Once aspirated it can cause obstruction of the airway and pulmonary air leak, chemical pneumonitis and secondary bacterial infection, secondary surfactant deficiency, and pulmonary hypertension of the newborn (PPHN) if hypoxemia persists. After birth, a depressed neonate with poor or no respiratory effort should be intubated and suctioned immediately after being placed under the radiant warmer. This action will clear the airway and prevent aspiration or any further aspiration. The key in preventing meconium aspiration in neonates who did not have in utero aspiration is suctioning of the airway at the perineum by the obstetrician as soon as the head is delivered. The severity of the disease varies. The arterial blood gas pictures vary from mild respiratory acidosis with mild hypoxemia to severe respiratory failure with marked hypoxemia. The classical radiographic finding of the lungs is that of patchy infiltrates throughout the lung fields; air leak is seen in 10% to 20% of these cases. Postnatal management consists of support to minimize all factors that will perpetuate asphyxia and trigger pulmonary hypertension. Decrease energy loss and oxygen consumption by providing warmth, oxygen, and glucose. Aggressive respiratory support is needed, providing high concentration of oxygen in a hood or through the ventilator. In cases associated with severe PPHN, inhaled nitric oxide (iNO [INO_{max}]), and ultimately extracorporeal membrane oxygenation (ECMO) may become part of the management.

PERSISTENT PULMONARY HYPERTENSION OF THE NEWBORN

Persistent pulmonary hypertension of the newborn is the result of severe hypoxemia because of right-to-left shunting through the foramen ovale and ductus arteriosus, without associated structural heart abnormality. The pulmonary hypertension results from increased pulmonary vasoreactivity and increased muscle mass of the pulmonary arterial vessels. The increase in pulmonary smooth arterial muscle mass seen in term infants is triggered by intrauterine stress or hypoxemia. The vasoreactive response seen after birth is caused by alteration of the balance between the circulating pulmonary vasodilator (endothelium-derived relaxing factor or endogenous nitric oxide) and pulmonary vasoconstrictors (endothelin). This vasoreactive response is seen also in preterm and term infants with primary lung disease, such as surfactant deficiency, pneumonia, or MAS. Tachypnea and cyanosis is the clinical presentation. The blood gas has severe hypoxemia and combine metabolic and respiratory acidosis. In primary PPHN, the chest radiograph is normal; in secondary PPHN, it will be characteristic of the disease in question. The diagnosis of PPHN is made with the aid of the echocardiogram, which will exclude structural heart disease, measure the pulmonary artery pressure and resistance and visualize the right-to-left shunts, and tricuspid regurgitation that is commonly present.

The management of neonates with PPHN can be challenging. The goal is to correct the hypoxemia and acidosis, both of which cause pulmonary vasoconstriction. The acidosis can be managed with hyperventilation using conventional or high-frequency ventilator (to achieve a $Paco_2$ close to 30 mm Hg) and/or infusion of sodium bicarbonate to maintain the arterial pH around 7.40. The hypoxemia is more difficult to manage because these infants do not always respond to high concentrations of oxygen with high ventilator support. The Pao_2 should be maintained above 80 mm Hg. Concurrent metabolic derangement, such as hypoglycemia and hypocalcemia, and polycythemia should be corrected. The systemic arterial BP should be maintained in the high range of normal. The use of vasopressor agents (dopamine [Intropin] or dobutamine [Dobutrex]) is recommended in achieving this goal, as opposed to volume expansion. The increase in the systemic BP may decrease the right-to-left shunt through the ductus arteriosus and improve pulmonary blood flow and in turn improve the hypoxemia.

When the previously described management fails, the use of iNO at a dose of 20 ppm or less will cause selective pulmonary vasodilatation. Because many infants respond to iNO, the need for ECMO has decreased. Extracorporeal membrane oxygenation is available only in a few medical centers for those cases that fail to respond to maximum ventilator support and iNO.

The Infant with Surgical Conditions

Infants before, during, or after surgery require special consideration regarding management and support of the cardiopulmonary system, thermoregulation, fluid and electrolyte management, nutritional support, and infection control.

GASTROSCHISIS

The combined incidence of omphalocele and gastroschisis is 1:4000 live births. Of these two abdominal wall defects, gastroschisis is the more common. It is a cleft in the abdominal wall to the right of the umbilical cord with herniation of the bowel. The association of other congenital and chromosomal anomalies is rare compared with omphalocele. Common associated problems seen in gastroschisis are malrotation of the bowel, undescended testes, stenosis, and atresia of the bowel, all of which are the result of vascular injury. In 20% of the patients, necrotizing enterocolitis has been reported postoperatively.

Gastroschisis can be diagnosed in the prenatal period. This will allow for proper counseling of the family as well as the plans for intrapartum and postnatal management. The intrapartum and postnatal management consist of preventing further injury to the bowel, temperature stabilization, fluid and electrolyte management, antibiotic therapy, nutritional support, and surgical correction. The exposed bowel is at risk for further circulatory compromise. This may be avoided by having the infant lie on his or her side. Because there is a large surface area exposed to the environment, heat and fluid losses are increased. The bowel should be wrapped in cephalexin (Keflex) soaked in warm normal saline, and then covered with a plastic barrier. The prolonged exposure of the bowel to the amniotic fluid causes a severe inflammatory response that results in ileus. In addition to the increased fluid losses through the exposed bowel, there is intraluminal loss of fluid and electrolyte because of the severe ileus. In these patients 1.5 to 2 times their fluid maintenance is needed for fluid resuscitation. The bowel should be decompressed using a nasogastric or orogastric tube connected to intermittent low suction. Close monitoring of vital signs, intake and output, and serum electrolytes will give indications of the fluid and electrolyte status of these infants.

Nutritional support in infants with gastroschisis is crucial for healing and to decrease morbidity and mortality. Prior to parenteral nutrition, the mortality in these infants was very high, malnutrition and complications associated with infection being major causes. These infants may go for several weeks before enteral feedings can be attempted or tolerated. Early placement of central venous access will facilitate the long-term nutritional support and the overall management. Long-term parenteral nutrition is the key for full recovery of these infants.

The surgical approach considers two options: primary or secondary closure. Secondary closure creates an enclosed hernia, a silo with the bowel content. The bowel is then slowly returned to the abdominal cavity over several days. Antibiotics are continued until the abdominal wall is closed. Primary closure returns the bowel into the abdominal cavity in one step. It is not uncommon, especially with large defects, to have respiratory compromise requiring ventilator support. Be conscious of the need for pain management in these infants, more so in those with respiratory compromise. Other complications seen with primary closure are further bowel compromise with bloody drainage, acidosis, and infection and increased intra-abdominal pressure that causes decrease renal and or central venous perfusion.

CONGENITAL DIAPHRAGMATIC HERNIA

The incidence of congenital diaphragmatic hernia (CDH) is 1:2000 to 5000 live births. This condition can be diagnosed in the prenatal period. When diagnosed in the prenatal period the plan of management begins. The infant should be delivered at a tertiary care center experienced in counseling and treatment of CDH. In these patients, further workup should be done to exclude other malformations of the heart, GI tract, GU system, and CNS and chromosomal anomalies. Associated malformations should be taken into account when counseling the family and when developing the postnatal plan of management. Plans to deliver at term, and at a center where there is a pediatric surgeon, capability for iNO (INO_{max}) and ECMO is desired. Once delivered, the infant should be intubated immediately, venous access obtained in case of needed circulatory support, and a nasogastric or orogastric tube placed to decompress the bowel. Bowel distention can further compromise respiration and cardiac function.

The infant should be transferred to the NICU, an arterial line should be placed and blood obtained for blood gas and crossmatch. Obtain a chest and abdominal radiograph to confirm the diagnosis and line placement. An echocardiogram should be done to assess for structural abnormalities of the heart and to estimate the degree of pulmonary hypertension. A head US should be obtained if the infant will be placed on ECMO, because of the risk of intracranial hemorrhage in patients on ECMO.

Skilled ventilator management is important because of the coexisting pulmonary hypertension. Barotrauma and volutrauma should be avoided in these patients. Permissive hypercapnia is permitted once there is adequate preductal oxygenation (preductal oxygenation is measured or obtained from the right upper extremity; the preductal blood perfuses the heart and brain). The highest rates of survival result in patients in whom barotrauma and volutrauma are avoided and permissive hypercapnia is allowed.

A patient is considered unstable or to have failed ventilator support when the pH is <7.25, a peak inspiratory pressure of >30 cm H_2O is needed, and preductal saturation is <90% on 60% oxygen. The use of iNO (INO_{max}) may be considered in these cases, but the direct effect on pulmonary vascular resistance and right heart function need to be monitored closely. Therapy should be discontinued if no response is demonstrated. Extracorporeal membrane oxygenation is a reasonable choice for patients that have received maximum medical intervention. A venous-venous shunt is preferred unless there is significant cardiac instability.

Surgical correction is done if the infant is stable after the honeymoon period (the first 24 hours). Achievement of 90% survival is possible in a nonselect group of patients with the combination of careful ventilator management, attention to the pulmonary hypertension, delayed surgery, and aggressive early nutrition support. Survival rates are also dependent on the presence or absence of associated abnormalities and their severity. Long-term follow-up beyond the neonatal period is necessary for accurate estimation of morbidity and mortality in patients who are placed on ECMO.

The Extremely Low Birth Weight Infant

A premature infant is a neonate who is delivered before 37 completed weeks of gestation. These infants can be further classified according to their birth weight:

- Low birth weight (LBW) if less than 2500 g
- Very low birth weight (VLBW) if less than 1500 g
- Extremely low birth weight (ELBW) if less than 1000 g

Within the ELBW infants is a subgroup called the micro-premie, if birth weight is less than 750 g. The need for intrapartum and postnatal intervention and support is inversely proportional to gestational age as well as the morbidity and mortality associated with these infants. The increased risks for asphyxia, heat and water loss, intraventricular hemorrhage, and respiratory distress increase with decreasing gestational age. In the delivery room, the initial steps of resuscitation will support transition by preventing heat

TABLE 4   Common Problems and Management of the Extremely Low Birth Weight Infant

Problems	Management
Delivery Room. It is anticipated that a complete team will be needed for resuscitation: neonatal nurse, respiratory therapist, and neonatologist.	Prevent heat loss, provide respiratory support, prevent asphyxia, and avoid trauma. Place under radiant warmer and dry well, use warm blankets and cap. Use bag and mask properly and prompt intubation when needed. Properly position the ETT; avoid high inspiratory pressure with overdistention of the lungs. Follow the ABCs of resuscitation.
NICU. The management in the delivery room and the first hours of life sets the stage for the rest of the NICU care.	In the NICU, the infant is placed under a radiant warmer for easy access and thermoregulation. Connect to all monitors, insert umbilical venous and arterial catheters for fluid management, BP monitoring, and to facilitate blood draw. Obtain chest and abdominal radiograph to assess the severity of lung disease and position of the ETT, venous, and arterial catheters. Cover infant with plastic wrap to decrease evaporative heat and fluid loss. Frequent weighing with a bed scale will estimate hydration status. There should be minimal handling and clustered care in the first week of life.
Fluid and Electrolytes. The high insensible water loss in the ELBW infant increases the risk for dehydration, hypernatremia, and hyperkalemia	Fluid requirements range from 100 to 150 mL/kg/d, given as D5W with no added electrolytes in the first 24-48 h. Monitoring of the electrolytes and strict I&O will estimate the hydration status. Monitor blood draw and replace with PRBC from a single donor, CMV negative, when 10% of blood volume is removed. Hypernatremia is caused by increased water loss and corrected with increased fluid intake. Risk of hyperkalemia is caused by water loss and increases if there is extravascular blood collection; this is corrected using insulin infusion with glucose, correcting acidosis with sodium bicarbonate, calcium gluconate to stabilize the myocardium, and a cation exchange resin per rectum—sodium polystyrene sulfonate (Kayexalate).
Nutrition. Long-term parenteral nutrition is required in these infants. Good nutritional support is necessary for growth and neurodevelopment.	Beginning early parenteral nutrition within the first 24 h in stable infants will provide a source of energy (glucose), protein to decrease the risk of negative nitrogen balance, calcium, vitamins, and trace minerals. Placement of percutaneous CVC should be done early in the course. Please refer to the section on nutrition in this article for further nutrition management.
CNS. There is an increased risk of developing IVH in unstable infants in the first few days of life.	To prevent IVH, stressful conditions like cold stress, hypoxemia, acidosis swing in BP, and increased intrathoracic pressure should be avoided. Initial US in the first 3 d if unstable and at the end of the first week if stable. Follow-up will depend on findings. Infants with no IVH should have a repeat at 36 weeks postmenstrual age. The use of sedation in the first week of life has not shown significant changes in the incidence of IVH.
Respiratory. HMD is the most common condition. Avoid complications associated with the disease (air leaks and pulmonary emphysema, pulmonary hemorrhage, ICH, and CLD).	Use of exogenous surfactant when indicated and rapid weaning of PIP and O_2 and close monitoring to avoid complications. Blood gas is obtained 10-15 min after each change. Use high ventilator rate and the lowest PIP to maintain saturation 93%-95%, permissive hypercapnia ($Paco_2$ 50-60), mild acidosis (pH 7.25-7.35), and Po_2 50-70 are the goal. When stable, extubate to NCPAP. Apnea is common in these infants; they are treated with caffeine citrate (Cafcit). An initial bolus of 20 mg/kg is given followed by maintenance of 5 mg/kg every 24 h.

TABLE 4 Common Problems and Management of the Extremely Low Birth Weight Infant—cont'd

Problems	Management
Cardiovascular. PDA occurs in >50% of ELBW infants. Appearing when the lung disease is improving, clinically there is increased need for respiratory support associated with desaturation, active precordium, bounding pulses, and wide pulse pressure. The diagnosis is confirmed by echocardiogram. The ductus arteriosus of the preterm responds less to the vasoconstrictive effect of oxygen.	Medical treatment consists of fluid restriction, maintenance of hematocrit around 40%, and the use of indomethacin (Indocin IV). Complications of indomethacin (Indocin IV) are decreased GFR causing fluid retention, and platelet dysfunction (contraindicated in renal failure, bleeding disorders, and low platelets). The dose is 0.2 mg/kg for four doses and a diuretic such as furosemide (Lasix) at 1 mg/kg/dose to try to prevent oliguria. If there is no response, additional dosing or courses can be given. The definitive treatment would be ligation of the ductus. Some centers use prophylactic indomethacin (Indocin IV).
Skin. Underdevelopment of the stratum corneum cause increase transepidermal water loss→dehydration→ electrolyte imbalance and evaporative heat loss. Traumatized skin is the port of entry for many infectious organisms. Acceleration of skin maturation occurs after birth over the next 10-14 d.	Use of plastic shields, increased humidity, and topical skin emollient will decrease heat and water loss and may be protective to the skin.
Glucose. Hyperglycemia is secondary to high glucose-infusion rates. When an infant becomes hyperglycemic on a stable glucose-infusion rate, consider infection and or IVH. Early hypoglycemia is common in this group of infants due to poor glycogen stores and immature hormonal adaptation of the endocrine system.	Glucose level should be >40 mg/dL in the first 48-72 h and >45 mg/dL after 72 h. When hypoglycemic, a bolus of D10W at 200 mg/kg (2 mL/kg) is given. Glucose level is obtained in 30 min, frequent monitoring is continued every 1-3 h, and further boluses are given as needed. Maintenance fluid provides 4-6 mg/kg/min of glucose infusion. This rate of infusion should be increased by 2 mg/kg/min with every need for D10W bolus. Refer to specific text for detailed management.
Calcium. The stores of calcium are limited and the reserves are rapidly depleted after birth.	Higher intake of calcium with adequate phosphorus intake is required for bone formation and growth.
Jaundice. These infants are at increased risk for brain toxicity from high bilirubin levels. High bilirubin level develops due to hepatic immaturity, shorter RBC life span, extravasation of blood, and increased enterohepatic circulation, coupled with lower serum albumin level.	The level that causes toxicity is lower in these infants. A crude method to determine the need for phototherapy at 50% the weight in kg: A 0.9 Kg infant is placed under phototherapy for a bilirubin level of 4.5 mg/dL. Exchange level is determined by the weight, in this case 9 mg/dL. The risk for toxicity increases in the unstable infant, the reason why lower levels should be used when managing. Fluid intake should be increased 15%-20% in infants under phototherapy.

Abbreviations: ABC = airway, breathing, and circulation; BP = blood pressure; CLD = chronic lung disease; CMV = cytomegalovirus; CVC = central venous catheter; ELBW = extremely low birth weight infant; ETT = endotracheal tube; GFR = glomerular filtration rate; HMD = hyaline membrane disease; I&O = intake and output; ICH = intracranial hemorrhage; IV = intravenous; IVH = intraventricular hemorrhage; NCPAP = nasal continuous positive airway pressure; NICU = neonatal intensive care unit; PDA = patent ductus arteriosus; PIP = peak inspiratory pressure; PRBC = packed red blood cells; RBC = red blood cell; US = ultrasound.

and water loss and asphyxia. The use of surfactant (Survanta) should be considered in ELBW infants. In infants more than 1000 g, surfactant replacement therapy should be done as soon as the neonate presents a clinical picture of surfactant deficiency (HMD). Surfactant should be given with the proper ventilator support and, it is not uncommon to require multiple doses. With delay in therapy the morbidity and mortality associated with HMD increases.

The ELBW infants are a special group within the premature infants because the advances in health care and technology seem to have had less of an impact on this group of infants. The overall morbidity and mortality continue to be comparatively high in these infants and more so in the micropremie or infants less than 27 weeks of gestation. Table 4 lists the common problems faced by the ELBW infants and their management.

Special Therapy

Although there are continued attempts to provide care for the ELBW infant, there are infants outside the scope of *viability*—infants with complex congenital malformations, including those labeled as *incompatible with life*, and those whose condition is irreversible and ultimately will lead to death. For such infants, we see the need for comfort care or palliative care. In these situations both the health care professional and parents find themselves in an awkward position. The family remains hopeful based on the perceived information that the health care professional gives, or the family goes through turmoil when interventions seem endless in a situation that they perceive as hopeless.

The decision for palliative care is made through collaboration between the health care team and the parents. The two factual considerations in making the decision for

CURRENT DIAGNOSIS

- Review of risk factors: antenatal, perinatal, and postnatal
- Assessment of infants in the delivery room: airway, breathing and circulation—respiration, heart rate, and color
- Continued assessment in the nursery: respirations, heart rate, color, temperature, and CNS
- Common problems: pulmonary, circulatory, gastrointestinal, metabolic, surgical, and temperature instability

Abbreviation: CNS = central nervous system.

palliative care are pertinent medical facts (diagnosis, response to treatment given, potential response to other treatments, and prognosis) and the human value (what the parents anticipate, expect, and desire for their infant) and what motivates these values in the parents. The values of the health care team involved in the care of the infant are also considered.

Palliative care, as defined by the World Health Organization (WHO), is care for patients for whom cure is no longer a reasonable expectation or possibility. It is an active and comprehensive management of the entire patient, and not abandonment of care.

Practical considerations that need to be taken into account, and specific components of the palliative care that are appropriate for each individual high-risk neonate, are considered before a specific plan can be put in place. The application of palliative care in the NICU is not only possible, but necessary.

CURRENT THERAPY

- Use functioning equipment and qualified personnel in the delivery room: initial steps and ABCs of neonatal resuscitation.
- Provide neutral thermal environment.
- Respiratory and cardiovascular support: oxygen, mechanical ventilation, vasopressor agent (dopamine).
- Infuse bolus of D10W and glucose at 6-8 mg/kg per minute or higher if needed.
- Use phototherapy for early jaundice and the bruised ELBW infant.
- Transfer to appropriate level of care when indicated.
- Monitor closely fluid and electrolytes and decreased IWL. Provide good nutritional support beginning in the first 24 hours and closely monitor for complications and tolerance.
- Provide family-centered care and appropriate environment to promote growth and development.
- Benefit special cases, especially those deemed futile, with a multidisciplinary approach.

Abbreviations: ABC = airway, breathing, and circulation; ELBW = extremely low birth weight; IWL = insensible water loss.

REFERENCES

Aly H: Respiratory disorders in the newborn: Identification and diagnosis. Pediatr Rev 2004;25:201-208.

Avery GB, Fletcher MA, Macdonald MG (eds): Neonatology: Pathophysiology and Management of the Newborn, 5th ed. Philadelphia, Lippincott Williams & Wilkins, 1999, pp 143-173.

Blackburn ST: Maternal, Fetal, and Neonatal Physiology: A Clinical Perspective, 2nd ed. Philadelphia, WB Saunders, 2003, pp 707-730.

Carter BS: Comfort care principles for the high-risk newborn. NeoReviews 2004;e484-e490.

Chescheir NC, Harsen WF: What's new in perinatology. Pediatr Rev 1999;20:57-63.

Downard CD, Wilson JM: Current therapy of infants with congenital diaphragmatic hernia. Semin Neonatol 2003;8:215-221.

Field TM: Stimulation of preterm infants. Pediatr Rev 2003;24:4-10.

Heird WC: Determination of nutritional requirements in preterm infants, with special reference to "catch-up" growth. Semin Neonatol 2001;6:365-375.

Klaus MH, Fanaroff MB: Care of the High-Risk Neonate, 5th ed. Philadelphia, WB Saunders, 2001, pp 195-215.

Kattwinkel J (ed): Neonatal Resuscitation Textbok, 5th ed. American Heart Association, American Academy of Pediatrics, Elk Grove Village, Ill.

Kleinman RE (ed): Pediatric Nutrition Handbook, 5th ed. American Academy of Pediatrics, Elk Grove Village, Ill, 2004, pp 23-55.

Thureen PJ, Deacon J, O'Neill P, Hernandez JA: Assessment and care of the well newborn. Philadelphia, WB Saunders, 1999, pp 83-113.

Welch KK, Malone FD: Advances in prenatal screening: Nuchal translucency ultrasonography in the first trimester. NeoReviews 2002;3:e202-e208.

Welch KK, Malone FD: Advances in prenatal screening: Maternal serum screening for Down syndrome. Neoreviews 2002;3:e209-e213.

Normal Infant Feeding

Method of
Meg Begany, RD, CSP, LDN, and Maria Mascarenhas, MBBS

Adequate and appropriate nutrition is especially critical during infancy. Infancy, defined as birth to 1 year of age, is characterized by the period of most rapid growth and development during the life cycle. In addition, recent research shows that nutrition during infancy can influence risk factors for disease at other stages of the life cycle.

Infant Feeding

For the healthy term infant, the suck-swallow and rooting reflexes are present at birth, and thus liquid feedings can be initiated almost immediately following delivery.

BREAST-FEEDING

The American Academy of Pediatrics (AAP) recommends human milk as the feeding of choice for nearly all infants whenever possible and mutually desirable for the mother and infant. Successful lactation and breast-feeding requires a supportive environment for the mother provided by the medical practitioner, including instruction and counseling. The World Health Organization (WHO) Expert Consultation on the Optimal Duration of Exclusive

Breastfeeding, which considered the results of a systematic review of the evidence, concluded that human milk is recommended as the exclusive source of nutrition for the first 6 months and continuing human milk in combination with complementary foods until at least 12 months of age. The nutrient needs of the full-term normal birth weight infant can be met by human milk alone, with few exceptions, for the first 6 months if the mother is well nourished. The benefits of breast-feeding over formula feeding are well established and include enhanced maturity and motility of the gastrointestinal tract; maternal–infant bonding; monetary savings; facilitated fat, protein, and carbohydrate digestion and absorption; passive immunity; improved cognitive development; and decreased incidence of otitis media and respiratory and gastrointestinal disease. Further potential benefits, such as lower risk of overweight in children and adults, as well as decreased risk of cardiovascular disease in adulthood, were demonstrated in recent research.

Breast-feeding should be offered as early as possible after birth and then every 2 to 3 hours until satiety for approximately 10 to 15 minutes per breast during the first few weeks. Less frequent feedings may occur once breast-feeding is established. Intervals of more than 5 hours in between breast-feeding should be avoided during the first few weeks, including at night. Adequacy of breast-feeding is demonstrated when the infant has feedings 8 to 12 times per day, at least 6 to 8 wet diapers per day, regular stooling pattern, and is growing along established growth curves.

The composition of breast milk varies from individual to individual, as well as within the same individual, with composition changes occurring with stage of lactation, time of day, maternal diet, and time elapsed since feeding began. Milk production tends to be higher during the daytime, and fat content is increased toward the end of a feeding. On average, breast milk provides approximately 20 calories per ounce.

Contraindications to breast-feeding include maternal infections by organisms known to be transmitted to the infant via breast milk (e.g., HIV); maternal exposure to drugs, foods, or environmental agents that are excreted in human milk and harmful to the infant; and inborn errors of metabolism that are exacerbated by components present in human milk (e.g., galactosemia).

INFANT FORMULA

When a mother chooses not to breast-feed or human milk is not an option, infant formula is an appropriate substitute. Although the composition of infant formula does not exactly duplicate that of breast milk, the composition of infant formulas continues to evolve in an effort to do so. The addition of docosahexaenoic acid (DHA) and arachidonic acid (ARA) is a recent modification to infant formula. Unlike breast milk, infant formulas prior to 2002 contained only the precursor essential fatty acids, linoleic and α-linolenic acids, from which DHA and ARA had to be synthesized. Multiple studies in both preterm and term infants have demonstrated significantly lower levels of DHA and ARA in the erythrocytes of formula-fed infants compared to their breast-fed counterparts. This suggested that infant formula containing only the precursors, α-linolenic acid and linoleic acid, could be ineffective in allowing adequate synthesis of DHA and ARA. Thus

multiple studies have been published comparing visual acuity, developmental outcomes, and growth of infants fed DHA and ARA supplemented and unsupplemented formula or breast milk. Some of these studies, but not all, found short-term improvements in visual and cognitive functions in both preterm and term infants. However, no long-term benefits were demonstrated. Although the single supplementation of DHA alone resulted in ARA deficiency status and poor growth in premature infants, the balanced supplementation of both DHA and ARA consistently do not show any adverse effect on growth.

Both iron-fortified and low-iron formulas are commercially available. The AAP has stated that there is no role for the use of low-iron formulas in infant feeding and recommends that all formulas fed to infants be fortified with iron. Well-controlled studies failed to show a benefit, in terms of feeding tolerance, related to the use of low-iron formula. The amount of iron present in iron-fortified formulas meets the iron requirements through the entire first year.

Infant formula should be prepared and stored with careful attention to the manufacturer's guidelines to prevent the risk of bacterial growth.

VITAMIN AND MINERAL SUPPLEMENTATION

The majority of vitamin and mineral requirements for infants are met in full by breast milk or infant formula. Guidelines for supplementation of vitamin K, vitamin D, iron, and fluoride are established. A single dose of vitamin K is typically given to all infants intramuscularly at birth to prevent hemorrhagic disease of the newborn.

For the breast-fed infant, the AAP recommends a supplement of 200 IU of vitamin D by 2 months of age. A multivitamin or tri-vitamin preparation can be used; solitary vitamin D supplements are not practical because of cost and dosing.

The iron requirements for formula-fed infants are met through iron-fortified formula. Although the iron content of human milk is minimal, its bioavailability is high. However, the iron body stores of the breast-fed infant diminish by 4 to 6 months of age, and thus an additional iron source is recommended at this age. Iron needs of the breast-fed infant can be met with the introduction of complementary foods when foods with good sources of iron are included (e.g., meat, fish, iron-fortified cereal, whole grains, and dark leafy green vegetables).

Fluoride supplementation is recommended at 6 months of age for both breast-fed infants and formula-fed infants who receive exclusively ready-to-feed formulas or whose water supply contains less than 0.3 ppm of fluoride.

INTRODUCTION OF COMPLEMENTARY FOODS

At approximately 6 months of age, human milk or infant formula can no longer supply all of an infant's nutrition requirements, and complementary foods are needed to ensure adequate nutrition and growth. It is the micronutrients, rather than energy and protein, which are likely to become lacking. The ability to digest and absorb carbohydrates, proteins, and fats is mature by 6 months of age. Trypsin and chymotrypsin activities increase during the first 4 months of life. Age should not be the only factor in

Infant Formula Composition and Indications

FORMULA	EXAMPLES	INDICATIONS	CHARACTERISTICS
Milk based	Enfamil LIPIL Similac Advance Enfamil LactoFree LIPIL Similac Lactose Free Enfamil AR LIPIL (prethickened) Good Start Supreme	Breast milk substitute for term infants	Ready to feed, powder, or liquid concentrate Variable whey: casein 20 kcal/oz Contain DHA/ARA
Soy based	ProSobee Isomil Good Start Supreme Soy Isomil DF	Breast milk substitute for infants with lactose intolerance or milk protein allergy*	Lactose free; some sucrose free Ready to feed, powder, or liquid concentrate 20 kcal/oz Contain DHA/ARA May contain fiber
Premature (hospital grade)	Enfamil Premature LIPIL Similac Special CareAdvance	Breast milk substitute for low birth weight hospitalized preterm infants	Low lactose 60:40 whey-to-casein ratio High calcium and phosphorus Contain MCT 20 and 24 cal/oz Contain DHA/ARA Ready to feed only
Human milk fortifiers	Similac HMF Enfamil HMF	Fortification of human milk for low birth weight preterm infants	Increase calorie, protein, and vitamin/mineral content of breast milk Contain MCT
Premature transitional	NeoSure Advance EnfaCare LIPIL	Breast milk substitute for preterm infants >2.5 kg or discharge formula for preterm infants (used until 6–12 mo corrected age or until catch-up growth is completed)	22 kcal/oz Ready to feed or powder Contain DHA/ARA Vitamin and mineral content between that of term and premature formulas
Hypoallergenic/protein hydrolysate	Nutramigen	Milk or soy protein allergy	Hydrolyzed protein Ready to feed, powder, or liquid concentrate Sucrose free Lactose free No MCT
Protein hydrolysate with MCT	Alimentum Pregestimil	Malabsorption Short bowel syndrome Allergy	Lactose free Hydrolyzed protein Contain MCT Ready to feed or powder
Amino acid based	Neocate EleCare	Malabsorption Short bowel syndrome Allergy	Lactose free Free amino acids Powder only
Fat modified	Portagen (no longer recommended for infants) Alimentum Pregestimil	Defects in digestion, absorption, or transport of fat	Contain increased % of kcal as MCT

Infant Formula Composition and Indications

FORMULA	EXAMPLES	INDICATIONS	CHARACTERISTICS
Carbohydrate modified	RCF Product 3232 A	Simple sugar intolerance	Requires addition of complex carbohydrate to be complete
Amino acid modified	Multiple products (e.g., Cyclinex, MSUD Analog, Phenyl-Free)	Inborn errors of metabolism	Low or devoid of specific amino acids that cannot be metabolized
Electrolyte modified	Similac PM 60/40	Renal or other disease state requiring low renal solute load	Decreased potassium content Decreased calcium and phosphorus content

*Children allergic to milk protein may also be allergic to soy protein.

Abbreviations: ARA = arachidonic acid; DHA = docosahexaenoic acid; HMF = human milk fortifier; MCT = medium chain triglycerides; MSUD = maple syrup urine disease.

determining the timing of introduction of complementary feeding, but rather the timing should be determined by individual physical and psychological readiness of the infant, as well as rate of maturation of the nervous system, intestinal tract, and kidneys. Before spoon feedings are introduced, the infant should exhibit trunk stability, head control, and disappearance of the extrusion reflex. At approximately 5 to 6 months, an infant is able to indicate a desire for food by leaning forward and opening his or her mouth to indicate hunger and leaning back and turning away to show disinterest or satiety. Muraro et al. state that introduction of complementary feedings prior to 4 months of age is associated with an increased risk of atopic eczema and cow's milk protein allergy. There are presently no controlled studies showing an allergy preventative effect of restrictive diets after 6 months of age. Studies suggest that introducing complementary foods prior to 6 months does not result in increased caloric intake and has no growth advantage because the infant will displace breast milk to maintain the same level of caloric intake. Although it is possible to meet the nutrition needs of the infant solely from infant formula through the entire first year, delay of introduction of solids can lead to feeding aversions and food refusal. All infants need exposure to a variety of tastes, textures, and foods to develop appropriate feeding practices and a wider acceptance of new foods. In addition to adequate nutrition, the feeding relationship between the infant and caregiver is vital for normal growth and development.

To observe for symptoms of intolerance, only one new food should be introduced every 3 days. Because of its hypoallergenicity, infant rice cereal is often introduced as the first feeding. However, if spoon feeding is initiated at 6 months of age, gastrointestinal and renal development is mature enough to allow feedings from multiple food groups. Despite enhanced bioavailability, breast milk is relatively low in iron and zinc. Because low liver reserves of zinc at birth may predispose some infants to zinc deficiency, similar to the situation for iron, meat may be the ideal first food to provide these nutrients at the levels needed. Dr. Samuel Fomon states that unless there is a strong family history of allergy, introduction of soft-cooked red meats is desirable by 5 to 6 months of age. Furthermore, the proportion of Dietary Reference Intakes that needs to be supplied by complementary foods is highest for iron, zinc, phosphorus, and magnesium. Regardless of the food choice for the first feeding, the consistency should be thin and liquid/pureed. Thinning foods with breast milk or infant formula can enhance acceptability of the food by the infant. Repeated exposure to a new food may be necessary before it is accepted.

By 9 months of age, finely chopped foods and finger foods can be added to the infant's diet. At 12 months of age, rotary chewing is well controlled, and many infants can progress to table foods. Choking hazards that are round and hard, such as grapes, nuts, popcorn, hot dogs, and hard candy, should be avoided.

For the average healthy infant, meals of complementary foods should be provided two to three times per day from 6 to 8 months of age and three to four times per day from 9 to 12 months of age, with addition of nutritious snacks once or twice per day as desired. Vegetarian diets cannot meet nutrient needs at this age unless fortified products or nutrient supplements are provided. Estimates of the energy gap that must be filled by complementary food in industrialized countries is approximately 130 kcal/day at 6 to 8 months, 310 kcal/day at 9 to 11 months and 580 kcal/day at 12 to 23 months of age.

Juice is not a necessary component of the diet and may displace the intake of nutrient-dense breast milk or formula. In addition, offering juice by bottle can contribute to dental caries. If juice is provided, it should be limited to 4 to 8 ounces per day and should not be given prior to 6 months of age.

Whole cow's milk should not be introduced before 12 months of age because of its low iron content, high renal solute load, potential for causing gastrointestinal bleeding, and increased risk of cow's milk protein allergy. Furthermore, cow's milk is a poor source of vitamin C, vitamin E, and essential fatty acids. Breast-fed infants weaned before 12 months of age should receive an iron-fortified infant formula rather than cow's milk.

Nutritional Requirements

Because of the rapid rate of growth and development during infancy, nutrient needs per unit of body weight are very high in comparison to that of the older child or adult. Energy needs for the healthy term infant are 108 kcal/kg from birth to 6 months of age. From 6 to 12 months of age, caloric needs are 98 kcal/kg. The Recommended Daily Allowance (RDA) for protein is 2.2 g/kg from birth to 6 months of age and 1.6 g/kg from 6 to 12 months of age. Caloric distribution during infancy is recommended to be 40% to 50% fat, 7% to 11% protein, and 40% to 55% carbohydrate. The water-to-energy ratio should be 1.5 mL/kcal. Both human milk and infant formulas are models of this distribution. Hydration requirements are met by breast milk or infant formula without further addition of water to the diet, except potentially during periods of illness with fever, diarrhea, or emesis.

Growth

Weight, length, and head circumference should be monitored serially during infancy and plotted on the gender-specific 2000 CDC (Centers for Disease Control and Prevention) Growth Charts. Breast-fed infants tend to gain less weight and usually are leaner than formula-fed infants in the second half of infancy. This difference does not seem to be the result of nutritional deficits but rather infant self-regulation of energy intake.

Obesity is increasing among children in the United States. High rates of weight gain during the first few months of life are associated with obesity in childhood and early adulthood. Optimal nutrition and growth during infancy should be promoted by encouraging healthy eating patterns in the infant to prepare for a healthy lifestyle later in life. Early identification and intervention may be a key component for establishing appropriate weight gain patterns.

Although no consensus exists on universal criteria to define failure to thrive, careful evaluation should occur when weight is less than the 5th percentile or falls more than two major percentiles from a previously established growth channel. In addition, relationship of weight to height must be considered. Prompt intervention with nutritional rehabilitation is essential to prevent illness, growth stunting, cognitive delay, and social and behavioral problems.

For the treatment of either over- or undernutrition, a multidisciplinary team approach involving the physician, dietitian, psychologist, and social worker, along with community services, can often be beneficial and necessary.

In conclusion, infant feeding during the first year of life is a complex process, and guidelines are based on developmental, nutritional, and social factors. Human milk is superior to infant formula and should be the feeding of choice for all infants. Although infant formulas do not exactly duplicate breast milk, the composition of infant formulas continues to evolve in an effort to do so. Complementary foods should be introduced at 6 months of age. Cow's milk should not be introduced until 1 year of age. Careful attention should be paid to growth and nutritional status throughout infancy, with prompt attention to any deviation from expected growth patterns.

REFERENCES

American Academy of Pediatrics, Committee on Nutrition: Iron fortification of infant formulas. Pediatrics 1999;104:119-123.
American Academy of Pediatrics, Section on Breastfeeding: Breastfeeding and the use of human milk. Pediatrics 2005;115:496-506.
Dewey KG: Nutrition, growth and complementary feeding of the breast-fed infant. Pediatr Clin North Am 2001;48:87-104.
Foman SJ: Feeding normal infants: Rationale for recommendations. J Am Diet Assoc 2001;101:1002-1005.
http://www.cdc.gov/growthcharts
Kleinman RE (ed): Pediatric Nutrition Handbook, 5th ed. Elk Grove Village, Ill, American Academy of Pediatrics, Committee on Nutrition, 2003.
Michaelsen KF: Cows' milk in complementary feeding. Pediatrics 2000;106:1302-1303.
Muraro A, Dreborg S, Halken S, et al: Dietary prevention of allergic diseases in infants and small children. Part III: Critical review of published peer-reviewed observational and interventional studies and final recommendations. Pediatr Allergy Immunol 2004;15:291-307.
PAHO and WHO: Guiding Principles for Complementary Feeding of the Breastfed Child. Washington, DC, Pan American Health Organization and World Health Organization, 2003.
Samour PQ, King K (eds): Handbook of Pediatric Nutrition, 3rd ed. Sudbury, Mass, Jones and Bartlett, 2005.
Slaughter CW, Bryant AH: Hungry for love: The feeding relationship in the psychological development of young children. Permanente J 2004;8:23-29.
WHO Working Group on the Growth Reference Protocol and the WHO Task Force on Methods for the Natural Regulation of Fertility: Growth of healthy infants and the timing, type, and frequency of complementary foods. Am J Clin Nutr 2002;76:620-627.

Diseases of the Breast

Method of
Paniti Sukumvanich, MD,
and Patrick Borgen, MD

Benign Diseases of the Breast

Benign diseases of the breast historically are subdivided into proliferative and nonproliferative lesions (Table 1). In a study by Dupont and Page, patients with breast biopsies yielding nonproliferative lesions had no increased risk of subsequent breast cancer. In contrast, proliferative lesions were associated with a minimal to a fivefold increased risk of breast cancer. In clinical practice, of the proliferative lesions, only atypical epithelial lesions increase breast cancer risk significantly. Appropriate treatment and counseling of patients depends on the risk of breast cancer associated with these benign breast diseases.

CURRENT DIAGNOSIS

Expected Growth Velocity during Infancy

AGE	WEIGHT GAIN (g/d)	LENGTH (cm/mo)	HEAD CIRCUMFERENCE (cm/wk)
0–3 mo	25–35	2.5–3.5	0.3–0.6
3–6 mo	15–21	1.6–2.5	0.2–0.5
6–12 mo	10–13	1.2–1.7	0.1–0.4

TABLE 1 Benign Diseases of the Breast

	Increase in Breast Cancer Risk
Nonproliferative Lesions	
Mild hyperplasia without atypia	None
Squamous or apocrine metaplasia	None
Duct ectasia	None
Mastitis	None
Cysts	None
Proliferative Lesions	
Fibroadenoma	None
Moderate or florid hyperplasia	Minimal
Microglandular adenosis	Minimal
Sclerosing adenosis	Minimal
Papilloma	Minimal
Atypical ductal hyperplasia	4- to 5-fold
Atypical lobular hyperplasia	5.8-fold

Nonproliferative Lesions

Nonproliferative lesions comprise mild hyperplasia without atypia, squamous or apocrine metaplasia, duct ectasia, mastitis, and cysts. In the study of 3303 patients by Dupont and Page, only 2.2% of patients with nonproliferative lesions had breast cancer following a benign breast biopsy with a mean follow-up time of 17 years (Figure 1).

BREAST CYSTS AND FIBROCYSTIC BREAST DISEASE

Fibrocystic breast disease is a benign process in which generalized microcystic formation with stromal proliferation

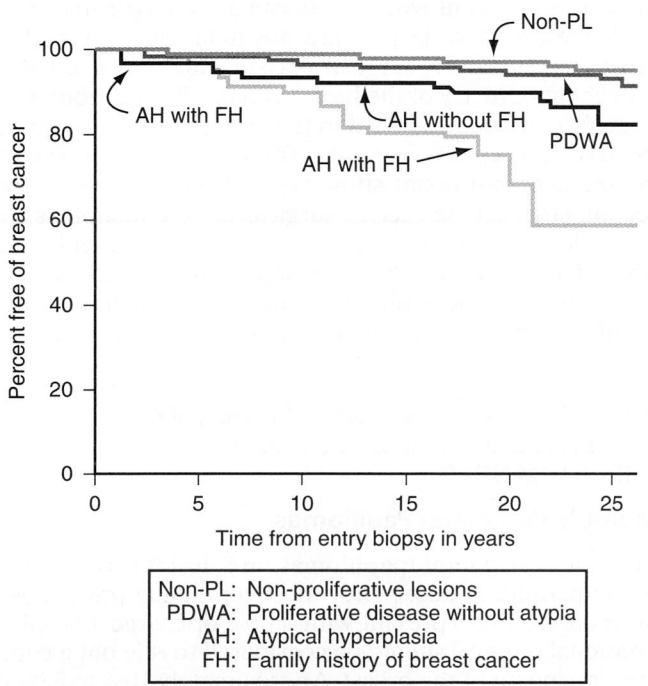

FIGURE 1. Nonproliferative lesions in breast cancer.

leads to increased breast nodularity. Cysts within the breast are most common in perimenopausal women 50 to 59 years of age as well as premenopausal women. Postmenopausal women not on hormone replacement therapy are unlikely to develop cysts in their breasts. Benign cysts are often tender and fluctuate in size with the menstrual cycle. Cysts may be detected either on physical examination as a palpable, smooth, mobile nodule or by breast ultrasound. They may appear as a solitary nodule or in a cluster. Ultrasonographic appearance of simple benign cysts is that of an anechoic, round or oval, well-circumscribed mass with posterior enhancement. If the mass has all four criteria, the accuracy of ultrasound is close to 100% for the diagnosis of a simple benign cyst. Cysts that appear complex, with internal echoes, thick septations, and irregular walls, are suspicious for breast carcinoma and should be examined surgically or with an ultrasound-guided biopsy. Confirmation of the diagnosis can be made by fine-needle aspiration (FNA) of the cystic fluid. Bloody fluid may be an indication for a biopsy. In a study of 6782 cyst aspirates, Ciatto and colleagues found that cytologic examination identified atypical cells in 1677 specimens. Of these specimens, only 0.3% of these cases had clinically and radiologically negative intracystic papillomas. Cytologic examination was positive in only 0.1% of these cases. Thus fluid from cyst aspirations are not sent routinely for cytologic examination. Figure 2 describes the management of suspected cysts.

MASTITIS AND DUCT ECTASIA

Mastitis is divided into lactational or nonlactational. Lactational mastitis can occur from the reflux of bacteria into the breast during breast-feeding. The causative bacteria are usually gram-positive cocci. Patients should be treated with antibiotics with the appropriate coverage and can continue to nurse or pump the breast to prevent engorgement. Nursing mothers can continue to breast-feed because the infant is not at risk for infection. Nonlactational (periductal) mastitis can be caused by duct ectasia, which occurs when the milk ducts become congested with secretions and debris, resulting in a periductal inflammation. These patients may present with greenish nipple discharge, nipple retraction, and subareolar noncyclical pain. The treatment of nonlactational mastitis includes broad-spectrum antibiotics to cover for gram-positive cocci and skin anaerobes. Total duct excision and eversion of the nipple may be necessary to treat recurrent periductal mastitis.

Proliferative Benign Breast Diseases

Proliferative breast diseases include moderate or florid hyperplasia, microglandular and sclerosing adenosis, papilloma, fibroadenoma, and atypical ductal and lobular hyperplasia. All proliferative lesions have an increased risk of subsequent breast cancer after biopsy except for fibroadenoma. Overall, with a median follow-up of 17 years, 5.3% of patients with proliferative lesions develop breast cancer. This percentage increases to 12.9% in the presence of atypia (see Figure 1). Patients with moderate or florid hyperplasia, sclerosing adenosis, and solitary papilloma without atypia carry a minimal increase in risk of developing breast cancer over the general population. These patients are not

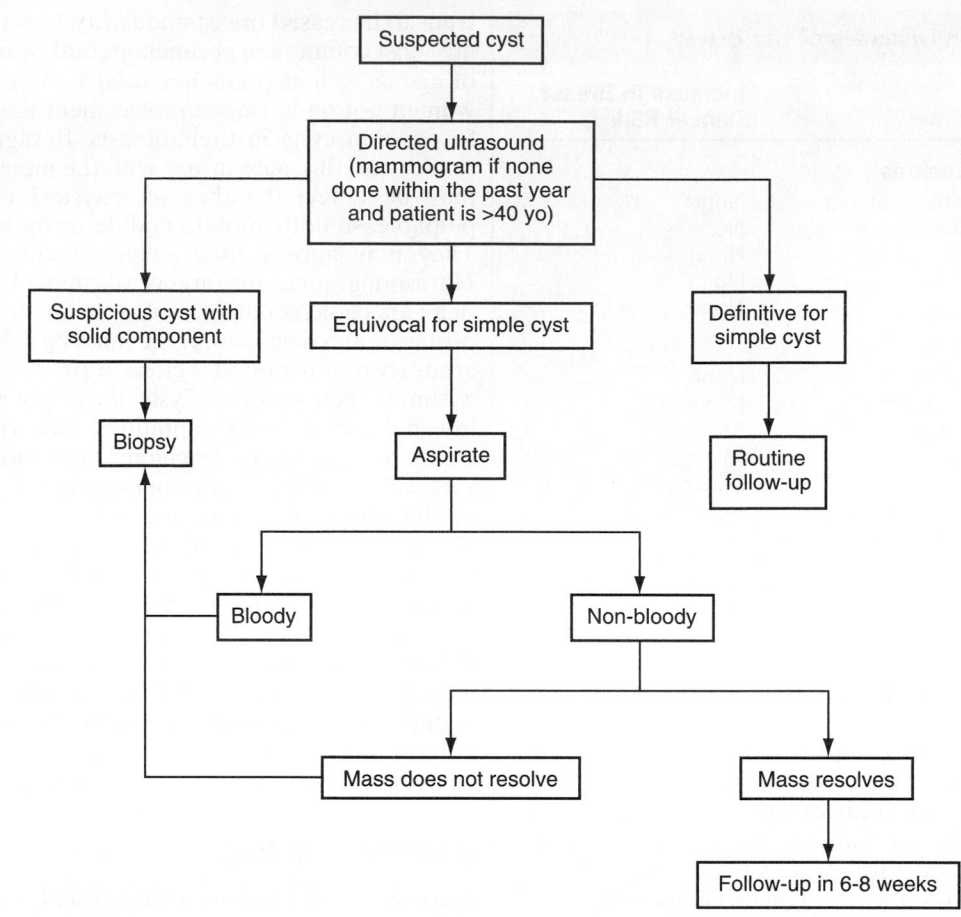

FIGURE 2. Algorithm for the management of suspected cysts.

classified as high risk. But the risk of subsequent breast cancer is increased by four- to fivefold in the presence of atypia. Atypical lobular hyperplasia carries a higher risk than atypical ductal hyperplasia, with a relative risk as high as 5.8. This increased risk applies to the contralateral breast because subsequent breast carcinomas are evenly divided between both breasts.

PROLIFERATIVE LESIONS WITH NO INCREASED RISK OF SUBSEQUENT CANCER: FIBROADENOMA

Fibroadenomas are benign tumors commonly found in young women (less than 30 years of age with a peak incidence at 21 to 25 years of age). They are characteristically detected on physical examination as well-circumscribed, rubbery, highly mobile, palpable masses. On mammograms, these lesions may appear as a well-circumscribed mass. Involution of fibroadenomas in the elderly can lead to hyalinization and dense popcorn-like calcification on mammograms. Fibroadenomas pose no increased risk of breast cancer and do not mandate surgical removal unless desired by the patient. Pregnancy can increase the size of these lesions; thus it may be reasonable to remove them prior to a planned pregnancy. Removal may facilitate follow-up, given the inability to follow breast masses adequately during pregnancy. Other types of fibroadenomas include juvenile and giant fibroadenomas. Juvenile fibroadenomas occur in adolescent women and can grow larger than 5 cm in diameter. These lesions are not malignant; given their large size, however, surgical excision may be needed to prevent asymmetry of the breasts. Giant fibroadenomas are large fibroadenomas found in the lactating breast or in the breasts of pregnant patients. These lesions may regress in size once hormonal stimulation subsides. Lesions that remain large can be excised surgically. Fibroadenomas and phyllodes tumors may be linked. Any rapidly enlarging fibroadenoma should be considered for surgical excision to rule out phyllodes tumor because it is difficult clinically to differentiate fibroadenoma from phyllodes tumor.

PROLIFERATIVE LESIONS WITH MINIMAL INCREASED RISK OF SUBSEQUENT BREAST CANCER

Multiple Peripheral Papillomas

Multiple peripheral papillomas are lesions that occur in the peripheral ducts. They most commonly present as a mass but may also present with nipple discharge. Complete excisional removal should be considered to rule out a papillary carcinoma of the breast. Approximately 10% to 33% of patients have subsequent breast cancer; thus close follow-up of these patients is warranted.

Sclerosing and Microglandular Adenosis

Sclerosing adenosis occurs as result of the proliferation of stromal tissue along with small terminal ductules. Often these lesions are picked up incidentally, but they may also present as microcalcifications on mammogram or as a mass (termed *adenosis tumor*). Sclerosing adenosis may be confused with a tubular carcinoma. Staining with immuno-histochemical (IHC) markers such as actin, smooth muscle myosin heavy chain p63, or calponin may be helpful in distinguishing between the two lesions because only sclerosing adenosis contains myoepithelial cells. Microglandular adenosis is an uncommon lesion that may be mistaken for tubular carcinoma on histologic examination, and it can increase the patient's subsequent breast cancer risk. Concomitant breast cancer has been reported, so complete surgical excision should be considered for these lesions.

PROLIFERATIVE LESIONS WITH A FOUR- TO FIVEFOLD RISK OF SUBSEQUENT BREAST CANCER: ATYPICAL DUCTAL AND LOBULAR HYPERPLASIA

Atypical ductal and lobular hyperplasia are very similar to their in situ counterparts. These lesions are termed *atypical hyperplasia* because they lack some of the microscopic features of in situ disease. The distinction between atypical hyperplasia and carcinoma in situ is sometimes hard to make. In a study by Rosai, five expert breast cancer pathologists reviewed 17 cases of ductal or lobular lesions. In no case did all five agree on a diagnosis. Four out of the five were able to agree on a diagnosis in three cases (18%). In one third of the patients, the diagnosis ran the gamut from hyperplasia without atypia to carcinoma in situ. Despite such difficulty, the diagnosis of atypical hyperplasia is on the rise as mammographic screening becomes more popular. Atypical hyperplasia, which is detected secondary to microcalcifications or by serendipity, carries the highest risk of subsequent breast carcinoma among all proliferative lesions of the breast, with a four- to fivefold increased risk over the general population. Atypical lobular hyperplasia carries a higher risk than atypical ductal hyperplasia, with a relative risk as high as 5.8. This risk applies to the contralateral breast as well as the ipsilateral breast. Surgical excision of atypical hyperplasia on a core biopsy is recommended because 20% of patients are found to have breast cancer at time of surgical excision for atypical hyperplasia. It is not necessary to achieve negative margins for these lesions.

OTHER BENIGN BREAST LESIONS: FAT NECROSIS, HAMARTOMA, MONDOR'S DISEASE, RADIAL SCARS, AND PSEUDOANGIOMATOUS STROMAL HYPERPLASIA

Other benign lesions of the breast include fat necrosis, hamartoma, Mondor's disease, radial scars, and pseudo-angiomatous stromal hyperplasia (PASH). Trauma to the breast may lead to fat necrosis and can be mistaken for carcinomas on clinical examination. Fat necrosis lesions present clinically as painless, irregular masses with or without associated skin changes such as skin thickening. These lesions can be normal or may have rim calcifications on mammograms. No further treatment is needed when a core biopsy definitively makes the diagnosis of fat necrosis.

Hamartomas are benign lesions that are often picked up on a mammogram. The fatty composition of the mass makes these lesions clinically occult. They can be mistaken for fibroadenomas on mammograms. Hamartomas can be left alone without histologic confirmation if diagnosed definitively on a mammogram.

Mondor's disease is a thrombophlebitis of the superficial breast veins that presents as a palpable tender cord leading to the axilla. In a study of 63 cases, 8 patients (25%) had an underlying malignancy; thus a mammogram should be done to rule out the presence of breast carcinoma.

Radial scars are benign lesions whose etiology is unknown. They are often mistaken for breast carcinoma on mammograms because of their stellate appearance. Radial scars may also mimic breast carcinoma histologically. Staining for myoepithelial cells can help distinguish between invasive carcinoma and a radial scar. Radial scars carry a 1.5-fold increase in risk of subsequent breast carcinoma, so these lesions should be considered markers of future disease.

First described in 1986, PASH is a benign proliferative lesion that may present as an incidental finding or a mobile breast mass. It can occur in all ages and also in men. On a mammogram, PASH appears as a round noncalcified mass. Histologically, PASH may be mistaken for low-grade angiosarcoma. Unlike angiosarcoma, however, there should be no evidence of mitosis or cytologic atypia in PASH specimens. The role of hormones in the pathogenesis of PASH is controversial. Although these lesions tend to occur in young patients or in elderly patients on hormone therapy, most cases tend to be negative for estrogen receptors. The treatment for PASH is complete surgical excision. Approximately 7% of cases recur despite adequate treatment.

Risk Factors for Breast Cancer

An estimated 80% of women in whom breast cancer develops have no documented risk factors or determinants. Risk factors cannot be changed, whereas risk determinants can be altered to decrease a person's risk of subsequent breast cancer. Common risk factors include a familial history of breast cancer, personal breast biopsy history, menarche before 12 years of age, menopause after 55 years of age, increasing age, geographical location, and mutations of the BRCA1 or BRCA2 genes. Women known to have the BRCA1 or BRCA2 genetic mutation have an 85% lifetime risk of breast cancer as well as an increased risk of ovarian cancer. BRCA1 carriers are at a higher risk for developing ovarian cancer than BRCA2 (60% versus 20%, respectively). The risk determinants for breast cancer include reproductive factors such as nulliparity and first pregnancy after the age of 30 years and previous radiation exposure. Previous therapy for lymphoma, especially during adolescence, elevates a woman's risk of subsequent breast cancer.

Screening Techniques

Screening for breast cancer includes mammography, ultrasound, breast self-examination (BSE), and physical examination by a physician. Multiple studies such as the Göthenborg and Malmö trials show a reduction in breast cancer mortality from 30% to 40% in patients 40 to 49 years of age who undergo screening mammograms. A meta-analysis of six randomized trials indicates a 30% reduction in breast cancer mortality in patients 50 to 69 years of age. The sensitivity of mammograms depends on the patient's age and ranges from 53% to 81% in women 40 to 49 years of age to 73% to 81% in patients 50 years of age or older. An estimated 10% to 15% of breast cancer cases are not detectable on screening mammography, thus emphasizing the importance of physical breast examination by a physician and BSE that include both visual inspection and manual examination of the breast. On inspection, signs of breast malignancy include skin or nipple retraction or discoloration, nipple discharge/crusting, or peau d'orange edema of the breast. On palpation, any asymmetric mass of the breast or axilla may be regarded as a potential malignancy that deserves further evaluation.

Current recommendations are for a woman to start performing BSE at 18 years of age, have a yearly physical exam, and initiate annual mammography at 40 years of age. Little data exist on what should be the upper age limit of mammogram screening. Given that breast density decreases with age and breast cancer increases with age, mammograms should be even more sensitive and specific in the older age group. For these reasons, mammograms may be continued in very elderly patients as long as the patient is not suffering from any major co-morbidities. In patients who have a very high risk of breast cancer, such as BRCA carriers, screening should start 10 years earlier than the age of onset of an affected relative or at the age of 35. Kriege screened 1909 patients (including 358 BRCA mutation carriers) who had more than a 15% lifetime risk of developing breast cancer. These patients had a biannual breast exam as well as annual mammogram and breast magnetic resonance imaging (MRI). In this population, mammograms had a sensitivity of 33% with a specificity of 95%. Breast MRI had significantly higher rates of sensitivity and specificity at 80% and 90%, respectively. Given these findings, breast MRI should be a part of the screening exam for these high-risk patients. MRI is recommended as a standard screening test in BRCA heterozygotes. Routine surveillance in high-risk patients includes a 6-month interval alternating between breast MRI and mammograms. Patients with a history of mantle radiation for lymphoma should start annual screening at 25 years of age and biannual screening 10 years after receiving radiation therapy.

Workup of a Breast Mass

DOMINANT PALPABLE MASS

The workup of a dominant palpable breast mass depends on the patient's menopausal status and the degree of suspicion. It is not unreasonable to follow a premenopausal patient with a nonsuspicious mass over one menstrual cycle and then reexamine her. Suspicious lesions present as a hard, nontender, irregular mass or as a mass in a high-risk patient. Palpable masses in postmenopausal patients may also warrant a workup. FNA should not be performed prior to diagnostic imaging because it may result in a hematoma that could obscure the image of the mass. Certain benign lesions on core biopsy should be excised, including lobular carcinoma in situ (LCIS), atypical ductal hyperplasia (ADH), radial scars, sclerosing papillary lesions, columnar cell hyperplasia with atypia, and PASH (Figure 3). Twenty percent of surgeries performed for atypical ductal hyperplasia have concurrent carcinoma in the specimen. Patients with a high-risk proliferative lesion should have close follow-up after surgery including physical examinations. Negative findings on a mammogram do not preclude the diagnosis of cancer because 10% of cancers are occult mammographically. This number drops to 3% when a lesion is occult both mammographically and ultrasonographically. An alternative to core biopsies in younger women is the use of the triple test: a physical exam in conjunction with breast imaging (mammogram or ultrasound) and FNA. When all three components indicate the mass is benign, the negative predictive value is 100%. In a study by Morris, a triple test score assigns points to each component of the test. One point is given for benign findings, 2 points for suspicious findings, and 3 points for malignant findings. When added together, masses with scores of 4 or less are found to be benign. The triple test should only be used in women 40 years of age or younger because the incidence of breast cancer increases dramatically after that cutoff.

MASSES REVEALED ON SCREENING MAMMOGRAMS

The American College of Radiology's classification lexicon, the Breast Imaging Reporting and Data System (BI-RADS), is used in breast imaging (Table 2). BI-RADS 0 means the assessment is incomplete and more workup is needed. BI-RADS 1 indicates a normal mammogram. Mammograms with BI-RADS 2 signify benign findings. Patients with BI-RADS 3 have a 1% to 2% risk of malignancy and should have short-term follow-up with another mammogram in 6 months. BI-RADS 4 indicates the presence of suspicious lesions with a 20% to 40% probability of a malignant lesion. BI-RADS 5 is highly suggestive of cancer with a greater than 95% chance of harboring an underlying malignant lesion. BI-RADS 6, recently added as a category, indicates known malignant disease. BI-RADS 4 and 5 both indicate a biopsy.

A core biopsy via ultrasound guidance may be attempted first. A stereotactic core biopsy should be considered if this is not possible. Stereotactic biopsies may be impossible in patients with lesions that are very superficial or close to the chest wall or in patients with very small breasts that compress to less than 3 cm or who are unable to lie still for the procedure. In such situations, surgical excision with needle localization is warranted. In studies comparing surgical excision to core biopsies, the concordance rate is close to 100%. The surgeon can obviate the need for multiple surgeries in the same patient by performing a core biopsy for diagnosis. High-risk proliferative lesions, such as LCIS, atypical ductal hyperplasia, radial scars, sclerosing papillary lesions, columnar cell hyperplasia with atypia, and PASH, should be considered for an excisional biopsy if the diagnosis is made by a core biopsy.

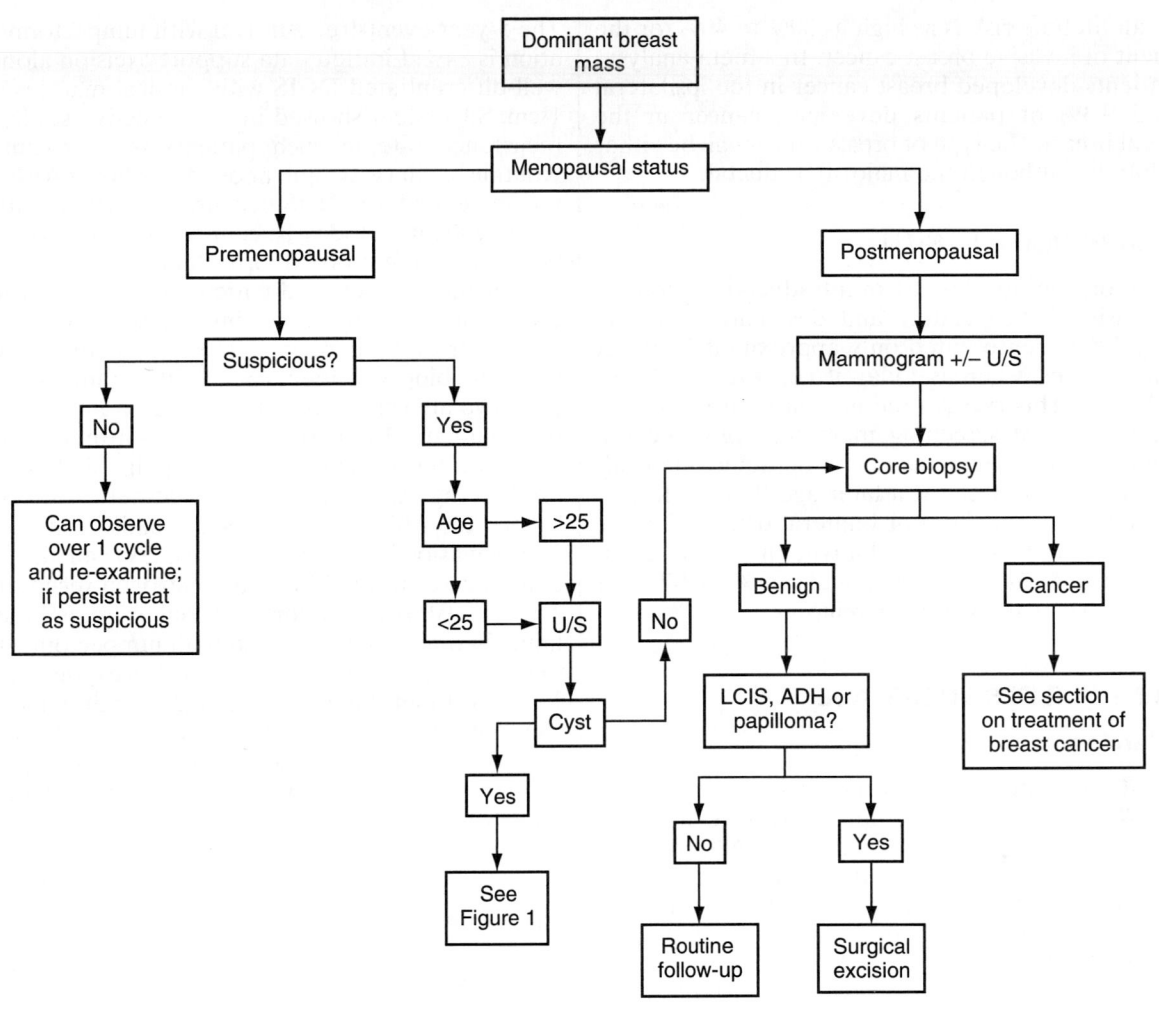

FIGURE 3. Algorithm for workup of a breast mass. ADH = atypical ductal hyperplasia; LCIS = lobular cancer in situ; U/S = ultrasound.

In Situ Diseases

LOBULAR CARCINOMA IN SITU

Lobular carcinoma in situ (LCIS) should be considered a marker for future breast cancer risk and not an early noninvasive lobular cancer. This disease is most commonly seen in premenopausal women, with a peak incidence in women 40 to 50 years of age. Only 10% of LCIS occurs in postmenopausal women. Unlike ductal carcinoma in situ, LCIS is often found incidentally because typically no clinical or radiologic abnormalities are seen at time of diagnosis. In 50% of patients, LCIS is a multifocal finding. In 30% of patients, it can be found in the contralateral breast. Patients with LCIS are at 8 to 10 times the risk of the general population for subsequent breast cancer.

TABLE 2 BI-RADS Mammography Classification

BI-RADS Category	Definition	Risk of Malignancy	Recommended Follow-Up
0	Incomplete assessment	N/A	Further workup
1	Negative study	N/A	Repeat mammogram in 1 y
2	Benign	N/A	Repeat mammogram in 1 y
3	Probably benign	<2%	Repeat mammogram in 6 mo
4	Suspicious	20%	Biopsy should be considered
5	Highly suggestive of malignancy	90%	Appropriate action should be taken
6	Known biopsy-proven malignancy	N/A	Appropriate action should be taken

Abbreviation: BI-RADS = Breast Imaging Reporting and Data System.

Their overall lifetime risk is as high as 30% to 40% for the development of invasive breast cancer. In a meta-analysis, 15% of patients developed breast cancer in the ipsilateral breast, and 9.3% of patients developed cancer in the contralateral breast. The type of breast cancer can be either ductal or lobular, although the majority is ductal.

DUCTAL CARCINOMA IN SITU

Ductal carcinoma in situ (DCIS), or intraductal carcinoma, is a noninvasive breast cancer and designated stage 0. Historically, DCIS represented only approximately 5% of breast cancer cases, whereas today it constitutes 20% to 30% of all cases. This rise is predominantly attributed to the increasing use of screening mammography because DCIS is most often detected as mammographic microcalcifications. It tends to occur at a later age than LCIS and is not considered a multifocal or bilateral disease. Unlike LCIS, DCIS should be considered a true precursor lesion because if left untreated, approximately 60% to 100% of DCIS cases progress to invasive carcinoma.

TREATMENT FOR IN SITU DISEASE

Lobular Carcinoma in Situ

LCIS should be treated as a marker for increased breast cancer risk. Surgery in an attempt to achieve negative margins is not warranted for LCIS. The NSABP P-1 (the National Surgical Adjuvant Breast and Bowel Project) randomized trial examined the role of tamoxifen (Nolvadex) as a chemopreventive agent in high-risk patients, including those with LCIS. Women taking tamoxifen had a 50% reduction in the subsequent risk of breast cancer without any improvement in overall survival. The main risks of tamoxifen include increased risk of thromboembolic disease and endometrial cancer. The rate of pulmonary embolism was 3 in 1000 patients in the tamoxifen group versus 1 in 1000 in the placebo group. The rate of deep-vein thromboembolism was 5 in 1000 patients in the tamoxifen group versus 3 in 1000 in the placebo group. Endometrial cancer was seen in 9 in 1000 patients in the tamoxifen group versus 3.5 in 1000 in the placebo group. The decision to use tamoxifen as a chemopreventive agent should be made on an individual basis given these side effects. The highest reduction in breast cancer occurred in the LCIS group with a 70% reduction in risk. Despite this, no difference in survival was seen between the tamoxifen and placebo group.

Ductal Carcinoma in Situ

Treatment of DCIS has evolved from simple mastectomy to lumpectomy with radiation therapy. A simple mastectomy is associated with a 1% local recurrence rate. Thus it is still considered a viable option in patients who do not desire or are ineligible for breast conservation therapy (BCT). No difference in survival is seen in patients treated with mastectomy versus BCT. The NSABP B-17 randomized trial examined the role of lumpectomy with and without radiotherapy for the treatment of DCIS. The addition of radiotherapy decreased the recurrence rate from 16.4% to 7% with 8 years of follow-up. More importantly, it decreased the rate of invasive carcinoma from 8% to 2%.

The 5-year event-free survival with lumpectomy and radiation is 84%. Limited data support excision alone in small well-differentiated DCIS with surgical margins of at least 1 cm. Silverstein showed in retrospective studies that the recurrence rate in such patients is approximately 4%. Routine axillary lymph node dissection (ALND) is not recommended for DCIS because only 1% of patients have positive axillary nodes. Recent studies, however, show that sentinel lymph node biopsy may have a role in the management of selected patients with DCIS. This is especially true in patients receiving a mastectomy as definitive treatment or if there is a question of microinvasion on the core biopsy. Patients with DCIS and microinvasion can have anywhere from a 3% to 20% incidence of nodal involvement. Indications for a sentinel node biopsy include extensive calcifications, a palpable lesion, patients undergoing mastectomy as treatment for DCIS, and lesions for which the pathology reads "can not rule out microinvasion." Tamoxifen (Nolvadex) can also be considered in cases of DCIS that are estrogen receptor positive. The NSABP B-24 randomized trial examined the utility of tamoxifen in patients treated with lumpectomy and radiotherapy. Ipsilateral tumor recurrences decreased from 13.4% without tamoxifen to 8.2% with tamoxifen. The incidence of invasive cancer was reduced by 47%. No difference in survival was observed between the placebo and the tamoxifen group. Side effects are similar to that of the NSABP P-1 trial.

Invasive Breast Cancer

INCIDENCE

An estimated 1 in 9 women living in the United States if they survive to 90 years of age will develop breast cancer. The average age at diagnosis is 64 years of age and increases along with age.

The American Joint Committee on Cancer TMN (tumor, metastasis, node) system designates breast cancer as stage 0, I, II, III, or IV. This system categorizes breast cancer by its invasive or noninvasive character, tumor size, axillary lymph node status, and the presence of metastatic disease (see Table 2). Overall survival with breast cancer is related to stage (Table 3).

HISTOLOGY

The most common type of infiltrating carcinoma is ductal carcinoma-not otherwise specified (IFDC-NOS), which represents 85% of all invasive breast cancer. Infiltrating lobular carcinoma originates from the lobular structures of the breast and accounts for 15% of all invasive breast cancer. Other less common subtypes represent less than 10% and include tubular, medullary, mucinous, and papillary carcinoma. Additional rare subtypes of breast cancer include inflammatory carcinoma, malignant phyllodes tumor, sarcoma, lymphoma, and Paget disease.

BREAST CANCER STAGING

In 2003 the American Joint Committee on Cancer (AJCC) revised their staging system on breast cancer. This latest revision stresses the importance of nodal status as a

TABLE 3 Overall Survival in
Breast Cancer Patients

Stage	10-Year Overall Survival	15-Year Overall Survival
I	74%-95%	64%
II	76%	62%
IIA	81%	72%
IIB	70%	52%
III	50%	40%
IIIA	59%	49%
IIIB	36%	18%
IIIC	36%	18%
IV	18%	18%

Adapted from Rosen PP, et al: J Clin Oncol 1989;355-366; Woodward WA, Strom EA, Tucker SL, et al: Changes in the 2003 American Joint Committee on Cancer staging for breast cancer, dramatically affect stage-specific survival. J Clin Oncol 2003;21:3244-3248.

prognostic factor by making several changes in how it is classified within the staging system. Major changes to the staging system include the following:

- Designation is made for isolated tumor cells (ITCs), which are differentiated from micrometastasis and defined as "single tumor cells or small cell clusters not greater than 0.2 mm, usually detected only by IHC (immunohistochemistry) or molecular methods, but which may be verified on H&E (hematoxylin-eosin) stains. ITCs do not usually show evidence of malignant activity, e.g., proliferation or stromal reaction." ITCs are designated as pN0 with modifiers for positive or negative IHC (i–, i+) and molecular findings (mol–, mol+).
- Internal mammary nodes (IMNs) are reclassified based on how they are detected and whether or not there is concomitant axillary lymph node metastasis. Detection of IMNs by sentinel node biopsy alone is classified as pN1b in the absence of positive axillary nodes or pN1c in the presence of positive axillary nodes. Internal mammary nodes detected by imaging studies (excluding lymphoscintigraphy) or by clinical exam are classified as pN2b in the absence of positive axillary nodes or pN3b in the presence of positive axillary nodes.
- Supraclavicular nodal involvement is now reclassified as N3 disease; thus a patient with supraclavicular nodal involvement does not automatically have stage IV disease.
- Infraclavicular nodal involvement is added as N3 disease.
- Axillary lymph node involvement is now classified by the number of nodes involved. Involvement of 1 to 3 axillary nodes is considered pN1 disease. Involvement of 4 to 9 axillary nodes is considered pN2 disease. Involvement of greater than 10 axillary nodes is considered pN3 disease.

Staging of breast cancer can be divided into clinical staging versus pathologic staging. Factors used for clinical staging include the size of the tumor within the breast, presence or absence of pathologically confirmed lymph nodes, and presence or absence of distant metastasis. There are five stages for breast cancer. Stage 0 is defined as the presence of in situ disease only, without evidence of nodal or distant metastasis. Stage I is considered breast cancer confined to the breast, regardless of tumor size. Exception to this general characterization includes tumors with extension to the chest wall or skin or inflammatory breast cancers. These tumors are at least stage IIIB. Stage II is considered a breast cancer of any size with pathologically positive ipsilateral mobile axillary nodes. Stage IIIA is considered a breast cancer of any size with pathologically positive ipsilateral fixed axillary nodes or clinically apparent internal mammary nodes in the absence of positive axillary nodes. Also any large tumors (bigger than 5 cm) with any type of positive axillary or internal mammary nodes are considered stage IIIA. Stage IIIB tumors are breast tumors with extension to the skin or chest wall or inflammatory breast cancer. Involvement of the pectoralis major or minor muscle does not constitute chest wall involvement. Stage IIIC tumors are breast cancers of any size with either positive infraclavicular or supraclavicular nodes or positive internal mammary nodes in the presence of positive axillary nodes. Stage IV connotes any breast cancers with distant metastasis (see Figure 3).

Pathologic staging of breast cancer is more complicated and differs from clinical staging in that the number of nodes involved as well as how nodal metastasis is detected are used in stage designation of nodal status (Figures 4 and 5).

SURGICAL TREATMENT OF THE BREAST

A significant paradigm shift in the treatment of breast cancer has occurred over the past several decades. The Halsted paradigm, popularized at the beginning of the 20th century, hypothesized that breast cancer spreads in a contiguous fashion from the breast to the axillary lymph nodes and then to distant sites elsewhere in the body. The Fisher paradigm, which views breast cancer as systemic from very early in the course of the disease, modified this theory; the axillary lymph nodes act not as a barrier but as indicators of disease aggressiveness. Both paradigms are correct and incorrect. At a certain point in the evolution of a breast cancer, the disease changes from a local disease to a systemic disease. The Halsted paradigm promotes more

	T1	T2	T3	T4
N0	I	IIA	IIB	IIIB
N1	IIA	IIB	IIIA	IIIB
N2	IIIA	IIIA	IIIA	IIIB
N3	IIIC	IIIC	IIIC	IIIC
M1	IV	IV	IV	IV

FIGURE 4. Pathologic staging of breast cancer.

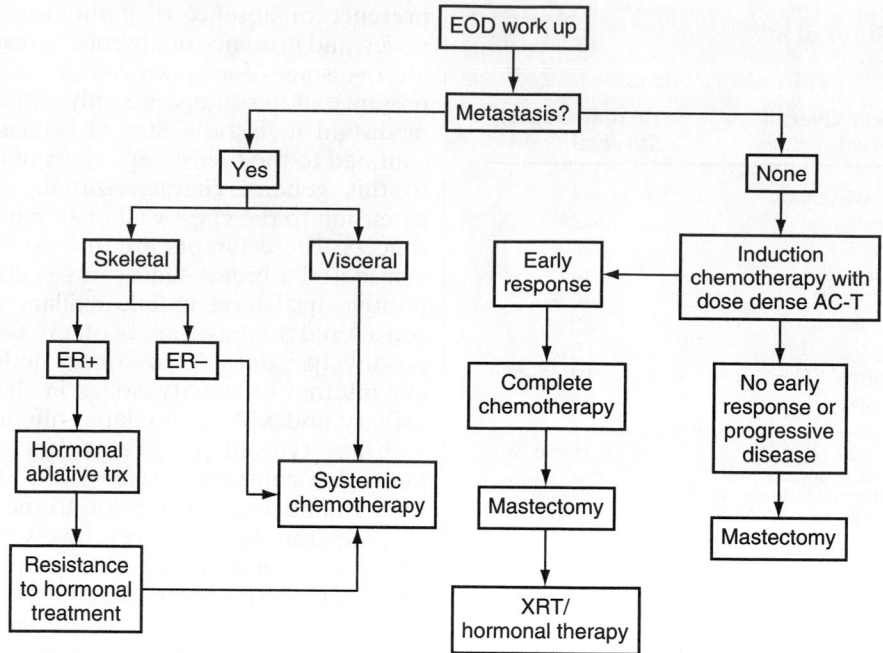

FIGURE 5. Algorithm for treatment of locally advanced breast cancer (LABC). AC-T = Adriamycyin and cyclophosphamide plus Taxol; EOD = extent-of-disease; trx = treatment; XRT = x-radiation therapy.

intensive local treatment to eradicate the cancer, whereas the Fisher paradigm promotes less aggressive local treatment with the addition of systemic treatment in most women, even with relatively early disease. Because of this philosophy change and the detection of earlier disease through diligent screening techniques, surgical treatment of breast cancer is progressing toward less radical surgery and more adjuvant therapy, with equal or better outcomes. Recent mammograms of both breasts should be reviewed for any other suspicious lesions. There may be a slight increase in synchronous breast cancer in patients with invasive lobular cancer, although the rate of contralateral breast cancer is equal to that of invasive ductal carcinoma over the lifetime of the patient. The risk of distant metastasis is 25% to 50% in patients with inflammatory breast cancer.

Breast Conservation Therapy

Most small noninvasive and invasive breast cancers are treated by BCT, which consists of wide local excision with negative surgical margins and irradiation of the breast. The NSABP B-06, Milan I and Milan II, as well as other clinical trials, show no statistically significant difference in patient survival with mastectomy or BCT.

The addition of radiation treatment to wide local excision in patients with noninvasive and invasive carcinoma is currently the standard of treatment. The NSABP B-06 randomized trial evaluated local recurrence of small invasive tumors with and without irradiation after lumpectomy. It found that patients who did not undergo radiation therapy had significantly higher rates of local recurrence. With BCT, incidence of recurrence in the treated breast is 7% at 5 years, 14% at 10 years, and 20% at 20 years.

Local recurrence rate is much lower in patients treated with mastectomy, with an overall incidence of 5% to 10%. The majority of recurrences occur in the first 3 years after surgery. Contraindications to BCT include tumor of any size that can not be adequately excised with significant deformity to the breast, multicentric disease, noncompliant patient, first- or second-trimester pregnant patient, history of significant collagen vascular disease, and history of previous radiation therapy to the chest wall. If both BCT and mastectomy are viable options, the patient's preference should also play a role in the decision to proceed with BCT versus a mastectomy.

MASTECTOMY

A patient with contraindications to breast conservation should have a mastectomy with or without immediate reconstruction. Total mastectomy surgically removes the breast parenchyma, pectoral fascia, nipple, and the areola complex. A modified radical mastectomy includes axillary dissection. A radical mastectomy, rarely done today, includes removal of the pectoralis major and minor muscles and axillary dissection.

BREAST RECONSTRUCTION

Any patient recommended to have a mastectomy should be offered the option of immediate or delayed reconstruction and referred to a plastic and reconstructive surgeon to discuss which techniques are appropriate. One commonly used method of breast reconstruction is a tissue expander breast implant. A tissue expander is placed beneath the pectoralis muscles, and expansions are performed over a period of several weeks to months to stretch the subpectoral pocket to accommodate the permanent implant. The permanent saline or silicone implant is then inserted as a secondary procedure.

Another method of breast reconstruction is the transverse rectus abdominis myocutaneous (TRAM) flap, which involves the transfer of skin, fat, and muscle from the lower part of the abdomen to create a reconstructed breast. This procedure can be performed as a free flap with the arterial and venous supply anastomosed to vessels in the axilla or as a pedicle flap with the arterial and venous supply from the superior epigastric vessels. Other types of flap reconstructions include latissimus dorsi or gluteal flaps. Reconstruction of the nipple and areola is often performed as a later procedure.

SURGICAL TREATMENT OF THE AXILLA

The status of the axilla should be assessed for metastases in any patient with invasive breast cancer for several reasons. The status of the axillary lymph nodes is important in determining the patient's stage of disease. The presence or absence of axillary lymph node metastases is predictive of the prognosis and facilitates decisions by the medical oncology team regarding adjuvant therapy. Relapse-free survival is closely related to the number of lymph nodes that are positive. In a study of 2873 patients, Hilsenbeck found that the relapse-free survival at 5 years was 80% in patients with node-negative disease. This number decreased to 70%, 60%, and 40% with 1 to 3 positive nodes, 4 to 9 positive nodes, and more than 10 positive nodes, respectively. Nodal status is now incorporated into the sixth revision of the AJCC staging system. Surgical removal of metastatic nodes in the axilla significantly decreases the possibility of axillary recurrence. ALND may improve overall survival, but this issue is debated in the medical literature.

Sentinel Lymph Node Biopsy

Axillary dissection traditionally was performed on all patients with invasive breast cancer. Today, sentinel lymphadenectomy, or sentinel lymph node (SLN) biopsy, identifies the first, or sentinel, lymph node or nodes in the axillary chain to receive drainage from the breast cancer and thus the most likely to contain metastases. The SLN biopsy is performed by injecting isosulfan blue dye and/or radioactive isotope to localize the sentinel lymph node.

The sentinel node can be identified in 95% of all cases. Multiple studies show that SLN biopsy can predict accurately the presence of axillary metastases in T1-2 breast cancer with a false-negative rate of 5% and an accuracy rate of 95%. The false-negative rate of SLN biopsy can be decreased to 1% to 3% if any palpable node is removed along with any hot or blue nodes. The SLN biopsy, a less invasive way to assess the status of the axilla, is associated with fewer complications than an axillary node dissection. Areas of controversy in SLN biopsy include T3, palpable suspicious axillary lymph nodes, and previous neoadjuvant therapy. In a study by Specht, 25% of palpable suspicious axillary lymph nodes proved benign on final pathology. Previous axillary dissection is not a strict contraindication per se because 75% of these patients can still have an identifiable sentinel node. The success rate depends on the number of nodes previously removed, with a success rate of 87% when fewer than 10 nodes are removed versus a success rate of 47% when more than 10 nodes are removed. Contraindications to SLN biopsy include T4 breast cancer and pregnancy. SLN biopsy is contraindicated in pregnancy because of the lack of data regarding fetal safety, although computer models suggest the amount of radiation exposure to the fetus is negligible.

Axillary Dissection

Patients who have metastatic cells on SLN biopsy typically undergo complete ALND. Alternatively, if a patient is not a candidate for SLN biopsy, ALND should be considered. Axillary dissection involves the removal of 10 to 30 lymph nodes from the axilla. The potential risk of axillary dissection includes the accumulation of a seroma, ipsilateral arm lymphedema, and numbness around the area of the intercostal brachial innervation if the nerve is sacrificed at the time of surgery. Because of the lifetime increased chance of arm lymphedema and possible infection, patients should avoid any trauma or procedures such as venipuncture or blood pressure measurements on the ipsilateral arm.

Adjuvant Therapy

Adjuvant therapy is used to treat patients with a demonstrable likelihood for the development of metastatic disease. Most medical oncologists consider this risk sufficient in node-negative patients with a tumor diameter of 1 cm or larger and in those with nodal metastases to justify adjuvant chemotherapy or hormonal therapy. Most commonly used cytotoxic regimens include CMF (cyclophosphamide [Cytoxan], methotrexate, and 5-FU [fluorouracil]) for 6 cycles or AC-T for 8 cycles (4 cycles of doxorubicin [Adriamycin] and cyclophosphamide followed by 4 cycles of paclitaxel [Taxol]). There appears to be a slight improvement of 3% in overall survival favoring the anthracycline-containing regimen over the CMF regimens. In the elderly population, the CMF regimen may be easier to tolerate than the AC-T regimens. In a recent study, a dose dense regimen of AC-T results in a slight improvement of disease-free and overall survival. Dose-dense regimen involves giving the chemotherapy in cycles every 2 weeks, with bone marrow support such as G-CSF (Neupogen), as opposed to the traditional cycles every 3 weeks. The improvement in survival is approximately 3%. In the Early Breast Cancer Trialists' Collaborative Group (EBCTCG) meta-analysis, adjuvant chemotherapy appears the most beneficial for women younger than 50 years of age. Combination chemotherapy resulted in the improvement of 10-year-overall survival from 71% in node-negative patients not receiving chemotherapy to 78% in those that did receive chemotherapy. This increase was even more dramatic in node-positive patients, with an improvement of overall survival from 42% to 53%. A much smaller effect was seen in patients older than 50 years of age. In this group of patients, survival was increased from 67% to 69% when node-negative patients not receiving chemotherapy were compared to those receiving chemotherapy. In node-positive elderly patients, improvement in overall survival was also minimal, with an increase of survival from 47% to 49% with chemotherapy.

Hormonal therapy, such as tamoxifen, is a commonly used adjuvant treatment in early breast cancer patients with estrogen receptor–positive tumors. The EBCTCG meta-analysis looking at the role of tamoxifen in the premenopausal patients found that tamoxifen results in an absolute improvement of 10-year overall survival of 5.6% in node-negative patients and 10.9% in node-positive patients. This effect is even greater in the postmenopausal population, with a 26% proportional reduction in 10-year mortality rates. The recommended length of treatment for node-negative patients is 5 years. Additionally, tamoxifen can be used as a chemopreventive agent to decrease the chance of an additional ipsilateral tumor developing in patients undergoing breast conservation or to decrease the possibility of contralateral breast cancer.

More recently, three large randomized trials of aromatase inhibitors, such as anastrozole (Arimidex), exemestane (Aromasin), and letrozole (Femara), was published. In the ATAC (Arimidex, Tamoxifen, Alone or in Combination) trial, patients on anastrozole had a statistically significant longer disease-free interval when compared with patients on tamoxifen alone (hazard ratio of 0.83). No difference in survival was seen between the two groups. In another large study, patients on tamoxifen for 2 to 3 years were randomized to continuing tamoxifen versus switching to exemestane for a total of 5 years of therapy. There appeared to be an improvement in disease-free survival in the aromatase inhibitor arm (hazard ratio of 0.68). No difference in survival was seen, and given the early stoppage and crossover of patients, no survival data will be obtainable from this study. Yet another large double-blinded randomized trial involved patients who had finished a 5-year course of tamoxifen and were then randomized to receiving letrozole versus placebo. The trial was stopped at a mean follow-up of 2.4 years secondary to a significant improvement in disease-free survival in the letrozole arm (hazard ratio of 0.57). Again, no difference in survival was seen. Aromatase inhibitors are useful only in postmenopausal patients. Premenopausal patients may benefit from an aromatase inhibitor only after ovarian ablation.

Recommendations regarding tamoxifen, aromatase inhibitors, and chemotherapy depend on the clinical judgment of the treating medical oncologist. In general, if adjuvant chemotherapy is given, it should take place prior to the initiation of radiotherapy. Consideration should be given to the likelihood of systemic recurrence based on nodal status, tumor size, and tumor grade. Estrogen receptor positivity of the tumor is predictive of a response to hormonal therapy, and *HER2-neu* may determine the type of appropriate chemotherapy. Another factor is the patient's age and any co-morbid diseases that would decrease the patient's tolerance to a course of chemotherapy.

Surveillance After a Diagnosis of Breast Cancer

Surveillance should continue alter diagnosis and treatment of breast cancer to detect local recurrence or a new primary breast cancer in either the ipsilateral or contralateral breast. The National Comprehensive Cancer Network guidelines recommend that patients continue diligent monthly self-examinations and that a physician perform a physical examination at 6-month intervals to assess for evidence of local recurrence and symptoms of metastatic disease. The ipsilateral arm should be evaluated to detect early signs of lymphedema and initiate appropriate management. Bilateral mammograms should be obtained every year. Bone and computed tomographic scans and other tumor markers should be performed only on patients with symptomatic systemic disease because of the lack of evidence of improved survival with early detection of distant metastases.

Special Topics in Breast Disease

PHYLLODES TUMOR

Phyllodes tumor (cystosarcoma phyllodes) is a fibroepithelial lesion that can be either benign or malignant. It is a rare tumor of the breast accounting for 1% of all cases. The mean age of patients is 54 years of age. These tumors often present as a breast mass on clinical and mammographic examination., and they are considered benign or malignant depending on stromal cellularity, mitotic activity, presence of necrosis, and type of borders. Treatment is complete excision without axillary node dissection. Metastases secondary to malignant phyllodes are hematogenous and primarily travel to the lungs. It is important to obtain negative margins. A mastectomy occasionally may be warranted for large lesions. Patients with malignant phyllodes have an 80% chance of 5-year survival as opposed to more than 95% for benign phyllodes.

NIPPLE DISCHARGE

Nipple discharge can occur at any age and presents as a bloody, serous, or milky discharge. Only 6% to 12% of patients with a nipple discharge are found to have an underlying malignancy. This risk is slightly elevated if the discharge is bloody. The most common cause of serous or serosanguineous nipple discharge is a benign intraductal papilloma. Numerous drugs can also cause nipple discharge, such as phenothiazine, tricyclic antidepressants, reserpine, butyrophenones, cimetidine (Tagamet), verapamil (Calan), metoclopramide (Reglan), thiazides, and hormone replacement therapy. The most common underlying malignancy is DCIS. Ductograms may be useful in locating the papilloma. When the nipple discharge is unilaterally persistent, spontaneous, or postmenopausal, further workup may be considered. Other suspicious nipple discharges are those confined to one duct or that are bloody or serous. In general, the evaluation of nipple discharge should begin with a clinical examination and a mammogram. Cytologic examination of the discharge has a low sensitivity for detection of underlying malignancy and should be not be used in the workup. Treatment consists of a major duct excision.

GYNECOMASTIA

Gynecomastia is the unilateral or bilateral benign enlargement of male breast tissue. The etiology is often related to various substances, including exogenous hormones, cimetidine (Tagamet), thiazides, digoxin, theophylline, phenothiazines, alcohol, and marijuana use; it may also be idiopathic. The main concern is to rule out the diagnosis of male breast cancer. Once breast cancer is excluded, no treatment is indicated. If medication and lifestyle etiologies are eliminated without remission of the gynecomastia, the excess breast tissue may be surgically removed for cosmetic considerations or for breast pain.

MALE BREAST CANCER

Carcinoma of the male breast represents 1% of all breast cancers. Because men are not routinely screened for breast cancer, the diagnosis is often delayed. The most common manifestation of male breast cancer is a painless, firm, subareolar breast mass. The differential diagnosis includes gynecomastia. Breast imaging with mammography and/or ultrasound may be helpful in rendering a diagnosis inasmuch as the appearance of male breast cancer is a stellate, irregular solid mass. Any suspicious breast mass in a male patient should undergo diagnostic biopsy. If a malignancy is diagnosed, standard treatment is mastectomy with assessment of the axillary nodes by SLN biopsy or ALND. Most cases of male breast cancer are estrogen receptor positive, and recommendations for adjuvant chemotherapy or hormonal therapy should be based on criteria similar to those for breast cancer in female patients.

BREAST CANCER IN PREGNANCY

Pregnancy-associated breast cancer represents less than 2% of all breast cancer diagnoses. The breast cancer frequently is diagnosed at a late stage because of the difficulty of examining the breast in pregnant women and the avoidance of mammography during pregnancy. Any suspicious lesion noted during pregnancy should be subjected to biopsy in the same fashion as in a nongravid woman. Radiation therapy should not be administered during pregnancy, so breast conservation is generally contraindicated unless the diagnosis is made within a few weeks of delivery. Surgical treatment with mastectomy and ALND is the standard treatment of breast cancer during pregnancy. Adjuvant chemotherapy can be delivered with selective agents during the second and third trimesters. The prognosis is similar to that of nongravid women in whom breast cancer is diagnosed at a comparable stage.

INFLAMMATORY BREAST CANCER

The classic manifestation of inflammatory breast cancer is erythema, edema, peau d'orange, and color of the breast resembling an infectious process. Malignant cells within the dermal lymphatic vessels of the breast confirm the diagnosis. The usual pathology of the associated carcinoma is IFDC-NOS. Inflammatory carcinoma is a very aggressive type of breast cancer, with over 90% of patients having positive axillary lymph nodes at diagnosis. The recommended treatment is multimodality therapy, with chemotherapy preceding surgery. Surgical treatment is mastectomy followed by radiation therapy and often additional chemotherapy.

LOCALLY ADVANCED BREAST CANCER

Patients with N2 or N3 nodal status or those with four or more positive axillary nodes, T3 or T4 tumors, or involvement of the pectoralis fascia have locally advanced breast cancer (LABC). The recommended treatment for patients is neoadjuvant chemotherapy, which is administered before surgical treatment, although it has no impact on overall survival. An extent-of-disease (EOD) workup should be done in patients with LABC and includes a computed tomography (CT) of the chest, abdomen, and pelvis along with a bone scan. Figure 5 provides an algorithm for the treatment of LABC.

Endometriosis

Method of
David L. Olive, MD

Endometriosis is one of the most common diseases encountered by the practicing gynecologist, yet it is also one of the most vexing. Researchers have been searching for answers to even the most fundamental questions regarding this disease for well over a century; even today huge gaps remain in the understanding of this disorder.

Definition

Endometriosis is defined as the presence of endometrial glands and stroma outside the endometrial cavity and uterine musculature. The requirement for both glands and stroma is an arbitrary standard, and it is unclear whether either component of endometrium alone, if placed ectopically, can result in the symptoms and signs of endometriosis.

Two related diseases are also frequently observed. Adenomyosis is the presence of endometrial glands and stroma within the myometrium. This disorder is epidemiologically and pathogenically distinct from endometriosis, but the resulting symptoms (and medical treatments) are similar. Endosalpingiosis is identical to endometriosis in location and appearance but histologically resembles tubal glands and stroma. This latter abnormality has been poorly studied, and to date, little is known regarding the distinction between endometriosis and endosalpingiosis.

Genetics

Evidence continues to accumulate that endometriosis has a genetic basis. Evidence for this includes familial clustering, concordance in monozygotic twins, and increased prevalence among first-degree relatives. A search was recently undertaken to identify the gene or genes responsible for susceptibility to endometriosis. Although suggestive linkages were discovered, no genes have been firmly identified as instrumental in this disorder. It is hoped, however, that genetic research will eventually uncover information critical to understanding the molecular and cellular basis of this disease.

Pathogenesis

The pathogenesis of endometriosis is a controversial subject inspiring many researchers to investigate it.

Over the last 25 years considerable advancement has been made, providing solid clues to the understanding of the disease process. Today, a clear picture is beginning to emerge regarding how women develop endometriosis.

HISTOGENESIS

Leading researchers in the field have proposed numerous theories of histogenesis. The primary theory of histogenesis is transplantation of shed uterine endometrium to ectopic locations. A number of routes of dissemination of the tissue are proposed, including lymphatic dissemination, vascular spread, iatrogenic transplantation, and retrograde menstruation.

A critical aspect of this theory is that cast-off endometrium cells remain viable and capable of implanting. Furthermore, it proposes that the tissue distribution has the capacity to sustain implantation. Considerable research has established that shed endometrial cells are viable in vitro. In vitro studies of endometrial attachment to peritoneum also support the concept of transplantation, attachment, and invasion.

Additional theories of histogenesis include coelomic metaplasia and induction of endometriosis. However, little scientific evidence indicates that either route is a viable etiology of the disease, much less a common method for development.

ETIOLOGY AND MAINTENANCE

Retrograde menstruation is a well-established phenomenon. Data available from women undergoing peritoneal dialysis and laparoscopy at the time of menses suggest that 76% to 90% of women have retrograde flow. This mechanism is considered a critical first step in the initiation of much if not most endometriosis by a wide variety of epidemiologic and anatomic data. However, the majority of women do not have endometriosis. The question that arises is "Why not?"

Because the placement of menstrual debris into the peritoneal cavity happens with each menses, a mechanism must exist to eliminate this tissue. The prime candidate for removal of endometrial cells is cell-mediated cytotoxicity. Deficient cytotoxic response to ectopic endometrium is suggested as a mechanism for allowing implantation and growth. It is also postulated that factors positively affecting growth and maintenance may be altered to enhance the risk of endometriosis. Current evidence suggests that a variety of cytokines, including monocyte chemotactic protein-1, interleukin-8, and regulated on activation, T-cell expressed and secreted (RANTES) are overexpressed in women with endometriosis, resulting in the attraction and activation of macrophages. The source of this cytokine increase could be one or more of several tissues: Endometrium, peritoneal mesothelium, and macrophages themselves could be the primary aberrancy by which this cascade is begun.

Other abnormalities are speculated to promote endometriosis. These include abnormal expression of matrix metalloproteinases and the enzyme aromatase, which could locally produce a hyperestrogenic proimplantation environment. The mechanisms by which these abnormalities may cause disease as well as the source of such alterations are under investigation.

> **BOX 1   Epidemiology of Endometriosis**
>
> Increased risk with:
> - Menses >6 d
> - More menses
>
> Decreased risk with:
> - Increased parity
> - Irregular menses
> - Oral contraceptives
> - Late menarche
> - Exercise
> - Smoking

Prevalence and Epidemiology

Endometriosis is a disease found almost exclusively in reproductive-age women. The mean age at diagnosis is reported to be from 25 to 29 years, although this figure depends on the diagnostic method. Because traditional diagnosis requires laparoscopy, it is likely that the disease is frequently present in even younger patients for whom many gynecologists do not readily schedule surgery.

Although rare in the premenarcheal female, adolescent endometriosis is a relatively common entity. Endometriosis is found in 47% to 65% of women younger than 20 years with chronic pelvic pain or dyspareunia.

Endometriosis is associated with increased exposure to menstruation typified by earlier menarche, more frequent menses, longer menses, fewer pregnancies, later initial pregnancy, and less breast-feeding. In addition, factors known to decrease the amount of menses or lower estrogen levels also reduce the risk: oral contraceptive use, irregular menses/oligomenorrhea, stress, exercise, and cigarette smoking (Box 1).

Postmenopausal endometriosis seldom occurs; this age group represents only 2% to 4% of all women requiring laparoscopy for endometriosis. The majority of such cases are a sequela to reactivation of disease by hormone replacement therapy; this is not true in all cases.

Clinical Presentation

Endometriosis is associated with a wide array of presenting signs and symptoms, although many women with physical manifestations of the disease remain completely asymptomatic. Commonly, the severity of symptoms does not correlate with the stage of endometriosis; extensive disease sometimes causes only minimal symptoms, and in others, minimal disease can be associated with severe symptoms. Some symptoms may strongly suggest the presence of endometriosis, but none are pathognomonic of this disorder. Because endometriosis most commonly involves the pelvis, infertility, dysmenorrhea, pelvic pain, dyspareunia, and menstrual dysfunction are common clinical presentations. When the ovary is severely involved, an ovarian cyst or pelvic mass may be the initial sign of endometriosis.

Pelvic pain is the most frequent complaint for endometriosis patients. This generally presents as secondary dysmenorrhea, worsening primary dysmenorrhea, dyspareunia, or even noncyclic lower abdominal pain, chronic pelvic pain, and backaches. In addition, pain may be site specific when endometriosis is found in unusual locations outside of the pelvis.

Only rarely are physical findings specific for endometriosis. Localized cul-de-sac and uterosacral ligament tenderness may frequently be detected. Thickened, nodular uterosacral ligaments or rectovaginal masses may be palpable. Adnexal enlargement or tenderness may reflect ovarian involvement. Retroverted fixation of the uterus may be noted with posterior cul-de-sac obliteration by the disease.

Cutaneous manifestations may be present, with apparent lesions on the perineum or vagina, or, less commonly, in the inguinal region, the umbilical area, or at the site of surgical scars. They should be suspected whenever a scar or lesion is associated with cyclical pain, tenderness, swelling, or bleeding.

Diagnosis

The current gold standard for the definitive diagnosis of endometriosis is laparoscopy. However, because of the heterogeneity in appearance of endometriosis lesions, the accuracy of laparoscopic diagnosis is variable and depends on the ability of the surgeon to recognize the disease. Although histologic confirmation would be ideal to ensure the presence of disease, this is infrequently accomplished because of the reticence of surgeons to excise endometriosis lesions.

Ultrasound is most useful for the detection of ovarian endometriomas, although the appearance of a cystic structure with heightened echogenicity is certainly not limited to this form of endometriosis. Structures often confused with endometriomas include corpora lutea, hemorrhagic cysts, unilocular dermoid cysts, and other benign cystic neoplasias. Ultrasound is not currently useful for identifying focal implants.

Magnetic resonance imaging (MRI) demonstrates significant potential in the diagnosis of endometriosis. MRI is clearly of value in diagnosing the ovarian endometrioma, and as technology improves, the potential for detecting peritoneal lesions will increase.

Treatment

MEDICAL THERAPY

The first drug to be approved for the treatment of endometriosis in the United States was danazol

CURRENT DIAGNOSIS

- Symptoms associated with endometriosis are primarily those of pain and infertility, although site-specific symptoms and signs may exist when the disease is in unusual locations.
- The standard for diagnosis is laparoscopic visualization; however, this method has a high false-positive and false-negative rate. The only method to confirm the disease absolutely is excisional biopsy.

CURRENT THERAPY

- Both medical and surgical therapies are efficacious in the treatment of endometriosis-associated pain. It is unclear which offers the better approach.
- Combined medical/surgical therapy may offer an advantage over surgery alone, if the medication is used at least 6 months postoperatively.
- Medical therapy has no role in the treatment of endometriosis-associated infertility.
- Surgical therapy for endometriosis-associated infertility appears to be of value for all stages of disease, but its relative value compared to assisted reproduction is not yet determined.

(Danocrine), a derivative of testosterone. It was originally thought to produce a pseudomenopause, but subsequent studies have revealed that the drug acts primarily by diminishing the midcycle luteinizing hormone (LH) surge, creating a chronic anovulatory state. The recommended dosage of danazol for the treatment of endometriosis is 600 to 800 mg/day; however, these doses have substantial androgenic side effects such as increased hair growth, mood changes, adverse serum lipid profiles, deepening of the voice (possibly irreversible), and, rarely, liver damage (possibly irreversible and life threatening) and arterial thrombosis. Studies of lower doses as primary treatment for endometriosis-associated pain have been uncontrolled or with small numbers and thus contain information of limited value.

Progestogens are a class of compounds that produce progesterone-like effects on endometrial tissue. A large number of progestogens exist, ranging from those chemically derived from progesterone (progestins), such as medroxyprogesterone acetate (MPA), to 19-nortestosterone derivatives such as norethindrone and norgestrel. The proposed mechanism of action of these compounds causes initial shedding of endometrial tissue followed by eventual atrophy. The most extensively studied progestational agent for the treatment of endometriosis is medroxyprogesterone (dep-subQ Provera 104), which is currently approved by the Food and Drug Administration (FDA) for use in treating endometriosis in a depot subcutaneous form. A common side effect is transient breakthrough bleeding, which occurs in 38% to 47% of patients. This is generally well tolerated and, when necessary, can be adequately treated with supplemental estrogen or an increase in the progestogen dose. Other side effects include nausea (0% to 80%), breast tenderness (5%), fluid retention (50%), and depression (6%). A recent approach to treating endometriosis with progestogen is the use of a progestogen-containing intrauterine contraceptive device[1] (Mirena).

The combination of estrogen and progestogen for therapy of endometriosis, the so-called pseudopregnancy regimen, has been used for 40 years. The most commonly used pseudopregnancy regimen today is the oral

---

[1]Not FDA approved for this indication.

contraceptive pill[1] (OCP); in fact, it is the most commonly prescribed treatment for endometriosis symptoms. Like progestational therapy, pseudopregnancy is believed to produce initial decidualization and growth of endometrial tissue, followed in several months by atrophy.

Gonadotropin-releasing hormone (GnRH) agonists are analogues of the hormone GnRH. This hypothalamic hormone is responsible for stimulating the pituitary gland to secrete follicle-stimulating hormone (FSH) and LH, two hormones necessary for normal ovarian function. GnRH is secreted in a pulsatile manner; the correct pulse results in stimulation of FSH and LH release, whereas too high or too low a pulse rate results in a decrease in pituitary hormone secretion. GnRH agonists are modified forms of GnRH that bind to the pituitary receptors and remain for a lengthy period. Thus, they are identified by the pituitary as rapidly pulsatile GnRH, and after initial stimulation of FSH and LH secretion, result in a shutdown (down-regulation) of the pituitary and no stimulation of the ovary. The result is a hypoestrogenic state similar to that of menopause, producing endometrial atrophy and amenorrhea. The agonist can be given intranasally (naferelin [Synarel]), subcutaneously (goserelin [Zoladex]), or intramuscularly (IM) (leuprolide acetate [Lupro Depot]), depending on the specific product, with frequency of administration ranging from twice daily to every 3 months. The side effects are those of hypoestrogenism such as transient vaginal bleeding, hot flashes, vaginal dryness, decreased libido, breast tenderness, insomnia, depression, irritability and fatigue, headache, osteoporosis, and decreased skin elasticity; these are dose dependent.

A recent modification of GnRH agonist treatment is to add back small amounts of steroid hormone in a manner similar to that used in the treatment of postmenopausal women. The theory is that the requirement for estrogen is greater for endometriosis than is needed by the brain (to prevent hot flashes), the bone (to prevent osteoporosis), and other tissues deprived of this hormone. With this approach there is an equivalent rate of pain relief with far fewer side effects than GnRH agonist alone. Estrogen as a solitary add-back, however, is less effective and thus not indicated.

SURGICAL THERAPY

Most surgeons performing surgery for endometriosis must choose one of two possibilities: conservative surgery, where the patient's future fertility remains an option, or definitive surgery. The latter procedure generally involves removal of the female gonads, a hysterectomy, or a combination of the two. The general perception is that definitive surgery is more effective over time than conservative treatment, but it must be reserved for patients in whom fertility or continued endocrine function is deemed less important than relief of pain symptoms.

When conservative surgery is desired, the first technical issue confronted is method of access. Traditionally, laparotomy was used for endometriosis surgery. However, recently, most surgeons performing extensive surgery for endometriosis have favored a laparoscopic approach because of improved magnification of disease with a resulting increase in surgical precision.

[1]Not FDA approved for this indication.

Surgical destruction of endometriosis lesions can be accomplished in a variety of ways: Excision, vaporization, and fulguration/desiccation have all been used. Excision is generally thought to be the most complete of these techniques, but no comparative trials have assessed the relative efficacy of each approach.

Endometriomas, or ovarian cysts formed from endometriosis, are commonly present in the patient with endometriosis. The ovaries should first be freed of all adhesions when operating on endometriomas. The endometrioma may open spontaneously during this process; if not, incision and drainage is indicated. At this point, the cyst wall may be stripped, excised, or drained.

TREATMENT RESULTS

Medical therapy is effective against endometriosis-associated pain. Placebo-controlled randomized clinical trials (RCTs) have proven that danazol and medroxyprogesterone reduce pain significantly better than no treatment for up to 6 months following discontinuation of the drug. No good data exist for longer follow-up periods. Numerous randomized trials have compared medical therapies to one another. In 15 RCTs comparing danazol to GnRH agonists, no difference was demonstrated between the two as first-line drugs. Similarly, little difference was seen when GnRH agonists were compared to oral contraceptives, progestogens, or gestrinone.

Several trials have addressed the efficacy of combined add-back therapy and GnRH agonist treatment during 6-month treatment periods. In general, pain was relieved as effectively with the combination as with GnRH agonist alone, and it significantly reduced the side effects of the GnRH agonist. The results were similar in three longer trials of approximately 1-year duration (Figure 1). The amelioration of side effects with maintenance of efficacy seems to be even when the add-back therapy is begun during the first month of treatment, suggesting that

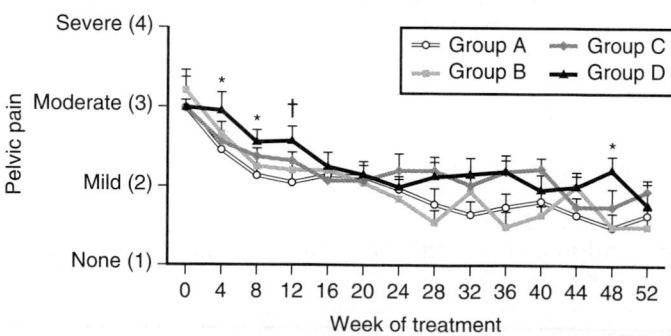

MEAN PELVIC PAIN SCORE AT EACH VISIT

* $P \le .05$ ⎫ Change from baseline
† $P \le .01$ ⎭ compared with Group A

FIGURE 1. Pain relief from gonadotropin-releasing hormone (GnRH) agonist (Group A) and three different add-back therapies. (High dose progestin, low dose estrogen/progestin, higher dose estrogen/progestin). No difference is seen among the groups in the amount of pain relief. (From Hornstein MD, Surrey ES, Weisberg GW, Casino LA: et al: Leuprolide acetate depot and hormonal add-back in endometriosis: A 12-month study. Lupron Add-Back Study Group. Obstet Gynecol 1998;91(1):16-24.

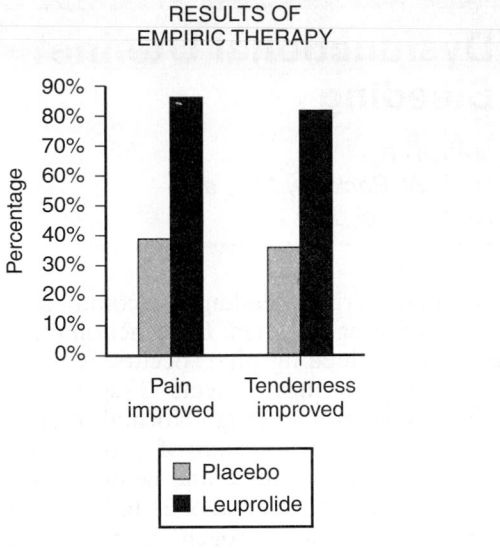

RESULTS OF
EMPIRIC THERAPY
Percentage
90%
80%
70%
60%
50%
40%
30%
20%
10%
0%
Pain
improved
Tenderness
improved
Placebo
Leuprolide

FIGURE 2. Patients with pain relief from empirical gonadotropin-releasing hormone (GnRH) agonist or placebo.

Study
Medical
No
treatment
Relative risk
(95% CL)
Bayer
11/37
17/36
0.63 (0.32–1.22)
Fedele
10/35
13/36
0.79 (0.36–1.68)
Telimaa
4/35
5/14
0.32 (0.08–1.24)
Thomas
4/20
4/17
0.85 (0.20–3.69)
Total
29/127
39/103
0.60 (0.39–0.93)
.1 .2
1
5 10

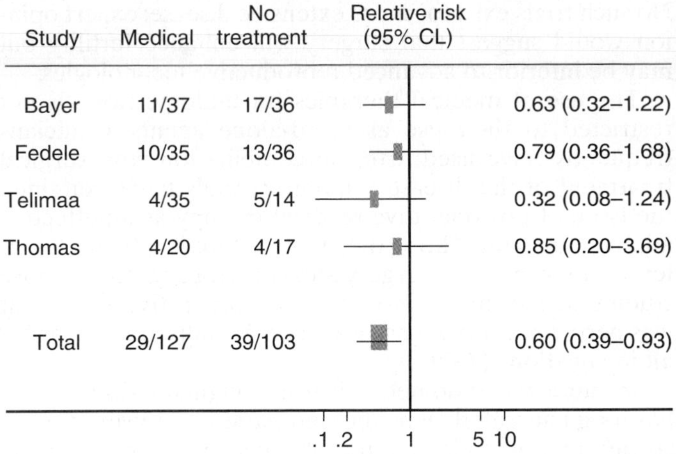

FIGURE 3. Meta-analysis of all randomized trials comparing medical therapy versus no treatment or placebo for endometriosis-associated infertility. Note that the untreated group has a significantly better pregnancy rate.

an add-back-free interval at the beginning of a treatment cycle is unnecessary.

Although the studies just described randomize patients for initial therapy of endometriosis-associated pain, one study examined the value of GnRH agonist in patients failing primary therapy. Ling and colleagues treated women having failed to obtain relief with OCPs with either GnRH agonist or placebo. Those treated with active drug responded significantly better than those given placebo, with more than 80% experiencing pain relief in 3 months (Figure 2). Of interest is the fact that the therapy seemed to be beneficial whether or not endometriosis was seen at laparoscopy.

Most of the established medical therapies used to treat endometriosis have been applied to the problem of subfertility in women with this disease. These medications inhibit ovulation, and thus they are used to treat the disease for a period of time prior to allowing an attempt at conception. Five randomized trials with six treatment arms have compared one of these medical treatments for endometriosis to placebo or no treatment with fertility as the outcome measure. Another eight RCTs compared danazol to a second medication. These latter trials were summarized by a meta-analysis by Hughes et al. and modified by Olive and Pritts to include loss of fertility while on the medications (Figure 3). The data clearly show that medical therapy for endometriosis has not proven to be of value, and in fact may be counterproductive, to the subfertile patient.

Only two studies have investigated surgery for endometriosis-associated pain versus sham surgery. Sutton and colleagues assessed the efficacy of laser laparoscopic surgery in the treatment of pain associated with minimal, mild, or moderate endometriosis. They found that there was no difference in pain at 3 months follow-up, but by 6 months a clear-cut advantage was seen for surgery. Abbott and colleagues evaluated excision of endometriosis versus diagnostic laparoscopy and had nearly identical results at 6 months. Thus, both techniques were proven better than no therapy.

Conservative surgery was used extensively in an attempt to enhance fertility. Most studies, however, are uncontrolled and of poor quality. Two randomized trials were performed to examine the value of ablation of early-stage endometriosis versus sham surgery, with contradictory results. When combined into a meta-analysis, surgical treatment of early-stage endometriosis still appears to provide a significant improvement in pregnancy rates.

TABLE 1 Postoperative Medical Therapy

Drug	Duration of Treatment	Studies	Findings
OCPs	6 mo	1	NS at 24, 36 mo
Medroxyprogesterone, 100 mg/d	6 mo	1	$p < 0.05$ at 6 mo
Danazol, 600 mg/d	3 mo	1	NS at 6 mo
Danazol, 600 mg/d	6 mo	1	$p < 0.05$ at 6 mo
Danazol, 100 mg/d	6 mo	1	$p < 0.05$ at 24 mo
GnRH-a	3 mo	1	NS at 6 mo
GnRH-a	6 mo	2	$p = 0.008$ at 12 mo

Abbreviations: GnRH = gonadotropin-releasing hormone; NS = no sample; OCP = oral contraceptive pill.

No such trials exist for more extensive disease; expert opinion would suggest that surgery will enhance fertility but may be inferior to advanced reproductive technologies.

The use of medical therapies for endometriosis is not restricted to their use as stand-alone agents. Clinicians frequently have used drugs in combination with surgical treatment of the disease. Numerous trials have examined the issue of postoperative medical therapy as an effective adjunct for pain. Those that have treated patients for at least 6 months after surgery showed efficacy, but in those studies where only 3 months of postoperative treatment was performed, no benefit was seen. Results are similar for all medications (Table 1).

In summary, endometriosis is an enigmatic disease that has long frustrated clinicians and patients. However, great strides in the understanding of this disorder are being made. The coming years are likely to produce a plethora of new treatment approaches targeting the biologic basis of this disease. In this regard, better understanding will undoubtedly result in renewed hope for the patient suffering from the ravages of endometriosis.

REFERENCES

Abbott JA, Hawe J, Hunter D, et al: Laparoscopic excision of endometriosis: A randomized, placebo controlled trial. Fertil Steril 2004;82:878-884.

Hornstein MD, Surrey ES, Weisberg GW, Casino LA, Lupron Add-Back Study Group: Leuprolide acetate depot and hormonal add-back in endometriosis: a 12-month study. Obstet Gynecol 1998;91:16-24.

Hughes E, Ferorkow D, Collins J, Vandekerckhone P: Ovulation suppression for endometriosis (Cochrane review). The Cochrane Library (issue 1): Oxford, England: Update Software, 2000.

Jacobson TZ, Barlow DH, Koninclex PR, et al: Laparoscopic surgery for subfertility associated with endometriosis. Cochrane Database Syst Rev 2002;(4):CD001398.

Jansen RPS, Russel P: Nonpigmented endometriosis: Clinical, laparoscopic and pathologic definition. Am J Obstet Gynecol 1986;155:1154.

Ling FW: Randomized controlled trial of depot leuprolide in patients with chronic pelvic pain and clinically suspected endometriosis. Obstet Gynecol 1999;93:51-58.

Moghissi KS, Schlaff WD, Olive DL, et al: Goserelin acetate (Zoladex) with or without hormone replacement therapy for the treatment of endometriosis. Fertil Steril 1998;69:1056-1062.

Olive DL, Pritts EA: The treatment of endometriosis: a review of the evidence. Ann NY Acad Sci 2002; 955:360-372.

Olive DL, Pritts EA: Treatment of endometriosis. N Engl J Med. 2001;345:266-275.

Sampson JA: Perforating hemorrhagic (chocolate) cysts of the ovary. Arch Surg 1921;3:245.

Sutton CJG, Ewen SP, Whitelaw N, Haines P: Prospective, randomized, double-blind, controlled trial of laser laparoscopy in the treatment of pelvic pain associated with minimal, mild, or moderate endometriosis. Fertil Steril 1994;62:696.

Dysfunctional Uterine Bleeding

Method of
Beth W. Rackow, MD, and
Aydin Arici, MD

Abnormal uterine bleeding is a common disorder among reproductive-age women. Dysfunctional uterine bleeding, defined as bleeding that occurs with no identifiable anatomic pathology, affects 33% to 50% of women with abnormal bleeding. Normal menstrual bleeding predictably occurs at the end of an ovulatory cycle because of estrogen and progesterone withdrawal, and lasts up to 7 days, with a cycle interval of 21 to 35 days. Any imbalance of either hormone, estrogen or progesterone, may lead to dysfunctional bleeding. Thus bleeding may occur from estrogen withdrawal because of bilateral oophorectomy or the midcycle fall in estrogen prior to ovulation; from estrogen breakthrough, such as with prolonged estrogen stimulation from chronic anovulation; from progesterone withdrawal after a short or long course of progestin therapy; and from progesterone breakthrough in the setting of a high ratio of progesterone to estrogen, such as with estrogen-progestin and progestin-based contraceptives. Dysfunctional uterine bleeding is a diagnosis of exclusion and requires eliminating other congenital and acquired abnormalities.

Evaluation of the patient with abnormal uterine bleeding must consider a broad differential diagnosis that includes a complication of pregnancy, cervical and uterine pathology (polyps, fibroids, adenomyosis, malignancies, chronic endometritis, congenital anomalies), infectious etiologies (sexually transmitted diseases, vaginitis), endocrinopathies (thyroid or androgen disorders, hyperprolactinemia), medications (exogenous hormonal therapy, anticoagulants, antibiotics, glucocorticoids, tamoxifen [Nolvadex], herbal supplements), bleeding diathesis, systemic illness (liver or renal disease), and genital trauma or foreign bodies. A thorough menstrual history is essential and should include details about past and present length of intermenstrual intervals, regularity of menses, volume and duration of bleeding during menses, onset of abnormal bleeding, factors associated with change in bleeding (postcoital, contraceptive method, postpartum, new medical diagnosis, change in weight), and associated symptoms (premenstrual symptoms, dysmenorrhea, dyspareunia, pelvic pain, hirsutism, galactorrhea). A complete medical history, list of medications, and review of systems helps identify any systemic illness or medication effect contributing to the abnormal bleeding. The physical exam should include careful inspection of the external genitalia, vagina, and cervix and a bimanual exam to palpate the uterus and adnexa to assess size, contour, and tenderness.

Laboratory evaluation provides further information. A pregnancy test (preferably quantitative) rules out bleeding because of a pregnancy complication. A complete blood count evaluates for anemia or thrombocytopenia and is important with prolonged or heavy bleeding. A serum progesterone timed to the luteal phase of the cycle determines if the patient is ovulatory; a level greater than 3 pg/mL is consistent with recent ovulation. Endocrine testing includes serum thyroid stimulating hormone, prolactin, and testosterone levels as indicated. Coagulation studies (prothrombin, partial thromboplastin, and bleeding times) should be performed in adolescents, patients with unexplained menorrhagia, and those with a personal or family history concerning for a bleeding disorder. In the setting of a systemic disorder such as chronic liver or renal disease, appropriate testing should be performed.

An endometrial biopsy should be performed in patients at high risk for hyperplasia and cancer based on age (35 years and older) and duration of unopposed estrogen exposure. Young patients (less than 35 years old) with chronic anovulation, thus prolonged estrogen exposure, should also have biopsies because they can develop endometrial hyperplasia and cancer. If the biopsy (preferably done in the luteal phase) reveals secretory, not proliferative, endometrium, ovulation has occurred. A pap smear, cervical cultures, and wet mount should also be performed as indicated.

A history of regular cycles with an increasing amount or duration of bleeding, or intermenstrual bleeding, is suggestive of an anatomic cause of abnormal bleeding. Transvaginal ultrasound provides a valuable assessment of the uterus and endometrium. Pathology such as fibroids and polyps can be identified, and size and location determined. Although an endometrial biopsy may not be necessary if the endometrium is thin (less than 5 mm), clinical suspicion of endometrial pathology takes precedence. Sonohysterography involves ultrasound assessment of the uterus and endometrium while sterile saline distends the uterine cavity. This test has high sensitivity and specificity for identifying uterine and endometrial pathology and is comparable to hysteroscopy. Hysteroscopy can diagnose and treat intrauterine pathology simultaneously, but it is a more invasive procedure. Regardless, it is important to recognize when anatomic abnormalities, such as fibroids, are present but not contributing to the bleeding.

Anovulatory Dysfunctional Uterine Bleeding

A menstrual history that reveals irregular, infrequent, unpredictable bleeding, a varying amount and duration of bleeding, and no reliable symptomatology is often sufficient to diagnose anovulatory bleeding. Considered a systemic disorder, anovulatory bleeding occurs because of a variety of endocrinologic, neurochemical, and pharmacologic processes. Estrogen breakthrough is the most common scenario: persistently high estrogen levels stimulate overgrowth of an endometrium that is fragile without the stabilizing, growth-limiting effects of progesterone, and focal areas of the endometrium breakdown, bleed, and subsequently heal because of estrogen effect. This dysfunctional bleeding is common in women with polycystic ovary syndrome or obesity, in postmenarchal adolescents, and in perimenopausal women. Other conditions associated with anovulatory states include thyroid disorders, hyperprolactinemia, androgen disorders, psychological or physical stress, eating disorders, dramatic weight changes, and insulin resistance.

Management of anovulatory bleeding involves treating both the cause of anovulation and the abnormal bleeding.

Progestins are the foundation of this medical therapy. Cyclic progestins stabilize the estrogen-stimulated endometrium and result in withdrawal bleeding after the progestin course. Medications used for a 10-day course every 4 to 6 weeks include medroxyprogesterone acetate (Provera), 5 to 10 mg, and norethindrone acetate (Aygestin), 5 mg. If bleeding does not occur after progestin withdrawal, the patient may also be hypoestrogenic, and further evaluation is indicated. Estrogen-progestin contraceptives are advantageous for patients with intermittent ovulation who require contraception, and they also effectively decrease the amount of bleeding. Combined contraceptives are available in pill, patch, and vaginal ring preparations. Medroxyprogesterone acetate (Depo-Provera),[1] 150 mg intramuscularly every 3 months, can also control anovulatory bleeding, especially if patients cannot take combined contraceptives. Treatment of prolonged heavy anovulatory bleeding can be achieved with either low-dose monophasic combined contraceptives,[1] one pill twice daily for 5 to 7 days until the bleeding slows or stops, followed by routine daily use if desired, or with a higher-dose course of progestin therapy. Once the heavy bleeding is controlled, further evaluation is warranted.

Estrogen therapy is indicated for the treatment of dysfunctional bleeding with a thinned endometrium because of low estrogen levels or after prolonged bleeding. This can be accomplished with conjugated estrogens (Premarin),[1] 1.25 mg, or micronized estradiol (Estrace),[1] 2 mg daily for 7 to 10 days. Similarly, estrogen (a 7- to 10-day course) can be used to treat progesterone breakthrough bleeding in the setting of low-dose combined contraceptives or long-acting progesterone therapy (medroxyprogesterone acetate [Depo-Provera]).

Ovulatory Dysfunctional Uterine Bleeding

Heavy or prolonged bleeding may occur during ovulatory cycles, and often no specific etiology is identified. Local defects in endometrial hemostasis are implicated. A number of medical and surgical therapies are effective in this situation. Nonsteroidal anti-inflammatory drugs (NSAIDs), such as ibuprofen (Motrin),[1] naproxen (Aleve),[1] or mefenamic acid (Ponstel),[1] decrease menstrual blood loss by inhibiting prostaglandin synthesis, an important component of endometrial hemostasis. NSAIDs may decrease blood loss by 20% to 40% and should be used for 3 to 5 days upon the onset of bleeding. Similarly, combined contraceptives can reduce menstrual flow by 40% to 60%. Another option is the levonorgestrel-releasing intrauterine system (Mirena)[1]; the local progestin effect on the endometrium is profound and can reduce menstrual blood loss by 75% to 90% in women with heavy bleeding. Although cyclic progestins are often ineffective in this setting, a course of progestin (norethindrone acetate, 5 mg three times daily) from days 5 to 26 of the cycle can suppress heavy ovulatory bleeding. Gonadotropin-releasing hormone agonists produce a hypoestrogenic state and thus cause amenorrhea as well as shrinkage of fibroids, if present. This therapy is best reserved for short-term management of heavy bleeding and severe anemia prior to a surgical procedure because of

---

[1]Not FDA approved for this indication.

expense and significant side effects such as menopausal symptoms and bone demineralization. Less commonly employed therapies include tranexamic acid (Cyklokapron),[1] an antifibrinolytic agent used in Europe to treat menorrhagia (1 g every 6 hours for the first few days of bleeding), and danazol (Danocrine),[1] a therapy that inhibits ovulation and decreases menstrual blood loss but involves androgenic side effects (200 mg daily).

Intermenstrual bleeding can also occur during ovulatory cycles. This dysfunctional bleeding may be caused by anatomic abnormalities, infection, or the preovulatory decline in estrogen. Similarly, breakthrough bleeding may be present during estrogen-progestin or progestin-only contraceptive therapy. Conjugated estrogens (Premarin),[1] 1.25 mg, or micronized estradiol (Estrace), 2 mg for 2 to 3 days midcycle or 7 to 10 days for persistent breakthrough bleeding, are effective.

For patients who fail medical therapy or for those who do not desire future fertility, surgical management is appropriate. The definitive procedure is hysterectomy, but this surgery carries a significant risk of complications and involves longer recovery time. Endometrial ablation by hysteroscopic, thermal, or cryosurgical techniques is a less invasive procedure for the management of abnormal bleeding. These techniques can result in significantly reduced bleeding and even amenorrhea, as well as less dysmenorrhea, but approximately 20% of patients require additional procedures. Patients with menorrhagia attributed to uterine fibroids can be managed with myomectomy (hysteroscopic, laparoscopic, or abdominal procedures as indicated) or uterine artery embolization. Pregnancy is not recommended after the latter option because little data are available on postprocedure pregnancy outcomes.

Uterine Hemorrhage

Acute heavy bleeding requires high-dose estrogen therapy. Patients who need inpatient management should receive conjugated estrogens (Premarin), 25 mg intravenously every 4 hours for 24 hours or until the bleeding decreases. A Foley catheter balloon can be placed in the uterine cavity to tamponade the bleeding. Additionally, dilation and curettage can be performed to help stop acute uterine hemorrhage. If stable for outpatient management, patients can receive conjugated estrogens (Premarin),[1] 1.25 mg, or micronized estradiol (Estrace),[1] 2 mg every

---

[1]Not FDA approved for this indication.

CURRENT DIAGNOSIS

- Detailed medical and menstrual history
- Thorough physical and gynecologic examination
- Pregnancy test for all reproductive-age women
- Determination of ovulatory status by history, laboratory tests
- Laboratory evaluation: complete blood count, endocrine studies, coagulation profile
- Endometrial sampling if high risk for hyperplasia or cancer
- Imaging studies to evaluate anatomy

CURRENT THERAPY

- Progestins
  Cyclic or intermittent use
  Prolonged therapy
  Progestin-releasing intrauterine device (IUD) (Mirena)[1]
- Estrogens[1]
  Intermittent use
  High-dose course for acute heavy bleeding
- Estrogen-progestin contraceptives[1]
  Cyclic use
  High-dose course with taper for heavy bleeding
- Other therapies
  Nonsteroidal anti-inflammatory drugs[1]
  Tranexamic acid (Cyklokapron)[1]
  Danazol (Danocrine)[1]
  Gonadotropin-releasing hormone agonists
- Surgical options
  Endometrial ablation
  Myomectomy
  Uterine artery embolization
  Hysterectomy

---

[1]Not FDA approved for this indication.

4 to 6 hours for 24 hours, and when the bleeding is controlled, the dose is tapered to once daily for 7 to 10 days. Another effective regimen uses high-dose combination contraceptives[1] (3 to 4 pills daily) until the bleeding is decreased, followed by a taper to 1 pill daily for several weeks. Estrogen therapy should be followed by progestins or combined contraceptives to stabilize the estrogen-stimulated endometrium.

Because dysfunctional uterine bleeding is a diagnosis of exclusion, a thorough history and evaluation, including determination of ovulatory status, is essential. A number of medical and surgical options exist for the management of dysfunctional bleeding. However, treatment failures require further evaluation.

REFERENCES

American College of Obstetricians and Gynecologists: Management of anovulatory bleeding. ACOG Practice Bulletin, no. 14, March 2000.

Berek JS (ed): Benign diseases of the female reproductive tract. In Berek JS, ed: Novak's Gynecology. Philadelphia, Lippincott Williams & Wilkins, 2002, pp 351-373.

Munro MG: Dysfunctional uterine bleeding: Advances in diagnosis and treatment. Curr Opin Obstet Gynecol 2001;13:475-489.

Munro MG: Medical management of abnormal uterine bleeding. Obstet Gynecol Clin North Am 2000;27:287-304.

Shwayder JM: Pathophysiology of abnormal uterine bleeding. Obstet Gynecol Clin North Am 2000;27:219-234.

Speroff L, Fritz M: Dysfunctional uterine bleeding. In Clinical Gynecologic Endocrinology and Infertility. Philadelphia, Lippincott Williams & Wilkins; 2005, pp 548-571.

---

[1]Not FDA approved for this indication.

Infertility

Method of
Steven R. Williams, MD

Absence of desired conception despite 12 months of unprotected intercourse generally defines infertility. Historical and physical factors allow the physician to adjust this definition to the individual patient. For example, women with longstanding amenorrhea or known distal hydrosalpinges should consider intervention before 12 months, time has elapsed. However, the couple, 22 years of age, with a negative history can be encouraged to try a bit longer than 12 months before evaluation begins. After 6 months of trying, approximately 45% of couples achieve pregnancy, and after 12 months of trying, approximately 85% will conceive. Pregnancy can occur with sex 6 days before ovulation, although one study found no pregnancies were conceived from sex the day after ovulation. Thus we recommend couples trying for a baby should plan to be active together every other day starting about 6 days before ovulation is expected (cycle day 8) until 2 to 3 days after ovulation has happened (cycle day 18). If the mood were to strike more often, that's fine with us; if the mood strikes less often, we can still be comfortable given the 6-day interval previously described. As in all of medicine, important historical points can guide the direction of the evaluation and treatment of the infertile couple.

Male-factor historical points include fathering past pregnancies or miscarriages, sexual function, urologic or hernia surgery, infections, medications, and tobacco use. Semen analysis remains the most important test for male factor evaluation. The World Health Organization (WHO) reports normal males to have more than 20 million sperm per cc with greater than 50% motility. It is probably best to advise 48 hours of abstinence before collection of the sample. A urologic exam and evaluation is indicated with abnormal counts. Modern in vitro fertilization (IVF) treatments can achieve pregnancies as long as any sperm at all can be isolated, even if that means surgical aspiration. Before pursuing assisted reproduction for severely low counts, genetic testing will be recommended because severely low counts can predict higher rates of cystic fibrosis carrier status, balanced translocation, and perhaps microdeletions of the Y chromosome.

A women's age has a strong correlation with fertility success. Figure 1 compares the live birth rate when IVF patients used their own eggs fertilized with their partner's sperm compared to the rate when young oocyte donor's eggs are fertilized with the IVF patient's partner's sperm and the resultant embryos transferred into the IVF patient's uterus. One must conclude from these data that the majority of the decline in success is related to oocyte quality, as anyone can expect the success of a woman 25 years of age who uses the oocytes from a woman 25 years of age! Follicle-stimulating hormone (FSH) measured on day 3 of the menstrual cycle correlates well with ovarian reserve and is commonly ordered for women more than 30 years of age with infertility. In our office, day-3 FSH values lower than 9 mU/mL are reassuring with respect to ovarian reserve, whereas values greater than 20 mU/mL

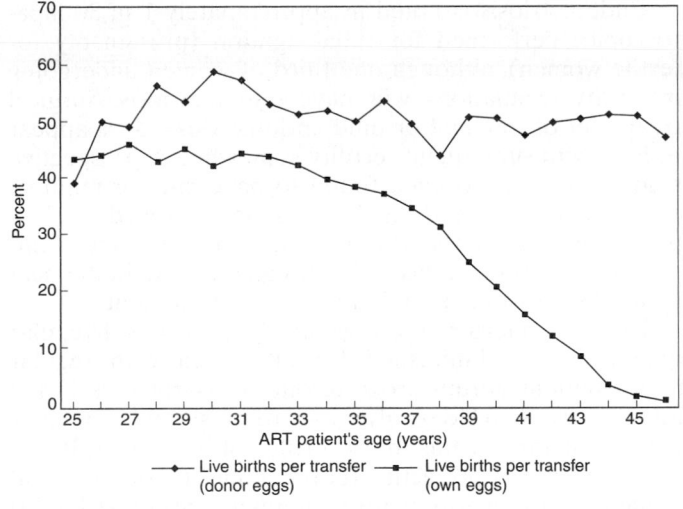

FIGURE 1. Live births per transfer for ART cycles using fresh embryos from own and donor eggs, by ART patient's age, 2002. ART = assisted reproductive technology.

are rarely associated with future fertility success using that patient's eggs.

Previous full-term deliveries are reassuring, whereas recurrent abortions or preterm deliveries can predict a uterine issue. Pelvic infections, intrauterine device (IUD) use, previous abdominal surgery, dysmenorrhea, or dyspareunia can predict tubal obstruction. This is explored with hysterosalpingography (HSG). After sterile preparation of the cervix, a sterile cannula is inserted, and under fluoroscopic guidance radiograph contrast is injected. The dye reveals the contour of the uterine cavity and displays uterine septa and intracavitary lesions such as fibroids or polyps. It then fills into the fallopian tubes and spills into the abdominal cavity. Most women describe the discomfort of the test as a severe menstrual cramp that lasts for several minutes. Pain is reduced by slow injection of the dye, gentle tissue handling, and pretreatment with nonsteroidal anti-inflammatory drugs (NSAIDs). Many authors suggest that the procedure itself has a fertility-enhancing effect. The American College of Obstetricians and Gynecologists (ACOG) suggests prophylaxis with doxycycline (Vibramycin)[1] 100 mg twice daily orally for 5 days after HSG if dilated tubes are demonstrated; no prophylaxis is indicated in a normal study. Abnormal uterine cavities can be further evaluated with saline infusion hysterograms or magnetic resonance imaging (MRI). Many uterine abnormalities can be treated completely with hysteroscopic surgery. Unilateral tubal disease noted on the HSG predicts subtle decreases in future fertility in these women compared with women with normal tubes. Bilateral tubal disease discovered on HSG predicts dramatic declines in fertility. Tubal patency established by HSG does not rule out peritubal adhesions that can affect fertility. Laparoscopy is an outpatient surgical procedure that can be used to further evaluate tubal abnormalities seen on HSG or to look for undetected peritubal adhesions. Laparoscopy also will detect endometriosis.

---

[1]Not FDA approved for this indication.

Endometriosis is noted in approximately 1 in 30 laparoscopies performed for tubal ligation (presumably for fertile women), although one third of women undergoing infertility evaluations will have endometriosis. Surgical treatment of minimal or mild endometriosis does appear to help with subsequent fertility somewhat. A prospective study of infertile women found to have mild or minimal endometriosis noted at laparoscopy showed a 31% preganancy rate in the next 9 months for patients randomized to treatment versus a 17% pregnancy rate in the next 9 months for women randomized to no treatment.

Irregular menstruation generally indicates irregular ovulation and diminished fertility. Even with regular menstruations, serum progesterone measurements in the luteal phase (6 to 8 days after ovulation) should be greater than 10 ng/mL for the "most fertile" of ovulations. If it is not, thyroid and prolactin studies should be ordered and induction of ovulation with clomiphene citrate (Clomid) considered. Clomiphene citrate in a 50-mg dose is taken orally for 5 days starting on menstrual day 3. Serum luteal phase progesterone is drawn 7 days after ovulation and is expected to be greater than 10 ng/dL. If it is, refills for 2 more months of treatment are written. If it is not, we recommend increasing the dose of clomiphene citrate to 100 mg daily for 5 days and repeating the luteal phase progesterone assay. If still not greater than 10 ng/dL, clomiphene citrate at 150 mg daily can be tried. If the patient is still anovulatory, referral to a gynecologist or reproductive endocrinologist is considered. For resistant patients, adjunctive treatments with the clomiphene citrate can include ultrasound monitoring with HCG injections when mature follicles are noted or adding insulin-sensitizing agents or glucocorticoids. Clomiphene ovulation induction yields approximately a 70% ovulation rate and, in young couples, approximately an 8% pregnancy rate per month. One in ten clomiphene citrate pregnancies are twins, although triplets and quadruplets are very rare on this therapy. Side effects of clomiphene citrate include hot flushes, emotional lability, mittelschmerz, headache, and sleep disturbance. Discontinue the drug if the patient experiences severe visual disturbance. Because the majority of clomiphene citrate pregnancies happen early in treatment, referral to reproductive specialists should be considered if the patients is not pregnant after 3 months of treatment.

Gonadotropin ovulation induction is available for women who failed to ovulate using clomiphene citrate or did not conceive on that therapy. This medication is the natural hormone used to initiate ovulation; therefore, response and pregnancy rates are better than with clomiphene citrate. Unfortunately, dramatic increases in multiple pregnancy are associated with these medications, and often they are quite expensive. One large study reviewed success and multiple pregnancy rates in patients treated with gonadotropin ovulation induction. The authors concluded the protocols

CURRENT DIAGNOSIS

- Medical history can guide fertility testing.
- Simple laboratory and radiograph tests can determine infertility causes.

CURRENT THERAPY

- Clomiphene citrate is a low risk treatment option when indicated.
- Assisted reproduction is delivering more and more babies with fewer multiples.

employed with gonadotropin ovulation induction lead to an unacceptably high incidence of higher-order multiple pregnancies and raised the question whether that treatment could be replaced by IVF.

IVF involves induction of ovulation with gonadotropin in hopes of retrieving multiple oocytes. Ovarian response is monitored with pelvic ultrasounds and serum estradiol measurements. When the oocytes are mature, HCG is given to trigger the completion of oocyte development. Then transvaginal ultrasound is used to guide an aspirating needle through the posterior cul-de-sac and into the ovaries for aspiration of the oocytes. The procedure takes approximately 15 minutes under local anesthesia and is often performed in an office setting. Oocytes are then inseminated in the lab with the husband's sperm and cultured. In certain circumstances (vey low sperm count, surgically aspirated sperm, previous failed fertilization) the oocytes can be directly injected with the sperm via intracytoplasmic sperm injection (ICSI). The resultant embryos are then cultured for 2 to 5 days and then transferred into the uterus via a simple transcervical approach. IVF thus allows embryo development without tubal ovarial interaction, making it a great choice for patients with tubal disease or endometriosis. In fact, nothing we can find at laparoscopy that was not discovered by pelvic ultrasound and HSG will affect IVF success (Figure 2). We are developing protocols that reduce the numbers of embryos transferred for couples at high risk for multiple pregnancy to one. I believe that in the future IVF will replace both gonadotropin ovulation induction and the need for laparoscopy for treatment of infertility. The 2001 Centers for Disease Control (CDC) report on assisted reproductive technology (ART) success reported national average live birth rates

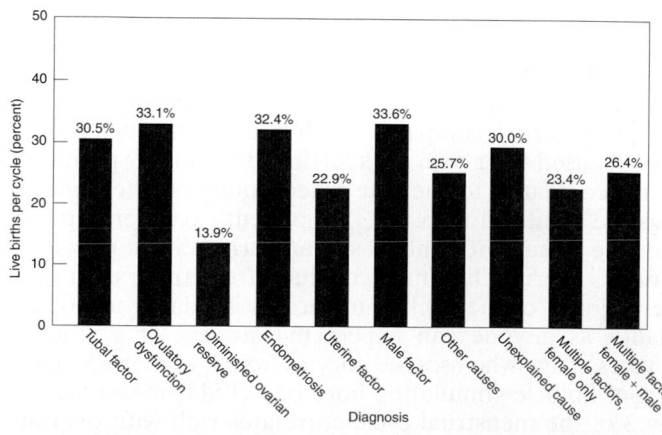

FIGURE 2. Live birth rates among women who had ART cycles using fresh nondonor eggs or embryos, by diagnosis, 2002. ART = assisted reproductive technology.

in the high 30% per cycle start for women younger than 35 years of age. Some individual centers are reporting live birth rates in the 50% range. IVF is a very effective and increasingly safer alternative to older treatments for refractory infertility.

REFERENCES

American College of Obstetrics and Gynecology: Antibiotic prophylaxis for gynecologic procedures. ACOG Practice Bulletin 2003;23.

Centers of Disease Control: 2002 Assisted reproductive technology success rates, National summary and fertility clinic reports. Atlanta, Center for Disease Control, 2002.

Gleicher N, Oleske DM, Tur-Kaspa I, et al: Reducing the risk of higher order multiple pregnancy after ovarian stimulation with gonadotropins. N Engl J Med 2000;343:2-7.

Jain T, Soules MR, Collins JA: Comparison of basal follicle-stimulating hormone versus the clomiphene citrate challenge test for ovarian reserve testing. Fertil Steril 2004;82:180-185.

Jordan J, Craig K, Clifton DK, et al: Luteal phase defect: The sensitivity and specificity of diagnostic methods in common clinical use. Fertil Steril 1995;63:427-428.

Marcoux S, Maheux R, Berube S: Laparoscopic surgery in infertile women with minimal or mild endometriosis. Canadian collaborative group on endometriosis. N Engl J Med 1997;337:217-222.

Mol BW, Swart P, Bossuyt BM, et al: Is hysterosalpingography an important tool in predicting fertility outcome? Fertil Steril 1997;67:663-669.

Schwabe MG. Shapiro SS, Haning RV Jr: Hysterosalpingography with oil contrast medium enhances fertility in patients with infertility of unknown etiology. Fertil Steril 1983;40:604-606.

Trimbos JB, Trimbos-Kemper GC, Peters AA, et al: Findings in 200 consecitive asymptomatic women, having a laparoscopic sterilization. Arch Gynecol Obstet 1990;247:121-124.

Wilcox AJ, Weinberg CR, Baird DD: Timing of sexual intercourse in relation to ovulation. Effects on the probability of conception, survival of the pregnancy, and sex of the baby. N Engl J Med 1995;333:1517-1521.

Amenorrhea

Method of
Carl A. Krantz, Jr., MD

Amenorrhea occurs in approximately 5% of all reproductive-age women and is defined as one of the following:

- No menstruation by age 14 years and the absence of secondary sexual characteristics
- No menstruation by age 16 years
- The absence of periods in a previously menstruating woman, with an interval of at least three times the length of the longest cycle or 6 months of amenorrhea

Although amenorrhea is classically described as primary (never had a menses) or secondary (cessation of menses in a once-menstruating woman), the two divisions can greatly overlap. Most importantly, the workup for amenorrhea is similar in either case and always should begin with a pregnancy test, which is by far the most common etiology.

Menstrual Cycle

A clear understanding of the normal menstrual cycle is necessary to understand the complexity of the differential diagnosis of amenorrhea. Cyclic menstruation is the result of a dynamic relationship known as the hypothalamic-pituitary-ovarian axis, which stimulates follicular development with the production of estrogen. This hormonal stimulation begins the proliferation of the endometrium, which is completed with luteinizing hormone (LH) release. Ovulation occurs and secretory endometrium is produced, which prepares the uterus for implantation or results in menstruation 14 days after ovulation if fertilization does not occur. Control of the cycle begins in the hypothalamus. Pulsatile gonadotropin-releasing hormone (GnRH) is secreted by the arcuate nucleus. This pulsatile release is critical. External environmental factors as well as neuro-hormonal factors from higher brain centers may interfere with the pulsatile release of GnRH.

The clinical manifestation of menstruation requires an intact hypothalamic-pituitary-ovarian axis as well as a functional uterus and patent outflow tract. The workup outlined here simplifies the identification of the malfunctioning compartment of the reproductive system.

Etiology of Amenorrhea

THYROID AND PROLACTIN

Thyroid abnormalities, hyperthyroidism or, more commonly, hypothyroidism, can cause menstrual irregularities or amenorrhea. High prolactin levels inhibit the pulsatile release of GnRH. Prolactin should be measured in all amenorrheic women because not all have galactorrhea as a clinical finding of hyperprolactinemia. Thyrotropin-releasing hormone stimulates both thyroid-stimulating hormone (TSH) and prolactin. In view of this relationship, those patients with an elevation in prolactin should have a TSH level drawn.

HYPOTHALAMUS

Amenorrhea associated with hypothalamic dysfunction is usually characterized by normal prolactin, low to low-normal follicle-stimulating hormone (FSH) and LH, as well as low estrogen levels. Both physical as well as psychological stress are common etiologies of hypothalamic amenorrhea. The elevation of corticotropin-releasing hormone associated with stress may inhibit GnRH pulsatility and thus cause amenorrhea. Extreme exercise may cause amenorrhea presumably because of decrease in body fat. Hormone supplementation should be considered in these patients to prevent osteoporosis and stress fractures.

Eating disorders, including bulimia and especially anorexia nervosa, are many times associated with amenorrhea. These patients are usually found to have low FSH, LH, estradiol, and 3,5,3'-triiodothyronine (T3), with normal prolactin, TSH, and cortisol.

Isolated FSH or LH deficiency is rare and probably caused by GnRH deficiency. Because of the lack of FSH and therefore estrogen production, these patients lack breast development. Hypogonadotropic hypogonadism associated with anosmia is known as Kallmann syndrome.

Pseudocyesis (false pregnancy) is a rare cause of amenorrhea and can be identified when a patient has pregnancy symptoms but a negative pregnancy test.

PITUITARY

Pituitary adenomas, usually prolactinomas, cause amenorrhea. Rarely, growth hormone and adrenalotropic hormone secreting pituitary adenomas may cause amenorrhea. If prolactin levels are elevated (more than 100 μg/mL), magnetic resonance imaging (MRI) or sella tomograms are indicated. Patients with empty sella syndrome may have elevated prolactin levels and thus menstrual disturbances. Finally, Sheehan's syndrome is panhypopituitarism, caused by postpartum hypovolemic shock.

OVARY

Polycystic ovarian (PCO) syndrome is the most common ovarian disorder causing oligorrhea or amenorrhea. Many times it is associated with hyperandrogenism and insulin resistance. Patients with chromosomal abnormalities, including Turner's syndrome (45,XO), have primary amenorrhea and sexual infantilism, but Turner mosaics (46,XX/45, XO), may develop sexually and have secondary amenorrhea. These mosaic patients rarely achieve pregnancy. Deletions in the short or long arms of the X chromosome may lead to ovarian failure. Those with pure gonadal dysgenesis have primary amenorrhea and may have a (46,XX) or (46,XY) karyotype. It is important to identify those with (46,XY) because these ovaries have a higher incidence of cancer and should be removed.

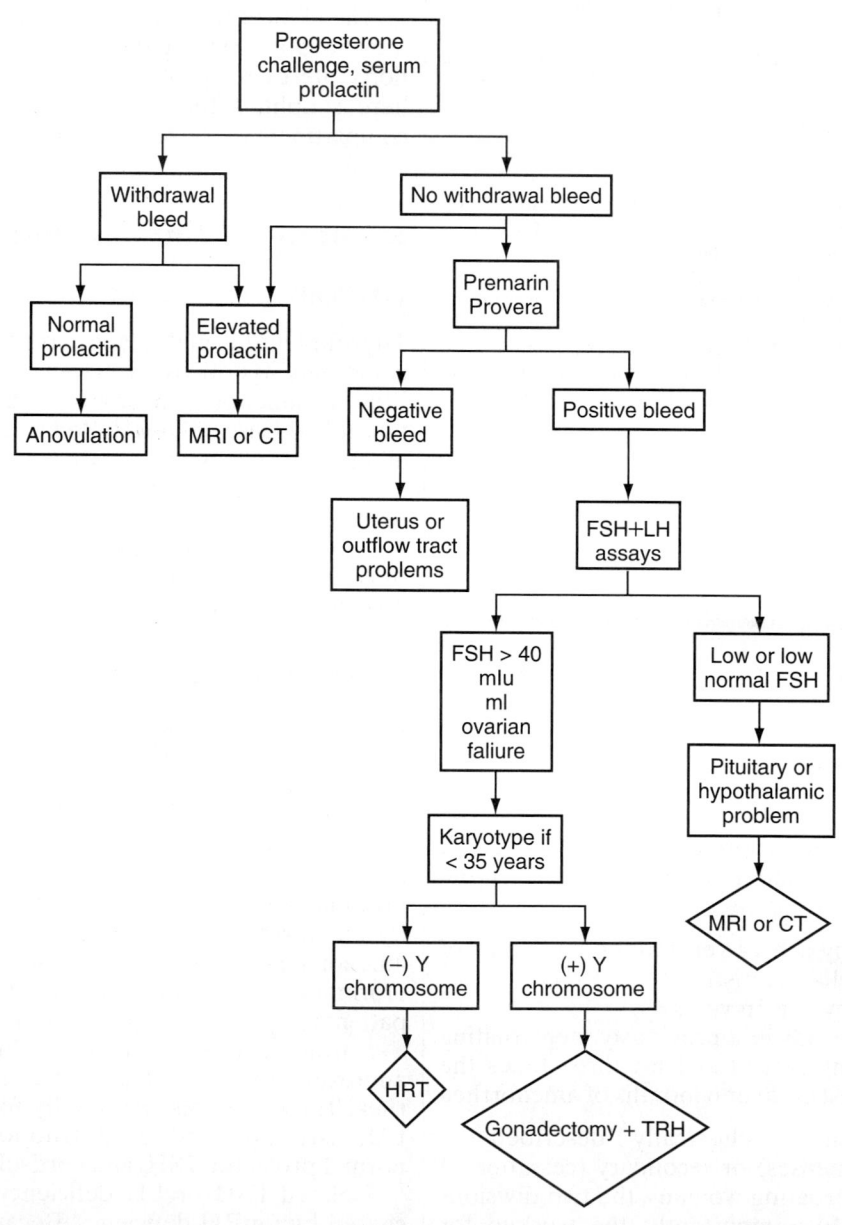

FIGURE 1. Workup for amenorrhea. CT = computed tomography; FSH = follicle-stimulating hormone; HRT = hormone replacement therapy; LH = luteinizing hormone; MRI = magnetic resonance imaging.

Because 50% of primary amenorrhea patients with elevated gonadotropin levels have chromosomal aberrations, a karyotype should be drawn. Many sources believe a woman under 35 years of age with an elevation of FSH should be included in karyotyping to rule out mosaics, although most are normal and simply have premature ovarian syndrome or resistant ovarian syndrome.

Androgen-secreting ovarian and, rarely, adrenal tumors may cause amenorrhea. These are associated with acne, temporal balding and hirsutism, and occasionally clitorimegaly. Adrenal tumors exhibit symptoms, including masculinization, rapidly, as compared to an androgen-secreting ovarian tumor that develops these symptoms over months. Patients with polycystic ovaries develop less significant changes over years. If the total testosterone level is greater than 200 µg/dL or DHEAS (sulfate salt of dehydroepiandrosterone) level is greater than 700 µg/dL, radiologic evaluation of ovaries and adrenals is indicated.

OUTFLOW TRACT

Complete agenesis of the müllerian ducts results in the absence of the uterus and cervix with a short blind vagina (Mayer-Rokitansky-Küster-Hauser syndrome). Cervical atresia, a transverse vaginal septum, and imperforate hymen present with amenorrhea and also with cyclic pain and sometimes endometriosis. These patients have normal ovarian function and therefore normal development of secondary sexual characteristics. Cervical stenosis may arise from cone, loop electrocautery excision procedure (LEEP), or cryosurgery and obstruct the outflow of menses from the uterus.

Uterine synechiae, resulting in obliteration of the endometrial cavity, may occur with dilation and curettage in conjunction with a recent pregnancy or missed abortion.

Testicular feminization (complete androgen insensitivity) presents with primary amenorrhea and a female phenotype. On exam, patients have a short blind vagina and scant pubic and axillary hair. The breasts are fibrous. These patients have normal male testosterone levels and one Barr body related to the (46,XY) karyotype. Because of a mutation in the androgen receptor, testosterone is rendered biologically inactive. The gonads should be removed after puberty to prevent gonadal tumors.

Diagnosis is made after a careful history and physical exam. Special attention to secondary sexual development is paramount because breasts develop with estrogen exposure. Hirsutism or more importantly, masculinization suggests androgen excess. The presence of galactorrhea suggests elevation of prolactin. A detailed pelvic exam identifies an imperforate hymen, transverse vaginal septum, cervical agenesis, or stenosis. Ultrasound identifies a uterus, cervix, and ovaries. After ruling out pregnancy, some simple steps that will elucidate the etiology of amenorrhea are (Figure 1):

- **Step I:** The first step involves drawing a prolactin and TSH level. If the prolactin level is more than 100 µg/mL, MRI or computed tomography of the pituitary should be ordered to rule out a pituitary adenoma. Many drugs elevate prolactin levels, so a detailed medication history is a necessity.

- **Step II:** If the prolactin is normal, a progestin, medroxyprogesterone acetate (Provera), 10 mg, should be taken for 5 to 10 days. Progesterone in oil, 200 mg intramuscularly, may be substituted. Menstrual bleeding should ensue 2 to 7 days after the completion of therapy. Menstrual flow (a positive challenge test) indicates an intact outflow tract and estrogen secretion, leaving anovulation as the etiology of the amenorrhea.
- **Step III:** A negative progesterone challenge test indicates an obstructed outflow tract or a non-estrogen-primed endometrium. Once obstruction of the outflow tract is eliminated as an etiology, conjugated estrogen (Premarin, 2.5 mg) should be given orally for 21 days, and Provera, 10 mg, should be added for the last 10 days. If menstruation does not follow, the regimen should be repeated a second time. With a second negative challenge test, the uterus is the etiology of the amenorrhea. An ultrasound with hysterosonogram or hysterosalpingogram with fluoroscopy can identify both cervical stenosis and Asherman's syndrome.
- **Step IV:** A positive response to estrogen and progesterone therapy identifies a nonestrogen-primed endometrium. FSH and LH levels should be measured. Premature ovarian failure is identified if the gonadotropins are elevated, especially the FSH. If the patient is under 35 years of age, a karyotype should be considered. These patients should have hormone replacement therapy to prevent osteoporosis and pathologic stress fractures.

If the gonadotropin levels are low to low normal, a pituitary or hypothalamic problem is identified. Hypothalamic dysfunction risk factors should be sought, including stress, weight loss, extreme exercise, or eating disorders. In the absence of these, a computed tomogram or MRI of the brain should be ordered to rule out a tumor or empty sella. Here again, hormone replacement is advisable.

REFERENCES

Berek J: Novak's Gynecology, 12th ed. Philadelphia, Williams & Wilkins, 1996, pp 809-830.
Braumuald F, Hauser K, Jameson L: Harrison's Principles of Internal Medicine, 15th ed. New York, McGraw-Hill, 2001.
Copeland L: Textbook of Gynecology. Philadelphia, WB Saunders, 1993.
Speroff L, Glass R, Kase N: Clinical Gynecologic Endocrinology and Infertility, 5th ed. Philadelphia, Williams & Wilkins, 1994.

Dysmenorrhea

Method of
Laeth S. Nasir, MBBS

Dysmenorrhea, or pain accompanying menses, is a leading cause of morbidity among women and accounts for substantial short-term disability. Prevalence rates among women of reproductive age are reported to be higher than 90%. In some women, dysmenorrhea is significant enough to impair their quality of life to the same extent as health conditions such as angina and osteoarthritis.

Prostaglandin production during menses, resulting in tetanic uterine contractions and ischemia, plays a central role in the production of symptoms. Menstrual fluid from women who suffer from dysmenorrhea contains much higher prostaglandin levels than those who do not. Evidence also suggests that increased stress and cognitive factors such as catastrophic pain are associated with greater menstrual pain intensity.

Primary dysmenorrhea is defined as pelvic pain not associated with macroscopic pelvic pathology; whereas secondary dysmenorrhea is the presence of menstrual pain coexisting with pelvic pathology.

Primary Dysmenorrhea

Primary dysmenorrhea typically presents with the onset of ovulatory cycles, which are present in 80% of adolescents by 4 to 5 years after menarche. The pain is often described as intermittent, cramping suprapubic pain, which may be severe and radiate to the back or inner thighs. Systemic symptoms such as fatigue, malaise, anxiety, dizziness, diarrhea, and nausea and vomiting are frequently present. Symptoms may persist for 48 to 72 hours.

DIAGNOSIS

In patients with primary dysmenorrhea, the history, including gynecologic review of systems, is usually unremarkable. Patients who present with a typical history and unremarkable past medical history do not generally require extensive evaluation at the initial visit. In sexually naive patients, a rectoabdominal exam may provide sufficient information if the clinician feels that an evaluation of the pelvic organs is in order. Patients with an atypical history or who may be at risk for conditions such as pelvic inflammatory disease (PID) should undergo a focused clinical examination, including a pelvic exam with

CURRENT DIAGNOSIS

- Colicky midline suprapubic pain radiates to lower back and thighs.
- Pain begins at onset of menses and lasts 12–72 h.
- May be accompanied by malaise, fatigue, diarrhea, vomiting, and other systemic symptoms.

microscopic examination of vaginal fluid. Microbiologic testing and other tests or procedures such as ultrasound or laparoscopy may be necessary if indicated by elements of the history or physical exam.

TREATMENT

The three major treatment approaches to the management of primary dysmenorrhea are nonsteroidal anti-inflammatory drugs (NSAIDs), hormonal treatment, and complementary therapies. Therapy can be initiated using any of these methods according to patient preferences or the clinical situation. In subsequent follow-up, incomplete response, side effects, or patient preference can lead to combining therapies or changing treatment modalities.

The majority of patients have tried self-care using NSAIDs before coming to the physician. Frequently, however, inappropriately low doses and irregular dose intervals of NSAID are used. The physician often supports patients' self-care efforts through reassurance and modifications of the patient's medication regimen. The goal of NSAID treatment of dysmenorrhea is aimed primarily at preempting the production of prostaglandins. The major principle of treatment is to start the medication prophylactically and use sufficient doses to maximally suppress prostaglandin production. Ideally, the NSAID should be started 24 to 48 hours prior to the onset of expected menses and continued for an additional 24 to 48 hours. Clinicians sometimes recommend an initial loading dose of NSAID, followed by regular doses for the subsequent 24 to 48 hours. In patients without special needs, it is often best to choose the least expensive, most readily available NSAID to start with (Table 1). Suboptimal response to a NSAID may necessitate a trial of a different NSAID class. Traditionally, clinicians have recommended to patients that three cycles be monitored prior to evaluation of regimen efficacy.

Patients who desire contraception and have no contraindications may be candidates for hormonal therapy of dysmenorrhea. Suppression of ovulation leads to a thinning of the endometrial lining of the uterus with subsequent reduction of fluid contents of the uterus during menses. Prostaglandin levels in menstrual fluid are also reduced. Hormonal therapy usually consists of oral

CURRENT THERAPY

- Nonsteroidal anti-inflammatory drugs
- Hormonal manipulation
- Complementary therapies

TABLE 1 Nonsteroidal Anti-inflammatory Drugs (NSAIDs) for Treatment of Dysmenorrhea

Drug	Formulation (mg)	Dosage
Propionic Acids		
Ibuprofen (Motrin, Advil)	200, 400, 600, 800	400 mg q4-6h; max 2400 mg/d
Ketoprofen (Orudis, Oruvail)	12.5, 25, 50, 75,100	25–50 mg PO q6–8h; max 300 mg/d
Naproxen (Naprosyn)	250, 375, 500	500 mg first dose, then 250 mg q6–8h prn; max 1250 mg/d
Naproxen sodium (Anaprox)	275, 550	550 mg PO first dose, then 275 mg PO q6–8h; max 1375 mg/d
Fenamates		
Mefenamic acid (Ponstel)	250	500 mg first dose, then 250 mg PO q6h prn; max 3 d
Meclofenamate	50, 100	100 mg PO tid; max 300 mg/d for 6 d
Cyclooxygenase-2 (COX-2) Selective Inhibitors		
Celecoxib (Celebrex)	100, 200, 400	400 mg PO first dose, then 200 mg PO bid; may take additional 200 mg on d 1

Abbreviations: max = maximum; PO = orally.

contraceptive pill[1] (OCP) or depot-medroxyprogesterone acetate[1] (Depo-Provera). Monophasic OCPs are believed to be more effective than triphasic formulations and hormonal patches in this regard. Women taking OCPs may elect to use the so-called long cycle method by skipping placebo pills and allowing menses to occur once every 3 months. The major disadvantage of this approach is the breakthrough bleeding that occurs in many women.

Rarely, therapies that suppress ovarian function more fully, such as the use of leuprolide acetate (Lupron[1]) or danazol (Danocrine[1]), may be considered. However, these have significant side effects and are very expensive. These should be considered once other causes of dysmenorrhea are ruled out and the cost-benefit ratio against other treatments is evaluated.

COMPLEMENTARY THERAPIES

Complementary therapies can be subdivided into pharmacologic methods, dietary modification or supplements, and physical modalities. Pharmacologic therapies that are efficacious in reducing symptoms but are infrequently used include nitroglycerin patches[1] (Nitro-Dur) and oral nifedipine[1] (Procardia).

Effective dietary or supplementation interventions are reported to include a low-fat vegetarian diet and an increased intake of omega-3 fatty acids as fish oil (one trial reported significant improvement with consumption of 2 g of fish oil daily). One study reported that 100 mg of thiamine[1] daily was highly effective in reducing dysmenorrhea, but 90 days of treatment was required before an effect was apparent. Two randomized controlled trials reported that 200 international units (IU) twice daily or 500 IU of vitamin E[1] once daily taken starting 48 hours before the onset of menses and continued for a total of 5 days were both effective in reducing symptoms.

A number of physical modalities are reported to be efficacious in the treatment of dysmenorrhea. A randomized, controlled, and blinded trial showed that acupuncture was highly effective in reducing symptoms. Acupressure and high-frequency transcutaneous electrical nerve stimulation (TENS) are also reported to reduce symptoms of cramping and pain significantly. A topically applied heating patch that maintained a temperature of approximately 38.9°C (102°F) for 12 hours a day was found to be as effective as ibuprofen (Advil) in reducing pain.

Although a Cochrane Review found insufficient evidence for benefit, invasive treatments such as nerve blocks, presacral neurectomy, uterosacral nerve ablation, and hysterectomy are rarely used in cases of severe primary dysmenorrhea resistant to conservative treatment.

Secondary Dysmenorrhea

Diagnosis of secondary dysmenorrhea may be made in patients who have significant pain with the onset of menses (when initial cycles are likely to be anovulatory), who develop increasingly severe dysmenorrhea after several years of stable menstrual symptoms, or those who fail to respond to conventional treatments such as NSAIDs or oral contraceptives. A history of atypical pelvic pain pattern such as the onset of pain several days before the onset of menses or persistence of pain after menses resolve is also suggestive of a secondary cause of dysmenorrhea. Common causes of secondary dysmenorrhea include endometriosis, pelvic inflammatory disease (PID), and anatomical abnormalities such as cervical stenosis, endometrial or endocervical polyps, or congenital obstructive müllerian anomalies.

Menstrually exacerbated nongenital causes of pelvic pain such as interstitial cystitis, irritable bowel syndrome, and psychogenic disorders seldom correspond to a history of symptoms in the menstrual cycle.

REFERENCES

ACOG Practice Bulletin Number 11. Medical Management of Endometriosis. December 1999.

Akin MD, Weingand KW, Hengehold DA, et al: Continuous low-level topical heat in the treatment of dysmenorrhea. Obstet Gynecol 2001;97:343.

Helms JM: Acupuncture for the management of primary dysmenorrhea. Obstet Gynecol 1987;69:51.

Proctor ML, Farquhar CM, Sinclair OJ, Johnson NP: Surgical interruption of pelvic nerve pathways for primary and secondary dysmenorrhea. In The Cochrane Library, Issue 3. Oxford, Update Software, 2003. Review.

[1]Not FDA approved for this indication.

Proctor ML, Roberts H, Farquhar CM: Combined oral contraceptive pill (OCP) as treatment for primary dysmenorrhoea. Cochrane Database Syst Rev 2001;(4):CD002120. Review.

Proctor ML, Smith CA, Farquhar CM, Stones RW: Transcutaneous electrical nerve stimulation and acupuncture for primary dysmenorrhea. Cochrane Database Syst Rev 2002;(1):CD002123. Review.

Smith RP: The dynamics of nonsteroidal anti-inflammatory therapy for primary dysmenorrhea. Obstet Gynecol 1987;70:785.

Sulak PJ, Cressman BE, Waldrop E, et al: Extending the duration of active oral contraceptive pills to manage hormone withdrawal symptoms. Obstet Gynecol 1997;89:179.

Wilson ML, Murphy PA: Herbal and dietary therapies for primary and secondary dysmenorrhoea. Cochrane Database Syst Rev 2001;(3):CD002124.

Ziaei S, Faghihzadeh S, Sohrabvand F, et al: A randomised placebo-controlled trial to determine the effect of vitamin E in treatment of primary dysmenorrhea. BJOG 2001;108:1181.

> **BOX 1 Symptoms of Premenstrual Syndrome**
>
> Affective
> - Irritability
> - Anxiety
> - Angry outbursts
> - Confusion
> - Social withdrawal
> - Depression
>
> Somatic
> - Bloating
> - Swelling
> - Breast tenderness
> - Headache
>
> From American College of Obstetricians and Gynecologists (ACOG) Practice Bulletin 15, 2001.

Premenstrual Syndrome

Method of
Ellen W. Freeman, PhD

The premenstrual syndromes (PMS) are characterized by mood, behavioral, and physical symptoms that occur from several days to 2 weeks before menses and remit with the menstrual flow. The term *PMS* as used by clinicians and the general public is generic, imprecise, and commonly applied to numerous symptoms. Included symptoms range from the mild and normal physiologic changes of the menstrual cycle to clinically significant symptoms that limit or impair normal functioning. In recent years, randomized controlled trials and other well-designed studies have defined diagnostic criteria for PMS and identified effective treatments for this disorder.

Based on scientific evidence at this time, serotonergic antidepressants are considered the primary treatment for clinically significant PMS, and particularly its severe form termed premenstrual dysphoric disorder (PMDD). This review focuses on PMS and its treatment with serotonergic antidepressants. It is not a comprehensive review of all treatments or associated literature. Other recent reviews may guide the reader to further information and other treatments for PMS and PMDD.

Symptoms

Numerous symptoms were traditionally attributed to PMS. This plethora is related in part to the absence of a clear diagnosis that distinguishes PMS from other co-morbid conditions. Many disorders, both physical and psychiatric, are exacerbated premenstrually or occur as a co-morbid disorder with PMS. When a careful diagnosis is made to distinguish PMS from other conditions, a much smaller group of symptoms appear to be typical of the disorder (Box 1).

Mood symptoms are usually the main complaint (irritability, anxiety, tension, mood swings, feeling out of control, depression), but behavioral symptoms (e.g., decreased interest, fatigue, poor concentration, poor sleep) and physical symptoms, most commonly breast tenderness and abdominal swelling, are also present. Several recent studies suggest that irritability is the cardinal symptom of PMS. Although depressive symptoms such as low mood, fatigue, sleep difficulties, and poor concentration are frequent complaints of women with PMS, the growing evidence indicates that PMS is not a simple variant of depression but has distinct mechanisms that differ from those of depressive disorders.

Prevalence

Surveys indicate that PMS is among the most common health problems reported by reproductive-age women. Current estimates from epidemiologic data indicate that approximately 25% of women experience severe and clinically significant premenstrual symptoms, although only 6% to 8% of menstruating women meet the stringent and predominantly dysphoric criteria for PMDD.

Morbidity

The morbidity of PMS is related to its severity, chronicity, and resulting distress that affect work, personal relationships, or daily activities. The level of impairment is significantly above community norms and similar to that of other health problems such as major depressive disorder. Studies consistently demonstrate that the greatest impairment or distress resulting from PMS is in relationships with the partner or children and in the effectiveness of work.

Etiology

The etiology of PMS remains undefined, although the monthly cycling of the reproductive hormones appears to have an essential role in the disorder. While circulating levels of the hormones are in normal range, the dominant theory is that some women have an underlying vulnerability to the normal fluctuations of one or more of these hormones. It is further believed that PMS involves central

CURRENT DIAGNOSIS

- Confirm that symptoms occur premenstrually and abate following menses.
- Confirm that symptoms are clinically significant and impair daily activities and/or cause problems for the woman.
- Obtain a medical history and conduct a physical examination to determine that other disorders are not causing the symptoms.
- Query depression, stress, substance abuse, and other diagnoses that could cause the symptoms.
- Ask the woman to maintain a daily symptom report for two or more menstrual cycles to confirm the reported symptoms and their relation to the menstrual cycle.
- Perform laboratory tests only as needed to confirm general good health or rule out other suspected conditions.

nervous system–mediated interactions of the reproductive steroids with neurotransmitters. The principal research evidence at this time supports the involvement of reproductive hormones, serotonergic dysregulation, and possibly dysregulation of GABAergic receptor functioning.

Diagnosis

A diagnosis of PMS is determined primarily by the *timing* and the *severity* of the symptoms. These factors, together with an assessment of whether other physical or psychiatric disorders may account for the symptoms, are more important for the diagnosis than the particular symptoms, which are typically nonspecific and must be assessed for their relationship to the menstrual cycle.

Box 2 lists the diagnostic criteria for PMS presented by the American College of Obstetricians and Gynecologists in 2000. These criteria indicate that PMS symptoms must be experienced during the 5 days before menses and abate during the menstrual flow. The symptoms should cause identifiable impairment or distress, be confirmed by prospective reports recorded daily by the woman for at least two menstrual cycles, and not be accounted for by other disorders.

BOX 2 Diagnosis of Premenstrual Syndrome

Presenting symptoms:
- Consistent with premenstrual syndrome
- Restricted to the luteal phase
- Cause impairment or distress
- Not an exacerbation of another disorder
- Confirmed by 2 cycles of daily symptom rating

From American College of Obstetricians and Gynecologists (ACOG) Practice Bulletin 15, 2001.

The diagnostic criteria for premenstrual dysphoric disorder (PMDD) are listed in the *Diagnostic and Statistical Manual of Mental Disorders, Fourth Edition (DSM-IV)*. Importantly, the Food and Drug Administration (FDA) has approved medications only for the indication of PMDD and not for the indication of PMS at the present time. The PMDD criteria are intended to diagnose a severe, dysphoric form of PMS and require 5 of 11 listed symptoms including at least one of the mood symptoms. Physical symptoms, regardless of the number, are considered a single symptom in meeting the diagnostic criteria. The 11 PMDD symptoms are depressed mood, anxiety or tension, mood swings, anger or irritability, decreased interest, concentration difficulties, fatigue, appetite change or food cravings, sleep disturbance, feeling overwhelmed, and physical symptoms. At least five of these symptoms must each be severe premenstrually and abate with the menstrual flow. The symptoms must markedly interfere with functioning, be confirmed by daily symptom reports for at least two menstrual cycles, and not be an exacerbation of another physical or mental disorder.

To diagnose PMS, a medical history should be obtained and a complete physical with gynecologic examination performed. PMS is understood to occur in ovulatory menstrual cycles; cycles that are irregular or outside the normal range are an indication for further gynecologic investigation. Co-morbid conditions such as dysmenorrhea, endometriosis, uterine fibroids, pelvic inflammatory disease, thyroid disorders, migraine, diabetes, mood disorders, substance abuse, and numerous other possibilities should be identified. It may be difficult to determine whether the symptoms under investigation are an exacerbation of a co-morbid condition or superimposed on another condition. In either case, the usual recommendation is to treat the ongoing condition first, then reassess and possibly add treatment for the symptoms that arise premenstrually.

No laboratory test identifies PMS and none should be routinely performed for diagnosis. Laboratory tests that indicate or confirm other possible disorders are useful if suggested by the individual woman's symptom presentation or medical findings.

The key diagnostic tool for evaluating premenstrual symptoms is the daily symptom report. The diagnostic criteria for both PMS and PMDD include a daily symptom report that is kept by the woman for at least two menstrual cycles to confirm that the woman's reported symptoms are linked to the menstrual cycle in the requisite pattern. Numerous symptom reports appropriate for this diagnosis are identified in the medical literature on PMS and PMDD. It is important that the ratings indicate the severity of each symptom (and not simply check the presence or absence of symptoms).

It is informative to use two visits for the diagnostic evaluation. Although counterintuitive, seeing the patient following menses when PMS symptoms have abated is instructive. If symptoms are absent, it provides strong evidence for the diagnosis. If symptoms are present in the follicular phase, the type and severity of the symptoms are important diagnostic information for identifying other physical or mental disorders that may be the primary focus of treatment.

CURRENT THERAPY

SSRI	Range Studied (mg)	Mean Dose (mg/d)
Escitalopram (Celexa[1])	10–30	20
Escitalopram (Lexapro[1])	10–20	15
Fluoxetine (Prozac,[1] Sarafem*)	10–60	20
Paroxetine (Paxil[1])	10–30	20
Paroxetine-CR* (Paxil-CR)	12.5, 25	NA[†]
Sertraline (Zoloft*)	50–150	75
SNRI		
Venlafaxine (Effexor[1])	37.5–200	112.5

[1]Not FDA approved for this indication
*FDA approved for the indication of premenstrual dysphoric disorder (PMDD).
[†]Not applicable because of fixed-dose study.

Treatment

SELECTIVE SEROTONIN REUPTAKE INHIBITORS

Serotonergic antidepressants are the primary treatment for severe PMS and PMDD at this time. Modulating serotonergic function is consistent with a leading theoretical view that the normal gonadal steroid fluctuations of the menstrual cycle are associated with an abnormal serotonergic response in vulnerable women. A meta-analysis of randomized controlled trials of selective serotonin reuptake inhibitors (SSRIs) in treatment of PMS and PMDD determined that these drugs were an effective first-line therapy, with both a statistically significant and clinically meaningful difference from placebo. The FDA has approved fluoxetine (Sarafem), sertraline (Zoloft), and paroxetine (Paxil) for the indication of PMDD. Other randomized, placebo-controlled, double-blind trials showed efficacy for citalopram (Celexa[1]), venlafaxine (Effexor[1]) (a selective serotonin-norepinephrine reuptake inhibitor [SNRI]), and clomipramine (Anafranil[1]) (a tricyclic antidepressant) for treatment of PMS and PMDD.

Effective doses of SSRIs are consistently at the low end of the dose range for depressive disorders in all reports of PMS and PMDD treatments. Significant response is often seen in the first menstrual cycle of treatment, with smaller increments with or without dose adjustments in the second and third treatment cycles. If there is not sufficient response in the first treated menstrual cycle, the dose should be increased in the next cycle unless precluded by side effects.

Side effects are common with the initiation of an SSRI but are usually transient and abate within 1 to 2 weeks of continued treatment. The most common side effects include headache, nausea, insomnia, fatigue or lethargy, diarrhea, decreased concentration, dizziness, and decreased libido or delayed orgasm. The sexual side effects of SSRIs have received considerable attention, although it is often difficult to determine the extent to which sexual effects are

[1]Not FDA approved for this indication.

related to the medication or to preexisting conditions. The incidence of decreased sexual interest or delayed orgasm in the few published reports of PMS patients is approximately 9% to 16%, which is notably lower than the rates reported with the use of SSRIs by depressed patients. Another important issue is the lack of any well-controlled clinical trials of SSRI treatment for PMS and PMDD in adolescents. Whether SSRIs are safe and effective for this indication in women younger than 18 years is not demonstrated.

Luteal Phase Dosing

The use of medication only in the symptomatic luteal phase of the menstrual cycle is particularly important in PMS because of the cyclic pattern of the symptoms, which occur only in the premenstrual phase and abate following menses. Efficacy of luteal phase administration of the SSRIs is demonstrated in multiple trials: three large multicenter, randomized, placebo-controlled trials that examined fluoxetine (Sarafem), paroxetine (Paxil), and sertraline (Zoloft); a trial that directly compared continuous and luteal phase administration of sertraline; and multiple preliminary studies.

Luteal phase administration of an SSRI is typically initiated 14 days prior to the expected onset of menstrual bleeding and concluded within several days of bleeding, using a taper for increased doses. As with continuous dosing, the SSRI doses are usually at the low end of the dose range.

One preliminary study compared symptom-onset dosing (mean of 6 days before menses) to luteal phase dosing and found no difference between the two dosing regimens in improvement overall, although there was suggestion that women with more severe symptoms may respond better to full luteal phase dosing.

Side effects may be less frequent with an intermittent dosing regimen because they may not occur when not taking the medication. However, some women experience recurring side effects when dosing is resumed, and discontinuation symptoms might also occur with the stop-start dosing pattern. At this time, no systematic data confirm discontinuation symptoms with the intermittent dosing regimen.

Insufficient Response to Selective Serotonin Reuptake Inhibitors

Approximately 60% of PMS and PMDD patients in controlled studies respond well to an SSRI. There are no clear predictors of response. An adequate trial of an SSRI for PMS and PMDD is at least two menstrual cycles at a dose level of demonstrated efficacy, with a third cycle when there is partial response. If a woman has an insufficient response or unacceptable side effects, it is reasonable to try another SSRI. Although the SSRIs are similar in their structure and have similar response rates and side-effect profiles, an individual patient may respond better to one SSRI versus another.

Other approaches to a poor treatment response include augmenting the SSRI with another medication to address the nonresponding symptoms, but there is no systematic information on this in PMS or PMDD treatment. Switching to another class of medication, such as anxiolytics, is suggested, but no data indicate whether nonresponders to SSRIs will respond to another class of medication. Nonresponse may also be related to other co-morbid disorders. A thorough review of the diagnosis and adjustments of the premenstrual doses of medication for both the primary disorder and PMS should be considered before pursuing other treatments.

OTHER TREATMENTS

Hormonal

In spite of the evidence for hormonal involvement in PMS and PMDD, traditional oral contraceptives (OCs) do not show efficacy for the disorder. However, preliminary data indicate that shortening or omitting the placebo week in the traditional OC pill pack may effectively treat PMS and PMDD.

Gonadotropin-releasing hormone (GnRH) agonists such as depot leuprolide[1] (Lupron) and buserelin[2] (Suprefact) are effective for PMS and PMDD but are of limited usefulness because of the risks associated with low estrogen levels that result from these treatments. Although add-back therapy using low-lose estrogen and progesterone together with the GnRH agonist did not appear to reduce efficacy in a meta-analysis, there are no definitive data on the safety and efficacy of this approach in long-term treatment. The historic use of progesterone has failed to show efficacy for the mood and behavioral symptoms of PMS in numerous controlled trials.

Anxiolytics

Alprazolam[1] (Xanax) and buspirone[1] (Buspar) showed modest efficacy for PMS in some studies but not others. Although these medications offer an alternative to antidepressants, the response rates appear much lower, and it is not known whether a PMS patient who does not respond to antidepressants will respond to an anxiolytic. The risk of dependency with alprazolam should be considered. Dosing should be strictly limited to the luteal phase, and the patient should have no history of substance abuse.

Nonpharmacologic

Calcium supplementation[1] (600 mg twice daily) reduced PMS symptoms significantly more than placebo. Calcium offers a dietary supplement approach that may be beneficial for some women with PMS, although there are no predictors of which women will respond well to this therapy. Other complementary and alternative therapies may be helpful for some women, but there is no convincing evidence of their efficacy for PMS.

Behavioral treatments that facilitate coping or reduce stress may reduce PMS symptoms. Cognitive-behavioral therapy is effective for PMS, and in one study it was as effective as the SSRI fluoxetine after 6 months of treatment.

TREATMENT DURATION

All published studies of treatment efficacy for PMS and PMDD are based on acute treatment of 2 to 3 months' duration. Several small pilot investigations suggest that PMS symptoms are likely to return within several months after medication is stopped. It also appears that PMS symptoms do not resolve spontaneously but continue for many years. These observations of PMS as a chronic condition and the swift return of symptoms following the cessation of medication suggest that treatment can be expected to be long term; notably, there are no data from long-term maintenance studies at this time.

The SSRIs are currently the first-line treatment for severe PMS and PMDD. Continuous dosing and luteal phase dosing regimens are similarly effective for these disorders when the symptoms are clearly limited to the luteal phase of the menstrual cycle. Hormonal treatments have lacked consistent scientific evidence of their efficacy or safety or both for PMS treatment. Several new oral contraceptives that decrease or omit the placebo interval may provide an effective alternative to antidepressant medications. Preliminary evidence indicates that long-term maintenance of the medication may be required for PMS and PMDD, but currently, there are no studies of the effectiveness, costs, and benefits of long-term treatment.

REFERENCES

ACOG Practice Bulletin: Premenstrual syndrome. Int J Gynecol Obstet 2001;73(2):183-190.
Dell DL: Premenstrual syndrome, premenstrual dysphoric disorder, and premenstrual exacerbation of another disorder. Clin Obstet Gynecol 2004;47(3):568-575.
Dimmock PW, Wyatt KM, Jones PW, O'Brien PM: Efficacy of selective serotonin-reuptake inhibitors in premenstrual syndrome: A systematic review. Lancet 2000;356(9236):1131-1136.
Freeman EW: Luteal phase administration of agents for the treatment of premenstrual dysphoric disorder. CNS Drugs 2004;18(7):453-468.
Girman A, Lee R, Kligler B: An integrative medicine approach to premenstrual syndrome. Am J Obstet Gynecol 2003;188(5 Suppl):S56-S65.
Grady-Weliky TA: Premenstrual dysphoric disorder. N Engl J Med 2003;348(5);433-438.
Halbreich U: The etiology, biology, and evolving pathology of premenstrual syndromes. Psychoneuroendocrinology 2003;28(Suppl 3):55-99.
Johnson SR: Premenstrual syndrome, premenstrual dysphoric disorder, and beyond: A clinical primer for practitioners. Obstet Gynecol 2004;104(4):845-859.
Stevinson C, Ernst E: Complementary/alternative therapies for premenstrual syndrome: A systematic review of randomized controlled trials. Am J Obstet Gynecol 2001;185(1):227-235.

Menopause

Method of
Jan L. Shifren, MD, and Isaac Schiff, MD

Menopause, the permanent cessation of menstruation, occurs at a mean age of 51 years. The age at menopause appears to be genetically determined and is unaffected by race, socioeconomic status, age at menarche, or number of prior ovulations. Factors that are toxic to the ovary often result in an earlier age of menopause; women who smoke experience an earlier menopause, as do many women exposed to chemotherapy or pelvic radiation. Despite a great increase in female life expectancy, the age

---

[1]Not FDA approved for this indication.
[2]Not available in the United States.

at menopause remains remarkably constant. A woman in the United States today will live approximately 30 years, or greater than a third of her life, beyond the menopause.

Options for caring for menopausal women have increased greatly since estrogen therapy (ET) was first introduced in the 1960s. With respect to hormone use, many choices of hormone type, dose, and method of administration are available. Not only have new forms of estrogens and progestins been introduced, but novel ways of combining the two hormones are available. In addition to hormones, selective estrogen receptor modulators (SERMs) and bisphosphonates are on the market. Women are requesting more information on complementary and alternative therapies, which are being studied more carefully. This chapter discusses health concerns after menopause and treatment options.

Vasomotor Symptoms

DIAGNOSIS

Vasomotor symptoms affect up to 75% of perimenopausal women. They last for 1 to 2 years after menopause in the majority of women but may continue for up to 10 years. Hot flashes are the primary reason women seek care at menopause and request hormone therapy (HT). Hot flashes not only disturb women at work and interrupt daily activities, but they also disrupt sleep. Many women complain of difficulty concentrating and emotional lability during the menopausal transition. Treatment of vasomotor symptoms should improve these cognitive and mood symptoms if they are secondary to sleep disruption and resulting daytime fatigue. The incidence of thyroid disease increases as women age, so thyroid function tests should be ordered if vasomotor symptoms are atypical or resistant to therapy.

TREATMENT

Systemic ET is the most effective treatment available for vasomotor symptoms and associated sleep disturbance. Vasomotor symptoms appear to be the result of estrogen withdrawal, rather than simply low estrogen levels. Abruptly stopping hormone treatment may result in a return of disruptive vasomotor symptoms. Thus, if cessation of HT is desired, the dose should be reduced slowly over several months. This recommendation is based on clinical experience because few controlled trials have examined the optimal way to cease HT use. When a woman chooses not to take estrogen or when it is contraindicated, progestin therapy alone is an option. Medroxyprogesterone acetate (Provera) and megestrol acetate (Megace) effectively treat vasomotor symptoms. Several drugs that alter central neurotransmitter pathways also are effective (Table 1). Clonidine (Catapres) may be used orally or as a weekly transdermal patch. Potential side effects include orthostatic hypotension and drowsiness.

Interestingly, selective serotonin reuptake inhibitors (SSRIs) and other antidepressants also are effective. Menopausal women experienced significant reductions in both hot flash frequency and severity in double-blind, randomized, placebo-controlled trials of paroxetine (Paxil CR) (12.5 and 25 mg per day), fluoxetine (Prozac)

TABLE 1 Alternative Treatments for Hot Flashes

Drug*	Suggested Dose
Venlafaxine (Effexor)	37.5–75 mg XR/d
Fluoxetine (Prozac)	20 mg/d
Paroxetine (Paxil)	10–20 mg/d or 12.5–25 mg CR/d
Clonidine (Catapres)	0.1 mg/wk patch
Gabapentin (Neurontin)	300–900 mg/d

*None of these medications is FDA approved for the treatment of hot flashes.
Abbreviations: CR = controlled release; XR = extended release.

(20 mg per day), and venlafaxine (Effexor) (75 mg per day). The improvement in vasomotor symptoms was independent of any significant change in mood symptoms. Possible side effects include fatigue, dry mouth, nausea, and decreased libido.

Many menopausal women are interested in trying nutritional and vitamin supplements for relief of hot flashes. Many of these therapies claim to relieve hot flashes, but they are rarely studied in controlled trials. Options include dietary soy and related compounds, vitamin E (800 IU per day), black cohosh, evening primrose oil, and others. Uncontrolled studies of acupuncture, exercise, and paced respiration demonstrate an improvement in vasomotor symptoms. Lifestyle interventions, including wearing light, layered clothing, avoiding hot beverages, and the liberal use of desk fans and air conditioners, should be encouraged.

Urogenital Atrophy

DIAGNOSIS

Urogenital atrophy results in vaginal dryness and pruritus, dyspareunia, dysuria, and urinary urgency. These are common complaints of menopausal women that respond well to therapy.

TREATMENT

Systemic ET is very effective for the relief of vaginal dryness, dyspareunia, and urinary symptoms. Another option

CURRENT THERAPY

Treatment options for urogenital atrophy:
- Systemic hormone therapy (if vasomotor symptoms also present)
- Vaginal estrogen cream (Estrace, Premarin): 0.5–1 g twice or 3 times weekly
- Vaginal estradiol tablet (Vagifem): 1 tablet twice weekly
- Vaginal estradiol ring (Estring): 1 ring q3mo
- Vaginal lubricants (e.g., Replens, KY Jelly): prior to intercourse as needed for dyspareunia

for women who should not or choose not to use standard ET is topical application. Low doses of estrogen cream (Estrace, Premarin) are effective when used only one to three times weekly. An estradiol vaginal tablet (Vagifem), inserted twice weekly, is available, as is an estrogen-containing vaginal ring (Estring) placed in the vagina every 3 months. Lubricants are a nonhormonal alternative for reducing discomfort with intercourse when urogenital atrophy is present.

Osteoporosis

DIAGNOSIS

Osteoporosis affects approximately 8 million women in the United States, with an additional 15 million women at risk for the disease. Because therapy is most likely to benefit those at highest risk, it is important to review a woman's risk factors for osteoporosis when making treatment decisions and to consider bone mineral density screening for high-risk women. Nonmodifiable risk factors include age, Asian or white race, family history, small body frame, early menopause, and prior oophorectomy. Modifiable risk factors include decreased intake of calcium and vitamin D, smoking, low body weight, excess alcohol use, and a sedentary lifestyle. Medical conditions associated with an increased risk of osteoporosis include hyperthyroidism, hyperparathyroidism, chronic renal disease, and diseases requiring systemic corticosteroid use.

TREATMENT

Counseling women to alter modifiable risk factors is important for both the prevention and treatment of osteoporosis. Many women have diets deficient in calcium and vitamin D and benefit from dietary changes and supplementation. Reducing the risk of osteoporosis is another of the many health benefits of smoking cessation

---

 CURRENT DIAGNOSIS

Risk Factors for Osteoporosis

Nonmodifiable:

- Age
- Race (white, Asian)
- Small body frame
- Early menopause
- Prior fracture
- Family history of osteoporosis

Modifiable:

- Inadequate intake of calcium and vitamin D
- Smoking
- Low body weight
- Excess alcohol use
- Sedentary lifestyle

Associated medical conditions:

- Hyperthyroidism
- Hyperparathyroidism
- Chronic renal disease
- Conditions requiring systemic corticosteroid use

---

and regular exercise. HT is very effective at both preventing and treating osteoporosis. The Women's Health Initiative (WHI) randomized controlled trial confirmed a significant 34% reduction in hip fractures in healthy women receiving HT after a mean follow-up of 5 years.

Bisphosphonates, including alendronate (Fosamax), risedronate (Actonel), and ibandronate (Boniva), specifically inhibit bone resorption and are very effective for both osteoporosis prevention and treatment. SERMs are compounds that act as both estrogen agonists and antagonists, depending on the tissue. Raloxifene (Evista) is a SERM approved for both the prevention and treatment of osteoporosis. Raloxifene has estrogen-like actions on bone and lipids, without stimulating the breast or endometrium. Calcitonin nasal spray (Miacalcin) and parathyroid hormone injections (Forteo) are other therapies for osteoporosis.

Cardiovascular Disease

DIAGNOSIS

Cardiovascular disease is the leading cause of death for women, accounting for approximately 45% of mortality. Nonmodifiable risk factors include age and family history. Modifiable risk factors include smoking, obesity, and a sedentary lifestyle. Medical conditions associated with an increased risk of heart disease include diabetes, hypertension, and hypercholesterolemia.

TREATMENT

Advising women to alter modifiable risk factors and adequately treating diabetes, hypertension, and hypercholesterolemia are important measures in reducing the risk of heart disease. In the past, prevention of heart disease was considered a potential benefit of HT use. Epidemiologic studies report an approximately 50% decrease in heart disease in women who use HT. Observational studies are prone to bias, however, and women who choose to use hormones are generally at lower risk for heart disease than those who do not.

However, the WHI randomized controlled trial of combination HT versus placebo showed that not only does HT not prevent heart disease in healthy women, it actually increases its risk slightly (Table 2). This trial enrolled approximately 16,000 women nationwide between 50 and 79 years of age. The average age of women in the study was 63 years. The trial's major goal was to determine whether combined estrogen and progestin HT (Prempro) prevent heart disease and fractures and whether there are associated risks. After an average of 5 years of follow-up, heart disease and stroke increased significantly in HT users by 29% and 41%, respectively. Venous thromboembolic events (VTEs) increased twofold.

Approximately 11,000 women without a uterus participated in a separate WHI study and were randomized either to estrogen alone (Premarin) or placebo. After an average follow-up of 7 years, no increased risk of heart disease was found in estrogen users. Estrogen use did have adverse vascular effects, though, increasing the risk of stroke by 39% and VTEs by 33%.

There is no role for ET in the prevention of coronary heart disease (CHD), not only in healthy women but also

TABLE 2 WHI and WHIMS Results: Risks per 10,000 Person-Years Attributable to Estrogen Plus Progestin

Excess Risk	Attributable Cases per 10,000 Person-Years
Coronary heart disease	+7
Stroke	+8
Pulmonary embolism	+8
Invasive breast cancer	+8
Dementia*	+23
Reduced Risk	
Colorectal cancer	−6
Hip fracture	−5

*Dementia was assessed in a subset of women from the WHI trial, 65 years or older. Increased risk of dementia was statistically significant when data from both estrogen plus progestin and estrogen alone trials were pooled.
Abbreviations: WHI = Women's Health Initiative; WHIMS = Women's Health Initiative Memory Study.
Adapted from Writing Group for the Women's Health Initiative Investigators: Risks and benefits of estrogen plus progestin in healthy postmenopausal women: Principal results from the Women's Health Initiative randomized, controlled trial. JAMA 2002;288:321-333; and Shumaker S, Legault C, Rapp S, et al: Estrogen plus progestin and the incidence of dementia and mild cognitive impairment in postmenopausal women. JAMA 2003;289:2651-2662.

in women with established heart disease. The Heart and Estrogen-Progestin Replacement Study (HERS), a randomized placebo-controlled trial of HT (Prempro) for secondary prevention of heart disease, also did not demonstrate any reduction in CHD events overall. The risk of cardiovascular events actually was greater in HT users during the first year of treatment.

Of note, the WHI trials and the HERS study examined only treatment with conjugated equine estrogens and medroxyprogesterone acetate. In addition, the majority of women in the trial initiated HT many years after the menopausal transition. The outcomes after initiating HT with the onset of menopausal symptoms and the effects of other oral estrogens, transdermal estradiol, cyclic HT, or therapy with other progestins may be different. Without data from randomized controlled trials, the conservative approach is to assume that the risks of various HT regimens in menopausal women are similar.

Raloxifene (Evista) has several beneficial effects on lipids, but had no significant effect on the risk of CHD in a large randomized, placebo-controlled trail in women with, or at increased risk for, heart disease.

Breast Cancer

DIAGNOSIS

Breast cancer is the most common cancer in women and the second leading cause of cancer death. The lifetime risk of developing invasive breast cancer is 12%, so any therapies that reduce or increase this risk have a major impact on women's health. Risk factors for breast cancer include age, early menarche, late menopause, family history, and prior breast disease, including epithelial atypia and cancer. Oophorectomy and a term pregnancy before 30 years of age are associated with reduced risk. Many of these risk factors are consistent with the hypothesis that prolonged estrogen exposure increases the risk of breast cancer.

Long-term use of HT is associated with an increased risk of breast cancer. Observational studies demonstrate a relative risk of approximately 1.3 with long-term HT use, generally defined as greater than 5 years. The WHI HT trial found a significant 26% increase in the risk of invasive breast cancer in women assigned to HT after approximately 5 years of use. Interestingly, the WHI trial of estrogen alone in women with prior hysterectomy demonstrated no increased risk of breast cancer after an average of 7 years of estrogen use.

The SERM tamoxifen (Nolvadex) is an estrogen antagonist in the breast, used in the treatment of estrogen receptor–positive breast cancer. Tamoxifen is also approved for the prevention of breast cancer in high-risk women, resulting in an approximately 50% reduction in the risk of disease. Raloxifene (Evista) is as effective as tamoxifen in reducing the risk of breast cancer in high-risk women, but is currently not approved for this indication. Compared to tamoxifen, raloxifene is associated with a lower risk of thromboembolic events and cataracts.

Risks are associated with SERM use. Tamoxifen and raloxifene increase the risk of VTEs approximately threefold, similar to the increased risk seen in HT users. Hot flashes are increased with raloxifene and tamoxifen use, and raloxifene is associated with leg cramps. Tamoxifen acts as an estrogen agonist in the endometrium, increasing the risk of endometrial polyps, hyperplasia, and cancer, whereas no endometrial stimulation is seen with raloxifene.

TREATMENT

Screening mammography annually for women older than 50 years is demonstrated to reduce breast cancer mortality in several large studies. Women at increased risk for breast cancer are advised not to use HT or to use it only short term. Women at high risk also may elect tamoxifen therapy.

Endometrial Cancer

The use of unopposed estrogen is associated with an increased risk of endometrial hyperplasia and cancer. Combination estrogen-progestin therapy, therefore, is recommended for all women with a uterus. Treatment may be provided in a sequential manner, with estrogen daily and progestin for 12 to 14 days of each month or in a continuous-combined fashion with estrogen and a lower dose of progestin daily. Sequential regimens result in regular, predictable vaginal bleeding. The benefit of continuous-combined regimens is that approximately 60% to 70% of women experience amenorrhea by the end of the first year of therapy; the problem is that the bleeding that does occur is irregular and unpredictable. Several combination therapies may have a lower incidence of bleeding, including norethindrone acetate (NETA), with either ethinyl estradiol (Femhrt) or estradiol (Activella), or low-dose conjugated equine estrogens and MPA (medroxyprogesterone acetate) (Prempro 0.45/1.5 or 0.3/1.5).

Alzheimer's Disease

Alzheimer's disease is the most common form of dementia. Women are at greater risk for developing the disease than men, and the number of affected Americans is expected to double to more than 8 million by 2010. Several small trials and observational studies, often of women who initiated HT early with the onset of menopausal symptoms, suggest HT use may decrease the risk of Alzheimer's disease. A randomized controlled study in women with mild to moderate Alzheimer's disease, however, demonstrated that 1 year of estrogen treatment did not slow disease progression or improve cognition. The effect of HT on cognitive function in women without dementia was studied in the WHI Memory Study (WHIMS), a randomized, double-blind, placebo-controlled trial of women 65 years or older enrolled in the WHI trial. In contrast to the findings of observational studies, women randomized to HT in WHIMS experienced a significant twofold increased risk of dementia.

Contraindications to Hormone Therapy Use

Contraindications to HT use include known or suspected breast or endometrial cancer, undiagnosed abnormal genital bleeding, active thromboembolic disorders, and active liver or gallbladder disease. Relative contraindications include heart disease, migraine headaches, a history of liver or gallbladder disease, previous breast or endometrial cancer, or prior thromboembolic events.

In conclusion, many options are available to address the quality of life and health concerns of menopausal women. The primary indication for HT currently is the alleviation of hot flashes and associated symptoms. Given the risks of HT, women should be advised to use the lowest dose for the shortest time that meets treatment goals. Women need to be informed of the potential benefits and risks of all therapeutic options, and care should be individualized based on a woman's needs and preferences.

REFERENCES

American College of Obstetricians and Gynecologists Task Force: Hormone therapy. Obstet Gynecol 2004;104(Suppl 4):S1-S129.

Cummings S, Black D, Thompson D, et al: Effect of alendronate on risk of fracture in women with low bone density but without vertebral fractures. JAMA 1998;280:2077-2082, 2119.

Cummings S, Eckert S, Krueger K, et al: The effect of raloxifene on risk of breast cancer in postmenopausal women: Results from the MORE randomized trial. JAMA 1999;281:2189-2197.

Fisher B, Costantino JP, Wickerham DL, et al: Tamoxifen for prevention of breast cancer: Report of the national surgical adjuvant breast and bowel project P-1 study. J Natl Cancer Inst 1998;90:1371-1388.

Laumann E, Paik A, Rosen R: Sexual dysfunction in the United States: Prevalence and predictors. JAMA 1999;281:537-544.

Shifren J, Braunstein G, Simon J, et al: Transdermal testosterone treatment in women with impaired sexual function after oophorectomy. N Engl J Med 2000;343:682-688.

Shumaker S, Legault C, Kuller L, et al: Conjugated equine estrogens and incidence of probable dementia and mild cognitive impairment in postmenopausal women: Women's Health Initiative Memory Study. JAMA 2004;291:2947-2958.

Stearns V, Beebe K, Iyengar M, Dube E: Paroxetine controlled release in the treatment of menopausal hot flashes. JAMA 2003;289:2827-2834.

Women's Health Initiative Steering Committee: Effects of conjugated equine estrogen in postmenopausal women with hysterectomy. JAMA 2004;291:1701-1712.

Writing Group for the Women's Health Initiative Investigators: Risks and benefits of estrogen plus progestin in healthy postmenopausal women: Principal results from the Women's Health Initiative randomized controlled trial. JAMA 2002;288:321-333.

Vulvovaginitis

Method of
David A. Baker, MD

Vulvovaginitis brings large numbers of women to see their health care provider. Over the last several decades with the availability of numerous over-the-counter preparations, most patients medicate themselves to treat their symptoms. However, it is clear that the majority of patients make the wrong diagnosis. They use the wrong medications and delay bringing their symptoms and complaints to the attention of the clinician; as a result, many women will experience complications from their vaginal infection. Therefore, the clinician needs to take this condition (vulvovaginitis) seriously and view the patient as one with a significant medical, physiologic, and social problem that may lead not only to significant medical conditions and complications but also to significant interpersonal problems.

An accurate diagnosis is required to provide proper and correct treatment of this condition. Symptoms presented to the health care provider by phone can be very nonspecific and may lead to an improper diagnosis and treatment. The three major categories of vaginitis in the United States (Figure 1) are those caused predominantly by candidiasis, trichomoniasis, and bacterial vaginosis (BV). Of these three abnormal symptomatic manifestations, BV is the most common in the United States. Many patients mistake BV for *Candida* infections and take over-the-counter antifungal preparations, which are costly and ineffective. Patients do not appreciate the significance of this most common condition: BV may lead to important medical complications not only during pregnancy but also when the patient is not pregnant. Of the three conditions, the only one that is considered a sexually transmitted disease (STD) is trichomoniasis. BV is associated with other STDs.

The goal of therapy is to not only treat or control the organism that is abnormally colonizing or growing in the vagina but also return the vagina to normal vaginal colonization. This objective may be difficult, and one of the major problems of recurrent vaginal infection is our inability to colonize the lower genital tract with healthy bacteria. The normal vagina has an acidic pH that is produced

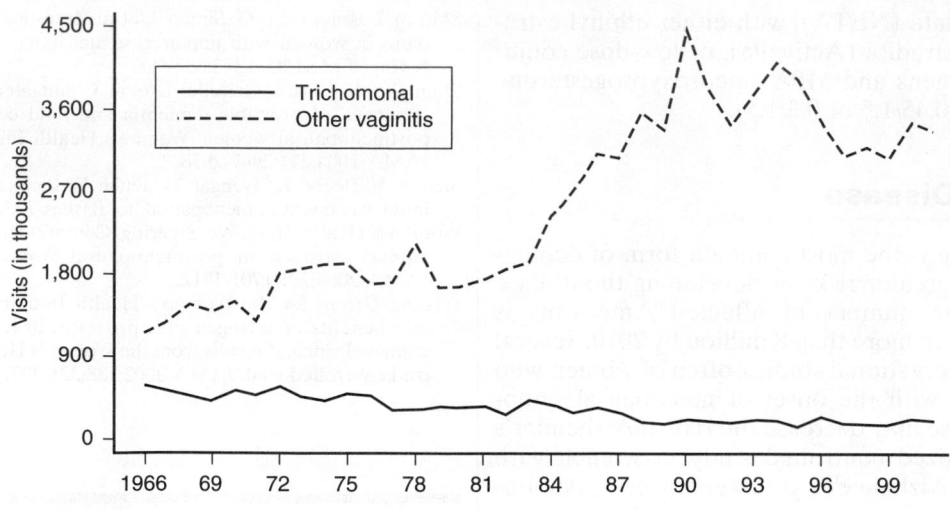

FIGURE 1. Major categories of vaginitis are candidiasis, trichomoniasis, and bacterial vaginosis.

by a combination of normal host flora and the genus *Lactobacillus*, which produces lactic acid. The importance of *Lactobacillus* strains that produce not only lactic acid but also hydrogen peroxide cannot be overemphasized; they maintain the lower genital tract flora and act as a protective barrier to the acquisition of certain STDs, including HIV. It is therefore the goal of the treating clinician to eradicate the patient's symptoms, control the abnormal vaginal colonization, and try to propagate normal lower genital tract flora. Women with normal lower genital tract flora containing lactobacilli producing lactic acid and hydrogen peroxide were less likely to contract chlamydiosis, trichomoniasis, and symptomatic candidiasis. In addition, the prevalence of gonorrhea, chlamydiosis, and trichomoniasis was significantly lower in women who had normal vaginal *Lactobacillus* flora during pregnancy.

Bacterial Vaginosis

The term given to abnormal colonization of the lower genital tract with anaerobic bacteria is bacterial vaginosis. However, a more meaningful definition of BV may be one that includes an inflammatory component of this anaerobic bacterial overgrowth. Currently, approximately 50% of women in the United States who visit a clinician for treatment of vaginitis have BV. It is a polymicrobial infection involving an increase in anaerobic bacteria, loss of the normal *Lactobacillus* flora, and consequently, an imbalance in the vaginal ecosystem. The absence or a decreased number of lactobacilli facilitates the overgrowth of pathogenic organism, which are predominantly anaerobic bacteria.

The exact factors that trigger the overgrowth of anaerobic bacteria are still not fully understood. Douching can lead to a disturbance in the delicate balance of lower genital tract organisms. Other risk factors for BV include trichomoniasis, other STDs, early sexual experience, multiple sexual partners, and the use of an intrauterine contraceptive device.

DIAGNOSIS

Proper diagnosis is important for the treatment and eradication of BV. The diagnosis can be made during vaginal examination and does not require expensive and elaborate techniques. The current 2002 Centers for Disease Control and Prevention (CDC) STD treatment guidelines require three of the following symptoms or signs for diagnosis: a homogeneous, white, noninflammatory discharge that coats the vaginal walls smoothly; the presence of clue cells on microscopic examination; a pH of vaginal secretions of less than 4.5; and a fishy odor of the vaginal discharge before or after the addition of 10% KOH (the whiff test). Gram stain is an acceptable laboratory method for diagnosing BV. However, culture is not recommended as a diagnostic tool. In addition, cervical Papanicolaou (Pap) tests have limited clinical utility for the diagnosis of BV because of low sensitivity. Other commercially available tests add to the cost and rarely aid the clinician in diagnosing this vaginal infection.

TREATMENT

The goal of therapy is to not only control this anaerobic infection but also relieve vaginal symptoms, lessen the risk of infectious complications after procedures, and reduce the risk of development of other infectious complications, HIV, and other STDs. All women who have symptomatic disease require treatment. Because of the increased risk of postoperative infectious complications associated with BV, it is suggested that before surgical procedures are performed on women, they be screened and treated for BV, in addition to undergoing other routine prophylactic measures.

BV during pregnancy has been associated with adverse pregnancy outcomes, including preterm labor, premature rupture of membranes, and postpartum infections. Therapy during pregnancy has the potential of reducing these potential risks, as well as reducing the risk of acquiring STDs and HIV during pregnancy. The CDC has given recommendations for the treatment of nonpregnant and

TABLE 1 Bacterial Vaginosis: Treatment Regimens

Recommended Regimens, Nonpregnant
Metronidazole (Flagyl), 500 mg orally twice a day for 7 d
or
Metronidazole (Metro-Gel), 0.75% gel, 1 full applicator (5 g) intravaginally once a day for 5 d
or
Clindamycin (Cleocin), 2% cream, 1 full applicator (5 g) intravaginally at bedtime for 7 d

Alternative Regimens, Nonpregnant
Metronidazole, 2 g orally in a single dose
or
Clindamycin, 300 mg orally twice a day for 7 d
or
Clindamycin ovules, 100 g intravaginally once at bedtime for 3 d

Recommended Regimens, Pregnant
Metronidazole, 250 mg orally three times a day for 7 d
or
Clindamycin, 300 mg orally twice a day for 7 d

Note: Patients should be advised to avoid consuming alcohol during treatment with metronidazole and for 24 hours thereafter. Clindamycin cream and ovules are oil based and might weaken latex condoms and diaphragms: Refer to condom product labeling for additional information.
From Centers for Disease Control and Prevention: Sexually transmitted diseases treatment guidelines 2002. MMWR Morb Mortal Wkly Rep 2002;51:42-48.

pregnant women with BV (Table 1). Patients need to be informed that clindamycin (Cleocin) cream and ovules are oil-based preparations that may interfere with the efficiency of latex condoms and diaphragms. In addition, oral and topical metronidazole (Flagyl) regimens are equally efficacious. Studies of vaginal clindamycin cream appear to demonstrate that it is less efficacious than metronidazole regimens. Short-course therapy for BV in the form of metronidazole, 2 g orally in a single dose, has been proposed. The clinician must recognize that metronidazole, 2 g in a single dose, is an alternative regimen because of its lower efficacy in the treatment of BV. Unfortunately, at the current time, no preparation, either intravaginal or oral, is able to induce reversion to the normal lower genital tract vaginal flora.

BV is not considered an STD, and therefore routine treatment of sex partners is not currently recommended. When using clindamycin and metronidazole, one must differentiate between side effects and allergic reactions. Metronidazole gel (MetroGel) may be appropriate for patients who have side effects with oral metronidazole, but it should not be used in a patient allergic to metronidazole.

Oral regimens are recommended (see Table 1) for pregnant women. Topical clindamycin (Cleocin vaginal cream) is contraindicated in pregnancy because of the potential overgrowth of gram-negative aerobic bacteria (Escherichia coli) in the vagina. Patients who have BV should be offered testing for HIV and other STDs. Patients with HIV should be screened and treated for BV with the same regimens as those who are HIV negative.

Trichomoniasis

The incidence of trichomoniasis has slowly declined in the United States since the mid 1960s and has remained at a low level over the past decade. Trichomoniasis is caused by the protozoan Trichomonas vaginalis. Women who are infected usually have a vaginal discharge and specific symptoms, in contrast to men, who are generally asymptomatic. T. vaginalis is a pear-shaped flagellated protozoon that is usually identified in wet mounts by a rapid swaying motion and the presence of polymorphonuclear leukocytes. Growth is typically enhanced by anaerobic conditions and an elevated pH. The incubation period ranges from 4 to 28 days. The clinician needs to recognize that infection with this organism occurs not only in the vagina but also in the urethra, Skene's glands, and the bladder. In men, the urethra is the most common site. However, the prostate and epididymis may also be infected, and the organism may be detected in semen and urine. Trichomoniasis is an STD transmitted through sexual contact, with infection documented in 85% of female partners of infected men. Risk factors for trichomoniasis are the presence of other STDS, an increased number of sexual partners, the presence of BV, smoking, and a vaginal pH over 4.5.

DIAGNOSIS

The patient usually has a discharge, odor, and vulvar itching with or without dysuria. The discharge is yellow-green with a frothy appearance. Further evaluation of the patient reveals that the pH of the vagina is over 4.5, the amine test may be positive, and on wet preparations, the organism and an increase in the white blood cell count (greater than 10 per high-power field) are usually found. Wet preparations and Pap smears have an approximately 50% to 60% sensitivity and greater than 90% specificity. Other techniques are in development that should better enable the clinician to diagnose this infection. Trichomoniasis in pregnant women has been associated with adverse pregnancy outcomes, specifically, preterm rupture of membranes, preterm labor, and preterm delivery. In addition, studies have shown that the presence of trichomoniasis is associated with an increased risk of acquiring HIV, so patients in whom trichomoniasis has been diagnosed should be screened for other STDs, and HIV testing should be encouraged.

TREATMENT

Current CDC treatment guidelines are presented in Table 2. The metronidazole regimen recommended has resulted in cure rates of approximately 90% to 95%. Because trichomoniasis is an STD, treatment of sexual partners is mandatory. Metronidazole gel has an efficacy of approximately 50% for the treatment of trichomoniasis. Because the organism may be found in locations other than the vagina, such treatment is less efficacious and not recommended. Women who fail oral therapy may repeat a 7-day course of therapy with topical metronidazole. Because metronidazole is currently the only approved therapy in the United States, patients with allergic reactions to metronidazole may be managed by desensitization.

TABLE 2   Trichomoniasis: Treatment Regimens

Recommended Regimen
Metronidazole (Flagyl), 2 g orally in a single dose

Alternative Regimen
Metronidazole, 500 mg twice a day for 7 d

From Centers for Disease Control and Prevention: Sexually transmitted diseases treatment guidelines 2002. MMWR Morb Mortal Wkly Rep 2002;51:42-48.

Tinidazole has been recently approved for the treatment of vaginal trichomoniasis. This newer medication may be of assistance in patients with the emerging problem of metronidazole-resistant trichomoniasis.

Candidiasis

Most patients think that their symptoms are associated with a yeast infection, but in reality, studies show that 75% of patients with chronic candidiasis have another etiologic agent responsible for their problems. However, candidiasis is still one of the most common vaginal infections and is usually treated initially with over-the-counter or alternative regimens. Patients who cannot control the infection or experience recurrent symptoms generally seek medical assistance. The CDC has classified vulvovaginal candidiasis (VVC) as uncomplicated VVC or complicated VVC (Table 3). This classification is based on clinical findings, microbiology, host factors, and response to therapy. Approximately 10% to 20% of women will have complicated VVC.

DIAGNOSIS AND TREATMENT

Pruritus and an inflammatory reaction suggest the diagnosis of candidal vaginitis. A white, cheesy discharge is usually what drives the patient to buy an over-the-counter antifungal preparation. The clinician needs to use additional modalities for diagnosis, including a wet preparation with 10% KOH, Gram stain or culture, and determination of vaginal pH (less than 4.5). Because a significant number of women are colonized with *Candida*, culture in the absence of symptoms is not clinically relevant. Most patients with uncomplicated VVC have no precipitating factor; however, VVC commonly develops after antibiotic use. The CDC has recommended numerous regimens (Table 4) for the treatment of uncomplicated VVC, including 14 topical regimens and 1 single-dose oral regimen. VVC is not acquired

TABLE 3   Classification of Vulvovaginal Candidiasis (VVC)

Uncomplicated	Complicated
Sporadic or infrequent VVC	Recurrent VVC
or	or
Mild-to-moderate VVC	Severe VVC
or	or
Likely to be *Candida albicans*	Non-*albicans* candidiasis
or	or
Nonimmunocompromised women	Women with uncontrolled diabetes, debilitation, or immunosuppression or those who are pregnant

From Centers for Disease Control and Prevention: Sexually transmitted diseases treatment guidelines 2002. MMWR Morb Mortal Wkly Rep 2002;51:42-48.

TABLE 4   Vulvovaginal Candidiasis: Recommended Treatment Regimens

Intravaginal Agents
Butoconazole (Mycelex), 2% cream, 5 g intravaginally for 3 d*
or
Butoconazole 2% cream, 5 g (butoconazole—sustained release), single intravaginal application
or
Clotrimazole (Gyne-Lotrimin), 1% cream, 5 g intravaginally for 7-14 d*
or
Clotrimazole, 100-mg vaginal tablet for 7 d
or
Clotrimazole, 100-mg vaginal tablet, 2 tablets for 3 d
or
Clotrimazole, 500-mg vaginal tablet, 1 tablet in a single application
or
Miconazole (Monistat), 2% cream, 5 g intravaginally for 7 d*
or
Miconazole, 100-mg vaginal suppository, 1 suppository for 7 d*
or
Miconazole, 200-mg vaginal suppository, 1 suppository for 3 d*
or
Nystatin, 100,000-U vaginal tablet, 1 tablet for 14 d or
Tioconazole (Vagistat), 6.5% ointment, 5 g intravaginally in a single application*
or
Terconazole (Terazol), 0.4% cream, 5 g intravaginally for 7 d
or
Terconazole, 0.8% cream, 5 g intravaginally for 3 d
or
Terconazole, 80-mg vaginal suppository, 1 suppository for 3 d

Oral Agent
Fluconazole (Diflucan), 150-mg oral tablet, 1 tablet in a single dose

Note: The creams and suppositories in these regimens are oil based and may weaken latex condoms and diaphragms. Refer to condom product labeling for further information.
*Preparations for intravaginal administration of butoconazole, clotrimazole, miconazole, and tioconazole are available over the counter (OTC). Self-medication with OTC preparations should be advised only for women in whom VVC has previously been diagnosed and who have a recurrence of the same symptoms. Any woman whose symptoms persist after using an OTC preparation or who has a recurrence of symptoms within 2 months should seek medical care. Unnecessary or inappropriate use of OTC preparations is common and can lead to a delay in treatment of other etiologies of vulvovaginitis that could result in adverse clinical outcomes.
From Centers for Disease Control and Prevention: Sexually transmitted disease treatment guidelines 2002. MMWR Morb Mortal Wkly Rep 2002;51:42-48.

through sexual activity, and therefore treatment of the partner is not usually recommended.

Complicated VVC is usually defined as four or more episodes of symptomatic VVC each year and should occur in only a small percentage of women. Most patients with recurrent VVC have no apparent predisposing or underlying conditions. Culture may be important in determining the appropriate treatment and management of these patients. Non-*albicans* species of *Candida* are found in only 10% to 20% of patients with recurrent VVC. Different therapeutic regimens for a longer duration may be of benefit in treating recurrent VVC. The use of antifungals for maintenance therapy or in specific daily or weekly recommended regimens can be considered for up to 6 months. However, side effects and the toxicity of oral medications need to be taken into account. Once maintenance therapy is discontinued, VVC will recur in upward of 40% of women.

Nonfluconazole azole drugs are recommended as first-line therapy for non-*albicans* VVC. In this specific clinical situation, 600 mg of boric acid* by capsule intravaginally once daily for 2 weeks may be beneficial.

Specific investigation to evaluate for pregnancy, HIV infection, and systemic immunocompromising conditions such as diabetes is important in managing vulvovaginitis.

REFERENCES

Sobel JD, Nyirjesy P, Brown W: Tinidazole therapy for metronidazole-resistant vaginal trichomoniasis. Clin Infect Dis 33(8):1341-1346, 2001.

---

*Not available in the United States. May be compounded by pharmacists.

Chlamydia trachomatis

Method of
Catherine Stevens-Simon, MD

The Scope of the Problem

Responsible for more than 3 million infections each year in the United States, *Chlamydia trachomatis* poses a public health problem of epidemic proportions. Because of the large reservoir of undiagnosed, asymptomatic infections, the number of reported cases significantly underestimates the true prevalence of this infection. Nonetheless, *C. trachomatis* is not only the most commonly reported bacterial sexually transmitted disease (STD) in the United States but also the nation's most commonly reported bacterial infection. It is difficult to give meaningful prevalence figures because the proportion of infected individuals depends on the characteristics of the population studied and how they are studied. In addition, whereas passive surveillance systems indicate that the prevalence of this infection has risen precipitously over the last decade, studies conducted at sentinel surveillance sites demonstrate a decline, which suggests that expanded screening, increased reporting, and improved test sensitivity mask a true decrease in prevalence in some sectors of American society. The epidemiologic characteristics and clinical manifestations of chlamydial infections in the United States reflect the fact that most infections are sexually transmitted and that prevalent stereotypes have an affinity for columnar epithelium. Teenage girls are most susceptible to these infections because of the following factors:

- At their age, the columnar epithelium is prominent on the ectocervix.
- Some experience a high level of unprotected, serially monogamous sexual activity with older men whose sexual risk profiles they rarely investigate.

With these two factors combined, teenage girls are at maximal biologic and social risk. Although the national prevalence of chlamydial infections in this population is unknown, school- and clinic-based studies suggest a range of 8% to 26% (compared to 3% to 5% in sociodemographically similar young adult women), with the highest age-specific prevalence reported among adolescents ages 14 to 15 years. Although readily eradicable, the economic and human costs of these infections are staggering. Annual expenditures are estimated to exceed $1.5 billion, with 75% of the cost devoted to treating sequelae of cervical infections that were initially uncomplicated. Because the majority of severe consequences of untreated infections occur in women, and as much as 66.6% of tubal factor infertility and 33.3% of ectopic pregnancies in the United States are attributed to chlamydial infections, it is estimated that every dollar spent on screening and treating asymptomatic young women and their sex partners saves approximately $12. Although this uniquely positions primary health care providers to prevent the costly sequelae of chlamydial infections, given their prevalence among teenagers, expansion of screening and treatment programs to nontraditional settings such as schools, juvenile detention centers, and drug treatment facilities is likely to be a critical component of any national strategy to ontrol this infection.

Clinical Presentation

Chlamydial infections are an excellent example of the dependence of the clinical manifestations of disease on the intrinsic properties of the pathogen and host. In Western industrialized countries, virtually all chlamydial infections are either sexually transmitted or vertically transmitted at birth. They are caused by nonlymphogranuloma venereum stereotypes that have an affinity for columnar epithelium and can only survive by a cytotoxic, replicative cycle that evokes a variable immune response in the host. Hence, in the United States, the endocervix, urethra, rectum, and conjunctiva are preferentially affected, and clinical manifestations range from asymptomatic to florid inflammatory conditions with severe reproductive consequences. *Chlamydia* should be suspected in these populations:

- Women and men with dysuria and pyuria
- Women with dyspareunia; abnormal vaginal discharge; postcoital, irregular menstrual, or breakthrough contraceptive bleeding; and lower abdominal or pelvic pain
- Infants with conjunctivitis or a staccato cough

These signs and symptoms are neither a sensitive nor a specific indication of infection, however. Indeed, because nearly 90% of chlamydial infections are asymptomatic and *C. trachomatis* is isolated from less than 33.3% of women with mucopurulent cervicitis and less than 50% of men with nongonococcal urethritis, such complaints are unreliable predictors of infection. In women, the most common sign is mucopurulent cervicitis, a nonspecific clinical syndrome characterized by erythema, edema, and friability of the ectocervix and purulent endocervical exudate. Mucopurulent cervicitis, however, is also caused by other STDs and noninfectious factors (i.e., cyclical fluctuations in gonadal hormones), which increase the size of the cervical ectropion or the resident population of cervical leukocytes. Other clinical manifestations of lower genital tract chlamydial infections in women include urethritis and bartholinitis. Although pelvic inflammatory disease (PID) is a polymicrobial infection, *C. trachomatis* is also often involved, and, conversely, PID is the most common complication of chlamydial cervicitis. The estimated incidence ranges from 10% to 40% in untreated women. Young age and prolonged or recurrent infection significantly increase, whereas treatment of asymptomatic infections significantly decreases both disease severity and sequelae, such as salpingo-oophoritis, perihepatitis (Fitz-Hugh-Curtis syndrome), infertility, ectopic pregnancy, and chronic pelvic pain. Adverse outcomes associated with chlamydial infections during pregnancy include preterm labor, premature rupture of the placental membranes, low-birth-weight delivery, neonatal death, postpartum or postabortal endometritis, and vertical transmission to infants. In the infected infants, 30% to 50% develop conjunctivitis, 15% to 20% develop nasopharyngitis, and 5% to 10% develop pneumonia.

In men, the most common clinical manifestation is urethritis, the symptoms of which typically commence 1 to 3 weeks after exposure and range from mild dysuria to frank penile discharge. Other clinical syndromes in men include epididymitis, prostatitis, acute proctocolitis, and Reiter syndrome (urethritis, conjunctivitis, arthritis, and mucocutaneous lesions). These suppurative complications rarely require inpatient therapy and are far less common than those encountered in women. Nonetheless, sequelae ranging from urethral strictures to infertility do occur. Nongenital clinical manifestations, such as conjunctivitis, tenosynovitis, and arthritis, are uncommon among adults in the United States.

Diagnosis and Screening

In the United States, testing for both symptomatic and asymptomatic chlamydial infections is done with ligase chain reaction (LCR), polymerase chain reaction (PCR), and other nucleic acid amplification techniques (NAATs) because they do not require the presence of intact organisms. Urine, cervical, vaginal, or urethral fluids can be used as the analyte for these tests; specimens are stable and easy to transport; and results can be obtained within a day. This is a major advantage over the stringent collection, transport, and 3-day growth period culturing requirements associated with this fastidious organism. Although nonculture assays, non-NAATs, and rapid diagnostic tests capable of making a diagnosis within 30 minutes

are available, these assays are too insensitive to be recommended for routine testing.

The signs and symptoms of chlamydial infection are nonspecific and often persist for weeks after documented eradication of the pathogen. Because of this, leukocyte, esterase-positive urine dipsticks, leukocyte-laden vaginal wet mounts, and endocervical Gram stains should be regarded as no more than a trigger for testing. Although concerns about the consequences of underdiagnosis and undertreatment typically overshadow concerns about the consequences of overdiagnosis and overtreatment, therapeutic decisions should not be based on these poorly standardized tests. Indeed, given their low positive predictive value for chlamydial infections, the adverse psychological effects of being diagnosed with an STD, and the serious public health problems that the indiscriminate use of antibiotics creates—even in settings where the prevalence of chlamydial infections is high and patient follow-up is uncertain and in resource-poor clinics where NAATs are unavailable—enthusiasm for the practice of diagnosing chlamydial infections empirically. This must be tempered by the knowledge that to prevent one individual from suffering the sequelae of an untreated infection, hundreds will needlessly suffer the adverse psychosocial consequences of an STD diagnosis. This is true even when the diagnosis is made based on characteristic symptom complexes, suggestive leukocyte esterase urine dipsticks, and/or vaginal wet mounts. Thus, with sensitivities and specificities fluctuating approximately 98% on male urethral and urine specimens as well as on female cervical specimens, NAATs are currently the best chlamydial tests available. However, because the sensitivity of these assays for detecting infections in women is significantly lower when urine (80% to 95%) or patient- or provider-collected vaginal fluid (70% to 85%) is the analyte, endocervical specimens should be used, except in screening situations where it is impractical to perform pelvic examinations. Thus every case diagnosed on a urine or vaginal specimen is a bonus.

Despite consensus about how to screen, uncertainty continues about whom to screen and how frequently to screen them. Pregnant women and sexually active women younger than 25 years of age are the only groups for whom there is good evidence that the benefits of screening outweigh the harms. Specifically, when prevalence rates exceed 2%, testing and treating these individuals for asymptomatic chlamydial infections is a cost-effective preventive measure that:

- Averts PID and associated medical complications.
- Reduces transmission to sex partners.
- Reduces the risk of acquiring HIV.
- Lowers the prevalence of *Chlamydia* in the community.

It is unlikely that these benefits reflect factors other than screening (i.e., increased condom use) because knowledge of sexual risk behavior adds nothing to predictive algorithms that include age and prior STD history. However, because of the highly infectious nature of this bacterium, the lack of a vaccine, and the failure of the human immune system to build up resistance to the bacteria, reinfection of effectively treated individuals tends to diminish short-term efficacy, making long-term periodic screening a prerequisite of cost efficacy.

The only other caveat is that most cost-effectiveness analyses are based on culture-proven disease and therefore may reflect a larger inoculum than infections diagnosed by NAAT assays, which can detect extremely low levels of viable and nonviable organisms. Thus further research is needed to determine if and how inoculum size affects disease presentation and to define the clinical and public health significance of NAAT-detectable infections. Specifically, studies comparing transmission rates and the clinical consequences of infections that are detected only by NAAT assay versus those that are detected by traditional assays are still needed to prove that routine, periodic, urine-based screening of asymptomatic individuals is a cost-effective way to control chlamydial infections at the population level. Moreover, because identifying infected individuals is only the first step in effective disease control, it is also important to demonstrate that once identified, the majority of these asymptomatically infected individuals and their sex partners can be contacted and treated. The randomized trial data that determine how frequently community members should be screened to lower chlamydial infections at the population level are lacking; however, observational studies consistently indicate that among sexually active teens the median time between first and repeat infections is approximately 6 months. Based on these data, biannual screening seems reasonable for women at this age (older than 25 years). Because the risk of reinfection is inversely related to age, it is unclear if this recommendation should be extended to young adults. Nevertheless, a history of prior infection predicts reinfection regardless of sexual risk behavior, and in women repeat infections are implicated in the pathogenesis of upper genital tract damage. It may be wise, therefore, to rescreen all women who were treated for chlamydial infections at 6-month intervals.

Developing selective screening criteria is a vigorously pursued public health goal. With the exception of age, however, no single demographic or behavioral risk factor or combination of risk factors consistently identifies a group of young, sexually active women who should not be screened. The utility of more selective screening is limited by the high proportion of missed infections.

Parallel evidence to support screening asymptomatic men may be lacking because before the introduction of urine screening men were not routinely tested for chlamydial infection. But because the cost of treating men is lower than the cost of treating women, a greater proportion of infected men are symptomatic than women, and the harm associated with misdiagnoses is not inconsequent, it will undoubtedly be more difficult to justify routine periodic male screening. However, false-negative test results create a reservoir of untreated disease that is likely to contribute disproportionately to the spread of *C. trachomatis*; but the psychosocial consequences of false-positive test results can range from dysphoric feelings and decreased self-esteem to the disruption of romantic relationships and domestic violence. Moreover, if treatment is initiated inappropriately, the adverse effects of drug reactions and bacterial resistance caused by antibiotic overuse must be taken into account. Thus, until more data become available, the United States Preventive Services Task Force recommends symptom-based screening for all men and for women older than 25 years of age who do not exhibit other characteristics associated with a high

CURRENT DIAGNOSIS

- Signs and symptoms are neither a sensitive nor a specific indication of chlamydial infection and often persist for weeks after documented eradication of the pathogen.
  Most chlamydial infections are asymptomatic.
  Chlamydia trachomatis is isolated from less than half of women and men with the most common signs and symptoms (mucopurulent cervicitis and urethritis).
- *Chlamydia* should be suspected in:
  Women and men with dysuria and pyuria.
  Women with dyspareunia, abnormal vaginal discharge, abnormal bleeding, and lower abdominal or pelvic pain; infants with conjunctivitis or a staccato cough
- Routine periodic screening with nucleic acid amplification techniques (NAATs) is the only reliable way to diagnose this infection.

prevalence of chlamydial infections (i.e., unmarried status, African American race, a history of STDs, a history of new or multiple sex partners, cervical ectopy, and inconsistent condom use).

Treatment

Recommendations for antibiotic treatment of chlamydial infections depend on the clinical syndrome. Box 1 summarizes the options for outpatient therapy of uncomplicated genital tract infections in men and women. However, because humans do not develop a natural immunity to chlamydia, treated patients remain at risk for reinfection. For this reason therapy should not be considered complete until all recent sexual contacts are treated and the patient is counseled about future disease prevention. An estimated 70% of the male partners of women with chlamydial cervicitis are infected, and, conversely, approximately 30% of the female partners of *Chlamydia*-infected men are infected. Treatment is recommended for the most recent sex partner and all other individuals who had sexual contact with the infected person during the 60 days preceding the onset of symptoms or diagnosis. Also, partners should abstain from sexual intercourse for a week after they complete treatment.

Although patient-delivered partner treatment is as effective as partner notification, partners are more likely to be treated if informed by physicians rather than by the patients. This is because only 65% (approximately) of women with known chlamydial infections refer their sex partners for therapy, and even fewer (approximately 45%) infected men do so. Because the cure rate for single-dose azithromycin (Zithromax) therapy is close to 100% and the medication can easily be administered under medical supervision, a test of cure 3 weeks after treatment—NAATs remain positive for this long despite successful eradication of infection—is only recommended for pregnant women (among whom antibiotic efficacy may be reduced) and when compliance is in doubt.

BOX 1 *Chlamydia trachomatis:* Recommended Treatment Regimens by Clinical Syndrome

Asymptomatic, cervicitis, urethritis*

- First-choice regimen
- Azithromycin (Zithromax), 1 g orally in a single dose

or

- Doxycycline (Vibramycin), 100 mg orally twice a day for 7 days

Alternative Regimens (One of the Following)

- Erythromycin base (E-Mycin), 500 mg orally four times a day for 7 days
- Erythromycin ethylsuccinate (EES), 800 mg orally four times a day for 7 days
- Ofloxacin (Floxin), 300 mg orally twice a day for 7 days
- Levofloxacin (Levaquin),[1] 500 mg orally for 7 days
- Epididymitis
- Ceftriaxone (Rocephin),[1] 250 mg intramuscularly (single dose)

or

- Doxycycline,[1] 100 mg orally twice a day for 7 days

Outpatient Pelvic Inflammatory Disease

- Ofloxacin, 400 mg orally twice a day for 14 days

or

- Levofloxacin,[1] 500 mg orally for 14 days

with or without

- Metronidazole (Flagyl), 500 mg orally twice a day for 14 days

Alternative Regimens

- Ceftriaxone, 250 mg intramuscularly (single dose)

or

- Cefoxitin (Mefoxin), 2 g intramuscularly (single dose)

plus

- Probenecid, 1 g orally

plus

- Doxycycline, 100 mg orally twice a day for 14 days

with or without

- Metronidazole, 500 mg orally twice a day for 14 days

Inpatient Pelvic Inflammatory Disease[†]

- Cefotetan (Cefotan), 2 g intravenously every 12 hours

or

- Cefoxitin, 2 g intravenously every 6 hours

plus

- Doxycycline,[1] 100 mg orally or intravenously every 12 hours

Alternative Regimens

- Clindamycin, 900 mg intravenously every 8 hours

plus

- Gentamicin,[1] 2 g/kg of body weight loading dose, then 1.5 mg/kg of body weight every 8 hours. Treatment should be continued for 24 to 48 hours after significant clinical improvement occurs and then should consist of oral therapy with doxycycline, 100 mg orally twice a day for 14 days, or clindamycin, 450 mg orally four times a day, for a total of 14 days.

---

[1]Not FDA approved for this indication.

*Pregnancy: Doxycycline, erythromycin estolate (Ilosone), and ofloxacin are contraindicated, and repeat testing 3 weeks after completion of therapy is recommended because antibiotics may be less efficacious. HIV infection: Patients who have chlamydial infection and who also are infected with HIV should receive the same treatment regimen as those who are HIV-negative.

[†]Studies indicate that the efficacy of inpatient and outpatient treatment is comparable in terms of fertility and other long-term health outcomes (e.g., ectopic pregnancy and chronic pelvic pain). Therefore, inpatient therapy is no longer recommended except for individuals who do not respond to outpatient regimes or develop tubo-ovarian abscesses or other manifestations of severe upper genital tract disease.

CURRENT THERAPY

- Antibiotic treatment is easy to summarize in tabular form but is ineffective if given in isolation of sexual network.

  Large reservoir of asymptomatically infected partners and potential partners undermines the effectiveness of individual treatments.

  Half of all chlamydial infections occur in previously treated persons.

- Therapy is not complete until all recent sexual contacts are treated and patient counseled about disease prevention.
- Prevalence of *Chlamydia trachomatis* in the sexual network is the best predictor of infection.
- Who an individual has sexual intercourse with puts them at higher risk for acquisition of this infection than how they do so.
- For disease prevention—condoms are plan B—plan A is choosing low-risk sexual partners.

Approximately 50% of all chlamydial infections occur in previously treated persons. Demographic characteristics, such as age and a past history of chlamydial infection, are better predictors of infection than behavioral risk factors, such as multiple sexual partners and the failure to use condoms consistently. Being involved with a sexual network in which *Chlamydia* is hyperendemic appears to put individuals at greater risk for infection than unsafe sexual behavior in the general population. Hence, to control the spread of *C. trachomatis*, it may be necessary to:

- Extend screening and treatment beyond recent partners to include the group of core transmitters in the infected individual's sexual network.
- Help STD patients learn to choose less risky sex partners by promoting sexual health communication within partnerships.

Although the debate about the content and duration of counseling necessary to achieve this goal is ongoing, there is a growing consensus that brief (5 minutes), personalized (provider-delivered and client-centered) counseling sessions—aimed at personal risk reduction and increasing awareness of partner risk behavior—are more effective than the conventional didactic approach to STD prevention education. They are certainly as effective as more prolonged sessions, which are difficult to conduct in busy public health clinics.

REFERENCES

Aral SO, Hughes JP, Stoner B, et al: Sexual mixing patterns in spread of gonococcal and chlamydial infections. Am J Pub Health 1999;89:825-833.

Biro F, Workowski K, Blythe MJ, Lara-Torre E: NASPAG/JPAG roundtable discussion annual clinical meeting 2003—Philadelphia, PA: Sexually transmitted diseases (STD) treatment guidelines 2002. J Pediatr Adolesc Gynecol 2004;17:143-146.

Cates W Jr: Contraception, unintended pregnancies, and sexually transmitted diseases: Why isn't a simple solution possible? Am J Epidemiol 1996;143:311-318.

Critchlow CW, Wolner-Hanssen P, Eschenbach DA, et al: Determinants of cervical ectopia and cervicitis: Age, oral contraception, specific cervical infection, smoking, and douching. Am J Obstet Gynecol 1995;173:534-543.

Duncan B, Hart G, Scoular A, Bigrigg A: Qualitative analysis of psychosocial impact of diagnosis of *Chlamydia trachomatis*: Implications for screening. BMJ 2001;322:195-199.

Ford CA, Viadro CI, Miller WC: Testing for chlamydial and gonorrheal infections outside of clinic settings. A summary of the literature. Sex Transm Dis 2004;31:38-51.

Kamb ML, Fishbein M, Douglas JM Jr, et al: Efficacy of risk-reduction counseling to prevent human immunodeficiency virus and sexually transmitted diseases: A randomized controlled trial for the Project RESPECT Study Group. JAMA 1998;280:1161-1167.

Peipert JF: Clinical practice. Genital chlamydial infections. N Engl J Med 2003;349:2424-2430.

Rietmeijer CA, Van Bemmelen R, Judson FN, Douglas JM: Incidence and repeat infection rates of *Chlamydia trachomatis* among male and female patients in an STD clinic. Sex Transm Dis 2002;29: 65-72.

U.S. Preventive Services Task Force. Screening for chlamydial infection: Recommendations and rationale. Am J Prev Med 2001; 20(3S):90-94.

Pelvic Inflammatory Disease

Method of
Adrianne Williams Bagley, MD,
and Maria Trent, MD, MPH

Pelvic inflammatory disease (PID) is a spectrum of disorders characterized by an infection of the female upper genital tract. Organs that may be affected include the uterus (endometritis, parametritis), fallopian tubes (salpingitis), and ovaries (oophoritis, tubo-ovarian abscesses [TOAs]), or the infection may involve the pelvic peritoneum.

Epidemiology

Approximately 800,000 women per year are diagnosed with PID. Up to 20% of cases occur in teenagers. Risk factors associated with development of PID mirror the risk factors that increase the likelihood of acquiring a sexually transmitted infection. These risk factors include having multiple sex partners and inconsistent or incorrect use of condoms. Douching and use of intrauterine devices are also associated with PID. Women with a prior diagnosis of PID are at higher risk of developing future episodes.

Pathophysiology

The infection of the female upper genital tract that characterizes PID is caused by the ascent of infectious organisms from the vagina and cervix. It is postulated that the ascent of organisms may occur more readily during menses because of reflux of blood in the fallopian tubes, and studies show a temporal relationship between menses and the subsequent diagnosis of PID.

The infectious agents most often implicated in PID are the sexually transmitted organisms *Neisseria gonorrhoeae* and *Chlamydia trachomatis*. However, PID may be a polymicrobial infection. Other contributing infectious etiologies include anaerobic bacteria such as *Bacteroides* and *Peptostreptococcus* species, *Gardnerella vaginalis*, *Haemophilus influenzae*, *Streptococcus* species, *Mycoplasma hominis*, *Ureaplasma urealyticum*, enteric gram-negative bacilli, and cytomegalovirus.

Diagnosis

The diagnosis of PID is made based on clinical assessment; therefore, a detailed history, careful examination, and the use of additional supportive diagnostic tests are warranted. Patients may present with varied nonspecific complaints including lower abdominal pain, vaginal discharge, and irregular menses or bleeding with sexual intercourse. Patients may or may not be febrile, experience vomiting or diarrhea, or have urinary symptoms. The differential diagnosis includes processes that affect not only the reproductive tract but also the gastrointestinal and urinary tracts. The differential diagnosis includes but is not limited to ovarian cyst, endometriosis, dysmenorrhea, ectopic pregnancy, septic or threatened abortion, gastroenteritis, appendicitis, diverticulitis, constipation, inflammatory bowel disease, irritable bowel syndrome, urethritis, cystitis, pyelonephritis, and nephrolithiasis.

The 2006 Centers for Disease Control and Prevention (CDC) guidelines recommend empirical treatment for PID in sexually active women with minimum diagnostic criteria of uterine tenderness, adnexal tenderness, or cervical motion tenderness, in whom no other cause can be identified. Additional supportive criteria may be used to increase the specificity of diagnosis; these criteria include oral temperature greater than 38°C (101°F), abnormal cervical or vaginal mucopurulent discharge, presence of white blood cells on saline wet mount of vaginal secretions, elevated erythrocyte sedimentation rate (ESR) or C- reactive protein (CRP), and documented cervical infection with *N. gonorrhoeae* or *C. trachomatis*. However, if cervical infection with *N. gonorrhoeae* or *C. trachomatis* is not found, these organisms can still be responsible for upper genital tract infection. Additional diagnostic tests may include complete blood cell count (CBC) with differential, urine dipstick or urinalysis, urine culture, and urine pregnancy test. Pelvic ultrasonography should be obtained if there is evidence of a pelvic mass on examination or if there is adnexal tenderness in the setting of high fever, elevated white blood cell count, or elevated CRP or ESR; this constellation of findings may suggest a TOA.

CURRENT DIAGNOSIS

- Pelvic inflammatory disease is a clinical diagnosis.
- The minimum diagnostic criterion is one or more of the following clinical findings: uterine tenderness, adnexal tenderness, *or* cervical motion tenderness in the patient in whom no other cause can be identified.
- The use of additional supportive criteria can increase the accuracy of the diagnosis.

CURRENT THERAPY

Inpatient Treatment for Pelvic Inflammatory Disease

Regimen A:

- Cefotetan (Cefotan), 2 g IV q12h, *or* cefoxitin (Mefoxin), 2 g IV q6h, *plus* doxycycline (Vibramycin), 100 mg PO or IV q12h

Regimen B:

- Clindamycin (Cleocin), 900 mg IV q8h,
- *Plus* gentamicin (Garamycin), loading dose: 2 mg/kg IV/IM, followed by maintenance dose: 1.5 mg/kg IV q8h.

Note: Parenteral therapy for PID should be continued for 24 h following clinical improvement, and patients should be discharged home on an oral course of doxycycline (Vibramycin), 100 mg PO bid, or clindamycin (Cleocin), 450 mg PO bid, to complete 14 d.

Outpatient Treatment for Pelvic Inflammatory Disease

Regimen A:

- Levofloxacin (Levaquin), 500 mg PO once daily for 14 d, *with or without* metronidazole (Flagyl), 500 mg PO bid for 14 d, *or*
- Ofloxacin (Floxin), 400 mg PO bid for 14 d

Regimen B:

- Ceftriaxone (Rocephin), 250 mg IM in a single dose, *or*
- Cefoxitin (Mefoxin), 2 g IM in a single dose, with probenecid, 1 g PO in a single dose, *or*
- Other parenteral third-generation cephalosporins (ceftizoxime [Cefizox] or cefotaxime [Claforan]) *plus* doxycycline (Vibramycin), 100 mg PO bid for 14 d, *with or without* metronidazole (Flagyl), 500 mg PO bid for 14 d.

Note: Recommendations from the Centers for Disease Control and Prevention 2006 Sexually Transmitted Diseases Treatment Guidelines are available at http://www.cdc.giv/std/treatment.
Abbreviations: IM = intramuscular; IV = intravenous; PO = orally.

Treatment

Treatment should be initiated promptly for the patient with suspected PID to prevent complications, which include chronic pelvic pain, ectopic pregnancy, and infertility. Antibiotic treatment is broad spectrum to ensure coverage of typical pathogens, namely *N. gonorrhoeae*, *C. trachomatis*, and anaerobes. With prompt appropriate medical treatment, the future reproductive ability of the patient may be protected.

The Current Therapy box outlines the 2006 CDC treatment guidelines for inpatient treatment. Hospitalization for parenteral treatment is reserved for patients for whom surgical causes of abdominal pain cannot be excluded, patients who are pregnant, patients who fail outpatient regimens (unable to follow or tolerate an outpatient regimen, no clinical response to oral antibiotics after 72 hours), patients with severe illness, nausea, vomiting, or high fever, and patients with a TOA. Patients younger than 16 years and those with extenuating social circumstances may also be candidates for inpatient treatment.

Outpatient treatment for PID is appropriate in most cases for patients who do not meet the criteria for hospitalization. Metronidazole (Flagyl) is often included as part of the treatment regimen to provide anaerobic coverage, and it is an appropriate adjunct medication in patients who also have evidence of bacterial vaginosis on saline wet mount.

FOLLOW-UP

Patients treated with outpatient therapy should be reevaluated in 48 to 72 hours to assess response to treatment. At this visit, the medical provider can review medication adherence, readdress partner notification, review the importance of safe sexual practices, discuss related family planning issues, answer questions that the patient may have about the diagnosis, and reexamine the patient to ensure that she is improving on the current therapeutic regimen. Patients who are not improving on oral antibiotics or who have been unable to adhere with the outpatient regimen may need additional diagnostic testing for complications and hospitalization for parental treatment.

Patients being treated for PID should be advised to abstain from sexual intercourse throughout the course of treatment. All sexual partners within the past 60 days should be tested and empirically treated for both *N. gonorrhoeae* and *C. trachomatis*.

Potential Complications

Short-term complications of PID include TOA and Fitz-Hugh-Curtis syndrome. Patients with TOA require hospitalization for parenteral treatment. Fitz-Hugh-Curtis syndrome is a perihepatitis that may result from spread of *N. gonorrhoeae* or *C. trachomatis* and is characterized by right upper quadrant pain.

Long-term complications of PID include chronic pelvic pain, tubal infertility secondary to scarring, and ectopic pregnancy. Patients with a history of PID have a 6- to 10-fold increased risk of ectopic pregnancy.

Prevention

Primary prevention of PID can be best accomplished by prevention of sexually transmitted infections. Sexually active women should undergo routine screening for gonorrhea and *Chlamydia* and be instructed about the importance of proper condom usage. Secondary prevention can be accomplished with partner notification and empirical treatment using antibiotics with adequate coverage for infections caused by *N. gonorrhoeae* and *C. trachomatis*.

REFERENCES

American Academy of Pediatrics: Pelvic inflammatory disease. In Pickering LK (ed): Red Book: 2003 Report of the Committee on Infectious Diseases, 26th ed. Elk Grove Village, Ill, American Academy of Pediatrics, 2003, pp 468-472.

Centers for Disease Control and Prevention: Sexually transmitted disease treatment guidelines 2002. MMWR 2002;51(No. RR-6):48-52.

Ness RB, Soper DE, Holley RL, et al: Effectiveness of inpatient and outpatient treatment strategies for women with pelvic inflammatory disease: Results from the pelvic inflammatory disease evaluation and clinical health (PEACH) randomized trial. Am J Obstet Gynecol 2002;186(5):929-937.

Rein DB, Kassler WJ, Irwin KL, et al: Direct medical costs of pelvic inflammatory disease and its sequelae: Decreasing, but still substantial. Obstet Gynecol 2000;95(3):397-402.

Shrier LA: Bacterial sexually transmitted infections: gonorrhea, chlamydia, pelvic inflammatory disease, and syphilis. In Emans SJ, Laufer MR, Goldstein DP (eds): Pediatric and Adolescent Gynecology, 5th ed. Lippincott-Raven, 2004, pp 583-598.

Trent MA, Ellen JM, Walker A: Pelvic inflammatory disease in adolescents—care delivery in pediatric ambulatory settings. Pediatr Emerg Care 2005;21(7):431-436.

Trent M, Judy SL, Ellen JM, Walker A: Use of an institutional intervention to improve quality of care for adolescents treated in pediatric ambulatory settings for pelvic inflammatory disease. J Adolesc Health 2006;39(1):50-56.

Uterine Leiomyomas

Method of
Tod C. Aeby, MD,
and Stella Dantas, MD

Epidemiology

Uterine leiomyomas are the most common pelvic tumor in women. They affect approximately 20% of women older than 35 years of age and 40% of women older than 50 years of age, although they are found any time from puberty through menopause. Survey studies involving histologic examination of the uterus suggest they are present in more than 80% of women. Nulliparity, early menarche, and African American ethnicity increase the risk of developing leiomyomas. The incidence among women of African descent is not as high in countries other than the United States, which suggests possible dietary, environmental, and genetic influences on development. Risk is also increased in women with a higher body mass index, presumably because of the increased estrogen production in adipocytes. Pregnancy reduces the risk of developing leiomyomas.

Pathophysiology

The etiology of uterine leiomyomas is not completely understood, but development is thought to be a multistep process. They are benign monoclonal tumors of the smooth muscle of the myometrium that presumably derive from a normal myocyte. Estrogen and progesterone, in concert with local growth factors, lead to a somatic mutation of normal myometrium to a leiomyoma. Some growth factors that cause leiomyoma proliferation are epidermal growth factors, insulin-like growth factors, heparin-binding growth factors, and transforming growth factor-β. Leiomyomas develop during the reproductive years and increase in size during pregnancy. Growth usually ceases in menopause, and leiomyomas then decrease in volume. This supports the theory that estrogen and progesterone promote growth.

Symptoms and Signs

Most uterine leiomyomas are asymptomatic. They are categorized into subgroups based on their anatomic relationship and position in the uterus, and symptoms usually depend on those relationships. They can be subserosal, intramural, submucosal, or pedunculated. The most common symptom is abnormal uterine bleeding, usually menorrhagia, occurring in 30% of women with leiomyomas. The cause of the abnormal bleeding is not totally clear but may be the result of abnormal growth and function of the endometrium near the leiomyoma and local interference with normal physiologic mechanisms for hemostasis.

Pelvic pain and increasing pelvic pressure occur in 30% of women with leiomyomas. Other symptoms include dysmenorrhea, postcoital bleeding, and dyspareunia. Pain can be caused by leiomyomas outgrowing their blood supply and becoming necrotic. This red degeneration is common in pregnancy. Patients may have an increasing abdominal girth and pressure symptoms as a result of large fibroids. Pressure on adjacent organs such as the bladder or bowel can cause urinary frequency and urgency or constipation. Rarely, an enlarged uterus causes a palpable kidney secondary to hydronephrosis from ureteral obstruction. Patients also may be lethargic from anemia secondary to menorrhagia. Leiomyomas may also be associated with infertility, although the relationship is controversial.

A rapidly enlarging uterus should raise concern for malignant transformation. But leiomyosarcomas are extremely rare, occurring in less than 0.1% of women operated on for presumed leiomyomas.

Diagnosis

Uterine leiomyomas are typically diagnosed at pelvic exam when an enlarged and irregularly shaped uterus is noted. Abdominal and transvaginal ultrasound is often helpful in making the diagnosis and in differentiating leiomyomas from adnexal masses or other pelvic pathology. Serial ultrasounds also can be used to monitor their growth. During a pelvic exam, it may not be possible to palpate ovaries next to an enlarged uterus, but an adnexal tumor can be suspected if the mass moves independently of the uterus. Submucosal leiomyomas are diagnosed using saline infusion sonohysterography and hysteroscopy. Definitive diagnosis requires histologic examination.

CURRENT DIAGNOSIS

- Abnormal uterine bleeding, postcoital spotting
- Pelvic pain, pressure, dysmenorrhea and dyspareunia
- Urinary frequency and urgency, constipation
- Lethargy
- Infertility
- Physical findings: Enlarged, irregular, and firm uterus
- Ultrasound: Diagnostic imaging modality of choice
- Saline infusion sonohysterography and/or hysteroscopy: Used to evaluate the uterine cavity

TABLE 1 Comparison of Various Procedures for the Treatment of Symptomatic Uterine Leiomyoma

Therapy	Success Rate	Complication Rate	Possibility of Future Childbearing	Comments
Hysterectomy	100%	40%	No	Recovery time varies depending on the route of removal.
Myomectomy and myolysis	75%	39%	Yes	Can be associated with significant blood loss and can result in an unplanned hysterectomy. Recurrent leiomyomas are common.
Myolysis			Yes	Several methods for myolysis are available, including bipolar electrocautery, laser energy, and cryotherapy.
Uterine artery embolization	77%-91%	5%	Not currently recommended	Complication rates are low but can be severe, including infection, sepsis, and nontarget tissue necrosis. A few deaths have been reported.
Hydrothermal endometrial ablation	91%*	1%-2%	No	Hysteroscopic resection of submucosal leiomyomas, prior to endometrial ablation, improves success rates. Pregnancies have occurred after these procedures, so contraception is still required.

*Best estimate based on limited studies.

Management

For the most part, asymptomatic leiomyoma should be managed expectantly. The approaches to the patient experiencing problems fall into the three general categories of medical management, conservative procedures, and hysterectomy. The choice should be individualized to the patient, based on the severity of her symptoms, her plans for future childbearing, and her personal interest in retaining her uterus. Other causes of abnormal bleeding should be considered.

Current medical therapy is limited to the use of gonadotropin-releasing hormone (GnRH) analogues and antagonists (i.e., leuprolide acetate [Lupron Depot], 3.75 mg monthly; nafarelin acetate [Synarel],[1] 200 µg intranasally twice a day; and goserelin acetate implant [Zoladex],[1] 3.6-mg implant monthly, cetrorelix [Cetrotide]).[1] These expensive medications are shown to decrease the

---

[1]Not FDA approved for this indication.

CURRENT THERAPY

- Only symptomatic leiomyomas require treatment.
- Medical therapy is for temporizing and making invasive procedures easier or more effective.
- Conservative procedures include myomectomy, myolysis, hydrothermal endometrial ablation, and uterine artery embolization.
- Hysterectomy is the only definitive therapy for leiomyomata.
- Choice of treatment should be made considering the severity of symptoms and respecting the patient's preferences.

uterine size by up to 65%, allowing for easier or more conservative surgical treatments. The progesterone antagonist mifepristone (Mifeprex)[1] is also effective but not currently available for this purpose in the United States. GnRH therapy has significant side effects, mostly related to the induced hypoestrogenic state. To preserve bone density the duration of therapy must be limited. Additionally, the uterus rapidly returns to its enlarged size when the therapy is discontinued. These medications are a very effective means of inducing amenorrhea to allow for correction of an anemia prior to surgery.

Conservative procedures include myomectomy or myolysis (surgical removal or destruction of the individual fibroids while preserving the uterus), uterine artery embolization, and endometrial ablation. Each of these approaches has different risks, benefits, and complications (Table 1).

Hysterectomy remains the most common treatment for women with symptomatic leiomyoma and offers the advantage of a complete and definitive cure. The uterus can be removed through the vagina (with or without the aid of laparoscopic techniques) or through an abdominal incision. The route of removal largely depends on the size of the uterus, the patient's medical and surgical history, and the experience and preference of her surgeon.

REFERENCES

Buttram VC Jr, Reiter RC: Uterine leiomyomata: Etiology, symptomatology, and management. Fertil Steril 1981;36:433-445.

Felberbaum RE, Germer U, Ludwig M, et al: Treatment of uterine fibroids with a slow-release formulation of the gonadotrophin-releasing hormone antagonist Cetrorelix. Hum Reprod 1998;13(6):1660-1668.

Goldfarb HA: Bipolar laparoscopic needles for myoma coagulation. J Am Assoc Gynecol Laparosc 1995;2(2):175-179.

Lethaby A, Vollenhoven B, Sowter M: Pre-operative GnRH analogue therapy before hysterectomy or myomectomy for uterine fibroids.

The Cochrane Database of Systematic Reviews 2001, Issue 2. Article CD000547. DOI: 10.1002/14651858.CD000547.

Parker WH, Fu YS, Berek JS: Uterine sarcoma in patients operated on for presumed leiomyoma and rapidly growing leiomyoma. Obstet Gynecol 1994;83:414.

Pron G, Bennett J, Common A, et al: Ontario Uterine Fibroid Embolization Collaboration Group. The Ontario Uterine Fibroid Embolization Trial: II. Uterine fibroid reduction and symptom relief after uterine artery embolization for fibroids. Fertil Steril 2003;79(1):120-127.

The Hydro ThermAblator system for management of menorrhagia in women with submucous myomas: 12- to 20-month follow-up. J Am Assoc Gynecol Laparosc 2003;10(4):521-527.

Ovarian Cancer

Method of
Lynne A. Eaton, MD, MS

Epithelial ovarian cancer accounts for 90% of all cases of ovarian cancer and is the leading cause of death from cancer of the female reproductive tract. Approximately 25,000 new cases and 16,000 deaths were reported in 2004 from this disease. The median age of patients with ovarian cancer is 60 years. There are few established risk factors for the disease, which include low parity, obesity, high-fat diet, and strong family history or genetic mutations. Preventative measures may include tubal ligation, hysterectomy, and breast-feeding. Oral contraceptive pills may decrease a woman's risk of developing the disease by as much as 50%, including those at highest risk for developing ovarian cancer.

Most ovarian cancers are acquired as a sporadic disease. A woman's lifetime risk of ovarian cancer increases with a family history of ovarian cancer (i.e., one first-degree relative, 4%; one-first- and one second-degree relative, 15%; and two first-degree relatives, 40%). Approximately 10% of epithelial ovarian cancers arise as a result of an inherited mutation. These cancers usually arise approximately 10 years earlier than previous generations, and most are linked to the presence of BRCA-1 or BRCA-2 gene mutation. These tumor suppressor genes have an autosomal dominant inheritance pattern and are found on chromosome 17 and 13, respectively. A woman may have up to an 80% chance of developing breast cancer and a 40% chance of developing ovarian cancer if she is BRCA-1 positive. In women who are BRCA-2 positive, their lifetime risk of developing breast and ovarian cancer is 50% to 85% and 15% to 20%, respectively. Ashkenazi Jewish women have a higher incidence of germ-line mutations in BRCA-1 or BRCA-2 genes. A second familial disorder with an increased risk of ovarian cancer is the Lynch II syndrome, or hereditary nonpolyposis colorectal cancer (HNPCC). It is caused by inherited germ-line mutations in DNA-mismatch repair genes. Women who present with a family history should be offered genetic counseling and testing for genetic mutations where appropriate. Oral contraceptives may be offered to those women who desire fertility, and oophorectomy may be considered in those who have completed their families because these measures decrease the risk of developing ovarian cancer.

Screening

Unfortunately, despite the high mortality rate of the disease, no effective screening method is available for ovarian cancer. CA-125 is an antigen found in structures derived from coelomic epithelium and in tubal, endometrial, and endocervical epithelium. The surface epithelium of the normal fetal and adult ovaries do not express CA-125, however, except in inclusion cysts, areas of metaplasia, and papillary excrescences. Serum CA-125 is quantified based on immunoradiometric assay of the monoclonal antibody OC-125. It is a serum with a low specificity and sensitivity. The elevation of the tumor marker often depends on the histology (most commonly elevated in serous histology) and can be elevated in other conditions that irritate the abdominal/pelvic cavity. These include but are not limited to endometriosis, pelvic inflammatory disease, endometrial cancer, appendicitis, liver disease, and pancreatitis. Only 50% of women with stage I disease have an elevated CA-125. Almost 80% of women with advanced disease have an elevated CA-125. This serum test is best used as a tumor marker to triage a patient with a known adnexal mass and to follow a woman postoperatively who is undergoing adjuvant chemotherapy to assess response to therapy. It can also be used as a surveillance marker, with an elevation indicating possible recurrent disease. Transvaginal ultrasonography has been examined as a screening tool. The sensitivity and specificity of this test is low in predicting ovarian cancer. Combining the two modalities may increase the screening statistical parameters. No effective screening modalities currently exist for the general population or for women at high risk of developing ovarian cancer.

Diagnosis

The symptoms of ovarian cancer are nonspecific. Many women present with abdomen pain, bloating, or fullness. They may feel their clothes are too tight or that they are gaining weight. Others complain of early satiety or dyspepsia. Some patients may present with pelvic pain because of abdominal distention from ascites or a pelvic mass. Unfortunately, at this point, 75% of women have stage III or IV disease. Diagnosis can often be made on physical examination with palpation of a mass either abdominally or on rectovaginal exam. Less frequently, the patient has a distended abdomen and a fluid wave may be present. If necessary, transvaginal ultrasound or computed tomography (CT) of the abdomen and pelvis may be performed to help establish the diagnosis. An ovarian mass that is complex in nature (i.e., having both solid and cystic components) is suspicious for ovarian cancer. This is especially true in postmenopausal women with an elevated CA-125. Women who present with a pleural effusion should also be assessed for the possibility of ovarian cancer. A CA-125 should be drawn if ovarian cancer is suspected so it may be followed postoperatively. If there is *any* suspicion a woman has an ovarian cancer, she should be referred to a gynecologic oncologist who specializes in the surgical and medical care of women with gynecologic cancers.

Management

Critical to the proper management decision in patients with ovarian cancer is the accurate staging of the disease. Comprehensive surgical staging is mandatory in this patient population. Approximately 30% to 40% of women with apparent stage I disease have occult disease outside the pelvis. Virtually every patient with ovarian cancer should undergo an exploratory laparotomy through a midline vertical incision that allows careful examination of the abdominal/peritoneal cavity. Usually a total abdominal hysterectomy with bilateral-salpingo-oophorectomy, pelvic and para-aortic lymph node dissection, and multiple peritoneal biopsies is performed. In instances of stage III or IV disease, these surgeries may additionally include rectosigmoid resections with reanastomosis, peritoneal and diaphragmatic stripping, splenectomy, and partial bladder cystectomy. The primary goal is cytoreduction of tumor nodules to less than 1.0 cm. Two large meta-analyses demonstrated that regardless of the initial tumor size, successful cytoreduction to small-volume disease increases the frequency of complete responses and enhanced survival. Cytoreductive surgery is thought to improve survival and response rates based on the following:

- Removal of resistant clones of tumor cells decreases the likelihood of early onset of drug resistance.
- Removal of large tumor volume increases vascularity and improves drug delivery.
- More vascularized tissue has a higher growth fraction, enhancing the effect of chemotherapy.
- Smaller masses of tumor may require fewer doses of chemotherapy and decrease the possibility of acquired drug resistance.
- Removal of bulky disease may enhance the immune system.

The standard of care for adjuvant therapy in the United States today is chemotherapy using a combination of intravenous (IV) paclitaxel (Taxol) and carboplatin (Paraplatin) as an outpatient regime. This combination is a result of four large randomized trials performed through the Gynecologic Oncology Group (GOG), OV-10 (Canadian-European consortium), and AGO (Arbeitsgemeinschaft Gynakologische Onkologie; Ovarian Cancer Study Group). These trials initially compared cisplatin/cyclophospamide to cisplatin (Platinol-AQ)/paclitaxel [Cytoxan]) and found the combination of cisplatin and paclitaxel superior in regard to overall response rate, clinical complete response rate, progression-free survival, and overall survival. Efficacy trials were then performed comparing cisplatin and carboplatin, and no major therapeutic differences were found between the two drugs. Thus paclitaxel and carboplatin are defined as the gold standard for treatment of ovarian cancer. More recently intraperitoneal (IP) chemotherapy was evaluated in a number of randomized trials in patients with small-volume disease. These trials showed significant improvement in progression-free and overall survival. The IP regimens have more toxicity then the IV routes of administration. In January 2006, an NCI announcement was issued recommending a combination of IV and IP chemotheraphy be utilized in women with advanced optimally cytoreduced ovarian cancer.

Adjuvant therapy depends on the stage and grade of the disease. In women with early-stage low-risk disease (stage IA-B, grades 1-2), no further therapy is warranted. In those women with stage IC or stage II disease, three to six cycles of paclitaxel and carboplatin are given. Patients with more advanced disease generally receive six cycles of IV paclitaxel and carboplatin. They have a CA-125 drawn with each cycle of chemotherapy in hopes of a rapid downward trend. Another important option for these women is participation in clinical trials. The GOG, as well as many other cooperative groups, are leaders in the research on ovarian cancer.

Despite an initial 80% response rate to chemotherapy, 75% of patients who achieve a clinical complete response eventually relapse and die of their disease. Patients who relapse greater than 6 months from their last course of chemotherapy are considered "platinum sensitive." These women have a 30% response to second-line agents, and depending on the length of remission, they may consider retreatment with paclitaxel and carboplatin. Second-line agents include topotecan (Hycamtin), liposomal doxorubicin (Doxil), gemcitabine (Gemzar),[1] ifosfamide (Ifex),[1] and hexamethylmelamine (Hexalen), as well as other agents.

Platinum-resistant patients have a recurrence within 6 months of their last treatment. Their prognosis is considered poor because platinum-based therapy is a key factor in treatment for ovarian cancer. Treatments with

---

[1]Not FDA approved for this indication.

CURRENT DIAGNOSIS

- Inherited gene mutation causes approximately 10% of ovarian cancers.
- No effective screening modalities are currently available.
- Symptoms of ovarian cancer are nonspecific.
- Physical examination and palpation of abdominal mass or fluid wave should be preformed.
- Rectovaginal exam and palpation of pelvic mass should be performed.
- Radiographic imaging demonstrates complex mass with cystic and solid components.
- Elevation of CA-125 occurs, especially in a post-menopausal woman.

CURRENT THERAPY

- Referral to gynecologic oncologist if ovarian cancer suspected based on CA-125 and/or radiographic imaging
- Adequate surgical staging of the disease by a gynecologic oncologist
- In patients with advanced disease, optimal cytoreductive surgery with tumor nodules less than 1 cm
- Adjuvant chemotherapy using IV and IP routes of administration or enrollment in a clinical trial if available.
- In patients with recurrent disease, second-line agents based on platinum sensitivity as well as consideration of convenience, toxicity, and quality of life issues

second-line agents can be initiated, but response rates are low. Treatment decisions should be made based on patient convenience, toxicity, and quality of life issues. Most women with ovarian cancer ultimately die from complications related to bowel obstruction or general deterioration. When signs of an obstruction occur in a patient with end-stage ovarian cancer, it is important to initiate conversations with the patient and family regarding symptomatic care, including gastric tube placement to relieve nausea and vomiting, pain management, and hospice.

Despite the ravages of ovarian cancer, progress is being made in the treatment of the disease. Since the 1970s and the introduction of cisplatin, and more recently of paclitaxel, the median survival has progressed from 6 to 12 months to 3 to 5 years. Knowledge gained in the genetics of the disease risk-reduction procedures can be offered to those at highest risk for developing ovarian cancer. There is hope for development of new screening tools in the future. Current clinical trials are using new cytotoxic agents as well as integrating biologic agents to front-line therapy to assess their role in the armamentarium for treating ovarian cancer. It is hoped these efforts will lead to a decrease in the mortality of this disease and one day a cure for ovarian cancer.

REFERENCES

Allen DG, Heintz APM, Touw FWMM: A meta-analysis of residual disease and survival in stage III and IV carcinoma of the ovary. Eur J Gynaecol Oncol 1995;16:349-356.

Armstrong DK, Bundy B, Wenzel L, et al: Intraperitoneal cisplatin and paclitaxel in ovarian cancer. N Engl J Med 2006;354:34-43.

Bristow RE, Tomacruz RS, Armstrong DK, et al: Survival effect of maximal cytoreductive surgery for advanced ovarian carcinoma during the platinum era: A meta-analysis. J Clin Oncol 2002;20:1248-1259.

Cannistra SA: Cancer of the ovary. N Engl J Med 2004;351:2519-2529.

Clinical Advisory: NCI Issues Clinical Announcement for Preferred Method of Treatment for Advanced Ovarian Cancer January 4, 2006.

Copeland LJ, Bookman M, Trimble E: Clinical trials of newer regimens for treating ovarian cancer: The rationale for Gynecologic Oncology Group Protocol GOG 182-ICON5. Gynecol Oncol 2003;90:S1-S57.

McGuire WP, Hoskins WJ, Brady MF, et al: Cyclophosphamide and cisplatin compared with paclitaxel and cisplatin in patients with stage III and stage IV ovarian disease. N Engl J Med 1996;334:1-6.

Ozols RF: Update on Gynecologic Oncology Group (GOG) trials in ovarian cancer. Cancer Invest 2004;22(Suppl 2):11-20.

Ozols RF, Bundy BN, Greer BE, et al: Phase III trial of carboplatin and paclitaxel compared with cisplatin and paclitaxel in patients with optimally resected stage III ovarian cancer: A Gynecologic Oncology Group study. J Clin Oncol 2003;21:3194-3200.

Rose PG, Nerenstone S, Brady MF, et al: Secondary surgical cytoreduction for advanced ovarian carcinoma. N Engl J Med 2004;351:2489-2497.

Thigpen T: First-line therapy for ovarian carcinoma: What's next? Cancer Invest 2004;22(Suppl 2):21-28.

Thigpen T: The if and when of surgical debulking for ovarian carcinoma. N Engl J Med 2004;351:2544-2546.

Endometrial Cancer

Method of
James J. Burke II, MD,
and Donald G. Gallup, MD

Endometrial cancer is the most common gynecologic cancer in the United States, with an estimated 40,100 new cases reported each year. Although approximately 80% of these cases are diagnosed as stage I disease, 6800 women will succumb to their disease annually.

Endometrial cancer is subdivided into two histologically and clinically separate groups. Type I endometrial cancer is directly related to an increased estrogenous state. This type of endometrial cancer is the most common and is usually found at an earlier stage, and treatment results in a more favorable outcome. Type II endometrial carcinoma is a more virulent type of carcinoma characterized by early metastasis, and it typically has a worse prognosis.

Epidemiology, Clinical Features, and Diagnosis

TYPE I ENDOMETRIAL CARCINOMA

Endometrial carcinoma is a heterogeneous mix of several histologic types with various clinical outcomes. This more common type of endometrial carcinoma represents approximately 90% of all endometrial cancers and is associated with a hyperestrogenic state. Table 1 lists risk factors associated with type I endometrial carcinoma. In the 1970s it was found that giving estrogen preparations without progestin for hormone replacement therapy led to at least a six times greater chance of endometrial carcinoma developing. Similarly, women who are obese have an increased risk of endometrial carcinoma as a result of peripheral conversion of androstenedione to estrone in peripheral adipose tissue by 5α-reductase enzyme activity. Finally, women who have untreated atypical endometrial hyperplasia, a well-known precursor to type I endometrial carcinoma, have a 29 times greater chance of endometrial carcinoma developing. Hence, intervention when this precursor is found can prevent endometrial cancer.

TABLE 1 Risk Factors for the Development of Endometrial Carcinoma

Risk Factor	RR
Overweight (age 50-59 y)	
By 20-50 pounds	3
By >50 pounds	10
Nulliparity versus multiparity	5
Menopause after age 52 y	2
Diabetes	3
Unopposed estrogen replacement	6
Combination OCP	0.5

Abbreviations: OCP = oral contraceptive preparation; RR = relative risk.

Although 90% of women with this type of carcinoma initially have painless, postmenopausal vaginal bleeding or some form of vaginal discharge, most postmenopausal vaginal bleeding is related to conditions other than malignancy. Nonetheless, all postmenopausal bleeding needs further evaluation. The gold standard is endometrial biopsy, usually carried out in the office with minimal patient discomfort. However, should the results of this type of in-office biopsy still be equivocal or performance of the biopsy not be possible because of cervical stenosis, formal fractional dilation and curettage should be performed. Another modality used for assessment of postmenopausal bleeding is transvaginal ultrasound (US) to measure the thickness of the endometrium. Endometrial stripes found to be thicker than 5 mm require endometrial sampling because of the higher likelihood of malignancy.

TYPE II ENDOMETRIAL CARCINOMA

Unlike type I endometrial carcinoma, type II is unrelated to an increased estrogenic state and encompasses several histologic variants that are quite aggressive. These carcinomas tend to have serous, papillary serous, or clear cell histology and typically occur in women older than age 70 years. Fortunately, carcinomas of these types account for less than 10% of all endometrial cancers; but unfortunately, they contribute the majority of deaths from endometrial cancer. Because of the aggressive nature of these cancers, most have metastasized before initial evaluation and diagnosis and spread in a fashion similar to ovarian carcinoma.

As with type I endometrial carcinoma, type II carcinomas are commonly manifested as painless, postmenopausal vaginal bleeding or vaginal discharge. However, patients may have no bleeding at all and instead have nonspecific gastrointestinal (GI) symptoms such as nausea and vomiting, constipation, early satiety, abdominal bloating, and abdominal pain. All these symptoms point to intra-abdominal metastasis, common with this type of endometrial carcinoma. In these patients, early computed tomography (CT) can aid in the diagnosis. Even when these carcinomas have not spread and are limited to the endometrium or endometrial polyps, the risk of recurrence is high.

Staging and Treatment

STAGING

Recognizing that clinical staging did not take into account pathologic or surgical prognostic information, the Gynecologic Oncology Group (GOG) conducted two large prospective surgical staging trials in the 1980s. In 1988 the Fédération Internationale de Gynécologie et d'Obstétrique (FIGO) adopted the surgical staging of endometrial cancer (Table 2). Surgical staging involves obtaining pelvic washings, extrafascial hysterectomy, bilateral salpingo-oophorectomy, and lymph node sampling from the pelvic and para-aortic regions. In addition, if high-risk histology or gross spread of disease is present at the time of surgery (common with type II endometrial cancers), removal of the omentum is recommended. Table 3 shows the typical stage distribution for endometrial carcinoma.

TABLE 2 Fédération Internationale de Gynécologie et d'Obstétrique (FIGO) Surgical Staging Classification for Endometrial Carcinoma

Stage IA	Tumor limited to the endometrium
Stage IB	Invasion to <50% myometrium
Stage IC	Invasion to ≥50% myometrium
Stage IIA	Endocervical glandular involvement only
Stage IIB	Cervical stromal invasion
Stage IIIA	Tumor invading the serosa of the corpus uteri and/or adnexa and/or positive cytologic findings
Stage IIIB	Vaginal metastases
Stage IIIC	Metastases to the pelvic and/or paraortic lymph nodes
Stage IVA	Tumor invasion of the bladder and/or bowel mucosa
Stage IVB	Distant metastases, including intra-abdominal metastasis and/or metastasis to the inguinal lymph nodes

ADJUVANT THERAPY

Radiotherapy is currently the mainstay of adjuvant therapy for early stage endometrial carcinoma at risk for recurrence. Several trials have examined hormonal therapy or chemotherapy in an adjuvant setting for early stage disease, but none has shown any benefit in reducing recurrences.

Although 75% of endometrial carcinomas are found to be confined to the uterus after surgical staging, some patients will be at risk for recurrence and failure with surgical treatment only (Figure 1). Patients found to be at high risk for recurrence are treated with whole-pelvic radiotherapy after surgery, whereas patients who are at *intermediate* risk usually do not need radiotherapy, provided that they have been surgically staged. However, any adjuvant therapy for this group of patients remains controversial.

ADVANCED-STAGE OR RECURRENT DISEASE

A study conducted by the GOG showed that 36% of patients who were found to have metastasis to the para-aortic lymph nodes (stage IIIC) and were treated with radiotherapy were tumor free after 5 years. Similarly, if only pelvic lymph node metastasis (stage IIIC) was found and treated with radiotherapy, 72% would be alive at 5 years.

For serous or clear cell carcinomas found to have extrauterine spread at the time of surgery, *debulking* the

TABLE 3 Distribution of Endometrial Cancer by Stage

Stage I	72.8%
Stage II	10.9%
Stage III	13.1%
Stage IV	3.2%

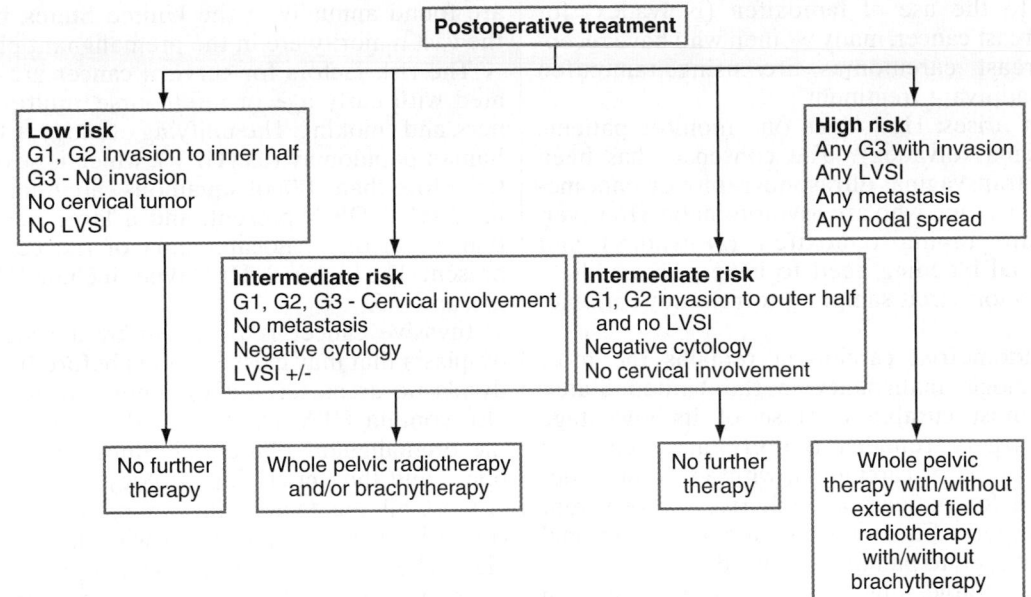

FIGURE 1. Postoperative treatment scheme at Memorial Health University Medical Center for surgical stage I endometrial carcinoma. G = grade; LVSI = lymphovascular space involvement.

metastasis and treating with chemotherapeutic regimens used for ovarian cancer have been shown to increase progression-free survival in several case series. Patients with gross intra-abdominal spread of endometrioid carcinoma generally have a grim prognosis and have not been shown to have prolonged survival with radiotherapy or chemotherapy. Therefore, these patients should be offered participation in clinical trials.

For most patients in whom cancer recurs, it will do so within 3 years of initial treatment. Unfortunately, if the recurrence is any place other than the pelvis (vaginal apex), the likelihood of long-term cure is poor. Depending on the location of the recurrence, radiotherapy, surgery, hormonal therapy, or chemotherapy can be used. Progestins have been studied for the treatment of recurrent disease but have demonstrated modest responses of limited duration.

FOLLOW-UP

Of the endometrial carcinomas that recur, most will do so within the first 3 years after treatment. Typically, the site of recurrence is in the pelvis, most commonly in the vaginal apex. Unfortunately a number of patients will have recurrence at distant sites such as the chest and upper part of the abdomen. Thus, patients treated for endometrial carcinoma are usually monitored closely for 5 years. At Memorial Health University Medical Center, we use an assessment program in which patients are seen every 3 months for the first year, every 4 months for the second year, and every 6 months until 5 years has elapsed since completion of treatment. In addition, a Papanicolaou (Pap) smear is performed at every visit, and chest radiographs are obtained annually for the first 2 years. Furthermore, annual mammography as well as counseling for screening colonoscopy is carried out. CT scanning is not generally used for surveillance in follow-up because of its high cost

and low yield of detection. However, patients with abdominal symptoms may be assessed with CT because the likelihood of finding pathology is greater. For patients with advanced disease or high-risk histologic features, serum measurement of cancer antigen (CA) 125 may be considered. Table 4 shows 5-year survival rates of patients with endometrial carcinoma by stage.

TAMOXIFEN (NOLVADEX)

The National Surgical Adjuvant Breast and Bowel Project (NSABP) conducted a prevention trial with tamoxifen (Nolvadex), known as the P-1 trial. In this randomized, double-blind, prospective trial, women with high-risk family histories were treated with tamoxifen (Nolvadex) or placebo for 5 years. The trial demonstrated a 49% reduced risk for breast cancer, but a 2.5 times greater risk for endometrial carcinoma. Most of the endometrial carcinomas detected were stage I carcinomas, were of endometrioid histology (type I endometrial carcinoma), and were successfully treated with surgery. Additionally, other nonmalignant endometrial abnormalities were detected.

TABLE 4 Endometrial Cancer: Five-Year Survival Rate by Stage

Stage	5-year Survival Rate
Stage IA	91%
Stage IB	88%
Stage IC	81%
Stage II	72%
Stage III	51%
Stage IV	9%

In addition to the use of tamoxifen (Nolvadex) for prevention of breast cancer, many women who have receptor-positive breast carcinomas are using tamoxifen (Nolvadex) for adjuvant treatment.

The question arises: How does one monitor patients taking tamoxifen (Nolvadex)? The consensus has been to not perform transvaginal ultrasonography or endometrial sampling in women who are asymptomatic. However, women who are taking tamoxifen (Nolvadex) and experience vaginal bleeding need to have an immediate evaluation by endometrial sampling to rule out endometrial carcinoma.

Although endometrial carcinoma remains the most common gynecologic malignancy in the United States, it is also the most curable because of its low stage at diagnosis. Surgery remains the primary treatment modality for this type of carcinoma, with adjuvant radiotherapy reserved for patients at high risk for recurrent disease after surgery. Chemotherapeutic and hormonal agents have been used to palliate advanced-stage or recurrent disease, but durable, long-term survival has not been demonstrated. Finally, women who are taking tamoxifen (Nolvadex) for prophylaxis or adjuvant treatment of breast carcinoma need no special surveillance for the development of endometrial carcinoma. However, should any postmenopausal or abnormal vaginal bleeding occur in this group of women, immediate evaluation by endometrial sampling is required.

Cancer of the Uterine Cervix

Method of
*Michael P. Hopkins, MD, MEd,
and Wilson Sawa, MD*

Epidemiology

Invasive cancer of the cervix in the United States has decreased in morbidity and mortality significantly over the past 50 years, in large part because of mass efforts with Papanicolaou (Pap) cytologic screening. Pap smears identify many with preinvasive disease, allowing treatment prior to the development of invasive disease. In the developing world, however, cervical cancer is the third most common malignancy and accounts for significant mortality. Whereas in the United States approximately 12,000 new cases of this disease occur annually, worldwide there are approximately 500,000 new cases with 200,000 deaths. It is five to eight times more common in women affected with AIDS or HIV and represents an enormous health problem in those countries most afflicted by the virus.

The probability of a woman in the United States developing a cervical cancer is approximately 1 in 120, but this statistic is age dependent, with the highest incidence between 40 and 49 years of age. Invasive cervical cancer in the United States is largely reduced because of cytologic screening. Approximately 2 million abnormal Pap smears are found annually in the United States, but fortunately the vast majority are in the premalignant phase.

The risk factors for cervical cancer are closely associated with early age of intercourse, multiple sexual partners, and smoking. The unifying etiology is linked with the human papillomavirus (HPV), which is sexually transmitted. More than 90% of squamous carcinomas of the cervix have HPV DNA present, and a large percentage (more than 90%) of adenocarcinoma of the cervix have HPV present. The high-risk HPV types include HPV-16, -18, -31, -33, and -35.

Invasive cancer is preceded by a process of cellular dysplasia that may exist for years before transitioning. The dysplastic areas termed *squamous intraepithelial lesions* also contain HPV DNA, providing strong evidence that the premalignant phase will transition into the invasive phase and the underlying etiology is also the HPV virus. Almost all the factors that increase a woman's risk of cervical cancer are associated with increased exposure to HPV. These include multiple sexual partners, early age of intercourse, contraceptive use, socioeconomic status, other venereal diseases (including herpes simplex), and cigarette smoking. Cigarette smoking may be related to cervical cancer not only because of indirect association with increased sexual activity but also because of carcinogenic cofactors found in the tobacco or possible mitigation of cervical mucosal immunologic factors that protect against HPV.

Pathophysiology

The best evidence suggests that HPV virus is the primary pathophysiologic etiology for premalignant and malignant disease of the cervix. The HPV family consists of more than 50 subtypes, classified as either low risk or high risk based on the ability to transform cells into malignancy. The high-risk cell types include HPV-16, -18, -31, -33, -35, and -51. The HPV produces an oncogenic DNA protein in E6 and E7. The epitome is incorporated into the cell that subsequently interferes with the normal cell tumor suppressor gene p53 and RB (retinoblastoma gene). This then produces a premalignant growth called squamous intraepithelial lesion or dysplasia. The cells most susceptible to infection and transformation are located in the transformation zone where the squamous epithelium is overriding the columnar epithelium, producing a metaplastic process. The dysplastic cells, especially low-grade changes, are confined to the lower level of the epithelium and may regress spontaneously in approximately 30% to 40% of patients. As transformation proceeds into a high-grade change, they are far less likely to regress spontaneously, and they eventually attain the potential to invade the basement membrane or become an invasive process. From this point on, the malignant cells invade the stroma of the cervix, eventually into the angiolymphatic spaces, and cause a local mass or ulcer through which they eventually metastasize. Hematogenous spread is less likely, but metastasis to the liver, lung, bone, and brain can occur.

Clinical Symptomatology

The symptoms of cervical cancer vary according to the extent of the disease. In the premalignant phase there are virtually no symptoms, although occasionally patients have some discharge. As a lesion begins to develop on the cervix, the hallmark symptom is postcoital bleeding, so any patient with postcoital bleeding should be investigated. As the disease progresses, the symptoms of advanced cervical cancer are sciatica and leg edema when the disease is extending into the side wall. Physical findings are usually confined to the pelvis with advanced disease, although adenopathy in the supraclavicular or inguinal region is a possibility. The cervix either develops an ulcerative exophytic-type lesion or if it is developing in the canal, an expanding so-called barrel-shaped cervix develops with an exocervix that can appear normal. When there is a lesion on the cervix, a watery, bloody, or purulent discharge is often present. The diagnosis of cervical cancer is made by a biopsy providing a tissue diagnosis. A Pap smear is a screening test, so even though it may come back from pathology as carcinoma, a tissue biopsy must be obtained. A gross lesion of the cervix, even in the presence of a normal Pap smear, should be biopsied to avoid the misdiagnosis from a false-negative Pap smear. When an abnormal Pap smear is discovered, a colposcopy is usually performed with directed biopsies followed by further diagnostic testing. A biopsy of a grossly visible lesion with the diagnosis of invasive cancer does not mandate a cone biopsy, which should be done if there is any diagnostic question or in the presence of a biopsy that shows microinvasion. The only way to diagnose microinvasion is to have a cone biopsy with negative margins. If the colposcopy suggests invasive cancer and the biopsy does not provide the finding, a cone biopsy is necessary for diagnosis.

Pathology

The most frequent histologic subtype of cervical cancer is squamous cell cancer, accounting for approximately 80% of cases. The other main subtype, which accounts for the other 20%, is adenoma carcinoma, which can take on a variety of forms including adenosquamous, clear cell, papillary, glassy cell, mucoid type, or adenoma malignum. The percentage of adenocarcinomas is increasing because of the decreasing number of squamous cell cancers and an apparent real increase in the number of adenocarcinomas. Other rare pathologic types that can involve the cervix include melanomas, sarcomas, and small cell neuroendocrine or metastatic lesions. The literature is divided on whether the squamous cell and adenocarcinoma cell types have a similar prognosis. When corrected for tumor differentiation and stage, the survival is approximate between the cell types. The most aggressive cell type is the small cell neuroendocrine type, but fortunately these are very rare on the cervix.

Staging

Staging is one of the most critical prognostic indicators for survival, largely because of the extent of the disease and the risk for lymph node metastasis. Cervical cancer is one of the few malignancies still staged clinically, mainly because beyond stage I disease, surgery is not the

treatment of choice. Rather, radiotherapy is the main therapy for any cervical cancer beyond stage I and also can be effective for stage I cervix cancer. The system employed for cervical cancer is the FIGO (International Federation of Obstetricians and Gynecologists) staging scheme. The stage is based on the natural route of cancer progression and the risk of lymph node metastasis. The latter relates directly to the depth of stromal invasion in stage I disease and then to the stage of disease afterward (Tables 1 and 2).

Under the FIGO system, the only acceptable diagnostic imaging studies that can be employed in addition to clinical exam are intravenous pyelogram, chest radiography, cystoscopy, and sigmoidoscopy because in developing countries further sophisticated imaging studies are not routinely available. In North America, sophisticated imaging studies are routinely performed for cervical cancer although not technically incorporated into the staging. These include computerized tomography (CT) and occasionally magnetic resonance imaging (MRI). In the absence of symptoms, bone scan for occult metastasis is rarely indicated. CT scans are a common pretreatment evaluation in patients with stages II to IV cancers. Their sensitivity in detecting lymph node metastasis is approximately 65%. Evaluation of suspicious lymph nodes may involve CT-guided percutaneous biopsy or retroperitoneal selective lymph node dissection. This information may alter or define treatment, but it does not change the clinical stage based on the accepted procedures. Surgical staging, employed in the past, is rarely used now except in selected institutions.

TABLE 1 International Federation of Obstetricians and Gynecologists (FIGO) Staging for Carcinoma of the Cervix (1995)

Stage 0	Carcinoma in situ, intraepithelial carcinoma
Stage I	Cancer confined to the cervix
Ia1	Microscopic invasion of stroma measuring 3 mm or less in depth and ≤7 mm in width
Ia2	Microscopic invasion of stroma measuring >3 mm in depth but not >5 mm in depth or >7 mm in width
Ib1	Lesions >Ia2 but not >4 cm
Ib2	Lesions >4 cm
Stage II	Cancer extends beyond the cervix
IIa	Cancer involves the upper two thirds of the vagina
IIb	Obvious parametrial extension
Stage III	Extension of cancer to pelvic wall or lower vagina
IIIa	Cancer involves lower third of vagina
IIIb	Cancer extends to pelvic wall or hydronephrosis or nonfunctioning kidney
Stage IV	
IVa	Cancer involves the bladder or rectal mucosa
IVb	Cancer metastasis to distant organs

Treatment

The treatment of cervical cancer is based on the stage of disease and the patient's age and medical condition. All three modalities—chemotherapy, radiation therapy, and surgery—are used to manage invasive cervical cancer. Patients with microinvasive disease with stromal invasion less than 3 mm can be treated by conservative measures. A cone biopsy with negative margins ensures that no disease remains in the cervix. When microinvasive disease is present, expectant observation is appropriate treatment, allowing patients to preserve childbearing should they desire. In those patients for whom preservation of fertility is not an issue, a standard extrafascial hysterectomy is employed. In patients with stages Ia2, Ib1, Ib2, and in selected patients with stage IIa, radical surgery can be used. These patients can also be treated with radiation therapy. Radical hysterectomy provides an excellent overall survival for patients with early-stage cervical cancer.

TABLE 2 Relationship between Stromal Invasion or Staging and the Incidence of Lymph Node Metastasis

Invasion or Stage	Pelvic Nodes (Positive)	Aortic Nodes (Positive)
<3 mm	0–1	
3–5 mm	2.5–5	
6–10 mm	4–8	
11–15 mm	10–25	
Ib1	15–25	5–10
Ib2	30–50	15–20
IIa	15–25	5–10
IIb	30–45	20
III	50	30

CURRENT THERAPY

- Treatment is based on the stage of the disease, patient's age, and her medical condition.
- Microinvasive disease (<3 mm stromal invasion) may be treated by cone biopsy in patients who desire to preserve fertility.
- An extrafascial total abdominal hysterectomy is recommended for those patients with microinvasive disease who do not desire future fertility.
- Radical surgery can be used in patients with stage Ia2, Ib1, Ib2, and selected cases of stage IIa.
- Radical hysterectomy provides excellent overall survival for patients with early stage disease, although radiation therapy can also be used for these stages.
- Preservation of the ovaries is an option for younger patients (cervical cancer almost never metastasizes to the ovaries).
- Patients with positive lymph nodes, positive resection margins, and deep invasion benefit from adjuvant radiation therapy.
- Treatment of stages IIb to IV consists of radiation therapy combined with chemotherapy.
- Radical trachelectomy is an alternative to radical abdominal or vaginal hysterectomy for patients with early-stage squamous cell cervical cancer who are interested in preserving fertility.

A radical hysterectomy is more extensive than its standard counterpart, removing lateral parametrium and a portion of the upper vagina. A lymph node dissection is also performed to identify those patients with lymph node metastasis who are at high risk of recurrence. Because cervical cancer, either adenocarcinoma or squamous cell, virtually never metastasizes to the ovaries, surgical treatment allows for preservation of ovarian function, making it the ideal operation in the patient younger than 40 years. Alternatively, in the population older than 80 years, the vagina is quite narrowed and atrophic with the cervix flush to the fornices, so radiation treatment is often inadequate. These patients occasionally benefit from radical surgeries if their medical condition permits it. Following radical surgery patients may require radiation therapy based on high-risk features such as positive lymph nodes, positive surgical margins, and deep invasion into the cervix. In patients who are at high risk for recurrence after radical hysterectomy because of these factors, radiotherapy reduces the risk of recurrence by approximately 50%. The standard therapy for advanced disease in stages IIb to IV is with radiation therapy, both external and internal, combined with chemotherapy. Concurrent weekly cisplatin (Platinol AQ)[1] is the usual regiment. Adjuvant chemotherapy with radiation is now routine and provides a significant improvement in survival of up to 15% to 20%. Radiation therapy typically consists of full-course external beam 45 to 50 Gy administered over 25 days by a high-energy linear accelerator, followed by intracavitary radiation with either one or two intracavitary tandem treatments or high dose after loading brachytherapy, which is now

[1]Not FDA approved for this indication.

done on an outpatient basis. This provides for an additional 30 to 35 Gy to point A (a point 2 cm lateral to the internal cervical os).

Radical trachelectomy is offered as an alternative to radical abdominal or vaginal hysterectomy for patients with early-stage squamous cell cervical cancer who are interested in preserving their reproductive function. This procedure consists of removal of the cervix and the parametrium, pelvic lymph node dissection, and placement of cervical cerclage. The selected patients are in stages Ia to Ib, with most of the reported cases in stage Ib1 or lower. In addition, patients must have negative lymph nodes. The survival rates are comparable to those achieved by radical hysterectomy for similar stage and grade cervical cancer, although the number of patients treated by this new technique is limited.

Survival

Survival is related to stage and lymph node status. Table 3 shows general 5-year survival rates without concurrent chemotherapy. The survival for stage I treated by radical hysterectomy and pelvic lymphadenectomy compared to radiotherapy is equal. The survival for stage I treated with either radiotherapy or radical surgery is approximately 90% when lymph nodes are negative. This statistic drops significantly depending on the lymph node status, with survival dropping down to 60% for unilateral lymph node positivity compared to approximately 40% when lymph nodes are involved bilaterally.

Patients with normal lymph nodes but high-risk cervical factors experience a 2-year disease-free survival of 88% when treated by postoperative pelvic radiation. In contrast, the prognosis for patients with positive nodes falls to approximately 65%. Because postoperative pelvic radiotherapy does not convincingly improve that survival, researchers are investigating postoperative chemoradiotherapy for these patients with positive pelvic nodes. This also reduces the risk of death by 45% as an alternative. The approximate 5-year survival for locally advanced disease with a combination of chemotherapy and radiation is approximately 60%.

Surveillance

After primary treatment by either surgery or radiotherapy, patients return every 3 to 4 months for 2 years, then semiannually for an additional 3 years, followed by annual visits afterward. Physical examination and a Pap smear are routine. Annual chest radiography is optional, and CT scan should be reserved for symptomatic or high-risk patients because the yield of routine follow-up with CT scans is minimal.

Recurrent Cancer

The sites of recurrence are local recurrence in the pelvis, liver, lung, bone, lymph nodes, and brain. Although 75% are diagnosed within the first 24 months and 90% within the first 3 years, late recurrences can occur. The treatment for localized recurring cancer in the pelvis following radiation primary radiation or chemoradiation is pelvic exenteration, which consists of removal of the entire pelvic viscera, including uterus, vagina, bladder, and rectum or some combination. This operation should only be reserved if metastatic disease is not present. Preoperative and intraoperative assessment for metastatic disease excludes nearly three fourths of the patients from having this operation either initiated or completed. Patients who do undergo exenteration experience a 40% to 60% 5-year survival when margins and lymph nodes are negative.

Pelvic recurrence following primary surgical treatment usually involves the pelvic wall or the central pelvis. These patients should receive radiation, including both external radiation and intracavitary or interstitial radiotherapy. Chemotherapy can be combined with it and is a well-accepted method for treating recurrence. The use of chemotherapy with radiation for recurrence is not as well studied as for primary treatment. The treatment of distant metastasis is limited to chemotherapy, whereas radiation can be used for palliative treatment for metastatic disease to the bone or the brain. Chemotherapy consists of cisplatin (Platinol AQ) alone or in combination with topotecan (Hycamtin),[1] which has a reported response rate of approximately 30% to 40%. Although this must be viewed as palliative, if the patient is willing it should be initiated for symptomatic relief and prolongation of life.

REFERENCES

Keys HM, Bundy BN, Stehman FB, et al: Cisplatin, radiation, and adjuvant hysterectomy compared with radiation and adjuvant hysterectomy for bulky stage IB cervical carcinoma. N Engl J Med 1999;340(15):1154-1161.

Peters WA III, Liu PY, Barrett RJ II, et al: Concurrent chemotherapy and pelvic radiation therapy compared with pelvic radiation therapy alone as adjuvant therapy after radical surgery in high-risk early-stage cancer of the cervix. J Clin Oncol 2000;18(8):1606-1613.

Rose PG, Bundy BN, Watkins EB, et al: Concurrent cisplatin-based radiotherapy and chemotherapy for locally advanced cervical cancer. N Engl J Med 1999;340(15):1144-1153.

TABLE 3 Five-Year Survival Rates Cervical Cancer by Stage

Stage	Survival: (%)
Ia1	99–100
Ia2	95
Ib1	85–90
Ib2	65–75
IIa	75–80
IIb	65
IIIa	45
IIIb	35
IV	15

[1]Not FDA approved for this indication.

Neoplasms of the Vulva

Method of
Susan A. Davidson, MD

The female external genitalia includes the mons pubis, labia majora, labia minora, clitoris, perineal body, and the structures of the vaginal introitus or vestibule. Whether benign or malignant, vulvar neoplasms are uncommon, occur at all ages, and have varying characteristics. Therefore liberal use of biopsies is usually required for diagnosis and to guide treatment.

Benign Cystic Neoplasms

Benign cystic lesions of the vulva include Bartholin's duct cyst, sebaceous and epidermal inclusion cysts, mucinous cysts, Skene duct cysts, and cysts of the canal of Nuck. Bartholin's duct cyst, located in the posterior labia near the vaginal introitus, is most common. Treatment is usually not required in asymptomatic young women (<40 years). If the cyst is symptomatic or infected, however, drainage by marsupialization or use of a Word catheter, is indicated. Bartholin's gland carcinomas are rare, especially in women younger than 40 years of age. But if the mass feels firm or nodular, it should be biopsied.

Sebaceous and epidermal inclusion cysts are also common. They are prone to infection but rarely malignant. If an infection develops, they should be incised and drained. Mucinous cysts are rare and possibly arise from the minor vestibular glands. They are located anteriorly on the vulva, typically on the inner labia minora. Skene duct cysts are located next to the urethra. Excision of these cysts is necessary only if symptomatic.

Cysts of the canal of Nuck are located in the anterior portion of the labia majora at the termination of the insertion of the round ligament. These cysts represent herniation of the peritoneum through the inguinal canal and contain peritoneal fluid. If symptomatic, excision must be accompanied by closure of the fascial defect to prevent recurrence.

Benign Solid Neoplasms

The benign solid tumors of the vulva include fibromas, myomas, lipomas, hidradenomas, syringomas, myoblastomas, vestibular adenomas, and angiomas, among others. Benign pigmented lesions, such as nevi and seborrheic keratoses, may occasionally be found. Malignancy is rare, but most should be excised for diagnostic and therapeutic purposes.

CONDYLOMA ACUMINATUM

Vulvar condyloma acuminatum is a sexually transmitted verrucous lesion of the vulva caused by human papilloma virus (HPV), most frequently types 6 and 11. These lesions are warty growths that frequently cover large areas of the vulva. Smoking and immunosuppression are risk factors. Representative biopsies should be obtained to document disease and rule out malignancy. Wide local excision can be used for small lesions, although these growths are usually best treated by ablation.

Chemical ablative techniques include topical application of trichloroacetic acid (Tri-Chlor), podofilox (0.5%, Condylox), 5-fluorouracil[1] (1%, Fluoroplex or 5%, Efudex),[1] or imiquimod (5%, Aldara). Podophyllin can be applied twice daily for 3 days, repeated weekly for 4 weeks. Imiquimod can be applied three times per week for up to 16 weeks. Podophyllin and 5-fluorouracil should not be used in women who could become pregnant. Surgical ablative therapies include CO_2 laser vaporization and use of the Cavitron ultrasonic aspirator (CUSA), especially for extensive disease.

Intraepithelial Neoplasms of the Vulva

VULVAR INTRAEPITHELIAL NEOPLASIA

Vulvar intraepithelial neoplasia (VIN) is a dysplastic condition of the squamous epithelium whose incidence is increasing, especially in younger women. Risk factors are HPV types 16 and 18, smoking, and immunosuppression. Symptoms include pruritus (most common), pain, a noticeable lesion, and discoloration. Most patients with HPV-related disease have multifocal lesions including vaginal and cervical dysplasia. The most common location is in the area of the posterior fourchette and perineal body. Typical findings are raised white, gray, red, or mottled lesions; application of 4% acetic acid for several minutes can help identify faint lesions and outline abnormal vascular patterns. Diagnosis of VIN is made by punch biopsies through full thickness of the epithelium to rule out invasion, present in 20% of patients with VIN III (full-thickness dysplasia or carcinoma in situ). Of those patients with invasion, half (10% of VIN III) have invasion more than 1 mm.

Treatment of VIN can be categorized into excisional and ablative therapies. Patients at risk for microinvasion (unifocal disease, raised lesions, older age, and prior radiation) should have the lesion excised completely if possible. Skinning vulvectomy is rarely used because of psychological and sexual consequences related to scarring and disfigurement.

The ablative therapies can be divided into mechanical and chemical. The mechanical method most commonly used is the CO_2 laser, although use of the CUSA is also described. Both can ablate large or multifocal lesions successfully with an excellent cosmetic and functional outcome. The chemical method most commonly used is topical 5-fluorouracil (5%, Efudex).[1] Because of its teratogenic potential, it should not be used in women who could become pregnant. It can be applied on two consecutive nights weekly for 10 weeks. An alternative ablative therapy is use of imiquimod[1] (Aldara), as described earlier. Because of the irritation caused by these topical therapies, many patients have problems with treatment compliance. Residual disease should be excised to rule out invasion.

---

[1]Not FDA approved for this indication.

TABLE 1 Recurrence of Vulvar Intraepithelial Neoplasia III

Treatment Method	% Recurrence
Chemical ablation	20-40
Mechanical ablation	20-40
Wide local excision	
Negative margin	15-25
Positive margin	30-45

Patients with VIN frequently have recurrent disease, regardless of the treatment method used (Table 1). Continued smoking increases this risk, so patients should be counseled in smoking cessation. In those patients whose cancers recur and are retreated, subsequent 5-fluorouracil prophylaxis, with a single application biweekly, is used successfully to minimize further recurrences.

PAGET'S DISEASE

Paget's disease of the vulva is an uncommon condition characterized by a patchy, eczematoid lesion that frequently covers much of the vulva. Most patients are postmenopausal and present with complaints of pruritus. Although Paget's disease is an in situ disease process, 15% to 25% of patients have an underlying malignancy, usually an adenocarcinoma of the apocrine glands but occasionally an invasive Paget's. In addition, up to 30% of patients have a synchronous adenocarcinoma of the breast, colon, rectum, or upper genital tract. Screening for these cancers is therefore recommended. To assess for invasion, the lesion should be excised via wide local excision or simple vulvectomy with at least 5 mm of the adjacent subcutaneous tissue. Achieving negative margin status is frequently difficult. However, the risk of recurrence is approximately 30% whether margins are negative or positive. Thus expectant management, reserving treatment for symptomatic recurrences, is usually recommended.

Invasive Vulvar Lesions

Less than 5% of gynecologic cancers arise on the vulva. Approximately 85% are squamous cell carcinomas. The etiology of this type appears mixed. Up to 50% evolve from VIN III and are usually associated with HPV-16. These women are slightly younger (age 45-52 years).

TABLE 2 Incidence of Regional Node Metastases by Tumor Diameter

Tumor Diameter (cm)	% Positive Inguinal Nodes
<1	0-15
5-20	
25-35	
35-50	
≥50	≥50

TABLE 3 Incidence of Regional Node Metastases by Depth of Tumor Invasion

Depth of Invasion (mm)	% Positive Inguinal Nodes
<1	1-5
1-3	10-15
3-5	15-30
5-10	30-45
>10	>40

Most arise in older women (mean age 60-69 years), and suggested risk factors include immunosuppression, hypertension, diabetes mellitus, obesity, and chronic vulvar inflammation. Other histologic types are melanomas (5% to 10%), basal cell carcinomas (2% to 3%), adenocarcinomas (1%), and sarcomas (1% to 2%) Most patients present with a combination of symptoms, including pruritus, discomfort, and complaints of a mass. Examination frequently reveals a suspicious lesion, which should be biopsied for diagnosis. Vulvar cancers typically spread by local extension and lymphatic dissemination. Factors that influence dissemination include tumor size (Table 2), depth of invasion (Table 3), lymphovascular space invasion, and tumor grade. Staging is surgical and classified using the tumor, nodes, and metastasis (TNM) system (Box 1) as well as the International Federation of Gynecology and Obstetrics (FIGO) system (Box 2).

SQUAMOUS CELL CARCINOMAS AND ADENOCARCINOMAS

Surgical management of squamous cell carcinomas and adenocarcinomas depends on the size, depth of invasion, and location of the lesion. The vulvar lesion is managed with a radical excision. Management of the groins is based on depth of invasion. Lesions with invasion of <1 mm have minimal risk of lymphatic spread and do not require lymphadenectomy. All others require surgical

BOX 1 TNM Classification of Vulvar Carcinoma

T	Primary tumor
Tis	Carcinoma in situ
T1	Confined to vulva, diameter ≤2 cm
T2	Confined to vulva, diameter >2 cm
T3	Adjacent spread to urethra, vagina, perineum, or anus (any size)
T4	Infiltration of upper urethral mucosa, bladder, rectum, or bone
N	Regional lymph nodes
N0	No lymph node metastases
N1	Unilateral regional lymph node metastasis
N2	Bilateral regional lymph node metastasis
M	Distant metastases
M0	No clinical metastases
M1	Distant metastasis (including pelvic lymph node metastasis)

Abbreviation: TNM = tumor, node, metastasis.

BOX 2 FIGO Classification (With Corresponding TNM Classification) for Vulvar Carcinoma

Stage I (T1N0M0)	Tumor confined to vulva and/or perineum, ≤2 cm in greatest dimension; nodes are negative
Stage IA	Stromal invasion no greater than 1 mm
Stage IB	Stromal invasion >1 mm
Stage II (T2N0M0)	Tumor confined to the vulva and/or perineum, >2 cm in greatest dimension; nodes are negative
Stage III	
T3N0M0	Tumor of any size with adjacent spread to the lower urethra and/or the vagina or the anus
T3N1M0	Unilateral regional lymph node metastasis
T2N1M0	
Stage IVA	
T1N2M0	Tumor invades any of the following: upper urethra, bladder mucosa, rectal mucosa, pelvic bone, and/or bilateral regional node metastasis
T2N2M0	
T3N2M0	
T4 any N M0	
Stage IVB	
Any T any N M1	Any distant metastasis including pelvic lymph nodes

Abbreviations: FIGO = International Federation of Gynecology and Obstetrics; TNM = tumor, node, metastasis.

CURRENT DIAGNOSIS

- Most cystic lesions are benign. Excision is reserved for symptomatic cysts and suspicious Bartholin's gland cysts, especially in women older than 40 years of age.
- All solid lesions should be biopsied for diagnostic purposes.
- Multifocal disease requires multiple biopsies to rule out invasive disease.
- Most premalignant and malignant lesions cause pruritus, discomfort, or a noticeable lesion.
- The vagina and cervix in women with dysplastic or malignant vulvar lesions should be evaluated.

MALIGNANT MELANOMA

Malignant melanoma is the second most common vulvar malignancy. Most patients have disease on the mucosal surfaces of the vulvar introitus, clitoris, and labia minora. The vulvar lesion is treated by radical excision, but management of the groins is controversial. The risk of spread is significant with a tumor thickness greater than 0.75 mm, but survival at 5 years is only approximately 10% with groin node metastases. Some argue against node dissection for this reason. However, given some long-term survivors with modern melanoma therapy, either lymphadenectomy or sentinel lymph node dissection, as is done for other cutaneous melanomas, appears indicated.

VERRUCOUS CARCINOMA

Verrucous carcinoma is a large exophytic tumor that resembles giant condyloma acuminatum. It is a variant of squamous carcinomas but has an excellent prognosis because of the lack of metastases. Verrucous carcinomas have a high tendency to recur and should be managed with radical local excision.

BASAL CELL CARCINOMA

Basal cell carcinomas typically occur in elderly white women, are commonly located on the labia majora, and have characteristics similar to basal cell carcinomas at other sites. Treatment is wide local excision only because

assessment of the lymph nodes. Lesions located in the midline structures require bilateral groin dissection, whereas lateral lesions are managed with ipsilateral groin dissection. This surgical approach is associated with significant morbidity including disfigurement, wound breakdown, and problems with lymphocysts and chronic lymphedema. For patients with very large lesions or lesions in sensitive areas such as the clitoris, preoperative radiation, followed by less radical excision of residual disease, may minimize problems with the vulvar wound. Current investigations are ongoing in the use of sentinel lymph node dissections as a method of minimizing the groin morbidity without sacrificing survival. Positive vulvar margins or metastases to lymph nodes are managed with postoperative radiation. Survival depends on stage at diagnosis (Table 4).

TABLE 4 Survival Rate by FIGO Stage for Patients With Invasive Squamous Cell Vulvar Cancer

FIGO Stage	% Surviving 5 years
I	70-90
II	50-80
III	30-50
IV	10-15

Abbreviation: FIGO = International Federation of Gynecology and Obstetrics.

CURRENT THERAPY

- Benign solid lesions should be excised.
- After ablative treatment of vulvar intraepithelial neoplasia (VIN), excise any residual lesions to rule out occult invasive disease.
- Avoid podophyllin and 5-fluorouracil in women of reproductive potential.
- Rule out synchronous neoplasms in women with Paget's disease.
- Invasion more than 1 mm requires radical excision and lymph node evaluation.

metastases are rare. Basal cell carcinomas are prone to local recurrence, however. A malignant squamous component must be ruled out because it should be managed as a squamous cell carcinoma.

SARCOMAS

Leiomyosarcoma is the most common vulvar sarcoma and usually arises in the labia majora. Malignant fibrous histiocytoma is the second most common. Management of these lesions is radical vulvar excision.

REFERENCES

Garland SM: Imiquimod. Curr Opin Infect Dis 2003;16:85-89.

Homesley HD, Bundy BN, Sedlis A, et al: Prognostic factors for groin node metastasis in squamous cell carcinoma of the vulva (a Gynecologic Oncology Group study). Gynecol Oncol 1993;49:279-283.

Krebs HB: The use of topical 5-fluorouracil in the treatment of genital condylomas. Obstet Gynecol Clin North Am 1987;14(2):559-568.

Modesitt SC, Waters AB, Walton L, et al: Vulvar intraepithelial neoplasia III: Occult cancer and the impact of margin status on recurrence. Obstet Gynecol 1998;92(6):962-966.

Phillips GL, Bundy BN, Okagaki T, et al: Malignant melanoma of the vulva treated by radical hemivulvectomy, a prospective study of the Gynecologic Oncology Group. Cancer 1994;73:2626-2632.

Tebes S, Cardosi R, Hoffman M: Paget's disease of the vulva. Am J Obstet Gynecol 2002;187:281-284.

Trimble CL, Trimble EL, Woodruff JD: Diseases of the vulva. In Hernandez E, Atkinson BF (eds): Clinical Gynecologic Pathology. Philadelphia, WB Saunders, 1995, pp 1-90.

Wright VC, Chapman WB: Colposcopy of intraepithelial neoplasia of the vulva and adjacent sites. Obstet Gynecol Clin North Am 1993;20(1):231-255.

Psychiatric Disorders

Alcohol Use Disorders

Method of
Richard L. Brown, MD, MPH

Alcohol use disorders are major public health problems in the United States. Alcohol consumption is linked to 75,000 deaths per year, with 30 years of lost life per death, and substantial numbers of acute injuries, chronic diseases, hospitalizations, emergency department visits, suicides, episodes of abuse and violence, and other crimes.

Health care professionals are in ideal positions to recognize and assist patients with risky and problem drinking. Despite recommendations by the U.S. Preventive Services Task Force, the National Institute on Alcohol Abuse and Alcoholism (NIAAA), and others, few health care professionals routinely provide alcohol screening, brief intervention, and referral services. With application of the medical counseling skills commonly used to manage other chronic health conditions, health care professionals can improve health and other outcomes for many patients with alcohol use disorders.

Diagnosis

Alcohol consumption is best considered as a continuum with five major guideposts. Current recommendations on low-risk drinking do not take into account long-term cardiovascular risk. Up to two standard drinks (Box 1) per day for men and one standard drink per day for women may be beneficial in reducing cardiovascular risk; more can increase cardiovascular risk through unfavorable effects on lipids and blood pressure.

For individuals with particular health problems, such as liver disease, pancreatitis, peptic ulcer disease, cardiomyopathy, dementia, encephalopathies, neuropathies, and current or prior alcohol and drug dependencies, any use of alcohol is risky. Alcohol should also be avoided completely by pregnant women and by individuals taking medicines such as certain antibiotics, anticoagulants, anticonvulsants, antidepressants, antihistamines, anti-inflammatories, anxiolytics, H_2 blockers, hypoglycemics, muscle relaxants, and opioid analgesics.

Individuals with at-risk drinking and abuse are by definition able to control their drinking without difficulty. They can readily decrease their drinking if they wish to do so.

Alcohol dependence is synonymous with alcoholism and alcohol addiction. The primary symptom is a consistent inability, or an inconsistent ability, to control one's drinking. Alcohol dependence may occur without any physical dependence, especially in those 18 years of age or under. Dependent individuals often suffer similar and more severe negative health and social consequences than seen with alcohol abuse (Table 1).

A key neurophysiologic lesion of alcoholism and other addictions occurs in the mesolimbic dopaminergic neural pathway in the brain's ventral tegmentum. In normal individuals, this pathway provides pleasurable reinforcement when hunger or sex drives are satisfied. In addicted individuals, neuronal function in this pathway is regulated by different DNA sequences. Thus the neurophysiologic basis of the disease of addiction involves a hijacking of the mesolimbic pathway such that it drives addictive behaviors along with or instead of adaptive eating and sexual behaviors. For alcoholics, the resulting cravings and impulses to drink make it difficult to avoid alcohol.

Alcohol Screening

Alcohol screening is recommended as a component of routine preventive care for several reasons. The combined prevalence of at-risk drinking, alcohol abuse, and alcohol dependence approaches or surpasses 20% in many practice settings. Most individuals with such drinking patterns lack obvious symptoms and signs. Such drinking often responds to intervention or treatment. Early identification and management of such drinking can avert more serious and sometimes irreversible health and social consequences. Screening, followed when warranted by brief interventions, saves nearly $1000 per patient in documented costs of health care utilization, motor vehicle crashes, and criminal justice system involvement; further undocumented cost savings are likely.

In most health care settings, the best source of information for screening and more detailed assessment is the history. Physical examination reveals signs of alcohol overuse only in the relatively few patients with advanced

1273

alcohol dependence. Laboratory studies, such as gamma-glutamyltransferase and mean corpuscular volume, are normal in most patients with alcohol use disorders. Carbohydrate-deficient transferrin, a newer blood test that can suggest alcohol overuse, lacks sensitivity, especially for episodic heavy drinkers. Self-reports of drinking usually match or exceed reports by family members. In emergency settings, blood alcohol levels can help document alcohol-related trauma and tolerance.

Several brief batteries of yes-or-no screening questions can identify most individuals with at-risk drinking and alcohol use disorders (Box 2). Such questions can be incorporated conversationally into routine histories. The CAGE (cut down, annoyed, guilty, eye-opener) questions are used most often and are most accurate in adult men. The TWEAK questions (tolerance, worried, eye-opener, amnesia, cut down) are more accurate in women, especially pregnant women. The CRAFFT (six questions include the words *Car, Relax, Alone, Friends, Forget,* and *Trouble*) is the best validated screen for adolescents. The SMAST-G (Short Michigan Alcoholism Screening Test–Geriatric Version) is useful for those over 65 years of age. The Two-Item Conjoint Screen (TICS) screens simultaneously for alcohol and drug problems; a conjoint screening approach has merit because one third of individuals who have substance use disorders have drug disorders.

The screens just cited are useful in identifying abuse and dependence. For patients with negative screens, questions on quantity and frequency of alcohol use can identify at-risk drinkers. Alternatively, the 10 multiple-choice questions of the AUDIT (Alcohol Use Disorders Identification Test) can be incorporated into written health history forms and can sensitively identify at-risk drinkers and patients with alcohol use disorders. An advantage of written questionnaires is they can save clinician time. A disadvantage is that they circumvent the opportunity to identify nonverbal responses to screening questions that may suggest an alcohol problem.

After Alcohol Screening

Alcohol screening provides a preliminary indication of where patients lie on the spectrum of alcohol use. Patients who abstain should be asked why. Some quit because of prior difficulties with alcohol. Others who abstain because of disillusionment about drinking by family members may be at high genetic risk for alcohol dependence. Endorsing moderate drinking for its cardioprotective benefit may be ill-advised for many abstainers, whose attempts at moderate drinking could trigger alcohol dependence.

TABLE 1 Common Negative Consequences of Alcohol Use

	Symptoms and Signs of Alcohol Use Disorders	
Category	Earlier, More Reversible	Later, Less Reversible
Biomedical	Gastritis, esophageal reflux, dyspepsia, peptic ulcer, hepatic inflammation, acute pancreatitis, diarrhea Hypertension Weight gain Mild traumatic injuries Sleep disturbance and fatigue Sexual dysfunction	Cirrhosis, esophageal varices, hepatic encephalopathy, chronic pancreatitis; cardiomyopathy, coronary artery disease, cardiac dysrhythmias; bone marrow and immune suppression; head, neck, and gastrointestinal cancers; cerebellar degeneration, dementia, malnutrition; major trauma-related disabilities
Psychological	Agitation, irritability, mood swings, dysphoria, anxiety disorders, depressive disorders, psychosomatic symptoms, hostility	Persistent, severe mental illness
Family	Marital and family dysfunction, childhood behavior and school problems, mental health problems in family members	Divorce, neglect, abuse, violence, estrangement
Other relationships	Alienation and loss of old friends, gravitation toward others who drink heavily	Social isolation
Work/school	Decline in performance, frequent job changes, frequent absences (especially on Mondays), requests for work excuses, initial preservation of work/school function in career-oriented individuals such as physicians	Chronic unemployment
Legal	Driving while intoxicated; various misdemeanors	Incarceration
Financial	Borrowing, debt	Insolvency, homelessness
Religious/spiritual	Shame, self-disgust, disconnection	Alienation

BOX 2 Alcohol Screening Instruments

CAGE Questions

1. Have you ever thought you should cut down on your drinking?
2. Have you ever felt Annoyed by others criticizing your drinking?
3. Have you ever felt bad or Guilty about your drinking?
4. Do you have a drink to help you get started in the morning (Eye-opener)?

One or more positive responses indicates the need for further assessment.

TWEAK

1. How many drinks does it take before you begin to feel the first effects of the alcohol? (Tolerance)
2. Have your friends or relatives Worried or complained about your drinking in the past year?
3. Do you sometimes take a drink in the morning when you first get up (Eye-opener)?
4. Are there times when you drink and afterward you can't remember what you said or did? (Amnesia)
5. Do you sometimes feel the need to cut (Kut) down on your drinking?

For item 1, more than two drinks scores 2 points.
For item 2, a positive response scores 2 points.
For items 3, 4, and 5, each positive response scores 1 point.
A total of 2 to 3 points indicates a possible alcohol problem.

CRAFFT

1. Have you ever ridden in a Car driven by someone (including yourself) who was high or had been using alcohol or drugs?
2. Do you ever use alcohol or drugs to Relax, feel better about yourself, or fit in?
3. Do you ever use alcohol or drugs while you are by yourself Alone?
4. Do you ever Forget things you did while using alcohol or drugs?
5. Do your Family or Friends ever tell you that you should cut down on your drinking or drug use?
6. Have you ever gotten into Trouble while you were using alcohol or drugs?

Two or more positive responses indicate the need for further assessment.

S-MAST-G

In the past year …
1. When talking with others, do you ever underestimate how much you actually drink?
2. After a few drinks, have you sometimes not eaten or been able to skip a meal because you didn't feel hungry?
3. Does having a few drinks help decrease your shakiness or tremors?
4. Does alcohol sometimes make it hard for you to remember parts of the day or night?
5. Do you usually take a drink to relax or calm your nerves?
6. Do you drink to take your mind off your problems?
7. Have you ever increased your drinking after experiencing a loss in your life?
8. Has a doctor or nurse ever said they were worried or concerned about your drinking?
9. Have you ever made rules to manage your drinking?
10. When you feel lonely, does having a drink help?

Two or more positive responses indicate a probable alcohol problem.

Two-Item Conjoint Screen

1. In the last year, have you ever drunk or used drugs more than you meant to?
2. Have you felt you wanted or needed to cut down on your drinking or drug use in the last year?

One or two positive responses indicate the need for further assessment.

AUDIT: Alcohol Use Disorders Identification Test

Q1. How often do you consume a drink containing alcohol?
0. Never
1. Monthly or less
2. 2 to 4 times a month
3. 2 or 3 times a week
4. 4 or more times a week

Q2. How many drinks containing alcohol do you have on a typical day when you are drinking?
0. 1 or 2
1. 3 or 4
2. 5 or 6
3. 7 to 9
4. 10 or more

Q3. How often do you have 6 or more drinks on one occasion?
0. Never
1. Less than monthly
2. Monthly
3. Weekly
4. Daily or almost daily

Q4. How often during the last year have you found that you were not able to stop drinking once you had started?
0. Never
1. Less than monthly
2. Monthly
3. Weekly
4. Daily or almost daily

Q5. How often during the last year have you failed to do what was normally expected from you because of drinking?
0. Never
1. Less than monthly
2. Monthly
3. Weekly
4. Daily or almost daily

Q6. How often during the last year have you needed a drink in the morning to get yourself going after a heavy drinking session the night before?
0. Never
1. Less than monthly
2. Monthly
3. Weekly
4. Daily or almost daily

Q7. How often during the last year have you had a feeling of guilt or remorse after drinking?
0. Never
1. Less than monthly
2. Monthly
3. Weekly
4. Daily or almost daily

Continued

BOX 2 Alcohol Screening Instruments—cont'd

Q8. How often during the last year have you been unable to remember what happened the night before because you had been drinking?
   0. Never
   1. Less than monthly
   2. Monthly
   3. Weekly
   4. Daily or almost daily

Q9. Have you or someone else been injured as a result of your drinking?
   0. No
   1. Yes, but not in the last year
   2. Yes, during the last year

Q10. Has a relative, a friend, or a physician or other health care worker been concerned about your drinking or suggested that you cut down?
   0. No
   1. Yes, but not in the last year
   2. Yes, during the last year

Add up the numbers to the left of each response.
   More than 8 points: Positive for an alcohol use disorder for both men and women.
   More than 4 points: May be positive for an alcohol use disorder for women.

Alcohol Case-Finding

Case-finding involves determining whether patients who exhibit possible negative consequences of drinking (see Table 1) truly have alcohol problems. Treating the consequences of excessive drinking without addressing the root cause usually fails. Case-finding can begin with screening questions and proceed with brief alcohol assessment.

Brief Alcohol Assessment

Brief alcohol assessment identifies where individuals lie on the spectrum of alcohol use. The objectives of assessment are to discern whether patients are suffering negative consequences of drinking and additional symptoms of alcohol dependence.

The negative consequences of drinking fall into eight categories (see Table 1). Clinicians should aim to identify alcohol use disorders before later, less reversible consequences occur. Psychological consequences often occur earliest. Full-fledged mood disorders and anxiety disorders may result from or lead to alcohol use disorders, but the earliest negative consequences are often subclinical anxiety and depressive symptoms.

Alcohol-related psychological symptoms often lead to dysfunction in significant relationships. An alcohol use disorder in one family member often produces stress, anxiety, depression, and psychosomatic symptoms in others. Such symptoms should therefore prompt questions on drinking by loved ones.

Health consequences of drinking may occur early or late in the course of alcohol abuse or dependence. Alcohol can produce blood pressure elevations by a direct pressor effect on arterioles and by autonomic instability of subclinical withdrawal syndromes. Individuals who engage in episodic heavy drinking may exhibit labile hypertension. Drinking may produce fatigue by interfering with deep, restorative stages of sleep.

To assess for the loss of control seen with alcohol dependence, ask whether patients set rules about drinking and have difficulty adhering to them. To assess for preoccupying thoughts, ask whether patients sometimes have difficulty getting thoughts of drinking out of their minds.

To assess for compulsive drinking, ask whether individuals have particular difficulty limiting their drinking after starting to drink. To assess for physical dependence, ask whether individuals experience shakiness hours after unusually heavy drinking. Alcohol-dependent patients may have just some of these symptoms.

Intervention

Brief interventions for alcohol problems involve counseling skills that clinicians routinely employ in managing other health problems. Recommended steps follow the FERNSS mnemonic:

- *Feedback*: Express concern that the patient's drinking may be linked with current consequences or future risks. When possible, provide authoritative medical opinion for alcohol-related health consequences. To avoid arguments, raise questions about the link between alcohol and social consequences rather than making definitive pronouncements. Emphasize risks and consequences that are important to the patient; for example, attempt to link drinking to chief complaints or to other difficulties that the patient wishes to avoid or resolve. Initially avoid alcohol-related diagnostic labels, which can elicit anger and shame. Finally, ask for the patient's point of view.
- *Education*: Explain how drinking can lead to medical or other concerns. For example, explain how alcohol can relax esophageal sphincters and cause reflux. To avoid arguments, when patients offer competing explanations for symptoms, acknowledge their possibility and affirm that alcohol is also a likely contributor.
- *Recommend*: Brief interventions are geared toward eliciting behavior change. Make a specific recommendation that the patient takes a particular action (Table 2). For patients with symptoms of alcohol dependence, initially recommend consultation with an alcohol specialist. Alternative recommendations could be a 1-month trial of abstinence to test for control and to assess whether possible consequences improve. Attendance at self-help meetings can help patients determine whether they have similarities to others who are committed to stop drinking.

TABLE 2 Recommendations to Make During Brief Interventions

Clinical Circumstances						
Alcohol Dependence Symptoms	Family History of Dependence	Health Issue or Alcohol/Medicine Incompatibility	Alcohol Abuse	At-Risk Drinking	Declined Recommendation Above	Recommendation
x						Consult with an alcohol treatment specialist or program.
					x	Attend self-help meetings.
	x	x			x	Abstain.
			x	x	x	Adhere to low-risk limits.
					x	Cut down as much as willing.

For patients with at-risk drinking or alcohol abuse and positive family histories of alcohol dependence, recommend abstinence as the safest option. As the first option for patients with alcohol abuse or at-risk drinking who have negative family histories of alcohol dependence, recommend adhering to limits for low-risk drinking.

- *Negotiate*: When patients decline recommendations, avoid arguments. Collaborate in identifying and attempting to work around barriers to adherence. Offer alternative recommendations. Express concern that continuing present drinking patterns may not allow them to attain their goals, such as more restful sleep, relief of gastric discomfort, or a better relationship. Support any commitment to decrease drinking.

- *Secure the agreement*: For patients who are willing to take action, secure concrete and specific agreement on what they will do by when. For example, for patients who are willing to set weekly and daily drinking limits, ask them to specify permissible ranges of numbers of standard drinks for each day of the week. Record the patient's agreement in writing and provide a copy for them. Written agreements are not binding but help ground discussions at follow-up visits.

- *Set follow-up*: Ask the patient to specify when follow-up contact would be useful, usually within 1 month. Provide two pieces of advice: (1) Seek immediate care for any symptoms of alcohol withdrawal, and (2) Reassure the patient that any difficulties they have implementing their plan will elicit concern and further discussion about what to do next but neither anger nor judgment.

- *At the follow-up visit*: Review the patient's progress. For patients who make positive changes, reinforce their success, and use the FERNSS approach in setting long-term plans for healthier drinking. For patients who had difficulty modifying their drinking, assess for difficulties with control; consider allowing for another try or referring for a consultation.

For patients who decline to address their risky or problem drinking, acknowledge that they are not ready to make a change. Let them know you are open to any future questions, or advise them where they can seek help if they change their minds. Although many physicians express frustration in managing alcohol use disorders, research shows that adherence to treatment recommendations on drinking is no worse than recommendations made for other chronic diseases.

Although some clinicians blame denial for patients' resistance to change, research shows that alcohol-dependent patients use denial as a defense mechanism no more frequently than non-alcohol-dependent patients. Clinicians who project warmth, empathy, respect, and partnership elicit more accurate information and adherence than those who project frustration, impatience, and judgment.

Detoxification and Withdrawal

Withdrawal from alcohol and other sedatives may be fatal. Goals are to maximize comfort, avoid oversedation and other complications, and engage patients in alcohol treatment.

Stage 1, or minor withdrawal, is characterized by tachycardia, hypertension, fever lower than 38.3°C (101°F), diaphoresis, nausea, vomiting, restlessness, agitation, and tremors. In stage 2, these symptoms and signs worsen, and hallucinations occur. Disorientation and mental clouding herald stage 3, also known as delirium tremens, or DTs. Seizures may complicate any of the three stages.

Risk factors for severe withdrawal include prior severe withdrawal, age older than 40 years, heavier and more regular drinking, higher tolerance to alcohol, poor health, and poor nutrition. Patients at low risk for severe withdrawal are best treated in supervised community settings, where favorable staffing and environmental conditions result in less need for pharmacologic treatment. Hospitalization is indicated for patients at high risk for severe withdrawal or seizures and for those with underlying medical conditions that can be aggravated by withdrawal, such as coronary artery disease or type I diabetes. Management includes ensuring appropriate hydration, restoring magnesium and other electrolyte balance, and administering thiamine and other vitamins.

Benzodiazepine loading is recommended for high-risk patients with recent and steady heavy drinking and blood alcohol levels of zero and for patients with any symptoms of withdrawal. Diazepam (Valium), 20 mg,[3] or lorazepam (Ativan),[1] 5 mg,[3] is repeated every 2 hours for a total of three doses. During loading and at any time during detoxification, sedatives should be withheld when patients become sleepy. Patients at low risk for withdrawal can be observed until symptoms begin. Long-acting benzodiazepines,[1] such as diazepam and chlordiazepoxide, provide the most comfortable detoxification. Short-acting benzodiazepines, such as lorazepam, should be reserved for patients with severe hepatic dysfunction (jaundice or elevated prothrombin times) or for patients who have already received large doses of long-acting benzodiazepines (e.g., 300 mg of diazepam). Obtain urine drug screens before administering any controlled substances.

Patients in alcohol withdrawal must be reassessed frequently. Avoid fixed, repeated doses of sedatives and imprecise "as needed" orders. Withdrawal treatment protocols that involve frequent scoring of withdrawal signs and symptoms, such as the CIWA-A (Clinical Institute Withdrawal Assessment for Alcohol), provide the most reliable guidance for continuing sedative administration.

Minor withdrawal can be treated with carbamazepine (Tegretol),[1] gabapentin (Neurontin),[1] or β-blockers. However, β-blockers can mask autonomic symptoms that herald severe withdrawal, which must be treated with a sedative. Withdrawal from alcohol or multiple sedatives can be treated with phenobarbital.[1]

Alcohol withdrawal seizures are treated with benzodiazepines and carbamazepine,[1] which should be discontinued after withdrawal. Avoid phenothiazines, which lower seizure thresholds; instead, use hydroxyzine (Atarax) for nausea and haloperidol (Haldol)[1] for agitation that does not respond to benzodiazepines.

Alcohol Treatment

According to authoritative, evidence-based reviews, treatment for alcohol dependence is effective. Although durable abstinence may elude many patients, those who receive treatment drink less, suffer fewer and less severe relapses, and exhibit better psychosocial function on average than those who do not.

A combination of professional and lay treatments is most effective. Next most effective is professionally administered treatment alone. Many patients can recover through lay-administered self-help groups, such as Alcoholics Anonymous or Rational Recovery. Physicians can facilitate referrals by arranging for escorts by other recovering patients and by suggesting that patients try several meetings and continue at those where they feel most comfortable.

[1]Not FDA approved for this indication.
[3]Exceeds dosage recommended by the manufacturer.

The mainstays of professionally administered alcohol treatment are nonpharmacologic. Psychoeducational, cognitive–behavioral, family, and network approaches are effective. A newer approach, motivational interviewing, is effective in changing drinking and other health-risk behaviors. Increasingly used in general medical settings, motivational interviewing can be used when brief interventions or referrals are ineffective.

Pharmacologic adjuncts can be helpful. Although disulfiram (Antabuse), an aversive agent, did not confer lasting benefit in a 1-year randomized controlled trial, it may facilitate abstinence in early recovery for patients who are prone to impulsive drinking. Naltrexone (ReVia), an opioid antagonist, reduces cravings by alcohol-dependent patients and facilitates receipt of nonpharmacologic treatment. Both medicines are safe for patients with transaminase levels less than three times normal. Approved in 2004 by the Food and Drug Administration (FDA), acamprosate (Campral) reduces cravings and bolsters abstinence for at least 12 months. Nalmefene (Revex),[1] a promising opioid antagonist, is now available in the United States. All pharmacologic treatments should supplement nonpharmacologic treatments.

[1]Not FDA approved for this indication.

 CURRENT DIAGNOSIS

Abstinence: No More Than a Few Drinks Per Year

Low-risk drinking

- For men, no more than 14 standard drinks per week and 4 per occasion
- For women, no more than 7 to 11 drinks per week and 3 per occasion
- For elders (65 years of age or older), no more than 7 drinks per week and 1 per occasion

At-risk drinking

- Exceeding above criteria for low-risk drinking
- Any alcohol use in the presence of certain health conditions or with certain medications
- Drinking that does not qualify for abuse or dependence

Abuse

- Continued drinking despite repeated adverse health and psychosocial consequences
- Repeated alcohol use in physically hazardous situations, such as while driving
- Dependence (synonymous with alcoholism or alcohol addiction)
- Difficulty controlling drinking
- Preoccupation with obtaining or drinking alcohol
- Difficulty stopping drinking, especially once started
- Physical dependence (propensity to suffer withdrawal with sudden cessation or diminution of alcohol use)

- Intervene or refer to treatment by giving feedback and education on risks and consequences, making a recommendation, negotiating for the most behavior change, securing a concrete and specific behavioral agreement, and setting follow-up for assessing progress.
- Provide or arrange for supervised detoxification, as necessary.
- For patients who cannot abstain or maintain low-risk drinking on their own, attempt referral to specialists and/or self-help groups. Also, consider naltrexone (ReVia), disulfiram (Antabuse), and acamprosate (Campral).
- In follow-up, help patients assess progress toward their substance use and other goals, revise their plan for attaining their goals as needed, and access resources.

Diagnosis

Nearly half of patients with addictive disorders have other psychiatric disorders. A common error is to treat the concomitant psychiatric disorder without recognizing or addressing the substance use disorder. All patients with psychiatric disorders should be assessed for substance use disorders. For those with both, a best first step, if the psychiatric symptoms do not demand immediate pharmacologic treatment, is to stop the substance use. For example, sometimes stopping alcohol is effective in treating symptoms of major depression.

For patients with alcohol dependence, it is best not to prescribe potentially addictive sedatives. Insomnia is expected during the first year of recovery and best treated nonpharmacologically or with noneuphoric agents, such as trazodone (Desyrel)[1] or doxepin (Sinequan).[1] For patients with alcohol dependence and anxiety disorders, clonazepam (Klonopin)[1] and clorazepate (Tranxene), long-acting agents that generate little euphoria, are the preferred benzodiazepines for patients who do not respond to, or cannot tolerate, other classes of pharmaceuticals. Patients with alcohol dependence and chronic psychosis need regular and coordinated care by primary care, mental health, and addictions professionals; again, for patients who require benzodiazepines, long-acting agents are best.

REFERENCES

American Psychiatric Association: Diagnostic and Statistical Manual of Mental Health Disorders, 4th ed. Washington, DC, Author, 1994.
Bayard M, McIntyre J, Hill KR, Woodside J Jr: Alcohol withdrawal syndrome. Am Fam Physician 2004;69:1443-1450.
Fleming MF, Mundt MP, French MT, et al: Brief physician advice for problem drinkers: Long-term efficacy and benefit-cost analysis. Alcohol Clin Exp Res 2002;26:36-43.
Miller WR, Rollnick S: Motivational Interviewing: Preparing People for Change. New York, Guilford Press, 2002.

[1]Not FDA approved for this indication.

National Institute on Alcohol Abuse and Alcohol: Helping Patients With Alcohol Problems: A Health Practitioner's Guide. Rockville, Md, Author, 2004.
Sullivan JT, Sykora K, Schneiderman J, et al: Assessment of alcohol withdrawal: The revised Clinical Institute Withdrawal Assessment for Alcohol scale (CIWA-As). Br J Addict 1989;84:1353-1357.
U.S. Preventive Services Task Force: Screening and Behavioral Counseling Interventions in Primary Care to Reduce Alcohol Misuse: Recommendation Statement. Rockville, Md, April 2004. Agency for Healthcare Research and Quality on line: Available at http://www.ahrq.gov/clinic/3rduspstf/alcohol/alcomisrs.htm

Drug Abuse

Method of
Joyce A. Tinsley, MD

The U.S. Department of Health and Human Services reported that in 2001 nearly 7% of the population, or 16 million Americans age 12 and older, were actively using illegal drugs. The combination of drug and alcohol use costs taxpayers a staggering sum; an estimated $143 billion per year is spent on associated health care costs, extra law enforcement, motor vehicle accidents, crime, and lost productivity. The president's fiscal year 2003 budget included $4.4 billion for all substance abuse–related activities, with $127 million earmarked for treatment services. The abuse of legal drugs, such as prescription medications and nicotine, is also a serious problem. Nicotine dependence is responsible for more morbidity and mortality than any other abused substance and is so highly addictive that quitting eludes many who try to stop.

Many addicts in need of treatment do not get it. Reasons for this include a lack of treatment and recovery resources, the stigma surrounding drug use, and pessimism about recovery from addictions. Unfortunately, much of the clinical pessimism about addiction treatment is based on an inadequate or outdated knowledge base. At a minimum, clinicians should be familiar with the common drugs of abuse; signs of intoxication, withdrawal, and overdose; management of simple detoxification; and contemporary treatment options.

Diagnosis

In the *Diagnostic and Statistical Manual of Mental Disorders, 4th ed., Text Revision* (*DSM-IV-TR*), published by the American Psychiatric Association, disorders are classified as either abuse or dependence (Box 1).

These criteria may be applied to any drug within the major classes of addictive substances. Inherent to the definition of dependence is the concept of impaired control. In other words, the addict cannot predictably control when or how much of a substance he or she will use. In both abuse and dependence, the individual continues to use the substance even though it causes problems in one or more important life areas. The diagnosis is based on behaviors

BOX 1 *DSM IV-TR* Diagnostic Criteria

Substance Abuse

A maladaptive pattern of use leading to clinically significant impairment and distress in at least one of the following areas within a 12-month period:

1. Failure to fulfill major role obligations at work, school, or home
2. Use in physically hazardous situations
3. Substance-related legal problems
4. Use despite social or interpersonal problems exacerbated by use of the substance

Substance Dependence

A maladaptive pattern of use leading to impairment and distress in at least three of the following areas within a 12-month period:

1. Tolerance—need for increasing amounts to achieve intoxication or desired effect or diminished effect with continued use of the same amount.
2. Withdrawal—development of characteristic withdrawal symptoms or use of the same or related substance to relieve or avoid withdrawal symptoms.
3. The substance is used in larger amounts or over longer time periods than intended.
4. Inability to cut down or control use.
5. Significant time is spent in activities related to obtaining the substance or recovering from its effects.
6. Social, occupational, or recreational activities are given up or reduced.
7. Use continues despite knowledge of harmful physical or psychological effects.

Adapted from: American Psychiatric Association: Diagnostic and statistical manual of mental disorders 4th ed., text revision (DSM-IV-TR). Washington, DC: Author, 2000. Used with permission.

---

surrounding the drug abuse rather than the amount consumed. Substance dependence, synonymous with addiction, is the more advanced disorder.

It is often challenging to diagnose drug abuse. Patients may be hesitant to reveal illegal drug abuse or the misuse of prescription drugs. Clinicians should ask questions that are perceived to be nonjudgmental. For instance, asking, "Has anyone ever been concerned about your drug use?" is less likely to be met with resistance than initial questions that ask about quantity or frequency of use. Supplemental history from significant others and objective data from urine drug screens can help clarify the diagnosis. Some addicts readily admit their addictions. For instance,

heroin users have been known to overestimate their use in order to receive a more generous opiate dose for detoxification or maintenance. Heroin and cocaine addicts with advanced dependence often acknowledge their addictions because of devastating social, legal, or physical consequences. In addition, a majority of cigarette smokers express a desire to stop smoking and attempt to get help.

Nicotine

Nicotine dependence is similar to other drug addictions in that it is best viewed as a chronic disease that requires ongoing attention. It is the addiction on which primary care clinicians may have the greatest impact. An estimated 25% of adults in the United States smoke cigarettes, and 70% of current smokers would like to quit. In view of the lethal nature of smoking, the high percentage of smokers who want to quit, and the number of individuals affected, the clinician should be prepared to encourage smoking cessation.

The nicotine withdrawal syndrome is a serious obstacle for patients who want to stop smoking. Withdrawal symptoms often begin within hours after the last cigarette, peak within 2 to 3 days, and may continue for several weeks. Nicotine cravings last much longer. Early abstinence is characterized by irritability, anxiety, restlessness, depressed mood, inattention, and insomnia. A nicotine replacement product is effective in ameliorating many of the withdrawal symptoms.

Brief counseling improves smoking cessation rates, especially when directed toward the patient's unique situation. The U.S. Public Health Service recommends easy-to-follow strategies that clinicians can use in counseling patients to quit smoking (Table 1). The "5 As" represent a strategy particularly helpful to the clinician who wants to initiate discussion about a patient's tobacco use. The "5 Rs" may be used if the patient lacks motivation to stop smoking. Finally, an action plan known by the mnemonic STAR is a guide for those ready to make a quit attempt.

There is solid evidence that several medications are effective in improving smokers' quit rates (Table 2). Unless there are contraindications to the use of these medications, a first-line agent, either a nicotine replacement product or bupropion (Zyban), should be recommended to patients who want to stop smoking. If initial agents are ineffective or contraindicated, the clinician should consider recommending a second-line agent,

---

TABLE 1 Office-Based Interventions for Smoking Cessation

Initial Intervention: 5 As	Motivational Intervention: 5 Rs	Action Plan: STAR
Ask about tobacco use.	Relevance: Why stop?	Set a quit date.
Advise the patient to quit.	Risks: Personalize them.	Tell others of plan.
Assess readiness to quit.	Rewards: Potential benefits.	Anticipate difficulties.
Assist in the quit attempt.	Roadblocks: Identify and address barriers.	Remove tobacco products.
Arrange follow-up.	Repetition: Repeat message at the next visit.	

Adapted from: U.S. Public Health Service: Treating tobacco use and dependence—clinician's packet. A how-to guide for implementing the Public Health Service clinical practice guideline. March 2003. http://www.surgeongeneral.gov/tobacco/clinpack.html

TABLE 2 Pharmacotherapy of Smoking Cessation

	Instructions	Dose	Advantages	Disadvantages
Nicotine gum/over-the-counter (Nicorette)	Chew until peppery taste, then park between cheek and gum.	2 or 4 mg per piece. Maximum 24 pieces per day. Use for up to 6 mo.	Flexibility with scheduled and/or prn doses to relieve cravings. Delivery is more rapid than the patch.	Incomplete absorption when chewed incorrectly. Cannot eat or drink while using. Caution with dental or jaw problems.
Transdermal nicotine patch/over-the-counter (Nicoderm)	Apply to skin daily. Available as 16-h or 24-h patch. Do not smoke while using.	Start 21 mg × 6 wk (14 mg if weight <100 lb or smoking <1/2 ppd). Taper to 14 mg, then 7 mg × 2-4 wk. Use for 2-3 mo total.	Easy to use. Few side effects. Releases steady dose of nicotine to reduce cravings. Can use in combination with gum.	Releases nicotine more slowly. No response for sudden cravings. Can cause skin irritation. Consider lower dosing in known cardiac disease.
Nasal spray/prescription (Nicotrol NS)	Use every 1-2 h. Take deep breath, spray into each nostril, and exhale through mouth.	From 8 to 40 times per day. Use for 3 mo with gradual taper.	Fastest delivery of nicotine. Good at reducing sudden cravings.	Nose and sinus irritation common at first. Caution with allergies or asthma.
Nasal inhaler/prescription (Nicotrol Inhaler)	Inhale nicotine by bringing inhaler to mouth when desired.	From 6 to 16 cartridges per day for first 3-6 wk. Use for 3 mo with gradual taper.	Delivers nicotine as quickly as gum. Satisfies hand-to-mouth habit. Few side effects.	May cause mouth or throat irritation. Caution with asthma or chronic lung disease.
Bupropion HCl/prescription (Zyban)	Take 1 pill in the morning, 1 in late afternoon. Start 2 wk before quit date.	150 mg SR bid. Continue for 7 to 12 weeks after quitting.	Easy to use, few side effects. May be more helpful when used with the patch.	Contraindicated in seizure, eating disorders, patients taking Wellbutrin or MAOIs, pregnancy, or breast-feeding.

Abbreviations: bid = twice daily; MAOIs = monoamine oxidase inhibitors; ppd = packs per day; prn = as needed; SR = slow release.
Adapted from: American Cancer Society: Set yourself free; deciding how to quit, a smoker's guide. 1999.

1281

specifically clonidine (Catapres)[1] or nortriptyline (Pamelor).[1] The Public Health Service provides additional information to clinicians who want to learn more about how to help patients stop smoking on their Web site http://www.surgeongeneral.gov/tobacco.

Marijuana

Marijuana, or cannabis, is the most commonly used illegal drug in the United States. Despite purported medical uses, it is not a benign substance. Individuals who become addicted often experience impairment in multiple life areas. The active ingredient in marijuana is tetrahydrocannabinol (THC). THC is classified as a hallucinogen, which it can be in large quantities or in highly sensitive individuals. More often intoxication brings relaxation, euphoria, a dreamy state, time-space distortion, and impaired attention. Perceptual disturbances may impair driving. Anxiety and paranoia are also common effects. Like other addictive substances, marijuana abuse can interfere with the assessment and treatment of psychiatric symptoms.

No specific medical management is warranted for either cannabis intoxication or withdrawal.

Teenagers are among the most vulnerable users. Common signs of problematic use during adolescence include changes in sleeping and eating habits, declining school performance, changes in the adolescent's peer group, and moodiness. Physical signs include increased appetite, dry mouth, and injected conjunctiva. The University of Michigan's Monitoring the Future survey of U.S. high school students has been tracking teenage substance use for the past 25 years. In 2000, they found that by the age of 18 years, 80% of U.S. youth had used alcohol and 54% had used illicit drugs. Their drug of choice was marijuana. One in five high school seniors and nearly as many tenth graders reported marijuana use during the previous month. Treatment for marijuana abuse and dependence in adolescents or adults consists of psychotherapeutic approaches.

Cocaine and Other Stimulants

Cocaine is a highly addictive drug that is extracted from the coca leaf. Amphetamine, which is structurally similar to cocaine, is a synthesized product used to suppress hunger,

[1]Not FDA approved for this indication.

improve energy or alertness, and improve mood. The euphoria that cocaine elicits is probably caused by increased dopamine activity. Physical effects include elevated heart rate and blood pressure, mediated by stimulation of the sympathetic nervous system. All stimulants possess these qualities, though in varying degrees and with variable risks. In overdose, these effects are intensified so that myocardial infarction, arrhythmia, stroke, and psychosis may occur. In those situations, therapeutic measures are supportive and aimed at reversing specific ill effects.

Physiologic withdrawal is not a major problem, and no medical management is indicated. However withdrawal from cocaine produces symptoms known as a *crash*. A crash may begin within hours of the last use and intensify over the next several days. During this time the addict feels extreme fatigue. Depression can be severe and carries a risk of suicidal ideation and behavior. Relapse is common during withdrawal because return to use provides quick and reliable relief.

The person who abuses cocaine may use it by snorting, injecting, or smoking. The rate at which the drug reaches the brain correlates with its addictive potential. Therefore, users with more advanced addictions commonly report a progression from snorting to intravenous use or the most rapid form of administration, smoking crack cocaine. Intravenous users are at risk for contracting hepatitis and HIV, as well as developing phlebitis and endocarditis. Treatment relies on psychotherapeutic approaches such as self-help, contingency management, and cognitive-behavioral therapy. Despite multiple medication trials, no drug effectively treats cocaine dependence.

Opiates

Among the opiates, heroin may be the most widely recognized drug of abuse. In 2000, there were an estimated 1,000,000 heroin addicts. There is concern that this number will increase because heroin has become less expensive in some parts of the country. All opiates have some abuse potential depending upon a specific drug's potency and its route of administration. Not only are illicit opiates abused, but the abuse of opiate analgesics such as methadone, hydromorphone (Dilaudid), oxycodone (OxyContin), and fentanyl (Duragesic) is also common.

Signs of intoxication include sedation, mild euphoria, pinpoint pupils, bradycardia, and low blood pressure. Overdose on drugs within the opiate class produces a reduced level of consciousness that may progress to coma and respiratory depression. When overdose is suspected, naloxone (Narcan), a synthetic opioid antagonist, can be administered to reverse the opiate's effects; the initial dose of 0.4 mg intravenously (IV) (0.01 mg/kg) can be repeated every 2 to 3 minutes as clinically indicated. Naloxone may be administered intramuscularly or subcutaneously if necessary. If the patient does not respond to a dose of 5 to 10 mg, opiate overdose is doubtful.

There is a well-defined withdrawal syndrome that occurs when an opiate is discontinued in one who is physiologically dependent (Table 3). Symptoms of withdrawal from a short-acting drug such as heroin begin within a few hours; withdrawal symptoms from a long-acting opiate such as methadone begin within 3 to 4 days. Opiate withdrawal

TABLE 3 Symptoms of Opiate Withdrawal

	Objective	Subjective
Early	Lacrimation	
	Rhinorrhea	
	Diaphoresis	
	Yawning	
Middle	Dilated pupils	Restlessness
	Piloerection	Irritability
		Insomnia
Late	Tachycardia	Bone pain
	Increased blood pressure	Nausea
	Vomiting	Abdominal cramps
	Diarrhea	Depression
	Mood lability	

is not a medical emergency in otherwise healthy adults. However, it is uncomfortable and may be a strong trigger for continued drug use.

There are several ways to address opiate withdrawal. In the context of a prescription medication being stopped too abruptly, the simplest approach is to restart the medication and reduce it more slowly. Planned detoxification is often accomplished by substituting methadone (Dolophine), a long-acting opioid agonist, for the shorter-acting opiate. With this method, the patient is stabilized on a methadone dose that blocks significant withdrawal. A dose of 40 mg given in divided doses during the day is adequate to block significant withdrawal symptoms in most patients. The stabilizing dose is tapered over several days. Clonidine (Catapres)[1] is a nonopiate that can be used to treat opiate withdrawal. It is a centrally acting a$_2$-agonist that reduces autonomic symptoms such as vomiting, diarrhea, and sweating (Table 4).

Methadone maintenance is the mainstay treatment for dependence on illicit opiates. The Food and Drug Administration (FDA) approved methadone for opioid maintenance therapy in 1972. Federal regulations placed tight restrictions on methadone programs that include special state and federal licensing. These restrictions have had an unintended effect of limiting treatment access for some opiate-addicted patients. Methadone maintenance treatment is criticized for a number of reasons:

- There is a risk that dispensed methadone will be sold on the street.
- Daily administration is inconvenient for patients.
- Some facilities offer inadequate adjunctive psychosocial or therapy services.

Despite concerns, methadone maintenance is effective in reducing criminal activity among heroin addicts, in decreasing the risk of HIV and hepatitis acquired through needle-sharing, and in returning some addicts to functional lifestyles.

Another synthetic opiate agonist, levomethadyl (Orlaam), is approved for maintenance therapy. This agent is also federally regulated. It has an advantage of a long

---

[1]Not FDA approved for this indication.

TABLE 4 Opioid Treatment Summary*

Treatment of Opioid Overdose

Drug	Administration
Naloxone (Narcan)	Initial dose 0.4 mg IV (0.01 mg/kg) Repeat every 2-3 minutes as indicated by symptoms Reevaluate diagnosis if no response to 5-10 mg Total

Sample Methadone Detoxification†

Day	Drug	Administration
Day 1	Methadone 40 mg (Dolophine)	Give initial dose of methadone 20 mg Additional doses of 10 or 20 mg may be given if withdrawal symptoms persist after 4 hours Maximum 40 mg total dose
Day 2-3	Methadone 25-30 mg	Reduce dose by 25% daily
Day 4	Methadone 20 mg	
Day 5	Methadone 10 mg	
Day 6	Methadone 5 mg	
Day 7	Discontinue	

Sample Clonidine Detoxification‡

Day	From Short-Acting Opioid	With or Without Naltrexone (ReVia) Induction	From Methadone
Day 1-2	0.3-0.6 mg	12.5 mg	0.3-0.6 mg
Day 3	0.3-0.8 mg	25 mg	0.4-0.6 mg
Day 4-5	0.6-1.2 mg Then reduce total daily dose by 50% each day, not to exceed 0.4 mg/d	50 mg Continue maintenance therapy	0.5-0.8 mg
Day 6-10			0.6-1.2 mg Then reduce total daily dose by 50% each day, not to exceed 0.4 mg/d

*All treatment must be individualized to meet specific patient needs and adjusted based on response to treatment.
†May be used in combination with clonidine (Catapres) or other as-needed medications. Catapres is not FDA approved for this indication.
‡Give a test dose of clonidine 0.1 mg. Continue only if blood pressure is >85/55. Clonidine 0.1-0.2 mg every 2-4 hours, hold for systolic blood pressure <85 or diastolic blood pressure <55.

half-life, allowing for less frequent dosing than methadone. However, it can prolong the QT interval, and this may account for the reluctance of some approved facilities to prescribe it.

Alternatively, an opiate antagonist may be useful for treatment of opiate addiction. Naltrexone (ReVia) blocks the euphoric effects of opiates. This medication should only be prescribed once a patient is opiate-free for 7 to 10 days, in order to avoid a precipitated withdrawal syndrome. The typical dose of naltrexone is 50 mg daily, often initiated at 25 mg daily to reduce the risk of sedation and nausea. One group that has benefited from naltrexone maintenance is health care professionals who participate in a comprehensive recovery plan and are carefully monitored by state licensing boards.

Buprenorphine (Subutex) is a mixed opioid agonist-antagonist that was recently approved for the treatment of opiate addiction. A product (Suboxone) that combines buprenorphine with the opioid-antagonist naloxone reduces the risk of medication diversion for intravenous use. Office-based clinicians, including primary care physicians, may prescribe buprenorphine for treatment of opiate addiction after taking an approved training course and receiving a special waiver from the Drug Enforcement Agency. It is unclear to what extent approval of this newest agent will improve the care of opiate addicts. The potential advantages include greater convenience for patients, decreased risk of drug diversion, additional options for less severely addicted individuals, and fewer federal regulations for practitioners.

Patients at greatest risk for prescription opiate dependence include those who abuse other substances and those with a history of illicit opiate abuse. Patients with chronic pain are at risk for opiate dependence when increasing doses of medication are needed to control pain. It is advisable for clinicians who are unsure about prescribing opiates to seek the opinions of other professionals, especially when treating patients with chronic, nonmalignant pain.

Benzodiazepines

Benzodiazepines are used most often in the outpatient setting for the treatment of anxiety and insomnia. They have replaced barbiturates as the sedative-hypnotic of choice because of a greater safety profile in overdose. Benzodiazepines act on the brain's γ-aminobutyric acid

(GABA) receptors, which results in relaxation and mild sedation. Signs of intoxication with benzodiazepines are similar to those experienced with alcohol, with higher doses producing greater sedation, slurred speech, and ataxia. However, benzodiazepines may be used as anesthetics, whereas alcohol is lethal in very high doses. In serious overdoses where benzodiazepines are suspected to play a role, the benzodiazepine antagonist flumazenil (Romazicon) may be administered at a dose of 0.2 mg IV over 30 seconds and repeated up to a 3-mg total dose. There is a risk of seizures in sedative-dependent individuals and in patients taking benzodiazepines as part of an antiepileptic regimen.

Benzodiazepines are effective in treating alcohol withdrawal. The symptoms of sedative withdrawal and alcohol withdrawal are similar—insomnia, anxiety, tachycardia, elevated blood pressure, and fever. In addition, seizures and delirium can be serious sequelae of an untreated alcohol- or sedative-withdrawal syndrome. Whereas opiate withdrawal is not a life-threatening condition unless it occurs in the context of medical frailty, untreated benzodiazepine withdrawal may result in death.

When a patient is addicted to a benzodiazepine and needs detoxification, it is common practice to substitute a long-acting benzodiazepine for a short-acting one. Table 5 gives an approximation of equivalent doses to ease the conversion from one medication to another. Once the patient is comfortable on the long-acting benzodiazepines, the dosage is gradually reduced and discontinued. However withdrawal does not always go smoothly and medication adjustments may be needed. The reduction schedule varies depending upon the severity of the addiction, the duration of benzodiazepine use, and the dosage used.

Hospitalized patients who are addicted to high doses of benzodiazepines often do well when converted to an equivalent dose of a long-acting agent such as clonazepam (Klonopin) or chlordiazepoxide (Librium). Then the dose may be reduced on a 10% per day schedule. In these patients it is necessary to monitor vital signs every 4 hours and have additional doses of benzodiazepine ordered for signs of withdrawal. Such signs include tremulousness, diaphoresis, blood pressure higher than 150/100,

and heart rate more than 100. Outpatients may require several weeks to months for detoxification. Some treatment centers use anticonvulsants, specifically valproic acid (Depakote)[1] and carbamazepine (Tegretol),[1] to prevent or minimize withdrawal symptoms.

Other Drugs of Abuse

Clinicians may deal with any number of abused substances. The popularity of particular drugs changes over time. However, there are several types of substances that come up frequently enough to warrant inclusion here. One example is the inhalants. The agents that make up this group are inexpensive and accessible in common household products such as glue, shoe polish, paint thinners, aerosols, and correction and cleaning fluids. Intoxication on these agents most resembles alcohol intoxication. Acute overdose is rare but can result in death from asphyxiation or cardiac arrhythmia. The brain, kidneys, and liver are susceptible to damage from repeated inhalant exposure. The result over the long term may be chronic delirium, psychosis, or renal failure. An estimated 15% of young adults have tried an inhalant. However, it is estimated that less than 1% are addicted to inhalant use.

Hallucinogens are another group of abusable drugs. Management of intoxication on these drugs is supportive in most cases. Lysergic acid diethylamide (LSD) is a well-known drug in this class. Like most hallucinogens it produces visual hallucinations and increases sensory awareness. Intoxication can also cause dilated pupils, facial flushing, tachycardia, and increased blood pressure. 3,4-Methylenedioxymethamphetamine (MDMA), or ecstasy, may be classified as either a hallucinogen or a stimulant because it has properties of both. It is generally considered a dangerous drug because of its potential for long-term brain damage. It may also be toxic to the heart and liver.

Phencyclidine (PCP) intoxication can have a frightening presentation. The patient may become agitated and unpredictable, requiring physical and chemical restraints to ensure the safety of the patient and those around him or her. Medication may not be necessary if the patient is placed in a quiet, supportive setting. If medications are used, benzodiazepines are typically chosen first. If antipsychotics are required, agents with low anticholinergic activity are preferred. Toxic doses of PCP can produce a life-threatening condition with severe autonomic instability in which hypertension, hyperthermia, convulsions, and coma may become serious medical management problems.

Treatment

While medication management is increasingly important in the treatment of alcohol and drug dependence, nonpharmacologic approaches are the mainstay of substance abuse treatment. Alcoholics Anonymous (AA) helped many alcoholics recover before physicians had treatment techniques to offer. AA remains a proven resource, and other self-help groups are modeled after it.

TABLE 5 Approximate Benzodiazepine Dose Equivalency

Generic Name (Trade Name)	Dose Equivalents (mg)*	Short- or Long-Acting
Alprazolam (Xanax)	1	Short
Chlordiazepoxide (Librium)	25	Long
Clonazepam (Klonopin)	0.5	Long
Diazepam (Valium)	10	Long
Flurazepam (Dalmane)	30	Long
Lorazepam (Ativan)	2	Short
Oxazepam (Serax)	30	Short
Prazepam (Centrax)	10	Long
Temazepam (Restoril)	20	Short
Triazolam (Halcion)	0.25	Short

*Doses are approximately equivalent to phenobarbital 30 mg.

---

[1]Not FDA approved for this indication.

TABLE 6 Benzodiazepine Treatment Summary*

Treatment of Overdose

Drug	Administration
Flumazenil (Romazicon)	Initial dose 0.2 mg IV over 30 seconds. Repeat every minute up to a 3-mg total dose. Re-evaluate diagnosis if no response after 3-5 minutes.

Detoxification Guidelines

Day	Action
Day 1	Long-acting benzodiazepine until symptom control is achieved. Common upper limits are clonazepam (Klonopin), 6-8 mg per 24 hours or chlordiazepoxide (Librium), 400 mg per 24 hours.
Day 2– Completion	Taper by 25% every 1-2 days Monitor vital signs every 4 hours Have PRN doses available, i.e., clonazepam, 1 mg, chlordiazepoxide, 25 mg, for signs or symptoms of withdrawal (tremulousness, diaphoresis, systolic blood pressure >150, diastolic blood pressure >100, or heart rate >100). Consider adding anticonvulsants.

*All treatment must be individualized to meet specific patient needs and adjusted based on response to treatment.

Narcotics Anonymous (NA) and Cocaine Anonymous (CA), similar to AA, are pivotal in the recovery of some drug abusers. The caveat is that one group may be very different from another.

There are significant problems in some self-help groups. Patients may have concerns about heavy cigarette-smoking in meetings, about attendees who actively use or sell drugs, and about criticism of prescribed psychotropic medications. Therefore, when a patient finds one group unsatisfactory for some reason, the clinician can suggest he or she try another group. Some patients object to the religious tone of traditional 12-step groups. For these individuals alternative groups such as Women for Sobriety and Rational Recovery may be more acceptable. In addition, self-help groups are free of charge, which is a factor for some patients.

Most professional addiction treatment occurs in an outpatient setting. However, higher levels of care are available in hospital, residential, or partial hospital programs if there are chaotic living situations, or pressing psychiatric or other medical needs. Social interventions are crucial for patients faced with unemployment, legal consequences, and housing dilemmas. Psychiatric disorders occur with a high frequency in drug-abusing populations, and both disorders should be treated to optimize the patient's chances for recovery. Therefore, a multidisciplinary approach to treatment often works best.

Psychiatric symptoms in patients who abuse drugs are easy to recognize. Mood lability, depression, and anxiety are common. The challenge lies in sorting out whether these symptoms are caused by the use of a mood-altering substance or represent a separate mood or anxiety disorder. Psychiatric expertise may be needed to assist in sorting out this diagnostic dilemma. Patients with schizophrenic and bipolar disorders are also at high risk for drug abuse, which can exacerbate psychoses.

The cognitive aspects of professional treatment often include educational, motivational, cognitive–behavioral, relapse prevention, and 12-step strategies. Most treatment programs try to get the patient to more fully recognize the problems associated with his or her drug use, identify reasons to change, acknowledge obstacles to sobriety, become aware of triggers to relapse, and consider ways to build a sober support network. Patients with addictive disorders do get better, and treatment of patients with drug abuse can be highly rewarding. It is important to recognize this problem as one of many chronic, relapsing conditions seen in medicine today.

Anxiety Disorders

Method of
Jacqueline Carinhas McGregor, MD

Anxiety disorders are the most common psychiatric disorders in the world among both children and adults. In the United States, 30 million people or approximately one of every four meet the criteria for an anxiety disorder in their lifetimes. It is estimated that the annual cost of anxiety disorders in 1998 dollars was more than $63 billion. More than half of these costs were due to nonpsychiatric direct medical costs, which include undiagnosed, misdiagnosed, or inadequately treated anxiety disorders. It is clear that much of the emotional and economic burden caused by these disorders could be alleviated by improving diagnosis and treatment.

Genetics, temperament, and life stressors can all be contributors to anxiety disorders. Norepinephrine and serotonin are thought to be the major neurotransmitters involved in mediating anxiety symptoms whereas the sympathetic nervous system also plays an important role. The onset of anxiety disorders can usually be traced to childhood, adolescence, or young adulthood. With the exception of obsessive-compulsive disorder, women are more likely than men to suffer from anxiety disorders. Anxiety disorders occur across racial groups without distinction.

Anxiety is characterized by subjective feelings of worry, dread, or anticipation and can include hypervigilance, excessive negativity, and a myriad of somatic symptoms. These symptoms can include diaphoresis, palpitations, shortness of breath, dizziness, chest pain, tremulousness, gastrointestinal complaints, fatigue, dry mouth, sleep problems, hot flashes, polyuria, and restlessness. Because of the wide variety of physical complaints, underlying organic causes and disorders secondary to substances use must first be ruled out (Box 1). A detailed history of present illness, past medical history, substance history, and review of symptoms is essential. If a patient initially presents with anxiety

BOX 1 Organic Causes of Anxiety Symptoms

Cardiopulmonary	Angina, mitral valve prolapse, pulmonary embolism, COPD, asthma
Endocrine	Hyperthyroidism, pheochromocytoma, Cushing's syndrome, menopause
Gastrointestinal	Gastroesophageal reflux, irritable bowel syndrome, gastritis
Neurologic	Dementia, substance intoxication or withdrawal, seizure disorder, migraine
Medications	Stimulants, herbal supplements, decongestants, steroids, antipsychotics, theophylline, calcium channel blockers, anticholinergics

Abbreviation: COPD = chronic obstructive pulmonary disease.

symptoms in middle or late adulthood, has no family history of anxiety disorders, has no temporally related stressors, and does not respond to psychiatric intervention, a closer investigation of organic causes of anxiety should be undertaken.

In patients describing chest pain, cardiovascular causes such as angina, mitral valve prolapse, arrhythmias, and pulmonary embolism should be ruled out. Pulmonary ailments such as asthma, chronic obstructive pulmonary disorder, and pneumonia should be considered in patients describing shortness of breath. Hyperthyroidism, pheochromocytoma, and Cushing's syndrome are examples of endocrine disorders that can mimic anxiety disorders. Other disorders to consider include anemia, delirium, menopause, and gastroesophageal reflux. Medications such as stimulants (including herbal supplements and caffeine), decongestants, antipsychotics, theophylline, steroids, calcium channel blockers, and anticholinergics should all be considered. Alcohol and illicit drug use or withdrawal are other possible causes of anxiety symptoms.

The most common diagnoses of anxiety disorders include generalized anxiety disorder (GAD), panic disorder, social anxiety disorder, obsessive-compulsive disorder (OCD), posttraumatic stress disorder (PTSD), and specific phobias. Those suffering from anxiety disorders are likely to have another co-morbid psychiatric disorder such as a mood disorder or substance dependence. These patients also have a higher risk for suicidal behaviors. It is important to distinguish anxiety disorders from each other, as well as from other psychiatric disorders because the specific diagnosis may have significant impact on treatment decisions. Simple phobias, for example, are not responsive to medication and require cognitive behavioral intervention. OCD requires significantly higher doses of antidepressants than other disorders. Patients with GAD and panic disorder need lower starting doses of antidepressants to avoid iatrogenically exacerbating their symptoms. In the case of patient with comorbid bipolar disorder, special care should be used with antidepressants to prevent the induction of a manic episode.

Psychotherapeutic interventions are often considered the first line of intervention in anxiety disorders, particularly for patients with mild symptoms, those who prefer nonpharmacologic treatment, and for children. Cognitive behavior therapy (CBT) is a specific type of psychotherapy that combines behavioral therapy with cognitive therapy and has the best evidence-based research supporting its use in anxiety disorders. The behavioral component of CBT includes exposure and ritual prevention whereas the cognitive aspect includes identifying false, irrational thoughts and the automatic responses to them. It is important to find skilled therapists with specialized training in these modalities in order to facilitate helpful referrals.

The pharmacologic treatment of most anxiety disorders usually includes selective serotonin reuptake inhibitors (SSRIs) serotonin-norepinephrine reuptake inhibitors (SNRIs), and/or benzodiazepines. The SSRIs fluoxetine (Prozac) and paroxetine (Paxil) are both potent inhibitors of cytochrome P450 2D6, and significant interactions can occur with other drugs that a patient may be taking. Escitalopram (Lexapro) has the most favorable SSRI side effect profile with the least protein-binding and cytochrome-P450 interactions. The most common side effects of SSRIs are nervousness, insomnia, restlessness, nausea, and diarrhea. Venlafaxine (Effexor) has a lower risk of significant drug interactions compared to the SSRIs; however, patients prescribed venlafaxine (Effexor) should have their blood pressure monitored as it can cause or worsen existing hypertension. Benzodiazepines should be used carefully because of their addictive potential and should be avoided in patients with a history of substance abuse.

As with any drug, it is important to discuss the risk and benefits of medication options with patients before coming to a treatment decision. The dosage of a medication should be carefully titrated to minimize side effects while providing adequate symptom response. The Food and Drug Administration (FDA) issued a labeling change request in October 2004 for a black box warning on antidepressant medications about the *possible* association of SSRIs with suicidality in the treatment of major depressive disorder. The antidepressant side effect of agitation has been known to trigger suicidal behavior in those with or without premorbid depression. A physician should exercise special care in using SSRI medications, especially with those younger than 18 years of age. Frequent follow-up visits are recommended to monitor side effects and treatment response. Three of the most prevalent and burdensome anxiety disorders are GAD, OCD, and panic disorder. The remainder of this article will focus on the diagnosis and treatment of GAD and OCD disorders. Panic disorder is discussed in another article.

Generalized Anxiety Disorder

DIAGNOSIS

According to the *Diagnostic and Statistical Manual of Mental Disorders IV-TR,* individuals with GAD suffer from uncontrollable, excessive anxiety and worry involving several areas of functioning on most days in a 6 month period. It must be associated with three or more of the following symptoms: restlessness, fatigue concentration difficulties, irritability, muscle tension, or sleep problems. The anxiety cannot be the result of another Axis I disorder; it must cause a significant impairment in functioning, and it cannot be due to substance abuse, a medical disorder, or occur exclusively in the context of a mood disorder, psychotic disorder, or pervasive developmental disorder.

The 12-month prevalence for GAD is 3.1%, and the lifetime prevalence is close to 5%. Women are twice as likely as men to suffer from GAD. GAD usually develops sometime during late adolescence or early adulthood, its symptoms tend to have a chronic duration, and there is a high incidence of comorbid psychiatric disorders (especially depression) associated with it.

GAD can be difficult for the physician to diagnose because patients can be reluctant to discuss their anxiety or be unable to identify it as the source of their concerns. Patient complaints of fatigue, insomnia, somatic symptoms, or chronic pain should be a signal for the physician to ask more about anxiety symptoms.

TREATMENT

Psychotherapy, pharmacotherapy, and their combination can be successfully used to treat GAD. Psychotherapy, particularly cognitive-behavior therapy and applied relaxation, are effective treatment strategies for GAD. Psychotherapy can be used concomitantly with pharmacotherapy, often with better result than if either were used alone.

There are a variety of psychopharmacologic interventions that can be used for patients with GAD (Table 1). An antidepressant or the 5-HT$_{1A}$ partial agonist, buspirone (BusPar), is considered the first line of drug treatment. Paroxetine (Paxil), escitalopram (Lexapro), and venlafaxine (Effexor) are the only antidepressants that have an FDA indication for GAD, although there is evidence that both imipramine (Tofranil)[1] and sertraline (Zoloft)[1] are effective drugs in the treatment of GAD. SSRIs are usually considered the antidepressant of choice because of their safety and relatively modest side effects. Use tricyclic antidepressants such as imipramine (Tofranil) with care

---

[1]Not FDA approved for this indication.

TABLE 1 Pharmacotherapy in the Treatment of Generalized Anxiety Disorder

Drug	Starting Dose	Target Dose
SSRIs		
Paroxetine (Paxil CR)*	10 mg qd	10-60 mg qd
Escitalopram (Lexapro)*	5-10 mg qd	10-20 mg qd
Sertraline (Zoloft)	12.5-25 mg qd	50-200 mg qd
Fluoxetine (Prozac)	10 mg qd	20-40 mg qd
SNRIs		
Venlafaxine (Effexor XR)*	37.5 mg qam	150-300 mg qam
OTHER		
Buspirone (BusPar)	5 mg bid-tid	10 mg bid to tid

*FDA indication for generalized anxiety disorder (GAD)
Abbreviations: bid = twice daily; qam = every morning; qd = every day; tid = three times daily.
SNRIs = serotonin-norepinephrine reuptake inhibitors; SSRIs = selective serotonin reuptake inhibitors.

because of their more troublesome side-effect profile, proarrhythmic properties, and potential lethality in overdose. The most commonly noted side effects of buspirone (BusPar) are dizziness, nausea, headache, nervousness, and insomnia. Benzodiazepines can play an important role in the treatment of GAD. It is important to keep in mind the addictive potential of these medications before using them. In the first weeks of treatment with SSRIs, it can be helpful to use benzodiazepines to address acute anxiety symptoms while allowing sufficient time for the SSRI to achieve its effect. As symptoms begin to respond, the physician should consider tapering and discontinuing the benzodiazepine.

After an 8- to 10-week course of treatment with an antidepressant, if there has been an insufficient response at an adequate dose, the clinician should consider switching to or augmenting with another drug (e.g., another antidepressant, buspirone [BusPar] or a benzodiazepine). Patients need significant support and encouragement from their physician to be compliant with daily medication regimes and to continue their medication once they begin to experience symptom relief. There is little data on the length of treatment or whether pharmacologic intervention can prevent future relapse. It is common practice to continue treatment for at least 6 to 12 months after resolution of symptoms before stopping medications. At that time a gradual tapering of the medication dose can be considered.

Obsessive Compulsive Disorder

DIAGNOSIS

The *Diagnostic and Statistical Manual of Mental Disorders IV-TR* outlines the criteria for OCD as having obsessions and/or compulsions. Obsessions are defined as recurrent, persistent thoughts, impulses, or images that are experienced as intrusive and inappropriate and cause significant distress. They cannot be excessive worries about realistic or reasonable concerns. The individual attempts to ignore the obsessions or counteract them with another thought or action and understands that the obsessions are a product of his or her own mind. Compulsions are defined as repetitive behaviors or mental acts that the individual feels compelled to perform in response to an obsession. The compulsion is aimed at reducing distress or preventing some dreaded event, but is not clearly connected to the distress or event or is clearly excessive. Except in the case of children, at some point in the course of the disorder the individual recognizes that the obsessions or compulsions are unreasonable. This last point is important in distinguishing OCD from obsessive compulsive personality disorder. The obsessions or compulsions must cause significant impairment and, if another Axis I disorder coexists, the obsessions and/or compulsions cannot be restricted only to the content of that disorder (e.g., preoccupations with food in the case of an eating disorder, hair pulling in the case of trichotillomania). As in the case of GAD, the symptoms cannot occur because of the effects of a substance or secondary to a general medical disorder.

It is not uncommon for OCD to occur with other psychiatric disorders including major depressive disorder, other anxiety disorders, eating disorders, and tic disorders. In children, streptococcal infections are associated with

CURRENT DIAGNOSIS

Generalized Anxiety Disorder

- Excessive anxiety and worry about multiple concerns
- Three additional anxiety symptoms (only one in children or adolescents)
- Difficulty controlling the anxiety and worry
- Symptoms last at least 6 months

Obsessive Compulsive Disorder

- Obsessions and/or compulsions
- Recognition that obsessions or compulsions are excessive or unreasonable (not necessary in children or adolescents)
- Causes significant impairment

Panic Disorder

- Repetitive, discrete periods of intense fear or discomfort
- At least four panic symptoms peaking within 10 minutes
- At least one panic attack followed by 1 month of anticipatory anxiety about having another panic attack

Social Phobia

- Marked and persistent fear of social or performance situations in which embarrassment can occur
- Exposure to the situation provokes anxiety
- Recognition that fear is excessive or unreasonable
- Feared situation is avoided
- Avoidance causes significant impairment
- Symptoms last at least 6 months in children or adolescents

Specific Phobia

- Intense fear reaction to a specific object or situation
- Level of fear in inappropriate to the situation
- Exposure to situation provokes an immediate anxiety response
- Recognition that fear is excessive or unreasonable (not necessary in children or adolescents)
- Situation is avoided or endured with significant distress

Post-Traumatic Stress Disorder

- Follows exposure to a traumatic event
- Event is re-experienced
- Leads to avoidance behavior and increased arousal
- Symptoms last longer than 1 month

Adapted from American Psychiatric Association: Diagnostic and Statistical Manual of Mental Disorders, 4th ed, text rev. Washington, DC, American Psychiatric Association, 2000.

the development of obsessions and compulsions. Psychotic disorders can have obsessive or compulsive behaviors, but these are typically much more bizarre, and the individual has little insight into his or her behavior. It is also important to consider illnesses that can have OCD-like symptoms such as basal ganglia disorders (e.g., Huntington's disease) or tic disorders.

OCD usually appears in late adolescence or early adulthood and has a waxing and waning course. Unlike other anxiety disorders there is an equal occurrence in males and females. The lifetime prevalence rate of OCD is 2% to 3% of the population. Neuroimaging studies of OCD suggest that there are structural and functional problems in the orbitofrontal-subcortical circuitry.

People with OCD often avoid seeking treatment for their illness. Diagnosis often requires explicit questioning regarding specific behaviors such as perfectionism, rituals, washing, counting, checking, or hoarding. The physicians should also be on the lookout for excessively red or raw hands, recurring request for reassurance about medical illnesses, frequent emergency room visits, or usual repetitive behaviors observed in the examining room such as tic-like motions or tapping.

TREATMENT

There are a variety of treatment approaches that can be used for OCD. As with GAD, psychotherapy can be utilized effectively. There is significant research that supporting cognitive behavioral therapy that incorporates exposure-response prevention is a successful treatment for obsessions and compulsions. In more severe cases of OCD, optimal treatment uses a combination of cognitive behavioral therapy and medication.

Several studies demonstrated the efficacy of SSRIs in OCD. A reasonable trial of SSRIs in OCD can be longer and requires higher doses than what would be expected in GAD or major depressive disorder. Setraline (Zoloft), fluoxetine (Prozac), paroxetine (Paxil), and fluvoxamine (Luvox) are SSRIs with FDA indications for OCD.

For those with an inadequate response to treatment with SSRIs, the clinician should consider changing SSRIs, switching to the tricyclic antidepressant, clomipramine (Anafranil), or to the SNRI, venlafaxine (Effexor).[1] The most common side effects of clomipramine (Anafranil)

---

[1]Not FDA approved for this indication.

TABLE 2 Pharmacotherapy in the Treatment of Obsessive-Compulsive Disorder

Drug	Starting Dose	Target Daily Dose
SSRI		
Sertraline (Zoloft)*	25-50 mg qd	100-300 mg[3]
Paroxetine (Paxil CR)*	12.5 mg qd	25-50 mg
Fluoxetine (Prozac)*	10 mg qd	20-60 mg
Fluvoxamine (Luvox)*	25-50 mg qd	100-300 mg
SNRI		
Venlafaxine (Effexor XR)	37.5 mg qam	150-300 mg
TCA		
Clomipramine* (Anafranil)	25 mg qhs	100-300 mg

*FDA indication for obsessive-compulsive disorder (OCD)
[3]Exceeds dosage recommended by the manufacturer.
Abbreviations: qam = every morning; qd = every day; qhs = at bed time.

CURRENT THERAPY

	First Intervention	Second Intervention	Third Intervention
GAD	CBT	SSRI OR venlafaxine (Effexor) OR buspirone (BusPar) OR	Change to different antidepressant or buspirone (BusPar) OR Augment with a different antidepressant class, buspirone (BusPar), or benzodiazepine
OCD	CBT	High dose SSRI (push to maximum dose in 4 to 8 weeks)	Change to another SSRI or clomipramine (anafranil) OR Augment with atypical antipsychotic

Abbreviations: CBT = cognitive behavior therapy; GAD = generalized anxiety disorder; OCD = obsessive-compulsive disorder; SSRI = selective serotonin reuptake inhibitor.

include dry mouth, sedation, dizziness, and weight gain, however, more serious, less common side effects include hypertension and cardiac arrhythmias. Augmentation with a dopamine agonist such as risperidone (Risperdal)[1] or olanzapine (Zyprexa) has been shown to be an effective treatment approach as has the addition of buspirone (BusPar)[1] or benzodiazepines (Table 2).

There is some evidence to support the use of monoamine oxidase inhibitors (MAOIs) in treatment-resistant OCD, but because of the significant side effects, potential drug and food interactions, and toxicity, they are considered an option only when other medication options have proven unsuccessful. For those who fail psychotherapy and psychopharmacology and continue to have significant functional impairment, transcranial magnetic stimulation and neurosurgery are considered treatments of last resort.

Treatment of OCD can usually be accomplished on an outpatient basis; however, in severe refractory cases, inpatient treatment at a facility that specializes in OCD may be necessary. Whatever treatment strategy is employed, the physician should be mindful of the fact that the patient's family often needs to be involved in the treatment. Families often unknowingly reinforce a patient's OCD behaviors by going along with their rituals or participating in excessive reassurance.

Anxiety disorders are quite common and cause a significant burden to individuals as well as to society. The differential diagnosis of anxiety disorders is quite extensive given that anxiety symptoms are often nonspecific. Anxiety disorders often go undiagnosed or are inadequately treated and are likely to occur together with other psychiatric disorders. Primary care physicians are more likely to have the opportunity to detect anxiety disorders and, in fact treat more of these disorders than mental health care practitioners. Effective treatments for anxiety including psychotherapeutic as well as psychopharmacologic interventions are shown in Box 2.

---

[1]Not FDA approved for this indication.

REFERENCES

American Psychiatric Association: Diagnostic and Statistical Manual of Mental Disorders, 4th ed, text rev. Washington, DC, American Psychiatric Association, 2000.

Baer L, Rauch SK, Ballantine T, et al: Cingulotomy for intractable obsessive-compulsive disorder. Arch Gen Psych 1995;52:384-392.

Borkovec T, Costello E: Efficacy of applied relaxation and cognitive-behavioral therapy in the treatment of generalized anxiety disorder. Journal of Consulting and Clinical Psychology 1993;61(4):611-619.

Food and Drug Administration: FDA labeling change request letter for antidepressant medications, 2004.

Greenberg BD, George MS, Martin DJ, et al: Effect of prefrontal repetitive transcranial stimulation in obsessive-compulsive disorder: A preliminary study. Am J Psychiatry 1997;154:867-869.

Greenberg PE, Sisitsky T, Kessler RC, et al: The economic burden of anxiety disorders in the 1990s. J Clin Psychiatry 1990;60:427-435.

Jenike MA, Baer L, Minichiello WE (eds): Obsessive-compulsive disorders: practical management 3rd ed. St Louis, Mosby, 1998.

Karno M, Golding JM, Sorenson SB, et al: The epidemiology of obsessive-compulsive disorder in five US communities. Arch Gen Psychiatry 1988;45(12):1094-1099.

Kessler RC, McGonagle KA, Zhao S: Lifetime and 12-month prevalence of DSM-III-R psychiatric disorders in the United States. Arch Gen Psychiatry 1994;51(1):8-19.

Kobak KA, Griest JH, Jefferson JW, et al: Behavioral versus pharmacologic treatment of obsessive compulsive disorder: A meta-analysis. Psychopharmacology (Berl) 1998;136:205-216.

Koran LM, Rinhold AL, Elliot MA: Olanzapine augmentation in obsessive compulsive disorder refractory to selective serotonin reuptake inhibitors: An open label case series. J Clin Psychiatry 2000;61:514-517.

Ladouceur R, Dugas MJ, Freeston MH, et al: Efficacy of a cognitive behavioral treatment for generalized anxiety disorder evaluation in controlled clinical trial. J Consult Clin Psychol 2000;68(6):957-964.

Liebowitz MR, DeMartinis NA, Weihs K, et al: Efficacy of sertraline in severe generalized social anxiety disorder: results of a double-blind, placebo-controlled study. J Clin Psychiatry 2003;64(7):785-792.

McDougle CJ, Epperson CN, Pelton GH, et al: A double blind placebo controlled study of risperidone addition in serotin reuptake inhibitor-refractory obsessive compulsive disorder. Arch Gen Psych 2000;57:794-801.

Rickels K, Downing R, Schweizer E, et al: Antidepressant for the treatment of generalized anxiety disorder: a placebo controlled comparison of imipramine, trrazodone, and diazepam. Arch Gen Psychiatry 1993;50:884-895.

Rickels K, Schweizer E: The spectrum of generalized anxiety in clinical practice: The role of short term intermittent treatment. Br J Psychiatry 1998;173(Suppl 34):49-54.

Saxena S, Bota RG, Brody AL: Brain-behavior relationships in obsessive-compulsive disorder. Semin Clin Neuropsychiatry 2001;6(2):82-101.

BOX 2 Helpful Resources for Anxiety Disorders

National Alliance for the Mentally Ill	www.nami.org
National Institute of Mental Health	www.nimh.org
Anxiety Disorders Association of America	www.adaa.org
Obsessive-Compulsive Foundation	www.ocfoundation.org

Bulimia Nervosa

Method of

David B. Herzog, MD, and Kamryn T. Eddy, MA

Bulimia nervosa is a prevalent eating disorder most commonly observed in late adolescent and young adult women and often associated with psychiatric co-morbidity and medical sequelae. The course of the disorder may be chronic and relapsing, and patients may demonstrate early ambivalence regarding treatment. There is often a considerable delay between onset of symptoms and presentation for treatment that may reflect shame, control issues, and fear of change (e.g., weight gain). Currently, psychosocial treatments—particularly cognitive behavioral therapy—are considered the first-line of treatment for the disorder, having demonstrated the most successful outcomes, but psychopharmacologic interventions are also promising.

Diagnosis and Clinical Features

DIAGNOSIS

Bulimia nervosa was first recognized formally as a clinical diagnosis in 1979 by Gerald Russell. The disorder is currently defined in the *Diagnostic and Statistical Manual of Mental Disorders, Fourth Edition* (*DSM-IV*) on the basis of recurrent binge eating and compensatory behaviors and related cognitions. Binge eating is defined as the consumption of a large amount of food (typically 2000 to 4000 calories) within a discrete period of time accompanied by loss of control overeating. Loss of control overeating involves the subjective experience of being unable to control what or how much one is eating and may be characterized by eating more rapidly than usual and consuming calorie-dense foods that are typically avoided outside of binge episodes. Compensatory behaviors are designed to counteract the effects of binge eating and can be classified as purging (self-induced vomiting, misuse of laxatives, diuretics, and enemas) and nonpurging (excessive exercise, fasting). The *DSM-IV* specifies that the binge eating and compensatory behaviors occur on average at least twice weekly during a 3-month period. In addition to the behavioral components, the *DSM-IV* indicates a cognitive component of overevaluation of the importance of weight and shape on sense of self. Weight is not part of the bulimia nervosa criteria; although most patients with bulimia nervosa are within an average weight range, patients may be overweight, obese, or even underweight.

Patients with bulimia nervosa can be grouped into purging and nonpurging types based on the compensatory behaviors used. Notably, purging type appears to be predominant; less research exists on the nonpurging type.

According to the *DSM-IV* hierarchy rules, a diagnosis of bulimia nervosa is not made if the binge and compensatory behaviors occur exclusively during a period of anorexia nervosa. Similarly, a diagnosis of binge eating disorder (currently recognized in the *DSM-IV* as an eating disorder not otherwise specified) can be appropriate if recurrent binge eating is present in the absence of any compensatory behaviors.

Although the current diagnostic system is useful, limitations exist. For example, there appears to be heterogeneity within the diagnostic category of bulimia nervosa on the basis of psychosocial functioning, personality style, and co-morbidity, which may have treatment implications. Furthermore, a large subset of patients present for treatment in clinical settings with symptom profiles that closely resemble that of a patient with bulimia nervosa but do not meet all of the diagnostic criteria. For example, although a formal diagnosis of bulimia nervosa stipulates a twice-weekly binge/compensatory behaviors frequency criterion, patients often present to eating disorder clinics for the treatment of bingeing and/or purging that occurs less frequently. Thus, this treatment review derives from the literature on bulimia nervosa but can be considered applicable across patients with a spectrum of bulimic symptoms.

DIFFERENTIAL DIAGNOSIS

Consideration of a range of conditions that may be characterized by features similar to bulimia nervosa is necessary in the initial assessment. Neurologic disorders impacting appetite regulation and eating behaviors (e.g., pituitary or hypothalamic brain tumors, Kleine-Levin or Klüver-Bucy syndromes), hormonal disorders relating to malnutrition and hypometabolism (e.g., adrenal disease, diabetes mellitus, pituitary dysfunction, hyperthyroidism), and gastrointestinal (GI) disorders (e.g., malabsorption, enteritis) should be considered. Psychiatric disorders including major depression and borderline personality disorder should be considered because they may be associated with binge eating even though compensatory behaviors and cognitive features of bulimia nervosa are absent.

MEDICAL COMPLICATIONS

Patients with bulimia nervosa are generally within the normal weight range, but they may show signs of malnutrition. Medical complications secondary to bingeing and purging behaviors and malnutrition are common. Patients often present with transient facial swelling, peripheral edema, weakness and fatigue, dental problems, and abrasions on the dorsal surface of the hand (Russell's sign). Medical assessment should be based on current symptom presentation and should include complete blood count, serum electrolytes, serum blood urea nitrogen (BUN)/creatinine levels, urinalysis, and an electrocardiogram (ECG). Electrolyte and acid-based complications secondary to purging are common and may include hypochloremia, hyponatremia, and hypokalemia. Hypokalemia is related to significant cardiac problems including arrhythmias. Long-term ipecac use may lead to cardiomyopathy. Edema may be present and related to laxative and diuretic abuse. Dental complications related to chronic regurgitation of gastric contents can include enamel erosion and caries. Swelling of the parotid glands is also common. GI difficulties ranging from constipation and bloating to esophageal disorders may also be present. Many of these symptom-related complications remit when the purging is discontinued, but additional treatment and monitoring can be warranted for some patients.

CO-MORBIDITY

Bulimia nervosa is often associated with psychiatric co-morbidity including mood, anxiety, and substance use disorders. Approximately half of patients with bulimia nervosa report a lifetime history of depression. Similarly, anxiety disorders including social phobia and obsessive-compulsive disorder are commonly reported. Although depression may precede the onset, have simultaneous onset, or follow the eating disorder onset, anxiety disorders most often precede the onset of the eating disorder. A substantial minority of patients with bulimia nervosa also reports a lifetime history of substance use disorders, with alcohol abuse being the most common.

Personality styles have received considerable attention in patients with bulimia nervosa. Research indicates that a subset of patients with bulimia can be characterized as multi-impulsive or dysregulated across multiple domains including eating, affect, interpersonal functioning, and sexuality, for example. Bulimic patients with dysregulated personality styles are more likely to present with co-morbid substance use disorders, cluster B axis II disorders, self-destructive and self-injurious behaviors, and kleptomania.

Epidemiology

Population surveys indicate a 1% to 4% lifetime prevalence rate for bulimia nervosa. However, subthreshold binge/purge symptoms and overvaluation of weight and shape are more common. Further, rates of bulimia nervosa are generally higher within given population subsets including college females, for example. Typical age of onset is in late adolescence or early adulthood and may occur during a time of transition (e.g., high school to college) or psychosocial stress. Approximately 90% of patients presenting for treatment of bulimia nervosa are female. Current research indicates that bulimia nervosa is prevalent across ethnicity and socioeconomic status. Notably, however, eating disorders are more commonly seen in industrialized nations where a thin female appearance is valued.

Etiology

A large body of research has considered the etiology of bulimia nervosa, implicating psychological, biological, and social factors. Psychological factors include general personality traits such as perfectionism and difficulty with emotion regulation, difficulty dealing with conflict, and pervasive low self-esteem. It is hypothesized that these variables represent vulnerability factors that are triggered by biological and environmental variables (e.g., transition, parent eating disorder, family conflict). The biological model of bulimia nervosa is supported by the higher concordance of monozygotic than dizygotic twins, which suggests genetic factors are implicated. Further, the biological model suggests that patient-induced dietary restraint leads to binge eating. The implication of social factors is supported by the increased prevalence of bulimia nervosa in industrialized nations. The images of ideal beauty portrayed by the media are inundating in Western society, and yet they are unrealistically thin for most women; women with a childhood history of overweight and obesity may be at particular risk. This leads to internalization of a thin body ideal and associated body dissatisfaction, both of which predict bulimic symptoms. It is likely that the confluence of multiple psychological, biological, and sociocultural factors predicts the development of bulimia nervosa. Early warning signs that may be observed by family members or primary care physicians are changes in eating behaviors and weight-related concerns (e.g., not eating with the family, nighttime eating, increased body concerns in normal or underweight females), physical changes (e.g., weight loss, amenorrhea), changes in social behaviors (e.g., avoidance of activities, isolation), and mood-related changes (e.g., loss of self-esteem, depressed mood, irritability).

Treatment Options

Treatment for bulimia nervosa often involves multiple components, the most common of which are psychosocial and pharmacologic. The primary aims of treatment for bulimia nervosa are to reduce and eliminate binge/purge behaviors, modify unhealthy attitudes toward weight and shape, and encourage healthier coping styles. Most patients with bulimia nervosa can be treated on an outpatient basis; however, hospitalization may be necessary for patients who are medically unstable (e.g., because of complications secondary to bulimia nervosa or medical morbidity such as diabetes), severely depressed, or treatment-refractory.

ASSESSMENT

A comprehensive assessment is needed to determine an appropriate and individualized treatment course. Assessment should provide detailed information regarding:

- Eating disorder symptom severity (i.e., frequency, type, history)
- Medical issues and bulimia-related complications
- Developmental history
- Psychiatric history
- Treatment history
- Family history

For a subset of patients bulimia nervosa may be complicated by a concomitant medical condition; in these cases prioritizing the severity of various medical problems is necessary as a piece of the assessment.

Patients with bulimia nervosa tend to manifest shame and embarrassment about their binge/purge symptoms. There is often considerable ambivalence in these patients who, on the one hand, describe feeling out of control with their eating behaviors and perhaps wish for immediate relief and therefore may be interested in beginning a treatment that will help them regain stability over their eating. Yet, they may be hesitant to implement recommendations, demonstrating significant fears that discontinuing the binge/purge cycle will result in weight gain, which they believe would be unbearable. Determining motivation and readiness to change is an important phase of the assessment process.

Psychosocial

Several psychosocial interventions have received empirical support for the treatment of bulimia nervosa, and currently psychotherapy is regarded as the first-line of treatment for the disorder.

Cognitive behavioral therapy (CBT) is one such approach that has received the strongest empirical support. CBT has been widely studied: in clinical trials it achieves 80% reductions in bingeing and purging behavior in patients and leads to full recovery in approximately 50% of patients. CBT for bulimia nervosa works on a model in which dietary restraint leads to binge eating and subsequent compensatory behaviors; both reinforce concern about eating, weight, and shape and in turn drive the bulimic cycle. CBT aims to intervene in this cycle by targeting dietary restraint to reduce and eliminate binge eating and purging and simultaneously address dysfunctional eating, weight, and shape cognitions. Core treatment components include psychoeducation around healthy eating and the implications of disordered eating behaviors, the prescription of *regular* eating, self-monitoring (in the form of daily food logs), and cognitive restructuring around eating, weight, and shape concerns. CBT is typically short-term focused treatment comprising 15 to 20 sessions held during a 4 to 5 month period. CBT can be delivered in an individual, group, or self-help manual format. Meta-analytic review indicates that individual treatment confers an advantage over group treatment. Additionally CBT-focused self-help and guided self-help approaches have also demonstrated efficacy. Although response rates with self-help are not as high as individual CBT, advantages include the wide availability and low cost.

Interpersonal psychotherapy (IPT) has also demonstrated efficacy in the treatment of bulimia nervosa, achieving rates of improvement and recovery comparable to those of CBT but somewhat less quickly. In the treatment of bulimia nervosa, IPT was first tested as a *viable control* treatment in clinical trials of CBT for bulimia nervosa. In contrast to CBT, which directly addresses the maladaptive eating disordered behaviors and cognitions, IPT focuses on interpersonal functioning. The IPT model of bulimia nervosa hypothesizes that interpersonal difficulties lead to low self-esteem and dysphoria and that bingeing and purging are used as coping mechanisms to regulate affect. The treatment focuses on addressing interpersonal difficulties in a short-term structured treatment, which leads to improvements in bulimic symptoms that often accrue even post-treatment.

In spite of the efficacy of CBT and IPT treatments, approximately 50% of patients in clinical trials do not achieve full recovery post-treatment. Presently treatment trials are aiming to deconstruct CBT and IPT approaches to identify mechanisms of change as well as understand why treatment does not work for all patients. Integrated therapies, which incorporate elements of different treatment modalities, are often used in clinical practice and attempts to study them in controlled treatment trials are underway. One such example is an enhanced version of CBT (CBT-E), which incorporates cognitive behavioral principles, interpersonal aspects, regulation strategies taken from dialectical behavior therapy, and other techniques all in an individualized approach as they apply to the patient. Preliminary findings suggest high rates of improvement and recovery for difficult-to-treat patients.

A limitation of these clinical trials for bulimia nervosa is that patient samples are most often adult; the generalizability of these findings to adolescents with the disorder is unclear. There is some evidence to suggest that a family therapy approach to the treatment of bulimia nervosa using the Maudsley model may be helpful, particularly for younger patients who are living with their parents. Multisite family therapy trials for adolescent bulimia nervosa are currently in progress.

These empirically supported treatments are described in detail in treatment manuals available for use by treating clinicians.

Pharmacotherapy

Psychotropic medication can be helpful for patients with bulimia nervosa in reducing bingeing and purging symptoms. Controlled trials have indicated that a range of antidepressants demonstrate efficacy in reducing bulimic symptoms, with the research finding post-treatment reductions in bingeing and purging symptoms for approximately 50% of patients and post-treatment abstinence rates of 30%. Currently, the only medication that has received FDA approval in the treatment of bulimia nervosa is fluoxetine (Prozac) at a recommended dose of 60 mg every day. Studies have suggested other selective serotonin reuptake inhibitors (SSRIs) may be equally effective but controlled clinical trials and long-term follow-up data are unavailable. In particular, patients with co-morbid anxiety disorders may benefit from paroxetine (Paxil)[1] or sertraline (Zoloft).[1] Additionally, earlier studies suggested tricyclic antidepressants, particularly desipramine (Norpramin),[1] were useful in reducing bulimic symptoms, but research indicates the SSRIs may be better tolerated. Monoamine oxidase inhibitors (MAOIs) are typically avoided because they may be dangerous in patients with erratic eating patterns and nutritional instability because of bingeing and purging. Similarly, bupropion (Wellbutrin) is contraindicated in patients with bulimia nervosa because of an increased risk of seizures.

Notably, the mechanism of action in the utility of antidepressant medication in reducing bulimic behaviors is unclear. Antidepressants seem to be equally effective in patients without depressive co-morbidity, arguing against an antidepressant effect. Given the role of serotonin in appetite regulation, it has been hypothesized that certain antidepressants may act on serotonin to reduce bingeing behaviors. Additionally, several other medications have been examined in patients with bulimia nervosa demonstrating moderate efficacy, including the opiate antagonist naltrexone (ReVia),[1] and the anticonvulsant Topiramate (Topamax).[1] There is also some indication that anxiolytic and sleep medications may also be useful for patients with bulimia nervosa.

Thus psychotropic medications, particularly antidepressants, can be helpful for patients with bulimia nervosa, but they are typically less effective than cognitive behavioral therapy. Further, there is some indication that medication in combination with psychotherapy confers an advantage,

---

[1]Not FDA approved for this indication.

CURRENT DIAGNOSIS

- *DSM-IV* defines bulimia nervosa on the basis of binge/compensatory behaviors and associated maladaptive cognitions.
- Binge eating is defined as the consumption of an objectively large amount of food within a discrete period of time accompanied by uncontrolled overeating.
- Compensatory behaviors include purging (self-induced vomiting, misuse of laxatives, diuretics, enemas) and nonpurging (excessive exercise, fasting).
- Binge/compensatory behaviors must occur on average twice weekly over a 3-month period.
- Cognitive component of overvaluation of weight and shape on sense of self.
- Differential diagnosis must consider medical and psychiatric conditions.

Abbreviations: DSM-IV = Diagnostic and Statistical Manual of Mental Disorders, Fourth Edition.

CURRENT THERAPY

- Goals of treatment for bulimia nervosa are to reduce and eliminate binge/compensatory behaviors, modify maladaptive eating- and body-related cognitions, and improve coping skills.
- Psychotherapy is considered first-line treatment. Psychotherapies receiving empirical support for the treatment of bulimia nervosa include CBT and IPT. Additional promising treatments include integrative psychotherapy approaches and family psychotherapy.
- Pharmacotherapy can also be helpful in targeting bulimic symptoms. Antidepressants have received the most empirical support. Fluoxetine (Prozac) at 60 mg qd is the only medication currently approved by the FDA in the treatment.
- CBT and IPT are effective in achieving reductions in binge/compensatory behaviors for the majority of patients and recovery in approximately 50% of patients. Antidepressant therapy leads to reductions in binge/compensatory behaviors for half of patients and recovery in approximately 30% of patients.
- Additional treatment research is warranted to address bulimic symptoms in the considerable subset of patients who remain ill following treatment.

Abbreviations: CBT = cognitive behavioral therapy; FDA = Food and Drug Administration; IPT = interpersonal psychotherapy.

but this finding is not consistent. Similar to the psychotherapy literature, however, clinical trials including adolescent patients are limited and the applicability of these findings to younger patients is unclear.

Adjunctive Treatments

A medical assessment is indicated in patients with bulimia nervosa, and ongoing medical management may be useful particularly to treat patients with complications or those discontinuing laxative and/or diuretic abuse. Nutritional counseling may also be helpful to provide additional structure, support, and education for patients who have difficulty meal planning and regulating their eating. Nutritional psychoeducation is often a component of psychotherapy (e.g., CBT), but additional support may be needed for some patients. Additionally, supportive group therapy can be useful for some patients, particularly in helping them feel less isolated by interacting with that others who experience similar feelings and symptoms.

Impact of Co-Morbidity on Treatment

The role of psychiatric co-morbidity in the treatment of bulimia nervosa is unclear. Generally, improvement of bulimic symptoms is associated with an improvement in mood and anxiety, but further treatment to target co-morbidity is often warranted. Pharmacologic intervention studies indicate that antidepressants improve mood in patients with bulimia who are depressed in addition to targeting bulimic symptoms.

Course and Outcome

The longitudinal course of bulimia nervosa is variable but can be chronic and relapsing. Long-term follow-up studies suggest that 50% to 75% of patients with bulimia nervosa will achieve full recovery from their eating disorder, but approximately 33% of them will go on to relapse. A small

minority of patients seem to present with chronic bulimia nervosa. It appears that a longer duration of illness, history of unsuccessful treatment attempts, co-morbid substance abuse, and cluster B personality disorders are predictive of a worse outcome for patients with bulimia nervosa.

Currently, viable psychosocial and pharmacologic treatments exist for the treatment of bulimia nervosa. Psychosocial approaches, particularly cognitive behavioral therapy, lead to substantial improvement in the majority of patients. Antidepressant therapy may also be useful for a subset of patients, but alone it does not seem to be as effective as psychotherapy. Self-help and guided self-help approaches with a cognitive behavioral focus may also be helpful for patients who have difficulty accessing care. Although these psychosocial and psychopharmacologic treatments are promising and helpful for most patients, approximately 50% of patients do not achieve full recovery even following treatment. Additional treatment research with adolescent and adults patients is needed.

REFERENCES

Agras WS, Walsh T, Fairburn CG, et al: A multicenter comparison of cognitive-behavioral therapy and interpersonal psychotherapy for bulimia nervosa. Arch Gen Psychiatry 2000;57(5):459-466.

Apple RF: Interpersonal therapy for bulimia nervosa. J Clin Psychol 1999;55:715-725.

Casper RC: How useful are pharmacological treatments in eating disorders? Psychopharmacol Bull 2002;36(2):88-104.

Fairburn CG, Cooper Z, Shafran R: Cognitive behaviour therapy for eating disorders: A "transdiagnostic" theory and treatment. Behav Res Ther 2003;41(5):509-528.

Fairburn CG, Marcus MD, Wilson GT: Cognitive-behavioral therapy for binge eating and bulimia nervosa: A comprehensive treatment manual. In Fairburn CG, Wilson GT (eds): Binge Eating: Nature, Assessment, and Treatment. New York, Guilford, 1993.

Fairburn CG, Wilson GT (eds): Binge eating: Nature, assessment and treatment. New York, Guilford Press, 1993, pp 361-404.

Kotler LA, Walsh BT: Eating disorders in children and adolescents: Pharmacological therapies. Eur Child Adolesc Psychiatry 2000; 9(Suppl 1):I108-I1016.

Mitchell JE, de Zwaan M, Roerig JL: Drug therapy for patients with eating disorders. Curr Drug Targets CNS Neurol Disord 2003; 2(1):17-29.

Peterson CB, Mitchell JE: Psychosocial and pharmacological treatment of eating disorders: A review of research findings. J Clin Psychol 1999;55:685-697.

Thompson-Brenner H, Westen D, Glass S: A multidimensional meta-analysis of psychotherapy for bulimia nervosa. Clin Psychol Rev 2003;10:269-287.

Wilson GT, Fairburn CC, Agras WS, et al: Cognitive-behavioral therapy for bulimia nervosa: Time course and mechanisms of change. J Consult Clin Psychol 2002;70:267-274.

Delirium

Method of
Marc E. Agronin, MD

A state of *delirium* is defined as an acute, transient, reversible brain syndrome characterized by fluctuating disturbances of consciousness, attention, perception, cognition, and neuropsychiatric function (e.g., sleep, appetite, psychomotor activity). Other common terms used for delirium include *acute confusional state*, *encephalitis*, *encephalopathy*, and *organic brain syndrome*. Delirium can present in both children and adults, but it is seen most frequently in older adults (>65 years of age) with preexisting brain disease. Although delirium is considered reversible, it can severely disrupt medical and rehabilitative recovery, unmask or even cause enduring cognitive impairment, and lead to long-standing functional decline. In addition, it is a particularly dangerous condition associated with mortality rates as high as 40% in the first year. For this reason, delirium should always be considered a medical emergency and treated aggressively.

Epidemiology

Delirium is most commonly seen in older individuals (>65 years of age), and in more women than men because of greater female-to-male ratios in late life. It is widely assumed that rates of delirium underestimate true prevalence because of delayed or missed diagnoses. Although an estimated 1% of individuals in the community suffer from delirium, prevalence rates increase dramatically in medical settings and with medical severity. Delirium is found in 10% of emergency room patients, in 10% to 30% of medical inpatients, and in up to 40% of hospitalized elderly individuals. It is seen in up to 30% of individuals after cardiac surgery, and in 30% to 40% of older individuals after hip and other orthopedic surgeries. Common factors that increase the risk of delirium across settings include the presence of multiple medical problems or medications, increased age, dementia, infection, fever, fractures, malnutrition, low albumin levels, sensory deprivation, recent surgery, alcohol or sedative dependence, physical restraints, and bladder catheters.

Clinical Presentation

Current diagnostic criteria in the *Diagnostic and Statistical Manual of Mental Disorders, Fourth Edition, Text Revision (DSM-IV-TR)*, focus on three primary presenting features of delirium:

1. A disturbance in consciousness, characterized by impairment in the ability to focus, sustain, and shift one's attention to the surrounding environment
2. A change in cognition, characterized by impairment in memory, orientation, language, or perception (for example, manifested by hallucinations)
3. A development of the symptoms over a relatively short period of time (hours to days) that may fluctuate throughout the course of the day

In addition to these defining symptoms of delirium, the clinical presentation frequently involves psychomotor agitation or retardation, sleep-wake cycle disturbances, mood lability (dysphoria, anxiety, euphoria), behavioral agitation, and psychosis (hallucinations, delusions, disorganized thinking). When they occur, delusions frequently involve paranoid themes or misidentification of individuals, and they tend to be fleeting. Hallucinations can occur in all sensory modalities, although they are most commonly visual. *DSM-IV-TR* identifies four basic categories of delirium: delirium because of a general medical condition, substance intoxication delirium, substance withdrawal delirium, and delirium because of multiple etiologies.

Delirious patients are at significant risk of harming themselves or others because their lack of insight and poor judgment impairs their ability to care for themselves independently, carry out activities of daily living, or fully cooperate with treatment. One subtype of delirium may involve psychomotor hyperactivity and agitation, leading to disruptive screaming, combativeness during caregiving, refusal to take medications or food, and pulling or picking at bandages, endotracheal tubes, or intravenous lines. Such symptoms are exacerbated by lack of sleep, overstimulating environments (such as a noisy and constantly lit intensive care unit) and lack of orientating cues to one's surroundings or time of day. Even with these symptoms, however, the delirious patient may have periods of lucidity and calm during the day.

The clinical presentation of delirium may mimic other acute psychiatric conditions such as mania, anxiety, depression, or psychosis. However, the cognitive changes that also accompany delirium are not typically seen in these conditions. Certain types of seizures or postictal states may also resemble delirium, although without ongoing symptoms beyond the day of the event. The main challenge is to distinguish delirium from dementia or to identify delirium within the setting of dementia. The diagnostic key lies in determining the individual's baseline cognition and functioning prior to the onset of more acute changes. Even though tremendous symptomatic overlap exists in terms of cognitive and neuropsychiatric impairment, the disturbance in consciousness and the fluctuating nature of symptoms that define delirium are not characteristic of most forms of dementia, with the exception of dementia with

Clinical Feature	Delirium	Dementia
Onset	Acute, over days to weeks	Chronic, over months to years
Course	Fluctuating symptoms	Stable symptoms with progressive decline
Duration	Days to weeks or months	Years until inevitable death
Awareness	Reduced	Clear
Attention	Impaired, fluctuating, distractible	Usually normal; able to focus on short, discrete tasks
Alertness	Fluctuates; lethargic or hypervigilant at times	Usually normal
Orientation	Impaired	Impaired
Memory	Immediate and recent memory impaired; remote memory intact	Recent and remote memory impaired
Perception	Hallucinations are common	Intact
Thinking	Fragmented, disorganized, with transient paranoid and other delusions	Impaired abstract thinking, vague or impoverished content; agnosia
Language	Speech slow or rapid, sometimes incoherent	Word-finding difficulty; aphasia
Psychomotor	Variable: hyper- or hypokinetic	Apraxia as dementia progresses; slowed in subcortical dementia
Sleep-wake cycle	Disrupted, reversed	Reversed or fragmented

*This table distinguishes between typical presentations of delirium and mild to moderate dementia (most consistent with Alzheimer's disease). Severe dementia is not described. Acute states of agitation and psychosis in dementia may obscure many of these clinical differences.

Lewy bodies. Table 1 outlines some of the main differences between dementia and delirium.

Etiology

Delirium always has a medical cause. Box 1 lists many of the medical conditions associated with delirium. Medications are the most common causes of delirium, especially when three or more medications are being administered simultaneously and one or more of them have anticholinergic, narcotic, antihistaminic, or sedative effects. Rapid discontinuation of some medications after extended use (months to years) can trigger a withdrawal delirium, particularly benzodiazepines, narcotics, stimulants, steroids, and selective serotonin reuptake inhibitor (SSRI) antidepressants. Anticholinergic medications can cause cognitive impairment or even frank delirium, and many commonly prescribed medications in the elderly have some degree of anticholinergic effects, including cimetidine, prednisolone, theophylline, digoxin, nifedipine, and furosemide. Anticholinergic delirium is the most extreme form of this impairment, caused by large doses of medications such as tricyclic antidepressants (e.g., imipramine, doxepin) or conventional antipsychotics (e.g., chlorpromazine, thioridazine).

Acute infections are common causes of delirium across all age groups, particularly infections that affect the central nervous system (CNS). Delirium secondary to CNS infection is often referred to as an *encephalitis*. Urinary tract infections are the most common cause of delirium in nursing home residents. Delirium can also result from an array of metabolic disturbances, including various endocrine diseases, renal and hepatic failure, and rapid alterations in sodium, calcium, or glucose levels. Cerebral injury because of stroke, trauma, and neoplasm can cause delirium. The increased rates of postoperative delirium may be related to factors such as anesthesia effects, dehydration, anemia,

and the use of narcotic analgesics. Older individuals undergoing orthopedic procedures and coronary artery bypass surgery are particularly susceptible.

Delirium is frequently caused by intoxication or withdrawal from substances of abuse such as alcohol and most street drugs. *Delirium tremens*, characterized by confusion, psychosis (including tactile hallucinations), agitation, and autonomic hyperactivity is a form of delirium seen in acute alcohol withdrawal, and it can be life-threatening without aggressive treatment. *Wernicke's encephalopathy* is a form of delirium resulting from thiamine deficiency. Core symptoms include confusion, nystagmus, gaze palsies, and ataxia. It is seen classically in chronic alcoholics with poor nutrition, but is less prevalent today because so many food products are vitamin fortified. *Wernicke-Korsakoff's syndrome* refers to an enduring form of learning and memory impairment that can result if the initial delirium is not treated rapidly.

It is not clear how medical problems trigger delirium, but several potential pathophysiologic mechanisms are proposed. Many conditions associated with delirium either reduce the flow of adequate blood, oxygen, or nutrients (e.g., glucose, vitamins) to the brain, increase the presence of circulating toxins in the central nervous system (either directly or indirectly by altering the blood–brain barrier), or lead to the release of endogenous mediators of infection, injury, inflammation, or stress (e.g., cytokines, cortisol). It is believed that delirium may result when one or more of these factors significantly disrupt cerebral neuronal oxidative metabolism. In addition, disruptions in several neurotransmitter systems are also implicated in delirium. Anticholinergic effects are most concerning given the central role of acetylcholine in learning, memory, and other cognitive functions. One study of hospitalized patients found a near-linear relationship between increasing serum anticholinergic activity and delirium. Dopaminergic agents can also cause delirium, and dopamine antagonists (i.e., antipsychotic medications) are used to treat delirium. Disturbances in the activity of the neurotransmitters glutamate, GABA (γ-aminobutyric acid), and serotonin are also associated with delirium.

Assessment and Treatment

Figure 1 presents a flow chart for the assessment and treatment of delirium. The first step is to identify the delirious patient, differentiating the symptoms of delirium from other psychiatric conditions that warrant attention. It is critical to obtain information from informants who have knowledge of the patient's baseline mental status prior to recent changes and who have observed the patient over time. The most salient features of delirium are the rapid change in mental status, even within the setting of advanced dementia, the disruption in the patient's attention level, and the sudden manifestation of behavioral changes, usually characterized by agitation. Sharon Inouye and colleagues developed the Confusion Assessment Method (CAM), a rating scale for delirium based on extensive research on hospitalized patients with delirium. Using this scale, a diagnosis of delirium should be considered if an acute onset and fluctuating course, inattention, and either disorganized thinking or an altered level of consciousness (rated as alert, vigilant, lethargic, stuporous, or comatose) are present. Other scales for delirium include the Delirium Rating Scale (DRS), the Delirium Symptom Interview, and the Memorial Delirium Assessment Scale (MDAS).

The clinician must simultaneously conduct a medical workup to identify reversible causes of delirium and make a judgment call whether disruptive behaviors require immediate treatment. This process requires intensive monitoring in a hospital or other medical setting that provides 24-hour care. The use of both chemical and physical restraints should be considered whenever there is imminent threat of self-harm or harm to others, such as from pulling out an endotracheal tube or physically fighting with staff. Although clinicians should always try to avoid the use of restraints because they can potentially worsen the delirium itself or lead to injury, they must also keep in mind that a highly agitated, delirious patient can easily extubate himself, fall out of bed and fracture a hip, or physically injure a nurse. For this same reason, a delirious patient must have 24-hour monitoring, either clearly visible from a nursing station or with a sitter. If physical restraints are needed, they must be reassessed every few hours and discontinued as soon as possible. Chemical restraints should be reevaluated daily to allow rapid titration and early discontinuation.

The medical evaluation flows from clinical suspicion but should always involve basic laboratory studies to rule out urinary tract and other infections that are common causes of delirium, as well as metabolic disturbances. A brain computed tomography (CT) or magnetic resonance imaging (MRI) scan should always be considered after any head injury or when focal neurologic symptoms are present. Such structural imaging helps identify potential causes of delirium but does not actually confirm a diagnosis. Lumbar puncture with cerebrospinal fluid (CSF) analysis and viral titers are indicated with suspected encephalitis. An electroencephalogram (EEG) is less frequently used but may help distinguish delirium from dementia or a seizure disorder. Typical EEG

BOX 1 Etiologies of Delirium

Medications (routine use, intoxication, or withdrawal)
Antibiotics (e.g., quinolones)
Anticholinergic properties (e.g., antispasmodics, conventional antipsychotics, tricyclic antidepressants, H₂ blockers, prednisolone, theophylline)
Anticonvulsants
Antihistamines (e.g., diphenhydramine, hydroxyzine)
Antipsychotics
Cardiovascular medications (e.g., antihypertensives, calcium channel blockers, digoxin, antiarrhythmics)
Chemotherapeutic medications
Corticosteroids
Diuretics
Dopaminergic agents (e.g., levodopa, amantadine)
Immunosuppressive agents
Lithium
Muscle relaxants
Narcotics/opiates
Nonsteroidal anti-inflammatory drugs (NSAIDs)
Sedative-hypnotics (e.g., benzodiazepines, barbiturates)
Serotonergic agents (e.g., selective serotonin reuptake inhibitor [SSRI] and other antidepressants)
Stimulants/sympathomimetics
Toxins (e.g., organophosphate insecticides, carbon monoxide, organic solvents)
Infection (e.g., central nervous system [CNS] encephalitis, urosepsis, pneumonia, cellulitis)
Endocrine disease (e.g., thyroid, parathyroid, or adrenal dysfunction, hyper- or hypoglycemia)
Metabolic disturbances (e.g., hypo- or hypernatremia, hypokalemia, hypo- or hypercalcemia, dehydration, thiamine deficiency/Wernicke's encephalopathy)
Organ failure (e.g., hepatic and uremic encephalopathy)
Neurological disease (e.g., seizure disorder, transient ischemic attacks, strokes, subdural hematoma, traumatic injury, cerebral neoplasm, vasculitis)
Cardiovascular disease (e.g., arrhythmias, myocardial infarction, congestive heart failure, severe hypertension)
Pulmonary disease (e.g., chronic obstructive pulmonary disease [COPD], exacerbation, pulmonary embolism, hypoxia)
Hematologic disease (e.g., anemia, malignancies, disseminated intravascular coagulation [DIC])
Occult malignancies (especially in CNS)
Occult bone fracture
Postoperative state (e.g., anesthetic effects, hip repair, coronary artery bypass graft [CABG])
Substance abuse or withdrawal (e.g., alcohol, cocaine, phencyclidine [PCP], hallucinogens, MDMA [methylenedioxymethamphetamine]/ecstasy, heroin, amphetamines, cannabis)
Sensory impairment (e.g., severe hearing or visual loss)
Severe burns
Severe pain
Sleep deprivation

---

findings in delirium are generalized slowing across alpha, theta, and delta frequencies.

The clinician must then address the potential causes of delirium, through active treatment of a specific condition (e.g., antibiotics for an infection) or the tapering and discontinuation of potentially offending medications. Attention must be given to maintaining adequate hydration, nutrition, pain control, sensory awareness, bowel and

DIAGNOSE DELIRIUM
- Identify core symptoms of delirium
- Obtain observations over time, using informant reports
- Use a delirium rating scale (e.g., CAM, DRS, MDAS)

IDENTIFY AND TREAT CAUSE(S)
- Comprehensive history and physical/neurologic examination (check vital signs)
- Identify relevant medications, substances, or toxic exposures, including problematic doses or amounts, sudden cessation, or combinations (obtain tox screen if warranted)
- Evaluate for pain, sensory deprivation, dehydration, malnutrition
- Psychiatric evaluation (rule out acute mania, anxiety or panic attacks, depression)
- Rule out infection (check urinalysis and complete blood count; consider relevant cultures, chest x-ray, lumbar puncture, HIV testing, viral titers)
- Rule out metabolic disturbance (electrolytes, glucose, calcium, liver, renal, and thyroid function, and ESR)
- Rule out cerebral damage or seizure (obtain brain CT or MRI; consider EEG)
- Rule out cardiovascular source (obtain ECG; echocardiogram, Doppler studies)
- Rule out pulmonary source (check O2 sat; consider arterial blood gas, V-Q scan, etc.)

TREAT AGITATION AND PSYCHOSIS
- Identify potential threat of harm to self or others
- 24-hour observation, with sitter if necessary
- Use physical restraints only in severe situations, with close monitoring and rapid discontinuation
- Use psychotropic medications for agitation and psychosis[1]:

Antipsychotic medications[2]
Haloperidol (Haldol) 0.25–0.5 mg PO BID and Q6–8 hrs PRN
  IM haloperidol for severe agitation
  IV haloperidol in ICU setting with cardiac monitoring
  (1 mg IV, repeated with dose doubled every 30 minutes until effect)
Risperidone (Risperdal) 0.25–0.5 mg PO QD or BID and Q6–8 hrs PRN
  Elixir and orally dissolving (Risperdal M-tab) preparations available
Olanzapine (Zyprexa) 2.5–5 mg PO QHS or BID and Q6–8 hrs PRN
  IM and orally dissolving (Zyprexa Zydis) preparations available
Quetiapine (Seroquel) 25–100 mg PO QHS or BID and Q6–8 hrs PRN
Ziprasidone (Geodon) 20 mg PO BID and Q6–8 hrs PRN
  IM preparation available
Aripiprazole (Abilify) 5–10 mg PO QHS and 5 mg Q8 hrs PRN

Benzodiazepines[3]
Lorazepam (Ativan) 0.25–0.5 mg PO QD or BID and Q6–8 hrs
Oxazepam (Serax) 15–30 PO QD or BID and Q6–8 hrs PRN
  Both agents can be given IM for severe agitation or refusal to take oral medications

[1]There are no FDA-approved psychotropic medications for the treatment of delirium or its complications. Recommended medications and doses are based on standard psychiatric practice guidelines, case studies, and small prospective studies. Doses listed here may be higher in certain individuals.

[2]Electrocardiagraphic monitoring is important before and during treatment with antipsychotic agents, specifically IV haloperidol and ziprasidone. According to APA guidelines, a QTc interval >450 ms or more than 25% over the baseline value warrants dose reduction, discontinuation, and/or cardiology consultation. High doses of IV haloperidol have been associated with torsades de pointes. Also, monitor for side effects including parkinsonism (haloperidol; risperidone in doses >2 mg/day), anticholinergic effects (olanzapine > other agents), and antihistamine effects (quetiapine + others).

[3]Benzodiazepines are preferred agents with alcohol withdrawal, and then should be used according to a specific detox protocol. Otherwise, their use should be restricted to patients who cannot take or tolerate antipsychotic medications, but their efficacy will be limited to agitation and not psychosis. Monitor for excess sedation or confusion, and paradoxical effects such as increased agitation or disinhibition.

FIGURE 1. An algorithm for the assessment and treatment of delirium. APA = American Psychiatric Association; BID = twice daily; CAM = confusion assessment method; CT = computed tomography; DRS = delirium rating scale; ECG = electrocardiogram; EEG = electroencephalogram; ESR = erythrocyte sedimentation rate; HIV = human immuno-deficiency virus; IV = intravenous; MDAS = Memorial delirium assessment scale; MRI = magnetic resonance imaging; PO = by mouth; PRN = as needed; QD = every day; QHS = at bedtime.

TREAT THE DELIRIUM ITSELF
- Provide adequate hydration, nutrition, and pain control
- Employ appropriate behavioral/environmental and pharmacologic approaches:

Behavioral/environmental strategies
- Maintain a consistent, structured environment and staffing
- Provide regular orientation clues (e.g., verbal reminders, large visible clock and calendar)
- Encourage personal effects in room and visits from family and friends
- Improve sensory deprivation (e.g., hearing aides, glasses)
- Encourage sleep hygiene (structure day and night, appropriate ambient lighting, avoid excess activity, food, or caffeine before bed, warm milk or tea before bed, relaxation techniques)
- Encourage early mobilization if bed-bound or post-op state
- Avoid over- or understimulation
- Provide regular bowel and bladder care
- Minimize use of physical restraints and bladder catheters

Pharmacologic strategies[4]
Antipsychotic medications (see above for dosing)
Acetylcholinesterase inhibitors (AChEIs)
  Donepezil (Aricept) 5 mg PO QD ×4 wks, then 10 mg
  Rivastigmine (Exelon) 1.5 mg PO BID ×4 wks, then 3 mg BID
  Galantamine (Razadyne ER) 8 mg PO QD ×4 wks, then 16 mg QD
NMDA-receptor antagonist
  Memantine (Namenda) 5 mg PO QD with 5 mg weekly increments
    in BID doses to total 10 mg BID at 4 weeks

For severe insomnia, consider short-term use of zolpidem (Ambien) 5–10 mg PO QHS, zaleplon (Sonata) 5–10 mg PO QHS, or trazodone (Desyrel) 25–100 mg PO QHS. Antipsychotic medications may also improve sleep in some individuals.

[4]There are no FDA-approved medications to treat delirium. The potential benefits of antipsychotic medications, AChEIs, and NMDA-receptor antagonists to treat delirium are based on small open-label studies and case series. There are no controlled trials to support their use. Further titration of AChEIs or NMDA-receptor antagonists is dependent on either persistent symptoms or underlying dementia.

FIGURE 1, cont'd.

bladder care, and treatment adherence. Medications believed to be causing delirium should be withdrawn expeditiously, although with a written taper schedule if possible, to avoid symptomatic withdrawal or rebound. Withdrawal from alcohol or benzodiazepines must be recognized and then treated with a detoxification protocol that involves close monitoring of physical symptoms of withdrawal and the administration of benzodiazepines such as lorazepam (Ativan) or oxazepam (Serax) as part of a standard taper. Narcotic analgesics can sometimes be replaced with other medications or modalities to relieve pain. In the postoperative state, potential dehydration, anemia, pain, and metabolic disturbances should be addressed.

Once the medical workup begins and the patient's safety is addressed, the next step is to consider environmental, behavioral, and pharmacologic interventions to treat the delirium. The goal is both to enhance the safety, comfort, and familiarity of the environment for the duration of the delirium and to minimize the impact of behavioral disturbances and/or psychotic and disorganized thinking. The delirious patient should be kept in a structured, familiar environment, with clear cues orienting them to person (e.g., personal photos and items), place (e.g., written sign, verbal reminders), and time (e.g., daytime lighting and nighttime darkness, visible calendar and clock, regular mealtimes, verbal reminders). Overstimulation should be avoided, although visits from family and other friendly faces can be helpful. Paranoid delusions, hallucinations, or anxiety attacks should be recognized but not given undue attention; rather, the patient should be reassured and then redirected in a warm but direct manner to more comfortable topics or simple activities. Again, family and familiar faces can play a critically supportive role here.

No FDA-approved medications for the treatment of delirium or its psychiatric complications are currently available. The acetylcholinesterase inhibitors (AChEIs) donepezil (Aricept),[1] rivastigmine (Exelon),[1] and galantamine (Razadyne ER)[1] are used to treat delirium, with anecdotal reports and small case series suggesting benefit. Theoretically, they might benefit some patients by enhancing cholinergic activity. Similarly, the NMDA [*N*-methyl-D-aspartate]-receptor antagonist memantine (Namenda)[1] is used, with theoretical benefit through the modulation of glutamate-induced excitotoxicity. Figure 1 lists dosing strategies.

Antipsychotic medications are used widely to treat delirium, particularly symptoms of agitation and psychosis.

[1]Not FDA approved for this indication.

Until recent years, haloperidol (Haldol)[1] was always the standard bearer, given its relatively good efficacy, versatility, and familiarity to nurses and physicians. However, the use of haloperidol carries a significant risk of extrapyramidal side effects (e.g., parkinsonism, akathisia), although interestingly enough the risk is less with intravenous (IV) preparations, even at high doses. The risk of tardive dyskinesia from extended haloperidol use is significant, with rates approaching 40% in elderly individuals after 9 months of treatment. Although ideally the use of haloperidol to treat delirium is short term, on the order of days to weeks, it is common for delirious patients to be discharged to an institutional setting where the medication is continued for months or longer.

Atypical antipsychotics are being used more widely as alternatives to haloperidol because they offer excellent efficacy with significantly lower risk of both extrapyramidal side effects and tardive dyskinesia. Small studies have found improvement in cognition, agitation, and psychosis associated with delirium in up to 90% of patients treated with risperidone (Risperdal),[1] olanzapine (Zyprexa),[1] and quetiapine (Seroquel).[1] All three agents are well tolerated with minimal side effects. The atypical antipsychotics ziprasidone (Geodon)[1] and aripiprazole (Abilify)[1] may carry similar benefits. Figure 1 lists dosing strategies and potential side effects.

For individuals who have failed or cannot tolerate antipsychotic agents, and for alcohol and benzodiazepine withdrawal, low-dose and short-term use of benzodiazepines can be considered. Both short and long half-life agents should be avoided because of risks of disinhibition, sedation, dizziness, respiratory depression, confusion, and falls. Although any benzodiazepine carries a risk of these side effects, the intermediate half-life agents lorazepam (Ativan)[1] and oxazepam (Serax)[1] are preferred agents

---

[1]Not FDA approved for this indication.

CURRENT DIAGNOSIS

- Delirium is an acute, transient brain syndrome characterized by fluctuating disturbances in consciousness, attention, cognition, perception, and behavior. Delirious patients may present with significant sleep-wake cycle disruptions, agitation, mood lability, and psychosis.
- Delirium is seen in 10% to 40% of individuals in medical settings. Key risk factors for delirium include advanced age, multiple medical problems, polypharmacy, dementia, infection, and recent surgery.
- Delirium always has a medical cause and is often multidetermined. Medications are the most common cause, followed by infection, substance intoxication or withdrawal, and metabolic disturbances.
- Delirium must be distinguished from dementia and other psychiatric disorders that involve mental status changes. Clinical history, observation over time, informant reports, and the use of a standardized instrument such as the Confusion Assessment Method can aid in diagnosis.

---

because of their simpler hepatic metabolism and lack of active metabolites. These same two benzodiazepines may be considered for short-term use in individuals with severe sleep-wake cycle disturbances; alternatively, clinicians may consider zolpidem (Ambien),[1] zaleplon (Sonata),[1] or trazodone (Desyrel).[1] Atypical antipsychotics may also improve sleep in some delirious individuals.

In general, all psychotropic medications used to treat delirium must be used cautiously and reevaluated frequently to determine if they are improving symptoms without worsening the delirium or introducing new side effects. Clinicians should consider tapering and then discontinuing these agents when symptoms abate while being vigilant for recurrence. The exception would be the use of AChEIs or memantine (Namenda)[1] in individuals with delirium and dementia; in those cases, long-term use is indicated for the treatment of the dementia itself after the delirium has abated.

Course and Prognosis

In two thirds of individuals with delirium, symptoms last from 2 days to a week. The delirium may persist for months in some individuals, and it is seen in up to 15% of

---

[1]Not FDA approved for this indication.

CURRENT THERAPY

- The treatment of delirium begins with identifying and treating underlying medical causes.
- Agitation and psychosis are common manifestations of delirium and can lead to self-harm, disruption of necessary medical treatment, and harm to caregivers. Affected individuals should be monitored 24 hours, with consideration of physical and/or chemical restraints for severe behavioral disturbances.
- Antipsychotic medications, including haloperidol (Haldol), risperidone (Risperdal),[1] olanzapine (Zyprexa),[1] quetiapine (Seroquel),[1] and others, are not FDA approved for the treatment of delirium, but in small studies they have demonstrated good efficacy and relative safety for treating symptoms of delirium, particularly agitation and psychosis.
- Benzodiazepines can be used to treat alcohol or benzodiazepine withdrawal or for individuals who cannot tolerate antipsychotic medications. They treat agitation but not psychosis.
- A nonpharmacologic approach to treat delirium involves providing a familiar, structured, and consistent environment with orientation cues and appropriate but not excessive stimulation. Pharmacologic agents that may provide some benefit for delirium include antipsychotic medications, the acetylcholinesterase inhibitors donepezil (Aricept),[1] rivastigmine (Exelon),[1] and galantamine (Razadyne ER),[1] and the NMDA [N-methyl-D-aspartate]-receptor antagonist memantine (Namenda).

---

[1]Not FDA approved for this indication.

sufferers after 6 months. The true efficacy of preventive strategies is unclear because several interventional studies do not demonstrate reduced rates of delirium. But one large comprehensive study of older hospitalized individuals at high risk for delirium found a lower rate, reduced duration, and fewer total episodes of delirium in individuals exposed to interventions for orientation, mobilization, sleep hygiene, sensory enhancement, and dehydration. Similar interventions that educate staff and provide adequate pain control and rapid attention to the inpatient environment and postoperative complications may help reduce both the severity and duration of delirium. Even with aggressive treatment, delirium delays functional improvement and increases the length of hospital stays, the degree of nursing care, the risk of cognitive and functional decline, and the need for home health services or nursing home placement. All of these factors are worse when there is underlying dementia and when underlying etiologies are not adequately treated. The rate of mortality ranges from 25% to 40% in the 6 to 12 months following an episode of delirium.

REFERENCES

American Psychiatric Association: Practice guideline for the treatment of patients with delirium. Am J Psychiatry 1999,156(Suppl 5):1-20.

Flacker JM, Cummings V, Mach JR Jr, et al: The association of serum anticholinergic activity with delirium in elderly medical patients. Am J Geriatr Psychiatry 1998;6:31-41.

Inouye SK. Bogardus ST Jr, Charpentier PA, et al: A multicomponent intervention to prevent delirium in hospitalized older patients. N Engl J Med 1999;340:669-676.

Inouye SK, Charpentier MP: Precipitating factors for delirium in hospitalized elderly patients. JAMA 1996;275:852-857.

Inouye SK, Rushing JT, Foreman MD, et al: Does delirium contribute to poor hospital outcome? A three-site epidemiologic study. J Gen Intern Med 1998;13:234-242.

Inouye SK, van Dyck CH, Alessi CA, et al: Clarifying confusion: The confusion assessment method: A new method for detection of delirium. Ann Intern Med 1990;113:941-948.

Liptzin B, Jacobson SA: Delirium. In BJ Sadock, VA Sadock (eds): Comprehensive Textbook of Psychiatry, 8th ed. Philadelphia, Lippincott Williams & Wilkins, 2005, pp 3693-3700.

Parellada E, Baeza I, de Pablo J, Martinez G: Risperidone in the treatment of patients with delirium. J Clin Psychiatry 2004;65(3):348-353.

Samuels SC, Neugroschl JA: Delirium. In BJ Sadock, VA Sadock (eds): Comprehensive Textbook of Psychiatry, 8th ed. Philadelphia, Lippincott Williams & Wilkins, 2005, pp 1054-1068.

Sasaki Y, Matsuyama T, Inoure S, et al: A prospective, open-label, flexible-dose study of quetiapine in the treatment of delirium. J Clin Psychiatry 2003;64(11):1316-1321.

Skrobik YK, Bergeron N, Dumont M, Gottfried SB: Olanzapine vs haloperidol: Treating delirium in a critical care setting. Intensive Care Med 2004;30(3):444-449.

Trepacz PT: Is there a final common pathway in delirium? Focus on acetylcholine and dopamine. Semin Clin Neuropsychiatry 2000; 5:132-148.

Mood Disorders

Method of
Melanie W. Conway, MD,
and Merry N. Miller, MD

Mood disorders are common. Depressed mood is the fourth most common presenting complaint in a primary care setting. Approximately 1 of 10 patients seen by a primary care physician has a major depressive disorder (MDD), with a 10% to 25% lifetime prevalence for women and a 5% to 12% lifetime prevalence for men. Prevalence for bipolar disorder ranges from 1% to 5%. Mood disorders worsen the morbidity and mortality rates of other medical disorders, and in fact, 68% of so-called service overutilizers of medical care have had a major depression diagnosis. Moreover, up to 15% of people with untreated depression kill themselves. Because nonpsychiatrists prescribe 80% of antidepressants, it is essential that the primary care physician be acquainted with the diagnosis and treatment of mood disorders.

Diagnosing Mood Disorders

As stated previously, mood disorders are very common, have high morbidity and mortality rates, and are highly treatable, but studies show that only a third to a half of those with major depressive episodes are properly recognized by practitioners, and fewer than a third of patients with bipolar disorder are in treatment. One reason might be that although mood disorders are not transitory reactions to external stressors, 70% of those who have a major depression could cite a stressor that preceded their depressive episode. A common occurrence is that both the patient and the physician focus on the stressor. This focus on the stressor generally elicits an internalized reaction from the physician, for example, "That is not bad enough

CURRENT DIAGNOSIS

- Look for symptoms (SIGECAPS) in patients with suspected depression regardless of the presence of stressors.
- Always screen for a history of mania in patients who present for depression.
- Always ask about suicidality, including the presence of thoughts, specific plans, intent, and a history of attempts.
- Be prepared to hospitalize, including involuntarily, if patients are actively suicidal.
- Look for medical conditions and medications that may precipitate or worsen depression.
- Check T4, TSH, and CBC in all patients with mood symptoms if not recently done.
- Always ask about use of alcohol and illicit drugs in patients presenting with depression.

Abbreviations: CBC = complete blood count; SIGECAPS = **S**leep, **I**nterest, **G**uilt, **E**nergy, **C**oncentration, **A**ppetite, **P**sychomotor, **S**uicide; T4 = thyroxine; TSH = thyroid-stimulating hormone.

TABLE 1 Diagnostic Criteria for Depressive and Manic Episodes

Major Depressive Episode	Manic Episode
Five or more of the following symptoms present most of the time for 2 weeks: ■ Depressed or irritable mood* ■ Diminished interest or pleasure (anhedonia)* ■ Disturbance of appetite ■ Insomnia or hypersomia ■ Psychomotor agitation or retardation ■ Fatigue or loss of energy ■ Feelings of worthlessness or guilt ■ Diminished ability to concentrate ■ Recurrent thoughts of death/suicidal ideation/suicide attempt	At least 3 (or 4 if mood is only irritable) of the following symptoms for at least a 1-wk period or any duration if hospitalization required: ■ Elevated, expansive, or irritable mood* ■ Inflated self-esteem or grandiosity ■ Decreased need for sleep ■ Hyperverbal ■ Racing thoughts/flight of ideas ■ Distractibility ■ Increased activity or psychomotor agitation ■ Excessive involvement with pleasurable activities with risk for painful consequences

*For a major depressive episode diagnosis, the symptom for either depressed mood or anhedonia must be present. For a manic episode diagnosis, the altered mood symptom must be present.

to get depressed about," or conversely, "If that were happening, I would be depressed, too"; both of these reactions decrease the probability that the physician will elicit depressive symptomatology and treat a possible mood disorder.

Also, many patients do not tell the physician that they are "depressed." In fact, a lot of men use the words "stressed out." Children and adolescents may commonly present with behavioral disturbances, and the elderly (65 years and older) with somatic complaints.

So key words that might clue the physician into a mood disorder are "irritated," short fused," "stressed," "not acting right," "not myself," "don't care," "no energy," "can't think, focus, or concentrate," or a plethora of vague physical complaints.

Table 1 summarizes the diagnostic criteria, and a decision-making algorithm can be followed as presented in Figure 1. First, the physician suspecting depression should ask about depressed mood and/or decreased interests and SIGE-CAPS (Sleep, Interest, Guilt, Energy, Concentration, Appetite, Psychomotor, Suicide*). Primary care physicians should routinely ask about sleep and appetite and consider depression when these are altered: With depression these may change in either direction, although it is more common for depressed patients to report decreased sleep and appetite. In addition, depressed patients report decreased interests (ability to enjoy usual activities, changes in energy (usually decreased), and difficulty concentrating. The latter symptom may cause the patient to develop problems with short-term memory, and it is not unusual for depressed patients to fear they are losing their mind or becoming demented owing to difficulty concentrating and remembering. They may show psychomotor slowing or alternatively, they may become agitated. Most seriously, patients with depression may develop suicidal ideation. They also may experience feelings of guilt about real or imagined sins, and may become preoccupied with feelings of worthlessness.

The physician must first address the management of any potential suicidal risk (see later discussion of suicide). Then

the physician answers this question: "Does this patient have depressed mood or loss of interests or pleasure in usual activities with four other neurovegetative symptoms most of the day, nearly every day, for at least 2 weeks or not?" If the answer is yes, the patient has a major depression regardless of the presence or absence of stressors.

If instead a patient reports a recent stressor but does not meet the full criteria for a major depression, the patient has an adjustment disorder. This distinction is important because first-line treatment recommendations differ between an adjustment disorder and MDD.

If a person is determined to have a major depressive episode, it is incumbent on the physician to ask about manic symptoms as well because the prevalence of bipolar disorder is now thought to be higher than previously documented. Antidepressants alone in a depressed patient with bipolar disorder can switch them into a mania even if they were never manic before. Useful screening questions include, "Have you ever felt the opposite of what you do now, like on top of the world?" or " Have you ever had a period in which you felt you did not need sleep, or very little sleep, and still had plenty of energy?" If they answer yes, then the rest of the mania answers can be elicited with the useful mnemonic DIGFAST (Distractibility, Insomnia, Grandiosity, Flight of ideas, Activities, Speech, Thoughtfulness*).

However, a word of caution: mania is very difficult to diagnose accurately retrospectively. It would not be difficult to get affirmative answers to such questions as "Have you ever spent more money than usual?" or "Have you ever had more energy than usual?" from most people asked the questions in the mania criteria. By definition (according to the *Diagnostic and Statistical Manual of Mental Disorders, Fourth Edition* [*DSM-IV*]), a mania has to be a distinctly different period than normal where "the mood disturbance is sufficiently severe to cause marked impairment in occupational functioning or in usual social activities or relationships with others" that must last at least 1 week (less if hospitalized) or with a hypomanic episode last at least 4 days and be "an unequivocal change

---

*Carey Gross, MD, originally developed this mnemonic for depression.

*William Falk, MD, originally developed this mnemonic for mania.

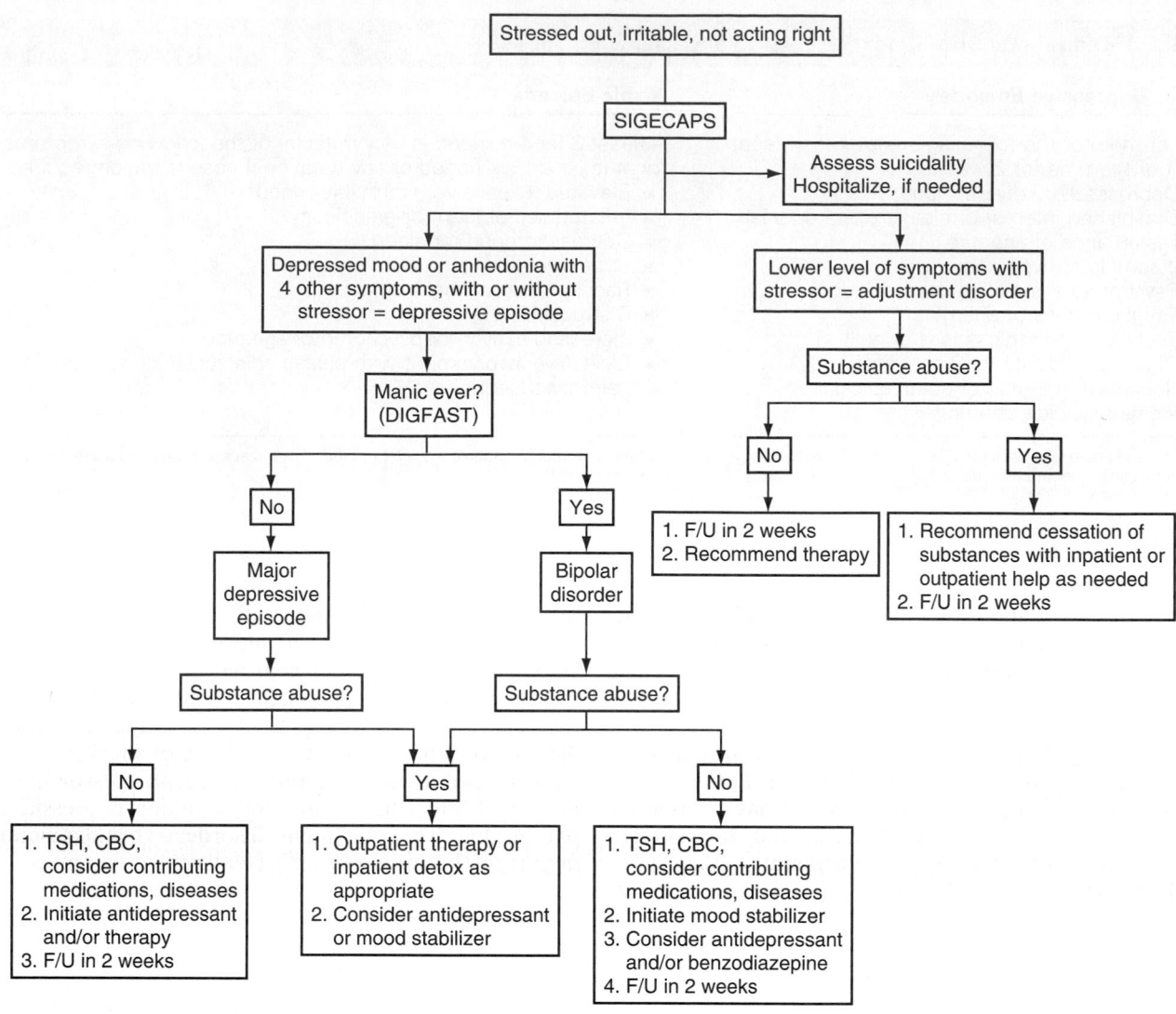

FIGURE 1. Basic algorithm for diagnosis and treatment of mood disorders. *Abbreviations:* CBC = complete blood count; DIGFAST = **D**istractibility, **I**nsomnia, **G**randiosity, **F**light of ideas, **A**ctivities, **S**peech, **T**houghtfulness; F/U = follow up; SIGE-CAPS = **S**leep, **I**nterest, **G**uilt, **E**nergy, **C**oncentration, **A**ppetite, **P**sychomotor, **S**uicide; TSH = thyroid-stimulating hormone.

in functioning that is uncharacteristic of the person when not symptomatic." The symptoms should occur together in the same 1-week period. Sometimes a severely depressed person answers yes to mania symptomatology when describing not a mania, but rather a baseline level of functioning as compared to the depression. The distinction is important because of its implications about treatment (see treatment discussion).

Other depressive disorders that should be screened for are dysthymic disorder and premenstrual dysphoric disorder (PMDD). In dysthymic disorder, patients have a chronic low-grade level of depression (not enough to qualify for MDD) that exists for more than 2 years. Women with PMDD experience depressive symptoms that occur exclusively during the premenstrual portion of the menstrual cycle and then resolve after the onset of menses. Another variation of depression is premenstrual exacerbation of depression in which women with MDD experience worsening of the mood premenstrually that does not fully resolve with the onset of menses.

These variations of depressive disorder may be treated with antidepressants, and PMDD responds to intermittent dosing (i.e., only during the premenstrual phase). A diagnostic and treatment review of other types of mood disorders is beyond the scope of this chapter.

SUICIDE

If you are considering a diagnosis of a mood disorder, and especially if you prescribe medications for a mood disorder, you must *always* ask about suicide because two thirds of all depressed patients contemplate suicide at some point. Studies show that 50% of all people who commit suicide see their primary care physician within 1 month of the suicide and 40% within 1 week of the suicide.

Suicidal ideation, just like radiating chest pain, is a medical emergency and should be treated as such, especially when being presented to the physician the first time. Critical considerations that increase the level of risk are these: (1) Does the patient have a plan and means?

How lethal is the plan? (Gunshots and hanging are the most lethal and most concerning plans.) Has the patient considered acting on the plan? (2) History of suicide attempts: Were high-risk methods used in the past, and how likely was the patient to be rescued? (3) Lack of social supports or recent losses (e.g., job, relationships); (4) Chronic medical illnesses; (5) Substances abuse, especially in the intoxicated or withdrawal state.

Consulting with a family member, with the patient's consent, is a very good way not only to elicit information but also to garner needed social support should the decision be made to treat the patient on an outpatient basis or to support an inpatient recommendation.

If the physician does not consider the patient's risk to be imminent and the decision is made to continue treatment on an outpatient basis, a psychiatric referral should be made and the physician should see the patient often; at least until the patient is seen by the psychiatrist. Contracting for safety with the patient has some psychological value, although doing so grants no legal protection to the physician.

In every area of the United States there is the equivalent of a mobile response team with a psychiatric backup that can be called in case no psychiatrist is available for consultation or if the patient or the patient's family is against an inpatient recommendation and you are very concerned about suicide risk. These telephone numbers should be readily available to the physician so during a time of crisis valuable time does not have to be spent searching for them.

Although there is some variation among the states, if the patient (and/or family) is unwilling for the patient to wait for the mobile crisis evaluation or go to the emergency department and the patient shows evidence of being dangerous to himself or others, he or she can be involuntarily committed. Every physician should know the commitment criteria for one's own state. If the patient's current symptoms meet these criteria, the police/security should be called to detain or apprehend the patient if necessary, and the patient should be held against his or her will until further evaluation by mobile crisis or an emergency department physician can be done. Although ideally rare, this set of events often garners extreme emotions and occasionally litigious threats. Most patients later are able to appreciate the concern that led to their hospitalization. Legal precedent tends to fall in favor of the physician who acted with due diligence rather than the physician whose patient was let go who went on to kill themselves. Regardless of the in/outpatient status of the patient, careful documentation of the symptoms, decision-making process, and plan is essential.

MEDICAL CONDITIONS AND DRUGS ASSOCIATED WITH MOOD DISORDERS

Fifty percent of those with psychiatric illness also have substance abuse problems. Substance use alone could cause mood disorders such as depression in chronic ethanol, benzodiazepine, barbiturate, and opiate use, cocaine withdrawal, or mania in methamphetamine or cocaine intoxication. However, many times it is difficult to separate which came first, the substance abuse or the mood disorder. Useful questions are these: (1) When did the mood disorder symptoms start? When did the

substance abuse start? (2) What has been your longest period of nonuse of any alcohol or illicit substances (drugs)? During that time (especially if it was more than 1 year), how was your mood?

Many prescribed substances can also evoke mood symptoms such as anesthetics, analgesics, anticholinergics, anticonvulsants, antihypertensives, antiparkinsonian medications, antiulcer medications, cardiac medications (especially β-adrenergic antagonists), isotretinoin (Accutane), oral contraceptives, muscle relaxants, anabolic steroids, corticosteroids, and sulfonamides. Heavy metals and toxins also can cause mood symptoms. This list is not exhaustive, and the patient's medication list always should be examined in search of temporal associations between newly prescribed agents and the onset or exacerbation of mood complaints.

Also, a long list of medical conditions can be associated with depression or mania, or a mood disorder can be the presenting symptom. The list is huge, but two deserve special mention. One medical condition is poststroke depression. At both 15-month and 10-year follow-ups, patients with poststroke major or minor depression are between four and eight times more likely to die than are nondepressed stroke patients. The second medical condition is cardiovascular disease. Even when one controls for smoking (depressed patients are more likely to smoke) and other factors, a large study showed that at 6 months, 17% of depressed patients had died versus 3% of the nondepressed patients. There was a 42% reduction in combined endpoint of death or recurrent myocardial infarction with antidepressant use.

LABORATORY TESTS

Again, although the list of medical illnesses that can cause or exacerbate a depression is extensive, two of the most common illnesses etiologically related to mood disorders are thyroid disease and anemia. Either hypothyroidism or hyperthyroidism can be associated with depressive symptoms. Therefore, obtaining a thyroxine/thyroid-stimulating hormone (T4/TSH) and a complete blood count (CBC) are standard in a mood disorder workup. Other laboratory tests may be indicated based on the medication chosen (see Treatment section).

Treatment

First, a physician must address any etiologic or contributing factors such as medical conditions or substance use. If substances are used, treatment for such must be addressed first because mood disorder symptoms may be related to their use alone, and even if mood disorder symptoms are primary (many substance abusers state they are "self-medicating"), the benefit of antidepressant or mood stabilizer pharmacotherapy will be reduced by continuing use. The standard used to be that clinicians waited to medicate until the patient had been sober many months, but recent studies show that pharmacotherapy does have a modest effect on abstinence rates.

For adjustment disorders, the recommended treatment is psychotherapy, and as with the other mood disorders, the patient is advised to return to see the physician within 2 weeks. At the later appointment, SIGECAPS should be

CURRENT THERAPY

- Choose an antidepressant based on how the side-effect profile fits with the symptoms of depression (e.g., a sedating medication for insomnia).
- Make sure to use an *adequate dose for an adequate duration* (at least 4–6 wk) before judging the effectiveness of an antidepressant.
- Watch for signs of antidepressant-induced switching to mania.
- If ineffective after an adequate trial, consider another antidepressant, possibly from another class.
- If still ineffective, consider augmentation of antidepressant with another class of medication; for example, lithium or thyroid hormone.
- For bipolar patients, start a mood stabilizer first. If the patient remains depressed, consider a possible antidepressant after the mood stabilizer dosage is therapeutic.
- When withdrawing antidepressants, taper the dose gradually to avoid the discontinuation syndrome.
- For patients with depression that does not respond to medication, consider electroconvulsive therapy (ECT).
- Always assess for suicidality throughout treatment for depression.

reevaluated for progressing to a major depressive episode, and the recommendation for psychotherapy is repeated if necessary.

The majority of patients with major depressive episodes, whether of the unipolar or bipolar type, are best treated with a combination of psychotherapy and medication. Cognitive-behavioral therapy and interpersonal therapy is as effective as medication in mild to moderate depression. In addition to individual psychotherapy, group and marital and family therapy may be useful depending on the patient's circumstances. It may be best to delay the use of marital or family therapy in a depressed patient until some improvement begins to occur. Psychotherapy produces longer lasting benefits than medication. Many patients have an individual preference for either psychotherapy or medication or may have logistical difficulty in participating in therapy, so the treatment plan should be developed in conjunction with the patient with mindfulness of patient preference. If the patient should initially choose medication management alone and does not garner the full benefits he or she expected from an adequate trial of medication(s), psychotherapy should definitely be reconsidered.

ANTIDEPRESSANTS

No particular antidepressant or class of antidepressants is more efficacious than the rest. However, effectiveness does differ because the older agents, tricyclic antidepressants (TCAs) and monoamine oxidase inhibitors (MAOIs), are less tolerable owing to side effects and lifestyle restrictions. Their use should not be ruled out because TCAs are generally inexpensive and are used to treat a variety of other medical conditions and MAOIs tend to work when other drugs have not.

Many factors need to be considered in picking an antidepressant, but there are three initial factors to consider in a treatment-naive patient. First, sleep-mood disorders do not get better if sleep does not improve, so, in treating someone who is not sleeping enough, one may consider a sedating antidepressant or a nonsedating one with a sleep agent. In treating someone who is sleeping too much or is anergic, the physician may consider a stimulating antidepressant. Second, side effects are one of the most common reasons for treatment failure because of lack of compliance. Two of the most common side effect concerns tend to be gender linked. Women are more likely to stop a drug if they feel it is making them gain weight. Therefore, in general, it is best to avoid antidepressants with higher rates of weight gain in the weight-conscious patient. Men may be more likely to stop a drug secondary to sexual side effects. Although they initially may not care about this possible side effect secondary to their depressive state, 2 or 3 months later they tend to change their mind, putting the clinician in the precarious position of either changing the antidepressant and risking relapse of the depressed state or adding agents such as yohimbine (Yocon) or sildenafil (Viagra) to help counter the sexual side effects. The third factor is cost because a minimum recommended duration of antidepressant treatment is approximately 1 year (see Patient Education section), and patients will not take or continue to take what they cannot afford to buy. That is why the TCAs are still useful to consider in some populations because of reduced cost. It is important to know your patient's resources and your sample closet. Also, many pharmaceutical companies have programs for those in need.

In the recurrent mood disorder patient, it is essential to obtain a more detailed history of what antidepressants the patient has tried, the length of treatment, the maximum dose, and the patient's view of the helpfulness of the agent. Many times antidepressant trials are not successful because of an inadequate length of treatment (generally 1 month or less) or inadequate dose. A partial response may have occurred in which the medication was not increased to a full therapeutic dose, or over time the effectiveness of the medication may have dwindled, which is common in selective serotonin reuptake inhibitors (SSRIs), and the dose not subsequently increased. In general, if it has worked before, it will probably work again with adjustments to dose. Another useful piece of information (in the treatment-naive patient as well) is family history of response to medication. A general rule of thumb is that if one family member has responded to a particular antidepressant agent, the patient seeking treatment may also respond to that agent. All that being said, with the wide selection of antidepressants available, there is no reason to fight the uphill battle of trying to get patients to take a medication they do not want to take regardless of their reasons. Convincing them in the short term will probably only lead to noncompliance later. Tables 2 through 5 summarize the currently available antidepressants.

Selective Serotonin Reuptake Inhibitors

The SSRIs (Table 2) are currently considered first-choice antidepressants for many patients with depression.

TABLE 2 Selective Serotonin Reuptake Inhibitors (SSRIs)

Drug	Effective Dose	Comments
Fluoxetine (Prozac, Prozac weekly, Sarafem)	20–80 mg/d; weekly capsule 90 mg	Longest half-life, good for noncompliant patients, many drug interactions
Sertraline (Zoloft)	50–200 mg/d	Least potential for cytochrome-related drug interactions of SSRIs
Paroxetine (Paxil)	20–50 mg/d	Benefit for anxious depression; discontinue slowly
(Paxil CR)	25–62.5 mg/d	
Citalopram (Celexa)	20–60 mg/d	Least highly protein bound so fewer drug interactions
Escitalopram (Lexapro)	10–20 mg/d	S-enantiomer of citalopram
Fluvoxamine (Luvox)	50–250 mg/d	Potentiates caffeine and theophyllines

These medications share the mechanism of blocking serotonin reuptake. As a group, they have the advantages of being relatively low in side effects, safer than the tricyclics (nonlethal in overdose), easy to administer, and efficacious. The most common side effects of the SSRIs are nausea and diarrhea during early treatment, and if these occur, they usually resolve within a week or two. Some patients experience increased energy or jitteriness soon after SSRIs begin, which can be desirable for patients with fatigue or can be uncomfortable but usually diminishes within a few weeks. Sexual dysfunction is another side effect sometimes seen with SSRIs and may include decreased libido, impotence, delayed ejaculation, or anorgasmia. Medication interactions are seen with certain SSRIs that inhibit the cytochrome P-450 liver enzyme systems, especially fluoxetine (Prozac) and paroxetine (Paxil), so caution should be used in patients taking other medications. A discontinuation syndrome is described that is most likely to occur with paroxetine and includes flulike symptoms such as nausea, vomiting, fatigue, headache, and myalgia. Slow tapering at discontinuation may prevent this syndrome.

Other Newer Antidepressants

A number of other antidepressants (Table 3) have been developed that differ in mechanism from the SSRIs.

Trazodone (Desyrel) and nefazodone (Serzone) block serotonin reuptake and also block 5-hydroxytryptamine 2 (5-HT2) receptors. Trazodone is often used for its sedative effect. The use of nefazodone has declined dramatically after being found to be the etiologic agent in some deaths secondary to hepatic failure.

Bupropion (Wellbutrin) is an effective antidepressant that acts to boost the neurotransmitters norepinephrine and dopamine. It has the potential benefits of being less likely to induce mania and less likely to cause sexual dysfunction than the SSRIs. It should be avoided in patients with a history of eating disorders because it can induce seizures in those patients.

Antidepressants with dual noradrenergic and serotonergic mechanisms include venlafaxine (Effexor) and duloxetine (Cymbalta). Venlafaxine actually has a mechanism that varies with its dose: At lower doses it blocks serotonin reuptake, whereas when the dose exceeds 150 mg/day, it blocks increasingly higher amounts of norepinephrine. Venlafaxine may increase blood pressure, especially at high doses, and should be monitored. Duloxetine is effective for major depression and also for pain that may coexist with depression.

Mirtazapine (Remeron) blocks α-2 and serotonin receptors. It has a low rate of sexual dysfunction, is sedating, and causes weight gain. It has the unusual feature of a decrease in side effects associated with increasing dose.

TABLE 3 Other Antidepressants (non-SSRIs)

Drug	Effective Dose	Comments
Bupropion (Wellbutrin, Zyban)	225–450 mg in 3 divided doses; do not give after 5 PM	Maximum single dose: 150 mg; seizure risk if dose excessive; contraindicated in bulimia and anorexia
Bupropion SR (Wellbutrin SR)	200–450 mg in 2 divided doses; do not give after 5 PM	Maximum single dose: 200 mg
Bupropion XL (Wellbutrin XL)	150–450 mg once daily	Less risk of sexual dysfunction than other antidepressants
Mirtazapine (Remeron)	15–45 mg at bedtime	Sedating, causes weight gain; low rates of sexual dysfunction
Venlafaxine (Effexor, Effexor XR)	75–225 mg/d once daily (extended release) or 2–3 doses (immediate release)	Monitor blood pressure; low protein binding so less drug interactions
Duloxetine (Cymbalta)	40–60 mg/d in 1–2 doses	Benefit for co-morbid pain

Abbreviations: SSRI = selective serotonin reuptake inhibitor.

TABLE 4 Tricyclic Antidepressants

Drug	Dosage Range (mg/d)
Amitriptyline	25–300
Clomipramine	50–250
Desipramine	25–300
Doxepin	25–300
Imipramine	25–300
Maprotiline	50–225
Nortriptyline	25–150
Protriptyline	20–60
Trimipramine	75–300

It may be especially helpful for patients with melancholic depression who have poor sleep and appetite.

Tricyclic Antidepressants

TCAs (Table 4) are as efficacious as the newer agents but less effective because of side effects. These side effects include antihistaminic effects (sedation and weight gain), anticholinergic effects (dry mouth, dry eyes, constipation), and antiadrenergic effects (orthostatic hypotension, which is a significant problem in the elderly (65 years and older) owing to increased fall risk). Cardiac conduction problems are of concern because the TCAs can provoke bradyarrhythmias, lengthen the QT interval, and induce symptomatic conduction delays in patients with conduction delays and bundle-branch block. The most serious problem with TCA therapy is lethality in overdose. As little as a 10-day supply can cause cardiac arrhythmias, seizures, and death. Other agents should also be considered in patients with narrow-angle glaucoma because of the TCA's anticholinergic properties. TCAs are also thought to switch depressed patients into mania at a higher rate than the other antidepressants.

All of this being said, TCAs have been used for decades for treatment of depression. Patients should receive a pretreatment electrocardiogram (ECG), and subsequent ECGs should be ordered, particularly with dosage increases. TCAs also have several other indications, including pain disorders, and sometimes simply increasing the TCA dose helps with pain and depression instead of adding a second antidepressant. This recommendation is especially important to keep in mind because TCA levels can increase two- to threefold with some SSRIs, especially fluoxetine (Prozac) and paroxetine (Paxil). Many TCAs also have the distinct advantage of the physician being able to obtain clinically relevant serum drug levels. Most TCAs show an onset of clinical effects occurring at serum levels between 150 and 200 µg/mL with little therapeutic benefit and increased side effects above these ranges. The exception is nortriptyline (Pamelor), which appears to have a therapeutic window of between 50 and 150 µg/mL.

Monoamine Oxidase Inhibitors

Although very effective, especially in cases of refractory or atypical depression, MAOIs are used very rarely, even in the hands of a specialist, owing to their medication interactions and dietary restrictions. However, physicians should be aware of this class, and drug interaction profiles should be run on any patient who is on a MAOI before another medication is prescribed.

Patient Education

The physician must spend a few minutes educating the patient for an antidepressant trial to be successful. As stated earlier, one of the major reasons for antidepressant trial failure is noncompliance. People stop taking antidepressants for a number of reasons including a so-called antibiotic view of medications: "Once I feel better I can stop." Anxious people, scared of initial side effects, may abruptly stop a medication. To address these, the physician needs to spend approximately 2 to 3 minutes saying something like this (tempered by the education and sophistication of the patient): "I am recommending that you take an antidepressant called _____. All antidepressants take

TABLE 5 Mood Stabilizers

Drug	Effective Dose	Comments
Lithium (Lithobid, Eskalith)	Start 300 mg bid–tid; maintain 900–1200 mg/d	See text.
Divalproex (Depakote, Depakote ER)	Titrate up to 20 mg/kg/d, usually 500 mg bid–tid or 1000 to 1500 mg extended release	See text.
Carbamazepine (Tegretol, Tegretol XR)	Start 200 mg bid up to maximum of 1600 mg/d	See text.
Lamotrigine (Lamictal)	25 mg qd × 2 wk, 50 mg qd × 2 wk, 50-mg increases weekly thereafter	Effective in depression. ½ dose for combination with Depakote (see text).
Aripiprazole (Abilify)	5–30 mg qd	Little sedation.
Olanzapine (Zyprexa, IM and Zydis forms)	5–20 mg/d (tab and Zydis) IM: 10 mg up to tid	More likely to cause weight gain, metabolic syndrome.
Quetiapine fumarate (Seroquel)	100–800 mg/d	Low rate of EPS, more effective at >300 mg/d.
Risperidone (Risperdal, Risperdal Consta)	2–3 mg qd initially, maximum 6 mg/d, Consta injection 25 mg IM q2wk in combination with oral for 2–3 mo	Slightly more likely to cause EPS, prolactinemia, especially at doses >6 mg/d.
Ziprasidone (Geodon)	20 mg bid with food; maximum dose: 160 mg	Discontinue if QTc >500 msec, less weight gain.

Abbreviations: EPS = extrapyramidal side effect; IM = intramuscular.

4 to 8 weeks to get a full effect, and you will not really know if this will work for you until you have been on it that long, although you may get a partial response sooner. Unfortunately, you may get side effects in the first few weeks before you get most of the good effects. Although there can be different side effects for different people, the most common ones for _____ are _____. I expect you to have at least one or two of these. If you have not had at least one side effect by 2 weeks, you need to call me. You can expect the side effects to be at their worst initially, then to decrease. The therapeutic benefit may not occur until a full month or more has passed, so it is important to keep taking it. If you respond to this medication, you will need to be on it at least a year to reduce your risk of a relapse." This short statement addresses two of the biggest obstacles to compliance: anxiety over side effects and duration of treatment.

It must be added, to the suicidal patient especially, that any emergence or worsening of suicidal ideation should be reported to the physician immediately because energy and concentration generally improve before mood, which would make the still depressed patient more capable of carrying out a plan. This explanation has been the historical reasoning for the tie between suicide and antidepressant treatment, and susceptible patients should be closely monitored, especially during the first month of treatment. In fact, the Food and Drug Administration (FDA) has now issued a black box warning for children and adolescents about the potential for emerging suicidal ideation with antidepressants and is considering extending this warning to all populations. Although this should not keep the clinician from prescribing needed treatment, it might lower the bar for specialist referral.

MOOD STABILIZERS

Although reliable data from well-designed randomized clinical trials are not available for mood-stabilizing actions of antimanic drugs other than lithium, a consensus panel involving 58 national experts produced strong agreement that antimanic drugs should be used in all phases of the treatment of bipolar disorder, including depression. For treatment of the manic phase, consensus guidelines suggested lithium (Eskalith) or divalproex (Depakote) as initial treatments, with carbamazepine (Tegretol)[1] as the next choice. Antipsychotic medications were recommended for psychotic bipolar disorder and as adjuncts for severe nonpsychotic mania and mixed states. Anticonvulsants were preferred over lithium for mixed and rapid-cycling states.

For bipolar depression, in view of the risk of antidepressant-induced mania, American Psychiatric Association Practice Guidelines and Expert Consensus Guidelines recommend that treatment of bipolar depression begin with an antimanic drug. Lithium and lamotrigine (Lamictal) are the two recommended bipolar depression agents. Lithium can be used alone or in conjunction with another mood stabilizer because it is effective in bipolar depression and mania. However, it is recommended that lamotrigine be used in conjunction with an antimanic agent because it is not effective alone for acute manic episodes.

---

[1]Not FDA approved for this indication.

In cases of refractory bipolar depression, antidepressants can be considered, but again, an antimanic drug needs to be continued. In contrast to unipolar depression, no evidence indicates that continuation of antidepressants after remission of bipolar depression prevents further depressive recurrences. In view of the risks of long-term antidepressant therapy, it seems prudent to attempt to withdraw the antidepressant once mood normalizes while continuing the mood-stabilizing regimen. Gradual discontinuation of antidepressants may reduce the risk of rebound of depression.

Lithium is generally started at 300 mg two to three times per day in the nonrenally impaired patient. An initial trough level can be obtained 4 to 5 days from initiation with a target blood level between 0.8 and 1.0 mEq/L. The effectiveness of lithium is decreased by its side effects, which include the following:

1. Tremor: Best evidenced when the patient's hands and fingers are outstretched; may benefit from mild dosage reduction or β-blockers.
2. Renal: Lithium is metabolized in the kidney and interactions with the kidney can cause polyuria with secondary polydipsia in 25% of cases. Also, certain diuretics, particularly thiazide diuretics, decrease the clearance of lithium, which could induce lithium toxicity and secondary renal failure.
3. Thyroid: 5% of patients (more often women) develop hypothyroidism during chronic lithium treatment.
4. Cardiac: Lithium can cause T-wave flattening or inversion owing to displacement of intracellular potassium.
5. Weight gain.
6. Cognitive: Mental slowing, memory problems, and apathy.
7. Hematologic: Benign leukocytosis that does not require intervention.
8. Birth defects: Not recommended in pregnancy, but only in the second or third trimester by a specialist if no other option is available.
9. Gastrointestinal: Initial nausea, vomiting, and diarrhea common.
10. Toxicity: Small therapeutic window; levels above 1.5 mEq/L are toxic.

Overdose, drug interactions, and dehydration can cause toxicity. Symptoms of toxicity include nausea, vomiting, tremor, diarrhea, confusion, and ataxia; at higher levels, toxicity can lead to seizures, coma, or death. Pretreatment, it is recommended that an ECG, blood urea nitrogen (BUN), creatinine, CBC, pregnancy test, and thyroid studies be done as well as an evaluation of the patient's medication list. Thyroid tests, renal tests, and trough (10 to 13 hours after the evening dose and before the morning dose) levels should be obtained every 2 to 3 months during the first 6 months of maintenance therapy and then every 6 months thereafter or when clinically indicated. A common practitioner mistake is to obtain random and not trough levels. Because this is relevant to lithium, divalproex (Depakote), and carbamazepine (Tegretol), it is important to understand that all therapeutic values are based on trough levels, so obtaining a random level is virtually useless.

Divalproex (Depakote) is generally started at 500 mg twice daily, but a loading dose of approximately 20 mg/kg can be given in acutely manic patients with an initial trough level obtained after 4 to 5 days with a target blood level between 50 and 125 µg/mL. Divalproex is generally thought to be better tolerated than lithium, but common dose-related side effects include sedation, nausea, vomiting, and diarrhea, especially upon initiation. Divalproex can cause thrombocytopenia and rarely can cause fatal hepatotoxicity, hemorrhagic pancreatitis, and agranulocytosis. Also, because divalproex is highly protein bound and only the free portion reaches the central nervous system (CNS), in cases of hypoalbuminemia or in combination with other highly protein-bound drugs, it is recommended that clinicians obtain free plasma levels. Divalproex can cause neural tube defects in pregnancy. Therefore, it is recommended hepatic functioning (divalproex metabolizes in the liver), pregnancy tests, and a CBC be obtained pretreatment. Trough level and CBC should be obtained every 2 to 3 months initially, with hepatic enzymes to be repeated or amylase if clinically indicated during the first 6 months of maintenance therapy and then every 6 months thereafter or when clinically indicated.

Carbamazepine (Tegretol) is generally started at 200 mg twice daily, with an initial trough level to be obtained after 4 to 5 days with a target blood level between 4 and 12 µg/mL. Most common dose-related side effects include gastrointestinal effects (nausea, vomiting, cramps, and diarrhea) and CNS effects (confusion, drowsiness, ataxia, hyperreflexia/clonus, and tremor). Uncommon, but potentially lethal, side effects include transient leukopenia and mild thrombocytopenia, which in rare cases can progress to aplastic anemia and agranulocytosis. From 10% to 30% of people develop an elevation of liver enzymes from chemical hepatitis, elevation of bilirubin and alkaline phosphatase, and hyponatremia and hypo-osmolality from an antidiuretic hormone-like effect. Therefore, patients should be warned to call their physician if they experience any symptoms of hepatitis such as malaise, anorexia, nausea/vomiting, edema, or abdominal pain. Of great importance is carbamazepine's propensity to speed up its own metabolism and that of a number of other drugs through induction of hepatic enzymes. This induction results in lowering of the serum drug levels and can cause it and particularly oral contraceptives not to work. Because carbamazepine can also cause neural tube defects, this interaction is of particular importance. Therefore, pretreatment hepatic functioning, a pregnancy test, and a CBC should be obtained with trough level and CBC every 2 to 3 months and hepatic enzymes when clinically indicated.

Lamotrigine (Lamictal) is started at 25 mg every day and increased to 50 mg after 2 weeks with 50-mg increment increases weekly up to 500 mg.[1] If combined with Depakote, the initial dosing is 25 mg every other day with 25-mg increments to a maximum dosage of 200 mg.[1] The slow dosage titration is related to the risk of Stevens-Johnson syndrome, especially when Lamictal is titrated up too quickly and/or combined with Depakote. Lamotrigine is considered more effective for treating and preventing the depressive phase of bipolar disorder than for manic episodes.

As stated earlier, most of the atypical antipsychotics have a second-line indication in nonpsychotic bipolar disorder. Because of their risk in inducing diabetes, a pretreatment fasting lipid and glucose level, body mass index (BMI), initial weight, and ECG should be performed with repeat of these in 3 months and then yearly thereafter while the patient is on the agent.

Other drugs commonly used in bipolar disorder are gabapentin (Neurontin) and topiramate (Topamax).[1] Although neither of these is indicated as monotherapy in bipolar disorder, gabapentin is used frequently for adjunct therapy for anxiety and pain complaints and topiramate for help with weight gain with antimanic agents.

Patient Education

Compliance is a major factor in treatment success. There are more suicides secondary to bipolar depressive episodes than unipolar depressive episodes. A major study found the prophylactic effects of lithium to be so great it added 7 years to the life expectancy. However, nonadherence rates range from 33% to 64% within 1 month from initiation of treatment, primarily because of denial of illness and need for treatment, especially in the substance-abusing population. With education, bipolar patients can learn to recognize the symptoms of an impending episode and avoid hospitalizations by working closely with their physician.

ELECTROCONVULSIVE THERAPY

Electroconvulsive therapy (ECT) is the most effective available treatment for mood disorders. It surpasses treatment efficacy of all the other modalities and is used in fragile populations such as pregnant women and the elderly (65 years and older). There are no absolute contraindications to ECT, and it is the treatment of choice when a patient is refractory to all other therapies.

REFERENCES

Bauer MS: Mood disorders: bipolar (manic-depressive) disorders. In Tasman A, Kay J, Lieberman JA (eds): Psychiatry, 2nd ed. Chichester, England, Wiley & Sons, 2003, pp 1237-1270.

Blazer G: Depression in Late Life. St. Louis, Mosby-Year Book, 1993.

Cohen BJ: Theory and Practice of Psychiatry. New York, Oxford University Press, 2003.

Dubovsky SL, Davies R, Dubovsky AN: Mood disorders. In Hales RE, Yudofsky SC (eds): Textbook of Clinical Psychiatry, 4th ed. Washington, DC, American Psychiatric Association, 2003, pp 439-542.

Ghaemi SN: Mood Disorders. Philadelphia, Lippincott Williams & Wilkins, 2003.

Greist JH, Jefferson JW: Depression and Its Treatment. Washington, DC, American Psychiatric Association, 1992.

Gruenberg AM, Goldstein RD: Mood disorders: Depression. In Tasman A, Kay J, Lieberman JA (eds): Psychiatry, 2nd ed. Chichester, England, Wiley & Sons, 2003, pp 1207-1236.

Mondimore FM: Depression: The Mood Disease. Baltimore, Md, Johns Hopkins University Press, 1993.

Pies RW: Handbook of Essential Psychopharmacology, 2nd ed. Washington, DC, American Psychiatric Association, 2005.

Sadock BJ, Sadock VA: Mood disorders. In Sadock BJ, Sadock VA (eds): Kaplan & Sadock's Synopsis of Psychiatry, 9th ed. Philadelphia, Lippincott Williams & Wilkins, 2003, pp 534-590.

Stahl SM: Essential Psychopharmacology: The Prescriber's Guide. Cambridge, England, Cambridge University Press, 2005.

U.S. Department of Health and Human Services: Depression in Primary Care. Vol 1: Detection and Diagnosis. Rockville, Md, Agency for Health Care Policy and Research, 1993.

---

[1]Not FDA approved for this indication.

---

[1]Not FDA approved for this indication.

Schizophrenia

Method of
Adriana Foster, MD, and Peter Buckley, MD

Schizophrenia is a chronic debilitating illness, affecting 1% of the population, with an economic burden of $32.5 billion per year in the United States. Its implications include lost human potential because of inability to function personally, socially, and professionally, disability, risk of suicide, and impact on families.

The etiology of schizophrenia is still elusive. The neurodevelopmental hypothesis prevails and postulates that illness starts in utero with abnormal neuronal development. The knowledge about potential genetic loci for schizophrenia is yet limited but it is known that dizygotic twins have a 12% chance of developing schizophrenia if one twin is affected, whereas for monozygotic twins the risk increases to 50%. Genetic predisposition is thus a major risk factor—but by no means the only risk factor—for schizophrenia. It is currently thought that individuals with genetic predisposition to schizophrenia are especially vulnerable to in utero factors like hypoxia, rubella, maternal influenza, birth during late winter and spring, and maternal malnutrition. The pathologic brain abnormalities thought to be resulting from this interaction (smaller prefrontal cortex and hippocampus, enlarged ventricles) appear to be static in nature and occur without evidence of gliosis, commonly found in neurodegenerative disorders. At the molecular level, it is thought that genetic factors converge, leading to abnormal neuronal connectivity and synaptic signaling, and they may alter the dopaminergic and the glutamatergic pathways of the brain. There is early evidence of altered gene expression profiles for a variety of neurotrophic factors involved in brain development and regulation. A causal relationship and a mechanism by which susceptibility genes can predispose to schizophrenia are still to be identified.

The neurodegenerative hypothesis of schizophrenia is based on longitudinal studies showing that morphologic brain changes progress, especially early, during the first 5 years of illness or in the prodromal period, even before the clinical manifestations of schizophrenia are apparent. A recent trend in schizophrenia research is the study of the prodromal period and family members of probands with schizophrenia, in an effort to understand the effect of brain changes thought to be induced by untreated illness. In parallel, we are trying to treat the illness as early as possible to avoid the potential for neuronal damage, which some claim may result from episodes of florid psychosis. However, this approach is contentious because it proposes treatment of a population in their early twenties with antipsychotic medications, associated with noxious side effects of abnormal movements or metabolic disturbances.

A summary of the recent knowledge about neurotransmitter changes in schizophrenia (Table 1) is necessary to understand the postulated mechanism of action for antipsychotic drugs.

Some patients may have a prodromal period, with peculiarities of thought and behavior, followed by onset of full-blown psychosis. The illness has a relapsing course. During acute episodes patients lose contact with reality and often attend and respond to internal stimuli (hallucinations).

CURRENT DIAGNOSIS

- Impairment in reality testing: delusions and hallucinations
- Negative symptoms: anhedonia, alogia, avolition, affective flattening
- Disorganized thought and behavior
- Cognitive and executive dysfunction
- Symptoms lasting >6 mo
- Significant impairment in professional, social function, and personal relationships
- Onset in early 20s in men and early 30s in women
- Psychosis because of drugs, general medical condition, or major mood disorder ruled out.

Behavior may be motivated by commands from voices or delusional beliefs. The patients' thought processes can be loose and disorganized leading to like behavior, with disregard to self-care, isolation and social withdrawal, sometimes aggression, and hostility. The course may become less acute as patients advance in age (residual type schizophrenia). However, deficits of attention and working memory, executive dysfunction with decrease in goal-directed behavior, planning, flexibility and self-monitoring, as well as poor insight and judgment, persist. Significant suicide risk is present, associated with delusions, command hallucinations, or superimposed depression. Co-morbidity with alcohol and drug abuse is significant. Noncompliance with medication is common and requires extensive psychosocial intervention. The patients have major difficulty accessing medical care, following recommendations, and complying with treatment for their psychiatric and medical conditions, as illustrated next.

Case 1

A man with schizophrenia was admitted after being forcefully evicted from his apartment. He maintained that he owned the place and referred to his relationship with God. He complained of difficulty urinating and squatted on the unit at times. As part of his routine laboratory tests, his prostate-specific antigen (PSA) value returned in the thousands. He invoked delusional beliefs when he refused a prostate biopsy. His family, after numerous attempts to care for him, was not available to do so any longer. An emergency guardianship was obtained, and a prostate biopsy was performed in the operating room under general anesthesia. The results showed cancer of the prostate, and the urologist offered treatment with hormone injections. The patient passively accepted the treatment but never agreed that he had cancer.

Case 2

A smoker with hypertension (HTN), chronic obstructive pulmonary disease (COPD), and paranoid schizophrenia requested to change doctors because he felt that his psychiatrist was part of a plot against him, along with people at his supported housing facility. He came in stating he felt "depressed" and demanded that his new psychiatrist

TABLE 1 Neurotransmitter Abnormalities in Schizophrenia

Neurotransmitter	Dysfunction	Localization	Normal Function	Antipsychotic Effect
Dopamine (DA)	Hyperactivity	Nigrostriatal tract	Extrapyramidal system, controlling movement.	Movement disorders.
		Mesolimbic tract	Memory, stimulus processing, motivation (internal and external stimuli are postulated to have exaggerated motivational and emotional relevance in psychosis).	Reduce psychosis.
		Mesocortical tract	Cognition, executive function.	Reduce psychosis. Can induce akathisia.
		Tuberoinfundibular tract	Controls prolactin release.	Increased prolactin, galactorrhea, sexual dysfunction.
Serotonin (5-HT)		Same distribution with dopaminergic neurons	Serotonergic stimulation in the striatum decreases DA release.	5-HT$_2$ antagonism reduces psychosis and decreases DA-related movement disorders.
Glutamate (excitatory neurotransmitter)	Corticostriatal glutamate hypoactivity leads to DA hyperactivity (e.g., psychosis related to phencyclidine, an antagonist of the NMDA glutamate receptor)	Widespread in the brain	Synaptic plasticity, learning, memory. Under traumatic or ischemic conditions, glutamate concentrations rise to excitotoxic levels (it is postulated that obstetric complications generate a toxic glutamatergic release and thus the brain development becomes abnormal in-utero).	Not a primary mechanism of action for any current antipsychotic.

be paged. He appeared somnolent and short of breath. The records showed visits to the emergency department (ED) twice in the past week, with vague complaints of fatigue; he was offered treatment for respiratory symptoms and left before any treatment was administered. At arrival in the ED, the patient's oxygen saturation was 79% and at a psychiatrist's insistence, he eventually agreed to be examined by the ED physician. He was admitted to the intensive care unit, intubated, and underwent treatment for community-acquired pneumonia. Upon discharge from the hospital he thanked the psychiatrist for "saving my life" but continued to refuse his antipsychotic medication.

Many patients with schizophrenia, after brief hospitalizations, become clients of state-sponsored and federal outpatient mental health systems, where case management, day treatment, substance rehabilitation, vocational and incentive therapy, employment, and housing programs are accessible. The most refractory and noncompliant patients may respond to assertive community treatment, an intensive outreach approach by multidisciplinary teams available around the clock. Often the relationships with their families are under strain because of the burden on caretakers or the patient's delusional mistrust. Counseling and peer support for families of patients with schizophrenia at illness onset is key and helps them maintain involvement for the patient's lifetime. The National Alliance for Mentally Ill (NAMI) is a remarkable resource for self-help, support, and advocacy for patients and families of people with severe mental illnesses. NAMI provides education, combats stigma, promotes increased funding for research, and advocates tirelessly at the local and national level for health insurance, housing, rehabilitation, and jobs for people with mental illnesses (www.nami.org). It is a challenge to integrate the broad range of outpatient services needed to fulfill the needs of the patients with schizophrenia. An innovative but yet untested approach is to include peer support specialists (trained individuals who are themselves in recovery from mental illness) to act as a support (analogous to the Alcoholics Anonymous [AA] sponsorship approach) and to help the patient focus on meaningful goals for his or her recovery. Table 2 presents the two classes of antipsychotics currently in clinical use.

Co-morbidity of schizophrenia with substance use disorders is common (estimated prevalence of 47%), nearly three times higher than in the general population, and can lead to frequent rate of relapse and hospitalization, treatment noncompliance, and poor overall response

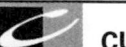 **CURRENT THERAPY**

- Lifelong approach
- Families involved as support system
- Complex psychosocial intervention
- Availability of crisis intervention and inpatient care
- Medication management customized for patient's co-morbid status and compliance level
- Ongoing monitoring of compliance and side effects in collaboration with primary care provider

TABLE 2 Summary of Antipsychotics in Clinical Use

First Generation	Mechanism of Action	Side Effects	Administration Forms
Chlorpromazine (Thorazine), thioridazine (Mellaril), perphenazine (Trilafon), trifluoperazine (Stelazine), haloperidol (Haldol), fluphenazine (Prolixin), pimozide (Orap)	Dopamine D2 receptor blockade	Extrapyramidal side effects (dystonia, parkinsonism treated with anticholinergics) Akathisia (treated with β-blocker or benzodiazepine), neuroleptic malignant syndrome (rare but life threatening), tardive dyskinesia (involuntary movements potentially irreversible) Hyperprolactinemia manifested as sexual dysfunction, menstrual irregularities, gynecomastia, galactorrhea, weight gain, and increased risk for diabetes; dyslipidemia and decreased bone mineral density; QT_c prolongation with thioridazine; anticholinergic effects for thioridazine and chlorpromazine	Oral for all; injectable forms available for haloperidol (can be given IM and IV) and fluphenazine. Haloperidol and fluphenazine available in long-acting injection form.
Second generation			
Risperidone (Risperdal)	D2 antagonism and 5-HT2 antagonism	Dose dependent EPS and Hyperprolactinemia; risk of CVA in elderly with dementia treated for behavioral symptoms	Oral (including rapid dissolving tablet Risperdal Soltab) and long acting injection (Risperdal Consta)
Olanzapine (Zyprexa)	D2 antagonism and 5-HT2 antagonism	Weight gain, abnormal glucose and lipid metabolism	Oral (including rapid dissolving tablet Zydis) and IM
Quetiapine (Seroquel)	Lowest D2 antagonism	Sedation and orthostatic hypotension at therapeutic dose	Oral
Ziprasidone (Geodon)	D2 antagonism and 5-HT2 antagonism, 5-HT1 agonist	QT prolongation, discontinue in patients with QTc > 500 ms	Oral and IM
Aripiprazole (Abilify)	Partial D2 agonist and antagonist	Warnings common to all atypical	Oral
Clozapine (Clozaril)	Low D2 antagonist and high 5-HT2 antagonist	Agranulocytosis, weight gain, seizures; fatalities due to myocarditis have been reported; highest risk in the first month of therapy	Oral (including rapid dissolving tablet FazaClo)

Abbreviations: IM = intramuscular; IV = intravenous.

to treatment. Alcohol has a prevalence rate of 33.7% and other substance use a rate of 27.5%, with cannabis and cocaine the most common. Patients with co-morbid substance abuse have an increased risk of violence and suicide and contribute to the increased overall economic burden of schizophrenia by extensive use of the social, institutional services, and EDs. Preliminary data exist about the possible role of second-generation antipsychotic drugs (clozapine [Clozaril], quetiapine [Seroquel], and olanzapine [Zyprexa]) in reducing the substance use in patients with schizophrenia. An estimated 58% to 90% of patients with schizophrenia smoke in comparison with the general population (28% to 30%).

Medical Co-morbidity

Patients with schizophrenia are at high risk for cardiovascular disease because of high rates of cigarette smoking, obesity, diabetes, and hypertriglyceridemia. Thioridazine, an older drug, has now only limited use because of its QT_c prolongation effect, which is associated with the development of torsades de pointes and sudden death. Dose-related QT_c prolongation with ziprasidone (Geodon) is reported, but it is not clinically relevant unless other risk factors occur, like hypokalemia, hypomagnesemia, or concomitant use of quinolone antibiotics (sparfloxacin [Zagam], moxifloxacin [Avelox], and gatifloxacin [Tequin]). Myocarditis can be associated with clozapine, especially in the first month of therapy.

Diabetes and obesity are 1.5 to 2 times more common in patients with schizophrenia than in the general population. Obesity (body mass index [BMI] = 30 kg/m) is common in patients with schizophrenia, especially women. Histamine-1 and serotonin-2C receptor antagonists and increased leptin levels may underlie the antipsychotic-induced weight gain. In addition to the common risks associated with obesity, coronary heart disease, and stroke, the patients with weight gain are more likely to face stigma and increased cost of health care. Treatment should include education of the patient and family or caregiver about nutrition, exercise, symptoms of diabetes, and results of neglecting one's medical care. Presently clinicians opt to switch antipsychotic if the weight gain is 5% over initial weight or if there is worsening of dyslipidemia or hyperglycemia, rather than adding antiobesity or lipid-lowering agents. Medications with additive weight gain effect should be avoided.

Patients with schizophrenia have an increased risk of abnormal glucose regulation with increased insulin resistance even without treatment with antipsychotics, which can further induce weight gain, reduce sensitivity to insulin, affect glucose transporters, and damage pancreatic islet cells.

Lipid abnormalities in schizophrenia occur as a result of antipsychotic treatment, with elevations in triglycerides and total cholesterol. Phenothiazine (chlorpromazine) and dibenzodiazepine (clozapine, olanzapine) derivatives increase serum triglycerides and total cholesterol. There is an intermediate effect from quetiapine. Risperidone (Risperdal) and ziprasidone lowered the baseline values of cholesterol and triglycerides in a landmark 18-month study comparing effectiveness of older agents with second-generation antipsychotics. The American Diabetes Association, American Psychiatric Association, and American Association of Clinical Endocrinologists developed monitoring guidelines for obesity, diabetes, and lipid abnormalities for patients on antipsychotic drugs. The patient's personal and family history should be taken before the treatment starts and annually; weight should be monitored monthly for the first 3 months and then quarterly; waist circumference, blood pressure, and fasting plasma glucose should be obtained at baseline, 3 months, then annually; and fasting lipid profile at baseline, 3 months, and then every 5 years.

Co morbidity with HIV affects 3.1% of patients with schizophrenia (eight times the prevalence in the general population). Hepatitis C affects 8.5% of psychiatric inpatients versus 1.8% of the general population. Some of the medications administered as part of the highly active antiretroviral treatment (HAART) may exacerbate psychosis. Interferon and ribavirin may induce or exacerbate depression. Cytochrome P450 2D6 and 3A4 interactions occur between antipsychotics and HAART (e.g., increased exposure to given doses of olanzapine and risperidone). Clozapine should be used with caution in patients with HIV because of possible agranulocytosis and seizures. Cognitive-behavioral therapy leads to lifestyle modifications in patients with schizophrenia; however, it has to be ongoing. Risk factors for noncompliance with treatment are poor insight, substance abuse, lack of social support, and poor therapeutic alliance. The coordination of care between medical and psychiatric staff is essential.

In using antipsychotics, psychiatrists have to bear in mind the characteristics of individual patients, appreciate the side-effect profile, and monitor carefully during the maintenance therapy. Their collaboration with primary care providers is vital in addressing the side effects when they occur. Algorithms were developed to guide the choice of antipsychotic and other somatic therapies (like electroconvulsive therapy [ECT]) at various stages of treatment.

Noncompliance is managed with long acting injectable and rapid dissolving forms of medication (Table 2) and through the psychiatrist's collaboration with the patient's family and caretakers. For refractory patients whose noncompliance exposes them at risk of hurting themselves or others, assertive community treatment and even involuntary treatment can be employed.

REFERENCES

American Diabetes Association, American Psychiatric Association, American Association of Clinical Endocrinologists, North American Association for Studies on Obesity: Consensus development conference on antipsychotic drugs and obesity and diabetes. J Clin Psychiatry 2004;65(2):267-272.

Cournos F, McKinnon K, Sullivan G: Schizophrenia and comorbid human immunodeficiency virus or hepatitis C virus. J Clin Psychiatry 2005;66(Suppl 6):27-33.

Glassman A: Schizophrenia, antipsychotic drugs and cardiovascular disease. J Clin Psychiatry 2005;66(Suppl 6):5-10.

Green A: Schizophrenia and comorbid substance use disorder: Effects of antipsychotics. J Clin Psychiatry 2005;66(Suppl 6):21-26.

Harrison PJ, Weinberger DR: Schizophrenia genes, gene expression, and neuropathology: On the matter of their convergence. Mol Psychiatry 2005;10(1):40-68.

Lieberman JA, Stroup TS, McEvoy JP, et al: Effectiveness of antipsychotic drugs in patients with chronic schizophrenia. N Engl J Med 2005;353(12):1209-1223.

Miller A, Hall CS, Buchanan RW, et al: The Texas Medication Algorithm Project Antipsychotic Algorithm for Schizophrenia, 2003 Update. J Clin Psychiatry 2004;65(4):500-508.

Practice Guideline for the Treatment of Patients with Schizophrenia, 2nd ed. Am J Psychiatry 2004;161(2)(Suppl).

Sadock BJ, Sadock VA: Schizophrenia and other psychotic disorders. In Sadock BJ, Sadock VA (eds): Kaplan and Sadock's Comprehensive Textbook of Psychiatry, 8th ed. Philadelphia, Lippincott Williams and Wilkins, 2005.

Panic Disorder

Method of
*Alexander Bystritsky, MD, PhD, and
Kira Williams, MD*

Diagnosis

Panic disorder (PD) and related agoraphobia (AG) are very prevalent and disabling conditions affecting 3% to 8% of the world population. Panic disorder is characterized by sudden episodes of acute apprehension or intense fear that occur *out of the blue* without any apparent cause-panic attacks. Intense panic usually lasts no more than a few minutes, but, in rare instances, can return in *waves* for a period of up to 2 hours. During the panic itself, any of the symptoms listed in Box 1 may occur.

The attack is spontaneous, unexpected, and occurs for no apparent reason. The word *agoraphobia* means fear of open spaces; however, under many instances agoraphobia is a fear of panic attacks. Patients suffering from agoraphobia are afraid of being in situations from which escape might be difficult, or in which help might be unavailable if they suddenly had a panic attack. Many agoraphobics not only fear having panic attacks but also fear embarrassment should they be seen having a panic attack. It is common for the agoraphobic to avoid a variety of situations (Box 2). The fear usually results in travel restrictions, or a need to be accompanied by others when leaving home. They may avoid certain situations such as waiting in a line, being in

BOX 1 Symptoms of Panic Attack

- Dizziness, unsteadiness, or faintness
- Fear of dying
- Fear of going crazy or losing control
- Feeling of choking
- Feeling of unreality—as if you're not all there
- Heart palpitations—pounding heart or accelerated heart rate
- Hot and cold flashes
- Nausea or abdominal distress
- Numbness, pain, or tingling in hands, feet, arms, legs, fingers, toes, lips, face
- Pain or discomfort in chest, upper back, shoulder blades
- Shortness of breath or a feeling of being smothered
- Sweating
- Trembling or shaking

crowded places (malls, theaters) and even using transportation, including driving a car. In the end, agoraphobic patients often end up completely housebound.

Impact and Cost

Panic attacks are very common events. Some studies show that lifetime prevalence of panic or panic-like episodes is somewhere from 15% to 45%. PD characterized by frequent, disturbing panic attacks accompanied by at least 1 month of persistent fear of having another attack is less frequent. Epidemiologic studies throughout the world indicate the lifetime prevalence of PD (with or without AG) ranges between 1.5% and 3.5%. Twice as many women as men suffer from panic disorder. Studies have suggested high co-morbidity, showing that 63% to 73% of PD patients have had at least one other mental health condition, including major depressive disorder, obsessive–compulsive disorder, or another anxiety disorder during their lifetime. Panic patients also tend to seek relief from their anxiety by self-medicating with alcohol and drugs (prescription and/or illicit). The professional life of a PD patient is also likely to suffer. The majority of these patients admit that the quality of their work diminished as a result of their anxiety. Those who are financially dependent and those who receive either welfare or disability benefits constitute a considerable 27% of all PD patients. Furthermore, there seems to be a lower life expectancy among PD patients because of an increased risk of developing some cardiovascular disease or because of suicidal behavior, although the evidence for this is not consistent. The actual costs of PD are difficult to evaluate because they are indirect and hidden, but it is estimated that they

BOX 2 Some of the More Common Situations Feared by Agoraphobics

- Being at home alone
- Crowded public places such as grocery stores, department stores, restaurants
- Enclosed or confined places such as tunnels, bridges, or the hairdresser's chair
- Public transportation such as trains, buses, subways, planes

BOX 3 Differential Diagnosis and Co-morbidity of Panic Disorder

1. Cardiac conditions
   a. Arrhythmias[a,c,d]
   b. Supraventricular tachycardia[a,c,d]
   c. Mitral valve prolapse[b,c,d]
2. Endocrine disorders
   a. Thyroid abnormality[a,b,c,d]
   b. Hyperparathyroidism[b,c,d]
   c. Pheochromocytoma[d]
   d. Hypoglycemia[a,c,d]
3. Vestibular dysfunctions[a,b,c,d]
4. Seizure disorders (temporal lobe epilepsy)[a,b,c,d]
5. Other psychiatric conditions
   a. Affective disorders
      (1) Major depression[d,e,f]
      (2) Bipolar disorder[b,d,e,f]
   b. Other anxiety disorders
      (1) Acute stress disorder[a,b,c,d,e,f]
      (2) Obsessive–compulsive disorder[a,b,c,d,e,f]
      (3) Post-traumatic stress disorder[a,b,c,d,e,f]
      (4) Social phobia[a,c,d,e,f]
      (5) Specific phobia[a,c,d,e,f]
   c. Psychotic disorders[a,d,e,f]
   d. Substance abuse and dependence
      (1) Withdrawal from central nervous system depressants[a,b,c,d,e,f]
         (a) Alcohol abuse (present in 40% of panic disorder patients)
         (b) Barbiturates
      (2) Stimulants[a,b,c,d,e,f]
         (a) Cocaine
         (b) Amphetamines
         (c) Caffeine
      (3) Cannabis[a,b,c,d,e,f]
      (4) Hallucinogens[a,b,c,d,e,f]

[a]The disorder can mimic panic disorder (PD).
[b]The disorder can cause or worsen PD through a variety of physiologic mechanisms.
[c]The disorder's symptoms could serve as triggers of panic attacks.
[d]The disorder could coexist with PD as an independent disorder.
[e]The disorder could be a co-morbid disorder with symptoms that intermingle with PD.
[f]The disorder could lead to PD or be a sequela of PD.

are quite extensive. Because of the physical nature of panic attack symptoms, most PD patients repeatedly consult their family physicians, internists or other health professionals. Current estimates of cost of these conditions in U.S. society are more than $44 billion per year, a figure comparable to the cost of cardiovascular disorders.

Differential Diagnoses

Box 3 summarizes the differential diagnoses for PD. The relationship between panic disorder and the other disorders listed in the table can be very complex, for example:

- Another disorder can mimic PD.
- Another disorder can cause or worsen PD through a variety of physiologic mechanisms.
- Another disorder's symptoms could serve as triggers of panic attacks.

- Another disorder could coexist with PD as an independent disorder.
- Another disorder could be a co-morbid disorder with symptoms that intermingle with PD.
- Another disorder could lead to PD or be a sequela of PD.

One such example of this interaction is cardiac arrhythmias. Although it is uncommon, an arrhythmia can coexist with panic disorder as an independent condition, and a sudden increase of heart rate could potentially provoke panic in a patient with PD. However, arrhythmia accompanied by fear could mimic a panic attack, and patients with potentially dangerous arrhythmias may receive inappropriate treatment as the result of misdiagnosis. Another possible association is mitral valve prolapse (MVP) in patients with PD, which is a frequent finding thought to be of doubtful clinical significance. However, recent research suggested that it is possible that these two disorders in some patients are linked genetically (via chromosome 13) in a syndrome characterized by β-adrenergic hyperactivity, MVP, panic, and kidney problems. Careful initial medical and psychiatric evaluation is recommended in panic patients. However, prolonged and repetitive testing should be discouraged.

Theoretical Framework

Different theories, including cognitive-behavioral and biomedical, have been used in an attempt to describe the biologic mechanisms of panic. A brief synthesis of these theories reveals that PD is likely a combination of:

- An increase in alarm reaction
- An error in information processing (catastrophic thinking)
- Abnormal coping strategies to relieve anxiety and provide a sense of security (safety rituals and avoidance)

The disorder represents a sequential process where the symptoms start with the physical symptoms of panic and progress through the stages of abnormal thinking, rituals, and, finally, avoidance (Table 1). These symptom clusters may be wired through different neuronal circuits and respond preferentially to different treatments. However, this theoretical frame work is incomplete, as the intricacy of the neuronal circuits and neurotransmitters is not fully understood.

Treatment Algorithm

The treatment of PD is a stepwise process that starts with treatments of proven efficacy that are capable of ameliorating symptoms and decreasing avoidance behaviors. Figure 1 provides an algorithm of the treatment steps.

Step 1 starts with a first-line medication of a selective serotonin reuptake inhibitor (SSRI) or a therapeutic approach with cognitive behavior therapy (CBT). Both treatments have demonstrated efficacy between 70% and 90% in multiple studies. The treatment choice is based on the initial patient session with the physician, in which patients usually express their preference for either medication or psychotherapy. When availability and cost of the therapy is an issue, medication is the simplest way of treating PD. If, after two trials, the SSRI is deemed unsuccessful, step 2 begins.

Step 2 should start with a discussion with the patient about his/her preference for adding another medication or switching to another treatment modality (e.g., psychotherapy).

Step 3 involves treatment with more intensive CBT or with medications or combinations of treatments that have not yet been tried. Unusual and alternative treatments may be considered at that point (an expert consultation is usually recommended).

BEHAVIORAL THERAPY

Behavior therapy can be effective in as few as four sessions and can significantly reduce a patient's distress. Box 4 gives the stages of CBT. The treatment is based on desensitizing patients to their internal sensations and external phobic situations via exposure, reduction of catastrophic thinking, and improvement in coping strategies. However, patients who have very severe anxiety accompanied by depression are frequently unable to follow the therapist's instructions and may need to be started on antidepressants early.

MEDICATION

Selection of medication depends on whether patients have received prior pharmacotherapy for the treatment of a mood or anxiety disorder, on their previous reaction to medication, and on the severity and acuity of their panic state. An SSRI is the treatment of choice for patients who have never received pharmacotherapy and have at least moderate

---

[1]Not FDA approved for this indication.

TABLE 1 Theory of Panic

Stages of Panic Disorder	Neuronal Circuits	Possible Treatments
Panic attacks (alarm reactions)	Periaqueductal gray amygdala, hippocampus	SSRI, SNRI, benzodiazepines, interoceptive exposure
Catastrophic thoughts (abnormal information processing)	Orbital frontal cortex, cingulum, hippocampus	SSRI, SNRI, cognitive restructuring, neuroleptics
Precaution rituals and avoidances	Prefrontal and temporal cortex	SSRI, SNRI, neuroleptics Exposure and response prevention

Abbreviations: SNRI = serotonin-norepinephrine reuptake inhibitor; SSRI = selective serotonin reuptake inhibitor.

Step 1

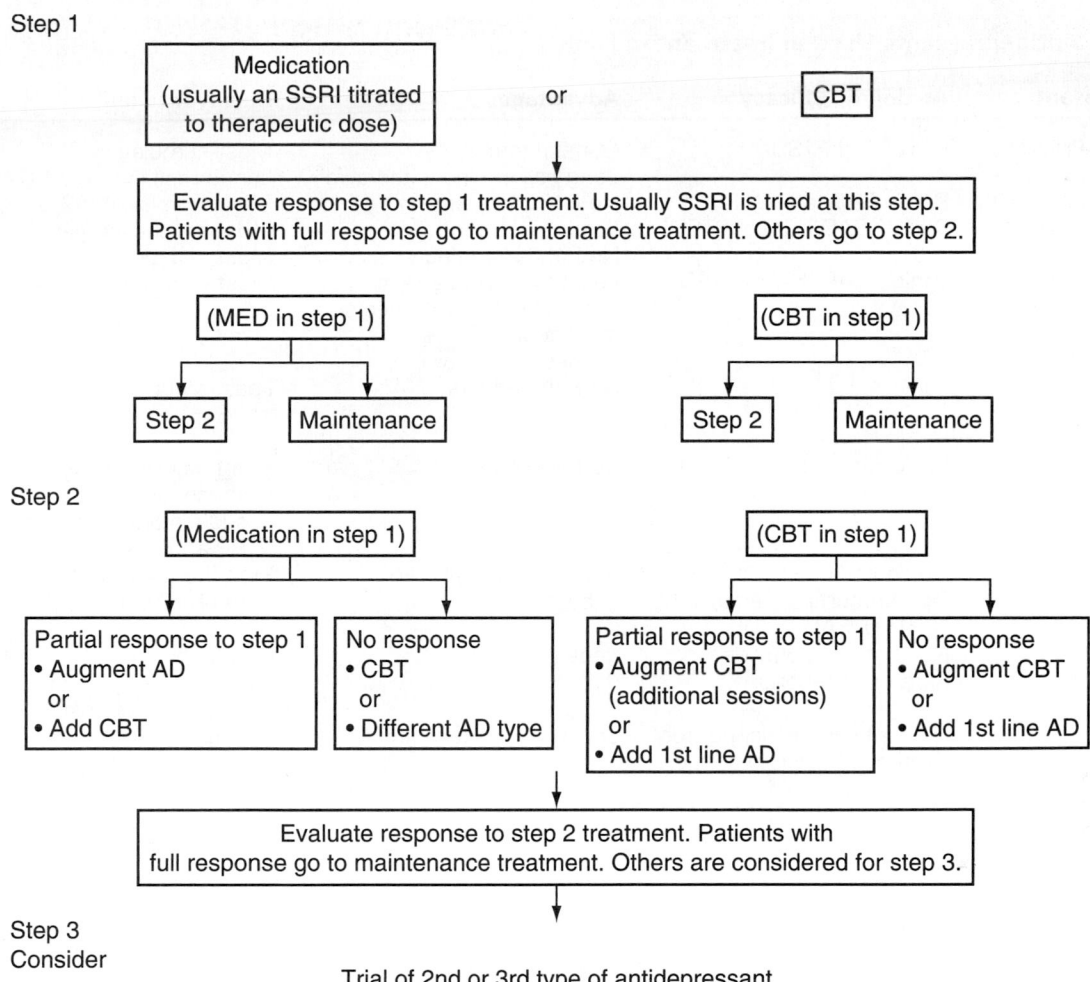

FIGURE 1. Treatment of panic disorder. AD = antidepressant; CBT = cognitive behavior therapy; MED = medication; PTSD = post-traumatic stress disorder; SSRI = selective serotonin reuptake inhibitor.

severity of illness. In addition to treating anxiety, SSRIs will treat a co-morbid major depressive episode (MDE) and lower the risk of future MDEs. All of the SSRIs are thought to be effective in the treatment of the four major anxiety disorders (including PD, obsessive–compulsive disorder, generalized anxiety disorder, and social anxiety disorder)

and have little differences except for subtle differences in side-effect profiles and differences in their effects on the cytochrome P450 liver enzyme system (Table 2). In general, selection among antidepressants should be based on the patient's anxiety symptom profile (one should avoid medications with side effects that mimic panic symptoms) and a history the side effects of medications previously taken. Table 3 can be used as a guide. For example, in the patient with severe insomnia, one might select a sedating tricyclic, such as nortriptyline (Pamelor),[1] or perhaps mirtazapine (Remeron).[1] Paroxetine (Paxil), fluvoxamine (Luvox),[1] or citalopram (Celexa)[1] would be the SSRI of choice for patients with prominent activation. For the patient with prominent gastrointestinal (GI) side effects, one would avoid sertraline (Zoloft), and paroxetine would be the SSRI of choice. For patients with prominent palpitations and

---

BOX 4 Cognitive Behavioral Therapy

- Assessment
- Cognitive restructuring (de-catastrophizing thinking)
- Coping enhancement
- Education
- Exposure and response prevention (to phobic situations)
- Interceptive exposure (exposure to internal sensation)
- Relapse prevention
- Self-monitoring

---

[1]Not FDA approved for this indication.

TABLE 2 Antidepressants Used in Treatment of Panic

Antidepressant	Anxiolytic Efficacy*	Advantages	Disadvantages
Fluoxetine (Prozac)	Panic[†] and PTSD	Generic form Long half-life (no withdrawal)	Most stimulating Longer half-life
Fluvoxamine (Luvox)[1]	Panic, GAD, and SAD	No P450 2D6 effects	Effects on P4501A2, 2C9, and 3A4
Paroxetine (Paxil)	Panic,[†] GAD,[†] SAD,[†] PTSD[†]	Least stimulating No P4503A4 effects	Most anticholinergic Most sedating
Sertraline (Zoloft)	Panic,[†] GAD, SAD,[†] PTSD[†]	Least P450-2D6 effects Minimal P450-3A4 effects Intermediate half-life (less withdrawal)	Most diarrhea
Citalopram (Celexa)[1] Escitalopram (Lexapro)[1]	Panic	No P450 effects	Least studied
Venlafaxine ER (Effexor XR)[1]	Panic, GAD,[†] SAD,[†] PTSD	No P450 effects	Short half-life Withdrawal with missed dose or sudden discontinuation—increased BP at >225 mg
Nefazodone (Serzone)[1]	No controlled studies Open reports in panic, PTSD, SAD	Sedation, can take at bedtime	Prominent P450 3A4 effects Rare reports of fatal hepatotoxicity
Mirtazapine (Remeron)[1]	No controlled studies Rare open reports	Sedation	Oversedation Increased appetite and weight gain Rare agranulocytosis
Nortriptyline (Pamelor)[1]	No controlled trials, but for other TCAs (imipramine), controlled evidence in panic, GAD, PTSD	Sedation, can take at bedtime	Too many SEs

[1]Not FDA approved for this indication.
*Data obtained from randomized clinical trials.
[†]FDA approved for this indication.
Abbreviations: BP = blood pressure; GAD = generalized anxiety disorder; PTSD = post-traumatic stress disorder; SAD = social anxiety disorder; SEs = side effects; TCAs = tricyclic antidepressants.

TABLE 3 Adverse Effects of the Antidepressants*

Adverse Effect	Fluoxetine (Prozac)	Sertaline (Zoloft)	Paroxetine (Paxil)	Fluvoxamine (Luvox)	Escitalopram (Lexapro)	Citalopram (Celexa) or Nortriptyline (Pamelor)	Venlafaxine[†]
Headache	↑	-	-	-		↓	-
Agitation/anxiety	↑↑	↑	-	-	↑	-	↑
Tremor	↑	↑	↑	-		↑↑	↑↑
Insomnia	↑↑	↑↑	-	-		↓	↑↑
Drowsiness	↑	↑	↑↑	↑↑		↑↑	↑↑
Fatigue	↑	-	↑↑	-		↑↑	↑
Confusion	-	-	-	-		-	-
Dizziness	-	-	↑	-		↑	↑
Anticholinergic[‡]	-	-	↑	-		↑↑↑	-
Sweating	-	-	↑	-		↑↑	↑↑
Weight gain	↑	↑	↑	↑		↑↑	↑
Gastrointestinal	↑	↑↑	-	↑↑		-	↑↑
Sexual	↑↑	↑↑	↑	↑	↑	↑	↑↑

*↑indicates the drug increases the occurrence of the adverse effect; ↓ indicates that it decreases the occurrence.
[†]Can increase blood pressure; must be monitored.
[‡]Anticholinergic side effects include dry mouth, constipation, urinary hesitancy or retention, blurred vision.

problems with weight gain, one would avoid tricyclics, paroxetine, and mirtazapine.

Benzodiazepines are not the first choice because of tolerance, dependency potential, and possible interference with CBT (especially with as-needed use). They should be reserved for emergency situations (initial panic attacks), for the reduction in extreme anxiety, or infrequent phobic situations (airplanes, elevators, etc.) before the beginning of the CBT. Finally, they can be used for maintenance of chronic patients with unremitting anxiety. If the benzodiazepines are used chronically, they should be prescribed using a pharmacokinetically appropriate schedule to minimize daily withdrawal or interdose anxiety. As-needed use of benzodiazepines should be avoided and history of alcohol and drug abuse should be assessed before beginning treatment.

TREATMENT RESISTANCE

If the patient is nonresponsive or has side effects to two prior SSRI trials, the choice is then between:

- A serotonin–norepinephrine reuptake inhibitor (SNRI)
- A newer antidepressant (e.g., venlafaxine [Effexor],[1] nefazodone [Serzone],[1] mirtazapine [Remeron][1])
- A tricyclic
- A γ-aminobutyric acid (GABA) agent (e.g., gabapentin [Neurontin][1]) (step 2)

A final consideration (step 3) involves the management of anxiety and other symptoms with a concomitant medication

---

[1]Not FDA approved for this indication.

that would not ordinarily be a first-line treatment choice for anxiety disorders. This involves the use of sedating atypical neuroleptics such as olanzapine (Zyprexa)[1] and quetiapine (Seroquel).[1] At this point one could consider the use of monoamine oxidase inhibitors (MAOIs), which boast very impressive data supporting their efficacy. These medications require dietary restrictions and stopping concomitant antidepressants. Combining intensive CBT (several times a week) with medication augmentation strategies may also bring a desired effect. Other strategies are under development for the treatment of this resistant population, but none of them have moved past an early experimental stage.

Long-Term Management

While in some patients panic attacks stop in the course of a few months, PD is usually a chronic, waxing and waning condition. Some patients may completely recover, while others may be left with symptoms of other disorders initially masked by the panic attacks. If CBT is initiated, it is important to coordinate the medication treatment with the therapy. Completely blocking anxiety may impair patients' learning in therapy and discourage them from developing new coping techniques. Gradual reduction and stopping medication can be attempted after 2 or 3 months of complete resolution of symptoms. Approximately 20% of patients will not respond to any treatment and need to be maintained in the most comfortable state with medication or therapy or a combination thereof.

---

[1]Not FDA approved for this indication.

Physical and Chemical Injuries

Burn Treatment Guidelines

Method of
Barbara A. Latenser, MD

The initial management of the severely burned patient follows guidelines established by the American College of Surgeons (ACS). It is crucial that the patient be managed properly in the early hours after injury because the initial management of a seriously burned patient can significantly affect the long-term outcome. Optimal burn-care criteria have been established and refined by the American Burn Association (ABA) over the past 20 years.

Because of regionalization, it is common for the initial care of the seriously burned patient to occur outside the burn center. Burns are a specialized form of trauma. Therefore, the ABCs (airway, breathing, circulation) are the same as for the trauma patient: airway with cervical spine immobilization if appropriate, breathing, circulation, disability, and exposure. Also, the burn patient could be a victim of associated trauma. It is easy to be sidetracked by the obvious thermal injury. Only after the primary and secondary surveys have been performed should you evaluate the severity of the burn injury. Obtain as much information as possible regarding the incident and about the patient. An easy way to remember the information is the mnemonic AMPLE:

- Allergies
- Medications
- Past medical history
- Last meal
- Events

Universal precautions appropriate for each burn patient must be implemented by every member of the health care team.

The most commonly used guide for making an initial estimate of the second- and third-degree burns is the Rule of Nines (Figure 1). Various anatomic regions are roughly 9% of the total body surface area (TBSA) or multiples thereof. To calculate scattered burn areas, the patient's palm, including fingers, represents approximately 1% of the TBSA. A much more precise estimate of TBSA burn is provided by the Lund-Browder Classification (Figure 2). By drawing in the areas that are burned, the TBSA burn necessary for calculating resuscitation requirements can be determined. The consensus formula for the first 24 hours postburn is:

$$\text{4 mL lactated Ringer's} \times \text{body weight in kg} \times \text{percent BSA burn}$$

Half the calculated amount is given in the first 8 hours and the rest over the remaining 16 hours. Patients with burns on more than 20% TBSA are prone to gastric dilatation and should have a nasogastric (NG) tube. To determine hourly urine output, a urinary catheter is necessary. Intravenous (IV) morphine sulfate is indicated for control of pain associated with burns. Intramuscular (IM) or subcutaneous (SC) routes of drug administration should not be used as absorption is erratic. To calculate fluid needs, weigh the patient or estimate the preinjury weight. Reliable peripheral veins should be used to establish an IV line. Use vessels underlying burned skin if necessary. If it is impossible to establish peripheral IV access, a central line may be necessary.

The burn wound should be covered with a clean, dry sheet to prevent air currents from causing pain in partial-thickness burns and to decrease fluid losses and hypothermia. Although there are many common topical antimicrobials in use, the optimal dressing prior to burn center transfer is plastic wrap such as Saran Wrap. Topical antimicrobials will just have to be washed off on arrival to the burn center, causing patient discomfort and mechanical trauma to the wound. Cold applications are appropriate only in small burns because they rapidly lead to hypothermia. Ice should never be applied because it will deepen the zone of ischemia in a thermal injury.

Escharotomies and/or fasciotomies are rarely required prior to burn center transfer, unless transfer is delayed beyond 24 hours. Patients most at risk are those with large TBSA burns, circumferential full-thickness burns, and those with electrical injury. Circumferential chest/abdominal burns may restrict ventilatory excursion. A child has a more pliable rib cage and may need an escharotomy earlier than an adult burn. If you are considering performing an escharotomy, confer with the accepting burn physician before proceeding.

So how do you know which patients should be referred to a burn center? To guide your decision making there are

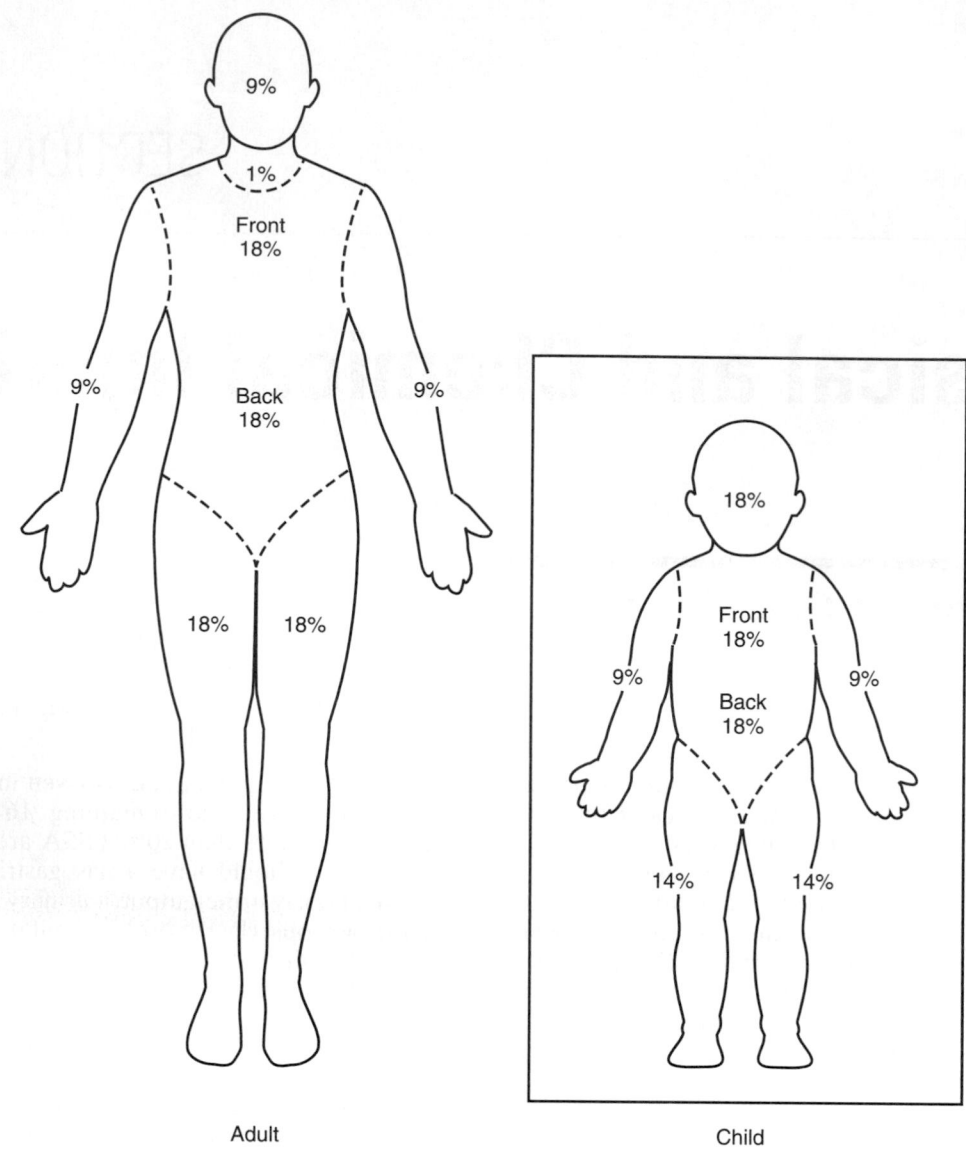

FIGURE 1. Rule of Nines.

currently 10 burn unit referral criteria. You should have a written transfer agreement in place with a referral burn unit. The agreement should specify which patients will be referred, what stabilization is expected, who arranges transportation, and what the patient will need during transport.

Partial-Thickness Burns on More Than 10% Total Body Surface Area

Second-degree or partial-thickness burns involve a variable portion of dermis. The skin may be red, blistered, and edematous. Because sensory nerves are damaged and/or exposed, these wounds are typically extremely painful. Healing time is proportional to the depth of dermal injury.

Scarring is minimal if healing occurs in 14 days or less. With closure time beyond 3 weeks, scarring will occur, the degree being greater in darker skinned individuals.

Proper fluid management is critical to the survival of patients with extensive burns. Fluid resuscitation is aimed at maintaining tissue perfusion and organ function while avoiding the complications of inadequate or excessive fluid therapy. Shock and organ failure, most commonly acute renal failure, may occur as a consequence of hypovolemia in a patient with an extensive burn who is inadequately resuscitated. The increase in capillary permeability caused by the burn is greatest in the immediate postburn period and diminution in effective blood volume is most rapid at that time. A marked increase in peripheral vascular resistance accompanied by a decrease in cardiac output occurs in the first 18 to 24 hours postinjury.

In the presence of increased capillary permeability, colloid content of the resuscitation fluid exerts little

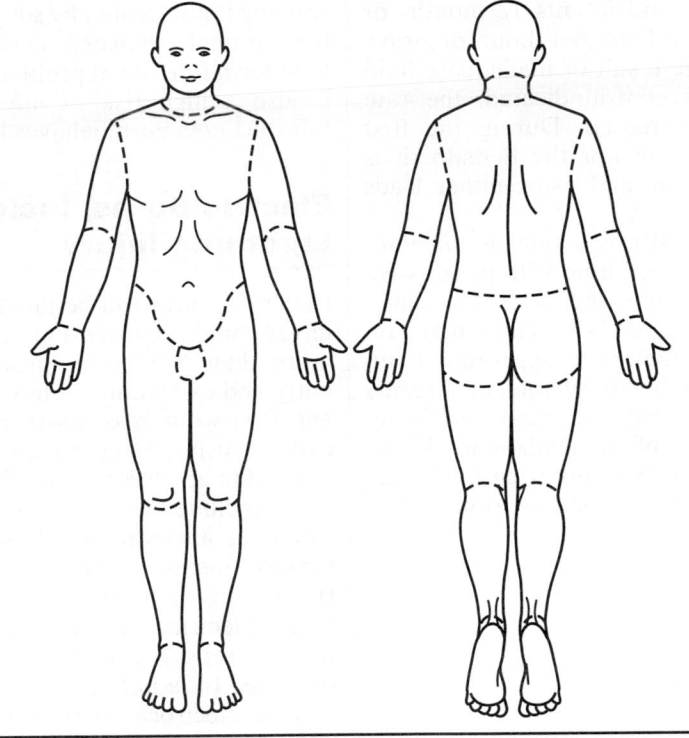

	Birth 1 yr.	1–4 yrs.	5–9 yrs.	10–14 yrs.	15 yrs.	Adult	Burn size estimate
Head	19	17	13	11	9	7	
Neck	2	2	2	2	2	2	
Anterior trunk	13	13	13	13	13	13	
Posterior trunk	13	13	13	13	13	13	
Right buttock	2.5	2.5	2.5	2.5	2.5	2.5	
Left buttock	2.5	2.5	2.5	2.5	2.5	2.5	
Genitalia	1	1	1	1	1	1	
Right upper arm	4	4	4	4	4	4	
Left upper arm	4	4	4	4	4	4	
Right lower arm	3	3	3	3	3	3	
Left lower arm	3	3	3	3	3	3	
Right hand	2.5	2.5	2.5	2.5	2.5	2.5	
Left hand	2.5	2.5	2.5	2.5	2.5	2.5	
Right thigh	5.5	6.5	8	8.5	9	9.5	
Left thigh	5.5	6.5	8	8.5	9	9.5	
Right leg	5	5	5.5	6	6.5	7	
Left leg	5	5	5.5	6	6.5	7	
Right foot	3.5	3.5	3.5	3.5	3.5	3.5	
Left foot	3.5	3.5	3.5	3.5	3.5	3.5	

Total BSAB _____

FIGURE 2. Lund-Browder Classification Burn Size and Diagram.

influence on intravascular retention during the initial hours postburn. Crystalloid fluid is the initial resuscitation of burn patients. *Always* remember, estimates are inexact. Each patient reacts differently to burn injury and resuscitation. The actual volume of fluid infused should be varied from the calculated volume as indicated by physiologic monitoring. The patient's general condition reflects the adequacy of fluid resuscitation and should be assessed and reassessed. Mental status, anxiety, and restlessness may be signs of hypoxemia, hypovolemia, or pain.

Although urine output does not guarantee tissue perfusion, it remains the most readily available and generally reliable guide to resuscitation. Adults should produce 0.5 mL/kg per hour of urine. Children should produce

1.0 mL/kg per hour of urine, and infants 12 months or younger should produce 2.0 mL/kg per hour of urine. Oliguria is most frequently the result of inadequate fluid administration. Diuretics are contraindicated; the rate of resuscitation should be increased. During the first 24 hours, neither the hemoglobin nor the hematocrit is a reliable guide to resuscitation, and using either leads to over-resuscitation.

Measuring blood pressure (BP) by a sphygmomanometer may be misleading in a burned limb with progressive edema formation. As the swelling increases, the signal becomes diminished. If fluid infusion is increased based on this finding, edema formation may be exaggerated. Even intra-arterial monitoring may be unreliable in patients with massive burns because of peripheral vasoconstriction secondary to marked elevation of catecholamines. Heart rate is also of limited usefulness in monitoring fluid therapy. The level of tachycardia depends on the normal heart rate in each child.

Burns That Involve the Face, Hands, Feet, Genitalia, Perineum, or Major Joints

Facial burns are considered a serious injury. The possibility of respiratory tract damage must be considered. Because of the rich blood supply and loose areolar tissue of the face, facial burns are associated with extensive edema formation. To minimize this edema, keep the head of the bed elevated at 30°. Cool saline compresses on the face may also help. Careful examination of the eyes should be completed as soon as possible because the rapid onset of eyelid swelling will make this difficult. Fluorescein should be used to identify corneal injury. Chemical burns to the eyes should be rinsed with copious amounts of saline. Burns of the ears require examination of the external auditory canal and ear drum before swelling occurs.

Minor burns of the hands may result in only temporary disability and inconvenience. More extensive thermal injury may cause permanent loss of function. Monitoring the digital and palmar pulses with an ultrasonic flowmeter is the most accurate means of assessing perfusion of the tissues in the hand. The burned extremity should be elevated above the heart to minimize edema formation. Digital escharotomies are not indicated prior to transfer to a burn center. Contact the accepting burn center physician if you are concerned about the extent of the digital injury. As with burns of the upper extremity, it is important to assess the circulation and neurologic function of the feet on an hourly basis.

Third-Degree Burns in Any Age Group

A full-thickness or third-degree burn occurs with destruction of the entire epidermis and dermis, leaving no dermal elements to repopulate. A characteristic initial appearance is a waxy white color. Full-thickness injuries require emergent management. In most cases, treatment of the wound requires surgical skin grafting. Deep partial-thickness and full-thickness burns heal with severe scarring if not treated by surgical excision and skin grafting for optimal recovery. Disfigurement is common, and long-term functional problems can persist for years. There is also a high risk of infection, because an unexcised full-thickness burn behaves like an undrained abscess.

Electric Burns, Including Lightning Injury

Electrical burns can be divided into flash (typical thermal injury) and high-tension injury. The latter, caused by more than 1000 volts, produces clinically characteristic entry and exit wounds. They are usually ischemic, painless, and dry; wounds of entry may appear charred and the exit explosive. Deep-muscle injury may be present even when skin appears normal. Findings that suggest electrical injury include loss of consciousness, paralysis or mummification of an extremity, loss of peripheral pulses, flexor surface burns, myoglobinuria, serum creatine kinase (CK) more than 1000, and cardiopulmonary arrest at the scene. Electrical injuries can produce vascular thrombosis, muscle tetany causing fractures, and internal organ damage. In addition to other interventions, obtain a 12-lead electrocardiogram (ECG), cardiac enzymes, and evaluate the urine for myoglobin. If there is evidence of myoglobin from muscle damage, the urine output should be maintained at 2 mL/kg per hour until the urine grossly clears to prevent acid hematin deposition in the kidney and irreversible renal damage. Compartment pressures must be monitored. If a compartment syndrome develops, contact your burn center physician because fasciotomy may be required. The most serious immediate problem associated with electrical injuries is ventricular fibrillation, asystole, or other dysrhythmias. Life-threatening arrhythmias are treated according to advanced cardiac life support (ACLS) protocols. Survival of contact with voltage greater than 70,000 volts is uncommon.

The approximate electrical potential of a lightning bolt is 20 million volts. Lightning injury can produce an enormous spectrum of clinical symptoms and signs ranging from common (cardiac asystole, respiratory arrest, arborescent markings) to the rare (disseminated intravascular coagulation [DIC], intracerebral hemorrhage). Immediate neurologic manifestations include agitation, amnesia, loss of consciousness, or motor disturbances. The eyes are particularly vulnerable to injury from electrical current, and symptoms closely correlate with the extent of the central nervous system (CNS) injury. Vitreous hemorrhage, iridocyclitis, retinal tear, macular puncture, and retinal detachment have been reported.

Lightning injuries are not usually associated with deep burns but most often with superficial injury to the skin and underlying soft tissue called *ferning*. The feathering type of burn appears as an arborescent, branching skin marking that disappears within a few days. Pathognomonic of lightning injury, they may be of great diagnostic value in a comatose patient. Often the respiratory arrest lasts longer than the cardiac arrest. Severely injured victims often present in asystole or ventricular fibrillation. Cardiac resuscitation may occasionally be successful; but direct brain trauma as well as blunt trauma, skull fracture, and intracranial injuries, are common in these patients. The prognosis for recovery in this group is usually poor.

Chemical Burns

Health care providers must wear protective clothing when caring for patients with potential chemical injury. The initial appearance of a chemical burn is usually deceptively benign. The severity of a chemical injury is related to the agent, concentration, volume, duration of contact, and mechanisms of action of the agent. Immediate irrigation decreases the concentration and duration of contact, reducing the severity of injury. If the agent is a powder, brush it off and irrigate with water. Irrigation should continue through emergency evaluation in the hospital and in general until evaluation in a burn center, especially for an alkali or if an unknown agent. Neutralizing agents are contraindicated because of the potential for heat generation, thereby giving the patient both a chemical and a thermal injury!

Acid burns are less severe than alkali burns. They are found in many household products including bathroom cleansers, drain cleaners, and swimming pool acidifiers. Tissue is damaged by coagulation necrosis and protein precipitation. Once a layer of eschar is formed, the burning process is self-limiting. The exception to this rule is hydrofluoric acid (HA), which is used to etch glass, make Teflon, and to remove rust. The pathogenesis of tissue damage in HA burns is distinct from other acids. HA readily crosses lipid membranes and has a potent diffusing capacity into the tissues. The molecule releases the freely dissociable fluoride ion, which produces extensive liquefactive necrosis of the soft tissues. Fluoride rapidly binds free calcium in the blood, and death from hypocalcemia may occur. Treatment is intra-arterial calcium gluconate[1] (or calcium chloride)[1] administered until the characteristic *pain out of proportion to the burn* has resolved. Even small areas of contact may result in profound hypocalcemia and death. Cardiac monitoring and frequent serum calcium determinations are indicated.

Alkalis damage tissue by liquefaction necrosis and protein denaturation. Tissue pH abnormalities may persist for 12 hours postburn, allowing deeper spread of the chemical and more severe burns. Examples would include the hydroxides, caustic sodas, and ammonium compounds found in oven cleaners, fertilizer, and cement. Wet cement damages skin in three ways: allergic dermatitis as a reaction to chromate ions, abrasions caused by the gritty nature of the cement, and as an alkali with a pH of 12.5. The ability of cement to cause such injury is not well recognized, even by professional users. With the increased media interest in do-it-yourself projects, it is likely this problem will increase.

Organic compounds such as creosote and petroleum products produce contact chemical burns as well as systemic toxicity. Gasoline and diesel fuel are petroleum products that may produce a full-thickness burn that initially appears as only partial thickness. Organic compounds cause cutaneous damage by delipidation because of their fat solvent action on cell membranes. After a motor vehicle crash involving petroleum products, always look for petroleum exposure in the lower extremities, back, and buttocks. Systemic effects include elevated liver enzymes and decreased urinary output.

[1]Not FDA approved for this indication.

Inhalation Injury

Smoke inhalation injuries are the leading cause of fatalities from burn injuries, accounting for some 80% of all fire-related deaths. The major forms of inhalation injuries are carbon monoxide (CO) toxicity, injury to the upper airway, and pulmonary parenchymal damage. Each has different symptoms and signs, treatment, and prognosis. The compromised airway is protected by tracheal intubation, and respiratory failure is treated with assisted ventilation. Inhalation injury is manifested by the pathology and dysfunction that rapidly become evident in the airways, lungs, and respiratory system after inhaling the products of incomplete combustion. Patients receiving massive fluid resuscitation can develop upper airway edema with subsequent asphyxiation.

Immediate medical attention and diagnosis depend on a high index of suspicion, an appropriate history, careful examination of the upper airway, the presence of clinical symptoms, and suggestive arterial blood gases. An inhalation injury is suspected in any patient with full-thickness facial burns or with any burns combined with a history of being confined within an enclosed space. Other classic signs are soot or carbonaceous sputum, stridor or hoarseness, or blistering of the pharynx or vocal cords. Late signs include grunting, nasal flaring, retractions, wheezes, and rales. Use of prophylactic antibiotics and steroids is discouraged.

The effect of CO poisoning may be exhibited by respiratory symptoms and CNS findings such as altered level of consciousness, seizures, or coma. Cardiovascular effects include diminished cardiac output evidenced by decreased perfusion and hypotension. There is much controversy regarding hyperbaric oxygen therapy, but there are no objective data proving the efficacy of hyperbaric oxygen in CO poisoning. At this time, hyperbaric oxygen treatment for acute CO toxicity should be restricted to randomized prospective studies. The correct treatment is administering 100% oxygen, thereby decreasing the CO half-life from 4 hours to 45 minutes.

Burn Injury in Patients with Preexisting Medical Disorders That Could Complicate Management, Prolong Recovery, or Affect Mortality

Peripheral vascular disease can lead to a decrease in wound blood flow. Diabetes, through high glucose, will impede capillary flow. Optimum control of the blood glucose is needed to optimize blood flow. A local decrease in wound-tissue oxygen tension is recognized to be a major wound-healing impediment because all phases of healing are oxygen dependent, including local infection control. Most common causes are a decrease in systemic blood volume and oxygen delivery, decrease in hemoglobin saturation, eschar on the wound surface, or infection. Treatment modalities need to focus first on correction of systemic abnormalities: correct cardiovascular and lung function, correct large vessel obstructive disease impeding wound flow, aggressive wound debridement, and eliminate tissue exudates. Patients with preexisting cardiac disease are particularly sensitive to fluids and may tolerate the necessary fluid resuscitation poorly.

Any Patient With Burns and Concomitant Trauma (Such as Fractures) in Which the Burn Injury Poses the Greatest Risk of Morbidity and Mortality

In such case, if the trauma poses the greater immediate risk, the patient may be initially stabilized in a trauma center before being transferred to a burn unit. Physician judgment will be necessary in such situations and should be in concert with the regional medical control plan and triage protocols.

Most burn-trauma publications cite a 5% frequency of burn-trauma patient. Because burn trauma is rare outside of a major conflict or disaster, most centers see only a few patients annually. By definition, child abuse falls into the burn-trauma category. It may be the burn injury that prompts relatives or neighbors to bring the child to the hospital or report the family to authority. The visibility of the injury may instigate corrective action. In a 44-month review we saw 120 cases of burns and trauma. Although motor vehicle crashes (MVCs) can result in fracture, soft tissue, and thermal injury, unique to this burn-trauma population was that the MVC injury was frequently a result of assault. With the graying of America, elder abuse may become a larger societal problem.

Burned Children in Hospitals Without Qualified Personnel or Equipment for the Care of Children

Each year more than 2500 children die and 10,000 more sustain permanent disability from thermal injury. Children are not just little adults! They respond differently than adults to severe trauma, maintaining normal vital signs longer but decompensating rapidly. Because of the smaller cross-sectional diameter of the pediatric airway, it takes much less edema to compromise a pediatric airway. If intubation is required, the most experienced pediatric airway manager should intubate the child because repeated attempts may create sufficient airway edema as

CURRENT DIAGNOSIS

- Maintain a high index of suspicion
- Remember the ABCs
- Rule out concomitant trauma
- Establish size and depth of burn
- Be wary of chemical and electrical burns, which may be misleading
- Establish resuscitation requirements

Abbreviations: ABC = airway with cervical spine immobilization if appropriate, breathing, circulation, disability, and exposure.

CURRENT THERAPY

- Communicate with your burn center early and often
- Remember the ABCs
- Cover the wound with Saran Wrap
- Prevent hypothermia
- Transport to the burn center

Abbreviations: ABC = airway with cervical spine immobilization if appropriate, breathing, circulation, disability, and exposure.

to cause obstruction. Anatomical airway differences make intubation by the inexperienced even more difficult.

The greater surface area per unit of body mass of children necessitates the administration of relatively greater amounts of resuscitation fluid. The surface area/body mass relationship of the child also defines a lesser intravascular volume per unit surface area burned. This makes the burned child more susceptible to fluid overload and hemodilution. Hypoglycemia may occur if the limited glycogen stores of the child are rapidly exhausted by the early postburn elevation of circulating levels of steroids and catecholamines. Infants should receive maintenance fluids with 5% dextrose in addition to the resuscitation fluids outlined in the consensus formula. Children younger than 2 years of age have disproportionally thin skin so that exposures that would produce only partial-thickness burns in older patients produce full-thickness injuries. Children have a relatively small muscle mass, hampering intrinsic heat generation. Children younger than 6 months of age are unable to shiver and thus are even more prone to develop hypothermia.

Stress for the burned child not only includes the body surface area (BSA) burn and the pain that is involved but also the separation from parents and loved ones. This escalates especially if the parents were also burned in the fire. Emergency management of each pediatric burn patient requires an individual care plan. Early consultation with the burn center physician is advised.

Burn Injury in Patients Who Will Require Special Social, Emotional, and/or Long-Term Rehabilitative Intervention

Failure to recognize the thermal manifestations of child abuse not only negates protection of the child but predicates potential lethal injury. Awareness of the patterns of abuse, the behavior patterns of the parents, and the physical manifestations will protect the child by early recognition and reporting. Physical child abuse victims frequently present with thermal injuries of varying degrees. The history of injury should correlate with the physical findings. The history also becomes important in identifying repetitive hospital visits for accidental injury. Not infrequently, the hospital visits will be made at different hospitals to avoid disclosure and identification.

The events leading to an injury are extremely important in the initial evaluation of an infant or child. *Always* consider the potential for child abuse. The incidence of child abuse is approximately 10% of all children presenting to an emergency department (ED), with a mortality rate less than 1%. Abused children present with a higher median Injury Severity Score, more severe injuries of the head and integument, longer hospital lengths of stay, and a high mortality rate.

A burn of any magnitude can be a serious injury. Health care providers must be able to assess the injuries rapidly and develop a priority-based plan of care. The plan of care is determined by the type, extent, and degree of burn as well as by available resources.

Burn care is complex. It involves a multisystem assessment and appropriate intervention. The first 24 hours of management are perhaps the most critical for patient survival. Burn centers provide optimal care in a cost-effective, multidisciplinary manner. Every health care provider must know how and when to contact the closest burn center. If the attending physician determines that the patient should be treated at the burn center, the extent of treatment provided at the referring hospital—and the method of transport to the burn center—should be decided in consultation with the burn center physician.

REFERENCES

Advanced Burn Life Support Course, American Burn Association, 625 N. Michigan Ave., Suite 1530, Chicago, IL. 60611. 2001.

American College of Surgeons Committee on Trauma: Resources for optimal care of the injured patient: 1999. Chicago, American College of Surgeons, 1999.

Andrews CJ, Cooper MA, Darveniza M, Mackerras D (eds): Lightning injuries: Electrical, medical, and legal aspects. Boca Raton, Fla, CRC Press, 1992, pp 62-63, 82-85, 88-98, 101-110.

Burd A: Hydrofluoric acid—revisited. Burns 2004;30(7):720-722.

Chang DC, Knight V, Ziegfeld S, et al: The tip of the iceberg for child abuse: The critical roles of the pediatric trauma service and its registry. J Trauma 2004;57(6):1189-1198.

Heimbach DM: Regionalization of burn care: A concept whose time has come. J Burn Care Rehabil 2003;24(3):173-174.

Latenser BA, Iteld L: Smoke inhalation injury. Seminars in Respiratory and Critical Care Medicine. 2001;22(1):13-22.

Luce EA (ed): Clinics in Plastic Surgery. An International Quarterly. Burn Care and Management. Philadelphia, WB Saunders, 2000; 27(1): 133-143.

Varghese TK, Kim AW, Kowal-Vern A, Latenser BA: Frequency of burn-trauma patients in an urban setting. Arch Surg. 2003;138:1292-1296.

High-Altitude Illness

Method of
James A. Litch, MD, DTMH

Decreased partial pressure of oxygen at high altitude results in pronounced physiologic responses that range from beneficial to pathologic. Slow ascent normally leads to acclimatization. High-altitude illness is a collective term for a cluster of acute clinical syndromes that are a direct consequence of rapid ascent to high altitude above 2500 m. The acute syndromes affecting the brain include acute mountain sickness (AMS) and high-altitude cerebral edema (HACE). The acute syndrome affecting the lung is high-altitude pulmonary edema (HAPE). All unacclimatized sojourners to high altitude are potentially at risk. The characteristic cerebral and pulmonary abnormalities are not subtle, but when unrecognized or ignored, they may progress to death. Each year millions travel to high-altitude locations on every continent, resulting in morbidity and mortality with associated economic consequences.

Normal Acclimatization

It is not uncommon for normal acclimatization of novice healthy visitors to high altitude to cause concern that they are experiencing a health problem. Normal acclimatization includes immediate hyperventilation, shortness of breath with moderate excursion, and a decreased work capacity. These are followed by diuresis, disturbed sleep (including periodic breathing), and peripheral/facial edema. It is important to recognize the signs of normal acclimatization so reassurance and education may be appropriately provided.

Incidence and Risk Factors

Determinants of whether high-altitude illness will occur are individual susceptibility, rate of ascent, altitude reached, and sleep altitude. Incidence rates of AMS reported in literature are difficult to compare because of variability in methodology and rates of ascent. Reported incident figures for AMS following ascent by hiking, vehicle, or flying range from 10% to 40% at 2700 to 3000 m, and from 40% to 95% at 3800 to 4000 m. HACE and HAPE are both far less common than mild AMS, but actual incident rates are unavailable. HAPE can occur as low as 2500 m. HACE is rare below 3600 m. Most cases of HACE and HAPE are preceded by AMS.

Risk factors for altitude illness include a history of previous high-altitude illness, residence at altitude below 1000 m, physical exertion, and preexisting cardiopulmonary conditions. Traveling in a large group presents a risk because a tight itinerary often does not allow time for acclimatization, and members are reluctant to declare symptoms for fear of being left behind. Children appear to carry the same risk for altitude illness as adults, but persons over 50 years of age seem less susceptible, possibly because of a more cautious ascent profile. There appears to be little or no gender difference for AMS, but women may be less susceptible to HAPE. Heavy physical exertion at exceedingly high altitude appears to be an important risk factor for HAPE. Rapid ascent, especially by flying or driving to altitude, places sojourners at risk for altitude illnesses.

Prevention of Altitude Illnesses

Gradual ascent to altitude over several days to allow for acclimatization reduces the likelihood of acute mountain sickness. Ascent rates of less than 300 m per day at altitudes of more than 2500 m is a common recommendation; but individuals will still experience altitude illness when abiding to this recommendation. However, the critical understanding to prevent serious life-threatening altitude illness (HAPE and HACE) is to halt further ascent until symptoms resolve.

Medications are available to help prevent the symptoms of AMS when rapid ascent (<24 hours) to altitudes more than 3000 m is anticipated, or for those with a past history of AMS with a similar ascent profile. These agents are started the evening before ascent and continued for 2 to 3 days. The most commonly used medications are acetazolamide (Diamox) (125 to 250 mg twice a day), acetaminophen[1] (325 mg four times a day), or aspirin[1] (325 mg three times a day). Acetazolamide (Diamox) is particularly useful because it actually improves oxygenation, has a positive impact on the quality of sleep at high altitude, and is effective for periodic breathing that occurs during sleep. However, these medications do not protect against the development of life threatening altitude illness: HAPE and HACE. Other medications have been suggested for use in preventing altitude illness. Randomized double blinded placebo-controlled trails of ginkgo biloba[1] and acetazolamide (Diamox) have shown no benefit from ginkgo biloba over placebo, and reduced incidence and severity of AMS symptoms from acetazolamide (Diamox). Dexamethasone (Decadron),[1] a potent steroid, is generally best avoided as a prevention measure against AMS during ascent so it may be used, if needed, for treatment of HACE along with descent.

Nifedipine (Adalat, Procardia)[1] has been studied for use in prevention of HAPE and found to be of benefit for persons with a history of recurrent HAPE. Studies are underway to evaluate sildenafil citrate (Viagra),[1] an agent that selectively lowers pulmonary artery pressure, in the prevention of HAPE. In addition, inhaled salmeterol (Serevent)[1] has been found effective for the prevention of HAPE in a small group of climbers who had previously shown susceptibility to HAPE. However, these high-risk individuals would do far better with cautious gradual ascent, rather than relying on a medication with limited effect for a life-threatening condition.

Several nonmedication measures that can prevent or ameliorate symptoms of high-altitude illness include the following:

- Begin a high-carbohydrate diet one or two days before the climb and maintain during the ascent
- Adapt plans to realistically reflect the decreased work capacity at high altitude
- Reschedule or slow the ascent should an upper respiratory or other active infection present
- Avoid overexertion during ascent by maintaining a reasonable pace and not overloading with nonessential gear
- Maintain adequate hydration on the climb to offset increased fluid loss at altitude
- Avoid nonessential medications and remedies
- Provide good ventilation for camp stoves used in confined places
- Allow for several days of altitude exposure the week prior to ascent to high altitude

Acute Mountain Sickness and High-Altitude Cerebral Edema

AMS is defined as a headache in the setting of recent altitude gain and typical symptoms which include

[1]Not FDA approved for this indication.

anorexia, nausea, vomiting, insomnia, dizziness, or fatigue (Current Diagnosis box). Symptoms are nonspecific, and there is an absence of physical findings. The differential diagnosis is extensive and other conditions should be considered (Box 1). Pulse oximetry values may be high, normal, or low for the altitude and do not correlate to severity of symptoms. A careful and detailed history is essential to steer diagnostic decision making. Often in outdoor settings multiple conditions can be present such as AMS and dehydration. Rapid resolution of symptoms during treatment with oxygen is very specific to AMS. Early recognition of AMS is a key principle in remote areas with limited support.

AMS is not life threatening, but ignoring it can be. Progressive neurologic deterioration may occur over hours or days as dangerous collections of fluid develop in the brain leading to HACE. HACE presents with truncal ataxia, confusion, and hallucination in the setting of recent altitude gain. The period of time from initial ataxia and confusion to onset of coma may be as little as 8 to 12 hours. If descent or oxygen supplementation is not accomplished within hours, coma and death can ensue from brain herniation. A presumptive and/or rigid diagnosis of HACE in the setting of progressive neurologic deterioration has led to tragic situations when other life-threatening

---

BOX 1 Differential Diagnosis of High-Altitude Illnesses

Acute Mountain Sickness and High-Altitude Cerebral Edema
- Alcohol intoxication
- Brain tumor
- CO inhalation
- CNS infection
- Cerebral vascular accident
- Dehydration
- Diabetic ketoacidosis
- Exhaustion
- Hypoglycemia and insulin shock
- Hyponatremia
- Hypothermia
- Migraine
- Narcotics
- Poisoning
- Psychosis
- Sedatives overdose
- Seizures
- Subarachnoid hemorrhage
- Transient ischemic attack

High-Altitude Pulmonary Edema
- Adult respiratory distress syndrome
- Asthma
- Bronchitis
- Congestive heart failure
- Myocardial infarction
- Pneumonia (infection or aspiration)
- Poisoning
- Pulmonary embolus
- Respiratory failure

Abbreviations: CNS = central nervous system; CO = carbon monoxide.

conditions were actually present (see Box 1). Details of the initial presentation, response to immediate descent/supplemental oxygen, and recognition of additional signs can guide clinical decision making while maintaining a high index of suspicion for other neurologic conditions. Patients with persistent symptoms after descent require prompt evacuation and thorough evaluation. In addition, HAPE may develop concurrently with HACE resulting in shortness of breath while at rest and a further reduction of oxygen delivery to the body.

Definitive diagnosis is available using imaging studies such as CT and MRI. However, these have limited application, because the condition should have greatly improved from oxygen/descent before the opportunity presents to obtain the study. Neuroimaging demonstrates vasogenic edema in individuals with moderate to severe AMS or HACE.

Management of AMS is directed at limiting further hypoxia by halting ascent, and providing additional oxygen should symptoms persist or progress to HACE. Acetazolamide (Diamox) is helpful for the treatment of AMS. For the management of HACE improved oxygenation is the definitive treatment. There are several methods of oxygen delivery: (1) descent, (2) supplemental oxygen via cylinder or concentrator, and/or (3) portable hyperbaric bag. These may be combined or applied in series depending on resources, location, and logistic support. Concomitant pharmacologic treatment with dexamethasone (Decadron)[1] and acetazolamide (Diamox) aid recovery. Persons with suspected HACE who do not rapidly recover during treatment or those with focal neurologic deficits should be hospitalized and undergo comprehensive neurologic evaluation including magnetic resonance imaging (MRI). The Current Therapy box summarizes management of HACE.

High-Altitude Pulmonary Edema

HAPE is defined as noncardiogenic edema resulting from hypoxia-induced changes in the pulmonary circulation. HAPE is commonly preceded by AMS, and 20% of individuals with HAPE develop HACE. Early symptoms of HAPE include decreased exercise performance beyond that expected for the altitude, often accompanied with a dry cough (see Current Diagnosis Box). Progression is rapid with even minimal continued physical activity without descent. The hallmark of progression requiring prompt action is dyspnea at rest. Rales are present at this stage. Resting pulse oximetry reveals below-normal oxygen saturation for the altitude. Tachypnea and tachycardia beyond that expected for the altitude also are present. Pink, frothy sputum develops late in the illness. Early diagnosis is important because progression of the illness further limits oxygenation and worsens the degree of hypoxemia causing the condition.

HAPE is a life-threatening emergency; immediate improvement in oxygenation is critical to arrest the progression and is the definitive treatment. In medical facilities high-flow supplemental oxygen while at rest and sitting in an upright position should be initiated immediately during the initial assessment of the patient. Response may

[1]Not FDA approved for this indication.

be assessed by pulse oximetry and resting respiratory rate. Despite prompt improvement during the first few hours of treatment, maintenance of oxygenation (oxygen saturation greater than 90%) with low-flow supplemental oxygen and rest is often required for 2 to 3 days unless descent is achieved. For vacationers to high-altitude resort areas, this oxygen requirement can be maintained outside the hospital using a cylinder or concentrator as an alternative to descent for informed individuals that wish to remain in the locale of family and friends. A continued requirement of high-flow oxygen of 4 to 5 L per minute or more to maintain oxygen saturation greater than 90%, or concurrent HACE, requires hospitalization. Antibiotics are indicated if infection is suspected. Endotracheal intubation and mechanical ventilation are rarely indicated. The differential diagnosis is extensive, and a high index of suspicion for other conditions should be maintained throughout the treatment course (see Box 1).

In remote areas oxygen may be administered by:

- Descent with minimal exertion
- Supplemental oxygen via cylinder or concentrator
- Portable hyperbaric bag placed on an incline to keep the head elevated

Because of a lack of equipment, immediate descent may be the only option available. In late stages more than one oxygen modality may need to be employed concurrently. These efforts place great strain on the limited resources of groups traveling in remote areas. It is common for the shared concern and cooperation among group members (tourists/staff/porters) to disintegrate or for groups to discover that they are woefully unequipped to handle HAPE. As a result fatal outcomes are common when HAPE presents in remote settings.

Pharmacologic treatment is directed at agents that reduce pulmonary artery pressure and thereby may improve oxygenation in HAPE. Medications including nifedipine (Adalat, Procardia),[1] nitric oxide (INO_max),[1] epoprostenol (Flolan),[1] and sildenafil (Viagra)[1] have been studied for

[1]Not FDA approved for this indication.

CURRENT DIAGNOSIS

- Acute Mountain Sickness—In the setting of a recent gain in altitude, the presence of headache and at least one of the following: GI symptoms (anorexia, nausea, or vomiting), fatigue or weakness, dizziness or lightheadedness, or difficulty sleeping
- High-Altitude Cerebral Edema—In the setting of a recent gain in altitude, the presence of a change in mental status and/or ataxia in a person with AMS, or the presence of both mental status change and ataxia in a person without AMS
- High-Altitude Pulmonary Edema—In the setting of a recent gain in altitude, the presence of at least two of the following symptoms: dyspnea at rest, cough, weakness or decreased exercise performance, chest tightness, or congestion; and two of the following signs: rales or wheezing in at least one lung field, central cyanosis, tachypnea, or tachycardia

*The Lake Louise Consensus on the Definition and Quantification of Altitude Illness.
Abbreviations: AMS = acute mountain sickness; GI = gastrointestinal.

CURRENT THERAPY

Acute Mountain Sickness

- Halt ascent, do not exceed light activity level, oral hydration.
- Administer acetazolamide (Diamox) 250 mg PO bid.
- Administer analgesics and antiemetics.
- If readily available, administer oxygen 1 to 2 L per minute as needed to resolve symptoms.
- If no improvement after 24 hours, descend to altitude where person last slept without symptoms until fully recovered.

High-Altitude Cerebral Edema

- Administer oxygen 2 to 4 L per minute.
- In remote mountain areas, prepare for immediate descent of at least 600 m by ground or aircraft, and if oxygen unavailable, use portable hyperbaric chamber.
- Monitor at all times, and replenish/maintain hydration as needed.
- Administer dexamethasone (Decadron) 8 mg IM, IV, or PO × 1 dose, then 4 mg q6h.
- Administer acetazolamide (Diamox) 250 mg PO bid.

High-Altitude Pulmonary Edema

- Administer oxygen initially 4 to 6 L per minute, then titrate to keep arterial oxygen saturation more than 90%.
- In remote mountain areas, prepare for immediate descent of at least 600 m by ground or aircraft; and if oxygen unavailable, use portable hyperbaric chamber on incline with head end elevated.
- Sit upright at 45 degree angle, strict rest, and monitor at all times.
- Administer nifedipine (Adalat, Procardia) 10 mg PO initially, then 30 mg extended release q12h *IF* oxygen unavailable *AND* IV fluid resuscitation immediately available.
- Administer salmeterol (Serevent) inhaler, 1 puff bid *OR* albuterol (Proventil) inhaler, 4 to 6 puffs q4h.
- Administer dexamethasone (Decadron) 8 mg IM, IV or PO × 1 dose, then 4 mg q6h *IF* suspect or unsure if HACE is also present.

Abbreviations: bid = twice daily; IM = intramuscular; IV = intravenous; PO = orally; q = every.

use in treatment of HAPE. Current clinical experience warrants consideration of nifedipine (Adalat, Procardia) as an adjunct treatment for HAPE when immediate supplemental oxygen is unavailable or descent is delayed. Vascular access and intravenous (IV) fluid should be immediately available if nifedipine (Adalat, Procardia) is administered because patients are often intravascularly depleted and risk a severe hypotensive event that could be devastating in the setting of concomitant HACE. Sildenafil citrate (Viagra)[1] can also selectively lower pulmonary artery pressure with less effect on systemic blood pressure, and is under study for the treatment of HAPE.

[1]Not FDA approved for this indication.

Inhaled β-agonists, salmeterol (Serevent),[1] and albuterol (Proventil)[1] are currently under study for treatment of HAPE because β-agonists increase the clearance of fluid from the alveolar space and might lower pulmonary artery pressure. The Current Therapy Box summarizes the management of HAPE.

Reascent After Altitude Illness

Mild AMS is common and indicative of an ascent rate that is too rapid for a given person. Further ascent should not resume until full resolution of all symptoms. Future trips with similar ascent profiles warrant consideration of prophylaxis with acetazolamide (Diamox).

After episodes of HACE and HAPE resolve fully, reascent has been successful for many patients, some reaching exceptionally high summits. Caution is warranted, however. Persons should be advised to ascend more slowly and to recognize and act appropriately for early signs of altitude illness. Persons with multiple episodes of HAPE may benefit during subsequent ascent from prophylaxis with nifedipine (Adalat, Procardia)[1] and potentially with salmeterol (Serevent)[1] while stressing the value of cautious gradual ascent over medication. Recurrent HAPE or HAPE occurring at altitudes below 3000 m should prompt evaluation to rule out cardiac or pulmonary shunts, valvular disease, or pulmonary hypertension.

REFERENCES

Bartsch P, Merki B, Hofstetter D, et al: Treatment of acute mountain sickness by simulated descent: A randomized controlled trial. BMJ 1993;306:1098-1101.

Chow T, Browne V, Heileson HL, et al: Ginkgo biloba and acetazolamide prophylaxis for acute mountain sickness: A randomized placebo-controlled trial. Arch Intern Med 2005;165:296-301.

Consensus Group: The Lake Louise Consensus on the Definition and Quantification of Altitude Illness. In JR Sutton, G Coates, CS Houston: Hypoxia and Mountain Medicine. Burlington, Vt, Queen City Printers, 1992, 327-330.

Litch JA: Endotracheal intubation and mechanical ventilation following respiratory arrest from high altitude pulmonary edema. West J Med 1999;170(3):174-176.

Litch JA, Basnyat B, Zimmerman M: Subarachnoid hemorrhage at high altitude. West J Med 1997;167(3):180-181.

Litch JA, Bishop RA: Re-ascent following resolution of high altitude pulmonary edema (HAPE). High Alt Med Biol 2001;2(1):53-55.

Litch JA, Bishop RA: Oxygen concentrators for the delivery of supplemental oxygen in remote high altitude areas. Wilderness Environ Med 2000;11(3):189-191.

Larson EB, Roach RC, Schoene RB, Hornbein TF: Acute mountain sickness and acetazolamide—Clinical efficacy and effect on ventilation. JAMA 1982;248:328-332.

Oelz O, Maggiorini M, Ritter M, et al: Prevention and treatment of high altitude pulmonary edema by a calcium channel blocker. Int J Sports Med 1992;13(Suppl 1):S65-S68.

Pollard AJ, Niermeyer S, Barry P, et al: Children at high altitude: An international consensus statement by an ad hoc committee of the International Society of Mountain Medicine. High Alt Med Biol 2001;2(3):389-403.

Rabold MB: Dexamethasone for prophylaxis and treatment of acute mountain sickness. West J Med 1992;3:54-60.

Sartori C, Allemann Y, Duplain H, et al: Salmeterol for the prevention of high-altitude pulmonary edema. N Engl J Med 2002;346(21):1631-1636.

[1]Not FDA approved for this indication.

Disturbances Caused by the Cold

Method of
Daniel F. Danzl, MD

Accidental Hypothermia

Accidental hypothermia occurs when the body's core temperature unintentionally drops below 35°C (95°F). At this temperature, the compensatory physiologic responses to conserve heat begin to fail. Primary hypothermia results from exposure in previously healthy patients, but the mortality is much higher when diseases or injuries result in secondary hypothermia, which is often underreported. Cold-induced tragedies continue to afflict both military and civilian populations. Urban indoor and outdoor settings produce the most cases in the United States.

PATHOPHYSIOLOGY

Humans are unable to generate sufficient heat to maintain thermoneutrality under a variety of conditions (Box 1). Significant cold exposure normally activates the preoptic anterior hypothalamus, which orchestrates thermoregulation. Physiologic responses to the cold include shivering thermogenesis as well as endocrinologic and autonomic nervous system activities. Adaptive behavioral responses include donning of more clothing and seeking a heat source. Radiation normally accounts for 55% to 65% of the heat loss. Conductive losses increase up to 5 times in wet clothing and 25 times in water. Compensatory responses to heat loss through radiation, conduction, convection, evaporation, and respiration eventually fail. As the core temperature continues to fall, the patient becomes poikilothermic and cools to the ambient temperature.

Each organ system is affected uniquely. Cerebral metabolism is progressively depressed. Cerebrovascular autoregulation remains intact until below 25°C (77°F), which helps maintain cortical blood flow. The electroencephalographic activity is clearly not prognostic and silences around 19°C to 20°C (66.2°F to 68°F). Cardiovascular effects are often pronounced. After the initial tachycardia, there is progressive bradycardia. The heart rate drops to half its normal rate at 28°C (82.4°F). Hypothermia also progressively depresses the mean arterial pressure and cardiac index. Core temperature

CURRENT DIAGNOSIS

- Obtain core temperature measurement.
- Anticipate atypical presentations.
- Identify predisposing factors that decrease heat production; increase heat loss, or impair thermoregulation.
- Decide whether to use passive or active rewarming.

afterdrop refers to the continual decline in core temperature after removal from the cold. This phenomenon results from temperature equilibration and reversal of circulatory arteriovenous shunting in the extremities.

All atrial arrhythmias are commonly encountered and should have a slow ventricular response; therefore they are considered innocent. The clinical significance of ventricular arrhythmias is more difficult to assess because suppressed preexistent ectopy may reappear during rewarming. The decreased ventricular fibrillation threshold is a real hazard below 28°C (82.4°F). Cardiac cycle prolongation is pronounced, as reflected in the corrected QT interval on the electrocardiogram (ECG). The characteristic J wave, or Osborn hypothermic hump, may be present at the junction of the QRS complex and ST segment. Because hypothermic ECG changes are not easily computer programmable, the misdiagnosis of a current injury can result in dangerous thrombolytic therapy.

Respiratory stimulation is followed by a progressive reduction in respiratory minute volume, which reflects the metabolic depression. Carbon dioxide production falls 50% for each 8°C drop in temperature. Although renal blood flow declines, there is a large initial diuresis.

CLINICAL PRESENTATION

Historical circumstances suggest the diagnosis when exposure is obvious. More subtle presentations predominate in urban settings. In such cases, the clinician may misfocus on a solitary diagnosis of a medical, toxicologic, neurologic, traumatic, or psychiatric emergency. Symptoms are often vague and physical findings nonspecific or deceptive. For example, if tachycardia is disproportionate for the temperature, the physician should consider a secondary cause of hypothermia, such as hypoglycemia, hypovolemia, or a drug overdose. Persistent hyperventilation suggests a central nervous system (CNS) lesion or an organic acidosis, such as lactic acidosis or diabetic ketoacidosis. A cold-induced ileus and rectus spasm can both mimic and mask an acute abdomen. When the level of consciousness is inconsistent with the temperature, an overdose or CNS trauma or infection should be suspected. Hypothermic areflexia can also obscure a spinal cord injury. Last, temporary psychiatric sequelae during hypothermia include maladaptive behavior such as paradoxical undressing, which is the inappropriate removal of clothes in response to cold stress.

Hypothermia is confirmed with a core temperature (e.g., rectal, esophageal, tympanic) measurement, preferably from two sites. Further heat loss should be gently prevented and cardiac monitoring initiated. Hypothermia adversely affects tissue oxygenation by numerous mechanisms, including the leftward shift of the oxyhemoglobin dissociation curve. Most patients are significantly dehydrated and benefit from a bolus crystalloid administration.

Routine hematologic evaluations should include arterial blood gases uncorrected for temperature. An uncorrected pH of 7.4 and $P\text{co}_2$ of 40 mm Hg reflect acid–base balance at any temperature. The hematocrit also increases 2% per 1°C drop in temperature, which can mask anemia. Leukopenia does not imply the absence of infection because bone marrow suppression and white blood cell sequestration are common. Unfortunately, there is no safe predictor of the electrolyte status. For example, hyperkalemic ECG changes are obscured by hypothermia. Hypokalemia is more common in chronic hypothermia. Finally, cold induces a renal glycosuria, which as a result does not imply normoglycemia.

A full clotting screen is necessary because cold hemagglutination and coagulation are aberrant. Platelet function is impaired. Cold also directly inhibits the enzymatic reactions of the coagulation cascade. Kinetic tests of coagulation are performed in the laboratory at 37°C (98.6°F). As a result, the observed in vivo coagulopathy is not reflected by a reported deceptively normal prothrombin time, activated partial thromboplastin time, or international normalized ratio (INR).

REWARMING STRATEGIES

The key clinical decision is choosing passive versus active rewarming. Passive external rewarming is noninvasive and ideal for mild cases in previously healthy persons. The patient should simply be covered with insulating materials. Active rewarming should be considered in the following situations: core temperature below 32°C (90°F), age extremes, CNS dysfunction, endocrine insufficiency, and cardiovascular instability.

Active external rewarming is best accomplished with forced-air heating blankets. There is a potential for thermal injury to vasoconstricted skin with the use of electric blankets. Limiting heat application to the trunk minimizes many of the physiologic concerns with heating the extremities. For example, heating the extremities after the occurrence of the diuresis and fluid sequestration common to chronic hypothermia causes a core temperature afterdrop.

Many techniques are available to deliver direct heat internally. Active core rewarming options include inhalation of heated humidified oxygen, heated intravenous fluids and irrigation of the peritoneum or thorax, and

---

 CURRENT THERAPY

Before thawing:
- Stabilize core temperature.
- Address medical or surgical conditions.
- Protect and do not massage frozen part.
- Avoid partial thawing and refreezing.
- Extricate from environment.
- Begin rehydration.

Thaw:
- Provide parenteral analgesia and hydration.
- Rapidly rewarm entire part in 38°C to 40°C (100.4°F to 104°F) circulating water until distal flush occurs (thermometer monitoring).
- Ask patient to spend 10–60 min moving part gently without friction massage; "partial thaw" should be avoided.

After thawing:
- For clear vesicles: aspirate if intact; débride if broken.
- For hemorrhagic vesicles: do not débride; may aspirate.
- Apply topical aloe vera (Dermaide Aloe)[1] or antibiotic ointment q6h.
- Use ibuprofen, 400 mg orally q8h.
- Consider tetanus diphtheria (Td) (toxoid) and streptococcal prophylaxis.
- Elevate part in protective cradle.
- Use whirlpool hydrotherapy three times daily (37°C [98.6°F]).
- Avoid vasoconstrictors, including nicotine.
- Consider phenoxybenzamine (Dibenzyline)[1] in severe cases.

[1]Not FDA approved for this indication.

extracorporeal rewarming. Airway rewarming 40°C to 45°C (104°F to 113°F) with a mask or endotracheal tube is a valuable adjunct in all cases because the access is simple. Preoxygenation and gentle technique prevent intubation arrhythmias. The inhalation eliminates respiratory heat loss. During massive volume resuscitations, administration of heated intravenous fluid and blood is helpful. The use of countercurrent heat exchangers is the most efficient method for heating and delivering the fluid.

Peritoneal lavage is another option for severely hypothermic patients. Peritoneal dialysate at 40°C to 45°C (104°F to 113°F) delivered by two catheters with outflow suction transfers heat efficiently. Thoracostomy tube irrigation with warm saline is also valuable. The sterile saline is warmed to 42°C (107.6°F), infused anteriorly, and then drained from the efferent midaxillary tube. Finally, irrigation of the gastrointestinal tract is of very limited value and should be reserved for use in combination with all available techniques in patients with cardiac arrest.

Extracorporeal rewarming is potentially indicated in patients with cardiac arrest, completely frozen extremities, or severe rhabdomyolysis. The standard circuit uses a mechanical pump with an oxygenator and heat exchanger. Other options are continuous arteriovenous, venovenous, and hemodialysis rewarming. Cardiopulmonary resuscitation is indicated unless:

- A do-not-resuscitate (DNR) status is documented and verified.
- Obviously lethal injuries are present.
- Chest wall depression is impossible.
- Any signs of life are present.
- Rescuers are endangered by evacuation delays or altered triage conditions.

The misdiagnosis of a cardiac arrest is a real concern. Palpation of peripheral pulses is difficult when an extreme bradycardia is coupled with peripheral vasoconstriction. The examiner should take a full minute to check for a central pulse, especially if no cardiac monitor is available. After *one* attempt to defibrillate with 2 watt-seconds/kg, active rewarming should be continued past 30°C to 32°C (86°F to 89.6°F). Successful defibrillation below that temperature is rare.

Resuscitation pharmacology usually reflects substandard therapeutic activity while the patient is cold, which progresses to toxicity after rewarming. Drug protein binding increases, and metabolism and excretion are impaired. Low-dosage infusions of catecholamines should be initiated in euvolemic patients who fail to rewarm and are disproportionately hypotensive. The treatment of ventricular arrhythmias is problematic. Class III agents possess direct antifibrillatory activity, but bretylium is unavailable and the safety of amiodarone (Cordarone) questionable. For severe bradydysrhythmias that do not resolve with rewarming, external noninvasive pacing with pads is preferable to transvenous pacing. The empirical use of levothyroxine (Synthroid)[1] and corticosteroids[1] is hazardous.

The clinical treatment of hypothermia should be predicated on the duration and extent of temperature depression and the severity of the predisposing factors. Outcome is difficult to predict. Indicators of a grave prognosis include evidence of cell lysis (hyperkalemia with potassium levels greater than 10 mmol/L), intravascular thrombosis (fibrinogen value below 50 mg/dL), a pH below 6.5, and a core temperature below 10°C to 12°C (50°F to 53.6°F). Recently, a physician was successfully resuscitated from 13.7°C (56.66°F) after 165 minutes of CPR followed by CPB.

Peripheral Cold Injuries

Peripheral local cold injuries include freezing and nonfreezing syndromes. Frostbite is the most common freezing injury. Trench foot and immersion foot are nonfreezing injuries resulting from exposure to wet cold. Nonfreezing injury after exposure to dry cold is called chilblain (pernio). With cold stress, the core temperature is maintained via a life-versus-limb mechanism at the expense of vasospasticity and shunting, which prevent heat distribution to the extremities.

PATHOPHYSIOLOGY

A unique aspect of peripheral cold injury is the pathogenesis of the freezing injury cascade. Tissue is initially damaged by the freeze-thaw insult and subsequently by progressive dermal ischemia. Before freezing, tissue cooling increases the viscosity of the vascular contents as the microvasculature constricts.

The freeze-thaw sequence begins during extracellular fluid crystallization. Water exits the cell, causing intracellular dehydration, hyperosmolality, cellular shrinkage, and collapse. Arachidonic acid breakdown products are then released from underlying damaged tissue into the vesicle fluid. Both prostaglandin $F_{2\alpha}$ and thromboxane A_2 produce platelet aggregation, leukocyte immobilization, and vasoconstriction. Endothelial cells are quite sensitive to cold injury, and the microvasculature becomes distorted and clogged.

After tissue thawing, progressive edema formation continues for 48 to 72 hours. Subsequent thrombosis and early superficial necrosis develop. This tissue eventually mummifies and demarcates. The incidence and severity of peripheral cold injury are determined by the duration and intensity of cutaneous cold exposure. Box 1 lists the factors predisposing to peripheral cold injuries.

CLINICAL PRESENTATION

The initial presentation of frostbite is often deceptively benign. Unlike in burns, classification of frostbite by degrees is often inaccurate prognostically and misleading therapeutically. The physical findings at 24 to 72 hours after completion of rewarming are more reliably used to classify frostbite. Superficial or mild frostbite does not entail eventual tissue loss, but deep or severe frostbite does. Frostnip is a superficial cold insult producing transient numbness or tingling that resolves after rewarming without tissue destruction.

All patients with frostbite have some initial sensory deficit in light touch, pain, or temperature. Acral areas and distal extremities are the usual insensate sites. Patients also complain of being clumsy or having a "chunk of wood" sensation in the extremity.

Deep frostbite may initially appear deceptively benign. Tissues remaining frozen can appear mottled,

---

[1]Not FDA approved for this indication.

violaceous, pale yellow, or waxy. Favorable presenting signs are warmth, normal color, and some sensation. If the subcutaneous tissue is soft and pliable or the dermis can be rolled over the bony prominences, the injury may be superficial.

Rapid rewarming produces an initial hyperemia, even in severe cases. A residual violaceous hue is ominous. Early formation of clear large blebs is a more favorable sign than smaller dark, hemorrhagic blebs, which imply cold damage to the subdermal vascular plexus.

Chilblain (pernio) is a form of dry cold injury often developing after repetitive exposures. These so-called cold sores typically involve facial areas and the dorsa of the hands and feet. Younger women under 50, especially those with a history of Raynaud's phenomenon, are at risk. Persistent vasospasticity and vasculitis result in pruritus, erythema, and mild edema. Plaques, blue nodules, and ulcerations eventually develop. Treatment of refractory perniosis is difficult; the physician should consider using nifedipine (Procardia)[1] at a dose of 20 to 60 mg daily. Limaprost, a prostaglandin E1 analogue, is also used.

Immersion (trench) foot is produced by prolonged exposure to wet cold at above-freezing temperatures. Feet often appear erythematous, edematous, or cyanotic. The bullae are indistinguishable from those seen in frostbite. This vesiculation proceeds to ulceration and liquefaction gangrene. In milder cases, hyperhidrosis, cold sensitivity, and painful ambulation persist for many years.

Warm-water immersion foot affects the soles of the feet and results from waterlogging of the thick stratum corneum. This commonly occurs in persons who lack shelter wearing wet shoes for prolonged periods.

Ancillary diagnostic adjuncts have limited value with peripheral cold injuries. Doppler ultrasonography, digital plethysmography, thermography, routine radiography, and angiography do not consistently predict tissue loss at presentation. Early scintigraphy may predict tissue loss and monitor the efficacy of treatment. Magnetic resonance angiography may predict eventual demarcation prior to clinical demarcation.

TREATMENT

Mills popularized rapid immersion rewarming after extensive experience with severe Alaskan frostbite cases. Before thawing, frozen parts should not be exposed to dry heat sources. Tissue refreezing is also disastrous; as an extreme example, it is preferable to ambulate to safety on frozen feet.

A circulating tank is ideal for rewarming the extremities, but a large container suffices for the hands and feet. The process starts with water at 38°C to 40°C (100.4°F to 104°F) and the temperature is gradually increased. Care should be taken to avoid thermal injury, which occurs if the water temperature markedly exceeds 45°C (113°F). A very common error is premature termination of rewarming because the establishment of reperfusion is quite painful and requires parenteral analgesia. Complete thawing may take up to 1 hour.

Extreme caution should be exercised in treating patients with completely frozen extremities because invariably they are hypothermic. Thawing produces significant core temperature, fluid, and electrolyte fluxes. Persistent cyanosis after a complete thaw should suggest elevated fascial compartment pressures.

Management of frostbite vesicles also varies. Large clear blisters should be sterilely aspirated. The débridement of hemorrhagic vesicles, however, can extend the injury by allowing secondary desiccation of deep dermal layers. There are two strategies for inhibition of prostaglandins. Topical aloe vera ointment (Dermaide Aloe)[1,*] is a specific thromboxane inhibitor but it is not proven to salvage tissue. An acceptable alternative is topical antibiotic ointment. Systemically, ibuprofen is preferable to the salicylates. Ibuprofen produces fibrinolysis in addition to limiting the accumulation of inflammatory mediators. Parenteral ketorolac (Toradol) is another antiprostaglandin option.

Multiple antithrombotic and vasodilatory treatment regimens are proposed. There is no conclusive evidence of enhanced tissue salvage with administration of dextran,[1] heparin,[1] steroids,[1] nonsteroidal anti-inflammatory drugs (NSAIDs),[1] dimethylsulfoxide (DMSO),[1] nonionic detergents,[1] dipyridamole (Persantine),[1] calcium channel blockers,[1] or hyperbaric oxygen.[1] Pentoxifylline (Trental),[1] 400 mg given orally every 8 hours, may facilitate small-vessel perfusion.

A long-acting α-blocker, phenoxybenzamine (Dibenzyline),[1] 10 mg/day up to 60 mg/day, may decrease the refractory vasospasm that develops during the clinical course in selected patients. Aggressive hydration is essential to minimize orthostatic hypotension. Chemical sympathectomy with intra-arterial reserpine could be helpful but is not available. Surgical sympathectomy does not enhance tissue salvage, although a sympathetic nerve block can relieve painful and refractory vasospasm.

SEQUELAE

Residual neuropathic symptoms are common and result from abnormal sympathetic tone and neuronal damage. Patients with chronic symptoms should be advised to avoid nicotine and cold exposure while using nonsteroidal anti-inflammatory agents and skin lubricants. Dermatologic findings include lymphedema, ulcerations, hair and nail deformities, and epidermoid or squamous carcinomas. Occult musculoskeletal injuries are most pronounced in children. Premature epiphyseal fusion and fragmentation can occur. Amputation decisions should be deferred unless there is supervening sepsis or gangrene. The ultimate tissue salvage after a spontaneous slough usually far exceeds the most optimistic initial estimates.

REFERENCES

American Heart Association 2005 Guidelines for CPR and Emergency Cardiovascular Care: Hypothermia. Circulation 2005;112:136.

Danzl DF: Hypothermia. Sem Resp Crit Care Med 2002;23:57.

Durrer B, Brugger H, Syme D: International Commision for Mountain Emergency Medicine: The medical on-site treatment of hypothermia: ICAR-MEDCOM recommendation. High Alt Med Biol 2003;4:99.

Giesbrecht GG: Cold stress, near drowning and accidental hypothermia: a review. Aviat Space Environ Med 2000;71:733.

Hildebrand F, Giannoudis PV, van Griensven M, et al: Pathophysiologic changes and effects of hypothermia on outcome in elective surgery and trauma patients. Am J Surg 2004;187:363.

---

[1]Not FDA approved for this indication.

---

[1]Not FDA approved for this indication.
*Available as alternative medicine.

Ittner KP, Bachfischer M, Zimmerman O, et al: Convective air warning is more effective than resistive heating in an experimental model with a water dummy. Eur J Emerg Med 2004;11:151.

Kempainen RR, Brunette DD: The evaluation and management of accidental hypothermia. Resp Care 2004;49:192.

Mallet ML, Pathophysiology of accidental hypothermia. OJM 2002;95:775.

Muszkat M, Durst RM, Ben-Yehuda A: Factors associated with mortality among elderly patients with hypothermia. Am J Med 2002;113:234.

Pedley DK, Paterson B, Morrison W: Hypothermia in elderly patients presenting to accident & emergency during the onset of winter. Scott Med J 2002;47:10.

Disturbances Caused by Heat

Method of
John F. Coyle II, MD

Exertional Heat Stroke

Heat stroke is an illness caused by failure of thermoregulation with elevation of core temperature to 40.6°C (105°F) or more, associated with central nervous system dysfunction. Heat stroke is traditionally subdivided into *exertional* and *classic* (or nonexertional) forms.

Exertional heat stroke is a sporadic illness triggered by exercise in warm environmental conditions that add to the thermal load produced by muscular contraction. It mainly strikes manual laborers, soldiers in training, and athletic competitors; indeed, it is the third leading cause of death among high school and college athletes in the United States. Exertional heat stroke may occur at moderate temperatures, especially if humidity is high, but both exertional and classic heat strokes most likely develop in conditions of high heat. The incidence of heat stroke increases exponentially when heat stress exceeds a boundary value. Appearance of the first case should sound an alarm that conditions have become dangerous, and more cases should be anticipated. The typical heat stroke victim is highly motivated, poorly conditioned, obese, and not acclimatized. Fatigue and sleep deprivation are commonly encountered, and recent or ongoing febrile or dehydrating illness increases risk. Dehydration may play a role, especially if severe. The use of certain medicines also increases risk, most notably those that decrease cardiac output (β-blockers), promote dehydration (diuretics), affect hypothalamic control (major tranquilizers, neuroleptics, alcohol), inhibit sweating (anticholinergics, tricyclic antidepressants, antihistamines), or increase thermogenicity (amphetamines, cocaine).

Prevention is the ideal treatment. Because behavior is the most powerful thermoregulatory mechanism, education and empowerment have the greatest preventive potential. To avoid exertional heat stroke, organizers should schedule vigorous exercise in the coolest hours of the day (shortly after dawn or after nightfall, in difficult seasons). Exercise level should be governed by athlete fitness, acclimatization, hydration status, and freedom from intercurrent illness. Clothing should be appropriate for exercise conditions. Medication use that might interfere with effective thermoregulation should be recognized, and medical personnel must be charged with the responsibility for stopping any participant who appears to be decompensating.

Triage of those with exertional heat stroke is highly variable. Runners who are plunged unconscious into an ice water bath at the end of a race often respond promptly to treatment, reawaken, and are sometimes sent home without hospitalization. A less-favorable response necessitates hospital admission.

Classic (Nonexertional) Heat Stroke

Classic (nonexertional) heat stroke usually occurs during heat waves that cause passive warming by exposure to unrelenting hot and humid conditions, afflicting urban dwellers who are elderly, infirm, solitary, and poor. Heat waves tend to be "silent and invisible killers of silent and invisible people." Their housing lacks air-conditioning or they do not use it because of expense or confusion. Alcoholism and chronic illness, especially mental illness, predispose people to heat stroke. Young children are susceptible, reflecting their high surface-to-volume ratio, relatively inefficient sweat glands, and dependent status. Classic heat stroke requires preventive measures at the community level. Those with chronic illness and substance abuse history are at highest risk, and they may be the most difficult to contact. Although ventilation fans are of little help in hot and humid conditions, a few hours spent in air-conditioned rooms each day can significantly reduce the likelihood of heat stroke. Whether this is primarily a physiologic or a sociologic effect is unclear. Patients with classic heat stroke usually respond slowly to treatment and require hospital admission.

Pathophysiology

The pathophysiology of heat stroke is incompletely understood. Although a vast number of runners in a marathon may develop dehydration and a high core temperature, very few proceed to heat stroke. Excessive heat is a noxious agent that causes direct cell injury. The severity of heat stroke is related to the degree and duration of temperature elevation above 41.6°C (106.9°F). Exercise lowers the thermal threshold for heat stroke because of hormonal effects and competing demands of organ systems as blood flow is directed away from the viscera to the active muscles and the skin. Gut ischemia may result in release of bacterial polysaccharides into the blood. What happens next is a complex interplay of factors including cytokines, bacterial polysaccharides, and heat shock proteins. As endothelial abnormalities accumulate, there is precipitation of a cascade of events including activation of the coagulation system and vascular dilation, resulting in hypotension and coagulation disorders. These events in many respects mimic sepsis.

Because the brain is extremely sensitive to heat stress, the first signs of heat stroke are neurologic. Judgment is impaired, and the chance for self-diagnosis is greatly reduced. After loss of consciousness, muscular activity is markedly diminished, but temperature may remain elevated for hours. Multisystem injury may follow, with the possibility of neurologic, pulmonary, cardiac, hepatic, renal, vascular, hematologic, and immunologic damage. A high percentage of classic heat stroke patients suffer infection within 36 hours of hospital admission.

Treatment

Treatment of heat stroke can be summarized easily:

- Lower rectal temperature immediately to 39°C (102.2°F).
- Support organ systems injured by heat, hypotension, inflammation, and coagulopathy.

There is a *golden hour* after the onset of heat stroke in which therapy can be extremely effective. When treating a patient outside of the hospital, the patient should be moved to a shaded area, clothes removed, and the person covered with water and fanned. When resources become available, the simplest treatment appears to be cold-water immersion in a shallow tub, with patient head, arms, and lower legs outside the tub. The high efficiency of this method comes from two properties of water: It has 25 times the thermal conductivity of air, and it makes perfect contact with all skin surfaces. In addition, the hydrostatic properties of water tend to reduce the risk of hypotension. Other methods of cooling include skin wetting with fanning, application of total-body ice packs (24 ice packs, with special emphasis on the neck, armpits, and groin), or use of a body-cooling unit (evaporation and convection).

Assessment of the patient with presumed heat stroke should be delayed pending initiation of cooling. Determination of rectal temperature, heart rate, and blood pressure can be carried out while the patient is

CURRENT DIAGNOSIS

- Heat stroke often occurs in the first 2 hours of exercise and may occur in so-called moderate heat stress conditions.
- Heat stroke may occur in sedentary urban dwellers during heat waves, especially in the presence of drug or alcohol use, senility, or in young children.
- Abnormal mental status (coma, delirium, agitation, confusion, combativeness) is a constant feature of heat stroke.
- Rectal temperature should be checked immediately. Axillary and aural temperatures may be misleadingly low. A rectal temperature of 40.6°C (105°F) or more is required for diagnosis of heat stroke, but delayed measurement may produce a misleadingly low temperature.
- The trap of proceeding with complex diagnostic procedures (such as computed tomographic scans) before core temperature is assessed and lowered to less than 39°C (102.2°F) should be avoided.
- After cooling measures are instituted, blood samples should be obtained to assess coagulation status, hepatic function, renal function, likelihood of infection, acid-base status, and muscle injury.

CURRENT THERAPY

- Injury because of heat stroke is related to both the magnitude and duration of core temperature elevation.
- After elevated rectal temperature is documented, treatment should not be delayed. In particular, it should not be delayed to start an intravenous line or to carry out advanced testing such as computed tomography or other radiograph study.
- Ideal treatment for heat stroke is cold-water immersion in a low tub, such as a child's wading pool, with the patient's arms, legs, and head hanging out of the tub.
- If low tub immersion is not available, constant flowing of cold water from a tap over the patient with drainage through a slotted Gurney cart in the presence of constant high-velocity electric fanning can be effective.
- Applying ice packs to the axillae, groins, trunk, and as many other skin surfaces as possible can be useful, but this method of cooling is not as efficient as cold-water immersion or constant cold-water flow because of reduced contact surface and limited thermal gradient.
- Rectal temperature should be checked every 5 minutes during cooling. Cooling measures are discontinued when rectal temperature reaches 39°C (102.2°F) to avoid excessive cooling. Clinicians should watch for rebound temperature elevation after cooling is discontinued.
- Clinicians should be prepared to support the patient through multisystem organ failure. Hemorrhage should be treated with transfusion of red blood cells, platelets, fresh-frozen plasma, and clotting factors. Heparin has no role in treatment of this consumptive coagulopathy. Volume expansion may be needed. Prolonged ventilator support and hemodialysis may be required.
- Medications that may be needed are diazepam (Valium), 5 mg intravenously (IV), for seizures; pressors; and mannitol, 0.25 g/kg IV, and furosemide (Lasix), 0.5 to 1.0 mg/kg IV, for renal protection from rhabdomyolysis, but only after adequate volume expansion is achieved.

being cooled. Oral and tympanic membrane temperatures cannot be used because they may be misleadingly low. Rectal temperature should be measured every 5 to 10 minutes, and the patient should be removed from cooling when 39°C (102.2°F) is reached, to avoid overshoot hypothermia. Hydration with normal saline or lactated Ringer's solution should be started after initiation of cooling, and most patients require 1 L in the first hour of treatment. Further rehydration needs to be guided by estimated water losses, and in difficult cases placement of a central venous monitoring catheter may be needed. Overhydration may promote cerebral edema, pulmonary edema, and hyponatremia.

Seizures, which occur commonly, should be managed with diazepam (Valium), 5 mg intravenously (IV).

Shivering may also be treated with diazepam. The patient must be monitored closely with use of this medication, which occasionally promotes hypotension. Hypotension should be treated with cooling and volume expansion. If blood pressure remains depressed, pressors may be needed. For patients with prolonged exertional heat stroke, mannitol, 0.25 g/kg, or furosemide (Lasix), 0.5 to 1 mg/kg, should be given after volume expansion is carried out to minimize the adverse effects of rhabdomyolysis on renal function.

In patients with severe multiorgan damage, disseminated intravascular coagulation (DIC) is a common finding. Bleeding in DIC should be treated with transfusion of fresh-frozen plasma, cryoprecipitate, and platelet concentrates as needed. There is no role for heparin or thrombolytics in DIC in this setting. Adult respiratory distress syndrome tends to occur in conjunction with DIC, and prolonged ventilator support may be required. Hepatic failure in heat stroke is usually transient. Renal failure may necessitate emergency hemodialysis. No evidence supports use of anti-inflammatory agents or antipyretic agents in heat stroke. Use of strategies that are helpful in sepsis may ultimately find a role in treatment of heat stroke, but such treatments should be considered experimental at this time.

Prognosis can be estimated by time to recovery of consciousness (shorter is better) and elevation of liver enzymes (lactate dehydrogenase [LDH] at 24 hours less than three times normal is a good prognostic sign).

Heat stroke should usually be regarded as an accident, like drowning. The population at highest risk is readily defined, but because of the rarity of this ailment it is difficult to maintain a high level of preparedness for its prevention and treatment. Once encountered, heat stroke must be treated with much the same urgency as cardiac arrest because prompt cooling can sometimes make the crisis little more than an inconvenience. After the process of systemic injury becomes established, heat stroke's cascade of microvascular dysfunction can take on a life of its own, eventuating in a desperate struggle against multisystem failure and a high mortality rate.

REFERENCES

Bouchama A, Knochel JP: Heat stroke. N Engl J Med 2002;346(25): 1978-1988.

Crandall CG, Vongpatanasin W, Victor RG: Mechanism of cocaine-induced hyperthermia in humans. Ann Intern Med 2002;136(11): 785-791.

Dematte JE, O'Mara K, Buescher J, et al: Near-fatal heat stroke during the 1995 heat wave in Chicago. Ann Intern Med 1998;129(3):173-181.

Eichner ER: Treatment of suspected heat illness. Int J Sports Med 1998;19(Suppl 2):S150-S153.

Epstein Y, Moran DS, Shapiro Y: Exertional heatstroke in the Israeli Defence Forces. In Pandolf KB, Burr RE (eds): Medical Aspects of Harsh Environments. U.S. Defense Dept., Army, Office of the Surgeon General, 2001, pp 281-292. Available free online: http://www.bordeninstitute.army.mil/medaspofharshenvrnmnts/

Gaffin SL, Hubbard RW: Pathophysiology of heatstroke. In Pandolf KB, Burr RE (eds): Medical Aspects of Harsh Environments. U.S. Defense Dept., Army, Office of the Surgeon General, 2001, pp 161-208. Available free online: http://www.bordeninstitute. army.mil/medaspofharshenvrnmnts/

Gardner JW, Kark JA: 2001. Clinical diagnosis, management and surveillance of exertional heat illness. In Pandolf KB, Burr RE (eds): Medical Aspects of Harsh Environments. U.S. Defense Dept., Army, Office of the Surgeon General, 2001, pp 221-279. Available free online: http://www.bordeninstitute.army.mil/medaspofharshenvrnmnts/

Klinenberg E: Review of heat wave: Social autopsy of disaster in Chicago. N Engl J Med 2003;348(7):666-667.

Shephard RJ, Shek PN: Immune dysfunction as a factor in heat illness. Crit Rev Immunol 1999;19(4):285-302.

Spider Bites and Scorpion Stings

Method of
Rachel Haroz, MD, and James R. Roberts, MD

Spider Bites

Most of the approximately 34,000 species of spiders are considered to be venomous, but their short and delicate jaws generally prevent significant human envenomation. Approximately 200 species, however, do possess the ability to envenomate humans, resulting in symptoms ranging from minor to occasionally serious skin lesions to neurotoxicity, systemic illness, multiorgan dysfunction, and death. Spider identification after a bite is desirable but usually impossible. Here we discuss features, symptoms of envenomation, and treatment for bites from the *Loxosceles, Latrodectus,* and tarantula spiders.

LOXOSCELES ENVENOMATION

Relatively small (approximately 1.5 cm in leg span), *Loxosceles* spiders are light brown in color with darker brown markings on their dorsal surface. The most distinctive identifying characteristic appears on the female brown recluse (*L. reclusa*), which is described as violin shaped. Eleven native species of *Loxosceles* exist in the United States in the southern, southwestern, and central states. Most confirmed necrotic arachnidism in the United States is caused by *L. reclusa. Loxosceles* spiders have six eyes, which differs from the typical eight eyes found in most other spiders. Females are usually larger than males, which are rarely considered venomous. Considered nonaggressive and nocturnal, most *Loxosceles* bites occur when the spider is inadvertently caught between clothing or bedding and the victim's skin. Perineal and genital bites can occur in outhouses. The bite may be minimally painful or go totally unnoticed.

CURRENT DIAGNOSIS

- *Loxosceles* spider bites generally result in local symptoms, whereas *Latrodectus* and scorpion stings have predominantly systemic manifestations, which may be severe.
- The spider or scorpion should be identified if at all possible.
- Not all necrotic wounds are spider bites; therefore a differential diagnosis should be entertained.

The initial skin manifestation is a small, erythematous, flat lesion surrounded by a light-colored ring. Within hours to days this lesion becomes bluish with a deepening of the color of the ring and progressing to a blister/bleb. A necrotic eschar with an ulcerative base may develop, which rarely becomes quite extensive. The lesion is minimally painful but often takes several weeks to heal, occasionally requiring extensive débridement or skin grafting. Some ulcerated wounds (approximately 10%) produce permanent scarring. *Loxosceles* venom contains various toxic enzymes, most notably sphingomyelinase D, that contribute to cellular destruction and tissue damage.

Systemic symptoms are rare (1% to 3% of all bites) but may include hemolysis, platelet aggregation, hemoglobinuria, myoglobinuria, maculopapular rash, nausea, vomiting, renal failure, disseminated intravascular coagulation, fever, seizures, coma, and death. These symptoms are more common in children and following South American *Loxosceles* bites.

There is little the clinician can do to affect favorably the course of a *Loxosceles* bite, with the ultimate outcome dependent on the amount and potency of the venom and host factors. Local wound care includes antisepsis, immobilization, and elevation of the affected extremity, cool compresses, appropriate analgesics, antihistamines for itching, and tetanus prophylaxis. Envenomation is difficult to differentiate from infection, but antibiotics may be necessary for secondarily infected wounds. Debridement of necrotic tissue is performed as needed. Delayed excision and wound grafting may be indicated. Once recommended, early wound excision and intrawound steroid injections should be avoided. Several other treatments to ameliorate tissue necrosis are advocated, including dapsone,[1] colchicine,[1] topical nitroglycerin,[1] high-dose vitamin C,[1] electric shock therapy, cyproheptadine (Periactin),[1] and hyperbaric oxygenation, but none has proven effective. Patients exhibiting systemic symptoms should be hospitalized and receive supportive care.

Absent a witnessed attack, a spider bite is usually a clinical diagnosis made by exclusion. *Loxosceles* and other spider bites are overreported and occur far less frequently than suspected by the lay public or diagnosed by clinicians. Outside of the endemic areas, *Loxosceles* bites are highly unlikely. Importantly, if the spider was not positively identified, a differential diagnosis should be entertained. Entities confused with a spider bite include clandestine drug injection (especially cocaine and amphetamines), methicillin-resistant *Staphylococcus aureus* (MRSA) skin infections, early shingles lesions, other bug bites, self-induced trauma, and infectious embolic lesions (such as endocarditis and gonococcemia).

NON-*LOXOSCELES* NECROTIC ARACHNIDISM

Several other species of spiders in the United States (*Cheiracanthium* species and *Tegenaria agrestis* [hobo] spiders) are associated with necrotic lesions. *Cheiracanthium* spiders are widespread and usually found indoors (e.g., in the folds of curtains or on warm windowsills). They are aggressive night foragers and produce painful, pruritic bites, usually resolving within several days. Their bites rarely

---

[1]Not FDA approved for this indication.

result in ulceration and necrosis. Hobo spiders inhabit the Pacific Northwest to where they recently emigrated from Western Europe. They are large, aggressive, and inhabit woodpiles, subfloors, and baseboards. Their bites are usually painless but may lead to multiple ruptured blisters within 1 to 2 days and a necrotic wound. Hobo spider bites are probably responsible for necrotic arachnidism in the colder areas of the United States where the brown recluse spider is not found. Treatment of hobo spider bites is similar to that of *Loxosceles* bites.

LATRODECTUS ENVENOMATION

Latrodectus species (widow spiders) are found worldwide. In the United States, five widow spiders are endemic. These spiders are generally dark with various ventral patterns; the most well known is the red hourglass figure found on the female black widow spider. Females are larger (16- to 20-mm leg span) and more venomous than males. *Latrodectus* spiders generally inhabit outdoor dark spaces and are nonaggressive, but they do bite if provoked. The initial bite may be mildly painful, resulting in a small raised wheal. The neurotoxicity associated with these bites results from α-latrotoxin in the venom that causes a large calcium-dependent presynaptic terminal release of neurotransmitters including norepinephrine, glutamate, acetylcholine, and dopamine. The reuptake of choline is simultaneously inhibited. Symptoms begin approximately 30 minutes to an hour after the bite, and patients can appear quite ill. Muscle cramps and pain spread from the bite site and can be severe. Facial contortion and periorbital swelling, *facies latrodectismica*, may occur. Abdominal rigidity mimicking an acute abdomen, thoracic muscle spasm leading to hypoventilation and respiratory failure, diaphoresis, hypertension, nausea, vomiting, diffuse skin erythema, tremor, priapism, headache, tachycardia, paresthesias, and coma have been described. Lower extremity pain and diaphoresis, even in upper extremity bites, seem to be characteristic features. Symptoms resolve over 3 to 7 days, and death is rare.

Local wound care includes thorough cleansing, appropriate analgesics, ice application, and tetanus prophylaxis. Severe pain and muscle spasms are treated with intravenous opioids and benzodiazepines. Intravenous calcium, although recommended in the past, is ineffective. *Latrodectus* antivenom (antivenin *Lactrodectus mactans*) is horse based and may cause anaphylaxis and serum sickness in allergic persons. It should be reserved for patients with severe systemic symptoms or those with potential for complications, such as the elderly, young children, pregnant patients, and patients with severe cardiovascular disease. Patients who manifest refractory pain, autonomic instability, respiratory distress, or significant neurologic changes should be treated with antivenom. The clinical response to antivenom can be dramatic even when administered 24 hours or more after envenomation.

TARANTULAS

Approximately 1500 species of tarantulas are found worldwide, with 40 species endemic to the southwestern United States. Tarantulas are also now popular household pets because many are considered harmless and nonvenomous. Relatively large spiders (18- to 24-cm leg span),

CURRENT THERAPY

- Conservative wound care is essential in all envenomations, particularly for a *Loxosceles* spider bite.
- Particular care should be given to the very young, elderly, and patients with co-morbidity. In the setting of significant systemic symptoms, the administration of antivenom, if available, should be considered.
- Patients with ocular symptoms after exposure to a tarantula spider must be promptly referred to an ophthalmologist.
- Supportive care is often more valuable than antivenom administration, particularly considering the relatively high rate of both immediate and delayed hypersensitivity reactions.

tarantulas live in underground burrows and are night foragers. Tarantula envenomations in humans often cause mild pain with some surrounding inflammation, but necrotic wounds and systemic symptoms are rare. Bites in dogs, however, are usually rapidly fatal.

Several tarantula species possess urticating hairs, which they launch to incapacitate their enemy. These hairs may penetrate the human skin and cause intense inflammation or lodge in the cornea leading to keratitis, uveitis, and ophthalmia nodosa, a condition characterized by granulomatous lesions in the cornea. Case reports generally describe patients who developed eye symptoms after cleaning tarantula cages or handling the tarantulas. Treatment involves wound care including cleansing, elevation, and immobilization of the affected extremity, tetanus prophylaxis, and appropriate analgesics. Hairs embedded in the cornea that are readily identified should be removed and the patient promptly referred to an ophthalmologist. Antihistamines and corticosteroids may be necessary for pruritus and inflammation. Patients with ophthalmia nodosa may require prolonged topical corticosteroids. Tarantula owners should be cautioned to wear gloves and eye protection when handling their pets and to wash their hands and avoid any eye rubbing after such interactions.

Scorpion Stings

Scorpions range in size from several millimeters to 15 cm. They have a lobster-like appearance with a small head, two front claws, eight paired legs, and a segmented abdomen ending in a venom-containing tail consisting of a storage vesicle and a stinger. Scorpions are typically night stalkers and often found hidden under rocks, in shallow burrows, and in shoes, clothing, and cooking pots. Most of the severe envenomations in the United States are caused by stings by *Centruroides exilicauda (sculpturata)*, a small (4 to 7 cm long) yellowish brown scorpion.

Scorpion stings are usually very painful, quickly causing local paresthesias and edema. In adults, this usually resolves in several hours. Systemic effects are usually seen in the elderly and in infants and children. Scorpion venom blocks sodium and potassium channels and causes marked acetylcholine and catecholamine release. This leads to an initial cholinergic toxidrome characterized by the SLUDGE

syndrome: salivation, lacrimation, urination, defecation, gastroenteritis, and emesis. Subsequently, catecholamine release leads to anxiety, tachycardia, hypertension, pulmonary edema, confusion, dystonic and myoclonic movements, seizures, ataxia, hyperglycemia, hyperpyrexia, and pancreatitis. Myocardial depression, myocardial infarctions without thrombosis, and ischemic strokes are rarely described.

Wound care should encompass thorough cleansing, elevation and immobilization of the affected extremity, cool compresses, tetanus prophylaxis, and appropriate analgesics. Patients should be observed for a period of 6 hours after the sting for the development of systemic symptoms.

Supportive care is the mainstay of treatment. Sympathetic symptoms should be blunted aggressively. Benzodiazepines, β-blockers, diuretics, digoxin (Lanoxin),[1] and nitroprusside (Nitropress) are successful. Dopamine (Intropin) and dobutamine (Dobutrex) may be necessary for the hypotensive patient, and mechanical ventilation may be required for respiratory failure. Angiotensin-converting enzyme inhibitors, opioids, and nifedipine may be detrimental and should be avoided.

Goat-derived antivenom use is controversial. It is not FDA approved and its availability is limited to the state of Arizona. The incidence of immediate and delayed hypersensitivity is relatively high (3% and 60%, respectively). The antivenom is species specific and must be administered within 1 hour of the exposure. Although helpful with pain, antivenom does not reverse cardiovascular and respiratory compromise because these are secondary to massive catecholamine release.

REFERENCES

Blaikie AJ, Ellis J, Sanders R, et al: Eye disease associated with handling pet tarantulas: Three case reports. BMJ 1997;314:1524-1525.

Clark RF, Wethern-Kestner S, Vance MV, et al: Clinical presentation and treatment of black widow spider envenomations: A review of 163 cases. Ann Emerg Med 1992;21:782-787.

Diaz HJ: The global epidemiology, syndromic classification, management, and prevention of spider bites. Am J Trop Med Hyg 2004;71:239-250.

Hered RW, Spaulding AG, Sanitato JJ, et al: Ophthalmia nodosa caused by tarantula hairs. Ophthalmology 1988;95:166-169.

LoVecchio F, Welch S, Klemens J, et al: Incidence of immediate and delayed hypersensitivity to Centruroides antivenom. Ann Emerg Med 1999;5:615-619.

Mazzei de Davila CA, Davila DF, Donis JH: Sympathetic nervous system activation, antivenin administration and cardiovascular manifestations of scorpion envenomation. Toxicon 2002;40:1339-1346.

Merchant ML, Hinton JF, Geren CR: Effect of hyperbaric oxygen on sphingomyelinase D activity of brown recluse spider (*Loxosceles reclusa*) venom as studied by ^{31}P nuclear magnetic resonance spectroscopy. Am J Trop Med Hyg 1997;56:335-338.

Mold JW, Thompson DM: Management of brown recluse spider bites in primary care. J Am Board Fam Pract 2004;17:347-352.

Saucier JR: Arachnid envenomation. Emerg Med Clin North Am 2004; 22:405-422.

Swanson DL, Vetter RS: Bites of brown recluse spiders and suspected necrotic arachnidism. N Engl J Med 2005;352:700-707.

---

[1]Not FDA approved for this indication.

Snakebite

Method of
Craig S. Kitchens, MD

The combination of fear of snakes and the unfamiliarity of most physicians with the management of snakebite often leads to an ill-founded perception of danger on the part of practitioners. It should be kept in mind that approximately 10,000 poisonous snakebites in the United States occur every year, yet fewer than 10 victims die.

In the past, treatment was often empirical and shrouded by folklore. Because survival is a near statistical certainty, various therapies including alcohol, application of ice, electric shock therapy, wide surgical débridement, or even providing no therapy have appeared efficacious. Treatment has now evolved from this disorganized state to a scientifically supported therapeutic regimen based on both the availability of antivenin and the experience garnered by large series of patients by clinical investigators. Morbidity and mortality are minimized by appropriate therapy.

Here we discuss care of patients bitten by North American poisonous snakes. In the United States, approximately 95% of poisonous snakebites are inflicted by pit vipers (family Crotalidae), which comprise multiple species of rattlesnakes as well as water moccasins and copperheads. Approximately 1% to 2% of all U.S. snakebites involve coral snakes (family Elapidae). Another 2% to 3% of snakebites are inflicted by exotic poisonous snakes that are either appropriately housed in zoos or owned by professional snake handlers or inappropriately kept as pets by amateurs. Treatment of persons bitten by exotic snakes is beyond the scope of this chapter. It is suggested that in such encounters a Poison Control Center should be consulted because antivenin to treat exotic snake bites is not commercially available in the United States; reputable handlers of such snakes usually have a supply of their own specific antivenin.

Diagnosis

It is of prime importance to know the species of the offending snake because prognosis and treatment both heavily depend on this information. Undue risk should not be assumed by either the victim or others, yet identification of the snake is important and, if possible, the snake should be brought to the treatment facility for identification. The species of snake is actually more important than is its size in terms of prognosis. Primary care practitioners and emergency department personnel should have at least a modicum of information for identification of local poisonous snakes. Bites from the pygmy rattlesnake (*Sistrurus miliarius*) have not resulted in a documented human death, and envenomations by the copperhead (*Agkistrodon contortrix*) and water moccasin (*A. piscivorus*) generally result in moderate envenomation syndromes with death rarely occurring. The Eastern diamondback (*Crotalus adamanteus*), Western diamondback (*C. atrox*), and Mojave rattlesnake (*C. scutulatus*) each have a higher

CURRENT THERAPY

- IV access and administer crystalloid as indicated.
- Obtain CBC, PT, PTT, platelet count q6–12h for 1 d, then daily if abnormal.
- Estimate severity of envenomation.
  - Species of snake
  - Age and health status of victim
  - Rate of progression of signs/symptoms
- Administer CroFab as per Table 2.
- Determine tetanus vaccination status.
- Seek consultation from experts or a Poison Control Center, especially if one is treating envenomation for the first few times.

Abbreviations: CBC = complete blood count; IV = intravenous; PT = prothrombin time; PTT = partial thromboplastin time.

degree of toxicity and indeed account for most of the fatalities in the United States.

The coral snake (*Micrurus fulvius*) accounts for only 1% to 2% of all snakebite cases in North America but has a higher than expected mortality based on its characteristic and severe neurotoxicity. Treatment of coral snake envenomation is not discussed further here. Suffice it to say that the neurotoxicity is the cause of morbidity and mortality from envenomation by the coral snake, usually through aspiration pneumonia and cessation of breathing. Accordingly, these severe manifestations can be attended by respiratory support and the natural history (i.e., without antivenin therapy), which usually is approximately a week before it reverses. Also important regarding coral snake envenomation is the absence of any signs of local pain, swelling, or discoloration, which are characteristic of pit viper envenomation. Patients cannot be assumed to have eluded envenomation by a coral snake because they lack these symptoms. That symptoms are often delayed for 8 to 24 hours must be anticipated, so 1 or 2 days of hospitalization for observation is frequently suggested.

The vast majority (approximately 80%) of envenomations by pit vipers are nonaccidental; that is, they are the result of poor judgment or senseless behavior, often in combination with intoxication with any of various substances. Most snakebite victims not only see and correctly identify the snake as poisonous but feel compelled to play with, taunt, or capture the animal and in the process may well be bitten. Fewer than 20% of snakebites are actually what most persons would call accidental.

Pit vipers are easily recognized by the so-called pit (an infrared heat-detection organ) approximately midway between the nostril and the eye. All North American pit vipers have pupils shaped like those of a cat, as opposed to round pupils characteristic of nonpoisonous snakes (with the exception of the coral snake). Pit vipers have large fangs through which a considerable volume of venom is injected, often deeply, into the victim. Because fangs are continually replaced, there may be one, two, three, or even four fangs at one time that may leave a similar number of puncture wounds.

Pit viper venom is extremely complex, containing a broad range of proteolytic enzymes designed to digest protein, fat, connective tissue, nucleic acids, and other biologic material. It also contains numerous small peptides, which probably accounts for autonomic symptoms such as tachycardia, diaphoresis, diarrhea, and vomiting. There is a great variability in this complex poison with variability not only between species but also within species, and even within a single specimen if it is observed over years. Variability of the venom most likely accounts for the variability of the signs, symptoms, and prognosis in envenomation syndromes because of various species of pit vipers.

For instance, the hematologic abnormalities seen in North American pit viper envenomation occur through certain principles in pit viper venom. The Eastern diamondback rattlesnake contains a thrombin-like enzyme that partially cleaves fibrinogen, clearing it from the circulation, with the concomitant production of huge amounts of fibrin degradation products with only modest thrombocytopenia. The venom of the Western diamondback rattlesnake contains a principle that directly activates plasminogen to plasmin with resulting hyperfibrinolysis. Although through differing mechanisms, bites of each of these rattlesnakes may result in dramatic alterations of the prothrombin time (PT) and partial thromboplastin time (PTT) but little bleeding. Whereas envenomation by the Eastern or Western diamondback rattlesnake produces a minimal elevation of serum creatinine kinase (CK), myonecrosis with marked CK elevations are the hallmark of the canebrake rattlesnake (*C. horridus atricaudatus*) to include a brisk elevation of the CK-MB band yet with negative assays for either troponin I or T consistent with the lack of cardiac muscle myonecrosis. The bite of the Mojave rattlesnake produces myonecrosis similar to that of the canebrake rattlesnake as well as neurologic symptoms but minimal coagulation abnormalities. Severe thrombocytopenia usually refractory to platelet transfusion is seen in envenomation by the timber rattlesnake (*C. horridus horridus*). Thus, one can see that many envenomations have a signature, so to speak, that is slowly being unraveled (Table 1).

Approximately 20% of persons bitten by a positively identified pit viper are fortunate enough not to be envenomated by the snake and are considered to have a "dry bite." For these fortunate victims, the administration of antivenin obviously is not indicated. Dry bites are often

CURRENT THERAPY

- Confirm patient was bitten by a venomous snake.
- Determine snake species if possible.
- Evaluate for local signs of envenomation:
    - Pain
    - Swelling
    - Discoloration
- Evaluate for systemic signs of envenomation:
    - Alterations in vital signs
    - Nausea, vomiting, diarrhea, and diaphoresis
    - Fasciculations
    - Coagulation abnormalities
    - Altered mental status

deduced by the normality of the patient with the near complete absence of any pain, swelling, or discoloration within 1 to 2 hours of the bite.

Treatment

It is most important to distinguish the severity of the bite to determine the need for and extent of antivenin therapy. Good supportive therapy should be instituted with the establishment of at least one large intravenous (IV) line and the infusion of saline or similar crystalloid for volume and blood pressure indications.

It is difficult to overestimate the importance of sensing the *rate of change of signs and symptoms* in determining the severity of bites. It is of more clinical significance that a patient bitten 20 minutes ago has a rapidly swelling arm than a patient bitten 3 hours ago has an even larger yet not still enlarging arm. Such a philosophy is also important in judging the efficacy of any administration of antivenin because one cannot expect prior damage to include swelling and discoloration to subside promptly, but rather one determines whether such symptoms cease to progress or progress at such a slow rate that continued therapy may not be indicated. It is clear that the efficacy

TABLE 1 Distinguishing Clinical Characteristics of Envenomation by Selected *Crotalus* Species

Common Name	Scientific Name	Distribution	Neurologic Symptoms	Coagulopathic Findings	Rhabdomyolysis
Eastern diamondback	*Crotalus adamanteus*	Southeastern United States	+	Prolonged PT/PTT	+
Canebrake	*C. horridus atricaudatus*	Eastern United States	—	—	++++
Mojave	*C. scutulatus*	Desert Southwest United States	+++	—	++++
Timber	*C. horridus horridus*	Eastern United States	—	Prolonged PT/PTT; moderate to severe thrombocytopenia	—

Abbreviations: PT = prothrombin time; PTT = partial thromboplastin time.
— = nil; + = mild; ++ = moderate; +++ = pronounced; ++++ = severe.

of the antivenin is a function of the time lapsed since the bite. It is ideal to treat bites that should be treated as soon as possible, and I prefer to initiate administration of antivenin prior to 6 or 12 hours after a bite, and essentially I never initiate treatment after 24 hours because what damage is going to be done is done and cannot be reversed.

Dry bites comprise approximately 20% of snakebites, and there is no evidence of any envenomation either locally or by laboratory evolutions. No treatment is indicated (Table 2).

Minimal envenomations are characterized by pain, swelling, and discoloration that are caused by the dissolution of underlying tissue. In general, there are no systemic signs, symptoms, or laboratory abnormalities, although anxiety is almost universal and, in the case of envenomation for rattlesnakes, notorious for their hematologic manifestations. Laboratory alterations of the coagulation system may be present, but in and of themselves they are not indications, in our experience, for the administration of antivenin.

The primary differentiation between minimal envenomations and *moderate envenomations* is not only the extent but particularly the rate of development and progression of pain, swelling, and discoloration because one may see a doubling of these symptoms within the initial hour of evaluation and care administered to the patient. Such patients should be administered antivenin to halt or lessen such progression. In general, these patients do not have severe alterations of vital signs or laboratory findings, although coagulation abnormalities may be quite dramatic with unclottable PTs and PTTs and modest thrombocytopenia on the order of 30,000 to 100,000/mm^3. Most of these patients are treated with antivenin, especially if they are children, elderly, or have significant co-morbidity.

Essentially all patients with *severe envenomation* are treated with antivenin. These are patients with severe alterations of vital signs, including hypotension, a peculiar unpleasant taste in the mouth, marked diaphoresis, universal diarrhea and vomiting, and frequently a stupor or inattention revealing alterations in mental status. Often the bite is in a highly vascular muscle (thenar, hypothenar, calf, or arm muscle) rather than the comparatively less vascular hand or foot. The coagulation abnormalities

may again be quite remarkable. In our experience, most severe envenomations are obviously severe soon after the bite (10 to 30 minutes) with only a very small minority progressing from lesser degrees to severe.

Clinically relevant bleeding is rarely seen despite the marked alterations in coagulation tests. The explanation for this is that with North American pit viper envenomations, thrombin generation is intact so what little fibrinogen and platelets are available are used to maintain effective hemostasis. In other words, this is not disseminated intravascular coagulation (DIC) but chiefly a syndrome whose laboratory values mimic DIC. Exotic snakes may directly activate prothrombin (*Echis* species and *Bothrops* species) and/or factor X (*Vipera* species and *Dispholidus* species) leading to a true DIC with marked organ dysfunction related to thrombosis of organs with subsequent death.

Bleb formation at the site of a bite is not an important sign in and of itself, although it generates much attention.

Compartment syndromes are seen quite rarely, with surgical intervention indicated in only 1% to 5% of envenomated patients. Of interest, marked swelling itself is not often a sign of a compartment syndrome because in a true compartment syndrome, swelling is limited owing to the anatomic restriction by fibrous tissue, such as seen in the lateral anterior compartment of the lower leg or in the palm of the hand. The chief sign for a true compartment syndrome is the intense hardness of these areas and dysfunction of muscles within the compartment.

The administration of fresh-frozen plasma (FFP), platelet concentrates, or other blood products is rarely necessary in North American pit viper envenomation. We advocate a permissive posture with regard to the prolongation of the PT and PTT as long as there is no clinical bleeding. Should bleeding be present, the lack of fibrinogen is best treated with infusions of 8 to 10 bags of cryoprecipitate and monitored by serial determination of the fibrinogen level. This maneuver typically corrects the PT and PTT. Severe thrombocytopenia, implying platelet counts of less than 10,000/mm^3, may well be an indication for platelet transfusion, particularly if an invasive or surgical procedure is planned. It has not been our experience that patients have significant hemorrhage. Leakage of blood into swollen tissues, dilution from crystalloid administration,

TABLE 2 Grades of Severity of Envenomation by Pit Vipers

Grade	Frequency (%)	Initial Findings	CroFab Vials in First 24 H
No envenomation	0–15	No local, systemic, or laboratory abnormalities 2 h after bite	0
Minimal envenomation	20–40	Local and slowly progressive swelling without systemic or severe laboratory abnormalities	0–6
Moderate envenomation	20–40	Rapidly progressive local swelling; systemic symptoms of nausea, vomiting, diarrhea, diaphoresis, fasciculations, moderate hypotension, and moderate hemostatic abnormalities but without bleeding	6–12
Severe envenomation	5–10	Severe systemic symptoms as above plus severe hypotension and lethargy; severe hemostatic abnormalities and possible bleeding	12—24 or more

and hemolysis of red blood cells from hemolysins in the venom account for most decreases in hematocrit values.

Emergency management in the field consists primarily of getting the patient to a medical facility. It is there that directed therapy should start. The use of tourniquets, cut-and-suck methodology, electric shock therapy, and the application of ice or administration of alcohol do not work and only serve to delay adequate evaluation and treatment. The victim should be kept calm and at rest during transport to the hospital. It is advised that should ice or tourniquets be in place on arrival at the hospital, it be documented in the report and removed.

The mainstay of treatment for North American pit viper envenomation is Crotalidae polyvalent immune Fab (ovine) antivenin (CroFab), which is an ovine-based preparation of immunoglobulins that is chemically treated so that only the Fab portion of the immunoglobulins is infused because the Fc fragment has been cleaved. Because the Fc fragment accounts for the majority of immunologic reactions, the Fab product appears to be much less allergenic than the prior equine-based product of intact immunoglobulins. Pretreatment skin or conjunctival testing is not required prior to administration of CroFab. Additionally, the smaller Fab molecule appears to give the advantage of facilitated penetration deep into affected tissues, but conversely, it has a rather short half-life of only several hours as opposed to several days with the previously available equine antivenin. This may be problematic in that an envenomation syndrome may appear by all accord to have been controlled with the cessation of the progression of swelling, normalization of vital signs, and the beginning of normalization of laboratory studies, only to have a relapse of these findings a few hours or days after antivenin administration. Readministration (as opposed to the initiation of antivenin administration) may very well be indicated. Because we hold that the defibrination syndrome is so benign in the first place, we do not regard the common reappearance of defibrination and secondary prolongation of the PT and PTT without evidence of clinical bleeding as an independent freestanding reason for antivenin readministration.

CroFab is administered as an IV solution starting slowly to alert for any possible adverse reaction. If such is not encountered, six vials are typically infused over 1 hour. If local and systemic findings cease or slow, the syndrome is deemed to be controlled. If not, two more vials, each over 6 hours, are suggested for a total of 12 vials in the first 24 hours. The rare severe and/or relapsing case may require up to 24 or more vials over several days.

Antibiotics are generally not employed but are indicated in wounds that were manipulated in the field, such as with a knife. Determination of which antibiotic to administer should include anaerobic bacterial coverage. Tetanus vaccination status should be determined and acted on appropriately. The extremities should be cleansed. Many find outlining the edges of the enlarging wound with a pen helpful in following the rate of change of progression of the swelling. We do not advocate determination of intercompartmental pressures routinely. The extremities should be slightly elevated above the level of the heart. The wound should not be covered or bound; it should be easily observable.

In-hospital therapy is usually given in closely monitored areas beginning with the emergency department and progressing to the intensive care unit (ICU), although ICU therapy is not necessarily a standard of care. Patients should be observed closely; particularly victims of coral snake bites or those who are deemed most likely to have dry bites. If signs, symptoms, or other evidence for envenomation do not occur within 24 to 36 hours, the patient can be discharged. We do not hold that all patients need admission to the hospital if it is very clear, within several hours, that envenomation did not occur, or if it did, it was minimal, such as with a pygmy rattlesnake bite. Because our patients typically are intoxicated, that in itself is more often than not a possible reason to keep the patient in the hospital for a day or so.

Nearly all swelling and tissue destruction is transient with North American pit viper envenomation. Edema that results from the dissolution of capillaries and particularly lymphatics may take as long as 1 to 2 months to resolve but may even be permanent in older or debilitated patients. In general, there is a total return of function to the bitten extremity, although a weakness or stiffness may be experienced by some patients for up to a year. A loss of tissue, to include fingers or limbs, is exceptionally rare and usually is accompanied by prehospital use of tourniquets and/or ice, extremely delayed therapy, overaggressive surgical procedures, or neural damage in rare cases where a fasciotomy may have been indicated. Unfortunately, patients who are bitten by snakes tend to retain those habits that led to this envenomation and therefore may be seen again.

REFERENCES

Bond RG, Burkhart KK: Thrombocytopenia following timber rattlesnake envenomation. Ann Emerg Med 1998;31:139-141.

Boyer LV, Seifert SA, Cain JS: Recurrence phenomena after immunoglobulin therapy for snake envenomations: Part 2. Guidelines for clinical management with Crotaline Fab antivenom. Ann Emerg Med 2001;37:196-201.

Carroll RR, Hall EL, Kitchens CS: Canebrake rattlesnake envenomation. Ann Emerg Med 1997;20:45-48.

Dart RC, Hurlbut KM, Garcia R, et al: Validation of a severity score for the assessment of crotalid snakebite in the United States. Ann Emerg Med 1996;27:321-326.

Farstad D, Thomas T, Chow T, et al: Mojave rattlesnake envenomation in southern California: A review of suspected cases. Wilderness Environ Med 1997;8:89-93.

Kitchens CS: Hemostatic aspects of envenomation by North American snakes. Hematol/Oncol Clin North Am 1992;6:1189-1195.

Kitchens CS: From ETOH to FAB: The medicalization of therapy for pit viper envenomation. Trans Am Clin Climatol Assn 2001;112:117-135.

Kitchens CS, van Mierop LHS: Mechanisms of defibrination in humans after envenomation by the eastern diamondback rattlesnake. Am J Hematol 1983;14:345-353.

Kitchens CS, van Mierop LHS: Envenomation by the Eastern coral snake (*Micrurus fulvius fulvius*). A study of 39 victims. JAMA 1987;258:1615-1618.

Marine Trauma, Envenomations, and Intoxications

Method of
John E. Gough, MD, FACEP

More than 70% of the Earth's surface is covered by water, and within these waters reside greater than 80% of the planet's living organisms. Many of these marine creatures have developed various systems for both attack and defense that can cause morbidity and mortality to humans. Although injuries and illnesses caused by marine creatures have been described since ancient times, many factors continue to contribute to frequent encounters. Some factors are the increased utilization of marine environments for both recreational and economic purposes, the popularity of seafood consumption, the growing interest in exotic animals in private and public aquariums, and the ability of air travel to make the movement of people and seafood to and from such environments more accessible.

Although there may be some overlap, for the purposes of this discussion, encounters with marine organisms are divided into the following general headings:

1. Nonvenomous trauma
2. Envenomations
3. Toxic ingestions

Nonvenomous trauma is mainly composed of bites. Treatment consists of the ABCs (airway, breathing, and circulation) of resuscitation, wound care, and prevention and treatment of infection. Envenomations may present with minor skin irritations or with life-threatening cardiovascular and respiratory compromise. Treatment is directed at resuscitation, supportive care, pain management, and administration of antidotes if available. Toxic ingestions often involve self-limited gastrointestinal conditions but, as with envenomations, may present with life-threatening symptoms. Treatment is mainly supportive.

Nonvenomous Trauma

SHARK ATTACKS

Sharks have existed for more than 400 million years, predating dinosaurs by more than 200 million years. Attacks on humans have been well documented in fiction and folklore. Although these attacks are often reported widely in the media, it is estimated that approximately 50 to 100 attacks occur annually worldwide. In the United States, fewer than 100 proven attacks have occurred over the past 8 years, with a dozen fatalities. The sharks most often implicated in human attacks are the great white, mako, bull, gray reef, and bull. Sharks have powerful crescent-shaped jaws with multiple (usually five or six) rows of sharp, triangular teeth that can cause significant soft tissue and bony injuries. Deaths from attacks are usually the result of exsanguinations and drowning.

Prevention of shark attacks involves avoiding shark-infested waters, not swimming at dusk or at night, and avoiding turbid waters, especially around waste outlets. Bright-colored bathing suits are believed to be attractants. Swimming with open wounds is not recommended. Although the majority of attacks occur in shallow waters, the most dangerous appear to occur in deeper waters.

The management of shark attacks is predicated on the ABCs of trauma care. Aggressive airway management, control of hemorrhage, and volume replacement are standards. Opiate medications may be necessary for pain control. Tetanus immunization including tetanus immunoglobulin (BayTet 250–500 U) as well as tetanus toxoid (Td; 0.5 cc IM) should be administered. Wound irrigation, débridement, and exploration for foreign bodies should be undertaken. Wounds are often packed and delayed primary closures performed. Organisms such as *Aeromonas, Vibrio,* and *Clostridia* are often encountered; therefore, antibiotics with activity against both aerobic and anaerobic organisms are often administered. Suitable choices of antibiotic agents are trimethoprim-sulfamethoxazole (Septra, Bactrim) 1 double-strength PO/400 mg IV; ciprofloxacin (Cipro) 500 to 750 mg PO/400 mg IV; imipenem-cilastatin (Primaxin) 500 to 750 mg IM; ceftriaxone (Rocephin) 1 to 2 g IV; and ceftazidime (Fortaz) 1 g IV or IM.

BARRACUDA

Barracuda may reach sizes of 2.5 m in length and 50 kg in weight; however, most are less than 1.5 m long. The great barracuda *(Sphyraena barracuda)* is the only one of the 22 species of barracuda implicated in attacks against humans. Attacks occur in tropical waters in the Atlantic from Brazil to Florida and in the Indo-Pacific from the Red Sea to Hawaii. Although barracuda attacks usually are from solitary fish, attacks from schools have been reported. Attacks are very quick and may be fierce. The barracuda possesses knifelike sharp teeth resulting in V-shaped injuries that are similar to shark bites but not as severe. Treatment priorities are the same as for shark bites.

MORAY EEL

Moray eels are bottom dwellers that typically reside in holes and crevices in rocks and corals. They inhabit tropical and temperate waters. Eels usually attack humans when they feel they are cornered or threatened. Attacks frequently occur when divers places their hand in one of the crevices and surprise the eel. Injuries have also been known to occur when the eel is accidentally entangled in fishing nets or when they are handled in an aquarium. The eel has powerful viselike jaws and sharp fangs that can cause significant soft tissue damage. The eel hangs on tenaciously, and further injury often occurs while the patient is struggling to remove the eel. Removal in some cases has required decapitation and breaking of the eel's jaws. Treatment strategies are similar to those for shark and barracuda bites.

Envenomations

INVERTEBRATES

Phylum Cnidaria (Coelenterates)

The phylum coelenterates consists of approximately 10,000 species of invertebrates, of which approximately

100 are dangerous to humans. Included in this phylum are organisms that may account for some of the most dangerous envenomations known. This phylum is typically divided into three classes: (1) Hydrozoa (fire corals, hydroids, Portuguese man-of-war), (2) Scyphozoa (jellyfish), and (3) Anthozoa (sea anemones)

Members of the coelenterates envenomate through the use of nematocysts. Nematocysts are venom-filled organelles located in specialized endothelial cells known as crinocytes. The nematocysts reside in these crindocytes and are located either in tentacles or around the mouth of the organism. Inside the nematocyst are crindoblasts, which contain venom and an eversible tube. The nematocyst responds to both physical and chemical triggers, which can cause ejection of the tube into the prey, with injection of the toxin. The toxin of the coelenterates varies among the species but is usually heat labile, with direct and indirect effects on the autonomic nervous system. The venom has been shown to destabilize cell membranes through interference with the sodium–potassium pump. Other effects of the venom may include hemolysis, cardiac toxicity, muscle paralysis, and dermatonecrosis. The venom can often be degraded by proteolytic substances.

Hydrozoa

The hydroids and stinging corals generally cause varying degrees of dermatitis and usually only require symptomatic local treatment. The most dangerous of the Hydrozoa is the Portuguese man-of-war *(Physalia physalis)* found in the Atlantic Ocean and the Gulf of Mexico. One species of Portuguese man-of-war is found in the Pacific Ocean *(Physalia utriculus)*. The Pacific variety is smaller and contains only one tentacle (approximately 15 m in length). Envenomations with the Pacific variety are not as severe as with the Atlantic varieties. Envenomations typically occur during the summer months.

The pneumatophore or float is the portion of the Portuguese man-of-war that is visible above the water. The pneumatophore acts like a sail that propels the animal through the water. Dangling from the pneumatophore are the tentacles that contain the nematocysts. The tentacles are numerous and may reach up to 30 m in length. The tentacles in a single animal may contain literally thousands of nematocysts. Envenomations often occur as a swimmer or diver becomes entangled in the tentacles; however, they can also occur from contact with a dead Portuguese man-of-war that is washed ashore.

The nematocysts respond to physical and chemical stimuli. Injection of the venom causes immediate stinging pain. Struggling to escape the tentacles frequently leads to entanglement and further envenomation. The pain is followed by the development of a local rash with papules in a linear pattern often described as "beaded." Over the next 2 hours and lasting for approximately 24 hours, the rash may then progress to erythematous welts. Systemic symptoms are nonspecific and include nausea, vomiting, myalgias, headache, respiratory distress, acute renal failure, anaphylaxis, cardiovascular collapse, and death.

Treatment is supportive. In addition to basic first aid measures, one of the initial goals is to prevent further envenomation. Undischarged nematocysts should be removed. Care should be taken while removing nematocysts to prevent accidental envenomation to the patient

or rescuer. Ideally the area should be washed with heated sea water, as fresh water may stimulate nematocysts to inject further venom. Heated water is preferable to help degrade the heat-labile toxin. Commercial preparations designed for salt water aquariums can be used. Acetic acid (vinegar) is also recommended to inactivate the venom. Alternatives that have been used include aluminum sulfate 20%/surfactant (Stingose), isopropyl alcohol, Adolph's Meat Tenderizer (papain), and even Pepsi-Cola. The nematocysts can be removed by using shaving cream or a paste made of baking soda and scraping the nematocysts off with a razor. Any object with a sharp edge can be used, including credit cards and cardboard. Once the nematocysts are removed, local anesthetics may be soothing. Application of a pressure immobilization dressing can also be used. The patient's tetanus status should be ascertained and updated as needed. Pain medications and antihistamines should be administered if necessary. Prophylactic antibiotics are not recommended.

Scyphozoa (Jellyfish)

Scyphozoa include many species of jellyfish, some of which are very dangerous to man. Jellyfish can vary in size from a few millimeters to 2 m across the main portion of the body, known as the bell. Some species have tentacles up to 40 m in length. They range from transparent to multicolored. As with the Portuguese man-of-war, the jellyfish are free-floating creatures that depend on the wind and tides for movement. Also as with the Portuguese man-of-war, envenomations can occur from both live and dead jellyfish. Scyphozoans are widely distributed through the Atlantic, Pacific, Caribbean, Indian, and even the Arctic oceans. Envenomations may be mild, limited to minimal skin irritation; moderate, which includes stinging, pruritus, and skin eruptions; and severe, which may manifest with varying degrees of systemic symptoms involving neurologic, gastrointestinal, ocular, and cardiovascular reactions. Chronic sequelae, such as keloids, hyperpigmentation, muscle spasms, contractures, and gangrene, have been reported.

The most dangerous of the jellyfish is the box jellyfish (*Chironex fleckeri*), which inhabits the South Pacific waters mainly off Australia. It is considered the most venomous of sea creatures. A much less lethal variety of the box jellyfish is found in the Chesapeake Bay off the U.S. Mid-Atlantic states. Envenomations by *Chironex fleckeri* can be fatal in as little as seconds to minutes. An adult box jellyfish contains enough venom (approximately 10 cc) to kill three adult humans. The box jellyfish is a large transparent jellyfish weighing approximately 6 kg and measuring up to 30 cm across its bell. The *Chironex* may possess as many as 60 tentacles, which can be up to 3 m in length and contain millions of nematocysts. Stings can occur at any time but most commonly in the summer months (September through May). Attacks usually occur in shallow water and often involve children.

Stings can be minor, but massive envenomations can be fatal. The venom is neurotoxic, and the action is not completely understood. Death can occur from respiratory failure, cardiotoxicity, or paralysis of the cardiac muscle. Often the victim becomes unconscious before he or she can leave the water. The venom also has dermatonecrotic actions that lead to patches of full-thickness skin necrosis and permanent scarring.

Symptoms include severe localized pain that may continue to increase even with the removal of the tentacles. Large erythematous areas occur where the skin has come in contact with the tentacles, and the size of the areas may give an indication as to the amount of envenomation. Systemic symptoms include difficulty breathing, swallowing, and speaking. In severe cases, the patient may become hypotensive, lose consciousness, and exhibit cardiac dysrhythmias or even cardiac arrest. First aid measures include removing the patient from the water, supporting the ABCs (including cardiopulmonary resuscitation if necessary), soaking the tentacles in vinegar for at least 30 seconds before removing them (in an attempt to inactivate the venom), applying a pressure immobilization dressing, administering analgesia (narcotics and muscle relaxers are recommended), and providing rapid transport. An antivenom from sheep immunoglobulin (box jellyfish antivenin) is available, and 20,000 U (one vial) should be administered as soon as possible for treatment of severe envenomations. Intravenous administration is the preferred route, but if intravenous access is not immediately available, the intramuscular route is acceptable so as not to delay administration. Indications for antivenom administration include cardiac dysrhythmias, cardiac arrest, difficulty with breathing or speaking, and severe pain. Even with apparent mild envenomations, the patient should be observed for at least 6 to 8 hours to ensure no progression of symptoms.

It is thought that many types of jellyfish may cause the Irukandji syndrome (rapid-onset pulmonary edema and respiratory failure); however, the one species known to cause this syndrome is *Carukia barnesi*. *Carukia barnesi* is a small (<2 cm in diameter across the bell) jellyfish found off North Queensland, Australia. Other similar species have been seen elsewhere in the Pacific and even

off the Florida coast. Symptoms of Irukandji syndrome include muscular chest and neck pain, sweating, anxiety, nausea, vomiting, headaches, tachycardia, hypotension, pulmonary edema, and cardiopulmonary collapse. Symptoms may persist for hours to days and are similar to those resulting from massive catecholamine release. Treatment is mainly supportive. Vinegar should be used acutely to aid in removal of tentacles and to prevent further envenomation. Analgesia should be given as needed. Box jellyfish antivenom does not appear to be effective.

Anthozoa

Sea anemones are flower-like, sessile creatures found in shallow waters and tidal pools. They range in size from a few millimeters to 0.5 m in diameter. Their multicolored appearance can attract unwary swimmers to handle them. They possess tentacles and have nematocysts similar to the Portuguese man-of-war. Envenomations are similar to the Portuguese man-of-war but generally not as severe. The "hell's fire anemone" (*Actinodendron plumosum*) produces significant local effects that have earned the animal its colorful name. Treatment is similar to that for the Portuguese man-of-war.

Echinodermata

Fire corals (*Millepora* species) are not true coral. They are found living on rocks and other corals. Fire corals are brushlike creatures that generally range from 5 to 10 cm in length but can reach up to 2 m. Syndromes after contact include pruritus, urticaria, and severe burning pain. The pain is usually short lived (1–2 hours); however, the urticarial wheals may become hyperpigmented and persist for several months. Treatment is similar to that of jellyfish stings. Long-term steroids can be used to treat the skin hyperpigmentation.

Sea urchins are free-living, hard-shelled creatures of the class *Echinoida*. They possess multiple, irregular, brittle spines that may or may not contain venom. Envenomation frequently occurs when the creature is handled by swimmers, fishermen, and divers. Sea urchins whose spines do not contain venom have jawed pedicellaria that may latch on so that venom can be injected. The venom causes an immediate local reaction that is marked by severe pain. The spines also contain a blue–black dye that may stain the skin but is of no medical significance. The brittle spines break off easily and contaminate the wound. Treatment consists of immersion in hot water to inactivate the venom and local débridement to clean the wound. Radiographs may be useful in detecting occult presence of spines. Care must be taken to remove the spines, which are brittle and crumble in the wound. Portions of spines remaining in the wound may lead to long-term dermatologic sequelae such as granulomas. Antibiotics and corticosteroids can be used for treatment of wounds.

STINGING VERTEBRATES

Stingrays

The stings and envenomations of stingrays have been recognized and recorded since ancient times. Aristotle referred

---

to them as "devilfish." It is reported that the spear Theolonius used to kill Odysseus had the barb of a stingray on its head. Stingrays, like sharks, are cartilaginous fish and usually range from a few millimeters to 1 to 2 m in length. Some species have attained lengths of 5 to 6 m. Although stingrays are one of the fishes most implicated in envenomations to humans (approximately 2000 stings annually worldwide), they are actually docile and only attack when startled or provoked. The most common mechanism of injury is a swimmer or fisherman accidentally stepping on the stingray while it is partially covered in sand at the bottom of shallow waters. The stingray reflexively whips its tail around and strikes the unsuspecting victim, usually in the lower leg but possibly also involving the upper extremities and torso. The venom-coated barb, which is located on the tail, is serrated and can cause significant lacerations. The venom is heat labile and composed of several compounds, including serotonin, phosphodiesterases, and 5'-nucleosidase. Symptoms include immediate intense stinging pain that is out of proportion to the apparent wound. The pain usually reaches maximal intensity in about 90 minutes. Systemic symptoms are not diagnostic and may include muscle weakness, cramping, nausea, vomiting, peripheral vasoconstriction, cardiac dysrhythmias, seizures, respiratory distress, coma, and even death.

Treatment of envenomations is focused on rapid stabilization, pain control, venom neutralization, and wound care. Initially the wound should be copiously irrigated with cool normal saline. Cool temperatures are thought to cause some vasoconstriction and to delay or decrease uptake of more venom. Local anesthesia applied to the wound site and potent narcotics are recommended for patient comfort. Once the initial irrigation has been completed, the wound should be immersed in hot water (113°F [45°C]) for 30 to 90 minutes to help destabilize the heat-labile venom. Care should be taken when attempting to débride and remove all pieces of the barb from the wound. The wound should not be closed primarily. Tetanus immunization should be administered if indicated. Prophylactic antibiotics are recommended.

Catfish

There are more than 1000 specifies of fresh and salt water catfish, many of which can envenomate humans. Catfish can introduce venom through glands on their dorsal and pectoral fins. In some cases, envenomations occur through crinotoxins present on the fish, with venom entering victims through abraded skin or puncture wounds inflicted by the catfish spines. The proteinaceous venom possesses dermonecrotic and vasoconstrictive factors. Symptoms of envenomation include pain and paresthesias that may last from minutes to several days. Erythema, edema, cyanosis, and hemorrhage are also seen. Rare systemic effects include weakness, fever, hypotension, syncope, and respiratory distress. Death from envenomations has been recorded but is rare.

Treatment includes pain control and wound management. The area should be immersed in hot water (110°F [43°C]) to inactivate the venom and reverse vasospasm and muscle cramping. Pain management can be accomplished with local anesthetics and possibly analgesia. Wounds should

be copiously irrigated. Radiographs should be obtained to rule out foreign bodies. Tetanus immunization should be administered as necessary. Antibiotics should be considered, especially for deep puncture wounds.

Scorpion Fish

Scorpion fish are divided into three groups based on their venom apparatus: (1) *Pterois* (zebrafish, lionfish*)*, (2) *Scorpaena* ("true" scorpion fish), and (3) *Synanceja* (stonefish). All have hard armor plating and are found in the shallow reef waters of the Florida Keys, Gulf of Mexico, southern California, and Hawaii. Envenomations have occurred when unsuspecting victims step on the scorpion fish. The venom glands are located on the dorsal, pectoral, and anal spines. Because of their beautiful colors, scorpion fish are now sought by many private aquariums, thus increasing the potential for envenomations. The venom has pronounced neurotoxic effects and has been likened to that of cobra venom.

Symptoms depend on the species, amount of venom injected, and underlying health of the victim. The most common initial symptom is intense pain that peaks at 90 minutes and persists for up to 12 hours. Other local symptoms include erythema, edema, and swollen lymph nodes. Paresthesias may occur and persist for weeks. Severe envenomations, particularly those seen with stonefish, may present with hypotension, cardiovascular collapse, and even death within hours. Treatment consists of immersion in hot water for 30 to 90 minutes, pain control, wound irrigation, and débridement. Tetanus immunizations should be administered when indicated. Prophylactic antibiotic use is recommended. An antivenin to stonefish venom is manufactured in Australia and is available from several sites in the United States.

Sea Snakes

There are at least 52 species of sea snakes (*Hydrophiidae*), with at least 11 implicated in human fatalities. Most are located in the Indo-Pacific waters off Australia, but an Atlantic species (*Pelamis platurus*) inhabits the coastal waters of South America. Sea snakes have two to four fangs associated with paired venom glands. The fangs are short and easily broken. Many bites do not result in envenomations. This is fortunate because the venom of sea snakes is considered to be more potent than that of most terrestrial snakes, including the cobra and krait.

Bites are not particularly painful, and onset of symptoms may be immediate or, more commonly, delayed by minutes to hours. Often multiple (up to 20) puncture wounds from fangs are seen. Initial symptoms may include muscle cramping, muscle spasms, myosis, papillary dilation, weakness of extraocular movements, slurred speech, and paralysis. Hemoglobinuria and myoglobinuria may occur and lead to acute renal failure. Death may result from respiratory failure. Treatment is similar to that of terrestrial snakebites, and the Australian pressure immobilization technique is recommended as with terrestrial elapids. A polyvalent antivenin (Sea Snake Antivenom) is produced in Australia. Antivenin administration as soon as possible is recommended, but delays at long as 36 hours have been reported but still associated with positive outcomes. If specific sea snake antivenin is not available, tiger snake antivenin can be used.

Blue-Ringed Octopus

The blue-ringed octopus (*Hapalochlaena* species) is found mainly off the waters of Australia. Its color is usually yellow-brown, with the striking blue rings appearing when the animal is disturbed. These animals are found in shallow tidal pools, and envenomations occur when the octopus is handled or stepped on. The venom contains tetrodotoxin and affects the neuronal sodium channels. Symptoms include weakness, paresthesias, respiratory distress, and possibly respiratory failure.

There is no specific treatment, although the pressure immobilization technique is recommended. No antivenin is available. The mainstay of treatment is supportive care. Endotracheal intubation may be necessary.

Toxic Ingestions

CIGUATERA

Ciguatera is the most common nonbacterial form of food poisoning. Furthermore, it is the most common poisoning associated with fish ingestion. Ciguatera has been associated with more than 500 different species of fish, many of which serve as food sources for man. Some of the more commonly implicated species are sea bass, grouper, barracuda, snapper, jack, parrot fish, and surgeon fish. The ciguatoxin is found in dinoflagellates, protozoa, and blue–green algae. This toxin is eaten by smaller fish, which in turn are eaten by larger fish, depositing the toxin in the flesh. The concentration of ciguatoxin increases as the fish moves up the food chain. The toxin does not appear to be harmful to the fish. The toxin is heat stable, is tasteless, and does not appear to be affected by refrigeration or cooking. The toxin has cholinergic and acetylcholinesterase properties. However, its main effect appears to be on calcium regulation through the sodium channels on the cell membranes.

Symptoms generally occur within 6 to 12 hours but may be delayed for more than 24 hours. Gastrointestinal symptoms are common and include nausea, vomiting, diarrhea, and abdominal cramping. The gastrointestinal symptoms tend to resolve more quickly than the neurologic complaints. Neurologic manifestations include pain, weakness, paresthesias, headaches, ataxia, and peripheral and central nerve palsies. An unusual complaint that these patients may volunteer is reversal of hot and cold sensations. These symptoms are generally self-limited, and there is no specific treatment other that symptomatic and supportive care.

SCOMBROID

Scombroid is the second most common poisoning associated with the ingestion of fish. Scombroid is most often seen with dark-meat fish, such as tuna, bluefish, mackerel, skipjack, and bonito. Unlike ciguatera, scombroid is related to improper refrigeration of the fish prior to eating.

Organisms on the surface of the fish, particularly *Klebsiella* species, *Aerobacter aerogenes*, *Escherichia coli*, and *Proteus morganii*, may elaborate histidine decarboxylase, which converts histidine to histamine. The presence of scombroid does not appear to affect the smell or taste of the fish, although a peppery taste has been described.

Symptoms usually occur within a few minutes to several hours. Because the symptoms are histamine regulated, they are often confused as allergic in origin. Nausea, vomiting, diarrhea, abdominal cramping, erythema, pruritus, and bronchospasm may occur. Treatment includes gastrointestinal decontamination, IV hydration, antihistamines, steroids, and epinephrine, and all may be used when appropriate. These symptoms are generally self-limiting; however, the severity may be affected by the underlying health of the patient.

TOXIC SHELLFISH

Humans who consume shellfish (mussels, oysters, clams, crabs) that have ingested dinoflagellates may contract toxic shellfish poisoning. The toxins do not appear to injure the shellfish, but ingestion by humans of as few as one to three of these infected animals may cause death. Symptoms may appear to be allergic, such as pruritus and respiratory distress. Gastrointestinal manifestations may include nausea, vomiting, diarrhea, and abdominal discomfort. Furthermore, saxitoxin, a potent neurotoxin, may be present and lead to respiratory failure. No specific antidote is available, and treatment is mainly supportive. The toxin is heat stable and water soluble, and it has curare-like properties. Symptoms may include headache, abnormal proprioception, paresthesias, and disturbance of deep tendon reflexes and may eventually progress to flaccid paralysis.

REFERENCES

Blomkalis AL, Otten EJ: Catfish spine envenomation: A case report and literature review. Wilderness Environ Med 1999;10:242-246.
Bonnet MS: The toxicology of Octopus maculosa: The blue-ringed octopus. Br Homeopath J 1999;88:166-171.
Currie BK: Marine antivenoms. J Toxicol Clin Toxicol 2003;41:301-308.
Isbister GK: Venomous fish stings in tropical northern Australia. Am J Emerg Med 2001;19:561-565.
Nimorakiotals B, Winkel KD: Marine envenomations. Part one. Aust Fam Physician 2003;32:969-974.
Nimorakiotals B, Winkel KD: Marine envenomations. Part two. Aust Fam Physician 2003;32:975-979.
O'Reily GM, Isbister GK, Lawrie PM, et al: Prospective study of jellyfish stings from tropical Australia including the major box jellyfish Chironex fleckeri. Med J Aust 2001;175:652-655.
Seymour J, Carrette T, Cullen P, et al: The use of pressure immobilization bandages in the first aid management of cubozoan envenomings. Toxicon 2002;40:1503-1505.
Sobel J, Painter J: Illnesses caused by marine toxins. Clin Infect Dis 2005;41:1290-1296.

---

[1]Not FDA approved for this indication

Medical Toxicology: Ingestions, Inhalations, and Dermal and Ocular Absorptions

Method of
Howard C. Mofenson, MD, Thomas R. Caraccio, PharmD, Michael McGuigan, MD, and Joseph Greensher, MD

Introduction and Epidemiology

According to the national Toxic Exposure Surveillance System (TESS), over 2.4 million potentially toxic exposures were reported last year to Poison Control Centers throughout the United States. Poisonings were responsible for 1183 deaths and more than 500,000 hospitalizations. Poisoning accounts for 2% to 5% of pediatric hospital admissions, 10% of adult admissions, 5% of hospital admissions in the elderly (>65 years of age), and 5% of ambulance calls. In one urban hospital, drug-related emergencies accounted for 38% of the emergency department visits. An evaluation of a medical intensive care unit and step-down unit over a 3-month period indicated that poisonings accounted for 19.7% of admissions.

The largest number of fatalities resulting from poisoning reported to the TESS are caused by analgesics. The other principal toxicologic causes of fatalities are antidepressants, sedative hypnotics/antipsychotics, stimulants/street drugs, cardiovascular agents, and alcohols. Less than 1% of overdose cases reaching the hospitals result in fatality. However, patients presenting in deep coma to medical care facilities have a fatality rate of 13% to 35%. The largest single cause of coma of inapparent etiology is drug poisoning.

Pharmaceutical preparations are involved in 50% of poisonings. The number one pharmaceutical agent involved in exposures is acetaminophen. The severity of the manifestations of acute poisoning exposures varies greatly depending on whether the poisoning was intentional or unintentional. Unintentional exposures make up 85% to 90% of all poisoning exposures. The majority of cases are acute, occurring in children younger than 5 years of age, in the home, and resulting in no or minor toxicity. Many are actually ingestions of relatively nontoxic substances that require minimal medical care. Intentional poisonings, such as suicides, constitute 10% to 15% of exposures and may require the highest standards of medical and nursing care and the use of sophisticated equipment for recovery. Intentional ingestions are often of multiple substances and frequently include ethanol, acetaminophen, and aspirin. Suicides make up 54% of the reported fatalities. About 25% of suicides are attempted with drugs. Sixty percent of patients who take a drug overdose use their own medication and 15% use drugs prescribed for close relatives. The majority of the drug-related suicide attempts involve a central nervous system (CNS) depressant, and coma management is vital to the treatment.

Assessment and Maintenance of the Vital Functions

The initial assessment of all patients in medical emergencies follows the principles of basic and advanced cardiac life support. The adequacy of the patient's airway, degree of ventilation, and circulatory status should be determined. The vital functions should be established and maintained. Vital signs should be measured frequently and should include body core temperature. The assessment of vital functions should include the rate numbers (e.g., respiratory rate) and indications of effectiveness (e.g., depth of respirations and degree of gas exchange). Table 1 gives important measurements and vital signs.

Level of consciousness should be assessed by immediate AVPU (Alert, responds to Verbal stimuli, responds to Painful stimuli, and Unconscious). If the patient is unconscious, one must assess the severity of the unconsciousness by the Glasgow Coma Scale (Table 2).

If the patient is comatose, management requires administering 100% oxygen, establishing vascular access, and obtaining blood for pertinent laboratory studies. The administration of glucose, thiamine, and naloxone, as well as intubation to protect the airway, should be considered. Pertinent laboratory studies include arterial blood gases (ABG), electrocardiography (ECG), determination of blood glucose level, electrolytes, renal and liver tests, and acetaminophen plasma concentration in all cases of intentional ingestions. Radiography of the chest and abdomen may be useful. The severity of a stimulant's effects can also be assessed and should be documented to follow the trend.

The examiner should completely expose the patient by removing clothes and other items that interfere with a full evaluation. One should look for clues to etiology in the clothes and include the hat and shoes.

Prevention of Absorption and Reduction of Local Damage

EXPOSURE

Poisoning exposure routes include ingestion (76.8%), dermal (8%), ophthalmologic (5%), inhalation (6%), insect bites and stings (4%), and parenteral injections (0.5%). The effect of the toxin may be local, systemic, or both.

Local effects (skin, eyes, mucosa of respiratory or gastrointestinal tract) occur where contact is made with the poisonous substance. Local effects are nonspecific chemical reactions that depend on the chemical properties (e.g., pH), concentration, contact time, and type of exposed surface.

Systemic effects occur when the poison is absorbed into the body and depend on the dose, the distribution, and the functional reserve of the organ systems. Shock and hypoxia are part of systemic toxicity.

DELAYED TOXIC ACTION

Therapeutic doses of most pharmaceuticals are absorbed within 90 minutes. However, the patient with exposure to a potential toxin may be asymptomatic at this time

TABLE 1 Important Measurements and Vital Signs

| Age | Body Surface Area (m²) | Weight (kg) | Height (cm) | Pulse (bpm) Resting | Blood Pressure | | | Respiratory Rate (rpm) |
| | | | | | Hypotension | Hypertension | | |
						Significant	Severe	
Newborn	0.19	3.5	50	70-190	<60/40	>96	>106	30-60
1 mo-6 mo	0.30	4-7	50-65	80-160	<70/45	>104	>110	30-50
6 mo-1 y	0.38	7-10	65-75	80-160	<70/45	>104	>110	20-40
1-2 y	0.50-0.55	10-12	75-85	80-140	<74/47	>112/74	>118/82	20-40
3-5 y	0.54-0.68	15-20	90-108	80-120	<80/52	>116/76	>124/84	20-40
6-9 y	0.68-0.85	20-28	122-133	75-115	<90/60	>122/82	>130/86	16-25
10-12 y	1.00-1.07	30-40	138-147	70-110	<90/60	>126/82	>134/90	16-25
13-15 y	1.07-1.22	42-50	152-160	60-100	<90/60	>136/86	>144/92	16-20
16-18 y	1.30-1.60	53-60	160-170	60-100	<90/60	>142/92	>150/98	12-16
Adult	1.40-1.70	60-70	160-170	60-100	<90/60	>140/90	>210/120	10-16

Data from Nadas A: Pediatric Cardiology, 3rd ed. Philadelphia, WB Saunders, 1976; Blumer JL (ed): A Practice Guide to Pediatric Intensive Care. St Louis, Mosby, 1990; AAP and ACEP: Respiratory Distress in APLS Pediatric Emergency Medicine Course, 1993; Second Task Force: Blood pressure control in children—1987, Pediatr 79:1, 1987; Linakis JG: Hypertension. In Fliesher GR, Ludwig S (eds); Textbook of Pediatric Emergency Medicine, 3rd ed. Baltimore, Williams & Wilkins, 1993.

TABLE 2 Glasgow Coma Scale

Scale	Adult Response	Score	Pediatric, 0-1 Years
Eye opening	Spontaneous	4	Spontaneous
	To verbal command	3	To shout
	To pain	2	To pain
	None	1	No response
Motor response			
To verbal command	Obeys	6	
To painful stimuli	Localized pain	5	Localized pain
	Flexion withdrawal	4	Flexion withdrawal
	Decorticate flexion	3	Decorticate flexion
	Decerebrate extension	2	Decerebrate flexion
	None	1	None
Verbal response: adult	Oriented and converses	5	Cries, smiles, coos
	Disoriented but converses	4	Cries or screams
	Inappropriate words	3	Inappropriate sounds
	Incomprehensible sounds	2	Grunts
	None	1	Gives no response
Verbal response: child	Oriented	5	
	Words or babbles	4	
	Vocal sounds	3	
	Cries or moans to stimuli	2	
	None	1	

Data from Teasdale G, Jennett B: Assessment of coma impaired consciousness. Lancet 2:83, 1974; Simpson D, Reilly P: Pediatric coma scale. Lancet 2:450, 1982; Seidel J: Preparing for pediatric emergencies. Pediatr Rev 16:470, 1995.

because a sufficient amount has not yet been absorbed or metabolized to produce toxicity at the time the patient presents for care.

Absorption can be significantly delayed under the following circumstances:

1. Drugs with anticholinergic properties (e.g., antihistamines, belladonna alkaloids, diphenoxylate with atropine [Lomotil], phenothiazines, and tricyclic antidepressants).
2. Modified release preparations such as sustained-release, enteric-coated, and controlled-release formulations have delayed and prolonged absorption.
3. Concretions may form (e.g., salicylates, iron, glutethimide, and meprobamate [Equanil]) that can delay absorption and prolong the toxic effects. Large quantities of drugs tend to be absorbed more slowly than small quantities.

Some substances must be metabolized into a toxic metabolite (acetaminophen, acetonitrile, ethylene glycol, methanol, methylene chloride, parathion, and paraquat). In some cases, time is required to produce a toxic effect on organ systems (*Amanita phalloides* mushrooms, carbon tetrachloride, colchicine, digoxin [Lanoxin], heavy metals, monoamine oxidase inhibitors, and oral hypoglycemic agents).

Initial Management

1. Stabilization of airway, breathing, and circulation and protection of same.
2. Identification of specific toxin or toxic syndrome.
3. Initial treatment: D50W; consider thiamine, naloxone (Narcan), oxygen, and antidotes if needed.
4. Physical assessment.
5. Decontamination: Gastrointestinal tract, skin, eyes.

DECONTAMINATION

In the asymptomatic patient who has been exposed to a toxic substance, decontamination procedures should be considered if the patient has been exposed to potentially toxic substances in toxic amounts.

Ocular exposure should be immediately treated with water irrigation for 15 to 20 minutes with the eyelids fully retracted. One should not use neutralizing chemicals. All caustic and corrosive injuries should be evaluated with fluorescein dye and by an ophthalmologist.

Dermal exposure is treated immediately with copious water irrigation for 30 minutes, not a forceful flushing. Shampooing the hair, cleansing the fingernails, navel, and perineum, and irrigating the eyes are necessary in the case of an extensive exposure. The clothes should be specially bagged and may have to be discarded. Leather goods can become irreversibly contaminated and must be abandoned. Caustic (alkali) exposures can require hours of irrigation. Dermal absorption can occur with pesticides, hydrocarbons, and cyanide.

Injection exposures (e.g., snake envenomation) can be treated with venom extracts. Venom extractors can be used within minutes of envenomation, and proximal lymphatic constricting bands or elastic wraps can be used to delay lymphatic flow and immobilize the extremity. Cold packs and tourniquets should not be used and incision is generally not recommended. Substances of abuse may be injected intravenously or subcutaneously. In these cases, little decontamination can be done.

Inhalation exposure to toxic substances is managed by immediate removal of the victim from the contaminated environment by protected rescuers.

Gastrointestinal exposure is the most common route of poisoning. Gastrointestinal decontamination historically has been done by gastric emptying: induction of emesis, gastric lavage, administration of activated charcoal, and the use of cathartics or whole bowel irrigation. No procedure is routine; it should be individualized for each case. If no attempt is made to decontaminate the patient, the reason should be clearly documented on the medical record (e.g., time elapsed, past peak of action, ineffectiveness, or risk of procedure).

Gastric Emptying Procedures

The gastric emptying procedure used is influenced by the age of the patient, the effectiveness of the procedure, the time of ingestion (gastric emptying is usually ineffective after 1 hour postingestion), the patient's clinical status (time of peak effect has passed or the patient's condition is too unstable), formulation of the substance ingested (regular release versus modified release), the amount ingested, and the rapidity of onset of CNS depression or stimulation (convulsions). Most studies show that only 30% (range, 19% to 62%) of the ingested toxin is removed by gastric emptying under optimal conditions. It has not been demonstrated that the choice of procedure improved the outcome.

A mnemonic for gathering information is STATS:

S—substance
T—type of formulation
A—amount and age
T—time of ingestion
S—signs and symptoms

The examiner should attempt to obtain AMPLE information about the patient:

A—age and allergies
M—available medications
P—past medical history including pregnancy, psychiatric illnesses, substance abuse, or intentional ingestions
L—time of last meal, which may influence absorption and the onset and peak action
E—events leading to present condition

The intent of the patient should also be determined.

The Regional Poison Center should be consulted for the exact ingredients of the ingested substance and the latest management. The treatment information on the labels of products and in the Physician's Desk Reference are notoriously inaccurate.

Ipecac Syrup

Syrup of ipecac–induced emesis has virtually no use in the emergency department. Although at one time it was considered most useful in young children with a recent witnessed ingestion, it is no longer advised in most cases. Current guidelines from the American Association of Poison Control Centers have significantly limited the indications for inducing emesis because the risk most often exceeds the benefit derived from this procedure.

The Poison Control Center should be called if inducting emesis is being considered.

Contraindications or situations in which induction of emesis is inappropriate include the following:

- Ingestion of caustic substance
- Loss of airway protective reflexes because of ingestion of substances that can produce rapid onset of CNS depression (e.g., short-acting benzodiazepines, barbiturates, nonbarbiturate sedative-hypnotics, opioids, tricyclic antidepressants) or convulsions (e.g., camphor [Ponstel], chloroquine [Aralen], codeine, isoniazid [Nydrazid], mefenamic acid, nicotine, propoxyphene [Darvon], organophosphate insecticides, strychnine, and tricyclic antidepressants)
- Ingestion of low-viscosity petroleum distillates (e.g., gasoline, lighter fluid, kerosene)
- Significant vomiting prior to presentation or hematemesis
- Age under 6 months (no established dose, safety, or efficacy data)
- Ingestion of foreign bodies (emesis is ineffective and may lead to aspiration)
- Clinical conditions including neurologic impairment, hemodynamic instability, increased intracranial pressure, and hypertension
- Delay in presentation (more than 1 hour postingestion)

The dose of syrup of ipecac in the 6- to 9-month-old infant is 5 mL; in the 9- to 12-month-old, 10 mL; and in the 1- to 12-year-old, 15 mL. In children older than 12 years and in adults, the dose is 30 mL. The dose can be repeated once if the child does not vomit in 15 to 20 minutes. The vomitus should be inspected for remnants of pills or toxic substances, and the appearance and odor should be documented. When ipecac is not available, 30 mL of mild dishwashing soap (not dishwasher detergent) can be used, although it is less effective.

Complications are very rare but include aspiration, protracted vomiting, rarely cardiac toxicity with long-term abuse, pneumothorax, gastric rupture, diaphragmatic hernia, intracranial hemorrhage, and Mallory-Weiss tears.

Gastric Lavage

Gastric lavage should be considered only when life-threatening amounts of substances were involved, when the benefits outweigh the risks, when it can be performed within 1 hour of the ingestion, and when no contraindications exist.

The contraindications are similar to those for ipecac-induced emesis. However, gastric lavage can be accomplished after the insertion of an endotracheal tube in cases of CNS depression or controlled convulsions. The patient should be placed with the head lower than the hips in a left-lateral decubitus position. The location of the tube should be confirmed by radiography, if necessary, and suctioning equipment should be available.

Contraindications to gastric lavage include the following:

- Ingestion of caustic substances (risk of esophageal perforation)
- Uncontrolled convulsions, because of the danger of aspiration and injury during the procedure

- Ingestion of low-viscosity petroleum distillate products
- CNS depression or absent protective airway reflexes, without endotracheal protection
- Significant cardiac dysrhythmias
- Significant emesis or hematemesis prior to presentation
- Delay in presentation (more than 1 hour post-ingestion)

Size of Tube

The best results with gastric lavage are obtained with the largest possible orogastric tube that can be reasonably passed (nasogastric tubes are not large enough to remove solid material). In adults, a large-bore orogastric Lavacuator hose or a No. 42 French Ewald tube should be used; in young children, orogastric tubes are generally too small to remove solid material and gastric lavage is not recommended.

The amount of fluid used varies with the patient's age and size. In general, aliquots of 50 to 100 mL per lavage are used in adults. Larger amounts of fluid may force the toxin past the pylorus. Lavage fluid is 0.9% saline.

Complications are rare and may include respiratory depression, aspiration pneumonitis, cardiac dysrhythmias as a result of increased vagal tone, esophageal-gastric tears and perforation, laryngospasm, and mediastinitis.

Activated Charcoal

Oral activated charcoal adsorbs the toxin onto its surface before absorption. According to recent guidelines set forth by the American Academy of Clinical Toxicology, activated charcoal should not be used routinely. Its use is indicated only if a toxic amount of substance has been ingested and is optimally effective within 1 hour of the ingestion. Because of the slow absorption of large quantities of toxin, activated charcoal may be beneficial after 1 hour postingestion.

Activated charcoal does not effectively adsorb small molecules or molecules lacking carbon (Table 3). Activated charcoal adsorption may be diminished by milk, cocoa powder, and ice cream.

There are a few relative contraindications to the use of activated charcoal:

1. Ingestion of caustics and corrosives, which may produce vomiting or cling to the mucosa and falsely appear as a burn on endoscopy.

TABLE 3 Substances Poorly Adsorbed by Activated Charcoal

C	Caustics and corrosives
H	Heavy metals (arsenic, iron, lead, mercury)
A	Alcohols (ethanol, methanol, isopropanol) and glycols (ethylene glycols)
R	Rapid onset of absorption (cyanide and strychnine)
C	Chlorine and iodine
O	Others insoluble in water (substances in tablet form)
A	Aliphatic hydrocarbons (petroleum distillates)
L	Laxatives (sodium, magnesium, potassium, and lithium)

2. Comatose patient, in whom the airway must be secured prior to activated charcoal administration.
3. Patient without presence of bowel sounds.

Note: Activated charcoal was shown not to interfere with effectiveness of *N*-acetylcysteine in cases of acetaminophen overdose, so it is no longer contraindicated as was thought in the past.

The usual initial adult dose is 60 to 100 g and the dose for children is 15 to 30 g. It is administered orally as a slurry mixed with water or by nasogastric or orogastric tube. *Caution:* Be sure the tube is in the stomach. Cathartics are not necessary.

Although repeated dosing with activated charcoal may decrease the half-life and increases the clearance of phenobarbital, dapsone, quinidine, theophylline, and carbamazepine (Tegretol), recent guidelines indicate there is insufficient evidence to support the use of multiple-dose activated charcoal unless a life-threatening amount of one of the substances mentioned is involved. At present there are no controlled studies that demonstrate that multiple-dose activated charcoal or cathartics alter the clinical course of an intoxication. The dose varies from 0.25 to 0.50 g/kg every 1 to 4 hours, and continuous nasogastric tube infusion of 0.25 to 0.5 g/kg/h has been used to decrease vomiting.

Gastrointestinal dialysis is the diffusion of the toxin from the higher concentration in the serum of the mesenteric vessels to the lower levels in the gastrointestinal tract mucosal cell and subsequently into the gastrointestinal lumen, where the concentration has been lowered by intraluminal adsorption of activated charcoal.

Complications of treatment with activated charcoal include vomiting in 50% of cases, desorption (especially with weak acids in intestine), and aspiration (at least a dozen cases of aspiration have been reported). There are many cases of unreported pulmonary aspirations and "charcoal lungs," intestinal obstruction or pseudoobstruction (three case reports with multiple dosing, none with a single dose), empyema following esophageal perforation, and hypermagnesemia and hypernatremia, which have been associated with repeated concurrent doses of activated charcoal and saline cathartics. Catharsis was used to hasten the elimination of any remaining toxin in the gastrointestinal tract. There are no studies to demonstrate the effectiveness of cathartics, and they are no longer recommended as a form of gastrointestinal decontamination.

Whole-Bowel Irrigation

With whole bowel irrigation, solutions of polyethylene glycol (PEG) with balanced electrolytes are used to cleanse the bowel without causing shifts in fluids and electrolytes. The procedure is not approved by the U.S. Food and Drug Administration for this purpose.

Indications

The procedure has been studied and used successfully in cases of iron overdose when abdominal radiographs reveal incomplete emptying of excess iron. There are additional indications for other types of ingestions, such as with body-packing of illicit drugs (e.g., cocaine, heroin).

The procedure is to administer the solution (GoLYTELY or Colyte), orally or by nasogastric tube, in a dose of

0.5 L per hour in children younger than 5 years of age and 2 L per hour in adolescents and adults for 5 hours. The end point is reached when the rectal effluent is clear or radiopaque materials can no longer be seen in the gastrointestinal tract on abdominal radiographs.

Contraindications

These measures should not be used if there is extensive hematemesis, ileus, or signs of bowel obstruction, perforation, or peritonitis. Animal experiments in which PEG was added to activated charcoal indicated that activated charcoal-salicylates and activated charcoal-theophylline combinations resulted in decreased adsorption and desorption of salicylate and theophylline and no therapeutic benefit over activated charcoal alone. Polyethylene solutions are bound by activated charcoal in vitro, decreasing the efficacy of activated charcoal.

Dilutional treatment is indicated for the immediate management of caustic and corrosive poisonings but is otherwise not useful. The administration of diluting fluid above 30 mL in children and 250 mL in adults may produce vomiting, reexposing the vital tissues to the effects of local damage and possible aspiration.

Neutralization is not proven to be either safe or effective.

Endoscopy and surgery have been required in the case of body-packer obstruction, intestinal ischemia produced by cocaine ingestion, and iron local caustic action.

Differential Diagnosis of Poisons on the Basis of Central Nervous System Manifestations

Neurologic parameters help to classify and assess the need for supportive treatment as well as provide diagnostic clues to the etiology. Table 4 lists the effects of CNS depressants, CNS stimulants, hallucinogens, and autonomic nervous system anticholinergics and cholinergics.

Central nervous system depressants are cholinergics, opioids, sedative-hypnotics, and sympatholytic agents. The hallmarks are lethargy, sedation, stupor, and coma. In exception to the manifestations listed in Table 4, (a) barbiturates may produce an initial tachycardia; (b) convulsions are produced by codeine, propoxyphene (Darvon), meperidine (Demerol), glutethimide, phenothiazines, methaqualone, and tricyclic and cyclic antidepressants; (c) benzodiazepines rarely produce coma that will interfere with cardiorespiratory functions; and (d) pulmonary edema is common with opioids and sedative-hypnotics.

The CNS stimulants are anticholinergic, hallucinogenic, sympathomimetic, and withdrawal agents. The hallmarks of CNS stimulants are convulsions and hyperactivity.

There is considerable overlapping of effects among the various hallucinogens, but the major hallmark manifestation is hallucinations.

Guidelines for In-hospital Disposition

Classification of patients as high risk depends on clinical judgment. Any patient who needs cardiorespiratory

support or has a persistently altered mental status for 3 hours or more should be considered for intensive care.

Guidelines for admitting patients older than 14 years of age to an intensive care unit, after 2 to 3 hours in the emergency department, include the following:

1. Need for intubation
2. Seizures
3. Unresponsiveness to verbal stimuli
4. Arterial carbon dioxide pressure greater than 45 mm Hg
5. Cardiac conduction or rhythm disturbances (any rhythm except sinus arrhythmia)
6. Close monitoring of vital signs during antidotal therapy or elimination procedures
7. The need for continuous monitoring
8. QRS interval greater than 0.10 second, in cases of tricyclic antidepressant poisoning
9. Systolic blood pressure less than 80 mm Hg
10. Hypoxia, hypercarbia, acid–base imbalance, or metabolic abnormalities
11. Extremes of temperature
12. Progressive deterioration or significant underlying medical disorders

Use of Antidotes

Antidotes are available for only a relatively small number of poisons. An antidote is not a substitute for good supportive care. Table 5 summarizes the commonly used antidotes, their indications, and their methods of administration. The Regional Poison Control Center can give further information on these antidotes.

Enhancement of Elimination

The acceptable methods for elimination of absorbed toxic substances are dialysis, hemoperfusion, exchange transfusion, plasmapheresis, enzyme induction, and inhibition. Methods of increasing urinary excretion of toxic chemicals and drugs have been studied extensively, but the other modalities have not been well evaluated.

In general, these methods are needed in only a minority of cases and should be reserved for life-threatening circumstances when a definite benefit is anticipated.

DIALYSIS

Dialysis is the extrarenal means of removing certain substances from the body, and it can substitute for the kidney when renal failure occurs. Dialysis is not the first measure instituted; however, it may be lifesaving later in the course of a severe intoxication. It is needed in only a minority of intoxicated patients.

Peritoneal dialysis uses the peritoneum as the membrane for dialysis. It is only 1/20 as effective as hemodialysis. It is easier to use and less hazardous to the patient but also less effective in removing the toxin; thus it is rarely used except in small infants.

Hemodialysis is the most effective dialysis method but requires experience with sophisticated equipment. Blood is circulated past a semipermeable extracorporeal membrane. Substances are removed by diffusion down a

Text continued on page 1362

TABLE 4   Agents with Central Nervous System (CNS) Effects

Agents	General Manifestations	Agents	General Manifestations

CNS Depressants
Alcohols and glycols (S–H)
Anticonvulsants (S–H)
Antidysrhythmics (S–H)
Antihypertensives (S–H)
Barbiturates (S–H)
Benzodiazepines (S–H)
Butyrophenones (Syly)
β-Adrenergic blockers (Syly)
Calcium channel blockers (Syly)
Digitalis (Syly)
Opioids
Lithium (mixed)
Muscle relaxants
Phenothiazines (Syly)
Nonbarbiturate/benzodiazepine
    glutethimide, methaqualone,
    methyprylon, sedative-hypnotics
    (chloral hydrate,ethchlorvynol, bromide)
Tricyclic antidepressants (late Syly)
	Bradycardia
	Bradypnea
	Shallow respirations
	Hypotension
	Hypothermia
	Flaccid coma
	Miosis
	Hypoactive bowel sounds
		Hallucinogens‡
		Amphetamines‡
		Anticholinergics
		Cardiac glycosides
		Cocaine
		Ethanol withdrawal
		Hydrocarbon inhalation (abuse)
		Mescaline (peyote)
		Mushrooms (psilocybin)
		Phencyclidine
			Tachycardia and dysrhythmias
			Tachypnea
			Hypertension
			Hallucinations, usually visual
			Disorientation
			Panic reaction
			Toxic psychosis
			Moist skin
			Mydriasis (reactive)
			Hyperthermia
			Flashbacks

CNS Stimulants Amphetamines (Sy) Anticholinergics*	Tachycardia Tachypnea and dysrhythmias	**Anticholinergics** Antihistamines Antispasmodic gastrointestinal preparations Antiparkinsonian preparations Atropine Cyclobenzaprine (Flexeril)	Tachycardia, dysrhythmias (rare) Tachypnea Hypertension (mild) Hyperthermia Hallucinations ("mad as a hatter")

Cocaine (Sy)
Camphor (mixed)
Ergot alkaloids (Sy)
Isoniazid (mixed)
Lithium (mixed)
Lysergic acid diethylamide (H)
Hallucinogens (H)
Mescaline and synthetic analogs
Metals (arsenic, lead, mercury)
Methylphenidate (Ritalin) (Sy)
Monoamine oxidase inhibitors (Sy)
Pemoline (Cylert) (Sy)
Phencyclidine (H)†
Salicylates (mixed)
Strychnine (mixed)
Sympathomimetics (Sy)
    (phenylpropanolamine,
    theophylline, caffeine, thyroid)
Withdrawal from ethanol,
    β-adrenergic blockers,
    clonidine, opioids,
    sedative–hypnotics (W)
	Hypertension
	Convulsions
	Toxic psychosis
	Mydriasis (reactive)
	Agitation and restlessness
	Moist skin
	Tremors
		Mydriatic ophthalmologic agents
		Over-the-counter sleep agents
		Plants (*Datura* sppl/mushrooms)
		
		Phenothiazines (early)
		Scopolamine
		Tricyclic/cyclic antidepressants (early)
			Mydriasis (unreactive)
			    ("blind as a bat")
			Flushed skin ("red as a beet")
			Dry skin and mouth ("dry as a bone")
			Hypoactive bowel sounds
			Urinary retention
			Lilliputian hallucinations ("little people")

		Cholinergics
		Bethanechol (Urecholine)
		Carbamate insecticides (Carbaryl)
		Edrophonium
		Organophosphate insecticides
		    (Malathion, parathion)
		Parasympathetic agents
		    (physostigmine, pyridostigmine)
		Toxic mushrooms (*Clitocybe* spp.)
			Bradycardia (muscarinic)
			Tachycardia (nicotinic effect)
			Miosis (muscarinic)
			Diarrhea (muscarinic)
			
			Hypertension (variable)
			
			Hyperactive bowel sounds
			Excess urination (muscarinic)
			Excess salivation (muscarinic)
			Lacrimation (muscarinic)
			Bronchospasm (muscarinic)
			Muscle fasciculations (nicotinic)
			Paralysis (nicotinic)

Abbreviations: H = hallucinogen; S–H = sedative–hypnotic; Sy = sympathomimetic; Syly = Sympatholytic; W = withdrawal.
*Anticholinergics produce dry skin and mucosa and decreased bowel sounds.
†Phencyclidine may produce miosis.
‡The amphetamine hybrids are methylene dioxymethamphetamine (MDMA, ecstasy,"ADAM") and methylene dioxyamphetamine (MDA, "Eve"), which are associated with deaths.

TABLE 5 Initial Doses of Antidotes for Common Poisonings

Antidote	Use	Dose	Route	Adverse Reactions/Comments
N-Acetyl Cysteine (NAC, Mucomyst): Stock level to treat 70 kg adult for 24 h: 25 vials, 20%, 30 mL	Acetaminophen, carbon tetrachloride (experimental)	140/mg/kg loading, followed by 70 mg/kg every 4 h for 17 doses.	PO	Nausea, vomiting. Dilute to 5% with sweet juice or flat cola.
		150 mg/kg in 200 mL of D$_5$W over 1 hr, then 50 mg/kg in 500 mL of D$_5$W over 4 hr, then 100 mg/kg in 1 liter D$_5$W over 16 hrs	IV	Useful for those who cannot tolerate oral route
Atropine: Stock level to treat 70 kg adult for 24 h: 1 g (1 mg/mL in 1, 10 mL)	Organophosphate and carbamate pesticides: bradydysrhythmics, β-adrenergics, calcium channel blockers/nerve agents	*Child:* 0.02-0.05 mg/kg repeated q5-10 min to max of 2 mg as necessary until cessation of secretions *Adult:* 1-2 mg q5-10 min as necessary. Dilute in 1-2 mL of 0.9% saline for ET instillation. *IV infusion dose:* Place 8 mg of atropine in 100 mL D$_5$W or saline. Conc. = 0.08 mg/mL; dose range = 0.02-0.08 mg/kg/h or 0.25-1 mL/kg/h. Severe poisoning may require supplemental doses of IV atropine intermittently in doses of 1-5 mg until drying of secretions occurs.	IV/ET	Tachycardia, dry mouth, blurred vision, and urinary retention. Ensure adequate ventilation before administration.
Calcium Chloride (10%): Stock level to treat 70 kg adult for 24 h: 10 vials 1 g (1.35 mEq/mL)	Hypocalcemia, fluoride, calcium channel blockers, β-blockers, oxalates, ethylene glycol, hypermagnesemia	0.1-0.2 mL/kg (10-20 mg/kg) slow push every 10 min up to max 10 mL (1 g). Since calcium response lasts 15 minutes, some may require continuous infusion 0.2 mL/kg/h up to maximum of 10 mL/h while monitoring for dysrhythmias and hypotension.	IV	Administer slowly with BP and ECG monitoring and have magnesium available to reverse calcium effects. Tissue irritation, hypotension, dysrhythmias from rapid injection. Contraindications: digitalis glycoside intoxication.
Calcium Gluconate (10%): Stock level to treat 70 kg adult for 24 h: 20 vials 1 g (0.45 mEq/mL)	Hypocalcemia, fluoride, calcium channel blockers, hydrofluoric acid; black widow envenomation	0.3-0.4 mL/kg (30-40 mg/kg) slow push; repeat as needed up to max dose 10-20 mL (1-2 g).	IV	Same comments as calcium chloride.
Infiltration of Calcium Gluconate	Hydrofluoric acid skin exposure	Dose: Infiltrate each square cm of affected dermis/subcutaneous tissue with about 0.5 mL of 10% calcium gluconate using a 30-gauge needle. Repeat as needed to control pain.	Infiltrate	

Antidote	Indication	Dose	Route	Comments
Intra-arterial Calcium Gluconate	Hydrofluoric acid skin exposure	Infuse 20 mL of 10% calcium gluconate (not chloride) diluted in 250 mL D5W via the radial or brachial artery proximal to the injury over 3-4 hours.		Alternatively, dilute 10 mL of 10% calcium gluconate with 40-50 mL of D5W.
Calcium Gluconate Gel: Stock level: 3.5 g	Hydrofluoric acid skin exposure	2.5 g USP powder added to 100 mL water-soluble lubricating jelly, e.g., K-Y Jelly or Lubifax (or 3.5 mg into 150 mL). Some use 6 g of calcium carbonate in 100 g of lubricant. Place injured hand in surgical glove filled with gel. Apply q4h. If pain persists, calcium gluconate injection may be needed (above).	Dermal	Powder is available from Spectrum Pharmaceutical Co. in California: 800-772-8786. Commercial preparation of Ca gluconate gel is available from Pharmascience in Montreal, Quebec: 514-340-1114.
Cyanide Antidote Kit: Stock level to treat 70 kg adult for 24 h: 2 Lilly Cyanide Antidote kits	Cyanide Hydrogen sulfide (nitrites are given only) Do not use sodium thiosulfate for hydrogen sulfide Individual portions of the kit can be used in certain circumstances (consult PCC)	Amyl nitrite: 1 crushable ampule for 30 secs of every min. Use new amp q3min. May omit step if venous access is established.	Inhalation	If methemoglobinemia occurs, do not use methylene blue to correct this because it releases cyanide.
	Cyanide Hydrogen sulfide (nitrites are given only) Do not use sodium thiosulfate for hydrogen sulfide Individual portions of the kit can be used in certain circumstances (consult PCC)	Sodium nitrite: *Child:* 0.33 mL/kg of 3% solution if hemoglobin level is not known, otherwise based on tables with product. *Adult:* up to 300 mg (10 mL). Dilute nitrite in 100 mL 0.9% saline, administer slowly at 5 mL/min. Slow infusion if fall in BP.	IV	If methemoglobinemia occurs, do not use methylene blue to correct this because it releases cyanide.
	Cyanide Hydrogen sulfide Do not use sodium thiosulfate for hydrogen sulfide Individual portions of the Kit can be used in certain circumstances (consult PCC)	Sodium thiosulfate: *Child:* 1.6 mL/kg of 25% solution, may be repeated every 30-60 min to a maximum of 12.5 g or 50 mL in adult. Administer over 20 min.	IV	Nausea, dizziness, headache. Tachycardia, muscle rigidity, and bronchospasm (rapid administration).
Dantrolene Sodium (Dantrium): Stock level to treat 70 kg adult for 24 h: 700 mg, 35 vials (20 mg/vial)	Malignant hyperthermia	2-3 mg/kg IV rapidly. Repeat loading dose every 10 minutes, if necessary up to a maximum total dose of 10 mg/kg. When temperature and heart rate decrease, slow the infusion	IV/PO	Hepatotoxicity occurs with cumulative dose of 10 mg/kg. Thrombophlebitis (best given in central line). Available as 20 mg lyophilized dantrolene powder for

Continued

TABLE 5   Initial Doses of Antidotes for Common Poisonings—cont'd

Antidote	Use	Dose	Route	Adverse Reactions/Comments
		1-2 mg/kg every 6 hours for 24-28 h until all evidence of malignant hyperthermia syndrome has subsided. Follow with oral doses 1-2 mg/kg four times a day for 24 h as necessary.		reconstruction, which contains 3 g mannitol and sodium hydroxide in 70-mL vial. Mix with 60 mL sterile distilled water without a bacteriostatic agent and protect from light. Use within 6 hours after reconstituting.
Deferoxamine (Desferal): Stock level to treat 70 kg adult for 24 h: 17 vials (500 mg/amp).	Iron	IV infusion of 15 mg/kg/h (3 mL/kg/h: 500 mg in 100 mL D$_5$W) max 6 g/d Rates of >45 µg/kg/h if conc >1000 µg/dL.	Preferred IV: avoid therapy >24 h	Hypotension (minimized by avoiding rapid infusion rates) DFO challenge test 50 mg/kg is unreliable if negative.
Diazepam (Valium): Stock level to treat 70 kg adult for 24 h: 200 mg, 5 mg/mL; 2,10 mL	Any intoxication that provokes seizures when specific therapy is not available, e.g., amphetamines, PCP, barbiturate and alcohol withdrawal.	Adult, 5-10 mg IV (max 20 mg) at a rate of 5 mg/min until seizure is controlled. May be repeated 2 or 3 times. Child, 0.1-0.3 mg/kg up to 10 mg IV slowly over 2 min.	IV	Confusion, somnolence, coma, hypotension. Intramuscular absorption is erratic Establish airway and administer 100% oxygen and glucose.
Digoxin-Specific Fab Antibodies (Digibind): Stock level to treat 70 kg adult for 24 h: 20 vials.	Chloroquine poisoning. Digoxin, digitoxin, oleander tea with the following: (1) Imminent cardiac arrest or shock, (2) hyperkalemia >5.0 mEq/L. (3) serum digoxin >5 ng/mL (child) at 8-12 h post ingestion in adults, (4) digitalis delirium, (5) ingestion over 10 mg in adults or 4 mg in child, (6) bradycardia or second- or third-degree heart block unresponsive to atropine, (7) life threatening digitoxin or oleander posioning.	(1) If amount ingested is known total dose × bioavailability (0.8) = body burden. The body burden + 0.6 (0.5 mg of digoxin is bound by 1 vial of 38 mg of FAB) = # vials needed. (2) If amount is unknown but the steady state serum concentration is known in ng/mL: Digoxin: ng/mL: (5.6 L/kg Vd) × (wt kg) = µg body burden. Body burden + 100 = mg body burden/0.5 = # vials needed. Digitoxin body burden = ng/mL × (0.56 L/kg Vd) × (wt kg) Body burden + 1000 = mg body burden/0.5 = # vials needed. (3) If the amount is not known, it is administered in life-threatening situations as 10 vials (400 mg) IV in saline over 30 min in adults. If cardiac arrest is imminent, administer 20 vials (adult) as a bolus.	IV	Allergic reactions (rare), return of condition being treated with digitalis glycoside. Administer by infusion over 30 min through a 0.22-µ filter. If cardiac arrest imminent, may administer by bolus. Consult PCC for more details.

Drug	Indication	Dose	Route	Adverse Effects/Precautions
Dimercaprol (BAL in Peanut Oil): Stock level to treat 70 kg adult for 24 h: 1200 mg (4 amps—100 mg/mL 10% in oil in 3 mL amp)	Chelating agent for arsenic, mercury, and lead.	3-5 mg/kg q4th usually for 5-10 d	Deep IM	Local infection site pain and sterile abscess, nausea, vomiting, fever, salivation, hypertension, and nephrotoxicity (alkalinize urine).
2,3 Dimercaptosuccinic Acid (DMSA Succimer): 100 mg/capsule: 20 capsules	Used as a chelating agent for lead, especially blood lead levels >45 µg/dL. May also be used for symptomatic mercury exposure	10 mg/kg 3 × daily for 5 days followed by 10 mg/kg 2 × daily for 14 days.	PO	Precautions: monitor AST/ALT; use with caution in G6PD-deficient patients. Avoid concurrent iron therapy. Relatively safe antidote, rarely severe, uncommon minor skin rashes may occur.
Diphenhydramine (Benadryl): Antiparkinsonian action. Stock level to treat a 70 kg adult for 24 h: 5 vials (10 mg/mL, 10 mL each)	Used to treat extrapyramidal symptoms and dystonia induced by phenothiazines, phencyclidine, and related drugs.	*Children:* 1-2 mg/kg IV slowly over 5 minutes up to maximum 50 mg followed by 5 mg/kg/24 h orally divided every 6 hours up to 300 mg/24h *Adults:* 50 mg IV followed by 50 mg orally four times daily for 5-7 days Note: Symptoms abate within 2-5 min after IV.	IV	Fatal dose: 20-40 mg/kg. Dry mouth, drowsiness.
Ethanol (Ethyl Alcohol): Stock level to treat 70 kg adult for 24 h: 3 bottles 10% (1 L each)	Methanol, ethylene glycol	10 mL/kg loading dose concurrently with 1.4 mL/kg (average) infusion of 10% ethanol (consult PCC for more details)	IV	Nausea, vomiting, sedation. Use 0.22 µm filter if preparing from bulk 100% ethanol.
Flumazenil (Romazicon): Stock level to treat 70 kg adult for 24 h: 4 vials (0.1 mg/mL, 10 mL)	Benzodiazepines (may also be beneficial in the treatment of hepatic encephalopathy)	Administer 0.2 mg (2 mL) IV over 30 sec (pediatric dose not established, 0.01 mg/kg), then wait 3 min for a response, then if desired consciousness is not achieved, administer 0.3 mg (3 mL) over 30 sec, then wait 3 min for response, then if desired consciousness is not achieved, administer 0.5 mg (5 mL) over 30 sec at 60-sec intervals up to a maximum cumulative dose of 3 mg (30 mL) (1 mg in children). Because effects last only 1-5 hours, if patient responds monitor carefully over next 6 hours for resedation. If multiple repeated doses, consider a continuous infusion of 0.2-1 mg/h.	IV	Nausea, vomiting, facial flushing, agitation, headache, dizziness, seizures, and death. It is not recommended to improve ventilation. Its role in CNS depression needs to be clarified. It should not be used routinely in comatose patients. It is **contraindicated** in cyclic antidepressant intoxications, stimulant overdose, long-term benzodiazepine use (may precipitate life-threatening withdrawal), if benzodiazepines are used to control seizures, in head trauma.

TABLE 5   Initial Doses of Antidotes for Common Poisonings—cont'd

Antidote	Use	Dose	Route	Adverse Reactions/Comments
Folic Acid (Folvite): Stock level to treat 70 kg adult for 24 h: 4 100-mg vials	Methanol/ethylene glycol (investigational)	1 mg/kg up to 50 mg q4h for 6 doses.	IV	Uncommon
Fomepizole (4-IMP, Antizol): Stock level to treat 70 kg adult for 24 h: 4 1.5-mL vials (1 g/mL)	Ethylene glycol Methanol	Loading dose: 15 mg/kg (0.015 mL/kg) IV followed by maintenance dose of 10 mg/kg (0.01 mL/kg) every 12h for 4 doses, then 15 mg/kg every 12h until ethylene glycol levels are <20 mg/dL.	IV	Suggested: co-administer folate 50 mg IV (child 1 mg/kg), thiamine 100 mg/d (child 50 mg), and pyridoxine 50 mg IV/IM q6h until intoxication is resolved. Monitor for urinary oxalate crystals. Adverse reactions include headache, nausea, and dizziness.
Glucagon: Stock level to treat 70 kg adult for 24 h: (10 vials, 10 units)	β-Blocker, calcium channel blocker	Fomipazole can be given to patients undergoing hemodialysis (dose q4h). 3-10 mg in adult, then infuse 2-5 mg/h (0.05-0.1 mg/kg in child, then infuse 0.07 mg/kg/h) Large doses up to 100 mg/24h used	IV	Antizole should be diluted in 100 mL 0.9% saline or D$_5$W and mixed well. Antizole should not be given undiluted. Use D$_5$W, not 0.9% saline, to reconstitute the glucagon (rather than diluent of Eli Lilly, which contains phenol). Vomiting precautions.
Magnesium Sulfate: Stock level to treat 70 kg adult for 24 h: approx 25 g (50 mL of 50% or 200 mL of 12.5%)	Torsades de pointes	*Adult:* 2 g (20 mL or 20%) over 20 min. If no response in 10 min, repeat and follow by continuous infusion 1 g/h. *Children:* 25-50 mg/kg initially and maintenance is (30-60 mg/kg/24h) (0.25-0.5 mEq/kg/24h) up to 1000 mg/24h. (Dose not studied in controlled fashion.)	IV	Use with caution if renal impairment is present.
Methylene Blue: Stock level to treat 70 kg adult for 24 h: 5 amps (10 mg/10 mL)	Methemoglobinemia	0.1-0.2 mL/kg of 1% solution, slow infusion, may be repeated every 30-60 min	IV	Nausea, vomiting, headache, dizziness.
Naloxone (Narcan): Stock level to treat 70 kg adult for 24 h: 3 vials (1 mg/mL, 10 mL)	Comatose patient; decreased respirations <12; opioids	In postoperative opioid depression reversal, IV 0.1-0.5 μg/kg every 2 min as needed and may repeat up to a total dose of 1 μg/kg In **suspected overdose**, administer IV 0.1 mg/kg in a child younger than 5 years of age up to 2 mg, in older children and adults administer 2 mg every 2 min up to a total of 10-20 mg. Can also be administered into the	IV, ET	**Larger doses** of naloxone may be required for more poorly antagonized synthetic opioid drugs: buprenorphine (Buprenex), codeine, dextromethorphan, fentanyl, pentazocine (Talwin), propoxyphene (Darvon), diphenoxylate, nalbuphine (Nubain), new potent "designer" drugs, or long-acting opioids such as methadone (Dolophine). **Complications.** Although naloxone is safe and effective, there are rare reports of

complications (<1%) of pulmonary edema, seizures, hypertension, cardiac arrest, and sudden death.

The infusions are titrated to avoid respiratory depression and opioid withdrawal manifestations.

Tapering of infusions can be attempted after 12h and when the patient's condition is stable.

endotracheal tube. If no response by 10 mg, a pure opioid intoxication is unlikely.

If opioid abuse is suspected, **restraints** should be in place before administration; **initial dose** 0.1 mg to avoid withdrawal and violent behavior. The initial dose is then doubled every minute progressively to a total of 10 mg.

A continuous infusion has been advocated because many opioids outlast the short half-life of naloxone (30-60 min). The **naloxone infusion hourly rate** to produce a response is equal to the effective dose required (improvement in ventilation and arousal). An additional dose may be required in 15-30 min as a bolus.

Physostigmine (Antilirium): Stock level to treat 70 kg adult for 24 h: 2-4 mg (2 mL each)

Anticholinergic agents (not routinely used, only indicated if life-threatening complications).

IV

Child: 0.02 mg/kg slow push to max 2 mg q30-60 min; Adult: 1-2 mg q5 min to max 6 mg.

Bradycardia, asystole, seizures, bronchospasm, vomiting, headaches. Do not use for cyclic antidepressants.

Pralidoxime (2PAM, Protopan): Stock level to treat 70 kg adult for 24 h: 12 vials (1 g per 20 mL)

Organophosphates/nerve agents

IV

Child ≤12 y, 25-50 mg/kg max (4 mg/min); >12 y, 1-2 g/dose in 250 mL of 0.9% saline over 5-10 min. Max 200 mg/min. Repeat q6-12h for 24-48h. Max adult 6 g/d. Alternative: Maintenance infusion 1 g in 100 mL, of 0.9% saline at 5-20 mg/kg/h (0.5-12 mL/kg/h) up to max 500 mg/h or 50 mL/h. Titrate to desired response. End point is absence of fasciculations and return of muscle strength.

Nausea, dizziness, headache; tachycardia. muscle rigidity, bronchospasm (rapid administration).

Pyridoxine (Vitamin B$_6$): Stock level to treat 70 kg adult for 24 h: 100 mg/mL 10% solution. For a 70 kg patient, 10 g = 10 vials

Seizures from isoniazid or *Gyromitra* mushrooms; ethylene glycol

IV

Isoniazid: Unknown amt ingested: 5 g (70 mg/kg) in 50 mL D$_5$W over 5 min + diazepam 0.3 mg/kg IV at rate of 1 mg/min in child or 10 mg dose at rate up to 5 mg/min in adults. Use different site (synergism). May repeat q5-20 min until seizure controlled.

After seizure is controlled, administer remainder of pyridoxine 1 g/1 g isoniazid total 5 g as infusion over 60 min. Adverse reactions uncommon; do not administer in same bottle as sodium bicarbonate. For *Gyromitra* mushrooms, some use PO 25 mg/kg/d early when mushroom ingestion is suspected.

TABLE 5 Initial Doses of Antidotes for Common Poisonings—cont'd

Antidote	Use	Dose	Route	Adverse Reactions/Comments
		Up to 375 mg/kg have been given (52 g). *Known amount:* 1 g for each gram isoniazid ingested over 5 min with diazepam (dose above) *Gyromitra mushroom:* Child 25 mg/kg or 2-5 g, adults IV over 15-30 min to max 20 g.		
Sodium Bicarbonate (NaHCO₃): Stock level to treat 70 kg adult for 24 h: 10 ampules or syringes (500 mEq)	Tricyclic antidepressant cardiotoxicity (QRS >0.12 sec; severe ventricular tachycardia, severe conduction disturbances); metabolic acidosis; phenothiazine toxicity *Salicylate:* to keep blood pH 7.5-7.55 (not >7.55) and urine pH 7.5-8.0. Alkalinization recommended if salicylate conc. >40 mg/dL in acute poisoning and at lower levels if symptomatic in chronic intoxication. 2 mEq/kg will raise blood pH 0.1 unit	*Ethylene glycol:* 100 mg IV daily. 1-2 mEq/kg undiluted as a bolus. If no effect on cardiotoxicity, repeat twice a few minutes apart

Adult with clear physical signs and laboratory findings of acute moderate or severe salicylism: Bolus 1-2 mEq/kg followed by infusion of 100-150 mEq NaHCO₃ added to 1 L of 5% dextrose at rate of 200-300 mL/h *Child:* Bolus same as adult followed by 1-2 mEq/kg in infusion of 20 mL/kg/h 5% dextrose in 0.45% saline. Add potassium when patient voids. Rate and amount of the initial infusion, if patient is volume depleted: 1 h to achieve urine output of 2 mL/kg/h and urine pH 7-8. | IV | Monitor sodium, potassium, and blood pH because fatal alkalemia and hyponatremia have been reported.

Monitor both urine and blood pH. Do not use the urine pH alone to assess the need for alkalinization because of the paradoxical aciduria that may occur. Adjust the urine pH to 7.5-8 by NaHCO₃ infusion. After urine output established, add potassium 40 mEq/L. |

In mild cases without acidosis and urine pH >6 administer 5% dextrose in 0.9% saline with 50 mEq/L or 1 mEq/kg NaHCO₃ as maintenance to replace ongoing renal losses. If acidemia is present and pH <7.2, add 2 mEq/kg as loading dose followed by 2 mEq/kg q3 to 4h to keep pH at 7.5–7.55. If acidemia is present, recommend isotonic NaHCO₃, 3 ampules to 1 L of D₅W @ 10–15 mL/kg/h or sufficient to produce normal urine flow and a urine pH of 7.5 or higher.

$Long\text{-}acting\ barbiturates:$ Phenobarbital and primidone (Mysoline) Note: Alkalinization is ineffective for the short- or intermediate-acting barbiturates

NaHCO₃: 2 mEq/kg during the first hour or 100 mEq in 1 L of D₅W with 40 mEq/L potassium at rate of 100 mL/h in adults. Adequate potassium is necessary to accomplish alkalinization
— IV — Additional sodium bicarbonate and potassium chloride may be needed. Adjust the urine pH to 7.5–8 by NaHCO₃ infusion.

Thiamine: 100 mg/mL, 2 vials — Thiamine deficiency, ethylene glycol poisoning, alcoholism — IV/IM — 100 mg IV followed with 100 mg V/IM for 5–7 days in an alcoholic and followed by 100 mg/d orally.

Vitamin K₁ (Aqua Mephyton): 10 mg/1–5 mL; 5 mg tablets — Warfarin anticoagulant or rodenticide toxicity — PO/SC, IV — Oral 0.4 mg/kg/dose child, 10–25 mg adults. If evidence of bleeding administer vitamin K₁, SC, IV 0.6 mg/kg/dose child and up to 25–50 mg adults for 6 hours depending on severity. — Give vitamin K daily until PT/INR are normal. Examine stools and urine for evidence of bleeding.

Abbreviations: ALT = alanine aminotransferase; amp = ampule; AST = aspartate aminotransferase; BAL = British anti-Lewisite; BP = blood pressure; Conc. = concentration; ECG = electrocardiogram; ET = endotracheal; G6PD = glucose-6-phosphate dehydrogenase; IM = intramuscular; IV = intravenous; PCC = poison control center; PO = oral; PT = prothrombin time; SC = subcutaneous.

concentration gradient. Anticoagulation with heparin is necessary. Flow rates of 300 to 500 mL/min can be achieved, and clearance rates may reach 200 or 300 mL/min.

Dialyzable substances easily diffuse across the dialysis membrane and have the following characteristics: (a) a molecular weight less than 500 daltons and preferably less than 350; (b) a volume of distribution less than 1 L/kg; (c) protein binding less than 50%; (d) high water solubility (low lipid solubility); and (e) high plasma concentration and a toxicity that correlates reasonably with the plasma concentration. Considerations for hemodialysis and hemoperfusion are cases of serious ingestions (the nephrologist should be notified immediately), and cases involving a compound that is ingested in a potentially lethal dose and the rapid removal of which may improve the prognosis. Examples of the latter are ethylene glycol 1.4 mL/kg 100% solution or equivalent and methanol 6 mL/kg 100% solution or equivalent. Common dialyzable substances include alcohol, bromides, lithium, and salicylates.

The patient-related criteria for dialysis are (a) anticipated prolonged coma and the likelihood of complications; (b) renal compromise (toxin excreted or metabolized by kidneys and dialyzable chelating agents in heavy metal poisoning); (c) laboratory confirmation of lethal blood concentration; (d) lethal dose poisoning with an agent with delayed toxicity or known to be metabolized into a more toxic metabolite (e.g., ethylene glycol, methanol); and (e) hepatic impairment when the agent is metabolized by the liver, and clinical deterioration despite optimal supportive medical management. Table 6 gives plasma concentrations above which removal by extracorporeal measures should be considered.

The contraindications to hemodialysis include the following: (a) substances are not dialyzable; (b) effective antidotes are available; (c) patient is hemodynamically unstable (e.g., shock); and (d) presence of coagulopathy because heparinization is required.

Hemodialysis also has a role in correcting disturbances that are not amenable to appropriate medical management. These are easily remembered by the "vowel" mnemonic:

A—refractory acid–base disturbances
E—refractory electrolyte disturbances
I—intoxication with dialyzable substances (e.g., ethanol, ethylene glycol, isopropyl alcohol, methanol, lithium, and salicylates)
O—overhydration
U—uremia

Complications of dialysis include hemorrhage, thrombosis, air embolism, hypotension, infections, electrolyte imbalance, thrombocytopenia, and removal of therapeutic medications.

HEMOPERFUSION

Hemoperfusion is the parenteral form of oral activated charcoal. Heparinization is necessary. The patient's blood is routed extracorporeally through an outflow arterial catheter through a filter-adsorbing cartridge (charcoal or resin) and returned through a venous catheter. Cartridges must be changed every 4 hours. The blood glucose,

TABLE 6 Plasma Concentrations Above Which Removal by Extracorporeal Measures Should Be Considered

Drug	Plasma Concentration	Protein Binding (%)	Volume Distribution (L/kg)	Method of Choice
Amanitin	NA	25	1.0	HP
Ethanol	500-700 mg/dL	0	0.3	HD
Ethchlorvynol	150 µg/mL	35-50	3-4	HP
Ethylene glycol	25-50 µg/mL	0	0.6	HD
Glutethimide	100 µg/mL	50	2.7	HP
Isopropyl alcohol	400 mg/dL	0	0.7	HD
Lithium	4 mEq/L	0	0.7	HD
Meprobamate (Equanil)	100 µg/mL	0	NA	HP
Methanol	50 mg/dL	0	0.7	HD
Methaqualone	40 µg/dL	20-60	6.0	HP
Other barbiturates	50 µg/dL	50	0-1	HP
Paraquat	0.1 mg/dL	poor	2.8	HP > HD
Phenobarbital	100 µg/dL	50	0.9	HP > HD
Salicylates	80-100 mg/dL	90	0.2	HD > HP
Theophylline		0	0.5	
Chronic	40-60 µg/mL			HP
Acute	80-100 µg/mL			HP
Trichlorethanol	250 µg/mL	70	0.6	HP

Abbreviations: HD = hemodialysis; HP = hemoperfusion; HP > HD hemoperfusion preferred over hemodialysis.
Note: Cartridges for charcoal hemoperfusion are not readily available anymore in most locations, so hemodialysis may be substituted in these situations.
   In mixed or chronic drug overdoses, extracorporeal measures may be considered at lower drug concentrations.
Data from Winchester JF: Active methods for detoxification. In Haddad LM, Winchester JF (eds). Clinical Management of Poisoning and Drug Overdose, 2nd ed. Philadelphia, WB Saunders, 1990; Balsam L, Cortitsidis GN, Fienfeld DA: Role of hemodialysis and hemoperfusion in the treatment of intoxications. Contemp Manage Crit Care 1:61, 1991.

electrolytes, calcium, and albumin levels; complete blood cell count; platelets; and serum and urine osmolarity must be carefully monitored. This procedure has extended extracorporeal removal to a large range of substances that were formerly either poorly dialyzable or nondialyzable. It is not limited by molecular weight, water solubility, or protein binding, but it is limited by a volume distribution greater than 400 L, plasma concentration, and rate of flow through the filter. Activated charcoal cartridges are the primary type of hemoperfusion that is currently available in the United States.

The patient-related criteria for hemoperfusion are (a) anticipated prolonged coma and the likelihood of complications; (b) laboratory confirmation of lethal blood concentrations; (c) hepatic impairment when an agent is metabolized by the liver; and (d) clinical deterioration despite optimally supportive medical management.

The contraindications are similar to those for hemodialysis.

Limited data are available as to which toxins are best treated with hemoperfusion. Hemoperfusion has proved useful in treating glutethimide intoxication, phenobarbital overdose, and carbamazepine, phenytoin, and theophylline intoxication.

Complications include hemorrhage, thrombocytopenia, hypotension, infection, leukopenia, depressed phagocytic activity of granulocytes, decreased immunoglobulin levels, hypoglycemia, hypothermia, hypocalcemia, pulmonary edema, and air and charcoal embolism.

HEMOFILTRATION

Continuous arteriovenous or venovenous hemodiafiltration (CAVHD or CVVHD, respectively) has been suggested as an alternative to conventional hemodialysis when the need for rapid removal of the drug is less urgent. These procedures, like peritoneal dialysis, are minimally invasive, have no significant impact on hemodynamics, and can be carried out continuously for many hours. Their role in the management of acute poisoning remains uncertain, however.

PLASMAPHERESIS

Plasmapheresis consists of removal of a volume of blood. All the extracted components are returned to the blood except the plasma, which is replaced with a colloid protein solution. There are limited clinical data on guidelines and efficacy in toxicology. Centrifugal and membrane separators of cellular elements are used. It can be as effective as hemodialysis or hemoperfusion for removing toxins that have high protein binding, and it may be useful for toxins not filtered by hemodialysis and hemoperfusion.

Plasmapheresis has been anecdotally used in treating intoxications with the following agents: paraquat (removed 10%), propranolol (removed 30%), quinine (removed 10%), L-thyroxine (removed 30%), and salicylate (removed 10%). It has been shown to remove less than 10% of digoxin, phenobarbital, prednisolone, and tobramycin. Complications include infection; allergic reactions including anaphylaxis; hemorrhagic disorders; thrombocytopenia; embolus and thrombus; hypervolemia and hypovolemia; dysrhythmias; syncope; tetany; paresthesia; pneumothorax; acute respiratory distress syndrome; and seizures.

Supportive Care, Observation, and Therapy for Complications

ALTERED MENTAL STATUS

If airway protective reflexes are absent, endotracheal intubation is indicated for a comatose patient or a patient with altered mental status. If respirations are ineffective, ventilation should be instituted, and if hypoxemia persists, supplemental oxygen is indicated. If a cyanotic patient fails to respond to oxygen, the practitioner should consider methemoglobinemia.

HYPOGLYCEMIA

Hypoglycemia accompanies many poisonings, including with ethanol (especially in children), clonidine (Catapres), insulin, organophosphates, salicylates, sulfonylureas, and the unripe fruit or seed of a Jamaican plant called ackee. If hypoglycemia is present or suspected, glucose should be administered immediately as an intravenous bolus. Doses are as follows: in a neonate, 10% glucose (5 mL/kg); in a child, 25% glucose 0.25 g/kg (2 mL/kg); and in an adult, 50% glucose 0.5 g/kg (1 mL/kg).

A bedside capillary test for blood glucose is performed to detect hypoglycemia, and the sample is sent to the laboratory for confirmation. If the glucose reagent strip visually reads less than 150 mg/dL, one administers glucose. Venous blood should be used rather than capillary blood for the bedside test if the patient is in shock or is hypotensive. Large amounts of glucose given rapidly to nondiabetic patients may cause a transient reactive hypoglycemia and hyperkalemia and may accentuate damage in ischemic cerebrovascular and cardiac tissue. If focal neurologic signs are present, it may be prudent to withhold glucose, because hypoglycemia causes focal signs in less than 10% of cases.

THIAMINE DEFICIENCY ENCEPHALOPATHY

Thiamine is administered to avoid precipitating thiamine deficiency encephalopathy (Wernicke-Korsakoff syndrome) in alcohol abusers and in malnourished patients. The overall incidence of thiamine deficiency in ethanol abusers is 12%. Thiamine 100 mg intravenously should be administered around the time of the glucose administration but not necessarily before the glucose. The clinician should be prepared to manage the anaphylaxis that sometimes is caused by thiamine, although it is extremely rare.

OPIOID REACTIONS

Naloxone (Narcan) reverses CNS and respiratory depression, miosis, bradycardia, and decreased gastrointestinal peristalsis caused by opioids acting through μ, κ, and δ receptors. It also affects endogenous opioid peptides (endorphins and enkephalins), which accounts for the variable responses reported in patients with intoxications from ethanol, benzodiazepines, clonidine (Catapres), captopril (Capoten), and valproic acid (Depakote) and in patients with spinal cord injuries. There is a high sensitivity for predicting a response if pinpoint pupils and circumstantial evidence of opioid abuse (e.g., track marks) are present.

In cases of suspected overdose, naloxone 0.1 mg/kg is administered intravenously initially in a child younger than 5 years of age. The dose can be repeated in 2 minutes, if necessary up to a total dose of 2 mg. In older children and adults, the dose is 2 mg every 2 minutes for five doses up to a total of 10 mg. Naloxone can also be administered into an endotracheal tube if intravenous access is unavailable. If there is no response after 10 mg, a pure opioid intoxication is unlikely. If opioid abuse is suspected, restraints should be in place before the administration of naloxone, and it is recommended that the initial dose be 0.1 to 0.2 mg to avoid withdrawal and violent behavior. The initial dose is then doubled every minute progressively to a total of 10 mg. Naloxone may unmask concomitant sympathomimetic intoxication as well as withdrawal.

Larger doses of naloxone may be required for more poorly antagonized synthetic opioid drugs: buprenorphine (Buprenex), codeine, dextromethorphan, fentanyl and its derivatives, pentazocine (Talwin), propoxyphene (Darvon), diphenoxylate, nalbuphine (Nubain), and long-acting opioids such as methadone (Dolophine).

Indications for a continuous infusion include a second dose for recurrent respiratory depression, exposure to poorly antagonized opioids, a large overdose, and decreased opioid metabolism, as with impaired liver function. A continuous infusion has been advocated because many opioids outlast the short half-life of naloxone (30 to 60 minutes). The hourly rate of naloxone infusion is equal to the effective dose required to produce a response (improvement in ventilation and arousal). An additional dose may be required in 15 to 30 minutes as a bolus. The infusions are titrated to avoid respiratory depression and opioid withdrawal manifestations. Tapering of infusions can be attempted after 12 hours and when the patient's condition has been stabilized.

Although naloxone is safe and effective, there are rare reports of complications (less than 1%) of pulmonary edema, seizures, hypertension, cardiac arrest, and sudden death.

AGENTS WHOSE ROLES ARE NOT CLARIFIED

Nalmefene (Revex), a long-acting parenteral opioid antagonist that the Food and Drug Administration has approved, is undergoing investigation, but its role in the treatment of comatose patients and patients with opioid overdose is not clear. It is 16 times more potent than naloxone, and its duration of action is up to 8 hours (half-life 10.8 hours, versus naloxone 1 hour).

Flumazenil (Romazicon) is a pure competitive benzodiazepine antagonist. It has been demonstrated to be safe and effective for reversing benzodiazepine-induced sedation. It is not recommended to improve ventilation. Its role in cases of CNS depression needs to be clarified. It should not be used routinely in comatose patients and is not an essential ingredient of the coma therapeutic regimen. It is contraindicated in cases of co-ingestion of cyclic antidepressant intoxication, stimulant overdose, and long-term benzodiazepine use (may precipitate life-threatening withdrawal) if benzodiazepines are used to control seizures. There is a concern about the potential for seizures and cardiac dysrhythmias that may occur in these settings.

Laboratory and Radiographic Studies

An electrocardiogram (ECG) should be obtained to identify dysrhythmias or conduction delays from cardiotoxic medications. If aspiration pneumonia (history of loss of consciousness, unarousable state, vomiting) or noncardiac pulmonary edema is suspected, a chest radiograph is needed. Electrolyte and glucose concentrations in the blood, the anion gap, acid–base balance, the arterial blood gas (ABG) profile (if patient has respiratory distress or altered mental status), and serum osmolality should be measured if a toxic alcohol ingestion is suspected. Table 7 lists appropriate testing on the basis of clinical toxicologic presentation. All laboratory specimens should be carefully labeled, including time and date. For potential legal cases, a "chain of custody" must be established. Assessment of the laboratory studies may provide a clue to the etiologic agent.

ELECTROLYTE, ACID-BASE, AND OSMOLALITY DISTURBANCES

Electrolyte and acid–base disturbances should be evaluated and corrected. Metabolic acidosis (usually low or normal pH with a low or normal/high $Paco_2$ and low HCO_3) with an increased anion gap is seen with many agents in cases of overdose.

The anion gap is an estimate of those anions other than chloride and HCO_3 necessary to counterbalance the

TABLE 7   Patient Condition/Systemic Toxin and Appropriate Tests

Condition	Tests
Comatose	Toxicologic tests (acetaminophen, sedative-hypnotic, ethanol, opioids, benzodiazepine), glucose.
Respiratory toxicity	Spirometry, FEV_1, arterial blood gases, chest radiograph, monitor O_2 saturation
Cardiac toxicity	ECG 12-lead and monitoring, echocardiogram, serial cardiac enzymes (if evidence or suspicion of a myocardial infarction), hemodynamic monitoring
Hepatic toxicity	Enzymes (AST, ALT, GGT), ammonia, albumin, bilirubin, glucose, PT, PTT, amylase
Nephrotoxicity	BUN, creatinine, electrolytes (Na, F, Mg, Ca, PO_4), serum and urine osmolarity, 24-hour urine for heavy metals if suspected, creatine kinase, serum and urine myoglobin, urinalysis and urinary sodium
Bleeding	Platelets, PT, PTT, bleeding time, fibrin split products, fibrinogen, type and match

Abbreviations: ALT = alanine aminotransaminase; AST = aspartate aminotransaminase; BUN = blood urea nitrogen; ECG = electrocardiogram; FEV₁ = forced expiratory volume at 1 second; GGT = γ-glutamyltransferase; PT = prothrombin time; PTT = partial thromboplastin time.

TABLE 8 Etiologies of Metabolic Acidosis

Normal Anion Gap Hyperchloremic	Increased Anion Gap Normochloremic	Decreased Anion Gap
Acidifying agents	Methanol	Laboratory error[†]
Adrenal insufficiency	Uremia*	Intoxication—bromine, lithium
Anhydrase inhibitors	Diabetic ketoacidosis*	Protein abnormal
Fistula	Paraldehyde,* phenformin	Sodium low
Osteotomies	Isoniazid	
Obstructive uropathies	Iron	
Renal tubular acidosis	Lactic acidosis[†]	
Diarrhea, uncomplicated*	Ethanol,* ethylene glycol*	
Dilutional	Salicylates, starvation solvents	
Sulfamylon		

*Indicates hyperosmolar situation. Studies have found that the anion gap may be relatively insensitive for determining the presence of toxins.
†Lactic acidosis can be produced by intoxications of the following: carbon monoxide, cyanide, hydrogen sulfide, hypoxia, ibuprofen, iron, isoniazid, phenformin, salicylates, seizures, theophylline.

positive charge of sodium. It serves as a clue to causes, compensations, and complications. The anion gap (AG) is calculated from the standard serum electrolytes by subtracting the total CO_2 (which reflects the actual measured bicarbonate) and chloride from the sodium: $(Na - [Cl + HCO_3]) = AG$. The potassium is usually not used in the calculation because it may be hemolyzed and is an intracellular cation. The lack of anion gap does not exclude a toxic etiology.

The normal gap is usually 7 to 11 mEq/L by flame photometer. However, there has been a "lowering" of the normal anion gap to 7 ± 4 mEq/L by the newer techniques (e.g., ion selective electrodes or colorimetric titration). Some studies have found anion gaps to be relatively insensitive for determining the presence of toxins.

It is important to recognize anion gap toxins, such as salicylates, methanol, and ethylene glycol, because they have specific antidotes, and hemodialysis is effective in management of cases of overdose with these agents.

Table 8 lists the reasons for increased anion gap, decreased anion gap, or no gap. The most common cause of a decreased anion gap is laboratory error. Lactic acidosis produces the largest anion gap and can result from any poisoning that results in hypoxia, hypoglycemia, or convulsions.

Table 9 lists other blood chemistry derangements that suggest certain intoxications.

Serum osmolality is a measure of the number of molecules of solute per kilogram of solvent, or mOsm/kg water. The osmolarity is molecules of solute per liter of solution, or mOsm/L water at a specified temperature. Osmolarity is usually the calculated value and osmolality is usually a measured value. They are considered interchangeable where 1 L equals 1 kg. The normal serum osmolality is 280 to 290 mOsm/kg. The freezing point serum osmolarity measurement specimen and the serum electrolyte specimens for calculation should be drawn simultaneously.

The serum osmolal gap is defined as the difference between the measured osmolality determined by the freezing point method and the calculated osmolarity. It is determined by the following formula:

$$(Sodium \times 2) + (BUN/3) + (Glucose/20)$$

(where BUN is blood urea nitrogen).

This gap estimate is normally within 10 mOsm of the simultaneously measured serum osmolality. Ethanol, if present, may be included in the equation to eliminate its influence on the osmolal gap (the ethanol concentration divided by 4.6; Table 10).

The osmolal gap is not valid in cases of shock and postmortem state. Metabolic disorders such as hyperglycemia, uremia, and dehydration increase the osmolarity but usually do not cause gaps greater than 10 mOsm/kg.

TABLE 9 Blood Chemistry Derangements in Toxicology

Derangement	Toxin
Acetonemia without acidosis	Acetone or isopropyl alcohol
Hypomagnesemia	Ethanol, digitalis
Hypocalcemia	Ethylene glycol, oxalate, fluoride
Hyperkalemia	β-Blockers, acute digitalis, renal failure
Hypokalemia	Diuretics, salicylism, sympathomimetics, theophylline, corticosteroids, chronic digitalis
Hyperglycemia	Diazoxide, glucagon, iron, isoniazid, organophosphate insecticides, phenylurea insecticides, phenytoin (Dilantin), salicylates, sympathomimetic agents, thyroid, vasopressors
Hypoglycemia	β-Blockers, ethanol, insulin, isoniazid, oral hypoglycemic agents, salicylates
Rhabdomyolysis	Amphetamines, ethanol, cocaine, or phencyclidine, elevated creatine phosphokinase

TABLE 10 Conversion Factors for Alcohols and Glycols

Alcohols/Glycols	1 mg/dL in Blood Raises Osmolality mOsm/L	Molecular Weight	Conversion Factor
Ethanol	0.228	40	4.6
Methanol	0.327	32	3.2
Ethylene glycol	0.190	62	6.2
Isopropanol	0.176	60	6.0
Acetone	0.182	58	5.8
Propylene glycol	not available	72	7.2

Example: Methanol osmolality. Subtract the calculated osmolality from the measured serum osmolarity (freezing point method) = osmolar gap × 3.2 (one-tenth molecular weight) = estimated serum methanol concentration.
Note: This equation is often not considered very reliable in predicting the actual measured blood concentration of these alcohols or glycols.

A gap greater than 10 mOsm/mL suggests that unidentified osmolal-acting substances are present: acetone, ethanol, ethylene glycol, glycerin, isopropyl alcohol, isoniazid, ethanol, mannitol, methanol, and trichloroethane. Alcohols and glycols should be sought when the degree of obtundation exceeds that expected from the blood ethanol concentration or when other clinical conditions exist: visual loss (methanol), metabolic acidosis (methanol and ethylene glycol), or renal failure (ethylene glycol).

A falsely elevated osmolar gap can be produced by other low molecular weight un-ionized substances (dextran, diuretics, sorbitol, ketones), hyperlipidemia, and unmeasured electrolytes (e.g., magnesium).

Note: A normal osmolal gap may be reported in the presence of toxic alcohol or glycol poisoning, if the parent compound is already metabolized. This situation can occur when the osmolar gap is measured after a significant time has elapsed since the ingestion. In cases of alcohol and glycol intoxication, an early osmolar gap is a result of the relatively nontoxic parent drug and delayed metabolic acidosis, and an anion gap is a result of the more toxic metabolites.

The serum concentration is calculated as mg/dL = mOsm gap × MW of substance divided by 10.

RADIOGRAPHIC STUDIES

Chest and neck radiographs are useful for suspected pathologic conditions such as aspiration pneumonia, pulmonary edema, and foreign bodies and to determine the location of the endotracheal tube. Abdominal radiographs can be used to detect radiopaque substances.

The mnemonic for radiopaque substances seen on abdominal radiographs is CHIPES:

C—chlorides and chloral hydrate
H—heavy metals (arsenic, barium, iron, lead, mercury, zinc)
I—iodides
P—PlayDoh, Pepto-Bismol, phenothiazine (inconsistent)
E—enteric-coated tablets
S—sodium, potassium, and other elements in tablet form (bismuth, calcium, potassium) and solvents containing chlorides (e.g., carbon tetrachloride)

TOXICOLOGIC STUDIES

Routine blood and urine screening is of little practical value in the initial care of the poisoned patient. Specific toxicologic analyses and quantitative levels of certain drugs may be extremely helpful. One should always ask oneself the following questions: (a) How will the result of the test alter the management? and (b) Can the result of the test be returned in time to have a positive effect on therapy?

Owing to long turnaround time, lack of availability, factors contributing to unreliability, and the risk of serious morbidity without supportive clinical management, toxicology screening is estimated to affect management in less than 15% of cases of drug overdoses or poisonings. Toxicology screening may look specifically for only 40 to 50 drugs out of more than 10,000 possible drugs or toxins and more than several million chemicals. To detect many different drugs, toxic screens usually include methods with broad specificity, and sensitivity may be poor for some drugs, resulting in false-negative or false-positive findings. On the other hand, some drugs present in therapeutic amounts may be detected on the screen, even though they are causing no clinical symptoms. Because many agents are not sought or detected during a toxicologic screening, a negative result does not always rule out poisonings. The specificity of toxicologic tests is dependent on the method and the laboratory. The presence of other drugs, drug metabolites, disease states, or incorrect sampling may cause erroneous results.

For the average toxicologic laboratory, false-negative results occur at a rate of 10% to 30% and false-positives at a rate of 0% to 10%. The positive screen predictive value is approximately 90%. A negative toxicology screen does not exclude a poisoning. The negative predictive value of toxicologic screening is approximately 70%. For example, the following benzodiazepines may not be detected by some routine immunoassay benzodiazepine screening tests: alprazolam (Xanax), clonazepam (Klonopin), temazepam (Restoril), and triazolam (Halcion).

The "toxic urine screen" is generally a qualitative urine test for several common drugs, usually substances of abuse (cocaine and metabolites, opioids, amphetamines, benzodiazepines, barbiturates, and phencyclidine). Results of these tests are usually available within 2 to 6 hours. Because these tests may vary with each hospital and community, the physician should determine exactly which substances are included in the toxic urine screen of his or her laboratory. Tests for ethylene glycol, red blood cell cholinesterase, and serum cyanide are not readily available.

For cases of ingestion of certain substances, quantitative blood levels should be obtained at specific times after the ingestion to avoid spurious low values in the distribution phase, which result from incomplete absorption. The detection time for drugs is influenced by many variables, such as type of substance, formulation, amount, time since ingestion, duration of exposure, and half-life. For many drugs, the detection time is measured in days after the exposure.

Common Poisons

ACETAMINOPHEN (PARACETAMOL, N-ACETYL-PARAAMINOPHENOL)

Toxic Mechanism

At therapeutic doses of acetaminophen, less than 5% is metabolized by P450-2E1 to a toxic reactive oxidizing metabolite, N-acetyl-p-benzoquinoneimine (NAPQI). In a case of overdose, there is insufficient glutathione available to reduce the excess NAPQI into nontoxic conjugate, so it forms covalent bonds with hepatic intracellular proteins to produce centrilobular necrosis. Renal damage is caused by a similar mechanism.

Toxic Dose

The therapeutic dose of acetaminophen is 10 to 15 mg/kg, with a maximum of five doses in 24 hours for a maximum total daily dose of 4 g. An acute single toxic dose is greater than 140 mg/kg, possibly greater than 200 mg/kg in a child younger than age 5 years. Factors affecting the P450 enzymes include enzyme inducers such as barbiturates and phenytoin (Dilantin), ingestion of isoniazid, and alcoholism. Factors that decrease glutathione stores (alcoholism, malnutrition, and HIV infection) contribute to the toxicity of acetaminophen. Alcoholics ingesting 3 to 4 g/d of acetaminophen for a few days can have depleted glutathione stores and require N-acetylcysteine therapy at 50% below hepatotoxic blood acetaminophen levels on the nomogram.

Kinetics

Peak plasma concentration is usually reached 2 to 4 hours after an overdose. Volume distribution is 0.9 L/kg, and protein binding is less than 50% (albumin).

Route of elimination is by hepatic metabolism to an inactive nontoxic glucuronide conjugate and inactive nontoxic sulfate metabolite by two saturable pathways; less than 5% is metabolized into reactive metabolite NAPQI. In patients younger than 6 years of age, metabolic elimination occurs to a greater degree by conjugation via the sulfate pathway.

The half-life of acetaminophen is 1 to 3 hours.

Manifestations

The four phases of the intoxication's clinical course may overlap, and the absence of a phase does not exclude toxicity.

- Phase I occurs within 0.5 to 24 hours after ingestion and may consist of a few hours of malaise, diaphoresis, nausea, and vomiting or produce no symptoms. CNS depression or coma is not a feature.
- Phase II occurs 24 to 48 hours after ingestion and is a period of diminished symptoms. The liver enzymes, serum aspartate aminotransferase (AST) (earliest), and serum alanine aminotransferase (ALT) may increase as early as 4 hours or as late as 36 hours after ingestion.
- Phase III occurs at 48 to 96 hours, with peak liver function abnormalities at 72 to 96 hours. The degree of elevation of the hepatic enzymes generally correlates with outcome, but not always. Recovery starts at about 4 days unless hepatic failure develops. Less than 1% of patients with a history of overdose develop fulminant hepatotoxicity.
- Phase IV occurs at 4 to 14 days, with hepatic enzyme abnormalities resolving. If extensive liver damage has occurred, sepsis and disseminated intravascular coagulation may ensue.

Transient renal failure may develop at 5 to 7 days with or without evidence of hepatic damage. Rare cases of myocarditis and pancreatitis have been reported. Death can occur at 7 to 14 days.

Laboratory Investigations

The therapeutic reference range is 10 to 20 μg/mL. For toxic levels, see the nomogram presented in Figure 1.

Appropriate and reliable methods for analysis are radioimmunoassay, high-pressure liquid chromatography, and gas chromatography. Spectroscopic assays often give falsely elevated values: bilirubin, salicylate, salicylamide, diflunisal (Dolobid), phenols, and methyldopa (Aldomet) increase the acetaminophen level. Each 1 mg/dL increase in creatinine increases the acetaminophen plasma level 30 μg/mL.

If a toxic acetaminophen level is reached, liver profile (including AST, ALT, bilirubin, and prothrombin time), serum amylase, and blood glucose must be monitored. A complete blood cell count (CBC); platelet count; phosphate, electrolytes, and bicarbonate level measurements; ECG; and urinalysis are indicated.

Management

Gastrointestinal Decontamination

Although ipecac-induced emesis may be useful within 30 minutes of ingestion of the toxic substance, we do not advise it because it could result in vomiting of the activated charcoal. Gastric lavage is not necessary. Studies have indicated that activated charcoal is useful within 1 hour after ingestion. Activated charcoal does adsorb N-acetylcysteine (NAC) if given together, but this is not clinically important. However, if activated charcoal needs to be given along with NAC, separate the administration of activated charcoal from the administration of NAC by 1 to 2 hours to avoid vomiting.

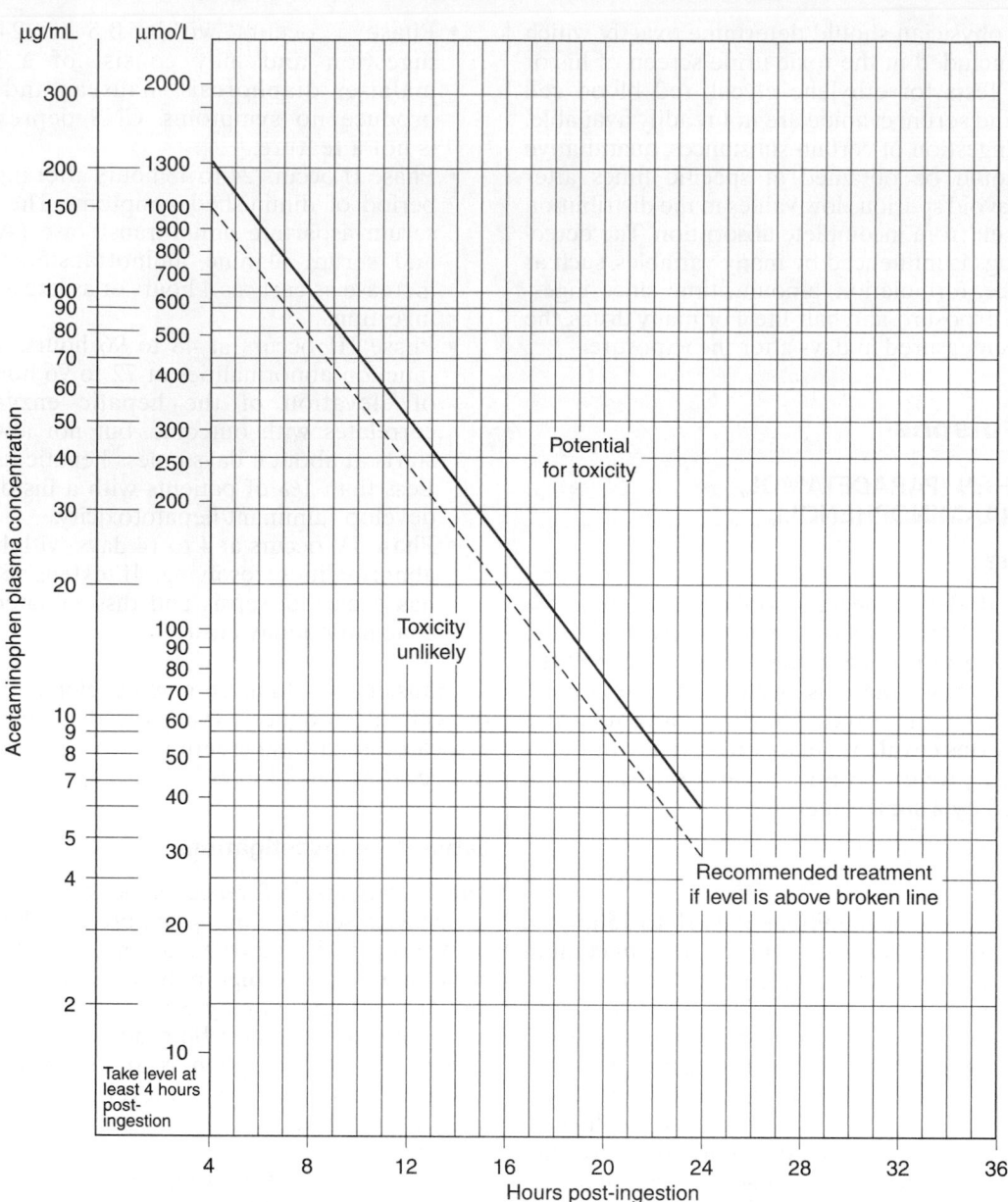

FIGURE 1. Nomogram for acetaminophen intoxication. *N*-acetylcysteine therapy is started if levels and time coordinates are above the lower line on the nomogram. Continue and complete therapy even if subsequent values fall below the toxic zone. The nomogram is useful only in cases of acute single ingestion. Levels in serum drawn before 4 hours may not represent peak levels. (From Rumack BH, Matthew H: Acetaminophen poisoning and toxicity. Pediatrics 55:871, 1975.)

N-Acetylcysteine (Mucomyst)

NAC (Table 11), a derivative of the amino acid cysteine, acts as a sulfhydryl donor for glutathione synthesis, as surrogate glutathione, and may increase the nontoxic sulfation pathway resulting in conjugation of NAPQI. Oral NAC should be administered within the first 8 hours after a toxic amount of acetaminophen has been ingested. NAC can be started while one awaits the results of the blood test for acetaminophen plasma concentration, but there is no advantage to giving it before 8 hours. If the acetaminophen concentration result after 4 hours following ingestion is above the upper line on the modified Rumack-Matthew nomogram (see Figure 1), one should continue with a maintenance course. Repeat blood specimens should be obtained 4 hours after the initial level is measured if it is greater than 20 mg/mL, which is below the therapy line, because of unexpected delays in the peak by food and co-ingestants. Intravenous NAC (see Table 11) is approved in the United States.

There have been a few cases of anaphylactoid reaction and death by the intravenous route.

Variations in Therapy

In patients with chronic alcoholism, it is recommended that NAC treatment be administered at 50% below the upper toxic line on the nomogram.

TABLE 11 Protocol for *N*-Acetylcysteine Administration

Route	Loading Dose	Maintenance Dose	Course	FDA Approval
Oral	140 mg/kg	70 mg/kg every 4 h	72 h	Yes
Intravenous	150 mg/kg over 15 min	50 mg/kg over 4 h followed by 100 mg/kg over 16h	20 h	Yes

If emesis occurs within 1 hour after NAC administration, the dose should be repeated. To avoid emesis, the proper dilution from 20% to 5% NAC must be used, and it should be served in a palatable vehicle, in a covered container through a straw. If this administration is unsuccessful, a slow drip over 30 to 60 minutes through a nasogastric tube or a fluoroscopically placed nasoduodenal tube can be used. Antiemetics can be used if necessary: metoclopramide (Reglan) 10 mg per dose intravenously 30 minutes before administration of NAC (in children, 0.1 mg/kg; maximum, 0.5 mg/kg/d) or ondansetron (Zofran) 32 mg (0.15 mg/kg) by infusion over 15 minutes and repeated for three doses if necessary. The side effects of these antiemetics include anaphylaxis and increases in liver enzymes.

Some investigators recommend variable durations of NAC therapy, stopping the therapy if serial acetaminophen blood concentrations become nondetectable and the liver enzyme levels (ALT and AST) remain normal after 24 to 36 hours.

There is a loss of efficacy if NAC is initiated 8 or 10 hours postingestion, but the loss is not complete, and NAC may be initiated 36 hours or more after ingestion. Late treatment (after 24 hours) decreases the rates of morbidity and mortality in patients with fulminant liver failure caused by acetaminophen and other agents.

Extended relief formulations (*ER* embossed on caplet) contain 325 mg of acetaminophen for immediate release and 325 mg for delayed release. A single 4-hour postingestion serum acetaminophen concentration can underestimate the level because ER formulations can have secondary delayed peaks. In cases of overdose of the ER formulation, it is recommended that additional acetaminophen levels be obtained at 4-hour intervals after the initial level is measured. If any level is in the toxic zone, therapy should be initiated.

It is recommended that pregnant patients with toxic plasma concentrations of acetaminophen be treated with NAC to prevent hepatotoxicity in both fetus and mother. The available data suggest no teratogenicity to NAC or acetaminophen.

Indications for NAC therapy in cases of chronic intoxication are a history of ingestion of 3 to 4 g for several days with elevated liver enzyme levels (AST and ALT). The acetaminophen blood concentration is often low in these cases because of the extended time lapse since ingestion and should not be plotted on the Rumack-Matthew nomogram. Patients with a history of chronic alcoholism or those on chronic enzyme inducers may also present with elevated liver enzyme levels and should be considered for NAC therapy if they have a history of taking acetaminophen on a chronic basis, because they are considered to be at a greater risk for hepatotoxicity despite a low acetaminophen blood concentration.

Specific support care may be needed to treat liver failure, pancreatitis, transient renal failure, and myocarditis.

Liver transplantation has a definite but limited role in patients with acute acetaminophen overdose. A retrospective analysis determined that a continuing rise in the prothrombin time (4-day peak, 180 seconds), a pH of less than 7.3 2 days after the overdose, a serum creatinine level of greater than 3.3 mg/dL, severe hepatic encephalopathy, and disturbed coagulation factor VII/V ratio greater than 30 suggest a poor prognosis and may be indicators for hepatology consultation for consideration of liver transplantation.

Extracorporeal measures are not expected to be of benefit.

Disposition

Adults who have ingested more than 140 mg/kg and children younger than 6 years of age who have ingested more than 200 mg/kg should receive therapy within 8 hours postingestion or until the results of the 4-hour postingestion acetaminophen plasma concentration are known.

AMPHETAMINES

The amphetamines include illicit methamphetamine ("Ice"), diet pills, and formulations under various trade names. Analogues include MDMA (3,4 methylenedioxymethamphetamine, known as "ecstasy," "XTC," "Adam") and MDA (3,4-methylenedioxyamphetamine, known as "Eve"). MDA is a common hallucinogen and euphoriant "club drug" used at "raves," which are all-night dances. Use of methamphetamine and designer analogues is on the rise, especially among young people between the ages of 12 and 25 years. Other similar stimulants are phenylpropanolamine and cocaine.

Toxic Mechanism

Amphetamines have a direct CNS stimulant effect and a sympathetic nervous system effect by releasing catecholamines from α- and β-adrenergic nerve terminals but inhibiting their reuptake.

Hallucinogenic MDMA has an additional hazard of serotonin effect (refer to serotonin syndrome in the SSRI section). MDMA also affects the dopamine system in the brain. Because of its effects on 5-hydroxytryptamine, dopamine, and norepinephrine, MDMA can lead to serotonin syndrome associated with malignant hyperthermia and rhabdomyolysis, which contributes to the potentially life-threatening hyperthermia observed in several patients who have used MDMA.

Phenylpropanolamine stimulates only the β-adrenergic receptors.

Toxic Dose

In children, the toxic dose of dextroamphetamine is 1 mg/kg; in adults, the toxic dose is 5 mg/kg. The potentially fatal dose of dextroamphetamine is 12 mg/kg.

Kinetics

Amphetamine is a weak base with pKa of 8 to 10. Onset of action is 30 to 60 minutes, and peak effects are 2 to 4 hours. The volume distribution is 2 to 3 L/kg.

Through hepatic metabolism, 60% of the substance is metabolized into a hydroxylated metabolite that may be responsible for psychotic effects.

The half-life of amphetamines is pH dependent—8 to 10 hours in acid urine (pH <6.0) and 16 to 31 hours in alkaline urine (pH >7.5). Excretion is by the kidney—30% to 40% at alkaline urine pH and 50% to 70% at acid urine pH.

Manifestations

Effects are seen within 30 to 60 minutes following ingestion.

Neurologic manifestations include restlessness, irritation and agitation, tremors and hyperreflexia, and auditory and visual hallucinations. Hyperpyrexia may precede seizures, convulsions, paranoia, violence, intracranial hemorrhage, psychosis, and self-destructive behavior. Paranoid psychosis and cerebral vasculitis occur with chronic abuse.

MDMA is often adulterated with cocaine, heroin, or ketamine, or a combination of these, to create a variety of mood alterations. This possibility must be taken into consideration when one manages patients with MDMA ingestions, as the symptom complex may reflect both CNS stimulation and CNS depression.

Other manifestations include dilated but reactive pupils, cardiac dysrhythmias (supraventricular and ventricular), tachycardia, hypertension, rhabdomyolysis, and myoglobinuria.

Laboratory Investigations

The clinician should monitor ECG and cardiac readings, ABG and oxygen saturation, electrolytes, blood glucose, BUN, creatinine, creatine kinase, cardiac fraction if there is chest pain, and liver profile. Also, one should evaluate for rhabdomyolysis and check urine for myoglobin, cocaine and metabolites, and other substances of abuse. The peak plasma concentration of amphetamines is 10 to 50 ng/mL 1 to 2 hours after ingestion of 10 to 25 mg. The toxic plasma concentration is 200 ng/mL. When the rapid immunoassays are used, cross-reactions can occur with amphetamine derivatives (e.g., MDA, "ecstasy"), brompheniramine (Dimetane), chlorpromazine (Thorazine), ephedrine, phenylpropanolamine, phentermine (Adipex-P), phenmetrazine, ranitidine (Zantac), and Vicks Inhaler (L-desoxyephedrine). False-positive results may occur.

Management

Management is similar to management for cocaine intoxication. Supportive care includes blood pressure and temperature control, cardiac monitoring, and seizure precautions. Diazepam (Valium) can be administered. Gastrointestinal decontamination can be undertaken with activated charcoal administered up to 1 hour after ingestion.

Anxiety, agitation, and convulsions are treated with diazepam. If diazepam fails to control seizures, neuromuscular blockers can be used and the electroencephalogram (EEG) monitored for nonmotor seizures. One should avoid neuroleptic phenothiazines and butyrophenone, which can lower the seizure threshold.

Hypertension and tachycardia are usually transient and can be managed by titration of diazepam. Nitroprusside can be used for hypertensive crisis at a maximum infusion rate of 10 µg/kg/minute for 10 minutes followed with a lower infusion rate of 0.3 to 2 mg/kg/minute. Myocardial ischemia is managed by oxygen, vascular access, benzodiazepines, and nitroglycerin. Aspirin and thrombolytics are not routinely recommended because of the danger of intracranial hemorrhage. It is important to distinguish between angina and true ischemia. Delayed hypotension can be treated with fluids and vasopressors if needed. Life-threatening tachydysrhythmias may respond to an α-blocker such as phentolamine (Regitine) 5 mg IV for adults or 0.1 mg/kg IV for children and a short-acting β-blocker such as esmolol (Brevibloc) 500 µg/kg IV over 1 minute for adults, or 300 to 500 µg/kg over 1 minute for children. Ventricular dysrhythmias may respond to lidocaine or, in a severely hemodynamically compromised patient, immediate synchronized electrical cardioversion.

Rhabdomyolysis and myoglobinuria are treated with fluids, alkaline diuresis, and diuretics. Hyperthermia is treated with external cooling and cool 100% humidified oxygen. More extensive therapy may be needed in severe cases. If focal neurologic symptoms are present, the possibility of a cerebrovascular accident should be considered and a CT scan of the head should be obtained.

Paranoid ideation and threatening behavior should be treated with rapid tranquilization using a benzodiazepine. One should observe for suicidal depression that may follow intoxication and may require suicide precautions.

Extracorporeal measures are of no benefit.

Disposition

Symptomatic patients should be observed on a monitored unit until the symptoms resolve and then observed for a short time after resolution for relapse.

ANTICHOLINERGIC AGENTS

Drugs with anticholinergic properties include antihistamines (H₁ blockers), neuroleptics (phenothiazines), tricyclic antidepressants, antiparkinsonism drugs (trihexyphenidyl [Artane], benztropine [Cogentin]), ophthalmic products (atropine), and a number of common plants.

The antihistamines are divided into the sedating anticholinergic types, and the nonsedating single daily dose types. The sedating types include ethanolamines (e.g., diphenhydramine [Benadryl], dimenhydrinate [Dramamine], and clemastine [Tavist]), ethylenediamines (e.g., tripelennamine

[Pyribenzamine]), alkyl amines (e.g., chlorpheniramine [Chlor-Trimeton], brompheniramine [Dimetane]), piperazines (e.g., cyclizine [Marezine], hydroxyzine [Atarax], and meclizine [Antivert]), and phenothiazine (e.g., Phenergan). The nonsedating types include astemizole (Hismanal), terfenadine (Seldane), loratadine (Claritin), fexofenadine (Allegra), and cetirizine (Zyrtec).

The anticholinergic plants include jimsonweed (*Datura stramonium*), deadly nightshade (*Atropa belladonna*), henbane (*Hyoscyamus niger*), and antispasmodic agents for the bowel (atropine derivatives).

Toxic Mechanism

By competitive inhibition, anticholinergics block the action of acetylcholine on postsynaptic cholinergic receptor sites. The toxic mechanism primarily involves the peripheral and CNS muscarinic receptors. H_1 sedating-type agents also depress or stimulate the CNS, and in large overdoses some have cardiac membrane–depressant effects (e.g., diphenhydramine [Benadryl]) and α-adrenergic receptor blockade effects (e.g., promethazine [Phenergan]). Nonsedating agents produce peripheral H_1 blockade but do not possess anticholinergic or sedating actions. The original agents terfenadine (Seldane) and astemizole (Hismanal) were recently removed from the market because of the severe cardiac dysrhythmias associated with their use, especially when used in combination with macrolide antibiotics and certain antifungal agents such as ketoconazole (Nizoral), which inhibit hepatic metabolism or excretion. The newer nonsedating agents, including loratadine (Claritin), fexofenadine (Allegra), and cetirizine (Zyrtec), have not been reported to cause the severe drug interactions associated with terfenadine and astemizole.

Toxic Dose

The estimated toxic oral dose of atropine is 0.05 mg/kg in children and more than 2 mg in adults. The minimal estimated lethal dose of atropine is more than 10 mg in adults and more than 2 mg in children. Other synthetic anticholinergic agents are less toxic, and the fatal dose varies from 10 to 100 mg.

The estimated toxic oral dose of diphenhydramine (Benadryl) in a child is 15 mg/kg, and the potential lethal amount is 25 mg/kg. In an adult, the potential lethal amount is 2.8 g. Ingestion of five times the single dose of an antihistamine is toxic.

For the nonsedating agents, an overdose of 3360 mg of terfenadine was reported in an adult who developed ventricular tachycardia and fibrillation that responded to lidocaine and defibrillation. A 1500-mg overdose produced hypotension. Cases of delayed serious dysrhythmias (torsades de pointes) have been reported with doses of more than 200 mg of astemizole. The toxic doses of fexofenadine (Allegra), cetirizine, and loratadine (Claritin) need to be established.

Kinetics

The onset of absorption of intravenous atropine is in 2 to 4 minutes. Peak effects on salivation after intravenous or intramuscular administration are at 30 to 60 minutes.

Onset of absorption after oral ingestion is 30 to 60 minutes, peak action is 1 to 3 hours, and duration of action is 4 to 6 hours, but symptoms are prolonged in cases of overdose or with sustained-release preparations.

The onset of absorption of diphenhydramine is in 15 minutes to 1 hour, with a peak of action in 1 to 4 hours. Volume distribution is 3.3 to 6.8 L/kg, and protein binding is 75% to 80%. Ninety-eight percent of diphenhydramine is metabolized via the liver by *N*-demethylation. Interactions with erythromycin, ketoconazole (Nizoral), and derivatives produce excessive blood levels of the antihistamine and ventricular dysrhythmias.

The half-life of diphenhydramine is 3 to 10 hours.

The chemical structure of nonsedating agents prevents their entry into the CNS. Absorption begins in 1 hour, with peak effects in 4 in 6 hours. The duration of action is greater than 24 hours.

These agents are metabolized in the gastrointestinal tract and liver. Protein binding is greater than 90%. The plasma half-life is 3.5 hours. Only 1% is excreted unchanged; 60% of that is excreted in the feces and 40% in the urine.

Manifestations

Anticholinergic signs are hyperpyrexia ("hot as a hare"), mydriasis ("blind as a bat"), flushing of skin ("red as a beet"), dry mucosa and skin ("dry as a bone"), "Lilliputian type" hallucinations and delirium ("mad as a hatter"), coma, dysphagia, tachycardia, moderate hypertension, and rarely convulsions and urinary retention. Other effects include jaundice (cyproheptadine [Periactin]), dystonia (diphenhydramine [Benadryl]), rhabdomyolysis (doxylamine), and, in large doses, cardiotoxic effects (diphenhydramine).

Overdose with nonsedating agents produces headache and confusion, nausea, and dysrhythmias (e.g., torsades de pointes).

Laboratory Investigations

Monitoring of ABG (in cases of respiratory depression), electrolytes, glucose, and the ECG should be undertaken. Anticholinergic drugs and plants are not routinely included on screens for substances of abuse.

Management

For patients in respiratory failure, intubation and assisted ventilation should be instituted. Gastrointestinal decontamination can be instituted. Caution must be taken with emesis in cases of diphenhydramine (Benadryl) overdose because of the drug's rapid onset of action and risk of seizures. If bowel sounds are present for up to 1 hour after ingestion, activated charcoal can be given. Seizures can be controlled with benzodiazepines (diazepam [Valium] or lorazepam [Ativan]).

The administration of physostigmine (Antilirium) is not routine and is reserved for life-threatening anticholinergic effects that are refractory to conventional treatments. It should be administered with adequate monitoring and resuscitative equipment available. The use of physostigmine should be avoided if a tricyclic antidepressant is present because of increased toxicity. Urinary retention should be relieved by catheterization to avoid reabsorption of the drug and additional toxicity.

Supraventricular tachycardia should be treated only if the patient is hemodynamically unstable. Ventricular dysrhythmias can be controlled with lidocaine or cardioversion. Sodium bicarbonate 1 to 2 mEq/kg IV may be useful for myocardial depression and QRS prolongation. Torsades de pointes, especially when associated with terfenadine and astemizole ingestion, has been treated with magnesium sulfate 4 g or 40 mL 10% solution intravenously over 10 to 20 minutes and countershock if the patient fails to respond.

Hyperpyrexia is controlled by external cooling. Hemodialysis and hemoperfusion are not effective.

Disposition

Antihistamine H₁ Antagonists

Symptomatic patients should be observed on a monitored unit until the symptoms resolve, then observed for a short time (3 to 4 hours) after resolution for relapse.

Nonsedating Agents

All asymptomatic children who acutely ingest more than the maximum adult dose and all symptomatic children should be referred to a health care facility for a minimum of 6 hours' observation as well as cardiac monitoring. Asymptomatic adults who acutely ingest more than twice the maximum adult daily dose should be monitored for a minimum of 6 hours. All symptomatic patients should be monitored for as long as there are symptoms present.

BARBITURATES

Barbiturates have been used as sedatives, anesthetic agents, and anticonvulsants, but their use is declining as safer, more effective drugs become available.

Toxic Mechanism

Barbiturates are γ-aminobutyric acid (GABA) agonists (increasing the chloride flow and inhibiting depolarization). They enhance the CNS depressant effect of GABA and depress the cardiovascular system.

Toxic Dose

The shorter-acting barbiturates (including the intermediate-acting agents) and their hypnotic doses are as follows: amobarbital (Amytal), 100 to 200 mg; aprobarbital (Alurate), 50 to 100 mg; butabarbital (Butisol), 50 to 100 mg; butalbital, 100 to 200 mg; pentobarbital (Nembutal), 100 to 200 mg; secobarbital (Seconal), 100 to 200 mg. They cause toxicity at lower doses than long-acting barbiturates and have a minimum toxic dose of 6 mg/kg; the fatal adult dose is 3 to 6 g.

The long-acting barbiturates and their doses include mephobarbital (Mebaral), 50 to 100 mg, and phenobarbital, 100 to 200 mg. Their minimum toxic dose is greater than 10 mg/kg, and the fatal adult dose is 6 to 10 g. A general rule is that an amount five times the hypnotic dose is toxic and an amount 10 times the hypnotic dose is potentially fatal. Methohexital and thiopental are ultrashort-acting parenteral preparations and are not discussed.

Kinetics

The barbiturates are enzyme inducers. Short-acting barbiturates are highly lipid-soluble, penetrate the brain readily, and have shorter elimination times. Onset of action is in 10 to 30 minutes, with a peak at 1 to 2 hours. Duration of action is 3 to 8 hours. The volume distribution of short-acting barbiturate is 0.8 to 1.5 L/kg; pKa is about 8. Mean half-life varies from 8 to 48 hours.

Long-acting agents have longer elimination times and can be used as anticonvulsants. Onset of action is in 20 to 60 minutes, with a peak at 1 to 6 hours. In cases of overdose, the peak can be at 10 hours. Usual duration of action is 8 to 12 hours. Volume distribution is 0.8 L/kg, and half-life is 11 to 120 hours. The pKa of phenobarbital is 7.2. Alkalinization of urine promotes its excretion.

Manifestations

Mild intoxication resembles alcohol intoxication and includes ataxia, slurred speech, and depressed cognition. Severe intoxication causes slow respirations, coma, and loss of reflexes (except pupillary light reflex).

Other manifestations include hypotension (vasodilation), hypothermia, hypoglycemia, and death by respiratory arrest.

Laboratory Investigations

Most barbiturates are detected on routine drug screens and can be measured in most hospital laboratories. Investigation should include barbiturate level; ABG; toxicology screen, including acetaminophen; glucose, electrolyte, BUN, creatinine, and creatine kinase levels; and urine pH. The minimum toxic plasma levels are greater than 10 µg/mL for short-acting barbiturates and greater than 40 µg/dL for long-acting agents. Fatal levels are 30 µg/mL for short-acting barbiturates and 80 to 150 µg/mL for long-acting agents. Both short-acting and long-acting agents can be detected in urine 24 to 72 hours after ingestion, and long-acting agents can be detected up to 7 days.

Management

Vital functions must be established and maintained. Intensive supportive care including intubation and assisted ventilation should dominate the management. All stuporous and comatose patients should have glucose (for hypoglycemia), thiamine (if chronically alcoholic), and naloxone (Narcan) (in case of an opioid ingestion) intravenously and should be admitted to the intensive care unit. Emesis should be avoided especially in cases of ingestion of the shorter-acting barbiturates. Activated charcoal followed by MDAC (0.5 g/kg) every 2 to 4 hours has been shown to reduce the serum half-life of phenobarbital by 50%, but its effect on clinical course is undetermined.

Fluids should be administered to correct dehydration and hypotension. Vasopressors may be necessary to correct severe hypotension, and hemodynamic monitoring may be needed. The patient must be observed carefully for fluid overload. Alkalinization (ion trapping) is used only for phenobarbital (pKa 7.2) but not for short-acting barbiturates. Sodium bicarbonate, 1 to 2 mEq/kg IV in 500 mL of 5% dextrose in adults or 10 to 15 mL/kg in children during the first hour, followed by sufficient bicarbonate to keep the urinary pH at 7.5 to 8.0, enhances excretion of phenobarbital and shortens the half-life by 50%. Diuresis is not advocated because of the danger of cerebral or pulmonary edema.

Hemodialysis shortens the half-life to 8 to 14 hours, and charcoal hemoperfusion shortens the half-life to 6 to 8 hours for long-acting barbiturates such as phenobarbital. Both procedures may be effective in patients with both long-acting and short-acting barbiturate ingestion. If the patient does not respond to supportive measures or if the phenobarbital plasma concentration is greater than 150 µg/mL, both procedures may be tried to shorten the half-life.

Bullae are treated as a local second-degree skin burn. Hypothermia should be treated.

Disposition

All comatose patients should be admitted to the intensive care unit. Awake and oriented patients with an overdose of short-acting agents should be observed for at least 6 asymptomatic hours; overdose of long-acting agents warrants observation for at least 12 asymptomatic hours because of the potential for delayed absorption. In the case of an intentional overdose, psychiatric clearance is needed before the patient can be discharged. Chronic use can lead to tolerance, physical dependency, and withdrawal and necessitates follow-up.

BENZODIAZEPINES

Benzodiazepines are used as anxiolytics, sedatives, and relaxants.

Toxic Mechanism

The GABA agonists produce CNS depression and increase chloride flow, inhibiting depolarization.

Flunitrazepam (Rohypnol; street name "roofies") is a long-acting benzodiazepine agonist sold by prescription in more than 60 countries worldwide, but it is not legally available in the United States.

Toxic Dose

The long-acting benzodiazepines (half-life >24 hours) and their maximum therapeutic doses are as follows: chlordiazepoxide (Librium), 50 mg; clorazepate (Tranxene), 30 mg; clonazepam (Klonopin), 20 mg; diazepam (Valium), 10 mg in adults or 0.2 mg/kg in children; flurazepam (Dalmane), 30 mg; and prazepam, 20 mg.

The short-acting benzodiazepines (half-life 10 to 24 hours) and their doses include the following: alprazolam (Xanax), 0.5 mg, and lorazepam (Ativan), 4 mg in adults or 0.05 mg/kg in children, which act similar to the long-acting benzodiazepines.

The ultrashort-acting benzodiazepines (half-life <10 hours) are more toxic and include temazepam (Restoril), 30 mg; triazolam (Halcion), 0.5 mg; midazolam (Versed), 0.2 mg/kg; and oxazepam (Serax), 30 mg.

In cases of overdose of short- and long-acting agents, 10 to 20 times the therapeutic dose (>1500 mg diazepam or 2000 mg chlordiazepoxide) have been ingested with resulting mild coma but without respiratory depression. Fatalities are rare, and most patients recover within 24 to 36 hours after overdose. Asymptomatic unintentional overdoses of less than five times the therapeutic dose can be seen. Ultrashort-acting agents have produced respiratory arrest and coma within 1 hour after ingestion of 5 mg of triazolam (Halcion) and death with ingestion of as little as 10 mg. Midazolam (Versed) and diazepam (Valium) by rapid intravenous injection have produced respiratory arrest.

Kinetics

Onset of CNS depression is usually in 30 to 120 minutes; peak action usually occurs within 1 to 3 hours when ingestion is by the oral route. The volume distribution varies from 0.26 to 6 L/kg (LA, 1.1 L/kg); protein binding is 70% to 99%. For flunitrazepam, the onset of action is in 0.5 to 2 hours, oral peak is in 2 hours, and duration 8 hours or more. The half-life of flunitrazepam is 20 to 30 hours, volume distribution is 3.3 to 5.5 L/kg, and 80% is protein bound. Flunitrazepam can be identified in urine 4 to 30 days after ingestion.

Manifestations

Neurologic manifestations include ataxia, slurred speech, and CNS depression. Deep coma leading to respiratory depression suggests the presence of short-acting benzodiazepines or other CNS depressants. In elderly persons, the therapeutic doses can produce toxicity and can have an additive effect with other CNS depressants. Chronic use can lead to tolerance, physical dependency, and withdrawal.

Laboratory Investigations

Most benzodiazepines can be detected in urine drug screens. Quantitative blood levels are not useful. Some of the immunoassay urinary screens cannot detect all of the new benzodiazepines currently available. A consultation with the laboratory analyst is warranted if a specific case occurs in which the test result is negative but benzodiazepine use is suspected by the patient's history. Situations in which benzodiazepines may not be detected include ingestion of a low dose (e.g., <10 mg), rapid elimination, and a different or no metabolite. Some immunoassay methods can produce a false-positive finding for the benzodiazepines when nonsteroidal anti-inflammatory drugs (tolmetin [Tolectin], naproxen [Aleve], etodolac [Lodine], and fenoprofen [Nalfon]) are used. If this is a concern, the laboratory analyst should be consulted.

In cases in which "date rape" drugs such as flunitrazepam are suspected, a police crime or reference laboratory should be consulted for testing.

Management

Emesis and gastric lavage should be avoided. Activated charcoal can be useful only if given early before the peak time of absorption occurs. Supportive treatment should be instituted but rarely requires intubation or assisted ventilation.

Flumazenil (Romazicon) is a specific benzodiazepine receptor antagonist that blocks the chloride flow and inhibitor of GABA neurotransmitters. It reverses the sedative effects of benzodiazepines, zolpidem (Ambien), and endogenous benzodiazepines associated with hepatic encephalopathy. It is not recommended to reverse benzodiazepine-induced hypoventilation. The manufacturer advises that flumazenil be used with caution in cases of overdose with possible benzodiazepine dependency (because it can precipitate life-threatening withdrawal), if cyclic antidepressant use is suspected, or if a patient has a known seizure disorder.

Disposition

If the patient is comatose, he or she must be admitted to the intensive care unit. If the overdose was intentional, psychiatric clearance is needed before the patient can be discharged.

β-ADRENERGIC BLOCKERS (β-BLOCKERS)

β-Blockers are used in the treatment of hypertension and of a number of systemic and ophthalmologic disorders. Properties of β-blockers include the factors listed in Table 12.

Lipid-soluble drugs have CNS effects, active metabolites, longer duration of action, and interactions (e.g., propranolol). Cardioselectivity is lost in overdose. Intrinsic partial agonist agents (e.g., pindolol) may initially produce tachycardia and hypertension. Cardiac membrane depressive effect (quinidine-like) occurs in cases of overdose but not at therapeutic doses (e.g., with metoprolol or sotalol). α-Blocking effect is weak (e.g., with labetalol or acebutolol).

Toxic Mechanism

β-Blockers compete with the catecholamines for receptor sites and block receptor action in the bronchi, the vascular smooth muscle, and the myocardium.

Toxic Dose

Ingestions of greater than twice the maximum recommended daily therapeutic dose are considered toxic (see Table 12). Ingestion of 1 mg/kg propranolol in a child may produce hypoglycemia. Fatalities have been reported in adults with 7.5 g of metoprolol. The most toxic agent is sotalol, and the least toxic is atenolol.

Kinetics

Regular-release formulations usually cause symptoms within 2 hours. Propranolol's onset of action is 20 to 30 minutes and peak is at 1 to 4 hours, but it may be delayed by co-ingestants. The onset of action with sustained-release preparations may be delayed to 6 hours and the peak to 12 to 16 hours. Volume distribution is 1 to 5.6 L/kg. Protein binding is variable, from 5% to 93%.

TABLE 12   Pharmacologic and Toxic Properties of β-Blockers

Blocker	Maximum Solubility	Therapeutic Plasma Level	Lipid Solubility	Intrinsic Sympathomimetic Activity (Partial Agonist)	Membrane Stabilizing Effect β-Selective β₁	β₂	Cardiac Selectivity α-Selective
Acebutolol (Sectral)	800 mg	200-2000 ng/mL	Moderate	+	+	+	+
Alprenolol[2]	800 mg	50-200 ng/mL	Moderate	2+	+	–	–
Atenolol (Tenormin)	100 mg	200-500 ng/mL	Low	–	–	2+	–
Betaxolol (Kerlone)	20 mg	NA	Low	+	–	+	–
Carteolol (Cartrol)	10 mg	NA	No	+	–	–	–
Esmolol (Brevibloc) (Class II antidysrhythmic, IV only)			Low	–	–	+	–
Labetalol (Trandate)	800 mg	50-500 ng/mL	Low	+	+/–	–	+
Levobunolol (AKBeta eyedrop) (Eye drops 0.25% and 0.5%)	20 mg	NA	No	–	–	–	–
Metoprolol (Lopressor)			Moderate	–	–	2+	–
Nadolol (Corgard)	320 mg	20-40 ng/mL	Low	–	–	–	–
Oxyprenolol[2]	480 mg	80-100 ng/mL	Moderate	2+	+	–	–
Pindolol (Visken)	60 mg	50-150 ng/mL	Moderate	3+	+/–	–	–
Propranolol (Inderal) (Class II antidysrhythmic)	360 mg	50-100 ng/mL	High	–	2+	–	–
Sotalol (Betapace) (Class II antidysrhythmic)	480 mg	500-4000 ng/mL	Low	–	–	–	–
Timolol (Blocadren)	60 mg	5-10 ng/mL	Low	–	+/–	–	–

[2]Not available in the United States.

Metabolism

Atenolol (Tenormin), nadolol (Corgard), and santalol (Betapace) have enterohepatic recirculation. The duration of action for regular-acting agents is 4 to 6 hours, but in cases of overdose it may be 24 to 48 hours. The duration of action for sustained-release agents is 24 to 48 hours.

The regular preparation with the longest half-life is nadolol, at 12 to 24 hours, and the one with the shortest half-life is esmolol, at 5 to 10 minutes.

Manifestations

See "Toxic Properties" and Table 12.

Highly lipid soluble agents produce coma and seizures. Bradycardia and hypotension are the major cardiac symptoms and may lead to cardiogenic shock. Intrinsic partial agonists initially may cause tachycardia and hypertension. ECG changes include atrioventricular conduction delay or asystole. Membrane-depressant effects produce prolonged QRS and QT interval, which may result in torsades de pointes. Sotalol produces a very prolonged QT interval. Bronchospasm may occur in patients with reactive airway disease with any β-blocker because the selectivity is lost in overdose. Other manifestations include hypoglycemia (because β-blockers block catecholamine counter-regulatory mechanisms) and hyperkalemia.

Laboratory Investigations

Measurements of blood levels are not readily available or useful. ECG and cardiac monitoring should be maintained, and blood glucose and electrolytes, BUN, and creatinine levels should be monitored, as well as ABG if there are respiratory symptoms.

Management

Vital functions must be established and maintained. Vascular access, baseline ECG, and continuous cardiac and blood pressure monitoring should be established. A pacemaker must be available. Gastrointestinal decontamination can be undertaken initially with activated charcoal up to 1 hour after ingestion. MDAC is no longer recommended, based on the latest guidelines. Whole-bowel irrigation can be considered in cases of large overdoses with sustained-release preparations, but there are no studies evaluating the efficacy of intervention.

If there are cardiovascular disturbances, a cardiac consultation should be obtained. Class IA antidysrhythmic agents (procainamide, quinidine) and III (bretylium) are not recommended. Hypotension is treated with fluids initially, although it usually does not respond. Frequently, glucagon and cardiac pacing are needed. Bradycardia in asymptomatic, hemodynamically stable patients requires no therapy. It is not predictive of the future course of the disease. If the patient is unstable (has hypotension or a high-degree atrioventricular block), atropine 0.02 mg/kg (up to 2 mg) in adults, glucagon, and a pacemaker can be used. In case of ventricular tachycardia, overdrive pacing can be used. A wide QRS interval may respond to sodium bicarbonate. Torsades de pointes (associated with sotalol) may respond to magnesium sulfate and overdrive pacing. Prophylactic magnesium for prolonged QT interval has been suggested, but there are no data. Epinephrine must not be used because an unopposed α effect may occur.

Hypotension and myocardial depression are managed by correction of dysrhythmias, Trendelenburg position, fluids, glucagon, or amrinone (Inocor), or a combination of these. Hemodynamic monitoring with a Swan-Ganz catheter or arterial line may be necessary to manage fluid therapy.

Glucagon is the initial drug of choice. It works through adenyl cyclase and bypasses catecholamine receptors; therefore, it is not affected by β-blockers. Glucagon increases cardiac contractility and heart rate. It is given as an intravenous bolus of 5 to 10 mg[C] over 1 minute and followed by a continuous infusion of 1 to 5 mg/h (in children, 0.15 mg/kg followed by 0.05 to 0.1 mg/kg/h). In large doses and in infusion therapy D_5W, sterile water, or saline should be used as a dilutant to reconstitute glucagon in place of the 0.2% phenol diluent provided with some drugs. Effects are seen within minutes. It can be used with other agents such as amrinone.

Amrinone (Inocor) inhibits phosphodiesterase enzyme, which metabolizes cyclic AMP. It is administered as a bolus of 0.15 to 2 mg/kg (0.15 to 0.4 mL/kg) intravenously, followed by infusion of 5 to 10 μg/kg/min.

Hypoglycemia should be treated with intravenous glucose. Life-threatening hyperkalemia is treated with calcium (avoid if digoxin is present), bicarbonate, and glucose or insulin. Convulsions can be controlled with diazepam or phenobarbital. If bronchospasm is present, $β_2$ nebulized bronchodilators are given.

Extraordinary measures such as intra-aortic balloon pump support can be instituted. Extracorporeal measures can be undertaken. Hemodialysis for cases of atenolol, acebutolol, nadolol, and sotalol (low volume distribution, low protein binding) ingestion may be helpful, particularly when there is evidence of renal failure. Hemodialysis is not effective for propranolol, metoprolol, and timolol.

Prenalterol[A] has successfully reversed both bradycardia and hypotension but is not currently available in the United States.

Disposition

Asymptomatic patients with history of overdose require baseline ECG and continuous cardiac monitoring for at least 6 hours with regular-release preparations and for 24 hours with sustained-release preparations. Symptomatic patients should be observed with cardiac monitoring for 24 hours. If seizures or abnormal rhythm or vital signs are present, the patient should be admitted to the intensive care unit.

CALCIUM CHANNEL BLOCKERS

Calcium channel blockers are used in the treatment of effort angina, supraventricular tachycardia, and hypertension.

Toxic Mechanism

Calcium channel blockers reduce influx of calcium through the slow channels in membranes of the myocardium, the

---

[A]Not available in the United States.
[C]Exceeds dosage recommended by the manufacturer.

atrioventricular nodes, and the vascular smooth muscles and result in peripheral, systemic, and coronary vasodilation, impaired cardiac conduction, and depression of cardiac contractility. All calcium channel blockers have vasodilatory action, but only bepridil, diltiazem, and verapamil depress myocardial contractility and cause atrioventricular block.

Toxic Dose

Any ingested amount greater than the maximum daily dose has the potential of severe toxicity. The maximum oral daily doses in adults and toxic doses in children of each are as follows: amlodipine (Norvasc), 10 mg for adults and more than 0.25 mg/kg for children; bepridil (Vascor), 400 mg for adults and more than 5.7 mg/kg for children; diltiazem (Cardizem), 360 mg for adults (toxic dose > 2 g) and more than 6 mg/kg for children; felodipine (Plendil), 40 mg for adults and more than 0.56 mg/kg for children; isradipine (DynaCirc), 40 mg for adults and more than 0.4 mg/kg for children; nicardipine (Cardene), 120 mg for adults and more than 0.85 mg/kg for children; nifedipine (Procardia), 120 mg for adults and more than 2 mg/kg for children; nimodipine (Nimotop), 360 mg for adults and more than 0.85 mg/kg for children; nitrendipine (Baypress),[A] 80 mg for adults and more than 1.14 mg/kg for children; and verapamil (Calan), 480 mg for adults and 15 mg/kg for children.

Kinetics

Onset of action of regular-release preparations varies: for verapamil it is 60 to 120 minutes, for nifedipine 20 minutes, and for diltiazem 15 minutes after ingestion. Peak effect for verapamil is 2 to 4 hours, for nifedipine 60 to 90 minutes, and for diltiazem 30 to 60 minutes, but the peak action may be delayed for 6 to 8 hours. Duration of action is up to 36 hours. The onset of action for sustained-release preparations is usually 4 hours but may be delayed, and peak effect is at 12 to 24 hours. In cases of massive overdose, concretions and prolonged toxicity can develop.

Volume distribution varies from 3 to 7 L/kg. Hepatic elimination half-life varies from 3 to 7 hours. Patients receiving digitalis and calcium channel blockers run the risk of digitalis toxicity, because calcium channel blockers increase digitalis levels.

Manifestations

Cardiac manifestations include hypotension, bradycardia, and conduction disturbances occurring 30 minutes to 5 hours after ingestion. A prolonged PR interval is an early finding and may occur at therapeutic doses. Torsades de pointes has been reported. All degrees of blocks may occur and may be delayed up to 16 hours. Lactic acidosis may be present. Calcium channel blockers do not affect intraventricular conduction, so the QRS interval is usually not affected.

Hypocalcemia is rarely present. Hyperglycemia may be present because of interference in calcium-dependent insulin release. Mental status changes, headaches, seizures, hemiparesis, and CNS depression may occur.

[A]Not available in the United States.

Laboratory Investigations

Specific drug levels are not readily available and are not useful. Monitor blood sugar, electrolytes, calcium, ABG, pulse oximetry, creatinine, and BUN, and also use hemodynamic monitoring, ECG, and cardiac monitoring.

Management

Vital functions must be established and maintained. Baseline ECG readings should be obtained and continuous cardiac and blood pressure monitoring maintained. A pacemaker should be available. Cardiology consultation should be sought.

Gastrointestinal decontamination with activated charcoal is recommended. If a large dose of a sustained-release preparation was ingested, whole-bowel irrigation can be considered, but its effectiveness has not been investigated.

If the patient is symptomatic, immediate cardiology consult must be obtained, because a pacemaker and hemodynamic monitoring may be needed. In the case of heart block, atropine is rarely effective and isoproterenol (Isuprel) may produce vasodilation. The use of a pacemaker should be considered early.

Hypotension and bradycardia can be treated with positioning, fluids, and calcium gluconate or chloride, glucagon, amrinone (Inocor), and ventricular pacing. Calcium salts must be avoided if digoxin is present. Calcium usually reverses depressed myocardial contractility but may not reverse nodal depression or peripheral vasodilation. Calcium chloride can be given in a 10% solution, 0.1 to 0.2 mL/kg up to 10 mL in an adult, or calcium gluconate in a 10% solution 0.3 to 0.4 mL/kg up to 20 mL in an adult. Administration is intravenous, over 5 to 10 minutes. One should monitor for dysrhythmias, hypotension, and the serum ionized calcium. The aim is to increase calcium 4 mg/dL to a maximum of 13 mg/dL. The calcium response lasts 15 minutes and may require repeated doses or a continuous calcium gluconate infusion 0.2 mL/kg/h up to maximum of 10 mL/h.

If calcium fails, glucagon can be tried for its positive inotropic and chronotropic effect, or both. Amrinone (Inocor), an inotropic agent, may reverse the effects of calcium channel blockers. An effective dose is 0.15 mg to 2 mg/kg (0.15 to 0.4 mL/kg) by intravenous bolus followed by infusion of 5 to 10 μg/kg/min.

In case of hypotension, fluids, norepinephrine (Levophed), and epinephrine may be required. Amrinone and glucagon have been tried alone and in combination. Dobutamine and dopamine are often ineffective.

Extracorporeal measures (e.g., hemodialysis and charcoal hemoperfusion) are not useful, but extraordinary measures such as intra-aortic balloon pump and cardiopulmonary bypass have been used successfully.

For cases of calcium channel blocker toxicity that fail to respond to aggressive management, recent studies demonstrate that insulin and glucose have therapeutic value. The suggested dose range for insulin is to infuse regular insulin at 0.5 IU/kg/h with a simultaneous infusion of glucose 1 g/kg/h, with glucose monitoring every 30 minutes for at least the first 4 hours of administration and subsequent glucose adjustment to maintain euglycemia (70 to 100 mg/dL). Potassium levels should be monitored regularly, as they may shift in response to the insulin.

Disposition

Patients who have ingested regular-release preparations should be monitored for at least 6 hours and those who have ingested sustained-release preparations should be monitored for 24 hours after the ingestion. Intentional overdose necessitates psychiatric clearance. Symptomatic patients should be admitted to the intensive care unit.

CARBON MONOXIDE

Carbon monoxide is an odorless, colorless gas produced from incomplete combustion; it is also an in vivo metabolic breakdown product of methylene chloride used in paint removers.

Toxic Mechanism

Carbon monoxide's affinity for hemoglobin is 240 times greater than that of oxygen. It shifts the oxygen dissociation curve to the left, which impairs hemoglobin release of oxygen to tissues and inhibits the cytochrome oxidase enzymes.

Toxic Dose and Manifestations

Table 13 describes the manifestations of carbon monoxide toxicity. Exposure to 0.5% for a few minutes is lethal. Sequelae correlate with the patient's level of consciousness at presentation. ECG abnormalities may be noted. Creatine kinase is often elevated, and rhabdomyolysis and myoglobinuria may occur.

The carboxyhemoglobin (CoHB) expresses in percentage the extent to which carbon monoxide has bound with the total hemoglobin. This may be misleadingly low in the anemic patient with less hemoglobin than normal. The patient's presentation is a more reliable indicator of severity than the CoHB level. The manifestations listed in Table 13 for each level are in addition to those listed at the level above. The CoHB may not correlate reliably with the severity of the intoxication, and linking symptoms to specific levels of CoHB frequently leads to inaccurate conclusions. A level of carbon monoxide greater than 40% is usually associated with obvious intoxication.

Kinetics

The natural metabolism of the body produces small amounts of CoHB, less than 2% for nonsmokers and 5% to 9% for smokers.

Carbon monoxide is rapidly absorbed through the lungs. The rate of absorption is directly related to alveolar ventilation. Elimination also occurs through the lungs. The half-life of CoHB in room air (21% oxygen) is 5 to 6 hours; in 100% oxygen, it is 90 minutes; in hyperbaric pressure at 3 atmospheres oxygen, it is 20 to 30 minutes.

Laboratory Investigations

An ABG reading may show metabolic acidosis and normal oxygen tension. In cases of significant poisoning, the ABG, electrolytes, blood glucose, serum creatine kinase and cardiac enzymes, renal function tests, and liver function tests should be monitored. A urinalysis and test for myoglobinuria should be obtained. Chest radiograph can be useful in cases of smoke inhalation or if the patient is being considered for hyperbaric chamber. ECG monitoring should be maintained, especially if the patient is older than 40 years, has a history of cardiac disease, or has moderate to severe symptoms. Which toxicology studies are used is based on symptoms and circumstances. CoHB should be monitored during and at the end of therapy. The pulse oximeter has two wavelengths and overestimates oxyhemoglobin saturation in carbon monoxide poisoning. The true oxygen saturation is determined by blood gas analysis, which measures the oxygen bound to hemoglobin. The co-oximeter measures four wavelengths and separates out CoHB and the other hemoglobin binding agents from oxyhemoglobin. Fetal hemoglobin has a greater affinity for carbon monoxide than adult hemoglobin and may falsely elevate the CoHB as much as 4% in young infants.

Management

The first step is to adequately protect the rescuer. The patient must be removed from the contaminated area, and his or her vital functions must be established.

The mainstay of treatment is 100% oxygen via a non-rebreathing mask with an oxygen reservoir or endotracheal tube. All patients receive 100% oxygen until the CoHB level is 5% or less. Assisted ventilation may be necessary. ABG and CoHB should be monitored and the present CoHB level determined. *Note:* A near-normal CoHB level does not exclude significant carbon monoxide poisoning, especially if the measurement is taken several hours after termination of exposure or if oxygen has been administered prior to obtaining the sample.

The exposed pregnant woman should be kept on 100% oxygen for several hours after the CoHB level is almost 0, because carbon monoxide concentrates in the fetus and oxygen is needed longer to ensure elimination of the carbon monoxide from fetal circulation. The fetus must be

TABLE 13 Carbon Monoxide Exposure and Possible Manifestations

CoHB Saturation (%)	Manifestations
3.5	None
5	Slight headache, decreased exercise tolerance
10	Slight headache, dyspnea on vigorous exertion, may impair driving skills
10-20	Moderate dyspnea on exertion, throbbing, temporal headache
20-30	Severe headache, syncope, dizziness, visual changes, weakness, nausea, vomiting, altered judgment
30-40	Vertigo, ataxia, blurred vision, confusion, loss of consciousness
40-50	Confusion, tachycardia, tachypnea, coma, convulsions
50-60	Cheyne-Stokes, coma, convulsions, shock, apnea
60-70	Coma, convulsions, respiratory and heart failure, death

monitored, because carbon monoxide and hypoxia are potentially teratogenic.

Metabolic acidosis should be treated with sodium bicarbonate only if the pH is below 7.2 after correction of hypoxia and adequate ventilation. Acidosis shifts the oxygen dissociation curve to the right and facilitates oxygen delivery to the tissues.

The decision to use the hyperbaric oxygen chamber must be made on the basis of the ability to handle other acute emergencies that may coexist in the patient and of the severity of the poisoning. The standard of care for persons exposed to carbon monoxide has yet to be determined, but most authorities recommend using the hyperbaric oxygen chamber under any of the following conditions:

- If the patient is in a coma or has a history of loss of consciousness or seizures
- If there is cardiovascular dysfunction (clinical ischemic chest pain or ECG evidence of ischemia)
- If the patient has metabolic acidosis
- If symptoms persist despite 100% oxygen therapy
- In a child, if the initial CoHB is greater than 15%
- In symptomatic patients with preexisting ischemia
- If there are signs of maternal or fetal distress regardless of CoHB level (infants and fetus are a special problem because fetal hemoglobin has greater affinity for carbon monoxide)

Although controversial, a neurologic-cognitive examination has been used to help determine which patients with low carbon monoxide levels should receive more aggressive therapy. Testing should include the following: general orientation memory testing involving address, phone number, date of birth, and present date; and cognitive testing, involving counting by 7s, digit span, and forward and backward spelling of three-letter and four-letter words. Patients with delayed neurologic sequelae or recurrent symptoms up to 3 weeks may benefit from hyperbaric oxygen chamber treatment.

Seizures and cerebral edema must be treated.

Disposition

Patients with no or mild symptoms who become asymptomatic after a few hours of oxygen therapy and have a carbon monoxide level less than 10%, and normal physical and neurologic-cognitive examination findings can be discharged, but they should be instructed to return if any signs of neurologic dysfunction appear. Patients with carbon monoxide poisoning requiring treatment need follow-up neuropsychiatric examinations.

CAUSTICS AND CORROSIVES

The terms *caustic* and *corrosive* are used interchangeably and can be divided into acids and alkalis. The U.S. Consumer Product Safety Commission Labeling Recommendations on containers for acids and alkalis indicate the potential for producing serious damage, as follows:

- Caution—weak irritant
- Warning—strong irritant
- Danger—corrosive

Some common acids with corrosive potential include acetic acid, formic acid, glycolic acid, hydrochloric acid, mercuric chloride, nitric acid, oxalic acid, phosphoric acid, sulfuric acid (battery acid), zinc chloride, and zinc sulfate. Some common alkalis with corrosive potential include ammonia, calcium carbide, calcium hydroxide (dry), calcium oxide, potassium hydroxide (lye), and sodium hydroxide (lye).

Toxic Mechanism

Acids produce mucosal coagulation necrosis and may be absorbed systemically; they do not penetrate deeply. Injury to the gastric mucosa is more likely, although specific sites of injury for acids and alkalis are not clearly defined.

Alkalis produce liquefaction necrosis and saponification and penetrate deeply. The esophageal mucosa is likely to be damaged. Oropharyngeal and esophageal damage is more frequently caused by solids than by liquids. Liquids produce superficial circumferential burns and gastric damage.

Toxic Dose

The toxicity is determined by concentration, contact time, and pH. Significant injury is more likely with a substance that has a pH of less than 2 or greater than 12, with a prolonged contact time, and with large volumes.

Manifestations

The absence of oral burns does not exclude the possibility of esophageal or gastric damage. General clinical findings are stridor; dysphagia; drooling; oropharyngeal, retrosternal, and epigastric pain; and ocular and oral burns. Alkali burns are yellow, soapy, frothy lesions. Acid burns are gray-white and later form an eschar. Abdominal tenderness and guarding may be present if perforation has happened.

Laboratory Investigations

If acid ingestion has taken place, the patient's acid–base balance and electrolyte status should be determined. If pulmonary symptoms are present, a chest radiograph, ABG measurement, and pulse oximetry are called for.

Management

It is recommended that the container be brought to the examination, as the substance must be identified and the pH of the substance, vomitus, tears, or saliva tested.

If the acid or alkali has been ingested, all gastrointestinal decontamination procedures are contraindicated except for immediate rinse, removal of substance from the mouth, and dilution with small amounts (sips) of milk or water. The examiner should check for ocular and dermal involvement. Contraindications to oral dilution are dysphagias, respiratory distress, obtundation, or shock. If there is ocular involvement one should immediately irrigate the eye with tepid water for at least 30 minutes, perform fluorescein stain of eye, and consult an ophthalmologist. If there is dermal involvement, one should immediately remove contaminated clothes and irrigate the skin with tepid water for at least 15 minutes. Consultation with a burn specialist is called for.

In cases of acid ingestion, some authorities advocate a small flexible nasogastric tube and aspiration within 30 minutes after ingestion.

Patients should receive only intravenous fluids following dilution until endoscopic consultation is obtained. Endoscopy is valuable to predict damage and risk of stricture. The indications are controversial, with some authorities recommending it in all cases of caustic ingestions regardless of symptoms, and others selectively using clinical features such as vomiting, stridor, drooling, and oral or facial lesions as criteria. We recommend endoscopy for all symptomatic patients or patients with intentional ingestions. Endoscopy may be performed immediately if the patient is symptomatic, but it is usually done 12 to 48 hours postingestion.

The use of corticosteroids is considered controversial. Some feel they may be useful for patients with second-degree circumferential burns. They recommend starting with hydrocortisone sodium succinate (Solu-Cortef) intravenously 10 to 20 mg/kg/d within 48 hours and changing to oral prednisolone 2 mg/kg/d for 3 weeks before tapering the dose. We do not usually recommend using corticosteroids because they have not been shown to be effective.

Tetanus prophylaxis should be provided if the patient requires it for wound care. Antibiotics are not useful prophylactically. Contrast studies are not useful in the first few days and may interfere with endoscopic evaluation; later, they can be used to assess the severity of damage.

Emergency medical therapy includes agents to inhibit collagen formation and intraluminal stents. Esophageal and gastric outlet dilation may be needed if there is evidence of stricture. Bougienage of the esophagus, however, has been associated with brain abscess. Interposition of the colon may be necessary if dilation fails to provide an adequate-sized passage.

Management of inhalation cases requires immediate removal from the environment, administration of humid supplemental oxygen, and observation for airway obstruction and noncardiac pulmonary edema. Radiographic and ABG evaluation should be obtained when appropriate. Intubation and respiratory support may be required.

Certain caustics produce systemic disturbances. Formaldehyde causes metabolic acidosis, hydrofluoric acid causes hypocalcemia and renal damage, oxalic acid causes hypocalcemia, phenol causes hepatic and renal damage, and picric acid causes renal injury.

Disposition

Infants and small children should be medically evaluated and observed. All symptomatic patients should be admitted. If they have severe symptoms or danger of airway compromise, they should be admitted to the intensive care unit. After endoscopy, if no damage is detected, the patient may be discharged when he or she can tolerate oral feedings. Intentional exposures require psychiatric evaluation before the patient can be discharged.

COCAINE (BENZOYLMETHYLECGONINE)

Cocaine is derived from the leaves of *Erythroxylum coca* and *Truxillo coca*. "Body packing" refers to the placement of many small packages of contraband cocaine for concealment in the gastrointestinal tract or other areas for illicit transport. "Body stuffing" refers to spontaneous ingestion of substances for the purpose of hiding evidence.

Toxic Mechanism

Cocaine directly stimulates the CNS presynaptic sympathetic neurons to release catecholamines and acetylcholine, while it blocks the presynaptic reuptake of the catecholamines; it blocks the sodium channels along neuronal membranes; and it increases platelet aggregation. Long-term use depletes the CNS of dopamine.

Toxic Dose

The maximum mucosal local anesthetic therapeutic dose of cocaine is 200 mg or 2 mL of a 10% solution. Although CNS effects can occur at relatively low local anesthetic doses (50 to 95 mg), they are more common with doses greater than 1 mg/kg; cardiac effects can occur with doses greater than 1 mg/kg. The potential fatal dose is 1200 mg intranasally, but death has occurred with 20 mg parenterally.

Kinetics

Cocaine is well absorbed by all routes, including nasal insufflation, and oral, dermal, and inhalation routes (Table 14). Protein binding is 8.7%, and volume distribution is 1.5 L/kg.

Cocaine is metabolized by plasma and liver cholinesterase to the inactive metabolites ecgonine methyl ester and benzoylecgonine. Plasma pseudocholinesterase is congenitally

TABLE 14 The Different Routes and Kinetics of Cocaine

Type	Route	Onset	Peak (min)	Half-life (min)	Duration (min)
Cocaine leaf	Oral, chewing	20-30 min	45-90	NA	240-360
Hydrochloride	Insufflation	1-3 min	5-10	78	60-90
	Ingestion	20-30 min	50-90	54	Sustained
	Intravenous	30-120 sec	5-11	36	60-90
Free base/crack	Smoking	5-10 sec	5-11	—	Up to 20
Coca paste	Smoking	Unknown	—	—	—

deficient in 3% of the population and decreased in fetuses, young infants, the elderly, pregnant people, and people with liver disease. These enzyme-deficient individuals are at increased risk for life-threatening cocaine toxicity.

Ten percent of cocaine is excreted unchanged. Cocaine and ethanol undergo liver synthesis to form cocaethylene, a metabolite with a half-life three times longer than that of cocaine. It may account for some of cocaine's cardiotoxicity and appears to be more lethal than cocaine or ethanol alone.

Manifestations

The CNS manifestations of cocaine ingestion are euphoria, hyperactivity, agitation, convulsions, and intracranial hemorrhage. Mydriasis and septal perforation can occur, as well as cardiac dysrhythmias, hypertension, and hypotension (with severe overdose). Chest pain is frequent, but only 5.8% of patients have true myocardial ischemia and infarction. Other manifestations include vasoconstriction, hyperthermia (because of increased metabolic rate), ischemic bowel perforation if the substance is ingested, rhabdomyolysis, myoglobinuria, and renal failure. In pregnant users, premature labor and abruptio placentae can occur.

Body cavity packing should be suspected in cases of prolonged toxicity.

Mortality can result from cerebrovascular accidents, coronary artery spasm, myocardial injury, or lethal dysrhythmias.

Laboratory Investigations

Monitoring of the ECG and cardiac rhythms, ABG, oxygen saturation, electrolytes, blood glucose, BUN, creatinine, and creatine kinase levels should be maintained. One should monitor cardiac fraction if the patient has chest pain, as well as the liver profile, and the urine for myoglobin. Intravenous drug users should have HIV and hepatitis virus testing.

Urine should be tested for cocaine and metabolites and other substances of abuse, and abdominal radiographs or ultrasonogram should be ordered for body packers. If the urine sample was collected more than 12 hours after cocaine intake, it will contain little or no cocaine. If cocaine is present, cocaine has been used within the past 12 hours. Cocaine's metabolite benzoylecgonine may be detected within 4 hours after a single nasal insufflation and for up to 114 hours. Cross-reactions with some herbal teas, lidocaine, and droperidol (Inapsine) may give false-positive results by some immunoassay methods.

Management

Supportive care includes blood pressure, cardiac, and thermal monitoring and seizure precautions. Diazepam (Valium) is the drug of choice for treatment of cocaine toxicity agitation, seizures, and dysrhythmias; doses are 10 to 30 mg intravenously at 2.5 mg per minute for adults and 0.2 to 0.5 mg/kg at 1 mg per minute up to 10 mg for a child.

Gastrointestinal decontamination should be instituted, if the cocaine was ingested, by administration of activated charcoal. MDAC may adsorb cocaine leakage in body stuffers or body packers. Whole-bowel irrigation with polyethylene glycol solution (PEG) has been used in body packers and stuffers if the contraband is in a firm container. If the packages are not visible on plain radiographs of the abdomen, a contrast study or CT scan can help to confirm successful passage. Cocaine in the nasal passage can be removed with an applicator dipped in a non–water-soluble product (lubricating jelly) if this is done within a few minutes after application.

In body packers and stuffers, venous access must be secured, and drugs must be readily available for treating life-threatening manifestations until the contraband is passed in the stool. Surgical removal may be indicated if the packet does not pass the pylorus, in an asymptomatic body packer, or in the case of intestinal obstruction.

Hypertension and tachycardia are usually transient and can be managed by careful titration of diazepam. Nitroprusside may be used for severe hypertension. Myocardial ischemia is managed by oxygen, vascular access, benzodiazepines, and nitroglycerin. Aspirin and thrombolysis are not routinely recommended because of the danger of intracranial hemorrhage.

Dysrhythmias are usually supraventricular (SVT) and do not require specific management. Adenosine is ineffective. Life-threatening tachydysrhythmias may respond to phentolamine (Regitine) 5 mg IV bolus in adults or 0.1 mg/kg in children at 5- to 10-minute intervals. Phentolamine also relieves coronary artery spasm and myocardial ischemia. Electrical synchronized cardioversion should be considered for patients with hemodynamically unstable dysrhythmias. Lidocaine is not recommended initially but may be used after 3 hours for ventricular tachycardia. Wide complex QRS ventricular tachycardia may be treated with sodium bicarbonate 2 mEq/kg as a bolus. β-Adrenergic blockers are not recommended.

Anxiety, agitation, and convulsions can be treated with diazepam. If diazepam fails to control seizures, neuromuscular blockers can be used. The EEG should be monitored for nonmotor seizure activity. For hyperthermia, external cooling and cool humidified 100% oxygen should be administered. Neuromuscular paralysis to control seizures will reduce temperature. Dantrolene and antipyretics are not recommended. Rhabdomyolysis and myoglobinuria are treated with fluids, alkaline diuresis, and diuretics.

If the patient is pregnant, the fetus must be monitored and the patient observed for spontaneous abortion.

Paranoid ideation and threatening behavior should be treated with rapid tranquilization. The patient should be observed for suicidal depression that may follow intoxication and may require suicide precautions. If focal neurologic manifestations are present, one should consider the possibility of a cerebrovascular accident and obtain a CT scan.

Extracorporeal clearance techniques are of no benefit.

Disposition

Patients with mild intoxication or a brief seizure that does not require treatment who become asymptomatic may be discharged after 6 hours with appropriate psychosocial follow-up. If cardiac or cerebral ischemic manifestations are present, the patient should be monitored in the intensive care unit. Body packers and stuffers require care in the intensive care unit until passage of the contraband.

CYANIDE

Hydrogen cyanide is a byproduct of burning plastic and wools in residential fires. Hydrocyanic acid is the liquefied form of hydrogen cyanide. Cyanide salts can be found in ore extraction. Nitriles, such as acetonitrile (artificial nail removers) are metabolized in the body to produce cyanide. Cyanogenic glycosides are present in some fruit seeds (such as amygdalin in apricots, peaches, and apples). Sodium nitroprusside, the antihypertensive vasodilator, contains five cyanide groups.

Toxic Mechanism

Cyanide blocks the cellular electron transport mechanism and cellular respiration by inhibiting the mitochondrial ferricytochrome oxidase system and other enzymes. This results in cellular hypoxia and lactic acidosis. *Note:* Citrus fruit seeds form cyanide in the presence of intestinal β-glucosidase (the seeds are harmful only if the capsule is broken).

Toxic Dose

The ingestion of 1 mg/kg or 50 mg of hydrogen cyanide can produce death within 15 minutes. The lethal dose of potassium cyanide is 200 mg. Five to 10 mL of 84% acetonitrile is lethal. Infusions of sodium nitroprusside in rates above 2 µg/kg per minute may cause cyanide to accumulate to toxic concentrations in critically ill patients.

Kinetics

Cyanide is rapidly absorbed by all routes. In the stomach, it forms hydrocyanic acid. Volume distribution is 1.5 L/kg. Protein binding is 60%. Cyanide is detoxified by metabolism in the liver via the mitochondrial thiosulfate-rhodanase pathway, which catalyzes the transfer of sulfur donor to cyanide, forming the less toxic irreversible thiocyanate that is excreted in the urine. Cyanide is also detoxified by reacting with hydroxocobalamin (vitamin B_{12a}) to form cyanocobalamin (vitamin B_{12}).

The cyanide elimination half-life from the blood is 1.2 hours. The elimination route is through the lungs.

Manifestations

Hydrogen cyanide has the distinctive odor of bitter almonds or silver polish. Manifestations of cyanide intoxication include hypertension, cardiac dysrhythmias, various ECG abnormalities, headache, hyperpnea, seizures, stupor, pulmonary edema, and flushing. Cyanosis is absent or appears late.

Laboratory Investigations

The examiner should obtain and monitor ABGs, oxygen saturation, blood lactate, hemoglobin, blood glucose, and electrolytes. Lactic acidemia, a decrease in the arterial-venous oxygen difference, and bright red venous blood occurs. If smoke inhalation is the possible source of cyanide exposure, CoHB and methemoglobin (MetHb) concentrations should be measured.

Cyanide levels in whole blood, red blood cells, or serum are not useful in the acute management because the determinations are not readily available. Specific cyanide blood levels are as follows: smokers have less than 0.5 µg/mL; a patient with flushing and tachycardia has 0.5 to 1.0 µg/mL, one with obtundation has 1.0 to 2.5 µg/mL, and one in coma or who has died has more than 2.5 µg/mL.

Management

If the cyanide was inhaled, the patient must be removed from the contaminated atmosphere. Attendants should not administer mouth-to-mouth resuscitation. Rescuers and attendants must be protected. Immediate administration of 100% oxygen is called for and oxygen should be continued during and after the administration of the antidote. The clinician must decide whether to use any or all components of the cyanide antidote kit.

The mechanism of action of the antidote kit is twofold: to produce methemoglobinemia and to provide a sulfur substrate for the detoxification of cyanide. The nitrites make methemoglobin, which has a greater affinity for cyanide than does the cytochrome oxidase enzymes. The combination of methemoglobin and cyanide forms cyanomethemoglobin. Sodium thiosulfate provides a sulfur substrate for the rhodanese enzyme, which converts cyanide into the relatively nontoxic sodium thiocyanate, which is excreted by the kidney.

The procedure for using the antidote kit is as follows:

Step 1: Amyl nitrite inhalant perles is only a temporizing measure (forms only 2% to 5% methemoglobin) and it can be omitted if venous access is established. Alternate 100% oxygen and the inhalant for 30 seconds each minute. Use a new perle every 3 minutes.

Step 2: Sodium nitrite ampule is indicated for cyanide exposures, except for cases of residential fires, smoke inhalation, and nitroprusside or acetonitrile poisonings. It is administered intravenously to produce methemoglobin of 20% to 30% at 35 to 70 minutes after administration. A dose of 10 mL of 3% solution of sodium nitrite for adults and 0.33 mL/kg of 3% solution for children is diluted to 100 mL 0.9% saline and administered slowly intravenously at 5 mL/min. If hypotension develops, the infusion should be slowed.

Step 3: Sodium thiosulfate is useful alone in cases of smoke inhalation, nitroprusside toxicity, and acetonitrile toxicity and should not be used at all in cases of hydrogen sulfide poisoning. The administration dose is 12.5 g of sodium thiosulfate or 50 mL of 25% solution for adults and 1.65 mL/kg of 25% solution for children intravenously over 10 to 20 minutes.

If cyanide symptoms recur, further treatment with nitrites or the perles is controversial. Some authorities suggest repeating the antidotes in 30 minutes at half of the initial dose, but others do not advise this for lack of efficacy. The child dosage regimen on the package insert must be carefully followed.

One hour after antidotes are administered, the methemoglobin level should be obtained and should not exceed 20%. Methylene blue should not be used to reverse excessive methemoglobin.

Gastrointestinal decontamination of oral ingestion by activated charcoal is recommended but is not very effective because of the rapidity of absorption. Seizures are treated with intravenous diazepam. Acidosis should be treated with sodium bicarbonate if it does not rapidly resolve with therapy. There is no role for hyperbaric oxygen or hemodialysis or hemoperfusion.

Other antidotes include hydroxocobalamin (vitamin B_{12a}) (Cyanokit), which has proven effective when given immediately after exposure in large doses of 4 g (50 mg/kg) or 50 times the amount of cyanide exposure with 8 g of sodium thiosulfate. Hydroxocobalamin has FDA orphan drug approval.

Disposition

Asymptomatic patients should be observed for a minimum of 3 hours. Patients who ingest nitrile compounds must be observed for 24 hours. Patients requiring antidote administration should be admitted to the intensive care unit.

DIGITALIS

Cardiac glycosides are found in cardiac medications, common plants, and the skin of the Bufo toad.

Toxic Mechanism

Cardiac glycosides inhibit the enzyme sodium/potassium-adenosine triphosphatase (NA^+, K^+, ATPase), leading to intracellular potassium loss and increased intracellular sodium, and producing phase 4 depolarization, increased automaticity, and ectopy. There is increased intracellular calcium and potentiation of contractility. Pacemaker cells are inhibited, and the refractory period is prolonged, leading to atrioventricular blocks. There is increased vagal tone.

Toxic Dose

Digoxin total digitalizing dose, the dose required to achieve therapeutic blood levels of 0.6 to 2.0 ng/mL, is 0.75 to 1.25 mg or 10 to 15 µg/kg for patients older than 10 years of age; 40 to 50 µg/kg for patients younger than 2 years of age; and 30 to 40 µg/kg for patients 2 to 10 years of age.

The acute single toxic dose is greater than 0.07 mg/kg or greater than 2 or 3 mg in an adult, but 2 mg in a child or 4 mg in an adult usually produces only mild toxicity. One to 3 mg or more may be found in a few leaves of oleander or foxglove. Serious and fatal overdoses are more than 4 mg in a child and more than 10 mg in an adult.

Acute digitoxin ingestion of 10 to 35 mg has produced severe toxicity and death. Digitoxin therapeutic steady state is 15 to 25 ng/mL. In cases of chronic or acute-on-chronic ingestions in patients with cardiac disease, more than 2 mg may produce toxicity; however, toxicity can develop within therapeutic range on chronic therapy.

Patients at greatest risk of overdose include those with cardiac disease, those with electrolyte abnormalities (low potassium, low magnesium, low T_4, high calcium), those with renal impairment, and those on amiodarone (Cordarone), quinidine, erythromycin, tetracycline, calcium channel blockers, and β-blockers.

Kinetics

Digoxin is a metabolite of digitoxin. In cases of oral overdose, the typical onset is 30 minutes, with peak effects in 3 to 12 hours. Duration is 3 to 4 days. Intravenous onset is in 5 to 30 minutes; peak level is immediate, and peak effect is at 1.5 to 3 hours.

Volume distribution is 5 to 6 L/kg. The cardiac-to-plasma ratio is 30:1. After an acute ingestion overdose, the serum concentration is not reflective of tissue concentration for at least 6 hours or more, and steady state is 12 to 16 hours after last dose.

Sixty percent to 80% of the parent compound is excreted unchanged in the urine. The elimination half-life is 30 to 50 hours.

Manifestations

Onset of manifestations is usually within 2 hours but may be delayed up to 12 hours.

Gastrointestinal effects of nausea and vomiting are frequently present in cases of acute ingestion but may also occur in cases of chronic ingestion. The "digitalis effect" on ECG is scooped ST segments and PR prolongation; in cases of overdose, any dysrhythmia or block is possible but none are characteristic. Bradycardia occurs in patients with acute overdose with healthy hearts; supraventricular tachycardia occurs in patients with existing heart disease or chronic overdose. Ventricular tachycardia is seen only in cases of severe poisoning.

The CNS effects include headaches, visual disturbances, and colored halo vision. Hyperkalemia occurs following acute overdose and correlates with digoxin level and outcome. Among patients with serum potassium levels of less than 5.0 mEq/L, all survive. If the level is 5 to 5.5, 50% survive, and if the level is greater than 5.5, all die. Hypokalemia is commonly seen with chronic intoxication. Patients with normal digitalis levels may have toxicity in the presence of hypokalemia.

Chronic intoxications are more likely to produce scotoma, color perception disturbances, yellow vision, halos, delirium, hallucinations or psychosis, tachycardia, and hypokalemia.

Laboratory Investigations

Continuous monitoring of ECG, pulse, and blood pressure is called for. Blood glucose, electrolytes, calcium, magnesium, BUN, and creatinine levels should also be monitored. An initial digoxin level should be measured on patient presentation and repeated thereafter. Levels should be measured more than 6 hours postingestion because earlier values do not reflect tissue distribution. Digoxin clinical toxicity is usually associated with serum digoxin levels of greater than 3.5 ng/mL in adults.

An endogenous digoxin-like substance cross-reacts in most common immunoassays (not with high-pressure liquid chromatography) and values as high as 4.1 ng/mL have been reported in newborns, patients with chronic renal failure, patients with abnormal immunoglobulins, and women in the third trimester of pregnancy.

Management

A cardiology consult should be obtained and a pacemaker should be readily available.

In undertaking gastrointestinal decontamination, excessive vagal stimulation should be avoided (e.g., emesis and gastric lavage). Activated charcoal should be administered, and if a nasogastric tube is required for the activated charcoal, pretreatment with atropine (0.02 mg/kg in children and 0.5 mg in adults) should be considered.

Digoxin-specific antibody fragments (Fab, Digibind) 38 mg binds 0.5 mg digoxin and then is excreted through the kidneys. The onset of action is within 30 minutes. Problems associated with Fab therapy are mainly from withdrawal of digoxin and worsening heart failure, hypokalemia, decrease in glucose (if the patient has low glycogen stores), and allergic reactions (very rare). Digitalis administered after Fab therapy is bound and may be inactivated for 5 to 7 days.

Absolute indications for Fab therapy include the following:

- Life-threatening malignant (hemodynamically unstable) dysrhythmias
- Ventricular dysrhythmias, unstable severe bradycardia, or second- or third-degree blocks unresponsive to atropine or rapid deterioration in clinical status
- Life-threatening digitoxin and oleander poisonings
- Relative indications for Fab therapy include the following:
- Ingestions greater than 4 mg in a child and 10 mg in an adult
- Serum potassium level greater than 5.0 mEq/L
- Serum digoxin level greater than 10 ng/mL in adults or greater than 5 ng/mL in children 6 hours after an acute ingestion
- Digitalis delirium and thrombocytopenia response

Digoxin-specific Fab fragments therapy can be administered as a bolus through a 22-μm filter if the case is a critical emergency. If the case is less urgent, then it can be administered over 30 minutes. An empiric dose is 10 vials in adults and 5 vials in a child for an unknown amount ingested in a symptomatic patient with history of a digoxin overdose.

To calculate the dose in the case of a known ingestion, the following equation is used:

$$\text{Amount (total mg)} \times (0.8) = \text{body burden}$$

If liquid capsules were taken or the substance was given intravenously the 80% bioavailability figure is not used. Instead, the body burden divided by 0.5 (0.5 mg digoxin is bound by 1 vial of 38 mg of Fab) equals the number of vials needed.

If the amount is unknown but the steady state serum concentration is known, the following equations are used:

For digoxin

$$\text{Digoxin ng/mL} \times (5.6 \text{ L/kg Vd}) \times (\text{wt kg}) = \text{mg body burden}$$

$$\text{Body burden} \div 1000 = \text{mg body burden}$$

$$\text{Body burden}/0.5 = \text{number of vials needed}$$

For digitoxin

$$\text{Digitoxin ng/mL} \times (0.56 \text{ L/kg Vd}) \times (\text{wt kg}) = \text{mg body burden}$$

$$\text{Body burden} \div 1000 = \text{mg body burden}$$

$$\text{Body burden}/0.5 = \text{number of vials needed}$$

Antidysrhythmic agents or a pacemaker should be used only if Fab therapy fails. For ventricular tachydysrhythmias, electrolyte disturbances should be corrected by the administration of lidocaine or phenytoin. For torsades de pointes, magnesium sulfate 20 mL 20% IV can be given slowly over 20 minutes (or 25 to 50 mg/kg in a child), titrated to control the dysrhythmia. Magnesium should be discontinued if hypotension, heart block, or decreased deep tendon reflexes are present. Magnesium is used with caution if the patient has renal impairment.

Unstable bradycardia and second-degree and third-degree atrioventricular block should be treated by Fab first. A pacemaker should be available if necessary. Isoproterenol should be avoided because it causes dysrhythmias. Cardioversion is used with caution, starting at a setting of 5 to 10 joules. The patient should be pretreated with lidocaine, if possible, because cardioversion may precipitate ventricular fibrillation or asystole.

Potassium disturbances are caused by a shift, not a change, in total body potassium. Hyperkalemia (>5.0 mEq/L) is treated with Fab only. Calcium must never be used, and insulin/glucose and sodium bicarbonate should not be used concomitantly with Fab because they may produce severe life-threatening hypokalemia. Sodium polystyrene sulfonate (Kayexalate) should not be used. Hypokalemia must be treated with caution because it may be cardioprotective. Treatment can be administered if the patient has ventricular dysrhythmias or a serum potassium level less than 3.0 mEq/L and atrioventricular block.

Extracorporeal procedures are ineffective. Hemodialysis is used for severe or refractory hyperkalemia.

One must never use antidysrhythmic types Ia (procainamide, quinidine, disopyramide [Norpace], amiodarone [Cordarone]), Ic (propafenone [Rythmol], flecainide [Tambocor]), II (β-blockers), or IV (calcium channel blockers). Class Ib drugs (lidocaine, phenytoin [Dilantin], mexiletine [Mexitil], and tocainide [Tonocard]) can be used.

Disposition

Consultation with a poison control center and a cardiologist experienced with digoxin-specific Fab fragments is warranted. All patients with significant dysrhythmias, symptoms, elevated serum digoxin concentration, or elevated serum potassium level should be admitted to the intensive care unit.

ETHANOL

Table 15 lists the features of alcohols and glycols.

Toxic Mechanism

Ethanol has CNS depressant and anesthetic effects. Ethanol stimulates the γ-aminobutyric acid (GABA) system. It promotes cutaneous vasodilation (contributes to hypothermia), stimulates secretion of gastric juice

TABLE 15 Summary of Alcohol and Glycol Features

	Methanol	Isopropanol	Ethanol	Ethylene Glycol
Principal uses	Gas line antifreeze, Sterno, windshield de-icer	Solvent jewelry cleaner, rubbing alcohol	Beverage, solvent	Radiator antifreeze, windshield de-icer
Specific gravity	0.719	0.785	0.789	1.12
Fatal dose	1 mL/Kg 100%	3 mL/kg 100%	5 mL/kg 100%	1.4 mL/kg
Inebriation	±	2+	2+	1+
Metabolic change		Hyperglycemia	Hypoglycemia	Hypocalcemia
Metabolic acidosis	4+	0	1+	2+
Anion gap	4+	±	2+	4+
Ketosis	Ketobutyric	Acetone	Hydroxybutyric	None
Gastrointestinal tract	Pancreatitis	Hemorrhagic gastritis	Gastritis	
Osmolality*	0.337	0.176	0.228	0.190

*1 mL/dL of substances raises freezing point osmolarity of serum. The validity of the correlation of osmolality with blood concentrations has been questioned.

(gastritis), inhibits the secretion of the antidiuretic hormone, inhibits gluconeogenesis (hypoglycemia), and influences fat metabolism (lipidemia).

Toxic Dose

A dose of 1 mL/kg of absolute ethanol (100% ethanol, or 200 proof) gives a blood ethanol concentration of 100 mg/dL. A potentially fatal dose is 3 g/kg for children or 6 g/kg for adults. Children are more prone to developing hypoglycemia than adults.

Kinetics

Onset of action is 30 to 60 minutes after ingestion; peak action is 90 minutes on empty stomach. Volume distribution is 0.6 L/kg. The major route of elimination (>90%) is by hepatic oxidative metabolism. The first step is by the enzyme alcohol dehydrogenase, which converts ethanol to acetaldehyde. Alcohol dehydrogenase metabolizes ethanol at a constant rate of 12 to 20 mg/dL/h (12 to 15 mg/dL/h in nondrinkers, 15 to 30 mg/dL/h in social drinkers, 30 to 50 mg/dL/h in heavy drinkers, and 25 to 30 mg/dL/h in children). At very low blood ethanol concentration (<30 mg/dL), the metabolism is by first-order kinetics. In the second step, acetaldehyde is metabolized by acetaldehyde dehydrogenase to acetic acid, which is metabolized by the Krebs cycle to carbon dioxide and water. The enzyme steps are nicotinamide adenine dinucleotide-dependent, which interferes with gluconeogenesis. Less than 10% of ethanol is excreted unchanged by the kidneys. The relationship between blood ethanol concentration (BEC) and dose (amount ingested) can be calculated as follows:

$$\text{BEC (mg/dL)} = \text{amount ingested (mL)} \times \% \text{ ethanol product} \times \text{SG (0.79)/Vd (0.6 L/kg)} \times \text{body wt (kg)}$$

$$\text{Dose (amount ingested)} = \text{BEC (mg/dL)} \times \text{Vd (0.6)} \times \text{body wt (kg)}/\% \text{ ethanol} \times \text{specific gravity (0.79)}$$

Manifestations

Table 16 lists the clinical signs of acute ethanol intoxication.

Chronic alcoholic patients tolerate higher blood ethanol concentration, and correlation with manifestations is not valid. Rapid interview for alcoholism is the CAGE questions:

- C—Have you felt the need to Cut down?
- A—Have others Annoyed you by criticism of your drinking?
- G—Have you felt Guilty about your drinking?
- E—Have you ever had a morning Eye-opening drink to steady your nerves or get rid of a hangover?

Two affirmative answers indicate probable alcoholism.

TABLE 16 Clinical Signs in the Nontolerant Ethanol Drinker

Ethanol Blood Concentration (mg/dL)*	Manifestations
>25	Euphoria
>47	**Mild incoordination,** sensory and motor impairment
>50	Increased risk of motor vehicle accidents
>100	Ataxia (legal toxic level in many localities)
>150	***Moderate incoordination,*** slow reaction time
>200	Drowsiness and confusion
>300	Severe incoordination, stupor, blurred vision
>500	***Flaccid coma,*** respiratory failure, hypotension; may be fatal

*Ethanol concentrations sometimes reported in %.
Note: mg% is not equivalent to mg/dL because ethanol weighs less than water (specific gravity 0.79). A 1% ethanol concentration is 790 mg/dL and 0.1% is 79 mg/dL. There is great variation in individual behavior at different blood ethanol levels. Behavior is dependent on tolerance and other factors.

Laboratory Investigations

The blood ethanol concentration should be specifically requested and followed. Gas chromatography or a breath-analyzer test gives rapid reliable results if no belching or vomiting is present. Enzymatic methods do not differentiate between the alcohols. ABG, electrolytes, and glucose should be measured, the anion and osmolar gaps determined (measure by freezing point depression, not vapor pressure), and a check for ketosis made.

Management

The examiner should inquire about trauma and disulfiram use. The patient must be protected from aspiration and hypoxia. Vital functions must be established and maintained. The patient may require intubation and assisted ventilation.

Gastrointestinal decontamination plays no role in the management of ethanol intoxication.

If the patient is comatose, glucose should be administered intravenously, 1 mL/kg 50% glucose in adults and 2 mL/kg 25% glucose in children. Thiamine, 100 mg intravenously, is administered if the patient has a history of chronic alcoholism, malnutrition, or suspected eating disorders to prevent Wernicke-Korsakoff syndrome. Naloxone (Narcan) has produced a partial inconsistent response but is not recommended for known alcoholics.

General supportive care includes administration of fluids to correct hydration and hypotension and correction of electrolyte abnormalities and acid–base imbalance. Vasopressors and plasma expanders may be necessary to correct severe hypotension. Hypomagnesemia is frequent in chronic alcoholics. In case of hypomagnesemia, a loading dose of 2 g magnesium sulfate 10% is administered by intravenous solution over 5 minutes in the intensive care unit with blood pressure and cardiac monitoring and calcium chloride 10% on hand in case of overdose. This is followed with constant infusion of 6 g of 10% solution over 3 to 4 hours. Caution must be taken with the use of magnesium if renal failure is present.

Hypothermic patients should be warmed. See the section on disturbances caused by cold.

Hemodialysis can be used in severe cases when conventional therapy is ineffective (rarely needed).

Repeated or prolonged seizures should be treated with diazepam (Valium). The brief "rum fits" do not need long-term anticonvulsant therapy. Repeated seizures or focal neurologic findings may warrant skull radiographs, lumbar puncture, and CT scan of the head, depending on the clinical findings. Withdrawal is treated with hydration and large doses of chlordiazepoxide (Librium) 50 to 100 mg or diazepam (Valium) 2 to 10 mg intravenously; these doses may be repeated in 2 to 4 hours. Very large doses of benzodiazepines may be required for delirium tremens. Withdrawal can occur in presence of elevated blood ethanol concentration and can be fatal if left untreated.

Chest radiograph is warranted to determine whether aspiration pneumonia is present. Renal and liver function tests and bilirubin level measurement should be made.

Disposition

Clinical severity (e.g., intubation, assisted ventilation, aspiration pneumonia) should determine the level of hospital care needed. Young children with significant unintentional exposure to ethanol (calculated to reach a blood ethanol concentration of 50 mg/dL) should have blood ethanol concentration obtained and blood glucose levels monitored for hypoglycemia frequently for 4 hours after ingestion. Patients with acute ethanol intoxication seldom require admission unless a complication is present. However, intoxicated patients should not be discharged until they are fully functional (can walk, talk, and think independently), have suicide potential evaluated, have proper disposition environment, and have a sober escort.

ETHYLENE GLYCOL

Ethylene glycol is found in solvents, de-icers, radiator antifreeze (95%), and air-conditioning units. Ethylene glycol is a sweet-tasting, colorless, water-soluble liquid with a sweet aromatic fragrance.

Toxic Mechanism

Ethylene glycol is oxidized by alcohol dehydrogenase to glycolaldehyde, which is metabolized to glycolic acid and glyoxylic acid. Glyoxylic acid is metabolized to oxalic acid via a pyridoxine-dependent pathway to glycine and by thiamine and magnesium-dependent pathways to α-hydroxy-ketoadipic acid. The metabolites of ethylene glycol produce a profound metabolic acidosis, increased anion gap, hypocalcemia, and oxalate crystals, which deposit in tissues (particularly the kidney).

Toxic Dose

The ingestion of 0.1 mL/kg 100% ethylene glycol can result in a toxic serum ethylene glycol concentration of 20 mg/dL. Ingestion of 3.0 mL (less than 1 teaspoonful or swallow) of a 100% solution in a 10-kg child or 30 mL of 100% ethylene glycol in an adult produces a serum ethylene glycol concentration of 50 mg/dL, a concentration that requires hemodialysis. The fatal amount is 1.4 mL/kg of 100% solution.

Kinetics

Absorption is via dermal, inhalation, and ingestion routes. Ethylene glycol is rapidly absorbed from the gastrointestinal tract. Onset is usually in 30 minutes but may be delayed by co-ingestion of food and ethanol. The usual peak level is at 2 hours. Volume distribution is 0.65 to 0.8 L/kg.

For metabolism, see *Toxic Mechanism*.

The half-life of ethylene glycol without ethanol is 3 to 8 hours; with ethanol, it is 17 hours, and with hemodialysis it is 2.5 hours. Renal clearance is 3.2 mL/kg/minute. About 20% to 50% is excreted unchanged in the urine. The relationship between serum ethylene glycol concentration (SEGC) and dose (amount ingested) can be calculated as follows:

$$0.12 \text{ mL/kg of } 100\% = \text{SEGC } 10 \text{ mg/dL}$$

Manifestations

Phase I

The onset of manifestations is 30 minutes to several hours longer after ingestion with concomitant ethanol ingestion.

The patient may be inebriated. Hypocalcemia, tetany, and calcium oxalate and hippuric acid crystals in urine can be seen within 4 to 8 hours but are not always present. Early, before metabolism of ethylene glycol, an osmolal gap may be present (see *Laboratory Investigations*). Later, the metabolites of ethylene glycol produce changes starting 4 to 12 hours following ingestion, including an anion gap, metabolic acidosis, coma, convulsions, cardiac disturbances, and pulmonary and cerebral edema. Because fluorescein is added to some antifreeze, the presence of fluorescence may be a clue to ethylene glycol exposure. However, it has been shown that fluorescent urine is not a reliable indicator of ethylene glycol ingestion and should not be used as a screen.

Phase II

After 12 to 36 hours, cardiopulmonary deterioration occurs, with pulmonary edema and congestive heart failure.

Phase III

Phase III occurs 36 to 72 hours after ingestion, with pulmonary edema and oliguric renal failure from oxalate crystal deposition and tubular necrosis predominating.

Phase IV

Neurologic sequelae may occur rarely, especially in patients who fail to receive early antidotal therapy. The onset ranges from 6 to 10 days after ingestion. Findings include facial diplegia, hearing loss, bilateral visual disturbances, elevated cerebrospinal fluid pressure with or without elevated protein levels and pleocytosis, vomiting, hyperreflexia, dysphagia, and ataxia.

Laboratory Investigations

Blood glucose and electrolytes should be monitored. Urinalysis should look for oxalate ("envelope") and monohydrate ("hemp seed") crystals. Urine fluorescence is not reliable as a screen. ABG, ethylene glycol, and ethanol levels, plasma osmolarity (using freezing point depression method), calcium, BUN, and creatinine should be measured. A serum ethylene glycol concentration of 20 mg/dL is toxic (ethylene glycol levels are very difficult to obtain). If possible, a glycolate level should be obtained. Cross-reactions with propylene glycol, a vehicle in many liquids and intravenous medications (phenytoin [Dilantin], diazepam [Valium]), other glycols, and triglycerides may produce spurious ethylene glycol levels. False-positive ethylene glycol values may occur with colorimetric or gas chromatography using an OV-17 column in the presence of propylene glycol.

The following equations can be used to calculate the osmolality, osmolal gap, and ethylene glycol level:

$$2(Na+ mEq/L) + (Blood\ glucose\ mg/dL)/20 + (BUN\ mg/dL)/3 = Total\ calculated\ osmolality\ (mOsmL/L)$$

$$Osmolar\ Gap = measured\ osmolality\ (by\ freezing\ point\ depression\ method) - calculated\ osmolality$$

A gap greater than 10 is abnormal. *Note:* if ethanol is involved, add ethanol level/4.6 to the calculated equation.

An increased osmolal gap is produced by the following common substances: acetone, dextran, dimethyl sulfoxide, diuretics, ethanol, ethyl ether, ethylene glycol, isopropanol, paraldehyde, mannitol, methanol, sorbitol, and trichloroethane. Table 10 gives the conversion factors for these substances.

Although a specific blood level of ethylene glycol in milligrams per deciliter can be estimated using the equation below, this is not considered to be a reliable method and should not take the place of obtaining a measured ethylene glycol blood concentration.

$$osmolar\ gap \times conversion\ factor = serum\ concentration$$

Caution: The accuracy of the ethylene glycol estimated decreases as the ethylene glycol levels decrease. The toxic metabolites are not osmotically active, and patients presenting late may show signs of severe toxicity without an elevated osmolar gap.

The anion gap can be calculated using the following equation:

$$Na - (Cl + HCO_3) = anion\ gap$$

The normal gap is 8 to 12. Potassium is not used because it is a small amount and may be hemolyzed. Table 8 lists factors that may account for an increased or a decreased anion gap.

Management

Vital functions should be established and maintained. The airway must be protected, and assisted ventilation can be used, if necessary. Gastrointestinal decontamination has a limited role. Only gastric aspiration can be used within 60 minutes after ingestion. Activated charcoal is not effective.

Baseline measurements of serum electrolytes and calcium, glucose, ABGs, ethanol, serum ethylene glycol concentration (may be difficult to obtain readily in some institutions), and methanol concentrations should be obtained. In the first few hours, the measured serum osmolality should be determined and compared to calculated osmolality (see osmolality equation, earlier). If seizures occur, one should measure serum calcium (preferably ionized calcium) and treat with intravenous diazepam. If the patient has hypocalcemic seizures, he or she should also be treated with 10 to 20 mL 10% calcium gluconate (0.2 to 0.3 mL/kg in children) slowly intravenously, with the dose repeated as needed. Metabolic acidosis should be corrected with intravenous sodium bicarbonate.

Ethanol therapy should be initiated immediately if fomepizole (Antizol) is unavailable (see next paragraph). Alcohol dehydrogenase has a greater affinity for ethanol than ethylene glycol. Therefore, ethanol blocks the metabolism of ethylene glycol. Ethanol therapy is called for if there is a history of ingestion of 0.1 mL/kg of 100% ethylene glycol, serum ethylene glycol concentration is greater than 20 mg/dL, there is an osmolar gap not accounted for by other alcohols or factors (e.g., hyperlipidemia), metabolic acidosis is present with an increased anion gap, or there are oxalate crystals in the urine. Ethanol should be administered intravenously (the oral route is less reliable) to produce a blood ethanol concentration of 100 to 150 mg/dL. The loading dose is 10 mL/kg of 10% ethanol intravenously, administered concomitantly with a maintenance dose of 10% ethanol of 1.0 mL/kg/h.

This dose may need to be increased to 2 mL/kg/h in patients who are heavy drinkers. The blood ethanol concentration should be measured hourly and the infusion rate should be adjusted to maintain a blood ethanol concentration of 100 to 150 mg/dL.

Fomepizole (Antizol, 4-methylpyrazole) inhibits alcohol dehydrogenase more reliability than ethanol and it does not require constant monitoring of ethanol levels and adjustment of infusion rates. Fomepizole is available in 1 g/mL vials of 1.5 mL. The loading dose is 15 mg/kg (0.015 mL/kg) IV; maintenance dose is 10 mg/kg (0.01 mL/kg) every 12 hours for four doses, then 15 mg/kg every 12 hours until the ethylene glycol levels are less than 20 mg/dL. The solution is prepared by being mixed with 100 mL of 0.9% saline or D_5W (5% dextrose in water). Fomepizole can be given to patients requiring hemodialysis but should be dosed as follows:

Dose at the beginning of hemodialysis:

- If <6 hours since last Antizol dose, do not administer dose
- If >6 hours since last dose, administer next scheduled dose

Dosing during hemodialysis:

- Dose every 4 hours

Dosing at the time hemodialysis is completed:

- If <1 hour between last dose and end of dialysis, do not administer dose at end of dialysis
- If 1 to 3 hours between last dose and end of dialysis, administer one half of next scheduled dose
- If >3 hours between last dose and end of dialysis, administer next scheduled dose

Maintenance dosing off hemodialysis:

- Give the next scheduled dose 12 hours from the last dose administered

Hemodialysis is indicated if the ingestion was potentially fatal; if the serum ethylene glycol concentration is greater than 50 mg/dL (some recommend at levels of >25 mg/dL); if severe acidosis or electrolyte abnormalities occur despite conventional therapy; or if congestive heart failure or renal failure is present. Hemodialysis reduces the ethylene glycol half-life from 17 hours on ethanol therapy to 3 hours. Therapy (fomepizole and hemodialysis) should be continued until the serum ethylene glycol concentration is less than 10 mg/dL, the glycolate level is nondetectable (not readily available), the acidosis has cleared, there are no mental disturbances, the creatinine level is normal, and the urinary output is adequate. This may require 2 to 5 days.

Adjunct therapy involving thiamine, 100 mg/d (in children, 50 mg), slowly over 5 minutes intravenously or intramuscularly and repeated every 6 hours and pyridoxine, 50 mg IV or IM every 6 hours, has been recommended until intoxication is resolved, but these agents have not been extensively studied. Folate, 50 mg IV (child 1 mg/kg), can be given every 4 hours for 6 doses.

Disposition

All patients who have ingested significant amounts of ethylene glycol (calculated level above 20 mg/dL), have a history of a toxic dose, or are symptomatic should be referred to the emergency department and admitted. If the serum ethylene glycol concentration cannot be obtained, the patient should be followed for 12 hours, with monitoring of the osmolal gap, acid–base parameters, and electrolytes to exclude development of metabolic acidosis with an anion gap. Transfer should be considered for fomepizole therapy or hemodialysis.

HYDROCARBONS

The lower the viscosity and surface tension of hydrocarbons or the greater the volatility, the greater the risk of aspiration. Volatile substance abuse has produced the "Sudden Sniffing's Death Syndrome," most likely caused by dysrhythmias.

Toxicologic Classification and Toxic Mechanism

All systemically absorbed hydrocarbons can lower the threshold of the myocardium to dysrhythmias produced by endogenous and exogenous catecholamines.

Aliphatic hydrocarbons are branched straight chain hydrocarbons. A few aspirated drops are poorly absorbed from the gastrointestinal tract and produce no systemic toxicity by this route. However, aspiration of very small amounts can produce chemical pneumonitis. Examples of aliphatic hydrocarbons are gasoline, kerosene, charcoal lighter fluid, mineral spirits (Stoddard's solvent), and petroleum naphtha. Mineral seal oil (signal oil), found in furniture polishes, is a low-viscosity and low-volatility oil with minimum absorption that never warrants gastric decontamination. It can produce severe pneumonia if aspirated.

Aromatic hydrocarbons are six carbon ring structures that are absorbed through the gastrointestinal tract. Systemic toxicity includes CNS depression and, in cases of chronic abuse, multiple organ effects such as leukemia (benzene) and renal toxicity (toluene). Examples are benzene, toluene, styrene, and xylene. The seriously toxic ingested dose is 20 to 50 mL in adults.

Halogenated hydrocarbons are aliphatic or aromatic hydrocarbons with one or more halogen substitutions (Cl, Br, Fl, or I). They are highly volatile and are abused as inhalants. They are well absorbed from the gastrointestinal tract, produce CNS depression, and have metabolites that can damage the liver and kidneys. Examples include methylene chloride (may be converted into carbon monoxide in the body), dichloroethylene (also causes a disulfiram [Antabuse] reaction known as "degreaser's flush" when associated with consumption of ethanol), and 1,1,1-trichloroethane (Glamorene Spot Remover, Scotchgard, typewriter correction fluid). An acute lethal oral dose is 0.5 to 5 mL/kg.

Dangerous additives to the hydrocarbons can be summed up with the mnemonic CHAMP: C, camphor (demothing agent); H, halogenated hydrocarbons; A, aromatic hydrocarbons; M, metals (heavy); and P, pesticides. Ingestion of these substances may warrant gastric emptying with a small-bore nasogastric tube.

Heavy hydrocarbons have high viscosity, low volatility, and minimal gastrointestinal absorption, so gastric decontamination is not necessary. Examples are asphalt (tar), machine oil, motor oil (lubricating oil, engine oil), home heating oil, and petroleum jelly (mineral oil).

Laboratory Investigations

The ECG, ABG, pulmonary function, serum electrolytes, and serial chest radiographs should be continuously monitored. Liver and renal function should be monitored in cases of inhalation of aromatic hydrocarbons.

Management

Asymptomatic patients who ingested small amounts of aliphatic petroleum distillates can be followed at home by telephone for development of signs of aspiration (cough, wheezing, tachypnea, and dyspnea) for 4 to 6 hours. Inhalation of any hydrocarbon vapors in a closed space can produce intoxication. The victim must be removed from the environment, have oxygen administered, and receive respiratory support.

Gastrointestinal decontamination is not advised in cases of hydrocarbon ingestion that usually do not cause systemic toxicity (aliphatic petroleum distillates, heavy hydrocarbons). In cases of ingestion of hydrocarbons that cause systemic toxicity in small amounts (aromatic hydrocarbons, halogenated hydrocarbons), the clinician should pass a small-bore nasogastric tube and aspirate if the ingestion was within 2 hours and if spontaneous vomiting has not occurred. Some toxicologists advocate ipecac-induced emesis under medical supervision instead of small-bore nasogastric gastric lavage; we do not.

Patients with altered mental status should have their airway protected because of concern about aspiration. The use of activated charcoal has been suggested, but there are no scientific data as to effectiveness and it may produce vomiting. Activated charcoal may, however, be useful in adsorbing toxic additives such as pesticides or co-ingestants.

The symptomatic patient who is coughing, gagging, choking, or wheezing on arrival has probably aspirated. The clinician should provide supportive respiratory care and supplemental oxygen, while monitoring pulse oximetry, ABG, chest radiograph, and ECG. The patient should be admitted to the intensive care unit. A chest radiograph for aspiration may be positive as early as 30 minutes after ingestion, and almost all are positive within 6 hours. Negative chest radiographs within 4 hours do not rule out aspiration.

Bronchospasm is treated with a nebulized β-adrenergic agonist and intravenous aminophylline if necessary. Epinephrine should be avoided because of susceptibility to dysrhythmias. Cyanosis in the presence of a normal arterial PaO_2 may be a result of methemoglobinemia that requires therapy with methylene blue. Corticosteroids and prophylactic antimicrobial agents have not been shown to be beneficial. (Fever or leukocytosis may be produced by the chemical pneumonitis itself.)

Most infiltrations resolve spontaneously in 1 week; lipoid pneumonia may last up to 6 weeks. It is not necessary to surgically treat pneumatoceles that develop because they usually resolve. Dysrhythmias may require α- and β-adrenergic antagonists or cardioversion.

There is no role for enhanced elimination procedures.

Methylene chloride is metabolized over several hours to carbon monoxide. See treatment of carbon monoxide poisoning. Halogenated hydrocarbons are hepatorenal toxins; therefore, hepatorenal function should be monitored. N-acetylcysteine therapy may be useful if there is evidence of hepatic damage.

Extracorporal membrane oxygenation (ECMO) has been used successfully for a few patients with life threatening respiratory failure. Surfactant used for hydrocarbon aspiration was found to be detrimental.

Disposition

Asymptomatic patients with small ingestions of petroleum distillates can be managed at home. Symptomatic patients with abnormal chest radiographic, oxygen saturation, or ABG findings should be admitted. Patients who become asymptomatic and have normal oxygenation and a normal repeat radiograph can be discharged.

IRON

There are more than 100 iron over-the-counter preparations for supplementation and treatment of iron deficiency anemia.

Toxic Mechanism

Toxicity depends on the amount of elemental iron available in various salts (gluconate 12%, sulfate 20%, fumarate 33%, lactate 19%, chloride 21% of elemental iron), not the amount of the salt. Locally, iron is corrosive and may cause fluid loss, hypovolemic shock, and perforation. Excessive free unbound iron in the blood is directly toxic to the vasculature and leads to the release of vasoactive substances, which produces vasodilation. In cases of overdose, iron deposits injure mitochondria in the liver, the kidneys, and the myocardium. The exact mechanism of cellular damage is not clear but is thought to be related to free radical formation.

Toxic Dose

The therapeutic dose is 6 mg/kg/d of elemental iron. An elemental iron dose of 20 to 40 mg/kg may produce mild self-limited gastrointestinal symptoms, 40 to 60 mg/kg produces moderate toxicity, more than 60 mg/kg produces severe toxicity and is potentially lethal, and more than 180 mg/kg is usually fatal without treatment. Children's chewable vitamins with iron have between 12 and 18 mg of elemental iron per tablet or 0.6 mL of liquid drops. These preparations rarely produce toxicity unless very large quantities are ingested and have never caused death.

Kinetics

Absorption occurs chiefly in the upper small intestine. Ferrous (+2) iron is absorbed into the mucosal cells, where it is oxidized to the ferric (+3) state and bound to ferritin. Iron is slowly released from ferritin into the plasma, where it binds to transferrin and is transported to specific tissues for production of hemoglobin (70%), myoglobin (5%), and cytochrome. About 25% of iron is stored in the liver and spleen. In cases of overdose, larger amounts of iron are absorbed because of direct mucosal corrosion. There is no mechanism for the elimination of iron (elimination is 1 to 2 mg/d) except through bile, sweat, and blood loss.

Manifestations

Serious toxicity is unlikely if the patient remains asymptomatic for 6 hours and has a negative abdominal radiograph. Iron intoxication can produce five phases of toxicity. The phases may not be distinct from one another.

Phase I

Gastrointestinal mucosal injury occurs 30 minutes to 12 hours postingestion. Vomiting starts within 30 minutes to 1 hour of ingestion and is persistent; hematemesis and bloody diarrhea may occur; abdominal cramps, fever, hyperglycemia, and leukocytosis may occur. Enteric-coated tablets may pass through the stomach without causing symptoms. Acidosis and shock can occur within 6 to 12 hours.

Phase II

A latent period of apparent improvement occurs over 8 to 12 hours postingestion.

Phase III

Systemic toxicity phase occurs 12 to 48 hours postingestion with cardiovascular collapse and severe metabolic acidosis.

Phase IV

Two to 4 days postingestion, hepatic injury associated with jaundice, elevated liver enzymes, and prolonged prothrombin time occur. Kidney injury with proteinuria and hematuria occur. Pulmonary edema, disseminated intravascular coagulation, and *Yersinia enterocolitica* sepsis can occur.

Phase V

Four to 8 weeks postingestion, pyloric outlet or intestinal stricture may cause obstruction or anemia secondary to blood loss.

Laboratory Investigations

Iron poisoning produces anion gap metabolic acidosis. Monitoring should include complete blood cell counts, blood glucose level, serum iron, stools and vomitus for occult blood, electrolytes, acid–base balance, urinalysis and urinary output, liver function tests, and BUN and creatinine levels. Blood type and match should be obtained.

Serum iron measurements taken at the proper time correlate with the clinical findings. The lavender top Vacutainer tube contains EDTA, which falsely lowers serum iron. One must obtain the serum iron measurement before administering deferoxamine. Serum iron levels of less than 350 µg/dL at 2 to 6 hours predict an asymptomatic course; levels of 350 to 500 µg/dL are usually associated with mild gastrointestinal symptoms; those greater than 500 µg/dL have a 20% risk of shock and serious iron toxicity. A follow-up serum iron measurement after 6 hours may not be elevated even in cases of severe poisoning, but a serum iron measurement taken at 8 to 12 hours is useful to exclude delayed absorption from a bezoar or sustained-release preparation. The total iron-binding capacity is not necessary.

Adult iron tablet preparations are radiopaque before they dissolve by 4 hours postingestion. A "negative" abdominal radiograph more than 4 hours postingestion does not exclude iron poisoning.

Patients who develop high fevers and signs of sepsis following iron overdose should have blood and stool cultures checked for *Yersinia enterocolitica*.

Management

Gastrointestinal decontamination should involve immediate induction of emesis in cases of ingestions of elemental iron of greater than 40 mg/kg if vomiting has not already occurred. Activated charcoal is ineffective. An abdominal radiograph should be obtained after emesis to determine the success of gastric emptying. Children's chewable vitamins and liquid iron preparations are not radiopaque. If radiopaque iron is still present, whole-bowel irrigation with polyethylene glycol solution should be considered. In extreme cases, removal by endoscopy or surgery may be necessary because coalesced iron tablets produce hemorrhagic infarction in the bowel and perforation peritonitis.

Deferoxamine (Desferal) in a dose of about 100 mg binds 8.5 to 9.35 mg of free iron in the serum. The deferoxamine infusion should not exceed 15 mg/kg/h or 6 g daily, but faster rates (up to 45 mg/kg) and larger daily amounts have been administered and tolerated in extreme cases of iron poisoning (>1000 mg/dL). The deferoxamine-iron complex is hemodialyzable if renal failure develops.

Indications for chelation therapy are any of the following:

- Very large, symptomatic ingestions
- Serious clinical intoxication (severe vomiting and diarrhea [often bloody], severe abdominal pain, metabolic acidosis, hypotension, or shock)
- Symptoms that persist or progress to more serious toxicity
- Serum iron level greater than 500 mg/dL

Chelation should be performed as early as possible within 12 to 18 hours to be effective. One should start the infusion slowly and gradually increase to avoid hypotension.

Adult respiratory distress syndrome has developed in patients with high doses of deferoxamine for several days; infusions longer than 24 hours should be avoided.

The endpoint of treatment is when the patient is asymptomatic and the urine clears if it was originally a positive "vin rosé" color.

For supportive therapy, intravenous bicarbonate may be needed to correct the metabolic acidosis. Hypotension and shock treatment may require volume expansion, vasopressors, and blood transfusions. The physician should attempt to keep the urinary output at greater than 2 mL/kg/h. Coagulation abnormalities and overt bleeding require blood products or vitamin K. Pregnant patients are treated in a fashion similar to any other patient with iron poisoning.

Hemodialysis and hemoperfusion are ineffective. Exchange transfusion has been used in single cases of massive poisonings in children.

Disposition

The asymptomatic or minimally symptomatic patient should be observed for persistence and progression of symptoms or development of toxicity signs (gastrointestinal bleeding, acidosis, shock, altered mental state). Patients with mild self-limited gastrointestinal symptoms who become asymptomatic or have no signs of toxicity for 6 hours are unlikely to have a serious intoxication and can be discharged after psychiatric clearance, if needed. Patients with moderate or severe toxicity should be admitted to the intensive care unit.

ISONIAZID

Isoniazid is a hydrazide derivative of vitamin B_3 (nicotinamide) and is used as an antituberculosis drug.

Toxic Mechanism

Isoniazid produces pyridoxine deficiency by increasing the excretion of pyridoxine (vitamin B_6) and by inhibiting pyridoxal 5-phosphate (the active form of pyridoxine) from acting with L-glutamic acid decarboxylase to form γ-aminobutyric acid (GABA), the major CNS neurotransmitter inhibitor, resulting in seizures. Isoniazid also blocks the conversion of lactate to pyruvate, resulting in profound and prolonged lactic acidosis.

Toxic Dose

The therapeutic dose is 5 to 10 mg/kg (maximum 300 mg) daily. A single acute dose of 15 mg/kg lowers the seizure threshold; 35 to 40 mg/kg produces spontaneous convulsions; more than 80 mg/kg produces severe toxicity. A fatal dose in adults is 4.5 to 15 g. The malnourished patients, those with a previous seizure disorder, alcoholic patients, and slow acetylators are more susceptible to isoniazid toxicity. In cases of chronic intoxication, 10 mg/kg/d produces hepatitis in 10% to 20% of patients but less than 2% at doses of 3 to 5 mg/kg/d.

Kinetics

Absorption from intestine occurs in 30 to 60 minutes, and onset is in 30 to 120 minutes, with peak levels of 5 to 8 μg/mL within 1 to 2 hours. Volume distribution is 0.6 L/kg, with minimal protein binding.

Elimination is by liver acetylation to a hepatotoxic metabolite, acetyl-isoniazid, which is then hydrolyzed to isonicotinic acid. In slow acetylators, isoniazid has a half-life of 140 to 460 minutes (mean 5 hours), and 10% to 15% is eliminated unchanged in the urine. Most (45% to 75%) whites and 50% of African blacks are slow acetylators, and, with chronic use (without pyridoxine supplements), they may develop peripheral neuropathy. In fast acetylators, isoniazid has a half-life of 35 to 110 minutes (mean 80 minutes), and 25% to 30% is excreted unchanged in the urine. About 90% of Asians and patients with diabetes mellitus are fast acetylators and may develop hepatitis on chronic use.

In patients with overdose and hepatic disease, the serum half-life may increase. Isoniazid inhibits the metabolism of phenytoin (Dilantin), diazepam, phenobarbital, carbamazepine (Tegretol), and prednisone. These drugs also interfere with the metabolism of isoniazid. Ethanol may decrease the half-life of isoniazid but increase its toxicity.

Manifestations

Within 30 to 60 minutes, nausea, vomiting, slurred speech, dizziness, visual disturbances, and ataxia are present. Within 30 to 120 minutes, the major clinical triad of severe overdose includes refractory convulsions (90% of overdose patients have one or more seizures), coma, and resistant severe lactic acidosis (secondary to convulsions), often with a plasma pH of 6.8.

Laboratory Investigations

Isoniazid produces anion gap metabolic acidosis. Therapeutic levels are 5 to 8 μg/mL and acute toxic levels are greater than 20 μg/mL. These levels are not readily available to assist in making decisions in acute overdose situations. One should monitor the blood glucose (often hyperglycemia), electrolytes (often hyperkalemia), bicarbonate, ABGs, liver function tests (elevations occur with chronic exposure), BUN, and creatinine.

Management

Seizures must be controlled. Pyridoxine and diazepam should be administered concomitantly through different IV sites. Pyridoxine (vitamin B_6) is given in a dose of 1 g for each gram of isoniazid ingested. If the dose ingested is unknown, at least 5 g of pyridoxine should be given intravenously. Pyridoxine is administered in 50 mL D_5W or 0.9% saline over 5 minutes intravenously. It must not be administered in the same bottle as sodium bicarbonate. Intravenous pyridoxine is repeated every 5 to 20 minutes until the seizures are controlled. Total doses of pyridoxine up to 52 g have been safely administered; however, patients given 132 and 183 g of pyridoxine have developed a persistent crippling sensory neuropathy.

Diazepam is administered concomitantly with pyridoxine but at a different site. They work synergistically. Diazepam should be administered intravenously slowly, 0.3 mg/kg at a rate of 1 mg/min in children or 10 mg at a rate of 5 mg/min in adults. After the seizures are controlled, the remainder of the pyridoxine is administered (1 g/1 g isoniazid) or a total dose of 5 g.

Phenobarbital or phenytoin is ineffective and should not be used.

In asymptomatic patients or patients without seizures, pyridoxine has been advised by some toxicologists prophylactically in gram-for-gram doses in cases of large overdoses (<80 mg/kg per dose) of isoniazid, although there are no studies to support this recommendation. In comatose patients, pyridoxine administration may result in the patient's rapid regaining of consciousness. Correction of acidosis may occur spontaneously with pyridoxine administration and correction of the seizures. Sodium bicarbonate should be administered if acidosis persists.

Hemodialysis is rarely needed because of antidotal therapy and the short half-life of isoniazid, but it may be used as an adjunct for cases of uncontrollable acidosis and seizures. Hemoperfusion has not been adequately evaluated. Diuresis is ineffective.

Disposition

Asymptomatic or mildly symptomatic patients who become asymptomatic can be observed in the emergency department for 4 to 6 hours. Larger amounts of isoniazid may warrant pyridoxine administration and longer periods of observation. Intentional ingestions necessitate psychiatric evaluation before the patient is discharged. Patients with convulsions or coma should be admitted to the intensive care unit.

ISOPROPANOL (ISOPROPYL ALCOHOL)

Isopropanol can be found in rubbing alcohol, solvents, and lacquer thinner. Coma has occurred in children sponged for fever with isopropanol. See Table 10 for ethanol features of alcohols and glycols.

Toxic Mechanism

Isopropanol is a gastric irritant. It is metabolized to acetone, a CNS and myocardial depressant. It inhibits gluconeogenesis. Normal propyl alcohol is related to isopropyl alcohol but is more toxic.

Toxic Dose

A toxic dose of 0.5 to 1 mg/kg of 70% isopropanol (1 mL/kg of 70%) produces a blood isopropanol plasma concentration of 70 mg/dL. The CNS depressant potency is twice that of ethanol.

Kinetics

Onset of action is within 30 to 60 minutes, and peak is 1 hour postingestion. Volume distribution is 0.6 kg/L. Isopropyl alcohol metabolizes to acetone. Its excretion is renal.

Note: The serum isopropyl concentration and amount ingested can be estimated using the same equation as is used in ethanol kinetics and substituting the specific gravity of 0.785 for isopropyl alcohol.

Manifestations

Ethanol-like inebriation occurs, with an acetone odor to the breath, gastritis, occasionally with hematemesis, acetonuria, and acetonemia without systemic acidosis.

Depression of the CNS occurs: lethargy at blood isopropyl alcohol levels of 50 to 100 mg/dL, coma at levels of 150 to 200 mg/dL, potentially death in adults at levels greater than 240 mg/dL.

Hypoglycemia and seizures may occur.

Laboratory Investigation

Monitoring of blood isopropyl alcohol levels (not readily available in all institutions), acetone, glucose, and ABG

should be maintained. The osmolal gap increases 1 mOsm per 5.9 mg/dL of isopropyl alcohol and 1 mOsm per 5.5 mg/dL of acetone. The absence of excess acetone in the blood (normal is 0.3 to 2 mg/dL) within 30 to 60 minutes or excess acetone in the urine within 3 hours excludes the possibility of significant isopropanol exposure.

Management

The airway must be protected with intubation, and assisted ventilation administered if necessary. If the patient is hypoglycemic, glucose should be administered. Supportive treatment is similar to that for ethanol ingestions.

Gastrointestinal decontamination has no role in the treatment of isopropanol ingestion. Hemodialysis is warranted in cases of life-threatening overdose but is rarely needed. A nephrologist should be consulted if the bloodisopropanol plasma concentration is greater than 250 mg/dL.

Disposition

Symptomatic patients with concentrations greater than 100 mg/dL require at least 24 hours of close observation for resolution and should be admitted. If the patient is hypoglycemic, hypotensive, or comatose, he or she should be admitted to the intensive care unit.

LEAD

Acute lead intoxication is rare and usually occurs by inhalation of lead, resulting in severe intoxication and often death. Lead fumes can be produced by burning of lead batteries or use of a heat gun to remove lead paint. Acute lead intoxication also occurs from exposure to high concentrations of organic lead (e.g., tetraethyl lead).

Chronic lead poisoning occurs most often in children 6 months to 6 years of age who are exposed in their environment and in adults in certain occupations (Table 17). In the United States, the prevalence in children aged 1 to 5 years with a venous blood lead greater than 10 µg/dL decreased from 88.2% in a 1976-1980 survey to 8.9% in a 1988-1991 survey as a consequence of measures to reduce lead in the environment, particularly leaded gasoline. However, an estimated 1.7 million children between 1 and 5 years of age and more than 1 million workers in over

---

TABLE 17 Occupations Associated with Lead Exposure

Lead production or smelting	Demolition of ships and bridges
Production of illicit whiskey	Battery manufacturing
Brass, copper, and lead foundries	Machining/grinding lead alloys
Radiator repair	Welding of old painted metals
Scrap handling	
Sanding of old paint	Thermal paint stripping of old buildings
Lead soldering	
Cable stripping	Ceramic glaze/pottery mixing
Worker or janitor at a firing range	

Modified from Rempel D: The lead-exposed worker. JAMA 262:533, 1989.

100 different occupations still have blood lead levels greater than 10 µg/dL.

Toxic Dose

In cases of chronic lead poisoning, a daily intake of more than 5 µg/kg/d in children or more than 150 µg/d in adults can give a positive lead balance. In 1991, the Centers for Disease Control and Prevention (CDC) recommended routine screening for all children younger than 6 years of age. In children a venous blood level greater than 10 µg/dL was determined to be a threshold of concern. The average venous blood level in the United States is 4 µg/dL. In cases of occupational exposure (see Table 17), a venous blood level greater than \40 µg/dL is indicative of increased lead absorption in adults.

Toxic Mechanism

Lead affects the sulfhydryl enzyme systems, the immature CNS, the enzymes of heme synthesis, vitamin D conversion, the kidneys, the bones, and growth. Lead alters the tertiary structure of cell proteins by denaturing them and causing cell death. Risk factors are mouthing behavior of infants and children and excessive oral behavior (pica), living in the inner city, a poorly maintained home, and poor nutrition (e.g., low calcium and iron). The CDC questionnaire given in Table 18 is recommended at every pediatric visit. If any answers to the CDC questionnaire are "positive," a blood screening test for lead should be administered. To be more accurate, however, identifying lead exposure studies have suggested that the questionnaire will have to be modified for each individual community because it has had poor sensitivity (40%) and specificity (60%) as it stands.

Table 19 lists sources of lead. The number one source is deteriorating lead-based paint, which forms leaded dust. Lead concentrations in indoor paint were not reduced to safer (0.06%) levels until 1978. Lead can also be produced by improper interior or exterior home renovation (scraping or demolition). It is found in pre-1960 built homes. The use of leaded gasoline (limited in 1973) resulted in residue from leaded motor vehicle emissions. Lead persists in the soil near major highways and in deteriorating

TABLE 18 CDC Questionnaire: Priority Groups for Lead Screening

1. Children age 6–72 months (was 12–36 months) who live in or are frequent visitors to older, deteriorated housing built before 1960.
2. Children age 6–72 months who live in housing built prior to 1960 with recent, ongoing, or planned renovation or remodeling.
3. Children age 6–72 months who are siblings, housemates, or playmates of children with known lead poisoning.
4. Children age 6–72 months whose parents or other household members participate in a lead-related industry or hobby.
5. Children age 6–72 months who live near active lead smelters, battery recycling plants, or other industries likely to result in atmospheric lead release.

TABLE 19 Sources of Lead

Product	Lead Content (%) by Dry Weight
Paint	0.06
Solder	0.6
Plastic additives	2.0
Priming inks	2.0
Plumbing fixtures	2.0
Pesticides	0.1
Stained glass cames	0.1
Wine bottle foils	0.1
Construction material	0.1
Fertilizers	0.1
Glazes, enamels	0.06
Toys/recreational games	0.1
Curtain weights	0.1
Fishing weights	0.1

homes and buildings. Vegetables grown in contaminated soil may contain lead.

Oil refineries and lead-processing smelters produce lead residue. Food cans produced in Mexico contain lead solder (95% do not in United States). Lead water pipes (until 1950) and lead solder (until 1986) deliver lead-containing drinking water (calcium deposits, however, may offer some protection). Water at a consumer's tap should contain less than 15 parts per billion (ppb) of lead (Table 20).

For occupational exposure, see Table 17. The Occupational Safety and Health Administration (OSHA) standards require employers to provide showering and clothes changing facilities for personnel working with lead; however, businesses with fewer than 25 employees are exempt from the regulation. The OSHA lead standard of 1978 set a limit of 60 µg/dL for occupational exposure to lead. At a blood lead level of 60 µg/dL, a worker should be removed from lead exposure and not allowed back until his or her lead level is below 40 µg/dL. Many authorities believe that this level should be lower. The lead residue on the clothes of the workers may represent a hazard to the family. Other occupations that are potential sources of lead exposure include plumbers, pipe fitters, lead miners, auto repairers, shipbuilders, printers, steel welders and cutters, construction workers, and rubber product manufacturers.

Leaded pots to make molds for "kusmusha" tea represent lead exposure. Imported pottery lined with ceramic glaze can leach large amounts of lead into acids (e.g., citrus fruit juices).

Hobbies associated with lead exposure are listed in Box 1. Some "traditional" folk remedies or cosmetics that contain lead include the following:

- "Azarcon por empacho" ("Maria Louisa" 90 to 95% lead trioxide): a bright orange powder used in Hispanic culture, especially Mexican, for digestive problems and diarrhea.
- "Greta" (4% to 90% lead): a yellow powder "por empacho" ("empacho" refers to a variety of gastrointestinal symptoms), used in Hispanic cultures, especially Mexican.
- "Pay-loo-ah": an orange-red powder used for rash and fever in Southeast Asian cultures, especially among Northern Laos Hmong immigrants.

TABLE 20 Agency Regulations and Recommendations Concerning Lead Content

Agency	Specimen	Level	Comments
CDC	Blood (child)	10 µg/dL	Investigate community
OSHA	Blood (adult)	60 µg/dL	Medical removal from work
OSHA	Air	50 µg/m³	PEL*
	Air	0.75 µg/m³	Tetraethyl or tetramethyl
ACGIH	Air	150 µg/m³	TWA†
EPA	Air	1.5 µg/m³	Three-month average
EPA	Water	15 µg/L (ppb)	5 ppb circulating
EPA	Food	100 µg/d	Advisory
FDA	Wine	300 ppm	Plan to reduce to 200 ppm
EPA	Soil/dust	50 ppm	
CPSC	Paint	600 ppm (0.06%) by dry weight	

Abbreviatons: ACGIH = American Conference of Governmental Industrial Hygienists; CDC = Centers for Disease Control and Prevention; CPSC = Consumer Product Safety Commission; EPA = Environmental Protection Agency; FDA = Food and Drug Administration; OSHA = Occupational Safety and Health Administration.
*PEL = permissible exposure limit (highest level over an 8-hour workday).
†TWA = time-weighted average (air concentration for 8-hour workday and 40 hour workweek).

- "Alkohl" (Al-kohl, kohl, suma 5% to 92% lead): a black powder used in Middle Eastern, African, and Asian cultures as a cosmetic and an umbilical stump astringent.
- "Farouk": an orange granular powder with lead used in Saudi Arabian culture.
- "Bint Al Zahab": used to treat colic in Saudi Arabian culture.
- "Surma" (23% to 26% lead): a black powder used in India as a cosmetic and to improve eyesight.
- "Bali goli": a round black bean that is dissolved in "grippe water," used by Asian and Indian cultures to aid digestion.

Cases of substance abuse involving lead poisoning have been reported, in which the patient sniffs leaded gasoline or uses improperly synthesized amphetamines.

Kinetics

Absorption of lead is 10% to 15% of the ingested dose in adults; in children, up to 40% is absorbed, especially in cases of iron deficiency anemia. With inhalation of fumes, absorption is rapid and complete. Volume distribution in blood (0.9% of total body burden) is 95% in red blood cells. Lead passes through the placenta to the fetus and is present in breast milk.

Organic lead is metabolized in the liver to inorganic lead. Its half-life is 35 to 40 days in blood; in soft tissue, the half-life is 45 days and in bone (99% of the lead), the half-life is 28 years. The major elimination route is the stool, 80% to 90%, and then renal 10% (80 g/d) and hair, nails, sweat, and saliva. Nine percent of organic lead is excreted in the urine per day.

Manifestations

Adverse health effects are given in Table 21 and include the following.

Hematologic

Lead inhibits γ-aminolevulinic acid dehydratase (early in the synthesis of heme) and ferrochelatase (transfers iron to ferritin for incorporation of iron into protoporphyrin to produce heme). Anemia is a late finding. Decreased heme synthesis starts at >40 µg/dL. Basophilic stippling occurs in 20% of severe lead poisoning.

Neurologic

Segmental demyelination and peripheral neuropathy, usually of the motor type (wrist and ankle drop), occurs in workers. A venous blood level of lead greater than 70 µg/dL (usually >100 µg/dL), produces encephalopathy in children (symptom mnemonic "PAINT": P, persistent forceful vomiting and papilledema; A, ataxia; I, intermittent stupor and lucidity; N, neurologic coma and refractory convulsions; T, tired and lethargic). Decreased cognitive abilities have been reported with a venous blood level of lead greater than 10 µg/dL, including behavioral problems, decreased attention span, and learning disabilities. IQ scores may begin to decrease at 15 µg/dL. Encephalopathy is rare in adults.

BOX 1 Hobbies Associated with Lead Exposure

Casting of ammunition
Collecting antique pewter
Collecting/painting lead toys (e.g., soldiers and figures)
Ceramics or glazed pottery
Refinishing furniture

Making fishing weights
Home renovation
Jewelry making, lead solder
Glass blowing, lead glass
Bronze casting

Print making and other fine arts (when lead white, flake white, chrome yellow pigments are involved)
Liquor distillation
Hunting and target shooting
Painting
Car and boat repair
Burning/engraving lead-painted wood
Making stained leaded glass
Copper enameling

TABLE 21 Summary of Lead-Induced Health Effects in Adults and Children

Blood Lead Level (µg/dL)	Age Group	Health Effect
>100	Adult	Encephalopathic signs and symptoms
>80	Adult	Anemia
	Child	Encephalopathy
		Chronic nephropathy (e.g., aminoaciduria)
>70	Adult	Clinically evident peripheral neuropathy
	Child	Colic and other gastrointestinal symptoms
>60	Adult	Female reproductive effects
		CNS disturbance symptoms (i.e., sleep disturbances, mood changes, memory and concentration problems, headaches)
>50	Adult	Decreased hemoglobin production
		Decreased performance on neurobehavioral tests
	Adult	Altered testicular function
		Gastrointestinal symptoms (i.e., abdominal pain, constipation, diarrhea, nausea, anorexia)
	Child	Peripheral neuropathy*
>40	Adult	Decreased peripheral nerve conduction
		Hypertension, age 40–59 years
		Chronic neuropathy*
>25	Adult	Elevated erythrocyte protoporphyrin in males
15-25	Adult	Elevated erythrocyte protoporphyrin in females
>10	Child	Decreased intelligence and growth
		Impaired learning
		Reduced birth weight*
		Impaired mental ability
	Fetus	Preterm delivery

*Controversial.
From Anonymous: Implementation of the Lead Contamination Control Act of 1988. MMWR Morb Mortal Wkly Rep 41:288, 1992.

Renal

Nephropathy as a result of damaged capillaries and glomerulus can occur at a venous blood level of lead greater than 80 µg/dL, but recent studies show renal damage and hypertension with low venous blood levels. A direct correlation between hypertension and venous blood level over 30 µg/dL has been reported. Lead reduces excretion of uric acid, and high-level exposure may be associated with hyperuricemia and "saturnine gout," Fanconi's syndrome (aminoaciduria and renal tubular acidosis), and tubular fibrosis.

Reproductive

Spontaneous abortion, transient delay in the child's development (catch up at age 5 to 6 years), decreased sperm count, and abnormal sperm morphology can occur with lead exposure. Lead crosses the placenta and fetal blood levels reach 75% to 100% of maternal blood levels. Lead is teratogenic.

Metabolic

Decreased cytochrome P450 activity alters the metabolism of medication and endogenously produced substances. Decreased activation of cortisol and decreased growth is caused by interference in vitamin conversion (25-hydroxyvitamin D to 1,25 hydroxyvitamin D) at venous blood levels of 20 to 30 µg/dL.

Other Manifestations

Abnormalities of thyroid, cardiac, and hepatic function occur in adults. Abdominal colic is seen in children at doses greater than 50 µg/dL. "Lead gum lines" at the dental border of the gingiva can occur in cases of chronic lead poisoning.

Laboratory Investigations

Serial venous blood lead measurements are taken on days 3 and 5 during treatment and 7 days after chelation therapy, then every 1 to 2 weeks for 8 weeks, and then every month for 6 months. Intravenous infusion should be stopped at least 1 hour before blood lead levels are measured. Table 22 gives a classification of blood lead concentrations in children.

One should evaluate CBC, serum ferritin, erythrocyte protoporphyrin (>35 µg/dL indicates lead poisoning as

TABLE 22 Classification of Blood Lead Concentrations in Children

Blood Lead (µg/dL)	Recommended Interventions
<9	None
10-14	Community intervention
	Repeat blood lead in 3 months
15-19	Individual case management
	Environmental counseling
	Nutritional counseling
	Repeat blood lead in 3 months
20-44	Medical referral
	Environmental inspection/abatement
	Nutritional counseling
	Repeat blood lead in 3 months
45-69	Environmental inspection/abatement
	Nutritional counseling
	Pharmacologic therapy
	DMSA succimer oral or CaNa$_2$EDTA parenteral
	Repeat every 2 weeks for 6-8 weeks, then monthly for 4-6 months
>70	Hospitalization in intensive care unit
	Environmental inspection/abatement
	Pharmacologic therapy
	Dimercaprol (BAL in oil) IM initial alone
	Dimercaprol IM and CaNa$_2$EDTA together
	Repeat every week

Abbreviations: BAL = British anti-Lewisite; CaNa$_2$EDTA = Edetate calcium disodium; DMS = dimercaptosuccinic acid; IM = intramuscular.

well as iron deficiency and other causes), electrolytes, serum calcium and phosphorus, urinalysis, BUN, and creatinine. Abdominal and long bone radiographs may be useful in certain circumstances to identify radiopaque material in bowel and "lead lines" in proximal tibia (which occur after prolonged exposure in association with venous blood lead levels greater than 50 µg/dL).

Neuropsychological tests are difficult to perform in young children but should be considered at the end of treatment, especially to determine auditory dysfunction.

Management

The basis of treatment is removal of the source of lead. Cases of poisoning in children should be reported to local health department and cases of occupational poisoning should be reported to OSHA. The source must be identified and abated, and dust controlled by wet mopping. Cold water should be let to run for 2 minutes before being used for drinking. Planting shrubbery (not vegetables) in contaminated soil will keep children away.

Supportive care should be instituted, including measures to deal with refractory seizures (continued antidotal therapy, diazepam, and possibly neuromuscular blockers), with the hepatic and renal failure, and intravascular hemolysis in severe cases. Seizures are treated with diazepam followed by neuromuscular blockers if needed.

Lead does not bind to activated charcoal. One must not delay chelation therapy for complete gastrointestinal decontamination in severe cases. Whole-bowel irrigation has been used prior to treatment. Some authorities recommend abdominal radiographs followed by gastrointestinal decontamination if necessary before switching to oral therapy. Chelation therapy can be used for patients in whom venous blood level of lead is greater than 45 µg/dL in children and greater than 80 µg/dL in adults or in adults with lower levels who are symptomatic or who have a "positive" lead mobilization test result (not routinely performed at most centers) (Table 23).

Succimer (dimercaptosuccinic acid, DMSA, Chemet), a derivative of British anti-Lewisite (BAL), is an oral agent for chelation in children with a venous blood level of greater than 45 µg/dL. The recommended dose is 10 mg/kg every 8 hours for 5 days, then every 12 hours for 14 days. DMSA is under investigation to determine its role in children with a venous blood level less than 45 µg/dL. Although not approved for adults, it has been used in the same dosage. Monitoring should be maintained by CBC, liver transaminases, and urinalysis for adverse effects.

D-Penicillamine (Cuprimine) is another oral chelator that is given in doses of 20 to 40 mg/kg/d not to exceed 1 g/d. However, it is not FDA approved and has a 10% adverse reaction rate. Nevertheless, D-penicillamine has been used infrequently in adults and children with elevated venous blood lead levels.

Edetate calcium disodium (ethylene diaminetetraacetic acid or CaNa$_2$EDTA Versenate) is a water-soluble chelator given intramuscularly (with 0.5% procaine) or intravenously. The calcium in the compound is displaced by divalent and trivalent heavy metals, forming a soluble complex, which is stable at physiologic pH (but not at acid pH) and enhances lead clearance in the urine. EDTA usually is administered intravenously, especially in severe cases. It must not be administered until adequate urine flow is established. It may redistribute lead to the brain; therefore, BAL may be given first at a venous blood lead level of greater than 55 µg/dL in children and greater than 100 µg/dL in adults. Phlebitis occurs at a concentration greater than 0.5 mg/mL. Alkalinization of the urine may be helpful. CaNa$_2$EDTA should not be confused with sodium EDTA (disodium edetate), which is used to treat hypercalcemia; inadvertent use may produce severe hypocalcemia.

Dimercaprol (BAL) is a peanut oil–based dithiol (two sulfhydryl molecules) that combines with one atom of lead to form a heterocyclic stable ring complex. It is usually reserved for patients in whom venous blood lead is greater than 70 µg/dL, and it chelates red blood cell lead, enhancing its elimination through the urine and bile. It crosses the blood–brain barrier. Approximately 50% of patients have adverse reactions, including bad metallic taste in

---

TABLE 23 Pharmacologic Chelation Therapy of Lead Poisoning

Drug	Route	Dose	Duration	Precautions	Monitor
Dimercaprol (BAL in oil)	IM	3-5 mg/kg q4-6h	3-5 days	G6PD deficiency Concurrent iron therapy	AST/ALT enzymes
CaNa$_2$EDTA (calcium disodium. versenate)	IM/IV	50 mg/kg per day	5 days	Inadequate fluid intake Renal impairment Penicillin allergy	Urinalysis, BUN Creatinine Urinalysis, BUN
D-Penicillamine (Cuprimine)	PO	10 mg/kg per day increase 30 mg/kg over 2 weeks	6-20 weeks	Concurrent iron therapy; lead exposure Renal impairment	Creatinine, CBC
2,3-Dimercaptosuccinic acid (DMSA; succimer)	PO	10 mg/kg per dose 3 times daily 10 mg/kg per dose twice daily for 14 days	19 days	AST/ALT Concurrent iron therapy G6PD deficiency lead exposure	AST/ALT

Abbreviations: ALT = alanine aminotransferase; AST = aspartate transaminase; BAL = British anti-Lewisite; bid = twice daily; BUN = blood urea nitrogen; CBC = complete blood count; G6PD = glucose-6-phosphate dehydrogenase; IM = intramuscular; IV = intravenous; PO = oral; tid = three times daily.

the mouth, pain at the injection site, sterile abscesses, and fever.

A venous blood lead level greater than 70 μg/dL or the presence of clinical symptoms suggesting encephalopathy in children is a potentially life-threatening emergency. Management should be accomplished in a medical center with a pediatric intensive care unit by a multidisciplinary team including a critical care specialist, a toxicologist, a neurologist, and a neurosurgeon. Careful monitoring of neurologic status, fluid status, and intracranial pressure should be undertaken if necessary. These patients need close monitoring for hemodynamic instability. Hydration should be maintained to ensure renal excretion of lead. Fluids, renal and hepatic function, and electrolyte levels should be monitored.

While waiting for adequate urine flow, therapy should be initiated with intramuscular dimercaprol (BAL) only (25 mg/kg/d divided into 6 doses). Four hours later, the second dose of BAL should be given intramuscularly, concurrently with CaNa$_2$EDTA 50 mg/kg/d as a single dose infused over several hours or as a continuous infusion. The double therapy is continued until the venous blood level is less than 40 μg/dL.

As long as the venous blood level is greater than 40 μg/dL, therapy is continued for 72 hours and followed by two alternatives: either parenteral therapy with two drugs (CaNa$_2$EDTA and BAL) for 5 days or continuation of therapy with CaNa$_2$EDTA alone if a good response is achieved and the venous blood level of lead is less than 40 μg/dL. If one cannot get the venous blood lead report back, one should continue therapy with both BAL and EDTA for 5 days. In patients with lead encephalopathy, parenteral chelation should be continued with both drugs until the patient is clinically stable before changing therapy. Mannitol and dexa-methasone can reduce the cerebral edema, but their role in lead encephalopathy is not clear. Surgical decompression is not recommended to reduce cerebral edema in these cases.

If BAL and CaNa$_2$EDTA are used together, a minimum of 2 days with no treatment should elapse before another 5-day course of therapy is considered. The 5-day course is repeated with CaNa$_2$EDTA alone if the blood lead level rebounds to greater than 40 μg/dL or in combination with BAL if the venous blood level is greater than 70 μg/dL. If a third course is required, unless there are compelling reasons, one should wait at least 5 to 7 days before administering the course.

Following chelation therapy, a period of equilibration of 10 to 14 days should be allowed and a repeat venous blood lead concentration should be obtained. If the patient is stable enough for oral intake, oral succimer 30 mg/kg/d in three divided doses for 5 days followed by 20 mg/kg/d in two divided doses for 14 days has been suggested, but there are limited data to support this recommendation. Therapy should be continued until venous blood lead level is less than 20 μg/dL in children or less than 40 μg/dL in adults.

Chelators combined with lead are hemodialyzable in the event of renal failure.

Disposition

All patients with a venous blood lead level of greater than 70 μg/dL or who are symptomatic should be admitted. If a child is hospitalized, all lead hazards must be removed

from the home environment before allowing the child to return. The source must be eliminated by environmental and occupational investigations. The local health department should be involved in dealing with children who are lead poisoned, and OSHA should be involved with cases of occupational lead poisoning. Consultation with a poison control center or experienced toxicologist is necessary when chelating patients. Follow-up venous blood lead concentrations should be obtained within 1 to 2 weeks and followed every 2 weeks for 6 to 8 weeks, then monthly for 4 to 6 months if the patient required chelation therapy. All patients with venous blood level greater than 10 μg/dL should be followed at least every 3 months until two venous blood lead concentrations are 10 μg/dL or three are less than 15 μg/dL.

LITHIUM (ESKALITH, LITHANE)

Lithium is an alkali metal used primarily in the treatment of bipolar psychiatric disorders. Most intoxications are cases of chronic overdose. One gram of lithium carbonate contains 189 mg (5.1 mEq) of lithium; a regular tablet contains 300 mg (8.12 mEq) and a sustained-release preparation contains 450 mg or 12.18 mEq.

Toxic Mechanism

The brain is the primary target organ of toxicity, but the mechanism is unclear. Lithium may interfere with physiologic functions by acting as a substitute for cellular cations (sodium and potassium), depressing neural excitation and synaptic transmission.

Toxic Dose

A dose of 1 mEq/kg (40 mg/kg) of lithium will give a peak serum lithium concentration about 1.2 mEq/L. The therapeutic serum lithium concentration in cases of acute mania is 0.6 to 1.2 mEq/L, and for maintenance it is 0.5 to 0.8 mEq/L. Serum lithium concentration levels are usually obtained 12 hours after the last dose. The toxic dose is determined by clinical manifestations and serum levels after the distribution phase.

Acute ingestion of twenty 300-mg tablets (300 mg increases the serum lithium concentration by 0.2 to 0.4 mEq/L) in adults may produce serious intoxication. Chronic intoxication can be produced by conditions listed below that can decrease the elimination of lithium or increase lithium reabsorption in the kidney.

The risk factors that predispose to chronic lithium toxicity are febrile illness, impaired renal function, hyponatremia, advanced age, lithium-induced diabetes insipidus, dehydration, vomiting and diarrhea, and concomitant use of other drugs, such as thiazide and spironolactone diuretics, nonsteroidal anti-inflammatory drugs, salicylates, angiotensin-converting enzyme inhibitors (e.g., captopril), serotonin reuptake inhibitors (e.g., fluoxetine [Prozac]), and phenothiazines.

Kinetics

Gastrointestinal absorption of regular-release preparations is rapid; serum lithium concentration peaks in 2 to 4 hours and is complete by 6 to 8 hours. The onset of toxicity may occur at 1 to 4 hours after acute overdose but usually is delayed because lithium enters the brain slowly. Absorption of sustained-release preparations and the development of toxicity may be delayed 6 to 12 hours.

Volume distribution is 0.5 to 0.9 L/kg. Lithium is not protein bound. The half-life after a single dose is 9 to 13 hours; at steady state, it may be 30 to 58 hours. The renal handling of lithium is similar to that of sodium: glomerular filtration and reabsorption (80%) by the proximal renal tubule. Adequate sodium must be present to prevent lithium reabsorption. More than 90% of lithium is excreted by the kidney, 30% to 60% within 6 to 12 hours.

Manifestations

The examiner must distinguish between side effects, acute intoxication, acute or chronic toxicity, and chronic intoxications. Chronic is the most common and dangerous type of intoxication.

Side effects include fine tremor, gastrointestinal upset, hypothyroidism, polyuria and frank diabetes insipidus, dermatologic manifestations, and cardiac conduction deficits. Lithium is teratogenic.

Patients with acute poisoning may be asymptomatic, with an early high serum lithium concentration of 9 mEq/L, and deteriorate as the serum lithium concentration falls by 50% and the lithium distributes to the brain and the other tissues. Nausea and vomiting may occur within 1 to 4 hours, but the systemic manifestations are usually delayed several more hours. It may take as long as 3 to 5 days for serious symptoms to develop. Acute toxicity and acute on chronic toxicity are manifested by neurologic findings, including weakness, fasciculations, altered mental state, myoclonus, hyperreflexia, rigidity, coma, and convulsions with limbs in hypertension. Cardiovascular effects are nonspecific and occur at therapeutic doses, flat T or inverted T waves, atrioventricular block, and prolonged QT interval. Lithium is not a primary cardiotoxin. Cardiogenic shock occurs secondary to CNS toxicity. Chronic intoxication is associated with manifestations at lower serum lithium concentrations. There is some correlation with manifestations, especially at higher serum lithium concentrations. Although the levels do not always correlate with the manifestations, they are more predictive in cases of severe intoxication. A serum lithium concentration greater than 3.0 mEq/L with chronic intoxication and altered mental state indicates severe toxicity. Permanent neurologic sequelae can result from lithium intoxication.

Laboratory Investigations

Monitoring should include CBC (lithium causes significant leukocytosis), renal function, thyroid function (chronic intoxication), ECG, and electrolytes. Serum lithium concentrations should be determined every 2 to 4 hours until levels are close to therapeutic range. Cross-reactions with green-top Vacutainer specimen tubes containing heparin will spuriously elevate serum lithium concentration 6 to 8 mEq/L.

Management

Vital function must be established and maintained. Seizure precautions should be instituted and seizures, hypotension,

and dysrhythmias treated. Evaluation should include examination for rigidity and hyperreflexia signs, hydration, renal function (BUN, creatinine), and electrolytes, especially sodium. The examiner should inquire about diuretic and other drug use that increase serum lithium concentration, and the patient must discontinue the drugs. If the patient is on chronic therapy, the lithium should be discontinued. Serial serum lithium concentrations should be obtained every 4 hours until serum lithium concentration peaks and there is a downward trend toward almost therapeutic range, especially in sustained-release preparations. Vital signs should be monitored, including temperature, and ECG and serial neurologic examinations should be undertaken, including mental status and urinary output. Nephrology consultation is warranted in case of a chronic and elevated serum lithium concentration (>2.5 mEq/L), a large ingestion, or altered mental state.

An intravenous line should be established and hydration and electrolyte balance restored. Serum sodium level should be determined before 0.9% saline fluid is administered in patients with chronic overdose because hypernatremia may be present from diabetes insipidus. Although current evidence supports an initial 0.9% saline infusion (200 mL/h) to enhance excretion of lithium, once hydration, urine output, and normonatremia are established, one should administer 0.45% saline and slow the infusion (100 mL/h) for all patients.

Gastric lavage is often not recommended in cases of acute ingestion because of the large size of the tablets, and it is not necessary after chronic intoxication. Activated charcoal is ineffective. For sustained-release preparations, whole-bowel irrigation may be useful but is not proven. Sodium polystyrene sulfonate (Kayexalate), an ion exchange resin, is difficult to administer and has been used only in uncontrolled studies. Its use is not recommended.

Hemodialysis is the most efficient method for removing lithium from the vascular compartment. It is the treatment of choice for patients with severe intoxication with an altered mental state, those with seizures, and anuric patients. Long runs are used until the serum lithium concentration is less than 1 mEq/L because of extensive re-equilibration. Serum lithium concentration should be monitored every 4 hours after dialysis for rebound. Repeated and prolonged hemodialysis may be necessary. A lag in neurologic recovery can be expected.

Disposition

An acute asymptomatic lithium overdose cannot be medically cleared on the basis of single lithium level. Patients should be admitted if they have any neurologic manifestations (altered mental status, hyperreflexia, stiffness, or tremor). Patients should be admitted to the intensive care unit if they are dehydrated, have renal impairment, or have a high or rising lithium level.

METHANOL (WOOD ALCOHOL, METHYL ALCOHOL)

The concentration of methanol in Sterno fuel is 4% and it contains ethanol, in windshield washer fluid it is 30% to 60%, and in gas-line antifreeze it is 100%.

Toxic Mechanism

Methanol is metabolized by alcohol dehydrogenase to formaldehyde, which is metabolized to formate. Formate inhibits cytochrome oxidase, producing tissue hypoxia, lactic acidosis, and optic nerve edema. Formate is converted by folate-dependent enzymes to carbon dioxide.

Toxic Dose

The minimal toxic amount is approximately 100 mg/kg. Serious toxicity in a young child can be produced by the ingestion of 2.5 to 5.0 mL of 100% methanol. Ingestion of 5-mL 100% methanol by a 10-kg child produces estimated peak blood methanol of 80 mg/dL. Ingestion of 15 mL 40% methanol was lethal for a 2-year-old child in one report. A fatal adult oral dose is 30 to 240 mL 100% (20 to 150 g). Ingestion of 6 to 10 mL 100% causes blindness in adults. The toxic blood concentration is greater than 20 mg/dL; very serious toxicity and potential fatality occur at levels greater than 50 mg/dL.

Kinetics

Onset of action can start within 1 hour but may be delayed up to 12 to 18 hours by metabolism to toxic metabolites. It may be delayed longer if ethanol is ingested concomitantly or in infants. Peak blood methanol concentration is 1 hour. Volume distribution is 0.6 L/kg (total body water).

For metabolism, see *Toxic Mechanism*.

Elimination is through metabolism. The half-life of methanol is 8 hours, with ethanol blocking it is 30 to 35 hours, and with hemodialysis 2.5 hours.

Manifestations

Metabolism creates a delay in onset for 12 to 18 hours or longer if ethanol is ingested concomitantly. Initial findings are as follows:

- 0 to 6 hours: Confusion, ataxia, inebriation, formaldehyde odor on breath, and abdominal pain can be present, but the patient may be asymptomatic. Note: Methanol produces an osmolal gap (early), and its metabolite formate produces the anion gap metabolic acidosis (see later). Absence of osmolar or anion gap does not always exclude methanol intoxication.
- 6 to 12 hours: Malaise, headache, abdominal pain, vomiting, visual symptoms, including hyperemia of optic disc, "snow vision," and blindness can be seen.
- More than 12 hours: Worsening acidosis, hyperglycemia, shock, and multiorgan failure develop, with death from complications of intractable acidosis and cerebral edema.

Laboratory Investigation

Methanol can be detected on some chromatography drug screens if specified. Methanol and ethanol levels, electrolytes, glucose, BUN, creatinine, amylase, and ABG should be monitored every 4 hours. Formate levels correlate more closely than blood methanol concentration with severity of intoxication and should be obtained if possible.

Management

One should protect the airway by intubation to prevent aspiration and administer assisted ventilation as needed. If needed, 100% oxygen can be administered. A nephrologist should be consulted early regarding the need for hemodialysis.

Gastrointestinal decontamination procedures have no role.

Metabolic acidosis should be treated vigorously with sodium bicarbonate 2 to 3 mEq/kg intravenously. Large amounts may be needed.

Antidote therapy is initiated to inhibit metabolism if the patient has a history of ingesting more than 0.4 mL/kg of 100% with the following conditions:

- Blood methanol level is greater than 20 mg/dL
- The patient has osmolar gap not accounted for by other factors
- The patient is symptomatic or acidotic with increased anion gap and/or hyperemia of the optic disc.

The ethanol or fomepizole therapy outlined below can be used.

Ethanol Therapy

Ethanol should be initiated immediately if fomepizole is unavailable (see *Fomepizole Therapy*). Alcohol dehydrogenase has a greater affinity for ethanol than ethylene glycol. Therefore, ethanol blocks the metabolism of ethylene glycol.

Ethanol should be administered intravenously (oral administration is less reliable) to produce a blood ethanol concentration of 100 to 150 mg/dL. The loading dose is 10 mL/kg of 10% ethanol administered intravenously concomitantly with a maintenance dose of 10% ethanol at 1.0 mL/kg/h. This dose may need to be increased to 2 mL/kg/h in patients who are heavy drinkers. The blood ethanol concentration should be measured hourly and the infusion rate should be adjusted to maintain a concentration of 100 to 150 mg/dL.

Fomepizole Therapy

Fomepizole (Antizol, 4-methylpyrazole) inhibits alcohol dehydrogenase more reliably than ethanol and it does not require constant monitoring of ethanol levels and adjustment of infusion rates. Fomepizole is available in 1 g/mL vials of 1.5 mL. The loading dose is 15 mg/kg (0.015 mL/kg) IV, maintenance dose is 10 mg/kg (0.01 mL/kg) every 12 hours for 4 doses, then 15 mg/kg every 12 hours until the ethylene glycol levels are less than 20 mg/dL. The solution is prepared by being mixed with 100 mL of 0.9% saline or D_5W. Fomepizole can be given to patients requiring hemodialysis but should be dosed as follows:

Dose at the beginning of hemodialysis:

- If less than 6 hours since last Antizol dose, do not administer dose
- If more than 6 hours since last dose, administer next scheduled dose

Dosing during hemodialysis:

- Dose every 4 hours

Dosing at the time hemodialysis is completed:

- If less than 1 hour between last dose and end dialysis, do not administer dose at end of dialysis
- If 1 to 3 hours between last dose and end dialysis, administer one half of next scheduled dose
- If more than 3 hours between last dose and end dialysis, administer next scheduled dose

Maintenance dosing off hemodialysis:

- Give the next scheduled dose 12 hours from the last dose administered

Hemodialysis increases the clearance of both methanol and formate 10-fold over renal clearance. A blood methanol concentration greater than 50 mg/dL has been used as an indication for hemodialysis, but recently some toxicologists from the New York City Poison Center recommended early hemodialysis in patients with blood methanol concentration greater than 25 mg/dL because it may be able to shorten the course of intoxication if started early. One should continue to monitor methanol levels and/or formate levels every 4 hours after the procedure for rebound. Other indications for early hemodialysis are significant metabolic acidosis and electrolyte abnormalities despite conventional therapy and if visual or neurologic signs or symptoms are present.

A serum formate level greater than 20 mg/dL has also been used as a criterion for hemodialysis, although this is often not readily available through many laboratories. If hemodialysis is used, the infusion rate of 10% ethanol should be increased 2.0 to 3.5 mL/kg/h. The blood ethanol concentration and glucose level should be obtained every 2 hours.

Therapy is continued with both ethanol and hemodialysis until the blood methanol level is undetectable, there is no acidosis, and the patient has no neurologic or visual disturbances. This may require several days.

Hypoglycemia is treated with intravenous glucose. Doses of folinic acid (Leucovorin) and folic acid have been used successfully in animal investigations to enhance formate metabolism to carbon dioxide and water. Leucovorin 1 mg/kg up to 50 mg IV is administered every 4 hours for several days.

An initial ophthalmologic consultation and follow-up are warranted.

Disposition

All patients who have ingested significant amounts of methanol should be referred to the emergency department for evaluation and blood methanol concentration measurement. Ophthalmologic follow-up of all patients with methanol intoxications should be arranged.

MONOAMINE OXIDASE INHIBITORS

Nonselective monoamine oxidase inhibitors (MAOIs) include the hydrazines phenelzine (Nardil) and isocarboxazid (Marplan), and the nonhydrazine tranylcypromine (Parnate). Furazolidone (Furoxone) and pargyline (Eutonyl)[2] are also considered nonselective MAOIs. Moclobemide,[2] which is available in many countries

_____
[2]Not available in the United States.

but not the United States, is a selective MAO-A inhibitor. MAO-B inhibitors include selegiline (Eldepryl), an antiparksonism agent, which does not have similar toxicity to MAO-A and is not discussed. Selectivity is lost in an overdose. MAOIs are used to treat severe depression.

Toxic Mechanism

Monoamine oxidase enzymes are responsible for the oxidative deamination of both endogenous and exogenous catecholamines such as norepinephrine. MAO-A in the intestinal wall also metabolizes tyramine in food. MAOIs permanently inhibit MAO enzymes until a new enzyme is synthesized after 14 days or longer. The toxicity results from the accumulation, potentiation, and prolongation of the catecholamine action followed by profound hypotension and cardiovascular collapse.

Toxic Dose

Toxicity begins at 2 to 3 mg/kg and fatalities occur at 4 to 6 mg/kg. Death has occurred after a single dose of 170 mg of tranylcypromine in an adult.

Kinetics

Structurally, MAOIs are related to amphetamines and catecholamines. The hydrazine peak levels are at 1 to 2 hours; metabolism is hepatic acetylation; and inactive metabolites are excreted in the urine. For the nonhydrazines, peak levels occur at 1 to 4 hours, and metabolism is via the liver to active amphetamine-like metabolites.

The onset of symptoms in a case of overdose is delayed 6 to 24 hours after ingestion, peak activity is 8 to 12 hours, and duration is 72 hours or longer. The peak of MAO inhibition is in 5 to 10 days and lasts as long as 5 weeks.

Manifestations

Manifestations of an acute ingestion overdose of MAO-A inhibitors are as follows:

Phase I

An adrenergic crisis occurs, with delayed onset for 6 to 24 hours, and may not reach peak until 24 hours. The crisis starts as hyperthermia, tachycardia, tachypnea, dysarthria, transient hypertension, hyperreflexia, and CNS stimulation.

Phase II

Neuromuscular excitation and sympathetic hyperactivity occur with increased temperature greater than 40°C (104°F), agitation, hyperactivity, confusion, fasciculations, twitching, tremor, masseter spasm, muscle rigidity, acidosis, and electrolyte abnormalities. Seizures and dystonic reactions may occur. The pupils are mydriatic, sometimes nonreactive with "ping-pong gaze."

Phase III

CNS depression and cardiovascular collapse occur in cases of severe overdose as the catecholamines are depleted.

Symptoms usually resolve within 5 days but may last 2 weeks.

Phase IV

Secondary complications occur, including rhabdomyolysis, cardiac dysrhythmias, multiorgan failure, and coagulopathies.

Biogenic interactions usually occur while the patient is on therapeutic doses of MAOI or shortly after they are discontinued (30 to 60 minutes), before the new MAO enzyme is synthesized. The following substances have been implicated: indirect acting sympathomimetics such as amphetamines, serotonergic drugs, opioids (e.g., meperidine, dextromethorphan), tricyclic antidepressants, specific serotonin reuptake inhibitors (SSRI; e.g., fluoxetine [Prozac], sertraline [Zoloft], paroxetine [Paxil]), tyramine-containing foods (e.g., wine, beer, avocados, cheese, caviar, chocolate, chicken liver), and L-tryptophan. SSRIs should not be started for at least 5 weeks after MAOIs have been discontinued.

In mild cases, usually caused by foods, headache and hypertension develop and last for several hours. In severe cases, malignant hypertension and severe hyperthermia syndromes consisting of hypertension or hyperthermia, altered mental state, skeletal muscle rigidity, shivering (often beginning in the masseter muscle), and seizures may occur.

The serotonin syndrome, which may be a result of inhibition of serotonin metabolism, has similar clinical findings to those of malignant hyperthermia and may occur with or without hyperthermia or hypertension.

Chronic toxicity clinical findings include tremors, hyperhidrosis, agitation, hallucinations, confusion, and seizures and may be confused with withdrawal syndromes.

Laboratory Investigations

Monitoring of the ECG, cardiac monitoring, CPK, ABG, pulse oximeter, electrolytes, blood glucose, and acid–base balance should be maintained.

Management

In the case of MAOI overdose, ipecac-induced emesis should not be used. Only activated charcoal alone should be used.

If the patient is admitted to the hospital and is well enough to eat, a nontyramine diet should be ordered.

Extreme agitation and seizures can be controlled with benzodiazepines and barbiturates. Phenytoin is ineffective. Nondepolarizing neuromuscular blockers (not depolarizing succinylcholine) may be needed in severe cases of hyperthermia and rigidity. If the patient has severe hypertension (catecholamine mediated), phentolamine (Regitine), a parenteral β-blocking agent, 3 to 5 mg intravenously, or labetalol (Normodyne), a combination of an α-blocking agent and a β-blocker, 20-mg intravenous bolus, should be given. If malignant hypertension with rigidity is present, a short-acting nitroprusside and benzodiazepine can be used. Hypertension is often followed by severe hypotension, which should be managed by fluid and vasopressors. *Caution:* Vasopressor therapy should be administered at lower doses than usual because of exaggerated pharmacologic response. Norepinephrine is preferred to dopamine, which requires release of intracellular amines.

Cardiac dysrhythmias are treated with standard therapy but are often refractory, and cardioversion and pacemakers may be needed.

For malignant hyperthermia, dantrolene (Dantrium), a nonspecific peripheral skeletal relaxing agent, is administered, which inhibits the release of calcium from the sarcoplasm. Dantrolene is reconstituted with 60 mL sterile water without bacteriostatic agents. Glass equipment must not be used, and the drug must be protected from light and used within 6 hours. Loading dose is 2 to 3 mg/kg intravenously as a bolus, and the loading dose is repeated until the signs of malignant hyperthermia (tachycardia, rigidity, increased end-tidal CO_2, and temperature) are controlled. Maximum total dose is 10 mg/kg to avoid hepatotoxicity.

When malignant hyperthermia has subsided, 1 mg/kg IV is given every 6 hours for 24 to 48 hours, then orally 1 mg/kg every 6 hours for 24 hours to prevent recurrence. There is a danger of thrombophlebitis following peripheral dantrolene, and it should be administered through a central line if possible. In addition one should administer external cooling and correct metabolic acidosis and electrolyte disturbances. Benzodiazepine can be used for sedation. Dantrolene does not reverse central dopamine blockade; therefore, bromocriptine mesylate (Parlodel) 2.5 to 10 mg should be given orally or through a nasogastric tube three times a day.

Rhabdomyolysis and myoglobinuria are treated with fluids. Urine alkalinization should also be treated.

Hemodialysis and hemoperfusion are of no proven value.

Biogenic amine interactions are managed symptomatically, similar to cases of overdose. For the serotonin syndrome cyproheptadine (Periactin), a serotonin blocker, 4 mg orally every hour for three doses, or methysergide (Sansert), 2 mg orally every 6 hours for three doses, should be considered. The effectiveness of these drugs has not been proven.

Disposition

All patients who have ingested more than 2 mg/kg of an MAOI should be admitted to the hospital for 24 hours of observation and monitoring in the intensive care unit because the life-threatening manifestations may be delayed. Patients with drug or dietary interactions that are mild may not require admission if symptoms subside within 4 to 6 hours and the patients remain asymptomatic. Patients with symptoms that persist or require active intervention should be admitted to the intensive care unit.

OPIOIDS (NARCOTIC OPIATES)

Opioids are used for analgesia, as antitussives, and as antidiarrheal agents and are illicit agents (heroin, opium) used in substance abuse. Tolerance, physical dependency, and withdrawal may develop.

Toxic Mechanism

At least four main opioid receptors have been identified. The μ receptor is considered the most important for central analgesia and CNS depression. The κ and δ receptors predominate in spinal analgesia. The σ receptors may mediate dysphoria. Death is a consequence of dose-dependent CNS respiratory depression or secondary to pulmonary aspiration or noncardiac pulmonary edema. The mechanism of noncardiac pulmonary edema is unknown.

Dextromethorphan can interact with MAOIs, causing severe hyperthermia, and may cause the serotonin syndrome (see *Selective Serotonin Reuptake Inhibitors*). Dextromethorphan inhibits the metabolism of norepinephrine and serotonin and blocks the reuptake of serotonin. It is found as a component of a large number of nonprescription cough and cold remedies.

Toxic Dose

The toxic dose depends on the specific drug, route of administration, and degree of tolerance. For therapeutic and toxic doses, see Table 24. In children, respiratory depression has been produced by 10 mg of morphine or methadone, 75 mg of meperidine, and 12.5 mg of diphenoxylate. Infants younger than 3 months of age are more susceptible to respiratory depression. The dose should be reduced by 50%.

Kinetics

Oral onset of analgesic effect of morphine is 10 to 15 minutes; the action peaks in 1 hour and lasts 4 to 6 hours. With sustained-release preparations, the duration is 8 to 12 hours. Opioids are 90% metabolized in the liver by hepatic conjugation and 90% excreted in the urine as inactive compounds. Volume distribution is 1 to 4 L/kg. Protein binding is 35% to 75%. The typical plasma half-life of opiates is 2 to 5 hours, but that of methadone is 24 to 36 hours. Morphine metabolites include morphine-3-glucuronide (inactive) and morphine-6-glucuronide (active) and normorphine (active). Meperidine (Demerol) is rapidly hydrolyzed by tissue esterases into the active metabolite normeperidine, which has twice the convulsant activity of meperidine. Heroin (diacetylmorphine) is deacetylated within minutes to 6-monacetylmorphine and morphine. Propoxyphene (Darvon) has a rapid onset of action, and death has occurred within 15 to 30 minutes after a massive overdose. Propoxyphene is metabolized to norpropoxyphene, an active metabolite with convulsive, cardiac dysrhythmic, and heart block properties. Symptoms of diphenoxylate overdose appear within 1 to 4 hours. It is metabolized into the active metabolite difenoxin, which is five times more active as a regular respiratory depressant agent. Death has been reported in children after ingestion of a single tablet.

Manifestations

Initially, mild intoxication produces miosis, dull face, drowsiness, partial ptosis, and "nodding" (head drops to chest then bobs up). Larger amounts produce the classic

TABLE 24 Doses and Onset and Duration of Action of Common Opioids

Drug	Adult Oral Dose	Child Oral Dose	Onset of Action	Duration of Action	Adult Fatal Dose
Camphored tincture of opium	25 mL	0.25-0.50 mL/kg (0.4 mg/mL)	15-30 min	4-5 h	NA
Codeine	30-180 mg	0.5-1 mg/kg	15-30 min	4-6 h	800 mg
	>1 mg/kg is toxic in a child, above 200 mg in adult >5 mg/kg fatal in a child				
Dextromethorphan	15 mg 10 mg/kg is toxic	0.25 mg/kg	15-30 min	3-6 h	NA
Diacetylmorphine; street heroin is less than 10% pure	60 mg	NA	15-30 min	3-4 h	100 mg
Diphenoxylate natiopine (Lomotil)	5-10 mg	NA	120-240 min	14 h	300 mg
	7.5 mg is toxic in a child, 300 mg is toxic in adult				
Fentanyl (Duragesic)	0.1-0.2 mg	0.001-0.002 mg/kg	7-8 min	Intramuscular: 1/2-2 h	1.0 mg
Hydrocodone with APAP (Lortab)	5-30 mg	0.15 mg/kg	30 min	3-4 h	100 mg
Hydromorphone (Dilaudid)	4 mg	0.1 mg/kg	15-30 min	3-4 h	100 mg
Meperidine (Demerol)	100 mg	1-1.5 mg/kg	10-45 min	3-4 h	350 mg
Methadone (Dolophine)	10 mg	0.1 mg/kg	30-60 min	4-12 h	120 mg
Morphine	10-60 mg	0.1-0.2 mg/kg	<20 min	4-6 h	200 mg
	Oral dose is 6 times parenteral dose, MS Contin sustained release prep				
Oxycodone APAP (Percocet)	5 mg	NA	15-30 min	4-5 h	NA
Pentazocine (Talwin)	50-100 mg	NA	15-30 min	3-4 h	NA
Propoxyphene (Darvon)	65-100 mg	NA	30-60 min	2-4 h	700 mg

triad of miotic pupils (exceptions below), respiratory depression, and depressed level of consciousness (flaccid coma). The blood pressure, pulse, and bowel activity are decreased.

Dilated pupils do not exclude opioid intoxication. Some exceptions to the miosis effect include dextromethorphan (paralyzes iris), fentanyl, meperidine, and diphenoxylate (rarely). Physiologic disturbances including acidosis, hypoglycemia, hypoxia, and postictal state, or a co-ingestant may also produce mydriasis.

Usually, the muscles are flaccid, but increased muscle tone can be produced by meperidine and fentanyl (chest rigidity). Seizures are rare but can occur with ingestion of codeine, meperidine, propoxyphene, and dextromethorphan. Hallucinations and agitation have been reported.

Pruritus and urticaria are caused by histamine release by some opioids or by sulfite additives.

Noncardiac pulmonary edema may occur after an overdose, especially with intravenous heroin abuse. Cardiac effects include vasodilation and hypotension. A heart murmur in an intravenous addict suggests endocarditis. Propoxyphene can produce delayed cardiac dysrhythmias.

Fentanyl is 100 times more potent than morphine and can cause chest wall muscle rigidity. Some of its derivatives are 2000 times more potent than morphine.

Laboratory Investigations

For patients with overdose, one should obtain and monitor ABG, blood glucose, and electrolyte levels; chest radiographs; and ECG. For drug abusers, one should consider testing for hepatitis B, syphilis, and HIV antibody (HIV testing usually requires consent). Blood opioid concentrations are not useful. They confirm diagnosis (morphine therapeutic dose, 65 to 80 ng/mL; toxic, <200 ng/mL), but are not useful for making a therapeutic decision. Cross-reactions can occur with Vick's Formula 44, poppy seeds, and other opioids (codeine and heroin are metabolized to morphine). Naloxone 4 mg IV was not associated with a positive enzyme multiplied immunoassay technique urine screen at 60 minutes, 6 hours, or 48 hours.

Management

Supportive care should be instituted, particularly an endotracheal tube and assisted ventilation. Temporary ventilation can be provided by a bag-valve mask with 100% oxygen. The patient should be placed on a cardiac monitor, have intravenous access established, and have specimens for ABG, glucose, electrolytes, BUN, and creatinine levels, CBC, coagulation profile, liver function, toxicology screen, and urinalysis taken.

For gastrointestinal decontamination, emesis should not be induced, but activated charcoal can be administered if bowel sounds are present.

If it is suspected that the patient is an addict, he or she should be restrained first and then 0.1 mg of naloxone (Narcan) should be administered. The dose should be doubled every 2 minutes until the patient responds or 10 to 20 mg has been given. If the patient is not suspected to be an addict, then 2 mg every 2 to 3 minutes to total of 10 to 20 mg is administered.

It is essential to determine whether there is a complete response to naloxone (mydriasis, improvement in ventilation), because it is a diagnostic therapeutic test. A continuous naloxone infusion may be appropriate, using the "response dose" every hour. Repeat doses of naloxone may be necessary because the effects of many opioids can last much longer than naloxone does (30 to 60 minutes). Methadone ingestions may require a naloxone infusion for 24 to 48 hours. Half of the response dose may need to be repeated in 15 to 20 minutes, after the infusion has been started.

Acute iatrogenic withdrawal precipitated by the administration of naloxone to a dependent patient should not be treated with morphine or other opioids. Naloxone's effects are limited to 30 to 60 minutes (shorter than most opioids) and withdrawal will subside in a short time.

Nalmefene (Revex), an FDA-approved long-acting (4 to 8 hours) pure opioid antagonist, is being investigated, but its role in cases of acute intoxication is unclear and it could produce prolonged withdrawal. It may have a role in place of naloxone infusion.

Noncardiac pulmonary edema does not respond to naloxone, and the patient needs intubation, assisted ventilation, positive end-expiratory pressure, and hemodynamic monitoring. Fluids should be given cautiously in patients with opioid overdose because opioids stimulate the antidiuretic hormone.

If the patient is comatose, 50% glucose (3% to 4% of comatose opioid overdose patients have hypoglycemia) and thiamine should be given prior to naloxone. If the patient has seizures that are unresponsive to naloxone, one administers diazepam and examines for metabolic (hypoglycemia, electrolyte disturbances) causes and structural disturbances.

Hypotension is rare and should direct a search for another etiology. If the patient is agitated, hypoxia and hypoglycemia must be excluded before opioid withdrawal is considered as a cause. Complications to consider include urinary retention, constipation, rhabdomyolysis, myoglobinuria, hypoglycemia, and withdrawal.

Disposition

If a patient responds to intravenous naloxone, careful observation for relapse and the development of pulmonary edema is required, with cardiac and respiratory monitoring for 6 to 12 hours. Patients requiring repeated doses of naloxone or an infusion, or those who develop pulmonary edema, require intensive care unit admission and cannot be discharged from the intensive care unit until they are symptom free for 12 hours. Intravenous overdose complications are expected to be present within 20 minutes after injection, and discharge after 4 symptom-free hours has been recommended. Adults with oral overdose have delayed onset of toxicity and require 6 hours of observation. Children with oral opioid overdose should be admitted to the hospital for observation because of delayed toxicity. Some toxicologists advise restraining a patient who attempts to sign out against medical advice after treatment with naloxone, at least until the patient receives psychiatric evaluation.

ORGANOPHOSPHATES AND CARBAMATES

Cholinergic intoxication sources are insecticides (organophosphates or carbamates), some medications, and some mushrooms. Examples of organophosphate insecticides are malathion (low toxicity, median lethal dose [LD_{50}] 2800 mg/kg), chlorpyrifos, which has been removed from market (moderate toxicity), and parathion (high toxicity, LD_{50} 2 mg/kg). Carbamate insecticides include carbaryl (low toxicity, LD_{50} 500 mg/kg), propoxur (moderate toxicity, LD_{50} 95 mg/kg), and aldicarb (high toxicity, LD_{50} 0.9 mg/kg). Pharmaceuticals with carbamate properties include neostigmine (Prostigmin) and physostigmine (Antilirium). Cholinergic compounds also include the "G" nerve war weapons tabun (GA), sarin (GB), soman (GB), and venom X (VX).

Toxic Mechanism

Organophosphates phosphorylate the active site on red cell acetylcholinesterase and pseudocholinesterase in the serum, neuromuscular and parasympathetic neuroeffector junctions, and in the major synapses of the autonomic ganglia, causing irreversible inhibition. There are two types of organophosphate intoxication: (a) direct action by the parent compound (e.g., tetraethylpyrophosphate), or (b) indirect action by the toxic metabolite (e.g., parathoxon or malathoxon).

Carbamates (esters of carbonic acid) cause reversible carbamylation of the active site of the enzymes. When a critical amount, greater than 50%, of cholinesterase is inhibited, acetylcholine accumulates and causes transient stimulation at cholinergic synapses and sympathetic terminals (muscarinic effect), the somatic nerves, the autonomic ganglia (nicotinic effect), and CNS synapses. Stimulation of conduction is followed by inhibition of conduction.

The major differences between the carbamates and the organophosphates are as follows: (a) carbamate toxicity is less and the duration is shorter; (b) carbamates rarely produce overt CNS effects (poor CNS penetration); (c) carbamate inhibition of the acetylcholinesterase enzyme is reversible and activity returns to normal rapidly; (d) pralidoxime, the enzyme regenerator, may not be necessary in the management of mild carbamate intoxication (e.g., carbaryl).

Toxic Dose

Parathion's minimum lethal dose is 2 mg in children and 10 to 20 mg in adults. The lethal dose of malathion is greater than 1375 mg/kg and that of chlorpyrifos is 25 g; the latter compound is unlikely to cause death.

Kinetics

Absorption is by all routes. The onset of acute ingestion toxicity occurs as early as 3 hours, usually before 12 hours and always before 24 hours. Lipid-soluble agents absorbed by the dermal route (e.g., fenthion) may have a delayed onset of more than 24 hours. Inhalation toxicity occurs immediately after exposure. Massive ingestion can produce intoxication within minutes.

Metabolism is via the liver. With some pesticides (e.g., parathion, malathion), the effects are delayed because they undergo hepatic microsomal oxidative metabolism to their toxic metabolites, the -oxons (e.g., paroxon, malaoxon).

The half-life of malathion is 2.89 hours and that of parathion is 2.1 days. The metabolites are eliminated in the urine and the presence of p-nitrophenol in the urine is a clue up to 48 hours after exposure.

Manifestations

Many organophosphates produce a garlic odor on the breath, in the gastric contents, or in the container. Diaphoresis, excessive salivation, miosis, and muscle twitching are helpful clues to diagnosis.

Early, a cholinergic (muscarinic) crisis develops that consists of parasympathetic nervous system activity. DUMBELS is the mnemonic for defecation, cramps, and increased bowel motility; urinary incontinence; miosis (mydriasis may occur in 20%); bronchospasm and bronchorrhea; excess secretion; lacrimation; and seizures. Bradycardia, pulmonary edema, and hypotension may be present.

Later, sympathetic and nicotinic effects occur, consisting of MATCH: muscle weakness and fasciculation (eyelid twitching is often present), adrenal stimulation and hyperglycemia, tachycardia, cramps in muscles, and hypertension. Finally, paralysis of the skeletal muscles ensues.

The CNS effects are headache, blurred vision, anxiety, ataxia, delirium and toxic psychosis, convulsions, coma, and respiratory depression. Cranial nerve palsies have been noted. Delayed hallucinations may occur.

Delayed respiratory paralysis and neurologic and neurobehavioral disorders have been described following certain organophosphate ingestions or dermal exposure. The "intermediate syndrome" is paralysis of proximal and respiratory muscles developing 24 to 96 hours after the successful treatment of organophosphate poisoning. A delayed distal polyneuropathy has been described with ingestion of certain organophosphates, such as triorthocresyl phosphate, bromoleptophos, and methomidophos.

Complications include aspiration, pulmonary edema, and acute respiratory distress syndrome.

Laboratory Investigations

Monitoring should include chest radiograph, blood glucose (nonketotic hyperglycemia is frequent), ABG, pulse oximetry, ECG, blood coagulation status, liver function, hyperamylasemia (pancreatitis reported), and urinalysis for the metabolite alkyl phosphate paranitrophenol. Blood should be drawn for red blood cell cholinesterase determination before pralidoxime is given. The red blood cell cholinesterase activity roughly correlates with clinical severity. Mild poisoning is 20% to 50% of normal, moderate poisoning is 10% to 20% of normal, and severe poisoning is 10% of normal (>90% depressed). A postexposure rise of 10% to 15% in the cholinesterase level determined at least 10 to 14 days after the exposure confirms the diagnosis.

Management

Protection of health care personnel with clothing (masks, gloves, gowns, goggles) and respiratory equipment or hazardous material suits, as necessary, is called for. General decontamination consists of isolation, bagging, and disposal of contaminated clothing and other articles. Vital functions should be established and maintained. Cardiac and oxygen saturation monitoring are needed.

Intubation and assisted ventilation may be needed. Secretions should be suctioned until atropinization drying is achieved.

Dermal decontamination involves prompt removal of clothing and cleansing of all affected areas of skin, hair, and eyes. Ocular decontamination involves irrigation with copious amounts of tepid water or 0.9% saline for at least 15 minutes. Gastrointestinal decontamination, if the ingestion was recent, involves the administration of activated charcoal.

Atropine sulfate can be given as an antidote. It is both a diagnostic and a therapeutic agent. Atropine counteracts the muscarinic effects but is only partially effective for the CNS effects (seizures and coma). Preservative-free atropine (no benzyl alcohol) should be used. If the patient is symptomatic (bradycardia or bronchorrhea), a test dose should be administered, 0.02 mg/kg in children or 1 mg in adults, intravenously. If no signs of atropinization are present (tachycardia, drying of secretions, and mydriasis), atropine should be administered immediately, 0.05 mg/kg in children or 2 mg in adults, every 5 to 10 minutes as needed to dry the secretions and clear the lungs. Beneficial effects are seen within 1 to 4 minutes and maximum effect in 8 minutes. The average dose in the first 24 hours is 40 mg, but 1000 mg or more has been required in severe cases. Glycopyrrolate (Robinul) can be used if atropine is not available. The maximum dose should be maintained for 12 to 24 hours, then tapered and the patient observed for relapse. Poisoning, especially with lipophilic agents (e.g., fenthion, chlorfenthion), may require weeks of atropine therapy. An alternative is a continuous infusion of atropine 8 mg in 100 mL 0.9% saline at rate of 0.02 to 0.08 mg/kg/h (0.25 to 1.0 mL/kg/h) with additional 1 to 5 mg boluses as needed to dry the secretions.

Pralidoxime chloride (Protopam) has both antinicotinic and antimuscarinic effects and possibly also CNS effects. Successful treatment with pralidoxime chloride may allow a reduction in the dose of atropine. Pralidoxime acts to reactivate the phosphorylated cholinesterases by binding the phosphate moiety on the esteritic site and displacing it. It should be given early before "aging" of phosphate bond produces tighter binding. However, recent reports indicate that pralidoxime chloride is beneficial even several days after the poisoning. Improvement is seen within 10 to 40 minutes. The initial dose of pralidoxime chloride is 1 to 2 g in 250 mL 0.89% saline over 5 to 10 minutes, maximum 200 mg/minute, in adults or 25 to 50 mg/kg, maximum 4 mg/kg/minute, in children younger than 12 years of age. The dose can be repeated every 6 to 12 hours for several days. An alternative is a continuous infusion of 1 g in 100 mL 0.89% saline at 5 to 20 mg/kg/h (0.5 to 12 mL/g/h) up to 500 mg/h and titrated to desired response. Maximum adult daily dose is 12 g. Cardiac and blood pressure monitoring are advised during and for several hours after the infusion. The end point is absence of fasciculations and return of muscle strength.

Contraindicated drugs include morphine, aminophylline, barbiturates, opioids, phenothiazine, reserpine-like drugs, parasympathomimetics, and succinylcholine.

Noncardiac pulmonary edema may require respiratory support. Seizures may respond to atropine and pralidoxime chloride but often require anticonvulsants. Cardiac dysrhythmias may require electrical cardioversion or antidysrhythmic therapy if the patient is hemodynamically unstable. Extracorporeal procedures are of no proven value.

Disposition

Asymptomatic patients with normal examination findings after 6 to 8 hours of observation may be discharged. In cases of intentional poisoning, the patients require psychiatric clearance for discharge. Symptomatic patients should be admitted to the intensive care unit. Observation of milder cases of carbamate poisoning, even those requiring atropine, for 6 to 8 hours symptom-free may be sufficient to exclude significant toxicity. In cases of workplace exposure, OSHA should be notified.

PHENCYCLIDINE (ANGEL DUST)

Phencyclidine is an arylcyclohexylamine related to ketamine and chemically related to the phenothiazines. Originally a "dissociative" anesthetic banned in United States since 1979, it is now an illicit substance, with at least 38 analogs. It is inexpensively manufactured by "kitchen chemists" and is mislabeled as other hallucinogens. Improper phencyclidine synthesis may release cyanide when heated or smoked and can cause explosions.

Toxic Mechanism

The mechanism of phencyclidine is complex and not completely understood. It inhibits some neurotransmitters and causes a loss of pain sensation without depressing the CNS respiratory status. It stimulates α-adrenergic receptors and may act as a "false neurotransmitter." The effects are sympathomimetic, cholinergic, and cerebellar.

Toxic Dose

The usual dose of phencyclidine mixed with marijuana joints is 100 to 400 mg of phencyclidine. Joints or leaf mixtures contain 0.24% to 7.9% of PCP, 1 mg of PCP/150 leaves. Tablets contain 5 mg (the usual street dose). CNS effects at doses of 1 to 6 mg include hallucinations and euphoria, 6 to 10 mg produces toxic psychosis and sympathetic stimulation, 10 to 25 mg produces severe toxicity, and more than 100 mg has resulted in fatalities.

Kinetics

Phencyclidine is a lipophilic weak base, with a pKa of 8.5 to 9.5. It is rapidly absorbed when smoked and snorted, poorly absorbed from the acid stomach, and rapidly absorbed from the alkaline middle small intestine. It has an enterogastric secretion and is reabsorbed in the small intestine. The onset of action when smoked is 2 to 5 minutes, with a peak in 15 to 30 minutes. With oral ingestion, the onset is in 30 to 60 minutes and when taken intravenously it is immediate. Most adverse reactions in cases of overdose begin within 1 to 2 hours. Its duration of action at low doses is 4 to 6 hours and normality returns in 24 hours; in large overdoses, fluctuating coma may last 6 to 10 days.

Volume distribution is 6.2 L/kg. Phencyclidine concentrates in brain and adipose tissue. Protein binding is 70%. The route of elimination is by gastric secretion, liver metabolism, and 10% urinary excretion of conjugates and free phencyclidine. Renal excretion may be increased 50% with urinary acidification. The half-life is 1 hour (in cases of overdose, it is 11 to 89 hours).

Manifestations

The classic picture is bursts of horizontal, vertical, and rotary nystagmus, which is a clue to diagnosis (occurs in 50% of cases), miosis, hypertension, and fluctuating altered mental state. There is a wide spectrum of clinical presentations.

Mild intoxication with 1 to 6 mg produces drunken and bizarre behavior, agitation, rotary nystagmus, and blank stare. Violent behavior and sensory anesthesia make these patients insensitive to pain, self-destructive, and dangerous. Most are communicative within 1 to 2 hours, are alert and oriented in 6 to 8 hours, and recover completely in 24 to 48 hours.

Moderate intoxication with 6 to 10 mg produces excess salivation, hypertension, hyperthermia, muscle rigidity, myoclonus, and catatonia. Recovery of consciousness occurs in 24 to 48 hours and complete recovery in 1 week.

Severe intoxication with 10 to 25 mg results in opisthotonus, decerebrate rigidity, convulsions, prolonged fluctuating coma, and respiratory failure. Patients in this category have a high rate of medical complications. Recovery of consciousness occurs in 24 to 48 hours, with complete normality in a month. Medical complications include apnea, aspiration pneumonia, cardiac arrest, hypertensive encephalopathy, hyperthermia, intracerebral hemorrhage, psychosis, rhabdomyolysis and myoglobinuria, and seizures. Loss of memory and "flashbacks" last for months. Phencyclidine-induced depression and suicide have been reported.

Fatalities occur with ingestions of greater than 100 mg and with serum levels greater than 100 to 250 ng/mL.

Laboratory Investigations

Marked elevation of creatine kinase level may occur. Values greater than 20,000 units have been reported. Urinalysis should be monitored and urine tested for myoglobin. One should monitor the blood for creatine kinase, uric acid (an early clue to rhabdomyolysis), BUN, creatinine, electrolytes (hyperkalemia), blood glucose (20% of patients have hypoglycemia), urinary output, liver function tests, ECG, and ABG if the patient has any respiratory manifestations. Measurement of phencyclidine in the gastric juice is called for because concentrations are 10 to 50 times higher than in blood or urine. Phencyclidine blood concentrations are not helpful. Phencyclidine may be detected in the urine of the average user for 10 days to 3 weeks after the last dose. In chronic users, it can be detected for over 1 month. The analogs of phencyclidine may not produce positive test results for phencyclidine in the urine. Cross-reactions with bleach and dextromethorphan may cause false-positive urine test results on immunoassay, and cross-reaction with doxylamine may produce a false-positive finding on gas chromatography.

Management

The patient should be observed for violent, self-destructive, bizarre behavior and paranoid schizophrenia.

Patients should be placed in a low sensory environment and dangerous objects should be removed from the area.

Gastrointestinal decontamination is not effective because phencyclidine is rapidly absorbed from intestines. Overtreating the mild intoxication should be avoided. There is insufficient evidence to support the use of MDAC. In cases of severe toxicity (stupor or coma), continuous gastric suction can be tried (with protection of the airway) because the drug is secreted into the gastric juice. The value of this procedure is controversial because of limited data.

The patient must be protected from harming himself or herself or others. Physical restraints may be necessary, but they should be used sparingly and for the shortest time possible because they increase risk of rhabdomyolysis. Metal restraints such as handcuffs should be avoided. For behavioral disorders and toxic psychosis, diazepam is the agent of choice. Pharmacologic intervention includes diazepam (Valium) 10 to 30 mg orally or 2 to 5 mg intravenously initially and titrated upward to 10 mg; however, up to 30 mg may be required. "Talk down" technique is usually ineffective and dangerous. Phenothiazines and butyrophenones should be avoided in the acute phase because they lower the convulsive threshold; however, they may be needed later for psychosis. Haloperidol (Haldol) administration has been reported to produce catatonia.

Seizures and muscle spasm are managed with diazepam, from 2.5 mg up to 10 mg. Hyperthermia (>38.5°C [101.3°F]) is treated with external cooling measures. Hypertension is usually transient and does not require treatment. In the case of emergent hypertensive crisis (blood pressure >200/115 mm Hg) nitroprusside can be used in a dose of 0.3 to 2 μg/kg/min. Maximum infusion rate is 10 μg/kg/min for only 10 minutes.

Acid ion trapping diuresis is not recommended because of the danger of myoglobin precipitation in the renal tubules. Rhabdomyolysis and myoglobinuria are treated by correcting volume depletion and insuring a urinary output of greater than 2 mL/kg/h. Alkalinization is controversial because of reabsorption of phencyclidine.

Hemodialysis is beneficial if renal failure occurs; otherwise, the extracorporeal procedures are not beneficial.

Disposition

All patients with coma, delirium, catatonia, violent behavior, aspiration pneumonia, sustained hypertension greater than 200/115, and significant rhabdomyolysis should be admitted to the intensive care unit until asymptomatic for at least 24 hours. If patients with mild intoxication are mentally and neurologically stable and become asymptomatic (except for nystagmus) for 4 hours, they may be discharged in the company of a responsible adult. All patients must be assessed for suicide risk before discharge. Drug counseling and psychiatric follow-up should be arranged. Patients should be warned that episodes of disorientation and depression may continue intermittently for 4 weeks or more.

PHENOTHIAZINES AND NONPHENOTHIAZINES (NEUROLEPTICS)

Toxic Mechanism

Neuroleptics have complex mechanisms of toxicity, including (a) block of the postsynaptic dopamine receptors;

(b) block of peripheral and central α-adrenergic receptors; (c) block of cholinergic muscarinic receptors; (d) quinidine-like antidysrhythmic and myocardial depressant effect in cases of large overdose; (e) lowering of the convulsive threshold; (f) effect on hypothalamic temperature regulation (Table 25).

Toxic Dose

Extrapyramidal reactions, anticholinergic effects, and orthostatic hypotension may occur at therapeutic doses. The toxic amount is not established, but the maximum daily therapeutic dose may result in significant side effects, and twice this amount may be potentially fatal. Chlorpromazine (Thorazine), the prototype, may produce serious hypotension and CNS depression at doses greater than 200 mg (17 mg/kg) in children and 3 to 5 g in an adult. Fatalities have been reported after 2.5 g of loxapine (Loxitane) and mesoridazine (Serentil) and 1.5 g of thioridazine (Mellaril).

Kinetics

These agents are lipophilic and have unpredictable gastrointestinal absorption. Peak levels occur 2 to 6 hours postingestion and have enterohepatic recirculation.

The mean serum half-life in phase 1 is 1 to 2 hours and the biphasic half-life is 20 to 40 hours. Volume distribution is 10 to 40 L/kg; protein binding is 92% to 98%. Chlorpromazine taken orally has an onset of action in 30 to 60 minutes, peak in 2 to 4 hours, and duration of 4 to 6 hours. With sustained-release preparations, the onset is in 30 to 60 minutes and duration is 6 to 12 hours.

Elimination is by hepatic metabolism, which results in multiple metabolites (some are active). Metabolites can be detected in urine months after chronic therapy. Only 1% to 3% is excreted unchanged in the urine.

Manifestations

In cases of phenothiazine overdose, anticholinergic symptoms may be present early but are not life-threatening. Miosis is usually present (80%) if the phenothiazine has strong α-adrenergic blocking effect (e.g., chlorpromazine), but anticholinergic activity mydriasis may occur. Agitation and delirium rapidly progress into coma. Major problems are cardiac toxicity and hypotension. The cardiotoxic effects are seen more commonly with thioridazine and its metabolite mesoridazine. These agents have produced the largest number of fatalities in patients with phenothiazine overdose. Cardiac conduction disturbances include prolonged PR, QRS, and QTc intervals, U- and T-wave abnormalities, and ventricular dysrhythmias, including

TABLE 25 Neuroleptics and Properties

Compound	Antipsychotic	Anticholinergic	Extrapyramidal	Hypotensive and Cardiotoxic	Sedative
Phenothiazine					
Aliphatic	1+	3+	2+	2+	3+
Chlorpromazine (Thorazine)					
Promethazine (Phenergan)					
Piperazine	3+	1+	3+	1+	1+
Fluphenazine (Prolixin)					
Perphenazine (Trilafon)					
Prochlorperazine (Compazine)					
Trifluoperazine (Stelazine)					
Piperidine	1+	2+	1+	3+	3+
Mesoridazine (Serentil)					
Thioridazine (Mellaril)					
Nonphenothiazine					
Butyrophenone	3+	1+	3+	1+	1+
Haloperidol (Haldol)					
Dibenzoxazepine	3+	1+	3+	1+	2+
Loxapine (Loxitane)					
Dihydroindolone	3+	1+	3+	1+	1+
Molindone (Moban)					
Thioxanthenes	3+	1+	3+	3+	1+
Thiothixene (Navane)					
Chlorprothixene (Taractan)					

1+ = very low activity; 2+ = moderate activity; 3+ = very high activity.

torsades de pointes. Seizures occur mainly in patients with convulsive disorders or with administration of loxapine. Sudden death in children and adults has been reported.

Idiosyncratic dystonic reactions are most common with the piperidine group. Reactions are not dose-dependent and consist of opisthotonos, torticollis, orolingual dyskinesia, or oculogyric crisis (painful upward gaze). These reactions are more frequent in children and women. Neuroleptic malignant syndrome occurs in patients on chronic therapy and is characterized by hyperthermia, muscle rigidity, autonomic dysfunction, and altered mental state. There is one case reported with acute overdose. The loxapine syndrome consists of seizures, rhabdomyolysis, and renal failure.

Laboratory Investigations

Monitoring should include arterial blood gases, renal and hepatic function, electrolytes, blood glucose, and creatine kinase and myoglobinemia in neurol-eptic malignant syndrome. Most of these agents are detected on routine screening. Quantitative serum levels are not useful in management. Cross-reactions with enzyme multiplied immunoassay technique tests occur with cyclic antidepressants. Phenothiazines give false-negative results on pregnancy urine tests using human chorionic gonadotropin as an indicator, and give false-positive results for urine porphyrins, indirect Coombs test, urobilinogen, and amylase.

Management

Vital functions must be established and maintained. All overdose patients require venous access, 12-lead ECG (to measure intervals), cardiac and respiratory monitoring, and seizure precautions. One should monitor core temperature to detect poikilothermic effect. If the patient is comatose, intubation and assisted ventilation may be required, as well as 100% oxygen, intravenous glucose, naloxone (Narcan), and thiamine.

Emesis is not recommended. Activated charcoal can be administered if ingestion was within 1 hour. MDAC has not been proven beneficial. A radiograph of the abdomen may be useful, if the phenothiazine is radiopaque. Haloperidol (Haldol) and trifluoperazine (Stelazine) are most likely to be radiopaque. Whole-bowel irrigation may be useful when a large number of pills are visualized on radiograph or if sustained-release preparations were taken, but whole-bowel irrigation has not been evaluated in patients with phenothiazine overdose.

Convulsions are treated with diazepam or lorazepam (Ativan). Loxapine (Loxitane) overdose may result in status epilepticus. If nondepolarizing neuromuscular blockade is required, pancuronium (Pavulon) or vecuronium (Norcuron) should be used (not succinylcholine [Anectine], which may cause malignant hyperthermia), and EEG should be monitored during paralysis.

Patients with dysrhythmias should be monitored with serial ECGs. Unstable rhythms can be treated with electrical cardioversion. Class 1a antidysrhythmics (procainamide, quinidine, and disopyramide [Norpace]) must be avoided.

Hypokalemia predisposes to dysrhythmias and should be corrected aggressively. Supraventricular tachycardia with hemodynamic instability is treated with electrical cardioversion. The role of adenosine has not been defined. Calcium channel and β-blockers should be avoided.

Prolongation of the QRS interval is treated with sodium bicarbonate 1 to 2 mEq/kg by intravenous bolus over a few minutes. Torsades de pointes is treated with magnesium sulfate IV 20% solution 2 g over 2 to 3 minutes. If there is no response in 10 minutes, the dose is repeated and followed by a continuous infusion of 5 to 10 mg/min or given as an infusion of 50 mg/minute for 2 hours followed by 30 mg/minute for 90 minutes twice a day for several days, as needed. The dose in children is 25 to 50 mg/kg initially and maintenance dose is 30 to 60 mg/kg per 24 hours (0.25 to 0.50 mEq/kg per 24 hours) up to 1000 mg per 24 hours. Serum magnesium levels should be monitored.

To treat ventricular tachydysrhythmias in a stable patient, lidocaine is used. If the patient is unstable, electrical cardioversion is used. Patients with heart block with hemodynamic instability should be managed with temporary cardiac pacing.

Hypotension is treated with the Trendelenburg position and 0.9% saline. If the condition is refractory to treatment or there is a danger of fluid overload, vasopressors are administered. The vasopressor of choice is α-adrenergic agonist norepinephrine (Levophed), titrated to response. Epinephrine and dopamine should not be used because β-receptor stimulation in the presence of α-receptor blockade may provoke dysrhythmias and phenothiazines are antidopaminergic.

Hypothermia and hyperthermia are treated with external warming and cooling measures, respectively. Antipyretic drugs must not be used.

Management of the neuroleptic malignant syndrome includes the following actions:

- Immediately discontinuing the offending agent
- Hyperventilating the patient, using 100% humidified, cooled oxygen at high gas flows (at least 10 L/min) because of rapid breathing
- Administering a benzodiazepine to control convulsions and facilitate cooling measures
- Initiating appropriate mechanical cooling measures, which may include intravenous cold saline (not lactated Ringer's), ice baths, cold lavage of the stomach, bladder, and rectum, and a hypothermic blanket
- Correcting acid–base and electrolyte disturbances and treating significant hyperkalemia with hyperventilation, calcium, sodium bicarbonate, intravenous glucose, and insulin; hemodialysis may be necessary

In addition, dysrhythmias usually respond to correction of the underlying acid–base disturbances and hyperkalemia. If antidysrhythmic agents are required, calcium channel blockers must be avoided because they may precipitate hyperkalemia and cardiovascular collapse. Dantrolene sodium (Dantrium), which is a phenytoin derivative, inhibits calcium release from the sarcoplasmic reticulum and results in decreased muscle contraction. Dantrolene acts peripherally and does not reverse the rigidity or psychomotor disturbances resulting from the central dopamine blockade; it therefore is often used in combination with bromocriptine. Bromocriptine mesylate (Parlodel) acts centrally as a dopamine agonist, as does amantadine hydrochloride (Symmetrel). Bromocriptine and dantrolene have been reported to be successful in combination with cooling and good supportive measures in malignant hyperthermia.

Dosing for these agents is as follows: dantrolene sodium at 2 to 3 mg/kg IV as a bolus, then 1 mg/kg/ minute to a maximum of 10 mg/kg or until the tachycardia, rigidity, increased end-tidal CO_2, and temperature elevation are controlled. *Note:* Hepatotoxicity occurs with doses greater than 10 mg/kg. To prevent symptom recurrence, 1 mg/kg should be administered every 6 hours for 24 to 48 hours after the episode. After that time, oral dantrolene can be used at a dose of 1 mg/kg every 6 hours for 24 hours as necessary. The patient should be observed for thrombophlebitis following intravenous dantrolene. It is best administered via a central line. Bromocriptine mesylate at 2.5 to 10 mg orally or via a nasogastric tube, three times a day, should be used in combination with dantrolene.

Idiosyncratic dystonic reaction can be treated with diphenhydramine (Benadryl) 1 to 2 mg/kg/dose intravenously over 5 minutes up to maximum of 50 mg intravenously; a response is noted within 2 to 5 minutes. This can be followed with oral doses for 4 to 6 days to prevent recurrence.

Extracorporeal measures (hemodialysis, hemoperfusion) are not effective in removing these agents.

Disposition

Asymptomatic patients should be observed for at least 6 hours after gastric decontamination. Symptomatic patients with cardiotoxicity, hypotension, and convulsions should be admitted to the intensive care unit and monitored for 48 hours.

SALICYLATES (ACETYLSALICYLIC ACID, SALICYLIC ACID)

Toxic Mechanism

The primary toxic mechanisms include (a) direct stimulation of the medullary chemoreceptor trigger zone and respiratory center; (b) uncoupling oxidative phosphorylation; (c) inhibition of the Krebs cycle enzymes; (d) inhibition of vitamin K dependent and independent clotting factors; (e) alteration of platelet function; and (f) inhibition of prostaglandin synthesis.

Toxic Dose

Acute mild intoxication occurs at a dose of 150 to 200 mg/kg, moderate intoxication at 200 to 300 mg/kg, and severe intoxication at 300 to 500 mg/kg. Acute salicylate plasma concentration greater than 30 mg/dL (usually >40 mg/dL) may be associated with clinical toxicity. Chronic intoxication occurs at ingestions greater than 100 mg/kg/d for more than 2 days because of accumulation kinetics. Methyl salicylate (oil of wintergreen) is the most toxic form of salicylate. A dose of 1 mL of 98% contains 1.4 g of salicylate. Fatalities have occurred with ingestion of 1 teaspoonful in children and 1 ounce in adults. It is found in topical ointments and liniments (18% to 30%).

Kinetics

Acetylsalicylic acid and salicylic acid are weak acids with a pKa of 3.5 and 3.0, respectively. Acetylsalicylic acid is absorbed from the stomach, from the small bowel, and dermally. Onset of action is within 30 minutes. Methyl salicylate and effervescent tablets are absorbed more rapidly. Salicylate plasma concentration is detectable within 15 minutes after ingestion and peaks in 30 to 120 minutes. The peak may be delayed 6 to 12 hours in cases of large overdose, overdose with enteric-coated or sustained-release preparations, and development of concretions. The therapeutic duration of action is 3 to 4 hours but is markedly prolonged in cases of overdose.

Volume distribution is 0.13 L/kg for salicylic acid but increases as the salicylate plasma concentration increases. Protein binding is greater than 90% for salicylic acid at pH 7.4 and a salicylate plasma concentration of 20 to 30 mg/dL, 75% at a salicylate plasma concentration greater than 40 mg/dL, 50% at a salicylate plasma concentration of 70 mg/dL, and 30% at a salicylate plasma concentration of 120 mg/dL.

The half-life for salicylic acid is 3 hours after a 300 mg dose, 6 hours after a 1 g overdose, and greater than 10 hours after a 10-g overdose. Elimination includes Michaelis-Menten hepatic metabolism by three saturable pathways: (a) glycine conjugation to salicyluric acid (75%); (b) glucuronyl transferase to salicyl phenol glucuronide (10%); and (c) salicyl aryl glucuronide (4%). Nonsaturable pathways are hydrolysis to gentisic acid (<1%). Ten percent is excreted unchanged.

Acidosis increases the severity of the intoxication by increasing the non-ionized salicylate that can cross membranes and enter the brain cells. In kidneys, the unionized salicylic acid undergoes glomerular filtration, and the ionized portion undergoes tubular secretion in proximal tubules and passive reabsorption in the distal tubules. Renal excretion of salicylate is enhanced by alkaline urine.

Manifestations

The ingestion of concentrated topical salicylic acid preparations (e.g., wart remover) can cause mucosal caustic injury to the gastrointestinal tract. Occult salicylate overdose should be considered in any patient with unexplained acid–base disturbance.

The manifestations of acute overdose of salicylates are as follows:

Minimal Symptoms

Tinnitus, dizziness, and deafness may occur at high therapeutic salicylate plasma concentrations of 20 to 30 mg/dL. Nausea and vomiting may occur immediately because of local gastric irritation.

Phase I. Mild manifestations occur at 1 to 12 hours after ingestion with a 6-hour salicylate plasma concentration of 45 to 70 mg/dL. Nausea and vomiting followed by hyperventilation are usually present within 3 to 8 hours after acute overdose. Hyperventilation, an increase in both rate (tachypnea) and depth (hyperpnea), is present but it may be subtle. It results in a mild respiratory alkalosis with a serum pH greater than 7.4 and urine pH greater than 6.0. Some patients may have lethargy, vertigo, headache, and confusion. Diaphoresis may be noted.

Phase II. Moderate manifestations occur at 12 to 24 hours after ingestion with a 6-hour salicylate plasma concentration of 70 to 90 mg/dL. Serious metabolic disturbances, including a marked respiratory alkalosis with anion gap metabolic acidosis, dehydration, and urine pH less than 6.0, may occur. Other metabolic disturbances include hypoglycemia or hyperglycemia, hypokalemia, decreased ionized calcium, and increased BUN, creatinine, and lactate. Mental disturbances (confusion, disorientation, hallucinations) may occur. Hypotension and convulsions have been reported.

Phase III. Severe intoxication occurs more than 24 hours after ingestion with a 6-hour salicylate plasma concentration of 90 to 130 mg/dL. In addition to the above clinical findings, coma and seizures develop and indicate severe intoxication. Pulmonary edema may occur. Metabolic disturbances include metabolic acidemia (pH <7.4) and aciduria (pH <6.0). In adults, alkalosis may persist until terminal respiratory failure.

In children younger than 4 years of age, a mixed metabolic acidosis and respiratory alkalosis develop earlier (within 4 to 6 hours) than in adults because children have less respiratory reserve and accumulate lactate and other organic acids. Hypoglycemia is more common in children.

Fatalities occur at 6-hour salicylate plasma concentrations greater than 130 to 150 mg/dL and result from CNS depression, cardiovascular collapse, electrolyte imbalance, and cerebral edema.

Chronic salicylism is more serious than acute intoxication and the 6-hour salicylate plasma concentration does not correlate well with the manifestations in both acute and chronic cases of intoxication. Chronic intoxication usually occurs with therapeutic errors in young children or the elderly with underlying illness, and the diagnosis is delayed because it is not recognized. Noncardiac pulmonary edema is a frequent complication in the elderly. The mortality rate is about 25%. Chronic salicylate poisoning in children may mimic Reye syndrome. It is associated with exaggerated CNS findings (hallucinations, delirium, dementia, memory loss, papilledema, bizarre behavior, agitation, encephalopathy, seizures, and coma). Hemorrhagic manifestations, renal failure, and pulmonary and cerebral edema may occur. The metabolic picture is hypoglycemia and mixed acid–base derangements. A chronic salicylate plasma concentration greater than 60 mg/dL with metabolic acidosis and an altered mental state is very serious.

Laboratory Investigations

All patients with intentional salicylate overdoses should have acetaminophen plasma level measured after 4 hours.

One should continuously monitor ECG, urine output, urine pH, and specific gravity. Every 2 to 4 hours in cases of severe intoxication, salicylate plasma concentration, glucose (in a case of salicylism, CNS hypoglycemia may be present despite normal serum glucose), electrolytes, ionized calcium, magnesium and phosphorous, anion gap, ABGs, and pulse oximeter should be monitored. Daily monitoring of BUN, creatinine, liver function tests, and prothrombin time should take place.

The therapeutic salicylate plasma concentration is less than 10 mg/dL for analgesia and 15 to 30 mg/dL for anti-inflammatory effect. Cross-reaction with diflunisal (Dolobid) will give a falsely high salicylate plasma concentration. The Done nomogram is not considered accurate in evaluating acute or chronic salicylate intoxications.

Management

Treatment is based on clinical and metabolic findings, not on salicylate levels. Continuous monitoring of the urine pH is essential for successful alkalinization treatment. One should always obtain an acetaminophen plasma level.

Vital functions must be established and maintained. If the patient is in an altered mental state, glucose, naloxone, and thiamine are administered in standard doses. Depending on the severity, the initial studies include an immediate and a 6-hour postingestion salicylate plasma concentration, ECG and cardiac monitoring, pulse oximeter, urine (analysis, pH, and specific gravity), chest radiograph, ABGs, blood glucose, electrolytes and anion gap calculation, calcium (ionized), magnesium, renal and liver profiles, and prothrombin time. Gastric contents and stool should be tested for occult blood. Bismuth and magnesium salicylate preparations may be radiopaque on radiographs. Consultation with a nephrologist is warranted in cases of moderate, severe, or chronic intoxication.

For gastrointestinal decontamination, activated charcoal is useful (each gram of activated charcoal binds 550 mg of salicylic acid) if a toxic dose was ingested up to 4 hours postingestion. MDAC is not recommended for salicylate intoxication.

Concretions may occur with massive (usually >300 mg/kg) ingestions. If blood levels fail to decline, prompt contrast radiography of the stomach may reveal concretions that have to be removed by repeated lavage, whole-bowel irrigation, endoscopy, or gastrostomy.

Fluids and electrolyte treatment of salicylate poisonings is given in Table 26. For shock, perfusion and vascular volume should be established with 5% dextrose in 0.9% saline, then the treatment can proceed with correction of dehydration and alkalinization.

For cases of acute moderate or severe salicylism (see Table 26), adults should receive a bolus of 1 to 2 mEq/kg of sodium bicarbonate ($NaHCO_3$) followed by an infusion of 100 to 150 mEq $NaHCO_3$ added to 500 to 1000 mL of 5% dextrose and administered over 60 minutes. Children should receive a bolus of 1 to 2 mEq/kg of $NaHCO_3$ followed by an infusion of 1 to 2 mEq/kg added to 20 mL/kg of 5% dextrose administered over 60 minutes. Potassium is added after the patient voids. The goal is to achieve a urine output of greater than 2 mL/kg/hr and a urine pH of greater than 8. The initial infusion is followed by subsequent infusions (two to three times normal maintenance) of 200 to 300 mL/h in adults or 10 mL/kg/h in children. If the patient is acidotic and has a serum pH of less than 7.15, an additional 1 to 2 mEq/kg of $NaHCO_3$ is given over 1 to 2 hours; persistent acidosis may require 1 to 2 mEq/kg of bicarbonate every 2 hours. The infusion rate, the amount of bicarbonate, and the electrolytes should be adjusted to correct serum abnormalities and to maintain the targeted urine output and urinary pH. Diuresis is not as important as the alkalinization. Careful monitoring for fluid overload should take place for patients at risk of pulmonary and cerebral edema (e.g., the elderly) and because of inappropriate secretion of the antidiuretic hormone.

In patients with mild intoxication who are not acidotic and have a urine pH greater than 6, 5% dextrose in 0.45% saline should be administered as maintenance to replace ongoing fluid loss. Some toxicologists may consider

TABLE 26 Fluid and Electrolyte Treatment of Salicylate Poisoning

Type of Salicylism	Metabolic Disturbance	Blood pH	Urine pH	Hydrating Solution	Amount of NaHCO$_3$ (mEq/L)	Amount of Potassium (mEq/L)
Mild	Respiratory alkalosis	>7.4	>6.0	5% Dextrose, 0.45% saline	50 (adult) 1 mEq/kg (child)	20
Moderate Chronic Child <4 Years	Respiratory alkalosis Metabolic acidosis	>7.4 or <7.4	<6.0	5% Dextrose in water	100 (adult) 1-2 mEq/kg (child)	40
Severe Chronic Child <4 years	Metabolic acidosis Respiratory alkalosis	<7.4	<6.0	5% Dextrose in water	150 (adult) 2m Eq/kg (child)	60
CNS Depressant Co-ingestant	Respiratory acidosis	<7.4	<6.0	5% Dextrose in water	100-150*	60

*Correct hypoventilation.
Modified from Linden CH, Rumack BH: The legitimate analgesics, aspirin and acetaminophen. In Hansen W Jr (ed): Toxic Emergencies. New York, Churchill Livingstone, 1984.

adding sodium bicarbonate 50 mEq/L or 1 mEq/kg in some cases.

To achieve alkalinization, sodium bicarbonate is administered to produce a serum pH 7.4 to 7.5 and a urine pH greater than 8. Carbonic anhydrase inhibitors (acetazolamide [Diamox]) should not be used. If the patient is acidotic, additional bicarbonate may be required. About 2 mEq/kg raises the blood pH 0.1. In children, alkalinization may be a difficult problem because of the organic acid production and hypokalemia. Hypokalemic and fluid-depleted patients cannot be adequately alkalinized. Alkalinization is usually discontinued in asymptomatic patients with a salicylate plasma concentration less than 30 to 40 mg/dL but is continued in symptomatic patients regardless of the salicylate plasma concentration. A decreased serum bicarbonate but normal or high blood pH indicates respiratory alkalosis predominating over metabolic acidosis, and the bicarbonate should be administered cautiously. An alkalemic pH of 7.40 to 7.50 is not a contraindication to bicarbonate therapy because these patients have a significant base deficit in spite of elevated blood pH.

Potassium is added, 20 to 40 mEq/L, to the infusion after the patient voids. In cases of severe, late, and chronic salicylism, 60 mEq/L of potassium may be needed. When the serum potassium is below 4.0 mEq/L, 10 mEq/L should be added over the first hour. If the patient has hypokalemia less than 3 mEq/L and flat T waves and U waves, 0.25 to 0.5 mEq/kg up to 10 mEq/h is administered. Potassium should be administered under ECG monitoring. Serum potassium is rechecked after each rapidly administered dose. A paradoxical urine acidosis (alkaline serum pH and acid urine pH) indicates that potassium is probably needed.

Convulsions are treated with diazepam or lorazepam, but hypoglycemia, low ionized calcium, cerebral edema, and hemorrhage should first be excluded with a CT scan. If tetany develops, the NaHCO$_3$ therapy is discontinued and calcium gluconate 0.1 to 0.2 mL/kg 10% administered.

Pulmonary edema management consists of fluid restriction, high FIO$_2$, mechanical ventilation, and positive end-expiratory pressure.

Cerebral edema management consists of fluid restriction, elevation of the head, hyperventilation, osmotic diuresis, and administration of dexamethasone. Vitamin K$_1$ is administered parenterally to correct an increased prothrombin time (>20 seconds) and coagulation abnormalities. If the patient has active bleeding, fresh plasma and platelets are administered as needed. Hyperpyrexia is managed by external cooling measures, not antipyretics.

Hemodialysis is the choice for removal of salicylates because it corrects the acid–base, electrolyte, and fluid disturbances as well. The indications for hemodialysis include the following:

- Acute poisoning with salicylate plasma concentration greater than 100 mg/dL without improvement after 6 hours of appropriate therapy
- Chronic poisoning with cardiopulmonary disease and a salicylate plasma concentration as low as 40 mg/dL with refractory acidosis, severe CNS manifestations (coma and seizures), and progressive deterioration, especially in elderly patients
- Impairment of vital organs of elimination
- Clinical deterioration in spite of good supportive care and alkalinization
- Severe refractory acid–base or electrolyte disturbances despite appropriate corrective measures

Disposition

There are limitations of salicylate plasma levels and patients are treated on the basis of clinical and laboratory findings. Patients who are asymptomatic should be monitored for a minimum of 6 hours, and longer if enteric-coated tablets or massive overdose was taken or if there is suspicion of concretions. Those who remain asymptomatic with a salicylate plasma concentration less than 35 mg/dL may be discharged following psychiatric evaluation, if indicated. Chronic salicylate-intoxicated patients with acidosis and an altered mental state should be admitted to the intensive care unit. Patients with acute ingestion and a salicylate plasma concentration less than 60 mg/dL and mild symptoms may be able to be treated in the emergency department. Patients with moderate and severe intoxications should be admitted to the intensive care unit.

SELECTIVE SEROTONIN REUPTAKE INHIBITORS

Selective serotonin reuptake inhibitors (SSRIs) are primarily prescribed as antidepressants. SSRIs include fluoxetine (Prozac), paroxetine (Paxil), and sertraline (Zoloft).

Toxic Mechanism

The SSRIs interfere with the neuron reuptake of serotonin (5-hydroxytryptamine) at the presynaptic ganglia sites in the brain, increasing the activity of serotonin. SSRIs should not be used within 5 weeks of when a MAOI is given, nor should MAOI therapy be initiated or discontinued within 5 weeks of SSRI therapy.

Toxic Dose

The therapeutic oral dose of fluoxetine is 20 to 80 mg/d. No toxicity is seen in children with up to 3.5 mg/kg/dose orally. A fatal dose for adults is 6 g. The therapeutic dose for paroxetine is 20 to 50 mg/d. In 35 adult patients, none developed serious side effects after the ingestion of 10 to 1000 mg, and a study involving 35 children failed to demonstrate serious adverse effects at doses less than 180 mg. The therapeutic dose for sertraline is 50 mg to 200 mg/d. Patients have ingested up to 2.6 g without serious side effects. Overdose involving children who ingested less than 100 mg failed to cause adverse events.

Kinetics

Fluoxetine is well absorbed from the gastrointestinal tract, and has a peak plasma concentration at 6 to 8 hours. Volume distribution is 20 to 42 L/kg; 95% is protein bound. The half-life is 4 days (for the demethylated active metabolite norfluoxetine, the half-life is 7 to 15 days). Elimination is 80% renal. Fluoxetine and other serotonin inhibitors are inhibitors of the cytochrome P450, CYP 2D6 enzyme. Therefore interactions may occur with many other medications, such as antidysrhythmic class IC drugs (quinidine), phenytoin (Dilantin), haloperidol, lithium, tricyclic antidepressants (TCAs), β-blockers, codeine, and carbamazepine (Tegretol).

Paroxetine is almost completely absorbed from the gastrointestinal tract, with a peak in 2 to 8 hours. Protein binding is greater than 90%; volume distribution is 13 L/kg. Paroxetine undergoes extensive first-pass liver metabolism by oxidation and methylation to inactive metabolites. It inhibits the P450 system (see fluoxetine metabolism). The average half-life is 21 hours.

Sertraline peaks in 8 to 12 hours. Its volume distribution is 20 L/kg and protein binding is 98%. The average half-life of sertraline is 26 hours. It is metabolized to form a less-active metabolite, *N*-desmethylsertraline (half-life of 62 to 104 hours).

Manifestations

All SSRIs may cause serotonin syndrome, a potentially life-threatening reaction, if they are administered concurrently with an MAOI. Serotonin syndrome is caused by cerebral serotonergic stimulation and can cause severe hyperthermia, myoclonus, rhabdomyolysis, confusion, tremors, and a variety of psychological disturbances. In addition, cardiovascular complications and extrapyramidal side effects, including akathisia, dyskinesia, and Parkinson-like syndromes may occur. Also, increased suicidal ideation, seizures, sexual disorders, and hematologic disorders (platelet serotonin activity blockade leading to prolonged bleeding times) may develop. Inappropriate secretion of antidiuretic hormone resulting in hyponatremia may occur when SSRIs are administered to the elderly. This effect is usually seen within the first week of therapy.

Overdose effects are similar to the serotonin syndrome.

Laboratory Investigations

One should obtain a complete blood count (CBC), electrolytes, glucose levels, a coagulation profile, liver function tests, creatine kinase level, and an ECG.

Management

There is no specific antidote to SSRI intoxication.

Initial management consists of stabilizing vital functions, including thermoregulation. Supportive therapy and anticipation of potential life-threatening manifestations (hypotension, hyperthermia, seizures, coma, disseminated intravascular coagulation, ventricular tachycardia, and metabolic acidosis), are essential. Vital signs, EEG, creatine kinase, and blood chemistry should be monitored.

Benzodiazepines are administered to prevent and control muscle hyperactivity (diazepam [Valium] for seizures, clonazepam [Klonopin] for myoclonus). If benzodiazepine therapy fails to control muscle activity or seizures, anesthesia or nondepolarizing neuromuscular blockade may be necessary.

Electrolyte abnormalities and acid–base balance should be corrected. Fluids are used to maintain a urine output of greater than 2 mL/kg/h if there is a risk of myoglobinuria.

There are no data to support the use of gastrointestinal decontamination, although activated charcoal may be used if an ingestion has occurred within 1 hour. Hemodialysis and charcoal hemoperfusion are unlikely to be beneficial. Haloperidol (Haldol), phenothiazines, and other highly protein-bound drugs are to be avoided.

Benzodiazepine and cooling therapy can be used for hyperthermia. Serotonin antagonists, such as cyproheptadine (Periactin), may be useful in treating serotonin syndrome, although there are no controlled data. Dantrolene (Dantrium) and bromocriptine (Parlodel) are not recommended and may actually precipitate serotonin syndrome.

Disposition

Cases of ingestions in children up to 5 years of age of less than 180 mg of paroxetine (Paxil), less than 3.5 mg/kg of fluoxetine (Prozac), or less than 100 mg of sertraline (Zoloft) can be observed at home. Symptomatic patients should be admitted to the intensive care unit until asymptomatic for 24 hours. Asymptomatic patients should be observed for 6 hours. All patients should be assessed for risk of suicide before discharge. When taken chronically, SSRIs may increase cholesterol and triglycerides and decrease uric acid, so these test results should be followed.

THEOPHYLLINE

Theophylline (Slo-Phyllin) is a methylxanthine alkaloid similar to caffeine and theobromine. Aminophylline is 80% theophylline. Theophylline is used in the acute treatment of asthma, pulmonary edema, chronic obstructive pulmonary disease, and neonatal apnea.

Toxic Mechanism

The proposed mechanisms of action include phosphodiesterase inhibition, adenosine receptor antagonism, inhibition of prostaglandins, and increase in serum catecholamines. Theophylline stimulates the central nervous, respiratory, and emetic centers and reduces the seizure threshold. It has positive cardiac inotropic and chronotropic effects, acts as a diuretic, relaxes smooth muscle, and causes peripheral vasodilation but cerebral vasoconstriction. Gastric secretions, gastrointestinal motility, lipolysis, glycogenolysis, and gluconeogenesis are all increased.

Toxic Dose

A single dose of 1 mg/kg produces a theophylline plasma concentration of approximately 2 µg/mL. The therapeutic range usually is 10 to 20 µg/mL. An acute, single dose greater than 10 mg/kg causes mild toxicity, a dose greater than 20 mg/kg causes moderate toxicity, and a dose greater than 50 mg/kg causes serious, possibly fatal toxicity. Fatalities occur at lower doses in patients with chronic toxicity, especially those with risk factors (see *Kinetics*).

Kinetics

The pKa is 9.5. Absorption from the stomach and upper small intestine is complete and rapid, with onset in 30 to 60 minutes. Peak theophylline plasma concentration occurs within 1 to 2 hours after ingestion of liquid preparations, 2 to 4 hours after ingestion of regular tablets, and 7 to 24 hours after ingestion of slow-release formulations. Volume distribution is 0.3 to 0.7 L/kg. Protein binding is 40% to 60% in adults, mainly to albumin (low albumin increases free active theophylline).

Elimination is 90% by hepatic metabolism to an active metabolite, 2-methyl xanthine. The half-life is 3.5 hours in a child and 4 to 6 hours in an adult. The half-life is shorter in smokers and patients taking enzyme-inducing drugs. Only 8% to 10% of the drug is excreted unchanged in the urine.

Risk factors that produce a longer half-life include age younger than 6 months or older than 60 years, use of enzyme-inhibitor drugs (calcium channel blockers, oral contraceptives, cimetidine [Tagamet], ciprofloxacin [Cipro], erythromycin, macrolide anti-biotics, isoniazid), illness (persistent fever >38.9°C [>102°F]), viral illness, liver impairment, heart failure, chronic obstructive pulmonary disease, and influenza vaccination.

Manifestations

Acute toxicity generally correlates with blood levels; chronic toxicity does not (Table 27).

In the case of an acute, single, regular-release overdose, vomiting and occasionally hematemesis occur at low theophylline plasma concentrations. CNS stimulation includes restlessness, muscle tremors, and protracted tonic–clonic seizures, but coma is rare. Convulsions are a sign of severe toxicity and usually are preceded by gastrointestinal symptoms (except with sustained-release and chronic intoxications). Cardiovascular disturbances include cardiac dysrhythmias (supraventricular tachycardia) and transient hypertension with mild overdoses, but hypotension and ventricular dysrhythmias with severe intoxications. Rhabdomyolysis and renal failure are occasionally seen. Children tolerate higher serum levels, and cardiac dysrhythmias and seizures occur at theophylline plasma concentrations greater than 100 µg/mL. Possible metabolic disturbances include hyperglycemia, pronounced hypokalemia, hypocalcemia, hypomagnesemia,

Table 27 Theophylline Blood Concentrations and Acute Toxicity

Plasma Concentration (µg/mL)	Toxicity Degree	Manifestations
8-10	None	Bronchodilation
10-20	Mild	Therapeutic range: nausea, vomiting, nervousness, respiratory alkalosis, tachycardia
15-25		35% have mild manifestations of toxicity
20-40	Moderate	Gastrointestinal complaints and central nervous system stimulation Transient hypertension, tachypnea, tachycardia; 80% will have some manifestations of toxicity
60	Severe	Convulsions, dysrhythmias
100		Hypokalemia, hyperglycemia Ventricular dysrhythmias, protracted convulsions, hypotension, acid–base abnormalities

Reprinted and modified from Linden CH, Rumack BH, In Toxic Emergencies (Honser W Jr [ed]): The legitimate analgesics, aspirin and acetaminophen, copyright 1984, with permission from Elsevier.

hypophosphatemia, increased serum amylase, and elevation of uric acid.

Chronic intoxication, defined as multiple doses of theophylline over 24 hours, or cases in which interacting drugs or illness interfere with theophylline metabolism are more serious and difficult to treat. Cardiac dysrhythmias and convulsions may occur at theophylline plasma concentrations of 40 to 60 µg/mL and there is no correlation with TPC. The seizures occur without warning and are protracted and repetitive and may produce status epilepticus. Vomiting and typical metabolic disturbances do not occur.

Differences with slow-release preparations are that few or no gastrointestinal symptoms occur, peak concentrations and convulsions may be delayed 12 to 24 hours postingestion, and convulsions occur without warning.

Laboratory Investigations

Monitoring includes vital signs, pulse oximeter, ABG, hemoglobin, hematocrit (for gastrointestinal hemorrhage), ECG and cardiac monitor, renal and hepatic function, electrolytes, blood glucose, acid–base balance, and serum albumin. Gastric contents and stools should be tested for occult blood. Samples for theophylline plasma concentration measurement should be drawn within 1 to 2 hours after ingestion of liquid preparations, 2 to 4 hours after ingestion of regular-release formulations, and 4 hours after ingestion of slow-release formulations. One should check the serum albumin level because a decrease in albumin levels may cause manifestations of toxicity despite normal theophylline plasma concentration. A single theophylline plasma concentration reading may be misleading; therefore, theophylline plasma concentration measurement should be repeated every 2 to 4 hours to determine the trend until a declining trend is reached and then monitored every 4 to 6 hours until it is below 20 µg/mL.

Management

Vital functions must be established and maintained. If the patient is in a coma or has convulsions or vomiting, he or she should be intubated immediately. The theophylline plasma concentration is obtained and repeated every 2 to 4 hours to determine peak absorption, and a theophylline bezoar should be considered if the theophylline plasma concentration fails to decline. Consultation with a nephrologist about charcoal hemoperfusion is recommended.

Gastrointestinal decontamination is warranted in the case of an acute overdose, but emesis must not be induced. Activated charcoal is the choice decontamination procedure in a dose of 1 g/kg to all patients, followed with MDAC 0.5 g/kg every 2 to 4 hours until the theophylline plasma concentration is less than 20 µg/mL. MDAC is effective in treating acute, chronic, and intravenous overdoses. Activated charcoal shortens the half-life of theophylline by about 50% and may be indicated up to 24 hours following ingestion.

Whole-bowel irrigation with polyethylene-electrolyte solution has been recommended for cases of massive overdose, possible concretions, and ingestion of sustained-release preparations. If intractable vomiting occurs, the antiemetic metoclopramide (Reglan) (0.1 mg/kg

adult dose), droperidol (Inapsine) (2.5 to 10 mg IV), or ondansetron (Zofran) (8 to 32 mg IV) is administered. Ondansetron, however, inhibits metabolism of theophylline after a few doses.

Convulsions are controlled with lorazepam (Ativan) or diazepam (Valium) and phenobarbital. Phenytoin (Dilantin) is ineffective. The convulsions in patients with chronic intoxication are often refractory and may require, in addition to anticonvulsants, neuromuscular paralyzing agents, sedation, assisted ventilation, and EEG monitoring.

Hypotension is treated with fluids and vasopressors, if necessary. Norepinephrine (Levophed) 0.05 µg/kg/min is preferred as the vasopressor over dopamine.

Supraventricular tachycardia with hemodynamic instability requires cardioversion. Low-dose β-blockers may be used but should not be used in patients with reactive airway disease or hypotension. Adenosine (Adenocard) is ineffective. For ventriculardys rhythmias, electrolyte disturbances should be corrected. Lidocaine is the treatment of choice but has the potential to cause seizures at toxic concentrations. Cardioversion may be needed.

Hematemesis is managed with sucralfate (Carafate) 1 g four times daily and/or Maalox TC 30 mL every 2 hours and blood replacement, if necessary. H_2 antihistamine blockers that are enzyme inhibitors are not used.

Fluid and metabolic disturbances should be corrected. Hyperglycemia does not require insulin therapy. Hypokalemia should be corrected cautiously, as it may be largely an intracellular shift and not total body loss. Usually adding 40 mEq potassium to a liter of fluid will suffice. The serum potassium level must be monitored closely.

Charcoal hemoperfusion is the management of choice for patients with serious intoxications. Hemoperfusion can increase the clearance twofold to threefold over hemodialysis, but hemodialysis can be used if hemoperfusion is not available. Criteria for charcoal hemoperfusion are as follows:

- Life-threatening events such as convulsions or dysrhythmias
- Intractable vomiting refractory to antiemetics
- Acute intoxications with a theophylline plasma concentration greater than 80 µg/mL or greater than 70 µg/mL 4 hours after overdose with a sustained-release formulation and greater than 40 µg/mL in the case of chronic intoxication
- Acute or chronic overdoses with a theophylline plasma concentration greater than 40 µg/mL, especially if the patient has risk factors that lengthen the half-life of the drug (see Kinetics).

Disposition

Patients with mild symptoms and a theophylline plasma concentration less than 20 µg/mL can be treated in emergency department and discharged when asymptomatic for a few hours. Any patient with acute ingestion and a theophylline plasma concentration greater than 35 µg/mL should be admitted to a monitored bed with seizure precautions and suicide precautions, if needed. If neurologic or cardiotoxic effects or a theophylline plasma concentration greater than 50 µg/mL is present, the patient should be admitted to the intensive care unit. A patient with an overdose of a sustained-release preparation, regardless of symptoms or initial theophylline plasma concentration, requires admission, monitoring, activated charcoal, and MDAC. In patients on chronic therapy, toxicity may occur at a lower theophylline plasma concentration, and these patients should not be discharged until they are asymptomatic for several hours.

TRICYCLIC AND CYCLIC ANTIDEPRESSANTS

Historically, tricyclic antidepressants are an important cause of pharmaceutical overdose fatalities. The mortality rate was reduced from 15% in the 1970s to less than 1% in the 1990s because of a better understanding of the pathophysiology of these agents and improvements in management (Table 28).

Toxic Mechanism

The major mechanisms of toxicity of the tricyclic antidepressants are (a) central and peripheral anticholinergic effects; (b) peripheral α-adrenergic blockade; (c) quinidine-like cardiac membrane stabilizing action blockade of the fast inward sodium channels; and (d) inhibition of synaptic neurotransmitter reuptake in the CNS presynaptic neurons. The tetracyclics, monocyclic aminoketones, and dibenzoxazepines possess convulsive activity and less cardiac toxicity in overdose than the older tricyclic antidepressants. Triazolopyridine has less serious cardiac and CNS toxicity.

Toxic Dose

The therapeutic dose of imipramine (Tofranil) is 1.5 to 5 mg/kg; a dose greater than 5 mg/kg may be mildly toxic; 10 to 20 mg/kg may be life threatening, although less than 20 mg/kg has produced few fatalities; greater than 30 mg/kg carries a 30% mortality rate; and at a dose greater than 70 mg/kg, patients rarely survive. In children 375 mg and in adults as little as 500 mg have been fatal. In adults, five times the maximum daily dose is toxic and 10 times is potentially fatal. Although major overdose symptoms are associated with plasma concentrations greater than 1 µg/mL (>1000 ng/mL), plasma tricyclic levels do not correlate well with toxicity; clinical signs and symptoms should guide therapy.

The relative dosage or potency equivalents are as follows: amitriptyline (Elavil) 100 mg = amoxapine (Asendin) 125 mg = desipramine (Norpramin) 75 mg = doxepin (Sinequan) 100 mg = imipramine (Tofranil) 75 mg = maprotiline (Ludiomil) 75 mg = nortriptyline (Pamelor) 50 mg = trazodone (Desyrel) 200 mg. This allows one to determine an equivalent dosage of an agent compared with another (see Table 28).

Kinetics

The tricyclic and cyclic antidepressants are lipophilic. They are rapidly absorbed from the alkaline small intestine, but absorption may be prolonged and delayed in cases of massive overdose owing to anticholinergic action. Onset varies from less than 1 hour (30 to 40 minutes) to,

TABLE 28 Cyclic Antidepressants, Daily Dose and Their Major Properties

Generic Name	Adult Daily Dose (mg)	Therapeutic Range (ng/mL)	Half-life (hours)	Toxicity* Antichol	CNS	Cardiac
Tertiary Amines						
Amitriptyline (Elavil)	75-300	120-250	31-46	3+	3+	3+
Imipramine (Tofranil)	75-300	125-250	9-24	3+	3+	2+
Doxepin (Sinequan)	75-300	30-150	8-24	3+	3+	2+
Trimipramine (Surmantil)	75-200	10-240	16-18	3+	3+	2+
Secondary Amines						
Nortriptyline (Pamelor)	75-150	50-150	18-93	2+	3+	3+
Desipramine (Norpramin)	75-200	75-160	14-62	1+	3+	3+
Protriptyline (Vivactil)	20-60	70-250	54-198	2+	3+	3+
Newer Cyclic Antidepressants						
Teracyclic			30-60	1+	2+	3+
Maprotiline (Ludiomil)	75-300	—	30-60	1+	2+	3+
Trizolopyridine, a noncyclic, produces less serious cardiac and CNS toxicity						
Trazodone (Desyrel)	50-600	700	4-7	1+	1+	1+
Monocyclic Aminoketones						
Bupropion (Wellbutrin)	200-400	—	8-24	1+	3+	1+
Dibenzazepine						
Clomipramine (Anafranil)	100-250	200-500	21-32	2+	2+	2+
Dibenoxazepine						
Amoxapine (Ascendin)	150-300	200-500	6-10	1+	3+	2+

*Antichol = anticholinergic effect; CNS = central nervous system effect primarily seizures; Cardiac = cardiac effect.
Other drugs with similar structures are cyclobenzaprine, a muscle relaxant (similar to amitriptyline), and carbamazepine, an anticonvulsant (similar to imipramine); however, they cause less cardiac toxicity.

rarely, 12 hours. The peak serum levels are reached in 2 to 8 hours and the peak effect is in 6 hours but may be delayed 12 hours because of erratic absorption. The clinical effects correlate poorly with plasma levels.

Cyclic antidepressants are highly protein-bound to plasma glycoproteins, 98% at a pH 7.5 and 90% at 7.0. Volume distribution is 10 to 50 L/kg. The elimination route is by hepatic metabolism. The tertiary amines are metabolized into active demethylated secondary amine metabolites. The active secondary amine metabolites undergo a 15% enterohepatic recirculation and are metabolized over a period of days into nonactive metabolites. The intestinal bacterial flora may reconstitute the metabolites, which are active.

The half-life varies from 10 hours for imipramine to 81 hours for amitriptyline and 100 hours for nortriptyline. The active metabolites have longer half-lives.

Only 3% of the ingested dose is excreted in the urine unchanged.

Manifestations

There are reports of asymptomatic patients who, upon arrival to an emergency department, suddenly have a seizure, develop hemodynamically unstable dysrhythmias, and die shortly thereafter from ingestion of a tricyclic antidepressant. Most patients with severe toxicity develop symptoms within 1 to 2 hours, but symptoms may be delayed 6 hours after overdose.

Small overdoses produce early anticholinergic effects, agitation, and transient hypertension, which are not life-threatening. Large overdoses produce depression of the CNS and myocardium, convulsions, and hypotension. Death can occur within the first 2 to 6 hours following ingestion.

Some ECG screening tools for predicting cardiac or neurologic toxicity from ingestion of a tricyclic antidepressant have been developed: (a) A QRS greater than 0.10 second may produce seizures, and if greater than 0.16 second, 50% of patients may develop ventricular dysrhythmias (20% of these may be life-threatening) and seizures; (b) a terminal 40 msec of the QRS axis greater than 120 degrees in the right frontal plane may be associated with toxicity; or (c) a large R wave greater than 3 mm in ECG lead aVR may predispose the patient to toxicity. The quinidine cardiac membrane stabilizing effect produces depression of myocardium, conduction, and ECG changes. The peripheral α-adrenergic blockade produces hypotension.

The secondary amines are metabolized to inactive metabolites. The tetracyclics produce a high incidence of cardiovascular disturbances and seizures. Monocyclic aminoketones produce seizures in doses greater than 600 mg. Dibenzoxazepines produce a syndrome of convulsions, rhabdomyolysis, and renal failure.

Laboratory Investigations

If the patient has altered mental status or ECG abnormalities, ABG, ECG, chest radiograph, blood glucose, serum electrolytes, calcium, magnesium, blood urea nitrogen, and creatinine levels, liver profile, creatine kinase level, urine output, and, in severe cases, hemodynamic monitoring are indicated. Levels of the tricyclic and cyclic antidepressants less than 300 ng/mL are therapeutic; levels greater than 500 ng/mL indicate toxicity, and levels greater than 1000 ng/mL indicate serious poisoning and are associated with QRS widening.

Management

Vital functions must be established and maintained. Even if the patient is asymptomatic, intravenous access should be established, vital signs and neurologic status monitored, and baseline 12-lead ECG and continuous cardiac monitoring obtained for at least 6 hours from admission or 8 to 12 hours postingestion. QRS interval should be measured on a limb lead ECG every 15 minutes for 6 hours postingestion.

For gastrointestinal decontamination, emesis should not be induced and gastric lavage should not be used. Activated charcoal is preferable. If the patient is in an altered mental state, the airway must be protected. Activated charcoal 1 g/kg is recommended up to 1 hour postingestion. Benefit from MDAC has not been demonstrated.

Alkalinization does not control seizures; diazepam or lorazepam should be used. Status epilepticus may require high-dose barbiturates or neuromuscular blockers with intravenous diazepam. If not successful, the patient can be paralyzed with short-term nondepolarizing neuromuscular blockers such as vecuronium (Norcuron), intubation, and assisted ventilation. A bolus of sodium bicarbonate is recommended as an adjunct to correct the acidosis produced by the seizures.

Sodium bicarbonate is administered in a dose of 1 to 2 mEq/kg undiluted as a bolus and repeated twice a few minutes apart, if needed, for "sodium loading" and alkalinization, which may increase protein binding from 90% to 98%. The sodium loading overcomes the sodium channel blockage and is more important than the alkalinization. Indications include (a) a QRS complex greater than 0.12 second, (b) ventricular tachycardia, (c) severe conduction disturbances, (d) metabolic acidosis, (e) coma, and (f) seizures. A continuous infusion of sodium bicarbonate is of limited usefulness for controlling dysrhythmias. Bolus therapy should be used as needed.

Hyperventilation alone has been recommended, but the pH elevation is not as instantaneous and there is compensatory renal excretion of bicarbonate; therefore, we do not recommend it. The combination of hyperventilation and sodium bicarbonate has produced fatal alkalemia and is not recommended. One should monitor serum potassium level (the sudden increase in blood pH can aggravate or precipitate hypokalemia), serum sodium, and ionized calcium levels (hypocalcemia may occur with alkalinization) and blood pH.

Specific cardiovascular complications should be treated as follows: Hypotension is treated with norepinephrine, a predominantly α-adrenergic drug, which is preferred over dopamine. Hypertension that occurs early rarely requires treatment. Sinus tachycardia usually does not require treatment. Supraventricular tachycardia in a patient who is hemodynamically unstable requires synchronized electrical cardioversion, starting at 0.25 to 1.0 watt-second per kg, after sedation. Ventricular tachycardia that persists after alkalinization requires intravenous lidocaine or countershock if the patient is hemodynamically unstable. Ventricular fibrillation should be treated with defibrillation.

Torsades de pointes is treated with magnesium sulfate IV 20% solution, 2 g over 2 to 3 minutes, followed by a continuous infusion of 1.5 mL 10% solution or 5 to 10 mg per minute. For the treatment of bradydysrhythmias, atropine is contraindicated because of the anticholinergic activity. Isoproterenol 0.1 μg/kg/minute, used with caution, may produce hypotension. If the patient is hemodynamically unstable, a pacemaker is used.

Extraordinary measures, such as aortic balloon pump and cardiopulmonary bypass, have been successful.

Investigational treatments include FAB fragments specific for tricyclic antidepressant, which have been successful in animals. Prophylactic $NaHCO_3$ to prevent dysrhythmias is also being investigated.

Physostigmine has produced asystole, and flumazenil has produced seizures. Both are contraindicated.

Disposition

A patient with an antidepressant overdose who meets any of the following criteria should be admitted to the intensive care unit for 12 to 24 hours: (a) ECG abnormalities except sinus tachycardia, (b) altered mental state, (c) seizures, (d) respiratory depression, and (e) hypotension. Low-risk patients include those in whom the above symptoms are absent at 6 hours postingestion, those who present with minor transient manifestations such as sinus tachycardia who subsequently become and remain asymptomatic for a 6-hour period, and asymptomatic patients who remain asymptomatic for 6 hours. These patients may be discharged if the ECG remains normal, they have normal bowel sounds, and they undergo psychiatric disposition.

Even if the patient is asymptomatic upon presentation to the health care facility, intravenous access should be established, vital signs and neurologic status monitored, a baseline 12-lead ECG obtained, and cardiac monitoring continued for at least 6 hours. *Caution:* in 25% of fatal cases, the patients were initially alert and awake at presentation. However, in most cases of fatality initially deemed as sudden cardiac death, the patient, upon reexamination, actually had symptoms that were missed.

Children younger than 6 years of age with non-intentional (accidental) exposures to amitriptyline (Elavil), desipramine (Norpramin), doxepin (Sinequan), imipramine (Tofranil), or nortriptyline (Aventyl) in a dose less than 5 mg/kg, who are asymptomatic and have what are deemed reliable caregivers, can be observed at home, with close poison control follow-up for 6 hours. Parents or caregivers should be given instructions regarding signs and symptoms to be alert for. Children who are symptomatic, or who ingested greater than 5 mg/kg, should be referred to the emergency department for monitoring, observation, and activated charcoal treatment.

Appendices and Index

Reference Intervals for the Interpretation of Laboratory Tests

Method of
William Z. Borer, MD, and
Laura J. McCloskey, PhD

Most of the tests performed in a clinical laboratory are quantitative; that is, the amount of a substance present in blood or serum is measured and reported in terms of concentration, activity (e.g., enzyme activity), or counts (e.g., blood cell counts). The laboratory must provide reference intervals to assist the clinician in the interpretation of laboratory results. These reference intervals represent the physiologic quantities of a substance (concentrations, activities, or counts) to be expected in healthy persons. Deviation above or below the reference range may be associated with a disease process, and the severity of the disease process may be associated with the magnitude of the deviation. Unfortunately, a sharp demarcation rarely exists to distinguish between physiologic and pathologic values, and the time of transition between the two is often gradual as the disease process progresses.

The terms *normal* and *abnormal* have been used to describe laboratory values that fall inside and outside the reference range, respectively. Use of these terms is inappropriate because no good definition of normality exists in the clinical sense and the term *normal* may be confused with the statistical term *gaussian*. Reference ranges are established from statistical studies in groups of healthy volunteers. These study subjects must be free of disease, but they may have lifestyles or habits that result in variations in certain laboratory values. Examples of these variables include diet, body mass, exercise, and geographic location. Age and gender may also affect reference values.

When the data from a large cohort of healthy subjects fit a gaussian distribution, the usual statistical approach is to define the reference limits as 2 standard deviations (SD) above and below the mean. By definition, the reference range excludes the 2.5% of the population with the lowest values and the 2.5% with the highest values. Nongaussian distributions are handled by different statistical methods, but the result is similar in that the reference range is defined by the central 95% of the population. In other words, the probability that a healthy person will have a laboratory result that falls outside the reference range is 1 in 20. If 12 laboratory tests are performed, the probability that at least one of the results will be outside the reference range increases to about 50%, which means that all healthy persons are likely to have a few laboratory results that are unexpected. The clinician must then integrate these data with other clinical information, such as the history and physical examination, to arrive at an appropriate clinical decision.

The reference intervals for many tests (especially enzyme and immunochemical measurements) vary with the method used. Accordingly, each laboratory must establish reference intervals that are appropriate for the methods used.

SI Units

During the 1980s, a concerted effort was made to introduce SI units (le Système International d'Unités). The rationale for conversion to SI units is sound. Laboratory data are scientifically more informative when the units are based on molar concentration rather than on mass concentration. For example, the conversion of glucose to lactate and pyruvate or the binding of a drug to albumin is more easily understood in units of molar concentration. Another example is illustrated as follows:

CONVENTIONAL UNITS

1.0 g of hemoglobin:

- Combines with 1.37 mL of oxygen
- Contains 3.4 mg of iron
- Forms 34.9 mg of bilirubin

SI UNITS

4.0 mmol of hemoglobin:

- Combines with 4.0 mmol of oxygen
- Contains 4.0 mmol of iron
- Forms 4.0 mmol of bilirubin

TABLE 1 Base SI Units

Property	Unit	Symbol
Length	Meter	m
Mass	Kilogram	kg
Amount of substance	Mole	mol
Time	Second	s
Thermodynamic temperature	Kelvin	K
Electrical current	Ampere	A
Luminous intensity	Candela	cd
Catalytic amount	Katal	kat

TABLE 3 Standard Prefixes

Prefix	Multiplication Factor	Symbol
yocto	10^{-24}	y
zepto	10^{-21}	z
atto	10^{-18}	a
femto	10^{-15}	f
pico	10^{-12}	p
nano	10^{-9}	n
micro	10^{-6}	μ
milli	10^{-3}	m
centi	10^{-2}	c
deci	10^{-1}	d
deca	10^{1}	da
hecto	10^{2}	h
kilo	10^{3}	k
mega	10^{6}	M
giga	10^{9}	G
tera	10^{12}	T

The use of SI units would also enhance the standardization of nomenclature to facilitate global communication of medical and scientific information. The units, symbols, and prefixes used in the international system are shown in Tables 1, 2, and 3.

Unfortunately, problems have arisen with the implementation of SI units in the United States. The introduction of this system in 1987 prompted many medical journals to report laboratory values in both SI and conventional units in anticipation of complete conversion to SI units in the early 1990s. The lack of a coordinated effort toward this goal forced a retrenchment on the issue. Physicians continue to think and practice with laboratory results expressed in conventional units, and few, if any, hospitals or clinical laboratories in the United States use SI units exclusively. Complete conversion to SI units is not likely to occur in the foreseeable future, but most medical journals will probably continue to publish both sets of units. For this reason, the values in the tables of reference ranges in this appendix are given in both conventional units and SI units.

Tables of Reference Intervals

Some of the values included in the tables that follow have been established by the Clinical Laboratories at Thomas Jefferson University Hospital in Philadelphia and have not been published elsewhere. Other values have been compiled from the sources cited in the suggested readings. These tables are provided for information and educational purposes only. Laboratory values must always be interpreted in the context of clinical data derived from other sources, including the medical history and physical examination. One must exercise individual judgment when using the information provided in this appendix.

SUGGESTED READINGS

Bick RL (ed): Hematology: Clinical and Laboratory Practice. St Louis, Mosby–Year Book, 1993.

Borer WZ: Selection and use of laboratory tests. In Tietz NW, Conn RB, Pruden EL (eds): Applied Laboratory Medicine. Philadelphia, WB Saunders, 1992, pp 1-5.

Campion EW: A retreat from SI units. N Engl J Med 327:49, 1992.

Drug Evaluations Annual. Chicago, American Medical Association, 1994.

Friedman RB, Young DS: Effects of Disease on Clinical Laboratory Tests, 3rd ed. Washington, DC, AACC Press, 1997.

Henry JB: Clinical Diagnosis and Management by Laboratory Methods, 19th ed. Philadelphia, WB Saunders, 1996.

Hicks JM, Young DS: DORA 97-99: Directory of Rare Analyses. Washington, DC, AACC Press, 1997.

Jacob DS, Demott WR, Grady HJ, et al (eds): Laboratory Test Handbook, 4th ed. Baltimore, Williams & Wilkins, 1996.

Kaplan LA, Pesce AJ: Clinical Chemistry: Theory, Analysis, and Correlation, 3rd ed. St Louis, Mosby-Year Book, 1996.

Kjeldsberg CR, Knight JA: Body Fluids: Laboratory Examination of Amniotic, Cerebrospinal, Seminal, Serous and Synovial Fluids, 3rd ed. Chicago, ASCP Press, 1993.

Laposata M: SI Unit Conversion Guide. Boston, NEJM Books, 1992.

Scully RE, McNeely WF, Mark EJ, McNeely BU: Normal reference laboratory values. N Engl J Med 327:718-724, 1992.

Speicher CE: The Right Test: A Physician's Guide to Laboratory Medicine, 3rd ed. Philadelphia, WB Saunders, 1998.

Tietz NW (ed): Clinical Guide to Laboratory Tests, 3rd ed. Philadelphia, WB Saunders, 1995.

Wallach J: Interpretation of Diagnostic Tests: A Synopsis of Laboratory Medicine, 6th ed. Boston, Little, Brown, 1996.

Young DS: Effects of Preanalytical Variables on Clinical Laboratory Tests, 2nd ed. Washington, DC, AACC Press, 1997.

Young DS: Effects of Drugs on Clinical Laboratory Tests, 4th ed. Washington, DC, AACC Press, 1995.

Young DS: Determination and validation of reference intervals. Arch Pathol Lab Med 116:704-709, 1992.

Young DS: Implementation of SI units for clinical laboratory data. Ann Intern Med 106:114-129, 1987.

TABLE 2 Derived SI Units and Non-SI Units Retained for Use with SI Units

Property	Unit	Symbol
Area	Square meter	m^2
Volume	Cubic meter	m^3
	Liter	L
Mass concentration	Kilogram/ cubic meter	kg/m^3
	Gram/liter	g/L
Substance concentration	Mole/cubic meter	mol/m^3
	Mole/liter	mol/L
Temperature	Degree Celsius	$C = K - 273.15$

Reference Intervals for Hematology

Test	Conventional Units	SI Units
Acid hemolysis (Ham test)	No hemolysis	No hemolysis
Alkaline phosphatase, leukocyte	Total score, 14-100	Total score, 14-100
Cell counts		
Erythrocytes		
Males	4.6-6.2 million/mm^3	4.6-6.2 × 10^{12}/L
Females	4.2-5.4 million/mm^3	4.2-5.4 × 10^{12}/L
Children (varies with age)	4.5-5.1 million/mm^3	4.5-5.1 × 10^{12}/L
Leukocytes, total	4500-11,000/mm^3	4.5-11.0 × 10^9/L
Leukocytes, differential counts*		
Myelocytes	0%	0/L
Band neutrophils	3-5%	150-400 × 10^6/L
Segmented neutrophils	54-62%	3000-5800 × 10^6/L
Lymphocytes	25-33%	1500-3000 × 10^6/L
Monocytes	3-7%	300-500 × 10^6/L
Eosinophils	1-3%	50-250 × 10^6/L
Basophils	0-1%	15-50 × 10^6/L
Platelets	150,000-400,000/mm^3	150-400 × 10^9/L
Reticulocytes	25,000-75,000/mm^3 (0.5-1.5% of erythrocytes)	25-75 × 10^9/L
Coagulation tests		
Bleeding time (template)	2.75-8.0 min	2.75-8.0 min
Coagulation time (glass tube)	5-15 min	5-15 min
D Dimer	<0.5 µg/mL	<0.5 mg/L
Factor VIII and other coagulation factors	50-150% of normal	0.5-1.5 of normal
Fibrin split products (Thrombo-Welco test)	<10 µg/mL	<10 mg/L
Fibrinogen	200-400 mg/dL	2.0-4.0 g/L
Partial thromboplastin time, activated (aPTT)	20-25 s	20-35 s
Prothrombin time (PT)	12.0-14.0 s	12.0-14.0 s
Coombs' test		
Direct	Negative	Negative
Indirect	Negative	Negative
Corpuscular values of erythrocytes		
Mean corpuscular hemoglobin (MCH)	26-34 pg/cell	26-34 pg/cell
Mean corpuscular volume (MCV)	80-96 µm^3	80-96 fL
Mean corpuscular hemoglobin concentration (MCHC)	32-36 g/dL	320-360 g/L
Haptoglobin	20-165 mg/dL	0.20-1.65 g/L
Hematocrit		
Males	40-54 mL/dL	0.40-0.54
Females	37-47 mL/dL	0.37-0.47
Newborns	49-54 mL/dL	0.49-0.54
Children (varies with age)	35-49 mL/dL	0.35-0.49
Hemoglobin		
Males	13.0-18.0 g/dL	8.1-11.2 mmol/L
Females	12.0-16.0 g/dL	7.4-9.9 mmol/L
Newborns	16.5-19.5 g/dL	10.2-12.1 mmol/L
Children (varies with age)	11.2-16.5 g/dL	7.0-10.2 mmol/L
Hemoglobin, fetal	<1.0% of total	<0.01 of total
Hemoglobin A$_{1C}$	3-5% of total	0.03-0.05 of total
Hemoglobin A$_2$	1.5-3.0% of total	0.015-0.03 of total
Hemoglobin, plasma	0.0-5.0 mg/dL	0.0-3.2 µmol/L
Methemoglobin	30-130 mg/dL	19-80 µmol/L
Erythrocyte sedimentation rate (ESR)		
Wintrobe:		
Males	0-5 mm/h	0-5 mm/h
Females	0-15 mm/h	0-15 mm/h
Westergren:		
Males	0-15 mm/h	0-15 mm/h
Females	0-20 mm/h	0-20 mm/h

*Conventional units are percentages; SI units are absolute cell counts.

Reference Intervals* for Clinical Chemistry (Blood, Serum, and Plasma)

Analyte	Conventional Units	SI Units
Acetoacetate plus acetone		
Qualitative	Negative	Negative
Quantitative	0.3–2.0 mg/dL	30-200 μmol/L
Acid phosphatase, serum (thymolphthalein monophosphate substrate)	0.1-0.6 U/L	0.1-0.6 U/L
ACTH (see Corticotropin)		
Alanine aminotransferase (ALT), serum (SGPT)	1-45 U/L	1-45 U/L
Albumin, serum	3.3-5.2 g/dL	33-52 g/L
Aldolase, serum	0.0-7.0 U/L	0.0-7.0 U/L
Aldosterone, plasma		
Standing	5-30 ng/dL	140-830 pmol/L
Recumbent	3-10 ng/dL	80-275 pmol/L
Alkaline, phosphatase (ALP), serum		
Adult	35-150 U/L	35-150 U/L
Adolescent	100-500 U/L	100-500 U/L
Child	100-350 U/L	100-350 U/L
Ammonia nitrogen, plasma	10-50 μmol/L	10-50 μmol/L
Amylase, serum	25-125 U/L	25-125 U/L
Anion gap, serum calculated	8-16 mEq/L	8-16 mmol/L
Ascorbic acid, blood	0.4-1.5 mg/dL	23-85 μmol/L
Aspartate aminotransferase (AST), serum (SGOT)	1-36 U/L	1-36 U/L
Base excess, arterial blood, calculated	0±2 mEq/L	0±2 mmol/L
Bicarbonate		
Venous plasma	23-29 mEq/L	23-29 mmol/L
Arterial blood	21-27 mEq/L	21-27 mmol/L
Bile acids, serum	0.3-3.0 mg/dL	0.8-7.6 mmol/L
Bilirubin, serum		
Conjugated	0.1-0.4 mg/dL	1.7-6.8 μmol/L
Total	0.3-1.1 mg/dL	5.1-19.0 μmol/L
Calcium, serum	8.4-10.6 mg/dL	2.10-2.65 mmol/L
Calcium, ionized, serum	4.25-5.25 mg/dL	1.05-1.30 mmol/L
Carbon dioxide, total, serum or plasma	24-31 mEq/L	24-31 mmol/L
Carbon dioxide tension (Pco_2), blood	35-45 mm Hg	35-45 mm Hg
β-Carotene, serum	60-260 μg/dL	1.1-8.6 μmol/L
Ceruloplasmin, serum	23-44 mg/dL	230-440 mg/L
Chloride, serum or plasma	96-106 mEq/L	96-106 mmol/L
Cholesterol, serum or EDTA plasma		
Desirable range	<200 mg/dL	<5.20 mmol/L
Low-density lipoprotein (LDL) cholesterol	60-180 mg/dL	1.55-4.65 mmol/L
High-density lipoprotein (HDL) cholesterol	30-80 mg/dL	0.80-2.05 mmol/L
Copper	70-140 μg/dL	11-22 μmol/L
Corticotropin (ACTH), plasma, 8 AM	10-80 pg/mL	2-18 pmol/L
Cortisol, plasma		
8:00 AM	6-23 μg/dL	170-630 μmol/L
4:00 PM	3-15 μg/dL	80-410 μmol/L
10:00 PM	<50% of 8:00 AM value	<50% of 8:00 AM value
Creatine, serum		
Males	0.2-0.5 mg/dL	15-40 μmol/L
Females	0.3-0.9 mg/dL	25-70 μmol/L
Creatine kinase (CK), serum		
Males	55-170 U/L	55-170 U/L
Females	30-135 U/L	30-135 U/L
Creatinine kinase MB isoenzyme, serum	<5% of total CK activity	<5% of total CK activity
	<5% of ng/mL by immunoassay	<5% of ng/mL by immunoassay
Creatinine, serum	0.6-1.2 mg/dL	50-110 μmol/L
Estradiol-17β, adult		
Males	10-65 pg/mL	35-240 pmol/L
Females		
Follicular	30-100 pg/mL	110-370 pmol/L
Ovulatory	200-400 pg/mL	730-1470 pmol/L
Luteal	50-140 pg/mL	180-510 pmol/L

Reference Intervals* for Clinical Chemistry (Blood, Serum, and Plasma)—cont'd

Analyte	Conventional Units	SI Units
Ferritin, serum	20-200 ng/mL	20-200 µg/L
Fibrinogen, plasma	200-400 mg/dL	2.0-4.0 g/L
Folate, serum	3-18 ng/mL	6.8-4.1 nmol/L
Erythrocytes	145-540 ng/mL	330-120 nmol/L
Follicle-stimulating hormone (FSH), plasma		
Males	4-25 mU/mL	4-25 U/L
Females, premenopausal	4-30 mU/mL	4-30 U/L
Females, postmenopausal	40-250 mU/mL	40-250 U/L
Gastrin, fasting, serum	0-100 pg/mL	0-100 mg/L
Glucose, fasting, plasma or serum	70-100 mg/dL	3.9-5.55 nmol/L
γ-Glutamyltransferase (GGT), serum	5-40 U/L	5-40 U/L
Growth hormone (hGH), plasma, adult, fasting	0-6 ng/mL	0-6 µg/L
Haptoglobin, serum	20-165 mg/dL	0.20-1.65 g/L
β-Hydroxybutyrate	0.2-2.8 mg/dL	20-280 µmol/L
Immunoglobulins, serum (see table of Reference Intervals for Tests of Immunologic Function)		
Iron, serum	75-175 µg/dL	13-31 µmol/L
Iron-binding capacity, serum		
Total	250-410 µg/dL	45-73 µmol/L
Saturation	20-55%	0.20-0.55
Lactate		
Venous whole blood	5.0-20.0 mg/dL	0.6-2.2 mmol/L
Arterial whole blood	5.0-15.0 mg/dL	0.6-1.7 mmol/L
Lactate dehydrogenase (LD), serum	110-220 U/L	110-220 U/L
Lipase, serum	10-140 U/L	10-140 U/L
Lutropin (LH), serum		
Males	1-9 U/L	1-9 U/L
Females		
Follicular phase	2-10 U/L	2-10 U/L
Midcycle peak	15-65 U/L	15-65 U/L
Luteal phase	1-12 U/L	1-12 U/L
Postmenopausal	12-65 U/L	12-65 U/L
Magnesium, serum	1.3-2.1 mg/dL	0.65-1.05 mmol/L
Osmolality	275-295 mOsm/kg water	275-295 mOsm/kg water
Oxygen, blood, arterial, room air		
Partial pressure (Pao$_2$)	80-100 mm Hg	80-100 mm Hg
Saturation (Sao$_2$)	95-98%	95-98%
pH, arterial blood	7.35-7.45	7.35-7.45
Phosphate, inorganic, serum		
Adult	3.0-4.5 mg/dL	1.0-1.5 mmol/L
Child	4.0-7.0 mg/dL	1.3-2.3 mmol/L
Potassium		
Serum	3.5-5.0 mEq/L	3.5-5.0 mmol/L
Plasma	3.5-4.5 mEq/L	3.5-4.5 mmol/L
Progesterone, serum, adult		
Males	0.0-0.4 ng/mL	0.0-1.3 mmol/L
Females		
Follicular phase	0.1-1.5 ng/mL	0.3-4.8 mmol/L
Luteal phase	2.5-28.0 ng/mL	8.0-89.0 mmol/L
Prolactin, serum		
Males	1.0-15.0 ng/mL	1.0-15.0 µg/L
Females	1.0-20.0 ng/mL	1.0-20.0 µg/L
Protein, serum, electrophoresis		
Total	6.0-8.0 g/dL	60-80 g/L
Albumin	3.5-5.5 g/dL	35-55 g/L
Globulins		
α$_1$	0.2-0.4 g/dL	2.0-4.0 g/L
α$_2$	0.5-0.9 g/dL	5.0-9.0 g/L
β	0.6-1.1 g/dL	6.0-11.0 g/L
γ	0.7-1.7 g/dL	7.0-17.0 g/L
Pyruvate, blood	0.3-0.9 mg/dL	0.03-0.10 mmol/L
Rheumatoid factor	0.0-30.0 IU/mL	0.0-30.0 kIU/L
Sodium, serum or plasma	135-145 mEq/L	135-145 mmol/L

Continued

Reference Intervals* for Clinical Chemistry (Blood, Serum, and Plasma)—cont'd

Analyte	Conventional Units	SI Units
Testosterone, plasma		
Males, adult	300-1200 ng/dL	10.4-41.6 nmol/L
Females, adult	20-75 ng/dL	0.7-2.6 nmol/L
Pregnant females	40-200 ng/dL	1.4-6.9 nmol/L
Thyroglobulin	3-42 ng/mL	3-42 µg/L
Thyrotropin (hTSH), serum	0.4-4.8 µIU/mL	0.4-4.8 mIU/L
Thyrotropin-releasing hormone (TRH)	5-60 pg/mL	5-60 ng/L
Thyroxine (FT$_4$), free, serum	0.9-2.1 ng/dL	12-27 pmol/L
Thyroxine (T$_4$), serum	4.5-12.0 µg/mL	58-154 nmol/L
Thyroxine-binding globulin (TBG)	15.0-34.0 µg/mL	15.0-34.0 mg/L
Transferrin	250-430 mg/dL	2.5-4.3 g/L
Triglycerides, serum, after 12-h fast	40-150 mg/dL	0.4-1.5 g/L
Triiodothyronine (T$_3$), serum	70-190 ng/dL	1.1-2.9 nmol/L
Triiodothyronine uptake, resin (T$_3$RU)	25-38%	0.25-0.38
Troponin I	0.05-0.50 ng/mL	0.05-0.50 ng/mL
Urate		
Males	2.5-8.0 mg/dL	150-480 µmol/L
Females	2.2-7.0 mg/dL	130-420 µmol/L
Urea, serum or plasma	24-49 mg/dL	4.0-8.2 nmol/L
Urea, nitrogen, serum or plasma	11-23 mg/dL	8.0-16.4 nmol/L
Viscosity, serum	1.4-1.8 × water	1.4-1.8 × water
Vitamin A, serum	20-80 µg/dL	0.70-2.80 µmol/L
Vitamin B$_{12}$, serum	180-900 pg/mL	133-664 pmol/L

*Reference values may vary, depending on the method and sample source used.

Reference Intervals for Therapeutic Drug Monitoring (Serum or Plasma)*

Analyte	Therapeutic Range	Toxic Concentrations	Proprietary Name(s)
Analgesics			
Acetaminophen	10-40 µg/mL	>150 µg/mL	Tylenol Datril
Salicylate	100-250 µg/mL	>300 µg/mL	Aspirin Bufferin
Antibiotics			
Amikacin	20-30 µg/mL	Peak >35 µg/mL Trough >10 µg/mL	Amkin
Gentamicin	5-10 µg/mL	Peak >10 µg/mL Trough >2 µg/mL	Garamycin
Tobramycin	5-10 µg/mL	Peak >10 µg/mL Trough >2 µg/mL	Nebcin
Vancomycin	5-35 µg/mL	Peak >40 µg/mL Trough >10 µg/mL	Vancocin
Anticonvulsants			
Carbamazepine	5-12 µg/mL	>15 µg/mL	Tegretol
Ethosuximide	40-100 µg/mL	>250 µg/mL	Zarontin
Phenobarbital	15-40 µg/mL	40-100 ng/mL (varies widely)	Luminal
Phenytoin	10-20 µg/mL	>20 µg/mL	Dilantin
Primidone	5-12 µg/mL	>15 µg/mL	Mysoline
Valproic acid	50-100 µg/mL	>100 µg/mL	Depakene
Antineoplastics and Immunosuppressives			
Cyclosporine	100-300 ng/mL	>400 ng/mL	Sandimmune
Methotrexate, high-dose, 48h	Variable	>1 µmol/L, 48h after dose	
Tacrolimus (FK-506), whole blood	3-20 µg/L	>15 µg/L	Prograf

Reference Intervals for Therapeutic Drug Monitoring (Serum or Plasma)*—cont'd

Analyte	Therapeutic Range	Toxic Concentrations	Proprietary Name(s)
Bronchodilators and Respiratory Stimulants			
Caffeine	3-15 ng/mL	>30 ng/mL	Elixophyllin
Theophylline (aminophylline)	10-20 µg/mL	>30 µg/mL	Quibron
Cardiovascular Drugs			
Amiodarone (obtain specimen more than 8h after last dose)	1.0-2.0 µg/mL	>2.0 µg/mL	Cordarone
Digoxin (obtain specimen more than 6h after last dose)	0.8-2.0 ng/mL	>2.4 ng/mL	Lanoxin
Disopyramide	2-5 µg/mL	>7 µg/mL	Norpace
Flecainide	0.2-1.0 µg/mL	>1 µg/mL	Tambocor
Lidocaine	1.5-5.0 µg/mL	>6 µg/mL	Xylocaine
Mexiletine	0.7-2.0 µg/mL	>2 µg/mL	Mexitil
Procainamide	4-10 µg/mL	>12 µg/mL	Pronestyl
Procainamide plus NAPA (N-acetyl procainamide)	8-30 µg/mL	>30 µg/mL	
Propranolol	50-100 ng/mL	Variable	Inderal
Quinidine	2-5 µg/mL	>6 µg/mL	Cardioquin Quinaglute
Tocainide	4-10 ng/mL	>10 ng/mL	Tonocard
Psychopharmacologic Drugs			
Amitriptyline	120-150 ng/mL	>500 ng/mL	Elavil Triavil
Bupropion	25-100 ng/mL	Not applicable	Wellbutrin
Desipramine	150-300 ngmL	>500 ng/mL	Norpramin
Imipramine	125-250 ng/mL	>400 ng/mL	Tofranil
Lithium (obtain specimen 12h after last dose)	0.6-1.5 mEq/L	>1.5 mEq/L	Lithobid
Nortriptyline	50-150 ng/mL	>500 ng/mL	Aventyl Pamelor

*Values may vary depending on the method and sample collection device used. Always consult the reference values provided by the laboratory performing the analysis.

1423

Reference Intervals* for Clinical Chemistry (Urine)

Analyte	Conventional Units	SI Units
Acetone and acetoacetate, qualitative	Negative	Negative
Albumin		
Qualitative	Negative	Negative
Quantitative	10-100 mg/24h	0.15-1.5 µmol/d
Aldosterone	3-20 µg/24h	8.3-55 nmol/d
δ-Aminolevulinic acid (δ-ALA)	1.3-7.0 mg/24h	10-53 µmol/d
Amylase	<17 U/h	<17 U/h
Amylase/creatinine clearance ratio	0.01-0.04	0.01-0.04
Bilirubin, qualitative	Negative	Negative
Calcium (regular diet)	<250 mg/24h	<6.3 nmol/d
Catecholamines		
Epinephine	<10 µg/24h	<55 nmol/d
Norepinephine	<100 µg/24h	<590 nmol/d
Total free catecholamines	4-126 µg/24h	24-745 nmol/d
Total metanephrines	0.1-1.6 mg/24h	0.5-8.1 µmol/d
Chloride (varies with intake)	110-250 mEq/24h	110-250 mmol/d
Copper	0-50 µg/24h	0.0-0.80 µmol/d
Cortisol, free	10-100 µg/24h	27.6-276 nmol/d

Continued

Reference Intervals* for Clinical Chemistry (Urine)—cont'd

Analyte	Conventional Units	SI Units
Creatine		
Males	0-40 mg/24h	0.0-0.30 mmol/d
Females	0-80 mg/24h	0.0-0.60 mmol/d
Creatinine	15-25 mg/kg/24h	0.13-0.22 mmol/kg/d
Creatinine clearance (endogenous)		
Males	110-150 mL/min/1.73 m^2	110-150 mL/min/1.73 m^2
Females	105-132 mL/min/1.73 m^2	105-132 mL/min/1.73 m^2
Cystine or cysteine	Negative	Negative
Dehydroepiandrosterone		
Males	0.2-2.0 mg/24h	0.7-6.9 µmol/d
Females	0.2-1.8 mg/24h	0.7-6.2 µmol/d
Estrogens, total		
Males	4-25 µg/24h	14-90 nmol/d
Females	5-100 µg/24h	18-360 nmol/d
Glucose (as reducing substance)	<250 mg/24h	<250 mg/d
Hemoglobin and myoglobin, qualitative	Negative	Negative
Hemogentisic acid, qualitative	Negative	Negative
17-Hydroxycorticosteroids		
Males	3-9 mg/24h	8.3-25 µmol/d
Females	2-8 mg/24h	5.5-22 µmol/d
5-Hydroxyindoleacetic acid		
Qualitative	Negative	Negative
Quantitative	2-6 mg/24 h	10-31 µmol/d
17-Ketogenic steroids		
Males	5-23 mg/24h	17-80 µmol/d
Females	3-15 mg/24h	10-52 µmol/d
17-Ketosteroids		
Males	8-22 mg/24h	28-76 µmol/d
Females	6-15 mg/24h	21-52 µmol/d
Magnesium	6-10 mEq/24h	3-5 mmol/d
Metanephrines	0.05-1.2 ng/mg creatinine	0.03-0.70 mmol/mmol creatinine
Osmolality	38-1400 mOsm/kg water	38-1400 mOsm/kg water
pH	4.6-8.0	4.6-8.0
Phenylpyruvic acid, qualitative	Negative	Negative
Phosphate	0.4-1.3 g/24h	13-42 mmol/d
Porphobilinogen		
Qualitative	Negative	Negative
Quantitative	<2 mg/24h	<9 µmol/d
Porphyrins		
Coproporphyrin	50-250 µg/24h	77-380 nmol/d
Uroporphyrin	10-30 µg/24h	12-36 nmol/d
Potassium	25-125 mEq/24h	25-125 mmol/d
Pregnanediol		
Males	0.0-1.9 mg/24h	0.0-6.0 µmol/d
Females		
Proliferative phase	0.0-2.6 mg/24h	0.0-8.0 µmol/d
Luteal phase	2.6-10.6 mg/24h	8-33 µmol/d
Postmenopausal	0.2-1.0 mg/24h	0.6-3.1 µmol/d
Pregnanetriol	0.0-2.5 mg/24h	0.0-7.4 µmol/d
Protein, total		
Qualitative	Negative	Negative
Quantitative	10-150 mg/24h	10-150 mg/d
Protein/creatinine ratio	<0.2	<0.2
Sodium (regular diet)	60-260 mEq/24h	60-260 mmol/d
Specific gravity		
Random specimen	1.003-1.030	1.003-1.030
24-h collection	1.015-1.025	1.015-1.025
Urate (regular diet)	250-750 mg/24h	1.5-4.4 mmol/d
Urobilinogen	0.5-4.0 mg/24h	0.6-6.8 µmol/d
Vanillylmandelic acid (VMA)	1.0-8.0 mg/24h	5-40 µmol/d

*Values may vary, depending on the method used.

Reference Intervals for Toxic Substances

Analyte	Conventional Units	SI Units
Arsenic, urine	<130 µg/24h	<1.7 µmol/d
Bromides, serum, inorganic	<100 mg/dL	<10 mmol/L
Toxic symptoms	140-1000 mg/dL	14-100 mmol/L
Carboxyhemoglobin, blood	Saturation, percent	
Urban environment	<5%	<0.05
Smokers	<12%	<0.12
Symptoms		
Headache	>15%	>0.15
Nausea and vomiting	>25%	>0.25
Potentially lethal	>50%	>0.50
Ethanol, blood	<0.05 mg/dL	<1.0 mmol/L
	<0.005%	
Intoxication	>100 mg/dL	>22 mmol/L
	>0.1%	
Marked intoxication	300-400 mg/dL	65-87 mmol/L
	0.3%-0.4%	
Alcoholic stupor	400-500 mg/dL	87-109 mmol/L
	0.4%-0.5%	
	>500 mg/dL	
Coma	>0.5%	>109 mmol/L
Lead, blood		
Adults	<20 µg/dL	<1.0 µmol/L
Children	<10 µg/dL	<0.5 µmol/L
Lead, urine	<80 µg/24h	<0.4 µmol/d
Mercury, urine	<10 µg/24h	<150 nmol/d

Reference Intervals for Tests Performed on Cerebrospinal Fluid

Test	Conventional Units	SI Units
Cells	<5 mm^3; all mononuclear	<5 × 10^6/L, all mononuclear
Protein electrophoresis	Albumin predominant	Albumin predominant
Glucose	50-75 mg/dL (20 mg/dL less than in serum)	2.8-4.2 mmol/L (1.1 mmol/L less than in serum)
IgG		
Children <14 y	<8% of total protein	<0.08 of total protein
Adults	<14% of total protein	<0.14 of total protein
IgG index		
$\dfrac{\text{CSF / serum IgG ratio}}{\text{CSF / serum albumin ratio}}$	0.3-0.6	0.3-0.6
Oligoclonal banding on electrophoresis	Absent	Absent
Pressure, opening	70-180 mm H$_2$O	70-180 mm H$_2$O
Protein, total	15-45 mg/dL	150-450 mg/L

Reference Intervals for Tests of Gastrointestinal Function

Test	Conventional Units
Bentiromide	6-h urinary arylamine excretion >57% excludes pancreatic insufficiency
β-Carotene, serum	60-250 ng/dL
Fecal fat estimation	
Qualitative	No fat globules seen by high-power microscope
Quantitative	<6 g/24h (>95% coefficient of fat absorption)
Gastric acid output	
Basal	
Males	0.0-10.5 mmol/h
Females	0.0-5.6 mmol/h
Maximum (after histamine or pentagastrin)	
Males	9.0-48.0 mmol/h
Females	6.0-31.0 mmol/h
Ratio: basal/maximum	
Males	0.0-0.31
Females	0.0-0.29
Secretin test, pancreatic fluid	
Volume	>1.8 mL/kg/h
Bicarbonate	>80 mEq/L
D-Xylose absorption test, urine	>20% of ingested dose excreted in 5h

Reference Intervals for Tests of Immunologic Function

Test	Conventional Units	SI Units
Complement, serum		
C3	85-175 mg/dL	0.85-1.75 g/L
C4	15-45 mg/dL	150-450 mg/L
Total hemolytic (CH_{50})	150-250 U/mL	150-250 U/mL
Immunoglobulins, serum, adult		
IgG	640-1350 mg/dL	6.4-13.5 g/L
IgA	70-310 mg/dL	0.70-3.1 g/L
IgM	90-350 mg/dL	0.90-3.5 g/L
IgD	0.0-6.0 mg/dL	0.0-60 mg/L
IgE	0.0-430 ng/dL	0.0-430 mg/L
Autoantibodies, serum, adult		
Antinuclear antibody	<1:40	
Anti dsDNA antibody		0-41 IU/mL
Anti CCP	0-19 units	
Rheumatoid factor	0-30 mg/dL	

Lymphocyte Subsets, Whole Blood, Heparinized

Antigen(s) Expressed	Cell Type	Percentage (%)	Absolute Cell Count
CD3	Total T cells	56-77	860-1880
CD19	Total B cells	7-17	140-370
CD3 and CD4	Helper-inducer cells	32-54	550-1190
CD3 and CD8	Suppressor-cytotoxic cells	24-37	430-1060
CD3 and DR	Activated T cells	5-14	70-310
CD2	E rosette T cells	73-87	1040-2160
CD16 and CD56	Natural killer (NK) cells	8-22	130-500

Helper/suppressor ratio: 0.8-1.8

Reference Values for Semen Analysis

Test	Conventional Units	SI Units
Volume	2-5 mL	2-5 mL
Liquefaction	Complete in 15 min	Complete in 15 min
pH	7.2-8.0	7.2-8.0
Leukocytes	Occasional or absent	Occasional or absent
Spermatozoa		
Count	$60\text{-}150 \times 10^6$ mL	$60\text{-}150 \times 10^6$ mL
Motility	>80% motile	>0.80 motile
Morphology	80-90% normal forms	>0.80-0.90 normal forms
Fructose	>150 mg/dL	>8.33 mmol/L

Toxic Chemical Agents Reference Chart: Symptoms and Treatment

Method of
James J. James, MD, DrPH, MHA, and
James M. Lyznicki, MS, MPH

Toxic chemical agents are poisonous vapors, aerosols, gasses, liquids, or solids that have toxic effects on people, animals, or plants. Most of these agents are liquid at room temperature and are disseminated as vapors and aerosols. They may be released as bombs, sprayed from aircraft and boats, or disseminated by other means to intentionally create a hazard to people and the environment. Some of these agents are highly toxic and persistent, features that can render a site uninhabitable and require costly and potentially hazardous decontamination and remediation. Health effects range from irritation and burning of skin and mucous membranes to rapid cardiopulmonary collapse and death.

Efficient deployment of hazardous materials (HazMat) teams is critical to control a chemical agent attack.

Although all major cities and emergency medical systems have plans and equipment in place to address this situation, physicians and other health professionals must be aware of principles involved in managing a patient or multiple patients exposed to these agents. Chemical weapon agents have a high potential for secondary contamination from victims to responders. This requires that medical treatment facilities have clearly defined procedures for handling contaminated casualties, many of whom will transport themselves to the facility. Precautions must be used until thorough decontamination has been performed or the specific chemical agent is identified. Health care professionals must first protect themselves (e.g., by using protective suits, respiratory protection, and chemical-resistant gloves) because secondary contamination with even small amounts of these substances (particularly nerve agents such as VX) may be lethal.

Primary detection of exposure to chemical agents will be based on the signs and symptoms of the potential victim (Table 1). Confirmation of a chemical agent, using detection equipment or laboratory analyses, will take considerable time and will not likely contribute to the early management of mass casualty victims. Several patients presenting with the same symptoms should alert physicians and hospital staff to the possibility of a chemical attack. If a chemical attack occurs, most victims will likely

TABLE 1 Quick Reference Chart on Chemical Weapon Agents

Chemical Agent	Diagnostic Considerations	Treatment Considerations*
Cyanides Cyanogen chloride (CK) Hydrogen cyanide (AC)	• Symptom onset: rapid, seconds to minutes • Odor: bitter almond, musty, or chlorine-like • Nonspecific hypoxic and hypoxemic symptoms • Binds cellular cytochrome oxidase causing chemical asphyxia • Respiratory: shortness of breath, chest tightness, hyperventilation, respiratory arrest • GI: nausea, vomiting • Cardiovascular: ventricular arrhythmias, hypotension, cardiac arrest, shock • CNS: anxiety, headache drowsiness, weakness, apnea, convulsions, seizure, coma • CNS effects may be confused with carbon monoxide and hydrogen sulfide poisoning • Metabolic acidosis and increased concentration of venous oxygen (patient also may present with cyanosis) • Laboratory testing: cyanide, thiocyanate, serum lactate levels; venous and arterial partial oxygen pressure	• Immediate treatment of symptomatic patients is critical • Antidote: sodium nitrite and sodium thiosulfate; repeat one-half initial doses of both agents in 30 minutes if there is inadequate clinical response • Amyl nitrate capsules are available for first aid until intravenous access is achieved • Cyanide antidone kits are commercially available • Investigational in the United States, available in Europe: hydroxycobalamin (vitamin B_{12a}) administered with thiosulfate • Activated charcoal[A] for oral exposure • Mechanical ventilation as needed • Circulatory support with crystalloids and vasopressors • Metabolic acidosis corrected with IV sodium bicarbonate • Seizures controlled with benzodiazepines • Antidote: physostigmine salicylate (Antilirium)[A] • Support, intravenous fluids
Incapacitating Agents Agent 15 3-quinuclidinyl benzilate (BZ)	• Symptom onset: hours 0-4 h: parasympathetic blockade and mild CNS effects 4-20 h: stupor with ataxia and hyperthermia 20-96 h: full-blown delirium Resolution phase: paranoia, deep sleep, reawakening, crawling, climbing automatisms, eventual reorientation	

Continued

TABLE 1   Quick Reference Chart on Chemical Weapon Agents—cont'd

Chemical Agent	Diagnostic Considerations	Treatment Considerations*
Nerve Agents Cyclohexyl sarin (GF) Sarin (GB) Soman (GD) Tabun (GA) VX	• Odorless • Competitive inhibitor of acetylcholine muscarinic receptor • Mydriasis, blurred vision, dry mouth, dry skin, possible atropine-like flush, initial rise in heart rate, decreased level of consciousness, confusion, disorientation, visual hallucinations, impaired memory • Symptom onset: vapor (seconds), liquid (minutes or hours); symptom onset may be delayed up to 18 hours particularly for localized exposures • Odor: none (GB, VX), fruity (GA), camphor-like (GD) • Most toxic of known chemical agents • Irreversible acetylcholinesterase inhibitors • Eyes: excessive lacrimation, miosis may be present • Respiratory: rhinorrhea, bronchospasm, respiratory failure • GI: hypersalivation, nausea, vomiting, diarrhea • Skin: localized sweating • Cardiac: sinus bradycardia • Skeletal muscles: fasciculations followed by weakness, flaccid paralysis • CNS: loss of consciousness, convulsions, apnea, seizures • May be confused with organophosphate and carbamate pesticide poisoning • Laboratory testing: erythrocyte or serum cholinesterase activity to confirm exposure	• Rapid establishment of patent airway • Antidote: Atropine[A] and pralidoxime[A] chloride (Protopam chloride, 2-PAM); additional doses until bronchial secretions are cleared and ventilation improved • Early administration of 2-PAM is critical to minimize permanent agent inactivation of acetylcholinesterase (i.e., "aging") • Benzodiazepines to control nerve agent-induced seizures • Airway and ventilatory support as needed • Atropine,[A] pralidoxime,[A] and diazepam[A] are available in autoinjector kits through the U.S. military
Pulmonary or Choking Agents Acrolein Ammonia (NH_3) Chlorine (CL) Choloropicrin (PS) Diphosgene (DP) Nitrogen oxides (NO_x) Perflouroisobutylene (PFIB) Phosgene (CG) Sulfur dioxide (SO_2)	• Symptom onset: rapid or delayed; 1-24 h (rarely up to 72 h) • Odor (CG): freshly mown hay or grass • Easily absorbed via mucous membranes of eyes, nose, oropharynx. Degree of water solubility of the agent influences onset and severity of respiratory injury. • Eye and airway irritation, dyspnea, chest tightness, rhinorrhea, hypersalivation, cough, wheezing • High dose inhalation may produce laryngospasm, pneumonitis, and acute lung injury with delayed onset (≤48 h) of acute respiratory distress syndrome • Chest radiograph: hyperinflation, noncardiogenic pulmonary edema • May be confused with inhalation exposure to industrial chemicals (e.g., HCl, Cl_2, NH_3)	• No specific antidote • Supportive measures; specific treatment depends on the agent • IV fluids for hypotension; no diuretics • Ventilation with or without positive airway pressure • Bronchodilators for bronchospasm • Methylprednisolone[A] may be effective in preventing noncardiogenic pulmonary edema
Riot Control Agents Mace (CN) Tear gas (CS)	• Symptom onset: immediate • Odor: apple blossom (CN); pepper (CS) • Metallic taste • SN_2 alkylating agents • Burning and pain on mucosal membranes and skin • Eyes: irritation, pain, tearing, blepharospasm	• Supportive care • Irrigation as necessary • Persons with asthma, emphysema may need oxygen, inhaled bronchodilators, steroids, assisted ventilation • Lotions, such as calamine,[A] for persistent erythema

TABLE 1 Quick Reference Chart on Chemical Weapon Agents—cont'd

Chemical Agent	Diagnostic Considerations	Treatment Considerations*
	• Airways: burning in nose and mouth, respiratory discomfort, bronchospam (may be delayed 36 h) • Skin: tingling, erythema • Nausea and vomiting common • CN can cause corneal opacification • No specific laboratory tests	
Vesicant or Blister Agents	• Symptoms onset: immediate (L, CX); delayed 2-48 h (H, HD) • Primary liquid hazard • May be confused with skin exposure to caustic irritants (e.g., sodium hydroxide, ammonia) • Intracellular enzyme and DNA alkylating agents • Clinical effects dependent on extent and route of exposure; effects may be delayed, appearing hours after exposure	• Immediate decontamination • Supportive care • Thermal burn-type treatment • Symptomatic management of lesions
Sulfur mustard (H) Distilled mustard (HD)	• Odor: garlic, horseradish, or mustard • Skin: erythema and blisters (may be delayed ≤8 h), pruritus • Eye: irritation, conjunctivitis, corneal damage, lacrimation, pain, blepharospasm • Respiratory: mild to marked acute airway damage, pneumonitis within 1-3 d, respiratory failure • GI effects (nausea, vomiting diarrhea) may be present • Bone marrow stem cell suppression leading to pancytopenia and increased susceptibility to infection • Fever, sputum production • Combination with Lewisite (called mustard-Lewisite or HL) results in rapid effects of Lewisite and delayed effects of mustard agents	• No specific antidote • Skin: silver sulfadiazine[A] • Eye: homatropine[A] ophthalmic ointment • Pulmonary: antibiotics, bronchodilators, steroids • Colony stimulating factor may be helpful for leukopenia • Systemic analgesic and antipruritics • Early use of positive-end expiratory pressure or continuous positive airway pressure • Maintain fluid and electrolyte balance (do not excessively fluid resuscitate as in thermal burns)
Lewisite (L)	• Odor: fruity or geranium • More volatile than mustard • Damages eyes, skin, and airways by direct contact • Skin: gray area of dead skin within 5 min, erythema within 30 min, blistering 2-3 h, immediate irritation or burning pain on contact, severe tissue necrosis • Eye: pain, blepharospasm, conjunctival and lid edema • Airway: pseudomembrane formation, nasal irritation • Intravascular fluid loss, hypovolemia, shock, organ congestion, leukocytosis	• Antidote: British Anti-Lewisite (BAL or Dimercaprol)
Phosgene Oxime (CX)	• Odor: freshly mown hay • Urticant, nonvesicant agent • Vapor extremely irritating; vapor and liquid cause tissue damage upon contact • Immediate burning, irritation, wheal-like skin lesions, eye and airway damage, conjunctivitis, lacrimation, lid edema, blepharospasm • No distinctive laboratory findings	• No antidote • Parenteral methylprednisolone[A] may be effective in preventing noncardiogenic pulmonary edema • Experimental: aerosolized dexamethasone[A] and theophylline[A] for pulmonary involvement

Continued

TABLE 1 Quick Reference Chart on Chemical Weapon Agents—cont'd

Chemical Agent	Diagnostic Considerations	Treatment Considerations*
Vomiting (Arsine-Based) Agents Adamsite (DM) Diphenylchlorarsine (DA) Diphenylcyanoarsine (DC)	• Symptom onset: All rapidly acting within minutes • Odor: none (DA), garlic (DC), burning fireworks (DM) • Primary route of absorption is through respiratory system • Arsine gas depletes erythrocyte glutathione and causes hemolysis • Eyes: conjunctival irritation, tearing, and blepharospasm • Airways: sneezing, mucosal lung irritation, edema, progressive cough, wheezing • Cardiac: tachypnea, tachycardia • GI: intestinal cramps, emesis, diarrhea • Skin: erythema, edema at the site of dermal contact • CNS: depression, syncope • Chest radiograph to rule out chemical pneumonitis	• Supportive care • Monitor for hemolysis • Wheezing or dyspnea; may need albuterol inhalation • Eye irrigation (water, normal saline, lactated Ringer's solution) in patients sustaining ocular exposure • Treat repetitive emesis with IV hydration and antiemetics • Blood transfusion may be required • Exchange transfusion may be required • Hemodialysis may be useful in decreasing arsenic level and treating renal failure

ANot FDA approved for this indication.

*Different situations may require different treatment and dosage regimens. Please consult other references as well as a regional poison control conter (1-800-222-1222), medical toxicologist, clinical pharmacologist, or other drug information specialist for definitive dosage information, especially dosages for pregnant women and children.

Abbreviations: CNS = central nervous system; GI = gastrointestinal.

arrive within a short time. This situation differentiates a chemical attack from a biological attack involving infectious microganisms. Additional diagnostic clues include:

• Unusual temporal or geographic clustering of illness
• Any sudden increase in illness in previously healthy persons
• Sudden increase in non-specific syndromes (e.g., sudden unexplained weakness in previously healthy persons; dimmed or blurred vision; hypersecretion, inhalation, or burn-like syndrome)

A coordinated communication network is critical for transmitting reliable information from the incident scene to treatment facilities. Any suspicious or confirmed exposure to a chemical weapons agent should be reported to the local health department, local Federal Bureau of Investigations office, and the Centers for Disease Control and Prevention (1-770-488-7100).

Biologic Agents Reference Chart—Symptoms, Tests, and Treatment

Method of
James J. James, MD, DrPh, MHA, and
James M. Lyznicki, MS, MPH

Biologic weapons are devices used intentionally to cause disease or death through dissemination of microorganisms or toxins in food and water, by insect vectors, or by aerosols. Potential targets include human beings, food crops, livestock, and other resources essential for national security, economy, and defense. Unlike nuclear, chemical, and conventional weapons, the onset of a biological attack will probably be insidious. For some infectious agents, secondary and tertiary transmission may continue for weeks or months after the initial attack.

Initial detection of an unannounced biological attack will likely occur when an astute health professional notices an unusual case or disease cluster and reports his or her concerns to local public health authorities. Physicians and other health professionals should be alert to the following:

• Unusual temporal or geographic clustering of illnesses
• Sudden increase of illness in previously healthy persons
• Sudden increase in non-specific illnesses (e.g., pneumonia, flulike illness; bleeding disorders; unexplained rashes, particularly in adults; neuromuscular illness; diarrhea)

To enhance detection and treatment capabilities, physicians and other health professionals in acute care settings should be familiar with the clinical manifestations, diagnostic techniques, isolation precautions, treatment, and prophylaxis for likely causative agents (e.g., smallpox, pneumonic plague, anthrax, viral hemorrhagic fevers). Table 1 provides a quick summary of diagnostic and treatment considerations for various infectious and toxic biological agents. For some of these agents, delay in medical response could result in a potentially devastating number of casualties. To mitigate such consequences, early identification and intervention are imperative. Front-line physicians must have an increased level of suspicion regarding the possible intentional use of biological agents as well as an increased sensitivity to reporting those suspicious to public health authorities, who, in turn, must be willing to evaluate a predictable increase in false positive reports.

Medical response efforts require coordination and planning with emergency management agencies, law enforcement, health care facilities, and social services agencies. Health care agencies should ensure that physicians know whom to call with reports of suspicious cases and clusters of infectious diseases, and should work to build a good relationship with the local medical community. Resource integration is absolutely necessary to:

- Establish adequate capacity to initiate rapid investigation of an outbreak

TABLE 1 Quick Reference Chart on Biological Weapon Agents

Disease/Agent	Diagnostic Considerations	Treatment Considerations[1]	Prophylaxis
Bacteria			
Anthrax *Bacillus anthracis*	Incubation period: 1-5 d (perhaps ≤60 d)[2] *Cutaneous:* • Evolving skin lesion (face, neck, arms), progresses to vesicle, dispressed ulcer, and black necrotic lesions • Lethality: 20% if untreated, otherwise rarely fatal *Gastrointestinal* • Nausea, vomiting, abdominal pain, bloody diarrhea, sepsis • Lethality: approaches 100% if untreated but data are limited; rapid, aggressive treatment may reduce mortality *Inhalational* • Abrupt onset of flu-like symptoms, fever with or without chills, sweats, fatigue or malaise, non- or minimally productive cough, nausea, vomiting, dyspnea, headache, chest pain, followed in 2-5 d by severe respiratory distress, mediastinitis, hemorrhagic meningitis, sepsis, shock.[3] • Widened mediastinum on chest radiograph is characteristic for inhalational and occasionally GI anthrax.[4] • Lethality: Once respiratory distress develops, mortality rates may approach 90%; begin treatment when inhalational anthrax is suspected, do not wait for confirmatory testing.[5]	Combination therapy of ciprofloxacin (Cipro) or doxycycline (Vibramycin) plus one or two other antimicrobials should be considered with inhalational anthrax[6] Penicillin[A] should be considered if strain is susceptible and does not possess inducible β-lactamases If meningitis suspected, doxycycline (Vibramycin) may be less optimal because of poor CNS penetration Steroids may be considered for severe edema and for meningitis.	Ciprofloxacin (Cipro) or doxycycline (Vibramycin) with or without vaccination If strain is susceptible, penicillin[A] or amoxicillin[A] (Amoxil) should be considered Inactivated vaccine (licensed but not readily available); six injections and annual booster

Continued

TABLE 1 Quick Reference Chart on Biological Weapon Agents—cont'd

Disease/Agent	Diagnostic Considerations	Treatment Considerations[1]	Prophylaxis
	Gram stain and culture of blood, pleural fluid, cerebrospinal fluid, ascitic fluid, vesicular fluid or lesion exudate; sputum rarely positive; confirmatory serological and PCR tests available through public health laboratory network		
Brucellosis *B. abortus* *B. canis* *B. mellitensis* *B. suis*	Incubation period: 5-60 d (usually 1-2 mo) • Non-specific flu-like symptoms, fever, headache, profound weakness and fatigue, GI symptoms such as anorexia, nausea, vomiting, diarrhea, or constipation • Osteoarticular complications common • Lethality: less than 5% even if untreated; tends to incapacitate rather than kill. Blood and bone marrow culture (may require 6 wk to grow *Brucella*); confirmatory culture and serological testing available through public health laboratory network	Doxycycline (Vibramycin) plus streptomycin or rifampin[A] (Rifadin) *Alternative therapies:* Ofloxacin (Floxin)[A] plus rifampin[A] (Rifadin) Doxycycline (Vibramycin) plus gentamicin (Garamycin) TMP/SMX (Bactrim,[A] Septra) plus gentamicin (Garamycin)	Doxycycline (Vibramycin) plus streptomycin or rifampin (Rifadin) No approved human vaccine
Inhalational (Pneumonic) Tularemia *Francisella tularensis*	Incubation period: 3-5 d (range of 1-21 d) • Sudden onset of acute febrile illness, weakness, chills, headache, generalized body aches, elevated WBCs • Pulmonary symptoms such as dry cough, chest pain or tightness with or without objective signs of pneumonia • Progressive weakness, malaise, anorexia, and weight loss occurs, potentially leading to sepsis and organ failure • Largely clinical diagnosis • Lethality: ≈30-60% fatal if untreated Culture of blood, sputum, biopsies, pleural fluid, bronchial washings (culture is difficult and potentially dangerous); confirmatory testing available through public health laboratory network	Streptomycin or gentamicin (Garamycin) *Alternative therapies:* Ciprofloxacin (Cipro)[A] Doxycycline (Vibramycin) Chloramphenicol[A] (Chloromycetin)	Tetracycline Doxycycline (Vibramycin) Ciprofloxacin (Cipro)[A] Live attenuated vaccine (USAMRIID, IND) given by scarification; currently under FDA review; limited availability
Pneumonic Plague *Yersinia pestis*	Incubation period: 1-10 d (typically 2-3 d) • Acute onset of flu-like prodrome: fever, myalgia, weakness, headache; within	Streptomycin; gentamicin (Garamycin) *Alternative therapies:* Doxycycline (Vibramycin) Tetracycline	Tetracycline Doxycycline (Vibramycin) Ciprofloxacin[A] (Cipro) Inactivated whole cell vaccine licensed but not

TABLE 1 Quick Reference Chart on Biological Weapon Agents—cont'd

Disease/Agent	Diagnostic Considerations	Treatment Considerations[1]	Prophylaxis
	24 h of prodrome, chest discomfort, cough with bloody sputum, and dyspnea. By day 2 to 4 illness, symptoms progressing to cyanosis, respiratory distress, and hemodynamic instability • Lethality: almost 100% if untreated; 20–60% if appropriately treated within 18-24 h of symptoms; begin treatment when diagnosis of plague is suspected; do not wait for confirmatory testing Gram stain and culture of blood, CSF, sputum, lymph node aspirates, bronchial washings; confirmatory serological and bacteriological tests available through public health laboratory network	Ciprofloxacin[A] (Cipro) Chloramphenicol[A] (Chloromycetin) is first choice for meningitis except for pregnant women	readily available; injection with boosters Vaccine not effective against aerosol exposure
Rickettsia **Q-Fever** *Coxiella burnetii*	Incubation period: 2-14 d (may be ≤40 days) • Nonspecific febrile disease, chills, cough, weakness and fatigue, pleuritic chest pain, pneumonia possible • Lethality: 1-3%. Fatalities are uncommon even if untreated but relapsing symptoms may occur Isolation of organism may be difficult; confirmatory testing via serology or PCR available through public health laboratory network	Tetracycline Doxycycline (Vibramycin)	Tetracycline Doxycycline (Vibramycin) Inactivated whole cell[B] vaccine (IND) Skin test to determine prior exposure to *C. burnetii* recommended before vaccination
Viruses **Smallpox** Variola major virus	Incubation period: 7-17 d • Prodrome of high fever, malaise, prostration, headache, vomiting, delirium followed in 2-3 d maculopapular rash uniformly progressing to pustules and scabs, mostly on extremities and face • Requires astute clinical evaluation; may be confused with chickenpox, erythema multiforme with bullae, or allergic contact dermatitis • Lethality: 30% in unvaccinated persons Pharyngeal swab, vesicular fluid, biopsies, scab material for electron microscopy and PCR testing through public health laboratory network Notify CDC Poxvirus Section at 1-404-639-2184	Supportive care Cidofovir (Vistide) shown to be effective in vitro and in experimental animals infected with surrogate orthopox virus	Live attenuated vaccinia vaccine derived from calf lymph; given by scarification (licensed, restricted supply) New vaccine being developed from tissue culture Vaccination given within 3-4 d following exposure can prevent or decrease the severity of disease

Continued

TABLE 1 Quick Reference Chart on Biological Weapon Agents—cont'd

Disease/Agent	Diagnostic Considerations	Treatment Considerations[1]	Prophylaxis
Viral Encephalitis Eastern (EEE) Western (WEE) Venezuelan (VEE)	Incubation period: 2-6 d (VEE); 7-14 d (EEE, WEE) • Systemic febrile illness, with encephalitis developing in some populations • Generalized malaise, spiking fevers, headache, myalgia • Incidence of seizures and/or focal neurologic deficits may be higher after biological attack • White blood cell count may show striking leukopenia and lymphopenia • Clinical and epidemiologic diagnosis • Lethality: <10% (VEE); 10% (WEE); 50-75% (EEE) Confirmatory test and viral isolation available through public health laboratory network	Supportive care Analgesics, anticonvulsants as needed	Several IND vaccines, poorly immunogenic, highly reactogenic
Viral Hemorrhagic Fevers (VHFs) Arenaviruses (Lassa, Junin, and related viruses) Bunyaviruses (Hanta, Congo-Crimean, Rift Valley) Filoviruses (Ebola, Marburg) Flaviviruses (yellow fever, dengue, various tick-borne disease viruses)	Incubation period: 4-21 d • Fever with mucous membrane bleeding, petechiae, thrombocytopenia and hypotension in patients without underlying malignancies • Malaise, myalgias, headache, vomiting, diarrhea possible • Lethality: Variable depending on viral strain; 15-25% with Lassa fever to ≤ 90% with Ebola Confirmatory testing and viral isolation available through public health laboratory network Call CDC Special Pathogens Office at 1-404-639-1115	Supportive therapy Ribavirin (Virazole)[A] may be effective for Lassa fever, Rift Valley fever, Argentine hemorrhagic fever, and Congo-Crimean hemorrhagic fever	Ribavarin (Virazole)[A] is suggested for Congo-Crimean hemorrhagic fever and Lassa fever Yellow fever vaccine is the only licensed vaccine available Vaccines for some of the other VHFs exist but are for investigational use only
Biological Toxins **Botulism** *Clostridium botulinum toxin*	Symptom onset: 1-5 d (typically 12-36 h) • Blurred vision, diploplia, dry mouth, ptosis, fatigue • As disease progresses, acute bilateral descending flaccid paralysis, respiratory paralysis resulting in death • Clinical diagnosis • Lethality: 60% without ventilatory support Serum and stool should be assayed for toxin by mouse neutralization bioassay, which may require several days	Intensive and prolonged supportive care; ventilation may be necessary Trivalent equine antitoxin (serotypes A,B,E, – licensed, available from the CDC) should be administered immediately after clinical diagnosis Anaphylaxis and serum sickness are potential complications of antitoxin Aminoglycosides and clindamycin (Cleocin)[A] must not be used	Pentavalent toxoid (A-E), yearly booster (IND, CDC) Not available to the public Antitoxin may be sufficient to prevent illness following exposure but is not recommended until patient is showing symptoms
Enterotoxin B *Staphylococcus aureus*	Symptom onset: 3-12 h • Acute onset of fever, chills headache, nonproductive cough	Supportive care	No vaccine available

TABLE 1 Quick Reference Chart on Biological Weapon Agents—cont'd

Disease/Agent	Diagnostic Considerations	Treatment Considerations[1]	Prophylaxis
	• Normal chest radiograph • Clinical diagnosis • Lethality: probably low (few data available for respiratory exposure) Serology on acute and convalescent serum can confirm diagnosis		
Ricin toxin *Ricinus communis*	Symptom onset: ≤6-24 h • Weakness, nausea, chest tightness, fever, cough, pulmonary edema, respiratory failure, circulatory collapse, hypoxemia resulting in death (usually within 36-72 h) • Clinical and epidemiological diagnosis • Lethality: mortality data not available but is likely to be high with extensive exposure Confirmatory serological testing available through public health laboratory network	Supportive care Treatment for pulmonary edema Gastric decontamination if toxin ingested	No vaccine available
T-2 Mycotoxins *Fusarium* *Myrothecium* *Trichoderma* *Stachybotrys*	Symptom onset: minutes to hours • Abrupt onset of mucocutaneous and airway irritation and pain • May include skin, eyes, and GI tract; systemic toxicity may follow	Clinical support Soap and water washing within 4-6 h reduces dermal toxicity; washing within 1 h may eliminate toxicity entirely	No vaccine available
Other filamentous fungi	• Lethality: severe exposure can cause death in hours to days Consult with local health department regarding specimen collection and diagnostic testing procedures; confirmation requires testing blood, tissue, and environmental samples	No effective medications or antidotes	

[A]Not FDA approved for this indication.

[B]Not available in the United States.

[1]Different situations may require different dosage and treatment regimens. Please consult other references and an infectious disease specialist for definitive dosage information, especially dosages for pregnant women and children.

[2]Data from 22 patients infected with anthrax in October and November 2001 indicate a median incubation period of 4 d (range 4-7 d) for inhalational anthrax and a mean incubation of 5 d (range 1-10 d) for cutaneous anthrax.

[3]Limited data from the October/November 2001 anthrax infections indicate hemorrhagic pleural effusions to be strongly associated with inhalational anthrax; rhinorrhea was present in only 1/10 patients.

[4]Chest radiograph abnormalities include paratracheal and hilar fullness and may be subtle. Consider chest computed tomography if diagnosis is uncertain.

[5]Limited data from the 2001 terrorist-related anthrax infections indicate that early treatment significantly decreased the mortality rate.

[6]Other agents with in vitro activity suggested for use in conjunction with ciprofloxacin (Cipro) or doxycycline (Vibramycin) for treatment of inhalational anthrax include rifampin (Rifadin), vancomycin (Vancocin), imipenem (Primaxin), chloramphenicol (Chloromycetin), penicillin and ampicillin, clindamycin (Cleocin), and clarithromycin (Biaxin).

Abbreviations: CDC = Centers for Disease Control and Prevention; CNS = central nervous system; CSF = cerebrospinal fluid; GI = gastrointestinal; IND = investigational new drug; PCR = polymerase chain reaction; TMP-SMX = trimethoprim-sulfamethoxazole; USAMRIID, U.S. Army Medical Research Institute of Infectious Diseases; WBC = white blood cell.

Adopted for *Biological Weapons: Quick Reference Guide*. American Medical Association; 2002. Available at http://www.amaassn.org/ama1/pub/upload/mm/415/quickreference0902.pdf.

- Educate the public
- Begin mass distribution of antibiotics and vaccines
- Ensure mass medical care
- Control public anger and fear

In an epidemic, overwhelming numbers of critically ill patients will require acute and follow-up medical care. Both infected persons and the *worried well* will seek medical attention, with a corresponding need for medical supplies, diagnostic tests, and hospital beds. The impact — or even the threat — of an attack can elicit widespread panic and civil disorder, overwhelm hospital resources, and disrupt social services.

Any suspicious or confirmed exposure to a biological weapons agent should be reported immediately to the local health department, local Federal Bureau of Investigation office, and the Centers of Disease Control and Prevention (1-770-488-7100).

Some Popular Herbs and Nutritional Supplements

Method of
Miriam M. Chan, RPh, PharmD

Herb/Nutritional Supplement	Common Uses	Reasonable Adult Oral Dosage*	Precautions and Drug Interactions
Bilberry fruit	Often used orally to improve visual acuity and to treat degenerative retinal conditions Also used orally to treat chronic venous insufficiency, varicose veins, and hemorrhoids Approved in Germany for use orally for acute diarrhea and topically for mild inflammation of the mucous membranes of mouth and throat	For eye conditions and circulation, 80–160 mg tid of the extract standardized to at least 25% anthocyanosides For diarrhea, 20–60 g/d of the dried, ripe berries or as a tea preparation (5–10 g of crushed dried berries in 150 mL water, brought to a boil for 10 min, then strained) For external use, 10% decoction	No known side effects reported with bilberry fruit and extract However, bilberry leaf taken in large quantities or used long term has been shown to cause wasting, anemia, jaundice, acute excitation, disturbances of tonus, and death in animals Anthocyanidin extracts from bilberry may increase the risk of bleeding in those taking warfarin or other blood thinners
Black cohosh root	Commonly used to relieve hot flashes and other menopausal symptoms Also used to treat premenstrual discomfort and dysmenorrhea	20 mg bid of the rhizome extract standardized to triterpene glycosides German guidelines do not recommend its use for >6 mo	Black cohosh may have an estrogen-like effect and should be avoided in women with breast cancer Large doses may induce miscarriage, so it is contraindicated during pregnancy May cause GI disturbances, headache, and hypotension International case reports of liver dysfunction suspected to be associated with its use

Herb/Nutritional Supplement	Common Uses	Reasonable Adult Oral Dosage*	Precautions and Drug Interactions
Chamomile flower	Used orally to calm nerves and treat GI spasms and inflammatory diseases of the GI tract Used topically to treat wounds, skin infections, and skin or mucous membrane inflammation	1 cup of freshly made tea 3–4 times daily (1 tbsp or 3 g of dried flower in 150 mL boiling water for 5–10 min)	Chamomile may cause an allergic reaction, especially in people with severe allergies to ragweed or other members of the daisy family (e.g., echinacea, feverfew, and milk thistle) Should not be taken concurrently with other sedatives, such as alcohol or benzodiazepines
Chaste tree berry (Chasteberry, Vitex)	For normalizing irregular menstrual periods and relieving premenstrual complaints For relieving menopausal symptoms For restoring fertility in women For treating acne associated with menstrual cycles Also for increasing breast milk production in lactating women	For menstrual irregularities and premenstrual complaints, 30–40 mg/d of the dried berries or an equivalent amount of aqueous-alcoholic extracts (50%–70% v/v) Dried fruit extract, standardized to 0.6% agnusides, is used in doses of 175–225 mg/d For other conditions, no established dosage documented	Chaste tree berry can have uterine stimulant properties and should be avoided in pregnancy Women with hormone-dependent conditions (e.g., breast, uterine, and ovarian cancer, and endometriosis and uterine fibroids) and men with prostate cancer should avoid chaste tree berry because it contains progestins Side effects include intermenstrual bleeding, dry mouth, headache, nausea, rash, alopecia, and tachycardia High doses (≥480 mg/d of extract) can paradoxically decrease lactation Chaste tree berry is thought to have dopaminergic effects and may interact with dopamine antagonists, such as antipsychotics and metoclopramide Chaste tree berry may decrease the effects of oral contraceptives and hormone replacement therapy
Chondroitin	Orally, used frequently in combination with glucosamine for osteoarthritis Topically, in combination with sodium hyaluronate, as a viscoelastic agent in cataract surgery	Oral: 200–400 mg tid	Occasional mild side effects include nausea, indigestion, and allergic reactions Chondroitin derived from bovine cartilage may carry a potential risk of contamination with diseased animals
Chromium	For diabetes For hypercholesterolemia Commonly found in weight-loss products Also promoted for bodybuilding	For diabetes, 100 µg bid for 4 mo or 500 µg bid for 2 mo For hypercholesterolemia, 200 µg tid or 500 µg bid for 2–4 mo For bodybuilding, 200–400 µg/d Chromium picolinate has been used in most studies, even though	Adverse effects are rare but may include headaches, insomnia, sleep disturbances, irritability and mood changes Some patients may experience cognitive, perceptual, and motor dysfunction

Continued

Herb/Nutritional Supplement	Common Uses	Reasonable Adult Oral Dosage*	Precautions and Drug Interactions
		the chloride form is also available	Long-term use of high doses (600–2400 μg/d) can cause anemia, thrombocytopenia, hemolysis, hepatic dysfunction, and renal failure Two case reports of interstitial nephritis A few studies suggest that chromium may cause DNA damage Chromium competes with iron for binding to transferrin and can cause iron deficiency Antacids, H_2 blockers, and proton pump inhibitors can decrease chromium absorption
Coenzyme Q10	As adjunctive treatment for congestive heart failure, angina, hypertension, and diabetes Also used to reduce cardiotoxicity associated with doxorubicin	For heart failure, 100 mg/d in two or three divided doses For angina, 50 mg tid For hypertension, 60 mg bid For diabetes, 100–200 mg/d	Mild adverse events include gastric distress, nausea, vomiting, and hypotension Doses >300 mg/d may cause elevated liver enzyme levels Coenzyme Q10 may reduce the anticoagulation effects of warfarin Oral hypoglycemic agents and HMG-CoA reductase inhibitors may reduce serum coenzyme Q10 levels
Creatine	To enhance muscle performance, especially during short-duration, high-intensity exercise	Loading dose of 20 g/d for 5–7 d followed by maintenance dose of ≥2 g/d Alternative dosing of 3 g/d for 28 d has been suggested	Creatine can cause gastroenteritis, diarrhea, heat intolerance, muscle cramps, and elevated serum creatinine levels Creatine is contraindicated in patients taking diuretics Concurrent use with cimetidine, probenecid, or nonsteroidal anti-inflammatory drugs increases the risk of adverse renal effects Caffeine may decrease creatine's ergogenic effects
Dehydroepian-drosterone (DHEA)	Replace low serum DHEA levels in adrenal insufficiency Treat SLE Reverse aging Used for many other conditions, including Alzheimer's disease, depression, diabetes, menopause, osteoporosis, impotence, and AIDS Used to promote weight loss Used by bodybuilders	For replacement therapy, 25–50 mg/d For SLE, 200 mg/d For antiaging and osteoporosis, 50 mg/d For other conditions, no established dosage documented	Most common side effects are androgenic in nature and include acne, hair loss, hirsutism, and deepening of the voice Cases of hepatitis have been reported When used in high doses, DHEA can cause insomnia, manic symptoms, and palpitations

Herb/Nutritional Supplement	Common Uses	Reasonable Adult Oral Dosage*	Precautions and Drug Interactions
	to increase muscle mass		DHEA at physiologic doses increases circulating androgen levels in women but not in men; it also increases circulating estrogen levels in both men and women Use of DHEA in individuals with a history of sex hormone–dependent malignancy should be avoided No information on the safety of DHEA in individuals <30 years old DHEA inhibits the cytochrome P-450 3A4 isoenzyme (CYP3A4) and can increase serum concentrations of drugs metabolized by this isozyme (e.g., lovastatin, ketoconazole, itraconazole, and triazolam)
Dong quai root	Commonly used for relief of premenstrual and menopausal symptoms Also used as a "blood tonic" and a strengthening treatment for the heart, spleen, liver, and kidneys	For premenstrual and menopausal symptoms, 3–4 g/d in three divided doses For other conditions, no established dosage documented	Dong quai should not be used in pregnant women because of its uterine stimulant and relaxant effects Women with hormone-sensitive conditions (e.g., breast, uterine, and ovarian cancer, and endometriosis and uterine fibroids) should avoid dong quai because of its estrogenic effects Drinking the essential oil of dong quai is not recommended because it contains a small amount of carcinogenic constituents Dong quai contains psoralens that can cause photosensitivity and photodermatitis Dong quai contains natural coumarin derivatives that can increase the risk of bleeding in those who are taking anticoagulant or antiplatelet drugs
Echinacea	As an immune stimulant, particularly for the prevention and treatment of the common cold and influenza Supportive therapy for lower urinary	300 mg tid of *Echinacea pallida* root or 2–3 mL tid of expressed juice of *Echinacea purpurea* herb Do not use for >8 wk because echinacea	Echinacea should not be used by transplant patients and those with autoimmune disease or liver dysfunction Allergic reactions have been reported

Continued

Herb/Nutritional Supplement	Common Uses	Reasonable Adult Oral Dosage*	Precautions and Drug Interactions
	tract infections Used topically to treat skin disorders and promote wound healing	may suppress immunity if used long term	Adverse events are rare and may include mild GI effects It should be discontinued as far in advance of surgery as possible Echinacea may decrease effectiveness of immunosuppressants
Ephedra (ma huang)	For diseases of the respiratory tract with mild bronchospasm Commonly found in weight-loss products Also marketed as a stimulant for performance enhancement	1 tsp or 2 g of dried herb (15–30 mg of ephedrine) in 240 mL boiling water for 10 min In Canada, the maximum allowable dosage of ephedrine is 8 mg per dose or 32 mg per day	Ephedra contains ephedrine, which has sympathomimetic activities; consequently, it should not be used in patients who have cardiovascular disease, diabetes, glaucoma, hypertension, hyperthyroidism, prostate enlargement, psychiatric disorders, or seizures Serious adverse effects, including seizures, arrhythmias, heart attack, stroke, and death, have been associated with the use of ephedra; as a result, the FDA has banned the sale of ephedra products in the United States Because of the cardiovascular effects of ephedrine, patients taking ephedra should discontinue use at least 24 h before surgery Concurrent use of ephedra and digitalis, guanethidine, monoamine oxidase inhibitors, and other stimulants, including caffeine, is not recommended
Evening primrose oil	For PMS, especially if mastalgia is present For treatment of atopic eczema Also used for other medical conditions, including rheumatoid arthritis, menopausal symptoms, Raynaud's phenomenon, Sjögren's syndrome, and diabetic neuropathy	For PMS, 2–4 g/d For atopic eczema, 6–8 g/d For rheumatoid arthritis, 2.8 g/d These doses are based on products standardized to 9% γ-linolenic acid Daily dose can be given in divided doses	Evening primrose oil may increase the risk of pregnancy complications Side effects may include indigestion, nausea, soft stools, and headache Seizures have been reported in patients with schizophrenia who were taking phenothiazines and evening primrose oil concomitantly Evening primrose oil may interact with anesthesia and cause seizures Concomitant use of evening primrose oil

Herb/Nutritional Supplement	Common Uses	Reasonable Adult Oral Dosage*	Precautions and Drug Interactions
			with anticoagulant and antiplatelet drugs can increase the risk of bleeding
Fenugreek seed	For diabetes and hypercholesterolemia Also for constipation, dyspepsia, gastritis, and kidney ailments Approved in Germany for use orally for loss of appetite and topically as a poultice for local inflammation	For loss of appetite, 1–2 g of the seed tid or 1 cup of tea (500 mg seed in 150 mL cold water for 3 h) several times a day Maximum 6 g/d For other conditions, no established dosage documented For topical use, 50 g powdered seed in ¼ L of hot water to form a paste	Fenugreek may cause uterine contractions and should be avoided in pregnancy Individuals who have allergies to peanuts or soybeans may also be allergic to fenugreek Fenugreek can cause diarrhea and flatulence; it may also make the urine smell like maple syrup Hypoglycemia may occur if fenugreek is taken in large amounts Repeated external applications can result in undesirable skin reactions Fenugreek contains small amounts of coumarins and may interact with anticoagulants and antiplatelet drugs High mucilage content of fenugreek can affect absorption of oral drugs; therefore, fenugreek should not be taken within 2 h of taking other drugs
Feverfew	For migraine headache prophylaxis For treatment of fever, menstrual problems, and arthritis	50–125 mg qd of the encapsulated dried leaf extract standardized to at least 0.2% parthenolide	Feverfew may induce menstrual bleeding and is contraindicated in pregnancy Fresh leaves may cause oral ulcers and GI irritation Sudden discontinuation of feverfew can precipitate rebound headache Feverfew may interact with anticoagulants and potentiate the antiplatelet effect of aspirin
Fish oils (omega-3 fatty acids)	Commonly used for treatment of hypertriglyceridemia Used to prevent CHD and stroke Also used in many noncardiac conditions, including depression, diabetes, dysmenorrhea, rheumatoid arthritis, and IgA nephropathy Used to reduce the risk of	For hypertriglyceridemia, 3–5 g/d For cardioprotection, 1 g/d for patients with CHD; oily fish at least twice per week, or about 0.5 g/d for people with no known heart disease For other conditions, no established dosage documented	Common side effects include fishy aftertaste, GI disturbances, belching, halitosis, and heartburn High doses can cause nausea and loose stools Doses >3 g/d can inhibit platelet aggregation, suppress immune function, worsen glycemia, and raise

Continued

Herb/Nutritional Supplement	Common Uses	Reasonable Adult Oral Dosage*	Precautions and Drug Interactions
	developing age-related maculopathy, Alzheimer's disease, and cancer Promote visual and mental development in children	Fish oils are composed of EPA and DHA. Fish oil capsules vary widely in amounts and ratios of EPA and DHA. The most common fish oil capsules in the United States provide 180 mg EPA and 120 mg DHA per capsule, and three capsules will provide about 1 g/d of omega-3 fatty acid	LDL cholesterol levels Long-term use may be associated with weight gain Less well-controlled preparations can contain appreciable amounts of organochloride contaminants Fish oil may increase the risk of bleeding in patients taking warfarin, an antiplatelet agent, or herbs that have antiplatelet constituents (e.g., garlic, ginkgo, and red clover) Fish oils can lower blood pressure and may have additive effects with antihypertensive agents Oral contraceptives may interfere with the triglyceride-lowering effects of fish oils
Garlic	To lower blood pressure and serum cholesterol level To prevent atherosclerosis	Fresh clove: 1 (4 g)/d Tablet: 300 mg bid to tid standardized to 0.6%–1.3% allicin	Intake of large quantities can lead to stomach complaints Garlic has antiplatelet effects, so patients should discontinue use of garlic at least 7 d before surgery Concomitant use of garlic and anticoagulants may increase the risk of bleeding
Ginger root	As an antiemetic For prevention of motion sickness	Fresh rhizome: 2–4 g/d Powdered ginger: 250 mg 3–4 times daily Tea: 1 cup tea tid (0.5–1 g dried root in 150 mL boiling water for 5–10 min)	Ginger should not be used by patients with gallstones because of its cholagogic effect May inhibit platelet aggregation; cases of postoperative bleeding have been reported Large doses of ginger may increase bleeding time in patients taking antiplatelet agents
Ginkgo biloba leaf	To slow cognitive deterioration in dementia To increase peripheral blood flow in claudication To treat sexual dysfunction associated with the use of SSRIs	60–120 mg bid of extract Egb761 standardized to 24% flavonoids and 6% terpenoids	Adverse effects are rare and may include mild stomach or intestinal upset, headache, and allergic skin reaction Ginkgo can inhibit platelet aggregation; reports of spontaneous bleeding have been published Patients should discontinue ginkgo at least 36 h before surgery Concurrent use of ginkgo and anticoagulants,

Herb/Nutritional Supplement	Common Uses	Reasonable Adult Oral Dosage*	Precautions and Drug Interactions
			antiplatelet agents, vitamin E, or garlic may increase the risk of bleeding
Ginseng root	As a tonic during times of stress, fatigue, disability, and convalescence To improve physical performance and stamina	Root: 1–2 g/d Tablet: 100 mg bid of extract standardized to 4%–7% ginsenosides A 2- to 3- wk period of using ginseng followed by a 1- to 2- wk "rest" period is generally recommended Ginseng is commonly adulterated, especially Siberian ginseng products	Ginseng has a mild stimulant effect and should be avoided in patients with cardiovascular disease Tachycardia and hypertension can occur Overdosages can lead to "ginseng abuse syndrome." characterized by insomnia, hypotonia, and edema Ginseng has estrogenic effects and may cause vaginal bleeding and breast tenderness Ginseng has been shown to inhibit platelets, so patients should discontinue ginseng use at least 7 d before surgery Ginseng should not be used with other stimulants Patients taking antidiabetic agents and ginseng should be monitored to avoid the hypoglycemic effects of ginseng Ginseng may interact with warfarin and cause a decreased international normalized ratio Siberian ginseng may increase digoxin levels Reports of a drug interaction between ginseng and phenelzine (a monoamine oxidase inhibitor) resulting in insomnia, headache, tremulousness, and manic-like symptoms
Glucosamine	For osteoarthritis	500 mg tid with meals Glucosamine is available in the form of sulfate, hydrochloride, or N-acetyl salt Glucosamine sulfate is the form that has been used in most clinical studies	Side effects are generally limited to mild GI symptoms, including stomach upset, heartburn, diarrhea, nausea, and indigestion Glucosamine derived from marine exoskeletons may cause reactions in people allergic to shellfish Glucosamine may raise blood glucose levels in patients with diabetes
Hawthorn leaf with flower	Commonly used in Germany to increase cardiac output in patients with New York Heart Association stage I and II heart failure	160–900 mg water-ethanol extract (30–169 mg procyanidins or 3.5–19.8 mg flavonoids) divided into 2–3 doses	Side effects include GI upset, palpitations, hypotension, headache, dizziness, and insomnia Concomitant use with CNS depressants may have additive CNS effects

Continued

Herb/Nutritional Supplement	Common Uses	Reasonable Adult Oral Dosage*	Precautions and Drug Interactions
			Hawthorn may potentiate effects of digoxin and vasodilators
Horse chestnut seed	To relieve symptoms of chronic venous insufficiency	250 mg bid of extract standardized to 50 mg aescin in delayed-release form Unsafe to ingest the raw seed, which contains significant amounts of the most toxic constituent esculin	Mild GI symptoms, headache, dizziness, and pruritus have been reported Ingestion of high doses may cause renal, hepatic, and hematologic toxicity Concomitant use with anticoagulants may increase the risk of bleeding Horse chestnut may potentiate the effects of hypoglycemic drugs
Kava kava	As an anxiolytic for nervous anxiety, stress, and restlessness As a sedative to induce sleep	Herb and preparations equivalent to 60–120 mg/d of kava pyrones Most clinical trials have used 100 mg tid of extract standardized to 70% kava pyrones for anxiety disorders	Kava should not be used by patients with depression Kava should not be taken by pregnant or nursing women Kava may affect motor reflexes and judgment, so it should not be taken while driving and/or operating heavy machinery Accommodative disturbances have been reported; kava may exacerbate Parkinson's disease Extended use can cause a temporary yellow discoloration of skin, hair, and nails Reports have linked kava use to at least 25 cases of severe liver toxicity; sale of products containing kava has been banned in Canada and several European countries Kava has been shown to have additive CNS depressant effects with benzodiazepines, alcohol, and herbal tranquilizers Kava may potentiate the sedative effects of anesthetics, so kava should be discontinued at least 24 h before surgery
Lutein	Commonly used to prevent AMD and cataracts Also used to prevent skin cancer, breast cancer, and colon cancer To protect against cardiovascular disease	For AMD and cataracts, 6–20 mg/d of lutein from diet For other uses, no established dosage documented Foods containing high concentrations of lutein include kale, spinach, broccoli, and romaine lettuce	No major adverse effects and drug interactions have been reported

Herb/Nutritional Supplement	Common Uses	Reasonable Adult Oral Dosage*	Precautions and Drug Interactions
		Not known if supplemental lutein is as effective as natural lutein	
		Supplemental lutein in the form of esters may require a higher fat intake for effective absorption than purified lutein	
Lycopene	Commonly used to prevent and treat prostate cancer Also used for cancer prevention, arthrosclerosis prevention, and reduction of asthma symptoms	For decreasing the growth of prostate cancer, 15 mg supplement bid For prostate cancer prevention, at least 6 mg/d from tomato products (or ≥10 servings per week) For other uses, no established dosage documented Heat processing converts lycopene in fresh tomatoes from the *trans-* to the *cis-*configuration. The *cis-*isomer has better bioavailability Lycopene supplements usually do not specify the type and amount of isomers in their product labeling	Lycopene, when consumed in amounts found in foods, is generally considered to be safe Concomitant ingestion of beta carotene may increase lycopene absorption Lycopene may reduce cholesterol levels and potentiate the effects of statins
Melatonin	For jet lag, insomnia, shift-work disorder, and circadian rhythm disorders Also for other medical conditions, including depression, multiple sclerosis, tinnitus, headache, and cancer	For jet lag, 5 mg at bedtime for 2–5 d beginning the day of return For sleep disorders, 0.3–5 mg taken 2 hr before bedtime Avoid melatonin from animal pineal gland because of possible contamination	Avoid use in pregnancy because melatonin decreases serum luteinizing hormone concentrations and increases serum prolactin levels Common adverse reactions include headache, transient depressive symptoms, daytime fatigue and drowsiness, dizziness, abdominal cramps, irritability, and reduced alertness Concomitant use of melatonin with alcohol, benzodiazepines, or other CNS depressants may cause additive sedation Melatonin can affect immune function and may interfere with immunosuppressive therapy Concomitant use with other herbs that have sedative properties (e.g., chamomile, goldenseal, hop, kava, valerian) may produce additive CNS-impairing effects

Continued

Herb/Nutritional Supplement	Common Uses	Reasonable Adult Oral Dosage*	Precautions and Drug Interactions
Milk thistle fruit	As a hepatoprotectant and antioxidant, particularly for treatment of hepatitis, cirrhosis, and toxic liver damage Used in Europe for treatment of hepatotoxic mushroom poisoning from *Amanita phalloides*	Average daily dose is 12–15 g of crude drug or formulations equivalent to 200–400 mg of silymarin	Adverse effects are rare but may include diarrhea and allergic reactions Milk thistle may potentiate the hypoglycemic effect of antidiabetic agents
Red clover flower	Commonly used for conditions associated with menopause, such as hot flashes, cardiovascular health, and osteoporosis Also used for PMS, benign prostate hyperplasia, and cancer prevention Used topically to treat psoriasis, eczema, and other rashes	For hot flashes, 40 mg/d of the isoflavones extract (Promensil) For other conditions, no established dosage documented	Red clover has estrogenic activity and should be avoided during pregnancy and lactation Women with hormone-dependent conditions (e.g., breast, uterine, and ovarian cancer, and endometriosis and uterine fibroids) and men with prostate cancer should avoid taking red clover Side effects include headache, myalgia, nausea, and rash Red clover contains coumarin derivatives and may increase the risk of bleeding in those who are taking anticoagulants or antiplatelet drugs Preliminary report suggests that red clover may antagonize the effects of tamoxifen Some evidence suggests that red clover can increase the levels of drugs metabolized by CYP3A4 (e.g., lovastatin, ketoconazole, itraconazole, fexofenadine, and triazolam)
SAMe (*S*-adenosyl-L-methionine)	For treatment of osteoarthritis, depression, fibromyalgia, and liver disease	For osteoarthritis, 200 mg tid For depression and fibromyalgia, 800 mg bid For liver disease, 600–800 mg bid	Common side effects include flatulence, nausea, vomiting, and diarrhea SAMe can cause anxiety in people with depression and hypomania in people with bipolar disorder Concurrent use of SAMe and other antidepressants may cause serotonin syndrome
Saw palmetto berry	To treat symptomatic benign prostatic hyperplasia and irritable bladder	160 mg bid of extract standardized to 85%–95% fatty acids and sterols	Adverse effects are rare but may include headache, nausea, and upset stomach High doses can cause diarrhea
Soy	Commonly used for cholesterol reduction in combination with a low-fat diet Also used for menopausal symptoms and for	For lowering cholesterol, 25–50 g/d of soy protein For hot flashes, 20–60 g/d of soy protein	Soy, when consumed as whole foods (e.g., tofu or soy milk), has minimal adverse effects Consumption of large

Herb/Nutritional Supplement	Common Uses	Reasonable Adult Oral Dosage*	Precautions and Drug Interactions
	prevention of osteoporosis and cardiovascular disease in postmenopausal women	For osteoporosis, 40 g/d of soy protein containing 90 mg isoflavones	amounts of soy may cause gastric complaints, such as constipation, bloating, and nausea Long-term use of soy tablets containing isoflavones (150 mg/d for 5 y) have been shown to cause endometrial hyperplasia
St. John's wort	Effective for treatment of mild to moderate depression May have anti-inflammatory and anti-infective activities	300 mg tid of hypericum extract standardized to 0.3% hypericin	St. John's wort should not be used in pregnancy Side effects include dry mouth, GI upset, dizziness, fatigue, and constipation St. John's wort may induce photosensitivity, especially in fair-skinned individuals It may cause serotonin syndrome if used with other antidepressants, including SSRIs, or other serotonergic drugs It has been shown to induce CYP3A4 and decrease blood levels of many drugs, such as indinavir, nevirapine, cyclosporine, digoxin, theophylline, simvastatin, oral contraceptive pills, and warfarin St. John's wort should be discontinued at least 5 d before surgery to avoid any potential drug interactions
Valerian root	Used as a mild sedative for insomnia and anxiety	2–3 g of dried root or 1–3 mL of tincture, qd to several times per day Two clinical trials found 400–450 mg of the root extract effective for insomnia	Valerian has a bad odor and can cause morning drowsiness Long-term administration may lead to paradoxical stimulation, including restlessness and palpitations Because of the risk of benzodiazepine-like withdrawal, valerian should be tapered over a period of several weeks before surgery It may potentiate the sedative effect of CNS depressants (e.g., benzodiazepines, alcohol) and other herbal tranquilizers

*Doses presented in the table are adapted from the German Commission E Monographs and/or data from clinical trials. Products from different manufacturers vary considerably. A reliable product should have a label clearly stating the botanical name of the herb and milligram amount contained in the product. Standardized extracts should be used whenever possible and are often disclosed on the label of quality products.

AMD = age-related macular degeneration; CHD = coronary heart disease; CNS = central nervous system; DHA = docosahexaenoic acid; EPA = eicosapentaenoic acid; FDA = Food and Drug Administration; GI = gastrointestinal; HMG-CoA = 3-hydroxy-3-methylglutaryl-coenzyme A; LDL = low-density lipoprotein; PMS = premenstrual syndrome; SLE = systemic lupus erythematosus; SSRI = selective serotonin reuptake inhibitor.

REFERENCES

Ang-Lee MK, Moss J, Yuan C: Herbal medicines and perioperative care. JAMA 2001;286:208-216.

Blumethal M (ed): Complete German Commission E Monographs: Therapeutic Guide to Herbal Medicines, 1st ed. Austin, Tx, American Botanical Council, 1998.

Cupp MJ: Herbal remedies: Adverse effects and drug interactions. Am Fam Phys 1999;59:1239-1244.

Ernst E: The risk-benefit profile of commonly used herbal therapies: Ginkgo, St. John's wort, ginseng, Echinacea, saw palmetto, and kava. Ann Intern Med 2002;136:42-53.

Jellin JM, Gregory P, Batz F, et al: Pharmacist's Letter/Prescriber's Letter Natural Medicines Comprehensive Database, 7th ed. Stockton, CA, Therapeutic Research Faculty, 2005.

Klepser TB, Klepser ME: Unsafe and potentially safe herbal therapies. Am J Health Syst Pharm 1999;56:125-38.

Kronenberg F, Fugh-Berman A: Complementary and alternative medicine for menopausal symptoms: A review of randomized controlled trials. Ann Intern Med 2002;137:805-813.

Mar C, Bent S: An evidence-based review of the 10 most commonly used herbs. West J Med 1999;171:168-171.

O'Hara MA, Kiefer D, Farrell K, Kemper K: A review of 12 commonly used medicinal herbs. Arch Fam Med 1998;7:523-536.

PDR for Herbal Medicines, 3rd ed. Montvale, NJ, Medical Economics Co., 2004.

Rotblatt MD: Cranberry, feverfew, horse chestnut, and kava. West J Med 1999;171:195-198.

Smet P: Herbal remedies. N Engl J Med 2002;347:2046-2056.

New Drugs in 2005 and Agents Pending FDA Approval

Method of
Miriam M. Chan, RPh, PharmD

Generic Name	Trade Name (Manufacturer)	Strength	Dosage Form	Normal Dosage Range	Pregnancy Rating*	FDA Approval Date	Indication	Classification
Abatacept	Orencia (Bristol-Myers Squibb)	250 mg in 15-mL vial	Injection	<60 kg: 500 mg. 60–100 kg: 750 mg. >100 kg: 1 g. Orencia is given as an IV infusion over 30 min. Repeat dose at 2 and 4 wk after first infusion, then q4wk thereafter.	C	12/26/05	For reducing signs and symptoms, inducing major clinical response, slowing progression of structural damage, and improving physical function in adult patients with moderately to severely active rheumatoid arthritis who have had an inadequate response to ≥1 DMARDs.	Biological, selective T cell costimulation modulator
Bromfenac sodium	Xibrom (ISTA Pharmaceuticals)	0.09%, 5 mL in 10-mL container	Ophthalmic solution	1 drop to affected eye(s) bid beginning 24 h after cataract surgery and continuing through first 2 wk of postoperative period.	C	03/24/05	Treatment of postoperative inflammation in patients who have undergone cataract extraction.	Ophthalmic, nonsteroidal anti-inflammatory drug

Continued

New Drugs Approved in 2005—cont'd

Generic Name	Trade Name (Manufacturer)	Strength	Dosage Form	Normal Dosage Range	Pregnancy Rating*	FDA Approval Date	Indication	Classification
Conivaptan hydro-chloride	Vaprisol (Astellas)	20 mg in 4-mL ampule	Injection	20 mg IV over 30 min, followed by 20 mg IV infusion over 24 h for additional 1–3 d. If serum sodium does not rise at desired rate, may titrate upward to daily dose of 40 mg IV infusion.	C	12/29/05	Treatment of euvolemic hyponatremia in hospitalized patients.	Nonpeptide, arginine vasopressin antagonist
Deferasirox	Exjade (Novartis)	125, 250, 500 mg	Tablet for oral suspen-sion	Starting dose: 20 mg/kg daily on an empty stomach. Maintenance: Monitor serum ferritin levels monthly and adjust dose q3mo–q6mo by 5 or 10 mg/kg based on ferritin trends; dose should not exceed 30 mg/kg/d and consider stopping therapy if serum ferritin level <500 mcg/L. Dose should be calculated to nearest whole tablet.	B	11/2/05	Treatment of chronic iron overload caused by blood transfusions (transfusional hemosiderosis) in patients ≥ 2 y.	Iron reduction drug, chelating drug
Drospire-none/ estradiol	Angeliq (Berlex)	0.5 mg/ 1 mg	Tablet	1 tablet daily.	X	09/28/05	Moderate to severe vasomotor	Hormones, progestin and estrogen

Generic Name	Brand (Manufacturer)	Strength / Supply	Dosage Form	Pregnancy Category	Approval Date	Dosing	Indication	Classification
							symptoms associated with menopause. Moderate to severe symptoms of vulvar and vaginal atrophy associated with menopause.	
Entecavir	Baraclude (Bristol-Myers Squibb)	0.5-, 1-mg film-coated tablet; 0.05 mg/mL oral solution in 260-mL bottle	Tablet, oral solution	C	03/29/05	Adults and adolescents ≥ 16 y who are nucleoside treatment-naive: 0.5 mg once daily Adults and adolescents ≥ 16 y who have viremia while receiving lamivudine or who have known lamivudine resistance mutations: 1 mg once daily. Baraclude should be administered on an empty stomach at least 2 h after meal or 2 h before next meal.	Treatment of chronic hepatitis B virus infection in adults with evidence of active viral replication and either evidence of persistent elevations in serum aminotransferases (ALT or AST) or histologically active disease.	Antiviral, nucleoside analogue
Exenatide	Byetta (Amylin Pharmaceuticals)	250 µg/mL in 1.2-, 2.4-mL prefilled pen	Injection	C	04/28/05	5 µg SC bid, within 60 min before morning and evening meals. May increase to 10 µg bid after 1 mo of therapy.	As adjunctive therapy to improve glycemic control in patients with type 2 diabetes mellitus who are taking metformin, a sulfonylurea, or a combination of metformin and a sulfonylurea but have not achieved adequate glycemic control.	Antidiabetic, incretin mimetic

New Drugs Approved in 2005 — cont'd

Generic Name	Trade Name (Manufacturer)	Strength	Dosage Form	Normal Dosage Range	Pregnancy Rating*	FDA Approval Date	Indication	Classification
Fluocinolone acetonide intravitreal implant	Retisert (Bausch & Lomb)	0.59 mg/ insert	Implantable tablet	One insert, surgically implanted into posterior segment of affected eye through a pars plana incision. Insert releases about 0.6 µg fluocinolone daily, decreasing over first mo to steady-state 0.3–0.4 µg/d over ≈ 30 mo. After implant is depleted, it may be replaced.	C	04/8/05	Treatment of chronic noninfectious uveitis affecting posterior segment of eye.	Ophthalmic, corticosteroid
Galsulfase	Naglazyme (Biomarin)	1 mg/mL in 5-mL vial	Injection	1 mg/kg once weekly as IV infusion over at least 4 h.	B	05/31/05	To improve walking and stair climbing in patients with mucopolysaccharidosis VI.	Mucopolysaccharidosis VI drug, glycoprotein recombinant enzyme
Hyaluronidase	Hydase (Prima Pharm)	150 U/mL in 2-mL vial	Injection	To increase absorption and dispersion of injected drug: Add 50–300 U to injection solution. Hypodermoclysis: Inject 150 U into tubing of infusion solution during clysis or SC prior to hypodermoclysis near infusion site. Adjunct in SC urography for improving resorption of radiopaque agents: Inject 75 units	C	10/25/05	An adjunct to increase absorption and dispersion of other injected drugs; for hypodermoclysis; and as an adjunct in SC urography for improving resorption of radiopaque agents.	Dispersion and absorption factor, protein enzyme

Drug	Brand (Manufacturer)	Strength	Form	Dosage	Preg.	Approval	Indication	Class
Insulin detemir (rDNA origin)	Levemir (Novo Nordisk)	100 U/mL in 10-mL vial and 3-mL prefilled pen	Injection	In insulin-naïve patients with type 2 diabetes, initially give 0.1–0.2 U/kg SC once daily in evening or 10 U SC once or twice daily; adjust dose to achieve glycemic target. Patients with type 1 or 2 diabetes receiving basal-bolus treatment or receiving only basal insulin can be switched to insulin detemir on a unit-to-unit basis with dosage adjusted to glycemic target.	C	06/16/05	Indicated for once- or twice-daily SC administration in treatment of adult patients with type 1 or type 2 diabetes mellitus who require basal insulin for control of hyperglycemia.	Antidiabetic, long-acting insulin analogue
Isosorbide dinitrate/hydralazine	BiDil (NitroMed)	20 mg/37.5 mg	Tablet	1 tablet tid; may increase, if needed, to maximum daily dose of 2 tablets tid.	C	06/23/05	Treatment of heart failure as an adjunct to standard therapy in self-identified black patients to improve survival, to prolong time to hospitalization for heart failure, and to improve patient-reported functional status.	Vasodilator, nitrate
Lenalidomide	Revlimid (Celgene)	5, 10 mg	Capsule	10 mg with water daily	X	12/28/05	Treatment of patients with transfusion-dependent anemia caused by low- or intermediate-risk myelodysplastic syndromes (MDS) associated with a deletion	Immunomodulator, thalidomide analogue

Continued

Note: SC over each scapula, followed by injection of contrast media at same sites.

New Drugs Approved in 2005—cont'd

Generic Name	Trade Name (Manufacturer)	Strength	Dosage Form	Normal Dosage Range	Pregnancy Rating*	FDA Approval Date	Indication	Classification
							5q cytogenetic abnormality with or without additional cytogenetic abnormalities.	
Mecasermin (rDNA origin)	Increlex (Tercica)	10 mg/mL in 4-mL vial	Injection	Start with 0.04–0.08 mg/kg SC bid. If well tolerated for at least 1 wk, may increase dose by 0.04 mg/kg per dose, to maximum dose of 0.12 mg/kg bid.	C	08/30/05	Long-term treatment of growth failure in children with severe primary IGF-1 deficiency or with growth hormone gene deletion who have developed neutralizing antibodies to growth hormone.	Growth factor, human insulin-like growth factor-1
Micafungin sodium	Mycamine (Fujisawa)	50-mg vial	Injection	Treatment of esophageal candidiasis: 150 mg once daily, given as IV infusion over 1 h. Prophylaxis of Candida infections: 50 mg once daily, given as IV infusion over 1 h.	C	03/16/05	Treatment of patients with esophageal candidiasis. Prophylaxis of Candida infections in patients undergoing hematopoietic stem cell transplantation.	Antifungal, echinocandin
Nelarabine	Arranon (Glaxo-SmithKline)	5 mg/mL in 50-mL vial	Injection	Adults: 1500 mg/m^2 IV over 2 h on 5 days 1, 3, and repeated q21d. Children: 650 mg/m^2 IV over 1 h for 5 consecutive days repeated q21d.	D	10/28/05	Treatment of patients with T cell acute lymphoblastic leukemia and T cell lymphoblastic lymphoma whose disease has not responded to or has relapsed following treatment with at least two chemotherapy regimens.	Antineoplastic, antimitotic
Nepafenac	Nevanac (Alcon)	0.1%, 3 mL in 4-mL bottle	Ophthalmic suspension	Instill 1 drop into affected eye(s) tid, beginning 1 d prior to	C	08/19/05	Treatment of pain and inflammation associated with cataract surgery.	Ophthalmic, nonsteroidal anti-inflammatory drug

Generic name	Brand (Company)	Strength	Form	Dose	Pregnancy category	Approval date	Indication	Classification
Paclitaxel protein-bound particles for injectable suspension	Abraxane (American BioScience)	100-mg vial	Injection	surgery, continuing on day of surgery and through first 2 wk of post-operative period. 260 mg/m² IV over 30 min q3wk.	D	01/7/05	Treatment of metastatic breast cancer after failure of combination chemotherapy or relapse within 6 mo of adjuvant anthracycline chemotherapy.	Antineoplastic, antimitotic
Pramlintide	Symlin (Amylin Pharmaceuticals)	0.6 mg/mL in 5-mL vial	Injection	Insulin-using type 2 diabetes: start at 60 μg SC and increase to 120 μg as tolerated. Type 1 diabetes: start at 15 μg SC and titrate at 15-μg increments to maintenance dose of 30 μg or 60 μg as tolerated. Symlin should be given immediately prior to major meals. Reduce rapid or short-acting insulin dose by 50%.	C	03/16/05	As an adjunct treatment in patients who use mealtime insulin therapy and who have failed to achieve desired glucose control despite optimal insulin therapy.	Antidiabetic agent, amylinomimetic
Ramelteon	Rozerem (Takeda)	8 mg	Tablet	8 mg taken within 30 min of bedtime.	C	07/22/05	Treatment of insomnia characterized by difficulty with sleep onset.	Hypnotic, melatonin receptor agonist
Sodium phenylacetate/sodium benzoate	Ammonul (Ucyclyd Pharma)	10%/10% in 50-mL vial	Injection	IV infusion through central line over 90–120 min as loading dose; then give an equivalent maintenance dose infusion over 24 h.	C	02/17/05	Adjunctive therapy for treatment of acute hyperammonemia and associated encephalopathy in patients with deficiencies in enzymes of urea cycle.	Ammonia reducer, metabolically active urea substitute

Continued

New Drugs Approved in 2005—cont'd

Generic Name	Trade Name (Manufacturer)	Strength	Dosage Form	Normal Dosage Range	Pregnancy Rating*	FDA Approval Date	Indication	Classification
				Dosage determined by weight in patients and patient's specific enzyme deficiency: carbamyl phosphate synthetase (CPS), ornithine transcarbamylase (OTC), argininosuccinate synthetase (ASS), or argininosuccinate lyase (ASL). Patients weighing <20 kg with CPS or OTC deficiency: 2.5 mL/kg Ammonul with 2 mL/kg arginine. Patients weighing <20 kg with ASS or ASL deficiency: 2.5 mL/kg Ammonul with 6 mL/kg arginine. Patients weighing >20 kg with CPS or OTC deficiency: 55 mL/m² Ammonul with 2 mL/kg arginine. Patients weighing >20 kg with ASS or ASL deficiency: 55 mL/m² Ammonul with 6 mL/kg arginine.				
Sorafenib tosylate	Nexavar (Bayer)	200 mg	Tablet	400 mg bid, without food.	D	12/20/05	Treatment of patients with advanced renal cell carcinoma.	Anticancer, multikinase inhibitor
Tigecycline	Tygacil (Wyeth)	50 mg powder in 5-mL vial	Injection	100 mg IV infusion over 30–60 min, followed by 50 mg IV q12h × 5–14 d,	D	06/15/05	Treatment of complicated skin and skin structure infections (cSSSI) and complicated	Antibacterial, glycylcycline

| | | | | based on patient response and bacterial progress. | | | intra-abdominal infections (cIAI). | |
| Tipranavir | Aptivus (Boehringer Ingelheim) | 250 mg | Capsule | 500 mg, co-administered with 200 mg of ritonavir, bid. | C | 06/22/05 | Aptivus, co-administered with 200 mg of ritonavir, is indicated for combination antiretroviral treatment of HIV-1 infected adult patients with evidence of viral replication, who are highly treatment experienced or have HIV-1 strains resistant to multiple protease inhibitors. | Antiviral, protease inhibitor |

*FDA Pregnancy Categories:

A—Adequate studies in pregnant women have not demonstrated a risk to the fetus in the first trimester of pregnancy, and there is no evidence of risk in later trimesters.

B—Animal studies have shown an adverse effect, but adequate studies in pregnant women have not demonstrated a risk to the fetus during the first trimester of pregnancy, and there is no evidence of risk in later trimesters.

C—Animal studies have shown an adverse effect on the fetus, but there are no adequate studies in humans; the benefits from the use of the drug in pregnant women may be acceptable despite its potential risks.

D—There is evidence of human fetal risk, but the potential benefits from the use of the drug in pregnant women may be acceptable despite its potential risks.

X—Adverse reaction reports indicate evidence of fetal risk; the risk of use in a pregnant woman clearly outweighs any possible benefit.

No drug should be administered during pregnancy unless it is clearly needed and potential benefit outweighs potential hazard to the fetus, regardless of the pregnancy category.

Abbreviations: DMARD = disease-modifying antirheumatic drug.

Agents Pending FDA Approval

Generic Name	Trade Name (Manufacturer)	Indication
Abetimus	Riquent (La Jolla Pharmaceutical)	Treatment of lupus kidney disease
Alvimopan	Entereg (Adolor Corp/GlaxoSmithKline)	Treatment of postoperative ileus in patients recovering from bowel surgery
Anecortave acetate	Retaane (Alcon)	Treatment of wet age-related macular degeneration
Anidulafungin	Eraxis (Pfizer)	Treatment of esophageal candidiasis
Armodafinil	Nuvigil (Cephalon)	To improve wakefulness in patients suffering from excessive sleepiness associated with narcolepsy, shift work sleep disorder, and obstructive sleep apnea/hypopnea syndrome
Ciclesonide	Alvesco (Sanofi-Aventis)	Treatment of persistent asthma (regardless of severity) in adults, adolescents, and children ≥4 y
Cilomilast	Ariflo (GlaxoSmithKline)	Treatment of patients with chronic obstructive pulmonary disease (COPD) who are poorly responsive to albuterol
Clodronate	Bonefos (Berlex Laboratories)	Adjuvant oral treatment for reducing occurrence of bone metastases in stage II/III breast cancer patients
Etonogestrel subdermal implant	Implanon (Organon)	Contraceptive
Everolimus	Certican (Novartis)	Prevention of rejection after heart and kidney transplantation
Febuxostat	No brand name (TAP)	For management of hyperuricemia in patients with chronic gout
Indiplon	No brand name (Neurocrine Biosciences/Pfizer)	Treatment of insomnia
Lubiprostone	Amitiza (Sucampo/Takeda)	Treatment of chronic idiopathic constipation in adults
Lucinactant	Surfaxin (Discovery Laboratories)	Treatment of respiratory distress syndrome in premature infants
Nebivolol	No brand name (Mylan)	Treatment of hypertension
Oxypurinol	Oxyprim (Cardiome)	Treatment of allopurinol-intolerant hyperuricemia
Paliperidone extended-release	No brand name (Janssen)	Treatment of schizophrenia
Ranolazine	Ranexa (CV Therapeutics)	Treatment of chronic stable angina
Selegiline transdermal system	EmSam Patch (Mylan Laboratories/Waston Pharmaceuticals)	Treatment of depression
Sunitnib	Sutent (Pfizer)	Treatment for patients with gastrointestinal stromal tumors (GISTs) and advanced kidney cancer
SnET2 (tin ethyl etiopurpurin)	No brand name (Miravent Medical Technologies)	Slow progression of wet age-related macular degeneration
Vapreotide	Sanvar IR (H3 Pharma)	Treatment of acute esophageal variceal bleeding secondary to portal hypertension
Varenicline	Champix (Pfizer)	Treatment of smoking cessation

Note: Page numbers followed by f, t, and b refer to illustrations, tables, and boxed material, respectively.